TOPIC INDEX

(continued on next page)

TOPIC INDEX

THE COLOR ATLAS OF INTERNAL MEDICINE

NOTICE

Medicine is an ever-changing science. As new research and clinical experience broaden our knowledge, changes in treatment and drug therapy are required. The authors and the publisher of this work have checked with sources believed to be reliable in their efforts to provide information that is complete and generally in accord with the standards accepted at the time of publication. However, in view of the possibility of human error or changes in medical sciences, neither the authors nor the publisher nor any other party who has been involved in the preparation or publication of this work warrants that the information contained herein is in every respect accurate or complete, and they disclaim all responsibility for any errors or omissions or for the results obtained from use of the information contained in this work. Readers are encouraged to confirm the information contained herein with other sources. For example and in particular, readers are advised to check the product information sheet included in the package of each drug they plan to administer to be certain that the information contained in this work is accurate and that changes have not been made in the recommended dose or in the contraindications for administration. This recommendation is of particular importance in connection with new or infrequently used drugs.

THE COLOR ATLAS OF INTERNAL MEDICINE

EDITORS

Richard P. Usatine, MD
Professor, Family and Community Medicine
Professor, Dermatology and Cutaneous Surgery
Assistant Director, Medical Humanities Education
University of Texas Health Science Center at San Antonio
Medical Director, Skin Clinic, University Health System
San Antonio, Texas

Gary Ferenchick, MD, MS
Professor of Internal Medicine
Division Chief, General Medicine
Internal Medicine Clerkship Director
Michigan State University, College of Human Medicine
East Lansing, Michigan

E.J. Mayeaux, Jr., MD
Professor and Chairman, Department of Family and Preventive Medicine
Professor of Obstetrics and Gynecology
University of South Carolina School of Medicine
Columbia, South Carolina

Mindy A. Smith, MD, MS
Clinical Professor
Department of Family Medicine
Michigan State University
East, Lansing, Michigan

Heidi S. Chumley, MD
Executive Dean and Chief Academic Officer
American University of the Caribbean

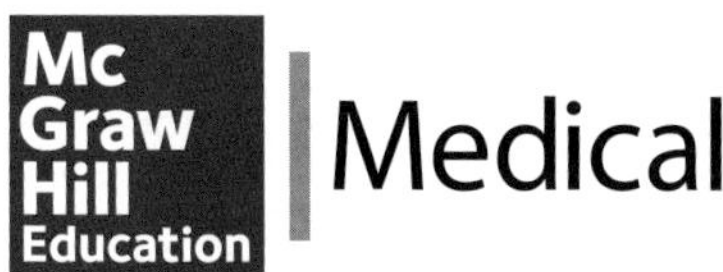

New York Chicago San Francisco Athens London Madrid Mexico City
Milan New Delhi Singapore Sydney Toronto

The Color Atlas of Internal Medicine

1 2 3 4 5 6 7 8 9 0 CTPS/CTPS 19 18 17 16 15 14

ISBN: 978-0-07-177238-9
MHID: 0-07-177238-3

This book was set in Perpetua by Cenveo® Publisher Services.
The editors were James Shanahan and Harriet Lebowitz.
The production supervisor was Rick Ruzycka.
Project management was provided by Hardik Popli, Cenveo Publisher Services.
The cover designer was Nancy McKeon.
China Translation & Printing Services was printer and binder.

This book is printed on acid-free paper.

Library of Congress Cataloging-in-Publication Data

Usatine, Richard, author.
The color atlas of internal medicine / Richard P. Usatine, Gary Ferenchick, Mindy A. Smith, E.J. Mayeaux Jr., Heidi S. Chumley.
p. ; cm.
Includes bibliographical references and index.
ISBN 978-0-07-177238-9 (alk. paper)— ISBN 0-07-177238-3 (alk. paper)
I. Ferenchick, Gary, author. II. Smith, Mindy A., author. III. Mayeaux, E. J., Jr., author. IV. Chumley, Heidi S., author. V. Title.
[DNLM: 1. Internal Medicine—methods—Atlases. WB 17]
RC46
616–dc23

2014029315

DEDICATION

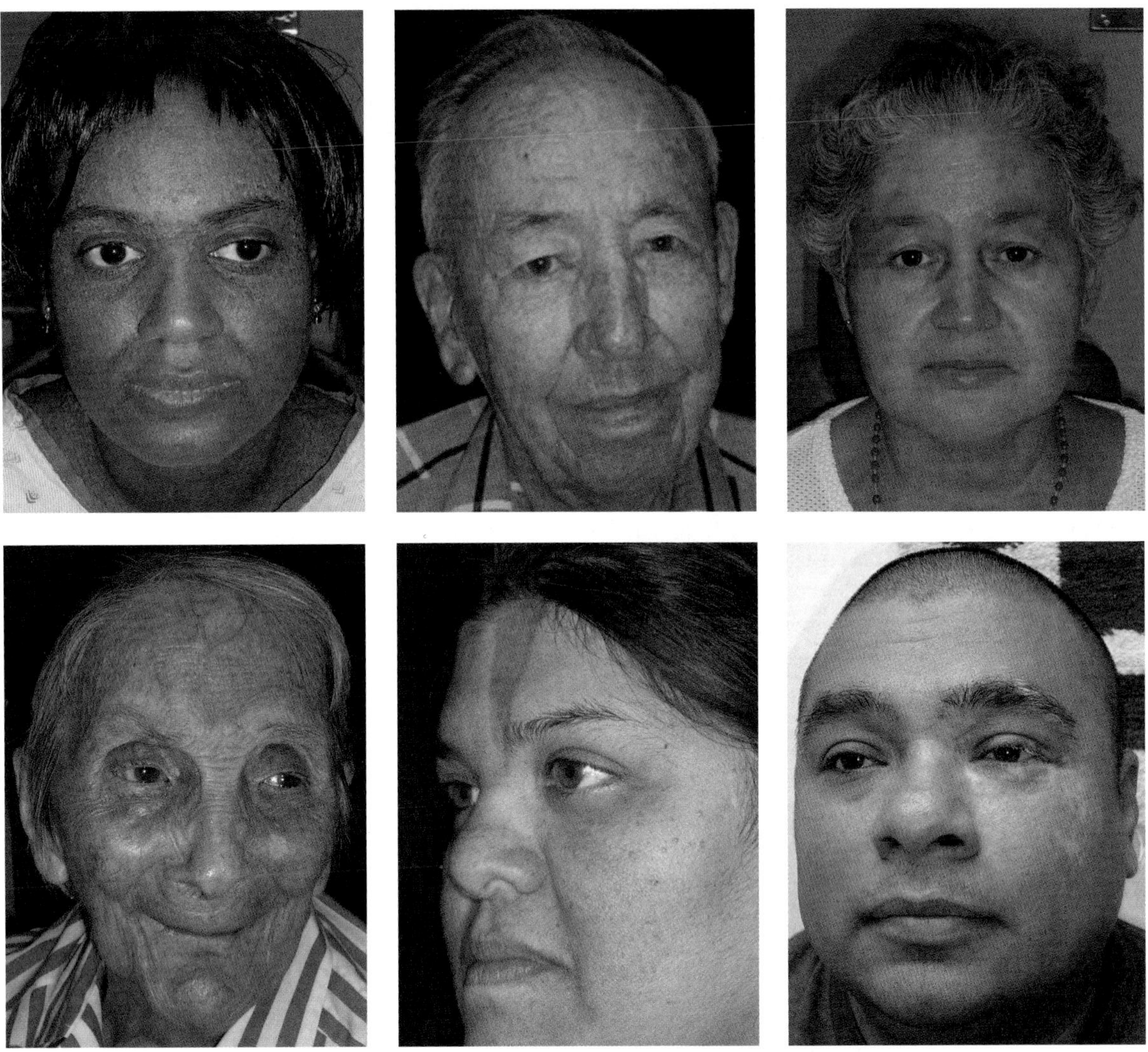

To our patients who unselfishly agreed to let us display their diseases and afflictions to the world to enhance the study and practice of medicine. We are honored by this trust. We have learned much from our patients as they continue to help us teach the next generation of health care providers.

COVER IMAGES

FRONT COVER

TOP ROW

Left: Nonproliferative diabetic retinopathy, with scattered intradot-blot, flame hemorrhages, and also macular exudates (*Figure 219-2; Reproduced with permission from Andrew Sanchez, COA*).

Middle: Sarcoidosis causing a lupus pernio pattern on the face of an African American woman (*Figure 63-3; Reproduced with permission from Richard P. Usatine, MD*).

Right: Rheumatoid arthritis with rheumatoid nodules over the PCP joints along with deformities of the digits (*Figure 97-7; Reproduced with permission from Ricardo Zuniga-Montes, MD*).

BOTTOM ROW

Left: Palmar patches and plaques in a young man with secondary syphilis and HIV/AIDS (*Figure 218-18B; Reproduced with permission from Jonathan B. Karnes, MD*).

Middle: Frontal chest radiograph of a primary pulmonary TB infection in a 20-year-old man, showing mediastinal and right hilar lymphadenopathy (black arrows) and right upper lobe consolidation (white arrow) (*Figure 64-1A; Reproduced with permission from Carlos Santiago Restrepo, MD*).

Right: Asymptomatic diverticulosis (*Figure 68-4; Reproduced with permission from John Rodney, MD*).

BACK COVER

Top: Multiple soft neurofibromas on the neck of a patient with neurofibromatosis (*Reproduced with permission from Richard P. Usatine, MD.*)

Middle: Localized bullous pemphigoid with large bulla on the thigh of a 91-year-old woman (*Figure 182-2; Reproduced with permission from Richard P. Usatine, MD*).

Bottom: Dactylitis (sausage fingers) in a woman with plaque psoriasis and psoriatic arthritis (*Figure 100-3; Reproduced with permission from Richard P. Usatine, MD*).

CONTENTS

CONTENTS

CONTENTS

PART 16

INFECTIOUS DISEASES

PART 17

ENDOCRINE

PART 18

NEUROLOGY

PART 19

SUBSTANCE ABUSE

APPENDICES

Cathy Abbott, MD
Assistant Professor
Department of Family Medicine
Michigan State University College of Human Medicine
East Lansing, Michigan

Oliver Abela, MD
Cardiovascular Fellow
University of Nevada
School of Medicine
Las Vegas, Nevada

Anna Allred, MD
Resident Physician
Department of Neurological Surgery
University of Texas South Western Medical Center
Dallas, Texas

Osama Alsara, MD
Chief Resident
Internal medicine program
Michigan State University
East Lansing, Michigan

Hend Azhary, MD
Assistant Professor
Department of Family Medicine
Michigan State University College of Human Medicine
East Lansing, Michigan

Michael Babcock, MD
Dermatologist
Colorado Springs Dermatology Clinic
Colorado Springs, Colorado

Yoon-Soo Cindy Bae-Harboe, MD
Boston University Hospital
Medical Center Department of Dermatology
Boston, Massachusetts

James C. Barrow, MD
Clinical Assistant Professor
Department of Obstetrics and Gynecology
Louisiana State University Health Center
Shreveport, Louisiana

Ruth E. Berggren, MD
Professor of Medicine
Division of Infectious Diseases
University of Texas Health Science Center
San Antonio, Texas

Margaret L. Burks, MD
Internal Medicine Resident
Vanderbilt University Medical Center
Nashville, Tennessee

Kevin J. Carter, MD
Assistant Professor
Department of Family Medicine
Louisiana State University Health Center
Shreveport, Louisiana

Gina R. Chacon, MD
Dermatology Resident
Marshfield Clinic - Marshfield Center
Marshfield, Wisconsin

Melissa M. Chan, MD
Family Practitioner
Sutter East Bay Medical Foundation
Albany, California

Satish Chandolu, MD
Hospitalist, Sparrow Hospital
Clinical Instructor
Michigan State University
East Lansing, Michigan

Pierre Chanoine, MD
Drexel University School of Medicine
Philadelphia, Pennsylvania
St. Christopher's Hospital for Children
Philadelphia, Pennsylvania

Thomas J. Corson, DO
Emergency Medicine
Banner Health Mckee Medical Center
Loveland, Colorado

John E. Delzell, Jr., MD, MSPH
Director, Medical Student Education
Associate Professor in Division of Family Medicine
Department of Humanities, Health, and Society
Herbert Wertheim College of Medicine
Florida International University
Miami, Florida

Rowena A. DeSouza, MD
Assistant Professor
Division of Urology
University of Texas Medical School at Houston
Houston, Texas

Lucia Diaz, MD
Chief Resident
Dermatology Department
University of Texas Medical School at Houston
MD Anderson Cancer Center
Houston, Texas

Hannah Ferenchick, MD
Resident, Emergency Medicine
Detroit Receiving Hospital
Detroit, Michigan

Lindsey B. Finklea, MD
Dermatologist
San Antonio, Texas

Javier LaFontaine, DPM, MS
Chief, Podiatry Section
Central Texas Veterans Health Care System
Temple, Texas

CONTRIBUTORS

Kelli Hejl Foulkrod, MS
Psychotherapist/Yoga Teacher
Psychology Center of Austin
Austin, Texas

Jeremy A. Franklin, MD
Director, Medical Sciences
MedImmune LLC
Lubbock, Texas

Radha Raman Murthy Gokula, MD, CMD
Geriatrician & Palliative Medicine Consultant
University of Toledo Medical Center
Assistant Professor
Department of Family Medicine
University of Toledo
Toledo, Ohio

Wanda C. Gonsalves, MD
Professor and Vice Chair
Department of Family and Community Medicine
University of Kentucky College of Medicine
Lexington, Kentucky

Venu Gourineni, MD
Cardiology fellow
Rush University Medical Center
Chicago, Illinois

Kelly Green, MD
Ophthalmology, Private Practice
Marble Falls, Texas
Clinical Assistant Professor
Department of Ophthalmology
University of Texas Health Science Center
San Antonio, Texas

Alfonso Guzman, MD
Family Physician
San Antonio, Texas

Churlson Han, MD
Assistant Professor of Internal Medicine
Michigan State University
East Lansing, Michigan

Meredith Hancock, MD
Preliminary Resident Internal Medicine
Loyola University Medical Center
Maywood, Illinois

Jimmy H. Hara, MD, FAAFP
Professor of Clinical Family Medicine
David Geffen School of Medicine at UCLA
Los Angeles, California

David Henderson, MD
Associate Professor, Department of Family Medicine
Associate Dean, Medical Student Affairs
University of Connecticut School of Medicine
Farmington, Connecticut

Nathan Hitzeman, MD
Faculty, Sutter Health Family Medicine Residency Program
Sacramento, California

Michaell A. Huber, DDS
Associate Professor
Oral Medicine Subject Expert
Department of Comprehensive Dentistry
University of Texas at San Antonio Health Science Center Dental School
San Antonio, Texas

Karen A. Hughes, MD, FAAFP
Associate Director
North Mississippi Center Family Medicine Residency Program
Tupelo, Mississippi

Khalilah Hunter-Anderson, MD
Assistant Professor
Department of Traumatology & Emergency Medicine
University of Connecticut Health Center
Farmington, Connecticut

Carlos Roberto Jaén, MD, PhD, MS
Professor and Chair of Family and Community Medicine
Professor of Epidemiology and Biostatistics
The Dr. and Mrs. James L. Holly Distinguished Professor
Scholar, ReACH (Research to Advance Community Health) Center
University of Texas Health Science Center at San Antonio
San Antonio, Texas

Natalia Jaimes, MD
Assistant Professor
Department of Dermatology
Universidad Pontificia Bolivariana
Attending Physician
Aurora Skin Cancer Center
Medellin, Colombia

Adeliza Jimenez, MD
Staff Physician
Southern California Permanente Medical Group
Downey, California

Anne E. Johnson, MD
Psychiatry Resident
University of Texas Southwestern
Dallas, Texas

Rajil M. Karnani, MD, MME
Assistant Professor of Internal Medicine
Michigan State University
East Lansing, Michigan

Jonathan B. Karnes, MD
Faculty
MDFMR Dermatology Services,
Main Dartmouth Family Medicine Residency
Augusta, Maine

Jennifer A. Keehbauch, MD, FAAFP
Director of Research, Graduate Medical Education
Florida Hospital
Assistant Director, Family Medicine, Residency, Florida Hospital
Director, Women's Medicine Fellowship, Florida Hospital
Orlando, Florida

Melanie Ketchandji, MD
Urology Resident
University of Texas Health Science Center
Houston, Texas

Amor Khachemoune, MD
Attending Physician, Dermatologist
Mohs Surgeon and Dermatopathologist
Veterans Affairs Medical Center
Brooklyn, New York

Joonseok Kim, MD
Fellow, Division of Cardiovascular Health and Disease
University of Cincinnati Medical Center
Cincinnati, Ohio

J. Michael King, MD
Otolaryngology, Head and Neck Surgery
Peak ENT and Voice Center
Boulder, Colorado

Robert Kraft, MD
Clinical Assistant Professor
Department of Family and Community Medicine
University of Kansas School of Medicine
Wichita, Kansas

Madhab Lamichhane, MD
Cardiovascular Diseases Fellow
Michigan State University
East Lansing, Michigan

Juanita Lozano-Pineda, DDS, MPH
Assistant Professor
Department of Comprehensive Dentistry
University of Texas at San Antonio Health Science
Center Dental School
San Antonio, Texas

Ashfaq A. Marghoob, MD
Associate Professor
Director, Skin Cancer Clinic, Hauppauge, Long Island
Memorial Sloan-Kettering Cancer Center
New York, New York

Angie Mathai, MD
Assistant Clinical Professor
East Carolina University
Greenville, North Carolina

Laura Matrka, MD
Assistant Professor
Department of Otolaryngology – Head and Neck Surgery
The Ohio State University Wexner Medical Center
Columbus, Ohio

Carolyn Milana, MD
Assistant Professor of Pediatrics
Stony Brook Long Island Children's Hospital
Stony Brook, New York

Shashi Mittal, MD
Family Physician
MedFirst Northeast Primary Care Clinic
San Antonio, Texas

Asad K. Mohmand, MD, FACP
VCU Pauley Heart Center
Medical College of Virginia
Virginia Commonwealth University
Richmond, Virginia

Melissa Muszynski, MD
Resident, Department of Dermatology
Georgetown University Hospital
Washington Hospital Center
Washington DC

Anjeli Nayar, MD
Assistant Professor of Medicine
Uniformed Services University of the Health Sciences Medical School
Staff Physician, Internal Medicine
Department of San Antonio Military Medical Center
San Antonio, Texas

Priyank Patel, MD
Hematology Oncology Fellow,
Roswell Park Cancer Institute,
University at Buffalo,
Buffalo, New York

Richard Paulis, MD
Emergency Medicine
Rochester General Hospital
Atlanta, Georgia

Deepthi Rao, MD
Fellow
Division of Endocrinology
Michigan State University
East Lansing, Michigan

Brian Z. Rayala, MD
Assistant Professor
Department of Family Medicine
University of North Carolina School of Medicine
Chapel Hill, North Carolina

Supratik Rayamajhi, MD
Assistant Professor of Internal Medicine
Director, Advanced Medicine Clerkship
Michigan State University
East Lansing, Michigan

Suraj Reddy, MD
Dermatology
Albuquerque Dermatology Associates
Albuquerque, New Mexico

CONTRIBUTORS

Katie Reppa, MD
Resident
University of Pittsburgh
Pittsburgh, Pennsylvania

Karl T. Rew, MD
Assistant Professor of Family Medicine and Urology
University of Michigan Medical School
Ann Arbor, Michigan

Michelle Rowe, DO
Family Medicine
San Joaquin General Hospital
French Camp, California

Khashayar Sarabi, MD
Internal & Integrative Medicine
Irvine, California

Shehnaz Zaman Sarmast, MD
Dermatologist, Skin Specialist
Allen/Addison, Texas

Ana Treviño Sauceda, MD
Assistant Clinical Professor
Dermatology and Cutaneous Surgery
University of Texas Health Science Center San Antonio
San Antonio, Texas

Andrew D. Schechtman, MD, FAAFP
Adjunct Clinical Assistant Professor
Stanford University School of Medicine
Division of General Medical Disciplines
Faculty, San Jose-O'Connor Hospital Family Medicine Residency Program
San Jose, California

Angela Shedd, MD
Dermatopathology Fellow
ProPath
Dallas, Texas

Maureen K. Sheehan, MD, MHA
Associate Professor, Division of Vascular Surgery
University of Texas Health Science Center San Antonio,
San Antonio, Texas

Naohiro Shibuya, DPM, MS, FACFAS
Associate Professor of Surgery
Texas A&M Health and Science Center
College of Medicine
Bryan, Texas

C. Blake Simpson, MD
Professor, Department of Otolaryngology, Head and Neck Surgery
University of Texas Health Science Center
San Antonio, Texas

Linda Speer, MD
Professor and Chair
Department of Family Medicine
University of Toledo College of Medicine and Life Sciences
Toledo, Ohio

Ernest Valdez, DDS
Assistant Professor
Department of Oral and Maxillofacial Surgery
University of Texas Health Science Center at San Antonio
San Antonio, Texas

Yu Wah, MD
Assistant Professor
Department of Family and Community Medicine
University of Texas Health Science Center at Houston
Houston, Texas

Mark L. Willenbring, MD
Founder and CEO, ALLTYR
Saint Paul, Minnesota

Brian Williams, MD
Brian J. Williams Dermatology, Private Practice
Midvale, Utah

Bonnie Wong, MD
Assistant Professor of Clinical Family Medicine
Indiana University, School of Medicine
Indianapolis, Indiana

Jana K. Zaudke, MD
Assistant Professor
Department of Family Medicine
University of Kansas School of Medicine
Kansas City, Kansas

Internists see a wide variety of diseases and conditions including cardiovascular, dermatologic, endocrine, gastrointestinal, and rheumatologic disorders. This comprehensive atlas that aids in diagnosis, using visible signs and internal imaging, can be of tremendous value. We have assembled more than 2000 outstanding clinical images for this very purpose, and are proud to present the first edition of a modern comprehensive atlas of Internal Medicine. Some photographs will amaze you; all will inform you about the various conditions that befall our patients.

It took a number of people many years to create the first edition of ***The Color Atlas of Internal Medicine***. For me (Dr. Usatine) as the lead editor, it is a lifelong work that started with little notebooks I kept in my white coat pocket to take notes during my residency. It then took on color when I began keeping a camera at work and taking photographs with my patient's permission of any interesting clinical finding that I might use to teach medical students and residents the art and science of medicine. I was inspired by many great physicians, including Dr. Jimmy Hara, who had the most amazing 35-mm slide collection of clinical images. His knowledge of medicine is encyclopedic and I thought that his taking photographs might have something to do with that. Also, I realized that these photographs would greatly enhance my teaching of others. As I began to expand my practice to see more dermatology cases, my photograph collection skyrocketed. Digital photography made it more affordable and practical to take and catalogue many new images.

The Color Atlas of Internal Medicine is written for internists and all health care providers involved in caring for adults. It can also be invaluable to medical students, residents, and dermatologists.

The Color Atlas of Internal Medicine is also available electronically for iPad, iPhone, iPod touch, all Android devices, Kindle, and on the web through Access Medicine. These electronic versions will allow health care providers to access the images and content rapidly at the point-of-care.

The Color Atlas of Internal Medicine is for anyone who loves to look at clinical photographs for learning, teaching, and practicing medicine. The first chapter begins with an introduction to learning with images and digital photography. The core of the book focuses on medical conditions organized by anatomic and physiologic systems. There are special sections devoted to the essence of Internal Medicine, physical/sexual abuse, women's health, and substance abuse.

The collection of clinical images is supported by evidence-based information that will help the health care provider to diagnose and manage common medical problems. The text is concisely presented with many easy-to-access bullets as a quick point-of-care reference. Each chapter begins with a patient story that ties the photographs to the real life stories of our patients. The photographic legends are also designed to connect the images to the people and their human conditions. Strength of recommendation ratings are cited throughout so that the science of medicine can be blended with the art of medicine for optimal patient care.

Because knowledge continues to advance after any book is written, use the online resources presented in many of the chapters to keep up with the newest changes in medicine. Care deeply about your patients and enjoy your practice, as it is a privilege to be a health care provider and healer.

ACKNOWLEDGMENTS

This book could not have been completed without the contributions of many talented physicians, health care professionals, and photographers. We received photographs from people who live and work across the globe. Each photograph is labeled and acknowledges the photographer and contributor. There are some people who contributed so many photographs; it is appropriate to acknowledge them upfront in the book. Paul Comeau was the professional ophthalmology photographer at University of Texas Health Science Center San Antonio (UTHSCSA). His beautiful photographs of the external and internal eye make the ophthalmology section of this book so rich and valuable. The dermatology division at UTHSCSA contributed much of their expertise in photography, writing, and reviewing the extensive dermatology section. During the last few years, I was fortunate to work closely with the dermatology faculty and residents and they contributed generously to our book. Dr. Eric Kraus, the program director, gave us many wonderful photographs, especially for the section on bullous diseases. He also gave us open access to the 35-mm slides collected by the Division of Dermatology. Dr. Jeff Meffert also contributed photographs to many chapters. Dr. Jack Resneck, Sr., from Louisiana, scanned his slides from more than 40 years of practice and gave them to Dr. E.J. Mayeaux, Jr., for use. Dr. Resneck's vast dermatologic experiences add to our atlas.

The UTHSCSA Head and Neck Department contributed many photographs for this book. We especially thank Dr. Frank Miller and Dr. Blake Simpson for their contributions. Dr. Dan Stulberg, a physician from New Mexico, with a passion for photography and dermatology, contributed many photographs throughout our book.

We thank our trainees, many of whom coauthored chapters with us. UTHSCSA medical students and residents and fellows from Michigan State University's Primary Care Faculty Development Fellowship program coauthored chapters and contributed photographs with great enthusiasm to the creation of this work. It was a pleasure to mentor these young writers and experience with them the rewards of authorship. Dr. Usatine is thankful for the contributions of his "Underserved Dermatology Fellows." Working closely with such brilliant and caring doctors in our Skin Clinic and free outreach clinics allowed me to learn from them while doing my best to advance their academic and humanistic careers.

Of course, we would have no book without the talented writing and editing of my coeditors, Drs. Gary Ferenchick, Mindy A. Smith, E.J. Mayeaux, and Heidi S. Chumley. They each bring years of clinical and educational experience to the writing of the *Atlas*. Dr. Mayeaux contributed many of his own photographs, especially in women's health care, to our *Atlas*.

Most of all we need to thank our patients who generously gave their permission for their photographs to be taken and published in this book. While some photos are not recognizable, we have many photos of the full face that are very recognizable and were generously given to us by our patients with full written permission to be published as is. For photographs that were taken decades ago in which written consents were no longer available, we have used bars across the eyes to make the photos less recognizable—verbal consent was always obtained for these images.

The last section of this book is dedicated to understanding substance abuse (chemical dependency) and its treatment. This could not have been done without the generous contributions of the dedicated staff and the women residents at Alpha Home, a nonprofit alcohol and drug treatment program in San Antonio. The medical students and faculty from UTHSCSA spend 2 to 3 evenings a week providing free health care to these women who are bravely facing their addictions and fighting to stay sober 1 day at a time. Their pictures have been generously added to our book with their permission.

I (Dr. Richard Usatine) thank my family for giving me the support to see this book through. It has taken much time from my family life and my family has supported me through the long nights and weekends it takes to write a book while continuing to practice and teach medicine. I am fortunate to have a loving wife, successful son, wonderful daughter, great son-in-law, and one very cute grandson who add meaning to my life and allowed me to work hard on the creation of this *Color Atlas*.

Dr Gary Ferenchick adds, "I want to acknowledge and thank my children Hannah Ferenchick, MD who contributed to this atlas and my son Jesse, both of whom are embarking on writing their own life stories. Also, I am grateful to my lovely wife Carol, whose support makes my life much easier and who is one of my life's bedrocks."

Dr. Mindy Smith adds, "I thank my late husband, Gary Crakes, and daughter, Jenny, for their support and willingness to listen when I struggle with phrasing and wording in my writing and editing. I also thank several colleagues who have helped me to establish myself as an editor and supported my continued growth in this field—Drs. Barry Weiss, Mark Ebell, Richard Usatine, Suzanne Sorkin, and Leslie Shimp."

Dr. E.J. Mayeaux adds, "I thank my wife and family for understanding the many hours of work and computer time it takes to produce this work. I would like to dedicate this work to Mr. Bob (Papa Bob) Mitchell who can always find the funny angle to any situation and who gave me my partner and love of my life. I would also like to thank my new work family at the Department of Family and Preventive Medicine at the University of South Carolina School of Medicine in Columbia. We are going to do great things!"

Dr. Heidi Chumley adds, "I want to thank my husband, John Delzell, who has brought love and peace to my often chaotic life, and my children, Cullen, Sierra, David, Selene, and Jack, who give me joy and provide the incentive to stay on task. Each one, in turn, has cheerfully pitched in to help a grumpy and tired mom who stayed up most of the night working on one of many chapters. I have been very blessed."

Finally, we all thank James Shanahan and Harriet Lebowitz from McGraw-Hill for believing in this project and guiding us through to completion. Our gratitude also extends to Hardik Popli for his dedicated work on this book.

PART 1

LEARNING WITH IMAGES AND DIGITAL PHOTOGRAPHY

Strength of Recommendation (SOR)	Definition
A	Recommendation based on consistent and good-quality patient-oriented evidence.*
B	Recommendation based on inconsistent or limited-quality patient-oriented evidence.*
C	Recommendation based on consensus, usual practice, opinion, disease-oriented evidence, or case series for studies of diagnosis, treatment, prevention, or screening.*

*See Appendix A on pages 1241-1244 for further information.

1 AN ATLAS TO ENHANCE PATIENT CARE, LEARNING, AND TEACHING

Richard P. Usatine, MD

People only see what they are prepared to see.

—Ralph Waldo Emerson

Whether you are viewing **Figure 1-1** in a book, in an aquarium, or in the sea, you immediately recognize the image as a fish. Those of you who are more schooled in the classification of fish might recognize that this is an angelfish with the tail resembling the head of the angel and the posterior fins representing the wings. If you are truly prepared to see this fish in all its splendor, you would see the blue circle above its eye as the crown of the queen angelfish.

Making a diagnosis in medicine often involves the kind of pattern recognition needed to identify a queen angelfish. This is much the same as recognizing a beautiful bird or the painting of a favorite artist. If you are prepared to look for the clues that lead to the identification (diagnosis), you will see what needs to be seen. How can we be best prepared to see these clues? There is nothing more valuable than seeing an image or a patient who has the condition in question at least once before you encounter it on your own. The memory of a powerful visual image can become hardwired into your brain for ready recall.

In medicine, it also helps to know where and how to look to find the clues you may need when the diagnosis cannot be made at a single glance. For example, a patient with inverse psoriasis may present with a rash under the breast that has been repeatedly and unsuccessfully treated with antifungal agents for candidiasis or tinea (**Figures 1-2** and **1-3**). The prepared clinician knows that not all erythematous plaques under the breast are fungal and looks for clues such as nail changes (**Figures 1-2** and **1-4**) or scaling erythematous plaques around the elbows, knees, or umbilicus (see **Figure 1-3**). Knowing where to look and what to look for is how an experienced clinician makes the diagnosis of psoriasis.

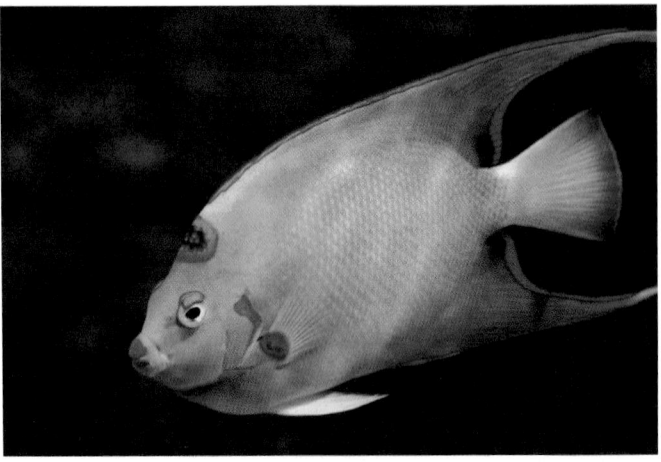

FIGURE 1-1 Queen angelfish (Holacanthus ciliaris). *(Reproduced with permission from Sam Thekkethil. http://www.flickr.com/photos/natureloving.)*

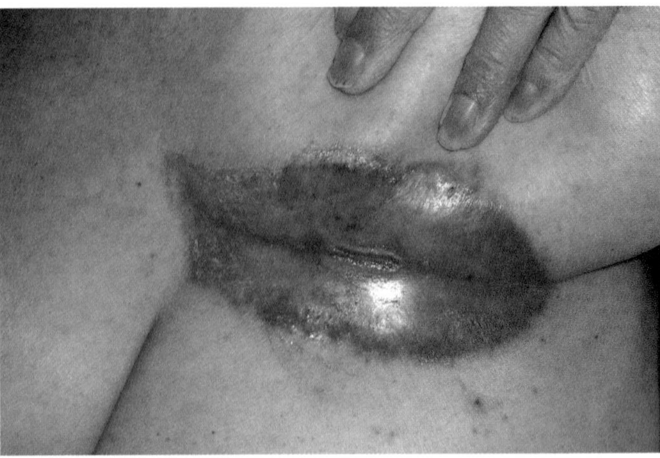

FIGURE 1-2 Inverse psoriasis under the breast that might appear to be a fungal infection to the untrained eye. Note the splinter hemorrhages in the nail of the third digit that provide a clue that the patient has psoriasis. *(Reproduced with permission from Richard P. Usatine, MD.)*

USING OUR SENSES

As physicians we collect clinical data through sight, sound, touch, and smell. Although physicians in the past used taste to collect data, such as tasting the sweet urine of a patient with diabetes, this sense is rarely, if ever, used in modern medicine. We listen to heart sounds, lung sounds, bruits, and percussion notes to collect information for diagnoses. We touch our patients to feel lumps, bumps, thrills, and masses. We occasionally use smell for diagnosis. Unfortunately, the odors of disease are rarely pleasant. Even the fruity odors of *Pseudomonas* are not like the sweet fruits of a farmers' market. Of course, we also use the patient's history, laboratory data, and more advanced imaging techniques to diagnose and manage patients' illnesses.

It was our belief in the value of visual imagery that led to the development of *The Color Atlas of Internal Medicine*. We are pleased to provide more than 2000 images to you and doctors around the world as a large, color textbook and as an interactive electronic application for easy use on the iPhone, iPod Touch, iPad, and all android devices.

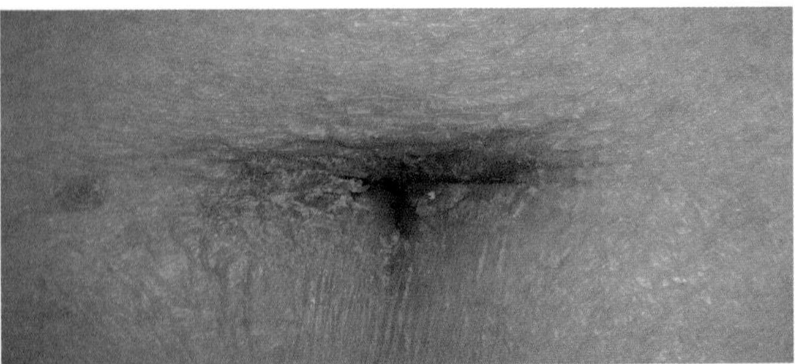

FIGURE 1-3 The patient in Figure 1-2 with inverse psoriasis had a typical psoriatic plaque in the umbilicus. This was the only other area involved besides the breasts and the nails but easily could have been missed without the knowledge of where to look for the clues needed to make the diagnosis. *(Reproduced with permission from Richard P. Usatine, MD.)*

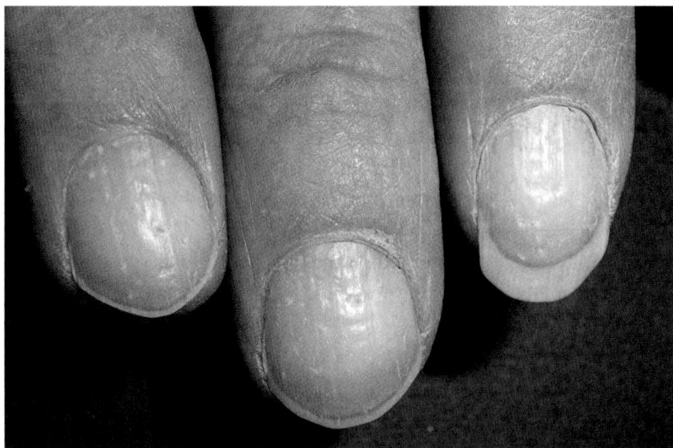

FIGURE 1-4 When the diagnosis of psoriasis is being considered, look at the nails for pitting or other nail changes such as splinter hemorrhages, onycholysis, or oil spots. This is a good example of nail pitting in a patient with psoriasis. (*Reproduced with permission from Richard P. Usatine, MD.*)

EXPANDING OUR INTERNAL IMAGE BANKS

The larger our saved image bank in our brain, the better clinicians and diagnosticians we can become. The expert clinician has a large image bank stored in memory to call on for rapid pattern recognition. Our image banks begin to develop in medical school when we view pictures in lectures and textbooks. We then begin to develop our own clinical image bank through our clinical experiences. Our references are printed color atlases, as well as those available on the Internet and electronically.

Studying and learning the patterns from any atlas can enhance your expertise by enlarging the image bank stored in your memory. An atlas takes the clinical experiences of clinicians over decades and gives it to you as a single reference. We offer you, for the first time in the United States, a modern, comprehensive internal medicine color atlas, which includes areas such as oral health, dermatology, podiatry, and the eye.

USING IMAGES TO MAKE A DIAGNOSIS

We all see visible clinical findings on patients that we do not recognize. When this happens, open this book and look for a close match. Use the appendix, index, or table of contents to direct you to the section with the highest-yield photos. If you find a direct match, you may have found the diagnosis. Read the text and see if the history and physical examination match your patient. Perform or order tests to confirm the diagnosis, if needed.

If you cannot find the image in our book try the Internet and the Google search engine. Try a Google image search and follow the leads. Of course this is easiest to do if you have a good differential diagnosis and want to confirm your impression. If you do not have a diagnosis in mind, you may try entering descriptive words and looking for an image that matches what you are seeing. If the Google image search does not work, try a Web search and look at the links for other clues.

Finally, there are dedicated atlases on the Internet for organ systems that can help you find the needed image. Most of these atlases have their own search engines, which can help direct you to the right diagnosis.

Table 1-1 lists some of the best resources currently available online.

USING IMAGES TO BUILD TRUST IN THE PATIENT–PHYSICIAN RELATIONSHIP

If you are seeing a patient with a mysterious illness that remains undiagnosed and you figure out the diagnosis, you can often bridge the issues of mistrust and anxiety by showing the patient the picture of another person with the diagnosis. Use our atlas for that purpose and supplement it with the Internet. This is especially important for a patient who has gone undiagnosed or misdiagnosed for some time. "Seeing is believing" for many patients. Ask first if they would want to see some pictures of other persons with a similar condition; most will be very interested. The patient can see the similarities between their condition and the other images and feel reassured that your diagnosis is correct. Write down the name of the diagnosis for your patient and use your patient education skills.

TABLE 1-1 Excellent Clinical Image Collections on the Internet

Derm Atlas	www.dermatlas.org	Johns Hopkins University
DermIS	www.dermis.net	Derm Information Systems from Germany
Dermnet	www.dermnet.com	Skin Disease Image Atlas
Interactive Derm Atlas	www.dermatlas.net	From Richard P. Usatine, MD
ENT	www.entusa.com	From an ENT physician
Eye	www.eyerounds.org	University of Iowa
Figure Search	http://figuresearch.askhermes.org	University of Wisconsin
Images of all types	http://commons.wikimedia.org	Wikimedia Commons
Infectious Diseases	www.phil.cdc.gov	CDC Public Health Image Library
Radiology	http://rad.usuhs.edu/medpix/	MedPix
Skinsight	http://www.skinsight.com/html	Logical Images

Do be careful when searching for images on the Web in the presence of patients. Sometimes what pops up is not pretty (or, for that matter, G- or PG-rated). I turn the screen away from the patient before initiating the search and then censor what I will show them.

If you teach, model this behavior in front of your students. Show them how reference books and the Internet at the point of care can help with the care of patients.

TAKING YOUR OWN PHOTOGRAPHS

Images taken by you with your own camera of your own patients complete with their own stories are more likely to be retained and retrievable in your memory because they have a context and a story to go with them. We encourage our readers to use a digital camera (within a smartphone or a stand-alone camera) and consider taking your own photos. Of course, always ask permission before taking any photograph of a patient. Explain how the photographs can be used to teach other doctors and to create a record of the patient's condition at this point in time. If the photograph will be identifiable, ask for written consent; for patients younger than age 18 years, ask the parent to sign. Store the photos in a manner that avoids any Health Insurance Portability and Accountability Act (HIPAA) privacy violations, such as on a secure server or on your own computer with password protection and data encryption. These photographs can directly benefit the patient when, for example, following nevi for changes.

Digital photography is a wonderful method for practicing, teaching, and learning medicine. You can show patients pictures of conditions on parts of their bodies that they could not see without multiple mirrors and some unusual body contortions. You can also use the zoom view feature on the camera or smartphone to view or show a segment of the image in greater detail. Children generally love to have their photos taken and will be delighted to see themselves on the screen of your camera.

The advent of digital photography makes the recording of photographic images less expensive, easier to do, and easier to maintain. Digital photography also gives you immediate feedback and a sense of immediate gratification. No longer do you have to wait for a roll of film to be completed and processed before finding out the results of your photography. Not only does this give you immediate gratification to see your image displayed instantaneously in the camera, but also alerts you to poor-quality photographs that can be retaken while the patient is still in the office. This speeds up the learning curve of the beginning photographer in a way that could not happen with film photography.

OUR GOALS

Many of the images in this atlas are from my collected works over the past 27 years of my practice in medicine. My patients have generously allowed me to photograph them so that their photographs would help the physicians and patients of the future. To these photos, we have added images that represent decades of experiences by other physicians and specialists. Physicians who have submitted their images to "Photo Rounds" in the *Journal of Family Practice* are also sharing their photos with you. Finally, 12 years of providing students with cameras during their clerkships at the University of California at Los Angeles (UCLA) and the University of Texas Health Sciences Center at San Antonio (UTHSCSA) have allowed our students to add their experiences to our atlas.

It is the goal of this atlas to provide you with a wide range of images of common and uncommon conditions and provide you with the knowledge you need to make the diagnosis and initiate treatment. We want to help you to be the best diagnostician you can be. We may aspire to be a clinician like Sir William Osler and have the detective acumen of Sherlock Holmes. The images collected for this atlas can help move you in that direction by making you prepared to see what you need to see.

PART 2

ISSUES IN INTERNAL MEDICINE

Strength of Recommendation (SOR)	Definition
A	Recommendation based on consistent and good-quality patient-oriented evidence.*
B	Recommendation based on inconsistent or limited-quality patient-oriented evidence.*
C	Recommendation based on consensus, usual practice, opinion, disease-oriented evidence, or case series for studies of diagnosis, treatment, prevention, or screening.*

*See Appendix A on pages 1241-1244 for further information.

2 DOCTOR–PATIENT RELATIONSHIP

Mindy A. Smith, MD, MS

Humor is one way through which patients and physicians relate to each other on a human level. Even politics is not off-limits in the doctor–patient relationship.

PATIENT STORY

Patient stories, particularly if we listen attentively and nonjudgmentally, provide us with a window into their lives and experiences. These stories help us to know our patients in powerful ways, and that knowledge about the patient, as someone special, provides the context, meaning, and clues about their symptoms and illnesses that can lead to healing. At our best, we serve as witness to their struggles and triumphs, supporter of their efforts to change and grow, and guide through the medical maze of diagnostic and therapeutic options. Sometimes, their stories become our own stories—those patients who we will never forget because their stories have changed our lives and the way we practice medicine (**Figure 2-1**).

WHAT PATIENTS WANT FROM THEIR PHYSICIAN

Based on 2002 telephone interviews of the general public ($N = 1031$),[1] most patients strongly agreed that they wanted to take an active role in their health care (82% and 91%, patients with family physicians and patients with general internists, respectively), they wanted

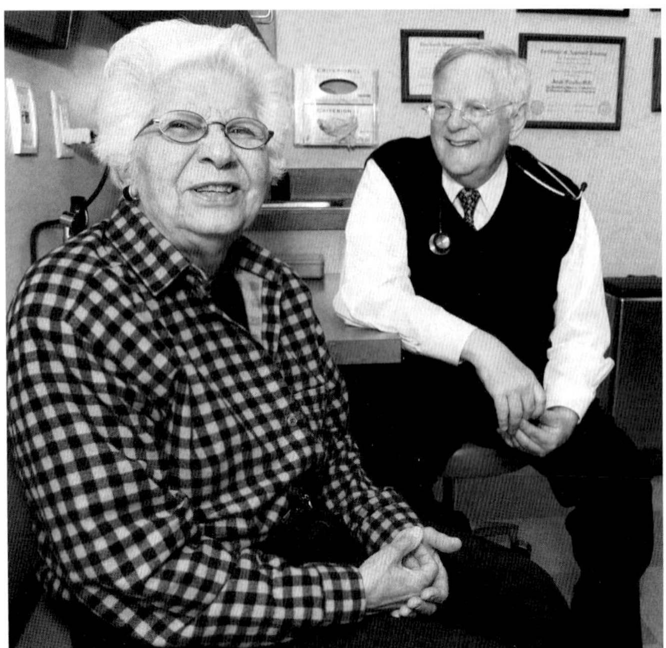

FIGURE 2-1 Dr. Jerry Winakur and Lydia Guild are enjoying a recent visit, one of many in their 30-year relationship as doctor and patient. They have each had their trials and joys over the decades and now find that they have grown old together. (*Reproduced with permission from Jeffrey M. Levine, MD*)

their physicians to treat a wide variety of medical problems but refer to a specialist when necessary (88% and 84%), and they wanted a physician who looks at the whole person—emotional, psychological, and physical (73% and 74%). In addition, of 39 possible attributes of physicians, most patients (68-97% stated extremely or very important) viewed the following as the most important attributes or services that drive overall satisfaction with their physician:

- Does not judge; understands and supports.
- Always honest, direct.
- Acts as partner in maintaining health.
- Treats both serious and nonserious conditions.
- Attends to emotional and physical health.
- Listens to me.
- Encourages healthier lifestyle.
- Tries to get to know me.
- Can help with any problem.
- Someone I can stay with as I get older.

WHAT PHYSICIANS WANT FROM AND FOR PATIENTS

Although the types and intensity of relationships with patients differ, our positive and negative experiences with patients shape us as clinicians, influence us in our personal relationships, and shape the character of our practices. Arthur Kleinman, in his prologue to *Patients and Doctors: Life-Changing Stories from Primary Care*, wrote, “We all seem to want (or demand) experiences that matter, but maybe what is foremost is that we want experiences in which *we* matter.” There is perhaps no greater satisfaction than the belief that what we do and who we are matters to those we care for in both our personal and professional lives.[2] A positive relationship with a patient is one of mutual growth. This concept of doctor–patient reciprocity is not new and can be found in the writings of Erasmus, more than 500 years ago, arising from a classical conception of friendship.[3]

As clinicians we want patients to be healthier and improved in some meaningful way after our encounter with them. Meaningful elements common to healing practices across cultures include the following[4]:

- Providing a meaningful explanation for the sickness
- Expressing care and concern
- Offering the possibility of mastery and control over the illness or its symptoms

Family physicians ($n = 300$) who were interviewed as part of the future of family medicine (FFM) initiative stated that the following things completely captured the essence of what they found as most satisfying about being a family physician[1]:

- The strong relationships developed with patients over the years (54%).
- The variety—no day is ever the same (54%).
- Offers me a strong sense of purpose because I can make a real difference in people’s lives (48%).
- Don’t spend their days taking care of illness, but take care of the whole patient (**Figure 2-2**) (46%).

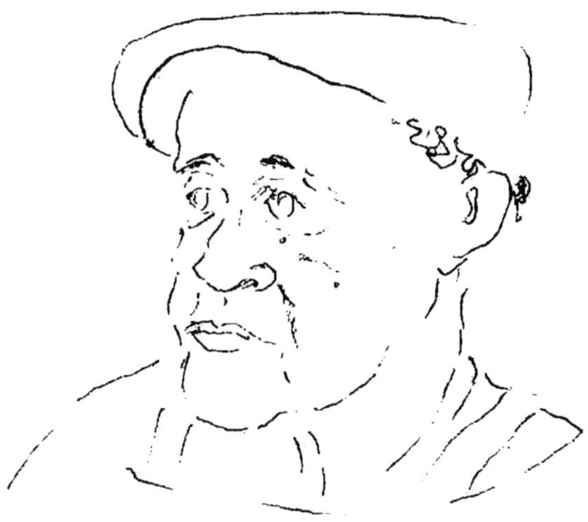

FIGURE 2-2 Dr. Alan Blum is a physician who has been doing sketches of his patients for decades now. When he presents his drawings, he reads his poetic stories that go with the drawings. Some of his drawings have been published in *JAMA*. Here is the poem that goes with this man's story:

"Gov'ment gave me a chance
to get a hearin' aid for free.
But when I went to th' doctor,
he say,
'Well, cap'n,
there gonna be a lot o' things
you don't want to hear!'"

LEARNING FROM PATIENTS

To learn from patients, clinicians must do the following:

- Move outside of their worldview and accept the patient's point of view and belief system.
- Let go of stereotypes, biases, and dogma.
- Use active empathic listening, see the patient in context, and adopt reflective and reflexive practices.[5]
- Emphasize patient dignity and control within a supportive team, which may include family, friends, aides, and community resources.
- Accept differences of opinion or patient refusal graciously without abandoning the patient.
- Look at each patient encounter as a cross-cultural event.[4] Western medical training acculturates clinicians into a world seen in large part as one of problems and solutions; this is often at odds with patients' need to find meaning in the illness episode, be heard and acknowledged, and learn to live a quality life with chronic illness.

BENEFITS OF A GOOD DOCTOR–PATIENT RELATIONSHIP

Beyond the benefit of enhancing the medical experience for both clinicians and patients, data that support developing a good doctor–patient relationship include the following:

- Patients who are satisfied with their physicians are 3 times more likely to follow a prescribed medical regimen.[6]
- Patients with diabetes cared for by physicians with high empathy scores (based on the physician's self-administered Jefferson Scale of Empathy) were significantly more likely to have good control based on hemoglobin A_{1C} than were patients of physicians with low empathy scores (56% and 40%, respectively).[7]
- Patients who reported an established relationship with a primary care provider (PCP) were less likely to currently smoke than those who lacked a PCP relationship (26.5% and 62.3%, respectively).[8]
- There is a direct link between patient satisfaction and the amount of information that physicians provide.[9,10]
- There is also a strong positive correlation between patient satisfaction, recall, and understanding and physician's partnership building (eg, enlisting patient input).[10]
- Provision of health information to patients influences patient decision making in important ways.

ESSENTIALS OF GOOD DOCTOR–PATIENT RELATIONSHIP

Although the doctor–patient relationship may be viewed as a contract for providing services, Dr. Candib argues that this view does not fit well with developing a healing relationship that must be based on "unconditional positive regard," beneficence, caring, and a moral basis of conduct.[11] Furthermore, contracts fail to deal with the unpredictable and fail to acknowledge the power inequality between physicians and patients. To counter this power imbalance, Candib emphasizes the need for clinicians to use that power to empower the patient. Following are the requirements of empowerment of patients[12]:

- Recognition of oppression—Acknowledging the patient's contextual problems (eg, poverty, race, religion, sexual preference) and the sources of inequality and oppression that contribute to their health status for the purpose of naming and supporting the patient's reality.
- Expressing empathy—A characteristic of being with the patient that leads to empowerment by confirming the worthiness of the other.
- Respecting the patient as a person (particularly those who are cognitively or otherwise impaired).
- Responding to the changing abilities of the patient—Using flexibility, timing, and a shifting of skills to advance the movement of the patient in a positive direction.
- Using language that increases patient's power—Solicit and legitimize the patient's explanations and experience. This may include using questions about what patients want from the encounter, what they think about their problem, what they think the clinician should do about the problem, and what they have tried that has worked for them in the past.
- Taking the patient seriously—This includes respecting the patients' fears, not trivializing their concerns, and allowing the truth to unfold over time to prevent harm or embarrassment to the patient.
- Supporting choice and control—Accepting patients' priorities, even if health is not the top one, and allowing patients to choose, even if their choice is to relinquish control.
- Eliciting the patient's story, often over time, to be able to put the illness experience into historical and social context.
- Providing patient education in a context in which the clinician asks what the patient already knows, what they want and need to know, and whether they have any questions. Health educators should discuss risks and benefits of a proposed diagnostic or treatment plan

that are meaningful to the patient and provide patients with the tools and information to make their own decisions.

Some patients prefer to delegate authority to the physician to make medical decisions; the challenge then is for the physician to find out the patient's preferences and values.

Caring is also an essential feature of a good doctor–patient relationship. Caring, as connectedness with a patient, evolves from the relationship. Within the context of this relationship, the clinician makes the patient feel known, pays attention to the meaning that a symptom or illness has in the patient's life, expresses real feeling (separate from reflecting back the patient's feelings), and practices devotion (eg, a willingness at times to do something extra for the patient).[13] To provide care to patients, clinicians must take care of themselves.

SKILLS FOR BUILDING GOOD DOCTOR–PATIENT RELATIONSHIPS

- One strategy for improving communication with patients is using the patient-centered interview.[14] This technique focuses on eliciting the patient's agenda in order to address their concerns more promptly.
- Incorporating the BATHE (Background, Affect, Trouble and Handling of their current situation, and Empathy) method into the standard patient interview was found to increase 8 of 11 measures of patient satisfaction.[15]
- Using self-disclosure for the purposes of role modeling and guiding, showing empathy, building trust, and developing a stronger relationship in the context of shared assumptions about the relationship are some of the other strategies. Self-disclosure, however, must be balanced with the obligation of not to take advantage of patients by using such disclosure as an appeal for help or intimacy.[16] In addition, it may be prudent to avoid disclosure of unresolved issues and to avoid repetitiousness (as when disclosure predominates over inquiry).

MAXIMIZING THE EFFECTIVENESS OF PATIENT EDUCATION

Steps for maximizing patient education for behavior change include the following[17]:

- Understanding the power of the clinician's expertise as a motivator toward behavior change.
- Being patient centered and patient responsive (eg, assess readiness to change, patient wishes for autonomy or assistance in decision making).
- Encouraging the patient to choose one or at most 2 behavior goals at a time.
- Being specific in the advice given.
- Obtaining commitment from the patient for change.
- Using multiple educational strategies, often over time and from a team of providers.
- Using social support when possible.
- Assuring appropriate follow-up.

Some guidance can be found in the literature for discussing clinical evidence with patients in the process of making medical decisions. Despite lack of clinical outcomes from this research, authors of a systematic review found the following[18]:

- Methods for communicating clinical evidence to patients include non-quantitative general terms, numerical translation of clinical evidence, graphical representations, and decision-making aids.
- Focus-group data suggested that clinicians present options and/or equipoise before asking patients about preferred decision-making roles or formats for information.
- Absolute risk reduction is preferred.
- The order of information presented and the time frame of outcomes can bias patient understanding.
- Limited evidence supports use of human stick figure graphics or faces for single probabilities and vertical bar graphs for comparative information.
- Less-educated and older patients preferred proportions to percentages and did not appreciate confidence intervals.

REFERENCES

1. American Academy of Family Physicians. *Future of Family Medicine Project*. http://www.aafp.org/online/en/home/membership/initiatives/futurefamilymed.html. Accessed March 2012.
2. Kleinman A. Prologue. In: Borkan J, Reis S, Steinmetz D, Medalie JH, eds. *Patients and Doctors: Life-Changing Stories from Primary Care*. Madison, WI: University of Wisconsin Press; 1999:ix.
3. Albury WR, Weisz GM. The medical ethics of Erasmus and the physician-patient relationship. *Med Humanit*. 2001;27(1):35-41.
4. Brody H. Family and community—reflections. In: Borkan J, Reis S, Steinmetz D, Medalie JH, eds. *Patients and Doctors: Life-Changing Stories from Primary Care*. Madison, WI: University of Wisconsin Press; 1999:67-72.
5. Medalie JH. Learning from patients—reflections. In: Borkan J, Reis S, Steinmetz D, Medalie JH, eds. *Patients and Doctors: Life-changing Stories from Primary Care*. Madison, WI: University of Wisconsin Press; 1999:50.
6. Rosenberg EE, Lussier MT, Beaudoin C. Lessons for clinicians from physician-patient communication literature. *Arch Fam Med*. 1997;6(3):279-283.
7. Hojat M, Louis DZ, Markham FW, et al. Physicians' empathy and clinical outcomes for diabetic patients. *Acad Med*. 2011;86(3):359-364.
8. DePew Z, Gossman W, Morrow LE. Association of primary care physician relationship and insurance status with reduced rates of tobacco smoking. *Chest*. 2010;138(5):1278-1279.
9. Blanchard CG, Labrecque MS, Ruckdeschel JC, Blanchard EB. Physician behaviors, patient perceptions, and patient characteristics as predictors of satisfaction of hospitalized adult cancer patients. *Cancer*. 1991;65(1):186-192.
10. Hall JA, Roter KL, Katz NR. Meta-analysis of correlates of provider behavior in medical encounters. *Med Care*. 1988;26(7):657-675.
11. Candib LM. *Medicine and the Family—A Feminist Perspective*. New York, NY: Basic Books; 1995:119-145.
12. Candib LM. *Medicine and the Family—A Feminist Perspective*. New York, NY: Basic Books; 1995:246-273.
13. Candib LM. *Medicine and the Family—A Feminist Perspective*. New York, NY: Basic Books; 1995:206-239.

14. Brown J, Stewart M, McCracken E, McWhinney IR, Levenstein J. The patient-centered clinical method. 2. Definition and application. *Fam Pract.* 1986;3(2):75-79.

15. Leiblum SR, Schnall E, Seehuus M, DeMaria A. To BATHE or not to BATHE: patient satisfaction with visits to their family physician. *Fam Med.* 2008;40(6):407-411.

16. Candib LM. *Medicine and the Family—A Feminist Perspective*. New York, NY: Basic Books; 1995:181-205.

17. Jaques LB, Curtis P, Goldstein AO. Helping your patients stay healthy. In: Sloane PD, Slatt LM, Ebell MH, Jacques LB, eds. *Essentials of Family Medicine*. Baltimore, MD: Lippincott Williams & Wilkins; 2002:117-125.

18. Epstein RM, Alper BS, Quill TE. Communicating evidence for participatory decision making. *JAMA*. 2004;291(19):2359-2366.

3 FAMILY PLANNING

E.J. Mayeaux Jr., MD
James Barrow, MD

PATIENT STORY

Your patient is a 25-year-old married woman who wants to postpone having children for another 2 years while she finishes graduate school. She and her husband are currently using condoms, but would like to change to something different. She is in good health and does not smoke. It is now your opportunity to discuss with her all the methods available to prevent pregnancy. First, you determine what she knows about the methods and if she has any preferences. She tells you that she is specifically interested in either the *hormonal vaginal ring* (NuvaRing) (**Figure 3-1**) or the newest *intrauterine device* (IUD) that releases a hormone (**Figure 3-2**). Then you participate in shared decision making as she comes up with the method that best fits her lifestyle and health issues.

INTRODUCTION

Contraception is like many other treatments in medicine. Each method has its risks and benefits. Each method has its barriers to use, such as compliance, cost, and social stigmas. By educating patients appropriately and letting them know beforehand of the potential side effects, we can greatly increase compliance and satisfaction.

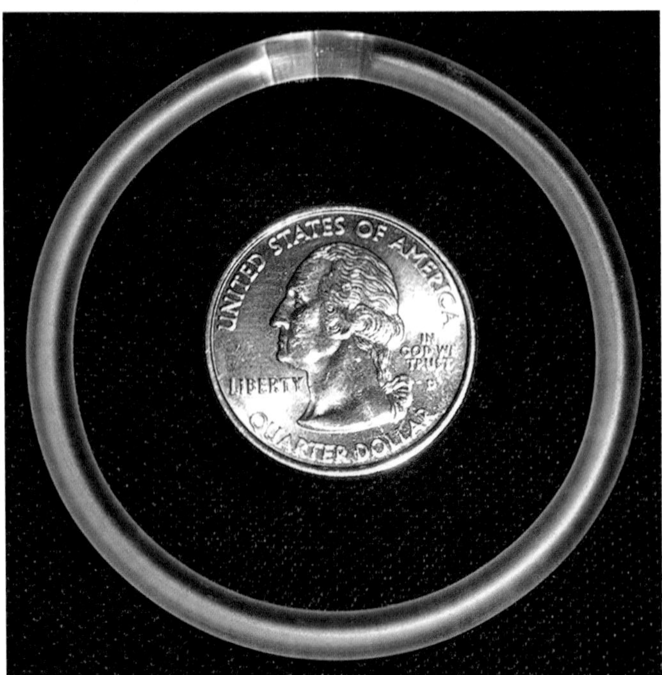

FIGURE 3-1 NuvaRing is a combined hormonal intravaginal contraceptive ring. The flexible material of the ring allows for easy insertion and removal. Note the size in comparison to a quarter. (*Reproduced with permission from Richard P. Usatine, MD.*)

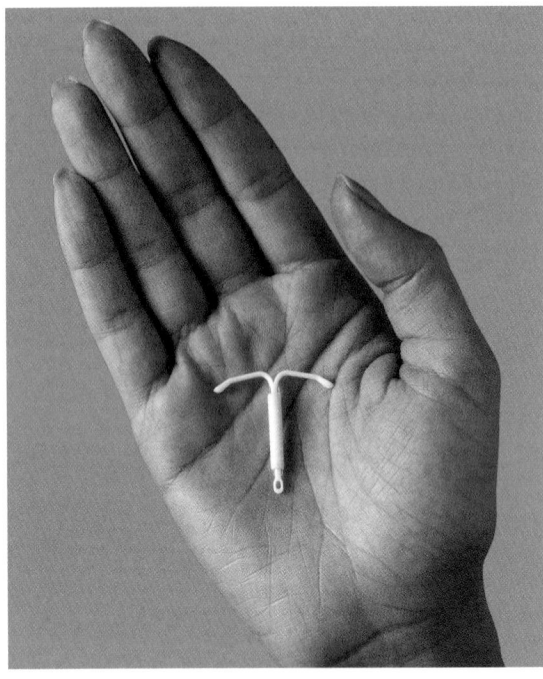

FIGURE 3-2 Mirena (levonorgestrel-releasing intrauterine system) provides effective contraception for at least 5 years. (*Reproduced with permission from Bayer HealthCare Pharmaceuticals Inc.*)

EPIDEMIOLOGY

- Approximately one-half of pregnancies in the United States are unintended[1] and approximately one-half of these occurred in women using reversible contraception.[2]
- The most commonly used contraceptive methods in the United States are oral contraceptive pills (OCPs), male condoms, and female sterilization.[3]
- Long-acting reversible forms of contraception are increasingly popular. Encouraging these methods may help lower the unintended pregnancy rate. Gaps or discontinuation of use of short-acting methods lead to unintended pregnancy.[4]
- Newer contraceptives often have improved side-effect profiles or have more convenient delivery systems that may not require daily patient adherence. Having a wide range of contraceptive options helps patients find a method that will work best for them.
- This chapter focuses on contraceptive methods available in the United States and the considerations one must address when counseling patients on their choice of method.

CONSIDERATIONS

- No contraception method is perfect. Each individual or couple must balance the advantages and disadvantages of each method and decide which offers the best choice. As the physician, one must help the patient make the appropriate decision based on many factors that are unrelated to their medical history or to the side-effect profile of the method, such as the likelihood of compliance and access to follow-up.
- Some important considerations in choosing a contraceptive method are its potential side effects, failure rates, and noncontraceptive benefits. See **Table 3-1**.

TABLE 3-1 Contraceptive Options Available in the United States in 2012

Method	Unintended Pregnancies With 1 Year of Use (%)		Noncontraceptive Benefits	Use With Breastfeeding
	Typical Use	Theoretical		
None	85	85	—	—
Spermicide	29	18	None	Yes
Withdrawal	27	4	None	Yes
Periodic abstinence (fertility awareness)	25	3-5	None	Yes
Diaphragm with spermicide	16	6	None	Yes
Female condom	21	5	Prevents STDs	Yes
Male condom	15	2	Prevents STDs	Yes
OCPs—combined and progestin-only	8	0.3	Regulation of menstrual cycle and dysmenorrhea, possible decrease in ovarian and endometrial cancer risk, decrease acne	No
Contraceptive patch	8	0.3	Same as OCPs	No
Vaginal ring	8	0.3	Same as OCPs	No
Depo-Provera	3	0.3	Same as OCPs	Yes
Copper-containing IUD	0.8	0.6	None	Yes
Levonorgestrel IUD	0.2	0.2	Regulation of menstrual cycles and dysmenorrhea	Yes
Female sterilization	0.5	0.5	None	Yes
Male sterilization	0.15	0.10	None	Yes
Etonogestrel implant	0.05	0.05	Same as OCPs	Safety conditional

IUD, intrauterine device; OCP, oral contraceptive pill; STD, sexually transmitted disease.
Data from Trussell J. Contraceptive efficacy. In: Hatcher RA, Trussell J, Nelson AL, et al, eds. *Contraceptive Technology,* 20th rev ed. New York, NY: Ardent Media; 2011:827-1010; Herndon EJ, Zieman M. New contraceptive options. *Am Fam Physician.* 2004;69:853-860; Herndon EJ, Zieman M. *Improving Access to Quality Care in Family Planning: Medical Eligibility Criteria for Contraceptive Use.* 2nd ed. Geneva, Switzerland: Reproductive Health and Research, World Health Organization; 2000. http://whqlibdoc.who.int/publications/2004/9241562668.pdf. Accessed July 4, 2006; Speroff L, Fritz MA. *Clinical Gynecologic Endocrinology and Infertility.* 7th ed. Philadelphia, PA: Lippincott Williams & Wilkins; 2005.

- Smoking increases the risks of the most dangerous side effects of estrogen-containing contraceptives. This is an important issue in helping a patient choose the safest and the best method. Encouraging smoking cessation is always a good intervention, but one might avoid prescribing an estrogen-containing contraceptive until the patient can truly quit smoking.
- Avoid estrogen-containing contraceptives in women with hypertension or migraine with aura. In both cases, the theoretical or proven risk of stroke outweighs the advantages.

NEWER CONTRACEPTIVE CHOICES

- In addition to the traditional 20 to 35 μg ethinyl estradiol (EE) OCPs, 30 and 20 μg EE in combination with the new progestogen *drospirenone* (Yasmin, YAZ) are available. Drospirenone has some antimineralocorticoid activity and has been shown to decrease the water retention, negative affect, and appetite changes that are commonly associated with menstrual cycle changes.[4] Serum potassium levels should be monitored when women are at a risk for hyperkalemia. The progesterone in these pills often helps in decreasing the severity of acne. Beyaz is a newer formulation of the above with the addition of folate. If a patient becomes pregnant while taking this pill, her folate levels would be adequate to prevent neural tube defects.
- *Extended OCP* regimens with 84 days of levonorgestrel-EE pills and 7 days of nonhormonal pills (Seasonale) are available. Seasonique has the same pills for the first 84 days but uses 10 μg EE pills for the last 7 days to make up the 91-day cycle. They have similar advantages to other OCPs except that the patient has only 4 periods a year. Another extended OCP regimen combining levonorgestrel and EE has been released in which there are no nonhormonal pills at all (Lybrel).

- The *hormonal vaginal ring* (NuvaRing) has similar active ingredients of OCPs, but it does not require daily attention (see **Figure 3-1**). It is placed in the vagina for 3 weeks at a time (with 1 week off) and releases EE and etonogestrel. Withdrawal bleeding occurs during the ring-free week. The vaginal ring is associated with a lower incidence of breakthrough bleeding than standard OCPs.
- There is a newer form of Depo-Provera given every 3 months, but is given subcutaneously (SQ) instead of intramuscularly (IM). The SQ version provides 30% less hormone, 104 versus 150 mg per injection. It works at least as well as Depo-Provera IM as a contraceptive, and also works as well as Lupron Depot for endometriosis pain with fewer hot flashes and less bone loss. If long-term use is considered, it may be prudent to select another contraceptive, discuss the risk of possible bone loss, or consider monitoring bone density in women using either version of Depo-Provera for more than 2 years. These medications can increase the incidence of acne and weight gain in some women as a result of the androgenic effects of the progesterone.
- The Mirena IUD releases levonorgestrel and provides effective contraception for at least 5 years (see **Figure 3-2**). Pregnancy rates are comparable with those occurring with surgical sterilization. Copper-containing IUDs are another long-term option lasting up to 10 years; however, it may be associated with dysmenorrhea and irregular vaginal bleeding some of the time. Twenty percent of women have amenorrhea after 1 year of use with Mirena, and as with the copper-containing IUDs, there is a risk of expulsion. The absolute risk of ectopic pregnancy with IUD use is extremely low because of the high effectiveness of IUDs. However, if a woman becomes pregnant during IUD use, the relative likelihood of ectopic pregnancy is greatly increased.[5]
- Nexplanon (etonogestrel implant) is an *etonogestrel-containing single rod implant* for subdermal use (**Figure 3-3**). It is a long-acting (up to 3 years), reversible, contraceptive method. It must be removed or replaced by the end of the third year. The implant is 4 cm in length with a diameter of 2 mm and contains 68 mg of the synthetic progestin etonogestrel (ENG). It does not contain estrogen or latex and is not radiopaque. The contraceptive effect of the ENG implant involves suppression of ovulation, increased viscosity of the cervical mucus, and alterations in the endometrium. In the first year of use, it had the lowest failure rate of any form of contraception, including tubal ligation.[7] The effectiveness of Nexplanon in women who weigh more than 130% of their ideal body weight has not been studied. Problems with Nexplanon are similar to other progestin-only contraceptives (acne and gaining weight).

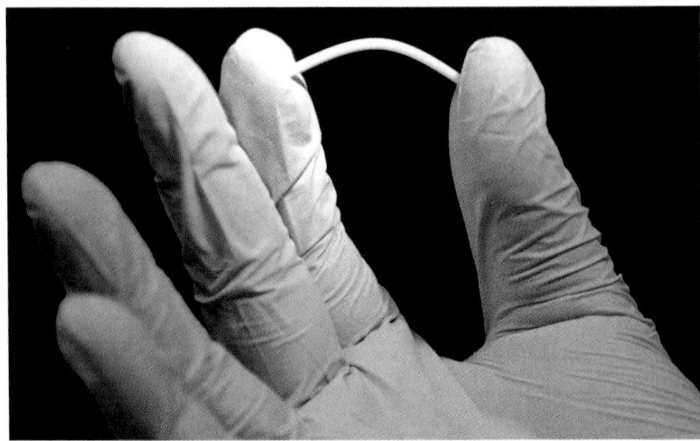

FIGURE 3-3 Nexplanon implantable subcutaneous contraceptive system. The insertion device is a sharp trochar and the implant is made of a soft silastic tube. (*Reproduced with permission from E.J. Mayeaux Jr., MD.*)

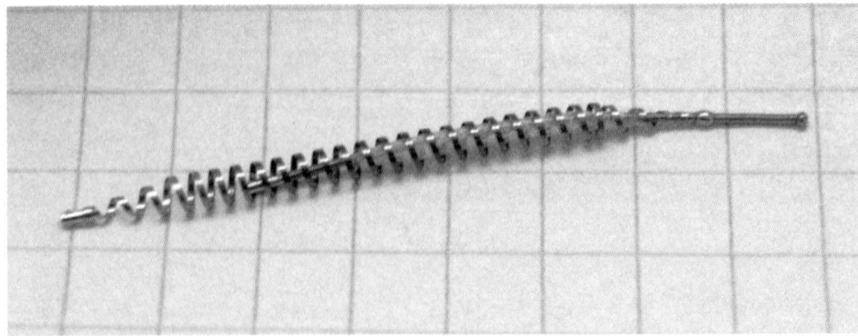

FIGURE 3-4 Essure tubal occlusion device for permanent sterilization. It is placed within the fallopian tubes using a vaginal approach and a hysteroscope. (*Reproduced with permission from Jay Berman, MD.*)

- Nexplanon sterilization is a common and very effective form of contraception that should be considered permanent.
- Hysteroscopic tubal occlusion (Essure) is a newer technique (**Figures 3-4** to **3-6**). The device is a flexible microcoil designed to promote tissue growth in the fallopian tubes. It does not require any incisions and can be performed without general anesthesia, typically in less than 30 minutes. There is a 3-month waiting period after the device is placed when an alternative birth control must be used. On the 3-month follow-up visit, a hysterosalpingogram (HSG) is performed to document that the tubes have been blocked.
- The *combination contraceptive patch* (Ortho Evra) releases EE and norelgestromin and has the same mechanism of action as OCPs (**Figure 3-7**). It is applied weekly for 3 weeks, followed by a patch-free week during which menses occur. Recommended application sites include the upper arm, buttocks, and torso (excluding the back and breasts). It has similar efficacy to OCPs but may be less effective in women weighing more than 90 kg (198 lb). In a rare instance of patch detachment, it must be replaced. The progesterone in the patch may decrease the severity of acne.

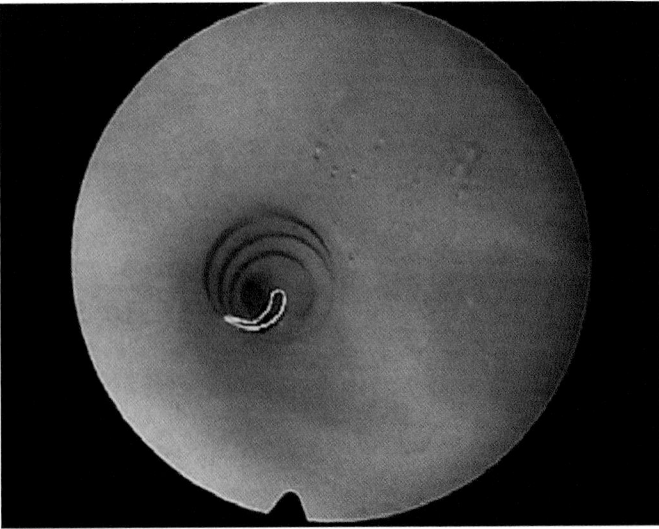

FIGURE 3-5 Hysteroscopic view showing the coiled Essure device within a fallopian tube immediately after it was implanted. (*Reproduced with permission from Jay Berman, MD.*)

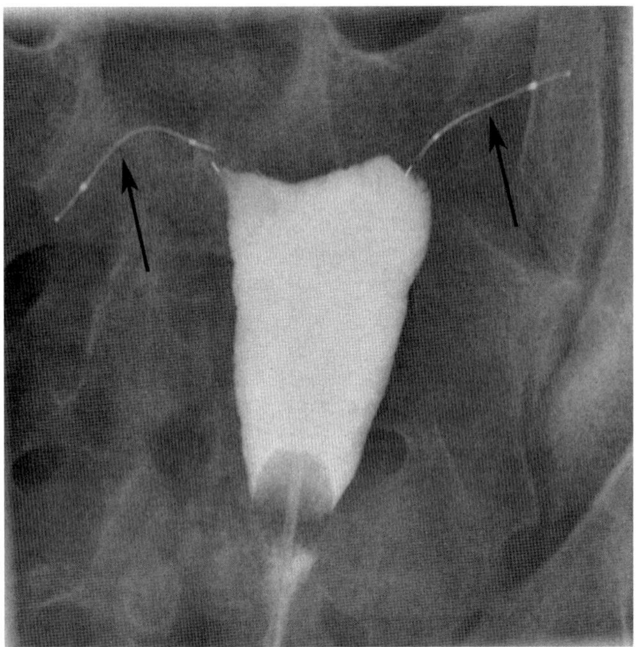

FIGURE 3-6 Hysterosalpingogram (HSG) with bilateral Essure devices within the fallopian tubes (arrows). Contrast material distends the uterine cavity but does not enter the cornua, fallopian tubes or peritoneal cavity, indicating successful occlusion. The black/gray bubble in the white-appearing uterus is the HSG catheter balloon. (*Reproduced with permission from E.J. Mayeaux Jr., MD.*)

PATIENT EDUCATION

For some contraceptive methods to be effective, the patient must be willing to use them consistently and correctly. Other methods do not require any action on the part of the patient. Patients will need to understand the benefits and risks of the method they choose and how to be best assured that the method is working for them. If patients are aware of the possible side effects, they can address any such effect with their physician if an adverse effect occurs.

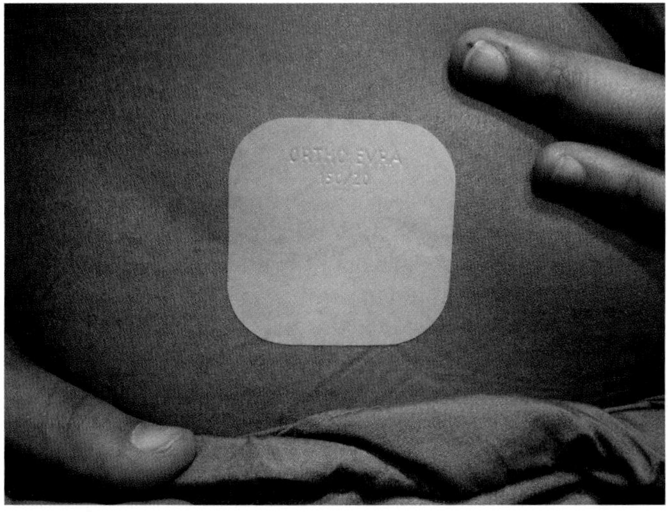

FIGURE 3-7 The Ortho Evra combined hormonal contraceptive patch. The patch is changed weekly for 3 weeks and then left off for 1 week per cycle. (*Reproduced with permission from E.J. Mayeaux, Jr., MD.*)

FOLLOW-UP

Monitor for side effects, level of usage, and tolerability. The contraceptive choice should be periodically reexamined as the patient may want to switch to a different method of contraception as needs and circumstances change.

PATIENT RESOURCES

- Managing Contraception Web site has a choices section that is good for patients—**http://managingcontraception.com/.**
- NuvaRing Web site—**http://www.nuvaring.com/.**
- Mirena Web site—**http://www.mirena-us.com/.**
- Essure Web site—**http://www.essure.com/.**
- Nexplanon Web site—**http://www.nexplanon-usa.com/.**
- CDC Web site—**http://www.cdc.gov/reproductivehealth/UnintendedPregnancy/Contraception.htm.**
- ACOG Web site—**http://www.acog.org/publications/patient_education/ab020.cfm.**

PROVIDER RESOURCES

- Contraceptive Technology Table of Contraceptive Efficacy—**http://www.contraceptivetechnology.org/table.html.**
- American Family Physician. *New Contraceptive Options*— **http://www.aafp.org/afp/20040215/853.html.**
- World Health Organization. Medical Eligibility Criteria for Contraceptive Use. 4th ed. 2009—**http://www.who.int/reproductivehealth/topics/en/.**

REFERENCES

1. Henshaw SK. Unintended pregnancy in the United States. *Fam Plann Perspect*. 1998;30:24-29, 46.
2. Kost K, Singh S, Vaughan B, et al. Estimates of contraceptive failure from the 2002 National Survey of Family Growth. *Contraception*. 2008;77:10.
3. Piccinino LJ, Mosher WD. Trends in contraceptive use in the United States: 1982-1995. *Fam Plann Perspect*. 1998;30:4-10, 46.
4. Raine TR, Foster-Rosales A, Upadhyay UD, et al. One-year contraceptive continuation and pregnancy in adolescent girls and women initiating hormonal contraceptives. *Obstet Gynecol*. 2011; 117(2 pt 1):363-371.
5. Herndon EJ, Zieman M. New contraceptive options. *Am Fam Physician*. 2004;69:853-860.
6. World Health Organization. *Medical Eligibility Criteria for Contraceptive Use*. 4th ed. 2009. http://www.who.int/reproductivehealth/topics/en/. Accessed May 21, 2012.
7. Trussell J. Contraceptive failure in the United States. *Contraception*. 2011;83;397-404.

4 END OF LIFE

Radha Ramana Murthy Gokula, MD
Mindy A. Smith, MD, MS

PATIENT STORY

An 89-year-old frail woman presents with Alzheimer disease, dementia, hypothyroidism, depression, congestive heart failure, and macular degeneration. Her functional status was gradually declining. It was difficult for her family to provide 24-hour care and she was admitted to a nursing facility. Her dementia worsened over a period of 2 years in the nursing facility and she became incontinent of urine and feces while developing limitations in speech and ambulation. She could not sit up without assistance and lost her ability to smile and hold her head up independently. The facility was very supportive and a hospice consult was initiated. **Figure 4-1** shows Dr. Gokula along with the hospice nurse visiting the patient for admission to hospice care.

INTRODUCTION

End-of-life care is care that is delivered to patients of all ages who have a very short life expectancy. This care is focused on meeting the patient's emotional and physical needs for symptom relief and general comfort care, and offering patient and family support.

Following are the 5 basic principles of palliative care[1]:

- Respect the goals, preferences, and choices of the person.
- Look after the medical, emotional, social, and spiritual needs.
- Support the needs of family members.
- Help patients and their families access needed health care providers and appropriate care settings.
- Provide excellence in care at the end of life (see **Figure 4-1**).

Following are the quality-of-care domains for a person at the end of life[2]:

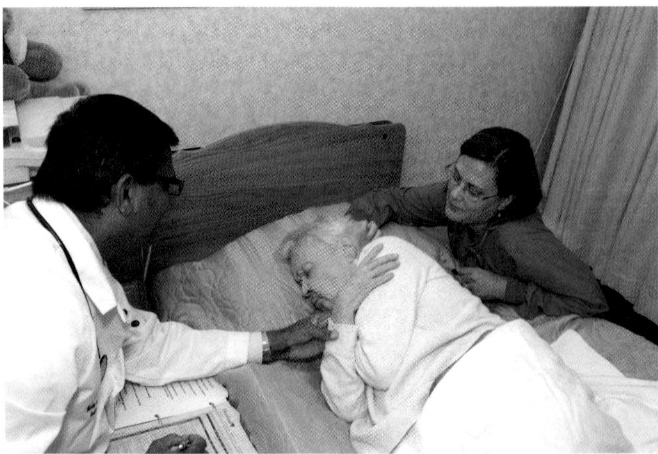

FIGURE 4-1 Family physician Dr. Murthy Gokula and hospice nurse Chris Emch are comforting and examining a terminally ill patient nearing the end of life in Heartland Hospice.

- Physical and emotional symptom management
- Support of function, autonomy, personal dignity, and self-respect
- Advanced care planning
- Aggressive symptom control near death
- Patient and family satisfaction
- Patient's assessment of overall quality of life and well-being
- Family burden—emotional and financial
- Survival time
- Provider continuity and skill
- Bereavement services

EPIDEMIOLOGY

- According to National Health Center statistics, there were approximately 2.42 million deaths in the United States in 2009, most were attributed to cardiovascular disease and cancer.[3]
- The major causes of death in the population aged 25 to 44 years were accidents, cancer, heart disease, suicide, homicide, and other causes.
- Among those aged 45 to 64 years, leading causes of death were cancer, heart disease, accidents, chronic respiratory diseases, and liver disease. The common causes of death in persons above age 65 years were heart disease, cancer, chronic lower respiratory disease, stroke, and Alzheimer disease.
- In 2009, heart disease, cancer, chronic lower respiratory diseases, stroke, and accidents accounted for almost 64% of all deaths in the United States.[4]
- Thirty-two percent of all deaths in the United States in 2007 were inpatient hospital deaths.[5] Average hospital costs for a stay ending in death were $23,000, about 2.7 times higher than for a patient discharged alive.

Hospice services were involved for approximately 20% of dying patients.[6] More than 70% of hospice patients had cancer and 90% of hospice patients died outside the hospital. The use of hospice and other end-of-life services varies among different racial groups in the United States[7]:

- Caucasians are more aware of advanced directives when compared to the non-white racial or ethnic groups.
- The use of life-sustaining treatments is more common among African Americans when compared to other racial groups.
- Cultural differences are also seen for disclosure of information about a terminal illness. Korean, Mexican, Japanese, and Native American populations are more likely to discourage discussion of terminal illness and patient prognosis and prefer families to be informed.
- The involvement of family in the decision-making process with end-of-life care was seen among all racial groups, but Asian and Hispanic Americans prefer family-centered decision making when compared to other racial and ethnic groups.

ETIOLOGY AND PATHOPHYSIOLOGY

Causes of death are multifactorial. Following are the major modifiable contributors:

- Tobacco use—20.6% of all the adults in the United States smoke cigarettes; the highest rates are among men (23.5%) and American Indians/Alaska Natives (23.2%).[8] It is estimated that nearly 1 of every 5 deaths each year in the United States is attributed to smoking.[9] Smoking increases the risk of developing emphysema (10- to 13-fold), heart and cardiovascular disease (2- to 4-fold), and many cancers (1.4- to 3-fold).

- Poor diet—Diets that are high in fat (>40% of calories consumed) are associated with increased risk of breast, colon, endometrial, and prostate cancer. Diet is important in controlling diabetes, heart disease, obesity, and chronic renal disease.
- Physical inactivity—Those who exercise regularly live longer and are healthier; exercise reduces the risk of cardiovascular disease and hypertension and improves function in those with depression, osteoarthritis, and fibromyalgia. Unfortunately less than 20% of adults met the 2008 federal guidelines for aerobic activity and muscle-strengthening.[10]
- Alcohol consumption—Alcohol is consumed by 80% of the population, and 10% to 15% of men and 5% to 8% of women are alcohol dependent. Excess alcohol consumption (>3 drinks per day) is associated with mood disorders (10-40%), cirrhosis (15-20%), and neuropathy (5-15%); it increases the risk of pancreatitis (3-fold) as well as cancers of the breast (1.4-fold), esophagus (3-fold), and rectum (1.5-fold).[11] In addition, based on data from 2009, an estimated 30.2 million people (12%) aged 12 years or older reported driving under the influence of alcohol at least once in the past year.[12]
- Injury—In 2004, 167,184 people died as a result of injury, accounting for 7% of all deaths.[13] The majority of injury-related deaths are unintentional. Falls are the leading mechanism of injury death for elderly people while for adults of 35 to 53 years, poisoning is the leading mechanism of injury death. Motor vehicles in traffic are the leading mechanism of injury death for all other age groups, except for children under age 2 years. Many of these deaths are preventable.
- Sexual behaviors—Sexually transmitted infections (STIs) are among the most common infectious diseases and affect approximately 13 million people in the United States each year; most of these people are younger than age 25 years. Sexually transmitted diseases (STDs) are associated with increased risk of HIV/AIDS; in 2007, there were approximately 455,636 persons living with AIDS in the United States.[14] Causes of death from AIDS include infections (especially, pulmonary and central nervous system), cancer (especially, Kaposi sarcoma and non-Hodgkin lymphoma), cardiomyopathy, and nephropathy.
- Illicit use of drugs—Drug addiction remains a major problem in the United States. According to data from the National Institute on Drug Abuse Monitoring the Future Survey of over 46,000 8th- to 12th-grade students, increases were seen in daily marijuana use (21.4% of high school seniors in the past 30 days) and lifetime ecstasy use in 8th graders (from 2.2% in 2009 to 3.3% in 2010) while decreases were noted in methamphetamine use (from 6.5% in 1999 to 2.2% in 2010) and current cocaine use (from 2.3 million in 2003 to 1.6 million in 2009).[12] Cocaine is associated with death from respiratory depression, cardiac arrhythmias, and convulsions; methamphetamine use is associated with life-threatening hypertension, cardiac arrhythmia, subarachnoid and intracerebral hemorrhage, ischemic stroke, convulsions, and coma.
- Microbial agents—Microbial agents remain a major cause of death and disability with continued discovery of new agents and increasing drug resistance. Although it is difficult to ascertain whether an infectious agent caused death or was incidental to death, the expert panel of investigators in New Mexico, on the basis of autopsy data, found that 85% (106/125) of the deaths (late 1994-mid 1996) were identified as infectious disease-related.[15]
- Toxic agents—Toxic agents include poisons and environmental toxins. In the United States in 2008, there were 36,500 poisoning deaths; the vast majority was unintentional.[16] Opioid pain medications were involved in over 40%. Poisoning was the third leading method of suicide from 2005 to 2007, with 75% owing to alcohol and/or drug overdose. The most commonly used drugs identified in drug-related suicides were prescription drugs in the opioid, benzodiazepine, and antidepressant classes.[17]

DIAGNOSIS

It is estimated that approximately 70% of all deaths are preceded by a disease or condition such that it is reasonable to plan for dying in the near future.[6] These diseases or conditions are as follows:

- Cancer that is widespread, aggressive or metastatic and for patients who no longer seek curative care. Other clues include a decline in performance status and/or significant unintentional weight loss.
- Dementia with an inability to ambulate, bathe, or dress without assistance; associated urinary or fecal incontinence; inability to meaningfully communicate; or associated with life-threatening infections, multiple stage 3 or 4 skin ulcers, inability to maintain sufficient fluid and calorie intake, or failure to thrive (including a temporal decline in functional status).
- Patients confined to bed or who require assistance with all the basic activities of daily living.
- Patients with a body mass index less than 22 and/or those who refuse or do not respond to enteral or parenteral nutritional support.
- Heart disease that is poorly responsive to optimal medical treatment, NYHA class IV, or congestive heart failure with poor ejection fraction (≤20%). Based on data from multiple studies including SUPPORT, Framingham, and IMPROVEMENT, 1-year mortality estimates are as follows: class II (mild symptoms), 5% to 10%; class III (moderate symptoms), 10% to 15%; class IV (severe symptoms), 30% to 40%. Independent predictors of poor prognosis in patients with heart failure include recent cardiac hospitalization, renal insufficiency (creatinine ≥1.4 mg/dL), systolic blood pressure less than 100 mm Hg and/or pulse greater than 100 bpm, treatment-resistant ventricular dysrhythmias, treatment-resistant anemia, hyponatremia, cachexia, reduced functional capacity, and comorbidities (eg, diabetes).[18]
- HIV/AIDS with CD4 count less than 25 or persistent viral load more than 100,000 copies/mL plus at least one of the following: wasting (loss of 33% of lean body mass), major AIDS-defining refractory infection (eg, cryptosporidium infection) or malignancy (eg, central nervous system or systemic lymphoma), progressive multifocal leukoencephalopathy, renal failure, Karnofsky performance status (KPS) less than 50%, advanced AIDS dementia complex, or significant functional decline in the activities of daily living.
- Neurologic disease (eg, Parkinson disease, amyotrophic lateral sclerosis, multiple sclerosis, muscular dystrophy, and myasthenia gravis) that is associated with rapid progression and/or critical nutritional state, life-threatening infections in the preceding 12 months, stage 3 or 4 skin ulcers, critically impaired breathing capacity and declined ventilator support, or life-threatening complication (eg, recurrent aspiration, sepsis).
- Pulmonary disease including disabling dyspnea at rest or with minimal exertion, increased emergency department visits and/or hospitalizations, hypoxemia on room air (oxygen saturation <88%), cor pulmonale, unintentional progressive weight loss, or resting tachycardia greater than 100 bpm.
- End-stage renal disease with progressive decline in those not seeking dialysis (or not a candidate), with a calculated creatinine clearance less

than 10 (<15 for patients with diabetes) or serum creatinine greater than 8 mg/dL (>6 mg/dL for patients with diabetes).

- End-stage liver disease with progressive decline in those with refractory ascites, spontaneous bacterial peritonitis, hepatorenal syndrome, hepatic encephalopathy, or recurrent variceal bleeding despite treatment.
- Stroke associated with coma in the acute phase; coma with abnormal brain stem response, absent verbal response, absent withdrawal response to pain, or serum creatinine greater than 1.5 mg/dL at day 3; dysphagia and insufficient intake of fluids and calories; poor functional status; or poststroke dementia.
- Nonspecific terminal illness characterized by a rapid decline, disease progression, or progressive weight loss; dysphasia with aspiration; increase in emergency department visits and/or hospitalizations; worsening pressure ulcers despite optimum care; or a decline in systolic blood pressure below 90 mm Hg.

Unfortunately, physicians are often reluctant to make this determination, resulting in palliative and hospice care not being offered until very late in the course of the illness. In addition, physicians often feel that they must be able to predict a life expectancy of less than 6 months with certainty to institute hospice care.

The National Hospice and Palliative Care Organization has evidence-based guidelines on determining prognosis for a number of noncancer conditions.[19] This information can assist clinicians in working with patients at the end of life on advanced care decisions and planning.

Two validated instruments that may help clinicians estimate prognosis are the palliative performance scale (PPS) and the KPS.

- The PPS (http://meds.queensu.ca/palliativecare/assets/pps_scale_tool.pdf) rates information on ambulation, activity and evidence of disease, self-care, intake, and consciousness level. The PPS was found to be a strong predictor of survival when applied at admission to patients in palliative care.[20] In this retrospective cohort study, median survival time at PPS of 10% was 1 day, survival with PPS of 20% was 2 days, at PPS of 30% survival was 9 days, while at PPS of 60% median survival was 40 days.
- The KPS (http://www.hospicepatients.org/karnofsky.html) is often used to follow the course of illness and is based on performance status ranging from normal (100%) to dead (0%).

CLINICAL FEATURES

Common physical symptoms reported by dying patients are as below[6]:

- Constipation (90%)
- Fatigue and weakness (90%)
- Dyspnea (75%) and other cardiopulmonary symptoms such as cough
- Pain (36-90%)
- Insomnia
- Other gastrointestinal symptoms, including dry mouth, anorexia, nausea, vomiting, constipation, diarrhea, and dysphagia
- Fecal and urinary incontinence
- Dizziness
- Swelling and numbness of the extremities

Following are the common mental and psychological symptoms reported by dying patients[6]:

- Depression (75% symptomatic; <25% with major depression) and feelings of hopelessness, anxiety, and/or irritability
- Confusion and delirium (up to 85% at the end stage)

A population-based survey of family members, friends, and caregivers in 6 US communities found the following[21]:

- Seventy-one percent of terminally ill patients had shortness of breath.
- Fify percent had moderate-to-severe pain.
- Thirty-six percent were incontinent of urine or feces.
- Eighteen percent were fatigued enough to spend more than 50% of their waking hours in bed.

MANAGEMENT

Management often begins with communicating bad news to patients and families about likely or imminent death. This task can be extremely difficult. In cases where the patient is not deemed legally competent, make sure that the legal decision maker is present. In addition, if the patient is a non-English speaker, consider obtaining a skilled medical interpreter rather than relying on a family member. Providers may find the following P-SPIKES approach useful[22]:

- Preparation—Review information to be presented and practice.
- Setting—Arrange time and place, ensure privacy, and include important support persons.
- Perception of patient—Inquire about the patient's and the family's understanding of the illness.
- Information needs—Find out about what the patient and family need to be told and in how much detail.
- Knowledge of the condition—Provide bad news sensitively and slowly, warning them that bad news is imminent and checking to see whether there is understanding.
- Empathy and exploration—Acknowledge the feelings expressed, give the patient and family time to react, and remind them that you are not abandoning them.
- Summary/strategic planning—Discuss next steps or schedule follow-ups to do this if more time is needed.

Roles for the primary care provider include consultation, providing anticipatory guidance, providing support and comfort, and assisting with identifying and managing symptoms (including pain control) (**Figure 4-2**).

In assisting dying patients and their families or caregivers with making decisions about their care, clinicians should be prepared to discuss the following:

- Realistic treatment options for cure or palliation of the primary disease process.
- Advance directives and withholding of life-sustaining treatment.
- Cultural beliefs and preferences (eg, truth-telling vs protecting the patient, religious beliefs).
- Preferences for place of care for those dying, involvement of others, and symptom management.

A number of factors are important in providing optimal care to the dying patient. In a study of factors considered important to seriously ill patients, recently bereaved family members, and physicians involved in end-of-life care, investigators found the following[23]:

- There was a general agreement on the items relating to having preferences in writing, symptom control, being kept clean, experiencing physical touch, good communication and knowing what to expect,

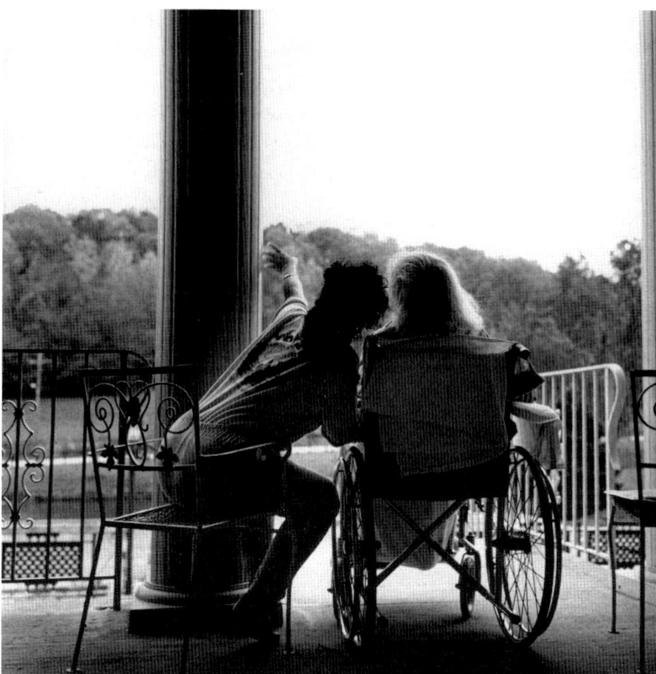

FIGURE 4-2 Photograph of Marjorie Clarke taken by her grandson. She suffered from Alzheimer disease that left her depressed and frustrated. In this picture, taken in 1996, Marjorie listens to her nurse describe the scene and explain that they are on the front porch of her home. She died in January, 1997. (*Reproduced with permission from Marshall Clarke.*)

getting one's affairs in order and achieving a sense of completion, and maintaining dignity and a sense of humor.

- Patients reported wanting to remain mentally aware, not be a burden, and noted the importance of prayer and being at peace with God. They were not as concerned about dying at home.
- Family members reported wanting to use all the treatment options and to help patients avoid pain, shortness of breath, and suffering.

ADVANCED DIRECTIVES

Advance directives and advance care planning continue to be poorly utilized. Clinicians should consider outpatient and inpatient opportunities to introduce these concepts with the goals of empowering the patient and understanding the patient's preferences if they are too sick to speak for themselves. Possible scenarios can be discussed such as recovery from an acute event (specifying acceptable interventions) and persistent vegetative state (preferences for life-sustaining interventions).

- The National POLST (physician orders for life-sustaining treatment) Paradigm task force is a new program designed to improve the quality of end-of-life care based on effective communication of patient wishes, documentation of medical orders, and a commitment by health care professionals to honor these wishes. Information can be found at http://closure.org and includes Web-based resources for patients and health providers.
- Advance directive documents are of 2 broad types—instructional directives and proxy designations.
    - Instructional directives such as living wills that describe decisions about care and health care. These can be general or specific. Although 80% of Americans endorse completing living wills, only 20% (and less than one-third of health care providers) have completed them.[6] Specific forms do not have to be used and oral directives may be enforceable.[24]
    - Proxy designations—Appointing an individual or individuals to make medical decisions (ie, durable power of attorney for health care).

Legal aspects—The US Supreme Court has ruled that patients have a right to decide about refusing or terminating medical interventions. Many states have their own statutory forms for living wills.

- The American College of Physicians and the American Society of Internal Medicine End-of-Life Care Consensus Panel note that life-sustaining treatment may be withheld for patients unable to speak for themselves if it is believed to be the patient's wish, the surrogate decision maker states that it is the patient's wish, and/or it is in the patient's best interests to do so.[25]
- The prescription of high-dose opioids to relieve pain in terminally ill patients that result in death will not lead to criminal prosecution provided it was the physician's intent to relieve suffering.[25]

HOSPICE CARE AND SERVICES

Hospice care refers to care when curative interventions have been judged to be no longer beneficial. This type of care can be delivered in many settings including home, hospital, or special residential facilities.

- The types of hospice services include physician and nursing care, home health aides, pastoral care, counseling, respite care, and bereavement programs (**Figure 4-3**).
- Hospice eligibility general guidelines include fulfilling the criteria for end-stage disease as outlined above and documenting both the patient's and family's decision on palliative care rather than curative care and rapid disease progression. In addition, documentation of significant functional decline is important using validated instruments like Functional Assessment Staging (FAST), PPS, basic activities of daily living (BADLs), and/or NYHA class IV heart disease. Other criteria include weight loss of 7.5% or 10% in the preceding 3 to 6 months, respectively, or serum albumin less than 2.5 g/dL.

Physicians should be aware of the Medicare hospice benefit (MHB) covered under Medicare Part A (physician services are billed under Medicare Part B).[25] In the United States, the MHB pays for 80% of all

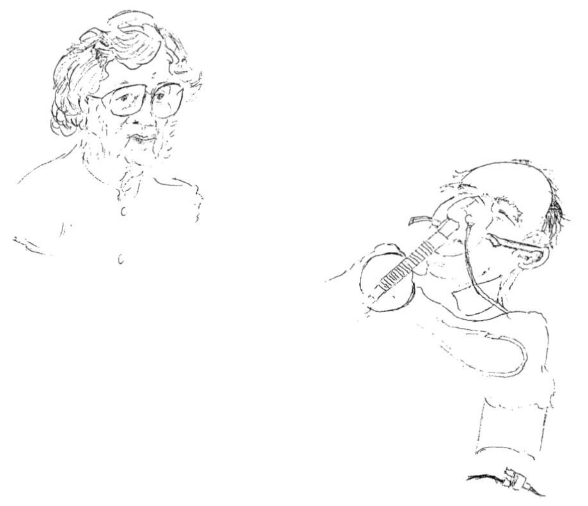

FIGURE 4-3 Dr. Alan Blum is a family physician who has been doing sketches of his patients for decades now. When he presents his drawings, he reads his poetic stories that go with the drawings. Some of his drawings have been published in *JAMA*.

hospice care including medical, nursing, counseling, and bereavement services to terminally ill patients and their families. Medicare beneficiaries who choose hospice care receive noncurative medical and support services for their terminal illness. Home care may be provided along with inpatient care if needed and a variety of other services that are not covered by Medicare. Eligibility criteria are listed below:

- Patient is eligible for Medicare Part A or Medicaid.
- Patient is terminally ill, that is, patient's physician and medical director of hospice certify that the patient is terminally ill and has a life expectancy of 6 months or less if the disease runs its normal course. If the medical director is the patient's physician only one signature is required.
- Patient chooses hospice care and signs a Medicare hospice benefits form. This process is reversible and patients may at a future time elect to return to Medicare Part A.
- Hospice care is provided by a Medicare-certified hospice program.
- Under Medicare, DNR status cannot be used as a requirement for admission.

Length of benefits

- Entitled to receive hospice care as long as he or she meets the eligibility criteria.
- Hospice benefit consists of two 90-day benefit periods, followed by an unlimited number of 60-day benefit periods.
- Benefit periods may be used consecutively or at intervals.
- Patient needs to be certified terminally ill at the beginning of each period.
- No life time limit to hospice care for Medicare beneficiaries.
- If patient experiences remission of the disease and is discharged from hospice, he or she can be eligible for hospice care in the future without any regard to the previous use of hospice services.
- The same rules apply for Medicaid patients.

Services covered include physician, nurse, dietician, and medical social services, medical supplies and equipment, outpatient drugs for symptom management and pain relief, and home care (eg, aids, physical, occupational, and speech therapy). Other services included are as follows:

- Short-term general inpatient care for problems that cannot be managed at home—most commonly intractable pain or delirium.
- Short-term respite care—up to 5 days to permit family caregivers to take a break (can incur a 5% copayment).
- Counseling in home for patient and family.
- Bereavement, pastoral, and spiritual support for patient and family.
- Payment of consulting physician fees at 100% of Medicare allowance.
- Physician, nurse, social worker, and counselor on-call availability 24 hours a day, 7 days a week.

Services not covered include active treatment of terminal illness (except for symptom management and pain control of the terminal illness), care provided by a physician or facility that has not contracted with the patient's hospice agency, and continuous nursing assistant or nursing home room and board charges.

PALLIATIVE CARE

Palliative care is care focused on preventing, relieving, reducing, or soothing symptoms of disease without affecting a cure.[26] As such, it is not restricted to patients who are dying but can be used along with a curative therapy. Many hospitals now have inpatient palliative care services to assist patients, families, and primary care providers in delivering this type of care.

General approach to palliative care focuses on 4 broad domains—managing physical symptoms, managing psychological symptoms, addressing social needs, and understanding spiritual needs.

- Needs assessment—Clinicians should focus on the 4 domains and try to understand the degree of difficulty and how much the identified problem interferes with the patient's life.
- Setting goals and continuous reassessment—Goals for care include improving symptoms, delaying disability, finding peace, and providing for the loved ones. Plan times to review these goals as the course of the illness changes or progresses.
- Pain management—There is no reason that patients need to suffer, particularly at the end of life. Barriers to managing pain successfully include limited ability of providers to assess pain severity, fear of sanction/prosecution, and lack of knowledge (including awareness of guidelines).
    - Assessment of pain—Important aspects include periodicity (eg, continuous), location, intensity, modifying factors, effects of treatments, and impact on the patient.
    - Intervention—This includes nonpharmacologic treatment (eg, massage, positioning, transcutaneous electrical nerve stimulation [TENS], physical therapy), pain medications, and other palliative procedures (eg, nerve blocks, radiotherapy, acupuncture).
    - Pain medications may be approached in a stepwise fashion from nonopioids (eg, acetaminophen [4 g/d], ibuprofen [1600 mg/d]), to mild opioids (eg, codeine [30 mg every 4 hours] or hydrocodone [5 mg every 4 hours]) to stronger opioids (eg, morphine 5-10 mg every 4 hours). Doses should be titrated as needed. Side effects (eg, constipation, nausea, and drowsiness) should be anticipated and prevented (eg, laxatives and antiemetic) or treated. Patients may become tolerant to these side effects after approximately 1 week. Specific pain syndromes may require additional consideration. These include the following:
        - Continuous pain, which requires round-the-clock dosing, rescue medication, and regular assessment and readjustment. If rescue medication has been needed, increase the daily opioid dose by the total dose of rescue medication the next day. For longer duration of action, transdermal fentanyl may be considered (100 μg/h is equianalgesic to morphine 4 mg/h and has a duration of 48-72 hours).
        - Neuropathic pain (arising from disordered, ectopic nerve signals) is typically shock-like or burning. Medications to consider in addition to opioids are gabapentin (100-300 mg daily or up to 3 times daily), 5% lidocaine patch (3 patches daily for a maximum of 12 hours), tramadol (50-100 mg 1-3 times daily), and tricyclic antidepressants (10-25 mg at bedtime titrated to 75-150 mg).[28]
        - Adjunctive analgesic medications are those that potentiate the effects of opioids. These include the above treatments for neuropathic pain, glucocorticoids (eg, dexamethasone once daily), clonidine, and baclofen.
        - Legal concerns—Physicians may be unwilling or uncomfortable providing high-dose opioids out of fear that they would be hastening the patient's death. However, the assumption that opioids appropriately titrated to control pain hasten death is not supported by medical evidence. In addition, as noted above, the physician's intent to relieve suffering, despite the risk of death, is ethical and unlikely to result in prosecution.

CONTROL OF COMMON SYMPTOMS

- Constipation[6]—Occurs due to medications, inactivity, and poor nutritional/hydration, limited fiber intake, confusion, and intestinal obstruction comorbidities such as diabetes mellitus, hypothyroidism, or hypercalcemia. The goal of treatment should be one bowel movement every 1 to 2 days. Constipation prophylaxis should be started for all patients taking regular opiate regimens. Options include increasing fiber, stool softeners (eg, sodium docusate [Colace] 300-600 mg/d oral), stimulant laxatives (eg, prune juice 1/2-1 glass/d, senna [Senokot] 2-4 tablet/d, bisacodyl 5-15 mg/d orally or per rectum), and osmotic laxatives (eg, lactulose 15-30 mL every 4-8 hours, magnesium hydroxide [milk or magnesia] 15-30 mL/d).
- Dyspnea—When possible, treat reversible causes (eg, infection, hypoxia). Options include opioids (eg, codeine 30 mg every 4 hours, morphine 5-10 mg every 4 hours) and anxiolytics (eg, lorazepam 0.5-2 mg oral/sublingual/intravenous [IV], diazepam 5-10 mg oral/IV). A parenteral infusion or long-acting opiate can also be tried, with bolus dosing for breakthrough pain; nebulized opiates are ineffective for dyspnea.[29] For patients with a history of respiratory disease consider bronchodilators and/or glucocorticoids. For those with excessive secretions, scopolamine may be considered, starting with a low dose every 2 hours or with worsening dyspnea, as needed. Oxygen is commonly prescribed although data do not support effectiveness in improving the sensation of breathlessness;[30] one crossover trial found ambient air delivered by nasal cannula was as effective as oxygen for dyspnea.[30] The inexpensive and simple practice of blowing ambient air on the patient's face may help relieve dyspnea.
- Fatigue—Occurs due to disease factors (eg, heart failure, tumor necrosis factor), cachexia, dehydration, anemia, hypothyroidism, and medications. Options include decreasing activity, increasing exercise as tolerated, changing medications, glucocorticoids (eg, dexamethasone once daily), or stimulants (eg, dextroamphetamine 5-10 mg oral). Modafinil, an analeptic drug, may also be considered (initial dose 200 mg).
- Depression—Because many of the somatic symptoms used to diagnose depression in healthy individuals are present in patients who are dying, psychological criteria become more important in making treatment decisions. Options include counseling, exercise, and medications (eg, selective serotonin reuptake inhibitor); low doses should be used initially (eg, fluoxetine 10 mg/d) and increased as needed. Psychostimulants (eg, dextroamphetamine or methylphenidate 2.5-5 mg twice daily) may be considered if rapid onset of action is needed; these may be used in conjunction with traditional antidepressants.
- Delirium—Occurs due to metabolic abnormalities (liver failure, electrolyte disturbance, vitamin B_{12} deficiency), infection, brain tumors, medications, and multiple other causes. Options include treating reversible causes and medications including neuroleptics (eg, haloperidol 0.5-5 mg oral/subcutaneous/intramuscular [IM]/IV every 1-4 hours, risperidone 1-3 mg every 12 hours), anxiolytics (eg, lorazepam 0.5-2 mg oral/IM/IV), and anesthetics (propofol 0.3-2 mg/h continuous infusion).

ADDRESSING SOCIAL NEEDS

Considerations include economic burden and caregivers:

- The US health insurance system is neither universal nor comprehensive and many patients and their families find themselves under tremendous financial strain.
- Twenty percent of terminally ill patients spend more than 10% of the family income on health care costs beyond insurance premiums.[6]
- Ten percent to thirty percent of families need to secure additional monies by means such as selling assets or taking out a second mortgage to cover health care costs.[6]
- Twenty percent of caregivers stop work to provide care for a terminally ill family member.[6]
- Families/caregivers often need outside help such as providing personal care for the patient such as bathing, psychological or spiritual counseling, respite care, or making arrangements for the body after death.
- Primary care providers can facilitate encounters with family and friends by offering their presence and suggestions about easing the visits (eg, reading to the patient, sharing music, or creating a videotape, audiotape, or scrapbook).
- Hospice and social workers can offer great assistance to patients and families in addressing these needs.

Understanding spiritual needs

- Approximately 70% of dying patients become more religious or spiritual at the end of life.
- As noted by Steinhauser et al., patients noted the importance of prayer and being at peace with God.[24]
- Physicians should ask about and support patient and family expressions of spirituality and consider encouraging pastoral care, as desired.

PATIENT AND FAMILY EDUCATION

It is very important to involve patients and their families in discussion at an early stage as most want to know their diagnosis and prognosis.

- The role of the primary care physician should be discussed, particularly if other providers are involved in the care of the patient. Possible roles include consultation about care needs, anticipatory guidance on prognosis and expected symptoms, provision of support and comfort, and assistance with managing symptoms.
- Families usually suffer emotionally, spiritually, and financially as they care for the patient.[21] Family members often experience a sense of hopelessness, anger, guilt, and powerlessness when they cannot relieve the suffering of their terminally ill family member.
- Families who need to provide care for a terminally ill patient should be made aware of community resources and the provisions in the Family Medical Leave Act.[31]
- It is not unusual to see hidden family conflicts resurface in the face of a terminal illness and any emotional tension that exists between the caregivers and patient can impede care. Physicians should be sensitive to the conflicts and cultural influences and closely observe how patients and their families are communicating so that they can better support them, allowing them to express their emotions and concerns and referring them to appropriate counselors or support groups when needed.[32,33]
- Children should not be excluded from this process and the physician, with permission, can help in determining what children already know about the illness and in providing accurate information about the diagnosis, prognosis, and treatment expectations for the dying family member. Also advise caregivers to try to maintain the children's daily schedule and routines of the family as much as possible, monitor for problems at school, encourage questions, and plan activities (eg, reading a story) when visiting ill family members. It may be helpful to inform teachers and counselors at school about the family situation and request that the teachers let the parent know if the child is having any difficulty or talks about worries.

- Consider counseling for the child if the child requests help or displays symptoms of depression or anxiety that interfere with school, home, or peers, risk-taking behavior, or significant discord with others.

The following are the processes that many dying people go through:

- Social withdrawal—Initial withdrawal is from the surroundings and then worldly interests decline and finally withdrawal from family, ultimately leading to loss of communication.
- Decreasing nutritional requirements—There is a decreased need for fluids and solids; fluids are usually preferred and should follow what the patient wants rather than force-feeding.
- Disorientation—There is increased confusion with time, place, and person. Usually patients talk about seeing people who have already died or state that their death is nearing. Redirecting the patient is necessary only if asked for or if the patient is distressed.
- Decreased senses—Hearing and vision decrease. Use soft lights that help with decreasing visual hallucinations. Speak softly and gently as patients hear even at the end of life. Hearing is the last of the 5 senses to be lost.
- Restlessness—Also called "terminal restlessness" is caused by the change in the body's metabolism. Reassurance is important and appropriate symptom management with medications may be helpful.
- Sleep—There is increased time spent in sleep that may be a result of changes in the body's metabolism or natural to the underlying disease process. Spending time at the bedside can help capture the time when the patient is most alert.
- Incontinence of urine and bowel movements is often not a problem until death is very near. Absorbent pads can be placed under the patient for greater comfort and cleanliness or a urinary catheter may be used for comfort care. The amount of urine will decrease and becomes darker at the end of life.

Expected physical changes include the following:

- Skin color changes include flushing, bluish hue to the skin, and cold sensation of the skin. Skin may have a jaundiced look when the patient is approaching death. The arms and legs of the body may become cool to the touch. The hands and feet become purplish. The knees, ankles, and elbows are blotchy. These symptoms are a result of decreased circulation.
- Blood pressure decreases; the pulse may increase or decrease.
- Body temperature can fluctuate; fever is common.
- Increased perspiration along with clamminess.
- Respirations may increase, decrease, or become irregular; there may be periods of cessation of breathing (apnea).
- Congestion can present as a rattling sound in the lungs and/or upper throat. This occurs because the patient is too weak to clear the throat or cough. The congestion can be affected by positioning, may be very loud, and sometimes just comes and goes. Elevating the head of the bed and swabbing the mouth with oral swabs may be helpful.
- The patient may enter a coma before death and not respond to verbal or tactile stimuli.

FOLLOW-UP

WITHDRAWAL OF LIFE-SUSTAINING TREATMENT

- Evidence-based criteria for guiding physicians through this process is lacking; however, general consensus exists based on ethical and clinical principles in the care of these patients.[34,35]
- Withdrawal of life-sustaining treatment can be considered when curative care is not possible and supportive or other treatment is no longer desired and does not provide comfort to the patient.
- Withholding life-sustaining treatment is morally, ethically, and legally equivalent to withdrawing life support. Any kind of treatment that is given to the patient can be withdrawn or withheld. In conducting these discussions with patients and their families, the physician needs to consider a patient's information-sharing preferences (eg, a preference for limited information), minimum acceptable quality of life and functional status, whether the patient is able to understand consequences of life-sustaining treatment, whether procedures offered conflict with the patient's values, and the patient's need for advice and guidance.[36]
- Treat withdrawal of life-sustaining treatment equivalent to a medical procedure and all formalities (eg, informed consent) should be fulfilled prior to the procedure.
- If withdrawal of one life-sustaining treatment is indicated, then consider withdrawing all existing treatments for the patient.
- A general consensus should be reached with the health care team and family members that is in the best interest of the patient. Following are the steps that should be taken for withdrawal of life support[36]:
  - Informed consent.
  - Appropriate setting and monitoring.
  - Sedation and analgesia.
  - Having a plan for withdrawal (information about the protocol can be found in fast facts at www.eperc.mcw.edu).
  - Pastoral, nursing, and emotional support.
  - Documentation.
  - Interventions to improve care during withdrawal of life-sustaining treatment that can be considered are consultation with an ethics committee, palliative care team, family conferences, and a standardized order form for withdrawing life-sustaining therapies.[37]

GRIEF AND BEREAVEMENT FOLLOW-UP

- Manifestations of grief consist of both psychological symptoms (eg, sadness, anxiety, emotional lability, apathy, impaired concentration) and physical symptoms (anorexia, change in weight, trouble initiating or maintaining sleep, fatigue, headache). In the first month following death, it is important to reassure surviving family members and friends that these manifestations of grief are normal and to offer support, suggestions for symptom management, and coping resources.
- Subsequent follow-up visits should be used to assess the progress of mourning and to identify depression; if the latter is identified, consider pharmacotherapy and counseling.
- Usually, the primary physician is notified of the death and may be required to make the pronouncement (based on lack of vital signs and lack of response to noxious stimulus) and complete the death certificate (noting cause of death and contributing medical conditions).
- Following the death of the patient, personal expressions of condolence from the primary care provider(s) and staff should be encouraged and range from cards to attending visitation and the funeral; based on personal experience, the latter can assist with grieving and closure for the physician.

SUGGESTED READINGS

- Callanan M, Kely P. *Final Gifts: Understanding the Special Awareness, Needs and Communications of the Dying.* Bantam Books; 1992.
- Ray MC. *I Am Here to Help: A Hospice Workers Guide to Communicating with Dying People and Their Loved Ones.* Hospice Handouts, McRay Company.

- Lattanzi-Licht M, Mahoney JJ, Miller GW. *The National Hospice Organization Guide to Hospice Care: The Hospice Choice: In Pursuit of A Peaceful Death*. Simon & Schuster.
- Hanson W. *The Next Place*. Waldman House Press; 1997.
- Baugher R, Calija M. *A Guide to the Bereaved Survivor*. Caring People Press. Newcastle, WA; 1998.
- Brown LK, Brown M. *When Dinosaurs Die: A Guide to Understanding Death*. Little Brown & Company. Boston; 1998.

PATIENT RESOURCES

- Caring Connections—**http://www.caringinfo.org.**
- Get Palliative Care—**www.getpalliativecare.org.**
- National Family Caregivers Association—**http://www.nfcacares.org/.**
- National Hospice and Palliative Care Organization—**http://www.nhpco.org.**

PROVIDER RESOURCES

- American Academy of Hospice and Palliative Medicine—**http://www.aahpm.org/.**
- National Hospice and Palliative Care Organization—**http://www.nhpco.org.**
- American Pain Society—**http://www.ampainsoc.org.**
- American Society for Bioethics and Humanities—**http://www.asbh.org.**
- American Society of Law, Medicine and Ethics—**http://www.aslme.org.**
- End-of-Life Care Consensus Panel—American College of Physicians-American Society of Internal Medicine—**http://www.acponline.org/running_practice/ethics/.**
- The EPEC Project (Education resource online)—**http://www.epec.net.**
- Palliative Care Matters—**http://www.pallcare.info.**

REFERENCES

1. Von Gunten CF. Interventions to manage symptoms at the end of life. *J Palliat Med*. 2005;8(suppl 1):S88-S94.
2. Lynn J. Measuring quality of care at the end of life: a statement of principles. *J Am Geriatr Soc*. 1997;45:526-527.
3. Xu J, Kochanek KD, Tejada-Vera B. Deaths: preliminary data for 2007. *National Vital Statistics Reports*. Hyattsville, MD: National Center for Health Statistics; 2009:58(1).
4. Kochanek KD, Xu JQ, Murphy SL, et al. Deaths: preliminary data for 2009. *National Vital Statistics Reports*. Hyattsville, MD: National Center for Health Statistics; 2011:59(4).
5. Zhao Y, Encinosa W. The cost of end-of-life hospitalizations, 2007. HCUP Statistical Brief #81. November 2009, revised April 2010. Rockville, MD: Agency for Healthcare Research and Quality. http://www.hcup-us.ahrq.gov/reports/statbriefs/sb81.pdf. Accessed March 2012.
6. Emanuel EJ, Emanuel LL. Palliative and end-of-life care. In: Kasper DL, Braunwald E, Fauci AS, Hauser SL, Longo DL, Jameson JL, eds. *Harrison's Principles of Internal Medicine*. 16th ed. New York, NY: McGraw-Hill Companies Inc.; 2005:53-66.
7. Kwak J, Healy WE. Current research findings on end-of-life decision making among racially or ethnically diverse groups. *Gerontologist*. 2005;45(5):634-641.
8. Centers for Disease Control and Prevention. Vital signs: current cigarette smoking among adults aged ≥18 years—United States, 2009. *MMWR Morb Mortal Wkly Rep*. 2010;59(35):1135-1140.
9. Centers for Disease Control and Prevention. State-specific smoking-attributable mortality and years of potential life lost—United States, 2000-2004. *MMWR Morb Mortal Wkly Rep*. 2009;58(02):29-33.
10. National Center for Health Statistics. Health, United States, 2010: in brief. Hyattsville, MD. 2011.
11. Schuckit MA. Alcohol and alcoholism. In: Kasper DL, Braunwald E, Fauci AS, Hauser SL, Longo DL, Jameson JL, eds. *Harrison's Principles of Internal Medicine*. 16th ed. New York, NY: McGraw-Hill Companies Inc.; 2005:2562-2566.
12. National Institute on Drug Abuse. InfoFacts: nationwide trends. http://www.drugabuse.gov/publications/infofacts/nationwide-trends. Accessed May 2013.
13. United States Department of Health and Human Services. Injury in the United States: 2007 Chartbook. http://www.cdc.gov/nchs/data/misc/injury2007.pdf. Accessed May 2013.
14. Centers for Disease Control and Prevention. AIDS in the United States by geographic distribution. http://www.cdc.gov/hiv/resources/factsheets/geographic.htm. Accessed May 2013.
15. Wolfe MI, Nolte KB, Yoon SS. Fatal infectious disease surveillance in a medical examiner database. http://www.cdc.gov/ncidod/eid/vol10no1/02-0764.htm. Accessed May 2013.
16. Centers for Disease Control and Prevention. Drug poisoning deaths in the United States, 1980-2008. http://www.cdc.gov/nchs/data/databriefs/db81.htm. Accessed May 2013.
17. Centers for Disease Control and Prevention. Suicides due to alcohol and/or drug overdose. http://www.cdc.gov/ViolencePrevention/pdf/NVDRS_Data_Brief-a.pdf. Accessed May 2013.
18. Reisfield GM, Wilson GR. Prognostication in heart failure. Fast facts and concepts. October 2005:143. http://www.eperc.mcw.edu/EPERC/FastFactsIndex/ff_143.htm. Accessed May 2013.
19. National Hospice and Palliative Care Organization. http://www.nhpco.org (for members). Accessed March 2012.
20. Lau F, Downing GM, Lesperance M, et al. Use of palliative performance scale in end-of-life prognostication. *J Palliative Med*. 2006;9(5):1066-1075.
21. Emanuel EJ, Fairclough DL, Slutsman J, et al. Assistance from family members, friends, paid care givers, and volunteers in the care of terminally ill patients. *N Engl J Med*. 1999;341(13):956-963.
22. Buckman R. *How to Break Bad News: A Guide for Health Care Professionals*. Baltimore, MD: Johns Hopkins University Press; 1992.
23. Steinhauser KE, Christakis NA, Clipp EC, et al. Factors considered important at the end of life by patients, family physicians, and other care providers. *JAMA*. 2000;284(19):1476-1482.
24. Meisel A, Snyder L, Quill T; American College of Physicians—American Society of Internal Medicine End-of-Life Care Consensus Panel. Seven legal barriers to end-of-life care: myths, realities and grains of truth. *JAMA*. 2000;284(19):2495-2501.

25. Turner R. Fast facts and concepts No. 82 and 83. Medicare hospice benefit Part 1. January 2003. End-of-Life Physician Education Resource Center. http://www.eperc.mcw.edu. Accessed March 2012.

26. Field MJ, Cassel CK, eds. *Approaching Death: Improving Care at the End of Life*. Washington, DC: National Academy Press; 1997.

27. World Health Organization. Pain ladder. http://www.who.int/entity/cancer/palliative/painladder/en/. Accessed March 1, 2007.

28. Dworkin RH, Backonja M, Rowbotham MC, et al. Advances in neuropathic pain: diagnosis, mechanisms, and treatment recommendations. Arch Neurol. 2003;60:1524-1534.

29. Clemens KE, Quednau I, Klaschik E. Use of oxygen and opioids in the palliation of dyspnea in hypoxic and non-hypoxic palliative care patients: a prospective study. *Support Care Cancer*. 2009;17:367-377.

30. Philip J, Gold M, Milner A, et al. A randomized, double-blind, crossover trial of the effect of oxygen on dyspnea in patients with advanced cancer. *J Pain Symptom Manage*. 2006;32:541-550.

31. Department of Labor. Wage and hour division. Family and Medical Leave Act. http://www.dol.gov/whd/fmla/. Accessed May 2013.

32. Larson DG, Tobin DR. End of life conversations: evolving practice and theory. *JAMA*. 2000;284:1573-1578.

33. Della Santina C, Bernstein RH. Whole patient assessment, goal planning, and inflection points: their role in achieving quality end-of life care. *Clin Geriatr Med*. 2004;20:595-620.

34. Jonsen AR, Seigler M, Winslade WJ. *Clinical Ethics: A Practical Approach to Ethical Decisions in Clinical Medicine*. 4th ed. New York, NY: McGraw-Hill; 1998.

35. Gordon DR. Principles and practice of withdrawing life-sustaining treatments. *Crit Care Clin*. 2004;20:435-451.

36. Billings JA, Krakauer EL. On patient autonomy and physician responsibility in end-of-life care. *Arch Intern Med*. 2011;171(9):849-853.

37. Curtis JR. Interventions to improve care during withdrawal of life-sustaining treatments. *J Palliat Med*. 2005;8(suppl 1):S116-S131.

5 SOCIAL JUSTICE

Mindy A. Smith, MD, MS
Richard P. Usatine, MD

Of all the forms of inequality, injustice in health care is the most shocking and inhumane.

—Martin Luther King, Jr.

The first question which the priest and the Levite asked was "If I stop to help this man, what will happen to me?" But ... the Good Samaritan reversed the question: "If I do not stop to help this man, what will happen to him?"

—Martin Luther King, Jr.

PATIENT STORIES

At only 5.5 lb (10 lb less than the fifth percentile for weight on the World Health Organization's growth chart), an 8-month-old infant boy suffered from severe malnutrition. In the summer of 2003, amid the height of Liberia's civil war, his aunt brought him to the Médecins sans Frontières/Doctors Without Borders hospital for treatment. Because of the war, his family had been forced to flee from their home, leaving behind their usual methods of getting food. Dr. Andrew Schechtman was there to help the day the child was brought to the clinic in Liberia **(Figure 5-1).** Despite the best available treatment for the malnutrition and concurrent pneumonia, the boy died on his third hospital day.

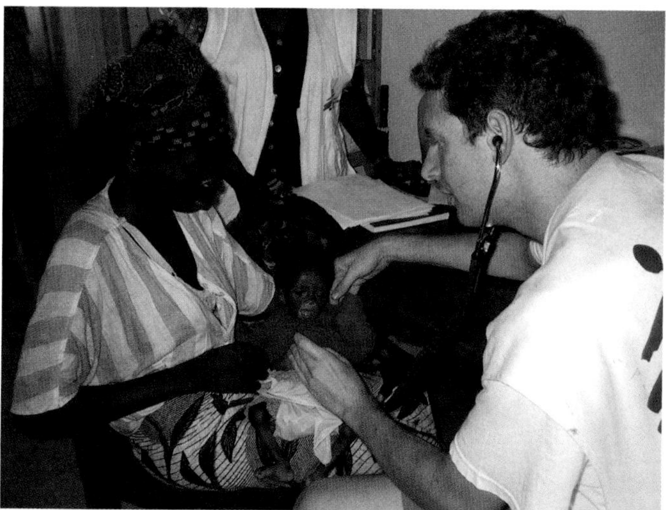

FIGURE 5-1 Dr. Andrew Schechtman was there to help the day a severely malnourished child was brought to the clinic in war-torn Liberia. Despite the best available treatment that could be provided in the Doctors Without Borders hospital, the child died of complications of malnutrition and pneumonia—a casualty of war and poverty. *(Reproduced with permission from Andrew Schechtman, MD.)*

OUR STORIES AS CARING CLINICIANS

Those of us who become physicians or other health care providers do so for many reasons. One reason is because of a desire to help someone else. Along the way, we sometimes lose ourselves in the day-to-day struggles, the disappointments, the obligations, the fatigue, and the profound helplessness that descends upon us after a particularly bad day. But we are still here and, if we listen with our hearts, we are still capable of great and small things.

We are privileged in so many ways and we must recognize our power over ourselves and over the communities that we serve. It is easy to become overwhelmed by the problems that we face as clinicians and as fellow human beings. Our health care system is in shambles, our natural world is being poisoned, our nations are continually at war, and yet, as this chapter highlights, there is so much that we can do—we can listen, we can observe, we can witness, we can bring aid, we can touch, we can love, and we can lead.

The text that follows highlights just a few examples of the ways in which our colleagues are challenging themselves to find creative solutions to the many problems faced by those who are underserved, displaced, or suffering.

DOCTORS WITHOUT BORDERS (ANDREW SCHECHTMAN, MD)

EPIDEMIOLOGY

The UN High Commissioner for Refugees reported that in 2011 there were 10.9 million refugees (those displaced across an international border) and 27.5 million internally displaced persons (IDPs, those displaced within their own country).[1] At the end of 2010, the UN refugee agency was caring for an estimated 14.7 million of these IDPs. During times of a complex humanitarian emergency (defined as a humanitarian crisis in a country, region, or society where there is a breakdown of authority resulting from internal or external conflict and which requires an international response that goes beyond the mandate or capacity of any single agency and/or the ongoing UN country program), the following usually occur[2]:

- Civilian casualties
- Populations besieged or displaced
- Serious political or conflict-related impediments to delivery of assistance
- Inability of people to pursue normal social, political, or economic activities
- High security risks for relief workers

ETIOLOGY

People can be displaced from their homes by man-made (war, persecution) or natural disasters (tsunami, earthquake, or hurricane). War is responsible for most of the displacement. Some of the source countries accounting for the most refugees are Afghanistan, Sudan, Somalia, the Palestinian territories, and Iraq.

- Communicable diseases usually cause the most illness and deaths in humanitarian emergencies in less-developed countries. Children younger than 5 years of age are the most vulnerable.[2] Other priority areas include provision of adequate safe water, food, shelter, and protection from violence.

- In addition to the usual causes of illness and death in emergency-affected populations in less-developed countries (measles, malaria, pneumonia, and diarrhea), crowded settlements may be prone to outbreaks of cholera, meningitis, and other diseases, which can be rapidly spread. Such outbreaks may be explosive and cause many deaths in a relatively short period of time.

PROBLEM IDENTIFIED

In times of stability, writes Dr. Andrew Schechtman, many of the poorest people in the world succeed in their struggle to meet basic needs for shelter, food, and water. When displaced from their homes by man-made or natural disaster, communities and extended families are disrupted, access to food and water are lost, and marginal circumstances become desperate. Displaced people are often dependent on the support of the international aid community to meet their basic needs.

BEING PART OF THE SOLUTION

When infrastructure collapses as a result of man-made or natural disasters, access to health care can be limited or nonexistent. Serving as a volunteer physician with Médecins sans Frontières (Doctors Without Borders) allowed Dr. Schechtman to provide medical care to people in desperate circumstances who had nowhere else to turn for assistance. Bearing witness to tragedies such as the case described in **Figure 5-1** gave him another means to help, that is, the authority to speak out on behalf of victims like this child, focus public attention on the situation, and encourage political pressure to bring the fighting to an end.

DISASTER RELIEF (RICHARD USATINE, MD)

EPIDEMIOLOGY

Hurricane Katrina was the deadliest hurricane to strike the United States since 1928. Katrina made initial landfall on August 25, 2005, in south Florida as a category 1 hurricane increasing rapidly in strength to category 5 upon reaching the Gulf of Mexico. On September 24, 2005, a second category 3 hurricane, Rita, forced the cessation of response activities in New Orleans and prompted the evacuation of Louisiana and Texas cities near the Gulf. In the days after the hurricane struck, displacement of people living in these areas resulted in more than 200,000 in evacuation centers in at least 18 states (**Figures 5-2** to **5-4**). There were more than 1800 deaths reported in Louisiana, Mississippi, Florida, Alabama, and Georgia.

- Eight hospitals and 9 acute care facilities in New Orleans reported on 17,446 visits (including 8997 [51.6%] for illness; 4579 [26.2%] for injury) during the days after hurricane Rita and during repopulation of the city.[3]
- Approximately 1500 people (10.9%) were admitted to a hospital. The most common reasons for hospital admission were heart disease (26.6%), gastrointestinal illness (12.3%), mental health condition (6.7%), and heat-related illness (6.1%).

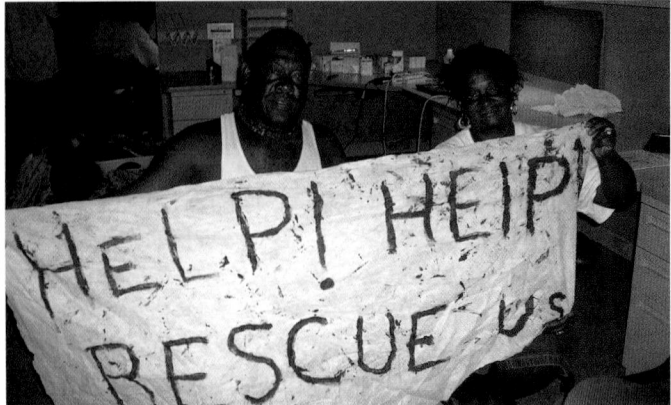

FIGURE 5-2 A husband and wife displaying the banner they made while being stranded on their roof during hurricane Katrina in New Orleans. The husband, who had an above-the-knee amputation, managed to climb with his crutches on to the roof of their flooded home. After 2 days they were saved from the floodwaters. In a shelter in San Antonio they displayed the sign that helped save their lives. (*Reproduced with permission from Richard P. Usatine, MD.*)

- Of the 25 deaths occurring in this period (0.2%), 23 occurred in patients who were seen for an illness (92%) and 2 occurred in patients seen for an injury (8%).
- About 1235 (9.1%) visits for injuries and illnesses were reported among relief workers (eg, paid military, paid civilian, self-employed, or volunteer).

ETIOLOGY

When hurricanes move onto land, the resulting storm surges, violent winds, heavy rains, and flooding can cause extensive damage. Hurricanes Katrina and Rita caused devastating storm-surge conditions for coastal

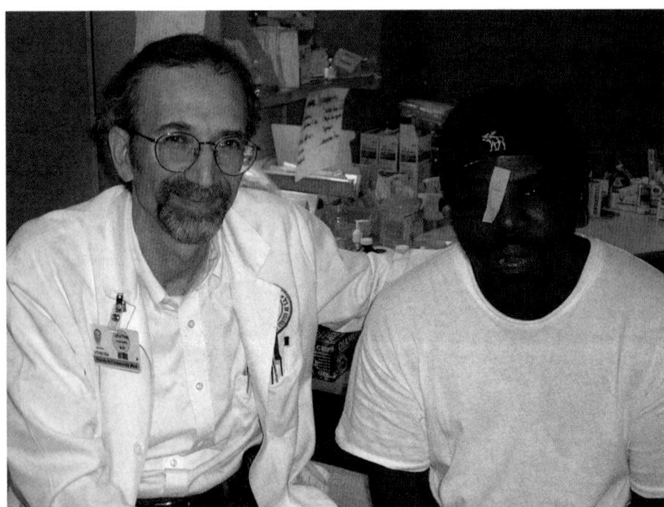

FIGURE 5-3 Dr. Usatine with a young man who was evacuated from New Orleans after hurricane Katrina. They are in a shelter in San Antonio and Dr. Usatine has just finished an incision and drainage of an abscess close to the eye (see Figure 123-1 for an image of the abscess prior to drainage). The San Antonio medical community mobilized quickly to provide medical care to the Katrina evacuees. (*Reproduced with permission from Richard P. Usatine, MD.*)

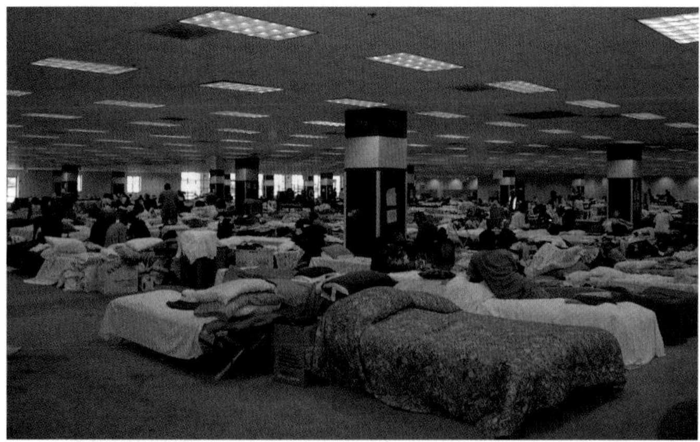

FIGURE 5-4 Thousands of people sleeping in a shelter in San Antonio after being evacuated from New Orleans and the Gulf Coast in 2005. The Katrina evacuees experienced the horrors of the hurricane, the flood, and the Super Dome. Some evacuees were added as hurricane Rita threatened the Gulf Coast. (*Reproduced with permission from Richard P. Usatine, MD.*)

Mississippi, Louisiana, and Alabama and damage as far east as the Florida panhandle. Storm-induced breaches in the New Orleans levee system resulted in the catastrophic flooding of approximately 80% of that city.[4] Hurricane Katrina disrupted basic utilities, food-distribution systems, health care services, and communications in large portions of Louisiana and Mississippi.

Before 1990, the majority of hurricane-related deaths in the United States resulted from drowning caused by sudden storm surges.[5] Since 1990, advances in warning technology and timely evacuation have increased the proportion of indirect causes of death and injury from hurricanes, such as electrocutions, cleanup injuries, and carbon monoxide poisonings. During and after hurricane Katrina, the majority of deaths resulted from storm surges along the Mississippi and Louisiana coastlines and flooding in the New Orleans area.

PROBLEM IDENTIFIED

Dr. Usatine, a professor of medicine at the University of Texas Health Science Center San Antonio watched the horror of hurricane Katrina comfortably from the safety of his home and work in San Antonio. On September 3, 2005 the first refugees (evacuees) from hurricane Katrina were brought to San Antonio. Dr. Usatine joined hundreds of other health care volunteers to provide free health care in the shelters that received these first evacuees (see **Figure 5-2**). Medical students also mobilized to be there to assist the local doctors in caring for these patients. Thousands of evacuees from New Orleans were transported directly to Kelly Air Force Base for food, shelter, social services, and medical care. Medications were donated from local pharmacies and doctors and nurses from the community and the universities came to provide services.

Many medical problems were identified and treated including skin infections from the unsanitary floodwaters. Common skin problems included cellulitis, skin abscesses, and impetigo (see **Figure 5-3**). Furthermore life-threatening conditions included patients with diabetes and hypertension out of control because they were evacuated without their medications, their medications were lost or their prescriptions ran out. One man began seizing in front of Dr. Usatine's eyes because he had been without his antiepileptic medicines for 1 week. Fortunately, he was stabilized and taken to a local hospital with EMT transport. The physical afflictions were the tip of the iceberg of the psychological trauma that the evacuees had suffered.

BEING PART OF THE SOLUTION

Every evacuee had a frightening story to tell and some were looking for family members and children from whom they had been separated. Providing shelter, food, medical and social services to thousands of people at once was a great challenge but with all the agencies and volunteers that could be mustered in San Antonio most would say that the effort was a success. The work of providing services and ultimately resettlement for these evacuees went on for months. Hurricane Rita threatened the Gulf Coast only 4 weeks after hurricane Katrina and this added additional evacuees to the people in San Antonio needing services (see **Figure 5-4**). As a physician, Dr. Usatine found it rewarding to be there at the time of need for his fellow human beings who had suffered immeasurably due to the natural disasters and the lack of preparedness for these disasters. To this day he finds it incredible that such a wealthy nation neglected the known risks of flooding in New Orleans and let the levees go unrepaired until the city of New Orleans had to pay the price of the disaster brought on by hurricane Katrina. He was proud to be part of the relief effort that was mounted in his hometown of San Antonio.

INTERNATIONAL HUMANITARIAN EFFORTS: ETHIOPIA (RICK HODES, MD)

EPIDEMIOLOGY

Chronic food deficits affect about 792 million people in the world, including 20% of the population in developing countries. Malnutrition greatly increases the risk of disease and early death, particularly in young children where protein-energy malnutrition plays a major role in half of all deaths of children under age 5 years annually in developing countries.[6] Worldwide, malnutrition affects 1 in 3 people and is especially common among the poor and those with inadequate access to health education, clean water, and good sanitation. About 26% of children with protein-energy malnutrition live in Africa. Severe forms of malnutrition include marasmus, iodine deficiency which can result in cretinism and irreversible brain damage, and vitamin A deficiency which can result in blindness and increased risk of infection and death.[6]

Worldwide, 2.4 billion people will remain without improved sanitation in 2015 and in 2011, 768 million people relied on unimproved drinking water sources. In most of Africa, sanitation coverage is less than 50%.[7] Ethiopia and its neighbor Somalia are among the few remaining countries in Africa with less than 50% of the population using improved sources of drinking water.[7] Piped drinking water supplies, associated with the best health outcomes, are present only for 1% to 10% of Ethiopia's population.

ETIOLOGY

Ethiopia has a population of over 91 million people. The gross national income per capita is $1100, making it one of the poorest nations in the world. The probability of dying under age 5 years is 68/1000 live births, in part due to the low percentage of women attending antenatal care and only 10% of births being attended by skilled health personnel.[8] The health workforce is nearly nonexistent with 0.3 physicians per 10,000 population and 2.5 nurses and midwives per 10,000 population. Health problems in Ethiopia include maternal mortality, malaria, tuberculosis (TB), and HIV/AIDS compounded by malnutrition and lack of access to clean water and sanitation.

PROBLEM IDENTIFIED

Rick Hodes is an internist who has lived and worked in Ethiopia for over 20 years. As an orthodox Jew, he always aspired to serve others and even as a child, his favorite books were about doctors who went to remote places to help people. He first went to Ethiopia in 1984 to do famine relief work. His experience of working at a mission in Ethiopia run by Mother Teresa changed his life. He returned to Ethiopia on a Fulbright Fellowship and in 1990 was hired by the American Jewish Joint Distribution Committee (JDC) as the medical adviser for the country. His original position was to care for 25,000 potential immigrants to Israel but he is continually drawn back to Ethiopia to provide care to patients. When asked once why he wouldn't prefer to work in the United States than Africa with its poverty and lack of resources, Hodes said, "It would be less frustrating—but it would also be less inspiring."

BEING PART OF THE SOLUTION

As senior consultant at a Catholic mission, Dr. Hodes helps patients with heart disease (rheumatic and congenital) (**Figure 5-5**), spinal disease (TB and scoliosis) (**Figure 5-6**), infectious disease and cancer. He has worked with refugees in Rwanda, Zaire, Tanzania, Somalia, and Albania in addition to Ethiopia. Dr. Hodes is part of a team at the American Jewish JDC, a Jewish humanitarian assistance organization founded in 1914 that provides needed services in more than 70 countries. One among his JDC duties has been providing medical care for thousands of Ethiopian Jews preparing to immigrate to Israel. In addition to its assistance to the Ethiopian Jewish community, the JDC has served tens of thousands of Ethiopians, Jews and non-Jews, through clinics, immunization, nutrition programs, family planning, and community health.

Dr. Hodes has worked primarily in Ethiopia for the JDC since 1990. In addition to providing direct patient care, he has arranged specialized care for hundreds of children in need with neurosurgeons and orthopedic surgeons in the United States and Ghana. He has fostered numerous orphaned children and adopted 4 children, providing needed medical care with his own insurance. Some of these children are now attending schools and colleges around the United States. He has also led teams of doctors, who come to work with him as volunteers (**Figure 5-7**). In one interview, Hodes said, "Getting free medical care in a Catholic hospital by a Jewish doctor is like the whole world coming together. It's the way the world should work."

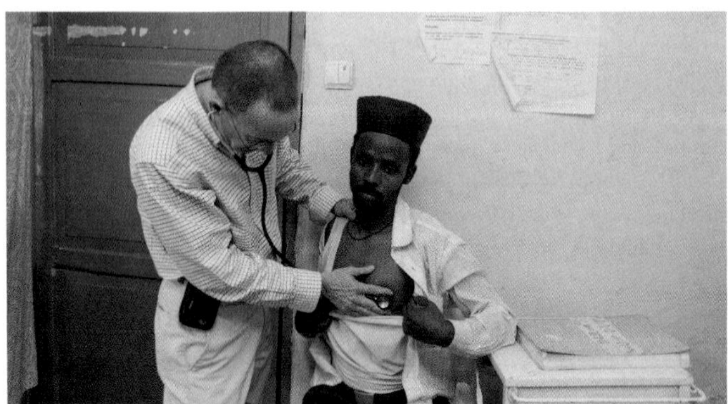

FIGURE 5-5 Examining an Ethiopian orthodox priest with rheumatic heart disease who has increasing congestive heart failure. (*Reproduced with permission from Rick Hodes, MD.*)

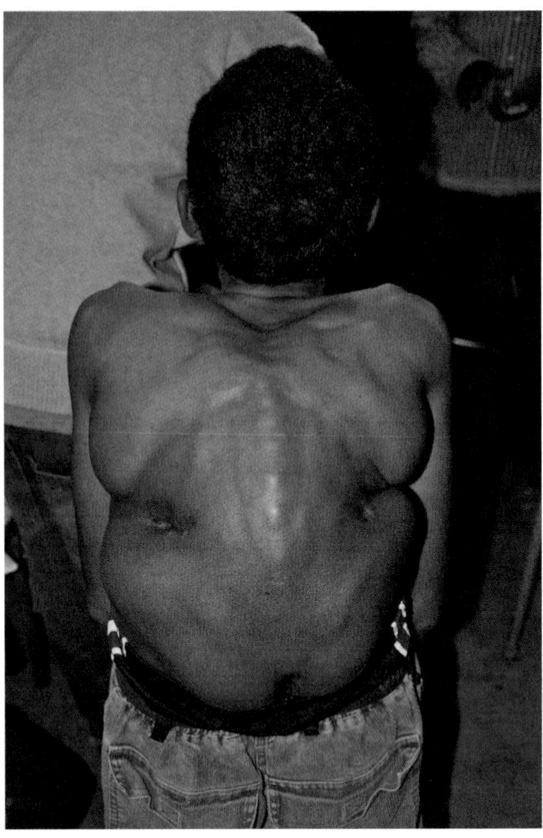

FIGURE 5-6 A patient of Dr. Hodes with severe kyphoscoliosis secondary to tuberculosis of the spine. (*Reproduced with permission from Richard P. Usatine, MD.*)

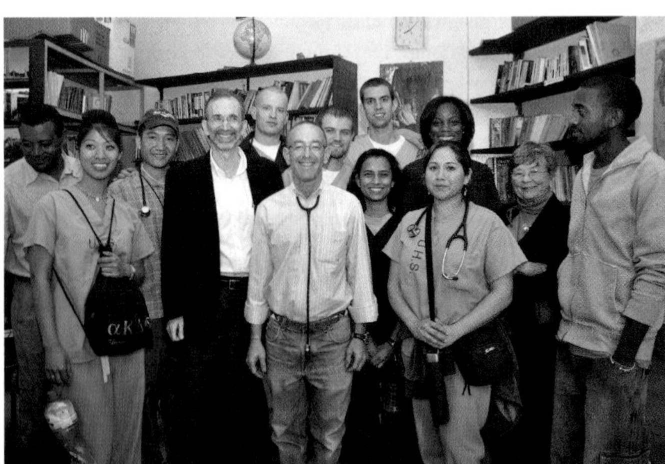

FIGURE 5-7 Dr. Hodes with American medical students and doctors visiting him at his clinic at Mother Teresa's mission in Addis Ababa, Ethiopia. (*Reproduced with permission from Richard P. Usatine, MD.*)

CARING FOR THOSE WITH DISABILITIES (LAURIE WOODARD, MD)

EPIDEMIOLOGY

Approximately 54 million Americans currently live with at least one disability and the vast majority (52 million) live in their communities (**Figure 5-8**).[9]

- According to data from 1999, the prevalence rate of disability was 24% among women and 20% among men.[10] Approximately 32 million adults had difficulty with one or more functional activities, and approximately 16.7 million adults had a limitation in the ability to work around the house. Two million adults used a wheelchair and 7 million used a cane, crutches, or a walker.
- Of children aged 3 to 17 years, 4.9 million were told that they had some type of learning disability and 12.8% (9.4 million) had special health care needs.[9]
- Racial and ethnic minorities have higher rates of disabilities than whites or Asian Americans; 7.3 million individuals (ages 15 to 65 years) with disabilities are of racial or ethnic minorities.
- In 2005, the surgeon general issued a Call to Action to improve the health and wellness of persons with disabilities underscoring the need in this population.[9]

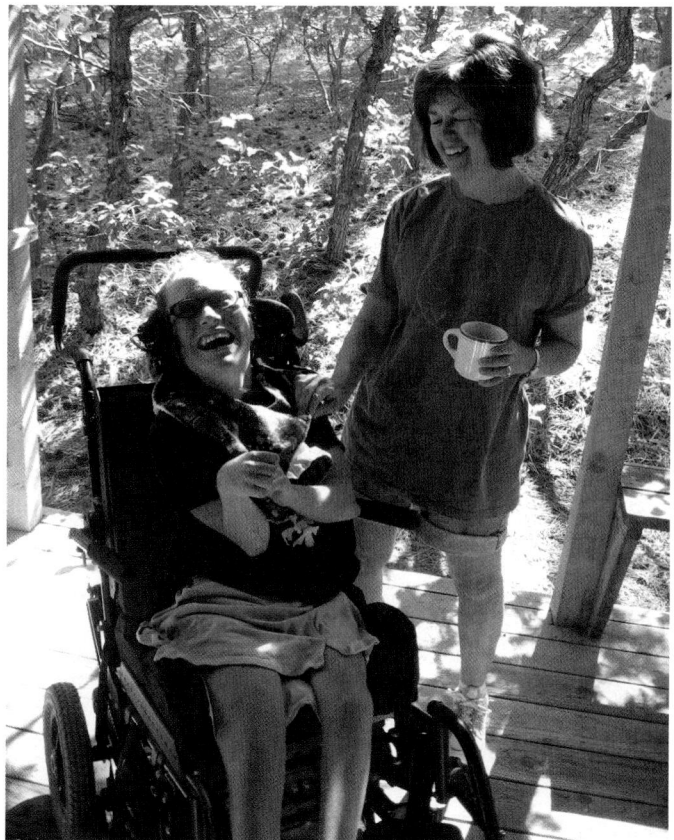

FIGURE 5-8 Dr. Laurie Woodard and her daughter Anika share a good laugh following breakfast while on vacation in New Mexico. Although Anika is dependent for all her activities of daily living and is nonverbal because of spastic quadriparetic cerebral palsy, she loves to travel and has a wonderful sense of humor.

ETIOLOGY

Challenges to a person's health can happen at any age and at any time. Disabilities are not illnesses, rather they are limitations related to a medical condition that have an influence on essential life functions such as walking, seeing, or working.[9] Furthermore, disabilities do not affect all people in the same way.

- Of all the adults with disabilities, 41.2 million (93.4%) reported that their disability was associated with a health condition including arthritis and rheumatism (17.5%), back or spine problems (16.5%), heart trouble or hardening of the arteries (7.8%), lung or respiratory problems (4.7%), deafness or hearing problems (4.2%), mental or emotional problems (3.7%), blindness or visual problems (3.4%), and intellectual disability (2%).[10]
- Rates of disability are increasing in part because of the aging population, better survival of catastrophic illnesses and trauma, and advances in preventing infant and child mortality.

PROBLEM IDENTIFIED

As a mother of a child with profound disabilities, Dr. Laurie Woodard found that her medical training did little to prepare her for caring for her child or finding help (see **Figure 5-8**). She became acutely aware that people with disabilities had great difficulty in finding physicians and those who provided care often seemed afraid of them. She said, "I couldn't imagine someone not wanting to care for her because she had a disability." Physicians tend to focus on the medical condition and not the whole person and their families; when confronted with the patient's health care needs and functional issues, the feeling of acting more like a social worker than a physician caused them to fall back into medical model framework. In addition, societal support for those with disabilities, particularly disabilities acquired as an adult, are fragmented and the primary care physician needs to become the link.

BEING PART OF THE SOLUTION

Dr. Woodard began to care for increasing numbers of patients with disabilities, training herself through reading, experience, and asking patients what worked. As she worked with individual students she planned for a time when she could break into the medical student curriculum to provide this training. Eight years ago, when the curriculum for third-year students underwent major reform, she saw her opportunity. Within the primary care 12-week experience, a curriculum on special populations was planned and Laurie made sure that it included teaching about people with disabilities. Her curriculum, implemented in 2005 with goals ranging from sensitivity training to understanding both the capabilities and needs of individuals with disabilities, contains the following components:

- Clinic-like experience with 8 to 10 patients with physical disabilities (eg, cerebral palsy, communication issues, wheelchair users) where pairs of students complete brief interview and physical examination under video monitoring. The session ends with a debriefing circle wrap up with students and patients.
- Panel discussion involves patients with varying abilities who usually represent an advocacy agency or organization. Special emphasis is placed on community services and opportunities including the arts and sports.

- Home visits where student pairs (2 medical students or a medical student and physical therapy student) receive a preparation sheet and checklist and learn how disability affects individuals and their family. Following the visit, students prepare reflection plus research reports that are posted on blackboard; part of the assignment is to read and comment on all the papers.
- Service learning project where students give presentations on health topics (eg, first aid, influenza) selected by staff at an adult daycare facility for individuals with intellectual disabilities or the high school group noted above, or assist in the recreational activities for individuals with disabilities (eg, free physicals for riders in therapeutic horseback riding program).
- An objective structured clinical examination (OSCE) case involving a manual wheelchair user with shoulder pain; the standardized patients are individuals who are wheelchair users.
- Sensitivity training session, run by Parks and Recreation where students are randomly assigned a disability (eg, using a wheelchair or other assistive device or blindfold) and complete tasks followed by watching the movie *Murderball* (an informative and proactive documentary about the Paralympics sport, quadriplegic rugby, and its players). A speech pathologist also provides a hands-on assistive/augment communication device tutorial.

"The students learn to see the patient first," she says, "that caring for these individuals requires recognizing the patient's expertise about their disability and problem solving together. For most students, even the most jaded, this is simply an eye-opening experience as the patients are usually quite physically impaired but lead full and active lives." (**Figure 5-9**)

Dr. Woodard has expanded this program and is coteaching with faculty from the School of Physical Therapy (PT) so that medical and PT students interview and examine patients together. In addition, she will begin providing training within the courses Doctoring 1 and Doctoring 2 to first- and second-year medical students (the home visit and panel discussion will be moved to the first year) allowing more complex and challenging issues to be addressed during the clerkship. Finally, she is also involved with Alliance for Disability in Health Education, a group mainly out of the Northeast whose mission is to get the American Association of Medical Colleges (AAMC) to require the topic of disability in the curriculum.

Dr. Woodard's daughter graduated from high school in June 2011. The family is working on helping her structure her day and move beyond the interminable wait list for services to which she is entitled. She is happy and healthy and the family members consider themselves lucky to have good, affordable caregivers, and companions to assist her.

CARING FOR THE HOMELESS (JIM WITHERS, MD)

EPIDEMIOLOGY

Throughout the United States and abroad there are growing numbers of people who are forced to sleep on the streets. In 2009, at least 643,000 people were homeless on any given night and 1 in every 200 Americans (approximately 1.56 million people) spent at least one night in a shelter during that year.[11] Even within homeless populations, the unsheltered homeless (or "rough sleepers"), have much greater challenges in terms of health, discrimination, environmental stress, and mental illness. The characteristics of the street homeless and the larger community conspire to create a disaffected, highly vulnerable subgroup for whom very little successful intervention is available. In many cases, even homeless health agencies view this population as either hopeless or "not ready" for services.

Coincident with the financial, moral, and social crisis associated with the growing street homeless population, systems of medical education are called upon to educate future clinicians that are capable of "bridging the reality gap" between the complex needs of individuals and the fairly rigid structure of modern health care. A classroom is needed in which we can "learn to learn" from those who are the most alienated and underserved **(Figure 5-10)**. Indeed, the skills thus learned have significant implications for how we approach health care that will meet the needs of all future populations. Creating a workable model for effectively including those living under the bridges, in the alleys, and along the rivers of our own communities can provide a template for bridging other such "reality gaps."

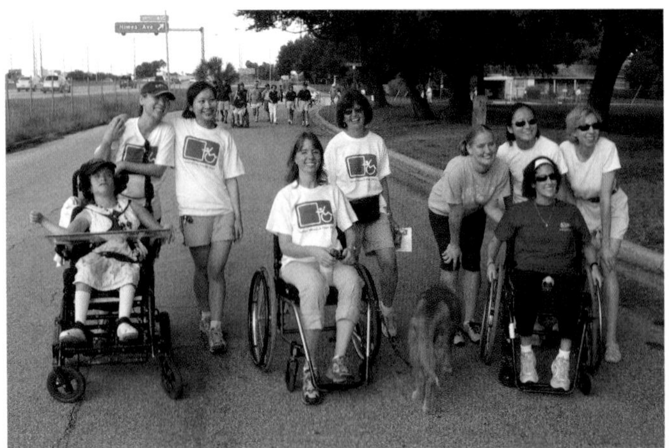

FIGURE 5-9 Dr. Woodard, daughter Anika, and dog Nikki are part of a team of University of South Florida (USF) medical students, faculty, and family who participated in a "wheel-a-thon" to raise money for Tampa's first fully accessible playground. Teaching medical students the therapeutic value of sports and recreation for people with disabilities is an important aspect of the USF curriculum.

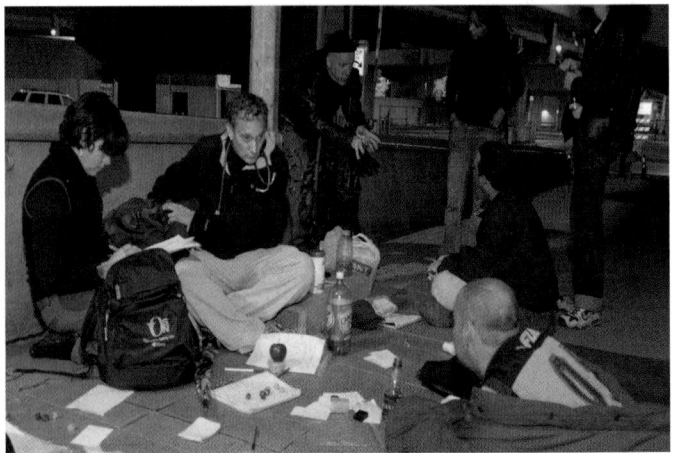

FIGURE 5-10 "Classroom of the streets." Dr. Withers with 2 medical students and 1 outreach guide (with black cap) working with homeless youth under a bridge on the north side of Pittsburgh. (*Reproduced with permission from Pittsburgh Mercy Health System and Operation Safety Net.*)

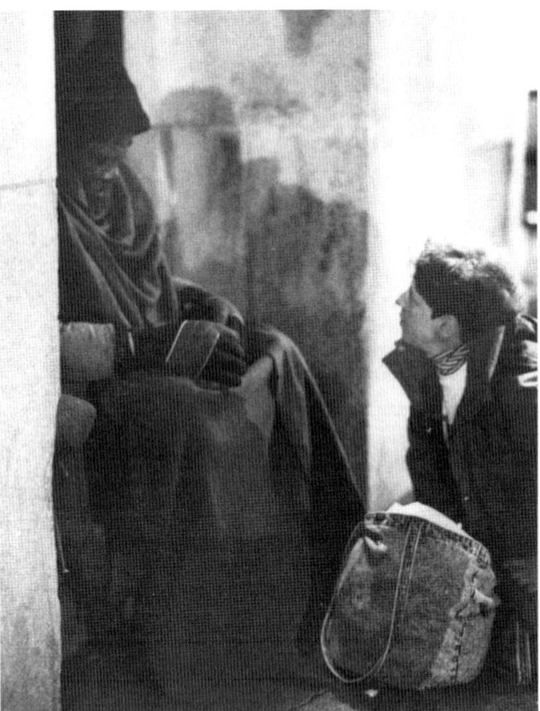

FIGURE 5-11 Volunteer nurse Carole trying to establish a relationship with a mentally ill homeless man in downtown Pittsburgh. This photo shows the importance of respect and meeting people where they are. (*Reproduced with permission from Sandy Marlin. © 2013 Pittsburgh Mercy Health System and Operation Safety Net.*)

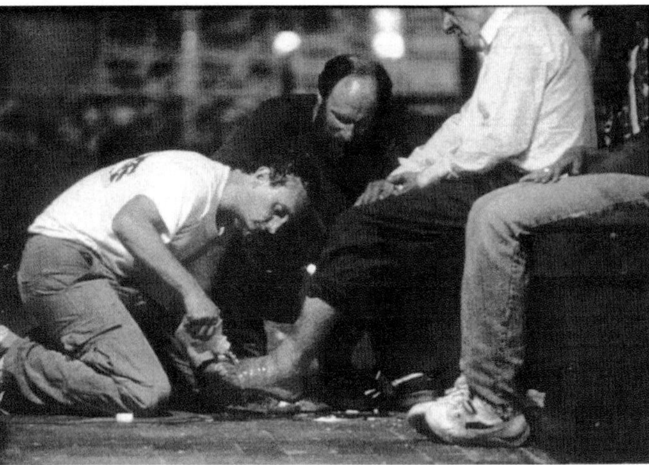

FIGURE 5-12 Dr. Withers is washing the feet of an older homeless man at Market Square, downtown Pittsburgh. A psychiatry nurse with the beard is watching. The man's feet needed care for moderate trench foot. Most importantly, this image demonstrates the concept of service. (*Reproduced with permission from Pittsburgh Mercy Health System and Operation Safety Net.*)

ETIOLOGY

The street homeless are a heterogeneous group, each with their own story that must be understood. However, there are a number of common factors that lead to street homelessness. These include mental illness, addiction, abuse, prejudice, and legal issues (**Figure 5-11**). They are paradoxically among the highest utilizers of costly emergency services and present for care only when forced to do so by crisis. By definition they do not engage preventive or primary care services, being largely alienated from mainstream society. As such, they present a unique challenge, but also an opportunity to learn how to recreate the health care response to meet the reality of those who have been excluded. In the final analysis, it is the health system itself that must be improved.

PROBLEM IDENTIFIED

Although there are notable models for health care delivery that "Go To The People," the vast majority of health care requires people to seek care on the terms of the system. Unable to do so, rough sleepers throughout the world are growing further alienated and resented by existing systems of care. This impasse is not only inefficient, but also results in mutual resentments—especially when the street homeless population contains disproportionate numbers of ethnic minorities. The ultimate cost of this situation is a lack of wholeness as a community leading to deeper fragmentation and fear.

Early in his career, Dr. Jim Withers (an Internal Medicine teaching physician for the Pittsburgh Mercy Health System in Pittsburgh) realized that a new approach to the care of disconnected populations could both provide much needed direct medical service and also act as a learning opportunity to explore the principles of effective medical-social connection. Experiences making "house calls" with his father as a child, international health work, and focused attention to the field of domestic violence stimulated his search for a suitable classroom that would force clinicians to work with people almost completely on their terms. In order to make this cognitive leap complete, he felt he needed to take a dramatic course of action.

In 1992, Dr. Withers began to dress as a homeless person and make nighttime visits to the street homeless of Pittsburgh. He was accompanied by a "street guide" who had been formerly homeless and was trusted by the street homeless community. His intention was to start as much as possible with no preconceptions or agenda in terms of medical solutions, but rather develop relationships with the street homeless that might lead to a shared path of healing (**Figure 5-12**). Of the first 119 unsheltered homeless he encountered, virtually none had any form of primary care despite the fact that there was a high prevalence of serious medical and mental health disease.

BEING PART OF THE SOLUTION

Dr. Withers began to bring medications in a backpack and then seek higher levels of care as each individual desired. Soon there were other medical volunteers and medical students working on the streets with their own formerly homeless guides (**Figure 5-10**). An electronic health record was created, an office established for follow-up issues and, by January of 1993, Operation Safety Net (OSN) was established as a part of the Pittsburgh Mercy Health System at Mercy Hospital.

Since the establishment of OSN (www.operationsafetynet.net), the program has had a significant impact on both health care delivery and medical education in Pittsburgh. Approximately 1200 individuals are seen each year on the streets. Most are now insured through targeted benefits counseling and are directed to a primary care office specifically tailored to their care. Street patients are managed within a "medical home" type model with a 24-hour on-call answering service and follow-up care.

Any homeless person, emergency department, or vested party can contact OSN as the "home care service for the streets." A city-wide hospital consult service serves to improve patient care and provide better discharge planning. With successful collaborations and grant support, OSN has housed over 900 chronically homeless individuals from 2004 to 2013. An increasingly comprehensive care system meets the specific needs of the recovering street homeless population and follows them at whatever stage of engagement they chose to participate. Over 100 students are trained within the OSN model each year and many go on to establish their own service-oriented programs throughout the world (see **Figure 5-10**).

Dr. Withers visited India in 1993 at which time he heard about the work of Dr. Jack Preger in Calcutta. Dr. Preger established the Calcutta Rescue program in 1979 which delivers medical care directly to the street homeless of that vast city (**Figure 5-13**). At that meeting, Dr. Withers had an epiphany and realized that a new field of medicine was being practiced in both their cities involving the same basic principles of care delivery. After many journeys to communities throughout the United States and abroad, Dr. Withers developed a network of grassroots organizations practicing what is now known as "street medicine." A number of established efforts in cities like Boston, Santiago Chile, and Dublin were linked and an even larger number of new programs have emerged being inspired by the street medicine movement.

In order to galvanize the street medicine movement, Dr. Withers established the first annual International Street Medicine Symposium in Pittsburgh in 2005. The symposium, held in a different city each year, has grown from the original meeting of 27 pioneers to 199 registrants from all over the United States and 12 other countries, spanning 5 continents, who came to the ninth International Street Medicine Symposium in Boston in 2013. Students also presented updates on their growing network and displayed 19 academic posters.

The Street Medicine Institute (www.streetmedicine.org) was established by Dr. Withers and other key partners in 2009 to be the global "home" of the street medicine movement. The vision is that one day every person forced to live on the streets will have direct access to medical care that is sensitive to their particular need. Also, it is envisioned that every possible health science school will have an elective "classroom of the streets" in which future clinicians can develop their service-oriented skills within their own communities (see **Figure 5-10**). The Street Medicine Institute is dedicated to assisting the development of new street medicine programs, improving the practice of street medicine, fostering the transformational value of the street medicine movement, and to create learning opportunities within the street medicine context. Dr. Withers believes that by serving the most vulnerable of our own communities, we learn to make health care an agent of positive change in ourselves and society at large.

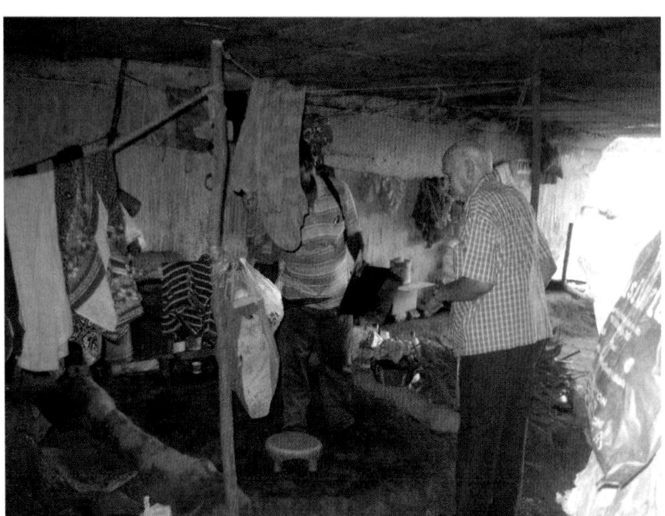

FIGURE 5-13 Dr. Jack Preger established the Calcutta Rescue program in 1979 which delivers medical care directly to the street homeless of that vast city. Dr. Preger is working under a bridge in Calcutta bringing medical care to a homeless man.

PROVIDER RESOURCES

International Humanitarian Efforts

- Doctors Without Borders—**http://www.doctorswithoutborders.org.**
- **http://www.globalcorps.com/jobs/ngolist.doc.**
- **http://www.exploringabroad.com/humanitarian-org.htm.**
- **http://www.internationalhealthvolunteers.org/.**
- Rick Hodes Web site—**http://rickhodes.org.**
- Calcutta Rescue—**http://www.calcuttarescue.org/**

Disabled Persons

- US Department of Justice—**http://www.usdoj.gov/crt/ada/cguide.htm.**
- Social Security Administration—**http://www.ssa.gov/disability/**(information on benefits).
- Information on Sports Events for the Disabled— http://**www.dsusa.org.**
- **http://www.disabilityinfo.gov.**

Homeless

- National Coalition for the Homeless—**http://www.nationalhomeless.org/.**
- National Alliance to End Homelessness—**http://www.naeh.org/.**
- US Department of Housing and Urban Development—**http://www.hud.gov/homeless/index.cfm.**
- Veterans Affairs—**http://www1.va.gov/homeless/.**
- The Society of Student-Run Free Clinics—**http://www.studentrunfreeclinics.org/.**
- Haven for Hope—**http://www.havenforhope.org/.**

REFERENCES

1. United Nations High Commissioner for Refugees (UNHCR). http://www.unhcr.org/pages/49c3646c11.html. Accessed November 2013.
2. Center for Disease Control (CDC). *Frequently Asked Questions About International Emergency and Refugee Health*. http://www.cdc.gov/globalhealth/gdder/ierh/FAQ.htm. Accessed November 2013.
3. Daley WR. *Public Health Response to Hurricanes Katrina and Rita—Louisiana, 2005*. http://www.cdc.gov/mmwr/preview/mmwrhtml/mm5502a1.htm. CDC. Accessed November 2013.
4. *Injury and Illness Surveillance in Hospitals and Acute-Care Facilities After Hurricanes Katrina and Rita—New Orleans Area, Louisiana, Sept 25 to Oct 15, 2005*. http://www.cdc.gov/mmwr/preview/mmwrhtml/mm5502a4.htm. Accessed November 2013.

5. Hanzlick R. Office of the Fulton County Medical Examiner. Surveillance and Programs Br, Div of Environmental Hazards and Health Effects, Center for Environmental Health, CDC. *MMWR Morb Mortal Wkly Rep*. 1987;36(19):297-299.

6. World Health Organization. Water-related diseases. *Malnutrition*. http://www.who.int/water_sanitation_health/diseases/malnutrition/en/. Accessed October 2013.

7. World Health Organization. *Progress on Sanitation and Drinking Water: 2013 Update*. http://apps.who.int/iris/bitstream/10665/81245/1/9789241505390_eng.pdf. Accessed October 2013.

8. *World Health Organization African Region: Ethiopia*. http://www.who.int/countries/eth/en/. Accessed November 2013.

9. Department of Health and Human Services. *The Surgeon General's Call to Action to Improve the Health and Wellness of Persons with Disabilities*. Rockville, MD: Public Health Service; 2005. http://www.surgeongeneral.gov/library/disabilities/calltoaction/calltoaction.pdf. Accessed April 25, 2007.

10. Prevalence of disabilities and associated health conditions among adults—United States, 1999. *MMWR Morb Mortal Wkly Rep*. 2001;50(07):120-125.

11 Centers for Disease Control and Prevention. *National Prevention Information Network*. http://www.cdcnpin.org/scripts/population/homeless.asp. Accessed May 1, 2012.

6 GLOBAL HEALTH

Ruth E. Berggren, MD
Richard P. Usatine, MD

COMMUNITY STORY

Common River is a US-based nongovernmental organization (NGO) implementing a community development program in Aleta Wondo, Ethiopia. This NGO is founded on the principle of positive deviance, in which local best practices are identified and replicated to maximize agricultural production (organically grown coffee is produced in this region), as well as to improve the nutritional status, health, and education of orphaned and vulnerable children. Since 2009, a group from the University of Texas School of Medicine in San Antonio has traveled annually to Aleta Wondo to provide school health screening and free health care, including treatment of endemic helminth infections, trachoma, and skin diseases, while collaborating with and supporting the local government-sponsored health clinic (**Figure 6-1A**). In **Figure 6-1B,** a University of Texas medical student helps an elderly man to a chair where he will be seen by the medical team working in Aleta Wondo. The people of Aleta Wondo will receive oral albendazole for the treatment of intestinal parasites and will undergo complete physical examinations for the detection and treatment of other common conditions, such as head lice, tinea capitis, trachoma, and foot infections. In **Figure 6-1C,** a group of women has just completed their woman's literacy class for the day. Improving women's literacy can improve the health of the entire community.

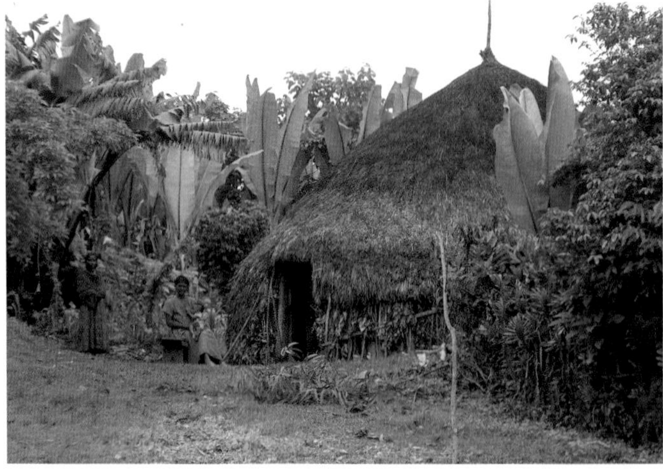

A

FIGURE 6-1 **A.** Many people still live in extreme poverty with no running water and electricity. This is a typical hut in Ethiopia. This one is inhabited by a grandmother, her grandchild, and a cow. The photograph was taken after a home visit to provide IM ceftriaxone to the child after her release from the local hospital where she was treated for a neck abscess and cellulitis. The medical team was staying at Common River and originated from the University of Texas. (*Reproduced with permission from Richard P. Usatine, MD.*)

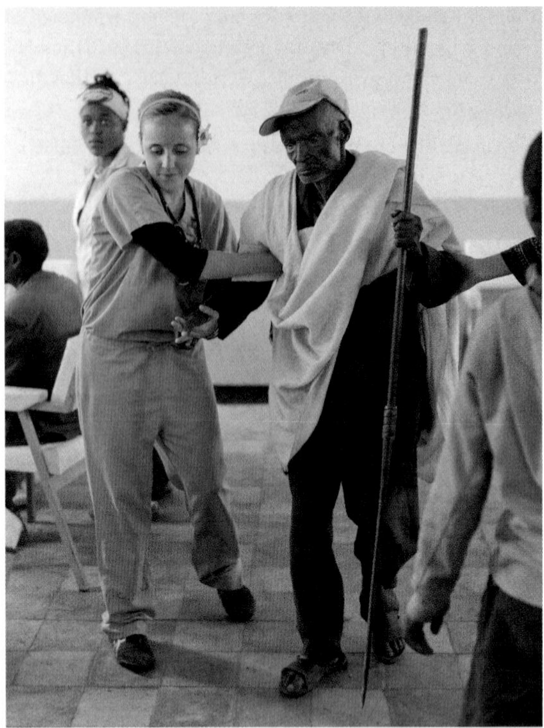

B

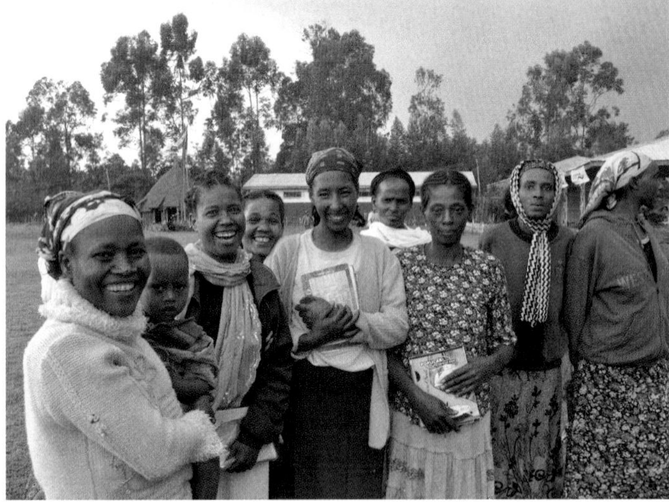

C

FIGURE 6-1 (Continued) **B.** A University of Texas medical student helps an elderly man to a chair where he will be seen by the medical team working in Aleta Wondo. One of the local nursing students is observing the clinical activity. (*Reproduced with permission from Lester Rosebrock.*) **C.** Smiling women who have just completed their woman's literacy class for the day. Improving woman's literacy is a great way to raise the health status of the community. (*Reproduced with permission from Richard P. Usatine, MD.*)

WHAT IS GLOBAL HEALTH?

For years, the term *international health* has described health work in resource-limited settings with an emphasis on tropical diseases, communicable diseases, and illness caused by poor nutrition and inadequate access to water, sanitation, and maternal care.[1] More recently, *global health* is commonly used to emphasize mutual sharing of experience and knowledge, in a bilateral exchange between industrialized nations and resource-limited countries, and the emphasis is expanding to include noncommunicable diseases and chronic illness.[2] One definition of global health, proposed by the Consortium of Universities for Global Health Executive Board, is "an area for study, research, and practice that places priority on improving health and achieving equity in health for all people worldwide."[1] This chapter focuses on a few conditions commonly encountered in developing nations, emphasizing communicable diseases and malnutrition.

Ethical dilemmas abound when professionals from resource-rich settings leave their familiar environment and apply their practices in a severely resource-limited setting. Consider, for example, breastfeeding guidelines in the setting of maternal-to-child HIV prevention. National protocols differ depending on resource availability. In some settings, telling an HIV-positive mother not to breast-feed (because breast-milk can transmit HIV) may sentence her infant to near-certain death from diarrhea. If a program overturns local teaching about exclusive breast-feeding, it must ensure a safe and sustainable alternative form of infant feeding. Imposing the standards of industrialized nations in a community that cannot afford to continue to provide these standards can undo years of program development. Care must be taken not to undermine the trust a community has placed in local health providers, as this can ultimately increase morbidity rather than relieve suffering. Working with local health providers is essential so that a short trip can result in extended benefits to the community.

This chapter briefly introduces some of the relevant subject areas with which global health providers should familiarize themselves when preparing for international work. Statistics that aid in understanding the state of a nation's health relative to other countries are the mortality rate of children younger than age 5 years and adult life expectancy. Least-developed countries report that as many as 112 of 1000 children die before age 5 years, compared to 8 per 1000 in developed countries,[3] and adult life expectancy ranges from 48 or 49 years at birth (Chad, Swaziland) to 88 or 89 years (Japan, Monaco).[3] Another important parameter by which to compare the health status of countries is that of maternal mortality, defined as the number of maternal deaths per 100,000 live births. These figures, together with basic epidemiology of disease, provide important insights into public health priorities for populations.

What statistics do not provide, however, is the level of importance ascribed to a particular health issue by a community. It is necessary to acknowledge and address the needs expressed by communities themselves, in order of their own priorities, so as to achieve sustained improvements in health outcomes. All health improvements ultimately rely on long-term behavioral changes, whether dietary, pill taking, physical activity, or hygiene related. Group behavioral change requires buy-in from the population with the approbation and influence of local leadership.

A useful method of creating a positive impact is to make use of ongoing peer-to-peer adult education techniques through the introduction of community health clubs. This can be effective for empowering resource-limited communities to develop their priorities, and to advocate their community health and development needs.[4] It is best to learn about and collaborate with the local and governmental community health activities before launching any intervention, be it clinical, infrastructural, or preventive.

WATER AND SANITATION

Many diseases in resource-poor settings are traceable to deficits in clean water supply and storage, lack of soap for bathing, and lack of functioning infrastructure to manage human waste (garbage collection, latrines)[5] (**Figure 6-2**). Some of the most important ones include typhoid fever, cholera, and intestinal parasites.

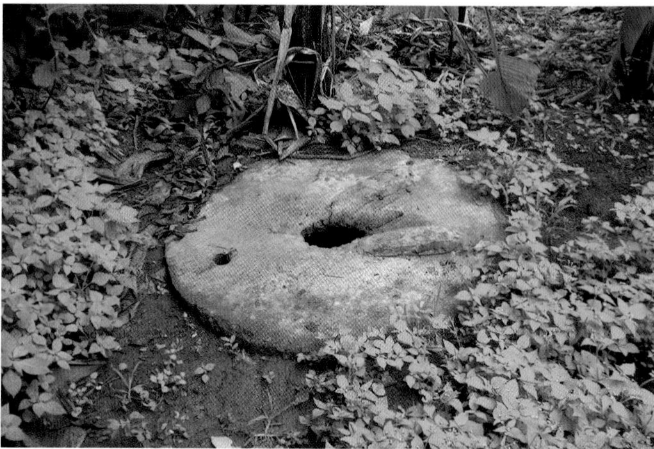

FIGURE 6-2 An Ethiopian pit latrine, which offers no mitigation for flies and is situated in proximity to the water table below. Heavy rains will lead to contamination of the water supply with fecal pathogens. *(Reproduced with permission from Richard P. Usatine, MD.)*

Lack of government and public health infrastructure in the developing world leads to large populations living without clean running water. The World Health Organization (WHO) and UNICEF estimate that 780 million people are without access to improved water sources and 2.5 billion (37% of the world's population) people are without access to improved sanitation sources.[6]

Water and sanitation deficiencies are responsible for most of the global burden of diarrheal disease. The most common diarrheal disease of returning travelers is caused by enterotoxigenic *Escherichia coli*. All over the world, young and malnourished children die of preventable diarrhea caused by rotavirus, *E. coli*, *Salmonella*, *Shigella*, and *Campylobacter*.

Diseases that are particularly deadly as a result of lack of access to clean water include typhoid fever and cholera. Intestinal parasites, while usually not deadly, do lead to chronic problems with malnutrition and anemia, which themselves contribute to cyclical poverty and disease because they lead to impaired learning, reduced productivity, and vulnerability to other infectious diseases.

TYPHOID FEVER

Typhoid fever, also known as enteric fever, is an acute systemic illness caused by the invasive bacterial pathogen, *Salmonella typhi*. *S. typhi* is ingested in contaminated water or food, invades the mucosal surface of the small intestine, and causes bacteremia, with seeding of the liver, spleen, and lymph nodes.

EPIDEMIOLOGY

Typhoid fever is mainly found in countries with poor sanitary conditions. Because most such countries do not routinely confirm the diagnosis with blood cultures, the disease is highly underreported. Outbreaks of typhoid are often seen in the rainy season, and in areas where human fecal material washes into sources of drinking water. Shallow water tables and improperly placed latrines are environmental risk factors for typhoid. Globally there are 16 to 33 million cases annually, with up to half a million deaths every year.[7]

CLINICAL PRESENTATION

Patients develop an acute systemic illness with prolonged fever, malaise, and abdominal pain after ingesting contaminated food or water. This truly nonspecific syndrome may include headache, mild cough, and constipation, with nausea and vomiting. Diarrhea may be present but it is not the rule. After a 10- to 20-day incubation period, there is a stepwise progression of fever over a period of 3 weeks, and the patient may display a transient rash described as rose spots (2- to 4-mm pink macules on the torso, which fade on pressure). Temperature pulse dissociation with relative bradycardia despite high fever may be noted in fewer than 25% of patients. In the second week, the patient becomes more toxic and may develop hepatosplenomegaly. Untreated, typhoid can progress to include delirium, neurologic complications, and intestinal perforation caused by a proliferation of *Salmonella* in the Peyer patches (lymphoid tissue) of the intestinal mucosa. Although the mortality rate for untreated typhoid is 20%, early antibiotic therapy can decrease mortality. Approximately 1% to 4% of those who recover from acute typhoid fever become carriers of the disease and continue to shed *Salmonella* in their stool despite not being ill.[7]

DIAGNOSIS

Culture of blood, stool, rectal swab, or bone marrow.[8]

DIFFERENTIAL DIAGNOSIS

- Malaria (often clinically indistinguishable from typhoid; empiric therapy for both malaria and typhoid may be warranted if diagnostic testing[9] is unavailable)
- Enteroinvasive *E. coli*
- *Campylobacter*
- Paratyphoid fever (*Salmonella para typhi*, other less virulent *Salmonellae*)
- Dengue fever (mosquito-borne arbovirus infection spread by *Aedes aegypti*)
- Rickettsial diseases (typhus, spotted fever, Q fever)
- Brucellosis
- Leptospirosis
- Heat stroke

MANAGEMENT

Prompt diagnosis and initiation of antibiotic therapy is essential and lifesaving. Oral rehydration therapy should be initiated first, followed by IV fluids if vomiting cannot be controlled and for patients with altered mental status or hypovolemic shock. Antibiotic resistance patterns differ with geographic location.

For Africa and resource-limited settings in the Americas, the first choice is chloramphenicol 1 g PO daily for 10 to 14 days, or ciprofloxacin. Historically, trimethoprim-sulfamethoxazole 960 mg PO twice daily for 10 to 14 days has been used,[8] but there has been increasing drug resistance to sulfa in these areas. In Asia, where multidrug resistant *S. typhi* strains are well described, ciprofloxacin (500-750 mg twice daily), ceftriaxone (60 mg/kg IV daily) or azithromycin (500 mg daily) may be used for 7 to 14 days.[8-10] Azithromycin should be used only in mild disease. Some guidelines advocate the use of dexamethasone 3 mg/kg IV followed by 1 mg/kg every 6 hours for 2 days in the setting of shock or altered mental status.[8] See vaccine information at the end of this chapter.

CHOLERA

Cholera is an acute, diarrheal disease caused by *Vibrio cholerae*. It is usually transmitted by contaminated water or food, and is associated with pandemics in countries that lack public health infrastructure and resources for sanitation. Although the infection is often mild or asymptomatic, in 5% to 10% of patients it can be severe and life threatening.[11]

EPIDEMIOLOGY

V. cholerae reservoirs occur in brackish and salt water, as well as estuaries. Although the organism occurs in association with copepods and zooplankton, its largest reservoir is in humans. Cholera pandemics have been reported in South Asia, Africa, and Latin America. Characteristically, cholera outbreaks occur in countries that have suffered destruction of public health infrastructure (collapse of water supplies, sanitation, and garbage collection systems). The 2010 outbreak in post-earthquake Haiti has been traced to UN peacekeeping soldiers, whose waste contaminated a major Haitian river used for bathing, irrigation, and drinking water. In just 10 months, 300,000 cases were reported, of whom 4500 died, and the outbreak has continued to wax and wane with the rainy seasons for years.[12] A large infective dose is necessary for infection, and although approximately only 10% of those infected fall ill, the infection can be fatal for young children, elderly, and malnourished individuals.

PATHOPHYSIOLOGY

V. cholerae is a motile, gram-negative rod. After ingestion via contaminated water or food, it must survive the acid environment of the stomach before colonizing the mucosal surface of the small intestine. The organism is noninvasive, and not associated with bloody diarrhea. Rather, it makes a potent toxin causing massive secretion of electrolyte-rich fluid into the gut lumen. Human-to-human contact spread virtually never occurs. Transmission through contaminated food or water is the rule.[13]

Clinical presentation ranges from mild watery diarrhea to acute, fulminant watery diarrhea that looks like rice water. After an incubation period of 18 to 40 hours, patients may lose up to 30 L of fluid daily, resulting in metabolic acidosis and electrolyte disturbances. Severe dehydration can lead to death in a matter of hours. Vomiting, when present, starts after the onset of diarrhea. Profoundly dehydrated patients present with decreased skin turgor, sunken eyes, and lethargy. Children, but not adults, may have mild fever. Cramping caused by loss of calcium and potassium is common.[13]

DIFFERENTIAL DIAGNOSIS AND LABORATORY TESTS

Early presentation may resemble enterotoxigenic *E. coli*; however, the syndrome is quickly distinguishable because of the extreme volume of "rice water" secretory diarrhea that is the result of the cholera toxin. *V. cholerae* may be confirmed by stool culture, polymerase chain reaction (PCR) for toxin genes, or dark-field microscopy with specific antisera, which will immobilize the *V. cholerae*.[14] The Centers for Disease Control and Prevention (CDC) recommends confirmation of cholera by stool specimen culture or rectal swab. For transport, Cary Blair media is used, and for identification, thiosulfate-citrate-bile-salts (TCBS) agar is recommended.[11]

MANAGEMENT

Water, sanitation, and hygiene education is essential, as is education about recognizing the symptoms and immediately seeking medical attention while initiating oral rehydration. Optimally, rehydration should commence with reconstitution of WHO-distributed oral rehydration salts (ORS), which is available in all but the most remote areas of the world. Hydration is the mainstay of therapy, and replacement of fluids should be calibrated to match losses. ORS should be prepared with previously boiled water and consumed within 24 hours of reconstitution.

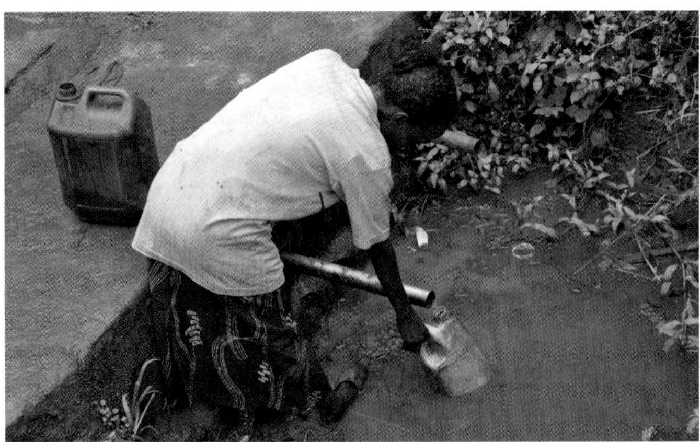

FIGURE 6-3 In this Ethiopian community without running water, water is collected in jerry cans. Thousands of women carry these heavy, filled cans for miles after filling them up from this single pipe. The local town has provided one single pipe as the water source for the community. Although there is muddy water below, the water coming from the pipe appears clear, although it is likely to harbor bacteria and parasites. (*Reproduced with permission from Richard P. Usatine, MD.*)

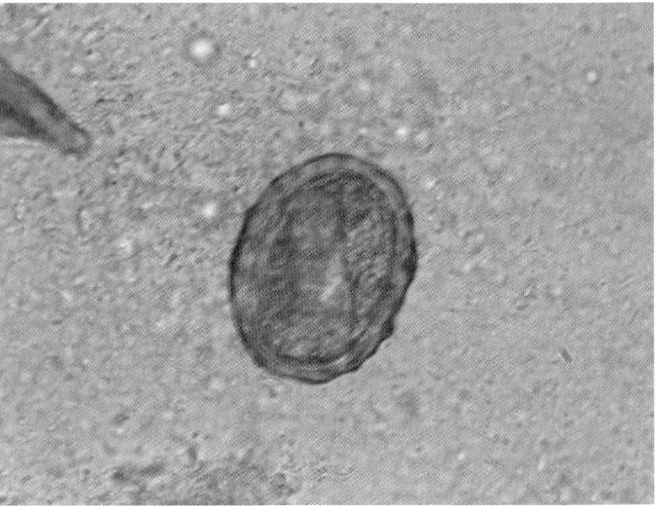

FIGURE 6-4 *Ascaris* egg found in the stool of a patient with intestinal parasites. In most developing countries *Ascaris* is treated empirically with albendazole; stool studies are not always available or may not be cost-effective. (*Reproduced with permission from Richard P. Usatine, MD.*)

IV or intraosseous hydration with Ringer lactate solution should be initiated if the patient is vomiting or in danger of hypovolemic shock. The volume needed to rehydrate a cholera patient is often underestimated; for this reason, collection and measurement of the watery stool in a bucket placed under the cholera cot is recommended.

Antibiotics are recommended for severe cases of cholera; the following are the options[15]:

1. Doxycycline 300 mg orally as single dose (contraindicated in pregnancy)
2. Azithromycin 1 g orally as single dose (more effective than either erythromycin or ciprofloxacin; appropriate first-line therapy for children and in pregnancy)
3. Ciprofloxacin
4. Furazolidone 100 mg orally

In pregnancy, erythromycin 250 mg PO daily for 3 days may also be used.

PREVENTION OF DISEASES SECONDARY TO CONTAMINATED WATER

Drinking purified or treated water, good handwashing practices, and avoidance of contaminated food are essential. Travelers should be reminded not to brush their teeth with tap water and to avoid having potentially contaminated ice added to their beverages. Carbonated beverages are safe as the carbonation process is bactericidal. Community education about handwashing and treatment of water is essential. In communities lacking running water (**Figure 6-3**), home storage of drinking water should be in containers with protective lids. Local guidelines regarding addition of chlorine to home-stored water containers should be followed.

INTESTINAL PARASITES

EPIDEMIOLOGY AND GEOGRAPHIC DISTRIBUTION

One-third of the world's population is infected with intestinal parasites, and although many parasitic infections are asymptomatic, some have serious health consequences. Especially affected are pregnant women and children, for whom hookworm-associated anemia results in maternal mortality, low-birth-weight babies, growth stunting, and impaired learning. The CDC recommends predeparture albendazole treatment as a single 600-mg dose for all refugees from sub-Saharan Africa and South Asia. While this treatment will eradicate most of the nematodes, it is insufficient for *Strongyloides stercoralis* and schistosomiasis.[16]

CLINICAL PRESENTATION

Abdominal pain, cramps, bloating, anorexia, anemia, fatigue, growth stunting of children, hepatomegaly (schistosomiasis)

DIAGNOSIS

Stool for ova and parasite studies (**Figure 6-4**) will not reliably detect *Strongyloides* or schistosomiasis; serologic testing is available for the latter. Eosinophilia is an important diagnostic clue for the presence of parasites; the finding of persistent eosinophilia warrants a careful diagnostic evaluation for parasitic infection.

TREATMENT

Adults

Albendazole 400 mg orally as single dose will eradicate hookworm, and *Ascaris*, but not *Trichuris* in most people.[17] Eradication of *Trichuris trichiura* requires 3 daily doses of albendazole or adding ivermectin to mebendazole.[18]

PREVENTION

Preventative measures include proper management of human waste, handwashing after defecation and before cooking, and wearing shoes (prevents hookworm and *Strongyloides*). WHO guidelines recommend mass treatment of school children in endemic areas with single-dose albendazole therapy once in every 6 months.

MALNUTRITION

A global shift is underway, from diseases of undernutrition to overnutrition in tandem with industrialization and advances in transportation and technology. In spite of this global shift, about a quarter of the world's preschool children demonstrate growth stunting caused by nutritional deficiencies. In resource-poor countries, adult obesity and childhood undernutrition may coexist within the same families. The causes of this seeming paradox include many factors associated with poverty: the vulnerability of preschool children to infection when sanitation is inadequate, lack of nutrition education, decreased physical activity with increasing availability of technology and transportation, and mass marketing of inexpensive, calorie-rich foods.

THE NUTRITION TRANSITION AND MICRONUTRIENT DEFICIENCIES

Obesity has become a leading global cause of death and disability,[19] and the term "nutrition transition" is used to describe the associated dietary change from one dominated by carbohydrates and fiber to a diet rich in sugar and animal fats.[20] Despite the surfeit of energy associated with the nutrition transition, global micronutrient deficiencies contribute importantly to developmental delays, reduced cognitive function, impaired immunity, obesity, and hypertension.[21] There are 4 micronutrient deficiencies of global importance, each with associated clinical syndromes that should be recognized. All can be associated with growth stunting in children, who may present with abnormally short stature but relatively normal weight for height. Growth stunting from micronutrient deficiency is associated with adult obesity,[22] and obese adults also demonstrate micronutrient deficiencies despite the fact that they appear overnourished.[23] Although many of the guidelines regarding micronutrient deficiencies are specific to children, the deficiencies persist and contribute to disease vulnerability and decreased productivity in adulthood, which in turn leads to the familiar cycle of disease and poverty.

VITAMIN A DEFICIENCY

Vitamin A is a critical regulator of immune function, which is required for maintaining the integrity of mucosal surfaces. Vitamin A supplementation in countries with malnutrition reduces blindness (from xerophthalmia) as well as the morbidity of infectious diseases (especially measles, diarrhea, and respiratory infections). In 2009, the WHO estimated that clinical vitamin A deficiency (night blindness) and biochemical vitamin A deficiency (serum retinol concentration <0.70 μmol/L) affected 5.2 and 190 million preschool-age children, respectively.[24] About 250,000 children develop blindness caused by vitamin A deficiency every year, and half of them die within 12 months of losing sight.[25]

Clinical Presentation

Pregnant women in vitamin A deficient communities may be among the first to signal the problem when they complain of night blindness. The earliest presentation of vitamin A deficiency is poor night vision, which may progress to night blindness, xerophthalmia, ulceration, and scarring of the cornea, with ultimate blindness. Vitamin A deficiency is also associated with anemia, and has been suggested as a preventable cause of maternal mortality.[26] However, a recent trial in Ghana involving more than half a million woman-years and over 2500 deaths concluded that weekly vitamin A administration did not reduce mortality in women of childbearing age.[27]

Management

While meta-analyses of large trials giving vitamin A supplements to hundreds of thousands of children under age 5 years reveal striking reductions in mortality and morbidity, the benefit of programmatic vitamin A supplementation for adults has not been demonstrated. In children, vitamin A reduces diarrhea and measles incidence as well as morbidity, mortality, and eye disease. In countries where vitamin A deficiency is problematic, pregnant women often report symptomatic night blindness. The most recent guidelines do not recommend vitamin A supplementation during pregnancy as part of routine antenatal care for preventing maternal mortality. WHO does state that for countries with significant public health problems from deficiency, vitamin A should be given to prevent night blindness. Pregnant women in these settings should get up to 10,000 IU vitamin A daily or 25,000 IU vitamin A weekly as an oral liquid, oil-based preparation. A single dose of vitamin A should never exceed 25,000 units, especially during the first trimester of pregnancy, to avoid teratogenicity. Supplementation is continued for 12 weeks during pregnancy until delivery. The WHO defines at-risk populations as those where the prevalence of night blindness is greater than or equal to 5% in pregnant women or greater than or equal to 5% in children aged 2 to 5 years.[28]

Treatment of active xerophthalmia is considered an emergency and management should include oral vitamin A. Current recommendations for xerophthalmia (night blindness and/or Bitot spots) are 10,000 units daily or 25,000 units weekly for 3 months. Active corneal lesions from vitamin A deficiency are rare, but should be treated with 200,000 units of vitamin A on days 1, 2, and 14.[29]

ZINC DEFICIENCY

Zinc plays a central role in cellular growth, differentiation, and metabolism. It is necessary for physical growth, gastrointestinal (GI), and immune function. Many zinc studies show improved growth of children and decreased infections when supplements are given to vulnerable populations. Studies suggest that the global prevalence of zinc deficiency approaches 31%, especially in Africa, the eastern Mediterranean, and South Asia.[30]

Clinical Presentation

The most common presentation of zinc deficiency is nonspecific and may include growth stunting, delayed sexual maturation, dermatitis, and defective immunity. Zinc deficiency is associated with decreased macrophage chemotaxis, decreased neutrophil activity, and decreased T-cell responses.[31] It is widely acknowledged that zinc deficiency contributes significantly to mortality from pneumonia, diarrhea, and malaria.

Diagnosis

Because there is no good biomarker for zinc deficiency, diagnosis must rest on clinical suspicion and documentation of therapeutic response to supplementation.

Management

WHO guidelines for diarrhea recommend use of low concentration ORS together with routine zinc supplementation for 10 to 14 days. While carefully studied in children, data regarding zinc supplementation for diarrhea in adults are lacking.[32] In children, zinc supplementation decreases the duration and volume of diarrheal stools by 25% and 30%, respectively, and brings an approximate 50% reduction in noninjury deaths in the year following the treatment.[33] Unfortunately, zinc supplementation benefits are still not widely known by health care workers in developing countries.[34]

IRON DEFICIENCY

Iron deficiency is the most common micronutrient deficiency in the world, and 2 billion people (nearly one-third of the global population) are anemic. In resource-limited countries, iron deficiency anemia is either caused or aggravated by malaria, intestinal parasites such as hookworm, and other chronic infections such as HIV, tuberculosis, or schistosomiasis. Iron deficiency causes enormous morbidity and contributes to 20% of global maternal mortality. Because the consequences include impaired cognition and physical development, increased risk of illness in children and reduced work productivity, iron deficiency is a real barrier to economic development in resource-poor countries.[35] As with zinc and vitamin A, iron deficiency can be detrimental to host immunity, causing decreased neutrophil chemotaxis.[31]

Interventions

The WHO has developed a 3-pronged strategy for addressing global iron deficiency: increasing iron uptake through dietary diversification and supplementation, improvement of nutritional status, and controlling infections, especially worms. In countries with significant iron deficiency anemia, malaria, and helminth infections, these interventions can restore individual health as well as raise national productivity levels, thereby interrupting the cycle of poverty and disease.[35]

IODINE DEFICIENCY

Insufficient dietary iodine can significantly lower the IQ of whole populations and is the leading preventable cause of brain damage. Although iodine deficiency is easily solved through food fortification costing 2 cents per person annually, prevalences of 60% to 90% iodine deficiency among school children are observed in multiple African, Asian, and eastern Mediterranean countries. There is tremendous variance of iodine deficiency within individual countries and deficiency is not linked to poor or disadvantaged districts.[36] Iodine deficiency occurs where the soil has low iodine content because of past glaciation or repeated leaching effects of precipitation. Food crops grown in iodine-deficient soil provide inadequate dietary iodine.[37]

Clinical Presentation

Because iodine is required for thyroid hormone synthesis, iodine deficiency results in hypothyroidism and goiter (**Figure 6-5**). Congenital iodine deficiency results in a form of profound cognitive impairment known as *cretinism*. Other consequences include stillbirths, deaf mutism, subclinical hyper- or hypothyroidism, impaired mental function, and retarded physical development.[37]

Interventions

Iodine may be supplied in tablets or liquid form and taken daily; in adults, 150 μg/d is sufficient for thyroid function and an adult multivitamin typically contains 150 μg of iodine per tablet, but this is impractical. Population-based interventions should include iodization of salt, and in some developing countries, eradication of iodine deficiency has been accomplished by adding iodine drops to well water.

VITAMIN B_3 (NIACIN) DEFICIENCY

Clinical niacin deficiency is a problem in severely resource-limited settings where diets rely heavily on corn or sorghum. Pellagra refers to a nutritional wasting disease that occurs when there is deficiency of nicotinic acid and/or tryptophan.[38]

Clinical Presentation

The term "pellagra" refers to a symptom complex of 4 Ds: diarrhea, dermatitis, dementia, and (sometimes) death, which is seen in niacin deficiency states. The dermatitis is a phototoxic rash, occurring primarily on sun-exposed skin of the neck and chest in a necklace-like distribution **(Figure 6-6),** as well as on the hands and forearms, or in a boot-like distribution sparing the heel. The rash is initially erythematous, and may be blistering or scaling with progression to hyperkeratosis and hyperpigmentation over bony prominences. Accompanying neurologic problems include disorientation, myoclonic jerks, tremors, depression, and in severe cases, central pontine myelinolysis.[39]

Diagnosis

Diagnosis requires clinical suspicion, recognition of the 4 Ds, and understanding of risk factors. In addition to poverty and maize diet, risk factors for pellagra include eating disorders, alcohol abuse, malabsorption, medications (especially INH, PZA, and phenytoin or phenobarbital), Crohn disease, and hypothyroidism. Oral niacin supplementation should ameliorate symptoms in 1 to 2 days, and can confirm the diagnosis.

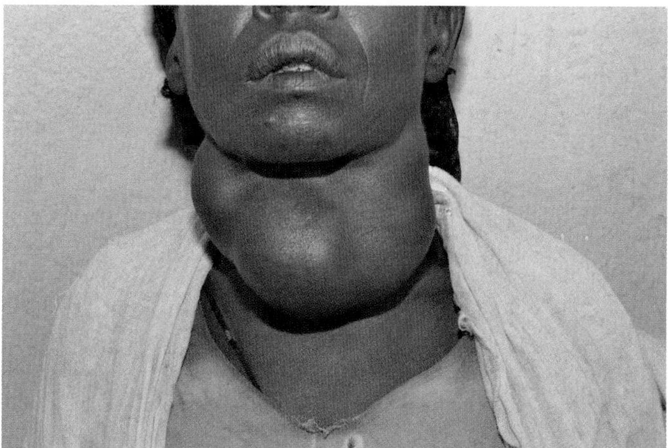

FIGURE 6-5 Massive goiter caused by iodine deficiency. This woman is from a country in Africa where iodine is not routinely supplemented in the diet and goiter is endemic. (*Reproduced with permission from Richard P. Usatine, MD.*)

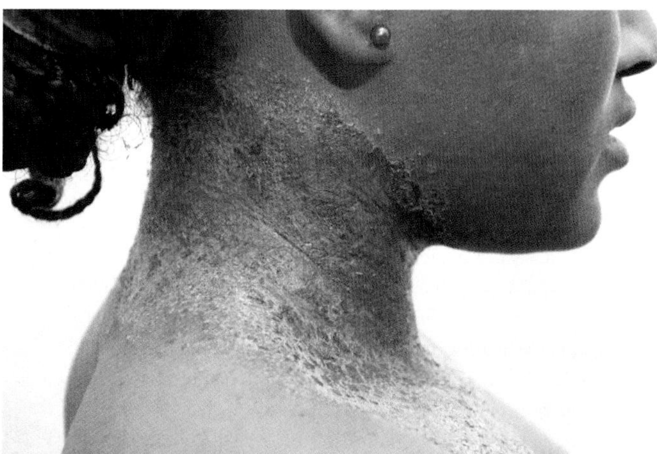

FIGURE 6-6 Pellagra from niacin deficiency causing the typical rash around the neck known as Casal necklace. (*Reproduced with permission from Rick Hodes, MD.*)

Management

On a population level, fortification of maize flour with niacin can be very effective. Patients should be educated about nutritional sources of niacin, which include eggs, peanuts, meat, poultry, fish, legumes, and beans. For clinical therapy in a symptomatic individual, niacin is dosed at 100 to 500 mg PO divided 2 to 3 times daily until complete recovery (3-4 weeks).[40] Because nutrient deficiencies generally do not occur in isolation, consider treating for other common deficiencies including protein, zinc, thiamine, and vitamin B_{12}. Although the dermatitis rarely leaves scars, residual hyperpigmentation may last for months. Hot flashes and headache from niacin may be diminished by pretreatment with aspirin, 325 mg about 30 minutes before the dose.[41]

VECTOR-BORNE DISEASES

MALARIA

Malaria is a protozoan infection spread by the Anopheles mosquito vector in endemic areas. Of the 4 species of malaria (*Plasmodium falciparum, Plasmodium ovale, Plasmodium malariae,* and *Plasmodium vivax*), *P. falciparum* is the most important to address, because if unrecognized and untreated, it can be rapidly fatal. Only *P. falciparum* exhibits high levels of parasitemia in blood, and it is the only type of malaria that causes sequestration of parasitized erythrocytes in microvasculature. This unique feature of *P. falciparum* is responsible for the severe end-organ damage, including renal failure, acute respiratory distress syndrome, and coma that is seen with untreated disease.[42]

Epidemiology and Geographic Distribution

There are more than 200 million cases of malaria in the world every year. According to the WHO, up to 1 million people worldwide die annually from malaria, with 89% of these deaths occurring in Africa. Most of the deaths caused by malaria occur in children younger than age 5 years. *P. falciparum*, *P. vivax, P. malariae*, and *P. ovale* are globally distributed in the tropics. *P. vivax* is more common in Asia, South America, Oceania, and India. *P. ovale* is found mainly in West Africa, and *P. malariae* is much less common than *P. vivax* or *P. falciparum*.

The risk for malaria varies greatly within a given country, and depends on altitude (higher altitudes have lower risk), season (greatest risk in rainy season), and urbanization (rural areas have greater risk than urban areas). Thus, travelers should be aware of these differences and plan for prophylaxis accordingly.

The CDC publication, *Health Information for International Travel*, is available online at http://www.cdc.gov/travel/ and should be consulted for updates about regional patterns of malaria risk, as well as drug resistance and guidelines, which are subject to frequent changes.[43]

Clinical Presentation

After a 1- to 3-week incubation period following the bite of an infected female mosquito, patients develop a nonspecific syndrome of high fever, headache, myalgia, and shaking chills. This syndrome is frequently accompanied by nausea, vomiting, and back pain, and occasional diarrhea. Splenomegaly and anemia (related to hemolysis) are common in all 4 types of malaria.

As untreated *P. falciparum* progresses, there is a risk of cerebral malaria, which is caused by parasitized erythrocytes sequestered in the capillaries of the brain, with secondary metabolic consequences. Cerebral malaria is characterized by severe headache and altered consciousness. These patients may also develop acute respiratory distress syndrome (ARDS), hypoglycemia, acidosis, and shock in the setting of hyperparasitemia. Untreated patients with cerebral malaria ultimately progress to coma, respiratory failure, and death.[44]

Differential Diagnosis

The initial presentation of malaria is so nonspecific that it mimics influenza (without the respiratory symptoms), enteric fever (see section on typhoid), dengue fever, rickettsial infections, brucellosis, and leishmaniasis. If hemolysis has been extensive, the patient may present with jaundice, and viral hepatitis or leptospirosis may also be on the differential diagnosis.[42]

Laboratory Diagnosis

Malaria is usually diagnosed by light microscopy of peripheral blood smears prepared with a Giemsa, Field, or modified Wright stain (**Figure 6-7A** and **B**). A thick-and-thin smear should be obtained

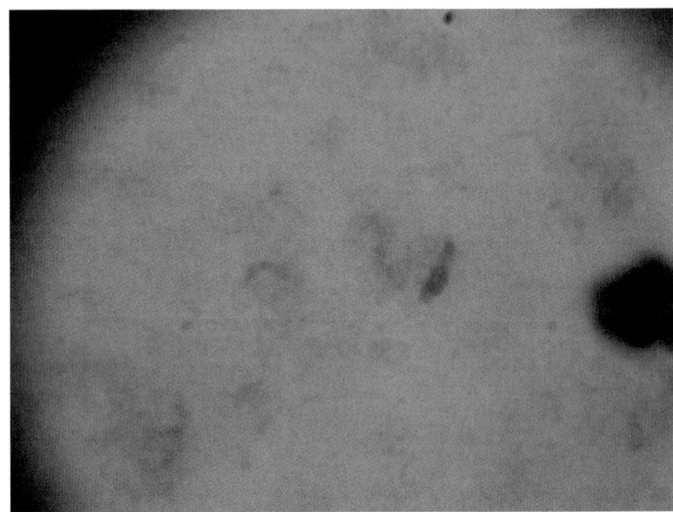

A

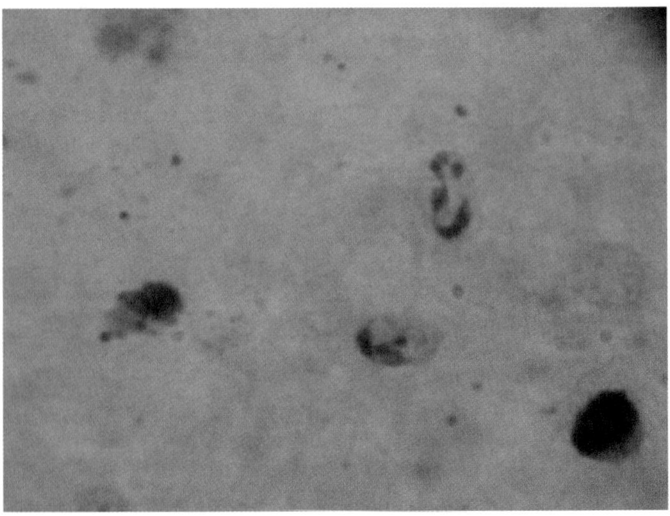

B

FIGURE 6-7 **A.** *Plasmodium falciparum* with a banana-shaped gametocyte. Of all the species of malaria, *P. falciparum* is most likely to cause severe morbidity and mortality. **B.** *P. falciparum* with chromatin in rings. (*Reproduced with permission from Richard P. Usatine, MD.*)

whenever possible for every febrile patient in whom malaria is suspected, especially from febrile travelers returning from malaria endemic areas. Thin smears allow relative quantification and speciation of parasites when the parasitemia is high; thick smears are useful to rule in malaria, especially when parasitemia is low. Because a single negative smear does not rule out malaria, the test must be repeated on at least 3 occasions at 12- to 24-hour intervals.[45] Patients with high levels of parasitemia (>5%) have a worse prognosis, and should be considered for inpatient care.

Other diagnostic modalities include the fluorochrome acridine orange stain for fluorescence microscopy and PCR (not yet widely available but helpful for very low levels of parasitemia). Rapid antigen assays using fingerstick blood samples on cards impregnated with specific antibodies are alternative methods for laboratory diagnosis of malaria. In the United States, the US Food and Drug Administration has approved the BinaxNOW Malaria test, which, although costly, is convenient for rapid field use. Unfortunately, this and other immunochromatographic strip assays are not able to determine parasite load.[43]

Treatment

Many cases of malaria can be treated effectively with oral medication, and parenteral therapy is reserved for severe disease or for patients who are vomiting. Before prescribing therapy, determine which species is most likely involved based on microscopy or rapid diagnostic test; consider the geographic area and local drug resistance patterns.

After the patient has been given the first dose of medication, the patient should be observed for an hour. Vomiting can be managed with metoclopramide, 10 mg orally, and if vomiting occurs within 30 minutes, the full initial dose can be repeated. The WHO recommends artemisinin-based combination treatments as first line for uncomplicated *P. falciparum*: artemether-lumefantrine 1 dose at hours 1, 8, 24, 36, 48, and 60 based on body weight: 5 to 14 kg: 1 tablet per dose; 15 to 24 kg: 2 tablets per dose; 25 to 34 kg: 3 tablets per dose; greater than 34 kg: 4 tablets per dose.

Other artemisinin combinations can be used as follows: artesunate plus amodiaquine, artesunate plus mefloquine, and artesunate plus sulfadoxine-pyrimethamine. The combination of choice depends on the level of resistance of the partner medication in a given region. Artemisinin and derivatives should not be given as monotherapy.

For US-returning travelers

- Quinine + doxycycline: quinine 10 mg/kg 3 times daily for 7 days and doxycycline twice daily for 7 days

  or

- Atovaquone-proguanil: atovaquone 20 mg/kg/d, proguanil 8 mg/kg/d for 3 days.

Treatment of Severe P. falciparum

All cases of severe malaria should be managed as medical emergencies. Give intravenous (IV) or intramuscular (IM) artesunate, artemether, or quinine dihydrochloride (not available in the United States).

In the United States give quinidine gluconate, 10 mg base/kg (up to 600 mg) in 0.9% saline by rate-controlled IV infusion over 1 to 2 hours, followed by a maintenance dose of 0.02 mg base/kg/min with electrocardiogram (ECG) monitoring until patient can take oral drugs. Quinine and quinidine must never be given by IV bolus because of the potential for fatal hypotension.

Patients with cerebral malaria should undergo lumbar puncture to rule out bacterial meningitis and their blood glucose should be checked every 4 hours because of the significant risk of hypoglycemia in severe malaria. Careful hemodynamic monitoring and management of seizures (with intravenous benzodiazepines) are essential.

Prevention

Prevention measures are a public health priority and should include mosquito control, elimination of standing water in households and gardens, insect repellant containing at least 10% to 50% diethyltoluamide (DEET; 30% DEET provides 6-8 hours of protection), and permethrin-impregnated bed nets. Since 2000, prevention and control measures have reduced malaria mortality by more than 25% globally and by 33% in Africa.[46]

Prevention for Travelers

Choice of chemoprophylaxis depends on drug-resistance patterns for *P. falciparum* in the country being visited. Generally, prophylaxis should start 1 week before arrival and should continue through 4 weeks after leaving the endemic area. In the case of atovaquone-proguanil, prophylaxis may start the day before arrival and end 7 days after departure. Drugs commonly used in prophylaxis include atovaquone-proguanil (Malarone, which is expensive in the United States), mefloquine (may cause central nervous system side effects), and doxycycline (causes photosensitivity). Chloroquine can be used only in a few areas; chloroquine-susceptible malaria is restricted to the Caribbean, Central America, and parts of the Middle East.

RESOURCES

- Centers for Disease Control and Prevention. *Malaria*—**http://www.cdc.gov/malaria.**
- World Health Organization. *Malaria*—**http://www.who.int/malaria/en/.**

LEISHMANIASIS

Leishmaniasis is a vector-borne disease transmitted by the sandfly. It can be divided into 2 major forms, a cutaneous form, which is the most common, and the visceral form. There is also a more rare mucocutaneous form that can cause significant facial disfigurement around the nose and mouth.

Synonyms

Kala-azar is another name for visceral leishmaniasis.

Epidemiology

- New World leishmaniasis is found in Mexico, Central America, and South America. Old World leishmaniasis is found in India, Africa, the Middle East, southern Europe, and parts of Asia.
- Most leishmaniasis diagnosed in the United States occurs in travelers returning from endemic areas including military personnel who served in Iraq or Afghanistan.
- Some cutaneous leishmaniasis cases acquired in the United States have been reported in Texas and Oklahoma.[47]
- Ninety percent of cutaneous leishmaniasis occurs in Afghanistan, Algeria, Iran, Saudi Arabia, Syria, Brazil, Colombia, Peru, and Bolivia.[47]
- Ninety percent of visceral leishmaniasis cases occur in parts of India, Bangladesh, Nepal, Sudan, Ethiopia, and Brazil.[47]

Etiology and Pathophysiology

- Leishmaniasis is caused by more than 20 species of the protozoan genus *Leishmania*.
- Leishmaniasis is transmitted to people through the bite of the sandfly.
- The intracellular amastigotes of *Leishmania* replicate within macrophages.
- The disease can also be transmitted like any blood-borne infection, but human-to-human transmission is rare.

Risk Factors

- Living in and traveling to endemic countries.
- Rural areas have a higher prevalence of disease in the endemic countries.
- Not protecting the skin from sandfly bites during the time from dusk to dawn.
- Blood transfusions, needle sharing in injection-drug users, needlestick injuries, and congenital transmission also are all reported risk factors for visceral leishmaniasis.[48]

Diagnosis

Clinical Features

- Six weeks after a sandfly bite, the cutaneous form may be localized to a single ulcer or nodule (**Figure 6-8**) or may be disseminated widely (**Figure 6-9**).
- After a 2- to 6-month incubation period, the visceral form can involve the liver, spleen, and bone marrow and causes systemic illness. The patient may present with fever, anemia, night sweats, weight loss, and an enlarged abdomen because of hepatosplenomegaly.[49]
- Mucocutaneous leishmaniasis affects the nose and mouth and may affect the nasal septum and palate (**Figure 6-10**). This form may occur months to years after what appears to be healing of cutaneous leishmaniasis.

Distribution

- A cutaneous form of leishmaniasis has a predilection for the nose and face (see **Figure 6-8**).
- Cutaneous leishmaniasis is also commonly seen on the extremities. Note that the sandfly would generally have more access to bite the face and extremities where clothing is less likely to be a protective barrier.
- Disseminated cutaneous leishmaniasis can be seen from the head to the toes (see **Figure 6-9**).

Laboratory Testing

- Cutaneous leishmaniasis may be diagnosed by clinical appearance and a biopsy or a scraping of the ulcer. A Giemsa stain will demonstrate parasites in the skin smears taken from the edge of an active ulcer.[49] In some centers, PCR is available and is considered as the method of choice.[50]
- Visceral leishmaniasis is diagnosed from a blood sample or a bone marrow biopsy. Several serologic agglutination tests (direct agglutination test [DAT] or fluorescent allergosorbent test [FAST]) are highly sensitive for the detection of *Leishmania* antibodies. Culture of a bone marrow aspirate or PCR improves diagnostic yield.[49]

Differential Diagnosis

- The differential diagnosis of cutaneous leishmaniasis includes leprosy, sarcoidosis, pyoderma gangrenosum, primary syphilis, and venous stasis ulcers.
- The differential diagnosis of visceral leishmaniasis includes malaria, typhoid fever, and lymphoma.

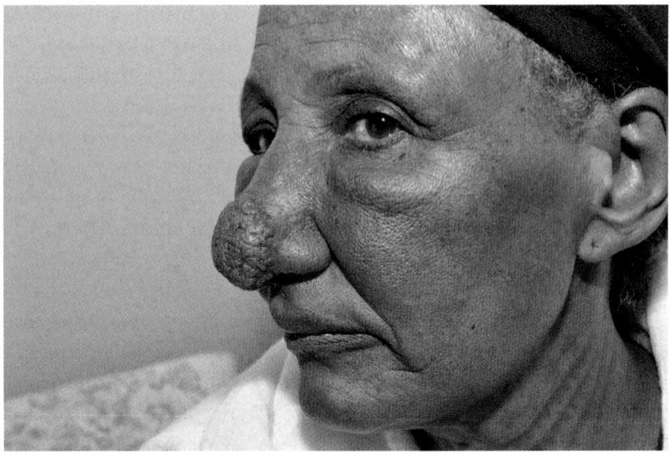

A

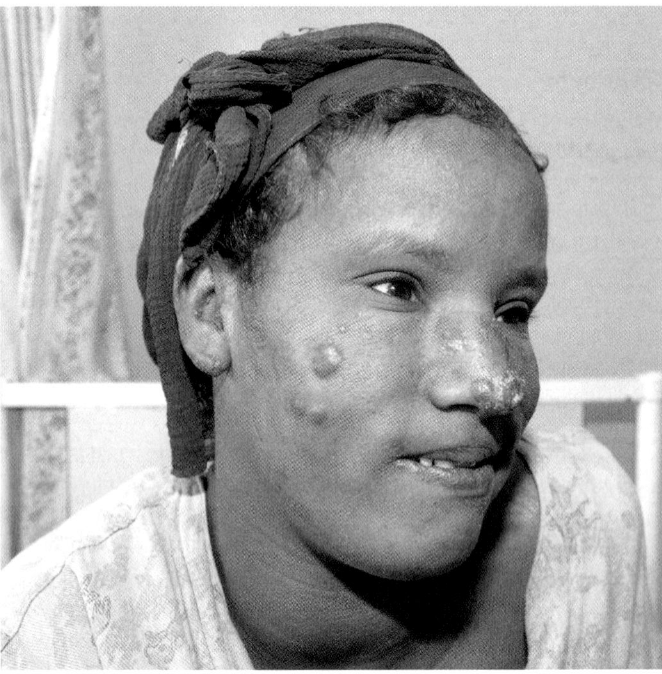

B

FIGURE 6-8 Examples of leishmaniasis on the face. Lesions emerge at the site of the sandfly bite; the nose is commonly affected as seen in the women in Figures **A** and **B** from Africa. (*Reproduced with permission from Richard P. Usatine, MD.*)

Management

Nonpharmacologic

Wound care for ulcers

Medications

The main drugs used to treat leishmaniasis include sodium stibogluconate (available from the CDC) and meglumine antimonate.[51,52] Other medications used include miltefosine (the only oral drug for leishmaniasis) fluconazole and liposomal amphotericin b (this is the only drug with FDA approval for visceral leishmaniasis in the United States).[51,52] Amphotericin b is the standard of care in India because of antimonial resistance.[50]

Surgery

Plastic surgery may be used to treat the disfigurement of mucocutaneous or cutaneous leishmaniasis.

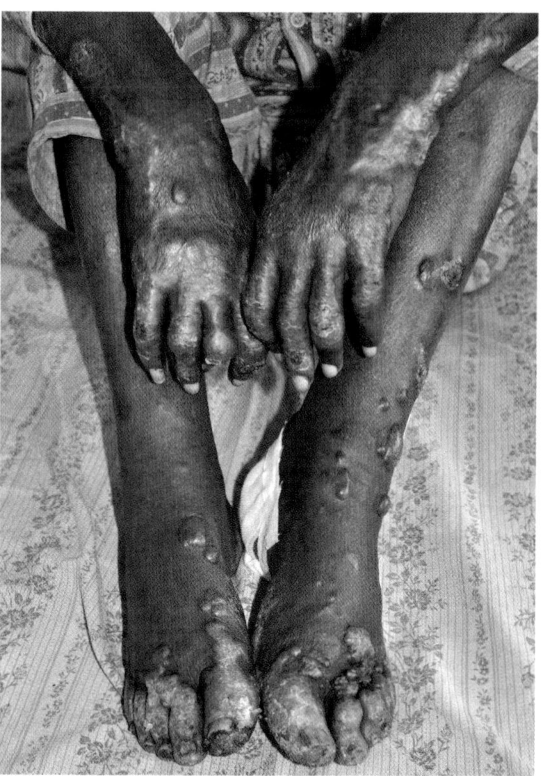

FIGURE 6-9 Diffuse leishmaniasis in an African man with involvement from the face to the toes. The multiple nodules look like lepromatous leprosy but by skin snip testing, the diagnosis of leishmaniasis was confirmed. (*Reproduced with permission from Richard P. Usatine, MD.*)

PREVENTION OF VECTOR-BORNE DISEASES

Prevention is a public health priority that must include vector (mosquito and sandfly) control, elimination of standing water in households and gardens, insect repellant containing 20% to 30% DEET, and permethrin-coated bednets. Sandflies and *Anopheles* mosquitoes bite from dusk to dawn, but the *A. aegypti* vector of dengue fever bites any time during the day making daytime use of mosquito repellant especially important in dengue-endemic areas.

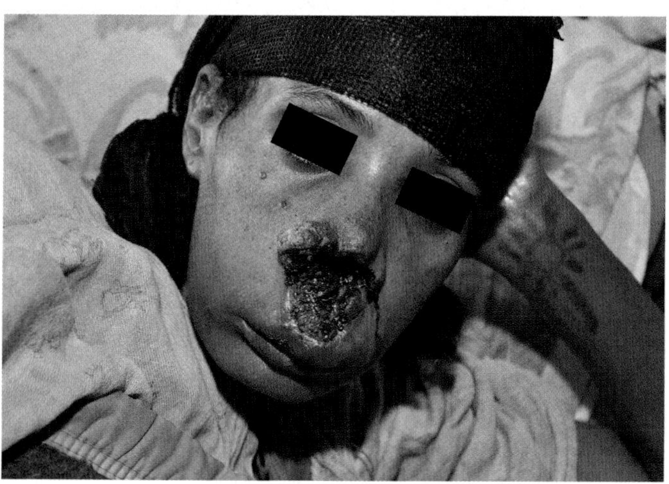

FIGURE 6-10 Severe mucocutaneous leishmaniasis causing destruction of the nose. (*Reproduced with permission from Richard P. Usatine, MD.*)

PROGNOSIS

- Cutaneous leishmaniasis does resolve spontaneously in some cases and in other cases it may persist and resist treatments. The prognosis is related to the severity of the case and the community of the host. Even in cases that resolve, scarring is frequent.
- Visceral leishmaniasis is fatal if not diagnosed and treated.

RESOURCES

- PubMed Health. *Leishmaniasis*—**http://www.ncbi.nlm.nih.gov/pubmedhealth/PMH0002362/.**
- Centers for Disease Control and Prevention. *Parasites–Leishmaniasis*—**http://www.cdc.gov/parasites/leishmaniasis/.**

EYES—TRACHOMA

EPIDEMIOLOGY AND GEOGRAPHIC DISTRIBUTION

Chlamydia trachomatis is the leading infectious cause of blindness, accounting for 3% of the world's blindness. Globally, 21.4 million people have trachoma, and of these, 1.2 million are blind.[53] Trachoma is associated with poor sanitation, inadequate water supply, and lack of personal hygiene. It is transmitted from person to person via unwashed fingers, flies, and close family contact (sharing of face towels and bedclothes). Trachoma is endemic in Africa (especially in the driest regions), India, South Asia, Australia, and parts of South America.

CLINICAL PRESENTATION

Patients experience inflammation of the eye with watery discharge, itching, burning, and blurry vision. Examination of the tarsal conjunctiva reveals follicles (round swellings that are paler than the surrounding conjunctiva, at least 0.5 mm in diameter). With progression, intense trachomatous inflammation develops, producing inflammatory thickening of the tarsal conjunctiva, which appears red and thickened with numerous follicles (**Figure 6-11**).

Eventually, trachoma causes scarring, with white lines or bands in the tarsal conjunctiva as well as trichiasis, in which eyelashes turn inward and

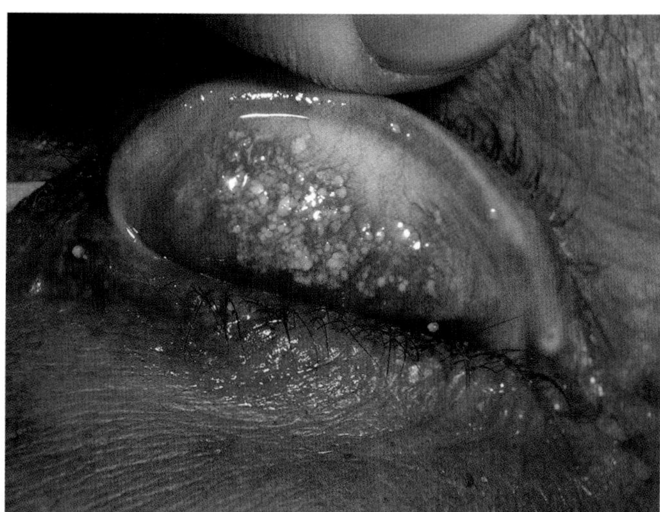

FIGURE 6-11 Trachoma causing prominent follicles on the upper eyelid in a person infected with *C. trachomatis*. Note how flipping the eyelid is needed to see the follicles under the upper eyelid. (*Reproduced with permission from Richard P. Usatine, MD.*)

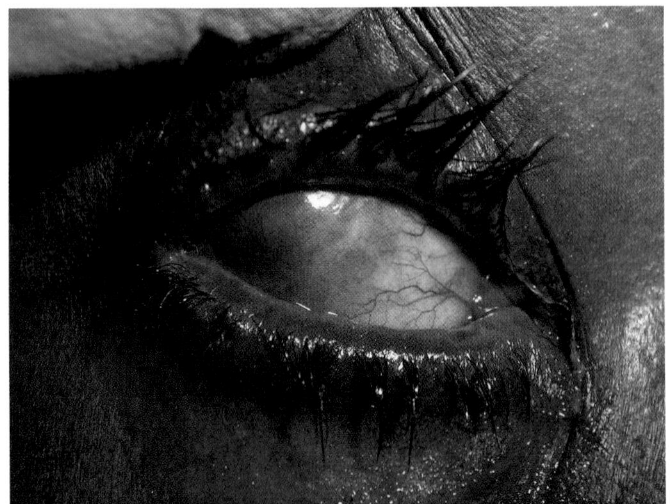

FIGURE 6-12 Blindness caused by untreated trachoma. Although this is one of the most common causes of blindness worldwide, trachoma is easily treatable with a single dose of oral azithromycin. Prevention is achieved through better access to water and soap, together with education about the three "Fs": flies, fingers, facial hygiene. (*Reproduced with permission from P. Usatine, MD.*)

begin to rub against the cornea, and entropion, or inward turning of the eyelid itself. With time, this chronic rubbing causes corneal opacity and blindness (**Figure 6-12**).

DIAGNOSIS

Although laboratory diagnostic testing is available for staining *C. trachomatis* in scrapings from the tarsal plate, most settings where trachoma is endemic do not offer this resource, and visual inspection of the everted upper eyelid must suffice. Each eye should be examined for trichiasis and corneal opacities. The upper eyelid is everted by asking the patient to look down, holding eyelashes between thumb and finger, and everting the lid using a cotton-tipped applicator. The everted lid is then checked for follicles, inflammation, and scarring. The differential diagnosis of trachoma includes allergic conjunctivitis (which can also produce follicles of the tarsal plate), and bacterial or viral conjunctivitis.

MANAGEMENT

- Azithromycin, 1 g single oral dose for adults and 20 mg/kg for children in a single dose.
- In pregnancy: erythromycin 500 mg twice daily for 7 days.
- Less effective: topical erythromycin and tetracycline.[10]
- In some settings, surgery is available to correct entropion and trichiasis.

PREVENTION

Preventive measures include community hygiene education, use of soap and water for washing hands and faces, and control of flies through use of ventilated improved pit (VIP) latrines. The WHO has developed the acronym "SAFE" for the global elimination of trachoma:

S Surgery for entropion and trichiasis

A Antibiotics for infectious trachoma

F Facial cleanliness to reduce transmission

E Environmental improvements such as control of disease-spreading flies and access to clean water[54]

SKIN

INFECTIOUS SKIN DISEASES

Many of the skin diseases encountered in resource-limited countries are secondary to crowded living conditions and lack of clean water and soap. Scabies mites and human lice are endemic in many populations that are unable to wash frequently. If clean water is scarce it is more likely to be used for drinking and cooking than bathing. In developed countries, we take clean running water (hot and cold), soap, and shampoo for granted. In developing countries, even if water is available, it may not be accessible as warm running water for showers or baths.

When an intervention as simple as mass distribution of free soap for personal hygiene draws enormous crowds to a mobile clinic, the vastness of inequality in access to basic health measures around the world becomes painfully obvious. Although people recognize the importance of access to soap and clean water, the absence of this luxury results in skin infections and infestations that are highly prevalent and spread from person to person.

We can divide skin diseases into infestations, bacterial, viral, and fungal infections. All of these skin infections are covered in the dermatology section of this book. Here we highlight some cases seen in developing countries.

Scabies (see Chapter 141, Scabies) is caused by a human mite that burrows under the skin causing itching and leading to scratching. The itching and scratching may keep the person awake at night and may lead to bacterial superinfections. Scabies is spread by direct skin contact (**Figure 6-13**), shared bedding and clothing, and occasionally by fomites.

Human lice (see Chapter 140, Lice) exist as 3 separate species that are known as head lice, body lice, and pubic lice. Schoolchildren are particularly at risk for head lice, and in areas with limited head washing, the majority of kids may be infested. Body lice live on clothing and feed on the blood of their host. Body lice are more prevalent in adults who bathe rarely and wear the same unwashed clothing day after day. Pubic lice are transmitted through sexual contact and are not known to be more prevalent in developing countries. Water and hygiene issues do predispose to increased head and body lice in developing countries.

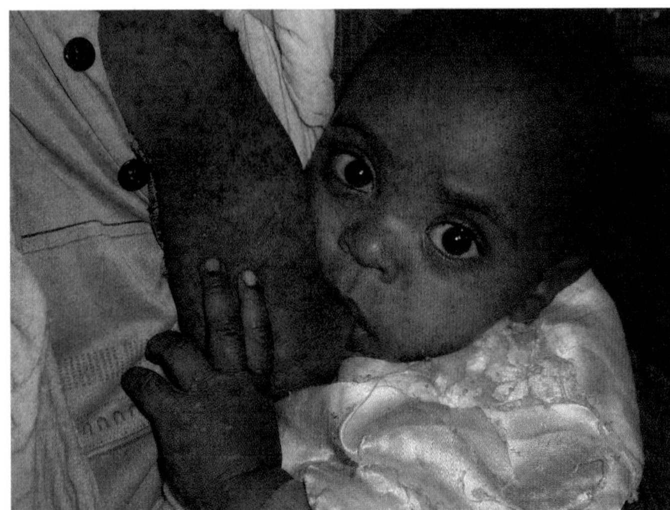

FIGURE 6-13 Scabies infestation covering the mother's breast and her baby's hand. With poor access to health care, this infestation would likely remain untreated, and could lead to bacterial superinfection and impetigo. (*Reproduced with permission from Richard P. Usatine, MD.*)

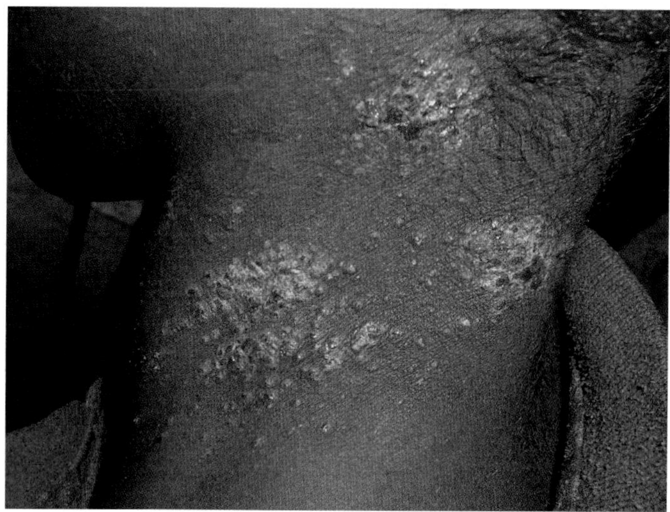

FIGURE 6-14 Impetigo caused by a bacterial infection on the neck with honey crusting. Impetigo is more prevalent when there is inadequate hygiene and lack of access to health care. (*Reproduced with permission from Richard P. Usatine, MD.*)

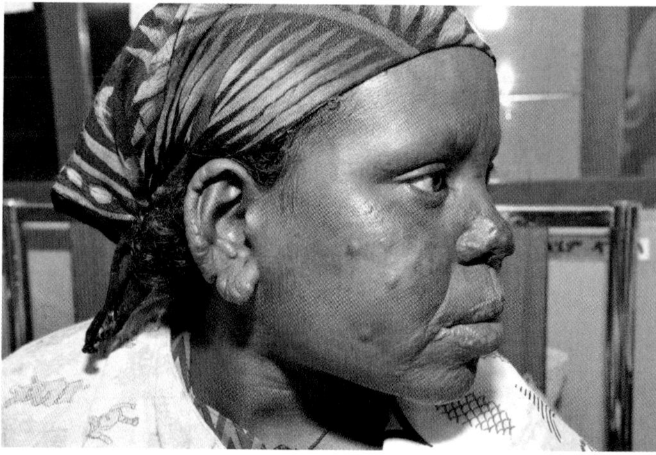

FIGURE 6-15 Lepromatous leprosy with leonine facies in a woman. Note the loss of eyebrows called madarosis and the prominent ear involvement. (*Reproduced with permission from Richard P. Usatine, MD.*)

Bacterial infections of the skin (see Chapter 118, Impetigo) are ubiquitous throughout the world. Impetigo is a superficial bacterial infection that presents with honey crusts (**Figure 6-14**) or bullae. Good hygiene can prevent impetigo and therefore it is not surprising that many cases of impetigo are seen in countries that lack access to soap and clean water. Impetigo is often secondary to other skin diseases such as scabies or fungal infections that create breaks in the skin barrier function. Cases of secondary infected scabies and tinea are seen commonly in developing countries.

Viral infections of the skin include herpes simplex, varicella zoster, molluscum contagiosum, and human papilloma virus infections. These infections are seen commonly in HIV-infected persons who are not receiving optimal antiretroviral therapy. In countries with a high prevalence of HIV-infected people, a severe case of molluscum, warts, or shingles in a young person should prompt a clinician to consider HIV testing, if possible. Molluscum infections and warts are so ubiquitous throughout the world that it is important to realize that healthy people with healthy immune systems can get these infections too. Viral exanthems caused by diseases such as varicella and measles may be more prevalent in countries where vaccinations are less available.

Fungal infections of the skin can occur from the head down to the toes. Heat, humidity, and lack of bathing are predisposing factors to fungal skin infections. Therefore, tropical developing countries provide good environments for tinea capitis, tinea corporis, and tinea pedis.

MYCOBACTERIUM (LEPROSY AND TUBERCULOSIS-HIV COINFECTION)

LEPROSY

Patient Story

A woman presents with significant changes to her face (**Figure 6-15**). A slit-skin examination is performed on the ear lobe of the woman and many acid-fast bacilli, characteristic of *Mycobacterium leprae*, are found. The woman is started on the WHO-standard multidrug therapy using rifampin, clofazimine, and dapsone.

Introduction

Leprosy (Hansen disease) is caused by *M. leprae* and is still endemic in many parts of the developing world where there is poverty and poor access to clean water. At one time, persons with leprosy were called "lepers" and isolated to leper colonies because the disease was disfiguring and the communities were afraid that it was highly contagious. Current science and epidemiology tell us that leprosy is transmitted via droplets from the nose and mouth during close and frequent contact over a period of years, and not by casual contact. Thus doctors working with patients who have leprosy are at no real risk of becoming infected. Issues related to stigma and discrimination still exist.

Epidemiology

- There were 219,075 new cases reported in the world by 105 countries in 2011.[55]
- The United States reported 173 new cases in 2011.[55]
- Since 1990, more than 14 million leprosy patients have been cured, about 4 million from 2000 to 2010.[56]

Etiology and Pathophysiology

- The clinical manifestations of leprosy depend on the immunologic reaction to the infection. The 2 opposite ends of the spectrum consist of the following:
  - Lepromatous leprosy in which there is a strong antibody response and a poor cell-mediated community resulting in larger amounts of *M. leprae* in the tissues (see **Figure 6-15**).
  - Tuberculoid leprosy in which there is a strong cell-mediated immunity and a poor antibody response resulting in less *M. leprae* in the tissues. This tends to present with hypopigmented anesthetic patches (**Figure 6-16**).
- There is also borderline leprosy in which there is a mixed cell-mediated immunity and antibody response showing features of both lepromatous leprosy and tuberculoid leprosy.
- Treatment regimens differ depending on whether the patient has paucibacillary (fewer organisms) or multibacillary leprosy. Lepromatous leprosy and borderline lepromatous leprosy are most likely to be multibacillary.

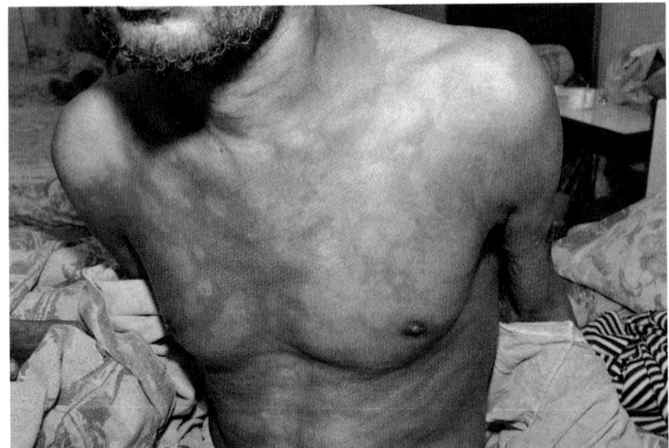

FIGURE 6-16 Multibacillary leprosy with hypopigmented patches. These patches are commonly numb due to cutaneous nerve damage from mycobacterial infection. (*Reproduced with permission from Richard P. Usatine, MD.*)

Risk Factors

- Poverty and living in an endemic area.
- Inadequate access to clean water and poor hygiene.
- Living in the household of an infected person.
- Eating or handling armadillos as these animals are natural hosts for *M. leprae.*

Diagnosis

Clinical Features

- Facial features include leonine facies, madarosis (loss of eyebrows as seen in **Figure 6-15**), elongated and dysmorphic earlobes, and saddle-nose deformities from destruction of the nasal cartilage and bone.
- Visible skin changes include nodules in lepromatous leprosy, hypopigmented patches in tuberculoid (see **Figure 6-16**) and borderline leprosy, and annular saucer-like lesions in borderline leprosy.
- Nerve involvement can cause a clawhand (flexion contractures of the fingers as seen in **Figure 6-17**), wristdrop, footdrop, Bell palsy, hammertoes, and sensory neuropathy leading to neurotropic ulcers and traumatic blisters.
- Eye involvement can cause corneal anesthesia, keratitis, episcleritis, lagophthalmos (the inability to close the eyelid completely), and blindness.
- Advanced untreated leprosy can lead to shortening and/or loss of fingers as a result of bone resorption in hands that have become anesthetic and not protected from repeated trauma (**Figure 6-18**).

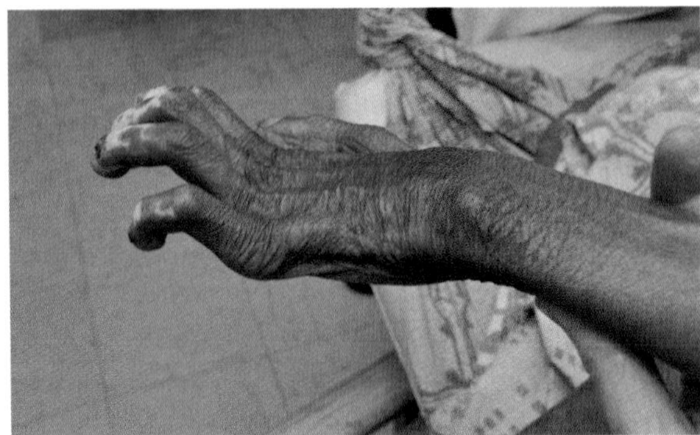

FIGURE 6-17 Clawhand caused by the neurologic damage of leprosy. This condition may be amenable to surgical intervention involving tendon transfer. (*Reproduced with permission from Richard P. Usatine, MD.*)

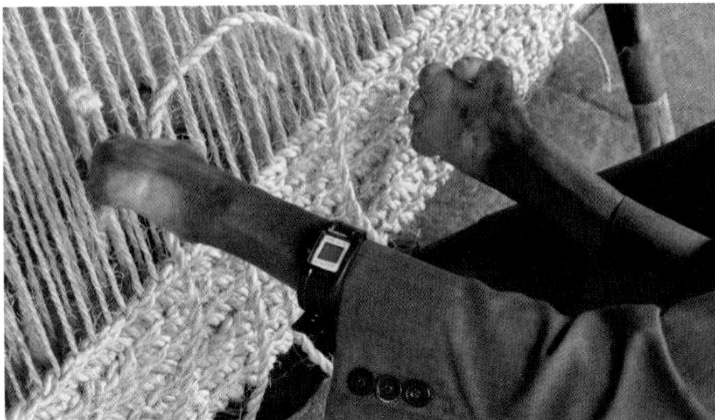

FIGURE 6-18 Leprosy has caused this old man to lose his fingers but he continues to lead a productive life weaving rugs for sale at a leprosy hospital. (*Reproduced with permission from Richard P. Usatine, MD.*)

Distribution

The nodules of lepromatous leprosy are mostly seen on the face and ears but can be seen in other areas. Hypopigmented patches can be seen anywhere on the body including the face.

Laboratory Testing

- In obvious cases of leprosy, the slit-skin examination done on the ear lobe for bacillary index is the most important test to determine if the patient has multibacillary or paucibacillary leprosy.
- In cases that are suspicious for leprosy (especially outside of endemic areas), a skin punch biopsy of a suspicious lesion is useful for finding *M. leprae* in the tissues.

Differential Diagnosis

Superficial mycoses, vitiligo, and cutaneous filariasis all cause changes in pigmentation similar to leprosy. Infiltrated lesions that resemble leprosy include those of leishmaniasis, psoriasis, and sarcoidosis.[57]

Management

Early diagnosis and multidrug therapy are essential for reducing the disease burden of leprosy worldwide. The WHO has supplied multidrug therapy free of cost to leprosy patients in all endemic countries.[58]

- Leprosy is curable and treatment at an early stage can prevent disability.
- Multidrug therapy is a combination of rifampin, dapsone, and clofazimine for multibacillary leprosy patients, and rifampin and dapsone for paucibacillary patients.
- Duration of multidrug therapy is 12 to 24 months for multibacillary and 6 months for paucibacillary patients.[57]
- Treatment with a single antileprosy drug will always result in development of drug resistance to that drug and is therefore an unethical practice.
- Strategies to increase early access to care and to provide easy-to-obtain free multidrug treatment are essential for eliminating leprosy in the world. Research on a preventive vaccine continues in tandem with *Mycobacterium tuberculosis* vaccine research.[59]
- Comprehensive treatment of advanced cases with neuropathy should include foot and hand care to prevent further damage to these insensitive limbs.[57]

- Surgical management for some leprosy-associated problems, such as tendon transfer to correct the clawhand, may be available in some centers.[60]

TUBERCULOSIS AND HIV

Epidemiology

Tuberculosis (TB) is a very common HIV-associated infection, and causes at least 13% of HIV-associated deaths worldwide.[61] In 2010 alone, the WHO estimated that there were 1.1 million HIV-associated new cases of TB, the majority of whom live in sub-Saharan Africa. Globally, about one-third of HIV-infected people are coinfected with TB (at least 11 million people).[62]

Pathogenesis

TB is transmitted by aerosolized respiratory droplet nuclei (see Chapter 64, Tuberculosis). Weakened cell-mediated immunity in HIV-infected individuals allows more rapid disease progression and causes higher mortality rates from TB. At the same time, untreated TB infection accelerates toward immunologic decline in HIV infection. Because these 2 diseases preferentially afflict populations with reduced access to medications and supportive care, the emergence of multidrug-resistant TB has become an increasing threat.

Clinical Presentation

The clinical presentation of TB in an HIV-infected person with a relatively preserved immune system (CD4+ T-cell count >350 cells/μL), is identical to that seen in HIV-negative patients. With increasing immunodeficiency, however, TB often presents atypically. Chest radiographs may not demonstrate classic findings of upper lobe fibronodular or cavitary disease, and extrapulmonary presentations (lymphadenitis, pleuritis, pericarditis, meningitis) are seen. Tuberculous lymphadenitis and cutaneous TB (designated scrofula when it affects the neck) are illustrated in **Figure 6-19.**

Diagnosis

HIV screening should be performed in all patients diagnosed with TB, and HIV-infected patients should be screened annually for *M. tuberculosis* with purified protein derivative (PPD) skin testing, chest x-ray, and/or blood test for interferon-γ release assay (IGRA) depending on availability.

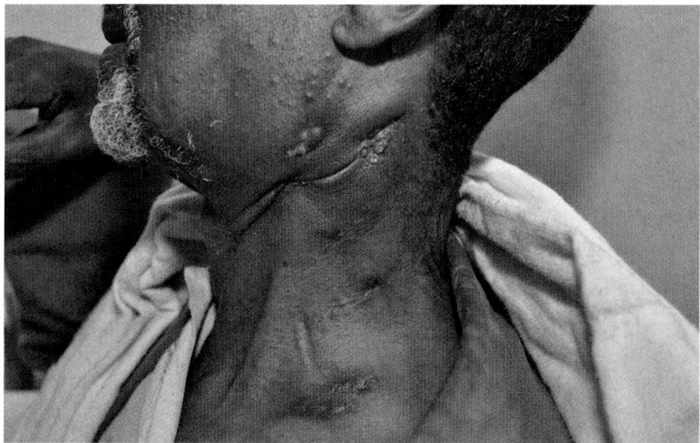

FIGURE 6-19 Scrofula of the neck caused by *M. tuberculosis* in an adult who did not complete his tuberculosis treatment. The long duration of therapy leads to challenges for adherence, and drug-resistant tuberculosis commonly results. (*Reproduced with permission from Richard P. Usatine, MD.*)

Patients with low CD4 cell counts (<200 cells/μL) commonly have poorly reactive skin tests for TB, and thus need a careful history of exposures, review of symptoms, and monitoring of the chest x-ray for evidence of active disease, with repeat TB screening when the CD4 cell count rises above 200 cells/μL.

Management

Latent TB Infection

HIV-positive patients with latent tuberculosis infection (LTBI) should have a chest x-ray and 3 sputum smears for acid-fast bacilli to rule out active disease. Once active TB is ruled out, isoniazid prophylaxis should be initiated regardless of age for any HIV-positive person with the following characteristics: (a) a positive diagnostic test for LTBI, or (b) a negative LTBI test but with evidence of old or poorly healed fibrotic lesions on chest x-ray, or (c) negative LTBI diagnostic test in a close contact of a person with infectious pulmonary TB.

Duration of LTBI prophylaxis: isoniazid 300 mg daily or twice weekly for 9 months given with vitamin B_6 (pyridoxine 25 mg daily). An alternative regimen of 12 doses of once weekly isoniazid-rifapentine has recently been validated. Pyridoxine prevents isoniazid-associated peripheral neuropathy.[63]

Active M. Tuberculosis *Disease*

Any HIV-positive patient with cough and pulmonary infiltrates should be placed in respiratory isolation until TB is ruled out by 3 separately obtained sputum smears (Ziehl-Neelsen) with cultures sent for acid-fast bacilli. This rule applies even when the chest radiograph does not demonstrate cavitary or upper lobe infiltrates. Smear-negative, culture-positive *M. tuberculosis* is not uncommon.

Treatment regimens for HIV-TB coinfected patients are largely identical to those of TB monoinfected patients. It is important not to start antiretroviral therapy (ART) and TB therapy simultaneously, to avoid confusion about drug allergies and side effects. In addition, there is a risk of immune reconstitution syndrome (immune reconstitution inflammatory reaction [IRIS]: inflammatory response that worsens manifestations of any opportunistic infection) when ART is started too soon after initiating TB medication.

Guidelines for ART in TB coinfection are specific. If the CD4 cell count is less than 50, ART should start within 2 weeks of TB therapy. If the CD4 count is greater than 50, ART should start within 8 to 12 weeks of TB therapy. If IRIS does occur, both ART and TB treatment should be continued while managing the IRIS.[64]

Directly observed therapy (DOT) for TB is strongly recommended for HIV-TB coinfected patients.

PROVIDER AND PATIENT RESOURCES

- Traveler's Health from the Centers for Disease Control and Prevention is a comprehensive site that includes information on more than 200 international destinations, travel vaccinations, diseases related to travel, illness and injury abroad, finding travel health specialists, insect protection, safe food and water, and a survival guide—**http://wwwnc.cdc.gov/travel/.**
- The *Yellow Book* 2012 is available online as a reference for those who advised international travelers about health risks—**http://wwwnc.cdc.gov/travel/page/yellowbook-2012-home.htm.**

- Detailed vaccine information for travel can be obtained at the CDC website on vaccinations. This includes information on yellow fever vaccine, typhoid vaccine, and routine vaccines—**http://wwwnc.cdc.gov/travel/page/vaccinations.htm.**
- Vaccine information can be looked up by specific destination on the traveler's health website—**http://wwwnc.cdc.gov/travel/.**
- US Department of State International Travel Site, including country specific information, travel alerts and travel warnings—**http://travel.state.gov/travel/travel_1744.html.**

CONCLUSION

Medical students and health professionals are being increasingly drawn to global health for reasons ranging from the desire for enhanced cultural understanding, to the mission to work for global health equity, to alleviate suffering, or to broaden medical experience beyond geographic boundaries. Whatever one's personal motivation, such experiences should never be undertaken without disciplined preparation. Medical professionals should learn in advance of their travels about the culture, language, and expressed needs and priorities of the local government and health providers and their service populations. In addition, they need to learn about the diagnoses and locally appropriate management of prevalent diseases in the population they plan to serve. Equally important, they should take appropriate preventive measures (vaccines, malaria prophylaxis) to protect their own health. Lack of personal and professional preparation can easily turn the tide from net benefit to major burdens for host country organizations. Ultimately, well-prepared medical educators and clinicians, wherever they may come from, are uniquely positioned to share knowledge that saves lives and leads to a more equitable world.

REFERENCES

1. Kaplan JP, Bond TC, Merson MH, et al. Towards a common definition of global health. *Lancet*. 2009;373:1993-1995.
2. Brown TM, Cueto M, Fee E. The World Health Organization and the transition from "international" to global" public health. *Am J Public Health*. 2006;96:62-72.
3. Central Intelligence Agency. *The World Factbook*. http://www.cia.gov/library/publications/the-world-factbood/geos/cy.html. Accessed September 20, 2012.
4. Waterkeyn J, Carincross S. Creating demand for sanitation and hygiene through community health clubs: a cost-effective intervention in two districts in Zimbabwe. *Soc Sci Med*. 2005;61(9): 1958-1970.
5. World Health Organization. *VIP and ROEC Latrines*. http://www.who.int/water_sanitation_health/hygiene/emergencies/fs3_5.pdf. Accessed September 21, 2012.
6. UNICEF and WHO. *Progress on Drinking Water and Sanitation 2012 Update*. http://www.wssinfo.org/fileadmin/user_upload/resources/JMP-report-2012-en.pdf. Accessed September 21, 2012.
7. Epstein J, Hoffman S. Typhoid fever. In: Guerrant, RL, Walker DH, Weller PF, eds. *Tropical Infectious Diseases: Principles, Pathogens & Practice*. 2nd ed. Philadelphia, PA: Elsevier; 2006:220-240.
8. Araujo-Jorge T, Callan M, Chappuis F, et al. Multisystem diseases and infections. In: Eddleston M, Davidson R, Brent A, Wilkinson R, eds. *Oxford Handbook of Tropical Medicine*. 3rd ed. New York, NY: Oxford University Press; 2008:665-739.
9. Boggild AK, Van Voorhis WC, Liles WC. Travel-acquired illnesses associated with fever. In: Jong E, Sanford E, eds. *Travel and Tropical Medicine Manual*. 4th ed. Philadelphia, PA: Saunders Elsevier; 2008.
10. Gilbert D, Moellering R, Eliopoulos G, Chambers H, Saag M. *The Sanford Guide to Antimicrobial Therapy*. 41st ed. Sperryville, VA: Antimicrobial Therapy; 2011.
11. Cravioto A, Lanata CF, Lantagne DS, Nair GB. *Final Report of the Independent Panel of Experts on the Cholera Outbreak in Haiti 2011*. http://www.un.org/News/dh/infocus/haiti/UN-cholera-report-final.pdf. Accessed September 21, 2012.
12. Levine MM, Gotuzzo E, Sow SO. Cholera infections. In: Guerrant RL, Walker DH, Weller PF, eds. *Tropical Infectious Diseases: Principles, Pathogens & Practice*. 2nd ed. Philadelphia, PA: Elsevier; 2006: 273-282.
13. Penny ME. Diarrhoeal diseases. In: Eddleston M, Davidson R, Brent A, Wilkinson R, eds. *Oxford Handbook of Tropical Medicine*. 3rd ed. New York, NY: Oxford University Press; 2008:213-267.
14. Centers for Disease Control and Prevention. *Cholera Diagnosis and Testing*. http://www.cdc.gov/cholera/diagnosis.html. Accessed September 21, 2012.
15. Centers for Disease Control and Prevention. *Recommendations for the Use of Antibiotics for the Treatment of Cholera*. http://www.cdc.gov/cholera/treatment/antibiotic-treatment.html. Accessed September 21, 2012.
16. Centers for Disease Control and Prevention. *Domestic Intestinal Parasite Guidelines*. http://www.cdc.gov/immigrantrefugeehealth/guidelines/domestic/intestinal-parasites-domestic.html. Accessed September 21, 2012.
17. Keiser J, Utzinger J. Efficacy of current drugs against soil-transmitted helminth infections: systematic review and meta-analysis. *JAMA*. 2008;299(16):1936-1948.
18. Knopp S, Mohammed K, Speich B, et al. Mebendazole administered alone or in combination with ivermectin against *Trichuris trichiura*: a randomized controlled trial. *Clin Infect Dis*. 2010;51(12):1420-1428.
19. World Health Organization. *Obesity and Overweight Factsheet, March 2013*. http://www.who.int/mediacentre/factsheets/fs311/en/. Accessed November 11, 2013.
20. Popkin BM. Nutritional patterns and transitions. *Pop Devel Rev*. 1993;19(1):138-157.
21. Branca F, Ferrari M. Impact of micronutrient deficiencies on growth: the stunting syndrome. *Ann Nutr Metab*. 2002;46(suppl 1): S8-S17.
22. Popkin BM, Richards MK, Montiero CA. Stunting is associated with overweight in children of four nations that are undergoing the nutrition transition. *J Nutr*. 1996;126(12):3009-3016.
23. Damms-Machado A, Weser G, Bischoff SC. Micronutrient deficiency in obese subjects undergoing low calorie diet. *Nutr J*. 2012;11:34. http://www.nutritionj.com/content/11/1/34. Accessed November 11, 2013.
24. World Health Organization. *Global Prevalence of Vitamin A Deficiency in Populations at Risk 1995-2005*. In: WHO Global Database on Vitamin A Deficiency. http://whqlibdoc.who.int/publications/2009/9789241598019_eng.pdf. Accessed September 21, 2012.

25. World Health Organization. *Micronutrient Deficiencies:Vitamin A Deficiency*. http://www.who.int/nutrition/topics/vad/en/index.html. Accessed September 21, 2012.

26. West KP. Vitamin A deficiency as a preventable cause of maternal mortality in undernourished societies: plausibility and next steps. *Int J Gynaecol Obstet*. 2004;85(suppl 1):S24-S27.

27. Hurt L, ten Asbroek A, Amenga-Etego S, et al. Effect of vitamin A supplementation on cause-specific mortality in women of reproductive age in Ghana: a secondary analysis from the ObaapaVitA trial. *Bull World Health Organ*. 2013;91(1):19-27.

28. McGuire S. WHO guideline: vitamin A supplementation in pregnant women. *Adv Nutr*. 2012;3(2):215-216.

29. Ross DA. Recommendation for vitamin A supplementation. *J Nutr*. 2002;132(9):S2902-S2906.

30. Brown K, Wuehler S, Peerson J. The importance of zinc in human nutrition and estimation of the global prevalence of zinc deficiency. *Food Nutr Bull*. 2001;22:113-169.

31. Kosek M, Black R, Keusch G. Nutrition and micronutrients in tropical infectious diseases. In: Guerrant, RL, Walker DH, Weller PF, eds. *Tropical Infectious Diseases: Principles, Pathogens & Practice*. 2nd ed. Philadelphia, PA: Elsevier; 2006:36-52.

32. World Health Organization. *Implementing the New Recommendations of the Clinical Management of Diarrhea. Guidelines for Policy Makers and Programme Managers*. Geneva, Switzerland: World Health Organization; 2006. http://whqlibdoc.who.int/publications/2006/9241594217_eng.pdf. Accessed September 21, 2012.

33. Baqui AH, Black RE, Shams EA, et al. Effect of zinc supplementation started during diarrhoea on morbidity and mortality in Bangladeshi children: community randomised trial. *BMJ*. 2002;325:1059.

34. Brown K, Wuehler S, Peerson J. The importance of zinc in human nutrition and estimation of the global prevalence of zinc deficiency. *Food Nutr Bull*. 2001. http://archive.unu.edu/unupress/food/fnb22-2.pdf. Accessed September 21, 2012.

35. World Health Organization. *Micronutrient Deficiencies. Iron Deficiency Anaemia*. http://www.who.int/nutrition/topics/ida/en/index.html. Accessed September 21, 2012.

36. Horton S, Miloff, A. Iodine status and availability of iodized salt: an across-country analysis. *Food Nutr Bull*. 2010;31:214-220.

37. World Health Organization. *Iodine Status Worldwide*. http://whqlibdoc.who.int.publications/2004/9241592001.pdf. Accessed September 21, 2012.

38. Prousky JE. Pellagra may be a rare secondary complication of anorexia nervosa: a systematic review of the literature. *Altern Med Rev*. 2003;8(2):180.

39. Lanska DJ. Historical aspects of the major neurological vitamin deficiency disorders: the water-soluble B vitamins. *Handbook of Clin Neurol*. 2010;95:445-476.

40. Tomkins A. Nutrition. In: Eddleston M, Davidson R, Brent A, Wilkinson R, eds. *Oxford Handbook of Tropical Medicine*. 3rd ed. New York, NY: Oxford University Press; 2008:652-653.

41. Tharp M, Shear N. *Drug Eruption: Pellagra*. http://www.visualdx.com/visualdx/visualdx6/getDiagnosisText.do?moduleId=14&diagnosisId=52131&view=text&topic=1. Accessed November 11, 2013.

42. Day N. Malaria. In: Eddleston M, Davidson R, Brent A, Wilkinson R, eds. *Oxford Handbook of Tropical Medicine*. 3rd ed. New York, NY: Oxford University Press; 2008:31-65.

43. Ashley E, White N. Malaria diagnosis and treatment. In: Jong E, Sanford E, eds. *Travel and Tropical Medicine Manual*. 4th ed. Philadelphia, PA: Saunders Elsevier; 2008:303-321.

44. Hoffman S, Campbell C, White N. Malaria. In: Guerrant, RL, Walker DH, Weller PF, eds. *Tropical Infectious Diseases: Principles, Pathogens & Practice*. 2nd ed. Philadelphia, PA: Elsevier; 2006:1024-1062.

45. Centers for Disease Control. *Treatment of Malaria (Guidelines for Clinicians)*. April 2011. http://www.cdc.gov/malaria/resources/pdf/clinicalguidance.pdf. Accessed September 21, 2012.

46. World Health Organization. *10 Facts on Malaria*. http://www.who.int/features/factfiles/malaria/en/index.html. Accessed September 21, 2012.

47. Centers for Disease Control and Prevention. *Parasites—Leishmaniasis*. http://www.cdc.gov/parasites/leishmaniasis/. Accessed September 15, 2012.

48. Singh S. New developments in diagnosis of leishmaniasis. *Indian J Med Res*. 2006;123:311-330.

49. Ryan T. Dermatology. In: Eddleston M, Davidson R, Brent A, Wilkinson R, eds. *Oxford Handbook of Tropical Medicine*. 3rd ed. New York, NY: Oxford University Press; 2008:566.

50. Schwartz E. Leishmaniasis. In: Jong E, Sanford E, eds. *Travel and Tropical Medicine Manual*. 4th ed. Philadelphia, PA: Saunders Elsevier; 2008:532-542.

51. Pub Med Health. *Leishmaniasis*. http://www.ncbi.nlm.nih.gov/pubmedhealth/PMH0002362/. Accessed September 15, 2012.

52. Pearson R, Weller P, Guerrant R. Chemotherapy of parasitic diseases. In: Guerrant, RL, Walker DH, Weller PF, eds. *Tropical Infectious Diseases: Principles, Pathogens & Practice*. 2nd ed. Philadelphia, PA: Elsevier; 2006:142-168.

53. World Health Organization. *Prevention of Blindness and Visual Impairment, Priority Eye Diseases: Trachoma*. http://www.who.int/blindness/causes/priority/en/index2.html. Accessed September 21, 2012.

54. Yorston D. Ophthalmology. In: Eddleston M, Davidson R, Brent A, Wilkinson R, eds. *Oxford Handbook of Tropical Medicine*. 3rd ed. New York, NY: Oxford University Press; 2008:523.

55. Global leprosy situation. *Wkly Epidemiol Rec*. 2012;87(34):316-328.

56. World Health Organization. *Leprosy; Fact Sheet No.101*. http://www.who.int/mediacentre/factsheets/fs101/en/index.html. Accessed August 26, 2012.

57. World Health Organization. *Leprosy Elimination.WHO Multidrug Therapy*. http://www.who.int/lep/mdt/en/index.html. Accessed August 26, 2012.

58. Meyers W. Leprosy. In: Guerrant, RL, Walker DH, Weller PF, eds. *Tropical Infectious Diseases: Principles, Pathogens & Practice*. 2nd ed. Philadelphia, PA: Elsevier; 2006:436.

59. Gormus BJ, Meyers WM. Under-explored experimental topics related to integral mycobacterial vaccines for leprosy. *Expert Rev Vaccines*. 2003;2(6):791-804.

60. Sapienza A, Green S. Correction of the claw hand. *Hand Clin*. 2012;28(1):53-66.

61. National Institutes of Health Clinical Guidelines Portal. *Federally Approved HIV/AIDS Medical Practice Guidelines*. http://www.aidsinfo.nih.gov/contentfiles/lvguidelines/adult_oi_041009.pdf. Accessed September 21, 2012.

62. World Health Organization. *TB/HIV FACTS 2011-2012*. http://www.who.int/tb/publications/TBHIV_Facts_for_2011.pdf. Accessed September 21, 2012.

63. Johnson J, Ellner J. Tuberculosis and atypical mycobacterial infections. In: Guerrant, RL, Walker DH, Weller PF, eds. *Tropical Infectious Diseases: Principles, Pathogens & Practice*. 2nd ed. Philadelphia, PA: Elsevier; 2006:411.

64. National Institutes of Health Clinical Guidelines Portal. *Considerations for Antiretroviral Use in Patients with Coinfections: Mycobacterium Tuberculosis Disease with HIV Coinfection*. http://www.aidsinfo.nih.gov/guidelines/html/1/adult-and-adolescent-treatment-guidelines/27/. Accessed December 9, 2013.

PART 3

PHYSICAL AND SEXUAL ABUSE

Strength of Recommendation (SOR)	Definition
A	Recommendation based on consistent and good-quality patient-oriented evidence.*
B	Recommendation based on inconsistent or limited-quality patient-oriented evidence.*
C	Recommendation based on consensus, usual practice, opinion, disease-oriented evidence, or case series for studies of diagnosis, treatment, prevention, or screening.*

*See Appendix A on pages 1241-1244 for further information.

7 INTIMATE PARTNER VIOLENCE

Mindy A. Smith, MD, MS

PATIENT STORY

A woman who fled her abusive boyfriend is observed sitting at a table with other women in a residential chemical dependency treatment program. Her bruised face could not be missed (**Figure 7-1**). The program physician was asked to speak with her and learned that her boyfriend beat her when she told him that she was voluntarily entering this program. The boyfriend was also an addict and had been physically abusive to her before. The violence escalated when she said that she needed help to stop the alcohol and drugs. She left him and did not believe that he would follow her. The program management assured her that they would not let him on the premises and would do all they could to keep her safe while she was recovering. **Figure 7-2** was taken 2 months later, when her face was healing along with her mind and spirit. She completed the 90-day program and is currently working and actively following a 12-step program.

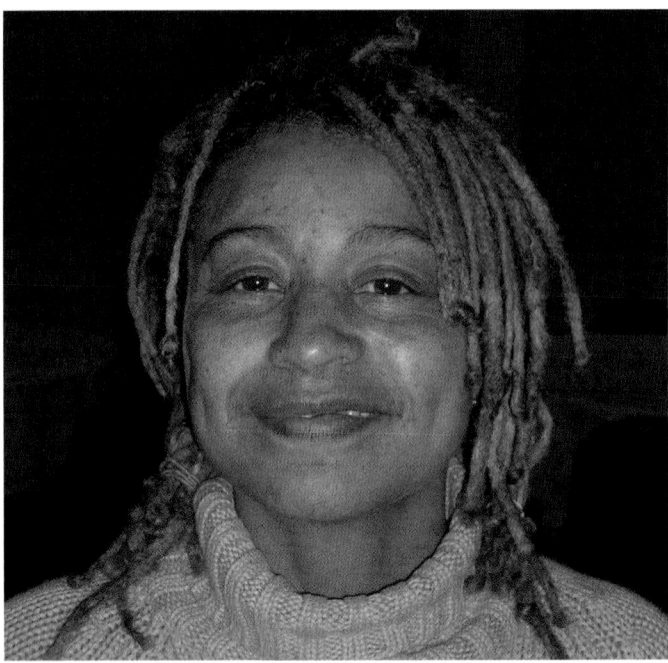

FIGURE 7-2 Photograph of the woman in Figure 7-1 taken 2 months later. Her facial and psychological wounds are healing. (*Reproduced with permission from Richard P. Usatine, MD.*)

INTRODUCTION

Intimate partner violence (IPV) is defined as an intimate partner's physical, emotional, or sexual abuse. Physical violence is the intentional use of physical force with the potential for causing death, disability, injury, or harm. Physical violence includes scratching; pushing; biting; punching; use of a weapon; and use of restraints or one's body, size, or strength against another person.[1]

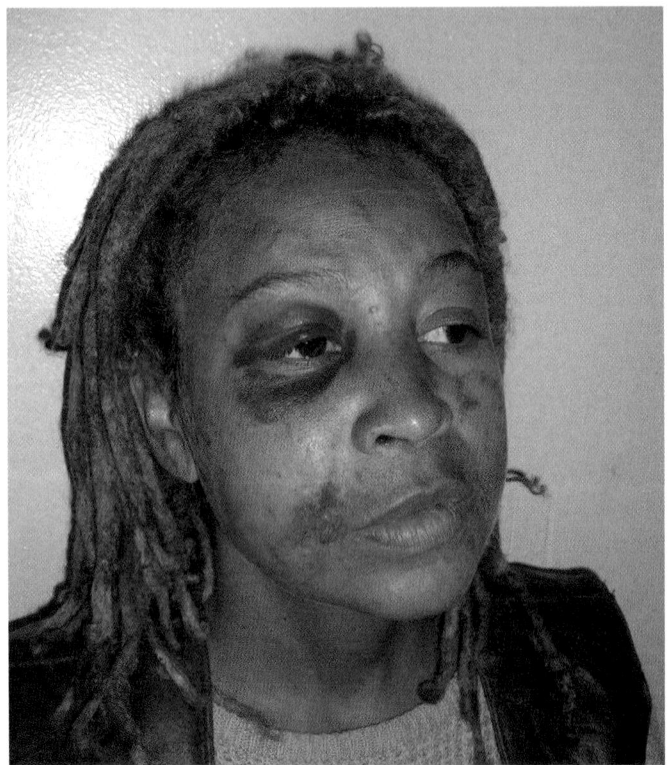

FIGURE 7-1 Bruising caused by intimate partner violence in a woman who fled her abusive boyfriend. (*Reproduced with permission from Richard P. Usatine, MD.*)

EPIDEMIOLOGY

IPV affects up to half of the women in the United States during their lifetime.[2]

- An estimated 4.9 million IPV rapes and physical assaults occur each year among US women (age 18 years and older) and 2.9 million assaults occur among US men. Most of these assaults include pushing, grabbing, shoving, slapping, and hitting and do not result in major injury.[3] In a national telephone survey of 8000 women and 8000 men, 41.5% of the women who were physically assaulted by an intimate partner were injured during their most recent assault, compared with 19.9% of men.[4]
- Physical violence by an intimate partner can result in direct injury including death (1181 women and 329 men in 2005; Bureau of Justice, 2007), adverse psychological, and social consequences, and impaired endocrine and immune systems through chronic stress and other mechanisms.[4]
- A national survey estimated that 503,485 women and 185,496 men are stalked by intimate partners each year.[4]
- Clinicians identify only a small number of victims (1.5-8.5%).[1] Only approximately 20% of IPV rapes or sexual assaults, 25% of physical assaults, and 50% of stalking directed toward women are reported; fewer events against men are reported.[4]
- Between 4% and 8% of women are battered during pregnancy.[5]
- According to the National Violence Against Women Survey, more than 200,000 women age 18 years and older were raped by intimate partners in the 12 months preceding the survey.[6]

RISK FACTORS

Risk factors for IPV include the following[7]:

- Individual factors—Individual factors include prior history of IPV, witnessing or experiencing violence as a child, being female, young, pregnant, less educated, unemployed, heavy user of alcohol or illicit drugs, mental health problems (eg, depression, borderline or antisocial personality traits), and engaging in aggressive or delinquent behavior as a youth.
- For women, having a greater education level than their partner, being American Indian/Alaska Native or African American, and having a verbally abusive, jealous, or possessive partner increased the risk. In addition, a risk of IPV by either a past or a new offender was almost double for women who had recently changed residence compared with those who had not moved.[8]
- For men, having a different ethnicity from their partner's increased the risk of IPV.
- Relationship factors—Relationship factors include couples with income, educational, or job status disparities or in which there is dominance and control of the relationship by one partner over the other, and marital conflict or instability.
- Community factors—Community factors include poverty and associated factors or weak community sanctions against IPV (eg, police unwilling to intervene).

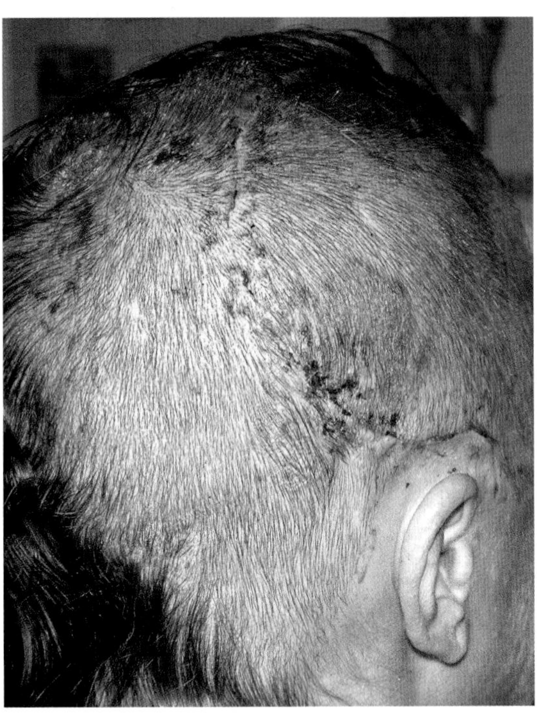

FIGURE 7-3 A woman with a large craniotomy wound that was needed to evacuate her intracranial bleeding secondary to being beaten over the head with a board by her fiancé. *(Reproduced with permission from Richard P. Usatine, MD.)*

DIAGNOSIS

Asking patients directly about violence at routine visits or when presenting with clues (as given below) is recommended for identifying patients suffering from IPV (see Screening and Prevention).[1,4] It is important to use patient-centered approaches.

- Questions that may be asked include general questions about how things are going at home or more specific questions about experiences of nonviolent (eg, insulting, threatening) or violent (eg, grabbing, punching, beating, forced sex) abusive acts.
- Several self-administered instruments are available for detecting IPV including the Woman Abuse Screening Tool (WAST).[9] In a study of screening tools, women preferred self-completed approaches (vs face-to-face), although no differences in prevalence was found for method or screening instrument.[10] In a predominantly Hispanic population, investigators found the Spanish version of the 4-question instrument HITS (Hurt-Insult-Threaten-Scream) to be moderately reliable with good validity compared with WAST for Spanish-speaking patients;[11] HITS has also been validated with male victims.[12]

CLINICAL FEATURES

Clues on patient history include the following:

- Chronic pain syndromes (eg, headache, backache, stomachache, or pelvic pain)
- Depression
- Drug and alcohol abuse

Up to 42% of women and 20% of men who were physically assaulted as adults sustained injuries during their most recent victimization.[3] Clues on physical examination include the following:

- Physical injury—Most physical injuries are minor (eg, contusions, lacerations, abrasions) but include broken bones, traumatic brain injury, and knife wounds (see **Figures 7-1** to **7-3**).

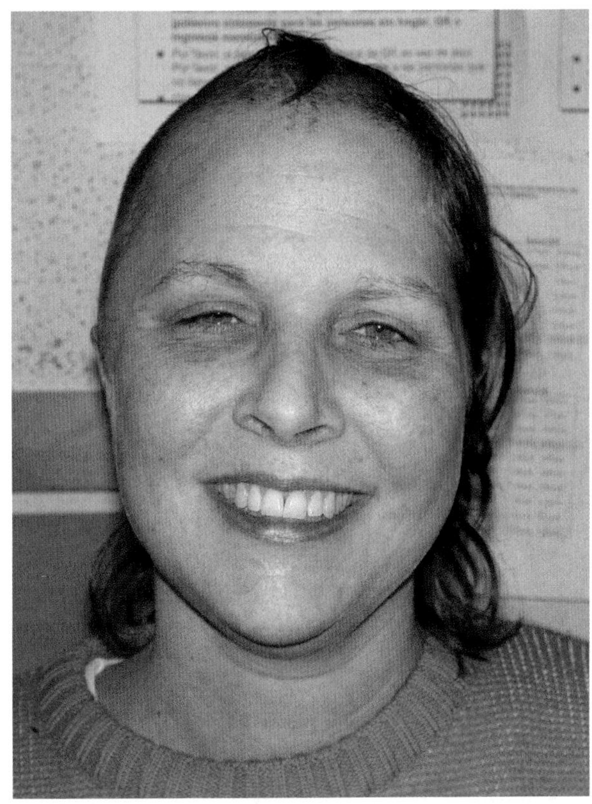

FIGURE 7-4 Frontal view of the woman in Figure 7-3 at a homeless shelter. She was putting her life back together again with the help of the shelter and the providers at the clinic. *(Reproduced with permission from Richard P. Usatine, MD.)*

- Ocular injuries can include soft tissue injuries, corneal abrasions, orbital fractures, lens dislocation, retinal detachment, visual field loss, double vision, and blindness (see **Figure 7-1**).
- Trauma to the mouth and lips may be accompanied by fractures, broken teeth, tongue lacerations, and altered taste and smell.
- Injuries suspicious for abuse are those only in areas covered by clothing, injuries in different stages of healing, and injuries that show a defensive wound pattern particularly on the hands or arms.
- Upper torso injury carries a high risk of injury to cervical spine, large vessels of the neck, chest, and lungs.

• Depression or symptoms of posttraumatic stress disorder (eg, emotional detachment, sleep disturbances, flashbacks, replaying assault in mind).
• Evidence of forced sexual assault.
• Presence of sexually transmitted infections.

MANAGEMENT

• Initial evaluation, following identification of abuse, is to assess for immediate danger to the woman and any children (eg, Do you feel it is safe to go home tonight? Where is your partner?). If danger is perceived, assist the woman in finding a safe place to go (**Figures 7-4** and **7-5**).
• Document all findings and include photographs (with date), if possible (**Figure 7-6**).
• Develop a safety plan. This should include the following:
  - A safe physical location that is not known to the abuser
  - Transportation to that location
  - A list of items to take or a packed suitcase—clothes, keys, cash, valuable documents, telephone numbers, prescriptions, something meaningful for each child
• Address the needs of any children—30% to 40% of children are also injured physically.[1]
• Data on effective intervention programs are scarce.
  - In a community intervention program in rural South Africa, providing loans to poor women combined with a participatory learning and action curriculum integrated into loan meetings every 2 weeks reduced IPV.[13]

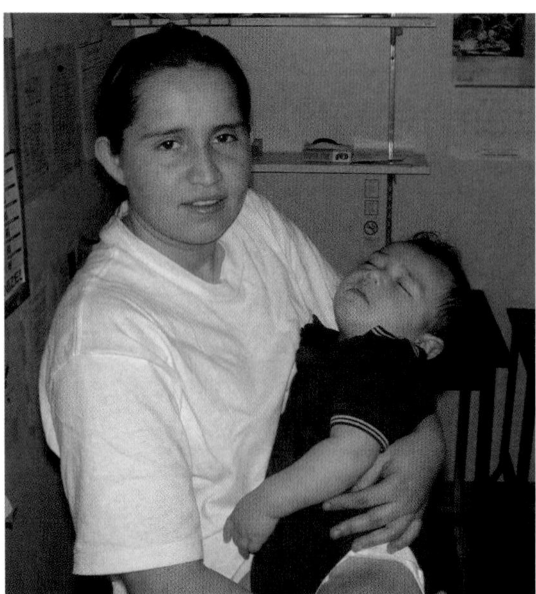

FIGURE 7-5 A young, Hispanic mom with her baby at a clinic in a homeless shelter. She had fled her abusive husband with her child. (*Reproduced with permission from Richard P. Usatine, MD.*)

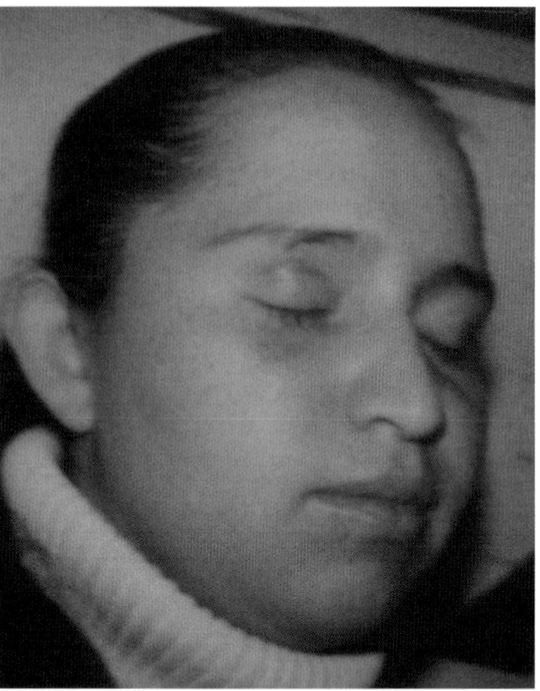

FIGURE 7-6 A copy of a photograph, which the woman had in her purse, showing her black eyes after being beaten by her husband the month before. Out of fear for her life and the well-being of her child, she left her husband. (*Reproduced with permission from Richard P. Usatine, MD.*)

  - Women residents in a domestic violence shelter showed improvement in psychological distress symptoms and less health care utilization following a social support intervention.[14]
  - An advocacy intervention for Chinese women who were victims of IPV did not reduce depression symptoms in a clinically meaningful way.[15]
  - In a Cochrane review of cognitive behavior therapy (CBT) for abusive men, only 4 small trials could be combined and no significant effect was found for reduced risk of violence (relative risk [RR], 0.86; 95% confidence interval [CI], 0.54, 1.38); the authors concluded that there were too few trials to determine the effectiveness.[16]

SCREENING AND PREVENTION

• With respect to screening, the US Preventive Services Task Force recommends screening women of childbearing age, including adolescents, for intimate partner violence and providing or referring women who screen positive to intervention services, SOR B.[17]
• In one randomized clinical trial (RCT), computer screening increased detection and opportunities to discuss IPV in a busy family medicine practice.[18]
• In an observational study of a convenience sample of 2134 patients presenting to an emergency room (25.7% screened positive), there were no harms identified from screening for IPV at 1 week postvisit and at 3 months; 35% of those screening positive reported having contacted community resources.[19]
• With respect to outcomes, a Canadian RCT (*N* = 6743 English-speaking women ages 18-64 years) conducted in 11 emergency departments,

12 family practices, and 3 obstetrics/gynecology clinics, screening for IPV did not significantly reduce IPV recurrence (46% vs 53% in screened vs unscreened patients [odds ratio [OR], 0.82; 95% CI, 0.32, 2.12]) or quality of life scores; loss to follow-up, however, was high (approximately 40%).[20]

PROGNOSIS

- Many women are not ready to leave an abusive relationship for a variety of reasons. In one study, duration of abuse was less than 1 year to 5 median years, and in 5% to 3% of the instances, IPV persisted for more than 20 years.[21]
- Women who are abused have a higher risk of posttraumatic stress disorder, depression (1 in 6 abused women will attempt suicide[1]), insomnia, nightmares, and alcohol (16-fold risk of alcohol use[1]) and drug abuse (9-fold risk over nonabused patient[1]).
- IPV for women also decreases the odds of completing substance abuse treatment.[22]

FOLLOW-UP

- Plan for the next visit and provide ongoing support as it often takes time for women to leave an abusive relationship.
- Monitor for depression, insomnia, nightmares, and alcohol and drug abuse.

PATIENT EDUCATION

- Assist patients in recognizing the cycle of abuse, that is, violence followed by remorse or apology, tension-building period (patient may experience fear, isolation, forced dependency, intermittent reward), followed by another episode of violence.
- Provide victim education and information on community resources (see Patient Resources below).
- Acknowledge that leaving may take time.
- Recovery from abuse may include shame and guilt, but often leads to an improved sense of self and self-worth.
- In a follow-up study of women exiting a shelter, women who were employed, reported higher quality of life, and had people in their networks who provided practical help and/or were available to talk about personal matters were less likely to be revictimized.[23]

PATIENT RESOURCES

- National Domestic Violence Hotline connects individuals to help in their area by using a nationwide database that includes detailed information about domestic violence shelters, other emergency shelters, legal advocacy and assistance programs, and social service programs. Help is more than 170 languages, 24 hours a day, 7 days a week—**www.ndvh.org.**

  Hotline: 800-779-SAFE (7233)

  TTY: 800-787-3224 available for the Deaf, Deaf-Blind and Hard of Hearing.

  Administrative phone: 512-453-8117
- National Coalition Against Domestic Violence is a membership organization that includes service programs, reading lists, advocacy, educational materials, and coordinates a national collaborative effort to assist battered women in removing the physical scars of abuse—**www.ncadv.org.**
- Centers for Disease Control and Prevention—**http://www.cdc.gov/ViolencePrevention/pdf/IPV_factsheet-a.pdf.**

PROVIDER RESOURCES

- Centers for Disease Control and Prevention. *Intimate Partner Violence*—**http://www.cdc.gov/ViolencePrevention/intimatepartnerviolence/index.html.**
- Futures without Violence—**http://www.futureswithoutviolence. org/.**
- Institute on Domestic Violence in the African American Community—**http://www.dvinstitute.org.**

REFERENCES

1. Centers for Disease Control. *Intimate Partner Violence: Definitions.* http://www.cdc.gov/ViolencePrevention/intimatepartnerviolence/definitions.html. Accessed August 2013.
2. Gilchrest VJ. Abuse of women. In: Smith MA, Shimp LA, eds. *20 Common Problems in Women's Health Care.* New York, NY: McGraw-Hill; 2000:197-224.
3. Tjaden P, Thoennes N. *Extent, Nature, and Consequences of Intimate Partner Violence: Findings from the National Violence Against Women Survey.* Washington, DC: Department of Justice (US); 2000. Publication No. NCJ 181867. Office of Justice Programs. http://www.ojp.usdoj.gov/nij/pubs-sum/181867.htm. Accessed August 2013.
4. Centers for Disease Control. *Intimate Partner Violence: Consequences.* http://www.cdc.gov/ViolencePrevention/intimatepartnerviolence/consequences.html. Accessed August 2013.
5. Centers for Disease Control. *Intimate Partner Violence During Pregnancy, A Guide for Clinicians: Download Instructions.* http://www.cdc.gov/reproductivehealth/violence/IntimatePartnerViolence/ipvdp_download.htm. Accessed August 2013.
6. Centers for Disease Control. *CDC Injury Fact Book.* www.cdc.gov/ncipc/fact_book/24_Sexual_Violence.htm. Accessed August 2013.
7. Centers for Disease Control. *Intimate Partner Violence: Risk and Protective Factors.* http://www.cdc.gov/ViolencePrevention/intimatepartnerviolence/riskprotectivefactors.html. Accessed August 2013.
8. Waltermaurer E, McNutt LA, Mattingly MJ. Examining the effect of residential change on intimate partner violence risk. *J Epidemiol Community Health.* 2006;60(11):923-927.
9. Fogarty CT, Burge S, McCord EC. Communicating with patients about intimate partner violence: screening and interviewing approaches. *Fam Med.* 2002;34(5):369-375.
10. MacMillan HL, Wathen CN, Jamieson E, et al. Approaches to screening for intimate partner violence in health care settings: a randomized trial. *JAMA.* 2006;296(5):530-536.

11. Chen PH, Rovi S, Vega M, et al. Screening for domestic violence in a predominantly Hispanic clinical setting. *Fam Pract*. 2005;22(6): 617-623.
12. Shakil A, Donald S, Sinacore JM, Krepcho M. Validation of the HITS domestic violence screening tool with males. *Fam Med*. 2005;37(3): 193-198.
13. Pronyk PM, Hargreaves JR, Kim JC, et al. Effect of a structural intervention for the prevention of intimate-partner violence and HIV in rural South Africa: a cluster randomised trial. *Lancet*. 2006;368(9551):1973-1983.
14. Contantino R, Kim Y, Crane PA. Effects of a social support intervention on health outcomes in residents of a domestic violence shelter: a pilot study. *Issues Ment Health Nurs*. 2005;26(6): 575-590.
15. Tiwari A, Fong DY, Yuen KH, et al. Effect of an advocacy intervention on mental health in Chinese women survivors of intimate partner violence: a randomized controlled trial. *JAMA*. 2010;304(5): 536-543.
16. Smedslund G, Dalsbø TK, Steiro AK, et al. Cognitive behavioural therapy for men who physically abuse their female partner. *Cochrane Database Syst Rev*. 2007 Jul 18;(3):CD006048.
17. United States Preventive Services Task Force. *Screening for Family and Intimate Partner Violence*. http://www.uspreventiveservicestaskforce.org/uspstf/uspsipv.htm. Accessed August 2013.
18. Ahmad F, Hogg-Johnson S, Stewart DE, et al. Computer-assisted screening for intimate partner violence and control: a randomized trial. *Ann Intern Med*. 2009;151(2):93-102.
19. Houry D, Kaslow NJ, Kemball RS, et al. Does screening in the emergency department hurt or help victims of intimate partner violence? *Ann Emerg Med*. 2008;51(4):433-442.
20. MacMillan HL, Wathen CN, Jamieson E, et al. Screening for intimate partner violence in health care settings: a randomized trial. *JAMA*. 2009;302(5):493-501.
21. Thompson RS, Bonomi AE, Anderson M, et al. Intimate partner violence: prevalence, types, and chronicity in adult women. *Am J Prev Med*. 2006;30(6):447-457.
22. Lipsky S, Krupski A, Roy-Bryne P, et al. Effect of co-occurring disorders and intimate partner violence on substance abuse treatment outcomes. *J Subst Abuse Treat*. 2010;38(3):231-244.
23. Bybee D, Sullivan CM. Predicting re-victimization of battered women 3 years after exiting a shelter program. *Am J Community Psychol*. 2005;36(1-2):85-96.

8 SEXUAL ASSAULT

Mindy A. Smith, MD, MS

PATIENT STORIES

CASE 1

A 19-year-old woman, a college student, presents to the office after being raped 3 weeks ago. She went out on a date and was forced to have sex against her will. She states that she had been a virgin and that he made her bleed by penetrating her vagina with his penis. She tried to stop him, but was afraid to fight too hard because he was a strong man and was drunk. She is in tears as she tells her story. She waited so long to come in for help because she did not know where to turn. She took emergency contraception (EC) immediately, and a home pregnancy test taken last night was negative. She wants to be checked for any sexually transmitted infections (STIs). Upon examination, there is a tear of her hymen at the 5-o'clock position that has healed (**Figure 8-1**). There are no signs of infection and STI screening is performed. She is afraid to prosecute but would like to be referred to a rape-counseling program.

CASE 2

A 47-year-old woman is seen in a follow-up for depression. She admits to being raped in a parking lot several months ago but did not report it to the police. She is continuing to have intrusive nightmares and flashbacks of the event. She is having difficulty concentrating at work and does not feel comfortable in social situations.

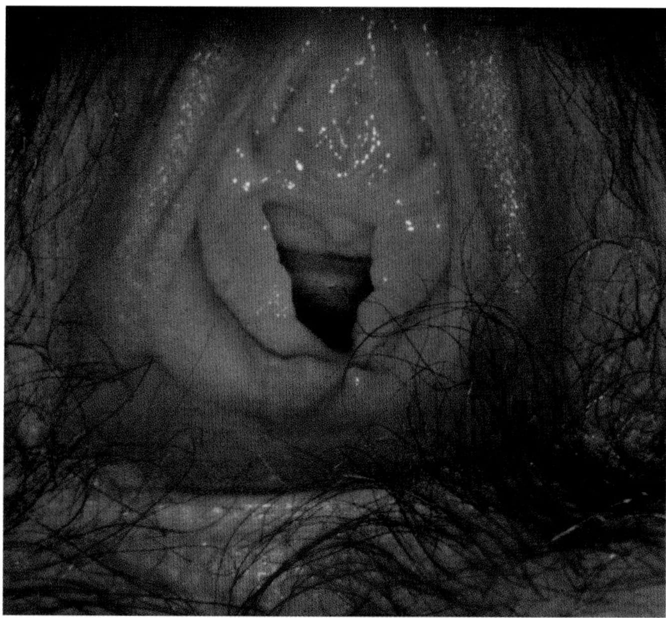

FIGURE 8-1 External genitalia of a 19-year-old woman, a college student, showing the tear of her hymen at approximately the 5-o'clock position. This was the result of date rape 3 weeks before the photograph was taken. *(Reproduced with permission from Nancy D. Kellogg, MD.)*

INTRODUCTION

Sexual violence is a sex act completed or attempted against a victim's will or when a victim is unable to consent because of age, illness, disability, or the influence of alcohol or other drugs.[1] It may involve actual or threatened physical force, use of guns or other weapons, coercion, intimidation, or pressure. Sexual violence includes unwanted intercourse (completed sex act defined as contact between the penis and the vulva or penis and anus involving penetration); an attempted sex act, abusive sexual contact (intentional touching either directly or through clothing of the genitals, anus, groin, breast, inner thigh, or buttocks against a victim's will or when a victim is unable to consent); and noncontact sexual abuse, such as voyeurism, intentional exposure to exhibitionism, undesired exposure to pornography, verbal or behavioral sexual harassment, threats of sexual violence, or taking nude photographs of a sexual nature of another person without his or her consent or knowledge or of a person unable to consent or refuse.

EPIDEMIOLOGY

- Based on the National Intimate Partner and Sexual Violence Survey (NISVS, 2010) of more than 16,000 adults, nearly 1 in 5 women (18.3%) and 1 in 71 men (1.4%) in the United States has been raped.[2] More than half of the women were raped by an intimate partner (see Chapter 7, Intimate Partner Violence) and 40.8% by an acquaintance. Among men, more than half were raped by an acquaintance and 15.1% by a stranger.[2]
- Unwanted sexual contact was reported in the NISVS by 27.2% of women and 11.7% of men.[2]
- Lifetime stalking victimization was reported by 1 in 6 women (16.2%) and 1 in 19 men (5.2%) in the NISVS.[2]
- Most victims of sexual assault are young:
    - In the NISVS, most women (79.6%) experienced their first completed rape before age 25 years and 42.2% before the age of 18 years.[2] More than one-quarter of male victims of completed rape (27.8%) experienced their first rape before they were 11 years of age.
    - Similar findings were reported in another national survey where 60.4% of female and 69.2% of male victims were first raped before age 18 years.[3] A quarter of females were first raped before age 12 years.
- In surveys of college students, annually 10% of women described a rape, 17% reported an attempted rape, 26% reported unwanted sexual coercion, and 63% experienced unwanted sexual contact.[4]
- Women in substance abuse treatment are a particularly high-risk group for having experienced violence. In one study, 89% reported a history of interpersonal violence and 70% reported a history of sexual assault.[5]
- Men are most often the perpetrators of sexual violence;[2] even among male victims, predominantly male perpetrators committed the rape or noncontact unwanted sexual experiences reported, and almost half of stalking victimizations of men were perpetrated by men.
- According to the FBI Uniform Crime Reports, there were an estimated 84,767 forcible rapes reported to law enforcement in 2010 or 54.2 per 100,000 women, a decrease of 5% from 2009 and 6.7% lower than 2001.[6] Most women, however, do not report being raped to the police:
    - As in the cases presented in this chapter, most cases of sexual assault go unreported (only about 1 in 5 women report their rape to police).[7] Reasons for failing to report include fear of reprisal, shame,

fear of the justice system, and failure to define the act as rape. Furthermore, according to victim accounts in the NISVS, only 37% of the rapes reported to police resulted in the rapist being criminally prosecuted, and of those prosecuted, less than half (46.2%) were convicted of a crime.[2]

ETIOLOGY AND PATHOPHYSIOLOGY

Two types of factors are believed to contribute to sexual violence—*Vulnerability factors* that increase the likelihood that a person will suffer harm and *risk factors* that increase the likelihood that a person will cause harm. Neither vulnerability nor risk factors are direct causes of sexual violence.[3]

RISK FACTORS

Vulnerability factors for sexual assault, in addition to young age and female gender, include the following[8,9]:

- Prior history of sexual violence
- Being disabled (physical, psychiatric illness, or cognitive impairment)
- Pregnancy
- Poverty, homelessness
- Having many sexual partners or involved in sex work
- Consuming alcohol or illicit drugs

Risk factors for perpetration include the following[8,10]:

- Alcohol and drug use
- Childhood history of physical or sexual abuse and/or witnessed family violence as a child
- Coercive sexual fantasies
- Preference for impersonal sex
- Hostility toward women
- Association with sexually aggressive and delinquent peers
- Family environment characterized by physical violence and few resources
- Poverty and lack of employment opportunities
- Societal norms that support sexual violence, male superiority, and sexual entitlement
- Weak laws and policies related to gender equity

DIAGNOSIS

It is recommended that patients are asked directly about violence during routine visits, when seen in the emergency department, or when presenting with substance abuse, depression, and/or physical clues (as listed below) so as to identify those who are suffering from the aftermath of sexual or physical violence (see Chapter 7, Intimate Partner Violence).

CLINICAL FEATURES

- Approximately 33% of women and 16% of men have physical injuries as a result of a rape; 36.2% of injured women received medical treatment.[1]

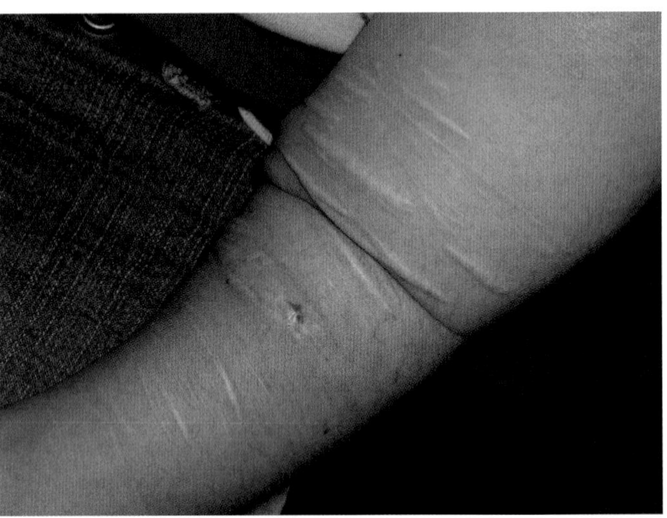

FIGURE 8-2 The mutilated arm of a 26-year-old woman who was raped 5 years before this photograph was taken. After being raped, she became suicidal and began cutting her arm repeatedly. The additional malformation of the arm is secondary to osteomyelitis from previous intravenous drug use. (*Reproduced with permission from Richard P. Usatine, MD.*)

- Women who are raped are significantly more likely than nonraped women to experience genital injuries and STIs, and have significantly greater difficulties with aspects of reproductive or sexual functioning, including dyspareunia, endometriosis, menstrual irregularities, and chronic pelvic pain.[11]
- Many women suffer psychological trauma following sexual assault such as posttraumatic stress disorder (PTSD) symptoms[1]:
    - Immediate psychological consequences include confusion, anxiety, withdrawal, fear, guilt, intrusive recollections, emotional detachment, and flashbacks.
    - Some victims may attempt suicide after being raped (**Figure 8-2**).

MANAGEMENT

NONPHARMACOLOGIC

Following a sexual assault, many women report that they thought they were going to be killed. The survivor may be terrified and unable to provide a complete history of the assault. It is important to provide support, reassurance of immediate safety, and obtain informed consent for examination, procedures, and contact of others. With permission, the clinician should contact a rape crisis worker and the police, although the survivor decides whether or not to file criminal charges; in general, notification of law enforcement is not required if the patient is an adult of age 18 years or older and is not disabled, mentally ill, or elderly. In these cases, reporting is done only if the patient gives his or her consent. Injury caused by any weapon or incidents involving life-threatening assault, however, must be reported to the law enforcement agency (per statute) irrespective of reporting the sexual assault.[12]

- A guideline developed for the state of Oregon is available from the US Department of Justice for the emergency medical evaluation of a sexual assault victim.[12] Steps in the evaluation are reviewed briefly below. A medical forensic evaluation is appropriate if the assault occurred within 84 hours of presentation. A Standard Sexual Assault Forensic Evidence (SAFE) Kit should be used for gathering forensic evidence.

- The patient should be assessed for safety and immediate mental health needs. The history includes details of the assault (eg, date, time, location, descriptors of assailant[s]), type of bodily and sexual contact (orifice[s] penetrated, objects used), and sexual activity or bathing or washing since the assault.[9,12] Laws in all 50 states strictly limit the evidentiary use of a survivor's previous sexual history, including evidence of previously acquired STIs, as part of an effort to undermine the credibility of the survivor's testimony.[13]
- Treat traumatic injuries—Physical examination should include observations of emotional state and descriptions of clothing and stains. Gently, and with permission, examine for lacerations, abrasions, ecchymoses, and bites. A body chart may be useful for documenting the size, type, color, and location of any injuries. A genital examination should be conducted by an experienced clinician in a way that minimizes further trauma to the survivor; examination is directed by history.
- Test and treatment for STI—A guideline for managing STI following sexual assault is available through the Centers for Disease Control and Prevention (CDC).[13]
  - Trichomoniasis, bacterial vaginosis (BV), gonorrhea, and chlamydial infection are the most frequently diagnosed infections following sexual assault. As the prevalence of these infections is high among sexually active women, their presence after an assault does not necessarily signify acquisition during the assault.
  - Nucleic acid amplification tests (NAATs) are recommended for *Neisseria gonorrhoeae* and *Chlamydia trachomatis*. These tests are preferred for the diagnostic evaluation of sexual assault victims, regardless of the sites of penetration or attempted penetration.[13]
  - Wet mount or point-of-care testing of a vaginal swab specimen for *Trichomonas vaginalis* infection is recommended. The wet mount also should be examined for evidence of BV and candidiasis, especially if vaginal discharge, malodor, or itching is present.
  - Collect a serum sample for immediate evaluation for HIV, hepatitis B, and syphilis, and obtain serum or urine for a pregnancy test in reproductive-aged women. Obtain toxicology and/or alcohol test if a patient has altered mental status, reports blackouts, or is concerned that he/she may have been drugged.[12]

MEDICATIONS

The following prophylactic regimen is suggested as preventive therapy:

- Hepatitis B vaccination, without hepatitis B immune globulin, is administered to sexual assault victims at the time of the initial examination if they have not been previously vaccinated. Follow-up doses of vaccine should be administered 1 to 2 and 4 to 6 months after the first dose.
- An empiric antimicrobial regimen for *Chlamydia*, gonorrhea, and *Trichomonas* is ceftriaxone 250 mg intramuscular (IM) in a single dose **or** cefixime 400 mg orally single dose **plus** metronidazole 2 g orally (single dose) **plus** azithromycin 1 g orally (single dose) **or** doxycycline 100 mg orally twice daily for 7 days. Clinicians should counsel patients about the possible benefits and toxicities associated with these treatment regimens, such as gastrointestinal (GI) side effects.
- HIV seroconversion has occurred in persons whose only known risk factor was sexual assault or sexual abuse, but the risk is probably low (in consensual sex, the risk for HIV transmission from vaginal intercourse is 0.1-0.2%, for receptive rectal intercourse the risk is 0.5-3%, and for oral sex the risk is substantially lower).[13]
- The health care provider should assess available information concerning HIV-risk behaviors of the assailant(s) (eg, a man who has sex with other men and/or injected drug or crack cocaine use), local epidemiology of HIV/AIDS, and exposure characteristics of the assault. Specific circumstances of an assault that might increase the risk for HIV transmission are trauma, including bleeding, with vaginal, anal, or oral penetration; exposure of mucous membranes to ejaculate; viral load in ejaculate (eg, multiple assailants); and the presence of an STI or genital lesions in the assailant or survivor.
- If HIV postexposure prophylaxis (PEP) is offered, the following information should be discussed with the patient: (a) the unproven benefit and known toxicities of antiretrovirals; (b) the close follow-up that will be necessary; (c) the benefit of adherence to recommended dosing; (d) the necessity of early initiation to optimize potential benefits (as soon as possible after and up to 72 hours after the assault). Providers should emphasize that PEP appears to be well-tolerated and that severe adverse effects are rare.
- Specialist consultation on PEP regimens is recommended. If the survivor and clinician decide that PEP is warranted, provide enough medication to last until the next return visit and reevaluate the survivor 3 to 7 days after initial assessment and assess tolerance of medications.[13]
- If PEP is started, perform a complete blood count (CBC) and serum chemistry at baseline (initiation of PEP should not be delayed, pending results).
- Collect samples for legal evidence. Most emergency departments have rape or sexual assault kits containing instructions for gathering material to support legal charges; all samples must be carefully labeled and kept under supervision. Details of these procedures may be found elsewhere.[12]
- Reproductive-age female survivors should be evaluated for pregnancy, if appropriate, and offered EC if desired. Providers might also consider anti-emetic medications, particularly if an EC containing estrogen is provided.
- Consider tetanus prophylaxis if skin wounds occur and the patient is not up-to-date on tetanus immunization. Offer hepatitis vaccine if the patient has not been previously fully immunized for hepatitis B, has a negative history for hepatitis B and secretion-mucosal contact occurred during the assault.[12]
- Arrange for safety.
- Provide written information about the visit and any instruction given to the patient.

REFERRAL

- If the victim is amenable, refer for advocacy or counseling.
- If you are not the primary health care provider, arrange for follow-up medical care.

PREVENTION

- Women who have been physically assaulted as adolescents are at greater risk for revictimization during their college years.[14] Although dating violence prevention–intervention programs have not been uniformly successful, women should be counseled about strategies for avoiding future victimization (eg, recognition of dangerous situations, limiting use of alcohol, safety with friends). One program, Safe Dates, has been shown in a randomized controlled trial (RCT) to be effective in preventing or interrupting sexual violence perpetration.[15]
- Life skills and educational programs are conducted to encourage men to take greater responsibility for their actions, relate better to others, have greater respect for women, and communicate more effectively. Although not many programs have been formally evaluated, there are

reports of reduced violence against women in communities in Cambodia, the Gambia, South Africa, Uganda, and the United Republic of Tanzania attributed to these programs.[8]

- Other prevention efforts include media campaigns, written materials, victim risk-reduction techniques (eg, self-defense, awareness), men's activism groups (eg, Men Can Stop Rape), school-based programs, and legal and policy responses (eg, encourage reporting, broadening the definition of rape and sexual assault).[8,16] In designing programs, information provided in documents prepared for the CDC may be useful.[16] Health providers can also become involved in prevention activities at multiple levels:
  - Strengthening individual knowledge and skills through skill-building programs in high schools or training bystanders to safely interrupt sexist and harassing behavior
  - Promoting community education by sponsoring activities such as plays that reinforce positive cultural norms and portray responsible sexual behavior or developing awards to recognize responsible media coverage
  - Educating other community leaders and providers, such as little league coaches, prison guards, nursing home providers
  - Fostering coalitions and networks to promote community understanding and strategies to prevent sexual violence
  - Changing organizational practices such as implementation and enforcement of sexual harassment policies in schools and workplaces, implementing environmental safety measures such as adequate lighting and emergency call boxes
  - Influencing policies and legislation such as offering comprehensive sex education programs in middle and high schools, including violence prevention

PROGNOSIS

- More than 32,000 pregnancies result yearly from rape (approximately 5% of rapes result in pregnancy).[8]
- Chronic psychological consequences—In a meta-analysis of 17 case-control and 20 cohort studies (N = 3,162,318 participants), there was an association between sexual abuse and a lifetime diagnosis of anxiety disorder (odds ratio [OR], 3.09; 95% confidence interval [CI], 2.43-3.94), depression (OR, 2.66; 95% CI, 2.14-3.30), eating disorders (OR, 2.72; 95% CI, 2.04-3.63), posttraumatic stress disorder (OR, 2.34; 95% CI, 1.59-3.43), sleep disorders (OR, 16.17; 95% CI, 2.06-126.76), and suicide attempts (OR, 4.14; 95% CI, 2.98-5.76).[17]
- Chronic somatic consequences—Authors of a meta-analysis of 23 studies found associations between sexual abuse and lifetime diagnosis of functional GI disorders (OR, 2.43; 95% CI, 1.36-4.31), nonspecific chronic pain (OR, 2.20; 95% CI, 1.54-3.15), psychogenic seizures (OR, 2.96; 95% CI, 1.12-4.69), and chronic pelvic pain (OR, 2.73; 95% CI, 1.73-4.30).[18] Significant associations with rape included lifetime diagnosis of fibromyalgia (OR, 3.35; 95% CI, 1.51-7.46), chronic pelvic pain (OR, 3.27; 95% CI, 1.02-10.53), and functional GI disorders (OR, 4.01; 95% CI, 1.88-8.57).

FOLLOW-UP

Follow-up visits provide an opportunity to (a) provide support and advocacy; (b) evaluate for resolution and healing of injury and current symptoms; (c) detect new infections acquired during or after the assault; (d) complete hepatitis B immunization, if indicated; (e) complete counseling and treatment for other STIs; and (f) monitor side effects and adherence to PEP, if prescribed.[12]

- Initial follow-up should be within 1 to 2 weeks following the assault.
- Provide ongoing support—Survivors of sexual abuse report strained relationships with family, friends, and intimate partners, including less emotional support and less frequent contact with friends and relatives.[8] In addition, only about half of the victims keep this appointment, so outreach efforts may be needed.
- Review results of tests and discuss the plan for redraw of Venereal Disease Research Laboratory (VDRL) 3 months after exposure and HIV in 6 weeks and 3 and 6 months (if initial test results were negative).
- Long-term support, monitoring, and treatment include the following:
  - For women suffering from PTSD, medications that may be useful include selective serotonin reuptake inhibitors and Risperdal.[19] Cognitive-Processing Therapy and Prolonged Exposure have been the most useful therapies for treating PTSD, depression, and anxiety in female rape victims.[20,21] However, more than one-third of women retain the diagnosis of PTSD or drop out of treatment.[21]
  - Imagery rehearsal therapy appears useful in decreasing chronic nightmares, improving sleep quality, and decreasing PTSD symptom severity.[22]

PATIENT EDUCATION

- Recovery from sexual assault is a slow process. In one study, one-third of survivors reported recovery within 1 year but one-quarter thought that they had not recovered after 4 to 6 years.[23]
- Counseling, and sometimes medication, is available to help control symptoms and treat depression and PTSD and patients should be encouraged to report and seek help for continuing difficulties.

PATIENT RESOURCES

- National Sexual Violence Resource Center serves as a comprehensive collection and distribution center for information, statistics, and resources related to sexual violence—**http://www.nsvrc.org.**
- Centers for Disease Control and Prevention. *Sexual Violence*—**http://www.cdc.gov/ViolencePrevention/sexualviolence/index.htm.**
- National Domestic Violence Hotline, 1-800-799-SAFE; National Sexual Assault Hotline, 1-800-656-HOPE.

PROVIDER RESOURCES

- *Recommended Medical Guideline Acute Sexual Assault Emergency Medical Evaluation for the State of Oregon*—**http://www.doj.state.or.us/crimev/pdf/guidelines05_000.pdf.**
- United States Department of Justice—Office on Violence Against Women, offers links to resources—**http://www.ovw.usdoj.gov/sexassault.htm.**
- Assistance with PEP decisions can be obtained by calling the National Clinician's Post-Exposure Prophylaxis Hotline **(PEPLine), 1-888-448-4911.**

- National Sexual Violence Resource Center serves as a comprehensive collection and distribution center for information, statistics, and resources related to sexual violence—**http://www.nsvrc.org.**
- The American College of Obstetricians and Gynecologists provides publications about violence against women, intimate partner violence, sexual violence, adolescent dating violence, and patient education materials in both English and Spanish—**http://www.acog.org.**
- A directory of sexual assault centers in the United States can be obtained from the following URL—**http://www.nsvrc.org/publications/nsvrc-publications/directory-sexual-assault-centers-united-states.**

REFERENCES

1. Centers for Disease Control and Prevention. *Sexual Violence. Scientific Information*. http://www.cdc.gov/ViolencePrevention/sexualviolence/index.html. Accessed August 2013.
2. Black MC, Basile KC, Breiding MJ, et al. *The National Intimate Partner and Sexual Violence Survey (NISVS): 2010 Summary Report*. Atlanta, GA: National Center for Injury Prevention and Control, Centers for Disease Control and Prevention; 2011. http://www.cdc.gov/ViolencePrevention/pdf/NISVS_Executive_Summary-a.pdf. Accessed August 2013.
3. Basile KC, Chen J, Lynberg MC, Saltzman LE. Prevalence and characteristics of sexual violence victimization. *Violence Vict*. 2007;22(4):437-448.
4. Koss MP. Detecting the scope of rape: a review of prevalence research methods. *J Interpers Violence*. 1993;8:198-222.
5. Lincoln AK, Liebschutz JM, Chernoff M, et al. Brief screening for co-occurring disorders among women entering substance abuse treatment. *Subst Abuse Treat Prev Policy*. 2006;1:26.
6. Federal Bureau of Investigation. *Uniform Crime Reports for the United States*. Washington, DC: U.S. Department of Justice; 2010. http://www.fbi.gov/about-us/cjis/ucr/crime-in-the-u.s/2010/crime-in-the-u.s.-2010/violent-crime/rapemain. Accessed August 2013.
7. National Institute of Justice. *Extent Nature and Consequences of Rape Victimization: Findings from the National Violence Against Women Survey (2006)*. https://www.ncjrs.gov/pdffiles1/nij/210346.pdf. Accessed August 2013.
8. World Health Organization. *World Report on Violence and Health, Sexual Violence*. Chapter 6. http://www.who.int/violence_injury_prevention/violence/global_campaign/en/chap6.pdf. Accessed August 2013.
9. Williams A. Managing adult sexual assault. *Aust Fam Physician*. 2004;33(10):825-828.
10. Centers for Disease Control and Prevention. *Sexual Violence. Risk and Protective Factors*. http://www.cdc.gov/ViolencePrevention/sexualviolence/riskprotectivefactors.html. Accessed August 2013.
11. Weaver TL. Impact of rape on female sexuality: review of selected literature. *Clin Obstet Gynecol*. 2009;52(4):702-711.
12. *Recommended Medical Guideline Acute Sexual Assault Emergency Medical Evaluation for the State of Oregon*. http://www.doj.state.or.us/crimev/pdf/guidelines05_000.pdf. Accessed August 2013.
13. Workowski KA, Berman S; Centers for Disease Control and Prevention. Sexual assault and STDs in sexually transmitted diseases treatment guidelines, 2010. *MMWR Recomm Rep*. 2010;59(RR-12):90-95. http://www.guideline.gov/content.aspx?id=25597&search=sexual+assault. Accessed August 2013.
14. Smith PH, White JW, Holland LJ. A longitudinal perspective on dating violence among adolescent and college-age women. *Am J Public Health*. 2003;93(7):1104-1109.
15. Foshee V, Bauman KE, Ennett ST, et al. Assessing the long-term effects of the Safe Dates program and a booster in preventing and reducing adolescent dating violence victimization and perpetration. *Am J Public Health*. 2004;94:619-624.
16. Centers for Disease Control and Prevention. *Sexual Violence: Prevention Strategies*. http://www.cdc.gov/ViolencePrevention/sexualviolence/prevention.html. Accessed August 2013.
17. Chen LP, Murad MH, Paras ML, et al. Sexual abuse and lifetime diagnosis of psychiatric disorders: systematic review and meta-analysis. *Mayo Clin Proc*. 2010;85(7):618-629.
18. Paras ML, Murad MH, Chen LP, et al. Sexual abuse and lifetime diagnosis of somatic disorders: a systematic review and meta-analysis. *JAMA*. 2009;302(5):550-561.
19. Padala PR, Madison J, Monnahan M, et al. Risperidone monotherapy for post-traumatic stress disorder related to sexual assault and domestic abuse in women. *Int Clin Psychopharmacol*. 2006;21(5):275-280.
20. Nishith P, Nixon RD, Resick PA. Resolution of trauma-related guilt following treatment of PTSD in female rape victims: a result of cognitive processing therapy targeting comorbid depression? *J Affect Disord*. 2005;86(2-3):259-265.
21. Vickerman KA, Margolin G. Rape treatment outcome research: empirical findings and state of the literature. *Clin Psychol Rev*. 2009;29:431-448.
22. Krakow C, Hollifield M, Johnston L, et al. Imagery rehearsal therapy for chronic nightmares in sexual assault survivors with posttraumatic stress disorder: a randomized controlled trial. *JAMA*. 2001;286(5):537-545.
23. Burgess AW, Holmstrom LL. Adaptive strategies and recovery from rape. *Am J Psychiatry*. 1979;136:1278-1282.

PART 4

OPHTHALMOLOGY

Strength of Recommendation (SOR)	Definition
A	Recommendation based on consistent and good-quality patient-oriented evidence.*
B	Recommendation based on inconsistent or limited-quality patient-oriented evidence.*
C	Recommendation based on consensus, usual practice, opinion, disease-oriented evidence, or case series for studies of diagnosis, treatment, prevention, or screening.*

*See Appendix A on pages 1241-1244 for further information.

9 PTERYGIUM

Heidi Chumley, MD

PATIENT STORY

A 50-year-old man had spent most of his adult life working outdoors in southern Texas near the Mexico border. He denies any problems with his vision, but wonders what is growing on his eye and if it should be removed (**Figure 9-1**). His eyes are often dry and irritated. He is diagnosed with a pterygium and instructed that it does not need to be removed unless it interferes with his vision in the future. Liquid tears are suggested for his dry and irritated eyes. He is also instructed to wear wraparound sunglasses to avoid ultraviolet (UV) exposure and irritation from wind and dust.

INTRODUCTION

A pterygium is a generally benign growth of fibroblastic tissue on the eye of an adult with chronic UV exposure. Pterygia can be unilateral or bilateral, are usually located on the nasal side, and extend to the cornea. Pterygia often require no treatment, but can be removed surgically if they interfere with vision. Patients with dry eyes are prone to the development and progression of pterygia.

EPIDEMIOLOGY

- Pterygium most often develops between the ages 20 and 50 years.
- The frequency of pterygium increases with sun exposure and age. In a population-based study (Indonesia), it was found that the prevalence ranged from 3% (in 21- to 29-year-olds) to 18% (older than 50 years of age).[1] In rural China, the prevalence was 3.76% and also increased with age.[2]
- In one study carried out in Australia, it was found that sun exposure is consistently the greatest risk factor, contributing 43% of the risk.[3]

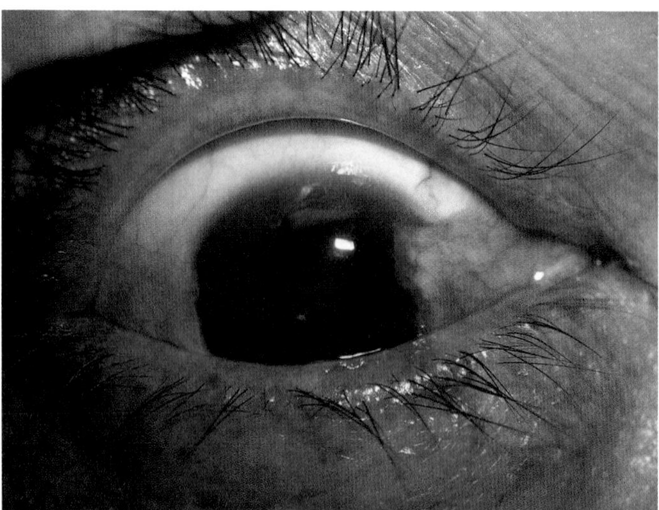

FIGURE 9-1 A nasal pterygium. (*Reproduced with permission from Richard P. Usatine, MD.*)

CHAPTER 9

ETIOLOGY AND PATHOPHYSIOLOGY

- A pterygium is a proliferation of fibrovascular tissue on the surface of the eye, which extends onto the cornea.
- The etiology of pterygium is incompletely understood; however, chronic UV exposure is accepted as a causative agent. Chronic inflammation and oxidative stress may also play a role in pathogenesis.
- Pterygia have features seen in malignant tissues, such as normal tissue invasion and high recurrence rate.[4] Pterygia can be associated with premalignant lesions.[4]

RISK FACTORS

Risk factors are related to chronic UV exposure:

- Living in low latitude, low precipitation area[2]
- Male gender[2]

DIAGNOSIS

CLINICAL FEATURES

- Redness, itching, and/or irritation of the involved eyes (some are symptom free).
- Visual blurring if the pterygium grows over the visual axis. Even if not obscuring the visual axis, the pterygium can cause poor vision by leading to irregular and high astigmatism.
- Pterygia are diagnosed clinically by their distinctive appearance (**Figures 9-1** to **9-4**).

TYPICAL DISTRIBUTION

- Unilateral or bilateral.

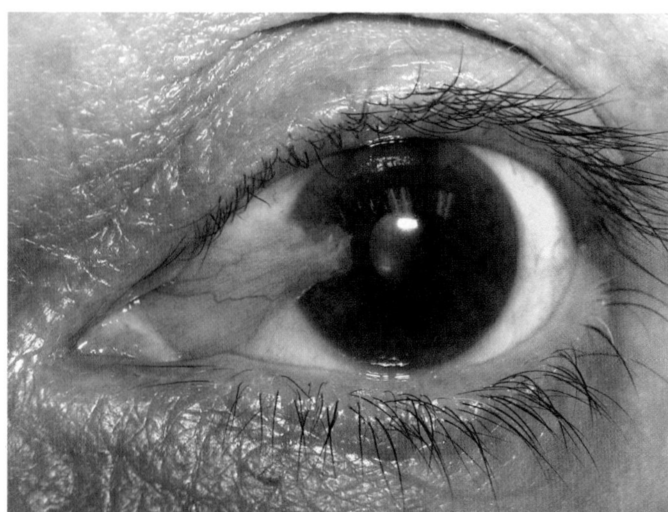

FIGURE 9-2 Pterygium that has grown onto the cornea but not covered the visual axis. This fibrovascular tissue has the shape of a bird's wing (literal definition of pterygium). The small vessels are prominent in this view. (*Reproduced with permission from Richard P. Usatine, MD.*)

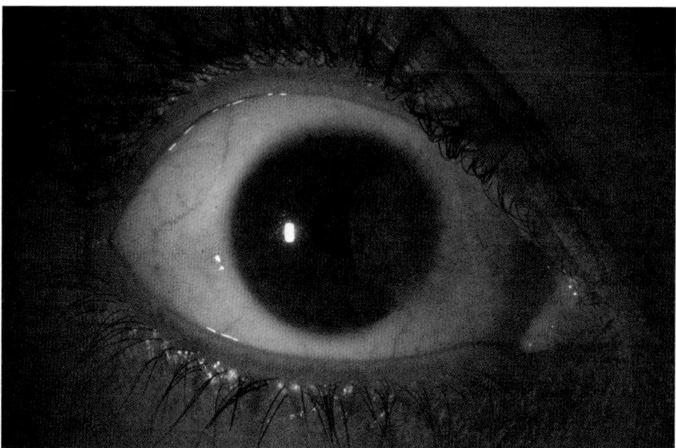

FIGURE 9-3 A pterygium that has grown over the visual axis and is interfering with this person's vision. The patient plans to undergo surgery. *(Reproduced with permission from Paul D. Comeau.)*

- Nasal or nasal and temporal.
- Consider another diagnosis with a unilateral temporal distribution.

BIOPSY

Biopsy is not indicated; however, excised pterygia are sent for histologic examination because of their association with premalignant lesions.[4]

DIFFERENTIAL DIAGNOSIS

- Pinguecula is a yellowish patch or nodule on the conjunctiva, and it does not extend onto the cornea (**Figure 9-5**).
- Conjunctivitis is conjunctival infection with discomfort and eye discharge (see Chapter 13, Conjunctivitis).
- Squamous cell carcinoma of the conjunctiva is rare. Consider carcinoma when a unilateral growth is noted on the temporal side. Also consider malignancy if there are grossly aberrant-appearing blood vessels on the surface of the eye. Patients with abnormal immune systems (eg, cancer, HIV) are at a particular risk for ocular surface malignancy.

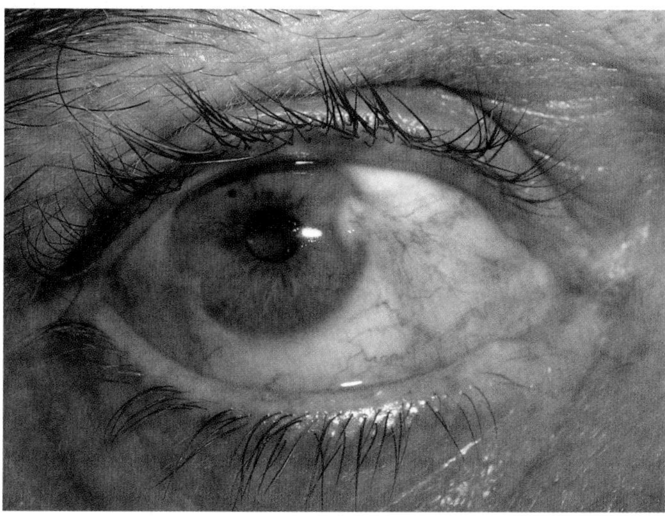

FIGURE 9-4 Bilateral pterygia growing over the cornea. *(Reproduced with permission from Richard P. Usatine, MD.)*

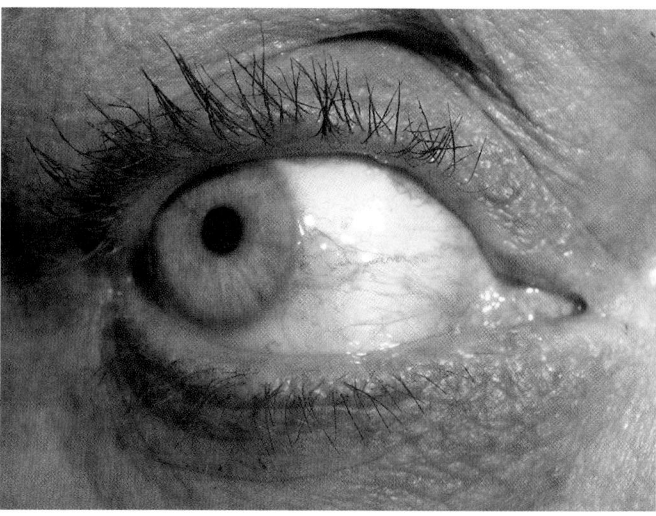

FIGURE 9-5 Pinguecula nodule on conjunctiva that does not extend to the cornea. Note the yellow color. *(Reproduced with permission from Richard P. Usatine, MD.)*

MANAGEMENT

NONPHARMACOLOGIC

Avoid sun exposure and use UV filtering sunglasses when sun exposure is unavoidable.

MEDICATIONS

Nonprescription artificial tears and/or topical lubricating drops are recommended to soothe the inflammation. Ophthalmologists will occasionally prescribe a short course of topical corticosteroid anti-inflammatory drops when symptoms of the pterygia are more intense.

SURGICAL

- Pterygia are usually treated when they interfere with vision or when they cause significant irritation or pain (see **Figure 9-3**). The standard therapy is surgical removal.
- Pterygia have a high rate of recurrence. Conjunctival autografting and an antifibrotic treatment (eg, mitomycin-C) can be used intraoperatively to lower the recurrence.[5]

ASSOCIATED RISKS

- Pterygia affect astigmatism[6,7] and are associated with increased rates of macular degeneration; however, it is unclear whether treatment reduces this risk.
- Eyes with a pterygium or previous pterygium surgery (but not pinguecula) have a higher risk of incident late age-related maculopathy (ARM) (odds ratio [OR] 3.3, 95% confidence interval [CI], 1.1-10.3) and early ARM (OR 1.8, 95% CI, 1.1-2.9).[8]

PREVENTION

Sunglasses with 100% UV protection should be used by everyone to protect the eyes from UV damage **(Figure 9-6)**. Sunglasses should fit close to the eye to block scattered or reflected light in addition to direct light.[9]

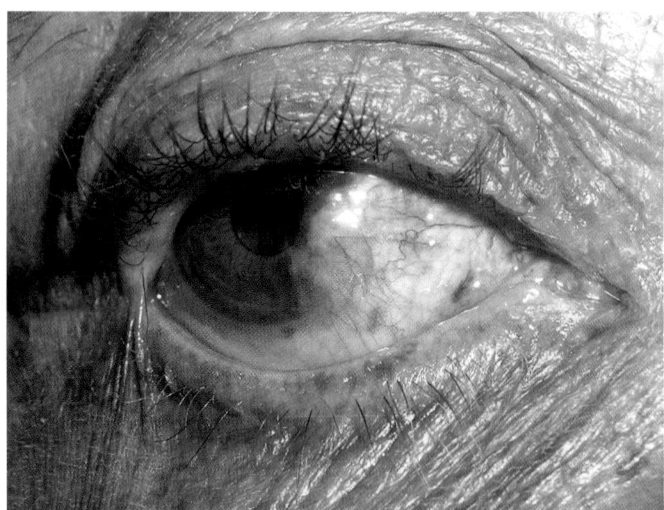

FIGURE 9-6 Nasal pterygium growing over the visual axis in a man living close to the equator. The patient did not use sunglasses. The melanosis within the pterygium is benign. (*Reproduced with permission from Richard P. Usatine, MD.*)

PROGNOSIS

Most pterygia do not require surgical treatment. Pterygia that interfere with vision and are removed have a high chance of recurrence.

FOLLOW-UP

No specific follow-up is needed; however, consider monitoring vision during annual examinations because of the increased risk of age-related macular degeneration.

PATIENT EDUCATION

Wraparound sunglasses are helpful to avoid UV exposure and irritation from wind and dust. Liquid tears are suggested for dry and irritated eyes.

PATIENT RESOURCES

- PubMed Health. *Pterygium*—**http://www.ncbi.nlm.nih.gov/pubmedhealth/PMH0002006/.**

PROVIDER RESOURCES

- Fisher JP. *Pterygium*—**http://emedicine.medscape.com/article/1192527.**

REFERENCES

1. Gazzard G, Saw SM, Farook M, et al. Pterygium in Indonesia: prevalence, severity and risk factors. *Br J Ophthalmol.* 2002;86(12):1341-1346.
2. Liang QF, Xu L, Jin XY, et al. Epidemiology of pterygium in aged rural population of Beijing, China. *Chin Med J (Engl).* 2010;123(13):1699-1701.
3. McCarty CA, Fu CL, Taylor HR. Epidemiology of pterygium in Victoria, Australia. *Br J Ophthalmol.* 2000;84(3):289-292.
4. Chui J, Coroneo MT, Tat LT, et al. Ophthalmic pterygium: a stem cell disorder with premalignant features. *Am J Pathol.* 2011;178(2):817-827.
5. Detorakis ET, Spandidos DA. Pathogenetic mechanisms and treatment options for ophthalmic pterygium: trends and perspectives. *Int J Mol Med.* 2009;23(4):439-447.
6. Ashaye AO. Refractive astigmatism and size of pterygium. *Afr J Med Med Sci.* 2002;31(2):163-165.
7. Kampitak K. The effect of pterygium on corneal astigmatism. *J Med Assoc Thai.* 2003;86(1):16-23.
8. Pham TQ, Wang JJ, Rochtchina E, Mitchell P. Pterygium/pinguecula and the five-year incidence of age-related maculopathy. *Am J Ophthalmol.* 2005;139(3):536-537.
9. Wang SQ, Balaqula Y, Osterwalder U. Photoprotection: a review of the current and future technologies. *Dermatol Ther.* 2010;23(1):31-47.

10 HORDEOLUM AND CHALAZION

Heidi Chumley, MD

PATIENT STORY

A 35-year-old woman presented with a tender nodule on the upper eyelid along with crusting and erythema to both eyelids (**Figure 10-1**). The upper eyelid had a large external hordeolum. When the lower eyelid was inverted, an internal hordeolum was also present. The physician recommended that she apply warm moist compresses to her eyelids 4 times a day. Her hordeola resolved within 7 days.

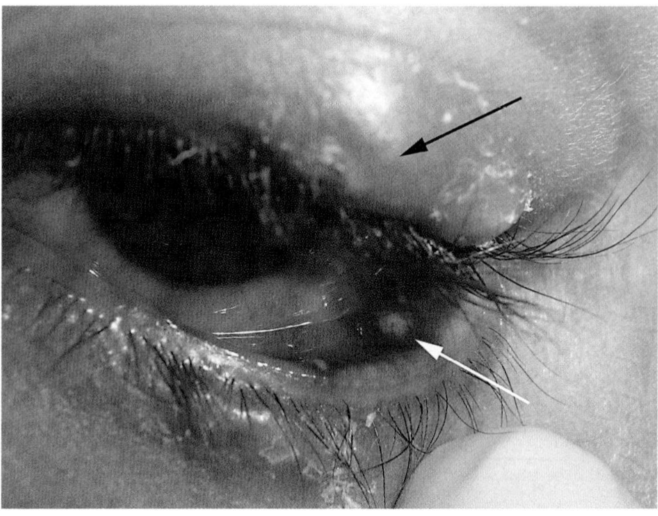

FIGURE 10-1 External hordeolum (*black arrow*) and an internal hordeolum (*white arrow*). (*Reproduced with permission from Richard P. Usatine, MD.*)

INTRODUCTION

A hordeolum is an acute painful infection of the glands of the eyelid, usually caused by bacteria. Hordeola can be located on the internal or external eyelid. Internal hordeola that do not completely resolve become cysts called chalazia. External hordeola are commonly known as styes.

SYNONYMS

External hordeolum is also known as stye.

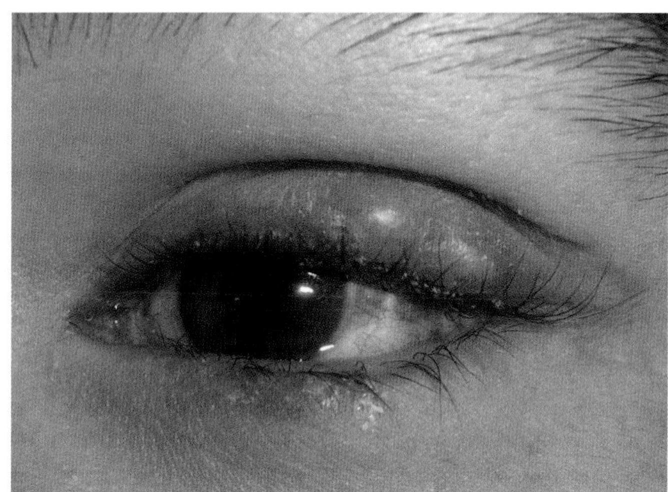

FIGURE 10-2 External hordeolum on upper lid with surrounding erythema. (*Reproduced with permission from Richard P. Usatine, MD.*)

EPIDEMIOLOGY

Unclear incidence or prevalence in the United States, but often stated to be more common in school-age children (0.2% chalazion and 0.3% hordeolum)[1] and in 30- to 50-year old adults.

ETIOLOGY AND PATHOPHYSIOLOGY

HORDEOLUM (ACUTELY TENDER NODULE IN THE EYE)

- Infection in the meibomian gland (internal hordeolum), often resolves into a chalazion (**Figure 10-1**).
- Infection in the Zeiss or Moll gland (external hordeolum) (**Figures 10-2** and **10-3**).
- *Staphylococcus aureus* is the causative agent in most cases.

CHALAZION

- Meibomian gland becomes blocked, often in a patient with blepharitis.
- Blocked meibomian gland's duct releases gland contents into the soft tissue of eyelid.
- Gland contents cause a lipogranulomatous reaction (**Figure 10-4**).
- Reaction can cause acute tenderness and erythema, which then resolves into a chronic nodule (**Figure 10-5**).

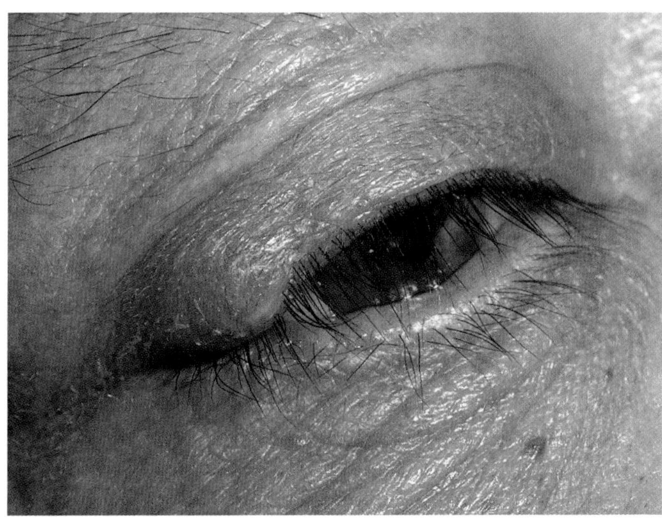

FIGURE 10-3 External hordeolum with visible purulence and the normal contour of the eyelid is disrupted. (*Reproduced with permission from Richard P. Usatine, MD.*)

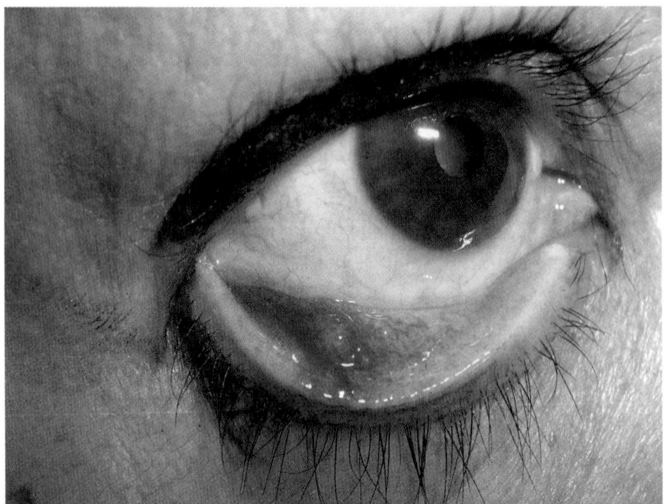

FIGURE 10-4 Chalazion viewed from internal eyelid showing the yellow lipogranulomatous material. (*Reproduced with permission from Richard P. Usatine, MD.*)

RISK FACTORS

- Hordeolum: *S. aureus* blepharitis, previous hordeolum
- Chalazion: Seborrheic blepharitis and rosacea

DIAGNOSIS

- Chalazion and hordeolum are clinical diagnoses.
- Chalazion is a nontender nodule on the eyelid.
- Hordeolum.
  - Tenderness and erythema are localized to a point on the eyelid (see **Figures 10-1** to **10-3**).
  - Conjunctival injection may be present.
  - Fever, preauricular nodes, and vision changes should be absent.
  - Laboratory tests are generally not indicated.

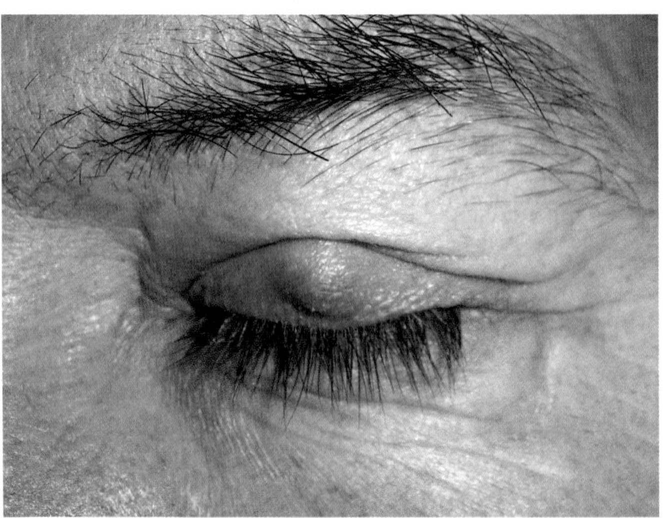

FIGURE 10-5 Chalazion present for 4 months with minimal symptoms but cosmetically unappealing. (*Reproduced with permission from Richard P. Usatine, MD.*)

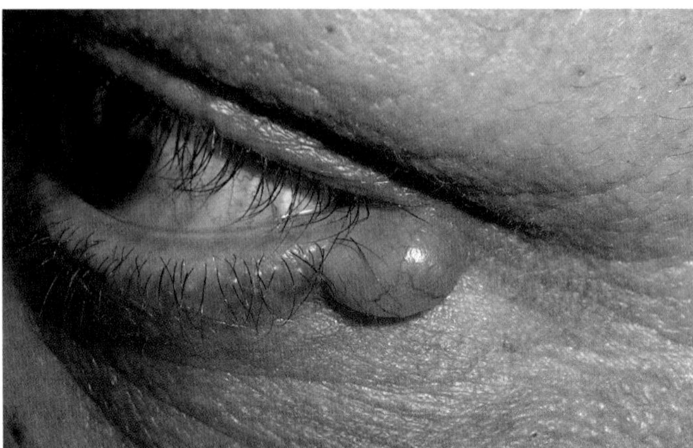

FIGURE 10-6 Hidrocystoma showing telangiectasias. The cyst was easily resected and the fluid was clear. (*Reproduced with permission from Richard P. Usatine, MD.*)

DIFFERENTIAL DIAGNOSIS

- Hidrocystoma—Benign cystic lesion that grows on the edge of the eyelids and is filled with clear fluid (**Figure 10-6**).
- Xanthelasma—Yellowish plaques, generally near medial canthus (see Chapter 223, Hyperlipidemia).
- Molluscum contagiosum—Waxy nodules with central umbilication, generally multiple (see Chapter 129, Molluscum Contagiosum).
- Sebaceous cell carcinoma—Rare cancer seen in middle-aged and elderly patients; difficult to distinguish from recurrent chalazion or unilateral chronic blepharitis without biopsy.
- Basal cell carcinoma—Pearly nodule, often with telangiectasias or central ulceration; more common on lower medial eyelid (see Chapter 168, Basal Cell Carcinoma).

MANAGEMENT

HORDEOLUM (INTERNAL)

- No studies of nonsurgical interventions (compresses, lid scrubs, antibiotics, steroids) met criteria for inclusion in a Cochrane study. No evidence for or against nonsurgical interventions for acute internal hordeolum.[1] SOR Ⓐ
- Treat as described below for external hordeolum.

HORDEOLUM (EXTERNAL)

- Warm soaks, 3 to 4 times a day for 15 minutes, will elicit drainage in most cases. SOR Ⓒ
- Topical antibiotics (eg, bacitracin ophthalmic ointment) may be beneficial for recurrent or spontaneously draining hordeolum. SOR Ⓒ
- Cases that do not respond to warm soaks or that are extremely painful and swollen may be incised and drained with a small incision using a #11 blade. Make the incision on either the internal or external eyelid depending on where the hordeolum is pointing. A chalazion clamp can be used to protect the globe from damage. SOR Ⓑ
- Antibiotics do not provide benefit after incision and drainage.[3] SOR Ⓑ
- Systemic antibiotics are usually not needed unless patient has preseptal cellulitis. SOR Ⓒ

CHALAZION

- Can be treated conservatively with lid hygiene and warm compresses. Warm compresses can be applied 2 to 3 times daily but may take weeks to months to work. SOR Ⓒ
- One study demonstrated a 58% response rate of 1% topical chloramphenicol with warm compresses.[3] SOR Ⓑ
- Higher percentages of resolution can be achieved with either incision and curettage or injection with steroid (eg, 0.3 mL triamcinolone acetonide) (80-92%).[4-6] SOR Ⓑ The chalazion is usually drained from the internal eyelid using a chalazion clamp to protect the globe. After anesthetizing the area, a #11 blade is carefully used to open the chalazion. A chalazion curette helps to scoop out the lipogranulomatous material. No suturing is needed.
- A study of 136 patients compared triamcinolone injection, incision and curettage, and warm compresses, and found resolution rates of 84%, 87%, and 46%, respectively.[6] SOR Ⓑ
- One study demonstrated a better response to incision and curettage in the following situations: patients 35.1 years of age or older, with lesion duration equal to or greater than 8.5 months and size equal to or greater than 11.4 mm.[5] SOR Ⓑ

REFERRAL

Refer to an ophthalmologist if the hordeolum or chalazion interferes with vision and does not respond to therapy. If a surgical intervention is needed and you lack experience doing such a procedure, refer to ophthalmology.

PREVENTION

Eyelid hygiene, keeping the area around the eyelid clean, may prevent hordeola.

PROGNOSIS

Chalazia can persist for years if untreated. Some patients are prone to recurrence of hordeola and chalazia.

FOLLOW-UP

A hordeolum with significant purulence and swelling should be reevaluated in 2 to 3 days or referred to an ophthalmologist. Warm compresses are slow to work for a chalazion, so follow-up should be no sooner than 1 month if nonsurgical treatment is prescribed.

PATIENT EDUCATION

Hordeolum commonly responds to warm soaks and topical antibiotics. It often recurs and can develop into a chronic chalazion, which may need to be treated with surgical removal or a steroid injection.

PATIENT RESOURCES

- The American Academy of Ophthalmology—**http://www.geteyesmart.org/eyesmart/diseases/chalazion-stye.cfm.**
- The American Academy of Family Physicians has a patient handout in English or Spanish on stye—**http://familydoctor.org/familydoctor/en/diseases-conditions/sty.html.**

PROVIDER RESOURCES

- *Hordeolum and Stye in Emergency Medicine*—**http://emedicine.medscape.com/article/798940.**
- *Chalazion*—**http://emedicine.medscape.com/article/1212709.**
- *Chalazion Injection Demonstration*—**http://www.youtube.com/watch?v=yYCCkDZwKgg.**
- *Chalazion Incision and Curettage*—**http://www.youtube.com/watch?v=tdKw_zjYCf8.**

REFERENCES

1. Garcia CA, Pinheiro FI, Montenegro DA, et al. Prevalence of biomicroscopic findings in the anterior segment and ocular adnexa among schoolchildren in Natal, Brazil. *Arq Bras Oftalmol.* 2005;68(2):167-170.
2. Lindsley K, Nichols JJ, Dickersin K. Interventions for acute internal hordeolum. *Cochrane Database Syst Rev.* 2010;9:CD00742.
3. Hirunwiwatkul P, Wachirasereechai K. Effectiveness of combined antibiotic ophthalmic solution in the treatment of hordeolum after incision and curettage: a randomized, placebo-controlled trial: a pilot study. *J Med Assoc Thai.* 2005;88(5):647-650.
4. Chung CF, Lai JS, Li PS. Subcutaneous extralesional triamcinolone acetonide injection versus conservative management in the treatment of chalazion. *Hong Kong Med J.* 2006;12(4):278-281.
5. Ahmad S, Baig MA, Khan MA, et al. Intralesional corticosteroid injection vs surgical treatment of chalazia in pigmented patients. *J Coll Physicians Surg Pak.* 2006;16(1):42-44.
6. Goawalla A, Lee V. A prospective randomized treatment study comparing three treatment options for chalazia: triamcinolone acetonide injections, incision and curettage and treatment with hot compresses. *Clin Experiment Ophthalmol.* 2007;35(8):706-712.
7. Dhaliwal U, Bhatia A. A rationale for therapeutic decision-making in chalazia. *Orbit.* 2005;24(4):227-230.

11 SCLERAL AND CONJUNCTIVAL PIGMENTATION

Heidi Chumley, MD

PATIENT STORY

A 40-year-old white man came to see his physician about a brown spot in his eye (**Figure 11-1**). He noticed this spot many years ago, but after recently reading information on the Internet about brown spots in the eye, became concerned about ocular melanoma. He thinks the spot has changed in size. He denies any eye discomfort or visual changes. He was referred for a biopsy, and the pathology showed a benign nevus that did not require further treatment.

INTRODUCTION

Scleral and conjunctival pigmentation is common and usually benign. Nevi can be observed and referred if they change in size. Primary acquired melanosis (PAM) must be biopsied because PAM with atypia has malignant potential, whereas PAM without atypia does not. Conjunctival melanoma is rare, but deadly.

EPIDEMIOLOGY

Although there is little information on the prevalence of ocular pigmentation other than physiologic (racial) melanosis, in a study of pigmented lesions referred for biopsy, investigators reported that 52% were nevi, 21% were PAM, and 25% were melanoma.[1]

- Scleral and conjunctival nevi (see **Figures 11-1** and **11-2**) are the most common causes of ocular pigmentation in light-skinned races. The pigmentation is generally noticeable by young adulthood, and is more common in whites.[2]
- Physiologic (racial) melanosis (**Figure 11-3**) is seen in 90% of black patients.[3] It can be congenital, and often presents early in life.
- PAM (**Figure 11-4**) is generally noted in middle-aged to older adults,[4,5] and is also more common in whites.
- Conjunctival melanoma (**Figures 11-5** to **11-7**) is rare, occurring in 0.000007% (7 per 1,000,000) of whites; it is even less common in other races.[5]

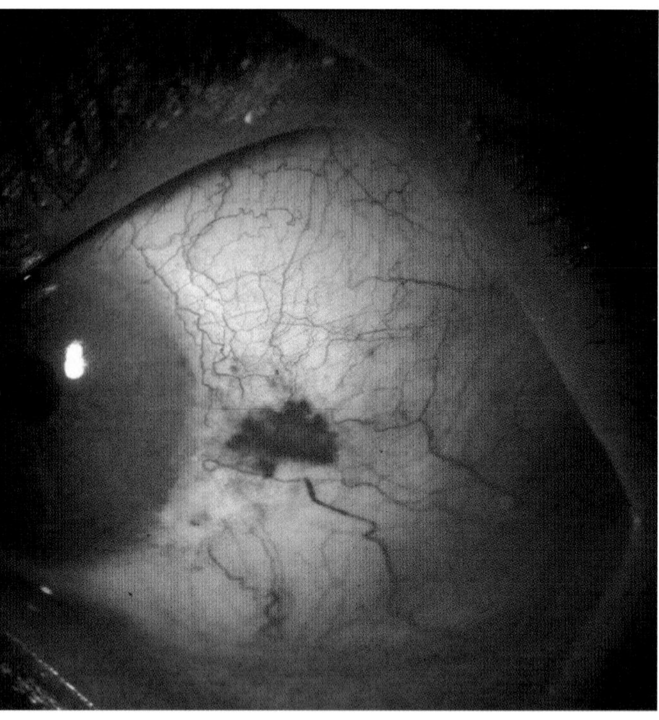

FIGURE 11-2 Conjunctival nevus. Unilateral localized distinct area of dark pigmentation on conjunctiva. (*Reproduced with permission from Paul D. Comeau.*)

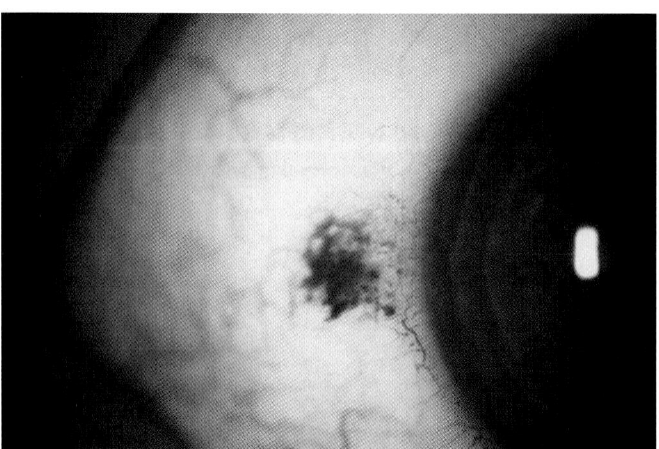

FIGURE 11-1 Scleral nevus. Unilateral localized distinct area of dark pigmentation on sclera. (*Reproduced with permission from Paul D. Comeau.*)

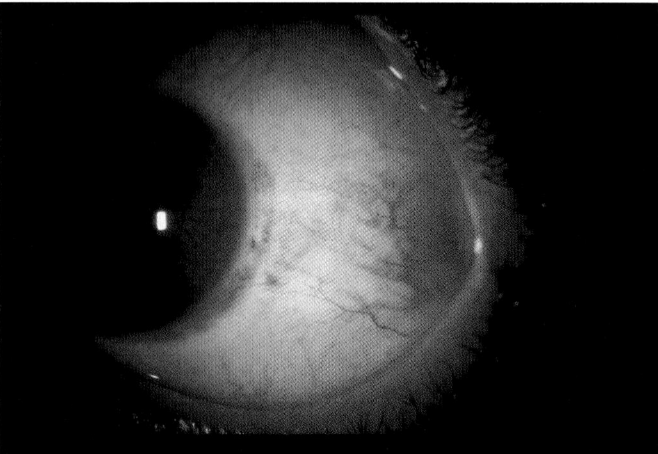

FIGURE 11-3 Physiologic (racial) melanosis. Flat conjunctival pigmentation that presents bilaterally starting at the limbus and most prominent in the interpalpebral zone is likely to be racial melanosis in a darkly pigmented patient. (*Reproduced with permission from Paul D. Comeau.*)

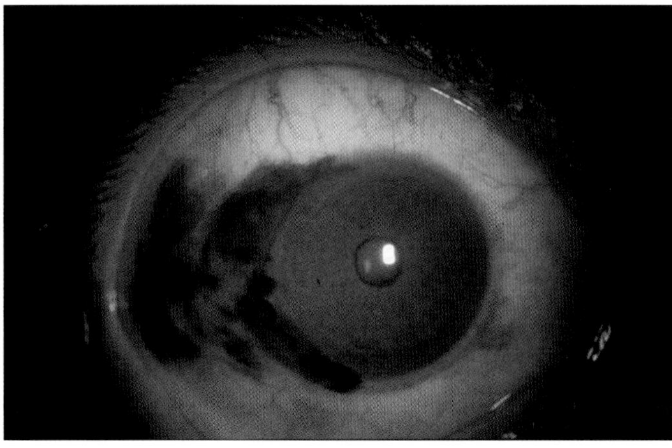

FIGURE 11-4 Primary acquired melanosis (PAM). Multiple unilateral indistinct areas of dark pigmentation. (*Reproduced with permission from Paul D. Comeau.*)

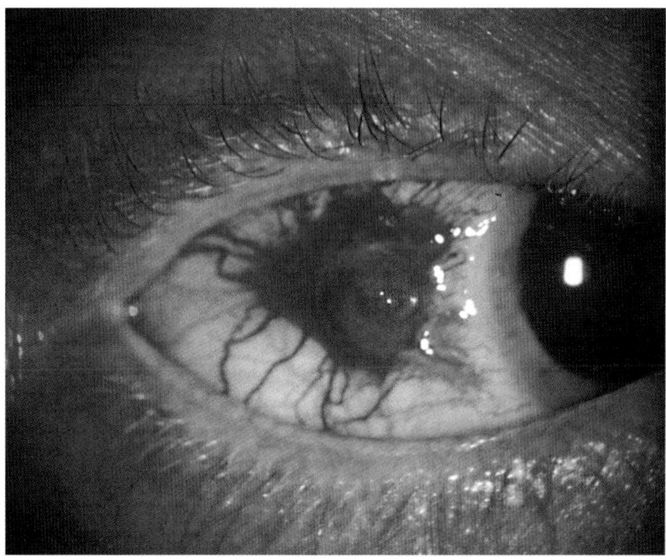

FIGURE 11-5 Conjunctival melanoma. Unilateral, nodular lesion with irregular contours and colors, and surrounded by hyperemic vessels. (*Reproduced with permission from Paul D. Comeau.*)

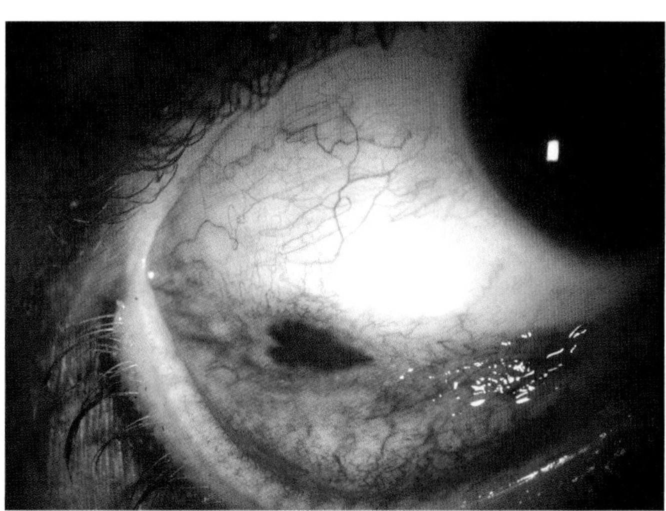

FIGURE 11-6 Early photo of conjunctival melanoma with irregular borders and variations in color. (*Reproduced with permission from Paul D. Comeau.*)

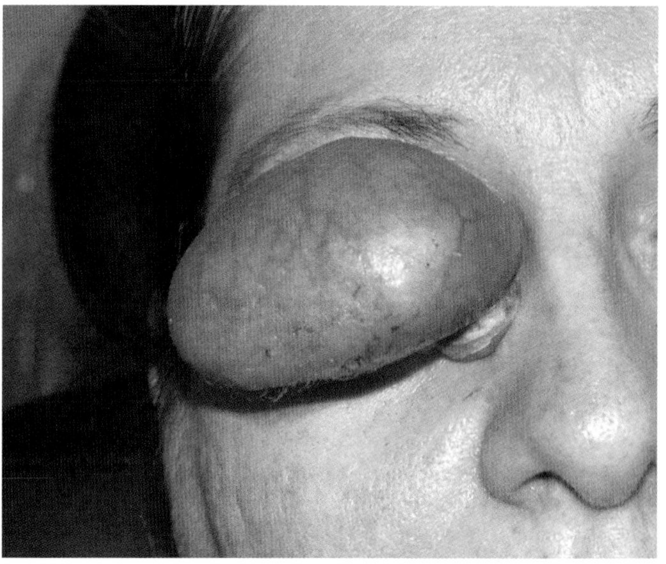

FIGURE 11-7 Conjunctival melanoma, 1 year after the previous photo, in a patient who initially declined treatment. (*Reproduced with permission from Paul D. Comeau.*)

ETIOLOGY AND PATHOPHYSIOLOGY

The etiology of scleral or conjunctival nevi is not well understood. Racial melanosis is genetically determined. Conjunctival melanoma can arise from PAM with severe atypia, nevi, or de novo.[6,7]

RISK FACTORS

- In non-Hispanic whites, the incidence of conjunctival melanoma increases as latitude decreases.[8]
- Fair-skinned individuals are at higher risk for conjunctival melanoma.

DIAGNOSIS

Definitive diagnosis of pigmented ocular lesions is made by biopsy.

CLINICAL FEATURES

- Benign nevi and physiologic or racial melanosis are stable over time, whereas PAM and melanoma change.
- Intrinsic cysts are common in conjunctival nevi and are rare in racial melanosis, PAM, and melanoma. They are seen with slit-lamp biomicroscopy.[9]

TYPICAL DISTRIBUTION

- Physiologic melanosis is typically bilateral and symmetrical.
- Nevi, PAM, and melanoma are typically unilateral; however, one study found that 13% of PAM cases were bilateral.[7]

LABORATORY TESTING

None indicated, other than biopsy.

IMAGING

- Often not helpful, as diagnosis is made by biopsy.
- Anterior segment coherence tomography is being studied as a diagnostic aid for conjunctival nevus because cysts are detectable. In one study, there was 100% positive predictive value (PPV) but only 60% negative predictive value (NPV).[9]

BIOPSY

- Eighty-seven percent of biopsy-proven nevi do not change over time.[4]
- Features seen more commonly in malignancy: ulceration, hemorrhage, change in color, and formation of new vessels around the lesion.
- Pathologic factors of conjunctival melanoma with a higher mortality rate include increased tumor thickness, location on the palpebral, caruncular or forniceal conjunctiva, increased mitotic activity, lymphocytic invasion, and association with PAM.[10]

DIFFERENTIAL DIAGNOSIS

Pigmented areas on the sclera or conjunctiva include the following:

- Benign nevi—Unilateral and stable over time (see **Figures 11-1** and **11-2**).
- Physiologic or racial melanosis—Bilateral and symmetric, most common circumlimbally, and relatively consistent throughout patient's life (see **Figure 11-3**).
- PAM—Typically unilateral, often multifocal indistinct areas of dark pigmentation, and can progress to malignancy over time (see **Figure 11-4**). This term is used clinically when the histology is not known.
- Secondary acquired melanosis—Seen with hormonal changes or after trauma to the conjunctiva with irradiation, chemical irritation, or chronic inflammation.
- Conjunctival melanoma—Unilateral, nodular, with variegated color and size changes (see **Figures 11-5** to **11-7**).
- Alkaptonuria—Rare disease accompanied by dark urine and arthritis.
- Nevus of Ota (also known as oculodermal melanocytosis)—Blue-gray scleral pigment involving the periorbital skin as well (see **Figure 11-8**).

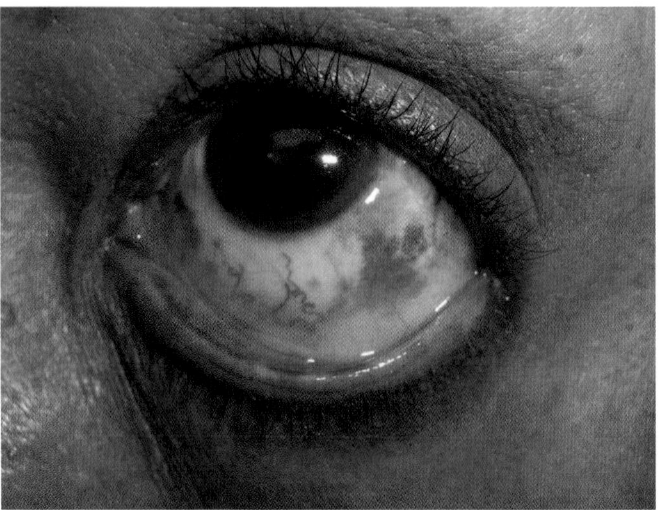

FIGURE 11-8 Nevus of Ota (also known as oculodermal melanocytosis). Unilateral blue-gray ocular pigmentation with periorbital hyperpigmentation. (*Reproduced with permission from Richard P. Usatine, MD.*)

It is more common in the Asian population but can be seen in any population. It can also be bilateral. Most importantly these people should be followed up by an ophthalmologist because they are at higher risk for glaucoma and possibly melanoma.

MANAGEMENT

- Racial melanosis and nevi are 2 lesions that can be monitored for changes without a biopsy.
- Refer any changing pigmented lesion in the eye to a specialist who can perform a biopsy.
- Biopsy-proven PAM without atypia does not require excision, but must be monitored for stability. SOR Ⓒ
- Melanosis with atypia is generally removed with large margins because of its potential for conversion into melanoma.[4] SOR Ⓒ
- The primary treatment for conjunctival melanoma is surgical removal. Cryotherapy, radiotherapy, and chemotherapy may be used as adjunct therapy. SOR Ⓒ

PREVENTION

To decrease risk of conjunctival melanoma, use sunglasses that protect the eye from ultraviolet (UV) radiation. SOR Ⓒ

PROGNOSIS

In one study, PAM without atypia or with mild atypia did not progress into melanoma. Thirteen percent of PAM cases with severe atypia did progress. The risk of melanoma increases as PAM covers more of the iris circumference (see **Figure 11-4**).[6] In one study, conjunctival melanoma arose from PAM, nevi, and de novo. Melanoma arising de novo had a worse prognosis. Other bad factors were fornix location and nodular tumor.[7]

FOLLOW-UP

Follow-up is based on the type of lesion. Nevi and physiologic melanosis that have not changed can be monitored without biopsy. PAM requires close follow-up because of its potential conversion to melanoma. Patients with nevus of Ota should be monitored for glaucoma and melanoma.

PATIENT EDUCATION

Most pigmentation in the eye is benign and does not change over time. Discuss the importance of reporting any changing pigmented lesion, even in the eye.

PATIENT RESOURCES

- American Academy of Ophthalmology—**http://www.aao.org**.
- Information on nevi and ocular melanoma. *What Is a Nevus?*—**http://www.geteyesmart.org/eyesmart/diseases/nevus.cfm.**
- Ocular Melanoma Foundation. *About Ocular Melanoma*—**http://www.ocularmelanoma.org/disease.htm.**

PROVIDER RESOURCES

- Medscape. *Conjunctival Melanoma*—**http://emedicine.medscape.com/article/1191840.**

REFERENCES

1. Shields CL, Demirci H, Karatza E, Shields JA. Clinical survey of 1643 melanocytic and nonmelanocytic conjunctival tumors. *Ophthalmology.* 2004;111(9):1747-1754.
2. Shields CL, Fasiudden A, Mashayekhi A, Shields JA. Conjunctival nevi: clinical features and natural course in 410 consecutive patients. *Arch Ophthalmol.* 2004;122(2):167-175.
3. Singh AD, Campos OE, Rhatigan RM, et al. Conjunctival melanoma in the black population [review]. *Surv Ophthalmol.* 1998;43(2):127-133.
4. Folberg R, Mclean IW, Zimmerman LE. Conjunctival melanosis and melanoma. *Ophthalmology.* 1984;91(6):673-678.
5. Seregard S, af Trampe E, Månsson-Brahme E, et al. Prevalence of primary acquired melanosis and nevi of the conjunctiva and uvea in the dysplastic nevus syndrome. A case-control study. *Ophthalmology.* 1995;102(10):1524-1529.
6. Shields CL, Markowitz JS, Belinsky I, et al. Conjunctival melanoma: outcomes based on tumor origin in 382 consecutive cases. *Ophthalmology.* 2011;118(2):389-395.
7. Shields JA, Shields CL, Mashayekhi A, et al. Primary acquired melanosis of conjunctiva: risks for progression to melanoma in 311 eyes. *Ophthalmology.* 2008;115(3):511-519.
8. Yu GP, Hu DN, McCormick SA. Latitude and incidence of ocular melanoma. *Photochem Photobiol.* 2006;82(6):1621-1626.
9. Shields CL, Belinsky I, Romanelli-Gobbi M, et al. Anterior segment optical coherence tomography of conjunctival nevus. *Ophthalmology.* 2011;118(5):915-919.
10. Shields CL, Shields JA, Gunduz K, et al. Conjunctival melanoma: risk factors for recurrence, exenteration, metastasis, and death in 150 consecutive patients [comment]. *Arch Ophthalmol.* 2000;118(11):1497-1507.

12 CORNEAL FOREIGN BODY AND CORNEAL ABRASION

Heidi Chumley, MD

PATIENT STORY

A 28-year-old man felt something fly into his eye while he was using a table saw without wearing protective eye gear. He presented with pain, tearing, photophobia, and thought that something was still in his eye. On examination with a slit lamp, the physician noted that he had a wood chip that had penetrated the cornea (**Figures 12-1** and **12-2**). He was referred to an ophthalmologist who successfully removed the foreign body. He was treated with a short course of topical nonsteroidal anti-inflammatory drugs (NSAIDs) for pain relief, and had complete healing.

INTRODUCTION

Corneal abrasions are often caused by eye trauma and can cause an inflammatory response. Corneal abrasions are detected using fluorescein and ultraviolet (UV) light. A corneal foreign body can be seen during a careful physical examination with a good light source or slit lamp. Non-penetrating foreign bodies can be removed by an experienced physician in the office using topical anesthesia. Refer all penetrating foreign bodies to an ophthalmologist.

SYNONYMS

Corneal abrasion is sometimes referred to as a corneal epithelial defect.

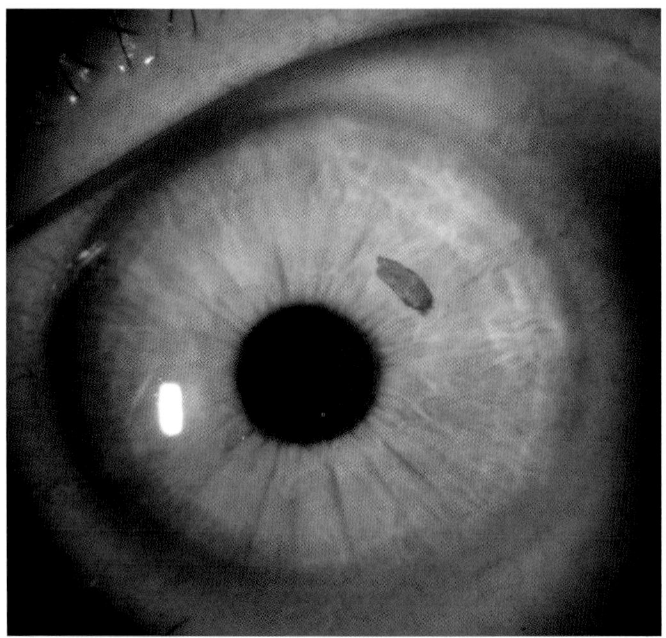

FIGURE 12-1 Wood chip is visible in the cornea on close inspection of the eye. *(Reproduced with permission from Paul D. Comeau.)*

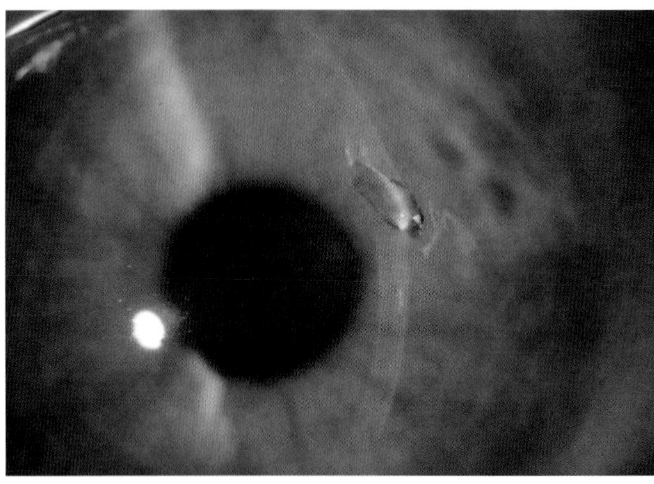

FIGURE 12-2 Slit-lamp examination reveals this wood chip has penetrated the cornea. *(Reproduced with permission from Paul D. Comeau.)*

EPIDEMIOLOGY

- Corneal abrasions with or without foreign bodies are common; however, the prevalence or incidence of corneal abrasions in the general population is unknown.
- Corneal abrasions accounted for 85% of closed-eye injuries in adults presenting to an emergency department.[1]

ETIOLOGY AND PATHOPHYSIOLOGY

- The cornea overlies the iris and provides barrier protection, filters UV light, and refracts light onto the retina.
- Abrasions in the cornea are typically caused by direct injury from a foreign body, resulting in an inflammatory reaction.
- The inflammatory reaction causes the symptoms and can persist for several days after the foreign object is out.

RISK FACTORS

- People occupied as metal workers, woodworkers, miners, and landscapers have an increased risk of corneal injuries from foreign bodies.[2]
- Participating in sports such as hockey, lacrosse, or racquetball raises the risk of corneal abrasions from ocular trauma.[2]
- Sedated patients (as a result of disruption of the blink reflex, and subsequent corneal exposure) are at increased risk for corneal abrasions.[2]

Contact lenses, especially soft, extended wear, increase the risk of developing an infected abrasion that ulcerates.[2]

DIAGNOSIS

CLINICAL FEATURES

History and physical

- History of ocular trauma or eye rubbing (although corneal abrasions can occur with no trauma history).

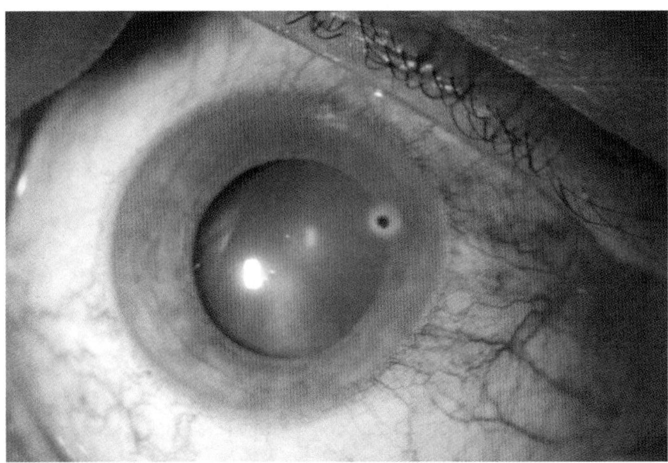

FIGURE 12-3 Metallic foreign body with rust ring within the corneal stroma and conjunctival injection. (*Reproduced with permission from Paul D. Comeau.*)

- Symptoms of pain, eye redness, photophobia, and a foreign-body sensation.
- Foreign body seen with direct visualization or a slit lamp (**Figure 12-3**).
- Fluorescein application demonstrates green area (which represents the disruption in the corneal epithelium) under cobalt-blue filtered light (**Figure 12-4**).
- History of contact lens wear.
- History of ocular or perioral herpes virus infection.

LABORATORY TESTING

Culture if an infection is suspected.

IMAGING

- If physical examination is equivocal, imaging may be useful to determine if a foreign body has perforated the cornea. An object that has fully perforated the cornea has passed through the cornea and will be located in the anterior or posterior segment of the eye, making it difficult to see without imaging technology.
- Computed tomography (CT) or spiral CT can detect nonmetallic and metallic foreign bodies.
- A metallic foreign body can be seen on an orbital radiograph. Avoid magnetic resonance imaging (MRI) if the history suggests the foreign body may be metallic.

Ultrasound and ultrasound biomicroscopy can also visualize intraocular foreign bodies and may be useful in some cases.

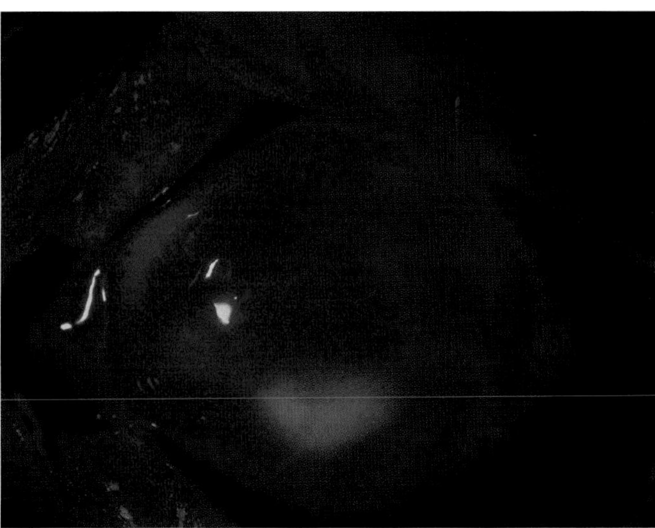

FIGURE 12-4 Fluorescein stains green, indicating corneal abrasion. (*Reproduced with permission from Paul D. Comeau.*)

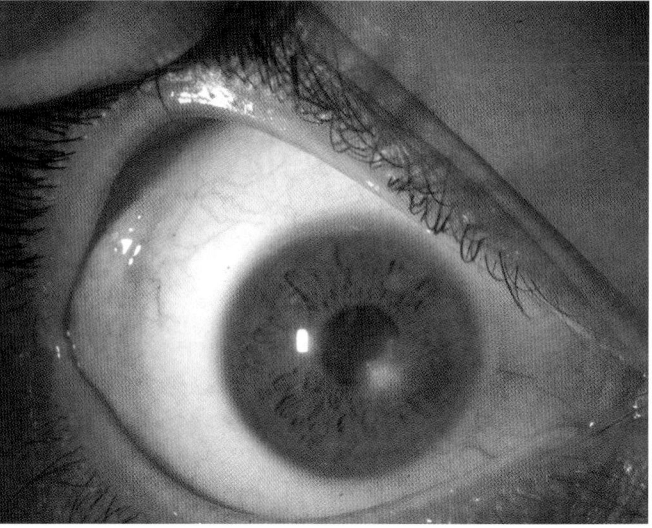

FIGURE 12-5 Small corneal ulcer in the visual axis. (*Reproduced with permission from Paul D. Comeau.*)

DIFFERENTIAL DIAGNOSIS

- Uveitis or iritis—Usually unilateral, 360-degree perilimbal injection, eye pain, photophobia, and vision loss (see Chapter 15, Uveitis and Iritis).
- Keratitis or corneal ulcerations—Diffuse erythema with ciliary injection often with miosis; eye discharge; pain, photophobia, and vision loss depending on the location of ulceration (**Figures 12-5** and **12-6**).

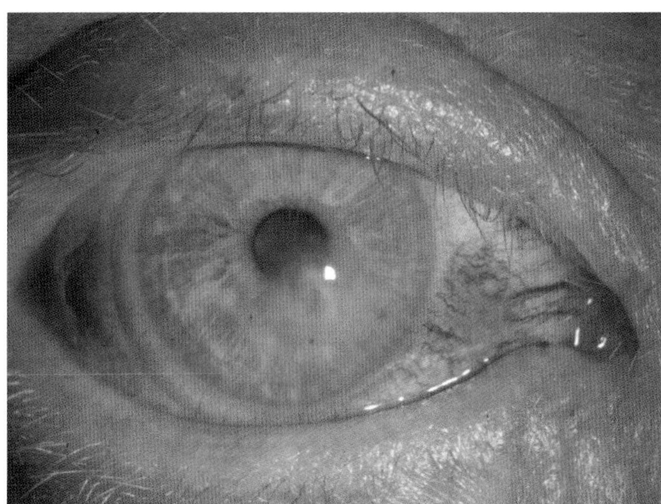

FIGURE 12-6 Larger corneal ulcer partially obscuring the visual axis. (*Reproduced with permission from Paul D. Comeau.*)

There is often a history of trauma, herpes simplex virus (HSV), or contact lens wear. Patients should see an ophthalmologist urgently.

- Conjunctivitis—Conjunctival injection; eye discharge; gritty or uncomfortable feeling; no vision loss, history of respiratory infection, or contacts with others who have red eyes (see Chapter 13, Conjunctivitis).
- Acute-angle closure glaucoma—Cloudy cornea and scleral injection; eye pain with ipsilateral headache; severe vision loss, acutely elevated intraocular pressure (see Chapter 16, Glaucoma).

MANAGEMENT

NONPHARMACOLOGIC

- Confirm diagnosis with fluorescein and UV light (for abrasion) if no foreign body is readily visible (see **Figure 12-4**).
- Carefully inspect for a foreign body. Invert the upper eyelid for full visualization. Slit-lamp visualization may be needed to determine if the cornea has been penetrated (see **Figure 12-2**).
- Remove (or refer for removal) nonpenetrating foreign bodies. Apply a topical anesthetic, such as proparacaine or tetracaine. Remove with irrigation, a wet-tipped cotton applicator, or a fine-gauge needle.
- Remove contact lenses until cornea is healed.[3] SOR Ⓒ
- Avoid patching in corneal abrasions smaller than 10 mm; it does not help.[4] SOR Ⓐ

MEDICATIONS

- Prescribe ophthalmic NSAIDs for pain if needed.[5] SOR Ⓐ
- Consider topical antibiotics. SOR Ⓒ Chloramphenicol ointment reduced the risk of recurrent ulcer in a prospective, nonplacebo, controlled trial.[6] Although chloramphenicol is rarely used in the United States, other ophthalmic antibiotics, such as erythromycin ointment, are used for corneal abrasions. SOR Ⓒ

REFERRAL

Refer penetrating foreign bodies to an experienced eye surgeon.

PREVENTION

Eye protection should be worn for high-risk occupational and recreational activities.

PROGNOSIS

Prognosis is generally good. Development of infection or a rust ring worsens prognosis.

FOLLOW-UP

See all patients in 24 hours for reassessment. If there is no improvement, look for an initially overlooked foreign body or a full-thickness injury. Do not hesitate to refer to ophthalmology if patient is not improving.

PATIENT EDUCATION

- Advise patients in specific professions (eg, woodworking, metal working) and those who play sports, such as racquetball or hockey, to wear eye protection for primary prevention.
- Advise patients with corneal abrasions that healing usually occurs within 2 to 3 days, and that they should report persistent pain, redness, and photophobia.
- Patients should be advised not to sleep wearing contact lenses, even if labeled "extended wear."

PATIENT RESOURCES

- FamilyDoctor.org. Patient handout on *Corneal Abrasions*—**http://familydoctor.org/familydoctor/en/prevention-wellness/staying-healthy/first-aid/corneal-abrasions.html.**

PROVIDER RESOURCES

- Medscape. Cao C. *Corneal Foreign Body Removal*—**http://emedicine.medscape.com/article/82717.**

REFERENCES

1. Oum BS, Lee JS, Han YS. Clinical features of ocular trauma in emergency department. *Korean J Ophthalmol.* 2004;18(1):70-78.
2. Wilson SA, Last A. Management of corneal abrasions. *Am Fam Physician.* 2004;1(70):123-128.
3. Weissman BA. *Care of the Contact Lens Patient: Reference Guide for Clinicians*. St Louis, MO: American Optometric Association; 2000.
4. Turner A, Rabiu M. Patching for corneal abrasion. *Cochrane Database Syst Rev.* 2006;(2):CD004764.
5. Weaver CS, Terrell KM. Evidence-based emergency medicine. Update: do ophthalmic nonsteroidal anti-inflammatory drugs reduce the pain associated with simple corneal abrasion without delaying healing [review]? *Ann Emerg Med.* 2003;41(1):134-140.
6. Upadhyaya MP, Karmacharyaa PC, Kairalaa S, et al. The Bhaktapur eye study: ocular trauma and antibiotic prophylaxis for the prevention of corneal ulceration in Nepal. *Br J Ophthalmol.* 2001;85:388-392.

13 CONJUNCTIVITIS

Heidi Chumley, MD
Richard P. Usatine, MD

PATIENT STORY

A 35-year-old woman presents with 2 days of redness and tearing in her eyes (**Figure 13-1**). She has some thin matter in her eyes, but neither eye has been glued shut when she awakens. She does not have any trouble seeing once she blinks to clear any accumulated debris. Both eyes are uncomfortable and itchy, but she is not having any severe pain. She does not wear contact lenses and has not had this problem previously. The patient was diagnosed with viral conjunctivitis and scored −1 on the clinical scoring system (see "Diagnosis" below). She was instructed about eye hygiene and recovered in 3 days.

INTRODUCTION

Conjunctivitis, inflammation of the membrane lining the eyelids and globe, presents with injected pink or red eye(s), eye discharge ranging from mild to purulent, eye discomfort or gritty sensation, and no vision loss. Conjunctivitis is most commonly infectious (viral or bacterial) or allergic, but can be caused by irritants. Diagnosis is clinical, based on differences in symptoms and signs.

SYNONYMS

Conjuctivitis is also known as pink eye.

EPIDEMIOLOGY

- Infectious conjunctivitis is common and often occurs in outbreaks, making the prevalence difficult to estimate.
- In the United States, the estimated annual incidence rate for bacterial conjunctivitis is 135 per 10,000 people.[1]
- Viral conjunctivitis is more common than bacterial conjunctivitis.
- Allergic conjunctivitis had a point prevalence of 6.4% and a lifetime prevalence of 40% in a large population study in the United States from 1988 to 1994.[2]

ETIOLOGY AND PATHOPHYSIOLOGY

Conjunctivitis in adults is predominately infectious (viral) or allergic.

- Adults and children of age 6 years or older are more likely to have viral or allergic causes for conjunctivitis.[3] Adenovirus is the most common viral cause.
- Coxsackie viruses have caused multiple large outbreaks in several Asian countries.
- Herpes simplex virus typically causes a keratitis, but may present as isolated conjunctivitis or as blepharoconjunctivitis.[4]
- Children younger than 6 years are more likely to have a bacterial than viral conjunctivitis (**Figure 13-2**) which can be transmitted to their adult caretakers. In the United States, the most common bacterial causes are *Haemophilus* species and *Streptococcus pneumoniae* accounting for almost 90% of cases in children.[3]

DIAGNOSIS

- To distinguish conjunctivitis from other causes of a red eye, ask about pain and check for vision loss. Patients with a red eye and intense pain or vision loss that does not clear with blinking are unlikely to have conjunctivitis and should undergo further evaluation.
- Always ask about contact lens use as this can be a risk factor for all types of conjunctivitis, including bacterial conjunctivitis (**Figure 13-3**).
- Typical clinical features of any type of conjunctivitis may include eye discharge, gritty or uncomfortable feeling, one or both pink eyes, and

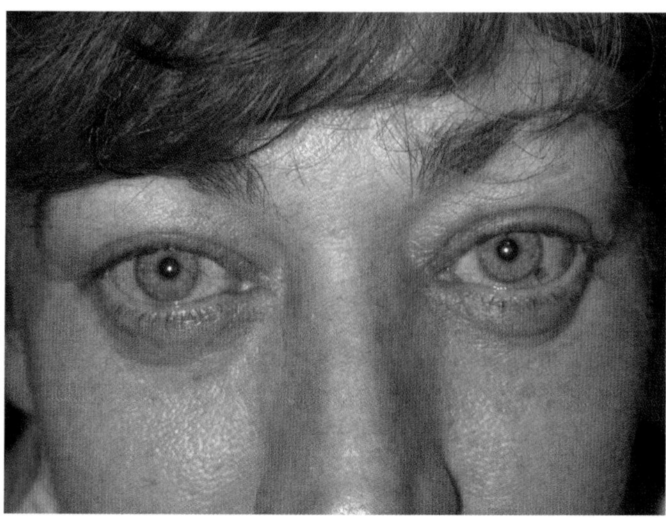

FIGURE 13-1 Viral conjunctivitis demonstrating bilateral conjunctival injection with little discharge. The patient has an incidental left eye conjunctival nevus. *(Reproduced with permission from Richard P. Usatine, MD.)*

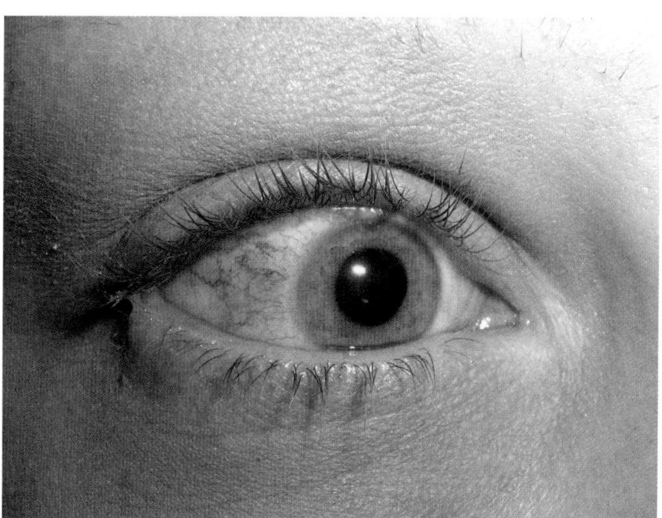

FIGURE 13-2 Bacterial conjunctivitis with visible purulent discharge. *(Reproduced with permission from Richard P. Usatine, MD.)*

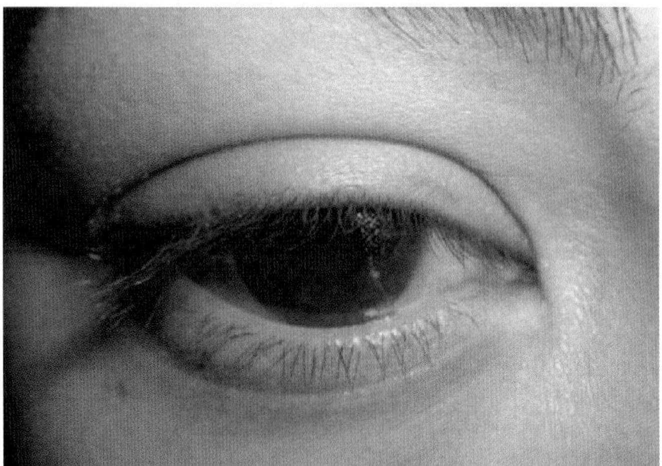

FIGURE 13-3 Bacterial conjunctivitis with a small amount of discharge. The patient was unable to clean her contacts while being evacuated from a hurricane-threatened Houston and the conjunctivitis was bilateral. (*Reproduced with permission from Richard P. Usatine, MD.*)

no vision loss. The infection usually starts in one eye, and progresses to involve the other eye days later.

- Bacterial conjunctivitis (see **Figures 13-2** to **13-4**) has a more purulent discharge than viral or allergic conjunctivitis.
- A clinical scoring system has been developed to distinguish bacterial from other causes of conjunctivitis in healthy adults who did not wear contact lenses. A score of +5 to –3 is determined as follows:
  - Two glued eyes (+5); one glued eye (+2); history of conjunctivitis (–2); eye itching (–1).
  - A score of +5, +4, or +3 is useful in ruling in bacterial conjunctivitis with specificities of 100%, 94%, and 92%, respectively.
  - Scores of –1, –2, or –3 are useful in ruling out bacterial conjunctivitis with sensitivities of 98%, 98%, and 100%, respectively.[5]

Allergic conjunctivitis is typically bilateral and accompanied by eye itching. Giant papillary conjunctivitis is a type of allergic reaction, most commonly to soft contact lenses (**Figure 13-5**).

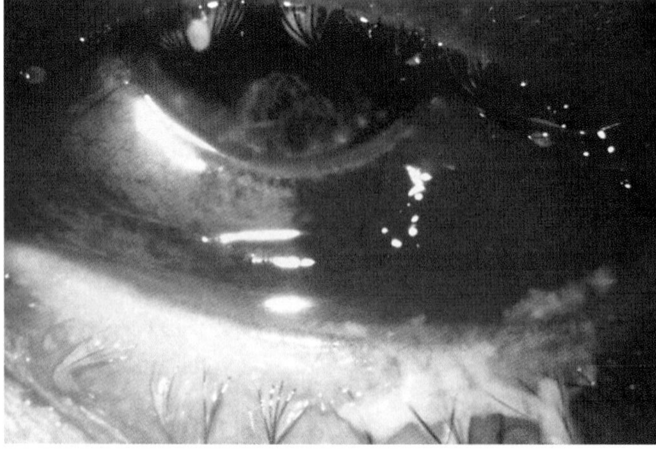

FIGURE 13-4 Gonococcus conjunctivitis has a copious discharge. This severe case resulted in partial blindness. (*Reproduced with permission from Centers for Disease Control and Prevention [CDC].*)

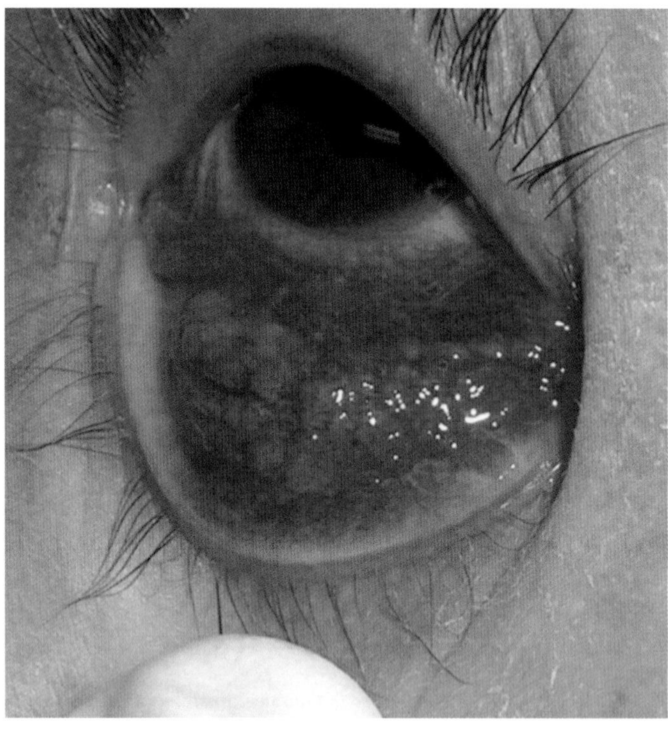

FIGURE 13-5 Giant papillary conjunctivitis in a contact lens wearer. (*Reproduced with permission from Richard P. Usatine, MD as contributed by Mike Johnson, MD.*)

LABORATORY TESTING

An in-office rapid test for adenoviral conjunctivitis (RPS adeno detector) has a sensitivity of 88% and a specificity of 91% compared to viral cell culture with confirmatory immunofluorescence staining.[6]

DIFFERENTIAL DIAGNOSIS

- Episcleritis—Segmental or diffuse inflammation of episclera (pink color), mild or no discomfort but can be tender to palpation, and no vision disturbance (see also Chapter 14, Episcleritis and Scleritis).
- Scleritis—Segmental or diffuse inflammation of sclera (dark red, purple, or blue color), severe boring eye pain often radiating to head and neck, and photophobia and vision loss (see also Chapter 14, Episcleritis and Scleritis).
- Uveitis or iritis—360-degree perilimbal injection, eye pain, photophobia, and vision loss. Frequently treated initially as conjunctivitis without resolution (see also Chapter 15, Uveitis and Iritis).
- Keratitis or corneal ulcerations—Diffuse conjunctival injection, often with miosis (constriction of pupil), eye discharge, pain, photophobia, and vision loss depending on the location of ulceration. Herpes keratitis is a diagnosis that should not be missed (**Figures 13-6** and **13-7**). The use of fluorescein and ultraviolet (UV) light can help identify dendritic ulcers or other corneal damage and prompt an emergent referral to an ophthalmologist (see **Figure 13-7**). Contact lens wearers should urgently see an ophthalmologist for keratitis.
- Acute-angle closure glaucoma—Cloudy cornea and scleral injection, eye pain with ipsilateral headache, elevated intraocular pressure, and severe vision loss (see also Chapter 16, Glaucoma).
- A foreign body in the eye can cause conjunctival injection and lead to a bacterial superinfection. If the foreign body is not easily dislodged with

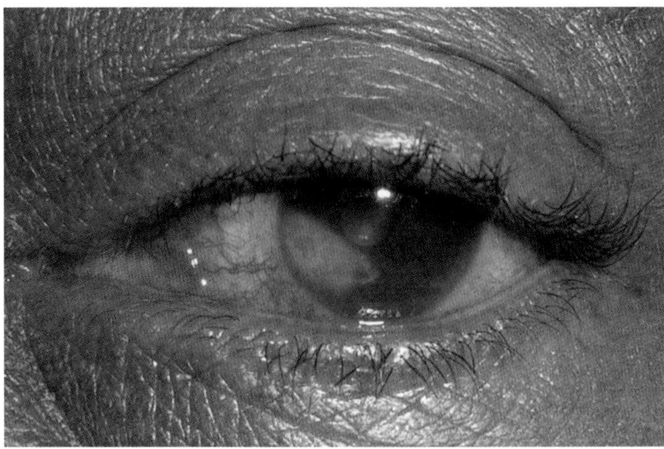

FIGURE 13-6 Herpetic keratitis in a 56-year-old woman staying in a shelter after hurricane Katrina. (*Reproduced with permission from Richard P. Usatine, MD.*)

conservative measures, or appears to be superinfected with ulceration or leukocyte infiltrate, prompt referral to an ophthalmologist is required (**Figure 13-8**).

Trachoma is an eye infection caused by *Chlamydia trachomatis* that is rare in the United States but common in the rural areas of some developing countries. It is a leading cause of blindness in the developing world. Poverty and poor hygiene are major risk factors. Once the eye is infected, follicles can be seen on the upper tarsal conjunctiva upon eyelid eversion (**Figure 13-9**). Superior tarsal conjunctival scarring leads to entropion that causes corneal scarring and ultimately blindness (**Figure 13-10**).

Vernal conjunctivitis is a severe recurrent form of allergic conjunctivitis that is more common in summer (not in spring). The term *vernal* refers to spring time, and therefore it is now referred to as "warm weather conjunctivitis" rather than "spring catarrh." Giant papillae that look like a cobblestone pattern may be seen in this condition. It occurs primarily in young boys, and typically ceases to recur seasonally with age.

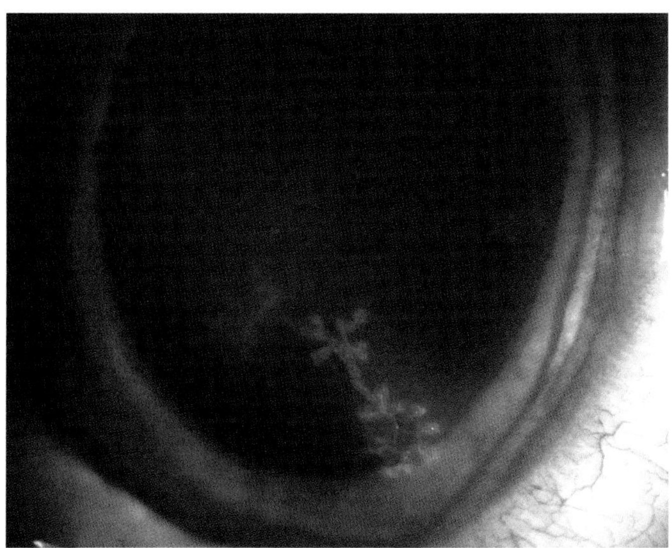

FIGURE 13-7 Slit-lamp view of a dendritic ulcer with fluorescein uptake from herpetic keratitis. (*Reproduced with permission from Paul D. Comeau.*)

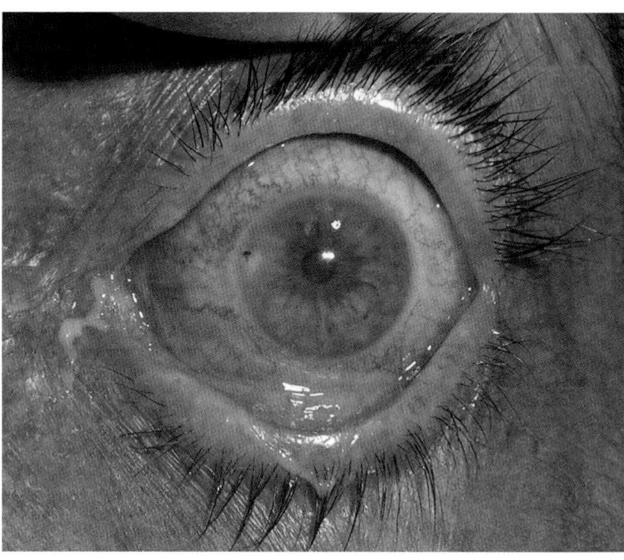

FIGURE 13-8 Conjunctivitis caused by a foreign body in the eye of a machinist. The ground metal speck is seen on the cornea, and the corneal infiltrate, along with a purulent discharge, indicate a bacterial superinfection. (*Reproduced with permission from Richard P. Usatine, MD.*)

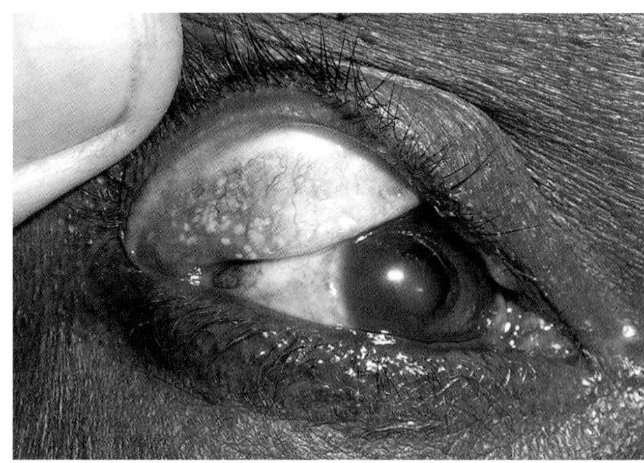

FIGURE 13-9 Trachoma showing many white follicles on the underside of the upper eyelid. (*Reproduced with permission from Richard P. Usatine, MD.*)

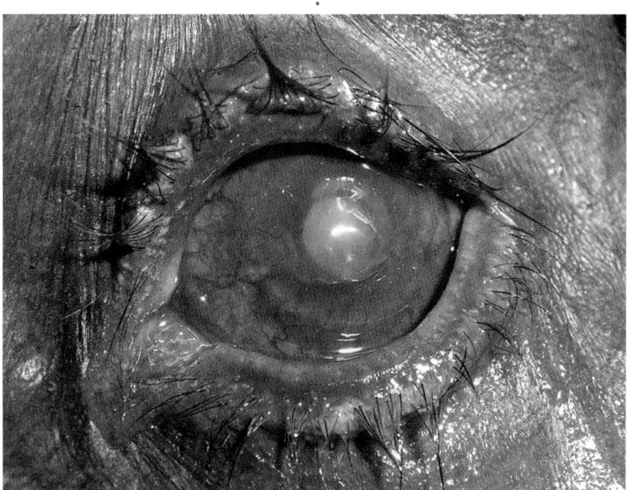

FIGURE 13-10 Advanced trachoma with blindness as a consequence of cornea opacities. Note the deep conjunctival injection and purulent discharge from the *C. trachomatis* infection. (*Reproduced with permission from Richard P. Usatine, MD.*)

MANAGEMENT

Hand hygiene can control the spread of infectious conjunctivitis.

Most acute conjunctival infections are viral and resolve without treatment. Adults who score +3 or above on the clinical scoring system for bacterial conjunctivitis are treated with topical antibiotics:

- Studies show that more than 80% of patients show improvements with 0.3% ciprofloxacin, tobramycin, norfloxacin, or gentamicin.[7,8]
- Levofloxacin 0.5% is dosed 3 times a day.[9]
- Delayed antibiotic prescription decreased antibiotic use by nearly 50% and provided similar symptom control compared to immediate antibiotics.[10]

Allergic conjunctivitis can be treated with antihistamines, mast-cell stabilizers, nonsteroidal anti-inflammatory agents, corticosteroids, and immunomodulatory agents.[11]

REFERRAL

- Refer patients who have vision loss, copious purulent discharge (this could represent gonococcal disease, which must be cultured, and which can cause vision loss), severe pain, lack of response to therapy, or a history of herpes simplex or zoster eye disease to an ophthalmologist.
- Any patient who may need ocular steroid should be seen by an ophthalmologist. There is a severe risk of complications with the use of ocular steroids.

PREVENTION

Good hygiene practices with washing of the hands and face with soap and water should be followed.

FOLLOW-UP

Routine follow-up is generally not needed if symptoms resolve in 3 to 5 days.

PATIENT EDUCATION

- Most adults (and children older than age 6 years) have a nonbacterial cause of conjunctivitis.
- Remove contact lenses until conjunctivitis has resolved.
- Avoid touching the face or rubbing the eyes and wash the hands immediately afterwards.
- Do not share face towels, eye makeup, or contact lens cases.
- Inform your physician immediately if you experience eye pain or vision loss.

PATIENT RESOURCES

- PubMed Health. *Conjunctivitis*—**http://www.ncbi.nlm.nih.gov/pubmedhealth/PMH0002005/.**
- American Academy of Ophthalmology has patient information under For Patients and the Public—**http://www.aao.org.**
- American Academy of Ophthalmology. *Conjunctivitis: What Is Pink Eye?*—**http://www.geteyesmart.org/eyesmart/diseases/conjunctivitis.cfm.**
- Centers for Disease Control and Prevention has patient information in English and Spanish—**http://www.cdc.gov.**
- Centers for Disease Control and Prevention. *Conjunctivitis (Pink Eye)*—**http://www.cdc.gov/conjunctivitis/index.html.**
- The Livestrong foundation has auditory patient information on YouTube. *Conjunctivitis Health Byte*—**http://www.youtube.com/watch?v=O8LkDfbLCaY**; and *A Healthy Byte: Pink Eye*—**http://www.youtube.com/watch?v=Hp28hS7XYCo&feature=relmfu.**

PROVIDER RESOURCES

- Agency for Healthcare Research and Quality. *Conjunctivitis guidelines*—**http://www.guidelines.gov/content.aspx?id=13501.**

REFERENCES

1. Smith AF, Waycaster C. Estimate of the direct and indirect annual cost of bacterial conjunctivitis in the United States. *BMC Ophthalmol.* 2009;9:13.
2. Singh K, Axelrod S, Bielory L. The epidemiology of ocular and nasal allergy in the United States, 1988-1994. *J Allergy Clin Immunol.* 2010;126(4):778-783.
3. Meltzer JA, Kunkov D, Crain EF. Identifying children at low risk for bacterial conjunctivitis. *Arch Pediatr Adolesc Med.* 2010;164:263-267.
4. Young RC, Hodge DO, Liesegang TJ, Baratz KH. Incidence, recurrence, and outcomes of herpes simplex virus eye disease in Olmsted County, Immesota, 1976-2007: the effect of oral antiviral prophylaxis. *Arch Ophthalmol.* 2010;128(9):1178-1183.
5. Rietveld RP. Predicting bacterial cause in infectious conjunctivitis: cohort study on informativeness of combinations of signs and symptoms. *BMJ.* 2004;329:206-210.
6. Sambursky R, Tauber S, Schirra F, et al. The RPS adeno detector for diagnosing adenoviral conjunctivitis. *Ophthalmology.* 2006;113(10):1758-1764.
7. Gross RD, Hoffman RO, Lindsay RN. A comparison of ciprofloxacin and tobramycin in bacterial conjunctivitis in children. *Clin Pediatr (Phila).* 1997;36(8):435-444.
8. Miller IM, Vogel R, Cook TJ, Wittreich J. Topically administered norfloxacin compared with topically administered gentamicin for the treatment of external ocular bacterial infections. The Worldwide Norfloxacin Ophthalmic Study Group. *Am J Ophthalmol.* 1992;113(6):638-644.

9. Szaflik J, Szaflik JP, Kaminska A. Clinical and microbiological efficacy of levofloxacin administered three times a day for the treatment of bacterial conjunctivitis. *Eur J Ophthalmol.* 2009;19(1):1-9.

10. Everitt HA, Little PS, Smith PW. A randomized controlled trial of management strategies for acute infective conjunctivitis in general practice. *BMJ.* 2006;333(7563):321.

11. Mishra GP, Tamboli V, Jwala J, Mitra AK. Recent patents and emerging therapeutics in the treatment of allergic conjunctivitis. *Recent Pat Inflamm Allergy Drug Discov.* 2011;5(1):26-36.

14 SCLERITIS AND EPISCLERITIS

Heidi Chumley, MD
Kelly Green, MD

PATIENT STORY

A 45-year-old woman presents with 1 day of increasing eye pain, eye redness, and difficulty in seeing. On examination there was scleral injection and exquisite globe tenderness (**Figure 14-1**). Her review of systems is positive for morning stiffness and swelling in both of her hands. The patient was urgently referred to an ophthalmologist who diagnosed her with scleritis. Her visual acuity was reduced minimally. A slit-lamp examination revealed injected sclera with a bluish hue in the affected eye and a rare anterior chamber cell. The posterior segment was normal.

The ophthalmologist prescribed an oral nonsteroidal anti-inflammatory drug (NSAID), specifically indomethacin, as it effectively crosses the blood-brain barrier and gets good levels in the eye.

Her rheumatoid factor was positive, so she was also referred to a rheumatologist.

INTRODUCTION

Episcleritis and scleritis are inflammation of the deeper layers of the eye, the vascular episclera, and the avascular sclera. Episcleritis presents with segmental eye redness, discomfort but not severe pain, and no vision loss. Scleritis can have overlying episcleritis, but also has a violaceous hue, is painful, and may cause vision loss. Scleritis typically has an associated underlying condition (autoimmune or infectious) that should be identified and treated. Scleritis is treated with NSAIDs, systemic glucocorticoids, or immunosuppressive medications. Patients with scleritis are often referred to an ophthalmologist as vision loss is common.

EPIDEMIOLOGY

Scleritis

- Scleritis usually presents between the ages of 30 and 50 years and is twice as common in women compared to men.[1]
- Forty-four percent of patients presenting with scleritis to specialty health centers were found to have an associated systematic disease (37% rheumatic, 7% infection), most commonly (15%) rheumatoid arthritis.[2]

Episcleritis

- Prevalence is unknown.
- Episcleritis usually presents between the ages of 20 and 50 years and may be more common in women.
- Nodular or recurrent episcleritis is more likely to be associated with an underlying systemic condition than is an isolated episode of simple episcleritis.

ETIOLOGY AND PATHOPHYSIOLOGY

- Scleritis and episcleritis are inflammatory conditions causing congestion of the deeper 2 of the 3 vascular layers (conjunctival, episcleral, and scleral plexuses) overlying the avascular sclera.
- Scleritis often occurs with episcleritis; episcleritis does not involve the sclera and does not progress to scleritis.
- Scleritis disrupts vascular architecture and may cause vision loss; whereas episcleritis does not.

Causes of scleritis

- Causes of scleritis include systemic autoimmune diseases such as rheumatoid arthritis, Wegener granulomatosis, seronegative spondyloarthropathies, relapsing polychondritis, systemic lupus erythematosus (SLE). **Figure 14-2** shows a young woman with SLE and scleritis.
- Infections (*Pseudomonas*, tuberculosis, syphilis, herpes zoster).
- Less common causes include gout and sarcoidosis.
- Idiopathic.

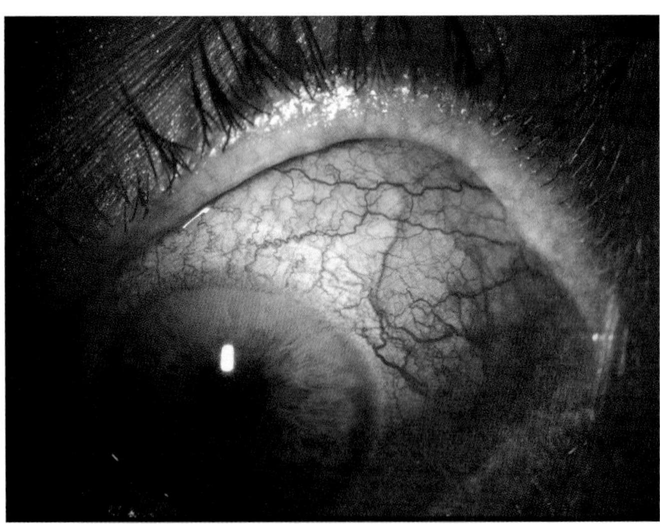

FIGURE 14-1 Scleritis in a patient with eye pain and exquisite globe tenderness. Untreated scleritis can result in loss of vision. (*Reproduced with permission from Paul D. Comeau.*)

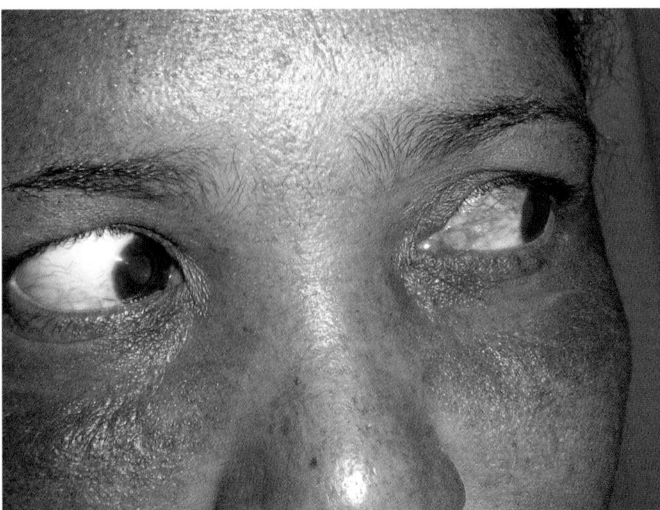

FIGURE 14-2 Scleritis in a young woman with systemic lupus erythematosus. Note the malar rash that is also present. (*Reproduced with permission from Richard P. Usatine, MD.*)

Causes of episcleritis

- Most often idiopathic.
- May be associated with any of the conditions listed above, especially if the presentation is nodular or recurrent.

DIAGNOSIS

CLINICAL FEATURES

Scleritis

- Segmental or diffuse inflammation of sclera (dark red, purple, or blue color), with overlying episclera and conjunctival inflammation (see **Figures 14-1** to **14-3**).
- Severe, boring eye pain often radiating to head and neck that worsens with eye movement. However, 20% of patients may not have pain, including those with the necrotizing type (scleromalacia perforans) and those taking immunosuppressive agents prior to the onset of scleritis.[1]
- Photophobia and vision loss.

Episcleritis

- Segmental or diffuse inflammation of episclera (pink color) and overlying conjunctival vessel injection (**Figures 14-4** and **14-5**).
- Mild, if any, discomfort but can be tender to palpation.
- No vision disturbance.
- Scleritis and episcleritis are often distinguished by history and physical examination features; however, when scleritis has extensive overlying episcleritis, the diagnosis becomes more difficult. Scleritis must be differentiated from episcleritis because scleritis requires treatment and an evaluation for underlying medical conditions.
- Ten percent phenylephrine blanches inflamed episcleral and conjunctival vessels, but not scleral vessels; in scleritis, this can reveal a focus of scleral engorgement covered by episcleral injection.
- Scleritis and episcleritis, as opposed to iritis with overlying episcleral injection, often have areas of focal tenderness to palpation. These can be elicited with a sterile cotton swab after applying a topical anesthetic.

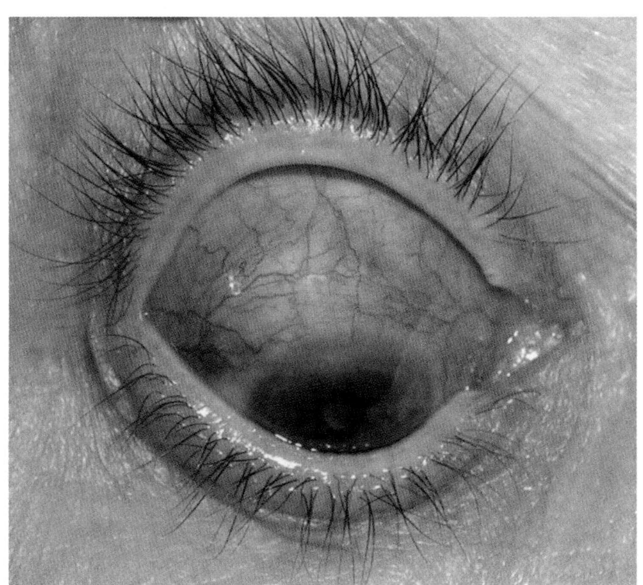

FIGURE 14-3 Scleritis in a patient with Wegener granulomatosis. Deep vessels are affected, giving the eye a purplish or blue hue. (*Reproduced with permission from Everett Allen, MD.*)

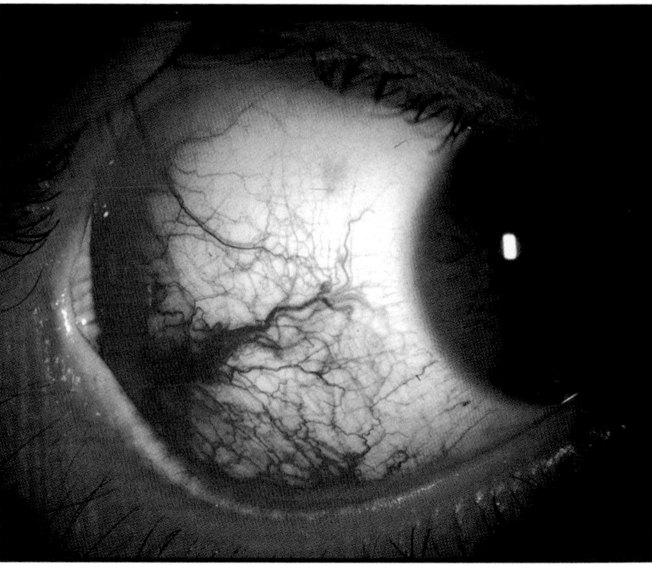

FIGURE 14-4 Episcleritis showing inflammation of the conjunctival and episcleral tissue with associated vascular engorgement. A sector of this eye is involved and that is typical. Vessels were blanched with 2.5% phenylephrine, which helped distinguish this from scleritis. (*Reproduced with permission from Paul D. Comeau.*)

Typical distribution

- Scleritis can be posterior (posterior to the medial and lateral rectus muscles) or anterior.
  - Posterior scleritis can produce retinal detachments and subretinal exudates and is often associated with uveitis (inflammation of the iris, ciliary body, or choroid).
  - Anterior scleritis can be diffuse, nodular, necrotizing with inflammation or necrotizing without inflammation.[1]
- Scleritis is bilateral in 50% of patients.[1]
- Episcleritis is often segmental, but can be diffuse, and is typically benign.

LABORATORY TESTING

In scleritis, if an associated systemic disease has not been previously diagnosed, consider ordering these tests: complete blood count, metabolic

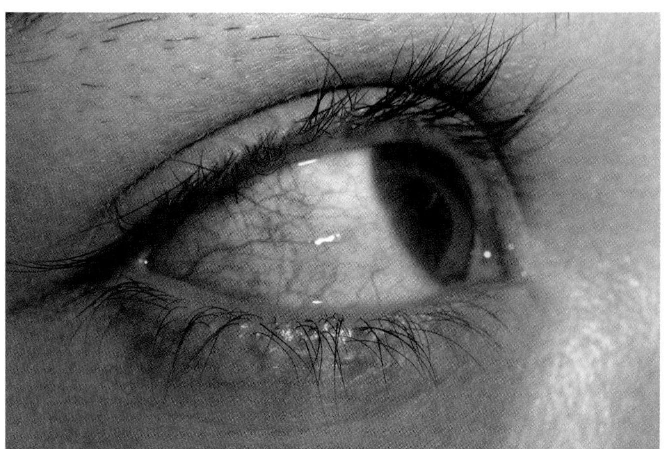

FIGURE 14-5 Episcleritis showing inflammation of only the conjunctival and episcleral tissue. Note the absence of violaceous color that is seen in scleritis. (*Reproduced with permission from Richard P. Usatine, MD.*)

panel, urinalysis, antineutrophil cytoplasmic antibody, antinuclear antibody, rheumatoid factor, anticyclic citrullinated peptide antibodies, rapid plasma reagin, and Lyme antibody in Lyme infested regions. Also consider tuberculin skin test, viral hepatitis panel, and cultures for bacteria, virus, and fungi.

IMAGING

In scleritis, if an associated systemic disease has not been previously diagnosed, consider the following: chest radiographs, sinus computed tomography (CT), or sacroiliac joint radiographs.

To diagnose posterior scleritis, ultrasound or orbital CT can demonstrate sclera thickening.

BIOPSY

An ophthalmologist may perform a biopsy when it is important to distinguish among scleritis caused by rheumatic diseases, infections, or sarcoidosis.

- Rheumatic—Zonal necrotizing granulomatous scleral inflammation with loss of anterior scleral tissue.
- Infectious—Necrotizing scleritis with microabscesses.
- Sarcoid—Sarcoidal granulomatous inflammation can be identified in cases of sarcoidosis.

DIFFERENTIAL DIAGNOSIS

Following are the causes of red eye, other than scleritis and episcleritis:

- Uveitis or iritis—360 degrees perilimbal injection, which is most intense at the limbus; eye pain, photophobia, and vision loss (see also Chapter 15, Uveitis and Iritis)
- Keratitis or corneal ulcerations—Diffuse erythema with ciliary injection often with pupillary constriction; eye discharge; pain, photophobia, and vision loss depending on location of ulceration
- Conjunctivitis—Conjunctival injection, eye discharge, gritty or uncomfortable feeling, no vision loss (see Chapter 13, Conjunctivitis)
- Acute-angle closure glaucoma—Cloudy cornea and scleral injection; eye pain with ipsilateral headache; severe vision loss (see Chapter 16, Glaucoma)

MANAGEMENT

For patients presenting with scleritis who do not have a previously diagnosed associated systemic condition, a search for an underlying cause is indicated.

- Evaluate for signs and symptoms of rheumatoid arthritis, Wegener granulomatosis (respiratory or renal symptoms), relapsing polychondritis (vasculitis around ear or nose cartilage or trachea; **Figure 14-6**), and seronegative spondyloarthropathies (inflammatory back pain, arthritis, and inflammatory bowel symptoms).
- Evaluate for signs, symptoms, and risk factors for infection including eye trauma, recent ocular surgery, recurrent herpes simplex or varicella zoster, or risk factors for tuberculosis.
- Evaluate for signs and symptoms of gout and sarcoidosis.

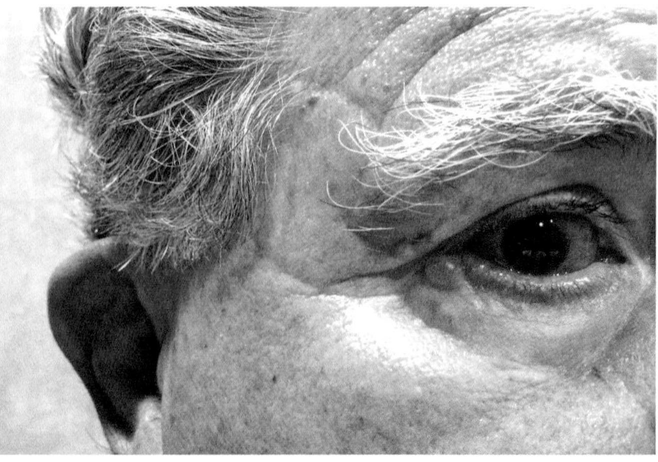

FIGURE 14-6 Scleritis associated with relapsing polychondritis. Note the floppy ear which is a classic finding in relapsing polychondritis (*Reproduced with permission from Everett Allen, MD.*)

MEDICATIONS

- Scleritis is initially treated with systemic NSAIDs and/or topical steroids; however, in one study only 47% of patients responded to 2 drops of 1% prednisolone every 2 hours for up to 2 weeks.[3] SOR B
- Scleritis that does not respond to NSAIDs and/or topical steroids may need systemic steroids, subconjunctival steroids, or immune modulators. SOR C
- Episcleritis often resolves spontaneously. Eye redness and irritation improve by 50% in less than a week. Treatment with topical NSAIDs was no better than artificial tears on measures of redness and comfort.[4] SOR B

REFERRAL

- If you suspect scleritis, refer the patient to an ophthalmologist immediately. This is especially important if there is any visual loss or eye pain.
- If episcleritis is not resolved, refer to an ophthalmologist.

PROGNOSIS

Simple episcleritis improves in 7 to 10 days. Episcleritis that is nodular or associated with an underlying disease may take 2 to 3 weeks to resolve.

Patients who smoke may take longer to recover from episcleritis or scleritis. One retrospective trial demonstrated that patients who smoked and had episcleritis or scleritis were 5.4 times more likely to have a delayed response of more than 4 weeks to any medication (95% confidence interval [CI] = 1.9-15.5).[5]

Vision loss with scleritis is common and the risk is dependent on the type of scleritis: diffuse anterior, 9%; nodular, 26%; necrotizing, 74%; posterior, 84%.[6]

FOLLOW-UP

- Advise patients with episcleritis to follow up for any increases in eye pain, changes in vision, or no improvement in 1 week.
- Advise patients with scleritis to follow up testing for underlying systemic illnesses. If none is found, consider retesting as patients with idiopathic scleritis develop a systemic illness at a 4% annual rate.[2]

PATIENT EDUCATION

- Reassure patients with episcleritis of its generally benign nature and that oral NSAIDs may be used for discomfort.
- Advise patients with scleritis of its association with systemic illnesses and the need for further workup.

PATIENT RESOURCES

- PubMed Health. *Scleritis*—**http://www.ncbi.nlm.nih.gov/pubmedhealth/PMH0001998/.**
- PubMed Health. *Episcleritis*—**http://www.ncbi.nlm.nih.gov/pubmedhealth/PMH0002014/.**

PROVIDER RESOURCES

- Patient.co.uk. *Scleritis and Episcleritis*—**http://www.patient.co.uk/doctor/Scleritis-and-Episcleritis.htm.**

REFERENCES

1. Galor A, Thorne JE. Scleritis and peripheral ulcerative keratitis. *Rheum Dis Clin North Am.* 2007;33(4):835-854.
2. Akpek EK, Thorne JE, Qazi FA, et al. Evaluation of patients with scleritis for systemic disease. *Ophthalmology*. 2004;111(3):501-506.
3. McMullen M, Kovarik G, Hodge WG. Use of topical steroid therapy in the management of nonnecrotizing anterior scleritis. *Can J Ophthalmol*. 1999;34(4):214-221.
4. Williams CP, Browning AC, Sleep TJ, et al. A randomised, double-blind trial of topical ketorolac vs artificial tears for the treatment of episcleritis. *Eye (Lond).* 2005;19(7):739-742.
5. Boonman ZF, de Keizer RJ, Watson PG. Smoking delays the response to treatment in episcleritis and scleritis. *Eye (Lond).* 2005;19(9):945-955.
6. Tuft SJ, Watson PG. Progression of sclera disease. *Ophthalmology*. 1991;98(4):467-471.

15 UVEITIS AND IRITIS

Heidi Chumley, MD

PATIENT STORY

A 28-year-old man presented with sudden onset of a right red eye, severe eye pain, tearing, photophobia, and decreased vision. He denied eye trauma. His review of systems was positive for lower back pain and stiffness over the past year. On examination, he had a ciliary flush (**Figure 15-1**) and decreased vision. He was referred to an ophthalmologist who confirmed the diagnosis of acute anterior uveitis. He was found to be HLA-B27 positive with characteristics of ankylosing spondylitis. His uveitis was treated with topical steroids.

INTRODUCTION

Uveitis is inflammation of any component of the uveal tract: iris (anterior), ciliary body (intermediate), or choroid (posterior). Most uveitis is anterior and is also called iritis. Uveitis is caused by trauma, inflammation, or infection and the most common etiologies vary by location in the uveal tract. Patients present with vision changes and, if uveitis is anterior, eye pain, redness, tearing, and photophobia. All patients with uveitis should be referred to an ophthalmologist.

SYNONYMS

Anterior uveitis includes iritis and iridocyclitis. *Iritis* is when the inflammation is limited to the iris. If the ciliary body is involved too, then it is called *iridocyclitis*. Posterior uveitis includes choroiditis and chorioretinitis.

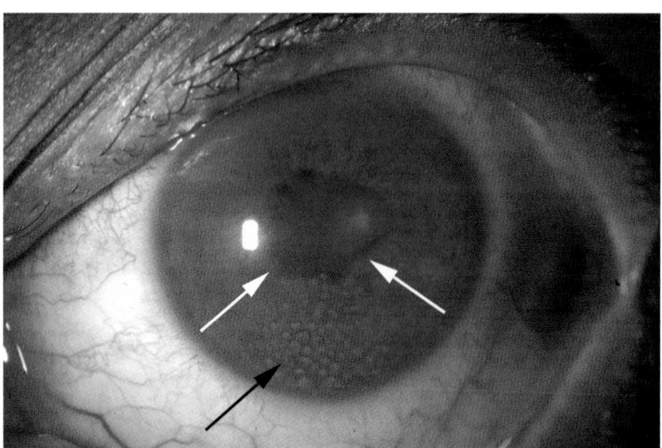

FIGURE 15-1 Acute anterior uveitis with corneal endothelial white cell aggregates (*black arrow*) and posterior synechiae formation (iris adhesions to the lens, *white arrows*). (*Reproduced with permission from Paul D. Comeau.*)

EPIDEMIOLOGY

- Annual incidence of uveitis is 17 to 52 per 100,000 population and prevalence is 38 to 714 per 100,000 population.[1]
- Occurs at any age, but most commonly between 20 and 59 years.[1]
- Anterior uveitis (iritis) accounts for approximately 90% of uveitis as seen in primary care settings.[1]
- In the United States, noninfectious uveitis accounts for 10% of legal blindness.[2]

ETIOLOGY AND PATHOPHYSIOLOGY

- Uveitis can be caused by trauma, infections, inflammation, or, rarely, neoplasms. Most likely causes differ by location.[3]
- Iritis—Trauma is common (**Figure 15-2**). In nontraumatic cases, causes include idiopathic (50%); seronegative spondyloarthropathies, that is, ankylosing spondylitis, reactive arthritis, psoriatic arthritis, inflammatory bowel disease (20%); and juvenile idiopathic arthritis (10%). Infections are less common and include herpes, syphilis, and tuberculosis.[3] Untreated HIV-positive patients may also develop iritis.
- Intermediate—Most are idiopathic[3] (**Figure 15-3**).
- Posterior—Toxoplasmosis is the most common, followed by idiopathic.[3]
- Panuveitis (affecting all layers)—Idiopathic (22-45%) and sarcoidosis (14-28%).[3] Unilateral panuveitis is often endophthalmitis (endogenous or related to trauma or surgery). Bilateral panuveitis can be caused by sarcoidosis or syphilis.

RISK FACTORS

Patients with Behçet disease and ankylosing spondylitis have uveitis more commonly than the general population (relative risk of 4-20) because of human leukocyte antigen (HLA) associations.[4]

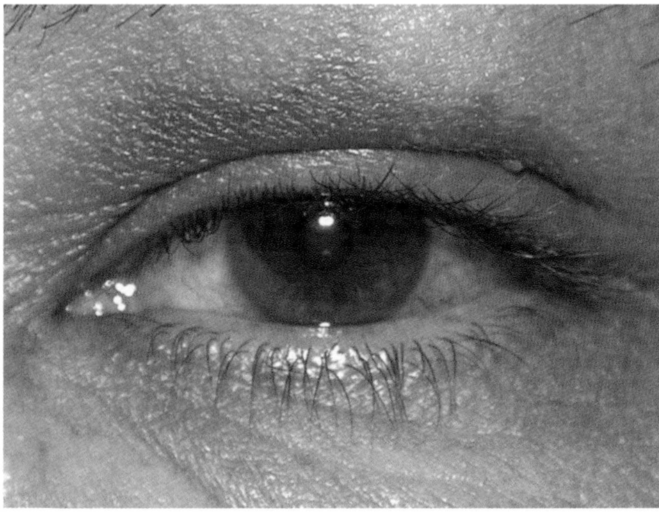

FIGURE 15-2 A young man with traumatic iritis (anterior uveitis) after being hit in the eye with a baseball. He has photophobia and eye pain. (*Reproduced with permission from Richard P. Usatine, MD.*)

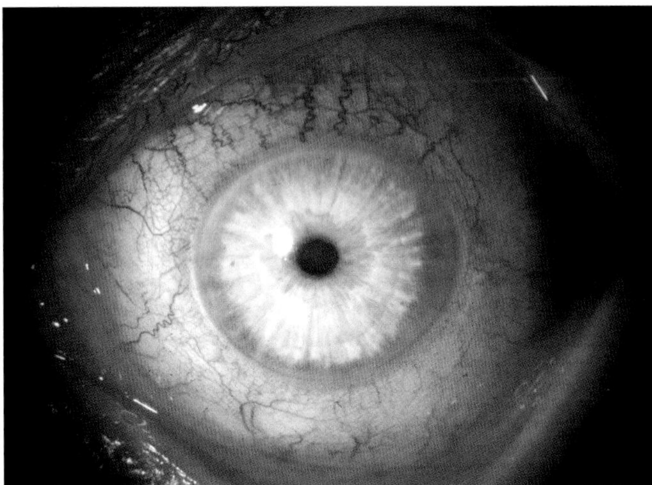

FIGURE 15-3 Idiopathic intermediate uveitis. The ciliary flush is perilimbal injection from dilation of blood vessels adjacent to the cornea, extending 3 mm into the sclera. Perilimbal injection may appear as a violet hue around the limbus with blurring of individual vessels. (*Reproduced with permission from Paul D. Comeau.*)

DIAGNOSIS

CLINICAL FEATURES

Anterior acute uveitis presents with the following symptoms:

- Usually unilateral eye pain, redness, tearing, photophobia, and decreased vision.
- 360-degree perilimbal injection, which is most intense at the limbus (see **Figures 15-1, 15-2**, and **15-4**).
- History of eye trauma, an associated systemic disease, or risk factors for infection.
- Severe anterior uveitis may cause a hypopyon from layering of leukocytes and fibrous debris in the anterior chamber (see **Figure 15-4**).

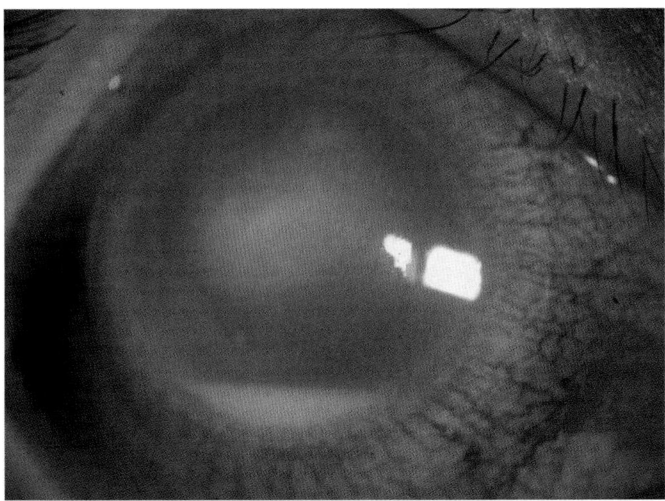

FIGURE 15-4 Hypopyon with severe anterior uveitis, showing layering of leukocytes and fibrinous debris in the anterior chamber, may be sterile or infectious. An intense ciliary flush is seen. Most commonly seen in HLA-B27-positive patients with uveitis. Hypopyon may also be a presenting sign of malignancy (retinoblastoma and lymphoma). (*Reproduced with permission from Paul D. Comeau.*)

Behçet syndrome and HLA-B27 disease are the only 2 common noninfectious causes of hypopyon.

Intermediate and posterior uveitis includes the following symptoms:

- Presents with altered vision or floaters.
- Often there is no pain, redness, tearing, or photophobia.

Sarcoid uveitis presents with the following symptoms:

- Panuveitis (anterior, intermediate, and posterior)
- Gradual and usually a bilateral onset
- Few vision complaints unless cataracts or glaucoma develops
- Characteristic findings on slit-lamp examination (ie, mutton-fat keratic precipitates, posterior iris synechiae)[5]

Typical distribution

Anterior uveitis is typically unilateral and sarcoid uveitis is typically bilateral.

DIFFERENTIAL DIAGNOSIS

Causes of red eye, other than uveitis

- Scleritis—Segmental or diffuse inflammation of sclera (dark red, purple, or blue color); severe, boring eye pain often radiating to head and neck; photophobia and vision loss (see Chapter 14, Scleritis and Episcleritis).
- Episcleritis—Segmental or diffuse inflammation of episclera (pink color), mild or no discomfort, but can be tender to palpation, and no vision disturbance (see Chapter 14, Scleritis and Episcleritis).
- Keratitis or corneal ulcerations—Diffuse erythema with ciliary injection often with constricted pupil; eye discharge; pain, photophobia, and vision loss depending on the location of ulceration. This is frequently associated with trauma, a history of herpes simplex virus (HSV) infection, or contact lens wear. Needs urgent evaluation by an ophthalmologist. There will be staining of the cornea with fluorescein.
- Conjunctivitis—Conjunctival injection, eye discharge, gritty or uncomfortable feeling, and no vision loss (see Chapter 13, Conjunctivitis). Recent history of red eye contacts or upper respiratory infection (URI) symptoms.
- Acute-angle closure glaucoma—Cloudy cornea and scleral injection, eye pain with ipsilateral headache, and severe vision loss (see Chapter 16, Glaucoma). May be a family history of the same.

MANAGEMENT

Refer patients for any red eye along with loss of vision to an ophthalmologist. Patients with uveitis warrant additional examinations by the ophthalmologist.

- Traumatic uveitis—Dilated funduscopy for other ocular trauma, measurement of intraocular pressure, gonioscopy to evaluate for angle recession and risk for future glaucoma, and treatment may include steroid and/or cycloplegics for comfort.
- Nontraumatic uveitis—Slit-lamp examination and laboratory tests to assist with diagnosis of underlying cause; treatment is based on underlying cause but is usually topical steroid drops with or without cycloplegia.
- Therapeutic dilation is used to break the posterior synechiae that can occur (**Figure 15-5**).

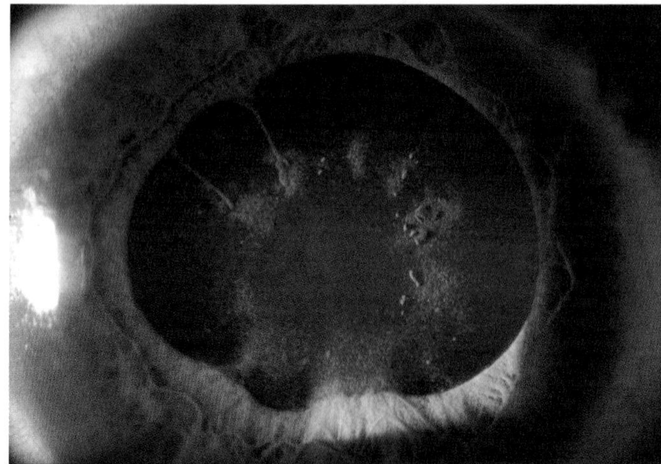

FIGURE 15-5 This patient with uveitis had posterior synechiae that are attachments of the iris to the anterior capsule of the lens. Therapeutic dilation broke the synechiae, but left residual pigment on the anterior capsule. *(Reproduced with permission from Paul D. Comeau.)*

PROGNOSIS

Uveitis causes vision loss, cataract, and often glaucoma if treatment is delayed or not provided. HLA-B27 disease is the most common etiology for anterior uveitis, and is associated with recurrent, bilateral, anterior uveitis.

FOLLOW-UP

Appropriate follow-up is based on the underlying cause.

PATIENT EDUCATION

- See a physician immediately for a red eye with loss of vision.
- A series of tests may be performed to determine the cause of the uveitis; however, the underlying cause is often elusive.

PATIENT RESOURCES

- PubMed Health. *Uveitis*—**http://www.ncbi.nlm.nih.gov/pubmedhealth/PMH0002000/.**

PROVIDER RESOURCES

- Medscape. *Iritis and Uveitis*—**http://emedicine.medscape.com/article/798323.**

REFERENCES

1. Wakefield D, Chang JH. Epidemiology of uveitis. *Int Ophthalmol Clin.* 2005;45(2):1-13.
2. Gritz DC, Wong IG. Incidence and prevalence of uveitis in northern California; the Northern California Epidemiology of Uveitis Study. *Ophthalmology.* 2004;111(3):491-500.
3. Brazis PW, Stewart M, Lee AG. The uveo-meningeal syndromes. *Neurologist.* 2004;10(4):171-184.
4. Capsi RR. A look at autoimmunity and inflammation in the eye. *J Clin Invest.* 2010;120(9):3073-3083.
5. Uyama M. Uveitis in sarcoidosis. *Int Ophthalmol Clin.* 2002;42(1):143-150.

16 GLAUCOMA

Heidi Chumley, MD

PATIENT STORY

A 50-year-old black man was noted to have a large cup-to-disc ratio during a funduscopic examination by his primary care provider (**Figure 16-1**). The patient reported no visual complaints. Further evaluation revealed elevated intraocular pressure (IOP) and early visual field defects. He was started on medication to lower his IOP. He remained asymptomatic, and his visual field defects did not progress for the next several years.

INTRODUCTION

Glaucoma is a leading cause of blindness in the United States and globally. Open-angle glaucoma is an acquired loss of retinal ganglion cells characterized by either normal or increased intraocular pressure, a large cup-to-disc ratio, and visual field defects. Open-angle glaucoma is treated by reducing intraocular pressure, most commonly with eye drops. Angle-closure glaucoma, which is much less common, is an acute increase in IOP from a mechanical obstruction that must be treated emergently to preserve vision.

EPIDEMIOLOGY

- Approximately 2.5 million people in the United States have glaucoma.
- Glaucoma is the second leading cause of blindness in the United States and the leading cause of blindness among African Americans.[1]
- Population studies predict there will be 60.5 million people worldwide with glaucoma by 2010, and of these, 74% will have open-angle glaucoma.[2]
- Women comprise approximately 60% of all glaucoma cases, but 70% of patients with acute angle-closure glaucoma.[2]
- Asians comprise approximately 47% of all glaucoma cases, but 87% of acute angle-closure glaucoma.[2]
- The incidence of primary open-angle glaucoma was 8.3 per 100,000 population in people older than 40 years in a Minnesota population study.[3]
- According to a population-based study, a family history of glaucoma increased the risk of having glaucoma (odds ratio [OR] = 3.08).[4]

ETIOLOGY AND PATHOPHYSIOLOGY

- Glaucoma pathophysiology is incompletely understood, but the end point is the acquired loss of retinal ganglion cells and axons with resulting irreversible vision loss.
- Increased IOP is a well-known risk factor; however, recent attention has turned to ocular perfusion pressure (OPP), the difference between blood pressure (BP) and IOP. OPP is essentially BP minus IOP. As such, OPP is decreased by either high IOP or low BP.[5] If a patient with apparently well-controlled IOP continues to have progressive visual field loss, it may be because of lack of perfusion of the optic nerve from aggressively lowered diastolic BPs. Therefore, the management of glaucoma requires attention to diastolic BP.
- Glaucoma is categorized as either open-angle glaucoma or angle-closure glaucoma.
  - Open-angle—Dysfunction of the aqueous humor drainage system with no visible pathology to the anterior chamber angle
  - Angle-closure—Occlusion of the anterior chamber angle
- Impaired outflow of aqueous humor elevates IOP in some patients, but many patients with open-angle glaucoma have normal IOPs.
- Optic nerve atrophy is seen as optic disc cupping and irreversible visual field loss. Compare **Figures 16-1** and **16-2** to see the difference between abnormal (see **Figure 16-1**) and normal (see **Figure 16-2**) optic disc cupping.

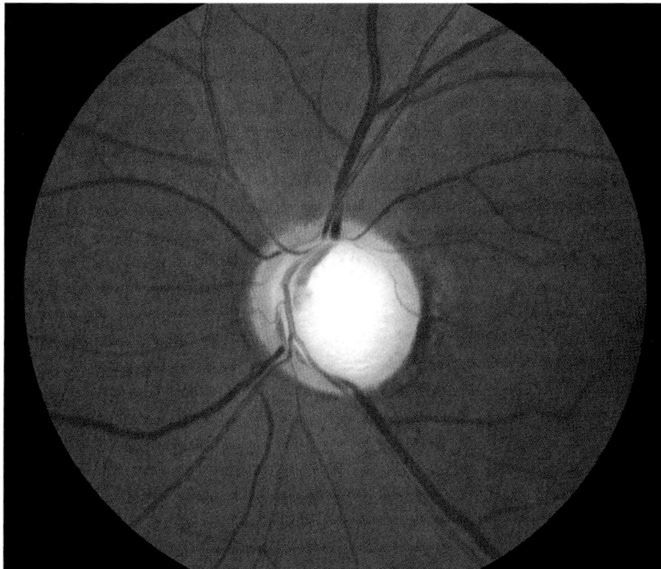

FIGURE 16-1 A 50-year-old man with glaucoma has an increased optic cup-to-disc ratio of 0.8. Median cup-to-disc ratio is 0.2 to 0.3, but varies considerably among individuals. (*Reproduced with permission from Paul D. Comeau.*)

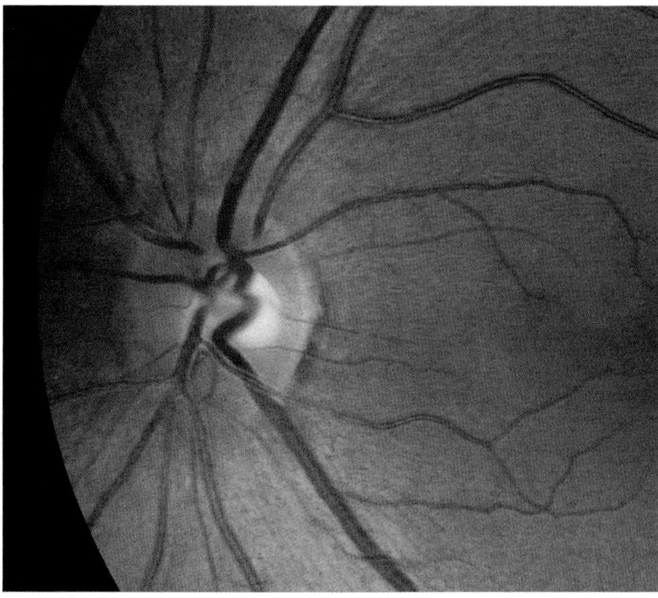

FIGURE 16-2 Normal eye with a normal cup-to-disc ratio of 0.4. A cup-to-disc ratio of more than 0.5 requires further evaluation. (*Reproduced with permission from Paul D. Comeau.*)

RISK FACTORS

Open-angle risk factors include the following:

- Nonmodifiable: age older than 50 years, first-degree family history, and African ancestry[6]
- Modifiable: high IOP, high or low BP, and maybe diabetes mellitus[6]

Acute closed-angle glaucoma is more common in people of Asian descent.

DIAGNOSIS

CLINICAL FEATURES

- Open-angle glaucoma
  - History—Usually asymptomatic, occasionally "tunnel vision"
  - Physical examination—Optic cupping and/or elevated IOP (glaucomatous changes can occur with IOPs in the normal range), loss of peripheral vision by automated perimetry (typically bilateral, but maybe asymmetric)
- Acute closed-angle glaucoma
  - History—Painful red eye (unilateral), vision loss, headache, nausea, halos around lights, and vomiting (**Figure 16-3**)
  - Physical examination—Shallow anterior chamber, optic cupping and elevated IOP, injection of the conjunctiva, and cloudy cornea (see **Figure 16-3**)

Typical distribution

- Open-angle glaucoma is typically bilateral.
- Closed-angle glaucoma is typically unilateral. However, there is a risk for the other eye to undergo the same process, as the abnormal anatomically narrow angle is usually present in the other eye too.

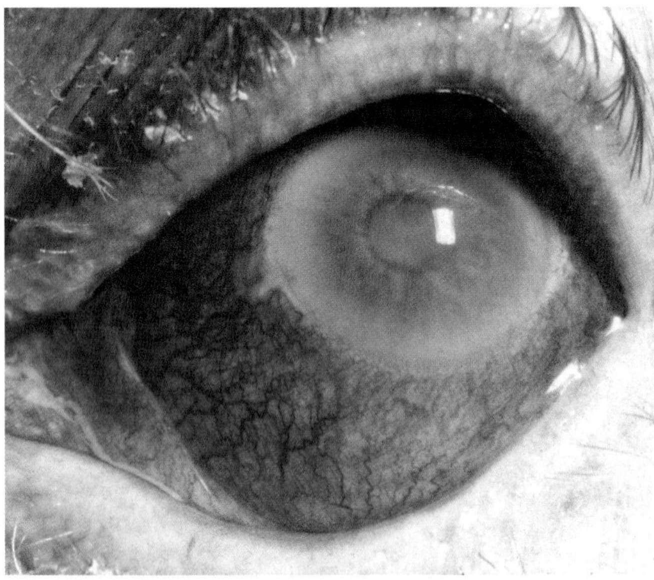

FIGURE 16-3 Acute closed-angle glaucoma with a painful red eye, vision loss, headache, nausea, and vomiting. This is a phacomorphic (ie, lens induced) secondary acute angle closure. The mature cataract increased in anteroposterior (AP) diameter, thus moving the lens-iris diaphragm forward and closing off the angle as well as the pupil thus resulting in high intraocular pressure (IOP), injected conjunctiva, and a cloudy cornea. *(Reproduced with permission from Gilberto Aguirre, MD.)*

DIFFERENTIAL DIAGNOSIS

Glaucoma is the most common cause of optic disc cupping and is sometimes accompanied by elevated IOP.

- Optic disc cupping without elevated IOP can be caused by the following[7]:
  - Physiologic cupping (see **Figure 16-2**)
  - Congenital optic disc anomalies (ie, coloboma or tilted discs)
  - Ischemic (ie, compression by tumors), traumatic (closed-head injury), or hereditary optic neuropathies
- Glaucomatous optic disc cupping compared to other causes has the following[7]:
  - Larger cup-to-disc ratios (compare **Figure 16-1** to **Figure 16-2**)
  - Vertical (as opposed to horizontal) elongation of the cup
  - Disc hemorrhages

MANAGEMENT

Treat with topical agents to decrease IOP by 20% to 40%, which has been demonstrated to decrease glaucoma progression.[8] SOR Ⓐ Many medications are available including the following:

- Nonspecific β-blockers (eg, timolol 0.5%, once or twice a day)
- Prostaglandin analogs (eg, latanoprost 0.005%, once a day)
- Carbonic anhydrase inhibitors (eg, dorzolamide 2%, 2-3 times a day)
- α-Agonists (eg, brimonidine 1.0%, 2-3 times a day)

REFERRAL

- Emergently refer patients with suspected angle-closure glaucoma to an ophthalmologist (see **Figure 16-3**).
- Evaluate (or refer for evaluation) patients with abnormal optic nerve cupping (cup-to-disc ratio >0.5; difference in cup-to-disc ratio of 0.2 or greater between eyes; asymmetric cup), or increased IOP measured by tonometry, or visual field deficits.
- Document the location and extent of visual field deficits with automated perimetry.
- Refer patients with shallow anterior chambers, severe farsightedness (hyperopia), or previous history of acute angle-closure glaucoma to an ophthalmologist.
- Refer for surgical evaluation if you are unable to medically reduce the IOP.

PREVENTION

Screening—According to the US Preventive Services Task Force update in 2005 (**http://www.ahrq.gov/clinic/uspstf/uspsglau.htm**) there is insufficient evidence to recommend for or against population screening for open-angle glaucoma. However, African Americans have been underrepresented in trials. Previously screening has been recommended for African Americans older than age 40 years, Caucasians older than age 65 years, and patients with a family history of glaucoma.[1] SOR Ⓒ

PROGNOSIS

Most patients with open-angle glaucoma, provided they are treated, will not lose vision.

Angle-closure glaucoma must be treated emergently to prevent vision loss.

FOLLOW-UP

Patients with glaucoma should have regular measurements of their IOP and visual fields to follow treatment efficacy.

PATIENT EDUCATION

Advise patients that glaucoma is a progressive disease requiring continued therapy to prevent vision loss.

PATIENT RESOURCES

- Glaucoma research foundation Web site has information on treatment, research progress, personal stories, and practical tips—**http://www.glaucoma.org.**
- PubMed Health. *Glaucoma*—**http://www.ncbi.nlm.nih.gov/pubmedhealth/PMH0002587/.**

PROVIDER RESOURCES

- Medscape. *Acute angle-closure glaucoma*—**http://emedicine.medscape.com/article/798811.**
- Medscape. *Primary open-angle glaucoma*—**http://emedicine.medscape.com/article/1206147.**

REFERENCES

1. Distelhorst JS, Hughes GM. Open-angle glaucoma. *Am Fam Physician.* 2003;67(9):1937-1944.
2. Quigley HA, Broman AT. The number of people with glaucoma worldwide in 2010 and 2020. *Br J Ophthalmol.* 2006;90(3):262-267.
3. Erie JC, Hodge DO, Gray DT. The incidence of primary angle-closure glaucoma in Olmsted County, Minnesota. *Arch Ophthalmol.* 1997;115(2):177-181.
4. Leske MC, Warheit-Roberts L, Wu SY. Open-angle glaucoma and ocular hypertension: the Long Island Glaucoma Case-control Study. *Ophthalmic Epidemiol.* 1996;3(2):85-96.
5. He Z, Vingrys AJ, Armitage JA, Bui BV. The role of blood pressure in glaucoma. *Clin Exp Optom.* 2011;94(2):133-149.
6. Leske MC, Wu SY, Hennis A, et al. Risk factors for incident open-angle glaucoma: the Barbados Eye Studies. *Ophthalmology.* 2008;115:85-93.
7. Piette SD, Sergott RC. Pathological optic-disc cupping. *Curr Opin Ophthalmol.* 2006;17(1):1-6.
8. Heijl A, Leske MC, Bengtsson B, et al. Reduction of intraocular pressure and glaucoma progression: results from the Early Manifest Glaucoma Trial. *Arch Ophthalmol.* 2002;120(10):1268-1279.

17 DIABETIC RETINOPATHY

Heidi Chumley, MD
Kelly Green, MD

PATIENT STORY

A 38-year-old man saw a physician for the first time in 10 years after noticing visual loss in his left eye. His history revealed many risk factors for and symptoms of diabetes mellitus (DM). On an undilated funduscopic examination, his physician was able to see some hemorrhages and hard exudates. A fingerstick in the office showed a blood glucose level of 420 mg/dL. He was treated for DM and referred to an ophthalmologist to be evaluated for diabetic retinopathy (**Figure 17-1**).

INTRODUCTION

Diabetic retinopathy (DR) is a leading cause of blindness in the United States. Nonproliferative DR is characterized by microaneurysms, macular edema, cotton-wool spots, superficial (flame) or deep (dot-blot) hemorrhages, and exudates. Proliferative DR also has neovascularization of the retina, optic nerve head, or iris. Because patients may be asymptomatic until vision loss occurs, screening is indicated in all diabetic patients. Excellent glycemic control lowers a patient's risk of developing DR.

EPIDEMIOLOGY

- In developed nations, DR is the leading cause of blindness among people younger than age 40 years.[1]
- In a community-based study, 29% of adults older than age 40 years with DM had DR. Prevalence in black patients was higher than in Caucasians patients (38.8% vs 26.4%).[2]
- Twenty-one percent of patients have retinopathy at the time type 2 diabetes is diagnosed.[3]
- More than 60% of patients with type 2 DM have retinopathy within 20 years of diagnosis.[3]
- After 40 years of type 1 DM, 84% of patients have retinopathy.[4]

ETIOLOGY AND PATHOPHYSIOLOGY

- Hyperglycemia results in microvascular complications including retinopathy.
- Several biochemical pathways linking hyperglycemia and retinopathy have been proposed.[3]
- In nonproliferative retinopathy, microaneurysms weaken vessel walls. Vessels then leak fluid, lipids, and blood resulting in macular edema, exudates, and hemorrhages (**Figures 17-1** and **17-2**).
- Cotton-wool spots result when small vessel occlusion causes focal ischemia to the superficial nerve fiber layer of the retina.
- In proliferative retinopathy, new blood vessels form in response to ischemia (**Figure 17-3**).

RISK FACTORS

- In type 1 DM, identified risk factors include longer diabetes duration, high hemoglobin (Hgb) A_{1c}, hypertension, smoking, and male gender.[4,5]
- In type 2 DM, identified risk factors include longer diabetes duration, high $HgbA_{1c}$, elevated systolic blood pressure, male gender, presence of albuminuria, and pharmacologic therapy.[6]

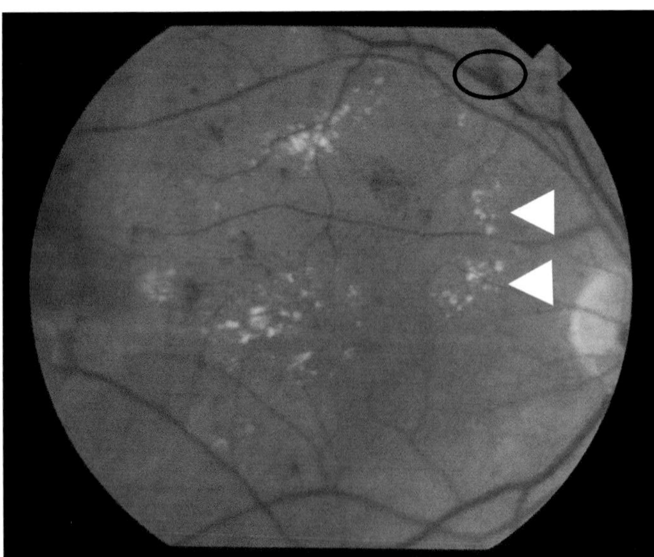

FIGURE 17-1 Dilated funduscopic photograph demonstrating microaneurysms (small red swellings attached to vessels), which are often the first change in diabetic retinopathy. Also present are flame hemorrhages (*black oval*) and hard exudates (*white arrowheads*). The hard exudates are yellow in color. This case is an example of diabetic nonproliferative retinopathy. (*Reproduced with permission from Paul D. Comeau.*)

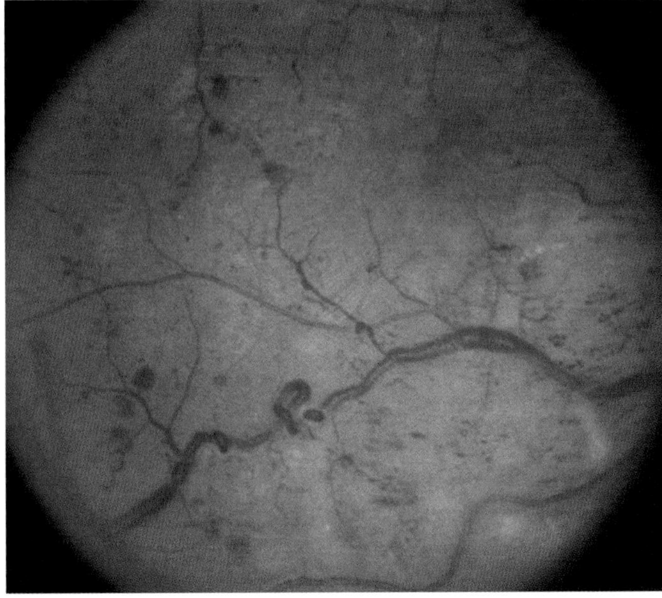

FIGURE 17-2 Very severe nonproliferative diabetic retinopathy with multiple deep dot-blot hemorrhages, venous beading, and looping. This patient may benefit from panretinal photocoagulation. (*Reproduced with permission from Paul D. Comeau.*)

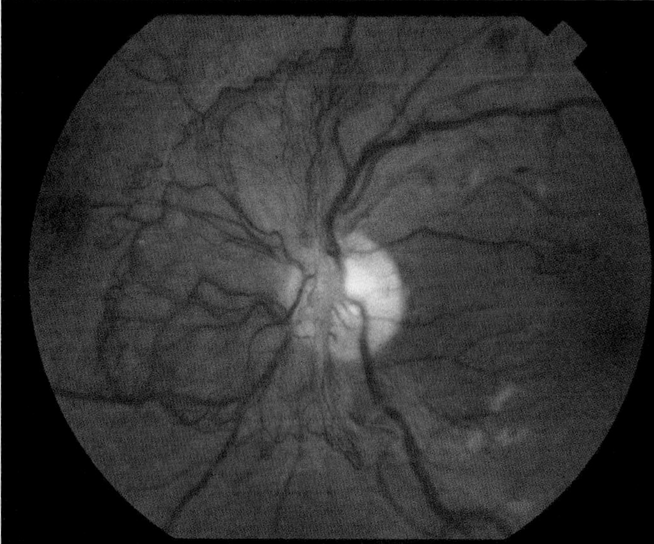

FIGURE 17-3 Proliferative diabetic retinopathy showing newly developed, porous, friable blood vessels. New vessels can be seen on the optic disc and peripheral retina. Panretinal photocoagulation may help prevent vitreous hemorrhage, retinal detachment, and neovascular glaucoma. (*Reproduced with permission from Paul D. Comeau.*)

DIAGNOSIS

Definitive diagnosis is made by an eye specialist.

- Gold standard is grading of stereoscopic color fundus photographs in seven standard fields.[3]
- In comparison with the gold standard, a single monochromatic digital photo through a nondilated eye is sufficient to determine the presence or absence of DR with a sensitivity and specificity of 71% and 96%, respectively.[7] SOR Ⓑ

CLINICAL FEATURES

- Central vision loss as a result of macular edema or macular ischemia.
- Nonproliferative retinopathy—Microaneurysms are seen initially (mild), followed by macular edema, cotton-wool spots, superficial (flame) or deep (dot-blot) hemorrhages, and exudates (**Figure 17-1** shows moderate, and **Figure 17-2** shows severe).
- Proliferative retinopathy—Neovascularization, that is, growth of new blood vessels on the optic disc (see **Figure 17-3**), the retina, or iris.

DIFFERENTIAL DIAGNOSIS

Retinopathy is also seen with other systemic illnesses and infections including the following:

- Hypertensive retinopathy—Arterial narrowing or atrioventricular nicking in addition to cotton-wool spots (see Chapter 18, Hypertensive Retinopathy)
- HIV retinopathy—Cotton-wool spots and infections such as cytomegalovirus

MANAGEMENT

Diabetes and vascular risk factors should be controlled.

- Glycemic control lowers the risk of retinopathy (35% risk reduction per 1 point $HgbA_{1C}$ reduction).[3] SOR Ⓐ
- Blood pressure control improves visual outcomes (34% risk reduction in retinopathy progression; 47% risk reduction for declines in visual acuity).[3] SOR Ⓐ
- Treatment with angiotensin-converting enzyme inhibitors (ACEIs) or angiotensin receptor blockers (ARBs) in type 1 DM or an ARB in type 2 DM have been shown to reduce retinopathy progression independent of blood pressure control.[8,9] SOR Ⓑ
- Patients with high lipids have more hard exudates and a higher risk of vision loss, but it is unclear if lipid control changes outcomes. SOR Ⓒ

REFERRAL

Work with an ophthalmologist to prevent vision loss.

- Complications of DR are vitreous hemorrhage (**Figure 17-4**), retinal detachment, and neovascular glaucoma. Each of these complications can result in devastating vision loss.
- Ophthalmologists will determine when peripheral retinal photocoagulation is indicated (**Figure 17-5**). Photocoagulation reduces the risk of severe visual loss by more than 50% with side effects of peripheral and night vision loss.[10] SOR Ⓐ Other surgical treatments, including vitrectomy, have been less successful.[3]

PREVENTION

Prevent DR by preventing development of type 2 DM or tightly controlling type 1 or type 2 DM.

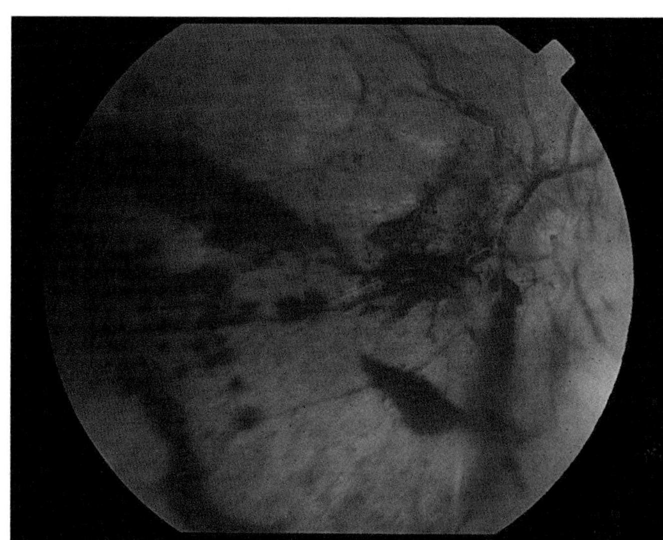

FIGURE 17-4 This vitreous hemorrhage occurred when friable neovascular membranes broke spontaneously. The patient described a "shower of red dots" obscuring the vision and then loss of vision in that eye. (*Reproduced with permission from Paul D. Comeau.*)

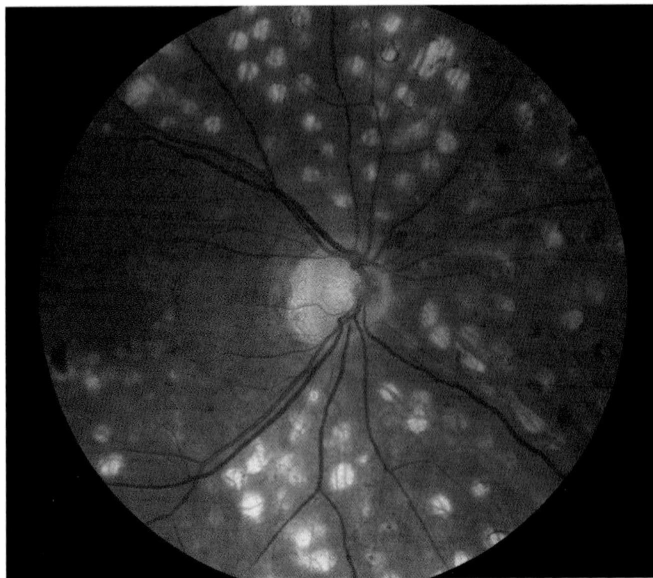

FIGURE 17-5 Panretinal photocoagulation is the application of laser burns to the peripheral retina. The ischemic peripheral retina is treated with thousands of laser spots to presumably eliminate vasogenic factors responsible for the development of neovascular vessels. Laser spots cause scarring of the retina and choroid. The scars may be hypotrophic (*white spots*) or hypertrophic (*black spots*). (*Reproduced with permission from Paul D. Comeau.*)

Screen patients with DM for DR based on national recommendations[11]:

- Type 1 DM—Adults and children older than age 10 years—Screen for retinopathy 5 years after diagnosis and at regular intervals as recommended by an eye specialist.
- Type 2 DM—Screen for retinopathy at diagnosis and then annually.

Patients can be referred to an eye specialist, or screened using telemedicine or retinal photographs taken during outreach screenings or in primary care offices.[12,13]

Mathematical models are being developed to individualize screening frequency. In one study, screening intervals ranged from 6 to 60 months (mean: 29 months). This resulted in 59% fewer visits than with fixed annual screening without compromising safety.[14]

FOLLOW-UP

Once DR is diagnosed frequency of examination is set by the ophthalmologist.

PATIENT EDUCATION

Preventing retinopathy by controlling diabetes and hypertension leads to better vision outcomes than any available treatment.[3,10]

PATIENT RESOURCES

- National Eye Institute—**http://www.nei.nih.gov/health/diabetic/**.

PROVIDER RESOURCES

- Medscape. *Diabetic Retinopathy*—**http://emedicine.medscape.com/article/1225122.**

REFERENCES

1. Congdon NG, Friedman DS, Lietman T. Important causes of visual impairment in the world today. *JAMA*. 2003;290(15):2057-2060.
2. Zhang X, Saaddine JB, Chou CF, et al. Prevalence of diabetic retinopathy in the United States, 2005–2008. *JAMA*. 2010;304(6):649-656.
3. Fong DS, Aiello LP, Ferris FL III, Klein R. Diabetic retinopathy. *Diabetes Care*. 2004;27(10):2540-2553.
4. Hammes HP, Kerner W, Hofer S, et al. Diabetic retinopathy in type 1 diabetes—a contemporary analysis of 8,784 patients. *Diabetologia*. 2011;54(8):1977-1984.
5. Romero-Aroca P, Baget-Bernaldiz M, Fernandez-Ballart J, et al. Ten-year incidence of diabetic retinopathy and macular edema. Risk factors in a sample of type 1 diabetes patients. *Diabetes Res Clin Pract*. 2011;94(1):126-132.
6. Semeraro F, Parrinello G, Cancarini A, et al. Predicting the risk of diabetic retinopathy in type 2 diabetic patients. *J Diabetes Complications*. 2011;25(5):292-297.
7. Vujosevic S, Benetti E, Massignan F, et al. Screening for diabetic retinopathy: 1 and 3 nonmydriatic 45-degree digital fundus photographs vs 7 standard early treatment diabetic retinopathy study fields. *Am J Ophthalmol*. 2009;148(1):111-118.
8. Chaturvedi N, Sjolie AK, Stephenson JM, et al. Effect of lisinopril on progression of retinopathy in normotensive people with type 1 diabetes. EURODIAB Controlled Trial of Lisinopril in Insulin-Dependent Diabetes Mellitus. *Lancet*. 1998;351:28-31.
9. Sjolie AK, Klein R, Porta M, et al. Effect of candesartan on progression and regression of retinopathy in type 2 diabetes (DIRECT-Protect 2): a randomised placebo-controlled trial. *Lancet*. 2008;372:1385-1393.
10. The Diabetic Retinopathy Study Research Group. Photocoagulation treatment of proliferative diabetic retinopathy: the second report of diabetic retinopathy study findings. *Ophthalmology*. 1978;85(1):82-106.
11. American Diabetes Association. Standards of medical care in diabetes—2009. *Diabetes Care*. 2009;32(suppl 1):S13-S61.
12. Sanchez CR, Silva PS, Cavallerano JD, et al. Ocular telemedicine for diabetic retinopathy and the Joslin Vision Network. *Semin Ophthalmol*. 2010;25(5-6):218-224.
13. Bragge P, Gruen RL, Chau M, et al. Screening for presence or absence of diabetic retinopathy: a meta-analysis. *Arch Ophthalmol*. 2011;129(4):435-444.
14. Aspelund T, Thornórisdóttir O, Olafsdottir E, et al. Individual risk assessment and information technology to optimise screening frequency for diabetic retinopathy. *Diabetologia*. 2011;54(10):2525-2532.

18 HYPERTENSIVE RETINOPATHY

Heidi Chumley, MD
Kelly Green, MD

PATIENT STORY

A 37-year-old man comes in for a physical examination and is noted to have a blood pressure of 198/142 mmHg. He has no symptoms at the time. The physician performs a dilated funduscopic examination and notes optic disc edema, cotton-wool spots, flame hemorrhages, dot-blot hemorrhages, arteriovenous nicking, and exudates (**Figure 18-1**). Fortunately, the remainder of the neurologic examination and the electrocardiography (ECG) are normal. The patient is sent to the emergency room to be evaluated further and treated for a hypertensive emergency.

INTRODUCTION

Hypertensive retinopathy (HR) develops from elevated blood pressure. HR is diagnosed clinically by the presence of classic retina findings seen on funduscopic examination or digital retinal photographs in a patient with hypertension. HR can result in vision loss. Treatment is control of blood pressure.

EPIDEMIOLOGY

- Prevalence of 7.7% (black) versus 4.1% (Caucasians) in a population study of men and women between 49 and 73 years of age without diabetes.[1]
- Multiple studies show that patients with moderate HR are 2 to 3 times more likely to have a stroke than those without HR at the same level of blood pressure control independent of other risk factors.[2]

ETIOLOGY AND PATHOPHYSIOLOGY

High blood pressure results in the following retinal findings[3]:

- Retinal vessels become narrow and straighten at diastolic blood pressure (DBP) of 90 to 110 mm Hg.
- Arteriovenous "nicking" (white oval in **Figure 18-1**) occurs when the arteriolar wall enlarges from arteriosclerosis, compressing the vein. Patients with hypertension are at risk for central and branch retinal vein occlusions, which can result in significant vision loss.
- Microaneurysms and flame hemorrhages (**Figures 18-1** and **18-2**) result from the increased intravascular pressure. Cotton-wool spots (dashed arrow in **Figure 18-2**) represent ischemia of the nerve fiber layer. Hard exudates indicate vascular leakage (see *white arrowheads* in **Figure 17-1**, Chapter 17).
- DBP 110 to 115 mmHg causes leakage of plasma proteins and blood products resulting in retinal hemorrhages and hard exudates (**Figures 18-1** to **18-4**).
- Optic nerve swelling occurs at DBP of 130 to 140 mmHg (see **Figure 18-3**).

DIAGNOSIS

The diagnosis is made clinically from typical retinal findings in a patient with hypertension. These findings can be seen using funduscopic examination or by viewing retinal digital images. Retinal digital images have a higher interobserver reliability than funduscopic examination.[4]

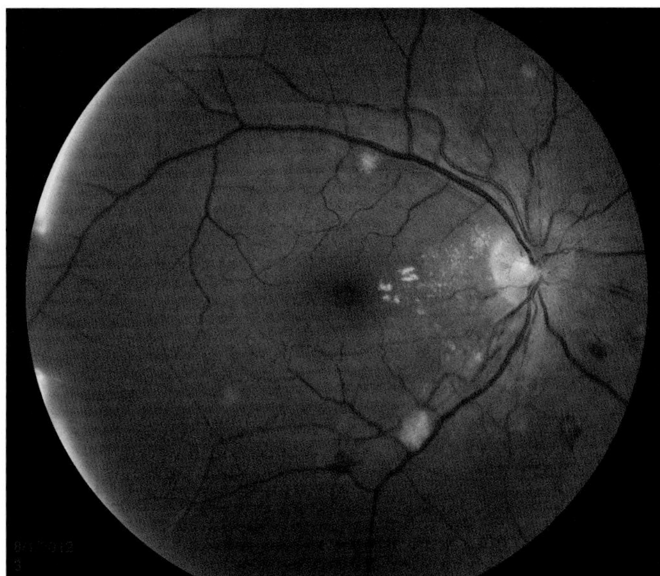

FIGURE 18-1 Hypertensive retinopathy with optic disc edema, cotton-wool spots, flame hemorrhages, dot-blot hemorrhages, arteriovenous nicking, and exudates. (*Reproduced with permission from EyeRounds.org and The University of Iowa.*)

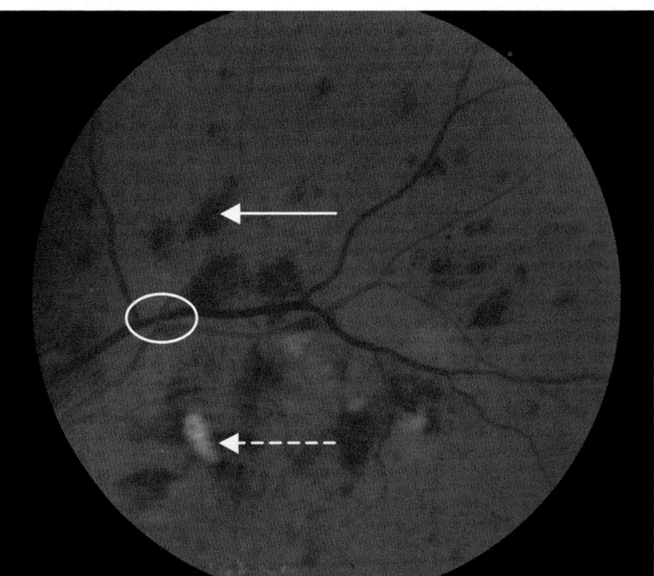

FIGURE 18-2 More advanced hypertensive retinopathy with flame hemorrhages (*white arrow*), arteriovenous nicking (*white oval*), and cotton-wool spots (*dashed arrow*). (*Reproduced with permission from Paul D. Comeau.*)

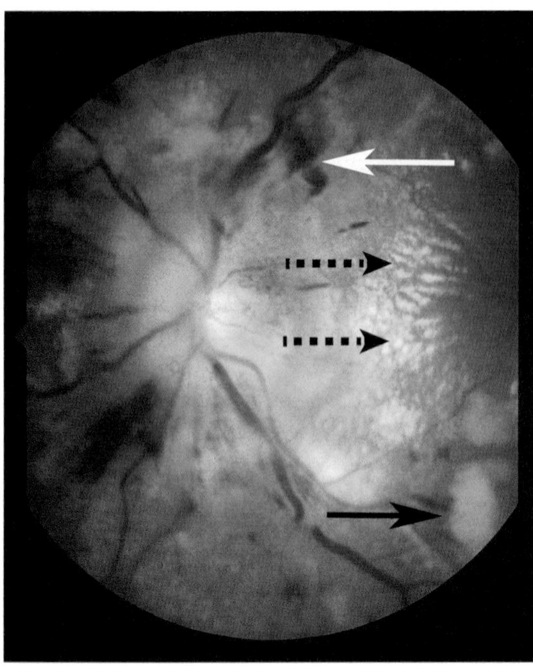

FIGURE 18-3 Malignant hypertensive retinopathy with optic nerve head edema (papilledema), flame hemorrhages (*white arrow*), cotton-wool spots (*black arrow*), and macular edema with exudates (*dashed arrows*). The patient was admitted to the hospital to treat malignant hypertension aggressively. (*Reproduced with permission from Paul D. Comeau.*)

CLINICAL FEATURES

Following are the clinical features in order of increasing severity:

- Mild arteriolar narrowing
- Severe arteriolar narrowing plus arteriovenous nicking
- Retinal hemorrhages, microaneurysms, hard exudation, cotton-wool spots
- Swelling of the optic nerve head and macular star, also called as accelerated or malignant HR

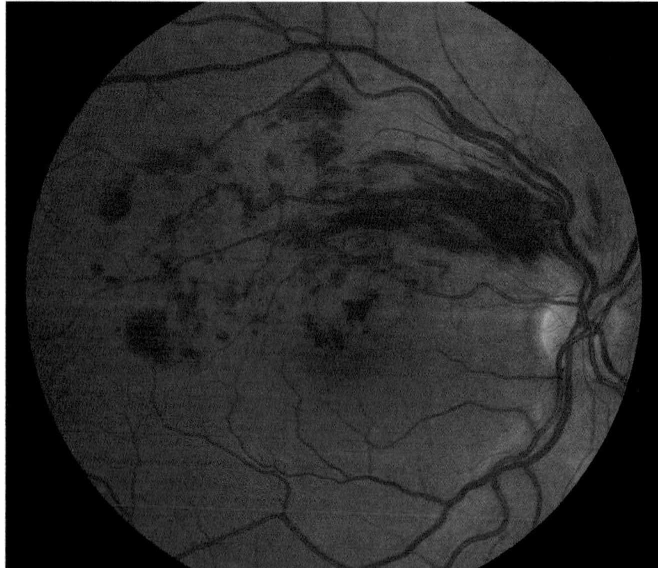

FIGURE 18-4 Branch retinal vein occlusion of a major retinal vein associated with hypertension. The patient noted new onset of blurred vision and visual field constriction. Flame hemorrhages are seen along the course of the obstructed vein. (*Reproduced with permission from Paul D. Comeau.*)

TYPICAL DISTRIBUTION

Bilateral and symmetrical

LABORATORY TESTING

- Laboratory tests are not needed to make the diagnosis.
- Recommended tests for patients with hypertension include urinalysis, blood glucose, hematocrit, serum potassium, creatinine, calcium, and a fasting lipid profile.
- 12-lead ECG is also recommended.[5]

DIFFERENTIAL DIAGNOSIS

Retinal vessel narrowing, atrioventricular nicking, microaneurysms, retinal hemorrhages, hard exudates, and cotton-wool spots are also seen in other conditions that impair blood flow, including the following:

- Diabetic retinopathy (see Chapter 17, Diabetic Retinopathy)
- Radiation retinopathy
- Venous or carotid artery occlusive disease
- Systemic illnesses such as collagen vascular disease
- Hematologic diseases such as anemia and leukemia
- Systemic infectious diseases such as HIV

Optic nerve swelling and a macular star (blurring of the macula in a star-like pattern) also occur in the following:

- Neuroretinitis
- Diabetic papillopathy
- Radiation optic retinopathy
- Optic neuritis
- Intracranial disease

MANAGEMENT

Patients with funduscopic findings of HR should have their blood pressure measured and treated to reduce the risk of heart and cerebrovascular disease.[5] SOR Ⓐ

Nonpharmacologic

- Assist patients in smoking cessation. This will result in the greatest benefit in morbidity and mortality.
- Reduce weight or maintain normal body mass index (BMI).
- Eat a diet rich in fruits and vegetables and low in saturated fats.
- Reduce sodium to less than 6 g of sodium chloride per day.
- Engage in regular physical activity for 30 minutes most days of the week.
- Limit alcohol to 2 drinks per day in men and 1 drink per day in women.

Medications

- Start a thiazide diuretic to achieve blood pressure of less than 140/90 mmHg unless contraindicated; a blood pressure goal of 130/80 mmHg should be used for patients with diabetes. Consider an angiotensin-converting enzyme inhibitor (ACEI) as an initial medication for patients with diabetes. Consider other medications only for patients with compelling indications.

- Although the largest benefit in outcomes is seen with the first medication, additional medications should be considered to achieve blood pressure less than 140/90 mmHg after weighing the risks and benefits with the patient.
- Evaluate and manage other risk factors for cardiovascular disease, including high cholesterol and diabetes.

REFERRAL

Patients experiencing acute visual disturbances should be referred for evaluation of hemorrhage or optic nerve edema (see **Figures 18-3** and **18-4**).

PREVENTION

- Maintain normal blood pressure through a healthy lifestyle and medications when needed.
- Patients with hypertension alone do not require routine funduscopic examination, unless they also have diabetes mellitus.[6] SOR Ⓐ
- Prevention is obtained by preventing and controlling high blood pressure.

PROGNOSIS

- Prognosis is associated with severity of hypertension retinopathy.
- Three-year survival in patients with mild arteriolar narrowing is 70% compared to 6% in patients with swelling of the optic nerve or macular star.[7]

FOLLOW-UP

Once diagnosed with hypertension, patients should be seen every month until blood pressure is controlled and then every 3 to 6 months.[4] SOR Ⓒ

PATIENT EDUCATION

- HR does not require treatment other than lowering blood pressure unless acute vision changes occur.
- Control of blood pressure typically reverses HR findings, except for optic nerve edema, which may result in permanent vision loss.
- Control of blood pressure also reduces the risk of heart attack and stroke.

PATIENT RESOURCES

- PubMed Health. *High blood pressure and eye disease*—**http://www.ncbi.nlm.nih.gov/pubmedhealth/PMH0001994/.**

PROVIDER RESOURCES

- Medscape. *Ophthalmologic Manifestations of Hypertension*—**http://emedicine.medscape.com/article/1201779.**
- The Eighth Report of the Joint National Committee on Prevention, Detection, Evaluation, and Treatment of High Blood Pressure (JNC 8), 2012—**http://www.nhlbi.nih.gov/guidelines/hypertension/jnc8/index.htm.**

REFERENCES

1. Wong TY, Klein R, Duncan BB, et al. Racial differences in the prevalence of hypertensive retinopathy. *Hypertension.* 2003;41(5):1086-1091.
2. Baker ML, Hand PJ, Wang JJ, Wong TY. Retinal signs and stroke: revisiting the link between the eye and brain. *Stroke.* 2008;39(4):1371-1379.
3. Luo BP, Brown GC. Update on the ocular manifestations of systemic arterial hypertension. *Curr Opin Ophthalmol.* 2004;15(3):203-210.
4. Castro AF, Silva-Turnes JC, Gonzalez F. Evaluation of retinal digital images by a general practitioner. *Telemed J E Health.* 2007;13(3):287-292.
5. NIH, NHLBI, and National High Blood Pressure Education Program. *The Seventh Report of the Joint National Committee on the Prevention, Detection, Evaluation, and Treatment of High Blood Pressure,* 2004. Washington, DC: U.S. Department of Health and Human Services; 2006.
6. van den Born BJ, Hulsman CA, Hoekstra JB, et al. Value of routine funduscopy in patients with hypertension: systematic review. *BMJ.* 2005;331(7508):73.
7. Keith NM, Wagener HP, Barker NW. Some different types of essential hypertension: their course and prognosis. *Am J Med Sci.* 1939;197:332-343.

19 PAPILLEDEMA

Heidi Chumley, MD

PATIENT STORY

A 29-year-old obese woman presented with chronic headaches that were worse in the morning or while lying down. She denied nausea or other neurologic symptoms. She had no other medical problems and took no medications. On examination, she had a visual acuity of 20/20 in both eyes, bilateral papilledema (**Figure 19-1**), no spontaneous venous pulsations (SVPs), and no other neurologic signs. She had a brain magnetic resonance imaging (MRI) showing no mass or hydrocephalus, and elevated intracranial pressure (ICP) measured by lumbar puncture. She was diagnosed with idiopathic intracranial hypertension (IIH) and was followed closely for any changes in her vision. She was started on acetazolamide and assisted with a weight loss program. Her symptoms resolved over the course of 18 months.

INTRODUCTION

The term *papilledema* refers specifically to optic disc swelling related to increased intracranial pressure. When no localizing neurologic signs or space-occupying lesion is present, IIH is a likely cause in patients younger than age 45 years, especially obese women. Patients with IIH usually present with daily pulsatile headache with nausea and often have transient visual disturbances and/or pulsatile tinnitus. Patients often report a "whooshing" sound that they hear. Bilateral papilledema and visual field defects on a perimetry test are found in almost all patients. Elevated opening pressure on lumbar puncture is required for the diagnosis.

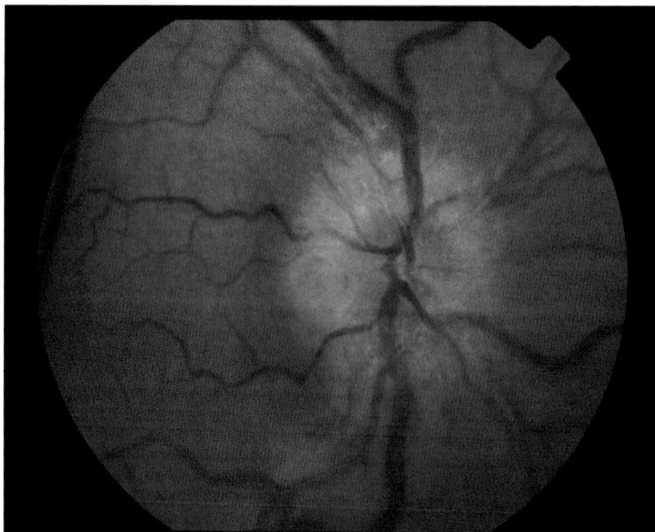

FIGURE 19-1 Papilledema from increased intracranial pressure (ICP). The optic disc is elevated and hyperemic with engorged retinal veins. The entire optic disc margin is blurred. Optic neuropathies can also have blurring of the entire disc margin, but often, only part of the disc is blurred. (*Reproduced with permission from Paul D. Comeau.*)

CHAPTER 19

SYNONYMS

Papilledema is also known as *pseudotumor cerebri* or *benign intracranial hypertension*.

EPIDEMIOLOGY

Idiopathic intracranial hypertension (IIH) occurs in the following:

- About 1 per 100,000 people.[1]
- About 20 per 100,000 obese females of ages 15 to 44 years.[1]
- Prevalence may be increasing with increasing obesity. A UK population study found a prevalence of 85.7 per 100,000 in obese women.[2]
- Mean age of diagnosis is approximately 30 years.

ETIOLOGY AND PATHOPHYSIOLOGY

The optic disc swells because of elevated intracranial pressure. In IIH, the cerebral spinal fluid pressure is increased. The cause of this increase in unknown, but a current hypothesis is that IIH is a syndrome of reduced cerebrospinal fluid (CSF) absorption.

RISK FACTORS

IIH is much more common in obese women of childbearing age.

DIAGNOSIS

Patients with papilledema should undergo imaging, preferably MRI, followed by lumbar puncture. IIH is a diagnosis of exclusion with the following criteria[3]:

- Signs and symptoms of increased ICP (headache, transient visual disturbances, papilledema) are present.
- Normal neurologic examination, except a sixth nerve palsy may be present. This will lead to a complaint of diplopia.
- Elevated ICP is present, as measured by lumbar puncture opening pressure greater than 250 mm of water in the lateral decubitus position, with normal CSF on microscopic examination.
- No evidence of mass, hydrocephalus, or vascular lesions is seen by MRI.
- No other identifiable cause of increased intracranial hypertension.

CLINICAL FEATURES

- More than 90% of patients with IIH are obese women of childbearing age. Look for a different diagnosis in children, men, and older patients.[3]
- Headaches and visual changes are the most common symptoms.
- Difficulty in thinking or concentrating is frequently reported. New studies indicate cognitive impairment, particularly in learning and memory.[4]
- SVP are retinal vein pulsations at the optic disc and are typically absent in IIH patients. SVP are seen in 90% of patients with normal intracranial pressure, and are absent when the CSF pressure is above 190 mmHg. As the CSF pressure may be transiently normal in IIH, the presence of SVP does not preclude IIH, but indicates that the CSF pressure is normal at that moment.[5]

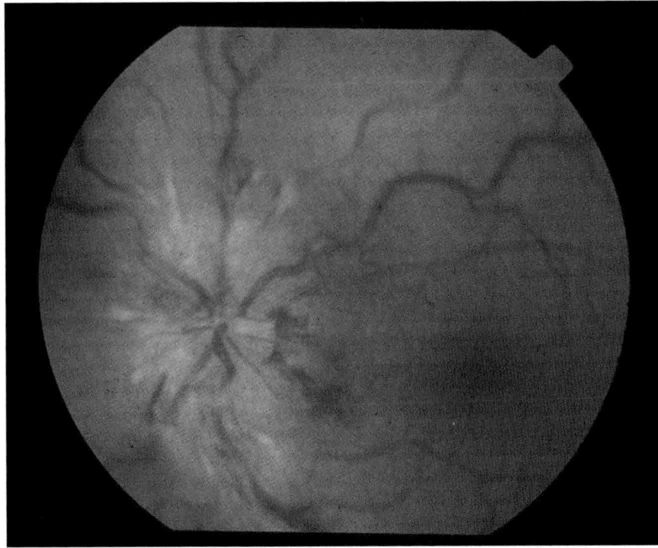

FIGURE 19-2 Severe acute papilledema with papillary flame hemorrhages and cotton-wool spots that obscure the disc vessels. The blurred edges of the optic disc appear as a starburst. (*Reproduced with permission from Paul D. Comeau.*)

TYPICAL DISTRIBUTION

Papilledema is bilateral in the overwhelming majority of cases (see **Figures 19-1** and **19-2**). Unilateral optic disc swelling has been rarely noted with elevated intracranial pressure.

LABORATORY TESTING

Cerebral spinal fluid is typically sent for cell count and culture.

IMAGING

- Traditionally, imaging was used to rule out intracranial mass or venus sinus obstruction; however, several imaging modalities show promise as tools that may mitigate the need for recurrent lumbar punctures to monitor pressures.
- Transorbital sonography measurements of optic nerve sheath diameter detected raised ICP with a sensitivity of 90% and a specificity of 84%.[6]
- Optical coherence tomography (OCT) is an imaging modality used in the ophthalmology office that can distinguish between a normal optic disc, moderate elevation, and papilledema in patients with IIH based on differences in retinal nerve fiber layer thickness.[7]
- MRI findings in IIH include optic nerve tortuosity, partial empty sella, and transverse sinus narrowing. These changes reverse after pressure is reduced and return if pressure increases.[8]

DIFFERENTIAL DIAGNOSIS

- Pseudopapilledema or optic disc drusen, an optic nerve anomaly that elevates the optic disc surface and blurs the disc margins, which can be caused by calcifications in the optic nerve head.
- Optic neuropathies, swelling of all or parts of one or both discs, which can be caused by ischemia or demyelination (as in multiple sclerosis), and may be seen in 1% to 2% of patients with diabetes mellitus type 1 or 2.[9]

Elevated ICP can also be caused by obstructing lesions, medical conditions, or medications[3]:

- Mass lesions, hydrocephalus, venus sinus or jugular venus thrombosis, and meningeal infections
- Addison disease, hypoparathyroidism, chronic obstructive pulmonary disease (COPD), sleep apnea, renal failure, pulmonary hypertension, and severe anemia
- Antibiotics in the tetracycline family, vitamin A, anabolic steroids, lithium, and corticosteroid withdrawal

MANAGEMENT

In many cases, IIH is self-limiting, presents without visual symptoms, and will resolve over several years without loss of vision. However, when patients present with persistent or worsening visual disturbances, treatment is required to lower the ICP to prevent optic nerve damage and irreversible loss of vision. Management of the headache is a key factor when choosing a therapeutic plan. Management includes the following:

- Nonpharmacologic
  - Careful observation (often by an ophthalmologist) with documentation of any visual changes. Formal visual field testing is indicated.
  - Weight loss of 15% of body weight is beneficial but will not decrease the ICP quickly enough if visual compromise is present.[1] SOR C
- Medications
  - Acetazolamide 1000 to 2000 mg/d; early studies indicate that topiramate may also be effective; other diuretics such as furosemide are less effective.[10] SOR C
  - High-dose corticosteroids for short time periods for rare cases of rapidly advancing vision loss.[1,10] SOR C
- Refer or hospitalize
  - Surgical interventions for severe, recalcitrant cases include optic nerve sheath fenestration and lumbar peritoneal shunt. Surgery is also considered in special populations such as pregnant women and dialysis patients.[1,10] SOR C
  - Transverse sinus stenting is a newer surgical technique that holds promise.[11]

PREVENTION

Maintenance of ideal body weight may prevent IIH.

PROGNOSIS

Although approximately two-thirds of patients with IIH present with visual impairment, the majority of patients improve. One study reported 9% of patients had permanent visual loss.[12]

FOLLOW-UP

Patients should be followed up every 3 to 6 months by a physician who can adequately view the entire optic disc and document visual acuity and visual field deficits. They should be seen immediately for any visual changes.

PATIENT EDUCATION

Advise patients with new papilledema of the need for an evaluation for dangerous causes of increased ICP, such as intracranial masses or underlying medical illnesses. Also advise patients that IIH often resolves spontaneously over several years, but they should report any visual changes immediately.

PATIENT RESOURCES

- The Intracranial Hypertension Research Foundation has information for patients—**http://www.ihrfoundation.org.**

PROVIDER RESOURCES

- The Intracranial Hypertension Research Foundation has information for medical professionals including ongoing research studies and information on patient registries—**http://www.ihrfoundation.org.**

REFERENCES

1. Mathews MK, Sergott RC, Savino PJ. Pseudotumor cerebri. *Curr Opin Ophthalmol.* 2003;14(6):364-370.
2. Raoof N, Sharrack B, Pepper IM, Hickman SJ. The incidence and prevalence of idiopathic intracranial hypertension in Sheffield, UK. *Eur J Neurol.* 2011;18(10):1266-1268.
3. Friedman DI, Jacobson DM. Diagnostic criteria for idiopathic intracranial hypertension. *Neurology.* 2002;59(10):1492-1495.
4. Kharkar S, Hernandez R, Batra S, et al. Cognitive impairment in patients with pseudotumor cerebri syndrome. *Behav Neurol.* 2011;24(2):143-148.
5. Jacks AS, Miller NR. Spontaneous retinal venous pulsation: aetiology and significance. *J Neurol Neurosurg Psychiatry.* 2003;74(1):7-9.
6. Bauerle J, Nedelmann M. Sonographic assessment of the optic nerve sheath in idiopathic intracranial hypertension. *J Neurol.* 2011;258(11):2014-2019.
7. Waisbourd M, Leibovitch I, Goldenberg D, Kesler A. OCT assessment of morphological changes of the optic nerve head and macula in idiopathic intracranial hypertension. *Clin Neurol Neurosurg.* 2011;113(10):839-843.
8. George U, Bansal G, Pandian J. Magnetic resonance "flip-flop" in idiopathic intracranial hypertension. *J Neurosci Rural Pract.* 2011;2(1):84-86.
9. Bayraktar Z, Alacali N, Bayraktar S. Diabetic papillopathy in type II diabetic patients. *Retina.* 2002;22(6):752-758.
10. Friedman DI, Jacobson DM. Idiopathic intracranial hypertension. *J Neuroophthalmol.* 2004;24(2):138-145.
11. Ahmed RM, Wilkinson M, Parker GD, et al. Transverse sinus stenting for idiopathic intracranial hypertension: a review of 52 patients and of model predictions. *AJNR Am J Neuroradiol.* 2011;32(8):1408-1414.
12. Baheti NN, Nair M, Thomas SV. Long-term visual outcome in idiopathic intracranial hypertension. *Ann Indian Acad Neurol.* 2011;14(1):19-22.

20 AGE-RELATED MACULAR DEGENERATION

Heidi Chumley, MD

PATIENT STORY

A 78-year-old white woman presents with loss of central vision that has gradually worsened over the last 6 months. Fully independent before, she can no longer drive and has difficulty with activities of daily living. Her peripheral vision remains normal. Funduscopic examination reveals macular depigmentation and drusen (yellowish-colored subretinal deposits on the macula) (**Figure 20-1**). She is diagnosed with dry, age-related macular degeneration (AMD). After her physician discusses the available information about antioxidants and therapeutic options, she decides to start antioxidants and see an ophthalmologist to discuss laser, surgical, or medical treatments.

INTRODUCTION

Age-related macular degeneration causes central vision loss in elderly patients. The pathophysiology of AMD is incompletely understood, but involves chronic changes in the retina and retinal pigment epithelium mediated by environmental and genetic factors. AMD is diagnosed by ophthalmoscopic detection of drusen. Healthy lifestyle decreases the risk of development and progression of AMD. Refer patients to an ophthalmologist to evaluate for intravitreal injections, laser photocoagulation or photodynamic therapy, or surgery.

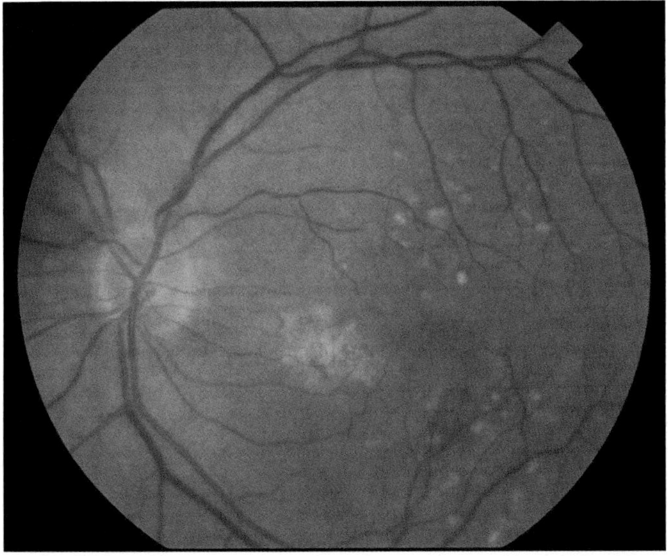

FIGURE 20-1 Intermediate, dry, age-related macular degeneration with macular depigmentation and drusen (yellowish-colored subretinal deposits on the macula). This patient has central vision distortion. (*Reproduced with permission from Paul D. Comeau.*)

EPIDEMIOLOGY

AMD is the leading cause of irreversible vision loss in the industrialized world.

- Prevalence of advanced AMD is 1.4% in patients older than 40 years of age and 15% in white women older than 80 years of age.[1]
- AMD that causes significant vision loss is more common in whites than blacks or Hispanics.[2]
- Smoking increases the risk in women (relative risk [RR] 2.5 for current smokers; 2.0 for former smokers).[2]
- AMD aggregates in families, but the specific genetic and familial risk factors are not clear.[2]

ETIOLOGY AND PATHOPHYSIOLOGY

AMD affects central but not peripheral vision. Environment and genetic attributes increase the risk of these pathologic changes with aging.[3]

- Oxidative stress from the buildup of free oxygen radicals causes retinal pigment epithelial (RPE) injury.
- RPE injury evokes a chronic inflammatory response. The complement system is involved and specific polymorphisms of complement genes are associated with advanced disease and progression.[4]
- RPE injury or inflammation forms an abnormal extracellular matrix (ECM), which alters diffusion of nutrients to the retina and RPE.
- The abnormal ECM and diffusion leads to retinal atrophy and new vessel growth.

RISK FACTORS

- For advanced AMD, strong risk factors are age, current cigarette smoking, previous cataract surgery (replaced lens provides less eye protection from sunlight), and family history of AMD.
- Moderate risk factors include higher body mass index, history of cardiovascular disease, hypertension, and high plasma fibrinogen.
- Weak or inconsistent risk factors include gender, ethnicity, diabetes, iris color, history of cerebrovascular disease, total cholesterol, high-density lipoprotein, and triglyceride levels.[5]

DIAGNOSIS

Diagnosis is made by ophthalmoscopy. AMD can be dry (early, intermediate, or advanced) or wet (always considered advanced).

- Early dry—May have no vision change; drusen present (**Figure 20-2**).
- Intermediate dry—Distortion in the center of vision; multiple medium-sized drusen (see **Figure 20-1**).
- Advanced dry—(Nonexudative) Significant central vision loss from breakdown of support tissues around the macula.
- Advanced wet—(Exudative) Gradual or sudden significant loss of vision; new onset of distortion in vision (straight lines appear wavy); abnormal blood vessels grow under the macula and can cause hemorrhage (**Figure 20-3**). Late changes include subretinal scarring and retinal atrophy (**Figure 20-4**).

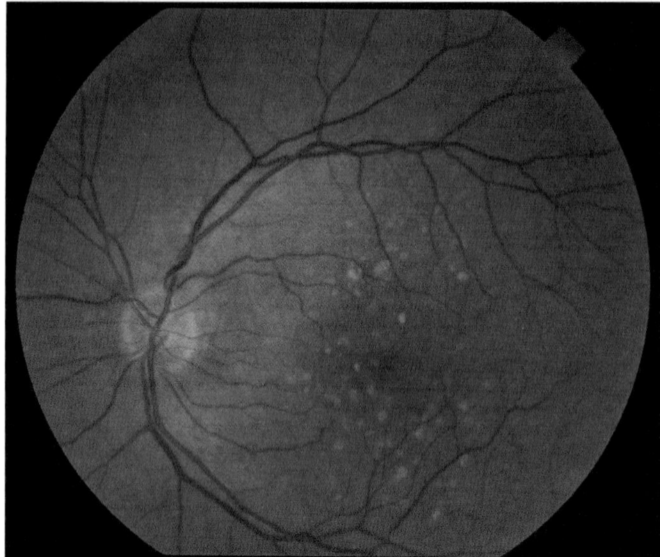

FIGURE 20-2 Early, dry, age-related macular degeneration demonstrating drusen, yellowish-colored subretinal deposits on the macula. Patients may have no visual complaints at this stage. (*Reproduced with permission from Paul D. Comeau.*)

CLINICAL FEATURES

- Symptoms that occur before vision loss include metamorphopsia (distorted vision) and central scotoma (impaired vision at the point of fixation).[6]
- Vision loss is central. Peripheral and night vision are generally not affected.
- Drusen is the classic physical examination finding (see **Figures 20-1** and **20-2**):
  - Hard: small, yellow punctuate nodules
  - Soft: large pale yellow or grayish white with less distinct borders

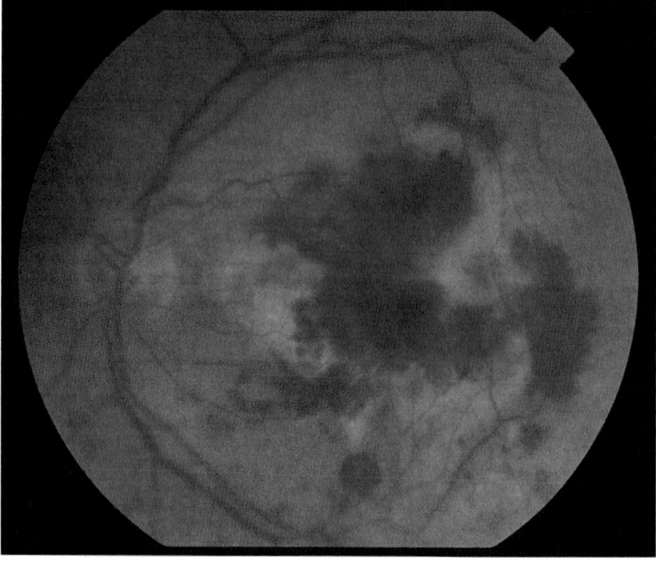

FIGURE 20-3 Late, wet, age-related macular degeneration (exudative) with subretinal hemorrhages. Patients usually have significant central vision loss. (*Reproduced with permission from Paul D. Comeau.*)

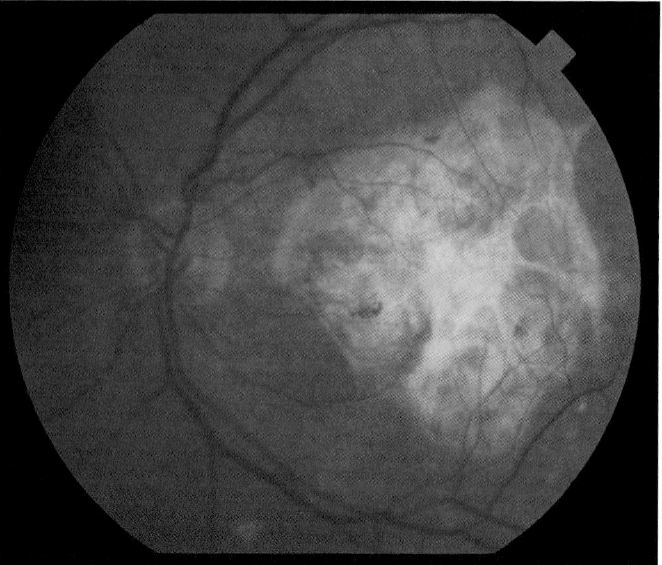

FIGURE 20-4 Late, wet, age-related macular degeneration (exudative) with subretinal scarring. Patients usually have significant central vision loss resulting from destruction of tissue around the macula. (*Reproduced with permission from Paul D. Comeau.*)

TYPICAL DISTRIBUTION

Bilateral, although usually one eye is affected before the other

ANCILLARY TESTING

Macular function is impaired before visual loss and can be detected by tests including macular recovery function and central visual field sensitivity.[7] Optical coherence tomography (OCT) and fluorescein angiography are most commonly used to assess for leakage from abnormal blood vessels. If leakage is present, this indicates that antivascular endothelial growth factor (anti-VEGF) treatment may help.

DIFFERENTIAL DIAGNOSIS

Vision loss in the elderly can also be caused by any of the following[8]:

- Glaucoma (open-angle)—Often asymptomatic until late in the disease, but then has visual field defects instead of central vision loss; funduscopic examination may reveal a large cup-to-disc ratio (see Chapter 16, Glaucoma).
- Diabetic retinopathy—May have central vision loss with macular edema; funduscopic examination demonstrates microaneurysms, cotton-wool spots, hemorrhages, and exudates (see Chapter 17, Diabetic Retinopathy).
- Cataracts—Blurred vision or glare; lens opacities seen when examining the red reflex.

Drusen can also be seen with the following:

- Pigmented nevi and choroidal malignant melanoma
- Retinal detachment
- Glomerulonephritis, particularly membranoproliferative glomerulonephritis type II[6]

MANAGEMENT

Refer to ophthalmologist to evaluate for treatments such as intravitreal injections, laser photocoagulation or photodynamic therapy, or surgery.

- Nonpharmacologic
  - Healthy lifestyle that includes diet, exercise, and no smoking.
- Medications
  - Intraocular injections of pegaptanib and ranibizumab (anti-VEGFs) reduce the risk of visual acuity loss in patients with advanced neovascular AMD, number needed to treat (NNT) 3-14.[9] SOR Ⓐ
  - Bevacizumab performs similarly to ranibizumab.[10]
  - Serious ocular or nonocular adverse events and mild ocular adverse events occur in 1% and 5% of injections, respectfully.[11]
- Complementary or alternative therapy
  - Consider antioxidants (vitamin C, 500 mg; vitamin E, 400 IU; and β-carotene, 15 mg) plus 80 mg zinc per day to decrease the risk of worsening vision loss in patients with intermediate to advanced AMD.[12] SOR Ⓑ These antioxidants are available in single-tablet formulations. Avoid β-carotene for smokers or people who have smoked in the last 10 years.

REFERRAL

- Most patients are treated by an ophthalmologist, and treatment may include intravitreal injections, laser photocoagulation or photodynamic therapy, or surgery.
- Urgently refer a patient with a history of dry AMD and acute changes in vision (distortion of lines, objects) to an ophthalmologist for evaluation and treatment.

PREVENTION

- Healthy diet—People with healthy diets, compared with nonhealthy diets, were 46% less likely to develop AMD.[13]
- Physical activity—Active people, compared to inactive people, were 54% less likely to develop AMD.[13]
- Healthy behaviors—People with a healthy diet who exercised and did not smoke, compared with people without these healthy behaviors, were 71% less likely to develop AMD.[13]
- Regular intake of age-related eye disease study (AREDS) formula (vitamins A, C, and E, and zinc) may reduce the risk of AMD.[14]

PROGNOSIS

Twenty-five percent to 33% of patients with early age-related maculopathy (ARM), a precursor to AMD, progressed over a 7-year period. Smoking, elevated C-reactive protein, and specific complement genotypes increase the risk of progression.[4]

FOLLOW-UP

Patients with ARM and AMD should have regular follow-up with an ophthalmologist.

PATIENT EDUCATION

- AMD can cause a loss of vision leading to an inability to read and drive, thereby affecting many activities of daily living.
- A healthy lifestyle may prevent development or progression of AMD.
- Treatment options are available that decrease the risk of vision loss.
- Most patients with AMD need to see an ophthalmologist regularly in addition to their primary care physician.

PATIENT RESOURCES

- The National Eye Institute has information for patients—**http://www.nei.nih.gov/health/maculardegen/index.asp.**

PROVIDER RESOURCES

- A tool for calculating the risk of advanced AMD—**http://caseyamdcalc.ohsu.edu/**.
- Medscape. *Exudative AMD*—**http://emedicine.medscape.com/article/1236030**.
- Medscape. *Nonexudative AMD*—**http://emedicine.medscape.com/article/1233154**.

REFERENCES

1. Friedman DS, O'Colmain BJ, Muñoz B, et al. Prevalence of age-related macular degeneration in the United States. *Arch Ophthalmol.* 2004;123:564-572.
2. Seddon JM, Chen CA. The epidemiology of age-related macular degeneration. *Int Ophthalmol Clin.* 2004;44(4):17-39.
3. Zarbin MA. Current concepts in the pathogenesis of age-related macular degeneration. *Arch Ophthalmol.* 2004;123(4):598-614.
4. Robman L, Baird PN, Dimitrov PN, et al. C-reactive protein levels and complement factor H polymorphism interaction in age-related macular degeneration and its progression. *Ophthalmology.* 2010;117(10):1982-1988.
5. Chakravarthy U, Wong TY, Fletcher A, et al. Clinical risk factors for age-related macular degeneration: a systematic review and meta-analysis. *BMC Ophthalmol.* 2010;10:31.
6. Kokotas H, Grigoriadou M, Petersen MB. Age-related macular degeneration: genetic and clinical findings. *Clin Chem Lab Med.* 2011;49(4):601-616.
7. Midena E, Degli Angeli C, Blarzino MC, et al. Macular function impairment in eyes with early age-related macular degeneration. *Invest Ophthalmol Vis Sci.* 1997;38(2):469-477.
8. Kroll P, Meyer CH. Which treatment is best for which AMD patient? *Br J Ophthalmol.* 2006;90(2):128-130.
9. Vedula SS, Krystolik MG. Antiangiogenic therapy with anti-vascular endothelial growth factor modalities for neovascular age-related macular degeneration. *Cochrane Database Syst Rev.* 2008;16(2):CD005139.
10. Fadda V, Maratea D, Trippoli S, Messori A. Treatments for macular degeneration: summarizing evidence using network meta-analysis. *Br J Ophthalmol.* 2011;95(10):1476-1477.

11. Van der Reis MI, La Heij EC, De Jong-Hesse Y, et al. A systematic review of the adverse events of intravitreal anti-vascular endothelial growth factor injections. *Retina.* 2011;31(8):1449-1469.
12. Age-Related Eye Disease Study Research Group. A randomized, placebo-controlled, clinical trial of high-dose supplementation with vitamins C and E, beta carotene, and zinc for age-related macular degeneration and vision loss: AREDS report no. 8. *Arch Ophthalmol.* 2001;119(10):1417-1436.
13. Mares JA, Voland RP, Sondel SA, et al. Healthy lifestyles related to subsequent prevalence of age-related macular degeneration. *Arch Ophthalmol.* 2011;129(4):470-480.
14. Wong IY, Koo SC, Chan CW. Prevention of age-related macular degeneration. *Int Ophthalmol.* 2011;31(1):73-82.

21 EYE TRAUMA—HYPHEMA

Heidi Chumley, MD

PATIENT STORY

A 22-year-old man was hit in the eye with a baseball and presented to the emergency department with eye pain and redness and decreased visual acuity. There was a collection of blood in his anterior chamber (**Figure 21-1**) and he was diagnosed with a hyphema. He was given an eye shield for protection, advised to take acetaminophen for pain, and counseled not to engage in sporting activities until his hyphema resolved. He was referred to ophthalmology urgently, but his eye was otherwise healthy. His hyphema resolved in 5 days.

INTRODUCTION

Hyphema, blood in the anterior chamber, can be seen following eye trauma or as a result of clotting disturbances, vascular abnormalities, or mass effects from neoplasms. Traumatic hyphema occurs more often in boys and men, often related to work or sports. Hyphema typically resolves in 5 to 7 days, but some cases are complicated by rebleeding.

EPIDEMIOLOGY

- Hyphema occurs in 17 to 20 per 100,000 persons per year in the United States.[1]
- Sixty percent of hyphemas result from sports injuries.[2] Sports with higher risk for eye injuries include paintball, baseball or softball, basketball, soccer, fishing, ice hockey, racquet sports, fencing, lacrosse, and boxing.

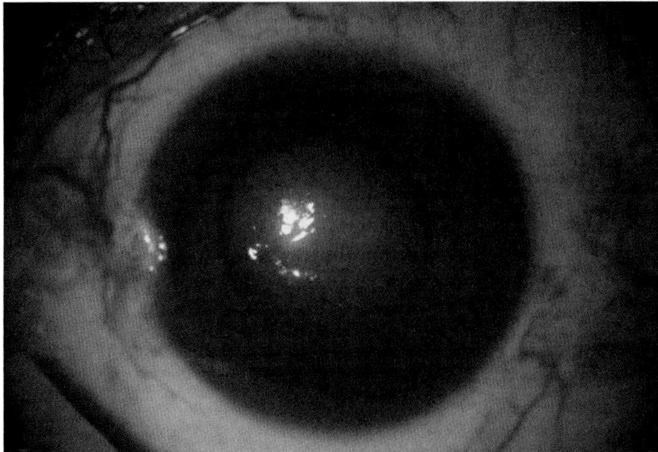

FIGURE 21-1 Layering of red blood cells in the anterior chamber following blunt trauma. This grade 1 hyphema has blood filling in less than one-third of the anterior chamber. *(Reproduced with permission from Paul D. Comeau.)*

ETIOLOGY AND PATHOPHYSIOLOGY

- A hyphema is a collection of blood, mostly erythrocytes, that layer within the anterior chamber.
- Trauma is the most common cause, often resulting from a direct blow from a projectile object such as a ball, air pellet or BB, rock, or fist.
- Direct force to the eye (blunt trauma) forces the globe inward, distorting the normal architecture.
- Intraocular pressure rises instantaneously causing the lens/iris/ciliary body to move posteriorly, thus disrupting the vascularization with resultant bleeding.
- Intraocular pressure continues to rise and bleeding stops when this pressure is high enough to compress the bleeding vessels.
- A fibrin-platelet clot forms and stabilizes in 4 to 7 days; this is eventually broken down by the fibrinolytic system and cleared through the trabecular meshwork.

DIAGNOSIS

The diagnosis of hyphema is clinical, depending on the classic appearance of blood layering in the anterior chamber.

CLINICAL FEATURES

History and physical

- Layered blood in the anterior chamber.
- History of eye trauma or risk factor for nontraumatic hyphema.
- Increased intraocular pressure (32%).
- Decreased vision.
- Hyphemas are classified according to the amount of blood in the anterior chamber[1]:
  - Grade 1: Less than one-third of the anterior chamber (see **Figure 21-1**); 58% of all hyphemas
  - Grade 2: One-third to one-half of the anterior chamber; 20% of all hyphemas
  - Grade 3: One-half to almost completely filled anterior chamber; 14% of all hyphemas
  - Grade 4: Completely filled anterior chamber; 8% of all hyphemas
- Eye trauma without hyphema (**Figures 21-2** and **21-3**) can lead to subconjunctival hemorrhage, anterior uveitis, and/or distortion of the normal architecture, including globe rupture.

LABORATORY TESTING (INCLUDE ANCILLARY TESTING, TOO)

Consider laboratory tests to evaluate for bleeding disorders: bleeding time, electrophoresis for sickle cell trait, platelet count, prothrombin and partial thromboplastin time, and liver tests.

IMAGING

Consider computed tomography (CT) imaging if a mechanism of injury suggests an associated orbital fracture or concern for orbital or intraocular foreign body.

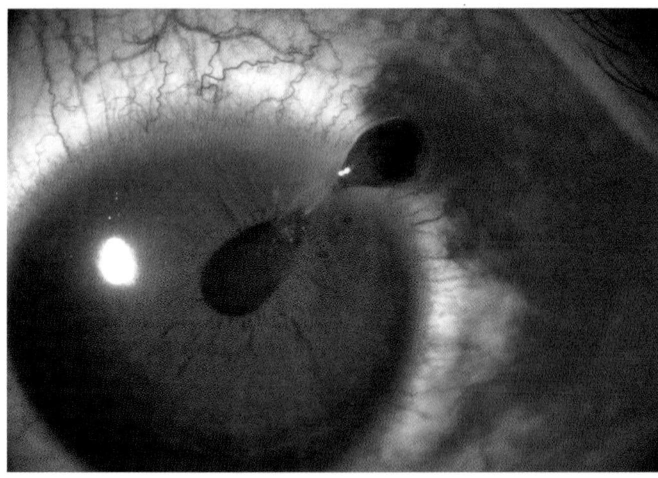

FIGURE 21-2 This patient was hit in the eye with the corner of a laminated name card. The sharp edge perforated the cornea and pulled a portion of the iris out of the wound. Note the abnormal configuration of the pupil (dyscoria). No hyphema noted. This patient required emergent surgical repair. *(Reproduced with permission from Paul D. Comeau.)*

DIFFERENTIAL DIAGNOSIS

Hyphema is an unmistakable physical examination finding that can be caused by any of the following:

- Trauma—History of trauma, including nonaccidental trauma (ie, child abuse).
- Blood clotting disturbances—Personal or family history of bleeding disorder, little or no trauma, and black race (increased incidence of sickle trait and disease).
- Medication-induced anticoagulation—Chronic use of aspirin or warfarin and little or no trauma.
- Neovascularization—Diabetes with diabetic retinopathy, history of other ocular disease (central retinal vein occlusion), or history of prior eye surgery (cataract); without trauma, often painless, sudden, blurry vision.

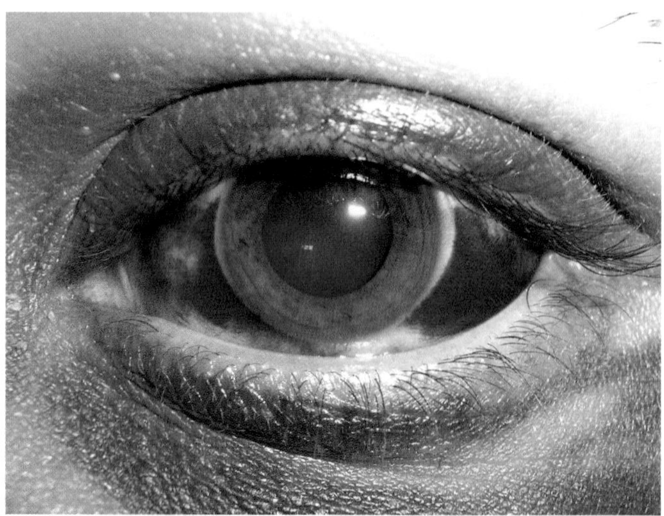

FIGURE 21-3 Subconjunctival hemorrhage and eyelid ecchymosis following accidental trauma. There was no hyphema present. *(Reproduced with permission from Richard P. Usatine, MD.)*

- Melanoma or retinoblastoma—Variety of presentations depending on the size and location; hyphema occurs when mass effect shears the lens/iris/ciliary body causing bleeding.
- Abnormal vasculature, that is, juvenile xanthogranuloma—Red to yellow papules and nodules in the eyes, skin, and viscera, most often present by 1 year of age.

MANAGEMENT

- Most hyphemas resolve in 5 to 7 days; management strategies protect the eye and decrease complications, including rebleeding.
- Evaluate or refer for evaluation for elevated intraocular pressure and other associated injuries. Urgent referral if concern for globe rupture.

A recent Cochrane review evaluated these interventions: antifibrinolytic agents, corticosteroids, cycloplegics, miotics, aspirin, conjugated estrogens, eye patching, head elevation, and bed rest.

- No interventions had a significant effect on visual acuity.
- Aminocaproic acid (antifibrinolytic) use resulted in a slower resolution of the primary hyphema.
- Antifibrinolytics: aminocaproic acid, tranexamic acid, and aminomethylbenzoic acid reduced the rate of secondary hemorrhage.[3]

NONPHARMACOLOGIC

Eye patching, head elevation, and bed rest do not independently affect visual acuity. However, experts recommend to patch and shield the injured eye and allow the patient to remain ambulatory as part of a comprehensive treatment plan.[1] SOR Ⓒ

MEDICATIONS

Although controversy remains about the best treatment, each of the following has been demonstrated to lower the risk of rebleeding in randomized-controlled trials:

- Oral antifibrinolytic agents (aminocaproic acid 50 mg/kg every 4 hours for 5 days, not to exceed 30 g/d, or tranexamic acid 75 mg/kg per day divided into 3 doses).[4] SOR Ⓒ
- Topical aminocaproic acid (30% in a gel vehicle 4 times a day) is as effective as oral.[4] SOR Ⓒ
- Avoid aspirin and nonsteroidal anti-inflammatory drugs (NSAIDs) which have been associated with higher rates of rebleeding.
- Use acetaminophen, if needed, for pain.

REFERRAL OR HOSPITALIZATION

- Signs of a violated globe, such as a perforation of the cornea, conjunctiva or sclera, distorted ocular architecture, or exposed and/or distorted uveal tissue such as the iris (causing a peaked pupil), require immediate surgical evaluation and repair (see **Figure 21-2**).
- Surgical intervention has been recommended for patients with persistent total hyphema or prolonged elevated intraocular pressure.
- Outpatient management is acceptable for adults if patient is likely to be able to follow treatment plan.[4,5] SOR Ⓑ

PREVENTION

Ninety percent of sports-related eye injuries can be prevented with appropriate eyewear.[6]

PROGNOSIS

The percentage of patients who regain 20/40 vision varies by severity of the hyphema: grade I, 80%; grade III, 60%; grade IV, 35%.[1]

FOLLOW-UP

Patients should be monitored daily for the first 5 or more days by a provider familiar with caring for hyphemas. Patient with a hyphema should be followed subsequently for signs of angle recession and high intraocular pressure, which predisposes the patient to traumatic glaucoma, an insidious cause of blindness in patients with a history of trauma.

PATIENT EDUCATION

- Complications include rebleeding, decreased visual acuity, posterior or peripheral anterior synechiae, corneal bloodstaining, glaucoma, and optic atrophy. Patients may need surgical or medical management for glaucoma.
- Patients who are more likely to rebleed include black patients (irrespective of sickle cell/trait status),[7,8] patients with a grade 3 or 4 hyphema, and patients with high initial intraocular pressure.
- Warn patients that they may have angle recession from traumatic causes of the hyphema. This will predispose the patient to a lifetime risk of traumatic glaucoma, which can cause blindness without any symptoms. These patients need to be monitored regularly by an ophthalmologist for increased pressure and glaucomatous nerve changes.

PATIENT RESOURCES

- Play Hard Play Safe Web site has recommended eye protection by sport—**http://www.lexeye.com.**
- The National Eye Institute has information for parents, teachers, and coaches—**http://www.nei.nih.gov/sports.**

PROVIDER RESOURCES

- Coalition to prevent eye injuries has a variety of handouts suitable for displaying or giving to patients—**http://www.sportseyeinjuries.com.**

REFERENCES

1. Sheppard J, Hyphema. *Medscape Reference.* http://emedicine.medscape.com/article/119016. Accessed June 15, 2012.
2. Schein OD, Hibberd PL, Shingleton BJ, et al. The spectrum and burden of ocular injury. *Ophthalmology*. 1988;95(3):300-305.
3. Gharaibeh A, Savage HI, Scherer RW, et al. Medical interventions for traumatic hyphema. *Cochrane Database Syst Rev.* 2011;19(1):CD005431.
4. Walton W, Von HS, Grigorian R, Zarbin M. Management of traumatic hyphema. *Surv Ophthalmol.* 2002;47(4):297-334.
5. Rocha KM, Martins EN, Melo LA Jr, Moraes NS. Outpatient management of traumatic hyphema in children: prospective evaluation. *J AAPOS*. 2004;8(4):357-361.
6. Harrison A, Telander DG. Eye injuries in the youth athlete: a case-based approach. *Sports Med.* 2002;l31(1):33-40.
7. Lai JC, Fekrat S, Barron Y, Goldberg MF. Traumatic hyphema in children: risk factors for complications. *Arch Ophthalmol.* 2001;119(1): 64-70.
8. Spoor TC, Kwitko GM, O'Grady JM, Ramocki JM. Traumatic hyphema in an urban population. *Am J Ophthalmol.* 1990;109(1):23-27.

22 DIFFERENTIAL DIAGNOSIS OF THE RED EYE

Heidi Chumley, MD
Richard P. Usatine, MD

PATIENT STORY

A 41-year-old man wakes up with eyes that are reddened bilaterally (**Figure 22-1**). He has some burning and itching in the eyes, but no pain. He describes minimal crusting on his eyelashes. Examination shows no loss of vision, no foreign bodies, and pupils that are equal, round, and reactive to light. He is diagnosed with viral conjunctivitis, which does not require antibiotic treatment. He is advised about methods to prevent spreading conjunctivitis to others and is asked to notify the physician immediately if he experiences eye pain or loss of vision. He recovers spontaneously without complications after a few days.

INTRODUCTION

A red eye signifies ocular inflammation. The differential diagnosis includes both benign and sight-threatening conditions. The pattern of redness; presence or absence of eye pain or photophobia, vision loss, or eye discharge; involvement of cornea; and visual acuity are helpful in differentiating among causes (**Table 22-1**). Although most red eyes seen in the primary care setting are a result of viral conjunctivitis, several causes of red eye require urgent referral.

EPIDEMIOLOGY

- An acute red eye or eyes is a common presentation in ambulatory and emergency departments.
- Conjunctivitis is the most common cause of a nontraumatic red eye in primary care.

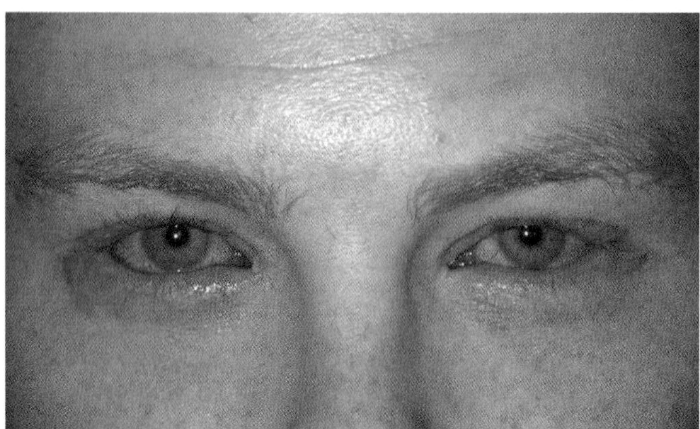

FIGURE 22-1 Bilateral viral conjunctivitis in a 41-year-old man. (*Reproduced with permission from Richard P. Usatine, MD.*)

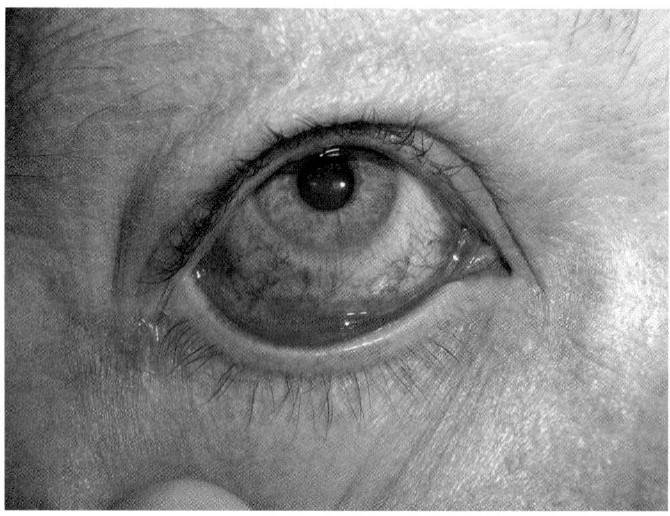

FIGURE 22-2 Bacterial conjunctivitis in a contact lens user. (*Reproduced with permission from Richard P. Usatine, MD.*)

ETIOLOGY AND PATHOPHYSIOLOGY

Red eye is caused by any of the following:

- Infectious or noninfectious inflammation of any layer of the eye (conjunctivitis, episcleritis, scleritis, uveitis, keratitis)
- Eyelid pathology (blepharitis, entropion, ie, inward turning of the eyelid, or other eyelid malposition)
- Acute glaucoma (usually angle-closure)
- Trauma
- Subconjunctival hemorrhage

DIFFERENTIAL DIAGNOSIS

An acute red eye can be caused by any of the following:

- Conjunctivitis[2]—Conjunctival injection, eye discharge, gritty or uncomfortable feeling, and no vision loss (**Figures 22-1** to **22-4**) (see Chapter 13, Conjunctivitis).

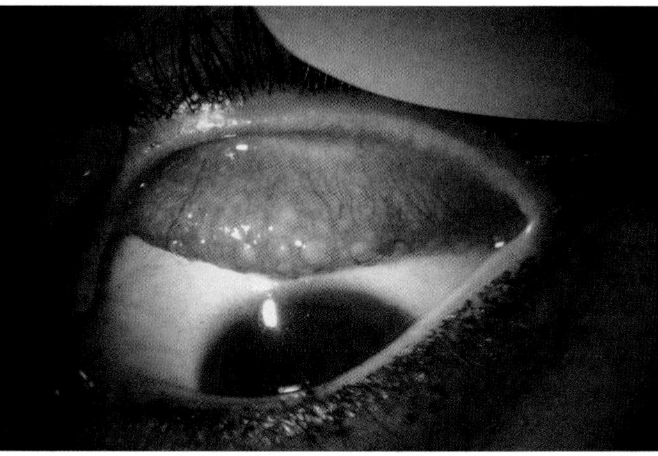

FIGURE 22-3 Giant papillary conjunctivitis secondary to contact lens use. (*Reproduced with permission from Paul D. Comeau.*)

TABLE 22-1 Clinical Features in the Diagnosis of Red Eye

	Conjunctivitis	Episcleritis	Scleritis	Uveitis	Keratitis	Closed-Angle Glaucoma	Subconjunctival Hemorrhage	Ocular Rosacea
Redness	Diffuse	Segmental; pink	Segmental or diffuse; dark red, purple, or blue	360-Degree perilimbal (worse at limbus)	Diffuse, ciliary injection	Diffuse, scleral	Blotchy, outside vessels	Diffuse
Eye pain	No	Mild, may be tender to touch	Severe, boring	Sometimes	Usually	Yes	No, unless caused by trauma	No
Vision loss	No	No	Sometimes	Sometimes	Maybe, depending on location	Yes	No	In severe cases
Discharge	Usually	No	No	No	Maybe	No	No	No
Photophobia*	No	No	Yes	Yes, if anterior	Yes	Yes	No	Sometimes
Pupil	Normal	Normal	Normal	Constricted	Normal to constricted	Mild dilation, less responsive	Normal; unless affected by trauma	Normal
Cornea	Clear	Clear	Clear	Clear to hazy	Hazy	Usually hazy	Clear	Clear or neovascularization, cloudy
Associated diseases	URI, allergy, exposure	Occasional systemic disease	Systemic disease	Systemic disease, idiopathic	Contact lenses, HSV or varicella, rosacea	Causes headaches, nausea, vomiting, GI symptoms	HTN, trauma, Valsalva, cough, blood thinners	Acne rosacea (can exist without also), blepharitis

HSV, herpes simplex virus; HTN, hypertension; URI, upper respiratory infection.
*For identifying serious causes of red eye, the presence of photophobia elicited with a penlight in a general practice had a positive predictive value of 60% and a negative predictive value of 90%.[1]

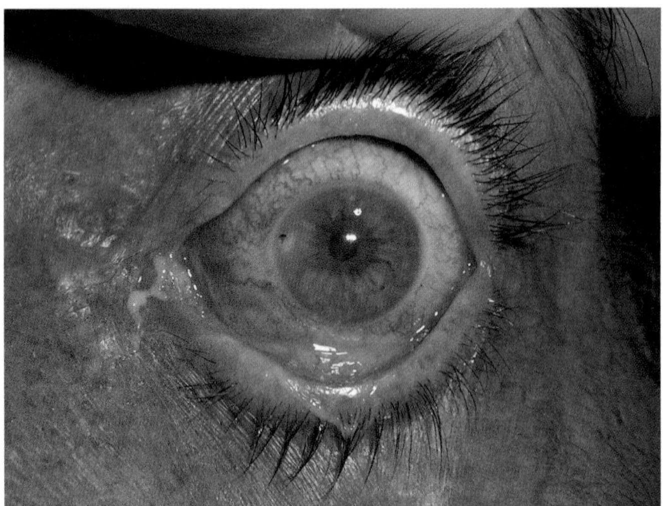

FIGURE 22-4 Conjunctival irritation caused by a fleck of metal (at 9-o'clock position) that was embedded in the eye of a man who was grinding steel. (*Reproduced with permission from Richard P. Usatine, MD.*)

- Episcleritis—Segmental or diffuse inflammation of episclera (pink color), mild or no discomfort, but can be tender to palpation, and no vision disturbance (**Figure 22-5**) (see Chapter 14, Episcleritis and Scleritis).
- Scleritis—Segmental or diffuse inflammation of sclera (dark red, purple, or blue color), severe boring eye pain often radiating to head and neck, and photophobia and vision loss (**Figure 22-6**) (see Chapter 14, Episcleritis and Scleritis).
- Keratitis or corneal ulcerations—Diffuse erythema with ciliary injection often with pupillary constriction; eye discharge; and pain, photophobia, vision loss depending on the location of ulceration (**Figure 22-7**). It is often associated with the use of contact lenses.
- Subconjunctival hemorrhage (**Figure 22-8**)—Bright red subconjunctival blood; usually not painful; can present after significant coughing or sneezing, after trauma, or in the setting of dry eyes with minor trauma from rubbing with a finger. Not vision-threatening.

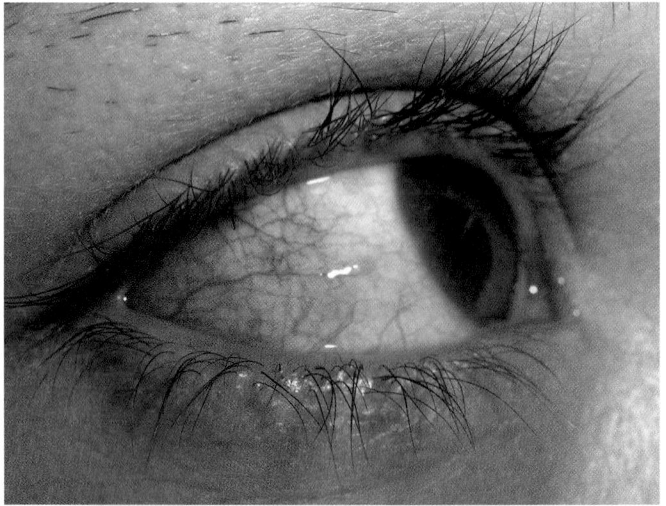

FIGURE 22-5 Episcleritis showing a sector of erythema. (*Reproduced with permission from Richard P. Usatine, MD.*)

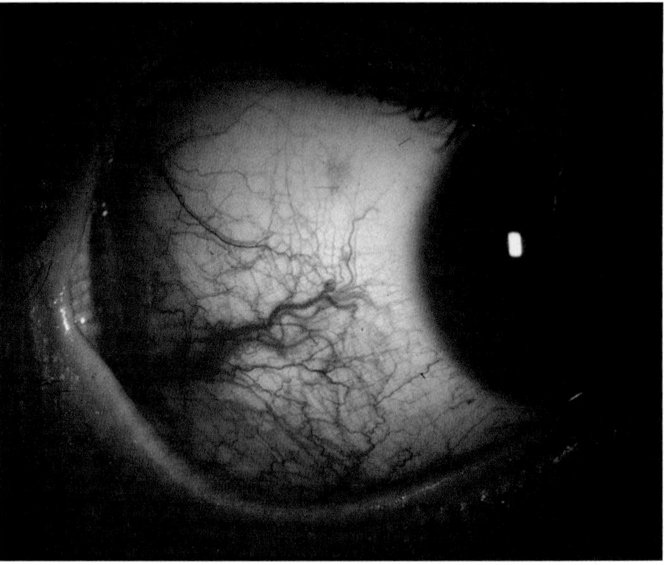

FIGURE 22-6 Scleritis with deeper, darker vessels than the episcleritis. (*Reproduced with permission from Paul D. Comeau.*)

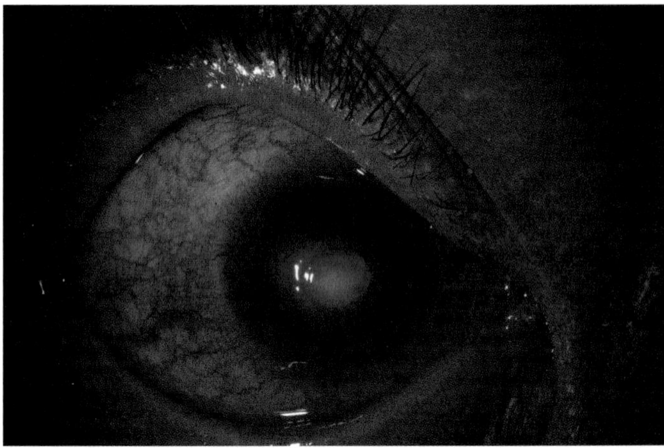

FIGURE 22-7 Diffuse ciliary injection and cloudy cornea demonstrating keratitis with corneal ulcer formation and a leucocyte infiltrate. (*Reproduced with permission from Paul D. Comeau.*)

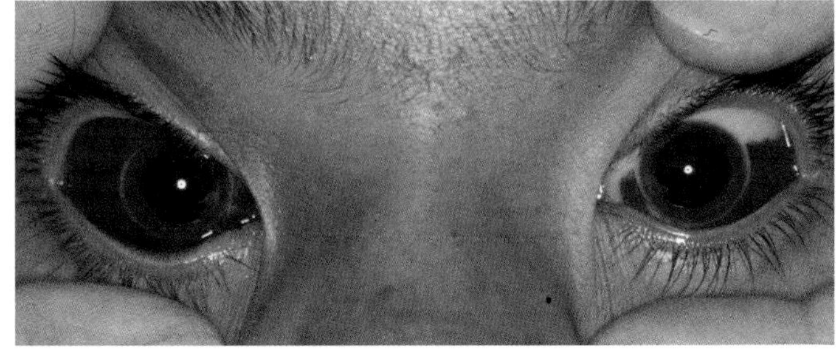

FIGURE 22-8 Subconjunctival hemorrhage secondary to trauma. (*Reproduced with permission from Paul D. Comeau.*)

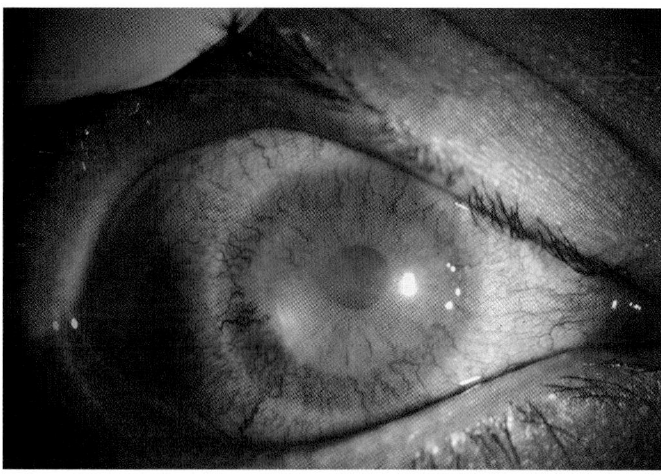

FIGURE 22-9 Ocular rosacea with new vessels growing onto the cornea. Many patients with rosacea have some ocular findings including blepharitis (inflammation of the eyelid), conjunctivitis (most common), episcleritis (rare), keratitis, or corneal ulceration/neovascularization. (*Reproduced with permission from Paul D. Comeau.*)

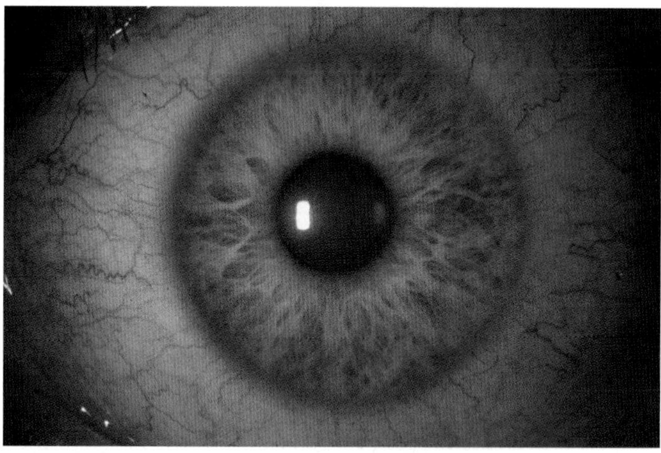

FIGURE 22-11 Iritis (anterior uveitis) with a limbal flush, red to purple perilimbal ring. For contrast, note the perilimbal area is not involved in conjunctivitis, as best seen in **Figure 22-2**. This patient has eye pain and vision loss, which are also absent in conjunctivitis. (*Reproduced with permission from Paul D. Comeau.*)

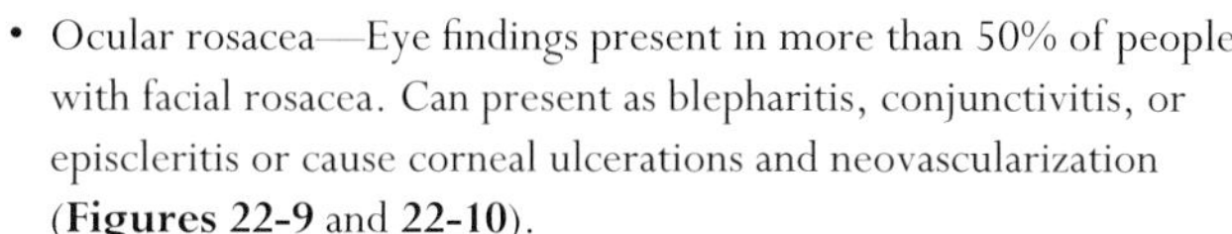

- Ocular rosacea—Eye findings present in more than 50% of people with facial rosacea. Can present as blepharitis, conjunctivitis, or episcleritis or cause corneal ulcerations and neovascularization (**Figures 22-9** and **22-10**).
- Uveitis or iritis—A 360-degree injection, which is most intense at the limbus, eye pain, photophobia, and vision loss (**Figure 22-11**) (see Chapter 15, Uveitis and Iritis).
- Trauma causing globe injury, or hemorrhage into the anterior chamber called hyphema (**Figures 22-12** and **22-13**) (see Chapter 21, Eye Trauma—Hyphema).
- Pterygium—Fibrovascular tissue on the surface of the eye extending onto the cornea (**Figure 22-14**) (see Chapter 9, Pterygium).
- Hypopyon is a term for visible white cells (pus) layered out in the anterior chamber. It may be caused by inflammation of the iris or an eye infection. The inflammation and/or infection also causes the conjunctiva and sclera to become red (**Figure 22-15**).
- Acute angle-closure glaucoma—Cloudy cornea and scleral injection, shallow anterior chamber (check other eye if difficult to assess chamber

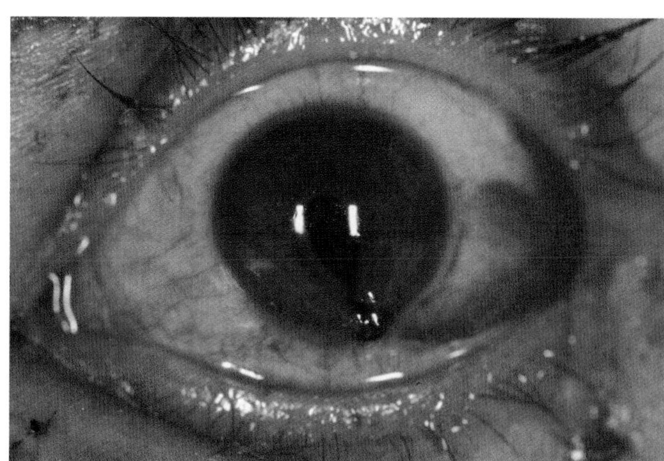

FIGURE 22-12 Trauma to the eye resulting in an open globe injury with extrusion of some of the iris through the cornea and an abnormal pupil. There is conjunctival injection and hemorrhage causing this red eye. (*Reproduced with permission from Paul D. Comeau.*)

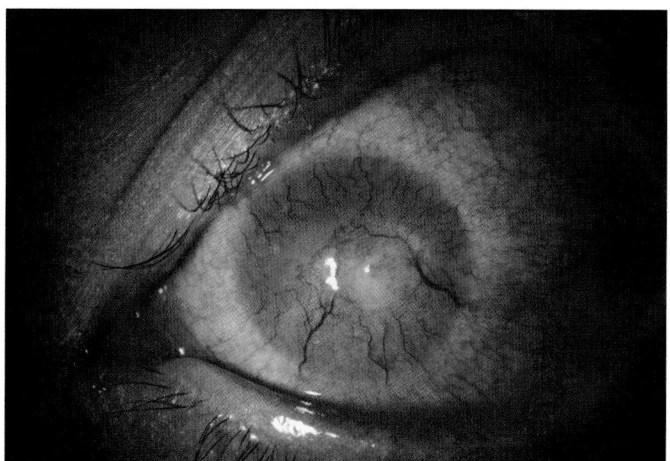

FIGURE 22-10 Severe ocular rosacea with blood vessels growing over the cornea leading to blindness. (*Reproduced with permission from Paul D. Comeau.*)

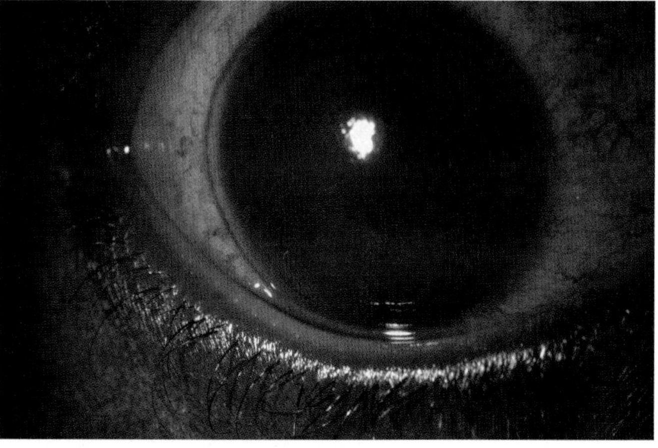

FIGURE 22-13 Hyphema with red cells in the anterior chamber and an inferior blood clot. (*Reproduced with permission from Paul D. Comeau.*)

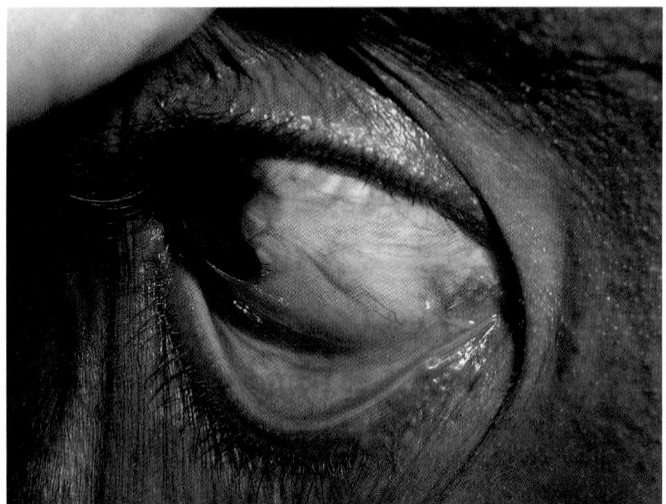

FIGURE 22-14 Pterygium that often becomes irritated and injected. (Reproduced with permission from Richard P. Usatine, MD.)

depth in the red eye), eye pain with ipsilateral headache, and severe vision loss (see Chapter 16, Glaucoma).

- Eyelid pathology—Blepharitis (inflammation of the eyelid) (**Figure 22-16**). Entropion is turning inward of the eyelid and can cause irritation to the conjunctiva and cornea.

MANAGEMENT

Treatment for specific causes is discussed in the corresponding chapters.

Refer patients with any of the following to an ophthalmologist[3]: SOR C

- Visual loss
- Moderate or severe pain
- Severe, purulent discharge
- Corneal involvement
- Conjunctival scarring
- Lack of response to therapy
- Topical steroid therapy
- Recurrent episodes
- Open globe or perforation

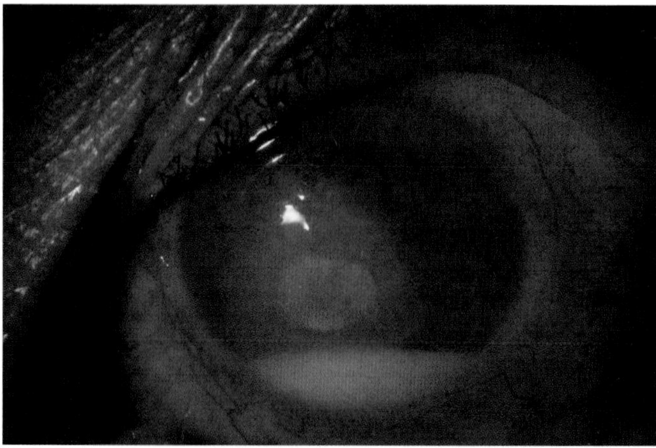

FIGURE 22-15 Hypopyon with white cells layered in the anterior chamber. (Reproduced with permission from Paul D. Comeau.)

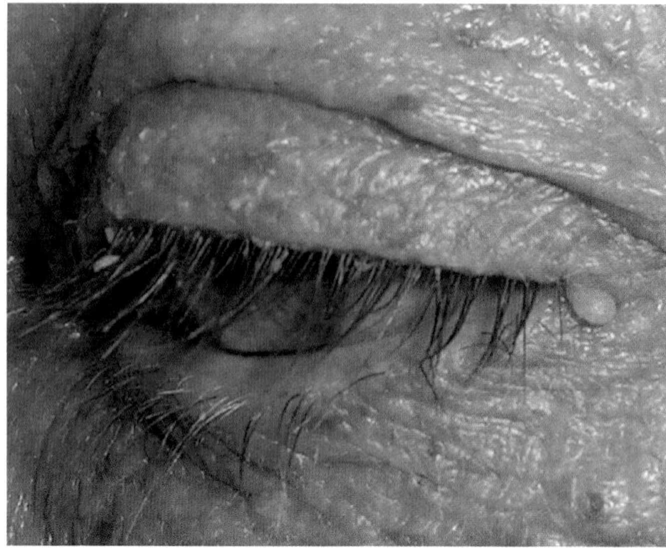

FIGURE 22-16 Blepharitis showing erythema of the eyelids and flaking in the eyelashes. Note the scale that has accumulated in the eyelashes. (Reproduced with permission from Richard P. Usatine, MD.)

- History of herpes simplex virus (HSV) eye disease
- History of contact lens wear

PROGNOSIS

Prognosis depends on underlying cause (see corresponding chapters).

FOLLOW-UP

Timing of follow-up and need for further testing is determined by the underlying cause (see corresponding chapters).

PATIENT EDUCATION

Advise patients to notify their physician immediately for eye pain (other than gritty discomfort) and/or loss of vision.

PATIENT RESOURCES

- Mayo Clinic. *Red Eye*—**http://www.mayoclinic.com/health/red-eye/MY00280.**

PHYSICIAN RESOURCES

- Medscape. *Red Eye*—**http://emedicine.medscape.com/article/1192122.**

REFERENCES

1. Yaphe J, Pandher K. The predictive value of the penlight test for photophobia for serious eye pathology in general practice. *Fam Pract*. 2003;20(4):425-427.
2. American Academy of Ophthalmology Cornea/External Disease Panel, Preferred Practice Patterns Committee. *Conjunctivitis*. San Francisco, CA: American Academy of Ophthalmology; 2003:25.
3. Cronau H, Kankanala RR, Mauger T. Diagnosis and management of red eye in primary care. *Am Fam Physician*. 2010;81(2):137-144.

PART 5

EAR, NOSE, AND THROAT

Strength of Recommendation (SOR)	Definition
A	Recommendation based on consistent and good-quality patient-oriented evidence.*
B	Recommendation based on inconsistent or limited-quality patient-oriented evidence.*
C	Recommendation based on consensus, usual practice, opinion, disease-oriented evidence, or case series for studies of diagnosis, treatment, prevention, or screening.*

*See Appendix A on pages 1241-1244 for further information.

SECTION 1 EAR

23 OTITIS MEDIA: ACUTE OTITIS AND OTITIS MEDIA WITH EFFUSION

Brian Z. Rayala, MD

PATIENT STORY

A 35-year-old business man comes to see his physician with left ear pain. He had been traveling for work and was fighting a cold all week. He experienced plugging of both ears on the airplane flight home 3 days ago. His right ear cleared quickly but his left ear remained plugged and from the last day he had been experiencing pain. On otoscopy, his left tympanic membrane (TM) appears retracted and slightly erythematous (**Figure 23-1**). His left TM fails to move on pneumatic otoscopy. The physician diagnoses acute otitis media and prescribes a 10-day course of amoxicillin.

INTRODUCTION

Acute otitis media (AOM) is characterized by middle-ear effusion in a patient with signs and symptoms of acute illness (eg, fever, otalgia). Otitis media with effusion (OME) is a disorder characterized by fluid in the middle ear in a patient without signs and symptoms of acute ear infection; it is very common in children.

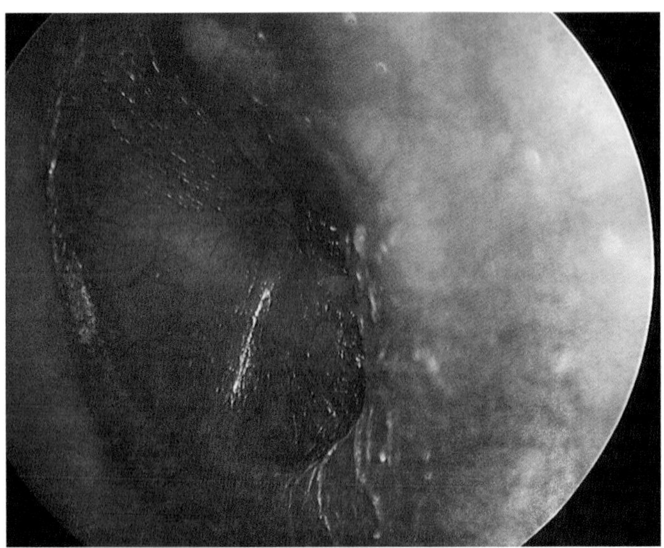

FIGURE 23-1 Early acute otitis media (AOM) at the stage of eustachian tube obstruction. Note the slight retraction of the TM, the more horizontal position of the malleus, and the prominence of the lateral process. *(Reproduced with permission from William Clark, MD.)*

EPIDEMIOLOGY

- AOM accounted for $5 billion of the total national health expenditure in 2000.[1]
- While the vast majority of children has had an episode of AOM by 2 to 3 years of age,[2] few adults experience purulent otitis media. In one retrospective study and literature review, the incidence was 0.25%.[3]
- Based on a study from the International Primary Care Network, adults make up fewer than 20% of patients presenting with AOM.[4]
- AOM is the most common reason for outpatient antibiotic treatment in the United States.[5]
- The combined direct and indirect health care costs of OME, diagnosed in over 2 million children, amount to $4 billion annually.[6]

ETIOLOGY AND PATHOPHYSIOLOGY

AOM is often preceded by upper respiratory symptoms such as cough and rhinorrhea.

- Pathogenesis of AOM includes the following[7]:
  - Eustachian tube dysfunction (usually a result of an upper respiratory infection) and subsequent tube obstruction
  - Increased negative pressure in the middle ear
  - Accumulation of middle-ear fluid
  - Microbial growth
  - Suppuration (that leads to clinical signs of AOM).
- Most common pathogens in the United States and United Kingdom are as below[8,9]:
  - Strains of *Streptococcus pneumoniae* not in the heptavalent pneumococcal vaccine (PCV7) (after introduction of PCV7 vaccine in 2000)
  - Nonencapsulated (nontypeable) *Haemophilus influenzae* (NTHi)
  - *Moraxella catarrhalis*
  - *Staphylococcus aureus*.
- In an older study of 34 adults with otitis media, *H. influenzae* and *S. pneumoniae* were cultured from 9 and 7 patients (26% and 21%), respectively.[10]
- Viruses account for 16% of cases. Respiratory syncytial viruses, rhinoviruses, influenza viruses, and adenoviruses have been the most common isolated viruses.[11]

OME most commonly follows AOM; it may also occur spontaneously.

- Fluid limits sound conduction through the ossicles and results in decreased hearing.
- Reasons for the persistence of fluid in otitis media remain unclear, although potential etiologies include allergies, biofilm, and physiologic features.
- "Glue ear" refers to extremely viscous mucoid material within the middle ear and is a distinct subtype of OME.

RISK FACTORS

The most important risk factor in adults is smoking.

DIAGNOSIS

CLINICAL FEATURES OF AOM

- To diagnose AOM, the clinician should confirm a history of acute onset, identify signs of middle-ear effusion (MEE), *and* evaluate for the presence of signs and symptoms of middle-ear inflammation.[6] SOR C
- Elements of the definition of AOM are *all* of the following[6]:
  1. Recent, usually abrupt, onset of signs and symptoms of middle-ear inflammation and MEE.
  2. The presence of MEE (**Figure 23-2**). Although MEE is often presumed by erythema of the TM (see **Figure 23-1**), bulging of the TM (**Figure 23-3**) or air–fluid level behind the TM (see **Figure 23-2**), the guideline stresses use of objective measures of confirming MEE such as the following[6]:
     a. Limited or absent mobility of the TM established by pneumatic otoscopy—The TM does not move during air insufflation; often initially seen as retraction of the TM (**Figures 23-1** and **23-4**).
     b. Objective measures such as tympanometry.
     c. Otorrhea.
  3. Signs or symptoms of middle-ear inflammation as indicated by either of the following:
     a. Distinct erythema of the TM (see **Figures 23-1** and **23-3**) in contrast to the normal TM (**Figure 23-5**), or
     b. Distinct otalgia (discomfort clearly referable to the ear[s] that results in interference with or precludes normal activity or sleep).

CLINICAL FEATURES OF OME

- The most common symptom, present in more than half of patients, is mild hearing loss.
- Absence of signs and symptoms of acute illness assists in differentiating OME from AOM.

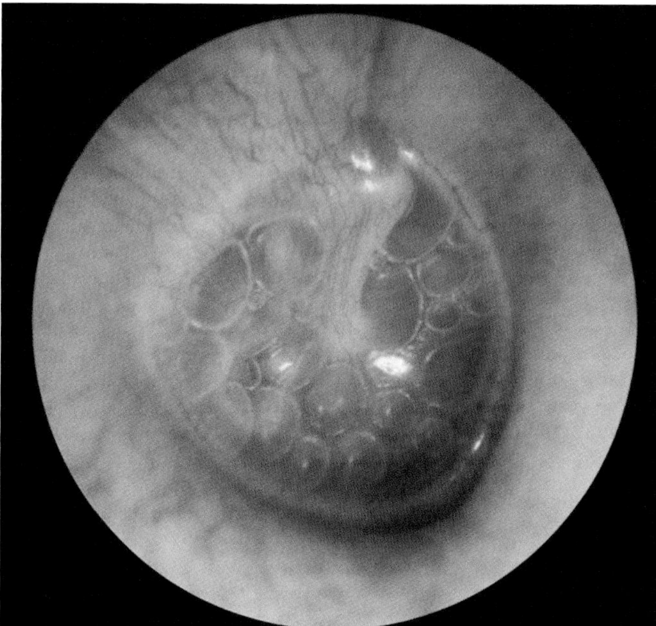

FIGURE 23-2 Otitis media with effusion (OME) in the right ear. Note multiple air–fluid levels in this slightly retracted, translucent, nonerythematous tympanic membrane. (*Reproduced with permission from Frank Miller, MD.*)

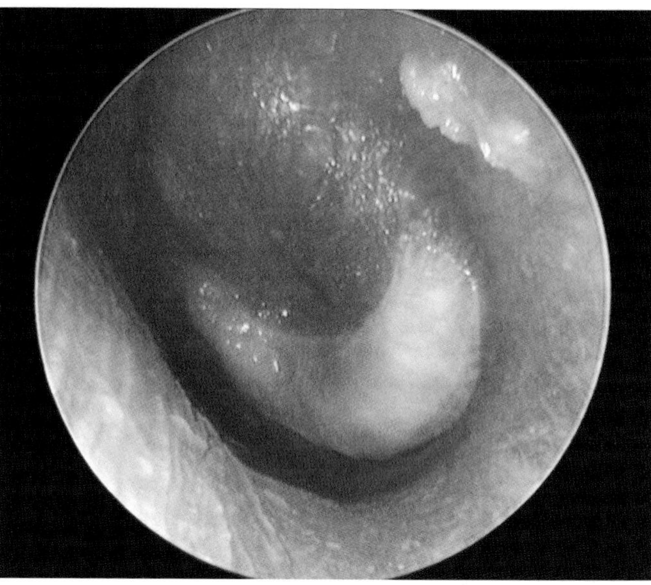

FIGURE 23-3 Acute otitis media, stage of suppuration. Note presence of purulent exudate behind the TM, the outward bulging of the TM, prominence of the posterosuperior portion of the drum, and generalized TM edema. The *white area* is tympanosclerosis from a previous infection. (*Reproduced with permission from William Clark, MD.*)

- Common otoscopic findings include the following:
  - Air–fluid level or bubble (see **Figure 23-2**).
  - Cloudy TM (see **Figure 23-1**) in contrast to the normal TM (see **Figure 26-5**).
  - Redness of the TM may be present in approximately 5% of ears with OME.

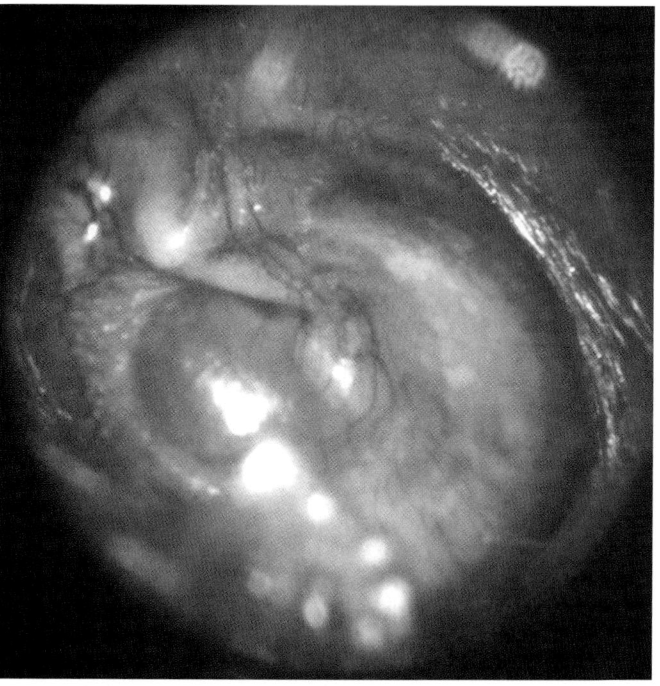

FIGURE 23-4 Otitis media with effusion in the left ear showing retraction of the TM and straightening of the handle of the malleus as the retraction pulls the bone upward. (*Reproduced with permission from Glen Medellin, MD.*)

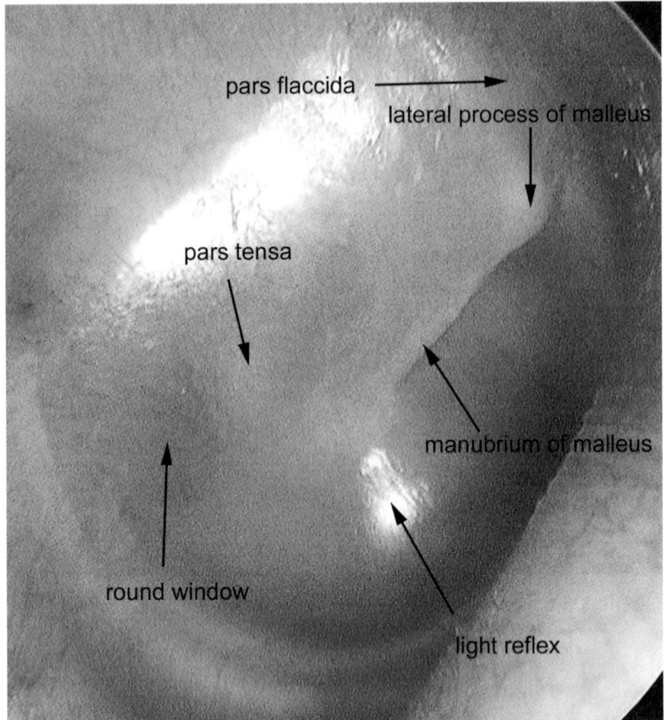

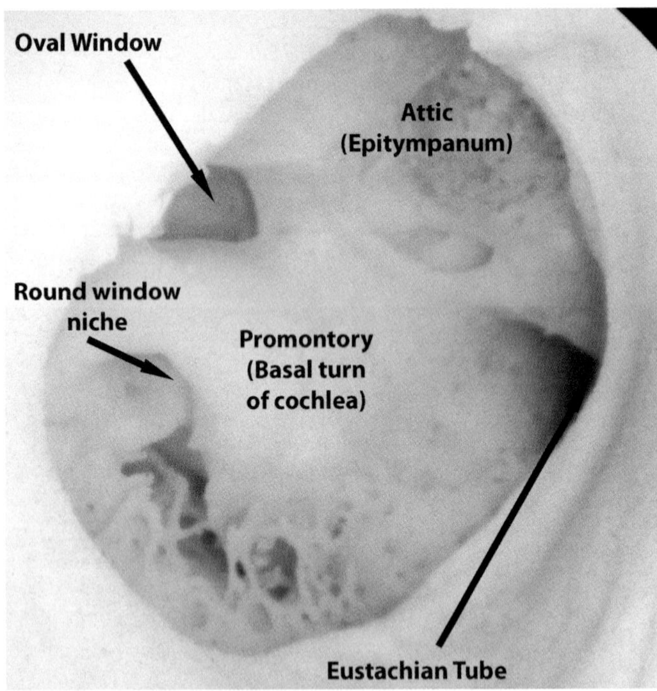

FIGURE 23-5 A. Normal right tympanic membrane with comparison using normal bony landmarks of the inner ear. B. The ossicles were removed in this dissection. (*Reproduced with permission from William Clark, MD.*)

- Clinicians should use pneumatic otoscopy as the primary diagnostic method for OME.[12] SOR A
  - Impaired mobility of the TM is the hallmark of MEE.
  - According to a meta-analysis, impaired mobility on pneumatic otoscopy has a pooled sensitivity of 94% and specificity of 80%, and positive likelihood ratio of 4.7 and negative likelihood ratio of 0.075.[12]

LABORATORY TESTS AND IMAGING

- Because AOM and OME are clinical diagnoses, diagnostic testing has a limited role. When clinical presentation and physical examination (including otoscopy) do not establish the diagnosis, the following can be used as adjunctive techniques:
  - Tympanometry—This procedure records compliance of the TM by measuring reflected sound. AOM and OME will plot as a reduced or flat waveform.
  - Acoustic reflectometry—This procedure, very similar to tympanometry, measures sound reflectivity from the middle ear. With this test, the clinician is able to distinguish air- or fluid-filled space without requiring an airtight seal of the ear canal.
  - Middle ear aspiration—For patients with AOM, aspiration may be warranted if patient is toxic, immunocompromised, or has failed prior courses of antibiotics.

DIFFERENTIAL DIAGNOSIS

The key differentiating feature between AOM and OME is the absence of signs and symptoms of acute illness in OME (eg, fever, irritability, otalgia). Otoscopic findings may be similar. Other clinical entities that may be confused with AOM and OME include the following:

- Otitis externa—Otitis externa presents with otalgia, otorrhea, and mild hearing loss, all of which can be present in AOM. Tragal pain on physical examination and signs of external canal inflammation on otoscopic examination differentiate it from AOM. Careful ear irrigation if tolerated may be helpful to visualize the TM to differentiate otitis externa from AOM (see Chapter 24, Otitis Externa).
- Otitic barotrauma—This often presents with severe otalgia. Key historical features include recent air travel, scuba diving, or ear trauma, preceded by an upper respiratory infection.
- Cholesteatoma—Unlike AOM, this is a clinically silent disease in its initial stages. Presence of white keratin debris in the middle ear cavity (on otoscopy) is diagnostic (**Figures 23-6** and **26-7**).

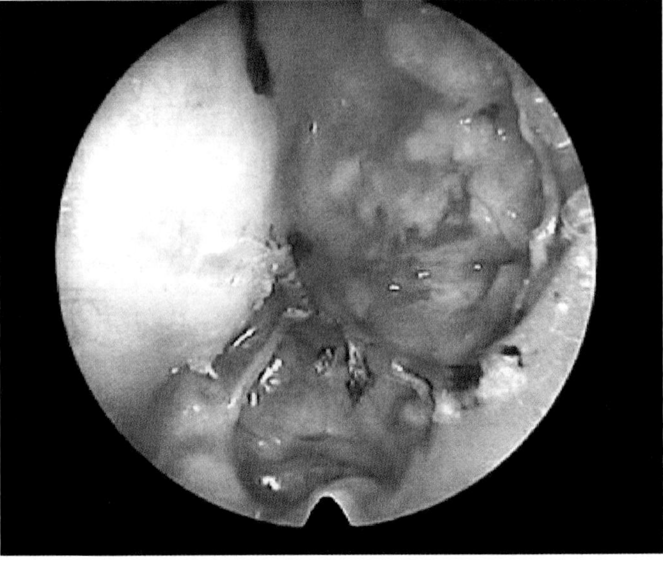

FIGURE 23-6 Cholesteatoma. (*Reproduced with permission from Vladimir Zlinsky, MD, in Roy F. Sullivan, PhD. Audiology Forum: Video Otoscopy, www.rcsullivan.com.*)

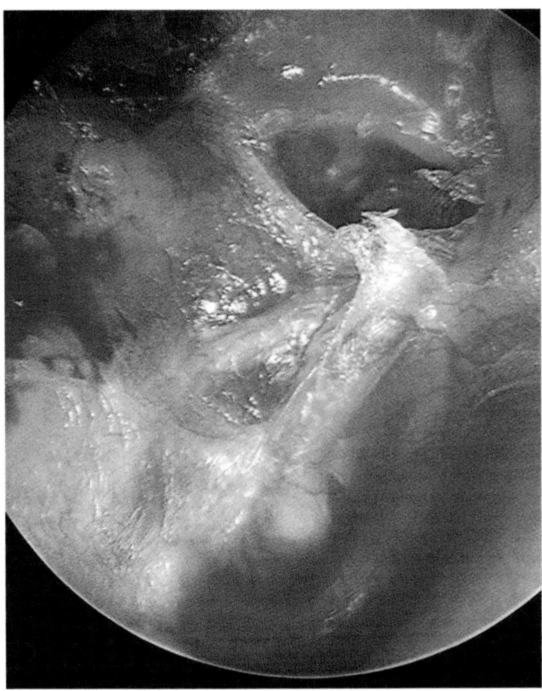

FIGURE 23-7 Primary acquired cholesteatoma with debris removed from the attic retraction pocket. (*Reproduced with permission from William Clark, MD.*)

- Foreign body—A foreign body may present with otalgia. Otoscopy reveals presence of foreign body (see Chapter 25, Ear: Foreign Body).
- Bullous myringitis—Bullous myringitis is often associated with viral or mycoplasma infection as well as usual AOM pathogens; in approximately one-third of patients, there is a component of sensorineural hearing loss. Otoscopy shows serous-filled bulla on the surface of the TM (**Figure 23-8**). Patients present with severe otalgia.

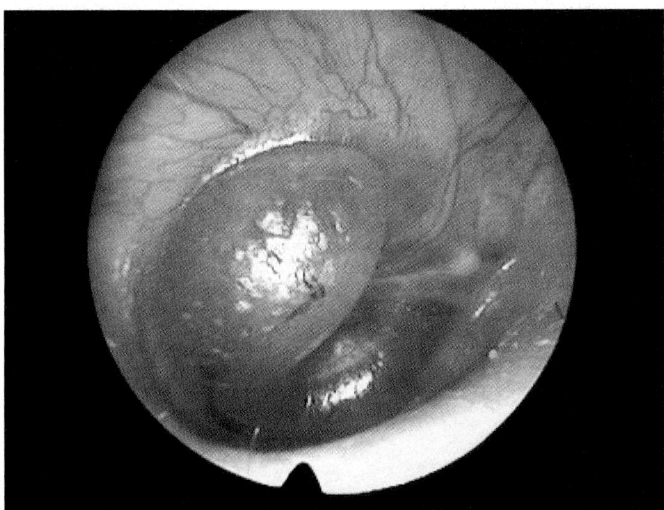

FIGURE 23-8 Bullous myringitis can be differentiated from otitis media with effusion by identifying serous-filled bulla on the surface of the TM. (*Reproduced with permission from Vladimir Zlinsky, MD, in Roy F. Sullivan, PhD. Audiology Forum: Video Otoscopy, www.rcsullivan.com.*)

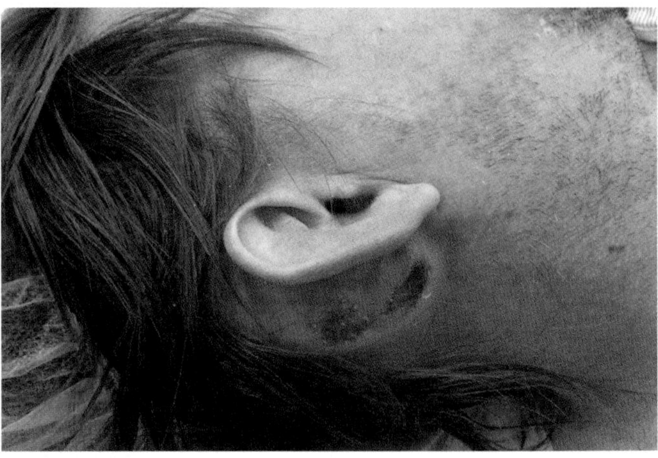

A

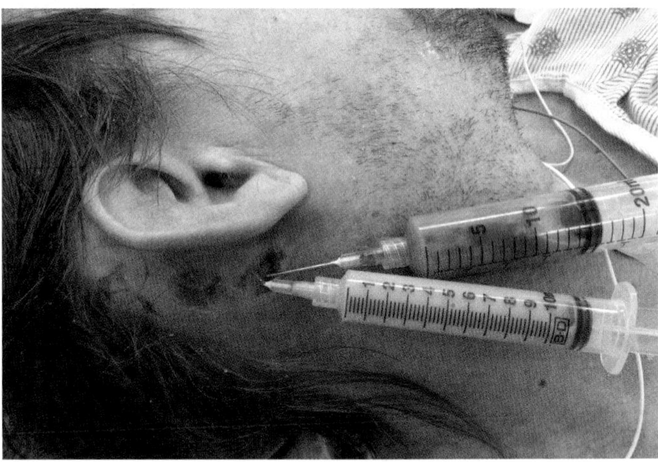

B

FIGURE 23-9 A. Mastoiditis in a man with 4 week history of an ear infection. The use of an inappropriate antibiotic without appropriate follow up resulted in "masked mastoiditis". CT scan showed bone erosion intracranially and laterally as a subperiosteal abscess. B. Needle aspiration of the abscess resulted in over 20 mL of pus being drained before a mastoidectomy was performed. The patient underwent mastoidectomy in the operating room to clean out the remaining infection. Fortunately he did not develop a brain abscess and he recovered fully after surgery. (*Reproduced with permission from Randal A. Otto, MD.*)

- Chronic suppurative otitis media (CSOM)—Otoscopy shows TM perforation and otorrhea; history reveals a chronically draining ear and recurrent middle-ear infections with or without hearing loss.
- Referred otalgia—This is rare in cases of bilateral otalgia, but should be considered in cases of otalgia that do not fit clinical features of AOM. Referred pain is usually from other head and neck structures (eg, teeth, jaw, cervical spine, lymph and salivary glands, nose and sinuses, tonsils, tongue, pharynx, meninges).
- Mastoiditis—Mastoiditis can be differentiated from simple AOM by presence of increasing pain and tenderness over mastoid bone in a patient with AOM who has not been treated with antibiotics, or recurrence of mastoid pain and tenderness in patients treated with antibiotics. Recurrence or persistence of fever, as well as progressive otorrhea, are other historical clues. The mastoid swelling may cause the pinna to protrude further than normal (**Figure 23-9**).
- Traumatic perforation of the TM (**Figure 23-10**)—A hole in the TM is seen without purulent drainage.

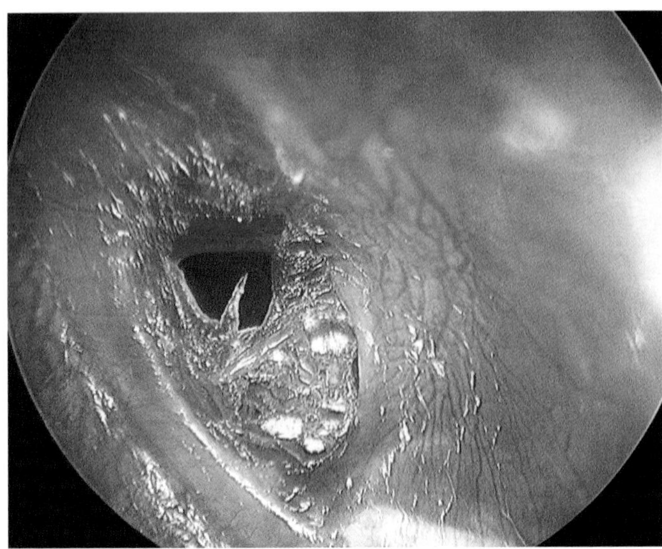

FIGURE 23-10 Traumatic perforation of the left tympanic membrane. (*Reproduced with permission from William Clark, MD.*)

MANAGEMENT

Most studies on management of AOM and OME have been performed with children. In the absence of data, the following is offered as likely to be useful in adults.

NONPHARMACOLOGIC

Antibiotics are not necessary to treat uncomplicated AOM.[13] SOR Ⓐ

Management of OME primarily consists of watchful waiting. Most cases resolve spontaneously within 3 months; only 5% to 10% last 1 year or longer. Treatment depends on duration and associated conditions. The following options should be considered:

- Document the laterality, duration of effusion, and presence and severity of associated symptoms.[6] SOR Ⓒ
- Hearing testing is recommended when OME persists in children for 3 months or longer[6] (SOR Ⓑ), but its role in adults is unclear.
- Autoinflation with a nasal balloon has been shown to provide short-term benefits in children, and adults can be taught to insufflate the ears by holding their nose, closing their mouth, and trying to blow their nose.

MEDICATIONS

- Oral acetaminophen (paracetamol) and ibuprofen may reduce earache.
  - There is insufficient data to evaluate the effectiveness of topical analgesics in AOM.[14] SOR Ⓑ
- Antibiotics may lead to more rapid reduction in symptoms of AOM, but increase the risk of adverse effects, including diarrhea, vomiting, and rash.[13] SOR Ⓑ
  - Antibiotics seem to reduce pain at 2 to 7 days, and may prevent development of contralateral AOM, but increase the risks of adverse effects compared with placebo.
  - There is insufficient effectiveness of data regarding which antibiotic regimen is better than another.[13]
  - Antibiotics found to be effective in AOM include amoxicillin, amoxicillin/clavulanic acid, ampicillin, penicillin, erythromycin, azithromycin, trimethoprim-sulfamethoxazole, and cephalosporins.
  - Longer (8- to 10-day) courses of antibiotics reduce short-term treatment failure but have no long-term benefits compared with shorter regimens (5-day courses).[13,15]
- Immediate antibiotic treatment (ie, given at initial consultation) may reduce the duration of symptoms of AOM, but increases the risk of vomiting, diarrhea, and rash compared with delayed treatment (ie, given after 72 hours).[13] SOR Ⓑ
- Treatment of AOM with decongestants and antihistamines is not recommended.[16] SOR Ⓑ
- Antihistamines and decongestants are not effective for OME.[6] SOR Ⓐ
- Antimicrobials and corticosteroids are not recommended for OME.[6] SOR Ⓐ

REFERRAL

- Refer to specialist (otolaryngologist, audiologist, or speech-language pathologist) for the following reasons[6]: SOR Ⓒ
  - Persistent fluid for 4 or more months with persistent hearing loss
  - Structural damage to TM or middle-ear

PREVENTION

- Xylitol chewing gum or syrup given 5 times daily has a small preventive effect on recurrence of AOM.[13] SOR Ⓑ
- Tympanostomy tubes lead to short-term reduction in the number of episodes of AOM in children but increase the risk of complications (ie, tympanosclerosis; **Figure 23-11**).[13] SOR Ⓑ

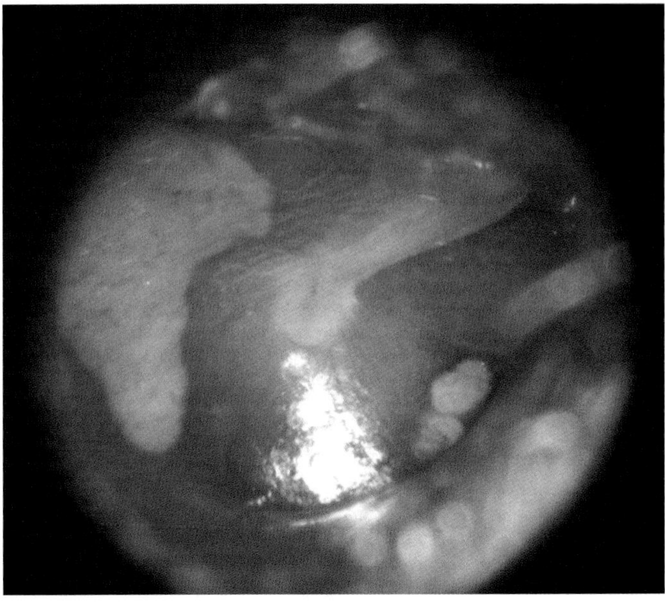

FIGURE 23-11 Tympanosclerosis as the result of previous recurrent episodes of otitis media and polyethylene (PE) tube placement. (*Reproduced with permission from Glen Medellin, MD.*)

PROGNOSIS

- Without antibiotics, AOM resolves within 24 hours in approximately 60% of children and within 3 days in approximately 80% of children. Rate of suppurative complications if antibiotics are withheld is 0.13%.[17]
- Most cases of OME resolve spontaneously within 3 months; only 5% to 10% last 1 year or longer. However, effusion will recur in 30% to 40% of patients.[6]

FOLLOW-UP

- If a patient with AOM fails to respond to the initial management option within 48 to 72 hours, the clinician should reassess the patient to confirm AOM and exclude other causes of illness. If AOM is confirmed in a patient initially managed with observation, the clinician should begin antibiotics. If the patient was initially managed with antibiotics, the clinician should change antibiotics.[6] SOR B
- Potentially serious complications of AOM, such as mastoiditis or facial nerve involvement, require urgent referral.
- There is no consensus in the medical community regarding timing of posttreatment follow-up of AOM or who should be receiving follow-up. There is some evidence that parents can be reliable predictors in the resolution or persistence of AOM following antibiotic treatment.[18]

PATIENT EDUCATION

- Smoking cessation should be recommended and assistance offered to smokers (see Chapter 237, Tobacco Addiction).
- Parents should be made aware of the high rates of spontaneous resolution of AOM and potential adverse effects of antibiotics. Providing a prescription for an antibiotic at the initial visit but advising delay of initiation of medication (ie, observational approach for up to 48 hours) is an alternative to immediate treatment and is associated with lower antibiotic use.[19]
- Patients should be informed that the natural history of OME is spontaneous resolution.
  - Periodic follow-up to monitor resolution of MEE is important and if MEE with hearing loss persists, additional treatment or referral may be considered.

PATIENT RESOURCES

Acute Otitis Media

- Medline Plus. *Ear infection-acute*—**http://www.nlm.nih.gov/medlineplus/ency/article/000638.htm.**
- NIDCD. *Ear Infections in Children*—**http://www.nidcd.nih.gov/health/hearing/earinfections.**
- FamilyDoctor.org. *Middle Ear Infections*—**http://www.kidshealth.org/PageManager.jsp?dn=familydoctor&lic=44&article_set=22743.**
- NHS. *Middle ear infection (otitis media)*—**http://www.nhs.uk/conditions/Otitis-media/Pages/Introduction.aspx.**

Otitis Media with Effusion

- Medline Plus. *Otitis Media with Effusion*—**http://www.nlm.nih.gov/medlineplus/ency/article/ 007010.htm.**

PROVIDER RESOURCES

Acute Otitis Media

- Guideline: diagnosis and management of acute otitis media. Clinical Practice Guideline by the American Academy of Family Physicians, American Academy of Otolaryngology-Head and Neck Surgery, and American Academy of Pediatrics Subcommittee on Management of Acute Otitis Media. *Pediatrics.* 2004;113:1451-1465.
- NHS. *Acute otitis media*—**http://www.npc.nhs.uk/merec/infect/commonintro/resources/merec_bulletin_vol17_no3_acute_otitis_media.pdf.**
- British Columbia Medical Association. *Acute Otitis Media (AOM)*—**http://www.bcguidelines.ca/pdf/otitaom.pdf.**
- General Practice Notebook. *Acute Otitis Media (AOM)*—**http://www.gpnotebook.co.uk/simplepage.cfm?ID=1926234161.**

Otitis Media with Effusion

- British Columbia Medical Association. *Otitis Media with Effusion (OME)*—**http://www.bcguidelines.ca/pdf/otitome.pdf.**

REFERENCES

1. Bondy J, Berman S, Glazner J, Lezotte D. Direct expenditures related to otitis media diagnoses: extrapolations from a pediatric medicaid cohort. *Pediatrics.* 2000;105(6):E72.
2. Paradise JL, Rockette HE, Colborn DK, et al. Otitis media in 2253 Pittsburgh-area infants: prevalence and risk factors during the first two years of life. *Pediatrics.* 1997;99(3):318-333.
3. Schwartz LE, Brown RB. Purulent otitis media in adults. *Arch Intern Med.* 1992;152(11):2301-2304.
4. Culpepper L, Froom J, Bartelds AI, et al. Acute otitis media in adults: a report from the International Primary Care Network. *J Am Board Fam Pract.* 1993;6:333-339.
5. Del Mar C, Glasziou P, Hayem M. Are antibiotics indicated as initial treatment for children with acute otitis media? A meta-analysis. *BMJ.* 1997;314:1526-1529.
6. Guideline: otitis media with effusion. Clinical practice guideline by the American Academy of Family Physicians, American Academy of Otolaryngology-Head and Neck Surgery, and American Academy of Pediatrics Subcommittee on Otitis Media With Effusion. *Pediatrics.* 2004;113:1412-1429.

7. Rovers MM, Schilder AG, Zielhuis GA, Rosenfeld RM. Otitis media. *Lancet.* 2004;363:465.

8. Casey JR, Adlowitz DG, Pichichero ME. New patterns in the otopathogens causing acute otitis media six to eight years after introduction of pneumococcal conjugate vaccine. *Pediatr Infect Dis J.* 2010;29(4):304-309.

9. McEllistrem MC. Acute otitis media due to penicillin-nonsusceptible *Streptococcus pneumoniae* before and after the introduction of the pneumococcal conjugate vaccine. *Clin Infect Dis.* 2005;40(12):1738-1744.

10. Celin SE, Bluestone CD, Stephenson J, et al. Bacteriology of acute otitis media in adults. *JAMA.* 1991;266(16):2249-2252.

11. Ruuskanen O, Arola M, Heikkinen T, Ziegler T. Viruses in acute otitis media: increasing evidence for clinical significance. *Pediatr Infect Dis J.* 1991;10:425.9.

12. Takata GS, Chan LS, Morphew T, et al. Evidence assessment of the accuracy of methods of diagnosing middle ear effusion in children with otitis media with effusion. *Pediatrics.* 2003;112:1379-1387.

13. Williamson I. Otitis media with effusion in children. *Clin Evid.* 2011;01:502-531.

14. Foxlee R, Johansson A, Wejfalk J, Dawkins J, Dooley L, Del Mar C. Topical analgesia for acute otitis media. *Cochrane Database Syst Rev.* 2006;3:CD005657.

15. Kozyrskyj AL, Hildes-Ripstein GE, Longstaffe SE, et al. Short-course antibiotics for acute otitis media. *Cochrane Database Syst Rev.* 2000;(2):CD001095.

16. Flynn CA, Griffin GH, Schultz JK. Decongestants and antihistamines for acute otitis media in children. *Cochrane Database Syst Rev.* 2004;3:CD001727.

17. Rosenfeld RM. Natural history of untreated otitis media. *Laryngoscope.* 2003;113:1645-1657.

18. Raimer PL. *Parents Can Be Reliable Predictors in the Resolution or Persistence of Acute Otitis Media Following Antibiotic Treatment.* University of Michigan Department of Pediatrics Evidence-based Pediatrics Web site. 2005. http://www.med.umich.edu/pediatrics/ebm/cats/omparent.htm. Accessed February 2012.

19. Spiro DM, Tay KY, Arnold DH, et al. Wait-and-see prescription for the treatment of acute otitis media: a randomized controlled trial. *JAMA.* 2006;296:1235-1241.

24 OTITIS EXTERNA

Brian Z. Rayala, MD

PATIENT STORY

A 40-year-old woman with type 2 diabetes presents to her family physician with a 2-day history of bilateral otalgia, otorrhea, and hearing loss. Symptoms started in the right ear and then rapidly spread to the left ear. She had a low-grade fever and was systemically ill. The external ear was swollen with honey-crusts (**Figures 24-1** and **24-2**). The external auditory canal (EAC) was narrowed and contained purulent discharge (**Figure 24-3**). Ear, nose, and throat (ENT) was consulted and she was admitted to the hospital for the presumptive diagnosis of malignant otitis externa. The magnetic resonance imaging (MRI) showed some destruction of the temporal bone. She was started on IV ciprofloxacin and the ear culture grew out *Pseudomonas aeruginosa* sensitive to ciprofloxacin. The patient responded well to treatment and was able to go home on oral ciprofloxacin 5 days later.

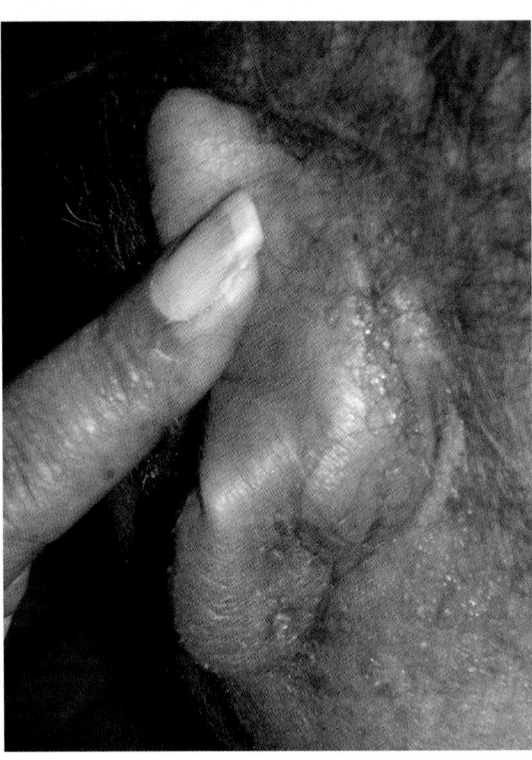

FIGURE 24-2 Another view of the malignant or necrotizing otitis externa. *(Reproduced with permission from E.J. Mayeaux, MD.)*

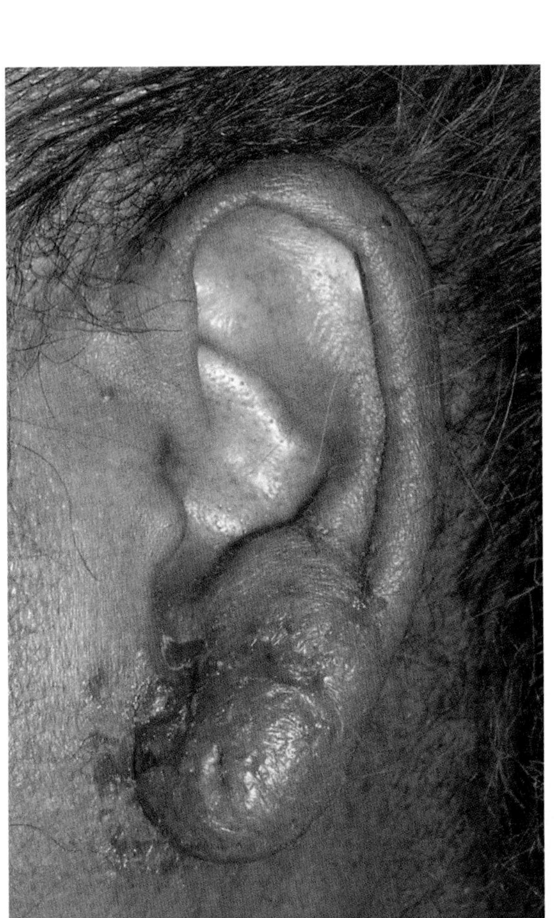

FIGURE 24-1 Malignant or necrotizing otitis externa in a 40-year-old woman with diabetes. Note the swelling and honey-crusts of the pinna. The EAC and temporal bone were involved. *(Reproduced with permission from E.J. Mayeaux, MD.)*

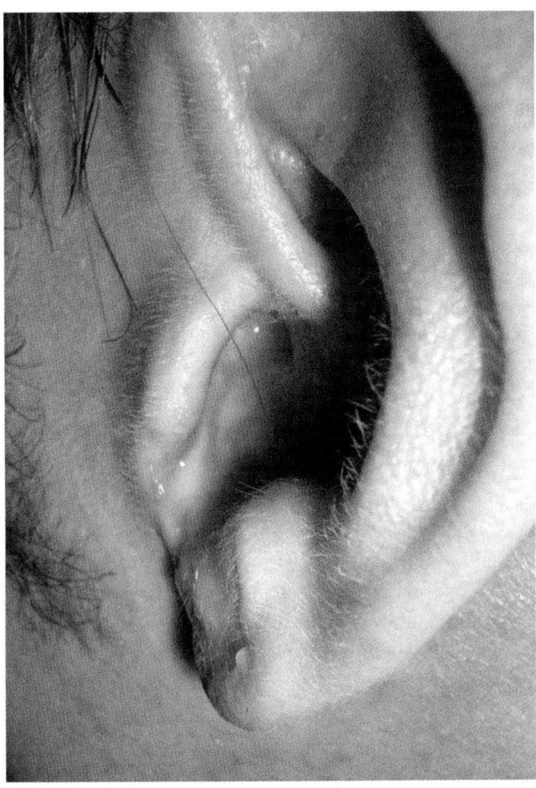

FIGURE 24-3 Chronic suppurative otitis media with purulent discharge chronically draining from the ear of this 25-year-old man. This image could be seen in acute otitis media with perforation of the tympanic membrane or in a purulent otitis externa. *(Reproduced with permission from Richard P. Usatine, MD.)*

INTRODUCTION

Otitis externa (OE) is common in all parts of the world. OE is defined as inflammation, often with infection, of the EAC.[1]

EPIDEMIOLOGY

- Incidence of OE is not known precisely; its lifetime incidence was estimated at 10% in one study.[2]
- Occurs more often in adults than in children.

ETIOLOGY AND PATHOPHYSIOLOGY

- Common pathogens, which are part of normal EAC flora, include aerobic organisms predominantly (*P. aeruginosa and Staphylococcus aureus*) and, to a lesser extent, anaerobes (*Bacteroides* and *Peptostreptococcus*). Up to a third of infections are polymicrobial. A small proportion (2-10%) of OE is caused by fungal overgrowth (eg, *Aspergillus niger* usually occurs with prolonged antibiotic use).[1]
- Pathogenesis of OE includes the following:
  - Trauma, the usual inciting event, leads to breech in the integrity of EAC skin.
  - Skin inflammation and edema ensue, which, in turn, lead to pruritus and obstruction of adnexal structures (eg, cerumen glands, sebaceous glands, and hair follicles).
  - Pruritus leads to scratching, which results in further skin injury.
  - Consequently, the milieu of the EAC is altered (ie, change in quality and quantity of cerumen, increase in pH of EAC, and dysfunctional epithelial migration).
  - Finally, the EAC becomes a warm, alkaline, and moist environment—ideal for growth of different pathogens.

RISK FACTORS

- Environmental factors[3]
  - Moisture—Macerates skin of EAC, elevates pH, and removes protective cerumen layer (from swimming, perspiration, high humidity).
  - Trauma—Leads to injury of EAC skin (from cotton buds, fingernails, hearing aids, ear plugs, paper clips, match sticks, mechanical removal of cerumen).
  - High environmental temperatures.
- Host factors
  - Anatomic—Wax and debris accumulate and lead to moisture retention (eg, a narrow ear canal, hairy ear canal).
  - Cerumen—Absence or overproduction of cerumen (leads to loss of the protective layer and moisture retention, respectively).
  - Chronic dermatologic disease (eg, atopic dermatitis, psoriasis, seborrheic dermatitis).
  - Immunocompromise (eg, chemotherapy, HIV, AIDS).

DIAGNOSIS

CLINICAL FEATURES

- OE can either be localized, like a furuncle, or generalized (**Figure 24-4**). The latter is known as "diffuse OE," or simply OE. Seborrheic dermatitis of the external ear and EAC can be diffuse or generalized (see **Figure 24-4**).

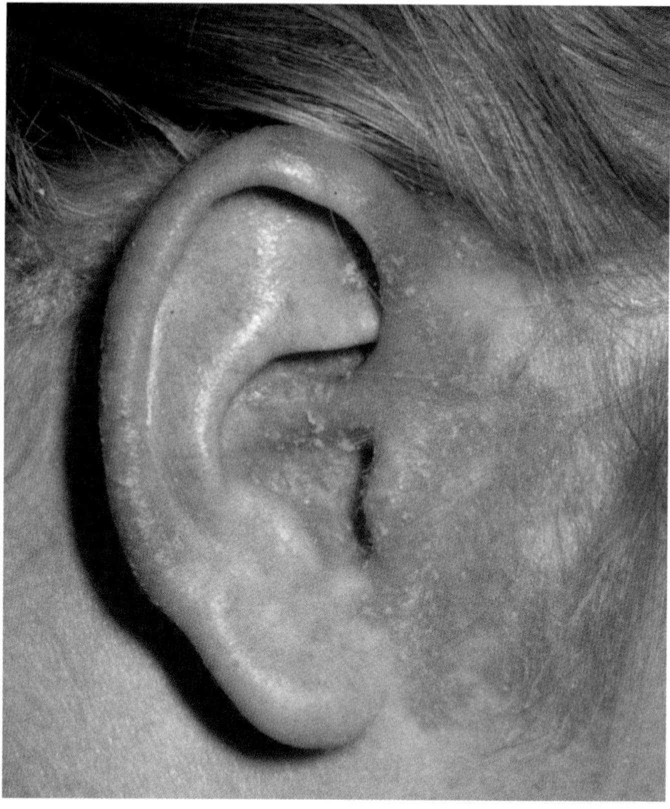

FIGURE 24-4 Seborrheic dermatitis causing erythema and greasy scale of the external ear and ear canal. The seborrheic dermatitis itself causes breaks in the skin and the coexisting pruritus may lead the patient to damage their own ear canal. This can become secondarily infected. *(Reproduced with permission from Eric Kraus, MD.)*

- Forms of (diffuse) OE[1]
  - Acute (<6 weeks; **Figures 24-5** and **24-6**).
  - Chronic (>3 months)—May cause hearing loss and stenosis of the EAC (**Figure 24-7**).
  - Necrotizing or malignant form—Defined by destruction of the temporal bone, usually in diabetic or immunocompromised people; often life threatening (see **Figure 24-1**).
- Key historical features
  - Otalgia, including pruritus
  - Otorrhea (see **Figure 24-3**)
  - Mild hearing loss
- Key physical findings
  - Pain with tragal pressure or pain when the auricle is pulled superiorly, this may be absent in very mild cases.
  - Signs of EAC inflammation (edema, erythema, aural discharge) (see **Figures 24-5** to **24-7**).
  - Fever, periauricular erythema, and lymphadenopathy point to severe disease.
  - Complete obstruction of EAC occurs in advanced OE.
- Establishing the integrity of the tympanic membrane (TM) (through direct visualization) and the absence of middle-ear effusion (through pneumatic otoscopy) is crucial in differentiating OE from other diagnoses (eg, suppurative otitis media, cholesteatoma).

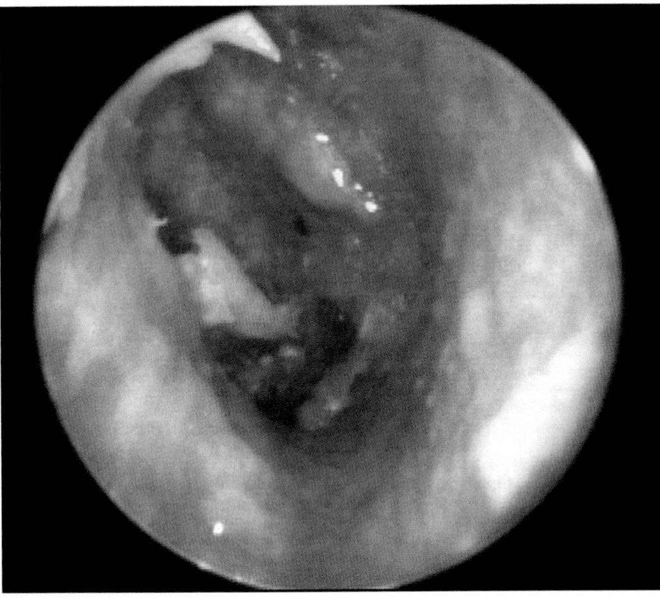

FIGURE 24-5 Acute otitis externa showing purulent discharge and narrowing of the ear canal. (*Reproduced with permission from Roy F. Sullivan, PhD. Audiology Forum: Video Otoscopy, www.rcsullivan.com.*)

LABORATORY AND IMAGING

- Because OE is mostly a clinical diagnosis, diagnostic testing has a limited role. When a patient fails to respond to empiric treatment, obtaining a culture of aural discharge may help guide proper choice of treatment (antibacterial vs antifungal agents).
- If necrotizing or malignant OE is suspected, computed tomography (CT) or MRI of the ear or skull base is warranted.

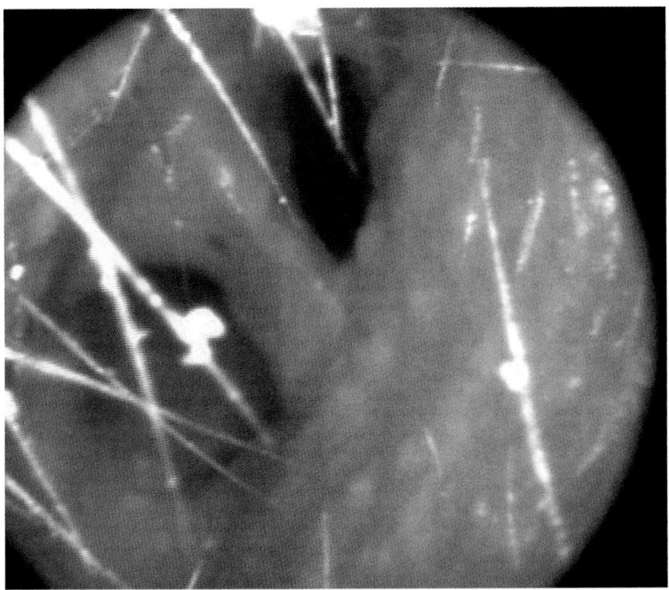

FIGURE 24-6 Acute otitis externa in an old man who wears a hearing aid. Note the viscous purulent discharge and narrowing of the ear canal. (*Reproduced with permission from Roy F. Sullivan, PhD. Audiology Forum: Video Otoscopy, www.rcsullivan.com.*)

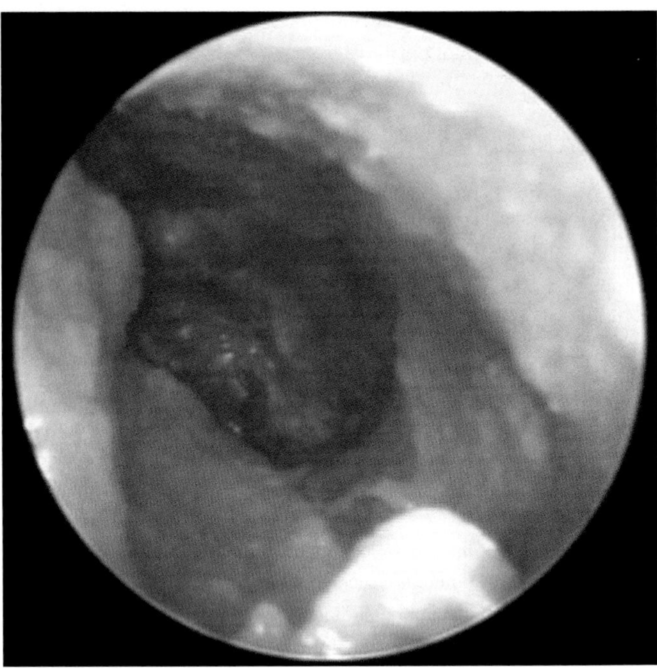

FIGURE 24-7 Chronic otitis externa in an old woman who wears a hearing aid. The ear canal is not narrowed but is coated with a purulent discharge. (*Reproduced with permission from Roy F. Sullivan, PhD. Audiology Forum: Video Otoscopy, www.rcsullivan.com.*)

DIFFERENTIAL DIAGNOSIS

- Chronic suppurative otitis media—Otoscopy shows TM perforation; history reveals a chronically draining ear and recurrent middle-ear infections with or without hearing loss (see **Figure 24-3**).
- Seborrheic dermatitis involving the external ear and EAC can lead to inflammation and breaks in the skin (see **Figure 24-4**). The coexisting pruritus may lead the patient to damage their own ear canal. This can all become secondarily infected and become an infected OE.
- Acute otitis media with perforated TM—Presents with purulent drainage from the canal in the setting of ear pain and clinical signs or symptoms of acute illness such as fever. If the TM is visible, it will be red with a perforation (see Chapter 23, Otitis Media: Acute Otitis and Otitis Media with Effusion).
- Foreign body in the EAC—Otoscopy, with or without aural toilet, confirms presence of foreign body (that incites an inflammatory response, leading to otalgia and otorrhea); see Chapter 25, Ear: Foreign Body.
- Otomycosis—Pruritus is generally more prominent and EAC inflammation (otalgia and otorrhea) is less pronounced; fungal organisms have a characteristic appearance in the EAC.
- Contact dermatitis—Usually caused by ototopical agents (eg, neomycin, benzocaine, propylene glycol); seen in patients with poor response to empiric OE treatment; prominent clinical features include pruritus, erythema of conchal bowl, crusting, and excoriations.

MANAGEMENT

NONPHARMACOLOGIC

- The effectiveness of ear cleaning is unknown.[3] SOR Ⓑ

- The effectiveness of specialist aural toilet (use of operating microscope to mechanically remove material from external canal) for treating OE is unknown.[1] SOR B

MEDICATIONS

- The management of acute OE should include an assessment of pain. The clinician should recommend analgesic treatment based on the severity of pain.[4] SOR B
- Topical treatments alone are effective for uncomplicated acute OE. Additional oral antibiotics are not required.[3] SOR B
- The evidence for steroid-only drops is very limited.[3] SOR B
- Given that most topical treatments are equally effective, it would appear that in most cases the preferred choice of topical treatment may be determined by other factors, such as risk of ototoxicity, risk of contact sensitivity, risk of developing resistance, availability, cost, and dosing schedule.[3] SOR B
  - Evidence from one trial of low quality found no difference in clinical efficacy between quinolone and nonquinolone drops. Quinolones are more expensive than nonquinolones.[3] SOR B
  - There is some evidence indicating that patients treated with topical preparations containing antibiotics and steroids benefit from reduced swelling, severe redness, secretion, and analgesic consumption compared to preparations without steroids. There is a suggestion that high-potency steroids may be more effective than low-potency steroids (in terms of severe pain, inflammation, and swelling).[3] SOR B
  - Acetic acid was effective and comparable to antibiotic or steroid at week 1. However, when treatment needed to be extended beyond this point it was less effective. In addition, patient symptoms lasted 2 days longer in the acetic acid group compared to antibiotic or steroid group.[3] SOR B
  - Topical aluminum acetate may be as effective as a topical antibiotic or steroid at improving cure rates in people with acute OE.[1] SOR B
- Patients prescribed with antibiotic or steroid drops can expect their symptoms to last for approximately 6 days after treatment has begun. Although patients are usually treated with topical medication for 7 to 10 days, it is apparent that this will undertreat some patients and overtreat others. It may be more useful when prescribing ear drops to instruct patients to use them for at least a week. If they have symptoms beyond the first week they should continue the drops until their symptoms resolve (and possibly for a few days after), for a maximum of an additional 7 days.[3] SOR B
- Evidence from one low-quality trial suggests a glycerine-ichthammol medicated wick may provide better pain relief in early severe acute OE than a triamcinolone/gramicidin/neomycin/nystatin medicated wick.[3] SOR B
- There is no evidence on the use of topical antifungal agents (with or without steroids) in OE.[1] SOR B

PREVENTION

Prophylactic treatments to prevent OE (topical acetic acid, topical corticosteroids, or water exclusion) have not been evaluated in clinical trials.[1] SOR B

PROGNOSIS

Acute OE often resolves within 6 weeks but can recur.

FOLLOW-UP

- If the patient fails to respond to empiric therapy within 48 to 72 hours, the clinician should reassess the patient to confirm the diagnosis of OE and to exclude other causes of illness.[4] SOR B
- Patients with persisting symptoms beyond 2 weeks should be considered treatment failures and alternative management should be initiated.[3] SOR B

PATIENT EDUCATION

- To avoid recurrent infections the following recommendations or suggestions should be followed[5]:
  - Recommend that patients not use cotton swabs inserted into the ear canal.
  - Avoid frequent washing of the ears with soap as this leaves an alkali residue that neutralizes the normal acidic pH of the ear canal.
  - Avoid swimming in polluted waters.
  - Ensure that the canals are emptied of water after swimming or bathing—This can be done by turning the head or holding a facial tissue on the outside of the ear to act as a wick.
- Consider ear drops for swimmers who get frequent OE. A combination of a 2:1 ratio of 70% isopropyl alcohol and acetic acid may be used after each episode of swimming to assist in drying and acidifying the ear canal.[5] SOR C
- Do not use earplugs while swimming because they may cause trauma to the ear canal leading to OE.[5]

PATIENT RESOURCES

- Patient.co.uk. *Otitis Externa*—**http://www.patient.co.uk/health/otitis-externa.**

PROVIDER RESOURCES

- Medscape. *Otitis Externa*—**http://emedicine.medscape.com/article/994550.**

REFERENCES

1. Hajioff D, MacKeith S. Otitis externa. *Clin Evid (Online)*. 2010 Aug 03;2010. pii:0510.
2. Raza SA, Denholm SW, Wong JC. An audit of the management of otitis externa in an ENT casualty clinic. *J Laryngol Otol*. 1995;109:130-133.
3. Kaushik V, Malik T, Saeed SR. Interventions for acute otitis externa. *Cochrane Database Syst Rev*. 2010 Jan 20;(1):CD004740.
4. Rosenfeld RM, Brown L, Cannon CR, et al; American Academy of Otolaryngology—Head and Neck Surgery Foundation. Clinical practice guideline: acute otitis externa. *Otolaryngol Head Neck Surg*. 2006;134(suppl 4):S4-S23.
5. Waitzman AA. *Otitis Externa*. Updated January 22, 2013. http://emedicine.medscape.com/article/994550-overview. Accessed on July 28, 2013.

25 EAR: FOREIGN BODY

Brian Z. Rayala, MD
Mindy A. Smith, MD, MS

PATIENT STORY

A 28-year-old woman comes to urgent care with left ear pain stating that, while hiking today, an insect flew into her ear. She tried rinsing her ear with water but nothing came out and she could hear the insect moving around in her ear. She is in obvious distress and on otoscopy you visualize a small live beetle near the tympanic membrane (TM). There is erythema in the external canal but the TM appears intact. The physician instills mineral oil into her ear which stops the movement. She then irrigates the ear and with suction removes the insect.

INTRODUCTION

Ear foreign bodies (FBs) can present with otalgia, otorrhea, or decreased hearing. At other times, patients may be asymptomatic.

EPIDEMIOLOGY

Ear FBs are commonly seen in children,[1] but can be seen in adults, both healthy and cognitively impaired.

ETIOLOGY AND PATHOPHYSIOLOGY

- In a retrospective case series from 2 Australian emergency departments, most patients presenting with ear FBs were adults (217/330).[2] Types of foreign bodies seen in adults included the following:
  - Inanimate objects such as cotton tips, cotton wool, and silicone ear plugs
  - Insects (**Figure 25-1**)
- Adults in this study were more likely to have associated otitis externa than children (see Chapter 24, Otitis Externa).[2] Following are some key elements of otitis externa in patients with ear foreign bodies:
  - Initial breakdown of the skin-cerumen barrier (caused by presence of FB).
  - Skin inflammation and edema leading to subsequent obstruction of adnexal structures (eg, cerumen glands, sebaceous glands, and hair follicles).
  - FB reaction leading to further skin injury.
  - In the case of alkaline battery electrochemical reaction, severe alkaline burns may occur.

RISK FACTORS

Silicone and wax ear plugs can become impacted in the ear canal when body temperature softens them to a dough-like consistency becoming effectively glued to the surrounding ear canal.[3]

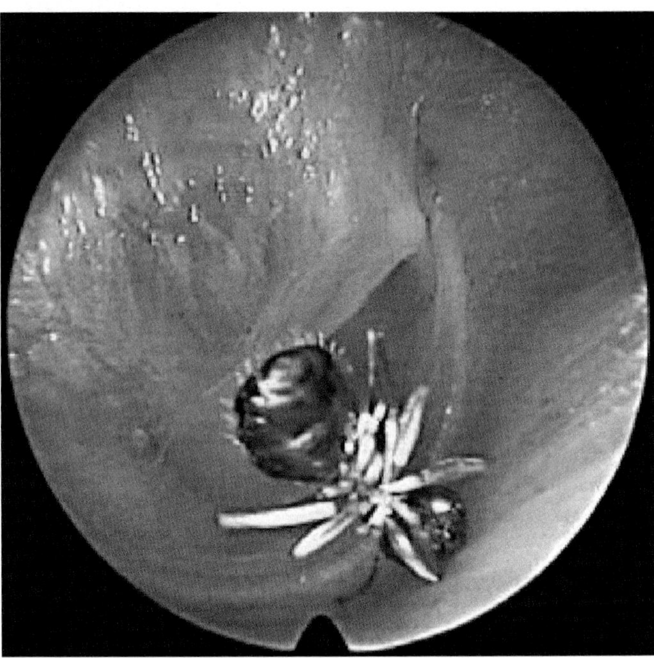

FIGURE 25-1 Ant in the ear canal. (*Reproduced with permission from Vladimir Zlinsky, MD in Roy F. Sullivan, PhD. Audiology Forum: Video Otoscopy, www.rcsullivan.com.*)

DIAGNOSIS

CLINICAL FEATURES

- Key historical features include the following:
  - Otalgia
  - Otorrhea or otorrhagia
  - Mild hearing loss
  - Ear itching or foreign body sensation
  - Tinnitus
  - History suspicious for FB insertion or witnessed FB insertion
- Patients may be asymptomatic.
- Hallmark of diagnosis includes visualization of FB on otoscopy (see **Figures 25-1** to **25-3**).
- Otoscopy may reveal signs of external auditory canal (EAC) inflammation (eg, edema, erythema, aural discharge) (see **Figure 25-2**).

LABORATORY AND IMAGING

Aural FB is a clinical diagnosis. Laboratory and imaging studies have very limited use.

DIFFERENTIAL DIAGNOSIS

- Otitis externa—Presents with otalgia, otorrhea, and mild hearing loss, all of which can be present in ear FB. Absence of FB (on otoscopic examination) is the key differentiating factor (see Chapter 24, Otitis Externa).
- Acute otitis media (with or without perforated TM)—Otoscopy shows absence of FB and presence of middle-ear inflammation and effusion (ie, bulging, erythematous, cloudy, immobile TM). Patients present with clinical signs or symptoms of acute illness like fever (see Chapter 23, Otitis Media: Acute Otitis and Otitis Media With Effusion).

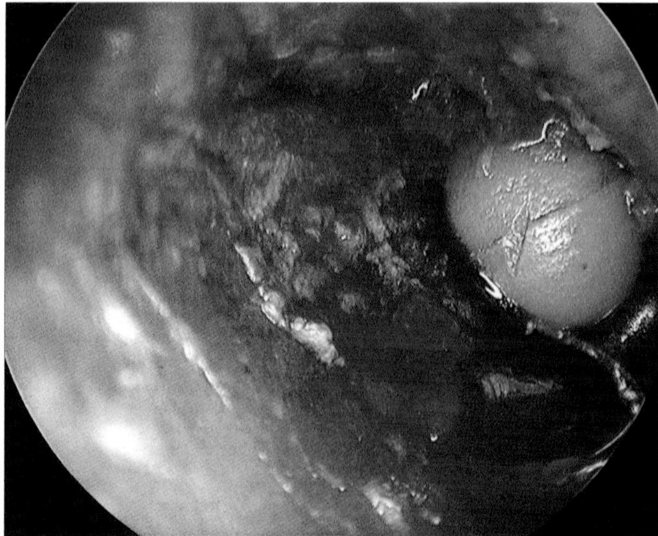

FIGURE 25-2 Foreign body (bead) in the ear canal of a 3-year-old girl with reactive tissue around it. (*Reproduced with permission from William Clark, MD.*)

- Chronic suppurative otitis media—Otoscopy shows absence of FB and presence of TM perforation; history reveals a chronically draining ear and recurrent middle-ear infections with or without hearing loss.

MANAGEMENT

MEDICATIONS

Topical treatment may be needed if there is accompanying otitis externa (see Chapter 24, Otitis Externa).

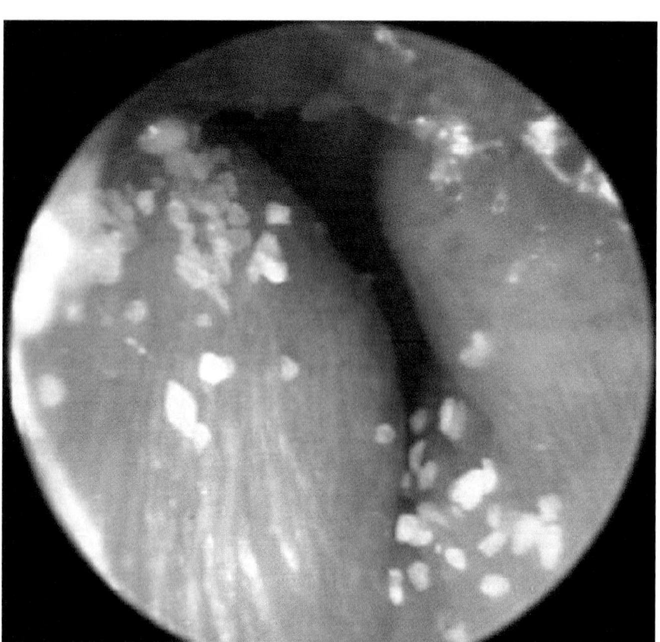

FIGURE 25-3 Beach sand granules with exostosis in the ear of a cold water surfer. The exostoses are common in cold water swimmers and surfers. (*Reproduced with permission from Roy F. Sullivan, PhD. Audiology Forum: Video Otoscopy, www.rcsullivan.com.*)

PROCEDURES

- Proper instrumentation allows the uncomplicated removal of many ear FBs. SOR C
  - The use of general anesthesia may be needed in some ear FBs whose contour, composition, or location predispose to traumatic removal in the ambulatory setting.[3] SOR C
- Ear FBs can be removed by irrigation, suction, or instrumentation. The type of procedure depends on the type of FB being removed.
  - Small inorganic objects can be removed from the EAC by irrigation. Contraindications to irrigation include the following:
    - Perforated TM.
    - Vegetable matter—Irrigation causes swelling of the vegetable matter which leads to further obstruction.
    - Alkaline (button) battery—Irrigation enhances leakage and potential for liquefaction necrosis and severe alkaline burns.
  - Objects with protruding surfaces or irregular edges can be removed with alligator forceps under direct visualization.
  - Objects that are round or breakable can be removed using a wire loop, a curette, or a right-angle hook that is slowly advanced beyond the object and carefully withdrawn.
  - Cyanoacrylate adhesive (eg, "superglue") has been used to remove tightly wedged, smooth, round FBs.
  - Live insects should be killed before removing them (by irrigation or forceps). Instilling alcohol or mineral oil into the auditory canal can kill them.

REFERRAL

Referral to otolaryngology should be considered in case of the following:

- More than one attempt has been carried out without success.[4]
- More than one instrument is needed for removal.[5]
- Patients who have firm, rounded FBs.[6]
- Patients who have FBs with smooth, nongraspable surfaces (see **Figure 25-1**).[7]

PREVENTION

- Efforts should focus on preventing small children or cognitively impaired adults from having access to tiny objects (eg, beads, small toys, etc).
- Adults should be instructed to avoid use of cotton swabs inserted into the ear canal and to use caution with silicone or wax ear plugs, avoiding prolonged placement.

PROGNOSIS

Several retrospective studies from urban emergency departments showed that emergency physicians successfully removed most FBs (53-80%) with minimal complications and no need for operative removal.[4-7] However, timely referral for difficult removal or following unsuccessful patient attempts at removal is prudent.

FOLLOW-UP

Follow-up is important in cases where EAC inflammation or infection is likely (eg, numerous attempts, use of numerous instruments, protracted exposure to the FB).

PATIENT EDUCATION

Parents should be informed that successful removal depends a great deal on the length of time the FB has remained in the EAC.

PATIENT RESOURCES

- eMedicine Health. *Foreign Body, Ear*—**http://www.emedicinehealth.com/foreign_body_ear/article_em.htm.**
- WebMD Pain Management Center. *Objects in the Ear*—**http://www.webmd.com/pain-management/tc/objects-in-the-ear-topic-overview.**

PROVIDER RESOURCES

- ENT USA. *External Ear Canal*—**http://www.entusa.com/external_ear_canal.htm.**
- Medline Plus. *Ear emergencies*—**http://www.nlm.nih.gov/medlineplus/ency/article/000052.htm.**
- Medscape. *Ear foreign body removal*—**http://emedicine.medscape.com/article/763712.**

REFERENCES

1. Baker MD. Foreign bodies of the ears and nose in childhood. *Pediatr Emerg Care*. 1987;3:67-70.
2. Ryan C, Ghosh A, Wilson-Boyd B, et al. Presentation and management of aural foreign bodies in two Australian emergency departments. *Emerg Med Australas*. 2006;18:372-378.
3. Shakeel M, Carlile A, Venkatraman J, et al. Earplugs presenting as an impacted foreign body in the ear canal. *Clin Otolaryngol*. 2013;38(3):280-281.
4. Marin JR, Trainor JL. Foreign body removal from the external auditory canal in a pediatric emergency department. *Pediatr Emerg Care*. 2006;22:630-634.
5. Ansley JF, Cunningham MJ. Response to O'Donovan. Glue ear and foreign body. *Pediatrics*. 1999;103(4):857.
6. Thompson SK, Wein RO, Dutcher PO. External auditory canal foreign body removal: management practices and outcomes. *Laryngoscope*. 2003;113:1912-1915.
7. DiMuzio J Jr, Deschler DG. Emergency department management of foreign bodies of the external ear canal in children. *Otol Neurotol*. 2002;23:473-475.

26 CHONDRODERMATITIS NODULARIS HELICIS AND PREAURICULAR TAGS

Linda Speer, MD

PATIENT STORY

A 44-year-old white man presents with a painful nodule on his right ear for 1 year (**Figure 26-1**). He has a long history of occupational sun exposure but no skin cancers. He states that it is too painful to sleep on his right side because of the ear nodule. He tried to remove it once with nail clippers but it bled too much. The patient is told that this is likely a benign condition called chondrodermatitis nodularis helicis. A shave biopsy is performed for diagnostic purposes. It is explained to the patient that this could be a skin cancer as a result of his sun exposure history. The biopsy confirms chondrodermatitis nodularis helicis, and the options for definitive treatment are described to the patient.

INTRODUCTION

Chondrodermatitis nodularis helicis is a benign neoplasm of the ear cartilage commonly believed to be related to excessive pressure, for example, during sleep, and sun exposure. The result is a localized overgrowth of cartilage, and subsequent skin changes. Preauricular tags are malformations of the external ear.

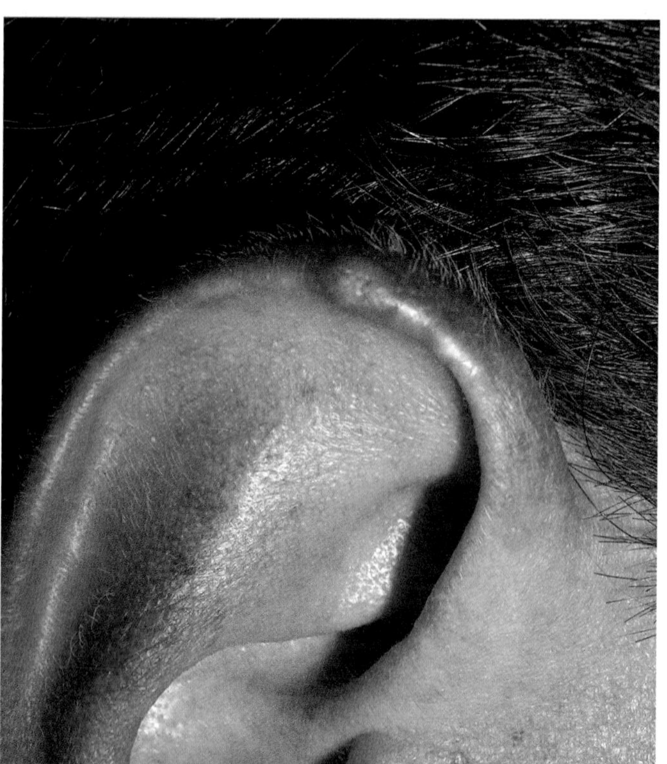

FIGURE 26-1 Chondrodermatitis nodularis helicis on the right ear of a 44-year-old man. (*Reproduced with permission from Richard P. Usatine, MD.*)

SYNONYMS

It is also known as chondrodermatitis nodularis chronica helicis.

EPIDEMIOLOGY

CHONDRODERMATITIS NODULARIS

- The incidence of chondrodermatitis nodularis has not been determined.
- Occurs most commonly in men older than 40 years of age, but older women can also be affected.

PREAURICULAR TAGS

Occur in approximately 1 of 10,000 to 12,500 births without predilection for gender or race. Several chromosomal abnormalities include preauricular tags[1] as one of the phenotypic expressions.

ETIOLOGY AND PATHOPHYSIOLOGY

CHONDRODERMATITIS NODULARIS HELICIS

In rare cases, especially when occurring at younger ages, the lesion may be related to an underlying disease associated with microvascular injury, such as vasculitis or other necrobiotic collagen disease.[2]

PREAURICULAR TAGS

- Arise from remnants of supernumerary branchial hillocks.[3]
- Early-stage embryology involves the formation of several slit-like structures on the side of the head, the branchial clefts. The 3 hillocks between the first 4 clefts eventually form the structure of the outer ear. Preauricular tags are generally minor malformations arising from remnants of supernumerary branchial hillocks.[4]

DIAGNOSIS

CLINICAL FEATURES OF CHONDRODERMATITIS

- Firm, painful nodule 3 to 20 mm in size (**Figures 26-1** to **26-4**).
- The helix is most often affected especially in men (see **Figures 26-1** and **26-2**). The antihelix is affected more often in women (see **Figures 26-3** and **26-4**).
- Overlying skin is normal in color or erythematous; a central ulcer may be present.

CLINICAL FEATURES OF PREAURICULAR TAGS

- Fleshy knob in front of the ear (**Figures 26-5** and **26-6**)
- Present from the time of birth
- Generally asymptomatic

TYPICAL DISTRIBUTION

- Chondrodermatitis is located at the helix or antihelix of the ear. The right ear is more often affected than the left.
- Preauricular tags may be unilateral or bilateral, more often present on the left.

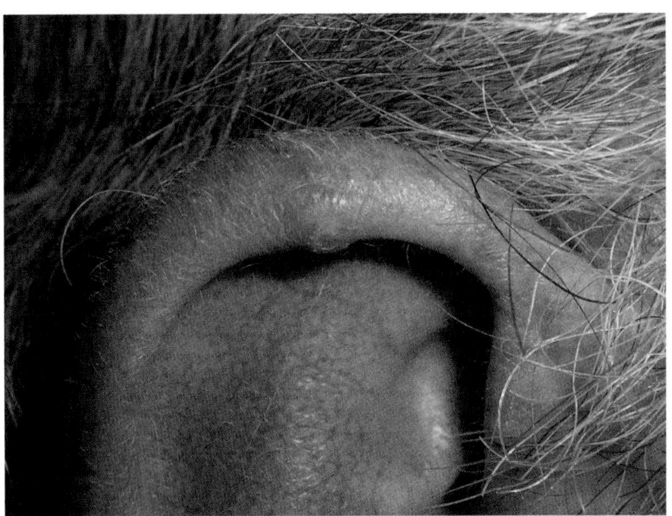

FIGURE 26-2 Chondrodermatitis nodularis on the helix of the right ear in a 62-year-old man. Note the pearly appearance, which may be seen with a basal cell carcinoma. (*Reproduced with permission from Richard P. Usatine, MD.*)

BIOPSY

- Often required for chondrodermatitis nodularis to rule out malignancy, especially when occurring in individuals with actinic damage and/or history of other skin cancers.
- Not indicated for preauricular tag.

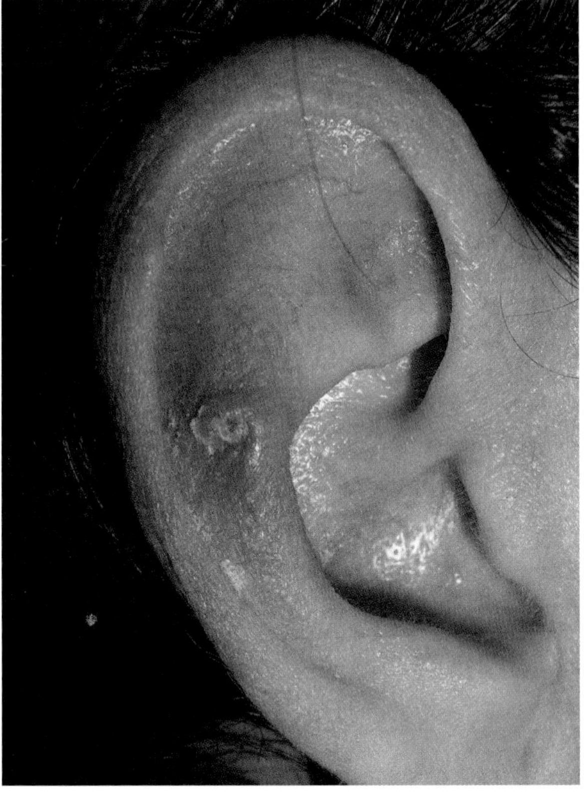

FIGURE 26-4 Chondrodermatitis nodularis on the antihelix of the right ear of a 52-year-old woman. Note the pearly nodule with central scale. A shave biopsy was performed to rule out basal cell carcinoma and squamous cell carcinoma. (*Reproduced with permission from Richard P. Usatine, MD.*)

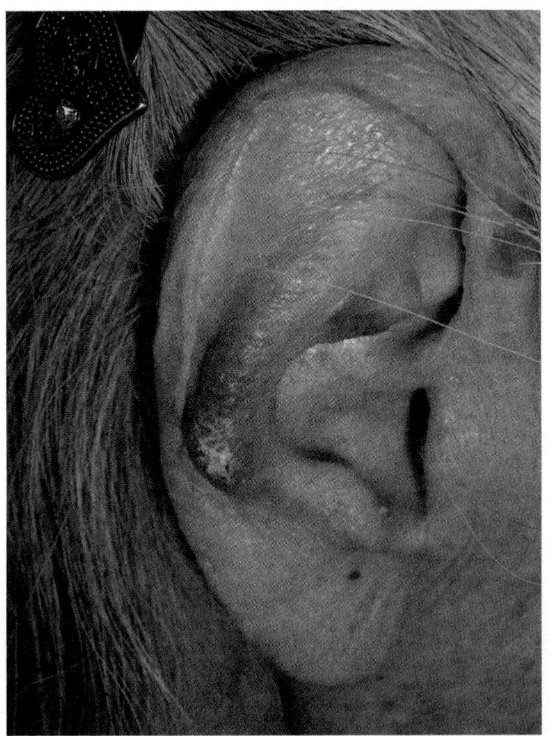

FIGURE 26-3 Chondrodermatitis nodularis on the antihelix of the right ear of an 86-year-old woman. Note the erythema and scale. A shave biopsy was performed to make sure this was not a squamous cell carcinoma. (*Reproduced with permission from Richard P. Usatine, MD.*)

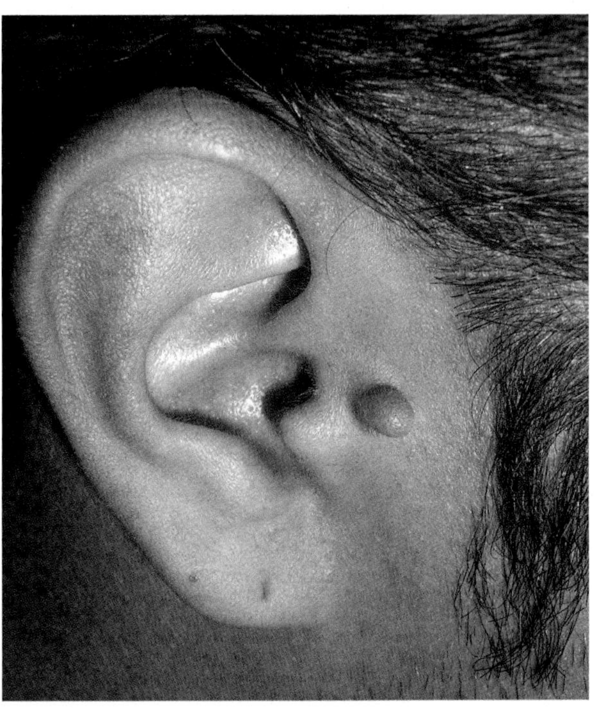

FIGURE 26-5 Preauricular tag in an adult man. (*Reproduced with permission from Richard P. Usatine, MD.*)

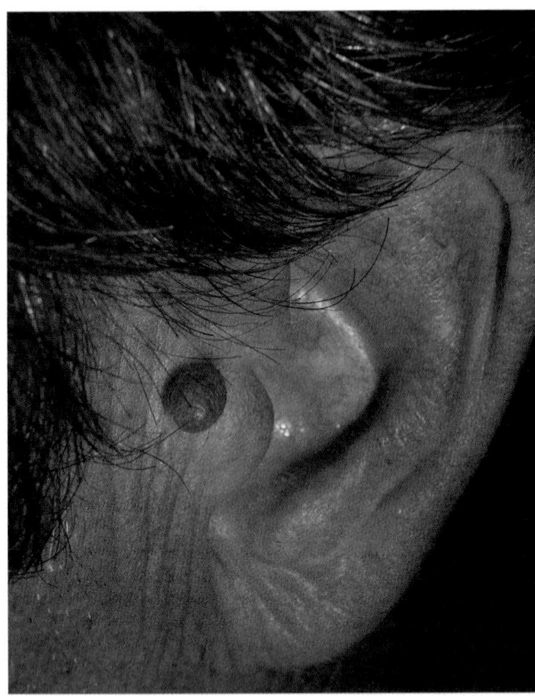

FIGURE 26-6 Preauricular tag present since birth in a 59-year-old man. The patient has never had any renal abnormalities or related medical problems. He wants it removed for cosmetic purposes. (*Reproduced with permission from Richard P. Usatine, MD.*)

DIFFERENTIAL DIAGNOSIS

- Chondrodermatitis nodularis helicis may be confused with skin cancer, especially squamous cell carcinoma (SCC; see Chapter 169, Squamous Cell Carcinoma). In SCC, the overlying skin is often ulcerated and the tumor has poorly defined margins.
- Preauricular tags can be an isolated anomaly or part of a syndrome involving vital organs, especially the kidneys. Skin lesions that could appear similar include basal cell carcinoma (**Figure 26-7**) and cysts (**Figure 26-8**).

MANAGEMENT

Chondrodermatitis nodularis is treated with the following:

NONPHARMACOLOGIC

A pressure-relieving prosthesis or donut-shaped pillow can be used.[4,5] SOR C This can also be created by cutting a hole from the center of a bath sponge. The sponge can then be held in place with a headband if needed. A special prefabricated pillow is available from **http://www.cnhpillow.com/.**

PROCEDURES

- Shave biopsy can be used to make the diagnosis and may relieve symptoms temporarily. SOR C
- Cryotherapy, intralesional steroids, or curettage and electrodesiccation can be performed after the result from the shave biopsy is known and there is no malignancy. SOR C

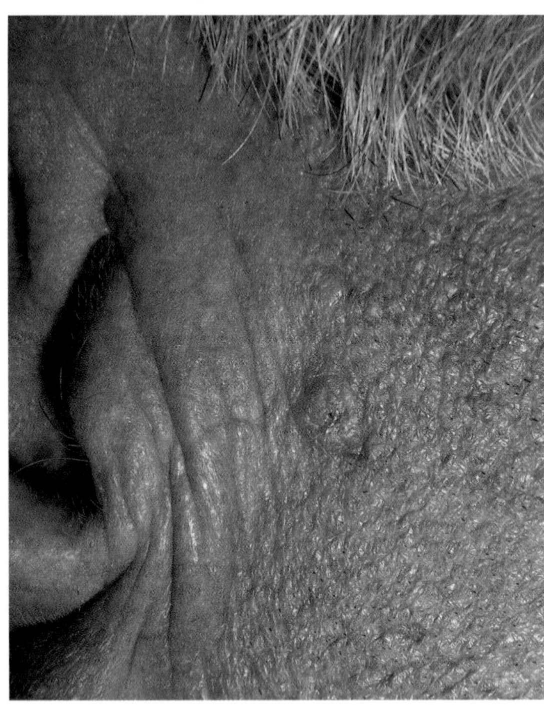

FIGURE 26-7 Basal cell carcinoma in a preauricular location. (*Reproduced with permission from Richard P. Usatine, MD.*)

- Photodynamic therapy (combines a photosensitizer with a specific type of light to kill nearby cells) has been reported to decrease pain in case reports.[6] SOR C
- A small elliptical excision of the nodule with removal of inflamed cartilage provides excellent results (**Figure 26-9**).[7,8] SOR C
- Preauricular tags can be left alone or surgically excised for cosmetic reasons. SOR C

FOLLOW-UP

Recurrences are common and may require further treatment.

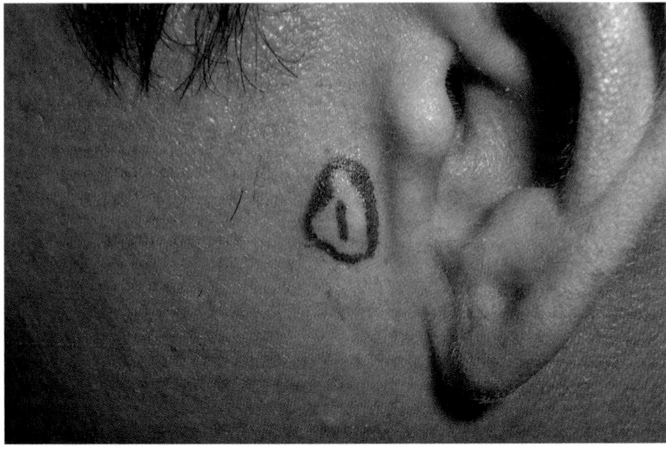

FIGURE 26-8 Preauricular cyst marked for excision. (*Reproduced with permission from Richard P. Usatine, MD.*)

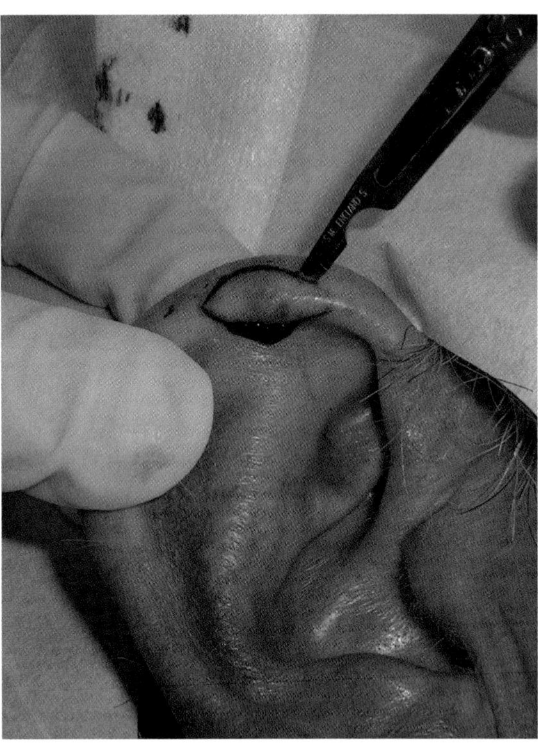

FIGURE 26-9 Elliptical excision of chondrodermatitis nodularis helicis. (*Reproduced with permission from Richard P. Usatine, MD.*)

PATIENT EDUCATION

Chondrodermatitis nodularis is a benign lesion that tends to recur; therapeutic options can be discussed.

PATIENT RESOURCES

- A special prefabricated pillow is available that helps relieve pressure on the ear. For more information, contact: CNH Pillow, PO Box 1247, Abilene, TX 79604; phone (800) 255-7487; **http://www.cnhpillow.com/.**
- Medline Plus. *Ear tag*—**http://nlm.nih.gov/medlineplus/ency/article/003304.htm.**

PROVIDER RESOURCES

- To learn how to perform an easy elliptical excision of chondrodermatitis nodularis helicis refer to the text and DVD: Usatine R, Pfenninger J, Stulberg D, Small R. *Dermatologic and Cosmetic Procedures in Office Practice*. Text and DVD. Philadelphia, PA: Elsevier; 2012.
- Medscape. *Chondrodermatitis Nodularis Helicis*—**http://emedicine.medscape.com/article/1119141-overview.**
- Medscape. *Preauricular Cysts, Pits, and Fissures*—**http://emedicine.medscape.com/article/845288-overview.**

REFERENCES

1. Roth DA, Hildesheimer M, Bardenstein S, et al. Preauricular skin tags and ear pits are associated with permanent hearing impairment in newborns. *Pediatrics.* 2008;122(4):e844-e890.
2. Magro CM, Frambach GE, Crowson AN. Chondrodermatitis nodularis helices as a marker of internal disease associated with microvascular injury. *J Cutan Pathol.* 2005;32:329-333.
3. Ostrower ST. *Preauricular Cysts, Pits, and Fissures*. http://emedicine.medscape.com/article/845288-overview#a05. Accessed July 20, 2011.
4. Sanu A, Koppana R, Snow DG. Management of chondrodermatitis nodularis chronica helicis using a “donut pillow”. *J Laryngol Otol.* 2007;121(11):1096-1098.
5. Moncrieff M, Sassoon EM. Effective treatment of chondrodermatitis nodularis chronica helices using a conservative approach. *Br J Dermatol.* 2004;150:892-894.
6. Pellegrino M, Taddeucci P, Mei S, et al. Chondrodermatitis nodularis chronics helicis and photodynamic therapy: a new therapeutic option? *Dermatol Ther.* 2011;24(1):144-147.
7. Rex J, Ribera M, Bielsa I, et al. Narrow elliptical skin excision and cartilage shaving for treatment of chondrodermatitis nodularis. *Dermatol Surg.* 2006;32:400-404.
8. Hudson-Peacock MJ, Cox NH, Lawrence CM. The long-term results of cartilage removal alone for the treatment of chondrodermatitis nodularis. *Br J Dermatol.* 1999;141:703-705.

SECTION 2 NOSE AND SINUS

27 NASAL POLYPS

Linda Speer, MD

PATIENT STORY

A 35-year-old man complains of unilateral nasal obstruction for the past several months of gradual onset. On examination of the nose, a nasal polyp is found (**Figure 27-1**).

INTRODUCTION

Nasal polyps are benign lesions arising from the mucosa of the nasal passages including the paranasal sinuses. They are most commonly semitransparent.

EPIDEMIOLOGY

- Prevalence of 1% to 4% of adults.[1]
- The male-to-female ratio in adults is approximately 2:1.
- Peak age of onset is between 20 and 40 years; rare in children younger than 10 years.
- Associated with the following conditions:
  - Nonallergic and allergic rhinitis and rhinosinusitis
  - Asthma—in 20% to 50% of patients with polyps
  - Cystic fibrosis
  - Aspirin intolerance—in 8% to 26% of patients with polyps
  - Alcohol intolerance—in 50% of patients with polyps

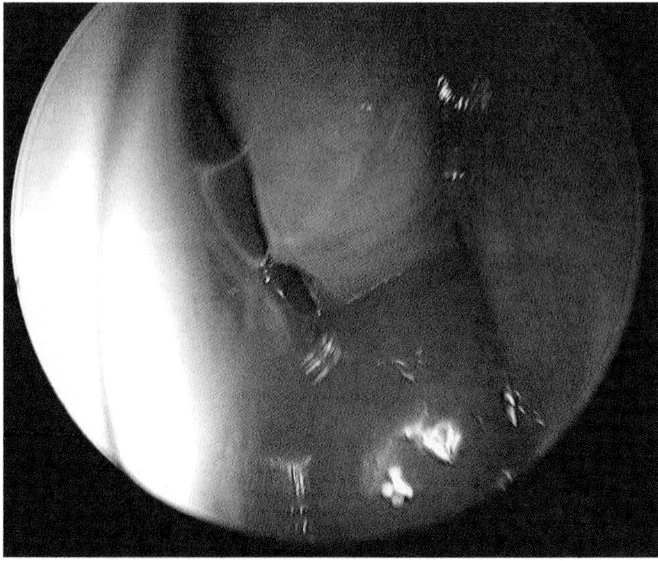

FIGURE 27-1 Nasal polyp in left middle meatus with normal surrounding mucosa. (*Reproduced with permission from William Clark, MD.*)

ETIOLOGY AND PATHOPHYSIOLOGY

- The precise cause of nasal polyp formation is unknown.
- Infectious agents causing desquamation of the mucous membrane may play a triggering role.
- Activated epithelial cells appear to be the major source of mediators that induce an influx of inflammatory cells, including eosinophils prominently; these in turn lead to proliferation and activation of fibroblasts.[2] Cytokines and growth factors play a role in maintaining the mucosal inflammation associated with polyps.
- Food allergies are strongly associated with nasal polyps.

DIAGNOSIS

CLINICAL FEATURES

- The appearance is usually smooth and rounded (see **Figure 27-1**).
- Moist and translucent (**Figure 27-2**).
- Variable size.
- Color ranging from nearly none to deep erythema.

TYPICAL DISTRIBUTION

The middle meatus is the most common location.

LABORATORY AND IMAGING

- Consider allergy testing.
- Computed tomography (CT) of the nose and paranasal sinuses may be indicated to evaluate extent of lesion(s) (**Figure 27-3**).

BIOPSY

Not usually indicated. Histology typically shows pseudostratified ciliary epithelium, edematous stroma, epithelial basement membrane, and pro-inflammatory cells with eosinophils present in 80% to 90% of cases.

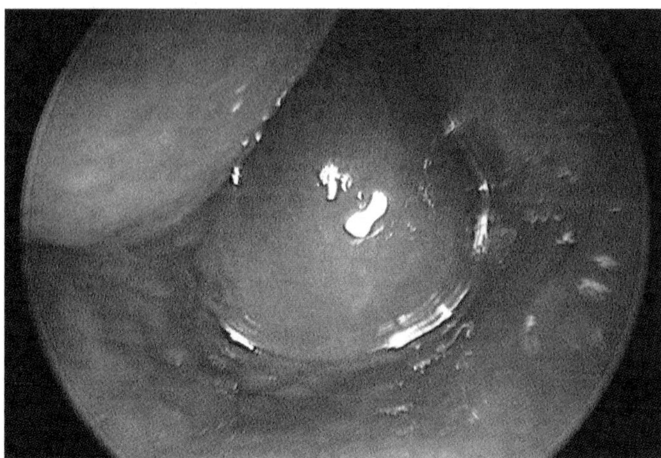

FIGURE 27-2 Nasal polyp in right nasal cavity in a patient with inflamed mucosa from allergic rhinitis. (*Reproduced with permission from William Clark, MD.*)

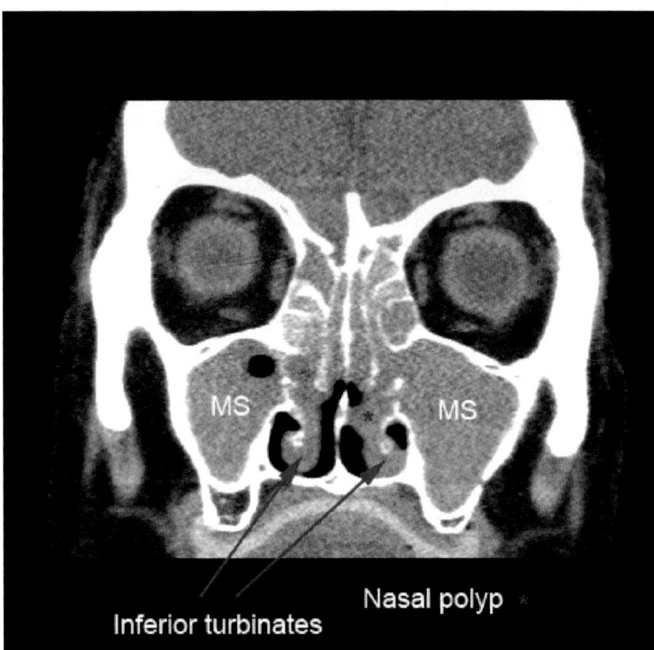

FIGURE 27-3 CT scan showing polyps (*asterisk*) and bilateral opacified maxillary sinuses (*MS*). Note the nasal polyp appears to be coming from the left maxillary sinus and is above the inferior turbinate. (*Reproduced with permission from Richard P. Usatine, MD.*)

DIFFERENTIAL DIAGNOSIS

Many relatively rare conditions can cause an intranasal mass including the following:

- Papilloma—About 1% of nasal tumors, affecting 1 in 100,000 adults per year. Locally invasive, these tend to recur especially if excision is not complete. Papillomas are of unknown etiology but are associated with chronic sinusitis, air pollution, and viral infections. They are irregular and friable in appearance and bleed easily.[3]
- Meningoencephalocele—Grayish gelatinous appearance.[4]
- Nasopharyngeal carcinoma—Firm, often ulcerated.
- Pyogenic granuloma—Relatively common benign vascular neoplasm of skin and mucous membranes (see Chapter 159, Pyogenic Granuloma).[5]
- Chordoma—Locally invasive neoplasms with gelatinous appearance that arise from notochordal (embryonic) remnants. Occurs in all age groups (mean age: 48 years).[6]
- Glioblastoma—Rare manifestation of the most common kind of brain tumor in adults.

MANAGEMENT

MEDICATIONS

- Medical treatment consists of intranasal corticosteroids.[7] SOR Ⓐ
- An initial short course (2-4 weeks) of oral steroids can be considered in severe cases.[8,9] SOR Ⓐ
- Steroid treatment reduces polyp size, but does not generally resolve them. Corticosteroid treatment is also useful preoperatively to reduce polyp size.
- Oral doxycycline 100 mg daily for 20 days was shown to decrease polyp size, providing benefit for 12 weeks in one randomized controlled trial.[10] SOR Ⓑ
- Topical nasal decongestants may provide some symptom relief, but do not reduce polyp size.[11] SOR Ⓑ
- Montelukast reduces symptoms when used as an adjunct to oral and inhaled steroid therapy in patients with bilateral nasal polyposis.[12] SOR Ⓑ

PROCEDURES

- Surgical excision is often required to relieve symptoms.
- Consider immunotherapy for patients with allergies.

PROGNOSIS

Lesions are benign and tend to recur.

FOLLOW-UP

Periodic reevaluation is recommended because recurrence rates are high.[13]

PATIENT EDUCATION

Patients should be informed about the benign nature of nasal polyps and their tendency to recur.

PATIENT RESOURCES

- Mayo Clinic. *Nasal Polyps*—**http://www.mayoclinic.com/health/nasal-polyps/DS00498.**
- Medline Plus. *Nasal Polyps*—**http://www.nlm.nih.gov/medlineplus/ency/article/ 001641.htm.**

PROVIDER RESOURCES

- Medscape. *Nasal Polyps*—**http://emedicine.medscape.com/article/994274.**
- Medscape. *Nonsurgical Treatment of Nasal Polyps*—**http://emedicine.medscape.com/article/861353.**

REFERENCES

1. McClay JE. *Nasal Polyps*. http://emedicine.medscape.com/article/994274. Accessed July 26, 2013.
2. Pawliczak R, Lewandowska-Polak A, Kowalski ML. Pathogenesis of nasal polyps: an update. *Curr Allergy Asthma Rep.* 2005;5:463-471.
3. Sadeghi N. *Sinonasal Papillomas*. http://emedicine.medscape.com/article/862677. Accessed July 26, 2013.
4. Kumar KK, Ganapathy K, Sumathi V, et al. Adult meningoencephalocele presenting as a nasal polyp. *J Clin Neurosci.* 2005;12:594-596.
5. Hoving EW. Nasal encephaloceles. *Childs Nerv Syst.* 2000;16:702-706.
6. Palmer CA. *Chordoma*. http://emedicine.medscape.com/article/250902. Accessed July 20, 2011.

7. Joe SA, Thambi R, Huang J. A systematic review of the use of intranasal steroids in the treatment of chronic rhinosinusitis. *Otolaryngol Head Neck Surg.* 2008;139(3):340-347.

8. Martinez-Devesa P, Patiar S. Oral steroids for nasal polyps. *Cochrane Database Syst Rev.* 2011;6(7):CD005232.

9. Vaidyanathan S, Barnes M, Williamson P, et al. Treatment of chronic rhinosinusitis with nasal polyposis with oral steroids followed by topical steroids: a randomized trial. *Ann Intern Med.* 2011;154(5):293-302.

10. Van Zele T, Gevaert P, Holtappels G, et al. Oral steroids and doxycycline: two different approaches to treat nasal polyps. *J Allergy Clin Immunol.* 2010;125(5):1069-1076.e4.

11. Johansson L, Oberg D, Melem I, Bende M. Do topical nasal decongestants affect polyps? *Acta Otolaryngol.* 2006:126:288-290.

12. Stewart RA, Ram B, Hamilton G, et al. Montelukast as an adjunct to oral and inhaled steroid therapy in chronic nasal polyposis. *Otolaryngol Head Neck Surg.* 2008;139(5):682-687.

13. Vento SI, Ertama LO, Hytonen ML, et al. Nasal polyposis: clinical course during 20 years. *Ann Allergy Asthma Immunol.* 2000;85:209-214.

28 SINUSITIS

Mindy A. Smith, MD, MS

PATIENT STORY

A 55-year-old woman complains of sinus pressure for the past 2 weeks along with headache, rhinorrhea, postnasal drip, and cough. This all started with a cold 3 weeks ago. She has chronic allergic rhinitis, but now the pressure on the right side of her face has become intense and her right upper molars are painful. The nasal discharge has become discolored and she feels feverish. She is diagnosed clinically with right maxillary sinusitis and is prescribed an antibiotic. Two weeks later when her symptoms have persisted, a computed tomography (CT) is ordered and she is found to have air-fluid levels in both maxillary sinuses and loculated fluid on the right side. (**Figures 28-1** and **28-2**.) The antibiotic is changed to amoxicillin/clavulanate and she is given information about nasal saline irrigation for symptom relief. If the symptoms do not improve the clinician plans to send her to ear, nose, and throat (ENT) for further evaluation.

INTRODUCTION

Rhinosinusitis is symptomatic inflammation of the sinuses, nasal cavity, and their epithelial lining.[1] Mucosal edema blocks mucous drainage, creating a culture medium for viruses and bacteria. Rhinosinusitis is classified by duration as acute (<4 weeks), subacute (4-12 weeks), or chronic (>12 weeks).

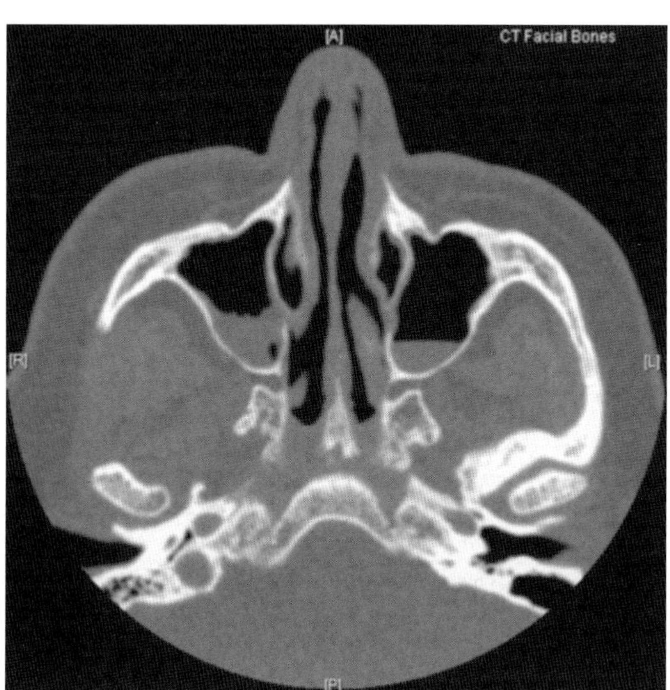

FIGURE 28-1 Bilateral maxillary sinusitis on axial CT. Note that fluid levels are greater on the right. (*Reproduced with permission from Chris McMains, MD.*)

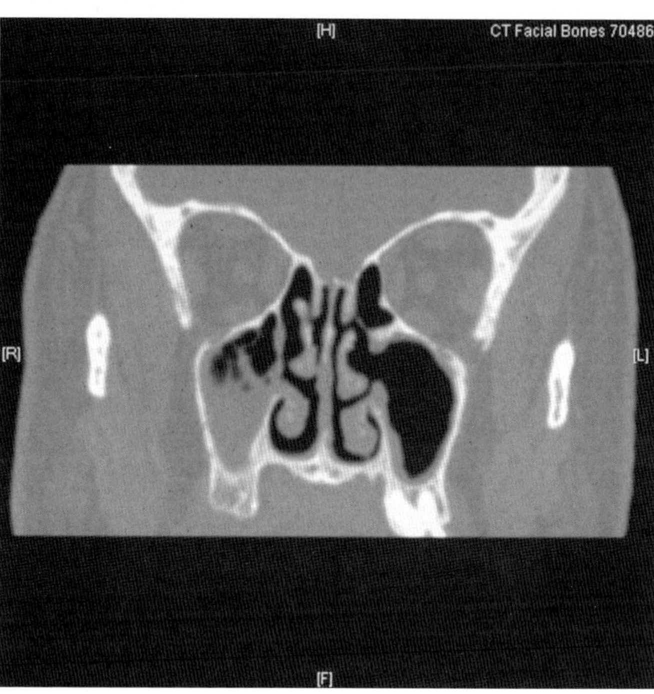

FIGURE 28-2 Maxillary sinusitis on coronal CT of same patient. (*Reproduced with permission from Chris McMains, MD.*)

EPIDEMIOLOGY

- Rhinosinusitis is common in the United States, with an estimated prevalence of 14% to 16% of the adult population annually.[1,2] The prevalence is increased in women and in individuals living in the southern United States.
- Only one-third to one-half of primary care patients with symptoms of sinusitis actually have bacterial infection.[3]
- Sinusitis is the fifth leading diagnosis for which antibiotics are prescribed in the United States.[1]
- This problem is responsible for millions of office visits to primary care physicians each year.[1]

ETIOLOGY AND PATHOPHYSIOLOGY

- Sinus cavities are lined with mucous-secreting respiratory epithelium. The mucus is transported by ciliary action through the sinus ostia (openings) to the nasal cavity. Under normal conditions, the paranasal sinuses are sterile cavities and there is no mucous retention.
- Bacterial sinusitis occurs when ostia become obstructed or ciliary action is impaired, causing mucus accumulation and secondary bacterial overgrowth.
- The causes of sinusitis include the following[4]:
  - Infection—Most commonly viral (eg, rhinovirus, parainfluenza, and influenza) followed by bacterial infection (eg, community-acquired acute cases—about half from *Streptococcus pneumoniae* and *Haemophilus influenzae* followed by *Moraxella catarrhalis*). In immunocompromised patients, fulminant fungal sinusitis may occur (eg, rhinocerebral mucormycosis—**Figure 28-3**).

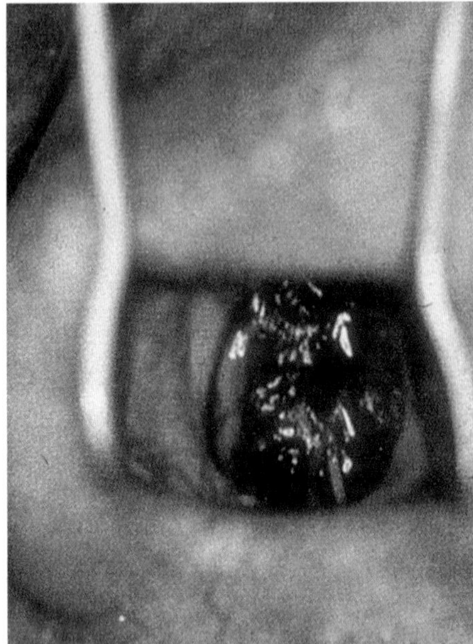

FIGURE 28-3 Mucormycosis sinusitis in a patient with diabetes showing the classic black nasal discharge. (*Reproduced with permission from Randal A. Otto, MD.*)

- Noninfectious obstruction—Allergies, polyposis, barotrauma (eg, deep-sea diving, airplane travel), chemical irritations, tumors (eg, squamous cell carcinoma, granulomatous disease, inverting papilloma), and conditions that alter mucous composition (eg, cystic fibrosis).

DIAGNOSIS

The diagnosis is based on the clinical picture with typical symptoms listed below. Symptoms arising from viral infection generally peak by day 5 or before. Acute bacterial rhinosinusitis is diagnosed when symptoms are present for 10 days or longer or when symptoms worsen after initial stability or improvement ("double worsening" or "double sickening"); it can also be presumed in patients with unusually severe presentations or extrasinus manifestations of infection.[1] Superimposed bacterial infection is estimated to occur in 0.5% to 2% of cases of viral rhinosinusitis.[1]

CLINICAL FEATURES

- Most cases are seen in conjunction with viral upper respiratory infections and represent sinus inflammation rather than infection.[3]
- Nonspecific symptoms include cough, sneezing, fever, nasal discharge (may be purulent or discolored), congestion, and headache.
- The American Academy of Otolaryngology guideline and the European Position Paper on Rhinosinusitis and Nasal Polyps recommend a diagnosis of rhinosinusitis with a combination (2 or more) of purulent nasal drainage associated with nasal obstruction, facial pain-pressure-fullness, or both; the latter also recognizes reduction or loss of smell as a cardinal feature.[1,5] There are no prospective trials that validate this approach.
- Other localizing symptoms include facial pain or pressure over the involved sinus when bending over or supine (ie, forehead in frontal sinusitis, cheek with maxillary sinusitis, between the eyes with ethmoid sinusitis, and neck and top of the head with sphenoid sinusitis) and maxillary tooth pain, most commonly the upper molars; the latter is seen more often with bacterial sinusitis. Halitosis is also attributed to bacterial causes.
- In a study of patients with chronic rhinosinusitis, diagnosis based on symptoms was problematic and only dysosmia (impairment in the sense of smell) and the presence of polyps could distinguish between normal and abnormal radiographs.[6]

TYPICAL DISTRIBUTION

Most sinus infections involve the maxillary sinus followed in frequency by the ethmoid (anterior), frontal, and sphenoid sinuses; however, most cases involve more than one sinus.

LABORATORY AND IMAGING

- Culture of nasal or nasopharyngeal secretions is not recommended as these have not been shown to differentiate between bacterial and viral rhinosinusitis.[1]
- If culture is needed because of suspected bacterial resistance or persistence of infection, a recent meta-analysis found endoscopically directed middle meatal cultures to be reasonably sensitive (80.9%), specific (90.5%), and accurate (87%; 95% confidence interval, 81.3-92.8%) compared with maxillary sinus taps.[7]
- Radiography should not be obtained for patients meeting diagnostic criteria for acute rhinosinusitis, unless a complication or alternate diagnosis is suspected.[1] If performed in cases of clinical uncertainty or for complications (eg, orbital, intracranial, or soft tissue involvement), plain sinus radiography is considered positive for acute sinusitis with the presence of air-fluid level, complete opacification, or at least 6 mm of mucosal thickening; it has a reported sensitivity of 76% and specificity 79%.[8] There are considerable limitations to the sensitivity of plain films, especially in diagnosing ethmoid and sphenoid disease.
- Nasal endoscopy, identifying purulent material within the drainage area of the sinuses, may be comparable to plain sinus radiography in diagnosing acute sinusitis.[7] In one case series of patients with suspected chronic rhinosinusitis, the addition of endoscopy to symptom criteria had similar sensitivity (88.7% vs 84.1%) but significantly improved specificity (66% vs 12.3%) using CT as the gold standard.[9]
- In acute disease, CT scanning is generally reserved for persistent or recurrent symptoms to confirm sinusitis, or to investigate infectious complications (**Figures 28-4** and **28-5**). Radiation dose (about 10 times that of plain radiography) can be lowered with careful choice of technical factors.[1]

REFER OR HOSPITALIZE

- Potentially life-threatening complications include subperiosteal orbital abscess, meningitis, epidural or cerebral abscess, and cavernous sinus thrombosis (**Figures 28-6** and **28-7**).
- The risks of frontal sinusitis includes eroding through the frontal bone forward and causing a Pott's puffy tumor, inward and spreading into the brain and cavernous sinuses (see **Figure 28-5**).
- Orbital abscess is highly dangerous and can be the result of spread from the frontal or ethmoid sinuses (see **Figure 28-6**).
- In immunocompromised patients, fulminant fungal sinusitis may cause orbital swelling, cellulitis, proptosis, ptosis, impairment of extraocular motion, nasopharyngeal ulceration, and epistaxis. Bony erosion may be evident.[5] Nasal mucosa may appear black (see **Figure 28-3**), blanched white, or erythematous.

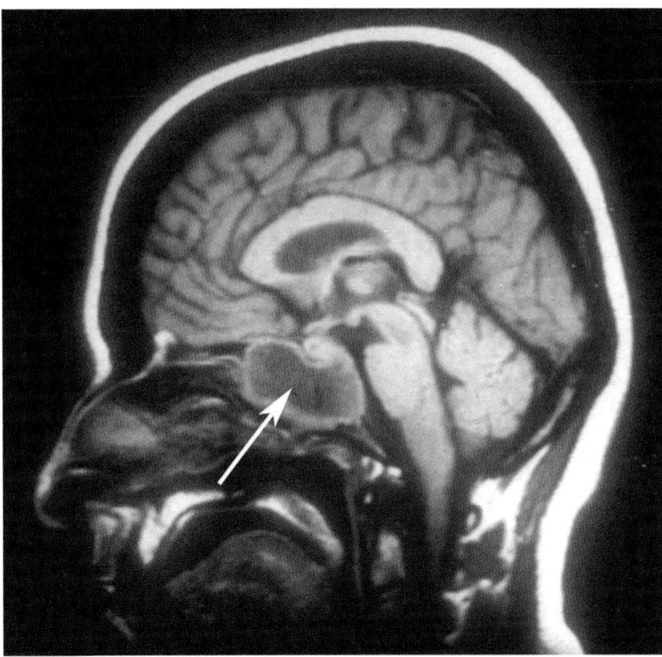

FIGURE 28-4 Mucopyocele in the sphenoid sinus (*arrow*) as a complication of bacterial sinusitis. (*Reproduced with permission from Randal A. Otto, MD.*)

- In hospitalized patients, patients may be critically ill and without localizing symptoms. Infections in these patients are often polymicrobial including *Staphylococcus aureus, Pseudomonas aeruginosa, Serratia marcescens, Klebsiella pneumoniae,* and *Enterobacter*.[5]

DIFFERENTIAL DIAGNOSIS

- Upper respiratory tract infections (URIs)—These are common infections, primarily viral (most commonly rhinovirus), that cause 2 to 4 infections per year in adults and 6 to 8 infections per year in children. Infections are self-limited (lasting approximately 7-10 days) and typical symptoms include rhinorrhea, nasal congestion, sore throat, and cough. URI often precedes acute sinusitis.
- Allergic rhinitis—Sneezing, itching, watery rhinorrhea.
- Tumor (usually squamous cell carcinoma)—Rare; unilateral epistaxis or discharge and obstruction, recurrent sinusitis, sinus pain.

Other causes of facial pain include the following:

- Migraine headache or cluster headache—Moderate-to-severe head pain that is usually deep seated, persistent, and pulsatile. There is a history of multiple occurrences and head pain may be associated with nausea, vomiting, photophobia, and scotomata. Attacks last for 4 to 72 hours.

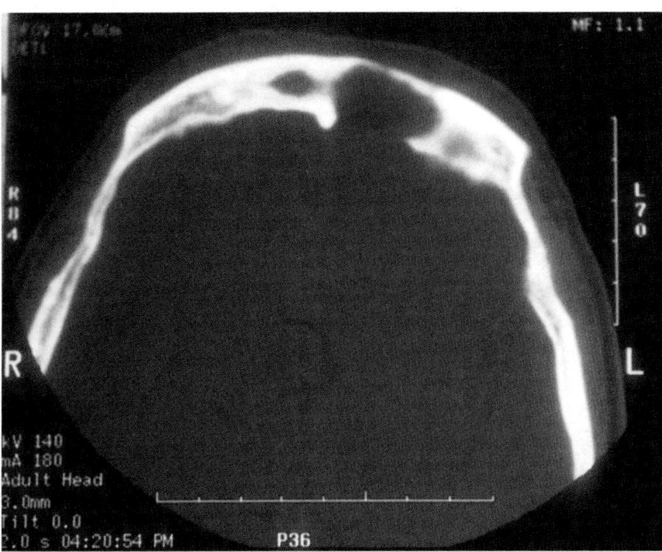

FIGURE 28-5 Frontal sinusitis eroded through the frontal bone inward toward the brain threatening such complications as a brain abscess and cavernous sinus thrombosis. Seen on CT scan. (*Reproduced with permission from Randal A. Otto, MD.*)

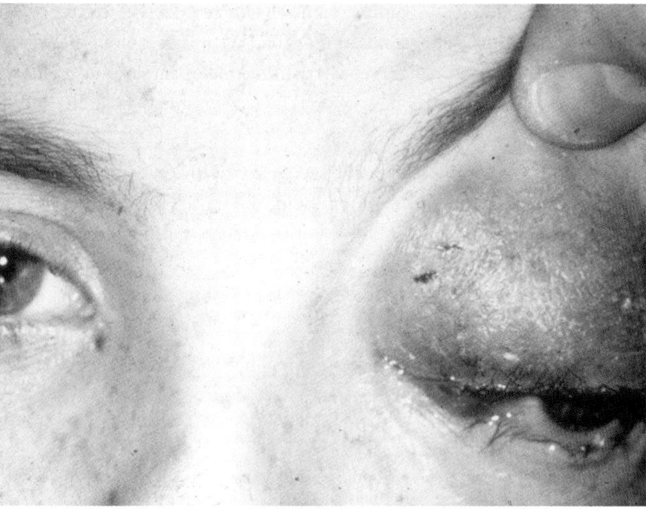

FIGURE 28-6 Right orbital abscess with proptosis as a complication of frontal sinusitis eroding through the superior orbital bones. (*Reproduced with permission from Randal A. Otto, MD.*)

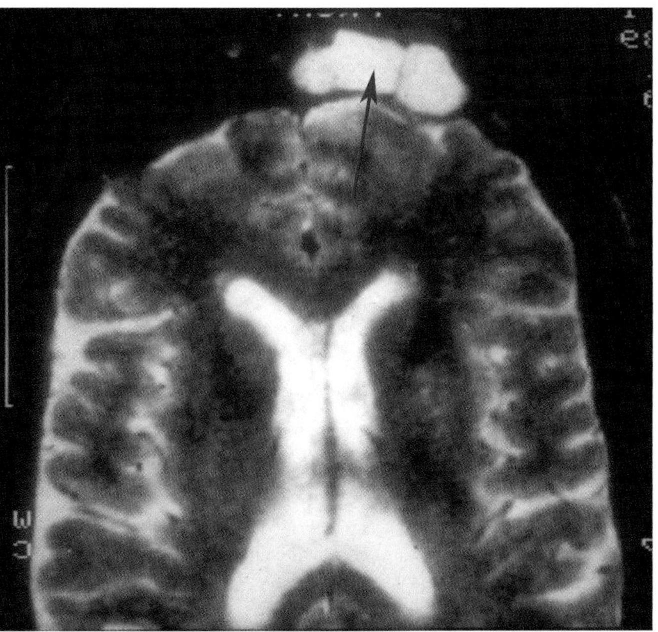

FIGURE 28-7 Mucopyocele (*red arrow*) in the right frontal sinus seen on magnetic resonance imaging (MRI) scan as a complication of frontal sinusitis. (*Reproduced with permission from Randal A. Otto, MD.*)

- Trigeminal neuralgia—Painful condition characterized by excruciating, paroxysmal, shock-like pain lasting seconds to minutes along the distribution of the trigeminal nerve (ophthalmic, maxillary and/or mandibular branches). Pain may be triggered by face washing, air draft, and chewing.
- Dental pain—Tooth pain may be secondary to caries or gingivitis. When caries extend into the tooth pulp, the tooth becomes sensitive to percussion and hot and cold food and beverages. If pulp necrosis occurs, pain becomes severe, sharp, throbbing, and often worse when supine. Abscess formation results in pain, swelling and erythema of the gum and surrounding tissue, and possibly purulent drainage.
- Temporal arteritis—Unilateral pounding headache that may be associated with visual changes and systemic symptoms (eg, fever, weight loss, muscle aches). Onset is usually in older adults (older than age 50 years) and laboratory testing reveals an elevated erythrocyte sedimentation rate (>50).

MANAGEMENT

Duration of illness assists in decision making as most patients improve without specific treatment; a period of watchful waiting for up to 7 days is consistent with guidelines.[1] Treatment of symptoms, including pain, is important.

NONPHARMACOLOGIC

Nasal saline irrigation for acute upper respiratory tract infection in adults is generally not helpful, although data are limited;[10] 2 trials suggested modest benefit from buffered hypertonic (3-5%) saline irrigation for acute rhinosinusitis.[1] SOR B In adults with chronic sinusitis, nasal saline irrigation provides symptom relief, both alone and as an adjunct to nasal steroids, and is well tolerated.[11] SOR B

MEDICATIONS

- Analgesics (acetaminophen or nonsteroidal anti-inflammatory drugs alone or in combination with an opioid) should be used for pain.[1]
- Oral and topical (nasal) decongestants may be offered for symptomatic relief; however, there are no randomized controlled trials (RCTs) demonstrating effectiveness for sinusitis and the effect is limited to the nasal cavity.[12] Topical agents are more potent but rebound nasal congestion may develop after discontinuation; use for 3 days only is suggested.[1]
- Topical corticosteroids appear to be of benefit in improvement and resolution of symptoms for acute sinusitis.[13] SOR B
- There have been no clinical trials of mucolytics reported in adults with acute bacterial sinusitis. However, they may be useful in preventing crust formation and liquefying secretions. SOR C
- Patients who fail to improve or have severe symptoms can be offered oral antibiotics. SOR A Although 10 days is usually recommended for adults, a shorter course (3-5 days) may be equally effective.[1]
    - Adults (after 7 days)—Amoxicillin (500 mg 3 times daily or 875 mg twice daily) for 10 days;[1] alternatives include trimethoprim-sulfamethoxazole (TMS-SMX) (1 DS twice daily) or a macrolide for 10 days.[1]
    - The Infectious Disease Society of America recommends use of amoxicillin-clavulanate rather than amoxicillin alone as empiric antimicrobial therapy for acute bacterial sinusitis in adults (low-quality evidence).[14]
- In a Cochrane review of 59 trials evaluating antibiotic treatment for acute maxillary sinusitis, antibiotics decreased clinical failure by approximately 10%.[15] Comparisons between classes of antibiotics showed no significant differences; therefore, narrow-spectrum antibiotics should be the first-line therapy.[15]
- Based on the Otolaryngology Head and Neck Surgery clinical guideline, the modest benefit of antibiotics for improving rates of clinical cure or improvement at 7 to 12 days (number needed to treat = 7) must be weighed against the risks of harm (primarily gastrointestinal, but also skin rash, vaginal discharge, headache, dizziness, and fatigue [number needed to harm = 9]).[1]

PROCEDURES

- Surgery and intravenous antibiotics are used for complications, including abscess and cases with orbital involvement.[4]
- Patients with fungal sinusitis are treated with aggressive debridement and adjunctive antifungals (eg, amphotericin).[4]
- Based on 3 RCTs, endoscopic sinus surgery is not superior to medical treatment; in one study there was a lower relapse rate (2.4% vs 5.6% without surgery).[16] SOR B Patients should be selected based on the severity of disease (frequency of antibiotics or oral steroid use), comorbidities (asthma, aspirin sensitivity, etc), and overall clinical picture (presence of polyps or fungal disease).

COMPLEMENTARY AND ALTERNATIVE MEDICINE

With respect to alternative therapy, there is limited evidence that Sinupret and bromelain may be effective adjunctive treatments in acute rhinosinusitis.[17] SOR B

PREVENTION

Smoking increases the risk for sinusitis; patients should be counseled about cessation.[1]

PROGNOSIS

- Based on a Cochrane review, cure or improvement rate for acute sinusitis within 2 weeks was high in both the placebo group (80%) and the antibiotic group (90%).[15]
- For patients with chronic sinusitis, a retrospective study of medical treatment reported treatment success in about half of patients (N = 74); 26 patients had partial resolution and 45 patients underwent surgery. Facial pressure or pain, mucosal inflammation, and higher endoscopic severity grade predicted treatment failure.[18]

FOLLOW-UP

For those adults who fail treatment after 7 days of antibiotic therapy,[1] a nonbacterial cause or resistant organism should be considered; amoxicillin-clavulanate (4 g per day amoxicillin equivalent) twice daily for 10 days, or a respiratory fluoroquinolone (eg, levofloxacin, 500 mg daily) for 7 days are alternatives.[1,4] SOR C

PATIENT EDUCATION

- Nasal congestion, purulent rhinitis, and facial pain following a cold may indicate a sinus infection. Symptoms due to a cold usually abate within 1 week.
- Methods to improve sinus drainage include oral and nasal decongestants and nasal saline irrigation. Patients should be cautioned against using nasal decongestants for more than 3 days to avoid rebound symptoms. For longer-term management, topical nasal steroids may prove useful.
- Patients should be encouraged to see their primary care provider if symptoms persist or worsen after 10 days, suggesting bacterial infection that may benefit from antibiotic treatment.

PATIENT RESOURCES

- National Institute of Allergy and Infectious Diseases. *Sinusitis*—**http://www.niaid.nih.gov/topics/sinusitis/Pages/Index.aspx.**
- MedlinePlus. *Sinusitis*—**http://www.nlm.nih.gov/medlineplus/sinusitis.html.**

PROVIDER RESOURCES

- Rosenfeld RM, Andes D, Neil B, et al. Clinical practice guideline: adult sinusitis. *Otolaryngol Head Neck Surg*. 2007;137:365-377.
- IDSA Clinical Practice Guideline for Acute Bacterial Rhinosinusitis in Children and Adults—**http://cid.oxfordjournals.org/content/54/8/1041.long.**

REFERENCES

1. Rosenfeld RM, Andes D, Neil B, et al. Clinical practice guideline: adult sinusitis. *Otolaryngol Head Neck Surg*. 2007;137:365-377.
2. Anand VK. Epidemiology and economic impact of rhinosinusitis. *Ann Otol Rhinol Laryngol*. 2004;193(suppl):3-5.
3. Holleman DR Jr, Williams JW Jr, Simel DL. Usual care and outcomes in patients with sinus complaints and normal results of sinus roentgenography. *Arch Fam Med*. 1995;4:246-251.
4. Rubin MA, Gonzales R, Sande MA. Infections of the upper respiratory tract. In: Kasper DL, Braunwald E, Fauci AS, Hauser SL, Longo DL, Jameson, JL, eds. *Harrison's Principles of Internal Medicine*. New York, NY: McGraw-Hill; 2005:185-188.
5. Daudia A, Jones NS. Sinus headaches. *Rhinology*. 2007;45:1-2.
6. Bhattacharyya N. Clinical and symptom criteria for the accurate diagnosis of chronic rhinosinusitis. *Laryngoscope*. 2006;116(7 pt 2 suppl 110):1-22.
7. Benninger MS, Payne SC, Ferguson BJ, et al. Endoscopically directed middle meatal cultures versus maxillary sinus taps in acute bacterial maxillary rhinosinusitis: a meta-analysis. *Otolaryngol Head Neck Surg*. 2006;134(1):3-9.
8. Berger G, Steinberg DM, Popoytzer A, Ophir D. Endoscopy versus radiography for the diagnosis of acute bacterial rhinosinusitis. *Eur Arch Otorhinolaryngol*. 2005;262(5):416-422.
9. Bhattacharyya N, Lee LN. Evaluating the diagnosis of chronic rhinosinusitis based on clinical guidelines and endoscopy. *Otolaryngol Head Neck Surg*. 2010;143(1):147-151.
10. Kassel JC, King D, Spurling GKP. Saline nasal irrigation for acute upper respiratory tract infections. *Cochrane Database Syst Rev*. 2010;(3):CD006821.
11. Harvey R, Hannan SA, Badia L, Scadding G. Nasal saline irrigations for the symptoms of chronic rhinosinusitis. *Cochrane Database Syst Rev*. 2007;(3):CD006394.
12. Shaikh N, Wald ER, Pi M. Decongestants, antihistamines and nasal irrigation for acute sinusitis in children. *Cochrane Database Syst Rev*. 2010;(12):CD007909.
13. Zalmanovici Trestioreanu A, Yaphe J. Intranasal steroids for acute sinusitis. *Cochrane Database Syst Rev*. 2009;(4):CD005149.
14. Chow AW, Benninger MS, Brook I, et al. IDSA clinical practice guideline for acute bacterial rhinosinusitis in children and adults. *Clin Infect Dis*. 2012;54(8):e72-e112.
15. Ahovuo-Saloranta A, Rautakorpi U-M, Borisenko OV, et al. Antibiotics for acute maxillary sinusitis. *Cochrane Database Syst Rev*. 2008;(2):CD000243.
16. Khalil HS, Nunez DA. Functional endoscopic sinus surgery for chronic rhinosinusitis. *Cochrane Database Syst Rev*. 2006;3:CD004458.
17. Guo R, Canter PH, Ernst E. Herbal medicines for the treatment of rhinosinusitis: a systematic review. *Otolaryngol Head Neck Surg*. 2006;135(4):496-506.
18. Lal D, Scianna JM, Stankiewicz JA. Efficacy of targeted medical therapy in chronic rhinosinusitis, and predictors of failure. *Am J Rhinol Allergy*. 2009;23:396-400.

SECTION 3 MOUTH AND THROAT

29 ANGULAR CHEILITIS

Linda Speer, MD
Richard P. Usatine, MD

PATIENT STORY

A middle-aged woman presents to your office with soreness at the right corner of her mouth for 4 months (**Figure 29-1**). On examination, she has cracking and fissures at the right corner of her mouth. She is diagnosed with angular cheilitis and treated with nonprescription clotrimazole cream and 1% hydrocortisone ointment twice daily. Within 2 weeks she was fully healed.

INTRODUCTION

Angular cheilitis is an inflammatory lesion of the commissure or corner of the lip characterized by scaling and fissuring.

SYNONYMS

Angular cheilitis is also known as perlèche, angular cheilosis, commissural cheilitis, and angular stomatitis.

EPIDEMIOLOGY

It is most common in the elderly. In one study of institutionalized elderly patients in Scotland, angular cheilitis was present in 25% of patients.[1]

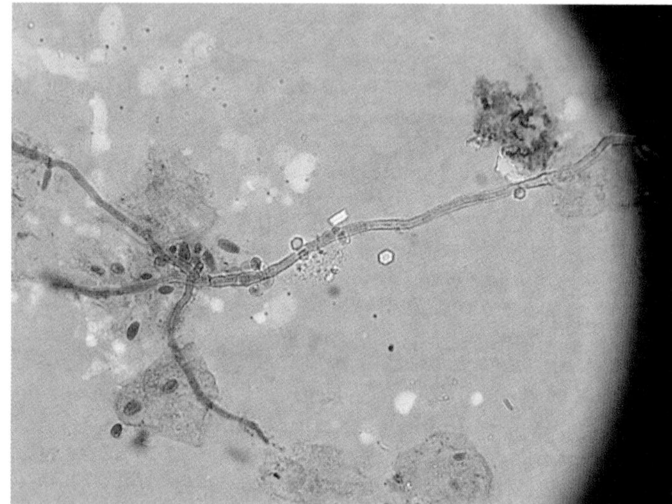

FIGURE 29-2 *Candida albicans* seen under the microscope after gently scraping a case of angular cheilitis and using KOH and blue ink on the slide. *(Reproduced with permission from Richard P. Usatine, MD.)*

ETIOLOGY AND PATHOPHYSIOLOGY

- Maceration is the usual predisposing factor. Microorganisms, most often *Candida albicans*, can then invade the macerated area (**Figure 29-2**).[2] Can also occur after use of antibiotics, especially in patients with risk factors described below (**Figure 29-3**).
- Lip licking can cause a contact dermatitis to the saliva along with perlèche (**Figure 29-4**). Perlèche is derived from the French word, "lecher," meaning to lick.
- Historically associated with vitamin B deficiency, which is rare in developed countries.

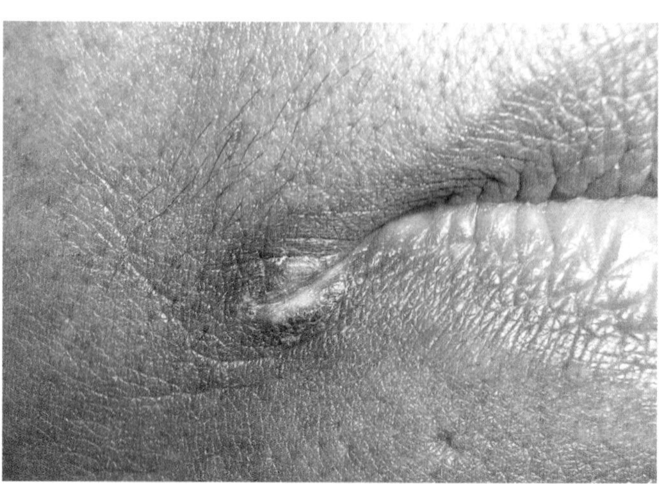

FIGURE 29-1 Angular cheilitis (perlèche). Note dry, erythematous, and fissured appearance. *(Reproduced with permission from Richard P. Usatine, MD.)*

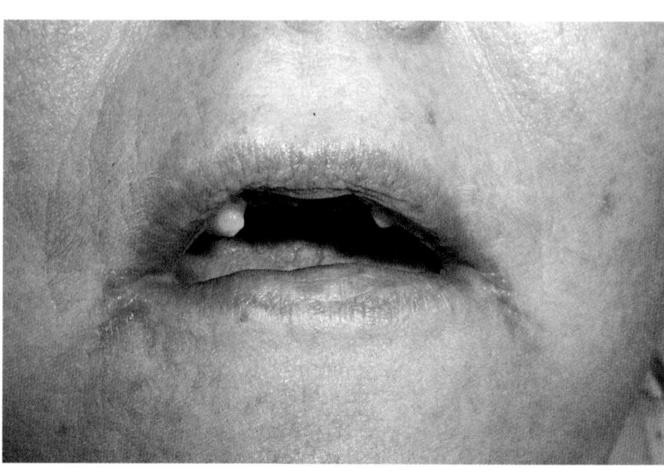

FIGURE 29-3 Angular cheilitis in a woman with poor dentition and thrush after receiving antibiotics for a urinary tract infection. *(Reproduced with permission from Richard P. Usatine, MD.)*

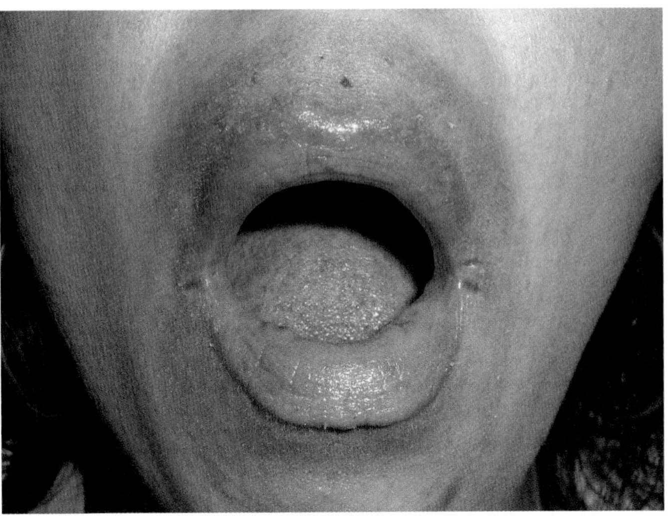

FIGURE 29-4 Perlèche in a woman with contact dermatitis related to lip licking. (*Reproduced with permission from Richard P. Usatine, MD.*)

RISK FACTORS

- Maceration can be related to poor dentition, deep facial wrinkles, orthodontic treatment, or poorly fitting dentures in the elderly (**Figure 29-5**).
- Other risk factors include incorrect use of dental floss causing trauma or diseases that enlarge the lips such as orofacial granulomatosis.
- Atopic dermatitis (**Figure 29-6**).
- HIV or other types of immunodeficiency may lead to more severe case of angular cheilitis with overgrowth of *Candida* (**Figure 29-7**).
- Use of isotretinoin dries the lips and predisposes to angular cheilitis.

DIAGNOSIS

CLINICAL FEATURES

Erythema and fissuring at the corners of the mouth, without exudates or ulceration (see **Figures 29-3** to **29-7**)

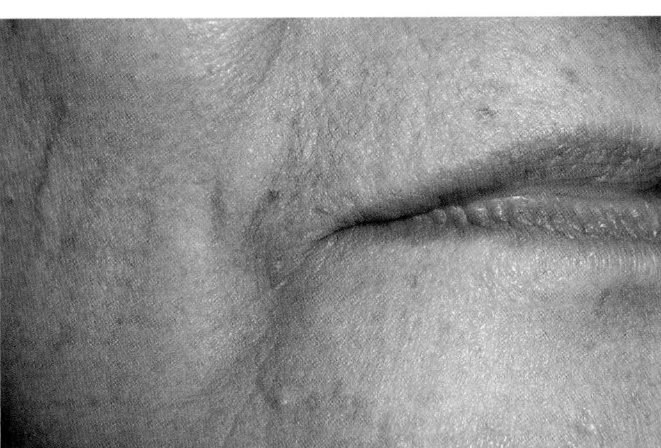

FIGURE 29-5 Angular cheilitis in an elderly woman. Note the wrinkle line extending downward from the corner of her mouth indicating some change in her facial anatomy that can predispose to this condition. The perlèche started while she was waiting for her dentures to be repaired. (*Reproduced with permission from Richard P. Usatine, MD.*)

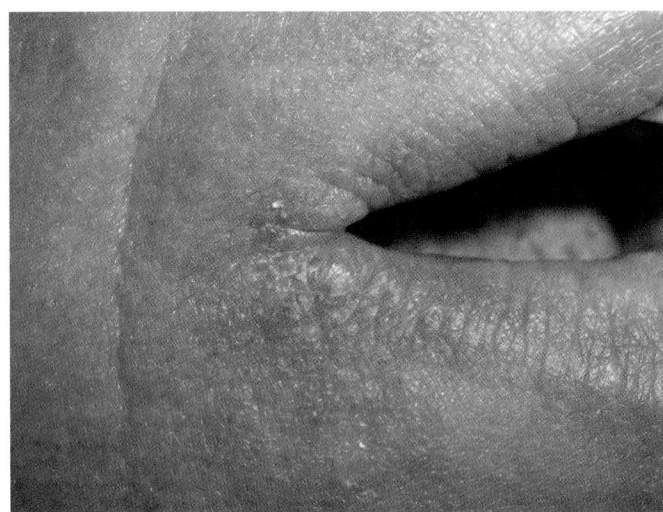

FIGURE 29-6 Angular cheilitis in a woman with atopic dermatitis. (*Reproduced with permission from Richard P. Usatine, MD.*)

TYPICAL DISTRIBUTION

Corners of the mouth (oral commissures or angles of the mouth), hence the names commissural cheilitis and angular cheilitis.

LABORATORY DIAGNOSIS

A light scraping of the corner of the mouth can be placed on a slide with potassium hydroxide (KOH) to look for *Candida* (see **Figures 29-2 and 29-3**).

BIOPSY

Not usually indicated.

DIFFERENTIAL DIAGNOSIS

- Impetigo—Yellowish crusts or exudates are characteristic of impetigo but not angular cheilitis (see Chapter 118, Impetigo).
- Herpes simplex (cold sores)—Initial blisters, followed by shallow ulcers, are characteristic of herpes simplex, but not angular cheilitis (see Chapter 128, Herpes Simplex).

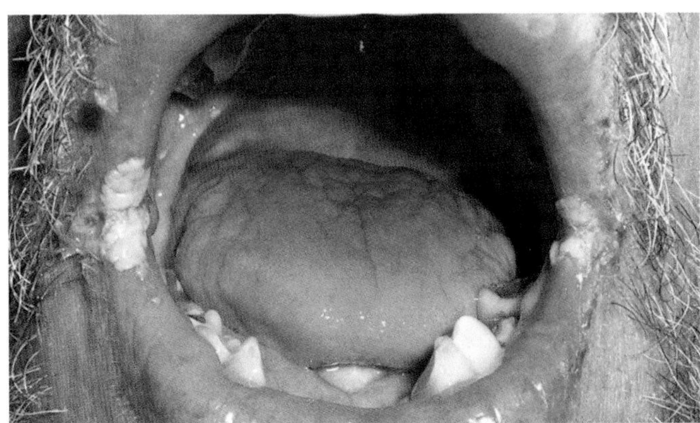

FIGURE 29-7 Severe angular cheilitis in an HIV-positive man with thrush. Note the white *Candida* growth on both corners of his mouth. (*Reproduced with permission from Richard P. Usatine, MD.*)

MANAGEMENT

NONPHARMACOLOGIC

- Attempt to relieve precipitating causes such as poorly fitting dentures.
- Counsel patients to stop licking their lips if this is part of the cause (see **Figure 29-4**).
- Recommend protective petrolatum or lip balm as needed.
- Counsel patients to stop using tobacco, either chewing or smoking.

MEDICATIONS

- Recommend topical antifungal creams or ointments, such as clotrimazole, to be applied twice daily.[3] SOR Ⓑ
- Low-potency topical corticosteroid, such as 1% hydrocortisone cream twice daily, may be added to treat the inflammatory component. SOR Ⓑ
- Nystatin lozenges work well but their use is limited because of their unpleasant taste.[3] SOR Ⓒ If thrush is also present, prescribe clotrimazole troches for treatment of both conditions.
- One randomized controlled study showed that medicated chewing gum can decrease the risk of angular cheilitis in older occupants of nursing homes. Consider recommending xylitol-containing gum to elderly patients with angular cheilitis.[4] SOR Ⓑ

PREVENTION

Attempt to identify predisposing factors and correct if possible, such as the following:

- Being edentulous
- Poorly fitting dentures
- Drooling
- Lip licking (see **Figure 29-4**)
- Atopic dermatitis (see **Figure 29-6**)

Protective lip balm may be helpful to prevent recurrences as long as the patient is not allergic to chemicals within the product. Plain petrolatum is often the safest product for dry lips.

PATIENT EDUCATION

Encourage patients to identify and correct predisposing factors (listed earlier). Protective lip balm may be helpful.

PATIENT AND PROVIDER RESOURCES

- Dr. Steven R. Pohlhaus' website. *Angular Chelitis*—**http://www.stevedds.com/toppage2.htm#Angular Cheilitis.**
- National Center for Emergency Medicine Informatics. *Perleche*—**http://www.ncemi.org/cse/cse0409.htm.**

REFERENCES

1. Samaranayake LP, Wilkieson CA, Lamey PJ, MacFarlane TW. Oral disease in the elderly in long-term hospital care. *Oral Dis*. 1995;1(3):147-151.
2. Sharon V, Fazel N. Oral candidiasis and angular cheilitis. *Dermatol Ther*. 2010;23(3):230-242.
3. Skinner N, Junker JA, Flake D, Hoffman R. Clinical inquiries. What is angular cheilitis and how is it treated? *J Fam Pract*. 2005 May;54(5):470-471.
4. Simons D, Brailsford SR, Kidd EA, Beighton D. The effect of medicated chewing gums on oral health in frail older people: a 1-year clinical trial. *J Am Geriatr Soc*. 2002 Aug;50(8):1348-1353.

30 TORUS PALATINUS

Linda Speer, MD
Mindy A. Smith, MD, MS

PATIENT STORY

An elderly woman is in the office for a physical examination. While looking in her mouth, a torus is seen at the midline on the hard palate (**Figure 30-1**). She states that she has had this for her whole adult life and it does not bother her. You explain to her that it is a torus palatinus and that nothing needs to be done. She is pleased to know the name of this lump and even happier to know that it is not harmful.

INTRODUCTION

Torus palatinus is a benign bony exostosis (bony growth) occurring in the midline of the hard palate. Torus mandibularis often presents as multiple benign bony exostoses on the floor of the mouth.

EPIDEMIOLOGY

- Most common bony maxillofacial exostosis, unclear origin.
- Usually in adults older than 30 years of age.
- Prevalence ranges from 9.5% to 26.9%; among ethnic groups, the range is wider (0.9% in Vietnamese to 30.8% among African Americans).[1]
- More common in women than men.
- Some populations seem to be more predisposed (eg, Middle Eastern).[2]

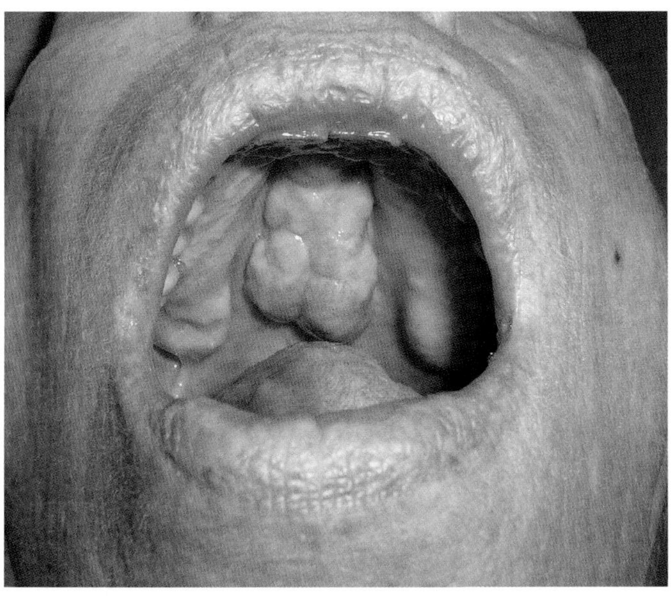

FIGURE 30-1 Torus palatinus in a 66-year-old woman. The patient was asymptomatic and this was an incidental finding. (*Reproduced with permission from Richard P. Usatine, MD.*)

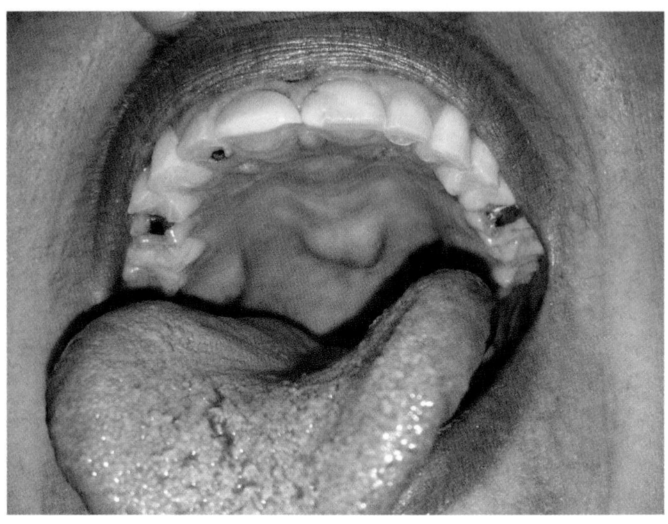

FIGURE 30-2 Torus palatinus in a 42-year-old woman. (*Reproduced with permission from Richard P. Usatine, MD.*)

DIAGNOSIS

CLINICAL FEATURES

- Hard lump protruding from the hard palate into the mouth covered with normal mucous membrane (**Figures 30-1** and **30-2**).
- Small size (<2 mm) appear most frequent (70% to 91%).[1]
- Shapes include flat, nodular, lobular, or spindle-shaped; nodular appears most common.[1] They may even by bifid (**Figure 30-3**).

TYPICAL DISTRIBUTION

Midline hard palate.

DIFFERENTIAL DIAGNOSIS

- Torus mandibularis is also a bony exostosis but is found under the tongue. These appear similar to a torus palatinus but are usually bilateral rather than midline (see **Figure 30-4**).

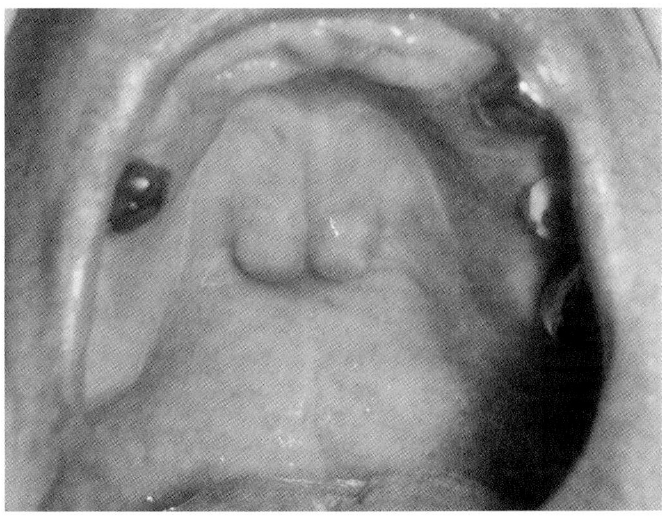

FIGURE 30-3 Bifid torus palatinus. (*Reproduced with permission from Richard P. Usatine, MD.*)

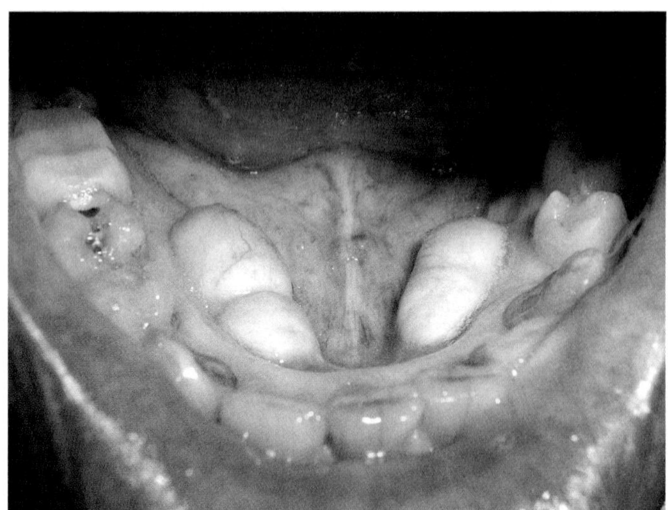

FIGURE 30-4 Torus mandibularis seen under the tongue caused by bony exostoses. Note these are bilateral and appear similar to a torus palatinus. The tori were asymptomatic and this was an incidental finding. (*Reproduced with permission from Richard P. Usatine, MD.*)

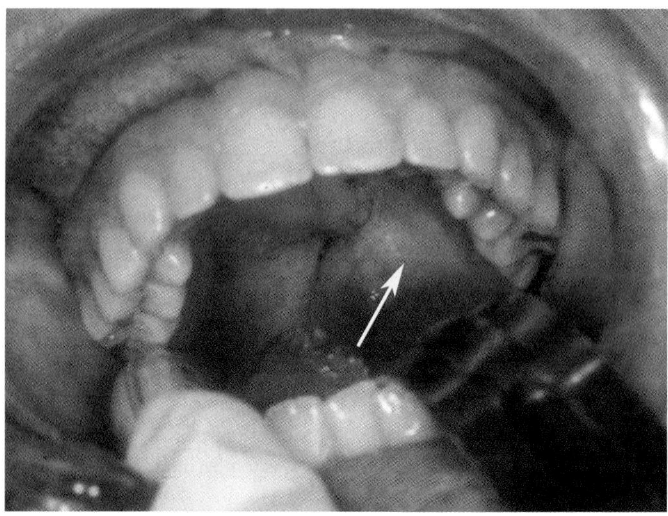

FIGURE 30-5 Adenoid cystic carcinoma in a 22-year-old woman. The arrow points to this unilateral tumor that should not be confused with a torus palatinus. (*Reproduced with permission from Randal A. Otto, MD.*)

- Squamous cell carcinoma is not as hard and the mucous membranes are usually ulcerated. Mucous membranes are normal in appearance with torus palatinus unless traumatized.
- Adenoid cystic carcinoma is a rare tumor that can start in a minor salivary gland over the hard palate. Note that this tumor will not be midline as found in the torus palatinus. If a suspected torus is not midline a biopsy is needed to rule out this potentially fatal carcinoma (**Figure 30-5**).

MANAGEMENT

- Excision can be considered if the lesion interferes with function, such as the fit of dentures. This is performed as an outpatient procedure.[3,4]
- Sometimes it needs to be removed because of disturbances of phonation, traumatic inflammation or ulcer, aesthetic reasons, or as source of autogenous cortical bone for grafts in periodontal surgery.[1]

PROGNOSIS

- Very slow growing; can stop growth spontaneously.[1]
- Surgical complications include perforation of nasal cavities, palatine nerve damage, bone necrosis, hemorrhage, and fracture of palatine bone.[1]

PATIENT EDUCATION

Patients should be informed about the benign nature of the lesion and that removal can be considered, if bothersome.

PATIENT RESOURCES

- Brea Dentistry. *Torus Palatinus*—**http://www.breadentistry.com/files/pdf/OPG_tor_pal.pdf.**

PROVIDER RESOURCES

- Otolaryngology Dr. T. Balasubramanian has posted information on his Web site including a video of surgical excision—**http://www.drtbalu.co.in/torus.html.**

REFERENCES

1. García-García AS, Martínez-González JM, Gómez-Font R, et al. Current status of the torus palatinus and torus madibularis. *Med Oral Patol Oral Cir Bucal*. 2010;15(2):e353-e360.
2. Yildiz E, Deniz M, Ceyhan O. Prevalence of torus palatinus in Turkish school children. *Surg Radiol Anat*. 2005;27:368-371.
3. Al-Quran FA, Al-Dwairi ZN. Torus palatinus and torus mandibularis in edentulous patients. *J Contemp Dent Pract*. 2006;7:112-119.
4. Cagirankaya LB, Dansu O, Hatipoglu MG. Is torus palatinus a feature of a well-developed maxilla? *Clin Anat*. 2004;17:623-625.

31 PHARYNGITIS

Brian Williams, MD
Richard P. Usatine, MD
Mindy A. Smith, MD

PATIENT STORY

A 27-year-old woman complains of 2 days of sore throat, fever, and chills. She is unable to swallow anything other than liquids because of severe odynophagia. She denies any congestion or cough. On examination, she has bilateral tonsillar erythema and exudate (**Figure 31-1**). Her anterior cervical lymph nodes are tender. Based on the presence of fever, absence of cough, tender lymphadenopathy, and tonsillar exudate, she is diagnosed with a high probability of group A β-hemolytic *Streptococcus* (GABHS) pharyngitis and prescribed antibiotics.

INTRODUCTION

Pharyngitis is inflammation of the pharyngeal tissues, and is usually associated with pain. The complaint of "sore throat" is a common one in the primary care office, and can be accompanied by other symptoms and signs including throat scratchiness, fever, headache, malaise, rash, joint and muscle pains, and swollen lymph nodes.

EPIDEMIOLOGY

- Pharyngitis accounts for 1% of primary care visits.[1]
- Viral infections account for an estimated 60% to 90% of cases of pharyngitis.
- Bacterial infections are responsible for between 5% and 30% of pharyngitis cases, depending on the age of the population and the season.
- The GABHS accounts for 5% to 10% of pharyngitis in adults and 15% to 30% in children.[2] Up to 38% of cases of tonsillitis are because of GABHS.
- Highest prevalence in winter.
- Acute rheumatic fever is currently rare in the United States.
- Up to 14% of deep neck infections result from pharyngitis.[3]

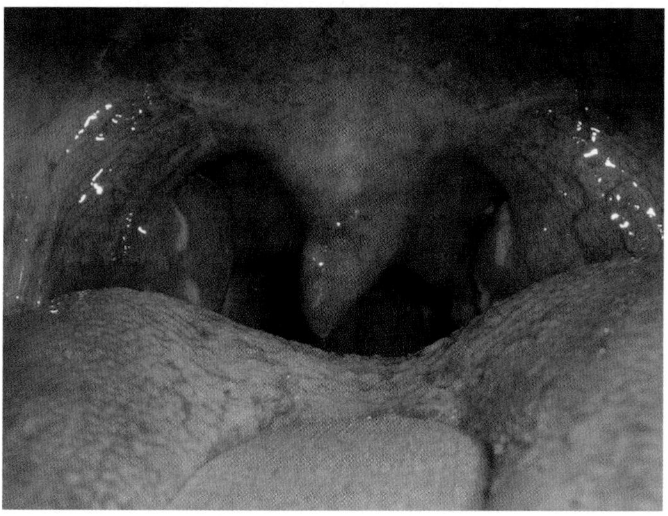

FIGURE 31-1 Strep pharyngitis showing tonsillar exudate and erythema. (*Reproduced with permission from Michael Nguyen, MD.*)

ETIOLOGY AND PATHOPHYSIOLOGY

- Some viruses, such as adenovirus, cause inflammation of the pharyngeal mucosa by direct invasion of the mucosa or secondary to suprapharyngeal secretions.[4] Other viruses, such as rhinovirus, cause pain through stimulation of pain nerve endings by mediators, such as bradykinin.
- The GABHS releases exotoxins and proteases. Erythrogenic exotoxins are responsible for the development of the scarlatiniform exanthem (**Figure 31-2**).[5] Secondary antibody formation because of cross-reactivity may result in rheumatic fever and valvular heart disease.[6] Antigen–antibody complexes may lead to acute poststreptococcal glomerulonephritis.
- Untreated GABHS pharyngitis can result in suppurative complications including bacteremia, otitis media, meningitis, mastoiditis, cervical lymphadenitis, endocarditis, pneumonia, or peritonsillar abscess formation (**Figure 31-3**). Nonsuppurative complications include rheumatic fever and poststreptococcal glomerulonephritis.

RISK FACTORS

- Immune deficiency
- Chronic irritation (eg, allergies, cigarette smoking)

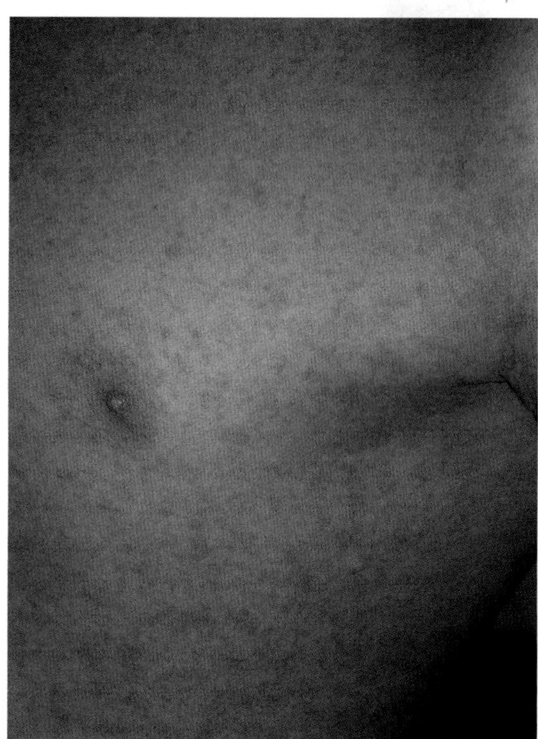

FIGURE 31-2 Scarlatiniform rash in scarlet fever. This 7-year-old boy has a typical sandpaper rash with his strep throat and fever. The erythema is particularly concentrated in the axillary area. (*Reproduced with permission from Richard P. Usatine, MD.*)

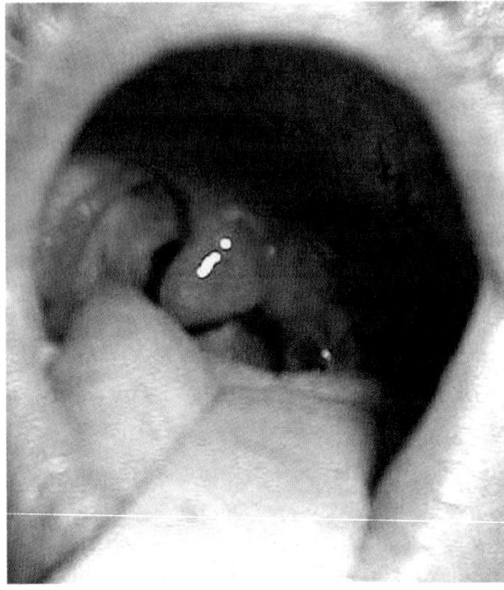

CHAPTER 31

A

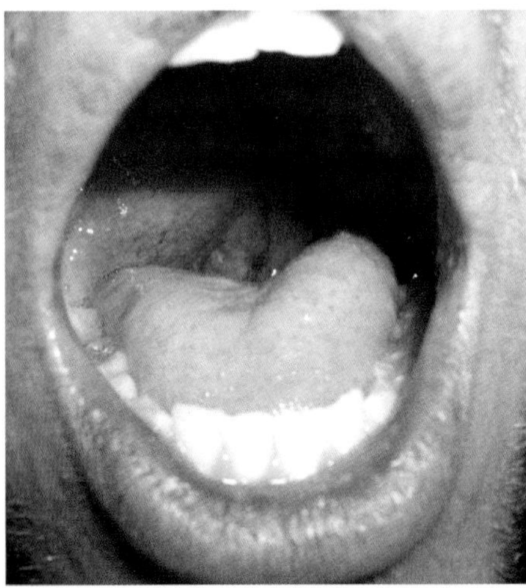

B

FIGURE 31-3 A. Peritonsillar abscess on the left showing uvular deviation away from the side with the abscess. B. Peritonsillar abscess with swelling and anatomic distortion of the right tonsillar region. (*Reproduced with permission from Charlie Goldberg, MD. Copyright © 2005 The Regents of the University of California.*)

DIAGNOSIS

CLINICAL FEATURES

- Rhinorrhea and cough are more consistent with viral etiology.
- Rapid-onset odynophagia, tonsillar exudates, anterior cervical lymphadenopathy, and fever are consistent with streptococcal pharyngitis.
- Not all tonsillar exudates are caused by streptococcal pharyngitis. Mononucleosis and other viral pharyngitis can cause tonsillar exudates (**Figures 31-4** and **31-5**). The positive predictive value for tonsillar exudate in strep throat is only 31%; that is, 69% of patients with tonsillar exudate will have a nonstreptococcal cause.
- Para- and supra-tonsillar edema with medial and/or anterior displacement of the involved tonsil and uvular displacement to the contralateral side suggest peritonsillar abscess (see **Figure 31-3**). Trismus and anterior cervical lymphadenopathy with severe tenderness to palpation are additional findings.
- Palatal petechiae can be seen in all types of pharyngitis (**Figure 31-6**).
- A sandpaper rash is suggestive of scarlet fever (see **Figure 31-2**).
- Lymphoid hyperplasia can cause a cobblestone pattern on the posterior pharynx or palate from viral infections, gastroesophageal reflux disease (GERD), or allergies (**Figure 31-7**). Although it usually is more suggestive of a viral infection or allergic rhinitis, lymphoid hyperplasia can be seen in strep pharyngitis (**Figure 31-8**).

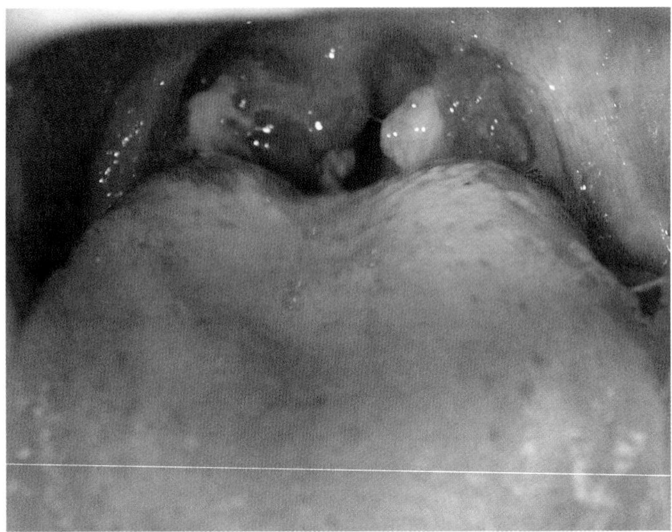

FIGURE 31-4 Mononucleosis in a young adult with considerable tonsillar exudate. (*Reproduced with permission from Tracey Cawthorn, MD.*)

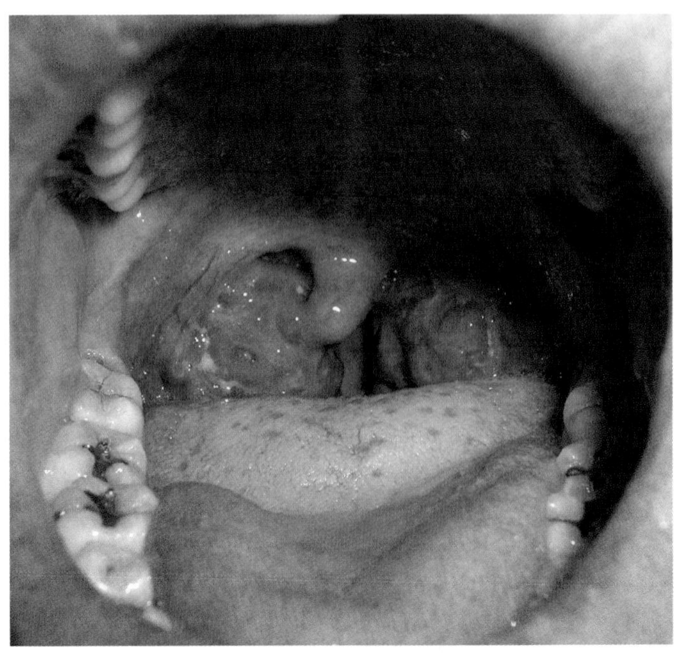

FIGURE 31-5 Viral pharyngitis in a young adult showing enlarged cryptic tonsils with some erythema and exudate. (*Reproduced with permission from Richard P. Usatine, MD.*)

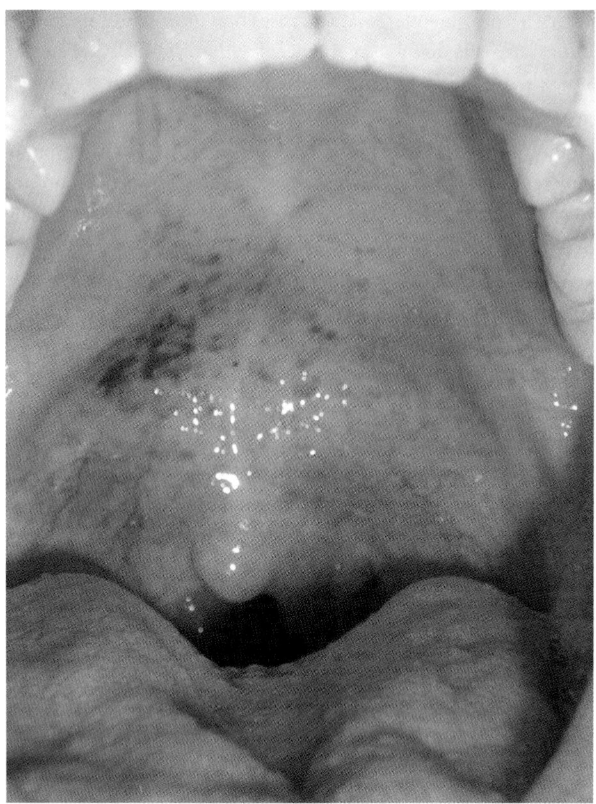

FIGURE 31-6 Viral pharyngitis with visible palatal petechiae. Palatal petechiae can be seen in all types of pharyngitis. (*Reproduced with permission from Richard P. Usatine, MD.*)

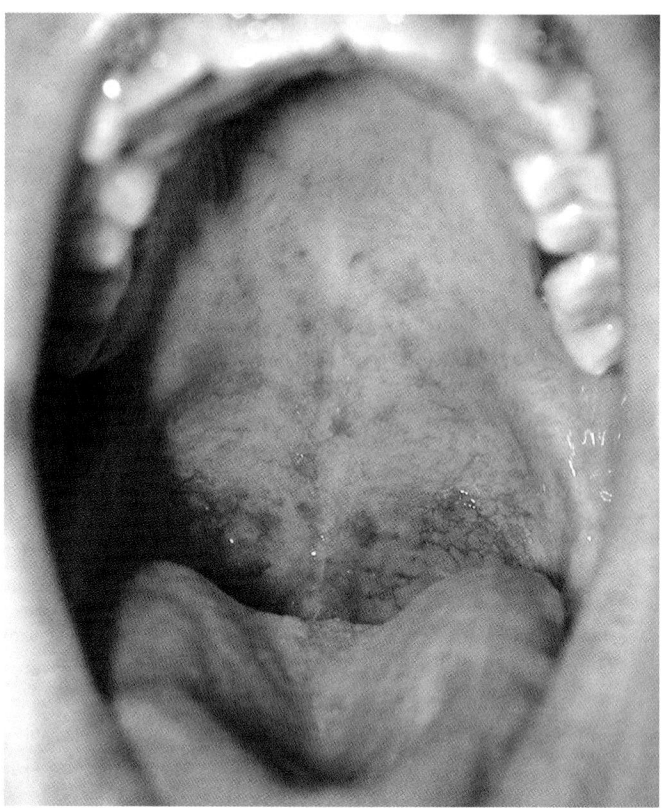

FIGURE 31-7 Viral pharyngitis with prominent vascular injection of the soft palate and lymphoid hyperplasia. (*Reproduced with permission from Richard P. Usatine, MD.*)

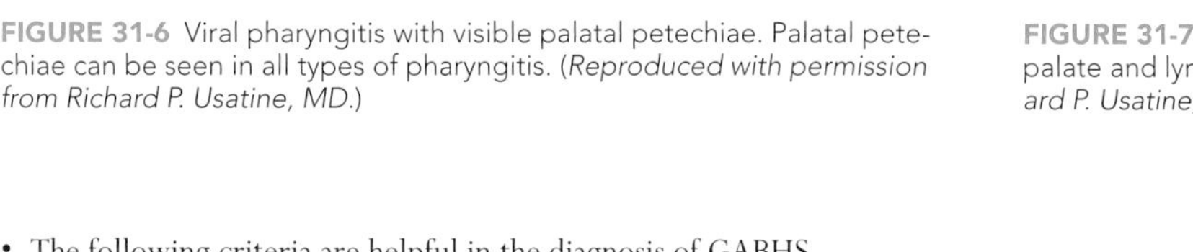

- The following criteria are helpful in the diagnosis of GABHS pharyngitis[7-10]:
  - History of fever or temperature of 38°C (100.4°F) (1 point)
  - Absence of cough (1 point)
  - Tender anterior cervical lymph nodes (1 point)
  - Tonsillar swelling or exudates (1 point)
  - Age
    - Less than 15 years (1 point)
    - 15 to 45 years (0 points)
    - Greater than 45 years (–1 point)

The probability of GABHS is approximately 1% with –1 to 0 points and approximately 51% with 4 to 5 points.[11]

LABORATORY TESTS AND IMAGING

- Rapid antigen detection is often used to diagnose GABHS. Test options include enzyme immunoassays, latex agglutination, liposomal method, and immunochromatograph assays; the latter has the highest reported sensitivity (0.97), specificity (0.97), and positive (32.3) and negative (0.03) likelihood ratios.[12]
- The gold standard for the diagnosis of streptococcal infection is a positive throat culture. However, GABHS is part of the normal oropharyngeal flora in many patients and the diagnosis of acute streptococcal pharyngitis must include both the clinical signs of acute infection and a positive throat culture.
- False-positive tests for streptococcal infection can occur when the patient is colonized with GABHS but it is not the cause of the acute disease.

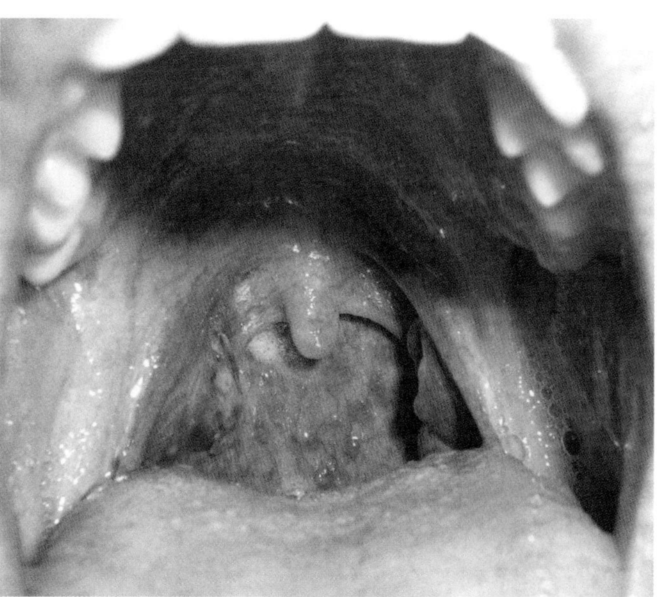

FIGURE 31-8 Strep pharyngitis with dark necrotic area on right tonsil and prominent lymphoid hyperplasia in a cobblestone pattern on the posterior pharynx. (*Reproduced with permission from Richard P. Usatine, MD.*)

- False-negative tests for streptococcal infection can occur when poor sampling technique with the throat swab fails to recover the streptococcal organism when it is the cause of the acute infection.
- A positive mono spot (likelihood ratio in the first week of illness 5.7) and/or greater than 40% atypical lymphocytes on the peripheral smear (likelihood ratio 39) indicate mononucleosis.[12]
- Viral cultures obtained from vesicles can be obtained in Coxsackievirus and herpes infections, but the diagnosis is usually based on clinical suspicion and findings.
- Head-neck computed tomography (CT) scan can assist in the diagnosis and localization of peritonsillar abscess and should be obtained if further extension into the deeper neck is suspected.[13]

DIFFERENTIAL DIAGNOSIS

- Infectious mononucleosis—Nausea, anorexia without vomiting, uvular edema, generalized symmetric lymphadenopathy, and lethargy particularly in teenagers and young adults, are more suggestive of acute mononucleosis (Epstein-Barr virus [EBV]) although the pharyngeal examination has a similar appearance to GABHS (see **Figure 31-4**). Hepatosplenomegaly is indicative of EBV in this group.
- Herpangina or Coxsackievirus infection—Oropharyngeal vesicles and ulcers on the palate indicate herpangina, which is caused by Coxsackievirus A16 in the majority of cases (**Figure 31-9**).
- Oral *Candida*—Whitish plaques of the oropharyngeal mucosa indicate oral *Candida* or thrush, which can be found in adults with immunosuppression (see Chapter 135, Candidiasis).
- Sexually transmitted infections—Primary human immunodeficiency virus, gonococcal and syphilitic pharyngitis can all present with the symptom of sore throat. Although uncommon, these diagnoses should be considered in high-risk populations.

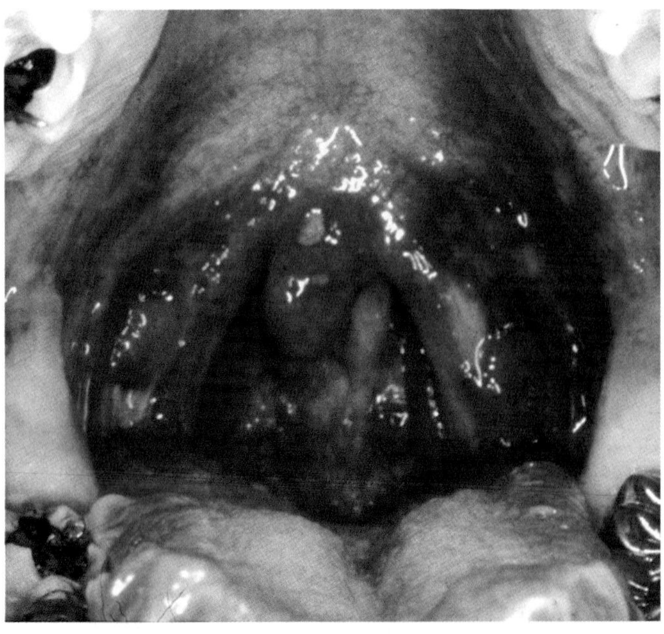

FIGURE 31-9 Herpangina caused by Coxsackievirus A16.

- Primary herpes gingivostomatitis causes oral ulcers and pain in the mouth. The wide distribution of ulcers with the first case of herpes simplex virus (HSV)-1 distinguishes this infection from other types of pharyngitis (see Chapter 128, Herpes Simplex).
- Cytomegalovirus (CMV)—Primary CMV infection in the immunocompetent host is usually asymptomatic. In the immunocompromised host, CMV may present with a mononucleosis-like syndrome clinically indistinguishable from EBV infection.
- Deep neck infections—Asymmetry of the neck, neck masses, and any displacement of the peripharyngeal wall should raise suspicion. Associated shortness of breath may be a warning sign of impending airway obstruction. Other complications include aspiration, thrombosis, mediastinitis, and septic shock.[13]
- Epiglottitis—Rapid-onset fever, malaise, sore throat, and drooling in the absence of coughing characterize acute epiglottitis; uncommon in adults. Progression of the disease can lead to life-threatening airway obstruction. Fortunately, this is a rare condition because of the preventive effect of the *Haemophilus influenzae* type b (HIB) vaccine.
- Supraglottitis—Symptoms are similar to epiglottitis. Sore throat and painful swallowing are the most common presenting symptoms, seen in more than 90% of cases. Muffled voice and drooling, dyspnea, stridor, and cough reported in less than 50% of cases. No definite organism is identified in the majority of cases. Unlike epiglottitis in children, HIB is responsible for less than 20% of adult cases but still accounts for the majority of positive cultures. Mortality rates have been reported up to 20%. Currently it is more common than epiglottitis, because of HIB vaccine.
- Diphtheria—A rare condition in the United States today, as most patients have been immunized. However, it needs to be considered, especially in unvaccinated and immigrant populations. Pharyngeal diphtheria presents with sore throat, low-grade fever, and malaise. The pharynx is erythematous with a grayish pseudomembrane that cannot be scraped off. Complications include myocarditis resulting in acute and severe congestive heart failure (CHF), endocarditis, and neuropathies.
- Other bacterial causes—Non–group A *Streptococcus*, *Fusobacterium necrophorum*, *Mycoplasma pneumoniae*, *Chlamydophila pneumoniae*, and *Arcanobacterium haemolyticum* have all been isolated as bacterial causes of pharyngitis; not as clinically significant, but all generally respond to treatments prescribed for strep pharyngitis.

MANAGEMENT

NONPHARMACOLOGIC

- Hydration with plenty of liquids
- Salt-water gargles
- Lozenges for comfort

MEDICATIONS

- Acetaminophen and ibuprofen can be used for symptomatic relief of fever and pain. Doses can be alternated as needed.
- Steroids (eg, dexamethasone single 10-mg injection) are indicated in severe tonsillitis in patients without immunocompromise.[12] SOR C However, there is no good evidence to recommend steroids in infectious mononucleosis.[14]

- In extreme cases of pharyngitis, 1 teaspoon of viscous lidocaine 2% in a half glass of water gargled 20 to 30 minutes before meals helps the odynophagia. This is typically only recommended in rare cases because of risk of aspiration, potential toxicity of lidocaine, and the risk for oral mucosal burns—consider hospitalization if symptoms are severe.
- Antibiotic use—Use the clinical prediction rule (given earlier [see "Clinical Features"]) for estimating the probability of GABHS[7-11]:
  - Low probability (no test, no treatment for GABHS): Patients scoring 0 points should be treated symptomatically and should not be given antibiotics.
  - Intermediate probability (test and treatment based on result): Patients with 1 to 3 points (probability of GABHS is approximately 18%) should undergo a rapid antigen test and be treated with antibiotics if positive.
  - High probability (no test, treatment for GABHS): Patients with 4 to 5 points should be considered for empiric antibiotic treatment.
- For suspected or proven GABHS, penicillin V 500 mg orally 2 to 3 times daily for 10 days continues to be the treatment of choice for adults.[15] Erythromycin 500 mg orally 4 times daily may be used in penicillin allergic patients. Penicillin G 1.2 million units intramuscular (IM) single dose may be used if unable to tolerate oral medication.
- Penicillin G (600 mg IV every 6 h for 24-48 h) in combination with metronidazole (15 mg/kg IV more than 1 h followed by 7.5 mg/kg IV more than 1 h every 6-8 h) is recommended for peritonsillar abscess.

REFERRAL

- If signs of airway impairment are present, the patient should be immediately transported to an emergency department. Intubation can be extremely difficult and risky.
- Refer patients with peritonsillar abscess to ear, nose, and throat (ENT). Incision and drainage is the treatment of choice in addition to using systemic antibiotics.
- Consider ENT referral for tonsillectomy in proven recurrent GABHS cases, or under certain other conditions (eg, antibiotic allergies or intolerances) with recurrence.[16] However, there is no evidence to support tonsillectomy for isolated cases.[17]

PROGNOSIS

- Sore throat, regardless of the cause, is typically self-limiting. Typical symptoms last for 3 to 4 days.
- Longer-term complications are rare but antibiotic treatment to prevent these sequelae remains justified for treatment. Antibiotics shorten the duration of illness by approximately 1 day and can reduce the risk of rheumatic fever by approximately two-thirds in communities where this complication is common.[15] However, gastrointestinal (GI) symptoms like mild diarrhea are common side effects of antibiotic therapy. The number needed to treat to prevent 1 sore throat at day 3 is less than 6; at week 1 it is 21.[15]

FOLLOW-UP

Follow up if clinically deteriorating, especially if swallowing or breathing becomes more difficult or severe headache develops.

PATIENT EDUCATION

- The treatment for most cases of non-GABHS pharyngitis is education. Explain to patients the difference between a viral and a bacterial infection to help them understand why antibiotics were prescribed or not prescribed. Antibiotic treatment for a patient with an obvious viral infection is inappropriate, despite patient requests. Studies demonstrate that spending time with the patient to explain the disease process is associated with greater patient satisfaction than prescribing an antibiotic.[18,19]
- Rest, liquids, and analgesics should be encouraged.
- Patients receiving antibiotics should be reminded to complete the entire course, even if symptoms improve. Common antibiotic side effects, like rash, nausea, and diarrhea should be reviewed.
- Patients with mononucleosis and splenomegaly should be warned to avoid contact sports because of the risk of splenic rupture.

PATIENT RESOURCES

- Healthline. *Pharyngitis*—**http://www.healthline.com/health/pharyngitis#Overview1.**
- MedlinePlus. *Strep throat*—**www.nlm.nih.gov/medlineplus/ency/article/000639.htm.**
- FamilyDoctor.org. *Mononucleosis*—**http://familydoctor.org/familydoctor/en/diseases-conditions/mononucleosis.html.**

PROVIDER RESOURCES

- Free clinical calculator online: Modified Centor Score for Strep Pharyngitis—**http://www.mdcalc.com/modified-centor-score-for-strep-pharyngitis.**

REFERENCES

1. *Vital Health and Statistics*. US Department of Health and Human Services, Series 13, Number 169 April 2011; *Ambulatory Medical Care Utilization Estimates for 2007*.
2. Bisno AL, Gerber MA, Gwaltney JM, et al. Practice guidelines for the diagnosis and management of group A streptococcal pharyngitis. *Clin Infect Dis*. 2002;35:(2):113-125.
3. Bottin R, Marioni G, Rinaldi R, et al. Deep neck infection: a present-day complication. A retrospective review of 83 cases (1998-2001). *Eur Arch Otorhinolaryngol*. 2003;260(10):576-579.
4. Aung K, Ojha A, Lo C. *Viral Pharyngitis*. http://emedicine.medscape.com/article/225362-overview. Accessed July 2013.
5. Halsey E. *Bacterial Pharyngitis*. http://emedicine.medscape.com/article/225243-overview. Accessed July 2013.
6. Guilherme L, Kalil J, Cunningham M. Molecular mimicry in the autoimmune pathogenesis of rheumatic heart disease. *Autoimmunity*. 2006;39(1):31-39.
7. Singh S, Dolan JG, Centor RM. Optimal management of adults with pharyngitis: a multi-criteria decision analysis. *BMC Med Inform Decis Mak*. 2006;6:14.
8. Choby BA. Diagnosis and treatment of streptococcal pharyngitis. *Am Fam Physician*. 2009;79(5):383-390.

9. Aalbers J, O'Brien KK, Chan WS, et al. Predicting streptococcal pharyngitis in adults in primary care: a systematic review of the diagnostic accuracy of symptoms and signs and validation of the Centor score. *BMC Med*. 2011 Jun 1;9:67.
10. Merrill B, Kelsberg G, Jankowski TA, Danis P. Clinical inquiries. What is the most effective diagnostic evaluation of streptococcal pharyngitis? *J Fam Pract*. 2004;53(9):734, 737-738, 740.
11. McIsaac WJ, Goel V, To T, Low DE. The validity of a sore throat score in family practice. *CMAJ*. 2000;163:811-815.
12. Ebell MH. Sore throat. In: Sloane PD, Slatt LM, Ebell MH, Jacques LB, eds. *Essentials of Family Medicine*. Baltimore, MD: Lippincott Williams & Wilkins; 2002:727-738.
13. Wang LF, Kuo WR, Tsai SM, Huang KJ. Characterizations of life-threatening deep cervical space infections: a review of one hundred ninety-six cases. *Am J Otolaryngol*. 2003;24(2):111-117.
14. Candy B, Hotopf M. Steroids for symptom control in infectious mononucleosis. *Cochrane Database Syst Rev*. 2006;3:CD004402.
15. Spinks A, Glasziou PP, Del Mar CB. Antibiotics for sore throat. *Cochrane Database Syst Rev*. 2006;(4):CD000023.
16. Baugh RF, Archer SM, Mitchell RB, et al. Clinical practice guideline: tonsillectomy in children. *Otolaryngol Head Neck Surg*. 2011;144(suppl 1):S1-S30.
17. Neill RA, Scoville C. Clinical inquiries. What are the indications for tonsillectomy in children? *J Fam Pract*. 2002;51(4):314.
18. Hamm RM, Hicks RJ, Bemben DA. Antibiotics and respiratory infections: are patients more satisfied when expectations are met. *J Fam Pract*. 1996;43(1):56-62.
19. Ong S, Nakase J, Moran GJ, et al. Antibiotic use for emergency department patients with upper respiratory infections: prescribing practices, patient expectations, and patient satisfaction. *Ann Emerg Med*. 2007;50(3):213-220.

32 THE LARYNX (HOARSENESS)

Laura Matrka, MD
C. Blake Simpson, MD
J. Michael King, MD

PATIENT STORY

A 47-year-old man with a 40 pack-year history of smoking presents with worsening hoarseness that began approximately 6 weeks ago. He complains of globus sensation and difficulty swallowing solid foods. He denies odynophagia, otalgia, hemoptysis, and hematemesis. There is no associated cough, and he has not had any constitutional symptoms such as fevers, chills, or recent weight loss.

Hoarseness in a middle-aged man with the above symptoms is very common, and the differential diagnosis is long (all the diseases discussed later are possibilities in this case scenario). The patient's smoking history and duration of symptoms should raise concern for a possible laryngeal malignancy. However, there is a higher incidence of laryngopharyngeal reflux (LPR) followed by benign vocal fold (cord) lesions.

INTRODUCTION

The evaluation of hoarseness typically involves first ruling out the most serious pathologies, such as laryngeal squamous cell carcinoma (SCC), in adults or recurrent respiratory papillomatosis in children, and then proceeding with a more focused and subtle evaluation to uncover any of the many benign pathologies that affect the larynx. Treatment of these benign pathologies must take into account the patient's lifestyle and voice needs. It also often incorporates education on vocal hygiene, which involves increasing hydration, decreasing mucus and vocal abuse, and reducing acid reflux if a factor.

SYNONYMS AND DEFINITIONS

- Hoarseness, dysphonia, vocal strain, breathiness, raspiness
- Vocal cords, true vocal cords, true vocal folds, glottis (**Figure 32-1**)
- False vocal folds, false vocal cords (mucosal folds in the supraglottis, just superior to the true vocal folds and separated from the true folds by the ventricle)
- Flexible fiberoptic laryngoscopy, direct laryngoscopy, nasopharyngeal scope (NP scope), transnasal fiberoptic laryngoscopy
- Stroboscopy, videolaryngostroboscopy (VLS), strobe examination

EPIDEMIOLOGY

- The most common cause of hoarseness in adults and children overall is viral infection causing laryngitis (**Figure 32-2**).
- LPR disease may be present in up to 50% of patients presenting with voice and laryngeal disorders.[1] It is less commonly the sole cause of hoarseness.

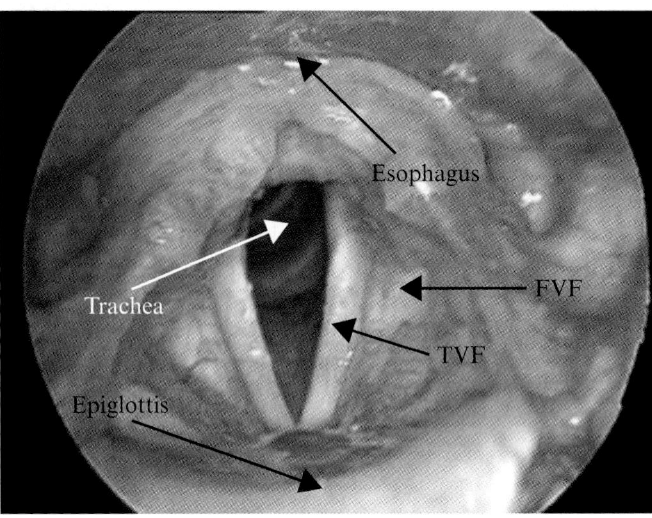

FIGURE 32-1 Normal larynx (true and false vocal folds). *FVF*, false vocal fold; *TVF*, true vocal fold (cord). (*Reproduced with permission from C. Blake Simpson, MD.*)

- Squamous cell carcinoma accounts for 95% of laryngeal cancer. Approximately 11,000 new cases are diagnosed in the United States each year. Peak incidence is in the sixth and seventh decades of life with a strong male predominance.[1]
- Recurrent respiratory papillomatosis (RRP) represents the most common benign neoplasm of the larynx among children and should be considered in children with chronic hoarseness. A known risk factor for juvenile onset is the triad of a firstborn child (75%), teenage mother, and vaginal delivery. The incidence is 4.3 per 100,000 children and 1.8 per 100,000 adults.[2] There is a known association between cervical human papillomavirus (HPV) infection in the mother and juvenile-onset RRP, but the precise mode of transmission is unclear. The risk of a child contracting RRP after delivery from an actively infected mother with genital HPV ranges from 0.25% to 3%.[3] Because cesarean section does not prevent RRP in all cases, routine prophylactic cesarean section in mothers with active condyloma acuminata is currently *not* recommended.

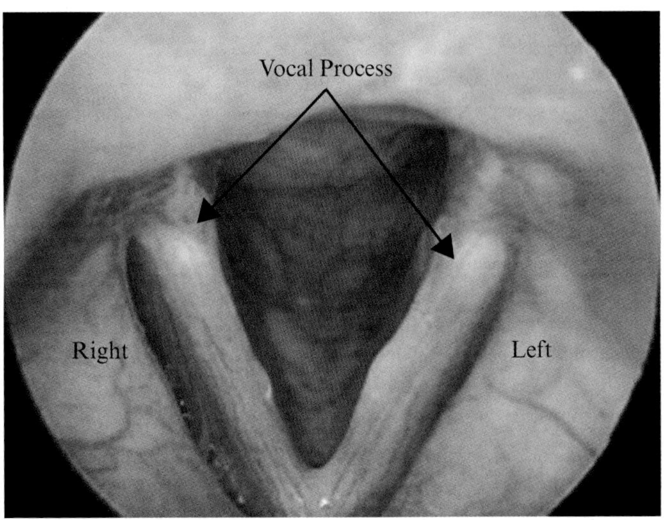

FIGURE 32-2 Laryngitis—diffuse erythema and inflammation, irregular vocal fold edges. (*Reproduced with permission from C. Blake Simpson, MD.*)

ETIOLOGY AND PATHOPHYSIOLOGY

- Laryngitis is a nonspecific term to describe inflammation of the larynx from any cause. Most commonly this is due to a viral upper respiratory infection. Compare the anatomy of the normal larynx (see **Figure 32-1**) with that of acute laryngitis (see **Figure 32-2**), with the primary differences being in the diffuse erythema and edema of the vocal folds and the often transient irregularities of the vocal fold medial edge as compared to the straight medial edge of the normal vocal fold. Laryngeal symptoms result from dry throat, mucous stasis, and recurrent trauma from coughing and throat clearing.
- LPR must be differentiated from gastroesophageal reflux disease (GERD), in which acid reflux is more likely to cause heartburn, indigestion, and regurgitation and does not necessarily reach the larynx or upper aerodigestive tract. LPR is more likely to present with frequent throat clearing, dry cough, hoarseness, and globus sensation and does not include heartburn in more than 60% of patients. The larynx is highly sensitive to even small amounts of acid or pepsin. Thus, patients who do not have severe enough reflux to cause esophagitis, with its associated symptoms of GERD, may still develop symptomatic laryngeal mucosal injury, with its associated symptoms of LPR.[1,4-6]
- SCC has a multifactorial etiology, but 90% of patients have a history of heavy tobacco and/or alcohol use. These risk factors have a synergistic effect. Other independent risk factors include employment as a painter or metalworker, exposure to diesel or gasoline fumes, and exposure to therapeutic doses of radiation.
- RRP is caused by HPV-6 and HPV-11. Onset is predominantly in young children, although an adult-onset variant exists. Its course is unpredictable and highly variable. Tracheal and bronchopulmonary spread can occur, as can malignant transformation to SCC; the latter is rare. Bronchopulmonary spread is uniformly fatal as a consequence of the lack of surgical options.
- Vocal cord nodules are benign lesions arising from mechanical trauma (vocal abuse or misuse) and are often described as a "callous" of the vocal folds. Vocal cord polyps or cysts can arise from vocal abuse, a blocked mucous gland, vocal fold hemorrhage, a background of polypoid corditis (see below), or idiopathic etiologies. They are a common cause of dysphonia in singers, teachers, and other professional voice users. Vocal cord granulomas are associated with LPR and/or intubation trauma and rarely require surgery.
- Causes of vocal cord paresis or paralysis are myriad:[1,7]
  - Iatrogenic surgical injury (anterior spine fusion, carotid endarterectomy, thyroidectomy) is most common (25%).
  - Nonlaryngeal malignancy (mediastinal, bronchopulmonary, and skull base) (24%).
  - No identifiable cause (idiopathic), often assumed to be viral (20%).
  - Nonsurgical trauma (penetrating or blunt injury and intubation injury) (10%).
  - Neurologic causes (stroke, central nervous system [CNS] tumors, multiple sclerosis [MS], and amyotrophic lateral sclerosis [ALS]) (8%).
  - Inflammatory or infectious disease (2-5%).
- Presbyphonia is a diagnosis of exclusion denoting vocal changes from aging of the larynx (gradually weakening voice, poor vocal projection, and vocal "roughness"). Hoarseness in patients older than 60 years of age is most commonly a result of benign vocal fold lesions followed by malignancy and vocal fold paralysis. Once a thorough evaluation has been done to rule out organic causes, presbyphonia is the cause of hoarseness in approximately 10% of elderly patients; it is characterized by atrophied vocal folds.[8]

DIAGNOSIS

CLINICAL FEATURES

- Key historical and physical examination findings can help differentiate benign pathology from potentially more serious problems:
  - Otalgia (ear pain)—Often a source of referred pain from primary laryngeal and pharyngeal carcinomas; it is not typically seen with benign pathologies.
  - Dysphagia and odynophagia (pain when swallowing)—Nonspecific complaints, but potentially worrisome for obstructing lesions or reactive pharyngeal edema.
  - Stridor or dyspnea—"Noisy breathing" with respiratory distress should be evaluated urgently to rule out impending airway obstruction. Less-severe dyspnea may be noted by patients with vocal cord paralysis caused by air escape during speech; a detailed history should reveal that it occurs only during speech or from the inability to perform adequate Valsalva maneuver as a result of loss of tight glottic closure.
  - Globus pharyngeus—The persistent or intermittent nonpainful sensation of a lump or foreign body in the throat. This is commonly associated with LPR.
  - Neck mass—Associated unilateral or bilateral lymphadenopathy is suspicious for a laryngeal neoplasm until proven otherwise.
  - Timing—Onset, duration, and frequency of symptoms are important.
- Red flags for laryngeal carcinoma include a history of smoking and/or alcohol abuse, associated neck mass, weight loss or severe dysphagia, presence of stridor (often initially noted with sleep or when lying flat), and otalgia.
- LPR symptoms include hoarseness, throat clearing, "postnasal drip," chronic cough, dysphagia, globus pharyngeus, and sore throat. "Heartburn" is *not* a requisite symptom!
- Hallmark of diagnosis is direct visualization of the larynx, often performed by an otolaryngologist with a flexible laryngoscopic examination. Stroboscopy is added to the evaluation when visualization of the mucosal wave of the vocal folds is necessary. Assessment of the mucosal wave aids in determining the depth of a lesion within the vocal fold and the severity of its effect on the voice.

LABORATORY AND IMAGING

- Laboratory studies are not usually helpful, except in the rare case that a previously undiagnosed rheumatologic disease presents with vocal complaints as the initial symptom.
- Plain films of the chest are useful to rule out bronchopulmonary or mediastinal masses as a cause of vocal cord paralysis, but are generally not helpful for primary laryngeal lesions.
- A computed tomography (CT) of the neck and chest with contrast is useful in ruling out pathology along the length of the recurrent laryngeal nerve in cases of unexplained vocal cord paralysis and in cases suspicious for carcinoma, especially if there is associated cervical lymphadenopathy. A chest X-ray is sometimes used to replace the chest CT.
- A magnetic resonance imaging (MRI) with and without gadolinium offers the best imaging for suspected primary CNS or skull base

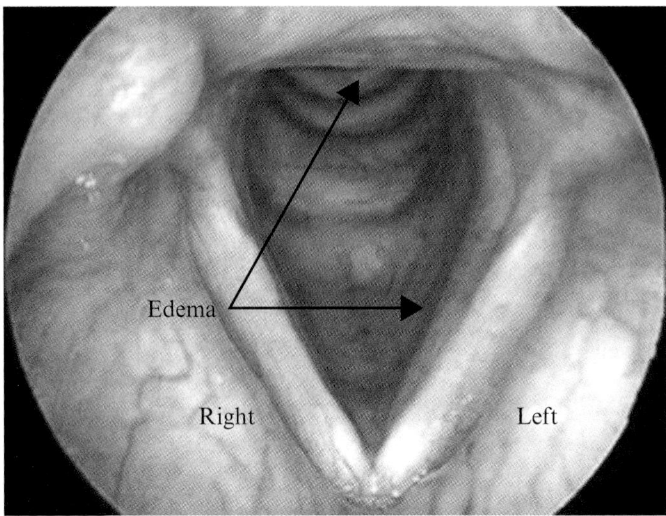

FIGURE 32-3 Laryngopharyngeal reflux. Postcricoid region edema (normal is less full and nearly concave) and edema just inferior to the true vocal fold edge (infraglottic edema) indicative of chronic inflammation from reflux, often called "pseudosulcus." Other findings of LPR not seen in this image include thick mucus and mucosal erythema. (*Reproduced with permission from C. Blake Simpson, MD.*)

lesions; this is typically added to the workup for vocal cord paralysis when evidence of high vagal injury such as weakness in palate elevation is present.

- Referral to a gastroenterologist for *dual-channel* 24-hour pH probe monitoring (*while on antireflux medications*) is a useful diagnostic tool for patients with suspected LPR.

DIFFERENTIAL DIAGNOSIS

- Laryngitis (see **Figure 32-2**)
- Laryngopharyngeal reflux (**Figures 32-3** and **32-4**)
- SCC (**Figure 32-5**)

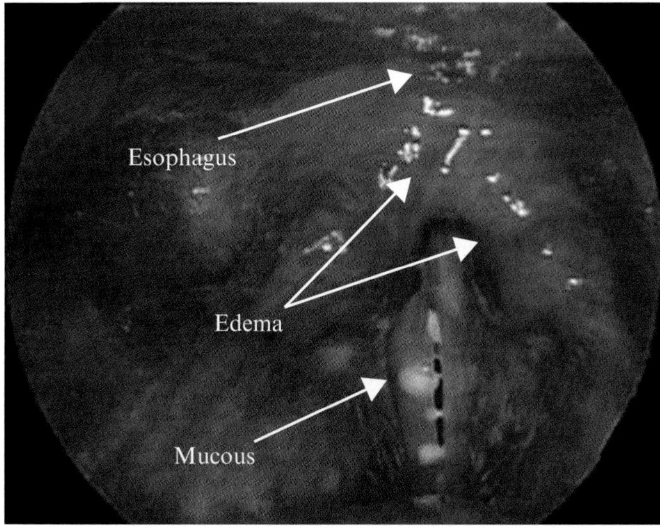

FIGURE 32-4 Laryngopharyngeal reflux during phonation with diffuse erythema, inflammation, and thick mucus. (*Reproduced with permission from C. Blake Simpson, MD.*)

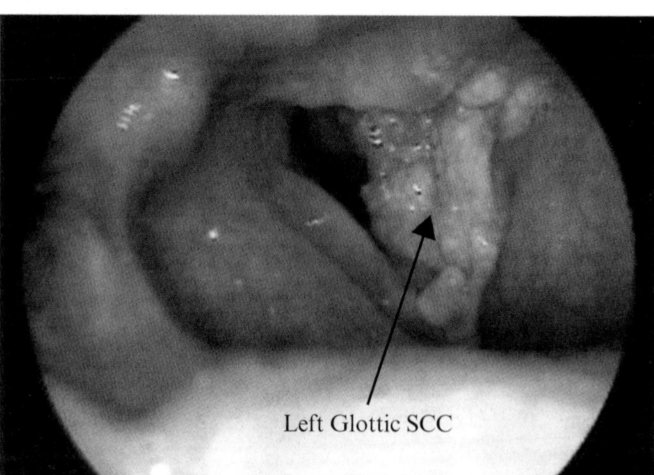

FIGURE 32-5 Squamous cell carcinoma, advanced stage with left true vocal cord paralysis. (*Reproduced with permission from C. Blake Simpson, MD.*)

- Laryngeal papillomatosis (**Figures 32-6** and **32-7**)
- Vocal cord nodule (**Figure 32-8**)
- Vocal cord polyp (**Figure 32-9**)
- Vocal cord cyst
- Vocal cord paresis or paralysis
- Presbyphonia
- Neurologic disorders (MS, Parkinson disease, ALS, and essential tremor)
- Systemic diseases (Wegener granulomatosis, sarcoidosis, rheumatoid arthritis)

MANAGEMENT

- Laryngitis—Empiric treatment is aimed at alleviating symptoms such as cough and thinning nasal or pharyngeal secretions. Hydration is critical for healing (increased water intake, steam showers, humidifiers,

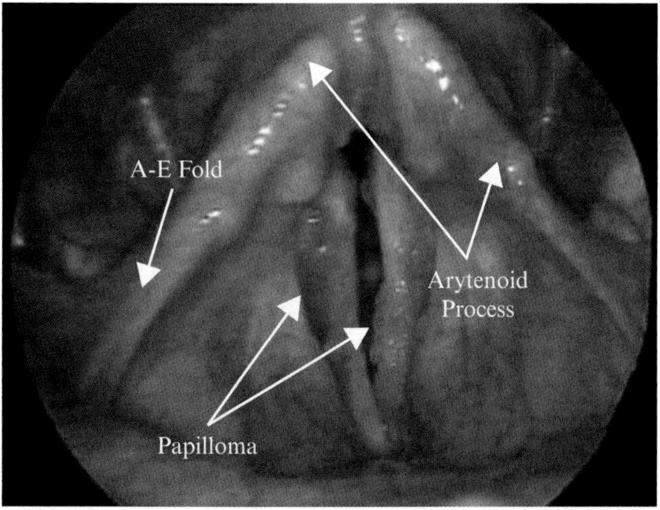

FIGURE 32-6 Adult recurrent respiratory papillomatosis. Aryepiglottic fold (A-E fold). (*Reproduced with permission from C. Blake Simpson, MD.*)

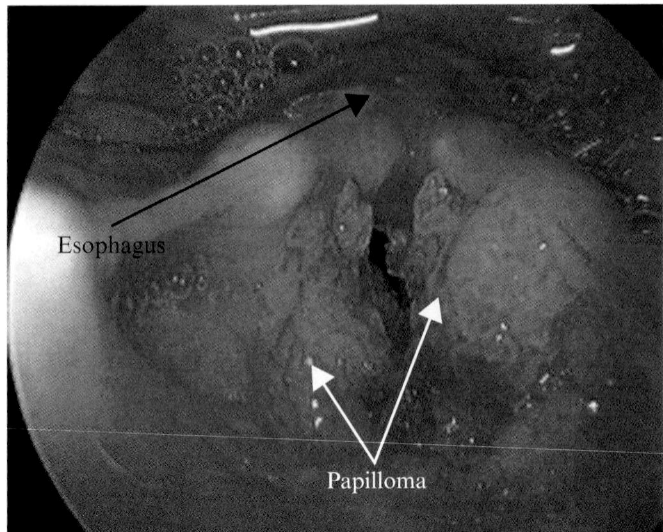

FIGURE 32-7 Recurrent respiratory papillomatosis in a 3-year-old child. The papillomas are nearly obstructing the airway and have required debridement. (*Reproduced with permission from C. Blake Simpson, MD.*)

and saunas may help). Throat clearing should be discouraged and voice rest encouraged. Talking should be conserved, not prohibited. Inform patients that whispering causes even more vocal strain than normal speech.

- Vocal cord nodules, polyps, and cysts—Initial management involves speech therapy accompanied by medical treatment of dehydration, allergies, sinonasal secretions (postnasal drip), and LPR. Refractory disease may require surgical excision.
- Laryngeal papillomatosis—Most children have a recalcitrant course that requires periodic surgical debridement by an otolaryngologist to prevent airway obstruction. Spontaneous remission may occur. Adjuvant therapy, such as intraepithelial injection of cidofovir at the time of surgery, is commonly utilized in more aggressive disease. It is hoped that the administration of the Gardasil vaccine will decrease the incidence of RRP over time. Some practitioners administer the Gardasil vaccine in a nonprophylactic manner to patients with existing RRP, although there is no strong evidence currently to support a treatment effect of the vaccine.[2,3]

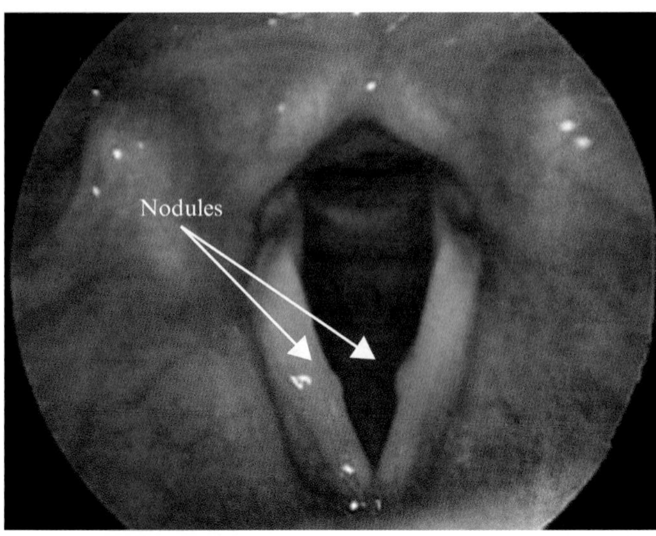

FIGURE 32-8 Vocal cord nodules. (*Reproduced with permission from C. Blake Simpson, MD.*)

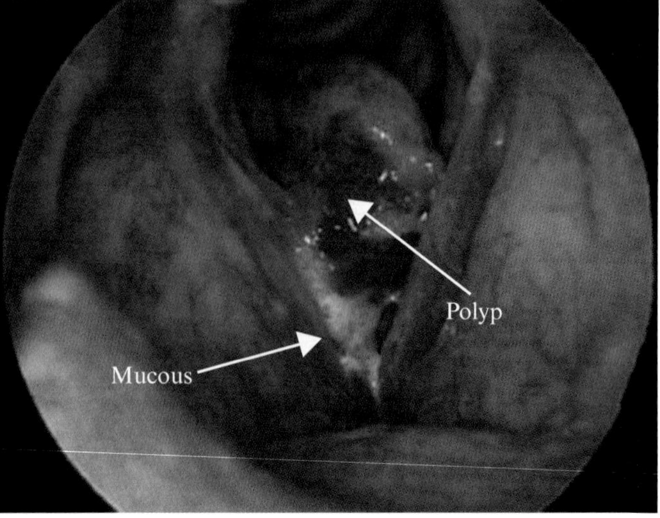

FIGURE 32-9 Large, obstructing laryngeal polyp with thick mucus collecting around it. (*Reproduced with permission from C. Blake Simpson, MD.*)

- LPR—Mainstay treatment involves patient education to modify diet and behavior (avoidance of acidic or greasy foods, tobacco cessation, limiting alcohol and caffeine, weight loss, and avoiding meals shortly before lying down). Medical therapy consists of *twice*-daily proton pump inhibitors (PPIs) 30 to 60 minutes before meals, which can often be weaned after several months of therapy. Some patients benefit from adding an H_2-blocker, such as ranitidine 300 mg, at bedtime.
- SCC—Multidisciplinary management is best. Depending on the staging and extent of disease, patients often receive one or more modalities of treatment including surgery, radiation, and chemotherapy.
- Vocal cord paresis or paralysis—Treatment is targeted at the underlying disorder. Some patients may be candidates for surgical intervention to reposition the paralyzed cord medially with an implant. With a mobile vocal fold on the contralateral side, airway is rarely compromised by medialization of the paralyzed vocal fold. These procedures restore voice quality and often alleviate chronic aspiration problems.
- Neurologic diseases—Laryngeal complaints can be associated with MS, myasthenia gravis, Parkinson disease, ALS, and essential tremor. In addition to managing the underlying disorder, a trial of voice therapy is sometimes useful.
- Systemic diseases—Diseases such as Wegener granulomatosis, sarcoidosis, relapsing polychondritis, and rheumatoid arthritis rarely may involve the larynx. Voice and swallowing problems in these patients should be evaluated by an otolaryngologist for possible therapies to improve the voice and to rule out associated airway stenosis.
- Presbyphonia—This is a diagnosis of exclusion. Once organic etiologies have been ruled out, a trial of voice therapy is recommended before considering surgical options, such as vocal fold injection augmentation to plump the atrophied vocal fold.

FOLLOW-UP

- Urgent referral to an otolaryngologist for flexible laryngoscopic examination of the larynx is advisable when the history and physical are suspicious for carcinoma.

- When symptoms worsen or fail to resolve, referral to an otolaryngologist (or laryngologist) is indicated (see "Provider Resources" below to find a laryngologist in your area).
- Patients suspected of having LPR should be seen approximately 6 to 8 weeks after initiating empiric therapy with a PPI and lifestyle measures. An otolaryngology and/or gastroenterology consultation is indicated when symptoms do not improve after optimized behavioral and medical management or for patients who require long-term PPI therapy (longer than 12 months). Some of these patients, particularly those with chronic cough or long-standing requirement for PPIs, may require transnasal esophagoscopy (performed in the otolaryngologist's office) or esophagogastroduodenoscopy (performed by a gastroenterologist in the endoscopy suite). Recent evidence has pointed to chronic cough as an independent indicator of esophageal adenocarcinoma, and Barrett esophagus should be ruled out in any patient requiring long-term PPI use.[9]

PATIENT EDUCATION

- In cases of nonmalignant pathology, vocal hygiene and other lifestyle measures often play an important role in treatment. Efforts should focus on increasing hydration, decreasing caffeine intake, tobacco cessation, and prevention of excessive alcohol use.
- Vocal cord nodules, polyps, and cysts typically occur in professional voice users (ministers, auctioneers, teachers, singers, etc). Speech therapists can be integral in preventing and healing lesions by teaching patients how to avoid vocal misuse.
- Benign laryngeal pathology may be improved, but not necessarily resolved, by controlling both gastroesophageal and LPR disease. Patients should be educated about GERD or LPR risk factors:
  - Spicy, acidic, or greasy foods
  - Tobacco and alcohol abuse
  - Caffeinated beverages (especially carbonated sodas)
  - Citric juices, tomato sauces, chocolate, mints
  - Obesity
  - Eating meals within 2 to 3 hours of lying down

PATIENT RESOURCES

- American Academy of Otolaryngology-Head and Neck Surgery—**http://www.entnet.org/healthinfo/index.cfm.**
- ENT USA—**http://www.entusa.com.**
- VoiceProblem.org—**http://www.voiceproblem.org.**

PROVIDER RESOURCES

- VoiceProblem.org—**http://www.voiceproblem.org.**
- Information about laryngeal pathology as well as an extensive list of laryngologists worldwide—**http://www.voicedoctor.net/links/physicians.html.**

REFERENCES

1. Ossoff R, Shapshay S, Woodson G, Netterville J. *The Larynx*. Philadelphia, PA: Lippincott Williams & Wilkins; 2003.
2. Derkay CS. Recurrent respiratory papillomatosis. *Laryngoscope*. 2001;111:57-69.
3. Gallagher TQ, Derkay CS. Recurrent respiratory papillomatosis: update 2008. *Curr Opin Otolaryngol Head Neck Surg*. 2008;16:532-542.
4. Simpson CB. Patient of the month program: breathy dysphonia. *American Academy of Otolaryngol Head Neck Surg*. 2002;31(7):19-28.
5. Koufmann JA, Amin MA, Panetti M. Prevalence of reflux in 113 consecutive patients with laryngeal and voice disorders. *Otolaryngol Head Neck Surg*. 2000;123:385-388.
6. Koufman JA, Aviv JE, Casiano RR, Shaw GY. Laryngopharyngeal reflux: position statement of the committee on speech, voice, and swallowing disorders of the American Academy of Otolaryngology-Head and Neck Surgery. *Otolaryngol Head Neck Surg*. 2002;127:32-35.
7. Benninger MS, Gillen JB, Altman JS. Changing etiology of vocal fold immobility. *Laryngoscope*. 1998;108:1346-1349.
8. Kendall K. Presbyphonia: a review. *Curr Opin Otolaryngol Head Neck Surg*. 2007;15:137-140.
9. Reavis KM, Morris CD, Gopal DV, et al. Laryngopharyngeal reflux symptoms better predict the presence of esophageal adenocarcinoma than typical gastroesophageal reflux symptoms. *Ann Surg*. 2004;239(6):849-858.

PART 6

ORAL HEALTH

Strength of Recommendation (SOR)	Definition
A	Recommendation based on consistent and good-quality patient-oriented evidence.*
B	Recommendation based on inconsistent or limited-quality patient-oriented evidence.*
C	Recommendation based on consensus, usual practice, opinion, disease-oriented evidence, or case series for studies of diagnosis, treatment, prevention, or screening.*

*See Appendix A on pages 1241-1244 for further information.

33 BLACK HAIRY TONGUE

Richard P. Usatine, MD
Wanda C. Gonsalves, MD

PATIENT STORY

A 60-year-old man who smokes presents to the physician's office smelling of alcohol. He complains of a black discoloration of his tongue and a gagging sensation on occasion. He admits to smoking 1 to 2 packs per day along with drinking at least 6 to 8 beers per day. The patient brushes his teeth infrequently and has not seen a dentist for a long time. On physical examination, his teeth are stained and his tongue shows elongated papillae with brown discoloration (**Figure 33-1**). Diagnoses include black hairy tongue (BHT), poor oral hygiene, and tobacco and alcohol addiction.

INTRODUCTION

BHT is a benign disorder of the tongue characterized by abnormally hypertrophied and elongated filiform papillae on the surface of the tongue.[1] In addition, there is defective desquamation of the papillae on the dorsal tongue resulting in a hair-like appearance.[2]

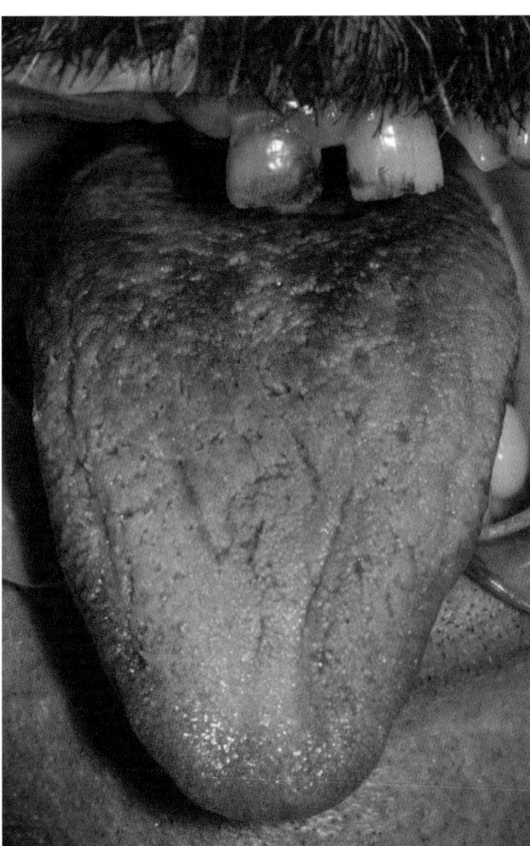

FIGURE 33-1 Black hairy tongue (BHT) showing elongated filiform papillae with brown discoloration in a man who is a heavy smoker and drinker. Note the tobacco-stained teeth. *(Reproduced with permission from Brad Neville, DDS.)*

SYNONYMS

BHT is also known as hyperkeratosis of the tongue, lingua villosa nigra.

EPIDEMIOLOGY

The prevalence of BHT varies depending on the risk factors in the population being studied.

- It can be as high as 57% in persons incarcerated or addicted to drugs.[3]
- The prevalence in Minnesota schoolchildren was 0.06%.[4]
- Turkish dental patients showed higher rates of BHT in men, smokers, and black tea drinkers. The highest prevalence was 54% in heavy smokers.[5]

ETIOLOGY AND PATHOPHYSIOLOGY

- BHT (see **Figure 33-1**) is a disorder characterized by elongation and hypertrophy of filiform papillae and defective desquamation of the papillae.[2,6]
- These papillae, which are normally about 1 mm in length, may become as long as 12 mm.
  - The elongated filiform papillae can then collect debris, bacteria, fungus, or other foreign materials.[1]
- In an extensive literature review of reported cases of drug-induced BHT, 82% of the cases were caused by antibiotics (**Figure 33-2**).[1]
- Dry mouth (xerostomia) from medications, tobacco, and radiation therapy can lead to BHT.[1]

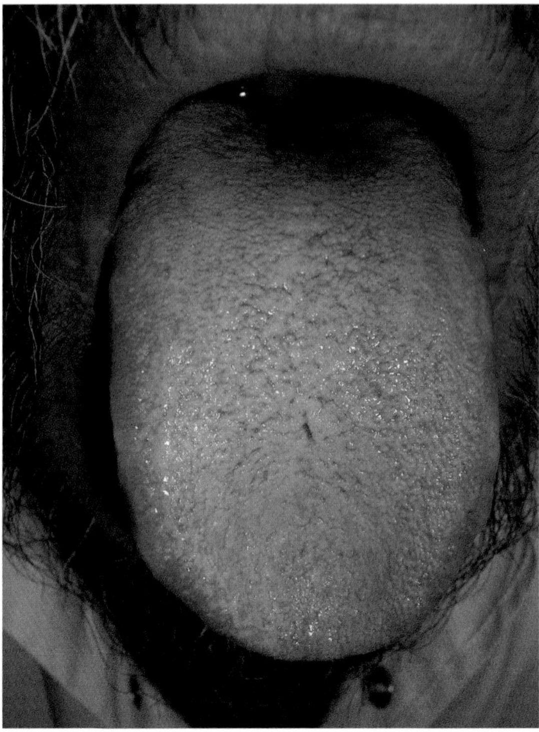

FIGURE 33-2 Drug-induced black hairy tongue (BHT) with yellowish-brown elongated filiform papillae in a patient taking a broad-spectrum antibiotic. *(Reproduced with permission from Richard P. Usatine, MD.)*

RISK FACTORS

- Tobacco (smoking and chewing)[1]
- Alcoholism and drug abuse (especially drugs that are smoked)
- Poor oral hygiene
- Medications (especially antibiotics and those causing xerostomia)
- Oxidizing mouthwashes (containing peroxide)
- Cancer, especially with radiation therapy
- Drinking black tea or coffee

DIAGNOSIS

CLINICAL FEATURES

- Patients may be asymptomatic. However, the accumulation of debris in the elongated papillae may cause taste alterations, nausea, gagging, halitosis, and pain or burning of the tongue.[1]

The diagnosis is made by visual inspection:

- BHT may exhibit a thick coating of black, brown, or yellow discoloration, depending on foods ingested, tobacco use, and amount of coffee or tea consumed (**Figure 33-3**).

TYPICAL DISTRIBUTION

The lesion is restricted to the dorsum of the tongue, anterior to the circumvallate papillae, rarely involving the tip or sides of the tongue.

LABORATORY TESTS

Consider performing a potassium hydroxide (KOH) preparation to rule out associated candidiasis.

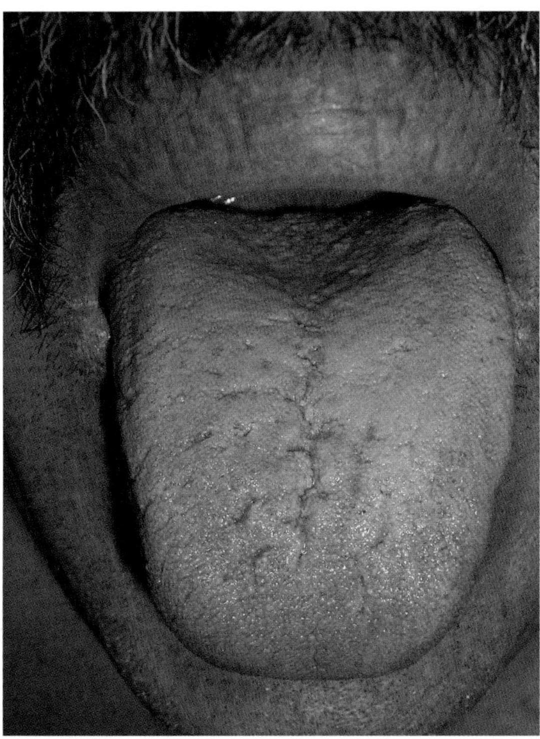

FIGURE 33-3 Black hairy tongue (BHT) that is also furrowed in a heavy smoker. Note this man also has angular cheilitis, poor dentition, and halitosis. (*Reproduced with permission from Richard P. Usatine, MD.*)

DIFFERENTIAL DIAGNOSIS

- Black tongue can occur with the ingestion of bismuth subsalicylate or minocycline. Although the tongue has a black coating, the papillae are not elongated. Without the hypertrophy of papillae this is not a BHT (**Figure 33-4**).
- Hairy leukoplakia—Appears as faint white vertical keratotic streaks typically on the lateral side of the tongue (**Figure 33-5**). Do not confuse BHT with oral hairy leukoplakia, an Epstein-Barr virus–related condition typically affecting the lateral tongue bilaterally in immunocompromised patients, especially those with HIV infection.
- Oral candidiasis—White plaques typically found on the buccal mucosa, tongue, and palate when removed has an erythematous base. The white color should make this easy to distinguish from BHT (see Chapter 135, Candidiasis).

MANAGEMENT

NONPHARMACOLOGIC

- Avoidance of predisposing risk factors (eg, tobacco, alcohol, and antibiotics). SOR Ⓒ
- Stop the offending medication in drug-induced BHT whenever possible.[1] SOR Ⓑ
- Regular tongue brushing using a soft toothbrush or tongue scraper. SOR Ⓒ

MEDICATIONS

If candidiasis is present, an oral antifungal is indicated. If there is no liver disease, the preferred regimen for oral candidiasis is fluconazole 100 mg daily for 14 days. An alternative is clotrimazole troches 5 times a day for 14 days. Nystatin is less effective. Fluconazole-treated HIV patients with oropharyngeal candidiasis were more likely to remain disease-free than those treated with other antifungal agents.[7] SOR Ⓐ

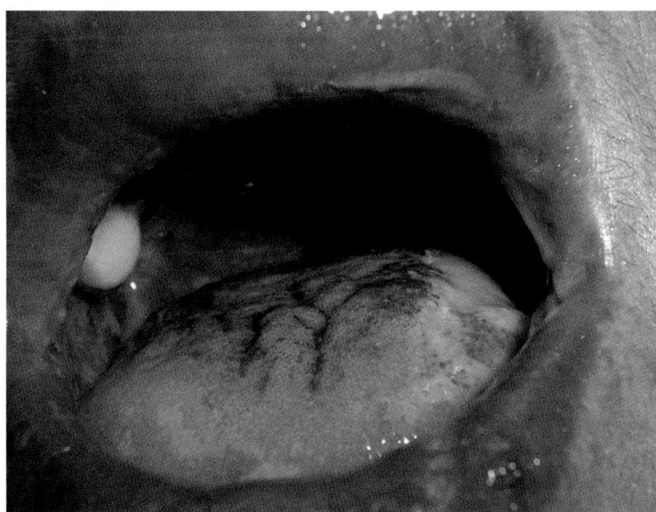

FIGURE 33-4 Black tongue without elongated papillae in a woman with untreated pemphigus vulgaris. Note the palatal erosions along with the black color of the tongue. The black color was gone in 2 days after prednisone was initiated and the patient was able to eat again. (*Reproduced with permission from Richard P. Usatine, MD.*)

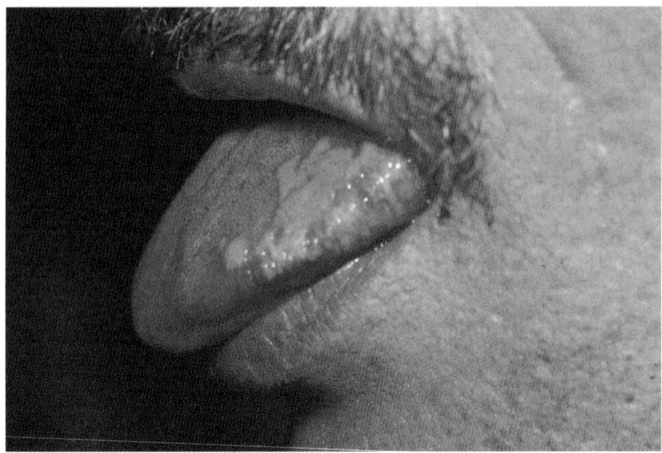

FIGURE 33-5 Oral hairy leukoplakia caused by Epstein-Barr virus on the tongue of a man with AIDS. (*Reproduced with permission from Richard P. Usatine, MD.*)

REFERRAL

Patients with poor oral hygiene should be referred to a dentist. All patients should be encouraged to see a dentist at least twice yearly.

PREVENTION

Good oral hygiene and avoidance of risk factors are essential.

PROGNOSIS

BHT is generally a self-limited disorder, so the prognosis should be excellent with good oral hygiene and treatment.

PATIENT EDUCATION

Tell the patients to brush their teeth and tongue twice a day or to use a tongue scraper. Address addictions and offer help to quit. Suggest that patients should eat firm foods, like fresh apples, that will help to clean the tongue.

PATIENT RESOURCES

- Mayo Clinic. *Black, Hairy Tongue*—**http://www.mayoclinic.com/health/black-hairy-tongue/DS01134.**

PROVIDER RESOURCES

- Medscape. *Hairy Tongue*—**http://emedicine.medscape.com/article/1075886.**

REFERENCES

1. Thompson DF, Kessler TL. Drug-induced black hairy tongue. *Pharmacotherapy.* 2010;30(6):585-593.
2. Harada Y, Gaafar H. Black hairy tongue. A scanning electron microscopic study. *J Laryngol Otol.* 1977;91:91-96.
3. Bouquot JE. Common oral lesions found during a mass screening examination. *J Am Dent Assoc.* 1986;112(1):50-57.
4. Redman RS. Prevalence of geographic tongue, fissured tongue, median rhomboid glossitis, and hairy tongue among 3,611 Minnesota schoolchildren. *Oral Surg Oral Med Oral Pathol.* 1970;30:390-395.
6. Sarti GM, Haddy RI, Schaffer D, Kihm J. Black hairy tongue. *Am Fam Physician.* 1990;41:1751-1755.
7. Albougy HA, Naidoo S. A systematic review of the management of oral candidiasis associated with HIV/AIDS. *SADJ.* 2002;57(11):457-466.

34 GEOGRAPHIC TONGUE

Ernest Valdez, DDS
Richard P. Usatine, MD
Wanda C. Gonsalves, MD

PATIENT STORY

A 23-year-old man presents to the physician's office complaining of his tongue's "strange appearance." He denies pain or discomfort and is unsure how long the lesions have been present. The lesions seem to change areas of distribution on the tongue. The examination reveals large, well-delineated, shiny and smooth, erythematous spots on the surface of the tongue (**Figure 34-1**). The diagnosis is geographic tongue (benign migratory glossitis). The physician explains that it is benign and that no treatment is needed unless symptoms develop.

INTRODUCTION

Geographic tongue is a recurrent, benign, usually asymptomatic, inflammatory disorder of the mucosa of the dorsum and lateral borders of the tongue. Geographic tongue is characterized by circinate, irregularly shaped erythematous patches bordered by a white keratotic band. The central erythematous patch represents loss of filiform papillae of tongue epithelium. Geographic tongue can, although rarely, present as symptomatic.

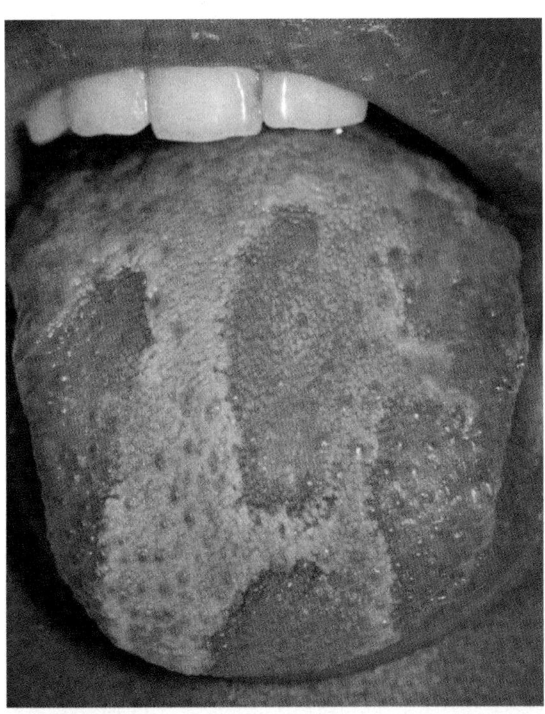

FIGURE 34-1 Geographic tongue (benign migratory glossitis). Note the pink continents among the white oceans. *(Reproduced with permission from Gonsalves WC, Chi AC, Neville BW. Common oral lesions: part II.* Am Fam Phys. *2007;75(4):501-508. Copyright © 2007 American Academy of Family Physicians. All rights reserved.)*

SYNONYMS

Geographic tongue is also known as benign migratory glossitis, geographic stomatitis.

EPIDEMIOLOGY

- Geographic tongue has an estimated prevalence of 1% to 3% of the population.[1]
- It may occur in either children or adults, and exhibits a female predilection.
- Geographic tongue in the United States has a greater prevalence among white and black persons than among Mexican Americans.[2]

ETIOLOGY AND PATHOPHYSIOLOGY

- Geographic tongue is a common oral inflammatory condition of unknown etiology.
- Some studies have shown an increased frequency in patients with allergies, pustular psoriasis, stress, type 1 diabetes, fissured tongue, and hormonal disturbances.[3]
- Histopathologic appearance resembles psoriasis.[4]
- Oddly, geographic tongue has an inverse association with cigarette smoking.[2,5]

DIAGNOSIS

CLINICAL FEATURES

- The diagnosis is made by visual inspection and history of the lesion. The lesions are suggestive of a geographic map (hence geographic tongue) with pink continents surrounded by whiter oceans (see **Figure 34-1**).
- Geographic tongue consists of large, well-delineated, shiny, and smooth, erythematous patches surrounded by a white halo (**Figure 34-2**).
- Tongue lesions exhibit central erythema because of atrophy of the filiform papillae and are usually surrounded by slightly elevated, curving, white-to-yellow elevated borders (see **Figures 34-1** and **34-2**).
- The condition typically waxes and wanes over time so the lesions appear to be migrating (hence migratory glossitis).
- Lesions may last days, months, or years. The lesions do not scar.
- Most patients are asymptomatic, but some patients may complain of pain or burning, especially when eating spicy foods.
- Suspect systemic intraoral manifestations of psoriasis or reactive arthritis if the patient has psoriatic skin lesions or has conjunctivitis, urethritis, arthritis, and skin involvement suggestive of reactive arthritis (see Chapter 153, Reactive Arthritis).

TYPICAL DISTRIBUTION

- The lesions are typically found on the anterior two-thirds of the dorsal tongue mucosa.
- Geographic tongue usually affects the tongue, although other oral sites may be involved such as the buccal mucosa, the labial mucosa and less frequently, the soft palate.[3]

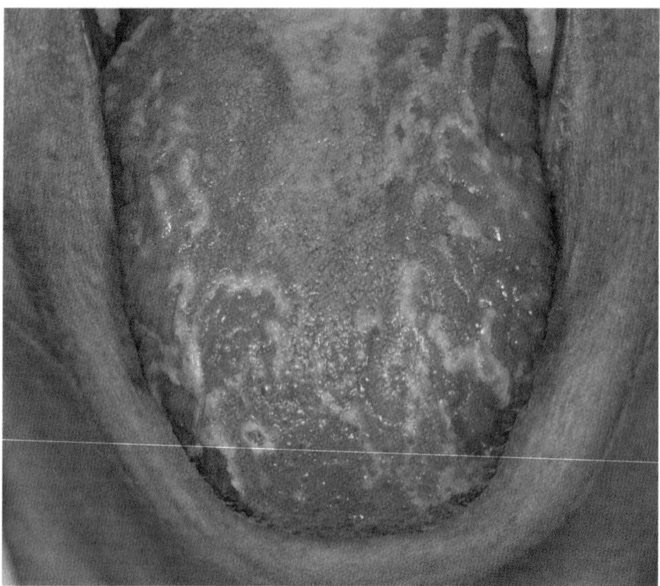

FIGURE 34-2 Geographic tongue lesions in a 71-year-old woman. Note the white halos around the pink areas of atrophy of filiform papillae. (*Reproduced with permission from Michaell Huber, DMD.*)

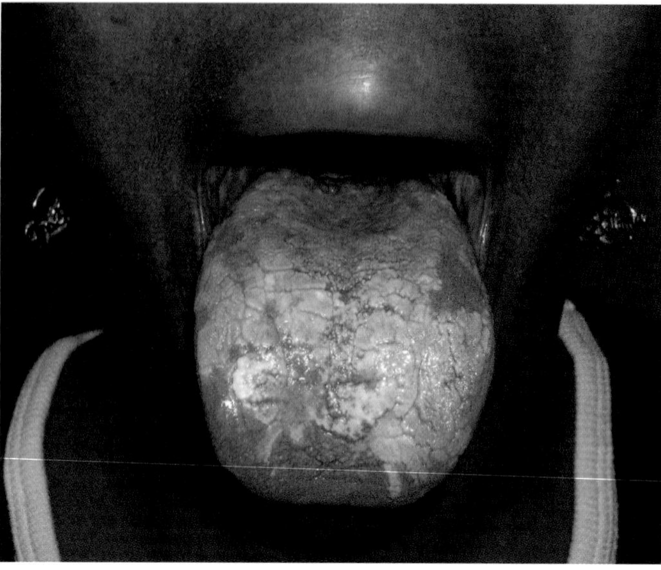

FIGURE 34-4 White plaques on the tongue of a black woman with severe cutaneous plaque psoriasis. A histologic specimen would appear similar to geographic tongue. (*Reproduced with permission from E.J. Mayeaux, Jr., MD.*)

DIFFERENTIAL DIAGNOSIS

- Erythroplakia or leukoplakia—May be suspected when lesions affect the soft palate (see Chapter 38, Leukoplakia).
- Lichen planus—Reticular forms are characterized by interlacing white lines commonly found on the buccal mucosa, or erosive forms, characterized by atrophic erythematous areas with central ulceration and surrounding radiating striae (see Chapter 152, Lichen Planus) (**Figure 34-3**).
- Psoriasis—Intraoral lesions have been described as red or white plaques associated with the activity of cutaneous lesions (see Chapter 150, Psoriasis) (**Figure 34-4**).
- Reactive arthritis—A condition characterized by the triad of "urethritis, arthritis, and conjunctivitis," may have rare intraoral lesions described as painless ulcerative papules on the buccal mucosa and palate (see Chapter 153, Reactive Arthritis).
- Fissured tongue—An inherited condition in which the tongue has fissures that are asymptomatic. Although it has been called a *scrotal tongue* in the past, the term *fissured tongue* is preferred by patients (**Figure 34-5**).

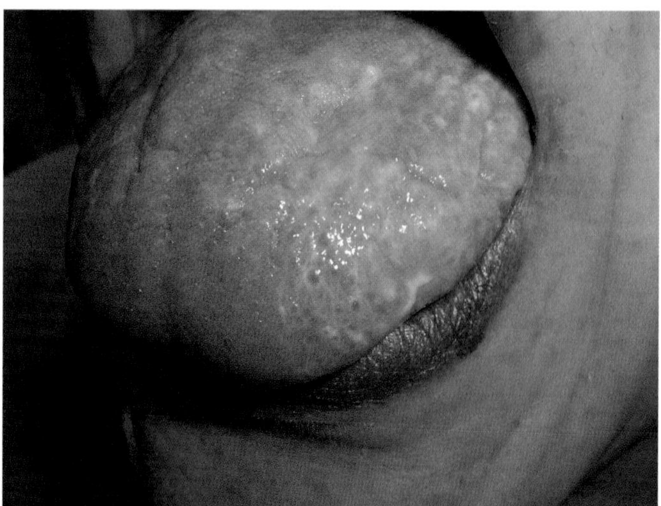

FIGURE 34-3 Lichen planus of the tongue. There are white striae; the surface is smooth in the affected area because of the loss of papillae. (*Reproduced with permission from Richard P. Usatine, MD.*)

MANAGEMENT

Most individuals are asymptomatic and do not require treatment (**Figure 34-6**).

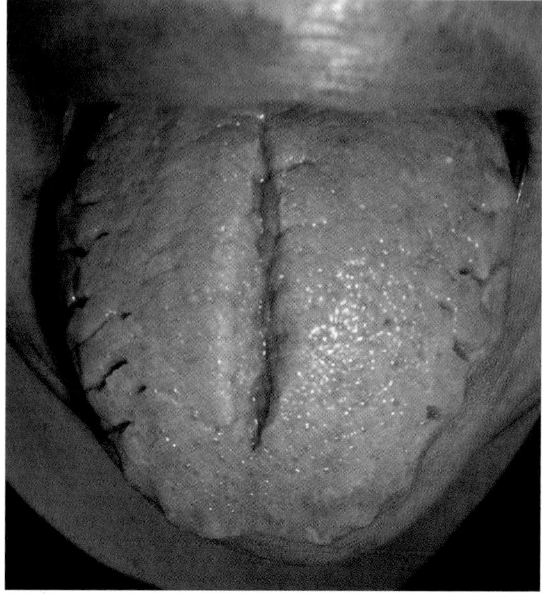

FIGURE 34-5 Fissured tongue present since birth. Although this has also been called a scrotal tongue, the preferred terminology is now fissured tongue, for obvious reasons. (*Reproduced with permission from Richard P. Usatine, MD.*)

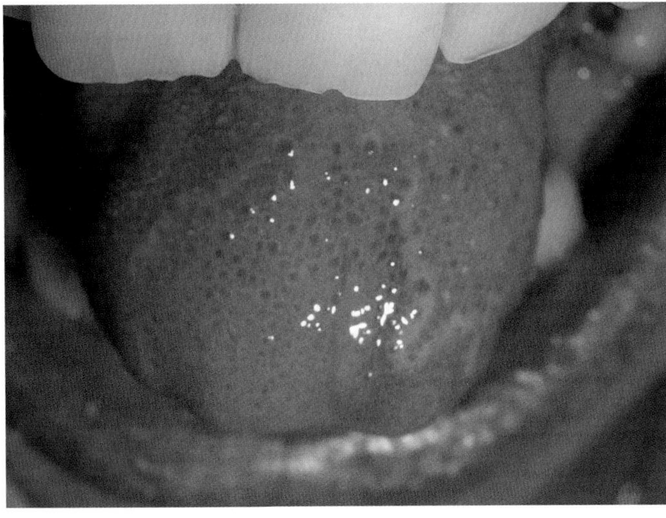

FIGURE 34-6 A mild asymptomatic case of geographic tongue. Note the atrophic filiform papillae and the subtle white halo. (*Reproduced with permission from Richard P. Usatine, MD.*)

- For symptomatic cases, several treatments have been proposed but not proven effective with good clinical trials[6,7]:
  - Topical steroids such as triamcinolone dental paste (Oralone or Kenalog in Orabase) SOR Ⓒ
  - Supplements such as zinc, vitamin B_{12}, niacin, and riboflavin SOR Ⓒ
  - Antihistamine mouth rinses (eg, diphenhydramine elixir 12.5 mg per 5 mL diluted in a 1:4 ratio with water) SOR Ⓒ
  - Topical anesthetic rinses[6,7] SOR Ⓒ

Geographic tongue can rarely present as persistent and painful (**Figure 34-7**). In one case report, 0.1% tacrolimus ointment was applied twice daily for 2 weeks with significant improvement of symptoms.[8] SOR Ⓒ

No treatment has been proven to be uniformly effective.[9]

FOLLOW-UP

Tell the patient to contact you if the symptoms continue from the past 10 days and to go to the emergency department immediately if the following conditions occur:

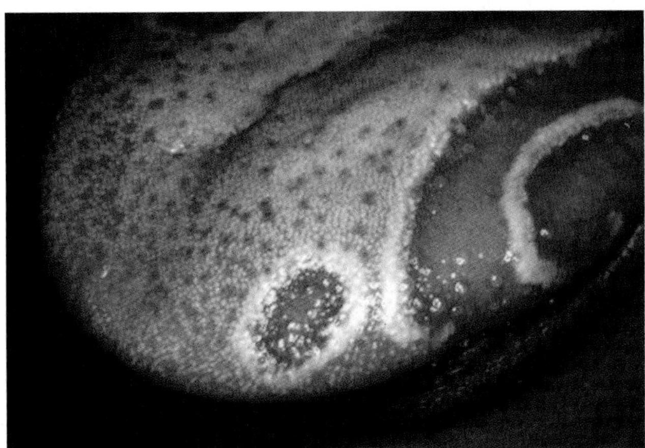

FIGURE 34-7 Geographic tongue with more severe symptomatology, including pain and a burning sensation when eating spicy foods. The contrast between the normal tongue tissue and the pink atrophic papillae is striking. (*Reproduced with permission from Ellen Eisenberg, DMD.*)

- The tongue swells significantly.
- The patient has trouble breathing.
- The patient has trouble talking or chewing/swallowing.

PATIENT EDUCATION

Patients should be reassured of the conditions that are benign in nature. Tell patients with geographic tongue to avoid irritating spicy foods and liquids.

PATIENT RESOURCES

- Medline Plus. *Geographic Tongue*—**http://www.nlm.nih.gov/medlineplus/ency/article/001049.htm.**

PROVIDER RESOURCES

- Medscape. *Geographic Tongue*—**http://emedicine.medscape.com/article/1078465.**
- Mayo Clinic. *Geographic Tongue*—**http://www.mayoclinic.com/health/geographic-tongue/DS00819.**

REFERENCES

1. Redman RS. Prevalence of geographic tongue, fissured tongue, median rhomboid glossitis, and hairy tongue among 3,611 Minnesota schoolchildren. *Oral Surg Oral Med Oral Pathol.* 1970;30:390-395.
2. Shulman JD, Carpenter WM. Prevalence and risk factors associated with geographic tongue among US adults. *Oral Dis.* 2006;12:341-346.
3. Assimakopoulos D, Patrikakos G, Fotika C, Elisaf M. Benign migratory glossitis or geographic tongue: an enigmatic oral lesion. *Am J Med.* 2002;113:751-755.
4. Espelid M, Bang G, Johannessen AC, et al. Geographic stomatitis: report of 6 cases. *J Oral Pathol Med.* 1991;20:425-428.
5. Darwazeh AM, Almelaih AA. Tongue lesions in a Jordanian population. Prevalence, symptoms, subject's knowledge and treatment provided. *Med Oral Patol Oral Cir Bucal.* 2011;16:e745-e749.
6. Abe M, Sogabe Y, Syuto T, et al. Successful treatment with cyclosporin administration for persistent benign migratory glossitis. *J Dermatol.* 2007;34:340-343.
7. Reamy BV, Derby R, Bunt CW. Common tongue conditions in primary care. *Am Fam Physician.* 2010; 81:627-634.
8. Ishibashi M, Tojo G, Watanabe M, et al. Geographic tongue treated with topical tacrolimus. *J Dermatol Case Rep.* 2010;4:57-59.
9. Gonsalves W, Chi A, Neville B. Common oral lesions: part 1. Superficial mucosal lesions. *Am Fam Physician.* 2007;75:501-507.

35 GINGIVITIS AND PERIODONTAL DISEASE

Richard P. Usatine, MD
Wanda C. Gonsalves, MD

PATIENT STORY

A 35-year-old woman presents to clinic for a routine physical examination. She says that for the last 6 months her gums bleed when she brushes her teeth. She reports smoking 1 pack of cigarettes per day. The oral examination finds generalized plaque and red swollen intradental papilla (**Figure 35-1**). The physician explains to her that she has gingivitis and that she should brush twice daily and use floss daily. The physician tells her that smoking is terrible for her health in all ways, including her oral health. The physician offers her help to quit smoking and refers her to a dentist for a cleaning and full dental examination.

INTRODUCTION

Gingivitis is the inflammation of the gingiva (gums). Gingivitis alone does not affect the underlying supporting structures of the teeth and is reversible (see **Figure 35-1**).

Periodontitis (periodontal disease) is a chronic inflammatory disease, which includes gingivitis along with loss of connective tissue and bone support for the teeth. It damages alveolar bone (the bone of the jaw in which the roots of the teeth are connected) and the periodontal ligaments that hold the roots in place. It is a major cause of tooth loss in adults (**Figures 35-2** to **35-4**).

EPIDEMIOLOGY

- Gingivitis and periodontal diseases are the most common oral diseases in adults.

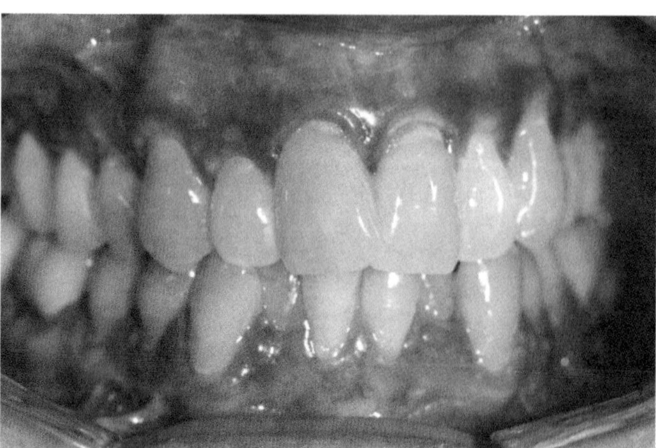

FIGURE 35-1 Chronic gingivitis in which the intradental papillae are edematous and blunted. There is some loss of gingival tissue. The gums bleed with brushing. (*Reproduced with permission from Gerald Ferretti, DMD.*)

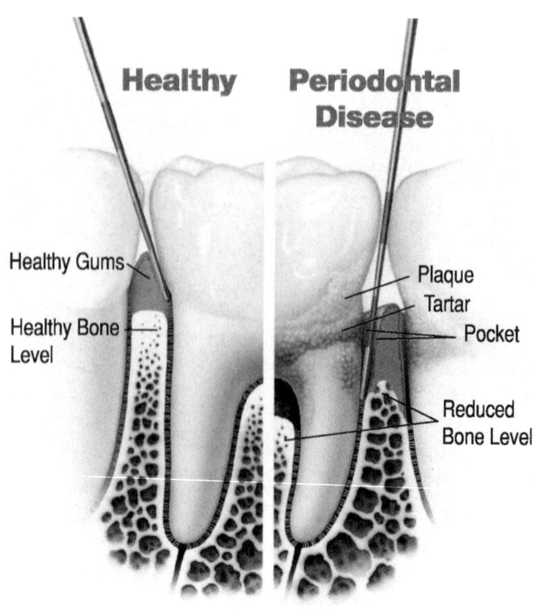

FIGURE 35-2 Healthy periodontal anatomy versus periodontal disease. (*Reproduced with permission from the American Academy of Periodontology; http://www.perio.org/consumer/2a.html. Copyright 2014, American Academy of Periodontology.*)

- It is estimated that 35% of adults of age 30 years or older in the United States have periodontal disease: 22% have a severe form and 13% have a moderate-to-severe form.[1]
- Homeless people are a very high-risk group for gingivitis, periodontitis, and all dental disease (see **Figure 35-4**).
- Periodontal disease has been shown in some studies to be an associated factor in coronary heart disease and chronic kidney disease.[2]
- Periodontal disease in pregnancy is associated with an increase in preterm birth.[3,4]

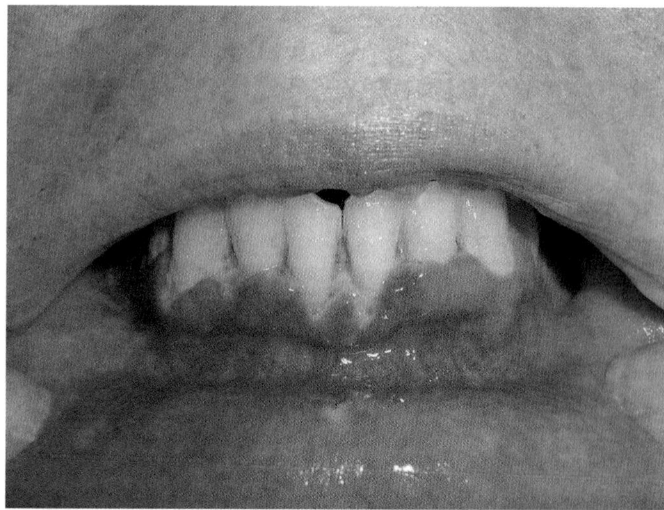

FIGURE 35-3 Severe periodontal disease in a woman who smokes and is addicted to cocaine. Note the blunting of the intradental papillae and the dramatic loss of gingival tissue. (*Reproduced with permission from Richard P. Usatine, MD.*)

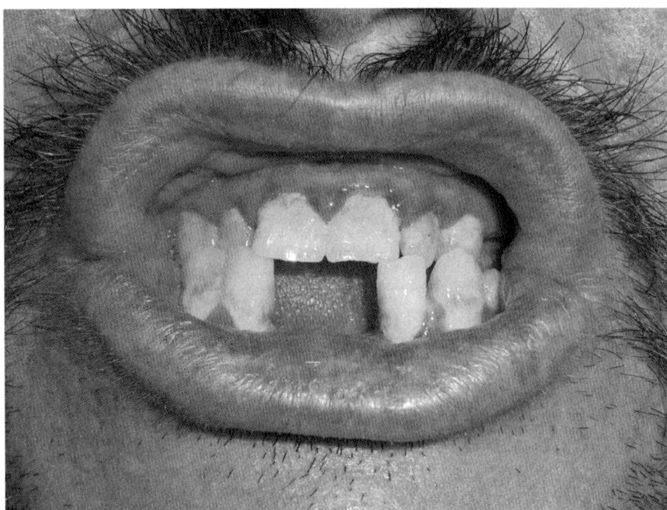

FIGURE 35-4 Severe periodontal disease in an alcoholic smoker with very edematous and blunted intradental papilla. This homeless man has already lost 2 teeth secondary to his severe periodontal disease. (*Reproduced with permission from Richard P. Usatine, MD.*)

ETIOLOGY AND PATHOPHYSIOLOGY

- Periodontal diseases are caused by bacteria in dental plaque that create an inflammatory response in gingival tissues (gingivitis) or in the soft tissue and bone supporting the teeth (periodontitis).
- The normal healthy gingival attachments form the gingival cuff around the tooth to help protect the underlying bone and teeth from the bacteria of the mouth.
- Gingivitis is caused by a reversible inflammatory process that occurs as the result of prolonged exposure of the gingival tissues to plaque and tartar (see **Figure 35-2**).
- Gingivitis may be classified by appearance (eg, ulcerative, hemorrhagic), etiology (eg, drugs, hormones), duration (eg, acute, chronic), or by quality (eg, mild, moderate, or severe).
- A severe form, acute necrotizing ulcerative gingivitis (ANUG) (**Figure 35-5**), also known as Vincent disease or trench mouth, is associated with α-hemolytic streptococci, anaerobic fusiform bacteria, and nontreponemal oral spirochetes. The term *trench mouth* was coined in World War I when ANUG was common among soldiers in the trenches. Predisposing factors now include diabetes, HIV, and chemotherapy.[2]

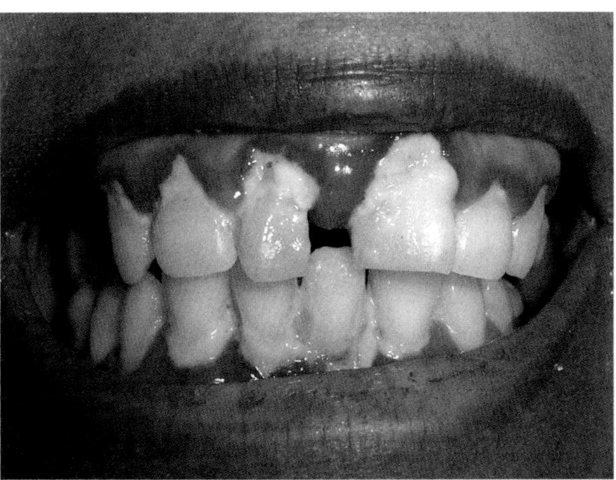

FIGURE 35-5 Acute necrotizing ulcerative gingivitis (ANUG) with intense erythema and ulcerations around the teeth. This is an acute infectious process. Note the destruction of the papillae between the teeth. (*Reproduced with permission from Richard P. Usatine, MD.*)

- The most common form of gingivitis is chronic gingivitis induced by plaque (see **Figure 35-1**). This type of gingivitis occurs in half of the population 4 years of age or older. The inflammation worsens as mineralized plaque forms calculus (tartar) at and below the gum surface (sulcus). The plaque that covers calculus causes destruction of bone (an irreversible condition) and loose teeth, which result in tooth mobility and tooth loss.
- Gingivitis may persist for months or years without progressing to periodontitis. This suggests that host susceptibility plays an important role in the development of periodontal disease.[5]

RISK FACTORS

Risk factors that contribute to the development of periodontal disease include poor oral hygiene, smoking, alcohol dependence, environmental factors (eg, crowded teeth and mouth breathing), and comorbid conditions, such as a weakened immune status (eg, HIV, steroids, or diabetes), low educational attainment, and low income.[6-8]

DIAGNOSIS

CLINICAL FEATURES

- Simple or marginal gingivitis first causes swelling of the intradental papillae and later affect the gingiva and dental interface (see **Figures 35-1** to **35-4**).
- Mild gingivitis is painless and may bleed when brushing or eating hard foods.
- ANUG (see **Figure 35-5**) is painful, ulcerative, and edematous, and produces halitosis and bleeding gingival tissue. Patients with ANUG may have systemic symptoms such as myalgias and fever.

TYPICAL DISTRIBUTION

Gingivitis begins at the gingival and dental margins and may extend onto the alveolar ridges.

LABORATORY STUDIES AND IMAGING

Radiographs of the mouth are used to evaluate for bone loss in periodontal disease.

DIFFERENTIAL DIAGNOSIS

- Gingivitis can be from poor dental hygiene only or secondary to conditions that affect the immune system such as diabetes, Addison disease, HIV, and pregnancy.
- Gingival hyperplasia is an overgrowth of the gingiva with various etiologies, including medications such as calcium channel blockers, phenytoin, and cyclosporine. This can occur with or without coexisting gingivitis (see Chapter 36, Gingival Overgrowth).

MANAGEMENT

- Recommend smoking cessation for all patients who smoke.[7] SOR A Offer help to support the patients' smoking cessation efforts with behavioral counseling and pharmacologic methods (see Chapter 237, Tobacco Addiction). SOR A
- Recommend alcohol cessation for patients with alcoholism and refer to Alcoholics Anonymous (AA) or another resource. For patients in whom alcohol use is heavy but addiction has not been diagnosed, at least recommend a decrease in alcohol use (see Chapter 238, Alcoholism).[8] SOR A
- Dental experts recommend tooth brushing twice a day and flossing daily. SOR C However, a Cochrane systematic review failed to show a benefit for daily flossing on plaque and clinical parameters of gingivitis.[9] SOR A
- Some experts suggest that electric toothbrushes may have additional benefit over manual brushing, but this remains unproven. SOR C In fact, one study of dental students showed that one electric toothbrush was no better than 2 different manual toothbrushes with respect to plaque control.[10] SOR B
- Systematic reviews indicate that there is strong evidence supporting the efficacy of chlorhexidine as an antiplaque, antigingivitis mouthrinse.[11] SOR A Mouthwashes should not be used as a replacement for tooth brushing. Chlorhexidine oropharyngeal 0.12% is available as a generic mouthrinse. Recommended dosing is 15 mL to swish (for 30 seconds) and spit twice daily.
- The treatments with chlorhexidine (gel and spray) achieved a significant reduction in plaque and gingival bleeding in children with special needs. The parents or caregivers preferred the administration of chlorhexidine in spray form.[12] SOR B
- In patients with ANUG, treatment involves antibiotics, nonsteroidal anti-inflammatory drugs (NSAIDs), and topical 2% viscous lidocaine for pain relief. Oral rinses with saline, hydrogen peroxide 3% solution, or chlorhexidine 0.12% may be of benefit. SOR C
- Antibiotics recommended for ANUG include penicillin VK, erythromycin, doxycycline, and clindamycin. SOR C
- Everyone should receive ongoing care from a dental professional for prevention and treatment of periodontal disease.

PREVENTION

- No smoking or tobacco use at all
- Avoid alcohol and drug abuse
- Good oral hygiene with tooth brushing and flossing
- Dental visits at least twice yearly even during pregnancy

PATIENT EDUCATION

- There is no safe level of smoking. Quitting is crucial to good health.
- Drink alcohol in moderation or do not drink at all.
- Practice good oral hygiene to remove plaque (ie, brush twice a day and use floss daily).
- Consider use of chlorhexidine-containing mouthrinse.
- Consult a dentist for regular checkups, especially when the condition does not improve after using good oral hygiene.
- Pregnancy is not a contraindication for dental visits and cleaning.

FOLLOW-UP

Follow up patients with ANUG closely. All patients need regular dental care and follow-up with their dentist.

PATIENT RESOURCES

- PubMed Health. *Gingivitis*—**http://www.ncbi.nlm.nih.gov/pubmedhealth/PMH0002051/.**
- The American Academy of Periodontology. *Types of Gum Disease*—**http://www.perio.org/consumer/2a.html.**

PROVIDER RESOURCES

- Stephen JM. *Gingivitis*—**http://emedicine.medscape.com/article/763801.**

REFERENCES

1. Albandar JM, Brunelle JA, Kingman A. Destructive periodontal disease in adults 30 years of age and older in the United States, 1988-1994. *J Periodontol.* 1999;70:13-29.
2. Fisher MA, Borgnakke WS, Taylor GW. Periodontal disease as a risk marker in coronary heart disease and chronic kidney disease. *Curr Opin Nephrol Hypertens.* 2010;19:519-526.
3. Corbella S, Taschieri S, Francetti L, et al. Periodontal disease as a risk factor for adverse pregnancy outcomes: a systematic review and meta-analysis of case-control studies. *Odontology.* 2012;100(2):232-240.
4. Chambrone L, Pannuti CM, Guglielmetti MR, Chambrone LA. Evidence grade associating periodontitis with preterm birth and/or low birth weight: II: a systematic review of randomized trials evaluating the effects of periodontal treatment. *J Clin Periodontol.* 2011;38:902-914.
5. Kornman KS, Crane A, Wang HY, et al. The interleukin-1 genotype as a severity factor in adult periodontal disease. *J Clin Periodontol.* 1997;24:72-77.
6. Boillot A, El Halabi B, Batty GD, et al. Education as a predictor of chronic periodontitis: a systematic review with meta-analysis population-based studies. *PLoS One.* 2011;6(7):e21508.
7. Hanioka T, Ojima M, Tanaka K, et al. Causal assessment of smoking and tooth loss: a systematic review of observational studies. *BMC Public Health.* 2011;11:221.
8. Amaral CS, Vettore MV, Leao A. The relationship of alcohol dependence and alcohol consumption with periodontitis: a systematic review. *J Dent.* 2009;37:643-651.
9. Berchier CE, Slot DE, Haps S, Van der Weijden GA. The efficacy of dental floss in addition to a toothbrush on plaque and parameters of gingival inflammation: a systematic review. *Int J Dent Hyg.* 2008;6:265-279.

10. Parizi MT, Mohammadi TM, Afshar SK, et al. Efficacy of an electric toothbrush on plaque control compared to two manual toothbrushes. *Int Dent J.* 2011;61:131-135.
11. Gunsolley JC. Clinical efficacy of antimicrobial mouthrinses. *J Dent.* 2010;38(suppl 1):S6-S10.
12. Chibinski AC, Pochapski MT, Farago PV, et al. Clinical evaluation of chlorhexidine for the control of dental biofilm in children with special needs. *Community Dent Health.* 2011;28:222-226.

36 GINGIVAL OVERGROWTH

Richard P. Usatine, MD
Wanda C. Gonsalves, MD

PATIENT STORY

A 31-year-old woman with a history of seizure disorder notices increasing gum enlargement (**Figure 36-1**). She is unemployed and does not have dental insurance. She has not been to a dentist in at least 10 years. She brushes her teeth only once a day and does not floss at all. She has been on phenytoin (Dilantin) since early childhood, and this does prevent her seizures. You talk to her about dental hygiene and refer her to a low-cost dental clinic that cares for people with limited resources.

INTRODUCTION

Gingival overgrowth (GO) (hyperplasia) can be hereditary or induced as a side effect of systemic drugs, such as phenytoin, cyclosporine, or calcium channel blockers. Besides the cosmetic effect it can make good oral hygiene more difficult to maintain.

SYNONYMS

It is also known as gingival hyperplasia, drug-induced gingival overgrowth (DIGO), hereditary gingival fibromatosis.

EPIDEMIOLOGY

- The prevalence of phenytoin-induced gingival hyperplasia is estimated at 15% to 50% in patients taking the medication[1,2] (**Figures 36-1** and **36-2**).

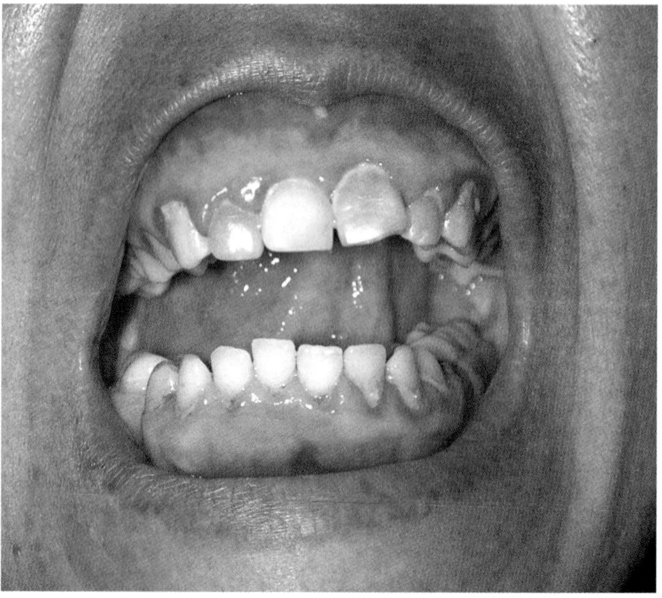

FIGURE 36-1 Gingival overgrowth secondary to phenytoin (Dilantin) in a woman with epilepsy. *(Reproduced with permission from Richard P. Usatine, MD.)*

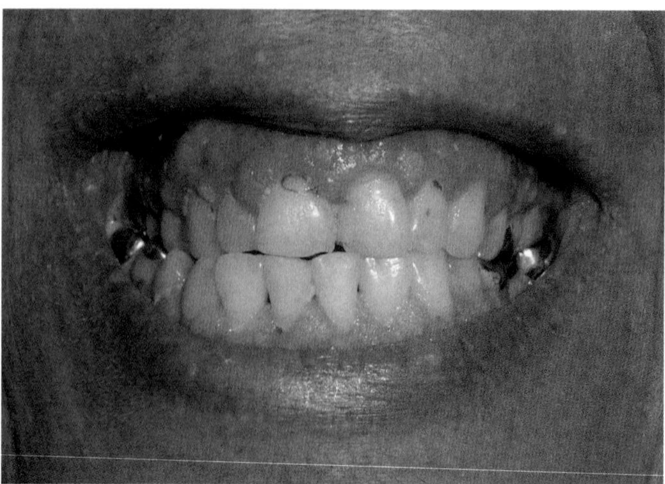

FIGURE 36-2 Multiple tiny hamartomas on the gums from Cowden disease with gingival overgrowth secondary to phenytoin. *(Reproduced with permission from Richard P. Usatine, MD.)*

- In patients receiving cyclosporine for more than 3 months, the incidence of GO can approach 70%[3] (**Figure 36-3**).
- The incidence of gingival hyperplasia has been reported as 10% to 20% in patients treated with calcium channel blockers in the general population.[2]

ETIOLOGY AND PATHOPHYSIOLOGY

- Although the etiology of GO is not entirely known, risk factors known to contribute to GO include the following: nonspecific chronic inflammation associated with poor hygiene, hormonal changes (pregnancy), medications (calcium channel blockers, phenytoin, and cyclosporine), and systemic diseases (leukemia, sarcoidosis, and Crohn disease).
    - Studies suggest that phenytoin, cyclosporine, and nifedipine interact with epithelial keratinocytes, fibroblasts, and collagen to lead to an overgrowth of gingival tissue in susceptible individuals.[2]

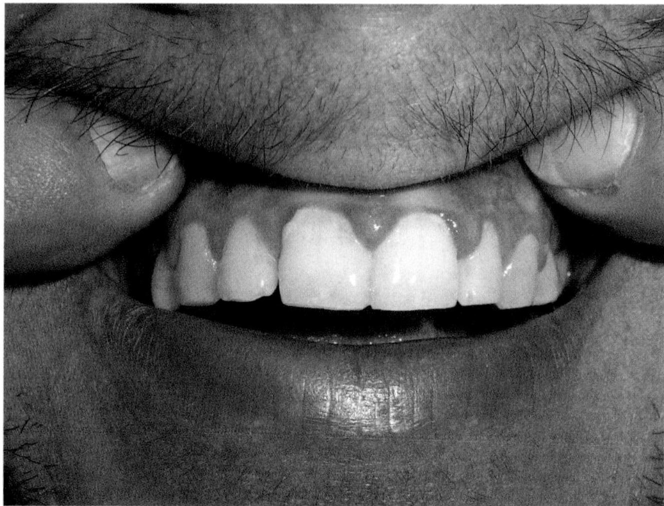

FIGURE 36-3 Gingival overgrowth secondary to cyclosporine use for 1 year to treat severe plaque psoriasis. Note the blunted and thickened interdental papillae. *(Reproduced with permission from Richard P. Usatine, MD.)*

- More than 15 drugs have been shown to cause GO.
- The most common nonreversible DIGO is caused by phenytoin (see **Figures 36-1** and **36-2**).

- Histopathologically, tissue enlargement is the result of proliferation of fibroblasts, collagen, and chronic inflammatory cells.

RISK FACTORS

- Prolonged use of phenytoin, cyclosporine, or calcium channel blockers (especially nifedipine)
- Pregnancy
- Systemic diseases (leukemia, sarcoidosis, and Crohn disease)
- Poor oral hygiene and the presence of periodontal disease

DIAGNOSIS

SIGNS AND SYMPTOMS

- The diagnosis is made by visual inspection and by obtaining a thorough history (see **Figures 36-1** to **36-3**).
- The gingiva appears edematous and bulky with loss of its stippling. It may be soft or firm.
- Nonspecific chronic inflammation, hormonal and systemic causes such as leukemia appear red and inflamed and may bleed.

TYPICAL DISTRIBUTION

Lobular gingiva enlargement occurs first at the interdental papillae and anterior facial gingiva approximately 2 to 3 months after starting the drug, and increases in maximum severity in 12 to 18 months (see **Figure 36-3**).

LABORATORY TESTS

Consider checking a complete blood count (CBC) with differential count to investigate for leukemia if there is not an obvious etiology.

IMAGING

The periodontist or oral medicine specialist may order bitewing radiographs and periapical films to evaluate for the presence of periodontal disease.

DIFFERENTIAL DIAGNOSIS

- Generalized gingivitis—Gums around the teeth become inflamed. This condition often occurs with poor oral hygiene (see Chapter 35, Gingivitis and Periodontal Disease).
- Pregnancy gingivitis—Inflamed gums. More than half of pregnant women will develop gingivitis during pregnancy because of hormonal changes.
- Pyogenic granuloma—A small red bump that may bleed and grow to approximately half an inch. These are most often found on the skin but can occur in the mouth secondary to trauma or pregnancy. When they occur in pregnancy, they are sometimes called pregnancy tumor. In reality, these are neither pyogenic nor granulomatous but are a type of lobular capillary hemangioma (see Chapter 159, Pyogenic Granuloma) (**Figure 36-4**).

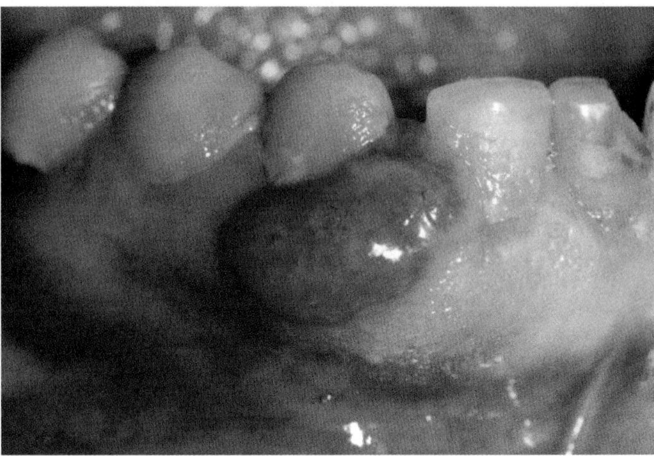

FIGURE 36-4 Pyogenic granuloma growing rapidly on the gums after minor trauma. (*Reproduced with permission from Gonsalves WC, Chi AC, Neville BW. Common oral lesions: part II. Masses and neoplasia.* Am Fam Physician. *2007;75(4):509-512. Copyright © 2007 American Academy of Family Physicians. All Rights Reserved.*)

- Leukemia—Leukemic cells may infiltrate the oral soft tissues producing a diffuse, boggy, nontender swelling of the gingiva that may ulcerate or bleed.

MANAGEMENT

NONPHARMACOLOGIC

- Teach and emphasize good oral hygiene including cleanings at least every 3 months to control plaque. SOR Ⓒ
- The use of a powered toothbrush, together with oral hygiene instruction, reduces GO for pediatric transplantation patients on cyclosporine. In one study, the sonic toothbrushing and oral hygiene instruction group had less severe GO after 12 months than did the control group.[4] SOR Ⓑ
- If possible, stop drugs that induce gingival hyperplasia as discontinuing the medications may reverse the condition in most cases (except phenytoin).
- If drugs cannot be stopped, try reducing the dose, if possible, as gingival hyperplasia can be dose dependent.

MEDICATIONS

- Tacrolimus is an alternative to cyclosporine to prevent transplant rejection; it causes less GO. In one study on the prevalence of gingival growth after renal transplantation, GO occurred in 29% of patients treated with tacrolimus and in 60% of patients treated with cyclosporine.[5] SOR Ⓑ In another study, switching patients from cyclosporine to tacrolimus reduced GO in the first month after the change was made.[6] SOR Ⓑ
- Case reports have reported regression of overgrowth with both oral metronidazole and azithromycin. In one randomized controlled trial (RCT), patients with GO were randomized to receive either 1 course of 5 days of azithromycin or 7 days of metronidazole. The extent of GO was measured at 0, 2, 4, 6, 12, and 24 weeks, and azithromycin was found to be more effective than metronidazole.[3] SOR Ⓑ

- Azithromycin with an oral hygiene program resulted in a reduction in cyclosporine-induced GO, whereas oral hygiene alone improved oral symptoms (pain, halitosis, and gum bleeding) but did not decrease cyclosporine-induced GO.[7] Patients were randomized into 2 groups, both receiving oral hygiene instructions, with the treatment group receiving 3 days of azithromycin 500 mg daily. They were evaluated after 15 and 30 days and only the azithromycin group had a reduction in GO.[7] SOR B
- Chlorhexidine 12% (Peridex) once before going to bed or Biotene mouthwash after meals is recommended for patients who are known to be at risk for gingivitis.[2] SOR C Warn patients that chlorhexidine 12% will taste bad and can stain the teeth. This staining can be removed with dental cleaning. This information should help improve adherence to the use of this mouthwash.

REFERRAL

For patients who do not respond to the above measures, refer to a dental health professional for possible gingivectomy. This can be done with a scalpel or a laser.

PREVENTION

Ensure healthy periodontal tissue prior to starting calcium channel blockers or phenytoin, or before any organ transplantation in which cyclosporine will be prescribed.

Folic acid supplementation, 0.5 mg per day, is associated with prevention of GO in children taking phenytoin monotherapy. Of patients in the folic acid arm, 21% developed GO, as compared with 88% receiving placebo.[1] SOR B

PATIENT EDUCATION

Advise patients to practice good oral hygiene (ie, brush at least twice a day and floss at least once a day) and have regular follow-up with their dental health professional to monitor for worsening periodontal disease.

FOLLOW-UP

Patients should be monitored by a periodontist or an oral medicine specialist as long as the patients are taking medicines that induce gingival hyperplasia.

PATIENT RESOURCES

- The Merck Manual of Health and Aging. *Periodontal Disease*—**http://www.merck.com/pubs/mmanual_ha/sec3/ch36/ch36c.html.**

PROVIDER RESOURCES

- Mejia L. *Drug-induced Gingival Hyperplasia*—**http://emedicine.medscape.com/article/1076264.**

REFERENCES

1. Arya R, Gulati S, Kabra M, et al. Folic acid supplementation prevents phenytoin-induced gingival overgrowth in children. *Neurology*. 2011;76:1338-1343.
2. Mejia L. *Drug-Induced Gingival Hyperplasia*. http://emedicine.medscape.com/article/1076264. Accessed January 23, 2012.
3. Chand DH, Quattrocchi J, Poe SA, et al. Trial of metronidazole vs. azithromycin for treatment of cyclosporine-induced gingival overgrowth. *Pediatr Transplant*. 2004;8:60-64.
4. Smith JM, Wong CS, Salamonik EB, et al. Sonic tooth brushing reduces gingival overgrowth in renal transplant recipients. *Pediatr Nephrol*. 2006;21:1753-1759.
5. Cota LO, Aquino DR, Franco GC, et al. Gingival overgrowth in subjects under immunosuppressive regimens based on cyclosporine, tacrolimus, or sirolimus. *J Clin Periodontol*. 2010;37:894-902.
6. Parraga-Linares L, Almendros-Marques N, Berini-Aytes L, Gay-Escoda C. Effectiveness of substituting cyclosporin A with tacrolimus in reducing gingival overgrowth in renal transplant patients. *Med Oral Patol Oral Cir Bucal*. 2009;14:e429-e433.
7. Ramalho VL, Ramalho HJ, Cipullo JP, et al. Comparison of azithromycin and oral hygiene program in the treatment of cyclosporine-induced gingival hyperplasia. *Ren Fail*. 2007;29:265-270.

37 APHTHOUS ULCER

Richard P. Usatine, MD

PATIENT STORY

A 58-year-old man presents with a 1-year history of painful sores in his mouth. (**Figures 37-1** to **37-3**). He has lost 20 lb over the past year because it hurts to eat. The ulcers come and go, but are found on his tongue, gums, buccal mucosa, and inner lips. Prior to the onset of these lesions the patient had been in good health and was not on any medications. The physician recognized his condition as recurrent aphthous ulcers with giant ulcers. No underlying systemic diseases were found on workup. The patient was started on oral prednisone and given dexamethasone oral elixir to swish and swallow. Within 1 week the patient was able to eat and drink liquids comfortably and began regaining his lost weight. Long-term management of his problem required the use of other medications so as to successfully taper him off prednisone without recurrences.

INTRODUCTION

Aphthous ulcers are painful ulcerations in the mouth which can be single, multiple, occasional, or recurrent. These ulcers can be small or large but are uniformly painful and may interfere with eating, speaking, and swallowing. Oral trauma, stress, and systemic diseases can contribute to the occurrence of these ulcers but no precise etiology is apparent. Recurrent aphthous stomatitis (RAS) is a frustrating condition that merits aggressive treatment aimed at pain relief and prevention.

SYNONYMS

Aphthous ulcers are also known as canker sores, aphthous stomatitis, aphthae, recurrent aphthous ulcer (RAU), RAS.

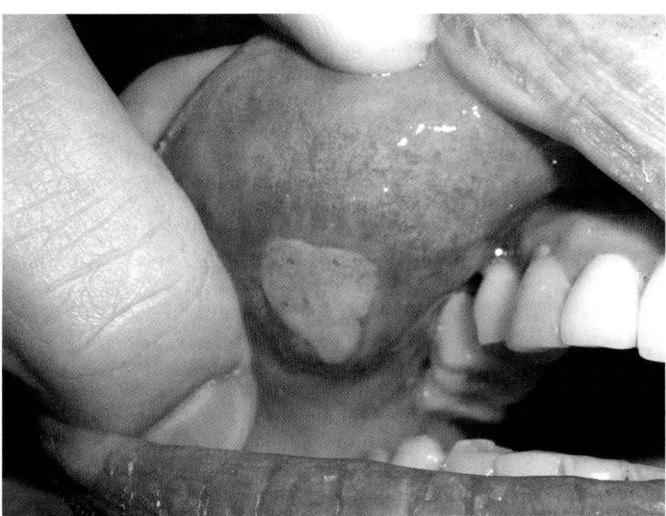

FIGURE 37-1 Major aphthous ulcer on the buccal mucosa of a 58-year-old man who has been suffering with recurrent aphthous stomatitis for the past year. (*Reproduced with permission from Richard P. Usatine, MD.*)

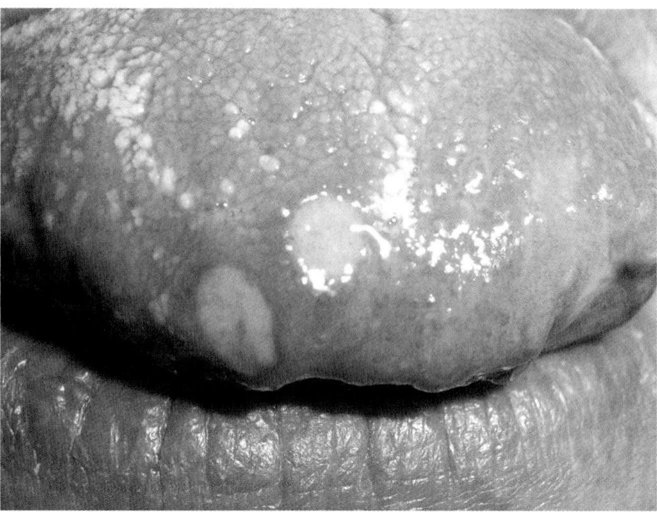

FIGURE 37-2 Two aphthous ulcers on the tongue of a 58-year-old man with recurrent aphthous stomatitis. (*Reproduced with permission from Richard P. Usatine, MD.*)

EPIDEMIOLOGY

- Twenty percent of general population are estimated to have aphthous ulcers.[1]
- Incidence rates of RAUs of 0.85% among adults and 1.5% among adolescents have been reported.[1]
- RAS is more common in women, in people younger than age 40 years, in whites, in nonsmokers, and in people of high socioeconomic status.[1]

ETIOLOGY AND PATHOPHYSIOLOGY

- The precise etiology and pathogenesis of this condition remains unknown, although a variety of host and environmental factors have been implicated.

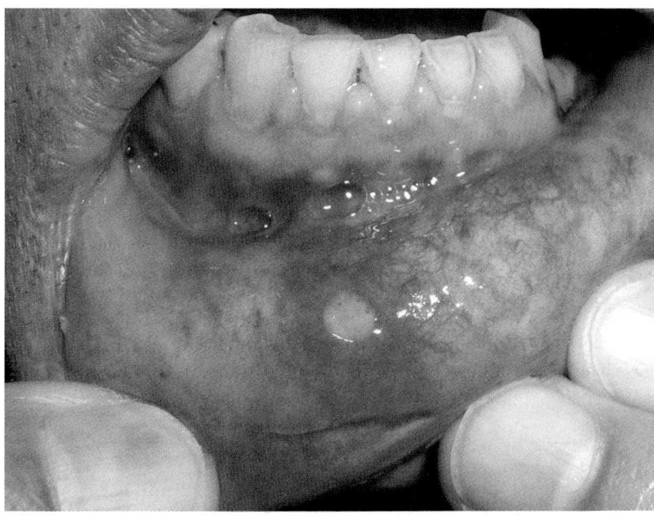

FIGURE 37-3 Minor aphthous ulcer occurring simultaneously with major aphthous ulcers on the buccal mucosa and tongue of a 58-year-old man with recurrent aphthous ulcers. (*Reproduced with permission from Richard P. Usatine, MD.*)

- A positive family history is seen in about one-third of RAS patients. A genetic predisposition is suggested by an increased frequency of human leukocyte antigen (HLA) types A2, A11, B12, and DR2.[1]
- In one study, Th1 (T-helper subtype 1) activation was more intense in the patients with RAUs. Many conditions that increase the incidence of RAUs, such as psychological stress, nonsteroidal anti-inflammatory drugs (NSAIDs), Crohn disease, and celiac disease, also shift the immune response toward the Th1 subtype. Conditions and medications that inhibit the Th1 immune response pathway, such as pregnancy, thalidomide, glucocorticoids, and tetracycline, decrease the incidence of RAUs.[2]
- Another study found significantly higher-than-normal serum level of tumor necrosis factor (TNF)-α in 20% to 39% of patients in the ulcerative stage of RAUs.[3] Medications that have anti–TNF-α effects, such as pentoxifylline, levamisole, and thalidomide, have also been found to be useful in the treatment of RAUs.[1-4]
- Although studies show that there are active immune mechanisms associated with RAUs, there is still much to learn regarding their etiology and pathogenesis.

RISK FACTORS

- Oral trauma
- Stress and anxiety
- Systemic diseases (celiac disease, Crohn disease, Behçet syndrome, HIV, reactive arthritis)
- Medications (NSAIDs, β-blockers, angiotensin-converting enzyme inhibitors [ACEIs])
- Vitamin deficiencies (zinc, iron, B_{12}, folate)
- Food and chemical sensitivities

DIAGNOSIS

CLINICAL FEATURES

History

- Symptoms may begin with a burning sensation and the pain is exacerbated by moving the area affected by the ulcer.
- Eating often hurts, especially foods and drinks with a high acid content.
- Ask about recurrences and onset in relation to the use of medications.
- Ask about gastrointestinal (GI) symptoms, genital ulcers, HIV risk factors, and joint pain.

Physical

- Three clinical variations are described based on the size of the ulcers:
  1. Minor (4-9 mm) (see **Figure 37-3**)—most common
  2. Major (>10 mm) (see **Figure 37-1**)
  3. Herpetiform (<3 mm)—least common
- The most common minor form appears as rounded, well-demarcated, single or multiple ulcers less than 1 cm in diameter that usually heal in 10 to 14 days without scarring (**Figure 37-4**).
- Herpetiform aphthae usually do not present until the second or third decade of life.
- The ulcers are solitary or multiple covered by a gray or tan pseudomembrane and surrounded by an erythematous halo (see **Figure 37-4**).

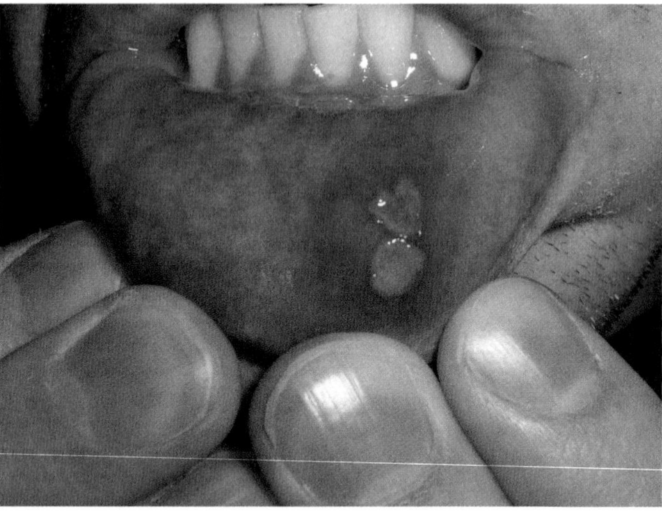

FIGURE 37-4 Two aphthous ulcers on the inside of the lower lip in a 27-year-old man with a history of recurrent aphthous ulcers. Note the gray necrotic centers and surrounding erythema on the labial mucosa. The aphthous ulcers tend to recur during times of stress. (*Reproduced with permission from Richard P. Usatine, MD.*)

TYPICAL DISTRIBUTION

Aphthous ulcers usually involve nonkeratinizing mucosa (eg, labial mucosa, buccal mucosa, ventral tongue). Aphthous ulcers spare the attached gingiva and the hard palate (nonmovable mucosa).

CLASSIFICATION

- Simple aphthosis—Aphthae are few at a time, not associated with systemic diseases, and occurs only 2 to 4 times per year.
- Complex aphthosis—Aphthae are associated with systemic diseases, or there are many lesions at one time, or include genital aphthous ulcers, or there is a continuous disease activity with new ulcers developing as older lesions heal or the ulcers recur more often than 4 times per year. Behçet disease is one example of a complex aphthosis.

LABORATORY TESTS

The diagnosis of a single episode of aphthous ulcers is usually based on history and physical examination. If there is RAS, consider complete blood count (CBC), ferritin, B_{12}, folate, erythrocyte sedimentation rate (ESR), viral culture, biopsy, and/or HIV testing, if indicated. If there is evidence of malabsorption consider testing for celiac disease.

DIFFERENTIAL DIAGNOSIS

- Primary oral herpes simplex virus (primary gingivostomatitis)—Begins as vesicular lesions, which quickly ulcerate on all mucosal lesions in the mouth. It is accompanied by systemic manifestations such as fever, malaise, anorexia, and sore throat. The ulcers are located on movable and nonmovable oral mucosa (includes attached gingiva and hard palate). Lesions may also appear on keratinized surfaces such as the lip (see Chapter 128, Herpes Simplex).
- Herpangina causes multiple ulcers in the mouth, especially on the soft palate and the anterior fauces (**Figure 37-5**). It is caused by Coxsackievirus A16 in most cases. The distribution of the ulcers is different than in aphthous ulcers.

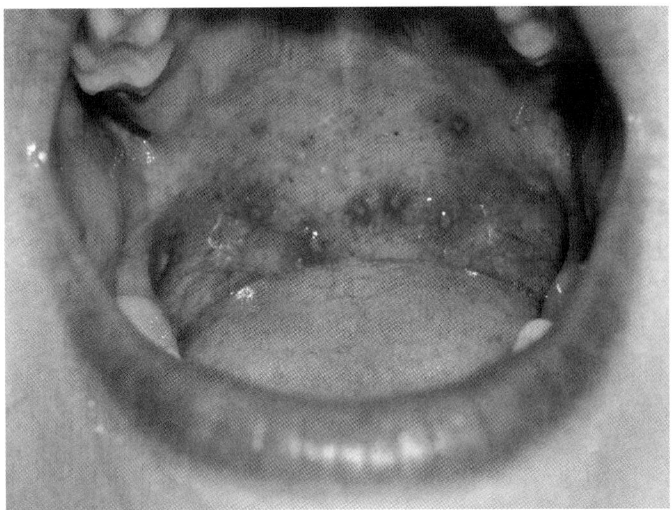

FIGURE 37-5 Herpangina with multiple ulcers on the soft palate. This is caused by Coxsackievirus A16 and the location and appearance of the ulcers differ from aphthous ulcers. (*Reproduced with permission from Emily Scott, MD.*)

- Candidiasis—White plaque, when removed, appears red (**Figure 37-6**). Scrape the white plaque with a tongue depressor and add potassium hydroxide (KOH) to the slide and the preparation will be positive for pseudohyphae and/or budding yeast (see Chapter 135, Candidiasis).
- Oral cancer—Ulcerative lesion that will not resolve by 2 weeks (see Chapter 39, Oropharyngeal Cancer).
- Erythema multiforme (EM)—Mucocutaneous lesion proceeded by infection of herpes simplex virus (HSV), *Mycoplasma pneumoniae*, or exposure to certain drugs or medications. Oral lesions begin as patches and evolve into large shallow erosions and ulcerations with irregular borders. Common sites include the lip, tongue, buccal mucosa, floor of the mouth, and soft palate. The presence of targetoid skin lesions should help differentiate EM from RAS (see Chapter 176, Erythema Multiforme).
- Erosive lichen planus—Erythematous ulcerative lesion with surrounding striae (see Chapter 152, Lichen Planus).

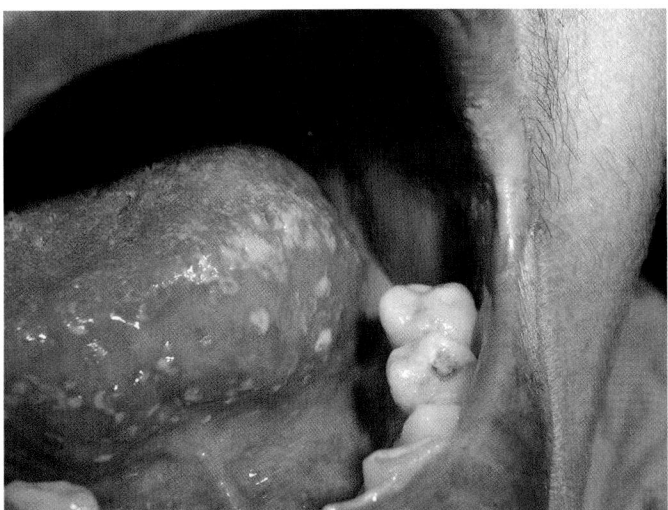

FIGURE 37-6 Oral candidiasis (thrush) in an immunosuppressed woman. Small white plaques under the tongue have a slight rim of erythema but appear different than aphthous ulcers in the same location. A KOH preparation will show evidence of Candida. (*Reproduced with permission from Richard P. Usatine, MD.*)

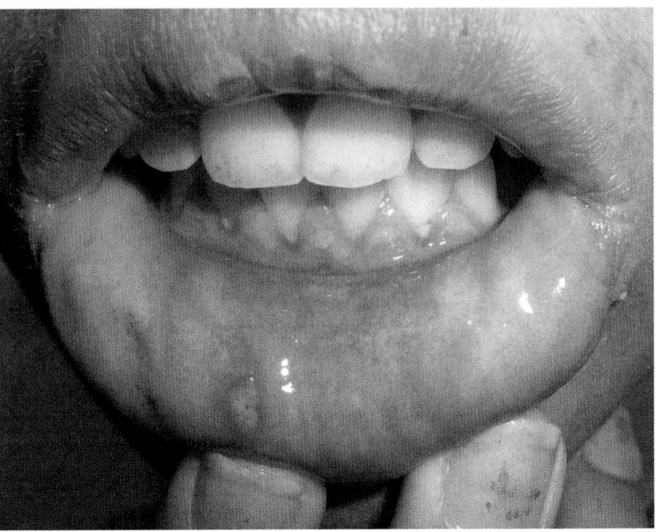

FIGURE 37-7 Behçet disease characterized by recurrent oral aphthous ulcers and recurrent painful genital ulcers in a young woman. The ulcers appear no different from aphthous ulcers in people without Behçet disease. (*Reproduced with permission from Richard P. Usatine, MD.*)

- Behçet disease was originally characterized by 3 conditions: (1) recurrent oral aphthous ulcers (**Figure 37-7**), (2) genital ulcers, and (3) uveitis. The aphthous ulcers appear no different from those found in people without Behçet disease. The recurrent genital ulcers are painful and heal with scarring (**Figure 37-8**). Diagnosis is now based on agreed clinical criteria that require recurrent oral ulcers and 2 of the following: recurrent genital ulcers, ocular inflammation, defined skin lesions, and pathergy.[5] If Behçet disease is suspected, refer the patient to an ophthalmologist to look for signs of uveitis or retinal vasculitis. Behçet disease is a multisystem vasculitis and referral to a rheumatologist may also be helpful.
- Hand, foot, and mouth disease presents as mucocutaneous lesions involving the hand, foot, and mouth caused by enterovirus. While it is much more common in children, adults sometimes get it from their children. Any area of oral mucosa may be involved. Lesions resolve within 1 week (see Chapter 128, Hand, Foot, and Mouth Disease).

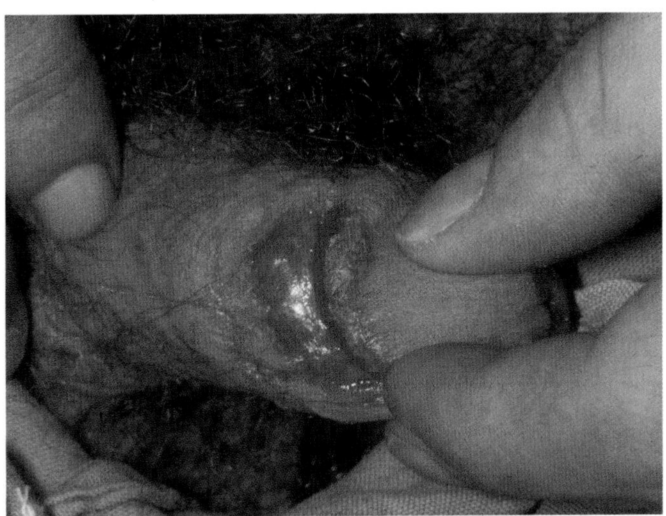

FIGURE 37-8 Painful ulcer on the penis of a patient with Behçet disease. This ulcer healed with scarring. (*Reproduced with permission from Richard P. Usatine, MD.*)

TABLE 37-1 Evidence-Based Summary of Treatments

Treatment	Route/Comparison	Total Patients Studied	Outcomes	Benefit
Amlexanox 5% paste[6]	Topical qid/placebo	1335	Pain-free by day 3	NNT = 5 (42% vs 22%; p <0.05)
			Ulcer resolution at prodromal stage	NNT = 1.6 (97% vs 35%; p <0.01)
			Ulcer healed by day 3	NNT = 7 (47% vs 21%; p <0.05)
Corticosteroids (various)[7]	Topical qid	116	Pain reduction	3 of 4 clinical trials show benefit
Silver nitrate[9]	One time topical application/placebo	97	Pain reduction by day 1	NNT = 1.7 (70% vs 10%; p <0.001)
Debacterol[10]	One time topical application/placebo	60	Complete ulcer resolution by day 6	NNT = 1.4 (100% vs 30%; p <0.01)
Chlorhexidine[14]	Mouthwash qid	77	Reduction in total days with ulcers	2 of 3 trials show benefit
Vitamin B_{12}[15]	Oral daily for prophylaxis	58	No new ulcers by 6 mo	NNT = 2.3 (74% vs 32%; p <0.01)

NNT, number needed to treat.
Data from Bailey J, McCarthy C, Smith RF. Clinical inquiry. What is the most effective way to treat recurrent canker sores? *J Fam Pract.* 2011;60:621-632. With permission.

MANAGEMENT

Identify and treat any vitamin deficiency, systemic disease, or recurrent oral trauma. Stress management is reasonable for all persons. See **Table 37-1** for an evidence-based summary of treatments.

NONPHARMACOLOGIC

Most isolated aphthae require no treatment or only periodic topical therapy.

MEDICATIONS

Topical

- Amlexanox 5% paste (Aphthasol) reduces ulcer size, pain duration, and healing time.[6] It is nonprescription medicine and the paste is applied directly to ulcers 4 times a day until ulcers heal.[6] SOR B
- Topical corticosteroids, such as clobetasol gel or fluocinonide gel, can promote healing and lessen the severity of RAS.[7] Patients should be instructed to dab the area of ulcer dry, apply the gel, paste, or cream after rinsing, and avoid eating or drinking for at least 30 minutes. SOR B
- Lidocaine 1% cream applied to aphthous ulcers was found to reduce pain intensity compared to the placebo cream.[8] SOR B
    - Silver nitrate cautery can lessen the pain of an aphthous ulcer with a single application. The application is painful and probably would only be acceptable to a teen wanting immediate relief from the pain. This must be performed by the physician in the office. The time for healing does not change.[9]
    - Debacterol is another topical agent that reduces pain in 1 day and requires a prescription. It is also painful on application, so its use is limited.[10]

Systemic

In severe RAS cases, systemic therapy with oral steroids, montelukast, colchicine may need to be considered:

- Both prednisone and montelukast were effective in reducing the number of aphthous ulcers and improving pain relief and ulcer healing when compared with placebo in a randomized controlled trial (RCT).[11] Prednisone was more effective than montelukast in pain cessation (p <0.0001) and in accelerating ulcer healing (p <0.0001). Montelukast may be useful in cases of RAS where pharmacologic therapy for long periods is needed and prednisone is to be avoided.[11] In this study, prednisone was given 25 mg daily for 15 days, 12.5 mg daily for 15 days, 6.25 mg daily for 15 days, and then 6.25 mg on alternate days for 15 days. Montelukast 10 mg daily was given every evening and then on alternate days for the second month.[11] SOR B
- In one RCT, 5 mg per day prednisolone was compared with 0.5 mg per day colchicine in the treatment of RAS. Both colchicine and prednisolone treatments significantly reduced RAS. No significant differences in size and number of lesions, recurrence and severity of pain, and duration of pain-free period were seen between the 2 treatment groups. Colchicine (52.9%) had significantly more side effects than prednisolone (11.8%), so the prednisolone seems to be a better alternative in reducing the signs and symptoms of RAS.[12] SOR B

COMPLEMENTARY AND ALTERNATIVE THERAPY

Vitamin C was shown to reduce the frequency of minor RAS and the severity of pain by 50% in a small group of teens. They were given 2000 mg/m^2 per day of ascorbate.[13]

PREVENTION

- Chlorhexidine mouth rinse was shown to reduce the total days with recurrent aphthous ulcers in 2 of 3 studies.[14] SOR B
- Oral vitamin B_{12} was studied in a RCT of adults. A sublingual dose of 1000 μg of vitamin B_{12} was used by patients in the intervention group for 6 months. During the last month of treatment more participants in the intervention group reached a status of "no aphthous ulcers" (74.1%

vs 32.0%; p <0.01). The treatment worked regardless of the serum vitamin B_{12} level.[15] SOR B This could be used as a treatment in older and/or adult-size teens.

PATIENT EDUCATION

Foods that are spicy or acidic worsen pain and should be avoided during outbreaks. Recommend the use of a soft bristled toothbrush as trauma from a firm toothbrush could precipitate an aphthous ulcer.

PATIENT RESOURCES

- MedicineNet.com. *Canker Sores (Aphthous Ulcers)*—**http://www.medicinenet.com/canker_sores/article.htm.**

PROVIDER RESOURCES

- Dermnet NZ. *Aphthous Ulcers*—**http://www.dermnetnz.org/site-age-specific/aphthae.html.**
- eMedicine. *Aphthous Ulcers*—**http://emedicine.medscape.com/article/867080.**
- eMedicine. *Aphthous Stomatitis*—**http://emedicine.medscape.com/article/1075570**.
- Keogan MT. Clinical Immunology Review Series: an approach to the patient with recurrent orogenital ulceration, including Behçet's syndrome. *Clin Exp Immunol*.2009. **http://www.ncbi.nlm.nih.gov/pmc/articles/PMC2673735/**

REFERENCES

1. Messadi DV, Younai F. Aphthous ulcers. *Dermatol Ther*. 2010;23:281-290.
2. Borra RC, Andrade PM, Silva ID, et al. The Th1/Th2 immune-type response of the recurrent aphthous ulceration analyzed by cDNA microarray. *J Oral Pathol Med*. 2004;33:140-146.
3. Sun A, Wang JT, Chia JS, Chiang CP. Levamisole can modulate the serum tumor necrosis factor-alpha level in patients with recurrent aphthous ulcerations. *J Oral Pathol Med*. 2006;35:111-116.
4. Casiglia JM. Recurrent aphthous stomatitis: etiology, diagnosis, and treatment. *Gen Dent*. 2002;50:157-166.
5. Keogan MT. Clinical Immunology Review Series: an approach to the patient with recurrent orogenital ulceration, including Behçet's syndrome. *Clin Exp Immunol*. 2009 Apr;156(1):1-11.
6. Bell J. Amlexanox for the treatment of recurrent aphthous ulcers. *Clin Drug Investig*. 2005;25:555-566.
7. Rodriguez M, Rubio JA, Sanchez R. Effectiveness of two oral pastes for the treatment of recurrent aphthous stomatitis. *Oral Dis*. 2007;13: 490-494.
8. Descroix V, Coudert AE, Vige A, et al. Efficacy of topical 1% lidocaine in the symptomatic treatment of pain associated with oral mucosal trauma or minor oral aphthous ulcer: a randomized, double-blind, placebo-controlled, parallel-group, single-dose study. *J Orofac Pain*. 2011;25:327-332.
9. Alidaee MR, Taheri A, Mansoori P, et al. Silver nitrate cautery in aphthous stomatitis: a randomized controlled trial. *Br J Dermatol*. 2005;153:521-525.
10. Rhodus NL, Bereuter J. An evaluation of a chemical cautery agent and an anti-inflammatory ointment for the treatment of recurrent aphthous stomatitis: a pilot study. *Quintessence Int*. 1998;29:769-773.
11. Femiano F, Buonaiuto C, Gombos F, et al. Pilot study on recurrent aphthous stomatitis (RAS): a randomized placebo-controlled trial for the comparative therapeutic effects of systemic prednisone and systemic montelukast in subjects unresponsive to topical therapy. *Oral Surg Oral Med Oral Pathol Oral Radiol Endod*. 2010;109:402-407.
12. Pakfetrat A, Mansourian A, Momen-Heravi F, et al. Comparison of colchicine versus prednisolone in recurrent aphthous stomatitis: a double-blind randomized clinical trial. *Clin Invest Med*. 2010;33: E189-E195.
13. Yasui K, Kurata T, Yashiro M, et al. The effect of ascorbate on minor recurrent aphthous stomatitis. *Acta Paediatr*. 2010;99: 442-445.
14. Meiller TF, Kutcher MJ, Overholser CD, et al. Effect of an antimicrobial mouthrinse on recurrent aphthous ulcerations. *Oral Surg Oral Med Oral Pathol*. 1991;72:425-429.
15. Volkov I, Rudoy I, Freud T, et al. Effectiveness of vitamin B12 in treating recurrent aphthous stomatitis: a randomized, double-blind, placebo-controlled trial. *J Am Board Fam Med*. 2009;22:9-16.

38 LEUKOPLAKIA

Michaell A. Huber, DDS
Wanda C. Gonsalves, MD

PATIENT STORY

A 57-year-old male smoker presents at the physician's clinic with a 7-month history of a nonpainful white patch below his tongue. He admits to drinking 2 to 3 beers in the evening and smoking 1 pack of cigarettes per day. Your examination reveals a painless white, thick lesion with fissuring below the tongue (**Figure 38-1**). A biopsy shows this to be premalignant and the patient is told that he must stop smoking and drinking. He is also referred to an oral surgeon for further evaluation of his dysplasia.

INTRODUCTION

The World Health Organization defines leukoplakia as a clinical term used to recognize "white plaques of questionable risk having excluded (other) known diseases or disorders that carry no increased risk for cancer."[1,2] For all types of leukoplakia (see "Clinical Features" later) the risk of malignant transformation is approximately 1%, with a much higher risk associated with leukoplakias manifesting a red and/or highly variable surface texture component.

The term *erythroplakia* is reserved for a purely red lesion, which is described as a "fiery red patch that cannot be characterized clinically or pathologically as any other definable disease."[1,2] It may be flat or slightly depressed and exhibits a smooth or granular surface texture. The majority of erythroplakias will undergo malignant transformation.

SYNONYMS

It is also known as homogenous leukoplakia, nonhomogenous leukoplakia, speckled leukoplakia, nodular leukoplakia, verrucous leukoplakia, erythroleukoplakia, erythroplakia, or erythroplasia.

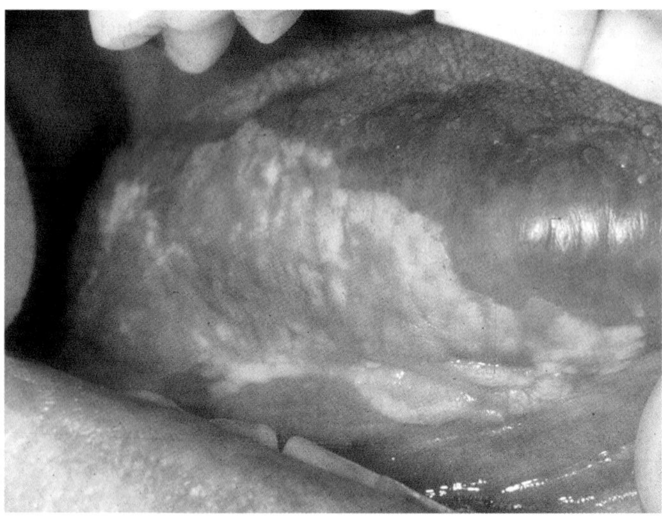

FIGURE 38-1 Homogenous leukoplakia on the lateral tongue presenting with a uniform surface plaque and surface cracks in a patient with a long smoking history. A 4-mm punch biopsy was performed and showed moderate dysplasia. *(Reproduced with permission from Richard P. Usatine, MD.)*

EPIDEMIOLOGY

- Leukoplakia occurs in 0.5% to 2% of adults and is most frequently seen in middle-aged and older men.[1]
- Erythroplakia occurs in approximately 0.02% to 0.83% of adults and is most commonly observed in middle-aged and elderly persons, with no gender distinction.[1]

ETIOLOGY AND PATHOPHYSIOLOGY

- Both leukoplakia and erythroplakia likely represent clinical changes associated with the underlying multistep progression of alterations at the molecular level underlying the development of dysplasia and subsequent carcinoma.
- For all types of leukoplakia, the risk of malignant transformation is approximately 1%, with a much higher risk associated with leukoplakias manifesting a red component.[1]
- For erythroplakia, the risk of malignant transformation is extremely high, with 85% of cases demonstrating either dysplasia or carcinoma in situ at the time of biopsy.[3]

RISK FACTORS

- Smoking and alcohol exposure are the most prominent risk factors for leukoplakia and erythroplakia, and create a synergistic effect when combined.[1]
- Human papillomavirus (HPV) is a recognized risk factor for oropharyngeal cancer, but its association with leukoplakia and erythroplakia is undetermined.[4]
- Up to 27% of leukoplakias are idiopathic.[4]

DIAGNOSIS

Both leukoplakia and erythroplakia are clinical working diagnoses of exclusion, to be applied when other conditions have been excluded.

CLINICAL FEATURES

- Leukoplakia may be characterized as either homogenous or nonhomogenous.[1,2]
- Homogenous leukoplakia (see **Figure 38-1**) presents uniformly as a thin surface plaque with possible shallow surface cracks.[2]
- Nonhomogenous leukoplakia (**Figures 38-2** and **38-3**) may be further characterized as speckled (white predominant with interspersed red component); nodular (small polypoid outcrops, may be red or white); or verrucous (corrugated or folded surface appearance).[2]
- Erythroplakia (**Figure 38-4**) presents as distinct flat or slightly depressed red lesion with a smooth or granular surface texture.[1,2]

TYPICAL DISTRIBUTION

- Both leukoplakia and erythroplakia may occur on any oropharyngeal mucosal site.[4]

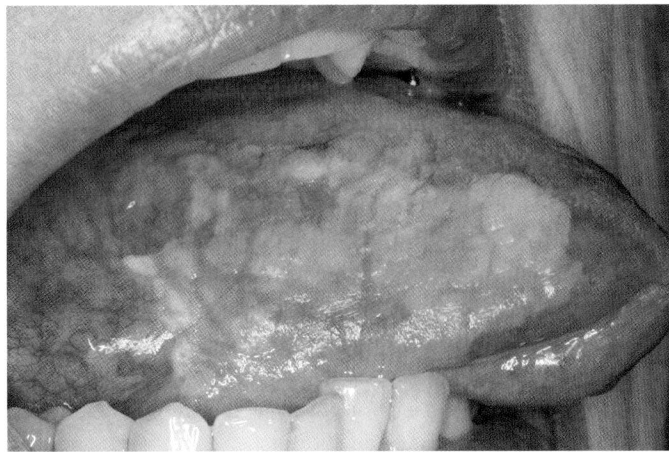

FIGURE 38-2 Nonhomogenous leukoplakia of the right ventral tongue in a 54-year-old white woman. Although she is a nonsmoker, she did have moderate alcohol exposure. Previous biopsy 6 years ago revealed hyperkeratosis. New biopsy indicated moderate-to-severe dysplasia. Patient was managed with total excision of the leukoplakia and an AlloDerm graft. *(Reproduced with permission from Michaell Huber, DDS.)*

- Lesions affecting the floor of the mouth, ventral or lateral tongue, and possibly the soft palatal complex, are associated with an increased risk for malignant transformation.[4,5]
- Idiopathic leukoplakias demonstrate a significantly higher risk of malignant transformation compared to risk-associated variants.[4]

LABORATORY

A biopsy is required to determine the histologic characterization of the lesion. Usually a 4-mm punch biopsy is a good start, but be wary of a false negative as a consequence of sampling error. If the lesion appears suspicious, refer to an oral surgeon, even with a negative result.

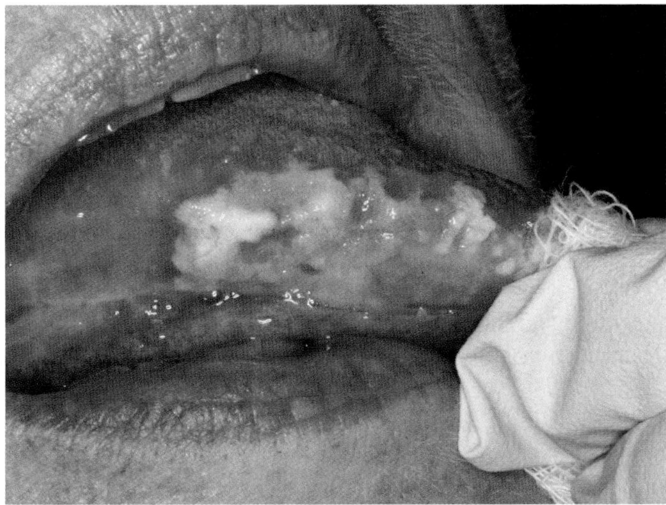

FIGURE 38-3 Leukoplakia (nonhomogenous) with moderate dysplasia on the lateral border of the tongue of a 65-year-old woman with a long history of smoking. She presented with discomfort and a noticeable white plaque on her tongue; a biopsy proved this to be moderate dysplasia. This was the third white dysplastic lesion she had developed in this area. A new excision will be performed and close follow-up is needed. Even though she quit smoking a few years ago, the damage done has led to a relentless dysplastic process. *(Reproduced with permission from Ellen Eisenberg, DMD.)*

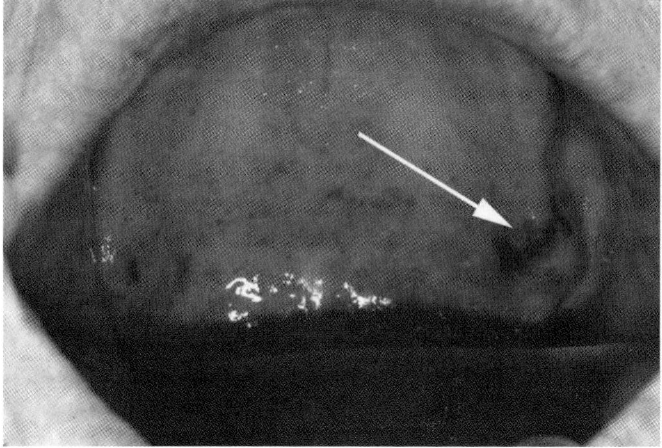

FIGURE 38-4 Erythroplakia with red patch (*arrow*) on the upper alveolar ridge of an edentulous person. *(Reproduced with permission from Gerald Ferritti, DMD.)*

DIFFERENTIAL DIAGNOSIS

- Aspirin/chemical burn—determined by history.[1,2]
- Candidiasis (thrush)—typically symmetrical and wipes off (see Chapter 135, Candidiasis).
- Discoid lupus—concurrent cutaneous lesions, circumscribed mucosal lesion with central erythema, radiating white lines, histopathology.
- Hairy leukoplakia—characteristic clinical presentation (bilateral tongue), histopathologic evidence Epstein-Barr virus (EBV).
- Lichen planus—presence of striations, symmetrical presentation (see Chapter 152, Lichen Planus).
- Lichenoid lesion—presence of striations, temporal association with trigger agent (eg, new drug, dental material, home care product).
- Linea alba—parallel to line of occlusion, often bilateral.
- Morsicatio—habitual chewing or biting habit of the oral mucosa, often bilateral (**Figure 38-5**).

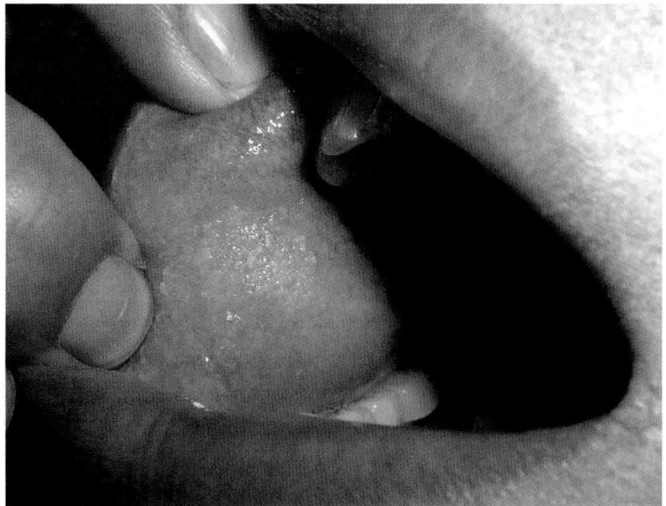

FIGURE 38-5 Morsicatio—leukoplakia caused by habitual chewing and biting of the oral mucosa. This young man only reluctantly acknowledged this habit upon further questioning of his bilateral leukoplakia. *(Reproduced with permission from Richard P. Usatine, MD.)*

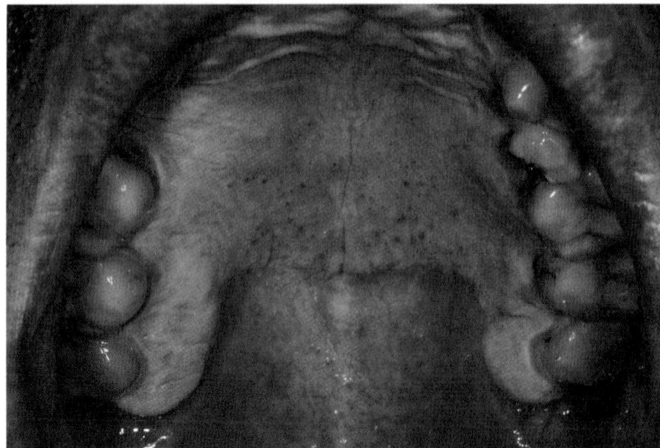

FIGURE 38-6 Nicotine stomatitis is observed in smokers. Note the hyperkeratosis affecting the hard palate and the erythematous minor salivary duct orifices. (*Reproduced with permission from Michaell Huber, DDS.*)

- Nicotine stomatitis—Smoking habit, characteristic appearance (**Figure 38-6**).
- Snuff patch—Characteristic folded, corrugated appearance at site of tobacco placement.
- White sponge nevus—Familial history, symmetrical pattern, and other mucosal sites often involved.

MANAGEMENT

MEDICATIONS

There are no pharmacologic regimens to manage either leukoplakia or erythroplakia.

SURGERY

- All leukoplakias and erythroplakias should be excised and biopsied to determine the presence of epithelia dysplasia, carcinoma in situ, or squamous cell carcinoma.[1,6,7] SOR C
- Watchful waiting is not recommended.

REFERRAL

Refer as appropriate to an oral and maxillofacial surgeon, an oral medicine expert, or an ear, nose, and throat (ENT) surgeon.

PREVENTION AND SCREENING

- Risk reduction measures are to be encouraged.
- Ensure a thorough and disciplined soft tissue examination is accomplished on a routine basis.

PROGNOSIS

- Prognosis is highly variable for leukoplakia; it may ultimately regress and disappear, persist, or progress to eventual carcinoma. Leukoplakia may recur after excision.[6-8]
- Erythroplakia almost always progresses to cancer.[1,3]

FOLLOW-UP

- Routine monitoring (eg, every 3-6 months) for recurrence should be done.[6-8] SOR C
- Risk factor elimination may reduce the risk of recurrence.[1,6,9]

PATIENT EDUCATION

Counsel patients who use tobacco (eg, smoke or smokeless tobacco) to quit. Ask if they are ready to quit at each visit, and sign a contract with them that specifies the date and time they will quit. Provide tools (see "Patient Resources" below) they can use to quit (see Chapter 237, Tobacco Addiction).

PATIENT RESOURCES

- American Lung Association. *Getting Help to Quit Smoking*—**http://www.lung.org/stop-smoking/how-to-quit/getting-help/.**
- QuitSmokingSupport.com—**http://www.quitsmokingsupport.com/.**
- Centers for Disease Control and Prevention. *Quit Smoking*—**http://www.cdc.gov/tobacco/quit_smoking/index.htm.**

PROVIDER RESOURCES

- Tobacco Use and Dependence Guideline Panel. *Treating Tobacco Use and Dependence: 2008 Update.* Rockville, MD: US Department of Health and Human Services; 2008. **http://www.ncbi.nlm.nih.gov/books/NBK63952/.**
- National Cancer Institute. *Cigarette Smoking: Health Risks and How to Quit (PDQ®)*—**http://www.cancer.gov/cancertopics/pdq/prevention/control-of-tobacco-use/HealthProfessional.**

REFERENCES

1. van der Waal I. Potentially malignant disorders of the oral and oropharyngeal mucosa; terminology, classification and present concepts of management. *Oral Oncol.* 2009;45:317-323.
2. Warnakulasuriya S, Johnson NW, van der Waal I. Nomenclature and classification of potentially malignant disorders of the oral mucosa. *J Oral Pathol Med.* 2007;36:575-580.
3. Scully C, Bagan JV, Hopper C, Epstein JB. Oral cancer: current and future diagnostic techniques. *Am J Dent.* 2008;21:199-209.
4. Napier SS, Speight PM. Natural history of potentially malignant oral lesions and conditions: an overview of the literature. *J Oral Pathol Med.* 2008;37:1-10.
5. Reibel J. Prognosis of oral pre-malignant lesions: significance of clinical, histopathological, and molecular biological characteristics. *Crit Rev Oral Biol Med.* 2003;14:47-62.
6. Lodi G, Porter S. Management of potentially malignant disorders: evidence and critique. *J Oral Pathol Med.* 2008;37:63-69.
7. Holmstrup P, Vedtofte P, Reibel J, Stoltze K. Oral premalignant lesions: is a biopsy reliable? *J Oral Pathol Med.* 2007;36:262-266.
8. Holmstrup P, Vedtofte P, Reibel J, Stoltze K. Long-term treatment outcome of oral premalignant lesions. *Oral Oncol.* 2006;38:461-474.
9. Vladimirov BS, Schiodt M. The effect of quitting smoking on the risk of unfavorable events after surgical treatment of oral potentially malignant lesions. *Int J Oral Maxillofac Surg* 2009;38:1188-1193.

39 OROPHARYNGEAL CANCER

Michaell A. Huber, DDS
Wanda C. Gonsalves, MD

PATIENT STORY

A 66-year-old man presents to the physician's office with a nonhealing painful lesion on the roof of his mouth (**Figure 39-1**). The lesion has increased in size recently and he is worried because his dad died from oral cancer. Your patient has smoked since he was 11 years old by getting cigarettes from his dad. He admits to being a heavy drinker. A biopsy shows squamous cell carcinoma and the patient is referred to a head and neck surgeon.

INTRODUCTION

In spite of the relative ease for the health care provider to accomplish a visual and tactile examination of the oropharyngeal cavity, fully two-thirds of oropharyngeal cancers (OPCs) will present with advanced disease at the time of diagnosis.[1] Ninety percent of OPCs are of the squamous cell type. Concern has been raised that practitioners are missing early disease by not accomplishing a thorough soft tissue examination on a routine basis.[2] However, the fact that more than 35% of patients do not see a dentist on a routine basis likely contributes to the diagnostic delay.[3] The 5-year survival rate is 62% for whites and 42% for blacks.[1]

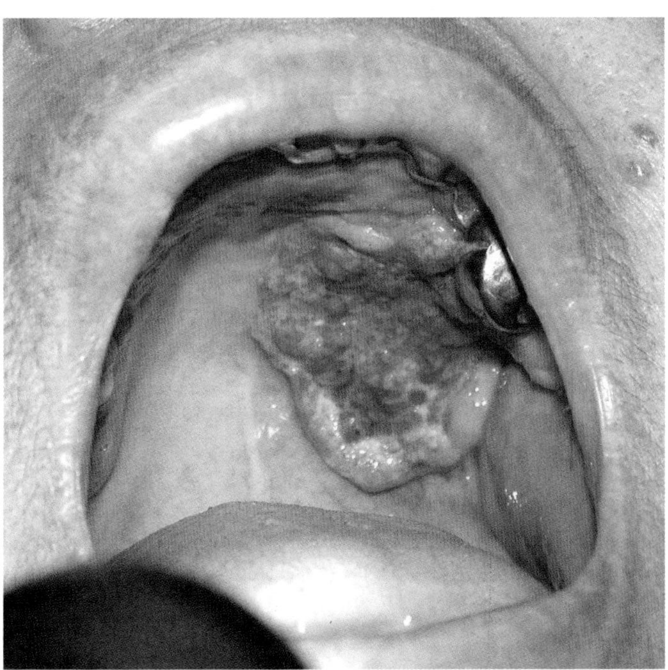

FIGURE 39-1 Squamous cell carcinoma of the palate of a 66-year-old man with a long history of smoking tobacco and alcohol abuse. (*Reproduced with permission from Frank Miller, MD.*)

SYNONYMS

Oropharyngeal cancer is also known as oral cancer, oral squamous cell carcinoma, mouth cancer, site specific (eg, gingival cancer, tongue cancer, lip cancer).

EPIDEMIOLOGY

- In the United States, an estimated 40,000 OPC cases occur annually, accounting for approximately 3.3% of malignancies among men and 1.5% of malignancies among women.[1]
- The median age at diagnosis is 62 years and more than 70% of cases occur after the age of 55 years.[4]
- Incidence rates vary from a low of 3.9 per 100,000 Hispanic women to a high of 16.1 per 100,000 white men.[4]
- Up to 35% of OPC patients will develop a new primary tumor within 5 years.[5]

ETIOLOGY AND PATHOPHYSIOLOGY

Typical OPC develops from a complex multistep progression marked by alterations at the molecular level, followed by phenotypic changes, and subsequent clinically observable changes affecting the squamous epithelium.[6]

RISK FACTORS

- Tobacco use is the major risk factor for OPC and is implicated in approximately 75% of cases.[7]
- Alcohol use is a major risk factor and the combined use of tobacco and alcohol increases the risk of OPC far more than either alone.[7]
- Human papillomavirus (HPV) (especially HPV-16) is a newly recognized major risk factor for carcinomas affecting the lingual and palatine tonsils.[8]
- Other risk factors include betel quid chewing, low intake of fruits and vegetables, immunosuppression, and maté drinking.[9]
- Excess sun exposure is the major risk factor for cancer of the lip.[7]

DIAGNOSIS

A scalpel biopsy is required to establish the diagnosis.[5,10]

CLINICAL FEATURES

- OPC may affect any area of the oropharyngeal cavity.
- Early OPC often presents as a leukoplakia or erythroplakia (see **Figure 39-1**). High-risk sites are the floor of the mouth and ventrolateral tongue (**Figure 39-2**).
- Features of more advanced disease include induration, persistent ulceration, tissue proliferation or erosion, pain or paresthesia, loss of function, and lymphadenopathy (**Figures 39-3** to **39-5**).[10]

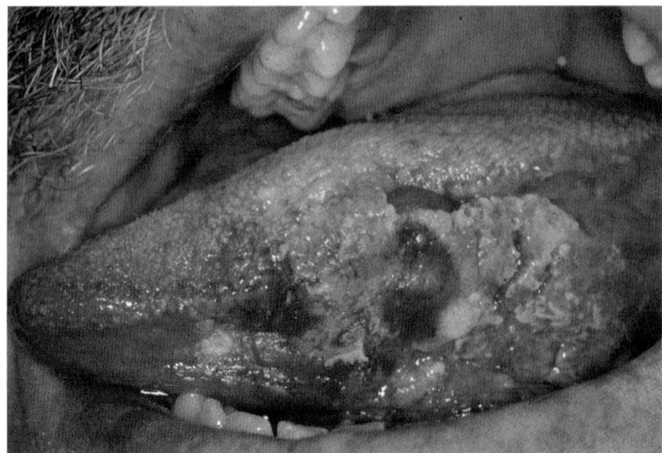

FIGURE 39-2 Squamous cell carcinoma on the lateral side of the tongue. This is a broad erythroleukoplakic plaque with surface ulcerations. (*Reproduced with permission from Ellen Eisenberg, DMD.*)

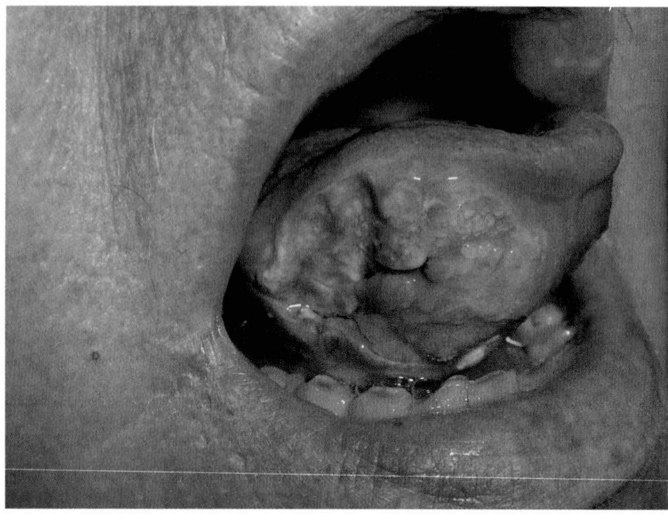

FIGURE 39-5 Squamous cell carcinoma manifesting chronic ulceration with induration on the right side of the tongue in a homeless woman with a long history of smoking tobacco and alcohol abuse. (*Reproduced with permission from Richard P. Usatine, MD.*)

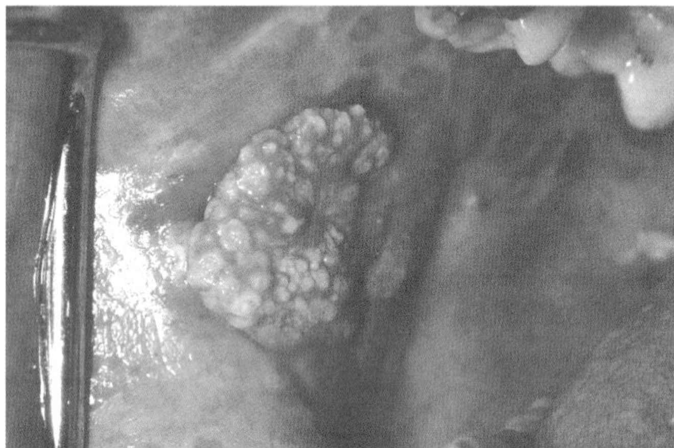

FIGURE 39-3 Squamous cell carcinoma arising on the buccal mucosa. (*Reproduced with permission from Gerald Ferritti, DDS.*)

- HPV-associated carcinomas are often less visible and share signs and symptoms (eg, sore throat, hoarseness, earaches, enlarged lymph nodes) of tonsillitis and pharyngitis. More advanced symptoms include dysphagia, hemoptysis, and weight loss.[10]
- Lip cancer typically presents as a relapsing or persistent chronic scab, plaque, crust, or ulceration (**Figure 39-6**). Antecedent actinic cheilosis is commonly observed.
- Nonsquamous-type cancers (eg, salivary gland tumors, melanoma, sarcomas) often present as a submucosal nodular swelling or mass (**Figures 39-7** and **39-8**).

TYPICAL DISTRIBUTION

OPCs occur most commonly (in order of frequency) on the tongue, floor of the mouth, and lower lip vermilion. The lymphoepithelial tissues of the Waldeyer ring (lateral tongue extending to the lateral soft palate and tonsillar area) has the greatest risk of developing an HPV-associated OPC.[8]

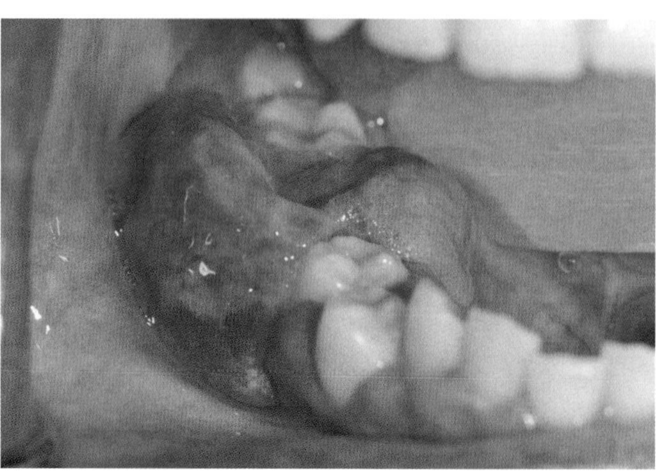

FIGURE 39-4 Exophytic cancer of the mouth. (*Reproduced with permission from Gerald Ferritti, DDS.*)

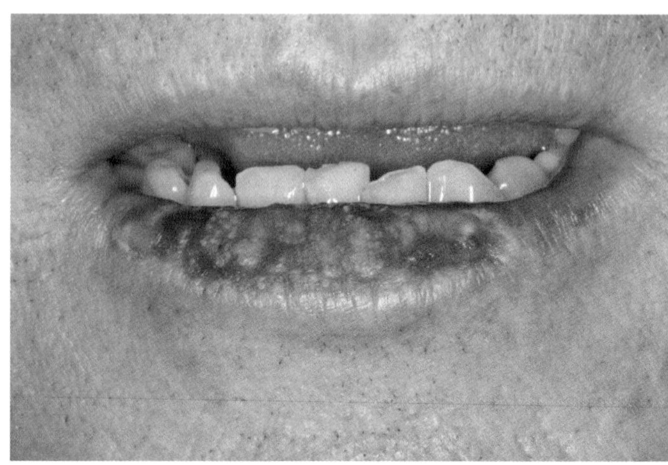

FIGURE 39-6 Squamous cell carcinoma of the lower lip in a 51-year-old man, managed with vermilionectomy. (*Reproduced with permission from Michaell Huber, DDS*).

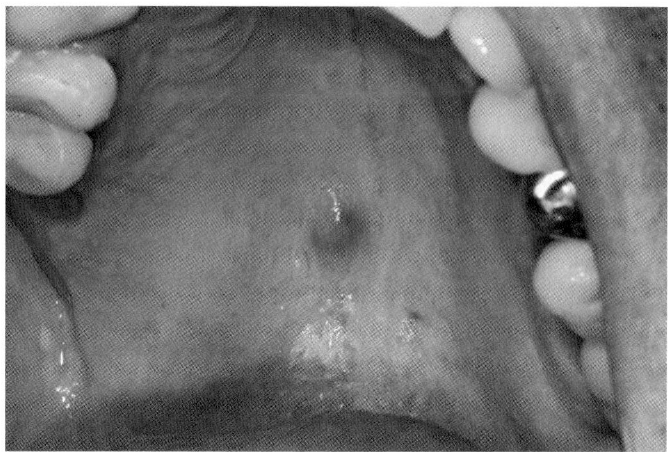

FIGURE 39-7 A 58-year-old man with well-defined soft, bluish diascopy positive nodule of unknown duration. Although a benign vascular lesion is the most likely diagnosis, a minor salivary gland tumor or a Kaposi sarcoma should also be considered. (*Reproduced with permission from Michaell Huber, DDS.*)

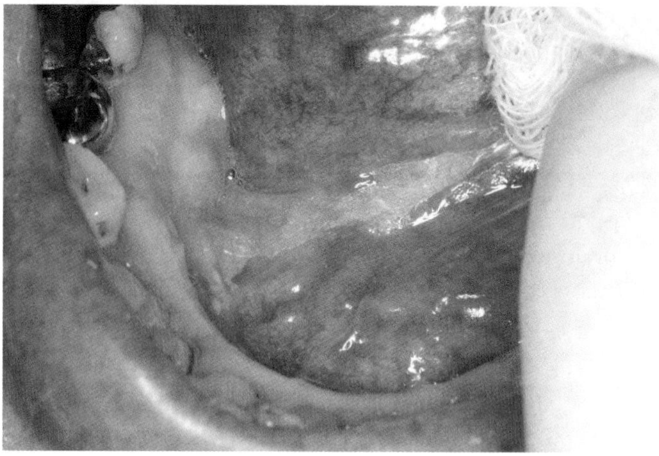

FIGURE 39-9 A 64-year-old woman with faint leukoplakia and a history of a hot coffee burn. Upon 2-week follow-up, the leukoplakia was still present and an excisional biopsy revealed carcinoma in situ completely excised. She was recommended for close monitoring. (*Reproduced with permission from Michaell Huber, DDS.*)

LABORATORY

A scalpel biopsy is required to establish the diagnosis. An excisional biopsy is preferred to better ensure all suspicious tissue is available for histologic assessment. Confirmed cases are staged utilizing the tumor, nodes, metastasis (TNM) scheme.

DIFFERENTIAL DIAGNOSIS

- OPC is capricious and may initially mimic any number of benign conditions such as aphthae, chronic ulcerative conditions, pharyngitis, and tonsillitis (see Chapter 31, Pharyngitis).
- Any lesion deemed suspicious or equivocal at discovery should be referred to an expert (oral and maxillofacial surgeon, an oral medicine expert, or an ear, nose, and throat [ENT] surgeon) for further assessment or immediate biopsy.
- Findings deemed innocuous should be reevaluated within 2 weeks for resolution and referred to an expert for further assessment or undergo biopsy if still present (**Figure 39-9**).

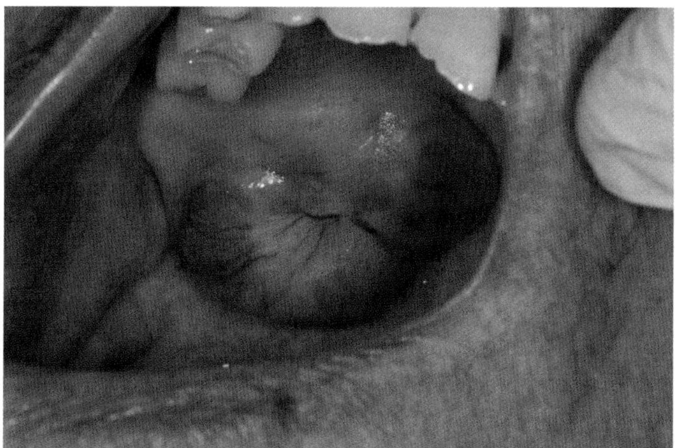

FIGURE 39-8 An 80-year-old Hispanic woman with a 25-year history of palatal mass, which she stated only recently started getting bigger. A low-grade adenocarcinoma of the palate was confirmed with biopsy. (*Reproduced with permission from Michaell Huber, DDS.*)

MANAGEMENT

- Confirmed OPC is best managed by the oncology team whose members deliver all indicated therapeutic antitumor modalities and provide appropriate adjunctive services such as dental care and nutritional, psychological, and social support. TNM staging is useful for treatment planning and prognostication.
- The principal therapeutic modalities are surgery, radiotherapy, and chemotherapy.[11,12]
- The use of one treatment over another depends on the size, location, and stage of the primary tumor, the patient's ability to tolerate treatment, and the patient's desires.[11,12]
- Surgical excision is the preferred modality for most well-defined and accessible solid tumors; however, it has its limitations for inaccessible or more advanced tumors demonstrating lymph node involvement and/or metastasis.[11,12]
- Radiotherapy may be either an effective alternative to surgery or a valuable adjunct to surgery and/or chemotherapy in the locoregional treatment of malignant head and neck tumors.[11,12]
- Protocols utilizing concomitant chemoradiotherapy improve both locoregional control and survival.[12]

PROGNOSIS

- Early OPCs (stage I and stage II) of the lip and oral cavity are highly curable with 5-year survival rates exceeding 90%.[11]
- Later-stage OPCs (stage III and stage IV) have a more guarded prognosis with 5-year survival rates ranging from 23% to 58%.[1]

FOLLOW-UP

- Vigilant posttherapy follow-up is required (every 6 months).
- Posttherapy OPC patients are at risk for developing a second primary tumor, 3% to 7% per year.[12]

PATIENT EDUCATION

Advise patients to discontinue smoking and/or drinking alcohol.

PATIENT RESOURCES

- The Oral Cancer Foundation—**http://www.oralcancerfoundation.org/.**
- Centers for Disease Control and Prevention, National Oral Health Surveillance System. *Cancer of the Oral Cavity and Pharynx*—**http://www.cdc.gov/nohss/guideCP.htm.**

PROVIDER RESOURCES

- National Cancer Institute. *Lip and Oral Cavity Cancer (PDQ®): Treatment*—**http://www.cancer.gov/cancertopics/pdq/treatment/lip-and-oral-cavity/HealthProfessional.**
- National Cancer Institute. *Oropharyngeal Cancer (PDQ®): Treatment*—**http://www.cancer.gov/cancertopics/pdq/treatment/oropharyngeal/HealthProfessional.**
- Medscape Reference. *Cancers of the Oral Mucosa*—**http://emedicine.medscape.com/article/1075729.**

REFERENCES

1. Siegel R, Naishadham D, Jemal A. Cancer statistics, 2012. *CA Cancer J Clin.* 2011;62:10-29.
2. Mignogna MD, Fedele S, Lo Russo L, et al. Oral and pharyngeal cancer: lack of prevention and early detection by health care providers. *Eur J Cancer Prev.* 2001;10(4):381-383.
3. Pleis JR, Ward BW, Lucas JW. Summary health statistics for U.S. adults: National Health Interview Survey, 2009. National Center for Health Statistics. *Vital Health Stat 10.* 2010;(249):1-207.
4. National Cancer Institute, Surveillance Epidemiology and End Results. *SEER Stat Fact Sheets: Oral Cavity and Pharynx.* http://seer.cancer.gov/statfacts/html/oralcav.html. Accessed February 17, 2012.
5. Lingen MW, Kalmar JR, Karrison T, Speight PM. Critical evaluation of diagnostic aids for the detection of oral cancer. *Oral Oncol.* 2008;44(1):10-22.
6. Haddad RI, Shin DM. Recent advances in head and neck cancer. *N Engl J Med.* 2008;359:1139-1154.
7. National Cancer Institute. *Oral Cancer Prevention (PDQ®).* http://www.cancer.gov/cancertopics/pdq/prevention/oral/HealthProfessional. Accessed February 27, 2012.
8. Cleveland JL, Junger ML, Saraiya M, et al. The connection between human papillomavirus and oropharyngeal squamous cell carcinomas in the United States. *J Am Dent Assoc.* 2011;142:915-924.
9. Warnakulasuriya S. Causes of oral cancer—an appraisal of controversies. *Br Dent J.* 2009;207:471-475.
10. Rethman MP, Carpenter W, Cohen EEW, et al. Evidence-based clinical recommendations regarding screening for oral squamous cell carcinomas. *J Am Dent Assoc.* 2010;141:509-520.
11. National Cancer Institute. *Lip and Oral Cancer Treatment (PDQ®).* http://www.cancer.gov/cancertopics/pdq/treatment/lip-and-oral-cavity/HealthProfessional. Accessed February 17, 2012.
12. National Cancer Institute. *Oropharyngeal Cancer Treatment (PDQ®).* http://www.cancer.gov/cancertopics/pdq/treatment/oropharyngeal/HealthProfessional. Accessed February 17, 2012.

40 ADULT DENTAL CARIES

Juanita Lozano-Pineda, DDS, MPH
Wanda C. Gonsalves, MD

PATIENT STORY

A 41-year-old homeless man presents to a clinic on "skid row" with a toothache (**Figure 40-1**). He has a history of alcoholism and smoking. Many of his teeth are loose and a number of his teeth have fallen out in the past year. He acknowledges that he does not floss or brush his teeth regularly. He has been sober for 60 days now and wants help to get his teeth fixed. He states that no one will hire him with his teeth as they are. He also has pain in a molar and wants something for the pain until he can see a dentist. On oral examination, you see missing teeth, generalized plaque, and teeth with multiple brown caries.

INTRODUCTION

Dental caries is a multifactorial disease that is primarily caused by an interaction between bacteria and fermentable carbohydrates producing acid that has potential to demineralize the tooth surface over time. Host factors, such as the plaque (biofilm) adherence, quality and quantity of saliva, immune system response, use of fluoride, and a diet that is caries-promoting, play a role in the formation of incipient demineralized lesions that progress to dental caries. Caries risk is impacted by factors that may be behavioral, biological, environmental, lifestyle-related, and physical. Age, diabetes, ethnic origin, gingival recession, smoking, and socioeconomic status are frequently associated with high caries prevalence.[1]

SYNONYMS

Dental decay, dental cavities, cavitated lesions are the synonyms of dental caries.

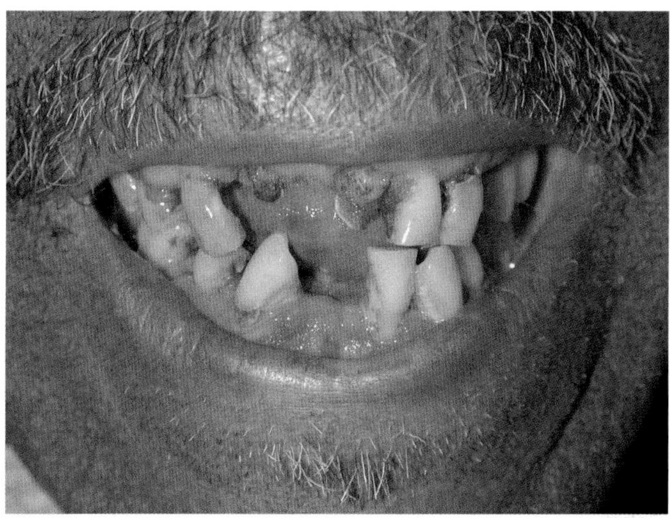

FIGURE 40-1 Severe caries in a homeless man. (*Reproduced with permission from Richard P. Usatine, MD.*)

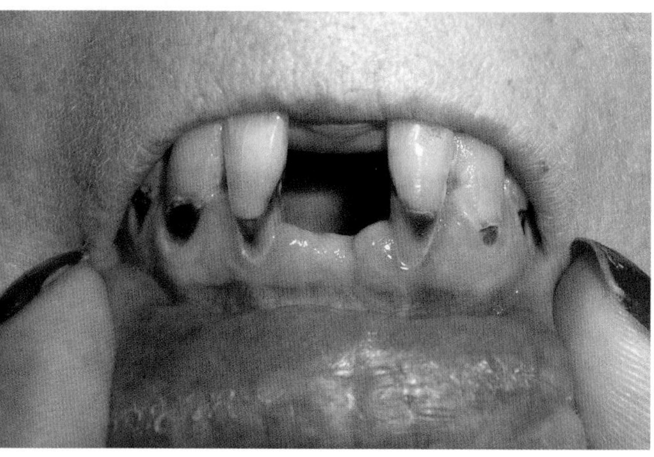

FIGURE 40-2 Root caries in a woman with a history of substance abuse. She has lost all of her upper teeth and is beginning to lose her lower teeth. Note the exposed and darkened roots. (*Reproduced with permission from Richard P. Usatine, MD.*)

EPIDEMIOLOGY

- Many adults (eg, 31% of those 20-34 years of age, 27% of those 35-49 years of age, 24% of those 50-64 years of age, and 20% of those 65 years of age and older) have untreated dental caries (see **Figure 40-1**).[2]
- Black and Hispanic adults, younger adults, and those with lower incomes and less education have more untreated decay.[3]
- Many older adults suffer from root caries (decay on the roots of their teeth) (**Figure 40-2**). The percentage of adults with root caries increased with age: 8% of adults 20 to 39 years of age had root decay, compared with 11% of adults 40 to 59 years of age, and 13% of adults 60 years of age and older. The prevalence is greater for black non-Hispanics (20%) and adults below 100% poverty level (19%).[4]
- More than twice as many current smokers (19%) as nonsmokers (7%) had root caries.[4]

ETIOLOGY AND PATHOPHYSIOLOGY

- Dental caries result from the activity of dental bacterial plaque, a complex biofilm containing microorganisms that demineralize and proteolyse tooth enamel and dentin through their action on the fermentation of sucrose and other sugars. The main organism is *Streptococcus mutans*.
- A caries-promoting diet that is high in sugar or acid increases the demineralization process. A cariostatic diet that contains calcium helps buffer the acidity and increases remineralization of the tooth's enamel surface.
- Low saliva flow and low pH also increase demineralization; the lack of saliva to buffer the acidity from plaque and diet increases caries risk.
- Dental caries progression or reversal depends on the balance between demineralization and remineralization. If caries is untreated and progresses, it eventually destroys enough tooth structure to either have the unsupported tooth fracture, or the caries reaches the tooth's pulp (nerve tissue) and leads to infection that can progress through the pulp to the tooth's root apex and surrounding bone.
- Plaque also impacts the gingival tissues; if it is not removed regularly, it may calcify with the minerals in the saliva and form calculus (tartar).

RISK FACTORS

The risk factors for adult caries include the following[5-7]:

- Increased acidic environment that may be a result of the following:
  - A diet that is high in fermentable carbohydrates and/or acid
  - High quantity of bacteria or poor oral hygiene
  - Physical and medical disabilities that often prevent proper oral hygiene
  - Medications that decrease pH[6]
  - Acid reflux
  - Bulimia
- Low saliva flow and dry mouth
  - Medications that decrease saliva flow (tricyclic antidepressants, antihistamines, steroids, diuretics).
  - Illicit drugs such as methamphetamine and cocaine dry the mouth (**Figure 40-3**).
  - Radiation to the head and neck that may damage salivary glands.
  - Sjögren syndrome affects saliva glands and decreases flow rate.
- The presence of existing restorations or oral appliances
- Gingival recession exposing root surfaces that demineralize at a higher pH
- Low socioeconomic status with limited or no access to medical or dental care

DIAGNOSIS

Caries can be diagnosed clinically through visual examination of the teeth, where lesions range from a white spot (incipient) to a large cavitated lesion. Radiographically, the carious lesion appears radiolucent (as a consequence of demineralization or cavitation) within a radiopaque, calcified tooth structure.

CLINICAL FEATURES

Dental caries, initially present as a painless white spot (demineralization of enamel) and if contributing risk factors are not modified, it progresses to a brownish discoloration, with eventual cavitation into the dentin. Pain is usually not felt until the caries progresses into the dentin and/or approximates the pulp. It presents only when stimulated with cold or sweets, and rarely with heat, subsiding shortly after stimulus removal. Once the caries infects the nerve, it leads to pulpal necrosis. The patient may present with pain that is spontaneous, triggered with heat and lingers, is more severe, and may be accompanied with soft tissue swelling.

TYPICAL DISTRIBUTION

It occurs on any enamel, exposed dentin or cementum surface, including occlusal, interproximal, and root surfaces.

LABORATORY AND IMAGING

An X-ray will show the extent of the cavity, but not all demineralized areas.

DIFFERENTIAL DIAGNOSIS

- Fluorosis—Mild fluorosis may be present as white-spot lesions with an appearance that is similar to the "white-spot" incipient carious lesions.
- Dark staining in the tooth's deep pits and fissures that may be a result of tobacco use or tartar buildup.
- Trauma—Usually involves maxillary incisors common in sports, accidents, violence, and epilepsy.
- Tooth erosion—Results from consumption of carbonated beverages and fruit drinks, repeated vomiting associated with eating disorders, gastroesophageal reflux, and alcoholism.
- Tooth attrition—Wearing down of teeth because of tooth grinding (bruxism) or an abrasive diet.
- Tooth abrasion—Caused by brushing with a hard toothbrush and using abrasive toothpaste.
- Bulimia can cause destruction of the teeth because of the gastric acids (**Figure 40-4**).

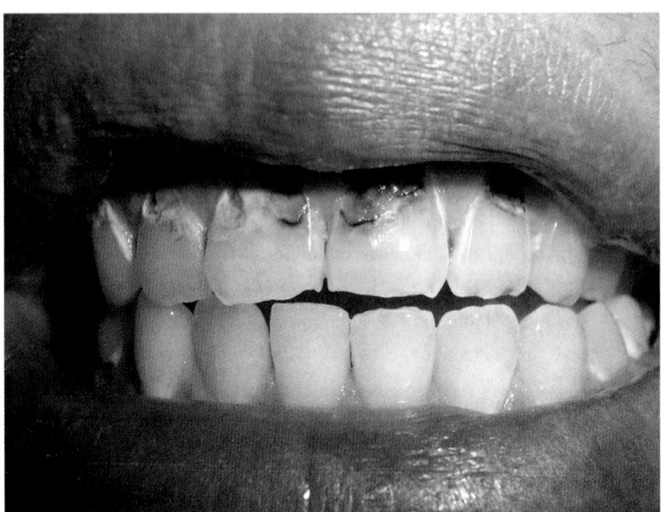

FIGURE 40-3 Gum line caries in a young woman with a history of illicit drug use including methamphetamine, cocaine, and heroin. She is now in recovery and would like to get dental care (*Reproduced with permission from Richard Usatine, MD*).

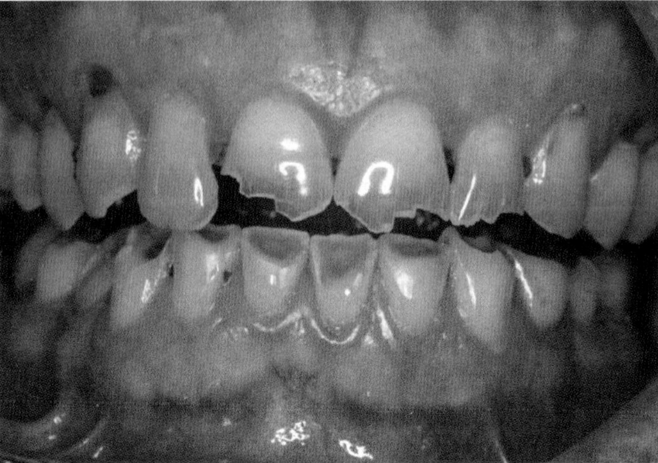

FIGURE 40-4 Destruction of the teeth in woman with bulimia. The gastric acids have dissolved the enamel. (*Reproduced with permission from Gerald Ferretti, DMD.*)

MANAGEMENT

- Demineralized lesions ("white spots") and caries—Topical fluorides such as varnishes (5% NaF; 23,000 parts per million [ppm] F^-) that are applied by dental health providers or the primary care physician twice a year have been shown to decrease dental caries by 21%.[7]
- Fluoride mouth rinses (0.2% NaF, 900 ppm F^-) are effective in controlling caries when used daily.[7]
- Refer to a dental health professional for sealant treatment of pits and fissures.[8]
- Refer patients with "white spots" and dental caries to a dental professional for treatment and/or restoration.[5]
- Patients with xerostomia may be treated with saliva substitutes such as Oralbalance in the Biotene product range.[5]

PREVENTION AND SCREENING

Most of the oral diseases, including cavities, are preventable. Proper oral hygiene (daily brushing and flossing), daily exposure to fluoride (systemic or topical), along with a healthy diet that is not high in sugar, can prevent the formation and/or progression of dental caries. Visual screening can detect caries at the early stages.

PROGNOSIS

The prognosis for lesions that are detected during their early stages or prior to approximating the tooth's nerve is very good. Removal of the carious portion of the tooth and placement of a filling will restore the tooth to function and prevent further progression of the cavity.

FOLLOW-UP

Remind adult patients who have incipient "white-spot" caries or active caries to go to a dentist for treatment. Patients with large caries should be referred for immediate treatment.

PATIENT EDUCATION

- Advise patients to maintain good oral hygiene by brushing their teeth twice daily with a small-headed, soft-to-medium hardness brush using a toothpaste that contains fluoride. Electric toothbrushes may be useful for those with poor manual dexterity. Counsel patients to floss once daily to remove plaque and food particles from between the teeth.
- Suggest that patients use antiplaque mouthwashes containing chlorhexidine to inhibit *S. mutans*, but caution coffee, tea, and red wine drinkers that such mouthwashes may increase dental staining.[5]
- Patients with xerostomia (dry mouth) should be advised to practice good oral hygiene, increase water intake, and avoid sugary foods. Chewing sugar-free gum will induce salivation.[5]
- Patients with xerostomia should also be advised to avoid alcohol-containing mouth rinses, as alcohol also dries the mouth.
- Advise patients that plaque formation may be reduced by chewing sugar-free gum and eating raw fruits and vegetables, which reduce bacteria through mechanical cleansing of the tooth surfaces.
- Patients who use asthma inhalers should be advised to rinse their mouth with water after inhaler use to decrease the amount of residue that is left in the oral cavity. Many inhalers contain lactose, a fermentable sugar.
- Eating calcium-containing foods, such as milk and cheese, helps buffer the acidic environment and helps with remineralization.
- Advise patients to visit a dental professional at least once a year for cleaning and examination.

PATIENT RESOURCES

- American Dental Association. *Public Resources*—**http://www.ada.org/public.aspx.**
- New York State Department of Health. *Oral Health Resources and Links*—**http://www.health.state.ny.us/prevention/dental/weblinks_oral_health.htm.**

PROVIDER RESOURCES

- Smiles for Life: A National Oral Health Curriculum—**http://www.smilesforlifeoralhealth.org/.**
- Centers for Disease Control and Prevention. *Preventing Cavities, Gum Disease, Tooth Loss, and Oral Cancers at a Glance 2011*—**http://www.cdc.gov/chronicdisease/resources/publications/AAG/doh.htm.**
- World Health Organization. *Oral Health*—**http://www.who.int/oral_health/en/.**

REFERENCES

1. Ritter AV, Preisser JS, Chung Y, et al; X-ACT Collaborative Research Group. Risk indicators for the presence and extent of root caries among caries-active adults enrolled in the Xylitol for Adult Caries Trial (X-ACT). *Clin Oral Investig.* 2012 Dec;16(6):1647-1657.
2. Griffin SO, Barker LK, Griffin PM, et al. Oral health needs among adults in the United States with chronic diseases. *J Am Dent Assoc.* 2009;140;1266-1274.
3. National Institute of Dental and Craniofacial Research. *Dental Caries (Tooth Decay) in Adults (Age 20 to 64).* http://www.nidcr.nih.gov/DataStatistics/FindDataByTopic/DentalCaries/DentalCariesAdults20to64.htm. Accessed July 22, 2013.
4. National Health and Nutrition Examination Survey (NHANES), 1999-2002. *NIDCR/CDC Oral Health Data Query System.* http://apps.nccd.cdc.gov/dohdrc/dqs/entry.html. Accessed July 22, 2013.
5. Johnson V, Chalmers J. *Oral Hygiene Care for Functionally Dependent and Cognitively Impaired Older Adults.* Iowa City, IA: University of Iowa College of Nursing, John A. Hartford Foundation Center of Geriatric Nursing Excellence; 2011 Jul:61. http://www.guideline.gov/content.aspx?id=34447. Accessed July 22, 2013.
6. Stookey GK. The effect of saliva on dental caries. *J Am Dent Assoc.* 2008;139(suppl):S11-S17.
7. Cappelli, DP, Mobley CC. *Prevention in Clinical Oral Health Care.* St. Louis, MO: Elsevier; 2008.
8. National Institutes of Health, Consensus Development Conference Statement, March 26-28, 2001. *Diagnosis and Management of Dental Caries Throughout Life.* http://consensus.nih.gov/2001/2001DentalCaries115html.htm. Accessed July 22, 2013.

PART 7

CARDIOVASCULAR

Strength of Recommendation (SOR)	Definition
A	Recommendation based on consistent and good-quality patient-oriented evidence.*
B	Recommendation based on inconsistent or limited-quality patient-oriented evidence.*
C	Recommendation based on consensus, usual practice, opinion, disease-oriented evidence, or case series for studies of diagnosis, treatment, prevention, or screening.*

*See Appendix A on pages 1241-1244 for further information.

41 AORTIC ANEURYSM

Deepthi Rao, MD
Venu Gourineni, MD

PATIENT STORY

A 72-year-old man presented to the emergency department complaining of dull abdominal pain in the umbilical area radiating to the back which started 2 days ago, after he had spent a day helping his daughter move. His pain was 5/10 in intensity, worse with movement, and not relieved with acetaminophen. He denied nausea, vomiting, diarrhea, melena, hematochezia, and heart burn. He stated that he had been healthy until then and had not seen a physician in more than 20 years. He had a 30 pack-year smoking history and was not on any medications. His initial vital signs were stable. Palpation of the abdomen revealed guarding, rigidity, and tenderness in the periumbilical area. Routing laboratory studies showed no evidence of infection. An abdominal X-ray revealed calcifications in the abdominal aortic area. This prompted a computed tomography (CT) of the abdomen, which showed a 6.5-cm ruptured abdominal aortic aneurysm (AAA) with fluid in the retroperitoneal area (**Figure 41-1A and 41-1B**). Meanwhile, the patient became hypotensive and was taken emergently to the operating room and underwent an open repair of the AAA. His postoperative course was uneventful and he had a successful recovery.

INTRODUCTION

Aortic aneurysm (AA) is defined as abnormal enlargement of the aorta when the diameter of the affected segment is more than one and a half times the normal size.[1] Normal size of the aorta varies with the segment of the aorta and depends on the age, gender, and body area.[1]

AA is classified on the basis of location and morphology. Based on *morphology* an aneurysm can be fusiform which is more common and involves the entire circumference of the aortic wall; and saccular which is a bulge from only a portion of the wall.[1] Classification by *location* is significant since the majority of treatment decisions are based on this. In terms of the location, AA can be classified as thoracic aortic aneurysm (TAA) which in turn can be ascending or descending. Ascending aortic aneurysm can be supra coronary (above the origin of the coronaries), annuloaortic (involving the annulus and proximal aorta), and tubular (uniform dilation of the entire ascending aorta).[1] Descending thoracic aneurysms are usually fusiform and associated with atherosclerosis.[1] AAAs occur most of the time in the infrarenal segment (**Figure 41-2**).

SYNONYMS

Other similar terms not to be confused with are as below:

- Aortic dissection
- Aortic transection
- Intramural hematoma

EPIDEMIOLOGY

- Aortic aneurysms (TAA and AAA) together constitute the 17th leading cause of mortality among all individuals in the United States.[1,2]
- The incidence of TAA is approximately 10.4 per 100,000 person per years and increases in frequency with age.[3]
- The prevalence of AAA varies due to asymptomatic course until a rupture. However, it is more commonly seen in men and elderly people. Many population studies have shown AAA prevalence of 4% to 8% in men aged between 65 and 80 years.[4]

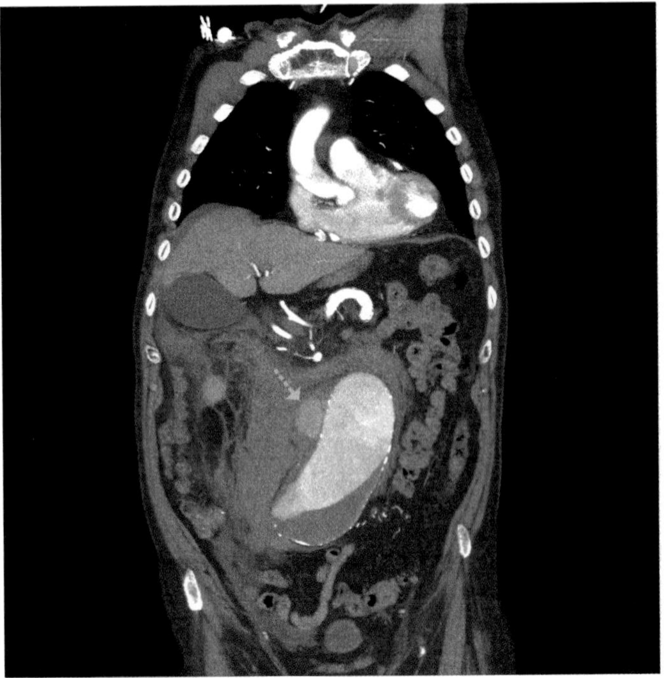

A

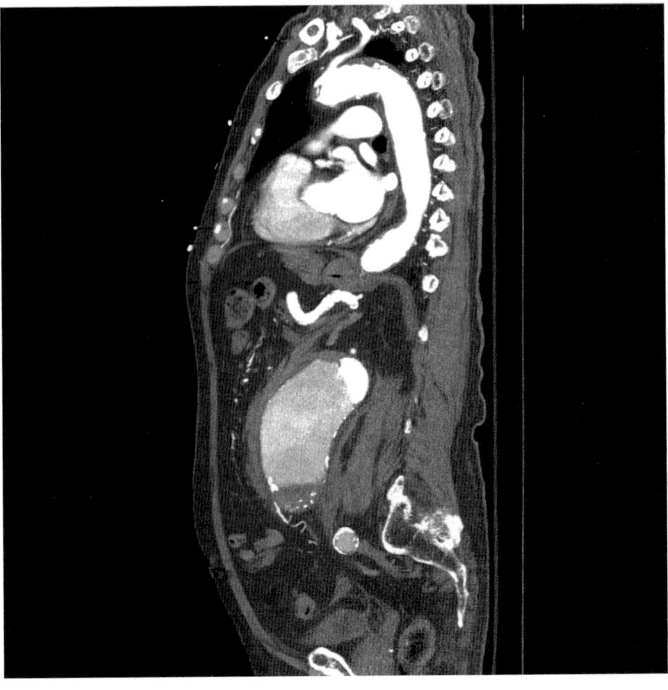

B

FIGURE 41-1 **A.** Sagittal view of a ruptured AAA. There is a subtle blush of contrast (yellow arrow) extending along the right wall of the large aneurysm creating a second pocket. **B.** The cross-sectional view of the same patient. (*Reproduced with permission from Gary Ferenchick, MD.*)

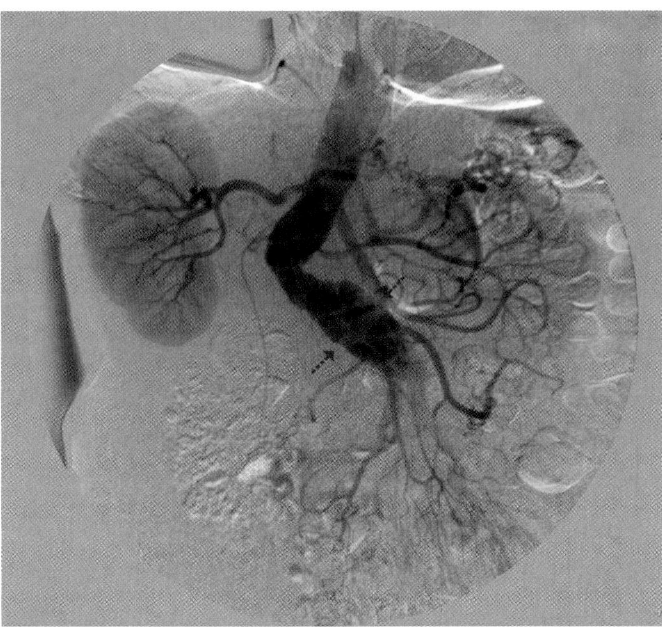

FIGURE 41-2 A large infrarenal fusiform aneurysm (arrows) is seen in this patient with diffuse atherosclerotic vascular disease in the arteriogram (*Reproduced with permission from Gary Ferenchick, MD.*)

- However, since majority of AAs are asymptomatic unless complicated, it is generally thought that the prevalence is underreported.
- TAA is distributed equally among men and women,[5] while AAA is more common in men.[4]

ETIOLOGY AND PATHOPHYSIOLOGY

TAA[7,8]

- Degeneration due to age-related changes which are accelerated by other factors like hypertension, smoking, hyperlipidemia, and genetic factors (**Table 41-1**). This accounts for majority of TAA and commonly involves the arch and descending aorta.[7]

TABLE 41-1 Causes of Aortic Aneurysm

TAA	AAA
Genetic[7] • Marfan • Ehlers-Danlos • Loeys-Dietz • Turner • Bicuspid • Familial nonsyndromic	Hereditary
Atherosclerosis /Degenerative • Smoking • Hyperlipidemia • Hypertension	Atherosclerosis/ Degenerative • Smoking • Age or hypertension • Hyperlipidemia
Aortitis • Infectious—syphilis, *Salmonella*	
Trauma	

- Atherosclerosis is also a frequent cause of descending TAA.[7,8]
- Genetics
  - Marfan syndrome—Inheritable autosomal dominant disorder due to mutation in one of the fibrillin genes which is part of elastin. This leads to alteration in the elastic properties of the aorta and increased stiffness and aortic dilation. Almost 75% of patients with Marfan have aortic dilation.[7,8]
  - Ehlers-Danlos syndrome is another inheritable connective tissue disorder predisposing to TAA, however, it is seen less frequently than Marfan.[7]
  - Familial nonsyndromic TAA syndrome—One of the significant causes of TAA with clustering among families and follows an autosomal dominant pattern of inheritance with reduced penetrance.[7]
  - Loeys-Dietz syndrome—Autosomal dominant disease involving the aorta as well as other systems with TGFBR1 or TGFBR2 mutation.[7]
  - Bicuspid aortic valve—Most of TAA in bicuspid aortic valve are tubular and have a higher growth rate compared to TAA in patients with trileaflet aortic valves.[7]
  - Turner syndrome—Typically involves the ascending aorta.[7]
- Aortitis
  - Causative agents include syphilis, *Salmonella*, and *Mycobacterium*.[7]
  - Noninfectious aortitis includes giant cell and Takayasu arteritis which are more common; other causes include Behçet, rheumatoid arthritis, relapsing polychondritis, and other granulomatous diseases.[7]
- Trauma

- AAA[6,8]:
  - Hereditary factors, although no gene defects have been identified, having a family history of AAA is an important risk factor for the occurrence of AAA, especially in males.
  - Eighty percent of AAA occurs between the renal arteries and the aortic bifurcation at the iliac arteries.
    - Atherosclerosis is a major cause of AAA.
    - Proteolysis and inflammation produce expansion of AAA.
      - The underlying pathology is medial degeneration which begins in a focal area and is executed by metalloproteinases (MMP) in susceptible patients.[9]
      - Elastin and collagen are 2 of the most important proteins of the tunica media. Degradation in these proteins by MMPs leads to stiffness, loss of elasticity, weakening and dilation of the aortic wall which is aggravated by a multitude of stresses including hypertension and smoking.[9] (**Figure 41-3**)
      - Inflammation also plays a role, especially in inflammatory AAAs, as evidenced by the presence of perianeurysmal fibrosis, cytokine, and macrophage accumulation.[6]
      - In accordance with Laplace law, the increasing radius of the aorta increases the wall tension which in turn causes worsening of the dilation, thereby causing propagation of the size of the aneurysm.
  - Note that AAA commonly coexists with disease in other arterial beds including iliac, femoral, popliteal, and the thoracic aorta.[6]
  - Rate of expansion of AAA is usually around 0.4 cm/y and is influenced to a major extent by the baseline size. Risk of rupture is greatest in smokers, hypertensives, and in women.[8]
  - The average rate of growth of a degenerative or idiopathic ascending TAA is about 0.1 cm/y with slightly higher rates for descending TAA.[1,7]
  - However, accelerated rate of growth can be seen in those with genetic predisposition for TAA and a higher baseline size at diagnosis.[1,7,8]

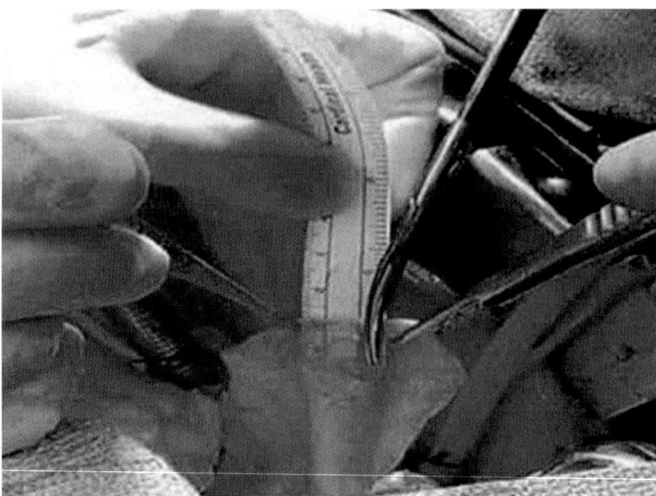

FIGURE 41-3 Ruler markings are easily seen through the aortic wall due to thinning of the wall from degradation of the proteins (presumably by matrix metalloproteinase-related activity). (*Reproduced with permission from Fuster V, Walsh RA, Harrington RA, et al.* Hurst's The Heart. *13th ed. New York, NY: McGraw-Hill; 2011.*)

RISK FACTORS

- Genetics.
- Atherosclerosis is the major cause of AAA, especially in the infrarenal area[7] (**Figure 41-4**).

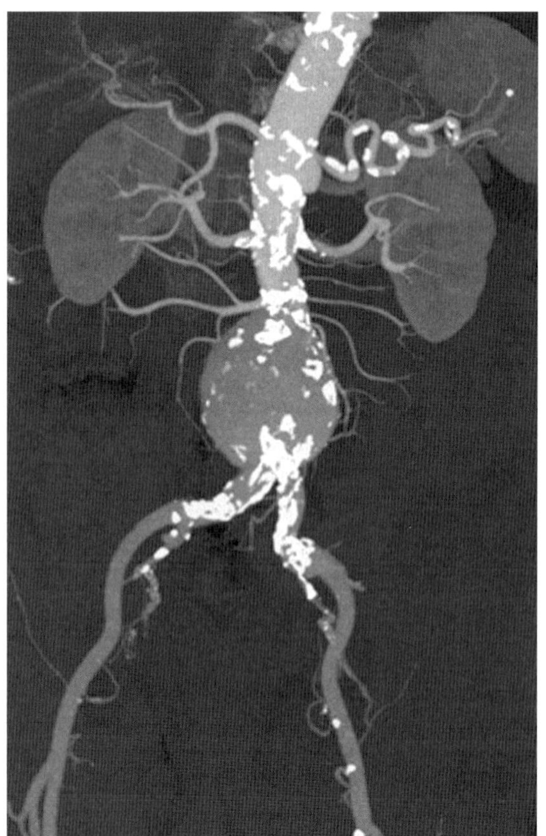

FIGURE 41-4 Extensive calcification and a large abdominal aortic aneurysm. (*Reproduced with permission from Pahlm O, Wagner GS.* Multimodal Cardiovascular Imaging: Principles and Clinics Applications. *New York, NY: McGraw-Hill; 2011.*)

- Smoking is the risk factor most strongly associated with AAA followed by age, dyslipidemia, and hypertension.
  - Smoking is the most important modifiable risk factor.
    - Ninety percent patients with AAA have a history of smoking.[10]
    - Five percent of all older men who have smoked have an AAA.[11]
    - Smokers are 5 times more likely than nonsmokers to develop AAA.[10-12]

SCREENING

See **Table 41-2.**

- TAA
  - Screening—First-degree relatives of patients with a gene mutation associated with TAA or dissection (FBN1, TGFBR1, TGFBR2, COL3A1, ACTA2, MYH11) should undergo genetic counseling and testing. Those relatives found to have the mutation should then undergo aortic imaging.[9] SOR C
  - For patients with TAA or dissection without a known mutation, aortic imaging is recommended for first-degree relatives to identify those with asymptomatic disease.[9] SOR B
  - If one or more first-degree relatives are found to have thoracic aortic dilatation, aneurysm, or dissection, then imaging of second-degree relatives is reasonable.[9] SOR C
- AAA
  - An AAA is defined as an aortic diameter of greater than 3 cm.[1,4,6]
  - Screening at age 65 will identify most with AAA and decreases the rate of aneurysm rupture by approximately 50% and the rate of aneurysm-related mortality by approximately 40% (however, overall mortality is not known to be decreased with screening).[10-12]
  - Following are the (USPSTF) recommendations[13]:
    - A onetime screening in 65- to 75-year-old men who have ever smoked (B recommendation).
    - No recommendation in men who never smoked (C recommendation).
    - Recommends against screening in women (D recommendation).

DIAGNOSIS

CLINICAL FEATURES—HISTORY AND PHYSICAL

- History and physical examination findings in cases of AA are neither sensitive nor specific.
- However, it is important to elicit any significant history of familial disorders or sudden or unexplained deaths which may suggest genetic predilection for AA.

TABLE 41-2 Screening for Aortic Aneurysm

TAA[9]	AAA[13]
Gene testing for first-degree relatives of patients with gene mutation causing TAA and aortic imaging for positive testers	Imaging by ultrasound for asymptomatic men aged 65-75 years with a smoking history
Aortic Imaging for first-degree relatives of patients with TAA and no known mutation	

- It is also vital to perform a thorough examination and to be able to recognize those patients with aortic disease who are at risk for a potential catastrophe.
- Most AAs are clinically silent except in rupture or dissection which can cause severe pain, shock, and other complications.
- It is imperative to examine all peripheral pulses for delay or widening, discrepancy of blood pressure between arms, signs of nonperfusion, and neurologic defects any of which, if present, can indicate that the AA is complicated by rupture or dissection.
- TAA
  - Pain or discomfort is the most common presenting symptom of TAA. Retrosternal, neck, or jaw pain may occur with ascending AA, whereas back, interscapular, or left shoulder pain may occur with descending TAA.[1,9]
  - Fever may be present in inflammatory causes of TAA.[9] A chronic leaking aneurysm may also cause fever and jaundice.
  - Patients can also present with compressive symptoms like hoarseness from left recurrent laryngeal nerve stretching; stridor, from tracheal or bronchial compression; dyspnea, from lung compression; dysphagia, from esophageal compression; and plethora and edema, from superior vena cava compression.[9]
  - Erosion into the lung parenchyma can cause hemoptysis and into the esophagus can cause hematemesis rarely.[1]
  - Aortic root dilatation can result in aortic valve regurgitation and result in heart failure.[9]
  - Most physical findings are not specific for thoracic aortic disease. Other findings may be related to genetic syndromes and connective tissue disorders or inflammatory diseases.
  - Ascending TAA is not detectible on physical examination unless it causes aortic regurgitation which can be heard as a diastolic blowing murmur in the left sternal area.
  - Descending TAAs are very rarely palpable except in cases of extreme enlargement.
- AAA
  - Symptomatic AAAs usually causes gnawing steady pain in the hypogastric area or low back.
  - Abrupt onset of new pain or acute worsening of existing pain can indicate expansion and impending rupture.[1]
  - AAA can be palpated as a pulsatile mass above the umbilicus, although this can be difficult in obese individuals.

LABORATORY TESTING

- No specific laboratory tests are available for AA.
- Genetic testing is available for the various clinical syndromes that cause TAA.
- Inflammatory markers are useful in cases of TAA due to inflammatory etiologies.
- Infectious laboratory workup can be pursued if such a cause is suspected in TAA.
- Routine laboratory tests including blood counts and serum chemistries can be done if a surgery is anticipated.

IMAGING

- TAA
  - Considering AA is typically asymptomatic and the high mortality of complicated AA, physicians should have a relatively lower threshold to order appropriate imaging studies for AA.
  - TAA may be evident on chest X-ray by mediastinal widening or enlargement of the aortic knob. However, the sensitivity is limited and enlarged aortic silhouette may also indicate tortuosity of the aorta rather than AA.[8]
    - Contrast-enhanced CT scanning (along with magnetic resonance angiography [MRA]) represent the preferred modality for TAA. SOR B
      - However, CT may not visualize the aortic root well. Also, in cases of tortuosity of the aorta, the measured diameter can be falsely high. A CT angiography can be done to accurately measure the size.[8]
  - MRA also accurately detects and sizes TAAs and is especially useful in aneurysms of the aortic root area.[8]
  - Transesophageal echocardiography (TEE) is usually used in evaluating for aortic root aneurysm in Marfan syndrome. However, TEE can be an important complementary test to evaluate the aortic valve anatomy and function.[7]
- AAA
  - Abdominal ultrasound (US) is an inexpensive diagnostic modality which does not involve radiation exposure and hence makes an excellent screening tool for AAA.[8] SOR B
  - CT imaging can better characterize the shape and size of an AAA. However, due to the ionizing radiation and contrast involved, it is used more often for monitoring the growth of AAA rather than as a screening tool.
  - MRA is an alternative option for imaging AAA in patients with contraindications to CT.

DIFFERENTIAL DIAGNOSIS

- Differential for TAA includes the following:
  - Pulmonary emboli—Pain is sudden onset, pleuritic and associated with hypoxia.
  - Pneumothorax—Sudden onset of pleuritic pain with decreased breath sounds on the affected side.
  - Myocardial infarction (MI)—Pain is mostly substernal and associated with injury patterns on the electrocardiography (ECG) and elevated cardiac biomarkers.
- Depending on the presenting clinical findings, ruptured AAA can be confused with acute gastrointestinal (GI) disease such as bowel ischemia and penetrating peptic ulcer, acute genitourinary disease such as renal stones or infection, or spinal disease such as herniated disc.

MANAGEMENT

- Surveillance
  - TAA (**Table 41-3**)
    - After the initial identification of a TAA, imaging should be repeated in 6 months. If the size of the TAA is stable, it can be safely monitored at annual intervals. Future screening intervals can be shortened if the rate of growth increases.[8]
    - TAA surveillance[7,9] SOR B
      - Ascending TAA due to degenerative causes and 3.5 to 4.4 cm in size obtain annual CT or MR.
      - Ascending TAA due to degenerative causes and 4.5 to 5.4 cm in size obtain semiannual CT or MR.
      - Ascending TAA due to Marfan bicuspid or other genetically mediated etiology and 3.5 to 4.4 cm in size obtain annual CT or MR.

TABLE 41-3 Surveillance of Asymptomatic TAA

TAA	Degenerative	Genetically mediated
Ascending[7,9]	3.5-4.4 cm—annual CT or MR 4.5-5.4 cm—semiannual CT or MR	3.5-4.4 cm—annual CT or MR 4.4-5 cm—semiannual CT or MR
Descending	3.5-4.4 cm—annual CT or MR 4.5-5.9 cm—semiannual CT or MR	3.5-4.4 cm—annual CT or MR 4.4-5.5 cm—semiannual CT or MR

- Ascending TAA due to Marfan bicuspid or other genetically mediated etiology and 4.4 to 5 cm in size obtain semiannual CT or MR.
- Descending TAA due to degenerative causes and 3.5 to 4.4 cm in size obtain annual CT or MR.
- Descending TAA due to degenerative causes and 4.5 to 5.9 cm in size obtain semiannual CT or MR.
- Descending TAA due to Marfan bicuspid or other genetically mediated etiology and 3.5 to 4.4 cm in size obtain annual CT or MR.
- Descending TAA due to Marfan bicuspid or other genetically mediated etiology and 4.4 to 5.5 cm in size obtain semiannual CT or MR.

- AAA (**Table 41-4**)
  - AAA surveillance[6] SOR B

    Infrarenal
    - AAA less than 4 cm in diameter obtain a biennial ultrasound.
    - AAA 4 to 5.4 cm in diameter obtains a semiannual ultrasound.

    AAA other than infrarenal
    - AAA less than 4 cm in diameter obtain annual CT or MR scan.
    - AAA 4 to 5.4 cm in diameter obtains CT or MR every 6 to 12 months.

- Medical Management (**Table 41-5**)
  - Blood pressure[8,14]
    - Aggressive management of blood pressure has been shown to reduce the complication rate from AA. SOR B
    - Blood pressure should be maintained in the low normal range.
  - Hyperlipidemia[8,14]
    - Patients with AA need to have their lipid status optimized especially in atherosclerotic AAs. SOR C
  - Smoking[8,14]
    - Smoking cessation needs to be encouraged in patients with AA. SOR B
  - β-Blockers[8,14]
    - β-Blockers have been shown to decrease the TAA dilatation rate in Marfan syndrome patients and can reduce the shear stress on the aortic wall. SOR B
    - β-Blockers are currently recommended in the treatment of all AA patients. SOR C
  - Statins[8,14]
    - It has been proposed that oxidative stress plays a role in aneurysm growth and hence, statins are being studied in AA.
    - Although they have not been proven to reduce AA growth at this time, statins are used for the control of hyperlipidemia.
  - Angiotensin II receptor blockers (ARB) or angiotensin-converting enzyme inhibitors (ACEI)[8,14]
    - ARBs are still being investigated for their potential to decrease the AA growth rate since they can inhibit growth factors as well as reduce oxidative stress.
  - Other drugs[8,14]
    - Doxycycline, an inhibitor of MMP as well as transforming growth factor antibodies are currently being researched for their role in AA.
- Surgical management (**Table 41-6**)
  - Indications for surgical intervention
    - TAA[7,9] SOR B
      - Ascending TAA due to degenerative causes consider surgery if size is greater than or equal to 5.5 cm, growth is greater than 0.5 cm/y, or if symptomatic at any size.
      - Descending TAA due to degenerative causes consider surgery if size is greater than or equal to 6 cm, growth is greater than 0.5 cm/y, or if symptomatic at any size.
      - Ascending TAA due to Marfan, bicuspid, or other genetically mediated etiologies consider surgery replacing aortic valve, if size is greater than 4.4 to 5 cm, growth is greater than 0.5 cm/y, or if symptomatic.
      - Descending TAA due to Marfan, bicuspid, or other genetically mediated etiologies consider surgery if size is greater than 5.5 cm, growth is greater than 0.5 cm/y, or if symptomatic.
    - AAA[6] SOR B
      - AAA considers surgery if size is greater than 5.5 cm or if symptomatic.

PROGNOSIS

- Mortality of an elective surgical ascending TAA is 3% to 5%; however, these rates are usually in large centers.[8] Similarly, elective surgical repair of descending TAAs is shown to have mortality rate from 5% to 14%.[8]

TABLE 41-4 Surveillance of Asymptomatic AAA

AAA[6]	Less Than 4 cm in Diameter	4-5.4 cm in Diameter
Infrarenal AAA	Biennial ultrasound, however, no clear consensus	Semiannual ultrasound or CT
AAA other than Infrarenal	Annual CT or MR	CT or MR every 6-12 months

TABLE 41-5 Management of Aortic Aneurysm

Medical Management[8,14]	Surgical Management
Blood pressure control • β-Blockers • ACEI/ARBs	Open surgical repair
Lipid control • Statins • Others	Endovascular repair
Aneurysm growth prevention • β-Blockers • ARBs • Statins • Transforming growth factor antibodies	

- Five-year survival from untreated TAAs has been variable and reported anywhere between 19% and 64% from various studies.[14]
- Most of AAA mortality occurs when these present with acute rupture. After an AAA repair, an estimated life expectancy for 65 year olds is 11 years and falls down to 8 years for 75 year olds, however, this varies with associated comorbid conditions.[10]
- Mortality after open or endovascular repair depends on several factors including location and type of aneurysm, patient's age and other comorbid conditions, hospital volume and surgeon experience, and the emergent need for surgery.
- Major complications including bleeding, stroke, spinal paraplegia, renal dysfunction necessitating renal replacement therapy have all been reported at varying rates in studies.
- Long-term mortality after AA repair is usually dependent on other coexisting cardiovascular conditions.

FOLLOW-UP

- Asymptomatic patients with AA should be monitored according to the surveillance guidelines given earlier.
- Patients being managed medically should be followed up at periodic intervals for optimization of their blood pressure and lipid levels.

TABLE 41-6 Indications for surgery in Aortic Aneurysm

	TAA[6,7,9]	
	Degenerative	Genetic
Ascending	If ≥5.5 cm, growth >0.5 cm/y, or if symptomatic at any size	If >4.4-5 cm, growth >0.5 cm/y, or if symptomatic at any size
Descending	If ≥6 cm, growth >0.5 cm/y, or if symptomatic at any size	If >5.5 cm, growth >0.5 cm/y, or if symptomatic at any size
	AAA	
AAA	If size >5.5 cm or if symptomatic at any size	

- Patients who undergo endovascular repair should be screened periodically by means of CT or MR imaging for complications from the procedure.

PATIENT EDUCATION

- Patients with AA should be instructed about limiting certain physical activities especially heavy lifting due to the risk of rupture.
- Patients with AA should also be informed about the symptoms which could suggest aneurysm rupture or bleeding and be educated about seeking medical attention immediately.
- Patients should be advised to inform medical personnel about their diagnosis at all times so that immediate attention would be given for any signs and symptoms of rupture.[6]

PATIENT RESOURCES

- AAA Patient Information—**http://www.uptodate.com/contents/patient-information-abdominal-aortic-aneurysm-beyond-the-basics.**
- Vascular Disease Foundation—**http://vasculardisease.org/thoracic-aortic-aneurysm/.**
- Vascular Disease Foundation—**http://vasculardisease.org/abdominal-aortic-aneurysm/.**
- Vascular Surgery Information—**http://www.vascularweb.org/Pages/default.aspx.**
- American Heart Association: Medical Treatment for Abdominal Aortic Aneurysm—**http://my.americanheart.org/idc/groups/ahamah-public/@wcm/@sop/@scon/documents/downloadable/ucm_323780.pdf.**

PROVIDER RESOURCES

- Screening for Abdominal Aortic Aneurysm—**http://annals.org/article.aspx?volume=142&issue=3&page=198.**

REFERENCES

1. Elefteriades JA. Thoracic aortic aneurysm: reading the enemy's playbook. *Curr Probl Cardiol*. 2008;33:203-277.
2. Center for Disease Control and Prevention. Aortic Aneurysm Fact Sheet. http://www.cdc.gov/dhdsp/data_statistics/fact_sheets/fs_aortic_aneurysm.htm. Accessed May 10, 2014.
3. Ramanath VS, Oh JK, Sundt TM, Eagle KA. Acute aortic syndromes and thoracic aortic aneurysm. *Mayo Clin Proc*. 2009;84(5):465-481.
4. Nordon IM, Hinchliffe RJ, Loftus IM, Thompson MM. Pathophysiology and epidemiology of abdominal aortic aneurysms. *Nat Rev Cardiol*. 2011;8:92-102.
5. Clouse WD, Hallett JW, Jr., Schaff HV, Gayari MM, Ilstrup DM, Melton LJ, 3rd. Improved prognosis of thoracic aortic aneurysms: a population-based study. *JAMA*. 1998;280(22):1926-1929.
6. Hirsch AT, Haskal ZJ, Hertzer NR, et al. 2006 ACC/AHA Guidelines for the management of PAD. *Circulation*. 2006 Mar 21;113(11):e463-e654.
7. Booher AM, Eagle KA. Diagnosis and management issues in thoracic aortic aneurysm. *Am Heart J*. 2011;162:38-46.e1.

8. Isselbacher EM. Thoracic and abdominal aortic aneurysms. *Circulation*. 2005;111:816-828.
9. Hiratzka LF, Bakris GL, Beckman JA, et al. ACCF/AHA/AATS/ACR/ASA/SCA/SCAI/SIR/STS/SVM guidelines for the diagnosis and management of patients with thoracic aortic disease. *Circulation*. 2010;121:e266-e369.
10. Powell JT, Greenhalgh RM. Clinical practice. Small abdominal aortic aneurysms. *N Engl J Med*. 2003;348:1895-1901.
11. Schermerhorn M. A 66-year-old man with an abdominal aortic aneurysm: review of screening and treatment. *JAMA*. 2009;302:2015-2022.
12. Lederle FA. In the clinic. Abdominal aortic aneurysm. *Ann Intern Med*. 2009;150:ITC5 1-15. quiz ITC5-16.
13. U.S. Preventive Services Task Force. *Screening for Abdominal Aortic Aneurysm*. http://www.uspreventiveservicestaskforce.org/uspstf/uspsaneu.htm. Accessed February 2005.
14. Danyi P, Elefteriades JA, Jovin IS. Medical therapy of thoracic aortic aneurysms. Are we there yet? *Circulation*. 2011;124:1469-1476.

42 ATRIAL FIBRILLATION

Venu Gourineni, MD

PATIENT STORY

A 66-year-old female with known history of coronary artery disease (CAD) is admitted with palpitations for the past 48 hours. She also complains of mild chest discomfort, associated shortness of breath, and mild dizziness. She was previously diagnosed with mild congestive heart failure (CHF) after an acute myocardial infarction 2 years ago and has been compliant with her medications since then. She denies a history of diabetes or stroke. Her medications include lisinopril, simvastatin, aspirin, and as needed furosemide. She denies alcohol intake and is a nonsmoker. On initial examination, her blood pressure is stable and her heart rate is 131 beats/min. Her electrocardiogram (ECG) at initial presentation shows atrial fibrillation (AF) with rapid ventricular rate (RVR) (**Figure 42-1**). She is admitted to a telemetry floor in stable condition with a diagnosis of new-onset AF. Her ECG at transfer shows rate-controlled AF. An echocardiogram is ordered, and she is started on b-blockers and intravenous heparin.

INTRODUCTION

- AF is the most common arrhythmia in clinical practice.[1-4] AF occurs in 1% to 2% of the general population, with nearly 2.2 million Americans having AF (paroxysmal or persistent).[1,2,4]
- With the rising prevalence of heart disease and the advances in detection of AF, there has been a nearly 60% increase of hospital admissions for AF over the last 2 decades.[3]
- It is estimated that by the year 2050 the number of persons in the United States with AF will increase to between 5.6 and 12.1 million.[2,5]

DEFINITION

- AF is a supraventricular arrhythmia characterized by uncoordinated atrial activation resulting in loss of normal atrial mechanical function and diminished atrial contraction.[1]
- ECG findings demonstrate absent p waves, replaced by fibrillatory waves, which are irregular and vary in amplitude, timing, and shape[1] (**Figure 42-1**).

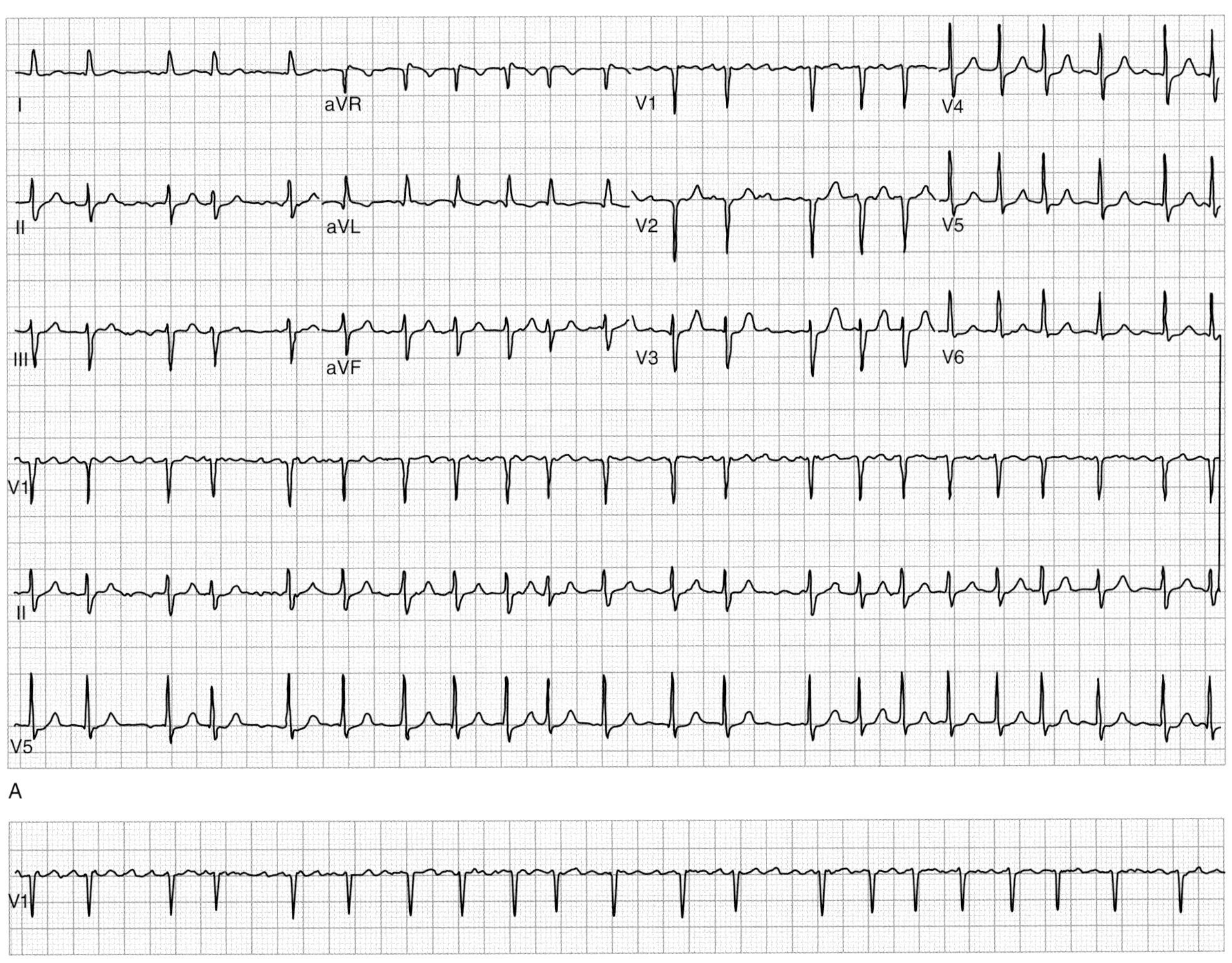

FIGURE 42-1 **A.** A 12-lead electrocardiogram (ECG) demonstrating atrial fibrillation with a rapid ventricular response. **B.** A rhythm strip from the same ECG demonstrating atrial fibrillation with an irregularly irregular rhythm and a ventricular rate of 131 beats/min. *(Reproduced with permission from Gary Ferenchick, MD.)*

CLASSIFICATION

- Several classifications have been proposed for AF, but the most commonly used one is the classification scheme recommended by the American College of Cardiology, American Heart Association, and European Society of Cardiology (ACC/AHA/ESC) practice guidelines[1,4,6] (**Table 42-1**).
- This classification replaces terms commonly used in the past, such as acute AF and chronic AF. The categories are not mutually exclusive. For example, a patient may have several episodes of paroxysmal AF and occasional persistent AF or vice versa.[1,4,6]
- Broadly, AF is divided into the categories or patterns shown in **Table 42-1**.

EPIDEMIOLOGY

AGE DIFFERENCES

- The median age of patients with AF is usually around 75 years, and approximately 70% of all such patients are between 65 and 85 years old.[1]
- In the Framingham Study, the incidence of AF increased from 0.4 per thousand at age younger than 40 years (30-39 years) to 45.9 per thousand at age older than 80 years (80-89 years) in men and from 0 to 35.8 per thousand in women, respectively.[7]
- Both the prevalence and the incidence of AF increase with advancing age and underlying cardiovascular disease.[1,7]

GENDER DIFFERENCES

- The age-adjusted prevalence rate of AF is higher in men.[8] But, because of the increased incidence of AF with age and the higher number of surviving women older than 75 years than men, the overall absolute number of men and women with AF is equal.[1,2,8]
- However, females with AF are more prone to thromboembolism and have a higher mortality than men with AF.[4,8]

OTHER FACTORS

- AF has a higher incidence of thrombus formation and increases stroke risk. Nearly 1 in 5 of all strokes is attributed to AF.[4]
- Age-adjusted stroke incidence was nearly 5-fold in a 34-year follow-up in the Framingham Study.[9]

TABLE 42-1 Classification of Atrial Fibrillation (AF) Based on ACC/AHA/ESC Practice Guidelines[1,4,6]

AF Based on Detection	Types of AF After Detection	Other Types of AF
First diagnosed or detected • Symptomatic or self-limited • Either paroxysmal or persistent AF • First-detected episode is not equivalent to new-onset AF	Paroxysmal • When episodes last less than 7 days (usually less than 24 hours) and terminate spontaneously	Secondary AF or "reversible" AF • Occurs in setting of other clinical conditions • Treatment of the underlying cause with management of acute episode of AF usually terminates the AF without recurrence • Does not reoccur after initial episode if it is truly a secondary AF; if AF reoccurs, then general principles of AF management apply Common conditions associated with secondary AF • Acute myocardial infarction • Myocarditis and pericarditis • Postcardiac or thoracic surgery • Heavy alcohol and caffeine intake • Pulmonary embolism • Hyperthyroidism • Pheochromocytoma
Recurrent AF • 2 or more episodes of AF	Persistent AF • Episodes last longer than 7 days and fail to self-terminate • Pharmacological or electrical cardioversion used to convert AF to sinus rhythm	Lone AF • Occurs in patients under 60 years old without any clinical or echocardiographic evidence of cardiopulmonary disease, including hypertension • Is not equivalent to secondary AF
	Permanent AF • AF lasts longer than 1 year and cardioversion failed or was not attempted • Term also used when the physician and patient have made a decision not to attempt rhythm control strategies and accept AF as a permanent condition	Nonvalvular • Occurs in "absence" of rheumatic mitral valve disease, any prosthetic heart valve, and mitral valve repair

- AF is associated with increased heart failure in dual ways: AF aggravates heart failure and vice versa, making this conjoint association challenging to treat.[1]
- Hence, it is essential to treat AF as untreated AF can result in significant complications and cardiovascular morbidity and mortality.

PATHOPHYSIOLOGY

- AF is associated with many structural cardiovascular conditions such as hypertension (HTN), CAD, and valvular heart disease, but the mechanisms by which these factors predispose to AF are not fully understood.[1,4,10-12]
- AF, like any tachyarrhythmia, needs a "trigger factor" for initiation and a "substrate" for its maintenance.[4]
- Trigger factors could be excessive sympathetic or parasympathetic stimulation, premature beats, and acute stretching of atria.[12]
- Structural heart diseases along with aging and other genetic and inflammatory processes cause atrial remodeling, dilation, and fibrosis, which make an electroanatomical substrate that further sustains AF.[1,4,10-12]
- Atrial dilation has "cause" and "effect" phenomenas on AF. Atrial dilation can cause AF, but at the same time AF can cause atrial dilation through increasing compliance and loss of atrial contraction.[12]
- When AF persists, it decreases the atrial refractory period and further perpetuates AF-AF, which begets AF.[13]
- The precise electrophysiological (EP) properties of AF are complicated; however, the focal mechanism and the multiple wavelet hypothesis are most commonly used to describe the EP mechanisms for AF.[1,4]

ETIOLOGY AND RISK FACTORS

- AF is common in patients with structural heart disease. Heart conditions associated with AF are valvular heart disease, especially of the mitral valve; heart failure; CAD; HTN (mostly when associated with left ventricular hypertrophy, LVH); cardiomyopathies (hypertrophic, dilated, and restrictive); congenital heart disease, especially atrial septal defect.[1]
- Other cardiac causes are cardiac tumors and pulmonary HTN.
- Wolf-Parkinson-White (WPW) syndrome has also been associated with AF, and careful attention must be paid to the management of this combination (**Figure 42-2**).

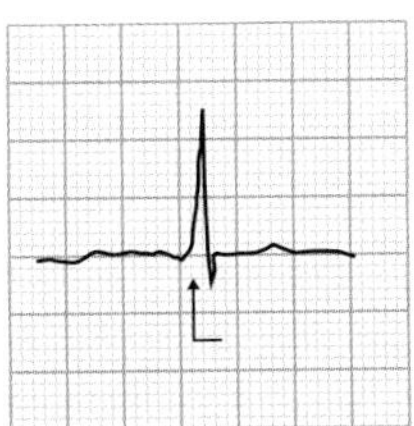

FIGURE 42-2 A delta wave pathognomonic of Wolf-Parkinson-White (WPW) syndrome, caused by early depolarization of the left ventricle from an accessory pathway (bundle of Kent) that bypasses normal physiological delay of the atrioventricular (AV) node. Most patients with WPW syndrome do not have other structural problems with their heart. *(Reproduced with permission from Gary Ferenchick, MD.)*

- There is also a familial form of AF without any underlying cardiomyopathy, but the underlying pathophysiological or molecular defects and transmission are unknown.[1,4]
- Obesity and sleep apnea are the other medical conditions associated with AF.[1]
- Autonomic influences have also been implicated in the initiation of AF (vagally mediated AF and adrenergically induced AF).[1,4]

DIAGNOSIS

HISTORY/PHYSICAL EXAMINATION

- AF can be asymptomatic or symptomatic.
- Symptoms are usually caused by RVR; the most common ones are palpitations, dizziness, lightheadedness, and fatigue.
- Complications of AF such as an embolic stroke or heart failure and the ensuing symptoms can sometimes be the first presentation of AF.
- A history inquiring about precipitating factors and underlying diseases should be obtained, and a complete cardiovascular examination should be performed (**Table 42-2**).

INITIAL DIAGNOSIS

- The initial workup and management process for AF is shown in **Figure 42-3**.
- AF is an ECG diagnosis and can be detected by a single-lead ECG, Holter monitor, or loop recorder.
- The diagnostic criteria for AF based on an ECG require the absence of a distinct p wave and the presence of irregularly irregular RR intervals (**Figure 42-4**); sometimes f waves (fibrillatory or oscillating waves) are present that vary continuously in amplitude/morphology and intervals.[1,4]
- The ECG will also help to identify any LVH, bundle branch block, left atrial (LA) enlargement, or WPW syndrome (abnormalities associated with AF).

DIFFERENTIAL DIAGNOSIS

- The diagnoses of AF can be challenging; AF can be confused with multifocal atrial tachycardia, a form of atrial tachycardia for which usually 3 forms of p waves are present, and p waves are separated by an isoelectric baseline in 1 or more ECG leads.
- AF is commonly associated with atrial flutter (**Figure 42-5**), which is usually regular and often has a classic 'sawtooth' pattern of regular flutter waves on the ECG, mostly the inferior leads.[1]
- Other differentials include atrial tachycardia and supraventricular tachycardia; however, these rhythms are commonly regular.

FURTHER TESTING

- All patients diagnosed with first-detected AF should undergo a transthoracic echocardiogram to assess LA size, left ventricular (LV) function, dimensions, and thickness and to exclude other cardiac conditions.[1,4] Additional workup may sometimes include chest X-ray to rule out any pulmonary causes (**Table 42-2**).
- Transesophageal echo (TEE) is rarely needed for initial workup, although it is used to guide cardioversion (CV) and is also helpful in identifying LA thrombus.

TABLE 42-2 Diagnostic Evaluation of Atrial Fibrillation (AF)

Initial Tests
• History and physical examination   ∘ Onset, duration, frequency, type of AF, associated symptoms, underlying cardiac or reversible conditions • Electrocardiogram • Transthoracic echocardiogram • Renal, hepatic, and thyroid function tests
Additional Tests
• Transesophageal echocardiogram • Chest X-ray • Exercise testing • Holter or implantable loop recorder monitoring • Additional blood tests such as evaluation of alcohol level, digoxin level (if the patient is on digoxin), hemoglobin A_{1c} (ruling out diabetes mellitus)

From Fuster V, Rydén LE, Cannom DS, et al. 2011 ACCF/AHA/HRS focused updates incorporated into the ACC/AHA/ESC 2006 Guidelines for the management of patients with atrial fibrillation: a report of the American College of Cardiology Foundation/American Heart Association Task Force on Practice Guidelines developed in partnership with the European Society of Cardiology and in collaboration with the European Heart Rhythm Association and the Heart Rhythm Society. *J Am Coll Cardiol*. 2011;57:e101-e198.

- Exercise tests or a stress test are not usually indicated but can be used to determine adequacy of rate control, especially in patients with permanent AF.[1,4]
- Sometimes a prolonged period of monitoring with an implantable loop recorder or ambulatory ECG is needed to diagnose asymptomatic AF, especially in patients with cryptogenic stroke.[1,4]
- An EP study is used only in rare scenarios, for which AF is a consequence of reentry tachycardia or WPW syndrome (detection of delta waves in ECG in a syncope patient should always prompt an EP study to rule out WPW syndrome).[1,4]
- Cardiac markers, both atrial natriuretic peptide (produced primarily in the atrium) and B-type natriuretic peptide (produced in the ventricle), are sometimes associated with AF.[1]

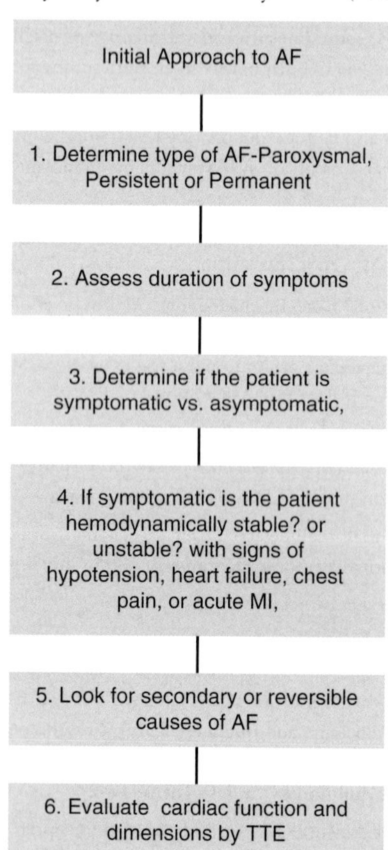

FIGURE 42-3 Initial workup and management of atrial fibrillation.[1-3]

MANAGEMENT

- The treatment of AF has 3 main objectives:
  1. Rate Control
  2. Rhythm control or restoration of normal sinus rhythm
  3. Anticoagulation or prevention of thromboembolism
- Goals of AF management should be directed to
  - Prevention of stroke
  - Treatment of AF rate-related consequences
  - Prevention of AF-related cardiac dysfunction
- **Figures 42-6** and **42-7** present approaches to acute and recurrent AF, respectively.

Rate control involves the following:

- Tachycardia in AF can cause rate-related ischemia and worsening hemodynamics and intraventricular conduction.[1]
- Current guidelines recommend achieving a lenient heart rate control of less than 110 beats/min at rest in patients with persistent AF or permanent AF with no symptoms and with no LV dysfunction; however, patients need close monitoring of LV function to prevent tachycardia-induced cardiomyopathy.[6,14]
- Criteria for rate control vary with age, and sometimes stress testing is indicated for assessing adequacy of rate control, especially in patients with permanent AF who have symptoms at appropriate rate control.[1,4]
- Medications for rate control
  - β-Blockers
    - β-Blockers are usually preferred in acute settings, especially in high-adrenergic situations (postoperatively) and for exercise-induced tachycardia.

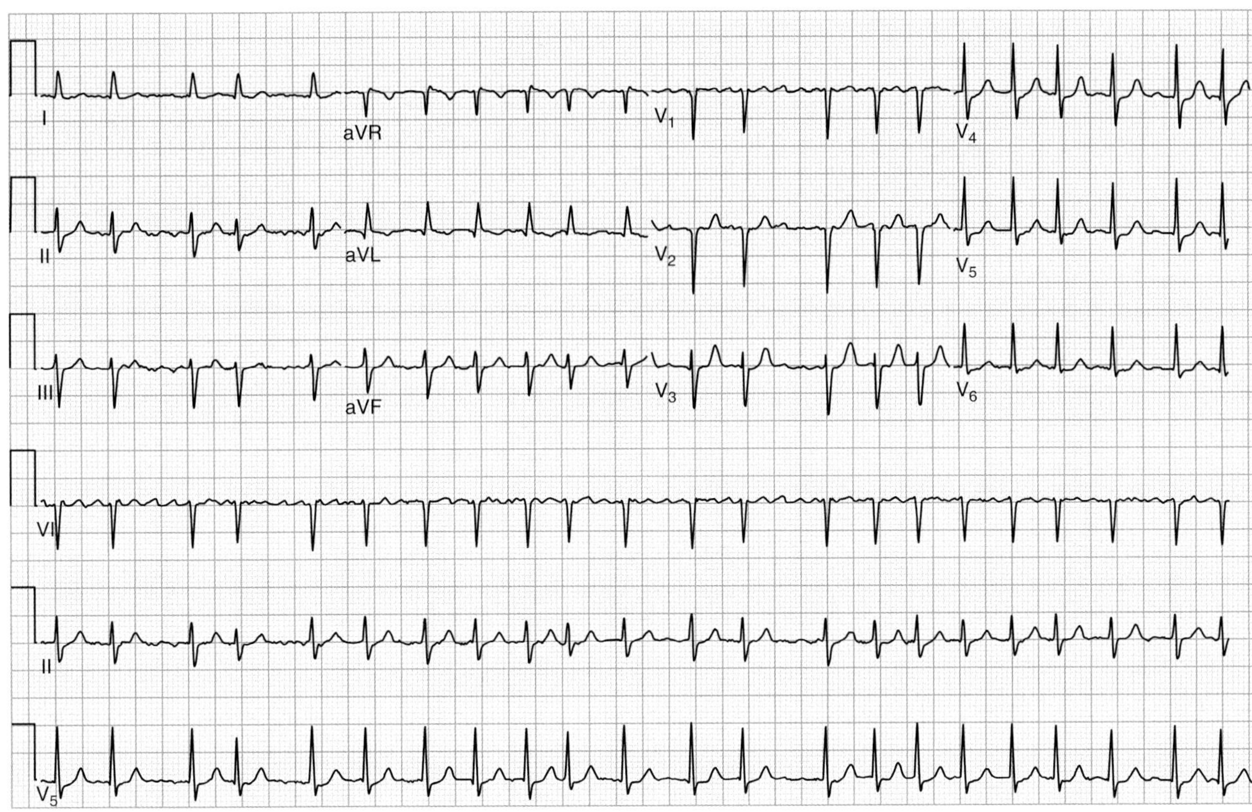

FIGURE 42-4 A 12-lead electrocardiogram demonstrating atrial fibrillation with a rapid ventricular response. Note the absence of p waves and an irregularly irregular rhythm. (*Reproduced with permission from Gary Ferenchick, MD.*)

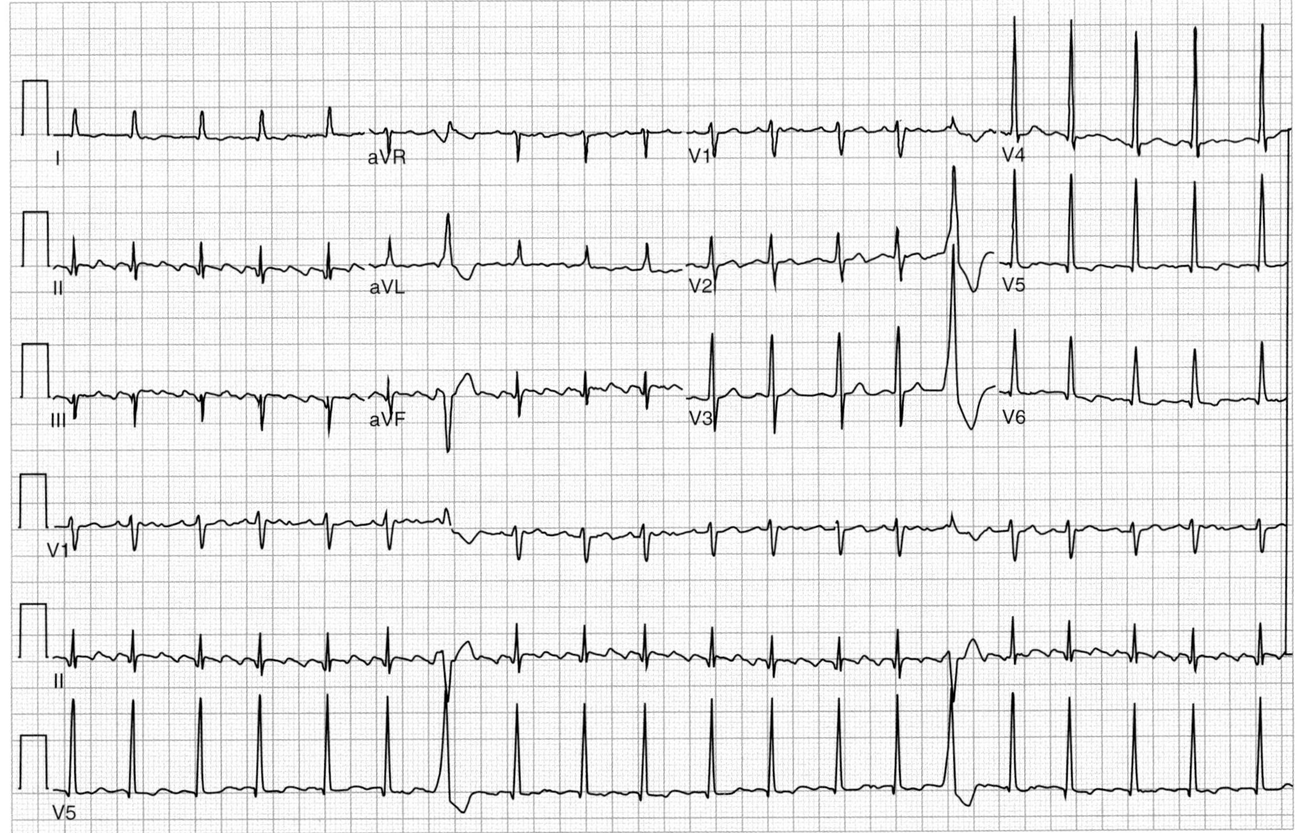

FIGURE 42-5 A 12-lead electrocardiogram demonstrating atrial flutter with an occasional premature ventricular contraction (PVC). In lead II of the rhythm strip, note the classic "sawtooth" pattern of the f or flutter waves. In this ECG, 2 f waves exist for every transmitted beat. (*Reproduced with permission from Gary Ferenchick, MD.*)

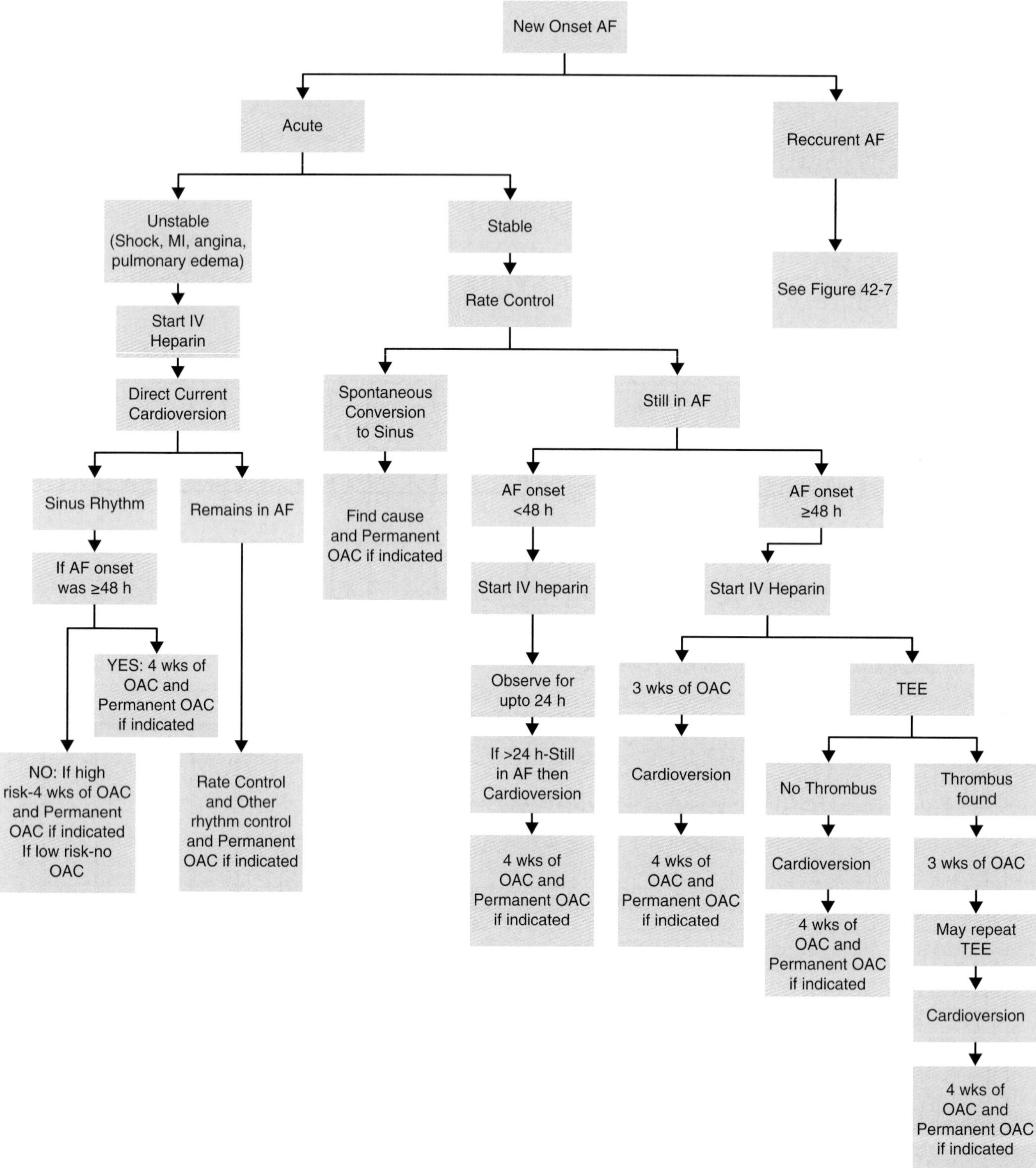

FIGURE 42-6 Approach to acute (new-onset) atrial fibrillation.

- Sotalol has shown excellent heart rate control when used to maintain sinus rhythm; however, it should not be used solely for heart rate control.[4]
  - Calcium channel blockers (CCBs)
    - Nondihydropyridine CCBs (verapamil and diltiazem) are equally effective rate control agents but should not be used in heart failure (systolic heart failure) because of their negative inotropic effects.[1]
  - Digoxin
    - Digoxin, which works via a vagotonic effect on the atrioventricular (AV) node, is less likely to be helpful in AF with high sympathetic tone and is not the first-line agent for rate control.[1]
    - Combinations of digoxin with β-blockers or CCBs are a reasonable choice to achieve adequate heart rate per ACC/AHA guidelines.[1] SOR B

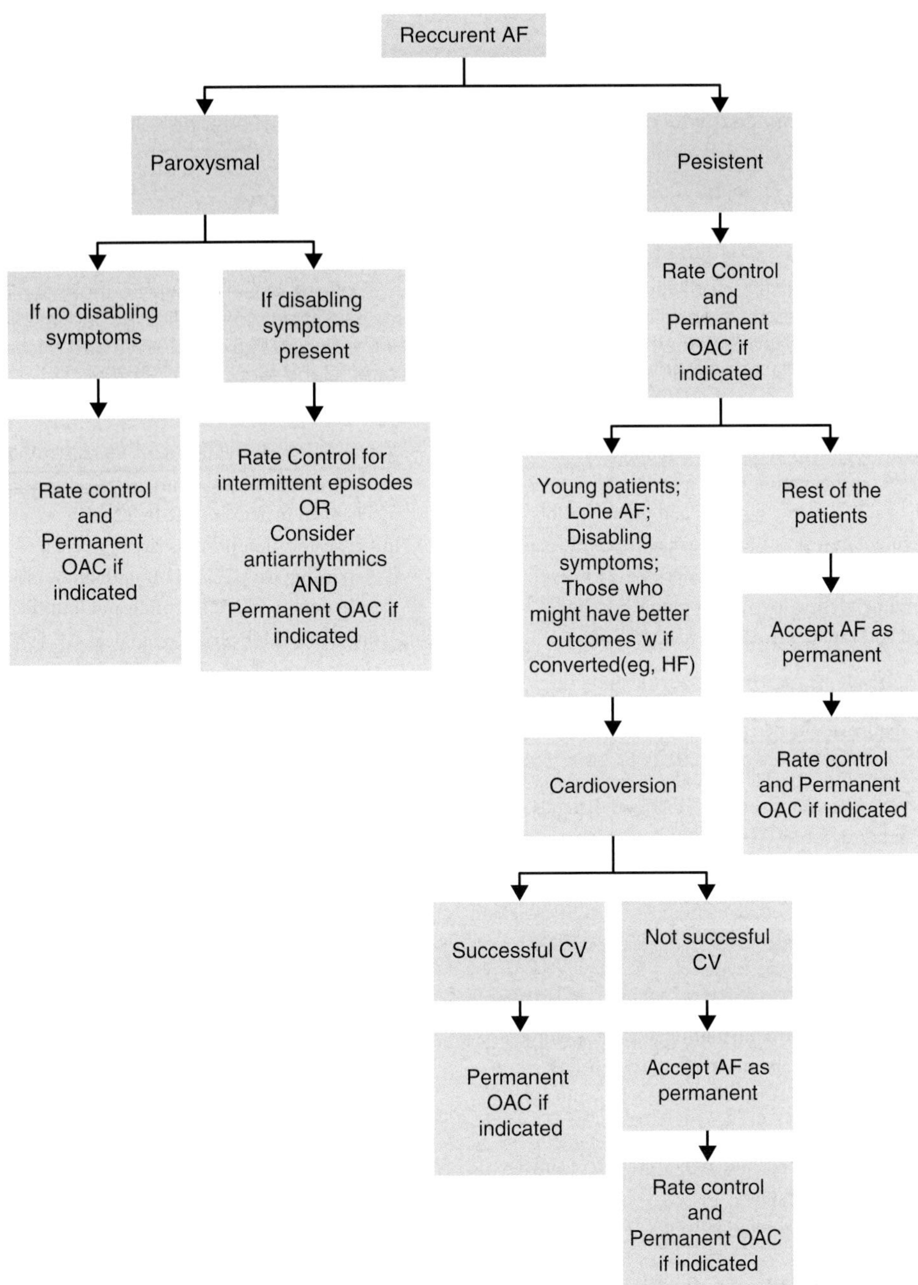

FIGURE 42-7 Approach to recurrent atrial fibrillation.

   - However, digoxin or amiodarone are recommended in AF with heart failure without an accessory pathway per ACC/AHA/ESC guidelines.[1] SOR B
  - Antiarrhythmic medications as rate control medications
    - Amiodarone is another medication that can be used for rate control if all other measures are unsuccessful; however, in view of the severe adverse effects, potential benefit must be weighed carefully against severe toxicity.[1] SOR C
- Other methods for rate control
  - AV node ablation and pacemaker placement
    - Drugs are usually the primary choice for rate control, but sometimes in patients who failed rate control with conventional medications or have tachycardia-induced cardiomyopathy, AV nodal ablation can be of benefit.[1,4]
    - AV node ablation needs to be followed by permanent pacemaker implantation. Anticoagulation is required for all patients who had AV node ablation depending on their risk score.[1]
  - Pacemaker without AV node ablation
    - In patients with AF and tachycardia-bradycardia syndrome, when rate control medications cause significant bradycardia, pacemakers are preferred.[1]
  - Rate control in WPW syndrome and preexcitation syndrome
    - AF with WPW syndrome can cause uncontrolled ventricular rate, ventricular fibrillation, and hypotension and shock; hence, common rate-limiting medications such as β-blockers and CCBs are contraindicated.[1,4]
    - Immediate direct current (DC) CV should be used for rate control in all AF patients with a preexcitation pathway and with

TABLE 42-3 Choosing Rate Control Drugs

AF Type	Drug Choice	Recommendation
Atrial fibrillation without accessory pathway or congestive heart failure (CHF)	β-Blockers/calcium channel blockers	Class I B
AF without accessory pathway with CHF	Digoxin/amiodarone	Class I B

From Fuster V, Rydén LE, Cannom DS, et al. 2011 ACCF/AHA/HRS focused updates incorporated into the ACC/AHA/ESC 2006 Guidelines for the management of patients with atrial fibrillation: a report of the American College of Cardiology Foundation/American Heart Association Task Force on Practice Guidelines developed in partnership with the European Society of Cardiology and in collaboration with the European Heart Rhythm Association and the Heart Rhythm Society. *J Am Coll Cardiol.* 2011;57:e101-e198 and Michelena HI, Powell BD, Brady PA, Friedman PA, Ezekowitz MD. Gender in atrial fibrillation: ten years later. *Gend Med.* 2010;7(3):206-217.

uncontrolled heart rate and hemodynamic instability[1] (level of evidence B, class of recommendation I).

- In hemodynamically stable patients with AF and preexcitation, per recent ACC/AHA guidelines, procainamide may be considered if electrical CV is not necessary[1] (level of evidence B). However, there is a weak recommendation for amiodarone if AF cannot be converted or ablated and rate control is needed[1] SOR C (**Table 42-3**).
- The definitive treatment remains the same: radiofrequency catheter ablation of the abnormal electric pathway.[1] SOR B

Rhythm Control

- Rhythm control is done to restore sinus rhythm in AF and depends on the patient's symptoms and duration of AF. Note that, irrespective of the rhythm control strategy, the rate should still be controlled and the need for anticoagulation be determined concurrently.
- CV (ie, converting AF to sinus rhythm) can be done both electively and emergently.
- Emergent CV is usually done in patients who are hemodynamically unstable and when arrhythmia is major contributing factor for worsening heart failure or chest pain or for ischemia in acute myocardial infarction.[1]
- Pharmacological CV
  - Pharmacological therapy entails 2 steps: initial restoration of sinus rhythm and maintenance of sinus rhythm.
  - New-onset AF has a high chance of spontaneous CV in 24-48 hours.[1,4]
  - The likelihood of spontaneous restoration to sinus rhythm decreases as the duration of AF increases, especially after 7 days. Thus, a pharmacological approach seems to be most efficacious if administered within 7 days of onset.[1]
  - According to the widely used Vaughan Williams classification,[15] antiarrhythmic medications are divided according to their primary mechanism of action (**Table 42-4**).
  - Initial restoration of sinus rhythm or CV
    - According to ACC/AHA guidelines, class Ic agents (flecainide and propafenone) and dofetilide and ibutilide (class III agents) are recommended for pharmacological CV SOR A for AF with a duration up to 7 days.[1] Flecainide and propafenone are contraindicated in patients with structural heart disease, CAD, or LV dysfunction.[1,4]
    - When AF has a duration of more than 7 days, dofetilide is usually recommended SOR A ahead of amiodarone and ibutilide.[1] SOR A
    - Amiodarone is recommended for AF duration of up to 7 days and more than 7 days SOR A; however, it is the drug of choice in patients with structural heart disease and LV dysfunction.[1,4]
    - Procainamide (class Ia antiarrhythmic agent) has been shown to be beneficial over placebo for conversion of AF with onset within 24 hours, but because of adverse effects, it has gone out of favor.[1]
    - β-Blockers and CCBs are used mainly for rate control, and there are no proven studies about the benefits of CV other than rate control; sotalol and digoxin should not be used for CV.[1,4]
  - Maintenance of sinus rhythm (**Table 42-5**)
    - Maintenance of the rhythm is an important consideration in patients after restoring sinus rhythm. The choice of drug is determined by the presence or absence of heart conditions.
    - Sotalol is the agent used only for maintenance of sinus rhythm rather than initial CV.[1]
    - Amiodarone is more effective than class I drugs, sotalol, or placebo in maintenance of sinus rhythm in patients with paroxysmal

TABLE 42-4 Classes of Antiarrhythmic Drugs

Class I—Sodium channel membrane-stabilizing medications
- Ia (disopyramide, procainamide, quinidine)
- Ib (lidocaine, mexiletine)
- Ic (flecainide, propafenone) depending on association and dissociation of sodium channel block, affecting length of action potential

Class II—β-Blockers
Class III—Potassium channel blockers (amiodarone, dronedarone, dofetilide, ibutilide, and bretylium)
Class IV—Calcium channel blockers (nondihydropyridine group)

From Vaughan Williams EM. A classification of antiarrhythmic actions reassessed after a decade of new drugs. *J Clin Pharmacol.* 1984;24:129-147.

TABLE 42-5 Choice of Antiarrhythmics to Maintain Sinus Rhythm

Health Status	Antiarrhythmics	Next-Line Agents
No heart disease (no CAD /HTN/heart failure)	Dronedarone, flecainide, propafenone, sotalol	Amiodarone, dofetilide
HTN		
• Without LVH	Dronedarone, flecainide, propafenone, sotalol	Amiodarone, dofetilide
• With LVH	Amiodarone	
CAD	Dronedarone, sotalol, dofetilide	Amiodarone
Heart failure	Amiodarone, dofetilide	

CAD, coronary artery disease; HTN, hypertension; LVH, left ventricular hypertrophy.
From Fuster V, Rydén LE, Cannom DS, et al. 2011 ACCF/AHA/HRS focused updates incorporated into the ACC/AHA/ESC 2006 Guidelines for the management of patients with atrial fibrillation: a report of the American College of Cardiology Foundation/American Heart Association Task Force on Practice Guidelines developed in partnership with the European Society of Cardiology and in collaboration with the European Heart Rhythm Association and the Heart Rhythm Society. *J Am Coll Cardiol.* 2011;57:e101-198; European Heart Rhythm Association, European Association for Cardio-Thoracic Surgery, Camm AJ, et al. Guidelines for the management of atrial fibrillation: the Task Force for the Management of Atrial Fibrillation of the European Society of Cardiology (ESC). *Eur Heart J.* 2010;31:2369-2429; and Wann LS, Curtis AB, January CT, et al. 2011 ACCF/AHA/HRS focused update on the management of patients with atrial fibrillation (updating the 2006 guideline): a report of the American College of Cardiology Foundation/American Heart Association Task Force on practice guidelines. *Circulation.* 2011;123:104-123.

or persistent AF refractory to other drugs.[1,16] But, because of serious adverse effects, it is less preferred than class Ic drugs in patients without any structural heart disease, LVH, or LV dysfunction.

- Dronedarone has similar EP properties as amiodarone, but it has a shorter half-life without the iodine moiety and has fewer side effects than amiodarone; however, dronedarone should not be used in class IV heart failure, class II-IV heart failure with recent decompensation or decreased LV systolic function (ejection fraction ≤ 35%), and it is absolutely contraindicated in permanent AF.[6,17]
- Promising results are being reported from trials of newer antiarrhythmic medications vernakalant, ranolazine, and tedisamil.[1]

- Nonpharmacological CV
  - DC cardioversion
    - DC CV involves delivery of electrical shock at the R wave of the ECG, synchronizing with intrinsic heart activity. This is different from defibrillation, in which asynchronous discharge of electric current is given.
    - DC CV can be performed both electively and emergently. This should be the primary method of CV in all hemodynamically unstable patients; in patients who failed to respond to pharmacological measures and are deemed unstable with ongoing myocardial infarction, symptomatic angina, or symptomatic heart failure; and in patients with preexcitation syndrome.[1] SOR Ⓐ
    - However, DC CV can also be an option in hemodynamically stable patients when symptoms of AF are unacceptable to the patient.
    - Pretreatment with antiarrhythmics can be useful, especially in patients who relapsed after an initial DC CV.[1]
    - Digitalis toxicity should be ruled out prior to attempting electrical CV.
    - Predictors for successful CV are in similar to those for pharmacological CV: younger patients, short duration of AF, and smaller LA size.[18]
  - Ablation
    - Surgical ablation—A surgical approach via a maze procedure is based on the hypothesis that reentry is the primary mechanism of AF, and incisions in the atrium can impede the conduction and stop sustained AF.[1,4] Despite the highly successful rate in patients undergoing mitral valve surgery, the need for cardiopulmonary bypass has prevented its widespread use.[1]
    - Catheter ablation
      - Uses either radiofrequency energy or freezing to ablate the foci of AF triggers to disconnect the pulmonary vein trigger and the atrial substrate.[1,4]
      - Has shown more potential recently, especially in a selective group of patients, hence there are updated guidelines and recommendations with caveats[6] (**Table 42-6**).

Anticoagulation/thromboembolism prevention

- Anticoagulation to reduce stroke should be considered in all AF patients irrespective of the rate or rhythm control strategy used for treatment of AF.
- Stroke risk assessment and scores
  - Many stroke risk classification schemes were developed to assess the risk of stroke and predictive factors.
  - The $CHADS_2$ score developed by Gage et al to assess the need for antithrombotics for nonrheumatic (nonvalvular) AF is the simplest and most widely used stroke risk assessment score[9] (**Table 42-7**).
  - Recommendations for OAC are based on the score attained by the patient on the $CHADS_2$ score, which predicts their risk of thromboembolism or stroke. Permanent oral anticoagulation (OAC) is recommended in those with a score of 2 or greater, while a score of 1 may be treated with aspirin or OAC19 (**Table 42-8**).
  - To further complement this score and to include additional stroke risk modifiers especially at the lower end of the risk stratum of CHADS2, European researchers developed the CHA2DS2-VASc score (**Table 42-9**).
  - Both $CHADS_2$ and CHA_2DS_2-VASc scores are only applicable for nonvalvular AF.

TABLE 42-6 Updated Guidelines Regarding Ablation

Type of Atrial Fibrillation (AF)	Prerequisites	Recommendation
Symptomatic paroxysmal	1. Failed at least one antiarrhythmic medication 2. Normal or mildly dilated left atrium 3. Normal or mildly reduced left ventricular function 4. No severe pulmonary disease 5. Experienced centers (≥50 cases/year)	Class I, level of evidence A
Symptomatic paroxysmal	With significant structural heart disease	Class IIb, level of evidence A
Symptomatic persistent	Failed at least one antiarrhythmic medication	Class IIa, level of evidence A

From Wann LS, Curtis AB, January CT, et al. 2011 ACCF/AHA/HRS focused update on the management of patients with atrial fibrillation (updating the 2006 guideline): a report of the American College of Cardiology Foundation/American Heart Association Task Force on practice guidelines. *Circulation*. 2011;123:104-123.

  - However, ACC/AHA recommend using "stroke risk factors" and the following risk factor stratification to anticoagulate patients with AF (**Tables 42-10** and **42-11**):
- Anticoagulation in patients undergoing CV
  - Thrombus formation depends on the duration of AF. Hence, anticoagulation recommendations for CV are divided according to duration of AF.
  - For AF of 48 hours or more
    - Any AF, if onset or duration is unknown or indeterminate, should be presumed as AF of 48 hours or longer.
    - Per ACC/AHA/ESC guidelines, anticoagulation is recommended for at least 3 weeks prior to and 4 weeks after elective electrical or chemical CV.[1]
    - If CV is needed for hemodynamically unstable patients, heparin should be administered prior to CV, and anticoagulation should be continued for 4 weeks after CV.[1,4]
    - After 4 weeks of anticoagulation post-CV, the decision to continue anticoagulation should be based on stroke risk scores mentioned previously.
    - TEE-based approach—For patients with AF of greater than 48-hour duration, instead of giving 3 weeks of anticoagulation prior to DC CV (conventional method), TEE can be used to rule out a thrombus in the LA or left atrial appendage, and immediate CV can be performed followed by 4 weeks of OAC.[1,4,21] Note that heparin should be given intravenously prior to CV.
    - If TEE shows a thrombus, then CV should be aborted, OAC should be given for at least 3 weeks, and then CV should be attempted.[1,21]
  - AF of duration less than 48 hours
    - For patients with AF duration less than 48 hours who are hemodynamically unstable (acute myocardial infarction, worsening angina, hypotension, heart failure), CV could be performed immediately without delaying for anticoagulation. SOR C
    - The need for anticoagulation before and after CV in patients with AF onset less than 48 hours may be based on a patient's risk score for thromboembolism.[1] SOR C However, most experts in clinical practice suggest the heparin intravenously in preparation for CV and then 4 weeks of OAC after CV.
- Medications for anticoagulation/antithrombotics
  - Warfarin
    - Warfarin is a potent oral vitamin K antagonist (VKA) used for anticoagulation.

TABLE 42-7 $CHADS_2$ Scoring

Clinical Parameter	Points
C—Congestive heart failure	1
H—History of hypertension	1
A—Age 75 or older	1
D—Diabetes mellitus	1
S_2—History of transient ischemic attack or prior ischemic stroke or systemic embolism	2

Data from Fuster V, Rydén LE, Cannom DS, et al. 2011 ACCF/AHA/HRS focused updates incorporated into the ACC/AHA/ESC 2006 Guidelines for the management of patients with atrial fibrillation: a report of the American College of Cardiology Foundation/American Heart Association Task Force on Practice Guidelines developed in partnership with the European Society of Cardiology and in collaboration with the European Heart Rhythm Association and the Heart Rhythm Society. *J Am Coll Cardiol*. 2011;57:e101-e198 and European Heart Rhythm Association, European Association for Cardio-Thoracic Surgery, Camm AJ, et al. Guidelines for the management of atrial fibrillation: the Task Force for the Management of Atrial Fibrillation of the European Society of Cardiology (ESC). *Eur Heart J*. 2010;31:2369-2429.

TABLE 42-8 Recommendations for Oral Anticoagulation (OAC) Based on $CHADS_2$ Scoring System

$CHADS_2$ Score	Recommendation
0	No OAC needed, but aspirin may be used
1	OAC preferred, aspirin may be substituted
≥2	OAC

From Guyatt GH, Akl EA, Crowther M, et al. Antithrombotic therapy and prevention of thrombosis, 9th ed: American College of Chest Physicians evidence-based clinical practice guidelines. *Chest*. 2012;141(2)(suppl):7S-47S.

TABLE 42-9 CHA_2DS_2-VASc Scoring

Clinical Parameter	Points
C—Congestive heart failure	1
H—History of hypertension	1
A_2—Age 75 or older	2
D—Diabetes mellitus	1
S_2—Two points for history of transient ischemic attack or prior stroke or systemic embolism	2
V—Vascular disease (old myocardial infarction, peripheral artery disease, or aortic plaque)	1
A—One point for age 65-74	1
Sc—Sex category—1 point for female gender	1

From European Heart Rhythm Association, European Association for Cardio-Thoracic Surgery, Camm AJ, et al. Guidelines for the management of atrial fibrillation: the Task Force for the Management of Atrial Fibrillation of the European Society of Cardiology (ESC). *Eur Heart J.* 2010;31:2369-2429 and Lip GY, Nieuwlaat R, Pisters R, Lane DA, Crijns HJ. Refining clinical risk stratification for predicting stroke and thromboembolism in atrial fibrillation using a novel risk factor-based approach: the euro heart survey on atrial fibrillation. *Chest.* 2010;137(2):263-272.

TABLE 42-10 ACC/AHA Stroke Risk Factor Classification

High-risk factors
1. Previous transient ischemic attack, stroke, or thrombus, or embolism
2. Mitral valve stenosis
3. Prosthetic heart valve

Moderate risk factors
1. Age ≥75
2. HTN
3. Heart failure
4. Cardiomyopathy, LV EF ≤35
5. DM

Weaker risk factors
1. Female gender
2. Age 65-74

From Fuster V, Rydén LE, Cannom DS, et al. 2011 ACCF/AHA/HRS focused updates incorporated into the ACC/AHA/ESC 2006 Guidelines for the management of patients with atrial fibrillation: a report of the American College of Cardiology Foundation/American Heart Association Task Force on Practice Guidelines developed in partnership with the European Society of Cardiology and in collaboration with the European Heart Rhythm Association and the Heart Rhythm Society. *J Am Coll Cardiol.* 2011;57:e101-e198.

    - ACC/AHA and ESC guidelines recommend use of oral VKA to target an international normalized ratio (INR) of 2 to 3 for stroke prevention in AF.[1,4]
    - Several studies have shown gross underutilization of OAC in AF patients, even in those with higher risk.[22]
    - Many factors play a role, particularly physicians' concern about bleeding in elderly patients and the need for frequent monitoring of INR, especially in noncompliant patients.
- Dabigatran
    - Newer anticoagulants without the need for frequent monitoring and variable dosing have emerged after extensive research (**Table 42-12**). These agents have a predictable effect with shorter half-lives, fixed dosing, fewer interactions, and rapid onset of action. Dabigatran, a direct thrombin inhibitor, is the first of the newer anticoagulants to become available for clinical use.[23,26]
    - Dabigatran is predominantly excreted by the kidneys; hence, caution is advised in patients with renal failure, and the dose should be adjusted.[19,23,26]
    - The new ACC, AHA, and Heart Rhythm Society focused update recommends dabigatran as an alternative for warfarin for stroke prevention in patients with AF without hemodynamically significant valvular disease, prosthetic valves, and severe renal and hepatic failure.[26] SOR B
    - In spite of some postmarket reports of increased bleeding risk that are under investigation, currently the Food and Drug Administration (FDA) guidelines recommend that when prescribed appropriately, the health benefits outweigh the risks of dabigatran in AF.[26]
- Rivaroxaban
    - Rivaroxaban is the first orally available direct factor Xa inhibitor approved by the FDA for stroke prevention in nonvalvular AF and

TABLE 42-11 ACC/AHA Recommendations for Oral Anticoagulation (OAC)

OAC Regime	Recommendation
1. OAC for any high risk or 2 or more moderate-risk factors	SOR A
2. Aspirin or OAC for 1 moderate-risk factor	SOR A
3. Aspirin or OAC for 1 or more less-validated risk factors, but patient's preference and bleeding risk should be assessed closely	SOR B
4. Aspirin only for no risk factors (but age 60-74 and lone atrial fibrillation excluded)	SOR A
5. Aspirin or no therapy for lone atrial fibrillation	SOR A

ACC/AHA recommendations from Fuster V, Rydén LE, Cannom DS, et al. 2011 ACCF/AHA/HRS focused updates incorporated into the ACC/AHA/ESC 2006 Guidelines for the management of patients with atrial fibrillation: a report of the American College of Cardiology Foundation/American Heart Association Task Force on Practice Guidelines developed in partnership with the European Society of Cardiology and in collaboration with the European Heart Rhythm Association and the Heart Rhythm Society. *J Am Coll Cardiol.* 2011;57:e101-e198.

TABLE 42-12 Newer Anticoagulants

Description	Anticoagulant		
	Dabigatran	Rivaroxaban	Apixaban
Type of drug	Direct thrombin inhibitor	Factor Xa inhibitor	Factor Xa inhibitor
Major trials	ReLY[23]	ROCKET-AF[24]	ARISTOTLE[25]
FDA approved for stroke prevention in nonvalvular AF	Yes	Yes	Yes
Other indications	VTE prevention in patients with knee replacement surgery (in Europe only)	VTE prevention in patients with knee or hip replacement surgery	N/A

AF, atrial fibrillation; FDA, Food and Drug Administration; VTE, venous thromboembolism.

for deep vein thrombosis prophylaxis for knee and hip replacement surgeries.[19,24,27] It is excreted by the kidneys and contraindicated in severe renal disease.[27]

- Apixaban
  - Apixaban is another factor Xa inhibitor that has shown promising results in recent studies.[25]
- Edoxaban
  - This is another factor X inhibitor currently under investigation.

FOLLOW-UP

- Regular follow-up is needed for patients treated for AF, and periodic ECG and Holter monitoring are needed, especially for those on rhythm control drugs.
- Patients with AF not on OAC should also be periodically reassessed for the need for OAC based on the development of new risk factors.
- Those on OAC therapy with VKA should be monitored with frequent assessment of INR levels.

PATIENT RESOURCES

- AF resources for patients—**http://www.a-fib.com/.**
- StopAfib.org—**http://www.stopafib.org/.**

PHYSICIAN RESOURCES

- Agency for Healthcare Research and Quality. *Antithrombotic Therapy for Atrial Fibrillation: American College of Chest Physicians Evidence-Based Clinical Practice Guidelines*—**http://www.guideline.gov/content.aspx?id=35270.**
- Wann LS, Curtis AB, January CT, et al. 2011 ACCF/AHA/HRS focused update on the management of patients with atrial fibrillation (updating the 2006 guideline). Circulation. 2011;123(1):104-123. **http://circ.ahajournals.org/content/123/1/104.full.**

REFERENCES

1. Fuster V, Rydén LE, Cannom DS, et al. 2011 ACCF/AHA/HRS focused updates incorporated into the ACC/AHA/ESC 2006 Guidelines for the management of patients with atrial fibrillation: a report of the American College of Cardiology Foundation/American Heart Association Task Force on Practice Guidelines developed in partnership with the European Society of Cardiology and in collaboration with the European Heart Rhythm Association and the Heart Rhythm Society. *J Am Coll Cardiol*. 2011;57:e101-e198.
2. Go AS, Hylek EM, Phillips KA, et al. Prevalence of diagnosed atrial fibrillation in adults: national implications for rhythm management and stroke prevention: the AnTicoagulation and Risk Factors in Atrial Fibrillation (ATRIA) Study. *JAMA*. 2001;285:2370-2375.
3. Friberg J, Buch P, Scharling H, et al. Rising rates of hospital admissions for atrial fibrillation. *Epidemiology*. 2003;14:666-672.
4. European Heart Rhythm Association, European Association for Cardio-Thoracic Surgery, Camm AJ, et al. Guidelines for the management of atrial fibrillation: the Task Force for the Management of Atrial Fibrillation of the European Society of Cardiology (ESC). *Eur Heart J*. 2010;31:2369-2429.
5. Miyasaka Y, Barnes ME, Gersh BJ, et al. Secular trends in incidence of atrial fibrillation in Olmsted County, Minnesota, 1980 to 2000, and implications on the projections for future prevalence. *Circulation*. 2006;114(2):119-125. Epub 2006 Jul 3.
6. Wann LS, Curtis AB, January CT, et al. 2011 ACCF/AHA/HRS focused update on the management of patients with atrial fibrillation (updating the 2006 guideline): a report of the American College of Cardiology Foundation/American Heart Association Task Force on practice guidelines. *Circulation*. 2011;123:104-123.
7. Wolf PA, Abbott RD, Kannel WB. Atrial fibrillation: a major contributor to stroke in elderly. The Framingham Study. *Arch Intern Med*. 1987;147:1561-1564.
8. Michelena HI, Powell BD, Brady PA, Friedman PA, Ezekowitz MD. Gender in atrial fibrillation: ten years later. *Gend Med*. 2010;7(3):206-217.
9. Wolf PA, Abbott RD, Kannel WB. Atrial fibrillation as an independent risk factor for stroke. The FraminghamStudy. *Stroke*. 1991;22:983-988.

10. Bailey GW, Braniff BA, Hancock EW, et al. Relation of left atrial pathology to atrial fibrillation in mitral valvular disease. *Ann Intern Med*. 1968;69:13-20.

11. Xu J, Cui G, Esmailian F, et al. Atrial extracellular matrix remodeling and the maintenance of atrial fibrillation. *Circulation*. 2004;109:363-368.

12. Allessie M, Ausma J, Schotten U. Electrical, contractile and structural remodeling during atrial fibrillation. *Cardiovasc Res*. 2002;54:230-246.

13. Lu Z, Scherlag BJ, Lin J, et al. Atrial fibrillation begets atrial fibrillation: autonomic mechanism for atrial electrical remodeling induced by short-term rapid atrial pacing. *Circ Arrhythm Electrophysiol*. 2008;1:184-192.

14. Van Gelder IC, Groenveld HF, Crijns HJ, et al. Lenient versus strict rate control in patients with atrial fibrillation. *N Engl J Med*. 2010;362:1363-1373.

15. Vaughan Williams EM. A classification of antiarrhythmic actions reassessed after a decade of new drugs. *J Clin Pharmacol*. 1984;24:129-147.

16. Naccarelli GV, Wolbrette DL, Khan M, et al. Old and new antiarrhythmic drugs for converting and maintaining sinus rhythm in atrial fibrillation: comparative efficacy and results of trials. *Am J Cardiol*. 2003;91:15D-26D.

17. Connolly SJ, Camm AJ, Halperin JL, et al. Dronedarone in high-risk permanent atrial fibrillation. *N Engl J Med*. 2011;365(24):2268-2276. Epub 2011 Nov 14.

18. Frick M, Frykman V, Jensen-Urstad M, et al. Factors predicting success rate and recurrence of atrial fibrillation after first electrical cardioversion in patients with persistent atrial fibrillation. *Clin Cardiol*. 2001;24:238-244.

19. Guyatt GH, Akl EA, Crowther M, et al. Antithrombotic therapy and prevention of thrombosis, 9th ed: American College of Chest Physicians evidence-based clinical practice guidelines. *Chest*. 2012;141(2)(suppl):7S-47S.

20. Lip GY, Nieuwlaat R, Pisters R, Lane DA, Crijns HJ. Refining clinical risk stratification for predicting stroke and thromboembolism in atrial fibrillation using a novel risk factor-based approach: the euro heart survey on atrial fibrillation. *Chest*. 2010;137(2):263-272.

21. Asher CR, Klein AL; ACUTE trial. Transesophageal echocardiography to guide cardioversion in patients with atrial fibrillation: ACUTE trial update. *Card Electrophysiol Rev*. 2003 Dec;7(4):387-391.

22. Lopes RD, Shah BR, Olson DM, et al. Antithrombotic therapy use at discharge and 1 year in patients with atrial fibrillation and acute stroke: results from the AVAIL Registry. *Stroke*. 2011;42(12):3477-3483.

23. Connolly SJ, Ezekowitz MD, Yusuf S, et al. Dabigatran versus warfarin in patients with atrial fibrillation. *N Engl J Med*. 2009;361:1139-1151.

24. Patel MR, Mahaffey KW, Garg J, et al. Rivaroxaban versus warfarin in nonvalvular atrial fibrillation. *N Engl J Med*. 2011;365:883-891.

25. Granger CB, Alexander JH, McMurray JJ, et al. ARISTOTLE Committees and Investigators. Apixaban versus warfarin in patients with atrial fibrillation. *N Engl J Med*. 2011;365(11):981-992.

26. Wann LS, Curtis AB, Ellenbogen KA, et al. 2011 ACCF/AHA/HRS focused update on the management of patients with atrial fibrillation (update on dabigatran): a report of the American College of Cardiology Foundation/American Heart Association Task Force on practice guidelines. *J Am Coll Cardiol*. 2011;57(11):1330-1337.

27. Vande Griend JP, Marcum ZA, Linnebur SA. A year in review: new drugs for older adults in 2011. *Am J Geriatr Pharmacother*. 2012;10(4):258-263.

43 CLUBBING

Heidi Chumley, MD

PATIENT STORY

A 31-year-old man with congenital heart disease has had these clubbed fingers since his childhood (**Figures 43-1** and **43-2**). A close view of the fingers shows a widened club-like distal phalanx. He has learned to live with the limitations from his congenital heart disease and his fingers do not bother him at all.

INTRODUCTION

Clubbing is a physical examination finding first described by Hippocrates in 400 BC. Clubbing can be primary (pachydermoperiostosis or hypertrophic osteoarthropathy) or secondary (pulmonary, cardiac, or gastrointestinal [GI] disease or HIV). Diagnosis is clinical based on nail fold angles and phalangeal depth ratios. The treatment is to correct the underlying cause, after which clubbing may resolve.

SYNONYMS

Clubbing is also known as hippocratic nails or fingers, drumstick fingers.

EPIDEMIOLOGY

Prevalence in the general population is unknown:

- Two percent of adult patients admitted to a Welsh general medicine or surgery service.[1]

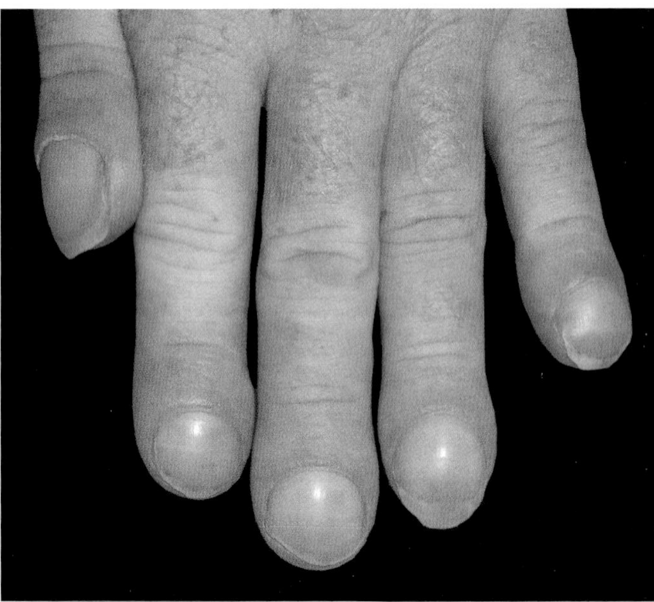

FIGURE 43-1 Clubbing of all the fingers in a 31-year-old man with congenital heart disease. Note the thickening around the proximal nail folds. (*Reproduced with permission from Richard P. Usatine, MD.*)

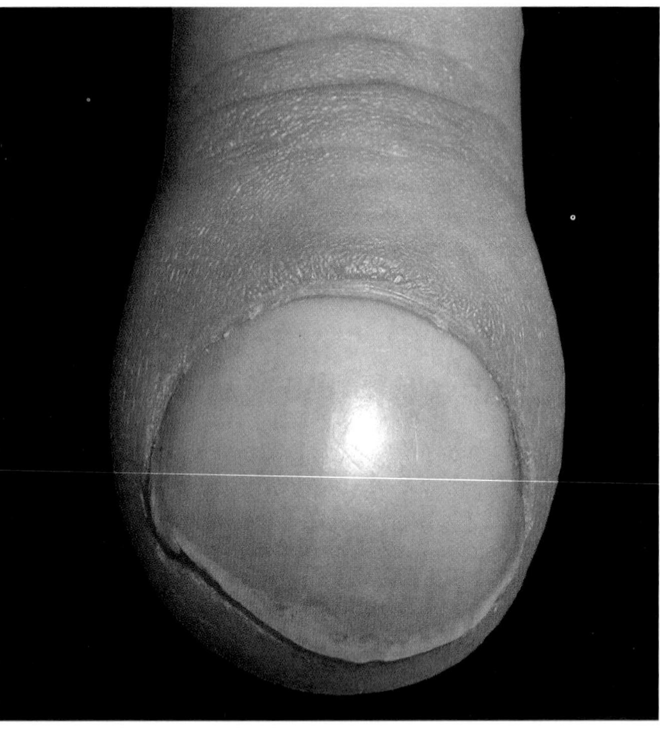

FIGURE 43-2 Close-up view of a clubbed finger. (*Reproduced with permission from Richard P. Usatine, MD.*)

- Thirty-eight percent and fifteen percent of patients deal with Crohn disease and ulcerative colitis, respectively.[2]
- Thirty-three percent and eleven percent of patients deal with lung cancer and chronic obstructive pulmonary disease (COPD), respectively.[3]

ETIOLOGY AND PATHOPHYSIOLOGY

- The etiology of clubbing is poorly understood.
- Increased connective tissue growth and angiogenesis in the nail bed result in the remodeling of the finger into a club shape.
- Current explanations include megakaryocyte release of platelet-activated growth factor, hypoxia, vasodilators in circulation, a neurocirculatory mechanism, and chronic activation of macrophages with production of profibrotic factors.[4]

RISK FACTORS

- Family history
- History of a disease associated with clubbing

DIAGNOSIS

CLINICAL FEATURES

- History of present illness: Gradual onset of painless enlargement at the ends of the fingers and toes
  - Family history suggests primary hypertrophic osteoarthropathy (HOA) or familial clubbing.

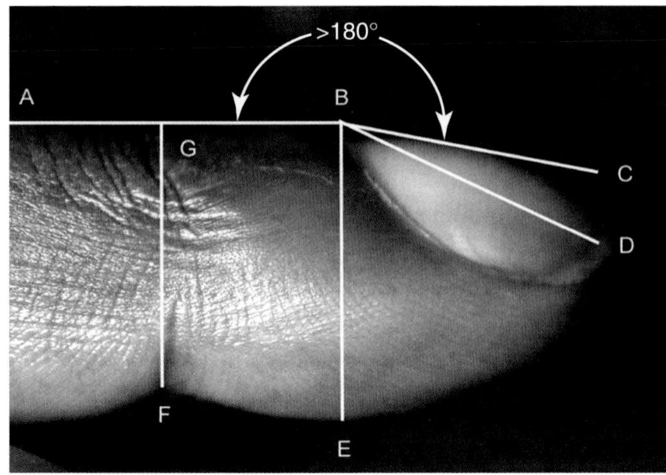

FIGURE 43-3 Clubbing of fingers in a 55-year-old man with chronic obstructive pulmonary disease (COPD). Abnormal profile angle (*ABC*) and hyponychial angle (*ABD*) are seen. Distal phalangeal depth (*BE*) is greater than interphalangeal depth (*GF*). (*Reproduced with permission from Richard P. Usatine, MD.*)

- Social history to identify exposure to asbestos, coal mine dust, and pigeons; tobacco use as risk factor for lung cancer; HIV, and tuberculosis risk factors.
- Review of systems: Constitutional, pulmonary, GI, and musculoskeletal symptoms for clues to an underlying disease[5]

PHYSICAL EXAMINATION

- Abnormal nail fold angles[6] (**Figure 43-3**).
  - Profile angle (*ABC*) greater than or equal to 180 degrees
  - Hyponychial (*ABD*) greater than or equal to 192 degrees
  - Phalangeal depth ratio (*BE:GF*) greater than or equal to 1[6] (see **Figure 43-3**)
- Schamroth sign, obliteration of the diamond shape, is normally created when dorsal surfaces of 2 corresponding fingers are opposed (**Figure 43-4**): LR+ (likelihood ratio) 7.60 to 8.40 and LR– 0.14 to 0.25.[7]

TYPICAL DISTRIBUTION

- Bilateral, involves all fingers and often toes
- Rarely unilateral or involves only one or some digits (consider neurologic or traumatic insult to extremity)

LABORATORY TESTING

Laboratory testing is useful to evaluate for secondary causes. Consider the following:

- HIV testing if risk factors present
- Complete blood count (CBC) and blood cultures if systemic symptoms (fever, night sweats, weight loss) are present
- Thyroid-stimulating hormone (TSH) or thyroxine (T_4) if exophthalmos or pretibial myxedema is present
- Liver function tests (LFTs), hepatitis serologies for right upper quadrant (RUQ) tenderness or jaundice

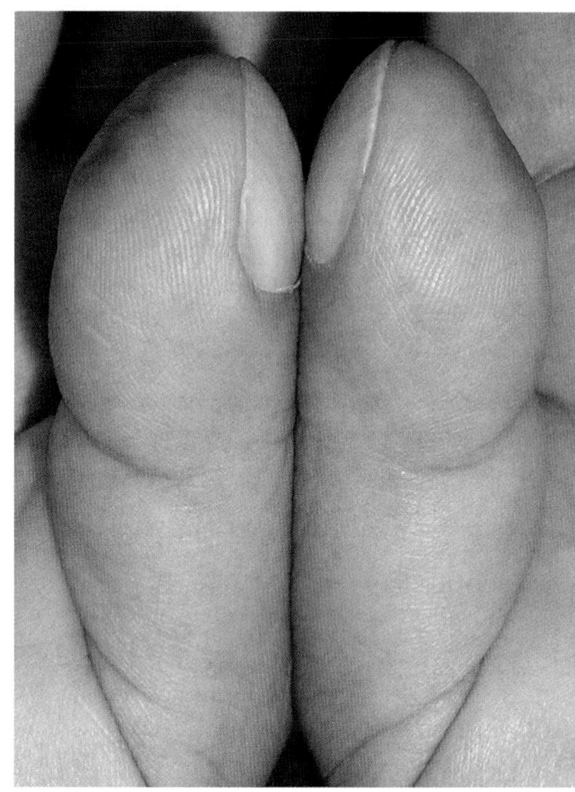

FIGURE 43-4 Schamroth sign. Loss of the normal diamond shape formed when right and left thumbs are opposed in a person with clubbing of the fingers. (*Reproduced with permission from Richard P. Usatine, MD.*)

IMAGING

- Screening chest radiograph if an underlying cause is not identified.
- Plain radiograph of the hand can distinguish clubbed from nonclubbed by measuring nail bed greater than or equal to 3 mm.[8]

DIFFERENTIAL DIAGNOSIS

PRIMARY CLUBBING

- Hypertrophic osteoarthropathy—Clubbing, periostosis, and arthritis or arthralgias
  - Primary HOA, also known as pachydermoperiostosis, is an autosomal dominant disorder.
  - Secondary HOA is often associated with pulmonary neoplasms.
- Familial clubbing, now thought to be an incomplete form of primary HOA

SECONDARY CLUBBING

Secondary clubbing can be caused by many conditions, including the following:[5]

- Pulmonary—Idiopathic pulmonary fibrosis, malignancy, asbestosis, COPD, and cystic fibrosis.
- Cardiac—Congenital heart disease, endocarditis, atrioventricular malformations, or fistulas.
- GI—Inflammatory bowel disease, cirrhosis, and celiac disease.
- HIV infection—Clubbing was found in 36% of patients with HIV in one study.[9]

MANAGEMENT

- Clubbing improves with the management of the underlying disease.[2]
- Evaluate patients without an obvious associated disease for lung cancer.[5] SOR C
- Evaluate patients with COPD and a phalangeal depth ratio greater than 1 for lung cancer.[3] (LR 3.9) SOR B

PROGNOSIS

Prognosis depends on the underlying process. Clubbing usually completely reverses after successful treatment of the underlying process.

FOLLOW-UP

Follow-up is dependent on the underlying disease process.

PATIENT EDUCATION

Clubbing may be secondary to many different types of diseases, some very serious.

PATIENT RESOURCES

- Medline Plus—**http://www.nlm.nih.gov/medlineplus/ency/article/003282.htm.**

PROVIDER RESOURCES

- Spicknall NE, Zirwas MJ, English JC. Provide an algorithm useful in identifying the underlying cause of clubbing.

REFERENCES

1. White HA, Alcolado R, Alcolado JC. Examination of the hands: an insight into the health of a Welsh population. *Postgrad Med J.* 2003;79(936):588-589.
2. Kitis G, Thompson H, Allan RN. Finger clubbing in inflammatory bowel disease: its prevalence and pathogenesis. *Br Med J.* 1979;2(6194):825-828.
3. Baughman RP, Gunther KL, Buchsbaum JA, Lower EE. Prevalence of digital clubbing in bronchogenic carcinoma by a new digital index. *Clin Exp Rheumatol.* 1998;16(1):21-26.
4. Toovy OT, Eisenhauer HJ. A new hypothesis on the mechanism of digital clubbing secondary to pulmonary pathologies. *Med Hypotheses.* 2010;759(6):511-513.
5. Spicknall NE, Zirwas MJ, English JC. Clubbing: an update on diagnosis, differential diagnosis, pathophysiology, and clinical relevance. *J Am Acad Dermatol.* 2005;52(6):1020-1028.
6. Myers KA, Farquhar DR. The rational clinical examination. Does this patient have clubbing [comment]? *JAMA.* 2001;286(3):341-347.
7. Pallares-Sanmartin A, Leiro-Fernandez V, Cebreiro TL, et al. Validity and reliability of the Schamroth sign for the diagnosis of clubbing. *JAMA.* 2010;304(2):159-161.
8. Moreira AL, Porto NS, Moreira JS, et al. Clubbed fingers: radiological evaluation of the nail bed thickness. *Clin Anat.* 2008;21(4):314-318.
9. Dever LL, Matta JS. Digital clubbing in HIV-infected patients: an observational study. *AIDS Patient Care STDS.* 2009;23(1):19-22.

44 HEART FAILURE

Heidi Chumley, MD

PATIENT STORY

A 60-year-old man presents to the emergency department with shortness of breath increasing in severity over the past several days, along with paroxysmal nocturnal dyspnea and orthopnea. He does not have a history of heart failure (HF) or previous myocardial infarction. On examination it was found that he had a third heart sound and an elevated jugular venous pressure. His chest radiograph showed cardiomegaly (**Figure 44-1**) and his B-type natriuretic peptide (BNP) was elevated at 600 pg/mL. He was diagnosed with heart failure, evaluated for underlying causes including coronary artery disease, and treated initially with an angiotensin-converting enzyme inhibitor (ACEI) and a diuretic. Later, he will be started on a β-blocker and an aldosterone inhibitor.

INTRODUCTION

Heart failure is common and increases with age. Multiple etiologies can cause the decrease in heart pumping capacity that leads to HF. ACEIs and β-blockers with or without aldosterone agonists and angiotensin II blockers are the main pharmacologic therapies.

SYNONYMS

HF is also known as congestive heart failure (CHF).

EPIDEMIOLOGY

- The prevalence of HF in the community increases with age: 0.7% (45-54 years), 1.3% (55-64 years), 1.5% (65-74 years), and 8.4% (75 years or older).[1]

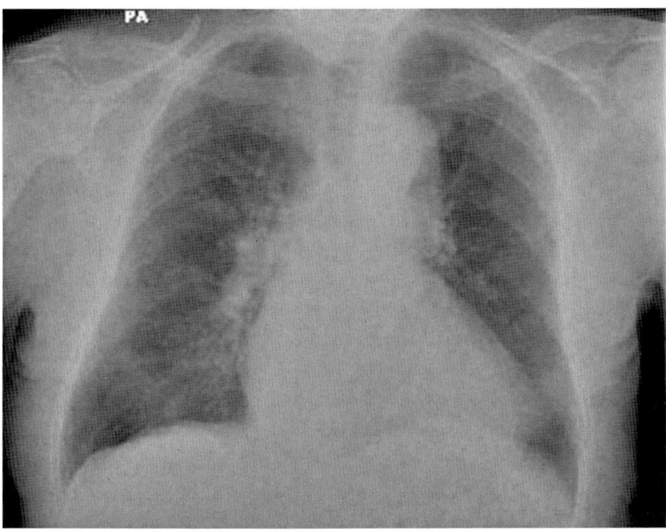

FIGURE 44-1 Cardiomegaly demonstrated in a posteroanterior (PA) view. The widest part of the heart is greater than 50% of the diameter of the chest. (*Reproduced with permission from Heidi Chumley, MD.*)

- More than 40% of patients in the community with HF have an ejection fraction greater than 50%.[1]
- At age 40 years, the lifetime risk for HF is 21% (95% confidence interval [CI] 18.7%-23.2%) for men and 20.3% (95% CI 18.2%-22.5%) for women.[2]

ETIOLOGY AND PATHOPHYSIOLOGY

- Heart pumping capacity declines from any cause (ie, myocardial infarction or ischemia, hypertension, valvular dysfunction, cardiomyopathy, or infections such as endocarditis or myocarditis).
- Cardiac dysfunction activates the adrenergic and renin-angiotensin-aldosterone systems.
- These systems provide short-term compensation, but chronic activation leads to myocardial remodeling and eventually worsening cardiac function.
- Norepinephrine, angiotensin II, aldosterone, and tissue necrosis factor each contributes to disease progression.
- Angiotensin II directly causes cell death through necrosis and apoptosis, as well as cardiac hypertrophy.

DIAGNOSIS

Many history, examination, radiography, electrocardiography (ECG), and laboratory features are helpful in making the diagnosis of HF for patients presenting with dyspnea in the emergency department.[3]

CLINICAL FEATURES

History and physical

- History of HF (likelihood ratio [LR+] = 5.8), myocardial infarction (LR+ = 3.1)[3]
- Symptoms of paroxysmal nocturnal dyspnea (LR+ = 2.6), orthopnea (LR+ = 2.2), edema (LR+ = 2.1)[3]
- Examination finding of third heart sound (LR+ = 11), hepatojugular reflex (LR+ = 6.4), jugular venous distention (LR+ = 5.1)[3]

LABORATORY AND ANCILLARY TESTING

- Laboratory value of BNP greater than or equal to 250 (LR+ = 4.6); BNP less than 100 decreases likelihood of HF.[3]
- ECG finding of atrial fibrillation (LR+ = 3.8), T-wave changes (LR+ = 3.0), any abnormality (LR+ = 2.2). A normal ECG lowers the likelihood (LR– = 0.640).[3]

IMAGING

Radiographic finding of pulmonary venous congestion (**Figure 44-2**) (LR+ = 12.0), interstitial edema (LR+ = 12.0), alveolar edema (LR+ = 6.0), cardiomegaly (see **Figures 44-1** to **44-3**) (LR+ = 3.3)[3]

DIFFERENTIAL DIAGNOSIS

Gradually increasing shortness of breath can also be caused by the following:

- Chronic obstructive pulmonary disease (COPD) may have dyspnea with exertion but does not have orthopnea; chest radiograph shows a

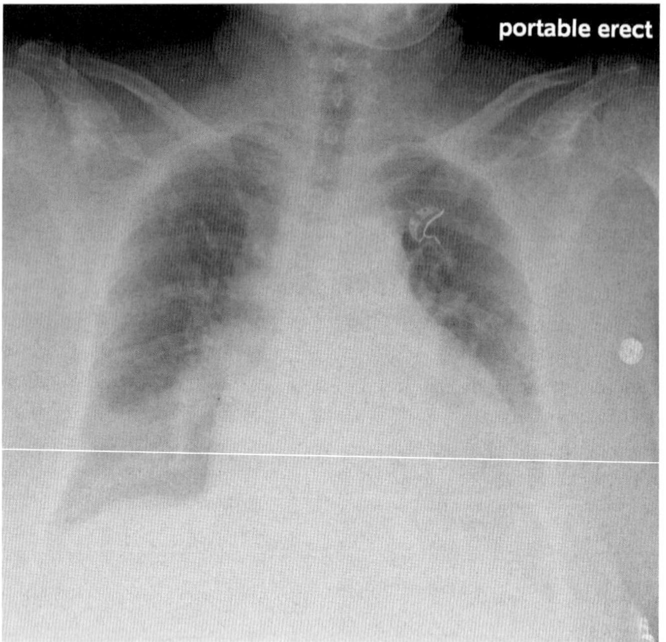

FIGURE 44-2 Cardiomegaly with pulmonary venous congestion and bilateral pleural effusions. (*Reproduced with permission from Heidi Chumley, MD.*)

normal-size heart, hyperinflated lungs, and flattened diaphragm; pulmonary function tests may be abnormal.

- Deconditioning has a normal chest radiograph.
- Metabolic acidosis from any cause can be differentiated with an arterial blood gas.
- Anxiety has episodic shortness of breath, not associated with exertion and a normal chest radiograph.
- Neuromuscular weakness may have abnormal pulmonary function tests and a normal chest radiograph.
- Pneumonia may have fever and an infiltrate on chest radiograph.

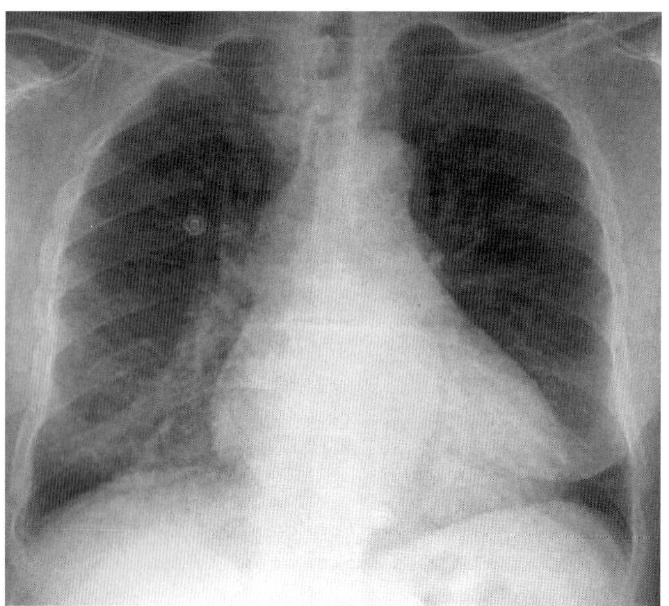

FIGURE 44-3 Cardiomegaly with increased pulmonary vasculature and Kerley B lines (2- to 3-cm horizontal lines in the lower lung fields). (*Reproduced with permission from Heidi Chumley, MD.*)

MANAGEMENT

NONPHARMACOLOGIC

- Telemonitoring of patients with known HF reduced all-cause mortality (relative risk [RR] 0.66). Telemonitoring and structure telephone support reduced HF-related hospitalization (RR 0.79 and 0.77, respectively).[4]
- Exercise rehabilitation increases quality of life and decreases hospital admissions in patients with left ventricular systolic dysfunction.[5]
- Salt restriction *increased* all-cause mortality in patients with HF (RR 0.84).[6]

MEDICATIONS

Individually, ACEIs, β-blockers, and aldosterone antagonists (AAs) lower mortality and should be considered for all patients without contraindications.

- Prescribe an ACEI. SOR Ⓐ ACEIs lower mortality rates by 23% overall. Use in patients with asymptomatic left ventricular dysfunction and all other stages of HF.[7]
- Prescribe a β-blocker. SOR Ⓐ β-Blockers reduce mortality by 32%.[8] Begin at a small dose and double the dose every 2 to 4 weeks until the target dose is reached or the patient cannot tolerate the increased dose. One study demonstrating a decrease in mortality had a large percentage of patients in the control and intervention groups already on an ACEI, indicating that the 2 together may decrease mortality more than an ACEI alone.[7] SOR Ⓑ
- Prescribe an AA when the creatinine is less than 2; monitor renal function and potassium.[7] SOR Ⓐ AAs lowered mortality in patients already on ACEI.[8] SOR Ⓑ
- Consider an angiotensin II receptor blocker (ARB) for patients who cannot tolerate an ACEI.[4] Patients with moderate, severe, or advanced HF may benefit from an ACEI plus an ARB or AA SOR Ⓑ, but the safety of all 3 is unknown.[7]
- After a myocardial infarction, an ARB has shown equivalent reductions in mortality to an ACEI, but the combination does not improve outcomes.

Nonpotassium-sparing diuretics, calcium channel blockers, and digoxin may improve symptoms but do not lower mortality.

- Nonpotassium-sparing diuretics (eg, furosemide) have been associated with worse outcomes, including higher mortality when used alone. Use for volume overload with ACEI, β-blocker, AA ± ARB as above.[8]
- Calcium channel blockers (verapamil and nifedipine) are avoided in systolic HF. Calcium channel blockers improve symptoms in diastolic HF, but do not lower mortality.[9] SOR Ⓐ
- Digoxin reduces hospitalizations and improves clinical symptoms, but does not lower mortality.[8] Consider adding digoxin when patients have symptoms despite adequate therapy with ACEI, β-blockers, AA ± ARB.

REFERRAL OR HOSPITALIZE

- Refer for evaluation for cardiac resynchronization therapy in patients with left ventricular ejection fraction (LVEF) less than 35% and QRS greater than 150 ms.[5] A recent meta-analysis demonstrated that cardiac resynchronization therapy decreased all-cause mortality and hospitalizations for HF in patients with New York Heart Association

(NYHA) class II. Number needed to treat (NNT) = 12 to prevent 1 hospitalization.[10]

- Refer for evaluation for implantable cardiac defibrillator (ICD) placement in patients with NYHA class II-IV and LVEF less than 35%. SOR Ⓒ ICDs have been shown to reduce mortality up to 30% and may offer greater risk reduction than antiarrhythmic medical therapy for some patients.[11]

PROGNOSIS

Absolute mortality is high in patients with HF.

- Patients with preserved ejection fraction (>50%) have a mortality rate of 121 per 1000 patient-years.[12]
- Patients with reduced ejection fraction (<40%) have a mortality rate of 141 per 1000 patient-years.[12]

FOLLOW-UP

Close follow-up in many forms, including telemedicine and structured telephone visits, can reduce hospitalizations and mortality.[4]

PATIENT EDUCATION

Fluid and sodium restriction are often advised, but a recent Cochrane review demonstrated an increased mortality with sodium restriction.

PATIENT RESOURCES

- PubMed Health. *Heart Failure Overview*—**http://www.ncbi.nlm.nih.gov/pubmedhealth/PMH0001211/.**
- The National Heart, Lung, and Blood Institute has patient information on HF—**http://www.nhlbi.nih.gov/health/health-topics/topics/hf/.**

PROVIDER RESOURCES

- The 2010 Heart Failure Society of America Comprehensive Heart Failure Practice Guideline—**http://www.heartfailureguideline.org/.**
- Management of Chronic Heart Failure. A National Clinical Guideline (Scottish)—**http://www.ngc.gov/content.aspx?id=10587.**

REFERENCES

1. Redfield MM, Jacobsen SJ, Burnett JC Jr, et al. Burden of systolic and diastolic ventricular dysfunction in the community: appreciating the scope of the heart failure epidemic [see comment]. *JAMA*. 2003;289(2):194-202.
2. Lloyd-Jones DM, Larson MG, Leip EP, et al. Lifetime risk for developing congestive heart failure: the Framingham Heart Study [see comment]. *Circulation*. 2002;106(24):3068-3072.
3. Wang CS, FitzGerald JM, Schulzer M, et al. Does this dyspneic patient in the emergency department have congestive heart failure [review]? *JAMA*. 2005;294(15):1944-1956.
4. Inglis SC, Clark RA, McAlister FA, et al. Which components of heart failure programmes are effective? A systematic review and meta-analysis of the outcomes of structured telephone support or telemonitoring as the primary component of chronic heart failure management in 8323 patients: abridged Cochrane Review. *Eur J Heart Fail*. 2011;139(9):1028-1040.
5. Mant J, Al-Mohammad A, Swain S, Laramée P; Guideline Development Group. Management of chronic heart failure in adults: synopsis of the national institute for health and clinical excellence guideline. *Ann Intern Med*. 2011;155(4):252-259.
6. Taylor RS, Ashton KE, Moxham T, et al. Reduced dietary salt for the prevention of cardiovascular disease. *Cochrane Database Syst Rev*. 2011;(7):CD009217.
7. Mielniczuk L, Stevenson LW. Angiotensin-converting enzyme inhibitors and angiotensin II type I receptor blockers in the management of congestive heart failure patients: what have we learned from recent clinical trials [review]? *Curr Opin Cardiol*. 2005;20(4):250-255.
8. Yan AT, Yan RT, Liu PP. Narrative review: pharmacotherapy for chronic heart failure: evidence from recent clinical trials [review]. *Ann Intern Med*. 2005;142(2):132-145. [Summary for patients in *Ann Intern Med*. 2005;142(2):I53.]
9. Haney S, Sur D, Xu Z. Diastolic heart failure: a review and primary care perspective [review]. *J Am Board Fam Pract*. 2005;18(3):189-198.
10. Adabag S, Roukoz H, Anand IS, Moss AJ. Cardiac resynchronization therapy in patients with minimal heart failure a systematic review and meta-analysis. *J Am Coll Cardiol*. 2011;58(9):935-941.
11. Kadish A, Mehra M. Heart failure devices: implantable cardioverter-defibrillators and biventricular pacing therapy [review]. *Circulation*. 2005;111(24):3327-3335.
12. Meta-analysis Global Group in Chronic Heart Failure. The survival of patients with heart failure with preserved or reduced left ventricular ejection fraction: an individual patient data meta-analysis. *Eur Heart J*. 2012;33(14):1750-1757.

45 CORONARY ARTERY DISEASE

Heidi Chumley, MD

PATIENT STORY

A 45-year-old man began having chest pressure with exertion that was relieved with rest. He did not have diabetes, high blood pressure, or high cholesterol, and never had a myocardial infarction (MI). His examination and resting electrocardiography (ECG) were normal. On the basis of the testing modalities available, he was scheduled for exercise stress testing. After a positive test, he underwent coronary angiography that demonstrated a significant stenosis in the left coronary artery (**Figure 45-1**). He underwent a stenting procedure and was placed on aspirin and cholesterol-lowering medication.

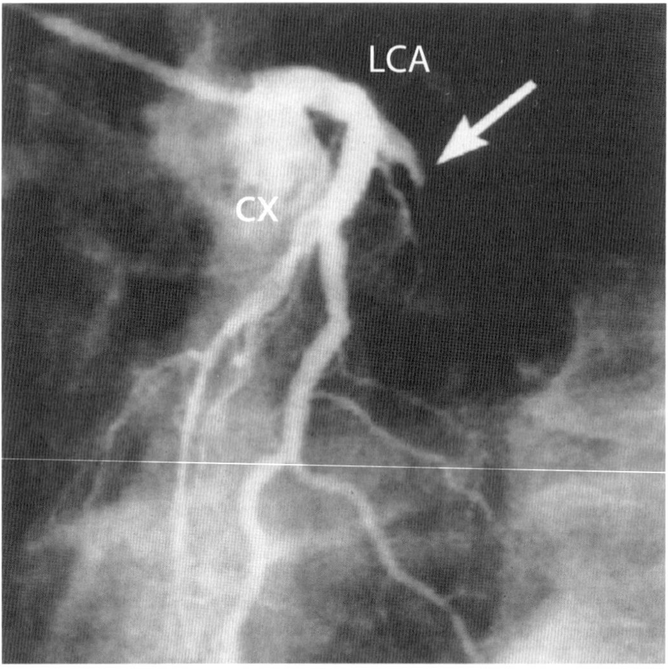

FIGURE 45-1 Coronary arteriogram demonstrating severe stenosis (*white arrow*) in the left coronary artery (LCA). Note that the circumflex artery (CX) is patent.

INTRODUCTION

In the United States, a person dies of coronary heart disease (CHD) every 39 seconds. CHD is a manifestation of atherosclerotic disease and has many modifiable risk factors. Patients with and without CHD should be advised to stop smoking, maintain normal blood pressure and cholesterol levels, exercise, achieve or maintain a normal weight, and control diabetes mellitus if present.

EPIDEMIOLOGY

- Coronary heart disease is the leading cause of death in the United States, responsible for approximately 400,000 deaths in 2008.[1]
- Each year, 1.5 million MIs occur (first and recurrent) with a 33% mortality rate.[1]
- In 2006 to 2010, the prevalence of CHD among US adults older than 18 years of age was higher in men than woman (7.8% vs 4.6%) and higher in people with a less-than-high-school-diploma education (9.2% vs 4.6% for college graduates).[2]
- The prevalence is higher in American Indian or Alaskan Natives (8.4%), than in Hispanic (5.3%), Black (5.9%), or White (4.2%) persons.[2]

ETIOLOGY AND PATHOPHYSIOLOGY

- CHD is one of several manifestations of atherosclerotic disease, which begins with endothelium dysfunction.[3]
- Endothelium, when normal, balances vasoconstrictors and vasodilators, impedes platelet aggregation, and controls fibrin production.
- Dysfunctional endothelium encourages macrophage adhesion, plaque growth, and vasoconstriction by recruiting inflammatory cells into the vessel walls, the initiating step of atherosclerosis.
- The vessel wall lesions develop a cap of smooth muscle cells and collagen to become fibroadenomas.
- The vessels with these lesions undergo enlargement, allowing progression of the plaque without compromising the lumen.
- Plaque disruption and thrombus formation, instead of progressive narrowing of the coronary artery lumen, is responsible for two-thirds of acute coronary events.[3]
- Plaques most likely to rupture (high-risk plaques) have a large core of lipids, many macrophages, decreased vascular smooth muscle cells, and a thin fibrous cap.
- After plaque rupture, the exposed lipid core triggers a superimposed thrombus that occludes the vessel.
- Increased thrombosis is triggered by known cardiac risk factors including elevated low-density lipoprotein (LDL) cholesterol, cigarette smoking, and hyperglycemia.
- The other one-third of acute coronary events occur at the site of very stenotic lesions (**Figure 45-2**).[3]

RISK FACTORS

- Family history of premature paternal or sibling MI increases risk of heart disease by 50%.[1]
- Tobacco use and secondhand smoke exposure increase the risk of CHD and smoking cessation reduces risk.[1]
- High total cholesterol, high LDL, and/or low high-density lipoprotein (HDL) are independent risk factors.
- Physical inactivity has a relative risk of CHD of 1.5 to 2.4.[1]
- Overweight and obesity increase the risk of heart disease by 20% (men and women) and (46% [men] and 64% [women], respectively).[1]
- Diabetes mellitus increases the risk of heart disease (hazard ratio 2.5).[1]

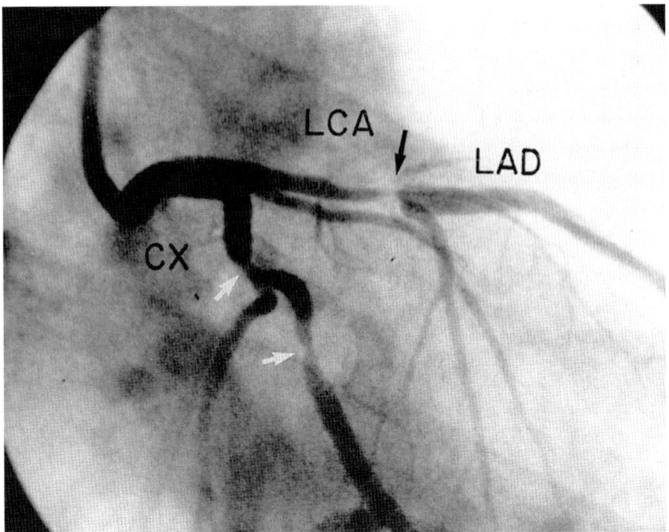

FIGURE 45-2 Coronary angiogram of a left coronary artery (*LCA*) with a tight stenosis in the proximal left anterior descending (*LAD*) artery (*black arrow*). The circumflex artery (*CX*) has 2 moderately severe stenoses (*white arrows*).

DIAGNOSIS

CLINICAL FEATURES

- Typical angina is chest pain or pressure, brought on by exertion or stress, and relieved with rest or nitroglycerin.
- Atypical angina has 2 of the 3 features of typical angina; however, women with coronary artery disease report more neck, throat, or jaw pain.[4]
- Noncardiac chest pain has zero to 1 of the 3 features of typical angina.

LABORATORY TESTING

- Risk factor assessment—Lipid profile and fasting blood glucose.
- Acute coronary syndrome—Cardiac-specific troponin is now preferred; when troponin cutoff is 0.1 g/L, sensitivity is 93%, specificity is 91%, positive likelihood ratio (LR+) is 10.33, and negative likelihood ratio (LR–) is 0.08.

COMMON NONINVASIVE TESTING

- Exercise treadmill testing[5]—Sensitivity 52% and specificity 71%, LR+ 1.79, LR+ 0.68
- Stress echocardiogram—Sensitivity 85% and specificity 77%, LR+ 3.70, LR– 0.19
- Stress thallium—Sensitivity 87% and specificity 64%, LR+ 2.42, LR– 0.20

Newer methods being tested include computed tomography (CT) for diagnosis[6]:

- A 4- or 16-slice study—Sensitivity 95% and specificity 84%, LR+ 5.94, LR– 0.06, for presence of stenosis, with 78% and 91% of segments evaluable.
- A 64-slice study—Sensitivity 100% and specificity 100%, for presence of stenosis, with 100% of segments evaluable.
- CT with noninvasive fractional flow reserve (measure of amount of flow in the presence of stenosis)—Sensitivity 90% and specificity 54%, for presence of ischemia.[7]

DIFFERENTIAL DIAGNOSIS

Chest pain can be caused by several conditions including the following:

- Cardiac—Pericarditis—slower onset of pain, pain aggravated by movement or inspiration, characteristic ECG changes
- Respiratory—Pneumothorax—acute onset with shortness of breath and characteristic radiographic findings; pneumonia—often accompanied by fever, cough, shortness of breath or hypoxia, and/or radiographic findings; pulmonary embolism—acute onset of shortness of breath, positive ventilation-perfusion scan, or spiral CT
- GI—Gastroesophageal reflux—related to eating, responds to H_2 blockers or proton pump inhibitor (PPI)
- Musculoskeletal—Costochondritis—chest muscles tender to palpation

MANAGEMENT

NONPHARMACOLOGIC

- Advise patients with coronary artery disease to stop smoking.[8] SOR A
- Recommend 30 minutes of physical activity 5 to 7 days per week.[1,8] SOR B
- Advise patients in weight management with a goal of body mass index (BMI) of 18.5 to 24.9.[8] SOR B

MEDICATIONS

Manage risk factors by the following ways:

- Lower LDL cholesterol using lifestyle modification and hydroxymethylglutaryl coenzyme A (HMG-CoA) reductase inhibitors (ie, statins) to decrease all-cause mortality (relative risk [RR] 0.90), cardiovascular mortality (RR 0.80), fatal and nonfatal MI (RR 0.82 and 0.74).[9] SOR A
- Lower blood pressure to 140/90; treat patients who are post-MI with a β-blocker, thiazide diuretic, or aldosterone antagonist.[10] SOR A
- Prescribe aspirin in patients with prior ST elevation or non-ST elevation acute coronary event or chronic stable angina. Prescribe clopidogrel alone in chronic stable angina or with aspirin in non-ST elevation acute coronary syndrome.[11] SOR A
- Prescribe a β-antagonist—Several trials demonstrate mortality decreases of 25% to 40% with various β-blockers used in the acute MI or post-MI period.[12]

Treat symptoms by the following ways:

- Nitroglycerin sublingual or spray for immediate relief of angina.[13] SOR B
- Long-acting nitrates or calcium antagonists if β-blockers are contraindicated; do not control symptoms, or have unacceptable side effects.[13] SOR B

REFERRAL OR HOSPITALIZATION

- Refer patients with positive noninvasive testing to be evaluated for cardiac catheterization.
- Consult with cardiologists and cardiothoracic surgeons to determine optimal management.

- Traditionally, patients with greater than 50% stenosis of left main, proximal stenosis of 3 major arteries, or significant stenosis of the proximal left anterior descending and one other major artery have been treated with coronary bypass surgery.[14] SOR A
- Advancements with drug-eluting stents may increase the numbers and types of patients who benefit from stenting.[14]

PREVENTION

Prevention of CHD is accomplished by risk factor control. In a study of older men that examined the risk factors of smoking, high LDL, high blood pressure, and no aspirin use, the number needed to treat (NNT) to prevent one cardiovascular outcome were 22, 8, 6, and 5 for 1, 2, 3, and 4 risk factors controlled, respectively.[15]

FOLLOW-UP

Follow-up frequency is based on the extent of illness and symptoms and may include primary care and subspecialty care. Patients should have ongoing evaluation of risk factors and symptoms every 4 to 12 months. Expert guidelines recommend annual exercise stress testing for patients with chronic stable angina.[13] SOR C

PATIENT EDUCATION

Advise patients in the importance of lifestyle modification and medications in the long-term management of CHD.

PATIENT RESOURCES

- PubMed Health. *Coronary Heart Disease*—**http://www.ncbi.nlm.nih.gov/pubmedhealth/PMH0004449/.**
- The American Heart Association has information about the warning signs of heart attacks and living a healthy lifestyle—**http://www.americanheart.org.**

PROVIDER RESOURCES

- Boudi FB. *Coronary Artery Atherosclerosis*—**http://emedicine.medscape.com/article/153647.**
- Online calculator for pre- and posttest probability of coronary artery disease based on history and physical—**http://www.soapnote.org/cardiovascular/chest-pain-evaluation/.**
- The National Heart, Lung, and Blood Institute—**http://www.nhlbi.nih.gov/index.htm.**

REFERENCES

1. Roger VL, Go AS, Lloyd-Jones DM, et al. Heart disease and stroke statistics—2012 update: a report from the American Heart Association. *Circulation*. 2012;125(1):188-197. http://circ.ahajournals.org/content/early/2011/12/15/CIR.0b013e31823ac046.citation. Accessed September 3, 2012.
2. Centers for Disease Control and Prevention. Prevalence of coronary heart disease—United States, 2006-2010. *MMWR Morb Mortal Wkly Rep*. 2011;60(40):1377-1381.
3. Viles-Gonzalez JF, Fuster V, Badimon JJ. Atherothrombosis: a widespread disease with unpredictable and life-threatening consequences. *Eur Heart J*. 2004;25(14):1197-1207.
4. Philpott S, Boynton PM, Feder G, Hemingway H. Gender differences in descriptions of angina symptoms and health problems immediately prior to angiography: the ACRE study. Appropriateness of Coronary Revascularisation study. *Soc Sci Med*. 2001;52(10):1565-1575.
5. Pryor DB, Shaw L, McCants CB, et al. Value of the history and physical in identifying patients at increased risk for coronary artery disease. *Ann Intern Med*. 1993;118(2):81-90.
6. Stein PD, Stein PD, Beemath A, et al. Multidetector computed tomography for the diagnosis of coronary artery disease: a systematic review. *Am J Med*. 2006;119(3):203-216.
7. Min JK, Leipsic J, Pencina MJ, et al. Diagnostic accuracy of fractional flow reserve from anatomical CT angiography. *JAMA*. 2012;308(12):1237-1245.
8. Smith SC Jr, Allen J, Blair SN, et al. AHA/ACC guidelines for secondary prevention for patients with coronary and other atherosclerotic vascular disease: 2006 update. *Circulation*. 2006;113:2363-2372.
9. Mills EJ, Wu P, Chong G, et al. Efficacy and safety of statin treatment for cardiovascular disease: a network meta-analysis of 170,255 patients from 76 randomized trials. *QJM*. 2011;104(2):109-124.
10. *The Seventh Report of the Joint National Committee on Prevention, Detection, Evaluation and Treatment of High Blood Pressure (JNC 7)*. http://www.nhlbi.nih.gov/guidelines/hypertension/index.htm. Accessed September 3, 2012.
11. Tran H, Anand SS. Oral antiplatelet therapy in cerebrovascular disease, coronary artery disease, and peripheral arterial disease. *JAMA*. 2004;292(15):1867-1874.
12. Ellison KE, Gandhi G. Optimising the use of beta-adrenoceptor antagonists in coronary artery disease. *Drugs*. 2005;65(6):787-797.
13. Gibbons RJ, Abrams J, Chatterjee K, et al. ACC/AHA 2002 guideline update for the management of patients with chronic stable angina: a report of the American College of Cardiology/American Heart Association Task Force on Practice Guidelines (Committee to Update the 1999 Guidelines for the Management of Patients with Chronic Stable Angina). 2002. http://www.acc.org/clinical/guidelines/stable/stable.pdf. Accessed September 3, 2012.
14. Schofield PM. Indications for percutaneous and surgical revascularization: how far does the evidence base guide us? *Heart*. 2003;89(5):565-570.
15. Robinson JG, Rahill-Tierney C, Lawler E, Gaziano JM. Benefits associated with achieving optimal risk factor levels for the primary prevention of cardiovascular disease in older men. *J Clin Lipidol*. 2012;6(1):58-65.

46 DEEP VENOUS THROMBOSIS

Rajil M. Karnani, MD, MME

PATIENT STORY

A 55-year-old man presents to his general internist with a 3-day history of swelling, redness, and pain in his left leg. The symptoms began shortly after a flight back to Boston from a vacation in Hawaii. He denies any dyspnea, chest pain, or lightheadedness. Physical examination reveals the left leg to be erythematous, swollen, and painful to palpation (**Figure 46-1**). Measurement of the circumference of the left calf reveals it to be 4 cm greater than the circumference of the right calf. Compression ultrasound of the left leg shows a noncompressible left femoral vein highly suspicious for a clot. The patient is diagnosed with a deep venous thrombosis (DVT) of the left thigh and started on enoxaparin (Lovenox) subcutaneously and warfarin (Coumadin) orally. Five days later, he discontinues the enoxaparin but continues with warfarin. Several weeks later, his international normalized ratio (INR) value is steady in the therapeutic range, and his left leg feels considerably better.

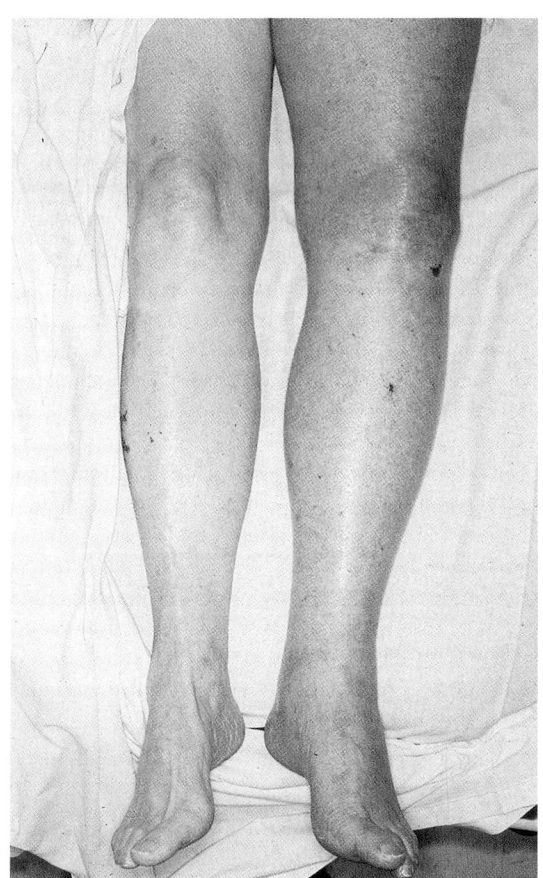

FIGURE 46-1 Deep venous thrombosis of the left leg with classic findings of swelling, erythema, pain, and tenderness. (*Reproduced with permission from Knoop KJ et al. The Atlas of Emergency Medicine, 3rd ed. McGraw-Hill, 2010; Photo contributor: Kevin J. Knoop, MD, MS*)

INTRODUCTION

A DVT is the result of pathologic intravascular clotting that produces a thrombus in any section of the venous system. DVT occurs most commonly in the deep venous system of the legs.

SYNONYMS

DVT is also known as deep venous thrombophlebitis or venous thromboembolism (VTE).

EPIDEMIOLOGY

- Occurs for the first time in approximately 100 persons per 100,000 population each year in the United States[1]
- Incidence of a first-time episode increases exponentially with age[1]
- Risk of VTE is 2.5- to 4-fold less in Asian-Pacific Islanders and Hispanics[1]
- More common occurrence in winter than summer[1]
- VTE recurrence rate approximately 7% in the first 6 months[1]
- Recurrence rates as high as about 19% in men after 3 years and about 10% in women after 3 years[1]

ETIOLOGY AND PATHOPHYSIOLOGY

Thrombogenesis begins with 1 or a combination of multiple factors relating to Virchow's triad:[2]

- Stasis resulting from inactivity from bed rest, prolonged travel, or a recent stroke.
- Endothelial injury resulting from trauma, surgery, or inflammation.
- Hypercoagulability from alterations in the blood that make it more likely to clot. Included among these are genetic mutations (protein C deficiency, protein S deficiency, prothrombin 20210A mutation, antithrombin III deficiency, factor V Leiden mutation), hyperviscosity, nephrotic syndrome, trauma, malignancy, late pregnancy, and medicines (hormone replacement therapy, tamoxifen, raloxifene, darbepoetin).
- Once thrombus has formed in a deep vein, it causes obstruction of venous outflow, leading to venous distention, which results in erythema, swelling, warmth, and pain. If the clot dislodges, it will pass through the venous circulation, into the heart, and wedge into the pulmonary circulation, causing a pulmonary embolus.

RISK FACTORS

In order of strength of risk[2,3]:

- Recent surgery (in previous 4 weeks)
- Recent trauma
- Immobility
- Cancer
- Neurological disease (with lower-extremity paralysis)
- Oral contraceptives
- Hormone therapy

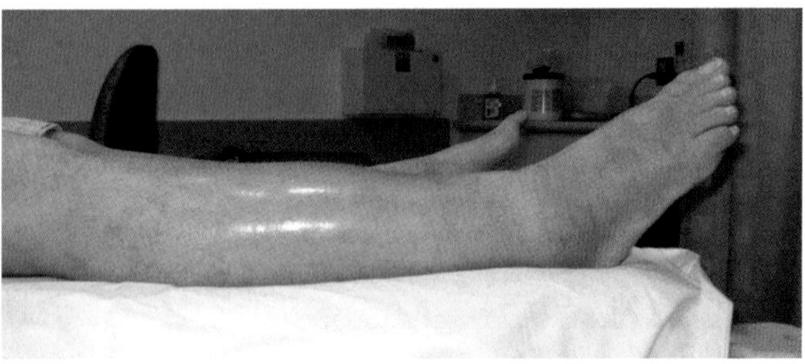

FIGURE 46-2 Right lower-extremity DVT with obvious swelling and erythema noted in the calf and foot. Duplex ultrasound revealed thrombosis in the peroneal and posterior tibial veins. (*Reproduced with permission from Dean S, Satiana B.* Color Atlas and Synopsis of Vascular Disease. *New York, NY:* McGraw-Hill; 2014.)

DIAGNOSIS

HISTORY

- Leg pain and/or swelling
- Previous history of DVT
- Risk factors including recent immobilization, cancer history, hormone therapy

PHYSICAL EXAMINATION

- There is unilateral swelling, erythema, and tenderness to palpation of the affected extremity (**Figure 46-2**).
- Increased calf diameter (>3 cm) in the symptomatic leg is consistent with DVT but not specific.

LABORATORY STUDIES

- Dimerized plasmin fragment D(D-dimer) assays are sensitive but not specific for VTE (a positive test does not "rule in" VTE; however, a negative test lowers the likelihood of VTE).
- A normal D-dimer in outpatients with low or intermediate probability of DVT is associated with a 0.4% to 0.5% 3-month incidence of DVT.

CLINICAL PREDICTION RULES

- The most widely accepted method for making the diagnosis of DVT is use of the modified Wells clinical score.
- The modified Wells clinical score (**Table 46-1**) assigns a specified point value for each patient characteristic present.[4]
  - History items—active cancer, immobilization of leg, recently bedridden, previous confirmed DVT.
  - Physical examination items—tenderness along the deep venous system, swelling of entire leg, calf swelling greater than 3 cm, pitting edema of involved leg, collateral superficial veins.

DIAGNOSTIC STEPS

The following diagnostic steps are used[3]:

1. If Wells score indicates low probability, measure the D-dimer.
   a. If D-dimer measurement is negative, DVT is effectively ruled out.
   b. If D-dimer measurement is positive, perform a compression ultrasound of the affected extremity.

TABLE 46-1 Modified Wells Clinical Score

Criteria	Points
Active cancer (treatment ongoing, within 6 months, or palliative)	1
Paralysis, paresis, or recent plaster immobilization of the legs	1
Recently bedridden >3 days or major surgery within 12 weeks requiring general/regional anesthesia	1
Localized tenderness along the distribution of the deep venous system	1
Entire leg swollen	1
Calf swelling 3-cm larger than asymptomatic side (measured 10 cm below the tibial tuberosity)	1
Pitting edema confined to the symptomatic leg	1
Collateral superficial veins (nonvaricose)	1
Previously documented DVT	1
Alternative diagnosis at least as likely as DVT	−2

Total score ≤0 indicates low probability for DVT.
Total score 1-2 indicates intermediate probability for DVT.
Total score ≥3 indicates high probability for DVT.

   i. If ultrasound is positive, begin treatment for DVT.
   ii. If ultrasound is negative, repeat the ultrasound in 1 week.
      (1) If repeat ultrasound is negative, DVT is effectively ruled out.
      (2) If repeat ultrasound is positive, begin treatment for DVT.
2. If Wells score indicates intermediate or high probability, perform a compression ultrasound of the affected extremity.
   a. If ultrasound is positive, begin treatment for DVT.
   b. If ultrasound is negative, measure the D-dimer.
      i. If D-dimer measurement is negative, DVT is effectively ruled out.
      ii. If D-dimer measurement is positive, repeat the ultrasound in 1 week.
         (1) If repeat ultrasound is negative, DVT is effectively ruled out.
         (2) If repeat ultrasound is positive, begin treatment for DVT.

DIFFERENTIAL DIAGNOSIS

The following entities may mimic the presentation of DVT[3]:

- Venous insufficiency from incompetent venous valves can be age related or caused by obesity.
- Superficial thrombophlebitis typically presents as a tender and firm varicose vein (**Figure 46-3**).
- Muscle strain/tear can be differentiated by pain that occurs with a particular range of motion of a muscle group, usually with an antecedent leg injury or trauma.
- A Baker cyst can lead to pain located in the popliteal portion of the posterior leg, typically diagnosed by ultrasound. Once a Baker cyst ruptures, the pain and inflammation can mimic a DVT.

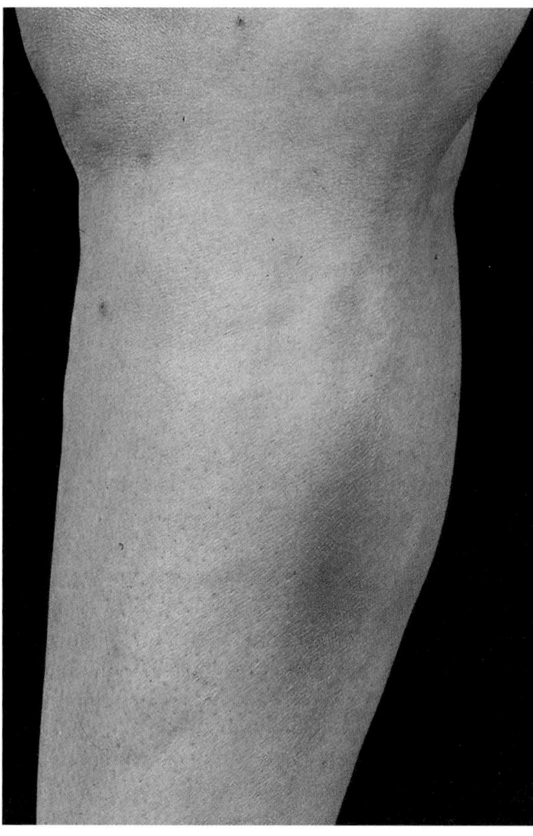

FIGURE 46-3 Superficial thrombophlebitis presenting with a linear inflammatory induration over the posterior aspect of this patient's leg. (*Reproduced with permission from Wolff K, Johnson RA.* Fitzpatrick's Color Atlas and Synopsis of Clinical Dermatology. *6th ed. New York, NY: McGraw-Hill; 2013.*)

- Cellulitis presents with erythema, warmth, and edema of the skin (**Figure 46-4**). There may also be an ascending lymphangitis, which would not be seen in a DVT. If a DVT is being considered, then an ultrasound will be negative for thrombosis.
- Lymphedema of the leg often causes more swelling in the foot than DVT. Lymphedema is most often chronic, causing long-standing changes in the tissues, which become brawny with a red-brown coloration. There may also be papules of lymphatic swelling and weeping of fluid (**Figure 46-5**).

MANAGEMENT

- The mainstay of treatment is anticoagulation. A DVT in the upper extremity is treated in the same manner as a DVT in the lower extremity. An upper extremity DVT caused by a catheter does not require that the catheter be removed if it is functioning properly and there is an ongoing need for the catheter.[2]
- Hospitalization is recommended in the following situations[3,5]:
    - Renal insufficiency (CrCl <30 mL/min)
    - Presence of pulmonary embolus
    - Presence of bilateral DVTs or recurrent DVTs
    - Severe pain requiring opioids
    - Increased risk of bleeding
    - Recent immobility
    - Chronic heart failure
    - Cancer

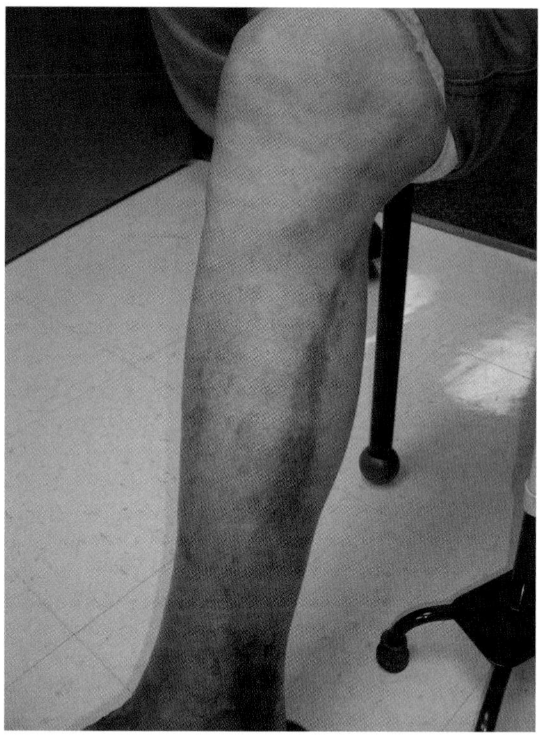

FIGURE 46-4 Cellulitis with lymphangitic spread up the leg. (*Reproduced with permission from Richard P. Usatine, MD.*)

    - A known hypercoagulable state
    - Pregnancy
    - Those not likely to be adherent to outpatient therapy
- Outpatient treatment for the treatment of DVT is safe and effective compared to inpatient treatment in selected patients.[5] (SOR A)
- Anticoagulation with one of the following should be started immediately once a DVT is strongly suspected (barring any contraindications)[3,5]:
    - Guidelines suggest the use of low molecular weight heparin (LMWH), not unfractionated heparin (UFH), as first-line therapy in patients with DVT (SOR A).[5]
        - The dose for LMWH is
            - Dalteparin—200 IU/kg SC once daily
            - Enoxaparin—1 mg/kg SC twice daily
            - Tinzaparin—175 IU/kg SC once daily
        - For patients not able to take heparin (eg, a history of heparin-induced thrombocytopenia), consider fondaparinux at 7.5 mg SC once daily.
        - If using UFH because of unavailability of LMWH, the dose is 80 U/kg bolus, followed by 18 U/kg/h titrated to a partial thromboplastin time (PTT) 1.5 to 2.5 times the upper limit of normal.
    - Long-term oral anticoagulation with warfarin should also be started on day 1, overlapping with one of the previously mentioned for at least 4 to 5 days and until the INR is in the therapeutic range of 2.0 to 3.0 for 2 consecutive days.
        - At this point, heparin/LMWH/fondaparinux can be discontinued and oral anticoagulation continued with warfarin.
        - The duration of warfarin therapy depends on the circumstances surrounding the diagnosis of DVT (**Table 46-2**).[3,5]
        - Extended-duration therapy with warfarin decreases the risk of recurrent DVT for as long as it is used; although the overall risk of recurrent DVT declines with time, the risk of bleeding remains.[5,6]

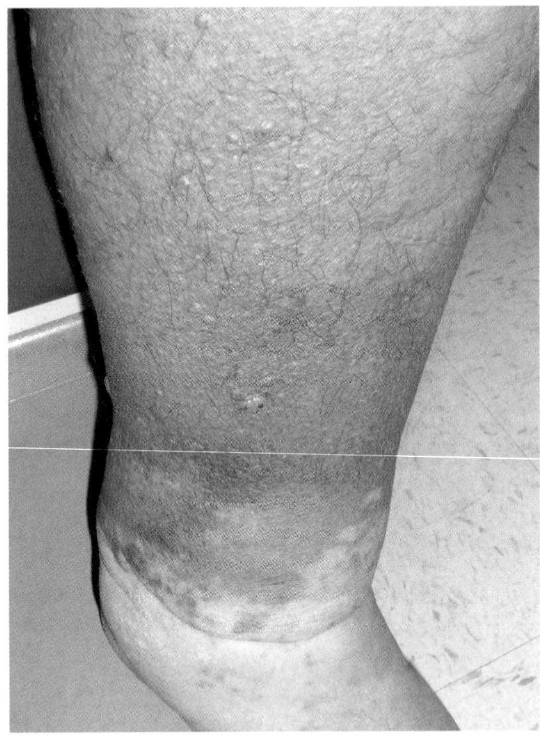

A

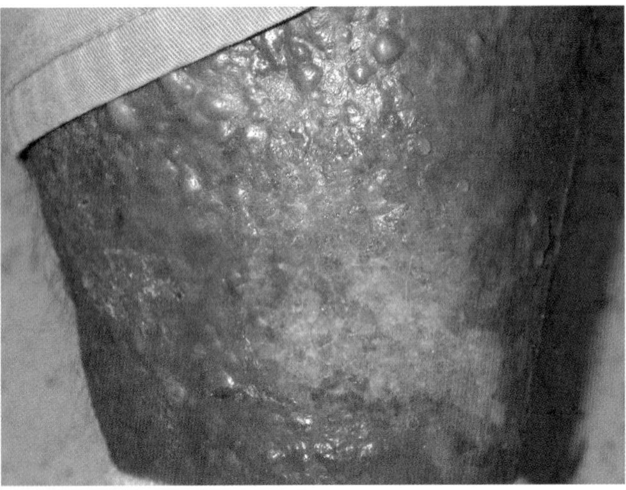

B

FIGURE 46-5 Lymphedema with leg swelling and red-brown coloration. Note the papules that represent dilation of the lymphatic tissue. A. The brown color is from hemosiderin deposition. B. Note the weeping of fluid and the dilated lymphatic tissue. (*Reproduced with permission from Richard P. Usatine, MD.*)

- Newer anticoagulants, including direct thrombin inhibitors (eg, dabigatran) and factor Xa inhibitors (eg, rivaroxaban) have shown promise in treating DVT (SOR B).[7,8]
- Other options[2]:
    - Inferior vena cava filter—should be placed if anticoagulation is contraindicated, if recurrent thrombosis occurs while on anticoagulants, or if patient is at high risk for a pulmonary embolus
    - Catheter-directed thrombolysis— used for a massive, limb-threatening ileofemoral DVT
    - IV tissue plasminogen activator (tPA)—used for a hemodynamically significant pulmonary embolus

TABLE 46-2 Recommended Duration of Treatment for DVT

Characteristic	Duration of Therapy
Transient risk factor (now resolved)	3 months
Transient risk factor (persistent)	Continue until 6 weeks after factor resolved
Idiopathic (1st event)—low suspicion for hypercoagulable state	6 months
Idiopathic (1st event)—high suspicion for hypercoagulable state	Indefinite
Recurrent idiopathic event	Indefinite
Recurrent thrombosis while on anticoagulants (whether caused by identified risk or idiopathic)	Indefinite
Thrombosis with malignancy	Indefinite

- Adjunctive measures[3,5]:
    - Early ambulation—highly recommended for an uncomplicated DVT while on anticoagulants.
    - Compression stockings—decrease the rate of postthrombotic syndrome by 50%. These should be worn at a pressure of 20 to 40 mm Hg for 6 to 12 months (SOR A).[5,9]

PROGNOSIS/CLINICAL COURSE

- Recurrence rate of VTE is approximately 7% in the first 6 months.[1]
- Within 3 years after an initial, unprovoked DVT, 19.7% of men will develop a recurrence, as will 9.1% of women.[10]
- Warfarin decreases the risk of recurrent DVT for as long as it is used, and although the overall risk of recurrent DVT declines with time, the risk of bleeding remains.
- In one study, the incidence of postthrombotic syndrome was 24.5%, 29.6%, and 29.8%, after 2, 5, and 8 years, respectively.[11]

FOLLOW-UP

- Patients on warfarin will need to have their INR monitored regularly to ensure that it is in the therapeutic range.
- If a hypercoagulable state is suspected, workup for this should be performed 2 weeks after the cessation of anticoagulation therapy.
- Monitor and treat patients for postthrombotic syndrome (presence of recurrent pain, swelling, and dermatologic signs of stasis).

PATIENT EDUCATION

- Anticoagulation can increase the risk of serious bleeding, and patients should avoid activities that predispose to potential bodily injury.
- Large amounts of dietary vitamin B_{12} will affect the quality of anticoagulation. The dose of warfarin needs to be adjusted in such cases to prevent suboptimal therapy.

PATIENT RESOURCES

- Agency for Healthcare Research and Quality (AHRQ): *Blood Thinner Pills*—**http://www.ahrq.gov/consumer/btpills.htm.**
- National Heart, Lung, and Blood Institute: *What Is Deep Venous Thrombosis?* **http://www.nhlbi.nih.gov/health/health-topics/topics/dvt/.**
- American Academy of Orthopaedic Surgeons. *Deep Vein Thrombosis*—**http://orthoinfo.aaos.org/topic.cfm?topic=A00219&return_link=0.**

PROVIDER RESOURCES

- *Antithrombotic and Thrombolytic Therapy, 8th Ed.: ACCP Guidelines*—**http://chestjournal.chestpubs.org/content/133/6_suppl.**

REFERENCES

1. White RH. The epidemiology of venous thromboembolism. *Circulation*. 2003;107(23)(suppl 1):I4-I8.
2. Blann AD, Lip GYH. Venous thromboembolism. *BMJ*. 2006;332(7535):215-219.
3. Goodacre S. In the clinic. Deep venous thrombosis. *Ann Intern Med*. 2008;149(5):ITC3-1.
4. Wells PS, Owen C, Doucette S, et al. The Rational Clinical Examination. Does this patient have deep venous thrombosis? *JAMA*. 2006;295(2):199-207.
5. Snow V, Qaseem A, Barry P, et al. Management of venous thromboembolism: a clinical practice guideline from the American College of Physicians and the American Academy of Family Physicians. *Ann Intern Med*. 2007;146:204.
6. Hutten BA, Prins MH. Duration of treatment with vitamin K antagonists in symptomatic venous thromboembolism [Cochrane Review]. *Cochrane Libr*. 2011 Issue 3. Chichester, UK: John Wiley and Sons, Ltd.
7. The EINSTEIN Investigators, Bauersachs R, Berkowitz SD, et al. Oral rivaroxaban for symptomatic venous thromboembolism. *N Engl J Med*. 2010;363(26):2499-2510.
8. Schulman S, Kearon C, Kakkar AK, et al, for the RE-COVER Study Group. Dabigatran versus warfarin in the treatment of acute venous thromboembolism. *N Engl J Med*. 2009;361(24):2342-2352.
9. Brandjes DP, Büller HR, Heijboer H, et al. Randomised trial of effect of compression stockings in patients with symptomatic proximal-vein thrombosis. *Lancet*. 1997;349(9054):759-762.
10. Douketis J, Tosetto A, Marucci M, et al. Risk of recurrence after venous thromboembolism in men and women: patient level meta-analysis. *BMJ*. 2011;342:d813.
11. Prandoni P, Villalta S, Bagatella P, et al. The clinical course of deep-vein thrombosis. Prospective long-term follow-up of 528 symptomatic patients. *Haematologica*. 1997;82(4):423-428.

47 BACTERIAL ENDOCARDITIS

Heidi Chumley, MD

PATIENT STORY

A 25-year-old man presented to the office because he had been feeling tired and feverish for several weeks. He admitted to injecting heroin regularly in the last 2 months. On examination, he was febrile and had a heart murmur of which he was previously unaware. His fingernails showed splinter hemorrhages (**Figure 47-1**). His funduscopic examination revealed Roth spots (**Figures 47-2** and **47-3**). An echocardiogram demonstrated vegetation on the tricuspid valve. He was hospitalized and treated empirically for bacterial endocarditis. After his blood cultures returned *Staphylococcus aureus*, his regimen was adjusted based on sensitivities and continued for 6 weeks.

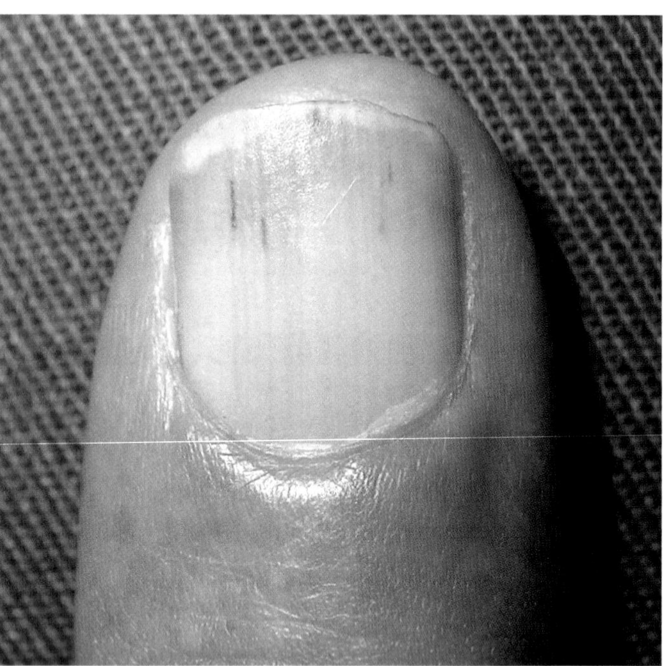

FIGURE 47-1 Splinter hemorrhages appearing as red linear streaks under the nail plate and within the nail bed. Although endocarditis can cause this, splinter hemorrhages are more commonly seen in psoriasis and trauma. *(Reproduced with permission from Richard P. Usatine, MD.)*

INTRODUCTION

Bacterial endocarditis is a serious infection seen most commonly in patients with prosthetic valves; injection drug users; patients with HIV, especially those who use intravenous (IV) drugs; and patients who are immunosuppressed. Diagnosis is made based on Duke criteria. Treatment is IV antibiotics. Mortality, despite treatment, is 26% to 37%.

EPIDEMIOLOGY

- About 5 to 7.9 cases per 100,000 patient-years.[1]
  - Historically it is more common in men; however, the incidence in women is increasing. Incidence in men and women 8.6 to 12.7 and 1.4 to 6.7 cases per 100,000 person-years, respectively.[1]
  - Average age has increased from 46.5 years (1980-1984) to 70 years (2001-2006).[1]
  - Incidence in IV drug users is 3 per 1000 person-years or 1% to 5% per year.[2]
  - Incidence in HIV-positive IV drug users is 13.8 per 1000 person-years.[2]
- Seen in immunosuppressed patients with central venous catheters or hemodialysis patients.
  - Fifty percent health care associated, 43% community acquired, and 7.5% nosocomial.[1]
  - Mortality ranges from 16% to 37%.[3]
- Prosthetic valve endocarditis makes up 10% to 15% of endocarditis cases.[4]
  - Incidence of 0.1% to 2.3% person-year.[4]
  - Can occur early (2 months after surgery) or late.

ETIOLOGY AND PATHOPHYSIOLOGY

- Endothelium is injured by mechanical or inflammatory processes.
- Microbes adhere to compromised endothelium during transient bacteremia.
- Common organisms include *S. aureus* (IV drug users, nosocomial infections, prosthetic valve patients), *Streptococcus bovis* (elderly patients), enterococci (nosocomial infections), and *Staphylococcus epidermis* (early infection in prosthetic valve patients).
- Blood contacts subendothelial factors, which promote coagulation.
- Pathogens bind and activate monocyte, cytokine, and tissue factor production, enlarging the vegetations on the heart valves.

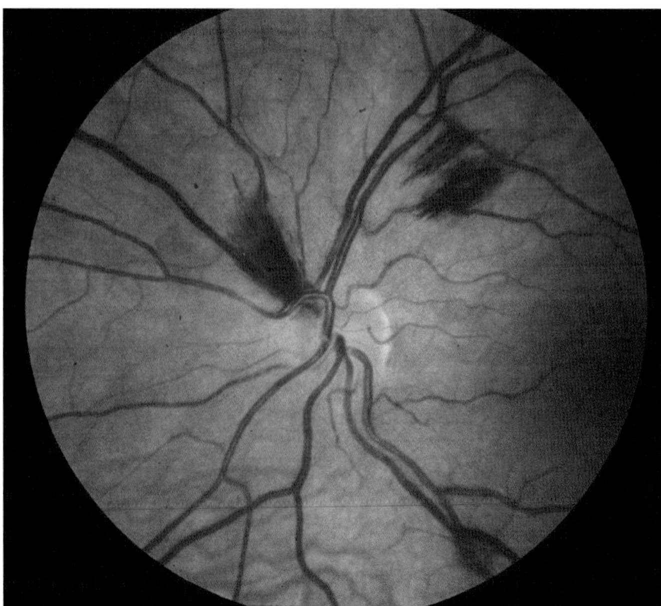

FIGURE 47-2 Roth spots that are retinal hemorrhages with white centers seen in bacterial endocarditis. These can also be seen in leukemia and diabetes. *(Reproduced with permission from Paul D. Comeau.)*

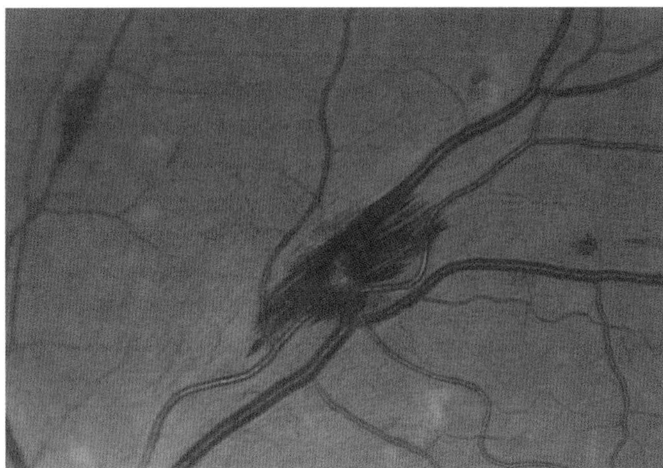

FIGURE 47-3 Close-up of a Roth spot, which is actually a cotton-wool spot surrounded by hemorrhage. The cotton-wool comes from ischemic bursting of axons and the hemorrhage comes from ischemic bursting of an arteriole. *(Reproduced with permission from Paul D. Comeau.)*

- The vegetations enlarge and damage the heart valves (**Figure 47-4**). This process can lead to death if not treated adequately in time.
- Septic emboli can occur, most commonly in the brain, spleen, or kidney.[4]

RISK FACTORS

- Prosthetic valve
- Injection drug use
- HIV infection
- Immunodeficiency

DIAGNOSIS

- Duke criteria use a combination of history, physical examination, laboratory, and echocardiogram findings, and have a sensitivity of approximately 80% across several studies.[5]
- Diagnosis is considered definite when patients have 2 major, 1 major and 3 minor, or 5 minor criteria.[5]

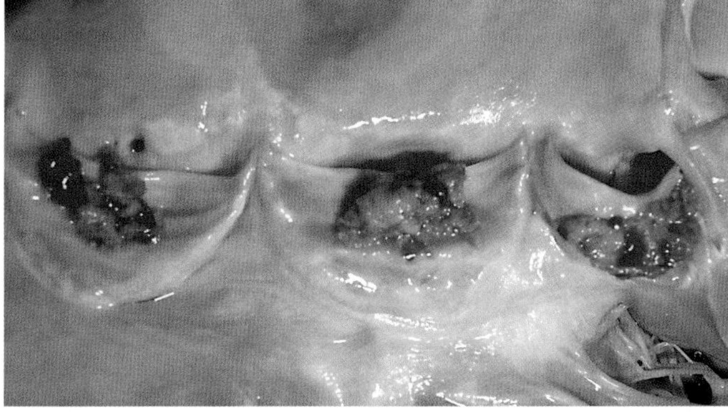

FIGURE 47-4 Pathology specimen of a patient who died of bacterial endocarditis. Bacterial growth can be seen on the 3 cusps of this heart valve. *(Reproduced with permission from Larry Fowler, MD.)*

- Diagnosis is considered possible with 1 major and 1 minor or 3 minor criteria.[5]
- Major criteria include the following[5]:
  - Two separate blood cultures positive with the following factors:
    - *Streptococcus viridans, S. bovis, Haemophilus, Actinobacillus, Cardiobacterium, Eikenella, Kingella*
    - Community-acquired *S. aureus* or *Enterococcus* without a primary focus
    - Microorganisms consistent with prior positive blood cultures in infective endocarditis
  - Endocardial involvement as evidenced by the following factors:
    - Echocardiogram evidence of vegetation, abscess, or new partial dehiscence of a prosthetic valve
    - New valvular regurgitation
  - Minor criteria include the following[5]:
    - Predisposition (eg, heart condition such as a congenital or acquired valvular defect, injection drug use, prior history of endocarditis)
    - Temperature greater than 38°C (100.4°F)
    - Clinical signs that include arterial emboli, septic pulmonary infarcts, mycotic aneurysms, intracranial hemorrhages, Janeway lesions (**Figures 47-5** and **47-6**)
    - Glomerulonephritis, Osler nodes, Roth spots, or positive rheumatoid factor (see **Figures 47-2, 47-3,** and **47-6)**
    - Positive blood culture not meeting major criteria
    - Echocardiographic findings consistent with infective endocarditis that do not meet major criteria

CLINICAL FEATURES

- Fever—Seen in 85% to 99% of patients, typically low grade, approximately 39°C (102.2°F)
- New or changing heart murmur—Seen in 20% to 80% of patients

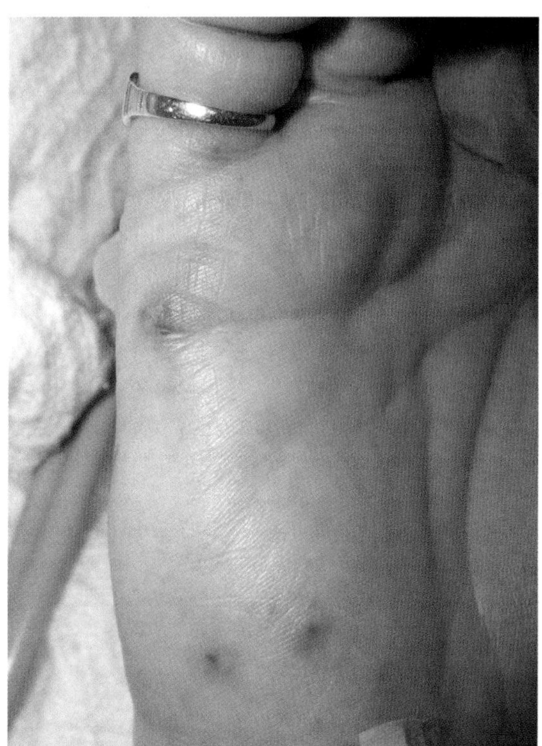

FIGURE 47-5 Janeway lesions on the palm of a woman hospitalized with acute bacterial endocarditis. These were not painful. *(Reproduced with permission from David A. Kasper, DO, MBA.)*

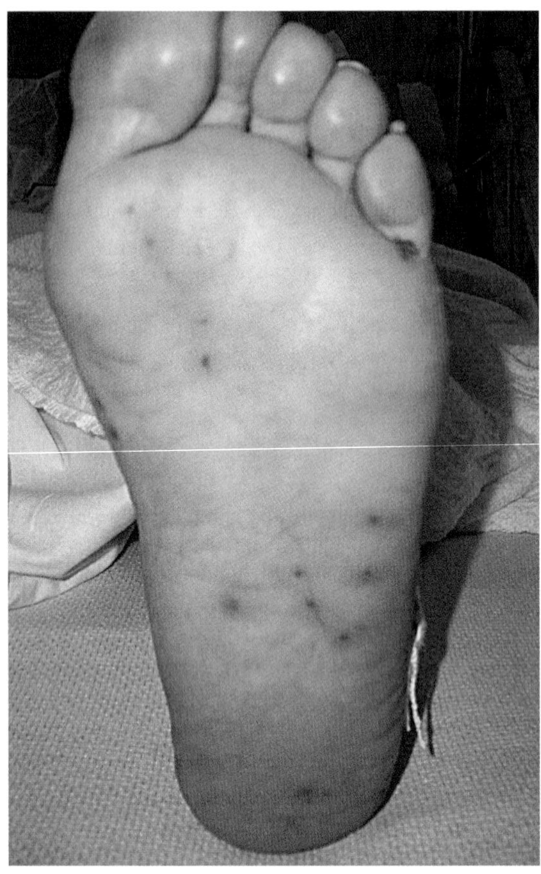

FIGURE 47-6 Osler node causing pain within pulp of the big toe in the same woman hospitalized with acute bacterial endocarditis. (Osler nodes are painful—remember "O" for Ouch and Osler.) Note the multiple painless flat Janeway lesions over the sole of the foot. (*Reproduced with permission from David A. Kasper, DO, MBA.*)

- Septic emboli—Seen in up to 60%, largely dependent on the size (>10 mm) and mobility of the vegetation
- Intracranial hemorrhages—Seen in 30% to 40% of patients, bleeding from septic emboli or cerebral mycotic aneurysms
- Mycotic aneurysms—Aneurysms resulting from infectious process in the arterial wall, most commonly in the thoracic aorta, also found in the cerebral arteries
- Janeway lesions—Very rare, flat, painless, red to bluish-red spots on the palms and soles (see **Figures 47-5** and **47-6**)
- Splinter hemorrhages—Red, linear streaks in the nail beds of the fingers or toes (see **Figure 47-1**)
- Glomerulonephritis—Immune mediated that can result in hematuria and renal insufficiency, occurs in approximately 15% of patients with endocarditis
- Osler nodes—Tender, subcutaneous nodules in the pulp of the digits (see **Figure 47-6**)
- Roth spots—Retinal hemorrhages from microemboli, seen in approximately 5% of endocarditis (see **Figures 47-2** and **47-3**)
- Positive rheumatoid factor—Seen in up to 50% of patients

TYPICAL DISTRIBUTION

- Native endocarditis—Mitral valve (prior rheumatic fever or mitral valve prolapse), followed by aortic (prior rheumatic fever, calcific aortic stenosis of bicuspid valve)
- Prosthetic valve endocarditis—Site of any prosthetic valve
- In IV drug users—Tricuspid valve, followed by aortic valve

LABORATORY AND ANCILLARY TESTING

In addition to blood cultures, consider a complete blood count for anemia and leukocytosis, erythrocyte sedimentation rate (ESR) (elevated in approximately 90%), and urinalysis for proteinuria or microscopic hematuria (seen in approximately 50%).

- Positive blood culture—First 2 sets of cultures are positive in 90%.[4]

IMAGING

- Abnormal echocardiogram in 85%.[5]
- If transthoracic echocardiogram is normal and endocarditis is still suspected, order a transesophageal echo.[6] SOR Ⓐ

DIFFERENTIAL DIAGNOSIS

Fever without a clear cause may be seen with the following:

- Connective tissue disorders—Typically with other signs depending on the disorder, negative blood cultures, normal echocardiogram
- Fever of unknown origin—Negative blood cultures or positive cultures with atypical organisms, normal echocardiogram in noncardiac causes
- Intra-abdominal infections—Fever and positive blood cultures, normal echocardiogram

Echocardiogram findings similar to bacterial endocarditis may be seen with the following:

- Noninfective vegetations—No fever and negative blood cultures
- Cardiac tumors—Embolic complications, right or left heart failure, often located off valves in cardiac chambers, negative blood cultures
- Cusp prolapse—No fever and negative blood cultures
- Myxomatous changes—Extra connective tissue in the valve leaflets
- Lamb excrescences—Stranding from wear and tear on the valve, most commonly aortic, no fever, and negative blood cultures

MANAGEMENT

- Draw blood cultures (2 to 3 sets) and admit suspected cases to the hospital for IV antibiotics.
- Start antibiotics empirically (SOR Ⓒ for specific regiments).

MEDICATIONS

- Cover *Streptococcus* in native valve endocarditis: penicillin G 12 to 18 million units divided every 4 hours and gentamicin 1.5 mg/kg loading dose, then 1 mg/kg every 8 hours.
- Cover *Staphylococcus* in IV drug abusers: nafcillin 2 g every 4 hours and gentamicin; use vancomycin instead of nafcillin when concerned about methicillin-resistant *S. aureus* (MRSA) (prior history of MRSA infection).
- Cover MRSA in prosthetic valve endocarditis: Vancomycin 30 mg/kg per day divided every 8 hours and gentamicin.

- Alter antibiotics based on culture results. SOR Ⓐ
- Treat gram-positive with a β-lactam; current evidence does not support adding an aminoglycoside.[7] SOR Ⓐ

SURGICAL CONSULTATION

- Surgical excision of infected tissue has a 10% to 16% mortality rate in the immediate post-op period.[8,9] Consider surgical consultation when the following occur:
  - Congestive heart failure is severe with mitral or aortic regurgitation.
  - Fever and/or bacteremia persist for 7 to 10 days despite adequate antibiotic therapy, abscesses or perivalvular involvement occurs, or fungal organisms are identified.
  - Embolic events recur on adequate antibiotic therapy or the risk of embolic events is high because of vegetations larger than 10 mm. SOR Ⓒ
- Early surgery in patients with large vegetations reduced the risk of embolic events, but did not affect all-cause mortality.[10]
- Anticoagulation and aspirin are not indicated for infective endocarditis and are contraindicated with cerebral complications or aneurysms.

PREVENTION

- Bacterial endocarditis is a serious life-threatening disease requiring long-term antibiotics and close follow-up.
- Educate patients with high risk for endocarditis of the importance of prophylactic antibiotics before certain procedures. Following are the 2007 American Heart Association recommendations[11]:
  - Prescribe prophylactic antibiotics only to patients at the highest risk: SOR Ⓑ
    - Patients with prosthetic cardiac valves
    - Patients with previous bacterial endocarditis
    - Cardiac transplant recipients with cardiac valvuloplasty
    - Patients with these congenital heart defects (CHDs): unrepaired cyanotic CHD, CHD repaired with prosthetic material within the last 6 months, repaired CHD with a residual defect at or adjacent to the site of a prosthetic device
  - Prophylactic antibiotics are *no longer recommended* for patients with mitral valve prolapse.
  - Prescribe prophylactic antibiotics only to patients undergoing one of the following:
    - Any dental procedure that involves manipulation of gingival tissue or the periapical region of teeth or perforation of the oral mucosa SOR Ⓒ
    - Respiratory procedures involving incision or biopsy of the respiratory mucosa such as a tonsillectomy or adenoidectomy SOR Ⓒ
    - Procedures on infected skin or musculoskeletal tissue
  - Endocarditis prophylaxis is *no longer recommended* for patients undergoing gastrointestinal or genitourinary procedures. SOR Ⓑ
  - Prescribe a one-dose regimen to be taken 30 minutes to 1 hour before the procedure[11]:
    - Amoxicillin 2 g orally.
    - Unable to take oral medications: ampicillin 2 g intramuscular (IM) *or* IV or cefazolin *or* ceftriaxone 1 g IM or IV.
    - Penicillin allergic: clindamycin 600 mg PO, IM, or IV; *or* azithromycin or clarithromycin 500 mg PO. If allergy to penicillin is *not* anaphylaxis, angioedema, or urticaria, may also use cephalexin 2 g PO; *or* cefazolin or ceftriaxone 1 g IM or IV.

PROGNOSIS

Bacterial endocarditis requires early detection and aggressive antibiotic therapy to decrease mortality.

- Thirty-day mortality is 16% to 25%.[3]
- Ninety-day mortality is 14.5%.[3]
- Greater than 6-month mortality is 20% to 37%.[3]

FOLLOW-UP

- Most patients with bacterial endocarditis will require 4 to 6 weeks of IV antibiotics.
- Depending on the antibiotics, some patients will need to have medication levels monitored.
- Repeat blood cultures to ensure response to therapy.
- An echocardiogram at the end of treatment provides baseline imaging, as patients with endocarditis are at risk for another episode.[6] SOR Ⓒ

PATIENT EDUCATION

- Bacterial endocarditis is a serious disease with a significant mortality rate.
- Finish all antibiotics and keep follow-up appointments to ensure adequate treatment.
- Mortality remains elevated even 6 months after an episode.
- Recurrence is common, especially if risk factors remain (ie, continued immunosuppression or IV drug use).

PATIENT RESOURCES

- The American Heart Association has information about who is at risk for bacterial endocarditis and a printable wallet card for at-risk patient, available in English or Spanish—**http://www.heart.org/HEARTORG/Conditions/CongenitalHeartDefects/TheImpactofCongenitalHeartDefects/Infective-Endocarditis_UCM_307108_Article.jsp.**

PROVIDER RESOURCES

- The American Heart Association guidelines on endocarditis prophylaxis—**http://circ.ahajournals.org/content/116/15/1736.full.pdf.**
- Guidelines on Infective Endocarditis: Diagnosis, Antimicrobial Therapy, and Management of Complications—**http://circ.ahajournals.org/content/111/23/e394.full.**
- MedCalc has an interactive Web site with Duke criteria for infective endocarditis—**www.medcalc.com/endocarditis.html.**

REFERENCES

1. de Sa DD, Tleyjeh IM, Anavekar NS, et al. Epidemiological trends of infective endocarditis: a population-based study in Olmsted County, Minnesota. *Mayo Clin Proc.* 2010;85(5):422-426.

2. Wilson LE, Thomas DL, Astemborski J, et al. Prospective study of infective endocarditis among injection drug users. *J Infect Dis.* 2002;185(12):1761-1766.

3. Nomura A, Omata F, Furukawa K. Risk factors of mid-term mortality of patients with infective endocarditis. *Eur J Clin Microbiol Infect Dis.* 2010;29(11):1355-1360.

4. Prendergast BD. The changing face of infective endocarditis. *Heart.* 2006;92(7):879-885.

5. Habib G. Management of infective endocarditis. *Heart.* 2006;92(1): 124-130.

6. Baddour LM, Wilson WR, Bayer AS, et al. American Heart Association Scientific Statement on Infective Endocarditis. *Circulation.* 2005;111:e394-e434.

7. Falagas ME, Matthaiou DK, Bliziotis IA. The role of aminoglycosides in combination with a beta-lactam for the treatment of bacterial endocarditis: a meta-analysis of comparative trials. *J Antimicrob Chemother.* 2006;57(4):639-647.

8. Fayad G, Leroy G, Devos P, et al. Characteristics and prognosis of patients requiring valve surgery during active infective endocarditis. *J Heart Valve Dis.* 2011;20(2):223-228.

9. Mokhles MM, Ciampichetti I, Head SJ, et al. Survival of surgically treated infective endocarditis: a comparison with the general Dutch population. *Ann Thorac Surg.* 2011;91(5):1407-1412.

10. Kang DH, Kim YJ, Kim SH, et al. Early surgery versus conventional treatment for infective endocarditis. *N Engl J Med.* 2012;366: 2466-2473.

11. Wilson W, Taubert KA, Gewitz M, et al. Prevention of infective endocarditis: a guideline from the American Heart Association. *Circulation.* 2007;116:1736-1754.

48 HYPERTENSION

Heidi Chumley

PATIENT STORY

A 40 year-old man presents after his blood pressure was measured as 180/100 mm Hg at a health screening. He has no complaints. His blood pressure today is 178/98 mm Hg. Based on these 2 readings, he is diagnosed with stage 2 hypertension (HTN). His family history is very positive for essential HTN. His examination is normal other than an enlarged and laterally displaced point of maximal impulse. His body mass index is normal. The provider sends him for a urinalysis, complete blood count (CBC), fasting lipid profile, and a chemistry panel that includes blood glucose, potassium, serum creatinine, and calcium. An electrocardiogram (ECG) shows left ventricular hypertrophy (**Figure 48-1**). He is counseled regarding lifestyle change, started on 2 medications, and asked to follow-up within a couple of weeks.

INTRODUCTION

Hypertension is a major risk factor for both myocardial infarction and stroke. Primary HTN constitutes 90% of HTN cases. Initial treatment includes lifestyle modifications and medications. Most patients require at least 2 medications to achieve control. Patients who are not controlled on 3 medications should undergo a workup for secondary causes.

EPIDEMIOLOGY

- Of US adults older than age 18 years, 30.4% have HTN.[1,2]
- Blood pressure is controlled in approximately 50% of adults with HTN.[1,2]
- Blood pressure control is lowest among those without health insurance (29%), Mexican Americans (37%), and adults ages 18 to 39 years (31%).[1,2]
- Ninety percent of patients with uncontrolled HTN have a usual source of care and health insurance.[2]
- In the United States, HTN contributes to 1 of every 7 deaths and to half of the cardiovascular disease-related deaths.[2]
- Cost of HTN to the US health care system is estimated to be $131 billion per year.[2]

ETIOLOGY AND PATHOPHYSIOLOGY

- Primary HTN (>90% of patients)—The specific cause is unknown, but environmental factors (ie, salt intake, excess alcohol intake, obesity) and genetics both play a role.
- Secondary HTN (5%-10% of patients)—Causes include medications, kidney disease, renal artery stenosis (**Figure 48-2**), thyroid disease, hyperaldosteronism, and sleep apnea. Rare causes include coarctation of the aorta, Cushing syndrome, and pheochromocytoma.

RISK FACTORS

- Family history or genetic predisposition
- Obesity
- High sodium chloride intake
- Medications, including oral contraceptives, nonsteroidal anti-inflammatory drugs (NSAIDs), decongestants, and some antidepressants
- Substances, including caffeine, licorice, amphetamines, cocaine, and tobacco

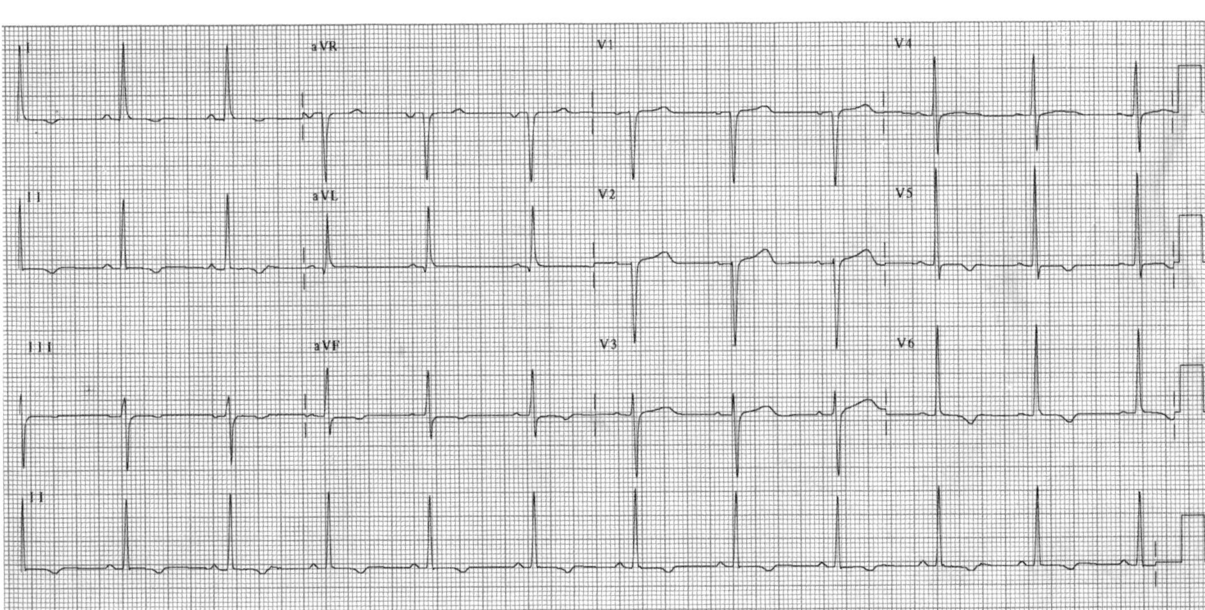

FIGURE 48-1 ECG showing left ventricular hypertrophy in this 58-year-old man with current blood pressure of 178/98. Note how S V_1 + R V_5 > 35 mm. Also his ECG shows left axis deviation and nonspecific ST changes in the high lateral leads (I and aVL). *(Reproduced with permission from Gary Ferenchick, MD.)*

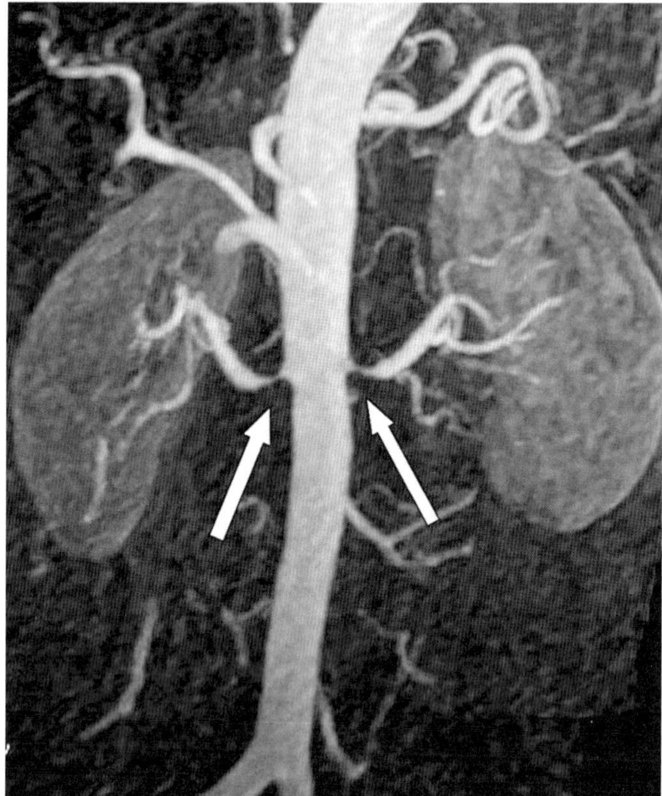

FIGURE 48-2 Angiogram revealing bilateral renal artery stenosis (arrows), one of the more common causes of secondary hypertension, most often a result of atherosclerotic disease in older patients. (*Reproduced with permission from Figure 111-15A in* Hurst's the Heart, *13th ed.*)

DIAGNOSIS

Average of 2 or more seated blood pressure readings on each of 2 or more office visits based on systolic (SBP) and diastolic (DBP) blood pressures.

- Prehypertension—SBP 120 to 139 mm Hg or DBP 80 to 89 mm Hg
- Stage 1 HTN—SBP 140 to 159 mm Hg or DBP 90 to 99 mm Hg
- Stage 2 HTN—SBP equal to or greater than 160 mm Hg or DBP equal to or greater than 100 mm Hg

CLINICAL FEATURES

- No symptoms may be present.
- When blood pressure is high, patients may have headaches, vision changes, confusion, chest pain or myocardial infarction, pulmonary edema, stroke, or hematuria.
- Hypertensive retinopathy may be present (**Figure 48-3** and Chapter 18, Hypertensive retinopathy).
- An S4 can be an early physical examination finding.
- Left ventricular hypertrophy may be manifest as an enlarged laterally displaced point of maximal impulse, abnormal ECG (see **Figure 48-1**), or abnormal chest radiograph.
- Abdominal bruits may be present with renal artery stenosis.

LABORATORY TESTING

- Before initiating therapy for presumed primary HTN perform the following tests: urinalysis, CBC, fasting lipid profile, and chemistry panel, including fasting blood glucose, potassium, creatinine, and calcium.

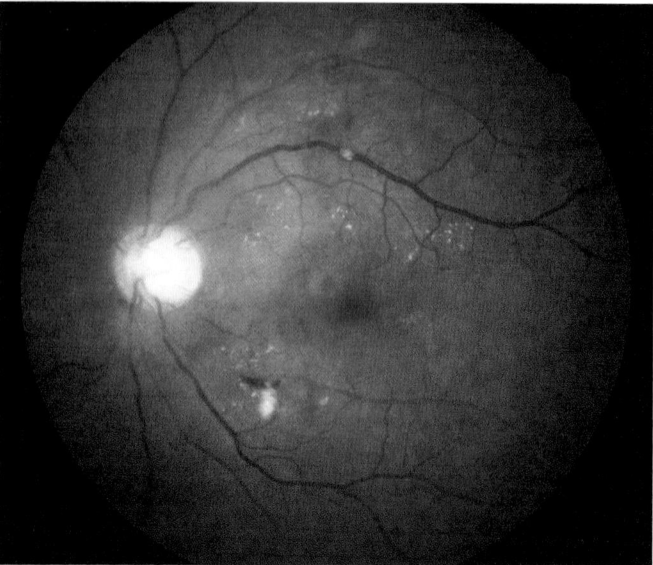

FIGURE 48-3 Hypertensive and diabetic retinopathy with dot-blot hemorrhages, a flame hemorrhage, and hard exudates. The arterioles are attenuated from the hypertension. (*Reproduced with permission from Carrie Cooke.*)

- Consider testing for thyroid disorders with a thyroid-stimulating hormone (TSH) if other signs or symptoms are present.
- For patients with abnormal screening tests, signs indicating a secondary cause, or inadequate control on 3 medications include the following:
    - Serum aldosterone and plasma renin activity are useful in patients with hypokalemia.
    - A 24-hour urine protein and creatinine for suspected renal disease.
    - A 24-hour urine-free cortisol or a dexamethasone suppression test for suspected Cushing syndrome.
    - Plasma and urine catecholamines or metanephrines for suspected pheochromocytoma.
    - Parathyroid hormone level for suspected hyperparathyroidism.

IMAGING AND ANCILLARY TESTS

- ECG on all patients with HTN.
- Chest radiograph is usually not ordered for primary HTN; however, if obtained, cardiomegaly may be present. If coarctation of the aorta is expected, rib notching may be present.
- Echocardiogram may also demonstrate left ventricular hypertrophy.
- Renal artery stenosis can be seen on magnetic resonance angiography or by angiography (see **Figure 48-2**).
- Renal ultrasound may demonstrate small or absent kidney.

DIFFERENTIAL DIAGNOSIS

- Falsely elevated blood pressure readings can be a result of improper cuff size (too small with a large-arm diameter) or method (patient not seated, arm in incorrect position, etc).
- Acute elevations in blood pressure may be caused by substances (eg, tobacco).
- White-coat HTN is defined as blood pressure that is consistently over 140/90 mm Hg in the presence of a health care provider with an ambulatory monitoring average of less than 135/85 mm Hg.

MANAGEMENT

NONPHARMACOLOGIC

- Weight reduction if overweight or obese.
- Dietary approaches to stop hypertension (DASH) diet, rich in fruits and vegetables, aimed at reducing sodium intake and eating a variety of foods rich in nutrients that help lower blood pressure, such as potassium, calcium, and magnesium.
- Low-fat diet.
- Low dietary sodium chloride.
- Regular aerobic exercise.
- Moderate alcohol intake: no more than 2 drinks per day for men and 1 drink per day for women.
- Smoking cessation for cardiovascular risk reduction (see Chapter 237, Tobacco Addiction).

MEDICATIONS

- Start a thiazide-type diuretic in most patients. An angiotensin-converting enzyme inhibitor (ACEI) may be the initial choice in white males.
- Consider starting 2 medications when blood pressure is 20/10 mm Hg higher than goal. Goal is 140/90 mm Hg or 130/80 mm Hg in patients with diabetes or chronic kidney disease.
- Add an ACEI, angiotensin receptor blocker (ARB), β-blocker (BB), or calcium channel blocker (CCB) if control is not achieved with initial agent.
- Specific medications have compelling indications in these situations:
    - Heart failure—Diuretic, BB, ACEI, ARB, aldosterone antagonist (AA)
    - Postmyocardial infarction—BB, ACEI, AA
    - Diabetes—Diuretic, BB, ACEI, ARB, CCB
    - Chronic kidney disease—ACEI, ARB
    - Recurrent stroke prevention—Diuretic, ACEI

REFERRAL OR HOSPITALIZATION

- Refer patients in whom adequate blood pressure control is not obtained.
- Women with HTN who are planning a pregnancy or who become pregnant should be referred to a provider with experience managing chronic HTN in pregnancy.

PREVENTION

Healthy lifestyle for all persons, including weight reduction (if overweight or obese), use of DASH, initiation and maintenance of adequate physical activity, and moderate alcohol intake.

PROGNOSIS

- Risk of cardiovascular disease increases as blood pressure increases.
- Between 115/75 and 185/115 mm Hg, every 20 mm Hg SBP or 10 mm Hg DBP doubles the risk of cardiovascular disease for adults ages 40 to 70 years.[3]

FOLLOW-UP

- Schedule visits monthly until blood pressure goal is obtained.
- Consider more frequent visits for patients with stage 2 HTN or significant comorbid conditions.
- See patients with controlled HTN every 3 to 6 months.

PATIENT EDUCATION

- HTN is a chronic disease requiring lifelong lifestyle modifications and one or more daily medications for most patients.
- Adequate control of HTN reduces the risk for heart attack and stroke.

PATIENT RESOURCE

- The National Heart Lung and Blood Institute. *What Is High Blood Pressure?*—**http://www.nhlbi.nih.gov/health/health-topics/topics/hbp/.**

PROVIDER RESOURCES

- The Seventh Report of the Joint National Committee on Prevention, Detection, Evaluation, and Treatment of High Blood Pressure (JNC 7)—**http://www.nhlbi.nih.gov/guidelines/hypertension/express.pdf.**
- The Eighth Report of the Joint National Committee on Prevention, Detection, Evaluation, and Treatment of High Blood Pressure (JNC 8)—**http://www.nhlbi.nih.gov/guidelines/hypertension/jnc8/index.htm.**

REFERENCES

1. Egan BM, Zhao Y, Axon RN. US trends in prevalence, awareness, treatment and control of hypertension, 1988-2008. *JAMA.* 2010;303(2):2043-2050.
2. Centers for Disease Control and Prevention. Vital signs: awareness and treatment of uncontrolled hypertension among adults—United States, 2003-2010. *MMWR Morb Mortal Wkly Rep.* 2012;61(35):703-709.
3. Lewington S, Clarke R, Qizilbash N, et al. Age-specific relevance of usual blood pressure to vascular mortality: a metaanalysis of individual data for one million adults in 61 prospective studies. *Lancet.* 2002;360:1903-1913.

49 PERICARDITIS AND PERICARDIAL EFFUSION

Heidi Chumley, MD

PATIENT STORY

A 50-year-old man presented to his physician with acute onset of pleuritic chest pain, which improved when he leaned forward, and shortness of breath. He did not take any medications, and had not had any recent trauma or surgery. He had a pericardial rub on examination. He had diffused ST changes on her electrocardiogram (ECG) (**Figure 49-1**). His chest radiograph showed a classic globular heart as demonstrated in **Figure 49-2.** An echocardiogram confirmed pericardial effusion (**Figure 49-3**) without cardiac tamponade. He was briefly hospitalized and treated with high-dose aspirin. The underlying etiology was not elucidated and he recovered over the next several months.

INTRODUCTION

Acute pericarditis typically presents with pleuritic chest pain and can be seen with or without a pleural effusion. Eighty-five percent of cases are idiopathic, but they can be caused by infections, neoplastic disease, autoimmune diseases, or following trauma or myocardial infarction. Diagnosis is made based on history, physical examination, and ECG. Treatment is with nonsteroidal anti-inflammatory drugs (NSAIDs).

Pericardial effusions are commonly found in the general population and the incidence increases with age. They can be caused by cardiac disease or surgery, connective tissue disorders, neoplasms, infections, renal disease, hypothyroidism, or medications; however, a cause is identified only 50% of the time. The definitive diagnosis is made by echocardiography.

EPIDEMIOLOGY

- Five percent of patients in the emergency department (ED) with noncardiac chest pain have pericarditis.[1]
- Six-and-a-half percent of adults (<1% with age 20-30 years; 15% older than 80 years of age) had echocardiogram findings consistent with pericardial effusion in a population-based study of 5652 adults and adult family members of participants in the Framingham Heart Study.[2]
- Seventy-seven percent of patients after cardiac surgery for valves or bypass have pericardial effusions, which rarely (<1%) require therapy.[3]

ETIOLOGY AND PATHOPHYSIOLOGY

Pericarditis is inflammation of the pericardium. Eighty-five percent of cases are idiopathic or presumed viral. Testing is low yield if history and physical examination does not reveal an associated underlying systemic disease or infection.

Pericardial effusion, acute or chronic, occurs when there is increased production or decreased drainage of pericardial fluid allowing accumulation in the pericardial space.

The underlying etiology is apparent clinically approximately 25% of the time and can be determined with testing in another 25% of cases, leaving 50% of cases idiopathic.[4] Most idiopathic cases have small effusions. Moderate-to-large pericardial effusions have an identifiable cause in 90%.[5]

RISK FACTORS

Eighty-five percent of acute pericarditis cases are idiopathic or presumed viral; other causes include the following[6]:

- Infections (identified viral, bacterial, tuberculosis, or rarely fungal or parasitic)
- Neoplastic disease
- Autoimmune disease
- Acute myocardial infarction
- Renal failure, especially in patients on dialysis

Underlying causes include the following:

- Congestive heart failure from other cardiac diseases, such as rheumatic heart disease, cor pulmonale, or cardiomyopathy[7]
- After cardiac surgery or after a myocardial infarction[3]

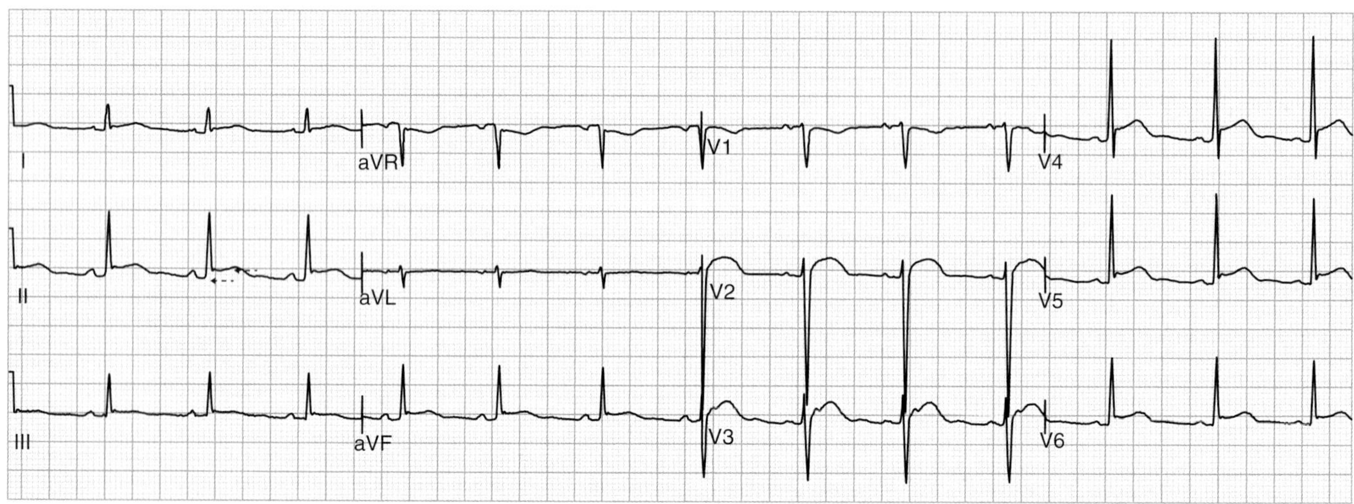

FIGURE 49-1 ECG of a 50-year-old man with acute pericarditis showing diffusely elevated ST segments in virtually all leads. (*Reproduced with permission from Gary Ferenchick, MD.*)

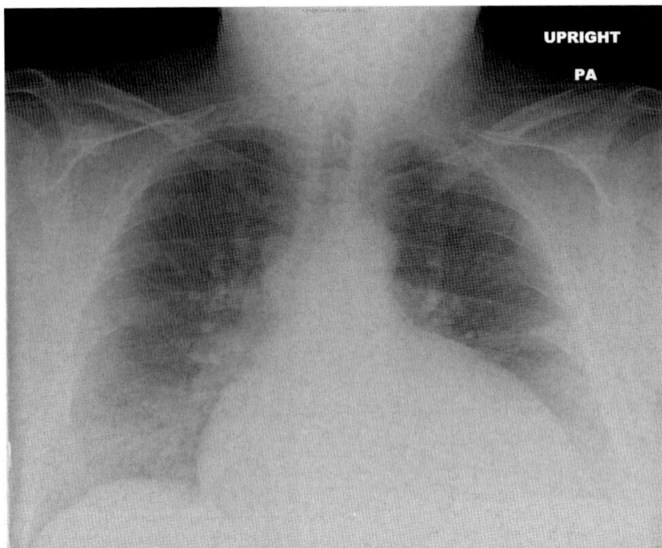

FIGURE 49-2 Globular cardiac silhouette in a 50-year-old man with acute pericarditis and pericardial effusion. A globular cardiac silhouette or classic "water-bottle heart" seen with a pericardial effusion can be difficult to distinguish from cardiomegaly on plain radiographs. (*Reproduced with permission from Heidi Chumley, MD.*)

- Connective tissue disorders (scleroderma, lupus erythematosus, rheumatoid arthritis)[7]
- Neoplasms: benign (atrial myxoma), primary malignant (mesothelioma), secondary malignant (ie, lung or breast cancer)[7]
- Chronic renal disease (uremia or hemodialysis) or other causes of hypoalbuminemia
- Infections: acute (enterovirus, adenovirus, influenza virus, *Streptococcus* pneumonia, *Coxiella burnetii*—responsible for Q fever) or chronic (tuberculosis, fungus, parasites)[4]
- Medications (procainamide, hydralazine) or after radiation[7]
- Severe hypothyroidism with myxedema[7]

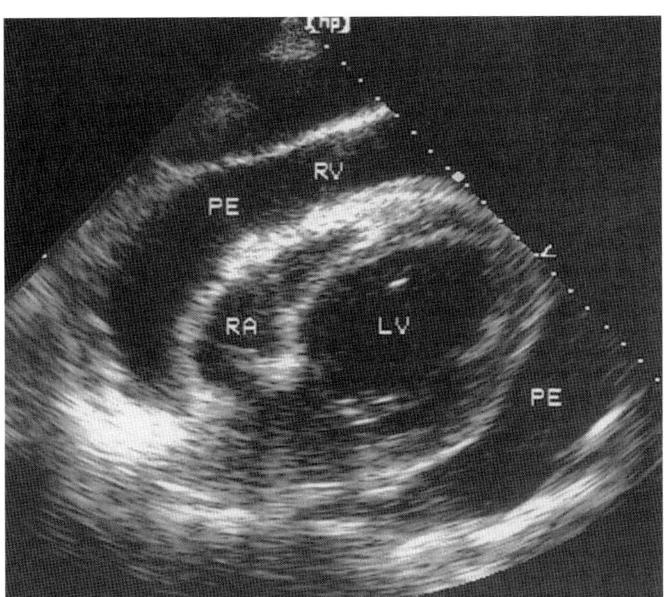

FIGURE 49-3 Echocardiogram showing right ventricular (RV) compression from a pericardial effusion (PE) in a 50-year-old man with acute pericarditis. LV, left ventricle; RA, right atrium. (*Reproduced with permission from Heidi Chumley, MD.*)

DIAGNOSIS

Acute pericarditis has at least 2 of 4 criteria: characteristic chest pain, pericardial friction rub, typical ECG changes, pericardial effusion.[6] Clinical features, chest radiograph, and ECG suggest pericardial effusion, which is confirmed by echocardiogram.

CLINICAL FEATURES

Acute pericarditis

- Pleuritic, retrosternal chest pain, that improves when patients lean forward
- Pericardial friction rub, heard in 85% of patients during the course of illness

Pericardial effusion

Signs and symptoms occur when the volume of fluid is large enough to affect hemodynamics. This occurs at 150 to 200 mL in acute pericardial effusion. Chronic pericardial effusion allows stretching overtime and may require up to 2 L to cause significant symptoms[7]:

- Hypotension, increased jugular venous pressure, and soft heart sounds form the classic triad of acute cardiac tamponade, but all 3 are present only in approximately 30% of cases.[7]
- Common symptoms include anorexia (90%), dyspnea (78%), cough (47%), and chest pain (27%).[7]
- Common physical examination findings include pulsus paradoxus (77% with acute tamponade, 30% with chronic effusions), sinus tachycardia (50%), jugular venous distention (45%), hepatomegaly, and peripheral edema (35%).[7]

LABORATORY AND ANCILLARY TESTING

Acute pericarditis

- Electrocardiogram initially shows diffuse ST segment elevation and PR segment depression (**see Figure 49-1**), followed by T-wave inversions.
- Laboratory tests rarely help to identify the underlying cause as follows[6]:
  - Complete blood count (CBC), sedimentation rate, and/or C-reactive protein are typically elevated.
  - If autoimmune is suspected, check antinuclear antibody (ANA).
  - If infection is suspected, test for TB and HIV, and collect blood cultures.
  - If myocardial infarction is considered, order troponin.
- Echocardiogram if pericardial effusion is suspected.

Pericardial effusion

Electrocardiogram is abnormal in 90%. Findings include low QRS voltage and nonspecific ST-T changes (59%-63%) and electrical alternans (0%-10%).[7]

When the diagnosis remains unclear, pericardial fluid can be sent for cell count and differential, protein, lactate dehydrogenase, glucose, Gram stain, bacterial cultures, fungal cultures, mycobacterial acid-fast stain and culture, and tumor cytology. Measure rheumatoid factor, ANA, and complement levels when collagen vascular disease is suspected.[7] Check HIV status in at-risk patients.

When there is no obvious cause, ordering this set of specific tests determined the underlying etiology more often than seen in historic controls (27.3% vs 3.9%; $p < 0.001$).[8]

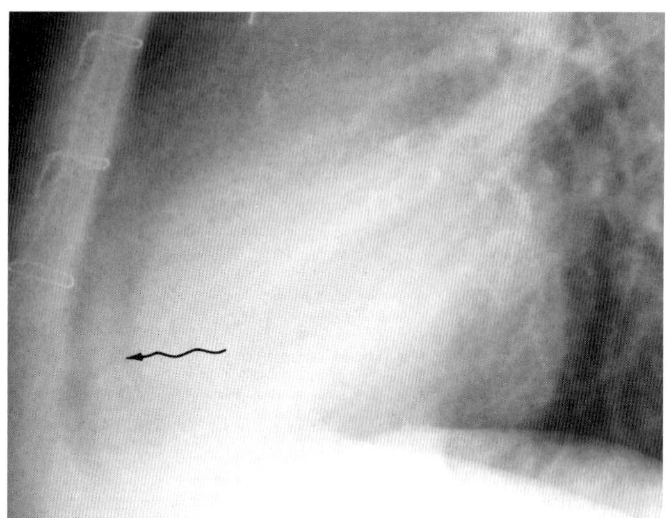

FIGURE 49-4 Moderate pericardial effusion is seen as a wide pericardium (arrow). (*Reproduced with permission from Heidi Chumley, MD.*)

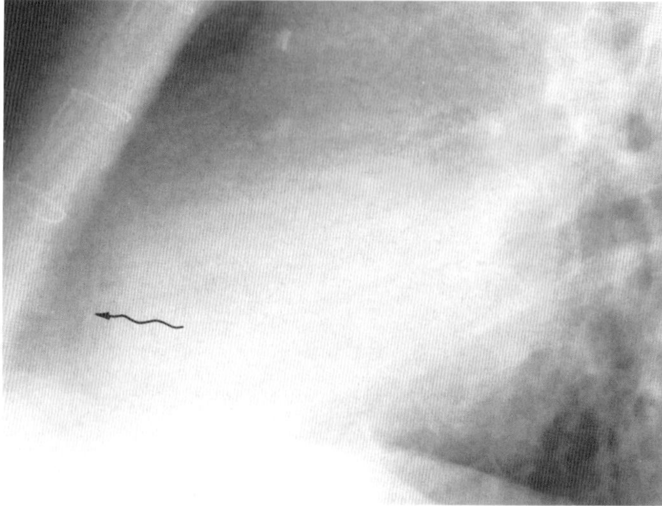

FIGURE 49-5 The lateral view demonstrates the normal thin pericardium (arrow), which should be less than 2 mm. (*Reproduced with permission from Heidi Chumley, MD.*)

- Aerobic and anaerobic blood cultures
- Throat swab cultures for influenza, adenovirus, and enterovirus
- Serologic tests for *Cytomegalovirus,* influenza, *C. burnetii, Mycoplasma pneumoniae, and Toxoplasma*
- Blood tests for ANA and thyroid-stimulating hormone (TSH)

IMAGING

Acute pericarditis

- Chest radiograph is often normal, unless a significant pericardial effusion is present.
- Cardiac computed tomography (CT) can detect a pericardial effusion and provide pericardial thickness.[6]
- Cardiac magnetic resonance imaging (MRI) shows delayed enhancement of the pericardium, a very sensitive finding, but generally not needed for the diagnosis.[6]

Pericardial effusion

- Chest radiograph shows a globular enlarged cardiac silhouette (**see Figure 49-2**) (sensitivity 78%, specificity 34% with moderate or severe effusions) and pericardial fat stripe (**Figure 49-4**) (sensitivity 22%, specificity 92%).[7]
- Echocardiography is the preferred imaging test. Echo can be used to quantify volume of pericardial effusion (correlation to amount of fluid withdrawn 0.7).[9] Echo-free, as opposed to echogenic fluid, is associated with a lower risk of constrictive pericarditis or recurrent pleural effusion.[10]
- CT scanning, typically done for another purpose, can demonstrate the presence of a pericardial effusion, but does not qualify volume as well as echocardiography (correlation to amount of fluid withdrawn 0.4).[9]

DIFFERENTIAL DIAGNOSIS

Acute pericarditis

- Myocardial infarction also presents with sudden onset of chest pain which is typically not pleuritic. Electrocardiogram findings are more localized. Troponin is often higher than the mild elevation seen with acute pericarditis.
- Pleurisy presents with pleuritic chest pain that is localized with an overlying friction rub.
- Costochondritis has reproducible chest pain and if ordered, inflammatory measures are normal.

Pericardial effusion

- Congestive heart failure has many similar signs and symptoms (dyspnea, jugular venous distention, hepatomegaly, and edema) but may have pulmonary rales, which are unusual in pericardial effusions. A lateral radiograph in a patient with congestive heart failure (without pleural effusion) should have a normal thin pericardium (**Figure 49-5**).
- Pleural effusions may also present with dyspnea, but have different physical examination and radiographic findings.
- Acute pericarditis (without pericardial effusion) can present with chest pain and nonspecific ECG changes also seen with pericardial effusion. In contrast, acute pericarditis often has elevated inflammatory markers and a normal chest radiograph.

MANAGEMENT

Acute pericarditis

- Treat underlying cause if identified.
- Prescribe NSAIDs (aspirin 800 mg every 6-8 hours for 7 days, then taper dose by 800 mg a week for 3 weeks). Add misoprostol or omeprazole for gastric protection. Indomethacin and ketorolac are also effective.[6]
- Consider colchicines for 4 to 6 weeks in patients without contraindications, especially those who did not respond after a week of NSAIDs.[6]
- Corticosteroids may be beneficial when pericarditis is due to autoimmune causes; however, they are an independent risk factor for recurrence. Consider only after no response to NSAIDs with colchicines.[6]
- Hospitalize patients with high-risk factors: fever, leukocytosis, large pericardial effusion, cardiac tamponade, trauma, immunosuppressed state, anticoagulation, failed NSAID therapy, or high troponin levels.[6]

Pericardial effusion

- Treat any identified underlying cause.
- When the diagnosis is unclear and the patient is hemodynamically stable, NSAIDs may be beneficial, especially if inflammatory markers are elevated.
- Pericardiocentesis is required when there is hemodynamic compromise. A pericardiocentesis is also useful when the pericardial effusion is large or suspected to be secondary to a bacterial infection or neoplastic process.
- Pericardiocentesis is performed by a specialist under local anesthesia as follows: Elevate the patient to a 45-degree angle. Insert a needle in the angle between the left costal arch and the xiphoid process, directed 15-degrees posterior, and angled toward the head or either shoulder. Complications are reduced when this procedure is guided by echocardiography. Fluid often reaccumulates. An indwelling catheter can be placed for up to 72 hours without increasing the risk of infection, until a more permanent procedure can be performed to decrease the likelihood of reaccumulation.
- Sclerosing therapy reduces the recurrence of symptoms from reaccumulation or the need for a repeat procedure for 30 days in more than 70% of patients. A caustic substance such as bleomycin or tetracycline is instilled into the pericardial space and held there for up to 4 hours.
- Other options to reduce recurrence include balloon pericardiotomy performed in a cardiac catheterization laboratory, radiation therapy, and surgery (ie, pericardial window).

PROGNOSIS

Prognosis depends on the underlying cause.

Acute pericarditis without high-risk features has an excellent prognosis.[11] Constrictive pericarditis rarely occurs with viral or idiopathic pericarditis, but can complicate pericarditis from other causes, especially bacterial etiologies.[12]

In a study of older adults undergoing echocardiography for reasons other than a pericardial effusion, patients with an incidental small pericardial effusion had a higher 1-year mortality (26%) than did patients without an effusion (11%).[13]

FOLLOW-UP

Follow-up is based on the underlying cause. Patients with acute pericarditis should be seen frequently to monitor for resolution of pericarditis and side effects of therapy. Pericardial effusions often disappear when the underlying illness resolves, and reappear when the underlying illness does not resolve (metastatic cancer).

PATIENT EDUCATION

- The cause of pericarditis is rarely identified; however, specific tests should be done to find causes which require a different treatment.
- Hospitalization is sometimes necessary, but many times pericarditis is effectively treated as an outpatient with anti-inflammatory medications.
- The underlying cause of a pericardial effusion is identified only 50% of the time; however, specific tests should be done to find treatable causes.
- In patients without an obvious underlying illness, infections (like the flu, Q fever, or tuberculosis) and cancer are the 2 most commonly identified causes of pericardial effusions.

PATIENT RESOURCES

- Mayo Clinic. *Pericarditis*—**http://www.mayoclinic.com/health/pericarditis/DS00505.**
- Mayo Clinic. *Pericardial Effusion*—**http://www.mayoclinic.com/health/pericardial-effusion/DS01124.**

PROVIDER RESOURCES

- Medscape. *Acute Pericarditis*—**http://emedicine.medscape.com/article/156951-overview.**
- Medscape. *Pericardial Effusion*—**http://emedicine.medscape.com/article/157325.**

REFERENCES

1. Spodick DH. Acute cardiac tamponade. *N Engl J Med.* 2003;349(7):684-690.
2. Savage DD, Garrison RJ, Brand F, et al. Prevalence and correlates of posterior extra echocardiographic spaces in a free-living population based sample (the Framingham study). *Am J Cardiol.* 1983;51(7): 1207-1212.
3. Ikaheimo MJ, Huikuri HV, Airaksinen KE, et al. Pericardial effusion after cardiac surgery: incidence, relation to the type of surgery, antithrombotic therapy, and early coronary bypass graft patency. *Am Heart J.* 1988;116(1 pt 1):97-102.
4. Levy PY, Corey R, Berger P, et al. Etiologic diagnosis of 204 pericardial effusions. *Medicine (Baltimore).* 2003;82(6):385-391.
5. Imazio M, Spodick DH, Brucato A, et al. Controversial issues in the management of pericardial diseases. *Circulation.* 2010;121(7):916-928.
6. Khandaker MH, Espinosa RE, Nishimura RA, et al. Pericardial disease: diagnosis and management. *Mayo Clin Proc.* 2010;85(6):572-593.
7. Karam N, Patel P, deFilippi C. Diagnosis and management of chronic pericardial effusions. *Am J Med Sci.* 2002;322(2):79-87.
8. Levy PY, Moatti JP, Gauduchon V, et al. Comparison of intuitive versus systematic strategies for aetiological diagnosis of pericardial effusion. *Scand J Infect Dis.* 2005;37(3):216-220.
9. Liebowitz D, Perlman G, Planer D, et al. Quantification of pericardial effusions by echocardiography and computed tomography. *Am J Cardiol.* 2011;107(2):331-335.
10. Kim SH, Song JM, Jung IH, et al. Initial echocardiographic characteristics of pericardial effusion determine the pericardial complications. *Int J Cardiol.* 2009;136(2):151-155.
11. Imazio M, Demichelis B, Parrini I, et al. Day-hospital treatment of acute pericarditis: a management program for outpatient therapy. *J Am Coll Cardiol.* 2004;43(6):1042-1046.
12. Imazio M, Brucato A, Maestroni S, et al. Risk of constrictive pericarditis after acute pericarditis. *Circulation.* 2011;124(11):1270-1275.
13. Mitiku TY, Heidenreich PA. A small pericardial effusion is a marker of increased mortality. *Am Heart J.* 2011;161(1):152-157.

50 PERIPHERAL ARTERIAL DISEASE

Madhab Lamichhane, MD

PATIENT STORY

A 51-year-old woman with a known history of hypertension, hyperlipidemia, and uncontrolled diabetes presents to the hospital with a nonhealing wound of the left second toe (**Figure 50-1**). She had partial amputation surgery of the left second toe 4 months ago. She has not been able to walk more than a block because of pain in the left foot for several months. She quit smoking 4 months ago after 20 years of smoking 2 packs per day. On examination, she has a foul-smelling, draining wound at the base of the second toe with mild tenderness around it. Left dorsalis pedis and left posterior tibial arteries are not palpable. Radiography of the foot shows focal osteopenia at the base of the proximal phalanx of the second toe. Doppler ultrasound shows monophasic waveforms in the left posterior tibial and dorsalis pedis artery segments. The ankle-brachial index (ABI) is 0.39 at the left dorsalis pedis and 0 at the great toe. A selective angiogram of the left lower extremity demonstrates 100% occlusion of the anterior tibial artery at its origin, occlusion of the peroneal artery in its proximal portion, and occlusion of the posterior tibial artery in its distal portion. The anterior tibial artery received collaterals at the level of the foot. Left posterior tibial angioplasty is performed. She receives wound debridement and is discharged on ertepenem based on wound culture growth of extended-spectrum β-lactamase-positive *Escherichia coli*.

INTRODUCTION

- Peripheral arterial disease (PAD) includes a broad range of noncoronary arterial diseases (non-CADs) caused by the altered structure and function of the arteries that supply the brain, visceral organs, and the limbs.[1]
- Altered structure or function leads to progressive stenosis or occlusion or aneurysmal dilation of the arteries supplying a tissue or organ, which manifest with a feature of acute or chronic ischemia.
- PAD is the preferred term to differentiate arterial disease from the broad term peripheral vascular diseases, which also include venous and lymphatic circulations.

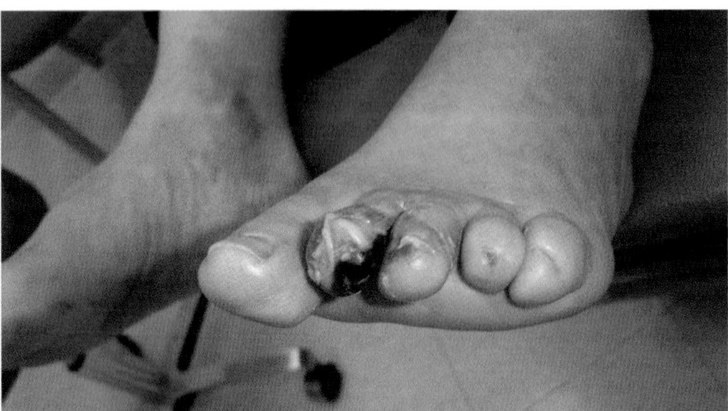

FIGURE 50-1 A necrotic second left toe in a patient with severe peripheral artery disease from uncontrolled diabetes. (*Reproduced with permission from Gary Ferenchick, MD.*)

SYNONYMS

- Peripheral arterial occlusive disease (excludes vasoreactive or aneurysmal PAD)
- Atherosclerotic vascular disease (includes only atherosclerotic PAD)

EPIDEMIOLOGY

- The prevalence of PAD increases with age.
- Its prevalence is 4.3% among adults 40 years or older and 14.5% among those 70 years or older.[2]
- About 5 million adults in the United States have PAD.[2]
- African Americans have a 2-fold higher incidence of PAD.[3]

ETIOLOGY/PATHOPHYSIOLOGY

- The pathophysiological processes that lead to PAD include atherosclerosis, dysplastic disorders, vasculitis, degenerative disease, and thromboembolism.[2]
- Atherosclerosis is the most common cause.
  - Risk factors are similar to classic atherosclerosis risk factors, including smoking, dyslipidemia, diabetes mellitus, hypertension, family history, postmenopausal state, hyperhomocysteinemia, and elevated C-reactive protein (CRP).[1]
  - PAD risk increases with the number of cigarettes smoked per day and the number of years smoked.
- Degenerative diseases such as Marfan and Ehlers-Danlos syndromes cause aneurysms or dissection of the arterial wall by affecting the structural integrity of the blood vessel.
- Dysplastic diseases such as fibromuscular dysplasia usually involve renal arteries, carotid arteries, and iliac arteries, causing progressive narrowing of the lumen.
- Vasculitis can affect arteries of any size.
  - Large vessel (aorta and its first- and second-order branches)—Giant cell arterial (Takayasu disease), Behçet syndrome, relapsing polychondritis, vasculitis associated with arthropathy
  - Medium-size vessels (conduit and muscular branches)—Temporal arteritis or polyarteritis nodosa
  - Small-vessel disease (arterioles and microvessels)—Rheumatoid arthritis, systemic lupus erythematosus (SLE), serum sickness, and other connective tissue or autoimmune diseases
- Thromboangitis obliterans (Buerger disease) is an arterial obliterative and thrombotic disorder, mostly seen in young individuals who smoke. It usually involves smaller distal limb arteries and superficial veins.[1]
- Primary prothrombotic disease is seen in abnormalities of the clotting system, such as protein C, protein S, or antithrombin III deficiencies; factor V Leiden; antiphospholipid syndrome; and prothrombotic state from malignancy and inflammatory bowel disease.
- Thromboembolic arterial occlusive disease
  - Macroemboli are usually cardiac in origin from the left atrial appendage, atrial fibrillation, or ventricular thrombus.
  - Microemboli can be from the heart (diseased native or thrombosed prosthetic heart valves) or an arterial source from rupture of cholesterol-containing plaque.

- Vasospastic diseases—Vasospasm occurs in primary Raynaud phenomenon or secondary to underlying connective tissue disease such as SLE or scleroderma.
- Other causes—Traumatic, entrapment syndromes, and external compression.

RISK FACTORS

- Diabetes
- Hypertension
- Hyperlipidemia
- Family history of atherosclerotic cardiovascular disease
- Elevated CRP[1]

DIAGNOSIS/SCREENING

- Guidelines vary in their recommendation for and against PAD screening.[3]
- The US Preventive Services Task Force recommends against routine screening for PAD in asymptomatic patients, a D recommendation.

HISTORY/SYMPTOMS

Specifically ask questions related to the following:

- The majority of the patients are asymptomatic, which is 2 to 5 times more prevalent than symptomatic lower-extremity PAD.[1]
- Symptomatic lower-extremity PAD is present in one-fifth of the population with objective evidence of lower-extremity PAD based on noninvasive tests.[1]
- Symptoms
  - Intermittent claudication—Claudication increases the likelihood of PAD (likelihood ratio [LR] 3.30-4.80).
  - Absence of claudication decreases the likelihood of moderate-to-severe PAD (LR 0.43-0.76) but does not lower the likelihood of any PAD.[4]
  - History of exertional limitation of activity or history of walking impairment.
  - Pain symptoms can help to localize the site of occlusion.
    - Iliac arteries involved—Pain occurs in hip, buttock, and thigh as well as calf.
    - Femoral and popliteal arteries involved—Calf pain.
    - Tibial artery involved—Calf pain or foot pain.
  - Poorly healing or nonhealing wounds of the legs or feet.
  - History of erectile dysfunction.
  - Family history of first-degree relative with an abdominal aortic aneurysm.
  - History of recent endovascular catheter procedure, symptoms of fatigue or muscle discomfort, symmetrical bilateral limb symptoms, livido reticularis, or rising creatinine values.
  - Critical limb ischemia (CLI)—The stenosis and impairment of blood flow is so severe that limb pain occurs at rest, and *symptoms are present for more than 2 weeks*.[5] Other manifestations like ulceration, nonhealing or poorly healing wounds, or gangrene in the extremities can develop with progression of disease.
    - CLI is present if an ankle pressure is less than 70 mm Hg and large toe pressure is less than 30 mm Hg in the presence of an ischemic lesion or gangrene and ankle pressure is less than 50 mm Hg in patients with resting pain.[6]
    - CLI is most frequently associated with 2 or more levels of stenosis or occlusion.
  - Acute limb ischemia (ALI)—It is an acute event with *symptoms up to 2 weeks*.
    - Rapid or sudden decrease in limb perfusion produces new or worsening symptoms and signs that threaten tissue viability.[5]
    - It is often associated with thrombosis in a ruptured atheromatous plaque, thrombosis of lower-extremity bypass graft, or lower-extremity embolism originating from the heart or proximal arterial aneurysm.
      - Embolism presents more abruptly than thrombosis.
      - Nonatherosclerotic causes of ALI—Arterial trauma, vasospasm (eg, ergotism), arteritis, hypercoagulable states, compartment syndromes, arterial dissection, and external arterial compression.

EXAMINATION

- Auscultation of neck, abdomen, and flank for bruits.
  - The presence of one bruit at rest (iliac, femoral, or popliteal) increases the likelihood of PAD (LR 5.60).[6]
  - Absence of femoral bruit was found to have little effect on the likelihood of PAD (LR 0.83).[4]
- If both dorsalis pedis and posterior tibial pulses are palpable in both lower limbs and there are no femoral bruits, the sensitivity, specificity, and negative predictive value for the absence of PAD are 58.2%, 98.3%, and 94.9%, respectively.[7]
- Palpation of pulses at the brachial, radial, ulnar, femoral, popliteal, dorsalis pedis, and posterior tibial sites.
  - Pulse intensity should be recorded as[2]
    - 0 = absent
    - 1 = diminished
    - 2 = normal
    - 3 = bounding
  - Absent or reduced pulses increase the likelihood of PAD (LR 4.70).[6]
  - Abnormal dorsalis pedis pulse (not palpable in 8.1% of healthy individuals) has lower specificity for identifying PAD compared with an abnormal femoral or posterior tibial artery pulse.[4]
  - Carotid bruit has not been shown to affect the LR of carotid stenosis.[8]
- Chronic ischemia—Dependent rubor, early pallor on elevation of the extremity, and reduced capillary refill; cool skin; ulceration; distal hair loss; trophic skin changes; and hypertrophic nails. Ulcers tend to be dry and painful and can progress to gangrene.
- ALI hallmark symptoms include 6 *P*'s: pain, pallor, paresthesia, pulselessness, paralysis, and poikilothermia.
- Peripheral manifestations of atheroemboli include livedo reticularis. Embolisms typically lodge at branch points because of the smaller caliber at the bifurcation.[2]
- Capillary refill time—Failure to return to normal skin color after 5 seconds of releasing the firm pressure to the plantar aspect of the great toe.[6] Abnormal capillary refill time is associated with moderate-to-severe disease.
- Buerger test
  - Examine for development of pallor with the patient's leg elevated to 45° and the patient in a supine position.

- The leg is then lowered slowly, and the angle at which the reddish hue returns is known as the *angle of circulatory sufficiency*.
- The result is positive[4] if the angle is less than 0 degree.

LABORATORY TESTING

- Risk factor identification—Hemoglobin A_{1c} (HbA_{1c}), lipid panel, fasting glucose level, CRP, homocysteine level.
- Other relevant tests depending on the clinical suspicion for less-common causes. Antinuclear antibody (ANA), rheumatoid factor for vasospastic diseases, antineutrophil cytoplasmic antibody (ANCA) panel for vasculitis, and hypercoagulability workup, and so on.

IMAGING

In patients with clinical suspicion for PAD based on symptoms and signs, one or more following studies are performed to localize the obstructive lesion and identify the severity of disease:

- ABI—Use to establish the diagnosis in patients with suspected lower-extremity PAD, including individuals with one or more of the following:
  - Exertional leg symptoms, nonhealing wounds, age 65 years and older (or 50 years and older with a history of smoking or diabetes). SOR B[9]
  - The ABI is calculated by taking the systolic blood pressure from both brachial arteries and from both the dorsalis pedis and posterior tibial arteries after the patient has been at rest in the supine position for 10 minutes.
    - A resting ABI should be used to establish the lower-extremity PAD diagnosis.
    - A falsely elevated ABI may be seen in patients with long-standing diabetes mellitus or chronic renal failure and in those who are very elderly.
    - Normal ankle pressure is 10 to 15 mm Hg higher than the brachial arterial systolic pressure because of pulse wave reflections.
    - The ABI is 79% sensitive and 96% specific to detect stenosis of 50% or more reduction in lumen diameter.[1]
  - ABI interpretation[10]
    - Normal values 1.00 to 1.40
    - Noncompressible—Less than 1.40, seen in calcified vessels; additional test required (eg, toe-brachial index [TBI]). If abnormal results on additional tests—PAD
    - Mild to moderate—Value is 0.41 to 0.9; often have claudication
    - Severely decreased if 0.40 or less; represents multilevel disease
  - Exercise treadmill tests with measurement of preexercise and postexercise ABI values
    - Used to assess the functional limitation of claudication and response to therapy for lower-extremity PAD[1] SOR B
    - Used when patient has claudication symptoms but resting ABI is normal
    - Helpful to differentiate nonarterial claudication (pseudoclaudication) from true arterial claudication SOR B
- Duplex ultrasound
  - Used to evaluate the location and degree of stenosis of PAD.[1] SOR A
  - Used for graft surveillance after femoral-popliteal or femoral tibial-pedal surgical bypass with venous conduit (not prosthetic). Minimal surveillance intervals are approximately 3, 6, and 12 months and then yearly after graft placement.[1] SOR A
  - May be considered for routine surveillance after femoral-popliteal bypass with a synthetic conduit.[1] SOR B
  - Velocity ratio at the suspected stenosis greater than 4.0 indicates 75% stenosis.
  - Sensitivity and specificity for the diagnosis of stenosis of more than 50% from the iliac to popliteal arteries are each 90% to 95%.[1]
  - Normal arterial Doppler velocity is triphasic. A flat waveform indicates severe obstruction.
  - Accuracy is diminished in aortoiliac arterial segments and if there is dense arterial calcification.
- Toe-brachial indices
  - Useful in patients with noncompressible posterior tibial or dorsalis pedis arteries.[1] SOR B
  - It can measure digital perfusion when small vessels are diseased, such as in diabetes.
  - TBI values less than 0.7 are considered diagnostic for lower-extremity PAD.[1] Absolute toe pressure greater than 30 mm Hg is favorable for wound healing.[11]
- Transcutaneous oxygen measurements[1]
  - Platinum oxygen electrodes are placed on the chest walls and the legs or feet.
  - Normal oxygen tension at the foot is 60 mm Hg, and the chest/foot ratio is 0.9. A wound is likely to heal if oxygen tension is greater than 40 mm Hg, except in those with diabetes, who require a higher value.
- Magnetic resonance angiography (MRA)
  - It is useful to diagnose anatomic locations and degree of stenosis and in selecting the patient for endovascular intervention SOR A and for surgical bypass SOR B.
  - Meta-analysis of MRA compared with catheter angiography[1] showed that sensitivity and specificity for diagnosis of stenosis greater than 50% were in the range of 90% to 100%.
  - It tends to overestimate the degree of stenosis and cannot be used if there is contraindication for magnetic resonance imaging (MRI).
- Computed tomographic angiography (CTA)
  - It is helpful to provide associated soft tissue diagnostic information and is contraindicated in renal failure because of the use of contrast medium. Small series show[1] that multidetector CTA has sensitivity for stenosis greater than 50% in the range of 89% to 100%, with specificity ranging from 92% to 100%.
  - It can be used when MRA is contraindicated.
  - Three-dimensional images help to visualize eccentric and ambiguous lesions.
- Contrast angiography
  - It is the gold standard for evaluation of PAD.
  - Angiography or combinations of angiography with noninvasive vascular techniques should be used to make a decision regarding the potential utility of invasive therapeutic interventions through complete anatomic assessment of the affected arterial territory, the lesion, and arterial inflow and outflow.[1] SOR B
  - Digital subtraction angiography is recommended as it provides enhanced imaging capabilities compared to conventional angiography.[1] SOR A
  - Use of noninvasive imaging modalities like duplex ultrasonography, MRA, or CTA prior to invasive diagnostic studies varies with the centers. These noninvasive imaging processes facilitate identification of lesions, preparation of appropriate equipment, and selection of the best access sites prior to an invasive procedure.[1]

- Monitor for complications such as contrast reaction, renal failure, atheroembolism, bleeding, infection, and vessel disruption after angiography.

DIFFERENTIAL DIAGNOSIS

- Spinal stenosis (pseudoclaudication)—Pain and weakness often involve bilateral buttocks, hip, and thighs; they follow the dermatome, and motor weakness is more prominent. Pain is relieved by lumbar spine flexion and is worse with standing and extension of the spine.
- Hip arthritis—Aching discomfort occurs in lateral hip or thigh. Pain is worse after weight bearing or exercise. Patient has a history of degenerative joint disease.
- Deep venous thrombosis (DVT) with phlegmasia cerulean dolens can mimic ALI.
- Chronic compartment syndrome—Tight or bursting pain is located in the calf muscle; it occurs after heavy exercise and is relieved with elevation.
- Venous claudication—Patient has history of iliofemoral DVT with signs of venous congestion or edema. Tight or bursting pain occurs after walking, and it is relieved by elevation of the limb.
- Nerve root compression—Sharp, lancinating pain radiates down the leg, often present at rest. There is a history of back problems.
- Symptomatic Baker cyst—Swelling and tenderness are present behind the knee; pain occurs at rest and with exercise.

MANAGEMENT

GOALS OF THERAPY

The following are therapy goals[5]:

- Relieve claudication/ischemic pain
- Heal ischemic ulcers
- Prevent limb loss
- Improve patient function and quality of life
- Prolong survival

RISK FACTOR MODIFICATION

- Smoking cessation SOR B[1]
  - Smoking cessation decreases the rate of PAD progression (see Chapter 237, Tobacco Addiction).
  - Based on observational studies, the amputation rate is higher and angioplasty and revascularization patency rates are lower in individuals who continue to smoke after intervention.[12]
- Treat risk factors such as diabetes, hypertension, hyperlipidemia.
  - Urgent evaluation in all diabetic patients with PAD.[1] SOR C
  - Low-density lipoprotein goal is less than 100 mg/dL, and for very-high-risk patients, the goal is less than 70 mg/dL. Statins are the drugs of choice.[1] SOR B
  - Statin use improves walking distance and speed, independent of cholesterol-lowering effects.[10]
  - Blood pressure should be controlled to 140/90 mm Hg or lower and less than 130/80 in those with diabetes and chronic kidney disease.[1] SOR A
- Exercise therapy—Patients should be referred to the supervised exercise training program. It is the initial modality of treatment for patients with intermittent claudication.[1,13] SOR A
  - Nonsupervised exercise is recommended when a supervised setting is not possible.[14] SOR C
  - A treadmill or track walking exercise session lasting longer than 30 minutes at least 3 times per week for a minimum of 3 months or longer and walking to near-maximal pain can decrease claudication pain and increase walking distance.[5] SOR A
    - Exercise training has been shown to improve treadmill walking distance to onset of pain by 115% and maximal walking distance by 65% after 6 months of exercise in a study.[13]
    - Proper foot care, including daily inspection, cleaning, appropriate footwear use and podiatric consultation in diabetic patients, and topical moisturizing cream use should be recommended to all patients.[1] SOR B

PHARMACOTHERAPY

- Antiplatelet agents SOR A
  - Aspirin 75 mg to 325 mg per day reduces the risk of myocardial infarction (MI), stroke, or vascular death in individuals with symptomatic atherosclerotic lower-extremity PAD.[9]
  - Clopidogrel (75 mg per day) is an alternative antiplatelet therapy to aspirin to reduce the risk of MI, ischemic stroke, or vascular death in individuals with symptomatic atherosclerotic lower-extremity PAD.[9] SOR B
- Combination antiplatelet therapy with aspirin plus clopidogrel for certain high-risk patients with PAD who are not considered at increased risk of bleeding[1] is reasonable based on the CHARISMA (Clopidogrel for High Atherothrombotic Risk and Ischemic Stabilization, Management, and Avoidance) trial.[9] SOR B
- In the absence of other proven indication for warfarin, its addition to an antiplatelet agent is not beneficial in reducing adverse cardiovascular events and is potentially harmful because of increased risk of bleeding based on evidence from the WAVE (Warfarin Antiplatelet Vascular Evaluation) trial.[9] SOR B
- Cilostazol
  - It is a phosphodiesterase type 3 inhibitor that increases cyclic adenosine monophosphate and has vasodilator and platelet inhibitory properties; its exact mechanism of action in intermittent claudication is not clear.[1,15]
  - A dose of 100 mg twice daily has been shown to improve walking distance by 50% and pain-free walking distance by 67% after 12 to 24 weeks of therapy.[6,15]
  - It is used in patients with lower-extremity PAD with intermittent claudication who failed exercise therapy. It should be used in patients with lifestyle-limiting claudication.[1] SOR A
  - It is contraindicated in patients with heart failure. Common side effects include headache, diarrhea, dizziness, and palpitations.
- Pentoxifylline 400 mg 3 times per day is a second-line agent when cilostazol is contraindicated or not tolerated.
  - It is a hemorheologic agent that decreases blood and plasma viscosity, increases erythrocyte and leukocyte deformability, inhibits neutrophil adhesion and activation, and lowers plasma fibrinogen concentration.[1]
  - Clinical benefits are questionable.[5]SOR C

- Naftidrofuryl—It is only available in Europe.
  - It is a 5-hydroxytryptamine type 2 antagonist that reduces red blood cells and platelet aggregation.
  - It has been shown to increase pain-free walking distance and quality of life.

TREATMENT OF INFECTION

- Infection should be diagnosed early and aggressively treated.
- Diabetics tend to have polymicrobial infection with gram-positive cocci, gram-negative rods, and anaerobic organisms.[5]
- Broad-spectrum antibiotic therapy is narrowed based on the organism identified from the wound culture. Deeper infection requires debridement of necrotic tissue and evaluation for osteomyelitis.

REVASCULARIZATION THERAPY

- Indication
  - Patients with severe lifestyle-limiting disability from claudication.[14] SOR C
  - Inadequate response to exercise or pharmacological therapy and there is a favorable risk/benefit ratio.[14] SOR C
  - CLI (**Figure 50-2A** and **50-2B**)
- In the absence of revascularization, 40% of patients with CLI will require amputation within 6 months. So, timely referral to a vascular specialist is important.
- Evaluate for cardiovascular risk preoperatively.[1]
- Risk of death, MI, and amputation is substantially greater and lower-extremity angioplasty and open surgical revascularization patency rates are lower in individuals with PAD who continue to smoke than in those who stop smoking.[9]
- Revascularization is indicated for limb salvage whenever technically feasible.[14] SOR A
- The multicenter BASIL (Bypass versus Angioplasty in Severe Ischemia of the Leg) trial involving 452 patients showed that outcomes like amputation-free survival and overall survival between bypass surgery first and balloon angioplasty first are similar when followed up over 2.5 years.[9]
- Endovascular treatment has lower morbidity and mortality (complication rates ranging from 0.5% to 4.0%, high technical success rates approaching 90%)[14] and acceptable short-term clinical outcome, but higher patency rates are seen with surgical treatment in those patients who survived for at least 2 years after randomization[9] (**Figure 50-3A and 50-3B**).
- Inflow disease should be treated first in patients with combined inflow and outflow disease.[9] SOR C
- Efficacy of revascularization may be reduced in patients with branch artery stenosis, and patients undergoing renal artery bypass may do best when surgery is performed in high-volume centers.[9]
- It is reasonable to perform bypass surgery with an autogenous vein conduit for patients with life expectancy of more than 2 years and balloon angioplasty for patients with life expectancy of 2years or less with limb-threatening ischemia.[1] SOR B

MANAGEMENT OF ACUTE LIMB ISCHEMIA

- Initiate immediate parenteral anticoagulant therapy in all patients to prevent thrombus propagation and worsening ischemia.[14] SOR C
- Provide immediate vascular specialist consultation.
- An irreversible or unsalvageable extremity that manifests with profound sensory loss and paralysis (rigor) will require amputation.[14]

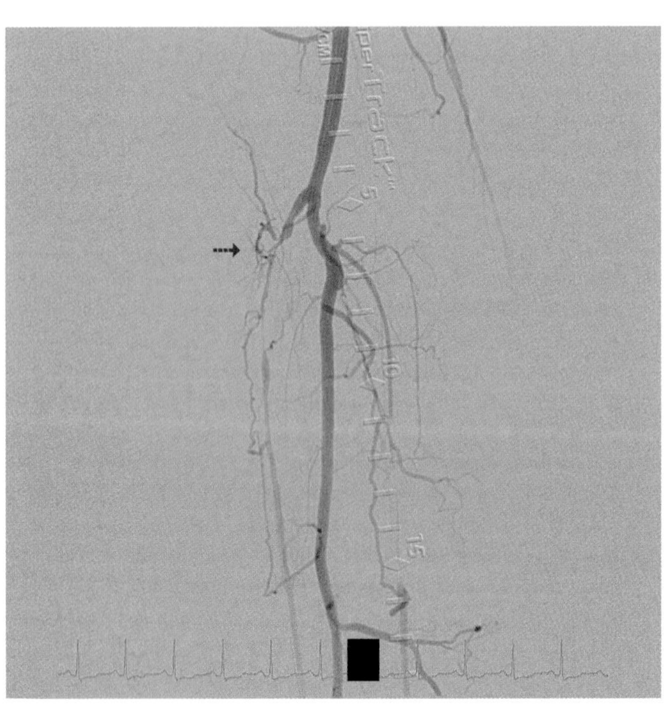
A

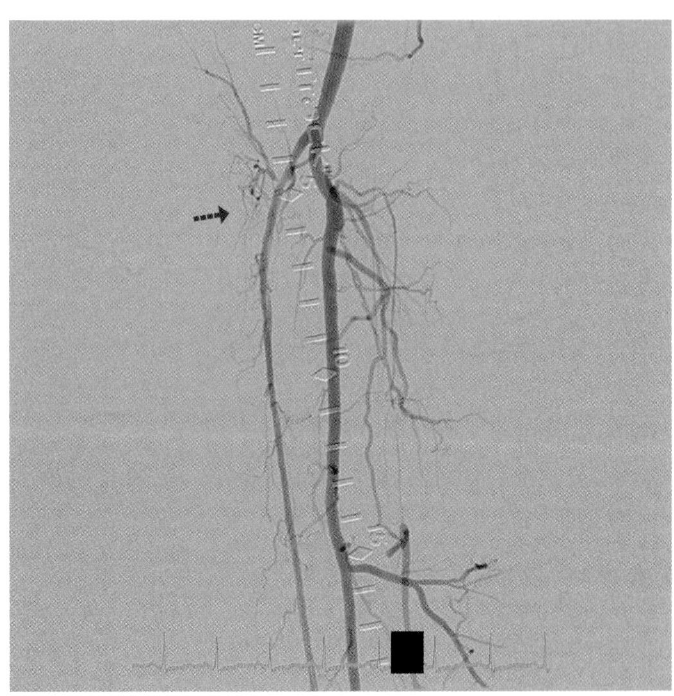
B

FIGURE 50-2 Posterior tibial artery angiography before (A) and after (B) stent placement showing improved distal perfusion after angioplasty. *(Reproduced with permission from Madhab Lamichhane, MD and Millind Karve, MD.)*

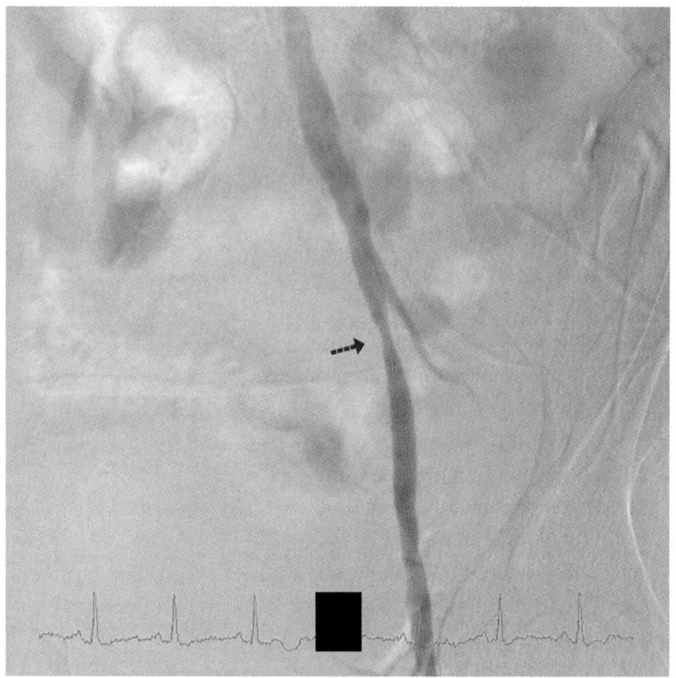

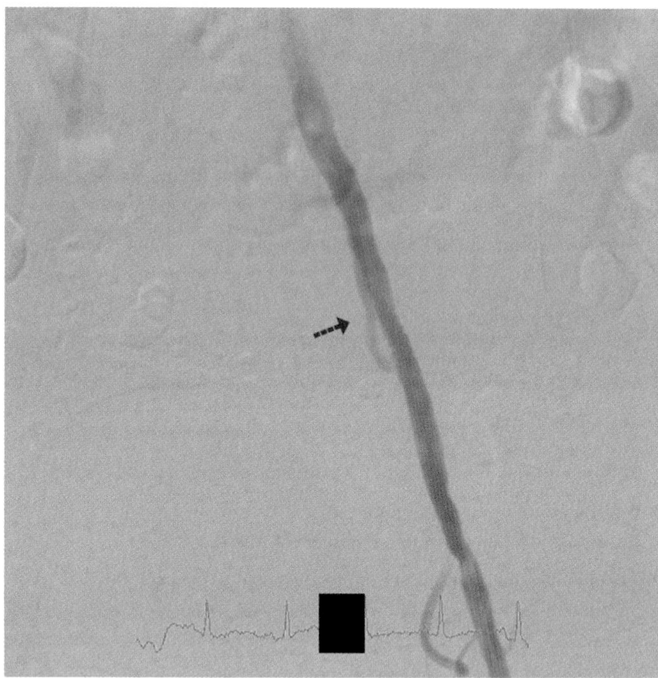

FIGURE 50-3 (A,B) Superficial femoral artery before and after stent placement. (*Reproduced with permission from Madhab Lamichhane, MD and Millind Karve, MD.*)

- A viable limb will require urgent imaging (duplex ultrasonography or angiography; **Figure 50-4**) and assessment of major comorbidities.
- Revascularization modalities depend on the type of occlusion (thrombus or embolus) and its location, duration of ischemia, comorbidities, type of conduit (artery or graft), and therapy-related risks and outcomes.[14]
- Reperfusion injury—Compartment syndrome—occurs in 5.3% in ALI after revascularization.[5]

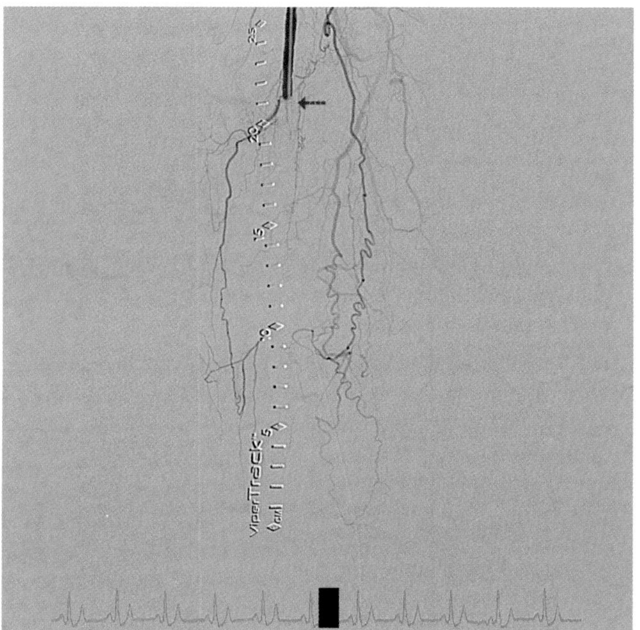

FIGURE 50-4 Acute occlusion of superficial femoral artery before thrombolytic therapy. (*Reproduced with permission from Madhab Lamichhane, MD and Millind Karve, MD.*)

 - Pain out of proportion to physical signs; presence of paresthesia and edema.
 - Compartment pressures 20 mm Hg or higher.
 - Treatment is 4-compartment fasciotomy.[5] SOR C. Rhabdomyolysis seen in 20% of patients; treatment is intravenous fluids and alkalinizing the urine.
- Amputation—If irreversible or unsalvageable extremity.
- Follow-up care—All patients should be treated with heparin in the immediate postoperative period, and warfarin is used for 3 to 6 months or longer.[5]
- Risk of recurrent ischemia is high in these patients, so long-term therapy may be considered.

PROGNOSIS

- In patients with lower-extremity PAD, 2- to 4-fold excess CAD and cerebrovascular disease are seen.
- CAD is the most common cause of death with PAD (40%-60%), and cerebral artery disease causes another 10% to 20% of deaths.[5]
- Patients with PAD, excluding CLI, have an annual 2% to 3% incidence of nonfatal MI.
- Those with chronic CLI have 20% mortality in the first year of presentation.[10]
- Twenty-five percent will require amputation.[5]
- Acute ischemia is related to short-term mortality of 15% to 20%. Major amputation occurs[5] in up to 25%.
- Reintervention within 3 months and readmission to the hospital within 6 months occur in half of patients who had acceptable patency and limb salvage following a revascularization intervention.[14]

PATIENT EDUCATION

- Risk factor modification such as to stop smoking and eating a healthy diet.
- Supervised exercise training. Keep a logbook to follow training and evolution of walking distance if unable to have supervised therapy.
- Seek early evaluation if there is pain at rest; wounds; cold, bluish feet; and infections.

FOLLOW-UP

- Follow up every year for PAD without any functional disability.[1]
- Follow up every 6 months after 4-6 months of exercise and cilostazol.[12]
- ABI and duplex ultrasonography at first office visit and every 6-12 months or whenever symptoms recur for iliac disease.[12]
- Patients who had angioplasty, stent placement, or surgical bypass: ABI and duplex ultrasonography at first office visit, then every 6 months for 24 months, and then yearly for infrailiac disease.[12]

PATIENT RESOURCES

- National Heart, Lung, and Blood Institute—*What Is Peripheral Arterial Disease?* **http://www.nhlbi.nih.gov/health/dci/Diseases/pad/pad_what.html.**
- American Heart Association—*About Peripheral Arterial Disease.* **http://www.heart.org/HEARTORG/Conditions/More/PeripheralArteryDisease/About-Peripheral-Artery-Disease-PAD_UCM_301301_Article.jsp.**
- Vascular Disease Foundation—*PAD and Related Vascular Diseases.* **http://vasculardisease.org/padcoalition/pad-and-related-vascular-diseases/.**
- Peripheral Arterial Disease (PAD) Coalition—**http://vasculardisease.org/padcoalition/.**

PROVIDER RESOURCES

- Rooke TW, Hirsch AT, Misra S, et al. 2011 ACCF/AHA focused update of the guideline for the management of patients with peripheral artery disease (updating the 2005 guideline): a report of the American College of Cardiology Foundation/American Heart Association Task Force on Practice Guidelines. *J Am Coll Cardiol. 2011;58(19):2020-2045.*

REFERENCES

1. Hirsch AT, Haskal ZJ, Hertzer NR, et al. ACC/AHA 2005 practice guidelines for the management of patients with peripheral arterial disease (lower extremity, renal, mesenteric, and abdominal aortic). *Circulation.* 2006;113:1474-1547.
2. Selvin E, Erlinger TP. Prevalence of and risk factors for peripheral arterial disease in the United States. Results from the National Health and Nutrition Examination Survey, 1999–2000. *Circulation.* 2004;110:738-743.
3. Ferket BS, Spronk S, Colkesen EB, et al. Systematic review of guidelines on peripheral artery disease screening. *Am J Med.* 2012;125(2):198-208.
4. Khan NA, Rahim SA, Anand SA, et al. Does the clinical examination predict lower extremity peripheral arterial disease? *JAMA.* 2006;295(5):536-546.
5. Norgren L, Hiatt WR, Dormandy JA, et al. Inter-society consensus for the management of peripheral arterial disease (TASC II). *J Vasc Surg.* 2007;45(suppl S):S5.
6. Thompson PD, Zimet R, Zhang P, et al. Meta-analysis of results from eight randomized, placebo-controlled trials on the effect of cilostazol on patients with intermittent claudication. *Am J Cardiol.* 2002;90:1314.
7. Armstrong DWJ, Tobin C, Matangi MF. The accuracy of the physical examination for the detection of lower extremity peripheral arterial disease. *Can J Cardiol.* 2010;26(10):e346-e350.
8. Cournot M, Boccalon H, Cambou JP, et al. Accuracy of the screening physical examination to identify subclinical atherosclerosis and peripheral arterial disease in asymptomatic subjects. *J Vasc Surg.* 2007;46(6):1215-1221
9. Rooke TW, Hirsch AT, Misra S, et al. 2011 ACCF/AHA focused update of the guideline for the management of patients with peripheral artery disease (updating the 2005 guideline): a report of the American College of Cardiology Foundation/American Heart Association Task Force on Practice Guidelines. *Circulation.* 2011;124:2020-2045.
10. McDermott MM, Guralnik JM, Greenland P, et al. Statin use and leg functioning in patients with and without lower-extremity peripheral arterial disease. *Circulation.* 2003;107:757-761.
11. Carter SA, Tate RB. Value of toe pulse waves in addition to systolic pressures in the assessment of the severity of peripheral arterial disease and critical limb ischemia. *J Vasc Surg.* 1996;24:258.
12. Olin JW, Sealove BA. Peripheral artery disease: current insight into the disease and its diagnosis and management. *Mayo Clin Proc.* 2010;85(7):678-692.
13. Stewart KJ, Hiatt WR, Regensteiner JG, Hirsch AT. Exercise training for claudication. *N Engl J Med.* 2002;347(24):1941-1951
14. European Stroke Organization; Tendera M, Aboyans V, et al. ESC guidelines on the diagnosis and treatment of peripheral artery diseases. *Eur Heart J.* 2011;32:2851-2906.
15. Sobel M, Verhaeghe R. Antithrombotic therapy for peripheral artery occlusive disease: American College of Chest Physicians evidence-based clinical practice guidelines (8th edition). *Chest.* 2008;133:815S.

51 VENOUS INSUFFICIENCY

Maureen K. Sheehan, MD

PATIENT STORY

A 45-year-old woman presents to her physician's office with complaints of heaviness and fatigue in her legs (**Figure 51-1**). She does not experience the symptoms in the morning but they become more noticeable as the day progresses and with prolonged standing. When she stands for many hours, she develops swelling in both of her legs. The symptoms are concentrated over her medial calf where she has prominent tortuous veins. She first noted the veins approximately 20 years ago when she was pregnant. Initially, they did not cause her any discomfort but have progressively enlarged now and over the past 10 years have become increasingly painful. She recalls that her mother had similar veins in her legs.

INTRODUCTION

Venous insufficiency, or improperly functioning valves in the venous system, can lead to variety of symptoms including, but not limited to, heaviness and/or swelling in the legs with prolonged standing, leg fatigue or aching, bleeding from leg varices, skin changes, and ulcerations. The prevalence is higher in industrialized nations and ranges from 15% to 30% of the US population.

SYNONYMS

Venous insufficiency is also known as varicose veins, venous stasis.

EPIDEMIOLOGY

- Varies by definition and region, but generally venous insufficiency affects 27% of the population.[1]
- Prevalence estimates vary by some reports, indicating a prevalence of 10.4% to 23% in men and 29.5% to 39% in women.[2,3]
- More frequent in women as compared to men.
- Symptomatic in more than two-thirds of those affected.
- Varicose veins are notable only in half of patients with venous insufficiency.[4]

ETIOLOGY AND PATHOPHYSIOLOGY

- Most frequently it is a result of valvular dysfunction.
- Valvular dysfunction may be primary or secondary (result of trauma, deep venous thrombosis [DVT], or May-Thurner syndrome).
- It may affect deep system (ie, femoral veins), superficial system (ie, saphenous vein), or both.
- The superficial system is involved in 88% of cases either alone or in conjunction with the deep system.
- Dysfunction leads to loss of compartmentalization of veins, leading to distention and increased pressure (**Figures 51-1** and **51-2**).
- Increased pressure in veins is transmitted to microvasculature leading to basement membrane thickening, increased capillary elongation, and visual skin changes (**Figures 51-3** and **51-4**).

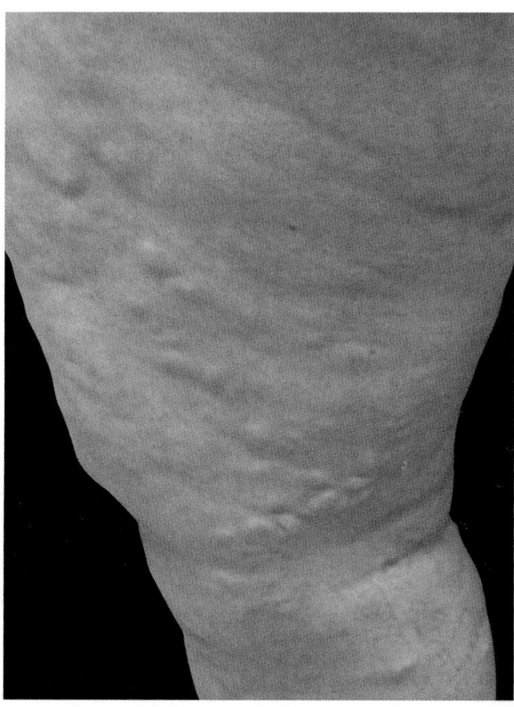

FIGURE 51-1 Uncomplicated varicose veins of thigh. (*Reproduced with permission from Maureen K. Sheehan, MD.*)

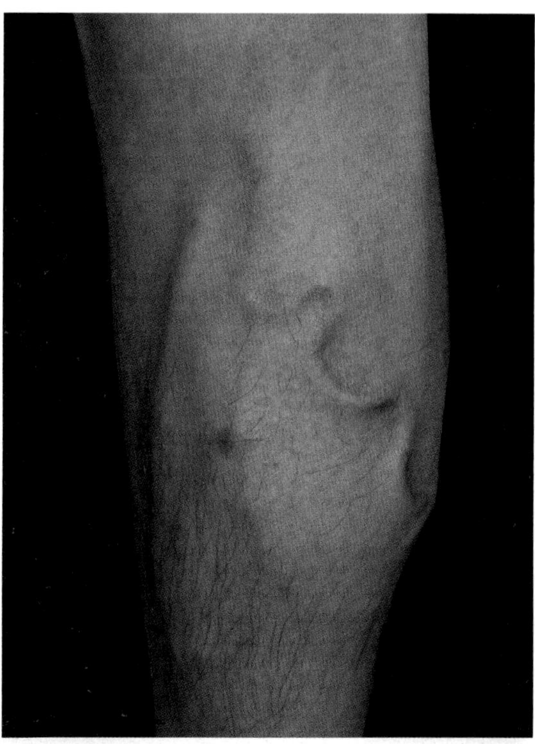

FIGURE 51-2 Varicose veins of posterior calf *without* hemosiderin deposition, lipodermatosclerosis, or ulceration. (*Reproduced with permission from Maureen K. Sheehan, MD.*)

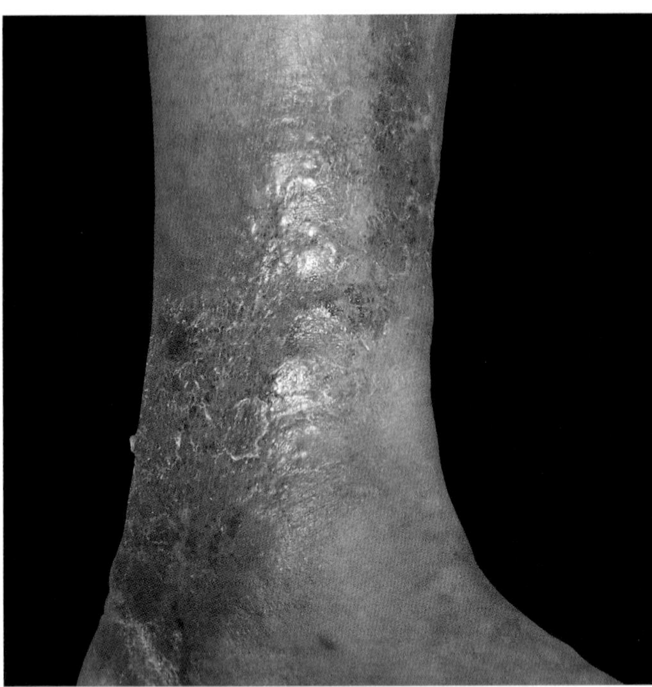

FIGURE 51-3 Lipodermatosclerosis with hemosiderin deposition. (*Reproduced with permission from Maureen K. Sheehan, MD.*)

RISK FACTORS

- Family history
- Deep venous thrombosis
- Female gender
- Estrogen increase (hormone replacement, pregnancy, oral contraceptive pills)
- Age
- Obesity
- Prolonged standing

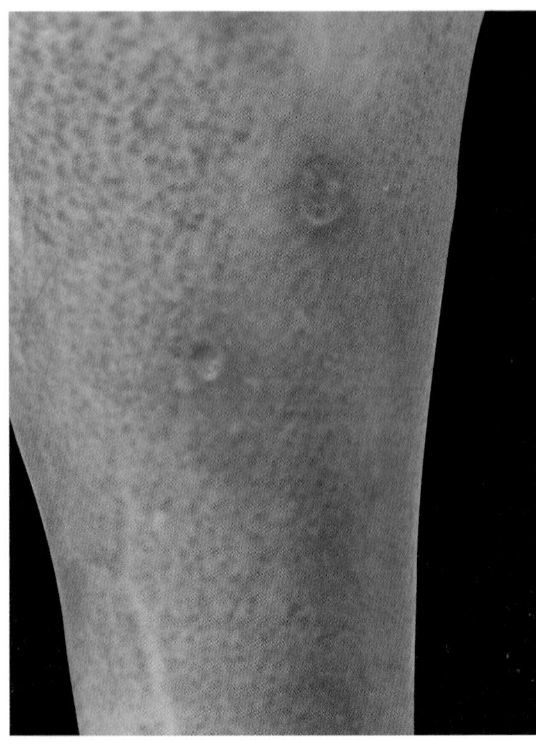

FIGURE 51-4 Healed ulcers with hemosiderin deposition. (*Reproduced with permission from Maureen K. Sheehan, MD.*)

DIAGNOSIS

SYMPTOMS

Heaviness, fatigue, and edema; not present immediately in the morning; gets worse with prolonged standing or walking; relieved with elevation

TYPICAL DISTRIBUTION

Varicose veins can be present anywhere on the leg depending on affected segments or branches; ulcers from venous disease tend to be near the medial malleoli (**Figure 51-5**).

TESTS

Duplex scanning is done to assess valve closure; normal valve closure takes 0.5 to 1 seconds.

DIFFERENTIAL DIAGNOSIS

- Arterial ulcers—Tend to be at toes, shin, and pressure points (heels or sides of feet)
- Diabetic ulcers—Occur at ambulatory pressure points, mostly at first metatarsal head
- Malignancy (basal cell or squamous cell carcinoma)
- Chronic infectious diseases (osteomyelitis, leprosy)
- Vasculitides—Irregular border, black necrosis, erythema, or bluish or purplish discoloration of adjacent tissue

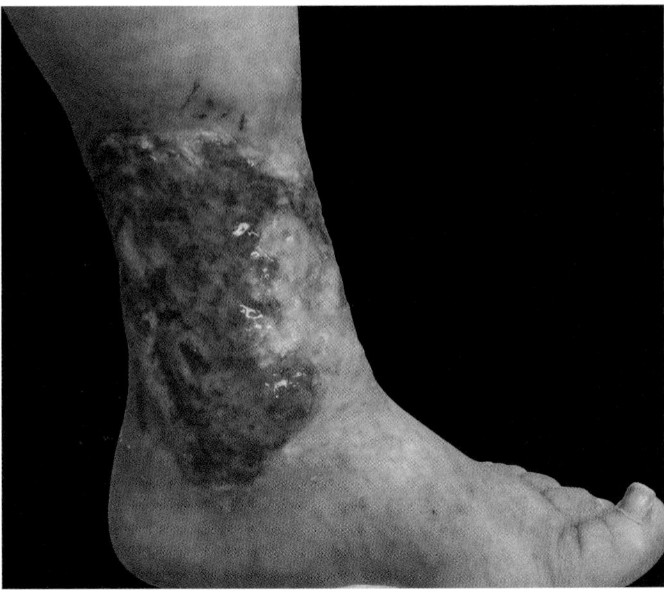

FIGURE 51-5 Venous stasis ulcer in the typical location around the medial malleolus. (*Reproduced with permission from Maureen K. Sheehan, MD.*)

MANAGEMENT

- Graduated compression hose for superficial or deep system insufficiency: SOR C
    - Fifteen to twenty mmHg—Minor reflux and minimal symptoms.
    - Twenty to thirty mmHg—Moderate-to-severe reflux and symptoms; moderate edema; postsurgical.
    - Thirty to forty mmHg—Severe reflux and symptoms; severe edema.
- Compression for open ulcer.[5] SOR B
- Compression hose treat symptoms, not underlying pathophysiology. It is effective only when being worn.
- Surgical intervention is available either with endovenous ablation or with stripping and ligation if superficial system is involved.
- If only deep system is involved, then compression hose is the mainstay of therapy. SOR C
- When superficial and deep systems are affected, treatment of superficial system leads to improvement of deep system reflux[6] in one-third of the patients.
- A study randomizing patients to stripping and ligation versus compression therapy demonstrated an improved quality of life in the surgical arm.[7] SOR A
- Endovenous therapy uses radiofrequency or laser energy to ablate vein. Because the vein is usually accessed with a needle under ultrasound guidance, an incision is avoided in most instances.
- Decreased postoperative pain and analgesic use in patients undergoing endovenous ablation compared to those undergoing stripping and ligation.[8] SOR A
- Adjunctive phlebectomies or sclerotherapy for branch varicosities may be necessary with either operative approach.

PREVENTION

Patients at risk for developing venous insufficiency (genetics, occupations with prolonged standing, etc) may benefit from compression hose use.

PROGNOSIS

Majority of patients with venous insufficiency live a full and complete life without significant sequelae. Those with only superficial involvement tend to have greater relief with treatment than those with superficial and deep or only deep system involvement. Most patients obtain relief from interventions such as compression hose or surgery.

FOLLOW-UP

- It depends on the treatment and severity of disease.
- Unna boots for ulceration need to be changed at least weekly.
- Compression hose needs to be replaced every 6 months.
- Following surgical intervention, follow-up depends on intervention. Stripping and ligation require wound checks, whereas endovenous ablations require ultrasound monitoring.

PATIENT EDUCATION

Venous insufficiency is not merely a cosmetic concern. Long-standing disease can give rise to skin changes (see **Figures 51-3** and **51-4**) and ulcers (see **Figure 51-5**). Compliance with compression hose is necessary. Compression hose only treats symptoms, not the underlying disease process. Even after surgical intervention, new varicose veins may appear as the process is chronic.

PATIENT RESOURCES

- MedlinePlus. *Venous Insufficiency*—**http://www.nlm.nih.gov/medlineplus/ency/article/000203.htm.**
- MedlinePlus. *Varicose Veins*—**http://www.nlm.nih.gov/medlineplus/ency/article/001109.htm.**
- MedlinePlus. *Stasis Dermatitis and Ulcers*—**http://www.nlm.nih.gov/medlineplus/ency/article/000834.htm.**

PROVIDER RESOURCES

- Medscape. *Venous Insufficiency*—**http://emedicine. medscape.com/article/1085412.**
- American College of Phlebology—**http://www.phlebology.org/.**

REFERENCES

1. White JV, Ryjewski C. Chronic venous insufficiency. *Perspect Vasc Surg Endovasc Ther*. 2005;17:319-327.
2. Beebe-Dimmer JL, Pfeifer JR, Engle JS, Schottenfeld D. The epidemiology of chronic venous insufficiency and varicose veins. *Ann Epidemiol*. 2005;15:175-184.
3. Mundy L, Merlin TL, Fitridge RA, Hiller JE. Systematic review of endovenous laser treatment for varicose veins. *Br J Surg*. 2005;92:1189-1194.
4. Reichenberg J, Davis M. Venous ulcers. *Semin Cutan Med Surg*. 2005;24:216-226.
5. Cullum N, Nelson EA, Fletcher AW, Sheldon TA. Compression for venous leg ulcers. *Cochrane Database Syst Rev*. 2000;3:CD000265.
6. Puggioni A, Lurie F, Kistner RL, et al. How often is deep venous reflux eliminated after saphenous vein ablation? *J Vasc Surg*. 2003;38:517-511.
7. Michaels JA, Brazier JE, Campbell WB, et al. Randomized clinical trial comparing surgery with conservative treatment for uncomplicated varicose veins. *Br J Surg*. 2006;93:175-181.
8. Rautio T, Ohinmaa A, Perala J, et al. Endovenous obliteration versus conventional stripping operation in the treatment of primary varicose veins: a randomized controlled trial with the comparison of the costs. *J Vasc Surg*. 2002;35:958-965.

PART 8

HEMATOLOGY

Strength of Recommendation (SOR)	Definition
A	Recommendation based on consistent and good-quality patient-oriented evidence.*
B	Recommendation based on inconsistent or limited-quality patient-oriented evidence.*
C	Recommendation based on consensus, usual practice, opinion, disease-oriented evidence, or case series for studies of diagnosis, treatment, prevention, or screening.*

*See Appendix A on pages 1241-1244 for further information.

52 IRON DEFICIENCY ANEMIA

Churlson Han, MD

PATIENT STORY

A 62-year-old woman with a history of acid reflux presents to her physician with complaints of fatigue and dyspnea on exertion, which have been progressively worsening over the past several months. Her examination reveals pallor, especially of the conjunctiva (**Figure 52-1**). Her pulmonary and cardiac examinations are normal. A digital rectal examination reveals positive occult blood. Laboratory examination shows a microcytic, hypochromic anemia, with a low serum ferritin level. She is diagnosed with iron deficiency anemia (IDA) caused by occult blood loss, and further testing for the source of blood loss is recommended.

EPIDEMIOLOGY

- IDA is the most common nutritional deficiency worldwide.
- The following are high-prevalence groups in the United States[1,2]:
  - Women, especially pregnant women
  - Mexican Americans
  - African Americans
  - Individuals of low socioeconomic status

ETIOLOGY AND PATHOPHYSIOLOGY

- Absorption and storage of iron cannot keep up with demand (negative iron balance).
- Causes[1]
  - Decreased absorption
    - Inadequate dietary intake
    - Acid suppression
    - Duodenal/jejunal gastrointestinal (GI) disease, gastric bypass surgery, malabsorption

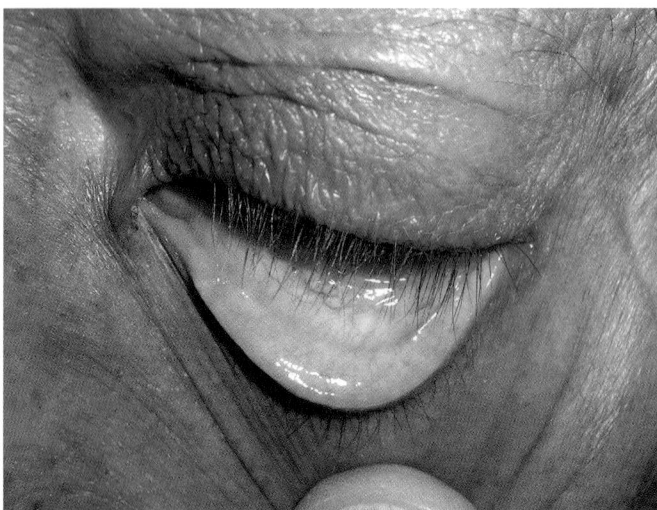

FIGURE 52-1 Severe conjunctival pallor in a 62-year-old woman with newly diagnosed iron deficiency anemia from gastrointestinal blood loss. (Reproduced with permission from Richard P. Usatine, MD.)

  - Increased loss
    - Menstruation
    - Pregnancy
    - Blood loss (occult or gross)
- Iron metabolism[3]
  - Iron is absorbed from GI lumen via enterocytes and bound to transferrin.
  - Plasma transferrin is utilized by erythroid and hepatic cells.
  - Iron is stored as ferritin intracellularly.
  - Stored iron is deposited in bone marrow.
- Stages of iron deficiency
  - Negative iron balance causes utilization of available transferrin-bound iron first.
  - Next, iron stored in the liver and bone marrow is utilized.
  - Once stores are exhausted, red blood cells (RBCs) are produced with decreased size (microcytic) and hemoglobin content (hypochromic).

RISK FACTORS

- Pregnancy
- Women of childbearing age who have heavy menses or who donate blood more than one time a year
- Frequent blood donors
- Patients who have had bariatric procedures, gastrectomy, or small-bowel resection
- Patients with celiac disease or inflammatory bowel disease

DIAGNOSIS/SCREENING

- The US Preventive Services Task Force (USPSTF) states that there is at least fair evidence that routine screening for iron deficiency in asymptomatic pregnant women improves health outcomes, but there is insufficient evidence to recommend for or against routine iron supplementation for nonanemic pregnant women.
  - The prevalence of IDA was noted to be 1.8%, 8.2%, and 27.4% in the first, second, and third trimesters among predominantly low-income and minority pregnant women.[4]
- Clinical features[1,5]
  - Clinical features can vary widely, but fatigue and pallor are common.
  - Historical findings
    - Fatigue
    - Exercise intolerance
    - Dyspnea
    - Pallor
    - Alopecia
    - Pica (eating nonfood items such as dirt, clay, or chalk)
    - Blood loss (hematemesis, hematochezia, heavy menstruation, hematuria, etc)
  - Physical findings
    - Pallor of skin and conjunctiva (**Figure 52-1**)
    - Systolic murmur
    - Identification of bleeding source
    - Positive stool guaiac
    - Koilonychia (spoon-shaped nails) (**Figure 52-2**)

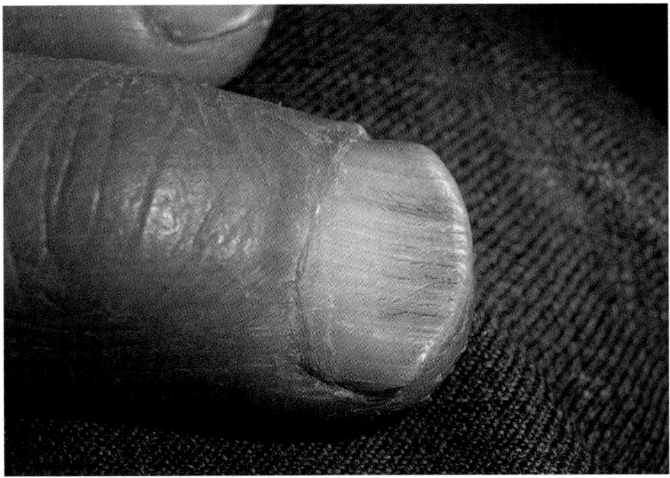

FIGURE 52-2 Koilonychia (spoon-shaped nails) is a manifestation of severe iron deficiency anemia and presents with brittle nails in the shape of spoons. Vertical stripes may also be present. (Reproduced with permission from Richard P. Usatine, MD.)

- Laboratory studies and imaging
  - Hemoglobin value is less than 13 g/dL in men or less than 12 g/dL in women.
    - RBC smears demonstrate hypochromia and microcytosis (**Figures 52-3** and **52-4**).
    - Results may be normal if the individual is not completely iron depleted.
  - Mean corpuscular volume (MCV) and mean corpuscular hemoglobin (MCH) will decrease only when iron depleted.
  - Ferritin[1,2,5-8]
    - Most accurate initial diagnostic test for iron deficit
    - Values less than 15 to 30 ng/mL—high probability of iron deficiency
    - Values above 100 ng/mL—low probability of iron deficiency
    - Negative: lack of consensus on cutoff values
    - Can be falsely normal or elevated in inflammatory states
  - Soluble transferrin receptor (sTfR)[3,6-8]
    - An increased sTfR value indicates increased tissue demand for iron.

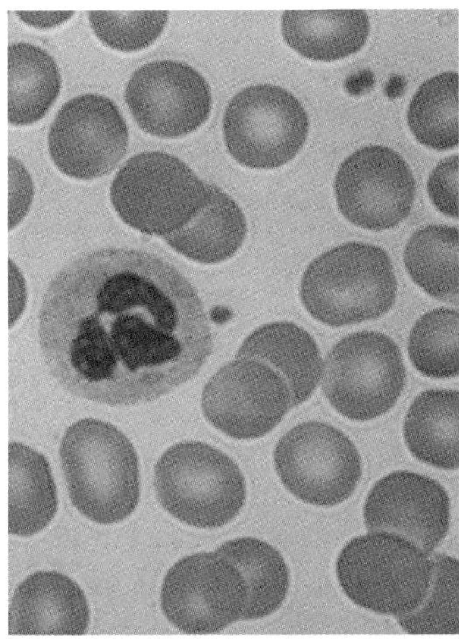

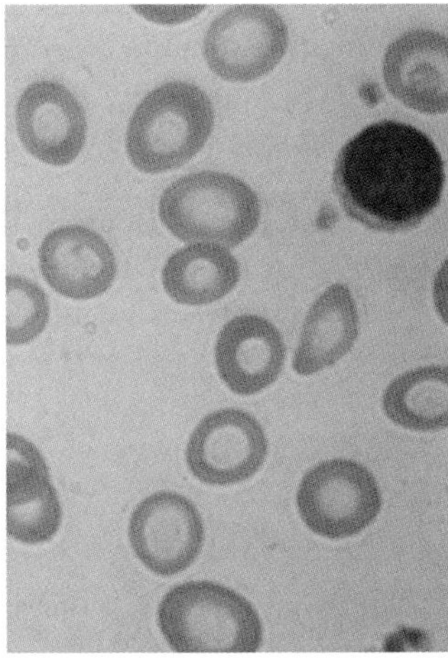

FIGURE 52-3 A normal blood smear (left panel) next to a smear indicating iron deficiency anemia. Note in the iron deficiency smear the central pallor, and the average size of the cells is smaller than the lymphocyte nucleus. The normal size of a red blood cell should be about the same as a lymphocyte nucleus. (Reproduced with permission from Longo DL, Fauci AS, Kasper DL, Hauser SL, Jameson JL, Loscalzo J. *Harrison's Principles of Internal Medicine.* 18th ed. New York, NY: McGraw-Hill.)

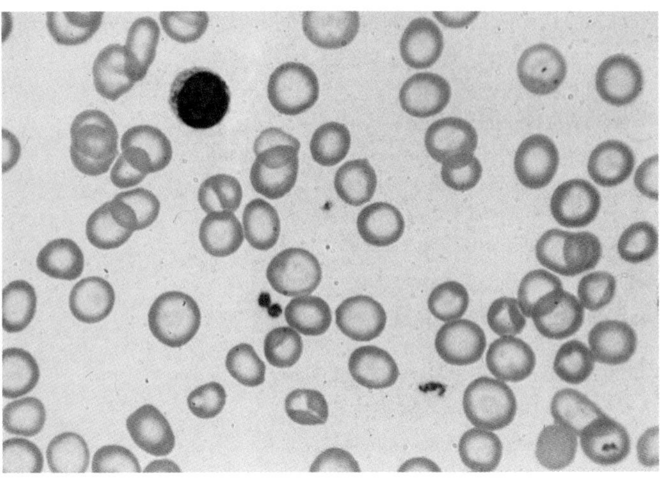

FIGURE 52-4 This blood smear demonstrates almost all hypochromic red blood cells (RBCs) with only a small peripheral rim of stainable hemoglobin noted. The RBCs are also generally smaller than the comparison lymphocyte nucleus in this smear, although there is considerable variation in the size of the RBCs here. (Reproduced with permission from Lichtman MA, Shafer MS, Felgar RE, Wang N. *Lichtman's Atlas of Hematology.* New York, NY: McGraw-Hill.)

    - The sTfR value is helpful in differentiating IDA from anemia of chronic disease (ACD).
    - This value can help differentiate equivocal ferritin levels caused by inflammation.
    - Negatives are lack of standardized values, slow turnaround time, and false positives with increased erythropoiesis.
    - The sTfR/log ferritin ratio may be a better discriminator, with values less than 1 suggestive of ACD.
  - Serum iron (SI), total iron-binding capacity (TIBC), and transferrin saturation[2]
    - SI is the plasma-bound iron level.
    - The TIBC is an analogue for unbound transferrin.
    - Transferrin saturation (TSAT) = SI/TIBC × 100.
    - Iron deficiency: SI low, TIBC high, causing low TSAT.
  - Red cell zinc protoporphyrin level (FEP)[8]
    - If iron is unavailable for heme synthesis, zinc substitutes.
    - Cannot differentiate iron deficiency and ACD.
  - Bone marrow biopsy
    - Considered the gold standard diagnostic test
    - Staining of marrow for iron
    - Invasive, expensive
  - Common diagnostic strategy[2,6,7]
    - Check ferritin: If value is less than 15 to 30, most likely the individual is iron deficient; if value is above 100, most likely the individual is not iron deficient.
    - If the ferritin value is 30 to 100, obtain further testing: SI/TIBC/TSAT; sTfR or sTfR/log ferritin.
    - If still equivocal (and further testing is warranted), perform a bone marrow biopsy.

DIFFERENTIAL DIAGNOSIS

- Thalassemia[9]
  - Both α and β types are hypochromic and microcytic.
  - The RBC count is usually elevated as a compensatory mechanism unless there is a coexisting iron deficiency.

- Family history is usually present.
- Normal or high ferritin is present.
- Hemoglobin electrophoresis may differentiate β-thalassemia.

- Anemia of chronic disease[3,6,9]
  - Like iron deficiency, can be normocytic or microcytic
  - Ferritin usually normal or high
  - SI and TIBC usually low with normal TSAT
  - sTfR/log ferritin ratio less than 1 in ACD
- Sideroblastic anemia
  - Abnormal number of sideroblasts is present in bone marrow (congenital or acquired).
  - This anemia is hypochromic and microcytic typically.
  - Acquired types are typically caused by alcohol, isoniazid, chloramphenicol.
  - Bone marrow biopsy may be needed for diagnosis.
- Lead poisoning[10]
  - Exposure to lead, typically by occupation
  - Microcytic and hypochromic, basophilic stippling
  - Diagnosed by blood lead level

MANAGEMENT

- Iron replacement—Management should involve replacement of iron stores.[1,3,6,8,10,11] SOR C
  - Oral iron
    - Ferrous sulfate, ferrous gluconate, ferrous fumarate, ferric bisglycinate
      - Sulfate and gluconate are preferred for cost and bioavailability.
      - For ferrous sulfate, use 325 mg 3 times daily (after the cause has been identified and treated).
    - Improved absorption in acidic gastric environment
      - Coadministration with ascorbic acid (vitamin C)
      - Avoidance of acid-neutralizing foods and therapies
    - Common GI side effects—nausea, epigastric pain, constipation
    - Safer, more convenient, and cost-effective than parenteral therapy
  - Parenteral iron
    - Iron sucrose, sodium ferric gluconate, iron dextran, ferric carboxymaltose
    - Indications
      - High-iron requirements caused by uncorrectable bleeding or hemodialysis
      - Iron malabsorption from GI pathology
      - Intolerance of oral therapy
    - Side effects of iron dextran include higher rates of anaphylaxis.
      - Test dosing of iron dextran required
  - Iron replacement not recommended in critical illness or infection[3,9]
- RBC transfusion reserved for acute or symptomatic anemia[1,6,8,11] SOR C
- Nutritional history and physical assessment[1] SOR C
  - Gastrointestinal evaluation for bleeding or malabsorption[11,12] SOR C
  - Upper and lower GI tract evaluations recommended in men 50 years or older and postmenopausal women
- Coadministration of recombinant human erythropoietin controversial[8,12]
  - Indicated in situations with low or ineffective endogenous erythropoietin[12]
  - Synergy only achieved with intravenous iron
  - In critical illness, does not improve morbidity and mortality[8]

PREVENTION AND SCREENING

- Do not screen the general population
- Screen those with conditions noted under risk factors.
- Provide iron supplementation to women who are pregnant to prevent iron deficiency and to women who are of childbearing age who donate blood more than one time yearly

PROGNOSIS AND FOLLOW-UP

- For oral iron replacement, expected trajectory of correction of anemia is 1-2 g/dL every 2 weeks and replacement of iron stores in 3-4 months.[1,12] SOR C
- Initial reexaminations of iron indices are recommended quarterly.[11] SOR C
- For refractory iron deficiency or undiagnosed cause, consider hematology referral.[12] SOR C

PATIENT EDUCATION

- Iron replacement is needed to correct iron deficiency.
- Treatment modalities for iron replacement can have significant side effects.
- The cause of iron deficiency should be determined.

PATIENT RESOURCES

- National Institutes of Health. *Understanding Your Complete Blood Count*—**http://www.cc.nih.gov/ccc/patient_education/pepubs/cbc97.pdf.**
- National Institutes of Health. *Understanding Your Complete Blood Count* (Spanish)—**http://www.cc.nih.gov/ccc/patient_education/pepubs_sp/cbcsp.pdf.**
- FamilyDoctor.org. *Anemia: Overview*—**http://familydoctor.org/familydoctor/en/diseases-conditions/anemia.html.**

PROVIDER RESOURCES

- Medscape. *Anemia*—**http://emedicine.medscape.com/article/198475.**

REFERENCES

1. Clark SF. Iron deficiency anemia. *Nutr Clin Pract.* 2008;23:128-141.
2. Killip S, Bennett JM, Chambers MD. Iron deficiency anemia. *Am Fam Physician.* 2007;75:671-678.
3. Munoz M, Garcia-Erce JA, Francisco Remacha A. Disorders of iron metabolism. Part II: iron deficiency and iron overload. *J Clin Pathol.* 2011;64:287-296.
4. Scholl TO. Iron status during pregnancy: setting the stage for mother and infant. Am J Clin Nutr. 2005;81(5):1218s-1222s.

5. Gisbert JP, Gomollon F. A guide to diagnosis of iron deficiency and iron deficiency anemia in digestive disease. *World J Gastroenterol.* 2009;15:4638-4643.

6. Pasricha SR, Flecknoe-Brown SC, Allen KJ, et al. Diagnosis and management of iron deficiency anaemia: a clinical update. *Med J Aust.* 2010;193:525-532.

7. Galloway MJ, Smellie SA. Investigating iron status in microcytic anaemia. *BMJ.* 2006;333:791-793.

8. Pieracci FM, Barie PS. Diagnosis and management of iron-related anemias in critical illness. *Crit Care Med.* 2006;34:1898-1905.

9. Van Vranken M. Evaluation of microcytosis. *Am Fam Physician.* 2010;82:1117-1122.

10. Brodin E, Copes R, Mattman A, Kennedy J, Kling R, Yassi A. Lead and mercury exposures: interpretation and action. *CMAJ.* 2007;176:59-63.

11. Goddard AF, James MW, McIntyre AS, Scott BB. Guidelines for the management of iron deficiency anaemia. *Gut.* 2011;60:1309-1316.

12. Zhu A, Kaneshiro M, Kaunitz JD. Evaluation and treatment of iron deficiency anemia: a gastroenterological perspective. *Dig Dis Sci.* 2010;55:548-559.

53 B_{12} DEFICIENCY

Priyank Patel, MD

PATIENT STORY

A 71-year-old woman presents with fatigue, pinprick sensations in the left leg, and "memory problems" that have gradually worsened over the last 3 to 4 months. Her medical history is significant only for hypothyroidism, for which she is on thyroid hormone supplementation. She lives with her husband in a house and is completely independent in terms of her daily activities. Her physical examination demonstrates an atrophic glossitis (**Figure 53-1**), paresthesias in the anterolateral left lower extremity below the knee, and diminished vibratory sensation in her ankles. Her Mini-Mental State Examination (MMSE) score is 26 out of 30, losing points for attention and calculation and a point for recall. Laboratory investigations show macrocytic anemia with a hemoglobin level of 11.0 g/dL and a mean corpuscular volume (MCV) of 122 fL. Her serum vitamin B_{12} is low at 184 ng/L. Further workup is negative for intrinsic factor (IF) antibody, but review of her peripheral smear reveals hypersegmented neutrophils and macro-ovalocytes (**Figure 53-2**). Therapy with intramuscular injections of vitamin B_{12} is started. In a return visit to clinic after 6 weeks, the patient reports an improvement in lower-limb paresthesias and some improvement in her cognition.

INTRODUCTION

Vitamin B_{12} or cyanocobalamin (Cbl) deficiency, which can be either clinical or subclinical, is defined as decreased body stores of vitamin B_{12} caused by either inadequate dietary intake or various gastrointestinal abnormalities in digestion or absorption of cyanocobalamin, classically including pernicious anemia but not limited to it. The clinical manifestations, if present, may be characterized as hematological, gastrointestinal, or neurological. Thomas Addison and Anton Biermer described pernicious anemia in the latter half of the nineteenth century, which led to subsequent discovery of IF, followed by discovery of vitamin B_{12} or Cbl in 1946. Cbl deficiency can be caused by multiple etiologies, pernicious anemia being one of them. Vitamin B_{12} deficiency is common in wealthier nations, especially in the elderly, but is significantly more prevalent in poorer countries.

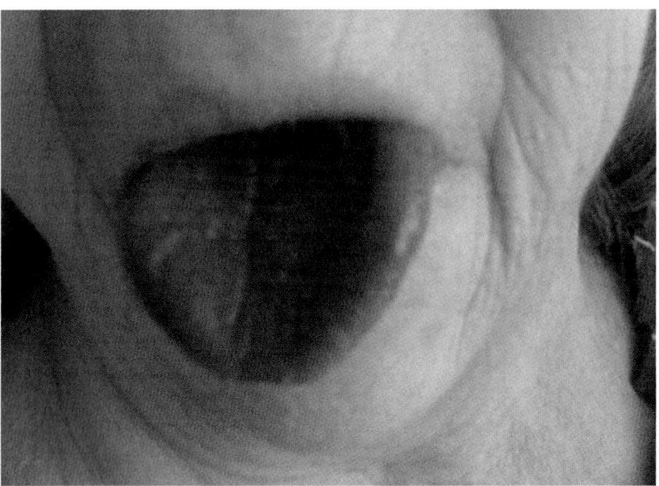

FIGURE 53-1 Atrophic (Hunter) glossitis secondary to B_{12} deficiency. Note how the tongue is a beefy red color, and the atrophic changes give it a smooth appearance. This 71-year-old woman presented with fatigue and was found to have a macrocytic anemia caused by her B_{12} deficiency. (Copyright Gary Ferenchick, MD.)

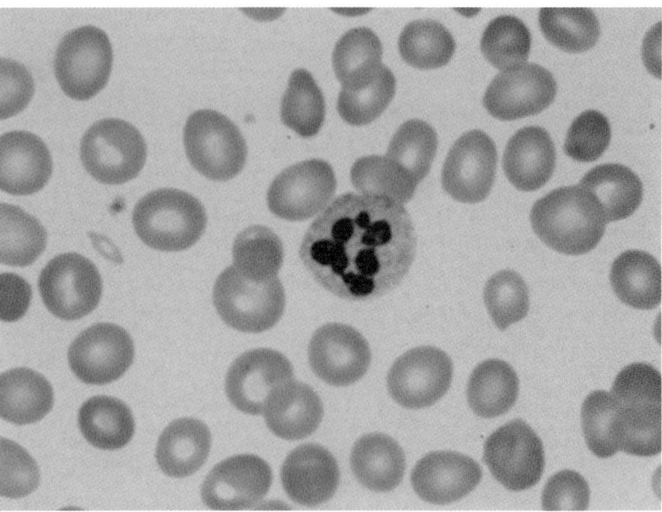

FIGURE 53-2 A hypersegmented neutrophil in a 71-year-old woman with a B_{12} deficiency. This neutrophil has 7 lobes, which is highly suggestive of B_{12} deficiency. The normal neutrophil nucleus has 3-5 lobes. (*Reproduced with permission from Gary Ferenchick, MD.*)

SYNONYMS

Vitamin B_{12} deficiency is also called cobalamin deficiency.

EPIDEMIOLOGY

- Prevalence of Cbl deficiency varies among age groups, socioeconomic conditions, and dietary preferences.
  - According to the National Health and Nutrition Examination Surveys (NHANES) from 1999 to 2002 in the United States, less than 3% of individuals between 20 and 39 years, approximately 4% between 40 and 59 years, and approximately 6% older than 70 years had low vitamin B_{12} levels (<148 pmol/L), but less than 1% of the entire population, including the elderly, had severe vitamin B_{12} deficiency (<74 pmol/L). Marginally low vitamin B_{12} levels (148-221 pmol/L) occurred in approximately 14% to16% between 20 and 59 years and more than 20% among those older than 60 years.[1]
- Prevalence of vitamin B_{12} deficiency in developing countries is far higher. Vitamin B_{12} levels less than 150 pmol/L were found in 68% of Asian-Indian men from a lower-middle-class background, with vegetarianism an independent risk factor.[2] Similarly, about 40% of Kenyan schoolchildren have been noted to have levels below 148 pmol/L.[3]

ETIOLOGY/PATHOPHYSIOLOGY

THE VITAMIN B_{12} PATHWAY

- Vitamin B_{12} absorption is a complex process, and its deficiency can be the result of any alterations in this mechanism.
  - Dietary sources of vitamin B_{12} are only through food of animal origin (eg, dairy products, fish, and meat).

- Stomach—Dietary vitamin B_{12} is protein bound, and it undergoes hydrolysis in an acidic environment, attaching to transcobalamin I (TC I), also known as the R-binder.
- Intestine—Under the influence of the pancreatic enzymes, the vitamin B_{12}-TC I complex dissociates to bind to IF, secreted by parietal cells of the gastric mucosa, to form a vitamin B_{12}-IF complex.
- Ileum—Vitamin B_{12}-IF complex is internalized via receptor-mediated endocytosis at the apical brush border membrane. The receptors responsible[4] are IF-vitamin B_{12} receptor cubilin encoded by the *CUBN* gene located on chromosome 10p12.33-p13 and amnionless protein encoded by the *AMN* gene located on human chromosome 14. The stability of the cubilin/*AMN* complex is ensured by megalin/gp330/LRP-2 receptor encoded by the *LRP-2* gene on chromosome 2q24-q31; this interaction is Ca^{2+} dependent.[5]
- Although most of the absorption of vitamin B_{12} is active as described, less than 1% of absorption is passive and occurs through mucosal surfaces.

- Blood—Vitamin B_{12} dissociates from IF and attaches to the carrier protein transcobalamin II (TC II).
- Cells—TC II-vitamin B_{12} is taken up into the target cells by TC II receptor and megalin/*LRP-2*-mediated endocytosis.
  - Lysosome—Vitamin B_{12}-TC II dissociates to form free Cbl and enters the cytoplasm.
  - Cbl serves as a cofactor for the enzyme methionine synthase, converting homocysteine to methionine and methyltetrahydrofolate reductase-mediated substrate 5-methyltetrahydrofolate to tetrahydrofolate.
  - Tetrahydrofolate is involved in synthesis of purines and pyrimidines and hence in DNA replication.
  - Vitamin B_{12} in the form of adenosyl-cobalamin in the mitochondria acts as a substrate for methylmalonyl-coenzyme A (CoA) mutase. This reaction converts methylmalonyl-CoA into succinyl-CoA, which is a product of odd-chain and some amino acid catabolism.
  - The deficiency of vitamin B_{12} hence causes elevated homocysteine and methylmalonyl-CoA levels.

NUTRITIONAL CAUSES

- Vegans and vegetarians are prone to vitamin B_{12} deficiency because they have no to low intake of animal source food, such as dairy products, fish, and meat.
- Alcoholics can have decreased dietary intake of nutritionally rich foods, leading to depletion of vitamin B_{12} levels.
- Developing countries or regions with lower socioeconomic standards are more prone to have lower vitamin B_{12} levels and other nutritional deficiencies, most likely secondary to lower animal source food intake.[2,3]

DIGESTIVE CAUSES

- Pernicious anemia
  - Although classically described as the cause of vitamin B_{12} deficiency and megaloblastic anemia, pernicious anemia affects only a limited proportion of elderly patients.
  - About 2% of elderly above age 60 have underlying undiagnosed pernicious anemia.[6]
  - It is an end result of type A gastritis, an autoimmune phenomenon resulting in loss of parietal cells in the gastric mucosa.
  - Antibodies to gastric parietal cells and IF are present.
  - About 20% of the relatives of patients with pernicious anemia are affected; however, a specific genetic linkage remains to be identified.[7]
- Food-cobalamin malabsorption
  - Leading cause of vitamin B_{12} deficiency, especially in the elderly, accounting for about 60% to 70% of cases.[8]
  - Caused by inability of the body to release vitamin B_{12} from food or binding proteins in the intestine, particularly in the setting of hypochlorhydria.
  - Characterized by low levels of vitamin B_{12} in the blood in the presence of normal food intake of the vitamin, normal Schilling test, and no anti-IF antibodies.
  - However, the absorption of the vitamin by a passive mechanism is intact.
- Gastrectomy
  - Occurs with total as well as partial gastrectomy, and the degree of vitamin B_{12} deficiency is directly related to proportion of stomach removed.
  - Can occur because of intrinsic factor deficiency (IFD), postsurgical malabsorption, and bacterial overgrowth.
  - Parenteral vitamin B_{12} should be commenced postoperatively.[9]

ABSORPTION

- Hereditary IFD
  - A rare cause of vitamin B_{12} deficiency in which children present with megaloblastic anemia, usually by second decade of life.
- Caused by mutation in the gene on chromosome 11 encoding for gastric intrinsic factor (GIF).[10]
- Imerslund-Gräsbeck syndrome (MGA1)
  - Presentation usually between 1 and 5 years with megaloblastic anemia.
  - Associated with tubular-type proteinuria.
  - Caused by mutations in either cubilin (*CUBN*) gene or amnionless (*AMN*) gene, which cause a defect in active absorption of vitamin B_{12}-IF complex in the enterocytes.[11]
  - Schilling test, although rarely done, can aid in the differentiation of MGA1 from IFD. It will show normal radiocobalamin absorption with IF in IFD, whereas in MGA1 it will be abnormal.[10]
- Malabsorption syndromes
  - Chronic pancreatitis, celiac disease, Crohn disease, tuberculosis of the intestine, Whipple disease, chronic graft-versus-host disease, bacterial overgrowth, and other diseases can cause varied degrees of vitamin B_{12} malabsorption.
  - Vitamin B_{12} levels may be low in such patients, but deficiency may not be severe enough to cause clinical manifestations.
- Ileal resection
  - The terminal ileum plays an important role in active absorption of vitamin B_{12}.
  - Removal of more than 60 cm of terminal ileum causes vitamin B_{12} deficiency and requires lifelong replacement.[12,13]
  - Resecting less than 20 cm is not a risk for developing vitamin B_{12} deficiency.
  - Over time, vitamin B_{12} absorption normalizes after ileal resection in children but not in adults.[13]
- Antacids
  - Proton pump inhibitors (PPIs) or histamine receptor antagonists can cause decreased stomach acidity and thereby bacterial overgrowth in the duodenum.

- Vitamin B_{12} dissociates from food proteins in the presence of gastric acidity.
- Short-term treatment with PPIs has not shown decreased vitamin B_{12} levels; however, long-term use may cause vitamin B_{12} deficiency, especially in the elderly.[14]

- Metformin
  - According to a study of 71 patients with diabetes on metformin, 30% had vitamin B_{12} malabsorption.[15]
  - Both dose and duration of metformin use are risk factors for developing vitamin B_{12} deficiency.[16]
  - Disruption of membrane charge at the luminal enterocytes causing calcium ion displacement can cause decreased absorption of vitamin B_{12}-IF complex, which is calcium dependent.[17]

TRANSPORT

- Congenital TC II deficiency
  - Congenital deficiency of TC II, which acts as a vitamin B_{12} transporter to the target cells, causes decreased cellular availability of vitamin B_{12} despite adequate dietary intake.
  - Presentation is usually in infancy with megaloblastic anemia with or without neurological manifestations.
  - Treatment with high doses (up to 2000 μg weekly) of parenteral vitamin B_{12} is required.

INBORN ERRORS OF INTRACELLULAR COBALAMIN DEFICIENCY

- Genetic abnormalities may cause abnormal intracellular processing of cobalamin, further leading to hyperhomocysteinemia or methylmalonyl acidemia.
- These disorders are classified into complementation groups *cblA-cblH* and *mut* based on complementation analysis in cultured human fibroblasts.[18]
- Presentation is usually in infancy or childhood, but cases presenting in adolescence and adulthood have been reported.
- Patients may present with developmental delay, megaloblastic anemia, or severe neuropsychiatric or thrombotic complications.

DIAGNOSIS/SCREENING

- Vitamin B_{12} deficiency is a laboratory diagnosis.
- A thorough history and physical examination, however, can help identify possible underlying etiology and clinical manifestation.
- No diagnostic gold standard exists.
- Deficiency for vitamin B_{12} can be classified into 2 broad categories—clinical and subclinical.
- Clinical deficiency of vitamin B_{12}
  - Clinical signs and symptoms are present (may be mild and can be related to only one organ system).
  - Vitamin B_{12} levels are below 148 pmol/L in 97% of cases.
  - Metabolic abnormalities are usually present in 99% of cases.
- Subclinical deficiency of vitamin B_{12}
  - Absent clinical symptoms
  - Vitamin B_{12} levels are usually marginally depleted (148-221 pmol/L) but can be low as well.
  - At least 1 metabolic abnormality may be present (elevated methylmalonic acid [MMA] or plasma total homocysteine [tHcy]).

HISTORY

Specifically ask about the following items:

- Nonspecific symptoms of paresthesias, tiredness, generalized apathy, memory, and mood problems such as irritability
- Dietary preference, because vegetarian and vegan meals have low to no animal source food and hence lower vitamin B_{12} intake
- Social history, such as alcoholism, family history of pernicious anemia
- Surgical history in case of abdominal surgeries

PHYSICAL EXAMINATION

A physical examination can provide information in several areas:

- Perform a general neurological examination, including strength testing and sensory testing to elucidate paresthesias or numbness.
- Ataxia, loss of balance, and other neurological findings may be present in case of subacute combined degeneration.
- Perform a neuropsychiatric examination, including cognition, using the MMSE and depression screening.

HEMATOLOGICAL INVESTIGATIONS

- Complete blood cell count (CBC) and peripheral smear
  - Anemia with megaloblasts (MCV > 100 fL) can be present; however, this is not always the case, and other causes of macrocytosis unrelated to vitamin B_{12} deficiency, such as alcohol abuse, liver disease, hypothyroidism, medications such as zidovudine, or antineoplastic drugs, should be included in the differential diagnosis.
  - Neutrophil hypersegmentation is a more sensitive marker and is present in about two-thirds of patients with low vitamin B_{12} (<150 pmol/L) compared to only 4% of controls[19] (**Figure 53-2**).
  - Patients with neurological symptoms may have a completely normal CBC.
- Bone marrow
  - Bone marrow examination is not routinely performed and is of average diagnostic utility considering the cost and morbidity.
  - Examination shows hypercellular bone marrow with an increased myeloid/erythroid ratio. Megakaryocytes are decreased in number and have abnormal morphology.[20]

LABORATORY INVESTIGATIONS

- Serum cobalamin
  - This is a widely available, cheap, and diagnostic assay of choice for vitamin B_{12} deficiency.
  - Vitamin B_{12} level below 74 pmol/L is severely low, less than 148 pmol/L is low, and 148-221 pmol/L is considered marginally low.
  - For clinical cobalamin deficiency, the sensitivity is 97%; however, it lacks specificity.
  - Levels can be falsely elevated in myeloproliferative disorders.
  - Levels can be falsely decreased in pregnancy, myelomatosis, folate deficiency, and TC deficiencies.[20]
  - Some drugs may cause aberrant results.
  - If there is a high index of clinical suspicion for vitamin B_{12} deficiency (neurological or psychiatric symptoms) and in patients at risk for deficiency (elderly, malnourished, alcoholics, vegans, etc), a marginally low level of vitamin B_{12} and normal hematological findings should not exclude the diagnosis. Further biochemical testing with tHcy and MMA should be considered.

- Plasma tHcy
  - This value has high sensitivity but poor specificity for clinical vitamin B_{12} deficiency.
  - An elevated level of serum homocysteine level is above 13 μmol/L.
  - Vitamin B_{12} deficiency represents only a small proportion of all causes of elevated tHcy levels.
  - Renal insufficiency, elevated creatinine, alcoholism, folate and vitamin B_6 deficiency, hypothyroidism, drugs (eg, isoniazid), and inborn errors of homocysteine metabolism are other important causes of elevated tHcy levels.[11]
- Plasma MMA
  - Plasma MMA levels above 0.4 μmol/L are considered elevated.
  - Plasma MMA is a highly sensitive and more specific marker than tHcy.
  - Elevated MMA in the presence of low or low normal serum cobalamin levels confirms the diagnosis of vitamin B_{12} deficiency.
  - Renal insufficiency and other poorly understood factors could cause falsely elevated MMA levels.
  - Major limitations are high cost, limited availability, and complexity of the assay itself.

ADDITIONAL TESTS FOR PERNICIOUS ANEMIA

- Antiparietal cell antibodies
  - Present in about 85% of patients with pernicious anemia and 3% to 10% of normal individuals.
- Anti-IF antibodies
  - These are more specific indicators and are positive in about 70% of patients.[7]
- Indicators for gastric atrophy
  - Elevated serum gastrin levels and low pepsinogen levels are indicators of gastric atrophy.
  - These levels along with anti-IF antibodies and low serum cobalamin levels are diagnostic of pernicious anemia.[20]

DIFFERENTIAL DIAGNOSIS

- Folate deficiency, whether dietary or from impaired intestinal absorption, can cause megaloblastic changes in the erythrocytes.
- Serum folate levels are low in this case. However, because of fortification of foods with folate, its deficiency is rare in the United States.
- Megaloblastosis can be one of the manifestations of myelodysplastic syndromes. It can be identified by examining the peripheral smear, which may contain dysplastic or Pelger-Huet cells, and confirmed by bone marrow aspiration and biopsy.
- Human immunodeficiency virus (HIV) can also cause megaloblastic features because of a direct effect on DNA synthesis; however, symptomatology may be different.

MANAGEMENT

PARENTERAL THERAPY

- Classically, vitamin B_{12} deficiency is treated with parenteral injections of Cbl given subcutaneously or intramuscularly.
- Dosage is usually as follows: 1000 μg Cbl every day for 1 week, followed by 1000 μg Cbl every week for 4 weeks and then once monthly for the rest of the patient's life.
- Usually, the therapy is lifelong, but if reversible conditions exist, such as dietary deficiency, alcoholism, and the like, the therapy can be discontinued after normalization of levels.

ORAL THERAPY

- High doses, ranging from 500 to 2000 μg/day, of vitamin B_{12} are given orally (more than 200 times the recommended dietary allowance); the vitamin B_{12} is absorbed by passive diffusion throughout the length of the small intestine. This mechanism accounts for 1% of total vitamin B_{12} absorption.
- Compliance can be an important issue with this modality.
- Intranasal and sublingual formulations are also available; however, studies showing the efficacy are lacking.
- Efficacy of oral B_{12} supplementation at 1000 to 2000 μg/day may be similar to intramuscular administration for improving hematologic and neurologic parameters in patients with vitamin B_{12} deficiency. SOR Ⓐ

SCREENING

- No established consensual guidelines for routine screening in any individuals exist; however, several authors recommend routine screening in the elderly population.[21]
- In patients with underlying conditions predisposing them to vitamin B_{12} deficiency (eg, those with chronic alcoholism, vegans, geriatric population, patients with gastric surgery), some authors recommend screening, irrespective of age.[22]
- Routine testing for vitamin B_{12} deficiency is clinically indicated in patients who present with anemia, cognitive impairment, and neurological symptoms.

PROGNOSIS/CLINICAL COURSE

Hematological manifestations may be as follows:

- These manifestations occur as a result of ineffective and dysplastic erythropoiesis, especially secondary to aberrant DNA replication in the form of megaloblastic anemia, thrombocytopenia, leukopenia, or pancytopenia.
- Hematological changes rapidly reverse and anemia improves after vitamin B_{12} therapy.

Gastrointestinal manifestations involve the following:

- Gastrointestinal changes occur as a result of changes in the metabolism of the mucosal epithelial cells, which have a very high rate of proliferation.
  - Atrophic (Hunter) glossitis in the form of beefy red and smooth tongue (**Figure 53-1**) may occur. The loss of normal papillae causes the tongue to become smooth.
  - Angular cheilitis (**Figure 53-3**), recurrent oral ulcerations, diarrhea, and so on may be present in a limited number of patients.
  - Elevated bilirubin and lactate dehydrogenase (LDH) can also occur.

Neurological manifestations may be seen.

- Demyelination of the nervous system tissue in the central nervous system (CNS) is the underlying pathophysiological process. Biochemically, it may be related to abnormal myelination and low levels of CNS S-adenosylmethionine.[23] Age-related lysosomal dysfunction is also one of the proposed mechanisms for decreased vitamin B_{12} processing in the elderly.[24]

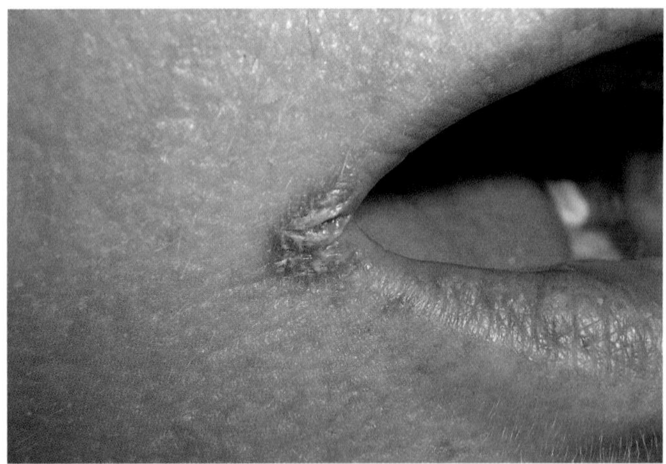

FIGURE 53-3 Angular cheilitis in a woman with B_{12} deficiency. (Reproduced with permission from Richard P. Usatine, MD.)

- This may manifest as follows:
  - Neuropathy and paresthesias
  - Ataxia
  - Subacute combined degeneration of spinal cord
  - Dementia
  - Stroke
  - Seizures
  - Optic atrophy
  - Urinary and fecal incontinence
- After treatment with vitamin B_{12}, neurological symptoms are reversible only in a few patients, with the majority having permanent neurological deficits, with the degree of improvement inversely related to duration and degree of deficiency. SOR B However, treatment with vitamin B_{12} prevents worsening.

Psychiatric manifestations may occur.

- Various psychiatric manifestations have been linked to vitamin B_{12} deficiency that may or may not be reversible with therapy.
  - Depression
  - Hallucinations
  - Personality changes
  - Abnormal behavior and psychosis

FOLLOW-UP

- At 6 to 10 days after starting vitamin B_{12} therapy, a CBC along with reticulocyte count and vitamin B_{12} levels should be undertaken to document a clinical response.
- This should be repeated after 8 weeks of therapy to confirm normal results.
- Long-term monitoring for vitamin B_{12} levels is not required in patients receiving replacement therapy.[25]

PATIENT EDUCATION

- Patients with a history of bariatric surgery, pernicious anemia, or resection of the terminal ileum should be advised that lifelong B_{12} supplementation is needed.
- Patients with neurological disease caused by B_{12} deficiency should be advised that the extent of neurological recovery is uncertain.
- Also, advise strict vegetarians that they are at risk for B_{12} deficiency and of the potential risk to newborns born to vegetarian mothers.

PATIENT RESOURCES

- Pernicious Anemia Society—**http://www.pernicious-anaemia-society.org.**

PROVIDER RESOURCES

- National Guideline Clearinghouse. *Dietary Guidelines for Americans, 2010*—**http://www.guideline.gov/content.aspx?id=34277&search=Diabetes+with+other+coma%2C+type+II+or+unspecified+type%2C+not+stated+as+uncontrolled.**

REFERENCES

1. Pfeiffer CM, Caudill SP, Gunter EW, Osterloh J, Sampson EJ. Biochemical indicators of B vitamin status in the US population after folic acid fortification: results from the National Health and Nutrition Examination Survey 1999-2000. *Am J Clin Nutr*. 2005;82(2):442-450.
2. Yajnik CS, Deshpande SS, Lubree HG, et al. Vitamin B_{12} deficiency and hyperhomocysteinemia in rural and urban Indians. *J Assoc Physicians India*. 2006;54:775-782.
3. McLean ED, Allen LH, Neumann CG, et al. Low plasma vitamin B-12 in Kenyan school children is highly prevalent and improved by supplemental animal source foods. *J Nutr*. 2007;137(3):676-682.
4. Fyfe JC, Madsen M, Højrup P, et al. The functional cobalamin (vitamin B_{12})-intrinsic factor receptor is a novel complex of cubilin and amnionless. *Blood*. 2004;103(5):1573-1579.
5. Korenberg JR, Argraves KM, Chen XN, et al. Chromosomal localization of human genes for the ldl receptor family member glycoprotein 330 (LRP2) and its associated protein rap (LRPAP1). *Genomics*. 1994;22(1):88-93.
6. Carmel R. Prevalence of undiagnosed pernicious anemia in the elderly. *Arch Intern Med*. 1996;156(10):1097-100.
7. Toh BH, van Driel IR, Gleeson PA. Pernicious anemia. *N Engl J Med*. 1997;337(20):1441-1448.
8. Andrès E, Affenberger S, Vinzio S, et al. Food-cobalamin malabsorption in elderly patients: clinical manifestations and treatment. *Am J Med*. 2005;118(10):1154-1159.
9. Beyan C, Beyan E, Kaptan K, Ifran A, Uzar AI. Post-gastrectomy anemia: evaluation of 72 cases with post-gastrectomy anemia. *Hematology*. 2007;12(1):81-84.
10. Tanner SM, Li Z, Perko JD, et al. Hereditary juvenile cobalamin deficiency caused by mutations in the intrinsic factor gene. *Proc Natl Acad Sci U S A*. 2005;102(11):4130-4133.
11. Carmel R, Green R, Rosenblatt DS, Watkins D. Update on cobalamin, folate, and homocysteine. *Hematology Am Soc Hematol Educ Program*. 2003;62-81.
12. Thompson WG, Wrathell E. The relation between ileal resection and vitamin B_{12} absorption. *Can J Surg*. 1977;20(5):461-464.
13. Behrend C, Jeppesen PB, Mortensen PB. Vitamin B_{12} absorption after ileorectal anastomosis for Crohn's disease: effect of ileal

resection and time span after surgery. *Eur J Gastroenterol Hepatol*. 1995;7(5):397-400.

14. Sheen E, Triadafilopoulos G. Adverse effects of long-term proton pump inhibitor therapy. *Dig Dis Sci*. 2011;56(4):931-950.
15. Tomkin GH, Hadden DR, Weaver JA, Montgomery DA. Vitamin-B_{12} status of patients on long-term metformin therapy. *BMJ*. 1971;2(5763):685-687.
16. Ting RZ-W, Szeto CC, Chan MH-M, Ma KK, Chow KM. Risk factors of vitamin B(12) deficiency in patients receiving metformin. *Arch Intern Med*. 2006;166(18):1975-1979.
17. Schäfer G. Some new aspects on the interaction of hypoglycemia-producing biguanides with biological membranes. *Biochem Pharmacol*. 1976;25(18):2015-2024.
18. Gravel RA, Mahoney MJ, Ruddle FH, Rosenberg LE. Genetic complementation in heterokaryons of human fibroblasts defective in cobalamin metabolism. *Proc Natl Acad Sci U S A*. 1975;72(8):3181-3185.
19. Metz J, Bell AH, Flicker L, et al. The significance of subnormal serum vitamin B_{12} concentration in older people: a case control study. *J Am Geriatr Soc*. 1996;44(11):1355-1361.
20. Klee GG. Cobalamin and folate evaluation: measurement of methylmalonic acid and homocysteine vs vitamin B(12) and folate. *Clin Chem*. 2000;46(8 Pt 2):1277-1283.
21. Clarke R, Refsum H, Birks J, et al. Screening for vitamin B-12 and folate deficiency in older persons. *Am J Clin Nutr*. 2003;77(5):1241-1247.
22. Dharmarajan TS, Adiga GU, Norkus EP. Vitamin B_{12} deficiency. Recognizing subtle symptoms in older adults. *Geriatrics*. 2003;58(3): 30-34, 37-38.
23. Metz J. Pathogenesis of cobalamin neuropathy: deficiency of nervous system s-adenosylmethonine? *Nutrition*. 1993;57(1):12-15.
24. Zhao H, Brunk UT, Garner B. Age-related lysosomal dysfunction: an unrecognized roadblock for cobalamin trafficking? *Cell Mol Life Sci*. 2011;3963-3969.
25. Galloway M, Hamilton M. Macrocytosis: pitfalls in testing and summary of guidance. *BMJ*. 2007;335(7625):884-886.

54 SICKLE CELL DISEASE

Gary Ferenchick, MD

PATIENT STORY

A 26-year-old patient with known sickle cell disease (SCD) presents with a sickle cell pain crisis affecting his hips and low back. His examination reveals tenderness to palpation at the low back and bilateral hip regions. His lower-extremity examination reveals a 12.5-cm superficial ulcer characterized by blistering and a shallow crater centrally on the medial surface of his left ankle, historically present for the previous 8 weeks (**Figure 54-1**). He is admitted to the hospital for management of his pain crisis and local care of his ulcer, including gentle debridement with wet-to-dry dressings and hydrocolloid dressings (DuoDERM) and the application of topical antibiotics and zinc oxide.

INTRODUCTION

SCD is inherited (autosomal recessive) and is a multisystem disease with 4 distinct sets of clinical manifestations: anemia, pain crises, chronic pain, and organ failure. Sickle cell anemia (SSA) is responsible for approximately 70% of SCD in the United States; other forms of SSD include sickle-hemoglobin C disease and sickle β-thalassemia disease.

SYNONYMS

Sickle cell anemia is a synonym for SSD.

EPIDEMIOLOGY

- The incidence of SCD is about 1 in 371 newborn African Americans, and fewer children with other ethnic backgrounds are affected.
- SCD affects approximately 80,000 patients in the United States; the majority of those affected are African American.[1]

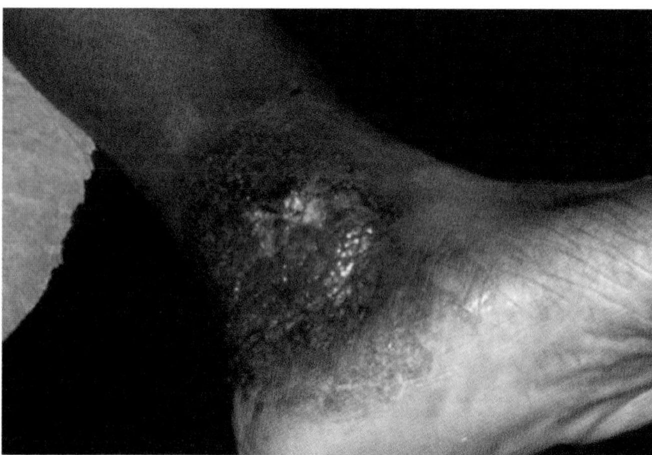

FIGURE 54-1 Leg ulcer in a patient with sickle cell disease. Approximately 10% of adult patients with SCD develop leg ulcers. (*Reproduced with permission from Lichtman MA, et al.* Lichtman's Atlas of Hematology. *New York, NY: McGraw-Hill; 2007. Copyright The McGraw-Hill Companies.*)

- Of African Americans, 8% have sickle cell trait, have normal hemoglobin concentrations, and do not have excess mortality.[2]
  - However, the risk of deep venous thrombosis and pulmonary embolism are increased by 2 to 4 times.

ETIOLOGY/PATHOPHYSIOLOGY

- The sickled red blood cells (RBCs) have a reduced life span caused by trapping in the reticuloendothelial system and from some intravascular hemolysis (**Figure 54-2**).
- Sickled RBCs are capable of occluding blood vessels of various sizes.

ANEMIA AND ITS SEQUELAE

- SCD occurs as a result of a single substitution of valine for glutamic acid in the β-globulin chain of hemoglobin A, which produces the sickle cell RBCs.
- SCD is characterized by normochromic normocytic indices with high reticulocyte, platelet, and leukocyte counts.
- The average hemoglobin level of patients with SSA is 7 to 8 g/dL.
- Hemoglobin electrophoresis at both alkaline pH (cellulose acetate) and acidic pH (citrate agar) distinguishes most different structural variants of hemoglobin. In addition, it establishes the relative percentage of sickle cell hemoglobin (HbS) and other hemoglobins.

RECURRENT EPISODES OF ACUTE PAIN (CRISES)

- Severe pain crises are the most common cause of hospital admission in most patients, especially in the adult population.
- In a cohort of 18,356 patients with SCD followed prospectively for approximately 5 years, the average rate of acute pain crises was 0.8 to 1.3 per year. The range of annual acute painful episodes was as follows:
  - Pain occurs rapidly and unexpectedly in patients with SCD.
  - Of patients with SCD, 39% did not seek medical attention for pain.

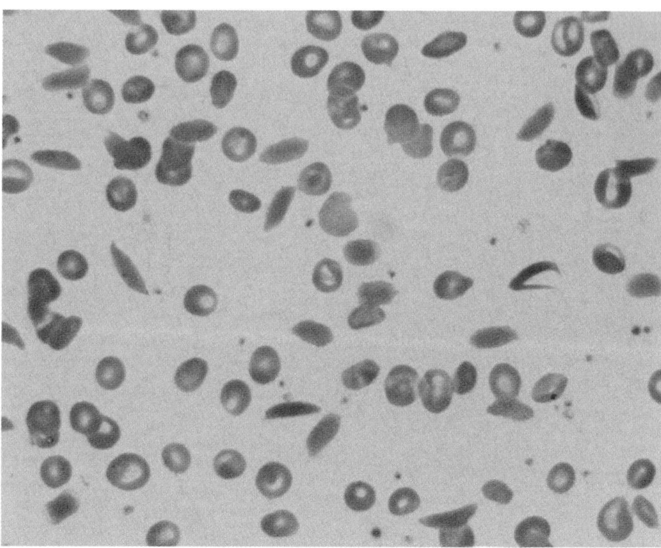

FIGURE 54-2 This blood smear show numerous sickle cells from patients with sickle cell anemia. Hemoglobin SS crystallizes when the oxygen tension is low, changing the red blood cell shape. The sickle forms decrease flow through the capillaries, leading to ischemia and infarction of the tissues supplied by the microcirculation. (*Reproduced with permission from Gary Ferenchick, MD.*)

- Of patients with SCD, 5.2% had 3 to 10 episodes.
  - This cohort accounted for approximately 33% of all acute painful episodes.
- Fewer than 6 episodes per year occurred for 1% of patients with SCD.[3]
- The rates of acute painful crises were higher for the 20- to 29-year-old age group than those aged 0 to 9 or older than 40 years.
- The mean duration of pain in patients with SCD with an acute painful crisis ranges from 10.1 hours to 9.6 days.[1]

- The frequency of SCD pain episodes is linked to mortality, with patients older than 20 years having more than 3 episodes per year experiencing a 2-fold higher rate of mortality compared to those with fewer episodes per year and compared to those younger than 20 years.[3]
- Patients with SCD with more severe anemia tend to have fewer episodes of acute pain; according to Platt, this is an example of divergence between the clinical and hematological severity of disease in these patients, possibly related to lower blood viscosity in those with more severe anemia.

CHRONIC PAIN SYNDROMES

- Among patients with SCD, at least 29% experience chronic pain (most frequent in those aged 25-44 years).
  - Chronic hip pain is manifested in 81%.
  - Chronic back pain affects 60%.
  - Chronic pain is experienced by 14% in multiple areas or bones simultaneously.
- A correlation between chronic pain and poor quality of life is present among patients with SCD.

ACUTE CHEST SYNDROME

- Acute chest syndrome is a lung injury syndrome of fever, respiratory distress (tachypnea, wheezing, or cough), and new infiltrates on a chest radiograph in a patient with SCD.
- Most patients who develop this have been in the hospital for an average of 2.5 days before developing acute chest syndrome, and approximately 9% of adults older than 20 years die as a result of acute chest syndrome.[4]

ORGAN FAILURE

Organ failure occurs with increasing age among patients with SCD and includes chronic renal failure, stroke, avascular bone necrosis, and pulmonary hypertension.[5]

DIAGNOSIS/SCREENING

The US Preventive Services Task Force recommends screening for SCD in all newborns, as do the American Academy of Family Physicians and the American Academy of Pediatrics.

HISTORY/SYMPTOMS

Specifically ask about the following in elucidating the history and symptoms:

- Frequent and unexplained pain episodes (back, chest, extremities, and joints) lasting 5 to 10 days on average.[6]
- History of cerebrovascular accident (CVA) at a younger age—About 10% of patients with SSA will have a CVA, and the risk of CVA is 3 times higher compared to age-matched African Americans without SCD.[7]
- Osteonecrosis of femur and humerus heads—This occurs in about 50% of adult patients with SSA.
- History of priapism, leg ulcers, infections—Acute chest syndrome is associated with fever, chest pain, cough, and pulmonary infiltrates (caused by infarction, infection, emboli, and atelectasis).

PHYSICAL EXAM

Specifically look for or establish the following:

- Pulmonary findings of acute chest syndrome (crackles, wheezing, signs of consolidation) may exist.
- Cardiomegaly and a systolic murmur are common.
- Untreated children may develop dactylitis (**Figure 54-3**), frontal bossing of the forehead, and a widened face along with short stature; these changes will persist into adulthood (**Figure 54-4**).

LABORATORY TESTING

- Complete blood cell count (CBC)—Normochromic, normocytic anemia is common.
- Reticulocyte count—Commonly, this is high unless an aplastic crisis is present.
- Lactate dehydrogenase (LDH) level—This is associated with the degree of hemolysis.
- Hemoglobin electrophoresis
  - Note that hemoglobin A (the normal hemoglobin in most of us) is comprised of 2 α chains and 2 β chains ($\alpha_2\beta_2$).
  - Most of the commonly encountered hemoglobinopathies are caused by alterations in the β-chain.
- Sickle cell anemia
  - SSA is the most common and severe form of SCD.
  - Genotype is HbSS (α_2/β_2^s), which means that both α chains are normal, and both β chains have HbS, which has a substitution of valine for glutamic acid in the β chain, changing hemoglobulin A (HbA) to HbS.

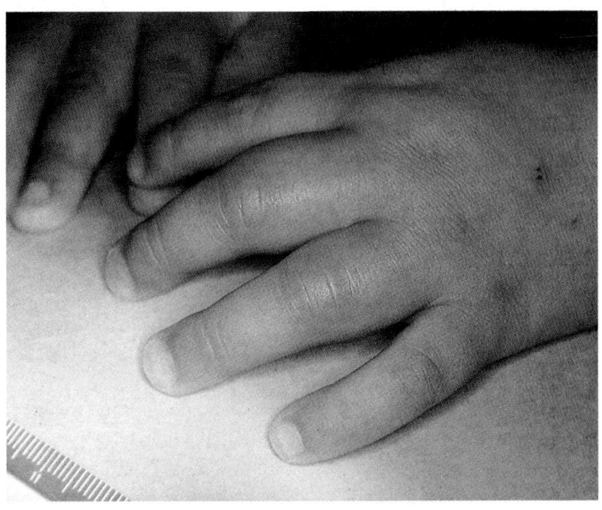

FIGURE 54-3 Acute sickle dactylitis caused by a vaso-occlusive crisis. Dactylitis represents swelling of the digits that can be seen in sickle cell disease in children (birth to 4 years) and is associated with marrow necrosis of the bones of the involved digits. (Reproduced with permission from Knoop K, Stack L, Storrow A, Thurman RJ. *The Atlas of Emergency Medicine*. 3rd ed. New York, NY: McGraw-Hill; 2010. Photo contributor: Donald L. Rucknagel, MD, PhD.)

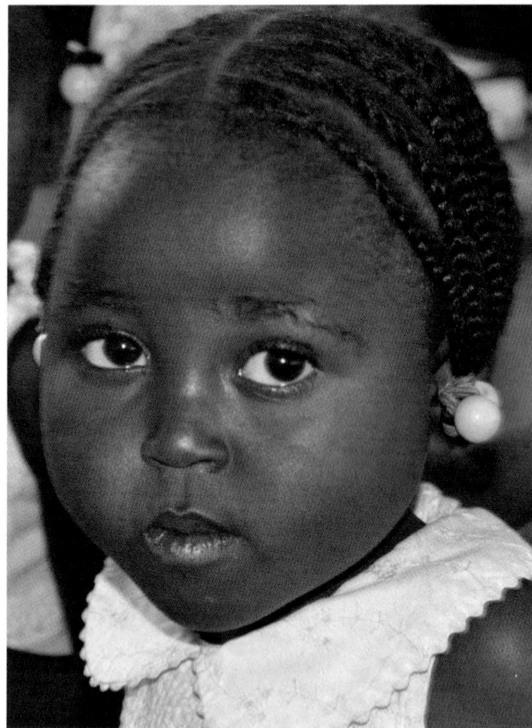

FIGURE 54-4 A young child from Haiti with untreated sickle cell disease that has led to frontal bossing and stunted growth. (Reproduced with permission from Richard P. Usatine, MD.)

- Hemoglobin electrophoresis shows the following:
  - HbS > 90%.
  - Fetal hemoglobin (HbF) = approximately 6%.
  - HbA_2 = approximately 3.5%.
  - HbA = 0% (unless the patient has received a blood transfusion in the past few months).
- Sickle cell trait
  - Approximately 10% of blacks have sickle cell trait; that is, they are heterozygous for the sickle cell gene, and their genotype is βS/βA.
  - Sickle cell trait is benign, and patients are essentially normal and protected against falciparum malaria, but they may have difficulty concentrating their urine (hyposthenuria).
  - Hemoglobin electrophoresis shows both HbA and HbS:
    - HbA is always greater than 50%, *and*
    - HbS percentage depends on the α genotype; *thus* HbS occurs in
      - 35% to 45% in patients with 4a genes
      - 30% to 35% with 3a genes
      - 25% to 30% with 2a genes
      - 17% to 25% with 1a gene
- Hemoglobin SC disease (one β chain has hemoglobin S and the other has hemoglobin C)
  - HbS approximately 50%
  - Hemoglobin C (HbC) approximately 50%
- Sickle-β^+-thalassemia
  - Thalassemia genes produce *normal hemoglobin but in reduced amounts.*
  - Differentiation among SSA and sickle-β-thalassemia (both β^+, in which there are some β chains, and β°, in which there are no β chains) may be difficult.
  - Microcytosis, elevated HbA_2, and the presence of a small amount of HbA with no history of recent blood transfusion favor the diagnosis of sickle-β^+-thalassemia.
- HbF is fetal hemoglobin and is a good predictor of the severity of SSA. It is followed for the efficacy of hydroxyurea treatment.

IMAGING

- Perform a transcranial Doppler ultrasound starting at age 2 to assess for stroke risk in children with SSA. Those who screen positive and start a long-term transfusion program experience a 92% reduction in risk of CVA.[8]
- Perform an echocardiogram to assess for pulmonary hypertension by checking the tricuspid regurgitant volume (TRV), although there is only a 25% positive predictive value for echocardiography.[9]

MANAGEMENT

ACUTE MANAGEMENT

- Simple transfusion is given when urgently needed; the goal is to restore hemoglobin and reduce HbS levels. SOR A
  - Urgent indications include aplastic crisis, acute chest syndrome or acute neurologic event, sepsis (including meningitis), multiple organ failure, acute hemorrhage, and sequestration in the liver or spleen.
  - Repeated transfusions are associated with iron overload and are not indicated as a primary treatment for acute painful crises.
  - Do not transfuse to a hemoglobin level of greater than 10 g/dL as blood viscosity increases.
- Consider a simple transfusion to a hemoglobin of 10 g/dL preoperatively.[2]
- Consider an urgent exchange transfusion in patients with SSA with acute CVA because this more rapidly decreases the HbS concentration. SOR A
- Analgesics (opioid and nonopioid) are given for pain. Patients may require large doses of narcotics for pain relief.
- Treatment of acute chest syndrome includes oxygen, adequate hydration, broad-spectrum antibiotics, bronchodilators/incentive spirometry, and transfusions to decrease the fraction of HbS to less than 30%.[2]
- Inhaled nitric oxide was not associated with resolution of the sickle cell crisis among 150 patients presenting with a sickle cell vaso-occlusive pain crisis.[10]

CHRONIC MANAGEMENT

- For newborns who screen positive, give a pneumococcal vaccine and provide prophylactic oral penicillin for 5 years to prevent serious infections. SOR A
- Hydroxyurea increases HbF and reduces long-term mortality in patients with SSA and decreases daily pain intensity. The decrease in pain intensity correlates with the amount of HbF increase in response to treatment.[11,12] SOR A
- Long-term use of hydroxyurea reduced mortality as measured over 17.5 years and was not associated with an increased risk of malignancy.[11]
  - HbF of 20% may be a threshold for the prevention of vaso-occlusive crisis.[6,12,13]

- Hydroxyurea was associated with a 44% reduction in pain crises and a 40% lower mortality rate.
- Exchange transfusions decrease the percentage of HbS.
- Omega-3 fatty acid supplements in 16 patients with SSA decreased the number of painful crises in a 6-month pilot study.[14] SOR B
- Bone marrow transplantation can cure patients, with a 95% disease-free survival.[15] SOR B
- Iron overload from multiple transfusions is a risk for patients with SSA. Guidelines suggest initiating iron chelation therapy in patients with a serum ferritin over 1000 ng/mL or patients with a cumulative transfusion of more than 120 packed RBCs. Patients with SSA treated with a once-daily oral iron chelator (deferasirox) decreased serum ferritin by 50%; this has a clinically acceptable safety profile in patients with SSA at risk for iron overload because of frequent transfusions.[16,17]

PROGNOSIS/CLINICAL COURSE

- Major complications of SCD include the following:
  - Cerebrovascular complications occur in 8.5% to 17% of patients with SSA in the United States.
  - Neurocognitive deficits are common in patients with SSA, including those relating to IQ, memory, processing speed, and measures of executive function.[18]
  - Proliferative retinopathy is more common in HbSCD than other sickle cell syndromes.
  - Cardiopulmonary complications, including acute chest syndrome, are the most frequent cause of death of patients with SSA, congestive heart failure, and pulmonary hypertension, which is associated with a 25% to 50% chance of death within 2 years.[19]
  - Cholelithiasis occurs in patients with SCD with symptomatic bilirubin stones.
  - Splenic sequestration can occur.
  - Renal complications
    - A "normal" creatinine in SCD is different from that for other patients; serum creatinine is very low (0.2 to 0.5 mg/dL) in patients with SCD.
    - A normal creatinine level of 1.2 mg/dL is associated with up to 40% loss of renal function in SCD.
    - Confirm with glomerular filtration rate and consider early therapy with angiotensin-converting enzyme (ACE) inhibitors.
  - Priapism—After major attacks of priapism, about one-third of the patients are completely impotent, one-third are partially impotent, and one-third recover normal function.
  - Leg ulcers—Approximately 5% to 10% of adult patients with SCD with SSA develop a leg ulcer at some time, especially near the malleoli. These are more common in male versus female patients with SCD[20] (**Figure 54-1**).
  - Avascular necrosis is a problem.
  - Infection—Patients with SSA have a compromised immune system that predisposes them to infection.
  - Blood pressure is generally lower than normal in patients with SSA. Patients with high values relative to this population are at an increased risk for increased morbidity and mortality.
  - Dactylitis (hand-foot syndrome) (**Figure 54-3**), splenomegaly, and splenic sequestration are common in children, especially before age 5 years.
  - Aplastic crises are commonly caused by coinfection with parvovirus B19.

FOLLOW-UP

- Stable patients should be followed every 4-6 months.
- Consider periodic retinal screening by an ophthalmologist and periodic echocardiography to assess for pulmonary hypertension.

PATIENT EDUCATION

Avoid extreme heat or cold and maintain adequate hydration.

PATIENT RESOURCES

- Sickle Cell Disease Association of America—**http://www.sicklecelldisease.org.**
- American Academy of Pediatrics. *Health Supervision for Children with Sickle Cell Disease*—**http://pediatrics.aappublications.org/content/109/3/526.full.**
- National Heart, Lung, and Blood Institute. *Sickle Cell Disease*—**http://ghr.nlm.nih.gov/condition/sickle-cell-disease.**

PROVIDER RESOURCES

- Geneva Foundation for Medical Education and Research. Clearinghouse for many articles and guidelines for SSA—**http://www.gfmer.ch/Guidelines/Anemia_and_hemoglobinopathies/Sickle_cell_anemia.htm.**
- Note that the SCDAA does not support the screening of athletes for sickle cell trait as a means to decrease heat- and exertion-related deaths among athletes—**http://www.sicklecelldisease.org/index.cfm?page=sickle-cell-trait-athletics.**
- Bender MA, Hobbs W. Sickle cell disease. *Gene Rev*. 2012, May. **http://www.ncbi.nlm.nih.gov/books/NBK1377/.**

REFERENCES

1. Taylor LE, Stotts NA, Humphreys J, et al. A review of the literature on the multiple dimensions of chronic pain in adults with sickle cell disease. *J Pain Symptom Manage*. 2010;40(3):416-435.
2. Steinberg MH. Sickle cell disease. *Ann Int Med*. 2011;155:ITC31.
3. Platt OS, Thorington BD, Brambilla DJ, et al. Pain in sickle cell disease. Rates and risk factors. *N Engl J Med*. 1991;325(1):11-16.
4. Laurie GA. Acute chest syndrome in sickle cell disease. *Intern Med J*. 2010;40(5):372-376.
5. Gladwin MT, Vichinsky E. Pulmonary complications of sickle cell disease. *N Engl J Med*. 2008;359(21):2254-2265.
6. Smith WR, Penberthy LT, Bovbjerg VE, et al. Daily assessment of pain in adults with sickle cell disease. *Ann Intern Med*. 2008;148:94-101.
7. Strouse JJ, Jordan LC, Lanzkron S, et al. The excess burden of stroke in hospitalized adults with sickle cell disease. *Am J Hematol*. 2009;84:548-552.
8. Adams RJ, McKie VC, Hsu L, et al. Prevention of a first stroke by transfusions in children with sickle cell anemia and abnormal results on transcranial Doppler ultrasonography. *N Engl J Med*. 1998;339:5-11.
9. Parent F, Bachir D, Inamo J, et al. A hemodynamic study of pulmonary hypertension in sickle cell disease. *N Engl J Med*. 2011;365:44-53.

10. Gladwin MT, Kato GJ, Weiner D, et al. Nitric oxide for inhalation in the acute treatment of sickle cell pain crisis: a randomized controlled trial. *JAMA*. 2011;305(9):893-902.
11. Steinberg MH, McCarthy WF, Castro O, et al. The risks and benefits of long-term use of hydroxyurea in sickle cell anemia: a 17.5 year follow-up. *Am J Hematol*. 2010;85:403-408.
12. Ware RE, Aygun B. Advances in the use of hydroxyurea. *Hematology Am Soc Hematol Educ Program*. 2009:62-69.
13. Smith WR, Ballas SK, McCarthy WF, et al. The association between hydroxyurea treatment and pain intensity, analgesic use, and utilization in ambulatory sickle cell anemia patients. *Pain Med*. 2011;12(5):697-705.
14. Okpala I, Ibegbulam O, Duru A, et al. Pilot study of omega-3 fatty acid supplements in sickle cell disease. *APMIS*. 2011;119(7):442-448.
15. Hsieh MM, Kang EM, Fitzhugh CD, et al. Allogeneic hematopoietic stem-cell transplantation for sickle cell disease. *N Engl J Med*. 2009;361:2309-2317.
16. Voskaridou E, Plata E, Douskou M, et al. Deferasirox effectively decreases iron burden in patients with double heterozygous HbS/β-thalassemia. *Ann Hematol*. 2011;90(1):11-15.
17. Vichinsky E, Bernaudin F, Forni GL, et al. Long-term safety and efficacy of deferasirox (Exjade) for up to 5 years in transfusional iron-overloaded patients with sickle cell disease. *Br J Haematol*. 2011;154(3):387-397.
18. Vichinsky EP, Neumayr LD, Gold JI, et al. Neuropsychological dysfunction and neuroimaging abnormalities in neurologically intact adults with sickle cell anemia. *JAMA*. 2010;303:1823-1831.
19. Gladwin MT, Sachdev V, Jison ML, et al. Pulmonary hypertension as a risk factor for death in patients with sickle cell disease. *N Engl J Med*. 2004;350:886-895.
20. Koshy M, Entsuah R, Koranda A, et al. Leg ulcers in patients with sickle cell disease. *Blood*. 1989;74(4):1403-1408.

PART 9

PULMONARY

Strength of Recommendation (SOR)	Definition
A	Recommendation based on consistent and good-quality patient-oriented evidence.*
B	Recommendation based on inconsistent or limited-quality patient-oriented evidence.*
C	Recommendation based on consensus, usual practice, opinion, disease-oriented evidence, or case series for studies of diagnosis, treatment, prevention, or screening.*

*See Appendix A on pages 1241-1244 for further information.

55 ASTHMA AND PULMONARY FUNCTION TESTING

Mindy A. Smith, MD, MS

PATIENT STORY

A 32-year-old Hispanic woman presents to your office with a chronic cough for 3 months. She states the cough is dry and started with a cold 3 months ago. She denies fever, chills, and night sweats. She has never been diagnosed with asthma or lung disease in the past. She does admit to having had persistent dry coughs that linger on after getting colds in the past. She is not sure what wheezing is but she has noticed a tight feeling in her chest at night with some whistling sound. On physical examination, her lungs are clear and she is moving air well. Her height is 5 ft and her weight is 220 lb giving her a body mass index (BMI) of 43. Her peak expiratory flow (PEF) in the office is at 80% of predicted. Even though she is not wheezing, her history and physical examination are highly suspicious for asthma. You prescribe a short-acting β_2-agonist (SABA) rescue inhaler with spacer and order pulmonary function tests (PFTs). You have your nurse provide asthma education (including proper use of an inhaler) and suggestions for weight loss.

The patient returns 1 week later and the cough is much improved. You review her PFTs (**Figure 55-1**) and note that she has reversible bronchospasm especially in the small airways (forced expiratory flow $[FEF]_{25\%-75\%}$ shows a 70% improvement with inhaled albuterol). See **Table 55-1** for the meaning of the typical abbreviations using with PFTs. Her lung volumes (**Figure 55-1B**) show hyperinflation with a high residual volume and her diffusing capacity is normal. The whole picture is consistent with asthma. An asthma action plan is created and a referral to a nutritionist is offered to help the patient with her obesity.

INTRODUCTION

Asthma is a chronic inflammatory airway disorder with variable airflow obstruction and bronchial hyperresponsiveness that is at least partially reversible, spontaneously or with treatment (eg, β_2-agonist treatment). Patients with asthma have recurrent episodes of wheezing, breathlessness, chest tightness, and cough (particularly at night or in the early morning).

EPIDEMIOLOGY

- Estimated prevalence of asthma in noninstitutionalized adults over age 18 years in the United States (2010) is approximately 8.2% (18.7 million cases).[1]
- The number of deaths from asthma in 2009 was 3388 (1.1/100,000 population).[1]
- Asthma accounts for 17 million visits per year (physician offices, emergency departments, and hospital outpatient sites).[1]
- Asthma was the first-listed diagnosis for 479,000 hospital discharges in 2009 with an average length of stay of 4.3 days.[1]
- Estimated direct costs associated with asthma in the United States grew from about $53 billion in 2002 to about $56 billion in 2007 (6% increase).[2]

ETIOLOGY AND PATHOPHYSIOLOGY

- Although the precise cause is unknown, early exposure to airborne allergens (eg, house–dust mite, cockroach antigens) and childhood respiratory infections (eg, respiratory syncytial virus, parainfluenza) are associated with asthma development.
- In addition to environmental factors, asthma has an inherited component, although the genetics involved remain complex.[3] The gene *ADAM 33* (a disintegrin and metalloproteinase) may increase the risk of asthma as metalloproteinases appear to effect airway remodeling.[4]
- The pulmonary obstruction characterizing asthma results from combinations of mucosal swelling, mucous production, constriction of bronchiolar smooth muscles, and neutrophils (the latter, particularly important in smokers or those with occupational asthma).[4] Over time, airway smooth muscle hypertrophy and hyperplasia, remodeling (thickening of the subbasement membrane, subepithelial fibrosis, and vascular proliferation and dilation), along with mucous plugging complicate the disease.[4]
- Allergen-induced acute bronchospasm involves immunoglobulin E (IgE)-dependent release of mast cell mediators.[4]

RISK FACTORS

- Family history of asthma.[5]
- Recurrent childhood chest infections or atopy.[5]
- Parental smoking.[5]
- Male gender.[5]
- Recent use of acetaminophen has also been associated with asthma symptoms in adolescents (odds ratio [OR], 1.43; 95% confidence interval [CI], 1.33-1.53 and OR, 2.51; 95% CI, 2.33-2.70 for at least once a year and at least once a month use vs no use, respectively).[6] One possible mechanism is through acetaminophen reducing the immune response and prolonging rhinovirus infection.[7]
- Modifiable risk factors include obesity (OR 3.3 for adult-onset asthma) and tobacco smoking; the latter also increases the risk of occupational asthma.[4]

DIAGNOSIS

The diagnosis of asthma is made on clinical suspicion (presence of symptoms of recurrent and partially reversible airflow obstruction and airway hyperresponsiveness) and confirmed with spirometry.[3] Alternative diagnoses should be excluded.

CLINICAL FEATURES

Asthma's most common symptoms are recurrent wheezing, difficulty breathing, chest tightness, and cough. An absence of wheezing or normal physical examination does not exclude asthma.[3] In fact, up to 25% of patients with asthma have normal physical examinations even though abnormalities are seen on pulmonary function testing.[4] As part of the diagnosis of asthma, ask about the following[3]:

- Pattern of symptoms and precipitating factors. Symptoms often occur or worsen at night and during exercise, viral infection, exposure to inhalant allergens or irritants (eg, tobacco smoke, wood smoke,

	Pre-Bronch			Post-Bronch		
	Pred	Actual	%Pred	Actual	%Pred	%Chng
---- SPIROMETRY ----						
FVC (L)	3.14	3.27	104	3.69	117	+12
FEV1 (L)	2.64	2.16	81	2.68	101	+24
FEV1/FVC (%)	85	66	77	73	85	+9
FEF 25-75% (L/sec)	3.14	1.44	45	2.47	78	+70
FEF Max (L/sec)	6.14	4.83	78	6.73	109	+39
FEF 25% (L/sec)	5.06	2.88	56	4.70	92	+62
FEF 50% (L/sec)	4.36	1.72	39	2.82	64	+64
FEF 75% (L/sec)	1.79	0.69	38	1.28	71	+86
FIVC (L)		3.24		3.75		+15
FIF 50% (L/sec)	4.18	5.09	121	5.45	130	+6

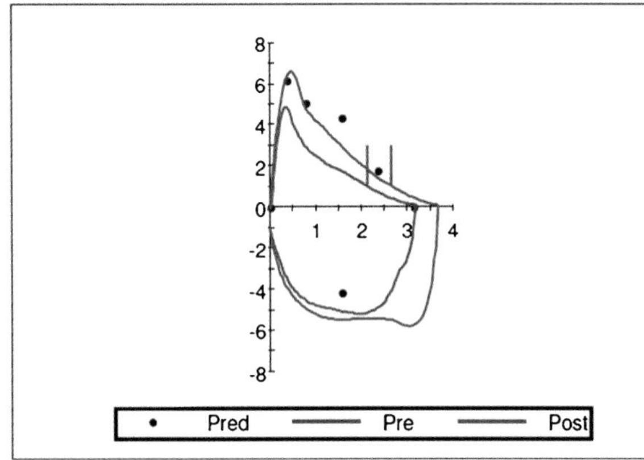

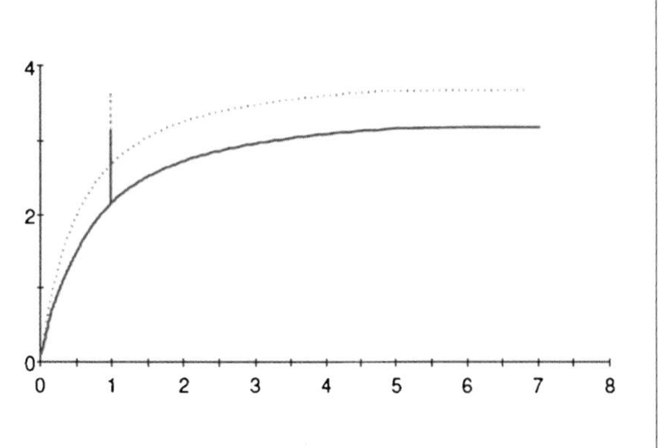

A

	Pre-Bronch			Post-Bronch		
	Pred	Actual	%Pred	Actual	%Pred	%Chng
---- LUNG VOLUMES --						
SVC (L)	3.14	3.17	101			
TLC (Pleth) (L)	4.30	5.12	119			
RV (Pleth) (L)	1.23	1.95	158			
RV/TLC (Pleth) (%)	29	38	131			
TGV (L)	2.32	3.33	143			
Raw (cmH2O/L/s)	1.86	3.71	199			
ERV (L)	1.16	1.38	118			
IC (L)	1.98	1.79	90			
---- DIFFUSION ----						
DLCOunc (ml/min/mmH	17.53	27.25	155			
DLCOcor (ml/min/mmH	17.53					
VA (L)	4.30	5.11	118			
DL/VA (ml/min/mmHg/	4.08	5.33	130			

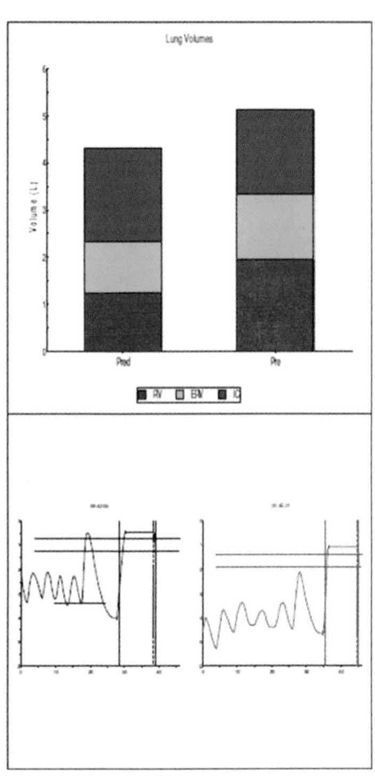

B

FIGURE 55-1 Pulmonary function tests (PFTs) in a woman with suspected asthma. A. Spirometry before and after bronchodilation with flow volume loops and graph of forced vital capacity (FVC). The FEV_1 is normal, but the FEV_1/FVC ratio and $FEF_{25\%-75\%}$ are reduced. Following administration of bronchodilators, there is a good response especially in the small airways as represented by $FEF_{25\%-75\%}$. B. Lung volumes are all increased (especially the residual volume) indicating overinflation and air trapping. The diffusing capacity is normal. Conclusions: minimal airway obstruction, overinflation, and a response to bronchodilators are consistent with a diagnosis of asthma. The patient has minimal obstructive airways disease of the asthmatic type. (*Reproduced with permission from Richard P. Usatine, MD.*)

TABLE 55-1 Pulmonary Function Tests, Key to Abbreviations

FVC (L)	Forced vital capacity
FEV_1(L)	Forced vital capacity at one second
FEV_1/FVC %	FEV_1 divided by FVC
$FEF_{25\%-75\%}$ (L/s)	Forced expiratory flow between 25% and 75% of capacity—same as maximal midexpiratory flow rate (MMFR)
FEF_{max} (L/s)	Forced expiratory flow maximum
$FEF_{25\%}$ (L/s)	Forced expiratory flow rate when 25% of the FVC has been exhaled (slope of FVC curve at 25% exhaled)
$FEF_{50\%}$ (L/s)	Forced expiratory flow rate when 50% of the FVC has been exhaled
$FEF_{75\%}$ (L/s)	Forced expiratory flow rate when 75% of the FVC has been exhaled
FITC (L)	Forced inspiratory vital capacity
$FIF_{50\%}$ (L/s)	Forced inspiratory flow at 50% capacity
SVC (L)	Slow vital capacity
TLC (L)	Total lung capacity
RV (L)	Residual volume
RV/TLC	Residual volume divided by total lung capacity
TGV (L)	Thoracic gas volume
Raw	Airway resistance
ERV (L)	Expiratory reserve volume
IC (L)	Inspiratory capacity
DLCO	Diffusing capacity of lung (using carbon monoxide measuring)
VA (L)	Alveolar volume
DL/VA	Diffusing capacity divided by alveolar volume

airborne chemicals), changes in weather, strong emotional expression (laughing hard or crying), menstrual cycle, and stress.[3]

- Family history of asthma, allergy or atopy in close relatives.
- Social history (eg, day care, workplace, social support).
- History of exacerbations (eg, frequency, duration, treatment) and impact on patient and family.

Findings on physical examination may include the following[3]:

- Upper respiratory tract—Increased nasal secretion, mucosal swelling, and/or nasal polyp.
- Lungs—Decreased intensity of breath sounds is the most common (33%-65% of patients).[4] Additional findings can include wheezing, prolonged phase of forced exhalation, use of accessory respiratory muscles, appearance of hunched shoulders, and chest deformity. During a severe exacerbation of asthma, minimal airflow can result in no audible wheezing.
- Skin—Atopic dermatitis and/or eczema (see Chapters 143, 145, and 146). There is a strong association between asthma, allergic rhinoconjunctivitis, and eczema (**Figure 55-2**), although the "atopic or allergic triad" with the coexistence of all 3 conditions at one time (**Figure 55-3**) is not very common. Data support a sequence of atopic manifestations beginning typically with atopic dermatitis in infancy followed by allergic rhinitis and/or asthma in later stages.[8]

Findings in patients with status asthmaticus (prolonged or severe asthma attack that is not responsive to standard treatment) may include the following[4]:

- Tachycardia (heart rate >120 beats/min) and tachypnea (respiratory rate >30 breaths/min)
- Use of accessory respiratory muscles
- Pulsus paradoxus (inspiratory decrease in systolic blood pressure >10 mm Hg)
- Mental status changes (due to hypoxia and hypercapnia)
- Paradoxical abdominal and diaphragmatic movement on inspiration

LABORATORY TESTING

- Spirometry is recommended by National Asthma Education Program (NAEP) for all adolescent and adult patients to determine airway obstruction that is at least partially reversible (**Figures 55-1, 55-4** and **55-5**).[3] SOR B

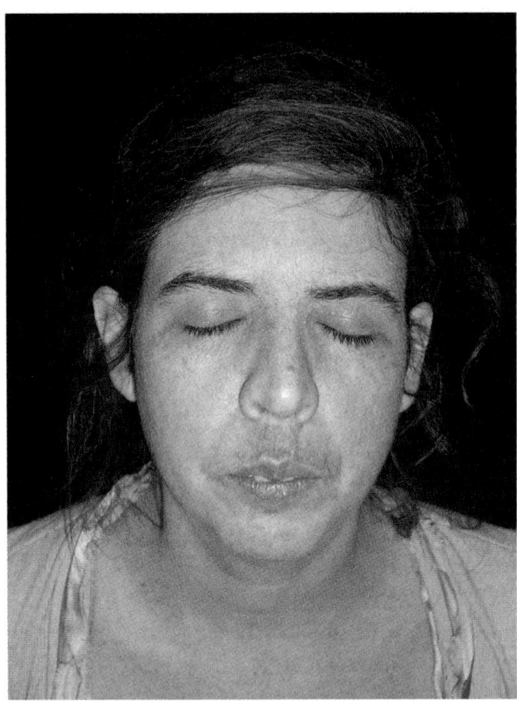

FIGURE 55-2 Patient with severe asthma, atopic dermatitis, and allergic rhinitis—atopic triad. (*Reproduced with permission from Richard P. Usatine, MD.*)

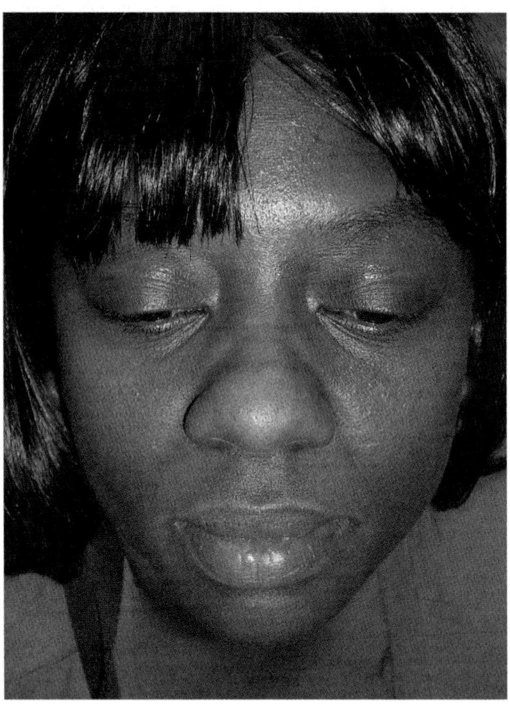

FIGURE 55-3 Patient with the "atopic triad" and a visible crease over her nose from the "allergic salute" secondary to allergic rhinitis. (*Reproduced with permission from Richard Usatine, MD.*)

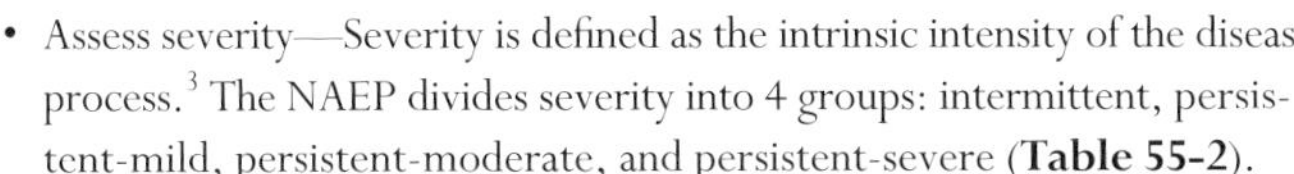

- Assess severity—Severity is defined as the intrinsic intensity of the disease process.[3] The NAEP divides severity into 4 groups: intermittent, persistent-mild, persistent-moderate, and persistent-severe (**Table 55-2**).
- Initially, severity can be assessed in the office, urgent or emergency care setting with predicted forced expiratory volume in 1 second (FEV_1) or PEF; a value of less than 40% indicates a severe exacerbation. A value of equal to or greater than 70% predicted FEV_1 or PEF is a goal for discharge from the emergency care setting.
- Once asthma control is achieved, severity can be assessed by the step of care required for control (ie, amount of medication) (see Medications).
- Additional tests that may be useful include the following[3]:
- Pulmonary function testing if a diagnosis of chronic obstructive pulmonary disease (COPD), restrictive lung disease, or vocal cord dysfunction is considered.
- Bronchoprovocation (using methacholine, histamine, cold air or exercise challenge) if spirometry is normal or near-normal and asthma is still suspected; a negative test is helpful in ruling out asthma.
- Pulse oximetry or arterial blood gas if hypoxia is suspected (eg, cyanosis, rapid respiratory rate).
- In the emergency room setting, B-type natriuretic peptide can help distinguish between heart failure and pulmonary disease.[4]

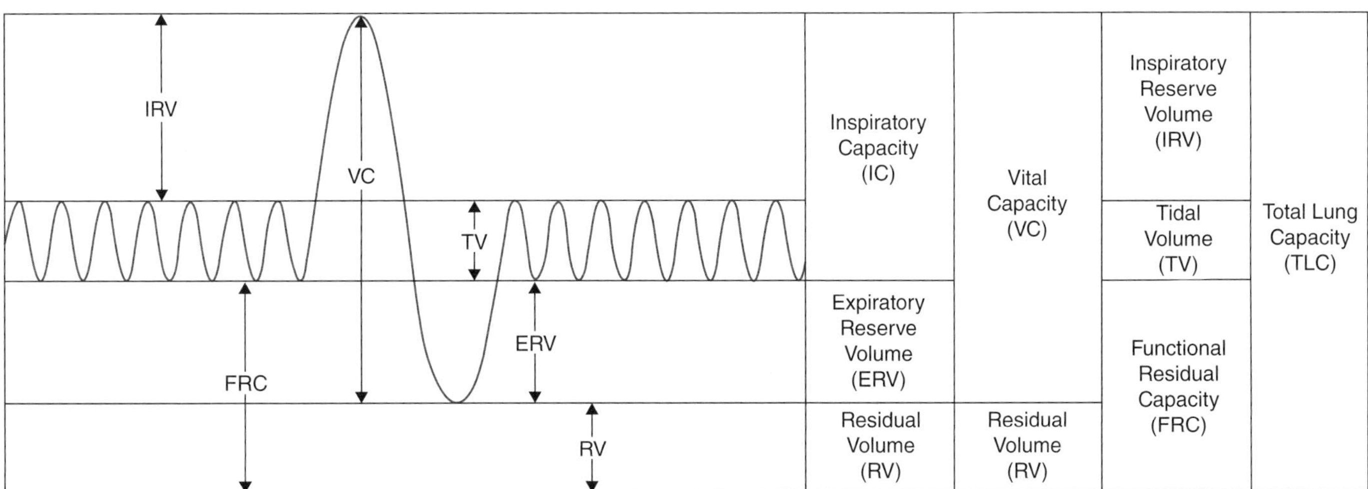

FIGURE 55-4 Graph of lung volumes showing the relationship of tidal volume to vital capacity and other important lung volumes.

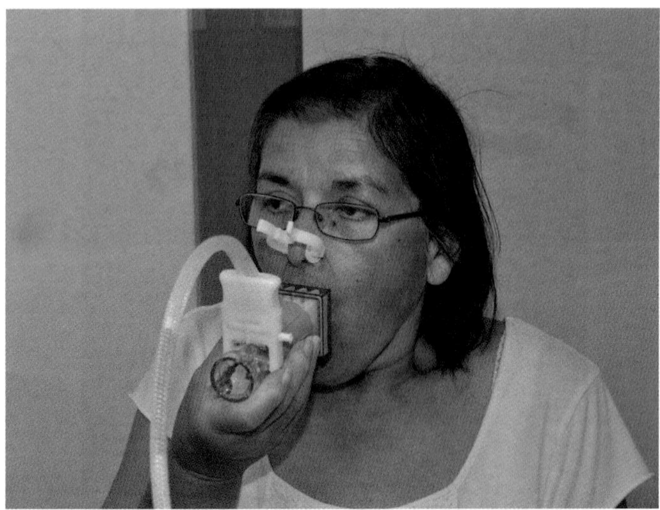

FIGURE 55-5 Patient having pulmonary function tests (PFTs). *(Reproduced with permission from Richard P. Usatine, MD.)*

IMAGING

A chest X-ray (CXR) is not useful for diagnosis but is helpful for excluding other diseases (eg, pneumonia) or identifying comorbidity (eg, heart failure). The main finding on CXR is hyperinflation (occurring in about 45% of patients with asthma).[4] Hyperinflation is manifested by the following:

- Increased anteroposterior (AP) diameter
- Increased retrosternal air space (**Figure 55-6**)
- Infracardiac air
- Low-set flattened diaphragms (best assessed in lateral chest)
- Vertical heart

Atelectasis is another finding seen during acute severe episodes (**Figure 55-7**).

DIFFERENTIAL DIAGNOSIS

The differential diagnosis of an adult with episodic wheezing, chest tightness, cough, and difficulty breathing includes the following:

- Chronic obstructive pulmonary disease—Usually begins after age 40 years with dyspnea (persistent or progressive or worse with exercise), chronic cough (even if intermittent or nonproductive) and/or sputum production, and/or a history of COPD risk factors including a family history of COPD (Chapter 56, Chronic Obstructive Pulmonary Disease).
- Chronic bronchitis—A clinical diagnosis defined as the presence of cough and sputum production of at least 3 months in 2 consecutive years[9]; although often seen in patients with COPD, chronic bronchitis can occur in patients with normal spirometry.
- Pneumonia—Symptoms include fever, chills, and pleuritic chest pain; physical findings include dullness to percussion, bronchial breathing, egophony (E-A change), and crackles with area of infiltrate or pneumonia usually confirmed on CXR (Chapter 59, Pneumonia).
- Tuberculosis—Any age, symptoms of chronic cough. CXR shows infiltrate, positive culture confirms (Chapter 64, Tuberculosis).
- Congestive heart failure—Nonspecific basilar crackles, CXR shows cardiomegaly, echocardiogram confirms (Chapter 44, Congestive Heart Failure).
- Cough secondary to drugs (eg, angiotensin-converting enzyme inhibitor), vocal cord dysfunction—identified on medication history or PFT.
- Asthma may occur in conjunction with these conditions.

MANAGEMENT

NAEP outlines 4 components of care: assessment and monitoring, provision of education, control of environmental factors and comorbid conditions, and use of medications.[3] The goals of asthma therapy are 2-fold[3]:

TABLE 55-2 Classification of Asthma Severity

	Intermittent	Mild Persistent	Moderate Persistent	Severe Persistent
Symptoms	2 or less days per week	More than 2 days per week	Daily	Throughout the day
Nighttime Awakenings	2 ×'s per month or less	3-4 ×'s per month	More than once per week but not nightly	Nightly
Rescue Inhaler Use	2 or less days per week	More than 2 days per week, but not daily	Daily	Several times per day
Interference With Normal Activity	None	Minor limitation	Some limitation	Extremely limited
Lung Function	FEV_1 >80% predicted and normal between exacerbations	FEV_1 >80% predicted	FEV_1 60%-80% predicted	FEV_1 less than 60% predicted

Data from National Heart, Lung and Blood Institute. Expert Panel Report 3: guidelines for the diagnosis and management of asthma.

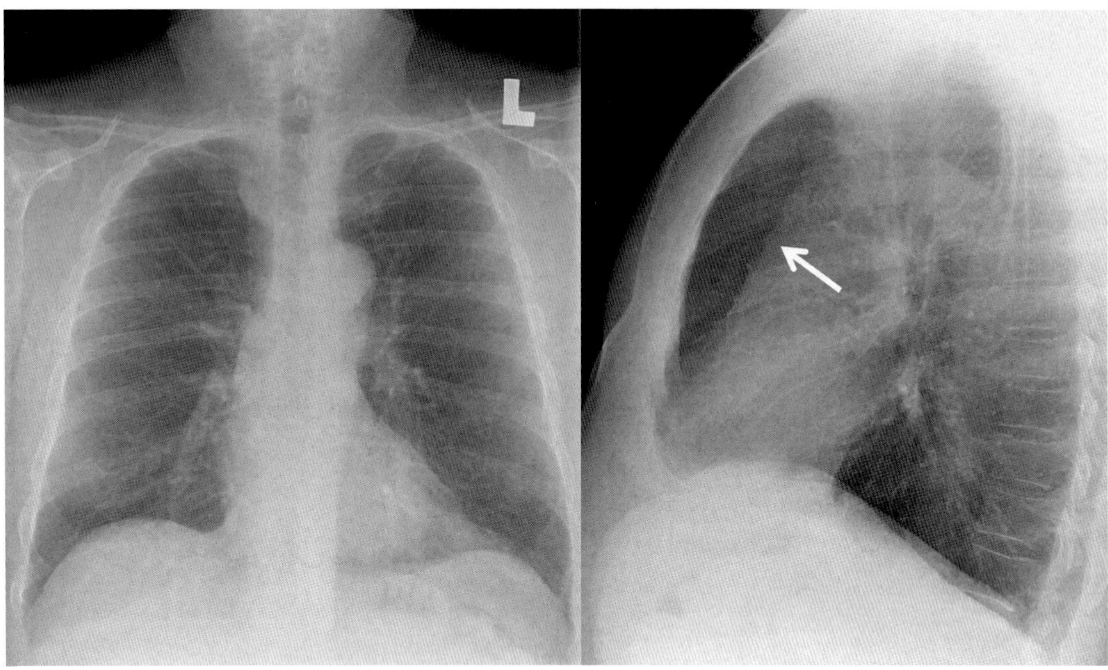

FIGURE 55-6 Acute asthma exacerbation with increased lung volumes on CXR. The lateral projection reveals enlargement of the retrosternal clear space (arrow). (*Reproduced with permission from Carlos Santiago Restrepo, MD.*)

- Reduce impairment—Prevent chronic symptoms, require infrequent (twice weekly or less) use of rescue inhaler, maintain near-normal pulmonary function, maintain normal activity levels, meet patient and family expectations and satisfaction with care.
- Reduce risk—Prevent recurrent exacerbations and minimize need for emergency or hospital care, prevent loss of lung function, and provide optimal pharmacotherapy while minimizing side effects and adverse effects.

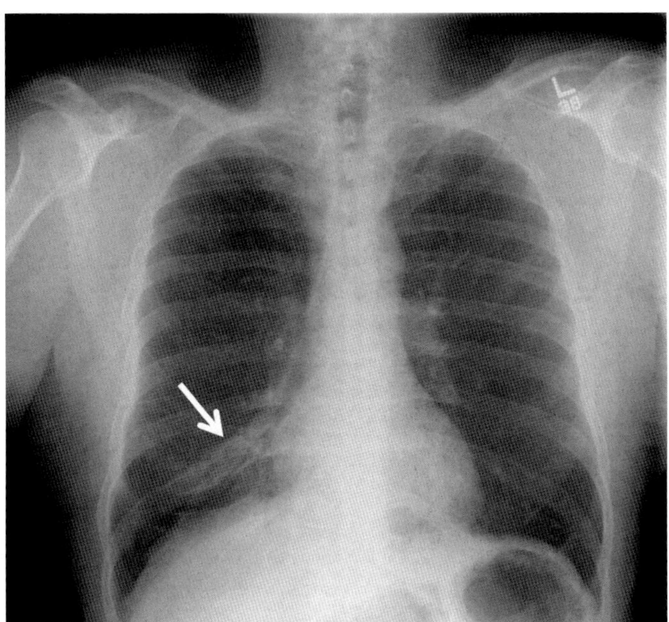

FIGURE 55-7 Acute asthma exacerbation in a 28-year-old man. Frontal chest radiograph demonstrates increased lung volumes and ill-defined opacity in the right infrahilar region consistent with middle lobe segmental atelectasis (arrow). (*Reproduced with permission from Carlos Santiago Restrepo, MD.*)

NONPHARMACOLOGIC

- Exercise should be encouraged. In a randomized clinical trial (RCT) of aerobic exercise in patients with persistent asthma, the group randomized to exercise showed significant improvements in physical limitations, frequency of symptoms, health-related quality of life, number of asthma-symptom-free days, and anxiety and depression levels over the control group (education and breathing exercises only).[10]
- For patients exposed to secondhand smoke in the home, use of high-efficiency, particulate-arresting (HEPA) air cleaners was shown in one RCT to decrease unscheduled asthma visits for children ages 6 to 12 years.[11]
- Dietary changes may also be useful. In a cross-sectional study, greater adherence to a Mediterranean-type diet was associated with a lower prevalence of asthma symptoms.[12]
- Provide patient education. SOR Ⓐ Reduction in hospital and emergency department (ED) visits and missed work or school has also been shown for self-management education with written asthma action plans and physician review.[4]
- Consider interventions to control home environmental triggers; comprehensive individual programs may reduce symptom days.[4] SOR Ⓑ
  - Many people who have asthma are allergic to dust mites (**Figure 55-8**). Two relatively easy interventions to decrease dust mite exposure are encase pillows and mattresses in special dust mite–proof covers and wash the sheets and blankets on the bed each week in hot water.[3]
  - Other suggestions for reducing environmental triggers can be found in the NAEP reference[3] at http://www.nhlbi.nih.gov/guidelines/asthma/asthsumm.pdf.

MEDICATIONS

To determine appropriate medication management, assess severity based on symptoms, medication usage, and lung function. In addition, assess risk based on number of exacerbations requiring systemic steroids.

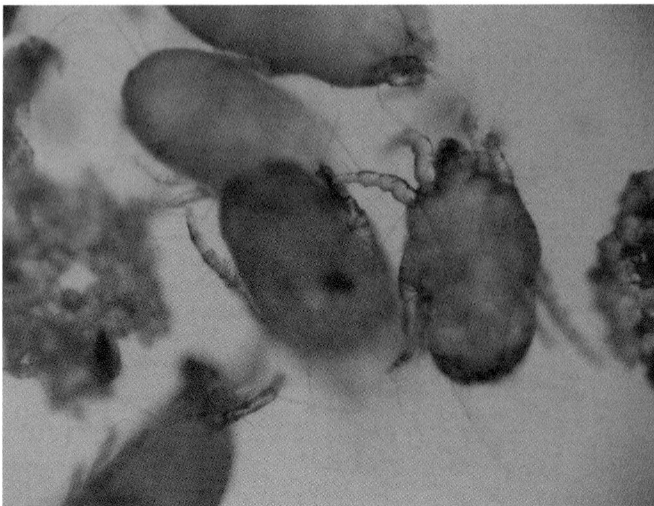

FIGURE 55-8 Dust mites under the microscope. Dust mites are a common allergen for patients who suffer from asthma and allergic rhinitis. Environmental control to minimize dust mite exposure can help control asthma for some individuals. (*Reproduced with permission from Richard P. Usatine, MD.*)

For youths (age 12 years and up) and adults, persistent asthma is divided into mild, moderate, or severe; these categories are matched to steps of medications described below. The NAEP 6 steps of care with respect to asthma medications are as below[3]:

- **Step 1:** For all aged patients with intermittent asthma, an inhaled SABA is recommended. SOR Ⓐ Metered-dose inhalers with spacers are at least as effective (with fewer side effects) as nebulized treatment for most patients.
- **Step 2:** Low-dose inhaled corticosteroids (ICS) are the preferred long-term control therapy for all ages with persistent asthma. SOR Ⓐ Alternatives include cromolyn inhaler, leukotriene receptor antagonist (LTRA), nedocromil, or theophylline. LTRAs are less effective than ICS but better than placebo.[3] SOR Ⓐ
- **Step 3:** Combination low-dose ICS and long-acting β_2-agonist (LABA) or medium-dose ICS are equally preferred options.[3] SOR Ⓐ Alternatives include low-dose ICS plus LTRA (less effective than ICS and LABA), theophylline, or zileuton. Theophylline requires monitoring serum concentration levels. Zileuton is less desirable due to limited supporting data and need to monitor liver function. Authors of a Cochrane review found the combination ICS-LABA modestly more effective in reducing the risk of exacerbations requiring oral corticosteroids than higher-dose ICS for adolescents and adults.[13]
- **Step 4:** Combination medium-dose ICS and LABA. Alternatives are combination medium-dose ICS plus LTRA, theophylline, or zileuton (see above).
- **Step 5:** Combination high-dose ICS and LABA.
- **Step 6:** Combination high-dose ICS and LABA plus oral corticosteroid.

Other drug options

- In a RCT, the addition of tiotropium bromide (a long-acting anticholinergic agent approved for the treatment of COPD but not asthma) to inhaled ICS was superior to doubling the ICS dose in improving lung function and symptoms and noninferior to the addition of a LABA to ICS (step 3).[14]
- Omalizumab should be considered for patients over 11 years of age who have allergies or for adults who require step 5 or 6 care (severe asthma).[3] In a RCT with inner-city children, adolescents, and young adults ($N = 419$) with persistent asthma, omalizumab reduced symptom days, and the proportion of subjects who had one or more exacerbations (30.3% vs 48.8% on placebo).[15]
- To assist with smoking cessation, consider nicotine replacement therapy (bupropion [150 mg, twice daily], varenicline [1 mg twice daily], nortriptyline [75-100 mg daily], or nicotine replacement [gum, inhaler, spray, patch]) and supportive counseling and follow-up; using these interventions improves rates of smoking cessation by up to 2-fold.[16-18] SOR Ⓐ (Chapter 237, Tobacco Addiction)
- In patients with persistent asthma attributed to allergies, consider allergy immunotherapy.[3] SOR Ⓑ One meta-analysis concluded that specific immunotherapy for patients with positive skin tests resulted in a reduction in need for increased medications (number needed to treat = 5) and another study in patients with high IgE found immunotherapy-reduced exacerbations.[4]
- The use of proton pump inhibitor therapy in adults with asthma is not likely to add significant benefit.[19]

For patients with an *exacerbation* of asthma (dyspnea with activity, PEF ≥70% predicted or personal best), SABAs and sometimes oral corticosteroids are used for home management of patients with a mild exacerbation, following their action plan. NAEP does not recommend doubling the dose of ICS for home management versus oral steroids for exacerbations.[3] A Cochrane review concluded that a short course of oral steroids was effective in reducing the number of relapses to additional care, hospitalizations, and use of SABA without an apparent increase in side effects.[20]

- Moderate exacerbation (dyspnea interferes with usual activity, PEF 40% to 69% predicted or personal best) usually requires an office or ED visit; SABA and oral corticosteroids (typically 40-60 mg prednisone for adults) are recommended for 3 to 10 days. SOR Ⓐ SABA can be administered every 20 minutes as needed and the addition of inhaled ipratropium bromide may reduce the need for hospitalization (0.68-0.75).[4] SOR Ⓐ Symptoms usually abate in 1 to 2 days.
- Severe exacerbation (dyspnea at rest, PEF <40% predicted or personal best) usually requires an ED visit and/or hospitalization; consider combination SABA and anticholinergic nebulized treatment hourly or continuously as needed, oral corticosteroids, and adjunctive treatment as needed (see below). Symptoms last for longer than 3 days after treatment begins.
- Life-threatening exacerbation (too dyspneic to speak, diaphoresis, PEF <25% predicted or personal best) requires an ED visit and likely hospitalization; consider intensive care unit, SABA or anticholinergic, intravenous corticosteroids, and adjunctive therapies.
- Oxygen therapy—Use to correct hypoxia in patients with moderate-to-life-threatening exacerbations; maintain O_2 saturation above 90%.[3,4] SOR Ⓒ
- Consider intravenous magnesium sulfate or heliox-driven albuterol nebulization if severe exacerbation and unresponsive to treatment after initial assessments.
- Monitor response to treatment with serial assessments of FEV_1 or PEF. Pulse oximetry may be useful for severe episodes or when unable to perform lung function testing; repeat assessments for hypoxia are useful for predicting need for hospitalization as are signs and symptoms at 1 hour posttreatment.
- Patients with severe or life-threatening exacerbation unresponsive to initial treatments may require intubation and mechanical ventilation. Drowsiness may be a symptom of impending respiratory failure.

- The following should not be used as they have no supporting evidence and may delay effective treatment: drinking large volumes of liquids; breathing warm, moist air; using nonprescription products, such as antihistamines or cold remedies, and pursed-lip and other forms of breathing.[3] In addition, NAEP does not recommend use of methylxanthines, antibiotics (except as needed for comorbid conditions), aggressive hydration, chest physical therapy, mucolytics, or sedation in the ED or hospital setting.[3]

REFERRAL

- Consider referral to an asthma specialist if signs and symptoms are atypical, there are problems in assessing other diagnoses, or if additional specialized testing is needed.
- Referral or consultation should also be considered if there are difficulties achieving or maintaining control of asthma, if the patient required greater than 2 bursts of oral systemic corticosteroids in 1 year or has an exacerbation requiring hospitalization, or if immunotherapy or omalizumab is considered.[3]
- Consultation with an asthma specialist should be conducted for patients with persistent asthma requiring step 4 care or higher and considered if a patient requires step 3 care.[3]

PREVENTION AND SCREENING

- Smoking cessation and avoidance of secondhand smoking, limiting occupational exposures and exposure to indoor air pollution may be preventive.
- Influenza and pneumococcal vaccination are recommended.[3] SOR Ⓑ
- Despite limited data, vitamins A, D, and E; zinc; fruits and vegetables; and a Mediterranean diet may be useful for the prevention of asthma.[21] In addition, cow's raw milk consumption appears protective (adjusted OR, 0.59; 95% CI, 0.46-0.74).[22]

PROGNOSIS

- More than half of children with asthma will no longer have symptoms by age 6 years.[4]
- In a meta-analysis, maternal asthma was associated with an increased risk of low birth weight (relative risk [RR], 1.46; 95% CI 1.22-1.75), small for gestational age (RR, 1.22; 95% CI 1.14-1.31), preterm delivery (RR, 1.41; 95% CI 1.22-1.61), and preeclampsia (RR, 1.54; 95% CI 1.32-1.81).[23] The RR of preterm delivery and preterm labor became nonsignificant by active asthma management. Pregnancy does not appear to increase asthma severity, provided women continue to use their prescribed medications.[24]
- For patients with an asthma exacerbation, the following factors place a patient at higher risk of asthma-related death; these patients should be advised to seek medical care early during an exacerbation[3]:
  - Previous severe exacerbation (eg, intubation or intensive care unit [ICU] admission for asthma)
  - Two or more hospitalizations or more than 3 ED visits in the past year
  - Use of more than 2 canisters of SABA per month
  - Difficulty perceiving airway obstruction or the severity of worsening asthma
  - Low socioeconomic status or inner-city resident

FOLLOW-UP

Many patients have asthma that is not well controlled. One of the new aspects of the NAEP 2007 guideline is the focus on monitoring asthma severity and control, the latter defined as the degree to which manifestations of asthma are minimized by therapeutic interventions and the therapy goals are met.

- At each visit ask about frequency and intensity of symptoms and functional limitations currently or recently experienced (impairment). A self-assessment sheet for follow-up visits is available in the NAEP document and a simple symptom checklist can be downloaded from http://www.qvar.com/asthma/asthma-symptoms-checklist.aspx (accessed June 2013). Severity can be measured by the step of care required to maintain control.[3] SOR Ⓒ
- In addition, at each visit, assess the likelihood of either asthma exacerbations, progressive decline in lung function, and risk of medication adverse effects. A patient's self-assessment sheet rating asthma control (eg, symptoms, PEF) and medication use is available in the NAEP reference.[3] Provision of a visually standardized, interpreted peak flow graph to assist in understanding when to add medication or contact a health provider may reduce need for oral steroids and urgent care visits.[25]
- For patients on medications, monitor treatment effectiveness ("have you noticed a difference, for example less breathlessness") and side effects. Observe inhaler technique at least once to ensure optimal delivery.
- For smokers, encourage cessation.
- Document exacerbations or hospitalizations—This may indicate a need for additional treatment.
- Monitor for comorbidities (eg, heart disease, chronic lung disease) and maximize control of those conditions.
- Measurement of fractional nitric oxide (NO) concentration in exhaled breath (FeNO) is a quantitative, noninvasive method of measuring airway inflammation.[26] It is under investigation as a complementary tool to other ways of assessing airways disease, including asthma.

PATIENT EDUCATION

- Smoking cessation should be strongly and repeatedly encouraged. Exercise should also be encouraged along with weight loss, if obese, or maintenance of a healthy weight.
- The NAEP suggests that key educational messages include basic facts about asthma, the role of medications (ie, rescue or short term vs control or long term), and patient skills (eg, correct inhaler technique, self-monitoring).
- Creation of an asthma action plan can be helpful in promoting self-management and greater understanding of warning signs of worsening asthma. An example of an action plan can be found in the NAEP document.[3] Asthma action plans usually use 3 zones, similar to traffic lights, with green zone representing good control (eg, few symptoms, PEF 80%-100%), yellow zone representing worsening or not well-controlled asthma (eg, mild-to-moderate symptoms, PEF 50%-80%), and red zone representing an alert or warning (severe symptoms, PEF <50%) with advice to seek emergency care if not better after 15 minutes of rescue medication use and unable to reach their care

provider. Each zone contains instructions for management which the primary care provider can modify.

PATIENT RESOURCES

- American Lung Association. *Asthma*—**http://www.lung.org/lung-disease/asthma/.**
- MedlinePlus. *Asthma*—**http://www.nlm.nih.gov/medlineplus/asthma.html.**

PROVIDER RESOURCES

- National Asthma Education and Prevention Program. *Guidelines for the Diagnosis and Management of Asthma*—**http://www.nhlbi.nih.gov/guidelines/asthma/asthsumm.pdf.**
- Centers for Disease Control and Prevention. *Asthma*—**http://www.cdc.gov/nchs/fastats/asthma.htm.**

REFERENCES

1. Centers for Disease Control and Prevention. *Asthma FastStats.* http://www.cdc.gov/nchs/fastats/asthma.htm. Accessed June 2013.
2. Centers for Disease Control and Prevention. *Asthma in the US.* http://www.cdc.gov/VitalSigns/Asthma/index.html. Accessed June 2013.
3. *National Asthma Education and Prevention Program Expert Panel Report 3 (2007).* http://www.nhlbi.nih.gov/guidelines/asthma/asthsumm.pdf. Accessed June 2013.
4. Roett MA, Gillespie C. Asthma. In: Sloane PD, Slatt LM, Ebell MH, Smith MA, Power D, Viera AJ, eds. *Essential of Family Medicine.* Philadelphia, PA: Lippincott Williams & Wilkins; 2011:607-623.
5. Arshad SH, Kurukulaaratchy RJ, Fenn M, Matthews S. Early life risk factors for current wheeze, asthma, and bronchial hyperresponsiveness at 10 years of age. *Chest.* 2005;127(2):502-508.
6. Beasley RW, Clayton TO, Crane J, et al. Acetaminophen use and risk of asthma, rhinoconjunctivitis, and eczema in adolescents: International Study of Asthma and Allergies in Childhood Phase Three. *Am J Respir Crit Care Med.* 2011;183(2):171-178.
7. Holgate ST. The acetaminophen enigma in asthma. *Am J Respir Crit Care Med.* 2011;183(2):147-151.
8. Spergel JM. From atopic dermatitis to asthma. *Ann Allergy Asthma Immunol.* 2010;105(2):99-106.
9. Global Initiative for Chronic Obstructive Lung Disease (GOLD). *Global Strategy for the Diagnosis, Management and Prevention of COPD, 2011.* http://www.goldcopd.org/. Accessed June 2013.
10. Mendes FA, Goncalves RC, Nunes MP, et al. Effects of aerobic training on psychosocial morbidity and symptoms in patients with asthma: a randomized clinical trial. *Chest.* 2010;138(2):331-337.
11. Lanphear BP, Hornung RW, Khoury J, et al. Effects of HEPA air cleaners on unscheduled asthma visits and asthma symptoms for children exposed to secondhand tobacco smoke. *Pediatrics.* 2011;127(1):93-101.
12. Arvaniti F, Priftis KN, Papadimitriou A, et al. Adherence to the Mediterranean type of diet is associated with lower prevalence of asthma symptoms, among 10-12 years old children: the PANACEA study. *Pediatr Allergy Immunol.* 2011;22(3):283-289.
13. Ducharme FM, Ni Chroinin M, Greenstone I, Lasserson TJ. Addition of long-acting beta2-agonists to inhaled steroids versus higher dose inhaled steroids in adults and children with persistent asthma. *Cochrane Database Syst Rev.* 2010;(4):CD005533.
14. Peters SP, Kunselman SJ, Icitovic N, et al. Tiotropium bromide step-up therapy for adults with uncontrolled asthma. *N Engl J Med.* 2010;363(18):1715-1726.
15. Busse WW, Morgan WJ, Gergen PJ, et al. Randomized trial of omalizumab (anti-IgE) for asthma in inner-city children. *N Engl J Med.* 2011;364(11):1005-1015.
16. Hughes JR, Stead LF, Lancaster T. Antidepressants for smoking cessation. *Cochrane Database Syst Rev.* 2007;(1):CD000031.
17. Stead LF, Perera R, Bullen C, Mant D, Lancaster T. Nicotine replacement therapy for smoking cessation. *Cochrane Database Syst Rev.* 2008;(1):CD000146.
18. Stead LF, Bergson G, Lancaster T. Physician advice for smoking cessation. *Cochrane Database Syst Rev.* 2008;(2):CD000165.
19. Chan WW, Chiou E, Obstein KL, et al. The efficacy of proton pump inhibitors for the treatment of asthma in adults: a meta-analysis. *Ann Intern Med.* 2011;171(7):620-629.
20. Rowe BH, Spooner CH, Ducharme FM, et al. Corticosteroids for preventing relapse following acute exacerbations of asthma. *Cochrane Database Syst Rev.* 2007;(3):CD000195.
21. Nurmatov U, Devereux G, Sheikh A. Nutrients and foods for the primary prevention of asthma and allergy: systematic review and meta-analysis. *J Allergy Clin Immunol.* 2011;127(3):724-733.e1-30.
22. Loss G, Apprich S, Waser M, et al. The protective effect of farm milk consumption on childhood asthma and atopy: the GABRIELA study. *J Allergy Clin Immunol.* 2011;128(4):766-773.e4.
23. Murphy VE, Namazy JA, Powell H, et al. A meta-analysis of adverse perinatal outcomes in women with asthma. *BJOG.* 2011;118(11):1314-1323.
24. Belanger K, Hellenbrand ME, Holford TR, Bracken M. Effect of pregnancy on maternal asthma symptoms and medication use. *Obstet Gynecol.* 2010;115(3):559-567.
25. Janson SL, McGrath KW, Covington JK, et al. Objective airway monitoring improves asthma control in the cold and flu season: a cluster randomized trial. *Chest.* 2010;138(5):1148-1155.
26. Dweik RA, Boggs PB, Erzurum SC, et al. An official ATS clinical practice guideline: interpretation of exhaled nitric oxide levels (FENO) for clinical applications. *Am J Respir Crit Care Med.* 2011;184(5):602-615.

56 CHRONIC OBSTRUCTIVE PULMONARY DISEASE

Mindy A. Smith, MD, MS

PATIENT STORY

A 74-year-old woman and longtime smoker presents with fatigue and shortness of breath. She has not seen a physician for many years and says she has been basically healthy. On physical examination, she is found to be pale, mildly cachectic, and her lips are cyanotic. Her breath sounds are distant, although crackles can be heard in both lung bases. Her heart sounds are best heard in the epigastrium; a third heart sound is present. She has mild peripheral edema. Her resting pulse oximetry is 74%. Her chest X-ray (CXR) shows emphysema (**Figure 56-1**) and her echocardiogram confirms heart failure.

INTRODUCTION

Chronic obstructive pulmonary disease (COPD) is defined as a disease state characterized by airflow limitation that is usually progressive and associated with an abnormal inflammatory response of the lung to noxious particles or gases.[1] COPD is preventable and treatable. Some patients have significant extrapulmonary effects (particularly cardiac) that may contribute to disease severity. Worldwide, tobacco smoke is the primary cause of COPD (**Figure 56-2**).

SYNONYMS

COPD is also known as emphysema (technically refers to destruction of the alveoli).

EPIDEMIOLOGY

- Estimated prevalence of COPD in adults older than age 18 years in the United States (2008) is about 13.2 million cases, or 4% of the population (95% confidence interval [CI], 3.8-4.1).[2]
- It is the fourth leading cause of death both in the United States and worldwide. Mortality rates have declined for men from 1999 to 2006 (57 per 100,000 to 46.4 per 100,000) and remained fairly stable for women (35.3 per 100,000 to 34.2 per 100,000).[3]
- In a study in Latin America, prevalence rates ranged from 7.8% to 19.7% of the population;[4] a prevalence of between 3% and 11% has been reported in never-smokers.[1] This high rate among never-smokers is most likely related to indoor cooking with open wood fires.
- In a Swedish study of COPD (birth cohorts from 1919-1950), the 10-year cumulative incidence rate of COPD was 13.5% using Global Initiative for Chronic Obstructive Lung Disease (GOLD) criteria (**Table 56-1**) based on 1109 patients with baseline respiratory symptoms (76.6% of the original symptomatic cohort and 16.7% of the total cohort).[5]
- Estimated direct costs associated with COPD in the United States are more than $29 billion with additional indirect costs of $20.4 billion.[1]

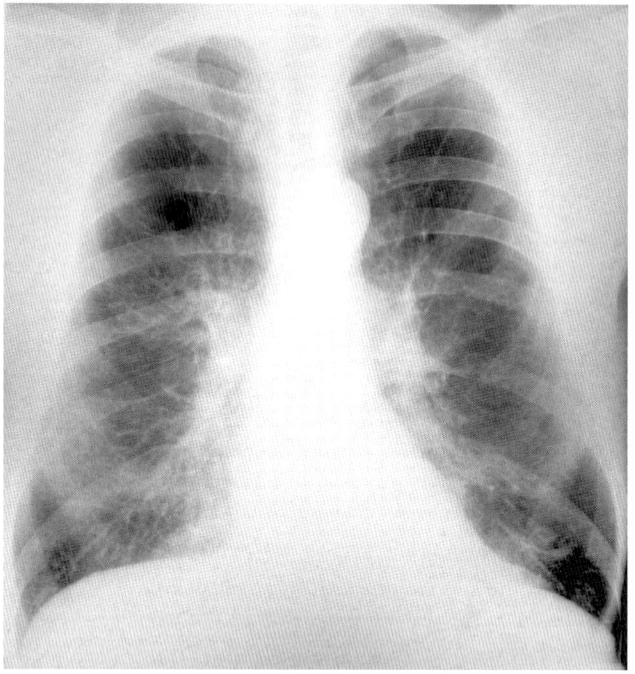

FIGURE 56-1 Emphysema with mild hyperinflation and increased interstitial markings. (*Reproducd with permission from Miller WT Jr. Diagnostic Thoracic Imaging. New York, NY: McGraw-Hill; 2006:106, Figure 3-37 A. Copyright 2006.*)

ETIOLOGY AND PATHOPHYSIOLOGY

- Mediated by chronic inflammatory responses to environmental factors, especially cigarette smoke, that results in recruitment of inflammatory cells in terminal airspaces and release of elastolytic proteases that damage the extracellular lung matrix and cause ineffective repair of elastin and other matrix components.
- Oxidative stress may be an important amplifying mechanism in COPD development and exacerbations.1 In addition, there appears to be an imbalance between proteases and antiproteases in the lungs of patients with COPD.

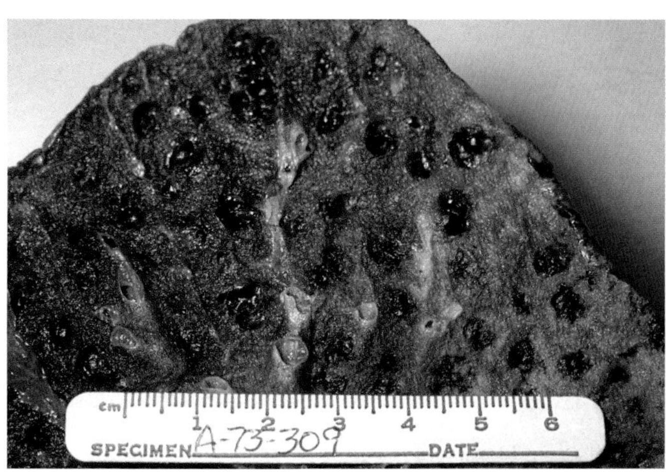

FIGURE 56-2 Gross pathology of lung showing centrilobular emphysema caused by tobacco smoking. Close-up of cut surface shows multiple cavities lined by heavy black carbon deposits. (*Reproduced with permission from Centers for Disease Control and Prevention [CDC] and Dr. Edwin P. Ewing, Jr.*)

TABLE 56-1 COPD Severity—GOLD Grade

Grade	FEV_1/FVC	FEV_1
Mild COPD (GOLD 1)	<0.7	≥80% predicted
Moderate COPD (GOLD 2)	<0.7	<80% but ≥50% predicted
Severe COPD (GOLD 3)	<0.7	<50% but ≥30% predicted
Very severe COPD (GOLD 4)	<0.7	<30% predicted or FEV_1 <50% with respiratory failure or right-sided heart failure

FEV_1, forced expiratory volume in 1 second; FVC, forced vital capacity.

- The inflammatory process leads to obstruction and later fibrosis of small airways and the destruction of lung parenchyma. Circulating inflammatory mediators may contribute to muscle wasting and cachexia and worsen comorbidities such as heart failure and diabetes.[1]
- Gas exchange abnormalities result in hypoxemia and hypercapnia.
- Pulmonary hypertension may occur as a result of hypoxic vasoconstriction of small pulmonary arteries.
- Genetic mutations (eg, α_1-antitrypsin deficiency [1%-2% of cases; affects 1 in 2000-5000 individuals]) are present in some patients. Suspect a genetic mutation when emphysema is found in a patient of age 45 to 50 years or younger, a positive family history of COPD, primarily basilar disease, or a minimal smoking history.[6] Single-nucleotide polymorphisms at 3 loci—TNS1, GSTCD, and HTR4—are associated with COPD, as is genetic variation in the transcription factor SOX5.[7,8]

RISK FACTORS

- Smoking (direct and passive)—COPD relative risk (RR) for ever smoking is 2.89 (95% CI, 2.63-3.17) and RR for current smoking is 3.51 (95% CI, 3.08-3.99).[9]
- Airway hypersensitivity (15% of the population attributable risk).[1]
- Occupational exposures (eg, gold and coal mining, cotton textile dust).1,2,6 The estimated fraction of COPD symptoms or functional impairment attributed to these exposures is 10% to 20%.[1]
- Indoor air pollution from burning wood and other biomass fuels, particularly with open fires, poorly functioning stoves, and poorly ventilated dwellings.[1]
- Reduced maximal attained lung function (eg, preterm vs full-term infants).[1]
- Infections (eg, early childhood infection, chronic bronchitis, HIV, tuberculosis).[1]
- Poverty.
- Parental history of COPD (odds ratio [OR] 1.73).[10]
- α_1-Antitrypsine deficiency (genetic disorder).

DIAGNOSIS

A diagnosis of COPD should be considered in a patient older than age 40 years with dyspnea (persistent or progressive or worse with exercise), chronic cough (even if intermittent or nonproductive) and/or sputum production, and/or a history of COPD risk factors including a family history of COPD.[1]

CLINICAL FEATURES

- COPD's 3 most common symptoms are cough, sputum production, and exertional dyspnea. In one study of newly diagnosed patients, most presented with cough (85%) and exertional dyspnea (70%); almost half (45%) reported increased sputum production.[11] Most patients were classified in GOLD stage 0 to 1 (42%) or 2 (46%) (see **Table 56-1**).
- Patients may also report chest tightness, often following exertion; fatigue, weight loss, and anorexia are symptoms later in the disease.
- Several validated questionnaires are available to assess symptoms in patients with COPD; GOLD recommends the Modified British Medical Research Council (MMRC) questionnaire (**Box 56-1**) or the 8-question COPD Assessment Test (CAT; http://catestonline.org).[1]
- Physical findings may include the following:
  - Tobacco odor and nicotine staining of fingernails
  - Increased expiratory phase or expiratory wheezing
  - Signs of hyperinflation—Barrel chest, poor diaphragmatic excursion
  - Use of accessory muscles of respiration—Intercostals, sternocleidomastoid, and scalene muscles
  - Late in illness—Cyanosis of the lips and nail beds, wasting, and cor pulmonale (right-sided heart failure—signs include increased jugular venous distention, right ventricular heave, third heart sound, ascites, and peripheral edema).

LABORATORY TESTING

Postbronchodilator spirometry secures the diagnosis and provides the severity classification[1,12]: SOR B

- At risk—Chronic cough and sputum production with normal spirometry

BOX 56-1 MMRC* Dyspnea Scale

0—Not troubled with breathlessness except with strenuous exercise.

1—Troubled by shortness of breath when hurrying on the level or walking up a slight hill.

2—Walks slower than people of the same age on the level because of breathlessness or has to stop for breath when walking at own pace on the level.

3—Stops for breath after walking about 100 yd or after a few minutes on the level.

4—Too breathless to leave the house or breathless when dressing or undressing.

*Modified British Medical Research Council

Additional tests that may be useful in management are sputum culture (in acute exacerbations to assist in confirming pneumonia), complete blood count (to identify anemia or polycythemia), and blood gases (confirms hypoxia when peripheral oxygen saturation is <92% or respiratory failure [P_{CO_2} >45]).[1,13]

- A serum level of α_1-antitrypsin should be measured if you suspect a genetic mutation (young age at presentation [≤45 years], lower lobe emphysema, family history, minimal smoking history).
- Exercise (walking) tests to assess disability or response to rehabilitation.[1]

IMAGING

A CXR is not useful for diagnosis but is helpful for excluding other diseases or identifying comorbidity (eg, heart failure). Findings on CXR include the following[3]:

- Hyperinflation is manifested by the following (**Figures 56-1 to 56-3**):
  - Increased anteroposterior (AP) diameter. (**Figure 56-4**).
  - Increased retrosternal air space.
  - Infracardiac air.
  - Low-set flattened diaphragms (best assessed in lateral chest).
  - Vertical heart.
  - Bullae are difficult to recognize in CXR but are easily seen on computed tomography (CT) (**Figures 56-5 to 56-8**).
  - Paucity of vascular markings in periphery (see **Figure 56-3**).
  - Pulmonary hypertension (CXR shows enlarged central pulmonary arteries).
- α_1-Antitrypsine deficiency leads to early COPD even in nonsmokers. See **Figure 56-9** for advanced pulmonary emphysema in a 30-year-old woman with α_1-antitrypsine deficiency. The CXR shows increased lung volumes, flattening of the diaphragms, and a vertical heart. A CT may show extensive panlobular emphysema of the mid and lower lung zones (**Figure 56-10**). The vascular markings are prominent in the upper lobes, demonstrating "cephalization" of flow.

A chest CT scan is the current definitive test for emphysema, but the findings do not influence treatment.[6] Cystic and bullous lesions are

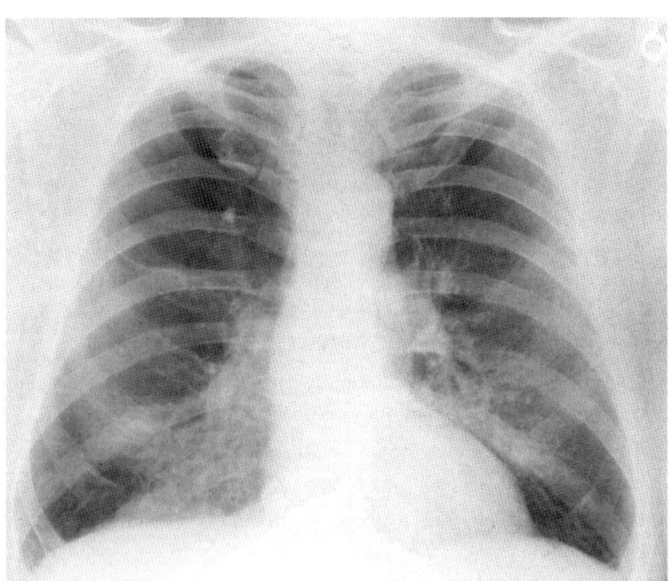

FIGURE 56-3 Posteroanterior (PA) radiograph showing flattened hemidiaphragms and decreased vascular markings from hyperinflation as a result of air trapping in a patient with COPD. (*Reproduced with permission from Miller WT Jr.* Diagnostic Thoracic Imaging. *New York, NY: McGraw-Hill; 2006:108, Figure 3-40 A. Copyright 2006.*)

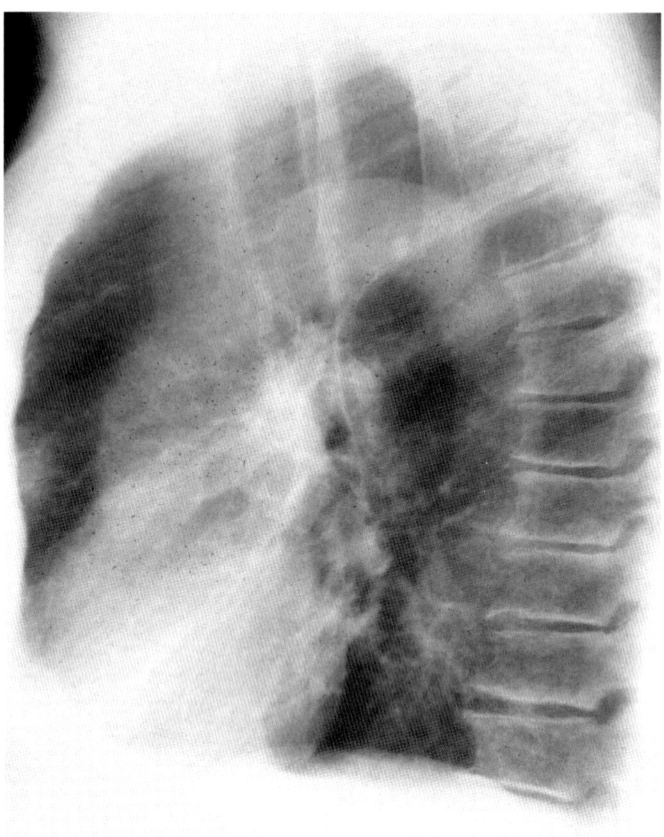

FIGURE 56-4 Lateral view in the patient in Figure 56-3 showing increased anteroposterior (AP) diameter from hyperinflation as a result of air trapping in a patient with COPD. (*Reproduced with permission from Miller WT Jr.* Diagnostic Thoracic Imaging. *New York, NY: McGraw-Hill; 2006:108, Figure 3-40 B. Copyright 2006.*)

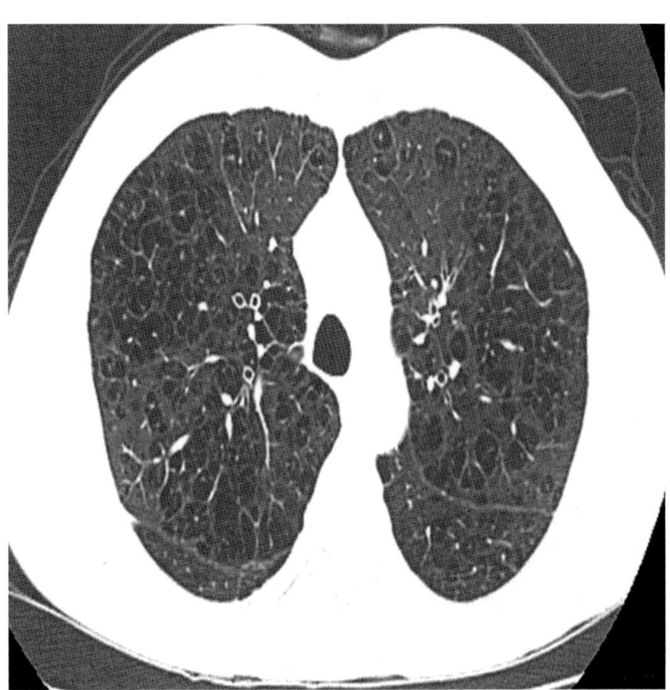

FIGURE 56-5 Centrilobular emphysema seen on high resolution CT of the chest. Diffuse emphysematous changes throughout both lungs are seen as darker round areas of cyst-like lesions. (*Reproduced with permission from Carlos S. Restrepo, MD.*)

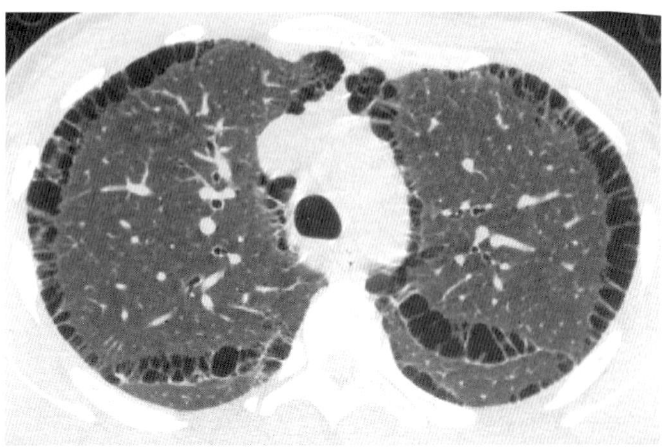

FIGURE 56-6 CT at the level of the aortic arch showing a pattern of cysts in the subpleural lung with an upper lung zone predominance characteristic of mild paraseptal emphysema. (*Reproduced with permission from Miller WT Jr. Diagnostic Thoracic Imaging. New York, NY: McGraw-Hill; 2006:110, Figure 3-41 D. Copyright 2006.*)

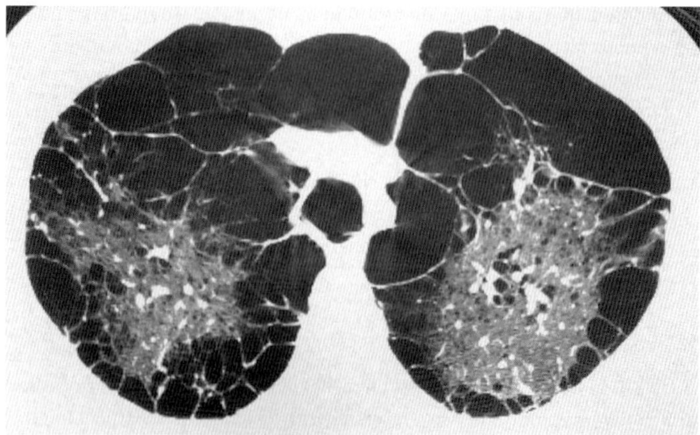

FIGURE 56-8 CT scan of the patient in **Figure 56-7** (at the level of the pulmonary veins) showing multiple large peripheral bullae; the patient was diagnosed with severe paraseptal emphysema. (*Reproduced with permission from Miller WT Jr. Diagnostic Thoracic Imaging. New York, NY: McGraw-Hill; 2006:111, Figure 3-42. Copyright 2006.*)

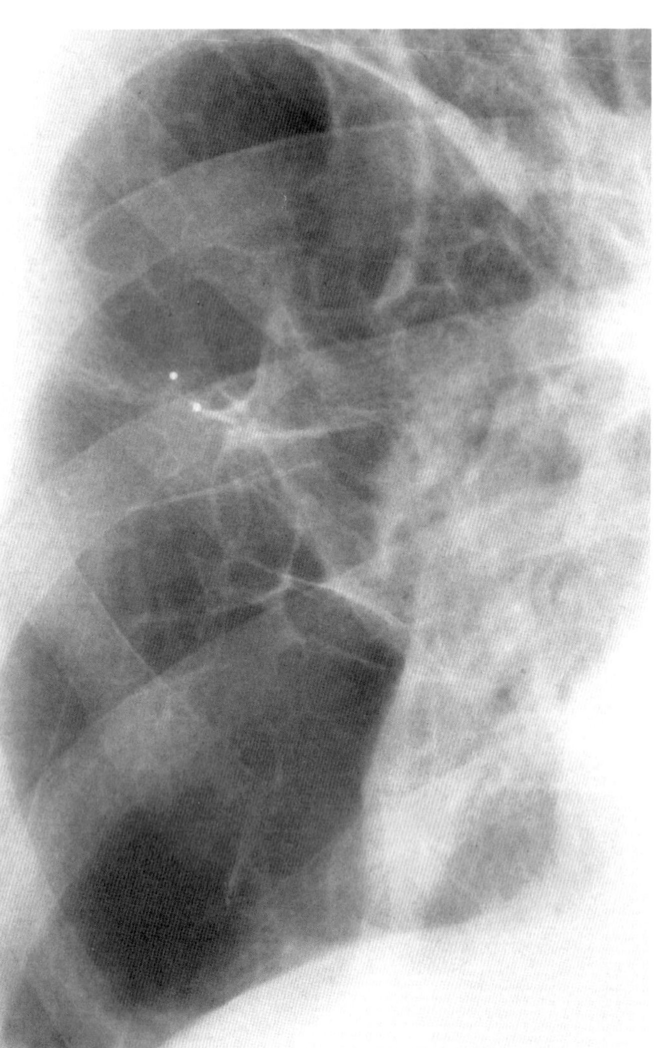

FIGURE 56-7 Close-up of CXR showing multiple large bullae in a patient with COPD. (*Reproduced with permission from Miller WT Jr. Diagnostic Thoracic Imaging. New York, NY: McGraw-Hill; 2006:111, Figure 3-42. Copyright 2006.*)

better delineated with CT scan (see **Figures 56-5, 56-6**, and **56-8**), and collapsing airways with inspiration and expiration can also be demonstrated with CT. Chest CT is recommended if surgery is contemplated.[1]

Echocardiography is suggested if features of cor pulmonale are present.[13]

DIFFERENTIAL DIAGNOSIS

The differential diagnosis of an individual with persistent productive cough and dyspnea includes the following:

- Asthma—Begins before age 40 years in most (often in childhood), usually episodic and characterized by increased responsiveness to stimuli (eg, allergens, occupational exposures). Nocturnal awakenings with symptoms are common. This condition is reversible with bronchodilators (see Chapter 55, Asthma).
- Chronic bronchitis—A clinical diagnosis defined as the presence of cough and sputum production of at least 3 months in 2 consecutive years;[1] although often seen in patients with COPD and associated with development and/or acceleration of fixed airflow limitation, chronic bronchitis can occur in patients with normal spirometry.
- Pneumonia—Symptoms include fever, chills, and pleuritic chest pain; physical findings include dullness to percussion, bronchial breathing, egophony (E-A change), and crackles with area of infiltrate, or pneumonia usually confirmed on CXR (see Chapter 59, Pneumonia).
- Tuberculosis—Any age; symptoms of chronic cough. CXR shows infiltrate; positive culture confirms (see Chapter 64, Tuberculosis).
- Congestive heart failure—Nonspecific basilar crackles; CXR shows cardiomegaly; echocardiogram confirms (see Chapter 44, Heart Failure).
- Lung cancer—Symptoms may occur with central or endobronchial growth of the tumor (eg, cough, hemoptysis, wheeze, stridor, dyspnea), collapse of airways from tumor obstruction (eg, postobstructive pneumonitis), involvement of the pleura or chest wall (eg, pleuritic chest pain), or from regional spread of the tumor (eg, dysphagia, hoarseness from recurrent laryngeal nerve paralysis, dyspnea, and elevated hemidiaphragm from phrenic nerve paralysis). Findings on CXR

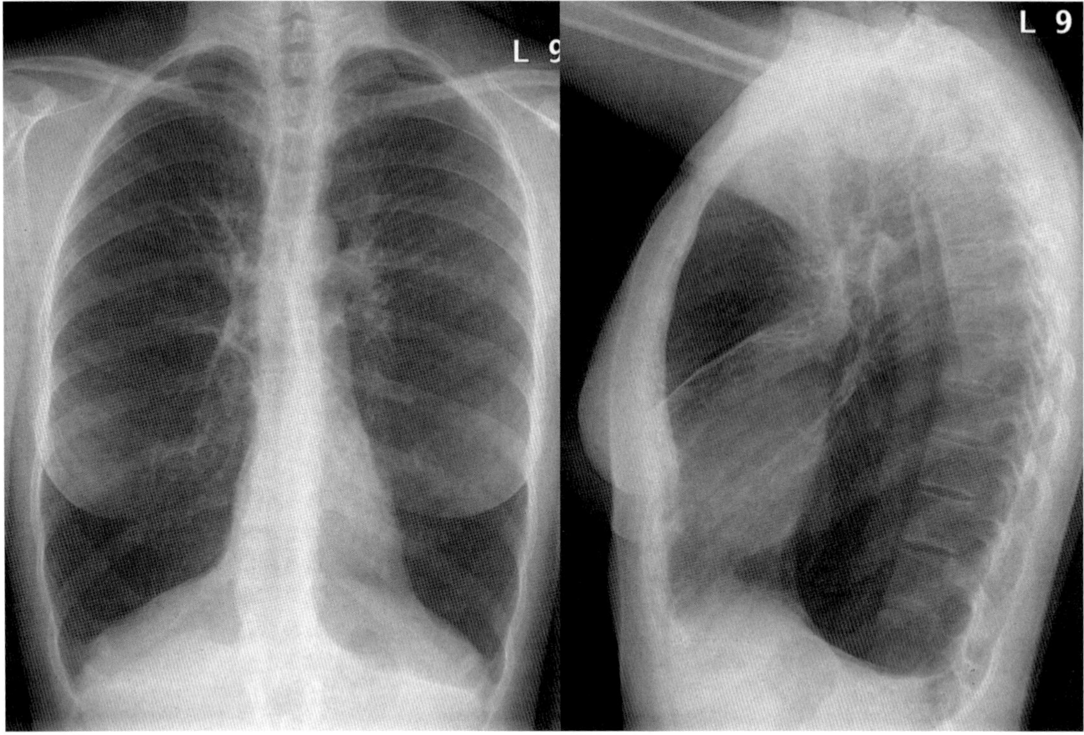

FIGURE 56-9 Advanced pulmonary emphysema in a 30-year-old woman with α_1-antitrypsine deficiency. The CXR shows increased lung volumes, flattening of the diaphragms, and a vertical heart. (*Reproduced with permission from Carlos S. Restrepo, MD.*)

or chest CT may be focal or unilateral and tissue confirms diagnosis (see Chapter 57, Lung Cancer).

Any of these processes or illnesses may occur in conjunction with emphysema.

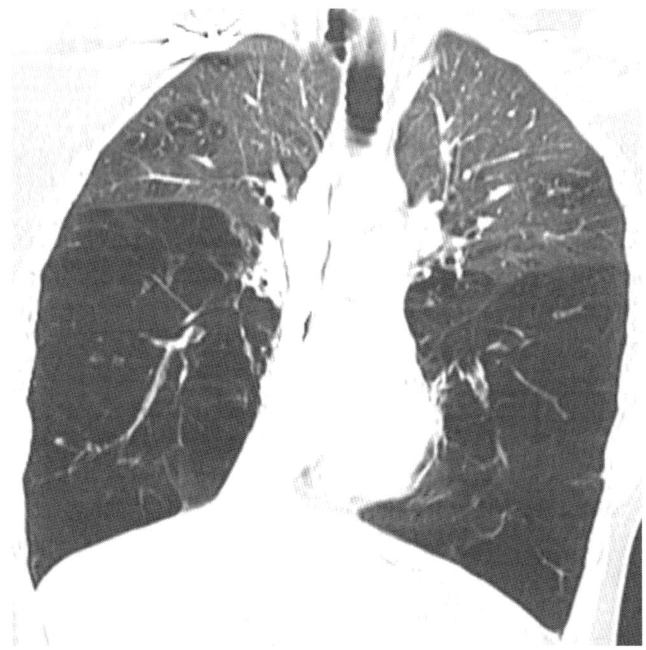

FIGURE 56-10 CT of the chest in the same 30-year-old woman with α_1-antitrypsine deficiency. Coronal reformation of the CT demonstrates extensive panlobular emphysema of the mid and lower lung zones, which is a typical distribution of this condition. The vascular markings are more prominent in the upper lobes showing "cephalization" of flow. (*Reproduced with permission from Carlos S. Restrepo, MD.*)

MANAGEMENT

Management of COPD is based on symptoms, risk or history of exacerbations, and severity or predicted survival. GOLD places patients into 4 categories as shown in **Table 56-2.**

NONPHARMACOLOGIC

Following are the nonpharmacologic therapies that should be considered for all patients[1,5]:

- Influenza and pneumococcal vaccination, which are most effective in the elderly. SOR B Also consider vaccination against herpes zoster as patients with COPD are at increased risk (adjusted hazard ratio [HR] 1.68, 95% CI, 1.45-1.95), especially if using inhaled steroids (adjusted HR 2.09, 95% CI, 1.38-3.16) or oral steroids (adjusted HR 3.00, 95% CI, 2.40-3.75).[14]
- Patient education (multidisciplinary and self-management training) improves patient outcomes and reduces costs and hospitalizations.[1,15] SOR A
- Pulmonary rehabilitation programs decrease hospitalization at 6 to 12 months, increase quality of life, and improve dyspnea and exercise capacity.[1,5] SOR A Pulmonary rehabilitation may increase survival and improve recovery following hospitalization.[1] SOR B
- There are no clear benefits of continuous positive pressure ventilation in patients with COPD unless they have coexisting sleep apnea, in which case there is an associated improvement in survival and decrease in risk of hospitalization.[1]

For patients with an *acute exacerbation* of COPD (defined as an increase in symptoms and change in the amount and character of the sputum and anticipated to occur about 1 to 3 times a year in patients with moderate

TABLE 56-2 Recommended Management of COPD Based on GOLD Grade and Exacerbation History

Patient Group	Description	Nonpharmacologic Treatment	(First Choice) Medications
A	Few symptoms (MMRC grade 0-1 or CAT score <10) and 0-1 exacerbations per year, and/or mild impairment (GOLD 1 or 2)*	Smoking cessation, physical activity, vaccinations	Short-acting bronchodilator (anticholinergic *or* β_2-agonist as needed)
B	More symptoms (MMRC ≥2 or CAT score ≥10) and 0-1 exacerbations per year; and/or mild impairment (GOLD 1 or 2)*	Smoking cessation, physical activity, vaccinations, pulmonary rehabilitation	Long-acting bronchodilator (anticholinergic or *or* β_2-agonist)
C	Few symptoms (MMRC grade 0-1 or CAT score <10) and ≥2 exacerbations per year, and/or severe impairment (GOLD 3 or 4)*	Smoking cessation, physical activity, vaccinations, pulmonary rehabilitation	Inhaled corticosteroid *and* long-acting bronchodilator (β_2-agonist *or* anticholinergic)
D	More symptoms (MMRC ≥2 or CAT score ≥10) and ≥2 exacerbations per year, and/or severe impairment (GOLD 3 or 4)*	Smoking cessation, physical activity, vaccinations, pulmonary rehabilitation	Inhaled corticosteroid and long-acting bronchodilator (β_2-agonist or anticholinergic)

CAT, COPD Assessment Test; GOLD, Global Initiative for Chronic Obstructive Lung Disease; MMRC, Modified British Medical Research Council.
*See laboratory testing.

or severe COPD), the following assessments and nonpharmacologic interventions are recommended[1,13]:

- Assess severity SOR C—Physical signs of a more severe exacerbation include use of accessory muscles of respiration, paradoxical chest wall movements, worsening (or new onset) cyanosis, new peripheral edema, hemodynamic instability, or worsening mental status. Consider pulse oximetry.
- Consider CXR for those with moderate-to-severe symptoms and focal lung findings to exclude other diagnoses.
- Consider an electrocardiography (ECG) if suspecting cardiac complication or comorbidity.
- Consider a complete blood count (to identify anemia, polycythemia, or leukocytosis) and a theophylline level if on theophylline at admission. Consider sputum or blood cultures if clinically appropriate (eg, purulent sputum, fever).
- Consider blood gas for those with moderate-to-severe symptoms, advanced COPD, history of hypercarbia, or mental status changes.
- Hospitalize—Based on clinical judgment; recommended in those with marked increase in symptom intensity or onset of new physical signs (eg, cyanosis); frequent exacerbations; older age; the presence of respiratory acidosis, hypercarbia, hypoxemia; severe underlying COPD or serious comorbidities (eg, heart failure); failure to respond to outpatient treatment; or poor home support.[1] SOR C

MEDICATIONS

For patients with *stable COPD*, only smoking cessation and oxygen therapy for those with hypoxia at rest have been shown to improve outcome.[1] SOR A

- To assist with smoking cessation, consider nicotine replacement therapy (bupropion [150 mg, twice daily], varenicline [1 mg twice daily], nortriptyline [75-100 mg daily], or nicotine replacement [gum, inhaler, spray, patch]) and supportive counseling and follow-up; using these interventions improves rates of smoking cessation by up to 2-fold (see Chapter 237, Tobacco Addiction).[1,16-18] SOR A
- Oxygen therapy is initiated for patients who have a resting O_2 saturation less than 89% (PaO_2 at or below 55 mm Hg [7.3 kPa], confirmed twice over a 3-week period or <89% in a patient with pulmonary hypertension or right-sided heart failure); chronic administration (<15 h/d) in patients with chronic respiratory failure is associated with greater survival.[1] SOR B

The following are recommended for symptomatic relief:

- Short-acting inhaled bronchodilators—β-Agonists (eg, albuterol) or anticholinergic agents (eg, ipratropium bromide)—intermittent use; SOR A these agents are comparable in efficacy and the choice of agent should be based on side effects, cost, and patient preference.[1]
- Inhaled long-acting β-agonists (eg, salmeterol, indacaterol)—Regular treatment is more effective, but more costly and may be associated with tachycardia and tremor.[1] SOR A Salmeterol reduces the risk of hospitalization but has no effect on mortality or the rate of lung function decline. Adverse effects include tachycardia, tremor.
- Combination long-acting β-agonists with inhaled anticholinergic agents can provide incremental benefit for symptoms.[1] SOR B They may also be used in combination with inhaled corticosteroids to improve health status and reduce exacerbations in patients with moderate- SOR B-to-severe COPD SOR A.[1]
- Inhaled long-acting anticholinergic (tiotropium)—Tiotropium has a duration of action of 24 hours and reduces exacerbations and improves symptoms.[1] SOR A Adverse effects include dry mouth;[1] a recent meta-analysis concluded that mortality was increased with use of this medication (2.4% vs 1.6% on placebo; number needed to harm over 1 year = 124).[19]
- Inhaled glucocorticoids—Regular use is associated with improved quality of life and a small decrease in the frequency of exacerbations (approximately half-a-day per month), but an increase in oral candidiasis, easy bruising, and bone loss (the latter shown for long-term triamcinolone acetonide).[1] SOR A These agents are recommended for patients with moderate-to-severe COPD or for frequent exacerbations. Parenteral steroids do not benefit patients with stable COPD. In a Cochrane review comparing inhaled glucocorticoids with long-acting

β-agonists, the authors concluded that effects were comparable on most outcomes, including reduced frequency of exacerbation, with β-agonists conferring a small additional benefit in lung function while inhaled corticosteroid therapy showed a small advantage in health-related quality of life but increased the risk of pneumonia.[20]

- Theophylline—Mildly effective for symptoms SOR Ⓐ and reduction in exacerbations SOR Ⓑ, but associated with nausea and risk of toxicity with high blood levels.[1,21]
- Mucolytic agents (eg, guaifenesin, carbocysteine, potassium iodide)—Produce a small decrease in the frequency of exacerbations (0.5 fewer exacerbations/y) and in disability days.[22] SOR Ⓐ GOLD does not recommend these medications for routine use.[1]
- Early investigation has begun on a phosphodiesterase-4 inhibitor (roflumilast) in patients with moderate-to-severe COPD already on an inhaled bronchodilator. There may be some improvement in exacerbations but other relevant patient outcome data are unevaluated; side effects include nausea, diarrhea, weight loss, and headache.[23]

For patients with *an acute exacerbation* of COPD, the 3 classes of medications commonly used are bronchodilators, corticosteroids, and antibiotics.

- Inhaled bronchodilators—Both β-agonist and anticholinergics can be used alone or in combination; metered-dose inhalers with proper patient instruction perform as well as nebulized treatments and are less expensive; nebulizers can be considered for sicker patients.[1] SOR Ⓐ
- Glucocorticoid—Use oral (prednisone 30-40 mg/d for 10-14 days) or intravenous (IV) glucocorticoids if the patient is unable to tolerate oral medication. Steroids decrease recovery time, hospital length of stay, and relapse rates.[1] SOR Ⓐ
- Antibiotics—Treating COPD with antibiotics is controversial. In a systematic review, investigators found 4 placebo-controlled clinical trials and a meta-analysis that demonstrated significant improvements in outcome for patients treated with an antibiotic versus placebo.[24] In contrast, 6 studies failed to demonstrate statistical differences. GOLD recommends the use of antibiotics for 5 to 10 days for patients with increased dyspnea, sputum volume, and sputum purulence, and for patients who require mechanical ventilation.[1] SOR Ⓑ Antibiotics should also be considered for patients with increased purulent sputum and either increased sputum volume or dyspnea.[1] SOR Ⓒ
- The choice of antibiotic does not appear to influence outcome and should be based on local bacterial resistance and severity of disease. For exacerbations of lesser severity, use narrow-spectrum antibiotics such as amoxicillin, doxycycline, or trimethoprim-sulfamethoxazole. For exacerbations of greater severity use broad-spectrum antibiotic such as azithromycin, amoxicillin-clavulanate, levofloxacin, cefuroxime axetil, or hospitalize for IV antibiotics. SOR Ⓒ
- Oxygen therapy—Use to maintain O_2 saturation above 88%.[1] SOR Ⓒ
- Noninvasive mechanical ventilation (NIV) decreases mortality, decreases the need for intubation, and reduces hospital length of stay.[1] SOR Ⓐ However, patients may find it difficult to tolerate. It should be considered for patients with moderate-to-severe dyspnea, moderate-to-severe acidosis (pH <7.35), hypercapnia ($Paco_2$ >6.0 kPa, 45 mm Hg), and respiratory rate greater than 25 breaths/min.[1]
- Mechanical ventilation support should be considered for patients with the above indications who are unable to tolerate NIV and for those with severe dyspnea, massive aspiration or inability to remove respiratory secretions, respiratory failure [life-threatening hypoxemia (Pao_2 <5.3 kPa, 40 mm Hg or Pao_2/Fio_2 <200 mm Hg), severe acidosis (pH <7.25) and hypercapnia ($Paco_2$ >8 kPa, 60 mm Hg)], heart rate less than 50 beats/min with loss of alertness, severe ventricular arrhythmias, and respiratory arrest.[1] SOR Ⓒ

COMPLEMENTARY AND ALTERNATIVE THERAPY

- There is supporting evidence for immunostimulant therapy (reduced hospital days), cineole (a constituent of eucalyptus oil on reducing severity and duration of exacerbations and improved lung function, dyspnea, and quality of life), and ginseng (on lung function and quality of life) in patients with COPD.[25-27] SOR Ⓑ
- Tai Chi and Qigong (twice weekly 60-minute sessions) significantly improved exercise tolerance and 3-month exacerbation rate compared with either exercise or no intervention in patients with COPD.[28] SOR Ⓑ

SURGERY

Two surgical therapies with the best supporting evidence may be considered for patients with severe disease despite optimal medical therapy:

- Lung volume reduction surgery (LVRS)—Patients with upper lobe predominant disease and low postrehabilitation exercise capacity appear to gain the most symptom benefit.[1] LVRS in contrast to medical treatment improves survival (54% vs 38.7%) in patients with severe upper lobe emphysema and low postrehabilitation exercise capacity.[1] SOR Ⓐ
- Lung transplantation—Considered for patients who are 65 years of age or younger with no comorbid disease. GOLD lists a BODE (body mass, obstruction, dyspnea, exercise index (see Prognosis) greater than 5 as an indication for transplantation.[1,29] However, investigators from Norway found no obvious survival benefit from lung transplantation in a cohort of 219 patients accepted onto the lung transplant waiting list.[30]

REFERRAL

Reasons to consider referral include diagnostic uncertainty; severe disease, including onset of cor pulmonale; assessment for oxygen, corticosteroid, or pulmonary rehabilitation therapy; surgical assessment (bullous lung disease, severe disease); rapid decline in forced expiratory volume in 1 second (FEV_1); early onset or family history of COPD; frequent infections; and hemoptysis.[13] There are new treatments for α_1-antitrypsine deficiency and these patients should be referred to a pulmonologist for evaluation and treatment.

PREVENTION AND SCREENING

- The best prevention for COPD is to not smoke or to quit smoking. Limiting occupational exposures and exposure to indoor air pollution is also preventive.
- GOLD recommends active case finding but not general population screening.[1] The US Preventive Services Task Force also recommends against screening adults for COPD using spirometry.[31]

PROGNOSIS

- In a longitudinal study of 227 patients with COPD in Japan, 5-year survival was 73%; level of dyspnea and not FEV_1 was correlated with survival rates.[32]
- Severity classification (see "Laboratory Testing" earlier) can be used in predicting risk of exacerbations (1.1-1.3 for severe and 1.2-2 for very

severe), hospitalizations per year (0.11-0.2 for moderate, 0.25-0.3 for severe, and 0.4-0.54 for very severe), or 3-year mortality (11% for moderate, 15% for severe, and 24% for very severe).[1]

- The BODE index is a composite measure using body mass, obstruction (FEV_1, % predicted), dyspnea (MMRC score), and exercise (6-minute walking distance) to predict mortality. The risk of death from respiratory causes increases by more than 60% for each 1 point increase in BODE score.[33] An online calculator is available at http://www.new-leaf.com/ns/c/calculator-bode.htm?storeID=j3qsseqx5cs92j2000akhmccqja05t39 (accessed January 2012).
- In-hospital mortality of patients admitted for hypercapnic exacerbation with acidosis is approximately 10% and mortality at 1-year postdischarge for those requiring mechanical ventilation is 40%.[1]

FOLLOW-UP

Patients should be followed regularly for disease progression or development of complications.

- At each visit ask about symptoms, activity, and sleep. For smokers, encourage cessation. Symptom questionnaires can be used (every 2-3 months suggested by GOLD) for monitoring.
- Spirometry is recommended by GOLD at least yearly.[1] SOR C
- For patients on medications, monitor treatment effectiveness ("have you noticed a difference, for example less breathlessness") and side effects. Observe inhaler technique at least once to ensure optimal delivery.
- Document exacerbations or hospitalizations; this may indicate a need for additional treatment.
- Monitor for comorbidities (eg, heart disease, hypertension, osteoporosis, anxiety or depression, lung cancer, infections, metabolic syndrome, and diabetes) and maximize control of those conditions. The GOLD reference provides information on management of these conditions in patients with COPD.[1]
- Additional concerns for patients with severe COPD include need for long-term oxygen, need for specialist referral, including social services; biyearly evaluation should be considered.[13] Hospice referral may also be appropriate.

PATIENT EDUCATION

Smoking cessation should be strongly and repeatedly encouraged. Progressive exercise should also be encouraged, activities that brace the arms and allow use of accessory muscles of respiration are better tolerated—these include pushing a cart, walker, or wheelchair, and use of a treadmill.

PATIENT RESOURCES

- American Lung Association—**http://www.lungusa.org/lung-disease/copd/.**
- Journal of the American Medical Association, Chronic Obstructive Pulmonary Disease, Patient Page with good diagram— **http://jama.ama-assn.org/content/300/20/2448.full.pdf.**
- The Family of COPD Support Programs, COPD Support, Inc. This Web site provides information and links to support groups—**http://www.copd-support.com.**

PROVIDER RESOURCES

- Several evidence-based guidelines are available—**http://www.guideline.gov/** and *search on COPD*.
- Evidence-based guidelines are also available on GOLD (GOLD)—**http://www.goldcopd.org/.**
- Another Web site that has links to National Heart, Lung, and Blood Institute, American Academy of Family Physicians, and others, patient education materials and an interactive tutorial—**www.nlm.nih.gov/medlineplus/copdchronicobstructivepulmonarydisease.html.**

REFERENCES

1. Global Initiative for Chronic Obstructive Lung Disease (GOLD). *Global Strategy for the Diagnosis, Management and Prevention of COPD, 2011*. http://www.goldcopd.org/uploads/users/files/GOLD_Report_2011_Feb21.pdf. Accessed January 2012.
2. Centers for Disease Control and Prevention. *Chronic Obstructive Pulmonary Disease Morbidity (Table 10.3)*. http://www2a.cdc.gov/drds/WorldReportData/FigureTableDetails.asp?FigureTableID=944&GroupRefNumber=T10-09. Accessed January 2012.
3. Centers for Disease Control and Prevention. *Chronic Obstructive Pulmonary Disease (COPD). Data and Statistics*. http://www.cdc.gov/copd/data.htm. Accessed January 2012.
4. Menezes AM, Perez-Padilla R, Jardim JR, et al. Chronic obstructive lung disease in five Latin American cities (the PLATINO study): a prevalence study. *Lancet*. 2005;366:1875-1881.
5. Lindberg A, Jonsson AC, Ronmark E, et al. Ten-year cumulative incidence of COPD and risk factors for incident disease in asymptomatic cohort. *Chest*. 2005;127:1544-1552.
6. Reilly JJ, Silverman EK, Shapiro SD. Chronic obstructive pulmonary disease. In: Kasper DL, Braunwald E, Fauci AS, Hauser SL, Longo DL, Jameson JL, eds. *Harrison's Principles of Internal Medicine*. 16th ed. New York, NY: McGraw-Hill; 2005:1547-1554.
7. Soler Artigas M, Wain LV, Repapi E, et al. Effect of five genetic variants associated with lung function on the risk of chronic obstructive lung disease, and their joint effects on lung function. *Am J Respir Crit Care Med*. 2011;184(7):786-795.
8. Hersh CP, Silverman EK, Gascon J, et al. SOX5 is a candidate gene for chronic obstructive pulmonary disease susceptibility and is necessary for lung development. *Am J Respir Crit Care Med*. 2011;183(11):1482-1489.
9. Forey BA, Thornton AJ, Lee PN. Systematic review with meta-analysis of the epidemiological evidence relating smoking to COPD, chronic bronchitis and emphysema. *BMC Pulm Med*. 2011;11:36.
10. Hersh CP, Hokanson JE, Lynch DA, et al. Family history is a risk factor for COPD. *Chest*. 2011;140(2):343-350.
11. Kornmann O, Beeh KM, Beier J, et al. Global Initiative for Obstructive Lung Disease. Newly diagnosed chronic obstructive pulmonary disease. Clinical features and distribution of the novel stages of the Global Initiative for Obstructive Lung Disease. *Respiration*. 2003;70:67-75.
12. Qaseem A, Wilt TJ, Weinberger SE, et al. Diagnosis and management of stable chronic obstructive pulmonary disease: a clinical practice guideline update from the American College of Physicians, American

College of Chest Physicians, American Thoracic Society, and European Respiratory Society. *Ann Intern Med.* 2011;155(3):179-191.

13. National Guideline Clearinghouse, Agency for Healthcare Research and Quality. *Chronic Obstructive Pulmonary Disease. Management of Chronic Obstructive Pulmonary Disease in Adults in Primary and Secondary Care.* http://www.guideline.gov/content.aspx?id=23801&search=chronic+obstructive+pulmonary+disease. Accessed January 2012.
14. Yang YW, Chen YH, Wang KH, et al. Risk of herpes zoster among patients with chronic obstructive pulmonary disease: a population-based study. *CMAJ.* 2011;183:E275-E280.
15. Gadoury MA, Schwartzman K, Rouleau M, et al. Chronic Obstructive Pulmonary Disease axis of the Respiratory Health Network, Fonds de la recherche en sante du Quebec (FRSQ). Self-management reduces both short- and long-term hospitalisation in COPD. *Eur Respir J.* 2005;26(5):853-857.
16. Hughes JR, Stead LF, Lancaster T. Antidepressants for smoking cessation. *Cochrane Database Syst Rev.* 2007;(1):CD000031.
17. Stead LF, Perera R, Bullen C, et al. Nicotine replacement therapy for smoking cessation. *Cochrane Database Syst Rev.* 2008;(1):CD000146.
18. Stead LF, Bergson G, Lancaster T. Physician advice for smoking cessation. *Cochrane Database Syst Rev.* 2008;(2):CD000165.
19. Singh S, Loke YK, Enright PL, Furberg CD. Mortality associated with tiotropium mist inhaler in patients with chronic obstructive pulmonary disease: systematic review and meta-analysis of randomised controlled trials. *BMJ.* 2011;342:d3215.
20. Spencer S, Evans DJ, Karner C, Cates CJ. Inhaled corticosteroids versus long-acting beta(2)-agonists for chronic obstructive pulmonary disease. *Cochrane Database Syst Rev.* 2011;(12):CD007033.
21. Ram FS. Use of theophylline in chronic obstructive pulmonary disease: examining the evidence. *Curr Opin Pulm Med.* 2006;12(2):132-139.
22. Poole P, Black PN. Mucolytic agents for chronic bronchitis or chronic obstructive pulmonary disease. *Cochrane Database Syst Rev.* 2010;(2):CD001287.
23. Rennard SI, Calverley PM, Goehring UM, et al. Reduction of exacerbations by the PDE4 inhibitor roflumilast—the importance of defining different subsets of patients with COPD. *Respir Res.* 2011;12:18.
24. Russo RL, D'Aprile M. Role of antimicrobial therapy in acute exacerbations of chronic obstructive pulmonary disease. *Ann Pharmacother.* 2001;35(5):576-581.
25. Collet JP, Shapiro P, Ernst P, et al. Effects of an immunostimulating agent on acute exacerbations and hospitalizations in patients with chronic obstructive pulmonary disease. The PARI-IS Study Steering Committee and Research Group. Prevention of Acute Respiratory Infection by an Immunostimulant. *Am J Respir Crit Care Med.* 1997;156:1719-1724.
26. Worth H, Schacher C, Dethlefsen U. Concomitant therapy with Cineole (Eucalyptole) reduces exacerbations in COPD: a placebo-controlled double-blind trial. *Respir Res.* 2009;10:69.
27. An X, Zhang AL, Yang AW, et al. Oral ginseng formulae for stable chronic obstructive pulmonary disease: a systematic review. *Respir Med.* 2011;105:165-176.
28. Chan AW, Lee A, Suen LK, Tam WW. Tai chi Qigong improves lung functions and activity tolerance in COPD clients: a single blind, randomized controlled trial. *Complement Ther Med.* 2011;19:3-11.
29. Puhan MA, Garcia-Aymerich J, Frey M, et al. Expansion of the prognostic assessment of patients with chronic obstructive pulmonary disease: the updated BODE index and the ADO index. *Lancet.* 2009;374:704-711.
30. Stavem K, Bjortuft O, Borgan O, et al. Lung transplantation in patients with chronic obstructive pulmonary disease in a national cohort is without obvious survival benefit. *J Heart Lung Transplant.* 2006;25(1):75-84.
31. United States Preventive Services Task Force. *Screening for Chronic Obstructive Pulmonary Disease Using Spirometry.* http://www.uspreventiveservicestaskforce.org/uspstf/uspscopd.htm. Accessed January 2012.
32. Nishimura K, Izumi T, Tsukino M, Oga T. Dyspnea is a better predictor of 5-year survival than airway obstruction in patients with COPD. *Chest.* 2002;121:1434-1440.
33. Celli BR, Cote CG, Martin JM, et al. The body-mass index, airflow obstruction, dyspnea, and exercise capacity index in chronic obstructive pulmonary disease. *N Engl J Med.* 2004;350(10):1005-1012.

57 LUNG CANCER

Mindy A. Smith, MD, MS

PATIENT STORY

A 60-year-old woman presents with a solid, nontender, movable mass on her upper chest that has been there for 6 months. It began as dime-sized and has been growing more rapidly over the past month (**Figure 57-1A**). She has lost 10 lb over the last year without dieting. She smoked one pack of cigarettes per day since age 18 years and gets short of breath easily. Her "smoker's cough" has gotten worse in the last few months and occasionally she coughs up some blood-tinged sputum. Her family physician excised the mass in the office and sent it to pathology (**Figure 57-1B**). When the result demonstrated squamous cell carcinoma of the lung, a chest X-ray (CXR) was ordered (**Figure 57-2A**). The radiologist suggested a computed tomography (CT) to confirm the diagnosis (**Figure 57-2B**). The patient chose to have no treatment and died 10 months later of her lung cancer.

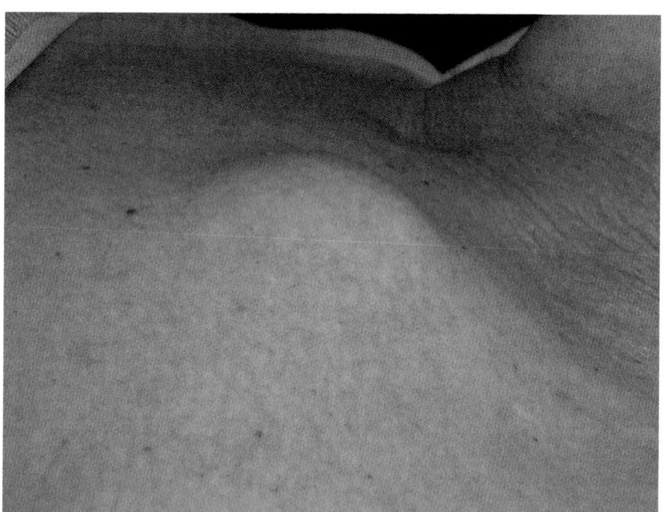

A

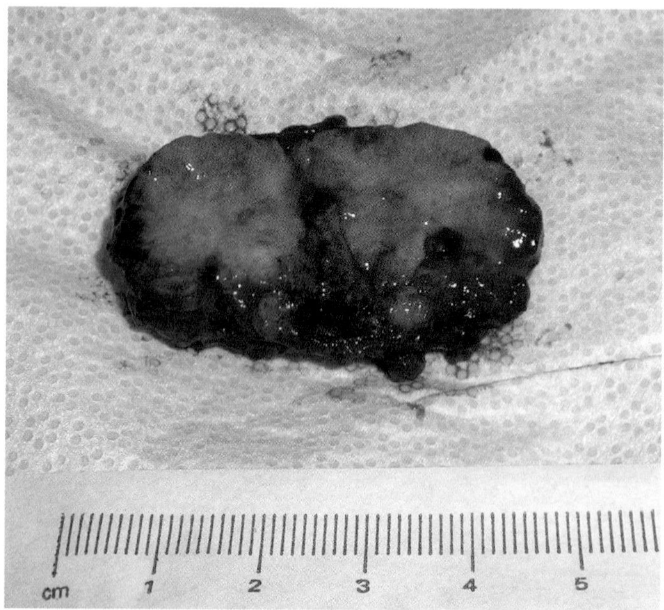

B

FIGURE 57-1 A. Growing chest nodule in a 60-year-old woman who smoked tobacco her whole adult life. The pathology demonstrated metastatic squamous cell carcinoma from the lung. B. The resected nodule was surgically removed in the office. (*Reproduced with permission from Leonard Chow, MD and Ross Lawler, MD.*)

INTRODUCTION

Lung cancer is a malignant neoplasm of the lung arising from respiratory epithelium (bronchi, bronchioles, or alveoli), most commonly adenocarcinoma or squamous cell carcinoma.

EPIDEMIOLOGY

- In 2007, lung cancer was diagnosed in 203,546 people in the United States (109,643 men and 93,893 women).[1] Both incidence and mortality rates have been decreasing since 1999 for men, but remain level for women.

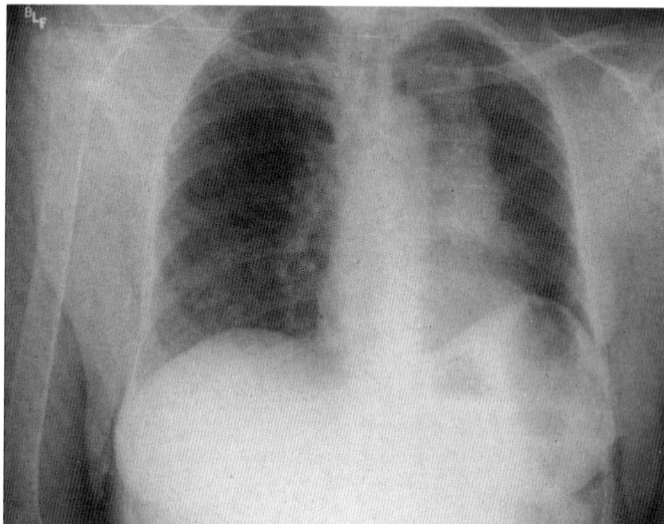

A

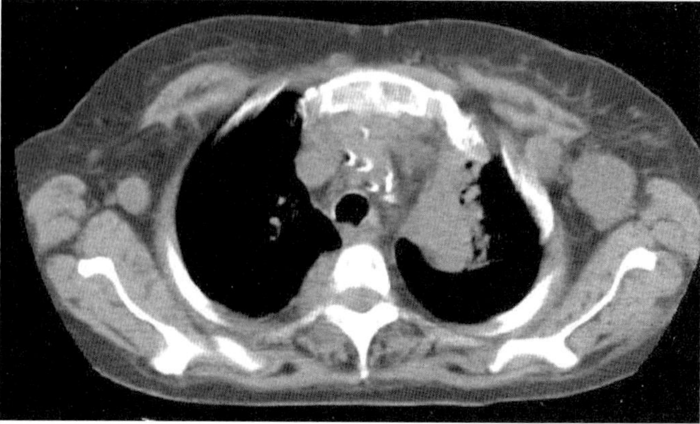

B

FIGURE 57-2 A. Chest X-ray showing squamous cell carcinoma of the lung. B. CT scan demonstrating the architecture of the squamous cell carcinoma of the lung. (*Reproduced with permission from David A. Kasper, DO, MBA.*)

- Black men have the highest age-adjusted incidence rates (99.8/100,000) followed by white men (75.3/100,000), and then black women (54.7/100,000) and white women (54.6/100,000); Hispanic men (41.5/100,000) and women (26.1/100,000) have the lowest incidence rates.[2]
- Risk increases with age; at age 60 years, 2.29% of men will develop lung cancer in 10 years and 5.64% in 20 years.[1] Among women at age 60 years, 1.74% will develop lung cancer in 10 years and 4.27% in 20 years. Median age at diagnosis is 71 years.[2]
- In 2007, lung cancer was the leading cause of cancer deaths accounting for 14% of all cancer diagnoses and 28% of all cancer deaths.[3]
- The 2011 estimate for new cases of lung cancer in the United States is 221,130 with 156,940 deaths from the disease.[4]

ETIOLOGY AND PATHOPHYSIOLOGY

- Lung cancer begins in the lungs spreading to regional lymph nodes and regional structures (eg, trachea, esophagus). Extrathoracic metastases are common (found at autopsy in 50%-95%) and sites include brain, bone, and liver.[5]
- Likely caused by a multistep process involving both carcinogens and tumor promoters; a number of genetic mutations (eg, epidermal growth factor receptor [EGFR] mutations) are present in lung cancer cells including activation of dominant oncogenes and inactivation of tumor suppressor oncogenes.[5]
- There are 2 main groupings of lung cancer—nonsmall-cell lung cancer (NSCLC; most common) and small-cell lung cancer (SCLC). The 4 major cell types responsible for 88% of cases[5] are the following:
  - Adenocarcinoma (including bronchoalveolar)—32% of cases
  - Squamous or epidermoid carcinoma—29% of cases
  - Small-cell (or oat cell) carcinoma—18% of cases
  - Large cell (or large-cell anaplastic)—9% of cases
- Adenocarcinoma, squamous carcinoma, and large cell are classified together under NSCLC because of similar diagnostic, staging, and treatment approaches.[4]
- Adenocarcinoma and squamous carcinoma have defined premalignant precursor lesions with lung tissue morphology ranging from hyperplasia to dysplasia and carcinoma in situ.[3]

RISK FACTORS

- Smoking is the major risk factor; a smoking history (current or former) is present in 90%, with a relative risk ratio of 13 (passive smoke exposure has a risk ratio of 1.5).[3] Currently 28% of men, 25% of women, and 38% of high school seniors smoke in the United States. Women have a higher susceptibility to the carcinogens in tobacco (Chapter 237, Tobacco Addiction).
- Occupations and exposures that increase the risk of lung cancer include asbestos mining and processing, welding, pesticide manufacturing (arsenic), metallurgy (chromium), polycyclic hydrocarbons (through coke oven emissions), iron oxide, vinyl chloride, and uranium.[3] Home exposure to asbestos or radon and diesel exhaust also increase risk.[2,6]
- Radiation therapy to the breast or chest.[4]
- Family history of lung cancer.
- β-Carotene supplementation in current smokers (small increased risk).
- Hormone therapy (women). In the Women's Health Initiative, although incidence of lung cancer was not significantly increased, death from lung cancer (primarily NSCLC) was increased (73 vs 40 deaths; 0.11% vs 0.06%).[7]

DIAGNOSIS

Signs and symptoms depend on location, tumor size and type, and the presence of local or distant spread.

- About 5% to 15% of patients are asymptomatic—the cancer is found on chest imaging performed for another reason.[5]
- Systemic symptoms (eg, anorexia, cachexia, weight loss [seen in 30% of patients]) may be seen but the cause is unknown.

The diagnosis of lung cancer requires tissue confirmation through the safest and least invasive procedure. Procedures include sputum cytology, bronchoscopy, lymph node biopsy, operative specimen, needle aspiration (eg, endobronchial ultrasound-guided transbronchial approach for mediastinal or hilar lymph nodes or CT-guided transthoracic approach for peripheral tumors), biopsy under CT guidance, or cell block from pleural effusion.[5,8]

- Immunohistochemistry (eg, thyroid transcription factor 1 for adenocarcinoma or P63 for squamous carcinoma) is now being used to help differentiate between cell types when morphologic criteria used in resections are not apparent.[8] Differentiation is important as different cell types respond differently to treatment.
- For suspicious central lung lesions, sputum cytology (at least 3 specimens) is a reasonable first step followed by bronchoscopy if needed.[5] SOR B
- In patients with a suspicious peripheral lung lesion (especially <2 cm), if sputum cytology fails to confirm the diagnosis, transthoracic needle aspiration has a higher sensitivity than bronchoscopy.[5] SOR A
- In patients with a lesion that is moderately suspicious for lung cancer who appear to have limited disease, excisional biopsy and subsequent lobectomy if a lung cancer is confirmed is recommended.[5] SOR B

CLINICAL FEATURES

- The most common symptoms at diagnosis are worsening cough or chest pain.[4] Symptoms may occur in the following situations[5]:
  - Central or endobronchial growth of the tumor can produce cough, hemoptysis, wheezing, stridor, and dyspnea.
  - Collapse of airways from tumor obstruction may cause postobstructive pneumonitis.
  - Involvement of the pleura or chest wall can cause pleuritic chest pain, dyspnea on a restrictive bases, or lung abscess from tumor cavitation.
  - Regional spread of the tumor may cause tracheal obstruction; dysphagia from esophageal spread; hoarseness from recurrent laryngeal nerve paralysis; dyspnea, and elevated hemidiaphragm from phrenic nerve paralysis; and Horner syndrome (enophthalmos, ptosis, miosis, ipsilateral loss of sweating from sympathetic nerve paralysis).
  - Spread to lymph nodes may be detected as firm masses in the supraclavicular area, axilla, or groin.
  - Extrathoracic metastases are common (found at autopsy in 50%-95%) and may cause neurologic symptoms with brain metastases; pain and fracture with bone metastases; cytopenias or

leukoerythroblastosis from bone marrow involvement; and liver dysfunction from metastases to the liver.
  - Paraneoplastic syndromes are common in SCLC and include endocrine syndromes (seen in 12%) such as hypercalcemia and hypophosphatemia from elevated parathyroid hormone or parathyroid hormone–related peptide, hyponatremia from secretion of antidiuretic hormone, electrolyte disturbances seen with secretion of adrenocorticotropic hormone, and Lambert-Eaton myasthenic syndrome (primarily proximal muscle weakness, abnormal gait, fatigue, autonomic dysfunction, paresthesias). The most common paraneoplastic syndromes in SCLC are the syndrome of inappropriate antidiuresis (15%-40% of patients with SCLC) and Cushing syndrome (2%-5% of patients with SCLC).[8]
  - Skeletal and connective tissue syndromes including clubbing (seen in 30%, especially with nonsmall-cell carcinoma) and hypertrophic pulmonary osteoarthropathy with pain and swelling from periostitis (1%-10%, especially with adenocarcinoma) can be seen.
  - Skin nodules from lung cancer metastases may not be painful but are a poor prognostic sign (see **Figures 57-1** and **57-2**).

LABORATORY TESTING

Molecular testing for mutational profiles is becoming more common for NSCLC with the rapid development of targeted therapies. Specifically, identification of activating EGFR mutations is the best predictor for response to EGFR–tyrosine kinase inhibitors.[9] In one multicenter study in Spain, EGFR mutations were found in 16.6% (350/2105) of patients and were more frequent in women (69.7%), never-smokers (66.6%), and in those with adenocarcinomas (80.9%).[10]

IMAGING

- For an incidental lung nodule not believed to be lung cancer, the American College of Radiology (ACR) recommends either percutaneous lung biopsy or whole body fluorine-18-2-fluoro-2-deoxy-D-glucose-positron emission tomography (FDG-PET); the latter if the patient has lung cancer risk factors.[11] Follow-up imaging only is recommended for selected patients with no lung cancer risk factors.
- If a tumor is associated with mediastinal adenopathy, endoscopic or bronchoscopic mediastinal biopsy is recommended.[11] In one study, endobronchial ultrasound-guided transbronchial needle aspiration was found to be comparable to mediastinoscopy for mediastinal staging in patients with potentially resectable NSCLC.[12]
- CXR may be useful as baseline, if not already performed, and a chest CT should be performed; these tests may show a nodule (**Figures 57-3** and **57-4**) or diffuse lung abnormalities often confused with pneumonia (**Figures 57-5** to **57-7**).

TYPICAL DISTRIBUTION

- Squamous and small-cell carcinoma tend to present as central masses with endobronchial growth.[5]
- Adeno- and large-cell carcinoma tend to present as peripheral masses, frequently with pleural involvement.

BIOPSY: HISTOLOGY

- SCLCs have scant cytoplasm, hyperchromatic nuclei with fine chromatin pattern, nucleoli that are indistinct, and diffuse sheets of cells.[5]
- NSCLCs have abundant cytoplasm, pleomorphic nuclei with coarse chromatin pattern, prominent nucleoli, and glandular or squamous architecture.

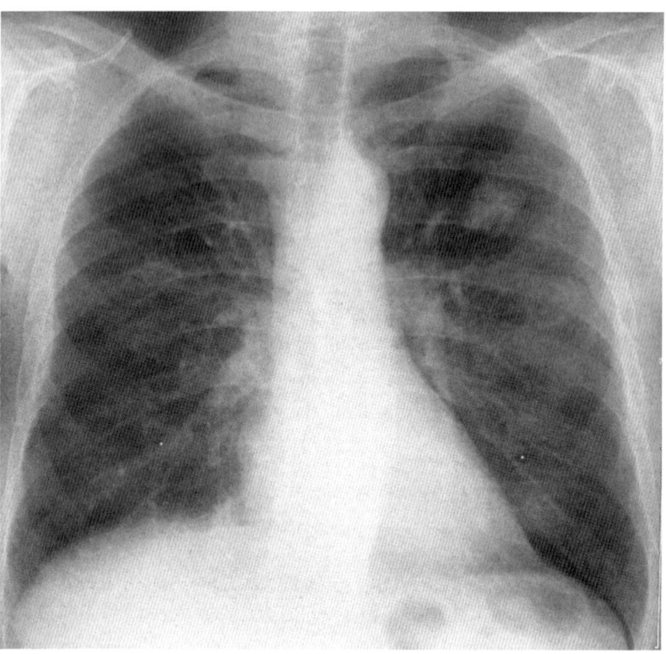

FIGURE 57-3 Chest X-ray demonstrating a 2.5-cm irregular nodule in the left upper lobe (*Reproduced with permission from Miller WT, Jr.* Diagnostic Thoracic Imaging. *New York, NY: McGraw-Hill; 2006.*)

DIFFERENTIAL DIAGNOSIS

The differential diagnosis of an individual with lung findings (eg, productive cough and dyspnea) includes the following:

- Chronic obstructive pulmonary disease—Most common symptoms are cough, sputum production, and exertional dyspnea. Although

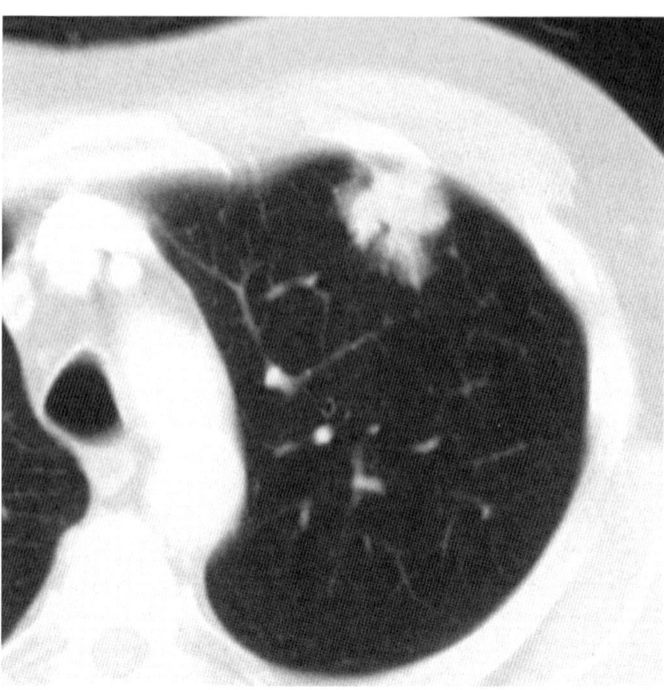

FIGURE 57-4 CT scan of the patient in **Figure 57-3** shows a spiculated mass confirmed at surgery to be an adenocarcinoma (*Reproduced with permission from Miller WT, Jr.* Diagnostic Thoracic Imaging. *New York, NY: McGraw-Hill; 2006.*)

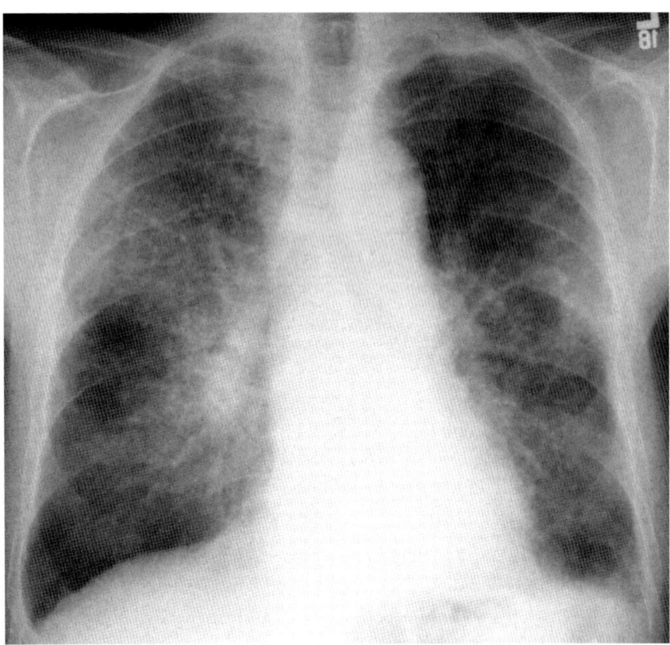

FIGURE 57-5 Diffuse lung abnormality seen on chest X-ray best characterized as ground-glass opacity, slightly worse in the right upper lobe. Open biopsy demonstrated bronchoalveolar carcinoma (*Reproduced with permission from Miller WT, Jr.* Diagnostic Thoracic Imaging. *New York, NY: McGraw-Hill; 2006.*)

hemoptysis may occur, imaging (chest CT is most definitive) will not show a tumor. There is an increased risk of lung cancer in these patients (Chapter 56, Chronic Obstructive Pulmonary Disease).

- Pneumonia—Symptoms include fever, chills, and pleuritic chest pain; physical findings include dullness to percussion, bronchial breathing, egophony (E-A change), and crackles with area of infiltrate (pneumonia usually confirmed on CXR; Chapter 59, Pneumonia).

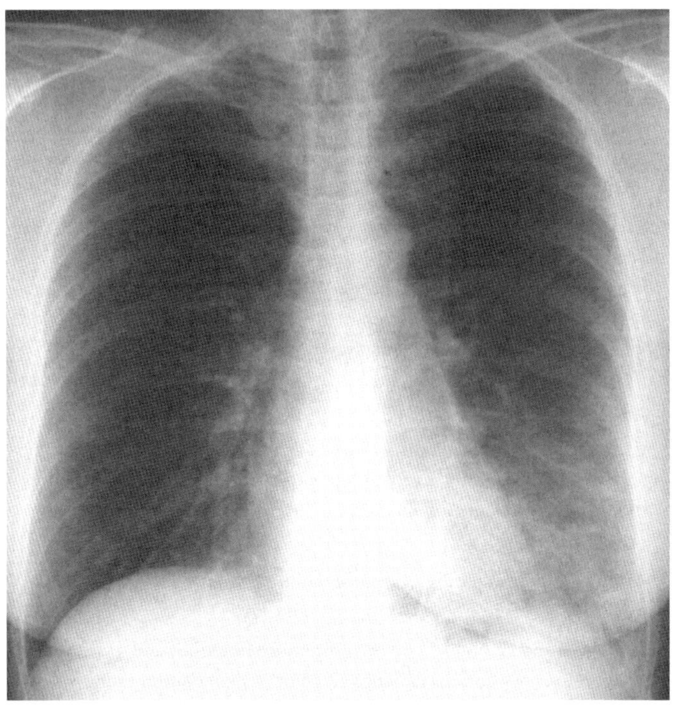

FIGURE 57-6 Chest X-ray showing local area of consolidation in the left lower lobe. Worsening consolidation for the subsequent 2 months despite antibiotic treatment leads to a surgical biopsy, which confirmed bronchoalveolar carcinoma (*Reproduced with permission from Miller WT, Jr.* Diagnostic Thoracic Imaging. *New York, NY: McGraw-Hill; 2006.*)

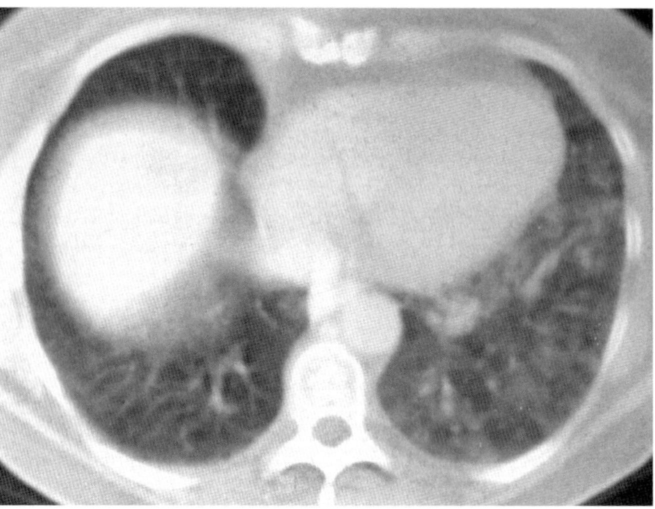

FIGURE 57-7 CT at the level of the bases in the patient in **Figure 57-6** showing areas of ground-glass opacification in the left lower lobe and lingula. Worsening consolidation for the subsequent 2 months despite antibiotic treatment leads to a surgical biopsy, which confirmed bronchoalveolar carcinoma. (*Reproduced with permission from Miller WT, Jr.* Diagnostic Thoracic Imaging. *New York, NY: McGraw-Hill; 2006.*)

Both these processes may occur in conjunction with lung cancer.

MANAGEMENT

Treatment is based on staging and cell type—both anatomic (eg, physical location of tumor) and physiologic (eg, patient's ability to withstand treatment) factors are considered. All patients should undergo the following[5,8]: SOR Ⓒ

- Complete history and physical
- Laboratory tests—Complete blood count with differential and platelets, electrolytes, glucose, calcium, phosphorus, and renal and liver function tests

For staging purposes for NSCLC, the ACR recommends the following imaging[13]:

- CT chest scan with contrast, if there are no strong contraindications, and a FDG-PET from skull base to midthigh. Use of FDG-PET has been shown to identify more patients with mediastinal and extrathoracic disease than conventional staging.[14] While this approach spares more patients from stage-inappropriate surgery, the strategy appears to incorrectly upstage disease in some patients and, in one RCT, did not affect overall mortality.[15]
- If a patient has neurologic symptoms or an adenocarcinoma greater than 3 cm or mediastinal adenopathy, a magnetic resonance imaging (MRI) of the head without and with contrast is recommended.[11]
- In addition, for patients with nonsmall-cell tumors who may be candidates for curative surgery or radiotherapy, obtain pulmonary function tests, coagulation tests, and possibly cardiopulmonary exercise testing.[5]

For staging of patients with SCLC, ACR recommends the following[11]:

- CT chest scan with contrast, if there are no strong contraindications, FDG-PET from skull base to midthigh, MRI of the head without and with contrast, and CT of the abdomen (liver metastases are common at diagnosis). The use of FDG-PET scanning is controversial for patients with SCLC as most chemoradiation studies were performed prior to use of this scan.[8]

Staging for patients with lung cancer is based on the TNM classification system where T describes the size of the tumor, N describes any regional lymph node involvement, and M notes the presence or absence of distant metastases (**Box 57-1**).[16] At diagnosis, approximately 15% have localized disease, 22% have regional disease (spread to regional lymph nodes), and 56% have distant metastases.[2]

NONPHARMALOGIC

Supportive care for the patient and family and palliative care of the patient should be provided, including adequate pain relief.

- Early palliative care was shown in one trial to improve quality of life and mood and increased median survival (11.6 months vs 8.9 months) for patients with metastatic NSCLC compared to those receiving standard care.[17]
- Smoking cessation—In a meta-analysis, continued smoking was associated with a significantly increased risk of all-cause mortality and recurrence in early-stage NSCLC and of all-cause mortality, development of a second primary tumour and recurrence in limited stage (all but stage IV) SCLC.[18] Using life table modeling, these investigators estimated that 5-year survival in 65-year-old patients with early-stage NSCLC who quit smoking would increase from 33% (for those who continued to smoke) to 70% and for those with limited-stage SCLC, from 29% (continued smokers) to 63% (quitters) (Chapter 237, Tobacco Addiction).

BOX 57-1 TNM Staging of Lung Cancer

- Stage 0—Carcinoma in situ (Tis N0 M0)
- Stage IA—Tumor size 2 cm or smaller (1a) or tumor size >2 cm but <3 cm (1b) (T1a,b N0 M0)
- Stage IB—Tumor size >3 cm but <5 cm (2a) and has any of the following: involves the main bronchus (>2 cm distal to the carina), invades visceral pleura, or associated with atelectasis or obstructive pneumonitis extending to the hilar region (T2a N0 M0)
- Stage IIA—Tumor size >5 cm but <7 cm (2b) (T2b N0 M0, T1a,b N1 M0, T2a N1 M0)
- Stage IIB—Tumor size >5 cm but <7 cm (2b) or tumor size >7 cm or directly invades the chest wall, diaphragm, phrenic nerve, mediastinal pleura, parietal pericardium; or tumor in the main bronchus <2 cm distal to the carina but without carina involvement; or associated atelectasis or obstructive pneumonitis of the entire lung or separate tumor nodule(s) in the same lobe as the primary (T3) (T2b N1 M0, T3 N0 M0)
- Stage IIIA—Any size tumor including a tumor that invades the mediastinum, heart, great vessels, trachea, recurrent laryngeal nerve, esophagus, vertebral body, carina, or separate tumor in a different ipsilateral lobe to that of the primary (T4) (T1a,b or T2a,b N2 M0, T3 N1or 2 M0, T4 N0 or 1 M0)

T, Tumor (size and extent); N, regional lymph nodes (N0 no regional lymph node metastasis, N1 metastasis in ipsilateral peribronchial and/or ipsilateral hilar lymph nodes and intrapulmonary nodes, including involvement by direct extension, N2 metastasis in ipsilateral mediastinal and/or subcarinal lymph node[s], N3 metastasis in contralateral mediastinal, contralateral hilar, ipsilateral or contralateral scalene, or supraclavicular lymph node[s]); M, metastases (M0 no distant metastasis, M1 distant metastasis).

MEDICATIONS

- Pain medication should be provided as needed (Chapter 4, End of Life). Opioids, such as codeine or morphine, may reduce cough.
- Adjuvant chemotherapy in patients with NSCLC, with or without postoperative radiotherapy, increases 5-year survival by about 4% to 5%.[8,19]
- Preoperative chemotherapy in patients with NSCLC increases survival by about 6% (absolute benefit) at 5 years.[20] Advantages of preoperative chemotherapy include early start on potential micrometastases and higher adherence to therapy.[8]
- Maintenance therapy with either cytotoxic agents or tyrosine kinase inhibitor agents (or switch therapy) can be considered as it appears to increase overall survival for patients with nonprogressive NSCLC.[21]
- Management of patients with SCLC includes combination, platinum-based chemotherapy (see later).[5,22] SOR Ⓐ Targeted therapies have not proven beneficial for patients with SCLC.[22]

COMPLEMENTARY OR ALTERNATIVE THERAPY

In a small RCT of patients with NSCLC on chemotherapy, nutritional intervention with 2.2 g of fish oil per day provided a benefit on maintenance of weight and muscle mass over standard care.[23] Fish oil also increased the response to chemotherapy in those with advanced NSCLC and may provide a survival benefit (trend).[24]

SURGERY AND RADIATION

Management of patients with NSCLC includes the following:

- Localized stage I and II—Pulmonary resection.[5,25,26] SOR Ⓐ Evidence is conflicting about whether video-assisted thoracoscopic surgery offers advantages over standard lobectomy; either technique can be used.[8,25,26]
- In patients undergoing resection, intraoperative systematic mediastinal lymph node sampling or dissection is recommended for accurate staging.[25] Although data are limited, a Cochrane review concluded that resection combined with complete mediastinal lymph node dissection is associated with a modest survival improvement compared with resection combined with systematic sampling of mediastinal nodes in patients with stage I to IIIA NSCLC.[27]
- For patients with stage I disease who are not surgical candidates, external beam radiotherapy is recommended;[28] stereotactic body radiation therapy or percutaneous ablation can be considered as a treatment option.[25,26] SOR Ⓑ
- Adjuvant chemotherapy is recommended for patients with stage II disease.[25,29]
- Stage IIIA and favorable age, cardiovascular function, and anatomy—Possible surgery and/or concurrent chemo- or radiation therapy.
- Stage IIIB—Concurrent chemo- or radiation therapy.[25]
- Stage IV—Options include radiation therapy to symptomatic local sites, chemotherapy or molecular targeted agents, chest tube for

malignant effusion, and consideration of resection of primary or isolated brain or adrenal metastases.[5,25] A Cochrane review concluded that chemotherapy improves overall survival in patients with advanced NSCLC (absolute improvement in survival of 9% at 12 months [20%-29%] or absolute increase in median survival of 1.5 months [from 4.5 months to 6 months]).[30]

- Curative radiotherapy should be considered for patients with good performance status and inoperable stage I to III disease.[25]

Management of patients with very limited (stage I) SCLC is surgical resection and adjuvant combined cisplatin-based chemotherapy, possibly with prophylactic cranial irradiation.[22]

- Other patients with limited-stage SCLC (stages II-III) should be offered thoracic irradiation concurrently with the first or second cycle of chemotherapy or following completion of chemotherapy if there has been at least a good partial response within the thorax.[5,22] Prophylactic cranial irradiation should be considered if nonprogressive after induction treatment.[22]
- For patients with extensive disease (stage IV), limited data support prolonged survival (added 63-84 days) using chemotherapy.[31] Supportive care plus palliative thoracic irradiation should be considered following chemotherapy (combination etoposide and cisplatin for non-Asian patients and irinotecan and cisplatin for Asian patients).[22]
- For patients who are not candidates for chemotherapy, palliative radiotherapy should be considered.[22] Palliative radiotherapy is associated with a modest increase in survival (5% at 1 year) in patients with better performance status who are given higher-dose radiotherapy.[32] Other targeted therapies, based on molecular testing of tumor mutational profiles (eg, erlotinib for mutant EGFR) should be considered.
- External beam radiotherapy could also be considered for the relief of breathlessness, cough, hemoptysis, or chest pain.[5]

PREVENTION

- Avoid smoking or smoking exposure or quit, if already smoking.
- Avoid workplace and home exposures (listed in risk factors).
- Daily aspirin appears to protect against lung adenocarcinoma.[33]
- Routine screening for lung cancer is not currently recommended; the US Preventive Services Task Force concluded insufficient evidence to support screening with any modality.[34] Results of the Prostate, Lung, Colorectal, and Ovarian (PLCO) Cancer Screening Trial (N = 154,901) demonstrated no benefit of annual CXR screening on reducing lung cancer mortality compared with usual care.[35]
- However, the National Lung Screening Trial (N = 53,454 patients at high risk for lung cancer) reported lower mortality from lung cancer after 3 annual screenings for patients randomized to low-dose CT versus single-view posteroanterior chest radiography (247 deaths from lung cancer per 100,000 person-years and 309 deaths per 100,000 person-years, respectively).[36] There was also reduced all-cause mortality in this group by 6.7%. As the risk of false positives with low-dose CT is high (33% after 2 screenings)[37] and there is potential for radiation-induced cancer, it is not clear that routine screening for high-risk patients should be conducted.

PROGNOSIS

- Perioperative mortality from a large database of over 18,000 lung cancer resections performed at 111 participating centers was 2.2% and composite morbidity and mortality occurred in 8.6%.[38] Predictive factors of mortality included pneumonectomy, bilobectomy, performance status, induction chemoradiation, steroids, age, and renal dysfunction among other factors.
- Adverse prognostic factors for NSCLC include presence of pulmonary symptoms, large tumor size (>3 cm), nonsquamous histology, metastases to multiple lymph nodes within a TNM-defined nodal station, and vascular invasion.[4]
- The overall 5-year relative survival from lung cancer (SEER data 2001-2007) was 15.6%. Five-year relative survival by race and sex was 18.3% for white women, 14.5% for black women, 13.7% for white men, and 11.6% for black men.[2]
- Five-year survival decreases by stage at diagnosis ranging from 52.2% for localized disease to 3.6% for those with distant metastases.[2] Estimates for 5-year survival by stage are stage IA 73%, stage IB 65%, stage IIA 46%, stage IIB 36%, stage IIIA 24%, stage IIIB 9%, and stage IV 13%.[16]
- For SCLC, median survival for patients with limited-stage disease is about 15 to 20 months (20%-40% survive to 2 years). For those with extensive-stage SCLC disease, median survival is about 8 to 13 months with 2-year survival of 5%.[8]
- Following lung cancer resection, there is a 1% to 2% risk per patient per year that a second lung cancer will occur.[5] One author reported higher risks of second tumors in long-term survivors, including rates of 10% for second lung cancers and 20% for all second cancers.[39] For patients with SCLC, second primary tumors are reported in 2% to 10% of patients per year.[22]

FOLLOW-UP

Surveillance for the recognition of a recurrence of the original lung cancer and/or the development of a metachronous tumor should be coordinated through a multidisciplinary team approach.

- This team should develop a lifelong surveillance plan appropriate for the individual circumstances of each patient immediately following initial curative-intent therapy.[5] SOR C
- In patients following curative-intent therapy for lung cancer, the use of blood tests, FDG-PET scanning, sputum cytology, tumor markers, and fluorescence bronchoscopy is not currently recommended for surveillance.[2]

PATIENT EDUCATION

- Smoking cessation, never initiating smoking, and avoidance of occupational and environmental exposure to carcinogenic substances are recommended to reduce the risk of recurrence or a second primary in curatively treated patients. In patients with metastatic disease, although smoking cessation has little effect on overall prognosis, it may improve respiratory symptoms.

- Information about local hospice services and support groups should be provided. The Lung Cancer Alliance Web site, listed in "Patient Resources" below, can be used to find support groups.

PATIENT RESOURCES

- Information for patients can be accessed at the Web site of National Cancer Institute—**http://www.cancer.gov/cancertopics/types/lung.**
- More information for patients can be accessed from—**http://www.mayoclinic.com/health/lung-cancer/DS00038.**
- American Lung Association—**http://www.lungusa.org.**
- Support groups for patients and families can be found at the following Web site—**http://www.lungcanceralliance.org/get-help-and-support/coping-with-lung-cancer/support-groups.html.**

PROVIDER RESOURCES

- Providers may find information on lung cancer and ongoing clinical trials at the following Web sites—**http://www.nlm.nih.gov/medlineplus/lungcancer.html** and **http://www.cancer.gov/cancertopics/types/lung.**

REFERENCES

1. Centers for Disease Control and Prevention. *Lung Cancer Statistics.* http://www.cdc.gov/cancer/lung/statistics/index.htm. Accessed January 2012.
2. National Cancer Institute. *SEER Stat Fact Sheets: Lung and Bronchus.* http://seer.cancer.gov/statfacts/html/lungb.html. Accessed January 2012.
3. Centers for Disease Control and Prevention. *Basic Information About Lung Cancer.* http://www.cdc.gov/cancer/lung/basic_info/index.htm. Accessed January 2012.
4. National Cancer Institute. *Non-Small Cell Lung Cancer Treatment (PDQ).* http://cancer.gov/cancertopics/pdq/treatment/non-small-cell-lung/healthprofessional. Accessed January 2012.
5. Minna JD. Neoplasms of the lung. In: Kasper DL, Braunwald E, Fauci AS, Hauser SL, Longo DL, Jameson, JL eds. *Harrison's Principles of Internal Medicine.* 16th ed. New York, NY: McGraw-Hill; 2005:506-516.
6. Olsson AC, Gustavsson P, Kromhout H, et al. Exposure to diesel motor exhaust and lung cancer risk in a pooled analysis from case-control studies in Europe and Canada. *Am J Respir Crit Care Med.* 2011;183(7):941-948.
7. Chlebowski RT, Schwartz AG, Wakelee H, et al. Oestrogen plus progestin and lung cancer in postmenopausal women (Women's Health Initiative trial): a post-hoc analysis of a randomised controlled trial. *Lancet.* 2009;374(9697):1243-1251.
8. Goldstraw P, Ball D, Jett JR, et al. Non-small-cell lung cancer. *Lancet.* 2011;378(9804):1727-1740.
9. Dacic S. Molecular diagnostics of lung carcinomas. *Arch Pathol Lab Med.* 2011;135(5):622-629.
10. Rosell R, Moran T, Queralt C, et al. Screening for epidermal growth factor receptor mutations in lung cancer. *N Engl J Med.* 2009;361(10):958-967.
11. Ray CE Jr, English B, Funaki BS, et al. Expert Panel on Interventional Radiology. ACR Appropriateness Criteria biopsies of thoracic nodules and masses. Reston, VA: American College of Radiology (ACR); 2011:7. http://www.guideline.gov/content.aspx?id=32616&search=lung+neoplasm. Accessed February 2012.
12. Yasufuku K, PierreA, Darling G, et al. A prospective controlled trial of endobronchial ultrasound-guided transbronchial needle aspiration compared with mediastinoscopy for mediastinal lymph node staging of lung cancer. *J Thorac Cardiovasc Surg.* 2011;142(6):1393-1400.e1.
13. Ravenel JG, Mohammed TH, Movsas B, et al., Expert Panel on Thoracic Imaging and Radiation-Oncology-Lung. ACR Appropriateness Criteria non-invasive clinical staging of bronchogenic carcinoma. Reston, VA: American College of Radiology (ACR); 2010:11. http://www.guideline.gov/content.aspx?id=32627&search=lung+neoplasm. Accessed February 2012.
14. Maziak DE, Darling GE, Inculet RI, et al. Positron emission tomography in staging early lung cancer: a randomized trial. *Ann Intern Med.* 2009;151(4):221-228, W-48.
15. Fischer B, Lassen U, Mortensen J, et al. Preoperative staging of lung cancer with combined PET-CT. *N Engl J Med.* 2009;361(1):32-39.
16. Goldstraw P, Crowley J, Chansky K, et al. The IASLC Lung Cancer Staging Project: proposals for revision of the TNM stage grouping in the forthcoming (seventh) edition of the TNM Classification of malignant tumours. *J Thorac Oncol.* 2007;2(8):706-714.
17. Temel JS, Greer JA, Muzikansky A, et al. Early palliative care for patients with metastatic non-small-cell lung cancer. *N Engl J Med.* 2010;363(8):733-742.
18. Parsons A, Daley A, Begh R, Aveyard P. Influence of smoking cessation after diagnosis of early stage lung cancer on prognosis: systematic review of observational studies with meta-analysis. *BMJ.* 2010 Jan 21;340:b5569.
19. NSCLC Meta-analysis Collaborative Group, Arriagada R, Auperin A, Burdett S, et al. Adjuvant chemotherapy, with or without postoperative radiotherapy, in operable non-small-cell lung cancer: two meta-analyses of individual patient data. *Lancet.* 2010;375(9722):1267-1277.
20. Burdett S, Stewart L, Rydzewska L. Chemotherapy and surgery versus surgery alone in non-small cell lung cancer. *Cochrane Database of Syst Rev.* 2007;(3):CD006157.
21. Zhang X, Zhang J, Xu J, et al. Maintenance therapy with continuous or switch strategy in advanced non-small cell lung cancer: a systematic review and meta-analysis. *Chest.* 2011;140(1):117-126.
22. vanMeerbeeck JP, Fennell DA, DeRuysscher DKM. Small-cell lung cancer. *Lancet.* 2011;378(9804):1741-1755.
23. Murphy RA, Mourtzakis M, Chu QS, et al. Nutritional intervention with fish oil provides a benefit over standard of care for weight and skeletal muscle mass in patients with nonsmall cell lung cancer receiving chemotherapy. *Cancer.* 2011;117(8):1775-1782.
24. Murthy RA, Mourizakis M, Chu QS, et al. Supplementation with fish oil increases first-line chemotherapy efficacy in patients with advanced nonsmall cell lung cancer. *Cancer.* 2011;117(16):3774-3780.
25. Carr LL, Finigan JH, Kern JA. Evaluation and treatment of patients with non-small cell lung cancer. *Med Clin North Am.* 2011;95(6):1041-1054.
26. Scott WJ, Howington J, Feigenberg S, et al. American College of Chest Physicians. Treatment of non-small cell lung cancer stage I and

stage II: ACCP evidence-based clinical practice guidelines (2nd ed). *Chest*. 2007 Sep;132(suppl 3): S234-S242. http://www.guideline.gov/content.aspx?id=11415&search=lung+cancer. Accessed February 2012.

27. Manser R, Wright G, Hart D, Byrnes G, Campbell D. Surgery for local and locally advanced non-small cell lung cancer. *Cochrane Database Syst Rev*. 2005;25(1):CD004699.
28. Gewanter RM, Movsas B, Rosenzweig KE, et al. Expert Panel on Radiation Oncology-Lung. ACR Appropriateness Criteria nonsurgical treatment for non-small-cell lung cancer: good performance status/definitive intent. Reston, VA: American College of Radiology (ACR); 2010:11. http://www.guideline.gov/content.aspx?id=23840&search=lung+cancer+acr. Accessed February 2012.
29. Decker RH, Langer CJ, Movsas B, et al., Expert Panel on Radiation Oncology-Lung. ACR Appropriateness Criteria postoperative adjuvant therapy in non-small-cell lung cancer. Reston, VA: American College of Radiology (ACR); 2010:10. http://www.guideline.gov/content.aspx?id=32607&search=lung+cancer+acr. Accessed February 2012.
30. Non-Small Cell Lung Cancer Collaborative Group. Chemotherapy and supportive care versus supportive care alone for advanced non-small cell lung cancer. *Cochrane Database Syst Rev*. 2010;(5):CD007309.
31. Pelayo Alvarez M, Gallego Rubio Ó, Bonfill Cosp X, Agra Varela Y. Chemotherapy versus best supportive care for extensive small cell lung cancer. Cochrane Database Syst Rev. 2009;(4):CD001990.
32. Lester JF, MacBeth F, Toy E, Coles B. Palliative radiotherapy regimens for non-small cell lung cancer. *Cochrane Database Syst Rev*. 2006;(4):CD002143.
33. Rothwell PM, Fowkes FG, Belch JF, et al. Effect of daily aspirin on long-term risk of death due to cancer: analysis of individual patient data from randomised trials. *Lancet*. 2011;377(9759):31-41.
34. United States Preventive Services Task Force. *Lung Cancer Screening*. http://www.uspreventiveservicestaskforce.org/uspstf/uspslung.htm. Accessed January 2012.
35. Oken NM, Hocking WG, Kvale PA, et al.; PLCO Project Team. Screening by chest radiograph and lung cancer mortality: the Prostate, Lung, Colorectal, and Ovarian (PLCO) randomized trial. *JAMA*. 2011;306(17):1865-1873.
36. National Lung Screening Trial Research Team, Aberle DR, Adams AM, Bery CD, et al. Reduced lung-cancer mortality with low-dose computed tomographic screening. *N Engl J Med*. 2011;365(5):395-409.
37. Croswell JM, Baker SG, Marcus PM, et al. Cumulative incidence of false-positive test results in lung cancer screening: a randomized trial. *Ann Intern Med*. 2010;152(8):505-512.
38. Kozower BD, Sheng S, O'Brien SM, et al. STS database risk models: predictors of mortality and major morbidity for lung cancer resection. *Ann Thorac Surg*. 2010;90(3):875-881.
39. Fry WA, Menck HR, Winchester DP. The National Cancer Data Base report on lung cancer. *Cancer*. 1996;77(9):1947-1955.

58 PLEURAL EFFUSION

Satish Chandolu, MD

PATIENT STORY

A 63-year-old woman with a 48 pack-year smoking history and lung cancer that was diagnosed 1 year ago with metastasis involving mediastinal lymph nodes presents with shortness of breath for the past 3 days. She also admits to experiencing cough with no sputum production and orthopnea. She was admitted 3 months previous for a similar problem, at which time she was diagnosed with a malignant pleural effusion and was treated with therapeutic thoracentesis. On examination, she is noted to have dullness to percussion on the right side of her chest, with the dullness extending from the right base to the apex, and decreased breath sounds and vocal fremitus on the same side. Chest radiography shows a pleural effusion extending to the apex of the lung on the right side of her chest (**Figure 58-1**). She is admitted to the hospital and is put on a PleurX catheter drain; within several hours, her dyspnea resolves.

INTRODUCTION

The pleural space exists between the visceral and parietal pleura, which normally has about 10 mL of fluid. A pleural effusion is the presence of an excess amount of fluid in the pleural space. Pleural fluid is formed by capillaries and drained by lymphatics in the same parietal pleura.[1] The lymphatics in parietal pleura have the capacity to drain 20 times more fluid than the capillaries in the periphery.

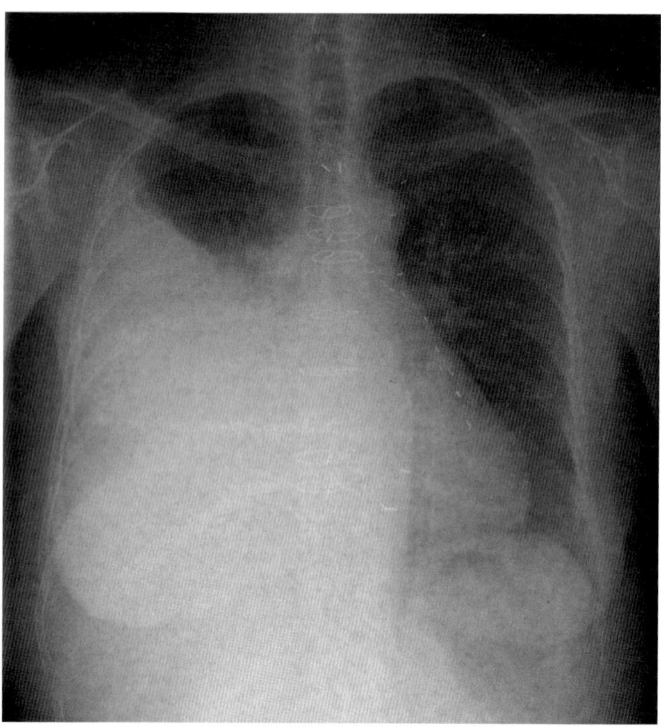

FIGURE 58-1 A posteroanterior chest radiograph demonstrating a large pleural effusion in the right hemithorax from a pulmonary malignancy. *(Reproduced with permission from Gary Ferenchick, MD.)*

SYNONYMS

- Hydrothorax
- Parapneumonic effusion
- Chylothorax—lymphatic fluid (chyle) accumulating in the pleural cavity
- Empyema—pus in the pleural cavity

ETIOLOGY/PATHOPHYSIOLOGY

- Conditions that can decrease the oncotic pressure, leading to a transudate, include the following:
  - Cirrhosis
  - Nephrotic syndrome
  - Peritoneal dialysis
  - Myxedema
- Conditions that can increase hydrostatic pressure, leading to a transudate, include the following:
  - Congestive heart failure (CHF)
  - Pulmonary embolism
  - Superior vena cava obstruction
- Conditions that can disrupt the vessel wall, leading to exudates, include the following:
  - Trauma (including esophageal rupture)
  - Any infection
  - Collagen vascular disorders
  - Malignancy
  - Iatrogenic
  - Lymphatic abnormalities
  - Treatments (certain drugs and chemotherapy)
  - Intra-abdominal conditions (exudate)
  - Pancreatic disease
  - Intra-abdominal abscesses
  - Diaphragmatic hernia
  - After abdominal surgery
  - Endoscopic variceal sclerotherapy
  - After liver transplant
- Fluid may also accumulate from visceral pleura or from the abdomen (through diaphragmatic openings).

DIAGNOSIS

HISTORY/SYMPTOMS

Based on the etiology, the patient may present with the following:

- shortness of breath,
- orthopnea,
- paroxysmal nocturnal dyspnea,
- chest pain,
- cough,
- fever,
- chills,
- weight loss, or
- abdominal distention

PHYSICAL EXAMINATION

- Inspection may show tracheal deviation to the opposite side of pleural effusion depending on the onset and severity of the effusion.
- Palpation, depending on the etiology, may show tenderness of the chest or abdomen.
- Percussion will show a stony dullness at the site of involvement. If the abdomen is involved, fluid thrill or shifting dullness may be present.
- Auscultation will reveal decreased breath sounds at the site of pleural involvement, and egophony may be heard at the air-fluid level.

IMAGING

- Chest radiography (both posteroanterior [PA] and lateral) is the most useful test for diagnosing a pleural effusion.
    - Based on the etiology, it can show bilateral or unilateral effusion.
    - Typically, about 300 mL of fluid are necessary to appreciate a pleural effusion in the PA film, but a lateral decubitus film can detect as little as 50 mL fluid.[2]
    - The other advantage of a decubitus radiograph is to differentiate loculated effusion from free fluid.
    - The typical radiographic signs of pleural effusion include blunting of the costophrenic (ie, the angle between pleura and diaphragm) and cardiophrenic (ie, the angle between heart borders and diaphragm) angles, opacity caused by fluid (**Figure 58-2**). Depending on the etiology, radiography also may show left atrial enlargement and prominent pulmonary vasculature (if the cause is cardiac), infiltrate or cavity changes (eg, parapneumonic effusions), or lymph node enlargement.
- Thoracic computed tomographic (CT) scanning is most sensitive in diagnosing fluid in the thorax and can detect as little as 10 mL of fluid (**Figure 58-3**). CT can also detect underlying lung infiltrate, suggesting parapneumonic effusion, thickened pleura, splitting of pleura, pleural calcifications, lung abscess, empyema, hemothorax, or liver cirrhosis and helps in guiding thoracentesis.[3]
- Thoracic ultrasound can help in identification of free fluid from loculated fluid and helps differentiating the latter with solid masses.[4]

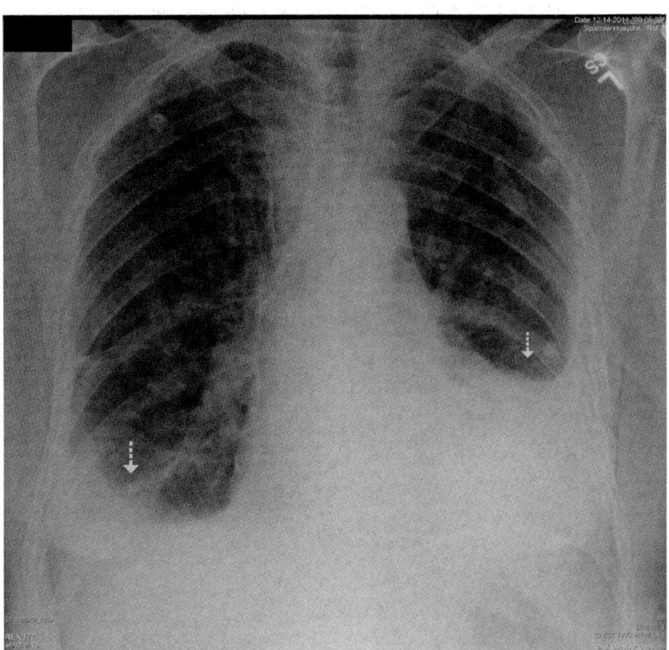

FIGURE 58-2 A chest radiograph demonstrating bilateral pleural effusion in a patient with cirrhosis. Note the meniscal sign at the costophrenic angle (yellow arrows). Also note the prominent horizontal fissure on the right from fluid in the fissure (*red arrow*). (*Reproduced with permission from Gary Ferenchick, MD.*)

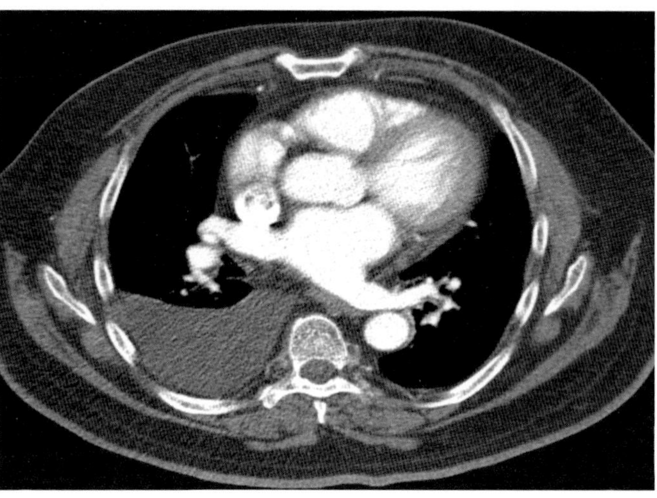

FIGURE 58-3 A chest computed tomographic scan demonstrating an effusion measuring more than 10 mm from the lung to the chest wall. (*Reproduced with permission from Gary Ferenchick, MD.*)

LABORATORY TESTING

- Thoracentesis is a procedure to remove fluid from the pleural space. It can be diagnostic or therapeutic.
- Diagnostic thoracentesis is indicated if the cause of effusion is not clear.
- Pleural fluid analysis may differentiate a transudate from an exudate. This differentiation and fluid analysis are crucial in planning a specific treatment.
- Light's criteria to differentiate transudate from exudative effusions include the following[5]:

Parameter	Transudate	Exudate
Pleural fluid protein/serum protein	<0.5	>0.5
Pleural fluid LDH/serum LDH	<0.6	>0.6
Pleural fluid LDH more than two-thirds of serum LDH	No	Yes

LDH, lactate dehydrogenase.

- A transudate should meet all three criteria.
- These criteria, however, may classify nearly 25% of transudates as exudates, and if the clinical suspicion of a transudate is high, measuring the protein gradient (a difference of protein level between serum and pleural fluid) may help.
- Although the fluid is exudate per the criteria, a gradient of more than 31 g/L is almost always a transudate.

- In an exudate, further fluid analysis, including Gram stain, acid-fast bacillus (AFB) stain, glucose, amylase, pH, cytology, differential cell count, triglycerides, cholesterol, and culture, may help identify the underlying diagnosis.

- New criteria have been proposed whose diagnostic accuracy is similar to Light's criteria. Presence of at least one criterion from this list qualifies the fluid as an exudate:
  - Two-test rule[6]
    - Pleural fluid cholesterol greater than 45 mg/dL
    - Pleural fluid LDH greater than 0.45 times the upper limit of the laboratory's normal serum LDH
  - Three-test rule[6]
    - Pleural fluid protein greater than 2.9 g/dL (29 g/L)
    - Pleural fluid cholesterol greater than 45 mg/dL (1.165 mmol/L)
    - Pleural fluid LDH greater than 0.45 times the upper limit of the laboratory's normal serum LDH

MANAGEMENT

- Transudates and exudates from nonmalignant pleural effusions (NMPF) often respond to treatment of underlying disease.
- But, if the symptoms are from the pleural fluid or if the fluid persists even after the treatment of an underlying condition, a therapeutic thoracentesis may be necessary.
- Reaccumulation of fluid—Repeat thoracentesis may be needed if the fluid accumulates slowly (nearly once in a month, but no specific guidelines) and if the procedure is not burdensome to the patient.
- Pleurodesis
  - This treatment involves obliterating the pleural space by injecting talc, bleomycin, or tetracyclines to create inflammation and then fibrosis. It is necessary for fibrosis to develop between the visceral and parietal pleural space without creating a gap where fluid can reaccumulate. Chemical pleurodesis may not be successful if the pleural fluid initially accumulated rapidly (eg, hepatic hydrothorax) or if any anatomical interference (eg, trapped lung) is present.[7]
  - The efficacy of pleurodesis is high in chronic ambulatory peritoneal dialysis, yellow nail syndrome, chylothorax, nephrotic syndrome, lupus pleuritis, heart failure, and malignant pleural effusions.
- Other treatment options
  - Chest tube placement to facilitate fluid drainage and to let the underlying lung expand during the acute episode is an option when the patient has significant dyspnea from pleural effusion.
  - Indwelling catheter drainage (commonly called a "pigtail" catheter or PleurX) in the dependent part of the fluid can be used to drain fluid out intermittently[8] (**Figure 58-4**).
  - Pleuroperitoneal shunts (internal drainage) are an option.[9]
  - Pleurovenous shunts (internal drainage) can be used.
  - Surgical pleurectomy can be a treatment option.[10]

COMPLICATIONS

- Untreated fluid may become infected.
- Fluid may prevent the underlying lung from expanding, causing atelectasis or pneumonia.
- Thoracentesis may rupture blood vessels and may cause bleeding and hemothorax.
- Thoracentesis may injure underlying lung parenchyma and cause pneumothorax (**Figure 58-5**).

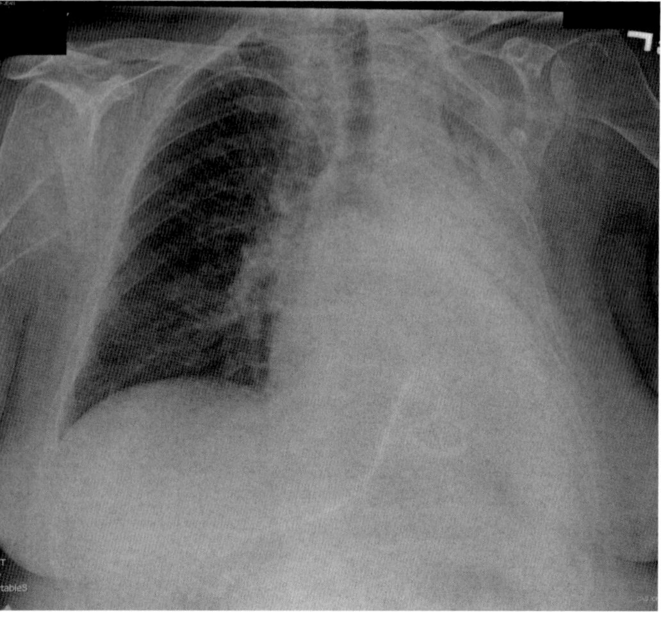

FIGURE 58-4 A chest radiograph demonstrating a massive left pleural effusion with a "whiteout" and a pigtail indwelling catheter at the bottom of the left lung (*arrow*). (*Reproduced with permission from Gary Ferenchick, MD.*)

- Pleurodesis from talc may cause an acute inflammatory reaction, including a systemic inflammatory response.
- Pleurodesis may fail if lungs are not well expanded during the process of sclerosis.

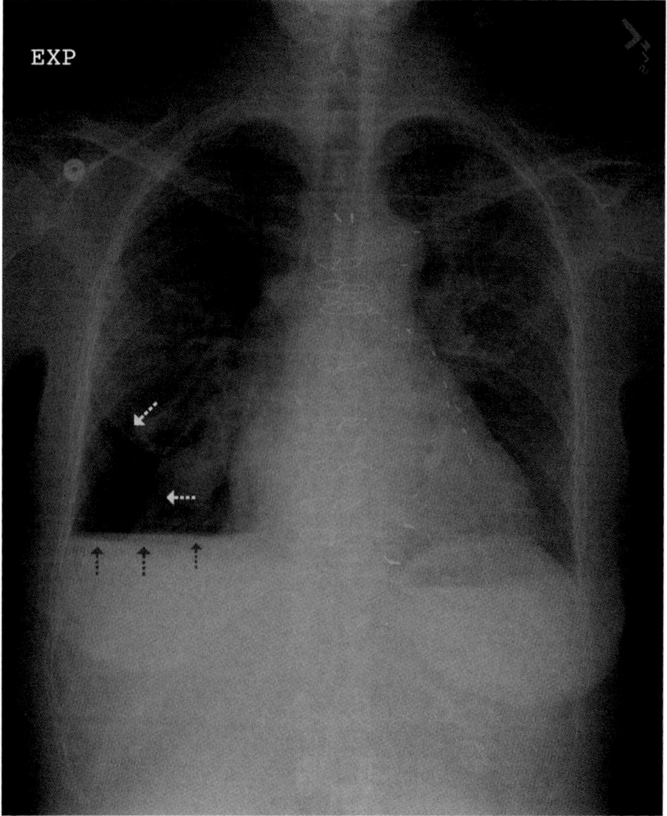

FIGURE 58-5 A chest radiograph demonstrating a combination of pneumothorax (*yellow arrows*) and a hydrothorax (*red arrows*) in a 62-year-old woman with an iatrogenic pneumothorax. (*Reproduced with permission from Gary Ferenchick, MD.*)

SPECIAL SITUATIONS

- Congestive heart failure
  - CHF commonly produces bilateral effusions.
  - If a unilateral effusion is present in a patient with CHF, perform thoracentesis and assess pleural fluid N-terminal pro-brain natriuretic peptide (NT-proBNP); if it is greater than 1500 pg/mL, this is virtually diagnostic of an effusion secondary to CHF.
- Parapneumonic effusions
  - The possibility of a parapneumonic effusion should be considered whenever a patient with bacterial pneumonia is initially evaluated.
  - If the free fluid separates the lung from the chest wall by more than 10 mm, a therapeutic thoracentesis should be performed. Consider the following factors for determining therapeutic thoracentesis in parapneumonic effusions[11]:
    - Loculated pleural fluid
    - Pleural fluid pH less than 7.20
    - Pleural fluid glucose less than 3.3 mmol/L (<60 mg/dL)
    - Positive Gram stain or culture of the pleural fluid
    - Presence of gross pus in the pleural space
  - If the fluid recurs after the initial therapeutic thoracentesis and if any of the characteristics outlined are present, a repeat thoracentesis should be performed. If the fluid cannot be completely removed with the therapeutic thoracentesis, consideration should be given to inserting a chest tube and instilling a fibrinolytic agent (eg, tissue plasminogen activator, 10 mg) or performing a thoracoscopy with the breakdown of adhesions. Decortication should be considered when these measures are ineffective.
  - Flat fluid level on radiograph—This gives a clue regarding the coexisting pneumothorax. It is commonly seen in motor vehicular accident pleural effusion, and it could be from injury to the underlying lung, chest wall injury, or a rib fracture.

FOLLOW-UP

The differential diagnosis for the cause of unilateral pleural effusions is wide; therefore, once the diagnosis is made. follow-up will be driven by the underlying etiology.

PATIENT EDUCATION

- The goal of treating a pleural effusion is to remove the fluid and determine the cause of the excess fluid collection to prevent the fluid from building up in the future.
- Effusions caused by infections are treated with antibiotics, and effusions caused by heart failure are treated with diuretics, whereas effusions caused by cancer are commonly treated with drainage with a chest tube and simultaneously treating the cancer.

PATIENT RESOURCES

- PubMed Health. *Pleural Effusion*—**http://www.ncbi.nlm.nih.gov/pubmedhealth/PMH0001150/.**
- Medline Plus. *Pleural Effusion*—**http://www.nlm.nih.gov/medlineplus/ency/article/000086.htm.**

PROVIDER RESOURCES

- BTS Guidelines. *Investigation of a Unilateral Pleural Effusion in Adults: British Thoracic Society Pleural Disease Guideline 2010*—**http://www.brit-thoracic.org.uk/Portals/0/Guidelines/PleuralDiseaseGuidelines/Pleural%20Guideline%202010/Pleural%20disease%202010%20investigation.pdf.**

REFERENCES

1. Broaddus VC, Everitt JI, Black B, Kane AB. Non-neoplastic and neoplastic pleural endpoints following fiber exposure. *J Toxicol Environ Health B Crit Rev.* 2011;14(1-4):153–178. Published online 2011 June 2. doi: 10.1080/10937404.2011.556049.
2. Stark P. The pleura. In: *Radiology. Diagnosis Imaging, Intervention,* Taveras JM, Ferrucci JT, eds. Philadelphia, PA: Lippincott Williams and Wilkins, 2000:1-29.
3. Moskowitz H, Platt RT, Schachar R, Mellins H. Roentgen visualization of minute pleural effusion. An experimental study to determine the minimum amount of pleural fluid visible on a radiograph. *Radiology.* 1973;109(1):33-35.
4. Moore CL, Copel JA. Point-of-care ultrasonography. *N Engl J Med.* 2011;364(8):749-757.
5. Light RW, Macgregor MI, Luchsinger PC, Ball WC Jr. Pleural effusions: the diagnostic separation of transudates and exudates. *Ann Intern Med.* 1972;77(4):507-513.
6. Heffner JE, Brown LK, Barbieri CA. Diagnostic value of tests that discriminate between exudative and transudative pleural effusions. Primary Study Investigators. *Chest.* 1997;111(4):970-980.
7. Huggins JT, Sahn SA, Heidecker J, Ravenel JG, Doelken P. Characteristics of trapped lung: pleural fluid analysis, manometry, and air-contrast chest CT. *Chest.* 2007;131(1):206-213.
8. Pollak JS. Malignant pleural effusions: treatment with tunneled long-term drainage catheters. *Curr Opin Pulm Med.* 2002;8(4):302-307.
9. Genc O, Petrou M, Ladas G, Goldstraw P. The long-term morbidity of pleuroperitoneal shunts in the management of recurrent malignant effusions. *Eur J Cardiothorac Surg.* 2000;18(2):143-146.
10. Nakas A, Martin Ucar AE, Edwards JG, Waller DA. The role of video assisted thoracoscopic pleurectomy/decortication in the therapeutic management of malignant pleural mesothelioma. *Eur J Cardiothorac Surg.* 2008;33(1):83-88.
11. Colice GL, Curtis A, Deslauriers J, et al. Medical and surgical treatment of parapneumonic effusions: an evidence-based guideline. *Chest.* 2000;118(4):1158-1171.

59 COMMUNITY-ACQUIRED PNEUMONIA

Mindy A. Smith, MD, MS

PATIENT STORY

A 65-year-old man presents with a "terrible cough" and fever for several days. He has just returned from a business trip and has been feeling quite run down. His cough is productive with rust-colored sputum. He is otherwise healthy and is a nonsmoker. His chest X-ray (CXR) is similar to the one shown in **Figure 59-1**. He is diagnosed with probable bacterial pneumonia and is placed on antibiotics. You note that he has never had vaccinations against influenza or pneumococcus and you offer these to him at a follow-up visit when he is well.

INTRODUCTION

Pneumonia refers to an infection in the lower respiratory tract (distal airways, alveoli, and interstitium of the lung). Community-acquired pneumonia (CAP) has traditionally referred to pneumonia occurring outside of the hospital setting. More recently, a subgroup of CAP has been identified that is associated with health care risk factors (eg, prior hospitalization, dialysis, nursing home residence, immunocompromised state); this form of pneumonia has been classified as a health care–associated pneumonia (HCAP) although definitions of HCAP vary. While severity and excess mortality is associated with HCAP as well as a slight increase in multidrug-resistant (MDR) pathogens, most studies do not support either a causal relationship between MDR and excess mortality or demonstrate benefit from broad-spectrum antibiotic coverage.[1] It is likely that excess mortality is due to underlying patient-related factors (eg, older age, comorbidities, higher initial severity).[1,2]

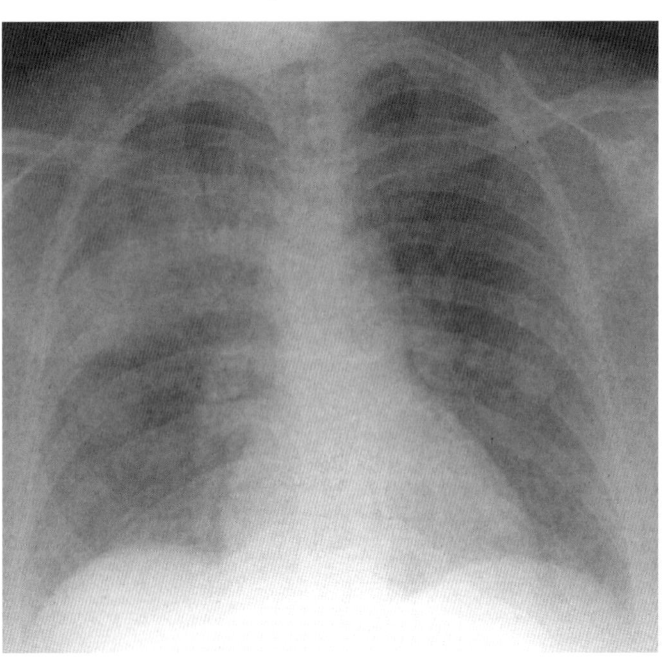

FIGURE 59-1 Chest X-ray (CXR) showing right upper lobe consolidation. *(Reproduced with permission from Miller WT Jr. Diagnostic Thoracic Imaging. New York, NY: McGraw-Hill; 2006:218, Figure 5-1 B. Copyright 2006.)*

EPIDEMIOLOGY

- Three to 4 million adults per year in United States are diagnosed with CAP (8-15/1000 persons/year).[3,4]
- Annual incidence rate of CAP requiring hospitalization is 267/100,000 population and 1014 individuals greater than 65 years of age.[5]
- About 10% to 20% of patients are admitted to the hospital.[3,4,6] Of those, 10% to 20% are admitted to the intensive care unit (ICU).[7]
- Increased incidence in men and blacks versus whites.[3]
- CAP is the most frequent cause of death due to infectious disease in the United States and the eighth leading cause of death overall (2007).[7,8]
- Economic burden associated with CAP is estimated at greater than $12 billion annually in the United States.[6]

ETIOLOGY AND PATHOPHYSIOLOGY

- In a single US hospital study, pathogens identified in adult patients with CAP separate from HCAP (N = 208) were *Streptococcus pneumoniae* (40.9%), *Haemophilus influenzae* (17.3%), *Staphylococcus aureus* (13.5%), and methicillin-resistant *S. aureus* (MRSA, 12%).[9] For HCAP, the most common pathogens were MRSA (30.6%) and *Pseudomonas aeruginosa* (25.5%). This distribution of pathogens for HCAP may be unique to this setting.[3]
- Most common route of infection is microaspiration of oropharyngeal secretions colonized by pathogens. In this setting, *S. pneumoniae* and *H. influenzae* are the most common pathogens.
- Pneumonia secondary to gross aspiration occurs postoperatively or in those with central nervous system disorders; anaerobes and gram-negative bacilli are common pathogens.
- Hematogenous spread, most often from the urinary tract, results in *Escherichia coli* pneumonia, and hematogenous spread from intravenous catheters or in the setting of endocarditis may cause S. aureus pneumonia.
- *Mycobacterium tuberculosis* (TB), fungi, *Legionella*, and many respiratory viruses are spread by aerosolization. Reported incidence rates of atypical pathogens vary greatly; for example *Legionella* species were identified in patients with CAP in 1.3% (defined as positive urine antigen),[9] 1.4% (defined as 4-fold rise in antibody titer or a single titer of ≥400),[10] and 18.9% (defined as 4-fold rise in antibody titer of 128),[11] with coinfection with another pathogen in about 10%.
- Etiology is unknown in up to 70% of cases of CAP.

RISK FACTORS

- Age greater than 70 years (relative risk [RR], 1.5 vs 60-69 year olds)[3,4,12]
- Smoking more than 20 cigarettes/d (odds ratio [OR], 2.77; 95% confidence interval [CI], 1.14-6.7)
- Alcohol consumption (RR, 9)
- Asthma (RR, 4.2), chronic bronchitis (OR, 2.22; 95% CI, 1.13-4.37) and other chronic lung diseases or pulmonary edema

- Previous respiratory infection (OR, 2.73; 95% CI, 1.75-4.26)
- Uremia
- Immune suppression (RR, 1.9)
- Malnutrition
- Acid-suppressing drugs (proton pump inhibitors and histamine-2 receptor antagonist; OR, 1.27; 95% CI, 1.11-1.46 and OR, 1.22; 95% CI, 1.09-1.36, respectively)[13]

DIAGNOSIS

The history can provide clues to the likely pathogen[3]:

- Alcoholism—Consider *S. pneumoniae, Klebsiella, S. aureus,* and anaerobes.
- Chronic obstructive pulmonary disease—Consider *S. pneumoniae, H. influenzae,* and *Moraxella*.
- Uncontrolled diabetes mellitus—Consider *S. pneumoniae* and *S. aureus*.
- Sickle cell disease—Consider *S. pneumoniae*.
- HIV with low CD4 count—*S. pneumoniae, Pneumocystis carinii, H. influenzae, Cryptococcus,* and TB.

CLINICAL FEATURES

- Constellation of symptoms includes cough, fever, chills, pleuritic chest pain, and sputum production. Patients may also complain of fatigue, myalgia, and headache.[4] Patients with viral or atypical pathogens (eg, *Mycoplasma, Chlamydia*) often present with fever, nonproductive cough, and constitutional symptoms developing over several days; patients with *Legionella* may present initially with gastrointestinal (GI) symptoms.[4]
- Signs include increased respiratory rate, dullness to percussion, bronchial breathing, egophony, crackles, wheezes, and pleural-friction rub. Lung findings in atypical pneumonia may be more diffuse.

LABORATORY STUDIES

- Sputum Gram stain may be helpful in determining the etiology in hospitalized patients. Pretreatment Gram stain and culture of expectorated sputum should be performed only if a good-quality specimen is obtained; indications are the same as for blood cultures listed below.[14] An adequate specimen has more than 25 white blood cells (WBCs) and fewer than 10 epithelial cells per high-powered field. For intubated patients with severe CAP, an endotracheal aspirate sample should be obtained.[14]
- Testing of induced sputum has established merit primarily for detection of TB and *P. carinii*. SOR Ⓐ Special stains are needed for detecting TB, *P. carinii,* and fungi.
- Routine diagnostic tests to identify an etiologic agent are optional for adult outpatients with CAP.[14] SOR Ⓒ Blood cultures should be considered in ambulatory patients with a temperature greater than 38.5°C or less than 36°C or in those who are homeless or abusing alcohol.[3] SOR Ⓒ
- Blood cultures (2 sets prior to administration of antibiotics) are suggested for hospitalized patients who meet clinical indications (ie, cavitary infiltrates, leukopenia, active alcohol abuse, chronic severe liver disease, asplenia, positive pneumococcal urinary antigen, or pleural effusion) or are admitted to the ICU.[14] SOR Ⓐ Blood cultures are positive in 6% to 20%.[3] Investigators in a Canadian study found that blood cultures had limited usefulness in the routine management of patients admitted to the hospital with uncomplicated CAP; only 1.97% (15 of 760 patients) had a change of therapy directed by blood culture results.[15]
- Urinary antigens can be useful in diagnosing Legionnaires' disease (*Legionella pneumophila*) and *S. pneumoniae* and are recommended in patients with severe CAP.[14] SOR Ⓑ
- Procalcitonin has been used in the emergency room setting to distinguish between pneumonia (increased level) and an exacerbation of asthma (area under the receiver operating characteristic curve 0.93 [95% CI, 0.88-0.98]).[16] In one study, use of guidelines including measurement of procalcitonin versus standard guidelines in patients with lower respiratory infection reduced exposure to antibiotics (mean duration 5.7 vs 8.7 days).[17]
- Pulse oximetry should be performed in patients with pneumonia and suspected hypoxemia. The presence of hypoxemia should guide decisions regarding site of care and further diagnostic testing. SOR Ⓑ

IMAGING

The diagnosis of pneumonia in adults based on clinical history and examination is only 47% to 69% sensitive and 58% to 75% specific and therefore CXR is considered a standard part of evaluation.[3,14] The presence of new infiltrate in conjunction with clinical features is diagnostic.[6] If the initial CXR is negative in a patient with clinical features of pneumonia, the CXR should be repeated in 24 to 48 hours or a chest computed tomography (CT) be considered. SOR Ⓒ Ultrasound may be useful for evaluation of pleural effusion.[18]

There are 4 general patterns of pneumonia seen on CXR[3]:

- Lobar—Consolidation involves the entire lobe (**Figures 59-1** to **59-5**). A cavity with an air-fluid level is sometimes seen within the area of consolidation representing abscess formation (see **Figure 59-5**).
- Bronchopneumonia—Patchy involvement of one or several lobes that may be extensive (**Figures 59-6** and **59-7**), usually in the dependent lower and posterior lungs (see **Figure 59-3**).
- Interstitial pneumonia—Inflammatory process involves the interstitium; usually patchy and diffuse (**Figure 59-8**). A nodular interstitial pattern is seen in patients with histoplasmosis (**Figure 59-9**), military TB, pneumoconiosis, and sarcoidosis.
- Miliary pneumonia—Numerous discrete lesions from hematogenous spread (see Chapter 64, Tuberculosis).

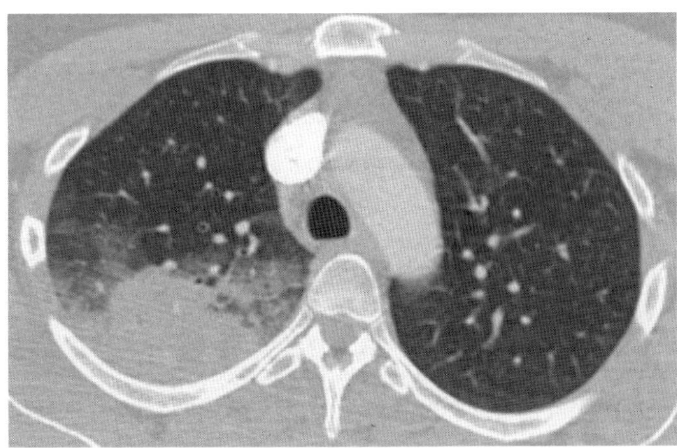

FIGURE 59-2 CT scan of the patient in **Figure 59-1** demonstrating a confluent region of lung consolidation with ground-glass opacification on the margins of the consolidated lung commonly seen in bacterial pneumonia. *(Reproduced with permission from Miller WT Jr. Diagnostic Thoracic Imaging. New York, NY: McGraw-Hill; 2006:218, Figure 5-1 C. Copyright 2006.)*

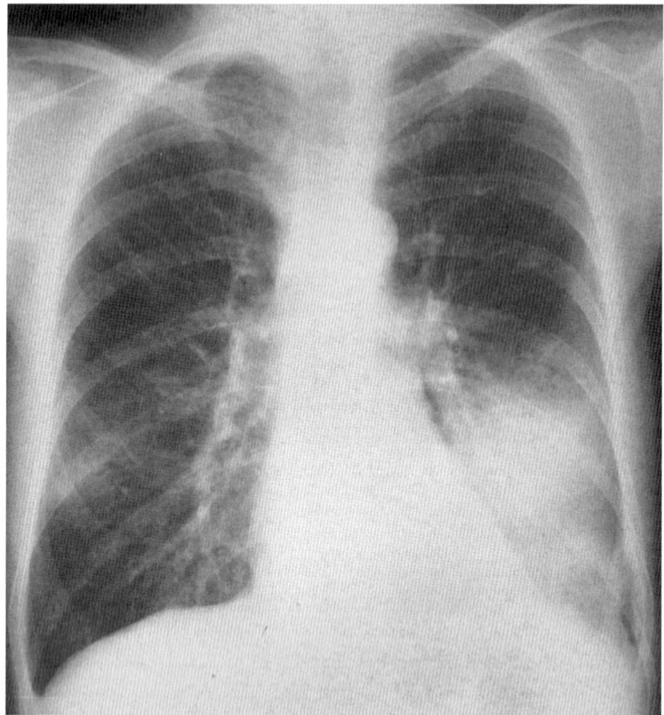

FIGURE 59-3 Posteroanterior CXR showing consolidation in the left lower lobe occupying all 3 basilar segments. There is blunting of the left costophrenic angle indicating a parapneumonic effusion. (*Reproduced with permission from Miller WT Jr.* Diagnostic Thoracic Imaging. *New York, NY: McGraw-Hill; 2006:219, Figure 5-2 C. Copyright 2006.*)

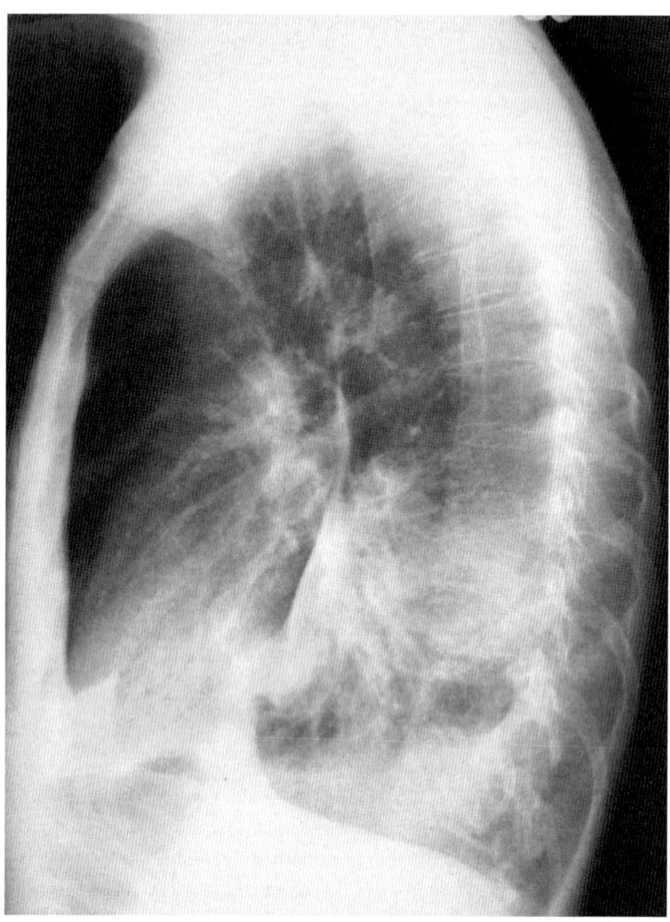

FIGURE 59-4 Lateral CXR of the patient in **Figure 59-3** showing posterior displacement of the major fissure indicating some atelectasis of the left lower lobe. (*Reproduced with permission from Miller WT Jr.* Diagnostic Thoracic Imaging. *New York, NY: McGraw-Hill; 2006:219, Figure 5-2 D. Copyright 2006.*)

DIFFERENTIAL DIAGNOSIS

- Upper respiratory illnesses, including bronchitis, can cause cough, fever, chills, and sputum production with a negative CXR.
- Pulmonary embolus should be considered in patients with pleuritic chest pain or hypoxia and a negative CXR (see Chapter 61, Pulmonary Embolus).
- Asthma can cause cough, wheezing, dyspnea, and hypoxia, whereas CXR is negative unless mucous plugging causes collapse of airways (see Chapter 55, Asthma).

MANAGEMENT

Initial determination of severity of illness is used to identify patients with CAP who may be candidates for outpatient treatment[14]:

- Respiratory rate (RR) greater than 30 breaths/min without underlying disease is the single best predictor.
- British Thoracic Society (BTS) rule—The presence of one or more of the following 4: confusion, blood urea nitrogen greater than 7 mmol/L, RR greater than 30/min, systolic blood pressure less than 90 mm Hg or diastolic blood pressure less than 60 mm Hg. If none are present, mortality rate is 2.4%; one present 8%; 2 present 23%; 3 present 33%; and all 4 present 80%.
- A number of other severity scores are available (eg, CURB-65 criteria [confusion, uremia, respiratory rate, low blood pressure, age 65 years or greater] and prognostic models such as the Pneumonia

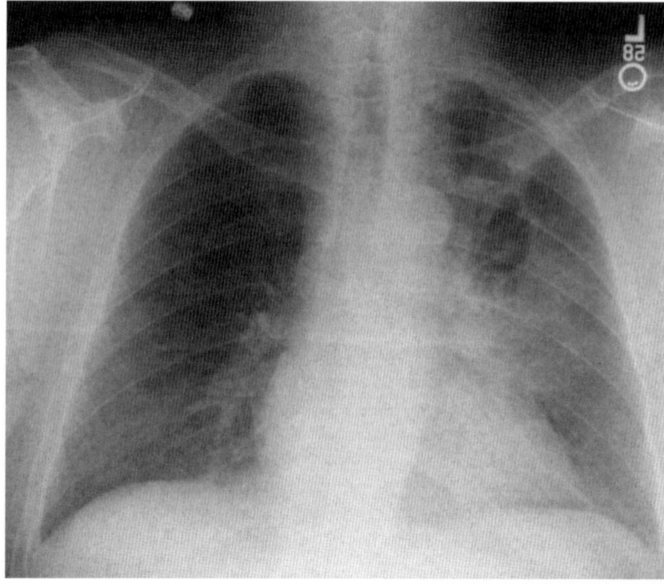

FIGURE 59-5 CXR showing a consolidation in the left upper lobe; note oval lucency that represents cavitation within the infiltrate. This patient had *Klebsiella pneumoniae*. (*Reproduced with permission from Miller WT Jr.* Diagnostic Thoracic Imaging. *New York, NY: McGraw-Hill; 2006:223, Figure 5-6 A. Copyright 2006.*)

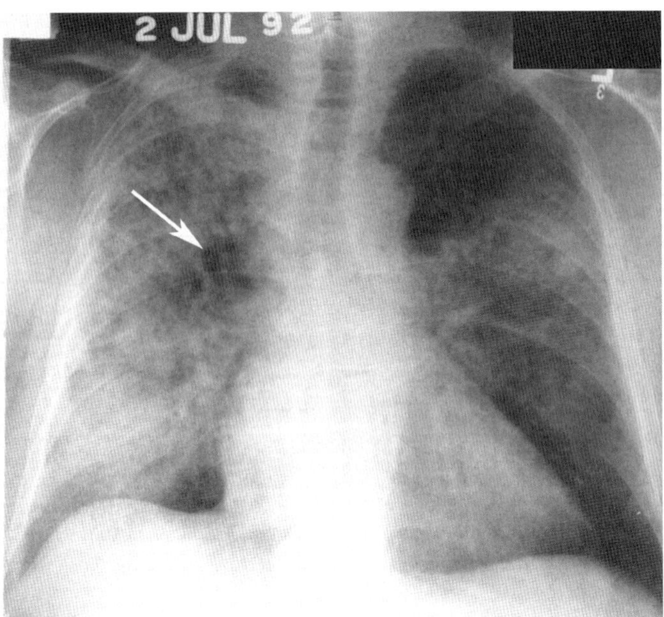

FIGURE 59-6 This patient has bilateral pulmonary infiltrates worsening despite antibiotics characteristic of severe bronchopneumonia. Note air bronchograms (arrow) on the right side. He was diagnosed with *Legionella* pneumonia. (*Reproduced with permission from Miller WT Jr.* Diagnostic Thoracic Imaging. *New York, NY: McGraw-Hill; 2006:221, Figure 5-4 B. Copyright 2006.*)

Severity Index),[4,14] but one study found that the modified BTS performed best, although they recommend validation in each clinical setting.[19]

- Assessment of oxygen consumption or hypoxia.

NONPHARMACOLOGIC

- Based on limited data, chest physiotherapy cannot be recommended as part of routine care for adults with pneumonia.[20] Positive expiratory pressure (vs no physiotherapy) and osteopathic manipulative treatment (OMT vs placebo therapy) appear to slightly reduce the duration of

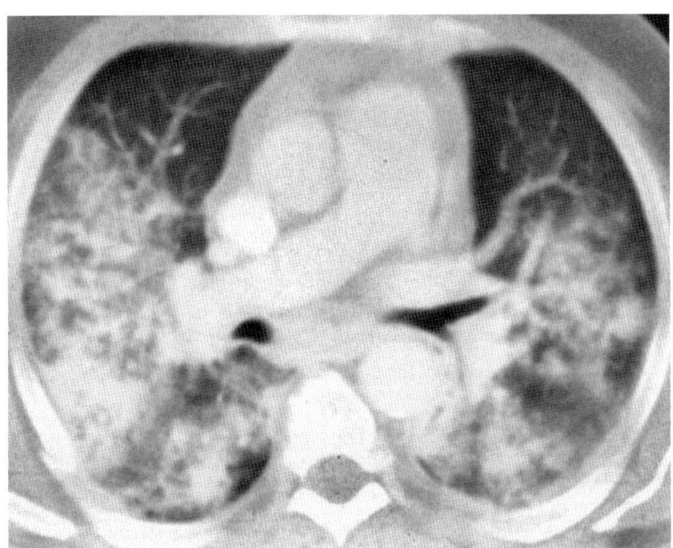

FIGURE 59-7 CT scan of the patient with *Legionella* pneumonia. In **Figure 59-6** at the level of the main pulmonary arteries showing extensive pulmonary consolidation in both lungs. (*Reproduced with permission from Miller WT Jr.* Diagnostic Thoracic Imaging. *New York, NY: McGraw-Hill; 2006:221, Figure 5-4 D. Copyright 2006.*)

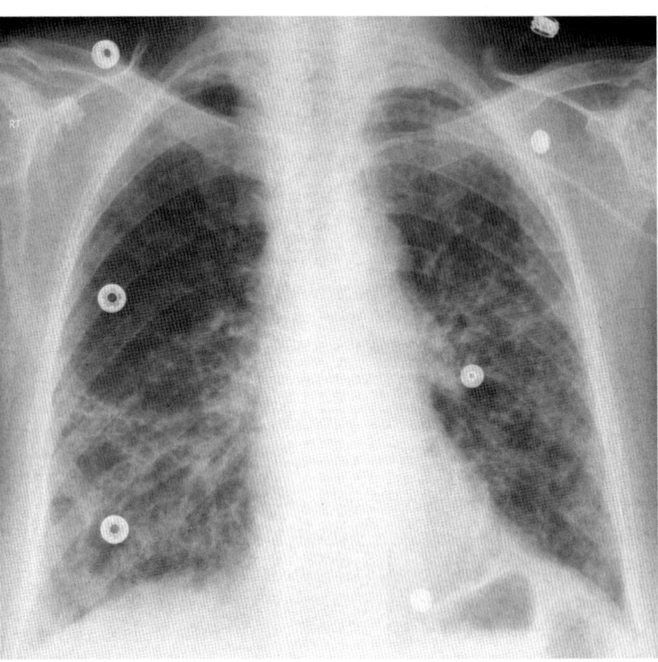

FIGURE 59-8 CXR showing basilar predominant interstitial lung disease in this 70-year-old woman; given her age, idiopathic pulmonary fibrosis is the most likely diagnosis. (*Reproduced with permission from Miller WT Jr.* Diagnostic Thoracic Imaging. *New York, NY: McGraw-Hill; 2006:81, Figure 3-10 A. Copyright 2006.*)

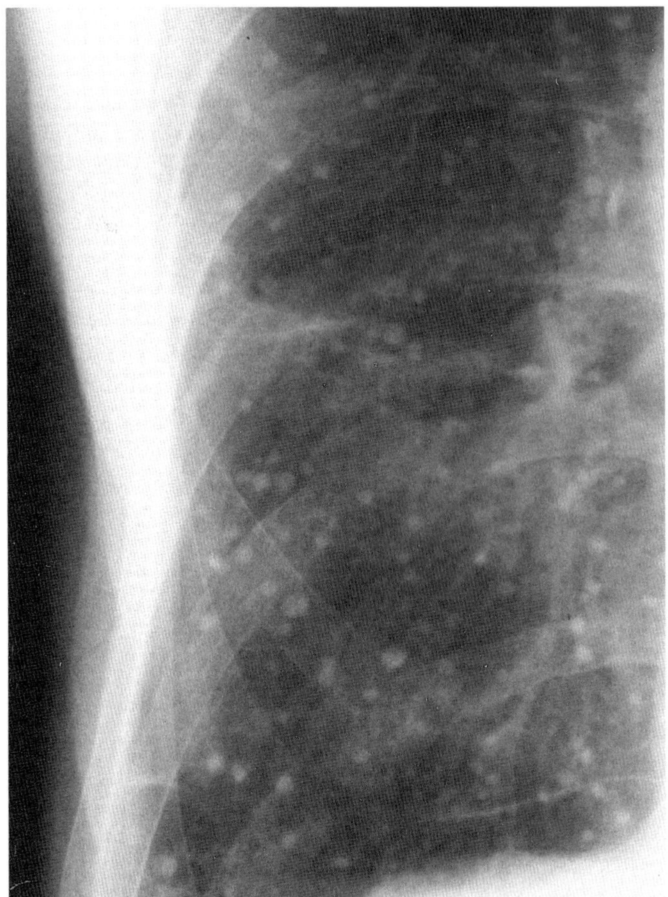

FIGURE 59-9 Nodular interstitial pattern with many calcified granulomas in a patient with histoplasmosis. (*Reproduced with permission from Schwartz DT, Reisdorff EJ.* Emergency Radiology. *New York, NY: McGraw-Hill; 2000:460, Figure 17-15. Copyright 2000.*)

hospital stay (by 2.02 and 1.4 days, respectively). OMT may also reduce duration of antibiotic use by 1 to 2 days.[20]

- The Infectious Diseases Society of America and American Thoracic Society recommend a cautious trial of noninvasive ventilation for patients with hypoxemia or respiratory distress unless they require immediate intubation because of severe hypoxemia (arterial oxygen pressure or fraction of inspired oxygen [PaO_2/FIO_2] ratio <150) and bilateral alveolar infiltrates.[14]
- One small RCT (N = 40) found continuous positive airway pressure (CPAP) delivered by helmet improved oxygenation more quickly than oxygen therapy alone (median 1.5 vs 48 hours, respectively) in patients with CAP and moderate hypoxemic acute respiratory failure.[21]

MEDICATIONS

Empiric antibiotic treatment for adults with CAP includes the following[14]:

- Outpatient, uncomplicated (previously healthy, no risk factors for drug-resistant *S. pneumoniae* [DRSP] infection)—Macrolide (erythromycin, azithromycin, or clarithromycin) SOR Ⓐ or doxycycline. SOR Ⓒ Authors of a Cochrane review did not find sufficient evidence to determine antibiotic choice for the treatment of CAP in ambulatory patients; individual study results did not demonstrate significant differences in efficacy between various antibiotics and antibiotic groups.[22]
- Outpatient with comorbidities (eg, cardiac disease, diabetes mellitus) or risk factors for DRSP—Respiratory fluoroquinolone (ie, levofloxacin [750 mg], moxifloxacin, and gemifloxacin) or β-lactam plus macrolide. SOR Ⓐ In regions with high rate (>25%) of macrolide-resistant *S. pneumoniae*, consider use of an alternate agent.
- Hospitalized patient (non-ICU)—Respiratory fluoroquinolone **or** β-lactam (preferred agents include cefotaxime, ceftriaxone, and ampicillin; ertapenem for selected patients) **plus** macrolide combination. SOR Ⓐ Doxycycline can be considered as an alternative to the macrolide. Treatment should be started in the emergency room for patients admitted from there. A Cochrane review, however, did not find benefit in survival or clinical efficacy using empirical atypical coverage (quinolone monotherapy to β-lactams or cephalosporins) in hospitalized patients with CAP.[23]
- Hospitalized patient in ICU—β-Lactam (cefotaxime, ceftriaxone, or ampicillin-sulbactam) **plus** either azithromycin SOR Ⓑ **or** a fluoroquinolone. SOR Ⓐ For penicillin-allergic patients, a respiratory fluoroquinolone and aztreonam are recommended. For *Pseudomonas* infection, an antipneumococcal, antipseudomonal β-lactam (piperacillin-tazobactam, cefepime, imipenem, or meropenem) **plus** either ciprofloxacin **or** levofloxacin (750-mg dose) **or** above β-lactam plus an aminoglycoside and azithromycin **or** above β-lactam plus an aminoglycoside and an antipneumococcal fluoroquinolone.
- If the etiology of CAP is identified on the basis of reliable microbiological methods, antimicrobial therapy should be directed at that pathogen.
- Early treatment (within 48 hours of the onset of symptoms) with oseltamivir or zanamivir is recommended for influenza A.[14]
- Duration—A minimum of 5 days. SOR Ⓐ The patient should be afebrile for 48 to 72 hours and have no more than one CAP-associated sign of instability (eg, temperature >37.8°C, tachycardia, respiratory rate >24 breaths/min, hypotension, oxygen saturation <90%, unable to maintain oral intake, altered mental status) before discontinuing antibiotics.[14]
- Dexamethasone reduced hospital length of stay (LOS) by about 1 day when added to antibiotic treatment in nonimmunocompromised patients with CAP.[24] There were no differences in in-hospital mortality or severe adverse events in this study. Steroid use increased LOS and readmission when used in patients who did not receive concomitant β-agonist therapy.

HOSPITALIZATION

For adults, severity-of-illness scores can be used to identify patients with CAP who may be candidates for outpatient treatment. SOR Ⓐ Consider hospitalization if the patients has severe CAP (CURB-65 ≥2 or BTS score >0) or has hypoxia, worsening symptoms, preexisting conditions that compromise safety of home care or for patients who fail to improve in more than 72 hours.[3,14]

PREVENTION

- Vaccination—Pneumococcal polysaccharide vaccine is recommended for persons greater than or equal to 65 years of age and for those with selected high-risk concurrent diseases.[14] SOR Ⓑ All adolescents, persons greater than or equal to 50 years of age, others at risk for influenza complications, and health care workers should be immunized annually with vaccines for influenza virus to prevent CAP.[14] SOR Ⓐ Vaccination status should be assessed at the time of hospital admission for all patients and appropriate vaccines should be offered at discharge.[14] SOR Ⓒ
- Smoking cessation assistance should be offered to patients who smoke.
- To prevent spread of respiratory pathogens, respiratory hygiene measures should be practiced.[14] These include the coughing into the elbow and use of hand hygiene and masks or tissues for patients with cough, particularly in outpatient settings and emergency departments.

PROGNOSIS

- Patients on adequate therapy for CAP should demonstrate clinical (and laboratory) signs of improvement within 48 to 72 hours.
- Outpatient mortality rate is 1%. The mortality rate for those who require admission to the hospital averages 12%, and the mortality rate for patients with severe CAP in the ICU setting approaches 40%.[3] In a multihospital study in Canada, 9% (N = 89) of patients died in hospital, 10% had died at 30 days, and 247 (26%) had died by 1 year. In-hospital mortality was higher among patients with admission hypoglycemia.[25]
- Using a large database, guideline concordant therapy for CAP (65% of cases) was associated with decreased in-hospital mortality (OR, 0.70; 95% CI, 0.63-0.77), sepsis (OR, 0.83; 95% CI, 0.72-0.96), and renal failure (OR, 0.79; 95% CI, 0.67-0.94), and reduced hospital LOS and duration of parenteral therapy (0.6 days for both).[26]

FOLLOW-UP

- Assess need and provide pneumococcal and influenza vaccination at hospital discharge and/or follow-up.
- Monitor improvement and treat comorbid illness (which may worsen).
- In adults, repeat CXR until clear if the patient is older than 40 years or smokes—2% of them may have underlying cancer.[3]

PATIENT EDUCATION

- Patients who smoke should be offered cessation assistance.
- Improvement is expected in healthy outpatients younger than 65 years in 48 to 72 hours with their returning to work or school in approximately 4 to 5 days and complete improvement within 2 weeks.
- In hospitalized patients, clinical stability is expected in 3 to 7 days; mortality is 8% with 70% developing a complication such as respiratory failure, congestive heart failure, shock, dysrhythmia, myocardial infarction, gastrointestinal bleeding, or renal insufficiency.[3]

PATIENT RESOURCES

- WebMD. *Pneumonia*—**http://www.webmd.com/lung/tc/pneumonia-topic-overview.**
- ALA. *Pneumonia*—**http://www.lung.org/lung-disease/pneumonia/.**

PROVIDER RESOURCES

- Medscape. *Bacterial Pneumonia*—**http://emedicine.medscape.com/article/300157.**

REFERENCES

1. Ewig S, Welte T, Torres A. Is healthcare-associated pneumonia a distinct entity needing specific therapy? *Curr Opin Infect Dis*. 2012 Apr;25(2):166-175.
2. Chalmers JD, Taylor JK, Singanayagam A, et al. Epidemiology, antibiotic therapy, and clinical outcomes in health care-associated pneumonia: a UK cohort study. *Clin Infect Dis*. 2011;53(2):107-113.
3. Marrie TJ, Campbell GD, Walker DH, Low DE. Pneumonia. In: Kasper DL, Braunwald E, Fauci AS, Hauser SL, Longo DL, Jameson JL, eds. Harrison's Principles of Internal Medicine. 16th ed. New York, NY: McGraw-Hill; 2005:1528-1541.
4. Butt S, Swiatlo E. Treatment of community-acquired pneumonia in an ambulatory setting. *Am J Med*. 2011;124(4);297-300.
5. Marston BJ, Plouffe JF, File TM Jr, et al; Community-Based Pneumonia Incidence Study Group. Incidence of community-acquired pneumonia requiring hospitalization: results of a population-based active surveillance study in Ohio. *Arch Intern Med*. 1997;157:1709-1718.
6. File TM Jr, Marrie TJ. Burdon of community-acquired pneumonia in North American adults. *Postgrad Med*. 2010;122(2):130-141.
7. File TM. Case studies of lower respiratory tract infections: community-acquired pneumonia. *Am J Med*. 2010;123(suppl 4):S4-S15.
8. Xu J, Kochanek MA, Murphy SL, Tejada-Vera B. Deaths: final data for 2007. *Natl Vital Stat Rep*. 2010;58(19):1-136.
9. Micek ST, Kollef KE, Reichley RM, et al. Health care-associated pneumonia and community-acquired pneumonia: a single-center experience. *Antimicrob Agents Chemother*. 2007;51(10):3568-3573.
10. Marrie TJ, Raoult D, La Scola B. Legionella-like and other amoebal pathogens as agents of community-acquired pneumonia. *Emerg Infect Dis*. 2001;7(6):1026-1029.
11. Benson RF, Drozanski WJ, Rowbatham TJ, Bialkowska I, Losos D, Butler JC. Serologic evidence of infection with 9 Legionella-like amoebal pathogens in pneumonia patients. Proceedings of the 95th ASM General Meeting. Washington, DC: USA; 1995 May 21-25:Abstract C-200. p. 35.
12. Almirall J, Bolibar I, Balanzo X, Gonzalez CA. Risk factors for community-acquired pneumonia in adults: a population-based case control study. *Eur Respir J*. 1999;13(2):349-355.
13. Eom CS, Jeon CY, Lim JW, et al. Use of acid-suppressive drugs and risk of pneumonia: a systematic review and meta-analysis. *CMAJ*. 2011;183(3):310-319.
14. Mandell LA, Wunderink RG, Anzueto A, et al. Infectious Diseases Society of America/American Thoracic Society consensus guidelines on the management of community-acquired pneumonia in adults. *Clin Infect Dis*. 2007;44(suppl 2):S27-S72.
15. Campbell SG, Marrie TJ, Anstey R, et al. The contribution of blood cultures to the clinical management of adult patients admitted to the hospital with community-acquired pneumonia: a prospective observational study. Chest. 2003;123(4):1142-1150.
16. Badfadhel M, Clark TW, Reid C, et al. Procalcitonin and C-reactive protein in hospitalized adult patients with community-acquired pneumonia or exacerbation of asthma or COPD. *Chest*. 2011;139(6):1410-1418.
17. Schuetz P, Christ-Crain M, Thomann R, et al. Effect of procalcitonin-based guidelines vs standard guidelines on antibiotic use in lower respiratory tract infections: the ProHOSP randomized controlled trial. *JAMA*. 2009;302(10):1059-1066.
18. Reynolds JH, McDonald G, Alton H, Gordon SB. Pneumonia in the immunocompetent patient, *Br J Radiol*. 2010;83(996):998-1009.
19. Buising KL, Thursky KA, Black JF, et al. Reconsidering what is meant by severe pneumonia: a prospective comparison of severity scores for community-acquired pneumonia. *Thorax*. 2006;61(5):419-424.
20. Yang M, Yan Y, Yin X, et al. Chest physiotherapy for pneumonia in adults. *Cochrane Database Syst Rev*. 2010;(2):CD006338.
21. Cosentini R, Brambilla AM, Aliberti S, et al. Helmet continuous positive airway pressure vs oxygen therapy to improve oxygenation in community-acquired pneumonia: a randomized, controlled trial. *Chest*. 2010;138(1):114-120.
22. Bjerre LM, Verheij TJM, Kochen MM. Antibiotics for community acquired pneumonia in adult outpatients. *Cochrane Database Syst Rev*. 2009;(4):CD002109.
23. Robenshtok E, Shefet D, Gafter-Gvili A, et al. Empiric antibiotic coverage of atypical pathogens for community-acquired pneumonia in hospitalized adults. *Cochrane Database Syst Rev*. 2008;(1):CD004418.
24. Meijvis SC, Hardeman H, Remmelts HH, et al. Dexamethasone and length of hospital stay in patients with community-acquired pneumonia: a randomised, double-blind, placebo-controlled trial. *Lancet*. 2011;377(9782):2023-2030.
25. Gamble JM, Eurich DT, Marrie TJ, Majumdar SR. Admission hypoglycemia and increased mortality in patients hospitalized with pneumonia. *Am J Med*. 2010;123(6):556.e11-e16.
26. McCabe C, Kirchner C, Zhang H, et al. Guideline-concordant therapy and reduced mortality and length of stay in adults with community-acquired pneumonia: playing by the rules. *Arch Intern Med*. 2009;169(16):1525-1531.

60 PNEUMOTHORAX

Joonseok Kim, MD

PATIENT STORY

A 25-year-old man with no significant past medical history presents with a sudden onset of chest pain and moderate dyspnea. His physical examination reveals normal vital signs and decreased breath sounds and hyperresonance percussion sounds on the right side. Chest radiography showed a right pneumothorax (**Figure 60-1**). He is admitted to the hospital for observation. The next day, the pneumothorax increases in size, and a chest tube is placed during hospitalization. After 3 days in the hospital, a follow-up chest radiograph reveals that his lung reexpanded, and the chest tube is removed. The patient is discharged the day after chest tube removal.

INTRODUCTION

Pneumothorax is defined as air collection in the pleural space preventing proper expansion of the lung. Spontaneous pneumothorax (SP) can occur without significant cause or with underlying lung disease.

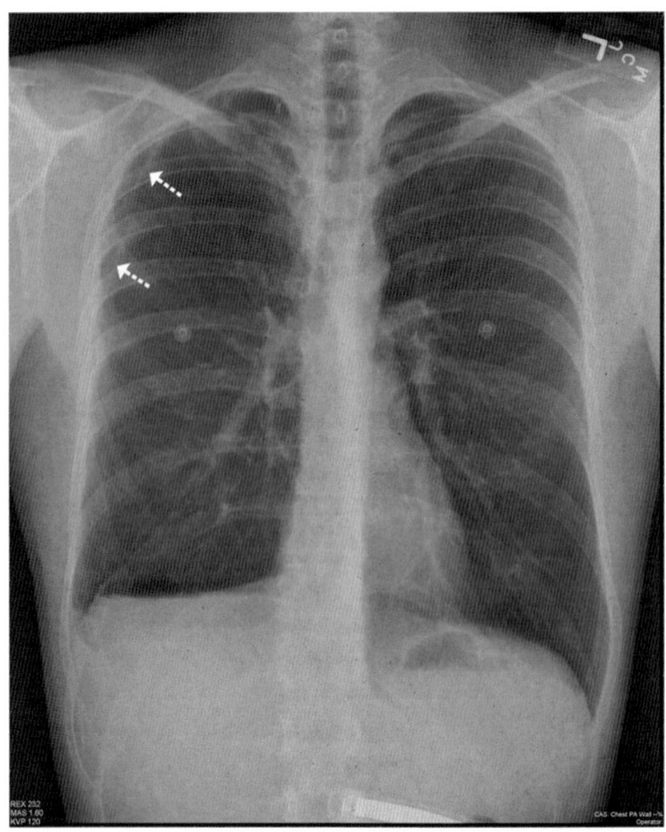

FIGURE 60-1 Primary spontaneous pneumothorax (arrows) is noted in a 25-year-old male who presented with chest pain and dyspnea. Also note the hydrothorax with fluid in the right costophrenic angle. (*Reproduced with permission from Gary Ferenchick, MD.*)

TERMINOLOGY

- Primary spontaneous pneumothorax (PSP) (without underlying lung disease)
- Secondary spontaneous pneumothorax (SSP) (with underlying lung disease)

EPIDEMIOLOGY

- Approximately 20,000 new cases of SP occur each year in the United States.
- The annual incidence of PSP is 7.4/100,000 in men and 1.2/100,000 in women.[1]
  - It is more common in younger persons, with a peak incidence between 20 and 40 years.[2]
- The annual incidence of SSP is 6.3/100,000 in men and 2.0/100,000 in women.[1]
  - The reason for these gender differences is unknown.

ETIOLOGY/PATHOPHYSIOLOGY

- PSP results from the rupture of subpleural emphysematous blebs, usually near the apex of the lungs in the upper lobes.
- The pathogenesis of PSP is attributed primarily to airway inflammation and secondarily to a hereditary predisposition to bleb formation.
- SSP is more likely to occur because of an underlying lung disease, and nearly every lung disease can be complicated by SSP.
  - Recent studies showed that chronic obstructive pulmonary disease (COPD) and *Pneumocystis carinii* pneumonia are the most common causes of SSP.
  - Other causes of SSP include asthma, cystic fibrosis, sarcoidosis, neoplasm, tuberculosis, and Marfan syndrome.
  - Less-common causes include ankylosing spondylitis, histiocytosis X, idiopathic pulmonary fibrosis, lymphangioleiomyomatosis, metastatic sarcoma, necrotizing pneumonia, and rheumatoid arthritis.
- Noniatrogenic traumatic pneumothorax may result from both penetrating and blunt trauma to the chest.
  - Pneumothorax caused by penetrating chest trauma is the result of the leakage of intrapulmonic air into the visceral pleura or the direct entry of atmospheric air into the pleural space through the injury site.
  - Pneumothorax caused by blunt chest trauma can result from rib fractures that result in visceral pleural injury.
  - Tension pneumothorax can occur in this type of pneumothorax because of a check-valve mechanism and is most common in patients on mechanical ventilation.
  - Tension pneumothorax is a medical emergency associated with hemodynamic instability and substantial mortality.
  - Of traumatic pneumothorax, 11% to 38% of cases are associated with scapular fractures.
- Iatrogenic pneumothorax may occur following various medical procedures, such as thoracentesis, central-line placement, and subacromial injections, in addition to other more invasive procedures. Reports showed that iatrogenic pneumothorax is the most common type of pneumothorax (**Figure 60-2**).

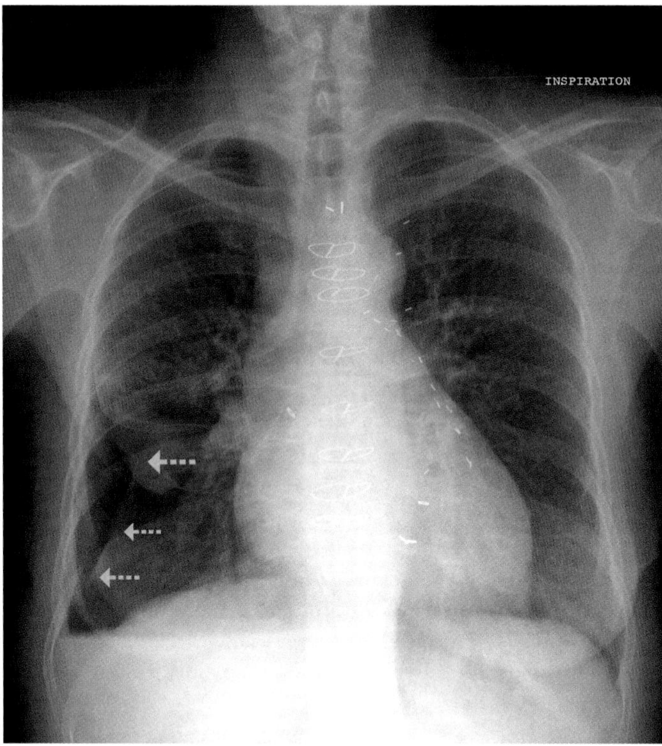

FIGURE 60-2 An example of iatrogenic pneumothorax (arrows) with collapse of the right lung and some pleural fluid remaining in the right pleural space; this occurred as a result of draining a large right pleural effusion. (*Reproduced with permission from Gary Ferenchick, MD.*)

RISK FACTORS

- Primary spontaneous pneumothorax
  - Smoking—Of PSPs, 90% occur in cigarette smokers, and the heaviest smokers have the greatest incidence. In men, heavy smokers have a 102 times higher relative risk of PSP compare to nonsmokers.[3]
  - Family history of pneumothorax is present in up to 11% of patients with PSP.
  - PSP is more common in tall, thin young males.
  - Marfan syndrome is a risk factor.
  - Thoracic endometriosis involves risk for PSP.
- SSP—Nearly every lung disease can be a risk factor.

DIAGNOSIS/CLINICAL FINDINGS

HISTORY AND PHYSICAL EXAMINATION

- Common symptoms of pneumothorax include dyspnea and pleuritic chest pain.
- PSP usually does not cause severe fluctuations in vital signs. Other than tachycardia, vital signs are usually normal.
- Patients with SSP are more likely to experience respiratory distress, cyanosis, and anxiety.

IMAGING

- The diagnosis of pneumothorax can be established by a chest radiograph showing a visceral pleural line in the lung area.

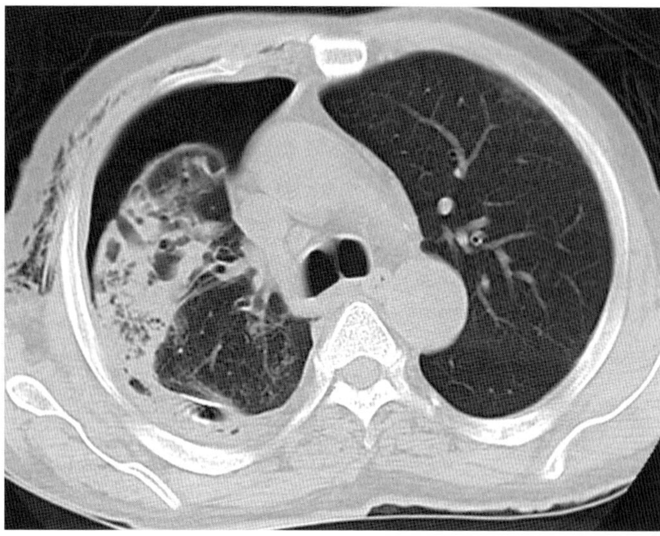

FIGURE 60-3 CT chest axial image demonstrates a spontaneous right side pneumothorax in a patient with necrotizing pneumonia and empyema secondary to *S. aureus*. (*Reproduced with permission from Carlos S. Restrepo, MD.*)

  - Additional radiographic signs include the absence of lung markings in the peripheral lung area and the presence of a white line on the inner border of that area marking the visceral pleural line.
  - The left lateral decubitus position is the most sensitive and the supine position is the least sensitive to SP. Small pneumothoraces are less than 15% or less than 2 cm from the chest wall to the outer edge of the lung as measured at the level of the hilum.
- A computed tomographic (CT) scan may be necessary in patients with a suspected pneumothorax that is difficult to visualize. The CT scan will help to differentiate pneumothorax from other problems, such as subpleural bullae. Patients with SSP especially require evaluation for underlying lung pathology (**Figure 60-3**).

MANAGEMENT

PRIMARY SPONTANEOUS PNEUMOTHORAX

According to guidelines from the British Thoracic Society[4]:

- Administration of 100% oxygen increases the rate of pneumothorax absorption by four times and should be administered to all pneumothorax patients. SOR C
- Unless there is progression of the pneumothorax, simple aspiration or insertion of a chest tube is not appropriate for most patients.
  - Up to 80% of patients who have small pneumothoraces and are not experiencing dyspnea have no persistent air leak and can be kept in the emergency department for observation for 6 hours.
  - They may be discharged if a repeat chest radiograph confirms that the pneumothorax has not progressed, and if they can easily obtain medical attention if their symptoms worsen. SOR B
- Patients who are clinically stable with large pneumothoraces should be hospitalized in most cases and undergo a procedure to have the lung reexpanded.
  - A small-bore needle (14-16 gauge) has a documented success rate from 50% to 69%. SOR A Stop the aspiration after 2.5 L of air have been aspirated as the presence of a persistent air leak is probable, and further reexpansion is unlikely.

- Seldinger chest drains (small bore < 14 F) have also been effective in reexpanding the lung.
- Finally, a 16-F to 22-F chest tube can be inserted.

- Unstable patients with large pneumothoraces should be hospitalized and have the lung reexpanded by inserting a chest catheter. SOR Ⓐ
- Patients who have persistent leakage of air lasting more than 4 days should be considered for surgery to close the air leak and a pleurodesis to prevent recurrence of pneumothorax. SOR Ⓐ
  - Open thoracotomy with pleurectomy is the procedure with the lowest recurrence rate.
  - Video-assisted thorascopic surgery (VATS) is associated with a 5% recurrence rate but is better tolerated than the open thoracotomy procedure.[4]
- The management of pain requires appropriate analgesics.

SECONDARY SPONTANEOUS PNEUMOTHORAX

- Patients who experience a pneumothorax and are older than 50 years and have a significant smoking history should be treated like patients with known lung disease.
- Patients with SSP should be hospitalized even if the SSP size is small and they are clinically stable. SOR Ⓒ Depending on their symptoms or course of pneumothorax, patients may be observed or have a chest tube inserted.
- Most patients who are clinically stable with large pneumothoraces (>2 cm from the edge of the lung to the thorax as measured at the level of the hilum) should be hospitalized and have a chest tube inserted to reexpand the lung. SOR Ⓑ
- Patients who are clinically stable with a smaller pneumothorax (1-2 cm from the edge of the lung to the thorax as measured at the level of the hilum) should be hospitalized and treated with aspiration with a 16- to 18-gauge needle cannula in an attempt to reexpand the lung, with the goal of achieving a pneumothorax of less than 1 cm. If this is not successful, then a chest tube should be inserted. SOR Ⓑ
- Unstable patients with pneumothoraces of any size should be hospitalized and have a chest tube inserted to reexpand the lung. SOR Ⓐ
- Because a secondary pneumothorax can be lethal, a procedure to prevent further pneumothorax recurrence is recommended. SOR Ⓐ Surgical thoracoscopy is the preferred method of recurrence prevention.
- Patients with persistent air leaks who refuse a surgical procedure can continue to be observed with prolonged chest tube drainage for 5 days. SOR Ⓐ
- Tension pneumothorax should always be treated by performing a large tube thoracostomy.

PROGNOSIS/CLINICAL COURSE

- The prognosis of patients with pneumothorax depends on the patient's underlying condition, severity of prior lung dysfunction, and physiological impairment from the pneumothorax itself.
  - PSP is seldom fatal.[4]
  - SSP is more dangerous than PSP and can be life threatening.
- Patients who are critically ill and those with a tension pneumothorax have the worst prognoses. Early studies showed mortality from tension pneumothorax to be 7%; delayed diagnosis increased mortality to 31%.
- The incidence of recurrent PSP is estimated to be 25% to more than 50%; most recurrences occur within 1 year of the initial event.
  - Risk factors for recurrence include male gender, tall stature, low body weight, and failure to stop smoking.[4]
  - Estimates of recurrence rates following SSP range from 39% to 47%.
- Complications associated with pneumothorax include bronchopleural fistula and pulmonary edema related to reexpansion.
  - Bronchopleural fistula is more commonly associated with SSP, traumatic pneumothorax, and pneumothorax in mechanically ventilated patients.
  - Pulmonary edema related to reexpansion is a rare complication characterized by unilateral pulmonary edema that occurs within 48 hours after lung reexpansion. Treatments include supportive management and mechanical ventilation for acute respiratory failure.

PATIENT EDUCATION

- Smokers have a higher risk of recurrence. Patients who smoke should be advised to stop smoking (see Chapter 237, Tobacco Addiction).[5] The patients who continued smoking had a higher recurrence rate (70%) than those patients who stopped smoking after the first pneumothorax (40%).[5]
- Patients are advised to avoid diving permanently unless the patient has a definite bilateral surgical pleurectomy.[4,6]
- A 1- to 2-month delay is recommended for air travelers who recovered from PSP.[7]

PATIENT RESOURCES

- Pneumothorax.org—**http://www.pneumothorax.org/.**

PROVIDER RESOURCES

- MacDuff A, Arnold A, Harvey J; BTS Pleural Disease Guideline Group. Management of spontaneous pneumothorax: British Thoracic Society pleural disease guideline 2010. Thorax. 2010;65(suppl 2): ii18-ii31. **http://thorax.bmj.com/content/65/Suppl_2/ii18.long.**

REFERENCES

1. Melton LJ III, Hepper NG, Offord KP. Incidence of spontaneous pneumothorax in Olmsted County, Minnesota: 1950 to 1974. *Am Rev Respir Dis.* 1979;120:1379-1382.
2. Abolnik IZ, Lossos IS, Gillis D, Breuer R. Primary spontaneous pneumothorax in men. *Am J Med Sci.* 1993;305:297-303.
3. Bense L, Eklund G, Wiman LG. Smoking and the increased risk of contracting spontaneous pneumothorax. *Chest.* 1987;92:1009-1012.
4. MacDuff A, Arnold A, Harvey J; BTS Pleural Disease Guideline Group. Management of spontaneous pneumothorax: British Thoracic Society pleural disease guideline 2010. *Thorax.* 2010;65(suppl 2):ii18-ii31.
5. Sadikot RT, Greene T, Meadows K, Arnold AG. Recurrence of primary spontaneous pneumothorax. *Thorax.* 1997;52:805-809.
6. Ziser A, Vaananen A, Melamed Y. Diving and chronic spontaneous pneumothorax. *Chest.* 1985;87:264-265.
7. Curtin SM, Tucker AM, Gens DR. Pneumothorax in sports: issues in recognition and follow-up care. *Phys Sportsmed.* 2000;28:23-32.

61 PULMONARY EMBOLISM

Mindy A. Smith, MD, MS

PATIENT STORY

A 52-year-old woman developed acute shortness of breath 3 weeks after a hysterectomy. She denied leg pain or swelling. She has no chronic medical problems and takes no medications. Her pulse is 105 beats/min, respiratory rate is 20 breaths/min, and the rest of her examination is unremarkable. She had an elevated hemidiaphragm on chest X-ray (CXR). These findings placed her at moderate risk for pulmonary embolism (PE) based on the Geneva score. Chest computed tomography (CT) demonstrated a moderate-sized PE similar to the one shown in **Figure 61-1**. She was treated with anticoagulation without complications.

INTRODUCTION

PE is a thromboembolic occlusion (total or partial) of one or more pulmonary arteries usually arising from a deep venous thrombosis (DVT).

EPIDEMIOLOGY

- Population estimate of the age- and sex-adjusted annual incidence of DVT is 48 per 100,000 and 69 per 100,000 for PE; the incidence increases with age.[1]

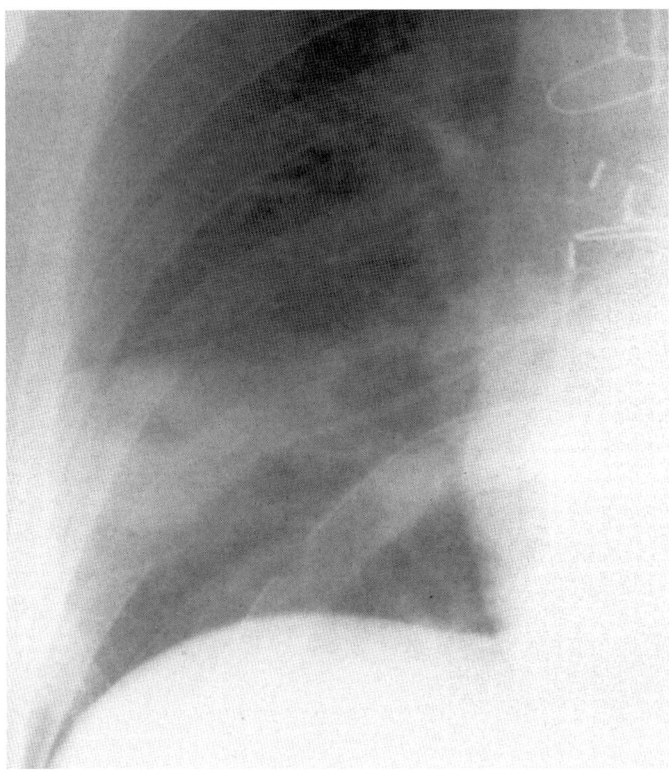

FIGURE 61-1 Chest X-ray showing a wedge-shaped pulmonary infarction with the base on the pleural surface and the apex at the tip of a pulmonary artery catheter; the catheter caused the occlusion of a peripheral artery. *(Reproduced with permission from Miller WT, Jr. Diagnostic Thoracic Imaging. New York, NY: McGraw-Hill; 2006:272, Figure 5-61, Copyright 2006.)*

- PEs are noted as incidental findings in 1% to 4% of chest CT studies.[2]
- One meta-analysis concluded that nearly 1 in every 4 to 5 patients presenting with an exacerbation of chronic obstructive pulmonary disease has a PE; presenting signs and symptoms did not distinguish patients with and without PE.[3]
- In a meta-analysis of randomized controlled trials (RCTs) of patients on venous thromboembolism (VTE) prophylaxis, the pooled rates of symptomatic DVT were 0.63% (95% confidence interval [CI], 0.47%-0.78%) following knee arthroplasty and 0.26% (95% CI, 0.14%-0.37%) following hip arthroplasty. The pooled rates for PE were 0.27% (95% CI, 0.16%-0.38%) following knee arthroplasty and 0.14% (95% CI, 0.07%-0.21%) following hip arthroplasty.[4]

ETIOLOGY AND PATHOPHYSIOLOGY

- PE is most commonly caused by embolization of a thrombus from a proximal leg or pelvic vein that enters the pulmonary artery circulation and obstructs a vessel. PE may also be caused by the following factors[1]:
    - An upper extremity thrombus (from indwelling catheters or pacemakers) (see **Figure 61-1**)
    - Fat embolus (following surgery or trauma)
    - Hair/talc/cotton embolus (from intravenous drug use)
    - Amniotic fluid embolus (from a tear at the placental margin in a pregnant woman)
- PE results from vascular endothelial injury which promotes platelet adhesion, blood flow stasis, and/or hypercoagulation causing more coagulants to accumulate than usual and resulting obstruction. Although most PEs are asymptomatic and do not alter physiology, PE can cause the following:
    - Increased pulmonary, vascular, and airway resistance (from obstruction of vessels or distal airways).
    - Impaired gas exchange (from increased dead space and right-to-left shunting).
    - Alveolar hyperventilation (from stimulation of irritant receptors).
    - Decreased pulmonary compliance (from lung edema, hemorrhage, or loss of surfactant).
    - Right ventricular (RV) dysfunction (from increased pulmonary vascular resistance, increased RV wall tension, and reduced right coronary artery flow).
    - Only about 10% of emboli cause pulmonary infarction; most PEs are multiple and involve the lower lobes.[5]

RISK FACTORS

In a population study, independent risk factors for DVT included the following[6]:

- Surgery (odds ratio [OR], 21.7; 95% CI, 9.4-49.9).
- Trauma (OR, 12.7; 95% CI, 4.1-39.7).
- Hospital or nursing home confinement (OR, 8.0; 95% CI, 4.5-14.2).
- Malignant neoplasm with (OR, 6.5; 95% CI, 2.1-20.2) or without (OR, 4.1; 95% CI, 1.9-8.5) chemotherapy.
- Central venous catheter or pacemaker (OR, 5.6; 95% CI, 1.6-19.6).
- Superficial vein thrombosis (OR, 4.3; 95% CI, 1.8-10.6). A recent study found a slightly higher OR, 6.3 (95% CI, 5-8) for DVT and 3.9 (95% CI, 3-5.1) for PE.[7]
- Neurologic disease with extremity paresis (OR, 3.0; 95% CI, 1.3-7.4).

- Other risk factors for PE include hormonal treatment (ie, combined estrogen/progestogen oral contraceptives [OCs] or menopausal hormone therapy), pregnancy, obesity, smoking, chronic obstructive pulmonary disease, immobility, bed rest for more than 3 days, and clotting disorders. In a Danish population study, the risk of venous thrombosis in current users of combined OCs decreased with duration of use (OR <1 year 4.17 [95% CI, 3.73-4.66]; OR 1-4 years 2.98 [95% CI, 2.73-3.26] and OR >4 years 2.76 [95% CI, 2.53-3.02]) and decreasing oestrogen dose.[8] OCs with desogestrel, gestodene, or drospirenone were associated with a significantly higher risk of venous thrombosis than those with levonorgestrel while progestogen-only pills and hormone-releasing intrauterine devices were not associated with an increased risk.
- Genetic predisposition includes factor V Leiden and prothrombin gene mutations.
- Use of an antipsychotic agent (particularly atypical antipsychotics) increased risk of DVT in a population nested case-control study (OR 1.32, 95% CI, 1.23-1.42).[9]

DIAGNOSIS

A history and physical examination should be completed to assess risk factors and determine whether the patient is clinically stable. If unstable (eg, hemodynamic instability [including systolic blood pressure <90 mm Hg, or a drop in 40 mm Hg], syncope, severe hypoxemia, or respiratory distress), thrombolytic therapy should be considered (**Figure 61-2**).[2,10]

Diagnostic strategy begins with the determination of a patient's (pretest) probability of PE using a clinical decision rule (see **Figure 61-2**). The 2 most frequently used rules are the Geneva and the Wells score.[11,12] Online calculators are available for the Wells score (http://www.mdcalc.com/wells-criteria-for-pulmonary-embolism-pe/. Accessed June 2013). The Geneva score appears to be the most consistent across experience of examiner;[13] and the revised Geneva scoring system performs as well as the Wells and also does not require laboratory testing or imaging.[14] A score of 0 to 3 indicates a low probability of PE (8%); 4 to 10 indicates intermediate probability of PE (28%); and greater than 10 indicates a high probability of PE (74%). The revised Geneva score is derived by summing the following points:

- Age older than 65 years (+1)
- Previous DVT or PE (+3)
- Surgery or fracture within 1 month (+2)
- Active malignant condition (+2)
- Unilateral lower limb pain (+3)
- Hemoptysis (+2)
- Heart rate 75 to 94 beats/min (+3) or greater than or equal to 95 beats/min (+5)
- Pain on lower limb deep venous palpation and unilateral edema (+4)

The Wells score is derived by summing the factors below; a score less than 2 indicates a low probability of PE (15%); 2 to 6 indicates intermediate

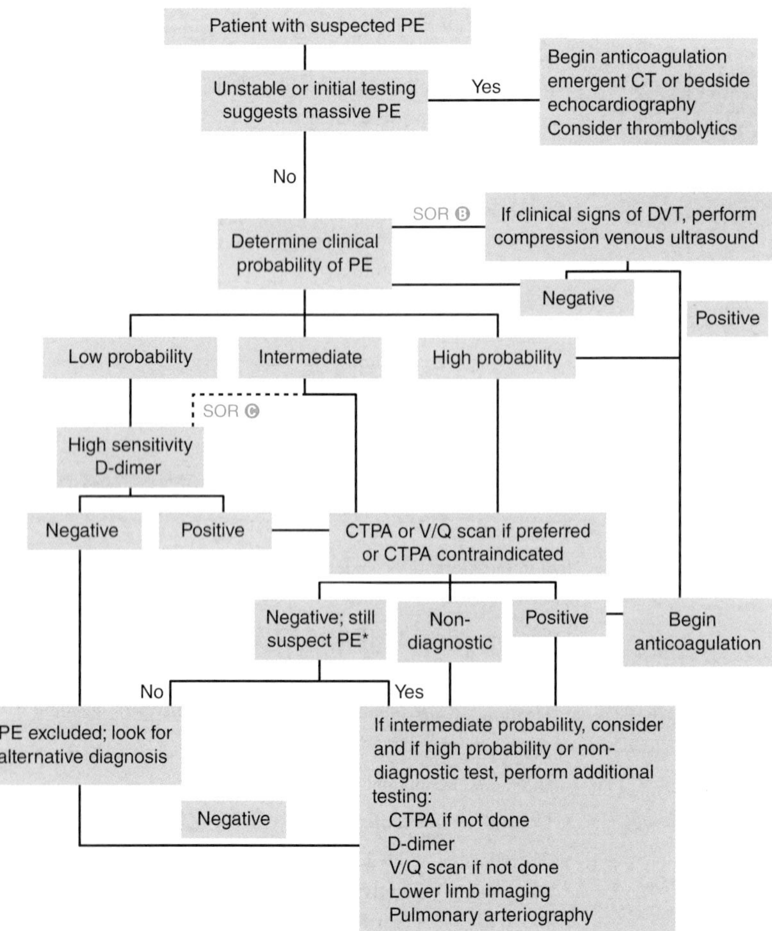

FIGURE 61-2 Approach to the patient with suspected pulmonary embolus.

probability of PE (29%); and greater than 6 indicates a high probability of PE (59%). Alternatively, the Wells score can be dichotomized as PE less likely or likely (the latter with score greater than 4)[2]:

- Clinically suspected DVT (+3)
- Alternative diagnosis is less likely than PE (+3)
- Tachycardia (+1.5)
- Immobilization or surgery in previous 4 weeks (+1.5)
- History of DVT or PE (+1.5)
- Hemoptysis (+1)
- Malignancy (treatment for within 6 months, palliative) (+1)

Patients with a high pretest probability of PE or high risk due to comorbidities (eg, pulmonary hypertension) should be started on anticoagulation during the workup.[2,10]

CLINICAL FEATURES

- Dyspnea—It is the most common symptom and tachycardia is the most common sign. Sudden onset of dyspnea is the best single predictor (positive likelihood ratio [LR+] 2.7).
- Chest pain—May be caused by a small, peripheral PE with pulmonary infarction.
- Other signs—Include fever, neck vein distention, and accentuated pulmonic component of the second heart sound.
- Massive PE—May present with shock, syncope, and cyanosis.

LABORATORY STUDIES AND ECG

- The combination of a clinical decision rule and sensitive plasma D-dimer is used to rule out PE (sensitive but not specific).[15,16] SOR B The test is suggested for patients with low or moderate probability of a PE; if low probability and negative (<500 ng/mL), there is only approximately a 0.4% chance that the patient has a PE.[14] If low or intermediate probability, a negative D-dimer concentration is associated with a posttest probability of PE below 5% (negative likelihood ratio [LR−] 0.08 [0.04-0.18]).[17] Of patients with a PE, 90% will have a value greater than 500 ng/mL. Use of an age-adjusted D-dimer (patient's age × 10 μg/L) was shown in one study to increase the percentage of patients in whom PE could be safely excluded (from 13% to 14% to 19% to 22%).[18] If the D-dimer is positive, further testing is needed (see **Figure 61-2**).[2]
- An electrocardiography (ECG) may be indicated to search for alternate diagnoses. The most frequent, sensitive, and specific ECG finding for PE is T-wave inversion in leads V_{1-4} indicative of RV strain. Other findings include tachycardia, new-onset atrial fibrillation or flutter, S in lead I, Q and inverted T in lead III, and a QRS axis greater than 90 degrees.
- An arterial blood gas is obtained if clinically indicated. A platelet count should be obtained prior to initiation of fondaparinux.[10]

IMAGING

- CXR is often nonspecific; dyspnea with a near-normal CXR should suggest PE. Findings that may be seen on CXR include the following:
  - Triad of basal infiltrate, blunted costophrenic angle, and elevated hemi-diaphragm.
  - Infiltrates similar to pneumonia (**Figure 61-3**) that may be diagnosed using CT (**Figure 61-4**).
  - A peripheral wedge-shaped density (see **Figure 61-1**).
  - Decreased vascular markings (**Figure 61-5**).
- When a patient has an intermediate or high PE probability score, PE is confirmed by a positive CT pulmonary angiography (CTPA) or high-probability lung scan and ruled out by a negative CTPA or normal lung scan (see **Figure 61-2**). The American College of Radiology (ACR) and Institute for Clinical Systems Improvement recommend CTPA over V/Q scan for patients with suspected PE, unless the former is contraindicated or nondiagnostic (see **Figure 61-2**).[2,19] CT (see **Figure 61-4**) can also provide evidence of alternate diagnoses.

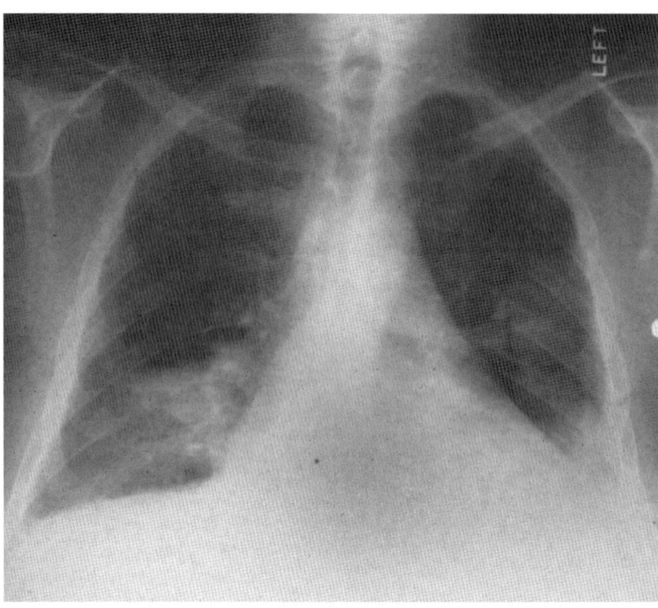

FIGURE 61-3 Chest X-ray showing bilateral pulmonary infiltrates thought to represent pneumonia. (*Reproduced with permission from Miller WT, Jr. Diagnostic Thoracic Imaging. New York, NY: McGraw-Hill; 2006:273, Figure 5-63 A, Copyright 2006.*)

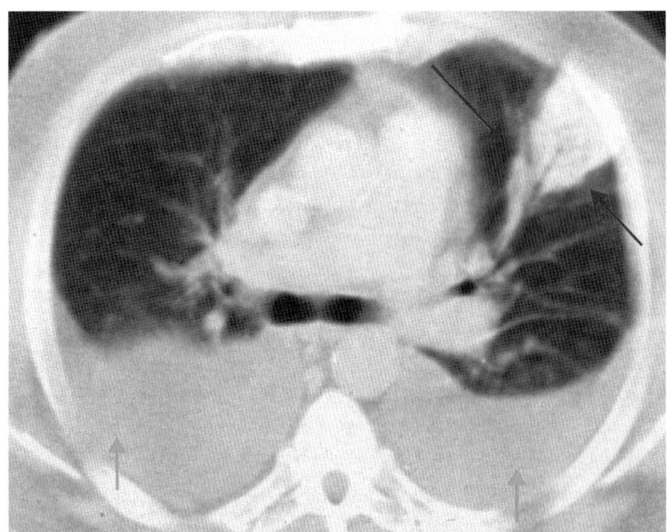

FIGURE 61-4 CT scan from the patient in Figure 61-3 demonstrates several large wedge-shaped pulmonary opacities with air bronchograms characteristic of pulmonary infarcts (red arrows). Incidentally noted is the presence of bilateral pleural effusions (green arrows). (*Reproduced with permission from Miller WT, Jr. Diagnostic Thoracic Imaging. New York, NY: McGraw-Hill; 2006:273, Figure 5-63 B, Copyright 2006.*)

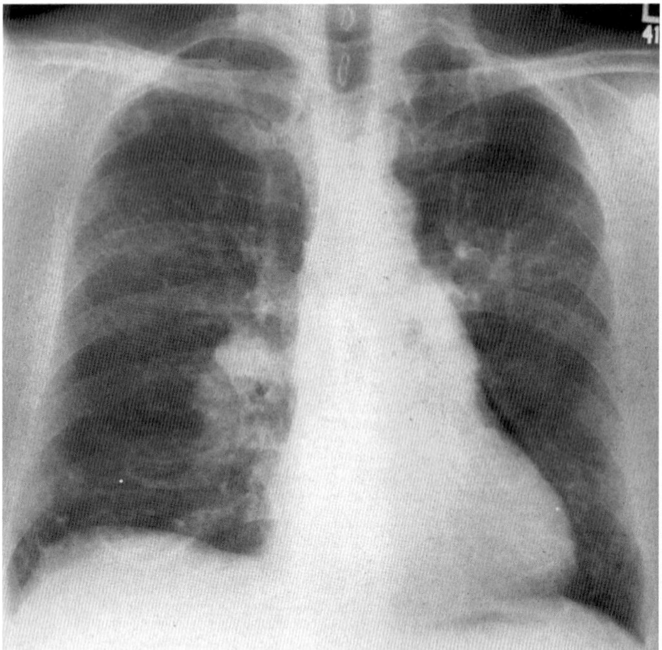

FIGURE 61-5 Pulmonary embolism: Westermark sign, an avascular zone because of obstructed vessel from a blood clot. In this patient, both lung apices and the mid-to-lower thorax have decreased vascular markings. Note the fusiform enlargement of both hila and the prominent pulmonary artery mediastinal shadow characteristic of pulmonary hypertension. (*Reproduced with permission from Miller WT, Jr. Diagnostic Thoracic Imaging. New York, NY: McGraw-Hill; 2006:748, Figure 14-19 A, Copyright 2006.*)

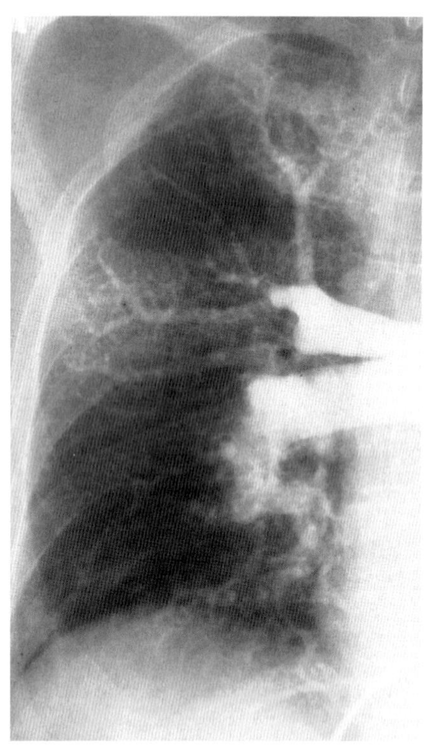

FIGURE 61-6 Pulmonary angiogram in the patient in **Figure 61-5** showing abruptly truncated pulmonary arteries associated with regions of diminished perfusion typical of chronic pulmonary emboli. (*Reproduced with permission from Miller WT, Jr. Diagnostic Thoracic Imaging. New York, NY: McGraw-Hill; 2006:748, Figure 14-19 B, Copyright 2006.*)

- A V/Q scan is considered the initial test for patients with high probability of PE who have renal insufficiency or dye allergy. A high-probability scan for PE (positive predictive value of 90%) has 2 or more segmental perfusion defects with normal ventilation.
- For pregnant women with suspected PE, the American Thoracic Society or Society of Thoracic Radiology recommend CXR as the initial study followed by lung scintigraphy (V/Q scan) if the CXR is normal and CTPA if the V/Q scan is nondiagnostic.[20]
- If the CTPA or lung scan is nondiagnostic, a leg ultrasound with compression is usually performed. If positive for a DVT, proceed with treatment as below. If normal or nondiagnostic, other testing such as a pulmonary angiogram is suggested (see **Figure 61-2**).
- Pulmonary angiography is generally reserved for patients with nondiagnostic CTPA, lung scans, or leg ultrasound and for patients who will undergo embolectomy or catheter-directed thrombolysis. ACR also recommends pulmonary angiography in circumstances where a specific diagnosis (ie, PE) is considered necessary for the proper patient management and before placement of an inferior vena cava (IVC) filter.[10] An intraluminal filling defect may be seen along with truncated arteries associated with regions of diminished perfusion (**Figure 61-6**).
- Although magnetic resonance imaging (MRI) is not indicated in the routine evaluation of suspected PE, magnetic resonance angiography (MRA) is used in certain centers with particular interest and expertise, and in patients in whom contrast administration for CTPA or pulmonary angiography is thought to be contraindicated because of renal failure, prior reaction to iodinated contrast, pulmonary hypertension or for other reasons.[19]

DIFFERENTIAL DIAGNOSIS

The differential diagnosis of a symptomatic PE includes the following:

- Pneumonia—Symptoms include chills, fever, and pleuritic chest pain (the latter 2 can occur with PE); physical findings include dullness to percussion, bronchial breathing, egophony (E-A change), and crackles with area of infiltrate or pneumonia usually confirmed on CXR (see Chapter 59, Pneumonia).
- Congestive heart failure—History of previous heart failure or myocardial infarction; symptoms of paroxysmal nocturnal dyspnea, orthopnea or the presence of bilateral lower extremity edema, third heart sound, hepatojugular reflex, and jugular venous distention. CXR may show pulmonary venous congestion, interstitial or alveolar edema, and cardiomegaly (see Chapter 44, Congestive Heart Failure).
- Pneumothorax—History of previous pneumothorax or chronic obstructive pulmonary disease, or current rib fracture; physical findings include absence of breath sounds and CXR may show free air, an elevated hemidiaphragm or a shift of the mediastinum to the contralateral side with a tension pneumothorax.

MANAGEMENT

NONPHARMACOLOGIC

- Knee-high compression stockings (30-40 mm Hg) are recommended to reduce recurrence and prevent postthrombotic syndrome.[10] SOR Ⓐ
- Psychological support may be needed.

MEDICATION

- Primary treatment of PE is considered for patients with hemodynamic instability, RV dysfunction, or infarct. In selected patients with massive PE, systemic administration of thrombolytic therapy (via a peripheral vein with a 2-hour infusion) is suggested.[2,10] SOR Ⓑ Brain natriuretic peptide and troponin testing, combined with echocardiography, can help identify patients at high risk of deterioration who would be candidates for thrombolytic therapy.[2]
- Moderate-to-large PE can be treated similarly or with anticoagulation only. In a recent Cochrane review, authors found no trials comparing thrombolytic therapy to surgical intervention and were unable to determine whether thrombolytic therapy was better than heparin for PE.[21]
- Acute PEs or proximal DVT are treated with oral anticoagulation to prevent future PE. In addition to beginning oral anticoagulation (eg, warfarin 5 mg daily, adjusted based on international normalized ratio [INR]), treatment options include intravenous unfractionated heparin (IV UFH) using a weight-based nomogram, subcutaneous (SC) low-molecular-weight heparin (LMWH; 1 mg/kg twice daily) or SC fondaparinux (a selective factor Xa inhibitor) for a minimum of 5 days.[2,10] SOR Ⓐ The American College of Chest Physicians (ACCP) recommends LMWH as first choice unless there is a massive PE, concern about SC absorption, severe renal insufficiency, or thrombolytic therapy is under consideration or planned; IV UFH is then the preferred agent.[10] If UFH is used, therapeutic levels (activated partial thromboplastin time [aPTT] 1.5-2.5 times normal) should be achieved within 24 hours.[22]
- Once the INR is therapeutic (range 2-3) (for at least 24 hours prior to discontinuing above treatment), oral anticoagulation is continued for a minimum of 3 to 12 months or indefinitely unless there is a known reversible or time-limited risk factor (eg, recent surgery) when oral anticoagulation may be discontinued after 3 months.[2,10] SOR Ⓐ For additional recommendations on duration of therapy, see the ACCP guideline.[10] A Cochrane review reported no excess recurrence of VTE after stopping therapy and while absolute risk of recurrence declines over time, the risk for major bleeding remains.[23]
- In another Cochrane review based on 15 RCTs, fixed-dose SC unfractionated heparin could not be proven noninferior to standard treatment with respect to DVT and PE at 3 months (trend favored standard arm), but was safe and effective with regard to rates of major bleeding and death.[24]
- Patients with a history of heparin-induced thrombocytopenia (HIT) should not be treated with either UFH or LMWH. Fondaparinux is an option although several cases of fondaparinux-associated HIT have been reported.[10]
- Direct thrombin inhibitors (eg, ximelagatran) appear to be as effective as LMWH in prevention of venous thromboembolism and treatment of PE, may have fewer side effects, and do not require routine monitoring. They are not considered initial therapy using current guidelines. In one trial, idraparinux was not as effective as heparin for PE treatment.[25] In another trial, oral ximelagatran was as effective as enoxaparin followed by warfarin in patients with PE.[26]

SURGERY AND PROCEDURES

Highly compromised patients who are unable to receive thrombolytic therapy or whose critical status does not allow sufficient time to infuse thrombolytic therapy may be treated with pulmonary embolectomy.[10] SOR Ⓒ In a Japanese case series of 19 patients undergoing embolectomy, most for massive or submassive PEs in the main pulmonary trunk or bilateral main pulmonary arteries, operative mortality was 5.3%.[27] No patients exhibited newly developed neurologic damage.

- IVC filter placement is reserved for patients with contraindications to anticoagulation or for failure of anticoagulation (ie, recurrence or progression of thromboembolism despite anticoagulation).[2,10] SOR Ⓒ While decreasing recurrent PE, they do not appear to improve long-term survival.
- Adjunctive therapy, if needed, includes pain relief and supplemental oxygen. RV failure or shock may be treated with dobutamine.

REFER OR HOSPITALIZE

- Consider consultation with a coagulation specialist for patients with recurrent VTE, if alternative anticoagulants are being considered, if there is an increased risk of bleeding, and for pregnant women.
- Patients with cardiovascular or respiratory compromise should be admitted to the intensive care unit. Patients with symptomatic PE are usually hospitalized due to decreased cardiopulmonary reserve.[10] One open label trial (N = 344) found no significant differences between inpatient and outpatient treatment with only 1 patient dying in each group.[28] However, 2 outpatients had major bleeding in the first 14 days and 3 by 90 days versus no patients in the inpatient group.

PREVENTION

- Mechanical methods (graduated compression stockings [GCS] and/or intermittent pneumatic compression) are recommended for thromboprophylaxis in hospitalized patients at high risk of bleeding or possibly as an adjunct to anticoagulant-based prophylaxis.[10] SOR Ⓐ For more detailed information on prophylaxis (eg, surgical or cancer patients), see the ACCP guidelines.
- A Cochrane review found GCS effective in reducing the risk of DVT in hospitalized patients from 26% without GCS to 13% with GCS and from 16% with another method of prophylaxis alone to 4% with GCS with another method of prophylaxis.[29]
- The American College of Physicians recommends assessment of thromboembolism and bleeding risk and pharmacologic prophylaxis with heparin or a related drug unless the assessed risk for bleeding outweighs the likely benefits for hospitalized nonsurgical patients. They recommend against use of GCS for routine hospitalized nonsurgical patients.[30]
- For long-distance travelers (eg, flights >8 hours) avoidance of constrictive clothing around the lower extremities or waist, maintenance of adequate hydration, and frequent calf muscle contraction are recommended.[10] SOR Ⓒ In high-risk individuals, consider use of GCS providing 15 to 30 mm Hg of pressure at the ankle or a single prophylactic dose of LMWH, injected prior to departure.[10] SOR Ⓒ

PROGNOSIS

- In a large multicenter study of patients with acute PE (N = 1880), mortality rate directly attributed to PE was 1% (95% CI, 0%-1.6%).[31] Mortality from hemorrhage was 0.2% and the all-cause 30-day mortality rate was 5.4% (95% CI, 4.4%-6.6%). Delay in initiating anticoagulation appeared to be a mortality factor as only 3 of 20 patients with fatal PE had systemic anticoagulation initiated before diagnostic confirmation; another 3 of these 20 received a fibrinolytic agent.

These figures were much improved over a 3-country registry of patients (N = 2110) with acute PE from 1999, where the 3-month mortality rate was 15.3%.[32]

- In a retrospective Japanese study of patients with PE treated surgically, the 10-year survival rate was 83.5% ± 8.7%.29.
- In one study with a rate of adverse events of 7.4% (N = 42) at 30 days following acute PE, factors associated with those events included altered mental state (OR 6.8; 95% CI, 2-23.3), shock on admission (OR 2.8; 95% CI, 1.1-7.5) and cancer (OR 2.9; 95% CI, 1.2-6.9).[33]
- In an Italian prospective cohort study of patients with DVT or PE following discontinuation of anticoagulation therapy (N = 1626), 22.9% had a recurrence of VTE.[34]
- Pulmonary hypertension develops in about 5% of patients following PE.[35]

FOLLOW-UP

- Patients on warfarin should be monitored using a standard protocol. Patients on LMWH do not require routine monitoring except for pregnant women where monitoring with anti-Xa levels is recommended.[10] SOR Ⓒ
- For patients with serious bleeding complications, management includes holding warfarin, giving vitamin K_1 10-mg slow IV plus fresh frozen plasma or prothrombin complex concentrate, and repeating vitamin K_1 every 12 hours as needed. SOR Ⓒ
- PE is slow to resolve; based on 4 imaging studies, the percentage of patients with residual pulmonary thrombi was 87% at 8 days after diagnosis, 68% after 6 weeks, 65% after 3 months, 57% after 6 months, and 52% after 11 months.[36]

PATIENT EDUCATION

- Patients taking warfarin should be instructed about the importance of remaining on oral anticoagulation for at least 3 months and use of compression stockings to decrease the likelihood of recurrence. Patients should also be counseled about the signs and symptoms of bleeding, to ask about potential drug interactions before starting a new medication, and the importance of laboratory monitoring.
- Use of an anticoagulation service or home self-monitoring[37] can be considered to improve adherence and reduce complications.
- Avoidance of periods of prolonged immobilization is suggested.

PATIENT RESOURCES

- National Heart, Lung, and Blood Institute. *Pulmonary Embolism*—**http://www.nhlbi.nih.gov/health/health-topics/topics/pe/.**

PROVIDER RESOURCES

- Medline Plus. *Pulmonary Embolism*—**www.nlm.nih.gov/medlineplus/pulmonaryembolism.html**.
- Agency for Healthcare Research and Quality. *Pulmonary Embolism*—**http://www.guideline.gov/content.aspx?id=34040.**
- Agency for Healthcare Research and Quality. *Thromboembolism in Pregnancy*—**http://www.guideline.gov/content.aspx?id=34439.**

REFERENCES

1. Silverstein MD, Heit JA, Mohr DN, et al. Trends in the incidence of deep vein thrombosis and pulmonary embolism. A 25-year population-based study. *Arch Intern Med*. 1998;158:585-593.
2. Institute for Clinical Systems Improvement (ICSI). *Venous Thromboembolism Diagnosis and Treatment*. Bloomington, MN: Institute for Clinical Systems Improvement (ICSI); 2011 Mar: 93. http://www.guideline.gov/content.aspx?id=32482&search=pulmonary+embolism. Accessed February 2012.
3. Rizkallah J, Man SF, Sin DD. Prevalence of pulmonary embolism in acute exacerbations of COPD: a systematic review and metaanalysis. *Chest*. 2009;135(3):786-793.
4. Januel JM, Chen G, Ruffieux C, et al. Symptomatic in-hospital deep vein thrombosis and pulmonary embolism following hip and knee arthroplasty among patients receiving recommended prophylaxis: a systematic review. *JAMA*. 2012;307(3):294-303.
5. Moser KM. Venous thromboembolism. *Am Rev Respir Dis*. 1990;141:235-249.
6. Heit JA, Silverstein MD, Mohr DN, et al. Risk factors for deep vein thrombosis and pulmonary embolism: a population-based case-control study. *Arch Intern Med*. 2000;160(6):809-815.
7. vanLangevelde K, Lijfering WM, Rosendaal FR, Cannegieter SC. Increased risk of venous thrombosis in persons with clinically diagnosed superficial vein thrombosis: results from the MEGA study. *Blood*. 2011;118(15):4239-4241.
8. Lidegaard Ø, Løkkegaard E, Svendsen AL, Agger C. Hormonal contraception and risk of venous thromboembolism: national follow-up study. *BMJ*. 2009 Aug 13;339:b2890.
9. Parker C, Coupland C, Hippisley-Cox J. Antipsychotic drugs and risk of venous thromboembolism: nested case-control study. *BMJ*. 2010 Sep 21;341:c4245.
10. Ansell J, Hirsh J, Hylek E, Jacobson A, Crowther M, Palareti G. Pharmacology and management of the vitamin K antagonists: American College of Chest Physicians Evidence-Based Clinical Practice Guidelines (8th ed). *Chest*. 2008;133(suppl 6):S160-S198.
11. Wicki J, Perneger TV, Junod AF, et al. Assessing clinical probability of pulmonary embolism in the emergency ward: a simple score. *Arch Intern Med*. 2001;161:92-97.
12. Wells PS, Anderson DR, Rodger M, et al. Derivation of a simple model to categorize patients probability of pulmonary embolism: Increasing the model's utility with the SimpliRED D-dimer. *Thromb Haemost*. 2000;83:416-420.
13. Iles S, Hodges AM, Darley JR, et al. Clinical experience and pretest probability scores in the diagnosis of pulmonary embolism. *Q J Med*. 2003;96:211-215.
14. Le Gal G, Righini M, Roy PM, et al. Prediction of pulmonary embolism in the emergency department: the revised Geneva score. *Ann Intern Med*. 2006;144(3):165-171.
15. American College of Emergency Physicians Clinical Policies Committee; Clinical Policies Committee Subcommittee on Suspected Pulmonary Embolism. Clinical policy: critical issues in the evaluation and management of adult patients presenting with suspected pulmonary embolism. *Ann Emerg Med*. 2003;41(2):257-270.
16. Lucassen W, Geersing GJ, Erkens PM, et al. Clinical decision rules for excluding pulmonary embolism: a meta-analysis. *Ann Intern Med*. 2011;155(7):448-460.

17. Roy PM, Colombet I, Durieux P, et al. Systematic review and meta-analysis of strategies for the diagnosis of suspected pulmonary embolism. *BMJ*. 2005 Jul 30;331(7511):259.

18. van Es J, Mos I, Douma R, et al. The combination of four different clinical decision rules and an age-adjusted D-dimer cut-off increases the number of patients in whom acute pulmonary embolism can safely be excluded. *Thromb Haemost*. 2012;107(1):167-171.

19. Bettmann MA, Lyders EM, Yucel EK, et al; Expert Panel on Cardiac Imaging. *Acute Chest Pain—Suspected Pulmonary Embolism*. Reston, VA: American College of Radiology (ACR); 2006:5. http://www.guideline.gov/content.aspx?id=35135. Accessed June 2013.

20. Leung AN, Bull TM, Jaeschke R, et al. An official American Thoracic Society/Society of Thoracic Radiology clinical practice guideline: evaluation of suspected pulmonary embolism in pregnancy. *Am J Respir Crit Care Med*. 2011;184(10):1200-1208.

21. Dong B, Hao Q, Yue J, et al. Thrombolytic therapy for pulmonary embolism. *Cochrane Database Syst Rev*. 2009;(3):CD004437.

22. Hull RD, Raskob GE, Brant RF, Pineo GF, Valentine KA. Relation between the time to achieve the lower limit of the APTT therapeutic range and recurrent venous thromboembolism during heparin treatment for deep vein thrombosis. *Arch Intern Med*. 1997;157: 2562-2568.

23. Hutten BA, Prins MH. Duration of treatment with vitamin K antagonists in symptomatic venous thromboembolism. *Cochrane Database Syst Rev*. 2006;(1):CD001367.

24. Vardi M, Zittan E, Bitterman H. Subcutaneous unfractionated heparin for the initial treatment of venous thromboembolism. *Cochrane Database Syst Rev*. 2009;(4):CD006771.

25. The van Gogh Investigators, Buller HR, Cohen AT, et al. Idraparinux versus standard therapy for venous thromboembolic disease. *N Engl J Med*. 2007;357:1094-1104.

26. Fiessinger JN, Huisman MV, Davidson BL, et al; THRIVE, Treatment Study Investigators. Ximelagatran vs low-molecular-weight heparin and warfarin for the treatment of deep vein thrombosis: a randomized trial. *JAMA*. 2005;293:681-689.

27. Fukuda I, Taniguchi S, Fukui K, et al. Improved outcome of surgical pulmonary embolectomy by aggressive intervention for critically ill patients. *Ann Thorac Surg*. 2011;91(3):728-732.

28. Aujesky D, Roy PM, Verschuren F, et al. Outpatient versus inpatient treatment for patients with acute pulmonary embolism: an international, open-label, randomised, non-inferiority trial. *Lancet*. 2011;378(9785):41-48.

29. Sachdeva A, Dalton M, Amaragiri SV, Lees T. Elastic compression stockings for prevention of deep vein thrombosis. *Cochrane Database Syst Rev*. 2010;(7):CD001484.

30. Qaseem A, Chou R, Humphrey LL, et al. Venous thromboembolism prophylaxis in hospitalized patients: a clinical practice guideline from the American College of Physicians. *Ann Intern Med*. 2011;155(9): 625-632.

31. Pollack CV, Schreiber D, Goldhaber SZ, et al. Clinical characteristics, management, and outcomes of patients diagnosed with acute pulmonary embolism in the emergency department: initial report of EMPEROR (Multicenter Emergency Medicine Pulmonary Embolism in the Real World Registry). *J Am Coll Cardiol*. 2011;57(6):700-706.

32. Goldhaber SZ, Visani L, De Rosa M. Acute pulmonary embolism: clinical outcomes in the International Cooperative Pulmonary Embolism Registry (ICOPER). *Lancet*. 1999;353:1386-1389.

33. Sanchez O, Trinquart L, Caille V, et al. Prognostic factors for pulmonary embolism: the prep study, a prospective multicenter cohort study. *Am J Respir Crit Care Med*. 2010;181(2):168-173.

34. Prandoni P, Noventa F, Ghirarduzzi A, et al. The risk of recurrent venous thromboembolism after discontinuing anticoagulation in patients with acute proximal deep vein thrombosis or pulmonary embolism. A prospective cohort study in 1,626 patients. *Haematologica*. 2007;92(2):199-205.

35. Kearon C. Natural history of venous thromboembolism. *Circulation*. 2003;107:I22-I30.

36. Nijkeuter M, Hovens MM, Davidson BL, Huisman MV. Resolution of thromboemboli in patients with acute pulmonary embolism: a systematic review. *Chest*. 2006;129:192-197.

37. Menendez-Jandula B, Souto JC, Oliver A, et al. Comparing self-management of oral anticoagulant therapy with clinic management. *Ann Intern Med*. 2005;142(1):1-10.

62 PULMONARY FIBROSIS

Gary Ferenchick, MD

PATIENT STORY

A 68-year-old man presents with dyspnea on exertion and mild intermittent cough for the previous 2 months. He is a nonsmoker and denies chronic exposure to organic or nonorganic dust. On examination, he has normal vital signs and a resting oximetry of 92%, which decreased to 87% with a 6-min walk test. His cardiac examination reveals an accentuated P2 and bilateral crackles on lung auscultation. Chest radiography reveals interstitial changes, and a high-resolution chest computed tomographic (CT) scan revealed extensive pulmonary fibrosis (**Figures 62-1** and **62-2**). Subsequent testing for connective tissue disease and hypersensitivity pneumonitis is negative. A diagnosis of idiopathic pulmonary fibrosis (IPF) is subsequently established after a lung biopsy.

INTRODUCTION

Idiopathic pulmonary fibrosis (IPF) is characterized by progressive dyspnea and a decline in lung function associated with progressive fibrosing interstitial pneumonia of unknown etiology, occurring primarily in older adults.[1] The diagnosis of IPF requires the exclusion of other causes of interstitial lung disease, including those associated with environmental exposures, medications, or connective tissue diseases.

SYNONYMS

Usual synonyms for IPF are interstitial pneumonia, cryptogenic fibrosing alveolitis, and idiopathic interstitial pneumonia.

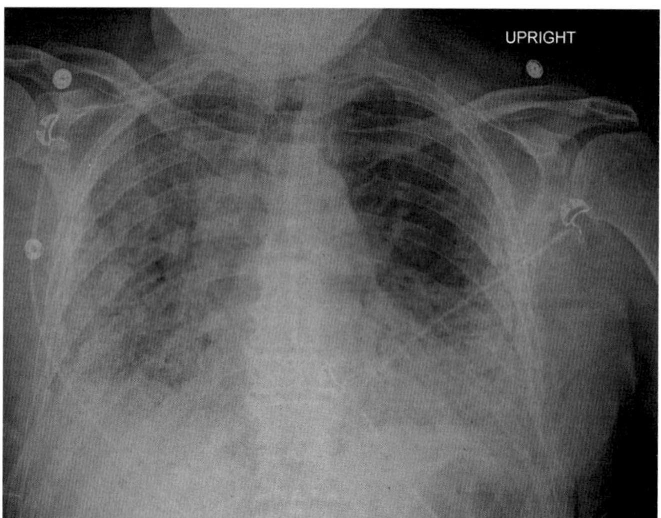

FIGURE 62-1 This chest radiograph demonstrates diffuse alveolar opacities throughout both lungs, with more consolidative changes at both bases. There is pulmonary fibrosis and a small pleural effusion on the right side. (*Reproduced with permission from Carlos Tavera, MD.*)

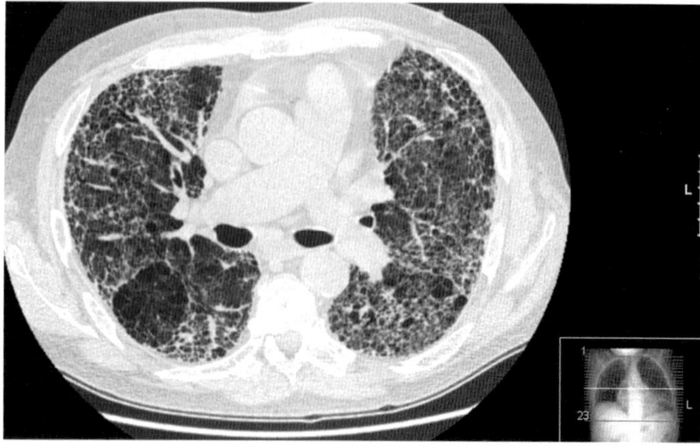

FIGURE 62-2 Chest computed tomographic scan of the same patient as in Figure 62-1 showing ground-glass consolidation of interstitial lung disease. However, the development of bilateral pleural effusions suggested a component of congestive cardiac failure. (*Reproduced with permission from Carlos Tavera, MD.*)

EPIDEMIOLOGY

The incidence of IPF is between 4.6 and 16.3 cases per 100,000 population, and prevalence is estimated to be up to 43 per 100,000 population.[1]

RISK FACTORS

- Genetic factors.
- Smoking (>20 pack-years) is strongly associated with IPF.
- Exposures to inorganic and organic particles, including metal, wood, vegetable, and animal dust may be associated with IPF.
- No definitive conclusions on the association between infectious agents (such as Epstein-Barr virus infection) and IPF can be made.
- Gastroesophageal reflux (GERD) may be a risk factor for IPF.

DIAGNOSIS

HISTORY

- A history of progressive dyspnea is the most common symptom and may be accompanied by cough.
- Symptoms are present for months to years and progress in varying degrees.
    - Wheezing and hemoptysis are unusual features.
- Evaluation for comorbid conditions and risk factors involves searching for occupational or environmental exposures, collagen vascular disease, human immunodeficiency virus (HIV) infection, use of drugs, or toxic exposures.
- A record of environmental exposure to smoking must be obtained as well as evaluation of current or previous malignancies and family history of lung disease.

PHYSICAL EXAMINATION

- Bibasilar inspiratory "Velcro" crackles are present; they may be widespread.
- Look for cor pulmonale signs with an accentuated second pulmonary sound.

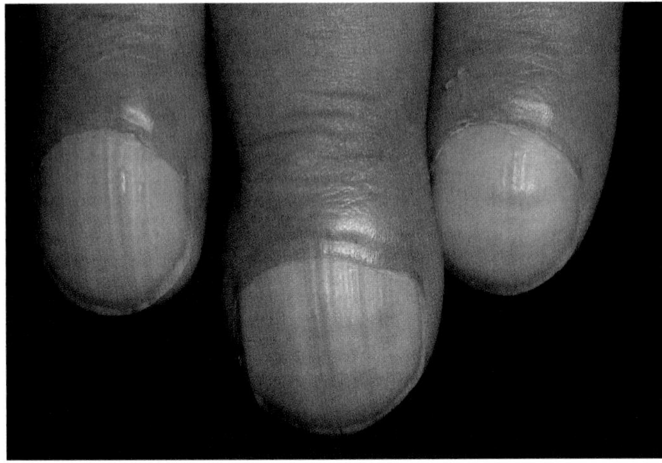

FIGURE 62-3 Clubbing showing soft-tissue swelling of the distal ends of the digits, associated with increased curvature of the nails and loss of the dorsal nail-fold angle. (*Reproduced with permission from Richard P. Usatine, MD.*)

- Clubbing is seen in 30% to35% of cases (**Figure 62-3**).
- Look for extrapulmonary findings of systemic disease (rash, joint deformities).

LABORATORY TESTING

- Serological testing to investigate for other diagnoses includes
  - Antinuclear antibody (ANA) titers, rheumatoid factor, and anticitrullinated protein antibodies (ACPA) to help identify lupus or rheumatoid arthritis as antecedent diseases. The two ACPAs include antibodies against anti-cyclic citrullinated protein (ACCP) and antimutated citrullinated vimentin (anti-MCV).
  - Elevated angiotensin-converting enzyme (ACE) levels are associated with sarcoidosis. Antibodies to organic antigens can be used to detect other explanations for fibrosis (eg, farmer's lung and bird fancier's disease).
- Spirometry is used to indicate restrictive lung disease (decreased vital capacity often with an increased ratio of forced expiratory volume in the first second of expiration and forced vital capacity [FEV1/FVC]) and impaired gas exchange (increased alveolar-arterial oxygen difference with rest or exercise or decreased lung diffusing capacity for carbon monoxide [DLCO]).
- Bronchoalveolar lavage (BAL) fluid may help to exclude infection, tumors, pulmonary alveolar proteinosis, Langerhans cell histiocytosis, hemosiderin-laden macrophages (suggesting alveolar hemorrhage), or lipid-laden macrophages (seen in aspiration from stomach or upper airway, lipid emboli, or amiodarone therapy).
- Surgical lung biopsy may establish a firm clinicopathological diagnosis that allows patients and clinicians to make informed decisions about therapy and its potential risks.

IMAGING

- Chest radiographs do not make the diagnosis of pulmonary fibrosis but are helpful in excluding other causes of breathlessness and in evaluating clinical deterioration by looking for cancer, superimposed infection, and superimposed pulmonary edema.

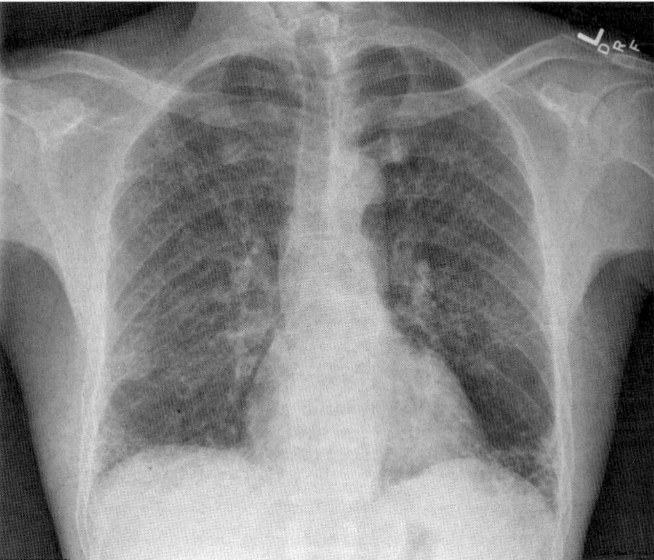

FIGURE 62-4 Note the coarsening of the interstitial marking at the lung bases (honeycombing noted in the costophrenic angles bilaterally) and upper lung fields. Also, note the large bullae at the left apex. This patient has interstitial fibrosis from rheumatoid arthritis. (*Reproduced with permission from Gary Ferenchick, MD.*)

  - A normal chest radiograph does not rule out pulmonary fibrosis in the presence of otherwise-unexplained dyspnea.
  - Typical chest radiographic changes, if present, in pulmonary fibrosis include coarse interstitial marking at the lung bases and upper lung fields (**Figure 62-4**).
- High-resolution CT (HRCT) scanning is an important test for patients with a suspected diagnosis of IPF and is highly accurate (90%-100% positive predictive value).[1] Findings include honeycombing (clusters of cystic air spaces between 3 mm and 2.5 cm) just below the pleural surface, reticular opacities, and ground-glass opacities.

DIFFERENTIAL DIAGNOSIS

- Chronic hypersensitivity pneumonitis is suggested with BAL findings of greater than 40% lymphocytosis.
- Collagen vascular diseases are associated with extrapulmonary signs and symptoms, including joint pain and positive serological studies.
  - Pulmonary fibrosis can precede other manifestations of connective tissue disease, so ordering rheumatoid factor, ACCP, and ANA studies is recommended by the American Thoracic Society (ATS).
  - Note that if the patient has established criteria for connective tissue disease, the patient does not have IPF. This should be suspected (even in the absence of established diagnostic criteria) in those younger than 50 years.
- Alveolar hemorrhage syndromes as seen in Goodpasture syndrome would be associated with a positive anti-GBM antibody.
- Occupational lung disease is suggested by exposures to dusts, silica, fumes, or radiation.
- Hypersensitivity pneumonitis is suggested by exposure to thermophilic bacteria or other animal proteins.
- Drug toxicity from drugs such as amiodarone, nitrofurantoin, and sulfasalazine, among others.

- Cryptogenic organizing pneumonia (COP)
  - The formal term is bronchiolitis obliterans obstructive pneumonia (BOOP).
  - The term *organizing pneumonia* is often used for both infectious and noninfectious etiologies.
  - There is equal gender distribution, and it can occur in nonsmokers.
  - The illness has a median presentation of less than 3 months, variable degrees of cough (may produce clear sputum), and dyspnea. Weight loss, chills, intermittent fever, and myalgias may be common.
  - On chest radiography, Bilateral or unilateral patchy peripheral consolidations and consolidations can be migratory.
  - CT—There are areas of air space consolidation in 90% of patients, and there are peribronchial distribution and bronchial dilation. Ground-glass attenuation occurs in 60% of cases.
  - The majority of patients recover on steroidal treatment: prednisone 1 to 1.5 mg/kg daily for 6 to 8 weeks.
- Acute Interstitial Pneumonia
  - Another term is Hamman-Rich syndrome, a rare fulminant form of lung injury.
  - Mean age at presentation is 50 years; there is no gender predominance, and it is not associated with smoking.
  - Onset is insidious, and there is a relentless progressive course; median time from first symptom to presentation is less than 3 weeks, often preceded by viral syndrome.
  - Consolidation and ground-glass opacification occur.
  - CT scan—Bilateral patchy areas of ground-glass attenuation sometimes occur with air space consolidation. Appearance is similar to adult respiratory distress syndrome (ARDS).
  - Most patients have moderate-to-severe hypoxia and develop respiratory failure.
  - Treatment is supportive.
  - Mortality rate is greater than 60%, with patients dying within 6 months of presentation.

MANAGEMENT

MEDICAL MANAGEMENT

- According to the ATS, "The predominance of evidence to date suggests that pharmacotherapy for IPF is without definitive, proven benefit."[1]
- The ATS strongly **recommends against** the following treatments: SOR Ⓐ
  - Corticosteroids (alone or in combination with azathioprine or cyclophosphamide), *but* note that the ATS does recommend the use of corticosteroids for acute exacerbations.
  - Colchicine
  - Cyclosporin A
  - Interferon-γ1b
  - Etanercept
- The ATS recommends against the following treatments for most patients, but these **may be reasonable in the minority of patients**: SOR Ⓒ
  - Corticosteroids in combination with azathioprine AND acetylcysteine
    - There was less decline in vital capacity and diffusing capacity at 12 months but no change in clinical outcomes in one study.
    - A recent study demonstrated an increased risk of death and hospitalization in patients with IPF treated with this combination.[2] SOR Ⓐ
  - Acetylcysteine monotherapy (as noted previously).
  - Anticoagulants (low-molecular-weight heparin followed by warfarin). Use was associated with a decrease in hospital mortality for those with acute exacerbations in one unblinded study.[3]
- Therapies without specific recommendations by the ATS include the following:
  - Sildenafil reduces pulmonary vasculature pressures in patients with IPF and pulmonary hypertension. In patients with IPF and reduced DLCO (<35% or predicted), at 12 weeks it was associated with improved dyspnea, quality of life, arterial oxygenation, and diffusing capacity.[1]
  - Imatinib is a tyrosine kinase growth factor inhibitor and is used as an antiproliferative agent. A recent study of an investigation with tyrosine kinase inhibitor (BIBF 1120) in patients with IPF was associated with a reduction in the decline of lung function, fewer acute exacerbations, and improved quality of life.[4]
- Long-term oxygen therapy in patients with IPF and resting hypoxia (saturation < 88%) is recommended.

SURGICAL MANAGEMENT

- The ATS recommends lung transplantation in selected patients as the 5-year survival after lung transplantation is about 55%.[1] SOR Ⓐ
  - There is progressive deterioration despite "optimal therapy."
  - Age is less than 60.
  - There is a diffusing capacity (DLCO) less than 39% of predicted, a decrement in FVC greater than 10% during 6 months of follow-up, a decrease in pulse oximetry below 88% saturation during a 6-min walk test, honeycombing on HRCT.

OTHER RECOMMENDATIONS

- Pulmonary rehabilitation ATS recommendations for most patients with IPF include the following[1]:
  - aerobic conditioning
  - strength and flexibility training
  - educational lectures
  - nutritional interventions
  - psychosocial support

PROGNOSIS

- The natural history of pulmonary fibrosis is unpredictable but is considered a fatal lung disease, with the majority of patients experiencing gradual worsening of symptoms and lung function.[1]
- Median survival is about 3 years from the time of diagnosis. However, other pulmonary disorders, such as chronic obstructive pulmonary disease (COPD) or pulmonary hypertension, have an impact on the course of the disease.
- Those with a worse prognosis have an increased level of dyspnea, desaturation of less than 89% during a 6-min walk test, pulmonary hypertension, and more extensive honeycombing on the HRCT at baseline and a greater than 10% decline in FVC in follow-up, among other features.[1]

FOLLOW-UP

- Patients with pulmonary fibrosis should be monitored for worsening symptoms and have resting and activity-associated oximetry tested at baseline and every 3 to 6 months.

- Other testing, including pulmonary function testing (with a change of > 10% in FVC indicating disease progression).
- A DLCO decline of 15% is also a marker of disease progression.

PATIENT RESOURCES

- American Lung Association. *Interstitial Lung Disease and Pulmonary Fibrosis*—**http://www.lung.org/lung-disease/pulmonary-fibrosis/.**
- Pulmonary Fibrosis Foundation—**http://www.pulmonaryfibrosis.org/.**
- PubMed Health. *Idiopathic Pulmonary Fibrosis*—**http://www.ncbi.nlm.nih.gov/pubmedhealth/PMH0001134/.**

PROVIDER RESOURCES

- Raghu G, Collard HR, Egan JJ, et al. An official ATS/ERS/JRS/ALAT statement: idiopathic pulmonary fibrosis: evidence-based guidelines for diagnosis and management. Am J Respir Crit Care Med. 2011;183(6):788-824. **http://ajrccm.atsjournals.org/content/183/6/788.long#content-block.**
- Medscape. *Idiopathic Pulmonary Fibrosis*—**http://emedicine.medscape.com/article/301226.**

REFERENCES

1. Raghu G, Collard HR, Egan JJ, et al. An official ATS/ERS/JRS/ALAT statement: idiopathic pulmonary fibrosis: evidence-based guidelines for diagnosis and management. Am *J Respir Crit Care Med*. 2011;183(6):788-824.
2. Idiopathic Pulmonary Fibrosis Clinical Research Network, Raghu G, Anstrom KJ, King TE Jr, Lasky JA, Martinez FJ. Prednisone, azathioprine, and N-acetylcysteine for pulmonary fibrosis. *N Engl J Med*. 2012;366(21):1968-1977.
3. Kubo H, Nakayama K, Yanai M, et al. Anticoagulant therapy for idiopathic pulmonary fibrosis. *Chest*. 2005;128(3):1475-1482.
4. Richeldi L, Costabel U, Selman M, et al. Efficacy of a tyrosine kinase inhibitor in idiopathic pulmonary fibrosis. *N Engl J Med*. 2011;365(12):1079-1087.

63 SARCOIDOSIS

Gina R. Chacon, MD

PATIENT STORY

A 39-year-old African-American woman presents with an acute onset of fever and new skin lesions on her shins that she noticed a week ago after she returned from a spring break trip. She also complains of dry cough, mild shortness of breath, feeling tired, and pain in her ankles. Her lungs are clear, and lower extremity examination reveals a number of tender 2-cm red nodules (**Figure 63-1**). Her physician recognized her leg lesions as erythema nodosum and was aware that this is found with sarcoidosis and tuberculosis. Therefore, a chest radiograph is ordered; it reveals bilateral hilar lymphadenopathy without parenchymal infiltrates. As this is consistent with sarcoidosis, workup and treatment is pursued with the provisional diagnosis of sarcoidosis. It is decided not to biopsy the erythema nodosum as the findings are nonspecific for the etiology and the leg lesions clinically support this finding.

INTRODUCTION

Sarcoidosis is a multisystem granulomatous disorder of yet unknown etiology; it predominantly involves the lungs in more than 90% of cases but can also involve any organ in the body, with the lymphatics, skin, eyes, and liver the most common.[1]

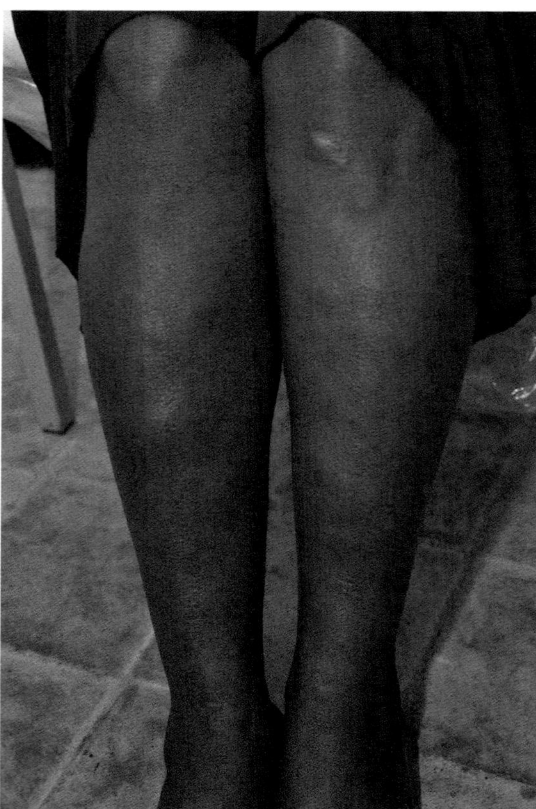

FIGURE 63-1 Erythema nodosum in a 40-year-old black woman newly presenting with sarcoidosis. Note how the erythema is less prominent because of the dark pigmentation. The nodules are clearly visible, palpable, and tender. *(Reproduced with permission from Richard P. Usatine, MD.)*

EPIDEMIOLOGY

- Sarcoidosis is a worldwide disease but with variable incidences, manifestations, and prognosis.[2]
- In the United States, the age-adjusted annual incidence rate in Caucasians is 10.9 in 100,000, and in African Americans, it is 35.5 in 100,000.[2]
- Sarcoidosis affects all ages and races and both sexes. The prevalence is slightly higher in women than in men.[3]
- Its onset is most often observed in adults under the age of 40 in both sexes, with a peak incidence between 20 and 29 years.[1]

ETIOLOGY/PATHOPHYSIOLOGY

The cause of this disease is still uncertain. Recent findings suggest that sarcoidosis may be caused by a chronic immune response produced by exposure of a genetically susceptible individual to an as-yet-undefined environmental antigenic stimulus.[4,5]

DIAGNOSIS

For an accurate diagnosis, the multimodality approach, including clinical, radiological, and histopathological evaluation is recommended.[2]

DIAGNOSTIC CRITERIA

- Sarcoidosis is characterized by the formation of well-formed, nonnecrotizing granulomas in affected organs. There are no formal diagnostic criteria for sarcoidosis, and the presence of noncaseating granulomas does not confirm the diagnosis of sarcoidosis on its own.[2]
- Sarcoidosis is a diagnosis of exclusion, and as such, other causes of granulomas, infectious and noninfectious, need to be evaluated for and ruled out.[6]

CLINICAL FEATURES

- Sarcoidosis is a multisystem disease that can affect any organ.[2]
- The clinical presentation can vary from asymptomatic organ involvement that is detected incidentally to a slowly progressive disease.
- An acute form of sarcoidosis, Löfgren syndrome, is defined as an acute onset of fever, erythema nodosum, polyarthritis, and chest radiograph showing bilateral hilar lymphadenopathy (**Figure 63-2**) with or without parenchymal infiltrates.
    - Lofgren syndrome typically portends an excellent course, with spontaneous resolution.[2,7]
    - The pulmonary system is involved in more than 90% of sarcoidosis cases followed by skin, lymph nodes, eyes, and liver.[2,8]
- In the ACCESS (A Case-Control Etiologic Study of Sarcoidosis) study, half of the sarcoidosis cohort had only 1 organ involved, 30% had 2 organs involved, 13% had 3 organs involved, and 7% had 4 or more organs involved with sarcoidosis.[8]

PULMONARY MANIFESTATIONS

- The lungs are the most common organs involved in sarcoidosis.[9]
- Patients can be asymptomatic, but more commonly they have nonspecific symptoms, such as cough, fatigue, and dyspnea on exertion.

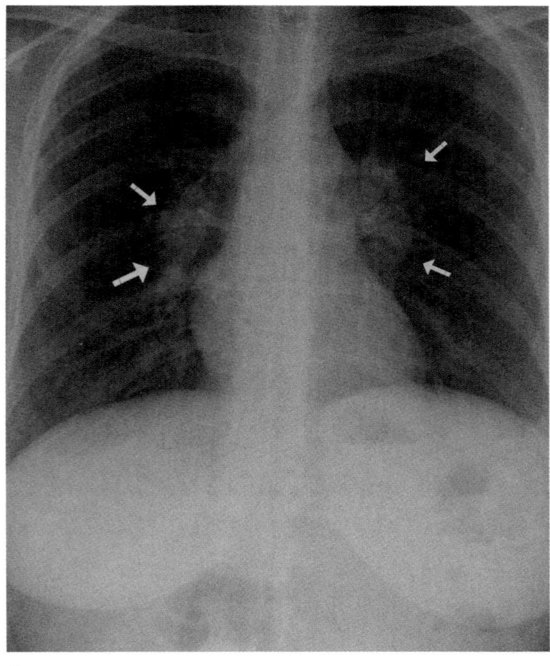

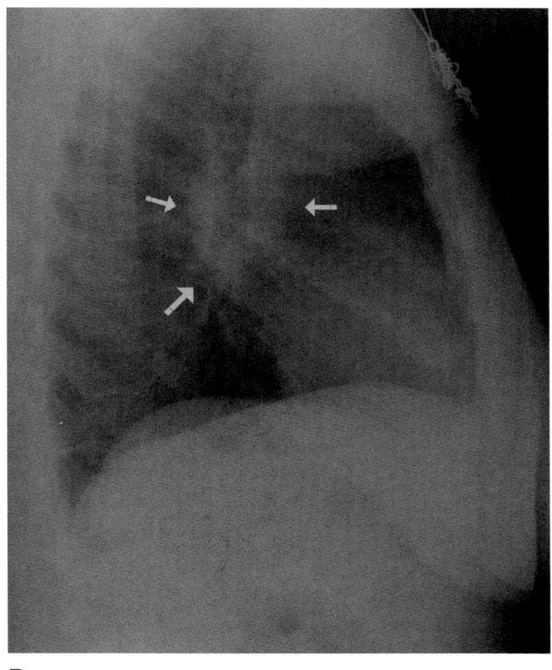

FIGURE 63-2 A. Posteroanterior and B. lateral chest radiograph showing bilateral hilar lymphadenopathy (*arrows*) without parenchymal infiltrates from a patient with sarcoidosis. (*Reproduced with permission from Gary Ferenchick, MD.*)

- On physical examination, findings can include normal pulmonary examination, dry inspiratory crackles or wheezes from airway involvement with sarcoidosis, or airway distortion from fibrotic changes.[2]

SKIN MANIFESTATIONS

- Skin is the second most common organ involved in sarcoidosis (see Chapter 173, Sarcoidosis).
- Cutaneous manifestations occur in 20%-35% of patients with sarcoidosis.[8-10]
- Sarcoidosis can present with reactive nonspecific lesions like erythema nodosum.[3,10]
- Specific lesions typically show noncaseating granulomas when biopsied.[11]
  - They include lupus pernio, papules, subcutaneous nodules, plaques, and infiltrated scars (**Figures 63-3** and **63-4**).
  - The nasal alae are common locations for the noncaseating granulomas to form (**Figure 63-5**).

EYE MANIFESTATIONS

- Ocular involvement can be seen in 10% to 80% of patients with sarcoidosis.
- The most common manifestation is anterior uveitis, but any part of the orbit or adnexa can be involved (**Figure 63-6**).[12]

GASTROINTESTINAL MANIFESTATIONS

- The liver is involved in about 30% to 80% of patients with sarcoidosis.
- Patients can be asymptomatic or complain of nonspecific abdominal pain or pruritus. Jaundice may be evident.[10,13]
- Hepatomegaly is detected clinically in 21% of cases and radiographically in more than 50% of patients.[13]

NEUROLOGIC MANIFESTATIONS

- Neurosarcoidosis affects 5% to 15% of patients.
- Any part of the nervous system can be affected, but cranial nerves are those most affected, the facial nerve being the most common, followed by the optic nerve.

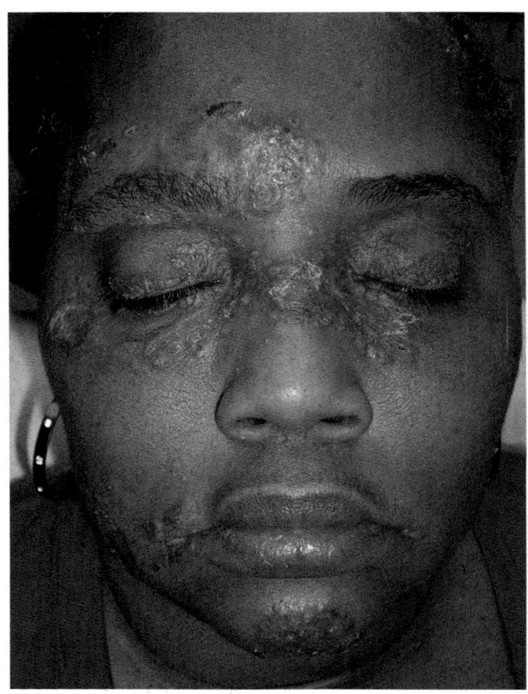

FIGURE 63-3 Sarcoidosis causing a lupus pernio pattern on the face of this African American woman with sarcoidosis. Note how some of the plaques have a malar distribution, as seen in lupus erythematosus. The patient does not have cutaneous lupus as this pattern is caused by sarcoidosis alone. (*Reproduced with permission from Richard P. Usatine, MD.*)

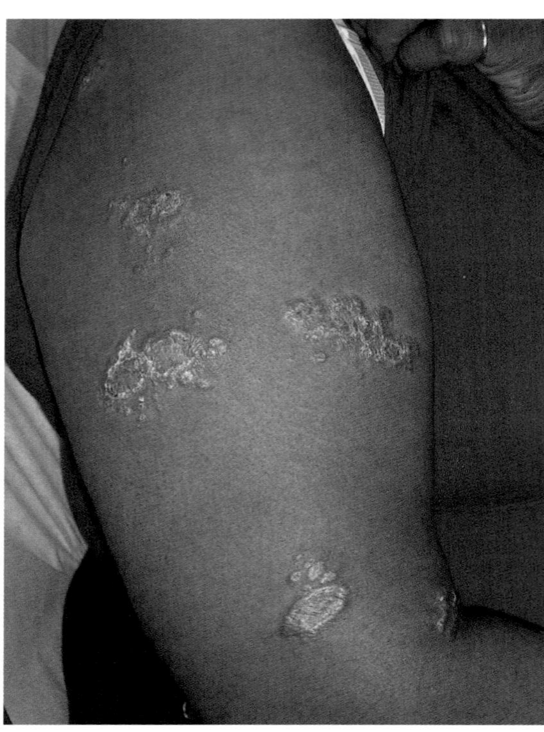

FIGURE 63-4 Cutaneous sarcoidosis on the arm with some annular patterns in the same patient with lupus pernio in Figure 63-3. (*Reproduced with permission from Richard P. Usatine, MD.*)

- Sometimes, the signs and symptoms are nonspecific and include cranial neuropathies, meningeal irritation, increased intracranial pressure, peripheral neuropathies, endocrine dysfunction, cognitive dysfunction, and personality changes.[14]

CARDIAC MANIFESTATIONS

- Cardiac sarcoidosis is detected clinically in about 5% of cases, but on autopsy in about 40% of cases.
- Cardiac involvement can be asymptomatic or present with palpitations, dyspnea, syncope or presyncopal episodes, or, rarely, sudden cardiac death.[15]

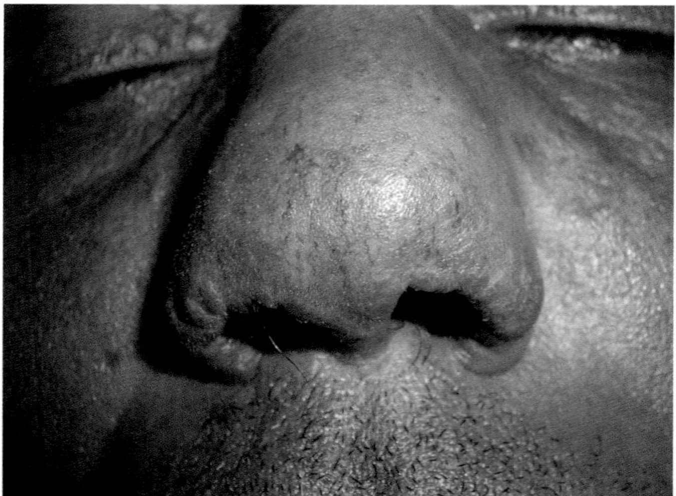

FIGURE 63-5 Sarcoidosis infiltrating the nasal alae of this 48-year-old African American man. Note the sarcoidosis is also on his cheeks and around his eyes. He also had pulmonary involvement. (*Reproduced with permission from Richard P. Usatine, MD.*)

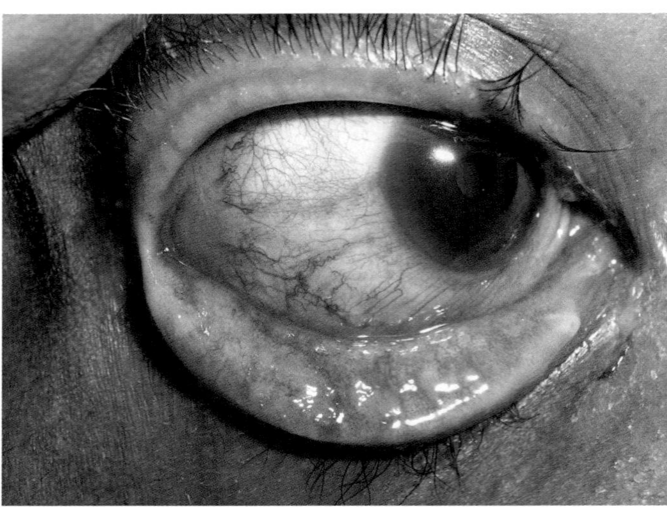

FIGURE 63-6 Ocular sarcoidosis with infiltration of the conjunctiva of the eyelids in this African American woman with extensive sarcoidosis of the skin and lungs. She has also had uveitis secondary to her sarcoidosis in the past. (*Reproduced with permission from Richard P. Usatine, MD.*)

MUSCULOSKELETAL MANIFESTATIONS

- Sarcoidosis can involve the articular, skeletal, and muscular systems (**Figure 63-7**).
- Early in the course of the disease, acute polyarthritis may be observed in up to 40% of patients, but this is often self-limited.
- Chronic or recurrent sarcoid arthritis is rare, affecting only 1% to 4% of patients.
- Asymptomatic involvement of muscles has been reported in 25% to 75% of patients in small series, but symptomatic involvement of muscles is rare (<0.5% of patients). Patterns of sarcoid muscle involvement include chronic, progressive myopathy; nodular or tumorous sarcoidosis affecting muscles; and an acute polymyositis-like syndrome. Similarly, clinically significant involvement of bone is rare (<2%-5%).[16]
- Acute arthritis is reactive.
- Bone involvement is usually asymptomatic. It most frequently affects the hands and feet and is associated with soft-tissue swelling, joint stiffness, and pain.
- The patient with bone sarcoidosis usually complains of polyarthralgia of the small joints of the hands and feet. Occasionally, the gait may become affected. Bone involvement reflects chronic irreversible progressive sarcoidosis and is common in conjunction with skin lesions, particularly lupus pernio.[16]

LABORATORY AND SELECTED STUDIES

- Once sarcoidosis is suspected, the workup will depend on the specific organ or system involved and generally advances from noninvasive to invasive methods.
- Complete blood cell count—Mild anemia occurs because of granulomatous bone marrow involvement or chronic disease state.
- The comprehensive metabolic panel and 24-hour urinary calcium level[2] demonstrate hypercalcemia in about 10% of patients with sarcoidosis and hypercalciuria (>300 mg/d) in about 30% of patients.

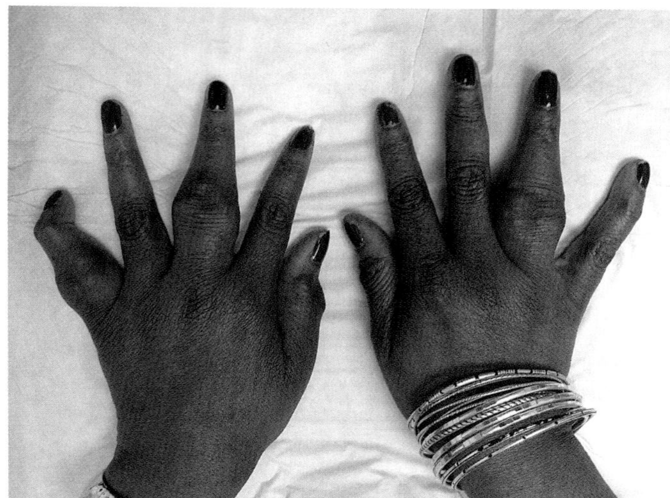

A

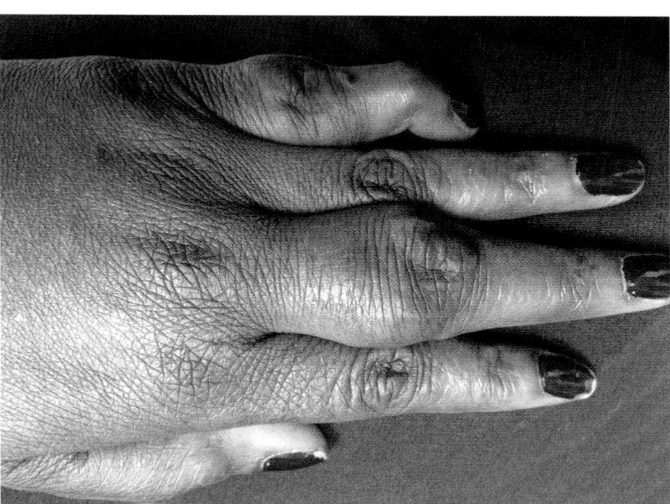

B

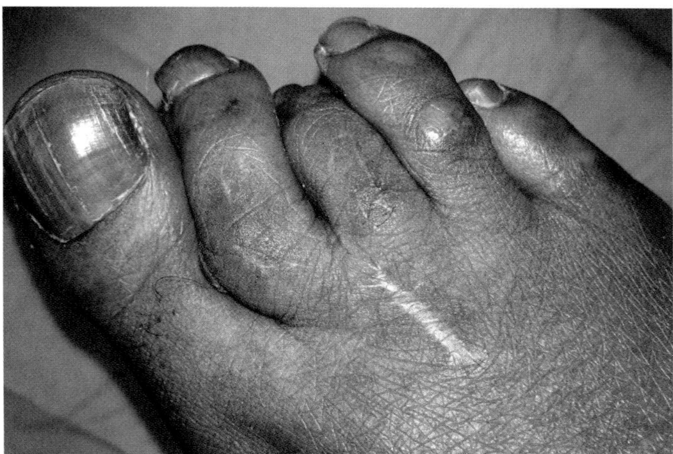

C

FIGURE 63-7 63-7 Musculoskeletal sarcoidosis in a 57-year-old woman who also has skin, eye, and pulmonary involvement. **A.** Both hands showing joint swelling and a swan neck deformity. **B.** Close-up of one hand. **C.** Close-up of sarcoidosis affecting the toes. (*Reproduced with permission from Richard P. Usatine, MD.*)

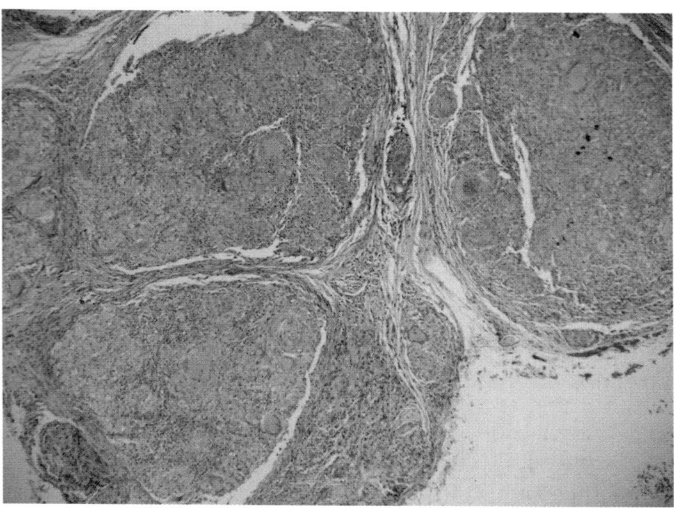

FIGURE 63-8 Biopsy image of sarcoidosis of the skin. There is a dense, noncaseating granulomatous infiltrate located within the dermis. The granulomatous inflammation is composed of circumscribed collections of epithelioid histiocytes with variable numbers of multinucleated giant cells. (*Reproduced with permission from Sandra Osswald, MD.*)

- Abnormal liver function tests often accompany sarcoidosis; most commonly, there is mild elevation of alkaline phosphatase levels. Alanine transaminase, aspartate transaminase, and bilirubin levels are usually normal.[17]
- Increased serum angiotensin-converting enzyme levels are elevated in 60% of patients at the time of diagnosis. Sensitivity and specificity as a diagnostic tests are 60% and 70%, respectively.
- Pulmonary function test—Granulomas and fibrosis of lung tissue reduce total lung capacity and decrease the carbon monoxide-diffusing capacity.
- Pathology study of biopsy—Noncaseating granulomas (**Figure 63-8**) can be used. Cutaneous lesions can provide an easily accessible source of tissue for histopathologic examination if present.
- Microscopic examination of specimens of lung tissue or other tissue of organs involved can show granulomas.[9]
- Echocardiogram and ambulatory electrocardiogram (ECG) (Holter and event monitors) are helpful in further investigating symptoms such as palpitations and dyspnea, which are suspicious for potential cardiac sarcoidosis.[15]

IMAGING

- Chest radiography—Bilateral hilar adenopathy can be the first indication of sarcoidosis.
- Cardiac magnetic resonance imaging (cMRI) and cardiac positron emission tomography (PET) imaging are new modalities used in the assessment of cardiac sarcoidosis.[18]
  - With cMRI and computed tomography (CT), the regions of sarcoid involvement produce a scar appearance with late gadolinium enhancement, which may be enough to establish the diagnosis in someone without other reasons for scar formation.
  - When additional confirmation is needed, PET can be used to show that these areas of the "scar" are actually hypermetabolic, consistent with sarcoid.

- Radiographs of the affected areas may show cystic or lytic lesions. Bone scans and PET can also detect increased activity in the involved bones.[16]

RISK FACTORS

- African American
- Female gender

DIFFERENTIAL DIAGNOSIS

Sarcoidosis is known as the "great imitator"; therefore, the differential diagnosis list is long (see the section on differential diagnosis in Chapter 173, Sarcoidosis of the Skin).

MANAGEMENT

- Management of patients with sarcoidosis is best accomplished in collaboration with a sarcoidosis center or expert and appropriate subspecialists as dictated by organ involvement.
- Immunosuppressive therapy is indicated when major organs are involved (neurologic, ophthalmologic, or cardiac) or when there is evidence of organ dysfunction or progressive disease in other organs.[2] SOR Ⓐ
- Corticosteroids are the basis of treatment of symptomatic sarcoidosis. Oral prednisone is often started to provide quick relief of symptoms.
- Methotrexate is an important steroid-sparing agent and may be used to taper patients off prednisone or to treat patients when corticosteroids are contraindicated.[1]
- Infliximab may be used.
- If patient has pain or fever, nonsteroidal anti-inflammatory drugs (NSAIDs), such as ibuprofen, may be taken. SOR Ⓐ

PROGNOSIS/CLINICAL COURSE

- In general, sarcoidosis appears briefly and resolves without relapse in most cases.
- Lofgren syndrome is the acute manifestation of sarcoidosis, typically presenting in the springtime with arthritis, erythema nodosum, uveitis, and enlarged hilar lymph nodes.[1]
- It usually has an excellent prognosis, with high rates of spontaneous remission.[2]
- Of these patients, 20% to 30% are left with some permanent lung damage, and 10% to 15% develop chronic sarcoidosis that may last for many years.
- In 5% to 10% of cases, the disease can become fatal if either granulomas or fibrosis seriously affects vital organs, such as the lungs, heart, nervous system, liver, or kidneys. End-stage lung disease may require lung transplantation.
- Cutaneous sarcoidosis usually has a prolonged course. Papules and nodules tend to resolve over months or years. Lupus pernio is often present in patients with chronic sarcoidosis and is associated with involvement of the upper respiratory tract, advanced lung fibrosis, bone cysts, and eye disease.
- With correct diagnosis and proper management, most patients with sarcoidosis continue to lead a normal life.

MAJOR COMPLICATIONS OF SARCOIDOSIS

- Hypercalcemia and hypercalciuria could be the initial manifestation of sarcoidosis, with patients presenting with symptoms of hypercalcemia, including lethargy, constipation, mental status changes, renal dysfunction, or nephrolithiasis.[19]
- High-grade conduction blocks and ventricular or atrial arrhythmias, left ventricular dysfunction, and wall motion abnormalities can occur.[15]
- Portal hypertension can be present with or without cirrhosis and can also develop from compression of the portal vein by enlarged lymph nodes in the hepatic hilum.[10,13]
- Eye damage such as asymptomatic uveitis may occur.

FOLLOW-UP

- If a patient fails to respond to corticosteroids, then the clinician should reassess the need for additional or different treatment.
- Stable patients should be followed every 4 to 6 months.
- Consider a periodic echocardiogram to assess for pulmonary hypertension if the patient presents symptoms like dyspnea and peripheral edema.
- Patients need ophthalmologic examination and to be monitored for ophthalmic side effects and toxicities from immunosuppressive agents, such as steroids and hydroxychloroquine.[2] SOR Ⓐ

PATIENT EDUCATION

- The patient should see a physician if any new symptoms appear or the medication is not working.
- Smoking should be avoided.

PATIENT RESOURCES

- Sarcoidosis support groups—**http://www.sarcoidosisonlinesites.com/index.html.**
- Sarcoid Networking Association—**http://www.sarcoidosisnetwork.org.**

PROVIDER RESOURCES

- American Lung Association. *Sarcoidosis*—**http://www.lungusa.org/lung-disease/sarcoidosis.**
- World Association for Sarcoidosis and Other Granulomatous Disorders—**http://www.wasog.org/.**
- MedlinePlus. *Sarcoidosis*—**http://www.nlm.nih.gov/medlineplus/sarcoidosis.html.**

REFERENCES

1. Costabel U. Sarcoidosis: clinical update. *Eur Respir J*. 2001;32:56s-68s.
2. Statement on sarcoidosis. Joint Statement of the American Thoracic Society (ATS), the European Respiratory Society (ERS) and the World Association of Sarcoidosis and Other Granulomatous Disorders (WASOG) adopted by the ATS Board of Directors and by the ERS Executive Committee, February 1999. *Am J Respir Crit Care Med*. 1999;160(2):736-755.
3. Ali MM, Atwan AA, Gonzalez ML. Cutaneous sarcoidosis: updates in the pathogenesis. *J Eur Acad Dermatol Venereol*. 2010;24(7):747-755.
4. Iannuzzi MC, Rybicki BA, Teirstein AS. Sarcoidosis. *N Engl J Med*. 2007;357(21):2153-2165.
5. English JC 3rd, Patel PJ, Greer KE. Sarcoidosis. *J Am Acad Dermatol*. 2001;44(5):725-743; quiz 44-46.
6. Newman LS, Rose CS, Maier LA. Sarcoidosis. *N Engl J Med*. 1997;336(17):1224-1234.
7. Keary PJ, Palmer DG. Benign self-limiting sarcoidosis with skin and joint involvement. *N Z Med J*. 1976;83(560):197-199.
8. Baughman RP, Teirstein AS, Judson MA, et al. Clinical characteristics of patients in a case control study of sarcoidosis. *Am J Respir Crit Care Med*. 2001;164(10 Pt 1):1885-1889.
9. Baughman RP, Lower EE. Evidence-based therapy for cutaneous sarcoidosis. *Clin Dermatol*. 2007;25(3):334-340.
10. Rose AS, Tielker MA, Knox KS. Hepatic, ocular, and cutaneous sarcoidosis. *Clin Chest Med*. 2008;29(3):509-524, ix.
11. Abu-Hilal M, Krotva J, Chichierchio L, Obeidat N, Madanat M. Dermatologic aspects and cutaneous manifestations of sarcoidosis. *G Ital Dermatol Venereol*. 2007;145(6):733-745.
12. Heiligenhaus A, Wefelmeyer D, Wefelmeyer E, Rosel M, Schrenk M. The eye as a common site for the early clinical manifestation of sarcoidosis. *Ophthalmic Res*. 2011;46(1):9-12.
13. Ebert EC, Kierson M, Hagspiel KD. Gastrointestinal and hepatic manifestations of sarcoidosis. *Am J Gastroenterol*. 2008;103(12):3184-3192; quiz 93.
14. Hoitsma E, Drent M, Sharma OP. A pragmatic approach to diagnosing and treating neurosarcoidosis in the 21st century. *Curr Opin Pulm Med*. 2010;16(5):472-479.
15. Mehta D, Lubitz SA, Frankel Z, et al. Cardiac involvement in patients with sarcoidosis: diagnostic and prognostic value of outpatient testing. *Chest*. 2008;133(6):1426-1435.
16. Zisman DA, Shorr AF, Lynch JP 3rd. Sarcoidosis involving the musculoskeletal system. *Semin Respir Crit Care Med*. 2002;23(6):555-570.
17. Sharma OP. Vitamin D, calcium, and sarcoidosis. *Chest*. 1996;109(2):535-539.
18. Ohira H, Tsujino I, Ishimaru S, et al. Myocardial imaging with 18F-fluoro-2-deoxyglucose positron emission tomography and magnetic resonance imaging in sarcoidosis. *Eur J Nuclear Med Mol Imaging*. 2008;35(5):933-941.
19. Burke RR, Rybicki BA, Rao DS. Calcium and vitamin D in sarcoidosis: how to assess and manage. *Semin Respir Crit Care Med*. 2010;31(4):474-484.

64 TUBERCULOSIS

Mindy A. Smith, MD, MS

PATIENT STORY

A 25-year-old man from Mexico presents to the emergency room in a South Texas hospital with a persistent cough for 3 weeks, low-grade fever, and night sweats. His chest X-ray (CXR) shows mediastinal and right hilar lymphadenopathy and right upper lobe consolidation concerning for primary tuberculosis (TB) (**Figure 64-1**). Upon review of the radiograph, the emergency room staff admits the patient to a single room with negative pressure. The patient is placed in respiratory isolation, sputum is sent for acid-fast bacillus (AFB) stain and cultures, and the results show AFB consistent with Mycobacterium spp. (**Figure 64-2**). While culture results are pending, the patient is started on 4 antituberculosis drugs. Fortunately the sputum culture result shows pan susceptible *Mycobacterium tuberculosis*, and his treatment continues with directly observed therapy (DOT) through the local city health department.

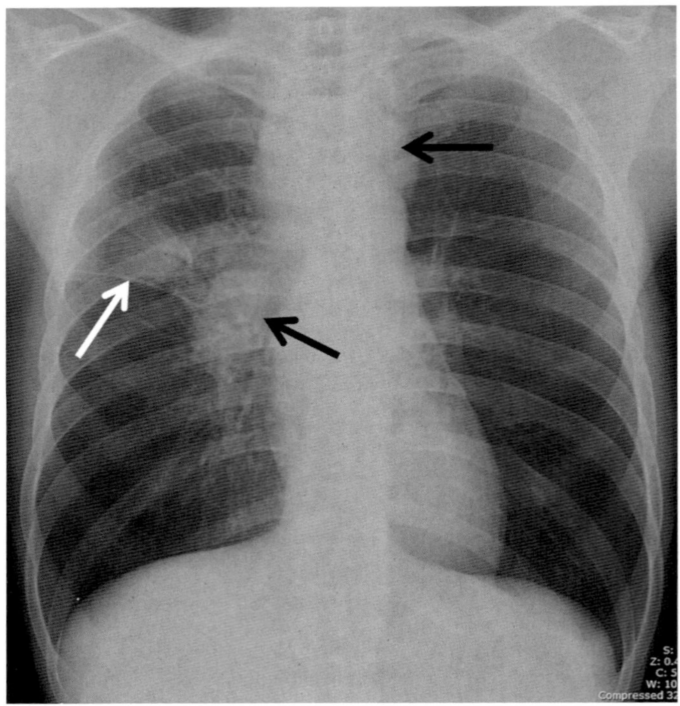

A

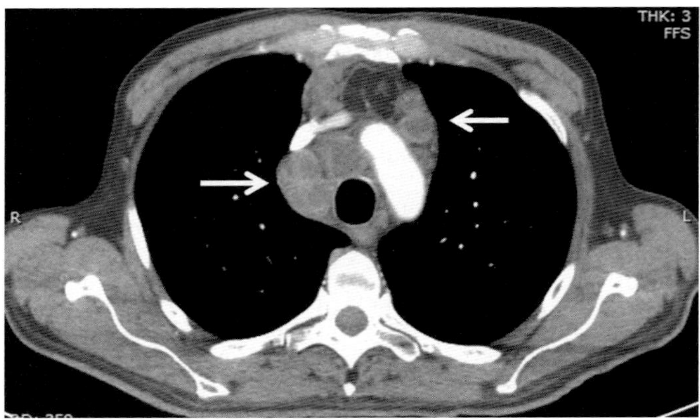

B

FIGURE 64-1 Typical presentation of a primary pulmonary TB infection in a 20-year-old man. **A.** Frontal chest radiograph shows mediastinal and right hilar lymphadenopathy (black arrows) and right upper lobe consolidation (white arrow). **B.** Contrast-enhanced CT demonstrates low-density enlarged mediastinal lymph nodes with peripheral rim enhancement consistent with necrotizing lymphadenopathy (arrows). (*Reproduced with permission from Carlos Santiago Restrepo, MD.*)

INTRODUCTION

Tuberculosis is a bacterial infection caused by *M. tuberculosis, an obligate intracellular pathogen that is aerobic, acid-fast, and nonencapsulated. TB* primarily involves the lungs, although other organs are involved in one-third of cases. Improvements in diagnostics, drugs, vaccines, and understanding of biomarkers of disease activity are expected to change future management of this devastating worldwide disease.

EPIDEMIOLOGY

- Over 8 million cases occur annually around the world, with nearly 2 million TB-related deaths;[1] 95% of TB deaths occur in low- and middle-income countries.
- A total of 11,182 TB cases (3.6/100,000 persons) were reported in the United States in 2010. This represents the lowest incidence rate since recording began in 1953.[2] An estimated 2 billion people worldwide have latent TB.[3]
- The multiple drug-resistant (MDR) TB rate in the United States was 1.2% (88 cases) in 2010; a rate which remains relatively stable in the United States.[1] MDR TB rates are highest in India, China, the Russian federation, South Africa, and Bangladesh.[3]
- Based on the 2010 data, 60% of reported US cases of *M. tuberculosis* occurred in foreign-born individuals (case rate 11 times higher than US-born individuals).[1]
- There were 547 reported deaths from TB in the United States in 2009 (a 7% decrease from 2008).[1]
- Prophylactic treatment of those with latent TB (infection without active disease—diagnosed by tuberculin skin test conversion from negative to positive or by an interferon-γ release assay performed on blood) can reduce the risk of active TB by 90% or more.[4] SOR Ⓐ

ETIOLOGY AND PATHOPHYSIOLOGY

- Infection is transmitted by aerosolized respiratory droplet nuclei.[4]
- About 10% of those infected develop active TB, usually within 1 to 2 years of exposure; risk factors for the development of active TB are listed later.
- There are 3 host responses to infection: immediate nonspecific macrophage and likely neutrophil ingestion of those bacilli reaching the alveoli, later tissue-damaging response (delayed-type hypersensitivity reaction), and specific macrophage activating and potentially

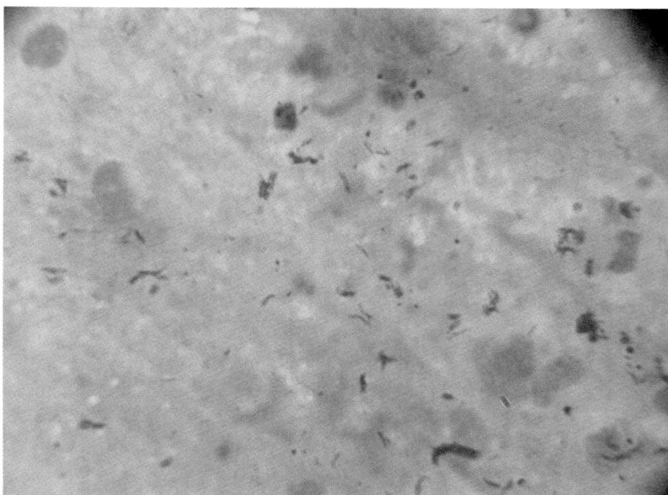

FIGURE 64-2 The acid-fast bacilli of *Mycobacterium tuberculosis* seen with acid-fast staining at 100 power with oil immersion microscopy. (*Reproduced with permission from Richard P. Usatine, MD.*)

neutrophil-related response—the latter, if effective, walling off infection into granulomas. Recent evidence suggests that mycobacteria themselves may promote granuloma formation and these granulomas are dynamic, blurring distinctions between latent and active TB.[3]

- In areas of high prevalence, TB is often seen in children. The disease process usually localizes to the middle and upper lung zones accompanied by hilar and paratracheal lymphadenopathy (as the tubercle bacilli spread from lung to lymphatic vessels). The primary focus usually heals spontaneously and may disappear entirely or, if encapsulated by fibroblasts and collagen fibers, be visible as a calcified lung nodule (Ghon complex) (**Figure 64-3**).

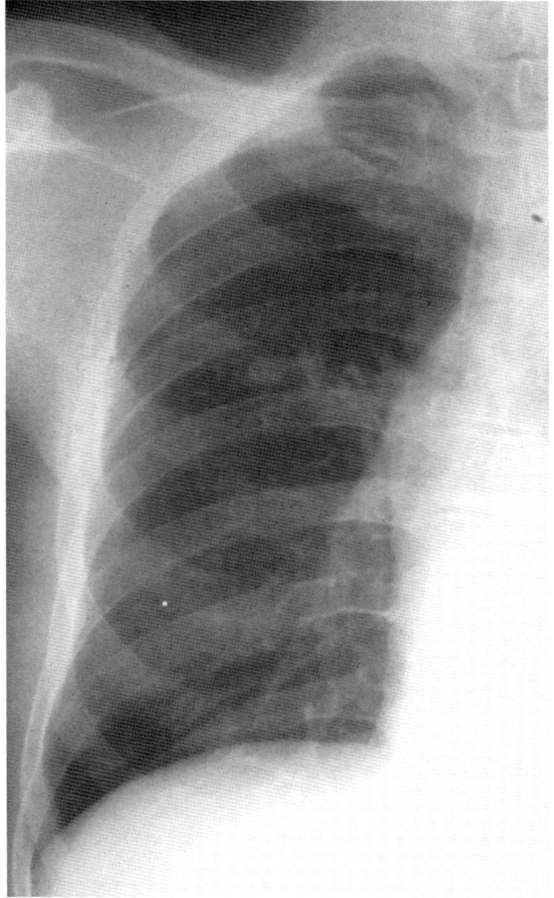

FIGURE 64-3 Primary TB may coalesce into a small granuloma in the upper lobe referred to as a Ghon complex. (*Reproduced with permission from Miller WT, Jr.* Diagnostic Thoracic Imaging. *New York, NY: McGraw-Hill; 2006:289, Figure 6-5 E.*.)

RISK FACTORS

Risk factors for infection or progression to active TB include the following[2,3,4]:

- Minority and foreign-born populations (subject to overcrowding and malnutrition).
- HIV (relative risk [RR] for progression to active TB 100) and other immunocompromised states (eg, cancer, treatment with tumor necrosis factor antagonists) (RR [progression to active TB] 10). As a result of the high susceptibility of HIV-infected patients, 12% of worldwide TB cases are HIV-associated with sub-Saharan Africa accounting for 4 out of every 5 of these cases.[3]
- Chronic diseases such as diabetes mellitus (RR 3) or chronic renal failure/hemodialysis (RR [infection and progression to active TB] 10-25 for renal failure).
- Malignancy.
- Genetic susceptibility.
- Bariatric surgery or jejunoileal bypass (RR [progression to active TB] 30-60) recipients.
- Injection drug users (RR [progression to active TB] 10-30).
- Smoking (RR 2 for progression and infection).
- Personnel who work or live in high-risk settings (eg, prisons, long-term care facilities, and hospitals).
- Adult women (ratio 2:1 adult man).
- Older age (both infection and progression).
- Children under 4 years of age who are exposed to high-risk individuals.
- Recent infection (<1 year) (RR [progression to active TB] 12.9 vs old infection).
- Fibrotic lung lesions (spontaneously healed) (RR [progression to active TB] 2-20).
- Silicosis (RR [infection] 3 and RR [progression to active TB] 30).
- Malnutrition (RR [progression to active TB] 2).
- In a study of hospital personnel, only the percentage of low-income persons within the employee's residential postal zone was independently associated with conversion (odds ratio [OR] 1.39, 95% confidence interval [CI], 1.09-1.78).[5]

DIAGNOSIS

The diagnosis of active TB requires a high index of suspicion. In addition, targeted testing for latent TB in vulnerable populations who would benefit from treatment (recent [<5 years] immigrants, immunosuppression, patients with diabetes mellitus and/or chronic renal disease, recent TB or close contact with someone with TB such as household members and health care workers) is suggested.[6] Manifestations of active TB can be classified as pulmonary or extrapulmonary. TB can affect any organ system.

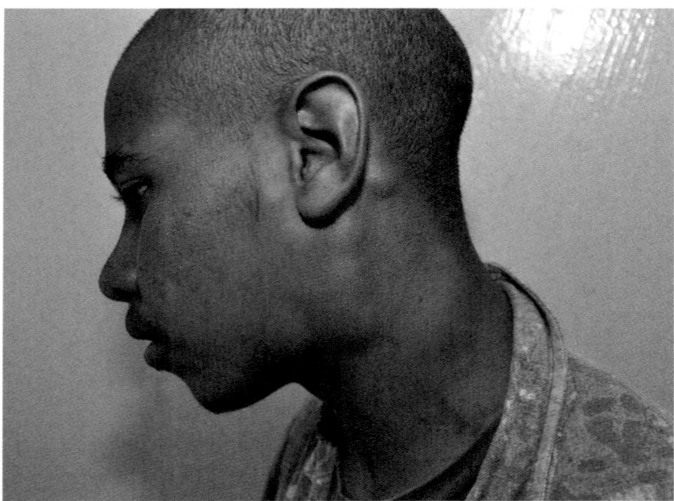

FIGURE 64-4 Scrofula of the neck with large cervical lymphadenopathy from tuberculosis. *(Reproduced with permission from Richard P. Usatine, MD.)*

CLINICAL FEATURES

The disease may be asymptomatic (one in 4 culture-confirmed cases from active case finding in Asia).[3]

Pulmonary

- Early nonspecific signs and symptoms include fever, night sweats, fatigue, anorexia, weight loss.
- Later nonproductive cough (lasting 2-3 weeks) or cough with purulent sputum.
- Patients with extensive disease may develop dyspnea or acute respiratory distress syndrome.
- Physical examination findings also nonspecific with crackles or rhonchi.

Extrapulmonary TB, caused by hematogenous spread, occurs in the following order of frequency[4]:

- Lymph nodes: painless swelling of cervical and supraclavicular nodes (scrofula) (**Figure 64-4**).
- Pleural effusion with exudates.
- Genitourinary tract: can cause urethral stricture, kidney damage or infertility (in women, affects the fallopian tubes and endometrium).
- Bones and joints: pain in the spine (Pott disease **[Figure 64-5]**), hips, or knees.
- Other less common sites are meninges, peritoneum, intestines, skin, eye, ear, and pericardium.
- TB of the skin (scrofuloderma) shows ulcerations of the skin (**Figures 64-4 and 64-6**) in the inguinal or cervical region along with lymphadenopathy.

SKIN TESTING AND RAPID TESTING

Positive results on either a tuberculin skin test (TST) or an interferon-γ release assay (IGRA) in the absence of active TB establish a diagnosis of latent TB infection.

- TST with purified protein derivative (PPD) is not useful in diagnosing active TB but is used to detect latent infection in exposed or high-risk individuals. A positive test is 10-mm induration at the inoculation site or 5-mm induration in a patient who is immunocompromised; evaluated in 48 to 72 hours after test placement.

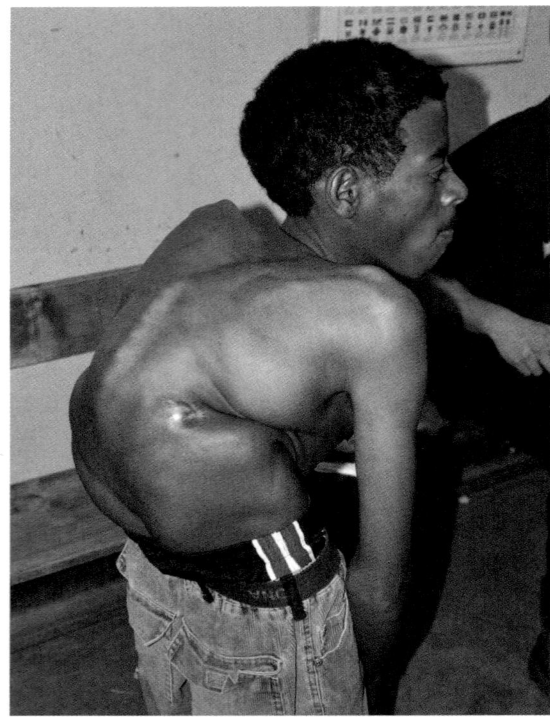

FIGURE 64-5 Pott disease from tuberculosis infection of the spine resulting in a severe kyphoscoliosis. Note the continued skin ulceration on the right and the severe deformity caused by this disease. *(Reproduced with permission from Richard P. Usatine, MD.)*

- Two commercially produced IGRAs are licensed for use in the United States and in many other countries: QuantiFERON-TB Gold (QFT-G, Cellestis Limited, Carnegie, Victoria, Australia) and TSPOT.TB (Oxford Immunotec, Inc; Oxford, England) as an aid for diagnosing *M. tuberculosis* infection.[3]
- IGRAs detect the release of interferon- in fresh heparinized whole blood from sensitized persons when it is incubated with mixtures of synthetic peptides using antigens present in *M. tuberculosis*. Advantages include no need for a return visit and greater specificity than skin testing. Disadvantages include cost, availability, and lack of supporting data that these tests improve patient outcomes.

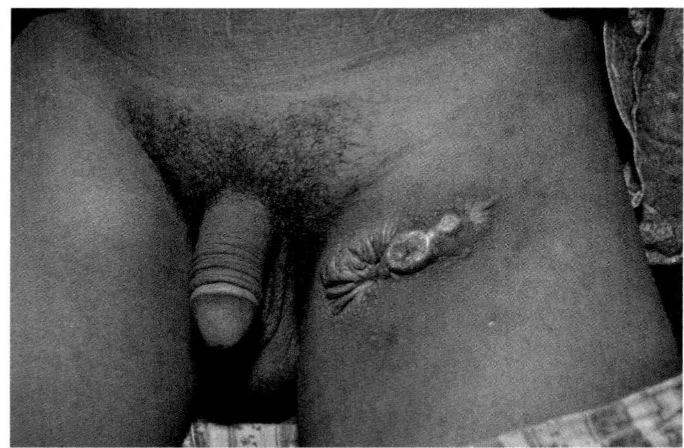

FIGURE 64-6 Young adult man in Africa with scrofuloderma showing an ulcerated lesion on one side and inguinal adenopathy on the other side. *(Reproduced with permission from Richard P. Usatine, MD.)*

- IGRAs have limited accuracy in diagnosing active TB in HIV-infected patients and should not be used alone to rule out or rule in disease.[7] In one study of children investigated for TB in 6 UK pediatric centers, TST had a sensitivity of 82%, QuantiFERON-TB Gold in tube (QFT-IT) had a sensitivity of 78% and TSPOT.TB of 66%; combining TST and IGRA results increased sensitivity for both tests (ability to rule out TB).[8] In practice, IGRA have become standard of care for MTB screening in some HIV clinics.
- Nucleic acid amplification tests (NAATs) on sputum specimens are under investigation and are being used to confirm diagnosis in some institutions.[3]

LABORATORY AND ANCILLARY TESTING

- Nonspecific findings include mild anemia and leukocytosis.
- Urinalysis may show "sterile" pyuria and hematuria with urinary tract involvement.
- Acid-fast bacilli may be seen on acid-fast staining from sputum or pleural or peritoneal fluid (see **Figure 64-2**). They may also be seen upon staining tissue from fine-needle aspiration or biopsy of lymph nodes or other tissues as above. Sputum processing with bleach or sodium hydroxide and centrifugation and use of fluorescent microscopy is associated with increased sensitivity of smear microscopy.[3]
- Definitive diagnosis is based on culture of sputum (3 sets of samples collected 8-24 hours apart), urine (3 morning specimens—positive in 90% with urinary tract infection), or from tissue or bone biopsy using automated liquid culture systems. *M. tuberculosis* is slow growing and can take 4 to 8 weeks to identify. Authors of a recent review note that one specimen should be tested with NAAT.[9] Once identified, testing for drug sensitivity should be performed.
- Obtaining baseline liver enzymes is recommended for patients older than age 35 years, or for those with a history of liver disease, HIV infection, pregnancy (or within 3 months postdelivery), concomitant hepatotoxic therapy, or regular alcohol use.
- Testing vision, including color vision, is suggested prior to initiating and throughout treatment with ethambutol, which can cause irreversible cumulative toxicity to the optic nerve.
- Biomarkers of disease activity are an area of active investigation; however, a simple, inexpensive point-of-care test is still not available.

IMAGING

- CXR is the diagnostic test of choice and classically shows upper lobe infiltrates with cavitation and/or lymphadenopathy (**Figures 64-1 and 64-7).**
- Other patterns of TB seen on CXR include a solitary nodule (Ghon complex) (see **Figure 64-3**) and diffuse infiltrates that may represent bronchogenic spread (**Figure 64-8**).
- CXR pattern in teens and young adults often shows an infiltrate with hilar and paratracheal lymphadenopathy (**Figures 64-1 and 64-9**).
- In disseminated (miliary) TB, innumerable tiny nodules are seen throughout both lungs on CXR, and computed tomography (CT) (**Figure 64-10**).
- Reactivation TB may show large cavities in both upper lobes associated with bronchiectasis and fibronodular opacities (**Figure 64-11**).
- X-ray, CT, or magnetic resonance imaging (MRI) of bone may show destructive lesions. Spinal MRI has a sensitivity of about 100% and specificity of 88% for detecting tuberculous lesions before deformity develops.[10]

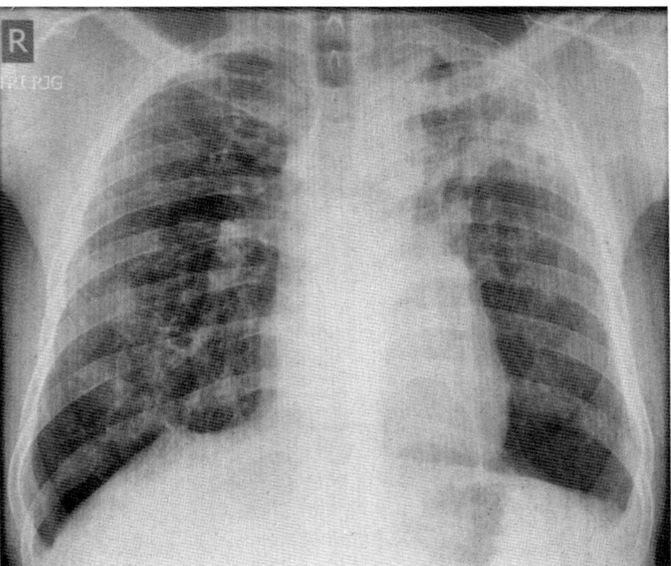

FIGURE 64-7 A 36-year-old man with pulmonary tuberculosis. There is an opacity in the left pulmonary apex associated with a cavity consistent with fibrosis and scarring changes of pulmonary tuberculosis. Also there is an infiltrate in the right lung. (*Reproduced with permission from Richard P. Usatine, MD.*)

BIOPSY

Histology reveals granulomas with caseating necrosis.

DIFFERENTIAL DIAGNOSIS

Because any pattern on CXR may be seen with active TB, the differential diagnosis includes the following:

- Bacterial or viral pneumonia—Sputum or blood culture may reveal the infecting organism, and the patient will usually respond to antibacterial drugs and/or time.

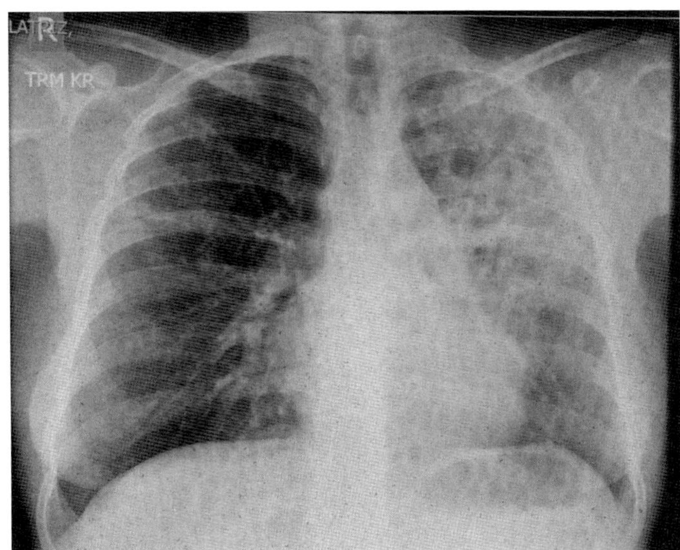

FIGURE 64-8 A 23-year-old woman with pulmonary tuberculosis. There is increased density of the lung parenchyma in the upper left lobe with a heterogeneous pattern showing areas of consolidation, fibrosis, and bullae. Other sections of the long show a micronodular pattern. There is a retraction of the mediastinum toward the left. This whole pattern is consistent with pulmonary tuberculosis. (*Reproduced with permission from Richard P. Usatine, MD.*)

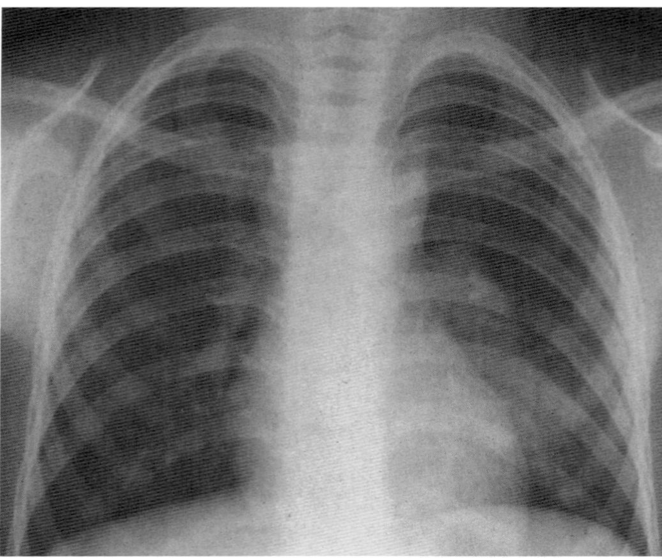

FIGURE 64-9 Primary TB in a child; note the left lower lobe infiltrate and the left hilar lymphadenopathy and right paratracheal adenopathy. (*Reproduced with permission from Schwartz DT and Reisdorff EJ.* Emergency Radiology. *New York, NY: McGraw-Hill; 2000:469, Figure 17-28.* .)

- Fungal respiratory infections—These patients will usually have a history of travel to or living in an area where histoplasmosis or coccidioidomycosis is endemic.
- Acute histoplasmosis is usually asymptomatic or causes only mild symptoms and CXR typically shows hilar adenopathy with or without pneumonitis (**Figure 64-12**); patients with chronic pulmonary histoplasmosis have gradually increasing cough, weight loss, and night sweats and CXR shows uni- or bilateral fibronodular, apical infiltrates; positive serology or culture, immunodiffusion test, or lung biopsy can be diagnostic.
- Coccidioidomycosis has similar clinical features to TB and CXR may show infiltrate, hilar adenopathy, and pleural effusion; serologic tests are useful in the diagnosis.
- Sarcoidosis—No TB contacts, dyspnea and cough, hilar adenopathy on CXR, skin lesions help differentiate along with serum angiotensin-converting enzyme (ACE) level or biopsy. Pathology shows noncaseating granulomata.(see Chapter 173, Sarcoidosis).

MANAGEMENT

Patients can be managed by their primary care provider, by public health departments, or jointly, but in all cases the health department is ultimately responsible for ensuring availability of appropriate diagnostic and treatment services and for monitoring the results of therapy.

NONPHARMACOLOGIC

- There are insufficient data to support use of free food or nutritional supplements on improving treatment outcome or quality of life in individuals with TB in the United States.[11] However, attention to nutrition has shown to be beneficial in a study of TB treatment in Haiti.[12]
- Vitamin D deficiency has been linked to TB susceptibility and there is evidence that vitamin D suppresses intracellular growth of *M. tuberculosis* in vitro. Data are insufficient to determine if vitamin D

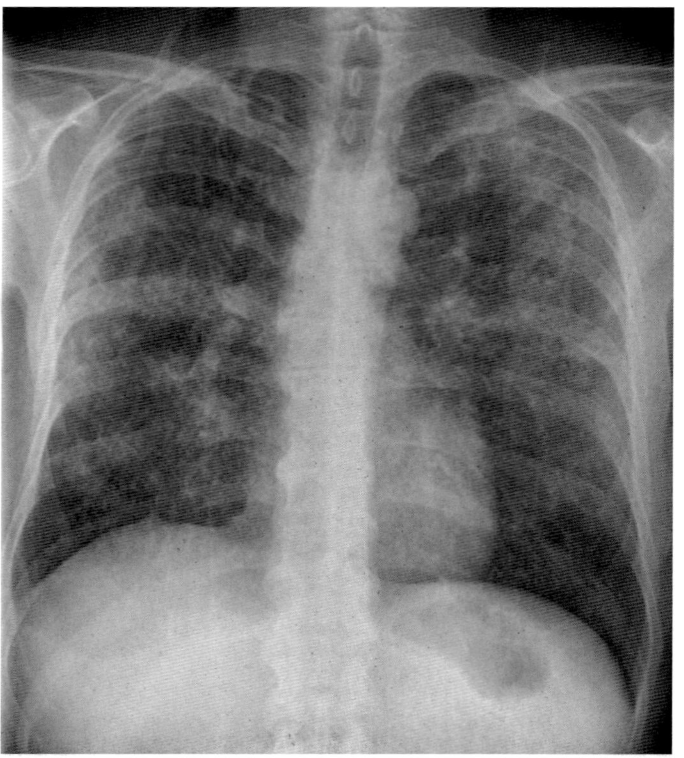

A

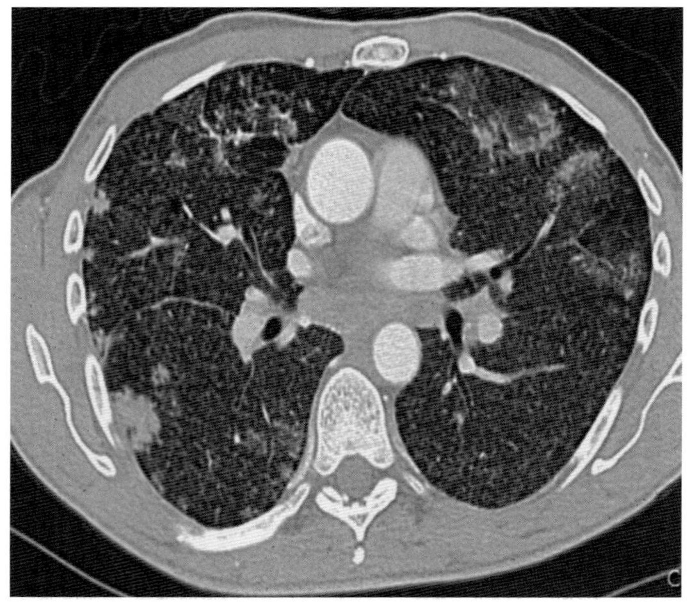

B

FIGURE 64-10 Disseminated (miliary) TB with tiny innumerable nodules throughout both lungs. A. CXR (*Reproduced with permission from Richard P. Usatine, MD.*) B. CT scan (*Reproduced with permission from Carlos Santiago Restrepo, MD.*)

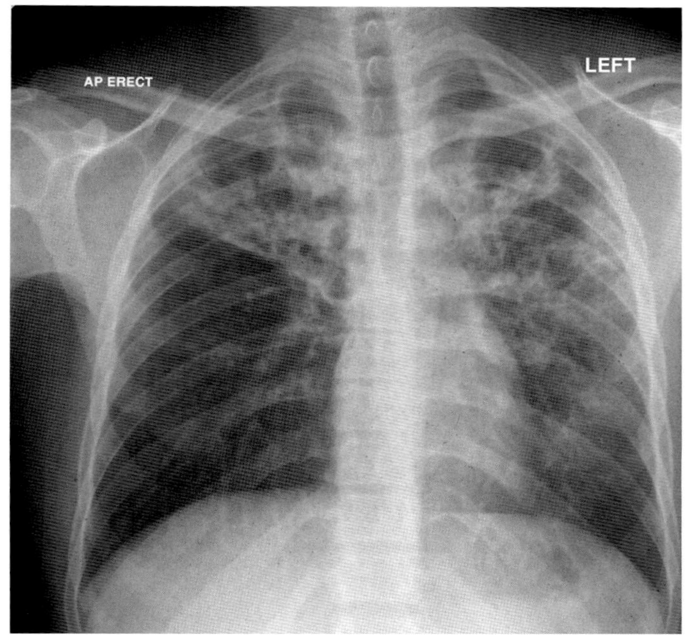

A

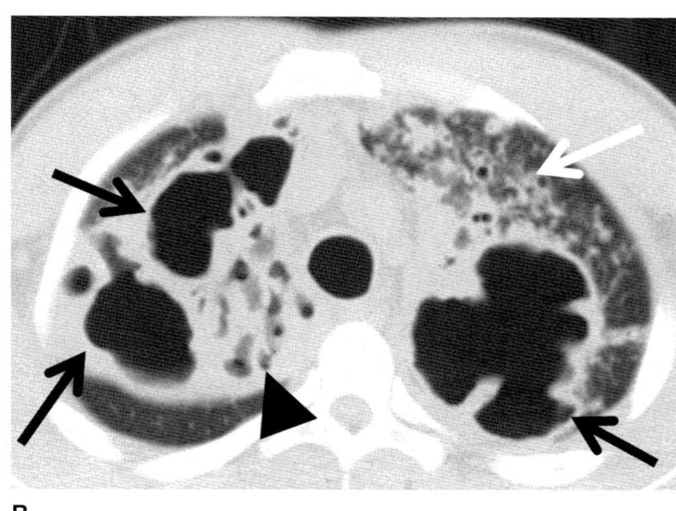

B

FIGURE 64-11 Reactivation TB with cavitary lesions in the upper lobes of a 35-year-old man. **A.** Frontal chest radiograph depicts large cavitary lesions in both upper lobes associated with bronchiectasis and fibronodular opacities. **B.** Noncontrast chest CT confirms the presence of irregular cavities in both upper lobes (black arrows), nodules (white arrow), and bronchiectasis (black arrowhead). (*Reproduced with permission from Carlos Santiago Restrepo, MD.*)

supplementation is useful as an adjunct to TB treatment. One randomized controlled trial (RCT) found no differences in time to sputum culture conversion with adjunctive vitamin D in the whole study population, but reported a significant hastening of sputum culture conversion in participants with the tt genotype of the TaqI vitamin D receptor polymorphism.[13] Many experts recommend screening and treatment for vitamin D deficiency in all TB patients. SOR C

FIGURE 64-12 Histoplasmosis in a 33-year-old man with a 6-month history of fatigue. Chest X-ray (CXR) shows a 4-cm mass overlying the right hilum and a lumpy contour of the left hilum that indicates lymphadenopathy. Histoplasmosis was diagnosed on bronchoscopy. (*Reproduced with permission from Miller WT, Jr. Diagnostic Thoracic Imaging. New York, NY: McGraw-Hill; 2006:357, Figure 7-54 A.*)

MEDICATIONS

For adult patients with *active TB* there are 4 major drugs used for treatment. The first-line anti-TB medications should be administered together; split dosing should be avoided. Review the patient's current medications to avoid drug interactions. A few combination medications are available but are more costly. The following regimen is suggested by the American Thoracic Society, Infectious Diseases Society of America, and the Center for Disease Control and Prevention (2003)[14]: SOR B

- Two-month initial-treatment phase with all 4 medications (isoniazid 5 mg/kg daily [maximum 300 mg] or 15 mg/kg thrice weekly [maximum 900 mg]; rifampin (10 mg/kg daily or thrice weekly [maximum 600 mg]; pyrazinamide (20-25 mg/kg daily [maximum 2 g] or 30-40 mg/kg thrice weekly [maximum 3 g]; and ethambutol (15-20 mg/kg daily or 25-30 mg/kg thrice weekly). A RCT found a fixed-dose 4-drug combination was noninferior to treatment with 4 drugs separately.[15]
- Four-month continuation phase with isoniazid (INH) and rifampin; treatment is extended to 7 months for patients with cavitary pulmonary TB who remain sputum-positive after initial treatment or if pregnant. The World Health Organization 2010 recommendations agree with continuing rifampin for 6 months and emphasize the importance of drug sensitivity testing to guide individual patient management.[16]
- To prevent INH-related neuropathy, pyridoxine 10 to 25 mg/d may be given, especially to those at risk for vitamin B_6 deficiency (ie, alcoholic, malnourished, pregnant or lactating women, HIV-positive, and those with chronic disease). SOR A

- Drug-resistant TB is treated with a variety of injectable drugs including streptomycin, kanamycin, and amikacin or oral drugs including fluoroquinolones, ethionamide, cycloserine, and *p*-aminosalicylic acid.[4] In a Cochrane review of 11 small trials on the use of fluoroquinolones in TB regimens, investigators found no difference in trials substituting ciprofloxacin, ofloxacin, or moxifloxacin for first-line drugs in relation to cure (416 participants, 3 trials), treatment failure (388 participants, 3 trials), or clinical or radiologic improvement (216 participants, 2 trials).[17] Substituting ciprofloxacin into first-line regimens in drug-sensitive TB led to a higher incidence of relapse in HIV-positive patients.
- Research into adjuvant immunotherapy (eg, antitumor necrosis factor therapies) is underway to determine whether this treatment will accelerate the response to treatment.
- In patients with HIV infection, treatment with antiretroviral therapy (ART) should be started during the first 2 to 8 weeks of TB treatment.[16] SOR B In a RCT of early ART treatment (2 weeks after initiating TB treatment) versus later (8 weeks after) in patients with TB and HIV, investigators found a significantly reduced risk of death in the earlier ART treatment group (18% vs 27% in delayed-treatment group).[18] Rates of immune reconstitution inflammatory syndrome, however, were higher when starting earlier.
- An open-label RCT in South Africa of patients with TB and HIV (plus CD4+ T-cell count <500 per cubic millimeter) found similar AIDS or death rates in the groups assigned to early ART (within 4 weeks) versus later ART (within the first 4 weeks of the continuation phase) (18 vs 19 cases, respectively) and also reported higher rates of immune reconstitution inflammatory syndrome when starting earlier (20.1 vs 7.7 cases/100 person-years).[19] AIDS and death rates were higher, however, for those with very low CD4 counts (<50 per cubic millimeter) randomized to later initiation of ART (26.3 vs8.5 cases/100 person-years).[19]
- Treatment can be given daily or intermittently (3 times a week throughout or twice weekly after the initial phase). For patients who are HIV-seronegative with noncavitary pulmonary TB and negative cultures at 2-months, treatment can be given once weekly.

For adult patients with *latent TB*, a treatment decision is made considering the benefits of treatment based on individual's risk for developing TB disease (see Risk Factors earlier) and the person's level of commitment to completion of treatment and resources available to ensure adherence.[20] Persons with no known risk factors for TB may be considered for treatment of latent TB if they have either a positive IGRA result ***or*** if their reaction to the TST is 15 mm or larger. The following options are used:

- INH 5 mg/kg daily (maximum 300 mg) for 9 months; SOR A twice-weekly regimens (15 mg/kg [maximum 900 mg]) may be considered if the patient is under direct observation therapy and 6-month therapy may be considered for adults who are not HIV-infected and have no fibrotic lesions on CXR. SOR B The standard treatment regimen is preferred for HIV-infected people taking antiretroviral therapy.
- Rifampin (10 mg/kg daily; maximum 600 mg) for 4 months if INH-resistant TB or allergy.
- Rifapentine (900 mg; a rifamycin derivative) plus INH (900 mg) for 3 months of directly observed once-weekly therapy. The Centers for Disease Control (CDC) recommends this regimen for otherwise healthy patients 12 years of age or older who have latent tuberculosis infection and factors that are predictive of TB developing (eg, recent exposure to contagious TB).[21] SOR A
- In an open-label, randomized noninferiority trial comparing 3 months of directly observed once-weekly therapy with rifapentine plus isoniazid with 9 months of self-administered daily isoniazid (300 mg) in subjects at high risk for tuberculosis, rates of TB were comparable (7 of 3986 subjects in the combination-therapy group [cumulative rate, 0.19%] and in 15 of 3745 subjects in the INH-only group [cumulative rate, 0.43%]) and completion rates were higher.[22] Three additional RCT (Brazil, South Africa, and International) have shown that this combination regimen administered weekly for 12 weeks as DOT is as effective for preventing TB as other regimens and is more likely to be completed than the US standard regimen of 9 months of INH daily without DOT.[21]
- Refusal of treatment for latent TB in another study at 32 clinics was 17.1% (95% CI, 14.5%-20%) and 52.7% (95% CI, 48.5%-56.8%) failed to complete the recommended course.[23]

PREVENTION

- There is no currently available vaccine with adequate effectiveness for the prevention of TB,[3] although about 10 vaccines are in the clinical trial phase.[24] Bacille Calmette-Guérin (BCG) vaccine, first released in 1921, can prevent up to 50% of TB cases.[25]
- BCG vaccine also has a protective effect against meningitis and disseminated TB in children, although it does not appear to prevent primary infection or reactivation of latent pulmonary infection, the principal source of bacillary spread in many communities.
- The Centers for Disease Control and Prevention recommend that BCG vaccine only be considered for very select persons who meet specific criteria and in consultation with a TB expert.[26]
- CDC consensus-based recommendations to prevent TB spread include not routinely hospitalizing patients with TB for diagnostic tests or care; separating patients with respiratory TB from immunocompromised patients; use of masks, gowns, or barrier nursing techniques if MDR TB is suspected or an aerosol-generating procedure is being performed; instructing patients with smear-positive pulmonary, laryngeal or respiratory tract disease to avoid unnecessary contact with people from outside the household (eg, avoid work, day care facilities, or schools) for the first 2 weeks of treatment, and considering chemoprophylaxis for young children who are close contacts to avoid parental separation.[27]

PROGNOSIS

- Without treatment, approximately one-third of individuals with active TB will die within 1 year and half within 5 years. Of those who survive 5 years, 60% will have undergone spontaneous remission and the remaining will continue to be infectious.[28]

FOLLOW-UP SOR C

- Patients are considered contagious until they have been on adequate chemotherapy for a minimum of 2 weeks, have 3 negative AFB sputum cultures (collected in 8- to 24-hour intervals with one early morning specimen), and show clinical improvement.[29]

- Monitor clinical recovery, medication adverse effects, and compliance with treatment monthly;[19] risk factors for noncompliance include lack of motivation, lack of perceived vulnerability, and poverty.
- Monitor response to treatment—Monthly sputum cultures should be obtained until culture negative (80% expected by 2 months). If culture positive at 3 or more months, consider drug resistance or treatment failure and institute additional evaluation and treatment. For those with extrapulmonary TB, monitor clinically.[4]
- CXR is not used for monitoring treatment as clearing lags behind clinical improvement. A CXR should be completed at the end of treatment for later comparison if reactivation is suspected.[4]
- Monitor drug toxicity.[4]
  - Gastrointestinal (GI) side effects and pruritus are common and can generally be managed without suspending treatment.
  - Hepatitis is the most common serious adverse event (symptoms include dark urine and decreased appetite); elevation of liver enzymes up to 3 times normal occurs in 20% and is of no clinical importance. Treatment (isoniazid, pyrazinamide, or rifampin) should be discontinued for elevations of 5 times or more or with symptoms, and drugs reintroduced one at a time after liver function has normalized.
  - Hypersensitivity reactions usually require discontinuing treatment.
  - Hyperuricemia and arthralgias can occur with pyrazinamide and can be managed with aspirin; the drug should be discontinued if the patient develops gouty arthritis.
  - Autoimmune thrombocytopenia may be caused by rifampin and requires discontinuing the drug.
  - Optic neuritis may occur with ethambutol and the drug should be discontinued. Visual acuity and color vision testing monthly if ethambutol is used for more than 2 months or in doses greater than 15 to 20 mg/kg.[29]
- Routine measurements of hepatic and renal function and platelet count are not necessary during treatment unless patients have baseline abnormalities or are at increased risk of hepatotoxicity (eg, hepatitis B or C virus infection, alcohol abuse).

PATIENT EDUCATION

- Identifying and testing household and other intimate contacts and maintaining follow-up are extremely important for preventing spread, insuring cure, and monitoring for drug toxicity (as below). The potential severity of TB should be emphasized.
- If available, patients should consider receiving treatment through a (DOT) short-course program comprised of 5 distinct elements: political commitment, microscopy services, drug supplies, surveillance and monitoring systems and use of highly efficacious regimens, and direct observation of treatment.[30] Although data are conflicting about the benefits of such programs, they may be better equipped to provide the intense services needed, especially in resource poor communities. DOT is recommended for the 3-month combination rifampin and INH treatment.
- TB is not spread through direct contact, sharing food, or kissing. The best prevention of progression and spread is to take the prescribed medications regularly for the recommended duration and to avoid unnecessary contact with people from outside the household (eg, avoid work, day care facilities, or schools) for the first 2 weeks of treatment and until you have 3 negative AFB sputum cultures and you feel better.

PATIENT RESOURCES

- Centers for Disease Control and Prevention—**http://www.cdc.gov/tb/.**
- MedlinePlus. *Tuberculosis*—**http://www.nlm.nih.gov/medlineplus/tuberculosis.html.**

PROVIDER RESOURCES

- Centers for Disease Control and Prevention—**http://www.cdc.gov/tb/.**
- Lawn SD, Zumla AI. Tuberculosis. Lancet. 2011;378(9785):57-72, **http://www.thelancet.com/journals/lancet/article/PIIS0140-6736(10)62173-3/abstract.**
- American Thoracic Society, CDC, and Infectious Diseases Society of America. Treatment of tuberculosis. MMWR Recomm Rep. 2003 Jun 20;54(RR-11):1-77, **http://www.cdc.gov/mmwr/preview/mmwrhtml/rr5211a1.htm.**
- Occupational Safety & Health Administration. *Occupational exposure and TB*—**http://www.osha.gov/SLTC/tuberculosis/index.html.**

REFERENCES

1. Centers for Disease Control and Prevention. *A Global Perspective on Tuberculosis (Fact Sheet)*. http://www.cdc.gov/tb/events/WorldTB-Day/resources_global.htm. Accessed January 2012.
2. Centers for Disease Control and Prevention. *Trends in Tuberculosis, 2010 (Fact Sheet)*. http://www.cdc.gov/tb/publications/factsheets/statistics/TBTrends.htm. Accessed January 2012.
3. Lawn SD, Zumla AI. Tuberculosis. *Lancet*. 2011;378(9785):57-72.
4. Escalante P. In the clinic. Tuberculosis. *Ann Intern Med*. 2009;150(11):ITC61-614.
5. Bailey TC, Fraser VJ, Spitznagel EL, Dunagan WC. Risk factors for a positive tuberculin skin test among employees of an urban, midwestern teaching hospital. *Ann Intern Med*. 1995;122(8):580-585.
6. Targeted tuberculin testing and treatment of latent tuberculosis infection. This official statement of the American Thoracic Society was adopted by the ATS Board of Directors, July 1999. This is a Joint Statement of the American Thoracic Society (ATS) and the Centers for Disease Control and Prevention (CDC). This statement was endorsed by the Council of the Infectious Diseases Society of America. (IDSA), September 1999, and the sections of this statement. *Am J Respir Crit Care Med*. 2000;161(4 pt 2):S221-S247.
7. Chen J, Zhang R, Wang J, et al. Interferon-gamma release assays for the diagnosis of active tuberculosis in HIV-infected patients: a systematic review and meta-analysis. *PLoS One*. 2011;6(11):e26827.
8. Bamford AR, Crook AM, Clark JE, et al. Comparison of interferon-gamma release assays and tuberculin skin test in predicting active tuberculosis (TB) in children in the UK: a paediatric TB network study. *Arch Dis Child*. 2010;95(3):180-186.
9. Sia IG, Wieland ML. Current concepts in the management of tuberculosis. *Mayo Clin Proc*. 2011;86(4):348-361.
10. Jain AK. Tuberculosis of the spine: a fresh look at an old disease. *J Bone Joint Surg Br*. 2010;92(7):905-913.
11. Sinclair D, Abba K, Grobler L, Sudarsanam TD. Nutritional supplements for people being treated for active tuberculosis. *Cochrane Database Sys Rev*. 2011;(11):CD006086.

12. Farmer P, Robin S, Ramilus SL, Kim JY. Tuberculosis, poverty, and "compliance": lessons from rural Haiti. *Semin Respir Infect*. 1991;6(4):254-260.

13. Martineau AR, Timms PM, Bothamley GH, et al. High-dose vitamin D(3) during intensive-phase antimicrobial treatment of pulmonary tuberculosis: a double-blind randomised controlled trial. *Lancet*. 2011;377(9761):242-250.

14. Centers for Disease Control and Prevention. Treatment of Tuberculosis, American Thoracic Society, CDC, and Infectious Diseases Society of America. *MMWR*. 2003;52(RR-11):1-77.

15. Lienhardt C, Cook SV, Burgos M, et al. Efficacy and safety of a 4-drug fixed-dose combination regimen compared with separate drugs for treatment of pulmonary tuberculosis: the Study C randomized controlled trial. *JAMA*. 2011;305(14):1415-1423.

16. WHO. *Treatment of Tuberculosis: Guidelines*. 4th ed. Geneva, Switzerland: World Health Organization; 2010. http://whqlibdoc.who.int/publications/2010/9789241547833_eng.pdf. Accessed January 2012.

17. Ziganshina LE, Squire SB. Fluoroquinolones for treating tuberculosis. *Cochrane Database of Syst Rev*. 2008;(1):CD004795.

18. Blanc FX, Sok T, Laureillard D, et al. Earlier versus later start of antiretroviral therapy in HIV-infected adults with tuberculosis. *N Engl J Med*. 2011;365(16):1471-1481.

19. Abdool Karim SS, Naidoo K, Grobler A, et al. Integration of antiretroviral therapy with tuberculosis treatment, *N Engl J Med*. 2011;365(16):1492-1501.

20. Centers for Disease Control and Prevention. *Treatment Options for Latent Tuberculosis Infection*. http://www.cdc.gov/tb/publications/factsheets/treatment/LTBItreatmentoptions.htm. Accessed January 2012.

21. Jereb JA, Goldberg SV, Powell K. Recommendations for use of an isoniazid-rifapentine regimen with direct observation to treat latent mycobacterium tuberculosis infection weekly. *MMWR*. 2011;60(48); 1650-1653.

22. Sterling TR, Villarino ME, Borisov AS, et al. Three months of rifapentine and isoniazid for latent tuberculosis infection. *N Engl J Med*. 2011;365(23):2155-2166.

23. Horsburgh CR Jr, Goldberg S, Bethel J, et al. Latent TB infection treatment acceptance and completion in the United States and Canada. *Chest*. 2010;137(2):401-409.

24. Kaufmann SH, Hussey G, Lambert PH. New vaccines for tuberculosis. *Lancet*. 2010;375(9731):2110-2119.

25. Colditz GA, Brewer TF, Berkley CS, et al. Efficacy of BCG vaccine in the prevention of tuberculosis. Meta-analysis of the published literature. *JAMA*. 1994;271(9):698-702.

26. Centers for Disease Control and Prevention. *Vaccine and Immunizations: TB Vaccine (BCG)*. http://www.cdc.gov/tb/topic/vaccines/default.htm. Accessed May 2012.

27. Harrison SW, Ganzhorn F, Radner A. Tuberculosis. In: Sloane P, Slatt L, Ebell M, et al, eds. *Essentials of Family Medicine*. 6th ed. Philadephia, PA: Lippencott, Williams & Wilkins. 2011.

28. Raviglione MC, O'Brien RJ. Tuberculosis. In: Kasper DL, Braunwald E, Fauci AS, Hauser SL, Longo DL, Jameson JL, eds. *Harrison's Principles of Internal Medicine*. 16th ed. New York, NY: McGraw-Hill; 2005:953-966.

29. Centers for Disease Control and Prevention. *Infection Control in Health-Care Settings (Fact Sheet)*. http://www.cdc.gov/tb/publications/factsheets/prevention/ichcs.htm. Accessed January 2012.

30. Davies PD. The role of DOTS in tuberculosis treatment and control. *Am J Respir Med*. 2003;2(3):203-209.

PART 10

GASTROINTESTINAL

Strength of Recommendation (SOR)	Definition
A	Recommendation based on consistent and good-quality patient-oriented evidence.*
B	Recommendation based on inconsistent or limited-quality patient-oriented evidence.*
C	Recommendation based on consensus, usual practice, opinion, disease-oriented evidence, or case series for studies of diagnosis, treatment, prevention, or screening.*

[a]See Appendix A on pages 1241-1244 for further information.

65 CLOSTRIDIUM DIFFICILE INFECTION

Rajil M. Karnani, MD

PATIENT STORY

A 78-year-old Caucasian male with a past history of hypertension, diabetes mellitus type 2, gastroesophageal reflux disease, and mild dementia presents to the hospital from an assisted-living facility with a fever, change in mental status, and lethargy. On workup, the patient is found to have a fever of 102.3°F, rhonchi in the right lung base, a white blood cell count of $15,500 \times 10^3$, and an elevated creatinine of 2.1 mg/dL. He is started empirically on broad-spectrum antibiotics and admitted to the general medicine ward. He gradually improves over the next several days, but on day 6, he starts to develop diarrhea and abdominal cramping. Subsequent stool testing reveals *Clostridium difficile* toxin, and the patient is started on oral metronidazole. The diarrhea improves, and the patient continues oral metronidazole therapy on discharge to treat his C. difficile infection (CDI) (**Figure 65-1**).

SYNONYM

- Pseudomembranous colitis
- Clostridium difficile colitis

EPIDEMIOLOGY

- CDI is the most common cause of hospital-acquired infectious diarrhea.
  - It complicates up to 1% of hospital admissions.[1]
  - It is the most commonly recognized etiology of health-care-associated infectious diarrhea.[2]
  - *Clostridium difficile* spores, which are highly resistant to drying and many antiseptic solutions, such as alcohol-based rubs, do not sufficiently kill the spores.[3]

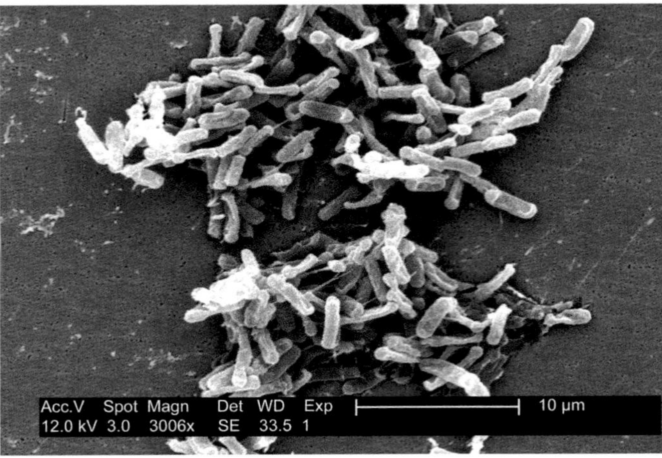

FIGURE 65-1 Electron micrograph of gram-positive *Clostridium difficile* bacteria from a stool culture. *(Reproduced with permission from the Centers for Disease Control and Prevention [CDC], Lois S. Wiggs, and Janice Carr.)*

- There is increased mortality associated with a hypervirulent strain that produces more toxin (B1/NAP1/O27) because of the absence of a gene (*tcdC*) that regulates toxin production.
- Rate of colonization
  - Of adult outpatients, 2% to 8% carry this organism.[1]
  - Of hospitalized adults, 20% are carriers (many are symptomless carriers of *C. difficile*, reflecting natural immunity).[1]

ETIOLOGY AND PATHOPHYSIOLOGY

- The normal route of transmission is fecal-oral, primarily within health care facilities.
- Estimated time between exposure to *C. difficile* and symptoms is 2 to 3 days.
- Normal colon flora confer "colonization resistance" against CDI by inhibiting overgrowth of *C. difficile* and other potential pathogens.[4]
- Loss of colonic resistance, most commonly caused by antibiotic use, predisposes to CDI.
- Most cases occur within 4 to 9 days of starting antibiotic use; however, CDI can occur several months after antibiotic exposure.
- Exotoxins (A and B) are produced by pathogenic strains, which produce mucosal injury and cell death in the colon, leading to an acute inflammatory reaction.
- The spectrum of CDI ranges from an asymptomatic carrier state → mild diarrhea → profuse diarrhea → colitis without pseudomembrane formation → colitis with pseudomembrane formation → fulminant colitis.

RISK FACTORS

- Age greater than 64 years[2]
- Duration of hospitalization
- Exposure to antimicrobial agents, with almost all antimicrobial agents implicated in CDI
- Cancer chemotherapy
- Gastrointestinal surgery
- Tube feeding
- Possible association of acid-suppressing medications with risk[2]

DIAGNOSIS

CLINICAL FEATURES

- Diarrhea (3 or more unformed stools in < 24 h)[5]
- Nausea, anorexia
- Fever, malaise
- Abdominal pain and cramping
- Signs of dehydration
- Peritoneal signs
- Abdominal distention

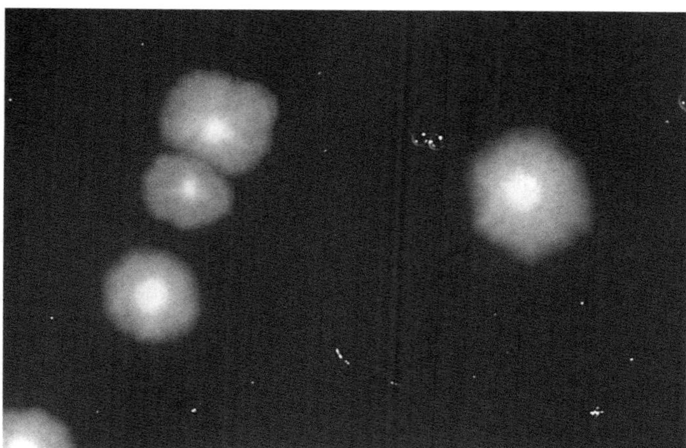

FIGURE 65-2 Stool culture positive for *Clostridium difficile*. This is a blood agar, cycloserine mannitol plate culture growing colonies of *C. difficile* after 48 h. (*Reproduced with permission from the Centers for Disease Control and Prevention [CDC] and Dr. Gilda Jones.*)

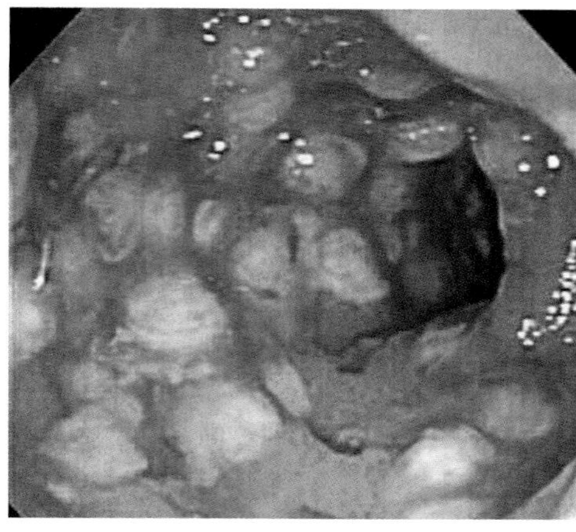

FIGURE 65-3 Yellow pseudomembranes noted in the colon of this patient with *Clostridium difficile* infection. (Reprinted with permission from Longo DL, Fauci A, Kasper D, Hauser S, Jameson J, Loscalzo J. *Harrison's Principles of Internal Medicine*. 18th ed. New York: McGraw-Hill, 2012.)

LABORATORY AND IMAGING STUDIES

- Enzyme immunoassays are the most widely used tests for CDI. They are fast and easy to perform but may carry a higher false-positive rate because some kits test only for toxin A, with some strains of *C. difficile* producing only toxin B.
    - Testing for toxins should only be done on unformed (diarrheal) stool.
    - Repeat testing for *C. difficile* toxin is not indicated to monitor response; following the clinical course, some patients will continue to shed *C. difficile* toxin in their stool weeks after complete clinical recovery.
- Stool culture (**Figure 65-2**) is the most sensitive test, although it is not clinically practical because of the slow turnaround time.
- Other blood tests to consider include a complete blood cell count (CBC) to check for leukocytosis and a serum urea nitrogen/creatinine ratio to check for prerenal azotemia as a sign of dehydration.
- Plain abdominal radiographs and computed tomography may reveal a thickened colonic mucosa, a dilated colon (which is indicative of toxic megacolon), or free air (indicative of perforation).
- Endoscopy can rapidly make the diagnosis of CDI with visualization of raised, yellow mucosal plaques (pseudomembranes) (**Figure 65-3**). This is not a first-line test when the diagnosis can be made by noninvasive testing.

DIFFERENTIAL DIAGNOSIS

- Other common causes of infectious diarrhea are the following:
    - *Salmonella*—Infection can be food-borne and community acquired; it is associated with fever, abdominal pain, and fecal leukocytes.
    - *Shigella*—Infection occurs via person-to-person spread; it is associated with fever, abdominal pain, vomiting. and fecal leukocytes.
    - *Campylobacter*—This is a community-acquired infection from undercooked poultry; fever, abdominal pain, and fecal leukocytes are common.
    - *Vibrio*—Infection results from seafood ingestion.
    - *Yersinia*—This infection is community acquired and food-borne; it can be associated with persistent abdominal pain, erythema nodosum, and mesenteric adenitis.
    - *Cryptosporidia*—Waterborne transmission, travel, or immunocompromised patients are associated with this infection; bloody stools are not characteristic. Consider cryptosporidia if diarrhea persists for more than 7 days.
    - *Giardia*—Infection can occur in relation to day care; consider this infection in a traveler or hiker who consumed untreated water. Transmission is waterborne. Consider if diarrhea persists for more than 7 days. Abdominal pain is common, but fever, bloody stool, and fecal leukocytes are not common. Check immunoglobulin A if diarrhea is refractory.
    - *Entamoeba*—Infection can result from travel from tropical areas; bloody or Hemoccult-positive stools are common.
    - Noroviruses (includes Norwalk virus)—These are the most common cause of viral gastroenteritis. Diarrhea and vomiting are common. Day care, nursing homes, cruise ships, undercooked shell fish are common means of transmission. Abdominal pain and nausea/vomiting are common. Bloody stools and fecal leukocytes are not common.
- Intestinal obstruction
- Ischemic bowel—Consider an ischemic bowel in patients older than 60 with established risk factors for thrombosis or emboli; signs and symptoms commonly are nonspecific, but the patient presents with a sudden onset of crampy abdominal pain and diarrhea and hematochezia within 24 h of symptom onset. Sudden onset of pain is from systemic emboli, and an insidious onset of pain results from atherosclerotic disease.
- Gastrointestinal malignancy.
- Noninfectious drug-associated diarrhea.
- Laxative use/abuse.

MANAGEMENT

- The Infectious Diseases Society of America guidelines in 2010 for CDI in adults recommend the following[2]:

- Stop the offending antibiotic unless it is necessary to treat the patient's underlying infection.[2] SOR Ⓐ
- Correct fluid and electrolyte abnormalities that are likely caused by the diarrhea.
- Avoid antiperistaltic agents as they may worsen the diarrhea and cause serious complications (eg, toxic megacolon). SOR Ⓒ
- Start enteric isolation precautions (use of gown and gloves by all health care workers in contact with the patient).
- Mild CDI: Metronidazole 500 mg three times a day for 10-14 days.[2] SOR Ⓐ
- Severe CDI (any 2 of the following: age > 60, temperature elevation above 101°F, serum albumin < 2.5 mg/dL, white blood cell count > 15,000).
  - Vancomycin 125 mg every 6 h orally for 10 to 14 days. SOR Ⓒ
  - Colonic levels if vancomycin are extremely high after an oral dose. It is *not* effective with intravenous dosing.
  - Use vancomycin per rectum as a retention enema if ileus is present.
- Intravenous immunoglobulin (IVIG) may be tried as more than 50% of the population has detectable antibodies to *C. difficile* toxins A and B; thus, IVIG has toxin-neutralizing capability (400 mg/kg).
- However, no controlled trials have been performed.[2]
- Perform a subtotal colectomy for severely ill patients or if there are signs of toxic megacolon.[2] SOR Ⓑ Monitor serum lactate levels; if greater than 5, there is an increase in perioperative mortality.

PROGNOSIS

- Complications of CDI include dehydration, electrolyte disturbance, toxic megacolon, bowel perforation, renal failure, systemic inflammatory response syndrome, sepsis, and death.[2]
- Recurrent episodes of CDI occur in 6% to 25% of patients with a first episode.[2]

FOLLOW-UP

- Patients should be followed for signs of clinical improvement, including resolution of fever, reduction in stool frequency, improvement in stool consistency, and rehydration.
- Repeated stool testing is not necessary in patients with resolved symptoms as treatment of asymptomatic carriers is not indicated.
  - If *C. difficile* diarrhea recurs, treat the second episode with the same regimen as the first episode.
  - Third and subsequent episodes should be treated with only vancomycin to avoid neurotoxicity associated with repeated administrations of metronidazole.
    - These recurrences should be treated with 10 to 14 days of oral vancomycin, followed by one of the following:
    - Tapering dose of vancomycin

      125 mg orally twice a day for 7 days, then

      125 mg orally every day for 7 days, then

      125 mg orally every 2 to 3 days for 2-8 weeks
    - Pulse dose course of vancomycin

      125, 250, or 500 mg every 3 days for 4 to 6 weeks

PATIENT EDUCATION

- Colonization with *C. difficile* is with fecal-oral transmission; therefore, hand hygiene is important.
- The use of antibiotics disrupts the balance of the intestinal flora, predisposing to CDI in patients colonized with *C. difficile*; therefore, limiting the unnecessary use and duration of antibiotic therapy is important.

PATIENT RESOURCES

- Kelly CP, LaMont JT. Patient information: antibiotic-associated diarrhea caused by Clostridium difficile (Beyond the Basics). UpToDate. **http://www.uptodate.com/contents/patient-information-antibiotic-associated-diarrhea-caused-by-clostridium-difficile-beyond-the-basics?source=search_result&search=clostridium+difficile&selectedTitle=1~2.**
- JAMA Patient Page: Clostridium difficile Colitis—**http://jama.ama-assn.org/content/301/9/988.full.pdf+html?sid=a210a6c7-b4e5-4dda-9891-b4209905ef90.**

PROVIDER RESOURCES

- *Clinical Practice Guidelines for Clostridium difficile Infection in Adults: 2010 Update by the Society for Healthcare Epidemiology of America (SHEA) and the Infectious Diseases Society of America (IDSA).* **http://www.jstor.org/stable/10.1086/651706.**

REFERENCES

1. Hessen MT. In the clinic. *Clostridium difficile* infection. *Ann Intern Med.* 2010;153(7):ITC41-15; quiz ITC416.
2. Cohen SH, Gerding DN, Johnson S, et al. Clinical practice guidelines for *Clostridium difficile* infection in adults: 2010 update by the Society for Healthcare Epidemiology of America (SHEA) and the Infectious Diseases Society of America (IDSA). *Infect Control Hosp Epidemiol.* 2010;31(5):431-455.
3. Oughton MT, Loo VG, Dendukuri N, et al. Hand hygiene with soap and water is superior to alcohol rub and antiseptic wipes for removal of *Clostridium difficile. Infect Control Hosp Epidemiol.* 2009;30:939-44.
4. Owens RC Jr, Donskey CJ, Gaynes RP, et al. Antimicrobial-associated risk factors for Clostridium difficile infection. *Clin Infect Dis.* 2008;46 Suppl 1:S19-31.
5. Bartlett JG and Gerding DN. Clinical recognition and diagnosis of *Clostridium difficile* infection. *Clin Infect Dis.* 2008;46 Suppl 1:S12-8.

66 COLON CANCER

Mindy A. Smith, MD, MS
Bonnie Wong, MD

PATIENT STORY

A 72-year-old man reports rectal bleeding with bowel movements over the past several months and the stool seems narrower with occasional diarrhea. He has a history of hemorrhoids but at this time is not experiencing rectal irritation or itching, as with previous episodes. His medical history is significant for controlled hypertension and a remote history of smoking. On digital rectal examination, his stool sample tests positive for blood but anoscopy fails to identify the source of bleeding. On colonoscopy, a mass is seen at 30 cm (**Figure 66-1**). A biopsy was obtained and pathology confirmed adenocarcinoma.

INTRODUCTION

Colon cancer is a malignant neoplasm of the colon, most commonly adenocarcinoma. With the establishment of screening programs and treatment improvements, there has been a slow decline in both the incidence and mortality from colon cancer, although it is still a leading cause of cancer death.[1]

EPIDEMIOLOGY

- Colon cancer is the third most common cancer in both men and women in the United States, second only to lung cancer as a cause of death.[1]
- The incidence and mortality have been slowly but steadily declining in the United States for the past decade.[2] The American Cancer Society estimated 142,570 new cases of colorectal cancer (102,900 colon cancer cases) and 51,370 deaths in 2010.[3]
- Onset is after age 50 years and peaks at around age 65 years.
- Proximal colon carcinoma rates in blacks are higher than in whites.[4]

ETIOLOGY AND PATHOPHYSIOLOGY

- Colon cancer appears to be a multipathway disease with tumors usually arising from adenomatous polyps or serrated adenomas; mutational events occur within the polyp including activation of oncogenes and loss of tumor-suppressor genes.[1,5]
- The probability of a polyp undergoing malignant transformation increases for the following cases[1]:
  - The polyp is sessile, especially if villous histology or flat.
  - Larger size—Malignant transformation is rare if smaller than 1.5 cm, 2% to 10% if 1.5 to 2.5 cm, and 10% if larger than 2.5 cm.
- Important genes involved in colon carcinogenesis include adenomatous polyposis gene mutations, *KRAS* oncogene, chromosome 18 loss of heterozygosity leading to inactivation of *SMAD4,* and *DCC* tumor suppression genes (deleted in colon cancer). Other mutations in genes such as *MSH2, MLH1,* and *PMS2* result in what is known as high-frequency microsatellite instability (H-MSI), which is found in cases of hereditary nonpolyposis colon cancer and in about 20% of sporadic colon cancers.[4]

RISK FACTORS

- Ingestion of red and processed meat[1,6]
- Hereditary syndromes—Polyposis coli and nonpolyposis syndromes (40% lifetime risk)[4]

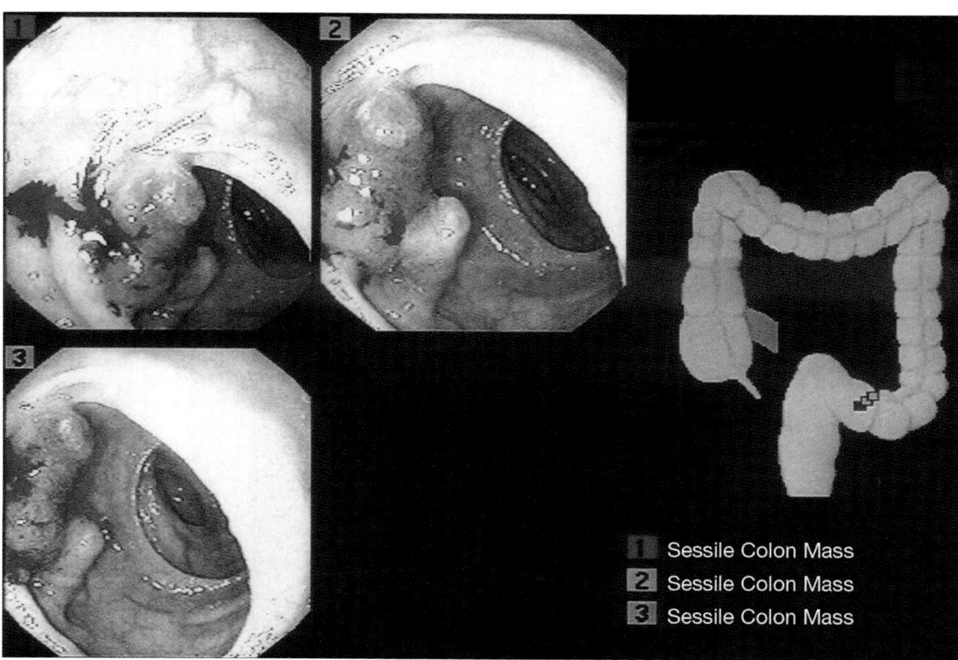

FIGURE 66-1 A sessile colon mass seen at 35 cm. At surgery, this was found to be a Duke stage A adenocarcinoma. (*Reproduced with permission from Michael Harper, MD.*)

- Inflammatory bowel disease
- Bacteremia with *Streptococcus bovis*—Increased incidence of occult tumors
- Following ureterosigmoidostomy procedures (5%-10% incidence over 30 years)
- Smoking
- Alcohol consumption
- Family history of colon cancer in a first-degree relative
- Obesity

DIAGNOSIS

The diagnosis of colon cancer is sometimes made following a positive screening test (ie, digital rectal examination, fecal occult blood testing [FOBT], sigmoidoscopy, colonoscopy, or barium enema). For patients who have symptoms and signs suggestive of colon cancer, the confirmative diagnostic test most commonly performed is colonoscopy with biopsy. Colonoscopy allows direct visualization of the lesion, examination of the entire large bowel for synchronous and metachronous lesions, and an ability to obtain tissue for histologic diagnosis.

CLINICAL FEATURES

Symptoms vary, primarily based on anatomic location, as follows[1]:

- Right-sided colon tumors more commonly ulcerate, occasionally causing anemia without change in stool or bowel habits.
- Tumors in the transverse and descending colon (**Figure 66-2**) often impede stool passage causing abdominal cramping, occasional obstruction, and rarely perforation.
- Tumors in the rectosigmoid region are associated more often with hematochezia, tenesmus (ie, urgency with a feeling of incomplete evacuation), narrow caliber stool, and uncommonly, anemia.

Physical signs often appear later in the course of the disease and can include the following[4]:

- Weight loss and cachexia
- Abdominal distention, discomfort, or tenderness
- Abdominal or rectal mass
- Ascites
- Rectal bleeding or occult blood on rectal examination

TYPICAL DISTRIBUTION

Colon cancers are approximately equally distributed between the right and left colon.[7]

IMAGING, ENDOSCOPY, AND WORKUP

- Colonoscopy of the entire colon is recommended to identify additional neoplasms or polyps (see **Figures 66-1** and **66-2**).
- Evaluation for metastatic disease includes the following[8]:
  - Local metastasis: Abdominal or pelvic computed tomography(CT) scans.
  - Lung metastasis: Chest X-ray (CXR) or chest CT.
  - Liver metastasis: magnetic resonance imaging (MRI) (pelvis), CT (abdomen and pelvis), or positron emission tomography (PET) CT scan (whole body).
  - The American College of Radiology also recommends transrectal rectum ultrasound for pretreatment staging for patients with rectal cancer and the addition of MRI of the abdomen for patients with large rectal tumors.[9]
  - Preoperative carcinoembryonic antigen (CEA)—An elevated pretreatment CEA (C-stage) has been shown to be an independent predictor of overall mortality (60% increased risk) in patients with colon cancer.[10] CEA may be elevated for reasons other than colon cancer, such as pancreatic or hepatobiliary disease; elevation does not always reflect cancer or disease recurrence. Post-treatment CEA levels can be used to monitor for recurrence.

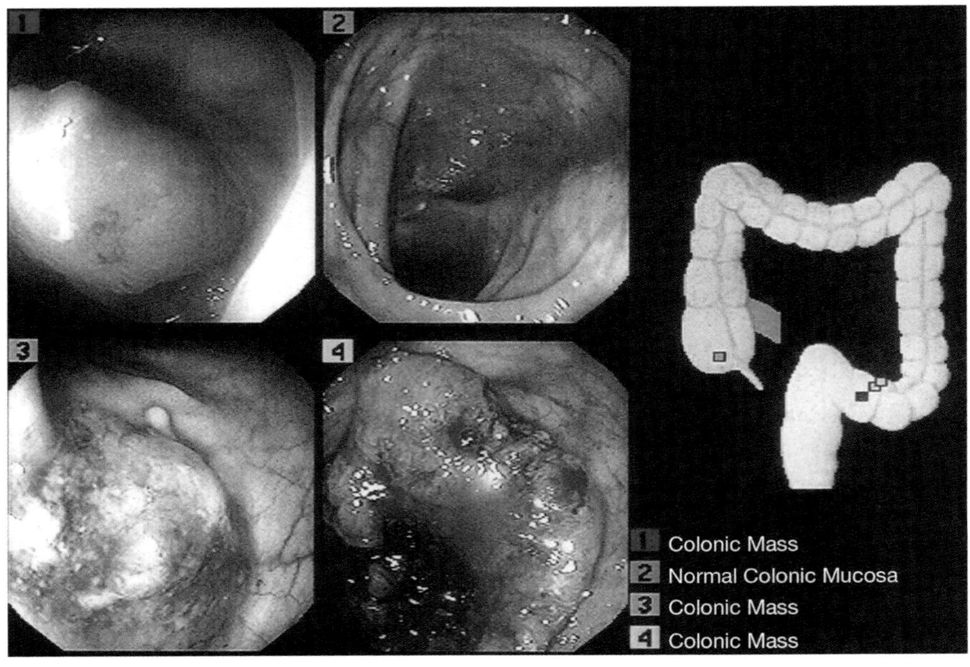

FIGURE 66-2 Plate 2 in this series shows normal cecum. The remaining frames show a large friable mass. Biopsy confirmed adenocarcinoma. The tumor was resected and determined to be Duke stage B adenocarcinoma. Colonoscopy 3 years later was negative. (*Reproduced with permission from Michael Harper, MD.*)

- At surgery, surgeons perform an examination of the liver, pelvis, hemidiaphragm, and full length of the colon for evidence of tumor spread.[1]

BIOPSY

Colonic adenocarcinomas can be microscopically well-differentiated or poorly differentiated glandular structures.[4] The addition of cytology brushings to forceps biopsies may increase the diagnostic yield, especially in the setting of obstructing tumors that cannot be traversed.[11]

DIFFERENTIAL DIAGNOSIS

Other causes of abdominal pain in patients in this age group are as follow:

- Inflammatory bowel disease, which includes ulcerative colitis and Crohn disease (see Chapter 77, Inflammatory Bowel Disease); symptoms include bloody diarrhea, tenesmus, passage of mucus, and cramping abdominal pain. Extraintestinal manifestations, more common in Crohn disease, include skin involvement (eg, erythema nodosum), rheumatologic symptoms (eg, peripheral arthritis, symmetric sacroiliitis), and ocular problems (eg, uveitis, iritis). Diagnosis can be made on the basis of endoscopy and biopsy.
- Diverticulitis—Patients present with fever, anorexia, lower left-sided abdominal pain, and diarrhea. Abdominal distention and peritonitis may be found on physical examination. Diagnosis is clinical or made on the basis of abdominal CT scan.
- Appendicitis—Initial symptoms include periumbilical or epigastric abdominal pain with time becoming more severe and localized to the right lower quadrant. Additional symptoms include fever, nausea, vomiting, and anorexia.

Following are other causes of rectal bleeding:

- Infectious agents—*Salmonella*, *Shigella*, certain *Campylobacter* species, enteroinvasive *Escherichia coli*, *Clostridium difficile*, and *Entamoeba histolytica* can cause bloody, watery diarrhea, and are identified by culture test. Bacterial toxins may be identified with *C. difficile*. Additional symptoms include fever and abdominal pain and the disease is often self-limited.
- Hemorrhoids (see Chapter 72, Hemorrhoids) and fissures—Bleeding is usually bright red and seen in the toilet or with wiping after bowel movements. Hemorrhoids can sometimes be visible as a protruding mass often associated with pruritus and fissures are identified as a cut or tear occurring in the anus. Hemorrhoidal pain is described as a dull ache but may be severe if thrombosed.
- Diverticula—Bleeding is usually abrupt in onset, painless, and can be massive, but often stops spontaneously. These may be seen on endoscopy or in radiographic study.
- Vascular colonic ectasias—Bleeding tends to be chronic resulting in anemia. Bleeding source may be identified during colonoscopy, but a radionuclide scan or angiography may be needed.
- Colon polyp (see Chapter 67, Colon Polyps)—Usually asymptomatic, although abdominal pain, diarrhea, or constipation can occur often with decreased stool caliber. Imaging studies often can distinguish and biopsy confirms absence of malignancy.

Other causes of intestinal obstruction include adhesions, peritonitis, inflammatory bowel disease, fecal impaction, strangulated bowels, and ileus.[2]

MANAGEMENT

MEDICATIONS

- Chemotherapy with fluorouracil (5-FU), irinotecan, with or without leucovorin (LV) is of marginal benefit with overall response in approximately 15% to 20% of patients.[1] For patients with stage II (Duke B) tumors (invasion into or through muscularis propria), authors of a systematic review found similar mortality rates with and without adjuvant chemotherapy.[12]
- Six months of postoperative treatment with 5-FU and LV decreased recurrence for stage III (Duke C) tumors (lymph node involvement) by 40% and increased survival;[1] the absolute survival benefit in one trial over LV alone was approximately 12% (49% vs 37%, respectively).[13] A reduction in relapse rate and a modest increase in 3-year disease-free survival were also seen in patients with Duke B and C colon cancer by adding oxaliplatin to 5-FU–leucovorin; however, overall survival is only improved for a subgroup of patients.[14]
- For patients with metastatic disease (stage IV/Duke D), first-line multiagent chemotherapy can be considered. Three randomized controlled trials (RCTs) have demonstrated improved response rates, progression-free survival, and overall survival when a biological agent (irinotecan or oxaliplatin) was combined with 5-FU–leucovorin.[15]

SURGERY OR OTHER TREATMENTS

- Total resection of the tumor is completed for attempted cure or for symptoms; open surgery or laparoscopic techniques can be used.[16]
- For superficial lesions, local excision or polypectomy with clear margins is performed; for other localized disease, wide surgical resection and reanastomosis is used.
- For patients with metastatic disease (stage IV/Duke D), treatment options include surgical resection, resection of liver metastases, palliative radiation or chemotherapy, first-line multiagent chemotherapy (see above) or participation in clinical trials.
- Total colonic resection is performed for patients with familial polyposis and multiple colonic polyps.
- For rectal carcinoma, sharp dissection is recommended (vs blunt) for rectal tumors to reduce recurrence to approximately 10%.[1] In addition, radiation therapy of the pelvis also decreases regional recurrence.[1] Postoperative treatment with 5-FU and radiation decreases recurrence for stage B2 and C tumors.[1]
- Preoperative radiation therapy can be used to shrink large tumors prior to resection.

PREVENTION AND SCREENING

- Primary prevention—Increased dietary fiber (conflicting evidence) and possibly increased ingestion of fruits, vegetables, fish, and milk.[6,17] High levels of physical activity also appear protective.[6,17] Low-dose aspirin is also associated with a lower risk of colon cancer and death from colon cancer.[18] Other medications possibly associated with a lower colon cancer risk include hormone therapy and oral contraceptives.
- Individuals who undergo at least one round of screening for colon cancer have a reduced risk of death from bowel cancer. In addition,

early polyp removal by colonoscopy with polypectomy is associated with a reduced risk for colorectal cancer in the population setting.[19] Of the screening tests, high-sensitivity fecal occult blood testing (FOBT), flexible sigmoidoscopy (FSG) with FOBT, and colonoscopy are recommended options.[20] The US Preventive Services Task Force (USPSTF) recommends screening for colorectal cancer in adults, beginning at age 50 years and continuing until age 75 years.[20] SOR Ⓐ

- FOBT—This test will be positive in 2% to 4% of asymptomatic patients; less than 10% will have colon cancer.[1] There is a good evidence that periodic FOBT reduces mortality from colorectal cancer; annual screening is recommended.[20]
- FSG—There is good evidence that sigmoidoscopy in combination with FOBT reduces mortality from colon cancer.[11] The ideal interval for surveillance is unknown but the USPSTF recommended a 5-year interval of surveillance by FSG combined with high-sensitivity FOBT every 3 years.[20]
- Colonoscopy—There is emerging evidence that screening colonoscopy is effective in reducing colorectal cancer mortality. Population-based observational study has shown a declining incidence of colon cancer and gains in life-years where colonoscopy screening programs are in place. Colonoscopy also allows inspection of the proximal colon and early removal of polyps.[11,21] Examples of colonoscopy pictures are shown in **Figures 66-1** to **66-3**.
- Double-contrast barium enema—This test offers an alternative means of whole-bowel examination, but is less sensitive than colonoscopy and there is no direct evidence that it is effective in reducing mortality rates. **Figures 66-4** and **Figure 66-5** display classic “apple-core deformities” of the colon from colon cancer.
- Other Tests—CT colonography and stool DNA test have been available for colorectal cancer screening. However, more research is needed to study their potential benefits and harms before widespread clinical use of these tests can be recommended as screening tools.[22]
- Secondary prevention—Low-dose aspirin (81 mg) has been shown to prevent adenomas in patients with previous colon cancer.[23]

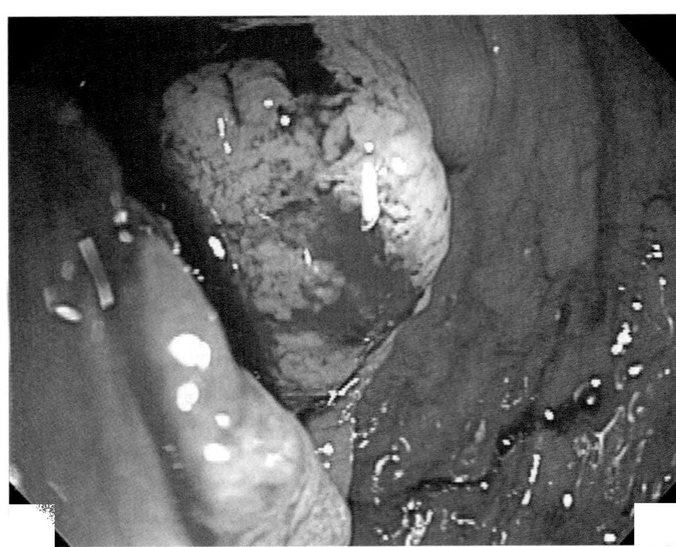

FIGURE 66-3 Adenocarcinoma in the cecum found on colonoscopy. (*Reproduced with permission from Marvin Derezin, MD.*)

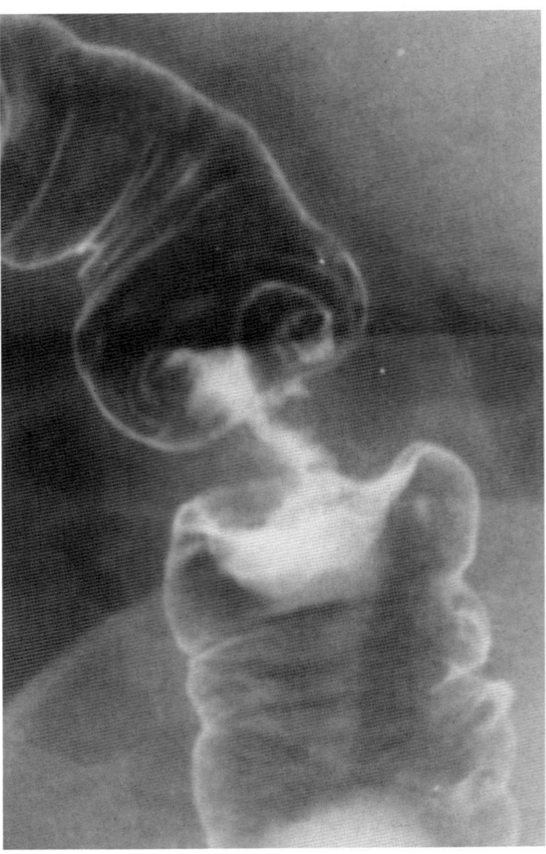

FIGURE 66-4 An “apple-core” lesion on barium enema consistent with colon cancer. The patient is a 72-year-old African American man who presented with weight loss. A complete blood count demonstrated moderate anemia and his Hemoccult cards were positive. (*Reproduced with permission from E.J. Mayeaux, Jr., MD.*)

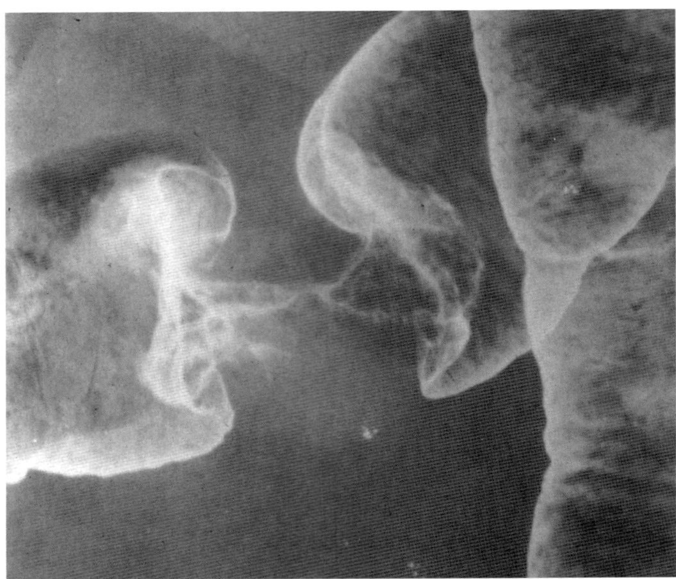

FIGURE 66-5 A barium enema reveals a large “apple-core” lesion consistent with colon cancer. The patient in a 64-year-old man who had a barium enema performed as part of the workup for weight loss and vague abdominal pain. (*Reproduced with permission from E.J. Mayeaux, Jr., MD.*)

PROGNOSIS

- Duke A (T1N0M0)—Cancer limited to mucosa and submucosa; 5-year survival: 90.1%.[1, 24]
- Duke B1 (T2N0M0)—Cancer extends into muscularis; 5-year survival: 85%.
- Duke B2 (T3N0M0)—Cancer extends into or through serosa; 5-year survival: 70% to 80%.
- Duke C (TxN1M0)—Cancer involves regional lymph nodes; 5-year survival: 35% to 69.2%.
- Duke D (TxNxM1)—Distant metastases (ie, lung, liver); 5-year survival: 5% to 11.7%.
- In addition to node involvement and metastases, poor outcome is associated with the following[1]:
  - Number of regional lymph nodes involved
  - Tumor penetration or perforation through the bowel wall
  - Histology of poor differentiation
  - Tumor adherence to adjacent organs
  - Venous invasion
  - Elevated preoperative CEA (ie, >5 ng/mL)
  - Aneuploidy
  - Specific chromosomal deletion (eg, allelic loss on chromosome 18q)

FOLLOW-UP

- Staging is based on tumor depth and spread and predicts survival as above[1]:
- Surveillance recommendations are as follows[25]:
  - Office visits and CEA evaluations should be performed at a minimum of 3 times per year for the first 2 years of follow-up. SOR Ⓐ
  - There is insufficient data to recommend for or against CXR as a part of routine colorectal cancer follow-up. SOR Ⓒ
  - Posttreatment colonoscopy should be performed at 3-year intervals. SOR Ⓐ
  - Periodic anastomotic evaluation is recommended for patients who have undergone resection/anastomosis or local excision of rectal cancer. SOR Ⓑ
  - Serum hemoglobin, Hemoccult II (FOBT), and liver function tests (hepatic enzymes tests) should not be routine components of a follow-up program. SOR Ⓐ
- For patients with progressive disease, options for further therapy must be discussed including discontinuing therapy, intrahepatic chemotherapy (if appropriate), and experimental (ie, phase I) therapy.

PATIENT EDUCATION

- Most recurrences occur within the first 3 to 4 years, so survival at 5 years is a good indication of cure.[1]
- Surveillance for recurrence should be conducted over the first 5 years following treatment as noted above. In addition to identifying recurrence, a second tumor is found in 3% to 5% and adenomatous polyps will be found in more than 15% of patients over that period.[1]

PATIENT RESOURCES

- Medline Plus. *Colon cancer*—**http://www.nlm.nih.gov/medlineplus/ency/article/000262.htm.**
- National Cancer Institute—**http://www.cancer.gov/cancertopics/pdq/treatment/colon/patient.**

PROVIDER RESOURCES

- National Cancer Institute—**http://www.cancer.gov/cancertopics/pdq/treatment/colon/HealthProfessional.**
- Medscape. *Colon Adenocarcinoma*—**http://emedicine.medscape.com/article/277496-overview.**

REFERENCES

1. Mayer R. Gastrointestinal tract cancer. In: Kasper DL, Braunwald E, Fauci AS, Hauser SL, Longo DL, Jameson JL, eds. *Harrison's Principles of Internal Medicine.* 16th ed. New York, NY: McGraw-Hill, 2005:523-533.
2. Edwards B, Ward E, Kohler B, et al. Annual report to the nation on the status of cancer, 1975-2006, featuring colorectal cancer trends and impact of interventions (risk factors, screening, and treatment) to reduce future rates. *Cancer.* 2010;116(3):544-573.
3. Jemal A, Siegel R, Xu J, Ward E. Cancer statistics, 2010. *CA Cancer J Clin.* 2010;60(5):277-300.
4. Dragovich T. *Colon Adenocarcinoma.* http://emedicine.medscape.com/article/277496-overview. Accessed June 2013.
5. Jass JR. Classification of colorectal cancer based on correlation of clinical, morphological, and molecular features. *Histopathology.* 2007;50:113-130.
6. Cancer Research UK. *Bowel Cancer.* http://info.cancerresearchuk.org/cancerstats/types/bowel/riskfactors/. Accessed June 2013.
7. Topazian M. Gastrointestinal endoscopy. In: Kasper DL, Braunwald E, Fauci AS, Hauser SL, Longo DL, Jameson JL, eds. *Harrison's Principles of Internal Medicine.* 16th ed. New York, NY: McGraw-Hill, 2005: 1730-1739.
8. Niekel MC, Bipat S, Stoker J. Diagnostic imaging of colorectal liver metastases with CT, MR imaging, FDG PET, and/or FDG PET/CT: a meta-analysis of prospective studies including patients who have not previously undergone treatment. *Radiology.* 2010;257(3):674-684.
9. Rosen MP, Bree RL, Foley WD, et al; Expert Panel on Gastrointestinal Imaging. *ACR Appropriateness Criteria® Pretreatment Staging of Colorectal Cancer.* http://www.guideline.gov/content.aspx?id=35139. Accessed June 2013.
10. Thirunavukarasu P, Sukumar S, Sathaiah M, et al. C-stage in colon cancer: implications of carcinoembryonic antigen biomarker in staging, prognosis, and management. *J Natl Cancer Inst.* 2011;103(8): 689-697.
11. Davila RE, Rajan E, Adler D, et al. ASGE guideline: The role of endoscopy in the diagnosis, staging, and management of colorectal cancer. *Gastrointest Endosc.* 2005;61(1):1-7.
12. Figueredo A, Charette ML, Maroun J, et al. Adjuvant therapy for stage II colon cancer: a systematic review from the Cancer Care Ontario Program in evidence-based care's gastrointestinal cancer disease site group. *J Clin Oncol.* 2004;22(16):3395-3407.

13. Laurie JA, Moertel CG, Fleming TR, et al. Surgical adjuvant therapy of large-bowel carcinoma: an evaluation of levamisole and the combination of levamisole and fluorouracil. The North Central Cancer Treatment Group and the Mayo Clinic. *J Clin Oncol.* 1989;7(10): 1447-1456.

14. André T, Boni C, Navarro M, et al. Improved overall survival with oxaliplatin, fluorouracil, and leucovorin as adjuvant treatment in stage II or III colon cancer in the MOSAIC trial. *J Clin Oncol.* 2009;27 (19):3109-3116.

15. National Cancer Institute. http://www.cancer.gov/cancertopics/pdq/treatment/colon/HealthProfessional/page9. Accessed June 2013.

16. National Cancer Institute. http://www.cancer.gov/cancertopics/pdq/treatment/colon/HealthProfessional/page4. Accessed June 2013.

17. National Cancer Institute. *Colorectal Cancer Prevention.* http://cancer.gov/cancertopics/pdq/prevention/colorectal/HealthProfessional. Accessed November 2011.

18. Rothwell PM, Wilson M, Elwin CE, et al. Long-term effect of aspirin on colorectal cancer incidence and mortality: 20-year follow-up of five randomised trials. *Lancet.* 2010;376(9754): 1741-1750.

19. Brenner H, Chang-Claude J, Seiler CM, et al. Protection from colorectal cancer after colonoscopy: a population-based, case-control study. *Ann Intern Med.* 2011;154(1):22-30.

20. U.S. Preventive Services Task Force. *Screeening for Colorectal Cancer.* http://www.uspreventiveservicestaskforce.org/uspstf08/colocancer/colosum.htm. Accessed June 2013.

21. Meza R, Jeon J, Renehan AG, Luebeck EG. Colorectal cancer incidence trends in the United States and United kingdom: evidence of right- to left-sided biological gradients with implications for screening. *Cancer Res.* 2010;70(13):5419-5429.

22. Zauber AG, Lansdorp-Vogelaar I, Knudsen AB, et al. Evaluating test strategies for colorectal cancer screening: a decision analysis for the U.S. Preventive Services Task Force. *Ann Intern Med.* 2008;149(9): 659-669.

23. Sandler RS, Halabi S, Baron JA, et al. A randomized trial of aspirin to prevent colorectal adenomas in patients with previous colorectal cancer. *N Engl J Med.* 2003;348(10):883-890.

24. National Cancer Institute. *Surveillance Epidemiology and End Results.* http://seer.cancer.gov/statfacts/html/colorect.html. Accessed June 2013.

25. Anthony T, Simmang C, Hyman N, et al. Practice parameters for the surveillance and follow-up of patients with colon and rectal cancer. *Dis Colon Rectum.* 2004;47(6):807-817.

67 COLON POLYPS

Cathy Abbott, MD
Mindy A. Smith, MD, MS

PATIENT STORY

A 62-year-old woman presents to her physician for routine annual examination. She has no known family history of colon disease and is asymptomatic. Stool cards and flexible sigmoidoscopy were recommended and on flexible sigmoidoscopy a 2.4-cm polyp was noted at 35 cm. A colonoscopy was performed and additional polyps were identified in the descending colon and cecum (**Figure 67-1**).

INTRODUCTION

Colon polyps are growths that arise from the epithelial cells lining the colon.

EPIDEMIOLOGY

- More than 30% of middle-aged and elderly patients are found to have adenomatous polyps on screening and based on autopsy surveys; fewer than 1% will become malignant.[1] The lifetime risk of colon cancer is 5.12%.[2]
- Patients with an adenomatous polyp have a 30% to 50% risk for developing another adenoma and are at higher risk for colon cancer. This risk is greatest in the first 4 years after diagnosis of the first polyp, and greater if a villous adenoma or more than 3 polyps were found.
- Familial adenomatous polyposis of the colon is a rare autosomal dominant disorder. Thousands of adenomatous polyps appear in the large colon, generally by age 25 years, and colorectal cancer develops in almost all of these patients by age 40 years.[1] Other hereditary polyposis syndromes include Gardner syndrome, Turcot syndrome, Peutz-Jeghers syndrome, Cowden disease, familial juvenile polyposis, and hyperplastic polyposis.[3]

ETIOLOGY AND PATHOPHYSIOLOGY

- Following are the several types of colon polyps:
  - Hyperplastic polyps—These contain increased numbers of glandular cells with decreased cytoplasmic mucus and an absence of nuclear hyperchromatism, stratification, or atypia. Traditionally thought to be benign, recent evidence suggests malignant potential particularly for right-sided polyps, especially proximal hyperplastic serrated polyps[1] and those associated with hyperplastic polyposis syndrome (a familial disorder with multiple [>30] hyperplastic polyps proximal to the sigmoid colon with 2 or more >10 mm).[3] The percentage of polyps reported to be in this category ranges from 12% to 90%.[3,4]
  - Adenomatous polyps—These may be tubular, villous (papillary), or tubulovillous. In a case series of 582 patients who had a polyp removed, 81% were adenomatous, including 65% that were tubular, 25.8% tubulovillous, 7.2% villous adenomas, and 0.5% mixed adenomatous hyperplastic polyps; 12 (1.4%) were invasive carcinomas.[4]
    - Adenomatous polyps may be pedunculated or sessile; cancers more frequently develop in sessile polyps.[1]
  - Villous polyps can cause hypersecretory syndromes characterized by hypokalemia and profuse mucous discharge; these more frequently harbor carcinoma in situ or invasive carcinoma than other adenomas.[3]
  - Nonneoplastic hamartoma (juvenile polyp)—These are benign cystic polyps with mucous-filled glands, most commonly found

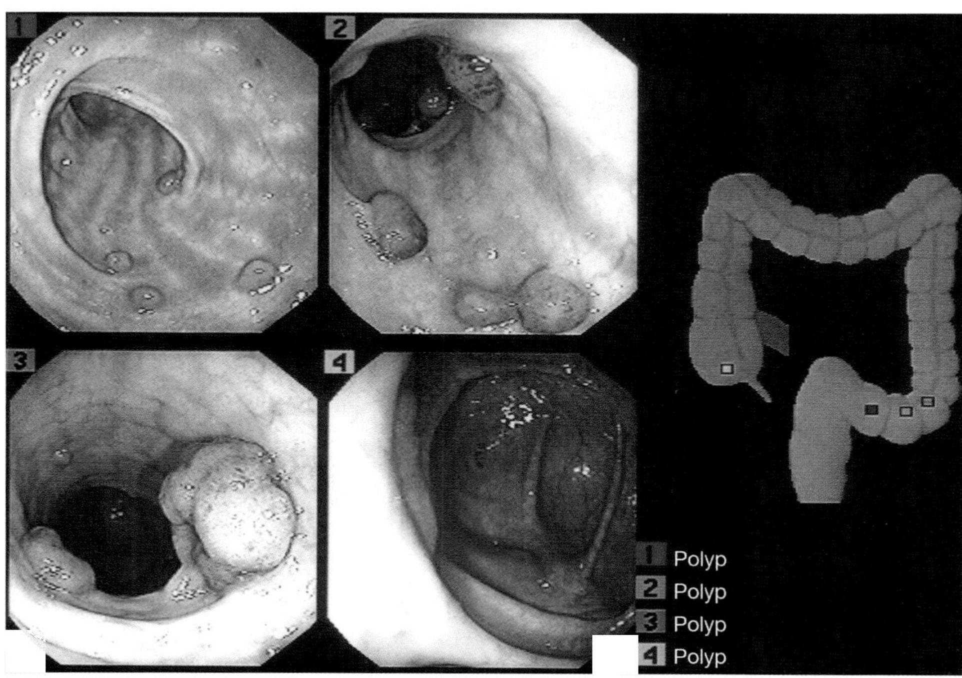

FIGURE 67-1 Colon polyps seen on colonoscopy. (*Reproduced with permission from Michael Harper, MD.*)

in male children, ages 2 to 5 years, and are often found as singular lesions, but additional polyps are found on panendoscopy in 40% to 50% of children. Juvenile polyps in adolescence may be associated with hereditary syndromes that carry malignant potential.[5]

- A series of genetic or molecular changes have been found that are thought to represent a multistep process from normal colon mucosa to malignant tumor.[3] These include the following:
  - Point mutations in the K-*ras* protooncogene lead to gene activation and deletion of DNA at the site of tumor-suppressor gene.
  - This results in an altered proliferative pattern and polyp formation.
  - Mutational activation of an oncogene, coupled with loss of tumor-suppressor genes, leads to malignant transformation.
  - Serrated polyps, which have in the past been characterized as hyperplastic polyps, are now known to have epigenetic alterations that may develop into colon cancers by another pathway—the CpG-island-methylation-phenotype pathway.[6]
  - Patients with familial polyposis inherit a germline alteration that leads into the above pathway.
- Insulin resistance, with increased concentrations of insulin-like growth factor type I, may also stimulate proliferation of the intestinal mucosa.

RISK FACTORS

- Older age—99% of cases occur in people older than age 40 years and 85% in those older than age 60 years.[7]
- Family history—Present in 10% to 20% of cases.[7]
- Diet appears to be associated with colon polyps and colon cancer. Animal fats may alter anaerobes in the gut microflora, increasing conversion of normal bile acids to carcinogens. Also, increased cholesterol is associated with an enhanced risk of development of adenomas.
- There may be an association between *Helicobacter* exposure and colonic polyps.[8,9]

DIAGNOSIS

CLINICAL FEATURES

- Usually asymptomatic.
- Patients may experience overt or occult rectal bleeding.
- Change in bowel habits—Diarrhea or constipation can occur, often with decreased stool caliber.
- Secretory villous adenomas can occasionally manifest as a syndrome of severe diarrhea with massive fluid and electrolyte loss.[3]

TYPICAL DISTRIBUTION

- Cancer distribution is approximately equal between the right and left colon. Juvenile polyps are usually found in the rectosigmoid region.

LABORATORY TESTING

- Occult blood in the stool is found in less than 5% of patients with polyps.[1] Of the 2% to 4% of asymptomatic patients who have heme positive stool on screening, 20% to 30% will have polyps.[1]
- For patients with a family history of familial adenomatous polyposis, DNA testing may be performed to detect the adenomatous polyposis coli *(APC)* gene mutation; this can lead to a definitive diagnosis before the development of polyps.[1] SOR Ⓒ A positive test finding only indicates susceptibility, not the actual presence of a polyp.[3]
- Genetic testing can also be considered for patients with a family history of hereditary nonpolyposis colorectal cancer (HNPCC), which is caused by germline mutation of the DNA mismatch repair genes (*hMLH1*, *hMSH2*, *hPMS1*, *hPMS2*, *hMSH6*).[10] SOR Ⓒ

IMAGING AND ENDOSCOPIC FEATURES

- Polyps may be identified on barium enema (**Figures 67-2** and **67-3**), flexible sigmoidoscopy, or colonoscopy (including virtual computer tomography colonoscopy) (**Figures 67-1** and **67-4**).
- A polyp is defined as a grossly visible protrusion from the mucosal surface, although adenomas can also be flat or even depressed.[11]
- Colonoscopy must be subsequently performed to identify additional lesions and remove all lesions.
- Synchronous lesions occur in one-third of cases (see **Figure 67-1**).

BIOPSY

- Polyps upon removal are sent for histology to determine type and whether dysplasia or carcinoma in situ is present (**Figure 67-5**).

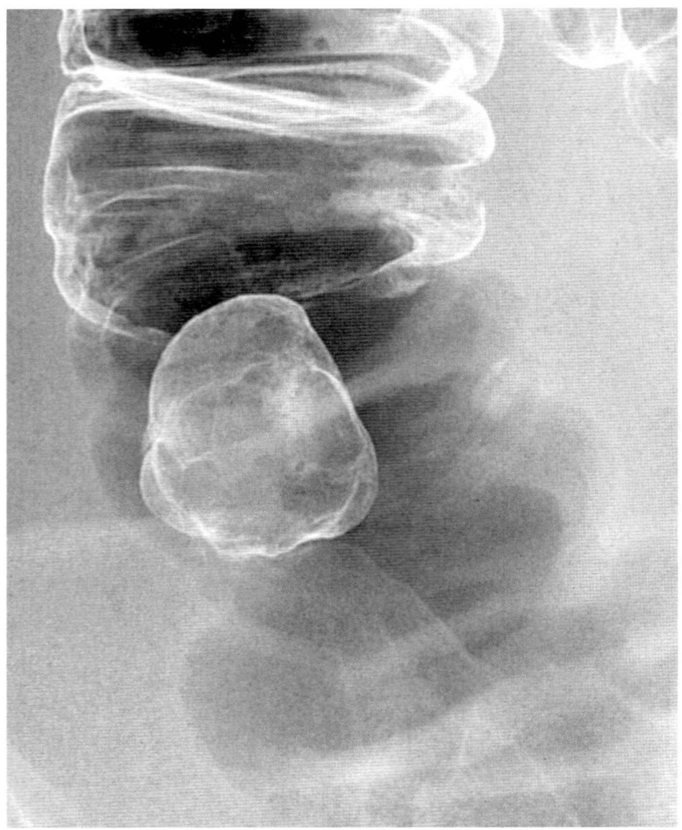

FIGURE 67-2 A 69-year-old woman with a family history of colon cancer presented for screening. Her Hemoccult test was positive. Her double-contrast barium enema (air contrast) demonstrated a large colonic polyp, which was found on surgery to be highly dysplastic. (*Reproduced with permission from E.J. Mayeaux, Jr., MD.*)

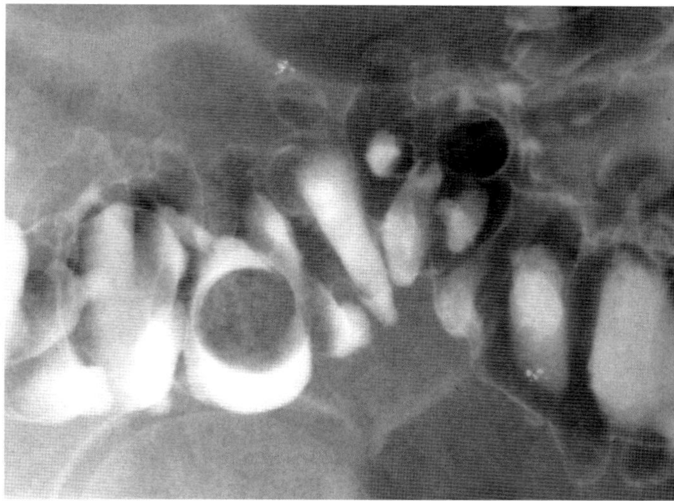

FIGURE 67-3 While getting a barium enema for other reasons, this patient was found to have a large colonic polyp. Biopsy of the polyp demonstrated early-stage colon cancer, which was treated by surgical resection. (*Reproduced with permission from E.J. Mayeaux, Jr., MD.*)

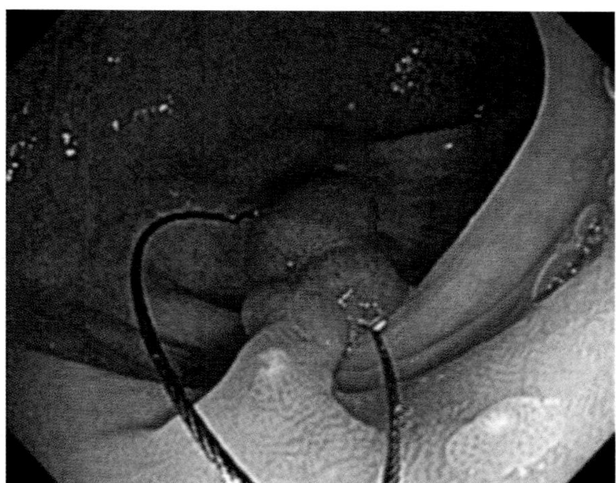

FIGURE 67-5 Polypectomy being performed through the colonoscope. (*Reproduced with permission from Marvin Derezin, MD.*)

DIFFERENTIAL DIAGNOSIS

Other causes of rectal bleeding include the following:

- Infectious agents—*Salmonella*, *Shigella*, certain *Campylobacter* species, enteroinvasive *Escherichia coli*, *Clostridium difficile*, and *Entamoeba histolytica* can cause bloody, watery diarrhea and are identified by culture. Bacterial toxins may be identified with *C. difficile* (see Chapter 65, *Clostridium difficile* Colitis). Additional symptoms include fever and abdominal pain, and the disease is often self-limited.
- Hemorrhoids and fissures—Bleeding is usually bright red blood and seen in the toilet or with wiping after bowel movements. Hemorrhoids can sometimes be visible as a protruding mass often associated with pruritus, and fissures are identified as a cut or tear occurring in the anus (see Chapter 72, Hemorrhoids). Hemorrhoidal pain is described as a dull ache, but may be severe if thrombosed.

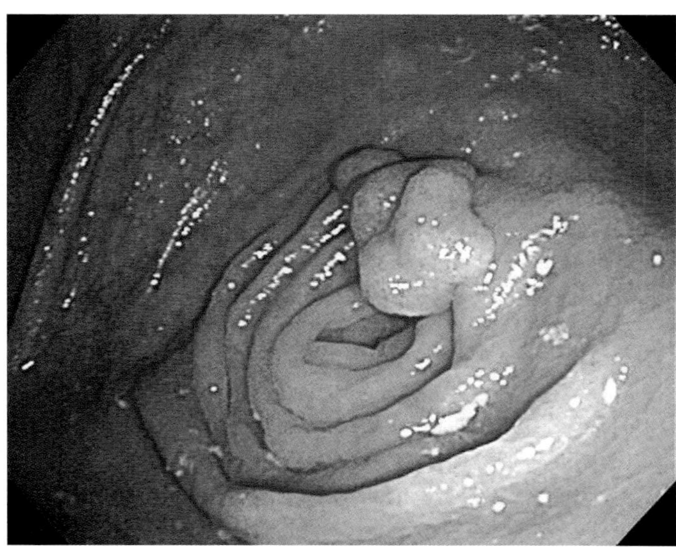

FIGURE 67-4 Polyp in the cecum seen on colonoscopy. (*Reproduced with permission from Marvin Derezin, MD.*)

- Diverticula—Bleeding is usually abrupt in onset, painless, and may be massive but often stops spontaneously. These may be seen on endoscopy or on radiographic study.
- Vascular colonic ectasias—Bleeding tends to be chronic, resulting in anemia. Bleeding source may be identified during colonoscopy but a radionuclide scan or angiography may be needed.
- Colon cancer—Other symptoms include abdominal cramping, tenesmus (ie, urgency with a feeling of incomplete evacuation), narrow caliber stool, occasional obstruction, and, rarely, perforation. Imaging studies often can distinguish and biopsy confirms malignancy (see Chapter 66, Colon Cancer).
- Inflammatory bowel disease—This includes ulcerative colitis and Crohn disease; symptoms include diarrhea, tenesmus, passage of mucus, and cramping abdominal pain (see Chapter 77, Inflammatory Bowel Disease). Extraintestinal manifestations are more common in Crohn disease and include skin involvement (eg, erythema nodosum), rheumatologic symptoms (eg, peripheral arthritis, symmetric sacroiliitis), and ocular problems (eg, uveitis, iritis). Diagnosis may be made on endoscopy.

MANAGEMENT

Removal of a solitary polyp can be completed during sigmoidoscopy or colonoscopy (see **Figure 67-5**).

PREVENTION

- Primary prevention of colon cancer should be encouraged.
  - Dietary alterations may be useful.
    - Decreasing animal fats as diets high in animal fats are thought to be a major risk factor based on epidemiologic studies. However, in the Women's Health Initiative study, a low-fat dietary intervention did not reduce the risk of colorectal cancer in postmenopausal women during 8.1 years of follow-up.[12]

- Additional dietary fiber has not shown to be helpful in controlled studies.[13]
- Increasing water consumption to 8 glasses per day may be helpful.
- Diets high in flavonols (fruits, vegetables, and tea) are associated with decreased risk of colon polyps, possibly by reducing serum interleukin (IL)-6, which is associated with inflammation and carcinogenesis.[14]

- Calcium supplements (1200 mg/d) have been shown to reduce the development of adenomatous polyps.[15] SOR Ⓐ
- Hormone therapy in women reduces colon cancer incidence.[16] SOR Ⓑ
- A meta-analysis failed to show that folic acid supplementation reduced the risk of recurrent colon adenomas.[17]
- Low-dose aspirin (81 mg/d) was found to decrease recurrent adenomas, including those containing advanced neoplasms.[18] SOR Ⓑ In patients with familial adenomatous polyposis, once-daily treatment with 25-mg rofecoxib significantly decreased the number and size of rectal polyps in one randomized trial.[19]
- Smoking cessation.[20]
- Increasing physical activity reduces the risk of advanced polyps and neoplasia, possibly by decreasing insulin resistance.[21]

PROGNOSIS

Patients with a polyp with tubulovillous features or with more than 3 polyps larger than 10 mm are at increased risk for further aggressive lesions on follow-up colonoscopy, and untreated patients with polyps larger than 10 mm are at increased risk for colon cancer both at the site of polyp and at other sites.[22]

FOLLOW-UP

- Secondary prevention of colon cancer should be maximized through screening and removal of additional or recurrent polyps or colon cancer in these patients (see Chapter 66, Colon Cancer). Although there is debate regarding the frequency of screening, the American Cancer Society, the US Multi-Society Task Force on Colorectal Cancer, and the American College of Radiology updated guideline recommends repeat colonoscopy at the following intervals:
  - Every 5 to 10 years for those with 1 to 2 small tubular adenomas with low-grade dysplasia after initial polypectomy.
  - Every 3 years for patients with 3 to 10 adenomas or 1 adenoma larger than 1 cm or any adenoma with villous features or high-grade dysplasia.
  - Less than every 3 years for patients with more than 10 adenomas.
  - At 2 to 6 months to verify complete removal in patients with sessile adenomas that are removed piecemeal.[23]
- Although screening options that enable detection of both adenomatous polyps and colon cancer include flexible sigmoidoscopy, colonoscopy, double-contrast barium enema, and computed tomography (CT) colonography (use of dyes or other visual enhancements during colonoscopy), authors of a Cochrane review found that chromoscopic colonoscopy enhances the detection of polyps in the colon and rectum.[24] This form of colonoscopy can be used to identify flat polyps, increasing the sensitivity of colonoscopy, and may allow for detection of high-risk polyps without the need for biopsy.

PATIENT EDUCATION

- Attention to lifestyle factors can contribute to decreasing the risk of colon polyps.
- Patients should be encouraged to undergo screening for colon cancer, including use of high-sensitivity Hemoccult cards, flexible sigmoidoscopy, or colonoscopy.[25] SOR Ⓐ
- Patients diagnosed with polyps should be encouraged to engage in continued surveillance for polyps and colon cancer. Those at increased risk for a subsequent advanced neoplasia (see earlier) should have a follow-up colonoscopy at 3 or fewer years.[23] SOR Ⓑ For other patients, follow-up is recommended at 5 to 10 years.[10] SOR Ⓒ

PATIENT RESOURCES

- National Digestive Diseases Information Clearinghouse. *Colon Polyps*—**http://digestive.niddk.nih.gov/ddiseases/pubs/colonpolyps_ez/index.htm.**
- Mayo Clinic. *Colon Polyps*—**http://www.mayoclinic.com/health/colon-polyps/DS00511/DSECTION=4.**

PROVIDER RESOURCES

- Medscape. *Colonic Polyps*—**http://emedicine.medscape.com/article/172674.**

REFERENCES

1. Mayer R. Gastrointestinal tract cancer. In: Kasper DL, Braunwald E, Fauci AS, Hauser SL, Longo DL, Jameson, JL, eds. *Harrison's Principles of Internal Medicine*, 16th ed. New York, NY: McGraw-Hill; 2005:523-533.
2. National Cancer Institute. http://seer.cancer.gov/statfacts/html/colorect.html. Accessed July 2013.
3. Enders GH. *Colon Polyps*. http://emedicine.medscape.com/article/172674-overview. Accessed July 2013.
4. Khan A, Shrier I, Gordon PH. The changed histologic paradigm of colorectal polyps. *Surg Endosc*. 2002;16(3):436-440.
5. Barnard J. Gastrointestinal polyps and polyp syndromes in adolescents. *Adolesc Med Clin*. 2004;15(1):119-129.
6. Noffsinger AE. Serrated polyps and colorectal cancer: new pathway to malignancy. *Annu Rev Pathol*. 2009;4:343-364.
7. Ballinger AB, Anggiansah C. Colorectal cancer. *BMJ*. 2007;335:715-718.
8. Mizuno S, Morita Y, Inui T, et al. *Helicobacter pylori* infection is associated with colon adenomatous polyps detected by high-resolution colonoscopy. *Int J Cancer*. 2005;117(6):1058-1059.
9. Abbass K, Gul W, Beck G, et al. Association of *Helicobacter pylori* infection with the development of colorectal polyps and colorectal cancer. *South Med J*. 2011;104(7):473-476.
10. American Gastroenterological Association medical position statement: hereditary colorectal cancer and genetic testing. *Gastroenterology*. 2001;121(1):195-197.
11. Anderson JC. Risk factors and diagnosis of flat adenomas of the colon. *Expert Rev Gastroenterol Hepatol*. 2011;5(1):25-32.
12. Beresford SA, Johnson KC, Ritenbaugh C, et al. Low-fat dietary pattern and risk of colorectal cancer: the Women's Health Initiative

Randomized Controlled Dietary Modification Trial. *JAMA.* 2006;295(6):643-654.

13. Asano TK., McLeod RS. Dietary fibre for the prevention of colorectal adenomas and carcinomas. *Cochrane Database Syst Rev.* 2002;(2): CD003430.
14. Bobe G, Albert PS, Sansbury LB, et al. Interleukin-6 as a potential indicator for prevention of high risk adenoma recurrence by dietary flavonols in the polyp prevention trial. *Cancer Prev Res (Phila).* 2010;3(6):764-775.
15. Weingarten MAMA, Zalmanovici Trestioreanu A, Yaphe J. Dietary calcium supplementation for preventing colorectal cancer and adenomatous polyps. *Cochrane Database Syst Rev.* 2008;(1):CD003548.
16. Nelson HS, Humphrey LL, Nygren P, et al. Postmenopausal hormone replacement therapy. *JAMA.* 2002;288(7):872-881.
17. Ibrahim EM, Zekri JM. Folic acid supplementation for the prevention of colorectal adenomas: metaanalysis of interventional trials. *Med Oncol.* 2010;27(3):915-918.
18. Baron JA, Cole BF, Sandler RS, et al. A randomized trial of aspirin to prevent colorectal adenomas. *N Engl J Med.* 2003;348(10):891-899.
19. Higuchi T, Iwama T, Yoshinaga K, et al. A randomized, double-blind, placebo-controlled trial of the effects of rofecoxib, a selective cyclooxygenase-2 inhibitor, on rectal polyps in familial adenomatous polyposis patients. *Clin Cancer Res.* 2003;9(13):4756-4760.
20. Botteri E, Iodice S, Raimondi S. Cigarette smoking and adenomatous polyps: a meta-analysis. *Gastroenterology.* 2008;134:388-395.
21. Wolin KY, Yan Y, Colditz GA. Physical activity and risk of colon adenoma: a meta-analysis. *Br J Cancer.* 2011;104(5):882-885.
22. Hassan C, Pickhardt PJ, Kim DH, et al. Systematic review: distribution of advanced neoplasia according to polyp size at screening colonoscopy. *Aliment Pharmacol Ther.* 2010;31(2):210-217.
23. Levin B, Lieberman DA, McFarland B, et al. Screening and surveillance for the early detection of colorectal cancer and adenomatous polyps, 2008: a joint guideline from the American Cancer Society, the US Multi-Society Task Force on Colorectal Cancer, and the American College of Radiology. *Gastroenterology.* 2008;134: 1570-1595.
24. Brown SR, Baraza W. Chromoscopy versus conventional endoscopy for the detection of polyps in the colon and rectum. *Cochrane Database Syst Rev.* 2010;(10):CD006439.
25. United States Preventive Services Task Force. *Colorectal Cancer Screening. Summary.* http://www.ahrq.gov/clinic/colorsum.htm. Accessed July 2013.

68 DIVERTICULITIS

Oliver Abela, MD

PATIENT STORY

A 68-year-old man presents with a 3-day history of constant pain in the left lower quadrant (LLQ) associated with nausea, fever, and chills. The pain is not relieved by bowel movement. He has never had abdominal pain in the past, and he has never had a colonoscopy. His past medical history is significant for hypertension and headaches, for which he takes hydrochlorothiazide and acetaminophen as needed. On physical examination, his temperature is 102.1°F, his blood pressure is 135/75 mm Hg, his pulse rate is 93/min, and his respiration rate is 16/min. There is tenderness to palpation of the LLQ without rebound or guarding, and his bowel sounds are decreased. His rectal examination is normal, and examination of his stool for occult blood is negative. His leukocyte count is 16,000/μL (16 × 109/L), and his contrast-enhanced computed tomographic (CT) scan of the abdomen and pelvis shows diverticula of the sigmoid colon with pericolic fatty infiltration and thickening of the bowel wall consistent with diverticulitis (**Figure 68-1**). The CT also shows a 1-cm abscess in association with the diverticulitis and a small amount of air in the abscess. There are no masses, strictures, obstructions, or fistula present. Patient is started on ciprofloxacin and metronidazole, clear liquids, intravenous fluids, and pain medications. He improves after 3 days of medical management; his diet is advanced, and he is sent home to finish a 14-day course of antibiotics.

INTRODUCTION

Diverticulitis is a disease in a spectrum that includes subclinical inflammation through a life-threatening inflammatory infectious condition. Diverticulitis is associated with acquired diverticulum. It rarely affects people in developing countries owing to the highly cultural risk factors of low-fiber diet and minimal physical activity found in industrialized cultures. In cultures in which diverticular disease is prevalent, it is highly correlated with increasing age.

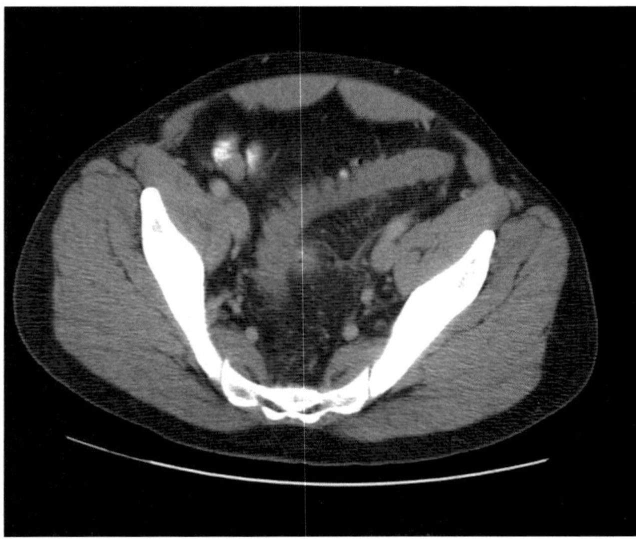

FIGURE 68-1 Abdominal computed tomographic scan demonstrating sigmoid diverticulitis. Note the inflammatory density outside the sigmoid colon, with a small amount of air suggesting perforation in this 45-year-old man, who presented with acute left lower quadrant abdominal pain. (*Reproduced with permission from Gary Ferenchick, MD.*)

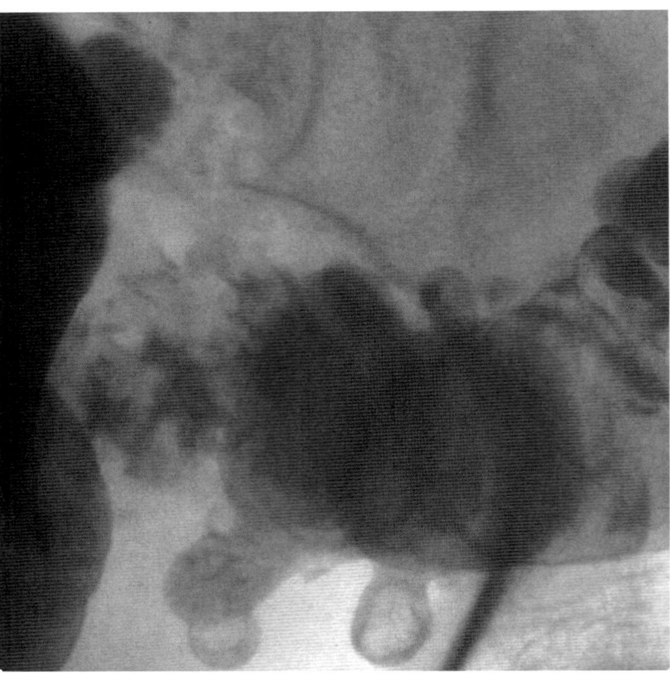

FIGURE 68-2 Multiple diverticuli are seen projecting off the sigmoid colon in this barium enema image. (*Reproduced with permission from Gary Ferenchick, MD.*)

TERMINOLOGY

- Diverticulosis is the presence of diverticula (outpouchings) that are asymptomatic (**Figure 68-2**).
- Diverticular disease is the presence of diverticula associated with symptoms (ie, hematochezia).
- Diverticulitis refers to evidence of diverticular inflammation commonly associated with symptoms of fever or tachycardia, with or without localized symptoms.
- Complicated diverticulitis includes perforation into the peritoneum, abscess, phlegmon, fistula formation, stricture, and obstruction.

EPIDEMIOLOGY

- Of the US population, 30% have diverticulosis by 60 years and 60% by 80 years.[1]
- Of the population with diverticulosis, 10% to 25% will develop diverticulitis, and 25% of these cases will be complicated.[1,2]
- Overall annual age-adjusted admissions for acute diverticulitis increased from 120,500 in 1998 to 151,900 in 2005, a 26% increase.[3]

ETIOLOGY/PATHOPHYSIOLOGY

- A low-fiber diet leads to less-bulky stools that retain less water and increase transit time, and these factors increase intracolonic pressure.
- Increased intracolonic pressure causes the mucosa and submucosa to protrude as pouches through the musculature.

- Such protrusions occur at locations of weakness, often where the vasculature travels through the layers of the colon.[4]
- Stasis or obstruction in the narrow-necked diverticulum by fecal material leads to increased mucus secretion, bacterial overgrowth, tissue inflammation, and ischemia, subsequently leading to translocation of bacteria into the peritoneum and perforation.[2,4]
- Inflammation and focal necrosis lead to micro- or macroscopic perforations.[5]
- An acute episode of diverticulitis ranges from subclinical inflammation to generalized peritonitis with abscess and fistula formation.[5]
- The sigmoid colon is less compliant than the ascending colon. This may predispose to the classic type of diverticulosis seen in Western countries characterized by increased intraluminal pressures, infectious complications, and perforation.[2]

RISK FACTORS

- Age—The risk of diverticulosis is 10% for those younger than 40 and up to 67% for those older than 80.[2]
- Low-fiber, high-fat diets.
- Chronic constipation.[4]

DIAGNOSIS

CLINICAL FEATURES

- Classic symptoms include LLQ abdominal pain and tenderness, nausea, constipation, and fever.
- Variable symptoms include right or central abdominal pain, vomiting, or diarrhea.
- Inquire about the presence or absence of a known history of diverticular disease, symptoms of prior hematochezia, constipation, and low-fiber diet.
- Because of the broad differential based on the symptoms described by the patient, many times the diagnosis is not confirmed until CT imaging is completed.

IMAGING

- CT scanning is 97% sensitive and 99% specific for diverticulitis.[4] SOR A
- CT can also assess for the presence of complications and their severity, such as abscess formation, and likelihood of responding to medical management.[5]
- Specific CT findings include the following:
  - Pericolonic fat stranding is present in 98% (**Figure 68-3**).
  - Diverticula are present in 84% (**Figure 68-3**).
  - Bowel wall thickening greater than 4 mm is present in 70% (**Figure 68-3B**).
  - Phlegmon/pericolic fluid is present in 35% (**Figure 68-3**).
- Contrast barium enema radiography (**Figure 68-2**), cystography, ultrasound, and endoscopy are sometimes helpful in the initial workup of suspected diverticulitis but are used less often because of the superiority of CT scanning.[5]

DIFFERENTIAL DIAGNOSIS

- Nephrolithiasis/ureteral calculi are differentiated by the presence of colicky pain associated with gross or microscopic hematuria and a positive CT scan for the presence of a stone.
- Cystitis/pyelonephritis can be differentiated by the presence of pyuria/bacteriuria and costovertebral angle tenderness.

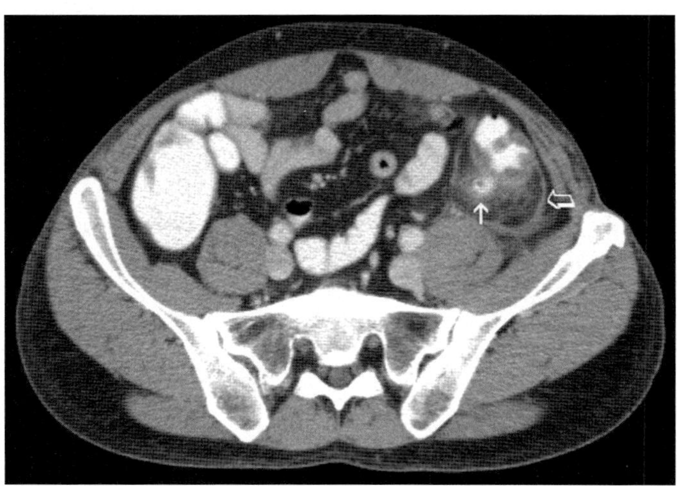
A

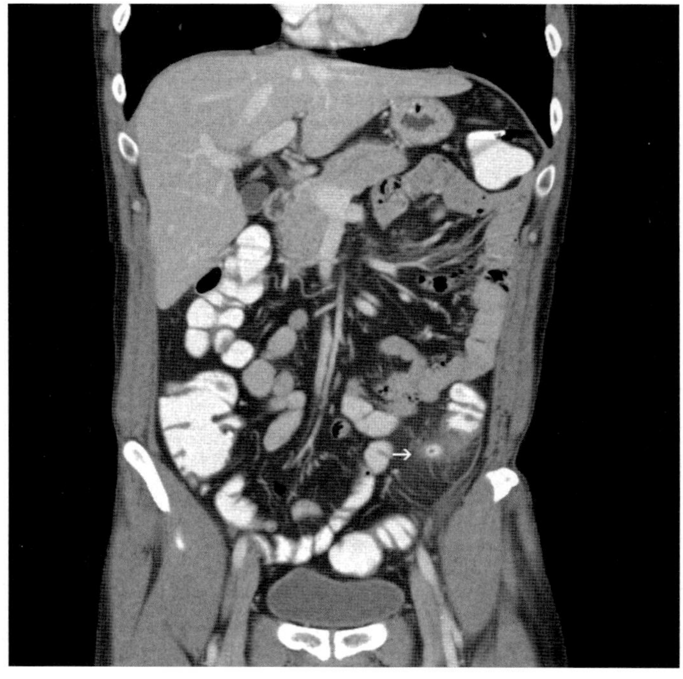
B

FIGURE 68-3 A. There is a hazy appearance to the pericolonic fat caused by edema (*open arrow* points to pericolonic fascia thickening). B. Contrast-filled diverticulum projects off thickened proximal sigmoid colon (*arrow*).

- Small-bowel obstruction (SBO) is associated with more prominent emesis plus obstipation and abdominal radiographs demonstrating dilated loops of bowel and air fluid levels.
- Colonic cancer presents with symptoms most likely from a secondary obstructive process, chronic anemia from stool occult bleeding, and no previous screening colonoscopy.
- Infectious colitis should be considered if the patient had recent antibiotic use, is presenting with frank hematochezia, and the microscopic examination of the stool reveals positive stool white blood cells.
- Inflammatory bowel disease (IBD) is associated with markedly elevated C-reactive protein/erythrocyte sedimentation rate (CRP/ESR), Hemoccult-positive stool, CT consistent with IBD, and a confirmatory biopsy on colonoscopy.
- Ovarian cyst or ectopic pregnancy should be considered in premenopausal women; the pregnancy test will be positive in an ectopic pregnancy, and a transvaginal ultrasound can confirm diagnosis of both.
- Appendicitis is commonly associated with early-onset epigastric pain migrating to the right lower quadrant (RLQ).

MANAGEMENT

- Factors to consider for admission include severity of pain, oral intake tolerance, older age, and comorbidities.[5]
- Provide bed rest, clear liquids if tolerated, and analgesics.[5]
  - Hospitalization is recommended if the patient cannot tolerate oral intake, needs better pain control, has complicated diverticulitis, failed outpatient treatment, or is immunocompromised.[4]
- Antibiotics are given to cover gram-negative rods and anaerobes (ie, typical dose in a patient without renal compromise includes metronidazole 500 mg orally or intravenously every 6 hours for 7-14 days plus ciprofloxacin 400 mg orally or intravenously every 8-12 hours for 7-14 days).[5]
- Indications for emergent surgery[1] SOR Ⓑ
  - Purulent or fecal peritonitis
  - Uncontrolled sepsis
  - Fistula
  - Obstruction
  - Inability to exclude carcinoma
  - Failure of medical management
- Abscess size greater than 2 cm is less likely to resolve; CT-guided drainage followed by one-stage primary anastomosis is an option.[1] SOR Ⓑ
- Operative treatment options include
  - Hartmann procedure, which is a sigmoid colectomy, descending colostomy, and rectal stump closure[1]
  - Primary anastomosis with or without intraoperative colonic lavage[1]
  - Resection with temporary diverting ileostomy
    - Laparoscopic approach is optimal in selected patients[1] SOR Ⓐ
- Hinchey classification[6]
  - Stage 1—Pericolic or mesenteric abscess (mortality $< 5\%$)
  - Stage 2—Walled-off or pelvic abscess (mortality $< 5\%$)
  - Stage 3—Generalized purulent peritonitis (mortality $< 13\%$)
  - Stage 4—Generalized fecal peritonitis (mortality $< 43\%$)
- The Hinchey classification provides mortality likelihoods and aids in the individualized decision making about which operative management options should be considered. Some studies showed stages I and II were reasonably managed with drainage and antibiotics and stages III and IV usually required surgery.[7] Other studies showed more often those with stages I and II having a sigmoid colectomy with a primary anastomosis and in stage III or IV having a colostomy and Hartmann pouch as the most commonly used procedure to avoid the risk of anastomosis leakage associated with primary anastomosis in overly inflamed colon.[8,9]

PROGNOSIS/CLINICAL COURSE

- Of patients with uncomplicated diverticulitis, 85% will resolve with medical management.[1]
- Abscesses are present in 16% of those with acute diverticulitis without peritonitis.[10]
- Purulent peritonitis mortality is 6%.
- Fecal peritonitis mortality is 35%.
- Of those affected, 33% will have a recurrent attack.[1]
- The likelihood of recurrence does not increase with frequency of attacks but with the severity of an attack and its complications.[1]
- Of all patients with a diagnosis of acute diverticulitis, 20% will require surgery at some point in their lifetime.[10]
- Approximately 2% to 11% of surgical patients may need repeat surgery for recurrent episode in the more proximal colon.[5]

FOLLOW-UP

- The standard of care is to recommend colonoscopy approximately 6 weeks after an episode (so that perforation risk is closer to baseline) to assess for other possible etiologies, including malignancy, IBD, and ischemia.[1] SOR Ⓒ Colonoscopy will commonly demonstrate a diverticulum (**Figure 68-4**).

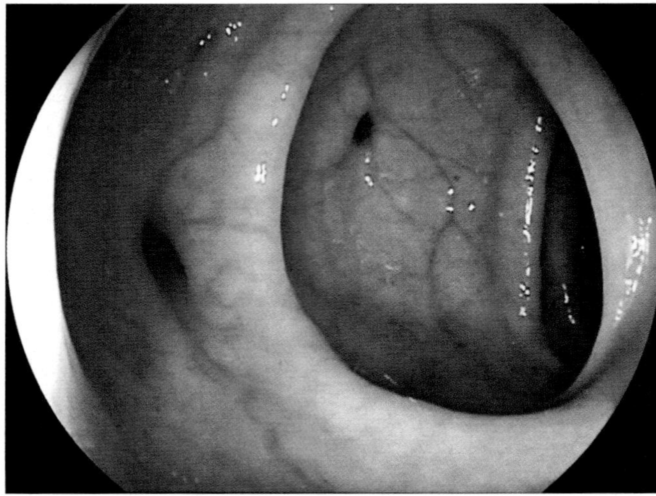

FIGURE 68-4 Asymptomatic diverticulosis. This is a common finding in screening colonoscopies and indicates precursor lesions for the development of diverticulitis. (*Reproduced with permission from John Rodney, MD.*)

- Elective surgery to prevent further attacks should be individualized. SOR B
  - Factors that should be considered include the patient's age; comorbidities (diabetes mellitus, collagenous disease, compromised immune system); severity of attacks (with complications); and persistent symptoms after acute attack.[5]
  - Young age is more likely a factor in elective resection preventing further attacks because of an inherent increased cumulative risk over time (not because of increased severity in younger individuals).[1]
  - Recurrence of diverticulitis is 36% at 5 years; complicated recurrence, which is defined by the presence of a fistula, perforation, or abscess formation, recurs in about 4% of patients.
    - Recurrent disease is more common in patients with a family history of diverticulitis, diverticulitis involving more than 5 cm of the sigmoid colon, or the presence of a retroperitoneal abscess. Patients with right-side diverticulitis (5% of total cases) are at low risk of recurrence.[11]

PATIENT EDUCATION

- Self-reported vegetarians are at a 31% lower risk of diverticular disease than meat eaters.[12]
- High dietary fiber is associated with a 41% lower risk of diverticular disease.[12]
- Nuts, corn, or popcorn consumption is not a risk factor in diverticulosis formation, diverticulitis, or complications.[13]

PATIENT RESOURCES

- National Digestive Diseases Information Clearinghouse (NDDIC). *Diverticulosis and Diverticulitis*— **http://digestive.niddk.nih.gov/ddiseases/pubs/diverticulosis/**

PROVIDER RESOURCES

- Medscape. *Diverticulitis*—**http://emedicine.medscape.com/article/173388.**

REFERENCES

1. Rafferty J, Shellito P, Hyman NH, Buie WD. Practice parameters for sigmoid diverticulitis. *Dis Colon Rectum*. 2006;49:939-944.
2. Janes SE, Meagher A, Frizelle FA. Management of diverticulitis. *BMJ*. 2006;332:271-275.
3. Etzioni DA, Mack TM, Beart RW Jr, Kaiser AM. Diverticulitis in the United States: 1998-2005: changing patterns of disease and treatment. *Ann Surg*. 2009;249:210-217.
4. Jacobs DO. Clinical practice. Diverticulitis. *N Engl J Med*. 2007;357: 2057-2066.
5. Szojda MM, Cuesta MA, Mulder CM, Felt-Bersma RJ. Review article: management of diverticulitis. *Aliment Pharmacol Ther*. 2007;26(suppl 2):67-76.
6. Schwesinger WH, Page CP, Gaskill HV 3rd, et al. Operative management of diverticular emergencies: strategies and outcomes. *Arch Surg*. 2000;135:558-562; discussion 62-63.
7. Hinchey EJ, Schaal PG, Richards GK. Treatment of perforated diverticular disease of the colon. *Adv Surg*. 1978;12:85-109.
8. Wong WD, Wexner SD, Lowry A, et al. Practice parameters for the treatment of sigmoid diverticulitis—supporting documentation. The Standards Task Force. The American Society of Colon and Rectal Surgeons. *Dis Colon Rectum*. 2000;43:290-297.
9. Schilling MK, Maurer CA, Kollmar O, Buchler MW. Primary vs. secondary anastomosis after sigmoid colon resection for perforated diverticulitis (Hinchey Stage III and IV): a prospective outcome and cost analysis. *Dis Colon Rectum*. 2001;44:699-703; discussion 705.
10. Chautems RC, Ambrosetti P, Ludwig A, Mermillod B, Morel P, Soravia C. Long-term follow-up after first acute episode of sigmoid diverticulitis: is surgery mandatory? A prospective study of 118 patients. *Dis Colon Rectum*. 2002;45:962-966.
11. Hall JF, Roberts PL, Ricciardi R, et al. Long-term follow-up after an initial episode of diverticulitis: what are the predictors of recurrence? *Dis Colon Rectum*. 2011; 54(3):283-288.
12. Crowe FL, Appleby PN, Allen NE, Key TJ. Diet and risk of diverticular disease in Oxford cohort of European Prospective Investigation into Cancer and Nutrition (EPIC): prospective study of British vegetarians and non-vegetarians. *BMJ*. 2011;343:d4131. doi:10.1136/bmj.d4131.
13. Strate LL, Liu YL, Syngal S, Aldoori WH, Giovannucci EL. Nut, corn, and popcorn consumption and the incidence of diverticular disease. *JAMA*. 2008;300:907-914.

69 GALLSTONES

Mindy A. Smith, MD, MS

PATIENT STORY

A 44-year-old woman reports frequent episodes of severe pain in the mid and upper right side of her abdomen that usually occurs shortly after her evening meal and sometimes at night. She is obese, but otherwise healthy. The pain lasts for several hours and is steady and often causes vomiting. On physical examination she complains of slight tenderness in the right upper quadrant (RUQ). An ultrasound confirms the presence of gallstones (**Figure 69-1**).

INTRODUCTION

Gallstones are inorganic masses usually composed of cholesterol that form in the gallbladder or bile duct. They are formed by concretion (joining together of adjacent parts and hardening) or accretion (growth by addition or adherence of parts normally separated) of normal and/or abnormal bile constituents.

EPIDEMIOLOGY

- Based on autopsy data, 20% of women and 8% of men have gallstones.[1]
- Approximately 20 million people in the United States are affected, with 1 million new cases each year.[1]
- In a Swedish incidence study of 621 randomly selected individuals ages 35 to 85 years, 42 (8.3%) of the 503 subjects available at 5 years developed gallstones; this yielded an incidence for newly developed gallstones of 1.39 per 100 person-years.[2]

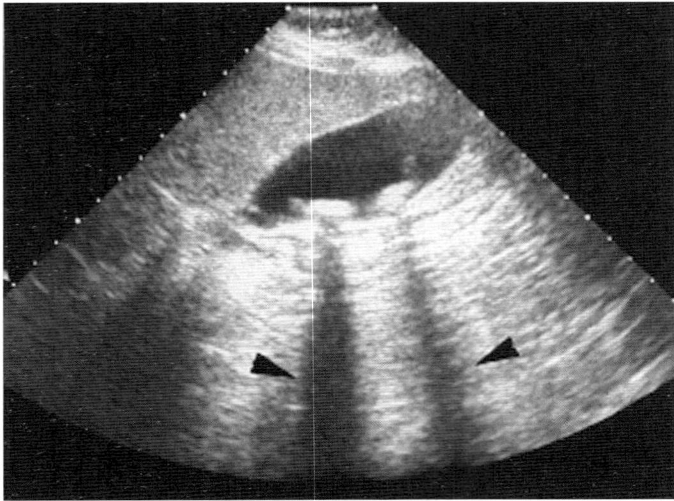

FIGURE 69-1 Ultrasound showing 2 echogenic gallstones in the gallbladder. Note the absence of echoes posterior to the gallstone called "shadowing" (arrowheads). (*Reproduced with permission from Schwartz's Principles of Surgery. 9th ed. New York, NY: McGraw-Hill; 2010:1141, Figure. 32-6. Copyright 2010, McGraw-Hill.*)

- Among pregnant women, 5% to 12% have gallstones and 20% to 30% have gallbladder sludge (thick mucus material containing cholesterol crystals and mucin thread or mucous gels). Gallbladder sludge is a possible precursor form of gallstone disease.[1]
- Patients with asymptomatic gallstones have a 1% to 2% risk per year of developing symptoms or complications of gallstones. Based on data primarily for men, this will occur in 10% by 5 years, 15% by 10 years, and 18% by 15 years following diagnosis.[1]
- Gallstone disease is responsible for approximately 10,000 deaths per year in the United States. Most (7000) of these deaths are attributable to acute gallstone complications (eg, cholecystitis, pancreatitis, cholangitis).[3]
- Although gallbladder cancers most often occur in the setting of stones (91% of 34 patients with gallbladder cancer in one study),[4] gallbladder cancer is rare. An incidence rate of 0.28% for incidental gallbladder carcinoma was reported in a Swiss database study of a population of more than 30,000 patients undergoing laparoscopic cholecystectomy.[5]

ETIOLOGY AND PATHOPHYSIOLOGY

- There are 2 types of gallstones: cholesterol stones (80%) and pigmented stones (primarily calcium bilirubinate, 20%).
- The solute components of bile include bile acids (80%), lecithin and other phospholipids (16%), and unesterified cholesterol (4%).[1] Cholesterol gallstones form when there is excess cholesterol or an abnormal ratio of cholesterol, bile acids, and lecithin.
- Excess biliary cholesterol can occur from a secondary increase in secretion of cholesterol caused by obesity, high cholesterol diet, clofibrate therapy, or a genetic predisposition to increased hydroxymethylglutaryl-coenzyme A reductase.
- The excess cholesterol becomes supersaturated and can precipitate out of solution in a process called *nucleation*, forming solid cholesterol monohydrate crystals that can become trapped in gallbladder mucus, producing sludge, and/or grow and aggregate to form cholesterol gallstones.
- Gallbladder hypomotility is a predisposing and possibly necessary factor in stone formation because of the failure to completely empty supersaturated or crystal-containing bile.[1] Situations associated with hypomotility include pregnancy, prolonged parenteral nutrition, surgery, burns, and use of oral contraceptives or estrogen therapy.
- Pigmented stones occur when increasing amounts of unconjugated bilirubin in bile precipitate to form stones. Bilirubin, a yellow pigment derived from the breakdown of heme, is actively secreted into bile by liver cells. In situations of high heme turnover such as chronic hemolytic states (eg, sickle cell anemia), calcium bilirubinate can crystallize from solution and form stones.
- Chronic gallstones may cause progressive fibrosis of the gallbladder wall and loss of function.

RISK FACTORS

- Genetic mutations can result in reduction of bile acids and lecithin that predispose some patients to stone formation. A high prevalence of gallstones is found in first-degree relatives of patients with gallstones and among Native Americans, Chilean Indians, and Chilean Hispanics.[1]

- In a case-control study, the prevalence of gallstones was 28.6% in first-degree relatives of subjects with gallstones versus 12.4% in first-degree relatives of subjects without gallstones (relative risk [RR] 1.80, 95% confidence interval [CI] 1.29-2.63).[3]
- Other risk factors for gallstones include rapid weight loss (10%-20% of these patients form stones),[1] increasing age, liver or ileal disease, and cystic fibrosis.

DIAGNOSIS

CLINICAL FEATURES

- Symptoms of gallstones are caused from inflammation or obstruction as stones migrate into the cystic or common bile duct (CBD).
  - Biliary colic is a steady, severe pain or ache, usually of sudden onset, located in the epigastrium or RUQ. Pain episodes last between 30 minutes and 5 hours and may radiate to the interscapular area, right scapula, or right shoulder.
  - Gallstone-related pain may be precipitated by a fatty meal, a regular meal, or a large meal followed by a prolonged fast.
  - Pain is recurrent and often nocturnal.
- RUQ tenderness may be elicited on physical examination.
- Nausea and vomiting are common.
- Accompanying fever and chills suggests a complication of gallstones. Complications are more common in patients with a calcified gallbladder or in those who have had a previous episode of acute cholecystitis.[1]

LABORATORY STUDIES

- No laboratory testing is usually indicated as the results are usually normal. However, an elevated γ-glutamyl transpeptidase suggests a CBD stone. In a study of patients with acute calculous gallbladder disease, investigators found a 1-in-3 chance of CBD stones when the γ-glutamyl transpeptidase level was above 90 U/L and a 1-in-30 chance when the level was less than 90 U/L.[6]

IMAGING

- Ultrasound is the diagnostic test of choice and is 95% accurate for stones as small as 2 mm in diameter (see **Figure 69-1**).[1] Shadowing, a discrete acoustic shadow caused by the absorption and reflection of sound by the stone that changes with patient positioning, is an important diagnostic feature that is shown in **Figures 69-1** and **69-2**.
- In one study, high-resolution ultrasound was more accurate than endoscopic ultrasonography or CT in differentiating benign disease from malignancy in cases with gallbladder polypoid lesions.[7]
- Gallstones may be seen on plain film, but only calcified stones are seen (**Figures 69-3** and **69-4**). This includes only 10% to 15% of cholesterol stones and 50% of pigmented stones.[1] Stones may be single or multiple and the gallbladder wall may be calcified (referred to as a *porcelain gallbladder*), indicating severe chronic cholecystitis or adenocarcinoma.
- CT is less sensitive and more expensive than ultrasound for the detection of gallstones (**Figures 69-5** and **69-6**). However, CT can detect both radiopaque stones and radiolucent stones.
- An oral cholecystogram can be used to assess cystic duct patency and emptying function. This test has largely been replaced by gallbladder ultrasound.

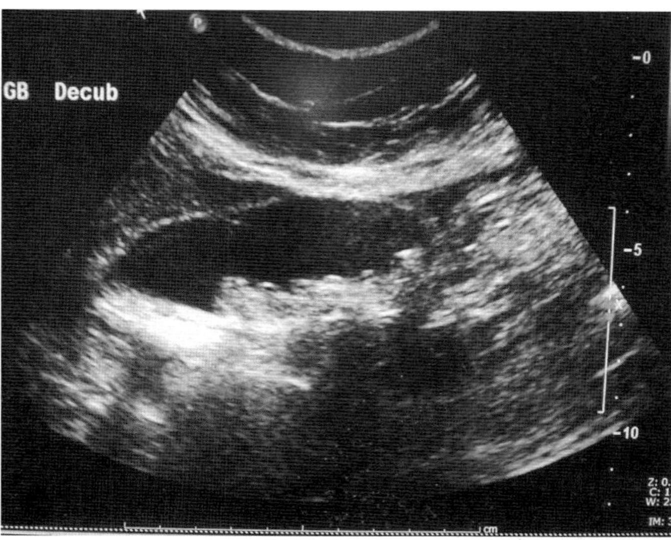

FIGURE 69-2 Gallstones visible in the gallbladder of a 43-year-old woman with right upper quadrant (RUQ) pain and a positive Murphy sign. (*Reproduced with permission from Richard P. Usatine, MD.*)

- Radioisotope scans (eg, technetium [Tc]-99m hepatoiminodiacetic acid [HIDA]) can be used to confirm acute cholecystitis (nonvisualizing gallbladder) and can be useful in evaluating functional abnormalities.
- Endoscopic retrograde cholangiopancreatography is used for imaging bile ducts. Stones in bile appear as filling defects in the opacified ducts. Endoscopic retrograde cholangiopancreatography is usually performed in conjunction with endoscopic retrograde sphincterotomy and gallstone extraction.

DIFFERENTIAL DIAGNOSIS

Severe epigastric and RUQ pain can be seen in the following conditions:

- Acute cholecystitis—Pain may radiate to the back, and fever is usually present. Physical examination can reveal RUQ rigidity and guarding with a positive Murphy sign (RUQ pain worsening with deep

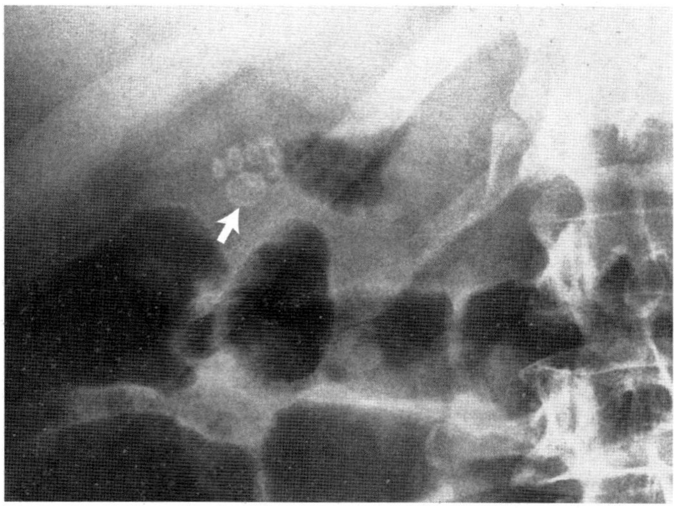

FIGURE 69-3 Plain film showing multiple gallstones (*white arrow*). (*Reproduced with permission from Schwartz DT, Reisdorff EJ.* Emergency Radiology. *New York, NY: McGraw-Hill; 2000:536, Figure. 19-37. Copyright 2000, McGraw-Hill.*)

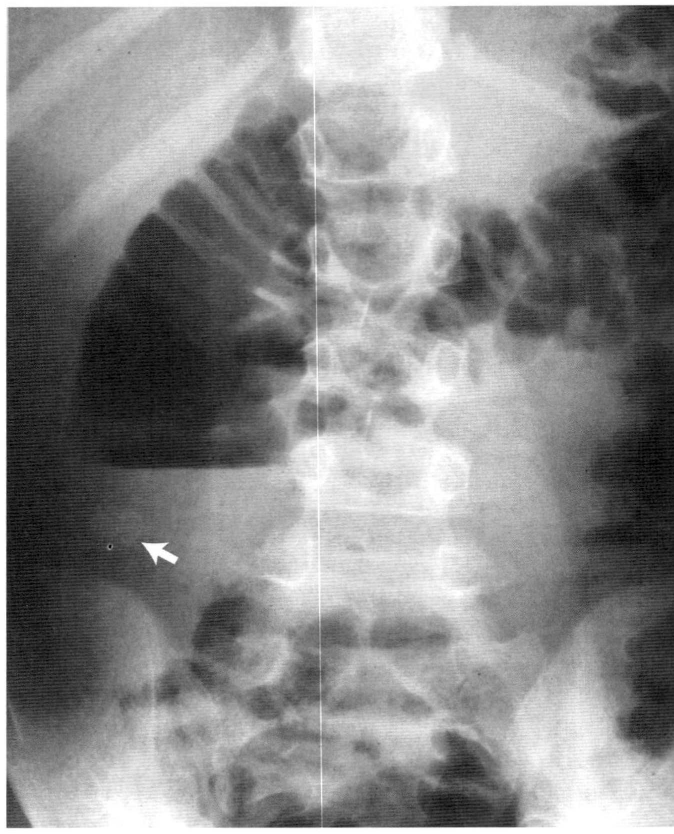

FIGURE 69-4 Gallstone ileus in an elderly patient with diabetes; note dilated loops of small bowel and an ectopic gallstone (*arrow*). (*Reproduced with permission from Schwartz DT, Reisdorff EJ.* Emergency Radiology. *New York, NY: McGraw-Hill; 2000:527, Figure. 19-21. Copyright 2000, McGraw-Hill.*)

inspiration while the examiner maintains steady pressure below the right costal margin). White blood count, serum amylase, aspartate transaminase, and alanine transaminase may all be elevated.

- Pancreatitis—Pain is located in the midepigastrium and left upper quadrant, but may radiate to the RUQ. Abdominal distention and diminished bowel sounds may be present. Elevations in lipase and

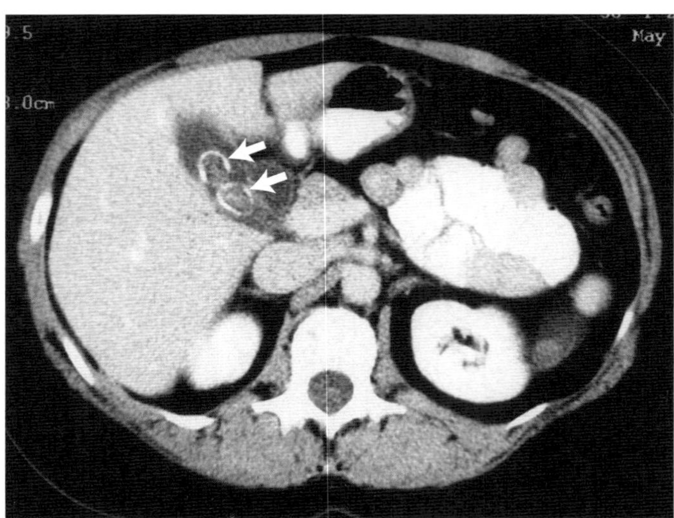

FIGURE 69-5 CT scan showing 2 large gallstones that have a rim of calcification (*large arrows*). (*Reproduced with permission from Schwartz DT, Reisdorff EJ.* Emergency Radiology. *New York, NY: McGraw-Hill; 2000:538, Figure. 19-41A. Copyright 2000, McGraw-Hill.*)

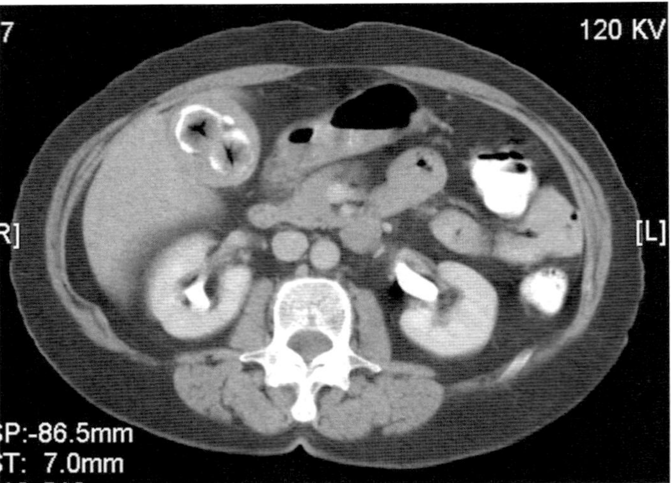

FIGURE 69-6 Radiographic Mercedes-Benz sign seen on a CT cut through the gallbladder (the gallstones produce a black pattern that resembles a Mercedes-Benz logo in the center). (*Reproduced with permission from Mike Freckleton, MD.*)

amylase are found and pancreatic pseudocysts or abscess may be present on ultrasound (see Chapter 75, Pancreatitis).

- Peptic ulcer disease—Pain may be described as burning and is usually epigastric and often relieved by antacids. Onset is 1 to 3 hours after meals or following nonsteroidal anti-inflammatory drug usage. Stool Hemoccult testing may be positive. An ulcer may be visualized on upper gastrointestinal (GI) barium swallow or endoscopy (see Chapter 76, Peptic Ulcer Disease).
- Hepatitis—Other symptoms and signs include malaise, anorexia, pruritus, tender liver, and low-grade fever. Jaundice may be present and urine may be dark (ie, bilirubinuria). Aspartate transaminase and alanine transaminase are elevated (see Chapter 74, Liver Disease).

MANAGEMENT

- Silent gallstones may be managed expectantly; prophylactic cholecystectomy is unwarranted based on the few who develop symptoms over time and the very low rate of complications (3%-4%).[8] There are no randomized controlled trials comparing cholecystectomy to watchful waiting for silent gallstones.[9] SOR C
- Cholecystectomy should be considered for patients with the following symptoms:[1]
    - Frequent symptoms that interfere with daily life
    - A prior complication of gallstone disease
    - The presence of an underlying condition (eg, calcified gallbladder) that predisposes the patient to increased risk of complications
- Laparoscopic cholecystectomy is the surgical treatment of choice because of the low rate of complications (4%) and mortality (<0.1%), shortened hospital stay, and reduced cost.[1] Conversion to an open laparotomy is infrequent (5%).[1] A Cochrane review found no differences in mortality or complications among open, small-incision, and laparoscopic cholecystectomy, but quicker recovery favors minimally invasive procedures; small-incision cholecystectomies appear to have shorter operative time and lower cost.[10]
- Early laparoscopic cholecystectomy (<7 days from symptom onset) during acute cholecystitis has comparable outcomes to delayed cholecystectomy and shortens hospital stay.[11]

- Single versus 4-port laparoscopic cholecystectomy may reduce postoperative pain.[12]
- For patients with gallbladder and CBD stones, intraoperative endoscopic sphincterotomy during laparoscopic cholecystectomy appears as safe and effective as preoperative endoscopic sphincterotomy followed by laparoscopic cholecystectomy and is associated with significantly shorter hospital stay.[13]
- Medical therapy with ursodeoxycholic acid may be considered for patients with functioning gallbladders and small stones (<10 mm).[1] Approximately 50% of these patients will have complete dissolution of stones in 6 to 24 months, but recurrences are common (see "Prognosis" below).[1]
- Medical therapy can also be used to prevent gallstone formation in patients with expected rapid weight loss caused by very-low-calorie diets or bariatric surgery. In one study, ursodeoxycholic acid at a dose of 500 mg daily for 6 months reduced the incidence of gallstones over placebo (3% vs 22%, respectively, at 12 months) and cholecystectomy (4.7% vs 12%, respectively).[14]
- Extracorporeal shock wave lithotripsy combined with medical therapy may be considered for patients with radiolucent, solitary stones less than 2 cm, and a functional gallbladder.[1]

PROGNOSIS

- Abdominal pain resembling biliary colic may persist in up to 30% of patients despite cholecystectomy (called postcholecystectomy syndrome).[15] In one follow-up survey of 1300 patients following cholecystectomy (44% response rate), preoperative pain resolved in 90% but postoperative pain was reported in 25%; in 10% of these patients the postoperative pain was the same quality and location as the preoperative pain, and in 17% a new abdominal pain developed, most often in the periumbilical area.[16] In a study of 100 consecutive patients, 13% had persistent pain following laparoscopic cholecystectomy.[17]
- In the follow-up survey noted above (N = 573), nonpain symptoms all decreased in prevalence following cholecystectomy, including indigestion (14%), fatty food intolerance (19%), and heartburn (13%). Diarrhea, however, was present in similar percentages pre- and postoperatively (19% and 21%, respectively).[16]
- Following medical therapy, recurrences are common (30%-50% at 3- to 5-year follow-up).[1]

FOLLOW-UP

- Approximately 5% to 10% of patients develop chronic diarrhea, attributed to increased bile salts reaching the colon, following cholecystectomy. Diarrhea is usually mild and can be managed with over-the-counter antidiarrheal agents (eg, loperamide).
- Postcholecystectomy pain may be related to recurrent stones, choledocholithiasis, biliary dyskinesia, inflammatory scarring or strictures involving the sphincter of Oddi or the CBD, and dilation of cystic duct remnants; ultrasound, CT, cholangiography, or magnetic resonance cholangiopancreatography can be useful in identification of the cause and some may be amenable to surgical management.[18,19]

PATIENT EDUCATION

- Patients with asymptomatic gallstones may be managed expectantly—The rates of developing symptoms and complications should be reviewed. They should be encouraged to report symptoms of biliary colic and acute cholecystitis or pancreatitis (described above).
- Laparoscopic cholecystectomy appears to be very successful for symptom resolution, although chronic diarrhea may occur and abdominal pain may persist or new pain develop in approximately one-quarter of patients.[15]

PATIENT RESOURCES

- National Digestive Diseases Information Clearinghouse (NDDIC). *Gallstones*—**http://digestive.niddk.nih.gov/ddiseases/pubs/gallstones/index.aspx.**
- Medline Plus. *Gallstones*—**http://www.nlm.nih.gov/medlineplus/gallstones.html.**

PROVIDER RESOURCES

- Ahmed A, Cheung RC, Keeffe EB. Management of gallstones and their complications—**http://www.aafp.org/afp/20000315/1673.html.**
- Heuman DM, Greenwald D, Soweid AM, et al. Cholelithiasis—**http://emedicine.medscape.com/article/175667-overview.**
- National Institute of Diabetes and Digestive and Kidney Diseases—**http://www2.niddk.nih.gov/Research/ScientificAreas/DigestiveDiseases/Gastrointestinal/GBBD.htm.**

REFERENCES

1. Greenberger NJ, Paumgartner G. Diseases of the gallbladder and bile ducts. In: Kasper DL, Braunwald E, Fauci AS, Hauser SL, Longo DL, Jameson JL, eds. *Harrison's Principles of Internal Medicine*, 16th ed. New York, NY: McGraw-Hill; 2005:1880-1884.
2. Halldestam I, Kullman E, Borch K. Incidence of and potential risk factors for gallstone disease in a general population sample. *Br J Surg.* 2009;96(11):1315-1322.
3. Attili AF, De Santis A, Attili F, et al. Prevalence of gallstone disease in first-degree relatives of patients with cholelithiasis. *World J Gastroenterol.* 2005;11(41):6508-6511.
4. Ishak G, Ribeiro FS, Costa DS, et al. Gallbladder cancer: 10 years of experience at an Amazon reference hospital. *Rev Col Bras Cir.* 2011;38(2):100-104.
5. Glauser PM, Strub D, Käser SA, et al. Incidence, management, and outcome of incidental gallbladder carcinoma: analysis of the database of the Swiss association of laparoscopic and thoracoscopic surgery. *Surg Endosc.* 2010;24(9):2281-2286.
6. Peng WK, Sheikh Z, Paterson-Brown S, Nixon SJ. Role of liver function tests in predicting common bile duct stones in acute calculous cholecystitis. *Br J Surg.* 2005;92(10):1241-1247.
7. Jang JY, Kim SW, Lee SE, et al. Differential diagnostic and staging accuracies of high resolution ultrasonography, endoscopic ultrasonography, and multidetector computed tomography for gallbladder polypoid lesions and gallbladder cancer. *Ann Surg.* 2009;250(6):943-949.

8. Gracie WA, Ransohoff DF. The natural history of asymptomatic gallstones: the innocent gallstone is not a myth. *N Engl J Med.* 1982;307:798-800.

9. Gurusamy KS, Samraj K. Cholecystectomy for patients with silent gallstones. *Cochrane Database Syst Rev.* 2007;(1):CD006230.

10. Keus F, Gooszen HG, van Laarhoven CJHM. Open, small-incision, or laparoscopic cholecystectomy for patients with symptomatic cholecystolithiasis. An overview of Cochrane Hepato-Biliary Group reviews. *Cochrane Database Syst Rev.* 2010;(1):CD008318.

11. Gurusamy KS, Samraj K. Early versus delayed laparoscopic cholecystectomy for acute cholecystitis. *Cochrane Database Syst Rev.* 2006;(4):CD005440.

12. Asakuma M, Hayashi M, Komeda K, et al. Impact of single-port cholecystectomy on postoperative pain. *Br J Surg.* 2011;98(7):991-995.

13. Gurusamy K, Sahay SJ, Burroughs AK, Davidson BR. Systematic review and meta-analysis of intraoperative versus preoperative endoscopic sphincterotomy in patients with gallbladder and suspected common bile duct stones. *Br J Surg.* 2011;98(7):908-916.

14. Miller K, Hell E, Lang B, Lengauer E. Gallstone formation prophylaxis after gastric restrictive procedures for weight loss: a randomized double-blind placebo-controlled trial. *Ann Surg.* 2003;238(5):697-702.

15. Gui GP, Cheruvu CV, West N, et al. Is cholecystectomy effective treatment for symptomatic gallstones? Clinical outcomes after long-term follow-up. *Ann R Coll Surg Engl.* 1998;80:25-32.

16. Lublin M, Crawford DL, Hiatt JR, Phillips EH. Symptoms before and after laparoscopic cholecystectomy for gallstones. *Am Surg.* 2004;70(10):863-866.

17. Luman W, Adams WH, Nixon SN, et al. Incidence of persistent symptoms after laparoscopic cholecystectomy: a prospective study. *Gut.* 1996;39(6):863-866.

18. Perera E, Bhatt S, Dogra VS. Cystc duct remnant syndrome. *J Clin Imaging Sci.* 2011;1:2.

19. Girometti R, Brondani G, Cereser L, et al. Post-cholecystectomy syndrome: spectrum of biliary findings at magnetic resonance cholangiopancreatography. *Br J Radiol.* 2010;83(988):351-361.

70 GASTRIC CANCER

Mindy A. Smith, MD, MS

PATIENT STORY

A 72-year-old Japanese immigrant was brought in by his family with complaints of difficulty in eating, vague abdominal pain, and weight loss. Endoscopy and biopsy confirmed gastric adenocarcinoma (**Figure 70-1**). Liver metastases were found on abdominal computed tomography (CT). The family and the patient chose only comfort measures and the patient died 6 months later.

INTRODUCTION

Gastric cancer is a malignant neoplasm of the stomach, usually adenocarcinoma.

EPIDEMIOLOGY

- Based on Surveillance Epidemiology and End Results (SEER) data, an estimated 12,730 men and 8270 women will be diagnosed with gastric cancer, and 10,570 men and women will die of this cancer in 2012 (2010).[1] The median age at diagnosis is 70 years and median age at death from gastric cancer is 73 years.[1]
- Stomach cancer occurs in 10.8 per 100,000 men and 5.4 per 100,000 women in a year. In 2008, the United States prevalence was 37,739 men and 28,271 women, with a lifetime risk of 0.88%.[1]
- High rates of stomach cancer occur in Japan, China, Chile, and Ireland.[2]

ETIOLOGY AND PATHOPHYSIOLOGY

- Eighty-five percent of stomach cancers are adenocarcinomas with 15% lymphomas and gastrointestinal (GI) stromal tumors.[2] Adenocarcinoma is further divided into the following 2 types:
  - Diffuse type—Characterized by absent cell cohesion, these tumors affect younger individuals infiltrating and thickening the stomach wall; the prognosis is poor. Several susceptibility genes have been identified for this type of cancer.[3]
  - Intestinal type—Characterized by adhesive cells forming tubular structures, these tumors frequently ulcerate.
- Tumor grade can be well (4.1%), moderate (23.1%), or poorly differentiated (54.9%), or undifferentiated (2.9%) (SEER data from 1988-2001; unknown type accounted for 15%).[4]
- Most tumors are thought to arise from ingestion of nitrates that are converted by bacteria to carcinogens. Exogenous and endogenous factors (see "Risk Factors" later) contribute to this process.[2]
  - Exogenous sources of nitrates—Sources include foods that are dried, smoked, and salted. *Helicobacter pylori* infection may contribute to carcinogenicity by creating gastritis, loss of acidity, and bacterial growth.
  - Oncogenic pathways identified in most gastric cancers are the proliferation or stem cell, nuclear factor-κB, and Wnt/β-catenin; interactions between them appear to influence disease behavior and patient survival.[5]
  - Gastric tumors are classified for staging using the T (tumor) N (nodal involvement) M (metastases) system. Two important prognostic factors are depth of invasion through the gastric wall (less than T2 [tumor invades muscularis propria]) and presence or absence of regional lymph node involvement (N0). Changes made to the classification system in the seventh edition of the American Joint Commission's *Cancer Staging Manual* for gastric cancer[6] demonstrate better survival discrimination.[7]
  - Gastric cancer spreads in by the following multiple ways[2]:

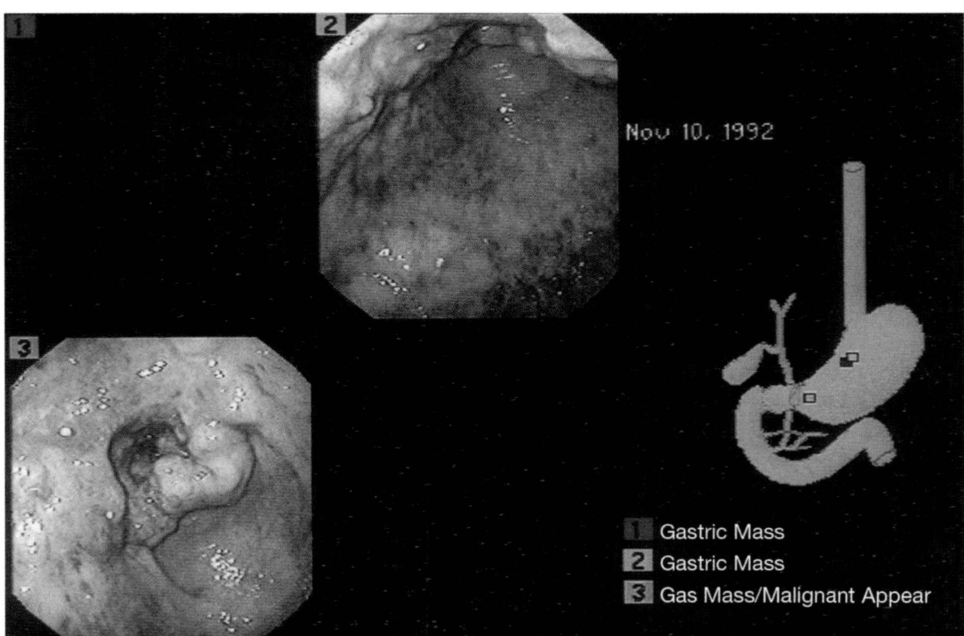

FIGURE 70-1 Endoscopy showing a raised and irregular mass in the antrum of the stomach deforming the pylorus. It fills the distal one-half of the antrum. The lesion was hard when probed with biopsy forceps. Biopsy indicated adenocarcinoma. (*Reproduced with permission from Michael Harper, MD.*)

- Local extension through the gastric wall to the perigastric tissues, omenta, pancreas, colon, or liver.
- Lymphatic drainage through numerous pathways leads to multiple nodal group involvement (eg, intra-abdominal, supraclavicular) or seeding of peritoneal surfaces with metastatic nodules occurring on the ovary, periumbilical region, or peritoneal cul-de-sac.
- Hematogenous spread is also common with liver metastases.

RISK FACTORS

- Previous gastric surgery—As a result of alteration of the normal pH or with biopsy showing high-grade dysplasia.[2,8]
- Other endogenous risk factors—Atrophic gastritis (including postsurgical vagotomized patients) and pernicious anemia are conditions that favor the growth of nitrate-converting bacteria. In addition, intestinal-type cells that develop metaplasia and possibly atypia can replace the gastric mucosa in these patients. Genetic polymorphisms (eg, interleukin-1B-511, interleukin-1RN, and tumor necrosis factor [TNF]-α) also appear to play a role. Familial adenomatous polyposis and hereditary nonpolyposis colorectal cancer are also risk factors.[8]
- Individuals infected with certain *H. pylori* bacteria (cytotoxin-associated gene A) are at increased risk of gastric adenocarcinoma (especially noncardia) and gastric mucosa-associated lymphoid tissue (MALT) lymphoma.[9]
- Additional risk factors—Smoking, low socioeconomic class, lower educational level, exposure to certain pesticides (eg, those who work in the citrus fruit industry in fields treated with 2,4-dichlorophenoxyacetic acid [2,4-D], chlordane, propargite, and triflurin[10]), radiation exposure, and blood type A.

DIAGNOSIS

CLINICAL FEATURES

- Asymptomatic, if superficial and/or early.
- Upper abdominal pain that ranges from vague to severe.
- Postprandial fullness.
- Anorexia and mild nausea are common.
- Nausea and vomiting occur with pyloric tumors.
- Late symptoms include weight loss and a palpable mass (regional extension).
- Late complications include peritoneal and pleural effusions; obstruction of the gastric outlet; bleeding from esophageal varices or postsurgical site; and jaundice.[11]
- Physical signs are also late features and include the following[11]:
  - Palpable enlarged stomach with succussion splash (splashing sound on shaking, indicative of the presence of fluid and air in a body cavity).
  - Primary mass (rare).
  - Enlarged liver.
  - Enlarged, firm to hard, lymph nodes (ie, left supraclavicular [Virchow]), periumbilical region (Sister Mary Joseph node), and peritoneal cul-de-sac (Blumer shelf; palpable on vaginal or rectal examination).

TYPICAL DISTRIBUTION

- Based on SEER data from 1988 to 2001, gastric tumors occur most often in the cardia (25.5%) and gastric antrum (20.7%), followed by the lesser curvature (9.9%), body (7.4%) and greater curvature (4.3%), and fundus (4.1%). Overlapping lesions were reported in 9.8% and no specific information was available in 15.2%.[4]
- Rates of noncardia gastric cancer appear to be decreasing.[9]

IMAGING AND ENDOSCOPY

- Diagnosis can be made on endoscopy (**Figures 70-1** and **70-2**) with biopsy of suspicious lesions. Confocal laser endomicroscopy may improve detection of early lesions.[12]
- Urgent referral for endoscopy (within 2 weeks) is recommended for patients with dyspepsia who also have GI bleeding, dysphagia, progressive unexplained weight loss, persistent vomiting, iron deficiency anemia, epigastric mass, family history of gastric cancer (onset <50 years), or whose dyspepsia is persistent and they are older than age 55 years.[13] SOR Ⓒ
- Double-contrast radiography is an alternative to endoscopy and can detect large primary tumors but distinguishing benign from malignant disease is difficult.[2]
- Although endoscopy is not necessary when radiography demonstrates a benign-appearing ulcer with evidence of complete healing at 6 weeks, some authors recommend routine endoscopy, biopsy, and brush cytology when any gastric ulcer is identified.[2]
- Some gastric polyps (adenomas, hyperplastic) have malignant potential and should be removed.[14]
- Workup for metastases includes the following[15]: SOR Ⓒ
  - Chest radiograph
  - CT scan or magnetic resonance imaging (MRI) of the abdomen and pelvis
- Endoscopic sonography is useful as a staging tool when the CT scan fails to find evidence of locally advanced or metastatic disease.[2]

LABORATORY STUDIES

- A hemoglobin or hematocrit can identify anemia, present in approximately 30% of patients.[11]
- Electrolyte panels and liver function tests can assist in assessing the patient's clinical state and any liver involvement.[11]
- Carcinoembryonic antigen (CEA) is increased in about half of cases.[11]

DIFFERENTIAL DIAGNOSIS

- Peptic ulcer—Typical symptoms include epigastric pain (described as a gnawing or burning), occurring 1 to 3 hours after meals and relieved by food or antacids. Patients may also have nausea and vomiting, bloating, abdominal distention, and anorexia. Endoscopy confirms diagnosis (see Chapter 76, Peptic Ulcer Disease).
- Nonulcer dyspepsia—Includes gastroesophageal reflux disease and functional dyspepsia. Classic symptoms of gastroesophageal reflux disease are heartburn (ie, substernal pain that may be associated with acid regurgitation or a sour taste) aggravated by bending forward or lying down, especially after a large meal; individual symptoms, however, do not help to distinguish these patients from those with peptic ulcer disease. Endoscopy is considered if symptoms fail to respond to treatment (eg, histamine-2 receptor agonist, proton pump inhibitor) or red flag signs/symptoms occur (eg, bleeding, dysphagia, severe pain, weight loss).
- Chronic gastritis—Includes autoimmune (body-predominant) and *H. pylori*–related (antral-predominant) types; mucosal inflammation

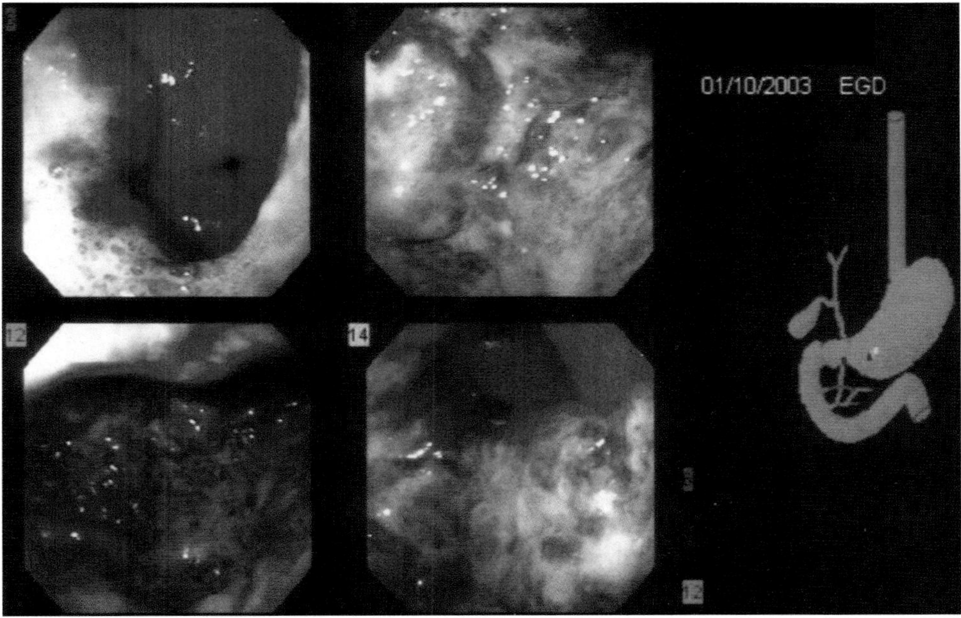

FIGURE 70-2 Endoscopy showing a deep ulcer with yellow-brown exudate in center of mass, consistent with cancer. Pathology confirmed a high-grade, diffuse, large B-cell lymphoma of the stomach. (*Reproduced with permission from Michael Harper, MD.*)

(primarily lymphocytes) may progress to atrophy and metaplasia. Abdominal pain and dyspepsia are common symptoms and patients may have pernicious anemia.

- Esophagitis—May be mechanical or infectious (primarily viral and fungal). Symptoms include heartburn (retrosternal wave-like pain that may radiate to the neck or jaw) and painful swallowing (odynophagia); regurgitation of sour or bitter tasting material may occur with obstruction. Barium swallow or esophagoscopy can be used to establish the diagnosis.
- Esophageal cancer—Relatively uncommon malignancy of 2 cell types: squamous cell cancers (largely related to smoking, excessive alcohol consumption, and other agents causing mucosal trauma) and adenocarcinomas (usually arising in the distal esophagus related to reflux disease). Symptoms include progressive dysphagia and weight loss; the diagnosis is confirmed on esophagoscopy and biopsy.

MANAGEMENT

Patients may be best managed by an experienced multidisciplinary team.[16] Based on SEER data from 1988 to 2001, only 20% of tumors had not spread beyond the stomach at diagnosis, one-third had spread to adjacent structures and lymph nodes, and another third had distant metastases.[4]

PHARMACOLOGIC

- Chemotherapy using 5-fluorouracil (FU) and doxorubicin with or without cisplatin or mitomycin C is somewhat helpful (partial response in 30%-50%).[2] The European Organization for Research and Treatment of Cancer (EORTC)-Gastrointestinal Cancer Group notes improved outcomes for resectable gastric cancer using a strategy of perioperative (pre- and postoperative) chemotherapy or postoperative chemoradiotherapy.[16] SOR Ⓐ
- In a meta-analysis, 3-drug regimens containing FU, an anthracycline, and cisplatin administered as adjunct therapy appeared to have the best survival rates,[17] and another meta-analysis confirmed that postoperative adjuvant chemotherapy based on FU regimens was associated with reduced risk of death from gastric cancer in patients with resectable cancer compared with surgery alone (hazard ratio [HR] 0.82; 95% CI 0.76-0.90) with an absolute 5-year survival benefit of 5.7%.[18] SOR Ⓒ
- EORTC-Gastrointestinal Cancer Group found no chemotherapy combination was an accepted gold standard and that in the treatment of unresectable, locally advanced, or metastatic gastric or gastroesophageal junction adenocarcinoma, response rates were poor.[16]

REFERRAL FOR SURGERY OR PROCEDURES

- Complete resection including adjacent lymph nodes is recommended.[3] For resectable gastric adenocarcinoma, EORTC-Gastrointestinal Cancer Group recommends free-margin surgery with at least D1 resection (perigastric lymph nodes) combined with removal of a minimum of 15 lymph nodes.[16]
- In a meta-analysis of 6 trials comparing D1 with D2 (extended lymph node dissection—hepatic, left gastric, celiac, and splenic arteries, as well as those in the splenic hilum) gastrectomy for patients with resectable gastric cancer, postoperative morbidity, and 30-day mortality rate were higher in the D2 group; 5-year survival was similar.[19]
- In a meta-analysis, laparoscopy-assisted distal gastrectomy compared to conventional distal gastrectomy was associated with lower morbidity, less pain, faster bowel function recovery, and shorter hospital stay; anastomotic and wound complications and mortality rates were similar.[20]
- Radiation is useful for palliation for pain.

PREVENTION

- Aspirin use reduces the risk of GI cancers (20-year cancer death HR 0.65; 95% CI 0.54-0.78); the latent period before an effect on death was seen for stomach cancer was more than 5 years.[21]
- Adherence to a relative Mediterranean diet is associated with a reduced risk of gastric cancer (HR 0.67; 95% CI 0.47-0.94).[22]

- Limited data are available regarding prevention of gastric cancer, but in a population of poorly nourished Chinese subjects, combined supplementation with β-carotene, α-tocopherol, and selenium reduced the incidence of and mortality rate from gastric cancer and the overall mortality rate from cancer by 13% to 21%.[23]
- In a meta-analysis, consumption of large amounts of allium vegetables (onions, garlic, shallots, leeks, chives) was associated with a reduced risk of gastric cancer (odds ratio [OR] 0.54; 95% CI 0.43-0.65).[24]
- Despite limited data, a meta-analysis of 6 studies conducted primarily in Asia found a reduced gastric cancer risk (0.6% absolute risk reduction) with eradication of *H. pylori* infection.[25]
- Screening for gastric cancer in Japan has led to a greater number of cases of gastric cancer being detected in an early stage.

PROGNOSIS

- Surgical morbidity (eg, anastomotic leaks, infection) occurs in approximately 25% of patients and operative mortality is approximately 3%.[26]
- Overall 5-year relative survival based on SEER 2001 to 2007 data was 26.3%. Five-year relative survival by race and gender was 23.2% for white men, 27.5% for white women, 22.5% for black men, and 29.4% for black women.[1]
- Five-year relative survival for localized disease is 61.5%, for spread to regional nodes is 27.8%, and for metastatic disease is 3%.[1]
- Median survival for grade of tumor decreases from well-differentiated tumors (22.6 months) to undifferentiated (7.6 months).[4]

FOLLOW-UP

- Recurrences occur in the first 8 years.
- Follow-up varies from evaluation based on clinical suspicion of relapse to intensive investigations to detect early recurrences; unfortunately there are no data to show that early detection of local recurrence by endoscopy or CT improves survival or quality of life because these recurrences are invariably incurable.[27]
- Isolated liver metastasis identified on CT, however, may be resectable.
- Tumor markers have been used with some success to detect subclinical recurrences and could be used to target more invasive or expensive procedures.[27,28] The National Academy of Clinical Biochemistry does not recommend the routine use of CEA or carbohydrate antigen 19-9 for postoperative monitoring of patients with gastric cancer.[29] SOR Ⓑ

PATIENT EDUCATION

- Surgery with perioperative chemotherapy is potentially curative; operative mortality is approximately 3%.[21]
- Early postoperative complications include anastomotic failure, bleeding, ileus, cholecystitis, pancreatitis, pulmonary infections, and thromboembolism. Further surgery may be required for anastomotic leaks.[11]
- Late mechanical and physiologic complications include dumping syndrome, vitamin B_{12} deficiency, reflux esophagitis, and bone disorders, especially osteoporosis.
- Postgastrectomy patients often are immunologically deficient.

PATIENT RESOURCES

- National Cancer Institute—**http://www.cancer.gov/cancertopics/types/stomach/.**
- Medline Plus. *Stomach Cancer*—**http://www.nlm.nih.gov/medlineplus/stomachcancer.html.**

PROVIDER RESOURCES

- National Cancer Institute. *Stomach Cancer*—**http://www.cancer.gov/cancertopics/types/stomach/.**

REFERENCES

1. Howlader N, Noone AM, Krapcho M, et al, eds. *SEER Cancer Statistics Review, 1975-2008*. Bethesda, MD: National Cancer Institute. http://seer.cancer.gov/csr/1975_2008/, based on November 2010 SEER data submission, posted to the SEER Web site, 2011. http://seer.cancer.gov/statfacts/html/stomach.html. Accessed October 2011.
2. Mayer R. Gastrointestinal tract cancer. In: Kasper DL, Braunwald E, Fauci AS, Hauser SL, Longo DL, Jameson JL, eds. *Harrison's Principles of Internal Medicine*, 16th ed. New York, NY: McGraw-Hill; 2005:523-533.
3. Saeki N, Saito A, Choi IJ, et al. A functional single nucleotide polymorphism in mucin 1, at chromosome 1q22, determines susceptibility to diffuse-type gastric cancer. *Gastroenterology*. 2011;140(3):892-902.
4. Key C, Meisner ALW. *Cancers of the Esophagus, Stomach, and Small Intestine*. http://seer.cancer.gov/publications/survival/surv_esoph_stomach.pdf. Accessed October 2011.
5. Ooi CH, Ivanova T, Wu J, et al. Oncogenic pathway combinations predict clinical prognosis in gastric cancer. *PLoS Genet*. 2009;5(10):e1000676.
6. American Joint Committee on Cancer. *Understanding the Changes from the Sixth to the Seventh Edition of the AJCC Cancer Staging Manual*. https://cancerstaging.org/references-tools/deskreferences/Documents/AJCCSummaryofChanges.pdf. Accessed May 2014.
7. Mcghan LJ, Pockai BA, Gray RJ, et al. Validation of the updated 7th edition AJCC TNM staging criteria for gastric adenocarcinoma. *J Gastrointest Surg*. 2012;16(1):53-61, discussion 61.
8. Layke JC, Lopez PP. Gastric cancer: diagnosis and treatment options. *Am Fam Physician*. 2004;69(5):1133-1141.
9. National Cancer Institute. *Cancer Topics Fact Sheet*. http://www.cancer.gov/cancertopics/factsheet/Risk/h-pylori-cancer. Accessed October 2011.
10. Mills PK, Yang RC. Agricultural exposures and gastric cancer risk in Hispanic farm workers in California. *Environ Res*. 2007;104(2):282-289.
11. Cabebe EC. Mehta VK, Fisher G. *Gastric Cancer*. http://emedicine.medscape.com/article/278744-clinical. Accessed October 2011.
12. Li WB, Zuo XL, Li CQ, et al. Diagnostic value of confocal laser endomicroscopy for gastric superficial cancerous lesions. *Gut*. 2011;60(3):299-306.
13. Gastrointestinal cancer. In: New Zealand Guidelines Group. *Suspected Cancer in Primary Care: Guidelines for Investigation, Referral and Reducing Ethnic Disparities*. Wellington, New Zealand: New Zealand Guidelines Group (NZGG); 2009:33-51. http://www.guideline

.gov/content.aspx?id=15447&search=gastric+cancer. Accessed October 2011.

14. Goddard AF, Badreldin R, Pritchard DM, et al. The management of gastric polyps. *Gut.* 2010;59(9):1270-1276.
15. Society for Surgery of the Alimentary Tract (SSAT). *Surgical Treatment of Gastric Cancer*. Manchester, MA: Society for Surgery of the Alimentary Tract (SSAT); 2004:15:4.
16. Van Cutsem E, Van de Velde C, Roth A, et al. Expert opinion on management of gastric and gastro-oesophageal junction adenocarcinoma on behalf of the European Organisation for Research and Treatment of Cancer (EORTC)—gastrointestinal cancer group. *Eur J Cancer.* 2008;44(2):182-194.
17. Wagner AD, Grothe W, Haerting J, et al. Chemotherapy in advanced gastric cancer: a systematic review and meta-analysis based on aggregate data. *J Clin Oncol.* 2006;24(18):2903-2909.
18. GASTRIC (Global Advanced/Adjuvant Stomach Tumor Research International Collaboration) Group, Paoletti X, Oba K, Burzykowski T, et al. Benefit of adjuvant chemotherapy for resectable gastric cancer: a meta-analysis. *JAMA.* 2010;303(17):1729-1737.
19. Memon MA, Subramanya MS, Khan S, et al. Meta-analysis of D1 versus D2 gastrectomy for gastric adenocarcinoma. *Ann Surg.* 2011;253(5):900-911.
20. Hosono S, Arimoto Y, Ohtani H, Kanamiya Y. Meta-analysis of short-term outcomes after laparoscopy-assisted distal gastrectomy. *World J Gastroenterol.* 2006;12(47):7676-7683.
21. Rothwell PM, Fowkes FG, Belch JF, et al. Effect of daily aspirin on long-term risk of death due to cancer: analysis of individual patient data from randomised trials. *Lancet.* 2011;377(9759):31-41.
22. Buckland G, Agudo A, Luján L, et al. Adherence to a Mediterranean diet and risk of gastric adenocarcinoma within the European Prospective Investigation into Cancer and Nutrition (EPIC) cohort study. *Am J Clin Nutr.* 2010;91(2):381-390.
23. Huang HY, Caballero B, Chang S, et al. The efficacy and safety of multivitamin and mineral supplement use to prevent cancer and chronic disease in adults: a systematic review for a National Institutes of Health state-of-the-science conference. *Ann Intern Med.* 2006;145(5): 372-385.57(1):69-74.
24. Zhou Y, Zhuang W, Hu W, et al. Consumption of large amounts of Allium vegetables reduces risk for gastric cancer in a meta-analysis. *Gastroenterology.* 2011;141(1):80-89.
25. Fuccio L, Zagari RM, Eusebi LH, et al. Meta-analysis: can *Helicobacter pylori* eradication treatment reduce the risk for gastric cancer? *Ann Intern Med.* 2009;151(2):121-128.
26. Zilberstein B, Abbud Ferreira J, Cecconello I. Management of postoperative complications in gastric cancer. *Minerva Gastroenterol Dietol.* 2011;57(1):69-74.
27. Whiting J, Sano T, Saka M, et al. Follow-up of gastric cancer: a review. *Gastric Cancer.* 2006;9(2):74-81.
28. Fareed KR, Kaye P, Soomro IN, et al. Biomarkers of response to therapy in oesophago-gastric cancer. *Gut.* 2009;58(1):127-143.
29. Sturgeon CM, Diamandis E, eds. *Use of Tumor Markers in Liver, Bladder, Cervical, and Gastric Cancers.* Washington, DC: National Academy of Clinical Biochemistry (NACB); 2010:57. http://www.guideline.gov/content.aspx?id=23861&search=gastric+cancer. Accessed October 2011.

71 GASTROESOPHAGEAL REFLUX DISEASE (GERD)

Osama Alsara, MD

PATIENT STORY

A 35-year-old woman with past medical history of hiatal hernia (**Figure 71-1**) presents to the clinic with a complaint of a burning sensation in the middle of her chest, especially when she lies down after meals. She has had this sensation many times this year, but it has been worsening in the last 2 weeks and will occasionally awaken her from sleep. She tried antacids without improvement. She smokes 1 pack a day and drinks alcohol occasionally. The physician diagnoses her with gastroesophageal reflux disease (GERD). She is instructed to stop smoking and not to eat for 3 hours prior to sleep; she is started on a proton pump inhibitor (PPI) to be taken on an empty stomach 45 minutes prior to her largest meal of the day. She returns in 3 weeks with her symptoms resolved.

INTRODUCTION

Gastroesophageal reflux disease (GERD) is a condition in which the stomach contents inappropriately reflux into the esophagus, causing troublesome symptoms or complications.[1]

SYNONYMS

Acid reflux and heartburn are synonyms.

EPIDEMIOLOGY

- In 2006, GERD was the most common gastrointestinal- (GI-) related diagnosis given in office visits in United States.[2]
- Roughly 7% to 10% of Americans complain of GERD symptoms on a daily basis, and about 25% to 40% of Americans experience symptoms of GERD at least once in their lives.[3]
- GERD occurs in all age groups, especially in middle-aged patients.[4]

PATHOLOGY

- The esophagus is normally protected from refluxed gastric acid by many mechanisms, including the following:
  - The lower esophageal sphincter (LES), which is a zone of elevated intraluminal pressure at the esophagogastric junction
  - Acid clearance by peristalsis, gravity, and neutralization from saliva and alkaline esophageal secretions
- Transient LES dysfunction is the pathophysiology of most GERD cases.[5] It may develop as a result of
  - Hiatal hernia—Although some patients with hiatal hernias do not have symptomatic reflux (**Figure 71-1**)
  - Pregnancy as progesterone decreases LES pressure
  - Obesity resulting from increased intra-abdominal pressure and incompetence of the LES
  - Medications with anticholinergic properties, such as tricyclic antidepressants
- Abnormal peristalsis of the esophagus may decrease acid clearance, which in turn irritates the esophageal mucosa. Abnormal motility was reported in almost half of patients with severe esophagitis.[6]

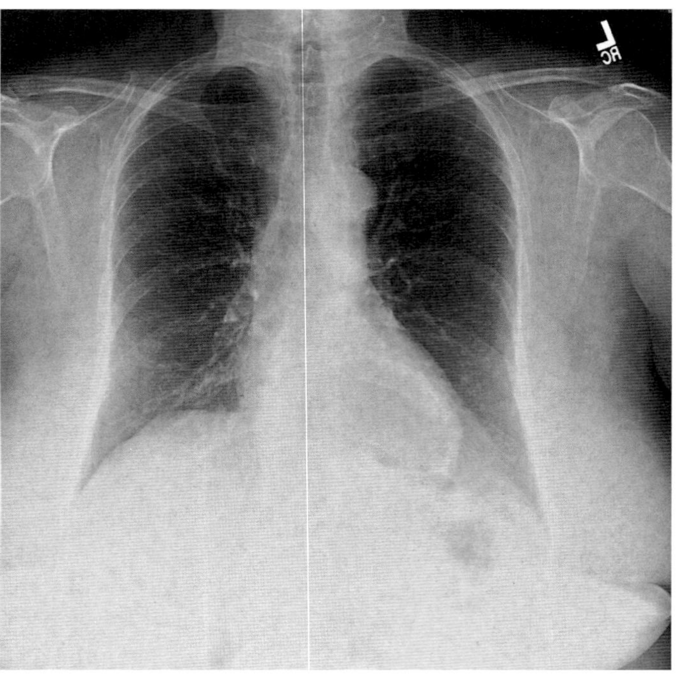

A

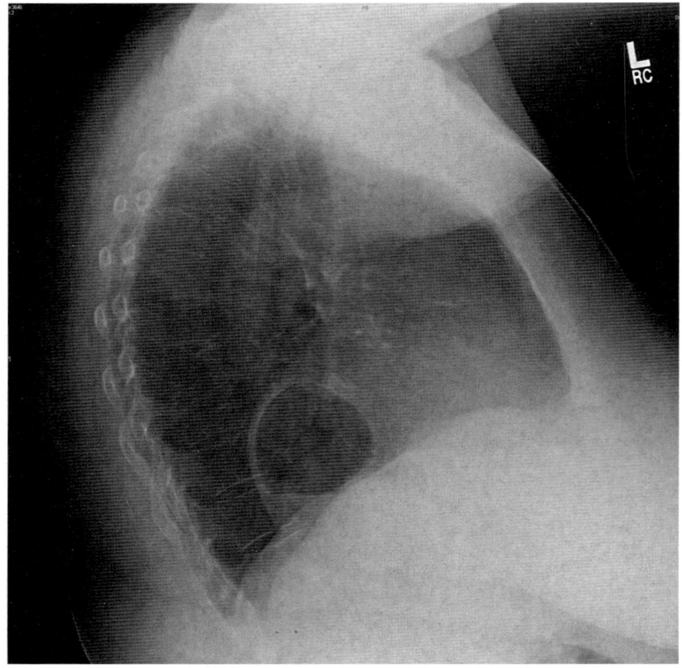

B

FIGURE 71-1 Posteroanterior (A) and lateral (B) chest radiograph of a patient presenting with substernal chest pain caused by reflux disease. Note the large hiatal hernia most prominent on the lateral chest radiograph. (*Reproduced with permission from Gary Ferenchick, MD.*)

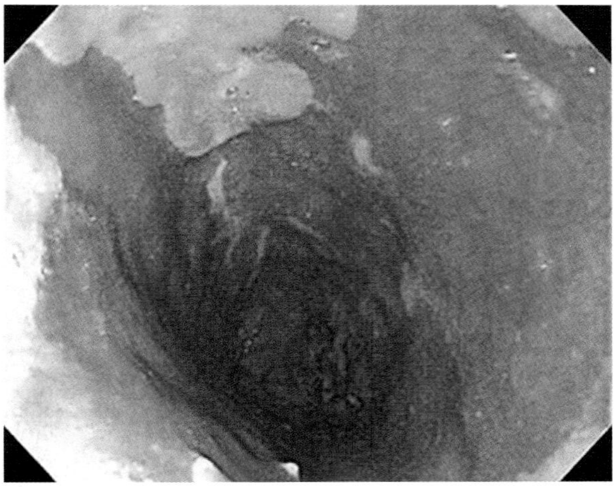

FIGURE 71-2 An endoscopic image of Barrett esophagus, which is a long-term consequence of chronic gastroesophageal reflux disease. Note the red area of columnar cells replacing the squamous cells that normally line the esophagus. Barrett esophagus is the major risk factor for adenocarcinoma of the esophagus. (*Reproduced with permission from Greenberger NJ, Blumberg R, Burakoff R.* Current Diagnosis and Treatment: Gastroenterology, Hepatology, and Endoscopy. *2nd ed. New York, NY: McGraw-Hill; 2012.*)

- GERD can manifest with either esophageal or extraesophageal symptoms:
  - Esophageal symptoms include reflux and regurgitation.
  - Extraesophageal symptoms involve noncardiac chest pain, nocturnal cough, asthma, laryngitis, dental erosions, and hoarseness.[7]
- Of patients with GERD symptoms, 50% to 70% have a normal esophagus on endoscopy, so those patient are known to have nonerosive reflux disease (NERD).[8-10]
- However, acid reflux can irritate the esophageal mucosa, causing several degrees of injury, including esophagitis, strictures, Barrett esophagus, or adenocarcinoma.
- Barrett esophagus is a change in the distal esophageal epithelium to a columnar-type mucosa as a result of long-term exposure to acid reflux. These changes can be recognized by endoscopy and confirmed by biopsy, which shows intestinal metaplasia[11] (**Figure 71-2**).

RISK FACTORS

- Being overweight
- In certain patients—coffee, chocolate, alcohol, peppermint, and fatty foods
- Smoking

DIFFERENTIAL DIAGNOSIS

- Myocardial pain (angina)—Retrosternal chest pain, worsening on exertion and relieved by rest
- Pericarditis—Sharp pain, worse with deep breathing, and relieved by sitting forward
- Aortic dissection—Sudden onset, tearing chest pain, radiates between shoulder blades
- Pulmonary embolism—Sudden onset of chest pain associated with tachycardia, tachypnea, and hypoxia
- Distal esophageal spasm—Chest pain after swallowing hot or cold food
- Peptic ulcer disease—Burning pain increase with hunger and relieved by eating certain foods that buffer stomach acid
- Other causes of esophagitis such as infectious esophagitis or pill esophagitis

DIAGNOSIS

HISTORY/SYMPTOMS

Specifically ask about the following:

- Burning sensation behind sternum, worse after meals or by lying down and relieved by antacids (reflux).
- Bringing gastric contents back up into mouth (regurgitation).
- Chest pain—GERD is the most frequent source of noncardiac chest pain.[12]
- History of nausea and vomiting, which may be a sign of delayed gastric emptying as a potential cause of acid reflux.
- History of blood in stool, anemia, anorexia, family history of peptic ulcer disease, weight loss, long duration of frequent symptoms, or dysphagia; these symptoms are considered alarm symptoms and need further workup as soon as they are identified.
- Asthma or nocturnal persistent nonproductive cough, especially with hoarseness, laryngitis, sore throat, or throat clearing.
- Dysphagia that results from esophageal stricture associated with the disease.
- Use of specific medications that may decrease LES pressure, including calcium channel blockers, anticholinergic drugs, theophylline, nitrates, sildenafil, albuterol.
- Consuming caffeine or alcohol or smoking, as they all decrease LES pressure.

PHYSICAL EXAMINATION

Specifically look for or establish the following:

- Dental erosions
- Pulmonary findings of asthma (wheezing)

IMAGING

- Perform barium studies of the esophagus to obtain an idea about the anatomy of the esophagus or to identify complications of gastroesophageal reflux.
- Perform upper GI endoscopy with or without biopsy to establish the diagnosis of GERD in patients with troublesome dysphagia or unresponsive to a trial of PPIs.
- Also, perform esophagogastroduodenoscopy (EGD) to assess GERD complications (esophagitis, strictures, Barrett esophagus) and to evaluate the anatomy (hiatal hernia, masses, strictures) (**Figure 71-2**).[13]
- Perform a biopsy only from endoscopically suspected lesions to make a histopathologic diagnosis and to rule out Barrett esophagus.[14]

- Perform manometry to determine the LES pressure and evaluate esophageal motility disorders, especially in patients with atypical symptoms in whom the EGD is normal or in whom surgical management is planned.[15]
- Perform 24-hour pH testing to confirm the diagnosis in patients with atypical symptoms, unclear history, symptoms not responsive to empiric trial of twice-daily PPIs, or with normal finding in endoscopy and manometry.[15]
- Perform a nuclear medicine gastric-emptying study in patients with symptoms suggesting inadequate gastric emptying as a cause of GERD.

MANAGEMENT

- Lifestyle modifications are the first line in management of GERD.[16] SOR B Effective strategies may include the following:
  - Losing weight (if overweight). SOR B
  - Avoiding alcohol, chocolate, citrus juice, peppermint, and coffee.[16]
  - Eating small, frequent meals.
  - Waiting at least 3 hours after a meal before lying down.
  - Elevating the head of the bed for patients who have regurgitation or heartburn when lying down. SOR B
  - Stopping smoking (see Chapter 237, Tobacco Addiction).
- Consider using antacids when needed. SOR C
- Consider PPIs or histamine-2 receptor blockers (H2RBs) for relieving both symptoms and esophagitis if the previous strategies are unsuccessful.[17] SOR A
  - Short-term use of a PPI is more effective than an H2RB in symptomatic patients with esophagitis SOR A and in patients without esophagitis.[17] SOR B
  - Consider further workup, including EGD, if the patient's symptoms remain after 2 weeks of medical therapy. SOR B
- Consider evaluation by EGD immediately if the patient had any alarm symptoms noted previously. SOR B
- Treatment of *Helicobacter pylori* does not improve or worsen symptoms of GERD.[18] SOR A
- Consider antireflux surgery in patients with refractory symptoms despite medical therapy. SOR B

LONG-TERM MANAGEMENT

- Most patients with GERD need long-term maintenance therapy to decrease recurrence of symptoms, which, once controlled, the dose of the antisecretory agent should be titrated down to the lowest effective dose.[17] SOR A
- Chronic use of PPIs is effective and may maintain remission more than H2 blockers.[17,19]

PROGNOSIS

- GERD can result in asthma, dental problems, Barrett esophagus, esophageal stricture (**Figure 71-3**), esophageal ulcer, and cancer.
- Without medical treatment, patients with mild esophagitis progress to more severe forms of reflux esophagitis (10.5%), relapse without disease progression (60%), or have no further episodes of esophagitis (29.5%).[20]

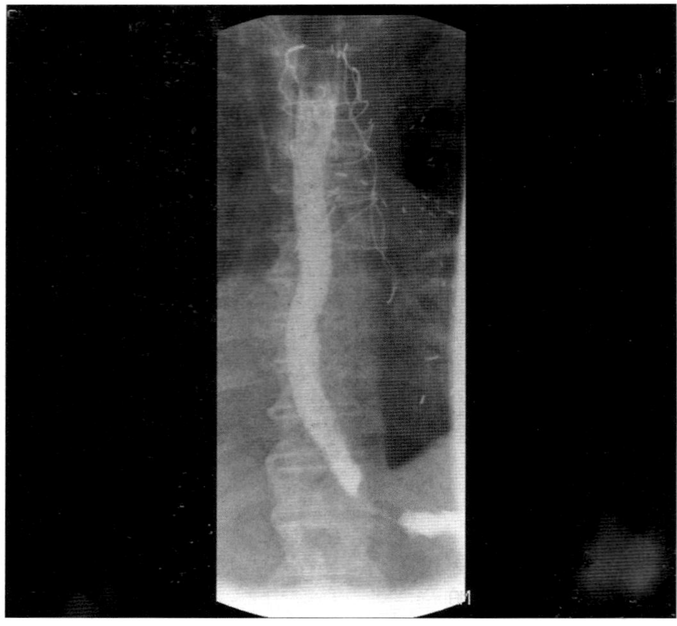

FIGURE 71-3 A barium swallow demonstrating distal esophageal stricture, in this case caused by severe esophagitis. (*Reproduced with permission from Gary Ferenchick, MD.*)

- Risk factors for progressive disease include increased age, female gender, and presence of symptoms at initial diagnosis by endoscopy, presence of hiatal hernia, absence of atrophic gastritis, and absence of *Helicobacter pylori* infection.[20]
- Barrett esophagus is the main cause of esophageal adenocarcinoma, which in turn leads to 2 deaths per million in the population.[21]
- Although antireflex surgery is as effective as medical therapy,[22] about half of patients undergoing antireflux surgery may still require GERD medications.[23]

PATIENT EDUCATION

- Smoking, and foods that may trigger heartburn, should be avoided.
- Weight should be controlled.

PATIENT RESOURCES

- Agency for Healthcare Research and Quality. *Treatment Options for GERD or Acid Reflux Disease: A Review of the Research for Adults*—**http://www.effectivehealthcare.ahrq.gov/ehc/products/165/756/gerd_consumer.pdf.**
- National Digestive Diseases Information Clearinghouse (NDDIC). *Heartburn, Hiatal Hernia, and Gastroesophageal Reflux Disease (GERD)*—**http://digestive.niddk.nih.gov/ddiseases/pubs/gerd/gerd.pdf.**

PROVIDER RESOURCES

- Kahrilas PJ, Shaheen NJ, Vaezi MF. American Gastroenterological Association medical position statement on the management of gastroesophageal reflux disease. *Gastroenterology*. 2008;135(4):1383-1391.e5—**http://www.gastrojournal.org/article/S0016-5085(08)01606-5/abstract.**
- National Digestive Diseases Information Clearinghouse (NDDIC). *GERD*—**http://digestive.niddk.nih.gov/ddiseases/pubs/gerd/#8.**

REFERENCES

1. Vakil N, Zanten SV, Kahrilas P, et al. The Montreal Definition and Classification of Gastroesophageal Reflux Disease: a global evidence-based consensus. *Am J Gastroenterol.* 2006;101(8): 1900-1920; quiz 1943.
2. Shaheen NJ, Hansen RA, Morgan DR, et al. The burden of gastrointestinal and liver diseases, 2006. *Am J Gastroenterol.* 2006;101(9): 2128-2138.
3. Herbella FA, Sweet MP, Tedesco P, et al. Gastroesophageal reflux disease and obesity. Pathophysiology and implications for treatment. *J Gastrointest Surg.* 2007;11(3):286-290.
4. Srinivasan R, Tutuian R, Schoenfeld P, et al. Profile of GERD in the adult population of a northeast urban community. *J Clin Gastroenterol.* 2004;38(8):651-657.
5. Hershcovici T, Mashimo H, Fass R. The lower esophageal sphincter. *Neurogastroenterol Motil.* 2011;23(9):819-830. doi:10.1111/j. 1365-2982.2011.01738.x. Epub 2011 Jun 29.
6. Kahrilas PJ, Dodds WJ, Hogan WJ, Kern M, Arndorfer RC, Reece A. Esophageal peristaltic dysfunction in peptic esophagitis. *Gastroenterology*. 1986;91(4):897-904.
7. Williams JL. Gastroesophageal reflux disease: clinical manifestations. *Gastroenterol Nurs.* 2003;26(5):195-200.
8. Winters C Jr, Spurling TJ, Chobanian SJ, et al. Barrett's esophagus: a prevalent, occult complication of gastroesophageal reflux disease. *Gastroenterology.* 1987;92:118–124.
9. Johansson KE, Ask P, Boeryd B, et al. Oesophagitis, signs of reflux, and gastric acid secretion in patients with symptoms of gastro-oesophageal reflux disease. *Scand J Gastroenterol.* 1986;21:837–847.
10. Lind T, Havelund T, Carlsson R, et al. Heartburn without oesophagitis: efficacy of omeprazole therapy and features determining therapeutic response. *Scand J Gastroenterol.* 1997;32:974–979.
11. Wang KK, Sampliner RE. Updated guidelines 2008 for the diagnosis, surveillance and therapy of Barrett's esophagus. *Am J Gastroenterol.* 2008;103(3):788-797.
12. Dimache M, Turcan E, Nătase M. Noncardiac chest pain and gastroesophageal reflux disease. *Rev Med Chir Soc Med Nat Iasi.* 2010;114(2):342-348.
13. Lichtenstein DR, Cash BD, Davila R, et al. Role of endoscopy in the management of GERD. *Gastrointest Endosc.* 2007;66(2):219-224.
14. Sharma P, McQuaid K, Dent J, et al. A critical review of the diagnosis and management of Barrett's esophagus: the AGA Chicago Workshop. *Gastroenterology.* 2004;127:310-330.
15. Lacy BE, Weiser K, Chertoff J, et al. The diagnosis of gastroesophageal reflux disease. *Am J Med.* 2010;123(7):583-592.
16. DeVault KR, Castell DO. Updated guidelines for the diagnosis and treatment of gastroesophageal reflux disease. *Am J Gastroenterol.* 2005;100(1):190-200.
17. Kahrilas PJ, Shaheen NJ, Vaezi M. American Gastroenterological Association medical position statement on the management of gastroesophageal reflux disease. *Gastroenterology.* 2008;135:1383-1391.
18. Yaghoobi M, Farrokhyar F, Yuan Y, et al. Is there an increased risk of GERD after *Helicobacter pylori* eradication? A meta-analysis. *Am J Gastroenterol.* 2010;105(5):1007-1013.
19. Hallerback B, Unge P, Carling L, et al. Omperazole or ranitidine in long term treatment of reflux esophagitis. *Gastroenterology.* 1994;107: 1305-1311.
20. Manabe N, Yoshihara M, Sasaki A, et al. Clinical characteristics and natural history of patients with low-grade reflux esophagitis. *Gastroenterol Hepatol.* 2002;17(9):949-954.
21. Sonnenberg A, El-Serag HB. Clinical epidemiology and natural history of gastroesophageal reflux disease. *Yale J Biol Med.* 1999;72 (2-3):81-92.
22. Lundell L, Miettinen P, Myrvold HE, et al. Continued (5-year) followup of a randomized clinical study comparing antireflux surgery and omeprazole in gastroesophageal reflux disease. *J Am Coll Surg.* 2001;192(2):172-179.
23. Dominitz JA, Dire CA, Billingsley KG, et al. Complications and antireflux medication use after antireflux surgery. *Clin Gastroenterol Hepatol.* 2006;4(3):299-305.

72 HEMORRHOIDS

Mindy A. Smith, MD, MS

PATIENT STORY

A 42-year-old woman presents to the office with rectal pressure and occasional bright red blood on the toilet paper when wiping after bowel movements (**Figure 72-1**). She has had difficulty with constipation off and on for many years and had large hemorrhoids during her last pregnancy. Physical examination confirms the diagnosis of external hemorrhoids.

INTRODUCTION

Hemorrhoids are cushions of highly vascular structures found within the submucosa of the anal canal. They become pathologic when swollen or inflamed.

SYNONYMS

Piles.

EPIDEMIOLOGY

- More than 1 million people in Western civilization suffer from hemorrhoids each year.[1]
- Estimated at 5% prevalence in the general population.[2]
- Approximately half of those older than age 50 years have experienced hemorrhoidal symptoms at some time.[2]
- More frequent in whites and in those of higher socioeconomic status.[2]

ETIOLOGY AND PATHOPHYSIOLOGY

- Three hemorrhoidal cushions (comprised of subepithelial connective tissue, elastic tissue, blood vessels, and smooth muscle) surround and support distal anastomoses between the terminal branches of the superior and middle rectal arteries and the superior, middle, and inferior rectal veins.[2] The hemorrhoidal cushions have several functions, including maintaining fecal continence by engorging with blood and closing the anal canal and by protecting the anal sphincter during defecation.
- Hemorrhoidal tissue provides important sensory information—enabling the differentiation between solid, liquid, and gas—and subsequent decision to evacuate.[2]
- Abnormal swelling of the anal cushions can occur from a number of causes (see "Risk Factors" below) resulting in increased pressure, with dilation and engorgement of the arteriovenous plexuses. Increased pressure can lead to stretching of the suspensory muscles, laxity of connective tissue, and eventual prolapse of rectal tissue through the anal canal.[2] The engorged anal mucosa is easily traumatized, leading to rectal bleeding. Prolapse predisposes to incarceration and strangulation.
- Hemorrhoids are classified with respect to their position relative to the dentate line.
  - Internal hemorrhoids (**Figure 72-2**) develop above the dentate line and are covered by columnar epithelium of anal mucosa. Internal hemorrhoids lack somatic sensory innervation.
  - External hemorrhoids (**Figure 72-1**) arise distal to the dentate line. They are covered by stratified squamous epithelium and receive somatic sensory innervation from the inferior rectal nerve.
- Hemorrhoids are further classified into 4 stages of disease severity[1,2]:
  - Stage I—Enlargement and bleeding
  - Stage II—Protrusion of hemorrhoids with spontaneous reduction
  - Stage III—Protrusion of hemorrhoids with manual reduction possible
  - Stage IV—Irreducible protrusion of hemorrhoids usually containing both internal and external components with or without acute thrombosis or strangulation

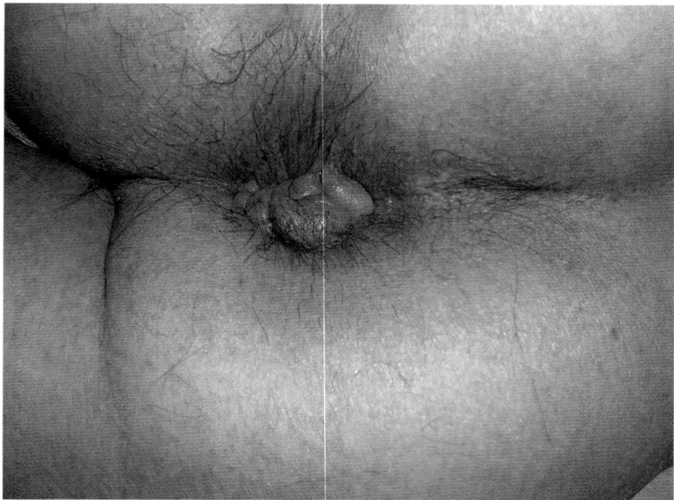

FIGURE 72-1 External hemorrhoid that is symptomatic. The patient had some bleeding with bowel movements. (*Reproduced with permission from Richard P. Usatine, MD.*)

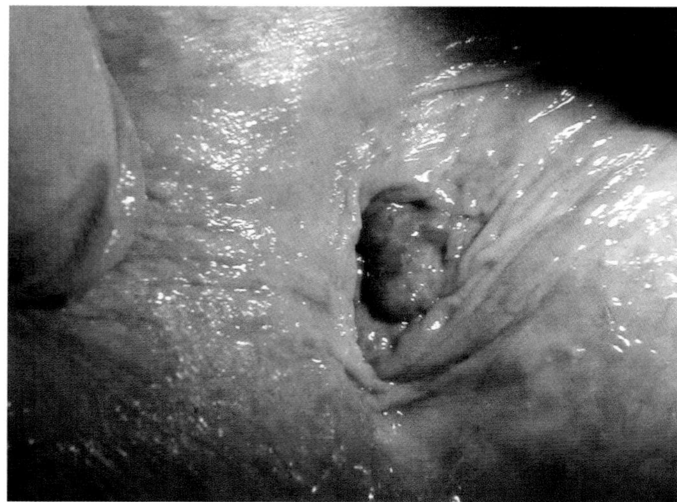

FIGURE 72-2 A large prolapsed internal hemorrhoid. (*Reproduced with permission from Charlie Goldberg, MD. Copyright © 2005 The Regents of the University of California.*)

RISK FACTORS

- Family history of hemorrhoids
- Personal history of constipation, diarrhea, and/or prolonged straining at stool
- Pregnancy
- Prolonged sitting or heavy lifting

DIAGNOSIS

CLINICAL FEATURES

- Bleeding described as bright red blood (a result of the high blood oxygen content within the arteriovenous anastomoses) seen in the toilet or with wiping after bowel movements.
- Protrusion/mass (**Figure 72-1**).
- Pain described as a dull ache or severe if thrombosed.
- Inability to maintain personal hygiene/staining/soiling secondary to prolapse.
- Pruritus, also secondary to prolapse.
- Diagnosis is made on visual inspection and anoscopy, with and without straining:
    - Physical findings of swollen blood vessels protruding from the anus (**Figure 72-1**).
    - Excoriations may also be seen on the skin surrounding the anus.
    - A thrombosed hemorrhoid will be tender and firm and appear as a circular purplish bulge adjacent to the anal opening (**Figure 72-3**). There may be a black discoloration if there is accompanying necrosis.
    - Internal hemorrhoids may be visualized on anoscopy as swollen purple blood vessels arising above the dentate line.
- Other physical findings that may accompany hemorrhoids are redundant tissue and skin tags (**Figure 72-4**) from old thrombosed external hemorrhoids.

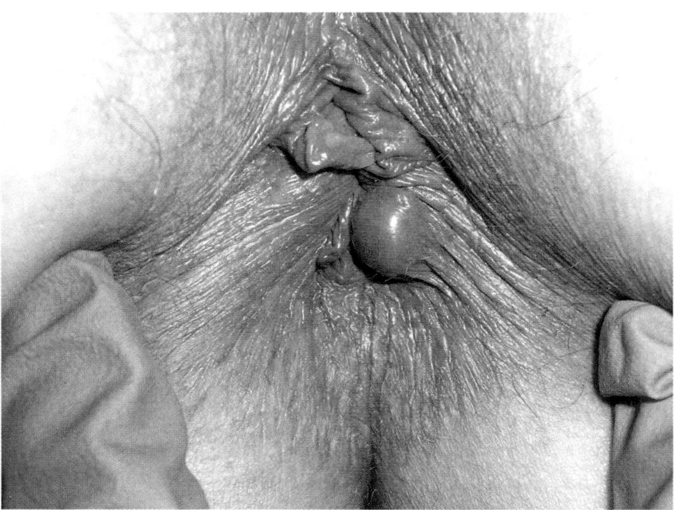

FIGURE 72-3 Thrombosed external hemorrhoid prior to elliptical excision and healing by secondary intention. Note how the hemorrhoid is at the typical 5 o'clock position. (*Reproduced with permission from Yu Wah, MD.*)

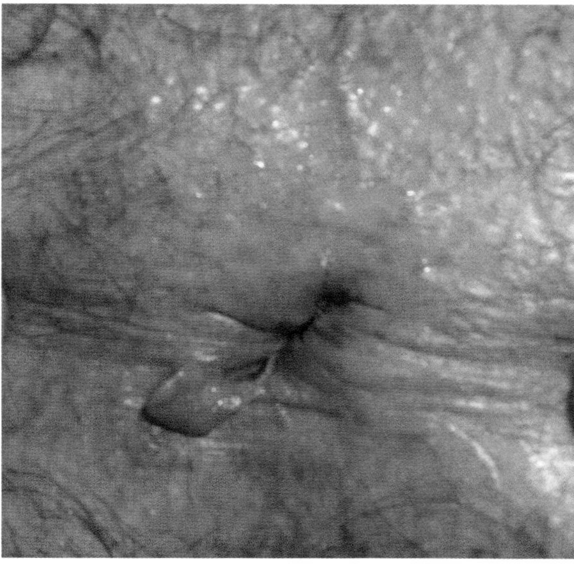

FIGURE 72-4 Rectal fissure with prominent skin tag. (*Reproduced with permission from Charlie Goldberg, MD. Copyright © 2005 The Regents of the University of California.*)

DIFFERENTIAL DIAGNOSIS

- Rectal prolapse—Full-thickness circumferential protrusion appearing as a bluish, tender perianal mass. More common in women (6-fold higher incidence) and associated with other pelvic-floor disorders (eg, cystocele, urinary incontinence). It can present as an anal mass with bleeding.[1]
- Condyloma acuminata (see Chapter 132, Genital Warts)—Appear as flesh-colored, exophytic lesions on perianal skin. They may be flat, verrucous, or pedunculated.
- Anal tumors—Tumors in the rectosigmoid region are associated with hematochezia, tenesmus (ie, urgency with a feeling of incomplete evacuation), and arrow-caliber stool; a firm mass may be found on rectal examination or seen outside the rectum.
- Inflammatory bowel disease (see Chapter 77, Inflammatory Bowel Disease)—Associated diarrhea, rectal bleeding, tenesmus, passage of mucus, and cramping abdominal pain.
- Signs of infection or abscess formation—Tender mass, sometimes feeling fluctuant, with overlying skin erythema (**Figure 72-5**). If cellulitis is also present, skin may have a woody, hard feel. Fistulas may also form, and an opening may be seen on the buttock.
- Fissures—A cut or tear occurring in the anus that extends upward into the anal canal. Common and occurring at all ages; fissures cause pain during bowel movements in addition to bleeding (**Figure 72-4**).

MANAGEMENT

NONPHARMACOLOGIC

- Patients with hemorrhoids should be encouraged to increase dietary fiber and/or add a fiber supplement to reduce severity and duration of symptoms. In a Cochrane review of 7 small randomized controlled trials (RCTs), fiber supplements decreased symptoms (eg, pain, itching, and bleeding) by 53% in the group receiving fiber.[3] SOR Ⓐ
- There are no data supporting use of sitz baths.

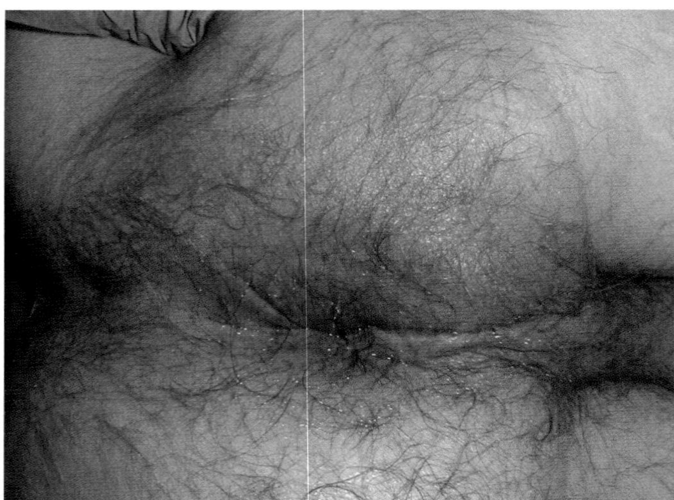

FIGURE 72-5 Perirectal abscess: Note surrounding erythema that extends onto the right buttock. *(Reproduced with permission from Charlie Goldberg, MD. Copyright © 2005 The Regents of the University of California.)*

MEDICATIONS

- Short course of a topical steroid cream or suppositories, twice daily. SOR Ⓒ
- For acute thrombosed external hemorrhoids, a small RCT of 98 patients treated nonsurgically found improved complete pain relief at 7 days with a combination of topical nifedipine 0.3% and lidocaine 1.5% compared with lidocaine alone (86% vs. 50%, respectively).[4] Resolution at 14 days was reported for 92% versus 45.8%, respectively.
- Use a stool softener and encourage adequate fluid intake if constipation is a factor. SOR Ⓒ

PROCEDURES

- Internal hemorrhoids:
  - Data are limited to retrospective studies and case series for most procedures.
  - Stages I and II hemorrhoids can be treated with sclerotherapy (1 to 5 mL of sclerosing agent such as sodium tetradechol sulfate injected via a 25-gauge needle into the submucosa of the hemorrhoidal complex).[1] Sclerotherapy, however, carries a high risk of postprocedure pain (70%). Urinary retention, abscess formation, and sepsis have also been reported; the author of a review recommends that only 2 sites should be sclerosed at 1 time to reduce risk.[2] Recurrence rates are as high as 30%.[2]
  - Stages II and III internal hemorrhoids can be treated with rubber band ligation. Two bands are placed around the engorged tissue producing ischemia and fibrosis of the hemorrhoid.
    - In a Cochrane review of 3 methodologically poor trials comparing excisional hemorrhoidectomy with banding for grade III hemorrhoids, results with hemorrhoidectomy were better than banding for resolution of symptoms but were associated with increased postprocedural pain, higher complication rate, and more time off work.[5]
    - Patients on anticoagulants may be better candidates for another procedure with less bleeding risk.[2]
    - Success rates of 50% to 100% are reported, depending on time to follow-up; there is a recurrence rate of 68% at 4 to 5 years.[2]
    - Complications are uncommon (<1%) and include pain, abscess formation, urinary retention, bleeding, band slippage, and sepsis.[2]
  - Lower-stage hemorrhoids can also be treated with infrared photocoagulation (IPC), bipolar electrocautery, laser therapy, or low-voltage direct current (the latter works for higher-grade hemorrhoids). IPC is initially successful in 88% to 100% of patients.[2]
- External hemorrhoids:
  - Based on retrospective studies, excision is the most effective treatment for thrombosed external hemorrhoids. This procedure is associated with lower recurrence rates (6.5% in one study) and faster symptom resolution.[6] SOR Ⓑ
  - Acutely thrombosed external hemorrhoids can also be safely excised in the office or emergency room for patients who present within 48 to 72 hours of symptom onset. A local anesthetic containing epinephrine is used followed by elliptical incision (not extending beyond the anal verge or deeper than the cutaneous layer) and excision of the thrombosed hemorrhoid and overlying skin. Simple incision and clot evacuation is inadequate therapy for complete resolution, although it may relieve pain. A pressure dressing is applied for several hours, after which time the wound is left to heal by secondary intention.
  - Intrasphincteric injection of botulinum toxin provided more effective pain relief at 24 hours than saline injection for patients with thrombosed external hemorrhoids not undergoing surgery.[7]

REFERRAL FOR SURGERY

- Surgeries for hemorrhoids include open and closed excision, harmonic scalpel, LigaSure tissue-sealing device, Doppler-guided transanal hemorrhoidal ligature, and stapled hemorrhoidopexy.[2] The ultimate need for surgical management is uncommon (5%-10%).[2] The major complication is postoperative pain that can delay work return for 2 to 4 weeks.[2]
- Indications for surgery include:
  - Failure of nonsurgical treatment (persistent bleeding or chronic symptoms)[6]
  - Grades III and IV hemorrhoids with severe symptoms[6]
  - Presence of other anorectal conditions (eg, anal fissure or fistula) requiring surgery
  - Patient preference
- Stage IV hemorrhoids can be treated with traditional excision or surgery using stapling. A Cochrane review of 12 RCTs comparing conventional hemorrhoidectomy with stapling hemorrhoidopexy in patients with grades I to III hemorrhoids found a lower long-term recurrence rate (9 out of 476 [1.9%] vs. 37 out of 479 [7.7%], respectively) in patients who had conventional hemorrhoidectomy (number needed to treat [NNT] = 17).[8] Another metaanalysis of 14 RCTs confirmed higher rates of prolapse recurrence with stapling (odds ratio [OR]: 5.5).[9]
- Use of perianal local anesthetic infiltration provides significant postoperative pain relief.[10] SOR Ⓐ
  - Combination acetaminophen and nonsteroidal antiinflammatory agents or cyclooxygenase (COX)-2–selective inhibitors should be used when possible for pain control as opioids may be constipating. There are no data supporting any particular drug over another.[8] SOR Ⓑ
  - Stapled hemorrhoidectomy reduces pain compared with other surgical techniques.[8] SOR Ⓐ
  - Other medications that can be considered as analgesic adjuncts are laxatives and metronidazole started before surgery.[8] SOR Ⓐ
- Complications of surgery include transient urinary retention (up to 34%), infection (rare), bleeding (2%), fecal incontinence (if sphincter muscle damage), anal stenosis, and rectal prolapse.

PROGNOSIS

Most hemorrhoids resolve spontaneously or with medical therapy alone. The recurrence rate with nonsurgical therapy is 10% to 50% (over a 5-year period), and for surgical treatment, less than 10%.

FOLLOW-UP

- After excision of a thrombosed hemorrhoid, patient instructions should include initial bed rest for several hours, sitz baths 3 times daily, stool softeners, and topical or systemic analgesia. SOR Ⓒ The patient should return in 48 to 72 hours for a wound check.
- Similar instructions are used for patients postoperatively with respect to bed rest (1 to 2 days), sitz baths, stool softeners, and adequate fluid intake. Pain control is discussed above.

PATIENT EDUCATION

- Patients should be counseled to avoid aggravating factors including constipation and prolonged sitting.
- Advise patients who elect rubber band ligation that complications, based on one follow-up study, include pain (at 1 week, 75% of patients were pain-free and 7% were still experiencing moderate-to-severe pain), rectal bleeding (in 65% on the day after banding, persisting in 24% at 1 week), and relatively low satisfaction (only 59% were satisfied with their experience and would undergo the procedure again).[11]
- Advise patients who elect or are recommended for surgery about potential complications of infection, thrombosis, ulceration, and incontinence.

PATIENT RESOURCES

- Medline Plus. *Hemorrhoids*—**http://www.nlm.nih.gov/medlineplus/hemorrhoids.html.**
- National Digestive Diseases Information Clearinghouse (NDDIC). *Hemorrhoids*—**http://digestive.niddk.nih.gov/ddiseases/pubs/hemorrhoids/index.aspx.**

PROVIDER RESOURCES

- Medscape. *Hemorrhoids*—**http://emedicine.medscape.com/article/775407.**
- Medscape. *Hemorrhoid surgery*—**http://emedicine.medscape.com/article/195401.**

REFERENCES

1. Gerhart SL, Bulkley G. Common diseases of the colon and anorectum and mesenteric vascular insufficiency. In: Kasper DL, Braunwald E, Fauci AS, Hauser SL, Longo DL, Jameson JL, eds. *Harrison's Principles of Internal Medicine*, 16th ed. New York: McGraw-Hill; 2005:1801-1802.
2. Sneider EB, Maykel JA. Diagnosis and management of symptomatic hemorrhoids. *Surg Clin North Am.* 2010;90(1):17-32.
3. Alonso-Coello P, Guyatt G, Heels-Ansdell D, et al. Laxatives for the treatment of hemorrhoids. *Cochrane Database Syst Rev.* 2005 Oct 19;(4):CD004649.
4. Perrotti P, Antropoli C, Molino D, et al. Conservative treatment of acute thrombosed external hemorrhoids with topical nifedipine. *Dis Colon Rectum.* 2001;44:405-409.
5. Shanmugam V, Thaha MA, Rabindranath KS, et al. Rubber band ligation versus excisional haemorrhoidectomy for haemorrhoids. *Cochrane Database Syst Rev.* 2005 Jul 20;3:CD005034.
6. Mounsey AL, Henry SL. Clinical inquiries. Which treatments work best for hemorrhoids? *J Fam Pract.* 2009;58(9):492-493.
7. Patti R, Arcara M, Bonventre S, et al. Randomized clinical trial of botulinum toxin injection for pain relief in patients with thrombosed external haemorrhoids. *Br J Surg.* 2008;95(11):1339-1343.
8. Jayaraman S, Colquhoun PH, Malthaner RA. Stapled versus conventional surgery for hemorrhoids. *Cochrane Database Syst Rev.* 2006 Oct 18;(4):CD005393.
9. Giordano P, Gravante G, Sorge R, et al. Long-term outcomes of stapled hemorrhoidopexy vs conventional hemorrhoidectomy: a meta-analysis of randomized controlled trials. *Arch Surg.* 2009; 144(3): 266-272.
10. Joshi GP, Neugebauer EA; PROSPECT Collaboration. Evidence-based management of pain after haemorrhoidectomy surgery. *Br J Surg.* 2010;97(8):1155-1168.
11. Watson NF, Liptrott S, Maxwell-Armstrong CA. A prospective audit of early pain and patient satisfaction following out-patient band ligation of haemorrhoids. *Ann R Coll Surg Engl.* 2006;88(3):275-279.

73 ISCHEMIC COLITIS

Supratik Rayamajhi, MD

PATIENT STORY

A 87-year-old woman is brought to the emergency center for altered mental status and is found to be in severe sepsis with no obvious source. She is admitted to the intensive care unit (ICU) and treated for septic shock. Because of persistent elevation in lactate despite florid fluid resuscitation, an abdominal source is suspected. Her abdomen is distended with absent bowel sounds, and radiography shows marked ileus with a massively dilated colon and pneumatosis coli. (**Figure 73-1**). After extensive discussion with family, exploratory laparotomy is performed. A gangrenous large bowel from severe ischemic colitis is resected. Unfortunately, she passes away from multiorgan failure within 6 hours of surgery.

INTRODUCTION

Ischemic colitis (**Figure 73-2**) is the most common form of intestinal ischemia. Colonic ischemia results from reduction in blood flow that is insufficient to meet the metabolic demands of the colon. The reduction in blood flow can result from an occlusion, vasospasm, or hypoperfusion of the mesenteric vasculature. Although uncommon in the general population, it carries potentially life-threatening consequences and is mostly seen in the elderly.

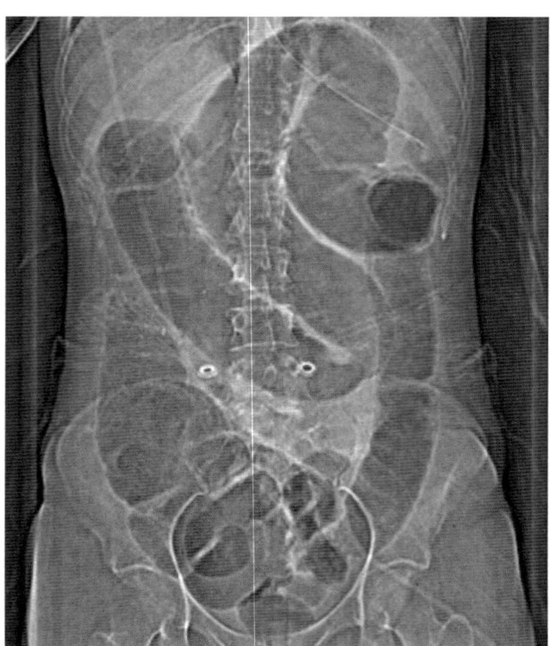

FIGURE 73-1 Dilated colon with pneumatosis coli in a patient with ischemic colitis. (*Used with permission from Jerry Aben, MD.*)

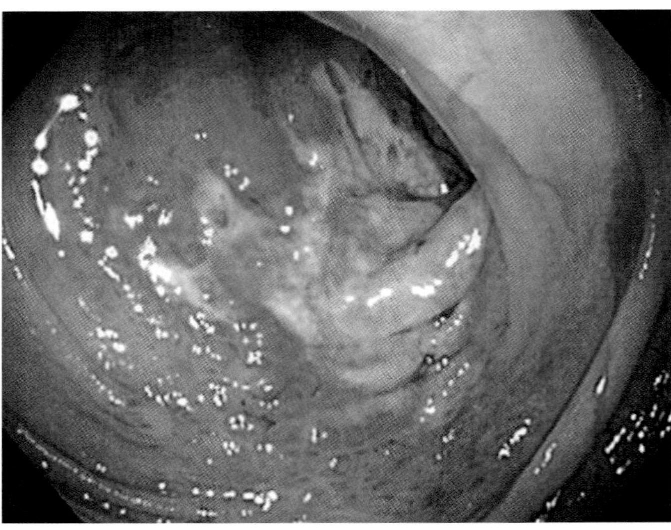

FIGURE 73-2 Endoscopic findings of moderate ischemic colitis. (*Reproduced with permission from McKean SC, Ross JJ, Dressler DD, Brotman DJ, Ginsberg JS. Principles and Practice of Hospital Medicine. New York, NY: McGraw-Hill; 2012.*)

EPIDEMIOLOGY

- The incidence of ischemic colitis in the general population in various studies ranged from 4.5 to 44 cases per 100 000 person-years.[1]
- Ischemic colitis accounts for 1 in 1000 hospitalizations.[2]

ETIOLOGY/PATHOPHYSIOLOGY

- Blood flow can be compromised by anatomic or functional changes in the local mesenteric vasculature.
- As compared with the small bowel, the colonic microvasculature plexus is not only less developed but also embedded in a relatively thicker wall, which makes the colon more susceptible to ischemic injuries.[3]
- The splenic flexure and rectosigmoid junction are the most vulnerable areas of the colon because of lack of collateral networks and are called "watershed" areas.

RISK FACTORS

- Common conditions that predispose to and are associated with ischemic colitis include shock, strenuous activity such as long-distance running or bicycling, aorto-iliac surgery, coronary artery bypass graft (CABG) surgery, hypercoagulable states, cardiac embolism, myocardial infarction, vasculitis, and hemodialysis.[4]
- The most common drugs that act as culprits are antihypertensive agents (especially in elderly patients because of vasodilation and decreased perfusion pressure); diuretics (from dehydration); nonsteroidal anti-inflammatory drugs (direct toxicity as well as by depleting cytoprotective prostaglandins and causing vasoconstriction); digoxin (causes mesentery bed vasoconstriction both directly and indirectly by the alpha-adrenergic pathway); oral contraceptives (because of hypercoagulable state); vasopressors (intense vasoconstriction); and

alosetron (vasoconstriction from serotonin receptor 5-HT_1 and 5-HT_2 activation and increased intraluminal pressure in severe constipation).[4]

DIAGNOSIS

HISTORY/SYMPTOMS

- The most common presentation is acute onset of mild cramping, abdominal pain, and tenderness over the affected bowel.[5]
- Tenesmus is common, and passage of bright red or maroon blood-mixed stool is seen within the next 24 hours.[5]
- Blood loss is usually minimal; actually, profuse bleeding goes against the diagnosis of colonic ischemia.
- Anorexia, nausea, vomiting, or abdominal distension may be present as the result of an associated ileus.

PHYSICAL EXAMINATION

- Nearly 15% of patients will have peritoneal signs caused by transmural infarction and necrosis and features of septic shock.[6]
- The diagnosis is usually established based on the history, physical examination, and radiological or endoscopic studies.

LABORATORY TESTING

- Markers of ischemia such as serum lactate, lactate dehydrogenase (LDH), alkaline phosphatase, and systemic acidosis may be present only late in the course.
- High levels of these markers (including elevated white blood cells [WBC]) suggest infarction.

IMAGING

- A plain radiograph is an insensitive and nonspecific test but is helpful in excluding other disorders, such as kidney stones, ileus, intestinal obstruction, volvulus, and pneumoperitonium.[7]
- Barium enema may show suggestive findings in 75% of patients, with thumbprinting (suggesting submucosal edema) as the most common finding, but it is nonspecific. Colonoscopy has replaced barium enema as the diagnostic modality of choice because of its higher sensitivity for detecting mucosal changes and the ability to obtain biopsy specimens if necessary.[5]
- CT findings are generally nonspecific and may initially be normal. The most common finding is segmental circumferential wall thickening. Pneumatosis suggests transmural ischemia or infarction.[8]
- Angiography is usually not indicated except when acute mesenteric ischemia is being considered (see the section on differential diagnosis).
- Colonoscopy is most sensitive in detecting mucosal lesions, permits biopsies to be obtained, and does not interfere with subsequent angiography.[5] Findings that favor ischemic colitis are segmental area of injury with abrupt transition between normal and affected mucosa and classic rectal sparing (**Figures 73-2** and **73-3**).

HISTOLOGY

- The histologic changes of ischemic colitis are nonspecific.
- These changes include edema, distorted crypts, mucosal and submucosal hemorrhage, inflammatory infiltration, granulation tissue, intravascular platelet thrombi, and necrosis.[9]

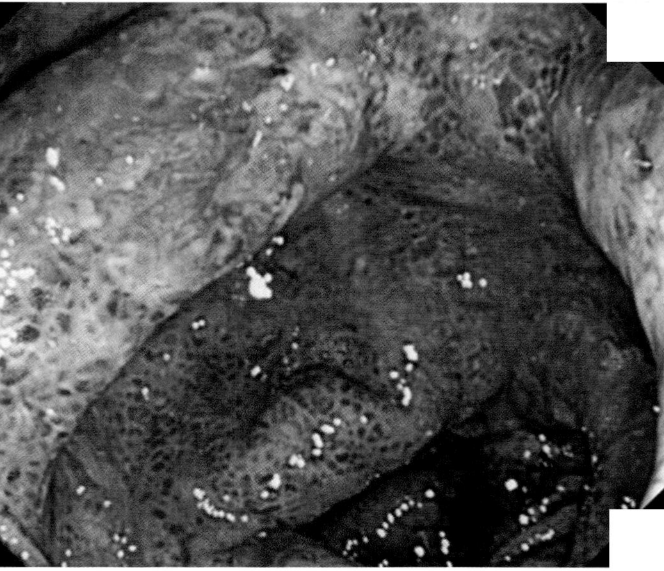

FIGURE 73-3 Endoscopic findings of severe ischemic colitis. (*Reproduced with permission from McKean SC, Ross JJ, Dressler DD, Brotman DJ, Ginsberg JS. Principles and Practice of Hospital Medicine. New York, NY: McGraw-Hill; 2012.*)

OTHER INVESTIGATIONS

- Although not routinely recommended by most authorities, an area of debate is the utility of searching for cardiac sources of embolization in patients with ischemic colitis.
- Potential cardiac sources are atrial fibrillation, left atrial or left ventricular thrombus, dilated cardiomyopathy, and valvular vegetations.[10]

DIFFERENTIAL DIAGNOSIS

- Infectious colitis commonly presents with profuse diarrhea and foul-smelling stool, which is not common in ischemic colitis, and the causative agent may be found using cultures from the stool.
- *Clostridium difficile* colitis has diarrhea as a predominant symptoms along with abdominal pain and cramping, with history of recent hospitalization, recent antibiotic use, or use of gastric acid-suppressive drugs or chemotherapy with positive toxin on stool test (see Chapter 65, *Clostridium difficile* Infection).
- Inflammatory bowel disease (IBD) such as ulcerative colitis (UC) is typically a chronic disease; therefore, a history of IBD is suggestive. UC is usually seen in younger people with diffuse involvement of the colon, as opposed to ischemic colitis, which is predominantly a disease of the elderly (see Chapter 77, Inflammatory Bowel Disease).
- Mesenteric ischemia should be suspected with the acute onset of severe abdominal pain in the absence of palpatory tenderness or abdominal peritoneal signs. The pain is typically out of proportion to examination, and auscultation of the abdomen may reveal a bruit. A history of bleeding is uncommon until very late.
- Diverticulitis commonly has pain and tenderness localized to the left lower quadrant of the abdomen and has characteristic findings on CT imaging, including inflammatory changes localized to the sigmoid colon (see Chapter 68, Diverticulitis).

- Colon carcinoma presents with a history of unintentional weight loss and iron deficiency anemia with painless lower gastrointestinal bleeding (see Chapter 66, Colon Cancer).

MANAGEMENT

SUPPORTIVE CARE

- Supportive care is appropriate in the absence of colonic gangrene or perforation. Elements of supportive care include the following:
  - Intravenous fluids should be given to ensure adequate colonic perfusion, and patients should receive nothing by mouth.
  - A nasogastric tube should be inserted if an ileus is present. SOR Ⓒ
  - Careful monitoring for persistent fever, leukocytosis, peritoneal irritation, protracted diarrhea, and bleeding is indicated.
  - Although there is a lack of prospective clinical data on humans, empiric broad-spectrum antibiotics are often administered in patients with moderate-to-severe colitis to minimize bacterial translocation and sepsis.[11] SOR Ⓒ
    - Consider antibiotics to cover the bowel flora, including gram-negative and anaerobic organisms.
    - Fluoroquinolones plus metronidazole or broad-spectrum penicillins, such as carbapenem alone or piperacillin-tazobactam alone, are appropriate choices.
  - Cathartics may rarely precipitate colonic perforation and therefore should be avoided.

SURGERY

- Approximately 20% of patients with ischemic colitis will require surgery because of peritonitis or clinical deterioration despite conservative management.[12]
- During laparotomy, all affected bowel should be resected, avoiding primary anastomosis, and a colostomy is formed.
- Despite resection, the mortality rates exceed 50% in those with infarcted bowel.[13]

PROGNOSIS

- The clinical course may progress from hyperactive (blood-mixed loose stool) to paralytic (ileus) phase and may end up in shock phase.
- The mortality rate is significantly different between nongangrenous colonic ischemia (approximately 6%) and gangrenous ischemia (as high as 50% to 75% with surgical resection and is almost always fatal if treated conservatively).[13,14]
- Severe ischemia may lead to segmental ulcerating colitis or strictures.
- Recurrence is unlikely if predisposing conditions can be prevented or treated, such as addressing the offending medications, atherosclerosis, hypercoagulable states, thromboembolism, severe exertion, and so on.

FOLLOW-UP

- Severe colitis should be monitored regularly with follow-up colonoscopies to document healing or the development of persistent colitis or stricture.
- Recurrent episodes of bacteremia or sepsis in patients with unhealed areas of segmental colitis are indications for segmental colon resection.

PATIENT EDUCATION

Exercise and intestinal ischemia—Extreme exercise (as occurs in marathon running or triathlon competition) has been associated with intestinal ischemia; therefore, adequate hydration is important.

PATIENT RESOURCES

- Mayo Clinic. *Ischemic Colitis*—**http://www.mayoclinic.com/health/ischemic-colitis/DS00794.**
- MedlinePlus. *Mesenteric artery ischemia*—**http://www.nlm.nih.gov/medlineplus/ency/article/001156.htm.**

PROVIDER RESOURCES

- American Gastroenterological Association (AGA). *Guidelines*—**http://www.gastro.org/practice/medical-position-statements.**

REFERENCES

1. Stoney RJ, Cunningham CG. Chronic visceral ischemia. In: Yao J, Pearce W, eds. *Long-term Results in Vascular Surgery.* Norwalk, CT: Appleton & Lange; 1993:305–316.
2. Higgins PD, Davis KJ, Laine L. Systematic review: the epidemiology of ischaemic colitis. *Aliment Pharmacol Ther.* 2004;19(7):729.
3. Gandhi SK, Hanson MM, Vernava AM, et al. Ischemic colitis. *Dis Colon Rectum.* 1996;39:88–100.
4. Longstreth GF, Yao JF. Diseases and drugs that increase risk of acute large bowel ischemia. *Clin Gastroenterol Hepatol.* 2010;8(1):49.
5. Green BT, Tendler DA. Ischemic colitis: a clinical review. *South Med J.* 2005;98(2):217-222.
6. Cappell MS. Intestinal (mesenteric) vasculopathy II. *Gastroenterol Clin North Am.* 1998;27:827–858.
7. Wolf EL, Sprayregen S, Bakal CW. Radiology in intestinal ischemia: plain film, contrast, and other imaging studies. *Surg Clin North Am.* 1992;72:107–124.
8. Balthazar EJ, Yen BC, Gordon RB. Ischemic colitis: CT evaluation of 54 cases. *Radiology.* 1999;211(2):381.
9. Price AB. Ischemic colitis. *Curr Top Pathol.* 1990;81:229–246.
10. Hourmand-Ollivier I, Bouin M, Saloux E, et al. Cardiac sources of embolism should be routinely screened in ischemic colitis. *Am J Gastroenterol.* 2003;98(7):1573-1577.
11. Saegesser F, Loosli H, Robinson JW, et al. Ischemic diseases of the large intestine. *Int Surg.* 1981;66:103–117.
12. Boley SJ. Colonic ischemia: twenty-five years later. *Am J Gastroenterol.* 1990;85:931–934.
13. Fitzgerald SF, Kaminski DL. Ischemic colitis. *Semin Colon Rectal Surg.* 1993;4:222–228.
14. Longo WE, Ballantyne GH, Gusberg RJ. Ischemic colitis: patterns and prognosis. *Dis Colon Rectum.* 1992;35(8):726.

74 LIVER DISEASE

Mindy A. Smith, MD, MS
Angie Mathai, MD

PATIENT STORY

A 64-year-old woman presents with complaints of itchy skin and fatigue. She is noted on physical examination to have scleral icterus and jaundice (**Figure 74-1**). Laboratory testing revealed elevated liver enzymes, particularly the serum alkaline phosphatase and γ-glutamyltranspeptidase, and positive antinuclear and antimitochondrial antibodies. A liver biopsy confirmed primary biliary cirrhosis. Two months later, she vomited up some blood and on endoscopy was found to have esophageal varices from her portal hypertension (**Figure 74-2**).

INTRODUCTION

Liver disease can be caused by any number of metabolic, toxic, microbial, circulatory, or neoplastic insults, resulting in direct liver injury or from obstruction of bile flow or both. Liver injury falls anywhere on the spectrum from transient abnormalities in biomarkers to life-threatening multiorgan failure.

SYNONYMS

The following terms refer to various types of liver diseases: hepatic failure, hepatic dysfunction, alcoholic hepatitis, viral hepatitis, cirrhosis, hepatocellular disease, cholestatic disease, and liver fibrosis.

EPIDEMIOLOGY

Common causes of liver disease include the following:

- Nonalcoholic fatty liver disease (NAFLD)—Present in 10% to 30% of adults in the general population; now the most common cause of chronic liver disease in Western countries.[1] NAFLD is believed responsible for 90% of cases of elevated liver enzymes without an identifiable cause (eg, viral hepatitis, alcohol, genetic, medications).[2]

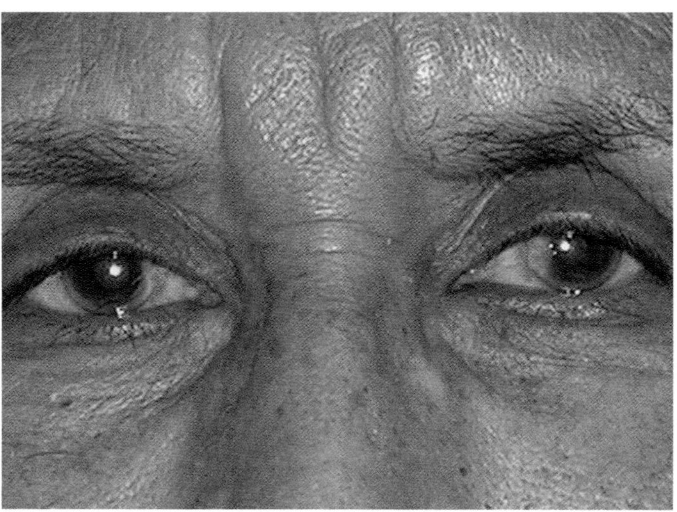

FIGURE 74-1 Scleral icterus in a 64-year-old Hispanic woman with primary biliary cirrhosis. (*Reproduced with permission from Javid Ghandehari, MD.*)

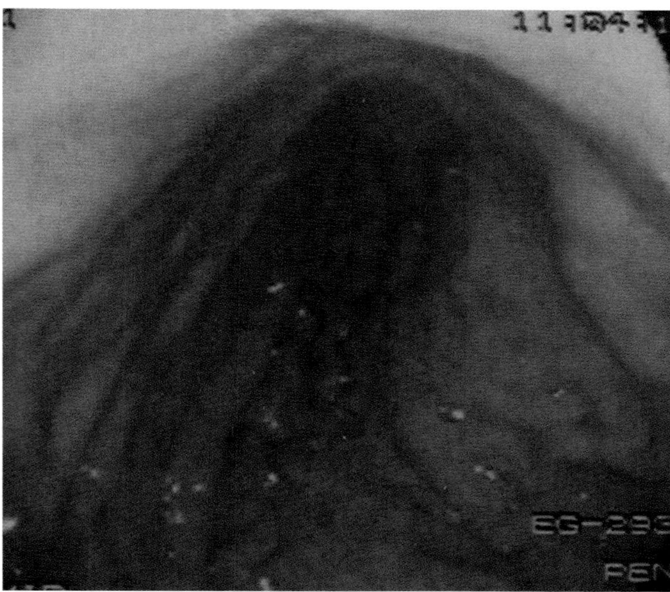

FIGURE 74-2 Esophageal varices in the patient in **Figure 61-1** secondary to her cirrhosis and portal hypertension. (*Reproduced with permission from Javid Ghandehari, MD.*)

- Alcohol, excessive use—Approximately 5% of the population are at risk; this includes women who drink more than 2 drinks per day and men who drink more than 3 drinks per day.[3]
- Drug-induced liver disease[4]:
  - Drugs causing hepatitis include phenytoin, captopril, enalapril, isoniazid, amitriptyline, and ibuprofen.
  - Drugs causing cholestasis include oral contraceptives, erythromycin, and nitrofurantoin.
  - Drugs causing both of the above include azathioprine, carbamazepine, statins, nifedipine, verapamil, amoxicillin/clavulanic acid, and trimethoprim-sulfamethoxazole.
- Infectious disease—Viral hepatitis, infectious mononucleosis, Cytomegalovirus, and coxsackievirus are most common. Viral hepatitis infections include the following:
  - Hepatitis A—Around 29% to 33% of patients have ever been infected with hepatitis A; there are no chronic infections.[5] Incidence rates in recent years have declined with approximately 1987 cases reported and 9000 estimated in 2009.[6]
  - Hepatitis B—In the United States, 5% to 10% of volunteer blood donors have evidence of prior infection, with 1% to 10% of those infected progressing to chronic hepatitis B virus (HBV) infection.[5] Up to 1.4 million people have chronic hepatitis B.[6]
  - Hepatitis C—In the United States, 1.8% of the general population have had hepatitis C, with 50% to 70% developing chronic hepatitis and 80% to 90% chronic infection.[5] Nearly 3.9 million have chronic hepatitis C.[6]
  - Hepatitis D—Transmitted through contact with infectious blood and can occur as a coinfection or as a superinfection in persons with HBV infection.[6]
  - Hepatitis E—Outbreaks are usually associated with contaminated water supply in countries with poor sanitation.[6]

Less common disorders include the following:

- Genetic inheritance—Wilson disease (defective copper transport with copper toxicity; autosomal recessive with 1 per 40,000 affected), hemochromatosis (disorder of iron storage; autosomal recessive—among individuals of northern European heritage, 1 in 10 individuals is a heterozygous carrier and 0.3%-0.5% have the disease), α_1-antitrypsin deficiency (autosomal recessive with 1%-2% of patients with chronic obstructive pulmonary disease affected).
- Autoimmune liver disease—Eleven percent to 23% of patients with chronic liver disease and accounts for approximately 6% of liver transplantations in the United States.[7]
- Primary biliary cirrhosis (approximately 5 per 100,000 persons worldwide)—A disease of unknown etiology characterized by inflammatory destruction of the small bile ducts and gradual liver cirrhosis (see **Figures 74-1** and **74-2**).

ETIOLOGY AND PATHOPHYSIOLOGY

To understand liver disease, the anatomy and key functions are briefly described here.

- The hepatic artery (20%) and the portal vein (80%) provide the vascular supply of the liver.[3] The liver is organized functionally into acini, which are divided into 3 zones[3]:
  - Zone 1—The portal areas where blood enters from both sources.
  - Zone 2—The hepatocytes and sinusoids where blood flows.
  - Zone 3—The terminal hepatic veins.
- Hepatocytes, the predominant cells in the liver, perform several vital functions, including the synthesis of essential serum proteins (eg, albumin, coagulation factors); production of bile and its carriers (eg, bile acids, cholesterol); regulation of nutrients (eg, glucose, lipids, amino acids); and metabolism and conjugation of lipophilic compounds (eg, bilirubin, various drugs) for excretion into the bile or urine.[3]
- There are 2 basic patterns of liver disease and 1 mixed pattern[3]:
  - Hepatocellular—Features of this type are direct liver injury, inflammation, and necrosis. Examples are alcoholic and viral hepatitis.
  - Cholestatic (obstructive)—It involves inhibition of bile flow. Examples are gallstone disease, malignancy, primary biliary cirrhosis, and some drug-induced disease.
  - Mixed pattern—Evidence of direct damage and obstruction. Examples are cholestatic form of viral hepatitis and some drug-induced diseases.
- Cirrhosis occurs following irreversible hepatic injury with hepatocyte necrosis resulting in fibrosis and distortion of the vascular bed. This, in turn, can cause portal hypertension.
- The spectrum of NAFLD ranges from hepatic steatosis (fat deposition in liver cells) to nonalcoholic steatohepatitis (NASH) and cirrhosis.[2] In NAFLD, steatosis occurs when free fatty acids, released in the setting of insulin resistance, are taken up by the liver; the same process can occur in alcoholism. The presence of these fatty acids leads to inflammation from other insults to the liver including oxidative stress, upregulation of inflammatory mediators, and dysregulated apoptosis, producing NASH, fibrosis, and sometimes cirrhosis (occurs in approximately 20% of patients with NASH).[2]

RISK FACTORS

- Risk factors for liver disease include the following[3]:
  - Alcohol and intravenous drug use
  - Drugs (eg, oral contraceptives)
  - Personal and sexual habits
  - Travel to underdeveloped countries
  - Exposure to contaminant in food (eg, shellfish) or individuals with liver disease (includes needle stick injuries)
  - Family history
  - Blood transfusion prior to 1992
- Obesity and the metabolic syndrome are risk factors for NAFLD and the more advanced form of NASH.

DIAGNOSIS

The goals of diagnosis are to determine the etiology and severity of the liver disease, and, where appropriate, the stage of the disease, including whether it is acute or chronic, early or late in the course of the disease, and whether there is cirrhosis present and to what degree.

CLINICAL FEATURES

- Patients with NAFLD are usually asymptomatic.
- Constitutional symptoms in patients with liver disease include fatigue (most common; especially following activity), weakness, anorexia, and nausea.
- Skin alterations[3]:
  - Jaundice (hallmark of obstructive pattern)—Best seen in the sclera or below the tongue; the latter is particularly useful in dark-skinned individuals. Not detected until serum bilirubin levels reach 2.5 mg/dL (43 μmol/L). Early, jaundice may manifest as dark (tea-colored) urine and later with light-colored stools. Jaundice without dark urine is usually from indirect hyperbilirubinemia, as seen in patients with hemolytic anemia or Gilbert syndrome.
  - Palmar erythema—Can be seen in both acute and chronic disease but also seen in normal individuals and during pregnancy (**Figure 74-3**).
  - Spider angiomas (superficial, tortuous arterioles that flow outward from the center)—Also seen in both acute and chronic disease, in normal individuals, and during pregnancy (**Figure 74-4**).
  - Excoriations—Pruritus is prominent in acute obstructive disease and chronic cholestatic diseases such as primary biliary cirrhosis.
  - Palpable purpura—Seen with hepatitis C and chronic HBV.

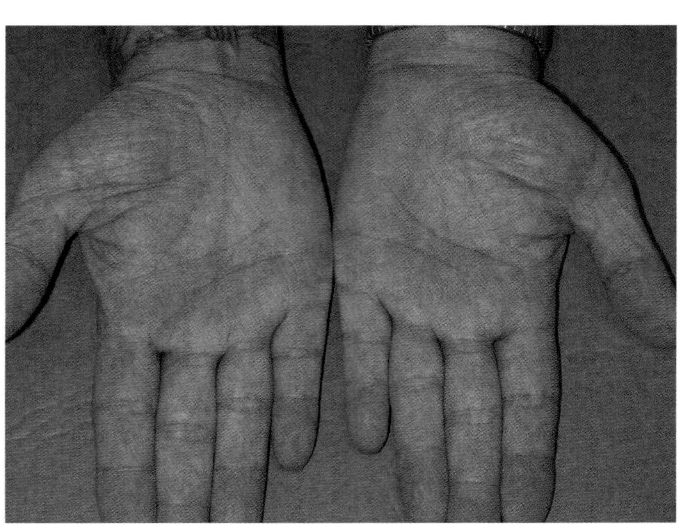

FIGURE 74-3 Palmar erythema in a man with cirrhosis secondary to alcoholism. (*Reproduced with permission from Richard P. Usatine, MD.*)

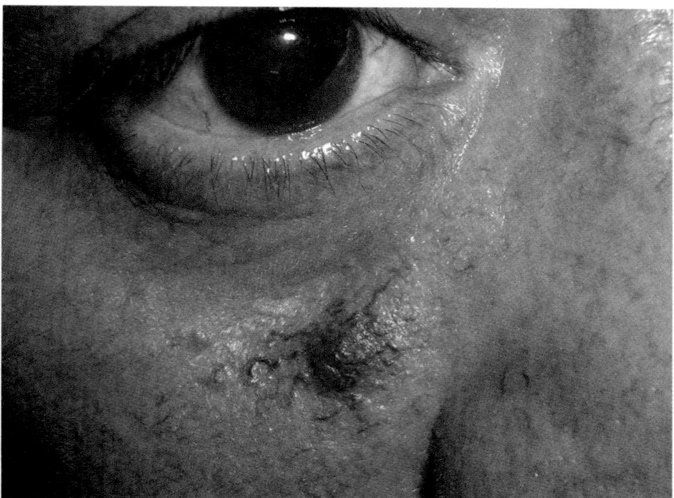

FIGURE 74-4 Spider angioma on the face of a woman with cirrhosis secondary to chronic hepatitis C. (*Reproduced with permission from Richard P. Usatine, MD.*)

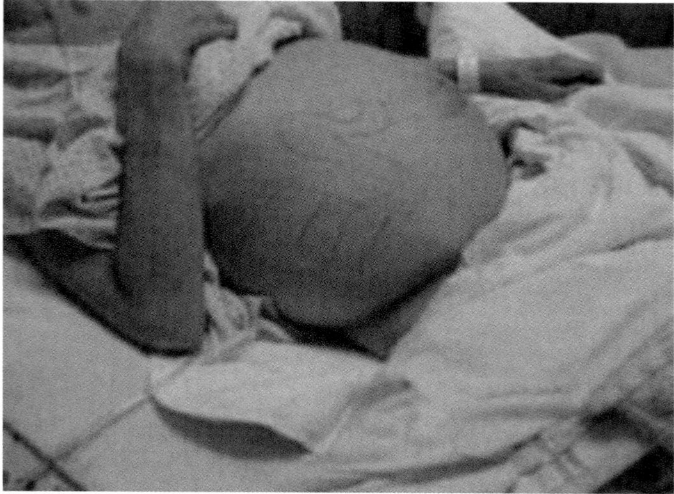

FIGURE 74-6 Patient with ascites and jaundice; lines drawn demonstrate the position of the fluid dullness to percussion (*solid stripes*), intestines (*tubular structure*), and the fluid intestine interface (*dotted line*). (*Reproduced with permission from Charlie Goldberg, MD. Copyright © 2005 The Regents of the University of California.*)

- Abdominal distention/bloating—Secondary to ascites (accumulation of excess fluid within the peritoneal cavity) (**Figure 74-5**).
    - Ascites may be detected on examination by shifting dullness on percussion (ascitic fluid will flow to the most dependent portions of the abdomen and the air-filled intestines will float on top of this fluid. The fluid–air interface is detected with the patient supine and then turned onto the side where the "line" shifts upward) (**Figures 74-6** and **74-7**).
- Pain in the right upper quadrant (caused by stretching or irritation of the Glisson capsule surrounding the liver) with tenderness on examination in the liver area. Pain and fever in a patient with ascites should suggest the diagnosis of spontaneous bacterial peritonitis (SBP).
- Hepatomegaly and splenomegaly (congestive splenomegaly from portal hypertension)—Seen in patients with cirrhosis, venoocclusive disease, malignancy, and alcoholic hepatitis.[3]
- Features of hyperestrogenemia in men including gynecomastia (**Figure 74-8**) and testicular atrophy.
- Physical signs of specific liver disease include the following:
    - Kayser-Fleischer rings—Brown copper pigment deposits around the periphery of the cornea seen in Wilson disease (**Figure 74-9**).
    - Excessive skin pigmentation (slate gray hue/bronzing), diabetes mellitus, polyarticular arthropathy, congestive heart failure, and hypogonadism can be seen in hemochromatosis.
    - Cachexia, wasting, and firm hepatomegaly can be seen in primary hepatocellular carcinoma or metastatic liver disease.
- Features of patients with advanced disease include muscle wasting, ascites, edema, dilated abdominal veins (eg, caput medusa—collateral veins seen radiating from the umbilicus), bruising, hepatic fetor (ie, sweet, ammonia odor), asterixis (ie, flapping of the hands when extended), and mental confusion, stupor, or coma.[3]
- Hepatic failure, defined as the occurrence of signs and symptoms of hepatic encephalopathy, may begin with sleep disturbance, personality

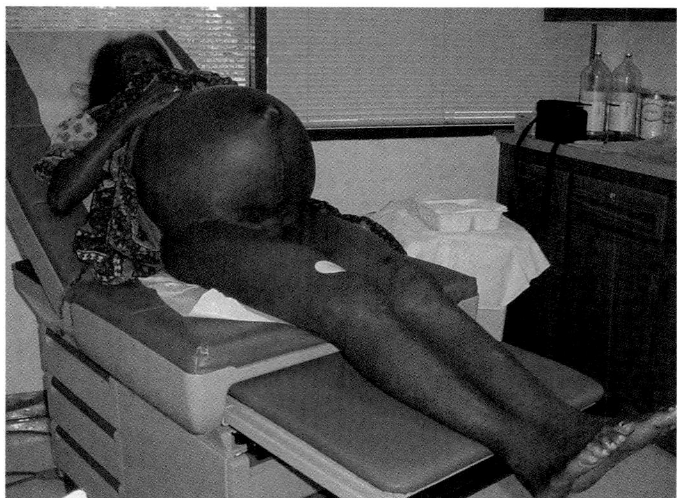

FIGURE 74-5 Tense ascites in a woman with cirrhosis from her alcoholism. An umbilical hernia is also seen from the increased intraabdominal pressure. (*Reproduced with permission from Richard P. Usatine, MD.*)

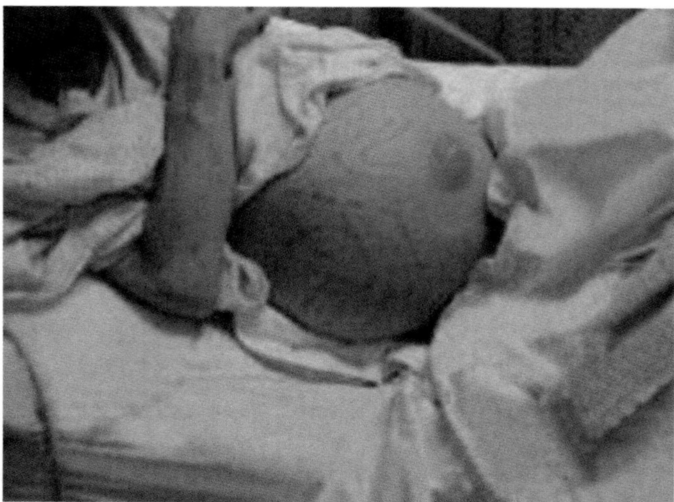

FIGURE 74-7 When patient is turned to the right side, the fluid intestine interface is shifted upward as shown; this is the sign called *shifting dullness*. (*Reproduced with permission from Charlie Goldberg, MD. Copyright © 2005 The Regents of the University of California.*)

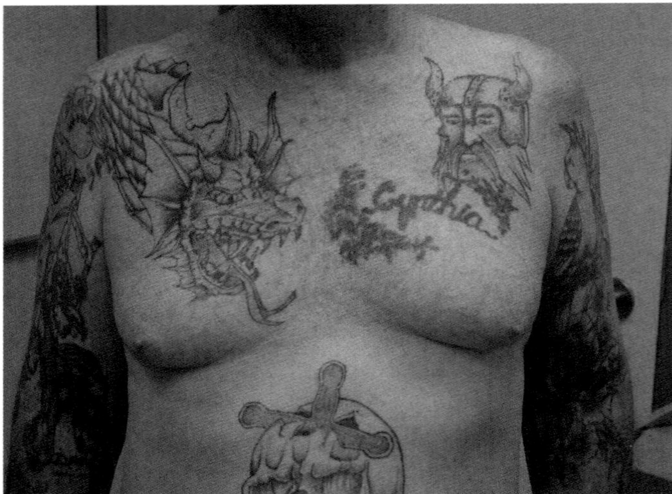

FIGURE 74-8 Gynecomastia in a man with cirrhosis secondary to alcoholism. *(Reproduced with permission from Richard P. Usatine, MD.)*

changes, irritability, and mental slowness.[3] Mental confusion, disorientation, or coma may occur later along with physical signs as above.

LABORATORY TESTING

- Initial evaluation with bilirubin, albumin, alanine aminotransferase (ALT), aspartate aminotransferase (AST), γ-glutamyl transpeptidase (GGT), and alkaline phosphatase (AlkP).[3] **Table 74-1** provides the diagnostic interpretation of the patterns of liver biochemical markers.
  - In acute disease (duration <6 months) with a hepatocellular pattern (see **Table 74-1**) consider infections, ingestions, or Wilson disease.
  - In acute disease with a cholestatic pattern (see **Table 74-1**) consider obstructing gallstones or masses, primary biliary cirrhosis, and cholangitis.
  - In chronic disease (duration >6 months) with hepatocellular pattern (see **Table 74-1**) or mixed pattern (↑ ALT, ↑ AlkP), consider hemochromatosis, Wilson disease, and α_1-antitrypsin deficiency. Because many of the acute processes can also cause a chronic picture, consider workup for hepatitis B or C, autoimmune hepatitis, alcoholic disease, chronic drug ingestion, or structural abnormalities.
  - In chronic disease with cholestatic pattern, consider primary sclerosing cholangitis (see **Table 74-1**).
  - In patients with NAFLD, elevations in ALT and AST are usually no more than 4 times the upper limit of normal; ALT usually predominates.[2]
  - Bilirubin, albumin, and prothrombin time along with the presence or absence of ascites and hepatic encephalopathy are part of the Child-Pugh classification of cirrhosis that has been used to estimate the likelihood of survival and complications of cirrhosis; it is also used to determine candidacy for liver transplantation.[8] Another scoring system, the model for end-stage liver disease (MELD), which uses the international normalized ratio, serum bilirubin, and serum creatinine, is a reliable measure of mortality risk in patients with end-stage liver disease and used to prioritize liver transplantations.[9] In 2007, the MESO index (MELD to Serum Sodium ratio) was published; it adjusts the MELD score by including serum sodium and may be more useful in determining prognosis in patients with decompensated cirrhosis than the MELD alone.[10]
- Suspected SBP can be confirmed following paracentesis of the ascitic fluid showing a polymorphonuclear leukocyte count greater than or equal to 250 cells/mm.[5]
- It may be possible to predict significant fibrosis and inflammation among patients with chronic hepatitis B using noninvasive markers, thereby limiting the number of biopsies needed. Serum microRNA profiles may serve as noninvasive biomarkers for HBV infection.[11] The aspartate aminotransferase-to-platelet ratio index (APRI) is a new marker that can identify hepatitis C-related fibrosis with a moderate degree of accuracy. This information may limit biopsies in patients with chronic hepatitis C.[12]
- In 1 study, significant liver fibrosis was predicted in patients who were hepatitis B e antigen (HBeAg)-negative using the HBV DNA levels, AlkP, albumin, and platelet counts with an area under receiver operating characteristic (ROC) curve of 0.91 for the training group and 0.85 for the validation group.[13]
- The best model for predicting significant inflammation included the variables age, HBV DNA levels, AST, and albumin with an area under the curve of 0.93 in the training and 0.82 in the validation group. In HBeAg-positive patients, no factor could accurately predict stages of liver fibrosis, but the best factor for predicting significant inflammation was AST with an area under the curve of 0.87.

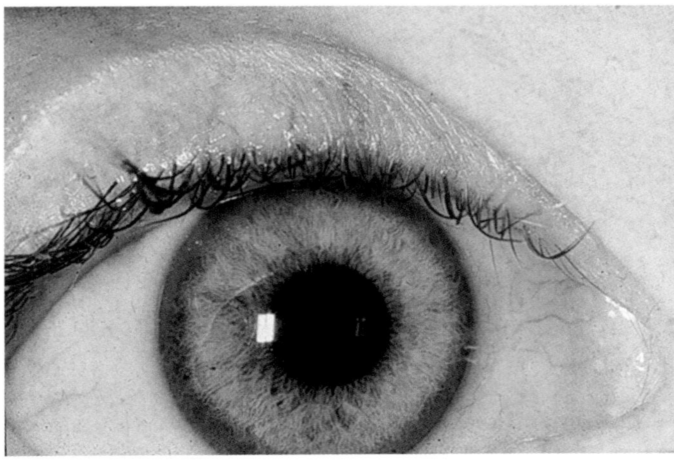

FIGURE 74-9 Kayser-Fleischer ring around the cornea in a patient with Wilson disease. *(Reproduced with permission from Marc Solioz, University of Berne.)*

IMAGING

Ultrasound is best for detection of NAFLD. It is most accurate when there is greater than 30% steatosis; use of liver elasticity can help distinguish severe from mild fibrosis.[2] MRI reliably detects lesser degrees of steatosis (down to 3%). NAFLD can usually be diagnosed by history, serologies, and abdominal imaging, although biopsy may be needed to judge severity.

BIOPSY

Liver biopsy is the gold standard for diagnosing those with acute disease where the etiology is unclear or for those with chronic disease (eg, chronic hepatitis B, hepatitis C) to assist in staging the disease and for prognosis.

TABLE 74-1 Patterns of Liver Disease with Usual Laboratory Features, Differential Diagnosis, and Key Components of Diagnostic Workup

Liver Pattern	AST	ALT	AlkP	GGT	TB	Differential Dx	Diagnostic Workup
Acute—Hepatocellular	↑	↑↑	Usually normal	↑	Usually normal	Hepatitis A/B/C	Hepatitis panel
						Autoimmune hepatitis	Antinuclear Ab Smooth muscle Ab
						Mononucleosis	Monospot
						Wilson disease	Ceruloplasmin screen Urinary copper
						Tylenol overdose	Tylenol level
						Alcoholic hepatitis	Ammonia level History of alcohol use
						Drug ingestion	Toxicology screen History of drug use
Acute—Cholestatic	Often normal	↑	↑↑	↑↑	↑	Gall stones	Ultrasound
						Mass, hepatic, or biliary	MRI MRCP
						Fatty infiltration	
						Biliary duct dilatation	
						Primary biliary cirrhosis	Antimitochondrial Ab
						Primary sclerosing cholangitis	ERCP with biopsies
Chronic—Hepatocellular	↑	↑↑	Usually normal	Usually normal	Usually normal	Hepatitis B/C	Hepatitis panel
						Hemochromatosis	Iron saturation and ferritin
						Wilson disease	Ceruloplasmin screen Urinary copper
						α_1-Antitrypsin deficiency	α_1-Antitrypsin serum level
Chronic—Cholestatic	Usually normal	↑	↑↑	↑↑	↑	Primary sclerosing cholangitis	Antimitochondrial Ab pANCA Ultrasound MRCP ERCP

Abbreviations: Ab, antibody; AlkP, alkaline phosphatase; ALT, alanine aminotransferase; AST, aspartate aminotransferase; dx, diagnosis; ERCP, endoscopic retrograde cholangiopancreatography; GGT, γ-glutamyl transferase; MRCP, magnetic resonance cholangiopancreatography; pANCA, peripheral antinuclear cytoplasmic antibody; TB, total bilirubin.

MANAGEMENT

Management decisions are based on the etiology, acuity, and severity of the disease.

- NAFLD/NASH—Diet and exercise have been shown to decrease liver enzymes, although it is not known if there is histologic improvement as well.[2] Other treatments for obesity, such as medication or bariatric surgery, may also be useful. Because NAFLD increases risk of cardiovascular disease,[1] treatment of other risk factors, such as hypertension and hyperlipidemia, should be undertaken. It is not known whether use of insulin sensitizers, such as metformin, and thiazolidinediones or statins specifically for NAFLD are beneficial.
- Alcoholic cirrhosis—Discontinue alcohol and provide supportive therapy. Alcoholic hepatitis is treated with either glucocorticoids or pentoxifylline based on Maddrey discriminant function (MDF).[14]
- Drug-induced disease—Withdrawal of agent. Routine screening of asymptomatic patients on statins is no longer recommended. Withdrawal of statins usually results in resolution of elevated transaminases within 2 months. The same statin could be continued at a lower dose or another statin could be started.[15]
- Viral hepatitis—Hepatitis A and acute hepatitis B are treated supportively; virtually all patients recover without specific treatment. Chronic hepatitis B may be treated with antiviral therapy (interferon) and the nucleoside analog lamivudine or the acyclic nucleotide analog adefovir.[5,16] Hepatitis C is currently treated with pegylated interferon and ribavirin.[5] All persons with chronic hepatitis B who are not immune to hepatitis A should receive 2 doses of hepatitis A vaccine 6 to 18 months apart.[15] Patients with hepatitis C should be vaccinated against hepatitis A and hepatitis B if they are seronegative for these other forms of hepatitis. SOR B Newborns of HBV-infected mothers should receive hepatitis B immunoglobulin and hepatitis B vaccine at delivery and complete the recommended vaccination series.[15] SOR A
- Wilson disease is treated with zinc acetate (50 mg 3 times daily) with or without trientine, a chelating agent (500 mg twice daily).[17]
- Hemochromatosis is treated with weekly or twice weekly phlebotomy.
- Primary biliary cirrhosis is managed with ursodiol (13 to 15 mg/kg per day) single dose in the presence of abnormal liver function tests regardless of histologic stage and eventual liver transplantation.[18,19] SOR A In a metaanalysis of 7 trials, ursodeoxycholic acid treatment resulted in a significant reduction of the incidence of liver transplantation (odds ratio [OR] 0.65, $p = 0.01$) and a marginally significant reduction of the rate of death or liver transplantation.[20] Bile acid sequestrants can be used for pruritis.[20]
- Autoimmune hepatitis is treated with glucocorticoid therapy with or without azathioprine. Oral budesonide, in combination with azathioprine, induces and maintains remission in patients with noncirrhotic autoimmune hepatitis, with a low rate of steroid-specific side effects.[21]

Management of the complications of cirrhosis includes the following:

- Control ascites with salt restriction (2 g per day of NaCl), fluid restriction if hyponatremic (1000 mL per day), and gentle diuresis to avoid electrolyte disturbance (spironolactone 100-400 mg per day) with or without furosemide (40-160 mg per day).[18] SOR A
- SBP is treated with empiric antibiotic therapy (eg, intravenous cefotaxime 2 g every 8 hours).[22] SOR A
- Portal hypertension may be managed with shunting.

PREVENTION AND SCREENING

- Maintaining normal weight and treating obstructive sleep apnea and diabetes may help prevent NAFLD.
- Screen for alcohol abuse using structured questionnaires (eg, CAGE [cutting, annoyance, guilt, eye-opener], Alcohol Use Disorders Identification Test [AUDIT]). Encourage abstinence and consider naltrexone or acamprosate in combination with counseling.[23]
- Risk for hepatitis A can be minimized by avoidance of susceptible foods in high-risk countries.
- For hepatitis B, recommendations include avoidance of high-risk behavior and blood contact, vaccination of risk groups, postexposure prophylaxis with anti–hepatitis B immunoglobulin, and cleaning of wound after exposure to infectious blood.[24]
- Screen for HBV infection in pregnant women at their first prenatal visit.[25] Patients with chronic liver disease should be vaccinated with hepatitis A and hepatitis B vaccines.[26]
- Hepatitis C risk can be decreased by avoidance of intravenous drug use, tattooing, and unprotected sexual intercourse. The Centers for Disease Control and Prevention now recommends one-time HCV-screening, independent of other risk factors, for anyone born during 1945 to 1965 based on a higher prevalence in this birth cohort.
- Screen patients with mild elevations of liver enzymes (above normal but <5 times the upper limit of normal) for hepatitis B and hepatitis C.[27]

PROGNOSIS

- Thirty percent of patients with NAFLD show histologic progression of fibrosis over 5 years and approximately 3% eventually develop cirrhosis.[2] Of those with NASH, 15% to 20% may develop cirrhosis. Leading causes of death appear to be cardiovascular disease, cancer (including hepatocellular carcinoma), and liver-related disease. Recurrence of hepatocellular carcinoma is higher in patients with NASH.[2]
- Patients presenting with a high clinical suspicion of alcoholic hepatitis should have their risk for poor outcome stratified using the MDF. Continued alcohol use is associated with disease progression.[23]
- Most cases of hepatitis B are self limiting. If the hepatitis B surface antigen (HBsAg) test remains positive 6 months after the disease onset, the patient is likely to have become a hepatitis B carrier. The carrier status is confirmed by a positive HBsAg test at 12 months.[24]
- Hepatitis C becomes chronic more often than hepatitis B; this occurs in approximately 50% to 80% of patients. The average time from primary infection to liver disease to cirrhosis is 21 years. Twenty percent to 30% develop cirrhosis as early as 5 to 7.5 years after contracting the disease. Treatment is more effective for genotypes 2 and 3 than for genotypes 1 and 4.[24]
- Approximately 50% of patients with autoimmune hepatitis will die within 5 years without treatment. Steroids can induce remission with survival rates similar to the general population.[7] The majority of patients with autoimmune hepatitis achieves complete remission within 3 months but requires long-term or permanent immunosuppressive therapy; such therapy is usually well tolerated. Long-term survival in well-managed patients is excellent.[28]
- In the absence of cirrhosis and diabetes, phlebotomy prevents further tissue damage and guarantees a normal life expectancy in patients with hemochromatosis.[29]

- Primary sclerosing cholangitis is a progressive process with a probability of transplant-free survival of 18 years in asymptomatic patients and of 8.5 years in symptomatic patients.[30]

FOLLOW-UP

- Hepatitis B virus carriers with high risk for hepatocellular carcinoma (HCC) (eg, men older than 45 years of age, those with cirrhosis, and individuals with a family history of HCC) should be screened periodically with both α-fetoprotein and ultrasonography.[16] SOR Ⓒ
- Patients who have survived an episode of SBP should receive long-term prophylaxis with daily norfloxacin or trimethoprim-sulfamethoxazole.[22] SOR Ⓐ

PATIENT EDUCATION

- Patients with liver disease should be counseled about avoidance of alcohol and medications that may cause liver injury. They should avoid aspirin use (coagulation impaired) and use acetaminophen at lower doses (2 g per day).
- For those with infectious causes of liver disease, prevention of the spread of disease should be emphasized including limiting alcohol, safe-sex practices, and avoiding needle sharing. Screening for sexual contacts and household members should be offered along with vaccination for hepatitis B, if nonimmune and noninfected.[16] SOR Ⓐ

PATIENT RESOURCES

- MedlinePlus has a wealth of information for patients with many kinds of liver diseases—**http://www.nlm.nih.gov/medlineplus/.**

PROVIDER RESOURCES

- A number of disease-specific evidence-based guidelines can be found through the National Guideline Clearinghouse—**http://www.guideline.gov.**
- O'Shea RS, Dasarathy S, McCullough AJ; Practice Guideline Committee of the American Association for the Study of Liver. Alcoholic liver disease. *Hepatology*. 2010;51(1):307-328.

REFERENCES

1. Targher G, Day CP, Bonora E. Risk of cardiovascular disease in patients with nonalcoholic fatty liver disease. *N Engl J Med*. 2010; 363(14):1341-1350.
2. Lewis JR, Mohanty SR. Nonalcoholic fatty liver disease: a review and update. *Dig Dis Sci*. 2010;55(3):560-578.
3. Ghany M, Hoofnagle JH. Approach to the patient with liver disease. In: Kasper DL, Braunwald E, Fauci AS, Hauser SL, Longo DL, Jameson JL, eds. *Harrison's Principles of Internal Medicine*, 16th ed. New York, NY: McGraw-Hill; 2005:1808-1813.
4. Dientag JL, Isselbacher KJ. Toxic and drug-induced hepatitis. In: Kasper DL, Braunwald E, Fauci AS, Hauser SL, Longo DL, Jameson JL, eds. *Harrison's Principles of Internal Medicine*, 16th ed. New York, NY: McGraw-Hill; 2005:1840.
5. Dienstag JL, Isselbacher KJ. Acute viral hepatitis. In: Kasper DL, Braunwald E, Fauci AS, Hauser SL, Longo DL, Jameson JL, eds. *Harrison's Principles of Internal Medicine*, 16th ed. New York, NY: McGraw-Hill; 2005:1822-1838.
6. Centers for Disease Control and Prevention. *Viral Hepatitis Statistics and Surveillance*. http://www.cdc.gov/hepatitis/Statistics/index.htm. Accessed November 2011.
7. Wolf DC, Raghuraman UV. *Autoimmune Hepatitis*. http://emedicine.medscape.com/article/172356-overview. Accessed November 2011.
8. Kamath PS, Wiesner RH, McDiarmid SV, et al. A model to predict survival in patients with end-stage liver disease. *Hepatology*. 2001;33(2): 464-470.
9. Asrani SK, Kim WR. Model for end-stage liver disease: end of the first decade. *Clin Liver Dis*. 2011;15(4):685-698.
10. Huo TI, Wang YW, Yang YY, et al. Model for end-stage liver disease score to serum sodium ratio index as a prognostic predictor and its correlation with portal pressure in patients with liver cirrhosis. Liver Int. 2007 May;27(4):498-506.
11. Li LM, Hu ZB, Zhou ZX, Chen X. Serum microRNA profiles serve as novel biomarkers for HBV infection and diagnosis of HBV-positive hepatocarcinoma. *Cancer Res*. 2010;70(23):798-807.
12. Lin ZH, Xin YN, Dong QJ, Wang Q. Performance of the aspartate aminotransferase-to-platelet ratio index for the staging of hepatitis C-related fibrosis: an updated meta-analysis. *Hepatology*. 2011;53(3): 726-736.
13. Mohamadnejad M, Montazeri G, Fazlollahi A, et al. Noninvasive markers of liver fibrosis and inflammation in chronic hepatitis B-virus related liver disease. *Am J Gastroenterol*. 2006;101(11):2537-2545.
14. Mailliard ME, Sorrell NF. Alcoholic liver disease. In: Kasper DL, Braunwald E, Fauci AS, Hauser SL, Longo DL, Jameson JL, eds. *Harrison's Principles of Internal Medicine*, 16th ed. New York, NY: McGraw-Hill; 2005:1855-1857.
15. Gillett RC Jr, Norrell A. Considerations for safe use of statins: liver enzyme abnormalities and muscle toxicity. *Am Fam Physician*. 2011; 83(6):711-716.
16. Lok AS, McMahon BJ. Chronic hepatitis B: update 2009. *Hepatology*. 2009;50(3):661-662. http://www.guideline.gov/content.aspx?id=15475&search=chronic+hepatitis+b. Accessed December 2011.
17. Brewer GJ. Wilson disease. In: Kasper DL, Braunwald E, Fauci AS, Hauser SL, Longo DL, Jameson JL, eds. *Harrison's Principles of Internal Medicine*, 16th ed. New York, NY: McGraw-Hill; 2005:2313-2315.
18. Chung RT, Podolsky DK. Cirrhosis and its complications. In: Kasper DL, Braunwald E, Fauci AS, Hauser SL, Longo DL, Jameson JL, eds. *Harrison's Principles of Internal Medicine*, 16th ed. New York, NY: McGraw-Hill; 2005:1808-1813.
19. Lindor KD, Gershwin ME, Poupon R, et al; American Association for Study of Liver Diseases. Primary biliary cirrhosis. *Hepatology*. 2009;50(1):291-308.
20. Shi J, Wu C, Lin Y, et al. Long-term effects of mid-dose ursodeoxycholic acid in primary biliary cirrhosis: a meta-analysis of randomized controlled trials. *Am J Gastroenterol*. 2006;101(7):1529-1538.
21. Manns MP, Woynarowski M, Kreisel W, Lurie Y. Budesonide induces remission more effectively than prednisone in a controlled trial of patients with autoimmune hepatitis. *Gastroenterology*. 2010; 139(4):1198-1206.
22. Runyon BA. Management of adult patients with ascites due to cirrhosis. *Hepatology*. 2004;39(3):841-856.

23. O'Shea RS, Dasarathy S, McCullough AJ. Practice Guideline Committee of the American Association for the Study of Liver. Alcoholic liver disease. *Hepatology*. 2010;51(1):307-328.

24. Finnish Medical Society Duodecim. *Viral Hepatitis*. http://www.guidelines.gov/content.aspx?id=12806&search=viral+hepatitis+b. Accessed November 2011.

25. U.S. Preventive Services Task Force. Screening for hepatitis B virus infection in pregnancy: U.S. Preventive Services Task Force reaffirmation recommendation statement. *Ann Intern Med*. 2009;150(12):869-873.

26. Kumar M, Herrera JL. Importance of hepatitis vaccination in patients with chronic liver disease. *South Med J*. 2010;103(12):1223-1231.

27. Senadhi V. A paradigm shift in the outpatient approach to liver function tests. *South Med J*. 2011;104(7):521-525.

28. Kanzler S, Löhr H, Gerken G, et al. Long-term management and prognosis of autoimmune hepatitis (AIH): a single center experience. *Z Gastroenterol*. 2001;39(5):339-341, 344-348.

29. Barton JC, McDonnell SM, Adams PC, Brissot P. Management of hemochromatosis. Hemochromatosis Management Working Group. *Ann Intern Med*. 1998;129(11):932-939.

30. Parés A. Primary sclerosing cholangitis: diagnosis, prognosis and treatment. *Gastroenterol Hepatol*. 2011;34(1):41-52.

75 ACUTE PANCREATITIS

Gary Ferenchick, MD

PATIENT STORY

A 45-year-old woman is admitted to the hospital with a 3-hour history of severe epigastric pain. The patient started to experience mild intermittent right upper quadrant (RUQ) abdominal pain 24 hours ago, followed by an acute onset of severe epigastric pain radiating to the midback. Her examination reveals normal vital signs and reproducible tenderness with voluntary guarding in the midepigastric area. Laboratory testing reveals a serum amylase of 1250 and a serum lipase of 1800. An ultrasound reveals a dilated common bile duct and an impacted stone at the ampulla of Vater. She is treated with intravenous hydration and intravenous morphine. Subsequent endoscopic retrograde cholangiopancreatography (ERCP) is performed and confirms an impacted stone, which is subsequently removed endoscopically. The patient has rapid relief of her pain, and her serum amylase and lipase are normalized.

INTRODUCTION

Pancreatitis is an inflammatory disease of the pancreas.

EPIDEMIOLOGY

- Acute pancreatitis is responsible for 200,000 hospital admissions in the United States per year.[1]
- Of the cases, 80% are mild; 20% of cases are complicated by increased morbidity/mortality.[1]
- Of the patients with acute pancreatitis, 4% die within 92 days of admission (2% within 14 days).[2]

ETIOLOGY/PATHOPHYSIOLOGY

- Gallstones (**Figure 75-1**) and alcohol are the most important risks (~80% of cases)[1]; other causes include the following:
  - Drug reaction (~1%, including tetracycline, furosemide, sulfonamides, thiazides, estrogens).
  - Pancreatic/ampulla tumors that produce duct obstruction.
  - Hypertriglyceridemia (usually > 1000 mg/dL).
  - Hypercalcemia caused by hyperparathyroidism.
  - Post-ERCP (~5% of patients have pancreatitis within 30 days of ERCP).
  - Congenital anomalies of pancreatic biliary system
    - Pancreatic divisum (absence of fusion between dorsal and ventral ductal systems, leading to stenosis, which prevents normal drainage of pancreatic secretions, leading to increased pressure within pancreatic ducts, eg, ductal hypertension).
    - Pancreatic divisum, however, occurs in about 5% of the healthy population, and only a small minority develop pancreatitis.
  - Consider genetic causes in unexplained recurrent pancreatitis.

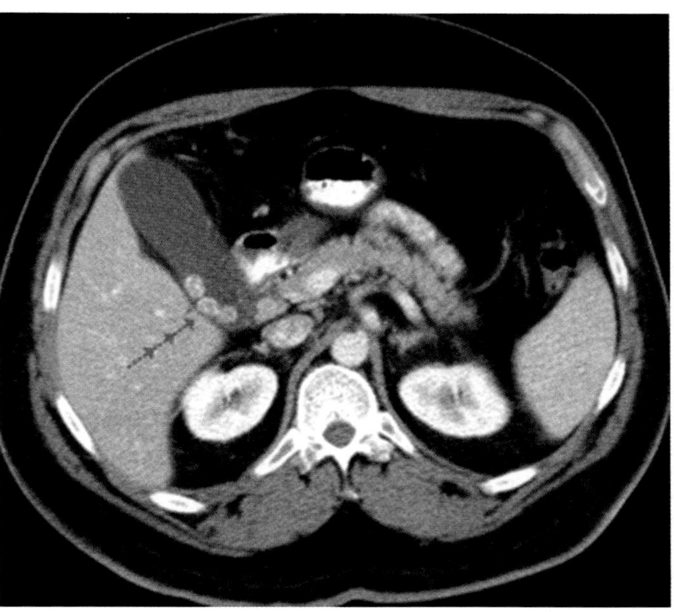

FIGURE 75-1 Three nonobstructing calcified gallstones are noted in the gall bladder (*green arrows*) in this patient's computed tomographic scan. Most gallstones are not calcified. (*Reproduced with permission from Gary Ferenchick, MD.*)

    Mutations in the *PRSS1* gene increase the function of trypsinogen, leading to premature trypsin activation. *PRSS1* mutations are autosomal dominant.
  - Idiopathic causes occur in 20% of cases.[1]
- The inappropriate activation of trypsin within the pancreatic cells and failure to eliminate active trypsin within the pancreas lead to autodigestion of pancreatic cells and inflammation.[2]
- Pancreatic enzymes are released into the bloodstream, and stimulation of cytokines and tumor necrosis factor can lead to systemic inflammatory response syndrome (SIRS).[2]
- With gallstones, obstruction leading to increased pressure within the pancreatic duct leads to activation of pancreatic enzymes.

DIAGNOSIS/SCREENING

HISTORY/SYMPTOMS

Specifically ask about the following:

- Location of pain—Pancreatitis causes epigastric or RUQ pain.
- Onset and duration of pain
  - Pain from gallstone pancreatitis is sudden in onset.
  - Pain from alcoholic pancreatitis is more gradual in onset.
  - Pancreatitis pain is usually acute in onset and constant in duration.
- Radiation of pain—pain radiates to the back.
- Nausea/vomiting—These are common with pancreatitis.

PHYSICAL EXAMINATION

specifically look for or establish the following:

- Tenderness in the epigastric area and RUQ.
- Ecchymoses in the flank (Turner sign or Grey-Turner sign as seen in **Figure 75-2**) or periumbilical area (Cullen sign as seen in **Figure 75-3**) are seen in less than 3% of patients, but their presence is associated with high mortality (~40%).

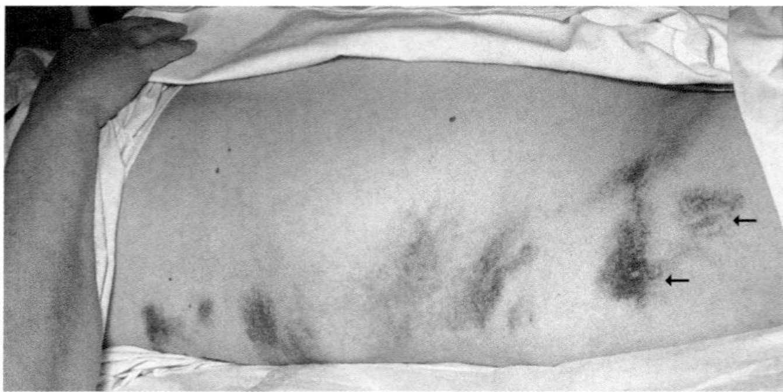

FIGURE 75-2 Turner sign seen in hemorrhagic pancreatitis. This 40-year-old woman had worsening epigastric pain of 5 days' duration. On examination, she had hypotension, a board-like abdomen, and extensive ecchymoses over her right loin. Emergency celiotomy disclosed a boggy pancreas, fat necrosis of the omentum, and reddish-brown peritoneal fluid. The ecchymotic discoloration of her loin (Turner's sign) is not specific for pancreatitis. In the absence of trauma or blood disorders, it is a manifestation of retroperitoneal or intra-abdominal hemorrhage. The image shown displays another indication of retroperitoneal hemorrhage: ecchymotic patches on the anterolateral surface of one or both thighs just below the inguinal ligament (Fox sign). The discoloration (*arrows*) presumably results from bloody fluid tracking extraperitoneally along the fascia of the psoas and iliacus muscles, becoming subcutaneous in the upper thigh. (*Reproduced with permission from Fred HL, van Dijk HA.* Images of Memorable Cases: 50 Years at the Bedside. *Houston, TX: Long Tail Press/Rice University Press; 2007.*)

LABORATORY TESTING

- Serum amylase that is more than 3 times normal supports the diagnosis.
  - Amylase values rise within several hours of symptom onset and returns to normal within 5 days.
  - Normal amylase values may be seen in about 20% of patients with acute pancreatitis on admission, possibly because of rapid urinary clearance.
  - False-positive increases in serum amylase are seen in macroamylasemia, renal insufficiency (because of decreased clearance of amylase), salivary gland diseases (ie, mumps and parotitis), and other inflammatory diseases in the abdomen, such as penetrating peptic ulcers and cholecystitis.
  - Macroamylasemia is the presence of high serum but low urine amylase.
- Serum lipase concentrations remain higher for longer than serum amylase concentrations.

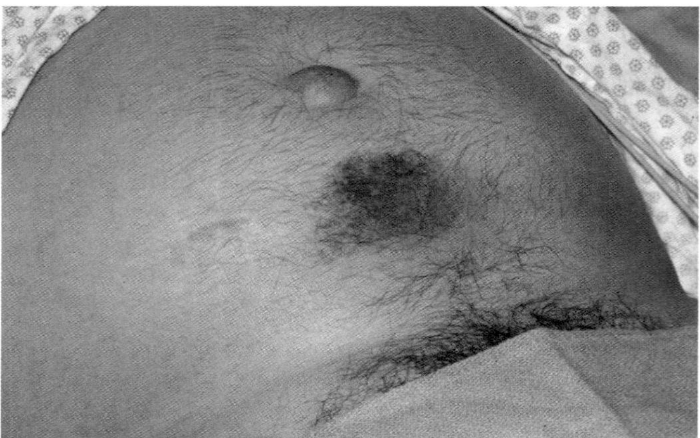

FIGURE 75-3 Cullen sign in acute pancreatitis. This 36-year-old man presented with a 4-day history of severe epigastric pain following an alcoholic binge. His serum amylase level was 821 U/L, and an abdominal computed tomographic scan showed marked inflammatory changes in his pancreas, omentum, and surrounding mesentery. In patients with acute pancreatitis, ecchymoses of the abdominal wall may appear near the midline anywhere from the umbilicus to the symphysis pubis (Cullen sign). These ecchymoses, however, are not specific for pancreatitis and, in the absence of trauma and blood disorders, merely signal retroperitoneal or intra-abdominal hemorrhage. (*Reproduced with permission from Fred HL, van Dijk HA.* Images of Memorable Cases: 50 Years at the Bedside. *Houston, TX: Long Tail Press/Rice University Press; 2007.*)

IMAGING

- Acute abdominal series might show a localized ileus.
- Abdominal computed tomographic (CT) scan is 90% sensitive and specific for the diagnosis of pancreatitis.
  - CT can also be helpful in identifying gallstones and ruling out other causes of pain.
- Ultrasound is more sensitive for identifying gallstones, gall bladder sludge, and bile duct dilation.

DIFFERENTIAL DIAGNOSIS

• Cholangitis	RUQ pain, fever, jaundice; bilirubin > 4; aspartate aminotransferase (AST) > 1000
• Acute cholecystitis and biliary colic	Pain in the epigastrium and RUQ radiates to right shoulder or shoulder blade; liver function tests (LFTs) increased
• Intestinal obstruction	Pain is colicky; obstructive pattern seen on imaging
• Dissecting aortic aneurysm	Sudden onset; pain may radiate to lower extremities
• Perforated peptic ulcer disease (PUD)	RUQ or midepigastric pain; sudden onset; free intraperitoneal air; perforation of PUD mimics cholecystitis
• Pulmonary/pleural disease	Consider if pleuritic pain is a dominant symptom
• Hepatitis	Malaise; alanine aminotransferase (ALT) > 1000
• Inferior wall myocardial infarction (MI)	Midepigastric pain; shortness of breath; abnormal electrocardiogram; MI should be in the differential diagnosis in all patients with upper abdominal pain
• Mesenteric ischemia	Abdominal pain severe, out of proportion to tenderness, with a fairly benign examination; look for postprandial abdominal pain, weight loss, and abdominal bruit
• Fitz-Hugh-Curtis syndrome	Gonococcal perihepatitis with RUQ pain, adnexal tenderness
• Pneumonia	Fever and respiratory symptoms (dyspnea, cough, sputum, chest pain) present
• Appendicitis	Pain may start in epigastrium but eventually moves to right lower quadrant (RLQ)

MANAGEMENT

ACUTE MANAGEMENT

- Determine the cause of pancreatitis.
- Studies have shown that ERCP for persistent biliary obstruction lowers the risk of pancreatitis-associated complications.[2] SOR Ⓑ
- Supportive
  - Intravenous fluids are given to maintain adequate intravascular volume to prevent hemoconcentration (250-500 cc/h if no renal or heart disease)[2]; a hematocrit value above 44 is a risk factor for pancreatic necrosis.
  - Pain medications.
  - Supplemental oxygen.
  - Antiemetics as needed.
  - Nothing by mouth—to avoid stimulation of the pancreas; begin feeding when pain is diminished and there is no small bowel ileus (usually 2-3 days).
  - Venous thromboembolism prophylaxis.
- Consider infection of pancreatic necrosis (usually occurs 1-2 weeks after onset of the symptoms) if there is fever, leukocytosis, failure to improve, or sudden deterioration (**Figure 75-4**).
  - This occurs during second week in about 50% of patients.
  - If suspected, give intravenous imipenem or meropenem for 14 days.
  - Consider prophylactic antibiotics in severe acute pancreatitis (>30% necrosis seen on CT) to prevent translocation of bacteria from gut to pancreatic bed.[2] SOR Ⓑ
  - Surgical consult is needed if there is biliary pancreatitis or infected necrosis, abscess, or pseudocyst.

LONG-TERM MANAGEMENT

- Pseudocysts develop over the course of weeks and are caused by pancreatic duct disruptions that lead to localized collection of fluid with high concentrations of pancreatic enzymes (**Figure 75-5**).

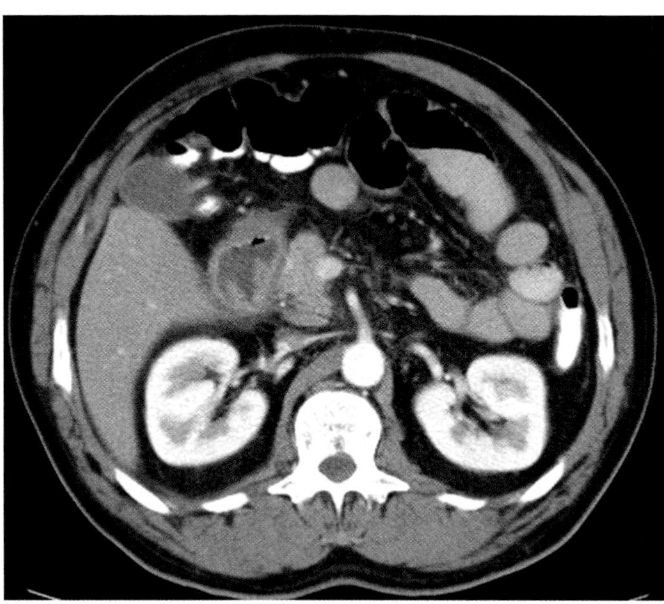

FIGURE 75-4 Acute pancreatitis with necrosis of pancreatic tissue (*red arrow*) on this computed tomographic scan. Note the edematous pancreas with evidence of air (*black*) within the necrotic mass. (*Reproduced with permission from Gary Ferenchick, MD.*)

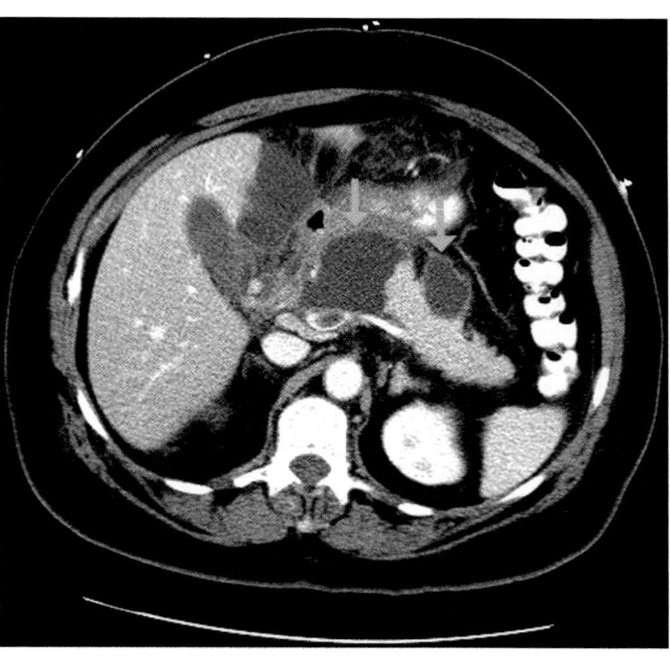

FIGURE 75-5 Two pseudocysts (*yellow arrows*) in the pancreas seen on this computed tomographic scan 4 weeks after an episode of acute gallstone pancreatitis. Disruption of the pancreatic duct from inflammation allows enzymes and fluid to collect in an area walled off by fibrous tissue and granulation tissue. Consider the diagnosis of pseudocyst when pain persists after an episode of acute pancreatitis. Most resolve with supportive care, but about 10% become infected. (*Reproduced with permission from Gary Ferenchick, MD.*)

- If there are no symptoms, treat conservatively.
- Obtain a surgical consult if the patient has pain unresponsive to medical treatment; especially if the disease is limited to the head or tail of the pancreas, the pancreatic duct is dilated.

PROGNOSIS/CLINICAL COURSE

- Severity is determined by the presence or absence or organ failure or the development of local complications.
- Of the cases, 80% are mild and self-limited.
- Severe disease associated with complications, such as multiple organ dysfunction, is seen in 20% of cases. Of the patients with severe pancreatitis, up to 30% will die; severe pancreatitis is commonly associated with the following:
  - Hypovolemia
  - Renal impairment
  - Pulmonary complications (mild → acute respiratory distress syndrome [ARDS])
- Pancreatic necrosis is the most severe local complication and is commonly associated with pancreatic infections (**Figure 75-4**).
- Markers of the risk of severe pancreatitis include
  - C-reactive protein (CRP) for predicting severity of pancreatitis—Useful marker of necrosis (> 150 mg/L) when measured 48 hours after admission
  - CT severity index[3] (**Table 75-1**)
  - Clinically with Ranson criteria, Acute Physiology and Chronic Health Evaluation II (APACHE II), or Sequential Organ Failure Assessment (SOFA) scores

TABLE 75-1 CT Severity Index (CSI)

Prognostic Indicator			Points
CT Grade			
Normal pancreas			0
Enlarged pancreas			1
Fat stranding			2
Single collection of fluid			3
Multiple collections of fluid or gas			4
Necrosis Score			
None			0
Necrosis 30%			2
Necrosis 50%			4
Necrosis > 50%			6
CSI Score			
Outcome	**0-3**	**4-6**	**7-10**
Complications (%)	8	35	92
Death (%)	3	6	17

- These measure injuries in extrapancreatic organs; the greater number of organs involved, the higher the score will be.
- The Bedside Index of Severity has recently been shown to be as accurate as the APACHE II score in predicting mortality in acute pancreatitis. Mortality is less than 1% for a score less than 2 and 20% for a score of 5.[4] One point is given for each of the following:
  - Serum urea nitrogen (BUN) greater than 25 mg/dL
  - Impaired mental status
  - SIRS
  - Age above 60
  - Presence of pleural effusion
- Obesity (body mass index [BMI] > 30) is associated with 3 times increased risk of severe clinical course.

PATIENT RESOURCES

- PubMed Health. *Acute pancreatitis*—**http://www.ncbi.nlm.nih.gov/pubmedhealth/PMH0001332/.**
- National Digestive Diseases Information Clearinghouse. *Pancreatitis*—**http://digestive.niddk.nih.gov/ddiseases/pubs/pancreatitis/index.aspx.**
- American Gastroenterological Association. *Understanding Pancreatitis*—**http://www.gastro.org/patient-center/digestive-conditions/pancreatitis.**

PROVIDER RESOURCES

- UK Working Party on Acute Pancreatitis. UK guidelines for the management of acute pancreatitis. *Gut*. 2005;54(suppl 3):iii1-iii9. doi:10.1136/gut.2004.057026. **http://www.ncbi.nlm.nih.gov/pmc/articles/PMC1867800/pdf/v054p0iii1.pdf.**

REFERENCES

1. Frossard JL, Steer ML, Pastor CM. Acute pancreatitis. *Lancet*. 2008;371(9607):143-152.
2. Tonsi AF, Bacchion M, Crippa S, Maleo G, Bassi C. Acute pancreatitis at the beginning of the 21st century. The state of the art. *World J Gastroenterol*. 2009;15:2945-2959.
3. Whitcomb DC. Clinical practice. Acute pancreatitis. *N Engl J Med*. 2006;354(20):2142-2150.
4. Wu BU, Johannes RS, Sun S, Tabak Y, Conwell DL, Banks PA. The early prediction of mortality in acute pancreatitis: a large population-based study. *Gut*. 2008;57(12):1698-1703.

76 PEPTIC ULCER DISEASE

Hend Azhary, MD
Mindy A. Smith, MD, MS

PATIENT STORY

A 41-year-old man presents with a 4-month history of epigastric pain. The pain is dull, achy, and intermittent; there is no radiation of the pain; and it has not changed in character since it began. Coffee intake seems to exacerbate the symptoms, whereas eating or drinking milk helps. Infrequently, he is awakened at night from the pain. He reports no weight loss, vomiting, melena, or hematochezia. On examination, there is mild epigastric tenderness with no rebound or guarding. The reminder of the examination is unremarkable. A stool antigen test is positive for *Helicobacter pylori*, and the patient is treated for peptic ulcer disease with eradication therapy.

INTRODUCTION

Peptic ulcer disease (PUD) is a disease of the gastrointestinal (GI) tract characterized by a break in the mucosal lining of the stomach or duodenum secondary to pepsin and gastric acid secretion; this damage is greater than 5 mm in size and with a depth reaching the submucosal layer.[1]

EPIDEMIOLOGY

- PUD is a common disorder affecting approximately 4.5 million people annually in the United States. It encompasses both gastric and duodenal ulcers (**Figures 76-1** and **76-2**).[2]
- One-year point prevalence is 1.8%, and the lifetime prevalence is 10% in the United States.[2]
- Prevalence is similar in both sexes, with increased incidence with age.[1] Duodenal ulcers most commonly occur in patients between the ages of 30 and 55 years, whereas gastric ulcers are more common in patients between the ages of 55 and 70 years.[2]
- PUD incidence in *H. pylori*-infected individuals is approximately 1% per year (6- to 10-fold higher than uninfected subjects).[1]
- Physician office visit and hospitalization for PUD have decreased in the last few decades.[1]
- The current U.S. annual direct and indirect health care costs of PUD are estimated at approximately $10 billion. However, the incidence of peptic ulcers keeps declining, possibly as a result of the increasing use of proton pump inhibitors and eradication of *H. pylori* infection.[3]

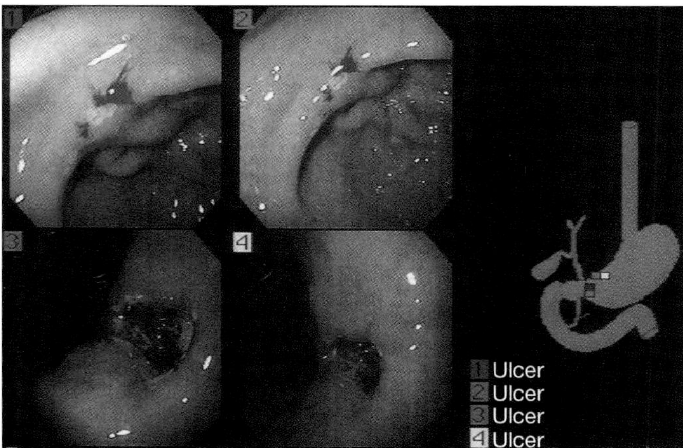

FIGURE 76-1 Endoscopic pictures of a gastric ulcer. Plates 1 and 2 show erosions. Note that the bleeding is from biopsy. Plates 3 and 4 show a large crater with evidence of recent bleeding. Both are consistent with severe ulcer disease. (*Reproduced with permission from Michael Harper, MD.*)

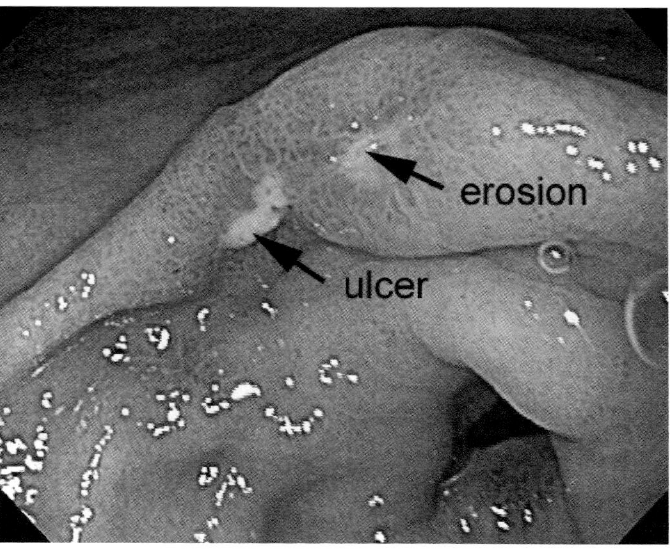

FIGURE 76-2 Endoscopic view of a pyloric ulcer and an erosion of the mucosa. The ulcer and erosion are benign peptic ulcer disease and not malignant. (*Reproduced with permission from Marvin Derezin, MD.*)

ETIOLOGY AND PATHOPHYSIOLOGY

- Causes of PUD include the following:
  - NSAIDs, chronic *H. pylori* infection, and acid hypersecretory states such as Zollinger-Ellison syndrome.[2]
  - Uncommon causes include *Cytomegalovirus* (especially in transplantation recipients), systemic mastocytosis, Crohn disease, lymphoma, and medications (eg, alendronate).[2]
  - Up to 10% of ulcers are idiopathic.[2]
- Infection with *H. pylori*, a short, spiral-shaped, microaerophilic gram-negative bacillus, is the leading cause of PUD. It is associated with up to 70% to 80% of duodenal ulcers.[2]
- *H. pylori* colonize the deep layers of the gel that coats the mucosa and disrupt its protective properties causing release of certain enzymes and toxins. These make the underlying tissues more vulnerable to damage by digestive juices and thus cause injury to the stomach (**Figures 76-1** to **76-3**) and duodenum cells.[1]
- NSAIDs are the second most common cause of PUD and account for many *H. pylori*-negative cases.
- NSAIDs and aspirin inhibit mucosal cyclooxygenase activity reducing the level of mucosal prostaglandin causing defects in the protective mucous layer.
- There is a 10% to 20% prevalence of gastric ulcers and a 2% to 5% prevalence of duodenal ulcers in long-term NSAID users.[2] The annual

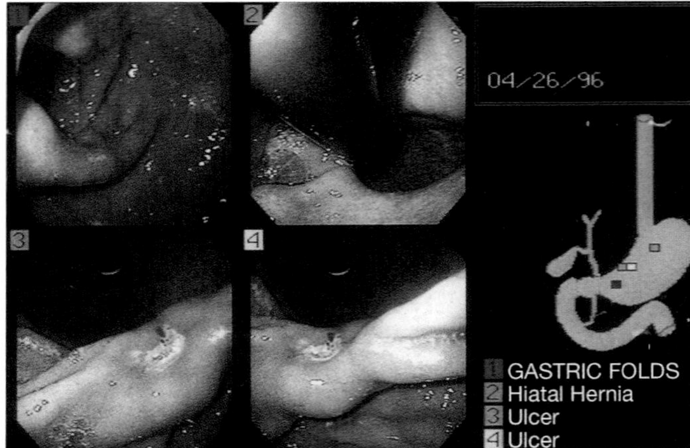

FIGURE 76-3 Stomach ulcer in a patient with a hiatal hernia. (*Reproduced with permission from Michael Harper, MD.*)

risk of a life-threatening ulcer-related complication is 1% to 4% in long-term NSAID users, with older patients having the highest risk.[4]

RISK FACTORS

- Severe physiologic stress—Burns, central nervous system trauma, surgery, and severe medical illness increase the risk for secondary (stress) ulceration.[5]
- Smoking—Evidence that tobacco use is a risk factor for duodenal ulcers in not conclusive, with several studies producing contradictory findings. However, smoking in the setting of *H. pylori* infection may increase the risk of relapse of PUD.[6]
- Alcohol use—Ethanol is known to cause gastric mucosal irritation and nonspecific gastritis. Evidence that consumption of alcohol is a risk factor for duodenal ulcer is inconclusive.[6]
- Medications—Corticosteroids alone do not increase the risk for PUD; however, they can potentiate ulcer risk in patients who use NSAIDs concurrently.[5]

DIAGNOSIS

CLINICAL FEATURES

- Epigastric pain (dyspepsia), the hallmark of PUD, is present in 80% to 90% of patients; however, this symptom is not sensitive or specific enough to serve as a reliable diagnostic criterion for PUD. Pain is typically described as gnawing or burning, occurring 1 to 3 hours after meals and relieved by food or antacids. It can occur at night, and sometimes radiates to the back.[2] Less than 25% of patients with dyspepsia have ulcer disease at endoscopy.[5]
- Other dyspeptic symptoms including belching, bloating, and distention are common but also not specific features of PUD as they are commonly encountered in many other conditions.
- Additional symptoms include fatty food intolerance, heartburn, and chest discomfort.
- Nausea and anorexia may occur with gastric ulcers.
- Significant vomiting and weight loss are unusual with uncomplicated ulcer disease and suggest gastric outlet obstruction or gastric malignancy.[2]
- Around 20% of patients with ulcer complications such as bleeding and nearly 61% of patients with NSAID-related ulcer complications have no antecedent symptoms.
- Rare and nonspecific physical findings include the following:
  - Epigastric tenderness
  - Heme-positive stool
  - Hematemesis or melena in cases of GI bleeding

TYPICAL DISTRIBUTION

- Duodenal ulcers occur most often in the first portion of the duodenum (>95%), with approximately 90% of ulcers located within 3 cm of the pylorus.[1]
- Benign gastric ulcers are located most commonly in the antrum (60%) and at the junction of the antrum and body on the lesser curvature (25%) (**Figure 76-3**).[1]

LABORATORY STUDIES

- In most patients with uncomplicated PUD, routine laboratory tests are not helpful.[5]
- Noninvasive tests include serum *H. pylori* antibody detection, fecal antigen tests, and urea breath tests; the latter 2, if positive, indicate active disease.[7]
- Serum enzyme-linked immunosorbent assay (ELISA) is the least accurate test and is useful only for diagnosing the initial infection.
- The stool antigen test is less convenient but is highly accurate and also can be used to confirm *H. pylori* eradication, as can the urea breath test.[7]
- Obtaining a serum gastrin may be useful in patients with recurrent, refractory, or complicated PUD and in patients with a family history of PUD to screen for Zollinger-Ellison syndrome.[1]

IMAGING

- Upper endoscopy is the procedure of choice for the diagnosis of duodenal and gastric ulcers (**Figures 76-1** to **76-3**).[2]
- Endoscopy provides better diagnostic accuracy than barium radiography and affords the ability to biopsy for the presence of malignancy and *H. pylori* infection. Endoscopy is usually reserved for the following situations:
  - Patients with red flag signs (eg, bleeding, dysphagia, severe pain, abdominal mass, recurrent vomiting, weight loss) or age older than 55 years
  - Patients who fail initial therapy
  - Patients whose symptoms recur after appropriate therapy
- Duodenal ulcers are virtually never malignant and do not require biopsy.[2]
- Gastric ulcers should be biopsied because 3% to 5% of benign-appearing gastric ulcers prove to be malignant.[2]
- Barium upper gastrointestinal (UGI) series is an acceptable alternative to endoscopy but is not as sensitive for the diagnosis of small ulcers (<0.5 cm) and does not allow for biopsy with gastric ulcer.[7]
- Patient's testing positive for PUD should undergo noninvasive testing for *H. pylori*.
- UGI series has limited accuracy in distinguishing benign from malignant gastric ulcers; therefore, all patients diagnosed this way should be reevaluated with endoscopy after 8 to 12 weeks of therapy.

DIFFERENTIAL DIAGNOSIS

Disease processes that may present with "ulcer-like" symptoms include the following:

- Nonulcer or functional dyspepsia (FD)—The most common diagnosis among patients seen for upper abdominal discomfort; it is a diagnosis of exclusion. Dyspepsia has been reported to occur in up to 30% of the U.S. population.
- Gastroesophageal reflux—Classic symptoms are heartburn (ie, substernal pain that may be associated with acid regurgitation or a sour taste) aggravated by bending forward or lying down, especially after a large meal. Endoscopy is considered if symptoms fail to respond to treatment (eg, histamine-2-receptor agonist, proton pump inhibitor [PPI]) or red flag signs and symptoms occur.
- Gastric cancer—Most patients do not become symptomatic until late in the disease; symptoms include upper abdominal pain, postprandial fullness, anorexia and mild nausea, vomiting (especially with pyloric tumors), weight loss, and a palpable mass. Endoscopic biopsy is used to make this diagnosis (see Chapter 60, Gastric Cancer).
- Biliary colic is characterized by discrete, intermittent episodes of pain that should not be confused with other causes of dyspepsia.
- Gastroduodenal Crohn disease—Symptoms include epigastric pain, nausea, and vomiting. On endoscopy, patients often have *H. pylori*-negative gastritis and may develop gastric outlet obstruction. Extraintestinal manifestations include erythema nodosum, peripheral arthritis, conjunctivitis, uveitis, and episcleritis. Endoscopy shows an inflammatory process with skip lesions, fistulas, aphthous ulcerations, and rectal sparing. Small bowel involvement is seen on imaging with longitudinal and transverse ulceration (cobblestoning) in addition to segmental colitis and frequent stricture (see Chapter 77, Inflammatory Bowel Disease).

MANAGEMENT

- The approach to patients with dyspepsia includes performing endoscopy for patients with red flag symptoms or who are older than age 55 years. For patients who have an ulcer identified on endoscopy, eradication of *H. pylori* is attempted (as below) and a PPI is continued for 4 to 8 weeks. For those without an ulcer on endoscopy, treatment with a PPI or H_2 blocker is provided.[4]
- For patients without red flag findings, testing and treating for *H. pylori*; counseling to avoid smoking, alcohol, and NSAIDs; and appropriate use of antisecretory therapy for 4 weeks will be successful in the majority of patients.[4]
- The goals of treatment of active *H. pylori*-associated ulcers are to relieve dyspeptic symptoms, to promote ulcer healing, and to eradicate *H. pylori* infection. Eradication of *H. pylori* is better than ulcer-healing drug therapy for duodenal ulcer healing[8] and greatly reduces the incidence of ulcer recurrence from 67% to 6% in patients with duodenal ulcers and from 59% to 4% in patients with gastric ulcers.[4]
- The worldwide empiric use of traditional triple therapy with PPI, clarithromycin, and amoxicillin no longer provides an acceptable cure rate (cure rate below 80%) because of the increasing prevalence of clarithromycin resistance.[9]
- Four drug combinations currently provide the best results and consist of 2 general combinations: (1) a PPI, amoxicillin, clarithromycin, metronidazole/tinidazole given either sequentially or concomitantly, or (2) a PPI, a bismuth, tetracycline HCL, and metronidazole/tinidazole.[9] SOR Ⓐ
- A PPI, levofloxacin, and amoxicillin for 10 days appears to be more effective and better tolerated than a PPI, bismuth, tetracycline, and metronidazole in patients with persistent *H. pylori* infection but requires validation in North America.[7]
- The European Helicobacter Study Group consensus guideline states that triple therapy (PPI-clarithromycin-amoxicillin/metronidazole) or Bismuth quadruple therapy remain first-line treatment in areas with low clarithromycin resistance. For areas with high clarithromycin resistance (>20%), Bismuth or non-Bismuth quadruple therapy are preferred.[10]
- Treat NSAID-induced ulcers with cessation of NSAIDs, if possible, and an appropriate course of standard ulcer therapy with an H_2-receptor antagonist or a PPI. If NSAIDs are continued, prescribe a PPI. SOR Ⓐ
- *H. pylori*-negative ulcers that are not caused by NSAIDs can be treated with appropriate antisecretory therapy, either H_2-receptor antagonist or PPI. SOR Ⓐ
- For patients with bleeding peptic ulcers, high-dose PPIs do not reduce rates of rebleeding, surgical intervention, or mortality after endoscopic treatment compared with non–high-dose PPIs.[11]

PREVENTION

- In a large randomized controlled trial (RCT) (N = 2426) of PUD prevention in patients taking low-dose acetylsalicylic acid who were at risk for ulcer development (eg, prior ulcer, GI symptoms and erosions, age older than 65 years), esomeprazole 40 mg or 20 mg reduced the rate of endoscopically confirmed peptic ulcer development (1.5% and 1.1%, respectively) versus placebo (7.4%).[12]
- Authors of a metaanalysis found the use of prophylactic H_2 blockers to prevent stress ulcers was not necessary in patients receiving enteral nutrition and that such therapy was associated with pneumonia and higher risk of hospital mortality.[13] In another metaanalysis, PPIs were similar to H_2-receptor antagonists in terms of stress-related UGI bleeding prophylaxis, pneumonia, and mortality among patients admitted to intensive care units.[14]

PROGNOSIS

- Hospitalization rate is approximately 30 per 100,000 cases.[5]
- Mortality rate is approximately 1 per 100,000 cases.[5]
- When the underlying cause is addressed, the prognosis is excellent.
- With the eradication of *H. pylori* infection, there has been a decrease in the ulcer recurrence rate from 60% to 90% to approximately 10% to 20% with the regard to NSAID-related ulcers.[5]
- The incidence of perforation is approximately 0.3% per patient year, and the incidence of obstruction is approximately 0.1% per patient year.[5]

FOLLOW-UP

- Endoscopy is required to document healing of gastric ulcers and to rule out gastric cancer; this is performed 6 to 8 weeks after the initial diagnosis.

- Confirmation of *H. pylori* eradication in patients with uncomplicated ulcers is not necessary.
- Confirmation of healing with endoscopy is required in all patients with ulcer complicated by bleeding, perforation, or obstruction.
- For patients without initial endoscopy who have persistent symptoms following initial treatment, the PPI or H_2 blocker can be continued for another 4 to 8 weeks.[4] If there is inadequate response to therapy, endoscopy and evaluation for hypersecretory states should be considered.

PATIENT EDUCATION

Patients with PUD should be encouraged to eat balanced meals at regular intervals, avoid heavy alcohol use, and avoid smoking (which has been shown to retard the rate of ulcer healing and increase the frequency of recurrences); stress-reduction counseling might be helpful in individual cases.

PATIENT RESOURCES

- National Digestive Diseases Information Clearing House—**http://digestive.niddk.nih.gov/ddiseases/pubs/pepticulcers_ez/index.htm.**
- Centers for Disease Control and Prevention—**http://www.cdc.gov/ulcer/.**

PROVIDER RESOURCES

- Medscape. *Peptic Ulcer Disease*—**http://emedicine.medscape.com/article/181753.**

REFERENCES

1. Del Valle J. Peptic ulcer disease and related disorders. In: Kasper DL, Braunwald E, Fauci AS, Hauser SL, Longo DL, Jameson JL, eds. *Harrison's Principles of Internal Medicine*, 16th ed. New York, NY: McGraw-Hill; 2005:1746-1762.
2. McPhee SJ, Papadakis MA, Tierney LW Jr. *Current Medical Diagnosis and Treatment*. New York, NY: McGraw-Hill; 2007.
3. University of Michigan Health System. *Peptic Ulcer Disease*. http://www.cme.med.umich.edu/pdf/guideline/PUD05.pdf. Accessed October 2011.
4. Ramakrishnan K, Salinas RC. Peptic ulcer disease. *Am Fam Physician*. 2007;76(7):1005-1012.
5. Anand BS, Bank S, Qureshi WA, et al. *Peptic Ulcer D* isease. http://emedicine.medscape.com/article/181753-overview. Accessed October 2011.
6. Aldoori WH, Giovannucci EL, Stampfer MJ, et al. A prospective study of alcohol, smoking, caffeine, and the risk of duodenal ulcer in men. *Epidemiology*. 1997;8(4):420-424.
7. Chey WD, Wong BCY; Practice Parameters Committee of the American College of Gastroenterology. American College of Gastroenterology guideline on the management of *Helicobacter pylori* infection. *Am J Gastroenterol*. 2007;102:1808-1825.
8. Ford AC, Delaney B, Forman D, Moayyedi P. Eradication therapy for peptic ulcer disease in *Helicobacter pylori* positive patients. *Cochrane Database Syst Rev*. 2006;(2):CD003840.
9. Graham DY, Rugge M. Diagnosis and evaluation of dyspepsia: clinical practice. *J Clin Gastroenterol*. 2010;44(3):167-172.
10. Malfertheiner P, Megraud F, O'Morain CA, et al; The European Helicobacter Study Group (EHSG). Management of *Helicobacter pylori* infection—The Maastricht IV/Florence Consensus Report. *Gut*. 2012;61:646-664.
11. Wang CH, Ma MH, Chou HC, et al. High-dose vs non-high-dose proton pump inhibitors after endoscopic treatment in patients with bleeding peptic ulcer: a systematic review and meta-analysis of randomized controlled trials. *Arch Intern Med*. 2010;170(9):751-758.
12. Scheiman JM, Devereaux PJ, Herlitz J, et al. Prevention of peptic ulcers with esomeprazole in patients at risk of ulcer development treated with low-dose acetylsalicylic acid: a randomised, controlled trial (OBERON). *Heart*. 2011;97(10):797-802.
13. Marik PE, Vasu T, Hirani A, Pachinburavan M. Stress ulcer prophylaxis in the new millennium: a systematic review and meta-analysis. *Crit Care Med*. 2010;38(11):2222-2228.
14. Lin PC, Chang CH, Hsu PI, et al. The efficacy and safety of proton pump inhibitors vs histamine-2 receptor antagonists for stress ulcer bleeding prophylaxis among critical care patients: a meta-analysis. *Crit Care Med*. 2010;38(4):1197-1205.

77 INFLAMMATORY BOWEL DISEASE

Mindy A. Smith, MD, MS

PATIENT STORY

A 30-year-old man presents with several days of diarrhea with a small amount of rectal bleeding with each bowel movement. This is his second episode of bloody diarrhea; the first seemed to resolve after several days and occurred several weeks ago. He has cramps that occur with each bowel movement, but feels fine between bouts of diarrhea. He has no travel history outside of the United States. He is of Jewish descent and has a cousin with Crohn disease. Colonoscopy shows mucosal friability with superficial ulceration and exudates confined to the rectosigmoid colon, and he is diagnosed with ulcerative colitis (**Figure 77-1**).

INTRODUCTION

Inflammatory bowel disease (IBD) comprises ulcerative colitis (UC) and Crohn disease. The intestinal inflammation in UC is usually confined to the mucosa and affects the rectum with or without parts or the entire colon (pancolitis) in an uninterrupted pattern. In Crohn disease, inflammation is often transmural and affects primarily the ileum and colon, often discontinuously. Crohn disease, however, can affect the entire GI tract from mouth to anus.

EPIDEMIOLOGY

- Incidence of UC in the West is 8 to 14 per 100,000 people and 6 to 15 per 100,000 people for Crohn disease.[1] Prevalence for UC and Crohn disease in North America (one of the highest rates in the world) is 37.5 to 238 per 100,000 people and 44 to 201 per 100,000 people, respectively; IBD, therefore, affects an estimated 1.3 million people in the United States.[1] Rates of IBD are increasing in both the West and in developing countries.[1]
- Age of onset is typically 30 to 40 years for UC and 20 to 30 years for Crohn disease. A bimodal distribution with a second peak at ages 60 to 70 years has been reported but not confirmed.[1]
- Predilection for those of Jewish ancestry (especially Ashkenazi Jews) followed in order by non-Jewish whites and African Americans, Hispanics, and Asians.[1]
- Inheritance (polygenic) plays a role with a concordance of 20% in monozygous twins and a risk of 10% in first-degree relatives of an incidence case.[2]

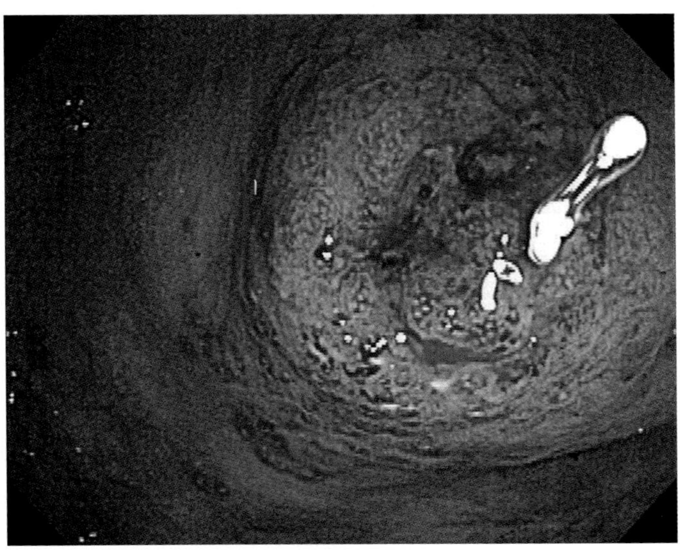

FIGURE 77-1 Ulcerative colitis in the rectosigmoid colon as viewed through the colonoscope. (*Reproduced with permission from Marvin Derezin, MD.*)

ETIOLOGY AND PATHOPHYSIOLOGY

- Unknown etiology—Current theory is that colitis is an inappropriate response to microbial gut flora or a lack of regulation of intestinal immune cells in a genetically susceptible host with failure of the normal suppression of the immune response and tissue repair.[2,3]
- Genetic regions containing nucleotide oligomerization domain 2 (NOD2; encodes an intracellular sensor of peptidoglycan), autophagy genes (regulate clearing of intracellular components like organelles), and components of the interleukin-23–type 17 helper T-cell (Th17) pathway are associated with IBD; the autophagy gene, *ATG16L1,* is associated with Crohn disease.[3]
- Multiple bowel pathogens (eg, *Salmonella, Shigella* species, and *Campylobacter*) may trigger UC. This is supported by a large cohort study where the hazard ratio of developing IBD was 2.4 (95% confidence interval [CI], 1.7 to 3.3) in the group who experienced a bout of infectious gastroenteritis compared with the control group; the excess risk was greatest during the first year after the infective episode.[4] People with IBD also have depletion and reduced diversity of some members of the mucosa-associated bacterial phyla, but it is not known whether this is causal or secondary to inflammation.[3]
- Other abnormalities found in patients with IBD include increased permeability between mucosal epithelial cells, defective regulation of intercellular junctions, infiltration into the lamina propria of innate (eg, neutrophils) and adaptive (B and T cells) immune cells with increased production of tumor necrosis factor α and increased numbers of CD4+ T cells, dysregulation of intestinal CD4+ T-cell subgroups, and the presence of circulating antimicrobial antibodies (eg, antiflagellin antibodies).[3] Many of the therapeutic approaches target these areas.
- Psychological factors (eg, major life change, daily stressors) are associated with worsening symptoms.
- Patients with long-standing UC are at higher risk of developing colon dysplasia and cancer; this is believed to be a developmental sequence (see "Prognosis" below).

RISK FACTORS

- Smokers are at increased risk for Crohn disease and tend to have more severe disease, whereas former smokers and nonsmokers are at greater risk for UC.[1,2]
- Environmental factors appear to be important triggers, especially of Crohn disease in children.[1]
- Appendectomy reduces the risk of UC.[1]

DIAGNOSIS

The diagnosis depends on the clinical evaluation, sigmoid appearance, histology, and a negative stool for bacteria, *Clostridium difficile* toxin, and ova and parasites.[2]

CLINICAL FEATURES

- Major symptoms of UC—Diarrhea, rectal bleeding, tenesmus (ie, urgency with a feeling of incomplete evacuation), passage of mucus, and cramping abdominal pain.
- Symptoms in patients with Crohn disease depend on the location of disease; patients become symptomatic when lesions are extensive or distal (eg, colitis), systemic inflammatory reaction is present, or when disease is complicated by stricture, abscess, or fistula. Gross blood and mucus in the stool are less frequent and systemic symptoms, extracolonic features, pain, perineal disease, and obstruction are more common.[2] There is no relationship between symptoms and anatomic damage.[1]
- UC is classified by severity based on the clinical picture and results of endoscopy[5]; treatment is based on disease classification.
    - Mild: Less than 4 stools per day, with or without blood, no signs of systemic toxicity, and a normal erythrocyte sedimentation rate (ESR).
    - Moderate: More than 4 stools per day but with minimal signs of toxicity.
    - Severe: More than 6 bloody stools per day, and evidence of toxicity demonstrated by fever, tachycardia, anemia, and elevated ESR.
    - Fulminant: May have more than 10 bowel movements daily, continuous bleeding, toxicity, abdominal tenderness and distention, a blood transfusion requirement, and colonic dilation on abdominal plain films.
- Extraintestinal manifestations are present in 25% to 40% of patients with IBD but are more common in Crohn disease than UC:[2,6]
    - Dermatologic (2%-34%)—Erythema nodosum (10%) that correlates with disease activity (see Chapter 176, Erythema Nodosum) and pyogenic gangrenosum (pustule that spreads concentrically and ulcerates surrounded by violaceous borders) in 1% to 12% of patients.[2]
    - Rheumatologic—Peripheral arthritis (5%-20%), spondylitis (1%-26%, but nearly all who are positive for human leukocyte antigen B27), and symmetric sacroiliitis (<10%).
    - Ocular—Conjunctivitis, uveitis, iritis, and episcleritis (0.3%-5%).[6]
    - Hepatobiliary—The most serious complication in this category is primary sclerosing cholangitis; although 75% of patients with this disease have UC, only 5% of those with UC and 2% of patients with Crohn disease develop it.[6] Hepatic steatosis (fatty liver) and cholelithiasis can also occur.
    - Cardiovascular—Increased risk of deep venous thrombosis, pulmonary embolus, and stroke (because of a hypercoagulable state from thrombocytosis and gut losses of antithrombin III among other factors); endocarditis; myocarditis; and pleuropericarditis.[2]
    - Bone—Osteoporosis and osteomalacia from multiple causes including medications, reduced physical activity, inflammatory-mediated bone resorption, vitamin D deficiency, and calcium and magnesium malabsorption. Fracture risk in patients with IBD is 1 per 100 patient-years (40% higher than the general population).[6]
    - Renal—Nephrolithiasis, obstructive uropathy, and fistulization of the urinary tract occur in 6% to 23%.[6]

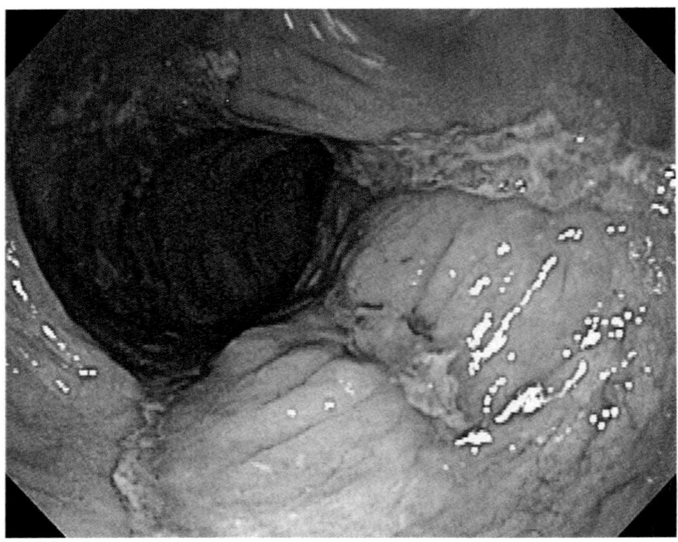

FIGURE 77-2 Crohn colitis with deep longitudinal ulcers and normal-appearing tissue between. The biopsies that showed normal tissue between the ulcers clinched the diagnosis for Crohn disease. Ulcerative colitis is diffuse whereas Crohn disease often skips areas as seen in this patient's colon. (*Reproduced with permission from Marvin Derezin, MD.*)

- Extraintestinal manifestations may occur prior to the diagnosis of IBD. For example, 10% to 30% of patients with IBD-related arthritis develop arthritis prior to IBD diagnosis.[6]
- Severe complications include toxic colitis (15% initially present with catastrophic illness), massive hemorrhage (1% of those with severe attacks), toxic megacolon (ie, transverse colon diameter >5-6 cm) (5% of attacks may be triggered by electrolyte abnormalities and narcotics), and bowel obstruction (caused by strictures and occurring in 10% of patients).[1]
- On endoscopy in patients with Crohn disease, rectal sparing is frequent and cobblestoning of the mucosa is often seen. Small bowel involvement is seen on imaging in addition to segmental colitis and frequent strictures (**Figure 77-2**).
- Diagnosis is changed from UC to Crohn disease over time in 5% to 10% of patients.[7]

TYPICAL DISTRIBUTION

- At presentation, about a third of patients with UC have disease localized to the rectum, another third have disease present in the colorectum distal to the splenic flexure, and the remainder with disease proximal to the splenic flexure; pancolitis is present in 1 quarter.[1] Adults appear to always have rectal involvement, which is not the case for children. Over time (20 years), half will have pancolitis (**Figure 77-1**).[8]
- In patients with Crohn disease, lesions occur in equal proportions in the ileum, colon, or both; 10% to 15% have upper GI lesions, 20% to 30% present with perianal lesions; and about half eventually develop perianal disease. Around 15% to 20% of patients have or have had a fistula.[1]

LABORATORY TESTS

- Acute disease can result in a rise of acute phase reactants (eg, C-reactive protein) and elevated ESR (rare in patients with just proctitis). C-reactive protein is elevated in nearly all patients with Crohn disease and in approximately half of the patients with UC.[9]

- Obtain hemoglobin (to assess for anemia) and platelets (to assess for reactive thrombocytosis).
- Of the biomarkers available to detect IBD, fecal calprotectin and lactoferrin are most commonly used.[9] The former is an indirect measure of neutrophil infiltrate in the bowel mucosa, and the later is an iron-binding protein secreted by mucosal membranes and found in neutrophil granules and serum. Although the optimal threshold value for calprotectin in detecting IBD is unknown, a study of adult patients suspected of having IBD based on clinical evaluation reported a sensitivity and specificity of the test of 93% and 96%, respectively.[10] Test characteristics for lactoferrin are lower at 80% and 82%.
- Stool should be examined to rule out infectious causes including *C. difficile*; the incidence of *C. difficile* is increasing in patients with UC and is associated with a more severe course in those with IBD.[11]

ENDOSCOPY AND IMAGING

Imaging has become more important for patients with IBD, not only for diagnosis in symptomatic patients but for early detection and treatment of inflammation in asymptomatic patients with Crohn disease and for monitoring inflammation and disease complications.[12]

- Colonoscopy with ileoscopy and mucosal biopsy should be performed in the evaluation of IBD and for differentiating UC from Crohn disease (**Figures 77-1** to **77-5**).[13] SOR Ⓑ It is the best test for detection of colonic inflammation.[5,10]
- Colonoscopy can show pseudopolyps in both active UC (**Figure 77-4**) and inactive UC (**Figure 77-5**). Risks of ileocolonoscopy include perforation, limited small bowel evaluation, and inability to stage penetrating disease.[12]
- Capsule endoscopy (CE) is a less-invasive technique for evaluating the small intestine in patients with Crohn disease and is more sensitive than radiologic and endoscopic procedures for detecting small bowel lesions and mucosal inflammation.[12,13] SOR Ⓑ CE should not be performed in patients with Crohn disease known or suspected to have a high-grade stricture. In that case, consider CT enterography.[13] The major risk is retention.[12]
- In patients with initial presentation of symptomatic Crohn disease, the American College of Radiology (ACR) recommends CT enterography.[14] Magnetic resonance (MR) enterography may be substituted based on institutional preference as this test appears to have similar test characteristics and avoids radiation exposure; it is the preferred test for investigating perianal disease.[13] In addition to radiation, risks of CT enterography are related to the iodine dye and for MR enterography, image quality can be suboptimal in some patients; both tests have limited ability to detect colonic cancer.[12]

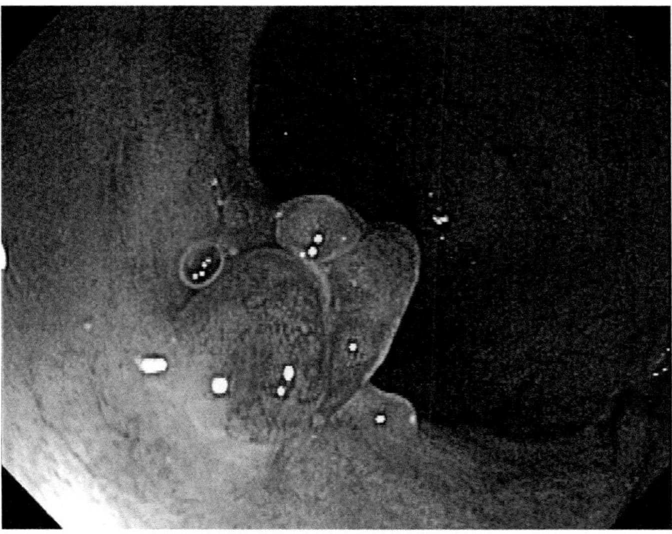

FIGURE 77-4 Pseudopolyps in "active" ulcerative colitis viewed through colonoscope. (*Reproduced with permission from Marvin Derezin, MD.*)

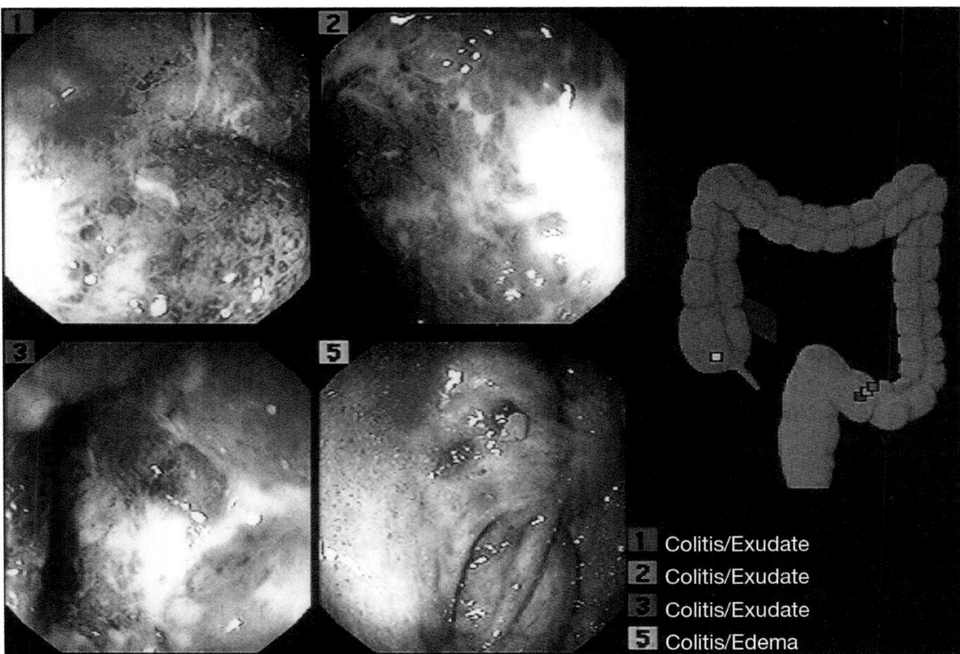

FIGURE 77-3 Ulcerative colitis. Endoscopic image showing friability and exudates over superficial ulceration in the sigmoid colon. There is edema in the cecum that, all together, indicates pan colitis. (*Reproduced with permission from Michael Harper, MD.*)

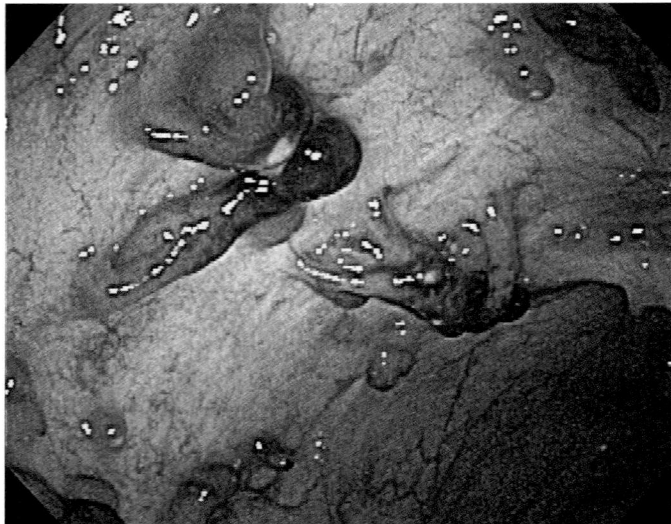

FIGURE 77-5 Pseudopolyps in "inactive" ulcerative colitis viewed through colonoscope. (*Reproduced with permission from Marvin Derezin, MD.*)

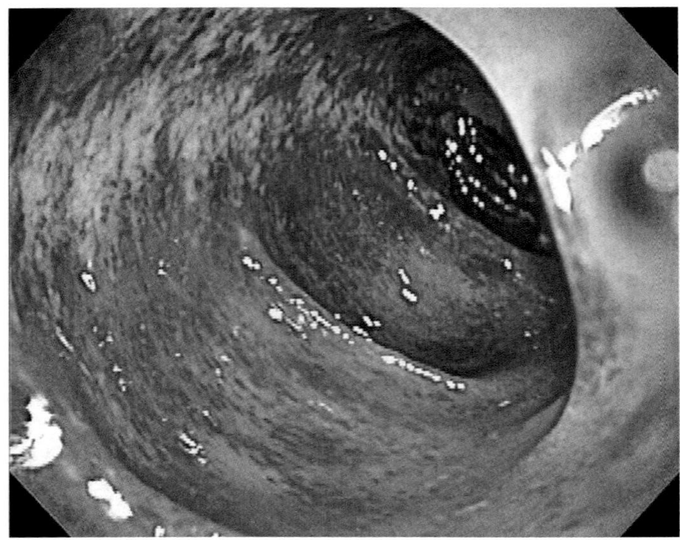

FIGURE 77-6 Ischemic colitis in an elderly patient. (*Reproduced with permission Marvin Derezin, MD.*)

- In patients with severe disease, a plain supine film may show edematous, irregular colon margins, mucosal thickening, and toxic dilation.[2]

DIFFERENTIAL DIAGNOSIS

- Infections of the colon—*Salmonella, Shigella* species, and *Campylobacter* have a similar appearance with bloody diarrhea and abdominal pain but disease is usually self-limited and stool culture can confirm the presence of these bacteria. *C. difficile* and *Escherichia coli* can also mimic IBD.
- Numerous infectious agents including *Mycobacterium*, *Cytomegalovirus*, and protozoan parasites can mimic UC in immunocompromised patients.
- Ischemic colitis—May present with sudden onset of left lower quadrant pain, urgency to defecate, and bright red blood via rectum (See Chapter 73, Ischemic Colitis). It can be chronic and diffuse and should be considered in elderly patients following abdominal aorta repair or when a patient has a hypercoagulable state. Endoscopic examination often demonstrates normal rectal mucosa with a sharp transition to an area of inflammation in the descending colon or splenic flexure (**Figure 77-6**).
- Colitis associated with NSAIDs—Clinical features of diarrhea and pain, but may be complicated by bleeding, stricture, obstruction, and perforation. History is helpful and symptoms improve with withdrawal of the agent.

MANAGEMENT

MEDICATION

Treatment of acute disease in patients with UC (treatment algorithms can be found in the reference provided) is based on disease activity as follows[15]:

- Mild to moderate distal disease—Oral aminosalicylates (ASAs), topical mesalamine, or topical steroids.[5] SOR Ⓐ An oral 5-ASA agent can be a prodrug (eg, sulfasalazine, 4-6 g/day), a drug with a pH-dependent coating (eg, Asacol, 2.4-4.8 g/day), or a slow-release agent (Pentasa, 2-4 g/day). Mesalamine suppositories (1 g/day) are the best way to induce remission in patients with proctitis.[15] Rectal suppositories or enemas should also be used to improve medication delivery when treating active distal colitis, and a combination of oral and rectal mesalamine is better than monotherapy for stopping rectal bleeding (89% vs. 46% [oral only] or 69% [rectal only]).[5,15] SOR Ⓐ Fifty percent to 75% of patients will show clinical improvement with 2 g/day of 5-ASA and a similar percentage will maintain remission with doses of 1.5 to 4 g/day.[2]
- For patients with mild to moderate active proctitis who do not respond to topical mesalamine, adding a topical corticosteroid should be considered. In patients refractory to oral ASAs or topical corticosteroids, mesalamine enemas or suppositories may still be effective.[5] SOR Ⓐ An oral steroid (eg, prednisone, 40-60 mg/day) or infliximab (induction regimen of 5 mg/kg at weeks 1, 2, and 6) can be added for patients with mild-moderate local disease who have an inadequate response to initial therapy; the latter is often reserved for patients who do not respond to or tolerate steroids.[5,13] SOR Ⓒ
- Mild to moderate extensive colitis—Oral sulfasalazine (titrated to 4-6 g/day) or 5-ASA (up to 4.8 g/day) with or without topical therapy. SOR Ⓐ Oral steroids are generally reserved for patients refractory to combined oral and topical ASA therapy or for those with severe symptoms requiring more prompt improvement.[5] SOR Ⓐ Immunomodulators (6-mercaptopurine and azathioprine) are effective for patients who do not respond to oral steroids and continue to have moderate disease.[5] SOR Ⓐ Patients who are steroid refractory, intolerant, or steroid-dependent despite adequate doses of a thiopurine can be considered for infliximab induction as above.[5] SOR Ⓐ Infliximab is contraindicated in patients with active infection, untreated latent tuberculosis, preexisting demyelinating disorder or optic neuritis, moderate to severe congestive heart failure, or current or recent malignancies.
- Severe colitis—Patients presenting with toxicity should be admitted to the hospital for IV steroids (methylprednisolone, 40 to 60 mg/day, or hydrocortisone, 200 to 300 mg/day) following hospitalization.[5,15] SOR Ⓒ Otherwise, treat with oral prednisone, oral ASA drugs, and

topical medications with the addition of infliximab (5 mg/kg) if refractory to treatment and urgent hospitalization is not necessary.[5] SOR Ⓐ If the patient fails to improve within 3 to 5 days, colectomy SOR Ⓑ or IV cyclosporine SOR Ⓐ should be considered. Antibiotics have no proven efficacy without proven infection and parenteral nutrition has not been shown to be of benefit as primary therapy for UC.[5]

- Fulminant disease—Patients should be treated as above with IV glucocorticoid and maintained without oral intake and with use of a decompression tube if small bowel ileus is present.[5] IV cyclosporine (2-4 mg/kg per day) or infliximab may be considered for patients who are not improving on maximal medical therapy as above.
- Patients with Crohn disease are treated similarly except that there is limited response to mesalamine or cyclosporin and better response to nutritional therapy. A research tool called the Crohn Disease Activity Index can be used to monitor disease activity (online calculator available at http://www.ibdjohn.com/cdai/. Accessed July 2013).
- Mild to moderate active ileocolic Crohn disease—Budesonide (9 mg) or prednisone if distal colonic disease is present.[15] Nutrition therapy is the first-line treatment for children. For patients who do not tolerate steroids or in cases where steroids are ineffective, biologic therapy with infliximab, adalimumab, or certolizumab pegol is appropriate. Methotrexate (up to 25 mg/week) is also effective.[15] Patients with weight loss or strictures may benefit from early introduction of biologic or immunomodulator therapy.[15]
- Severe Crohn disease in any location-Initial treatment with oral or intravenous steroids; antitumor necrosis factor therapy is reserved for patients who do not respond to initial therapy. In a single-center cohort study of 614 patients treated with infliximab, only 10.9% were not primary responders by 12 weeks, and sustained benefit was seen in 63% who received long-term treatment (mean follow-up: 55 months).[16] Management also includes nutritional support and treatment of iron deficiency.
- Side effects of biologic therapy include serious infections, induction of autoimmune phenomena, and neurotoxicity.[17] However, in a report of a cohort of 734 patients with IBD treated with infliximab, the most commonly observed systemic side effects were skin eruptions including psoriasiform eruptions in 20%; 2 patients developed tuberculosis but none of the 16 patients with positive skin tests who received prophylaxis.[18]

SURGERY

Surgery—Total proctocolectomy with ileostomy or continence-preserving operation (ie, ileal pouch-anal anastomosis [IPAA]) is performed in approximately half of patients with UC within 10 years of disease onset. Indications for surgery include the following[2,5]: SOR Ⓒ

- Intractable or fulminant disease
- Toxic megacolon
- Massive hemorrhage
- Colonic obstruction or perforation
- Colon cancer or dysplasia in flat mucosa,[8] SOR Ⓑ or for cancer prophylaxis.

PROGNOSIS

- In UC (**Figure 77-7**), disease flares and remissions with mucosal healing occur; remission is seen in about half of the patients within a year of onset.[1] Those who have complete clinical and endoscopic remission have a significantly decreased risk of colectomy.[1] Disease activity lessens over time with longer periods of remission. In a population study of 1575 patients with UC in Denmark, 13% had no relapse, 74% had 2 or more relapses, and 13% had active disease every year for 5 years after diagnosis.[19]

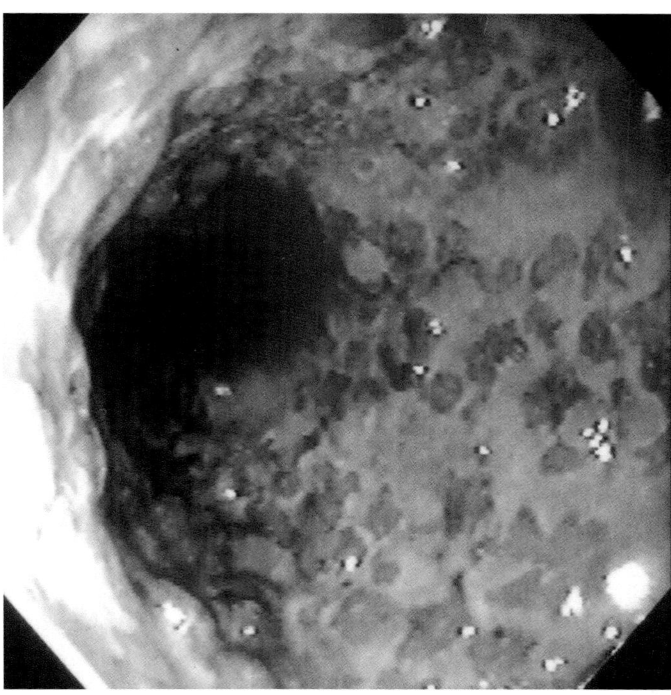

FIGURE 77-7 Ulcerative colitis in a 27-year-old man presenting with rectal bleeding. (*Reproduced with permission from Mark Koch, MD.*)

- The probability of colectomy over 25 years for those with UC is 20% to 30%.[1] Colectomy is not necessarily curative as pouchitis episodes occur in half of these patients by 5 years postoperatively, and in up to 10% of cases, pouchitis is chronic and often refractory to antibiotic treatment.[1]
- Overall mortality is not increased for patients with UC, unless there is severe disease.[1] Although UC-related mortality from liver disease or colorectal cancer is increased, there is a decreased rate of death from pulmonary cancer and other tobacco-related diseases.[1]
- Recurrence postoperatively is the norm for patients with Crohn disease; only 5% have normal endoscopy at 10 years follow-up and symptoms occur about 2 to 3 years after anatomic lesions are found.[20] Natural progression of the disease with or without surgery is variable with spontaneous and treatment-related remissions, especially of more superficial lesions. Only approximately 10% to 15% of patients have chronic continuous disease.[1]
- Most patients with Crohn disease (60%-80%) require surgery by the time they have had the disease for 20 to 30 years (estimated at 3%-5% per year) and greater than 10% eventually require fecal diversion, especially in patients with colorectal disease or anal stenosis.[1]
- Factors associated with poor prognosis in IBD are younger age and more extensive disease. Other factors associated with poor prognosis are pouchitis and extraintestinal manifestations at surgery (IPAA) for UC and need for steroids at presentation for Crohn disease.[1]
- Mortality rate for Crohn disease is slightly increased (standardized mortality ratio = 1.52); most deaths are connected to malnutrition, postoperative complications, and intestinal cancer.

- Both patients with UC and Crohn disease are at increased risk for colorectal cancer. The risk increases with duration and extent of disease and decreases following successful treatment.[21] Colorectal cancer is rare within the first 7 years of colitis onset and increases at a rate of approximately 0.5% to 1% per year thereafter, which is likely associated with histologic disease activity.[9] It is not clear if anti-inflammatory medications reduce this risk.[9]
- Patients with cholestasis should be evaluated for primary sclerosing cholangitis and subsequent cholangiocarcinoma.[5]

FOLLOW-UP

- Support and patient education should be provided to address medication side effects, the uncertain nature of the disease, and potential complications. Discuss medication adherence in patients with apparent inadequate response to treatment.
- For maintenance of remission of mild to moderate distal disease—Mesalamine suppositories (proctitis) or enemas (distal colitis) can be dosed as infrequently as every third night.[5] SOR Ⓐ Patients, however, prefer oral therapy.[15] Sulfasalazine, mesalamine compounds, and balsalazide are also effective in maintaining remission; the combination of oral and topical mesalamine is more effective than either one alone.[5] SOR Ⓐ If these fail, thiopurines and infliximab may be effective.[5] SOR Ⓐ
- For maintenance of remission of mild to moderate extensive colitis—Sulfasalazine, olsalazine, mesalamine (2.4 g/day), and balsalazide are effective in reducing relapses; chronic steroid use should be avoided.[5] SOR Ⓐ Infliximab can be used for maintenance of remission in patients who respond to infliximab induction.[5] SOR Ⓐ For patients who relapse despite therapy, azathioprine or 6-mercaptopurine can be used (number needed to treat to prevent 1 recurrence is 5).[15]
- For patients with severe colitis, long-term remission is significantly enhanced with the addition of maintenance 6-mercaptopurine.[5] SOR Ⓑ
- Periodic bone mineral density assessment is recommended for patients on long-term corticosteroid therapy (>3 months).[22] SOR Ⓐ
- Annual ophthalmologic examinations are recommended for patients on long-term corticosteroid therapy.[22] SOR Ⓒ
- Patients with long-standing IBD are at higher risk of developing colon dysplasia and cancer. For patients with pancolitis, the risk is 0.5% to 1% per year after 8 to 10 years of disease.[1,2] Surveillance colonoscopy with multiple biopsies should be performed every 1 to 2 years beginning after 8 to 10 years of disease.[5] SOR Ⓑ There is evidence that cancers are detected at an earlier stage in patients who are undergoing surveillance.[23]
- In the near future, it may be possible to monitor patients for intestinal ulcerations or thickening using noninvasive techniques (assays for C-reactive protein, fecal calprotectin, and lactoferrin; videocapsule and magnetic resonance imaging) and treat them as early as possible to prevent disease progression.[1,12] In addition, biomarkers may be useful for assessing mucosal healing, predicting relapse, and making therapeutic adjustments.[9]

PATIENT EDUCATION

- Patients should be informed about the unpredictable course of IBD and the need for frequent contact with an experienced provider for medical management, support, and surveillance.
- Smoking cessation should be stressed, particularly for patients with Crohn disease.[2]

PATIENT RESOURCES

- National Digestive Diseases Information Clearinghouse, *Ulcerative Colitis*—**http://digestive.niddk.nih.gov/ddiseases/pubs/colitis/.**
- National Digestive Diseases Information Clearinghouse, *Crohn Disease*—**http://digestive.niddk.nih.gov/ddiseases/pubs/crohns/.**
- Crohn's and Colitis Foundation of America—**www.ccfa.org.**

PROVIDER RESOURCES

- Kornbluth A, Sachar D; Practice Committee of the American College of Gastroenterology. Ulcerative colitis practice guidelines in adults: American College of Gastroenterology, Practice Parameters Committee. *Am J Gastroenterol*. 2010;105:501-523.
- Burger D, Travis S. Conventional medical management of IBD. *Gastroenterology*. 2011;140(6):1827-1837.

REFERENCES

1. Cosnes J, Gower-Rousseau C, Seksik P, Cortot A. Epidemiology and natural history of inflammatory bowel diseases. *Gastroenterology*. 2011;140(6):1785-1794.
2. Friedman S, Blumberg RS. Inflammatory bowel disease. In: Kasper DL, Braunwald E, Fauci AS, Hauser SL, Longo DL, Jameson JL, eds. *Harrison's Principles of Internal Medicine*, 16th ed. New York, NY: McGraw-Hill; 2005:1776-1789.
3. Abraham C, Cho J. Inflammatory bowel disease. *N Engl J Med*. 2009;361:2066-2078.
4. Garcia Rodriguez LA, Ruigomez A, Panes J. Acute gastroenteritis is followed by an increased risk of inflammatory bowel disease. *Gastroenterology*. 2006;130(6):1588-1594.
5. Kornbluth A, Sachar D; Practice Committee of the American College of Gastroenterology. Ulcerative colitis practice guidelines in adults: American College of Gastroenterology, Practice Parameters Committee. *Am J Gastroenterol*. 2010;105:501-523.
6. Levine JS, Burakoff R. Extraintestinal manifestations of inflammatory bowel disease. *Gastroenterol Hepatol (NY)*. 2011;7(4):235-241.
7. Langholz E, Munkholm P, Davidsen M, et al. Course of ulcerative colitis: analysis of changes in disease activity over years. *Gastroenterology*. 1994;107:3-11.
8. Langholz E, Munkholm P, Davidsen M, et al. Changes in extent of ulcerative colitis: a study on the course and prognostic factors. *Scand J Gastroenterol*. 1996;31:260-266.
9. Lewis JD. The utility of biomarkers in the diagnosis and therapy of inflammatory bowel disease. *Gastroenterology*. 2011;140(6):1817-1826.
10. van Rheenen PF, Van de Vijver E, Fidler V. Faecal calprotectin for screening of patients with suspected inflammatory bowel disease: diagnostic meta-analysis. *BMJ*. 2010;341:c3369.
11. Ananthakrishnan AN, McGinley EL, Binion DG. Excess hospitalization burden associated with Clostridium difficile in patients with inflammatory bowel disease. *Gut*. 2008;57:205-210.
12. Fletcher JG, Fider JL, Bruining DH, Huprich JE. New concepts in intestinal imaging for inflammatory bowel disease. *Gastroenterology*. 2011;140(6):1795-1806.
13. Leighton JA, Shen B, Baron TH, et al; Standards of Practice Committee, American Society for Gastrointestinal Endoscopy.

ASGE guideline: endoscopy in the diagnosis and treatment of inflammatory bowel disease. *Gastrointest Endosc.* 2006;63(4):558-565.

14. *ACR Appropriateness Criteria Crohn's Disease*. http://www.guideline.gov/content.aspx?id=35137. Accessed July 2013.
15. Burger D, Travis S. Conventional medical management of inflammatory bowel disease. *Gastroenterology.* 2011;140(6):1827-1837.
16. Schnitzler F, Fidder H, Ferrante M, et al. Long-term outcome of treatment with infliximab in 614 patients with Crohn's disease: results from a single-centre cohort. *Gut.* 2009;58:492-500.
17. Van Assche G, Vermeire S, Rutgeerts P. Safety issues with biological therapies for inflammatory bowel disease. *Curr Opin Gastroenterol.* 2006;22(4):370-376.
18. Fidder H, Schnitzler F, Ferrante M, et al. Long-term safety of infliximab for the treatment of inflammatory bowel disease: a single-centre cohort study. *Gut.* 2009;58(4):501-508.
19. Jess T, Riis L, Vind I, et al. Changes in clinical characteristics, course, and prognosis of inflammatory bowel disease during the last 5 decades: a population-based study from Copenhagen, Denmark. *Inflamm Bowel Dis.* 2007;13:481-489.
20. Olaison G, Smedh K, Sjodahl R. Natural course of Crohn's disease after ileocolic resection: endoscopically visualized ileal ulcers preceding symptoms. *Gut.* 1992;33:331-335.
21. Ullman TA, Itzkowitz SH. Intestinal inflammation and cancer. *Gastroenterology.* 2011;140(6):1807-1816.
22. Lichtenstein GR, Abreu MT, Cohen R, Tremaine W. American gastroenterological association institute medical position statement on corticosteroids, immunomodulators, and infliximab in inflammatory bowel disease. *Gastroenterology.* 2006;130(3): 935-939.
23. Collins PD, Mpofu C, Watson AJ, Rhodes JM. Strategies for detecting colon cancer and/or dysplasia in patients with inflammatory bowel disease. *Cochrane Database Syst Rev.* 2006;(2): CD000279.

PART 11

GENITOURINARY/ RENAL

Strength of Recommendation (SOR)	Definition
A	Recommendation based on consistent and good-quality patient-oriented evidence.*
B	Recommendation based on inconsistent or limited-quality patient-oriented evidence.*
C	Recommendation based on consensus, usual practice, opinion, disease-oriented evidence, or case series for studies of diagnosis, treatment, prevention, or screening.*

*See Appendix A on pages 1241-1244 for further information.

78 BLADDER CANCER

Mindy A. Smith, MD, MS

PATIENT STORY

A 68-year-old man, who is a retired painter and in good health, comes to the office at the insistence of his wife. He reports that his urinary stream is smaller and he has occasional dysuria. He has no major medical problems, although he continues to smoke one pack of cigarettes per day. His urinalysis in the office shows microscopic hematuria, and an irregular mass is seen in the bladder on CT scan (**Figure 78-1**). Cystoscopy shows a bladder tumor (**Figure 78-2**). Complete endoscopic resection is performed and confirms transitional cell carcinoma.

INTRODUCTION

Bladder cancer is a malignant neoplasm of the bladder, almost exclusively urothelial (transitional cell) carcinoma.

EPIDEMIOLOGY

- In 2008, there were approximately 398,329 men and 139,099 women alive in the United States who had a history of cancer of the urinary bladder.[1]
- Almost 70,000 new cases (52,020 men and 17,230 women) were diagnosed and approximately 14,990 deaths occurred from bladder cancer in 2011.[1] Mean age at diagnosis is 73 years.
- The age-adjusted incidence rate (based on 2004-2008 data) was 21.1 per 100,000 men and women per year with a male-to-female ratio of approximately 4:1. Among men, bladder cancer is more prevalent in whites than in blacks or Hispanics (ratio of 2:1) and more prevalent in whites than in Asian/Pacific Islander or American Indian/Alaska Natives (ratio 2.4:1); for white women, incidence rates are also higher but the differences are not as great.[1]

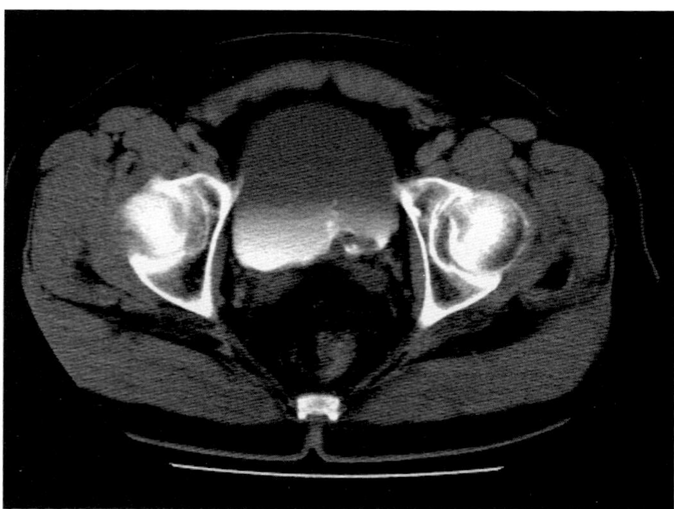

FIGURE 78-1 CT with contrast reveals a bladder cancer in a 68-year-old man with hematuria. (*Reproduced with permission from Michael Freckleton, MD.*)

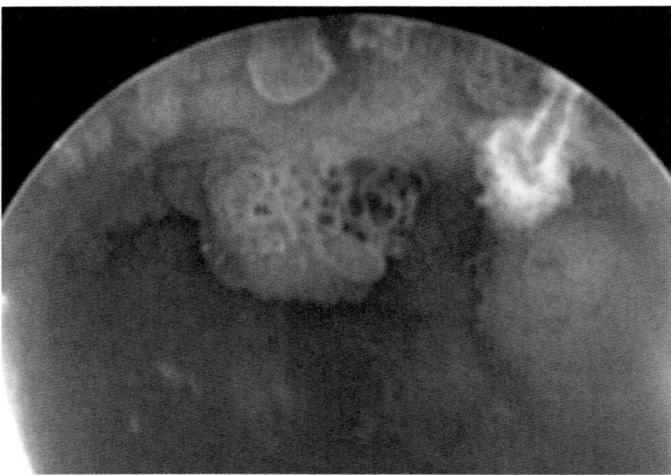

FIGURE 78-2 Cystoscopic view of the transitional cell carcinoma in the man in **Figure 72-1**. (*Reproduced with permission from Carlos Enrique Bermejo, MD.*)

ETIOLOGY AND PATHOPHYSIOLOGY

- Around 90% to 95% are transitional cell cancers and the remainder are nonurothelial neoplasms, including primarily squamous cell, adenocarcinoma, and small cell carcinoma[2,3] (**Figures 78-1** to **78-4**). Rare forms include nonepithelial neoplasms (approximately 1%), including benign tumors, such as hemangiomas or lipomas, and malignant tumors, such as angiosarcomas.[3]
- Transitional cells line the urinary tract from the renal pelvis to the proximal two-thirds of the urethra. Ninety percent of transitional cell tumors develop in the bladder, and the others develop in the renal pelvis, ureters, or urethra.[2]

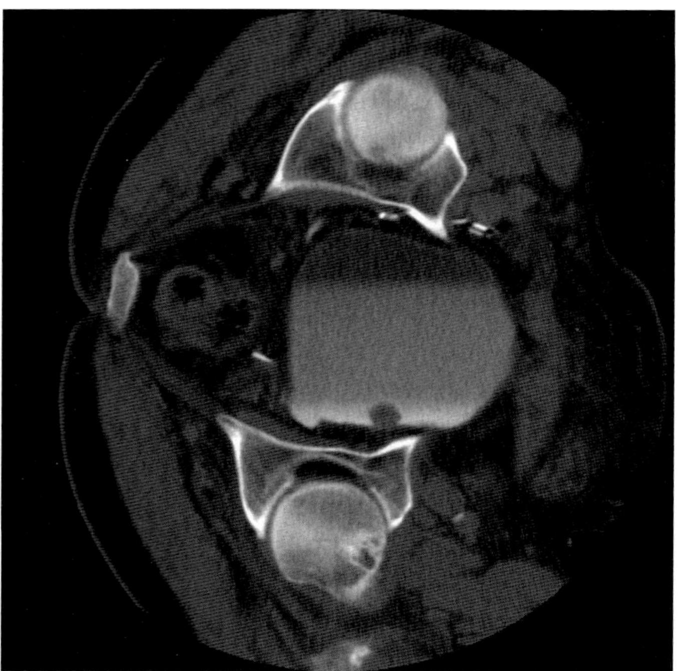

FIGURE 78-3 CT with contrast of a small transitional cell carcinoma of the bladder that was barely visible until the patient was scanned on side. A small bladder diverticulum is visible as well. (*Reproduced with permission from Michael Freckleton, MD.*)

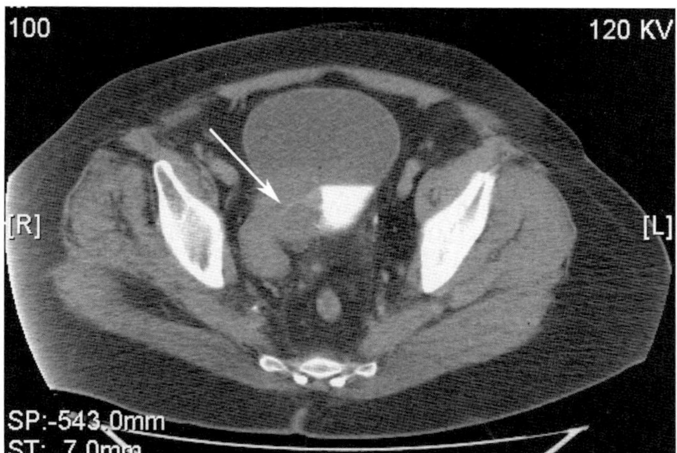

FIGURE 78-4 CT of locally invasive transitional cell carcinoma (arrow) of the bladder extending outside of the bladder in a 71-year-old man. The carcinoma on the patient's right is displacing the contrast toward the left side of the patient's bladder. (*Reproduced with permission from Michael Freckleton, MD.*)

- Most tumors are superficial (75%-85%).[4] At diagnosis, approximately 51% are in situ and 35% are localized (confined to primary site) with an additional 7% of cases having regional spread and 4% having distant metastases at diagnosis (3% unknown).[2]
- Multiple tumors are seen in 30% of cases.[4]
- Bladder tumor cells are also graded based on their appearance and behavior into well differentiated or low grade (grade 1), moderately well differentiated or moderate grade (grade 2), and poorly differentiated or high grade (grade 3).
- The most common sites of hematogenous spread are lung, bone, liver, and brain. Superficial lesions do not metastasize until they invade deeply and may remain indolent for years.[2]

RISK FACTORS

- Risk factors include smoking (odds ratio increased by 3-4 fold; 50% attributable risk) and exposure to pelvic radiation,[5] the drugs phenacetin and chlornaphazine, external-beam radiation, and chronic infection, including *Schistosoma haematobium* and genitourinary tuberculosis.[2,3]
- There is an increased risk in certain occupations, particularly those involving exposure to metals (eg, aluminum), paint and solvents, polycyclic aromatic hydrocarbons, diesel engine emissions, aniline dyes (eg, workers in chemical plants exposed to benzidine or *o*-toluidine),[2] and textiles.[6]
- An increased risk was also seen with drinking tap water (odds ratio [OR] for >2 L/day vs. ≤0.5 L/day was 1.46 [1.20-1.78]), with a higher risk among men (OR = 1.50, 1.21-1.88).[7]
- Familial cases indicate a genetic predisposition.[8]

DIAGNOSIS

CLINICAL FEATURES

- Hematuria in 80% to 90%; with microscopic hematuria approximately 2% have bladder cancer and with gross hematuria approximately 20% have bladder cancer.[3]
- Irritative symptoms (ie, dysuria, frequency) are the most common presentation.
- Obstructive symptoms may occur if the tumor is located near the urethra or bladder neck.

LABORATORY

- Urine microscopy and culture to rule out bladder infection.[3]
- Urine cytology (high specificity [90%-95%] but low sensitivity [23%-60%]), CT scan of the pelvis (**Figures 78-1**, **78-3**, and **78-4**) or intravenous urography (IVU), and cystoscopy with biopsy (**Figure 78-2**) comprise the basic work-up.[2] Fluorescence cystoscopy (use of photosensitizer instilled into the bladder), can enhance detection of flat neoplastic lesions like carcinoma in situ (CIS).[4] When CIS is found in a cystectomy specimen, 9% to 13% of patients have upper urinary tract disease.[4]
- Bladder wash cytology during cystoscopy detects most CIS.[3]
- A complete blood count, blood chemistry tests (including alkaline phosphatase tests), liver function tests, CT or MRI of the chest or abdomen, and a bone scan may be needed for suspected metastatic disease.[2,3] Bone scanning may be limited to patients with bone pain and/or elevated levels of serum alkaline phosphatase.[4]
- Tumor markers such as fluorescence in situ hybridization (FISH) analysis and nuclear matrix protein (NMP) 22 identify changes in cells in the urine and are more sensitive than urine cytology for low-grade tumors with equivalent sensitivity for high-grade tumors and CIS.[9] As specificity is low, tumor markers should not be used for diagnosis.

IMAGING

- For pretreatment staging of invasive bladder cancer, the American College of Radiology (ACR) recommends a chest X-ray (with chest CT if equivocal), CT of the abdomen and pelvis (without and with contrast) or MRI of the pelvis (especially in cases where patients are unable to undergo contrast injection), and possibly IVU; contrast-enhanced MRI is preferred over CT for local staging.[4] SOR Ⓒ
- The European Association of Urology (EAU) recommends multidetector-row CT (MDCT) of the chest, abdomen, and pelvis as the optimal form of staging for patients with confirmed muscle-invasive bladder cancer, including MDCT urography for examination of the upper urinary tracts.[9] If MDCT is not available, alternatives are excretory urography and a chest X-ray. SOR Ⓑ
- EAU recommends renal and bladder ultrasonography, and IVU or CT prior to transurethral resection for presumed invasive bladder cancer.[10] SOR Ⓑ ACR agrees that ultrasound is useful for local tumor staging.[4] For patients with verified invasive bladder cancer, EAU recommends either MRI with fast dynamic contrast-enhancement or MDCT with contrast enhancement for patients considered suitable for radical treatment. SOR Ⓑ

BIOPSY

Diagnosis is made by cystoscopy, biopsy, and histology.

DIFFERENTIAL DIAGNOSIS

- Among adult patients with microscopic hematuria, most patients have benign pathology, such as urinary tract infection, with 25% having prostate cancer and only 2% having bladder cancer.[2]

- Among adult patients with gross hematuria, 22% have benign cystitis and 15% to 20% have bladder cancer.[2]

MANAGEMENT

MEDICATIONS

Neoadjuvant cisplatin-containing combination chemotherapy (administered prior to main treatment) improves overall 5-year survival by 5% to 7% and should be considered in muscle-invasive bladder cancer irrespective of definitive treatment.[9,11] SOR Ⓐ It is not recommended for patients with performance status of 2 or more and impaired renal function or for primary therapy for localized bladder cancer.[9]

- The role of adjuvant chemotherapy (usually administered after surgery) for invasive bladder cancer is under debate. A Cochrane review based on 6 small trials (N = 491) found a 25% relative reduction in the risk of death for chemotherapy compared to control patients (hazard ratio for survival 0.75; 95% CI 0.60, 0.96), suggesting a benefit for these patients.[12]
- Cisplatin-containing combination chemotherapy is first-line therapy for patients with metastatic disease, and treated patients can achieve a median survival of up to 14 months.[9,13] SOR Ⓐ

SURGICAL

It depends on the extent (depth and grade) or spread of the disease (**Table 78-1**). Recommendations have been provided by the American Urological Association (AUA, 2007)[13] and the EAU (2009)[9] as given below:

- Non–muscle-invasive disease (70%-75% of cases)—Complete endoscopic resection with or without intravesical treatment (bacille Calmette-Guérin [BCG] weekly for 6 weeks or interferon or mitomycin C). SOR Ⓒ Low-grade tumors (Ta tumors) can be treated with resection alone or with a single postoperative dose of intravesical chemotherapy. SOR Ⓑ In a metaanalysis of 3 trials, tumor recurrence was significantly lower with intravesical BCG, but there was no difference in disease progression or survival.[14] SOR Ⓑ BCG treatment causes urinary frequency (71%), cystitis (67%), hematuria (23%), fever (25%),[15] and, rarely, systemic granulomatous infection requiring antituberculosis treatment.

TABLE 78-1 Bladder Cancer Categories, Stage, and 5-Year Survival Rate

Tumor Category	Stage of Tumor*	Description	5-Year Survival
Non–muscle-invasive disease			
Ta	Stage 0 (N0,M0)	Nonmuscle-invasive papillary carcinoma	90%
Tis	Stage 0 (N0,M0)	Carcinoma in situ	96.6%
T1	Stage I (N0,M0)	Tumor invading the lamina propria	
Muscle-invasive disease			
T2a	Stage II (N0,M0)	Tumor grown into inner half of muscle layer	70.7%
T2b	Stage II (N0,M0)	Tumor grown into outer half of muscle layer	
T3†	Stage III (N0,M0)	Tumor through muscle layer into fatty tissue	
T4a	Stage III (N0,M0)	Tumor beyond fatty tissue into nearby organs‡	
T4b	Stage IV (N0,M0)	Tumor beyond into pelvic or abdominal wall‡	
Lymph node			
N0	Stage IV	No lymph node involvement	34.6%
N1	Stage IV	Spread to single lymph node in true pelvis	
N2	Stage IV	Spread to 2 or more lymph nodes in true pelvis	
N3		Spread to nodes along the common iliac artery	
Metastatic disease			
M0	Stage IV	No distant spread	5.4%
M1		Cancer has spread to distant sites*	

*Determined by combining the tumor category with presence or absence and number of lymph nodes involved (N), and presence or absence or distant spread (eg, distant lymph nodes, bones, lungs, and liver).
†Also divided into *a* (microscopic spread into fatty tissue) and *b* (visible spread on imaging or to the eye).
‡ Also divided into *a* (spread to prostate or uterus/vagina) and *b* (spread to pelvic or abdominal wall).
Information based on SEER data. http://seer.cancer.gov/statfacts/html/urinb.html. Accessed June 2014.

- For Ta, Tis, or T1 tumors that are initially histologically confirmed as high grade, the AUA recommends repeat resection and additional intravesical therapy (induction course of BCG followed by maintenance therapy).[13] SOR Ⓐ A Cochrane review based on 5 small trials found that immunotherapy with intravesical BCG following surgery benefits patients with medium/high risk Ta or T1 bladder cancer on delaying tumor recurrence.[15] Additional Cochrane reviews found intravesical BCG more effective than intravesical epirubicin or mitomycin C in reducing tumour recurrence (the latter only for patients at high risk of recurrence) [16,17]; mitomycin C, however, was equivalent to BCG for disease progression and survival. SOR Ⓐ
- Persistent or recurrent superficial disease—Repeat resection with an induction course of BCG; maintenance BCG or mitomycin C is recommended or consideration of intravesical chemotherapy (valrubicin or gemcitabine). SOR Ⓑ For treatment failure of patients with non–muscle-invasive bladder tumors, EAU recommends radical cystectomy for those with high-grade tumors and cystectomy for other patients with T1 tumors.[9] SOR Ⓑ Delay in cystectomy for these patients increases the risk of progression and cancer-specific death.[9]
- Recurrent high-grade T1 tumors or invasive-muscle disease (extends to muscle or lymph nodes)—Radical cystectomy and pelvic lymphadenectomy with or without systemic chemotherapy.[2,9] SOR Ⓒ In men, radical cystectomy includes removal of the prostate, seminal vesicles, and proximal urethra resulting in impotence. In women, the uterus, ovaries, and anterior vaginal wall are removed. Most patients receive cutaneous reservoirs (bowel or orthotopic neobladder) drained by intermittent self-catheterization.
- Chemotherapy is not used for nonurothelial cancers, such as squamous cell carcinoma or adenocarcinoma, which are primarily treated with cystectomy.[2]
- Upper urinary tract recurrence—Radical nephroureterectomy. SOR Ⓑ

OTHER THERAPY

- In a Cochrane review of 3 trials comparing radical radiotherapy followed by surgery (salvage cystectomy) versus radical cystectomy, overall survival was better with radical cystectomy.[18] SOR Ⓐ
- External-beam radiotherapy alone is considered an option for patients unfit for cystectomy or to stop the bleeding from a tumor when local control can't be achieved by transurethral manipulation because of extensive local tumor growth.[9] SOR Ⓒ

PREVENTION

Eliminate active and passive smoking.[9] SOR Ⓒ

PROGNOSIS

- Most recurrences are also superficial tumors with only approximately 10% to 15% of tumors progressing to invasive disease.[4]
- Performance status, ranging from 0 (fully active) to 4 (completely disabled), and the presence or absence of visceral metastases are independent prognostic factors for survival.
- The EAU working group suggests use of a weighted scoring system to estimate recurrence and progression risk.[19] Factors include number, size, category, and grade of tumors; recurrence; and concomitant CIS. Scores range from 0 to 17 for recurrence and 0 to 23 for progression. These scores are translated into probabilities for 1-year and 5-year recurrence (15% and 31%, respectively, for a score of 0, and 61%-78%, respectively, for a score of 10-17) and 1-year and 5-year progression (0.2% and 0.8%, respectively, for a score of 0, and 17%-45%, respectively, for a score of 14-23).
- Risk of disease progression by tumor grade: 10% to 15% progress with grade 1 tumors, 14% to 37% with grade 2, and 33% to 64% with grade 3 tumors.[20]
- Five-year survival rates for superficial disease are 90%; infiltrating (stage II or III), 35% to 70%; metastatic disease (stage IV), 5.4% to 20% (see **Table 78-1**).[1] Long-term disease-free survival is reported in approximately 15% of patients with nodal disease and good performance status.

FOLLOW-UP

- Recurrence rates overall are 50% with a median recurrence at 1 year (0.4 to 11 years), and 5% to 20% progress to a more advanced stage. Patients should be seen every 3 months for the first year. SOR Ⓒ The ACR and EAU recommend stopping oncologic surveillance after 5-years of normal follow-up to be replaced by functional surveillance (eg, renal function).[4,9]
- For patients with high-grade Ta and T1 disease, cystoscopy, urinalysis, and urine cytology are recommended every 3 months for 2 years, then every 6 months for 2 years, then annually. Imaging of the upper tract collecting system is performed every 1 to 2 years.[2,4]
- For patients with muscle-invasive disease, laboratory tests (liver function test, creatinine clearance, electrolyte panel) in addition to a chest X-ray are recommended every 6 to 12 months with imaging of upper urinary tract, abdomen, and pelvis for recurrence every 3 to 6 months for 2 years, and then as clinically indicated.[3]
- For patients undergoing bladder-sparing surgery, urine cytology with or without biopsy is conducted every 3 months for 1 year, then at increasing intervals.[3]
- For patients undergoing cystectomy, urine cytology is conducted every 6 to 12 months, and for those undergoing cystectomy and cutaneous diversion, urethral wash cytology is recommended every 6 to 12 months.[3]
- For patients with cystectomy and continent orthotopic diversion, vitamin B_{12} level should be checked annually.[3,21]
- Bladder tumor markers from voided urine will likely improve detection of recurrence in the future, but data are still insufficient to warrant substitution of cystoscopic follow-up.[4,22]

PATIENT EDUCATION

- The most important primary prevention for muscle-invasive bladder cancer is to eliminate active and passive smoking.
- Tumor recurrence and progression risk can be estimated from clinical and pathologic factors;[4] this information may help in joint decision-making for primary treatment and follow-up intervals.

PATIENT RESOURCES

- Medline plus. *Bladder Cancer*—**www.nlm.nih.gov/medlineplus/bladdercancer.html.**
- Cancer Research, UK. *Bladder Cancer*—**http://cancerhelp.cancerresearchuk.org/type/bladder-cancer/about/.**
- Macmillan Cancer Support. *Bladder Cancer*—**http://www.macmillan.org.uk/Cancerinformation/Cancertypes/Bladder/Bladdercancer.aspx.**

PROVIDER RESOURCES

- *SEER Cancer Statistics Review*—**http://seer.cancer.gov/statfacts/html/urinb.html.**

REFERENCES

1. *SEER Cancer Statistics Review.* http://seer.cancer.gov/statfacts/html/urinb.html. Accessed November 2011.
2. Scher HI, Motzer RJ. Bladder and renal cell carcinomas. In: Kasper DL, Braunwald E, Fauci AS, Hauser SL, Longo DL, Jameson JL, eds. *Harrison's Principles of Internal Medicine*, 16th ed. New York, NY: McGraw-Hill; 2005:539-540.
3. Sharma S, Ksheersagar P, Sharma P. Diagnosis and treatment of bladder cancer. *Am Fam Physician.* 2009;80(7):717-723.
4. American College of Radiology (ACR), Expert Panel on Urologic Imaging. *ACR Appropriateness Criteria® Pretreatment Staging of Invasive Bladder Cancer (2009).* http://www.guideline.gov/content.aspx?id=43878&search=bladder+cancer. Accessed July 2013.
5. Quilty PM, Kerr GR. Bladder cancer following low or high dose pelvic irradiation. *Clin Radiol.* 1987;38(6):583-585.
6. Band PR, Le ND, MacArthur AC, et al. Identification of occupational cancer risks in British Columbia: a population-based case-control study of 1129 cases of bladder cancer. *J Occup Environ Med.* 2005;47(8):854-858.
7. Villanueva CM, Cantor KP, King WD, et al. Total and specific fluid consumption as determinants of bladder cancer risk. *Int J Cancer.* 2006;118(8):2040-2047.
8. Aben KK, Witjes JA, Schoenberg MP, et al. Familial aggregation of urothelial cell carcinoma. *Int J Cancer.* 2002;98(2):274-278.
9. Gutiérrez Baños JL, Rebollo Rodrigo MH, Antolín Juárez FM, Martín García B. NMP 22, BTA stat test and cytology in the diagnosis of bladder cancer: a comparative study. *Urol Int.* 2001;66(4):185-190.
10. European Association of Urology. *Guidelines on Bladder Cancer: Muscle-Invasive and Metastatic.* http://www.guidelines.gov/content.aspx?id=12524&search=bladder+cancer. Accessed July 2013.
11. Advanced Bladder Cancer Meta-analysis Collaboration. Neoadjuvant chemotherapy for invasive bladder cancer. *Cochrane Database Syst Rev.* 2005 Apr 18;(2):CD005246.
12. Vale CL, Advanced Bladder Cancer Meta-analysis Collaboration. Adjuvant chemotherapy for invasive bladder cancer (individual patient data). *Cochrane Database Syst Rev.* 2006 Apr 19;(2):CD006018.
13. American Urological Association guideline. http://www.guidelines.gov/content.aspx?id=11795&search=bladder+cancer. Accessed July 2013.
14. Shelley MD, Wilt TJ, Court J, et al. Intravesical bacillus Calmette-Guerin is superior to mitomycin C in reducing tumour recurrence in high-risk superficial bladder cancer: a meta-analysis of randomized trials. *BJU Int.* 2004;93(4):485-490.
15. Shelley M, Court JB, Kynaston H, et al. Intravesical bacillus Calmette-Guérin in Ta and T1 bladder cancer. *Cochrane Database Syst Rev.* 2000;(4):CD001986.
16. Shang PF, Kwong J, Wang ZP, et al. Intravesical Bacillus Calmette-Guérin versus epirubicin for Ta and T1 bladder cancer. *Cochrane Database Syst Rev.* 2011 May 11;(5):CD006885.
17. Shelley M, Court JB, Kynaston H, et al. Intravesical bacillus Calmette-Guérin versus mitomycin C for Ta and T1 bladder cancer. *Cochrane Database Syst Rev.* 2003;(3):CD003231.
18. Shelley M, Barber J, Wilt T, Mason M. Surgery versus radiotherapy for muscle invasive bladder cancer. *Cochrane Database Syst Rev.* 2002;(1):CD002079.
19. European Association of Urology. *Guidelines on TaT1 (Non-Muscle Invasive) Bladder Cancer.* http://www.guideline.gov/content.aspx?id=34059. Accessed July 2013.
20. Canadian Cancer Society. http://www.cancer.ca/?Val=E. Accessed July 2013.
21. Ganesan T, Khadra MH, Wallis J, Neal DE. Vitamin B12 malabsorption following bladder reconstruction or diversion with bowel segments. *ANZ J Surg.* 2002;72(7):479-482.
22. Lokeshwar VB, Habuchi T, Grossman HB, et al. Bladder tumor markers beyond cytology: International consensus panel on bladder tumor markers. *Urology.* 2005;66:35-63.

79 HYDRONEPHROSIS

Mindy A. Smith, MD, MS

PATIENT STORY

A 74-year-old man presented with a 2-day history of severe, steady pain radiating down to the lower abdomen and left testicle. He has had urinary frequency, nocturia, hesitancy, and urinary dribbling for several years with slight worsening with time. CT scan revealed left-sided hydronephrosis (**Figure 79-1**). In this patient, an irregular mass was seen at the left ureterovesical junction compressing the bladder. Prostate cancer was found on biopsy.

INTRODUCTION

Hydronephrosis refers to distention of the renal calyces and pelvis of 1 or both kidneys by urine. Hydronephrosis is not a disease but a physical result of urinary blockage that may occur at the level of the kidney, ureters, bladder, or urethra. The condition may be physiologic (eg, occurring in up to 80% of pregnant women) or pathologic.

EPIDEMIOLOGY

- Of acquired causes in adults, pelvic tumors, renal calculi, and urethral stricture predominate.[1] If renal colic is present, renal stone is likely present (90% in 1 study).[2]

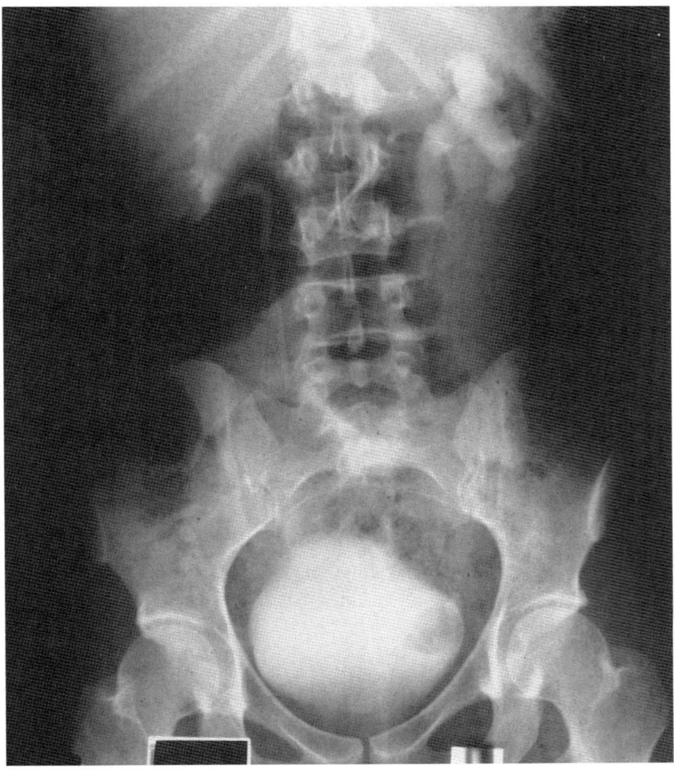

FIGURE 79-1 Intravenous urogram showing left hydronephrosis and hydroureter. (*Reproduced with permission from Schwartz DT, Reisdorff EJ. Emergency Radiology. New York: McGraw-Hill; 2000:540, Figure. 19-45. Copyright 2000.*)

- Hydronephrosis is common in pregnancy because of the compression from the enlarging uterus and functional effects of progesterone.

ETIOLOGY AND PATHOPHYSIOLOGY

- Bilateral hydronephrosis is caused by a blockage to urine flow occurring at or below the level of the bladder or urethra.
- Unilateral hydronephrosis is caused by a blockage to urine flow occurring above the level of the bladder.
- Multiple causes result in this condition including congenital (eg, vesicoureteral reflux [VUR]), acquired intrinsic (eg, calculi, inflammation, and trauma), and acquired extrinsic (eg, pregnancy or uterine leiomyoma, retroperitoneal fibrosis). Within these groupings, obstruction may be a result of mechanical (eg, benign prostatic hypertrophy) or functional (eg, neurogenic bladder) defects.
- Urinary obstruction causes a rise in ureteral pressure leading to declines in glomerular filtration, tubular function (eg, ability to transport sodium and potassium or adjust urine concentration), and renal blood flow.
- If obstruction persists, tubular atrophy and permanent nephron loss can occur.

DIAGNOSIS

A work-up for hydronephrosis in adults is often triggered by the discovery of azotemia (caused by impaired excretory function of sodium, urea, and water). Sudden or new onset of hypertension (because of the increased renin release with unilateral obstruction) may also trigger an investigation. A first step in the evaluation is to perform bladder catheterization. If diuresis occurs, the obstruction is below the bladder neck.

CLINICAL FEATURES

- Pain is the symptom that most commonly leads an adult patient to seek medical attention. This is caused by distention of the collecting system or renal capsule. The pain is often described as severe, steady, and radiating down to the lower abdomen, testicles, or labia. Flank pain with urination is pathognomonic for VUR.
- Disturbed excretory function or difficulty in voiding: Oliguria and anuria are symptoms of complete obstruction whereas polyuria and nocturia occur with partial obstruction (impaired concentrating ability causes osmotic diuresis).
- Fever or dysuria can occur with associated urinary tract infection (UTI).
- The physical examination may reveal distention of the kidney or bladder. Rectal examination may show an enlarged prostate, or rectal/pelvic mass and pelvic examination may reveal an enlarged uterus or pelvic mass.

LABORATORY TESTING

- Urinalysis may show hematuria, pyuria, proteinuria, or bacteruria but the sediment is often normal.[3]
- Assess renal function (blood urea nitrogen [BUN], creatinine).
- Urodynamic testing may be indicated for patients with neurogenic bladder or other suspected bladder causes of hydronephrosis.

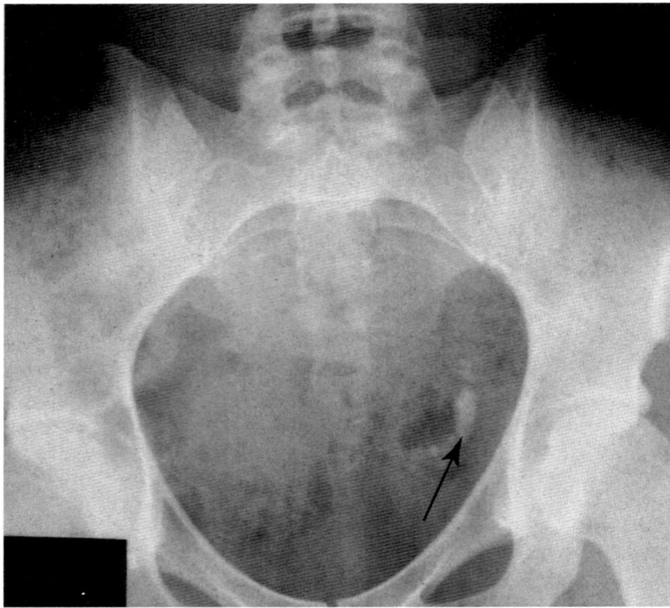

FIGURE 79-2 Large irregular calcification (*arrow*) representing ureterolithiasis in the left side of the pelvis in the patient in **Figure 69-1**. (*Reproduced with permission from Schwartz DT, Reisdorff EJ.* Emergency Radiology. *New York: McGraw-Hill; 2000:539, Figure. 19-43. Copyright 2000.)*

IMAGING

- Ultrasound imaging has a sensitivity and specificity of 90% for identifying the presence of hydronephrosis if no diuresis occurs following bladder catheterization.[4]
- If a source remains unidentified, an IV urogram (**Figures 79-1** and **79-2**) and/or CT scan (**Figure 79-3**) should be obtained to diagnose intraabdominal or retroperitoneal causes.

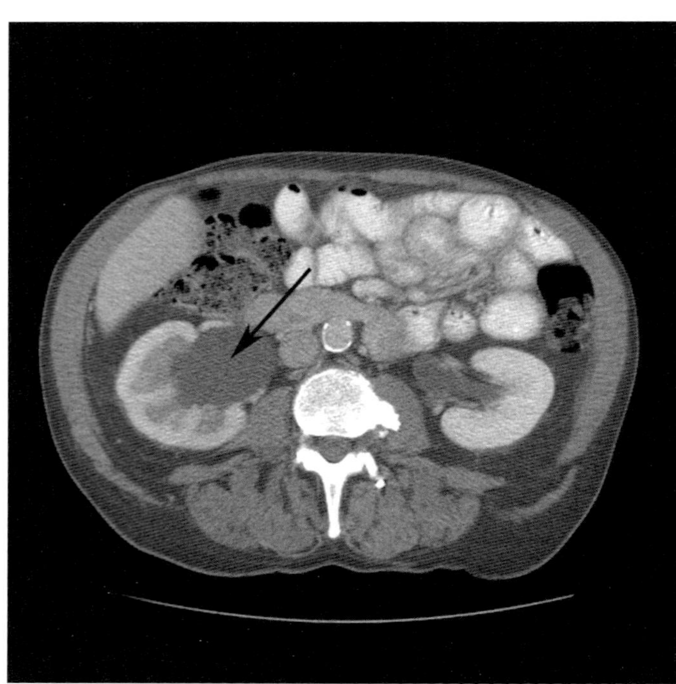

FIGURE 79-3 Right-sided hydronephrosis (arrow) seen on CT. (*Reproduced with permission from Karl T. Rew, MD.)*

- One study of magnetic resonance (MR) pyelography (vs. ultrasound and urography) reported a sensitivity in detecting stones, strictures, and congenital ureteropelvic junction obstructions of 68.9%, 98.5%, and 100%, respectively, with a specificity of 98%.[3] Accuracy regarding the level of obstruction was high (100%).
- Antegrade urography (percutaneous placement of ureteral catheter) or retrograde urography (cystoscopic placement of ureteral catheter) may be needed in patients with azotemia and poor excretory function or in those at high risk of acute renal failure from IV contrast (ie, diabetes, multiple myeloma).
- A voiding cystourethrogram is useful in the diagnosis of VUR and bladder neck and urethral obstructions.

DIFFERENTIAL DIAGNOSIS

Hydronephrosis is usually found during an investigation for symptoms such as flank pain or renal failure. Following are other causes of flank pain:

- Pyelonephritis—Fever, chills, nausea, vomiting, and diarrhea often occurring with or without symptoms of cystitis.
- Cholelithiasis—Pain is more typical in the epigastrium and right upper quadrant (biliary colic) and often nausea and vomiting occurs (see Chapter 69, Gallbladder Disease).
- Other urologic disorders include ureteropelvic junction obstruction, renal subcapsular hematoma, and renal cell carcinoma (see Chapter 85, Renal Cell Carcinoma).

Causes of unexplained renal failure in adults:

- Hypoperfusion (prerenal failure) (see Chapter 86, Renal Failure).
- Acute tubular necrosis (ATN), interstitial, glomerular, or small vessel disease (intrarenal failure).
- Hypoperfusion and ATN account for the majority of cases of acute renal failure.

MANAGEMENT

NONPHARMACOLOGIC

Functional causes can be treated by frequent voiding or catheterization (intermittent preferred). SOR B

MEDICATIONS

- Adult patients with hydronephrosis, complicated by infection, should be treated with appropriate antibiotics for 3 to 4 weeks. Chronic or recurrent unilateral infections may require nephrectomy. SOR A
- Anticholinergic drugs (eg, oxybutynin, tolterodine) are recommended for patients with neurogenic bladder. SOR B

PROCEDURES AND SURGERY

- Hydronephrosis with infection is a urologic emergency that can be treated by prompt drainage using retrograde stent insertion or percutaneous nephrostomy.[4]
- Pyeloplasty is a surgical technique for repairing an obstruction between the ureter and kidney that involves excising the obstructing segment with reanastomosis of the ureter. In 1 review of largely retrospective

data, both open and laparoscopic pyeloplasty had higher success rates than endopyelotomy (94.1% and 95.9%-97.2% vs. 62%-83%, respectively).[5]

- Treatment for VUR includes surgical repair (ureteral reimplantation or ureteroneocystostomy) or endoscopic injection of a bulking agent. Surgical repair reduces rates of pyelonephritis compared to medical treatment, but not UTI or renal scarring.[6]
- Stenting (conventional and metallic) is also used for bypassing ureteral obstruction to alleviate hydronephrosis.[7] The American College of Radiology (ACR) recommends percutaneous antegrade ureteral stenting or percutaneous nephrostomy for afebrile nonanuric patients with acute hydronephrosis.[8] In a septic patient with acute obstruction, ACR recommends urgent percutaneous nephrostomy (preferred) or urgent retrograde ureteral stenting.[8]
- Patients with renal failure can be treated with dialysis (see Chapter 86, Renal Failure). SOR Ⓐ
- Elective surgery for drainage is performed for persistent pain or progressive loss of renal function. SOR Ⓒ

PREVENTION AND SCREENING

The prevalence of VUR in siblings of an index case is 27.4% and in offspring 35.7%; severe reflux is identified in approximately 10% of screened patients.[9] Because of the lack of randomized controlled trials of treated versus untreated screened siblings with VUR regarding health outcomes, the best screening strategy is not known.

PROGNOSIS

Prognosis depends on the underlying etiology.

FOLLOW-UP

- Prognosis for an adult patient depends on the duration and completeness of the obstruction and associated complications like infection; complete obstruction for 1 to 2 weeks may be followed by partial return of renal function, but after 8 weeks, recovery is unlikely.[1]
- Postobstructive diuresis can cause loss of sodium, potassium, and magnesium that may require replacement in the setting of hypovolemia, hypotension, or electrolyte imbalance.

PATIENT EDUCATION

Education regarding VUR should include a discussion of the treatment rationale, treatment approaches, and likely adherence with the care plan.

PATIENT RESOURCES

- National Kidney Foundation (800-622-9010) or **www. kidney.org.**
- National Institutes of Health, MedlinePlus. *Bilateral Hydronephrosis*—**http://www.nlm.nih.gov/medlineplus/ency/article/000474.htm.**

PROVIDER RESOURCES

- Lusaya DG, Lerma EV. *Hydronephrosis and Hydroureter*—**http://emedicine.medscape.com/article/436259.**
- Vatakencherry G, Funaki BS, Ray CE Jr, et al; Expert Panel on Interventional Radiology. *ACR Appropriateness Criteria® Treatment of Urinary Tract Obstruction*. [online publication]. Reston, VA: ACR; 2010. 7 p. **http://www.guideline.gov/content.aspx?id=23819**.

REFERENCES

1. Seifter JL, Brenner BM. Urinary tract obstruction. In: Kasper DL, Braunwald E, Fauci AS, Hauser SL, Longo DL, Jameson JL, eds. *Harrison's Principles of Internal Medicine*, 16th ed. New York, NY: McGraw-Hill; 2005:1722-1724.
2. Pepe P, Motta L, Pennisi M, Aragona F. Functional evaluation of the urinary tract by color-Doppler ultrasonography (CDU) in 100 patients with renal colic. *Eur J Radiol.* 2005;53(1):131-135.
3. Blandino A, Gaeta M, Minutoli F, et al. MR pyelography in 115 patients with a dilated renal collecting system. *Acta Radiol.* 2001;42(5): 532-536.
4. Ramsey S, Robertson A, Ablett MJ, et al. Evidence-based drainage of infected hydronephrosis secondary to ureteric calculi. *J Endourol.* 2010;24(2):185-189.
5. Gallo F, Schenone M, Giberti C. Ureteropelvic junction obstruction: which is the best treatment today? *J Laparoendosc Adv Surg Tech A.* 2009; 19(5):657-652.
6. Estrada CR, Cendron M. *Vesicoureteral Reflux Treatment and Management*. http://emedicine.medscape.com/article/439403-treatment#a1128. Accessed January 2012.
7. Modi AP, Ritch CR, Arend D, et al. Multicenter experience with metallic ureteral stents for malignant and chronic benign ureteral obstruction. *J Endourol.* 2010;24(7):1189-1193.
8. Vatakencherry G, Funaki BS, Ray CE Jr; Expert Panel on Interventional Radiology. *ACR Appropriateness Criteria®; Treatment of Urinary Tract Obstruction* [online publication]. Reston, VA: American College of Radiology; 2010. 7 p. http://www.guideline.gov/content.aspx?id=23819&search=hydronephrosis. Accessed January 2012.
9. Skoog SJ, Peters CA, Arant BS Jr, et al. Pediatric Vesicoureteral Reflux Guidelines Panel summary report: clinical practice guidelines for screening siblings of children with vesicoureteral reflux and neonates/infants with prenatal hydronephrosis. *J Urol.* 2010;184(3): 1145-1151.

80 KIDNEY STONES

Karl T. Rew, MD
Mindy A. Smith, MD, MS

PATIENT STORY

A 55-year-old woman presents with severe pain in the right flank. The pain began suddenly after supper and increased dramatically over the next hour. Urinalysis shows blood but no signs of infection. Abdominal X-ray reveals bilateral renal stones (**Figure 80-1**). A noncontrast CT scan confirms multiple bilateral renal stones, with an obstructing right distal ureteral stone and enlargement of the right kidney (**Figure 80-2**). She is subsequently found to have hyperparathyroidism, which is the cause of her multiple stones.

INTRODUCTION

A kidney stone is a solid mass that forms when minerals crystallize and collect in the urinary tract. Kidney stones can cause pain and hematuria and may lead to complications such as urinary tract obstruction and infection.

SYNONYMS

Kidney stone, nephrolithiasis, renal calculus, renal stone, urinary tract stone, ureterolithiasis, and urolithiasis.

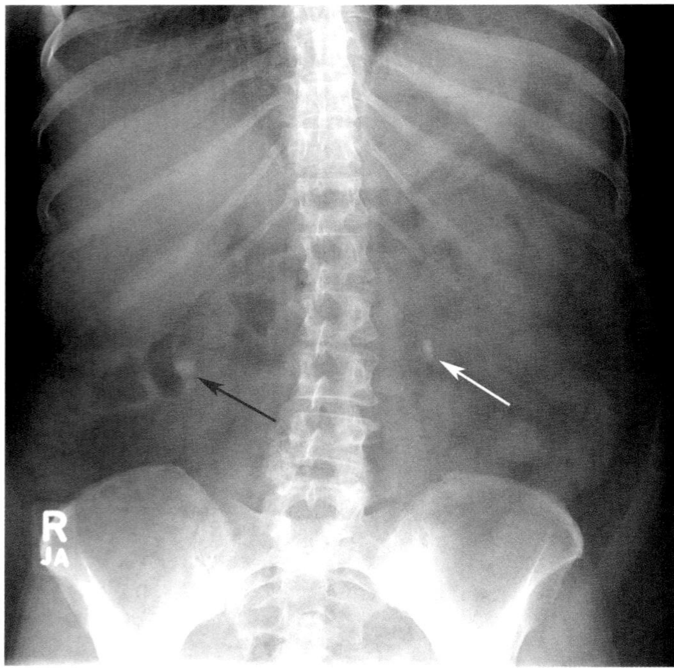

FIGURE 80-1 Plain X-ray of the abdomen in a 55-year-old woman showing several stones in the right kidney (*red arrow*) and a large left ureteral stone (*white arrow*) adjacent to the L2-L3 disc space. (*Reproduced with permission from Karl T. Rew, MD.*)

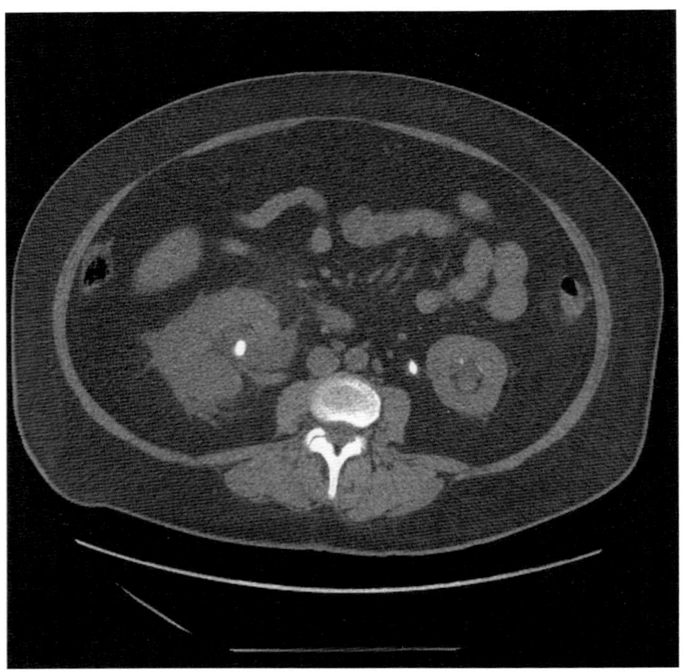

FIGURE 80-2 Noncontrast CT of the abdomen and pelvis of the same woman showing several of the stones seen in **Figure 80-1**, including a nonobstructing stone in the interpolar region of the right kidney. Because the right ureter is obstructed by a distal stone (not visible on this image), the right kidney is enlarged, with collecting system dilation and perinephric stranding. The large left proximal ureteral stone seen in this image is only partially obstructing, causing mild dilation in the left kidney collecting system. Several small stones are visible in the left kidney, and the left kidney is somewhat atrophied from chronic obstruction. (*Reproduced with permission from Karl T. Rew, MD.*)

EPIDEMIOLOGY

- The prevalence of kidney stones is increasing in the United States.[1] More than 5% of adults have kidney stone disease, with a lifetime risk of 13% for men and 7% for women.
- Men between the ages of 40 and 60 years have the highest risk of stones; for women, the risk peaks in their 50s.[2]
- African Americans have a lower rate of kidney stones than white Americans.[1]
- Calcium oxalate and calcium phosphate stones are the most common, occurring in 75% to 85% of patients. Struvite (magnesium ammonium phosphate) stones occur in 5% of cases. Uric acid stones occur in 5% to 10% of patients and cystine stones occur in 1% of cases. Other types of stones are less common.[3]
- Calcium stones are more common in men than in women (ratio 2:1), whereas struvite stones are more common in women than in men (ratio 3:1).[3]

ETIOLOGY AND PATHOPHYSIOLOGY

- Kidney stones form when there is supersaturation of otherwise soluble materials, usually from increased excretion of these compounds or dehydration. Urine pH is a factor in stone formation because urinary phosphate increases in alkaline urine, whereas uric acid predominates in acidic urine (pH <5.5). Higher urine citrate can decrease stone formation.

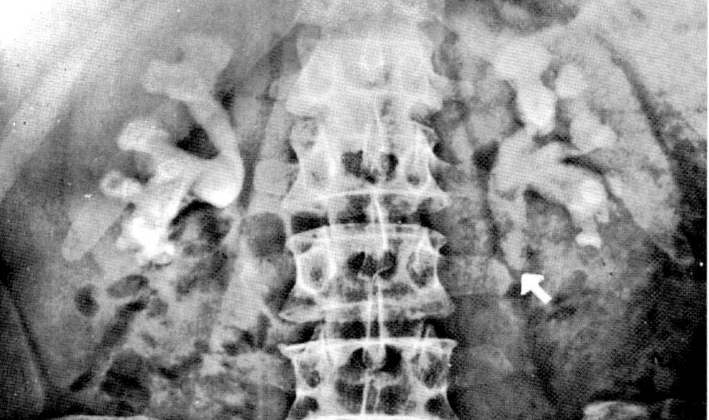

FIGURE 80-3 Bilateral staghorn calculi. (*Reproduced with permission from Doherty GM. Current Surgical Diagnosis and Treatment; Figure 40-17, p. 1023. Copyright 2006, McGraw-Hill.*)

- Struvite stones are caused by infection with urea-splitting bacteria, mainly *Proteus*.
- Uric acid stones form in patients with gout or hyperuricemia caused by other causes, including myeloproliferative disorders, chemotherapy, and Lesch-Nyhan syndrome.
- Cystine stones occur in patients with an inherited defect of dibasic amino acid transport.
- Struvite, cystine, and uric acid stones can grow large, filling the renal pelvis, and extending into the calyces to form staghorn calculi (see **Figure 80-3**).

RISK FACTORS

Infections, genetic defects, and certain drugs can increase the risk of stones, but most stones are idiopathic. Risk factors vary with type of stone, which are as follows:

- Calcium stones are more likely in patients who are obese[4] and in those with diets higher in animal protein, salt, and oxalate-containing foods. Contrary to popular belief, calcium in the diet does not lead to calcium stones; in fact, calcium supplementation can prevent calcium stones by trapping oxalate in the gastrointestinal (GI) tract.
- Patients with poor urinary drainage or indwelling catheters are at risk for *Proteus* urinary tract infections (UTIs) and struvite stones.
- Uric acid stones are associated with acidic urine, which is more common in obese patients with metabolic syndrome and insulin resistance, and in patients with chronic diarrhea.

DIAGNOSIS

CLINICAL FEATURES

- Kidney stones are often asymptomatic. Stone passage into the ureter usually causes pain and hematuria. The pain of renal colic typically begins suddenly in the ipsilateral flank or abdomen and progresses in waves, gradually increasing in intensity over the next 20 to 60 minutes. As the stone moves downward, pain may be felt in the ipsilateral groin, testis, or vulva.
- Obstructing stones cause hydronephrosis, with an associated constant dull flank pain. Stones in the bladder may cause frequency, urgency, dysuria, or recurrent UTIs.

LABORATORY

- Urinalysis usually reveals microscopic hematuria and limited pyuria. Gross hematuria is possible.
- Because treatment depends on stone type, stone capture and analysis is recommended SOR Ⓒ.
- Additional work-up is recommended for adults with recurrent stones and for children with a first stone.[1] This includes a 24-hour urine collection for pH, volume, oxalate, and citrate, with simultaneous serum tests for calcium, uric acid, electrolytes, and creatinine. In patients with elevated serum calcium, parathyroid hormone (PTH) should be measured.

IMAGING

- Plain abdominal X-ray will demonstrate most calcium, struvite, and cystine stones. It is recommended for patients with a prior radiopaque stone (**Figure 80-1**).
- Noncontrast helical CT (**Figures 80-4** and **80-5**) has largely replaced intravenous urography for patients with a suspected urinary tract stone because it is rapid, exposes patients to less radiation, requires no contrast, and may provide clues to diagnoses outside the urinary system. Although uric acid stones are radiolucent, they often can be detected with CT.
- Ultrasound can be used to monitor uric acid stones (typically radiolucent), to assess hydronephrosis, or to avoid using X-rays in pregnant women. Ultrasound also may provide clues to diagnoses outside the urinary system.

DIFFERENTIAL DIAGNOSIS

Other causes of flank and lower pelvic/groin pain include the following:

- Gynecologic conditions in women (ovarian torsion, cyst, or ectopic pregnancy)—These can often be distinguished on ultrasound. Pelvic

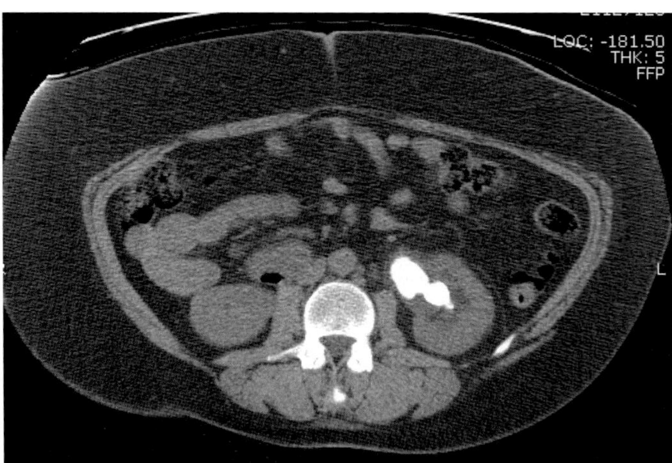

FIGURE 80-4 An unenhanced CT performed on a 49-year-old woman with known renal stones reveals a large left staghorn calculus. The striated appearance of the left renal cortex is seen in obstruction, infection, and ischemia. (*Reproduced with permission from Michael Freckleton, MD.*)

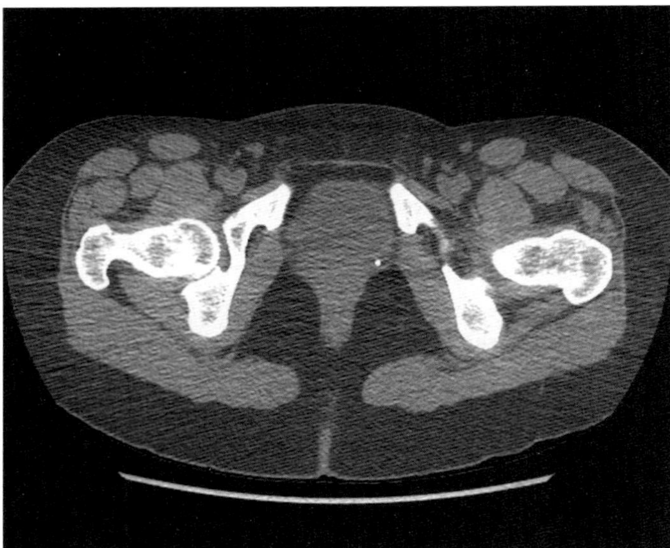

FIGURE 80-5 Noncontrast CT of the abdomen and pelvis in a 33-year-old woman showing a 3-mm obstructing stone in the distal ureter, just proximal to the ureterovesical junction. (*Reproduced with permission from Karl T. Rew, MD.*)

inflammatory disease can also present with pain and is diagnosed based on clinical examination and culture.

- In men, epididymitis, prostatitis, or testicular torsion may cause pain that can be confused with kidney stones. Testicular tumors rarely cause pain. Physical examination can help differentiate these conditions.
- Cholelithiasis—Biliary colic is usually described as a steady, severe pain or ache, usually of sudden onset, located in the epigastrium or right upper quadrant (RUQ) (see Chapter 69, Gallbladder Disease). RUQ tenderness may be elicited on physical examination and ultrasound usually shows stones in the gallbladder.
- Urologic disorders include ureteropelvic junction obstruction, renal subcapsular hematoma, and renal cell carcinoma (see Chapter 85, Renal Cell Carcinoma). Imaging assists in differentiating these from kidney stones.

Abdominal pain from renal stones may be confused with the following:

- Colitis, appendicitis, and diverticulitis—Systemic symptoms such as fever are often seen. Symptoms of colitis include diarrhea, rectal bleeding, tenesmus (ie, urgency with a feeling of incomplete evacuation), passage of mucus, and cramping abdominal pain (see Chapter 77, Inflammatory Bowel Disease). GI symptoms with kidney stones are limited to nausea and vomiting from stimulation of the celiac plexus.
- Peptic ulcer disease—Epigastric pain is the hallmark, along with dyspeptic symptoms (see Chapter 76, Peptic Ulcer Disease). Stool antigen test can confirm *Helicobacter pylori* infection. Upper endoscopy is the preferred procedure for diagnosing ulcers.
- Abdominal aortic aneurysm—Peak incidence is later, usually in the sixth and seventh decades (see Chapter 41, Aortic Aneurysms). Pain is described as severe and tearing localized to the front or back of the chest and associated with diaphoresis. Syncope and weakness may also occur.

Stones within the bladder may mimic UTI. Helpful indictors of UTI are a urine dipstick positive for nitrates (positive likelihood ratio [LR+] 26.5) and urinary sediment showing 10 or more bacteria/high-power field (LR+ 85).

Hematuria is also seen in patients with infection (eg, UTI, sexually transmitted infection, schistosomiasis), cancer of the bladder (see Chapter 78, Bladder Cancer) or kidney (see Chapter 85, Renal Cell Carcinoma), renal disease (glomerulonephritis, immunoglobulin [Ig] A nephropathy, lupus nephritis, hemolytic uremic syndrome), in men with prostatitis, benign prostatic hypertrophy, or prostate cancer (see Chapter 83, Prostate Cancer), or following trauma.

MANAGEMENT

NONPHARMACOLOGIC

- Adequate fluid intake is essential—2 to 3 L of water per day for most patients.[5] SOR B
- Stones smaller than 5 mm are likely to pass spontaneously. About three-fourths of distal ureteral stones and about half of proximal ureteral stones will pass spontaneously. The 3-mm distal ureteral stone shown in **Figure 80-3** passed spontaneously.

MEDICATIONS

- Medical expulsive therapy with α-adrenergic blockers (such as tamsulosin) or calcium-channel blockers can increase the chance of stone passage.[6] SOR B
- Effective pain control should be provided using NSAIDs and narcotics if needed. NSAIDs may need to be avoided if planning lithotripsy because of increased risk of perinephric bleeding.

COMPLEMENTARY AND ALTERNATIVE THERAPY

For prevention of struvite stones, urine can be acidified with cranberry juice.[5] Other supplements have been suggested as potentially protective against renal stones, but study results are conflicting.

PROCEDURES

Stones that do not pass spontaneously or with medical expulsive therapy can be treated with lithotripsy or removed via ureteroscopy. Large stones may require percutaneous nephrolithotomy (PCNL) or open surgery.

REFERRAL

Urgent urologic consultation is recommended for patients with stones and urosepsis, anuria, or renal failure. Urologic consultation is recommended for patients with refractory pain and nausea, extremes of age, major comorbidities, and stones larger than 5 mm. SOR C

Indications for operative intervention:

- Infection
- Persistent symptoms of flank pain, nausea, and vomiting
- Failure to pass a ureteral stone after an appropriate trial of observation (2-4 weeks)

PREVENTION

- Foods high in oxalate should be avoided by those who form calcium oxalate stones, including Rhubarb, Spinach, Swiss Chard, Beets, Apricots, Figs, Kiwi, many soy products, chocolate, and many nuts and seeds.

- Uric acid stones are prevented with allopurinol and a low-purine diet. High-purine foods to avoid include most fish, shellfish, and meats (especially game meats and organ meats), and protein supplements such as brewer's yeast.
- Low-calcium diets should not be used in patients with calcium stones. A low-calcium diet can increase stone formation and lower bone mineral density.

Additional treatments may be warranted based on the type of stone:

- Patients with recurrent calcium-containing stones caused by idiopathic hypercalciuria can be treated with a thiazide diuretic (reduces recurrence by 50% over 3 years). Hypokalemia should be avoided; low potassium reduces urinary citrate.
- Idiopathic stone disease can be treated with fluids and potassium citrate (2 g/day).
- For cystine stones, increasing fluid intake, alkalinizing the urine to a pH ≥7.5, and a low-sodium diet are recommended. D-Penicillamine has also been used.

PROGNOSIS

- Half of the patients with a first calcium-containing stone have a recurrence within 10 years. Twenty-five percent of struvite stones recur if there was incomplete removal of the stone.
- Long-term complications are uncommon. The proportion of nephrolithiasis-related end-stage renal disease (ESRD) appears small (3.2%).

FOLLOW-UP

A follow-up consultation to discuss kidney stone prevention is important for all patients with an initial stone. Patients started on medical therapy should be reevaluated with a 24-hour urine in 3 months. Those with a history of recurrent stones should be seen at least annually.

PATIENT EDUCATION

Maintaining water intake of at least 2 to 3 L/day (to keep urine specific gravity around 1.005) is recommended for most patients as this fluid level has been shown to reduce recurrences by half. Dietary information is available (see "Patient Resources" box).

PATIENT RESOURCES

- National Kidney and Urologic Diseases Information Clearinghouse. *Kidney Stones in Adults*—**http://kidney.niddk.nih.gov/Kudiseases/pubs/stonesadults/.**
- National Kidney and Urologic Diseases Information Clearinghouse. *Diet for Kidney Stone Prevention*—**http://kidney.niddk.nih.gov/kudiseases/pubs/kidneystonediet/.**
- *The Oxalate Content of Food*—**http://www.ohf.org/docs/Oxalate2008.pdf.**

PROVIDER RESOURCES

- American Urologic Association. *2007 Guideline for the Management of Ureteral Calculi*—**http://www.auanet.org/education/guidelines/ureteral-calculi.cfm.**
- European Association of Urology. *Guidelines on Urolithiasis*, update March 2011—**http://www.uroweb.org/gls/pdf/18_Urolithiasis.pdf.**

REFERENCES

1. Worcester EM, Coe FL. Calcium kidney stones. *N Engl J Med*. 2010; 363:954-963.
2. Curhan GC. Epidemiology of stone disease. *Urol Clin North Am*. 2007; 34(3):287-293.
3. Asplin JR, Coe FL, Favus MJ. Nephrolithiasis. In: Longo DL, Fauci AS, Kasper DL, Hauser SL, Jameson JL, Loscalzo J, eds. *Harrison's Principles of Internal Medicine*, 18th ed. New York, NY: McGraw-Hill; 2012. http://www.accessmedicine.com/content.aspx?aID=9131116. Accessed December 28, 2011.
4. Taylor EN, Stampfer MJ, Curhan GC. Obesity, weight gain, and the risk of kidney stones. *JAMA*. 2005;293(4):455-462.
5. Frasetto L, Kohlstadt I. Treatment and prevention of kidney stones: an update. *Am Fam Physician*. 2011;84(11):1234-1242.
6. Hollingsworth JM, Rogers MA, Kaufman SR, et al. Medical therapy to facilitate urinary stone passage: a metaanalysis. *Lancet*. 2006;368: 1171-1179.

81 NEPHROTIC SYNDROME

Gary Ferenchick, MD

PATIENT STORY

A 45-year-old male with a long-standing history of type 1 diabetes mellitus (DM) presents to the hospital with a 40-pound weight gain and new onset of peripheral edema over the past 5 weeks. He denies dyspnea, orthopnea, and all cardiorespiratory symptoms. His examination reveals a blood pressure of 154/92 mm Hg, 4+ peripheral edema, and anasarca as manifested by pitting edema when palpating his abdominal wall and leg (**Figures 81-1** and **81-2**). His urinalysis reveals 4+ proteinuria, his serum albumin is 1.8 mg/dL, and his creatinine clearance is calculated at 28 mL/min. A subsequent renal biopsy reveals glomerulosclerosis attributable to diabetic nephropathy.

INTRODUCTION

Nephrotic syndrome (NS) represents the end result of many conditions of complex and diverse etiology that are all characterized by significant albuminuria, leading to edema, hypoalbuminemia, and commonly hyperlipidemia.

EPIDEMIOLOGY

The incidence of NS is approximately 3 new cases per 100,000 per year.

ETIOLOGY/PATHOPHYSIOLOGY

- Increased glomerular permeability to albumin (among other plasma proteins) is the primary pathological process regardless of the etiology of NS.
- Edema is the manifestation of hypoalbuminemia caused by renal albumin losses that exceed the liver's capacity to compensate with increased albumin synthesis.
- Primary NS
    - Idiopathic membranous nephropathy (33% overall, but the most common etiology in white patients and the most important cause of NS in patients > 65 years old)
    - Focal segmental glomerulosclerosis (35% overall, but up to 57% of NS cases among patients of African descent)
    - Minimal-change disease and immunoglobulin (Ig) A nephropathy (25%)
- Secondary NS
    - Diabetes (the most common cause of NS in the United States)
    - Amyloid (consider in older patients with otherwise-unexplained NS)
    - Systemic lupus erythematosus (SLE)
    - Myeloma
    - Medications (eg, nonsteroidal anti-inflammatory drugs [NSAIDs], lithium, interferon-alfa)

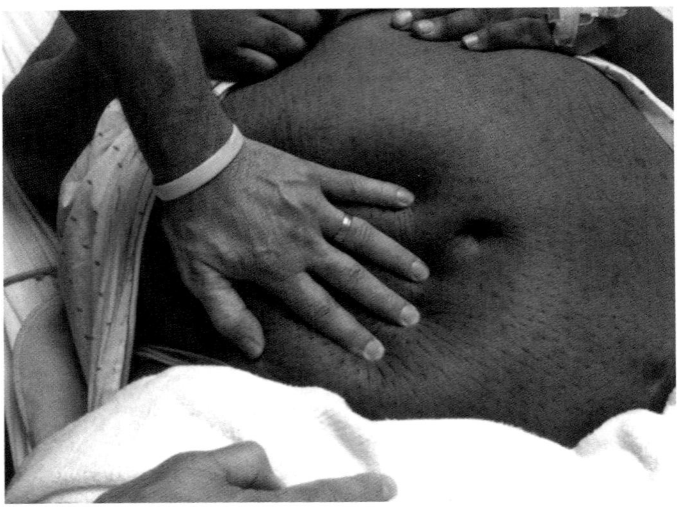

A

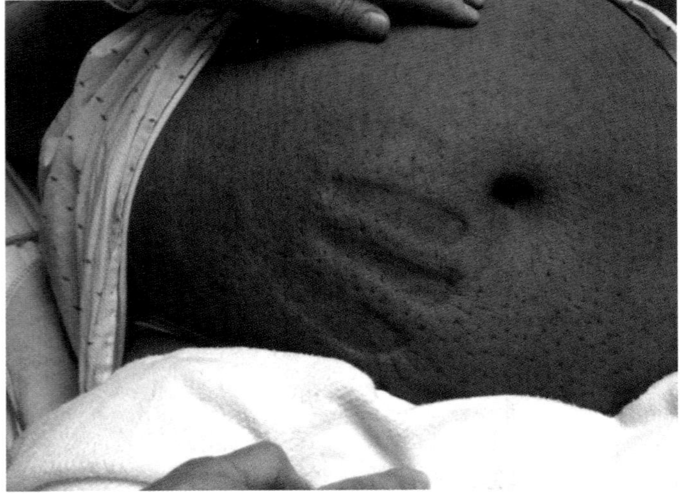

B

FIGURE 81-1 Palpation of this patient's abdominal wall (A) during the course of an abdominal examination resulted in abdominal wall pitting edema as exemplified by the examiner's hand imprint (B). This patient presented with a several-month history of increasing lower-extremity edema and a several-year history of untreated and poorly controlled type II diabetes mellitus. In the course of his workup, a renal biopsy confirmed a diagnosis of diabetic renal disease. Also, note the peau d'orange change of the skin of the abdominal wall caused by the massive subcutaneous edema from this patient's nephrotic syndrome. (*Reproduced with permission from Gary Ferenchick, MD.*)

    - Infections (eg, human immunodeficiency virus [HIV], hepatitis B and C, syphilis)
    - Congenital etiologies (eg, Alport syndrome)

DIAGNOSIS/SCREENING

HISTORY/SYMPTOMS

Specifically ask about the following:

- New onset of edema (the key clinical feature of NS)
    - Periorbital edema
    - Lower-extremity edema
    - Abdominal wall edema (**Figures 81-1** and **81-2**)

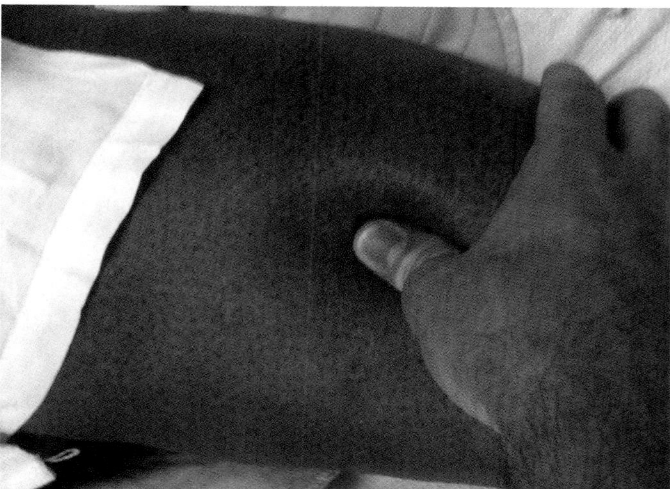

A

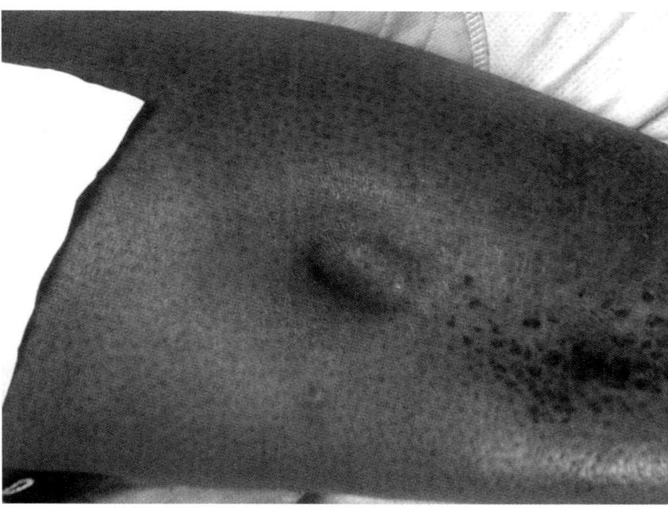

B

FIGURE 81-2 These photos show the severe peripheral edema in the left pretibial area of the same patient as in Figure 81-1 presenting with nephrotic syndrome from diabetic nephropathy. Compression with the thumb (A) leaves an impressive thumbprint in the edematous tissue (B). (*Reproduced with permission from Gary Ferenchick, MD.*)

- Ascites
- Scrotal edema

• Weight gain and fatigue

• Medications (including NSAIDs)

• Symptoms of, or risk factors for, acute or **chronic infections** (eg, HIV, hepatitis B and C, syphilis), including being rejected as a blood donor, known history of a sexually transmitted disease, high-risk sexual behavior, injection drug use, mild right upper quadrant pain, fatigue

• Symptoms suggestive of **systemic disease**
  - Neuropathy or visual changes of DM—Diabetic retinopathy is present in the majority of type 1 diabetic patients with nephropathy; therefore, if a diabetic patient presents with NS and has no retinopathy, a nondiabetic cause of NS should be sought.[1]
  - Photosensitivity rash and arthralgias which might suggest SLE.
  - Symptoms or signs of chronic infectious hepatitis, including a recognized history of jaundice or elevated liver tests.
  - Symptoms and signs of malignancy (especially bowel and lung as these have an association with membranous nephropathy).

PHYSICAL EXAMINATION

Specifically look for or establish the following:

• The presence of periorbital or lower-extremity edema (**Figures 81-3** and **81-4**); in severe cases, anasarca may be present with edema of the scrotum and abdominal wall and the presence of ascites.

• The presence of xanthomas or xanthelasma (**Figures 81-3** and **81-4**, respectively). Xanthelasma consists of yellow lipid-laden deposits on the eyelids in some patients with hyperlipidemia. However, 50% of people with xanthelasma have normal lipids.
  - Xanthomas are yellow, pink, or brown papules and plaques that can erupt on the skin of people with very high lipid levels.
  - Although the NS causes hyperlipidemia, it does not necessarily lead to xanthomas and xanthelasma.
  - NS should be considered in the differential diagnosis of any patient with the skin findings and hyperlipidemia (see Chapter 223, Hyperlipidemia).
  - Cardiomyopathy, peripheral neuropathy, and hepatomegaly suggesting amyloidosis.
  - Pulmonary findings of a pleural effusion.
  - Cutaneous findings of chronic liver disease.

LABORATORY TESTING

• Proteinuria above 3 g in a 24-hour period or spot urine protein:creatinine (mg/mg) ratio of 3 represents nephrotic-range proteinuria. Note that recent iodinated contrast studies interfere with urinary protein determination.

• Urinalysis is used to assess for hematuria, which if present would suggest *glomerulonephritis*, and to assess for the presence of a urinary tract infection.

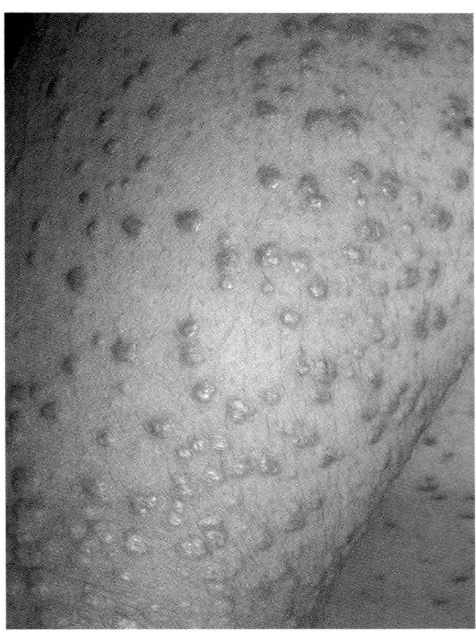

FIGURE 81-3 Eruptive xanthomas in a man with very high triglycerides and cholesterol. Although nephrotic syndrome can cause this, there are other causes of severe hyperlipidemia than can lead to eruptive xanthomas. (*Reproduced with permission from Richard P. Usatine, MD.*)

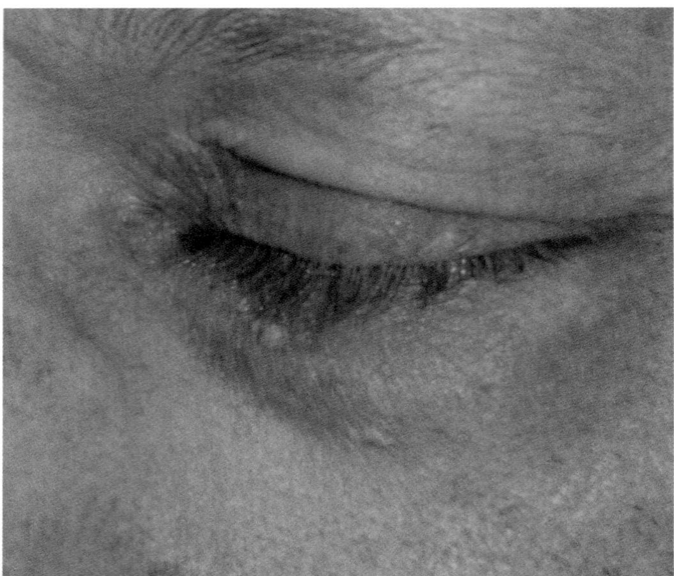

FIGURE 81-4 Xanthelasma in a patient with marked hypercholesterolemia. Hypercholesterolemia is not specific for nephrotic syndrome; however, most patients with nephrotic syndrome have hypercholesterolemia, and most should be strongly considered for statin therapy. (*Reproduced with permission from Gary Ferenchick, MD.*)

- Serum albumin less than 2.5 gm/dL is common is patients with NS.
- Serum lipids should be evaluated as total cholesterol levels above 300 mg/dL are present in 53% of patients.[2]
- Serum urea nitrogen (BUN), creatinine level, and glomerular filtration rate (GFR) assess for renal failure.
- Tests can assess for potential systemic etiologies of NS, including
  - Urine microscopy for red blood cells (which, if present, suggest glomerulonephritis) and to assess for the presence of infection
  - Liver function tests to help identify the presence of hepatitis
  - Specific tests for hepatitis B and C and HIV
  - Glucose and hemoglobin A_{1c} (HbA_{1c}) to assess for the presence, or degree, of glucose intolerance
  - C-reactive protein and sedimentation rate, although nonspecific, to screen for the presence of systemic inflammatory conditions
  - Antinuclear antibodies (ANA) (and follow-up anti-Smith antibody and anti-double-stranded DNA (anti-dsDNA) if the ANA value is positive)
  - Serum and urine electrophoresis to identify multiple myeloma or amyloid
- Renal biopsy alters management 85% of the time.[3]

IMAGING

- Chest radiography to assess for the presence of a pleural effusion
- Echocardiogram to assess for the presence of a pericardial effusion
- Renal ultrasound for renal size and shape
- Doppler of renal veins if flank pain and hematuria are present to assess for renal vein thrombosis

DIFFERENTIAL DIAGNOSIS

- Congestive heart failure (CHF) is a primary differential diagnosis in patients presenting with edema. Commonly, such patients have a history of known cardiovascular disease and other findings of cardiac compromise, such as pulmonary congestive symptoms and signs of reduced ventricular compliance, such as and S_3 or S_4 and abnormal echocardiogram.
- Hypoalbuminemia can be a manifestation of severe chronic liver disease and can be differentiated from NS by other stigmata of chronic liver disease, the presence of portal hypertension, abnormal tests of liver function, and abnormal hepatic imaging.

MANAGEMENT

LONG-TERM MANAGEMENT

- Edema management (goal weight loss of 0.5 kg per day).
  - Sodium restriction (<3 g a day).
  - Restricted fluid intake (<1.5 L a day).
  - Loop diuretics initiated in a stepwise slow fashion to limit the potential for hypovolemia.
  - Sequential nephron blockade may be appropriate for patients resistant to the use of a loop diuretic (combination of a loop diuretic and aldosterone antagonist with or without addition of thiazide).[4]
  - Diuretics may need to be given intravenously initially as gut wall edema may limit absorption of oral diuretics.
- The majority of patients with NS, regardless of etiology, face the prospect of continued heavy protein loss, which can be associated with metabolic and immunologic disorders.[4]
- Treat proteinuria with angiotensin-converting enzyme (ACE) inhibitors or angiotensin II receptor antagonists.[4-6] SOR Ⓐ
  - Aggressive antihypertensive treatment in patients with type 2 diabetes with nephrotic-range albuminuria with ACE inhibitors or angiotensin II receptor blockers is associated with a 66% improved survival rate and 66% decreased risk of progression to end-stage renal disease in patients achieving a decrease in albuminuria from 2.5 g per day to less than 600 mg per day in response to therapy.[7] SOR Ⓒ
- Treat hyperlipidemia with a statin.[8] SOR Ⓒ
- Advise normal protein intake.[4] SOR Ⓒ
- Assess bone mineral density and treat if osteoporosis is present (T < -2.5) or if the patient is osteopenic with a 10-year risk of hip fracture greater than 3% or a 10-year risk of any osteoporotic fracture of greater than 10%.
- Consider corticosteroids.[9] SOR Ⓑ

PROGNOSIS/CLINICAL COURSE

Major complications of NS

- Venous thrombosis is a result of antithrombotic factors being filtered through the glomeruli, producing an imbalance between procoagulant and anticoagulant factors.
  - Greatest risk for venous thrombosis is within the first 6 months of NS diagnosis.
  - NS is associated with elevated procoagulant fibrinogen and factors V and VII and is associated with a decrease in fibrinolysis and anticoagulant factor antithrombin III.[4]
  - Greatest risk is in patients with a serum albumin of <2.5 mg/dl
    - Lower-extremity deep vein thrombosis (DVT) occurs in 1.5% of patients with NS.

- Renal vein thrombosis occurs in 0.5% of patients with NS.
- However, rates of thromboembolism as high as 35% have been reported, with the highest risk in patients with membranous nephropathy.[10]
- Patients with NS at high risk for thromboembolism (albumin <2.5 mg/dL, bed rest, membranous nephropathy, and clinical hypovolemia) should be considered for prophylactic anticoagulation with heparin during periods of enforced bed rest or systemic anticoagulation[11] if serum albumin is persistently less than 2 g/dL.

- Infection (cellulitis, bacterial pneumonia) occurs partly as a result of loss of protective IgG and complement levels and reduced T-cell function.
- Patients with NS should be given the pneumococcal vaccine.
- Loss of vitamin D produces bone disease.

FOLLOW-UP

- Assess the patient's GFR and the amount of proteinuria using the protein-creatinine ratio every 3 months initially, then every 4 to 6 months thereafter in stable patients.
- Monitor patients for worsening GFR, infections, venous thromboembolism, cytopenias in patients on immunosuppressive therapy, and bone mineral density in patients on glucocorticoids.

PATIENT EDUCATION

Educate patients on the potential adverse effects of their medications, the potential complications of NS, and their expected clinical course.

PATIENT RESOURCES

- National Institute of Diabetes and Digestive and Kidney Diseases. *Nephrotic Syndrome in Adults.*—**http://kidney.niddk.nih.gov/kudiseases/pubs/nephrotic/.**
- National Kidney Foundation. *Nephrotic Syndrome*—**http://www.kidney.org/atoz/content/nephrotic.cfm.**

PROVIDER RESOURCES

- Medscape. *Nephrotic Syndrome*—**http://emedicine.medscape.com/article/244631.**

REFERENCES

1. Parving HH, Hommel E, Mathiesen E, et al. Prevalence of microalbuminuria, arterial hypertension, retinopathy and neuropathy in patients with insulin dependent diabetes. *Br Med J (Clin Res Ed).* 1988;296(6616):156-160.
2. Radhakrishnan J, Appel AS, Valeri A, Appel GB. The nephrotic syndrome, lipids, and risk factors for cardiovascular disease. *Am J Kidney Dis.* 1993;22(1):135-142.
3. Richards NT, Darby S, Howie AJ, Adu D, Michael J. Knowledge of renal histology alters patient management in over 40% of cases. *Nephrol Dial Transplant.* 1994;9(9):1255-1259.
4. Charlesworth JA, Gracey DM, Pussell BA. Adult nephrotic syndrome: non-specific strategies for treatment. *Nephrology (Carlton).* 2008;13(1):45-50.
5. Korbet SM. Angiotensin antagonists and steroids in the treatment of focal segmental glomerulosclerosis. *Semin Nephrol.* 2003;23(2):219-228.
6. Ruggenenti P, Mosconi L, Vendramin G, et al. ACE inhibition improves glomerular size selectivity in patients with idiopathic membranous nephropathy and persistent nephrotic syndrome. *Am J Kidney Dis.* 2000;35(3):381-391.
7. Rossing K, Christensen PK, Hovind P, et al. Remission of nephrotic-range albuminuria reduces risk of end-stage renal disease and improves survival in type 2 diabetic patients. *Diabetologia.* 2005;48(11):2241-2247.
8. Thomas ME, Harris KP, Ramaswamy C, et al. Simvastatin therapy for hypercholesterolemic patients with nephrotic syndrome or significant proteinuria. *Kidney Int.* 1993;44(5):1124-1129.
9. Crook ED, Habeeb D, Gowdy O, et al. Effects of steroids in focal segmental glomerulosclerosis in a predominantly African-American population. *Am J Med Sci.* 2005;330(1):19-24.
10. Ponticelli C, Passerini P. Treatment of the nephrotic syndrome associated with primary glomerulonephritis. *Kidney Int.* 1994;46(3):595-604.
11. Kayali F, Najjar R, Aswad F, Matta F, Stein PD. Venous thromboembolism in patients hospitalized with nephrotic syndrome. *Am J Med.* 2008;121(3):226-230.

82 POLYCYSTIC KIDNEYS

Mindy A. Smith, MD, MS

PATIENT STORY

A 43-year-old woman with newly diagnosed hypertension reports persistent bilateral flank pain. She has a family history of "kidney problems." On urinalysis, she is noted to have microscopic hematuria. An ultrasound and abdominal CT scan show bilateral polycystic kidneys (**Figure 82-1**).

INTRODUCTION

Polycystic kidney disease (PKD) is a manifestation of a group of inherited disorders resulting in renal cyst development. In the most common form, autosomal-dominant polycystic kidney disease (ADPKD), extensive epithelial-lined cysts develop in the kidney; in some cases, abnormalities also occur in the liver, pancreas, brain, arterial blood vessels, or a combination of these sites.

EPIDEMIOLOGY

- Most common tubular disorder of the kidney, affecting 1 in 300 individuals.
- Autosomal dominant in 90% of cases, rarely as an autosomal recessive trait.[1]
- Sporadic mutation in approximately 1:1000 individuals.
- ADPKD accounts for approximately 5% to 10% of cases of end-stage renal disease (ESRD) in the United States.
- Most frequently seen in the third and fourth decades of life, but can be diagnosed at any age.

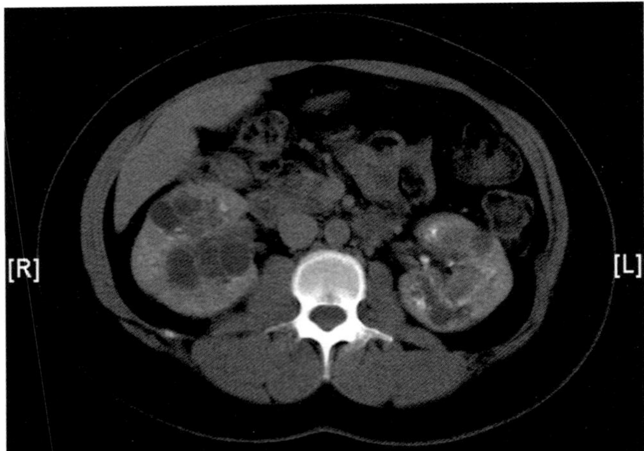

FIGURE 82-1 Bilateral polycystic kidneys seen on CT scan in a 43-year-old woman with hypertension, hematuria and flank pain. (*Reproduced with permission of Michael Freckleton, MD.*)

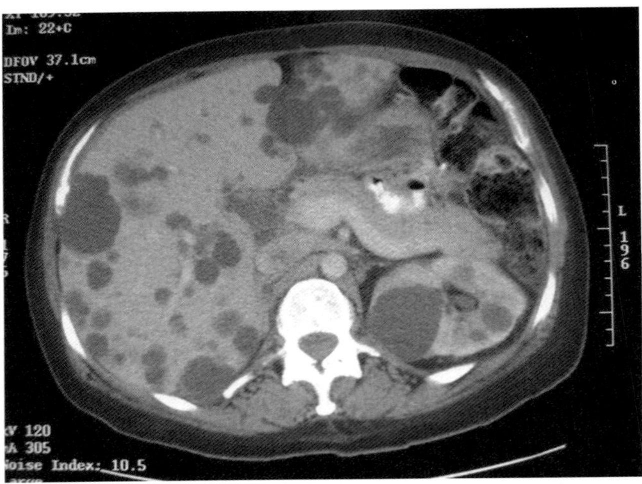

FIGURE 82-2 CT scan showing multiple liver cysts and multiple cysts in both kidneys in a patient with polycystic kidney disease. (*Reproduced with permission of Ves Dimov, M.D., Section of Allergy, Asthma and Immunology, Department of Pediatrics, Department of Medicine, University of Chicago, ClinicalCases.org*)

ETIOLOGY AND PATHOPHYSIOLOGY

- ADPKD results from mutations in either of 2 genes that encode plasma membrane–spanning polycystin 1 (PKD1) and polycystin 2 (PKD2).[2] Polycystins regulate tubular and vascular development in the kidneys and other organs (liver, brain, heart, and pancreas). PKD1 and PKD2 are colocalized in primary cilia and appear to mediate Ca^{2+} signaling as a mechanosensor, essential for maintaining the differentiated state of epithelia lining tubules in the kidney and biliary tract.[3] These mutations result in many abnormalities including increased proliferation and apoptosis and loss of differentiation and polarity.[4]
- Few (1%-5%) nephrons actually develop cysts.
- Remaining renal parenchyma shows varying degrees of tubular atrophy, interstitial fibrosis, and nephrosclerosis.
- Cysts are also found in other organs such as liver (**Figure 82-2**), spleen, pancreas, and ovaries. Liver cysts are found in up to 80% of patients with ADPKD.[2] There is also an increased incidence of intracranial aneurysms (5%-12%).
- Autosomal-recessive PKD (ARPKD) is the neonatal form of PKD that is associated with enlarged kidneys and biliary dysgenesis.[3]
- Rare syndromic forms of PKD include defects of the eye, central nervous system, digits, and/or neural tube.[3]
- A variant of PKD is glomerulocystic kidney (GCK), which refers to a kidney with greater than 5% cystic glomeruli.[5] This condition is usually diagnosed in young patients. Although PKD-associated gene mutations have been excluded in many cases, there is a familial form of GCK presenting with cystic kidneys, hyperuricemia, and isosthenuria (concentration similar to plasma).[5]

DIAGNOSIS

Family history is a useful tool for diagnosing early ADPKD.

CLINICAL FEATURES

- Chronic flank pain as a result of the mass effect of enlarged kidneys.
- Acute pain with infection, obstruction, or hemorrhage into a cyst.

- Enlarged liver.
- Hypertension is common in adults (75%) and may be present in 10% to 30% of children.
- Kidney stones (calcium oxalate and uric acid) develop in 15% to 20% of affected individuals because of urinary stasis from distortion of the collecting system, low urine pH, and low urinary citrate.
- Nocturia may also be present from impaired renal concentrating ability.

LABORATORY TESTING

Gross or microscopic hematuria (60%).[2] Obtain a urinalysis to document hematuria and a complete blood count or hemoglobin to identify anemia.

IMAGING

- Diagnosis often made with ultrasound. More than 80% of patients have cysts present by age 20 years and 100% by age 30 years. In one study, the sensitivity of ultrasound in at-risk individuals younger than age 30 years was 70% to 95%, depending on the type of PKD present.[6] For younger patients or those with small cysts, CT scan (**Figures 82-1** and **82-2**) or MRI may be preferred.
- Cysts are commonly found in the liver (50%-80%) (**Figure 82-2**), spleen, pancreas, and ovaries.
- The diagnosis of PKD can usually be made from ultrasound characteristics, the presence or absence of extrarenal abnormalities, and screening of parents older than 40 years of age.[7] Age-dependent ultrasound criteria have been established for both diagnosis and disease exclusion in subjects at risk of PKD1 (the more severe disorder).[8]
- If the diagnosis is uncertain, genetic testing is available for both ADPKD and ARPKD.

DIFFERENTIAL DIAGNOSIS[2]

- Simple cyst—Diagnosed at any age; few cysts seen; benign features.
- Acquired cystic disease—Diagnosed in adulthood; few to many cysts; cyst development preceded by renal failure.
- Tuberous sclerosis—Diagnosed at any age; few to many renal angiomyolipomas; inherited nonmalignant tumors grow in the skin, brain/nervous system, kidneys, and heart.

MANAGEMENT

The current role of therapy in PKD is to slow the rate of progression of renal disease and minimize symptoms. However, specific treatments are on the horizon.

NONPHARMACOLOGIC

- Neither protein restriction nor tight blood pressure control decreased the decline in glomerular filtration rate (GFR) in clinical trials.[9,10] However, in a UK population study, increasing coverage (from 7% to 46% of the population prescribed an antihypertensive agent) showed a trend toward decreasing mortality and increased intensity of antihypertensive therapy was associated with decreasing mortality in people with ADPKD.[11]
- For episodes of gross hematuria, one author recommends bed rest, analgesics, and hydration sufficient to increase the urinary flow rate to 2 to 3 L/day; hematuria generally declines to microscopic levels in a few days.[2] SOR C

MEDICATIONS

- Control blood pressure to reduce the risk of associated cardiovascular disease. SOR A
- In 1 randomized controlled trial (RCT) of 46 patients with ADPKD and hypertension, no differences in renal function, urinary albumin excretion, or left ventricular mass index were detected between those treated with ramipril versus metoprolol, during 3 years of follow-up.[12] Renal function declined significantly in both groups. Angiotensin-converting enzyme inhibitors and angiotensin receptor blockers are the traditionally used agents for patients with chronic kidney disease and hypertension. SOR A
- Treat infection as early as possible. If pyocyst is suspected, agents that penetrate cysts such as trimethoprim-sulfamethoxazole, chloramphenicol, and ciprofloxacin are used. SOR C
- Future therapies focus on exploiting signaling mechanisms underlying disease pathogenesis. Experimental and observational studies suggest that the mammalian target of rapamycin (mTOR) pathway plays a critical role in cyst growth.
- A 2-year RCT of the mTOR inhibitor everolimus for 46 patients with ADPKD demonstrated a slowing of the increase in total kidney volume over placebo but not the progression of renal impairment.[13] An open-label trial (N = 100 patients with ADPKD and early chronic kidney disease) of the mTOR inhibitor sirolimus did not show slowing of kidney growth or improved function over standard care.[14]
- In an RCT of octreotide (a long-acting somatostatin analog) versus placebo for patients with polycystic liver disease (some of whom had ADPKD), patients with ADPKD randomized to octreotide had a stabilization of kidney volume (versus an increase in the control group) and all patients randomized to treatment showed a reduced liver volume; there was no difference between groups in GFR.[15]

SURGERY AND OTHER PROCEDURES

- Cyst puncture and a sclerosing agent (ie, ethanol) can be used in painful cysts. SOR C
- For painful liver enlargement, partial hepatectomy can be performed, with good outcomes reported at experienced centers.[2] SOR C
- For patients with ESRD as a result of PKD, transplantation and dialysis are options.
- In a nationwide study of 15-year outcomes following renal transplantation (N = 534 patients with ADPKD and 4779 patients without ADPKD), patients with ADPKD had better graft survival and no difference in infections, but more thromboembolic complications, more metabolic complications, and increased incidence of hypertension.[16]

REFERRAL

- Patients with PKD with progressive renal failure and/or ESRD should be managed by a team of providers as they often require dialysis or kidney transplantation and can develop multiple complications; other considerations include anemia management, aneurysm screening pretransplantation, and nephrectomy of the native ADPKD kidneys.[17] SOR C
- Consider hospitalization for patients with PKD who develop acute pyelonephritis and symptomatic cyst infection.[2]

PROGNOSIS

- Approximately 50% of patients with ADPKD progress slowly to ESRD; kidney failure requiring renal-replacement therapy typically develops in the fourth to sixth decade of life.[2] Patients with ADPKD and ESRD may have more favorable outcomes compared to those with other causes of kidney failure.[16]
- The following are the characteristics that predict a faster rate of decline in GFR in persons with ADPKD[18]:
  - Greater serum creatinine (independent of GFR).
  - Greater urinary protein excretion.
  - Higher mean arterial pressure (MAP).
  - Young age.
  - Increased kidney volume (>1500 mL).[2]
  - Disease caused by PKD1 mutation.[19]
  - The presence of tubulointerstitial fibrosis.[20]
- Patients with ADPKD are also more prone to kidney stones (Chapter 80, Kidney Stones).[21]

FOLLOW-UP

- Monitor patients renal function and watch for hypertension and post-transplantation diabetes mellitus; imaging to assess the rate of increased kidney and total cyst volume may be useful in prognosis.[22]
- Avoid exogenous estrogen use for women with ADPKD and liver cystic enlargement; consider limiting use in women with liver cysts.[2]
- For all patients with PKD with renal dysfunction, review medications to adjust for level of kidney function and avoid nephrotoxic drugs if possible. SOR C
- The prognosis for patients following renal transplant is fairly good. In a follow-up study of patients with ADPKD, adult cadaveric renal transplant survival at 5 years was found to be 79%.[23]
- In the absence of a family history of aneurysm, screening is not routinely recommended for asymptomatic patients; diagnostic testing should be considered in patients with ADPKD and new-onset or severe headache or other central nervous system symptoms or signs.[2]
- Posttransplantation, patients with ADPKD may be more prone to the development of diabetes mellitus (odds ratio 2.3, 95% confidence interval, 1.008 to 5.14).[24]

PATIENT EDUCATION

- Explain the genetics (among patients with ADPKD disease will develop in half of their offspring) and prognosis to patients. Referral to a genetic counselor may be useful for patients considering childbearing.
- Hypertension is common and should be treated.
- Kidney dysfunction is also common and should be monitored.
- Avoid high-impact sports in which abdominal trauma may occur (eg, boxing).[2]
- In otherwise healthy women with ADPKD, pregnancy is usually uncomplicated but the risks of severe hypertension and preeclampsia are higher than those in the general population when elevated blood pressure or renal insufficiency is present before conception.[25]

PATIENT RESOURCES

- National Kidney Foundation (800-622-9010)—**http://www.kidney.org.**
- National Kidney Disease Education Program—**http://www.nkdep.nih.gov.**
- PubMed Health. *Polycystic Kidney Disease*—**http://www.ncbi.nlm.nih.gov/pubmedhealth/PMH0001531/.**

PROVIDER RESOURCES

- Roser T. *Polycystic Kidney Disease*—**http://emedicine.medscape.com/article/244907.**

REFERENCES

1. Asplin JR, Coe FL. Tubular disorders. In: Kasper DL, Braunwald E, Fauci AS, Hauser SL, Longo DL, Jameson JL, eds. *Harrison's Principles of Internal Medicine*, 16th ed. New York, NY: McGraw-Hill; 2005:1694-1696.
2. Grantham JJ. Autosomal dominant polycystic kidney disease. *Ann Transplant*. 2009;14(4):86-90.
3. Harris PC, Torres VE. Polycystic kidney disease. *Annu Rev Med*. 2009;60:321-337.
4. Park EY, Woo YM, Park JH. Polycystic kidney disease and therapeutic approaches. *BMB Rep*. 2011;44(6):359-368.
5. Lennerz JK, Spence DC, Iskandar SS, et al. Glomerulocystic kidney: one hundred-year perspective. *Arch Pathol Lab Med*. 2010;134(4):583-605.
6. Nicolau C, Torra R, Bandenas C, et al. Autosomal dominant polycystic kidney disease types 1 and 2: assessment of US sensitivity for diagnosis. *Radiology*. 1999;213(1):273-276.
7. Sweeney WE Jr, Avner ED. Diagnosis and management of childhood polycystic kidney disease. *Pediatr Nephrol*. 2011;26(5):675-692.
8. Barua M, Pei Y. Diagnosis of autosomal-dominant polycystic kidney disease: an integrated approach. *Semin Nephrol*. 2010;30(4):356-365.
9. Klahr S, Breyer JA, Beck GJ, et al. Dietary protein restriction, blood pressure control, and the progression of polycystic kidney disease. Modification of Diet in Renal Disease Study Group. *J Am Soc Nephrol*. 1995;6(4):1318.
10. Schrier R, McFann K, Johnson A, et al. Cardiac and renal effects of standard versus rigorous blood pressure control in autosomal-dominant polycystic kidney disease: results of a seven-year prospective randomized study. *J Am Soc Nephrol*. 2002;13(7):1733-1739.
11. Patch C, Charlton J, Roderick PJ, Gulliford MC. Use of antihypertensive medications and mortality of patients with autosomal dominant polycystic kidney disease: a population-based study. *Am J Kidney Dis*. 2011;57(6):856-862.
12. Zeltner R, Poliak R, Stiasny B, et al. Renal and cardiac effects of antihypertensive treatment with ramipril vs metoprolol in autosomal dominant polycystic kidney disease. *Nephrol Dial Transplant*. 2008;23(2):573-579.
13. Walz G, Budde K, Mannaa M, et al. Everolimus in patients with autosomal dominant polycystic kidney disease. *N Engl J Med*. 2010;363(9):830-840.
14. Serra AL, Poster D, Kistler AD, et al. Sirolimus and kidney growth in autosomal dominant polycystic kidney disease. *N Engl J Med*. 2010;363(9):820-829.

15. Hogan MC, Masyuk TV, Page LJ, et al. Randomized clinical trial of long-acting somatostatin for autosomal dominant polycystic kidney and liver disease. *J Am Soc Nephrol.* 2010;21(6):1052-1061.

16. Jacquet A, Pallet N, Kessler M, et al. Outcomes of renal transplantation in patients with autosomal dominant polycystic kidney disease: a nationwide longitudinal study. *Transpl Int.* 2011;24(6):582-587.

17. Alam A, Perrone RD. Management of ESRD in patients with autosomal dominant polycystic kidney disease. *Adv Chronic Kidney Dis.* 2010;17(2):164-172.

18. Klahr S, Breyer JA, Beck GJ, et al. Dietary protein restriction, blood pressure control, and the progression of polycystic kidney disease. Modification of Diet in Renal Disease Study Group. *J Am Soc Nephrol.* 1995;6(4):1318.

19. Pei Y. Practical genetics for autosomal dominant polycystic kidney disease. *Nephron Clin Pract.* 2011;118(1):c19-c30.

20. Norman J. Fibrosis and progression of autosomal dominant polycystic kidney disease (ADPKD). *Biochim Biophys Acta.* 2011;1812(10): 1327-1336.

21. Nishiura JL, Neves RF, Eloi DR, et al. Evaluation of nephrolithiasis in autosomal dominant polycystic kidney disease patients. *Clin J Am Soc Nephrol.* 2009;4(4):838-844.

22. Bae KT, Grantham JJ. Imaging for the prognosis of autosomal dominant polycystic kidney disease. *Nat Rev Nephrol.* 2010;6(2):96-106.

23. Johnston O, O'Kelly P, Donohue J, et al. Favorable graft survival in renal transplant recipients with polycystic kidney disease. *Ren Fail.* 2005;27(3):309-314.

24. Gonclaves S, Guerra J, Santana A, et al. Autosomal-dominant polycystic kidney disease and kidney transplantation: experience of a single center. *Transplant Proc.* 2009;41(3):887-890.

25. Vora N, Perrone R, Bianchi DW. Reproductive issues for adults with autosomal dominant polycystic kidney disease. *Am J Kidney Dis.* 2008;51(2):307-318.

83 PROSTATE CANCER

Rowena DeSouza, MD
Melanie Ketchandji, MD

PATIENT STORY

A 65-year-old man in good health comes to the office having had a prostate specific antigen (PSA) test performed at a local health fair. He reports a normal voiding pattern and normal erectile function with no evidence of weight loss or bone pain. He has no major medical problems but does have a strong family history of prostate cancer. His PSA is 9.3 ng/mL, and he chooses to have a prostate biopsy. Pathology demonstrates prostate cancer with a Gleason score of 6 (**Figure 83-1**).

INTRODUCTION

Prostate cancer is a very common cancer in men. Secondary to widespread testing, we have seen a stage migration in prostate cancer. Most patients are diagnosed with asymptomatic, clinically localized disease. Multiple factors—such as Gleason score, PSA level, stage at diagnosis, and life expectancy—are all applied to risk stratify patients associated with varying possibilities of achieving a cure. It is especially important to consider life expectancy prior to offering PSA screening.

EPIDEMIOLOGY

- In United States, prostate cancer (**Figure 83-2**) is the leading cancer in men and the second leading cause of cancer deaths in men.[1]
- It is the second most common cancer in men worldwide, with an estimated 900,000 cases and 258,000 deaths in 2008.[2]
- Incidence is increased with age.

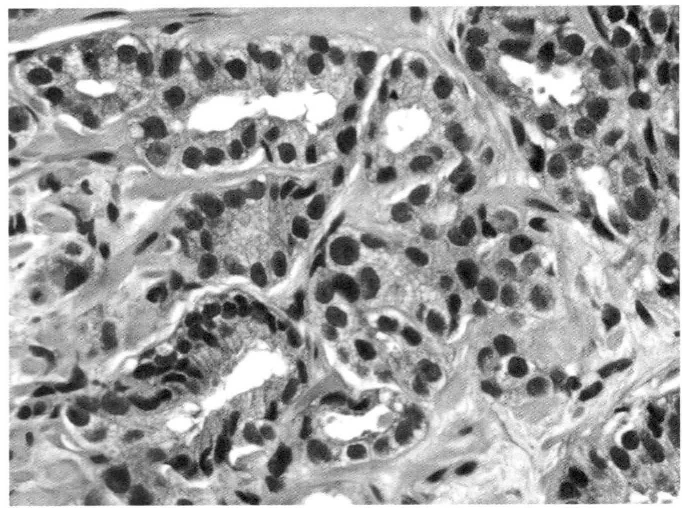

FIGURE 83-1 Microscopic image of biopsy demonstrating glands with enlarged nuclei and prominent nucleoli (hematoxylin and eosin [H&E] staining). The patient was diagnosed with prostate cancer with a Gleason score of 6. (*Reproduced with permission of E.J. Mayeaux Jr, MD.*)

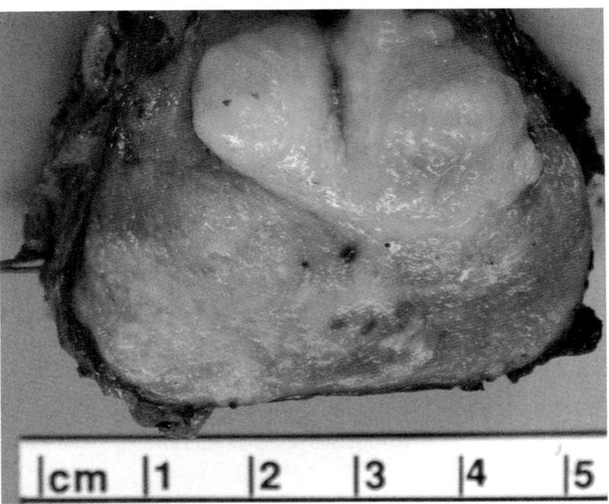

FIGURE 83-2 Photograph showing adenocarcinoma on the left lower side of the specimen and bilateral benign prostatic hypertrophy toward the top. (*Reproduced with permission of E.J. Mayeaux, Jr., MD.*)

- The risk of developing prostate cancer increases at age 40 years in black men and in those who have a first-degree relative with prostate cancer.
- The risk of developing prostate cancer begins to increase at age 50 years in white men who have no family history of the disease.[3]
- There is no peak age or modal distribution.
- The highest incidence of prostate cancer in the world is found in African American men, who have approximately a 9.8% lifetime risk of developing prostate cancer. This is accompanied by a high rate of prostate cancer mortality (**Figure 83-3**).
- The lifetime risk of prostate cancer for white men in the United States is 8%.[3]
- Japanese and mainland Chinese populations have the lowest rates of prostate cancer.
- Socioeconomic status appears to be unrelated to the risk of prostate cancer.

ETIOLOGY AND PATHOPHYSIOLOGY

- Greater than 95% of prostate cancers are adenocarcinomas.
- Histologic variants include ductal or endometrioid carcinoma, mucinous adenocarcinoma, signet cell carcinoma, small cell carcinoma, squamous and adenosquamous carcinoma, basaloid, and adenoid cystic carcinoma.
- Of prostate adenocarcinomas, 70% occur in the peripheral zone, 20% in the transitional zone, and approximately 10% in the central zone (**Figure 83-4**).
- Biologic behavior is affected by histologic grade as described by the Gleason grade and Score (**Figure 83-5**). The Gleason grade is based on the architectural pattern of prostate cancer cells. Based upon the growth pattern and differentiation, tumors are graded from 1 to 5, with grade 1 being the most differentiated and grade 5 the least differentiated. One grade is assigned to the most common tumor pattern, and a second grade to the next most common tumor pattern. The Gleason Score is obtained by adding the two grades together and ranges from 2 to 10. A higher score indicates a greater likelihood of having non–organ-confined disease, as well as a worse outcome after treatment of localized disease.

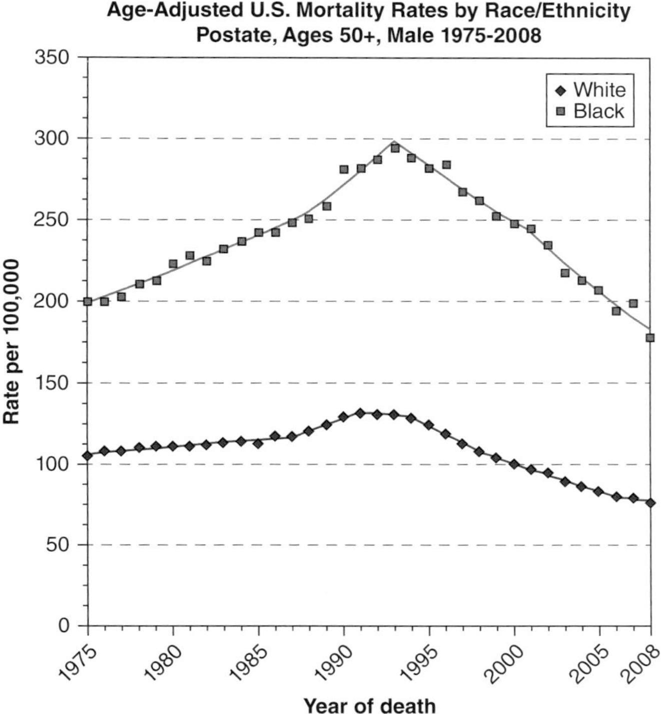

Cancer sites include invasive cases only unless otherwise noted. Mortality source: US Mortality Files, National Center for Health Statistics, CDC. Rates are per 100,000 and are age-adjusted to the 2000 US Std Population (19 age groups-Census P25–1130). Regression lines are calculated using the Joinpoint Regression Program Version 3.5, April 2011, National Cancer Institute.

FIGURE 83-3 Age-adjusted US prostate cancer mortality rates by race and ethnicity in males older than the age of 50 years. Note the higher mortality in blacks.

- Patterns of spread include direct extension, hematogenous, and lymphatic.
- Lymphatic spread occurs to the hypogastric, obturator, external iliac, presacral, common iliac, and paraaortic nodes.[4]
  - Of distant metastases, 90% are osseous.
  - Visceral metastases to lung, liver, and adrenals are less commonly seen without bone involvement.[4]

RISK FACTORS

- Men who have a first-degree relative with prostate cancer have approximately a 2-fold increased risk of developing prostate cancer during their lifetime.
- African American ethnicity.

DIAGNOSIS

CLINICAL FEATURES

- Prostate cancer can be associated with urinary obstructive symptoms or hematuria, but these are usually a result of other causes.
- Rarely, bone pain can be an initial symptom, but it generally represents very advanced disease. Prior to PSA screening, men commonly presented with this symptom.

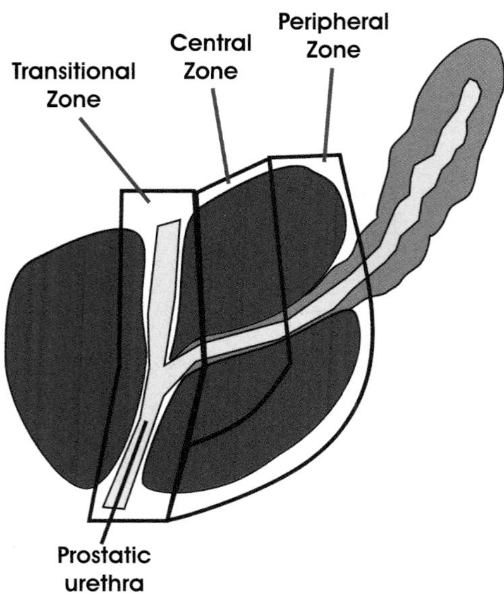

FIGURE 83-4 Diagram of prostate zones. Most prostate adenocarcinomas occur in the peripheral zone. (*Reproduced with permission of E.J. Mayeaux, Jr., MD.*)

- A prostatic nodule on digital rectal examination (DRE) is not always specific for a carcinoma and can underestimate the extent of disease when it does represent a carcinoma.

LABORATORY TESTING

PSA Screening

- PSA is a glycoprotein produced primarily by the epithelial cells that line the acini and ducts of the prostate gland.
- PSA is concentrated in prostatic tissue, and serum PSA levels are normally very low.
- Disruption of the normal prostatic architecture, such as by prostatic disease, inflammation, or trauma, allows greater amounts of PSA to enter the general circulation.[5]
- The sensitivity and specificity for PSA as a detection tool is 80% and 65%, respectively.[5] After treatment PSA is the primary tool used to evaluate for persistent disease or metastatic disease before imaging is employed.
- The American Urological Association guidelines support screening from age 40 years old to 75 years old.[6]
- The U.S. Prevention Task Force (USPSTF) has published final recommendations against PSA-based screening for prostate cancer in asymptomatic men.[7] They gave the guidance a D recommendation, which means there is moderate or high certainty that the service has no net benefit or that the harms outweigh the benefits, and the task force discourages use of the service. In May 2012, they concluded that many men are harmed as a result of prostate cancer screening [with PSA] and few, if any, benefit. A better test and better treatment options are needed. Until these are available, the USPSTF has recommended against screening for prostate cancer.[7]

IMAGING

Transrectal Ultrasound

- Transrectal ultrasound (TRUS) is a sensitive but nonspecific method of detecting prostate cancer.

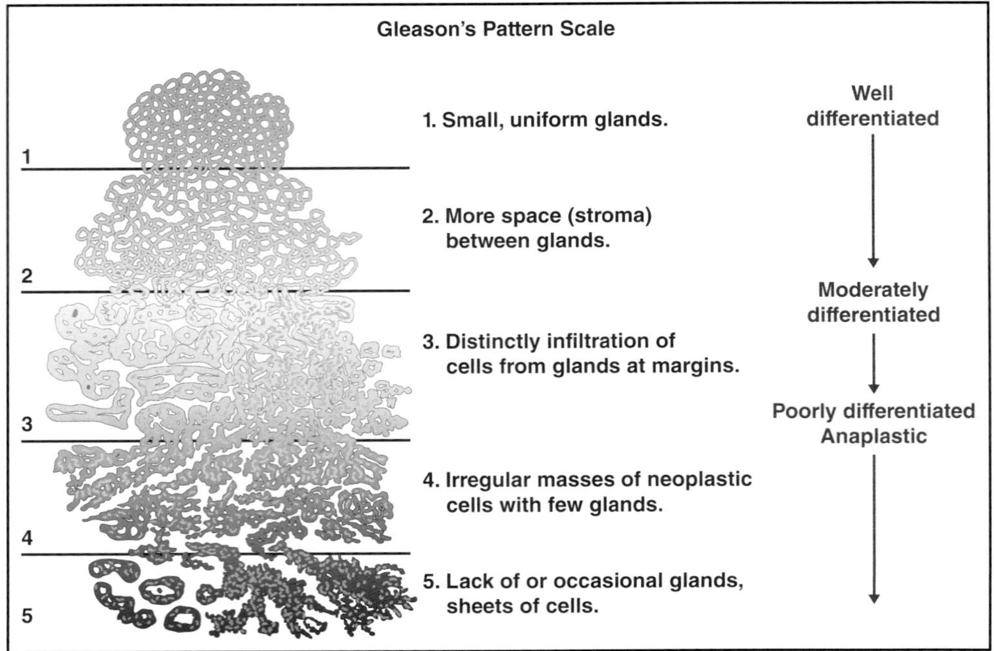

FIGURE 83-5 Gleason scoring of prostate cancer. (*From Gleason, DF. Histologic grading and clinical staging of prostatic carcinoma. In Tannenbaum M. Urologic Pathology: The Prostate. Philadelphia, PA: Lea and Febiger; 1977:171–197.*)

- A hypoechoic lesion as seen on TRUS has a 30% chance of being carcinoma.
- TRUS should not be used as a screening tool.
- The most important use of TRUS is in combination with 12-core prostate needle biopsy.[3]

Bone Scan

- Radionuclide imaging is routinely used to evaluate for disseminated disease.
- Recent studies show that the likelihood of a positive bone scan in patients with a PSA value less than 10 ng/mL and no bone symptoms is 1 per 1000.[8]

CT Scan and MRI

- CT scans and body-surface-coil MRI of the pelvis have poor performance characteristics for assessing metastatic disease and are not part of standard screening or staging.
- MRI with an endorectal coil is sometimes used to evaluate disease beyond the capsule, in focal therapy, and for surgical planning.

Prostate Biopsy

- Performed with local anesthesia and ultrasound guidance using a spring-loaded biopsy needle to obtain 12 prostate biopsy specimens. The patient may experience significant discomfort despite the anesthetic.
- There is an estimated false negative rate of 0% to 9.3% and an estimated false positive rate of 0% to 3.8% amongst pathologists.[9]
- The percentage of positive cores, length, or percentage of cancer per core can provide predictive information.
- Lower GI tract cleansing enemas and prophylactic antibiotics are routinely used.

DIFFERENTIAL DIAGNOSIS

- Prostatitis—Infection or inflammation of the prostate. This is often associated with perineal or suprapubic pain, dysuria frequency while prostate cancer is often asymptomatic.
- Benign prostatic hyperplasia—Enlarged prostate that may cause obstructive symptoms. There is no relative increase in the risk of developing prostate cancer.
- Prostatic intraepithelial neoplasia (PIN)—High-grade PIN has been noted as a precursor to prostate carcinoma.[10]
- Atypical glands on biopsy—The probability of detecting cancer following an atypical diagnosis is approximately 40%. Often a repeat biopsy is recommended with increased sampling of the atypical site.

MANAGEMENT

- General considerations include age and general performance status, Gleason score, initial serum PSA, estimated tumor volume, tumor stage, and patient life expectancy.
- Options should be explained to patients so that patients can make an informed decision about which treatment best fits their values and goals.
- Active surveillance—Monitoring for disease progression over time in low-risk individuals who are likely to die with the disease rather than from the disease. Treatment is considered if significant disease progression is detected. This involves PSA testing and periodic rebiopsy.[11] SOR B
- Radical prostatectomy—Treatment of choice for patients with organ-defined disease and a life expectancy of more than 10 years. Walsh has shown that the cavernosal nerves that mediate erectile function can be identified and avoided, reducing postoperative erectile dysfunction. Rarely, significant urinary incontinence may be encountered.[3]

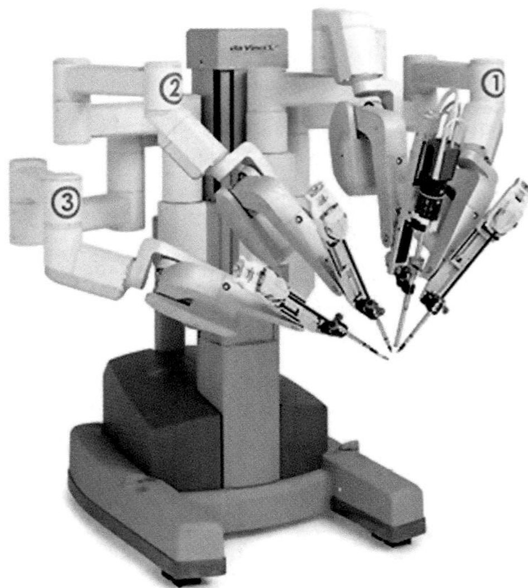

FIGURE 83-6 The DaVinci robot: three working arms and a camera. The robot allows for better visualization of the pelvic anatomy. (*Reproduced with permission of Intuitive Surgical.*)

  - Robotic-assisted laparoscopic radical prostatectomy (RALRP)—RALRP was developed to overcome of the difficulties of the standard laparoscopic prostatectomy. The robotic technique allows for magnified high definition 3-dimensional visualization of the operative field and wider range of motion. The majority of men opting for radical prostatectomy in the United States are having RALRP (**Figure 83-6**).[12] SOR B
- External beam radiation therapy (EBRT)—EBRT is also a viable treatment option for localized disease and is the choice treatment option for T3 disease. EBRT utilizes high-energy electrons to destroy cancer cells by damaging cellular DNA. Side effects can include rectal and bladder symptomatology. Short-term androgen deprivation therapy (1-3 years) may increase efficacy.[13,14] SOR B
- Brachytherapy—Outpatient, ultrasound-guided, transperineal placement of ^{125}I or Pd radioactive seeds into the prostate. Optimal candidates have low-risk prostate cancer. Many centers utilize short-term neoadjuvant hormonal blockade given the difficulty in treated glands larger than 50 gs.[15] SOR B
- Androgen ablation in combination with EBRT—There may be some synergy between the apoptotic response induced by androgen deprivation and radiotherapy. Androgen deprivation results in an average 20% decrease in prostate volume to reduce the number of target cells, and thereby improve tumor treatment. Shrinking the prostate can decrease side effects by diminishing the volume of rectum and bladder irradiated.[13,16] SOR B
- For recurrent or advanced disease—Docetaxel (Taxotere)-based regimens can be included among the most effective treatment options for the management of patients with advanced, androgen independent prostate cancer. Results with docetaxel as a single agent and in combination regimens with estramustine (Emcyt) have provided patient benefit through an improved palliative response and improvement in quality of life as assessed through quality of life questionnaires. In addition, treatment with Docetaxal-based regimens have produced objective responses such as reduced serum PSA levels by 50%, reduction in measurable disease on imaging, pain, and health-related quality of life. Progression-free survival was significantly increased in patients receiving docetaxel plus estramustine compared to those receiving mitoxantrone and prednisone (6.3 vs. 3.2 months).[17,18] SOR B

PREVENTION

- The Prostate Cancer Prevention Trial (PCPT) aimed to determine the prevalence of histologically proven prostate cancer among men randomized to receive daily finasteride or placebo.[19]
- The authors described a 24.8% reduction in the prevalence of prostate cancer among men taking finasteride; however, the cancers detected in these men were significantly higher risk cancers.[19]
- More recently, the Selenium and Vitamin E Cancer Prevention Trial (SELECT) found that although selenium does not prevent prostate cancer, vitamin E is associated with a significantly increased risk of prostate cancer.[20]

PROGNOSIS

The optimal management of patients with prostate cancer varies widely and is highly dependent upon a patient's age, overall health, and tumor risk assessment.

PATIENT EDUCATION

- Patients should be provided balanced and objective information about the risks and benefits of PSA screening, prostate biopsies, and the various options for prostate cancer treatment. This is challenging as there are conflicting opinions and interpretations of existing data. New studies are published frequently, which can change evidence-based recommendations and expert opinions. It is the physician's job to help patients navigate through the vast data and varied opinions to find a course of prevention and treatment that fits their individual needs. Although some patients will want the physician to make decisions about whether or not to get a PSA test or which cancer treatment is best; many others will appreciate balanced information so they may decide for themselves. See Patient and Provider Resources below to help inform patient–doctor discussions on these matters.
- Risk assessment calculations can be useful in discussions with patients to help them decide about screening, biopsy, and treatment. Links to prostate cancer online prediction tools are listed under Provider Resources below.

PATIENT RESOURCES

- National Alliance of State Prostate Cancer Coalitions—**http://www.naspcc.org.**
- Men's Health Network—**http://www.menshealthnetwork.org.**
- Links to prostate cancer online prediction tools are listed under Provider Resources below and are useful for patients in their discussions with physicians.

PROVIDER RESOURCES

- The Prostate Cancer Prevention Trial Prostate Cancer Risk Calculator (PCPTRC) provides a person's estimated risk of biopsy-detectable prostate cancer and high grade prostate cancer—**http://deb.uthscsa.edu/URORiskCalc/Pages/uroriskcalc.jsp.**

- Prostate cancer gene 3 (PCA3) data and use of finasteride can be entered into a more advanced version of this calculator on the same site.
- Prostate cancer online prediction tools are available from Memorial Sloan-Kettering Cancer Center. They can be used to in conjunction with patients to decide which treatment approaches will result in the greatest benefit at various stages of prostate cancer. The four nomograms are found at **http://www.mskcc.org/mskcc/html/10088.cfm.**
  1. Pretreatment (Diagnosed with Cancer But Not Yet Begun Treatment)
  2. Postradical Prostatectomy (Recurrence After Surgery)
  3. Salvage Radiation Therapy (Considering Radiation Therapy After Surgery)
  4. Hormone Refractory (Progression of Metastatic Prostate Cancer That Can No Longer Be Controlled by Hormones Alone)
- Additional tools for measuring PSA doubling time, male life expectancy and tumor volume are found at: **http://nomograms.mskcc.org/Prostate/index.aspx.**
- National Cancer Institute (NCI). *Prostate Cancer*—**http://www.cancer.gov/cancertopics/types/prostate.**
- National Comprehensive Cancer Network (NCCN)— **http://www.nccn.org/professionals/physician_gls/f_guidelines.asp.**
- National Prostate Cancer Coalition (NPCC)—**http://www.4npcc.org.**
- Screening for Prostate Cancer: A Review of the Evidence for the U.S. Preventive Services Task Force—**http://www.uspreventiveservicestaskforce.org/uspstf12/prostate/prostateart.htm.**

REFERENCES

1. Lim LS, Sherin K. Screening for prostate cancer in U.S. men ACPM position statement on preventive practice. *Am J Prev Med*. 2008;34(2):164-170.
2. Jemal A, Bray F, Center MM, et al. Global cancer statistics. *CA Cancer J Clin*. 2011;61:69.
3. Morey A, Shoskes D. *The American Urological Association Educational Review Manual in Urology*. 1st ed. New York, NY: Castle Connolly Graduate Medical Publishing; 2007.
4. Wein A. *Clinical Manual of Urology*. 3rd ed. New York, NY: McGraw Hill; 2001.
5. Greene KL, Albertsen PC, Babaian RJ, et al. Prostate specific antigen best practice statement: 2009 update. *J Urol*. 2009;182(5):2232-2241.
6. Williams SB, Salami S, Regan MM, et al. Selective detection of histologically aggressive prostate cancer: an Early Detection Research Network Prediction model to reduce unnecessary prostate biopsies with validation in the Prostate Cancer Prevention Trial. *Cancer*. 2012;118(10):2651-2658. http://www.ncbi.nlm.nih.gov/pubmed/22006057. Accessed October 25, 2011.
7. U.S. Preventive Services Task Force. Screening for Prostate Cancer. Current Recommendation. May 2012. http://www.uspreventiveservicestaskforce.org/prostatecancerscreening.htm. Accessed September 1, 2012.
8. Oxley JD, Sen C. Error rates in reporting prostatic core biopsies. *Histopathology*. 2011;58(5):759-765.
9. Tanaka N, Fujimoto K, Shinkai T, et al. Bone scan can be spared in asymptomatic prostate cancer patients with PSA of < = 20 ng/ml and Gleason Score of < = 6 at the initial stage of diagnosis. *Jpn J Clin Oncol*. 2011;41(10):1209-1213. http://www.ncbi.nlm.nih.gov/pubmed/21862505. Accessed September 12, 2011.
10. Epstein JI, Herawi M. Prostate needle biopsies containing prostatic intraepithelial neoplasia or atypical foci suspicious for carcinoma: implications for patient care. *J Urol*. 2006;175(3 Pt 1): 820-834.
11. Albertsen PC, Hanley JA, Fine J. 20-year outcomes following conservative management of clinically localized prostate cancer. *JAMA*. 2005;293(17):2095-2101.
12. Parsons JK, Bennett JL. Outcomes of retropubic, laparoscopic, and robotic-assisted prostatectomy. *Urology*. 2008;72(2):412-416.
13. Payne H, Mason M. Androgen deprivation therapy as adjuvant/neo-adjuvant to radiotherapy for high-risk localised and locally advanced prostate cancer: recent developments. *Br J Cancer*. 2011;105(11):1628-1634. http://www.ncbi.nlm.nih.gov/pubmed/22009028. Accessed October 25, 2011.
14. Potosky AL, Davis WW, Hoffman RM, et al. Five-year outcomes after prostatectomy or radiotherapy for prostate cancer: the prostate cancer outcomes study. *J Natl Cancer Inst*. 2004;96(18):1358-1367.
15. Merrick GS, Butler WM, Wallner KE, Galbreath RW, Adamovich E. Permanent interstitial brachytherapy in younger patients with clinically organ-confined prostate cancer. *Urology*. 2004;64(4):754-759.
16. Bolla M, Collette L, Blank L, et al. Long-term results with immediate androgen suppression and external irradiation in patients with locally advanced prostate cancer (an EORTC study): a phase III randomised trial. *Lancet*. 2002;360(9327):103-106.
17. Logothetis CJ. Docetaxel in the integrated management of prostate cancer. Current applications and future promise. *Oncology (Williston Park, N.Y.)*. 2002;16(6 Suppl 6):63-72.
18. Machiels J-P, Mazzeo F, Clausse M, et al. Prospective randomized study comparing docetaxel, estramustine, and prednisone with docetaxel and prednisone in metastatic hormone-refractory prostate cancer. *J Clin Oncol*. 2008;26(32):5261-5268.
19. Crawford ED, Andriole GL, Marberger M, Rittmaster RS. Reduction in the risk of prostate cancer: future directions after the Prostate Cancer Prevention Trial. *Urology*. 2010;75(3):502-509.
20. Klein EA, Thompson IM Jr, Tangen CM, et al. Vitamin E and the risk of prostate cancer: the Selenium and Vitamin E Cancer Prevention Trial (SELECT). *JAMA*. 2011;306(14):1549-1556.

84 RENOVASCULAR HYPERTENSION

Madhab Lamichhane, MD

PATIENT STORY

A 50-year-old woman is admitted to the medical intensive care unit with complaints of severe shortness of breath that requires mechanical ventilation for acute respiratory failure related to pulmonary edema. She has a history of dyslipidemia and a 20-pack-year history of smoking, but she denies any past medical history of hypertension, diabetes, or family history of heart disease, hypertension, and stroke. Electrocardiogram is suggestive of left ventricular hypertrophy (LVH). She has a mild troponin elevation with normal electrolytes. Her echocardiogram shows a normal ejection fraction of 60% with no regional wall motion abnormality. Lisinopril is added for a newly diagnosed blood pressure (BP) elevation of 190/100 mm Hg. Her creatinine increased to 1.6 mg/dL from her baseline of 1.2 mg/dL after starting lisinopril, and her renal function normalized with its discontinuation. She subsequently underwent diagnostic cardiac catheterization with renal angiogram to evaluate the etiology of her acute pulmonary edema and hypertension; she is found to have a hemodynamically significant stenosis of her right renal artery, for which she had percutaneous renal artery angioplasty with stent placement (**Figure 84-1**).

INTRODUCTION

Renovascular hypertension (RVH) is a type of secondary systemic hypertension caused mainly by occlusive disease of the renal arteries. Renal artery stenosis (RAS) is one cause of RVH that, when treated, can partially or completely cure hypertension.

SYNONYMS

Renovascular hypertension is also called renovascular disease.

EPIDEMIOLOGY

- Renovascular hypertension is the most common cause of secondary hypertension and accounts for hypertension in 1% to 5% of all patients with hypertension.[1]
- Incidence is higher in patients with severe or refractory hypertension.
- The prevalence of RAS was 6.8% in individuals 65 years or older in a community-based sample of subjects.[2]
- Atherosclerotic RAS is seen in about 18% to 20% of individuals undergoing coronary angiography and 35% to 70% of those undergoing peripheral vascular angiography.[3]
- Of normotensive individuals, 3% to 6% have RAS.[4]

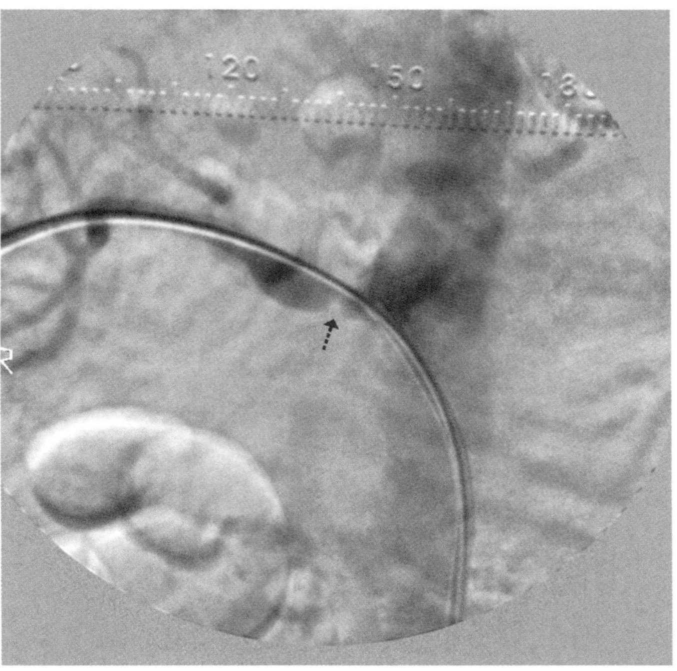

A

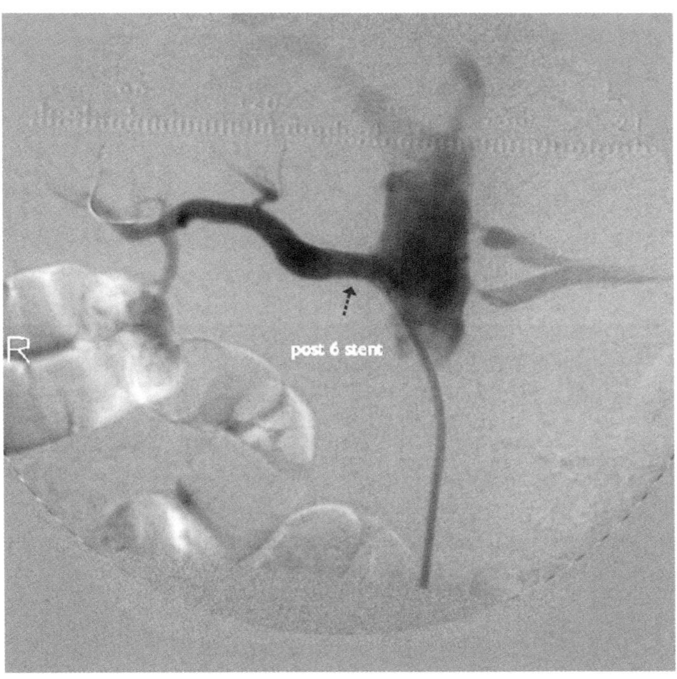

B

FIGURE 84-1 High-grade right renal artery stenosis demonstrating improved flow after stent placement. **A.** Before stent. **B.** Improved flow after stent placement. (*Reproduced with permission from Milind Karve, MD, FACC.*)

ETIOLOGY

Renovascular hypertension is most commonly caused by atherosclerotic disease and fibromuscular dysplasia (FMD). Renovascular hypertension etiology can be classified as follows[2]:

- Atherosclerotic RAS
- Fibromuscular disease from medial, perimedial, intimal hyperplasia (**Figure 84-2**)
- Extrinsic fibrous band
- Renal trauma: arterial dissection, segmental renal infarction, Page kidney (perirenal fibrosis)[2]
- Aortic dissection
- Aortic endograft occluding the renal artery
- Arterial embolus
- Other medical disorders
  - Hypercoagulable state with renal infarction
  - Takayasu arteritis
  - Radiation-induced fibrosis
  - Tumor encircling the renal artery
  - Polyarteritis nodosa
- Atherosclerosis RAS
  - Atherosclerosis is the major cause involving 90% of all cases of RVH and usually involves the ostium and proximal third of the main renal and perirenal aorta.[4]
  - It is a progressive disease, and total occlusion occurs in 39% over 12 to 60 months follow-up when RAS is greater than 75% at the time of diagnosis.[5]
- Fibromuscular dysplasia
  - Fibromuscular dysplasia is the second-most-common cause of RAS and accounts for about 10% of the cases of RVH; it predominantly affects younger females.[6]
  - It is a nonatherosclerotic and noninflammatory disease of unclear etiology. A genetic factor may play a role, as suggested by a higher incidence in first-degree relatives.[5]
  - Medial fibroplasia is the histological finding in most cases (80%-85%), and perimedial fibroplasia makes up most of the remaining 10% to 15%. Other mechanisms include intimal fibroplasia, medial fibrodysplasia, and adventitial fibroplasia. Renal arteries are the most commonly affected arterial bed; however, other arteries can be affected and include the carotid, vertebral, iliac, and mesenteric arteries.[5]
  - Bilateral disease is seen in about 60% of patients with renal vascular bed involvement.[5]
  - It usually involves the middle and distal two-thirds of main renal artery and may involve renal artery branches.[5]
  - About 28% of individuals with FMD have involvement of multiple vascular beds.[6]
  - There is good response to revascularization.

PATHOPHYSIOLOGY

- Based on experimental models, RVH is caused by activation of the renin-angiotensin-aldosterone system (RAAS) in patients with unilateral RAS with a normal contralateral kidney.
- The nonstenotic kidney receives higher perfusion pressure, which leads to "pressure natriuresis" to lower the BP by excreting sodium. However, the fall in BP decreases the perfusion to the stenotic kidney, which in turn stimulates more renin release. The stenotic kidney fails to lower the BP with the pressure natriuresis because of angiotensin-II-mediated aldosterone secretion, distal sodium reabsorption, and renal vasoconstriction. Renal vasoconstriction decreases renal plasma flow, which promotes sodium reabsorption in both proximal and distal tubules.[3]
- In bilateral renal arterial disease, or stenosis to a solitary functioning kidney, angiotensin II increases the BP, but the kidney is unable to excrete sodium by natriuresis. This leads to volume-expansion-related hypertension from sodium and water retention.[3]

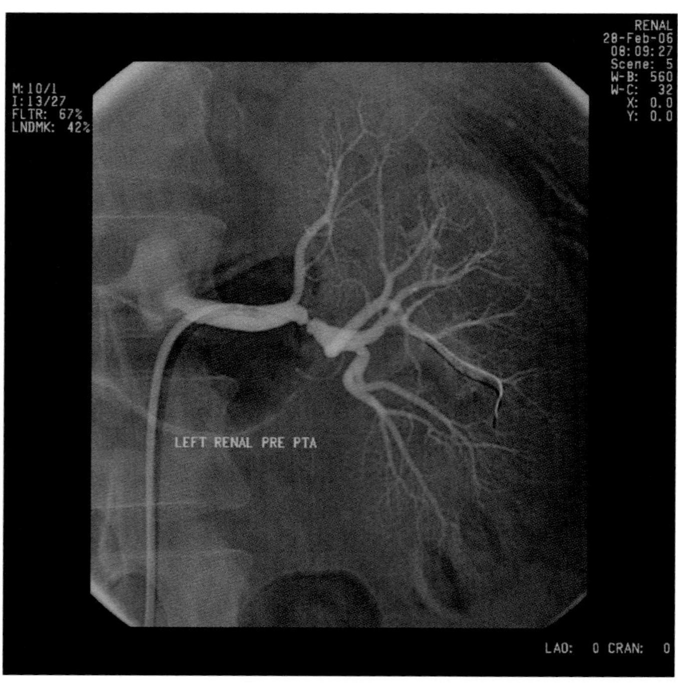

A

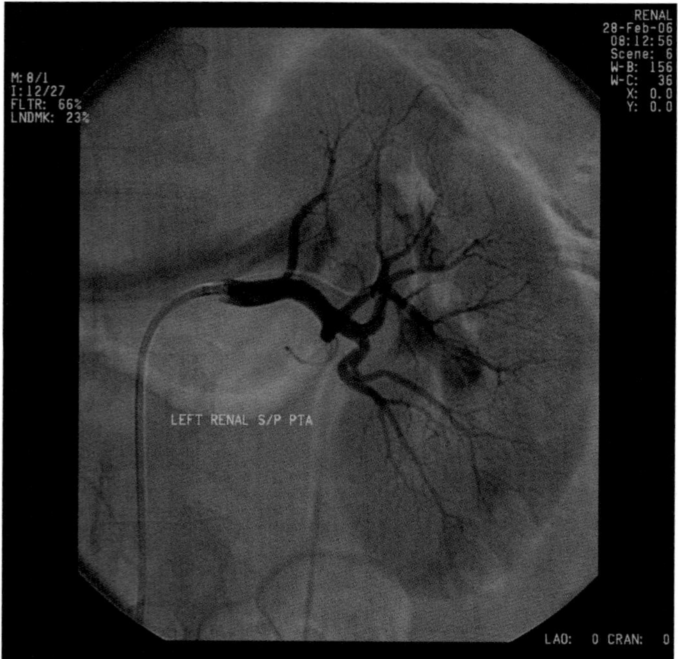

B

FIGURE 84-2 Angiographic images of intimal fibroplasia variant of fibromuscular dysplasia in the mid/distal rena artery before (**A**) and after (**B**) angioplasty. (*Reproduced with permission from Dean S, Satiani B.* Color Atlas and Synopsis of Vascular Disease. *New York, NY: McGraw-Hill; 2014.*)

- The activation of renin release occurs when the pressure gradient is above 10 to 20 mm Hg between the aorta and poststenotic segments, which is seen with greater than 70% to 75% lumen obstruction.[2]
- Increased sympathetic activity is common in this disorder, possibly from the altered afferent signals from the underperfused kidney or augmentation of nerve signals in the presence of angiotensin II.[2,3]
- Endothelial dysfunction with impaired relaxation also develops in RVH.[2]
- The aldosterone level is higher in RVH. It has an important role in regulation of tissue fibrosis, LVH, and sodium retention.

DIAGNOSIS/SCREENING

- The US Preventive Services Task Force has made no recommendations with regard to screening individuals for RVH.
- The American Heart Association recommends screening with Doppler ultrasound in the appropriate clinical settings mentioned in the diagnostic section of this chapter.

HISTORY/SYMPTOMS

Specifically ask about the following:

- Onset of hypertension before 35 years of age, which is suggestive of FMD
- Severe hypertension (systolic BP ≥ 180 or diastolic pressure of 120 mm Hg) after the age of 55 years, which is suggestive of atherosclerotic RAS
- Accelerated and resistant hypertension
- Sudden and unexplained pulmonary edema, such as in the introductory case
- Absent family history of hypertension (except in FMD)

PHYSICAL EXAMINATION

Specifically look for or establish the following:

- High BP—Note that wider variability in BP compared to essential hypertension during 24-hour ambulatory BP monitoring is seen because of increased sympathetic activity.[2]
- Palpate and listen for carotid and peripheral pulse bruit. Positive findings increase the possibility of a renovascular cause of hypertension.
  - Epigastric area bruit—The presence of an abdominal bruit has sensitivity of 20% to 77.7% and specificity of about 63% to 90% for renovascular disease.
  - Bruits are found in 77.7% to 86.9% of RVH cases with angiographically proven RAS.[7] A systolic-diastolic bruit (audible in systolic phase with extension to the diastole) is more common in those with renovascular disease than in healthy people. Location, intensity, and pitch have questionable value.
- Severe hypertension with signs of end-organ damage such as papilledema, retinal hemorrhage, heart failure, or neurological deficits can occur.
- Look for xanthomas and xanthelasma, which favor underlying hyperlipidemia and atherosclerotic disease (see Chapter 223, Hyperlipidemia).
- Target organ damage findings like LVH is more severe than that seen in essential hypertension for the same level of BP.[3] The apical impulse is sustained in LVH.
- Some patients can have refractory fluid retention often out of degree of myocardial pump failure.

LABORATORY TESTING

- Complete blood cell count (CBC)—Values are normal in FMD, but anemia and thrombocytopenia can occur in arteritis-associated disease.
- Baseline renal function—Worsening renal function after initiation of angiotensin-converting enzyme (ACE) inhibitor or angiotensin receptor blocking agent can occur. Renin angiotensin inhibitors block angiotensin-II-induced efferent arteriolar vasoconstriction, which results in a decrease in transglomerular hydrostatic pressure and fall in glomerular filtration rate (GFR). Use of these medications in patients with bilateral RAS or stenosis to a solitary kidney results in renal failure.
- Examination of urine for proteinuria assesses the severity of renal damage.
- Screening for atherosclerosis risk factors—Use fasting glucose, fasting lipid panel, level of hemoglobin A1C (HbA1C).

IMAGING

- Diagnostic imaging studies are recommended to evaluate for RAS in the following clinical settings:
  - Onset of hypertension before 30 years of age[4,5] SOR B
  - Severe hypertension after the age of 55 years[4,5] SOR B
  - Accelerated and resistant hypertension (sudden and persistent worsening of previously controlled hypertension)[4,5] SOR C
  - Malignant hypertension (hypertension with coexistent end-organ damage)[4,5] SOR C
  - Significant azotemia (greater than 50% rise in creatinine that persists or worsens even after correction of hypoperfusion state[5] after initiation of ACE inhibitor or angiotensin receptor blocking agent)[4,5] SOR B
  - Unexplained atrophic kidney or discrepancy in size between 2 kidneys of 1.5 cm[4,5] SOR B
  - Sudden and unexplained pulmonary edema[4,5] SOR B
- **Specific imaging studies**—The choice of diagnostic imaging technique depends on the availability of the diagnostic procedure, the operator's experience, and the patient's characteristics, such as body size, renal function, contrast allergy, and presence of previous stents or metallic objects in the body.
  - Duplex ultrasonography is recommended as a screening test.[5] SOR B
    - It has a sensitivity of 84% to 98% and specificity of 62% to 99% for detecting RAS.[5]
    - It is also used to monitor renal artery patency after endovascular treatment or surgical vascularization of RAS.
    - Limitations include operator skill, less visualization of accessory renal arteries, or inadequate images in obese patients or intervening bowel gas.
    - Parameters for diagnosis of RAS are (1) peak systolic velocity in the renal artery exceeding 1.8 or 2.0 m/s and a renal artery/aortic velocity ratio exceeding 3.5, with sensitivities varying from 85% to 90% and about 90% specificity[8]; (2) an end diastolic velocity of greater than 150 cm/s predicts more than 80% RAS.[5]
  - Computed tomographic angiography (CTA) can be used. SOR B
    - Sensitivity and specificity for detecting RAS vary from 59% to 96% and 82% to 99%, respectively.[2]
    - Metal stents and in-stent restenosis can be diagnosed.
    - Computed tomographic angiography is not indicated in patients with renal insufficiency caused by iodinated contrast.
    - Secondary signs on CTA—Poststenotic dilatation, renal parenchymal changes of atrophy, and decreased cortical enhancement.[8]

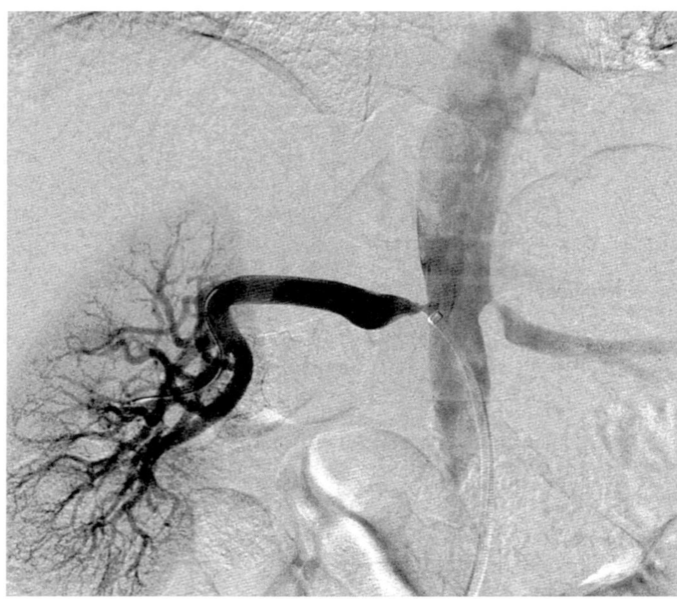

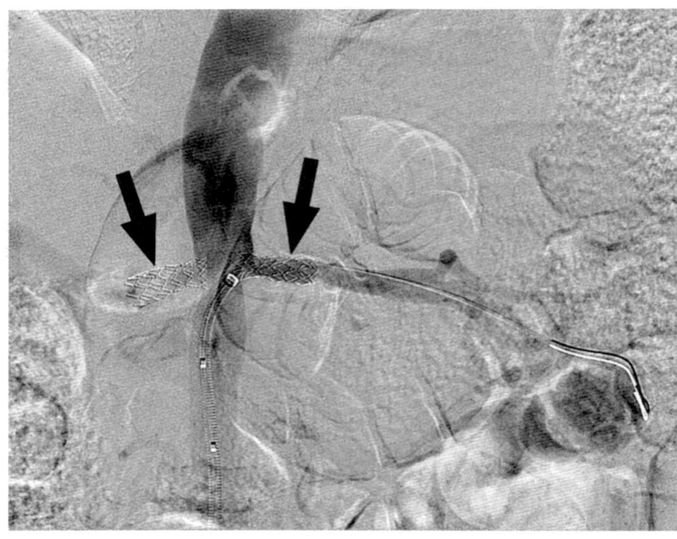

FIGURE 84-3 Angiograms in a 70-year-old man with a history of coronary artery disease, previous coronary artery bypass graft surgery, and hypertension; the man was taking 2 antihypertensive agents and developed sudden worsening of blood pressure control, requiring 4 antihypertensive agents with blood pressure still greater than 190/100 mm Hg. **A.** Angiogram revealing bilateral renal artery stenosis. **B.** After stenting (*arrows*) of bilateral renal ostial stenotic lesions. Blood pressure control improved markedly, and the patient now requires only one antihypertensive agent. (*Reproduced with permission from Fuster V, Walsh R, Harrington R.* Hurst's The Heart. *13th ed. New York, NY: McGraw-Hill; 2011.*)

- Gadolinium-enhanced magnetic resonance angiography (MRA)[2] SOR B
  - Magnetic resonance angiography has a sensitivity of 90% to 100% and specificities of 76% to 94% for detection of RAS.[2]
  - It is less effective in assessment of patients with more subtle beading and changes of FMD in the medial and distal segments.[3]
  - It is not useful in patients with metallic stents.
  - Magnetic resonance angiography is contraindicated in patients with GFR less than 30% because of the enhanced risk of nephrogenic systemic fibrosis, which is seen in 1% to 6% of dialysis patients given gadolinium.[3]
- Catheter angiography (**Figures 84-3** and **84-4**)
  - It is the gold standard for diagnosis of RAS.
  - It is used mostly as a confirmatory diagnostic test when other noninvasive diagnostic procedures are inconclusive and concomitant angioplasty or stent placement is planned. SOR B
  - String-of-beads appearance with the diameter of the bead larger than the diameter of the artery is seen in medial fibroplasia. Long tubular areas of stenosis are seen in intimal fibroplasia or periadventitial fibroplasia.
  - Contrast-induced acute kidney injury incidence is seen in fewer than 3% of patients without diabetes or chronic kidney disease (CKD), 5% to 10% in diabetes, 10% to 20% in CKD, 20% to 50% in those with diabetes and CKD.[5]
  - Iso-osmolar nonionic contrast is associated with fewer nephrotoxic effects.
  - The translesional pressure gradient can be measured across the stenosis to determine its significance in doubtful cases.
- Captopril renography SOR C provides scintigraphic images and information about renal size, perfusion, and excretory capacity.
  - This is of limited value in patients with azotemia, bilateral RAS, or RAS to a single functioning kidney.
  - Sensitivity is 74%, and specificity is about 59%.[5]
  - It is not helpful except in cases of RAS of borderline angiographic severity of unclear clinical significance.[2]
- Selective renal vein renin studies—These have limited value in diagnosis of RAS compared to noninvasive methods, which are highly reliable. SOR B

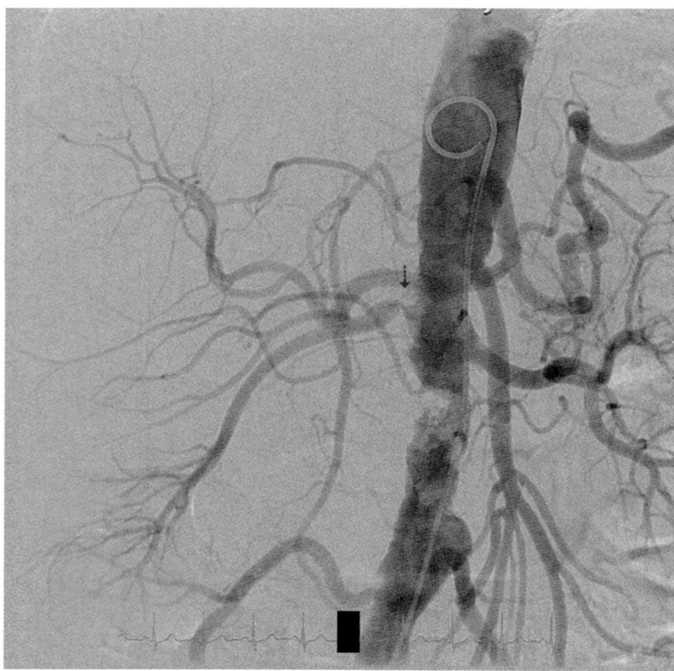

FIGURE 84-4. Right renal artery stenosis from atherosclerosis. It usually involves ostium and the proximal segment of the artery (*red arrow*). (*Reproduced with permission from Milind Karve, MD, FACC.*)

- Plasma renin activity
  - Plasma renin level is measured at baseline and 60 minutes after a 50-mg dose of oral captopril administration.
  - Elevated plasma renin activity is seen in about 15% of patients with essential hypertension.
  - This test has sensitivity of 61% and specificity of 86% for the detection of renal artery disease.[5]
  - It is not recommended as a screening test for diagnosis of RAS. SOR B

DIFFERENTIAL DIAGNOSIS

CAUSES OF SECONDARY HYPERTENSION

- Pheochromocytoma—Commonly associated with paroxysmal BP changes, palpitations, sweating, and headache
- Primary aldosteronism—Associated with hypokalemia and adrenal adenomas
- Cushing syndrome—Associated with moon-shaped facies, central obesity, striae, and easy bruising
- Hyperthyroidism—Associated with heat intolerance, palpitations, weight loss (see Chapter 227, Hyperthyroidism)
- Hyperparathyroidism—Associated with renal stones, hypercalcemia, and elevated parathyroid hormone levels
- Coarctation of aorta—Causes pulse delay between radial and femoral artery, diminished pulse and BP distal to coarctation; may be associated with Turner syndrome
- Parenchymal renal diseases—Associated with decreased GFR and protein or cellular elements in the urinalysis

MANAGEMENT

- Antiplatelet agents based on the known benefit in atherosclerotic disease.
- Antihypertensive therapy to optimize BP control—BP goal is 130/80 mm Hg in those with diabetes and CKD, 140/90 mm Hg in other patients.
- Control BP
  - Angiotensin-converting enzyme inhibitors, angiotensin II receptor blockers (ARBs), and calcium channel blockers slow the progression of renal disease.[4] SOR B
  - RAAS blockers decrease the GFR and elevate the creatinine temporarily and require close monitoring. The GFR fall of 30% or greater and a creatinine rise of more than 0.5 mg/dL may be an indication for renal revascularization.
  - Angiotensin-converting enzyme inhibitors are contraindicated in bilateral RAS and in RAS in a single functional kidney.[3] SOR B
  - Thiazide diuretics, hydralazine, and β-blockers are also effective.
  - Usually, multiple medications are required.
  - No randomized controlled study has been done to evaluate different medical regimens.
- Treat atherosclerotic risk factors (including tobacco abuse, dyslipidemia) and attain appropriate glycemic control in diabetic patients (see respective Chapters 237, Tobacco Addiction; 223, Hyperlipidemia; and 219, Diabetes).
- Medical therapy is preferred to revascularization for atherosclerotic RAS and advanced renal disease.
- Two recent randomized trials (**A**ngioplasty and **ST**ent for **R**enal **A**rtery **L**esions [ASTRAL] and **ST**ent placement and blood pressure and lipid-lowering for the prevention of progression of renal dysfunction caused by **A**therosclerotic ostial stenosis of the **R**enal artery [STAR]) compared stent angioplasty combined with medical therapy or medical therapy alone for atherosclerotic renovascular disease. Both trials did not show any difference in renal events, cardiovascular morbidity, and mortality.[4,9,10]
- Revascularization therapy
  - It is controversial because of evolving information and lack of clear benefit from recent randomized controlled trials.
  - Based on meta-analysis of 47 angioplasty studies (1616 patients) and 23 surgery studies (1014 patients), cure rates (BP of 140/90 mm Hg without treatment) are only 36% and 54% after angioplasty and surgery, respectively, in RAS caused by FMD.[11]
  - In the ASTRAL study, no significant benefit in systolic BP reduction was seen in 806 patients with atherosclerotic renovascular disease who either underwent revascularization in addition to receiving medical therapy or received medical therapy alone.[12]
  - Recommendations to consider revascularization should be based on the patient's life expectancy, comorbidities, quality of BP control, and renal function.[4]
  - Percutaneous revascularization is indicated in anatomically and functionally significant RAS with the following presentation SOR B :
    - Recurrent, unexplained congestive heart failure or sudden, unexplained pulmonary edema.[5]
    - Percutaneous revascularization is reasonable for hemodynamically significant RAS with any of the following: accelerated hypertension, resistant hypertension, malignant hypertension, hypertension with unexplained unilateral small kidney, and hypertension with intolerance to drug treatment. SOR B
    - Balloon angioplasty with stent placement is superior to balloon angioplasty in atherosclerotic lesions.[4]
    - Drug-eluting stents have not shown any better outcomes.[4]
  - Balloon angioplasty with or without bailout stent placement is recommended for FMD lesions.[4,13]
    - Medical therapy is the preferred treatment in well-controlled individuals who are compliant patients.[6] High rates of BP improvement are noted after angioplasty in FMD, unlike atherosclerotic RAD, for which it is less effective.[12]
    - Meta-analysis of 7 studies (207 patients) did not show any difference between baseline renal function and follow-up after revascularization.[9]
    - The rate of restenosis is 7% to 27% at 6-month to 2-year follow-up.[6]
  - Complications of angioplasty include renal atheroembolization.
    - This occurs during diagnostic and direct manipulation of the renal artery during angioplasty or stenting.
    - The patient develops subacute renal failure or features of embolization like blue toes and livedo reticularis (see Chapter 198, Erythema Ab Igne).
    - Preexisting renal insufficiency and long-standing hypertension are predictors of progression to end-stage renal disease (ESRD). No specific therapy is available. Distal occlusion balloons or filter may reduce incidence.[14]
  - Surgical revascularization is considered for patients requiring surgical repair of the aorta and patients with complex disease of renal arteries (eg, aneurysms or failed endovascular procedures).[4] SOR C
    - Surgical procedures include aortorenal bypass grafting using saphenous vein or a prosthesis, aortic implantation, resection anastomosis, and autotransplantation.
    - Surgical revascularization has a 30-day mortality of 3.7% to 9.4%.[4]

PROGNOSIS

- Renal artery stenosis is associated with a significantly increased rate of CKD, 25% versus 2% among those without renal RAS, coronary artery disease (67% vs 25%), stroke (37% vs 12%), and peripheral vascular disease (56% vs 13%).[13]
- Increased risk of cerebrovascular disease (CVD) in atherosclerotic RAS occurs from activation of the RAAS and sympathetic nervous system and concomitant atherosclerotic disease in other organs.[4]
- Of those with RAS, 80% die from cardiovascular events.
- Prevalence of LVH is 79% in RAS versus 46% in essential hypertension. LVH is associated with increased morbidity and mortality.[4]
- Progression to high-grade stenosis or occlusion occurs in 1.3% to 11.1% of patients.[4]
- Atherosclerotic RAS leads to progressive renal function loss, and 27% of patients will develop chronic renal failure within 6 years. Patients with atherosclerotic RAS who progress to ESRD have high mortality rates.[2]
- The 2-, 5-, and 10-year survival rates are 56%, 18%, and 5%, respectively, in atherosclerotic RAS.[5]
- Patients with FMD who achieve hypertension cure with angioplasty include those younger than 40 years at diagnosis, those with a duration of hypertension less than 5 years, and those with a systolic BP less than 160 mm Hg.[13]

FOLLOW-UP

- Close follow-up is indicated until adequate BP control is achieved.
- Check creatinine and electrolytes values every 3 to 6 months and 2 to 4 weeks after adjustment of antihypertensive therapy, especially when using ACE inhibitors, ARBs, and diuretics.
- For patients who are managed with medical therapy,
  - Monitor serum creatinine level and BP every 3 months.
  - Noninvasive imaging (such as duplex ultrasonography) should be obtained every 6 to 12 months to assess the progression of the disease or assess loss of renal volume.
- Patients who have undergone revascularization need follow-up with duplex ultrasonography soon after the procedure to assess the adequacy of intervention, then after 6 months and 12 months and yearly thereafter or whenever there is worsening of hypertension or unexplained elevation in creatinine.[6]

PATIENT EDUCATION

- Emphasize adherence to medical therapy.
- Educate the patient on home BP monitoring and reporting to the physician if a significant increase in BP is noted.
- Emphasize the continued need for risk factor reduction: diabetes, hypertension, dyslipidemia.

PATIENT RESOURCES

- Vascular Disease Foundation. *Renovascular Hypertension*—**http://vasculardisease.org/renovascular-hypertension-ras/.**
- Vascular Disease Foundation. *Fibromuscular Dysplasia*—**http://www.vdf.org/diseaseinfo/fmd/.**

PROVIDER RESOURCES

- National Heart Lung and Blood Institute. *Your Guide to Lowering High Blood Pressure*—**http://www.nhlbi.nih.gov/hbp/index.html.**
- Society for Vascular Surgery: VascularWeb. *Renovascular Conditions*—**http://www.vascularweb.org/vascularhealth/Pages/renovascular-conditions.aspx.**

REFERENCES

1. Bloch MJ, Basile J. The diagnosis and management of renovascular disease: a primary care perspective. Part II. Issues in management. *J Clin Hypertens (Greenwich)*. 2003;5(4):261-268.
2. Stephen C, Textor, MD Textor SC. Current approaches to renovascular hypertension. *Med Clin N Am*. 2009;93:717-732.
3. Garovic V, Textor SC. Renovascular hypertension and ischemic nephropathy. *Circulation*. 2005;112:1362-1374.
4. European Stroke Organization; Tendera M, Aboyans V, et al. ESC guidelines on the diagnosis and treatment of peripheral artery diseases. *Eur Heart J*. 2011;32:2851-2906.
5. Hirsch AT, Haskal ZJ, Hertzer NR, et al. ACC/AHA 2005 practice guidelines for the management of patients with peripheral arterial disease (lower extremity, renal, mesenteric, and abdominal aortic). *Circulation*. 2006;113:e463.
6. Slovut DP, Olin JW. Fibromuscular dysplasia. *N Engl J Med*. 2004;350:1862-1871.
7. Turnbull JM. The rational clinical examination. Is listening for abdominal bruits useful in the evaluation of hypertension? *JAMA*. 1995;274:1299.
8. Hartman RP, Kawashima A. Radiologic evaluation of suspected renovascular hypertension. Department of Radiology, Mayo Clinic, Rochester, Minnesota. *Am Fam Physician*. 2009;80(3):273-279.
9. ASTRAL Investigators; Wheatley K, Ives N, et al. Revascularization versus medical therapy for renal-artery stenosis. *N Engl J Med*. 2009;361:1953-1962.
10. Bax L, Woittiez AJ, Kouwenberg HJ, et al. Stent placement in patients with atherosclerotic renal artery stenosis and impaired renal function: a randomized trial. *Ann Intern Med*. 2009;150:840.
11. Trinquart L, Mounier-Vehier C, Sapoval M, Gagnon N, Plouin PF. Efficacy of revascularization for renal artery stenosis caused by fibromuscular dysplasia: a systematic review and meta-analysis. *Hypertension*. 2010;56:525-532.
12. Wheatley K, Ives N, Gray R, Kalra PA, et al. Revascularization versus medical therapy for renal-artery stenosis. *N Engl J Med*. 2009;361:1953-1962.
13. Dworkin LD, Cooper CJ. Renal-artery stenosis. *N Engl J Med*. 2009;361:1972-1978.
14. Rocha-Singh KJ, Eisenhauer AC, Textor SC, et al. Atherosclerotic Peripheral Vascular Disease Symposium II: intervention for renal artery disease. *Circulation*. 2008;118:2873-2878.

85 RENAL CELL CARCINOMA

Mindy A. Smith, MD, MS

PATIENT STORY

A 56-year-old man with hypertension presents with a 2-week history of left-sided flank pain. Urinalysis shows microscopic hematuria and, a CT scan (**Figures 85-1** and **85-2**) demonstrates a solid left renal mass. Work-up for metastatic disease was negative. A biopsy confirmed renal cell carcinoma and a radical nephrectomy was performed.

INTRODUCTION

Renal tumors are a heterogeneous group of kidney neoplasms derived from the various parts of the nephron. Each type of tumor possesses distinct genetic characteristics, histologic features, and, to some extent, clinical phenotypes that range from benign (approximately 20% of small masses) to high-grade malignancy. Around 90% to 95% of kidney neoplasms are renal cell carcinomas (RCCs).[1,2]

EPIDEMIOLOGY

- RCC comprises 2% to 3% of all malignant diseases in adults and is the seventh most common cancer in men and ninth most common cancer in women.[2]
- An estimated 60,920 cases were diagnosed and approximately 13,120 deaths occurred in 2011 from kidney and renal pelvis cancer.[3] The age-adjusted incidence rate was 14.6 per 100,000 persons with a median age at diagnosis of 64 years.[3]
- Lifetime risk of kidney and renal pelvis cancer is 1.56% (1 in 63 people will be diagnosed during their lifetime).[3] These cancers are more common in men than women (approximately 2:1).
- Approximately 2% to 3% of cases are familial (eg, von Hippel-Lindau syndrome).[2]

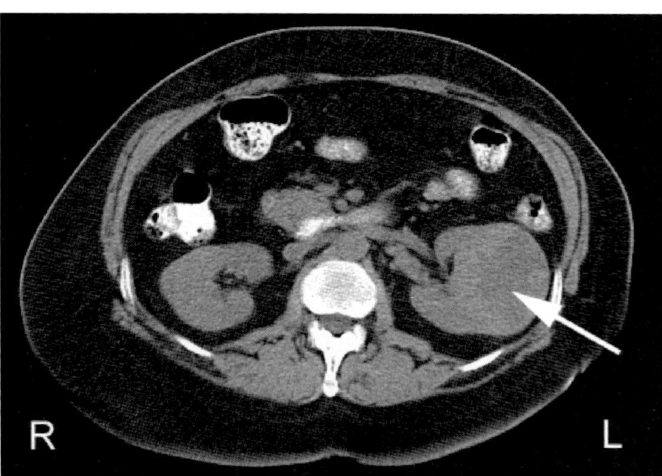

FIGURE 85-1 Renal cell carcinoma. CT shows solid mass in the left kidney (*arrow*). (*Reproduced with permission of Michael Freckleton, MD.*)

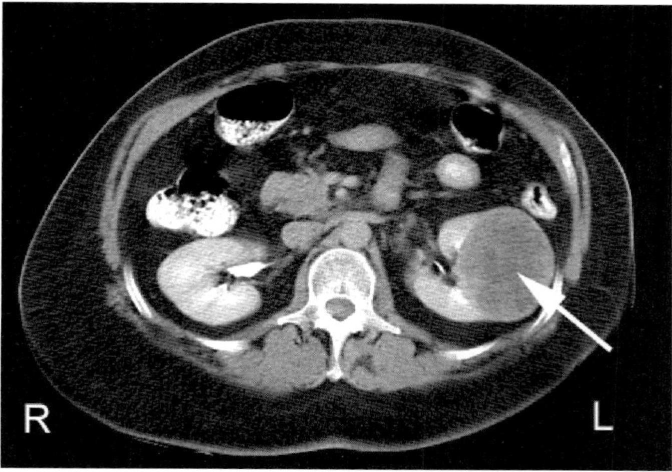

FIGURE 85-2 CT with contrast in the same patient shows the solid hypodense renal cell carcinoma mass (*arrow*) in the left kidney and contrasting normal parenchyma. The contrast is taken up better by the remaining normal kidney tissue and the tumor becomes more visible. (*Reproduced with permission of Michael Freckleton, MD.*)

- Metastatic disease at presentation occurs in 23% to 33%; the most common sites of distant metastases (in descending order) are lung (with or without mediastinal or hilar nodes), bone, upper abdomen (including the tumor bed, adrenal gland, contralateral kidney, and liver), brain, and other sites (eg, skin, spleen, heart, diaphragm, gut, connective tissue, and pancreas).[4]

ETIOLOGY AND PATHOPHYSIOLOGY

The majority of renal tumors fall into the following categories[1,2]:

- Clear cell carcinoma (from high lipid content) (60%-80%).
- Papillary carcinoma (5%-15%), further delineated into type 1 and the more aggressive type 2.
- Chromophobic tumors (3%-10%) and other rare subtypes, such as medullary, which occurs almost exclusively in patients with sickle cell trait.

RISK FACTORS[1,2]

- Smoking (relative risk 2-3)
- Obesity
- Hypertension
- Acquired cystic disease and end-stage renal disease, including dialysis treatment
- Family history of the disease

DIAGNOSIS

Most presentations are incidental (identified during other tests) and, consequently, although the incidence has increased, more cancers are diagnosed at early stages.[2] Despite this fact, mortality rates have also increased.

CLINICAL FEATURES

- Hematuria (40%) and flank pain (40%).
- Weight loss and anemia (approximately 33%).
- Flank mass (approximately 25%).
- The classic triad of hematuria, flank pain, and flank mass occurs in 5% to 10% of patients.[1]
- Other reported symptoms include night sweats, bone pain, fatigue, and sudden onset of left varicocele.
- Systemic symptoms may be caused by metastases or paraneoplastic syndromes, such as parathyroid hormone-related protein (causing hypercalcemia and renal stones), renin (causing hypertension), or erythropoietin (causing erythrocytosis).[2]

LABORATORY TESTING

Potentially useful studies: SOR Ⓒ

- Hemoglobin (anemia).
- Liver chemistries (metastatic disease or paraneoplastic syndrome).
- Urinalysis (hematuria—gross or microscopic).
- Urine cytology (neoplastic cells).
- The National Comprehensive Cancer Network (NCCN) also suggests a metabolic panel including lactate dehydrogenase (LDH) as part of the initial work-up.[5]

IMAGING

- The work-up for indeterminate renal masses suggested by the American College of Radiology (ACR) includes either CT scan of the abdomen (**Figures 85-1** to **85-3**) (solid renal mass; signs suggestive of renal vein or caval thrombus include filling defects, enlargement of the vessel, and rim enhancement) or abdominal MRI (slightly more sensitive and tends to upgrade cystic lesions; **Figure 85-4**); either scan should be done without and with contrast.[6]

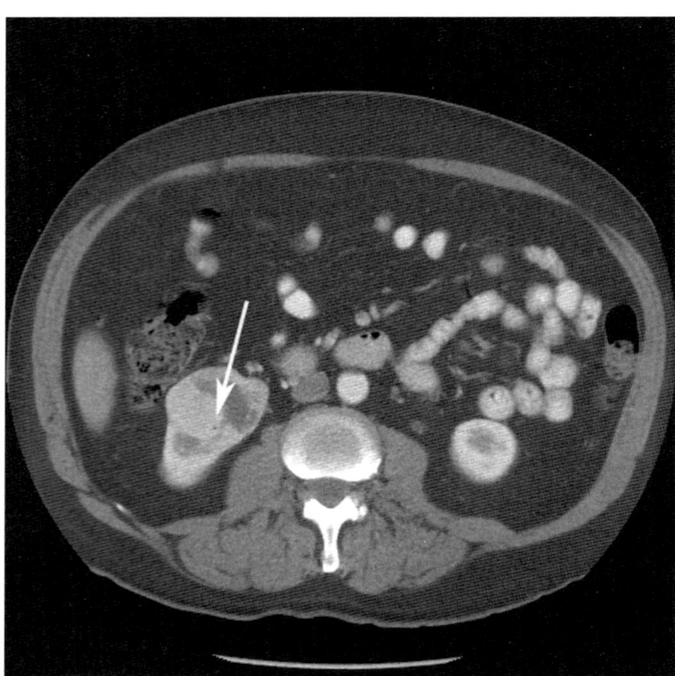

FIGURE 85-3 CT in a 70-year-old man demonstrating a heterogeneous solid mass in the midportion to lower pole of the right kidney (arrow), consistent with a primary renal cancer. The mass contains low-attenuation, likely necrotic, components and is exophytic. (*Reproduced with permission of Karl T. Rew, MD.*)

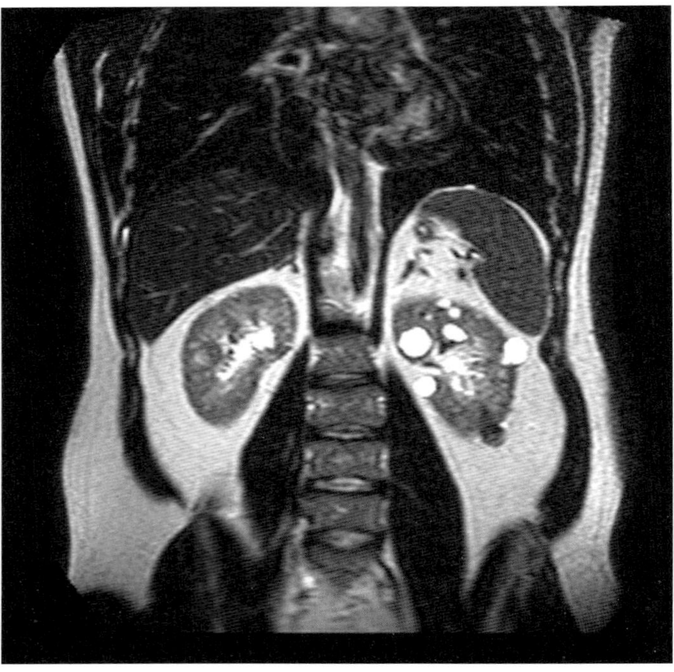

FIGURE 85-4 Patient with tuberous sclerosis. MRI shows multiple angiomyolipomas in the kidneys with several lesions suspicious for renal cancer. (*Reproduced with permission of Karl T. Rew, MD.*)

- An ultrasound (US) of the kidney retroperitoneal may help to clarify a mass that is probably a hyperdense cyst (the most common renal mass).
- Angiography can be used to define vascular anatomy before nephron-sparing surgery.[6]

For the purpose of staging an RCC, ACR recommends[6]:

- Multidetector CT without and with contrast.
- Chest X-ray (CXR, tumor may extend into the hilar lymph nodes) or chest CT.
- MRI if patient is unable to undergo CT with contrast.
- Bone scans and brain MRI should be reserved for patients with abnormal blood chemistries, symptoms, or large and locally aggressive or metastatic primary renal cancers.

BIOPSY

A renal biopsy is only needed on occasion based on the appearance and size of the mass; US, CT, or MRI can be used for image guidance.[4] ACR indications for biopsy include the following:

- Confirming an infected cyst
- Identifying lymphoma
- Determining a metastasis
- Confirming RCC in certain circumstances, including prior to ablative therapies

DIFFERENTIAL DIAGNOSIS

The differential diagnosis of a renal mass includes the following:

- Simple cysts.
- Renal calculi/nephrolithiasis (see Chapter 80, Kidney Stones).
- Benign neoplasms (infrarenal hematoma, adenoma, angiomyolipoma [see **Figure 85-4**], and oncocytoma).
- Inflammatory lesions (focal bacterial nephritis, abscess, pyelonephritis, and renal tuberculosis); patients often present with systemic signs and symptoms of infection such as fever and chills.
- Other primary or metastatic tumors (neoplastic tumors involving the kidney include squamous cell carcinoma of the collecting system, transitional cell carcinomas of the renal pelvis or collecting system, sarcoma, lymphoma, nephroblastoma, and melanoma).

These can frequently be differentiated from RCC on CT scan, but biopsy may be necessary.

MANAGEMENT

Because an increasing number of tumors are identified early (tumor size <4 cm) and may be slow growing with low risk of early progression, some authors are advocating initial active surveillance.[7]

MEDICATIONS

- Investigational therapy should be considered for patients with advanced disease because chemotherapy and immunotherapy are not known to be effective.
- There is some evidence that high-dose intravenous interleukin-2 results in complete remission in 7% to 8% of patients with metastatic RCC; interferon-α has also conferred minimal improvement in overall survival (3.8 months) versus control group.[2]
- The NCCN recommends high-dose interleukin-2 as first-line therapy for predominantly clear cell carcinoma.[5]
- Similar improvement in survival (4-5 months), but not cure, has been reported for targeted therapies, primarily those using antivascular epithelial growth factor agents (bevacizumab, sorafenib, sunitinib, pazopanib, tivozanib, or axitinib) or mammalian target of rapamycin (mTOR) inhibitors (temsirolimus or everolimus) usually compared to interferon-α.[8] No placebo-controlled trial has reported a benefit on health-related quality of life.
- The European Society of Medical Oncologists recommends either sunitinib or combination of bevacizumab and interferon in good-risk and intermediate-risk patients, and temsirolimus in patients with poor-risk features and clear cell renal carcinoma.[9] The NCCN recommends any of these as first-line therapy for predominantly clear cell carcinoma and enrollment in a clinical trial as the preferred strategy for non–clear cell cancers, although temsirolimus has shown some promise.[5]
- Presurgical treatment with sunitinib was reported in 1 case series; the drug decreased the size of primary RCC in 17 of 20 patients treated.[10]

SURGERY

- For localized disease, partial nephrectomy for small tumors and radical nephrectomy (complete removal of the kidney and Gerota fascia) for large tumors is the gold standard.[2,9] SOR Ⓑ For T1 tumors (**Table 85-1**), the NCCN recommends either partial (preferred) or radical nephrectomy, active surveillance for selected patients, or thermal ablation for nonsurgical candidates.[5]
- Similar to lumpectomy for localized breast cancer, partial nephrectomy for small tumors in the presence of a normal contralateral kidney appears to have similar outcomes to radical nephrectomy, based on observational data.[11] Complications are uncommon and include urinary leak (3%-5%) and hemorrhage (1%).[2] Advantages include better preservation of renal function, which is associated with fewer hospitalizations and lower risk of cardiac events and mortality.[2] In 1 long-term follow-up study, 5- and 10-year cancer-specific survival for nephron-sparing surgery in these cases was 98.5% and 96.7% for tumors less than 4 cm, respectively, and for imperative indications (solitary kidney) they were 89.6% and 76%, respectively. Chronic renal failure requiring dialysis was reported in 9 patients (11.2%) with a solitary kidney.[12]
- Percutaneous cryoablation or radiofrequency ablation of smaller (≤3.5 cm) renal masses is an alternative treatment[13,14]; outcomes for the 2 methods appear comparable, but the procedures have not been compared in a randomized trial.[15] Limitations of thermoablation include

TABLE 85-1 Stages of Renal Cell Carcinoma

Stage	Characteristics	TNM* Staging System
I	Tumor size 7 cm or smaller and found only in the kidney	T1 N0 M0
II	Tumor size larger than 7 cm and found only in the kidney	T2 N0 M0
III	Any size tumor and cancer is found only in the kidney and in 1 or more nearby lymph nodes OR Cancer is found in the main kidney blood vessels or in the fatty tissue around the kidney; cancer may be found in 1 or more nearby lymph nodes	T1 or T2 N1 M0 T3 N0 or N1 M0
IV	Tumor has spread to distant sites	T4 and N M0 Any T and N M1

*T, tumor (size and extent; T4 tumors invade beyond Gerota fascia); N, regional lymph nodes (NX unable to assess, N0 no regional lymph node metastasis, N1 metastasis in a single regional lymph node); M, metastases (M0 no distant metastasis, M1 distant metastasis).[5]

high local recurrence compared to surgery, lack of long-term data, and subsequent fibrosis that may compromise subsequent surgery if needed.

- For patients with larger tumors or local extension, radial nephrectomy offers a 40% to 60% chance of cure.[2] Laparoscopic approaches are used more recently, but there are no RCTs supporting this approach.[16]
- For patients with metastatic disease, cytoreductive nephrectomy (similar to radical nephrectomy with removal of the kidney and possibly other surrounding structures) should be considered.[9] NCCN recommends nephrectomy and surgical metastasectomy for a potentially surgically resectable solitary metastatic site.[5]
- In a combined analysis of trials, survival was longer in patients with metastatic RCC randomized to radical nephrectomy followed by interferon versus interferon alone (13.6 vs. 7.8 months, respectively).[17]
- Regional lymphadenectomy is controversial.
- Resection of solitary metastasis should be considered.[18] In a systematic review of data on 311 surgically and 73 nonsurgically treated patients with RCC metastatic to pancreas, metastases were single in approximately 60% of both groups. Surgery appeared to improve overall survival at 2 and 5 years (80.6% and 72.6%, respectively, for the surgical group, and 41% and 14%, respectively, in unresected patients).[19]

FOLLOW-UP

There is no standardized follow-up regimen based on evidence. The ACR recommends a follow-up CXR and CT of the abdomen without and with contrast for patients who have been treated for RCC by radical nephrectomy or nephron-sparing surgery.[4] The NCCN recommends chest and abdominal imaging at 2 to 6 months.[5] An MRI can be used for patients unable to undergo CT with contrast.[4] Most recurrences occur within 2 to 3 years after initial resection.[4]

- For patients with T1 tumors, most surveillance protocols recommend a history, physical examination, laboratory tests, and CXR be obtained every 6 to 12 months for 3 years and then yearly until year 5.[4] Others have suggested no imaging if the tumor is less than 2.5 cm. Most protocols do not recommend surveillance with abdominal CT for patients with T1 tumors.
- For patients with T2 primary tumors, a history, physical examination, laboratory tests, and CXR are recommended annually or every 6 months for 3 years, then annually thereafter until year 5.[4] Protocols vary widely with some not recommending abdominal CT at all, while others recommend CT at intervals ranging from annually for 3 years to once in year 2 and year 5.
- For patients with T3 or T4 primary tumors, most protocols recommend a history, physical examination, laboratory tests, and CXR be obtained every 6 months for a few years, then annually thereafter.[4] Most also recommend abdominal CT every 3 to 6 months for 3 years after surgery and less frequently (yearly or every other year) thereafter.

PROGNOSIS

- The clinical course is highly variable and spontaneous remissions have occurred.
- In a metaanalysis of 300 cases, small tumors had an average growth rate of 0.28 cm per year.[20] Although follow-up for most patients was only 2 to 3 years, only 1% of these patients developed metastases.
- Among patients initially treated with partial or radical nephrectomy, local or metastatic recurrences develop in approximately 20% to 50% of them.
- Five-year survival rates are 90.8% for localized disease (stage I, confined to the kidney), 63.1% for regional disease (spread to regional lymph nodes), and 11% for metastatic disease (stage IV).[3]
- In 1 retrospective study across 5 European centers (N = 1124), prognostic factors for survival following nephrectomy for RCC on univariate analysis were TNM (tumor, nodes, metastases) stage, Fuhrman grade (based on cell morphology), symptoms, Eastern Cooperative Oncology Group performance status, tumor size, and urinary collecting system invasion.[21]
- For papillary RCC, 1 study found incidental detection, T classification, M classification, vascular invasion, and tumor necrosis extent were independent prognostic factors of disease-specific survival.[22]
- For advanced RCC, a multivariate analysis with 246 patients found performance status 1 versus 0 (hazard ratio [HR] 1.95, $p < 0.0001$), high alkaline phosphatase (HR 1.5, $p = 0.002$), and lung metastasis only (HR 0.73, $p = 0.028$) were overall survival predictors.[23]

PATIENT EDUCATION

Several prognostic algorithms, or nomograms, for RCC survival are available that may be useful in counseling patients about their probable clinical course and facilitating treatment planning.[22,24]

PATIENT RESOURCES

- National Kidney Foundation—**http://www.kidney.org/.**
- National Institutes of Health, MedlinePlus. *Kidney Cancer*—**http://www.nlm.nih.gov/medlineplus/kidneycancer.html.**

PROVIDER RESOURCES

- National Cancer Institute Surveillance Epidemiology and End Results. *SEER Stat Fact Sheets: Kidney and Renal Pelvis*—**http://seer.cancer.gov/statfacts/html/kidrp.html.**
- Kidney Cancer Trial Search Tool, (800) 850-9132—**http://www.kidneycancer.org/knowledge/clinical-trials/about-clinical-trials.**

REFERENCES

1. Scher HI, Motzer RJ. Bladder and renal cell carcinomas. In: Kasper DL, Braunwald E, Fauci AS, Hauser SL, Longo DL, Jameson JL, eds. *Harrison's Principles of Internal Medicine*, 16th ed. New York, NY: McGraw-Hill; 2005:541-543.
2. Rini BI, Campbell SC, Escudier B. Renal cell carcinoma. *Lancet.* 2009;373:1119-1132.
3. National Cancer Institute. *SEER Stat Fact Sheets: Kidney and Renal Pelvis.* http://seer.cancer.gov/statfacts/html/kidrp.html. Accessed January 2012.
4. Casalino DD, Francis IR, Arellano RS, et al; Expert Panel on Urologic Imaging. *ACR Appropriateness Criteria® Follow-Up of Renal Cell Carcinoma* [online publication]. Reston, VA: American College of

Radiology; 2009:6. http://www.guideline.gov/content.aspx?id=15762&search=renal+cell+carcinoma. Accessed July 2013.

5. Motzer RJ, Agarwal N, Beard C, et al. NCCN clinical practice guidelines in oncology: kidney cancer. *J Natl Compr Canc Netw.* 2009;7(6):618-630.

6. Israel GM, Casalino DD, Remer EM, et al; Expert Panel on Urologic Imaging. *ACR Appropriateness Criteria® Indeterminate Renal Masses* [online publication]. Reston, VA: American College of Radiology; 2010:7. http://www.guideline.gov/content.aspx?id=32641&search=renal+cell+carcinoma. Accessed July 2013.

7. Jewett MA, Zuniga A. Renal tumor natural history: the rationale and role for active surveillance. *Urol Clin North Am.* 2008;35(4):627-634.

8. Coppin C, Kollmannsberger C, Le L, et al. Targeted therapy for advanced renal cell cancer (RCC): a Cochrane systematic review of published randomised trials. *BMJ (Int Ed).* 2011;108(10):1556-1563.

9. Escudier B, Kataja V; ESMO Guidelines Working Group. Renal cell carcinoma: ESMO clinical practice guidelines for diagnosis, treatment and follow-up. *Ann Oncol.* 2010;21 Suppl 5:v137-v139.

10. Hellenthal NJ, Underwood W, Penetrante R, et al. Prospective clinical trial of preoperative sunitinib in patients with renal cell carcinoma. *J Urol.* 2010;184(3):859-864.

11. Butler BP, Novick AC, Miller DP, et al. Management of small unilateral renal cell carcinomas: radical versus nephron-sparing surgery. *Urology.* 1995;45:34-40.

12. Roos FC, Pahernik S, Brenner W, Thuroff JW. Imperative and elective indications for nephron-sparing surgery for renal tumors: long-term oncological follow-up. *Aktuelle Urol.* 2010;Suppl 1:S70-S76.

13. Uppot RN, Harisinghani MG, Gervais DA. Imaging-guided percutaneous renal biopsy: rationale and approach. *AJR Am J Roentgenol.* 2010;194(6):1443-1449.

14. Venkatesan AM, Wood BJ, Gervais DA. Percutaneous ablation in the kidney. *Radiology.* 2011;261(2):375-391.

15. Pirasteh A, Snyder L, Boncher N, et al. Cryoablation vs. radiofrequency ablation for small renal masses. *Acad Radiol.* 2011;18(1):97-100.

16. Nabi G, Cleves A, Shelley M. Surgical management of localised renal cell carcinoma. *Cochrane Database Syst Rev.* 2010;(3):CD006579.

17. Flanigan RC, Mickisch G, Sylvester R, et al. Cytoreductive nephrectomy in patients with metastatic renal cancer: a combined analysis. *J Urol.* 2004;171:1071-1076.

18. Karam JA, Rini BI, Varella L, et al. Metastasectomy after targeted therapy in patients with advanced renal cell carcinoma. *J Urol.* 2011; 185(2):439-444.

19. Tanis PJ, van der Gaag NA, Busch OR, et al. Systematic review of pancreatic surgery for metastatic renal cell carcinoma. *Br J Surg.* 2009;96(6):579-592.

20. Chawla SN, Crispen PL, Hanlon AL, et al. The natural history of observed enhancing renal masses: meta-analysis and review of the world literature. *J Urol.* 2006;175:425-431.

21. Verhoest G, Avakian R, Bensalah K, et al. Urinary collecting system invasion is an independent prognostic factor of organ confined renal cell carcinoma. *J Urol.* 2009;182(3):854-859.

22. Klatte T, Remzi M, Zigeuner RE, et al. Development and external validation of a nomogram predicting disease specific survival after nephrectomy for papillary renal cell carcinoma. *J Urol.* 2010;184(1): 53-58.

23. Lars PN, Tangen CM, Conlon SJ, et al. Predictors of survival of advanced renal cell carcinoma: long-term results from Southwest Oncology Group Trial S8949. *J Urol.* 2009;181(2):512-516.

24. Lane BR, Kattan MW. Predicting outcomes in renal cell carcinoma. *Curr Opin Urol.* 2005;15(5):289-297.

86 CHRONIC KIDNEY DISEASE

Gary Ferenchick, MD

PATIENT STORY

A 75-year-old male with a known history of chronic kidney disease (CKD) and nephrotic syndrome caused by focal glomerular sclerosis and hypertension (HTN) treated with sodium restriction, protein restricted diet, and angiotensin II receptor blockers presents with worsening renal function. His most recent glomerular filtration rate was 13 mL/min. He has recently been going to dialysis education classes. His hemoglobin is 10.8 g/dL, and his parathyroid hormone level is 286 (pg/mL). Given his worsening renal function and the complication of anemia and secondary hyperparathyroidism, he is started on peritoneal dialysis. Within 1 month, the patient's blood pressure (BP) improved, as did his quality of life.

INTRODUCTION

According to the National Kidney Foundation, CKD includes glomerular filtration rate (GFR) less than 60 mL/min per 1.73 m^2 for more than 3 months with or without kidney damage and/or damage of the kidneys that can lead to decreased function. Markers of CKD include changes in the urinary sediment, such as albuminuria (which is a marker of glomerular damage), or changes on imaging studies that persist for more than 3 months, with or without a decrease in GFR. Damage can be detected on biopsy or in the blood or urine (eg, the presence of persistent proteinuria) or via imaging studies.[1]

Note that elderly patients can have a GFR below 60 but without evidence of kidney damage. Also, end-stage renal disease (ESRD) exists in patients who require dialysis or transplant to stay alive.

EPIDEMIOLOGY

- In the United States 26 million adults have CKD.
- About 5% of community-living persons[2] have an estimated GFR less than 60.
- More than 6 million persons older than 12 have a serum creatinine greater than 1.5 mg/dL.
- The incidence and prevalence of ESRD has increased twice in the United States since 2002.
- Microalbuminuria is present in about 10% of the US adult population, and about 1% have overt albuminuria.

ETIOLOGY

- Other than kidney damage, the most important factor affecting the GFR is the age of the patient. Therefore, mild decreases in the GFR are normal in the aging patient in the absence of kidney damage.
- Risk factors for the development of CKD
  - Most common is diabetes (44% of all dialysis patients) and HTN (27% or fewer of all dialysis patients).
  - Less common
    - Glomerular disease (10%)
    - Cystic disease (2%)
    - Autoimmune disease (<10%)
    - Urinary tract or systemic infections (<5%)
    - Lower urinary tract obstruction
    - Other: Family history of kidney disease, older age, black race, smoking
  - Risk factors for the progression of CKD
    - Poor control of diabetes mellitus (DM)
    - Poor BP control
    - Volume depletion
    - Intravenous contrast
    - Medications (antibiotics, nonsteroidal anti-inflammatory drugs [NSAIDs], angiotensin-converting enzyme [ACE] inhibitors, angiotensin II receptor blockers [ARBs])
- Urinary tract obstruction

PATHOGENESIS

Chronic HTN leads to renal disease by inducing glomerular ischemia by damaging glomerular arterioles.

- Structural damage to the glomeruli is induced by the loss of arteriole autoregulation, giving rise to high systemic arterial pressure transmitted to the glomeruli.[3]

CLINICAL MANIFESTATION

HISTORY/SYMPTOMS

Specifically ask about the presence or absence of the following:

- Patients with CKD are commonly without symptoms
- DM or HTN history
- Established diagnosis or risk factors for hepatitis B, hepatitis C, or human immunodeficiency virus (HIV) (can lead to CKD and proteinuria)
- Family history of renal disease (ie, polycystic disease, Alport syndrome, medullary kidney)
- Urinary symptoms suggestive of infection (eg, dysuria) or obstruction (eg, nocturia, hesitancy)
- Established diagnosis of or symptoms of connective tissue disease (eg, rash, arthralgias)
- Medications (eg, NSAIDs)

PHYSICAL EXAM

Specifically look for or establish the presence or absence of the following:

- Elevated BP and orthostatic changes
- Use a funduscopic examination to look for hypertensive or diabetic changes
- Uremic frost (**Figure 86-1**). This is rarely seen now.
- Signs of volume overload (eg, pretibial edema, JVD, pulmonary edema)
- Anasarca (total body pitting edema) (**Figure 86-2**)
- Renal bruit (suggesting renal artery stenosis)

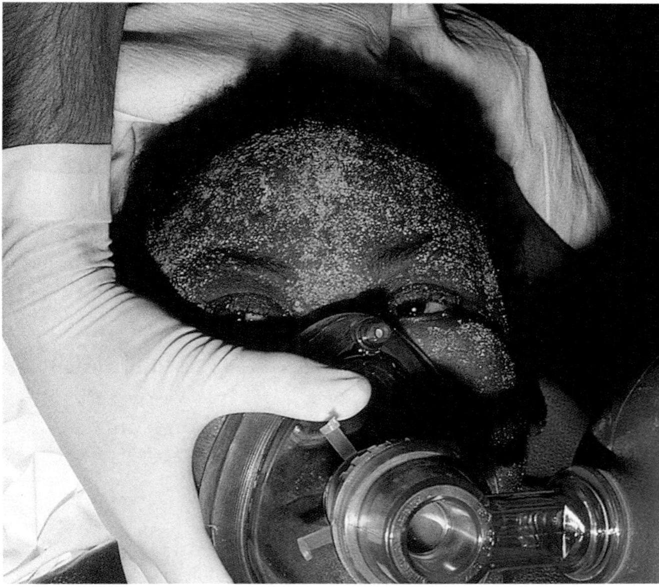

FIGURE 86-1 Uremic frost—the white crystalline material on the skin surface of a patient with profound azotemia caused by urea and other nitrogenous waste products that appear in sweat and crystallize on the skin. (*Used with permission from Knoop KJ, et al. The Atlas of Emergency Medicine, 3rd ed. McGraw-Hill, 2010. Photographer: Kevin J. Knoop, MD*)

OTHER FEATURES

Complications of CKD include the following:

- HTN is a consequence *and* a cause of CKD.
- Anemia is common in patients with a GFR less than 60.
- Bone disease may be present.
- There may be electrolyte abnormalities.

DIAGNOSIS

- Urine for protein
  - Normal daily urinary albumin excretion in adults is 10 mg per day and for total protein is about 50 mg per day.

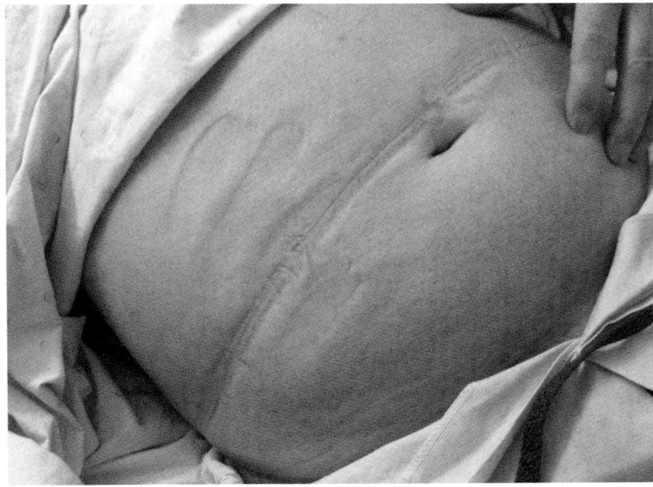

FIGURE 86-2 Anasarca—abdominal wall pitting edema in a patient with nephrotic syndrome and chronic renal failure caused by focal glomerular sclerosis. (*Reproduced with permission from Gary Ferenchick, MD.*)

  - Physiological variables such as fever, upright position, pregnancy, and exercise increase albumin excretion.
  - Persistently elevated urinary protein is a marker of CKD.
  - Persistently elevated excretion of albumin is a marker of CKD from DM, HTN, or glomerular disease.
  - According to the National Kidney Foundation
    - Proteinuria is the increased excretion of total protein (eg, albumin and globulins).
    - Albuminuria is the increased urinary excretion of albumin.
    - Microalbuminuria is albumin excretion greater than normal but below the range commonly detected by dipstick testing.
  - If the dipstick test is positive, quantitatively assess for increased urinary protein by checking protein-to-creatinine ratio or albumin-to-creatinine ratio in urine. If positive times 2, at least 2 weeks apart, then the diagnosis of persistent proteinuria should be made.
  - The normal spot urine albumin-to-creatinine ratio is less than 17 mg/g in men and less than 25 mg/g in women.
- Other urinary markers of CKD include dysmorphic red blood cells (RBCs) or RBC casts (suggests glomerulonephritis) and white blood cells (WBCs).
- Complete blood cell count (CBC), basic metabolic profile, uric acid, serum albumin
  - Anemia is a common complication in patients with CKD because of a decline in erythropoietin.
  - This is commonly normochromic and normocytic with a low reticulocyte count.
  - Assess for iron deficiency in patients with CKD; if present, consider a gastrointestinal (GI) source of blood loss.
- Others: calcium, phosphorus, vitamin D, serum parathyroid hormone level.
- Certain circumstances: hepatitis B and C serology, HIV, antinuclear antibodies (ANA; ie, lupus), antineutrophil cytoplasmic antibody (ANCA) (ie, vasculitis), serum and urine protein electrophoresis (ie, multiple myeloma)
- Structural abnormalities of the kidney can be identified with
  - Renal ultrasound—most commonly ordered as there is no risk for further renal damage; look for increased echogenicity, small kidneys, scarring, cysts, masses
  - Intravenous pyelogram (IVP) (asymmetry, stones, or medullary sponge changes)
  - Computed tomographic (CT) scan (cysts, tumors, stones)
  - Magnetic resonance imaging (MRI) (arterial disease or thrombosis)
  - Nuclear imaging (asymmetry, scars)

PROGNOSIS AND COMPLICATIONS

- Atherosclerotic cardiovascular disease (ASCVD)—Among patients with moderate-to-severe reduction of GFR, the 6-year rates of development of ESRD are 6% versus about 15% for coronary heart disease development. A GFR below 53 is associated with 32% higher 6-year risk of cardiovascular heart disease (CHD) compared to those with GFR above 104.
- Patients aged 25 to 35 on dialysis have an increase in CV mortality that is 500 times normal.

DIFFERENTIAL DIAGNOSIS

MANAGEMENT

- Goal BP is less than 130/80 for all patients with chronic renal disease (CRD).
  - Use ACE inhibitors or angiotensin receptor blockers if diabetic kidney disease is present or nondiabetic kidney disease with spot urine total protein-to-creatinine ratio greater than 200 mg/g; add diuretic as needed (thiazide if GFR > 30, loop diuretic if GFR < 30).
  - A diuretic is the first agent in nondiabetic kidney disease and when spot urine total protein-to-creatinine ratio is greater than 200 mg/g; add amlodipine as needed.
- Goal glycemic control is about 7.5%.
- Other risk factor modifications
  - Smoking cessation
  - Statin therapy to lower low-density lipoprotein (LDL) less than 100 mg/dL
  - Limit salt intake to less than 2.4 g/day
- Limit protein intake to less than 0.6 g/kg/day in patients with stage 4 or 5 CKD.
- Correct **phosphorus and vitamin D abnormalities**—Provide dietary phosphate restriction and phosphate-binding agents, vitamin D supplementation to maintain serum calcium, phosphorus (2.7-4.6 mg/dL) and parathyroid hormone levels (35-70 stage 3 or 70-110 stage 4) at goal range.
- Correct **acidosis** with oral sodium bicarbonate therapy to maintain serum bicarbonate above 22 mmol/L.
- Correct **hyperkalemia**—Chronic correction with sodium polystyrene sulfonate resin (Kayexalate) may be used.
- **Anemia**—Once a GI source of blood loss is ruled out, provide iron to maintain adequate iron stores (ferritin levels > 100 mg/dL, transferrin saturation > 20%).
- Giving erythropoietin to achieve a hemoglobin level of about 13 is associated with worse outcomes than achieving about an 11 for the hemoglobin level.[4]
- If a contrast study is needed, give 0.45% normal saline before and after the procedure. Also, consider intravenous N-acetylcysteine or sodium bicarbonate.[5,6]
- Avoid MRI scans with gadolinium in patients with stage 4 or stage 5 CKD because of the enhanced risk of nephrogenic systemic fibrosis.[7]
- Provide a nephrology consult for all patients with a GFR less than 30.
- Dialysis indications include
  - Volume overload not responsive to diuretics
  - Pericarditis
  - Uremic encephalopathy
  - HTN not responsive to treatment
- Others can include metabolic abnormalities noted previously not responsive to treatment; fatigue, nausea, and vomiting not otherwise responsive to treatment.

PATIENT RESOURCES

- National Kidney Foundation. Clinical practice guidelines for CKD—**http://www.kidney.org/professionals/kdoqi/guidelines_ckd/toc.htm.**

PROVIDER RESOURCES

- *KDIGO 2012 Clinical Practice guideline for the Evaluation and Management of Chronic Kidney Disease*—**http://www.kdigo.org/clinical_practice_guidelines/pdf/CKD/KDIGO_2012_CKD_GL.pdf.**

REFERENCES

1. National Kidney Foundation. *KDOQI Clinical Practice Guidelines for Chronic Kidney Disease*. 2002. http://www.kidney.org/professionals/kdoqi/guidelines_ckd/toc.htm.
2. Hallan SI, Dahl K, Oien CM, et al. Screening strategies for chronic kidney disease in the general population: follow-up of cross sectional health survey. *BMJ*. 2006;333(7577):1047. Epub 2006 Oct 24.
3. Ruzicka M, Burns KD, Culleton B, et al. Treatment of hypertension in patients with nondiabetic chronic kidney disease. *Can J Cardiol*. 2007;23(7):595-601.
4. Drüeke TB, Locatelli F, Clyne N, et al; and CREATE Investigators. Normalization of hemoglobin level in patients with chronic kidney disease and anemia. *N Engl J Med*. 2006;355(20):2071-2084.
5. Kelly AM, Dwamena B, Cronin P, et al. Meta-analysis: effectiveness of drugs for preventing contrast-induced nephropathy. *Ann Intern Med*. 2008;148(4):284-294.
6. Merten GJ, Burgess WP, Gray LV, et al. Prevention of contrast-induced nephropathy with sodium bicarbonate: a randomized controlled trial. *JAMA*. 2004;291(19):2328-2334.
7. Agarwal R, Brunelli SM, Williams K, et al. Gadolinium-based contrast agents and nephrogenic systemic fibrosis: a systematic review and meta-analysis. *Nephrol Dial Transplant*. 2009;24(3):856-863. doi:10.1093/ndt/gfn593. Epub 2008 Oct 24.

87 URINARY SEDIMENT

Mindy A. Smith, MD, MS
Richard P. Usatine, MD

PATIENT STORY

A 47-year-old woman presents to the office with severe right flank pain that does not radiate. Dipstick urinalysis shows hematuria, and microscopic examination confirms the presence of many red blood cells per high-power field (**Figure 87-1**). There is no pyuria or bacteriuria. The physician gives her some pain medication and sends her to get a CT urogram. The CT urogram shows a stone in the right ureter and some mild hydronephrosis. Fortunately, the patient passes the stone when urinating after the imaging study is complete.

INTRODUCTION

Examination of the urinary sediment is a test frequently done for evaluation of patients with suspected genetic/intrinsic (eg, systemic lupus nephritis, renal sarcoidosis, sickle cell disease, glomerulonephritis, interstitial nephritis), anatomic (eg, arteriovenous malformation), obstructive (eg, kidney or bladder stones, benign prostatic hypertrophy), infectious, metabolic (eg, coagulopathy), traumatic, or neoplastic disease of the urinary tract. Potential findings of red or white blood cells, casts, bacteria, or neoplastic cells help in directing further evaluation.

EPIDEMIOLOGY

- A finding of hematuria (2-5 red blood cells [RBCs]/high-power field [HPF]) on a single urinalysis in an asymptomatic person is common and most often a result of menses, allergy, exercise, viral illness, or mild trauma.[1]

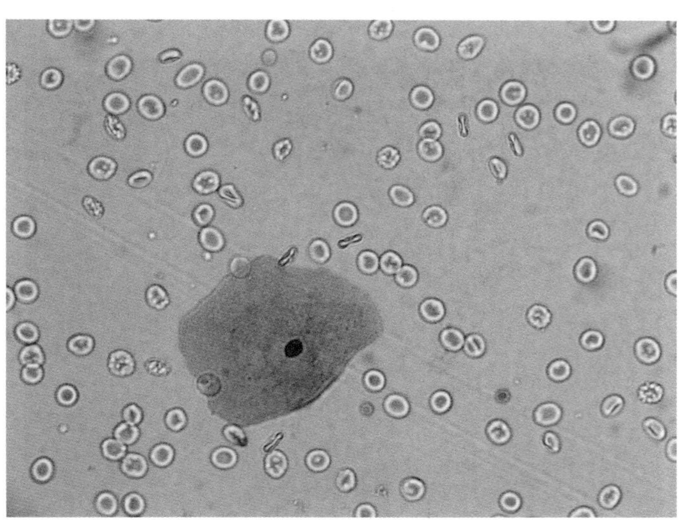

FIGURE 87-1 Red blood cells (RBCs) seen in the urine of a woman passing a kidney stone. Some of the RBCs are crenated, and there is 1 epithelial cell visible. (*Reproduced with permission of Richard P. Usatine, MD.*)

- One study of servicemen, conducted for a period of 10 years, found an incidence of 38%.[1]
- In 1 UK population study, first episode of hematuria resulted in a noncancer or cancer diagnosis within 90 days in 17.5% of women (95% confidence interval [CI], 16.4%-18.6%) and 18.3% of men (95% CI, 17.4%-19.3%).[2]
- Persistent (>3 RBCs/HPF over 3 specimens) and significant hematuria (>100 RBCs/HPF or gross hematuria) was associated with significant lesions in 9.1% of more than 1000 patients.[1]
- In a review of hematuria, approximately 5% of patients with significant microscopic hematuria (>3 RBCs/HPF on 2 of 3 properly collected specimens during a 2- to 3-week period)[3] and up to 40% of patients with gross hematuria have a neoplasm.[4]
- Isolated pyuria (>2-10 white blood cells per high-power field [WBCs/HPF]) is uncommon, as inflammatory processes in the urinary tract are usually associated with hematuria.[1]
- In a laboratory study from 88 institutions, 62.5% of urinalysis tests received a manual microscopic evaluation of the urinary sediment, usually triggered by an abnormal urinalysis. New information was obtained 65% of the time as a result of the manual examination.[5]

ETIOLOGY AND PATHOPHYSIOLOGY

- Hematuria (**Figure 87-1**) has many causes including the following:[1]
  - Idiopathic (increasing incidence in the young)
  - Stones
  - Neoplasms (increasing incidence with increase in age)
  - Trauma
  - Infection/inflammation including acute cystitis, urethritis, pyelonephritis, and prostatitis
  - Benign prostatic hypertrophy
  - Metabolic abnormalities, including hypercalcemia and hyperuricemia
  - Glomerular diseases such as immunoglobulin (Ig) A nephropathy, hereditary nephritis, and thin basement membrane disease
- Hematuria with dysmorphic RBCs or RBC casts (**Figure 87-2**) and excess protein excretion (>500 mg/dL) indicates glomerulonephritis.
- Gross hematuria suggests a postrenal source in the collecting system.
- Pyuria (**Figure 87-3**) is often the result of urinary tract infection.
  - The presence of bacteria (>10^2 organisms per mL or >10^5 using a midstream urine specimen) suggests infection. A urinalysis with 10 bacteria per HPF is highly suggestive (specificity 99%) of infection (positive likelihood ratio [LR+] 85).[2]
  - Asymptomatic bacteruria is found in 4% to 15% of pregnant women, usually *Escherichia coli*.
  - The presence of WBC casts (**Figure 87-4**) with bacteria indicates pyelonephritis.
- WBCs and/or WBC casts can be seen in tubulointerstitial processes like interstitial nephritis, systemic lupus erythematosus, or transplant rejection.
- Urinary casts are formed only in the distal convoluted tubule (DCT) or in the collecting duct (distal nephron).
- Hyaline casts are formed from mucoprotein secreted by the tubular epithelial cells within the nephrons. These translucent casts are the most common type of cast and can be seen in normal persons after vigorous exercise or with dehydration. Low urine flow and concentrated

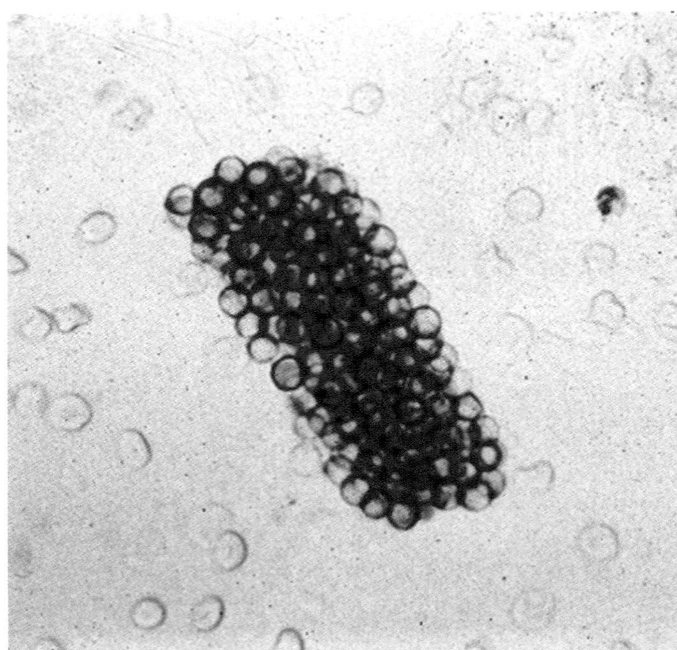

FIGURE 87-2 An RBC cast caused by bleeding into the tubule from the glomerulus. These casts are seen in glomerulonephritis, IgA nephropathy, lupus nephritis, Goodpasture syndrome, and Wegener granulomatosis. RBC casts are always pathologic. (*Reproduced with permission of Agnes B. Fogo, MD, Vanderbilt University.*)

urine from dehydration can contribute to the formation of hyaline casts (**Figure 87-5**).

- Granular casts are the second most common type of cast seen (**Figure 87-6**). These casts can result from the breakdown of cellular casts or the inclusion of aggregates of albumin or immunoglobulin light chains. They can be classified as fine or coarse based on the size of the inclusions. There is no diagnostic significance to the classification of fine or coarse.

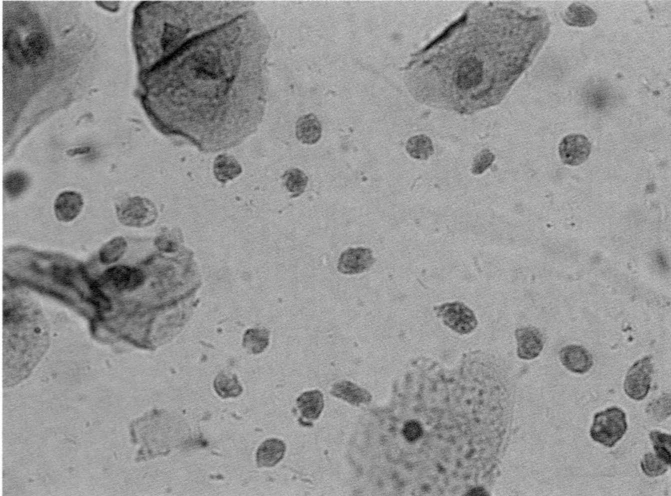

FIGURE 87-3 Pyuria and bacteriuria in a woman with a urinary tract infection. A simple stain was added to the wet mount of spun urine. Although there are epithelial cells present, the culture demonstrated a true urinary tract infection (UTI) and not merely a contaminated urine. (*Reproduced with permission of Richard P. Usatine, MD.*)

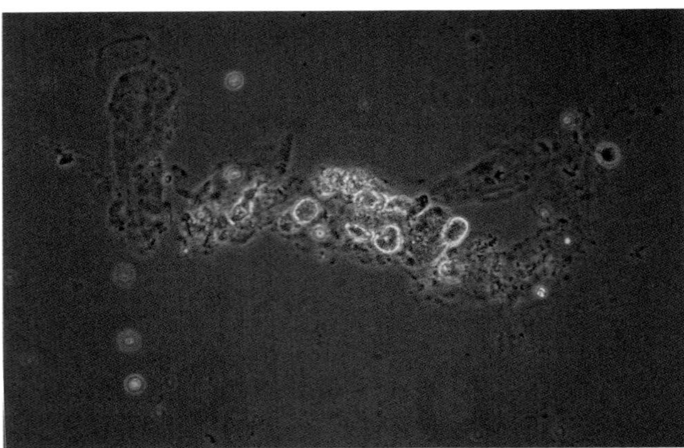

FIGURE 87-4 WBC casts seen in pyelonephritis. These can be differentiated from a clump of WBCs by their cylindrical shape and the presence of a hyaline matrix. (*Reproduced with permission of Agnes B. Fogo, MD, Vanderbilt University.*)

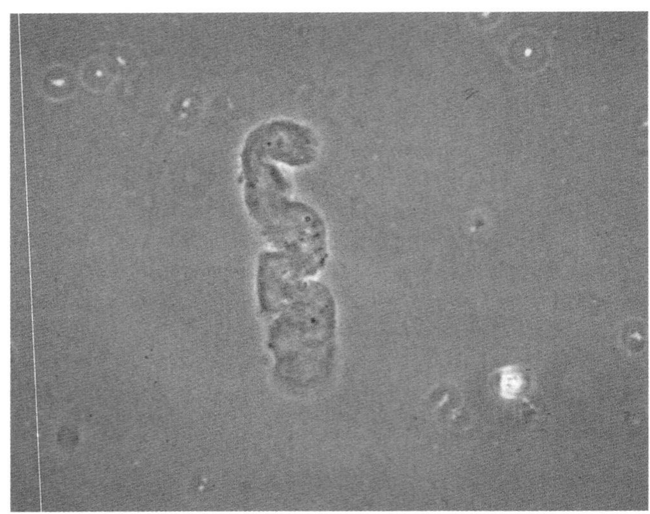

FIGURE 87-5 Hyaline casts are translucent and proteinaceous. These are the most common casts found in the urine and can be seen in normal individuals. Concentrated urine with low flow, usually caused by dehydration, exercise, and/or diuretics, can lead to hyaline cast formation. (*Reproduced with permission of Agnes B. Fogo, MD, Vanderbilt University.*)

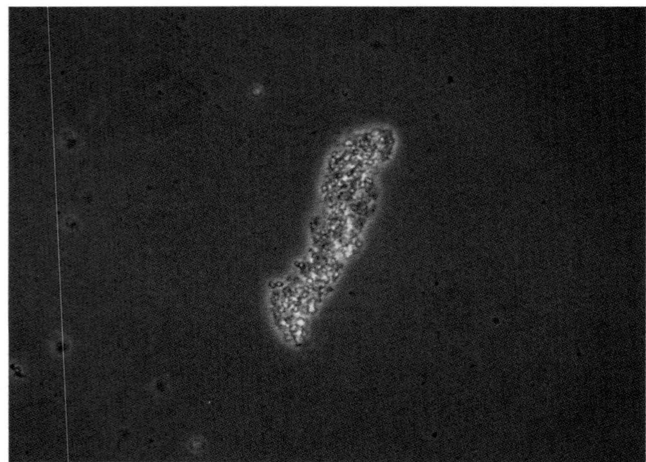

FIGURE 87-6 Coarse granular cast. All granular casts indicate underlying renal disease. These are nonspecific and may be seen in diverse renal conditions. (*Reproduced with permission of Agnes B. Fogo, MD, Vanderbilt University.*)

RISK FACTORS

- Constipation (for urinary tract infection [UTI] in elderly).
- Risk factors for cancer in patients with microscopic hematuria include the following[4]:
  - Smoking
  - Age older than 40 years
  - Medical history of gross hematuria, urologic disease, or pelvic radiation
  - Occupational history of exposure to chemicals or dyes
  - Analgesic abuse

DIAGNOSIS

CLINICAL FEATURES

- Other signs and symptoms of glomerular disease include various degrees of renal failure, edema, oliguria, and hypertension.
- Hematuria is often asymptomatic in patients with glomerular disease or metabolic abnormalities. Renal stones can cause pain in the ipsilateral flank and/or abdomen with radiation to the ipsilateral groin, testicle or vulva or irritative symptoms of frequency, urgency, and dysuria, if located in the bladder.
- Symptoms of UTI include dysuria, nocturia, urgency, frequency, offensive odor of urine, or a combination of these; positive likelihood ratios, however, are low (1.3-2.3).[6]
- Symptoms of pyelonephritis include chills and rigor, fever, nausea and vomiting, and flank pain; positive likelihood ratios are 1.5 to 2.5.
- Family history of renal failure or microscopic hematuria or history of trauma, weight loss, and changes in urine volume may be useful.

LABORATORY TESTING AND IMAGING

The work-up for persistent or significant hematuria includes the following[1]:

- Urinary sediment looking for dysmorphic cells or RBC casts (**Figure 87-2**) and a 24-hour urine sample for proteinuria.
  - If positive, suspect glomerular disease and consider blood cultures, antiglomerular basement membrane (GBM) antibody, antineutrophil cytoplasmic antibody (ANCA), complement, cryoglobulins, hepatitis serologies, Venereal Disease Research Laboratory (VDRL), HIV, and antistreptolysin O; a renal biopsy may be indicated.
  - If negative and the sediment contains WBCs (**Figure 87-3**) or WBC casts (**Figure 87-4**), suspect infection and obtain a urine culture and susceptibility test if pyelonephritis is suspected; *E. coli* is the most common organism (more than 80%) in uncomplicated cystitis. WBCs seen in conjunction with many epithelial cells, particularly in women, can indicate a contaminated specimen; and a new clean catch urine specimen should be obtained if possible.
  - If negative and no WBCs, obtain a hemoglobin electrophoresis, urine cytology, urinalysis (UA) from family members looking for hematuria or signs of glomerular disease, and a 24-hour urine for calcium and uric acid.
- In all adult patients with hematuria (except for those with generalized renal parenchymal disease or young women with hemorrhagic cystitis), the American College of Radiology (ACR) recommends obtaining CT urography.[7] In patients with generalized renal parenchymal disease, ultrasound of the kidneys and bladder is recommended. For painful hematuria, a CT of the abdomen and pelvis without contrast and/or an ultrasound of the kidneys and bladder is most appropriate.[7] For hematuria associated with trauma, obtain a CT of the abdomen and pelvis with contrast.
  - If the above is negative or high risk for cancer, perform cystoscopy.
  - If the above is positive, an open renal biopsy may be indicated.
  - If the above is negative, consider periodic follow-up (6, 12, 24, and 36 months).
- If RBC casts (**Figure 87-2**) are seen on UA in addition to proteinuria, also consider nephrotic syndrome caused by diabetes or amyloidosis.
- Note that RBC casts are fragile and are best seen in a fresh urine specimen (Figure 87-2).

MANAGEMENT

Treatment will depend on the underlying etiology:

- Cystitis is treated with appropriate antibiotics based on knowledge of the sensitivities of *E. coli* in your practice location (nitrofurantoin [100 mg twice daily for 5 days], trimethoprim-sulfamethoxazole [1 double-strength tablet twice-daily for 3 days], or fosfomycin [3-g single dose] are first-line agents).[8] Symptoms usually improve within 24 to 36 hours.
- Uncomplicated pyelonephritis is treated with appropriate antibiotics as an outpatient (oral ciprofloxacin [500 mg twice daily] for 7 days with or without an initial 400-mg intravenous dose when resistance is not known to exceed 10%).[8] The urine should always be cultured in pyelonephritis to help guide therapy. Pregnant women may need hospitalization.
- See Chapter 80 (Kidney Stones) for management of patients with kidney stones, Chapter 85 (Renal Cell Carcinoma) for renal cell carcinoma, and Chapter 78 (Bladder Cancer) for bladder cancer.

PREVENTION AND SCREENING

The United States Preventive Services Task Force concluded that there was insufficient evidence to assess the balance of benefits and harms of screening for bladder cancer in asymptomatic adults.[9] The positive predictive value of screening is less than 10% in asymptomatic persons, including higher-risk populations.

PROVIDER RESOURCES

- *Urinalysis*—**http://library.med.utah.edu/WebPath/TUTORIAL/URINE/URINE.html**
- Urine Sediment Atlas—**https://ahdc.vet.cornell.edu/clinpath/modules/ua-sed/ua-intro.htm**

REFERENCES

1. Denker BM, Brenner BM. Azotemia and urinary abnormalities. In: Kasper DL, Braunwald E, Fauci AS, Hauser SL, Longo DL, Jameson JL, eds. *Harrison's Principles of Internal Medicine*, 16th ed. New York, NY: McGraw-Hill; 2005:250-251.
2. Jones R, Charlton J, Latinovic R, Gulliford MC. Alarm symptoms and identification of non-cancer diagnoses in primary care: cohort study. *BMJ*. 2009;339:b3094. doi: 10.1136/bmj.b3094.

3. Grossfeld GD, Litwin MS, Wolf JS, et al. Evaluation of asymptomatic microscopic hematuria in adults: the American Urological Association best practice policy—part I: definition, detection, prevalence, and etiology. *Urology.* 2001;57(4):599-603.
4. Margulis V, Sagalowsky AI. Assessment of hematuria. *Med Clin North Am.* 2011;95:153-159.
5. Tworek JA, Wilkinson DS, Walsh MK. The rate of manual microscopic examination of urine sediment: a College of American Pathologists Q-Probes study of 11,243 urinalysis tests from 88 institutions. *Arch Pathol Lab Med.* 2008;132(12):1868-1873.
6. Bergus GR. Dysuria. In: Sloane PD, Slatt LM, Ebell MH, Smith MA, Power D, Viera AJ, eds. *Essentials of Family Medicine*, 6th ed. Baltimore, MD: Lippincott Williams & Wilkins; 2012:327-336.
7. Ramchandani P, Kisler T, Francis IR, et al; Expert Panel on Urologic Imaging. *ACR Appropriateness Criteria® Hematuria*. Reston, VA: American College of Radiology; 2008 [online publication]. http://www.guideline.gov/content.aspx?id=15763&search=hematuria. Accessed July 2013.
8. Gupta K, Hooton TM, Naber KG, et al; Infectious Diseases Society of America, European Society for Microbiology and Infectious Diseases. International clinical practice guidelines for the treatment of acute uncomplicated cystitis and pyelonephritis in women: a 2010 update by the Infectious Diseases Society of America and the European Society for Microbiology and Infectious Diseases. *Clin Infect Dis.* 2011;52(5):e103-e120.
9. Moyer VA; U.S. Preventive Services Task Force. Screening for bladder cancer: U.S. Preventive Services Task Force recommendation statement. *Ann Intern Med.* 2011;155(4):246-251.

PART 12

WOMEN'S HEALTH

Strength of Recommendation (SOR)	Definition
A	Recommendation based on consistent and good-quality patient-oriented evidence.*
B	Recommendation based on inconsistent or limited-quality patient-oriented evidence.*
C	Recommendation based on consensus, usual practice, opinion, disease-oriented evidence, or case series for studies of diagnosis, treatment, prevention, or screening.*

*See Appendix A on pages 1241-1244 for further information.

SECTION 1 VAGINITIS/CERVICITIS

88 OVERVIEW OF VAGINITIS

E.J. Mayeaux Jr, MD

PATIENT STORY

A 39-year-old woman presented to her physician with a malodorous vaginal discharge. On examination, a thin white discharge was seen covering the introitus (**Figure 88-1**). A speculum examination revealed a thin whitish gray discharge and a distinct fishy odor. The pH of the discharge was 4.6, and 40% of the epithelial cells on her wet prep were clue cells (**Figure 88-2**). She was diagnosed with bacterial vaginosis and treated with oral metronidazole.

INTRODUCTION

Vaginal discharge is a frequent presenting complaint in primary care. The 3 most common causes are bacterial vaginosis, candidiasis, and trichomoniasis. However, a significant number of patients with vaginal discharge will have some other condition, such as atrophic vaginitis. Providers must refrain from "diagnosing" a vaginitis based solely on the color and consistency of the discharge, as this may lead to misdiagnosis and may miss concomitant infections.[1]

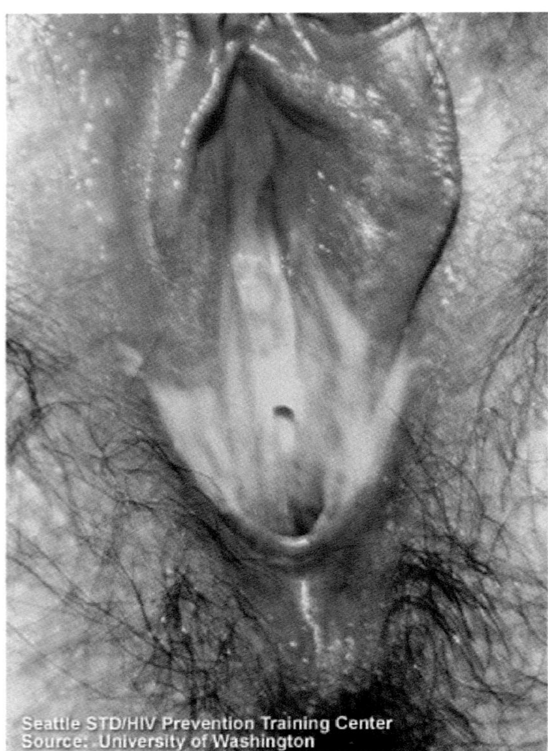

FIGURE 88-1 Thin white discharge from bacterial vaginosis seen covering the introitus prior to speculum examination. (*Reproduced with permission of Seattle STD/HIV Prevention Training Center, University of Washington.*)

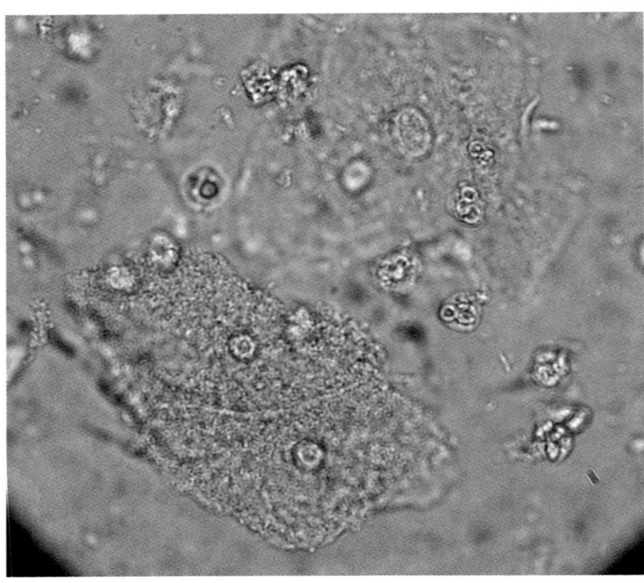

FIGURE 88-2 A wet mount of vaginal discharge in saline under high-power light microscopy. Note the presence of vaginal epithelial cells, smaller white blood cells (polymorphonucleocytes), and bacteria. The bacteria are the coccobacilli of *Gardnerella vaginalis* covering the cell membranes of the 2 vaginal epithelial cells near the lower end of the field. These are clue cells seen in patients with bacterial vaginosis. (*Reproduced with permission of Richard P. Usatine, MD.*)

EPIDEMIOLOGY

The reported rates of chlamydia and gonorrhea are highest among females ages 15 to 19 years. Adolescents are at greater risk for sexually transmitted diseases (STDs) because they frequently have unprotected intercourse, are biologically more susceptible to infection, are often engaged in partnerships of limited duration, and face multiple obstacles to utilization of health care.[1]

ETIOLOGY AND PATHOPHYSIOLOGY

- The quantity and quality of normal vaginal discharge in healthy women vary. Physiologic leukorrhea refers to generally nonmalodorous, mucousy, white, or yellowish vaginal discharge in the absence of a pathologic cause. It is not accompanied by signs and symptoms such as pain, pruritus, burning, erythema, or tissue friability. However, slight malodor and irritative symptoms can be normal for some women at certain times.[2] Physiologic leukorrhea is usually a result of estrogen-induced changes in cervicovaginal secretions.
- Noninfectious causes of vaginitis include irritants (eg, scented panty liners, spermicides, povidone-iodine, soaps and perfumes, and some topical drugs) and allergens (eg, latex condoms, topical antifungal agents, chemical preservatives) that produce hypersensitivity reactions.
- Before starting an examination, determine whether the patient douched recently, because this can lower the yield of diagnostic tests and increase the risk of pelvic inflammatory disease.[3] Patients who have

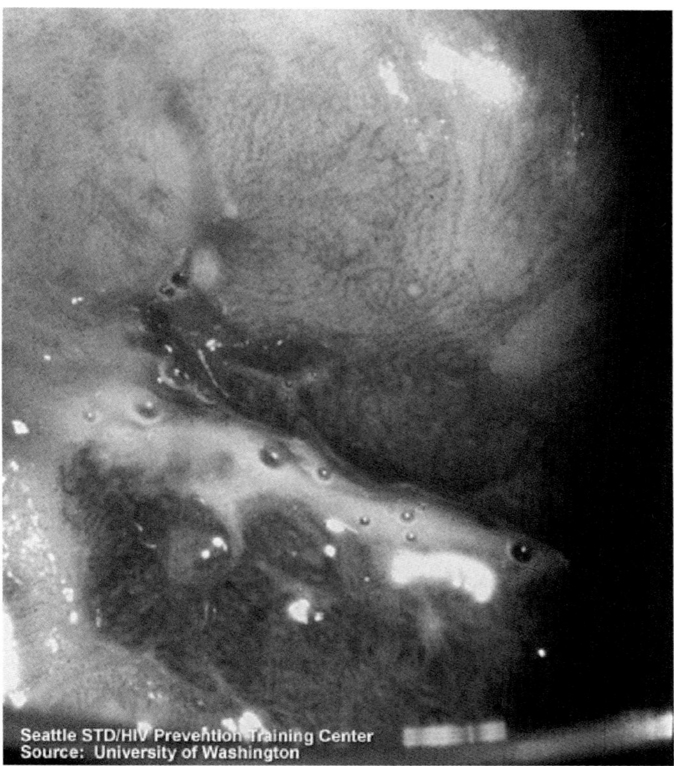

FIGURE 88-3 Colposcopic view of the cervix in a patient infected with trichomonas vaginalis. Note the frothy discharge with visible bubbles and the cervical erythema. (*Reproduced with permission of Seattle STD/HIV Prevention Training Center, University of Washington.*)

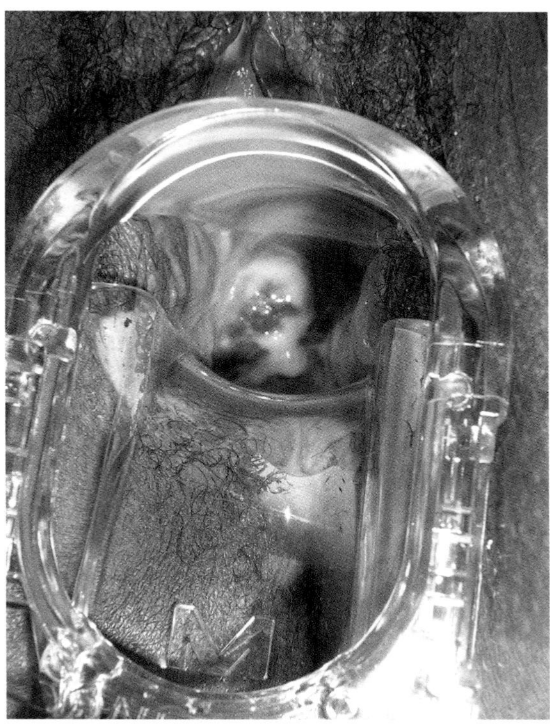

FIGURE 88-4 Speculum examination showing mucopurulent discharge with a friable appearing cervix. (*Reproduced with permission of Richard P. Usatine, MD.*)

been told not to douche will sometimes start wiping the vagina with soapy washcloths, which also irritates the vagina and cervix and may cause a discharge. Douching is associated with increases in bacterial vaginosis and acquisition of sexually transmitted infections when exposed. However, recent studies indicate that douching with plain water once a week or less did not disturb normal flora.[4,5]

- There are many causes of vaginitis in humans. Infectious causes include bacterial vaginosis (40%-50% of cases) (see **Figures 88-1 and 88-2**), vulvovaginal candidiasis (20%-25%), and trichomonas (15%-20%) (**Figure 88-3**).[6] Less common causes include atrophic vaginitis, foreign body (especially in children), cytolytic or desquamative inflammatory vaginitis, streptococcal vaginitis, ulcerative vaginitis, and idiopathic vulvovaginal ulceration associated with HIV infection.
- Rarer noninfectious causes include chemicals, allergies, hypersensitivity, contact dermatitis, trauma, postpuerperal atrophic vaginitis, erosive lichen planus, collagen vascular disease, Behçet syndrome, and pemphigus syndromes.

DIAGNOSIS

CLINICAL FEATURES

- Examine the external genitalia for irritation or discharge (see **Figure 88-2**). Speculum examination is done to determine the amount and character of the discharge (**Figure 88-4**). A chlamydia and gonorrhea test should always be done in sexually active females with a vaginal discharge. Look closely at the cervix for discharge and signs of infection, dysplasia, or cancer (**Figure 88-3**). Bimanual examination may show evidence of cervical, uterine, or adnexal tenderness. **Table 88-1** shows diagnostic values for examination of vaginitis.
- Vaginal pH testing can be helpful in the diagnosis of vaginitis. The pH can be checked by applying pH paper to the vaginal sidewall. Do not place the pH paper in contact with the cervical mucus. A pH above 4.5 is seen with menopausal patients, trichomonas infection, or bacterial vaginosis.
- Wet preps are obtained by applying a cotton-tipped applicator to the vaginal sidewall and placing the sample into normal saline. A drop of the suspension is then placed on a slide and examined for the presence and number of white blood cells (WBCs), trichomonads, candidal hyphae, or clue cells (**Figure 88-1**).
- A KOH prep is made by adding a drop of KOH solution to a drop of saline suspension of the discharge. The KOH lyses epithelial cells in 5 to 15 minutes (faster if the slide is warmed briefly) and allows easier visualization of candidal hyphae. The use of KOH with DMSO allows for quicker lyses of the epithelial cells and immediate examination of the smear.
- Another diagnostic procedure is the "whiff" test, which is performed by placing a drop of KOH on a slide of the wet prep and smelling for a foul, fishy odor. The odor is indicative of anaerobic overgrowth or infection. The "whiff" test is positive if the fishy amine odor is detected during the examination and it is then not necessary to add KOH and "whiff" again.

LABORATORY TESTING

- Nucleic acid amplification tests are highly sensitive tests for *Neisseria gonorrhoeae*, *Chlamydia*, and *Chlamydia trachomatis* that can be performed on genital specimens or urine. Urine screening for gonorrhea, chlamydia, or both using nucleic acid amplification test can be used successfully in difficult-to-reach adolescents.[7]

TABLE 88-1 Diagnostic Values for Vaginal Infections

Diagnostic Criteria	Normal	Bacterial Vaginosis	Trichomonas Vaginitis	Candida Vulvovaginitis
Vaginal pH	3.8-4.2	>4.5	4.5	<4.5 (usually)
Discharge	White, thin, flocculent	Thin, white, gray	Yellow, green, or gray, frothy	White, curdy, "cottage cheese"
Amine odor "whiff" test	Absent	Fishy	Fishy	Absent
Microscopic	Lactobacilli, epithelial cells	Clue cells, adherent cocci, no white blood cells	Trichomonads, white blood cells >10/hpf	Budding yeast, hyphae, Pseudohyphae

Data from E.J. Mayeaux Jr, MD.

MANAGEMENT

- Management is based on the identification of the causative agent.
- Treatment for physiologic leukorrhea is unnecessary.
- Management of vaginal irritants and allergens involves identifying and eliminating the offending agents. However, irritants and allergens can often be difficult to identify.
- Health food store lactobacilli are the wrong strain and do not adhere well to the vaginal epithelium. Ingestion of live-culture, nonpasteurized yogurt does not significantly change the incidence of candidal vulvovaginitis or bacterial vaginosis.[8]

PATIENT RESOURCES

- Centers for Disease Control and Prevention. *Sexually Transmitted Diseases* page—**http://www.cdc.gov/std/.**
- Planned Parenthood—**http://www.plannedparenthood.org/cameron-willacy/images/South-Texas/What_Every_Woman_Needs_to_Know_English.pdf.**
- Illinois Department of Public Health. *Vaginitis*—**www.idph.state.il.us/public/hb/hbvaginitis.htm.**

PROVIDER RESOURCES

- Centers for Disease Control and Prevention. *2010 Guidelines for Treatment of Sexually Transmitted Diseases*—**http://www.cdc.gov/std/treatment/2010/STD-Treatment-2010-RR5912.pdf.**
- Centers for Disease Control and Prevention. *Self-Study STD Module–Vaginitis*—**http://www2a.cdc.gov/STDTraining/Self-Study/vaginitis/default.htm**
- Centers for Disease Control and Prevention. Vaginitis slides—**http://www2a.cdc.gov/stdtraining/ready-to-use/Manuals/Vaginitis/vaginitis-slides-2010.pdf.**
- eMedicine. *Vaginitis*—**http://emedicine.medscape.com/article/257141-overview.**
- American Family Physician. *Diagnosis of Vaginitis*—**http://www.aafp.org/afp/20000901/1095.html.**

REFERENCES

1. Centers for Disease Control and Prevention. *Sexually Transmitted Disease Surveillance 2001*. Atlanta, GA: U.S. Department of Health and Human Services, CDC, 2002.
2. Anderson M, Karasz A, Friedland S. Are vaginal symptoms ever normal? A review of the literature. *Med Gen Med*. 2004;6:49.
3. Zhang J, Thomas AG, Leybovich E. Vaginal douching and adverse health effects: a meta-analysis. *Am J Public Health*. 1997;87:1207-1211.
4. Hassan S, Chatwani A, Brovender H, et al. Douching for perceived vaginal odor with no infectious cause of vaginitis: a randomized controlled trial. *J Low Genit Tract Dis*. 2011;15(2):128-133.
5. Zhang J, Hatch M, Zhang D, et al. Frequency of douching and risk of bacterial vaginosis in African-American women. *Obstet Gynecol*. 2004;104(4):756-760.
6. Sobel JD. Vaginitis. *N Engl J Med*. 1997;337:1896-1903.
7. Monroe KW, Weiss HL, Jones M, Hook EW 3rd. Acceptability of urine screening for *Neisseria gonorrheae* and *Chlamydia trachomatis* in adolescents at an urban emergency department. *Sex Transm Dis*. 2003;30:850-853.
8. Pirotta M, Gunn J, Chondros P, et al. Effect of lactobacillus in preventing post-antibiotic vulvovaginal candidiasis: a randomised controlled trial. *BMJ*. 2004;329:548.

89 ATROPHIC VAGINITIS

E.J. Mayeaux Jr, MD

PATIENT STORY

A 60-year-old woman with vaginal dryness and irritation is seen to follow-up on an inflammatory Pap smear. She denies discharge, odor, douching, and sexually transmitted disease (STD) exposure. She does admit to some postcoital bleeding. Her cervix has atrophic changes and an endocervical polyp (**Figure 89-1**). The polyp was removed easily with a ring forceps and no dysplasia was found on pathology.

INTRODUCTION

Vaginal atrophy caused by estrogen deficiency is common and usually is asymptomatic except for vaginal dryness.

SYNONYMS

Vaginal atrophy, vulvovaginal atrophy, urogenital atrophy, senile vaginitis.

EPIDEMIOLOGY

- The average age of menopause is 51 years in the United States.
- Approximately 5% of women experience menopause after age 55 years (late menopause), and another 5% experience the transition between the ages of 40 and 45 years (early menopause). This means that in the United States, most women will live a significant portion of their lives during menopause. Women who in menopause have surgical menopause or have ovarian suppression without estrogen supplementation (progestin-only contraceptives) are susceptible to atrophic changes in their lower genital tract.
- Vaginal dryness occurs in approximately 3% of women of reproductive age, 4% to 21% of women in the menopausal transition, and 47% of women 3 years postmenopause.[1] Internationally, 39% of women experience menopause-related vaginal discomfort.[2]

ETIOLOGY AND PATHOPHYSIOLOGY

- After menopause, circulating estrogen levels dramatically decrease to a level at least one-sixth their premenopausal levels.[3] Changes that occur in the vaginal and cervical epithelium include proliferation of connective tissue, loss of elastin, thinning of the epithelium (**Figure 89-2**), and hyalinization of collagen.
- A long-term decrease in estrogen is generally necessary before symptoms become apparent. Genital symptoms include decreased vaginal lubrication, dryness, burning, dyspareunia, leukorrhea, itching, and yellow malodorous discharge.
- Urinary symptoms, such as frequency, hematuria, urinary tract infection, dysuria, and stress incontinence, are usually late symptoms. Over time, the lack of vaginal lubrication often results in sexual dysfunction.
- Cervical polyps (**Figure 89-1**) are pedunculated tumors that usually arise from the endocervical canal mucosa, and are common in patients with atrophic vaginitis. Many will show squamous metaplasia, and they may develop squamous dysplasia. Polyps are most commonly asymptomatic unless they bleed.
- Menopause is the most common cause of atrophic vaginitis. In premenopausal women, radiation therapy, chemotherapy, immunologic disorders, and oophorectomy may greatly decrease production of ovarian estrogen and lead to atrophic vaginitis. Antiestrogen medications may also result in atrophic vaginitis. Women who are naturally premenopausally estrogen deficient, smoke cigarettes, or have not given vaginal birth tend to have more severe symptoms.[3]

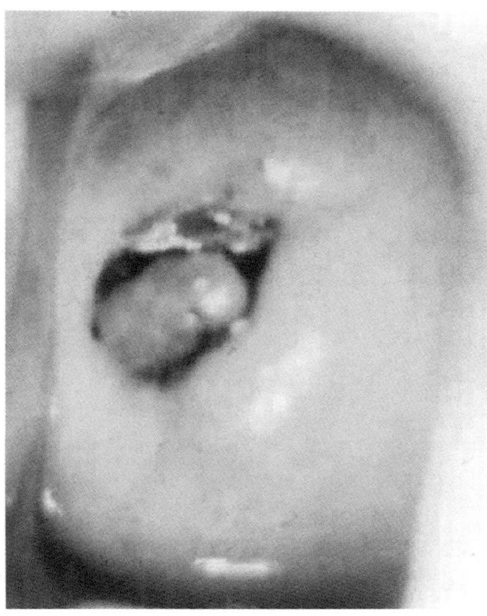

FIGURE 89-1 Colposcopic photograph (scanning objective with 10× eyepiece) demonstrating atrophic vaginitis. Note thinned white epithelium, friable epithelium with bleeding, and a cervical polyp. (*Reproduced with permission of E.J. Mayeaux Jr, MD.*)

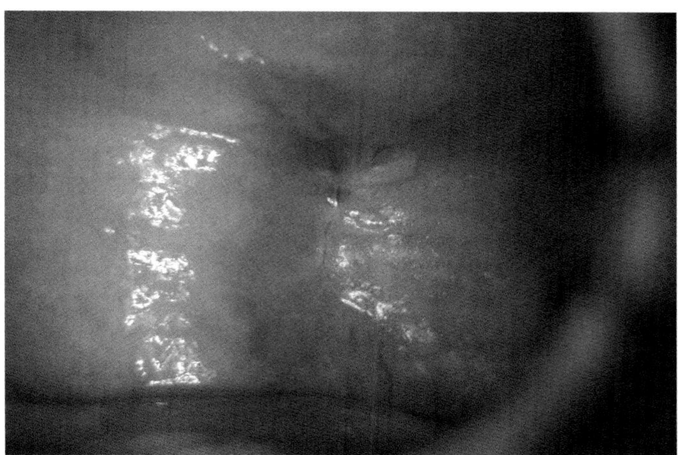

FIGURE 89-2 Colposcopic photograph (scanning objective with 10× eyepiece) demonstrating atrophic cervicovaginitis. Note thin white epithelium, relative dryness, and a barely visible cervical os. (*Reproduced with permission of E.J. Mayeaux Jr, MD.*)

RISK FACTORS

- Age
- Family history of early menopause
- Bilateral oophorectomy
- Spontaneous premature ovarian failure
- Antiestrogenic medications effects, such as tamoxifen, danazol, medroxyprogesterone acetate
- Gonadotropin-releasing hormone agonists (leuprolide, nafarelin, goserelin), or antagonists (ganirelix)
- Prolactin elevation as a result of hypothalamic-pituitary disorders with secondary reduction of estrogen secretion
- Certain chemotherapeutic agents
- Pelvic radiation therapy
- Severe systemic lupus erythematosus or rheumatoid arthritis (because of hypothalamic hypogonadism or primary ovarian insufficiency) combined with glucocorticoid therapy cause combined suppression of ovarian and adrenal activity

DIAGNOSIS

CLINICAL FEATURES

- Diagnosis is clinical, based upon characteristic symptoms and findings. Many women with symptoms of vaginal atrophy do not discuss their condition with a health care provider because they believe their symptoms are a normal part of the aging process.[4]
- Atrophic vaginal and cervical epithelium appears pale, smooth, relatively dry, and shiny (**Figure 89-2**). Inflammation with patchy erythema, petechiae, and friability is common in more advanced cases. The external genitalia may demonstrate diminished elasticity, turgor of skin, sparsity of pubic hair, dryness of labia, erythema (**Figure 89-3**), and fusion of the labia minora.[5]

LABORATORY TESTING

- Laboratory tests to confirm hypoestrogenic findings are typically not necessary.

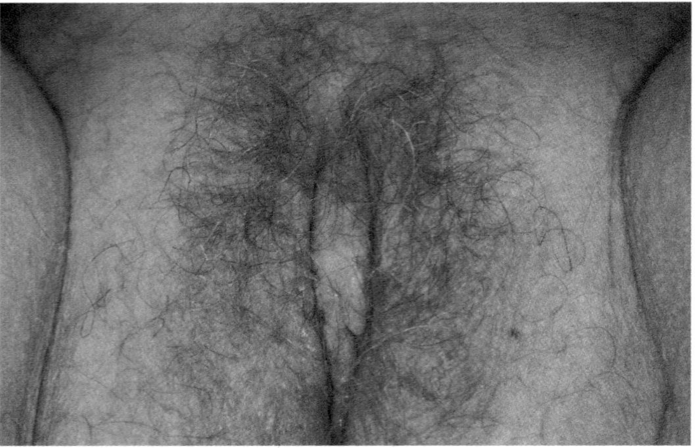

FIGURE 89-3 The vulva of a postmenopausal woman demonstrating thinning of the hair and thinning and erythema of vulvar skin associated with atrophic vulvitis. *(Reproduced with permission of Gordon Davis, MD, Arizona Vulva Clinic, Inc.)*

- Serum estradiol levels of less than 20 pg/mL support a clinical diagnosis of a low-estrogenic state. However, values are very laboratory dependent, and most assays are neither sufficiently sensitive nor reliable for diagnosis of hypoestrogenic states without clinical signs and symptoms.
- A serum follicle-stimulating hormone (FSH) level greater than 40 mIU/mL is diagnostic of menopause.
- A Papanicolaou smear can confirm the presence of urogenital atrophy. Cytologic examination of smears from the upper one-third of the vagina shows an increased proportion of parabasal cells and a decreased percentage of superficial cells.
- An elevated vaginal pH level (>5), monitored by a pH strip in the vaginal vault, may also be a sign of vaginal atrophy.[3]

IMAGING

- Testing for associated osteoporosis should be considered if not previously performed.

DIFFERENTIAL DIAGNOSIS

- Atrophic vaginitis symptoms can be mimicked or exacerbated by coinfection of candidiasis, trichomoniasis, or bacterial vaginosis. These can be identified by wet prep, pH, and whiff test (see Chapter 90, Bacterial Vaginosis).
- Sexually transmitted diseases, including gonorrhea, trichomonas, and chlamydia, also may coexist with or mimic atrophic vaginitis. Cultures or nucleic acid amplification tests can identify these infections. It is important not to assume a diagnosis of solely atrophic vaginitis in the postmenopausal patient who presents with urogenital complaints. (Chapter 88, Overview of Vaginitis).
- Contact dermatitis because of environmental agents (eg, perfumes, deodorants, soaps, panty liners, perineal pads, spermicides, lubricants, or tight fitting/synthetic clothing) may cause erythema, itching, burning, or pain. (Chapter 144, Contact Dermatitis).
- Vulvovaginal lichen planus may produce labial fusion. (Chapter 154. Lichen Planus).
- Lichen sclerosus (LS) appears to cause atrophy of the vulva and can be mistaken for the atrophy of estrogen deficiency. It can be recognized by the hour-glass configuration of the involvement around the vulva and perianal region **(Figure 89-4)**. LS is treated with a high-potency steroid ointment rather than estrogen.

MANAGEMENT

NONPHARMACOLOGIC

- Nonhormonal local vaginal moisturizers and lubricants may be used to help maintain natural secretions and comfort during intercourse. Sexual activity has been shown to encourage vaginal elasticity and pliability, and the lubricative response to sexual stimulation. An open-label study indicated that Replens, a bioadhesive vaginal moisturizer, was a safe and effective alternative to estrogen vaginal cream, with both therapies exhibiting statistically significant increases in vaginal moisture, vaginal fluid volume, and vaginal elasticity.[6] SOR Ⓐ
- Water-based vaginal lubricants include the following:
  - Slippery Stuff (polyoxyethylene, methylparaben, propylene glycol, isopropanol)

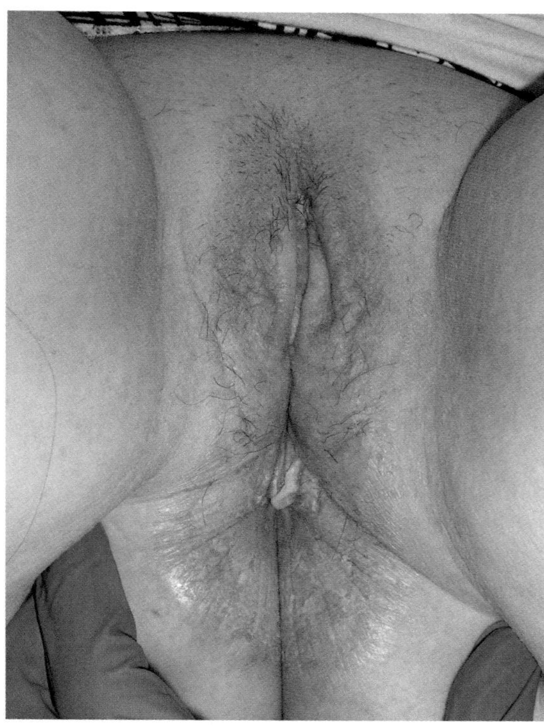

FIGURE 89-4 Lichen sclerosus of the vulva in this 53-year-old woman. Lichen sclerosus can be recognized by the hour-glass configuration of involvement around the vulva and perianal region. The term "et atrophicus" was dropped from the name because the condition is actually sclerotic, not atrophic. (*Reproduced with permission of Richard P. Usatine, MD.*)

- Astroglide (glycerin, methylparaben, propylparaben, polypropylene glycol, polyquaternium, hydroxyethylcellulose)
- K-Y Jelly (glycerin, hydroxyethylcellulose, parabens, and chlorhexidine)
- Pre-Seed (hydroxyethylcellulose, arabinogalactan, paraben, and Pluronic copolymers), which is promoted for women who are trying to conceive

- Silicone-based are as follows:
  - ID Millennium (cyclomethicone, dimethicone, and dimethiconol)
  - Pjur Eros (cyclopentasiloxane, dimethicone, and dimethiconol)
  - Pink (dimethicone, vitamin E, aloe vera, dimethiconol, and cyclomethicone)
- Oil-based are as follows:
  - Elégance Women's Lubricant
  - Natural oils (such as olive oil)
- Water-based and silicone-based vaginal lubricants are compatible with condom use. Oil-based lubricants may damage latex-based condoms.
- Patients should stop smoking, as women who smoke cigarettes are relatively estrogen-deficient.[7] SOR Ⓐ

MEDICATIONS

- Estrogen replacement therapy relieves menopausal symptoms including atrophic vaginitis.[8] SOR Ⓐ Routes of administration include oral, transdermal, and intravaginal. Risks associated with estrogen use include breast cancer, coronary heart disease, stroke, and venous thromboembolism.
- A Cochrane review found that estrogen creams, pessaries, vaginal tablets, and the estradiol vaginal ring appeared to be equally effective for the symptoms of vaginal atrophy.[8] SOR Ⓐ One trial found significant side effects following conjugated equine estrogen cream administration when compared to tablets causing uterine bleeding, breast pain, and perineal pain. Another trial found significant endometrial overstimulation following use of the conjugated equine estrogen cream when compared to the estrogen vaginal ring. Women appeared to favor the estradiol-releasing vaginal ring for ease of use, comfort of product, and overall satisfaction.[8] SOR Ⓐ
- The amount of estrogen and the duration of time required to eliminate symptoms depend on the degree of vaginal atrophy, and varies among patients. Progestin therapy should be considered in any woman with an intact uterus to avoid causing endometrial cancer. When oral estrogen is used at typical doses, atrophic symptoms will persist in 10% to 25% of patients.[9]
- Topical administration of estrogen is an excellent treatment for genitourinary symptoms of atrophy, because exposure of other organs can be minimized if low doses of topical estrogens are used. Absorption rates with topical therapy increase with treatment duration because of the enhanced vascularity of the epithelium.
- Vaginal estrogen therapy available in the United States are conjugated estrogens cream (0.625 mg conjugated estrogens/g, 0.5 g of cream intravaginally twice weekly) and estradiol cream (100 mcg estradiol/g of cream, 2-4 g of cream intravaginally administered daily for 2 weeks, then decreased to 1 g of cream 1-3 times per week), tablet (10 mcg estradiol/tablet intravaginally daily for 2 weeks then twice weekly), and ring (0.5 mcg estradiol/day, released over 90 days). In Europe and some other countries, estriol cream is also available.
- Vaginal estrogen therapy results in some estrogen absorption into the circulation, although to a lesser degree than oral or transdermal estrogen treatment. In 1 study, systemic absorption was 30% lower in a study of vaginal versus conjugated estrogen therapy.[10] SOR Ⓑ
- Progestin therapy is probably not necessary to protect against endometrial hyperplasia in women treated with the low-dose ring or intravaginal tablet when used as approved. The systemic estrogen absorption with use of the vaginal creams is difficult to quantify, so some experts recommend use of an opposing progestin for women treated with vaginal estrogen cream.[11] SOR Ⓒ

FOLLOW-UP

Follow-up is needed for all patients placed on estrogen therapy to monitor for estrogen-related side effects. Otherwise, follow-up can be as needed.

PATIENT EDUCATION

Discuss the risks and benefits of estrogen replacement therapy with patients interested in the use of estrogens. Vaginal lubricants (nonprescription) may safely help prevent pain during intercourse.

PATIENT RESOURCES

- NCBI. *Atrophic Vaginitis*—**www.ncbi.nlm.nih.gov.**
- MedlinePlus. *Atrophic Vaginitis*—**www.nlm.nih.gov/medlineplus/ ency/article/000892.htm.**
- Harvard Medical School. *Atrophic Vaginitis*—**www.health.harvard.edu/fhg/updates/update0703c.shtml.**

PROVIDER RESOURCES

- eMedicine. *Vaginitis*—**http://emedicine.medscape.com/article/257141.**
- eMedicine. *Vulvovaginitis in Emergency Medicine*—**http://emedicine.medscape.com/article/797497.**
- Bachmann GA, Nevadunsky NS. Diagnosis and treatment of atrophic vaginitis. *Am Fam Physician*. 2000;61(10):3090-3096.—**http://www.aafp.org/afp/2000/0515/p3090.html.**
- American Family Physician. *Diagnosis and Treatment of Atrophic Vaginitis*—**http://www.aafp.org/afp/20000515/3090.html.**

REFERENCES

1. Dennerstein L, Dudley EC, Hopper JL, et al. A prospective population-based study of menopausal symptoms. *Obstet Gynecol.* 2000;96:351.
2. Nappi RE, Kokot-Kierepa M. Women's voices in the menopause: results from an international survey on vaginal atrophy. *Maturitas.* 2010;67:233.
3. Pandit L, Ouslander JG. Postmenopausal vaginal atrophy and atrophic vaginitis. *Am J Med Sci.* 1997;314:228-231.
4. Bachmann GA, Nevadunsky NS. Diagnosis and treatment of atrophic vaginitis. *Am Fam Physician.* 2000;61:3090.
5. Johnston SL, Farrell SA, Bouchard C, et al. The detection and management of vaginal atrophy. *J Obstet Gynaecol Can.* 2004;26:503.
6. Nachtigall Le. Comparative study: Replens versus local estrogen in menopausal women. *Fertil Steril.* 1994;61:178.
7. Tansavatdi K, McClain B, Herrington DM. The effects of smoking on estradiol metabolism. *Minerva Ginecol.* 2004;56:105.
8. Suckling J, Lethaby A, Kennedy R. Local oestrogen for vaginal atrophy in postmenopausal women. *Cochrane Database Syst Rev.* 2006 Oct 18;(4):CD001500.
9. Smith P, Heimer G, Lindskog M, Ulmsten U. Oestradiol-releasing vaginal ring for treatment of postmenopausal urogenital atrophy. *Maturitas.* 1993;16:145-154.
10. Dorr MB, Nelson AL, Mayer PR, et al. Plasma estrogen concentrations after oral and vaginal estrogen administration in women with atrophic vaginitis. *Fertil Steril.* 2010;94:2365.
11. Bachmann G, Bouchard C, Hoppe D, et al. Efficacy and safety of low-dose regimens of conjugated estrogens cream administered vaginally. *Menopause.* 2009;16:719.

90 BACTERIAL VAGINOSIS

E.J. Mayeaux Jr, MD
Richard P. Usatine, MD

PATIENT STORY

A 31-year-old woman presents with a malodorous vaginal discharge for 3 weeks. There is no associated vaginal itching or pain. She is married and monogamous. She admits to douching about once per month to prevent odor but it is not working this time. On examination, her discharge is visible (**Figure 90-1**). It is thin and off-white. Wet prep examination shows that more than 50% of the epithelial cells are clue cells (**Figure 90-2**). The patient is treated with oral metronidazole 500 mg bid for 7 days with good results.

INTRODUCTION

Bacterial vaginosis (BV) is a clinical syndrome resulting from alteration of the vaginal ecosystem. It is called a vaginosis, not a vaginitis, because the tissues themselves are not actually infected, but only have superficial involvement. Women with BV are at increased risk for the acquisition of HIV, *Neisseria gonorrhoeae*, *Chlamydia trachomatis*, and herpes simplex virus (HSV)-2, and they have increased risk of complications after gynecologic surgery.[1]

BV is associated with adverse pregnancy outcomes, including premature rupture of membranes, preterm labor, preterm birth, intraamniotic infection, and postpartum endometritis. However, the only established benefit of BV therapy in pregnant women is the reduction of symptoms and signs of vaginal infection.[1]

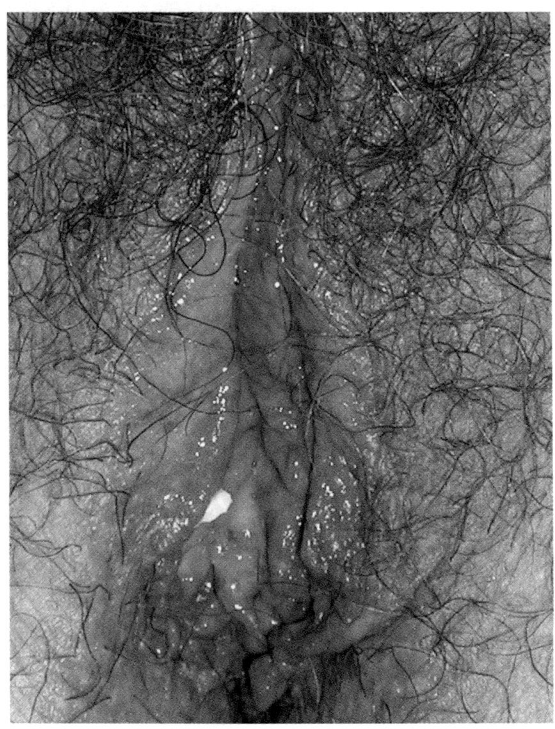

FIGURE 90-1 A 31-year-old woman with homogeneous, thin white malodorous vaginal discharge. (*Reproduced with permission of Richard P. Usatine, MD.*)

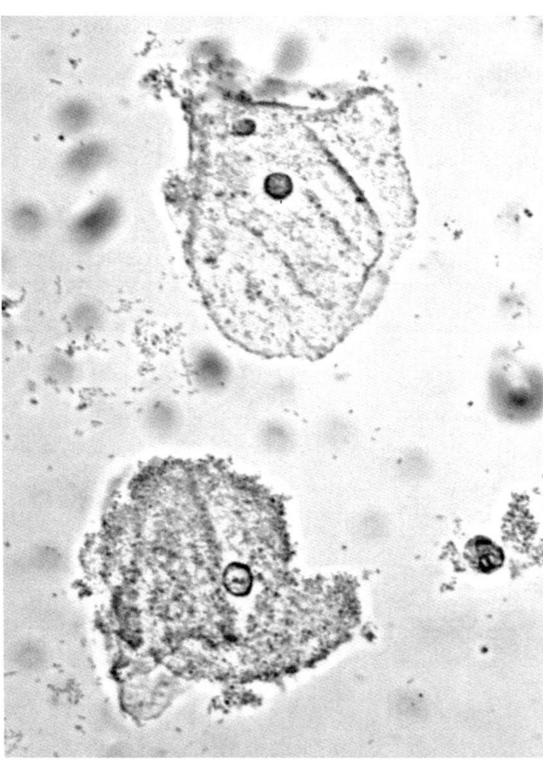

FIGURE 90-2 Clue cell and bacteria seen in bacterial vaginosis. The lower cell is a clue cell covered in bacteria while the upper cell is a normal epithelial cell. Light microscope under high power. (*Reproduced with permission of E.J. Mayeaux Jr, MD.*)

SYNONYMS

- Vaginal bacteriosis
- *Corynebacterium* vaginosis/*vaginalis*/*vaginitis*
- *Gardnerella vaginalis*/vaginosis
- *Haemophilus vaginalis*/vaginitis
- Nonspecific vaginitis
- Anaerobic vaginosis

EPIDEMIOLOGY

BV is estimated to be the most prevalent cause of vaginal discharge or malodor in women presenting for care in the United States. However, more than 50% of women with BV are asymptomatic.[1] It accounts for more than 10 million outpatient visits per year.[2] The worldwide prevalence is unknown.

ETIOLOGY AND PATHOPHYSIOLOGY

- Hydrogen peroxide-producing *Lactobacillus* is the most common organism composing normal vaginal flora.[1] In BV, normal vaginal lactobacilli are replaced by high concentrations of anaerobic bacteria such as *Mobiluncus*, *Prevotella*, *Gardnerella*, *Bacteroides*, and *Mycoplasma* species.[1,2]

- The hydrogen peroxide produced by the *Lactobacillus* may help in inhibiting the growth of atypical flora.
- The odor of BV is caused by the aromatic amines produced by the altered bacterial flora in the vagina. These aromatic amines include putrescine and cadaverine—aptly named to describe their foul odor.

RISK FACTORS

- Multiple male or female partners[1,3]
- A new sex partner[1]
- Douching[4]
- Lack of condom use[1]
- Lack of vaginal lactobacilli[1]
- Prior BV infection[1]

DIAGNOSIS

CLINICAL FEATURES

- Symptomatic patients present with an unpleasant, "fishy smelling" discharge that is more noticeable after coitus (the basic pH of seminal fluid is like doing the whiff test with KOH). There may be pruritus but not as often as seen with *Candida* vaginitis. The physical examination should include inspection of the external genitalia for irritation or discharge. Speculum examination is done to determine the amount and character of the discharge. A nucleic acid amplification test for *N. gonorrhoeae*, *Chlamydia*, and/or *C. trachomatis* (or similar test) should be performed on genital specimens (urethral or cervical) or urine.
- BV is usually clinically diagnosed by finding 3 of the following 4 signs and symptoms:
    - Homogeneous, thin, white discharge that smoothly coats the vaginal walls (**Figure 90-3** and **90-4**).
    - Presence of clue cells on microscopic examination (**Figure 90-2**).
    - pH of vaginal fluid >4.5.
    - A fishy odor of vaginal discharge before or after addition of 10% KOH (ie, the whiff test).[1]

LABORATORY TESTING

- Vaginal pH testing can be very helpful in the diagnosis of vaginitis. The normal vaginal pH is usually 3.5 to 4.5. A pH above 4.5 is seen with menopausal patients, *Trichomonas* infection, or BV. A small piece of pH paper is touched to the vaginal discharge during the examination or on the speculum. Do not test a wet-prep sample if saline has been added because the saline alters the pH.
- Wet preps are obtained using a cotton-tipped applicator applied to the vaginal sidewall, placing the sample of discharge into normal saline (not water). Observe for clue cells, number of white blood cells, trichomonads, and candidal hyphae. Clue cells are squamous epithelial cells whose borders are obscured by attached bacteria. More than 20% to 25% of epithelial cells seen in BV should be clue cells (**Figure 90-2**).
- A proline aminopeptidase test card (Pip Activity Test Card), a DNA probe-based test for high concentrations of *G. vaginalis* (Affirm VP III), and the OSOM BVBLUE test have shown acceptable performance

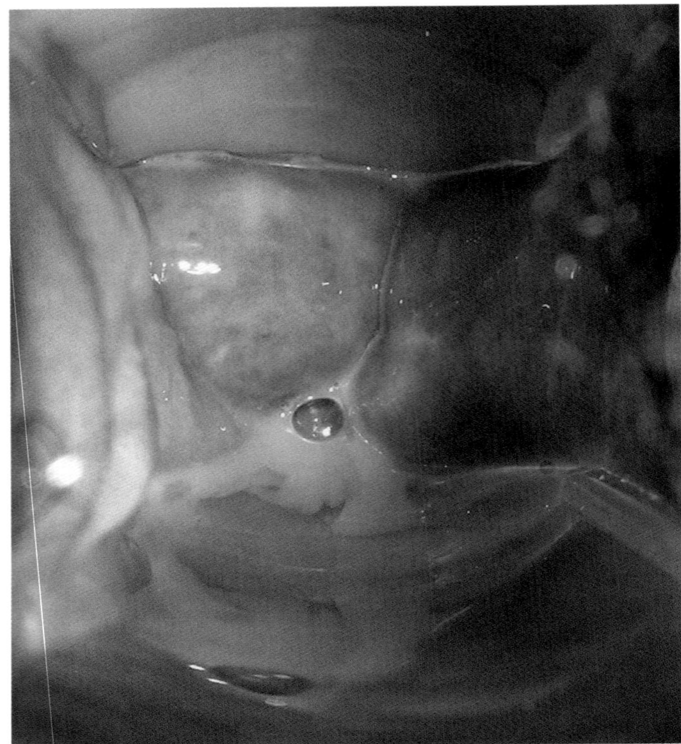

FIGURE 90-3 A homogeneous, off-white creamy malodorous discharge that adheres to the vaginal walls and pools in the vaginal vault in a woman with bacterial vaginosis. (*Reproduced with permission of Richard P. Usatine, MD.*)

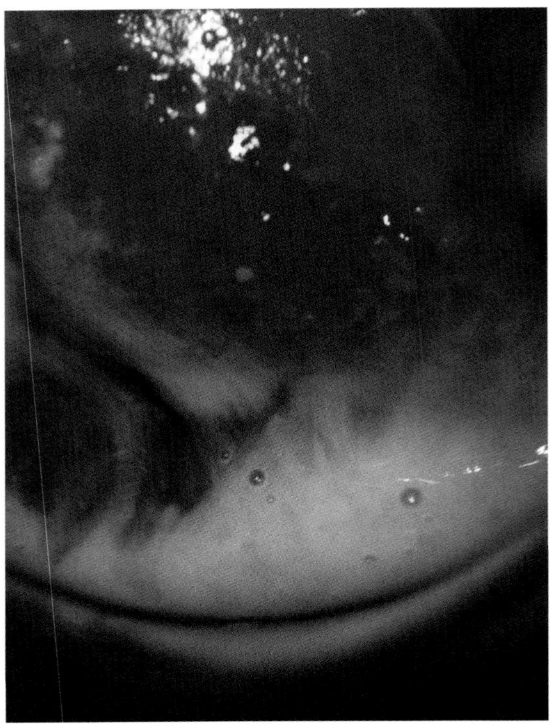

FIGURE 90-4 Close-up view of the cervix showing a yellowish white homogeneous discharge in a woman with bacterial vaginosis. Note the lack of clumping or "cottage-cheese" appearance usually found with *Candida* infections. (*Reproduced with permission of E.J. Mayeaux Jr, MD.*)

characteristics compared with Gram stain (gold standard).[1] However, they are more costly than traditional testing without clear advantages.

- Although a test card is available for the detection of elevated pH and trimethylamine, it has low sensitivity and specificity and is not recommended by the Centers for Disease Control and Prevention (CDC).[1]
- Culture of *G. vaginalis* is not recommended as a diagnostic tool because it is not specific.
- Pap tests are not useful for the diagnosis of BV because of their low sensitivity.[1]

DIFFERENTIAL DIAGNOSIS

- *Trichomonas* also may have the odor of aromatic amines and, therefore, easily confused with BV at first glance. Look for the strawberry cervix on examination and moving trichomonads on the wet prep (Chapter 84, Trichomonas Vaginitis).
- *Candida* vaginitis tends to present with a cottage-cheese-like discharge and vaginal itching (Chapter 83, *Candida* Vulvovaginitis).
- Gonorrhea and chlamydia should not be missed in patients with vaginal discharge. Consider testing for these sexually transmitted diseases (STDs) based on patients' risk factors and the presence of purulence clinically and white blood cells on the wet prep (Chapter 85, Chlamydia Cervicitis).

MANAGEMENT

- Treatment is recommended for women with symptoms.
- Treatment of male sex partners has not been beneficial in preventing the recurrence of BV.[1] SOR Ⓐ

MEDICATIONS

- The established benefits of therapy for BV in nonpregnant women are to (a) relieve vaginal symptoms and signs of infection and (b) reduce the risk for infectious complications after abortion or hysterectomy.[1] SOR Ⓐ Other potential benefits might include a reduction in risk for other sexually transmitted infections (STIs).[1] SOR Ⓑ **Table 90-1** shows CDC recommended treatments.
- Metronidazole, a 2-g single-dose therapy has the lowest efficacy for BV and is no longer a recommended or alternative regimen. Clindamycin cream is oil-based and might weaken latex condoms and diaphragms for 5 days after use. Topical clindamycin preparations should not be used in the second half of pregnancy.[1] Multiple studies and metaanalyses have not demonstrated an association between metronidazole use during pregnancy and teratogenic or mutagenic effects in newborns.[1] SOR Ⓐ
- The only established benefit of therapy for BV in pregnant women is to relieve vaginal symptoms and signs of infection.[1] SOR Ⓐ Additional potential benefits of therapy include (a) reducing the risk for infectious complications associated with BV during pregnancy and (b) reducing the risk for other infections (eg, other STDs or HIV). Multiple studies and metaanalyses have not demonstrated an association between metronidazole use during pregnancy and teratogenic or mutagenic effects in newborns.[5]
- One randomized trial for persistent BV indicated that metronidazole gel 0.75% twice per week for 6 months after completion of a recommended regimen was effective in maintaining a clinical cure for 6 months.[6] SOR Ⓑ
- Limited data suggest that oral nitroimidazole followed by intravaginal boric acid and suppressive metronidazole gel for those women in remission might be an option in women with recurrent BV.[7] SOR Ⓑ
- Intravaginal clindamycin cream has been associated with adverse outcomes if used in the latter half of pregnancy.[1]

TABLE 90-1 CDC Recommended Regimens SOR Ⓐ

Metronidazole 500 mg orally twice a day for 7 days
OR
Metronidazole gel 0.75%, 1 full applicator (5 g) intravaginally, once a day for 5 days
OR
Clindamycin cream 2%, 1 full applicator (5 g) intravaginally at bedtime for 7 days
CDC Alternative Regimens SOR Ⓐ
Tinidazole 2 g orally once daily for 3 days
OR
Tinidazole 1 g orally once daily for 5 days
OR
Clindamycin 300 mg orally twice a day for 7 days
OR
Clindamycin ovules 100 mg intravaginally once at bedtime for 3 days
OR
Metronidazole 750-mg extended-release tablets once daily for 7 days
CDC Recommended Regimens for Pregnant Women SOR Ⓐ
Metronidazole 500 mg orally twice a day for 7 days
OR
Metronidazole 250 mg orally three times a day for 7 days
OR
Clindamycin 300 mg orally twice a day for 7 days

Data from Centers for Disease Control and Prevention.[1]

COMPLEMENTARY AND ALTERNATIVE THERAPY

- Extended ingestion of live culture, nonpasteurized yogurt may theoretically increase colonization by lactobacilli and decrease the episodes of BV.[8] SOR Ⓒ However, health food store lactobacilli are the wrong strain and are not well-retained by the vagina.
- The efficacy of exogenous lactobacillus recolonization with probiotic lactobacilli vaginal gelatin capsules has been reported in 2 small trials.[9,10]

PREVENTION

- Avoidance of risk factors is recommended, although asymptomatic BV is common.
- The evidence is insufficient to assess the impact of screening for BV in pregnant women at high risk for preterm delivery.[1]

FOLLOW-UP

- Follow-up visits are unnecessary in nonpregnant women if symptoms resolve.[1]
- Treatment of BV in asymptomatic pregnant women who are at high risk for preterm delivery might prevent adverse pregnancy outcomes. Therefore, a follow-up evaluation 1 month after completion of treatment should be considered to evaluate whether therapy was effective.[1] SOR Ⓒ
- If symptoms do recur, consider a treatment regimen different from the original regimen to treat recurrent disease.[1] SOR Ⓒ

PATIENT EDUCATION

Avoid consuming alcohol during treatment with metronidazole and for 24 hours thereafter. Women should be advised to return for additional therapy if symptoms recur because recurrence of BV is not unusual.

PATIENT RESOURCES

- Centers for Disease Control and Prevention. *Bacterial Vaginosis Fact Sheet*—**http://www.cdc.gov/std/BV/STDFact-Bacterial-Vaginosis.htm.**
- MedicineNet.com. *Bacterial Vaginosis*—**http://www.medicinenet.com/bacterial_vaginosis/article.htm.**

PROVIDER RESOURCES

- Centers for Disease Control and Prevention. *2010 Guidelines for Treatment of Sexually Transmitted Diseases*—**http://www.cdc.gov/std/treatment/2010/STD-Treatment-2010-RR5912.pdf.**

REFERENCES

1. Centers for Disease Control and Prevention. *Guidelines for Treatment of Sexually Transmitted Diseases*. http://www.cdc.gov/std/treatment/2010/STD-Treatment-2010-RR5912.pdf. Accessed December 24, 2011.
2. Martius J, Krohn MA, Hillier SL, et al. Relationships of vaginal lactobacillus species, cervical chlamydia trachomatis, and bacterial vaginosis to preterm birth. *Obstet Gynecol.* 1988;71:89-95.
3. Gorgos LM, Marrazzo JM. Sexually transmitted infections among women who have sex with women. *Clin Infect Dis.* 2011;53(3):S84-S91.
4. Klebanoff MA, Nansel TR, Brotman RM, et al. Personal hygienic behaviors and bacterial vaginosis. *Sex Transm Dis.* 2010;37:94.
5. Burtin P, Taddio A, Ariburnu O, et al. Safety of metronidazole in pregnancy: a meta-analysis. *Am J Obstet Gynecol.* 1995;172 (2 Pt 1):525-529.
6. Sobel JD, Ferris D, Schwebke J, et al. Suppressive antibacterial therapy with 0.75% metronidazole vaginal gel to prevent recurrent bacterial vaginosis. *Am J Obstet Gynecol.* 2006;194:1283-1289.
7. Reichman O, Akins R, Sobel JD. Boric acid addition to suppressive antimicrobial therapy for recurrent bacterial vaginosis. *Sex Transm Dis.* 2009;36:732-734.
8. Baylson FA, Nyirjesy P, Weitz MV. Treatment of recurrent bacterial vaginosis with tinidazole. *Obstet Gynecol.* 2004;104 (5 Pt 1):931-932.
9. Anukam KC, Osazuwa E, Osemene GI, et al. Clinical study comparing probiotic Lactobacillus GR-1 and RC-14 with metronidazole vaginal gel to treat symptomatic bacterial vaginosis. *Microbes Infect.* 2006;8:2772.
10. Ya W, Reifer C, Miller LE. Efficacy of vaginal probiotic capsules for recurrent bacterial vaginosis: a double-blind, randomized, placebo-controlled study. *Am J Obstet Gynecol.* 2010;203:120.

91 CANDIDA VULVOVAGINITIS

E.J. Mayeaux Jr, MD
Richard P. Usatine, MD

PATIENT STORY

A 35-year-old woman presents with severe vaginal and vulvar itching. She also complains of a thick white discharge. **Figure 91-1** demonstrates the appearance of her vulva and introitus and **Figure 91-2** shows her cervix. **Figure 91-3** shows the wet prep with pseudohyphae. Treatment with a nonprescription intravaginal preparation was successful.

INTRODUCTION

Vulvovaginal candidiasis (VVC) is a common fungal infection in women of childbearing age. Pruritus is accompanied by a thick, odorless, white vaginal discharge. VVC is not a sexually transmitted disease. On the basis of clinical presentation, microbiology, host factors, and response-to-therapy, VVC can be classified as either uncomplicated or complicated.[1] Uncomplicated VVC is characterized by sporadic or infrequent symptoms, mild-to-moderate symptoms, and the patient is nonimmunocompromised. Complicated VVC is characterized by recurrent (4 or more episodes in 1 year) or severe VVC, non-albicans candidiasis, or the patient has uncontrolled diabetes, debilitation, or immunosuppression.[1]

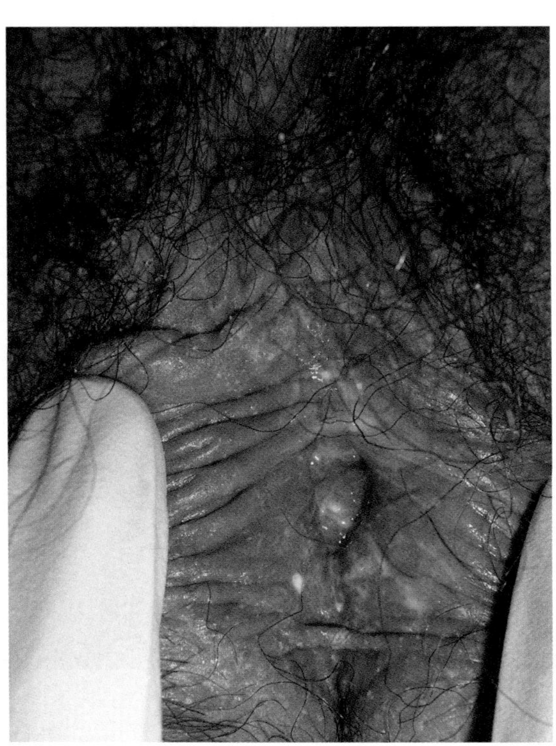

FIGURE 91-1 *Candida* on the vulva and introitus showing whitish patches with erythema. (*Reproduced with permission from Richard P. Usatine, MD.*)

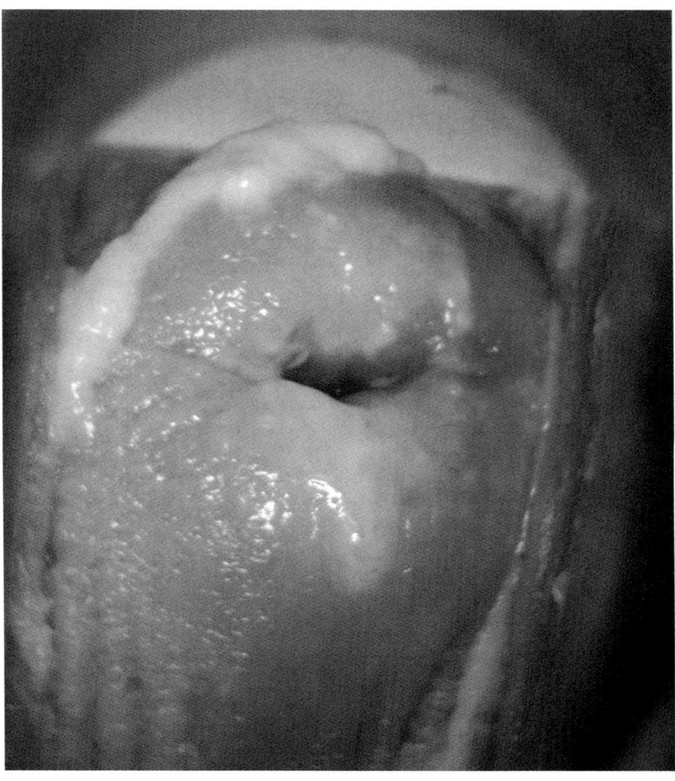

FIGURE 91-2 *Candida* vaginitis visible on the cervix. Note the thick, white, adherent, "cottage-cheese-like" discharge. (*Reproduced with permission from EJ Mayeaux Jr, MD.*)

SYNONYMS

Yeast vaginitis, yeast infection, candidiasis, and moniliasis.

EPIDEMIOLOGY

- VVC accounts for approximately one-third of vaginitis cases.[1]
- *Candida* species are part of the lower genital tract flora in 20% to 50% of healthy asymptomatic women.[2]
- Around 75% of all women in the United States will experience at least 1 episode of VVC. Of these, 40% to 45% will have 2 or more episodes within their lifetime.[3] Approximately 10% to 20% of women will have complicated VVC that necessitates diagnostic and therapeutic considerations.
- It is a frequent iatrogenic complication of antibiotic treatment, secondary to altered vaginal flora (**Figure 91-4**).
- Nearly half of all women experience multiple episodes, and up to 5% experience recurrent disease.[1]
- Recurrent vulvovaginal candidiasis (RVVC) is defined as 4 or more episodes of symptomatic VVC in 1 year. It affects a small percentage of women (<5%).[4] Recurrent yeast vaginitis is usually caused by relapse, and less often by reinfection. Recurrent infection may be caused by *Candida* recolonization of the vagina from the rectum.[5]

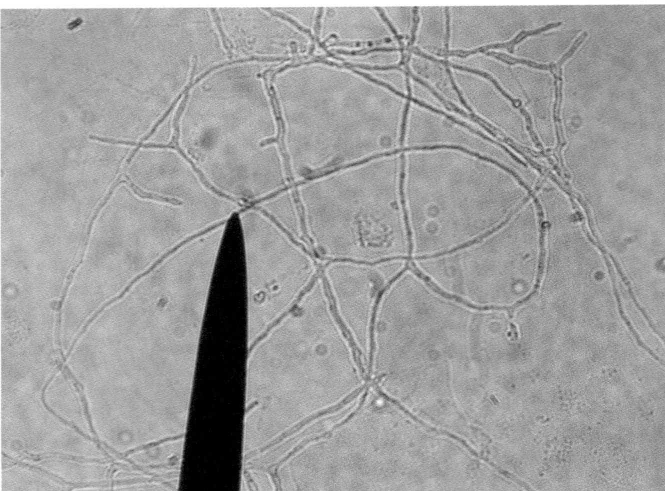

CHAPTER 91

FIGURE 91-3 Wet mount with KOH of *Candida albicans* in a woman with *Candida* vaginitis. Seen under high power demonstrating branching pseudohyphae and budding yeast. (*Reproduced with permission from Richard P. Usatine, MD.*)

ETIOLOGY AND PATHOPHYSIOLOGY

- Most vulvovaginal Candidiasis is caused by *Candida albicans* (**Figure 91-3**).[1,6] *Candida glabrata* now causes a significant percentage of all *Candida* vulvovaginal infections. This organism is resistant to the nonprescription imidazole creams. It can mutate out of the activity of treatment drugs much faster than *albicans* species.[7]
- The disease is suggested by pruritus in the vulvar area, together with erythema of the vagina and vulva (**Figures 91-1, 91-2, and 91-4**). The familiar reddening of the vulvar tissues is caused by an ethanol by-product of the *Candida* infection. This ethanol compound also produces pruritic symptoms. A scalloped edge with satellite lesions is characteristic of the erythema on the vulva.
- VVC can occur concomitantly with sexually transmitted diseases (STDs).

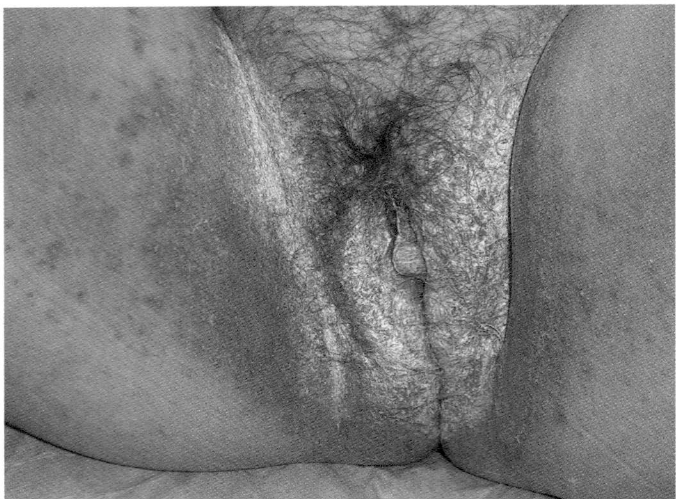

FIGURE 91-4 Red pruritic rash in the vulva and inguinal areas of this 46-year-old woman who suffered a stroke with significant residual hemiparesis. Diagnosis was confirmed with a KOH microscopic examination. The case was particularly severe secondary to her use of an adult diaper for incontinence and a preceding course of antibiotics. (*Reproduced with permission from Richard P. Usatine, MD.*)

- The pathogenesis of recurrent VVC is poorly understood, and most women with these recurrences have no apparent predisposing or underlying conditions.[1]

RISK FACTORS[8,9]

- Diabetes mellitus
- Recent antibiotic use (**Figure 91-4**)
- Increased estrogen levels
- Immunosuppression (**Figure 91-5**)

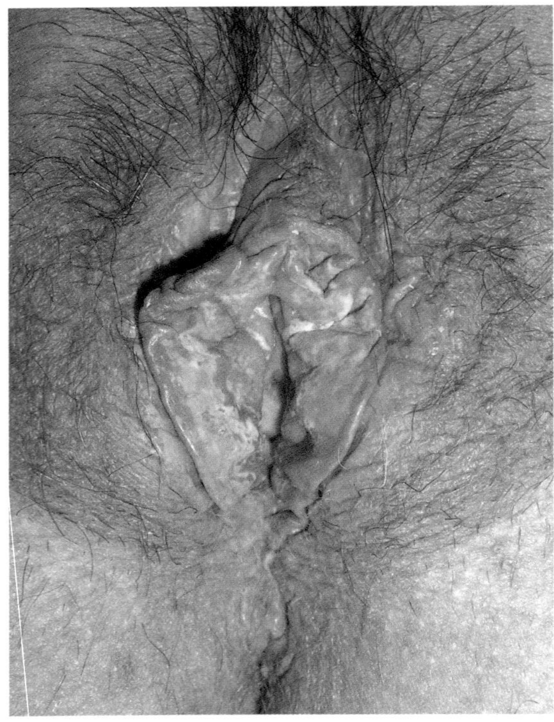

A

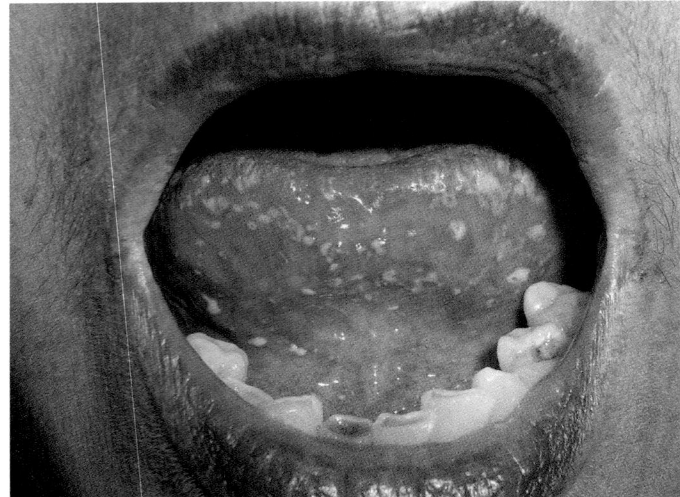

B

FIGURE 91-5 **A.** Candida vulvovaginitis in a 52-year-old woman with pemphigus vulgaris on prednisone and mycophenolate to control her immunobullous disease. **B.** The patient also has Candida thrush in her mouth secondary to her immunosuppression. (*Reproduced with permission from Richard P. Usatine, MD.*)

- Incontinence and adult diapers (**Figure 91-4**)
- Contraceptive devices (vaginal sponges, diaphragms, and intrauterine devices)
- Genetic susceptibility
- Behavioral factors—VVC may be linked to orogenital and, less commonly, anogenital sex
- Spermicides are **not associated** with *Candida* infection
- There is no high-quality evidence showing a link between VVC and hygienic habits or wearing tight or synthetic clothing

DIAGNOSIS

CLINICAL FEATURES

The diagnosis is usually suspected by characteristic findings (**Figures 91-1, 91-2,** and **91-4**). Typical symptoms include pruritus, vaginal soreness, dyspareunia, and external dysuria. Typical signs include vulvar edema, fissures, excoriations, or thick, curdy vaginal discharge.[1]

LABORATORY TESTING

- Vaginitis solely caused by *Candida* generally has a normal vaginal pH of less than 4.5.
- The wet prep, KOH smear, or Gram stain may demonstrate yeast and/or pseudohyphae (**Figures 91-3** and **91-6**). Wet preps may also demonstrate white blood cells, trichomonads, candidal hyphae, or clue cells.
- The KOH prep is made by adding a drop of KOH solution to a drop of saline suspension of the discharge. The KOH lyses epithelial cells in 5 to 15 minutes (faster if the slide is warmed) and allows easier visualization of candidal hyphae or yeast.[1] Swartz-Lamkins stain (potassium hydroxide, a surfactant, and blue dye) may facilitate diagnosis by staining the yeast organisms a light blue.[10]
- Rapid antigen testing is also available for *Candida*. The detection of vaginal yeast by rapid antigen testing is feasible for office practice and more sensitive than wet mount. A negative test result, however, was not found to be sensitive enough to rule out yeast and avoid a culture.[6] SOR Ⓐ
- Fungal culture with Sabouraud agar, Nickerson medium, or Microstix-*Candida* medium should be considered in patients with symptoms and a negative KOH because *C. glabrata* does not form pseudohyphae or hyphae and is not easily recognized on microscopy. If the wet mount is negative and *Candida* cultures cannot be done, empiric treatment can be considered for symptomatic women with any sign of VVC on examination.[1] SOR Ⓒ Asymptomatic women should not be cultured as 10% to 20% of women harbor *Candida* species and other yeasts in the vagina.[1] SOR Ⓐ
- Vaginal cultures should be obtained from patients with RVVC to confirm the clinical diagnosis and to identify unusual species, including non-*albicans* species, particularly *C. glabrata* (*C. glabrata* does not form pseudohyphae or hyphae and is not easily recognized on microscopy).[1] SOR Ⓑ *C. glabrata* and other non-*albicans Candida* sp. are observed in 10% to 20% of patients with RVVC.[1]
- Given the frequency at which RVVC occurs in the immunocompetent healthy population, the occurrence of RVVC alone should not be considered an indication for HIV testing.[1] SOR Ⓒ

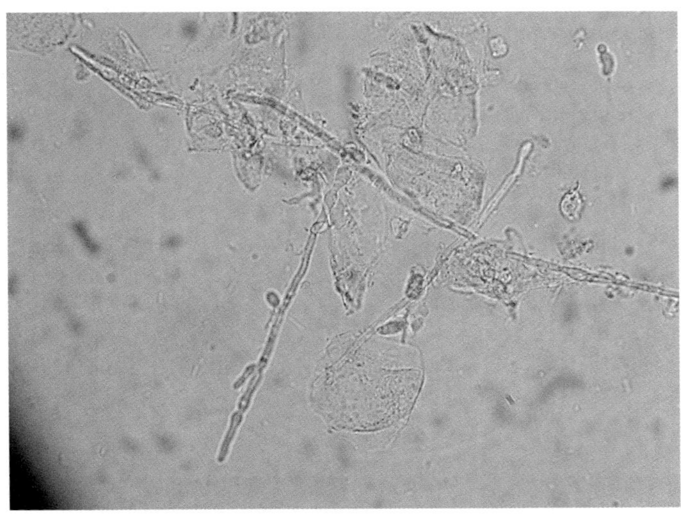

FIGURE 91-6 Wet mount with saline showing *Candida* in a woman with *Candida* vaginitis. Note how the branching pseudohyphae and budding yeast can be seen even though the epithelial cells have not been lysed by KOH. *(Reproduced with permission from Richard P. Usatine, MD.)*

DIFFERENTIAL DIAGNOSIS

- Trichomoniasis can be confused with candidiasis because patients may report itching and a discharge in both diagnoses. Look for the strawberry cervix on examination and moving trichomonads on the wet prep (Chapter 92, *Trichomonas* Vaginitis).
- Bacterial vaginosis can be confused with candidiasis because patients may report a discharge and an odor in both diagnoses. The odor is usually much worse in bacterial vaginosis, and the quality of the discharge can be different. The wet prep should allow for differentiation between these 2 infections (Chapter 90, Bacterial Vaginosis).
- Gonorrhea and *Chlamydia* should not be missed in patients with vaginal discharge. Consider testing for these STDs based on patients' risk factors and the presence of purulence clinically and white blood cells on the wet prep (Chapter 93, *Chlamydia* Cervicitis).
- Cytolytic vaginosis, or Döderlein cytolysis, can be confused with candidiasis. Cytolytic vaginosis is produced by a massive desquamation of epithelial cells related to excess lactobacilli in the vagina. The signs and symptoms are similar to *Candida* vaginitis, except no yeast are found on wet prep. The wet prep will show an overgrowth of lactobacilli. The treatment is to discontinue all antifungals and other agents or procedures that alter the vaginal flora.

MANAGEMENT

NONPHARMACOLOGIC

- VVC is not usually acquired through sexual intercourse; treatment of sex partners is not recommended but may be considered in women who have recurrent infection. Some male sex partners might have balanitis (Chapter 135, Candidiasis) and might benefit from treatment.[1] SOR Ⓐ
- Any woman whose symptoms persist after using a nonprescription preparation or who has a recurrence of symptoms within 2 months should be evaluated with office-based testing as they are not necessarily

more capable of diagnosing themselves even with prior diagnosed episodes of VVC, and delay in the treatment of other vulvovaginitis etiologies can result in adverse clinical outcomes.[1] SOR Ⓐ

MEDICATIONS

- Women with typical symptoms and a positive test result should receive treatment. Short-courses of topical formulations effectively treat uncomplicated VVC (**Table 91-1**).[1] SOR Ⓐ Topical azole drugs are more effective than nystatin, and result in clinical cure and negative cultures in 80% to 90% of patients who complete therapy. SOR Ⓐ The creams and suppositories in **Table 91-1** are oil-based and might weaken latex condoms and diaphragms.[1]
- The cure rates with single-dose oral fluconazole and all the intravaginal treatments are equal.[11] Fluconazole (Diflucan) 150-mg single dose has become very popular, but may have clinical cure rates of approximately only 70%. SOR Ⓐ Systemic allergic reactions are possible with the oral agents.
- The oral agents fluconazole, ketoconazole, and itraconazole also appear to be effective.[1] SOR Ⓑ
- VVC frequently occurs during pregnancy. Only topical azole therapies, applied for 7 days, are recommended for use among pregnant women.[1] SOR Ⓒ
- The optimal treatment of non-*albicans* VVC remains unknown. Options include longer duration of therapy (7-14 days) with topical therapy or a 100-mg, 150-mg, or 200-mg oral dose of fluconazole every third day for a total of 3 doses.[1] SOR Ⓒ

TABLE 91-1 Centers for Disease Control and Prevention Recommended Treatment Regimens

Intravaginal Agents:

- **Butoconazole** 2% cream 5 g intravaginally for 3 days
- **Butoconazole** 2% cream 5 g (Butaconazole1-sustained release), single intravaginal application*
- **Clotrimazole** 1% cream 5 g intravaginally for 7-14 days
- **Clotrimazole** 2% cream 5 g intravaginally for 3 days
- **Clotrimazole** 100 mg vaginal suppositories, one intravaginally for 3 days
- **Miconazole** 2% cream 5 g intravaginally for 7 days
- **Miconazole** 100 mg vaginal suppositories, 1 suppository for 7 days
- **Miconazole** 200 mg vaginal suppositories, 1 suppository for 3 days
- **Miconazole** 1200 mg vaginal suppositories, 1 suppository for 1 day
- **Nystatin** 100,000-U vaginal tablet, 1 tablet for 14 days*
- **Tioconazole** 6.5% ointment 5 g intravaginally in a single application
- **Terconazole** 0.4% cream 5 g intravaginally for 7 days*
- **Terconazole** 0.8% cream 5 g intravaginally for 3 days*
- **Terconazole** 80 mg vaginal suppositories, 1 suppository for 3 days*

Oral Agent:

- **Fluconazole** 150-mg oral tablet, 1 tablet in single dose*

*Prescription only in the United States.
Data from the Centers for Disease Control and Prevention.[1]

- Severe VVC (ie, extensive vulvar erythema, edema, excoriation, and fissure formation) is associated with lower clinical response rates in patients treated with short courses of topical or oral therapy. Either 7 to 14 days of topical azole or 150 mg of fluconazole in 2 sequential doses (second dose 72 hours after initial dose) is recommended.[1] SOR Ⓒ

COMPLEMENTARY AND ALTERNATIVE THERAPY

- If recurrence VVC occurs, 600 mg of boric acid in a gelatin capsule is recommended, administered vaginally once daily for 2 weeks. This regimen has clinical and mycologic eradication rates of approximately 70%.[1] SOR Ⓑ
- *Lactobacillus acidophilus* does not adhere well to the vaginal epithelium, and it does not significantly change the incidence of candidal vulvovaginitis.[5,12]
- There is no evidence from randomized trials that other complementary and alternative medicine (CAM) therapies, such as garlic, tea tree oil, yogurt, or douching, are effective for the treatment or prevention of VVC caused by *C. albicans*.[13,14]

PREVENTION

MAINTENANCE REGIMENS

- Oral fluconazole (ie, 100-mg, 150-mg, or 200-mg dose) weekly for 6 months is the first line of treatment. If this regimen is not feasible, some specialists recommend topical clotrimazole 200 mg twice a week, clotrimazole (500-mg dose vaginal suppositories once weekly), or other topical treatments used intermittently.[1] SOR Ⓒ
- Suppressive maintenance antifungal therapies are effective in reducing RVVC.[1] SOR Ⓐ However, 30% to 50% of women will have recurrent disease after maintenance therapy is discontinued. Routine treatment of sex partners is controversial. *C. albicans* azole resistance is rare in vaginal isolates, and susceptibility testing is usually not warranted for individual treatment guidance.

PROGNOSIS

- Women with underlying debilitating medical conditions (eg, those with uncontrolled diabetes or those receiving corticosteroid treatments) do not respond as well to short-term therapies. Efforts to correct modifiable conditions should be made, and more prolonged (ie, 7-14 days) conventional antimycotic treatment is necessary.[1] SOR Ⓒ
- Symptomatic VVC is more frequent in HIV-seropositive women and correlates with severity of immunodeficiency. In addition, among HIV-infected women, systemic azole exposure is associated with the isolation of non–*C. albicans* species from the vagina. According to the available data, therapy for VVC in HIV-infected women should not differ from that for seronegative women.[1] SOR Ⓒ

FOLLOW-UP

Patients should be instructed to return for follow-up visits only if symptoms persist or recur within 2 months of onset of initial symptoms.[1]

PATIENT EDUCATION

Studies show that women who were previously diagnosed with VVC are not necessarily more likely to be able to diagnose themselves.[1] Any woman whose symptoms persist after using a nonprescription preparation, or who has a recurrence of symptoms within 2 months, should be evaluated with office-based testing. Explain that unnecessary or inappropriate use of nonprescription preparations can lead to a delay in the treatment of other vulvovaginitis etiologies, which can result in adverse clinical outcomes.[1]

PATIENT RESOURCES

- FamilyDoctor.org from AAFP. *Yeast Infections*—**http://familydoctor.org/online/famdocen/home/women/reproductive/vaginal/206.htm.**
- MedicineNet. *Vaginal Yeast Infection (Yeast Vaginitis)*—**http://www.medicinenet.com/yeast_vaginitis/article.htm.**
- WebMD. *Vaginal Yeast Infections*—**http://women.webmd.com/tc/vaginal-yeast-infections-topic-overview.**
- Womenshealth.gov. *Vaginal Yeast Infections Fact Sheet*—**http://www.womenshealth.gov/publications/our-publications/fact-sheet/vaginal-yeast-infections.cfm.**
- MedLinePlus. *Yeast Infections*—**http://www.nlm.nih.gov/medlineplus/yeastinfections.html.**
- eMedicine Health. *Candidiasis*—**http://www.emedicinehealth.com/candidiasis_yeast_infection/article_em.htm.**

PROVIDER RESOURCES

- Centers for Disease Control and Prevention. *2010 Guidelines for Treatment of Sexually Transmitted Diseases*—**http://www.cdc.gov/std/treatment/2010/STD-Treatment-2010-RR5912.pdf.**
- American Family Physician. Management of vaginitis. *Am Fam Physician.* 2004;70:2125-2132.—**http://www.aafp.org/afp/20041201/2125.html.**
- eMedicine. *Candidiasis*—**http://emedicine.medscape.com/article/213853-overview.**
- eMedicine. *Vulvovaginitis in Emergency Medicine*—**http://emedicine.medscape.com/article/797497-overview.**

REFERENCES

1. Centers for Disease Control and Prevention. *2010 Guidelines for Treatment of Sexually Transmitted Diseases.* http://www.cdc.gov/std/treatment/2010/STD-Treatment-2010-RR5912.pdf. Accessed November 2, 2011.
2. Goldacre MJ, Watt B, Loudon N, et al. Vaginal microbial flora in normal young women. *Br Med J.* 1979;1:1450.
3. Hurley R, De Louvois J. *Candida* vaginitis. *Postgrad Med J.* 1979;55:645.
4. Sobel JD. Epidemiology and pathogenesis of recurrent vulvovaginal candidiasis. *Am J Obstet Gynecol.* 1985;152:924.
5. Shalev E, Battino S, Weiner E, et al. Ingestion of yogurt containing acidophilus compared with pasteurized yogurt as prophylaxis for recurrent candidal vaginitis and bacterial vaginosis. *Arch Fam Med.* 1996;5:593-596.
6. Cohen DA, Nsuami M, Etame RB, et al. A school-based chlamydia control program using DNA amplification technology. *Pediatrics.* 1998;(1):101.
7. Horowitz BJ, Giaquinta D, Ito S. Evolving pathogens in vulvovaginal candidiasis: implications for patient care. *J Clin Pharmacol.* 1992;32:248.
8. Foxman B. The epidemiology of vulvovaginal candidiasis: risk factors. *Am J Public Health.* 1990;80:329.
9. Sobel JD. *Candida* vaginitis. *Infect Dis Clin Pract (Baltim Md).* 1994;3:334.
10. Swartz JH, Lamkins BE. A rapid, simple stain for fungi in skin, nail scrapings, and hair. *Arch Dermatol.* 1964 Jan;89:89-94.
11. Sobel JD, Brooker D, Stein GE, et al. Single oral dose fluconazole compared with conventional clotrimazole topical therapy of candida vaginitis. *Am J Obstet Gynecol.* 1995;172:1263-1238.
12. Pirotta M, Gunn J, Chondros P, et al. Effect of lactobacillus in preventing post-antibiotic vulvovaginal candidiasis: a randomised controlled trial. *BMJ.* 2004;329:548.
13. Van Kessel K, Assefi N, Marrazzo J, Eckert L. Common complementary and alternative therapies for yeast vaginitis and bacterial vaginosis: a systematic review. *Obstet Gynecol Surv.* 2003;58(5):351-358.
14. Boskey ER. Alternative therapies for bacterial vaginosis: a literature review and acceptability survey. *Altern Ther Health Med.* 2005;11(5):38-43.

92 TRICHOMONAS VAGINITIS

E.J. Mayeaux Jr, MD
Richard P. Usatine, MD

PATIENT STORY

A 27-year-old woman presents with a vaginal itching, odor, and discharge for 1 week. She has one partner who is asymptomatic. Speculum examination shows a strawberry cervix seen with *Trichomonas* infections (**Figure 92-1**). This strawberry pattern is caused by inflammation and punctate hemorrhages on the cervix. There is a scant white discharge with a fishy odor. Wet mount shows trichomonads swimming in saline (**Figures 92-2** and **92-3**). The trichomonads are larger than white blood cells (WBCs) and have visible flagella and movement. She is diagnosed with trichomoniasis and treated with 2 g of metronidazole in a single dose. The patient is tested for other sexually transmitted diseases (STDs), and her partner is treated with the same regimen.

INTRODUCTION

Trichomonas vaginitis is a local infection caused by the protozoan *Trichomonas vaginalis* that is associated with vaginal discharge. The woman often has an itch and an odor along with the discharge but may be asymptomatic.

SYNONYMS

Trichomoniasis, trich, tricky monkeys.

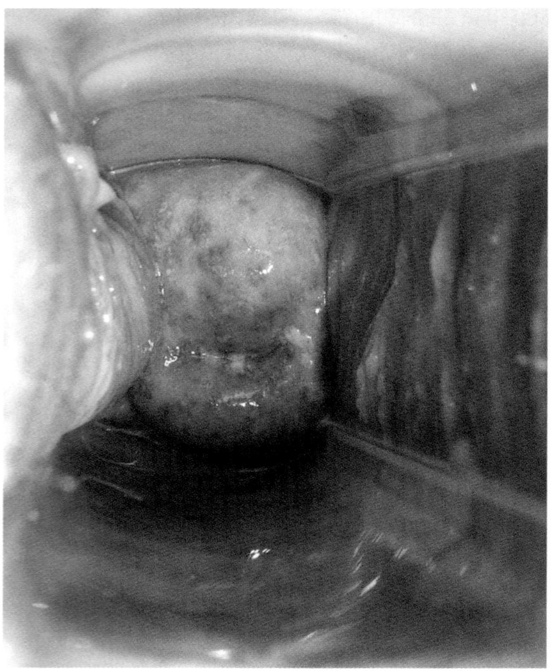

FIGURE 92-1 Speculum examination showing the strawberry cervix pattern seen with *Trichomonas* infections. This strawberry pattern is caused by inflammation and punctate hemorrhages on the cervix. There is a scant white discharge. *(Reproduced with permission from Richard P. Usatine, MD.)*

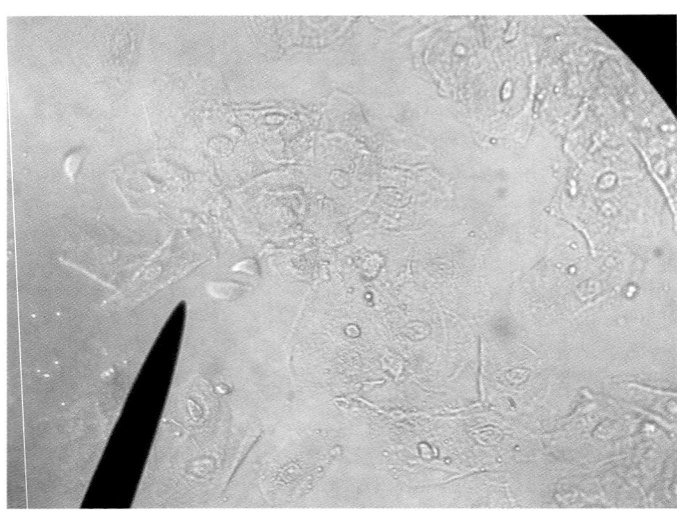

FIGURE 92-2 Wet mount showing *Trichomonas* in saline under low power. There are 2 visible trichomonads to the right and above the tip of the pointer. The largest cells are vaginal epithelial cells with visible nuclei. *(Reproduced with permission from Richard P. Usatine, MD.)*

EPIDEMIOLOGY

- An estimated 3 to 5 million cases of trichomoniasis occur each year in the United States.[1]
- The worldwide prevalence of trichomoniasis is estimated to be 180 million cases per year; and these cases account for 10% to 25% of all vaginal infections.[2]

ETIOLOGY AND PATHOPHYSIOLOGY

- *Trichomonas* infection is caused by the unicellular protozoan *T. vaginalis*.[3]
- The majority of men (90%) infected with *T. vaginalis* are asymptomatic, but many women (50%) report symptoms.[4]

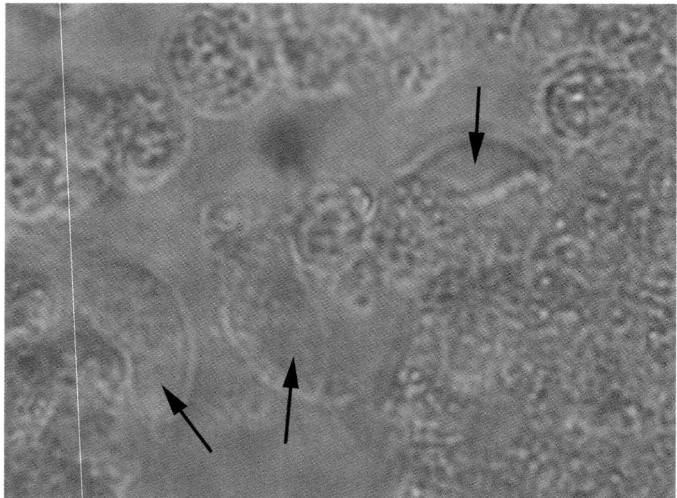

FIGURE 92-3 Wet mount showing *Trichomonas* (*arrows*) in saline under high power. The smaller more granular cells are white blood cells. *(Reproduced with permission from Richard P. Usatine, MD.)*

- The infection is predominantly transmitted via sexual contact. The organism can survive up to 48 hours at 10°C (50°F) outside the body, making transmission from shared undergarments or from infected hot spas possible although extremely unlikely.
- *Trichomonas* infection is associated with low-birth-weight infants, premature rupture of membranes, and preterm delivery in pregnant patients.[5]
- In a person coinfected with HIV, the pathology induced by *T. vaginalis* infection can increase HIV shedding. *Trichomonas* infection may also act to expand the portal of entry for HIV in an HIV-negative person. Studies from Africa have suggested that *T. vaginalis* infection may increase the rate of HIV transmission by approximately 2 fold.[6]

RISK FACTORS[3]

- New or multiple partners
- A history of STDs
- Exchanging sex for payment or drugs
- Injection drug use

DIAGNOSIS

CLINICAL FEATURES

- The physical examination should include inspection of the external genitalia for irritation or discharge. Speculum examination is done to determine the amount and character of the discharge and to look for the characteristic strawberry cervix (**Figures 92-1** and **92-4**).
- Typically, women with trichomoniasis have a diffuse, malodorous, yellow-green or white discharge (**Figure 92-5**) with vulvar irritation (**Figure 92-6**).[3] Vaginal and vulvar itching and irritation are common.[3]

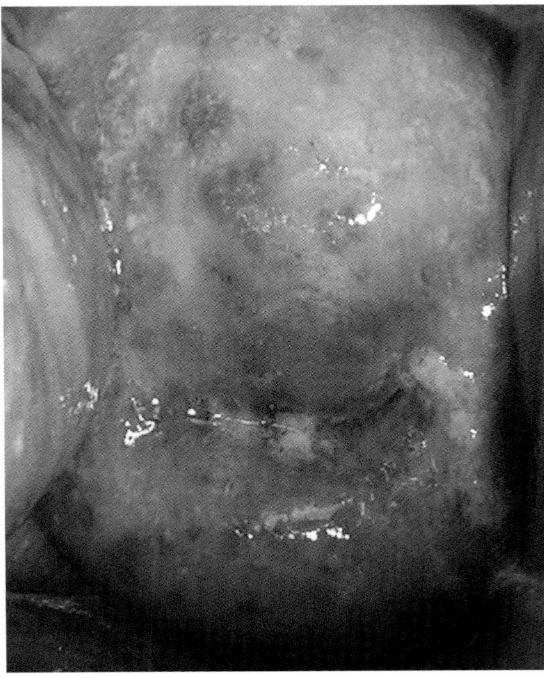

FIGURE 92-4 Close-up of strawberry cervix in a *Trichomonas* infection demonstrating inflammation and punctate hemorrhages. (*Reproduced with permission from Richard P. Usatine, MD.*)

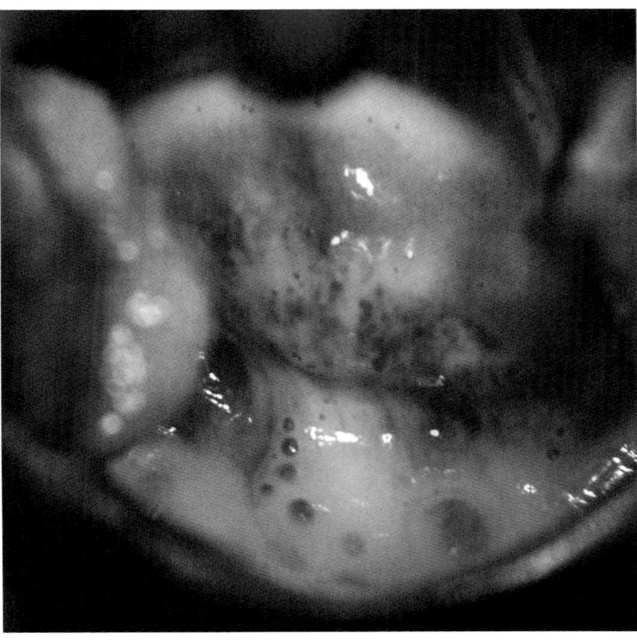

FIGURE 92-5 Speculum examination demonstrating the thick yellow-green discharge that may be seen in *Trichomonas* infection. The discharge can also be frothy white. (*Reproduced with permission from E.J. Mayeaux Jr, MD.*)

- It should be determined whether the patient douched recently, because this can lower the yield of diagnostic tests. Patients who have been told not to douche will sometimes start wiping the vagina with soapy washcloths to "keep clean" as an alternative. This greatly irritates the vagina and cervix, lowers test sensitivity, and may cause a discharge.

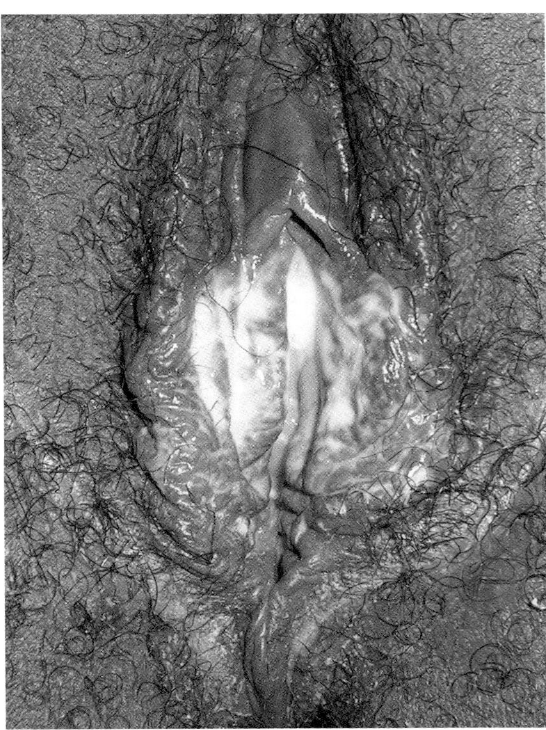

FIGURE 92-6 *Trichomonas* infection in a 28-year-old woman showing copious white discharge and vulvar irritation. The woman had worked as an "escort" and fortunately her other tests for sexually transmitted infections were negative. (*Reproduced with permission from Richard P. Usatine, MD.*)

TYPICAL DISTRIBUTION

In women, *T. vaginalis* may be found in the vagina, urethra, and paraurethral glands of infected women. Other sites include the cervix and Bartholin and Skene glands.

LABORATORY TESTING

- Because of the high prevalence of trichomoniasis, testing should be performed in women seeking care for vaginal discharge. Screening should be considered for women with risk factors.[3]
- Wet preps are obtained using a cotton-tipped applicator applied to the vaginal side-wall, placing the sample of discharge into normal saline (not water). A drop of the suspension is then placed on a slide, covered with a coverslip, and carefully examined with the low-power and high-dry objective lenses. Under the microscope, observe for motile trichomonads, which are often easy to visualize because of their lashing flagella (**Figure 92-2**).
- Wet prep has a sensitivity of only approximately 60% to 70% and requires immediate evaluation of wet preparation slide for optimal results.[3]
- The OSOM Trichomonas Rapid Test and the Affirm VP III are FDA cleared for trichomoniasis in women. Both tests are performed on vaginal secretions at the point of care and have a sensitivity greater than 83% and a specificity greater than 97%. The results of the OSOM Trichomonas Rapid Test are available in approximately 10 minutes, and results of the Affirm VP III are available within 45 minutes. False-positive tests might occur, especially in populations with a low prevalence of disease.[3]
- An FDA-approved polymerase chain reaction (PCR) assay for detection of gonorrhea and chlamydial infection (Amplicor, manufactured by Roche Diagnostic Corp.) has been modified to test for *T. vaginalis* in vaginal or endocervical swabs and in urine from women and men, with sensitivity ranges from 88% to 97% and specificity from 98% to 99%.[7]
- APTIMA *T. vaginalis* Analyte Specific Reagents (ASR; manufactured by Gen-Probe, Inc.) also can detect *T. vaginalis* RNA using the same instrumentation platforms available for the FDA-cleared APTIMA Combo 2 assay for diagnosis of gonorrhea and chlamydial infection. Published validation studies found sensitivity ranging from 74% to 98% and specificity from 87% to 98%.[8]
- A vaginal pH above 4.5 is seen with menopausal patients, *Trichomonas* infection, or bacterial vaginosis.[4]
- Culture is a sensitive and highly specific method of diagnosis. In women in whom trichomoniasis is suspected but not confirmed by microscopy, vaginal secretions should be cultured for *T. vaginalis*.[3]
- A nucleic acid amplification test for *Neisseria gonorrhoeae*, and/or *Chlamydia trachomatis* should be performed on all patients with *Trichomonas*.

DIFFERENTIAL DIAGNOSIS

- Bacterial vaginosis and *Trichomonas* may have the odor of aromatic amines, and therefore may easily be confused with each other. Look for clue cells and trichomonads on the wet prep to differentiate between the 2 (Chapter 90, Bacterial Vaginosis).
- *Candida* vaginitis tends to present with a cottage-cheese-like discharge and vaginal itching (Chapter 91, Candida Vaginitis).
- Gonorrhea and *Chlamydia* should not be missed in patients with vaginal discharge. Consider testing for these STDs based on patients' risk factors and the presence of purulence clinically and WBCs on the wet prep (Chapter 93, Chlamydia Cervicitis).

MANAGEMENT

MEDICATIONS

- **Table 92-1** shows treatments for *T. vaginalis* infections. Metronidazole 2 g orally as a single dose, or 500 mg bid for 7 days (including pregnant patients) are the best treatments by Cochrane analysis.[9] SOR Ⓐ
- Tinidazole (Tindamax), a second-generation nitroimidazole, is indicated as a 1-time dose of 2 g for the treatment of trichomoniasis (including metronidazole-resistant trichomoniasis).[3] SOR Ⓐ It is effective therapy in nonresistant and resistant *T. vaginalis*.[10,11] The contraindications (including ethyl alcohol [ETOH]) to the use of tinidazole are similar to those for metronidazole.
- Pregnant women may be treated with 2 g of metronidazole in a single dose. Metronidazole is pregnancy category B. Vaginal trichomoniasis is associated with adverse pregnancy outcomes, particularly premature rupture of membranes, preterm delivery, and low birth weight. Unfortunately, data do not suggest that metronidazole treatment results in a reduction in perinatal morbidity and treatment may even increase prematurity or low birth weight.[3] Treatment of *T. vaginalis* might relieve symptoms of vaginal discharge in pregnant women and might prevent respiratory or genital infection of the newborn and further sexual transmission. The Centers for Disease Control and Prevention (CDC) recommends that clinicians counsel patients regarding the potential risks and benefits of treatment during pregnancy.[3]
- Some strains of *T. vaginalis* can have diminished susceptibility to metronidazole. Low-level metronidazole resistance has been identified in 2% to 5% of cases of vaginal trichomoniasis. These infections should respond to tinidazole or higher doses or longer durations of metronidazole. High-level resistance is rare.
- Metronidazole gel is 50% less efficacious for the treatment of trichomoniasis than oral preparations and is not recommended.[3]

PREVENTION

- Patients should be instructed to avoid sex until they and their sex partners are cured (ie, when therapy has been completed and patient and partner[s] are asymptomatic).[3]
- Spermicidal agents such as nonoxynol-9 reduce the rate of transmission of *Trichomonas*.[12]
- The risk of acquiring infection can be reduced by consistent use of condoms and limiting the number of sexual partners.

TABLE 92-1 Centers for Disease Control and Prevention Recommended Regimens for Pregnant and Nonpregnant Patients. SOR Ⓐ

Metronidazole 2 g orally in a single dose
OR
Tinidazole 2 g orally in a single dose
CDC Alternative Regimen SOR Ⓐ
Metronidazole 500 mg orally twice a day for 7 days

Data from Centers for Disease Control and Prevention.[2,3]

FOLLOW-UP

Because of the high rate of reinfection among patients in whom trichomoniasis was diagnosed, rescreening at 3 months following initial infection can be considered for sexually active women.[3]

PATIENT EDUCATION

Sexual partners of patients with *Trichomonas* should be treated. Patients can be sent home with a dose for a partner when it is believed that the partner will not come in on his own.

PATIENT RESOURCES

- Centers for Disease Control and Prevention information—**http://www.dpd.cdc.gov/dpdx/HTML/Trichomoniasis.htm.**
- MedlinePlus. *Trichomoniasis*—**http://www.nlm.nih.gov/medlineplus/ency/article/001331.htm.**
- Centers for Disease Control and Prevention. *STDs: Trichomoniasis*—**http://www.cdc.gov/std/trichomonas/default.htm.**
- PubMed Health. *Trichomoniasis*—**http://www.ncbi.nlm.nih.gov/pubmedhealth/PMH0002307/.**
- MedLinePlus. *Trichomoniasis*—**http://www.nlm.nih.gov/medlineplus/trichomoniasis.html.**
- eMedicine Health. *Trichomoniasis*—**http://www.emedicinehealth.com/trichomoniasis/article_em.htm.**

PROVIDER RESOURCES

- Medscape. *Trichomoniasis*—**http://emedicine.medscape.com/article/230617.**
- eMedicine. *Trichomoniasis*—**http://emedicine.medscape.com/article/787722.**
- Centers for Disease Control and Prevention. *2010 Guidelines for Treatment of Sexually Transmitted Diseases*—**http://www.cdc.gov/std/treatment/2010/STD-Treatment-2010-RR5912.pdf.**

REFERENCES

1. Sutton M, Sternberg M, Koumans EH, et al. The prevalence of *Trichomonas vaginalis* infection among reproductive-age women in the United States, 2001-2004. *Clin Infect Dis.* 2007;45:1319.
2. Weinstock H, Berman S, Cates W Jr. Sexually transmitted diseases among American youth: incidence and prevalence estimates, 2000. *Perspect Sex Reprod Health.* 2004;36(1):6-10.
3. Centers for Disease Control and Prevention. *2010 Guidelines for Treatment of Sexually Transmitted Diseases.* http://www.cdc.gov/std/treatment/2010/STD-Treatment-2010-RR5912.pdf. Accessed 1 December, 2011.
4. Gjerdngen D, Fontaine P, Bixby M, et al. The impact of regular vaginal pH screening on the diagnosis of bacterial vaginosis in pregnancy. *J Fam Pract.* 2000;49:3-43.
5. Cotch MF, Pastorek JG 2nd, Nugent RP, et al. Trichomonas vaginalis associated with low birth weight and preterm delivery: the Vaginal Infections and Prematurity Study Group. *Sex Transm Dis.* 1997;24:353-360.
6. Sorvillo F, Smith L, Kerndt P, Ash L. *Trichomonas vaginalis*, HIV, and African-Americans. *Emerg Infect Dis.* 2001;7(6):927-932.
7. Van Der PB, Kraft CS, Williams JA. Use of an adaptation of a commercially available PCR assay aimed at diagnosis of chlamydia and gonorrhea to detect *Trichomonas vaginalis* in urogenital specimens. *J Clin Microbiol.* 2006;44:366-373.
8. Nye MB, Schwebke JR, Body BA. Comparison of APTIMA *Trichomonas vaginalis* transcription-mediated amplification to wet mount microscopy, culture, and polymerase chain reaction for diagnosis of trichomoniasis in men and women. *Am J Obstet Gynecol.* 2009;200:188-197.
9. Epling J. What is the best way to treat trichomoniasis in women? *Am Fam Physician.* 2001;64:1241-1244.
10. Mammen-Tobin A, Wilson JD. Management of metronidazole-resistant *Trichomonas vaginalis*—a new approach. *Int J STD AIDS.* 2005;16(7):488-490.
11. Hager WD. Treatment of metronidazole-resistant *Trichomonas vaginalis* with tinidazole: case reports of three patients. *Sex Transm Dis.* 2004;31(6):343-345.
12. d'Oro LC, Parazzini F, Naldi L, La Vecchia C. Barrier methods of contraception, spermicides, and sexually transmitted diseases: a review. *Genitourin Med.* 1994;70:410.

93 CHLAMYDIA CERVICITIS

E.J. Mayeaux Jr, MD
Richard P. Usatine, MD

PATIENT STORY

A young woman presents to her primary care physician with a vaginal discharge. On physical examination, there is cervical ectopy, inflammation, and some mucoid discharge (**Figure 93-1**). The cervix bled easily while obtaining discharge and cells for a wet mount and genetic probe test. The wet mount showed many white blood cells (WBCs) but no visible pathogens. She was sent to the laboratory for rapid plasma reagin (RPR) and HIV tests and given a follow-up appointment in 1 week. The genetic probe test was positive for *Chlamydia* and all the other examinations were negative. The patient was treated with 1 g of azithromycin taken in front of a clinic nurse. She was also counseled to discuss the result with her male partners and the importance of safe sex was emphasized.

INTRODUCTION

Chlamydia trachomatis causes genital infections that can result in pelvic inflammatory disease (PID), ectopic pregnancy, and infertility. Asymptomatic infection is common among both men and women so health care providers must rely on screening tests to detect disease. The Centers for Disease Control and Prevention (CDC) recommends annual screening of all sexually active women ages 25 years and younger, and of older women with risk factors, such as having a new sex partner or multiple sex partners.[1]

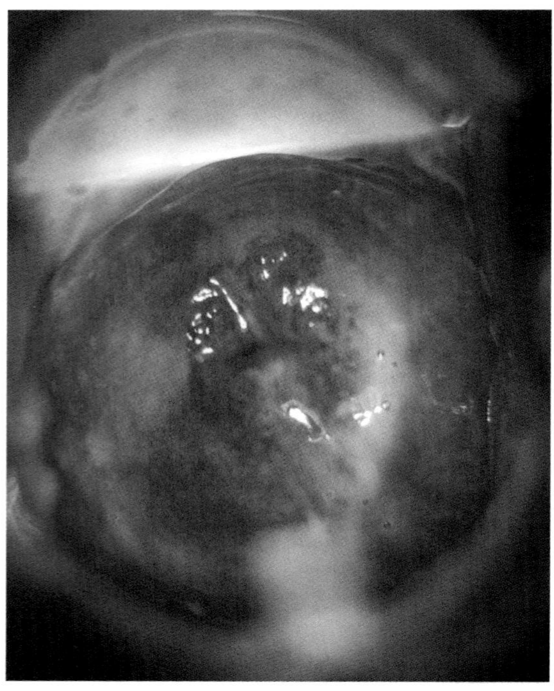

FIGURE 93-1 Chlamydia cervicitis in a patient with a vaginal discharge. A NAAT test was positive for *Chlamydia*. The rest of her work-up was negative. (*Reproduced with permission from E.J. Mayeaux Jr, M.D.*)

EPIDEMIOLOGY

- A very common STD, *Chlamydia* is the most frequently reported infectious disease in the United States (excluding human papillomavirus [HPV]).[1] An estimated 1.2 million cases are reported to the CDC annually in the United States.[2]
- The World Health Organization (WHO) estimates there are 140 million cases of Chlamydia trachomatis infection worldwide every year.[3]
- The CDC estimates screening and treatment programs can be conducted at an annual cost of $175 million. Every dollar spent on screening and treatment saves $12 in complications that result from untreated *Chlamydia*.[4]
- It is common among sexually active adolescents and young adults.[5] As many as 1 in 10 adolescent girls tested for *Chlamydia* is infected. Based on reports to the CDC provided by states that collect age-specific data, teenage girls have the highest rates of chlamydial infection. In these states, 15- to 19-year-old girls represent 46% of infections and 20- to 24-year-old women represent another 33%.[4]

ETIOLOGY AND PATHOPHYSIOLOGY

- *C. trachomatis* is a small gram-negative bacterium with unique biologic properties among living organisms. *Chlamydia* is an obligate intracellular parasite that has a distinct life-cycle consisting of 2 major phases: The small elementary bodies attach and penetrate into cells, and the metabolically active reticulate bodies that form large inclusions within cells.
- It has a long growth cycle, which explains why extended courses of treatment are often necessary. Immunity to infection is not long lived, so reinfection or persistent infection is common.
- The infection may be asymptomatic and the onset often indolent. It can cause cervicitis, endometritis, PID, urethritis, epididymitis, neonatal conjunctivitis, and pediatric pneumonia. Of exposed babies, 50% develop conjunctivitis and 10% to 16% develop pneumonia.[1]
- *Chlamydia* infections may lead to reactive arthritis, which presents with arthritis, conjunctivitis, and urethritis (Chapter 155, Reactive Arthritis). Past or ongoing *C. trachomatis* infection may be a risk factor for ovarian cancer.[6,7]
- Up to 40% of women with untreated *Chlamydia* will develop PID. Undiagnosed PID caused by *Chlamydia* is common. Of those with PID, 20% will become infertile; 18% will experience debilitating, chronic pelvic pain; and 9% will have a life-threatening tubal pregnancy. Tubal pregnancy is the leading cause of first-trimester, pregnancy-related deaths in American women.[4]

RISK FACTORS[1,2,8]

- Adolescents and young adults
- Nonwhite populations
- Multiple sexual partners
- Poor socioeconomic conditions
- Single marital status
- Nonbarrier contraceptive use
- History of prior STD

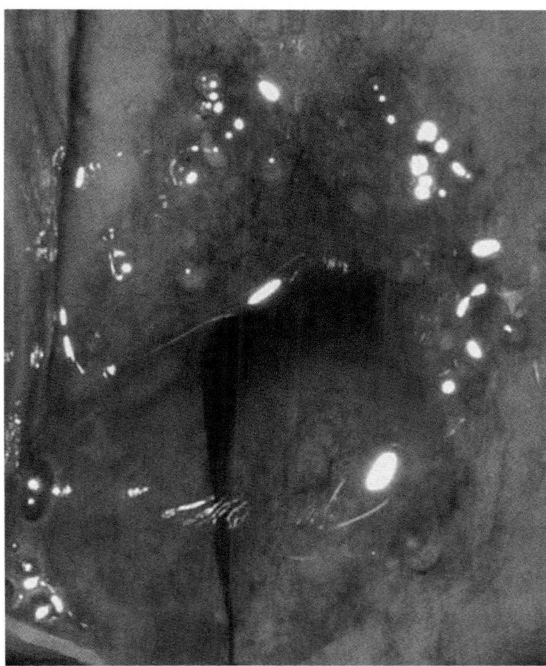

FIGURE 93-2 Chlamydial cervicitis with ectopy, mucoid discharge, and bleeding. The cervix is inflamed and friable. (*Reproduced with permission from Connie Celum and Walter Stamm, Seattle STD/HIV Prevention Training Center, University of Washington.*)

DIAGNOSIS

CLINICAL FEATURES

- The cervix is inflamed, friable, and may bleed easily with manipulation. The cervix may show ectopy (columnar cells on the ectocervix). The discharge is usually mucoid or mucopurulent (**Figure 93-2**).
- In many cases, the infected cervix may appear normal or mildly friable (**Figure 93-3**).

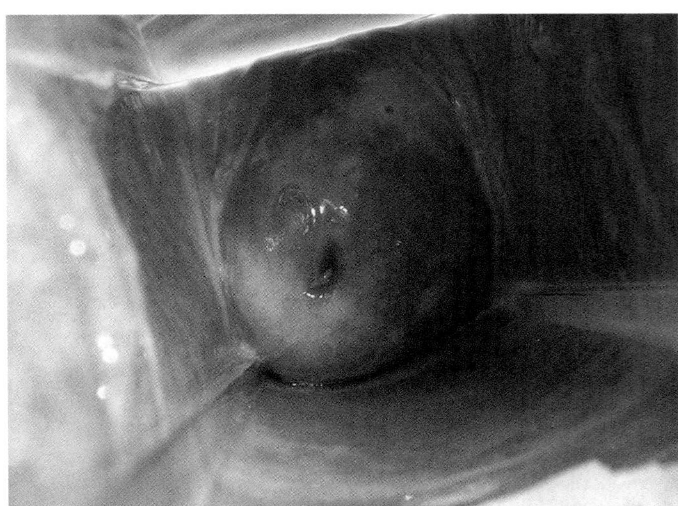

FIGURE 93-3 A normal appearing cervix with minimal discharge in a patient found to have gonorrhea and chlamydia through lab testing at the time of her Pap test. She was enrolled in a residential drug rehabilitation program and had a history of unprotected sex with multiple partners. High risk patients should be tested for chlamydia and gonorrhea regardless of the findings on physical exam. (*Reproduced with permission from Richard P. Usatine, MD.*)

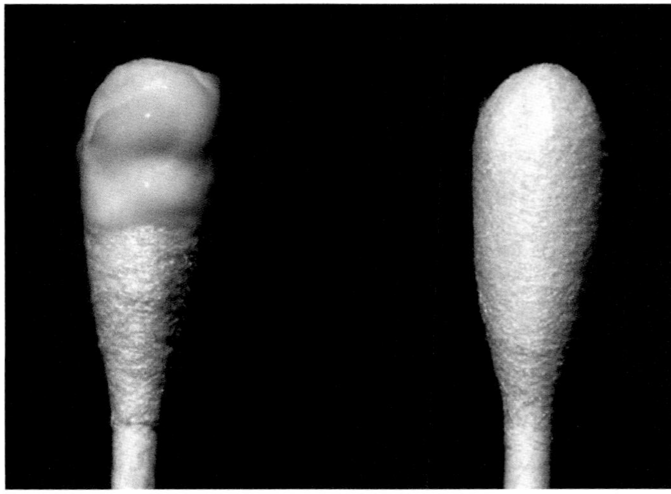

FIGURE 93-4 Mucopurulent discharge on the left swab from a cervix infected with *Chlamydia* (positive swab test). (*Reproduced with permission from Connie Celum and Walter Stamm, Seattle STD/HIV Prevention Training Center, University of Washington.*)

- Swab test—A white cotton-tip applicator is placed in the endocervical canal and removed to view. A visible mucopurulent discharge constitutes a positive swab test for *Chlamydia* (**Figure 93-4**). This is not specific for *Chlamydia* as other genital infections can cause a mucopurulent discharge, and it is not recommended for diagnosis.

LABORATORY TESTING

- A significant proportion of patients with *Chlamydia* are asymptomatic, providing a reservoir for infection. All pregnant women and sexually active women younger than 25 years of age should be screened with routine examinations. A wet prep is usually negative for other organisms. Only WBCs and normal flora are seen.
- *Chlamydia* cannot be cultured on artificial media because it is an obligate intracellular organism. Tissue culture is required to grow the live organism. When testing for *Chlamydia*, a wood-handled swab must not be used, as substances in wood may inhibit *Chlamydia* organism. Culture has sensitivity of 70% to 100% and a specificity of almost 100%, which makes it the gold standard.[1]
- The enzyme-linked immunosorbent assay (ELISA) technique (Chlamydiazyme) has a sensitivity of 70% to 100% and a specificity of 97% to 99%.[5] Fluorescein-conjugated monoclonal antibodies test (MicroTrak) has a sensitivity of 70% to 100% and a specificity of 97% to 99%.[5]
- *C. trachomatis* can be detected using nucleic acid amplification techniques (NAATs) on swabs or voided urine specimens. These tests are often used for testing to detect gonorrhea and *Chlamydia*. Nucleic acid amplification tests have been used successfully in difficult-to-reach adolescents ("street kids") as well as in pediatric emergency departments and school-based settings.[9,10] Screening in school-based settings was associated with significant reduction in *Chlamydia* rates during a 1-year period. Self-collected vaginal swab specimens perform at least as well as with other approved specimens using NAATs.[11]
- Rectal and oropharyngeal *C. trachomatis* infection in persons engaging in anal or oral intercourse can be diagnosed by testing at the site of exposure. Although not FDA cleared for this use, NAATs have demonstrated improved sensitivity and specificity compared with culture for the detection at rectal sites[12] and at oropharyngeal sites in men.[13]

- Certain NAATs have been FDA-cleared for use on liquid-based cytology specimens, although test sensitivity using these specimens might be lower.[14]
- Persons who undergo testing for *Chlamydia* should be tested for other STDs as well.[1]

DIFFERENTIAL DIAGNOSIS

- Gonorrhea frequently coexists with *Chlamydia* and should be tested for when a patient is thought to have *Chlamydia*. The discharge of gonorrhea may be more purulent but this is not always the case (Chapter 213, Gonococcal Urethritis)
- Bacterial vaginosis—The aromatic amine odor and clue cells help to distinguish between these infections (Chapter 90, Bacterial Vaginosis).
- Trichomoniasis—Look for the strawberry cervix and *Trichomonas* on the wet prep. There may also be a positive whiff test (see Chapter 92, *Trichomonas* Vaginitis).

MANAGEMENT

NONPHARMACOLOGIC

Patients diagnosed with *Chlamydia* cervicitis should be tested for other STDs.[1]

MEDICATIONS

- **Table 93-1** shows CDC-recommended treatments for *Chlamydia*. Azithromycin (Zithromax) 1000 mg 1-time dose is easy and may be directly observed in the clinic.[1] SOR Ⓐ It is the first-line therapy for *Chlamydia* during pregnancy.
- Other treatments include doxycycline 100 mg PO bid × 7 days.[1] SOR Ⓐ Avoid dairy products around time of dosing.
- Erythromycin might be less efficacious than either azithromycin or doxycycline, mainly because of the frequent occurrence of GI side effects that can lead to nonadherence.
- Ofloxacin (Floxin) 300 mg PO bid × 7 days is an alternative that should be taken on an empty stomach.[1] SOR Ⓐ It is contraindicated in children or pregnant and lactating women, but may also cover *Neisseria gonorrhoeae* infection. Levofloxacin 500 mg PO for 7 days is another fluoroquinolone alternative.[1] SOR Ⓐ
- A metaanalysis of 12 randomized clinical trials of azithromycin versus doxycycline for the treatment of genital chlamydial infection demonstrated that the treatments were equally efficacious, with microbial cure rates of 97% and 98%, respectively.[15]
- Partners need treatment. If concern exists that sex partners will not seek evaluation and treatment, then delivery of antibiotic therapy (either a prescription or medication) to their partners is an option.[1]
- Medications for chlamydial infections should be dispensed on site and the first dose directly observed to maximize medication adherence.[1]

REFERRAL OR HOSPITALIZATION

With evidence of complications such as a tuboovarian abscess or severe PID.

TABLE 93-1 Centers for Disease Control and Prevention Recommended Regimens SOR Ⓐ

Azithromycin 1 g orally in a single dose
OR
Doxycycline 100 mg orally twice a day for 7 days
CDC Alternative Regimens
Erythromycin base 500 mg orally 4 times a day for 7 days
OR
Erythromycin ethylsuccinate 800 mg orally 4 times a day for 7 days
OR
Ofloxacin 300 mg orally twice a day for 7 days
OR
Levofloxacin 500 mg orally once daily for 7 days
CDC Recommended Regimens in Pregnancy
Azithromycin 1 g orally in a single dose
OR
Amoxicillin 500 mg orally 3 times a day for 7 days
Alternative Regimens in Pregnancy
Erythromycin base 500 mg orally 4 times a day for 7 days
OR
Erythromycin base 250 mg orally 4 times a day for 14 days
OR
Erythromycin ethylsuccinate 800 mg orally 4 times a day for 7 days
OR
Erythromycin ethylsuccinate 400 mg orally 4 times a day for 14 days

Data from the Centers for Disease Control and Prevention.[1]

PREVENTION

Individuals who are sexually active should be aware of the risk of STDs and that ways of avoiding infection include mutual monogamy and appropriate barrier protection.

PROGNOSIS

Treatment failures with full primary therapies are quite rare. Reinfection is very common and is related to nontreatment of sexual partners or acquisition from a new partner.

FOLLOW-UP

Test of cure (repeat testing 3-4 weeks after completing therapy) is not recommended for persons treated with the recommended or alterative regimens, unless therapeutic compliance is in question, symptoms persist, or reinfection is suspected. However, test of cure is recommended in pregnant women.[1]

PATIENT EDUCATION

- To minimize transmission, persons treated for *Chlamydia* should be instructed to abstain from sexual intercourse for 7 days after single-dose therapy or until completion of a 7-day regimen.
- To minimize the risk for reinfection, patients also should be instructed to abstain from sexual intercourse until all their sex partners are treated.[1]

PATIENT RESOURCES

- eMedicine Health. *Cervicitis*—**http://www.emedicinehealth.com/cervicitis/article_em.htm.**
- eMedicine Health. *Chlamydia*—**http://www.emedicinehealth.com/chlamydia/article_em.htm.**
- CDC. *Chlamydia*—**http://www.cdc.gov/std/Chlamydia/STDFact-Chlamydia.htm.**

PROVIDER RESOURCES

- CDC. *Sexually Transmitted Diseases (STDs) 2010: Diseases Characterized by Urethritis and Cervicitis*—**http://www.cdc.gov/std/treatment/2010/urethritis-and-cervicitis.htm.**
- Medscape. *Chlamydial Genitourinary Infections*—**http://emedicine.medscape.com/article/214823-overview.**
- Medscape. *Cervicitis*—**http://emedicine.medscape.com/article/253402.**

REFERENCES

1. Centers for Disease Control and Prevention. *Sexually Transmitted Diseases (STDs) 2010: Diseases Characterized by Urethritis and Cervicitis*. http://www.cdc.gov/std/treatment/2010/urethritis-and-cervicitis.htm. Accessed December 2, 2011.
2. Centers for Disease Control and Prevention. *Sexually Transmitted Disease Surveillance, 2009—Chlamydia*. http://www.cdc.gov/std/stats09/default.htm. Accessed December 25, 2011.
3. World Health Organization. *Chlamydia Trachomatis. Initiative for Vaccine Research*. http://www.who.int/vaccine_research/diseases/soa_std/en/index.html. Accessed December 2, 2011.
4. Centers for Disease Control and Prevention. http://www.cdc.gov/std/Chlamydia/STDFact-Chlamydia.htm. Accessed December 2, 2011.
5. Skolnik NS. Screening for *Chlamydia trachomatis* infection. *Am Fam Physician*. 1995;51:821-826.
6. Martius J, Krohn MA, Hillier SL, et al. Relationships of vaginal lactobacillus species, cervical *Chlamydia trachomatis*, and bacterial vaginosis to preterm birth. *Obstet Gynecol*. 1988;71:89-95.
7. Ness RB, Goodman MT, Shen C, Brunham RC. Serologic evidence of past infection with *Chlamydia trachomatis*, in relation to ovarian cancer. *J Infect Dis*. 2003;187:1147-1152.
8. Datta SD, Sternberg M, Johnson RE, et al. Gonorrhea and *Chlamydia* in the United States among persons 14 to 39 years of age, 1999 to 2002. *Ann Intern Med*. 2007;147:89.
9. Monroe KW, Weiss HL, Jones M, Hook EW 3rd. Acceptability of urine screening for *Neisseria gonorrheae* and *Chlamydia trachomatis* in adolescents at an urban emergency department. *Sex Transm Dis*. 2003;30:850.
10. Rietmeijer CA, Bull SS, Ortiz CG, et al. Patterns of general health care and STD services use among high-risk youth in Denver participating in community-based urine *Chlamydia* screening. *Sex Transm Dis*. 1998;25:457.
11. Doshi JS, Power J, Allen E. Acceptability of chlamydia screening using self-taken vaginal swabs. *Int J STD AIDS*. 2008;19:507-509.
12. Bachmann LH, Johnson RE, Cheng H, et al. Nucleic acid amplification tests for diagnosis of *Neisseria gonorrhoeae* and *Chlamydia trachomatis* rectal infections. *J Clin Microbiol*. 2010;48:1827-1832.
13. Bachmann LH, Johnson RE, Cheng H, et al. Nucleic acid amplification tests for diagnosis of *Neisseria gonorrhoeae* oropharyngeal infections. *J Clin Microbiol*. 2009;47:902-907.
14. Chernesky M, Freund GG, Hook E, 3rd, et al. Detection of *Chlamydia trachomatis* and *Neisseria gonorrhoeae* infections in North American women by testing SurePath liquid-based Pap specimens in APTIMA assays. *J Clin Microbiol*. 2007;45:2434-2438.
15. Lau C-Y, Qureshi AK. Azithromycin versus doxycycline for genital chlamydial infections: A meta-analysis of randomized clinical trials. *Sex Transm Dis*. 2002;29:497-502.

SECTION 2 BREAST

94 MASTITIS AND BREAST ABSCESS

E.J. Mayeaux, Jr., MD

PATIENT STORY

A 23-year-old woman, who is currently breast-feeding and 6 weeks postpartum presents with a hard, red, tender, indurated area medial to her right nipple (**Figure 94-1**). She also has a low-grade fever. There is a local area of fluctuance and so incision and drainage is recommended. The area is anesthetized with 1% lidocaine and epinephrine and drained with a No. 11 scalpel. A lot of purulence is expressed and the wound is packed. The patient is started on cephalexin 500 mg qid for 10 days to treat the surrounding cellulitis and seen in follow-up the next day. The patient was already feeling better the next day and went on to full resolution in the following weeks.

EPIDEMIOLOGY

The prevalence of mastitis is estimated to be at least 1% to 3% of lactating women (**Figure 94-2**). Risk factors include a history of mastitis with a previous child, cracks and nipple sores, use of an antifungal nipple cream in the same month, and use of a manual breast pump.[1]

Breast abscess is an uncommon problem in breast-feeding women with an incidence of approximately 0.1%.[2] Risk factors include maternal age more than 30 years of age, primiparity, gestational age of 41 weeks, and mastitis.[2,3] Breast abscess develops in 5% to 11% of women with mastitis, often caused by inadequate therapy.[3]

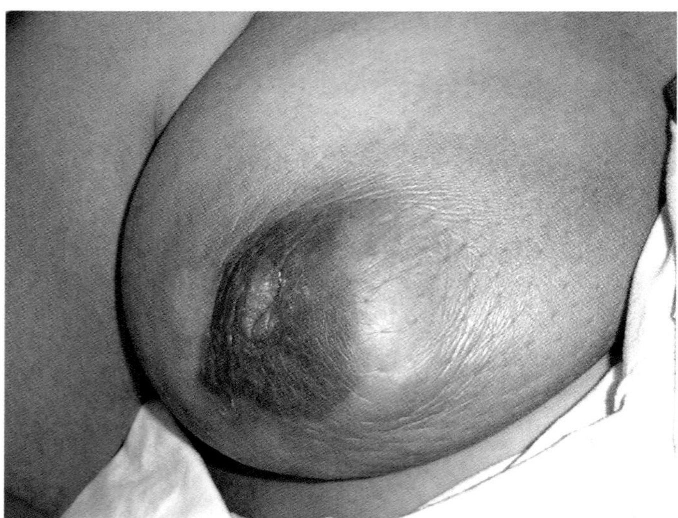

FIGURE 94-1 Localized cellulitis and breast abscess in a breast-feeding mother. Note the Peau d' orange appearance of the edematous breast tissue. (*Reproduced with permission from Nicolette Deveneau, MD.*)

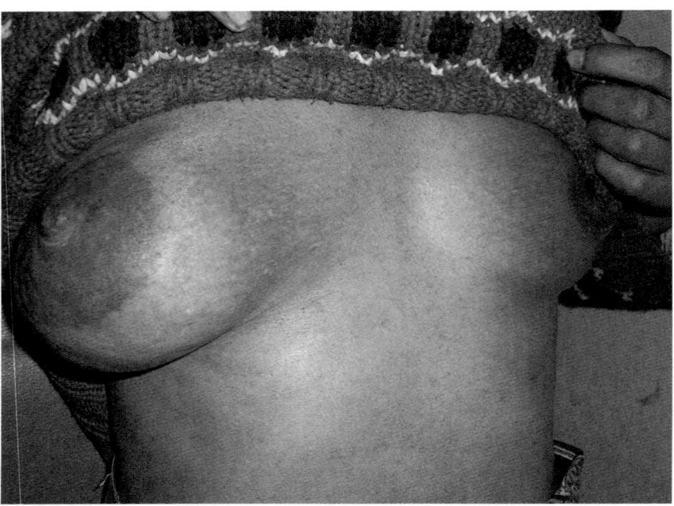

FIGURE 94-2 Mastitis in a postpartum breast-feeding woman. The right breast was warm, tender, enlarged, and painful. Erythema is barely visible on the areola because of the naturally darker pigmentation of the skin. (*Courtesy of Richard P. Usatine, MD.*)

ETIOLOGY AND PATHOPHYSIOLOGY

Mastitis, defined as an infection of the breast, and breast abscesses are typically found in breast-feeding women (**Figures 94-1 and 94-2**). A breast abscess can occur in older women unrelated to pregnancy and breast-feeding (**Figure 94-3**).

Mastitis is most commonly caused by *Staphylococcus aureus*, Streptococcus species, and *Escherichia coli*.

Recurrent mastitis can result from poor selection or incomplete use of antibiotic therapy, or failure to resolve underlying lactation management problems. Mastitis that repeatedly recurs in the same location, or does not respond to appropriate therapy, may indicate the presence of breast cancer.[3]

DIAGNOSIS

CLINICAL FEATURES

- Mastitis causes a hard, red, tender, swollen area on the breast (**Figures 94-1** and **94-2**).
- Fever is common.
- Pain usually extends beyond the indurated area.
- It is often associated with other systemic complaints including myalgia, chills, malaise, and flu-like symptoms.
- Breast abscess can occur with mastitis, except a fluctuant mass is palpable. (In **Figure 94-3**, the fluctuant mass is close to the midline with 2 openings of spontaneous drainage. The remainder of the erythema is cellulitis.)
- Breast abscesses, especially in the inframammary area, may also be associated with hydradenitis suppurativa (**Figure 94-4**).[4]
- Typical distribution is usually unilateral.

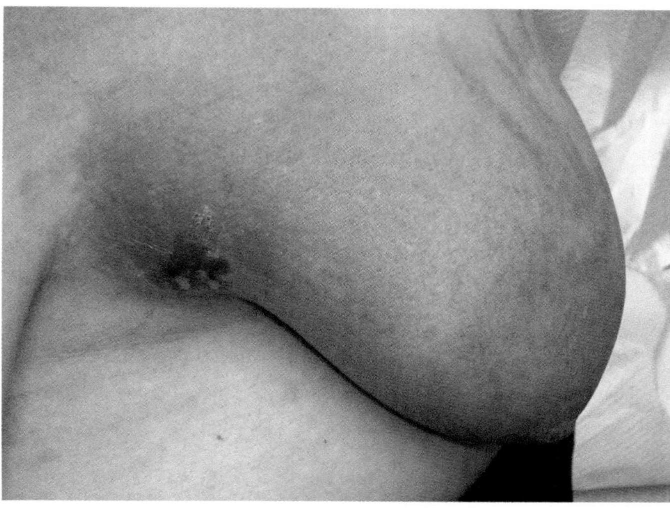

FIGURE 94-3 Breast abscess and cellulitis in a 40-year-old woman. Pus was already draining at the time of presentation, but a further incision and drainage through the openings yielded another 30 cc of pus. The patient was treated with oral antibiotics and scheduled to get a mammogram when the infection is cleared. (*Courtesy of Richard P. Usatine, MD.*)

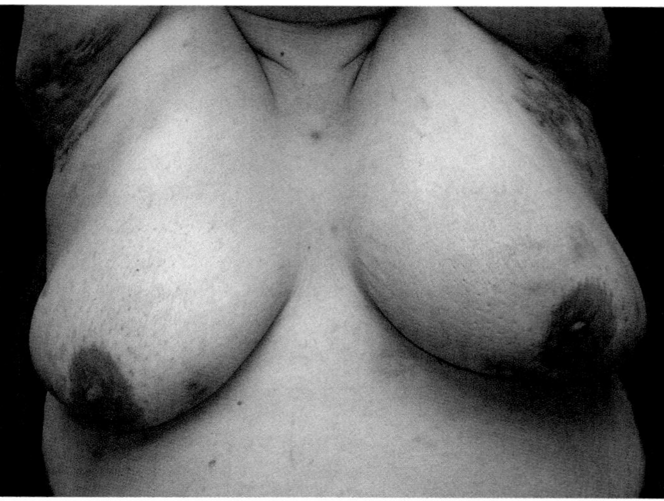

FIGURE 94-4 A breast abscess in the left breast of a 43-year-old women with hidradenitis suppurativa. Note the peau d'orange appearance of the left breast before the abscess was drained. Both breasts and axillae have multiple old scars from previous incisions to drain abscesses and hidradenitis in the past. Her axillae have active chronic disease but her acute problem is the breast abscess. (*Reproduced with permission from Richard P. Usatine, MD.*)

- Biopsy is unnecessary, but in persistent cases, a midstream milk sample may be cultured and antibiotics prescribed based upon the identification and sensitivity of the specific pathogen.

DIFFERENTIAL DIAGNOSIS

- Mastitis should be distinguished from plugged lacrimal ducts, which present as hard, locally tender, red areas without associated regional pain or fever.
- Tinea corporis can cause erythema and scaling on any part of the body including breast. It is often annular and pruritic (see Chapter 132, Tinea Corporis).

MANAGEMENT

- Management of mastitis includes supportive measures such as continued breast-feeding and bed rest. SOR Ⓒ If the infant cannot relieve breast fullness during nursing, breast massage during nursing or pumping afterward may help reduce discomfort.
- Acetaminophen or an anti-inflammatory agent such as ibuprofen may be used for pain control.
- Antibiotic treatment should be initiated with dicloxacillin or cephalexin (500 mg PO 4 times daily) for 10 to 14 days.[5] SOR Ⓐ Consider clindamycin if the patient is allergic to penicillin and/or cephalosporins.[5] Clindamycin may be a good choice if methicillin-resistant *S. aureus* (MRSA) is suspected. All of the antibiotics recommended are safe for the baby during pregnancy and lactation. Trimethoprim/sulfamethoxazole is an alternative for MRSA and/or penicillin allergic patients but it should be avoided near term pregnancy and in the first 2 months of breast-feeding because of a risk to the baby of kernicterus. Shorter courses of antibiotic therapy may be associated with higher relapse rates. SOR Ⓒ
- The management of a breast abscess consists of drainage of the abscess.[5] SOR Ⓐ Antibiotic therapy should be considered and is especially important if there is surrounding cellulitis (**Figures 94-2** and **94-3**).
- Drainage can usually be performed by needle aspiration, with the addition of ultrasound guidance if necessary.
- If needle aspiration is not effective, incision and drainage should be performed. Incision and drainage is often preferred because it allows for continued drainage through the opening. In many cases a cotton wick is placed to keep the abscess open while the purulence drains in the following days.
- Breast-feeding may continue on both breasts if the incision isn't too painful and it does not interfere with the baby latching on. Otherwise a breast pump may be used on the affected breast for 3 to 4 days until nursing can resume.

PATIENT EDUCATION

- The patient may take acetaminophen or ibuprofen for pain since these medications are safe while breast-feeding and are indicated for use in children.
- Warm compresses applied before and after feedings can provide some pain relief. A warm bath may also help.
- Instruct the patient to finish the antibiotic prescription, even if they feel better in a few days, to lower the risk of bacterial resistance or relapse.
- Continue feedings and use a breast pump to completely empty the breast if necessary.
- Educate the parents that the mastitis or the antibiotics will not harm the baby, and that the source of the infection was probably the baby's own mouth.
- Continue to drink plenty of water and eat well-balanced meals.

FOLLOW-UP

- If no response is seen within 48 hours or if MRSA is a possibility, antibiotic therapy should be switched to trimethoprim/sulfamethoxazole 1 double strength PO twice a day, or Clindamycin 300 mg orally every 6 hours. Avoid trimethoprim/sulfamethoxazole in near-term pregnancy and in the first 2 months of breast-feeding.
- Hospitalization and intravenous antibiotics are rarely needed but should be considered if the patient is systemically ill and not able to tolerate oral antibiotics.

PATIENT RESOURCES

- MedlinePlus. *Breast infection*—**http://www.nlm.nih.gov/medlineplus/ency/article/001490.htm.**
- National Health Service (Brittan) Direct Online Health Encyclopaedia—**http://www.nhsdirect.nhs.uk/articles/article.aspx?articleId=62.**

PROVIDER RESOURCES

- eMedicine. *Breast Abscess and Masses*—**http://www.emedicine.com/EMERG/topic68.htm.**
- Andolsek KM and Copeland JA. Benign breast conditions and disease: Mastitis. In: Tayor RB ed. *Family Medicine Principles and Practice.* 6th ed. New York, NY: Springer, 2003:898.

REFERENCES

1. Foxman B, D'Arcy H, Gillespie B, et al. Lactation mastitis: Occurrence and medical management among 946 breastfeeding women in the United States. *Am J Epidemiol.* 2002;155:103.
2. Kvist LJ, Rydhstroem H. Factors related to breast abscess after delivery: a population-based study. *BJOG.* 2005;112:1070.
3. Berens PD. Prenatal, intrapartum, and postpartum support of the lactating mother. *Pediatr Clin North Am.* 2001;48:365.
4. Dixon JM. ABC of breast diseases. Breast infection. *BMJ.* Oct 8 1994;309(6959):946-949.
5. Stevens DL, Bisno AL, Chambers HF, et al. Practice guidelines for the diagnosis and management of skin and soft-tissue infections. *Clin Infect Dis.* 2005;41:1373-1406.

95 BREAST CANCER

E.J. Mayeaux Jr, MD

PATIENT STORY

A 55-year-old woman presents for routine screening mammogram. The patient does not have any complaints but has a family history of breast cancer in a sister at age of 40 years. Her mammogram demonstrates an irregular mass with possible local spread (**Figures 95-1** and **95-2**). She is referred to a breast surgeon and the biopsy confirms the diagnosis of breast cancer.

INTRODUCTION

Breast cancer is a major health concern for all women. It is the most common female cancer in the United States, and the second most common cause of cancer death in women after lung cancer.[1]

EPIDEMIOLOGY

- In 2007, approximately 178,000 women in the United States were diagnosed with breast cancer.[1] Breast cancer incidence in the United States has doubled over the past 60 years. Since the early 1980s, most of the increase has been in early stage and in situ cancers because of mammogram screening (**Figures 95-1** to **95-4**).
- Approximately 232,620 new cases of invasive breast cancer were expected to be diagnosed in the United States in 2011, and 39,970 were expected to die from the disease.[1]

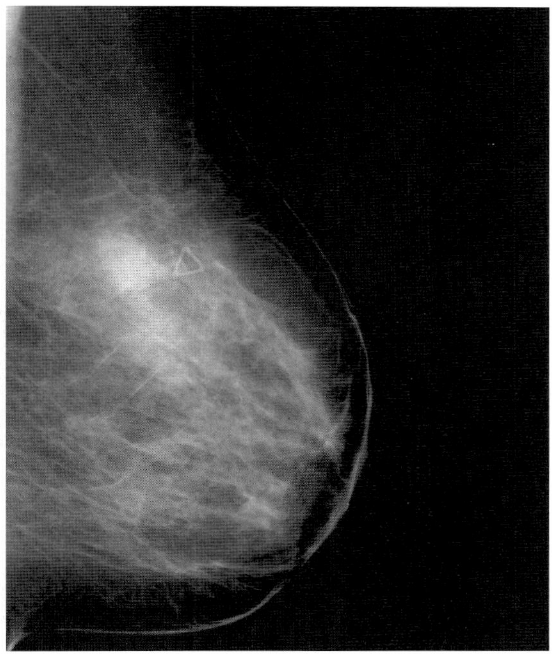

FIGURE 95-1 A mammogram that demonstrates an irregular mass with possible local spread. Biopsy confirmed this to be breast cancer. *(Reproduced with permission from John Braud, MD.)*

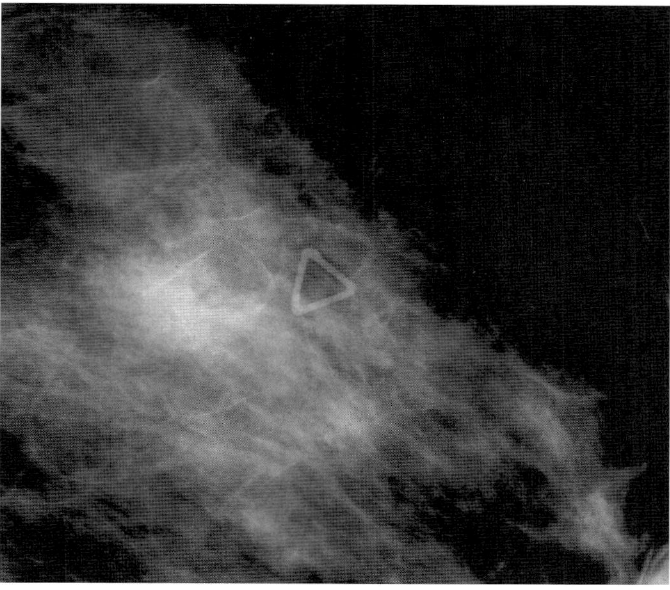

FIGURE 95-2 A close-up mammographic view of the breast cancer lesion shown in Figure 95-1. *(Reproduced with permission from John Braud, MD.)*

- Globally, breast cancer is the most common cancer and the leading cause of cancer death in females. Breast cancer incidence rates are highest in North America, Australia-New Zealand, and Europe and lowest in Asia and sub-Saharan Africa.[2]
- Locally advanced breast cancer (LABC) has been decreasing in frequency over the past several decades, at least partially as a result of

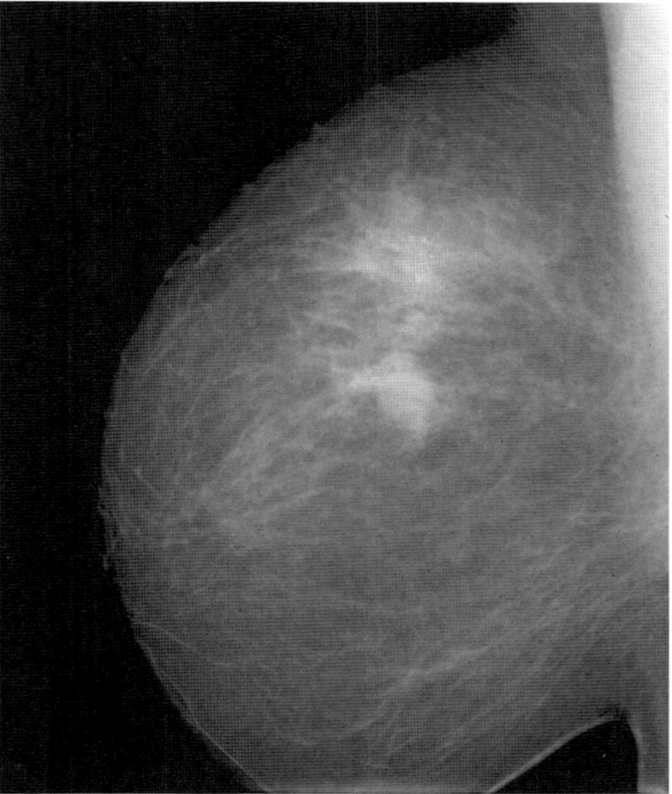

FIGURE 95-3 A screening mammogram of a 55-year-old woman who is without breast complaints. The mammogram demonstrates a significant mass with speculations. Biopsy confirmed this to be breast cancer. *(Reproduced with permission from John Braud, MD.)*

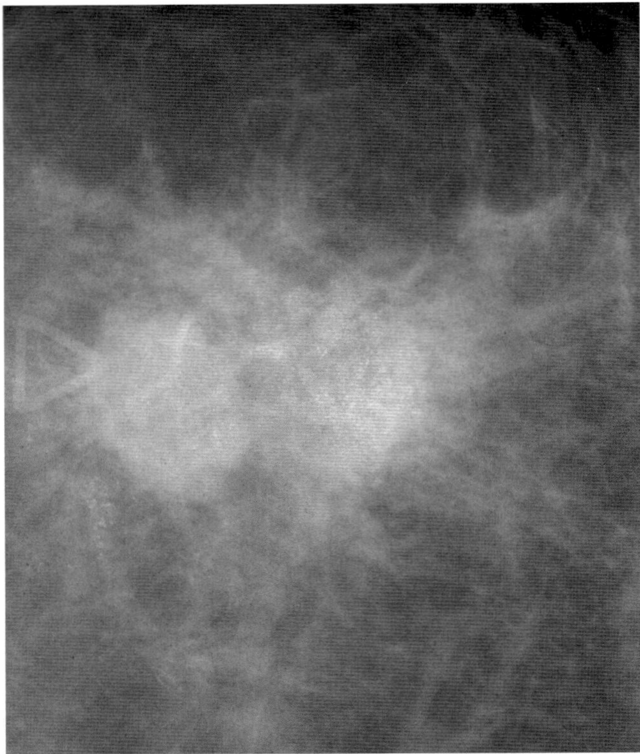

FIGURE 95-4 Close-up mammographic view of the breast cancer shown in Figure 95-3 demonstrating clear spiculations and microcalcifications. (*Reproduced with permission from John Braud, MD.*)

earlier diagnosis because of better screening (**Figures 95-5** to **95-8**). It represents 30% to 50% of newly diagnosed breast cancers in medically underserved populations.[3]

- Primary inflammatory breast cancer (IBC) is relatively rare, accounting for 0.5% to 2% invasive breast cancers.[4] However, it accounts for a greater proportion of cases presenting with more advanced disease. IBC is a clinical diagnosis. At presentation, almost all women with primary IBC have lymph node involvement and approximately one-third have distant metastases.[5]

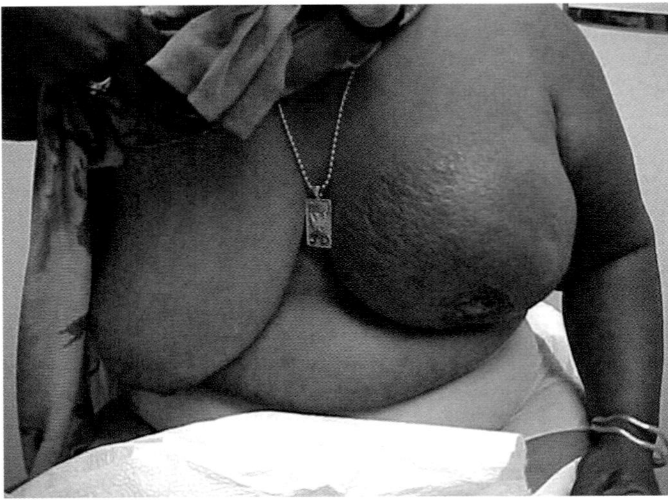

FIGURE 95-6 The woman with breast cancer in Figure 95-5 showing breast retraction and brawny edema of the breast and arm. (*Reproduced with permission from Richard P. Usatine, MD.*)

ETIOLOGY AND PATHOPHYSIOLOGY

- The incidence of breast cancer increases with age. White women are more likely to develop breast cancer than black women. One percent of breast cancers occur in men.
- Primary risk factors for the development of breast cancer include age older than 50 years, female sex, increased exposure to estrogen (including early menarche and late menopause), and a family history in a first-degree maternal relative (especially if diagnosed premenopausally).
- Approximately 8% of breast cancers are hereditary and of these one-half are associated with mutations in genes BRCA1 and BRCA2. It is more common in premenopausal women, multiple family generations, and bilateral breasts.[6] Typically, several family members are affected over at least 3 generations and can include women from the paternal side of the family.
- A history of a proliferative breast abnormality, such as atypical hyperplasia, may increase a woman's risk for developing breast cancer.

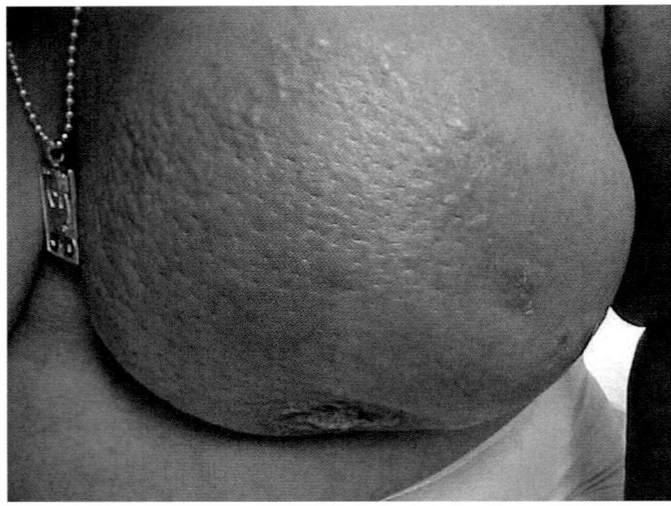

FIGURE 95-5 Woman with advanced breast cancer and peau d'orange sign. The skin looks like the skin of an orange as a consequence of lymphedema. (*Reproduced with permission from Richard P. Usatine, MD.*)

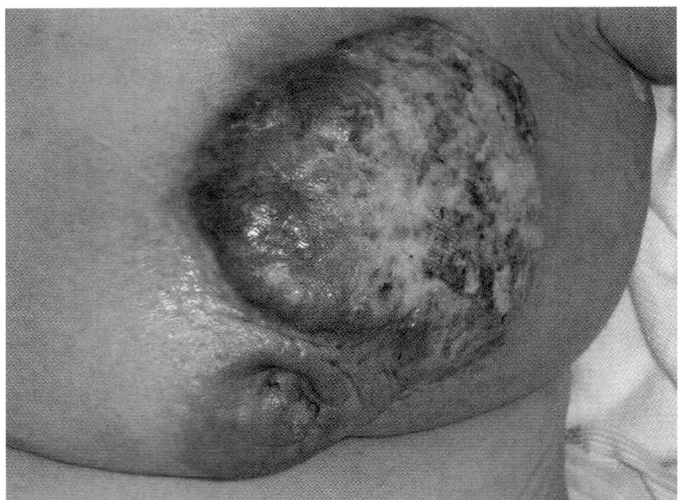

FIGURE 95-7 Advanced breast cancer with fungating mass and distortion of the normal breast anatomy. (*Reproduced with permission from Kristen Sorensen, MD.*)

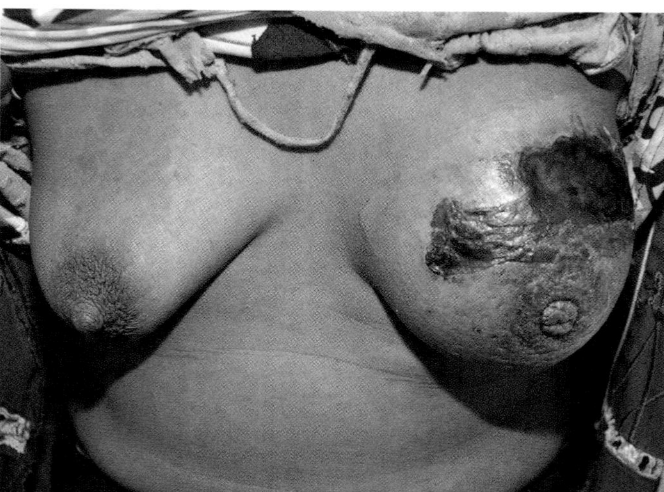

FIGURE 95-8 Ethiopian woman with breast cancer and 5 enlarged firm left axillary lymph nodes. Note the breast asymmetry and the peau d'orange skin on the left breast. The dark black area was caused by a "traditional healer" who burned the skin. Unfortunately the woman could not afford to get care at the local hospital, making her prognosis very grave. (*Reproduced with permission from Richard P. Usatine, MD.*)

- The selective estrogen receptor modulator tamoxifen (and possibly raloxifene) reduces the risk of developing breast cancer.
- The American Cancer Society, American College of Radiology, American Medical Association, and American College of Obstetrics and Gynecology all recommend starting routine screening at age 40 years.[7]
- The United States Preventive Services Task Force and the 2002 statement by the American Academy of Family Physicians recommend screening mammography every 1 to 2 years for women ages 40 years and older.[8]
- Women who have a family history of BRCA mutation should begin annual mammography between 25 and 35 years of age.[9] SOR Ⓐ
- MRI screening is more sensitive for detecting breast cancers than mammography and is being used to screen women with BRCA mutations.[10] It is not proven that surveillance regimens that include MRI will reduce mortality from breast cancer in high-risk women.[10]
- Although the sensitivity of MRI is higher than that of conventional imaging. MRI has a lower specificity. One study suggests that unnecessary biopsies can be avoided with second-look ultrasound when MRI is positive and mammography is not. Second-look ultrasound can be used to recognize false-positive MRI results and guide biopsies.[11]

RISK FACTORS

- Positive family history of breast and/or ovarian cancer (especially with BRCA mutations).
- Personal history of breast cancer.
- Increasing age in women.
- Early age at menarche and late menopause.
- Prolonged exposure to and higher concentrations of endogenous or exogenous estrogen.
- Exposure to ionizing radiation.
- Dense breast tissue and atypical hyperplasia.
- Women who have had no children or who had their first child after age 30 have a slightly higher breast cancer risk.
- Low physical activity levels.
- High-fat diet.
- Alcohol intake of 2 or more drinks daily.

DIAGNOSIS

CLINICAL FEATURES

- Detection of a breast mass is the most common presenting breast complaint. However, 90% of all breast masses are caused by benign lesions. Breast pain is also a common presenting problem. Physical examination of the breast should be performed in the upright (sitting) and supine positions. Inspect for differences in size, retraction of the skin or nipple (**Figures 95-5** and **95-6**), prominent venous patterns, and signs of inflammation (**Figures 95-5** and **95-6**). Palpate the breast tissue, axillary area, and supraclavicular areas for masses or adenopathy. Gently squeeze the nipple to check for discharge.
- Most LABCs are both palpable and visible (**Figures 95-7** and **95-8**). Careful palpation of the skin, breasts, and regional lymph nodes is the initial step in diagnosis. The patient in **Figure 95-8** had 5 palpable lymph nodes at the time of presentation.
- IBC usually presents clinically as a diffuse brawny induration of the skin of the breast with an erythematous edge, and usually without an underlying palpable mass. Patients with de novo IBC typically present with pain and a rapidly enlarging breast. The skin over the breast is warm, and thickened, with a "peau d'orange" (skin of an orange) appearance (**Figures 95-5** and **95-6**). The skin color can range from a pink flushed discoloration to a purplish hue.

TYPICAL DISTRIBUTION

A mass that is suspicious for breast cancer is usually solitary, discrete, hard, unilateral, and nontender. It may be fixed to the skin or the chest wall.

IMAGING

More than 90% of breast cancers are identified mammographically.[12] When an abnormality is found, supplemental mammographic views and possibly ultrasound are usually done. Diagnostic mammography is associated with higher sensitivity but lower specificity as compared to screening mammography.[13]

BIOPSY

Fine-needle aspiration biopsy generally uses a 20- to 23-gauge needle to obtain samples from a solid mass for cytology. Ultrasound or stereotactic guidance is used to assist in collecting a fine-needle aspiration from a nonpalpable lump. Core biopsy uses a 14-gauge or similar needle to remove cores of tissue from a mass. Excisional biopsy is done as the initial procedure or when needle biopsies are negative when the clinical suspicion is high. Guided biopsy and nonguided biopsy are also commonly used to make a definitive diagnosis.

DIFFERENTIAL DIAGNOSIS

- Fibroadenoma usually present as smooth, rounded, rubbery masses in women in their 20s and 30s. A clinically suspicious mass should be biopsied even if mammography findings are normal.

- Benign cysts are rubbery and hollow feeling in women in their 30s and 40s. A cyst can be diagnosed by ultrasound imaging. A simple cyst can be aspirated, but a residual mass requires further evaluation. Ultrasound is useful to differentiate between solid and cystic breast masses, especially in young women with dense breast tissue.
- Bilateral mastalgia is rarely associated with breast cancer, but it does not eliminate the possibility. It is usually related to fibrocystic changes in premenopausal women that are associated with diffuse lumpy breasts. A unilateral breast lump with pain must be evaluated for breast cancer.
- Nipple discharge may be from infection which is usually purulent, and from pregnancy, stimulation, or prolactinoma which produces a thin, milky, often bilateral discharge. A pregnancy test may be helpful. A suspicious discharge from a single duct can be evaluated with a ductogram.
- Infectious mastitis and breast abscess, which typically occur in lactating women, appear similar to IBC but are generally associated with fever and leukocytosis (see Chapter 92, Breast Abscess and Mastitis).
- Ductal ectasia with inflammation appears similar but is usually localized.
- Leukemic involvement of the breast may mimic IBC, but the peripheral blood smear is typically diagnostic.

MANAGEMENT

NONPHARMACOLOGIC

- Surgical resection is required in all patients with invasive breast cancer. Oncologic outcomes are similar with mastectomy and breast-conserving therapy (lumpectomy plus breast radiation therapy) in appropriately selected patients. For women undergoing mastectomy, breast reconstruction may be performed at the same time as the initial breast cancer surgery, or deferred to a later date.[14] SOR Ⓐ
- Long-term survival can be achieved in approximately 50% of women with LABC who are treated with a multimodality approach.[15] Prognostic factors include age, menopausal status, tumor stage and histologic grade, clinical response to neoadjuvant therapy, and estrogen receptor status.
- In general, women with IBC are approached similarly to those with noninflammatory LABC except that breast conservation therapy is generally considered inappropriate for these women.[16] SOR Ⓐ

MEDICATIONS

- Adjuvant systemic therapy consists of administration of hormone therapy, chemotherapy, and/or trastuzumab (a humanized monoclonal antibody directed against HER-2/neu) after definitive local therapy for breast cancer. It benefits most women with early stage breast cancer, but the magnitude of benefit is greatest for those with node-positive disease.[17] SOR Ⓐ
- The most common approach for advanced breast cancer is preoperative chemotherapy followed by surgery and radiotherapy. Questions regarding sequencing and choice of specific chemotherapy regimens and extent of surgery (including the utility of the sentinel node biopsy) persist. SOR Ⓐ
- Preoperative (as opposed to postoperative) chemotherapy has several advantages for advanced breast cancer (**Figure 95-7**) treatment. It can reduce the size of the primary tumor, thus allowing for breast-conserving surgery, permits assessing an identified mass to determine the sensitivity of the tumor cells to drugs with discontinuation of ineffective therapy (thus avoiding unnecessary toxicity), and enables drug delivery through an intact tumor vasculature.[18] SOR Ⓐ
- Tamoxifen and aromatase inhibitors may be used in selective patients as neoadjuvant hormone therapy of decrease overall tumor volume. SOR Ⓐ

REFERRAL OR HOSPITALIZATION

With the emergence of breast-conserving therapy (BCT), many women now have the option of preserving a cosmetically acceptable breast without sacrificing survival for early stage invasive breast cancer.

PREVENTION

- Healthy lifestyle choices can decrease the risk of breast cancer, including a low-fat diet, regular exercise, and no more than 1 drink daily.
- Having children before age 30 years and prolonged breast-feeding may be of help in primary prevention, but will not be a commonly used strategy for most women.
- Secondary prevention involves screening for breast cancer with physical examinations and mammography. There is a strong consensus based on consistent findings from multiple randomized trials that routine screening mammography should be offered to women ages 50 to 69 years. Consensus is less strong for routine screening among women ages 40 to 49 years, women older than age 70 years, or for how frequently to screen.
  - The American Cancer Society,[19] the National Cancer Institute,[20] the American College of Obstetricians and Gynecologists,[21] and the National Comprehensive Cancer Network[22] recommend starting routine screening at age 40 years.
  - The United States Preventive Services Task Force (USPSTF)[23] and the Canadian Task Force on the Periodic Health Examination[24] recommend beginning routine screening at age 50 years.
- Prophylactic mastectomy is an effective and accepted method by some BRCA-positive women after childbearing when their risk of lifetime breast cancer without this intervention is high (eg, over 60%).
- Chemoprevention with tamoxifen or raloxifene is an option for women who are at high risk for breast cancer.

FOLLOW-UP

Regular follow-up will usually be maintained during treatment. After treatment, life-long regular follow-up for surveillance should be maintained. Metastases can present in many ways including difficulty breathing, back pain, or a new skin nodule (**Figure 95-9**). These complaints should be taken seriously and worked up carefully in any patient with a history of breast cancer.

PATIENT EDUCATION

The contralateral breast is at increased risk of breast cancer and should be monitored. Patients on tamoxifen should be monitored for endometrial hyperplasia or cancer.

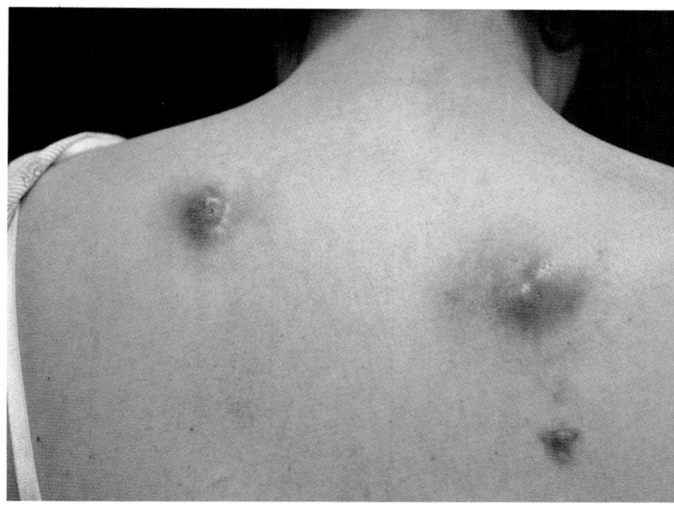

FIGURE 95-9 Metastatic breast cancer with firm palpable nodules on the back. (*Reproduced with permission from Richard P. Usatine, MD.*)

PATIENT RESOURCES

- Breast cancer support group for survivors—**http://bcsupport.org/.**
- Breastcancer.org—**http://www.breastcancer.org/.**

PROVIDER RESOURCES

- American Academy of Family Physicians. *Breast Cancer*—**http://www.aafp.org/online/en/home/clinical/exam/breastcancer.html.**
- U.S. Preventive Services Task Force. *Screening for Breast Cancer*—**http://www.uspreventiveservicestaskforce.org/uspstf/uspsbrca.htm.**
- National Cancer Institute. *Breast Cancer*—**http://www.cancer.gov/cancertopics/types/breast.**

REFERENCES

1. Siegel R, Ward E, Brawley O, Jemal A. Cancer statistics, 2011: the impact of eliminating socioeconomic and racial disparities on premature cancer deaths. *CA Cancer J Clin.* 2011;61(4):212-236.
2. Jemal A, Bray F, Center MM, et al. Global cancer statistics. *CA Cancer J Clin.* 2011;61(2):69-90.
3. Hortobagyi GN, Sinigletary SE, Strom EA. Treatment of locally advanced and inflammatory breast cancer. In: Harris JR, Lippman ME, Morrow M, Osborne CK, eds. *Diseases of the Breast*, 2nd ed. Philadelphia: Lippincott Williams & Wilkins; 2000:645-660.
4. Hance KW, Anderson WF, Devesa SS, et al. Trends in inflammatory breast carcinoma incidence and survival: The surveillance, epidemiology, and end results program at the national cancer institute. *J Natl Cancer Inst.* 2005;97(13):966-975.
5. Kleer CG, van Golen KL, Merajver SD. Molecular biology of breast cancer metastasis: inflammatory breast cancer: Clinical syndrome and molecular determinants. *Breast Cancer Res.* 2000;2(6):423-429.
6. Krainer M, Silva-Arrieta S, FitzGerald MG, et al. Differential contributions of BRCA1 and BRCA2 to early-onset breast cancer. *N Engl J Med.* 1997;336(20):1416-1421.
7. Smith RA, Saslow D, Sawyer KA, et al. American Cancer Society guidelines for breast cancer screening: update 2003. *CA Cancer J Clin.* 2003;53(3):141-169.
8. U.S. Preventive Services Task Force. *Guide to Clinical Preventive Services*, 3rd ed. http://www.ahrq.gov/clinic/uspstfix.htm. Accessed February 24, 2012.
9. Burke W, Daly M, Garber J, et al. Recommendations for follow-up care of individuals with an inherited predisposition to cancer. II. BRCA1 and BRCA2. *JAMA.* 1997;277(12):997-1003.
10. Warner E, Plewes DB, Hill KA, et al. Surveillance of BRCA1 and BRCA2 mutation carriers with magnetic resonance imaging, ultrasound, mammography, and clinical breast examination. *JAMA.* 2004;292(11):1317-1325.
11. Trecate G, Vergnaghi D, Manoukian S, et al. MRI in the early detection of breast cancer in women with high genetic risk. *Tumori.* 2006;92(6):517-523.
12. Smart CR, Hartmann WH, Beahrs OH, Garfinkel L. Insights into breast cancer screening of younger women. Evidence from the 14-year follow-up of the Breast Cancer Detection Demonstration Project. *Cancer.* 1995;72(4 Suppl):1449-1456.
13. Barlow WE, Lehman CD, Zheng Y, et al. Performance of diagnostic mammography for women with signs or symptoms of breast cancer. *J Natl Cancer Inst.* 2002;94(15):1151-1159.
14. Vandeweyer E, Hertens D, Nogaret JM, Deraemaecker R. Immediate breast reconstruction with saline-filled implants: No interference with the oncologic outcome? *Plast Reconstr Surg.* 2001;107(6):1409-1412.
15. Brito RA, Valero V, Buzdar AU, et al. Long-term results of combined-modality therapy for locally advanced breast cancer with ipsilateral supraclavicular metastases: The University of Texas M.D. Anderson Cancer Center experience. *J Clin Oncol.* 2001;19(3):628-633.
16. Lyman GH, Giuliano AE, Somerfield MR, et al. American Society of Clinical Oncology. American Society of Clinical Oncology guideline recommendations for sentinel lymph node biopsy in early-stage breast cancer. *J Clin Oncol.* 2005;23(30):7703-7720.
17. Goldhirsch A, Glick JH, Gelber RD, et al. Meeting highlights: international expert consensus on the primary therapy of early breast cancer 2005. *Ann Oncol.* 2005;16(10):1569-1583.
18. Fisher B, Gunduz N, Saffer EA. Influence of the interval between primary tumor removal and chemotherapy on kinetics and growth of metastases. *Cancer Res.* 1983;43(4):1488-1492.
19. Smith RA, Cokkinides V, Brawley OW. Cancer screening in the United States, 2009: a review of current American Cancer Society guidelines and issues in cancer screening. *CA Cancer J Clin.* 2009;59(1):27-41.
20. National Cancer Institute. *Breast Cancer Screening (PDQ).* http://www.cancer.gov/cancertopics/pdq/screening/breast/HealthProfessional/page2. Accessed February 24, 2012.
21. American College of Obstetricians-Gynecologists. Practice bulletin no. 122: breast cancer screening. *Obstet Gynecol.* 2011;118(2 Pt 1):372-382.

22. Bevers TB, Anderson BO, Bonaccio E, et al. National Comprehensive Cancer Network. NCCN clinical practice guidelines in oncology: breast cancer screening and diagnosis. *J Natl Compr Canc Netw.* 2009;7(10):1060-1096.
23. US Preventive Services Task Force. Screening for breast cancer: U.S. Preventive Services Task Force recommendation statement. *Ann Intern Med.* 2009;151(10):716-726, W-236.
24. Canadian Task Force on the Periodic Health Examination. *Screening for Breast Cancer*. http://www.canadiantaskforce.ca/recommendations/2011_01_eng.html. Accessed February 24, 2012.

96 PAGET DISEASE OF THE BREAST

E.J. Mayeaux, Jr., MD

PATIENT STORY

A 62-year-old woman presents with a 6-month history of an eczematous, scaly, rash near her nipple. It is mildly pruritic. On physical examination, the nipple and the areola are involved (**Figure 96-1**). Also, a hard mass is present in the lateral lower quadrant of the same breast. A 4-mm punch biopsy of the affected area including the nipple demonstrates Paget disease. The mammogram is suspicious for breast cancer at the site of the mass and the patient is referred to a breast surgeon.

INTRODUCTION

Paget disease of the breast is a low-grade malignancy of the breast that is often associated with other malignancies. It is an important consideration when working up a chronic persistent abnormality of the nipple.

SYNONYMS

Paget's disease, Mammary Paget disease.

EPIDEMIOLOGY

- The incidence of Paget disease of the breast is approximately 0.6% in women in the United States, according to National Cancer Institute Surveillance, Epidemiology, and End Results (SEER) data.[1] Paget disease, like all breast cancers, is rare in men.
- The peak incidence is between 50 and 60 years of age.[2]
- It is associated with underlying in situ and/or invasive breast cancer 85% to 88% of the time.[3]

ETIOLOGY AND PATHOPHYSIOLOGY

- Most patients delay presentation, assuming the abnormality is a benign condition of some sort. The median duration of signs and symptoms prior to diagnosis is 6 to 8 months.[2]
- Presenting symptoms are sometimes limited to persistent pain, burning, and/or pruritus of the nipple (**Figures 96-1** and **96-2).**
- A palpable breast mass is present in 50% of cases, but is often located more than 2 cm from the nipple–areolar complex.[4]
- Twenty percent of cases will have a mammographic abnormality without a palpable mass, and 25% of cases will have neither a mass nor abnormal mammogram, but will have an occult ductal carcinoma.
- In less than 5% of cases, Paget disease of the breast is an isolated finding.[4]
- There are 2 theories regarding the pathogenesis of Paget disease of the breast, the choice of which affects treatment choices.
  - The more widely accepted epidermotropic theory proposes that the Paget cells arise from an underlying mammary adenocarcinoma that migrates through the ductal system of the breast to the skin of the nipple. It is supported by the fact that Paget disease is usually associated with an underlying ductal carcinoma, and both Paget cells and mammary ductal cells usually express similar immunochemical staining patterns and molecular markers. This could mean that there is a common genetic alteration and/or a common progenitor cell for both Paget cells and the underlying ductal carcinoma.
  - The less widely accepted transformation theory proposes that epidermal cells in the nipple transform into malignant Paget cells, and that Paget disease of the breast represents an independent epidermal carcinoma in situ. It is supported by the fact that there is no parenchymal cancer identified in a small percentage of cases, and underlying breast carcinomas are often located at some distance to the nipple. Most pathologists disagree with the transformation theory.

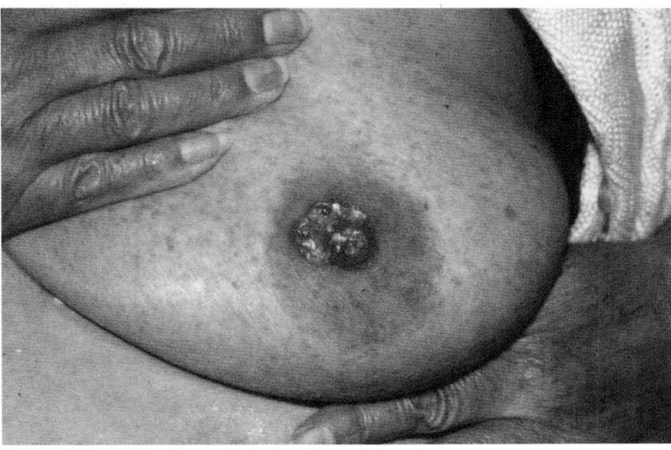

FIGURE 96-1 Paget disease of the breast of a 62-year-old woman that presented as a persistent eczematous lesion. (*Reproduced with permission from the University of Texas Health Sciences Center, Division of Dermatology.*)

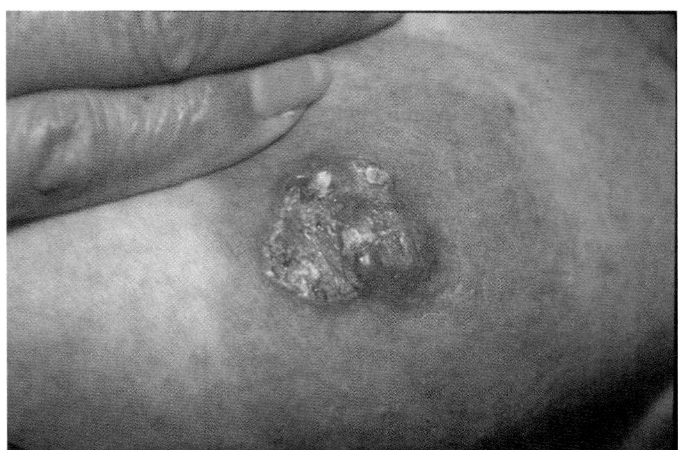

FIGURE 96-2 Close-up of Paget disease of the breast. Note the erythematous, eczematous, scaly appearance of the lesion. (*Reproduced with permission from the University of Texas Health Sciences Center, Division of Dermatology.*)

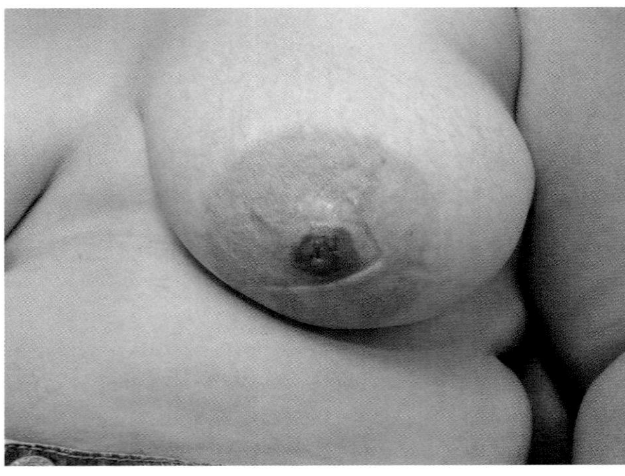

FIGURE 96-3 Paget disease of the breast in a 29-year-old woman that presented as a persistent eczematous lesion for 8 months prior to biopsy. The patient did not have a palpable breast mass. (*Reproduced with permission from Richard P. Usatine, MD.*)

DIAGNOSIS

CLINICAL FEATURES

- Paget disease of the breast presents clinically in the nipple–areolar complex as a dermatitis that may be erythematous, eczematous, scaly, raw, vesicular, or ulcerated (**Figures 96-1** to **96-4**). The nipple is usually initially involved, and the lesion then spreads to the areola. Spontaneous improvement or healing of the nipple dermatitis can occur and should not be taken as an indication that Paget disease is not present. The diagnosis is made by finding malignant, intraepithelial adenocarcinoma cells on pathology. Rarely, nipple retraction is found.
- Pain, burning, and/or pruritus may be present or even precede clinically apparent disease develops on the skin.

TYPICAL DISTRIBUTION

- Paget disease of the breast is almost always unilateral, although bilateral cases have been reported.
- Work-up must also be directed toward identifying any underlying breast cancer.

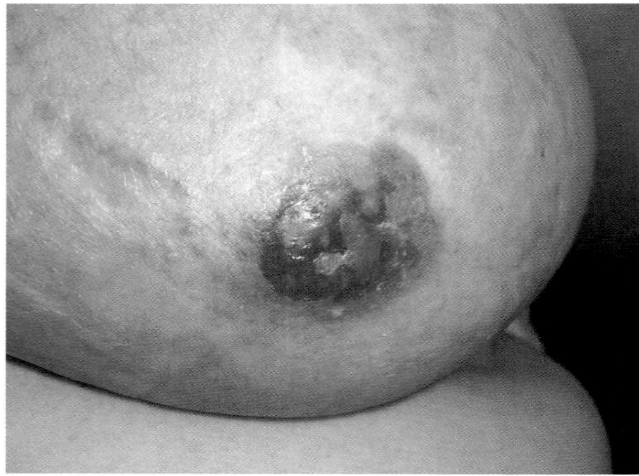

FIGURE 96-4 Close-up of Paget disease of the breast in the young woman in Figure 96-3. Note the erythematous, scaly, and ulcerated appearance of the lesion. (*Reproduced with permission from Richard P. Usatine, MD.*)

LABORATORY TESTING

The diagnosis is made by finding intraepithelial adenocarcinoma cells (Paget cells) either singly or in small groups within the epidermis of the nipple complex.

IMAGING

- Bilateral mammography is mandatory to asses for associated cancers. MRI may disclose occult cancer in some women with Paget disease of the breast and normal mammography and/or physical examination.[5]
- Polarized dermoscopy may also be useful in diagnosis, especially in cases of pigmented mammary Paget disease.[6]

BIOPSY

The diagnosis is usually made by full-thickness punch or wedge biopsy that shows Paget cells. Nipple scrape cytology can diagnose Paget disease and may be considered for screening eczematous lesion of the nipple.

DIFFERENTIAL DIAGNOSIS

- Eczema of the areola is the most common cause of scaling of the breast (**Figure 96-5**). If the patient (**Figure 96-5**) had new nipple inversion with the onset of skin changes, this would be more suspicious for Paget disease.
- Bowen disease is squamous cell carcinoma in situ and can differentiate from Paget disease by histology. Also, Bowen disease expresses high-molecular-weight keratins, whereas Paget disease expresses low-molecular-weight keratins (see Chapter 166, Actinic Keratosis and Bowen Disease and Chapter 169, Squamous Cell Carcinoma).
- Superficial spreading malignant melanoma may be confused with Paget disease but histologic study and immunohistochemical staining can separate the 2 (**Figure 96-6**) (see Chapter 170, Melanoma).

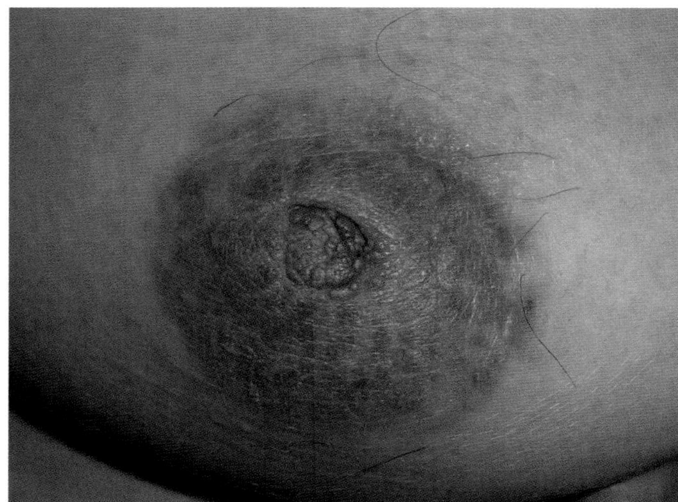

FIGURE 96-5 Eczema of the areola in a 43-year-old woman who has had an inverted nipple her whole adult life. She remembers having difficulty breastfeeding her children. The current eczema has been present on the areola on and off for more than 10 years and always responds to topical corticosteroids. Breast examination and mammography are negative. (*Reproduced with permission from Richard P. Usatine, MD.*)

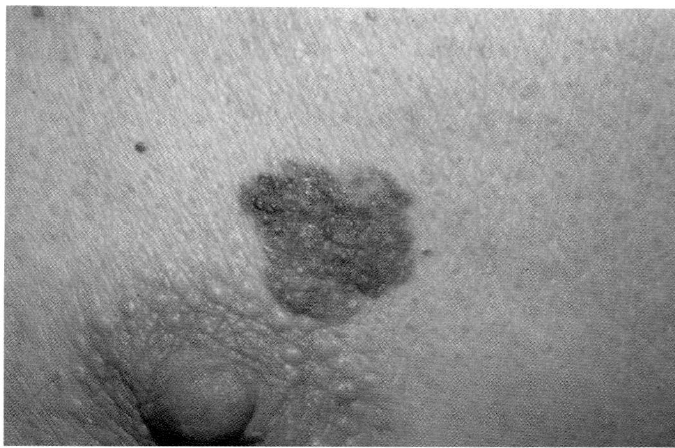

FIGURE 96-6 Superficial spreading melanoma adjacent to the areola. (*Reproduced with permission from the University of Texas Health Sciences Center, Division of Dermatology.*)

- Seborrheic keratoses and benign lichenoid keratoses can occur on and around the areola and be suspicious for Paget disease (**Figure 96-7**). A biopsy is the best way to make the diagnosis (see Chapter 156, Seborrheic Keratosis).
- Nipple adenoma, which usually presents as an isolated mass with redness, can be diagnosed with biopsy.

MANAGEMENT

SURGICAL

The treatment and prognosis of Paget disease of the breast is first based on the stage of any underlying breast cancer. Simple mastectomy has traditionally been the standard treatment for isolated Paget disease of the breast, but breast-conserving treatment is being used more often. Breast-conserving surgery combined with breast irradiation is gaining wider acceptance. The surgically conservative approaches include excision of the complete nipple–areolar complex with margin evaluation. Sentinel lymph node biopsy should be performed to evaluate axillary lymph node status.[7] SOR Ⓑ

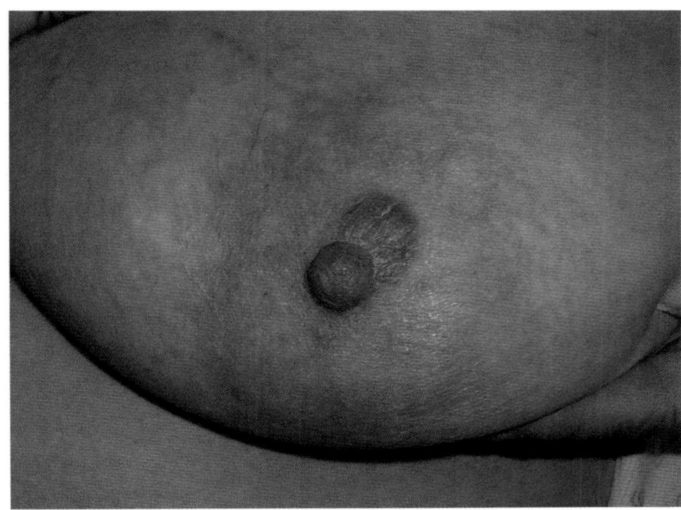

FIGURE 96-7 Benign lichenoid keratosis on the areola proven by biopsy. (*Reproduced with permission from Richard P. Usatine, MD.*)

PROGNOSIS

Patients with only noninvasive Paget disease of the nipple have excellent cancer outcome with conservative surgery, with survival rates similar to those achieved with mastectomy.[8,9] SOR Ⓑ The prognosis of Paget disease with synchronous cancer is dependent upon the tumor stage of the underlying cancer.

PATIENT EDUCATION

- All lesions of the breast that do not heal should be checked for cancer.
- The patient's prognosis is based on the underlying cancer, if present, not the Paget disease itself.

PATIENT RESOURCES

- Breastcancer.org. *Paget Disease of the Nipple*—**www.breastcancer.org/symptoms/types/pagets/.**
- Imaginis. *Paget Disease of the Nipple*—**http://imaginis.com/breasthealth/pagets_disease.asp.**
- Macmillan Cancer Support. *Paget Disease of the Breast*—**http://www.macmillan.org.uk/Cancerinformation/Cancertypes/Breast/Aboutbreastcancer/Typesandrelatedconditions/Pagetsdisease.aspx.**

PROVIDER RESOURCES

- Medscape. *Mammary Paget Disease*—**http://emedicine.medscape.com/article/1101235-overview.**
- National Cancer Institute. *Paget Disease of the Nipple*—**http://www.cancer.gov/cancertopics/factsheet/Sites-Types/pagets-breast.**

REFERENCES

1. SEER Brest Cancer. *Cancer Statistics Review 1975-2008. Table 4.1. Cancer of the Female Breast (Invasive)*. http://seer.cancer.gov/csr/1975_2008/results_merged/sect_04_breast.pdf. Accessed January 7, 2012.
2. Chaudary MA, Millis RR, Lane EB, Miller NA. Paget's disease of the nipple: a ten year review including clinical, pathological, and immunohistochemical findings. *Breast Cancer Res Treat*. 1986;8(2):139-146.
3. Chen CY, Sun LM, Anderson BO. Paget disease of the breast: changing patterns of incidence, clinical presentation, and treatment in the U.S. *Cancer*. 2006;107(7):1448-1458.
4. Ashikari R, Park K, Huvos AG, Urban JA. Paget's disease of the breast. *Cancer*. 1970;26(3):680-685.
5. Morrogh M, Morris EA, Liberman L, et al. MRI identifies otherwise occult disease in select patients with Paget disease of the nipple. *J Am Coll Surg*. 2008;206(2):316-321.

6. Crignis GS, Abreu Ld, Buçard AM, Barcaui CB. Polarized dermoscopy of mammary Paget disease. *An Bras Dermatol.* 2013;88(2): 290-292.
7. Caliskan M, Gatti G, Sosnovskikh I, et al. Paget's disease of the breast: the experience of the European institute of oncology and review of the literature. *Breast Cancer Res Treat.* 2008;112(3):513-521. http://www.springerlink.com/content/6270v27346461v08/. Accessed February 25, 2008.
8. Marshall JK, Griffith KA, Haffty BG, et al. Conservative management of Paget disease of the breast with radiotherapy: 10- and 15-year results. *Cancer.* 2003;97(9):2142-2149.
9. Pezzi CM, Kukora JS, Audet IM, et al. Breast conservation surgery using nipple-areolar resection for central breast cancers. *Arch Surg.* 2004;139(1):32-37.

PART 13

MUSCULOSKELETAL/ RHEUMATOLOGIC

Strength of Recommendation (SOR)	Definition
A	Recommendation based on consistent and good-quality patient-oriented evidence.*
B	Recommendation based on inconsistent or limited-quality patient-oriented evidence.*
C	Recommendation based on consensus, usual practice, opinion, disease-oriented evidence, or case series for studies of diagnosis, treatment, prevention, or screening.*

*See Appendix A on pages 1241-1244 for further information.

97 ARTHRITIS OVERVIEW

Heidi Chumley, MD
Richard P. Usatine, MD

PATIENT STORY

A 50-year-old woman presents with new complaint of pain in several fingers. She has had psoriasis for many years; however, she only developed joint pain last year. Her examination is significant for swelling and tenderness at the distal interphalangeal (DIP) joints of her second, third, and fourth fingers (**Figure 97-1, A**). She had an elevated erythrocyte sedimentation rate (ESR) and radiographs with erosive changes (**Figure 97-1, B**). Choices for therapy include methotrexate and the new biologic anti-tumor necrosis factor (TNF)-α medications.

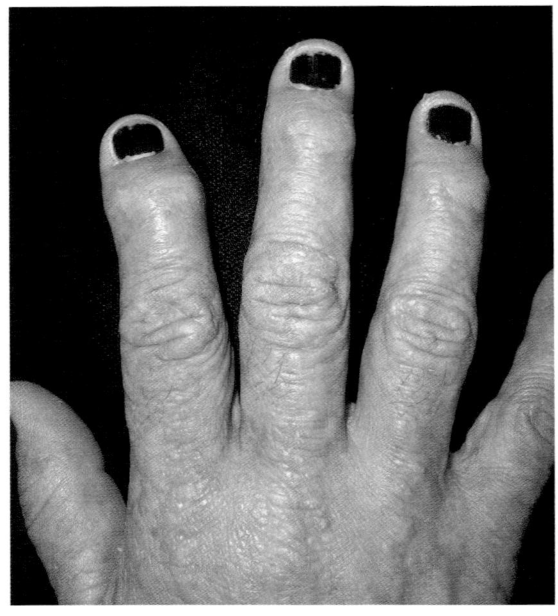

A

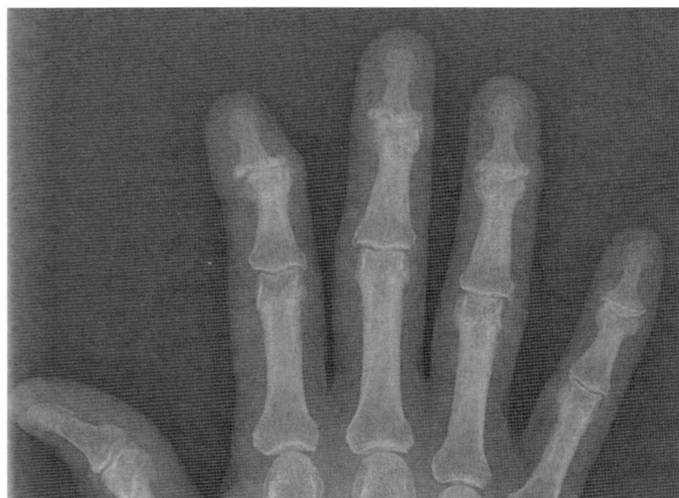

A

FIGURE 97-1 Psoriatic arthritis at initial presentation in a 50-year-old woman with psoriasis and new-onset hand pain. **A.** Note the prominent involvement of the distal interphalangeal joints. **B.** Radiography showing early psoriatic arthritis changes with periarticular erosions seen at the distal interphalangeal joints. (*Reproduced with permission from Richard P. Usatine, MD.*)

INTRODUCTION

Arthritis means inflammation of the joints; however, the term is used for any disease or condition that affects joints or the tissues around the joints. Joint pain can be classified as monoarticular or polyarticular and inflammatory or noninflammatory. Diagnosis is based on a combination of clinical presentation, synovial fluid analysis, other laboratory tests, and radiographic findings. Management goals include minimizing joint damage, controlling pain, maximizing function, and improving quality of life.

EPIDEMIOLOGY

- Fifty million adults in the United States (22%) report doctor-diagnosed arthritis.[1]
- Arthritis is the most common cause of disability in the United States. Twenty-one million adults have functional limitations because of arthritis.[1]
- Fifty percent of adults age 65 years or older have been diagnosed with arthritis.[1]
- In 2003, the total cost attributable to arthritic conditions was $128 billion.[2]

ETIOLOGY AND PATHOPHYSIOLOGY

Arthritis can be caused by 1 of several mechanisms.

- Noninflammatory arthritis (ie, osteoarthritis) is caused by bony overgrowth (osteophytes) and degeneration of cartilage and underlying bone (**Figures 97-2** and **97-3**).
- Autoimmune arthritis (ie, rheumatoid arthritis, systemic lupus erythematosus [SLE], psoriatic arthritis) is caused by an inappropriate immune response.
- Crystalline arthritis (ie, gout, calcium pyrophosphate dehydrate deposition disease) is caused by deposition of uric acid crystals (gout) or calcium pyrophosphate dehydrate crystals (CPPD) resulting in episodic flares with periods of remission.
- Septic arthritis is most commonly caused by bacteria (*Neisseria gonorrhoeae*, *Staphylococcus*, or *Streptococcus*; also gram-negative bacilli in immunocompromised patients and *Salmonella* in patients with sickle cell disease). Several viral illnesses may also have an associated arthritis.
- Postinfectious (reactive) arthritis is caused by an immune reaction several weeks after a urethritis or enteric infection.
- Fibromyalgia has an unknown etiology but includes abnormal pain perception processing.

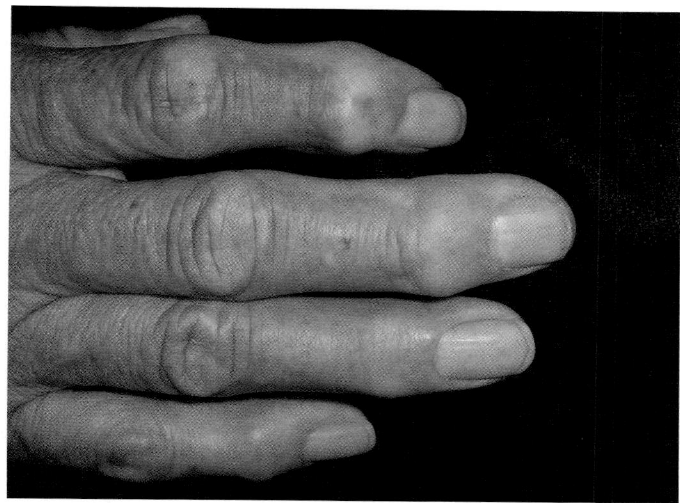

FIGURE 97-2 Osteoarthritis in an elderly woman with Heberden nodes at the distal interphalangeal joints. There is some swelling beginning at the proximal interphalangeal joints creating Bouchard nodes. (*Reproduced with permission from Richard P. Usatine, MD.*)

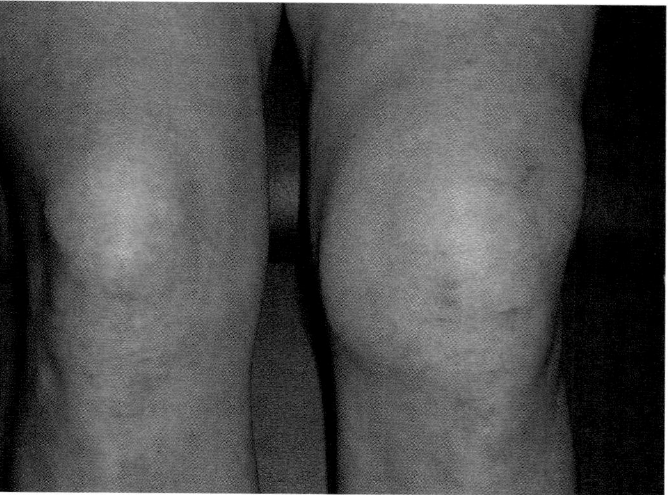

FIGURE 97-4 Osteoarthritis with visible unilateral knee effusion. The effusion was tapped and the synovial fluid was consistent with osteoarthritis. An intraarticular steroid injection was given and provided great relief to the pain and stiffness. (*Reproduced with permission from Richard P. Usatine, MD.*)

DIAGNOSIS

CLINICAL FEATURES

- Two features help limit the differential diagnosis: mono- or polyarticular and inflammatory or noninflammatory.
  - Monoarticular noninflammatory—Osteoarthritis, trauma, avascular necrosis
  - Monoarticular inflammatory—Infectious (gonococcal, nongonococcal, Lyme disease) or crystalline (gout or CPPD)
  - Polyarticular noninflammatory—Osteoarthritis
  - Polyarticular inflammatory—Rheumatologic (rheumatoid arthritis [RA], SLE, psoriatic, ankylosing spondylitis [AS], and others) or infectious (bacterial, viral, postinfectious) or crystalline later in the disease

TYPICAL DISTRIBUTION

- Most commonly affected joints
  - Osteoarthritis (see Chapter 98, Osteoarthritis)—Knees, hips, hands (DIP and proximal interphalangeal [PIP]), and spine (**Figures 97-2** to **97-4**).

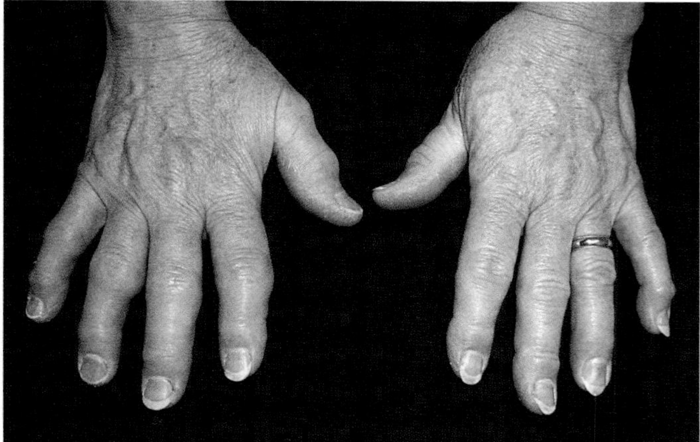

FIGURE 97-3 Osteoarthritis with visible Heberden (DIP) and Bouchard (PIP) nodes. (*Reproduced with permission from Ricardo Zuniga-Montes, MD.*)

  - RA (see Chapter 99, Rheumatoid Arthritis)—Wrists, metacarpophalangeal (MCP), PIP, metatarsophalangeal (MTP) early in the disease with larger joints affected later in the disease (**Figures 97-5** and **97-6**). Rheumatoid nodules may be found over the fingers, hands, wrists, or elbows (**Figures 97-6** and **97-7**).
  - SLE—Hands, wrists, and knees (see Chapter 178, Lupus: Systemic and Cutaneous) (**Figure 97-8**).
  - AS—Lower back and hips, costosternal junctions, shoulders (see Chapter 101, Ankylosing Spondylitis).
  - Psoriatic arthritis—Hands, feet, knees, spine, sacroiliac; typically with a personal or family history or psoriasis (**Figures 97-9** to **97-11**); (see Chapter 100, Psoriatic arthritis).
  - Gonococcal—Migratory with a single joint affected, such as knee, wrist, ankle, hand, or foot.
  - Lyme disease—Knee and/or other large joints.

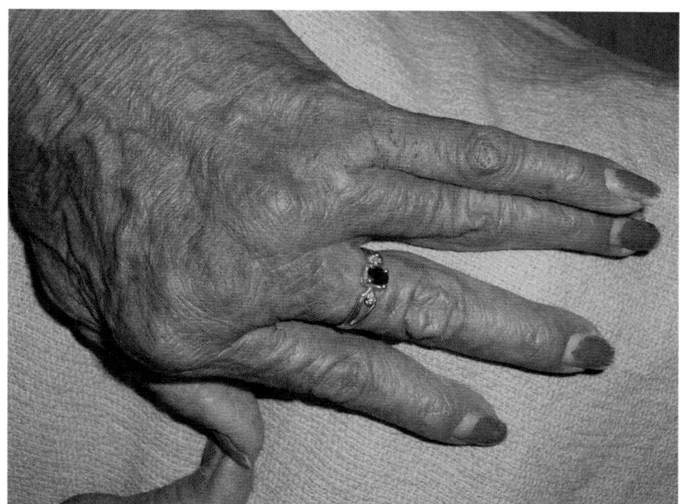

FIGURE 97-5 Rheumatoid arthritis showing typical ulnar deviation at the metacarpophalangeal joints. (*Reproduced with permission from Richard P. Usatine, MD.*)

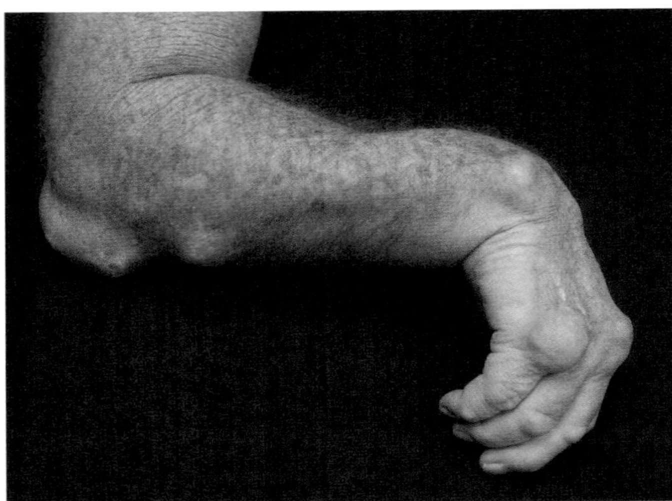

FIGURE 97-6 Rheumatoid arthritis involving the whole upper-extremity joints with nodules on the elbow, wrist, and hand joints. (*Reproduced with permission from Ricardo Zuniga-Montes, MD.*)

- Gout (see Chapter 105, Gout)—Begins as monoarticular with MTP joint of the first toe; hands, ankles, tarsal joints, and knee may also be affected (**Figures 97-12** to **97-14**); gout may be present with tophi over any joint; olecranon bursitis can also be the result of gout (**Figure 97-15**).
- CPPD—Knee, but also seen in shoulder, elbow, wrist, hands, and ankle joints; most patients have polyarticular disease.
- Septic arthritis can involve any joint; acute onset of pain, swelling, and joint immobility; fever may be present; must be recognized and treated immediately as joint destruction occurs within days (**Figure 97-16**).

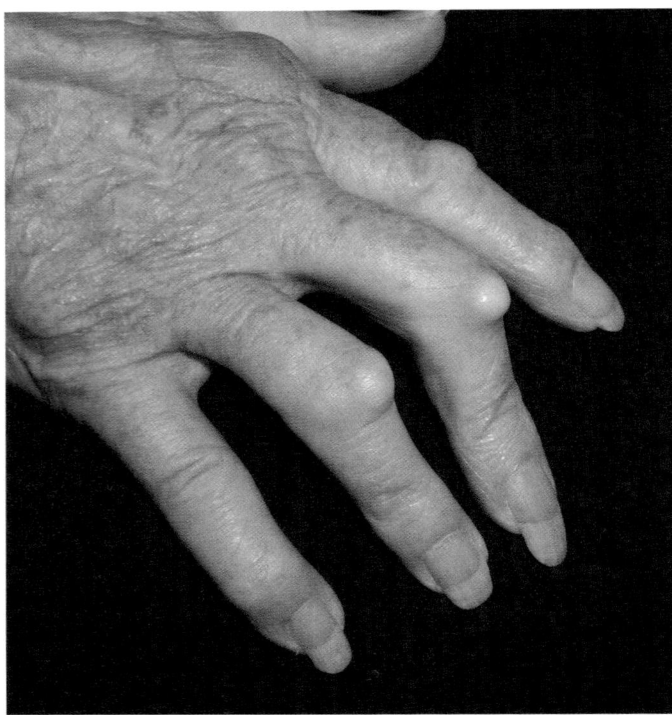

FIGURE 97-7 Rheumatoid arthritis with rheumatoid nodules over the PCP joints along with deformities of the digits. (*Reproduced with permission from Ricardo Zuniga-Montes, MD.*)

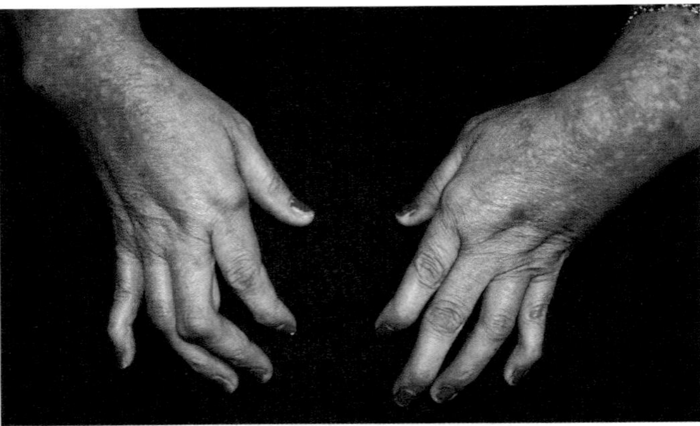

FIGURE 97-8 Long-standing lupus erythematosus has caused swan-neck deformities without bone erosions. This is called Jaccoud arthropathy and is caused by synovitis and inïammatory capsular fibrosis. (*Reproduced with permission from Everett Allen, MD.*)

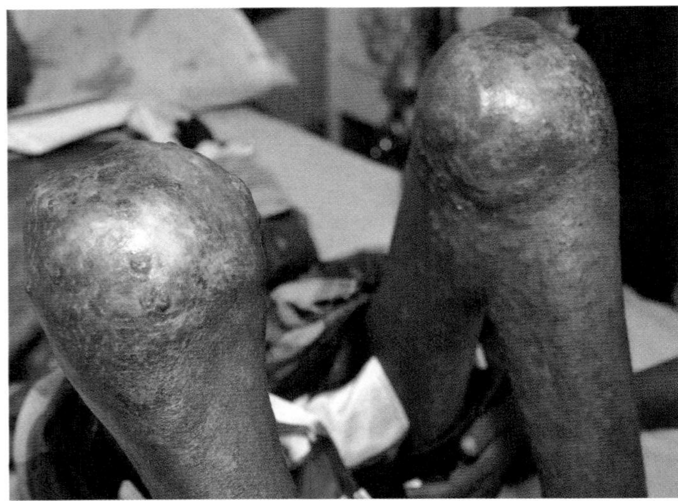

FIGURE 97-9 Psoriatic arthritis of both knees. This patient has asymmetric psoriatic arthritis in his hands. (*Reproduced with permission from Richard P. Usatine, MD.*)

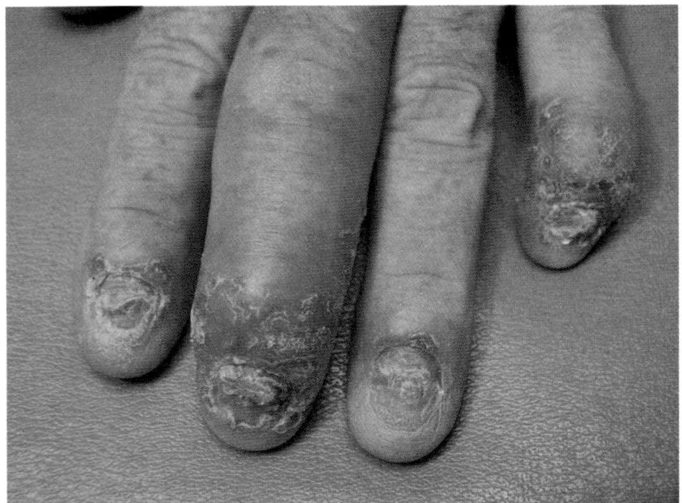

FIGURE 97-10 Psoriatic arthritis with dactylitis and significant distal interphalangeal joint involvement. Note the destruction of the nails. Almost all patients with psoriatic arthritis have nail involvement. (*Reproduced with permission from Ricardo Zuniga-Montes, MD.*)

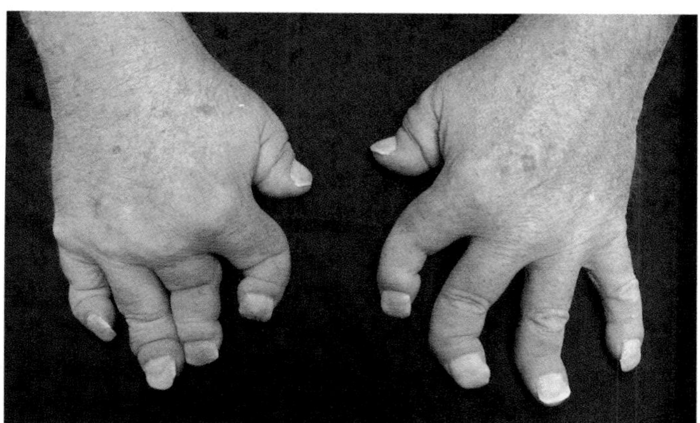

FIGURE 97-11 Psoriatic arthritis mutilans with severe destruction of the fingers. (*Reproduced with permission from Ricardo Zuniga-Montes, MD.*)

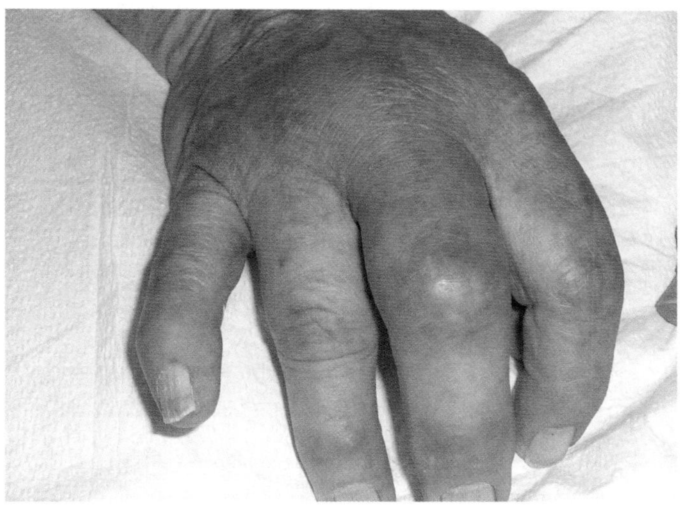

FIGURE 97-12 An acute gouty arthritis attack of multiple finger joints in a 75-year-old man with gout. His joints have been painful for 3 weeks. The erythema of the acute inflammation is evident. (*Reproduced with permission from R. Treadwell, MD.*)

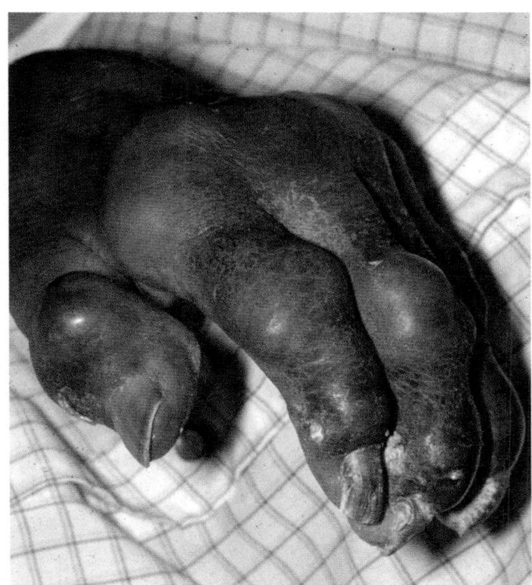

FIGURE 97-13 Severe tophaceous gout with chronic gouty arthritis causing hand deformities and disabilities. (*Reproduced with permission from Jack Resneck, Sr., MD.*)

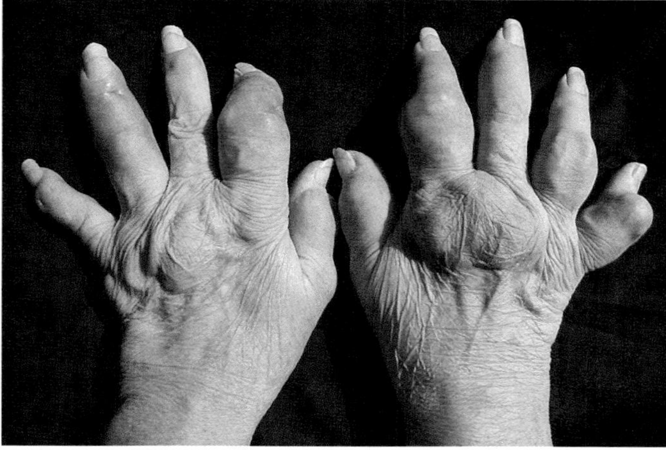

FIGURE 97-14 Severe tophaceous gout with large tophi and joint destruction of the hands. (*Reproduced with permission from Ricardo Zuniga-Montes, MD.*)

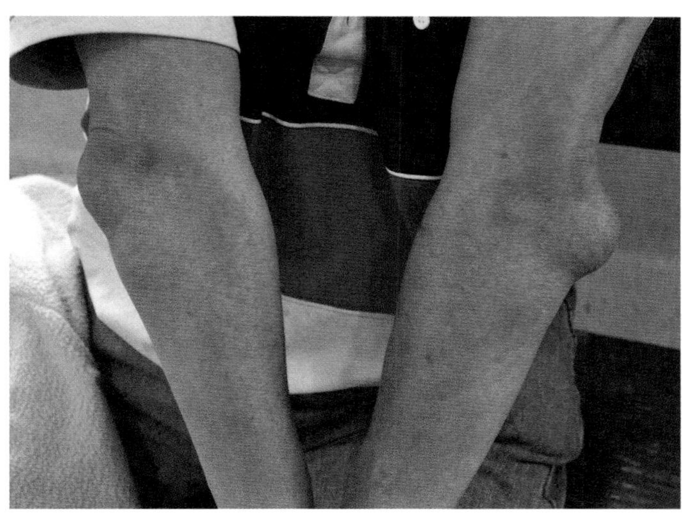

FIGURE 97-15 Olecranon bursitis bilaterally in a man with gout. (*Reproduced with permission from Richard P. Usatine, MD.*)

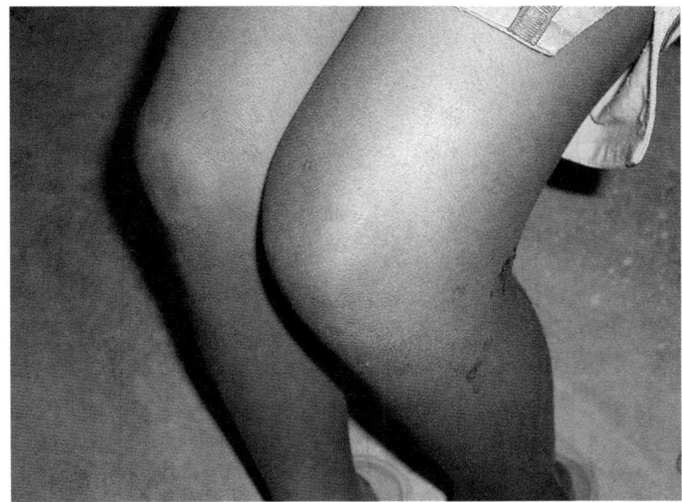

FIGURE 97-16 Septic left knee joint in a girl who presented with knee pain, fever, and limited ability to ambulate. (*Reproduced with permission from Richard P. Usatine, MD.*)

LABORATORY TESTING

- Not indicated for noninflammatory arthritis.
- Inflammatory polyarthritis: Use laboratory tests to supplement the clinical impression. Initial tests to consider include the following:
  - ESR or C-reactive protein as a nonspecific measure of inflammation.
  - Rheumatoid factor or anti-CCP (anti-cyclic citrullinated peptide) antibody when RA is expected. Anti-CCP antibody is more sensitive and specific than rheumatoid factor.
  - Antinuclear antibody (ANA), anti–double-stranded DNA (dsDNA) and anti-Ro when SLE is expected.
  - Human leukocyte antigen (HLA)-B27 when AS is expected.
  - Serum uric acid can be used, especially to follow hypouricemic therapy in patients with gout; levels can be normal or low during an attack.
- Joint aspiration:
  - Synovial fluid analysis is critical when septic or crystalline arthritis are suspected.
  - Assess for clarity/color, cell count, crystals, and culture. Gram stain may give quick information, but a culture should also be done. If there is clinical suspicion for septic arthritis, empiric antibiotics should be started even if the Gram stain is negative.
  - White blood cell (WBC)—Normal <200 cells/μL; noninflammatory arthritis <2000 cells/μL; inflammatory, crystalline, or septic arthritis >2000 cells/μL, often 30,000 to 50,000 cells/μL.
  - Crystals—Monosodium urate (gout) are needle shaped and negatively birefringent; CPPD are rhomboid-shaped positively birefringent.
  - Culture—Gonococcal arthritis synovial fluid cultures can be negative in two-thirds of cases (synovial biopsy is positive); tuberculosis, fungal, and anaerobic infections may also be difficult to identify on culture.

IMAGING

- Osteoarthritis—Osteophytes, sclerosis, narrowed joint space (**Figure 97-17**).
- Rheumatoid arthritis—Soft-tissue swelling, erosions, and loss of joint space; severe destruction and subluxation in advanced disease. MRI changes may appear first and include synovitis, effusions, and bone marrow changes.
- SLE—Soft-tissue swelling; erosions are rare and joint deformities are uncommon.
- AS—Symmetric sacroiliitis, erosions, sclerosis; active sacroiliitis is best seen on MRI.
- Psoriatic arthritis—Erosions with adjacent proliferation, "pencil-in-cup" deformity, osteolysis, digit telescoping, asymmetric sacroiliitis.
- Gout—Only soft-tissue swelling until advanced disease when erosions with sclerotic margins may be present.
- CPPD—Can mimic other types of arthritis; chondrocalcinosis, linear, or punctate radiodense deposits in cartilage or menisci may be present.

Table 97-1 provides a comparison of psoriatic arthritis with RA, osteoarthritis, and AS.

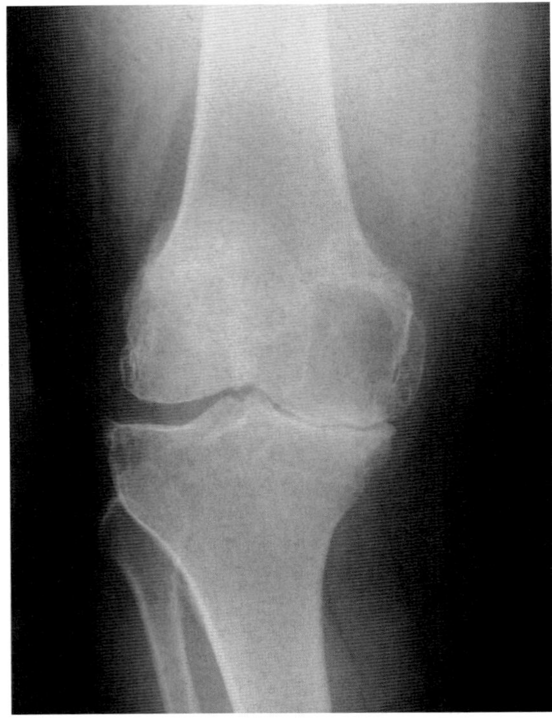

FIGURE 97-17 Radiograph showing osteoarthritis of the knee with asymmetric joint space narrowing. (*Reproduced with permission from Ricardo Zuniga-Montes, MD.*)

DIFFERENTIAL DIAGNOSIS

- Bursitis is inflammation of a bursa. Pain and tenderness is localized to the bursa. Common locations include subdeltoid, trochanteric, and olecranon.
- Tendinitis is inflammation of a tendon that produces a localized pain aggravated by stretching of the affected tendon.
- Inflammatory myopathy or myositis is inflammation of the muscle most commonly caused by an autoimmune or infectious process. Pain is in the muscles instead of the joints.
- Polymyalgia rheumatica is a systemic inflammatory disease with aching and stiffness in the torso and proximal extremities. Pain is in the muscles, but synovitis or tenosynovitis may also be present. Passive joint range of motion is preserved. ESR is elevated. Normocytic anemia and thrombocytosis can be present.
- Fibromyalgia—Widespread pain not limited to joints. Joint swelling is absent. Laboratory tests and imaging if obtained are normal.

MANAGEMENT

The goals of treatment are to control pain, maximize function, improve quality of life, and, for inflammatory causes, minimize joint damage.

NONPHARMACOLOGIC

- Recommend an exercise program. Aerobic exercise, strength training, or both improves pain and function in arthritis and other rheumatic diseases.[3] SOR Ⓐ

TABLE 97-1 Comparison of Psoriatic Arthritis with Rheumatoid Arthritis, Osteoarthritis, and Ankylosing Spondylitis

	PsA	RA	OA	AS
Peripheral disease	Asymmetric	Symmetric	Asymmetric	No
Sacroiliitis	Asymmetric	No	No	Symmetric
Stiffness	In morning and/or with immobility	In morning and/or with immobility	With activity	Yes
Female-to-male ratio	1:1	3:1	Hand/foot more common in female patients	1:3
Enthesitis	Yes	No	No	No
High-titer rheumatoid factor	No	Yes	No	No
HLA association	CW6, B27	DR4	No	B27
Nail lesions	Yes	No	No	No
Psoriasis	Yes	Uncommon	Uncommon	Uncommon

Abbreviations: *AS*, ankylosing spondylitis; *OA*, osteoarthritis; *PsA*, psoriatic arthritis; *RA*, rheumatoid arthritis.

Adapted from Gottlieb A, Korman NJ, Gordon KB, et al. Guidelines of care for the management of psoriasis and psoriatic arthritis: Section 2. Psoriatic arthritis: overview and guidelines of care for treatment with an emphasis on the biologics. *J Am Acad Dermatol*. 2008;58(5):851-864.

- Splints or braces may be used to offload stress on a particular joint.
- Weight loss reduces joint load for weight-bearing joints.

REFERRAL OR HOSPITALIZATION

- Hospitalize patients with suspected septic arthritis and begin empiric therapy with appropriate intravenous antibiotics.
- Refer patients in whom the diagnosis is unclear, especially if RA is suspected as early diagnosis and treatment improves outcomes.
- Refer patients in whom surgical management is indicated.

PROGNOSIS

Prognosis depends on the type of arthritis as well as psychosocial factors and socioeconomic status.

FOLLOW-UP

Acute arthritis should be followed closely until resolution. Chronic arthritis is managed as other chronic diseases with the frequency of follow-up dependent upon the type of arthritis and the severity of the disease.

PATIENT EDUCATION

For chronic arthritic conditions, the goals of treatment are to control pain, maximize function, improve quality of life, and minimize joint damage. Self-management is an important part of chronic arthritic conditions.

PATIENT RESOURCES

- Centers for Disease Control and Prevention: Information on the Arthritis Self-Management Program is available in English and Spanish—**http://www.cdc.gov/arthritis/interventions/self_manage.htm#1.**

PROVIDER RESOURCES

- Centers for Disease Control and Prevention: Information on arthritis and other rheumatologic conditions—**http://www.cdc.gov/arthritis/.**
- American College of Rheumatology: Clinical support, including practice guidelines, classification criteria, and clinical forms—**http://www.rheumatology.org/practice/clinical/index.asp.**

REFERENCES

1. Centers for Disease Control and Prevention (CDC). Prevalence of doctor-diagnosed arthritis and arthritis-attributable activity limitation—United States, 2007-2009. *MMWR Morb Mortal Wkly Rep*. 2010;59(39):1261-1265. http://www.cdc.gov/mmwr/preview/mmwrhtml/mm5939a1.htm?s_cid=mm5939a1_w. Accessed May 1, 2014.
2. Yelin E, Murphy L, Cisternas MG, et al. Medical care expenditures and earnings losses among persons with arthritis and other rheumatic conditions in 2003, and comparisons to 1997. *Arthritis Rheum*. 2007;56(5): 1397-1407.
3. Kelley GA, Kelley KS, Hootman JM, Jones DL. Effects of community-deliverable exercise on pain and physical function in adults with arthritis and other rheumatic diseases: a meta-analysis. *Arthritis Care Res (Hoboken)*. 2011;63(1):79-93.

98 OSTEOARTHRITIS

Jana K. Zaudke, MD
Heidi Chumley, MD

PATIENT STORY

A 70-year-old woman presents with pain and swelling in the joints of both hands, which impedes her normal activities. Her pain is better in the morning after resting and worse after she has been working with her hands. She denies stiffness. On examination, you find bony enlargement of some distal interphalangeal (DIP) and proximal interphalangeal (PIP) joints on both hands (**Figure 98-1**). Radiographs confirm the presence of Heberden and Bouchard nodes. She begins taking 1 g of acetaminophen twice a day and has significant improvement in her pain and function.

INTRODUCTION

Osteoarthritis is the most common type of arthritis. It involves degeneration of the articular cartilage accompanied by osteophytes (hypertrophic bone changes) around the joints. Osteoarthritis leads to pain in the joints with movement and relief with rest.

SYNONYMS

Degenerative joint disease.

EPIDEMIOLOGY

- Osteoarthritis is the most common type of arthritis, affecting 10% of men and 13% of women age 60 years or older.[1,2]
- Incidence and prevalence will likely increase given the obesity epidemic and the aging of the population.[2]

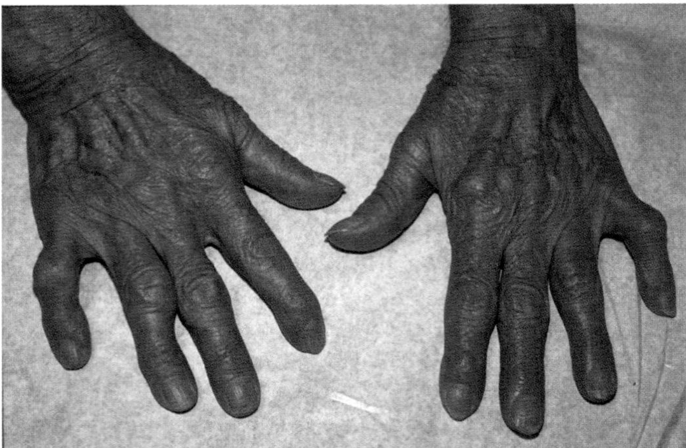

FIGURE 98-1 Bony enlargement of some distal interphalangeal (DIP) and proximal interphalangeal (PIP) joints consistent with Heberden (DIP) and Bouchard (PIP) nodes. (*Reproduced with permission from Richard P. Usatine, MD.*)

- In the Framingham cohort (mean age 71 years at baseline), women and men developed symptomatic knee osteoarthritis at the rate of 1% and 0.7% per year, respectively.[1]
- Risk of developing osteoarthritis increases with knee injury in adolescence or adulthood (relative risk [RR] = 2.95) and obesity (RR = 1.51-2.07).[1]
- Occupational physical activity and abnormal joint loading also increase the risk.[1,2]

ETIOLOGY AND PATHOPHYSIOLOGY

- Biomechanical factors and inflammation upset the balance of articular cartilage biosynthesis and degradation.
- Chondrocytes attempt to repair the damage; eventually, however, enzymes produced by the chondrocytes digest the matrix and accelerate cartilage erosion.
- Inflammatory molecules related to cytokine production, prostaglandin, and arachidonic acid metabolism may be involved in susceptibility to osteoarthritis.[3]

RISK FACTORS

- Advanced age
- Female gender
- Genetics
- Obesity
- Knee injury in adolescence and adulthood
- Abnormal joint loading
- Occupational history

DIAGNOSIS

The American College of Rheumatology uses the following criteria for the most common joints involved in osteoarthritis.

- Knee—Knee pain, osteophytes on radiograph, and 1 of 3: age older than 50 years, stiffness less than 30 minutes, or crepitus on physical examination (sensitivity = 91%, specificity = 86%).[4]
- Hip—Hip pain and 2 of 3: erythrocyte sedimentation rate (ESR) less than 20 mm/h; femoral or acetabular osteophytes by radiograph; superior, axial, or medial joint space narrowing by radiograph (sensitivity = 89%, specificity = 91%).[5]
- Hand—Hand pain, aching, or stiffness and 3 of 4: hard tissue enlargement of 2 or more DIP joints, fewer than 3 swollen metacarpophalangeal (MCP) joints, hand tissue enlargement of 2 or more selected joints, deformity of 1 or more selected joints. Selected joints include second and third DIP, second and third PIP, first carpometacarpal (CMC) on both hands (sensitivity = 94%, specificity = 87%).[6]

CLINICAL FEATURES

- Typically, joint pain is worsened with movement and relieved by rest. A small subset may demonstrate inflammatory symptoms including prolonged stiffness.
- Loss of function (ie, impaired gait with knee or hip osteoarthritis, impaired manual dexterity with hand osteoarthritis).

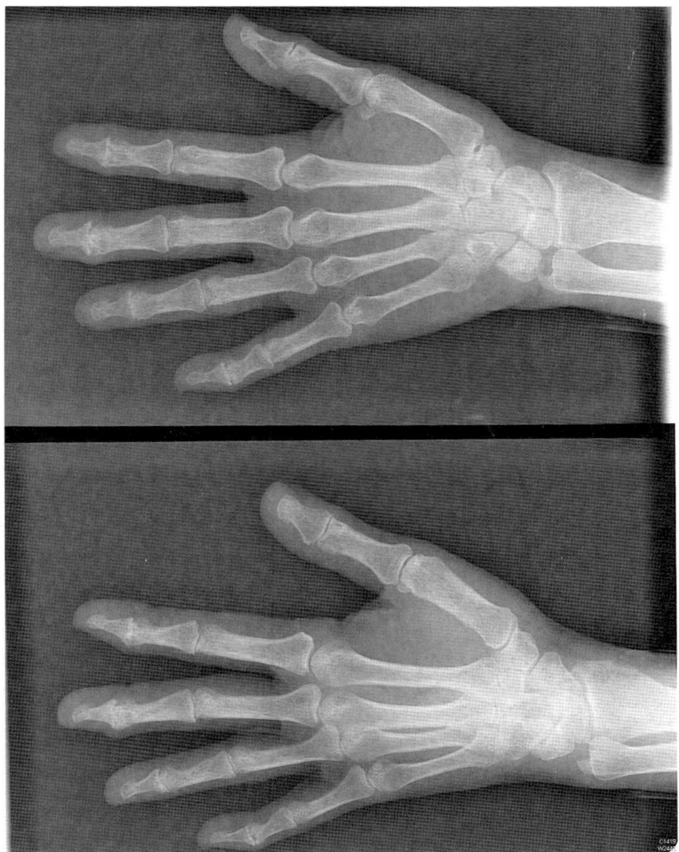

FIGURE 98-2 Joint space narrowing, marginal osteophytes, and Heberden nodes at the distal interphalangeal joints of the second through fifth fingers. (*Reproduced with permission from Heidi Chumley, MD.*)

- Radicular pain when vertebral column osteophytes impinge nerve roots.
- Bony enlargement of the DIP joints (Heberden nodes) or PIP joints (Bouchard nodes) (**Figure 98-1**).

TYPICAL DISTRIBUTION

Most common joints affected include knees, hands, hips, and back.

LABORATORY TESTING

Not typically indicated. Normal ESR and synovial fluid white blood cell (WBC) count less than 2000/mm.[3,4]

IMAGING

Loss of joint space or osteophytes on radiographs (**Figures 98-2** to **98-5**).

DIFFERENTIAL DIAGNOSIS

Musculoskeletal pain can also be caused by:

- Connective tissue diseases (scleroderma and lupus) that have other specific systemic signs.
- Fibromyalgia—Pain at trigger points instead of joints.
- Polyarticular gout—Erythematous joints and crystals in joint aspirate (see Chapter 105, Gout).
- Polymyalgia rheumatica—Proximal joint pain without deformity, elevated ESR. (see Chapter 113, Polymyalgia rheumatic).

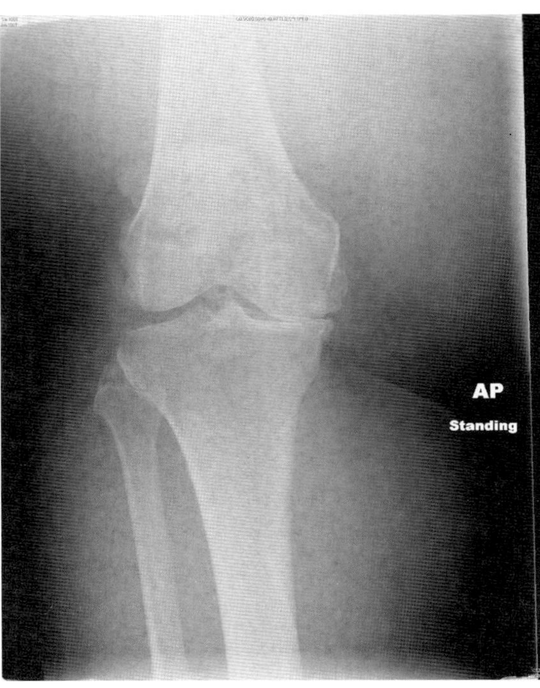

FIGURE 98-3 Osteoarthritis of the knee causing joint space narrowing, sclerosis, and bony spurring in all 3 compartments of the right knee, most pronounced in the medial compartment. (*Reproduced with permission from Heidi Chumley, MD.*)

- Seronegative spondyloarthropathies—Asymmetric joint involvement, spine often involved (see Chapter 101, Ankylosing Spondylitis).
- Reactive arthritis—History of infection, sexually transmitted disease, or bowel complaints. The patient may have conjunctivitis, iritis, urethritis in addition to joint pain and arthritis (see Chapter 153, Reactive Arthritis).
- Rheumatoid arthritis—Symmetric soft-tissue swelling in distal joints, stiffness after inactivity, positive rheumatoid factor. Ulnar deviation of the fingers at the MCP joints is a distinct finding in rheumatoid arthritis (**Figure 98-6**; Chapter 99, Rheumatoid Arthritis).
- Bursitis—Pain at 1 site, often increased with direct pressure.

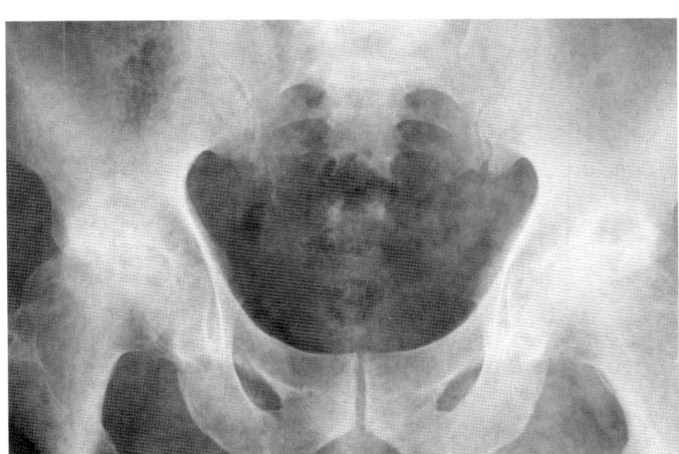

FIGURE 98-4 Articular space narrowing, sclerosis, and subchondral cyst formation of both hips because of osteoarthritis. (*Reproduced with permission from Chen MYM, Pope TL Jr, Ott DJ. Basic Radiology. McGraw-Hill; 2004:189, Figure 7-34.*)

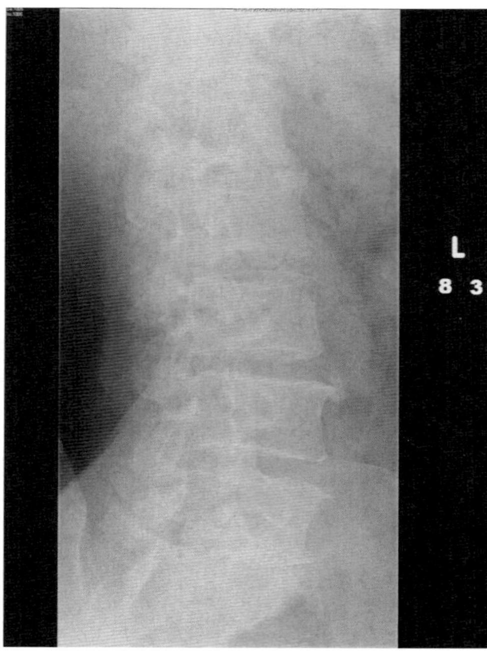

FIGURE 98-5 Loss of disc space and facet arthropathy at L5-S1 and small osteophytes, best seen on L4 and L5. These changes are caused by osteoarthritis. (*Reproduced with permission from Heidi Chumley, MD.*)

MANAGEMENT

NONPHARMACOLOGIC

Table 98-1 lists the nonpharmacologic options for management of osteoarthritis.

- Recommend therapeutic land-based or aquatic exercise to maintain range of motion and strengthen muscles surrounding affected joints.[7,8] SOR A

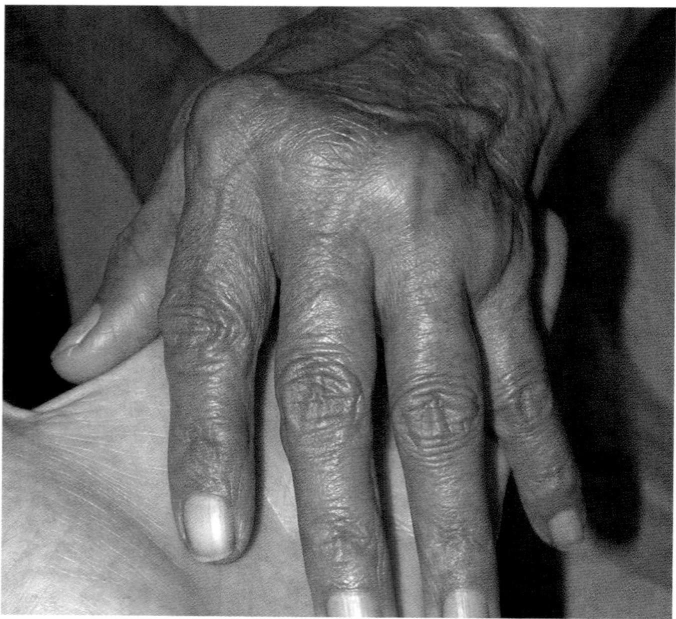

FIGURE 98-6 Rheumatoid arthritis showing ulnar deviation of the fingers at the metacarpophalangeal joints. (*Reproduced with permission from Richard P. Usatine, MD.*)

TABLE 98-1 Nonpharmacologic Options for Osteoarthritis

Weight loss (if overweight)
Aerobic exercise
Range-of-motion exercises
Muscle strengthening
Assistive devices for walking
Yoga and Tai Chi
Safe shoes
Lateral-wedged insoles (for genu varum) bracing
Physical and occupational therapy
Joint protection such as braces
Assistive devices for activities of daily living
Arthritis Foundation Self-Management Program
Social support

- Recommend weight loss for knee or hip osteoarthritis. Weight loss may not improve current pain, but may slow progression and can be recommended for numerous other health reasons.[8] SOR C
- Consider a knee brace that alters knee mechanics (ie, Counterforce brace).[9] SOR B

MEDICATIONS

Table 98-2 lists the pharmacologic therapy for osteoarthritis.

- Prescribe acetaminophen (2-4 g/day) for pain relief in patients at higher risk for GI complications. In a pooled analysis, acetaminophen improved pain by 5%, number needed to treat (NNT) 4 to 14.[10] SOR A
- Prescribe an NSAID for moderate-to-severe hip or knee osteoarthritis in patients who are at low risk for GI complications. GI bleeding is a significant risk to many elderly patients with osteoarthritis (see **Table 98-3**). A 2006 Cochrane review found NSAIDs were slightly more effective than acetaminophen, although more likely to produce adverse GI events.[10] SOR A
- If NSAIDs are to be used in patients with risk factors (see **Table 98-3**), consider giving misoprostol or a proton pump inhibitor for protection.[8] Note that H_2-blockers may decrease gastric symptoms from NSAIDs but are not protective against GI bleeding.
- Consider opioid analgesics for patients with severe osteoarthritis who have not responded to NSAIDs (be careful to not prescribe narcotics to patients in recovery from substance abuse).[8] SOR C

TABLE 98-2 Pharmacologic Options for Osteoarthritis

Oral
- Acetaminophen
- COX-2-specific inhibitor
- NSAID plus a proton pump inhibitor
- Opioids (eg, hydrocodone)
- Salsalate
- Tramadol

Topical
- Methylsalicylate
- Topical NSAID (eg, diclofenac gel)

Intraarticular
- Glucocorticoids (eg, triamcinolone)
- Hyaluronic acid

TABLE 98-3 Risk Factors for Upper GI Adverse Effects in Persons Taking NSAIDs

- Age 65 years or older
- Anticoagulants
- Comorbid medical conditions
- History of peptic ulcer disease
- History of upper gastrointestinal bleeding
- Oral steroids
- Taking NSAIDs with an empty stomach

- Consider a topical NSAID rather than an oral NSAID for hand or knee osteoarthritis, especially in patients 75 years of age or older. SOR Ⓒ There is not yet enough data to recommend topical NSAID for hip osteoarthritis.[8]
- Consider topical capsaicin 0.025% cream 4 times a day for hand osteoarthritis.[2] SOR Ⓑ
- Consider an intraarticular corticosteroid injection for acute pain related to knee or hip osteoarthritis.[8,11] SOR Ⓑ
- Consider an intra-articular hyaluronic injection for symptomatic chronic knee osteoarthritis. A 2006 Cochrane review of 76 clinical trials concluded that these injections were effective for treating knee osteoarthritis.[11] SOR Ⓐ

COMPLEMENTARY AND ALTERNATIVE THERAPY

- Consider participation in tai chi programs for knee or hip osteoarthritis.[8]
- Consider traditional Chinese acupuncture or transcutaneous electrical stimulation for patients with knee osteoarthritis who choose not to have or are not candidates for a total-knee arthroplasty.[8]
- In their newest guidelines, the American College of Rheumatology does not recommend use of chondroitin sulfate and glucosamine for osteoarthritis.[8]

REFERRAL

Refer patients who do not respond to conservative therapy to

- Any physician with experience doing joint injections if this is not within your skill set
- Rheumatologist for evaluation and treatment
- Orthopedic surgeon for evaluation for arthroplasty or joint replacement

FOLLOW-UP

There are no recommended intervals for follow-up; however, it is reasonable to see patients periodically to assess pain management and function.

PATIENT EDUCATION

Osteoarthritis is a chronic, progressive disease. Nonpharmacologic and pharmacologic therapies can reduce pain and preserve function.

PATIENT RESOURCES

- Arthritis Foundation. *Osteoarthritis*—**http://www.arthritis.org/osteoarthritis.php.**
- PubMed Health. *Osteoarthritis*—**http://www.ncbi.nlm.nih.gov/pubmedhealth/PMH0001460/.**
- FamilyDoctor.org. *Osteoarthritis*—**http://familydoctor.org/familydoctor/en/diseases-conditions/osteoarthritis.html.**

PROVIDER RESOURCES

- American College of Rheumatology Subcommittee on Osteoarthritis Guidelines. *Recommendations for the Medical Management of Osteoarthritis of the Hip and Knee*—**http://www.rheumatology.org/practice/clinical/guidelines/oa-mgmt.asp.**

REFERENCES

1. Sharma L, Kapoor D, Issa S. Epidemiology of osteoarthritis: an update [review]. *Curr Opin Rheumatol*. 2006;18(2):147-156.
2. Zhang Y, Jordan JM. Epidemiology of osteoarthritis. *Clin Geriatr Med*. 2010;26(3):355-369.
3. Valedez AM, Spector TD. The clinical relevance of genetic susceptibility to osteoarthritis. *Best Pract Res Clin Rheumatol*. 2010;24(1):3-14.
4. American College of Rheumatology. http://www.rheumatology.org/practice/clinical/classification/oaknee.asp. Accessed April 6, 2012.
5. http://www.rheumatology.org/practice/clinical/classification/oa-hip/oahip.asp. Accessed April 6, 2012.
6. http://www.rheumatology.org/practice/clinical/classification/oa-hand/oshand.asp. Accessed April 6, 2012.
7. Ottawa panel evidence-based clinical practice guidelines for therapeutic exercises and manual therapy in the management of osteoarthritis [review] [178 refs]. *Phys Ther*. 2005;85:907-971.
8. Hochberg MC, Altman RD, April KT, et al. American College of Rheumatology 2012 recommendations for the use of nonpharmacologic and pharmacologic therapies in osteoarthritis of the hand, hip and knee. *Arthritis Care Res*. 2012;64(4):465-474.
9. Barnes CL, Cawley PW, Hederman B. Effect of CounterForce brace on symptomatic relief in a group of patients with symptomatic unicompartmental osteoarthritis: a prospective 2-year investigation. *Am J Orthop*. 2002;31:396-401.
10. Towheed TE, Maxwell L, Judd MG, et al. Acetaminophen for osteoarthritis. *Cochrane Database Syst Rev*. 2006 Jan 25;(1):CD004257.
11. Sinusas, K. Osteoarthritis: diagnosis and treatment. *Am Fam Physician*. 2012;85(1):49-56.

99 RHEUMATOID ARTHRITIS

Heidi Chumley, MD

PATIENT STORY

A 79-year-old woman with late-stage rheumatoid arthritis comes for routine follow-up (**Figures 99-1** to **99-3**). She began having hand pain and stiffness approximately 40 years ago. She took nonprescription medications for pain for approximately 10 years before seeing a physician. She was diagnosed with rheumatoid arthritis on the basis of combination of clinical, laboratory, and radiograph findings. She was treated with prednisone and tried most of the disease-modifying agents as they became available; however, her disease progression continued. Approximately 10 years ago, she began having increased foot pain and difficulty walking. Today, she works with a multidisciplinary team to control pain and preserve hand function and independence.

INTRODUCTION

Rheumatoid arthritis (RA) is a progressive chronic illness that causes significant pain and disability. RA is a polyarticular inflammatory arthritis that causes symmetrical joint pain and swelling and typically involves the hands. Early recognition and treatment with nonbiologic and/or biologic disease-modifying antirheumatologic agents (DMARDs) can induce remission and preserve function.

EPIDEMIOLOGY

- RA is found in 0.8% of the adult population worldwide.[1]
- It is more than twice as common in women as compared to men (54 per 100,000 vs. 25 per 100,000).[1]
- Typical age of onset is 30 to 50 years.[1]

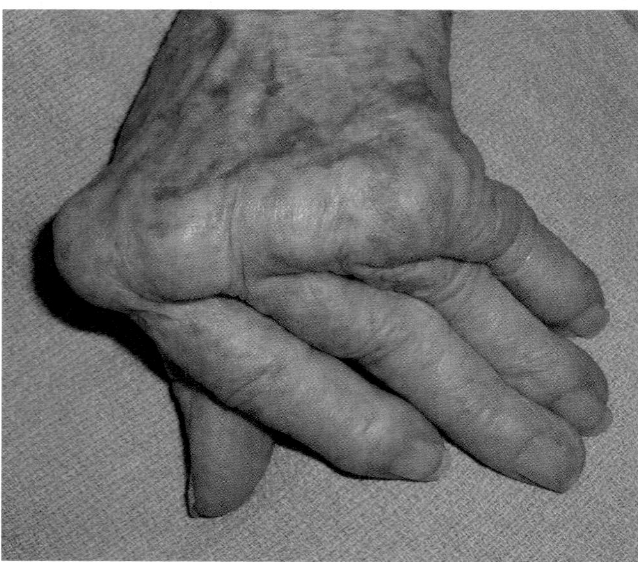

FIGURE 99-1 Ulnar deviation at metacarpophalangeal joints in advanced rheumatoid arthritis. Also note the swelling at the distal interphalangeal joints, seen best on the first finger. (*Reproduced with permission from Richard P. Usatine, MD.*)

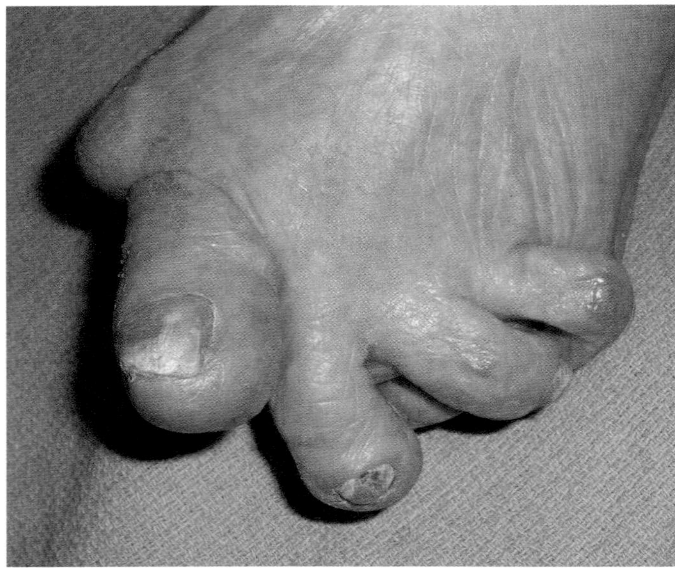

FIGURE 99-2 Rheumatoid arthritis in the foot of a 79-year-old woman with subluxation of the first metatarsophalangeal joint. (*Reproduced with permission from Richard P. Usatine, MD.*)

ETIOLOGY AND PATHOPHYSIOLOGY

- Genetic predisposition coupled with an autoimmune or infection-triggering incident.
- Synovial macrophages and fibroblasts proliferate, leading to increased lymphocytes and endothelial cells.
- Increased cellular material occludes small blood vessels, causing ischemia, neovascularization, and inflammatory reactions.
- Inflamed tissue grows irregularly, causing joint damage.
- Damage causes further release of cytokines, interleukins, proteases, and growth factors, resulting in more joint destruction and systemic complications including a higher risk for cardiovascular disease

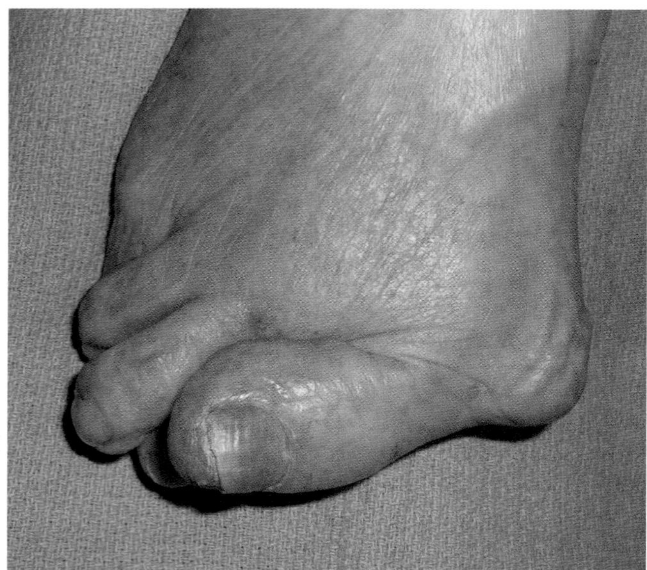

FIGURE 99-3 Deviation at the metatarsophalangeal joints from bony destruction in advanced rheumatoid arthritis. (*Reproduced with permission from Richard P. Usatine, MD.*)

RISK FACTORS

Genetic predisposition signified by a positive family history.

DIAGNOSIS

The 2010 American College of Rheumatology/European League Against Rheumatism classification criteria uses a scoring system to designate patients as definite RA. A score of 6 or greater out of 10 meets criteria for definite RA.[2]

- Joint involvement—1 large joint (0 points); 2 to 10 large joints (1 point); 1 to 3 small joints with or without large joints (2 points); 4 to 10 small joints with or without large joints (3 points); more than 10 joints with at least 1 small joint (5 points).
- Serology—Negative rheumatoid factor (RF) and anti-cyclic citrullinated peptide (anti-CCP) (0 points); low positive RF or anti-CCP (2 points); high positive RF or ACPA (3 points).
- Acute-phase reactants—Normal C-reactive protein (CRP) and erythrocyte sedimentation rate (ESR) (0 points); abnormal CRP or ESR (1 point).
- Duration of symptoms—Less than 6 weeks (0 points); 6 or more weeks (1 point).

American Rheumatism Association criteria (with positive likelihood ratio abbreviated as LR+):[3]

- Stiffness around joint for 1 hour after inactivity (LR+1.9).
- Three or more of these have soft-tissue swelling—Wrist, proximal interphalangeal (PIP), metacarpophalangeal (MCP), elbow, knee, ankle, metatarsophalangeal (MTP) (LR+1.4).
- Hand joints involved (LR+1.5) (**Figures 99-1, 99-4,** and **99-5**).

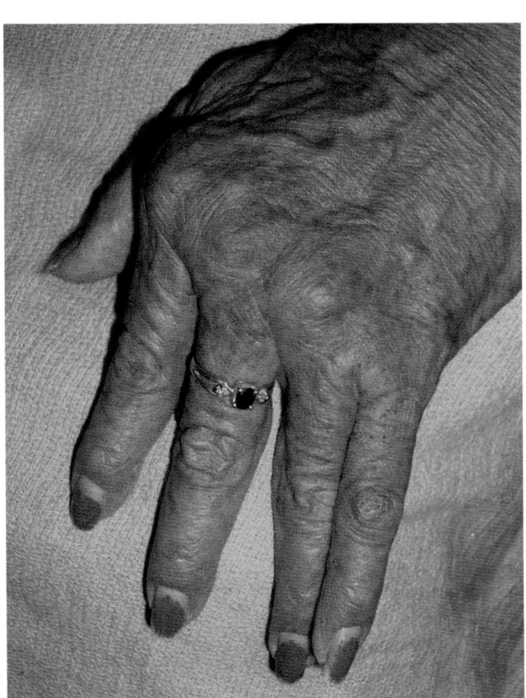

FIGURE 99-4 Ulnar deviation at metacarpophalangeal joints seen in a 64-year-old woman with rheumatoid arthritis. (*Reproduced with permission from Richard P. Usatine, MD.*)

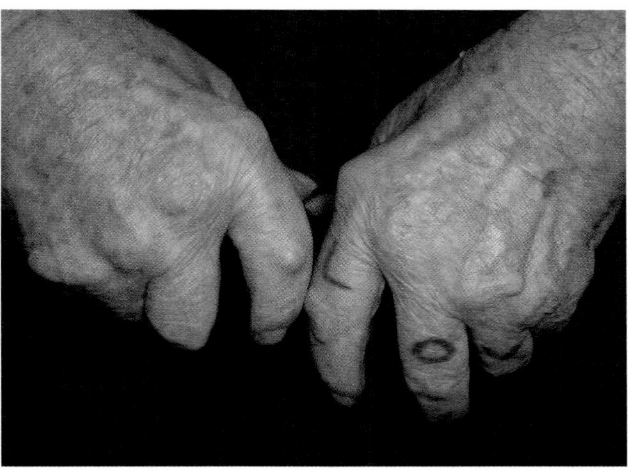

FIGURE 99-5 Rheumatoid nodules in the hands. (*Reproduced with permission from Richard P. Usatine, MD.*)

- Symmetrical involvement of 1 of these: wrist, PIP, MCP, elbow, knee, ankle, MTP (LR+1.2).
- Subcutaneous nodules (LR+3.0) (**Figures 99-5** and **99-6**).
- Positive serum RF (LR+8.4).
- Osteopenia or erosion of surrounding joints on hand or wrist films (LR+11) (**Figures 99-7** and **99-8**).

CLINICAL FEATURES

Joint pain and swelling, polyarticular and symmetrical.

TYPICAL DISTRIBUTION

- Hands are typically involved (**Figures 99-1, 99-4,** and **99-5).**
- Commonly involved joints include wrist, PIP, MCP, elbow, knee, ankle, and MTP.
- Subcutaneous nodules (**Figures 99-5** and **99-6**).

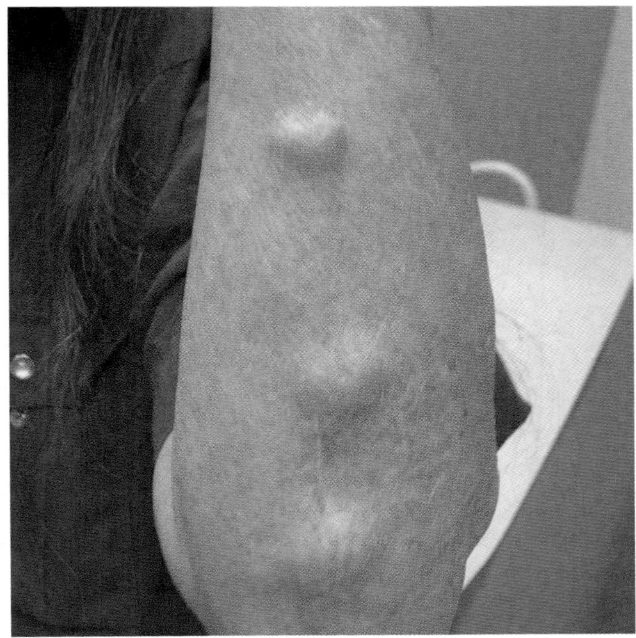

FIGURE 99-6 Rheumatoid nodules on the arm of a patient with rheumatoid arthritis. (*Reproduced with permission from Richard P. Usatine, MD.*)

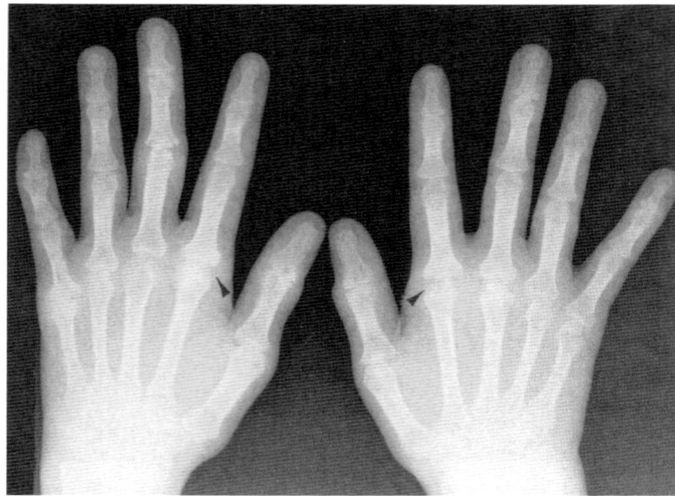

FIGURE 99-7 Hand radiographs in long-standing rheumatoid arthritis demonstrating carpal destruction, radiocarpal joint narrowing, bony erosion (arrowheads), and soft-tissue swelling. (*From Chen MYM, Pope TL Jr, Ott DJ. Basic Radiology. New York: McGraw-Hill; 2004:194, Figure 7-42. Copyright 2004.*)

LABORATORY TESTING

- RF (negative in 30% of patients; positive in many connective tissue, neoplastic, and infectious diseases).
- Anti-CCP, high specificity, often presents before definitive diagnosis can be made; presence predicts arthritis development.
- CRP (>0.7 pg/mL) or ESR (>30 mm/h).
- Complete blood count (normocytic or microcytic anemia, thrombocytosis).

IMAGING

Hand or wrist radiographs may show soft tissue swelling, osteopenia, erosions, subluxations, and deformities (**Figures 99-7** and **99-8**).

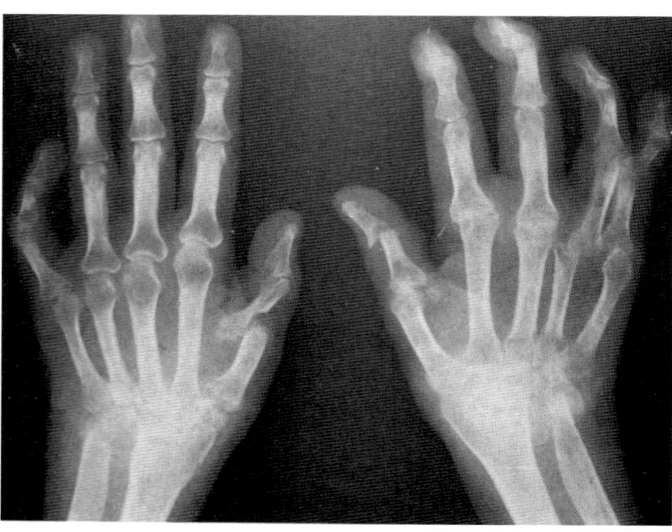

FIGURE 99-8 Severe changes of late rheumatoid arthritis including radiocarpal joint destruction, ulnar deviation, erosion of the ulnar styloid bilaterally, dislocation of the left thumb PIP joint, and dislocation of the right fourth and fifth MCP joints. (*Reproduced with permission from Brunicardi CF, Andersen DK, Billiar TR, et al. Schwartz's Principles of Surgery. New York: McGraw-Hill; 2005:1666, Figure 42-40. Copyright 2005.*)

DIFFERENTIAL DIAGNOSIS

RA can mimic many systemic diseases and should be differentiated from the following:[1]

- Connective tissue diseases (scleroderma and lupus), which have other specific systemic signs.
- Fibromyalgia—Pain at trigger points instead of joints.
- Hemochromatosis—Abnormal iron studies and skin changes.
- Infectious endocarditis—Heart murmurs, high fever, risk factors, such as IV drug use.
- Polyarticular gout—Erythematous joints and crystals in joint aspirate.
- Polymyalgia rheumatica—Proximal joint pain without deformity.
- Seronegative, spondyloarthropathies—Asymmetric joint involvement, spine often involved.
- Reactive arthritis—History of infection, sexually transmitted disease, or bowel complaints.

MANAGEMENT

Target outcome is remission through use of disease-modifying agents. Monitor for complications:

- Patients with RA are twice as likely to have serious GI complications; monitor carefully.
- Anemia—25% will respond to iron therapy.
- Cancer—Two-fold increase risk of lymphomas and leukemias.
- Cardiac complications such as pericarditis or pericardial effusion (30% at diagnosis).
- Cervical spine disease—Atlas instability; careful with intubation and avoid flexion films after trauma until atlas visualized.

NONPHARMACOLOGIC

- Use of multidisciplinary team improves outcomes.[4] SOR B
- Exercise improves aerobic capacity and strength without increases in pain or disease activity.[5] SOR B

MEDICATIONS

- NSAIDs can be used for pain control,[5] SOR A but do not alter disease progression and should not be used alone.
- Systemic corticosteroids relieve pain and slow progression,[5] SOR A but have serious side effects and should be used at lowest dose possible with added bone protection (eg, calcium and vitamin D or a bisphosphonate).
- Nonbiologic DMARDs such as methotrexate, leflunomide, hydroxychloroquine, sulfasalazine, and minocycline reduce disease progression and should be considered in all patients without contraindications. SOR A
- Biologic DMARDs, such as antitumor necrosis factor (TNF) drugs, rituximab, abatacept, adalimumab, etanercept, and infliximab, reduce disease progression and should be considered in patients with high disease activity and poor prognostic features. SOR C

COMPLEMENTARY AND ALTERNATIVE THERAPY

Diet modifications—Omega-3 polyunsaturated fatty acids may decrease anti-inflammatory medication use.[1] SOR B

REFERRAL

- Refer patients with new diagnosis of or with a suspicion of RA to a physician experienced in the use of nonbiologic and biologic DMARDs.

Recommendations for initiating DMARDs are based on[6]

- Disease duration
- Presence of poor prognostic factors (functional limitations, extraarticular disease, positive RF and/or anti-CCP bony erosions)
- Classification of low, moderate, or high disease activity, based on one of several validated instruments (eg, Rheumatoid Arthritis Disease Activity Index)

DMARDs reduce disease progression, but have several contraindications and must be followed closely.

- Do not start nonbiologic or biologic DMARDs when the patient has an active bacterial infection, active or latent (before preventive therapy is initiated) tuberculosis (TB), acute hepatitis B or C, active herpes zoster, or a systemic fungal infection.[6]
- Avoid DMARDs if white blood cell (WBC) count is less than 3000/mm^3 or platelets are under 50,000/mm^3, New York Heart Association class III or IV heart failure, or liver transaminases more than twice the normal value.[6]
- Start methotrexate or leflunomide monotherapy for any disease duration, with or without poor prognostic factors, and any classification of disease activity.[6]
- Combination DMARD therapy (eg, methotrexate [MTX] and sulfasalazine) may be used in patients with any duration of disease, poor prognostic features, and moderate or high disease activity.[6]
- Consider biologic DMARDs for patients with any disease duration, high disease activity, and poor prognostic features. Etanercept, infliximab, and adalimumab improve function and quality of life as monotherapy or in combination with nonbiologic DMARDs.[6]

PROGNOSIS

- Poor prognostic features include functional limitations, extraarticular disease, positive RF and/or anti-CCP, and bony erosions.[6]
- RA patients have an increased risk of cardiovascular disease.

FOLLOW-UP

Multidisciplinary follow-up with primary care, rheumatologist, occupational and physical therapists, and patient educators improves outcomes.

PATIENT EDUCATION

RA is a chronic illness. Twenty to 40 percent of patients will have remission with therapy. Early treatment can prevent complications and allow the person to maintain function. It is best to stay active and exercise to the best of your ability.

PATIENT RESOURCES

- Information on RA is available at **http://www.rheumatoidarthritis.com/ra/** and **http://www.ra.com/.**
- American College of Rheumatology. *Rheumatoid Arthritis*—**http://www.rheumatology.org/practice/clinical/patients/diseases_and_conditions/ra.asp.**

PROVIDER RESOURCES

- Saag KG, Teng GG, Patkar NM, et al. American College of Rheumatology 2008 recommendations for the use of nonbiologic and biologic disease-modifying antirheumatic drugs in RA. *Arthritis Rheum* 2008;59(6):762-784—**http://www.rheumatology.org/practice/clinical/guidelines/recommendations.pdf.**

REFERENCES

1. Rindfleisch JA, Muller D. Diagnosis and management of rheumatoid arthritis. *Am Fam Physician*. 2005;72(6):1037-1047, 1049-1050.
2. American College of Rheumatology/European League Against Rheumatism. 2010 Rheumatoid arthritis classification criteria. *Arthritis Rheum*. 2010;62(9):2569-2581.
3. Saraux A, Berthelot JM, Chales G, et al. Ability of the American College of Rheumatology 1987 criteria to predict rheumatoid arthritis in patients with early arthritis and classification of these patients two years later. *Arthritis Rheum*. 2001;44(11):2485-2491.
4. Vliet Vlieland TP, Breedveld FC, Hazes JM. The 2-year follow-up of a randomized comparison of in-patient multidisciplinary team care and routine out-patient care for active rheumatoid arthritis. *Br J Rheum*. 1997;36(1):82-85.
5. American College of Rheumatology Subcommittee on Rheumatoid Arthritis Guidelines. Guidelines for the management of rheumatoid arthritis: 2002 Update. [see comment]. *Arthritis Rheum*. 2002;46(2):328-346.
6. Saag KG, Teng GG, Patkar NM, et al. American College of Rheumatology 2008 recommendations for the use of nonbiologic and biologic disease-modifying antirheumatic drugs in rheumatoid arthritis. *Arthritis Rheum*. 2008;59(6):762-784.

100 PSORIATIC ARTHRITIS

Gina R. Chacon, MD
Richard P. Usatine, MD

PATIENT HISTORY

A 19-year-old man presents with psoriatic plaques covering his body from head to lower legs; he reports pain in his fingers, wrists, ankles, and feet for the past month. He states that it is painful to walk. On physical examination, it is noted that he has plaques covering 80% of his body surface area, nail pits, and swelling of his ankles and some fingers (**Figure 100-1**). There is no question that the patient has plaque psoriasis, so a skin biopsy is not needed. Plain films of the hands, ankles, and feet show nothing more than soft-tissue swelling. The patient still has psoriatic arthritis (PsA) even though it is too early to see bone changes in the radiographs. The patient is initially treated with topical steroid ointments while baseline laboratory tests are made, and a purified protein derivative (PPD) antigen is used to test for tuberculosis. Methotrexate is started when the laboratory tests show no liver disease and there is a negative PPD test. The joint pains and plaque psoriasis improved over time.

INTRODUCTION

Psoriatic arthritis (PsA) is common in patients with psoriasis and is associated with significant morbidity and decreased quality of life.[1] PsA can be disabling, with radiographic damage noted in 7% to 47% of patients at a median interval of 2 years despite clinical improvement with standard disease-modifying antirheumatic therapy.[2]

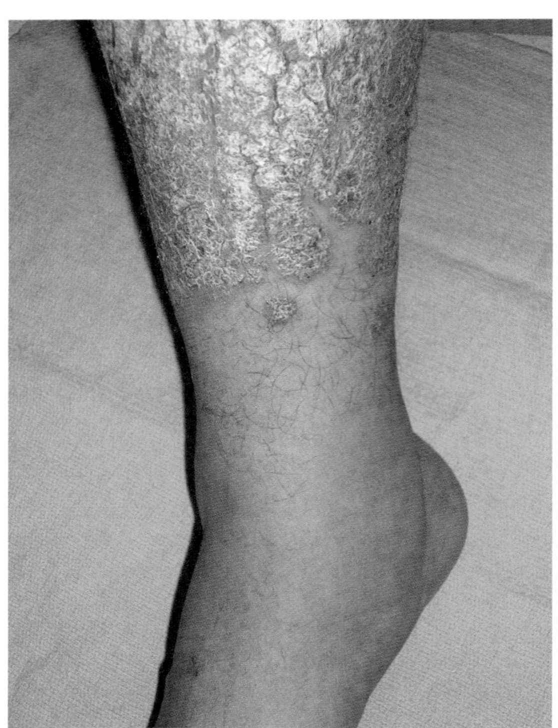

B

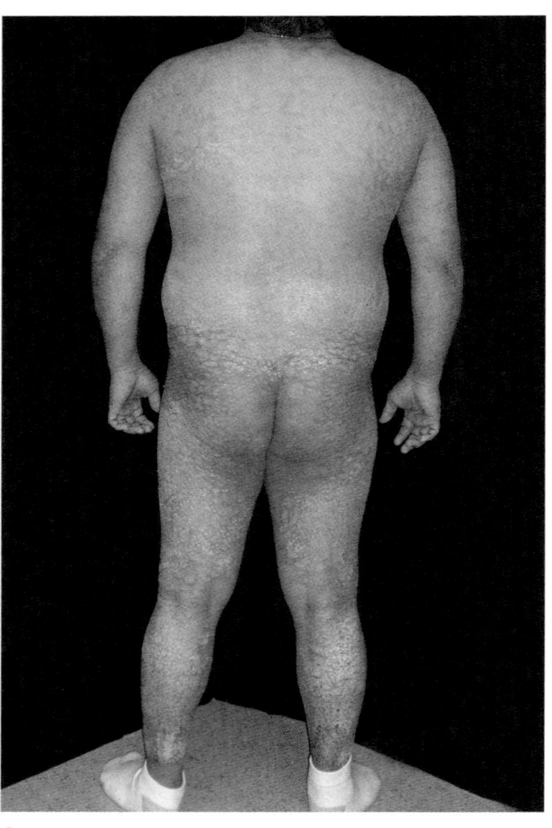

A

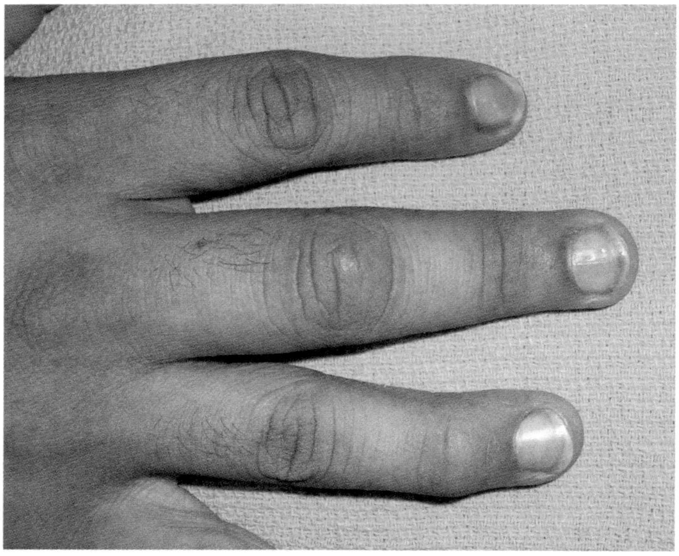

C

FIGURE 100-1 A. New-onset plaque psoriasis in a 19-year-old man. B. He has significant ankle and foot pain with minimal joint swelling on examination. C. There is tenderness and swelling in the finger joints even though the radiographs do not show psoriatic arthritis changes. (*Reproduced with permission from Richard P. Usatine, MD.*)

EPIDEMIOLOGY

- Psoriasis affects approximately 2% to 3% of the population in the United States and over 125 million people worldwide.[3]
- The exact proportion of patients with psoriasis who will develop PsA is an area of significant controversy, with studies demonstrating a range from 6% to 10% in broadly representative population-based studies to as high as 42% of patients with psoriasis in clinic-based populations.[4]
- The prevalence of PsA increases in patients with more extensive skin disease. In the general population of the United States,[5] it has been estimated to be 0.1% to 0.25%.
- PsA can develop at any time from childhood on, but for the majority of patients, it presents between the ages of 30 and 50 years.[4]
- Caucasians are more frequently affected with PsA than any other racial or ethnic groups.[6]
- PsA affects men and women equally.[7]

ETIOLOGY/PATHOPHYSIOLOGY

Psoriasis is an inflammatory immune-based disorder with a genetic predisposition.[8,9]

DIAGNOSIS

- Clinicians can often diagnose psoriasis and PsA based on clinical history, physical examination, and radiography of joints (see Chapters 97, Arthritis Overview; 150, Psoriasis; 193, Psoriatic Nails).
- In challenging cases, skin histopathology can be helpful in distinguishing psoriasis from other types of skin diseases.
- Full-body skin examination should include the nails and scalp. Common features of psoriasis may include the following:
  - characteristic morphology of erythema, scaling, and induration
  - scalp involvement
  - nail involvement (pitting, onycholysis, crumbling, or oil spots)
  - involvement of the intertriginous folds
  - family history of psoriasis[7]

HISTORY/SYMPTOMS

- Affected individuals with plaque psoriasis often present with chronic, recurrent, erythematous, scaly patches and plaques. PsA tends to persist for months to years, and intermittent flares are common.[4,10]
- Common skin symptoms associated with psoriasis include pruritus, irritation, burning, sensitivity, and pain.[7]
- PsA is characterized by early morning stiffness lasting longer than 30 minutes, pain, swelling, and tenderness of the joints and the surrounding ligaments and tendons (eg, the Achilles tendons) (**Figure 100-2**) and ligamentous attachments to the ribs, spine, and pelvis.[4]
- PsA may start slowly with mild symptoms and, on occasion, may be preceded by a joint injury. The course is variable and unpredictable, ranging from mild and nondestructive to severe, debilitating, erosive arthropathy.[4]
- Flares and remissions usually characterize the course of PsA. Left untreated, patients with PsA can have persistent inflammation, progressive joint damage, severe physical limitations, and disability.[4]

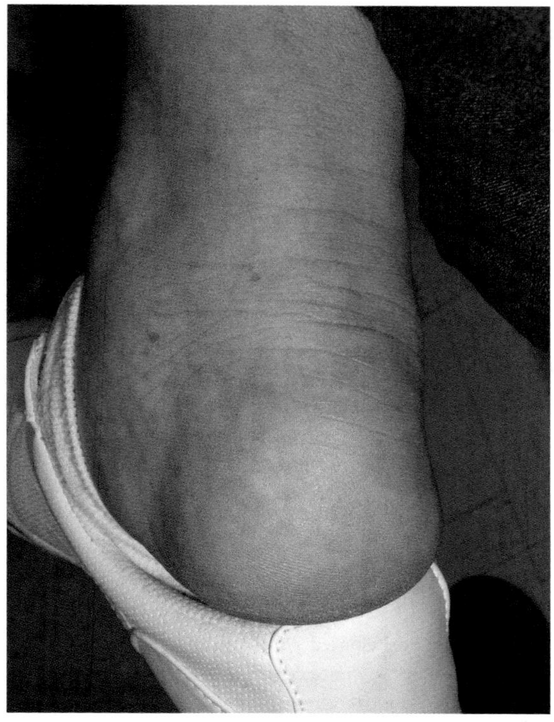

FIGURE 100-2 Achilles enthesopathy in a middle-aged woman with long-standing psoriasis. She presented with pain, swelling, and tenderness over the Achilles tendon. (*Reproduced with permission from Richard P. Usatine, MD.*)

PHYSICAL EXAMINATION

- Examine those joints that are reported to be painful or stiff. Patients with PsA show tender and swollen joints.[4]
- Dactylitis, or "sausage digit," is a combination of enthesitis of the tendons and ligaments along with synovitis involving a whole digit (**Figure 100-3**).[4]
- Plaque psoriasis appears as sharply marginated, erythematous patches or plaques with a characteristic silvery-white scale.[11] Lesions may initially manifest as erythematous, scaly papules that coalesce to form plaques.

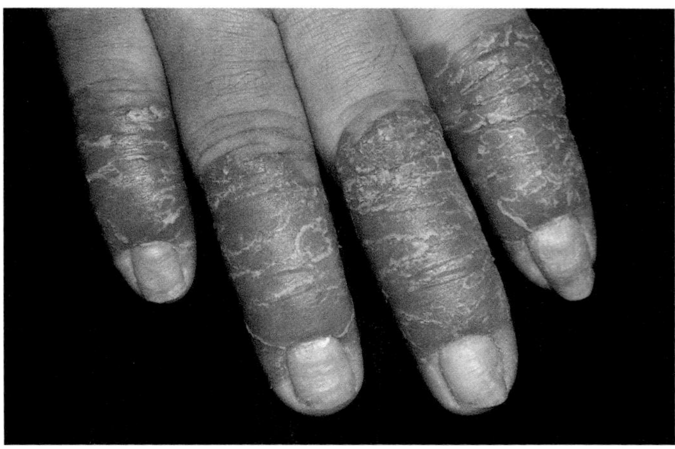

FIGURE 100-3 Dactylitis (sausage fingers) in a woman with plaque psoriasis and psoriatic arthritis. (*Reproduced with permission from Richard P. Usatine, MD.*)

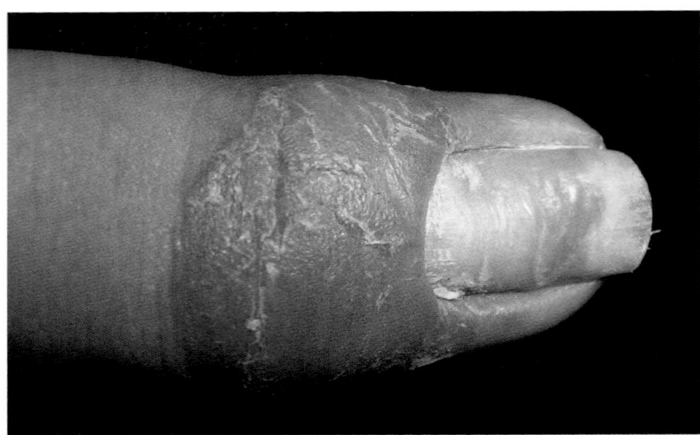

FIGURE 100-4 Psoriatic arthritis of the distal interphalangeal predominant (DIP) joint with psoriatic nail changes and psoriatic skin changes of the distal digit. (*Reproduced with permission from Richard P. Usatine, MD.*)

- New psoriasis lesions can form at sites of trauma, which is termed the Koebner phenomenon. Removal of scale often reveals pinpoint bleeding, which is called the Auspitz phenomenon.[7]
- Psoriatic lesions are distributed symmetrically and can affect any part of the body. The most commonly affected sites are the scalp, torso, and extensor surfaces of the extremities, such as the knees and elbows.[12]

There are five types of PsA:

1. Symmetric arthritis—Involves multiple symmetric pairs of joints in the hands and feet; resembles rheumatoid arthritis. It affects approximately 15% of patients with PsA.[12]
2. Asymmetric arthritis—Involves only 1 to 3 joints in an asymmetric pattern and may affect any joint (eg, knee, hip, ankle, and wrist). Hands and feet may have enlarged sausage digits caused by dactylitis **(Figure 100-4)**. As the most common type, it is found in approximately 80% of patients.[12]
3. Distal interphalangeal predominant (DIP)—Involves the distal joints of the fingers and toes. It may be confused with osteoarthritis, but nail changes are common in this type of PsA. The fingers with DIP involvement are most likely to have psoriatic nail changes, such as pitting **(Figure 100-4)**. This "classic type" occurs in approximately 5% of patients.[12]
4. Spondylitis (axial)—Inflammation of the spinal column causes a stiff neck and pain in the lower back and sacroiliac area. The arthritis may involve peripheral joints in the hands, arms, hips, legs, and feet.[12]
5. Arthritis mutilans—A severe, deforming type of arthritis that usually affects a few joints in the hands and feet **(Figure 100-5)**. It has been associated with pustular psoriasis. It affects fewer than 5% of patients with PsA.[12]

NAIL PSORIASIS

See Chapter 193, Psoriatic Nails, for more information on the subject.

- Nail disease is commonly found in patients with PsA, especially those with distal interphalangeal joint involvement **(Figure 100-4)**.[4]
- Psoriatic nail disease occurs more commonly in the fingernails than the toenails and manifests as pitting, onycholysis, oil spots, hyperkeratosis, or nail grooving.[3]

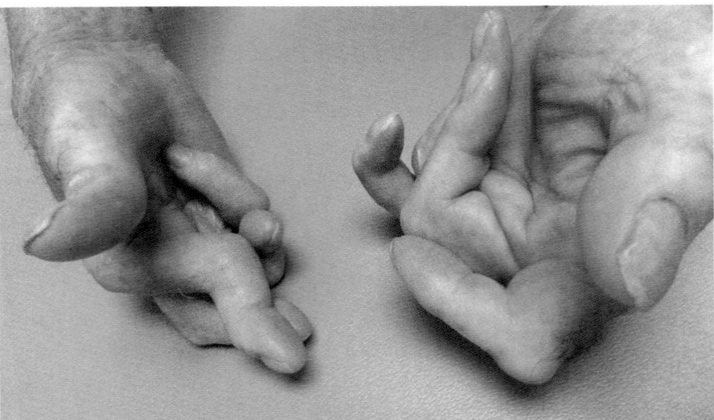

FIGURE 100-5 Arthritis mutilans in both hands in a man with long-standing psoriasis and arthritis. (*Reproduced with permission from Robert Gilson, MD.*)

- Nail pitting occurs as a result of psoriasis affecting the nail matrix. Yellowish-brown nail discoloration or oil spots on the nail result from psoriasis involvement of the nail bed.
- Onycholysis occurs at the distal nail plate at the point of separation from the hyponychium.[7]

DIAGNOSTIC TESTS

- The erythrocyte sedimentation rate or the C-reactive protein level can be used to measure signs of systemic inflammation.[4]
- Skin biopsy is not routinely required for diagnosis of psoriasis. Histological findings vary depending on the age of the lesions.[3]

IMAGING

Radiographs may show juxta-articular erosions **(Figure 100-6)**, "pencil-in-cup" deformity, osteolysis, digit telescoping, or asymmetric sacroiliitis.

MANAGEMENT

- Inflammation driven by T cells is responsible for keratinocyte growth and angiogenesis in the psoriatic plaque.[13] Many of the therapies for skin psoriasis are therefore devised to target T cells or their inflammatory mediators.[13,14]
- Indeed, many of the topical and systemic therapies and phototherapies also act at least in large part by interfering with this same immune response.
- For patients with moderate-to-severe skin psoriasis and PsA, systemic therapies should be used **(Figure 100-7)**.[15] SOR Ⓐ
- Patients with PsA may have skin psoriasis at the same time, and treatment should be for the joints and the skin at the same time.

THERAPY FOR SKIN PSORIASIS

- Corticosteroids are the mainstay of treatment for symptomatic skin psoriasis.[9]
- Topical steroids as monotherapy give fast relief of inflammation and itching. Small, chronic plaques may be treated with intralesional steroid.[16] SOR Ⓐ
- Vitamin D derivative–corticosteroid combination therapy is more effective than vitamin D derivative monotherapy.[16] SOR Ⓐ

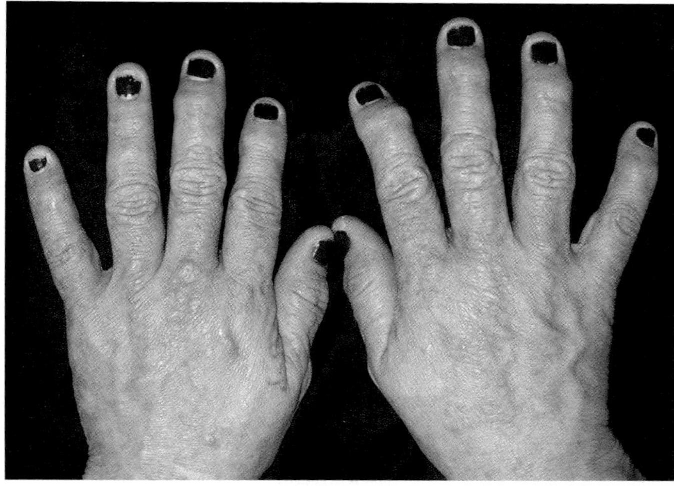

A

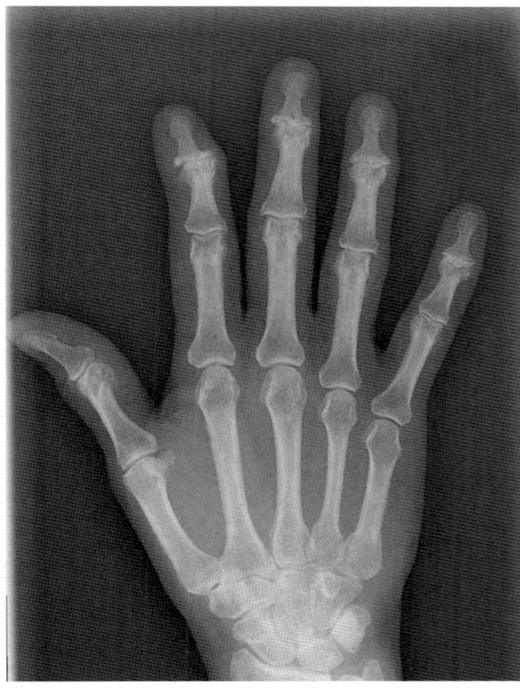

B

FIGURE 100-6 A. Symmetrical psoriatic arthritis in both hands of a 50-year-old woman. B. This radiograph of her right hand shows juxta-articular erosions. (*Reproduced with permission from Richard P. Usatine, MD.*)

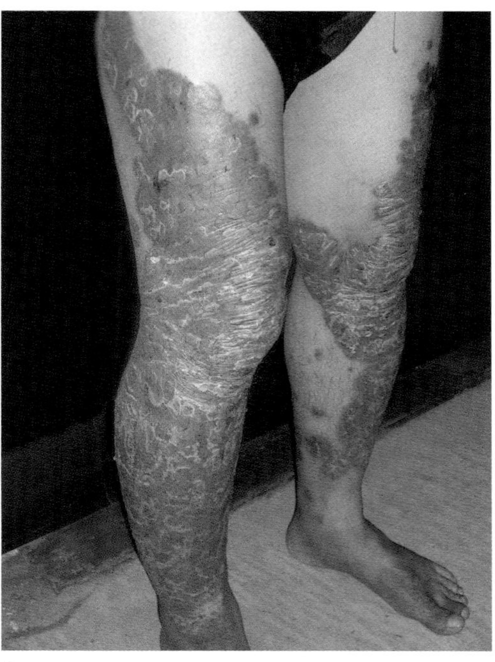

A

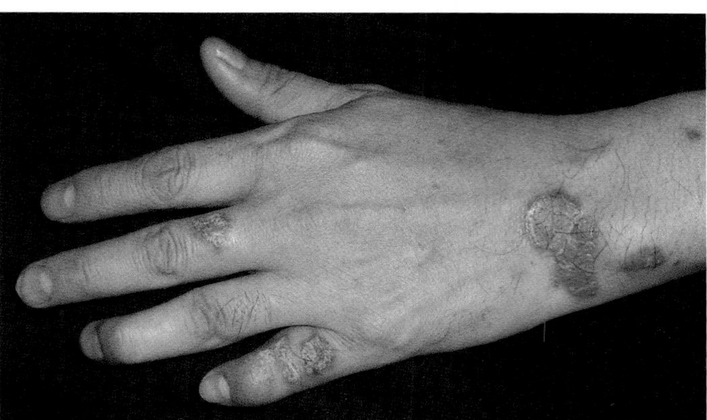

B

FIGURE 100-7 A. Plaque psoriasis on both legs in a 41-year-old man with right knee pain and psoriatic arthritis. B. The skin psoriasis is seen on the dorsum of his left hand along with joint deformities of the fingers from the advanced psoriatic arthritis. The fourth digit shows a swan-neck deformity. He is a good candidate for systemic therapy to treat the skin and joints in an attempt to prevent further joint deformities. (*Reproduced with permission from Richard P. Usatine, MD.*)

- Acitretin is an antipsoriatic retinoid. The combination of acitretin with topical vitamin D, biological therapy, or phototherapy may increase rates of clearance but does not treat PsA.[16] SOR Ⓐ

SYSTEMIC THERAPY

- Patients with both chronic psoriasis and PsA may find a major improvement in their quality of life with systemic treatment.[16] SOR Ⓐ
- Mild PsA is most often managed with nonsteroidal anti-inflammatory drugs (NSAIDs) alone. If the PsA is unresponsive after 2 to 3 months of therapy with NSAIDs, treatment with methotrexate (MTX) should be considered.[4] SOR Ⓐ
- Methotrexate is an inhibitor of folate biosynthesis and therefore impairs DNA replication. It is an anti-inflammatory because of its effects on T-cell gene expression patterns. It can be used continuously for many years with durable benefits.
- For patients with moderate-to-severe PsA, MTX, tumor necrosis factor α (TNF-α) blockade, or the combination of these therapies is considered first-line treatment.[4] SOR Ⓐ
- The combination of orally administered MTX and cyclosporine can also be effective in the treatment of PsA.[4] SOR Ⓐ

BIOLOGICAL AGENTS

- Immunomodulatory therapy interacts with specific molecular targets in T-cell-mediated inflammatory processes and exerts an anti-inflammatory effect, decreasing the progression of the disease.[15] SOR Ⓐ
- All TNF-α inhibitors show similar efficacy for the signs and symptoms of PsA. There are, however, observed differences in the efficacy of

these agents for the treatment of cutaneous psoriasis. Infliximab clears cutaneous psoriasis in the highest proportion of patients and with the greatest rapidity.[4] SOR Ⓐ

- All of the TNF-α inhibitors appear to diminish the likelihood of radiographic progression of PsA compared with MTX, but these findings are derived from comparing several different studies rather than one large comparator study.[4] SOR Ⓐ
- Etanercept is a recombinant soluble TNF-α receptor fused to the Fc portion of a human immunoglobulin G molecule. Etanercept binds soluble TNF-α, thus blocking its pro-inflammatory effects. SOR Ⓐ
- Adalimumab is a TNF inhibitor that binds to TNF-α, preventing it from activating TNF receptors. It offers effective control of plaque psoriasis. SOR Ⓐ
- Infliximab is a chimeric monoclonal antibody that blocks the pro-inflammatory effect of TNF-α. It offers rapid and thorough suppression of psoriasis. SOR Ⓐ
- Ustekinumab is a human monoclonal antibody to interleukin 12 (IL-12) and IL-23 that inhibits T-cell subsets involved in plaque psoriasis. SOR Ⓐ
- In general, it is appropriate to initiate MTX treatment for patients with moderate-to-severe PsA who have no contraindications to MTX therapy. Check PPD first and make sure that, if the test was positive, the patient has had at least 2 months of isoniazid (INH).
    - If after 12 to 16 weeks of MTX therapy with appropriate dose escalation (maximum 25 mg/week) there is minimal improvement in the signs and symptoms of PsA, it is appropriate to either add or switch to a TNF-α inhibitor, with all of the TNF-a inhibitors equally reasonable choices.[4] SOR Ⓐ

PROGNOSIS/CLINICAL COURSE

- The manifestations of PsA can be severe and widespread, with signs and symptoms that greatly affect patients' quality of life.[7]
- Some patients may have PsA involving only their hands, but it may have a devastating effect on their ability to work and socialize **(Figure 100-8)**.

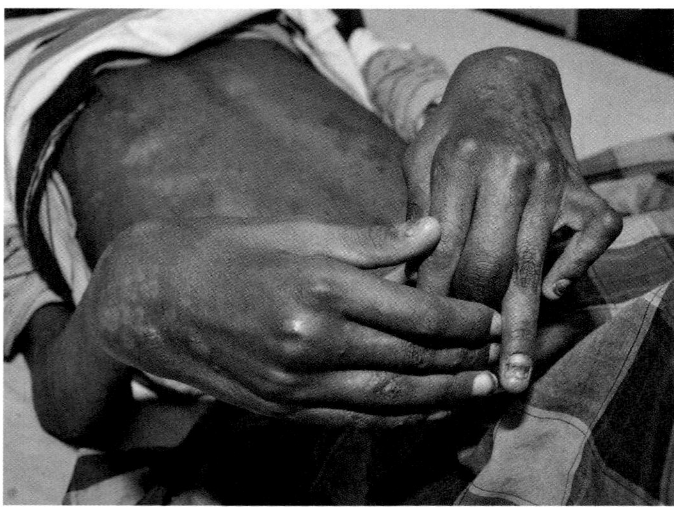

FIGURE 100-8 Psoriatic arthritis in the hands of a man with widespread psoriasis. Multiple metacarpophalangeal (MCP) and proximal interphalangeal (PIP) joints are involved. He also has psoriatic arthritis of the knees. He is a good candidate for systemic therapy. *(Reproduced with permission from Richard P. Usatine, MD.)*

- It is expected that control of the underlying inflammatory process in patients with extensive psoriasis will make a significant difference to their morbidity.[9]
- With correct diagnosis and proper management, most patients with psoriasis continue to lead a normal life.

MAJOR COMPLICATIONS OF PSORIASIS

- Psoriasis is associated with a number of serious systemic comorbidities, including PsA, anxiety, depression, obesity, hypertension, diabetes, hyperlipidemia, metabolic syndrome, smoking, cardiovascular disease, alcoholism, Crohn disease, lymphoma, and systemic multiple sclerosis.[17]
- The associated comorbidities, which can be severe and debilitating, may complicate management and increase the risk of early death.[17,18]

FOLLOW-UP

- If a patient fails to respond to steroid therapy, then the clinician should reassess the need for additional or different treatment. SOR Ⓐ
- Stable patients should be followed every 4 to 6 months.

PATIENT EDUCATION

- Patients should see a physician if any new symptoms appear or the medication is not working.
- Skin care measures—Psoriasis is made worse by scratching, rubbing, and picking; by excessively hot water; and by skin dryness.
- Patients should avoid smoking.
- Patient education is essential for optimizing psoriasis treatment for all categories of disease severity. A good physician-patient relationship fosters confidence and trust, likely improving adherence to treatment.[4]
- Patients should be fully informed of the benefits and risks of their treatments and believe that they have significant input into their treatment plan.[4]

PATIENT RESOURCES

- The National Psoriasis Foundation—**http://www.psoriasis.org.**
- The Psoriasis Association—**https://www.psoriasis-association.org.uk/.**

PROVIDER RESOURCES

- American Academy of Dermatology—**http://www.aad.org.**
- International Federation of Psoriasis Associations—**http://www.ifpa-pso.org.**
- Geneva Foundation for Medical Education and Research. Clearing house for many articles and guidelines for psoriasis—**http://www.gfmer.ch.**
- US National Library of Medicine. *Psoriasis*—**http://www.nlm.nih.gov.**

REFERENCES

1. Gottlieb AB, Lebwohl M, Totoritis MC, et al. Clinical and histologic response to single-dose treatment of moderate to severe psoriasis with an anti-CD80 monoclonal antibody. *J Am Acad Dermatol.* 2002;47(5):692-700.
2. Kane D, Stafford L, Bresnihan B, FitzGerald O. A prospective, clinical and radiological study of early psoriatic arthritis: an early synovitis clinic experience. *Rheumatology (Oxford).* 2003;42(12):1460-1468.
3. Kurd SK, Gelfand JM. The prevalence of previously diagnosed and undiagnosed psoriasis in US adults: results from NHANES 2003-2004. *J Am Acad Dermatol.* 2009;60(2):218-224.
4. American Academy of Dermatology Work Group; Menter A, Korman NJ, Elmets CA, et al. Guidelines of care for the management of psoriasis and psoriatic arthritis: section 6. Guidelines of care for the treatment of psoriasis and psoriatic arthritis: case-based presentations and evidence-based conclusions. *J Am Acad Dermatol.* 2011;65(1):137-174.
5. Shbeeb M, Uramoto KM, Gibson LE, O'Fallon WM, Gabriel SE. The epidemiology of psoriatic arthritis in Olmsted County, Minnesota, USA, 1982-1991. *J Rheumatol.* 2000;27(5):1247-1250.
6. Koo J. Population-based epidemiologic study of psoriasis with emphasis on quality of life assessment. *Dermatol Clin.* 1996;14(3):485-496.
7. Johnson MA, Armstrong AW. Clinical and histologic diagnostic guidelines for psoriasis: a critical review. *Clin Rev Allergy immunol.* 2013;44(2):166-172.
8. Ayala F. Clinical presentation of psoriasis. *Reumatismo.* 2007;59(suppl 1): 40-45.
9. Clarke P. Psoriasis. *Aust Fam Physician.* 2011;40(7):468-473.
10. Nevitt GJ, Hutchinson PE. Psoriasis in the community: prevalence, severity and patients' beliefs and attitudes towards the disease. *Br J Dermatol.* 1996;135(4):533-537.
11. Meier M, Sheth PB. Clinical spectrum and severity of psoriasis. *Curr Probl Dermatol.* 2009;38:1-20.
12. Van Voorhees A, Feldman SR, Koo JYM, et al.; National Psoriasis Foundation. *The Psoriasis and Psoriatic Arthritis Pocket Guide: Treatment Algorithms and Management Options.* 3rd ed. http://www.psoriasis.org/document.doc?id=354. Accessed March 1, 2014.
13. Lowes MA, Kikuchi T, Fuentes-Duculan J, et al. Psoriasis vulgaris lesions contain discrete populations of Th1 and Th17 T cells. *J Invest Dermatol.* 2008 May;128(5):1207-1211.
14. Marble DJ, Gordon KB, Nickoloff BJ. Targeting TNFalpha rapidly reduces density of dendritic cells and macrophages in psoriatic plaques with restoration of epidermal keratinocyte differentiation. *J Dermatol Sci.* 2007;48(2):87-101.
15. Hsu S, Papp KA, Lebwohl MG, et al. Consensus guidelines for the management of plaque psoriasis. *Arch Dermatol.* 2012;148(1): 95-102.
16. Bailey EE, Ference EH, Alikhan A, Hession MT, Armstrong AW. Combination treatments for psoriasis: a systematic review and meta-analysis. *Arch Dermatol.* 2012;148(4):511-522.
17. Guenther L, Gulliver W. Psoriasis comorbidities. *J Cutan Med Surg.* 2009;13(suppl 2):S77-S87.
18. Han C, Lofland JH, Zhao N, Schenkel B. Increased prevalence of psychiatric disorders and health care-associated costs among patients with moderate-to-severe psoriasis. *J Drugs Dermatol.* 2011;10(8):843-850.

101 ANKYLOSING SPONDYLITIS

Heidi Chumley, MD
Richard P. Usatine, MD

PATIENT STORY

A 43-year-old man falls and presents with acute back and diffuse abdominal pain. He has had back pain on and off for years. Also, his wife notes that he has become "stooped" forward in the last few years. The radiographs show flowing ligamentous ossification and syndesmophyte formation about the cervical, thoracic, and lumbar spine consistent with ankylosing spondylitis (bamboo spine) (**Figure 101-1**). The KUB (kidneys, ureters, bladder) view film also shows fusion of the sacroiliac (SI) joints consistent with ankylosing spondylitis (**Figure 101-2**). No fracture, dislocation, or abdominal pathology is identified. The patient's symptoms are treated and nonsteroidal anti-inflammatory drugs (NSAIDs) are started. On follow-up a blood test reveals that he is human leukocyte antigen (HLA)-B27–positive.

INTRODUCTION

Ankylosing spondylitis is an inflammatory disease of the axial spine associated with the HLA-B27 genotype. Symptoms of low back and/or hip pain begin in late adolescence or early adulthood. Diagnosis is based on clinical features and radiographic findings.

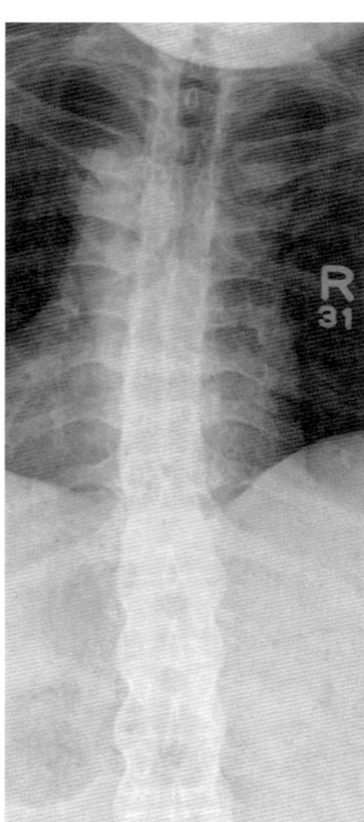

A

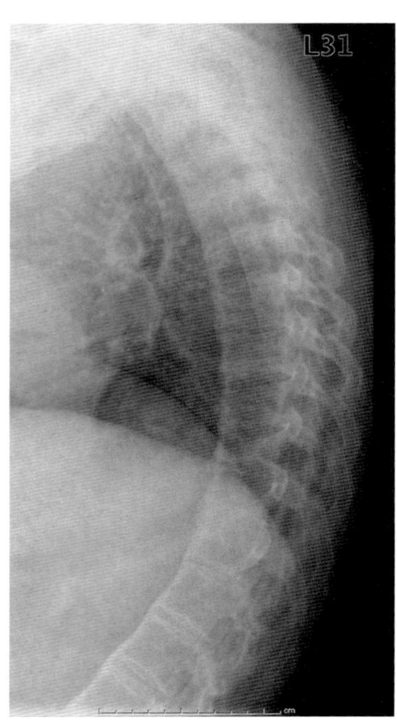

B

FIGURE 101-1 A. Fusion of the vertebral bodies and posterior elements gives the spine the classic "bamboo" appearance seen in ankylosing spondylitis. B. Note the marked kyphosis and the syndesmophytes that are the thin vertical connections between the anterior aspects of the vertebral bodies. They are located in the outer layers of the annulus fibrosis. *(Reproduced with permission from Richard P. Usatine, MD.)*

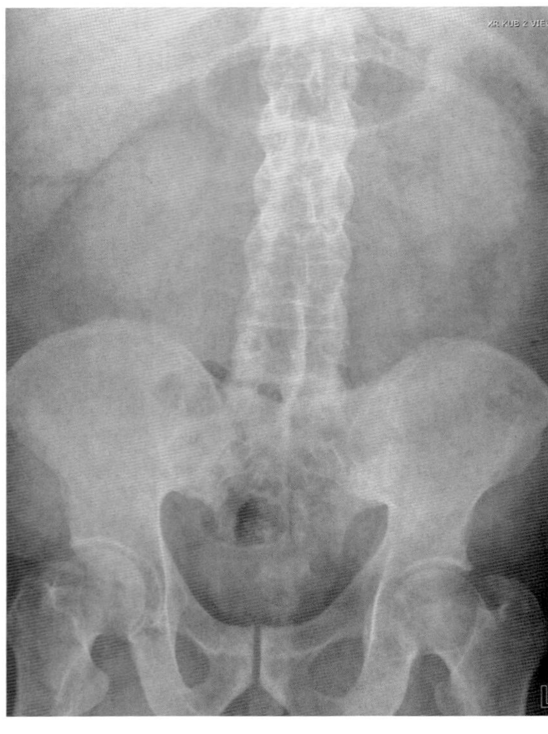

FIGURE 101-2 KUB view showing bamboo spine and fusion of both sacroiliac (SI) joints. *(Reproduced with permission from Richard P. Usatine, MD.)*

EPIDEMIOLOGY

- Prevalence in general population is approximately 0.2% to 0.5%.
- Five percent of patients in primary care with low back pain have a spondyloarthritis, a spectrum of diseases that includes ankylosing spondylitis.[1]
- More common in males than in females (approximate ratio: 4:1).
- Ninety percent of patients are HLA-B27–positive.[2] However, many people with HLA-B27 do not develop the disease.

ETIOLOGY AND PATHOPHYSIOLOGY

- Inflammatory arthritis with a poorly understood pathology.
- Environment and genetic factors result in inflammation.
- Chronic inflammation causes extensive new bone formation.

RISK FACTORS

- Male gender
- HLA-B27–positive genotype

DIAGNOSIS

Mean delay of 7 to 8 years until diagnosis. Consider screening patients younger than 45 years of age with chronic low back pain for more than 3 months.[3]

CLINICAL FEATURES

- Younger patient (younger than 40 years of age at start of disease).
- Inflammatory (pain and stiffness worsen with immobility and improve with motion; symptoms are worse at night or early morning).
- Good response to NSAIDs—Sensitivity = 77%, specificity = 85%, positive likelihood ratio (LR+) 5.1.[1]
- Symptoms of inflammatory back pain have fair sensitivity (75%) and specificity (75%). LR+ is 3.1. Number needed to screen is 7.[1,3]

PHYSICAL EXAMINATION

- Limited range of motion of the spine.
- Tenderness over the spine and sacroiliac joints.
- In the advanced stages, kyphosis may occur with a stooped posture (see **Figure 101-1**).
- Uveitis of the eye is the most common extra-articular manifestation occurring in 20% to 30% of patients. This can present with a red painful eye along with photophobia. The involved eye may have an irregular pupil and a 360-degree perilimbal injection (see Chapter 15, Uveitis and Iritis).

TYPICAL DISTRIBUTION

Pain in lower back and/or sacroiliac joints

LABORATORY TESTING

- HLA-B27 has good sensitivity (90%) and specificity (90%). LR+ is 9. Number needed to screen is 3. Test is expensive.[1,3]
- May also consider HLA-B27 for patients with inflammatory back pain only.[1]

IMAGING

- Radiologic findings confirm the diagnosis; however, these may occur years after the onset of symptoms.
- Plain films—Typical spinal features include erosions, squaring, sclerosis, syndesmophytes, and fractures; may also see sacroiliac joint fusion (**Figure 101-3**). Flowing ligamentous ossification and syndesmophyte formation about the cervical, thoracic, and lumbar spine form the classic bamboo spine described in ankylosing spondylitis (see **Figures 101-1** and **101-2**).
- Magnetic resonance imaging (MRI)—Detects inflammation, such as acute sacroiliitis, which occurs prior to bony change visible by radiographs.

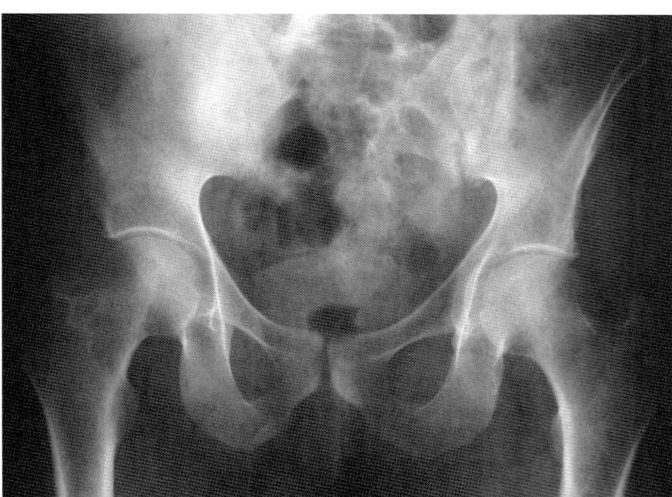

FIGURE 101-3 Ankylosing spondylitis with near fusion of right sacroiliac (SI) joint and pseudowidening (from erosive changes) of the left SI joint. *(Reproduced with permission from Everett Allen, MD.)*

DIFFERENTIAL DIAGNOSIS

The following are causes of back pain in patients younger than age 45 years:

- Lumbar strain or muscle spasm—Acute onset often with precipitating event.
- Herniated disc—Acute onset with pain radiating below the knee into lower leg or foot with numbness, weakness, and/or loss of ankle jerk reflex.
- Vertebral fractures—Risk factors are osteoporosis or significant trauma.
- Abdominal pathology such as pancreatitis—Associated with gastrointestinal (GI) symptoms.
- Kidney diseases—Nephrolithiasis (pain radiating into groin); pyelonephritis (fever, nausea, and urinary symptoms).
- Osteoarthritis—Worse after working; less commonly has inflammatory symptoms (see Chapter 98, Osteoarthritis).
- Other spondyloarthritis (SpA) include psoriatic spondyloarthritis (**Figure 101-4**), SpA associated with inflammatory bowel disease, reactive SpA, and undifferentiated SpA.

MANAGEMENT

- NSAIDs and physical therapy reduce pain. Continuous NSAIDs reduce radiographic progression.[4] SOR Ⓑ
- Disease-modifying antirheumatic drugs (methotrexate, leflunomide) have not been demonstrated to have patient-oriented outcomes.[4] SOR Ⓑ
- Tissue necrosis factor blockers are recommended for patients who fail NSAIDs and physical therapy. Consider treating or referring for treatment with shorter duration of symptoms, elevated acute phase reactants (ie, C-reactive protein), or rapid radiographic progression. SOR Ⓒ

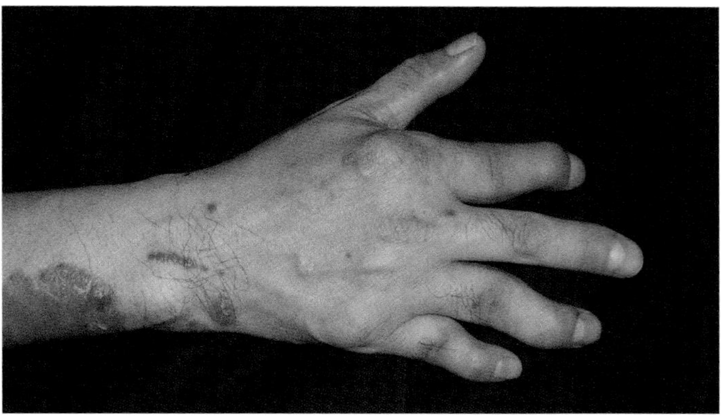

FIGURE 101-4 Psoriatic arthritis showing swan-neck deformities, involvement of proximal interphalangeal (PIP) and distal interphalangeal (DIP) joints and skin plaques. *(Reproduced with permission from Richard P. Usatine, MD.)*

- Infliximab improves pain scores and quality of life within 2 weeks (61% vs 19% placebo).[4] SOR B Many relapse; high cost, but economic analysis is favorable compared to estimated cost of loss of function.[4]
- Adalimumab improves quality of life and function scores by 12 weeks. Improvement continues for up to a year and remains stable through 3 years.[5] SOR B
- Etanercept improves pain scores (60% vs 12%).[4] SOR B Relief comes within 2 weeks. Many relapse; reinitiation works.[4] Seventy-six percent of patients treated with etanercept, compared to 53% of patients treated with sulfasalazine, improved by 20% within 4 months.[6] Improvements in pain, function, and mobility were sustained at 5 years.[7]

PROGNOSIS

Mortality is increased in male patients with ankylosing spondylitis. Leading cause of death was cardiovascular. Risk factors for reduced survival include absence of NSAID use (odds ratio [OR] 4.35), work disability (OR 3.65), increased C-reactive protein (OR 2.68), and diagnostic delay (OR 1.05).[8]

FOLLOW-UP

Follow patients for progression of pain or decreased function using standard ankylosing spondylitis, such as the Ankylosing Spondylitis Disease Activity Score or the Bath Ankylosing Spondylitis Disease Activity Index or Functional Index.

PATIENT EDUCATION

Ankylosing spondylitis is a chronic disease. NSAIDs and physical therapy and exercise are important in controlling pain and slowing progression of disease. If these are ineffective, tissue necrosis factor blockers are effective; however, these are expensive and pain recurs when they are stopped.

PATIENT RESOURCES

- American College of Rheumatology. Patient education handout: *Spondyloarthritis (Spondyloarthropathy)*—**http://www.rheumatology.org/practice/clinical/patients/diseases_and_conditions/spondyloarthritis.asp.**
- The Spondylitis Association of America—**http://www.spondylitis.**org.
- PubMed Health. *Ankylosing Spondylitis*—**http://www.ncbi.nlm.nih.gov/pubmedhealth/PMH0001457/.**

PROVIDER RESOURCES

- Assessment of SpondyloArthritis International Society. *Ankylosing Spondylitis Disease Activity Score Information and Online Calculator*—**http://www.Asas-Group.Org/Research.Php?Id=01#Null.**
- Medscape. Brent LH. *Ankylosing Spondylitis and Undifferentiated Spondyloarthropathy*—**http://emedicine.medscape.com/article/332945.**
- Assessment of SpondyloArthritis International Society (ASAS) and European League Against Rheumatism (EULAR); Zochling J, van der Heijde D, Burgos-Vargas R, et al. ASAS/EULAR recommendations for the management of ankylosing spondylitis. *Ann Rheum Dis.* 2006;65(4):442-452.—**http://www.ncbi.nlm.nih.gov/pmc/articles/PMC1798102/.**

REFERENCES

1. Rudwaleit M, van der HD, Khan MA, et al. How to diagnose axial spondyloarthritis early. *Ann Rheum Dis.* 2004;63(5):535-543.
2. Kim Th, Uhm WS, Inman RD. Pathogenesis of ankylosing spondylitis and reactive arthritis [review] [73 refs]. *Curr Opin Rheumatol.* 2005;17(4):400-405.
3. Sieper J, Rudwaleit M. Early referral recommendations for ankylosing spondylitis (including pre-radiographic and radiographic forms) in primary care [review]. *Ann Rheum Dis.* 2005;64(5):659-663.
4. Zochling J, Braun J. Management and treatment of ankylosing spondylitis [review]. *Curr Opin Rheumatol.* 2005;17(4):418-425.
5. Kimel M, Revicki D, Rao S, et al. Norms-based assessment of patient-reported outcomes associated with adalimumab monotherapy in patients with ankylosing spondylitis. *Clin Exp Rheumatol.* 2011;29(4):624-632.
6. Braun J, van der Horst-Bruinsma IE, Huang F, et al. Clinical efficacy and safety of etanercept versus sulfasalazine in patients with ankylosing spondylitis: a randomized, double-blind trial. *Arthritis Rheum.* 2011;63(6):1543-1551.
7. Martin-Mola E, Sieper J, Leirisalo-Repo M, et al. Sustained efficacy and safety, including patient-reported outcomes, with etanercept treatment over 5 years in patients with ankylosing spondylitis. *Clin Exp Rheumatol.* 2010;28(2):238-245.
8. Bakland G, Gran JT, Nossent JC. Increased mortality in ankylosing spondylitis is related to disease activity. *Ann Rheum Dis.* 2011;70(11):1921-1925.

102 BACK PAIN

Heidi Chumley, MD

PATIENT STORY

A 60-year-old woman presents with chronic low back pain (LBP) that began many years ago. Her back pain waxes and wanes and she has taken acetaminophen and ibuprofen with some relief. About 3 months ago, she began to have daily pain. She recalls no trauma. Her examination is unremarkable other than some decreased flexion. Straight leg raise test is negative. As the patient is older than 55 years of age, radiographs are ordered and they demonstrate degenerative changes in her lumbar spine (**Figure 102-1**). She is started on scheduled acetaminophen and ibuprofen along with an exercise program.

INTRODUCTION

Back pain is one of the most common reasons that adults see their physician. Most acute back pain is a result of mechanical causes. Serious pathology can be recognized by the presence of red flags. Acute back pain is treated with reassurance, returning to activities, and acetaminophen with or without a nonsteroidal anti-inflammatory drug (NSAID). Psychological factors increase the risk of development of chronic pain. Chronic back pain is difficult to treat and the best outcomes are typically achieved by an interprofessional team.

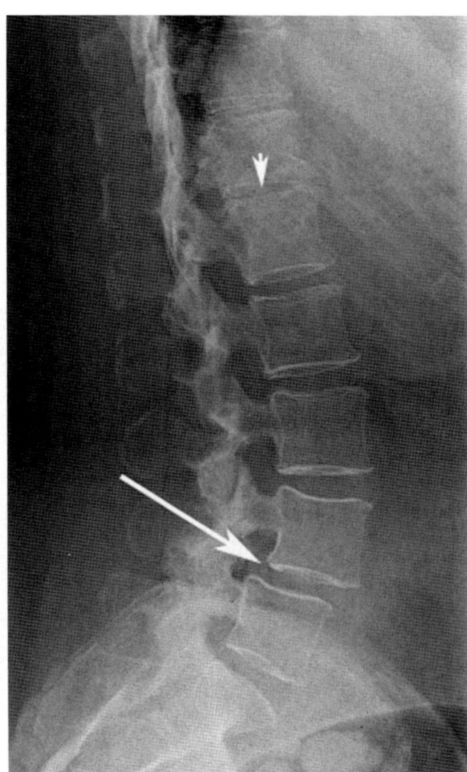

FIGURE 102-1 Lateral view shows grade 1 degenerative spondylolisthesis at L4-L5 (*arrow*), moderate facet osteoarthritis of L5-S1. Marked T12-L1 disc degeneration (*arrowhead*) and mild L4-L5 disc degeneration.

EPIDEMIOLOGY

- Six percent of visits to primary care physicians are for back pain.[1]
- Low back pain 1-year incidence is 20% and 1-year prevalence is 40% in adults.[2]
- Thoracic back pain 1-year prevalence is 15% to 27% in adults.[3]
- Treatment for back and neck problems accounted for approximately $86 billion in health care expenditures in the United States in 2005.[4]
- Prevalence of malignancy in patients with LBP presenting to a primary care office or emergency room is 0.1% to 1.5%.[5]

ETIOLOGY AND PATHOPHYSIOLOGY

- LBP can be caused by pain in the muscles, ligaments, joints, bones, discs, nerves, or blood vessels.[2]
- In 90% of cases, the specific cause of LBP is unclear.[2]
- In 10% of cases, a specific cause such as an infection, fracture, or cancer is identified.

RISK FACTORS

- Older age—Prevalence of LBP increases with age into the sixth decade.[2]
- Low educational status.[2]
- Occupational factors—Manual labor, bending, twisting, and whole-body vibration.[2]
- Psychosocial factors increase the risk of transition from acute to chronic pain.[2]
- Risk factors for cancer—Previous history of cancer (positive likelihood ratio [LR+] 23.7), elevated erythrocyte sedimentation rate (ESR) (LR+ 18), reduced hematocrit (LR+ 18.3).[5]

DIAGNOSIS

The diagnosis can be classified into 3 categories:

1. Nonspecific back pain—Pain for less than 6 weeks (acute), 6 to 12 weeks (subacute), or more than 12 weeks (chronic); negative straight leg raise test; absence of red flags.
2. Radicular syndrome—LBP with radiation down leg; positive straight leg raise test; absence of red flags.
3. Serious pathology—Further workup required for presence of red flags, including age younger than 20 or older than 55 years; significant trauma; fever; unexplained weight loss; neurologic signs of cauda equina; progressive neurologic deficit.

TYPICAL DISTRIBUTION

Lumbar pain is about twice as common as thoracic pain.

LABORATORY TESTING

It is helpful in the presence of red flags:

- Complete blood count (CBC) to evaluate for anemia (malignancy) or leukocytosis (infection).

- Consider human leukocyte antigen (HLA)-B27 in younger patients with inflammatory symptoms.

IMAGING

- In acute back pain without red flags, imaging can be delayed for 6 weeks.
- Radiographs may show degenerative joint disease changes in osteoarthritis; vertebral fractures; malignancies; and findings of ankylosing spondylitis including erosions, sclerosis, syndesmophytes (see Chapter 101, Ankylosing Spondylitis).
- Magnetic resonance imaging (MRI) is the best imaging test for disc herniation and imaging of the spinal cord. Emergent MRI is indicated in patients with suspected spinal cord compromise or cauda equina syndrome.
- Computerized tomography (CT) myelogram is a useful alternative to evaluate disc herniation in patients who cannot undergo MRI.

DIFFERENTIAL DIAGNOSIS

- Osteoporotic vertebral fracture—Acute onset of pain, typically seen in older patients or those at risk for osteoporosis, point tenderness at the level of the fracture, confirmation by plain radiographs demonstrating compression or burst fracture (**Figure 102-2**).
- Spinal stenosis—Pain worse with extension, presence of unilateral or bilateral leg symptoms worse with walking and better with sitting, confirmation by CT or MRI.
- Herniated disc—Radicular pain that is worse with flexion or sitting, may be accompanied by numbness or weakness of foot plantar flexion (L5/S1) or dorsiflexion (L4/L5), MRI confirms the level and shows the type of herniation (**Figures 102-3** and **102-4**).
- Spinal infection/abscess—Most commonly seen in patients who use intravenous (IV) drugs, have diabetes mellitus, have cancer, or have a transplant; symptoms include fever, night pain, night sweats, and elevated ESR. MRI is the study of choice. If neurologic deficit is present, obtain an urgent MRI to evaluate for an abscess, which would require hospitalization and consultation with a spinal surgeon.
- Ankylosing spondylitis (see Chapter 101, Ankylosing Spondylitis)—Pain, most commonly in the low back or sacroiliac joints, usually begins in late adolescence or early adulthood. Pain and stiffness worsen with immobility and improve with motion. HLA-B27 may be positive. Radiographic findings confirm the diagnosis, but occur years after symptoms.

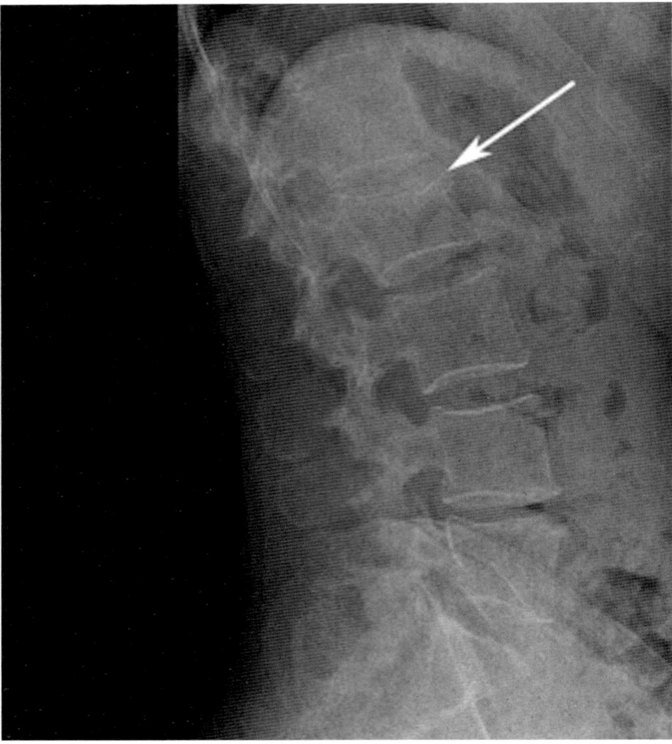

FIGURE 102-2 Lateral view demonstrating the loss of vertebral body height seen with a compression fracture deformity (*arrow*) of the superior end plate of the L2 vertebral body. There is also a mild concave compression deformity of the superior end plate of the L5 vertebral body.

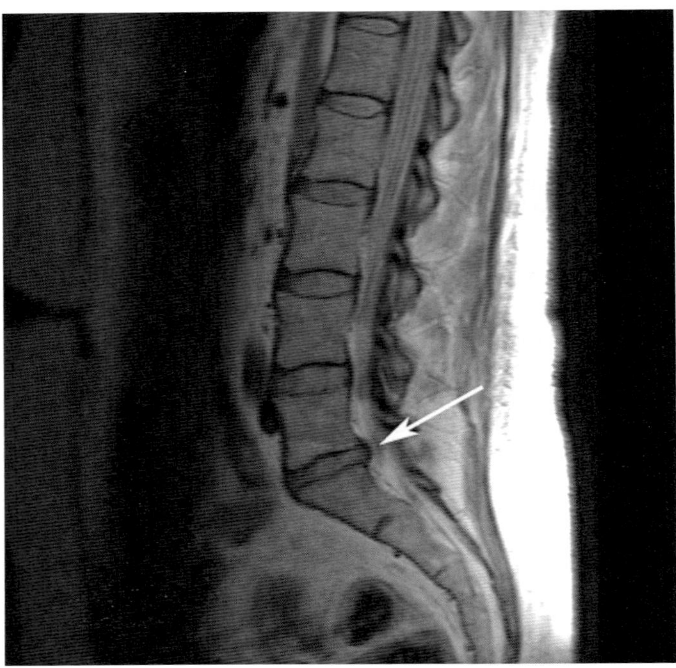

FIGURE 102-3 MRI showing herniated nucleus pulposus (*arrow*) at L5-S1 in a patient with radicular pain and a poor response to 6 weeks of conservative therapy.

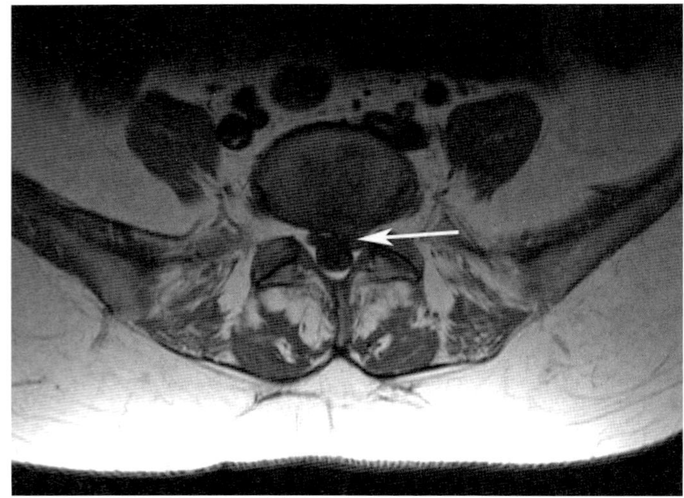

FIGURE 102-4 MRI cross-section demonstrates that the herniated disc (*arrow*) is compressing S1 nerve root.

- Malignancy—Typically seen in an older patient; symptoms of weight loss and night pain; significant anemia; history of cancer; nonresponse to therapy. Often seen on plain radiographs. Bone scan is the most sensitive test.
- Abdominal pathology such as pancreatitis, pyelonephritis, and cholecystitis can present as back pain or pain radiating to the back.

MANAGEMENT

ACUTE BACK PAIN

Most national guidelines agree on the following factors[6]:

- Nonpharmacologic
  - Reassure patients without red flags that they do not have a serious condition, advise them to remain active, discourage bed rest, and encourage an early return to work while back pain is still present.
  - Exercise is considered no more effective than return to normal activities for LBP within the first 4 to 6 weeks.[6]
- Medications
  - Acetaminophen.
  - Add NSAID if needed (ask about gastrointestinal [GI] problems and protect against ulcers as needed).
  - Consider a short course of opiates or muscle relaxers if pain is severe and inadequately treated with acetaminophen and NSAIDs.
  - Consider amitriptyline or gabapentin for radicular pain.
- Complementary and alternative therapy
  - National guidelines differ; some recommend and some do not recommend spinal manipulative therapy for acute back pain.
  - Spinal manipulative therapy has a similar effect on pain relief and functional status as other interventions.[7]
- Referral or hospitalization
  - Patients with cauda equina syndrome should have expedient imaging and urgent referral to a spinal surgeon.
  - Refer patients with serious pathology such as infection, tumor, or fracture to appropriate consultants.

SUBACUTE (6-12 WEEKS) OR CHRONIC (>12 WEEKS) BACK PAIN

Most national guidelines agree on the following recommendations[6]:

- Nonpharmacologic
  - Encourage an exercise program.
  - Recommend cognitive-behavioral therapy.
  - Discourage ultrasound or electrotherapy.
- Medications
  - National guidelines vary on medication recommendations.
  - Start with acetaminophen, then add NSAIDs if needed.
  - Consider adding one of these medications: tramadol, an antidepressant, a benzodiazepine, or an opiate.
- Complementary and alternative therapy
  - Yoga—There have been a number of randomized controlled trials (RCTs) and meta-analyses that have found yoga to be an excellent treatment for chronic and recurrent LBP.[1-4] SOR Ⓐ A 12-week yoga program for adults with chronic or recurrent LBP led to greater improvements in back function than did usual care.[4] Yoga classes were more effective than a self-care book, but not more effective than stretching classes, in improving function and reducing symptoms caused by chronic LBP, with lasting benefits.[3]
- Referral or hospitalization
  - Chronic pain is difficult to treat. Use an interdisciplinary team to maximize effectiveness if possible.
  - Consider referring patients who do not respond to conservative therapy to a pain management specialist or a spine surgeon.

PREVENTION

Good posture, appropriate lifting techniques, maintaining a healthy weight, and enjoying an active lifestyle may help prevent back pain. Adding yoga to an active lifestyle has the potential to prevent recurrent back pain and diminish the pain of chronic back pain.[1-4] SOR Ⓐ

PROGNOSIS

- Patients with nonradicular acute back pain—By 12 months, 40% recover fully.[8]
- Patients with acute back pain who have psychological factors at baseline are more likely to develop chronic LBP.[9]

FOLLOW-UP

Follow-up is determined by etiology. Patients with acute back pain, without red flags, especially those at risk to develop chronic pain, should be followed closely. Patients with chronic pain benefit from ongoing treatment by an interprofessional team.

PATIENT EDUCATION

- Reassure patients without red flags that most acute back pain is not a result of a serious cause and can be treated conservatively.
- Advise patients with chronic back pain that a comprehensive approach to pain management is more likely to result in pain improvement than medications alone.
- Yoga and stretching can be a valuable adjunct to other treatments.[1-4]

PATIENT RESOURCES

- Written and auditory patient information is available in English and Spanish at Family Doctor.org—**http://familydoctor.org/familydoctor/en/diseases-conditions/low-back-pain.html.**
- Yoga therapy for back pain. Audio and visual instructions for patients wanting to use yoga—**http://www.samata.com/video4.php.**
- YouTube. *Gentle yoga routine for lower back relief*—**http://www.youtube.com/watch?v=u0BLxSY2L3Y.**

PROVIDER RESOURCES

- A comprehensive list of red flags for back pain can be found in family practice notebook—**http://www.fpnotebook.com/Ortho/Sx/LwBckPnRdFlg.htm.**
- WebMD Back Pain Health Center. Useful for patients and providers—**http://www.webmd.com/back-pain/default.htm.**

REFERENCES

1. Jordan KP, Kadam UT, Hayward R, et al. Annual consultation prevalence of regional musculoskeletal problems in primary care: an observational study. *BMC Musculoskelet Disord.* 2010;11:144.
2. Hoy D, Brooks P, Blyth F, Buchbinder R. The epidemiology of low back pain. *Best Pract Res Clin Rheumatol.* 2010;24(6):769-781.
3. Briggs AM, Smith AJ, Straker LM, Bragge P. Thoracic spine pain in the general population: prevalence, incidence and associated factors in children, adolescents and adults. A systematic review. *BMC Musculoskelet Disord.* 2009;10:77.
4. Martin BI, Deyo RA, Mirza SK, et al. Expenditures and health status among adults with back and neck problems. *JAMA.* 2008;299:656-664.
5. Henschke N, Maher CG, Refshauge KM. Screening for malignancy in low back pain patients: a systematic review. *Eur Spine J.* 2007;16(10):1673-1679.
6. Koes BW, van Tulder M, Lin CW, et al. An updated overview of clinical guidelines for the management of non-specific low back pain in primary care. *Eur Spine J.* 2010;19(12):2075-2094.
7. Rubinstein SM, van Middelkoop M, Assendelft WJ, et al. Spinal manipulative therapy for chronic low-back pain. *Cochrane Database Syst Rev.* 2011:CD008112.
8. Costa Lda C, Maher CG, McAuley JH, et al. Prognosis for patients with chronic low back pain: inception cohort study. *BMJ.* 2009;339:b3829.
9. Mello M, Elfering A, Egli Presland C, et al. Predicting the transition from acute to persistent low back pain. *Occup Med (Lond).* 2011;61(2):127-131.

103 LUMBAR SPINAL STENOSIS

Gary Ferenchick, MD

PATIENT STORY

An 82-year-old man presents with a 12-month history of lower-back, bilateral buttock, and leg pain, which was worse with walking. The leg pain extended to the knees and was felt both posteriorly and anteriorly. The pain was only present while ambulating and with prolonged standing and was not present at rest. The pain was described as an achy quality, which made it difficult for the patient to carry objects, perform house- or yard work, or climb and descend stairs. His physical examination reveals negative straight-leg raising (SLR) bilaterally, and his range-of-motion at the lumbosacral (LS) spine reveals pain with lumbar extension and lateral motion. His lower-extremity reflexes and muscle strength are normal as are his pedal pulses. A magnetic resonance imaging (MRI) scan reveals spinal stenosis at L2-3, L3-4, and L4-5 with normal lordotic curvature, patent foramina, and the absence of spondylolisthesis (**Figure 103-1**).

INTRODUCTION

- According to the North American Spine Society, degenerative lumbar spinal stenosis (LSS) is "a condition in which there is diminished space available for the neural and vascular elements in the lumbar spine secondary to degenerative changes in the spinal canal. When symptomatic, this causes a variable clinical syndrome of gluteal and/or lower extremity pain and/or fatigue which may occur with or without back pain. Symptomatic lumbar spinal stenosis has certain characteristic provocative and palliative features … including upright exercise such as walking or positionally-induced neurogenic claudication. Palliative features commonly include symptomatic relief with forward flexion, sitting and/or recumbency."[1]

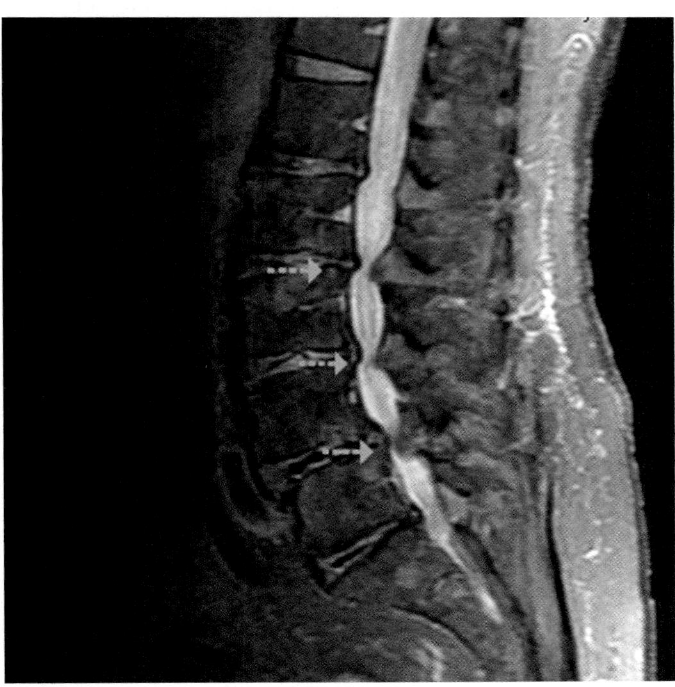

FIGURE 103-1 Spinal canal stenosis with moderate diffuse disk bulging at L2-3, L3-4, and L4-5 (*arrows*). The anteroposterior diameter of the spinal canal measures 6.5 mm. (*Reproduced with permission from Gary Ferenchick, MD.*)

SYNONYMS

Synonyms for LSS are lumbar degenerative spinal stenosis and central canal stenosis.

EPIDEMIOLOGY

- For patients over 65, LSS is the most frequent indication for spinal surgery.[2]
- Lower-extremity pain coexisting with low-back pain occurs in 12% to 21% of older adults.[3]

ETIOLOGY/PATHOPHYSIOLOGY

- Compression of nerve roots from congenital (less common) or degenerative (more common) changes leads to symptoms of LSS.
  - Short pedicles lead to a narrow canal in congenital disease, whereas loss of disk height, changes in the ligamentum flavum, and osteophyte formation lead to canal narrowing in degenerative disease.
- Less-common causes of LSS include the following[3]:
  - Spondylolisthesis
  - Prior spinal surgery
  - Paget disease
  - Cushing syndrome

DIAGNOSIS/SCREENING

HISTORY/SYMPTOMS

Gluteal or lower-extremity symptoms are exacerbated with walking, prolonged standing, or spinal extension and show improvement with sitting or forward flexion (eg, neurogenic claudication).[1]

- If symptoms are not worsened with ambulation, there is a low likelihood of LSS.[1]
- Some patients have more subtle symptoms, such as subjective weakness or fatigue of the legs or gait disturbances and sensory loss.[3]
- Low-back pain is present in the majority of patients with LSS.

PHYSICAL EXAMINATION

- Unsteadiness and a wide-based gait
- Wide-based stance with the Romberg test
- Discomfort with extension and relief with flexion at the LS spine
  - Note that lower-extremity weakness that interferes with normal activity is uncommon[3]

IMAGING

- Order an MRI of the LS spine[1] (**Figures 103-1** and **103-2**). SOR B
  - Sensitivity of MR imaging for LSS is greater than 70%.
    - Up to 19% to 47% of patients between the ages of 60 and 69 have radiographic LSS (depending on the degree of stenosis, < 12 mm vs < 10 mm); however, most of these patients have no symptoms.[4]
    - Computed tomography (CT) or CT myelography is an alternative test in patients in whom an MRI cannot be accomplished or is inconclusive.[1] SOR B

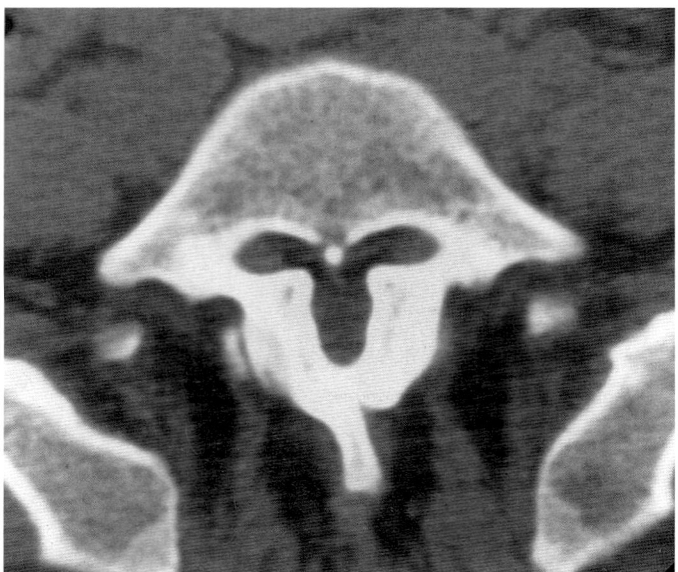

FIGURE 103-2 Severe spinal stenosis seen on computed tomographic scan of the lumbosacral spine in a patient with achondroplasia. (*Reproduced with permission from Skinner HB.* Current Diagnosis and Treatment in Orthopedics. *4th ed. New York, NY: McGraw Hill; 2006.*)

- In patients in whom LSS is clinically suspected but not confirmed with MRI or CT scanning, axial loading of the spine (imaging upright or imaging in both flexion and extension) will increase the sensitivity of the image.[1] SOR B
- Plain films of the LS spine are not as useful as CT or MRI, but they may show predisposing pathology, such as loss of height of the disk space, osteophyte formation, and spondylolisthesis.[3]
- Electromyography is not commonly needed in the diagnosis of LSS but may be helpful in patients with neuropathy (eg, diabetes).[1,2]

DIFFERENTIAL DIAGNOSIS

- Vascular claudication is not altered by changes in position such as flexion and will be associated with an abnormal ankle-brachial index (ABI).
- Compression fracture of the LS spine causes pain that is more acute in onset and is not associated with lower-extremity pain unless there is secondary nerve root impingement.
- Radicular pain from a herniated disk is commonly unilateral and associated with a positive SLR test.

MANAGEMENT

NONOPERATIVE MANAGEMENT

- Nonoperative management includes exercises that occur during flexion (including bicycling) and strengthening of the abdominal musculature.[2]
- Lumbar support corsets worn for short periods may help with posture and provide some pain relief.[1,2]
- Acetaminophen or nonsteroidal anti-inflammatory drugs (NSAIDs) are given for pain treatment.
- Physical therapy (stretching, strengthening, and cycling at low intensities and ultrasound) may improve pain and disability scores.[1] SOR C
- There is insufficient evidence to recommend for or against spinal manipulation, education, traction, or electrical stimulation (transcutaneous electrical nerve stimulation, TENS) for LSS.[1]
- Epidural corticosteroid injections may be helpful for up to 6 months for symptom relief in patients with LSS.[1] SOR B
- After 2 to 10 years, 50% to 70% of patients managed nonoperatively will have their symptoms improved, and 20% to 40% of patients will require surgery to manage symptoms.[1]

OPERATIVE MANAGEMENT

- Decompressive surgery to eliminate pressure on the spinal nerve roots improves outcomes in patients with moderate-to-severe symptoms of LSS and is associated with good or excellent results at 4 years.[1] SOR B
    - Up to 80% of patients with LSS have symptomatic relief with surgery; after 7 to 10 years, a third of these patients have recurrent symptoms, and reoperation rates of 23% have been reported.[2]
- In patients with spondylolisthesis, decompression and fusion are more effective than decompression alone.[2]

PROGNOSIS/CLINICAL COURSE

- The natural history of mild-to-moderate LSS is "favorable" in 33% to 50%, and there are no reports of "rapid or catastrophic" neurological decline in such patients.[1]
- The majority of patients followed for 1 year report no major change in the characteristics of their pain.[5]

PATIENT RESOURCES

- American Association of Neurological Surgeons (AANS). *Lumbar Spinal Stenosis*—**http://www.aans.org/Patient%20Information/Conditions%20and%20Treatments/Lumbar%20Spinal%20Stenosis.aspx.**
- MedlinePlus. *Lumbar Spinal Stenosis*—**http://www.nlm.nih.gov/medlineplus/spinalstenosis.html.**

PROVIDER RESOURCES

- The North American Spine Society. *Evidence-Based Clinical Guidelines for Multidisciplinary Spine Care*— **https://www.spine.org/Documents/ResearchClinicalCare/Guidelines/LumbarStenosis.pdf.**

REFERENCES

1. The North American Spine Society. *Evidence-Based Clinical Guidelines for Multidisciplinary Spine Care*. http://www.spine.org/Documents/LumbarStenosis11.pdf. Accessed September 12, 2012.
2. Katz JN, Harris MB. Lumbar spinal stenosis. *N Engl J Med*. 2008;358:818-825.
3. Suri P, Rainville J, Kalichman L, Katz JN. Does this older adult with lower extremity pain have the clinical syndrome of lumbar spinal stenosis? *JAMA*. 2012;304:2628-2636
4. Kalichman L, Cole R, Kim DH, et al. Spinal stenosis prevalence association with symptoms: the Framingham Study. *Spine J*. 2009;9:545-950.
5. Benoist M. The natural history of lumbar degenerative spinal stenosis. *Joint Bone Spine*. 2002;69:450.

104 COMPRESSION FRACTURES

Gary Ferenchick, MD

PATIENT STORY

A previously healthy 75-year-old woman presents with a 3-day history of midthoracic back pain. The pain started shortly after she bent over to pick up her grandchild. The pain was not relieved with one gram of acetaminophen 3 times daily. Her examination reveals percussion tenderness over the thoracic spine, and a subsequent thoracic spine radiograph reveals compression fractures of T5 and T8 (**Figure 104-1A** and **104-1B**). She is started on 600 mg ibuprofen three times daily (with food) and 200 IU of calcitonin nasal spray to treat her pain. A subsequent bone mineral density study (dual-energy X-ray absorptiometry [DXA] scan) reveals a spinal T score of -2.9, consistent with osteoporosis. Her physician chooses to start her on oral ibandronate (a bisphosphonate) 2.5 mg daily to treat her osteoporosis.

INTRODUCTION

Compression fractures refer to vertebral collapse, often at the midthoracic (T7-T12) or lumbar (L1) spine regions, resulting from osteoporosis. About 66% of osteoporotic vertebral compression fractures (OVCFs) are asymptomatic and are often discovered on chest or abdominal radiographs obtained for other reasons or because of the self-report of loss of height. The remaining 33% of compression fractures are discovered as a result of a sudden onset of back pain, commonly from atraumatic events such as bending, lifting, coughing, or falling from a standing height or less.

SYNONYMS

Other terms for compression fraction are fragility fracture, insufficiency fracture, and low-trauma fracture.

EPIDEMIOLOGY

- Of Americans, 10 million are estimated to have osteoporosis.[1]
- Among Canadians, 1 in 4 women and 1 in 8 men have a lifetime risk of a vertebral compression fracture.[2]
- More than 70% of fractures in those over the age of 70 are caused by osteoporosis.[1]
- In Rochester, Minnesota, the incidence of vertebral compression fractures in women is 145 and in men 73 per 100,000 adults per year.[3]

ETIOLOGY/PATHOPHYSIOLOGY

- Osteoporosis (see Chapter 225, Osteoporosis and Osteopenia).
- Paget disease.
- Celiac disease prevalence is increased in patients with compression fractures.

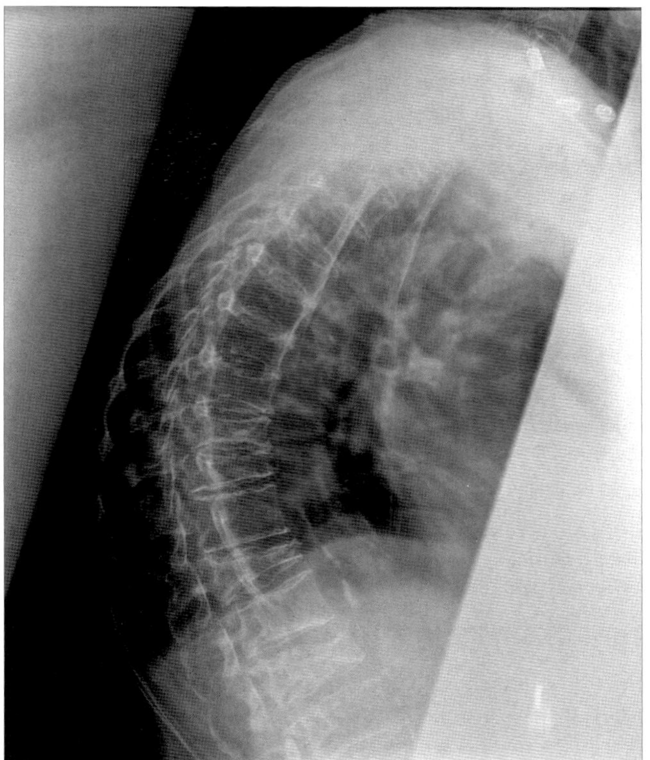

A

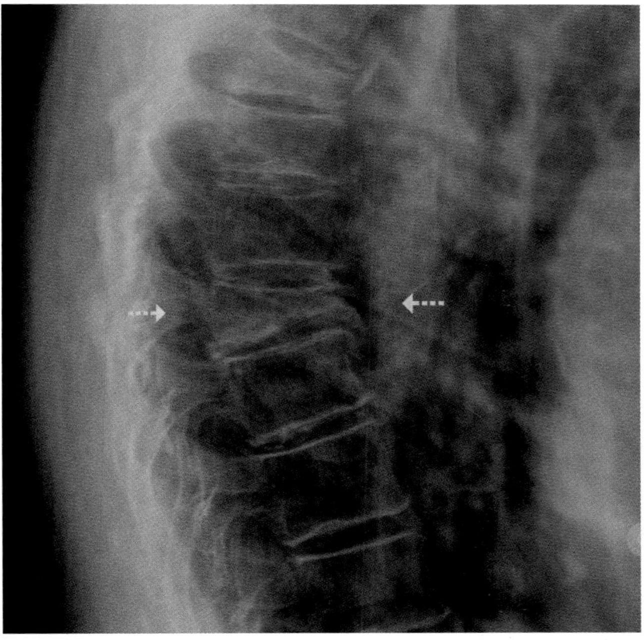

B

FIGURE 104-1 **A.** Compression fractures of T5 and T8 in a postmenopausal woman with osteoporosis. **B.** Close-up of compression fracture (*yellow arrow*) in the same patient. (*Reproduced with permission from Gary Ferenchick, MD.*)

- Risk factors include the following:
  - Age greater than 50
  - Trauma
  - Corticosteroid use
  - Previous fracture
  - Low body weight (<127 pounds)

- Current smoking
- Low calcium intake
- Frailty and fall risk

DIAGNOSIS/SCREENING

HISTORY/SYMPTOMS

- Back pain radiating bilaterally into the anterior abdomen
- Loss of height

PHYSICAL EXAMINATION

- Kyphosis can be found on physical examination; however, this finding does occur independently in the absence of a vertebral compression fracture.[4]
- Loss of height—With 1-cm loss for each vertebral compression fracture.
- The presence or absence of neurological findings that might suggest the presence of spinal canal impingement, requiring neurosurgical intervention.

LABORATORY TESTING

Up to 32% of patients with osteoporosis have a secondary cause.[5] To establish the presence of risk factors or identify secondary causes of osteoporosis, consider ordering the following:

- Serum calcium, phosphate, and parathyroid hormone (if calcium elevated)
- Serum creatinine to screen for chronic kidney disease, which may be associated with secondary hyperparathyroidism
- Complete blood cell count—May be helpful in identifying a nutrition-related anemia or malignancy
- Serum protein electrophoresis (SPEP)—If multiple myeloma is suspected
- Thyroid-stimulating hormone (TSH)—To check for hyperthyroidism or over-replacement, both of which can produce bone loss
- Liver function testing
- Serum testosterone levels in men
- 24-hour cortisol if hypercortisolism is suspected
- Tests for celiac disease if clinical suspicion is present, including serum antigliadin, endomysial and tissue transglutaminase antibodies
- 25-Hydroxy-vitamin D levels

IMAGING

- Order plain radiographs of the thoracic and lumbosacral spine.
  - Common abnormalities include anterior wedge deformities (**Figure 104-1**).
  - Computed tomography (CT), magnetic resonance imaging (MRI), or a radionuclide bone scan may be helpful if the results of the plain film are inconclusive or if malignancy or an infection are suspected (**Figures 104-2** and **104-3**).
- Order a bone mineral density study to establish the presence and severity of osteoporosis (see Chapter 225, Osteoporosis and Osteopenia).

DIFFERENTIAL DIAGNOSIS

- Back pain caused by nonspecific musculoskeletal etiologies such as degenerative joint disease will fail to reveal the presence of a compression fracture in the spine (see Chapter 102, Back Pain).

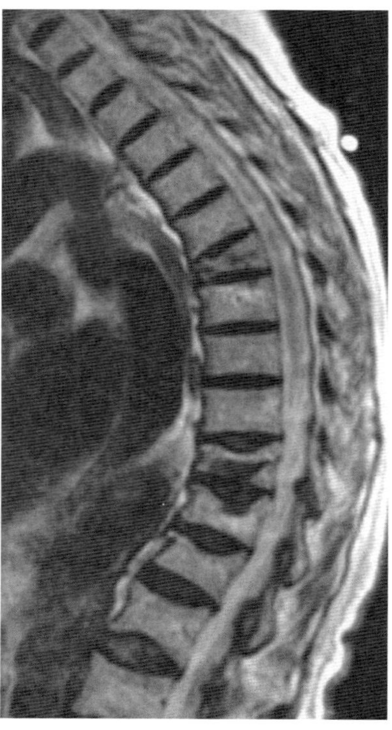

FIGURE 104-2 On this sagittal T1-weighted magnetic resonance image, note the multiple wedge-shaped compressions of the vertebral bodies caused by osteoporosis. (*Reproduced with permission from Tehranzadeh J.* Musculoskeletal Imaging Cases. *New York, NY: McGraw-Hill; 2009.*)

- Other causes of back pain could be considered in the appropriate setting, including the following:
  - Multiple myeloma—This is seen in elderly patients and is associated with anemia and a monoclonal spike on SPEP.

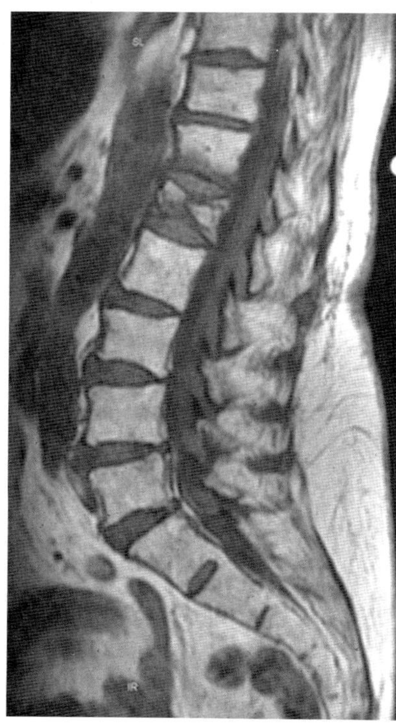

FIGURE 104-3 A compression fracture of L1 is noted on this magnetic resonance image of a 72-year-old postmenopausal woman with osteoporosis. (*Reproduced with permission from Tehranzadeh J.* Musculoskeletal Imaging Cases. *New York, NY: McGraw-Hill; 2009.*)

- Osteomyelitis or discitis—These are associated with fever and destructive changes on imaging studies.
- Metastatic cancer can present with a pathologic fracture.

MANAGEMENT

The American Academy of Orthopedic Surgeons (AAOS) clinical practice guidelines for the treatment of acute symptomatic osteoporotic spinal compression fractures recommends the following[2]:

- Neurologically intact patients who develop a symptomatic spinal compression fracture should be treated with calcitonin for 4 weeks if it can be started within 5 days of symptom onset. SOR B
  - Note that calcitonin provides no added benefit for rest pain experienced by patients with chronic (>3 months) pain from a remote OVCF and only a slight decrease in pain with mobility at 6 months.[6]
  - Calcitonin may be given as an intranasal spray, injectable (subcutaneous or intramuscular), or a rectal suppository.
- Use an L2 nerve root block in a patient who presents with a symptomatic acute L3 or L4 osteoporotic fracture. SOR C
- Kyphoplasty (placement of inflatable bone tamp to restore height of collapsed vertebral body followed by injection of bone cement into the vertebral body) is an option for treating symptomatic but neurologically intact osteoporotic spinal compression fractures. SOR C
- The following have neither a positive nor a negative recommendation:
  - Bed rest
  - Complementary and alternative medicines
  - Opioids
  - Bracing
  - Exercise programs
  - Electrical stimulation
  - Any specific treatment in patients with an osteoporotic fracture who are not neurologically intact
- The AAOS recommends against vertebroplasty (percutaneous injection of bone cement in fractured vertebral body).[7] SOR A
- Ibandronate can be given for the prevention of additional osteoporotic fractures. SOR C

PROGNOSIS/CLINICAL COURSE

- Acute episodes of pain resolve in 4 to 6 weeks; mild pain may last longer.
- About 75% of patients with an OVCF have chronic pain.
- A single osteoporotic fracture is a strong risk factor for subsequent osteoporotic fractures.
  - Of women who develop a single OVCF, 19.2% will have another OCVF within 1 year.[8]
  - The presence of an OVCF increases the risk of subsequent OVCF by 5-fold and the risk of hip and nonvertebral fractures 2.8-fold over 8 years.[9]
- OVCFs are associated with a decreased quality of life and functional impairments and mortality similar to those with hip fractures.[10]

PATIENT EDUCATION

- Treatment with bisphosphonates is commonly required to prevent future osteoporotic fractures, and adequate intake of vitamin D and calcium should be maintained.
- Following a precise dosing regimen for bisphosphonates is important, including reinforcing that the medications should be taken on an empty stomach and the patient should remain upright for at least 30 minutes.
- Adequate weight-bearing exercises are also important in preventing further fractures.

PATIENT RESOURCES

- MedlinePlus. *Compression Fractures of the Back*—**http://www.nlm.nih.gov/medlineplus/ency/article/000443.htm.**

PROVIDER RESOURCES

- American Academy of Orthopaedic Surgeons. *The Treatment of Symptomatic Osteoporotic Spinal Compression Fractures: Guideline and Evidence Report.* 2010. **http://www.aaos.org/research/guidelines/SCFguideline.pdf.**
- National Guideline Clearinghouse. *ACR Appropriateness Criteria Management of Vertebral Compression Fractures.*—**http://guidelines.gov/content.aspx?id=32646.**

REFERENCES

1. Holroyd C, Cooper C, Dennison E. Epidemiology of osteoporosis. *Best Pract Res Clin Endocrinol Metab.* 2008;22(5):671-685.
2. Esses SI, McGuire R, Jenkins J, et al. The treatment of symptomatic osteoporotic spinal compression fractures. *J Am Acad Orthop Surg.* 2011;19(3):176-182.
3. Cooper C, Atkinson EJ, O'Fallon WM, Melton LJ. Incidence of clinically diagnosed vertebral fractures: a population-based study in Rochester, Minnesota, 1985-1989. *J Bone Miner Res.* 1992;7(2):221-227.
4. Bartynski WS, Heller MT, Grahovac SZ, Rothfus WE, Kurs-Lasky M. Severe thoracic kyphosis in the older patient in the absence of vertebral fracture: association of extreme curve with age. *AJNR Am J Neuroradiol.* 2005;26(8):2077-2085.
5. Tannenbaum C, Clark J, Schwartzman K, et al. Yield of laboratory testing to identify secondary contributors to osteoporosis in otherwise healthy women. *J Clin Endocrinol Metab.* 2002;87(10):4431-4437.
6. Knopp-Sihota JA, Newburn-Cook CV, Homik J, Cummings GG, Voaklander D. Calcitonin for treating acute and chronic pain of recent and remote osteoporotic vertebral compression fractures: a systematic review and meta-analysis. *Osteoporos Int.* 2012;23(1):17-38.
7. American Academy of Orthopaedic Surgeons. *The Treatment of Symptomatic Osteoporotic Spinal Compression Fractures: Guideline and Evidence Report.* 2010. http://www.aaos.org/research/guidelines/SCFguideline.pdf. Accessed August 24, 2012.
8. Lindsay R, Silverman SL, Cooper C, et al. Risk of new vertebral fracture in the year following a fracture. *JAMA.* 2001;285(3):320-323.
9. Black DM, Arden NK, Palermo L, Pearson J, Cummings SR. Prevalent vertebral deformities predict hip fractures and new vertebral deformities but not wrist fractures. Study of Osteoporotic Fractures Research Group. *J Bone Miner Res.* 1999;14(5):821-828.
10. Papaioannou A, Watts NB, Kendler DL, Yuen CK, Adachi JD, Ferko N. Diagnosis and management of vertebral fractures in elderly adults. *Am J Med.* 2002;113(3):220-228.

105 GOUT

Mindy A. Smith, MD
Heidi Chumley, MD

PATIENT STORY

A 91-year-old woman arrives by ambulance to the emergency department because she was experiencing severe pain in her right middle finger (**Figure 105-1**). History reveals that she has had swelling of her finger for approximately 1 year. Palpation of the distal interphalangeal joint demonstrated firmness rather than fluctuance. A radiograph of the finger was ordered (**Figure 105-2**). The radiograph and physical examination are consistent with acute gouty arthritis superimposed on tophaceous gout. The diagnosis was confirmed by an aspirate of the finger that demonstrated negatively birefringent, needle-like crystals, both intracellularly and extracellularly. She was given 1.2 mg of colchicine followed by a second dose of 0.6 mg after 1 hour. Her pain was markedly decreased in 4 hours. Her serum uric acid level was determined to be 10.7 mg/dL. The colchicine was used in this case because the risk of using nonsteroidal anti-inflammatory drugs (NSAIDs) was considered to be high because of her previous history of gastric bleeding secondary to NSAIDs.

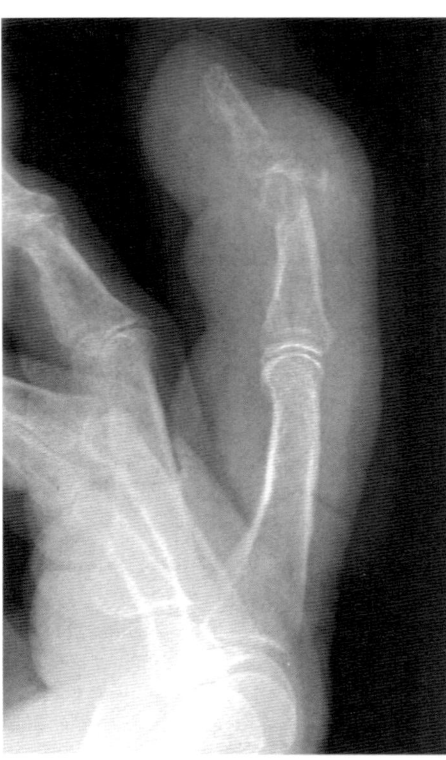

FIGURE 105-2 This X-ray of the finger in **Figure 105-1** shows several tophi (monosodium urate [MSU] deposits) in the soft tissue over the third distal interphalangeal joint. Note the typical punched out lesions under the tophi. This is subchondral bone destruction. (*Reproduced with permission from Geiderman JM. An elderly woman with a warm, painful finger.* West J Med. *2000;172(1):51-52.*)

INTRODUCTION

Gout is an inflammatory crystalline arthritis. Elevated uric acid leads to deposition of monosodium urate (MSU) crystals in the joints resulting in a red, hot, swollen joint. Gout typically begins as a monoarthritis, but can become polyarthritic. Treatment of acute episodes includes NSAIDs, colchicine, or intra-articular steroids. Chronic therapy includes lowering the uric acid level using dietary modifications and urate-lowering drugs.

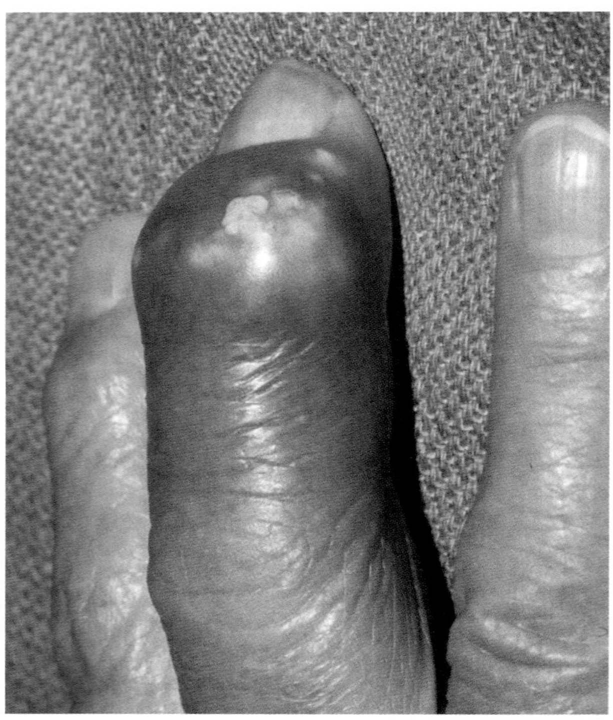

FIGURE 105-1 Acute gouty arthritis superimposed on tophaceous gout. (*Reproduced with permission from Geiderman JM. An elderly woman with a warm, painful finger.* West J Med. *2000;172(1):51-52.*)

EPIDEMIOLOGY

- Gout affects 1% to 2% of the US population and approximately 6% of men older than 80 years of age.[1]
- Gout is more prevalent in men than women.
- Gout usually begins after age 30 years in men and after menopause in women; it is familial in approximately 40% of patients.[1]

ETIOLOGY AND PATHOPHYSIOLOGY

- Defective uric acid metabolism with inefficient renal urate excretion leads to underexcretion of uric acid and an elevated serum uric acid level.
- Overproduction of uric acid, instead of underexcretion, occurs in approximately 10% of patients with gout, and also leads to elevated serum uric acid levels.
- Elevated serum uric acid leads to deposition of MSU crystals in the joints and the kidneys.
- Crystals trigger proinflammatory cytokines, which cause local inflammation, tissue necrosis, fibrosis, and subchondral bone destruction.

RISK FACTORS

- Medications that cause hyperuricemia—Thiazide diuretics, cyclosporine, aspirin (<1 g/d).[2]
- Conditions associated with gout—Insulin resistance, obesity, hypertension, hypertriglyceridemia, hypercholesterolemia, congestive heart failure, renal insufficiency, early menopause, organ transplant.[2,3]
- Dietary—Increased intake of meat and seafood, alcohol, soft drinks, and fructose.[2]

DIAGNOSIS

Following are the diagnostic characteristics useful in predicting gout, based on the 1977 criteria developed by the American College of Rheumatology:

- Monoarthritis
- Redness over the joints
- First metatarsophalangeal (MTP) joint involved (**Figure 105-3**)
- Unilateral first MTP joint attack
- Unilateral tarsal joint attack
- Tophi identified (**Figures 105-1**, **105-4**, and **105-5**)
- Hyperuricemia
- Asymmetric swelling in joint on radiograph
- Subcortical cysts on radiograph
- MSU crystals in joint fluid (**Figure 105-6**)
- Joint fluid culture negative

The presence of 6 of these 11 criteria helps confirm gout (positive likelihood ratio [LR+] 20, negative likelihood ratio [LR−] 0.02).[4]

CLINICAL FEATURES

- Gout usually begins at night as an acute attack over several hours.
- Fever, chills, and arthralgias sometimes precede gout.
- The affected joint is swollen, red, hot, and painful to touch and movement (see **Figures 105-1**, **105-3**, and **105-6**). Symptoms subside in 3 to 10 days.
- Dietary or alcohol excess, trauma, surgery, and serious medical illness can precipitate gout attacks.

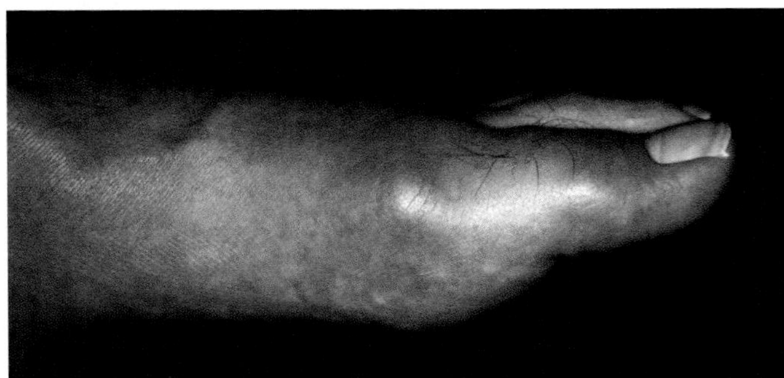

FIGURE 105-3 Podagra. Typical inflammatory changes of gout at first MTP joint. *(Reproduced with permission from Richard P. Usatine, MD.)*

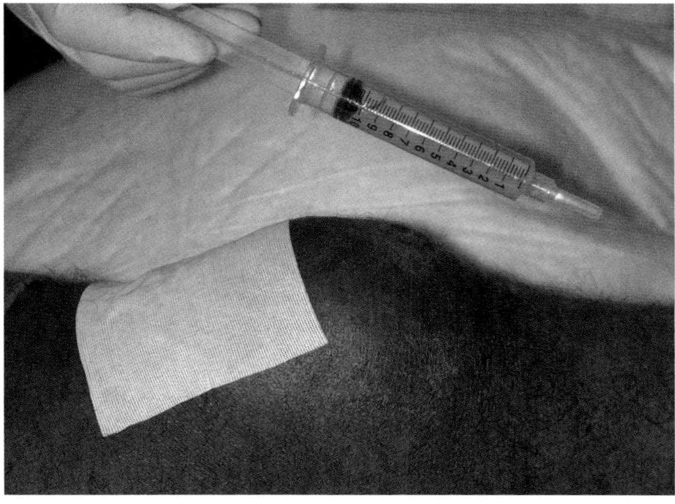

A

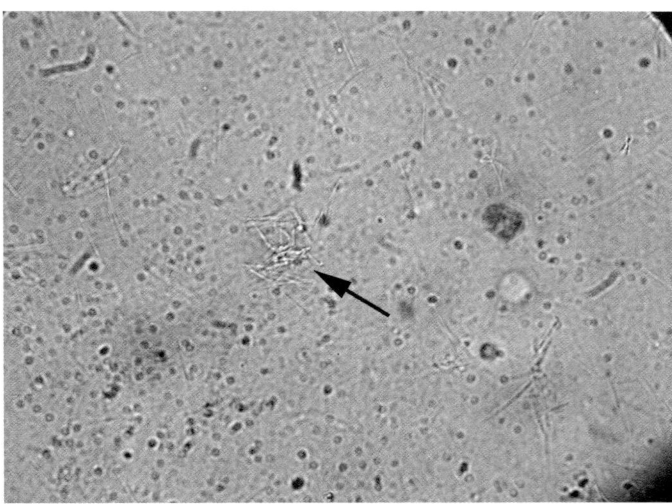

B

FIGURE 105-4 **A.** A 52-year-old homeless man with acute monoarticular gouty arthritis presenting with knee pain and swelling. Knee aspiration revealed a straw-colored effusion. **B.** With light microscopy numerous refractile needle-shaped crystals of uric acid were visualized in the joint fluid. The *arrow* points to a cluster of needle-shaped uric acid crystals. (*Top: Reproduced with permission from Usatine RP, Sacks B, Sorci J. A swollen knee.* J Fam Pract. *2003;52(1):53-55. Bottom: Reproduced with permission from Frontline Medical Communications.*)

TYPICAL DISTRIBUTION

Initially, only one joint may be affected, but other joints commonly involved are fingers and toes (75%) and knees and ankles (50%).

- The most common site is the first MTP joint and the name for gout at this site is podagra (see **Figure 105-3**).
- Joint involvement is often asymmetric.
- Tophi may be seen at the MTP joint, elbow, hands, and ears (see **Figures 105-1**, **105-4**, and **105-5**).

LABORATORY TESTING

- Serum uric acid is often elevated, but is variable from week to week and normal in 25% of patients with gout.
- Measure 24-hour urine for excretion of uric acid.

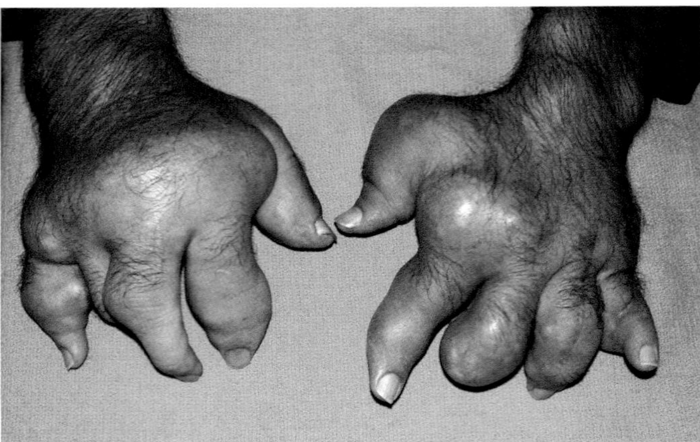

FIGURE 105-5 Severe tophaceous gout causing major deformities in the hands. (*Reproduced with permission from Eric Kraus, MD.*)

- On microscopy, the presence of MSU crystals from synovial fluid or a tophus that are negatively birefringent in polarized light (yellow against a red background) helps to confirm the diagnosis, but there are limited data on the accuracy of crystal identification.
- Even with light microscopy refractile needle-shaped crystals of uric acid can be visualized in the joint fluid (see **Figure 105-6**).

IMAGING

Although radiographs are negative early in the disease, punched-out erosions ("rat bites") are seen later and can be diagnostic, especially if seen adjacent to tophi (see **Figure 105-2**).

DIFFERENTIAL DIAGNOSIS

In addition to gout, the differential diagnosis of inflammatory monoarthritis includes the following:

- Cellulitis—Joint motion is not painful; synovial culture is negative (see Chapter 122, Cellulitis).
- Septic arthritis—Fever; painful motion; synovial fluid has many white blood cells and a positive culture.

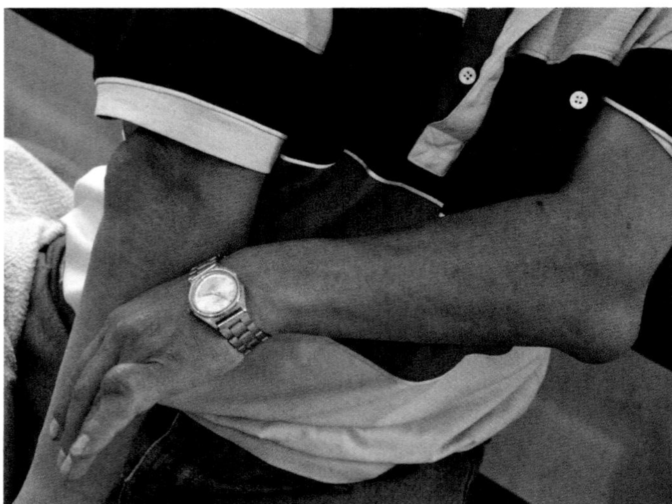

FIGURE 105-6 Tophaceous deposits on both elbows and one finger in a man with gout. (*Reproduced with permission from Richard P. Usatine, MD.*)

- Rheumatic arthritis—Symmetric joint involvement (usually hands); slow onset; synovial culture is negative (see Chapter 99, Rheumatoid Arthritis).
- Pseudogout—Findings like gout; synovial fluid with short rods; crystal refraction blue on red background (calcium pyrophosphate dihydrate).

MANAGEMENT

ACUTE GOUT

- Prescribe an NSAID, such as indomethacin 50 to 75 mg every 6 to 8 hours, in patients without renal impairment (serum creatinine should be <2) or peptic ulcer disease.[5] SOR Ⓑ
- Colchicine can be used in patients who cannot take NSAIDs. Colchicine 1.2 mg followed by 0.6 mg after 1 hour has equivalent efficacy and lower side effects compared to a high dose of 4.8 mg given over 6 hours. One-third of patients will respond.[6] SOR Ⓑ
- In monoarticular gout, consider an intra-articular injection with long-acting steroid (eg, triamcinolone acetonide, 10-40 mg, depending on the size of the joint).[5] SOR Ⓒ

CHRONIC GOUT

The treatment of chronic gout includes modifications in diet and existing medications (if possible) and lowering urate levels.

Treatment measures include the following[1]:

- Nonpharmacologic
  - Reduce the intake of purine-rich foods (eg, organ meats, red meats, and seafood).
  - Increase fluid intake to 2000 mL/d.
  - Lower alcohol intake.
  - Consume dairy products as these may be protective against gout.[1]
- Medications
  - Change medications—Discontinue aspirin (low dose up to 2 g/d causes uric acid retention) and consider stopping a thiazide diuretic. Calcium channel blockers and losartan are associated with a lower risk of gout in patients with hypertension.[7]
  - Lower urate levels with xanthine oxidase inhibitors (eg, allopurinol), uricosuric agents (eg, probenecid), or uricase agents (eg, pegloticase).
  - The level of urinary uric acid helps to determine which medication should be used with levels greater than or equal to 600 mg/24 h indicating a need to halt production with xanthine oxidase inhibitors and levels less than 600 mg/24 h indicating a need for uricosuric drugs.
  - Allopurinol (100-300 mg/d for mild gout; for patients with moderate-to-severe tophaceous gout give 400-600 mg/d with a maximum daily dose of 800 mg/d). Titrate allopurinol to a serum uric acid level less than 6.[8] SOR Ⓑ
  - Give colchicine (0.6 mg twice daily for the first 6 months of therapy) concomitantly during initiation of allopurinol to reduce the frequency and severity of acute flares.[9] SOR Ⓑ
  - Consider uricosuric agents (probenecid, 250 mg twice daily increasing to 2-3 g/d or sulfinpyrazone, 50-100 mg twice daily increasing to 200-400 twice daily) in patients with uric acid excretion of less than 600 mg/24 h, with normal renal function, younger than age 60 years, and no history of renal calculi.[5] SOR Ⓒ

- Consider oral potassium citrate (10-20 mEq 3-4 times a day) to prevent crystal precipitation in the urine as uricosuric agents increase urinary uric acid excretion.
- Pegloticase, a mammalian recombinant uricase, is a medication that degrades urate when administered by intravenous infusion. Early randomized controlled trials show improvements in pain and quality of life; however, adverse events are high. This may be an option for patients with severe gout, allopurinol intolerance or refractoriness, and serum uric acid greater than 8 mg/dL despite conventional therapy.[10]

- Complementary and alternative therapy
  - A number of Chinese and Vietnamese medicinal plants and herbs have xanthine oxidase inhibitory activity, but few have been tested for clinical effectiveness.

PREVENTION

- Intake of dairy products, folate, and coffee lowers the risk of gout.[3]
- In a patient with a prior episode of gout, avoid medications that cause hyperuricemia—Thiazide diuretics, cyclosporine, aspirin (<1 g/d).[2]

PROGNOSIS

- Untreated, recurrent, and more severe attacks are common with 60% of patients experiencing a recurrence in the first year and 25% in the second year.
- Colchicine 0.5 mg up to 3 times a day decreases attacks, but may not decrease joint destruction.[8] SOR B

FOLLOW-UP

Follow patients with an acute flare through resolution and initiation of prophylactic therapy if indicated.

PATIENT EDUCATION

Advise patients to lose weight, minimize alcohol use, eat less meat and seafood, and obtain more protein from dairy.[5]

PATIENT RESOURCES

- The Arthritis Foundation. *Gout Living*—**http://www.arthritis.org/goutliving-basics.php.**
- MedlinePlus. *Gout*—**http://www.nlm.nih.gov/medlineplus/goutandpseudogout.html.**
- The American College of Rheumatology. *Gout*—**http://www.rheumatology.org/practice/clinical/patients/diseases_and_conditions/gout.asp.**

PROVIDER RESOURCES

- Medscape. *Gout and Pseudogout*—**http://emedicine.medscape.com/article/329958.**

REFERENCES

1. Choi HK, Curhan G. Gout: epidemiology and lifestyle choices. *Curr Opin Rheumatol.* 2005;17(3):341-345.
2. Neogi T. Gout. *N Engl J Med.* 2011;362:443-452.
3. Singh JA, Reddy SG, Kundukulam J. Risk factors for gout and prevention: a systematic review of the literature. *Curr Opin Rheumatol.* 2011;23(2):192-202.
4. Silman AJ, Hochberg MC. *Epidemiology of the Rheumatic Diseases.* New York, NY: Oxford University Press; 1993.
5. Wortmann RL. Recent advances in the management of gout and hyperuricemia. *Curr Opin Rheumatol.* 2005;17(3):319-324.
6. Terkeltaub RA, Furst DE, Bennett K, et al. High versus low dosing of oral colchicine for early acute gout flare: twenty-four-hour outcome of the first multicenter, randomized, double-blind, placebo-controlled, parallel-group, dose-comparison colchicine study. *Arthritis Rheum.* 2010;62(4):1060-1080.
7. Choi HK, Soriano LC, Zhang Y, Rodriguez LA. Antihypertensive drugs and risk of incident gout among patients with hypertension: population based case-control study. *BMJ.* 2012;344:d8190.
8. Winklerprins VJ, Weismantel AM, Trinh TH. Clinical inquiries. How effective is prophylactic therapy for gout in people with prior attacks? *J Fam Pract.* 2004;53(10):837-838.
9. Borstad GC, Bryant LR, Abel MP, et al. Colchicine for prophylaxis of acute flares when initiating allopurinol for chronic gouty arthritis. *J Rheumatol.* 2004;31(12):2429-2432.
10. Sundy JS, Baraf HS, Yood RA, et al. Efficacy and tolerability of pegloticase for the treatment of chronic gout in patients refractory to conventional treatment. *JAMA.* 2011;306(7):711-720.

106 OLECRANON BURSITIS

Heidi Chumley, MD

PATIENT STORY

A 60-year-old man presents with swelling in his elbow for the last 2 months. He does not have pain unless he leans on his elbow. He denies any trauma. **Figure 106-1** demonstrates a "goose egg" swelling over the olecranon bursa that is not warm and is tender only to palpation. He has full range of motion. His olecranon bursitis was treated with ice, rest, and nonsteroidal anti-inflammatory drugs (NSAIDs) and he was told to avoid leaning on his elbow.

INTRODUCTION

Olecranon bursitis can be aseptic, from repetitive trauma or systemic disease, or septic, most commonly from gram-positive bacteria. Differences in clinical presentation help differentiate aseptic from septic olecranon bursitis; however, analysis of fluid may be necessary. Aseptic olecranon bursitis is treated with an elbow pad, NSAIDs, and ice. Septic olecranon bursitis is treated with drainage and antibiotics.

SYNONYMS

Olecranon bursitis is also known as popeye elbow, student elbow, or baker elbow.

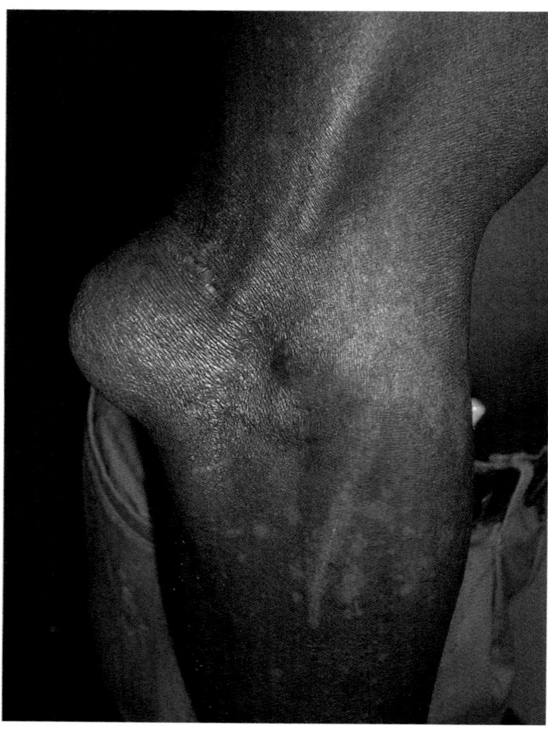

FIGURE 106-1 Chronic aseptic olecranon bursitis in a 60-year-old man showing typical swelling over the olecranon. There is no erythema or tenderness. *(Reproduced with permission from Richard P. Usatine, MD.)*

EPIDEMIOLOGY

Prevalence of aseptic olecranon bursitis is unknown, but is estimated to be twice as common as septic olecranon bursitis.[1]

- Prevalence of septic olecranon bursitis is at least 10 per 100,000 in the general population.[2]
- Peak age of onset is 40 to 50 years.
- Eighty-one percent are male.
- Fifty percent have antecedent trauma.

ETIOLOGY AND PATHOPHYSIOLOGY

Inflammation or degeneration of the sac overlying the olecranon bursa occurs because of the following factors:

- Repetitive motion or trauma, such as direct pressure on the elbow
- Systemic diseases such as gout, pseudogout, and rheumatoid arthritis
- Infection, typically by *Staphylococcus aureus* or another gram-positive organism

RISK FACTORS

- Aseptic bursitis—Occupation-related activities such as leaning on the elbow
- Septic bursitis—Immunocompromised state

DIAGNOSIS

The diagnosis of olecranon bursitis is made clinically, by its typical appearance (**Figures 106-1** and **106-2**). When necessary, joint aspiration verifies the diagnosis and separates septic from aseptic bursitis.

CLINICAL FEATURES OF SEPTIC BURSITIS

- Common symptoms[2]—Pain (87%), redness (77%), and subjective fever or chills (45%)
- Common signs—Erythema (92%), swelling (85%), edema (75%), tenderness (59%), and fluctuance (50%)
- Less common signs—Decreased range of motion (27%) and temperature greater than or equal to 37.8°C (100.04°F) (20%)

CLINICAL FEATURES OF ASEPTIC BURSITIS

- Swelling with minimal pain and tenderness.
- Erythema may be present (see **Figure 106-2**).
- Fever is typically absent.

LABORATORY TESTING

- Erythrocyte sedimentation rate (ESR) and C-reactive protein may be elevated in both septic and aseptic presentations.[3]
- Bursal fluid findings that help differentiate septic from aseptic olecranon bursitis are as below[3]:
  - White blood cell (WBC) count is greater than 30,000 in septic bursitis and less than 28,000 in aseptic bursitis; however, elevated WBC count is also seen in rheumatoid arthritis or gout.

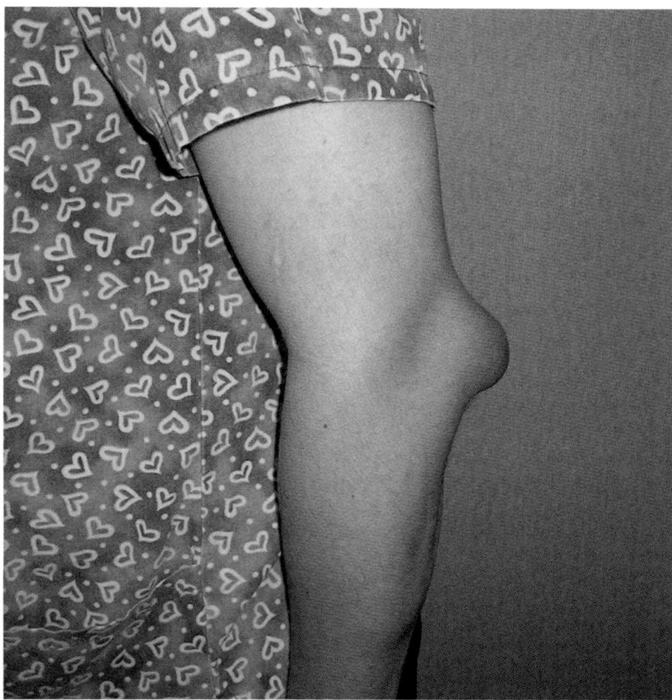

FIGURE 106-2 Aseptic olecranon bursitis secondary to repetitive elbow leaning in this computer programmer. There is some erythema and minimal tenderness. The aspirated fluid was clear. Most patients (70%) retain full extension in the elbow despite swelling over the olecranon. (*Reproduced with permission from Richard P. Usatine, MD.*)

- Neutrophils are seen in septic bursitis; monocytes are seen in aseptic bursitis.
- Glucose less than 50% of serum glucose is found in septic bursitis and greater than 70% of serum glucose is found in aseptic bursitis.
- Gram-positive organisms are seen on Gram stain in septic bursitis.

IMAGING

- Usually not indicated.
- In traumatic bursitis, radiographs may identify a foreign body.
- In atypical cases, magnetic resonance imaging (MRI) may be needed to determine the extent of soft tissue involvement.

ASPIRATION

Aspirate when there is suspicion of infection or crystal disease (moderate pain, fever, warmth over the olecranon)[4] or for discomfort caused by extensive swelling (**Figures 106-3 and 106-4**).[5]

DIFFERENTIAL DIAGNOSIS

Pain and swelling around the elbow joint may be caused by the following factors:

- Gout or pseudogout (acute pain with signs of inflammation), prior history of gout (pseudogout)
- Rheumatoid arthritis (pain, inflammation, loss of range of motion, often involves other joints)
- Septic joint (acute pain, loss of range of motion, fever)
- Hemorrhage into the bursa (history of trauma, bruising)

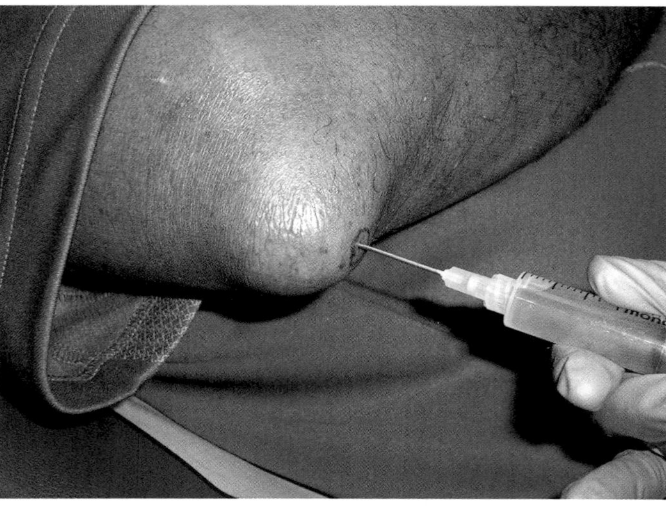

FIGURE 106-3 Aspiration of an olecranon bursitis produced straw-colored fluid with no WBCs or bacteria seen under a microscope. This confirmed the clinical impression that the patient did not have a septic olecranon bursitis. He also had relief of symptoms with the fluid aspiration. (*Reproduced with permission from Richard P. Usatine, MD.*)

Other causes of elbow pain typically without swelling include the following factors:

- Lateral or medial epicondylitis (pain lateral or medial, not over olecranon)
- Ulnar nerve entrapment (concurrent numbness in fingers)

MANAGEMENT

SEPTIC BURSITIS

- Identify organism using Gram stain and culture (**Figure 106-4**).
- If the WBC is slightly elevated and no organisms are seen on Gram stain, treat empirically with oral antibiotics active against gram

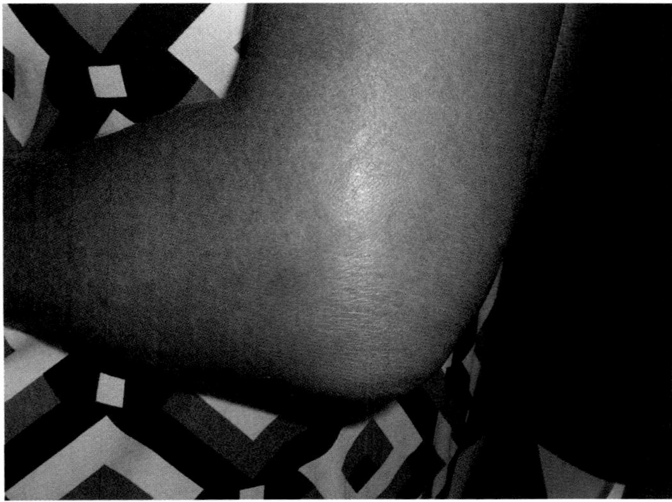

FIGURE 106-4 Septic olecranon bursitis in an immunosuppressed patient with pemphigus vulgaris. Aspiration showed gram-positive cocci on Gram stain and MRSA grew out of the culture. Patient was treated in the hospital with IV vancomycin and then discharged on oral doxycycline when the sensitivities were available and the patient was stable. (*Reproduced with permission from Richard P. Usatine, MD.*)

positives until culture results are available (ie, cephalexin 500 mg twice a day or levofloxacin 500 mg/d).[6] SOR C

- If WBCs are moderately elevated and organisms are seen on Gram stain, use intravenous (IV) medications such as oxacillin or nafcillin 2 g every 6 hours or cefazolin 1 to 2 g every 8 hours.[6] SOR C
- Vancomycin can be considered for penicillin- or cephalosporin-allergic patients or in communities with high rates of methicillin-resistant *S. aureus* (MRSA).[6] SOR C
- Home IV therapy is safe and effective for immunocompetent patients.[2] SOR B
- Hospitalize immunosuppressed patients or those who do not respond to therapy.[6] SOR C
- Aspirate after several days of treatment and continue antibiotics for 5 days after fluid is sterile.[6] SOR C
- Refer to an orthopedic specialist if incision and debridement of the bursa is needed. SOR C

ASEPTIC BURSITIS

- The first line of treatment should be wearing an elbow pad at all times in addition to modification of activities (no leaning on elbows) and NSAIDs as tolerated.
- Patient education about aggravating factors.
- Ice and rest.
- Consider corticosteroid injection for severe pain, persistent, or recurrent fluid accumulation.[6] SOR C Because there is a risk of converting an aseptic olecranon bursitis to a septic one with aspiration and steroid injection, the treatment options noted above should be exhausted prior to consideration of steroid injection.
- Consider surgical referral for recalcitrant fluid accumulation.

ASPIRATION

When indicated, aspirate fluid as follows[5]:

- Flex elbow to 45 degrees.
- Locate triangle formed by lateral olecranon, the head of the radius, and the lateral epicondyle.
- Using sterile technique, insert needle into the soft tissue in the middle of the triangle, pointing toward the medial epicondyle. (If there is a significant amount of fluid, it is hard to miss the fluid regardless of the direction of the needle as long as the needle gauge is sufficient for aspiration. Consider a 20- to 22-gauge needle, and if an 18-gauge needle is to be used, give the patient some local anesthetic first.
- Aspirate fluid and send for complete blood count (CBC), Gram stain, culture, and evaluate for crystals if gout or pseudogout is expected.
- Consider injecting with steroid (see below) only if aspirate is clear and history does not suggest infection.

PROGNOSIS

- Aseptic olecranon bursitis often resolves with conservative therapy.[7]
- Septic bursitis has a recurrence rate of 15% in hospitalized patients treated with surgical interventions and antibiotics.[7]

FOLLOW-UP

Follow septic bursitis until fluid is sterile. Reaspirate after 4 to 5 days of antibiotics and continue antibiotics for 5 days after fluid is sterile.

PATIENT EDUCATION

Limit bursa aggravation by not leaning on elbows or pushing off on elbows when arising. Aseptic and septic bursitis may require multiple aspirations.

PATIENT RESOURCES

- Patient.co.uk. *Olecranon Bursitis*—**http://www.patient.co.uk/health/Olecranon-Bursitis.htm.**

PROVIDER RESOURCES

- American Academy of Family Physicians. *Diagnostic and Therapeutic Injection of the Elbow Region* (includes a description of aspiration technique)—**http://www.aafp.org/afp/2002/1201/p2097.html.**

REFERENCES

1. Stell IM. Septic and non-septic olecranon bursitis in the accident and emergency department–an approach to management. *J Accid Emerg Med.* 1996;13(5):351-353.
2. Laupland KB, Davies HD. Calgary home parenteral therapy program study group. Olecranon septic bursitis managed in an ambulatory setting. The Calgary home parenteral therapy program study group. *Clin Invest Med.* 2001;24:171-178.
3. Wasserman AR, Melville LD, Birkhahn RH. Septic bursitis: a case report and primer for the emergency clinician. *J Emerg Med.* 2009;37(3):269-272.
4. Work Loss Data Institute. *Elbow (Acute and Chronic). National Guidelines Institute.* http://guidelines.gov/content.aspx?id=33179. Updated April 28, 2011. Accessed November 21, 2011.
5. Cardone DA, Tallia AF. Diagnostic and therapeutic injection of the elbow region. *Am Fam Physician.* 2002;66(11):2097-2100.
6. Sheon RP, Kotton CN. *Septic Bursitis. UpToDate.* http://www.utdol.com/utd/content/topic.do?topicKey=skin_inf/12648. Accessed February 24, 2008.
7. Perez C, Huttner A, Assal M, et al. Infectious olecranon and patellar bursitis: short-course adjuvant antibiotic therapy is not a risk factor for recurrence in adult hospitalized patients. *J Antimicrob Chemother.* 2010;65(5):1008-1014.

107 CLAVICULAR FRACTURE

Heidi Chumley, MD

PATIENT STORY

A 22-year-old man presents after falling and landing directly on his lateral shoulder. He had immediate pain and swelling in the middle of his clavicle. His examination revealed a bump in the middle of his clavicle. A radiograph confirmed a midclavicular fracture (**Figure 107-1**). He was treated conservatively with a sling, which he wore for approximately one of the recommended 3 weeks. A follow-up radiograph demonstrated good healing. The bump on his clavicle is still palpable; however, this does not bother him.

INTRODUCTION

Clavicular fractures are common and are usually caused by accidental trauma. The clavicle most commonly fractures in the midshaft (**Figures 107-1** to **107-3**), but can also fracture distally (**Figure 107-4**). Many fractures can be treated conservatively. Refer patients with significant displacement or distal fractures for surgical evaluation.

EPIDEMIOLOGY

Clavicular fractures account for 2.6% of all fractures in adults, with an overall incidence of 64 per 100,000 people per year; midshaft fractures account for approximately 69% to 81% of all clavicle fractures.[1,2]

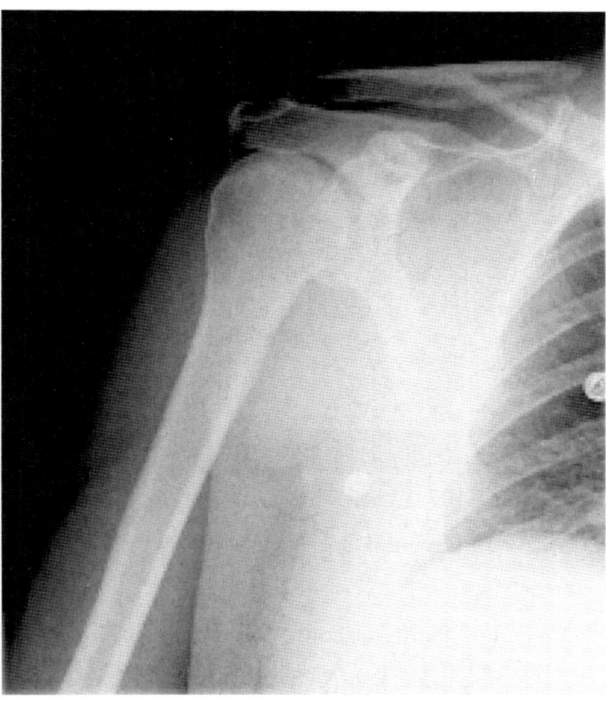

FIGURE 107-1 Midshaft clavicle fracture. Clavicle fractures are designated midshaft (in the middle third), distal (distal third), or medial (medial third). (*Reproduced with permission from John Delzell, MD.*)

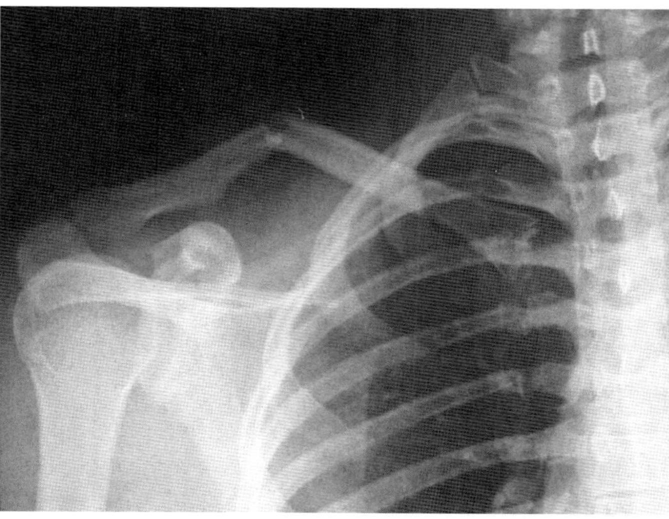

FIGURE 107-2 Midshaft clavicle fracture with angulation. (*Reproduced with permission from John Delzell, MD.*)

ETIOLOGY AND PATHOPHYSIOLOGY

- Most are caused by accidental trauma from fall against the lateral shoulder or an outstretched hand or direct blow to the clavicle; however, stress fractures in gymnasts and divers have been reported.
- Pathologic fractures (uncommon) can result from lytic lesions, bony cancers, or metastases, or radiation.
- Physical assaults or intimate partner violence can cause clavicular fractures.

DIAGNOSIS

CLINICAL FEATURES

- History of trauma with a mechanism known to result in clavicle fractures (ie, fall on an outstretched hand or lateral shoulder, or direct blow)

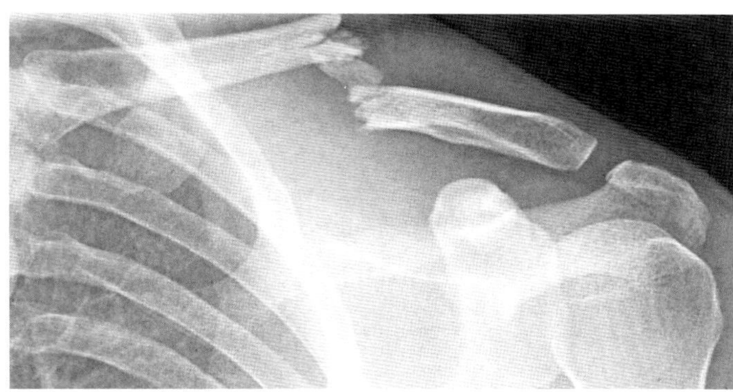

FIGURE 107-3 Midshaft clavicular fracture with proximal fragment displaced superiorly from the pull of the sternocleidomastoid muscle. (*Reproduced with permission from Simon RR, Sherman SC, Koenigsknecht SJ. Emergency Orthopedics the Extremities. New York, NY: McGraw-Hill; 2007:283, Figure 11-32. Copyright 2007.*)

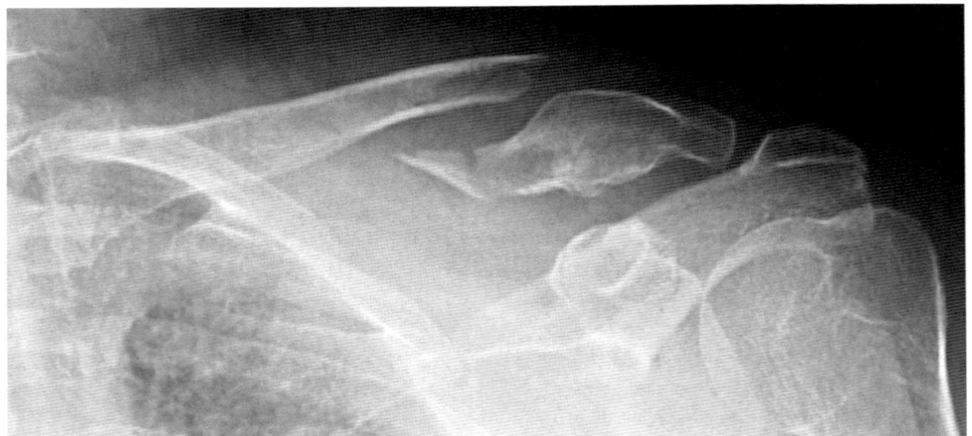

FIGURE 107-4 Distal clavicular fracture. (*Reproduced with permission from Simon RR, Sherman SC, Koenigsknecht SJ.* Emergency Orthopedics the Extremities. *New York, NY: McGraw-Hill; 2007:286, Figure 11-35. Copyright 2007.*)

- Pain and swelling at the fracture site
- Gross deformity at the site of fracture

TYPICAL DISTRIBUTION

For the typical distribution and classification of clavicular fractures, see **Table 107-1**.

IMAGING

Obtain plain films of the clavicle for radiographic evidence of fracture.

DIFFERENTIAL DIAGNOSIS

- Acromioclavicular (AC) separation (**Figure 107-5**)—Fall directly on the "point" of the shoulder or a direct blow, pain with overhead movement, tenderness at the AC joint, and AC joint separation on radiographs
- Sternoclavicular dislocation—Fall on the shoulder, chest and shoulder pain exacerbated by arm movement or when lying down, and a prominence from the superomedial displacement of the clavicle (uncommon)
- Pseudoarthrosis of the clavicle—Painless mass in the middle of the clavicle from failure of the central part of the clavicle to ossify (extremely rare)

MANAGEMENT

Initial assessment includes the following:

- Assess neurovascular status of injured extremity.
- Assess for damage to lungs (pneumothorax or hemothorax).
- Determine the classification and amount of displacement by radiograph (see **Figure 107-1**; see also **Table 107-1**).

NONPHARMACOLOGIC

Most clavicular fractures can be treated nonoperatively, other options include fixation with plates or pins.

Midclavicular fractures

- Treat adults with non- or minimally displaced midshaft clavicular fractures nonoperatively. SOR B
- Place adults in a sling instead of a figure-of-8 bandage. Patients treated with a sling had higher treatment satisfaction than those treated with a figure-of-8 bandage.[3] SOR B
- Midclavicular fractures can be treated with a clavicle brace; treat until radiographic evidence of healing has occurred. SOR C Wearing the brace frees the upper extremities for activities of daily living. The clavicle brace may improve the alignment of the midclavicular fracture.

TABLE 107-1 Typical Distribution/Classification

Group (Approx. %)	Fracture Location	Radiographic Appearance
Group I (80%)	Middle third	Upward displacement (see **Figures 107-1 to 107-3**)
Group II (15%)	Distal third	Medial side of fragment is displaced upward (see **Figure 107-4**)
Type I		Minimal displacement
Type II		Fracture medial to coracoclavicular ligaments; some overlapping of fragments
Type III		Fracture at the articular surface of the acromioclavicular (AC) joint; can look like AC separation
Group III (5%)	Medial third	Medial side of fragment up; distal side down

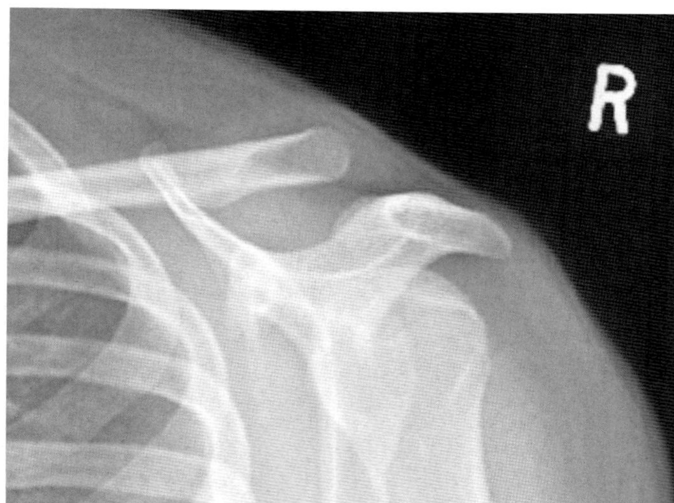

FIGURE 107-5 Acromioclavicular (AC) joint separation (third degree) with a wide AC joint and the clavicle displaced from the acromion. (*Reproduced with permission from Simon RR, Sherman SC, Koenigsknecht SJ.* Emergency Orthopedics the Extremities. *New York, NY: McGraw-Hill; 2007:297, Figure 11-54. Copyright 2007.*)

- Refer patients with initial fracture shortening over 2 cm to discuss operative and conservative options. SOR Ⓑ These patients have a higher risk of a nonunion associated with poor functional outcomes.[4]

Distal clavicular fractures

- Treat patients with nondisplaced distal clavicle fractures conservatively.
- Distal clavicle fractures are commonly treated by wearing a sling for 6 weeks to minimize the weight of the arm pulling on the distal clavicle fragment.
- Some patients with displaced distal clavicle fracture may benefit from surgery. Refer patients, other than the very elderly, to discuss risks and benefits of operative and nonoperative options.[5]

MEDICATIONS

Treat pain as needed with acetaminophen or nonsteroidal anti-inflammatory drugs (NSAIDs).

REFERRAL

- Refer for surgical evaluation, patients with impingement of soft tissue/muscle, instability of shoulder girdle, displacement with skin perforation/necrosis, or risk to mediastinal structures.[2] SOR Ⓒ
- Consider referring patients with displaced fractures. Nonoperative treatment has a 15.1% nonunion rate, whereas operative rates are 0% to 2%.[1]
- Consider consulting with a physician skilled in managing clavicular fractures in patients with a distal clavicle fracture. These fractures have a high rate of nonunion; however, only a portion of nonunions are painful or inhibit function. If the patient continues to have a symptomatic nonunion after many months, surgery may be considered.

PROGNOSIS

- Midclavicular displaced fractures treated nonoperatively have a nonunion rate of up to 15% and a poor functional outcome in up to 5%. Operative nonunion rates are 0% to 2%.[1]
- Patients with distal clavicle fractures treated nonoperatively had nonunion rates of 21%; however, there was no difference in function between those who healed and those with a nonunion.[6] SOR Ⓑ

FOLLOW-UP

Monitor with examination and radiographs until pain has resolved, any lost function has returned, and there is radiographic evidence of healing. Initially, repeat X-ray every 1 to 2 weeks to evaluate for any change in alignment. If the fracture is stable, repeat X-ray every 4 to 6 weeks until the clavicle has healed. If there is no evidence of healing after 2 to 3 months, referral should be considered.

PATIENT EDUCATION

Most clavicle fractures heal without surgery, especially if the fracture is not displaced. Fractures in adults take 6 to 8 weeks to heal. Often, there will be a bump at the site of the healed fracture, which typically does not interfere with any activities.

PATIENT RESOURCES

- American Academy of Orthopedic Surgeons. Patient information handout under *Broken Collarbone*—**http://orthoinfo.aaos.org/topic.cfm?topic=A00072.**

PROVIDER RESOURCES

- Medscape. *Clavicle Fractures*—**http://emedicine.medscape.com/article/1260953.**
- Duke University online. *Wheeless' Textbook of Orthopaedics*—**http://www.wheelessonline.com/ortho/clavicle_fractures.**

REFERENCES

1. Zlowodzki M, Zelle BA, Cole PA, et al; Evidence-Based Orthopaedic Trauma Working Group. Treatment of acute midshaft clavicle fractures: systematic review of 2144 fractures: on behalf of the Evidence-Based Orthopaedic Trauma Working Group. *J Orthop Trauma.* 2005;19(7):504-507.
2. Kubiak R, Slongo T. Operative treatment of clavicle fractures in children: a review of 21 years. *J Pediatr Orthop.* 2002;22:736-739.
3. Andersen K, Jensen PO, Lauritzen J. Treatment of clavicular fractures. Figure-of-eight bandage versus a simple sling. *Acta Orthop Scand.* 1987;58(1):71-74.
4. Preston CF, Egol KA. Midshaft clavicle fractures in adults. *Bull NYU Hosp Jt Dis.* 2009;67(1):52-57.
5. Khan LA, Bradnock TJ, Scott C, Robinson CM. Fractures of the clavicle. *J Bone Joint Surg Am.* 2009;91(2):447-460.
6. Robinson CM, Cairns DA. Primary nonoperative treatment of displaced lateral fractures of the clavicle. *J Bone Joint Surg Am.* 2004;86-A(4):778-782.

108 DISTAL RADIUS FRACTURE

Heidi Chumley, MD
Richard P. Usatine, MD

PATIENT STORY

A 65-year-old woman tripped on a rug in her home and fell on her outstretched hand with her wrist dorsiflexed (extended). She felt immediate pain in her wrist and has difficulty in moving her wrist or hand. She has been postmenopausal for 15 years and has never taken hormone replacement therapy or bisphosphonates. She presented with pain and swelling in her wrist. Her arm had a "dinner-fork" deformity. Radiographs showed a distal radius fracture with dorsal angulation on the lateral view (**Figure 108-1**).

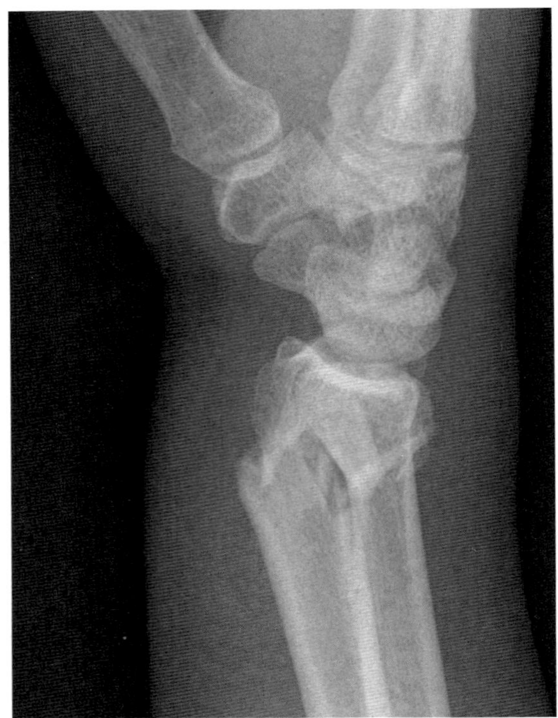

A

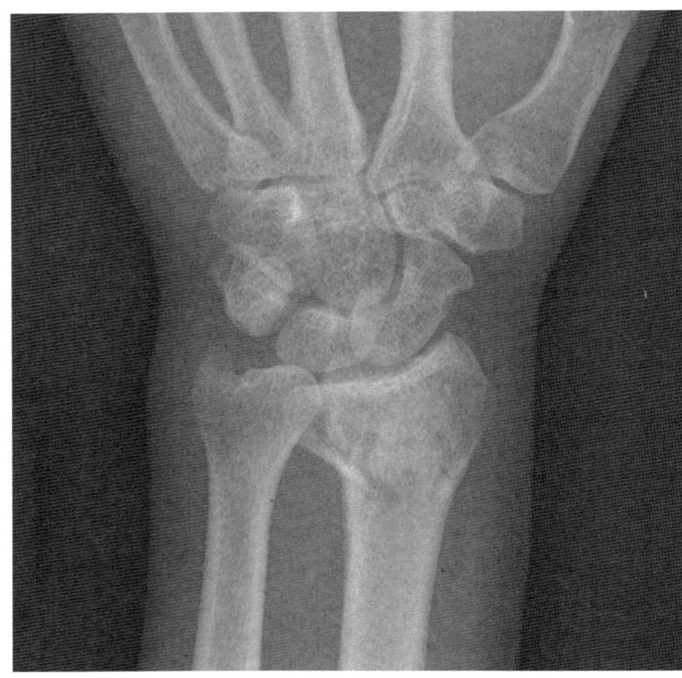

B

FIGURE 108-1 Colles fracture. This occurred after a fall on an extended wrist. A. Lateral view shows a distal radius fracture with dorsal angulation. B. Anterior-posterior view demonstrating a transverse distal radius fracture. *(Reproduced with permission from Rebecca Loredo-Hernandez, MD.)*

INTRODUCTION

Distal radius fractures are common, especially in postmenopausal women. Patients present with wrist pain and a "dinner-fork" deformity. Diagnosis is confirmed by radiographs. Treatment is either operative or nonoperative, based on the degree of displacement and the age of the patient.

SYNONYMS

Colles fracture is the most common type. Other types of distal radius fractures include Smith fracture, Barton fracture, and Hutchinson fracture.

EPIDEMIOLOGY

- More common in older women—Female-to-male ratio of 3.2:1.[1]
- Prevalence—In a community study of 452 people older than age 40 years in the United Kingdom, 10.8% of women and 2.6% of men had a prior distal radius fracture.[2]
- Incidence—In Sweden, the incidence is 115 per 100,000 women and 29 per 100,000 men.[1]

ETIOLOGY AND PATHOPHYSIOLOGY

- Classic history is a fall on an outstretched hand.
- In patients older than 40 years of age, there is a strong association with osteoporosis. Patients with low-impact distal radius fractures have higher rates of osteoporosis than age-matched controls without fractures by bone density measured at the wrist (60% vs 35%; p <0.001; odds ratio [OR], 5.7; 95% confidence interval [CI], 1.2-27.2) and lumbar spine (47% vs 20%; p <0.005; OR, 3.9; 95% CI, 1.1-14.3).[3]
- Postmenopausal women and older men with distal radius fractures have an increased risk for a future hip fracture (relative risk [RR] = 1.53; 95% CI, 1.34-1.74; p <0.001; RR = 3.26; 95% CI, 2.08-5.11; p <0.001, respectively).[4]

RISK FACTORS

Osteoporosis is the risk factor for both men or women.[5]

DIAGNOSIS

Diagnosis is suspected by a compatible history, such as falling on a dorsiflexed wrist and confirmed with a plain radiograph showing the fracture of the distal radius (see **Figure 108-1**).

CLINICAL FEATURES

Patients present with wrist pain and are not able to use the wrist or hand. The distal radius typically angles dorsally, creating the "dinner-fork" deformity (see **Figure 108-1**). Swelling is usually present.

IMAGING

Wrist radiographs (2 views) confirm the fracture and demonstrate the degree of displacement and angulation.

While Colles fracture is the most common distal radius fracture, there are 3 other types that can be classified based on their radiographic appearance, history, and physical examination:

1. Smith fracture is a reverse Colles fracture in which the angulation is in the palmar direction. It usually occurs after a fall on a flexed wrist or a direct blow to the dorsal wrist. The distal radial metaphysis is displaced and angulated in the palmar direction and an associated ulnar styloid fracture may be seen (**Figure 108-2**).
2. Barton fracture is an intra-articular dorsal or volar rim fracture. It occurs with forced wrist dorsiflexion and pronation. A triangular fragment of the distal radial styloid occurs as seen in **Figure 108-3**.

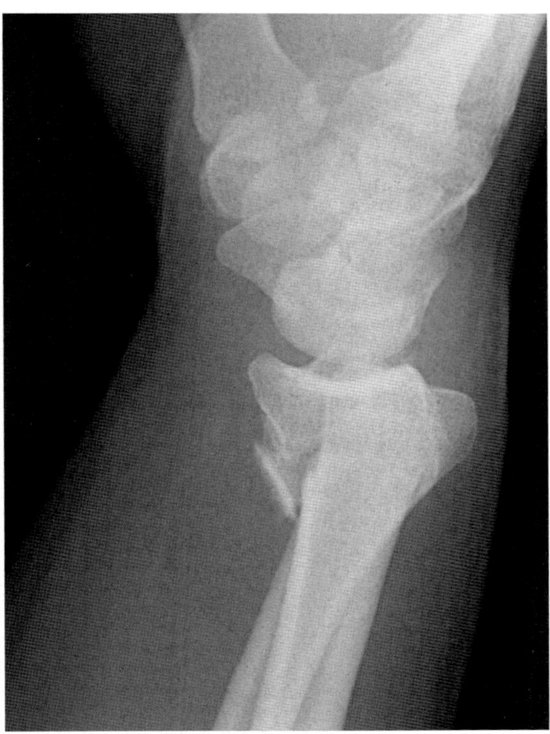

FIGURE 108-2 Smith fracture (Reverse Colles fracture). Lateral view of a fracture of the distal radial metaphysis that is displaced and angulated in the palmar direction. This occurred after a fall on a flexed wrist. *(Reproduced with permission from Rebecca Loredo-Hernandez, MD.)*

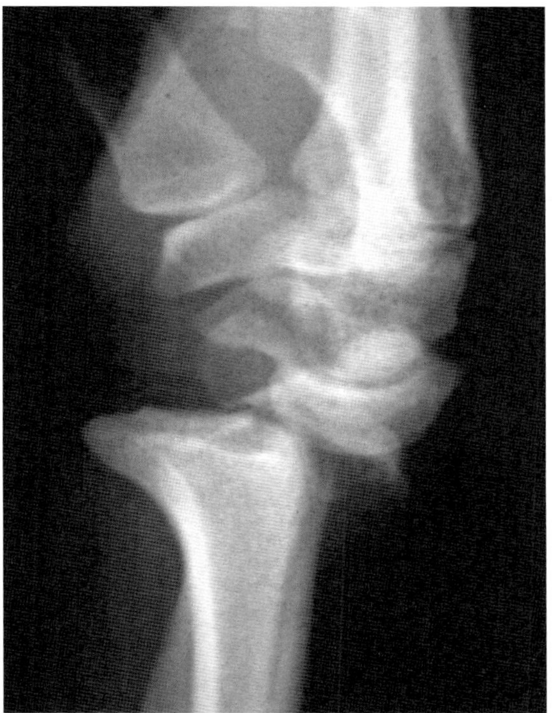

A

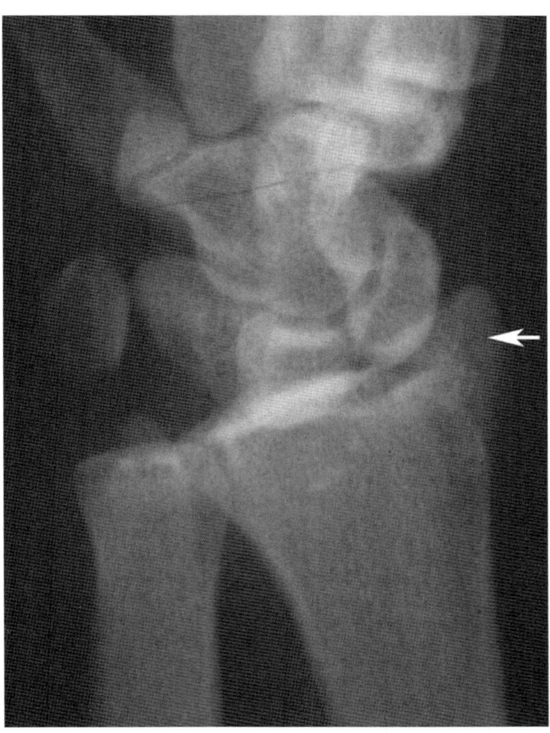

B

FIGURE 108-3 Barton fracture. **A.** Lateral view showing a marginal fracture of the dorsal rim of the radius that is displaced along with the carpus producing a fracture-subluxation. **B.** AP view showing the triangular fragment of the radial styloid (*arrow*). *(Reproduced with permission from Rebecca Loredo-Hernandez, MD.)*

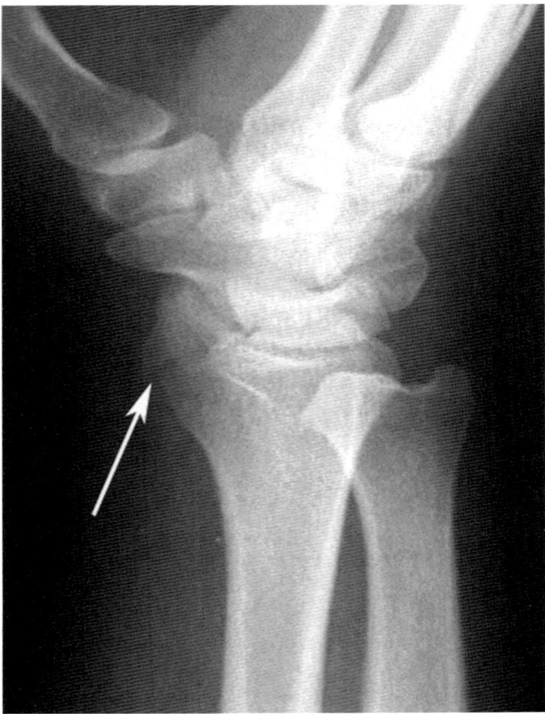

FIGURE 108-4 Hutchinson fracture or chauffeur's fracture. This oblique view demonstrates a fracture through the base of the radial styloid (*arrow*). (*Reproduced with permission from Rebecca Loredo-Hernandez, MD.*)

3. Hutchinson fracture (chauffeur's fracture) is a fracture through the base of the radial styloid. It occurs with forced hyperextension of the wrist. There will be tenderness at the radial styloid on examination and the radiograph indicates a radial styloid fracture (**Figure 108-4**). It is also named a chauffeur's fracture from the past when a chauffeur would crank a car manually and the kick back could break the wrist in this pattern.

DIFFERENTIAL DIAGNOSIS

Other causes of pain at the wrist include the following:

- Scaphoid fracture—Forced hyperextension, tenderness in anatomic snuffbox. Radiograph demonstrates scaphoid fracture (70%).
- de Quervain tenosynovitis—No acute injury, pain on radial side of wrist from abductor pollicis longus and extensor pollicis brevis involvement, pain over the tendon when the thumb is placed into the patient's fist and the wrist is deviated to the ulnar side. Radiographs (not usually done) are normal.

MANAGEMENT

Examine patients for the following associated complications:

- Flexor tendon injuries
- Median and ulnar nerve injuries

Examine radiographs for the following associated injuries:

- Ulnar styloid or neck fractures
- Carpal fractures
- Distal radioulnar subluxation

Management is based on whether the fracture is nonarticular or articular, displaced or nondisplaced, reducible or irreducible (**Figure 108-5**). Although there are multiple accepted classification schemes, the Universal classification of radial fractures, shown in **Table 108-1**, is the most straightforward when determining management.[6] See **Figure 108-6** for

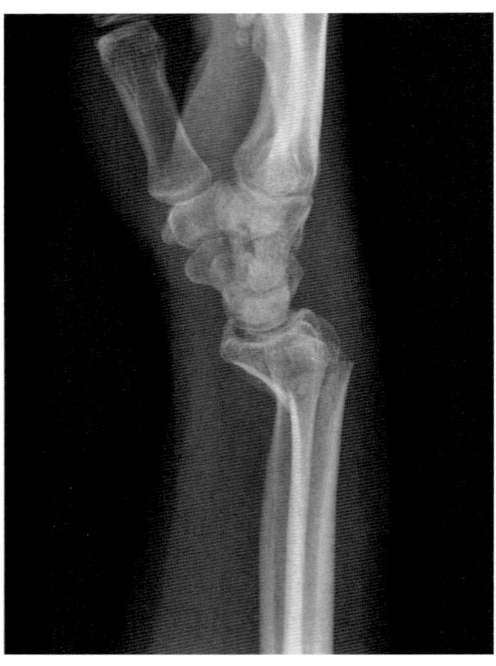

A

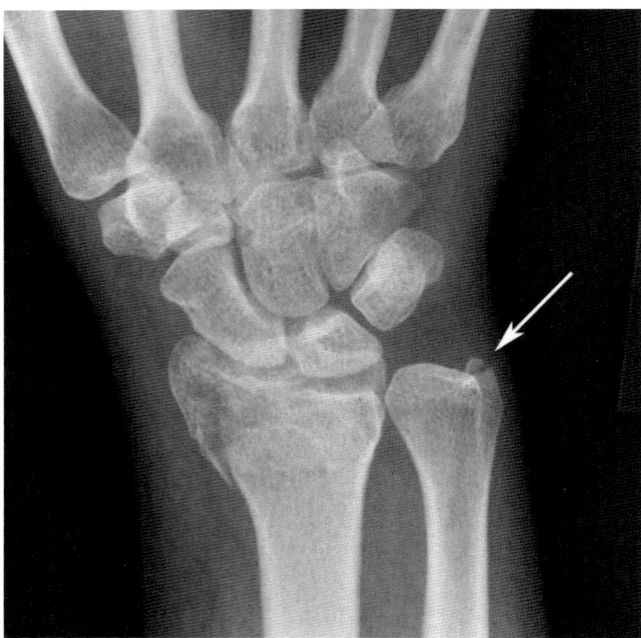

B

FIGURE 108-5 A 31-year-old woman fell on a flexed wrist. **A.** Lateral view shows a distal radius comminuted intra-articular fracture with palmar displacement and volar angulation occurred (Smith fracture). This type IV fracture is best managed with surgery. **B.** Posterior-anterior (PA) view shows an associated ulnar styloid process fracture that is mildly displaced (*arrow*). (*Reproduced with permission from Richard P. Usatine, MD.*)

TABLE 108-1 Universal Classification of Radial Fractures

Fracture Classification	Management
I Nonarticular, nondisplaced	Immobilization with cast or splint[6] for 4-6 weeks
II Nonarticular, displaced	Reduction with cast or splint immobilization; surgical management if irreducible or unstable fracture
III Articular, nondisplaced	Immobilization; pinning if unstable
IV Articular, displaced	Surgical management (see Figures 108-5 and 108-6)

a successful open reduction and internal fixation on a distal radial fracture. Note that this fracture was articular with displacement (see **Figure 108-5**).

- The patient's wrist in most cases is splinted for the first few days after injury to allow swelling to decrease prior to casting.
- On the basis of the type of fracture, the patient's wrist is typically cast from 4 to 6 weeks and followed with serial radiographs.
- The patient should be referred to a musculoskeletal or orthopedic specialist if a fracture requires reduction. Management of displaced fractures is controversial, with surgical and nonsurgical treatments demonstrating similar outcomes.
  - External fixation, compared to cast immobilization, reduces displacement, but does not result in an improved functional outcome in adults.[7]
  - Open reduction and internal fixation was compared to closed reduction and cast fixation in patients older than age 65 years with an unstable displaced radial fracture. At 12 months, there was no difference in range of motion, pain, or function.[8]
- All patients with a low-impact distal radius fracture are at a higher risk for osteoporosis and clinicians should consider screening for osteoporosis.

PREVENTION

Screening for and treatment of osteoporosis may reduce fractures, including distal radial fractures.

PROGNOSIS

Most patients recover adequate function and do not have chronic pain, whether treated nonsurgically or surgically. In nonsurgically treated patients, higher degree of displacement leads to increased risk of poor function or pain 10 years after fracture.[9]

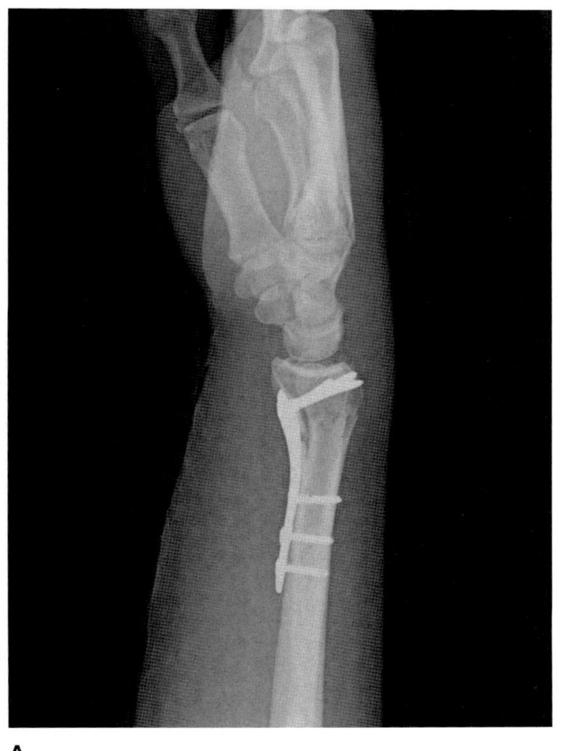

A

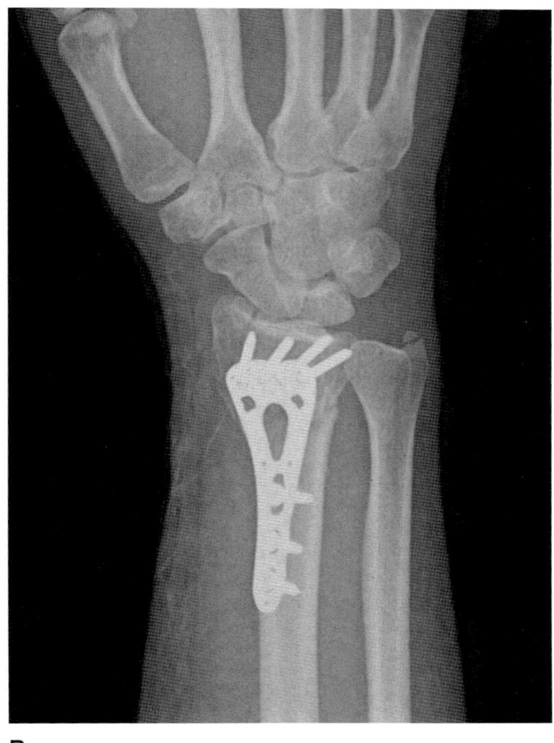

B

FIGURE 108-6 Open reduction and internal fixation of the distal radius fracture in **Figure 108-5**. Volar plate and screw fixation has placed the wrist in anatomic alignment for healing. **A.** Lateral view. **B.** Oblique view. (*Reproduced with permission from Richard P. Usatine, MD.*)

FOLLOW-UP

- Management and follow-up often involve a physician with expertise in managing distal radial fractures.
- Evaluate for osteoporosis.

PATIENT EDUCATION

- Distal radial fractures may result in limitations of wrist function.
- Nontraumatic fractures, in patients older than 40 years of age, may indicate osteoporosis.

PATIENT RESOURCES

- WebMD. *Colles' Fracture*—**http://www.webmd.com/a-to-z-guides/colles-fracture.**

PROVIDER RESOURCES

- *Wheeless' Textbook of Orthopaedics* has additional information about the types of distal radius fractures, classification systems, and radiographic findings—**http://www.wheelessonline.com/ortho/12591.**

REFERENCES

1. Masud T, Jordan D, Hosking DJ. Distal forearm fracture history in an older community-dwelling population: the Nottingham Community Osteoporosis (NOCOS) Study. *Age Ageing.* 2001;30:255-258.
2. Mallmin H, Ljunghall S. Incidence of Colles' fracture in Uppsala. A prospective study of a quarter-million population. *Acta Orthop Scand.* 1992;63(2):213-215.
3. Kanterewicz E, Yanez A, Perez-Pons A, et al. Association between Colles' fracture and low bone mass: age-based differences in post-menopausal women. *Osteoporos Int.* 2002;13(10):824-828.
4. Haentjens P, Autier P, Collins J, et al. Colles fracture, spine fracture, and subsequent risk of hip fracture in men and women. A meta-analysis. *J Bone Joint Surg Am.* 2003;85-A(10):1936-1943.
5. Oyen J, Brudvik C, Gjesdal CG, et al. Osteoporosis as a risk factor for distal radial fractures: a case-control study. *J Bone Joint Surg Am.* 2011;93(4):348-356.
6. Newport ML. Upper extremity disorders in women. *Clin Orthop.* 2000;(372):85-94.
7. Handoll HH, Huntley JS, Madhok R. External fixation versus conservative treatment for distal radial fractures in adults. *Cochrane Database Syst Rev.* 2007;18(3):CD006194.
8. Arora R, Lutz M, Deml C, et al. A prospective randomized trial comparing nonoperative treatment with volar locking plate fixation for displaced and unstable distal radial fractures in patients sixty-five years of age and older. *J Bone Joint Surg Am.* 2011;93(23):2146-2153.
9. Foldhazy Z, Törnkvist H, Elmstedt E, et al. Long-term outcome of nonsurgically treated distal radial fractures. *J Hand Surg Am.* 2007;32(9):1374-1384.

109 METATARSAL FRACTURE

Heidi Chumley, MD

PATIENT STORY

A 37-year-old man inverted his ankle while playing basketball with his teenagers in their driveway. He felt a pop and had immediate pain. He had tenderness over the base of his fifth metatarsal. Having met the Ottawa ankle rules for radiographs (see later), a radiograph was obtained, which revealed a nondisplaced fracture at the base of the fifth metatarsal (**Figure 109-1**).

INTRODUCTION

Most metatarsal fractures involve the fifth metatarsal and include avulsion fractures at the base, acute diaphyseal fractures (Jones fracture), and diaphyseal stress fractures. Fractures of the first through fourth metatarsals are less common but can be associated with a Lisfranc injury. Diagnosis is based on the mechanism of injury or type of overuse activity and radiographic appearance. Treatment depends on the type of fracture. Most metatarsal fractures have a good prognosis; however, Jones fractures have a high rate of nonunion and Lisfranc injuries can result in chronic symptoms.

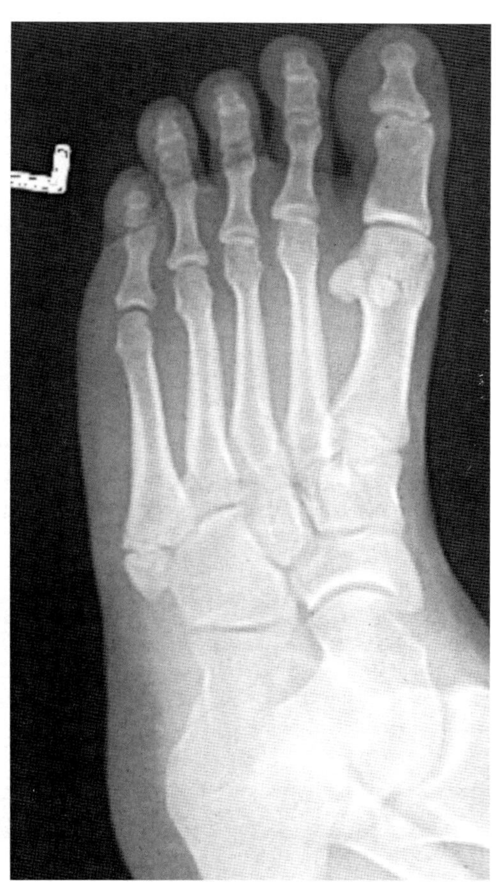

FIGURE 109-1 Fifth metatarsal tuberosity avulsion fracture (dancer fracture). *(Reproduced with permission from Simon RR, Sherman SC, Koenigsknecht SJ.* Emergency Orthopedics, The Extremities. *5th ed. New York, NY: McGraw-Hill; 2007:488, Figure 18-21B. Copyright 2007.)*

SYNONYMS

Avulsion fracture at base of fifth metatarsal: fifth metatarsal tuberosity fracture, dancer fracture, pseudo-Jones fracture.

Jones fracture—Acute diaphyseal fracture of the fifth metatarsal.

EPIDEMIOLOGY

- Foot fractures are common injuries among recreational and serious athletes; however, incidence and prevalence in most populations is unknown.
- In women older than age 70 years, the incidence of foot fractures is 3.1 per 1000 woman-years, and more than 50% of these are fifth metatarsal fractures.[1]
- Fifty percent of metatarsal fractures in adults ages 16 to 75 years involve the fifth metatarsal.[2]
- The majority of fifth metatarsal fractures are avulsion injuries (see **Figure 109-1**).
- Twenty-three percent of elite military personnel sustain metatarsal stress fracture, most of these occur after 6 months of training.[3]

ETIOLOGY AND PATHOPHYSIOLOGY

- Avulsion fractures result when the peroneus brevis tendon and the lateral plantar fascia pull off the base of the fifth metatarsal, typically during an inversion injury while the foot is in plantar flexion.
- Jones (acute diaphyseal) fracture results from landing on the outside of the foot with the foot plantar flexed.
- Diaphyseal stress fractures are caused by chronic stress from activities such as jumping and marching.
- Fractures of the first through fourth metatarsals are caused by direct blows or falling forward over a plantar-flexed foot. These fractures may be associated with a Lisfranc injury.

DIAGNOSIS

The diagnosis of avulsion or Jones fractures is made on plain radiographs in a patient with a history of injury and acute lateral foot pain. Diaphyseal stress fractures may require computed tomography (CT) imaging.

CLINICAL FEATURES

- Avulsion injury—Sudden onset of pain (and tenderness on examination) at the base of the fifth metatarsal after forced inversion with the foot and ankle in plantar flexion
- Acute Jones fracture—Sudden pain at the base of the fifth metatarsal, with difficulty bearing weight on the foot, after a laterally directed force on the forefoot during plantar flexion of the ankle
- Stress fracture—History of chronic foot pain with repetitive motion

IMAGING

- Avulsion fracture—Fracture line at base of fifth metatarsal oriented perpendicularly to the metatarsal shaft (see **Figure 109-1**).

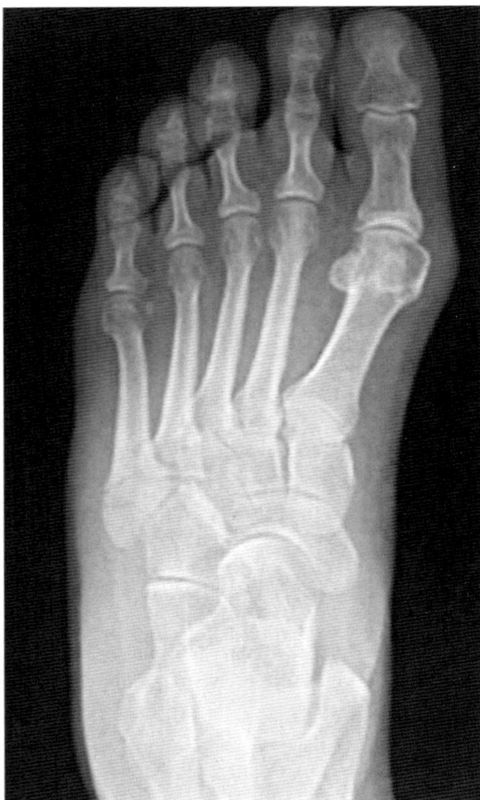

FIGURE 109-2 Jones fracture, a transverse fracture at the junction of the diaphysis and metaphysis. (*Reproduced with permission from Simon RR, Sherman SC, Koenigsknecht SJ.* Emergency Orthopedics, The Extremities. *5th ed. New York, NY: McGraw-Hill; 2007:488, Figure 18-21A. Copyright 2007.*)

May extend into joint with cuboid bone, but does not extend into the intermetatarsal joint.

- Acute Jones fractures (**Figure 109-2**) and stress fractures both have a fracture line through the proximal 1.5 cm of the fifth metatarsal shaft. These should be classified into type I, II, or III as below[4]:
  - Type I fractures have a sharp, narrow fracture line, no intramedullary sclerosis, and minimal cortical hypertrophy.
  - Type II fractures (delayed unions) have a widened fracture line with radiolucency, involve both cortices, and have intramedullary sclerosis.
  - Type III fractures (nonunions) have a wide fracture line, periosteal new bone and radiolucency, and obliteration of the medullary canal by sclerotic bone.
- Early stress fractures may have normal radiographs and can be seen on CT, magnetic resonance imaging (MRI), or bone scan. Ultrasound may be a less expensive option—sensitivity 83%, specificity 76%, positive predictive value 59%, and negative predictive value 92% in one small study.[5]

DIFFERENTIAL DIAGNOSIS

Pain at the fifth metatarsal can also be caused by the following:

- Diaphyseal stress fracture—May be radiographically similar to Jones fracture but is often seen more distally in the shaft; occurs in patients with no injury and history of overuse (eg, ballet dancing, marching).
- Lisfranc injury—Disruption of the tarsal metatarsal joints. This pain is typically in the midfoot and more commonly medial, may be associated with fractures in the first through fourth metatarsals.

X-ray findings that can be confused with foot fractures include the following:

- Accessory ossicles (ie, os peroneum, located at the lateral border of the cuboid) have smooth edges, whereas avulsion fractures have rough edges.

MANAGEMENT

Apply the Ottawa ankle rules to determine which patients with an injury and ankle/foot pain should have an X-ray.[6] SOR Ⓐ Ottawa rules include X-ray patients who cannot walk 4 steps immediately after the injury or who have localized tenderness at the posterior edge or tip of either malleolus, the navicular, or the base of the fifth metatarsal.[6]

- Treat nondisplaced avulsion fractures with an ankle splint or walking boot with ambulation for 3 to 6 weeks.[7] SOR Ⓑ Refer displaced avulsion fractures.
- Consider referring Jones fractures because of the high rate of nonunion caused by the poor blood supply. Type I or II may be treated with immobilization for at least 6 to 8 weeks. Type II can also be treated with surgery. Type III requires surgical repair. Elite athletes or patients needing a faster recovery are often surgically treated.[8] SOR Ⓑ
- Treat stress fractures with elimination of the causative activity for 4 to 8 weeks. Immobilization is often not required. If walking is painful, partial or non–weight bearing for 1 to 3 weeks may be necessary.[9]

Refer patients with the following symptoms[9]:

- Neurovascular compromise, compartment syndrome or open fractures
- First metatarsal fracture, multiple metatarsal fractures, displaced fracture, intra-articular fracture, or Lisfranc injury
- Inadequate response to treatment

PROGNOSIS

Metatarsal fractures have an excellent outcome, with most patients symptom free at 33 months. Patients with higher body mass index (BMI), diabetes mellitus, women, and a dislocation with the fracture have less positive outcomes.[2]

FOLLOW-UP

Patients should be followed every 1 to 3 weeks to evaluate for appropriate clinical and radiographic response to treatment.

PATIENT EDUCATION

Patients with nondisplaced avulsion fractures require a splint or boot, but can remain ambulatory. Jones fractures have a poor blood supply and often do not reconnect, even with immobilization. Surgery may result in a faster return to activities in some cases.

PATIENT RESOURCES

- Patient.co.uk. *Metatarsal Fractures*—**http://www.patient.co.uk/health/Metatarsal-Fractures.htm.**

PROVIDER RESOURCES

- MD+CALC. *Ottawa Ankle Rules*—**http://www.mdcalc.com/ottawa-ankle-rules.**

REFERENCES

1. Hasselman CT, Vogt MT, Stone KL, et al. Foot and ankle fractures in elderly white women. Incidence and risk factors. *J Bone Joint Surg Am.* 2003;85-A(5):820-824.
2. Cakir H, Van Vliet-Koppert ST, Van Lieshout EM, et al. Demographics and outcome of metatarsal fractures. *Arch Orthop Trauma Surg.* 2011;131(2):241-245.
3. Finestone A, Milgrom C, Wolf O, et al. Epidemiology of metatarsal stress fractures versus tibial and femoral stress fractures during elite training. *Foot Ankle Int*. 2011;32(1):16-20.
4. Lehman RC, Torg JS, Pavlov H, Delee JC. Fractures of the base of the fifth metatarsal distal to the tuberosity: a review. *Foot Ankle.* 1987;7:245-252.
5. Banal F, Gandjbakhch F, Foltz V, et al. Sensitivity and specificity of ultrasonography in early diagnosis of metatarsal bone stress fractures: a pilot study of 37 patients. *J Rheumatol.* 2009;36(8):1715-1719.
6. Stiell IG, Greenberg GH, Mcknight RD, et al. Decision rules for the use of radiography in acute ankle injuries. Refinement and prospective validation. *JAMA.* 1993;269:1127-1132.
7. Konkel KF, Menger AG, Retzlaff SA. Nonoperative treatment of fifth metatarsal fractures in an orthopaedic suburban private multi-speciality practice. *Foot Ankle Int*. 2005;26:704-707.
8. Portland G, Kelikian A, Kodros S. Acute surgical management of Jones' fractures. *Foot Ankle Int.* 2003;24:829-833.
9. Hatch RL, Alsobrook JA, Clugston JR. Diagnosis and management of metatarsal fractures. *Am Fam Physician.* 2007;76(6):817-826.

110 HIP FRACTURE

Heidi Chumley, MD

PATIENT STORY

A 60-year-old woman comes to the emergency room for hip pain. She felt a pop in her hip accompanied by the immediate onset of pain that prohibited her from walking. She had fallen 2 days prior. **Figure 110-1** shows a transcervical left femoral neck fracture with varus angulation and superior offset of the distal fracture fragment. She was evaluated by an orthopedic surgeon and underwent surgery the next day (**Figure 110-2**). After many months of rehabilitation, she was able to walk again.

EPIDEMIOLOGY

- Approximately 300,000 hip fractures per year occur in the United States.[1]
- Seventy percent to 80% of hip fractures occur in women.[1]
- Average age is 70 to 80 years; risk increases with age.[1]
- Half of the patients with a hip fracture have osteoporosis.[2]

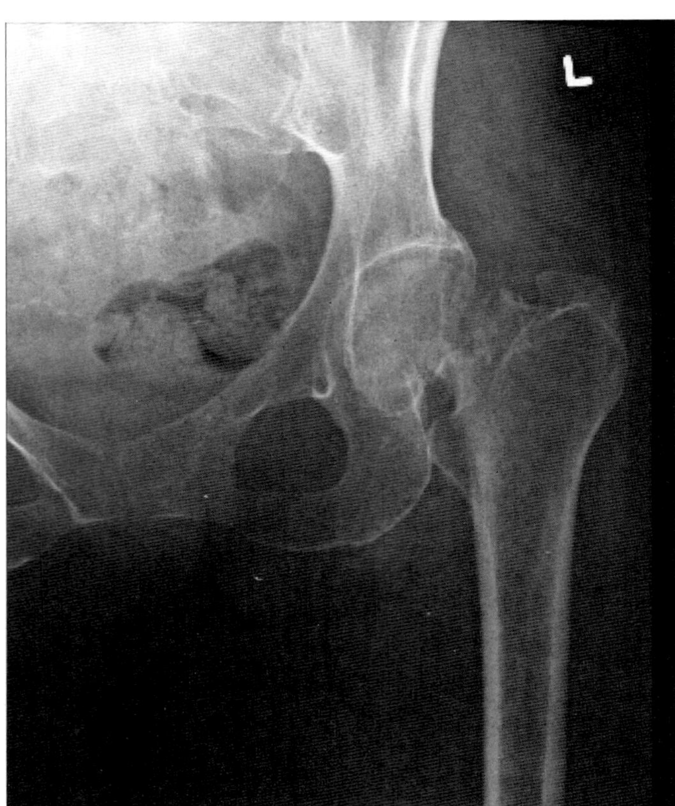

FIGURE 110-1 Transcervical left femoral neck fracture with varus angulation and superior offset of the distal fracture fragment. The femoral head is within the acetabular cup. Degenerative changes of the left hip are also present. (*Reproduced with permission from John E. Delzell Jr, MD.*)

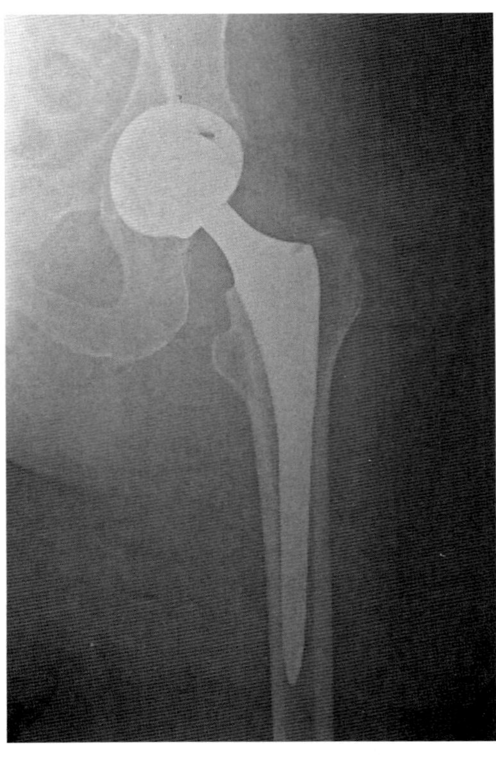

CHAPTER 110

FIGURE 110-2 Postsurgical portable radiograph demonstrating good positioning of artificial hip. (*Reproduced with permission from John E. Delzell Jr, MD.*)

ETIOLOGY AND PATHOPHYSIOLOGY

Approximately 95% of hip fractures are caused by a fall.

RISK FACTORS

- Low body mass index (BMI) and low physical activity in postmenopausal women[3]
- Low physical activity[3]

Long-term use of proton pump inhibitor (PPI) is associated with increased risk of any fracture, including hip fracture.[4]

In patients with diabetes mellitus over 70 years of age, hemoglobin A_{1C} (HbA_{1C}) less than 7% compared to greater than 8%, is associated with a 2- to 3-fold higher risk of hip fracture.[5]

DIAGNOSIS

CLINICAL FEATURES: HISTORY AND PHYSICAL

In a population study, major risk factors for hip fracture include the following:

- Low bone mineral density (3.6-fold [95% confidence interval (CI), 2.6-4.5] in women and 3.4-fold [95% CI, 2.5-4.6] in men for each standard deviation [SD] [0.12 g/cm^2] reduction in bone mineral density).[6]

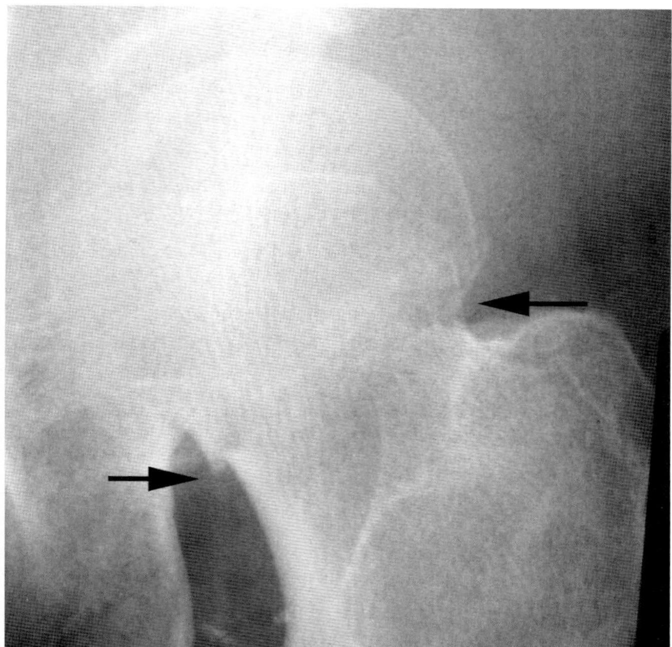

FIGURE 110-3 Nondisplaced, complete, femoral neck fracture (*black arrows*). Nondisplaced fractures can be incomplete (fracture through part of the femoral neck) or complete (fracture through the entire femoral neck). (*Reproduced with permission from Simon RR, Sherman SC, Koenigsknecht SJ.* Emergency Orthopedics, The Extremities. *5th ed. New York, NY: McGraw-Hill; 2007:358, Figure 13-8. Copyright 2007.*)

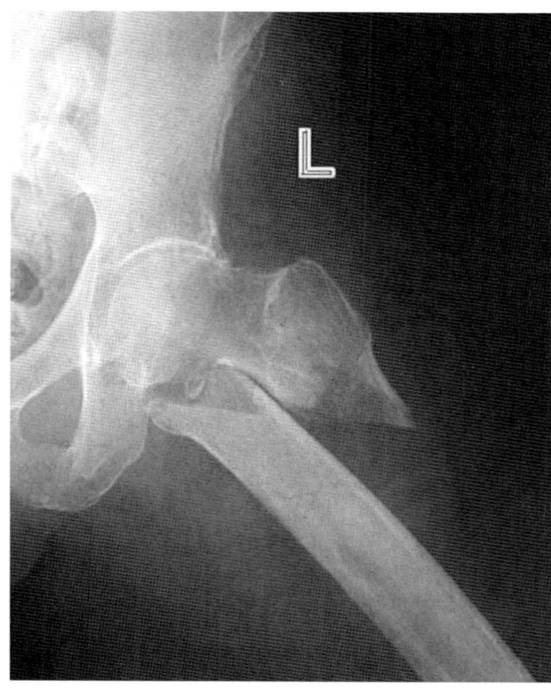

FIGURE 110-4 Unstable intertrochanteric fracture demonstrating displacement and a reverse oblique fracture line. Intertrochanteric fractures are unstable when there are multiple fracture lines, displacement between the femoral shaft and neck, or when the fracture line runs in an oblique reverse direction, with the most superior part of the fracture on the medial surface of the femur. The patient experiences severe pain, hip swelling, and shortening of the involved leg. (*Reproduced with permission from Simon RR, Sherman SC, Koenigsknecht SJ.* Emergency Orthopedics, The Extremities. *5th ed. New York, NY: McGraw-Hill; 2007:361, Figure 13-12. Copyright 2007.*)

- Postural instability and/or quadriceps weakness.
- A history of falls.
- Prior hip fracture.[6]
- Other factors associated with increased risk include dementia, tobacco use, physical inactivity, impaired vision, and alcohol use.

Physical examination—Abducted and externally rotated hip; limp or refusal to walk.

TYPICAL DISTRIBUTION

Hip fractures are classified according to anatomic location.[7]

- Intracapsular (femoral neck fracture; **Figures 110-1** and **110-3**)
- Extracapsular (intertrochanteric or subtrochanteric fracture; **Figure 110-4**)

IMAGING

- Radiographs—Plain radiographs show most hip fractures.
- Consider magnetic resonance imaging (MRI), bone scan, or computed tomography (CT) for indeterminate radiographs.

DIFFERENTIAL DIAGNOSIS

Hip pain can be caused by bone or joint pathology, soft tissue injuries, spine pathology, or can be referred. Some causes include the following[7]:

- Pelvic fractures, bone cancers, or metastases; osteoarthritis, inflammatory, crystal, or septic arthritis
- Iliotibial band syndrome, trochanteric bursitis, iliopsoas bursitis, piriformis syndrome, muscle strain
- Lumbar disc herniation, lumbar spinal stenosis, sciatica
- Hernia, abdominal or pelvic pathology

MANAGEMENT

Preventing hip fracture is important; 50% of patients with a hip fracture do not regain previous level of function; 20% die within a year.

Lower risk of hip fracture can be prevented by the following:

- Screen for osteoporosis.[8] SOR B
- Treat osteoporosis with bisphosphonates. SOR A
- Prevent falls by monitoring vision; assessing gait, strength, and balance; and minimizing the use of psychotropic medications in the elderly. SOR C
- Encourage exercise, such as tai chi, for lower-body strengthening and balance.
- Calcium and vitamin D supplementation do not decrease risk of hip fracture, but should be part of an osteoporosis prevention and treatment strategy.[9] SOR A
- Providing hip protectors to older residents of nursing home facilities may reduce the number of hip fractures; however, the clinical significance of the intervention is unclear.[10] SOR A
- Consider modifying the HbA_{1C} goal to 8% in patients over the age of 70.[5] SOR C

Refer to an orthopedic surgeon if the patient is not healthy enough to withstand surgery.

PREVENTION

- Thiazide diuretics may reduce the risk of hip fracture by 24%, based on meta-analysis of observational studies.[11]
- β-Blockers decrease the risk of hip fracture by 17%.[12]
- Population interventions are effective. Kaiser Permanente decreased hip fractures by 40% by identifying patients who had not received recommended bone density screening and treating as appropriate.[13]

PROGNOSIS

- One-year postoperation mortality of 27.3%.[14]
- All-cause mortality is 3 times higher in patients with a hip fracture than in the general population.[14]

FOLLOW-UP

Patients with hip fracture may benefit from multidisciplinary follow-up, including monitoring for complications such as avascular necrosis, identifying and treating osteoporosis, modifying risk factors for further falls, and maximizing function through therapy.

PATIENT EDUCATION

It is much easier to prevent hip fractures than to treat hip fractures. After a hip fracture, patients often need prolonged time (months) in a nursing care facility. Physical therapy is crucial in regaining as much function as possible.

PATIENT RESOURCES

- FamilyDoctor.org has written and auditory information in English and Spanish—**http://familydoctor.org/familydoctor/en/diseases-conditions/hip-fractures.html.**
- The American Academy of Orthopedic Surgeons (**http://www.aaos.org/**) has a patient handout called "Live it Safe—Prevent Broken Hips"—**http://orthoinfo.aaos.org/topic.cfm?topic=A00305.**
- Mayo Health on hip fractures with the option to view with larger type—**http://www.mayoclinic.com/health/hip-fracture/DS00185.**

PROVIDER RESOURCES

- eMedicine article: Davenport M. *Hip Fracture in Emergency Medicine*—**http://emedicine.medscape.com/article/825363-overview.**
- Validated hip fracture risk assessment tools
  - FRAX, the World Health Organization fracture risk assessment tool—**http://www.shef.ac.uk/FRAX/.**
  - QFracture, a United Kingdom tool—**http://www.qfracture.org/.**

REFERENCES

1. National Center for Health Statistics. *Center for Disease Control. Department of Health and Human Services. National Health and Nutrition Examination Survey (NHANES) 2005-2006*. http://www.cdc.gov/nchs. Accessed June 2, 2008.
2. Robbins JA, Schott AM, Garnero P, et al. Risk factors for hip fracture in women with high BMD: EPIDOS study. *Osteoporos Int.* 2005;16(2):149-154.
3. Armstrong ME, Spencer EA, Cairns BJ, et al. Body mass index and physical activity in relation to the incidence of hip fracture in postmenopausal women. *J Bone Miner Res.* 2011;26(6):1330-1338.
4. Eom Cs, Park SM, Myung DK, et al. Use of acid-suppressive drugs and risk of fracture: a meta-analysis of observational studies. *Ann Fam Med.* 2011;9(3):257-267.
5. Puar Th, Khoo JJ, Cho LW, et al. Association between glycemic control and hip fracture. *J Am Geriatr Soc.* 2012;60(8):1493-1497.
6. Nguyen ND, Pongchaiyakul C, Center JR, et al. Identification of high-risk individuals for hip fracture: a 14-year prospective study. *J Bone Miner Res.* 2005;20(11):1921-1928.
7. Brunner LC, Eshilian-Oates L, Kuo TY. Hip fractures in adults. *Am Fam Physician.* 2003;67(3):537-542.
8. Kern LM, Powe NR, Levine MA, et al. Association between screening for osteoporosis and the incidence of hip fracture. *Ann Intern Med.* 2005;142(3):173-181.
9. Porthouse J, Cockayne S, King C, et al. Randomised controlled trial of calcium and supplementation with cholecalciferol (vitamin D3) for prevention of fractures in primary care. *BMJ.* 2005;330(7498):1003.
10. Gillespie WJ, Gillespie LD, Parker MJ. Hip protectors for preventing hip fractures in older people. *Cochrane Database Syst Rev.* 2010;(10):CD001255.
11. Aung K, Htay T. Thiazine diuretics and the risk of hip fracture. *Cochrane Database Syst Rev.* 2011;(10):CD005185.
12. Yang S, Nguyen ND, Eisman JA, Nguyen TV. Association between beta-blockers and fracture risk: a Bayesian meta-analysis. *Bone.* 2012;51(5):969-974.
13. Dell R. Fracture prevention in Kaiser Permanente Southern California. *Osteoporos Int.* 2011;22(suppl 3):457-460.
14. Panula J, Pihlajamäki H, Mattila VM, et al. Mortality and cause of death in hip fracture patients aged 65 or older: a population-based study. *BMC Musculoskelet Disord.* 2011;12:110.

111 THE KNEE

Heidi Chumley, MD

PATIENT STORY

A 33-year-old woman felt a pop in her knee while skiing around a tree. She felt immediate pain and had difficulty walking when paramedics removed her from the slopes. Within a couple of hours, her knee was swollen. On examination the next day, she was able to walk 4 steps with pain. She had a moderate effusion without gross deformity and full range of motion. She had no tenderness at the joint line, the head of the fibula, over the patella, or over the medial or lateral collateral ligaments. She had a positive Lachman test, a negative McMurray test, and no increased laxity with valgus or varus stress. The physician suspected an anterior cruciate ligament (ACL) tear, placed her in a long leg range of motion brace, and advised her to use crutches until an evaluation by her physician within the next several days. She was treated with acetaminophen for pain and advised to rest, apply ice, and keep her leg elevated. Later, a magnetic resonance imaging (MRI) confirmed an ACL tear (**Figure 111-1**).

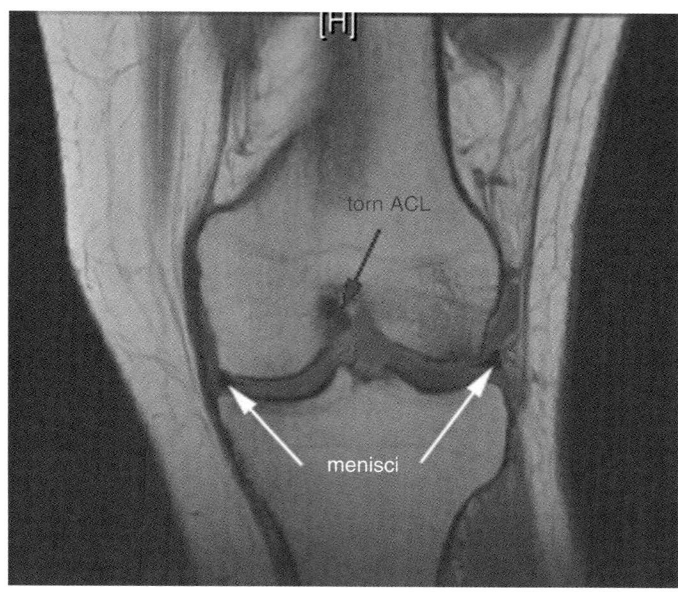

FIGURE 111-1 MRI of ACL tear in the frontal view. Note the normal menisci, which are black throughout. (*Reproduced with permission from John E. Delzell Jr, MD, MSPH.*)

INTRODUCTION

Knee injuries are common. Women have a greater risk of knee injuries because of body mechanics. Most knee injuries involve the ACL, meniscus, or medial or lateral collateral ligaments. The mechanism of injury and physical examination findings suggest the type of injury, which can be confirmed by MRI. Treatment includes rest, ice, compression, elevation, and referral to an orthopedic surgeon.

EPIDEMIOLOGY

- Knee injuries are common in adults engaging in sports or in the military. **Figure 111-2** shows the normal anatomy of the knee.
- The risk of ACL injury while playing soccer, is 2 to 3 times higher in woman than in men.[1]
- Incidence of ACL injuries was approximately 3 per 1000 person-years in US active military personnel, with no difference in gender.[2]
- Meniscal injuries commonly occur with ACL tears (23%-65%).[3]
- Meniscal tears were seen on MRI in 91% of patients with symptomatic osteoarthritis, but also seen in 76% of age-matched controls without knee pain.[4]
- Collateral ligament injuries account for approximately 25% of acute knee injuries.

ETIOLOGY AND PATHOPHYSIOLOGY

- ACL injuries occur with sudden deceleration with a rotational maneuver, usually without contact.
- ACL injuries are thought to occur more commonly in women because of decreased leg strength, increased ligamentous laxity, and differences in lumbopelvic core control.
- Acute meniscal injuries occur with a twisting motion on the weight-bearing knee.
- Chronic meniscal tears occur from mechanical grinding of osteophytes on the meniscus in older patients with osteoarthritis.
- Medial collateral and lateral collateral injuries occur from valgus and varus stress, respectively.

RISK FACTORS

Women are at higher risk for ACL injuries.

DIAGNOSIS

CLINICAL FEATURES ON HISTORY

ACL

- Rotational injury
- "Pop" reported by patient
- Unable to bear full weight
- Effusion within the first few hours

Meniscal injury

- Foot planted with femur rotated internally with valgus stress (medial) or femur rotated externally with varus stress (lateral)
- Joint line pain
- Effusion over the first several hours
- Usually ambulatory with instability or locking (mechanical) symptoms

Collateral injury

- Valgus or varus stress injury
- Usually ambulatory without instability or locking symptoms

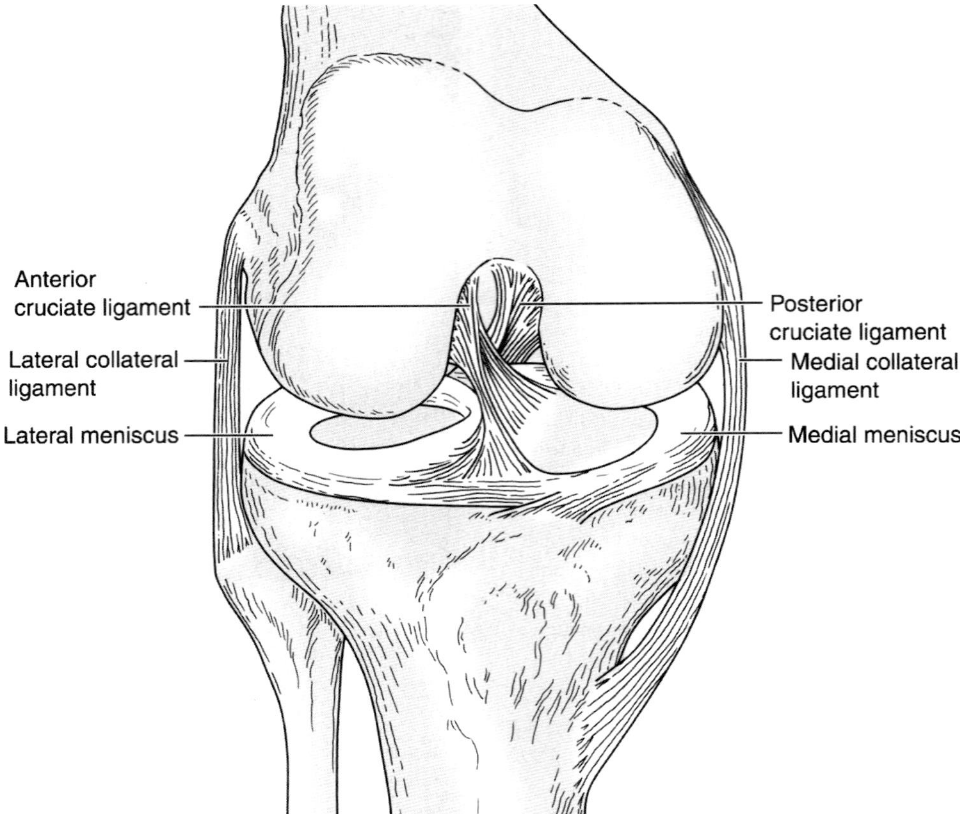

FIGURE 111-2 Anatomy of a normal knee. (*Reproduced with permission from Simon RR, Sherman SC, Koenigsknecht SJ.* Emergency Orthopedics, The Extremities. *5th ed. New York, NY: McGraw-Hill; 2007:392, Figure 15-5. Copyright 2007.*)

PHYSICAL EXAMINATION

A complete physical examination of the knee is demonstrated online from the University of British Columbia at **http://www.youtube.com/user/BJSMVideos.**

- Inspect the knee for effusions—Usually present for an ACL tear.
- Test range of motion—Often normal, inability to extend fully can indicate either a medial meniscal tear or an ACL tear displaced posteriorly.
- Palpate for tenderness—Joint line tenderness may indicate a meniscal tear (positive likelihood ratio [LR+] = 1.1; negative likelihood ratio [LR–] = 0.8).[5] Tenderness at the head of the fibula or at the patella are 2 of the 5 Ottawa rules for obtaining radiographs; tenderness along the medial or lateral collateral ligament may indicate damage to those ligaments.
- Perform tests for ACL tear—Lachman test (LR+ = 12.4; LR– = 0.14),[5] anterior drawer test (LR+ = 3.7; LR– = 0.6),[5] pivot shift test (LR+ = 20.3; LR – = 0.4).[5]
- Patients with ACL tears typically have a history of rotational injury; inability to bear weight; positive provocative tests; normal plain radiographs; and abnormal MRI.
- Perform tests for meniscal tears—McMurray test (LR+ = 17.3; LR– = 0.5).[5]
- Patients with meniscal tears typically have history of rotational injury with valgus/varus stress or history of osteoarthritis; able to bear weight, commonly with instability or locking; positive McMurray test; normal plain radiographs; and abnormal MRI.
- Perform varus and valgus stress to test the lateral and medial collateral ligaments.
- Patients with injuries to the collateral ligaments typically have a history of valgus/varus stress to extended knee; able to bear weight without instability or locking; laxity with valgus or varus stress testing; normal plain radiographs and abnormal MRI.

IMAGING

- Determine whether or not to obtain plain radiographs (anteroposterior, lateral, intercondylar notch, and sunrise views) to assess for a fracture based on either the Pittsburgh or Ottawa knee rules (the Ottawa rules may be less sensitive in children).
  - Pittsburg (99% sensitivity, 60% specificity; tested in population ages 6-96 years)[5]—Obtain X-ray for the following:
    - Recent significant fall or blunt trauma
    - Age younger than 12 years or older than 50 years
    - Unable to take 4 unaided steps
  - Ottawa (98.5% sensitivity, 48.6% specificity; LR– = 0.05; tested in 6 studies of 4249 adult patients)[6]—Obtain X-ray for the following:
    - Age 55 years or older
    - Tenderness at the head of the fibula
    - Isolated tenderness of the patella
    - Inability to flex knee to 90 degrees
    - Inability to bear weight for 4 steps both immediately and in the examination room regardless of limping
- MRI is 95% and 90% accurate in identifying ACL tears and meniscal injuries, respectively (**Figures 111-2** to **111-4**).[7]

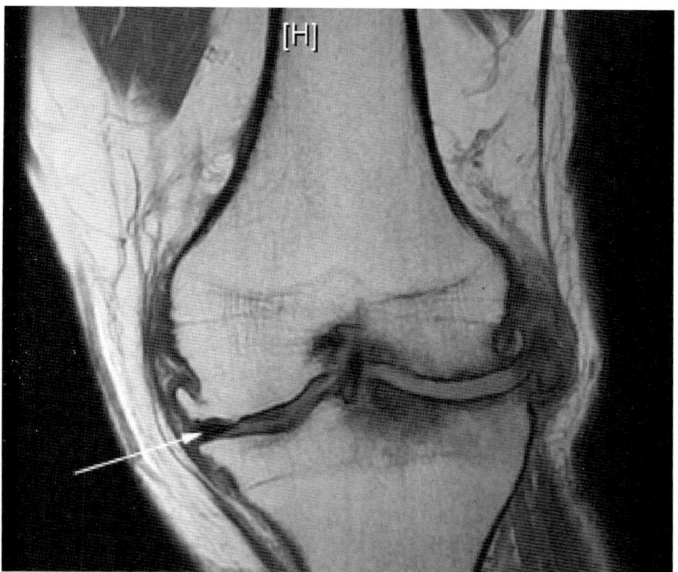

FIGURE 111-3 Medial meniscal tear on the frontal view, seen as a small white line through the black meniscus (*arrow*). (*Reproduced with permission from Heidi Chumley, MD.*)

DIFFERENTIAL DIAGNOSIS

Acute knee pain can be caused by trauma affecting structures of the knee other than ligaments and menisci, arthritis, infection, or tumors including the following:

- Trauma
- Intra-articular fractures (patella, femoral condyles, tibial eminence, tibial tuberosity, and tibial plateau)—history of trauma or chronic overuse; edema, ecchymosis, point tenderness, or deformity may be present; visible on plain radiographs (**Figures 111-5** and **111-6**)
- Patellar dislocation—Severe hyperextension (anterior dislocation), fall on a bent knee or knee hitting the dashboard (posterior dislocation), valgus or varus stress (medial or lateral dislocation); visible deformity; effusion and immobility; neurovascular complications (peroneal nerve and popliteal artery); visible on plain radiographs
- Arthritis—No history of trauma (see Chapter 97, Arthritis Overview)
- Reactive arthritis—Fever/malaise; oligoarthritis involving the knee, ankle, feet and/or wrist involvement, urethritis, conjunctivitis or iritis;

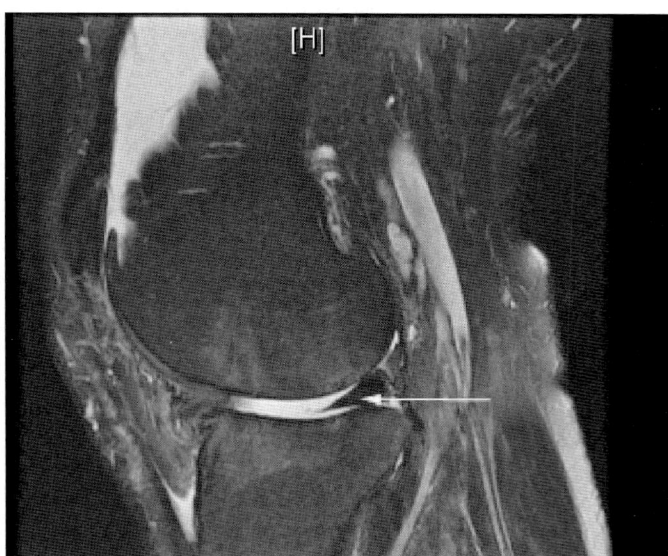

FIGURE 111-4 Lateral meniscal tear on a sagittal view, seen as a small white line in the black meniscus (*arrow*). (*Reproduced with permission from Heidi Chumley, MD.*)

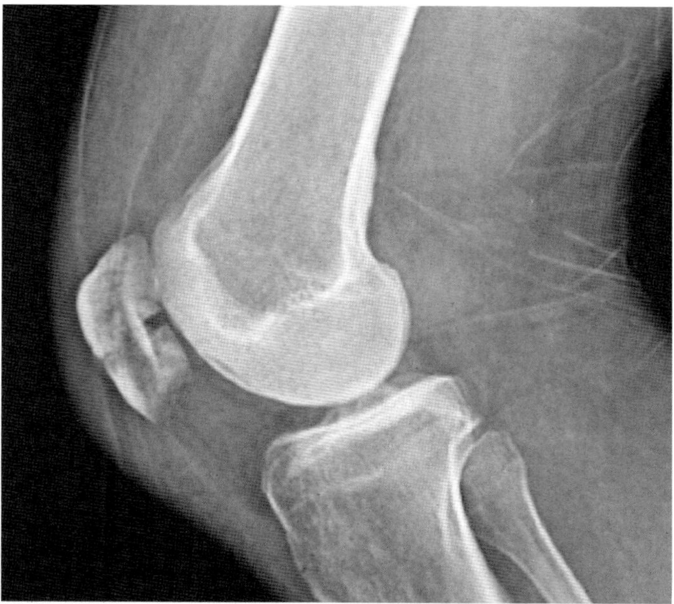

FIGURE 111-5 Nondisplaced patellar fracture seen best on the lateral view. (*Reproduced with permission from Simon RR, Sherman SC, Koenigsknecht SJ.* Emergency Orthopedics, The Extremities. *5th ed. New York, NY: McGraw-Hill; 2007:405, Figure 15-26, bottom photo only. Copyright 2007.*)

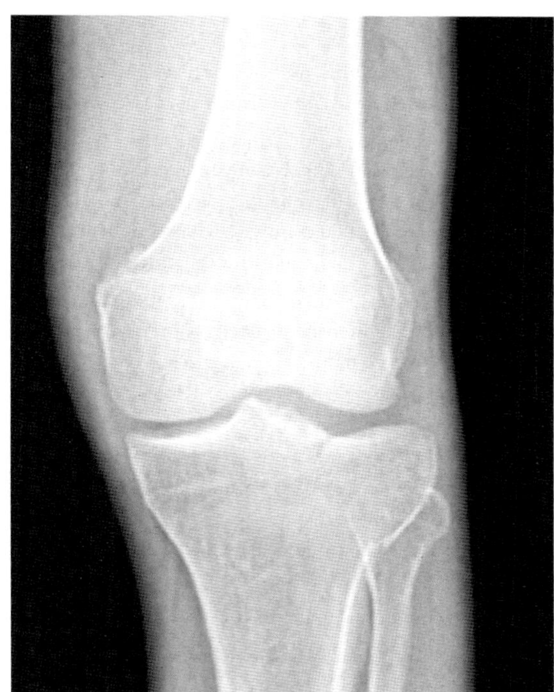

FIGURE 111-6 Lateral condylar split fracture (type 1) has no depression of the articular surface and is usually the result of low-impact trauma. More common in children. (*Reproduced with permission from Simon RR, Sherman SC, Koenigsknecht SJ.* Emergency Orthopedics, The Extremities. *5th ed. New York, NY: McGraw-Hill; 2007:398, Figure 15-14. Copyright 2007.*)

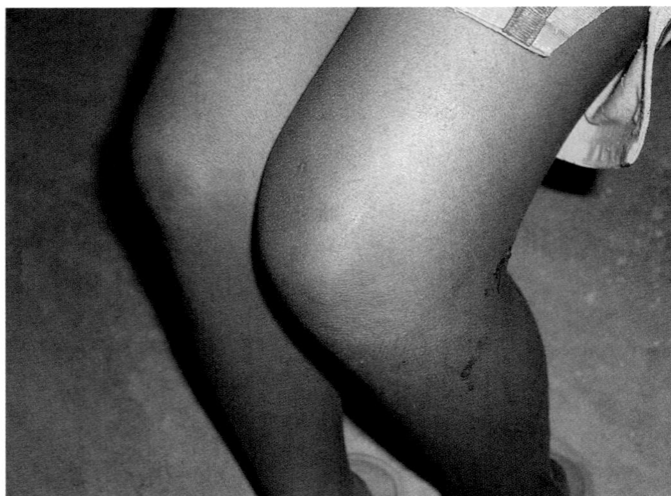

FIGURE 111-7 Septic arthritis in a girl who presented with a painful swollen left knee, decreased range of motion and difficulty walking. A knee aspiration revealed turbid fluid with elevated leukocytes. The joint fluid culture grew Staphylococcus aureus. (*Reproduced with permission from Richard P. Usatine, MD.*)

elevated C-reactive protein or erythrocyte sedimentation rate (ESR); arthritic changes on radiographs (see Chapter 153, Reactive Arthritis)

- Rheumatoid arthritis—Adults ages 30 to 50 years, more commonly women; polyarthritis involving hands, wrists, feet, and knees; fever/malaise; positive rheumatoid factor; erosive arthritis changes on radiographs (see Chapter 99, Rheumatoid Arthritis)
- Gout or pseudogout—Adults ages 30 to 60 years, more commonly men; single joint erythema, warmth and tenderness without trauma; abnormal joint fluid with elevated white blood cell count (WBC); radiographs may be normal or abnormal (sclerotic regions, degenerative changes, or soft tissue calcifications) (see Chapter 105, Gout)
- Osteoarthritis—Older adults; gradual onset; symptoms worse after use; radiographic osteophytes (see Chapter 98, Osteoarthritis)
- Infections such as cellulitis, septic arthritis (**Figure 111-7**), osteomyelitis—May have history of skin break by bite or puncture wound; fever; erythema, warmth with cellulitis; decreased range of motion, inability to walk, abnormal fluid aspirate with septic arthritis; chronic symptoms and abnormal radiograph with osteomyelitis
- Malignant tumors (eg, osteosarcoma, chondroblastoma) or benign tumors (eg, bone cysts, osteochondroma)—No (or insignificant) history of trauma; chronic symptoms or acute symptoms caused by pathologic fracture; abnormal radiographs and MRI

MANAGEMENT

Initial management for traumatic knee pain includes rest, ice, compression, and elevation.

- Provide pain relief with acetaminophen. Add a nonsteroidal anti-inflammatory medication if needed.[8] SOR C
- Prevent further injury (eg, limit activities to toe-touch weight bearing and place in a long leg range of motion brace)[7] until evaluation by a provider trained to manage acute knee injuries. SOR C
- Obtain plain radiographs if indicated by the Pittsburg or Ottawa rules.[6] SOR A
- Consider an MRI for suspected ACL, meniscal, or collateral ligament tear based on the mechanism of injury and physical examination findings.[7] SOR C

FOR ACL TEARS

- Refer young, active adults to a physician trained in surgical repair as repair results in 80% to 95% return to normal activity in 4 to 6 months.[8] SOR C
- Refer less active adults and adults over the age of 50 to a physician trained in surgical repair to discuss the advantages and disadvantages of surgical repair.[9]
- Surgical repair is typically done at least 3 weeks after the injury. Repair within the first 3 weeks results in a high incidence of arthrofibrosis.
- Refer to physical therapy if available to institute early knee range of motion (before surgery).[8] SOR C

FOR MENISCAL TEARS

- Refer to a physician for discussion of nonsurgical and surgical treatments as rates of healing vary by location of meniscal tear and associated injuries.[10] SOR C
- Adults of age 45 to 65 with knee pain, nontraumatic meniscal tears, and osteoarthritis11 may benefit from the following factors:
  - Most likely to benefit from arthroscopic surgery: displaced tear, mechanical symptoms, and acute increase in pain
  - Least likely to benefit from arthroscopic surgery: oblique tear, no mechanical symptoms, and no acute change in pain

FOR COLLATERAL TEARS

- The treatment is based on the severity of the tear. SOR C
- For all grades, instruct in early range of motion exercises (or refer to physical therapy).
- Grade I medial collateral ligament (MCL) or lateral collateral ligament (LCL) (≤5 cm laxity on valgus or varus stress), weight bearing as tolerated with early ambulation.
- Grade II MCL or LCL (5-10 cm laxity), place in a brace blocking the last 20 degrees of flexion, weight bearing as tolerated.
- Grade III MCL (>10 cm laxity), place in a hinged brace, initially non–weight bearing, advancing to weight bearing over 4 weeks. Grade III LCL tears often require surgery.

PREVENTION

- Neuromuscular retraining programs reduce the incidence of ACL injuries in female basketball, soccer, and volleyball players.[12]
- Structured warm-up program to improve cutting, jumping, balance and strength decreased acute knee injuries, number needed to treat was 43 over 8 months.[13]

PROGNOSIS

Most young active adults have an excellent prognosis from knee injuries. Nonsurgical management of ACL tears has a good prognosis from 1 to 5 years, but patients reduce their activity level by 21%.[14]

FOLLOW-UP

Timing of follow-up is determined by the orthopedic surgeon, sports medicine specialist, or other provider skilled in acute knee injury management.

PATIENT EDUCATION

- ACL tears often require surgery, take 4 to 6 months to heal, and require a commitment to rehabilitation for the best results.
- Meniscal tears may require surgery when mechanical symptoms are present. The location of the tear determines how likely surgical repair is to be effective because of the blood supply available for healing.
- Meniscal tears are commonly seen on MRI in patients with osteoarthritis who do not have pain and meniscal tears seen on MRI may not be contributing to arthritic pain.
- Collateral tears can often be treated conservatively, while protecting the knee in a brace and preserving range of motion. Complete tears to the LCL often require surgery.

PATIENT RESOURCES

- The American Academy of Family Physicians has a patient algorithm for knee pain—**http://familydoctor.org/familydoctor/en/health-tools/search-by-symptom/knee-problems.html.**
- The National Institute of Health through the National Institute for Arthritis and Musculoskeletal and Skin Diseases has patient information on several types of knee problems—**http://www.niams.nih.gov/Health_Info/Knee_Problems/default.asp.**

PROVIDER RESOURCES

- The Ottawa and Pittsburgh Knee Rules are available in an online calculator—**http://www.mdcalc.com/ottawa-and-pittsburg-knee-rules.**
- Dr. Hutchinson's Knee Exam from the University of British Columbia—**http://www.youtube.com/user/BJSMVideos.**

REFERENCES

1. Walden M, Hagglund M, Werner J, Ekstrand J. The epidemiology of anterior cruciate ligament injury in football(soccer): a review of the literature from a gender-related perspective. *Knee Surg Sports Traumatol Arthrosc*. 2011;19(1):3-10.
2. Owens BD, Mountcastle SB, Dunn WR, et al. Incidence of anterior cruciate ligament injury among active duty U.S. military servicemen and servicewomen. *Mil Med*. 2007;172(1):90-91.
3. Cimino PM. The incidence of meniscal tears associated with acute anterior cruciate ligament disruption secondary to snow skiing accidents. *Arthroscopy*. 1994;10(2):198-200.
4. Bhattacharya T, Gale D, Dewire P, et al. The clinical importance of meniscal tears demonstrated by magnetic resonance imaging in osteoarthritis of the knee. *J Bone Joint Surg Am*. 2003;85-A:4-9.
5. Ebell MH. Evaluating the patient with a knee injury. *Am Fam Physician*. 2005;71(6):1169-1172.
6. Bachmann KM, Haberzeth S, Steurer J, Ter Riet G. The accuracy of the Ottawa knee rule to rule out knee fractures: a systematic review. *Ann Intern Med*. 2004;140(2):121-124.
7. David K, Frank B. Anterior cruciate ligament rupture. *Br J Sports Med*. 2005;39:324-329.
8. New Zealand Guidelines Group (NZGG). *The Diagnosis and Management of Soft Tissue Knee Injuries: Internal Derangements*. Wellington, NZ: New Zealand Guidelines Group (NZGG), 2003:100.
9. Legnani C, Terzaghi C, Borgo E, Ventura A. Management of anterior cruciate ligament rupture in patients aged 40 years and older. *J Orthop Traumatol*. 2011;12(4):177-184.
10. Greis PE, Bardana DD, Holmstrom MC, Burks RT. Meniscal injury I: basic science and evaluation. *J Am Acad Orthop Surg*. 2002;10(2):168-176.
11. Suter LG, Fraenkel L, Losina E, et al. Medical decision making in patients with knee pain, meniscal tear, and osteoarthritis. *Arthritis Rheum*. 2009;61(11):1531-1538.
12. Barber-Westin SD, Noyes FR, Smith ST, Campbell TM. Reducing the risk of noncontact anterior cruciate ligament injuries in the female athlete. *Phys Sportsmed*. 2009;37(3):49-61.
13. Olsen OE, Myklebust G, Engebretsen L, Holme I, Bahr R. Exercises to prevent lower limb injuries in youth sports: cluster randomised controlled trial. *BMJ*. 2005;330(7489):449.
14. Muaidi QI, Nicholson LL, Refshauge KM, et al. Prognosis of conservatively managed anterior cruciate ligament injury: a systematic review. *Sports Med*. 2007;37(8):703-716.

112 DUPUYTREN DISEASE

John E Delzell Jr, MD, MSPH
Heidi Chumley, MD

PATIENT STORY

A 53-year-old man presented with stiffness in his hands. He said his hands began to feel stiff several years ago, and now he finds that he cannot straighten many of his fingers (**Figure 112-1**). He delayed seeing a physician because he did not feel any pain in his hands. He recently began having difficulty holding his woodworking tools and wants to regain the function he has lost in his hands. The physician diagnosed him with Dupuytren contracture and discussed the disease with him along with his options for treatment.

INTRODUCTION

Dupuytren contracture is a flexion contracture of one or more of the fingers in the hand. Patients develop a progressive thickening of the palmar fascia, which causes the fingers to bend in toward the palm and limits extension. Diagnosis is clinical and the palpable nodules in the palm are considered diagnostic. Treatment has historically been surgical, but a new nonsurgical treatment with a collagenase has been approved.

SYNONYMS

Dupuytren disease is also known as Dupuytren contractures, palmar fibromatosis, morbus Dupuytren, or Ledderhose disease.

EPIDEMIOLOGY

- Dupuytren contracture is an autosomal dominant disease with incomplete penetrance (**Figure 112-2**).

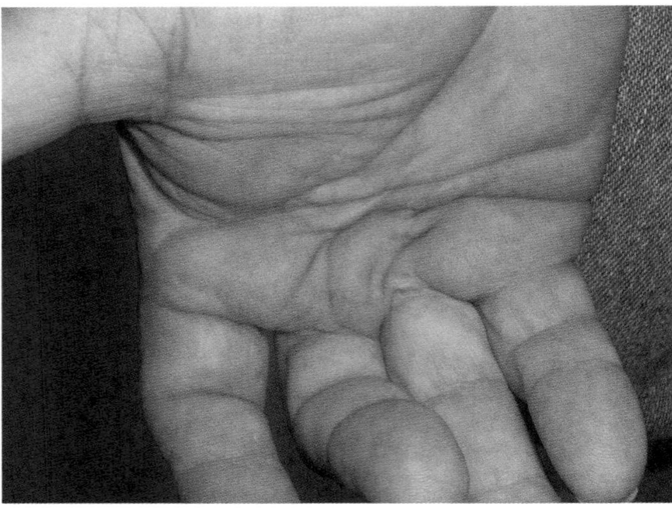

FIGURE 112-1 Dupuytren contracture in a 53-year-old man showing flexion contractures at the proximal interphalangeal joints of the third digit and a palmar cord. (*Reproduced with permission from Richard P. Usatine, MD.*)

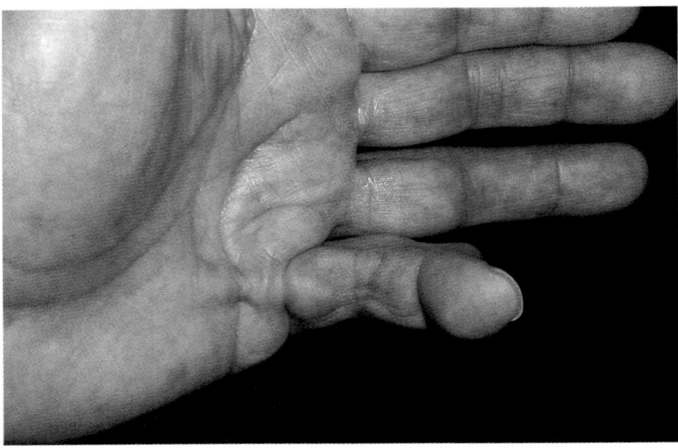

FIGURE 112-2 Dupuytren contracture in a 60-year-old man showing a flexion contracture of the fifth digit and a palmar cord. All of his brothers have Dupuytren contractures. (*Reproduced with permission from Richard P. Usatine, MD.*)

- Higher prevalence is among whites, particularly of Northern European descent. There is an increasing incidence related to aging.[1]
- It is more common in men than women (approximately 6:1).[2,3]
- Incidence in the United States is estimated to be approximately 3 per 10,000 adults with an estimated prevalence of 7%.
- Higher incidence is found in people who use tobacco and alcohol or who have diabetes mellitus or epilepsy.[4]

ETIOLOGY AND PATHOPHYSIOLOGY

Dupuytren contractures form in following 3 stages:

- Myofibroblasts in the palmar fascia proliferate to form nodules.
- Myofibroblasts then align along the lines of tension, forming cords.
- Tissue becomes acellular leaving thick cords of collagen that tighten resulting in flexion contractures at the metacarpal phalangeal joint, the proximal interphalangeal joint, and, occasionally, the distal interphalangeal joint.

RISK FACTORS

- Tobacco use
- Alcohol consumption
- Epilepsy
- Diabetes mellitus
- Carpal tunnel syndrome
- History of manual labor
- History of hand injury

DIAGNOSIS

CLINICAL FEATURES

- Clinical diagnosis is based on the history and physical examination.
- Patients complain of a slowly progressive tightness in the hands and a lack of the ability to fully extend their fingers.

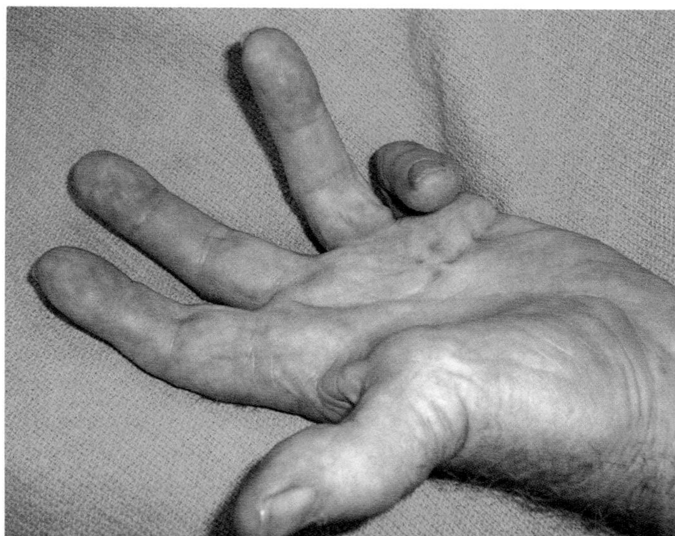

FIGURE 112-3 Dupuytren contracture in a 58-year-old man showing flexion contractures of the fourth and fifth digits and a palmar cord. (*Reproduced with permission from Richard P. Usatine, MD.*)

- Typically painless.
- Examination findings—Nodules with flexion contractures are considered diagnostic, particularly in older white males; however, nodules may disappear late in the disease.[4]

TYPICAL DISTRIBUTION

- Either hand can be affected
- More commonly seen in the fourth and fifth digits (**Figure 112-3**)

LABORATORY TESTING

Not indicated

IMAGING

Magnetic resonance imaging (MRI) of the contractures may be helpful prior to surgical intervention, but is not needed to confirm a clinical diagnosis.

BIOPSY

- Typically not indicated.
- Early diagnosis or diagnosis in atypical populations, such as children, may require histologic confirmation.

DIFFERENTIAL DIAGNOSIS

Consider the other causes of hand contractures and palmar nodules including the following:

- Intrinsic joint contractures—Loss of range of motion from any primary joint disease.
- Trigger finger, stenosing tenosynovitis—Localized swelling of the flexor tendon limits movement within the sheath with resulting "triggering"; digit catches, but can be straightened.
- Rheumatoid arthritis—Bony deformities resulting in ulnar deviation at the metacarpophalangeal joints and/or the wrist.
- Ganglion cysts and palmar nodules.
- Occupational hyperkeratosis and callous formation.
- Hand tumors including epithelioid sarcomas and soft tissue giant cell tumors.

MANAGEMENT

The treatment goal of Dupuytren contracture is to maintain or restore hand function by increasing range of motion at involved joints.

NONPHARMACOLOGIC

- Physical therapy with splinting does not seem to be helpful as a sole treatment. SOR Ⓒ
- Radiation therapy has been used but there is little evidence to support it and significant potential side effects of the treatment. SOR Ⓒ
- Hyperbaric oxygen is being studied with mixed results. SOR Ⓒ

MEDICATIONS

- Intralesional injection of corticosteroids is only mildly successful and may place the patient at risk for tendon rupture. SOR Ⓒ
- Collagenase injection, a nonsurgical treatment, reduced contractures to 0 to 5 degrees in 44% to 64% of patients. Thirty-five percent of contractures recur by 3 years and most contractures will recur by 8 years.[5,6]

REFERRAL FOR SURGERY

- Surgical correction is considered when there is at least 30 degrees of contracture at the metacarpophalangeal (MCP) joint. SOR Ⓒ
- Surgical fasciotomy decreases the degree of flexion deformity and results in modest improvements in hand function. Studies indicated that improvements in function are best correlated to changes at the proximal interphalangeal joint.[1] SOR Ⓑ

PROGNOSIS

- Recurrence rate is related to the amount of fascia that is removed on surgery.
- There is an increased risk for recurrence with time.

FOLLOW-UP

Postoperative follow-up should include hand therapy with a goal of increasing extension in the affected digits.

PATIENT EDUCATION

- Modifying risk factors (eg, smoking, alcohol intake) that are known to contribute to the development of Dupuytren contracture is prudent, but are not shown to alter the course of the disease.
- After surgery, postoperative hand therapy may improve function and use of the hand. However, initial decreases in joint deformity and improvements in hand function may be lost over time.

PATIENT RESOURCES

- PubMed Health. *Dupuytren's Contracture*—**http://www.ncbi.nlm.nih.gov/pubmedhealth/PMH0002213/.**
- American Family Physician (AAFP). *Dupuytren's Disease: What You Should Know*—**http://www.aafp.org/afp/2007/0701/p90.html.**

PROVIDER RESOURCES

- Mayo Clinic. *Dupuytren's Contracture*—**http://www.mayoclinic.com/health/dupuytrens-contracture/DS00732.**
- American Family Physician (AAFP). Trojian TH, Chu SM. Dupuytren's disease: diagnosis and treatment *Am Fam Physician.* 2007;76(1):86-89—**http://www.aafp.org/afp/2007/0701/p86.html.**
- Medscape. *Dupuytren Contracture*—**http://emedicine.medscape.com/article/329414.**

REFERENCES

1. Draviaraj KP, Chakrabarti I. Functional outcome after surgery for Dupuytren's contracture: a prospective study. *J Hand Surg Am.* 2004;29(5):804-808.
2. Gudmundsson KG, Arngrimsson R, Sigfusson N, et al. Epidemiology of Dupuytren's disease: clinical, serological, and social assessment. The Reykjavik study. *J Clin Epidemiol.* 2000;53(3):291-296.
3. Hindocha S, McGrouther DA, Bayat A. Epidemiological evaluation of Dupuytren's disease incidence and prevalence rates in relation to etiology. *Hand (NY).* 2009;4(3):256-269.
4. Saar JD, Grothaus PC. Dupuytren's disease: an overview. *Plast Reconstr Surg.* 2000;106(1):125-134.
5. Lo S, Pickford M. Current concepts in Dupuytren's disease. *Curr Rev Musculoskeletal Med.* 2013;6(1):26-34.
6. Peimer CA, Blazar P, Coleman S, et al. Dupuytren contracture recurrence following treatment with collagenase clostridium histolyticum (CORDLESS study): 3-year data. *J Hand Surg Am.* 2013;38(1):12-22.

113 POLYMYALGIA RHEUMATICA AND TEMPORAL ARTERITIS

Gary Ferenchick, MD

PATIENT STORY

A 65-year-old male presents to the clinic with fatigue and a slowly progressive onset of pain in his shoulders for the past 3 months. The shoulder pain is worse in the morning and while working with his arms over his head. Over the past 2 weeks, he required help from his wife getting dressed in the morning. He also described pain in his calves and buttock muscles. He denies any symptoms in his small joints and denies headache or visual disturbance. Blood tests reveal a platelet count of 411 and an erythrocyte sedimentation rate (ESR) of 54 mm/h. A diagnosis of polymyalgia rheumatica (PMR) is made based on the clinical picture (**Figure 113-1**). The patient is started on 15 mg of prednisone daily. Within 7 days, he is 95% improved, and a follow-up sedimentation rate is 10 mm/h 4 weeks later. Over several months, he is weaned off prednisone and remains asymptomatic.

INTRODUCTION

Polymyalgia rheumatica is a condition of unknown etiology associated with bilateral shoulder, pelvic girdle, and neck aching along with morning stiffness in patients over 50 years of age. It may be associated with more systemic symptoms of low-grade fever, weight loss, and fatigue and is commonly associated with an elevated sedimentation rate or elevated C-reactive protein (CRP).[1]

Temporal arteritis (TA) is chronic vasculitis of unknown etiology of medium and large vessels. TA should be considered a medical emergency because of increased risk of stroke and vision loss.

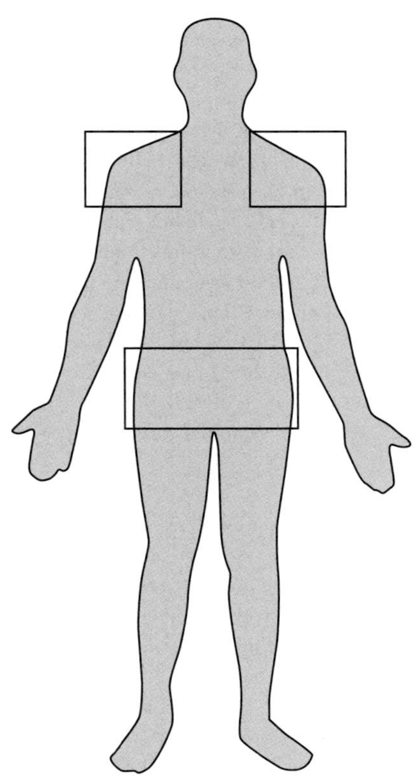

FIGURE 113-1 Typical areas of pain and stiffness in patients presenting with PMR.

SYNONYMS

Temporal arteritis is also known as giant cell arteritis (GCA).

EPIDEMIOLOGY

- Polymyalgia rheumatica is the most common systemic inflammatory problem faced by the elderly and a common reason for long-term corticosteroid therapy. It is 3 times more common than TA.
- Temporal arteritis is the most common medium-/large-vessel vasculitis and may cause acute blindness (20% of patients with TA experience visual loss).[2]
- Mean age of onset for TA is 70, and it is rare before age 50.
- Temporal arteritis is more common in Caucasians.
- Temporal arteritis is accompanied by PMR about 50% of the time.

ETIOLOGY/PATHOPHYSIOLOGY

- Temporal arteritis mostly involves the proximal cranial vessels arising from the aortic arch and is associated with granulomatous inflammation with multinucleated giant cells on histology[3] (**Figures 113-2** and **113-3**).

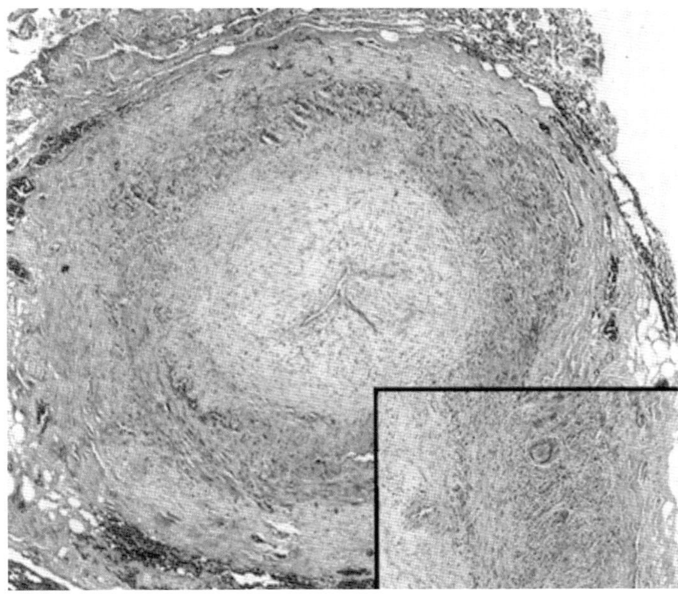

FIGURE 113-2 Giant cell arteritis. Temporal artery biopsy showing endothelial proliferation, fragmentation of internal elastic lamina, and infiltration of the adventitia and media by inflammatory cells. Giant cells show especially well in the inset. (*Reproduced with permission from Hellmann DB. Vasculitis. In: Stobo J, Traill TA, Hellmann DB, Ladenson PW, Petty BG.* Principles and Practice of Medicine. *New York, NY: Appleton & Lange; 1996:215.*)

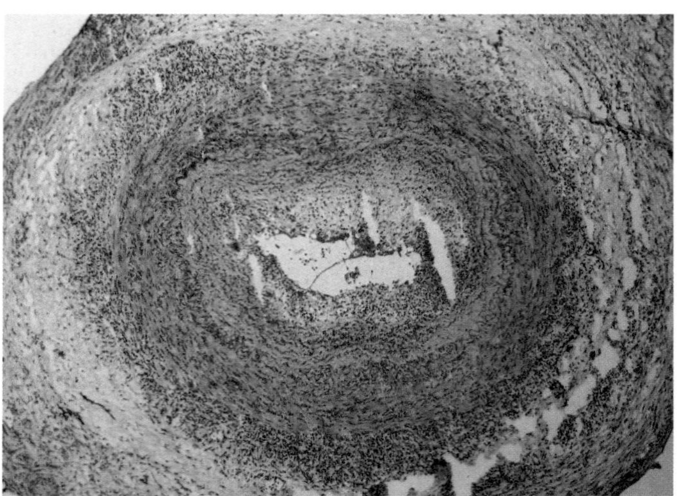

CHAPTER 113

FIGURE 113-3 Temporal artery biopsy in giant cell arteritis. This temporal artery biopsy demonstrates a panmural infiltration of mononuclear cells and lymphocytes that are particularly seen in the media and adventitia. Scattered giant cells are also present. *(Reproduced with permission from Longo DL, Fauci A, Kasper D, Hauser S, Jameson J, Loscalzo J.* Harrison's Principles of Internal Medicine. *18th ed. New York, NY: McGraw-Hill.)*

- The arteritis may involve the aorta and its branches and be complicated by dissection and occlusion (**Figures 113-4** and **113-5**, respectively).
- Polymyalgia rheumatica is associated with a synovitis that includes vascular proliferation along with macrophage and T-lymphocyte infiltration on histology.[4]

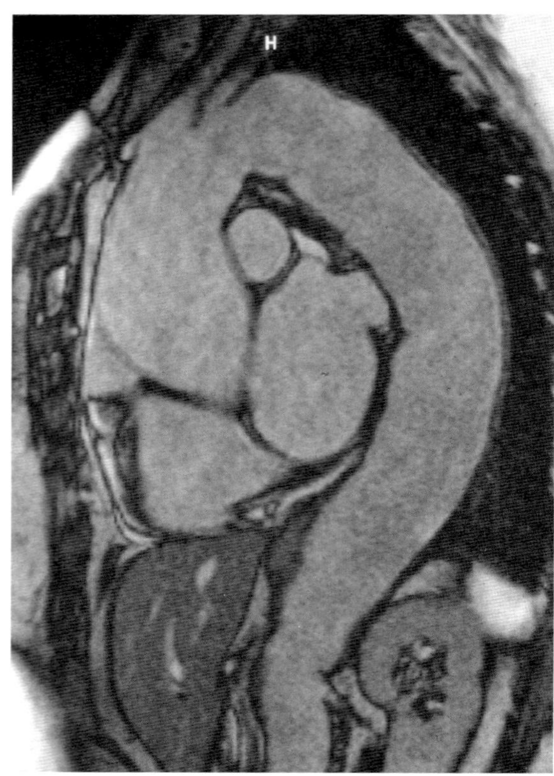

FIGURE 113-4 Magnetic resonance imaging demonstrating extensive aneurysmal disease of the thoracic aorta in an 80-year-old female. The patient had been diagnosed with biopsy-proven giant cell arteritis 10 years prior to presenting with this aneurysm. *(Reproduced with permission from Longo DL, Fauci A, Kasper D, Hauser S, Jameson J, Loscalzo J. Harrison's Principles of Internal Medicine. 18th ed. New York, NY: McGraw-Hill.)*

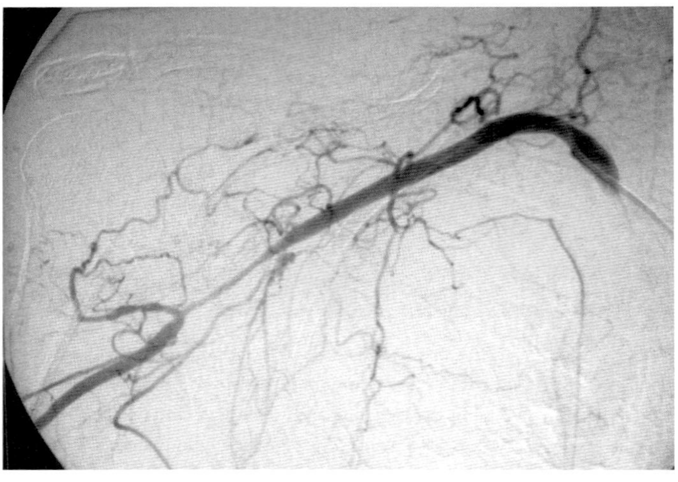

FIGURE 113-5 Upper-extremity arteriogram demonstrating a long stenotic lesion of the axillary artery in a 75-year-old female with giant cell arteritis. *(Reproduced with permission from Longo DL, Fauci A, Kasper D, Hauser S, Jameson J, Loscalzo J.* Harrison's Principles of Internal Medicine. *18th ed. New York, NY: McGraw-Hill.)*

RISK FACTORS

- Age greater than 50
- Female gender
- Northern European ancestry

DIAGNOSIS/SCREENING

CLINICAL FEATURES—HISTORY AND PHYSICAL

- Diagnostic criteria for PMR—Guidelines are not specific on the number of these "core inclusion criteria" that are required to make the diagnosis.[5]
  - Age greater than 50; symptoms present for more than 2 weeks.
  - Bilateral shoulder or pelvic girdle aching or both.
  - Morning stiffness lasting longer than 45 minutes.
  - Evidence of an acute-phase response (elevated ESR or CRP).
  - The diagnosis of PMR can be made in the absence of an elevated ESR (or CRP) if there are classic symptoms and there is a rapid response to corticosteroids (initial dose commonly 15 mg/day).
    - A 70% clinical response within 7 days is consistent with PMR.
  - Normalization of ESR or CRP within 4 weeks of starting prednisone.
  - Hips are involved in up to 70% of patients with PMR.
  - Up to 30% of patients with PMR lack shoulder symptoms.
  - Peripheral/constitutional symptoms occur in up to 50% of patients with PMR.
  - Exclude
    - Active infection or cancer as the management of PMR typically includes corticosteroids
    - Temporal arteritis as the management of this condition is different from that of PMR
    - Other inflammatory rheumatic diseases, such as rheumatoid arthritis
    - Drug-induced myalgias, such as that seen with statins
    - Chronic pain syndromes, such as fibromyalgia
    - Endocrine disease, such as hypothyroidism, which may present with myopathy
    - Parkinson disease

- Clinical manifestations of TA vary from subtle to dramatic.
  - For the diagnosis of TA, use 3 of the following 5 (93% sensitivity and 91% specificity)[6]:
    - Age of onset past 50 years (mean age 70)
    - Abrupt onset of a new headache (temporal is common) and temporal tenderness, but tenderness can occasionally be diffuse or bilateral
    - Temporal artery tenderness (and prominent beading or diminished pulse on the temporal artery not related to atherosclerosis) or decreased pulsation
    - Erythrocyte sedimentation rate more than 50 mm/h
    - Temporal artery biopsy (showing vasculitis with granulomatous inflammation and multinucleated giant cells)
  - Other features that may be associated with TA include jaw or tongue claudication, blurring or diplopia, scalp tenderness, fever, fatigue, weight loss, cranial nerve palsies, and bruits over the upper-limb arteries. A high index of suspicion for TA is needed in the presence of jaw/tongue claudication or visual symptoms in the absence of headache.

LABORATORY TESTING

- A complete blood cell count (CBC), although nonspecific, may help identify a systemic disease or infection.
- Core diagnostic tests for the presence of both TA and PMR are ESR and CRP.
- Complete a comprehensive profile prior to starting corticosteroids to assess for glycemic control and liver and renal function.
- Parathyroid hormone and 25-hydroxy-vitamin D level—Vitamin D deficiency and hyperparathyroidism are secondary causes of osteopenia and osteoporosis, which can be worsened with the anticipated prednisone therapy for both PMR and TA.
- Bence-Jones protein (in urine and plasma) helps to exclude the presence of multiple myeloma, which can present with musculoskeletal pain and is a disease primarily of the elderly.
- Thyrotropin (TSH)—Hypothyroidism can be associated with myopathy.
- Testing for creatine kinase should be ordered to help exclude the presence of inflammatory muscle disease, such as polymyositis.
- Rheumatoid factor (RF) testing (a blood test for anti-cyclic citrullinated peptide [anti-CCP] antibody should be considered as it is more sensitive) will help exclude the diagnosis of rheumatoid arthritis.
- Antinuclear antibody (ANA) will evaluate for systemic lupus erythematosus (SLE) or overlap syndromes.

IMAGING

- Ultrasound, demonstrating edema in the temporal artery along with stenosis has 69% sensitivity and 82% specificity for the diagnosis of TA. However, it is not a replacement for TA biopsy.[7]
- Chest radiography can check for aortic aneurysm in patients with TA (consider an echocardiogram or computed tomographic [CT] angiography).
- Biopsy of the temporal artery for a diagnosis of TA should be completed within 1 week of starting corticosteroids. However, do not delay the initiation of corticosteroid therapy while arranging for the biopsy.[8]

DIFFERENTIAL DIAGNOSIS

- Differential diagnosis of PMR includes the following:
  - Rheumatoid arthritis, lupus, or other vasculidities—Stiffness, pain swelling, tenderness, and warmth are more common in the distal joints (hands and feet) (see Chapters 99, Rheumatoid Arthritis; and 178, Lupus: Systemic and Cutaneous).
  - Inflammatory myopathies—Dermatomyositis and polymyositis are associated with muscle weakness and an increase in serum muscle enzymes. In addition, dermatomyositis is associated with a rash (see Chapter 179, Dermatomyositis).
  - Osteoarthritis—Pain is worse with use and better with rest (see Chapter 98, Osteoarthritis).
  - Primary shoulder disease, including rotator cuff lesions or capsulitis—Pain is worse with use and better with rest and is more commonly unilateral.
  - Fibromyalgia—This is commonly associated with widespread pain in the musculoskeletal system and multiple trigger points and is most common in women.
- Differential diagnosis of TA includes the following:
  - Headache differential (see Chapter 230, Headache)
    - Migraine—Onset of migraine after the age of 50 is unusual, and migraine is associated with pulsatile pain, nausea/vomiting, and photophobia and phonophobia.
    - Cluster headache—This is most common in males, and the pain of cluster headaches has a typical duration of 15 minutes to 3 hours with symptom-free intervals of up to 2 days.
    - Herpes zoster (shingles)—Localized pain, including a headache, is followed by a vesicular rash in a dermatomal distribution (see Chapters 126, Zoster; and 127, Zoster Ophthalmicus).
    - Cervical spine disease—Pain of cervical spine disease is commonly worse with movement of the cervical spine.
    - Sinus disease—This presents with pain over the sinus, rhinorrhea, and pus in the nasal cavity (see Chapter 28, Sinusitis).
  - Acute vision loss.
    - Transient ischemic attack (TIA) (for acute vision loss)—This causes abrupt onset of visual loss in the absence of headache.
  - Jaw claudication.
    - Temperomandibular joint (TMJ) pain may be confused with jaw claudication but is commonly associated with audible clicking and crepitus during jaw movement.

MANAGEMENT

MEDICATIONS

- Polymyalgia rheumatica—Urgently starting corticosteroids is *not necessary in PMR* (as opposed to TA) and can be delayed to initiate a complete assessment.
  - Prednisone 15 mg daily for 3 weeks, then 12.5 mg for 3 weeks, then 10 mg for 4 to 6 weeks, then reduction by 1 mg every 4 to 8 weeks until discontinuation.[1,9] SOR Ⓐ
    - Less than 1% of patients initially treated with 15 mg prednisone subsequently required higher doses to control symptoms; therefore, a 15-mg starting dose is an effective initial dose in most patients.[1]
    - Follow-up 3 times in the first 4 months; the first visit should be within several weeks, then every 3 months for 1 year.
    - Some patients benefit from a more rapid steroid-tapering regimen.
  - Duration of treatment is commonly 1 to 2 years (discontinue when asymptomatic from their inflammatory condition and ESR and CRP levels normalize).
  - In the case of a relapse, increase corticosteroid to the previous higher dose (or use intramuscular injections of methylprednisolone 120 mg every 3-4 weeks, decreasing by 20 mg every 2-3 months).[5]

- *For TA, begin corticosteroid therapy immediately.*[3,10] SOR A
  - Prednisone 1 mg/kg/d or 40 to 60 mg daily until symptoms disappear and laboratory abnormalities (eg, ESR) normalize, commonly 4 weeks.
  - Reduce dose by 10 mg every 2 weeks to 20 mg, then by 2.5 mg every 2 to 4 weeks to 10 mg, then 1 mg every 1 to 2 months.[3]
  - If visual evolving loss or amaurosis fugax, use methylprednisolone 500 mg to 1 g intravenously daily for 3 days.[3]
- Osteoporosis prevention—Start a bisphosphonate with vitamin D and calcium to prevent osteoporosis in patients with high-fracture risk (age >65 and prior fragility fracture). In patients without a high-fracture risk start calcium and vitamin D when starting steroid therapy; in these patients, obtain a dual-energy X-ray absorptiometry (DXA) scan and if the T score is less than −1.0, start a bisphosphonate.[11]
- Initiate low-dose aspirin 160 mg/d in patients with TA in the absence of contraindications.[3] SOR C
  - The aspirin decreases visual loss and cerebrovascular ischemic events by about 20%.
- Consider a proton pump inhibitor for gastrointestinal protection in those on corticosteroids. SOR C
- Steroid-sparing drugs (to reduce the potential risk of long-term steroid use) have been studied in PMR.
  - Methotrexate (10 mg/week) added to 10 mg of prednisone per day appears to have an effect on decreasing relapses, reducing prednisone requirements, and decreasing prednisone-related adverse effects and may be of most benefit in those at high risk of steroid complications.[1,12] SOR B
- Infliximab demonstrated no beneficial effect (and possible harm) in newly diagnosed patients with PMR treated with prednisone.[13] SOR B

REFER OR HOSPITALIZE

- Refer patients with atypical features such as lack of shoulder involvement, prominent systemic symptoms, or normal or very high acute-phase reactants.
- Refer patients with therapeutic dilemmas, including nonresponse or inability to reduce corticosteroids or contraindications to corticosteroids.

PROGNOSIS

- Risk of vision loss is up to 50% in the contralateral eye in the presence of vision loss in one eye.
- About 27% of patients with TA are at risk for the late complications of aortic aneurysm, dissection, or stenosis.[14]

FOLLOW-UP

- For PMR, follow up patients in 1 to 3 weeks, then 4 to 6 weeks depending on the response to treatment.
- Assess for proximal muscle pain (hips and shoulders), morning stiffness, and fatigue.
- For TA, follow up more frequently, including within 1 week, 4 times within the first 3 months, and every 3 months afterward within the first year.

PATIENT EDUCATION

- Educate patients on features of relapse, including new fever, headache, scalp tenderness, visual symptoms, jaw or tongue claudication, PMR, or cerebrovascular symptoms.
- Osteoporosis prevention is more than taking medications. Other lifestyle issues should be discussed, including diet and exercise (see Chapter 225, Osteoporosis and Osteopenia).

PATIENT RESOURCES

- American College of Rheumatology
  - *Giant Cell Arteritis*—**http://www.rheumatology.org/practice/clinical/patients/diseases_and_conditions/giantcellarteritis.asp.**
    - Spanish version—**http://www.rheumatology.org/practice/clinical/patients/diseases_and_conditions/giantcellarteritis-esp.asp.**
  - *Polymyalgia Rheumatica*—**http://www.rheumatology.org/practice/clinical/patients/diseases_and_conditions/polymyalgiarheumatica.asp.**
    - Spanish version—**http://www.rheumatology.org/practice/clinical/patients/diseases_and_conditions/polymyalgiarheumatica-esp.asp.**

PROVIDER RESOURCES

- Dasgupta B, Borg FA, Hassan N, et al. BSR and BHPR guidelines for the management of polymyalgia rheumatica. *Rheumatology*. 2010;49(1):186-190. **http://rheumatology.oxfordjournals.org/content/49/1/186.long.**
- Dasgupta B, Borg FA, Hassan N, et al. BSR and BHPR guidelines for the management of giant cell arteritis. *Rheumatology*. 2010;49(8):1594-1597. **http://rheumatology.oxfordjournals.org/content/49/8/1594.long.**
- Grossman JM, Gordon R, Ranganath VK, et al. American College of Rheumatology 2010 recommendations for the prevention and treatment of glucocorticoid-induced osteoporosis. *Arthritis Care Res (Hoboken)*. 2010;62(11):1515-1526. **http://www.rheumatology.org/practice/clinical/guidelines/GIOP_Guidelines_Nov_2010.pdf.**

REFERENCES

1. Hernandez-Rodriguez J, Cid MC, Lopez-Soto A, Espigol-Frigole G, Bosch X. Treatment of polymyalgia rheumatic: a systematic review. *Arch Intern Med*. 2009;169:1839-1850.
2. Smeeth L, Cook C, Hall AJ. Incidence of diagnosed polymyalgia rheumatica and temporal arteritis in the United Kingdom, 1990-2001. *Ann Rheum Dis*. 2006;65(8):1093-1098. Epub 2006 Jan 13.
3. Dasgupta B, Borg FA, Hassan N, et al. for the BHPR Standards, Guidelines and Audit Working Group. BSR and BHPR guidelines for the management of giant cell arteritis. *Rheumatology (Oxford)*. 2010;49(8):1594-1597. Epub 2010 Apr 5.
4. Meliconi R, Pulsatelli L, Uguccioni M, et al. Leukocyte infiltration in synovial tissue from the shoulder of patients with polymyalgia rheumatica. Quantitative analysis and influence of corticosteroid treatment. *Arthritis Rheum*. 1996;39(7):1199-1207.

5. Dasgupta B, Borg FA, Hassan N, et al. for the BSR and BHPR Standards, Guidelines and Audit Working Group. BSR and BHPR guidelines for the management of polymyalgia rheumatica. *Rheumatology (Oxford).* 2010;49(1):186-190. Epub 2009 Nov 12.
6. Hunder GG, Bloch DA, Michel BA, et al. The American College of Rheumatology 1990 criteria for the classification of giant cell arteritis. *Arthritis Rheum.* 1990;33(8):1122-1128.
7. Karassa FB, Matsagas MI, Schmidt WA, Ioannidis JP. Meta-analysis: test performance of ultrasonography for giant-cell arteritis. *Ann Intern Med.* 2005;142(5):359-369.
8. Mukhtyar C, Guillevin L, Cid MC, et al. for the European Vasculitis Study Group. EULAR recommendations for the management of large vessel vasculitis. *Ann Rheum Dis.* 2009;68(3):318-323. Epub 2008 Apr 15.
9. Salvarani C, Cantini F, Hunder GG. Polymyalgia rheumatic and giant-cell arteritis. *Lancet.* 2008;372:234.
10. Mukhtyar C, Guillevin L, Cid MC, et al. EULAR recommendations for the management of large vessel vasculitis. *Ann Rheum Dis.* 2009;68:318-323.
11. Grossman JM, Gordon R, Ranganath VK, et al. American College of Rheumatology 2010 recommendations for the prevention and treatment of glucocorticoid-induced osteoporosis. *Arthritis Care Res (Hoboken).* 2010;62(11):1515-1526.
12. Ferraccioli G, Salaffi F, De Vita S, et al. Methotrexate in polymyalgia rheumatica: preliminary results of an open, randomized study. *Rheumatology.* 1996;23(4):624-628.
13. Salvarani C, Macchioni P, Manzini C, et al. Infliximab plus prednisone or placebo plus prednisone for the initial treatment of polymyalgia rheumatica: a randomized trial. *Ann Intern Med.* 2007;146(9):631-639.
14. Nuenninghoff DM, Hunder GG, Christianson TJ, et al. Incidence and predictors of large-artery complication (aortic aneurysm, aortic dissection, and/or large-artery stenosis) in patients with giant cell arteritis: a population-based study over 50 years. *Arthritis Rheum.* 2003;48(12):3522-3531.

PART 14

DERMATOLOGY

Strength of Recommendation (SOR)	Definition
A	Recommendation based on consistent and good-quality patient-oriented evidence.*
B	Recommendation based on inconsistent or limited-quality patient-oriented evidence.*
C	Recommendation based on consensus, usual practice, opinion, disease-oriented evidence, or case series for studies of diagnosis, treatment, prevention, or screening.*

*See Appendix A on pages 1241-1244 for further information.

SECTION 1 ACNEIFORM DISORDERS

114 ACNE VULGARIS

Richard P. Usatine, MD

PATIENT STORY

A 20-year-old man (**Figure 114-1a**) with severe nodulocystic acne and scarring presents for treatment. After trying oral antibiotics, topical retinoids, and topical benzyl peroxide with no significant benefit, the patient requests isotretinoin. After 6 months of isotretinoin, the nodules and cysts cleared (**Figure 114-1b**). He is much happier and more confident about his appearance.

INTRODUCTION

Acne is an obstructive and inflammatory disease of the pilosebaceous unit that can occur at any age. While it is typically associated with the teenage years, many adults suffer with acne severe enough to affect their self-esteem and well-being (**Figure 114-2**).

EPIDEMIOLOGY

Acne vulgaris affects more than 80% of teenagers, and persists beyond the age of 25 years in 3% of men and 12% of women.[1]

ETIOLOGY AND PATHOPHYSIOLOGY

The 4 most important steps in acne pathogenesis are as below:

1. Sebum overproduction related to androgenic hormones and genetics
2. Abnormal desquamation of the follicular epithelium (keratin plugging)
3. Propionibacterium acnes proliferation
4. Follicular obstruction, which can lead to inflammation and follicular disruption

Acne can be precipitated by medications such as phenytoin and lithium (**Figure 114-3**).

There are some studies that suggest that consumption of large quantities of milk (especially skim milk) increase the risk for acne in teenagers and young adults.[2,3] Recent studies suggest that a high glycemic load diet contributes to acne and changing to a low glycemic load diet can reduce acne lesions.[3-5]

DIAGNOSIS

CLINICAL FEATURES

Morphology of acne includes comedones, papules, pustules, nodules, and cysts.

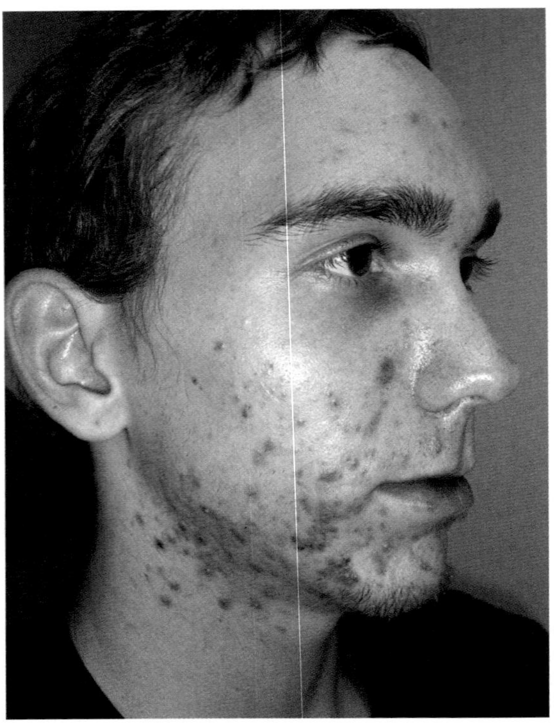

A

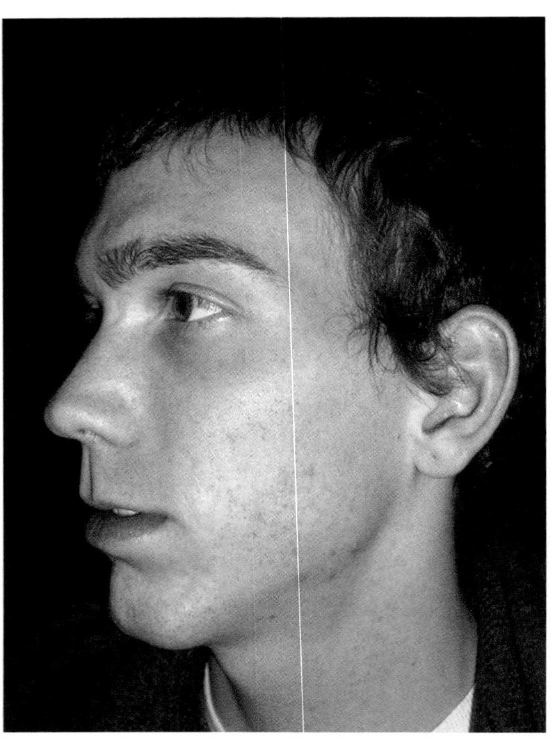

B

FIGURE 114-1 A. Severe nodulocystic acne with scarring in a 20-year-old man. B. Excellent results after 6 months of isotretinoin. (*Reproduced with permission from Richard P. Usatine, MD.*)

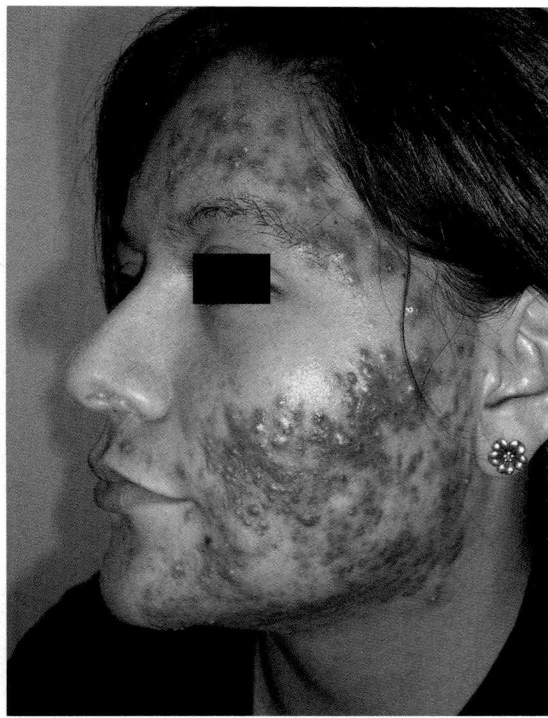

FIGURE 114-2 Severe inflammatory acne in a 24-year-old woman who has failed all topical treatments and oral antibiotics. She is a perfect candidate for isotretinoin as long as she has no contraindications and will adhere to the use of 2 contraceptive methods or abstinence. (*Reproduced with permission from Richard P. Usatine, MD.*)

- Obstructive acne = comedonal acne = noninflammatory acne and consists of only comedones (**Figure 114-4**).
- Open comedones are blackheads and closed comedones are called whiteheads and look like small papules.
- Inflammatory acne has papules, pustules, nodules, and cysts in addition to comedones (**Figures 114-5** and **114-6**).

TYPICAL DISTRIBUTION

The parts affected with acne vulgaris are face, back, chest, and neck.

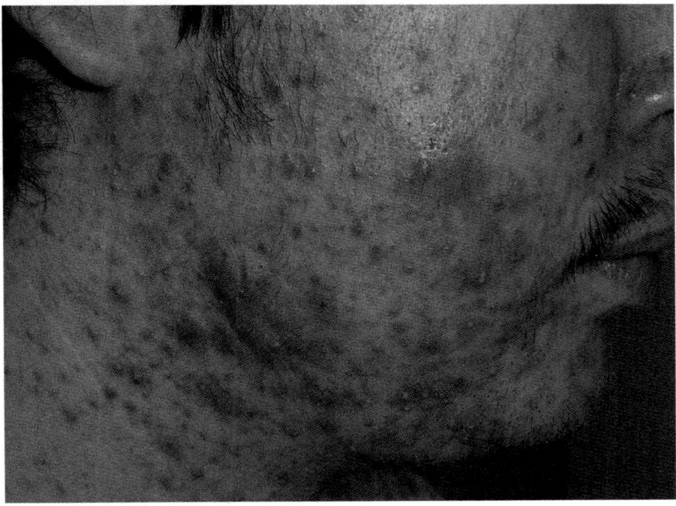

FIGURE 114-3 Severe inflammatory acne in a young adult. His acne worsened when he was started on phenytoin for his seizure disorder. (*Reproduced with permission from Richard P. Usatine, MD.*)

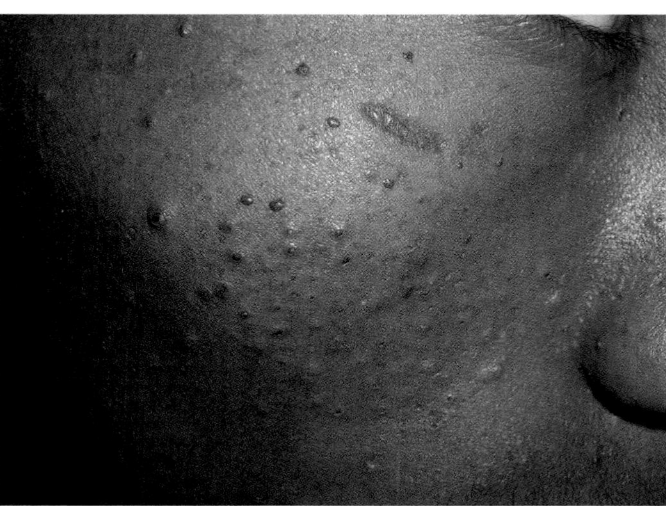

FIGURE 114-4 Comedonal acne with large open comedones. (*Reproduced with permission from Richard P. Usatine, MD.*)

LABORATORY STUDIES

None unless you suspect androgen excess and/or polycystic ovarian syndrome (PCOS).[6] SOR Ⓐ Obtain testosterone and dehydroepiandrosterone sulfate (DHEA-S) levels if you suspect androgen excess and/or PCOS.

Consider follicle-stimulating hormone (FSH) and luteinizing hormone (LH) levels if you suspect PCOS.

DIFFERENTIAL DIAGNOSIS

- Acne conglobata is an uncommon and unusually severe form of acne characterized by multiple comedones, cysts, sinus tracks, and

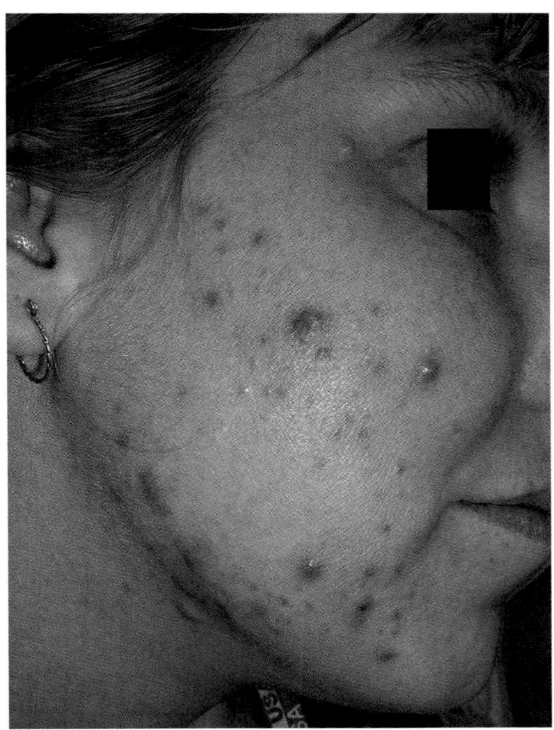

FIGURE 114-5 Inflammatory acne in a 20-year-old woman. It is very common for the jaw line to be involved in women suffering with acne at this age. (*Reproduced with permission from Richard P. Usatine, MD.*)

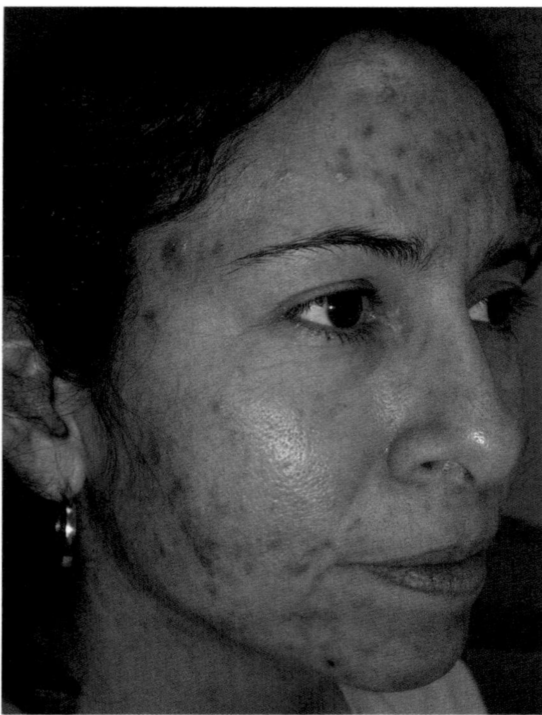

FIGURE 114-6 Inflammatory acne in an older woman. She is tired of having painful cysts on her face and chooses to have some acne injections that day. Knowing this is only a temporary treatment, isotretinoin is discussed. (*Reproduced with permission from Richard P. Usatine, MD.*)

abscesses. The inflammatory lesions and scars can lead to significant disfigurement.[7] Sinus tracks can form with multiple openings that drain foul-smelling purulent material (**Figures 114-7, 114-8,** and **114-9**). The comedones and nodules are usually found on the chest, the shoulders, the back, the buttocks, and the face. In some cases acne conglobata is part of a follicular occlusion triad including hidradenitis and dissecting cellulitis of the scalp (see **Figure 114-9**).

- Acne fulminans is characterized by sudden-onset ulcerative crusting cystic acne, mostly on the chest and back (**Figures 114-10** and **114-11**).[8] Fever, malaise, nausea, arthralgia, myalgia, and weight loss are common. Leukocytosis and elevated erythrocyte sedimentation rate are usually found. There may also be focal osteolytic lesions. The term *acne fulminans* may also be used in cases of severe aggravation of acne without systemic features.[8]
- Rosacea can resemble acne by having papules and pustules on the face. It is usually seen in older adults with prominent erythema and telangiectasias. Rosacea does not include comedones and may have ocular or nasal manifestations (see Chapter 115, Rosacea). Rosacea fulminans or pyoderma faciale has features of severe acne and rosacea (**Figure 114-12**).
- Folliculitis on the back may be confused with acne. Look for hairs centrally located in the inflammatory papules of folliculitis to help distinguish it from acne. Acne on the back usually accompanies acne on the face as well (see Chapter 119, Folliculitis).
- Acne keloidalis nuchae consists of papules, pustules, nodules, and keloidal tissue found at the posterior hairline. It is most often seen in men of color after shaving the hair at the nape of the neck (see Chapter 116, Pseudofolliculitis and Acne Keloidalis Nuchae).
- Actinic comedones (blackheads) are related to sun exposure and are seen later in life (**Figure 114-13**).

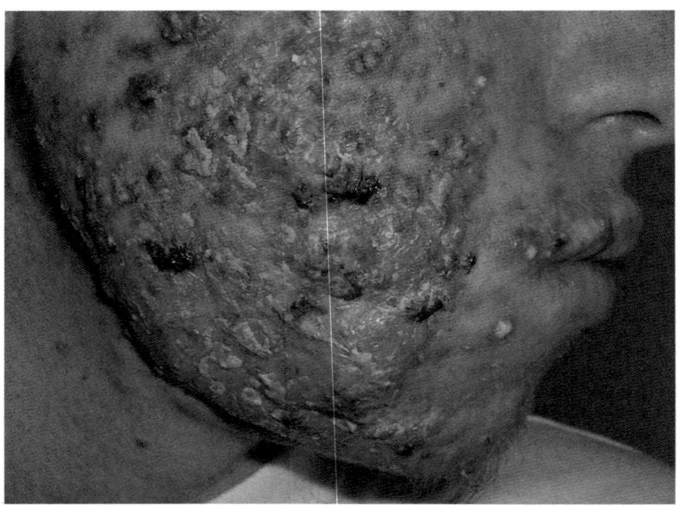

A

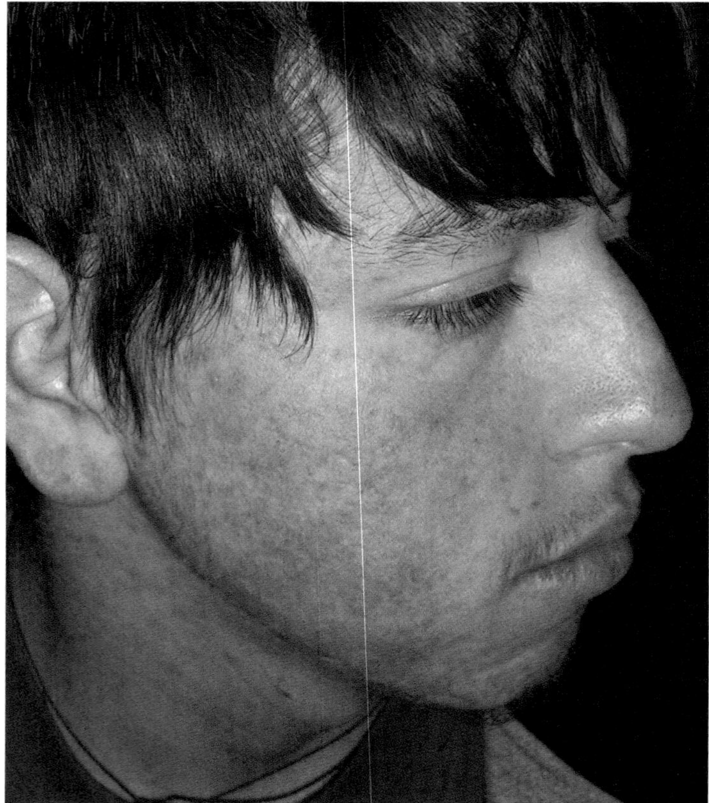

B

FIGURE 114-7 **A.** Acne conglobata in a 16-year-old boy. He has severe cysts on his face with sinus tracks between them. He required many weeks of oral prednisone before isotretinoin was started. His acne cleared completely with his treatment. **B.** Acne conglobata cleared with minimal scarring after oral prednisone and 5 months of isotretinoin therapy. (*Reproduced with permission from Richard P. Usatine, MD.*)

MANAGEMENT

Treatment is based on type of acne and severity. Medical therapy categories to choose from are topical retinoids, topical antimicrobials, systemic antimicrobials, hormonal therapy, oral isotretinoin, and injection therapy.

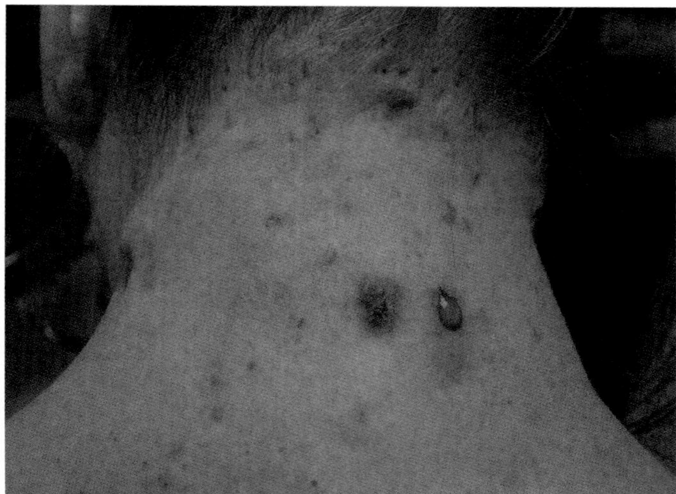

FIGURE 114-8 Acne conglobata in a 42-year-old woman showing communicating sinus tracks between cysts. There is pus draining from one of the sinus tracts on the right side of the neck. (*Reproduced with permission from Richard P. Usatine, MD.*)

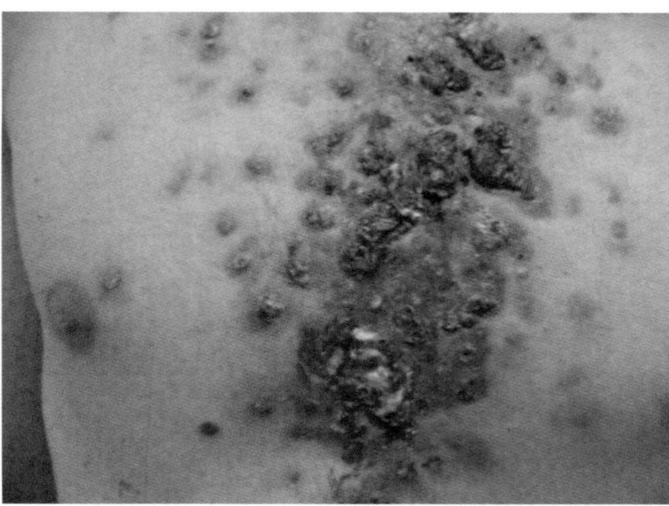

FIGURE 114-10 Acne fulminans in a 17-year-old boy. He was on isotretinoin when he developed worsening of his acne with polymyalgia and arthralgia. He presented with numerous nodules and cysts covered by hemorrhagic crusts on his chest and back. (*Reproduced with permission from Grunwald MH, Amichai B. Nodulocystic eruption with musculoskeletal pain.* J Fam Pract. *2007;56:205-206, reproduced with permission from Frontline Medical Communications.*)

Discussion of diet is reasonable for all patients as a low glycemic load diet and weight loss may be beneficial for many patients.

DIETARY CHANGES

- Take a brief diet history asking about milk intake and whether the diet contains high glycemic load foods such as simple sugars.
- Suggest that excessive milk intake be decreased.[2,3] SOR Ⓑ
- Discuss the role a healthy lower glycemic load diet substituting foods with more complex carbohydrates (eg, whole-grain bread, pasta, and fruit) for those with simple sugars. Also including more foods higher in protein (eg, lean meat, poultry, beans, or fish) and not relying on a high carbohydrate diet alone.[4,5] SOR Ⓑ
- In one randomized controlled trial (RCT) of a low glycemic load diet in 43 male patients with acne, total lesion counts and weight decreased more in the experimental group compared with the control group.[5] Part of the benefit may have been secondary to weight loss. Certainly, suggesting that obese patients lose weight as part of their acne treatment can only be beneficial for the skin and general health of the patients.[5] SOR Ⓑ

MEDICATIONS FOR ACNE THERAPY

In a review of 250 comparisons, the Agency for Healthcare Research and Quality found 14 had evidence of level A.[9] These comparisons demonstrated the efficacy over vehicle or placebo control of topical clindamycin, topical erythromycin, benzoyl peroxide, topical tretinoin, oral tetracycline, and norgestimate/ethinyl estradiol.[9] Level A conclusions demonstrating equivalence include benzoyl peroxide at various strengths was equally efficacious in mild or moderate acne; adapalene and tretinoin were equally efficacious.[9] SOR Ⓐ

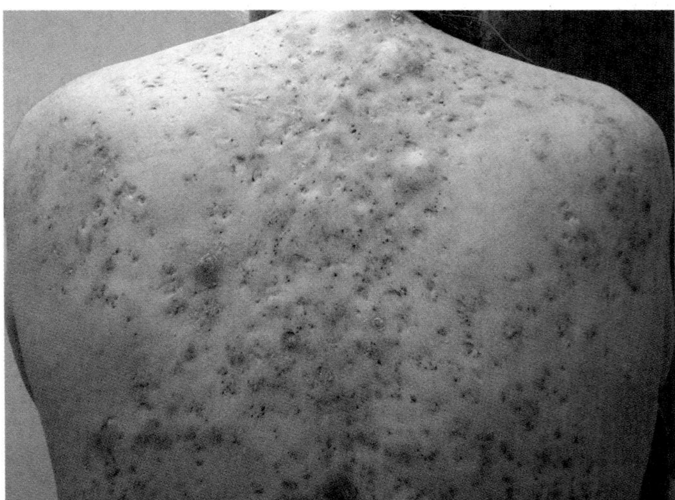

FIGURE 114-9 Acne conglobata in a 53-year-old man covered with open comedones and cysts on his back. He has the follicular occlusion triad including hidradenitis, dissecting cellulitis of the scalp, and acne conglobata. (*Reproduced with permission from Richard P. Usatine, MD.*)

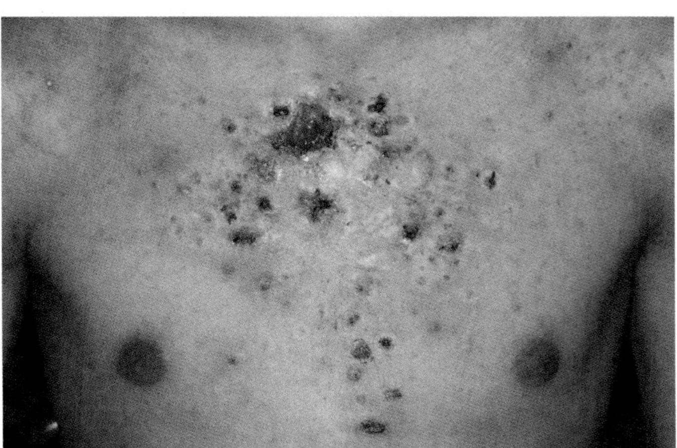

FIGURE 114-11 Acne fulminans with severe rapidly worsening truncal acne in a 15-year-old adolescent boy. He did not have fever or bone pain but had a white blood cell count of 17,000. He responded rapidly to prednisone and was started on isotretinoin. The ulcers and granulation tissue worsened initially on isotretinoin but prednisone helped to get this under control. (*Reproduced with permission from Richard P. Usatine, MD.*)

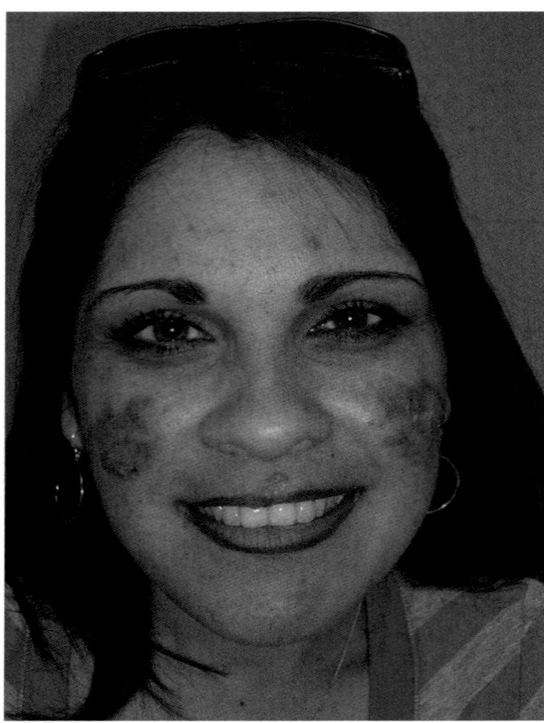

FIGURE 114-12 Pyoderma faciale is almost exclusively seen in adult women. It can present with severe cystic facial acne often in a malar distribution. It also is called rosacea fulminans. It started abruptly 6 months before and her antinuclear antibody was normal. (*Reproduced with permission from Richard P. Usatine, MD.*)

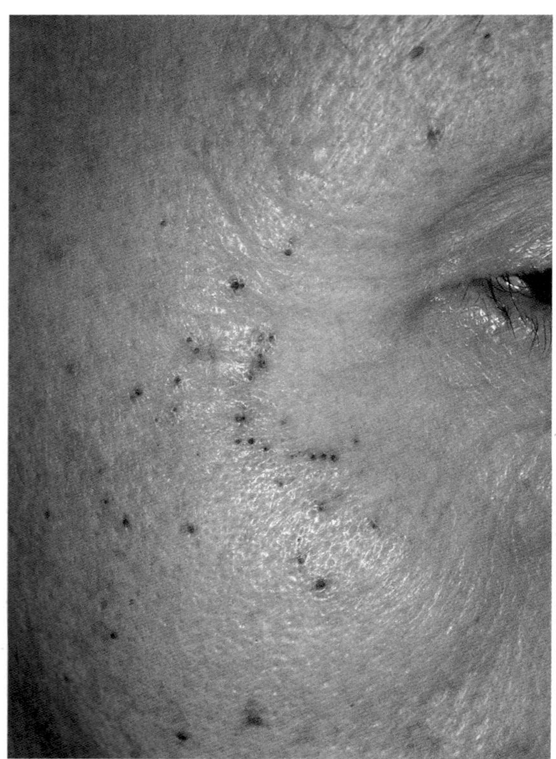

FIGURE 114-13 Actinic comedones related to sun exposure in an older man. These are typically seen on the side of the face clustering around the eyes. (*Reproduced with permission from Richard P. Usatine, MD.*)

Topical

- Benzoyl peroxide—Antimicrobial effect (gel, cream, lotion) (2.5%, 5%, 10%) 10% causes more irritation and is not more effective.[1] SOR Ⓐ
- Topical antibiotics—Clindamycin and erythromycin are the mainstays of treatment.
- Erythromycin—Solution, gel.[6] SOR Ⓐ
- Clindamycin—Solution, gel, lotion.[6] SOR Ⓐ
- Benzamycin gel—Erythromycin 3%, benzoyl peroxide 5%.[6] SOR Ⓐ
- BenzaClin gel—Clindamycin 1%, benzoyl peroxide 5%.[6] SOR Ⓐ
- Dapsone 5% gel.[10] SOR Ⓑ

Retinoids

- Tretinoin (Retin-A) gel, cream, liquid, micronized.[1] SOR Ⓐ
- Adapalene gel—Less irritating than tretinoin.[1] SOR Ⓐ
- Tazarotene—Strongest topical retinoid with greatest risk of irritation.[11] SOR Ⓐ

Topical retinoids will often result in skin irritation during the first 2 to 3 months of treatment, but new systematic reviews do not demonstrate that they worsen acne lesion counts during the initial period of use.[2]

- Azelaic acid—Useful to treat spotty hyperpigmentation and acne (**Figure 114-14**).[6] SOR Ⓑ

Systemic

- Oral antibiotics.
- Tetracycline 500 mg qd bid—Inexpensive, absorbed best on an empty stomach.[6] SOR Ⓐ
- Doxycycline 40 to 100 mg qd bid—Inexpensive, well tolerated, can take with food and increases sun sensitivity.[6] SOR Ⓐ
- Minocycline 50 to 100 mg qd bid—More expensive, not proven to be better than other systemic antibiotics including tetracycline.[6,12] SOR Ⓐ
- Erythromycin 250 to 500 mg bid—Inexpensive, frequent gastrointestinal (GI) disturbance but can be used in pregnancy.[6] SOR Ⓐ
- Trimethoprim/sulfamethoxazole DS bid—Effective but risk of Stevens-Johnson syndrome is real. Reserve for short courses in particularly severe and resistant cases.[6] SOR Ⓐ

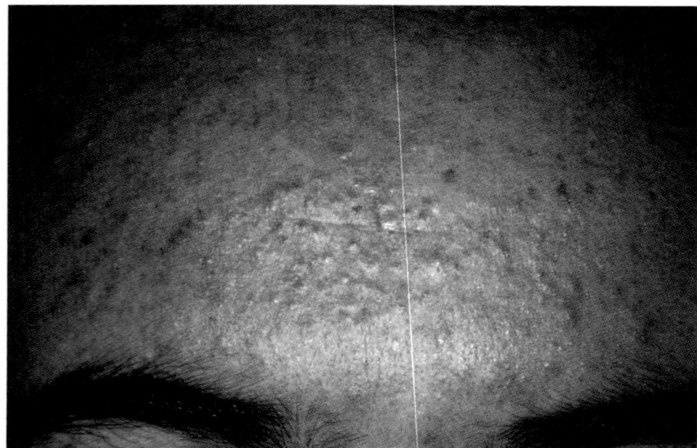

FIGURE 114-14 Obstructive or comedonal acne with spotty hyperpigmentation. Azelaic acid was helpful to treat the acne and the hyperpigmentation. (*Reproduced with permission from Richard P. Usatine, MD.*)

Oral azithromycin has been prescribed in pulse dosing for acne in a number of small poorly done studies and has not been found to be better than oral doxycyline.[13]

- Isotretinoin (often referred to as Accutane even though this brand name is off the market) is the most powerful treatment for acne. It is especially useful for cystic and scarring acne that has not responded to other therapies.[6] SOR Ⓐ Dosed at approximately 1 mg/kg per day for 5 months. Women of childbearing age must use 2 forms of contraception. Monitor for depression.
- The US Food and Drug Administration (FDA) requires that prescribers of isotretinoin, patients who take isotretinoin, and pharmacists who dispense isotretinoin all must register with the iPLEDGE system (**www.ipledgeprogram.com**).
- Hormonal treatments
  - Oral contraceptives only for females—Choose ones with low androgenic effect.[6] SOR Ⓐ FDA-approved oral contraceptives are Ortho Tri-Cyclen, Yaz, and Estrostep. Other oral contraceptives with similar formulations also help acne in women even though these have not received FDA approval for this indication. Note Yaz and Yasmin have progestin drospirenone, which is derived from 17α-spironolactone. It shares an antiandrogenic effect with spironolactone. There may be an increased risk of venous thromboembolism with drospirenone versus other progestins.[14]
  - Spironolactone may be used for adult women when other therapies fail.[3,15,16] This may be especially useful if the patient has hirsutism. Standard dosing is 50 to 200 mg/d. May start with 50 mg daily and monitor for hyperkalemia. The risk of hyperkalemia increases with a higher dose. Titrate up as needed and tolerated.[6] SOR Ⓑ A recent systematic review failed to show a benefit for spironolactone in acne even though it was found to decrease hirsutism.[17] Note that acne is not an FDA-approved indication for spironolactone.
  - One small prospective study of 27 women with severe papular and nodulocystic acne used a combination of EE/DRSP (Yasmin) and spironolactone 100 mg daily. Eighty-five percent of subjects were entirely clear of acne lesions or had excellent improvement and there was no significant elevation of serum potassium.[18]

STEROID INJECTION THERAPY

This therapy is used for painful nodules and cysts. SOR Ⓒ Be careful to avoid producing skin atrophy by diluting the steroid and following the directions below:

- Dilute 0.1 cc of 10 mg/cc triamcinolone acetonide (Kenalog) with 0.4 cc of sterile saline for a 2 mg/cc suspension.
- Inject 0.1 cc with a 1-cc tuberculin syringe into each nodule using a 30-gauge needle (**Figure 114-15**).

COMPLEMENTARY AND ALTERNATIVE THERAPY

Tea tree oil 5% gel[19] SOR Ⓑ

ACNE THERAPY BY SEVERITY

Comedonal acne (see Figure 114-6)

- Topical retinoid or azelaic acid.
- Consider benzoyl peroxide as a wash or leave-on product.
- No need for antibiotics—No need to kill Propionibacterium acnes.

Mild papulopustular

- Topical antibiotics and benzoyl peroxide.
- Topical retinoid or azelaic acid.

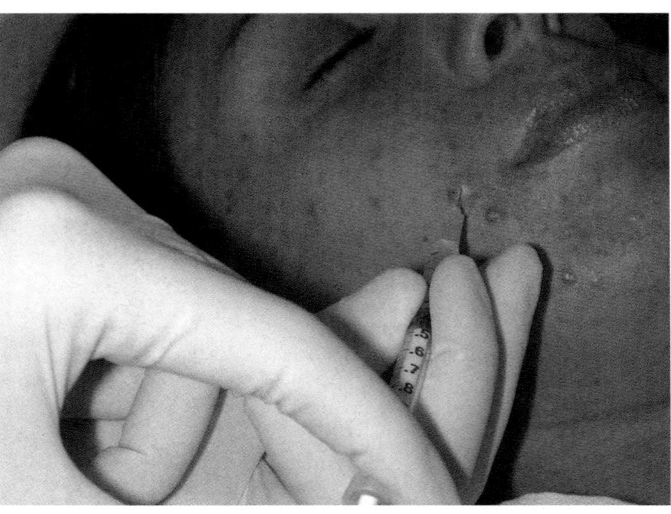

FIGURE 114-15 Injection of acne nodules with 2 mg/cc triamcinolone acetonide. (*Reproduced with permission from Richard P. Usatine, MD.*)

- May add oral antibiotics if topical agents are not working.

Papulopustular or nodulocystic acne—moderate to severe—inflammatory

- Topical antibiotic, benzoyl peroxide, and oral antibiotic.
- Oral antibiotics are often essential at this stage.
- Topical retinoid or azelaic acid (titrate up to more potent retinoids as needed)
- Steroid injection therapy—For painful nodules and cysts.

Severe cystic or scarring acne

- Isotretinoin if there are no contraindications. This is the most effective therapy **(Figure 114-16).**
- Steroid injection therapy—For painful nodules and cysts.

Acne fulminans (see Figures 114-9 to 114-11)

- Start with systemic steroids (prednisone 40-60 mg/d—approximately 1 mg/kg per day).[20] SOR Ⓒ
- Systemic steroid treatment rapidly controls the skin lesions and systemic symptoms. The duration of steroid treatment in one Finnish series was 2 to 4 months to avoid relapses.[20] SOR Ⓒ
- Therapy with isotretinoin, antibiotics, or both was often combined with steroids, but the use of these agents combined is not proven.[20] SOR Ⓒ If an antibiotic is used with isotretinoin, avoid any in the tetracycline class as the combination of the 2 increases the risk of pseudotumor cerebri.
- One British series used oral prednisolone 0.5 to 1 mg/kg daily for 4 to 6 weeks (thereafter slowly reduced to zero).[21] SOR Ⓒ
- Oral isotretinoin was added to the regimen at the fourth week, initially at 0.5 mg/kg daily and gradually increased to achieve complete clearance.[21] SOR Ⓒ
- Consider introducing isotretinoin at approximately 4 weeks into the oral prednisone if there are no contraindications. SOR Ⓒ

Acne conglobata and pyoderma faciale may be treated like acne fulminans but the course of oral prednisone does not need to be as long. SOR Ⓒ

COMBINATION THERAPIES

- Combination therapy with multiple topical agents can be more effective than single agents.[6] SOR Ⓑ

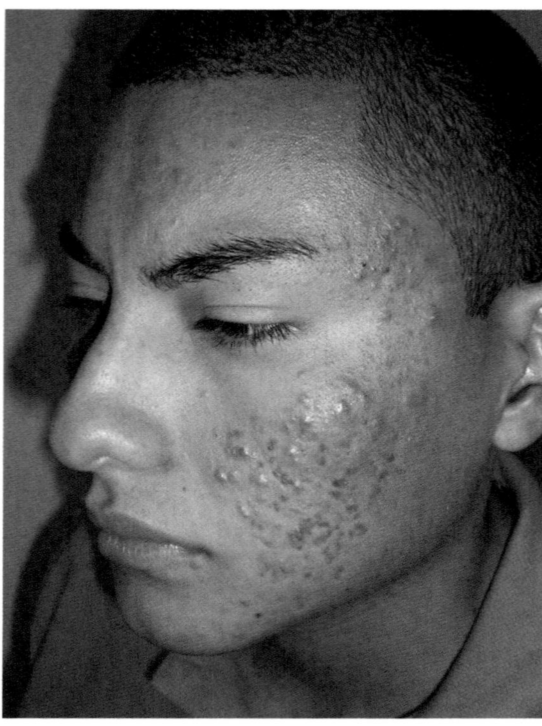

A

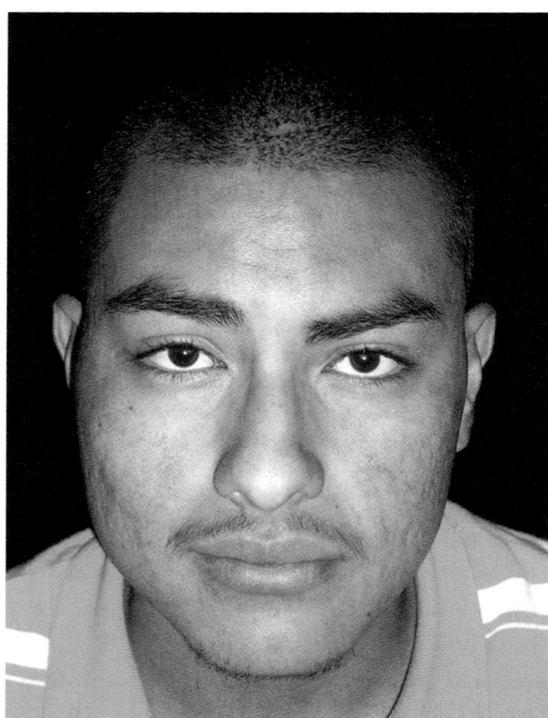

B

FIGURE 114-16 A. A young man presents with severe cystic acne unresponsive to topical medicines and oral antibiotics. He is started on isotretinoin. B. Excellent cosmetic results lead to a happy patient 6 months later. (*Reproduced with permission from Richard P. Usatine, MD.*)

- Topical retinoids and topical antibiotics are more effective when used in combination than when either is used alone.[6] SOR Ⓑ
- Benzoyl peroxide and topical antibiotics used in combination are effective treatment for acne by helping to minimize antibiotic resistance.[6] SOR Ⓑ
- The adjunctive use of clindamycin/benzoyl peroxide gel with tazarotene cream promotes greater efficacy and may also enhance tolerability.[22]
- Combination therapy with topical retinoids and oral antibiotics can be helpful at the start of acne therapy. However, maintenance therapy with combination tazarotene and minocycline therapy showed a trend for greater efficacy but no statistical significance versus tazarotene alone.[23]

MEDICATION COST

The most affordable medications for acne include topical benzoyl peroxide, erythromycin, clindamycin, and oral doxycycline. The most expensive acne medications are the newest brand name combination products of existing topical medication. These medications are convenient for those with insurance that covers them (Epiduo contains benzoyl peroxide and adapalene; Ziana contains clindamycin and tretinoin).

NEWER EXPENSIVE MODES OF THERAPY

Intense pulsed light and photodynamic therapy (PDT) use lasers, special lights, and topical chemicals to treat acne.[24-26] These therapies are very expensive and the data do not suggest that these should be first-line therapies at this time. Light and laser treatments have been shown to be of short-term benefit if patients can afford therapy and tolerate some discomfort. These therapies have not been shown to be better than simple topical treatments.[2]

One comparative trial demonstrated that PDT was less effective than topical adapalene in the short-term reduction of inflammatory lesions.[2]

FOLLOW-UP

Isotretinoin requires monthly follow-up visits but other therapies can be monitored every few months at first and then once to twice a year. Keep in mind that many treatments for acne take months to work, so quick follow-up visits may be disappointing.

PATIENT EDUCATION

Adherence with medication regimens is crucial to the success of the therapy. Adequate face washing twice a day is sufficient. Do not scrub the face with abrasive physical or chemical agents. If benzoyl peroxide is not being used as a leave-on product, it can be purchased to use for face washing.

PATIENT RESOURCES

- PubMed Health. *Acne*—**http://www.ncbi.nlm.nih.gov/pubmedhealth/PMH0001876/**.

PROVIDER RESOURCES

- Usatine R, Pfenninger J, Stulberg D, Small R. *Dermatologic and Cosmetic Procedures in Office Practice*. Philadelphia, PA: Elsevier; 2012—Covers how to do acne surgery, steroid injections for acne, chemical peels, PDT and laser treatment for acne. It is also available as an app at **www.usatinemedia.com.**

REFERENCES

1. Purdy S, de Berker D. Acne vulgaris. *Clin Evid (Online)*. 2011;2011:1714.
2. Smith EV, Grindlay DJ, Williams HC. What's new in acne? An analysis of systematic reviews published in 2009-2010. *Clin Exp Dermatol*. 2011;36:119-122.
3. Ismail NH, Manaf ZA, Azizan NZ. High glycemic load diet, milk and ice cream consumption are related to acne vulgaris in Malaysian young adults: a case control study. *BMC Dermatol*. 2012;12:13.
4. Kwon HH, Yoon JY, Hong JS, Jung JY, Park MS, Suh DH. Clinical and histological effect of a low glycaemic load diet in treatment of acne vulgaris in Korean patients: a randomized, controlled trial. *Acta Derm Venereol*. 2012;92(3):241-246.
5. Smith RN, Mann NJ, Braue A, Mäkeläinen H, Varigos GA. The effect of a high-protein, low glycemic-load diet versus a conventional, high glycemic-load diet on biochemical parameters associated with acne vulgaris: a randomized, investigator-masked, controlled trial. *J Am Acad Dermatol*. 2007;57(2):247-256.
6. Strauss JS, Krowchuk DP, Leyden JJ, et al. Guidelines of care for acne vulgaris management. *J Am Acad Dermatol*. 2007;56:651-663.
7. Shirakawa M, Uramoto K, Harada FA. Treatment of acne conglobata with infliximab. *J Am Acad Dermatol*. 2006;55:344-346.
8. Grunwald MH, Amichai B. Nodulo-cystic eruption with musculo-skeletal pain. *J Fam Pract*. 2007;56:205-206.
9. AHRQ. *Management of Acne*. http://www ahrq gov/clinic/epcsums/acnesum htm [serial online]. 2001.
10. Draelos ZD, Carter E, Maloney JM, et al. Two randomized studies demonstrate the efficacy and safety of dapsone gel, 5% for the treatment of acne vulgaris. *J Am Acad Dermatol*. 2007;56:439-410.
11. Webster GF, Guenther L, Poulin YP, et al. A multicenter, double-blind, randomized comparison study of the efficacy and tolerability of once-daily tazarotene 0.1% gel and adapalene 0.1% gel for the treatment of facial acne vulgaris. *Cutis*. 2002;69(suppl 2):4-11.
12. Garner SE, Eady EA, Popescu C, Newton J, Li WA. Minocycline for acne vulgaris: efficacy and safety. *Cochrane Database Syst Rev*. 2003;(1):CD002086.
13. Maleszka R, Turek-Urasinska K, Oremus M, et al. Pulsed azithromycin treatment is as effective and safe as 2-week-longer daily doxycycline treatment of acne vulgaris: a randomized, double-blind, non-inferiority study. *Skinmed*. 2011;9:86-94.
14. Wu CQ, Grandi SM, Filion KB, Abenhaim HA, Joseph L, Eisenberg MJ. Drospirenone-containing oral contraceptive pills and the risk of venous and arterial thrombosis: a systematic review. *BJOG*. 2013;120(7):801-810.
15. Shaw JC. Low-dose adjunctive spironolactone in the treatment of acne in women: a retrospective analysis of 85 consecutively treated patients. *J Am Acad Dermatol*. 2000;43:498-502.
16. Sato K, Matsumoto D, Iizuka F, et al. Anti-androgenic therapy using oral spironolactone for acne vulgaris in Asians. *Aesthetic Plast Surg*. 2006;30:689-694.
17. Brown J, Farquhar C, Lee O, et al. Spironolactone versus placebo or in combination with steroids for hirsutism and/or acne. *Cochrane Database Syst Rev*. 2009;CD000194.
18. Krunic A, Ciurea A, Scheman A. Efficacy and tolerance of acne treatment using both spironolactone and a combined contraceptive containing drospirenone. *J Am Acad Dermatol*. 2008;58:60-62.
19. Enshaieh S, Jooya A, Siadat AH, Iraji F. The efficacy of 5% topical tea tree oil gel in mild to moderate acne vulgaris: a randomized, double-blind placebo-controlled study. *Indian J Dermatol Venereol Leprol*. 2007;73:22-25.
20. Karvonen SL. Acne fulminans: report of clinical findings and treatment of twenty-four patients. *J Am Acad Dermatol*. 1993;28:572-579.
21. Seukeran DC, Cunliffe WJ. The treatment of acne fulminans: a review of 25 cases. *Br J Dermatol*. 1999;141:307-309.
22. Tanghetti E, Dhawan S, Green L, et al. Randomized comparison of the safety and efficacy of tazarotene 0.1% cream and adapalene 0.3% gel in the treatment of patients with at least moderate facial acne vulgaris. *J Drugs Dermatol*. 2010;9:549-558.
23. Leyden J, Thiboutot DM, Shalita AR, et al. Comparison of tazarotene and minocycline maintenance therapies in acne vulgaris: a multicenter, double-blind, randomized, parallel-group study. *Arch Dermatol*. 2006;142:605-612.
24. Yeung CK, Shek SY, Bjerring P, et al. A comparative study of intense pulsed light alone and its combination with photodynamic therapy for the treatment of facial acne in Asian skin. *Lasers Surg Med*. 2007;39:1-6.
25. Wiegell SR, Wulf HC. Photodynamic therapy of acne vulgaris using 5-aminolevulinic acid versus methyl aminolevulinate. *J Am Acad Dermatol*. 2006;54:647-651.
26. Horfelt C, Funk J, Frohm-Nilsson M, et al. Topical methyl aminolaevulinate photodynamic therapy for treatment of facial acne vulgaris: results of a randomized, controlled study. *Br J Dermatol*. 2006;155:608-613.

115 ROSACEA

Richard P. Usatine, MD

PATIENT STORY

A 34-year-old woman with extensive papulopustular rosacea (**Figures 115-1** to **115-3**) has a history of easy facial flushing since her teen years. Her face has been persistently redder in the past 5 years and she is bothered by this. She acknowledges that her mom has similar redness in her face and that she is from northern European heritage. In the last 6 months, since her daughter was born, she has developed many "pimples." Physical examination reveals papules, pustules, and telangiectasias. No comedones are seen. She knows that the sun makes it worse but finds that many sunscreens are irritating to her skin. The patient is started on oral tetracycline daily and 0.75% metronidazole cream to use once daily. She agrees to wear a hat and stay out of the sun during the middle of the day. She will continue to look for a sunscreen she can tolerate. She knows that precipitating factors for her include hot and humid weather, alcohol, hot beverages, and spicy foods. She will do her best to avoid those factors.

INTRODUCTION

Rosacea is an inflammatory condition of the face and eyes that mostly affects adults. Most commonly the face becomes reddened over the cheeks and nose and this is often accompanied by telangiectasias and a papulopustular eruption.

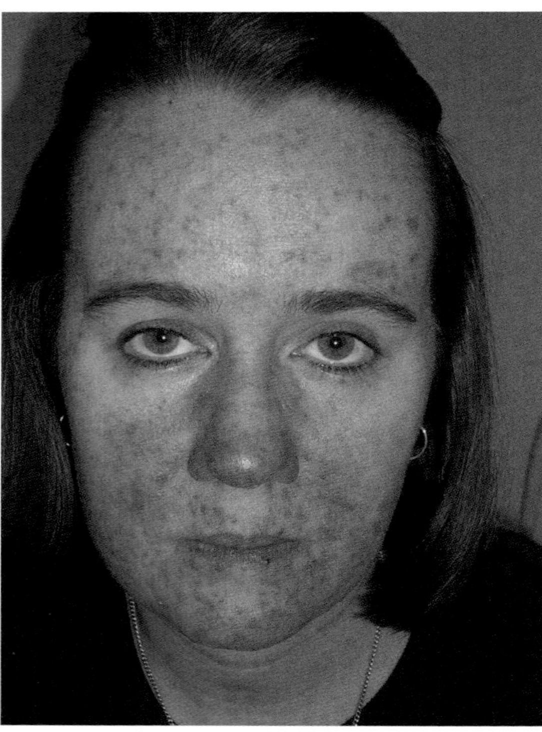

FIGURE 115-1 Rosacea in a 34-year-old woman showing erythema, papules, and pustules covering much of the face. Note her fair skin and blue eyes from her northern European heritage. *(Reproduced with permission from Richard P. Usatine, MD.)*

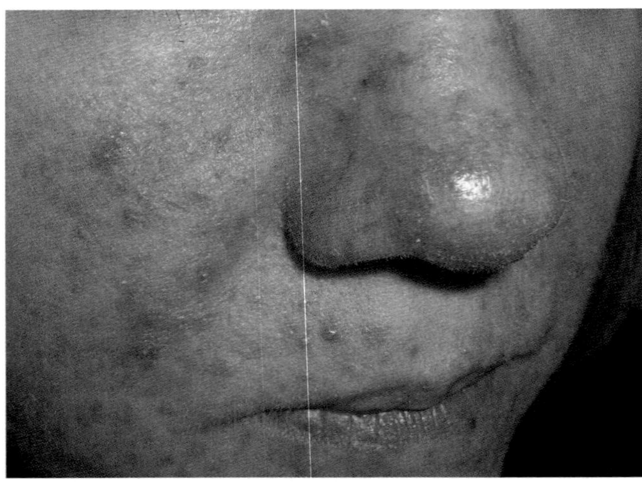

FIGURE 115-2 Close-up of papules and pustules in the same woman. Note the absence of comedones. This is not acne. This is papulopustular rosacea. *(Reproduced with permission from Richard P. Usatine, MD.)*

SYNONYMS

Rosacea is also called acne rosacea.

EPIDEMIOLOGY

- Rosacea is common in fair-skinned people of Celtic and northern European heritage.
- Women are more often affected than men.

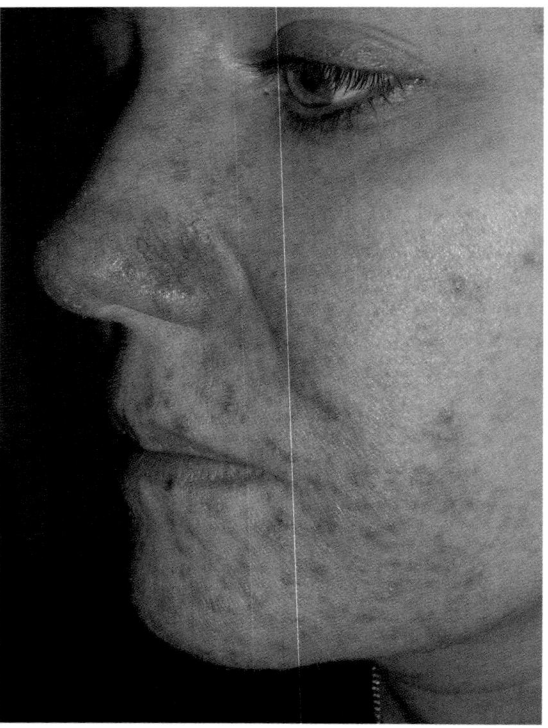

FIGURE 115-3 Close-up showing telangiectasias on the nose and papules around the mouth and chin. *(Reproduced with permission from Richard P. Usatine, MD.)*

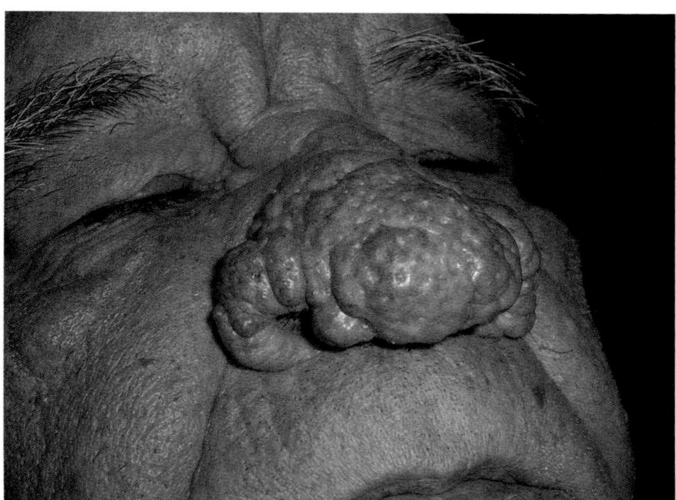

FIGURE 115-4 Rhinophymatous rosacea with hypertrophy of the skin of the nose of a 51-year-old Hispanic man. The patient acknowledges previous heavy alcohol intake. (*Reproduced with permission from Richard P. Usatine, MD.*)

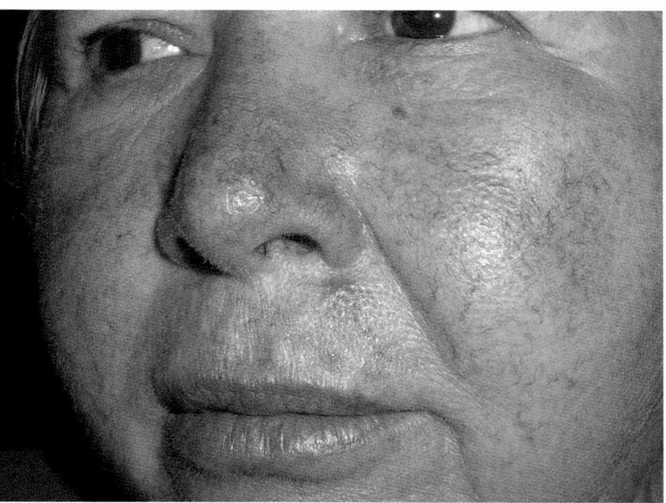

FIGURE 115-6 Erythematotelangiectatic subtype of rosacea in a middle-aged Hispanic woman. (*Reproduced with permission from Richard P. Usatine, MD.*)

- Men are more prone to the extreme forms of hyperplasia, which causes rhinophymatous rosacea (**Figures 115-4** and **115-5**).

ETIOLOGY AND PATHOPHYSIOLOGY

- Although the exact etiology is unknown, the pathophysiology involves nonspecific inflammation followed by dilation around follicles and hyperreactive capillaries. These dilated capillaries become telangiectasias (**Figures 115-6** and **115-7**).

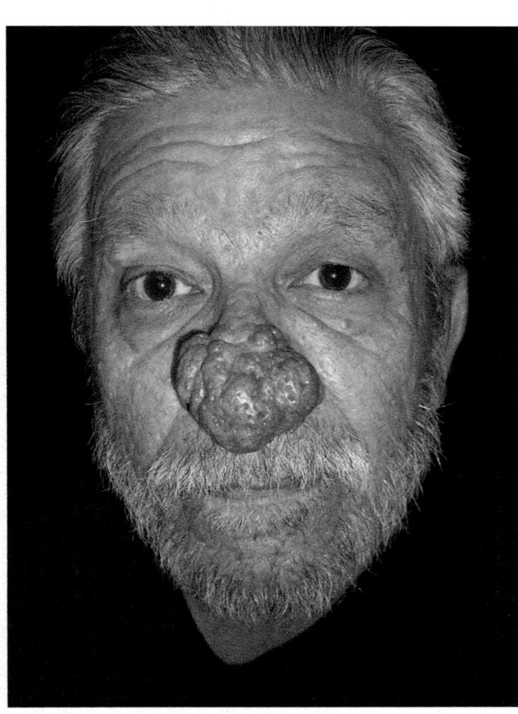

FIGURE 115-5 Rhinophymatous rosacea in an older man who does not drink alcohol. Although this is often called a W. C. Field nose, it is not necessarily related to heavy alcohol use. (*Reproduced with permission from Richard P. Usatine, MD.*)

- As rosacea progresses, diffuse hypertrophy of the connective tissue and sebaceous glands ensues (see **Figures 115-4** and **115-5**).
- Alcohol may accentuate erythema, but does not cause the disease. Rosacea runs in families.
- Sun exposure may precipitate an acute rosacea flare, but flare-ups can happen without sun exposure.
- A significant increase in the hair follicle mite Demodex folliculorum is sometimes found in rosacea.[1] It is theorized that these mites play a role because they incite an inflammatory or allergic reaction by mechanical blockage of follicles.

RISK FACTORS

Risk factors include genetics, *Demodex* infestation,[1] sun exposure.

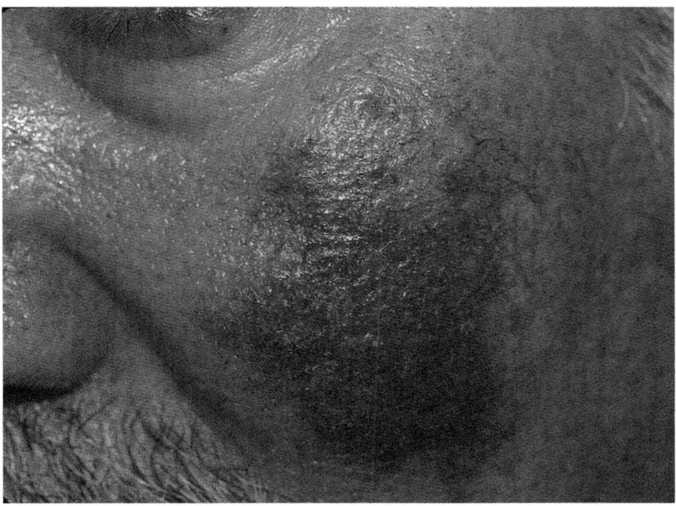

FIGURE 115-7 Rosacea in a middle-aged man showing deep erythema and many telangiectasias. (*Reproduced with permission from Richard P. Usatine, MD.*)

DIAGNOSIS

CLINICAL FEATURES

Rosacea has following 4 stages or subtypes:

1. ***Erythematotelangiectatic rosacea*** (see **Figures 115-6** and **115-7**)—This stage is characterized by frequent mild-to-severe flushing with persistent central facial erythema.
2. ***Papulopustular rosacea*** (see **Figures 115-1** to **115-3, 115-8** and **115-9**)—This is a highly vascular stage that involves longer periods of flushing than the first stage, often lasting from days to weeks. Minute telangiectasias and papules start to form by this stage, and some patients begin having very mild ocular complaints such as ocular grittiness or conjunctivitis. These patients may have many unsightly pustules with severe facial erythema. They are more prone to develop a hordeolum (stye) (see Chapter 10, Hordeolum and Chalazion).
3. ***Phymatous or rhinophymatous rosacea*** (see **Figures 115-4** and **115-5**)—Characterized by hyperplasia of the sebaceous glands that form thickened confluent plaques on the nose known as rhinophyma. This hyperplasia can cause significant disfigurement to the forehead, eyelids, chin, and nose. The nasal disfiguration is seen more commonly in men than women. W. C. Fields is famous for his rhinophyma and intake of alcohol. Rhinophyma can occur without any alcohol use, as seen in the patient in **Figure 115-5**.
4. ***Ocular rosacea*** (**Figures 115-10** to **115-12**)—An advanced subtype of rosacea that is characterized by impressive, severe flushing with persistent telangiectasias, papules, and pustules. The patient may complain of watery eyes, a foreign-body sensation, burning, dryness, vision changes, and lid or periocular erythema. The eyelids are most commonly involved with telangiectasias, blepharitis, and recurrent hordeola and chalazia (see **Figures 115-10** and **115-11**). Conjunctivitis may be chronic. Although corneal involvement is least common, it can have the most devastating consequences. Corneal findings may include punctate erosions, corneal infiltrates, and corneal neovascularization. In the most severe cases, blood vessels may grow over the cornea and lead to blindness (see **Figure 115-12**).

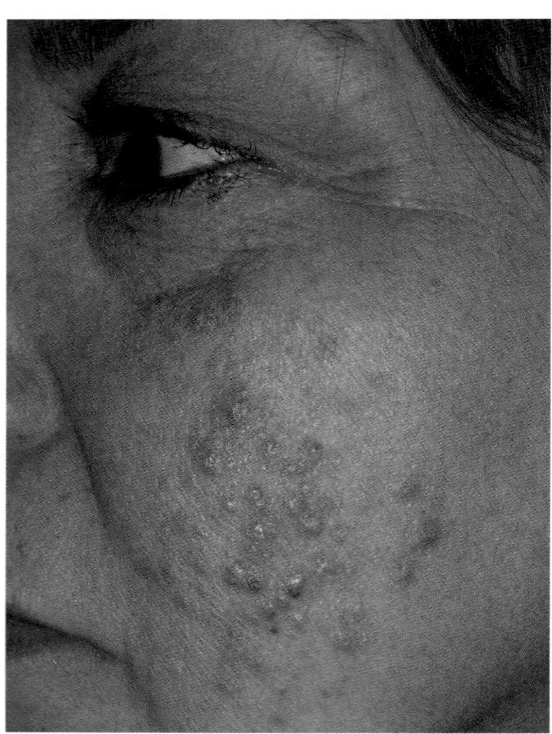

FIGURE 115-8 Papulopustular rosacea in a middle-aged woman. (*Reproduced with permission from Richard P. Usatine, MD.*)

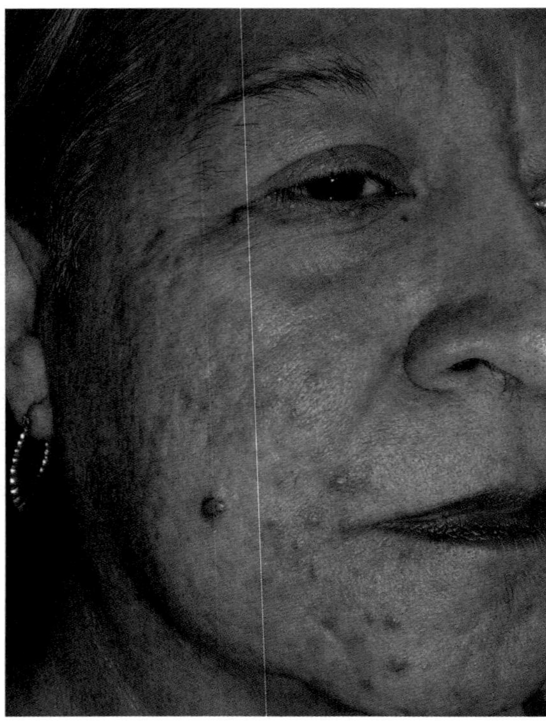

FIGURE 115-9 Papulopustular rosacea in a woman who has a history of recurrent hordeola. (*Courtesy of Richard P. Usatine, MD.*)

TYPICAL DISTRIBUTION

Rosacea occurs on the face, especially on the cheeks and nose. However, the forehead, eyelids, and chin can also be involved (**Figure 115-13**).

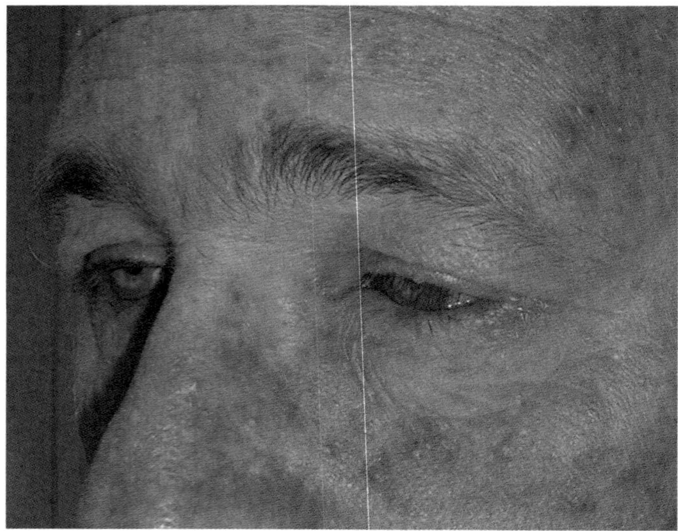

FIGURE 115-10 Ocular rosacea showing blepharitis, conjunctival hyperemia, and telangiectasias of the lid. (*Reproduced with permission from Richard P. Usatine, MD.*)

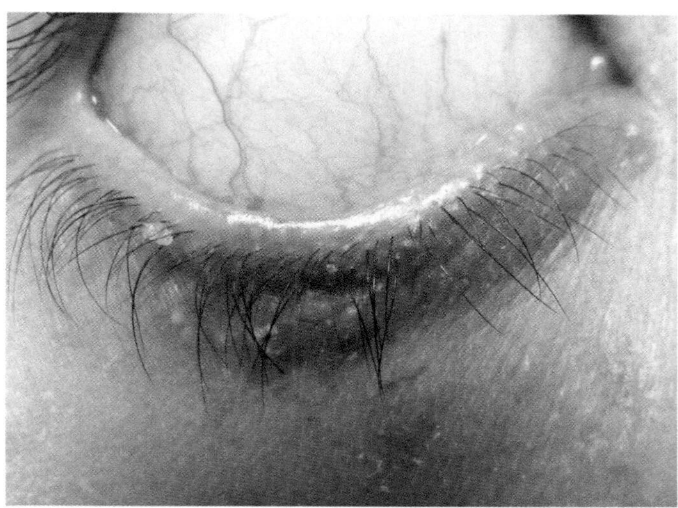

FIGURE 115-11 Ocular rosacea with blepharitis, conjunctivitis, and crusting around the eyelashes. This patient has meibomian gland dysfunction. (*Reproduced with permission from Richard P. Usatine, MD.*)

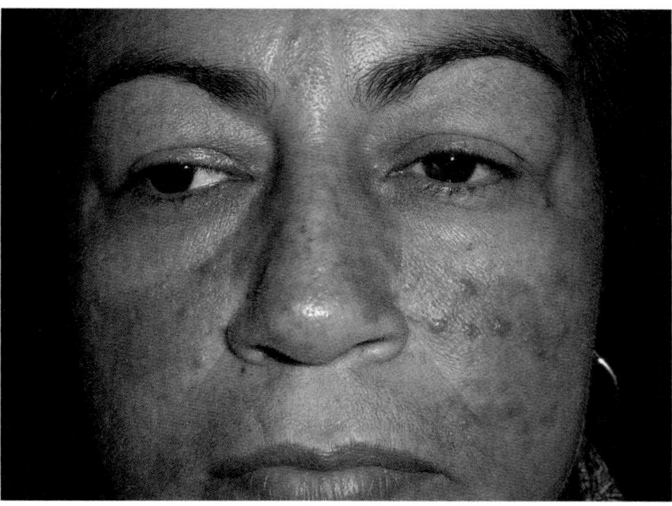

FIGURE 115-13 Rosacea in a young woman with a butterfly pattern along with chin involvement. This is not lupus. (*Reproduced with permission from Richard P. Usatine, MD.*)

LABORATORY STUDIES

It is not needed when the clinical picture is clear. If you are considering lupus or sarcoid, an antinuclear antibody (ANA), chest X-ray, or punch biopsy may be needed.

DIFFERENTIAL DIAGNOSIS

- Acne–The age of onset for rosacea tends to be 30 to 50 years, much later than the onset for acne vulgaris. Comedones are prominent in most cases of acne and generally absent in rosacea (see Chapter 114, Acne Vulgaris).
- Sarcoidosis on the face is much less common than rosacea, but the inflamed plaques can be red and resemble the inflammation of rosacea (see Chapter 173, Sarcoidosis of the skin).

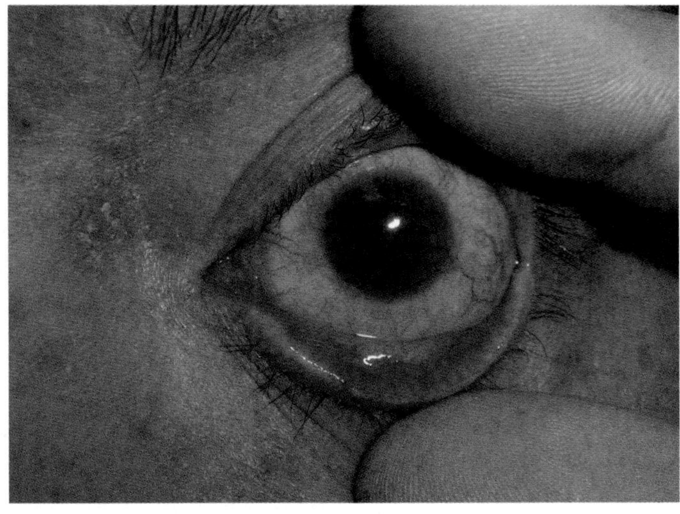

FIGURE 115-12 Neovascularization involving the cornea in a 30-year-old woman with severe ocular rosacea. This type of corneal involvement has caused a decrease in vision. The woman is hoping for a corneal transplant in the future. (*Reproduced with permission from Richard P. Usatine, MD.*)

- Seborrheic dermatitis tends to produce scale, whereas rosacea does not. Although both cause central facial erythema, papules and telangiectasias are present in rosacea and are not part of seborrheic dermatitis (see Chapter 149, Seborrheic Dermatitis).
- Systemic lupus erythematosus (SLE) can be scarring, does not usually produce papules or pustules, and it spares the nasolabial folds and nose (see Chapter 178, Lupus: Systemic and Cutaneous). The patient in **Figure 115-13** has a butterfly distribution of her rosacea, but her right nasolabial fold is involved along with her chin.

The following 3 diagnoses were once considered variants of rosacea but a recent classification system identified these as separate entities[2]:

- Rosacea fulminans (known as pyoderma faciale) is characterized by the sudden appearance of papules, pustules, and nodules, along with fluctuating and draining sinuses that may be interconnecting. The condition appears primarily in women in their 20s, and intense redness and edema also may be prominent (**Figure 115-14**).[2]
- Steroid-induced acneiform eruption is not a variant of rosacea and can occur as an inflammatory response in any patient during or after chronic corticosteroid use. The same inflammatory response may also occur in patients with rosacea (**Figure 115-15**).
- Perioral dermatitis without rosacea symptoms should not be classified as a variant of rosacea. Perioral dermatitis is characterized by microvesicles, scaling, and peeling around the mouth (**Figure 115-16**).

MANAGEMENT

- A Cochrane Database systematic review examined the efficacy of rosacea interventions.[3] Oral doxycycline appeared to be significantly more effective than placebo and there was no statistically significant difference in effectiveness between the 100-mg and 40-mg doses.[3] SOR Ⓐ They found some evidence to support the effectiveness of topical metronidazole (0.75% or 1%), azelaic acid (15% or 20%) for the treatment of moderate-to-severe rosacea.[3] SOR Ⓐ Cyclosporine ophthalmic emulsion was significantly more

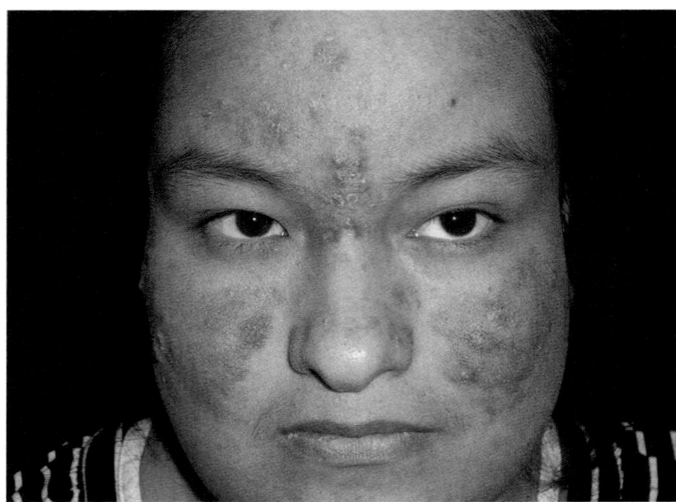

FIGURE 115-14 Rosacea fulminans (known as pyoderma faciale) is characterized by the sudden appearance of papules, pustules, and nodules. (*Reproduced with permission from Richard P. Usatine, MD.*)

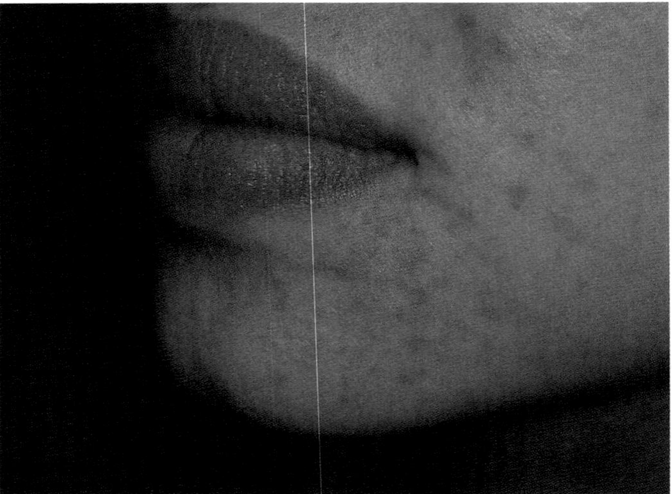

FIGURE 115-16 Perioral dermatitis in this 23-year-old woman with microvesicles, scaling, and peeling around the mouth. Note the sparing of the skin immediately around the lips. (*Reproduced with permission from Richard P. Usatine, MD.*)

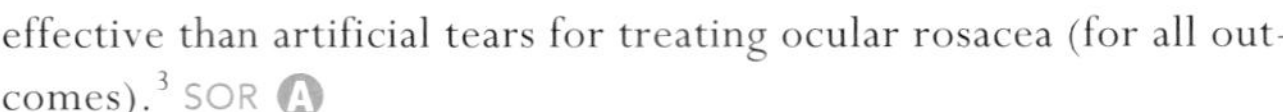

effective than artificial tears for treating ocular rosacea (for all outcomes).[3] SOR A

- When there are a limited number of papules and pustules, start with topical metronidazole (0.75% or 1%) or topical azelaic acid (15% or 20%).[3]
    - There are no substantial differences between topical metronidazole of 0.75% and 1%, or between once daily and twice daily regimens.[4] Metronidazole cream, gel, and lotion have similar efficacies as well.[4]

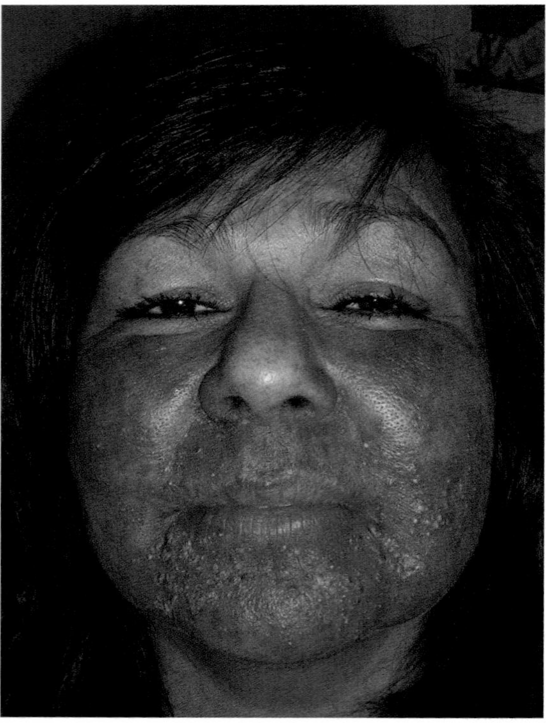

FIGURE 115-15 Steroid-induced acneiform eruption caused by the use of topical fluocinonide daily in this woman who probably had some underlying rosacea. (*Reproduced with permission from Richard P. Usatine, MD.*)

- Azelaic acid in a 15% gel applied bid appeared to offer some modest benefits over 0.75% metronidazole gel in a manufacturer-sponsored study.[4] Azelaic acid was not as well tolerated, so both medications are reasonable options with the choice depending on patient preference and tolerance.[3] SOR B One study found that once-daily azelaic acid 15% gel was as effective as twice-daily application, which can translate into a significant cost saving.[5]
- If the skin lesions are more extensive, oral antibiotics, such as doxycycline (40 mg or 100 mg daily) is recommended.[3] SOR A When attempting to avoid the photosensitivity side effects of doxycycline it is reasonable to prescribe oral tetracycline (250-500 mg daily) or oral metronidazole (250-500 mg daily). SOR C
- Patients who are started on oral antibiotics alone and improve may be switched to topical agents such as metronidazole or azelaic acid for maintenance.
- The *Demodex* mite may be one causative agent in rosacea. One study found permethrin 5% cream to be as effective as metronidazole 0.75% gel and superior to placebo in the treatment of rosacea.[5] SOR B
- Severe papulopustular disease refractory to antibiotics and topical treatments can be treated with oral isotretinoin at a low dose of 0.3 mg/kg per day.[6] SOR B
- Simple electrosurgery or laser without anesthesia can be used to treat the telangiectasias associated with rosacea. SOR C
- Rhinophyma can be excised with radiofrequency electrosurgery or laser. Isotretinoin is also used to treat rhinophyma.[6] SOR B
- Traditional therapies for mild ocular rosacea include oral tetracyclines, lid hygiene, and warm compresses.[1] SOR C Topical ophthalmic cyclosporine 0.05% (Restasis) is more effective than artificial tears for the treatment of rosacea-associated lid and corneal changes.[7] SOR B Ocular rosacea that involves the cornea should be immediately referred to an ophthalmologist to prevent blindness (see **Figure 115-12**).

FOLLOW-UP

Follow-up can be done in 1 to 3 months as needed.

PATIENT EDUCATION

Sun protection, including use of a hat and daily application of sunscreen, should be emphasized. Choose a sunscreen that is nonirritating and protects against UVA and UVB rays. Advise patients to keep a diary to identify and avoid precipitating factors such as hot and humid weather, alcohol, hot beverages, spicy foods, and large hot meals.

PATIENT RESOURCES

- National Rosacea Society. Its mission is to improve the lives of people with rosacea by raising awareness, providing public health information, and supporting medical research—**http://www.rosacea.org/**.

PROVIDER RESOURCES

- The National Rosacea Society also has an excellent set of materials that are geared for physicians—**http://www.rosacea.org/**.

REFERENCES

1. Zhao YE, Wu LP, Peng Y, Cheng H. Retrospective analysis of the association between Demodex infestation and rosacea. *Arch Dermatol*. 2010;146:896-902.
2. Wilkin J, Dahl M, Detmar M, et al. Standard classification of rosacea: report of the National Rosacea Society Expert Committee on the Classification and Staging of Rosacea. *J Am Acad Dermatol*. 2002;46:584-587.
3. van Zuuren EJ, Kramer S, Carter B, et al. Interventions for rosacea. *Cochrane Database Syst Rev*. 2011;(3):CD003262.
4. Yoo J, Reid DC, Kimball AB. Metronidazole in the treatment of rosacea: do formulation, dosing, and concentration matter? *J Drugs Dermatol*. 2006;5:317-319.
5. Kocak M, Yagli S, Vahapoglu G, Eksioglu M. Permethrin 5% cream versus metronidazole 0.75% gel for the treatment of papulopustular rosacea. A randomized double-blind placebo-controlled study. *Dermatology*. 2002;205:265-270.
6. Gollnick H, Blume-Peytavi U, Szabo EL, et al. Systemic isotretinoin in the treatment of rosacea- doxycycline- and placebo-controlled, randomized clinical study. *J Dtsch Dermatol Ges*. 2010;8:505-515.
7. Schechter BA, Katz RS, Friedman LS. Efficacy of topical cyclosporine for the treatment of ocular rosacea. *Adv Ther*. 2009;26:651-659.

116 PSEUDOFOLLICULITIS AND ACNE KELOIDALIS NUCHAE

E.J. Mayeaux, Jr, MD

PATIENT STORY

A young African American man comes to the office because he has been bothered by the uncomfortable bumps on the back of his neck and scalp. (**Figure 116-1**). He likes to wear his hair short but notices that every times he shaves his scalp the bumps on his scalp get irritated. He is diagnosed with acne keloidalis nuchae. It was suggested that he minimize shaving the scalp and let the hair grow out a bit longer. Additional treatment consisted of 0.025% tretinoin cream and 0.1% triamcinolone cream once to twice daily to the involved area.

INTRODUCTION

Pseudofolliculitis is a common skin condition affecting the hair-bearing areas of the body that are shaved (**Figures 116-2** to **116-4**). Potential complications include postinflammatory hyperpigmentation, bacterial superinfection, and keloid formation.

SYNONYMS

- Pseudofolliculitis—Razor bumps, shave bumps
- Acne keloidalis nuchae—Folliculitis keloidalis

EPIDEMIOLOGY

- Pseudofolliculitis is most common in black men, with at least 50% of black men who shave being prone to the condition.[1] In the beard area it is called *pseudofolliculitis barbae*, and when it occurs after pubic hair is shaved, it is referred to as *pseudofolliculitis pubis*. It may also occur in the neck area.
- Acne keloidalis nuchae occurs most often in black men but can be seen in all ethnicities (**Figures 116-1, 116-5,** and **116-6**). The lesions are often painful and cosmetically disfiguring.
- Both conditions are seen in women but far less often than in men (**Figure 116-7**).

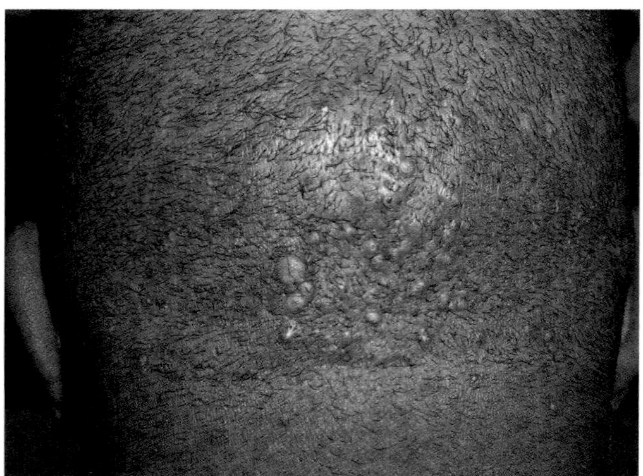

FIGURE 116-1 Acne keloidalis nuchae in a young African American man. He likes to wear his hair short but notices that every times he shaves his scalp the bumps on his scalp get irritated. (*Reproduced with permission from Richard P. Usatine, MD.*)

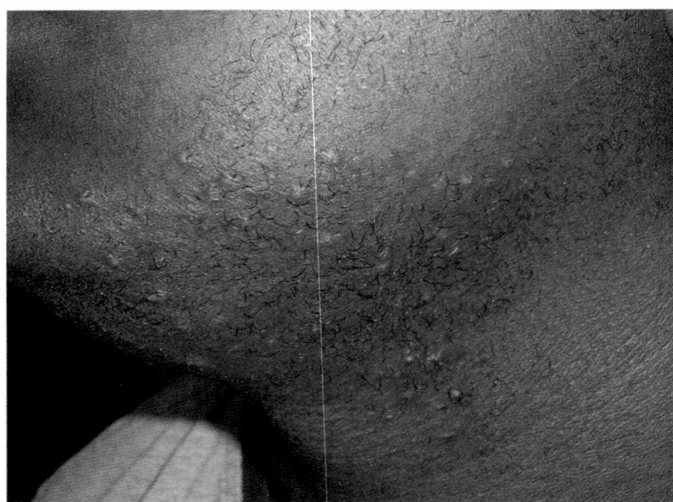

FIGURE 116-2 Pseudofolliculitis barbae along the jawline and neck in a young man. (*Reproduced with permission from Richard P. Usatine, MD.*)

ETIOLOGY AND PATHOPHYSIOLOGY

- Pseudofolliculitis develops when, after shaving, the free end of tightly coiled hair reenters the skin, causing a foreign-body–like inflammatory reaction. Shaving produces a sharp free end below the skin surface. Tightly curled hair has a greater tendency for the

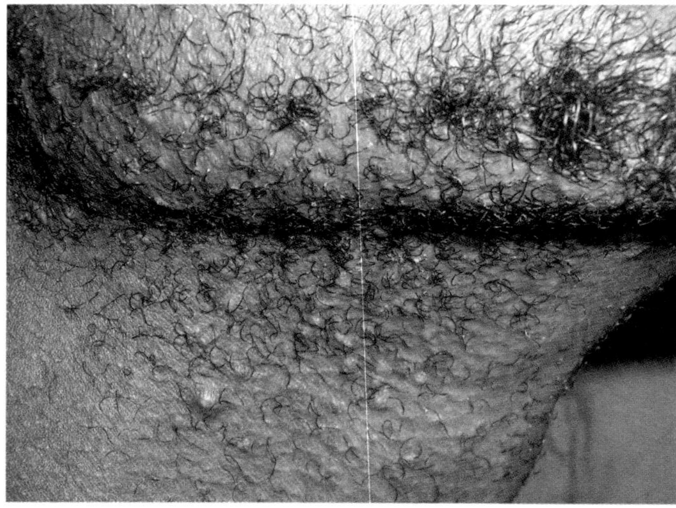

FIGURE 116-3 Pseudofolliculitis barbae in a Dominican man. Note the active pustules on the neck. (*Reproduced with permission from Richard P. Usatine, MD.*)

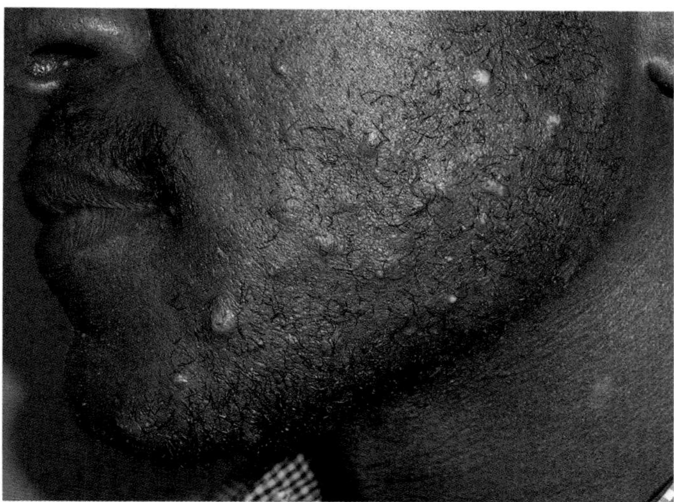

FIGURE 116-4 Pseudofolliculitis barbae on the face of a 28-year-old African man who works providing aid to Darfur refugees. The painful nodules become worse every time he shaves. (*Reproduced with permission from Richard P. Usatine, MD.*)

tip to pierce the surface of the skin and form ingrown hairs. This explains the relative predominance of this condition in patients of African ethnicity. The hair eventually forms a loop and if the embedded tip is pulled out there may be spontaneous resolution of symptoms.

- The exact cause of acne keloidalis is uncertain. It often develops in areas of pseudofolliculitis or folliculitis. It may be associated with haircuts where the posterior hairline is shaved with a razor and with tightly curved hair shafts. Other possible etiologies include irritation from shirt collars, chronic bacterial infections, and an autoimmune process. It is a form of primary scarring alopecia.[2] As such, multiple hairs can be seen growing from single follicle (hair tufts) in the midst of the keloidal scarring (see **Figure 116-6**).

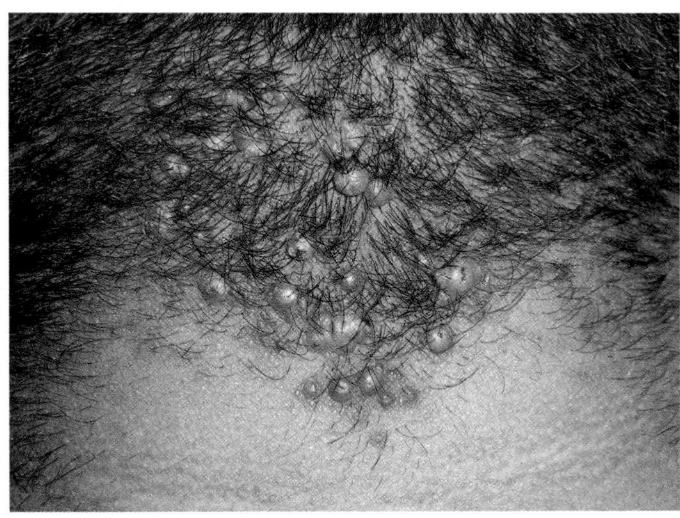

FIGURE 116-5 Acne keloidalis with multiple firm keloidal papules in a Hispanic man who prefers to keep his hair short. (*Reproduced with permission from Richard P. Usatine, MD.*)

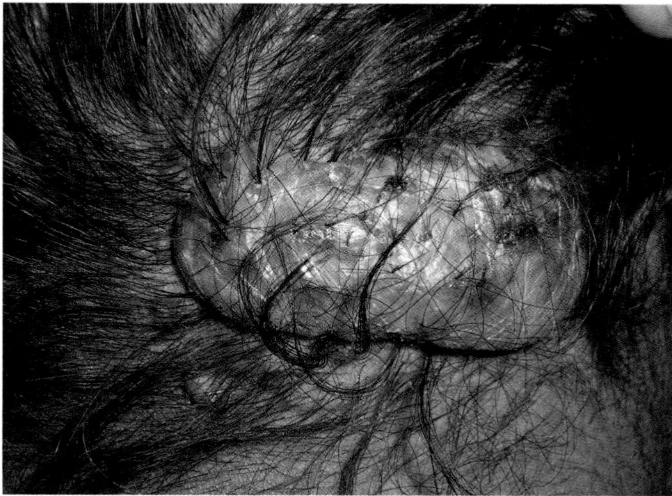

FIGURE 116-6 Acne keloidalis nuchae with large keloidal mass in a Hispanic man. Note multiple hairs can be seen growing from single follicles (hair tufts). Surgery is the only treatment that can remove this keloidal mass. (*Reproduced with permission from Richard P. Usatine, MD.*)

RISK FACTORS

- Pseudofolliculitis
  - African ethnicity
  - Curly hair
- Acne keloidalis nuchae
  - Shaving the hair on the neck
  - Pseudofolliculitis

DIAGNOSIS

CLINICAL FEATURES

- The diagnosis of pseudofolliculitis is based on clinical appearance. A piece of hair often may be identified protruding from a lesion. Inflammation results in the formation of firm, skin-colored, erythematous or hyperpigmented papules that occur after shaving (see **Figures 116-2** to **116-4**). Pustules may develop secondarily. The severity varies from a few papules or pustules to hundreds of lesions.
- Patients with acne keloidalis initially develop a folliculitis or pseudofolliculitis, which heals with keloid-like lesions, sometimes with discharging sinuses. It starts after puberty as 2- to 4-mm firm, follicular papules (see **Figure 116-2**). More papules appear and enlarge over time (see **Figure 116-5**). Papules may coalesce to form keloid-like plaques, which are usually arranged in a band-like distribution along the posterior part of the hairline (**Figures 116-6** and **116-8**).

TYPICAL DISTRIBUTION

- Pseudofolliculitis affects the hair-bearing areas of the body that are shaved, especially the face, neck, and pubic area (see **Figures 116-2** to **116-4**).
- Acne keloidalis occurs on the occipital scalp and the posterior part of the neck (see **Figures 116-1**, **116-5**, and **116-6**).

BIOPSY

Histologic evaluation of a biopsy may confirm either diagnosis but is usually not necessary.

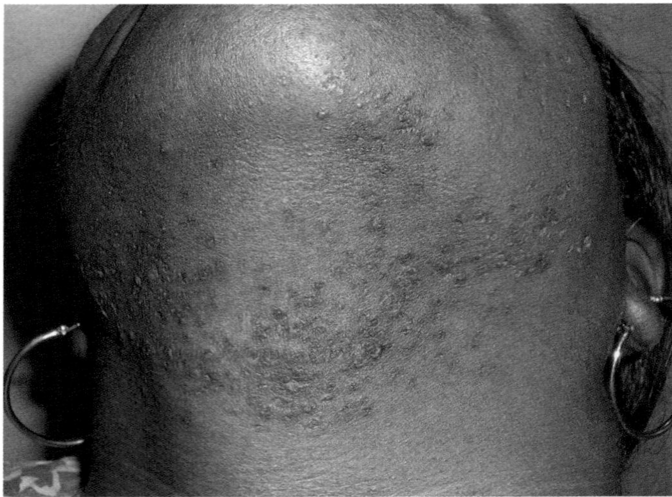

FIGURE 116-7 Pseudofolliculitis barbae in a black woman with hirsutism. The scarring is related to plucking and shaving the hairs on the neck. (*Reproduced with permission from Richard P. Usatine, MD.*)

DIFFERENTIAL DIAGNOSIS

- True folliculitis, which is an acute pustular infection of a hair follicle with more localized inflammation (see Chapter 119, Folliculitis)
- Impetigo, which presents with yellowish pustules or bullae that rupture and develop honey crusts, sometimes with adenopathy (see Chapter 118, Impetigo)
- Acne vulgaris, which presents with comedones and pustules usually including the forehead (see Chapter 114, Acne Vulgaris)

MANAGEMENT

NONPHARMACOLOGIC

- Avoid close shaving, avoid all shaving, or permanently remove hair.[3] Some occupations, however, such as the military and law enforcement, require facial shaving. Occasionally, a doctor's note will allow these men to go without shaving. In mild cases, shaving should be discontinued for a month. The beard can be coarsely trimmed with scissors or electric clippers during this time. Shaving should not resume until all inflammatory lesions have resolved. Warm Burow solution compresses may be applied to the lesions for 10 minutes, 2 times per day. Instruct the patient to search for ingrown hairs each day using a magnifying mirror and release them gently using a sterilized needle or tweezers. The hairs should not be plucked as this may cause recurrence of symptoms with hair regrowth (see **Figure 116-7**). SOR C
- Chemical depilatories (Ali, Royal Crown, Magic Shave, and others) cause fewer symptoms than shaving.[4] SOR B However, these creams can cause severe irritation, so testing a small amount on the forearm is important. They work by breaking the disulfide bonds in hair, which results in the hair being bluntly broken at the follicular opening instead of sharply cut below the surface. They should be used every second or third day to avoid skin irritation, although this can be controlled with hydrocortisone cream. Barium sulfide 2% powder depilatories can be made into a paste with water, applied to the beard, and removed after 3 to 5 minutes. Calcium thioglycolate preparations are left on 10 to 15 minutes, but the fragrances can cause an allergic reaction and chemical burns can result if it is left for too long.
- People who have acne keloidalis nuchae should avoid anything that causes folliculitis or pseudofolliculitis, such as getting their neck or hairline shaved with a razor.

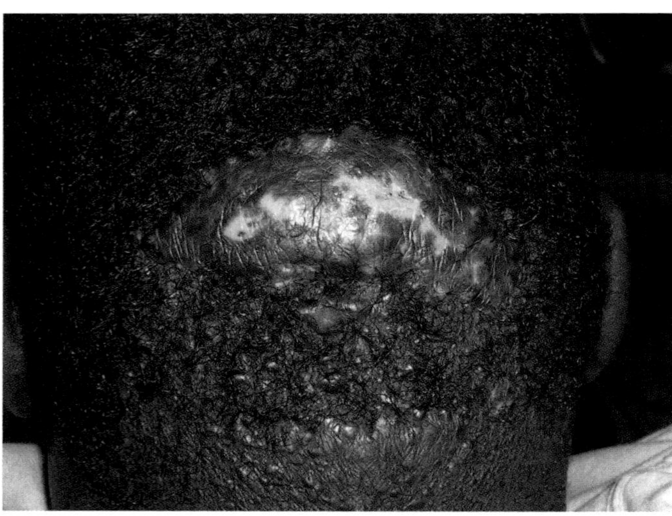

FIGURE 116-8 Acne keloidalis nuchae after injection with intralesional triamcinolone. Although the keloid is smaller and softer, some hypopigmentation has occurred. (*Reproduced with permission from Richard P. Usatine, MD.*)

MEDICATIONS

- Topical eflornithine HCL 13.9% cream (Vaniqa; by prescription only) may be used to inhibit hair growth. It decreases the rate of hair growth and may make the hair finer and lighter. Unfortunately, this medication is expensive and requires daily application for continued efficacy. SOR C
- Twice-daily treatment with a class 2 or 3 corticosteroid may be sufficient to shrink pseudofolliculitis lesions and relieve symptoms (see Appendix B: Topical and Intralesional Corticosteroids). SOR C
- When pustules, crust formation, or drainage is present, use topical clindamycin or erythromycin. Unresponsive patients may be changed to a systemic antibiotic. SOR C
- Topical erythromycin, clindamycin, and combination clindamycin–benzoyl peroxide (BenzaClin, Duac) and erythromycin–benzoyl peroxide (Benzamycin) may be used once or twice daily.[5] SOR B
- Oral doxycycline 100 mg bid, tetracycline 500 mg bid, or erythromycin 500 mg bid may be used for patients with more severe secondary inflammation. SOR C
- Tretinoin cream, 0.025%, may be useful in patients with mild disease, but is rarely helpful in moderate-to-severe cases.[6] It is applied nightly for a week then reduced to every second or third night. Tretinoin may be used in conjunction with a mid-potency topical corticosteroid applied each morning. The mechanism of action is thought to be by relieving hyperkeratosis and "toughening" the skin. Topical combination cream (tretinoin 0.05%, fluocinolone acetonide 0.01%, and hydroquinone 4%) (Tri-Luma) adds an additional postinflammatory hyperpigmentation treatment. SOR C
- Intralesional steroid injections (10-20 mg/mL) may be used to soften and shrink keloids. Warn patients that this therapy may cause hypopigmentation (see **Figure 116-8**). SOR C

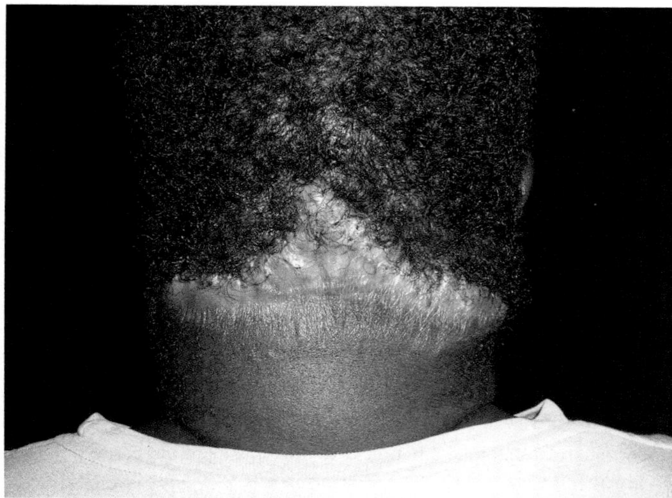

FIGURE 116-9 Hypertrophic scarring after the excision of acne keloidalis nuchae. (*Reproduced with permission from Richard P. Usatine, MD.*)

SURGICAL

- The only definitive cure for pseudofolliculitis is permanent hair removal. Electrolysis is expensive, painful, and sometimes unsuccessful. Laser hair removal is fairly successful for treating pseudofolliculitis.[7] SOR Ⓑ Diode laser (810 nm) treatments have been proven safe and effective in patients with skin phototypes I to IV.[8]
- Excision of acne keloidalis lesions may be attempted. Recalcitrant keloidal lesions may be treated with removing individual papules with a small punch, or large keloids (**Figure 116-9**) with an elliptical excision closed with sutures. After removal, the wound edges should be injected with a mixture of equal amount of triamcinolone acetonide 40 mg/mL and sterile saline. Remove the sutures in 1 to 2 weeks and inject the edges every month with the above mixture for 3 to 4 times. SOR Ⓒ Excision should extend into the subcutaneous tissue and the wound edges can be injected with 10 to 40 mg/mL of triamcinolone acetonide and be reapproximated. SOR Ⓒ Recurrence is common, especially with shallow excisions or not treating with steroids.
- Other therapies that may be considered are laser therapy (carbon dioxide or Nd:YAG [neodymium:yttrium-aluminum-garnet]) followed by intralesional triamcinolone injections or cryotherapy for two 20-second bursts that are allowed to thaw and are then applied again a minute later. These methods may produce more pain and hypopigmentation. SOR Ⓒ

PREVENTION

Termination of shaving prevents the development of pseudofolliculitis.

PROGNOSIS

No specific cure exists. If the patient is able to stop shaving, the problem usually disappears (except for any scar formation).

FOLLOW-UP

Instruct patients to return if any complications occur. Otherwise have them return for possible initiation of intralesional steroid injections or topical steroid/retinoic acid therapy once the area has healed.

PATIENT EDUCATION

- For those who must shave, have the patient clip hairs no shorter than needed for maintenance. Use fine scissors or facial hair clippers if possible. When shaving, have the patient rinse with warm tap water for several minutes, use generous amounts of a highly lubricating shaving gel, and allow it to soften the skin for 5 to 10 minutes before shaving. The patient should always use sharp razors and shave in the direction of hair growth. Specialized guarded razors (eg, PFB Bump Fighter) are available in pharmacies and by mail order. After shaving rinse the face with tap water, and then apply cold water compresses.
- With acne keloidalis, instruct males who play football to make sure their helmets fit properly and do not cause irritation on the posterior part of the scalp. They should avoid having the posterior part of the hairline shaved with a razor as part of a haircut, and discontinue wearing garments that rub or irritate the posterior parts of the scalp and the neck.

PATIENT RESOURCES

- American Osteopathic College of Dermatology. *Pseudofolliculitis*—**http://aocd.org/skin/dermatologic_diseases/pseudofolliculitis.html.**
- Skin Channel. *Acne Keloidalis Nuchae*—**http://skinchannel.com/acne/acne-keloidalis-nuchae/.**

PROVIDER RESOURCES

- eMedicine. *Pseudofolliculitis*—**http://emedicine.medscape.com/article/1071251.**
- eMedicine. *Acne Keloidalis*—**http://emedicine.medscape.com/article/1072149.**
- DermNet NZ. *Acne Keloidalis*—**http://dermnetnz.org/acne/keloid-acne.html.**

REFERENCES

1. Coquilla BH, Lewis CW. Management of pseudofolliculitis barbae. *Mil Med.* 1995;160(5):263-269.
2. Sperling LC, Homoky C, Pratt L, Sau P. Acne keloidalis is a form of primary scarring alopecia. *Arch Dermatol.* 2000;136(4):479-484.
3. Chui CT, Berger TG, Price VH, Zachary CB. Recalcitrant scarring follicular disorders treated by laser-assisted hair removal: a preliminary report. *Dermatol Surg.* 1999;25(1):34-37.
4. Hage JJ, Bowman FG. Surgical depilation for the treatment of pseudofolliculitis or local hirsutism of the face: experience in the first 40 patients. *Plast Reconstr Surg.* 1991;88:446-451.
5. Cook-Bolden FE, Barba A, Halder R, Taylor S. Twice-daily applications of benzoyl peroxide 5% clindamycin 1% gel versus vehicle in the treatment of pseudofolliculitis barbae. *Cutis.* 2004;73(suppl 6):18-24.
6. Brown LA Jr. Pathogenesis and treatment of pseudofolliculitis barbae. *Cutis.* 1983;32(4):373-375.
7. Ross EV, Cooke LM, Timko AL, et al. Treatment of pseudofolliculitis barbae in skin types IV, V, and VI with a long-pulsed neodymium: yttrium aluminum garnet laser. *J Am Acad Dermatol.* 2002;47(2): 263-270.
8. Kauvar AN. Treatment of pseudofolliculitis with a pulsed infrared laser. *Arch Dermatol.* 2000;136(11):1343-1346.

117 HIDRADENITIS SUPPURATIVA

Richard P. Usatine, MD

PATIENT STORY

A 25-year-old woman presents with new tender lesions in her axilla (**Figure 117-1**). She admits to years of similar outbreaks in both axilla and occasional painful bumps in the groin. She states that it is painful to have them opened and just wants to get some relief without surgery. We elected to inject the nodules with triamcinolone and start the patient on doxycycline 100 mg twice daily. Smoking cessation was emphasized and the patient agreed to start on a nicotine patch that evening. She had relief within 24 hours from the steroid injection.

INTRODUCTION

Hidradenitis suppurativa (HS) is an inflammatory disease of the pilosebaceous unit in the apocrine gland-bearing skin. HS is most common in the axilla and inguinal area, but may be found in the inframammary area as well. It produces painful inflammatory nodules, cysts, and sinus tracks with mucopurulent discharge and progressive scarring.

SYNONYMS

It is called acne inversa because it involves intertriginous areas and not the regions affected by acne (similar to inverse psoriasis).

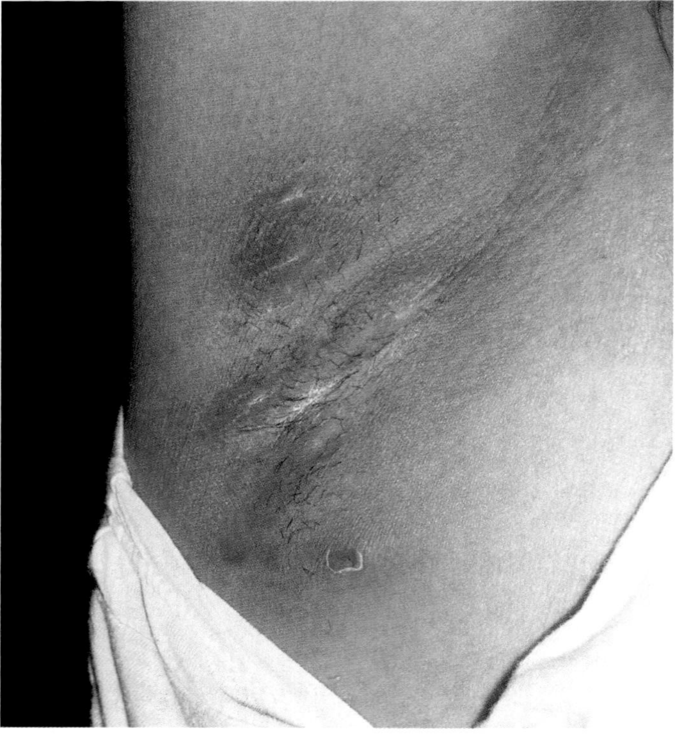

FIGURE 117-1 Mild hidradenitis suppurativa in the axilla of a young woman. She has a history of recurrent lesions in her axilla. (*Reproduced with permission from Richard P. Usatine, MD.*)

EPIDEMIOLOGY

- Occurs after puberty in approximately 1% of the population.[1]
- Incidence is higher in females, in the range of 4:1 to 5:1. Flare-ups may be associated with menses.[1]

ETIOLOGY AND PATHOPHYSIOLOGY

- Disorder of the terminal follicular epithelium in the apocrine gland-bearing skin[1]
- Starts with occlusion of hair follicles that lead to occlusion of surrounding apocrine glands
- Chronic relapsing inflammation with mucopurulent discharge (**Figures 117-2** to **117-7**)
- Can lead to sinus tracts, draining fistulas, and progressive scarring (see **Figures 117-2** to **117-7**)

RISK FACTORS

Obesity, smoking, and tight-fitting clothing are the risk factors of HS.

DIAGNOSIS

CLINICAL FEATURES

- Most common presentation is painful, tender, firm, nodular lesions in axillae (see **Figures 117-1** to **117-3**).
- Nodules may open and drain pus spontaneously and heal slowly, with or without drainage, over 10 to 30 days.[1]
- Nodules may recur several times yearly, or in severe cases new lesions form as old ones heal.
- Surrounding cellulitis may be present and require systemic antibiotic treatment.

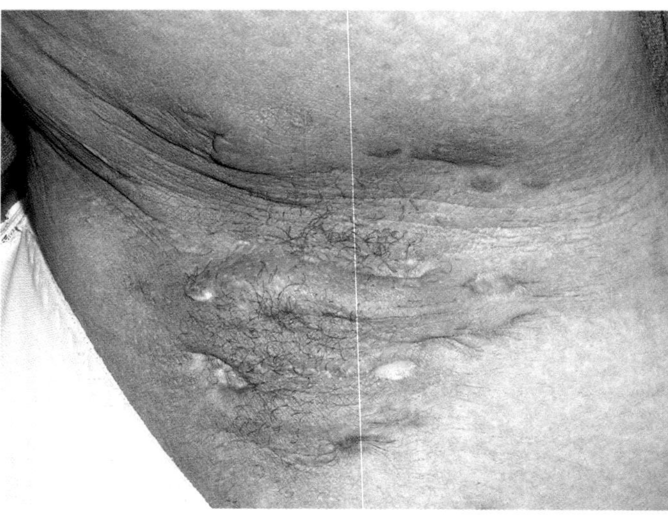

FIGURE 117-2 Moderate hidradenitis suppurativa in a young woman. The lesions are deeper and there have been some chronic changes with scarring and fibrosis from previous lesions. (*Reproduced with permission from Richard P. Usatine, MD.*)

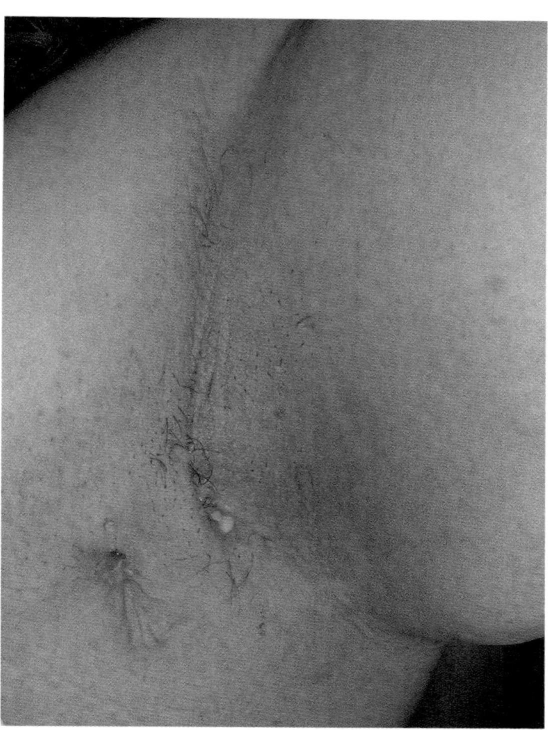

FIGURE 117-3 A 33-year-old Hispanic woman with sinus tracts, draining fistulas, and scarring secondary to her chronic hidradenitis suppurativa. Note the mucopurulent discharge. (*Reproduced with permission from Richard P. Usatine, MD.*)

- Chronic recurrences result in thickened sinus tracts, which may become draining fistulas (see **Figures 117-3** to **117-7**).
- HS can cause disabling pain, diminished range of motion, and social isolation (see **Figure 117-5**).

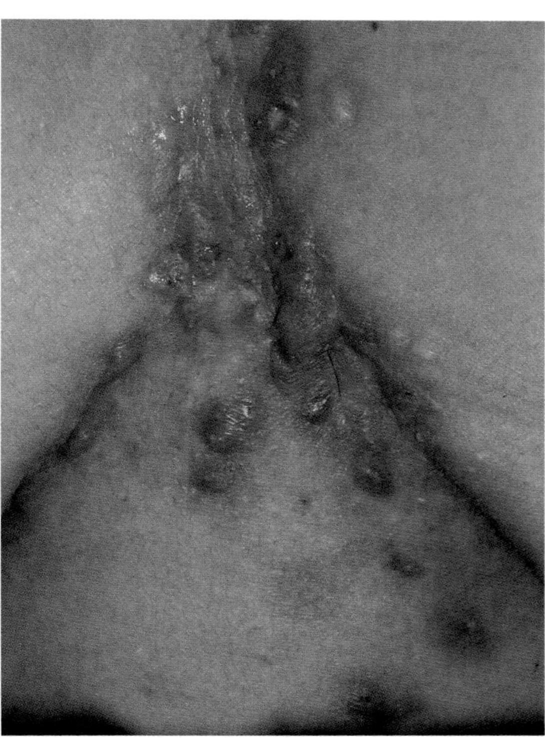

FIGURE 117-4 Long-standing painful severe hidradenitis suppurativa between the breasts of a 45-year-old woman. (*Reproduced with permission from Richard P. Usatine, MD.*)

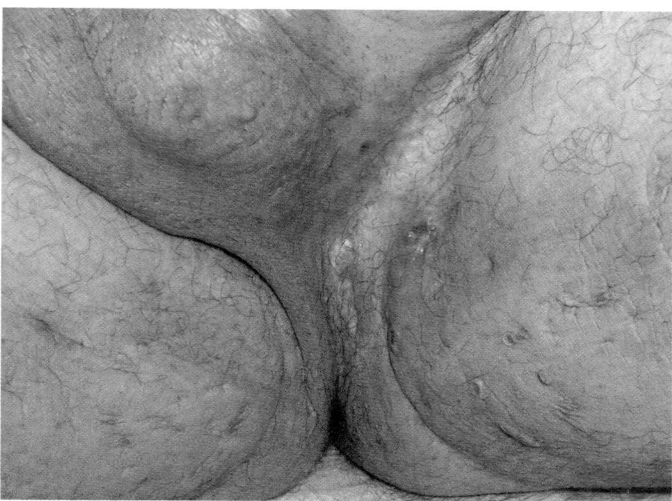

FIGURE 117-5 Severe disabling hidradenitis suppurativa in a 34-year-old white man who is morbidly obese. He finds it painful to walk. (*Reproduced with permission from Richard P. Usatine, MD.*)

TYPICAL DISTRIBUTION

Axillary, inguinal, periareolar, intermammary zones, pubic area, infraumbilical midline, gluteal folds, top of the anterior thighs, and the perianal region.[1]

LABORATORY STUDIES

Culture of purulence is likely to yield staphylococci and streptococci and is usually unnecessary to determine treatment. Culture may be useful if you suspect methicillin-resistant *Staphylococcus aureus* (MRSA).

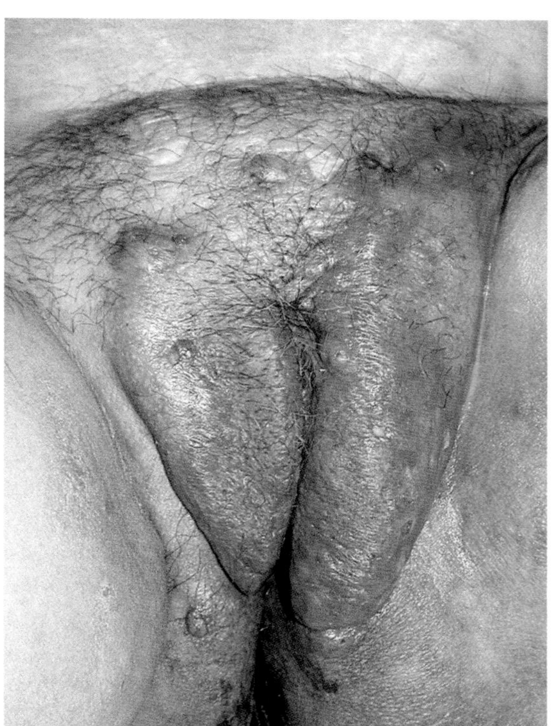

FIGURE 117-6 Severe hidradenitis suppurativa in the vulva and on the mons pubis. The skin is thickened and hyperpigmented from the ongoing inflammatory lesions present in the area. (*Reproduced with permission from Suraj Reddy, MD.*)

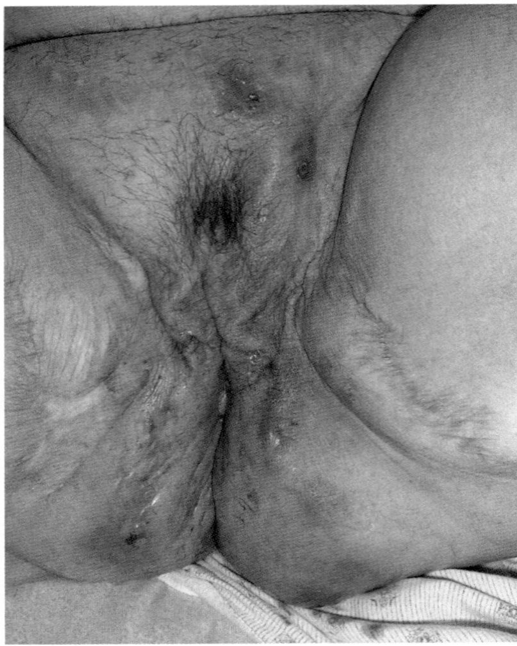

FIGURE 117-7 Thirty-year history of severe hidradenitis in a 54-year-old woman. Note the scars from previous plastic surgeries. Note the draining cysts, fistulas, and the acute abscess on her left buttocks. (*Reproduced with permission from Richard P. Usatine, MD.*)

DIFFERENTIAL DIAGNOSIS

- Bacterial infections, including folliculitis, carbuncles, furuncles, abscess, and cellulitis, may resemble HS but are less likely to be recurrent in the intertriginous areas.
- Epidermal cysts in the intertriginous regions may resemble HS. Theses cysts contain malodorous keratin contents.
- Granuloma inguinale and lymphogranuloma venereum are sexually transmitted infections that can produce inguinal ulcers and adenopathy that could be mistaken for HS.

MANAGEMENT

- Lifestyle changes are recommended, including weight loss if obesity is present. SOR Ⓒ
- Smoking is a risk factor for HS and cessation is highly recommended for many reasons.[1] See SOR Ⓑ for HS and SOR Ⓐ for other health reasons.
- Frequent bathing and wearing loose-fitting clothing may help.

Medical treatment is similar to acne treatment.

- Oral antibiotics are used in acute and chronic treatment. Oral tetracyclines, clindamycin, rifampin, and dapsone have been touted as beneficial. If MRSA is present there, trimethoprim/sulfamethoxazole or clindamycin should be used.
- Tetracycline 500 mg bid and doxycycline 100 mg bid can be used acutely and to prevent new lesions in the mildest of cases. Many patients do not find these antibiotics to be of great help. SOR Ⓒ
- Topical clindamycin bid may be used in the mildest of cases. In one randomized controlled trial (RCT), systemic therapy with tetracyclines did not show better results than topical therapy with clindamycin.[1] SOR Ⓑ
  - Combination of systemic clindamycin (300 mg twice daily) and rifampin (600 mg daily) is recommended for patients with more severe HS.[2,3] In a series of 116 patients, parameters of severity improved, as did the quality-of-life score.[2] In another study, 28 of 34 patients (82%) experienced at least partial improvement, and 16 (47%) showed a total remission.[3] The maximum effect of treatment appeared within 10 weeks. Following total remission, 8 of 13 (61.5%) patients experienced a relapse after a mean period of 5 months. Nonresponders were predominantly patients with severe disease. The most frequent side effect is diarrhea.[2,3]
  - Oral dapsone may be considered in milder cases. In one study, only 38% of patients experienced improvement.[4] SOR Ⓑ Rapid recurrence after stopping treatment suggests that anti-inflammatory effects may predominate over antimicrobial effects. The total effect appears to be smaller than that reported with combination therapy using clindamycin and rifampicin.
- Isotretinoin can reduce the severity of attacks in some patients but is not a reliable cure for HS.[5] SOR Ⓒ
- Acitretin can be an effective treatment for refractory HS. In one study, all 12 patients achieved remission and experienced a significant decrease in pain. Long-lasting improvement was observed in 9 patients, with no recurrence of lesions after 6 months (n = 1), 1 year (n = 3), more than 2 years (n = 2), more than 3 years (n = 2), and more than 4 years (n = 1).[5] SOR Ⓑ
- Antitumor necrosis factor (TNF) agents are being studied for severe, recalcitrant HS (**Figure 117-8**). In one series, infliximab therapy (weight based) was shown to be effective and well tolerated in 6 of 7 patients with HS who were resistant to previous therapy.[6] This was in agreement with preexisting literature showing that 52 of 60 patients (87%) were improved after infliximab therapy.[6] SOR Ⓑ Adalimumab helps in the short term, but no long-term curative effect was uniformly seen.[7]
- Intense pulsed light (IPL) with laser may be worth considering for patients who can afford the cost and time for treatment. In one study of 18 patients who were randomized to treatment of one axilla, groin, or inframammary area with IPL 2 times per week for 4 weeks, there was a significant improvement in the mean examination score, which was maintained at 12 months. Patients reported high levels of satisfaction with the IPL treatment.[8] SOR Ⓑ

Surgical treatments include the following:

- Intralesional steroids with 5 to 10 mg/mL of triamcinolone may help to decrease inflammation and pain within 24 to 48 hours. SOR Ⓒ
- Incision and drainage of acute lesions are suggested for the large fluctuant abscesses that can occur in HS. Although this may give some relief of the pressure, the surgical treatment and repacking of the wound is painful, and there is no evidence that it speeds healing. SOR Ⓒ
- Lancing small nodules is more painful than helpful and is not recommended.
- Surgical excision of affected area with or without skin grafting is used for recalcitrant disabling disease and should be individualized based on the stage and location of the disease.[9] SOR Ⓑ One surgical group has been using a medial thigh lift for immediate defect closure after radical excision of localized inguinal hidradenitis.[10]

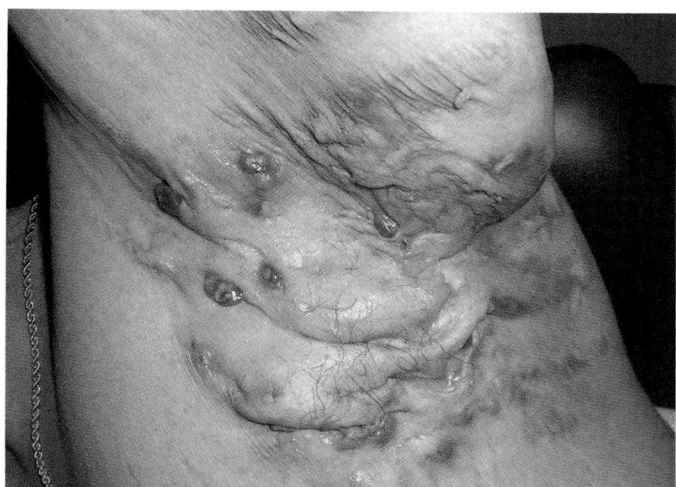

A

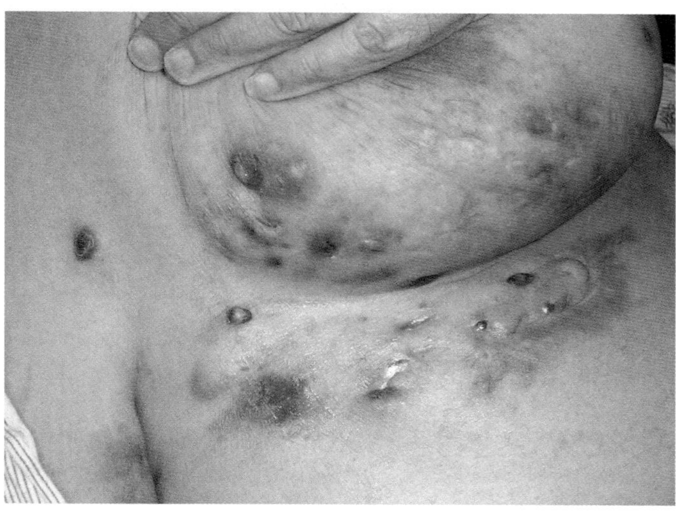

B

FIGURE 117-8 Severe recalcitrant hidradenitis in this 42-year-old woman with sinus tracts and scarring. She has experienced significant symptomatic relief with infliximab infusions. A. Axillary involvement. B. Inframammary involvement. (*Reproduced with permission from Richard P. Usatine, MD.*)

FOLLOW-UP

If there is cellulitis or a large abscess was drained, follow-up should be within days. Chronic relapsing disease can ultimately be managed with appointments every 3 to 6 months depending on the treatment and its success.

PATIENT EDUCATION

Smoking cessation, weight loss if overweight, and avoidance of tight-fitting clothes should be emphasized.

PATIENT RESOURCES

- Medline Plus. *Hidradenitis Suppurativa*—**http://www.nlm.nih.gov/medlineplus/hidradenitissuppurativa.html.**

PROVIDER RESOURCES

- Medscape. *Hidradenitis Suppurativa*—**http://emedicine.medscape.com/article/1073117-overview.**

REFERENCES

1. Jemec GB, Wendelboe P. Topical clindamycin versus systemic tetracycline in the treatment of hidradenitis suppurativa. *J Am Acad Dermatol.* 1998;39:971-974.
2. Gener G, Canoui-Poitrine F, Revuz JE, et al. Combination therapy with clindamycin and rifampicin for hidradenitis suppurativa: a series of 116 consecutive patients. *Dermatology.* 2009;219:148-154.
3. van der Zee HH, Boer J, Prens EP, Jemec GBE. The effect of combined treatment with oral clindamycin and oral rifampicin in patients with hidradenitis suppurativa. *Dermatology.* 2009;219:143-147.
4. Yazdanyar S, Boer J, Ingvarsson G, et al. Dapsone therapy for hidradenitis suppurativa: a series of 24 patients. *Dermatology.* 2011;222(4):342-346.
5. Boer J, Nazary M. Long-term results of acitretin therapy for hidradenitis suppurativa. Is acne inversa also a misnomer? *Br J Dermatol.* 2011;164:170-175.
6. Delage M, Samimi M, Atlan M, et al. Efficacy of infliximab for hidradenitis suppurativa: assessment of clinical and biological inflammatory markers. *Acta Derm Venereol.* 2011;91:169-171.
7. Miller I, Lynggaard CD, Lophaven S, et al. A double-blind placebo-controlled randomized trial of adalimumab in the treatment of hidradenitis suppurativa. *Br J Dermatol.* 2011;165:391-398.
8. Highton L, Chan WY, Khwaja N, Laitung JK. Treatment of hidradenitis suppurativa with intense pulsed light: a prospective study. *Plast Reconstr Surg.* 2011;128:459-466.
9. Kagan RJ, Yakuboff KP, Warner P, Warden GD. Surgical treatment of hidradenitis suppurativa: a 10-year experience. *Surgery.* 2005;138:734-740.
10. Rieger UM, Erba P, Pierer G, Kalbermatten DF. Hidradenitis suppurativa of the groin treated by radical excision and defect closure by medial thigh lift: aesthetic surgery meets reconstructive surgery. *J Plast Reconstr Aesthet Surg.* 2009;62:1355-1360.

SECTION 2 BACTERIAL

118 IMPETIGO

Richard P. Usatine, MD

PATIENT STORY

A young woman presented to the office with a 3-day history of an uncomfortable rash on her lip and chin (**Figure 118-1**). She denied any trauma or previous history of oral herpes. This case of impetigo resolved quickly with oral cephalexin.

INTRODUCTION

Impetigo is the most superficial of bacterial skin infections. It causes honey crusts, bullae, and erosions.

EPIDEMIOLOGY

- It is most frequent in children ages 2 to 6 years, but it can be seen in patients of any age.
- It is common among homeless people living on the streets.
- It is often seen in third world countries in persons living without easy access to clean water and soap.
- Contagious and can be spread within a household.

ETIOLOGY AND PATHOPHYSIOLOGY

- Impetigo is caused by *Staphylococcus aureus* and/or group A β-hemolytic *Streptococcus* (GABHS).

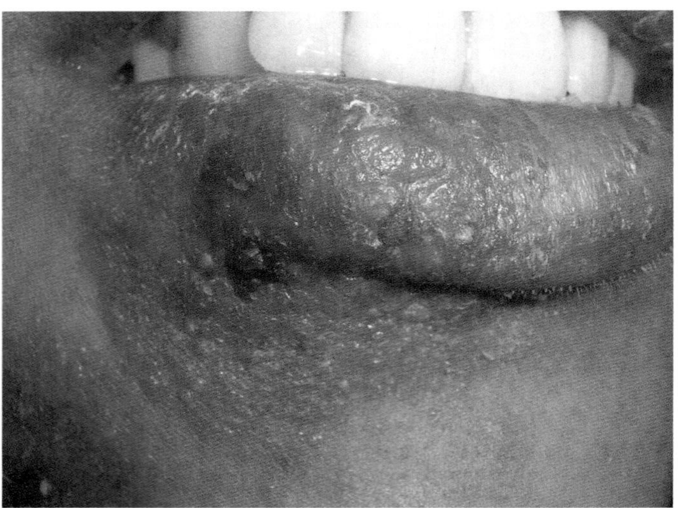

FIGURE 118-1 Typical honey-crusted plaque on the lip of an adult with impetigo. (*Reproduced with permission from Richard P. Usatine, MD.*)

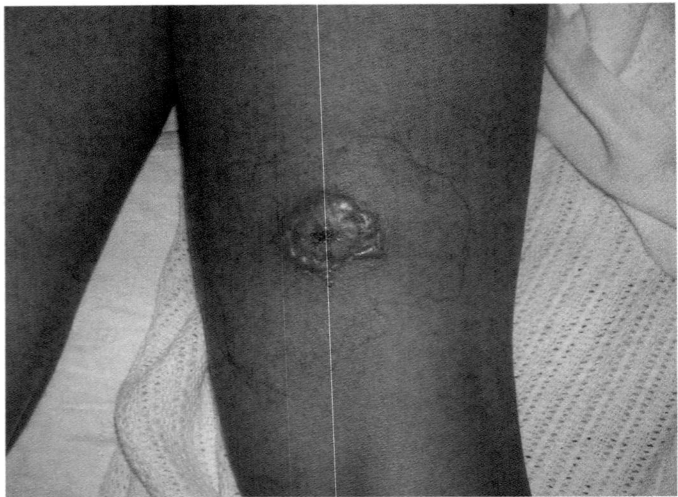

FIGURE 118-2 Bullous impetigo secondary to methicillin-resistant *Staphylococcus aureus* (MRSA) on the leg. Note the surrounding cellulitis. (*Reproduced with permission from Studdiford J, Stonehouse A. Bullous eruption on the posterior thigh 1. J Fam Pract. 2005;54:1041-1044. Reproduced with permission from Frontline Medical Communications.*)

- Bullous impetigo (**Figure 118-2**) is almost always caused by *S. aureus* and is less common than the typical crusted impetigo.[1]
- Impetigo may occur after minor skin injury, such as an insect bite, abrasion, or dermatitis.

DIAGNOSIS

CLINICAL FEATURES

Vesicles, pustules, honey-colored (see **Figure 118-1**), brown or dark crusts, erythematous erosions (**Figure 118-3**), ulcers in ecthyma (**Figure 118-4**), and bullae in bullous impetigo (**Figures 118-5 to 118-7**)

TYPICAL DISTRIBUTION

Face (see **Figures 118-1, 118-4** to **118-6**, and **118-8**) is most common, followed by hands, legs (see **Figure 118-2**), trunk, and buttocks.

CULTURE

Culture should be considered in severe cases because of the rising incidence of methicillin-resistant *S. aureus* (MRSA)-causing impetigo.

DIFFERENTIAL DIAGNOSIS

Many of the conditions below can become impetigo after being secondarily infected with bacteria. This process is called impetiginization.

- Atopic dermatitis—A common inflammatory skin disorder characterized by itching and inflamed skin. It can become secondarily infected with bacteria (**Figure 118-9**) (see Chapter 143, Atopic Dermatitis).

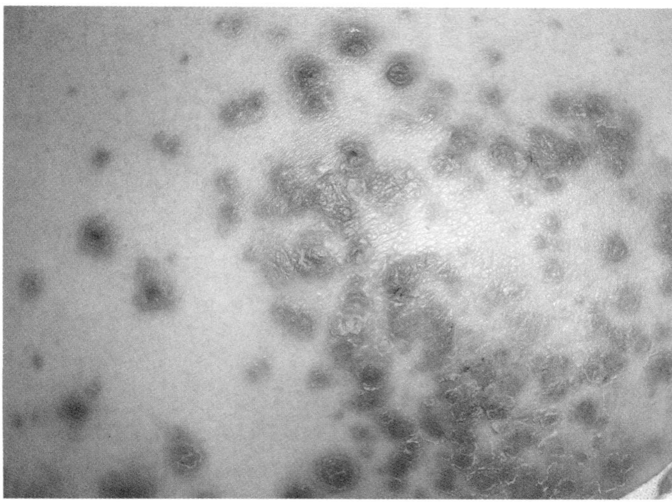

FIGURE 118-3 Widespread impetigo with honey-crusted erythematous lesions on the back. (*Reproduced with permission from Richard P. Usatine, MD.*)

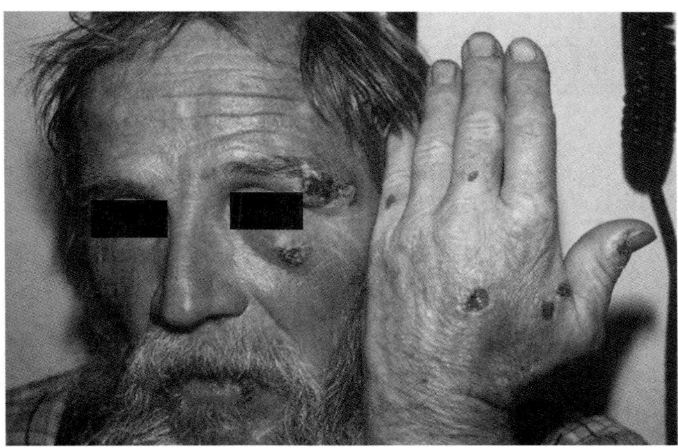

FIGURE 118-4 Impetigo on the face and hand of a homeless man. Note the ecthyma (ulcerated impetigo) on the dorsum of the hand. (*Reproduced with permission from Richard P. Usatine, MD.*)

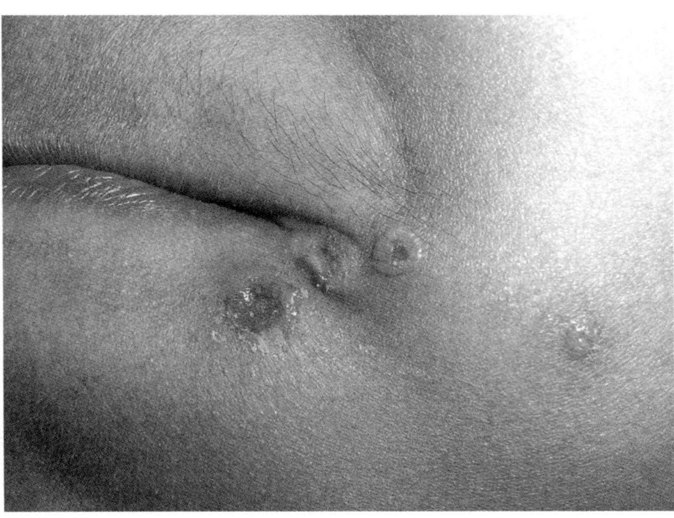

FIGURE 118-5 Bullous impetigo around the mouth that progressed to desquamation of the skin of the hands and feet. (*Reproduced with permission from Richard P. Usatine, MD.*)

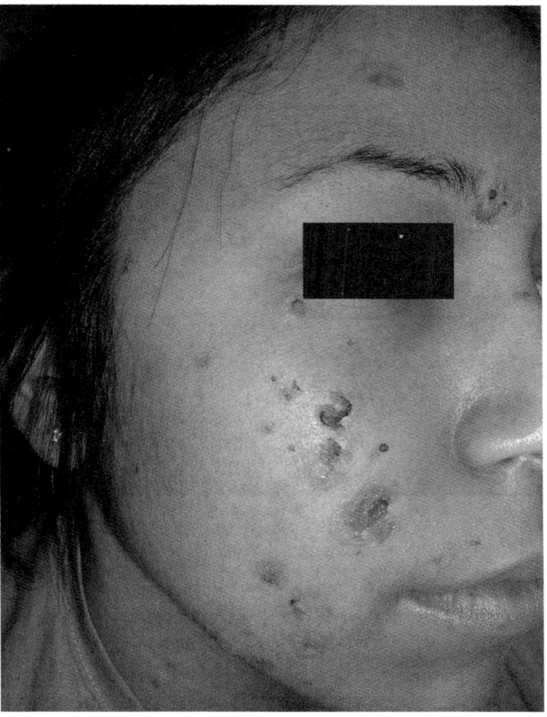

FIGURE 118-6 Bullous impetigo on the face. Methicillin-resistant *Staphylococcus aureus* (MRSA) was cultured from the impetigo. (*Reproduced with permission from Richard P. Usatine, MD.*)

- Herpes simplex virus infection anywhere on the skin or mucous membranes can become secondarily infected (see Chapter 128, Herpes Simplex).
- Eczema herpeticum is eczema superinfected with herpes rather than bacteria.
- Scabies—Pruritic contagious disease caused by a mite that burrows in skin (see Chapter 141, Scabies).
- Folliculitis—Inflammation and/or infection of hair follicles that may be bacterial (see Chapter 119, Folliculitis).
- Tinea corporis—A cutaneous fungal infection caused by dermatophytes, frequently with ring-like scale (see Chapter 136, Tinea Corporis).

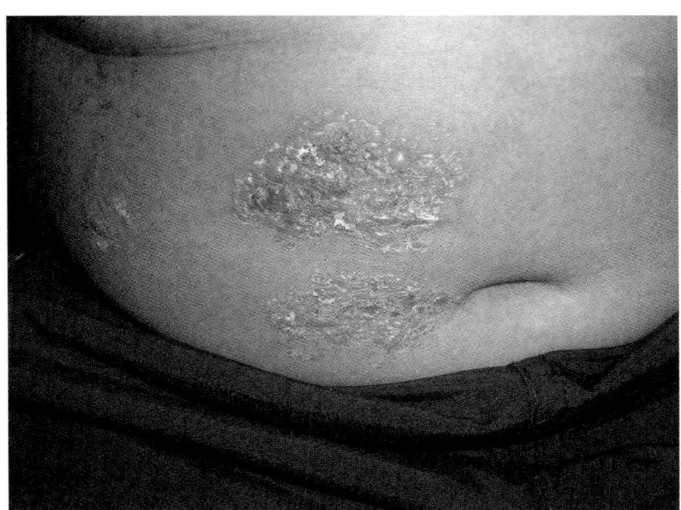

FIGURE 118-7 Bullous impetigo on the abdomen. (*Reproduced with permission from Richard P. Usatine, MD.*)

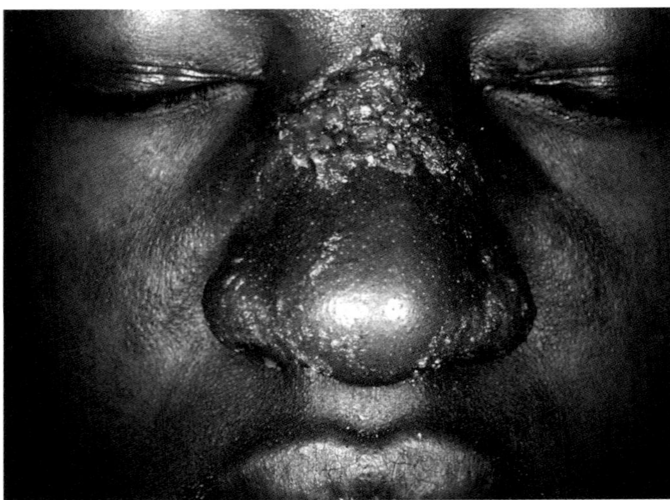

FIGURE 118-8 Impetigo on the nose of a young woman as part of the initial presentation of systemic lupus erythematosus. Note the subtle butterfly hyperpigmentation on the cheeks. (*Reproduced with permission from Richard P. Usatine, MD.*)

- Pemphigus vulgaris—Somewhat rare bullous autoimmune condition with flaccid vesicles and bullae that rupture easily, affecting people between 40 and 60 years of age (see Chapter 183, Pemphigus).
- Bullous pemphigoid—An autoimmune condition with multiple tense bullae that primarily affects people older than 60 years of age (see Chapter 182, Bullous Pemphigoid).
- Acute allergic contact dermatitis—Dermatitis from direct cutaneous exposure to allergens such as poison ivy. Acute lesions are erythematous papules and vesicles in a linear pattern (see Chapter 144, Contact Dermatitis).
- Insect bites—Scratched, open lesions can become secondarily infected with bacteria (impetiginized).
- Second-degree burn or sunburn—The blisters when opened leave the skin susceptible to secondary infection (**Figure 118-10**).
- Staphylococcal scalded skin syndrome—Life-threatening syndrome of acute exfoliation of the skin caused by an exotoxin from a staphylococcal infection. This condition is seen almost entirely in infants and young children.

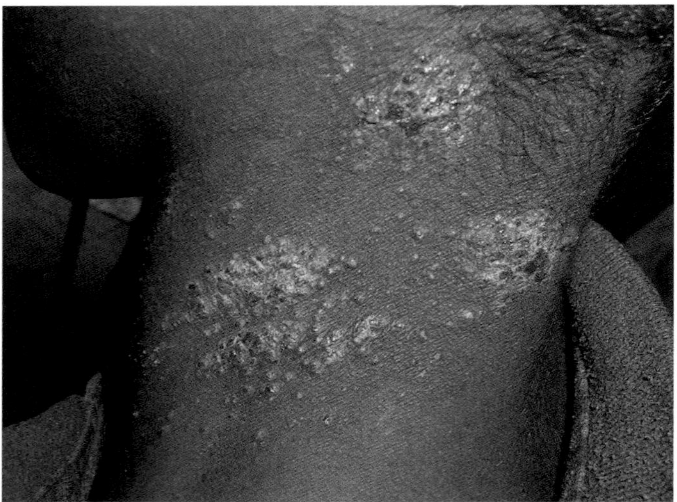

FIGURE 118-9 Impetigo secondary to papular eczema on the neck. Note the honey crusting of the lesions close to the hairline. (*Reproduced with permission from Richard P. Usatine, MD.*)

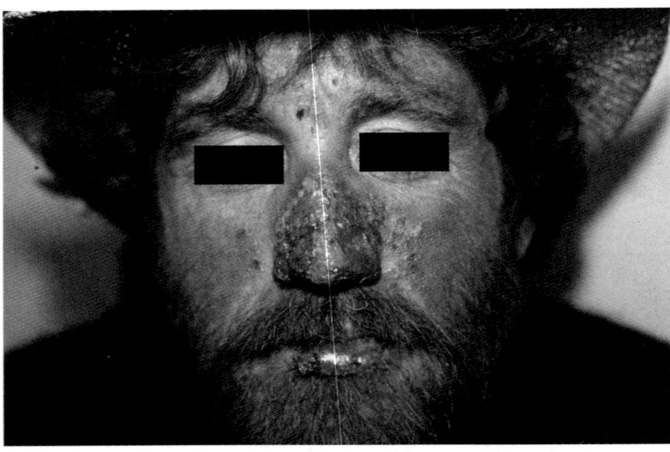

FIGURE 118-10 Secondary impetiginization of a second-degree sunburn in a homeless man. (*Reproduced with permission from Richard P. Usatine, MD.*)

MANAGEMENT

- There is good evidence that topical mupirocin is equally or more effective than oral treatment for people with limited impetigo. SOR Ⓐ Mupirocin also covers MRSA.[2]
- Extensive impetigo could be treated for 7 days with antibiotics that cover GABHS and *S. aureus*, such as cephalexin or dicloxacillin.[3] SOR Ⓐ
- Community-acquired MRSA can present as bullous impetigo (see **Figures 118-2** and **118-6**).
- If you suspect MRSA, culture the lesions and start one of the following oral antibiotics: trimethoprim-sulfamethoxazole, clindamycin, tetracycline, or doxycycline.[4] SOR Ⓐ Trimethoprim-sulfamethoxazole achieved 100% clearance in the treatment of impetigo in children cultured with MRSA and GABHS in one small randomized controlled trial (RCT).[5]
- If there are recurrent MRSA infections, one might choose to prescribe intranasal mupirocin ointment and chlorhexidine bathing to decrease MRSA colonization.[6] SOR Ⓑ

PREVENTION

Practice good hygiene with soap and water. Avoid sharing towels and wash clothes.

FOLLOW-UP

Arrange follow-up based on severity of case and the age and immune status of the patient.

PATIENT EDUCATION

Discuss hygiene issues and how to avoid spread within the household or other living situations such as homeless shelters.

REFERENCES

1. Studdiford J, Stonehouse A. Bullous eruption on the posterior thigh 1. *J Fam Pract*. 2005;54:1041-1044.
2. Koning S, Verhagen AP, van-Suijlekom-Smit LWA, et al. Interventions for impetigo. *Cochrane Database Syst Rev*. 2012;CD003261.
3. Stevens DL, Bisno AL, Chambers HF, et al. Practice guidelines for the diagnosis and management of skin and soft-tissue infections. *Clin Infect Dis*. 2005;41:1373-1406.
4. Naimi TS, LeDell KH, Como-Sabetti K, et al. Comparison of community- and health care-associated methicillin-resistant *Staphylococcus aureus* infection. *JAMA*. 2003;290:2976-2984.
5. Tong SY, Andrews RM, Kearns T, et al. Trimethoprim-sulfamethoxazole compared with benzathine penicillin for treatment of impetigo in aboriginal children: a pilot randomised controlled trial. *J Paediatr Child Health*. 2010;46(3):131-133.
6. Wendt C, Schinke S, Württemberger M, et al. Value of whole-body washing with chlorhexidine for the eradication of methicillin-resistant *Staphylococcus aureus:* a randomized, placebo-controlled, double-blind clinical trial. *Infect Control Hosp Epidemiol*. 2007;28(9):1036-1043.

119 FOLLICULITIS

Richard P. Usatine, MD
Khalilah Hunter-Anderson, MD

PATIENT STORY

A 42-year-old woman is seen for multiple papules and pustules on her back (**Figure 119-1**). Further questioning demonstrates that she was in a friend's hot tub twice over the previous weekend. The outbreak on her back started after she went into the hot tub the second time. This is a case of *Pseudomonas* folliculitis or "hot tub" folliculitis. The patient avoided this hot tub and the folliculitis disappeared spontaneously. Another option is to treat with an oral fluoroquinolone that covers *Pseudomonas*.

INTRODUCTION

Folliculitis is an inflammation of hair follicles usually from an infectious etiology. Multiple species of bacteria have been implicated, as well as fungal organisms.

EPIDEMIOLOGY

- Folliculitis is a cutaneous disorder that affects all age groups and races, and both genders.

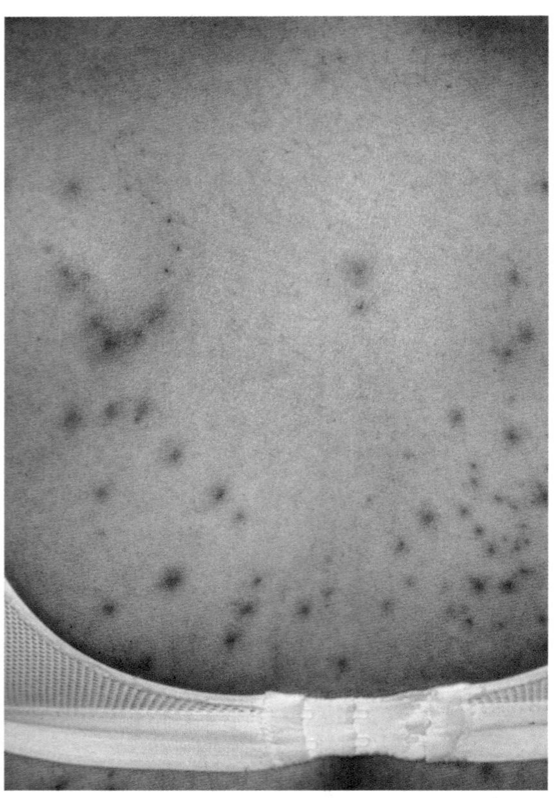

FIGURE 119-1 "Hot-tub" folliculitis from *Pseudomonas aeruginosa* in a hot tub. (*Reproduced with permission from Richard P. Usatine, MD.*)

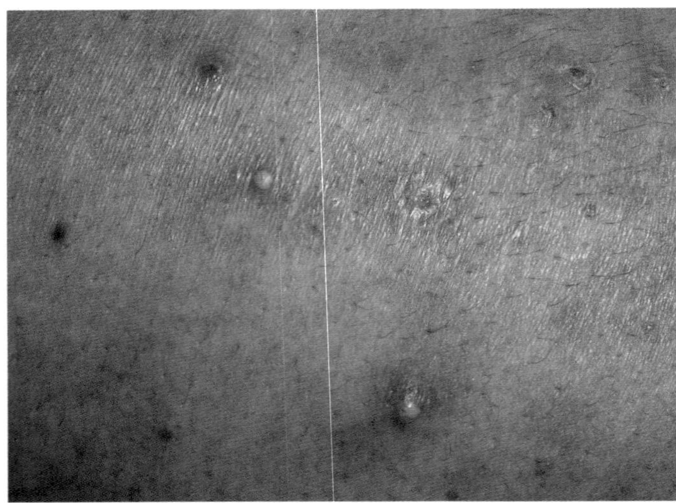

FIGURE 119-2 Close-up of bacterial folliculitis showing hairs coming through pustules. (*Reproduced with permission from Richard P. Usatine, MD.*)

- It can be infectious or noninfectious. It is most commonly of bacterial origin (**Figures 119-2** and **119-3**).
- Pseudofolliculitis or sycosis barbae is most frequently seen in men of color and made worse by shaving (**Figure 119-4**).[1]
- Acne keloidalis nuchae or keloidal folliculitis is commonly seen in black patients, but can be seen in patients of any ethnic background (**Figures 119-5** and **119-6**).[2]
- Eosinophilic folliculitis is described in patients with HIV infection (**Figure 119-7**).
- Methicillin-resistant *Staphylococcus aureus* (MRSA) can pose a challenge to the treatment of folliculitis (**Figure 119-8**).

ETIOLOGY AND PATHOPHYSIOLOGY

- Folliculitis is an infection of the hair follicle and can be superficial, in which it is confined to the upper hair follicle, or deep, in which inflammation spans the entire depth of the follicle.

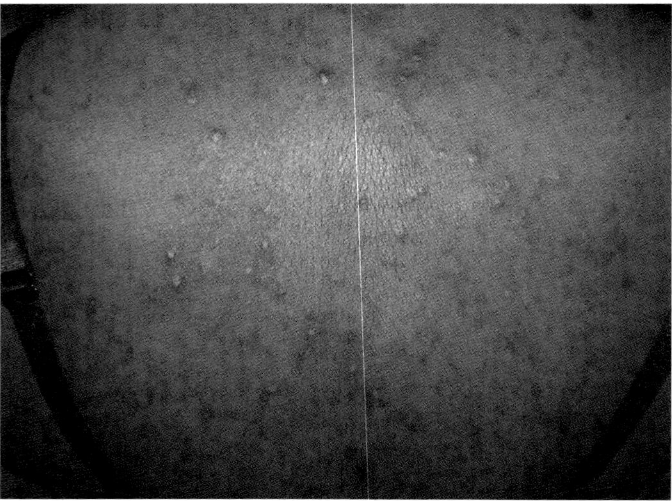

FIGURE 119-3 Chronic bacterial folliculitis on the back with scarring and hyperpigmentation. (*Reproduced with permission from E.J. Mayeaux, Jr, MD.*)

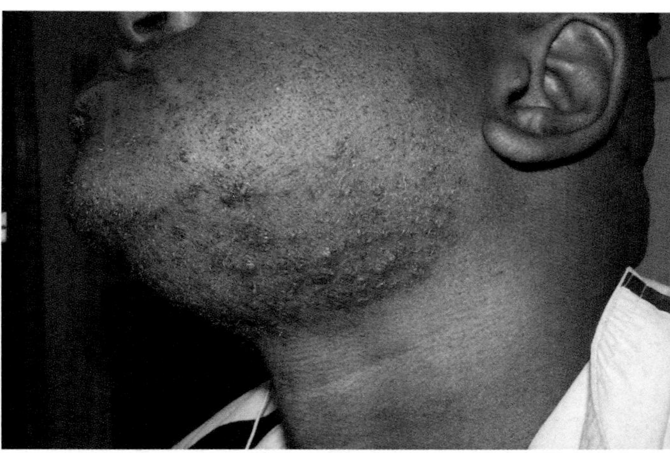

FIGURE 119-4 Pseudofolliculitis barbae in a black man. Shaving makes it worse and he notes many problems with ingrown hairs. (*Reproduced with permission from Jonathan Karnes, MD.*)

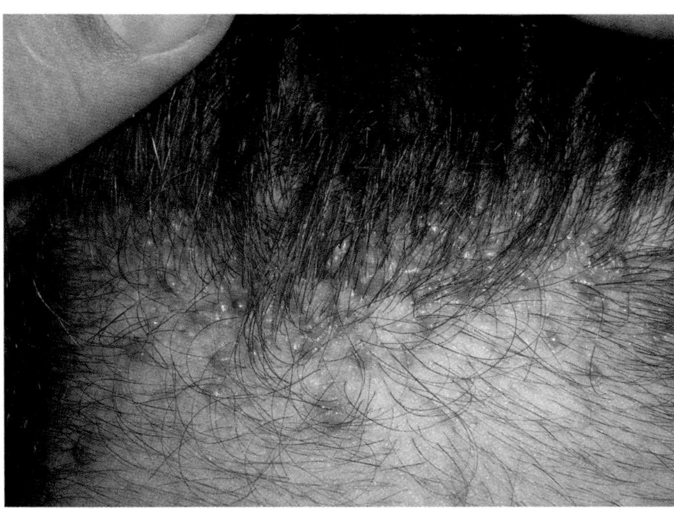

FIGURE 119-5 Acne keloidalis nuchae with inflamed papules and pustules on the back of the neck of a young Hispanic man. (*Reproduced with permission from Richard P. Usatine, MD.*)

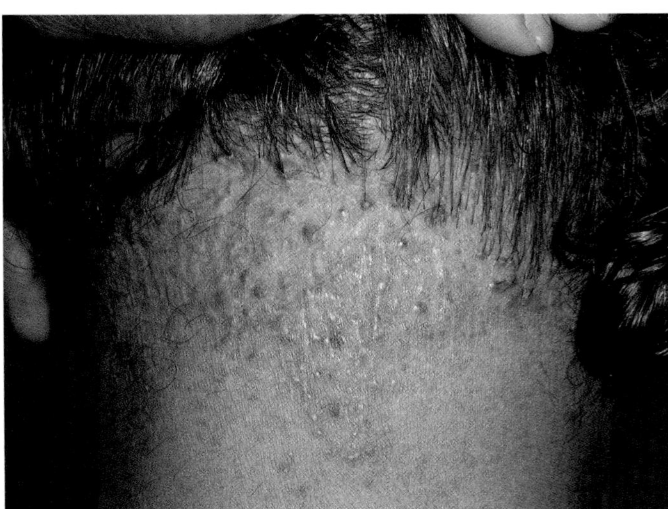

FIGURE 119-6 Acne keloidalis nuchae in a woman demonstrating the folliculitis around the hair follicles and the scarring alopecia that has occurred. (*Reproduced with permission from Richard P. Usatine, MD.*)

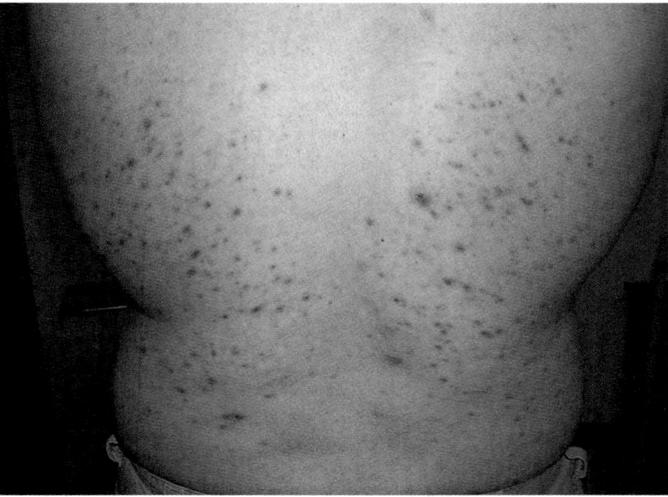

FIGURE 119-7 Eosinophilic folliculitis on the back of an HIV-positive man. (*Reproduced with permission from Richard P. Usatine, MD.*)

- Infection can be of bacterial, viral, or fungal origin. *S. aureus* is by far the most common bacterial causative agent.
- The noninfectious form of folliculitis is often seen in adolescents and young adults who wear tight-fitting clothes. Folliculitis can also be caused by chemical irritants or physical injury.
- Topical steroid use, ointments, lotions, or makeup can swell the opening to the pilosebaceous unit and cause folliculitis.
- Bacterial folliculitis or *Staphylococcus* folliculitis typically presents as infected pustules most prominent on the face, buttocks, trunk, or extremities. It can progress to a deeper infection with the development of furuncles or boils (**Figure 119-9**). Infection can occur as a result of mechanical injury or via local spread from nearby infected wounds. An area of desquamation is frequently seen surrounding infected pustules in *S. aureus* folliculitis.[1-3]
- Parasitic folliculitis usually occurs as a result of mite infestation (*Demodex*). These are usually seen on the face, nose, and back and typically cause an eosinophilic pustular-like folliculitis.[1]

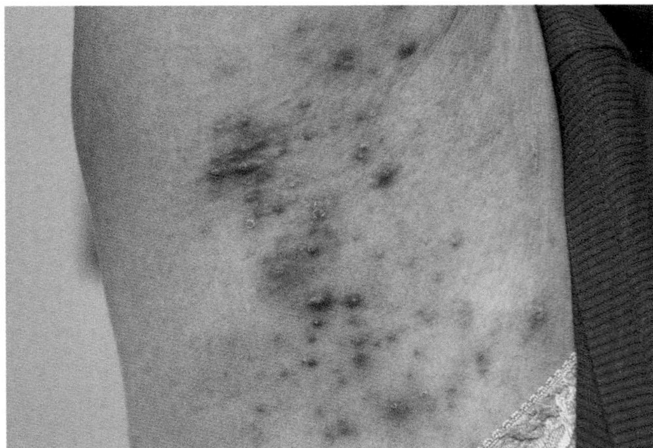

FIGURE 119-8 MRSA folliculitis in the axilla of a 29-year-old woman. The lesions were present for 4 weeks in the axilla, left forearm, and right thigh. The MRSA was sensitive to tetracyclines and resolved with oral doxycycline. (*Reproduced with permission from Alisha N. Plotner, MD, and Robert T. Brodell, MD, and used with permission from Plotner AN, Brodell RT. Bilateral axillary pustules.* J Fam Pract. *2008;57(4):253-255. Reproduced with permission from Frontline Medical Communications.*)

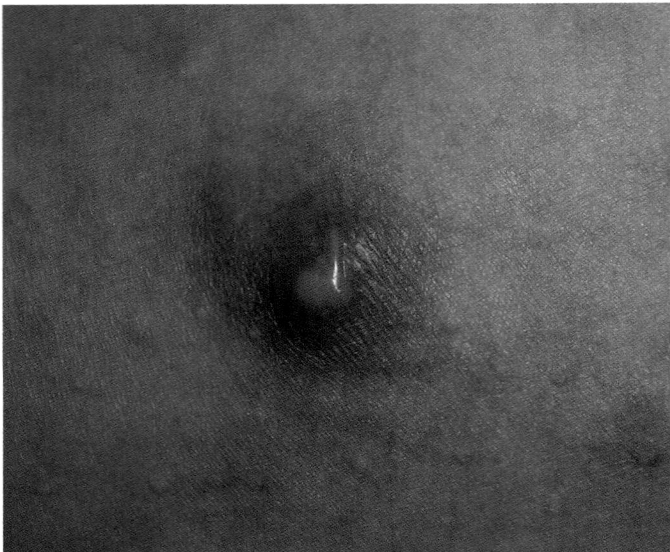

FIGURE 119-9 Isolated single furuncle in an adult woman. (*Reproduced with permission from Richard P. Usatine, MD.*)

- Folliculitis decalvans is a chronic form of folliculitis involving the scalp, leading to hair loss or alopecia (**Figure 119-10**). Staphylococci infection is the usual causative agent, but there also has been a suggested genetic component to this condition.[1] It is also called tufted folliculitis because some of the hair follicles will have many hairs growing from them simultaneously (**Figure 119-11**) (see Chapter 187, Scarring Alopecia).
- Acne keloidalis nuchae is a chronic form of folliculitis found on the posterior neck that can be extensive and lead to keloidal tissue and alopecia.[1-3] Although it is often thought to occur almost exclusively in black men, it can be seen in men of all ethnic backgrounds and occasionally in women (see **Figures 119-5** and **119-6**) (see Chapter 116, Pseudofolliculitis and Acne Keloidalis Nuchae).
- Fungal folliculitis is epidermal fungal infections that are seen frequently. Tinea capitis infections are a form of dermatophytic folliculitis. *Pityrosporum* folliculitis is caused by yeast infection (*Malassezia* species) and is seen in a similar distribution as bacterial folliculitis on the back, chest, and shoulders (**Figure 119-12**) (see Chapter 139, Tinea Versicolor). Candidal infection is less common and is usually seen in individuals who are immunosuppressed, present in hairy areas that are moist, and unlike most cases of folliculitis, may present with systemic signs and symptoms.[1-4]

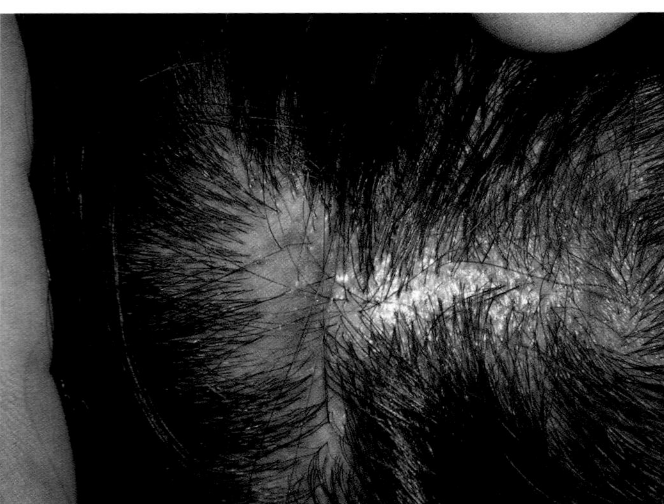

FIGURE 119-10 Early folliculitis decalvans showing scalp inflammation, pustules around hair follicles, and scarring alopecia. (*Reproduced with permission from Richard P. Usatine, MD.*)

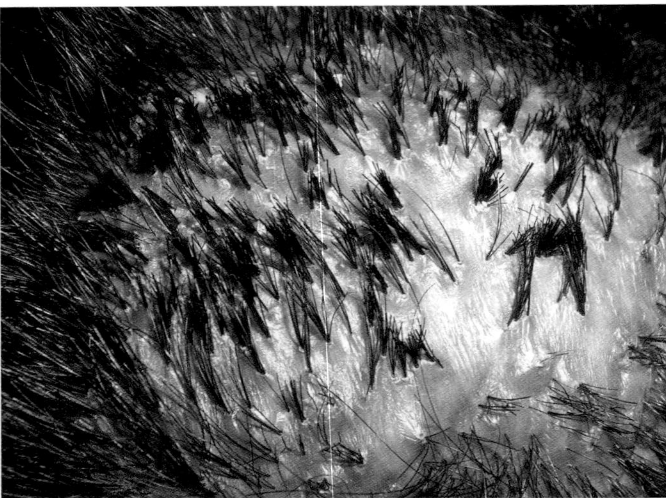

FIGURE 119-11 Tufted folliculitis with visible tufts of hair (multiple hairs from one follicle) growing from a number of abnormal follicles. This is one example of scarring alopecia. (*Reproduced with permission from Richard P. Usatine, MD.*)

- *Pseudomonas* folliculitis or "hot tub" folliculitis is usually a self-limited infection that follows exposure to water or objects that are contaminated with *Pseudomonas aeruginosa* (see **Figure 119-1**). This occurs when hot tubs are inadequately chlorinated or brominated. This also occurs when loofah sponges or other items used for bathing become a host for pseudomonal growth. Onset of symptoms is usually within 6 to 72 hours after exposure, with the complete resolution of symptoms in a couple of days, provided that the individual avoids further exposure.[4]
- Gram-negative folliculitis is an infection with gram-negative bacteria that most typically occurs in individuals who have been on long-term antibiotic therapy, usually those taking oral antibiotics for acne. The most frequently encountered infective agents include *Klebsiella*, *Escherichia coli*, *Enterobacter*, and *Proteus*.[5]
- Pseudofolliculitis barbae (razor bumps) is most commonly seen in black males who shave. Papules develop when the sharp edge of the hair shaft reenters the skin (ingrown hairs), and is seen on the cheeks and neck as a result of curled ingrown hair.[2] It can also occur in women with hirsutism who shave or pluck their hairs (see **Figure 119-4**) (see Chapter 116, Pseudofolliculitis and Acne Keloidalis Nuchae).[6]
- Viral folliculitis is primarily caused by herpes simplex virus and molluscum contagiosum.[4] Herpetic folliculitis is seen primarily in individuals with a history of herpes simplex infections type I or II. But most notably, it may be a sign of immunosuppression, as is the case with HIV infection.[7] The expression of herpes folliculitis in HIV infection ranges from simple to necrotizing folliculitis and ulcerative lesions. Molluscum is a pox virus and molluscum contagiosum has been well documented in similar patient populations (ie, HIV and AIDS) and in children (see Chapters 128, Herpes Simplex and 129, Molluscum Contagiosum).[7-9]
- Actinic superficial folliculitis is a sterile form of folliculitis seen predominantly in warm climates or during hot or summer months. Pustules occur primarily on the neck, over the shoulders, upper trunk, and upper arms, usually within 6 to 36 hours after sun exposure.[10]

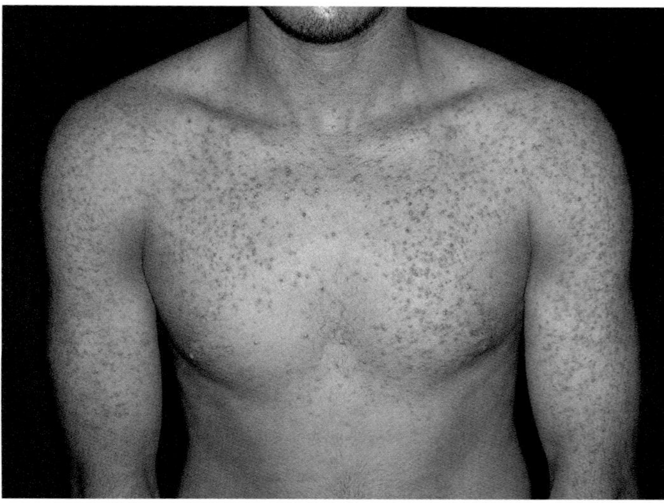

A

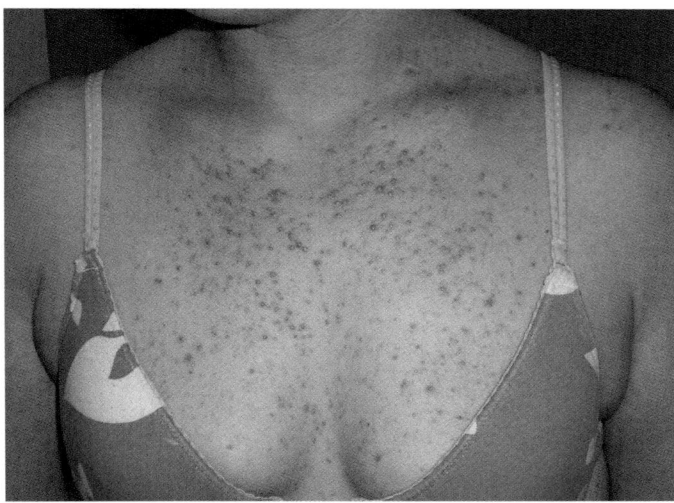

B

FIGURE 119-12 A. *Pityrosporum* folliculitis on the chest, shoulders, and arms of a young man; biopsy proven. B. *Pityrosporum* folliculitis on the chest of a young woman. KOH preparation showed *Pityrosporum* looking like ziti and meatballs. (*Reproduced with permission from Richard P. Usatine, MD.*)

- Eosinophilic folliculitis is associated with HIV infection and can occur as a result of the viral infection itself, in which case the exact mechanism by which this occurs is uncertain (though thought to be autoimmune) (see **Figure 119-7**).[9,11-14] It is associated with diminished CD4 cell counts. Eosinophilic folliculitis generally improves with the initiation of highly active antiretroviral therapy (HAART), but can occur during the restoration of immune function with HAART.[12]

DIAGNOSIS

Often the diagnosis of folliculitis is based on a good history and physical.

CLINICAL FEATURES

Folliculitis has its characteristic presentation as the development of papules or pustules that are thin-walled and surrounded by a margin of erythema or inflammation. Look for a hair at the center of the lesions (see **Figure 119-2**). There is usually an absence of systemic signs and patients' symptoms range from mild discomfort and pruritus to severe pain with extensive involvement.

TYPICAL DISTRIBUTION

Any area of the skin may be affected and often location may be related to the pathogen or cause of folliculitis. The face, scalp, neck, trunk, axillae, extremities, and groin are some of the more common areas affected.

LABORATORY TESTS

Laboratory testing may be unnecessary in simple superficial folliculitis and where the history is clear and quick resolution occurs. Clinical diagnosis of herpes and fungal folliculitis may be difficult and diagnosis may be made based on strong clinical suspicion or as a result of failed antimicrobial therapy. Potassium hydroxide (KOH) preps can be used to look for tinea versicolor or other fungal organisms. Herpes culture or a quick test for herpes can be used when herpes is suspected.[1] SOR Ⓐ

DIFFERENTIAL DIAGNOSIS

- *Grover disease* is a very pruritic condition of unknown cause that produces reddish papules and slight scale on the backs of middle-aged men. It is also called "transient acantholytic dermatosis" and may resolve spontaneously in a period of years. It resembles folliculitis but the papules are not centered on hair follicles (**Figure 119-13**).
- *Miliaria* is blockage of the sweat glands that can resemble the small papules of folliculitis. The eccrine sweat glands become blocked so that

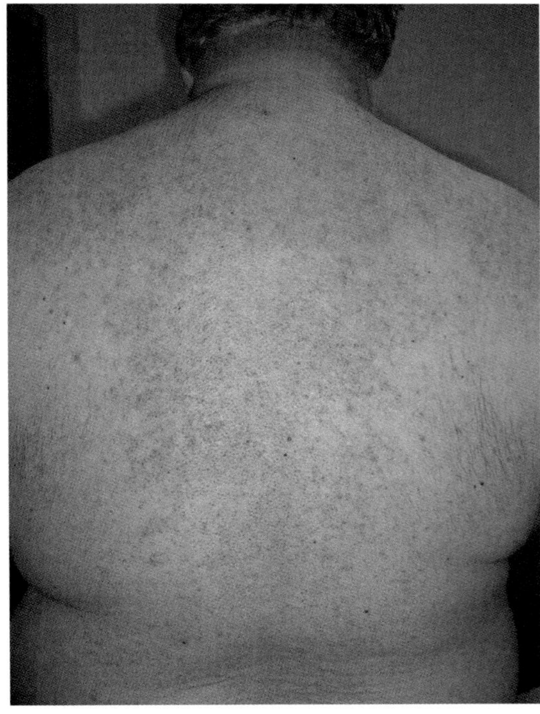

FIGURE 119-13 Grover disease on the back of a middle-aged man. This is also called "transient acantholytic dermatosis." It is very pruritic with reddish papules and slight scale. (*Reproduced with permission from Richard P. Usatine, MD.*)

sweat leaks into the dermis and epidermis. Clinically, skin lesions may range from clear vesicles to pustules. These skin lesions primarily occur in times of increased heat and humidity, and are self-limited.[1]

- *Impetigo* is a bacterial infection of the skin that affects the superficial layers of the epidermis as opposed to hair follicles. It is contagious, unlike folliculitis. It has a bullous and nonbullous form, and honey-crusted lesions frequently predominate as opposed to the usual pustules seen in folliculitis (see Chapter 118, Impetigo).[4,6]
- *Keratosis pilaris* consists of papules that occur as a result of a buildup of keratin in the openings of hair follicles, especially on the lateral upper arms and thighs. It is not an infection but can develop into folliculitis if lesions become infected (see Chapter 143, Atopic Dermatitis).[1,6]
- *Acne vulgaris* is characterized by the presence of comedones, papules, pustules, and nodules that are a result of follicular hyperproliferation and plugging with excessive sebum. Inflammation occurs when Propionibacterium acnes and other inflammatory substances get extruded from the blocked pilosebaceous unit.[15] Although acne on the face is rarely confused with folliculitis, acne on the trunk can resemble folliculitis. To distinguish between them look for facial involvement and comedones seen in acne (see Chapter 114, Acne Vulgaris).

MANAGEMENT

- Management of folliculitis varies by causative agent and underlying pathophysiology.
- Antivirals, antibiotics, and antifungals are used as topical and/or systemic agents. Approaches to nonpharmacologic therapy include patient education on the prevention of chemical and mechanical skin irritation.[16] Glycemic control in diabetic patients may help treat folliculitis.[1-3] Good hygiene helps to control symptoms and prevent recurrence.
- With superficial bacterial folliculitis, treatment with topical preparations such as mupirocin (Bactroban) or fusidic acid may be sufficient.[1] SOR Ⓐ Additionally, topical clindamycin may be considered in the mildest cases in which MRSA is involved.[1] SOR Ⓐ
- Deep or extensive bacterial folliculitis warrants oral therapy with first-generation cephalosporins (cephalexin), penicillins (amoxicillin/clavulanate and dicloxacillin), macrolides, or fluoroquinolones.[1,4,6] SOR Ⓐ
- *Pseudomonas* or "hot tub" folliculitis usually resolves untreated within a week of onset (see **Figure 119-1**). For severe cases, treatment with ciprofloxacin provides adequate antipseudomonal coverage.[1,4] SOR Ⓑ Application of a warm compress to affected areas also provides symptomatic relief.
- *Pityrosporum* folliculitis and/or tinea versicolor can be treated with systemic antifungals, topical azoles, and/or with shampoos containing azoles, selenium, or zinc (see **Figur**e **119-12**) (see Chapter 139, Tinea Versicolor).
- Candidal folliculitis in immunosuppressed persons may be treated with oral itraconazole (see Chapter 135, Candidiasis).[1] SOR Ⓐ
- *Demodex* folliculitis can be treated with ivermectin or topically with 5% permethrin cream.[4] SOR Ⓑ
- Herpes folliculitis can be treated with acyclovir, valacyclovir, and famciclovir. Regimens may frequently include acyclovir 200 mg 5 times a day for 5 days (see Chapter 128, Herpes Simplex).[1] SOR Ⓐ
- Eosinophilic folliculitis associated with HIV is treated with HAART, topical steroids, antihistamines, itraconazole, metronidazole, oral retinoids, and UV light therapy.[11] Topical steroids and nonsteroidal anti-inflammatory drugs (NSAIDs) and isotretinoin are treatments of choice for HIV-associated eosinophilic folliculitis.[9-13] SOR Ⓑ Relief with systemic antihistamines are variable and UV therapy is time consuming and expensive.[11,12] SOR Ⓒ

FOLLOW-UP

Most cases of folliculitis are superficial and resolve easily with treatment. Dermatologic and surgical consultation may be required in cases of chronic folliculitis with scarring.

PATIENT EDUCATION

Prevention is most important, and centers on good personal hygiene and proper laundering of clothing. Patients should be encouraged to avoid tight-fitting clothing. Hot tubs should be properly cleaned and the chemicals should be maintained appropriately. Electric razors for shaving can help prevent pseudofolliculitis barbae and should be cleaned regularly with alcohol. Patients with acne keloidalis nuchae should avoid shaving the hair in the involved area.

PATIENT RESOURCES

- PubMed Health. *Folliculitis*—**http://www.ncbi.nlm.nih.gov/pubmedhealth/PMH0001826/.**

PROVIDER RESOURCES

- Medscape. *Folliculitis.*—**http://emedicine.medscape.com/article/1070456.**

REFERENCES

1. Luelmo-Aguilar J, Santandreu MS. Folliculitis recognition and management. *Am J Clin Dermatol.* 2004;5(5):301-310.
2. Habif T. *Clinical Dermatology*. 5th ed. Philadelphia, PA: Saunders Elsevier; 2010.
3. Levy AL, Simpson G, Skinner RB Jr. Medical pearl: circle of desquamation, a clue to the diagnosis of folliculitis and furunculosis caused by *Staphylococcus aureus*. *J Am Acad Dermatol.* 2006;55(6):1079-1080.
4. Stulberg DL, Penrod MA, Blatny RA. Common bacterial skin infections. *Am Fam Physician.* 2002;66(1):119-124.
5. Neubert U, Jansen T, Plewig G. Bacteriologic and immunologic aspects of Gram-negative folliculitis: a study of 46 patients. *Int J Dermatol.* 1999;38(4):270-274.
6. Ferri FF. *Ferri's Clinical Advisor 2012.* , Philadelphia, PA: Elsevier; 2012.
7. Boer A, Herder N, Winter K, Falk T. Herpes folliculitis: clinical histopathological, and molecular pathologic observations. *Br J Dermatol.* 2006;154(4):743-746.
8. Weinberg JM, Mysliwiec A, Turiansky GW, et al. Viral folliculitis. Atypical presentations of herpes simplex, herpes zoster, and molluscum contagiosum. *Arch Dermatol.* 1997;133(8):983-986.
9. Fearfield LA, Rowe A, Francis N, et al. Itchy folliculitis and human immunodeficiency virus infection: clinicopathological and immunological features, pathogenesis and treatment. *Br J Dermatol.* 1999;141(1):3-11.

10. Labandeira J, Suarez-Campos A, Toribio J. Actinic superficial folliculitis. *Br J Dermatol.* 1998;138(6):1070-1074.

11. Nervi SJ, Schwartz RA, Dmochowski M. Eosinophilic pustular folliculitis: a 40 year retrospect. *J Am Acad Dermatol.* 2006;55(2):285-289.

12. Rajendran PM, Dolev JC, Heaphy MR Jr, Maurer T. Eosinophilic folliculitis: before and after the introduction of antiretroviral therapy. *Arch Dermatol.* 2005;141(10):1227-1231.

13. Jang KA, Kim SH, Choi JH, et al. Viral folliculitis on the face. *Br J Dermatol.* 2000;142(3):555-559.

14. Toutous-Trellu L, Abraham S, Pechère M, et al. Topical tacrolimus for effective treatment of eosinophilic folliculitis associated with human immunodeficiency virus infection. *Arch Dermatol.* 2005;141(10):1203-1208.

15. Strauss JS, Krowchuk DP, Leyden JJ, et al. Guidelines of care for acne vulgaris management. *J Am Acad Dermatol.* 2007;56(4):651-663.

16. Gupta AK, Batra R, Bluhm R, et al. Skin diseases associated with *Malassezia* species. *J Am Acad Dermatol.* 2004;51(5):785-798.

120 PITTED KERATOLYSIS

Michael Babcock, MD
Richard P. Usatine, MD

PATIENT STORY

A young man comes to the office with a terrible foot odor problem. He is wearing cowboy boots and he says that his feet are always sweaty. He is embarrassed to remove his boots, but when his mother convinces him to do so the odor is unpleasant. The clinician sees the typical pits of pitted keratolysis and notes that the boy's socks are moist. His foot has many crateriform pits on the heel (**Figure 120-1**). He is prescribed topical erythromycin solution for the pitted keratolysis and topical aluminum chloride for the hyperhidrosis. It is suggested that he wear a lighter and more breathable shoe until this problem improves.

INTRODUCTION

Pitted keratolysis is a superficial foot infection caused by gram-positive bacteria. These bacteria degrade the keratin of the stratum corneum leaving visible pits on the soles of the feet.

EPIDEMIOLOGY

- Seen more commonly in males.
- Often a complication of hyperhidrosis.
- Seen more often in hot and humid climates.
- Prevalence can be as high as 42.5% among paddy field workers.[1]
- May be common in athletes with moist, sweaty feet.[2]

ETIOLOGY AND PATHOPHYSIOLOGY

- *Kytococcus sedentarius* (formerly *Micrococcus* spp.), *Corynebacterium* species, and *Dermatophilus congolensis* have all been shown to cause pitted keratolysis.[3]

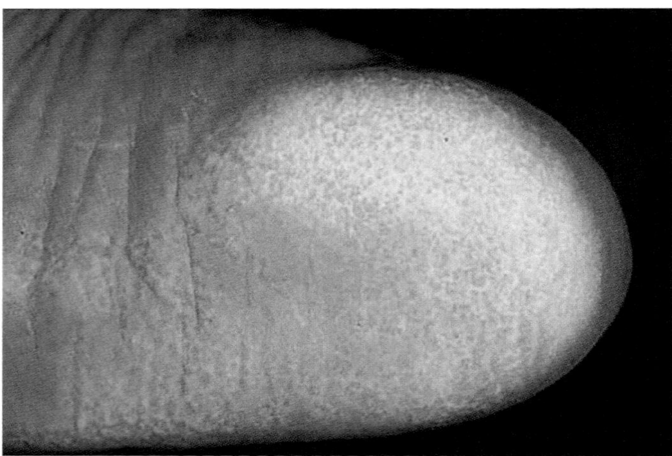

FIGURE 120-1 Many crateriform pits on the heel of the foot with pitted keratolysis and hyperhidrosis. (*Reproduced with permission from Richard P. Usatine, MD.*)

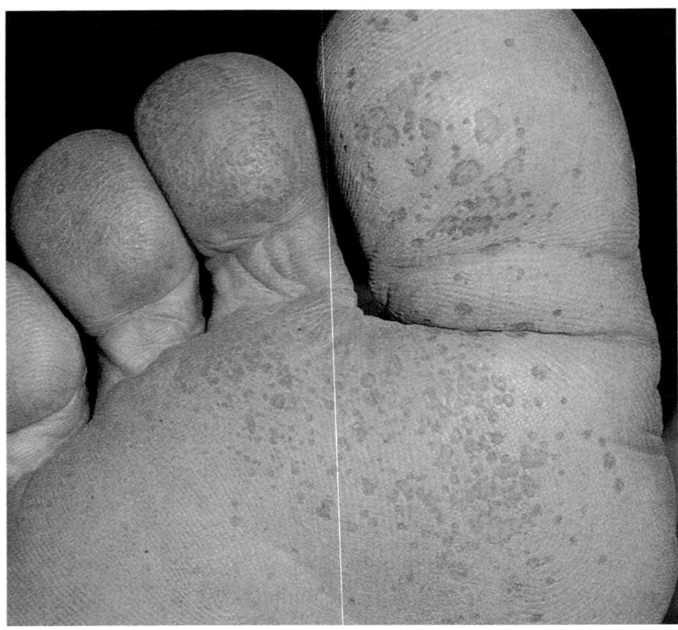

FIGURE 120-2 Pitted keratolysis on the pressure-bearing areas of the toes and the ball of the foot. (*Reproduced with permission from Richard P. Usatine, MD.*)

- Proteases produced by the bacteria degrade keratins to give the clinical appearance.[4]
- The associated malodor is likely secondary to the production of sulfur by-products.[3]

DIAGNOSIS

CLINICAL FEATURES

Pitted keratolysis usually presents as painless, malodorous, crateriform pits coalescing into larger superficial erosions of the stratum corneum (**Figures 120-1** to **120-4**). It may be associated with itching and a burning sensation in some patients (see **Figure 120-3**).

TYPICAL DISTRIBUTION

Pitted keratolysis usually involves the callused pressure-bearing areas of the foot, such as the heel, ball of the foot, and plantar great toe. It can also be found in friction areas between the toes.[5]

LABORATORY STUDIES

Typically a clinical diagnosis but biopsy will reveal keratin pits lined by bacteria.

DIFFERENTIAL DIAGNOSIS

- Characteristic clinical features make the diagnosis easy, but it is possible to have other diseases causing plantar pits, which can be included in the differential. These other diseases include plantar warts, basal cell nevus syndrome, and arsenic toxicity.
- Plantar warts are typically not as numerous. They have a firm callus ring around a soft core with small black dots from thrombosed capillaries (see Chapter 133, Plantar Warts).

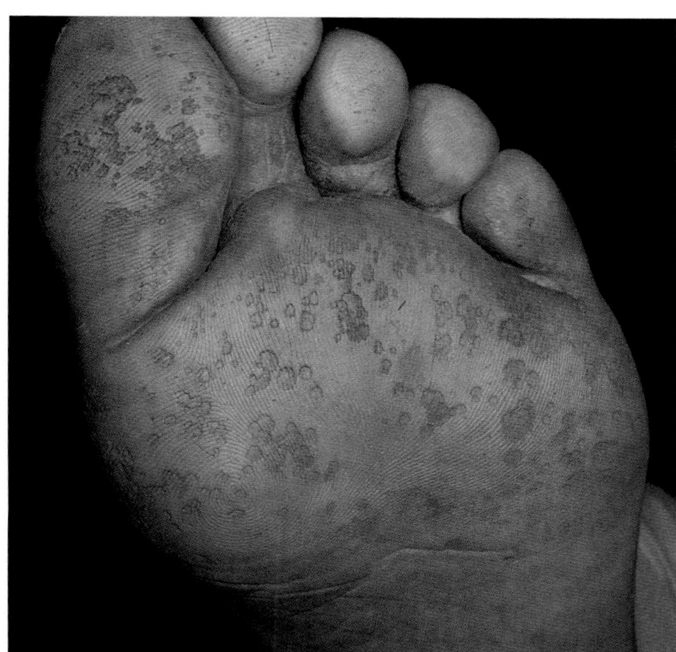

FIGURE 120-3 Pitted keratolysis with hyperpigmented crateriform pits on the pressure-bearing areas of the foot. The patient complained of itching and burning on the feet. (*Reproduced with permission from Richard P. Usatine, MD.*)

- Basal cell nevus syndrome typically has pits involving the palms and soles, bone abnormalities, a history of many basal cell carcinomas, and a characteristic facies with frontal bossing, hypoplastic maxilla, and hypertelorism (wide-set eyes) (see Chapter 168, Basal Cell Carcinoma).

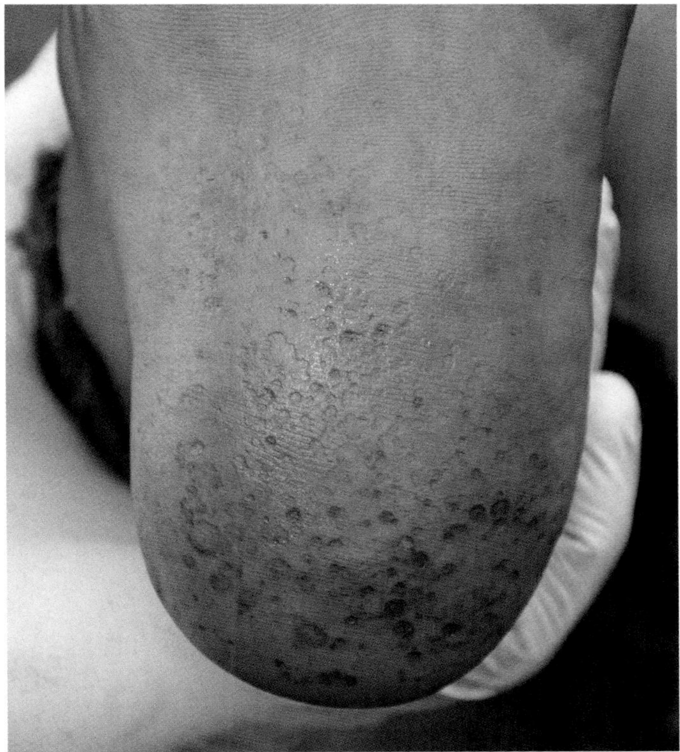

FIGURE 120-4 Pitted keratolysis with many crateriform pits on the heel. (*Reproduced with permission from Richard P. Usatine, MD.*)

- Arsenic toxicity can result in pits on the palms and soles, but it can also have hyperpigmentation, many skin cancers, Mees lines (white lines on the fingernails), or other nail disorders.

MANAGEMENT

- Treatment is based on bacterial elimination and reducing the moist environment in which the bacteria thrive. Various topical antibiotics are effective for pitted keratolysis.
- Topical erythromycin or clindamycin solution or gel can be applied twice daily until the condition resolves. SOR Ⓒ Generic 2% erythromycin solution with an applicator top is a very inexpensive and effective preparation. It may take 3 to 4 weeks to clear the odor and skin lesions.
- Topical mupirocin is more expensive but also effective. SOR Ⓒ
- Oral erythromycin is effective and may be considered if topical therapy fails. SOR Ⓒ
- Treating underlying hyperhidrosis is also important to prevent recurrence. This can be done with topical aluminum chloride of varying concentrations. SOR Ⓒ Drysol is 20% aluminum chloride solution and can be prescribed with an applicator top.
- Botulinum toxin injection is an expensive and effective treatment for hyperhidrosis.[6] SOR Ⓒ It should be reserved for treatment failures because of the cost, the discomfort of the multiple injections, and the need to repeat the treatment every 3 to 4 months.

FOLLOW-UP

Follow-up is needed for treatment failures, recurrences, and the treatment of underlying hyperhidrosis if present. Follow-up can be performed annually for prescription aluminum chloride or approximately every 4 months for botulinum toxin injections.

PATIENT EDUCATION

Patients should be taught about the etiology of this disorder to help avoid recurrence. Helpful preventive strategies include avoiding occlusive footwear and using moisture-wicking socks or changing sweaty socks frequently.

PATIENT RESOURCES

- International Hyperhidrosis Society—**http://www.sweathelp.org.**

PROVIDER RESOURCES

- Medscape. *Pitted Keratolysis*—**http://emedicine.medscape.com/article/1053078-overview.**

REFERENCES

1. Shenoi SD, Davis SV, Rao S, et al. Dermatoses among paddy field workers—a descriptive, cross-sectional pilot study. *Indian J Dermatol Venereol Leprol.* 2005;71:254-258.
2. Conklin RJ. Common cutaneous disorders in athletes. *Sports Med.* 1990;9:100-119.

3. Bolognia J, Jorizzo J, Rapini R. *Dermatology*. 2nd ed. Philadelphia, PA: Mosby; 2008:1088-1089.
4. Takama H, Tamada Y, Yano K, et al. Pitted keratolysis: clinical manifestations in 53 cases. *Br J Dermatol.* 1997;137(2):282-285.
5. Longshaw C, Wright J, Farrell A, et al. Kytococcus sedentarius, the organism associated with pitted keratolysis, produces two keratin-degrading enzymes. *J Appl Microbiol.* 2002;93(5):810-816.
6. Vadoud-Seyedi J. Treatment of plantar hyperhidrosis with botulinum toxin type A. *Int J Dermatol.* 2004;43(12):969-971.

121 ERYTHRASMA

Richard P. Usatine, MD
Anna Allred, MD
Mindy A. Smith, MD, MS

PATIENT STORY

A 59-year-old woman (with obesity and type 2 diabetes) presents with a 6-month history of a brown, somewhat pruritic, rash in both axillae (**Figure 121-1a**). She has been seen by multiple physicians and many antifungal creams and topical steroids have been tried with no results. She had stopped wearing deodorant for fear that she was allergic to all deodorants. The rash demonstrated the classic coral red fluorescence of erythrasma (**Figure 121-1b**). The patient was given a prescription for oral erythromycin and the erythrasma cleared to the great delight of the patient.

INTRODUCTION

Erythrasma is a chronic superficial bacterial skin infection that usually occurs in a skin fold.

EPIDEMIOLOGY

- The incidence of erythrasma is approximately 4%.[1]
- Both sexes are equally affected.
- The inguinal location is more common in men.

ETIOLOGY AND PATHOPHYSIOLOGY

- *Corynebacterium minutissimum*, a lipophilic gram-positive non–spore-forming rod-shaped organism, is the causative agent.
- Under favorable conditions, such as heat and humidity, this organism invades and proliferates the upper one-third of the stratum corneum.
- The organism produces porphyrins that result in the coral red fluorescence seen under a Wood lamp (**Figures 121-1 and 121-2**).

RISK FACTORS

- Warm climate[1]
- Diabetes mellitus
- Immunocompromised states

A

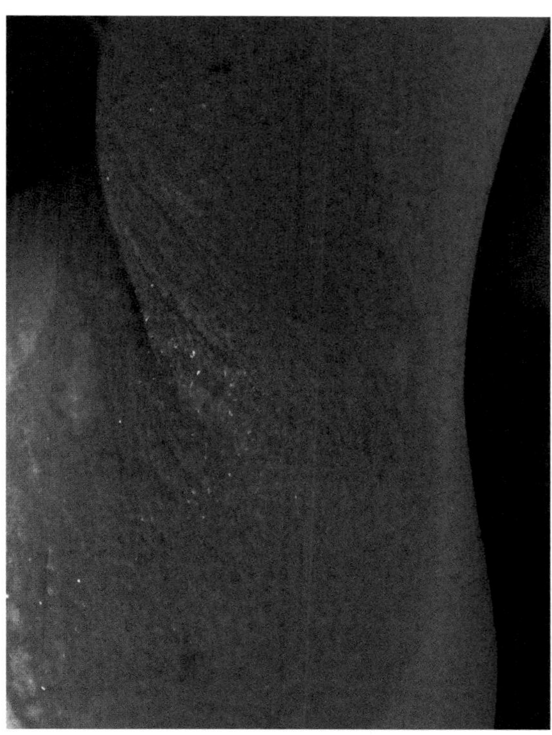

B

FIGURE 121-1 A. Erythrasma in the axilla of 59-year-old woman with obesity and diabetes. B. Coral red fluorescence seen with a Wood lamp. (*Reproduced with permission from Richard P. Usatine, MD.*)

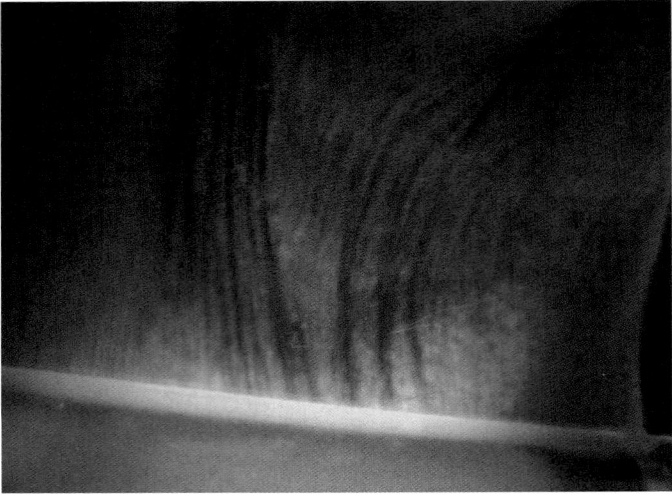

FIGURE 121-2 Coral red fluorescence seen with a Wood lamp held in the axilla of a patient with erythrasma. (*Reproduced with permission from the University of Texas Health Sciences Center, Division of Dermatology.*)

- Obesity
- Hyperhidrosis
- Poor hygiene
- Advanced age

DIAGNOSIS

CLINICAL FEATURES

- Erythrasma is a sharply delineated, dry, red-brown patch with slightly scaling patches. Some lesions appear redder, whereas others have a browner color (**Figures 121-3** and **121-4**).

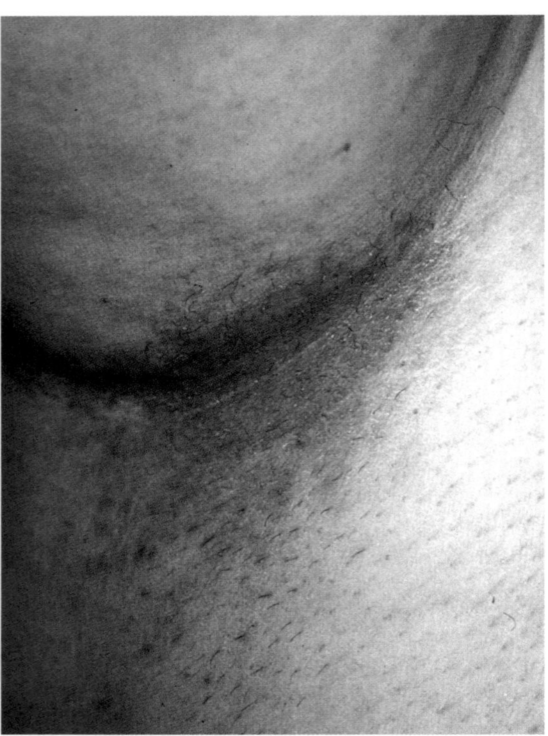

FIGURE 121-3 Reddish brown erythrasma in the axilla of an obese woman with diabetes. (*Reproduced with permission from Richard P. Usatine, MD.*)

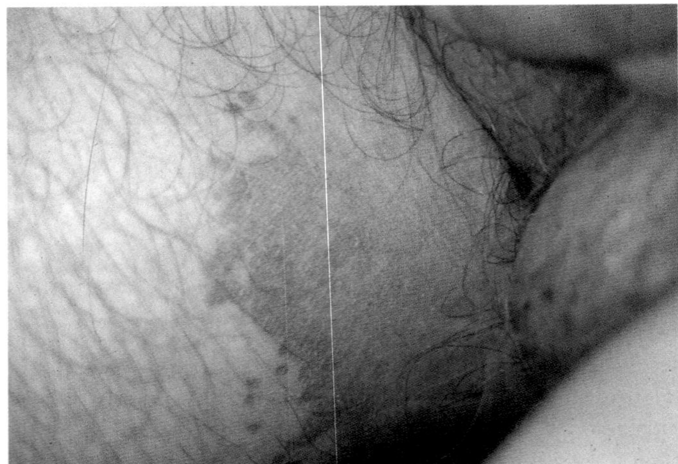

FIGURE 121-4 Brown erythrasma in the groin of a man with diabetes. (*Reproduced with permission from the University of Texas Health Sciences Center, Division of Dermatology.*)

- The lesions may appear with central clearing and be slightly raised from the surrounding skin (**Figure 121-5**).
- The lesions are typically asymptomatic; however, patients sometimes complain of itching and burning when lesions occur in the groin (**Figure 121-6**).

TYPICAL DISTRIBUTION

Erythrasma is characteristically found in the intertriginous areas, especially the axilla and the groin (**Figure 121-7**). Patches of erythrasma may also be found in the interspaces of the toes, intergluteal cleft, perianal skin, and inframammary area.

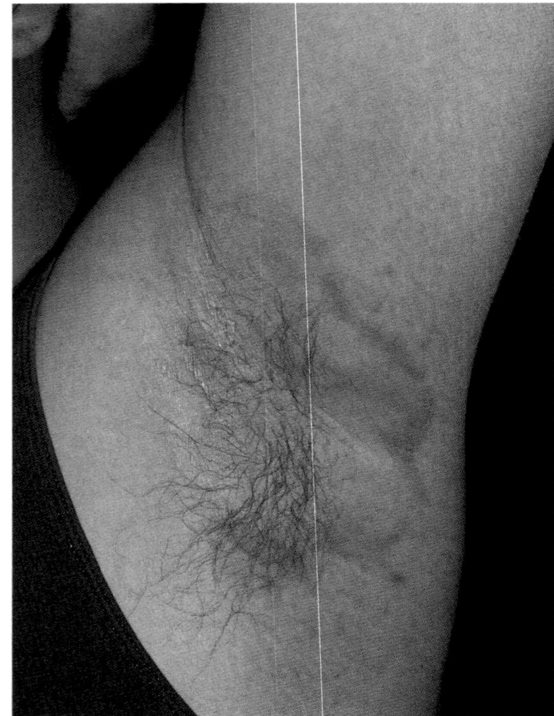

FIGURE 121-5 Pinkish erythrasma in the axilla of a 32-year-old man with some central clearing and elevated borders. (*Reproduced with permission from Richard P. Usatine, MD.*)

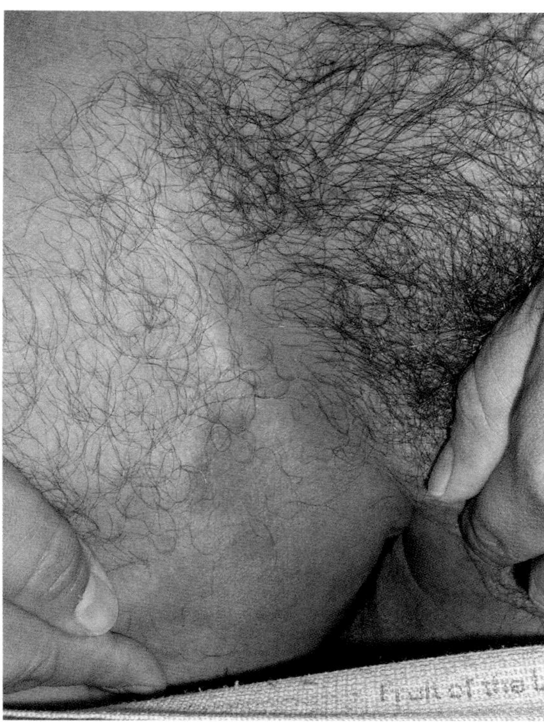

FIGURE 121-6 Pinkish erythrasma in the groin of the man in Figure 121-5. Men are more likely to have erythrasma in the crural region. (*Reproduced with permission from Richard P. Usatine, MD.*)

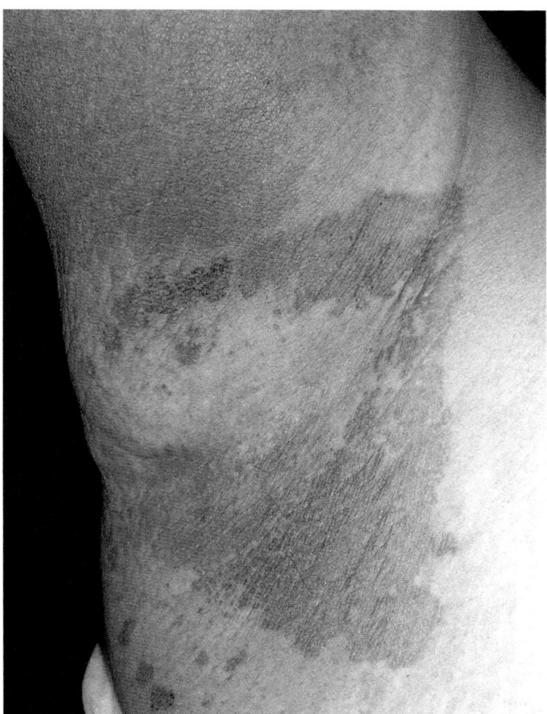

A

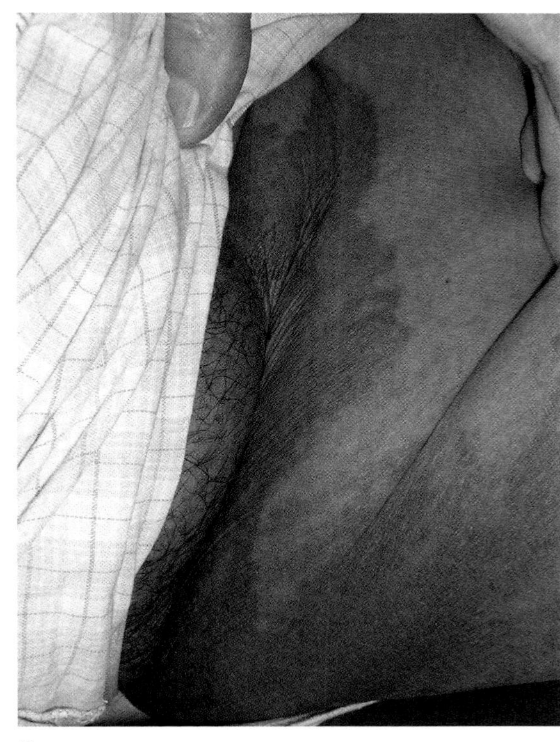

B

FIGURE 121-7 Erythrasma in the axilla and groin of a middle-aged woman with diabetes. **A.** Axilla **B.** Groin. (*Reproduced with permission from Richard P. Usatine, MD.*)

LABORATORY STUDIES

- Illumination of the plaque with a Wood lamp reveals coral red fluorescence (**Figure 121-8**). It should be noted that washing the area before examination may eliminate the fluorescence.
- The diagnosis may be confirmed by applying Gram stain or methylene blue stain to scrapings from the skin to reveal gram-positive rods and dark blue granules, respectively. However, if the presentation is typical and the plaque reveals fluorescence then microscopic examination and cultures are not needed.
- Microscopic examination is useful if erythrasma is suspected but the plaque does not fluoresce.

DIFFERENTIAL DIAGNOSIS

- Psoriasis—Inverse psoriasis occurs in the same areas as erythrasma and also causes pink-to-red plaques with well-demarcated borders. The best way to distinguish psoriasis from erythrasma is to look for other clues of psoriasis in the patient, including nail pitting or onycholysis and hyperkeratotic plaques on the elbows, knees, or scalp. Also, inverse psoriasis may be seen in the intergluteal cleft as well as below the breasts or pannus in overweight individuals (see Chapter 150, Psoriasis). The Wood lamp may help differentiate between these diagnoses.
- Dermatophytosis—Cutaneous fungal infections also closely resemble erythrasma when they occur in the axillary and inguinal areas. Tinea infections also have well-demarcated borders that can be raised with central clearing. This distinctive ringworm look is more obvious with tinea than erythrasma but a scraping for microscopic examination should be able to distinguish between the 2 conditions. Examination of the feet will frequently show tinea pedis and onychomycosis when there are tinea infections elsewhere on the body (see Chapters 136, Tinea Corporis and 137, Tinea Cruris).

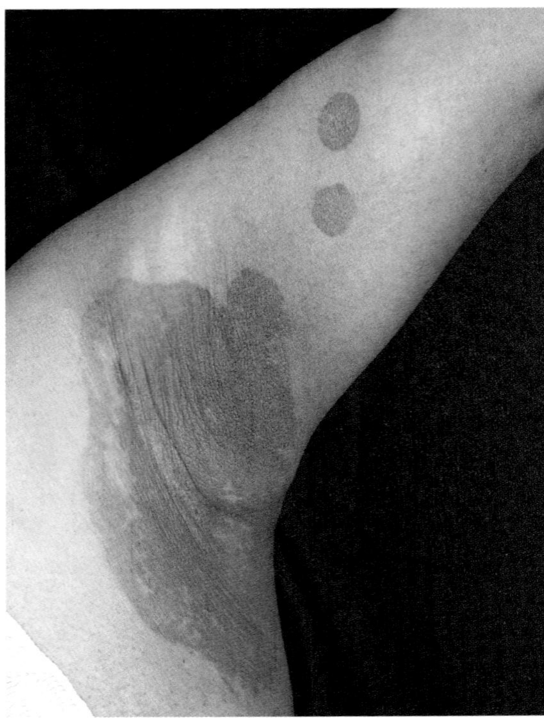

A

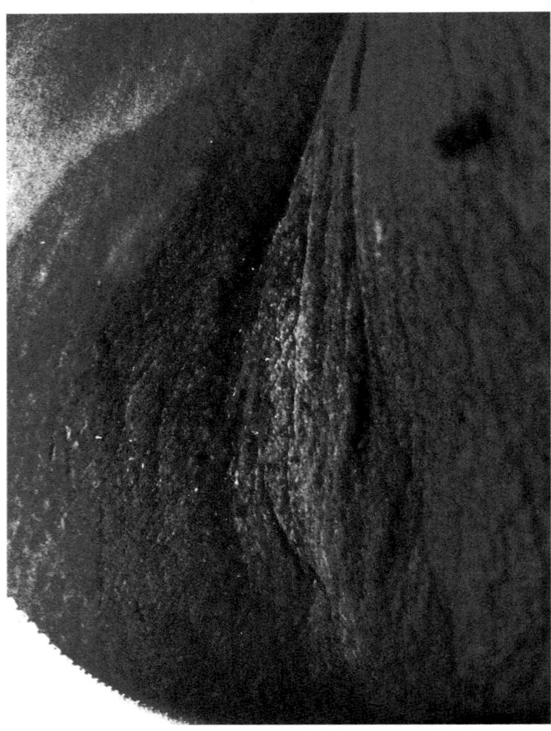

B

FIGURE 121-8 A. Erythrasma in the axilla with 2 satellite areas of involvement on the upper arm. B. Close-up of coral red fluorescence with Wood lamp in the same patient. (*Reproduced with permission from Richard P. Usatine, MD.*)

- Candidiasis—Look for satellite lesions to help distinguish candidiasis from erythrasma. Candidiasis will not fluoresce and a microscopic examination of a *Candida* infection should show branching pseudohyphae (see Chapter 135, Candidiasis).
- Intertrigo—This is a term for inflammation in intertriginous areas (skin folds). It is caused or exacerbated by heat, moisture, maceration, friction, and lack of air circulation. It is frequently made worse by infection with *Candida*, bacteria, or dermatophytes, and therefore overlaps with the erythrasma, *Candida*, and dermatophytosis. Obesity and diabetes especially predispose to this condition. All efforts should be made to find coexisting infections and treat them.
- Contact dermatitis to deodorants can mimic erythrasma. The history and Wood lamp should help to differentiate the 2 conditions (see Chapter 144, Contact Dermatitis).

MANAGEMENT

NONPHARMACOLOGIC

- It has been advocated that the areas should be vigorously washed with soap and water prior to application of topical antibiotics. SOR C
- Consider loose-fitting cotton undergarments during treatment and to help prevent recurrence. SOR C

MEDICATIONS

- Although the bacteria responds to a variety of antibacterial agents (eg, penicillins, first-generation cephalosporins), the treatment of choice is oral erythromycin 250 mg 4 times a day for 14 days. Erythromycin shows cure rates as high as 100%.[2-4] SOR B
- However, some advocate that oral erythromycin is only required for the treatment of extensive or resistant cases and topical antibiotic treatment may be sufficient.[5] SOR C
- Topical therapy (antibacterial, antifungal, and benzoic acid 6%) has been recommended in addition to oral therapy in patients with hidden reservoirs of infection (ie, interdigital involvement). SOR C
- Topical clindamycin may be applied once daily during the course of oral erythromycin therapy and for 2 weeks after physical clearance of the lesions for treatment and prophylaxis.[3,6] SOR C
- Topical erythromycin 2% solution applied twice daily for 2 weeks is one option.[4,5,7] SOR C
- In a Turkish study, topical fusidic acid was more effective than erythromycin or single-dose clarithromycin based on Wood light reflection scores.[8]
- Optimal blood glucose control is recommended in the management of a diabetic patient with erythrasma.[2] SOR C

PROGNOSIS

- Usually it is a benign condition; however, in immunocompromised individuals, *Corynebacterium* can cause abscess formation, bacteremia, endocarditis, pyelonephritis, cellulitis, and meningitis.[1]
- The condition tends to recur if the predisposing condition is not addressed.

FOLLOW-UP

Have the patient to follow up in 2 to 4 weeks as needed to determine if erythrasma has resolved.

PATIENT EDUCATION

Reassure the patient that erythrasma is curable with antibiotic treatment.

PATIENT RESOURCES

- PubMed Health. *Erythrasma*—**http://www.ncbi.nlm.nih.gov/pubmedhealth/ PMH0002441/.**
- Dermnet NZ. *Erythrasma*—**http://www.dermnetnz.org/bacterial/erythrasma.html.**

PROVIDER RESOURCES

- Medscape. *Erythrasma*—**http://emedicine.medscape.com/article/1052532.**

REFERENCES

1. Kibbi AG, Bahhady RF, Saleh Z, Haddad FG. *Erythrasma*. http://emedicine.medscape.com/article/1052532-overview#a0199. Accessed April 2, 2012.
2. Ahmed I, Goldstein B. Diabetes mellitus. *Clin Dermatol.* 2006;24(4):237-246.
3. Holdiness MR. Management of cutaneous erythrasma. *Drugs.* 2002;62(8):1131-1141.
4. James WD, Berger TG, Elston DM. *Andrew's Diseases of the Skin Clinical Dermatology*. 10th ed. London, UK: Saunders/Elsevier; 2006.
5. Karakatsanis G, Vakirlis E, Kastoridou C, Devliotou-Panagiotidou D. Coexistence of pityriasis versicolor and erythrasma. *Mycoses.* 2004;47(7):343-345.
6. Holdiness MR. Erythrasma and common bacterial skin infections. *Am Fam Physician.* 2003;15:67(2):254.
7. Miller SD, David-Bajar K. Images in clinical medicine. A brilliant case of erythrasma. *N Engl J Med.* 2004;14:351(16):1666.
8. Avci O, Tanyildizi T, Kusku E. A comparison between the effectiveness of erythromycin, single-dose clarithromycin and topical fusidic acid in the treatment of erythrasma. *J Dermatolog Treat.* 2013;24(1):70-74.

122 CELLULITIS

Richard P. Usatine, MD

PATIENT STORY

A 63-year-old man presents to his internist with a painful red swollen left leg for 3 days. He has a known history of venous stasis and stasis dermatitis. He ran out on his topical steroid and could not resist scratching the very itchy lower leg. On physical examination the patient is noted to have a temperature of 100.4°F and significant erythema from his foot up to his knee. The left leg is swollen and there is scaling of the skin consistent with the stasis dermatitis. There are excoriations in the skin where the bacteria may have entered to initiate the cellulitis. Because of his coexisting diabetes it was decided to admit the patient to the hospital and treat him with intravenous (IV) antibiotics.

INTRODUCTION

Cellulitis is an acute infection of the skin that involves the dermis and subcutaneous tissues.

EPIDEMIOLOGY

- Facial cellulitis occurs more often in adults ages 50 years or older, or in children ages 6 months to 3 years.
- Perianal cellulitis occurs more commonly in young children but can be seen in adults as well.

ETIOLOGY AND PATHOPHYSIOLOGY

- Often begins with a break in the skin caused by trauma, a bite, or an underlying skin disease (eg, tinea pedis, stasis dermatitis, psoriasis) (**Figures 122-1** to **122-4**).
- It is most often caused by group A β-hemolytic *Streptococcus* (GABHS) or *Staphylococcus aureus*. The most common etiology of cellulitis with intact skin, when it has been determined through needle aspiration and/or punch biopsy, is *S. aureus*, outnumbering GABHS by a ratio of nearly 2:1.[1]

There are increasing concerns about the role of community-acquired methicillin-resistant *S. aureus* (CAMRSA) in all soft tissue infections including cellulitis.[2-5]

- After a cat or dog bite, cellulitis is often caused by *Pasteurella multocida*.
- Cellulitis can be secondary to *Vibrio vulnificus* found in saltwater and seafood. A *V. vulnificus* infection can start with raw oyster ingestion in an immunosuppressed person leading to sepsis and secondary cutaneous involvement (**Figure 122-5**).
- Erysipelas is a specific type of superficial cellulitis with prominent lymphatic involvement and leading to a sharply defined and elevated border (**Figure 122-6**).

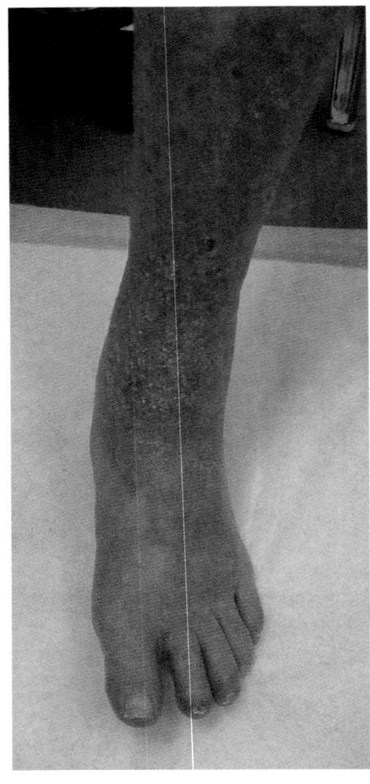

FIGURE 122-1 Cellulitis in an older man with venous stasis dermatitis. *(Reproduced with permission from Richard P. Usatine, MD.)*

DIAGNOSIS

CLINICAL FEATURES

The clinical features include rubor (red), calor (warm), tumor (swollen), and dolor (painful).

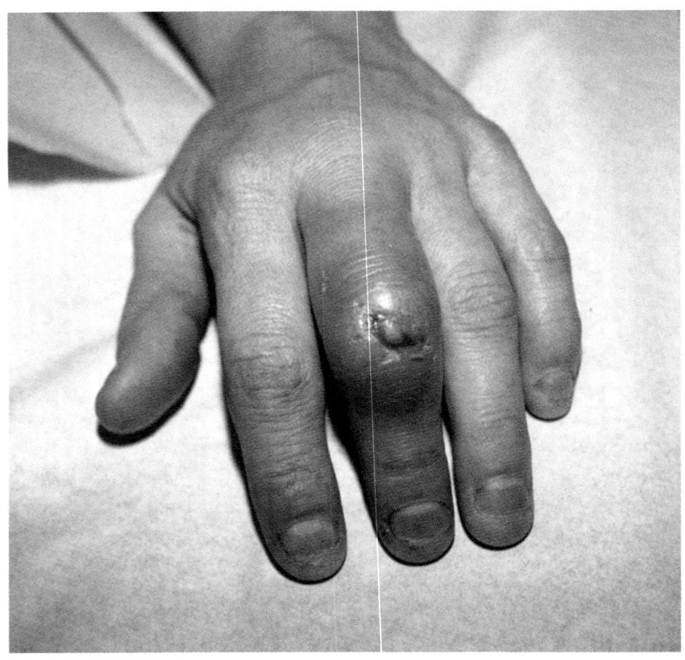

FIGURE 122-2 Cellulitis and abscess of the finger after a clenched fist injury in which the patient cut his finger on the tooth of the man he assaulted. *(Reproduced with permission from Richard P. Usatine, MD.)*

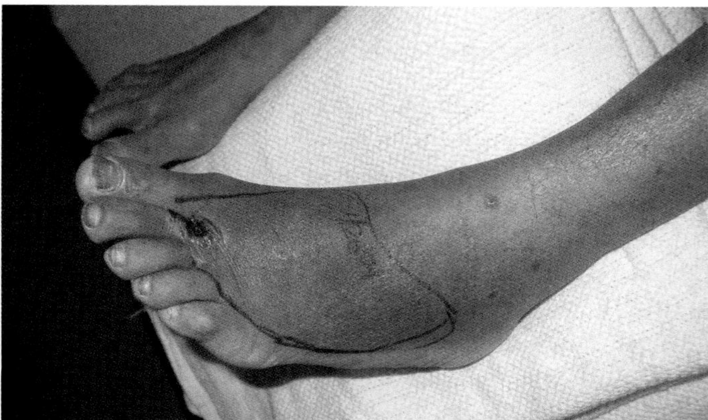

FIGURE 122-3 Cellulitis of the foot of a diabetic person in which there is possible necrosis and gangrene of the second toe, requiring hospitalization and a podiatry consult. (*Reproduced with permission from Richard P. Usatine, MD.*)

TYPICAL DISTRIBUTION

Can occur on any part of the body, but is most often seen on the extremities and face (**Figures 122-1** to **122-8**). Periorbital cellulitis can be life threatening (**Figure 122-9**). Cellulitis can also occur around the anus. This is called perianal cellulitis (**Figure 122-10**).

LABORATORY TESTS

- Aspiration—If there is fluctuance within the area of erythema, a needle aspiration or incision and drainage should be performed. If pus is aspirated, perform a culture to guide antibiotic use.
- Blood cultures—Results are positive in only 5% of cases and the results of culture of needle aspirations of the inflamed skin are variable and not recommended.[4]

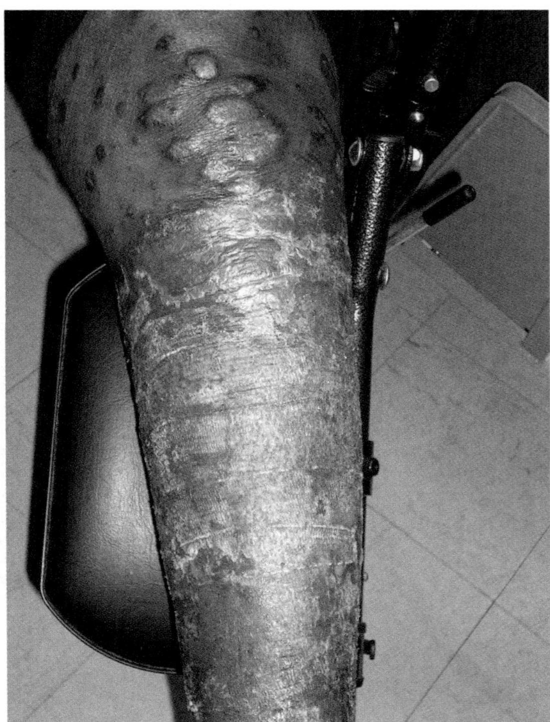

FIGURE 122-4 Cellulitis that occurred on the leg of a 50-year-old woman with severe psoriasis being treated with methotrexate and adalimumab. (*Reproduced with permission from Richard P. Usatine, MD.*)

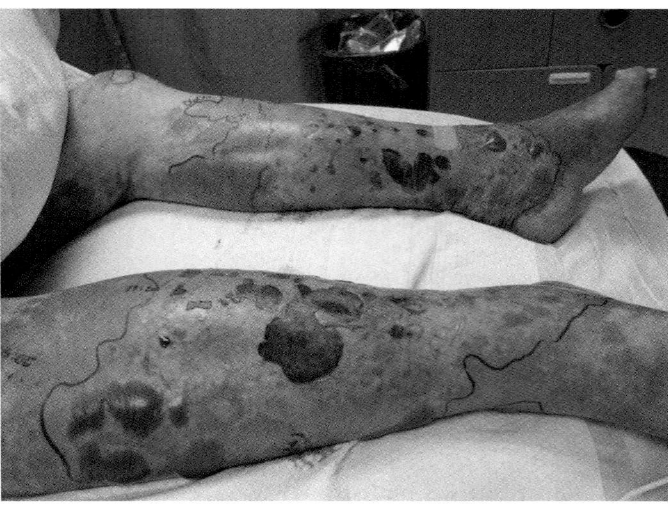

FIGURE 122-5 Fatal *Vibrio vulnificus* sepsis in a man with cirrhosis who ate raw oysters. The bacteremia led to widespread cellulitis and cutaneous bullae. The violaceous bullae should be a red flag for this infection and/or necrotizing fasciitis. Even though the infection was identified early, the overwhelming sepsis resulted in death. (*Reproduced with permission from Donna Nguyen, MD.*)

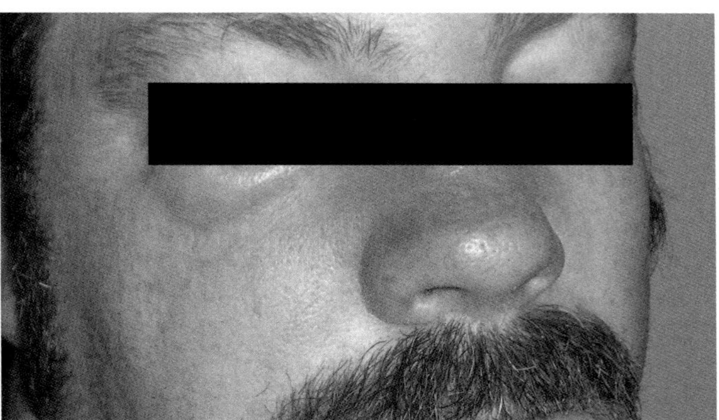

FIGURE 122-6 Erysipelas of the central face that responded well to oral antibiotic therapy. (*Reproduced with permission from Ernesto Samano Ayon, MD.*)

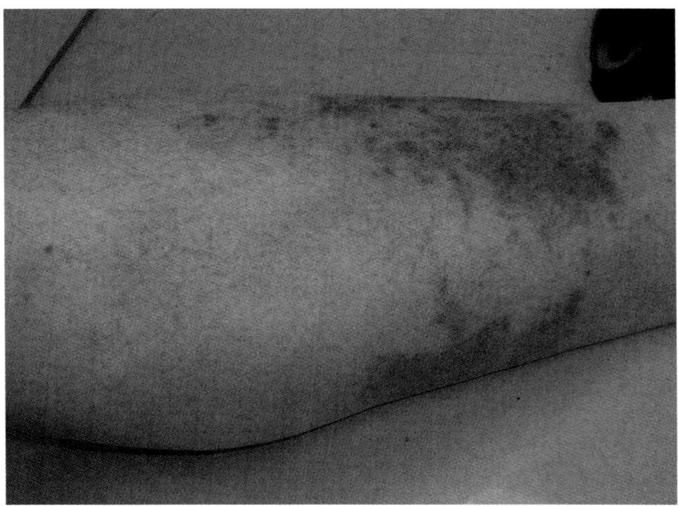

FIGURE 122-7 Cellulitis of the leg in a 55-year-old man that developed after a minor abrasion and a long plane flight. Petechiae and ecchymoses are visible and not infrequently seen in cellulitis. (*Reproduced with permission from Richard P. Usatine, MD.*)

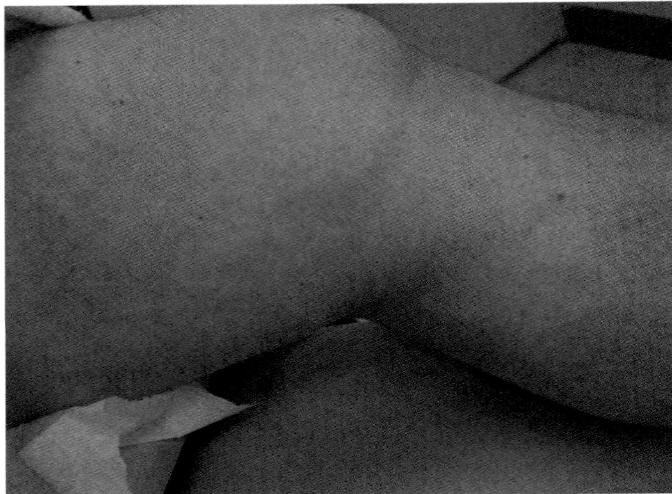

FIGURE 122-8 Ascending lymphangitis characterized by lymphatic streaking up the leg in the patient of Figure 122-7. (*Reproduced with permission from Richard P. Usatine, MD.*)

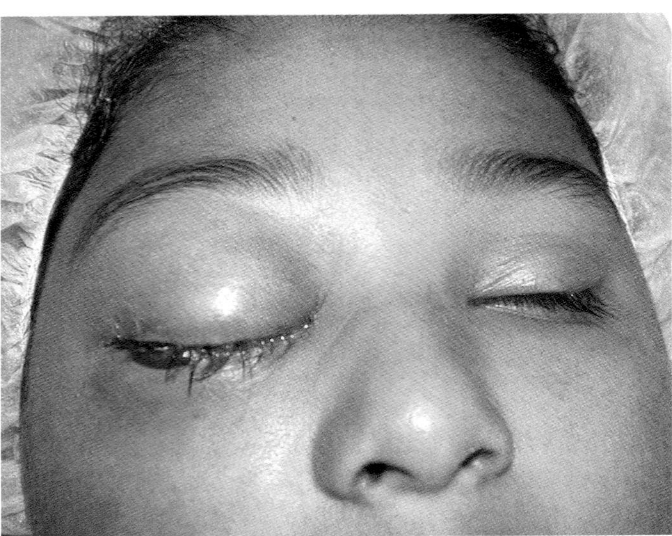

FIGURE 122-9 Life-threatening staphylococcal periorbital cellulitis requiring operative intervention. (*Reproduced with permission from Frank Miller, MD.*)

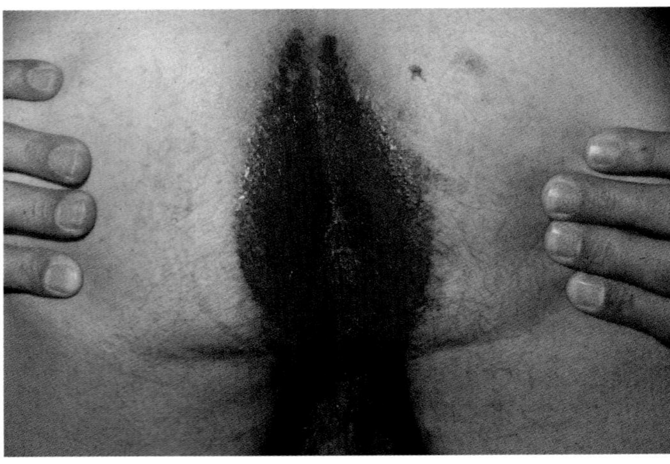

FIGURE 122-10 Severe perianal cellulitis in an adult man. (*Reproduced with permission from Jack Resneck Sr., MD.*)

DIFFERENTIAL DIAGNOSIS

- Thrombophlebitis—Inflammation of a vein caused by a blood clot. The pain and tenderness are over the involved vein.
- Venous stasis—Swelling, discoloration, and pain of the lower extremities that can lead to cellulitis. Venous stasis dermatitis can add erythema and scaling to the picture and resemble cellulitis (see **Figure 122-4**) (see Chapter 51, Venous Stasis).
- Allergic reactions—Allergic reactions to vaccines or bug bites may resemble cellulitis because of the erythema and swelling (**Figure 122-11**).
- Acute gout—May resemble cellulitis if there is significant cutaneous inflammation beyond the involved joint (see Chapter 105, Gout).
- Necrotizing fasciitis—Deep infection of the subcutaneous tissues and fascia with diffuse swelling, severe pain, and bullae in a toxic-appearing patient. It is important to recognize the difference between standard cellulitis and necrotizing fasciitis. Imaging procedures can detect gas in the soft tissues. Rapid progression from mild erythema to violaceous or necrotic lesions and/or bullae in a number of hours is a red flag for necrotizing fasciitis. The toxicity of the patient and the other physical findings should encourage rapid surgical consultation (see Chapter 124, Necrotizing Fasciitis).

MANAGEMENT

- The first decision is whether or not the patient needs hospitalization and IV antibiotics. It is often best to hospitalize any immunocompromised patients (eg, HIV, transplant recipient, chronic renal or liver disease, on prednisone, diabetes out of control) with cellulitis because they may decompensate quickly. SOR C
- Evidence comparing different durations of treatment, oral versus intravenous antibiotics is lacking.[6] Randomized controlled trials (RCTs) comparing different antibiotic regimens found clinical cure in 50% to 100% of people, but provided insufficient information on differences between regimens.[6] SOR A

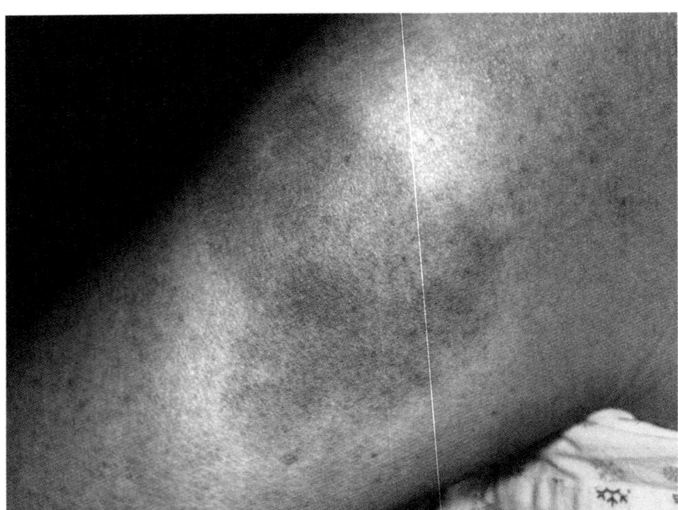

FIGURE 122-11 Redness and swelling after a pneumococcal vaccine the day before in a 66-year-old woman. This allergic reaction looks like bacterial cellulitis. It resolved with oral diphenhydramine. (*Reproduced with permission from Richard P. Usatine, MD.*)

- One quasi-randomized trial in 73 hospitalized people with erysipelas, but excluding patients with clinical signs of septicemia, compared oral versus intravenous penicillin and found no significant difference in clinical efficacy.[6] SOR Ⓑ
- Standard oral therapy for cellulitis not requiring hospitalization (in the pre-MRSA era) involves covering GABHS and *S. aureus* with cephalexin or dicloxacillin.[4] SOR Ⓐ The standard dose is 500 mg orally every 6 hours for each antibiotic and the typical duration is 7 to 10 days. SOR Ⓒ
- Penicillin-allergic patients may be treated with clindamycin rather than erythromycin because of macrolide resistance and increasing MRSA prevalence.[4] SOR Ⓐ
- Parenteral treatment is usually done with penicillinase-resistant penicillins or first-generation cephalosporins such as cefazolin, or, for patients with life-threatening penicillin allergies, clindamycin, or vancomycin.[4] SOR Ⓐ
- In cases of uncomplicated cellulitis, 5 days of antibiotic treatment with levofloxacin is as effective as a 10-day course.[7] SOR Ⓑ This is not a good choice if MRSA is suspected.

Two recent studies (published in 2009 and 2010) addressed concerns over CAMRSA in cellulitis and came up with different conclusions:

- An electronic chart review of patients seen in a Texas emergency department with cellulitis in 2000 and 2005 was performed. Exclusion criteria were incision and drainage, surgery, or admission on initial visit. Treatment failure was defined as a repeat visit in the subsequent 30 days and a change in antibiotics, admission to the hospital, incision and drainage of abscess, or surgical intervention. There was a significant decrease in β-lactam antibiotics and an increase in CAMRSA-effective antibiotics prescribed in 2005 versus 2000. The difference in treatment failure rates of the β-lactams and CAMRSA antibiotics was statistically insignificant. The β-lactam antibiotics performed as well as "CAMRSA antibiotics" in their setting.[5] SOR Ⓑ
- A 3-year retrospective cohort study of outpatients with cellulitis empirically treated in Hawaii was performed. Exclusion criteria included patients who received more than one oral antibiotic or were hospitalized. The overall treatment success rate of trimethoprim-sulfamethoxazole was significantly higher than the rate of cephalexin (91% vs 74%; $p < 0.001$). Clindamycin success rates were higher than those of cephalexin in patients who had subsequently culture-confirmed MRSA infections ($p = 0.01$), had moderately severe cellulitis ($p = 0.03$), and were obese ($p = 0.04$). MRSA was recovered in 72 of 117 positive culture specimens from 405 included patients. The researchers concluded that trimethoprim-sulfamethoxazole and clindamycin are preferred empiric therapy for outpatients with cellulitis in the CAMRSA-prevalent setting.[2] SOR Ⓑ
- Although MRSA is increasing in its prevalence in skin and soft tissue infections,[3] the difficulty in obtaining microbiologic cultures for cellulitis still makes it difficult to know how much MRSA is a problem in cellulitis with intact skin. If there is a coexisting abscess or crusting lesion, it is best to obtain a culture to guide therapy and start empiric therapy with trimethoprim-sulfamethoxazole and clindamycin.[2] SOR Ⓑ
- Do not miss necrotizing fasciitis. Patients with severe pain, bullae, crepitus, skin necrosis, or significant toxicity merit imaging and immediate surgical consultation (see Chapter 124, Necrotizing Fasciitis).
- Treat underlying conditions (eg, tinea pedis, lymphedema) that predispose the patient to the infection. SOR Ⓒ

PATIENT EDUCATION

Recommend that the patient should take rest and elevate the involved extremity. If outpatient therapy is followed, then provide precautions (eg, vomiting and unable to hold medicine down) for which the patient should seek more immediate follow-up.

FOLLOW-UP

If prescribing oral outpatient therapy, consider follow-up in 1 to 2 days to assess response to the antibiotic and to determine the adequacy of outpatient therapy.

PATIENT RESOURCES

- Medline Plus for patients—**http://www.nlm.nih.gov/medlineplus/cellulitis.html.**

PROVIDER RESOURCES

- Guidelines on the management of cellulitis in adults from Ireland—**http://www.gain-ni.org/Library/Guidelines/cellulitis-guide.pdf.**
- Practice Guidelines for the Diagnosis and Management of Skin and Soft Tissue Infections from the Infectious Diseases Society of America—**http://cid.oxfordjournals.org/content/41/10/1373.full.**

REFERENCES

1. Chira S, Miller LG. *Staphylococcus aureus* is the most common identified cause of cellulitis: a systematic review. *Epidemiol Infect.* 2010;138:313-317.
2. Khawcharoenporn T, Tice A. Empiric outpatient therapy with trimethoprim-sulfamethoxazole, cephalexin, or clindamycin for cellulitis. *Am J Med.* 2010;123:942-950.
3. Moran GJ, Krishnadasan A, Gorwitz RJ, et al. Methicillin-resistant *S. aureus* infections among patients in the emergency department. *N Engl J Med.* 2006;355:666-674.
4. Stevens DL, Bisno AL, Chambers HF, et al. Practice guidelines for the diagnosis and management of skin and soft-tissue infections. *Clin Infect Dis.* 2005;41:1373-1406.
5. Wells RD, Mason P, Roarty J, Dooley M. Comparison of initial antibiotic choice and treatment of cellulitis in the pre- and post-community-acquired methicillin-resistant *Staphylococcus aureus* eras. *Am J Emerg Med.* 2009;27:436-439.
6. Morris AD. Cellulitis and erysipelas. *Clin Evid (Online).* 2008 Jan 2;2008:1708.
7. Hepburn MJ, Dooley DP, Skidmore PJ, et al. Comparison of short-course (5 days) and standard (10 days) treatment for uncomplicated cellulitis. *Arch Intern Med.* 2004;164:1669-1674.

123 ABSCESS

Richard P. Usatine, MD

PATIENT STORY

A young man is seen in a shelter in San Antonio after being evacuated from New Orleans after the devastating floods of hurricane Katrina (**Figure 123-1**). He has facial pain and swelling and noticeable pus near the eye. His vision is normal. The area is anesthetized with lidocaine and epinephrine. The abscess is drained with a #11 blade. The patient is started on an oral antibiotic because of the proximity to the eye and the local swelling that could represent early cellulitis. A culture to look for methicillin-resistant *Staphylococcus aureus* (MRSA) was not available in the shelter, but close follow-up was set for the next day and the patient was doing much better.

INTRODUCTION

An abscess is a collection of pus in the infected tissues. The abscess represents a walled-off infection in which there is a pocket of purulence. In abscesses of the skin the offending organism is almost always *S. aureus*.

EPIDEMIOLOGY

- MRSA was the most common identifiable cause of skin and soft tissue infections among patients presenting to emergency departments in 11 US cities. *S. aureus* was isolated from 76% of these infections and 59% were community-acquired MRSA (CAMRSA).[1]
- Risk factors for MRSA infection and other abscesses—Intravenous drug abuse, homelessness, dental disease, contact sports, incarceration, and high prevalence in the community (**Figure 123-2**).

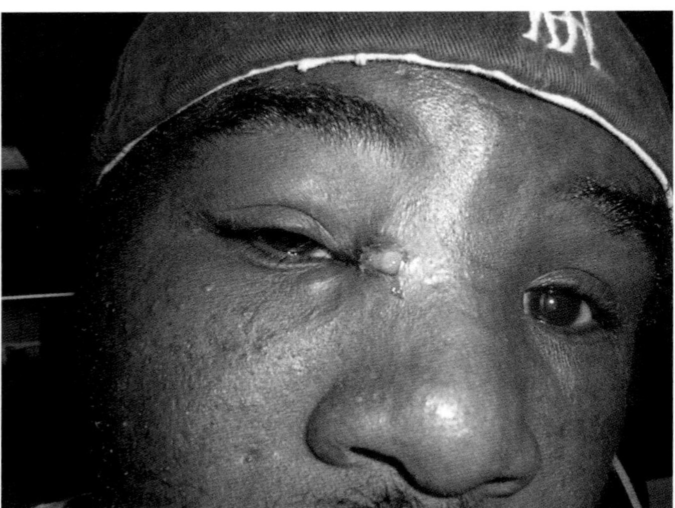

FIGURE 123-1 Abscess seen on the face of a man after evacuation from the flood waters of New Orleans following hurricane Katrina. (*Reproduced with permission from Richard P. Usatine, MD.*)

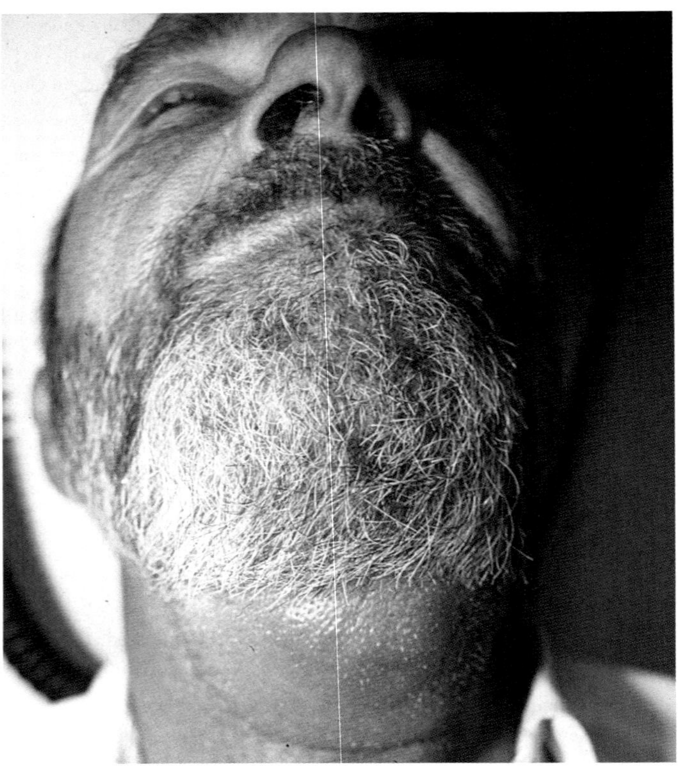

FIGURE 123-2 Neck abscess secondary to dental abscess in a homeless man. This was drained in the operating room by an ENT specialist. (*Reproduced with permission from Richard P. Usatine, MD.*)

ETIOLOGY AND PATHOPHYSIOLOGY

- Most cutaneous abscesses are caused by *S. aureus*.
- Risk factors for developing an abscess with MRSA include patients who work or are exposed to a health care system, intravenous drug use, previous MRSA infection and colonization, recent hospitalization, being homeless, African American, and having used antibiotics within the last 6 months.[2]
- CAMRSA has become so prevalent in our community that both the patients shown in **Figures 123-3** and **123-4** had no special risk factors and both had abscesses that grew out MRSA. One study that evaluated management of skin abscesses drained in the emergency department showed that there was no significant association between amount of surrounding cellulitis or abscess size with the likelihood of MRSA-positive cultures.[2]
- A dental abscess can spread into tissue outside the mouth, as in the homeless person in **Figure 123-2**.

DIAGNOSIS

CLINICAL FEATURES

Clinical feature indicates collection of pus in or below the skin. Patients often feel pain and have tenderness at the involved site. There is swelling, erythema, warmth, and fluctuance in most cases (**Figures 123-1** to **123-5**). Determine if the patient is febrile and if there is surrounding cellulitis.

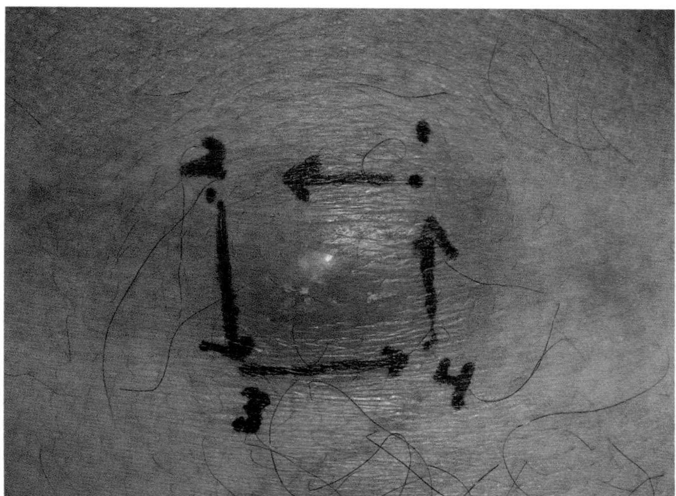

FIGURE 123-3 MRSA abscess on the back of the neck that patient thought was a spider bite. Note that a ring block was drawn around the abscess with a surgical marker to demonstrate how to perform this block. (*Reproduced with permission from Richard P. Usatine, MD.*)

TYPICAL DISTRIBUTION

Skin abscesses can be found anywhere from head to feet. Frequent sites include the hands, feet, extremities, head, neck, buttocks, and breast (see **Figure 123-5**).

LABORATORY STUDIES

Clinical cure is often obtained with incision and drainage alone so the benefits of pathogen identification and sensitivities are low in low-risk patients.[2] Most clinical studies have excluded patients who were immunocompromised, diabetic, or had other significant comorbidities.[2] Consequently, it may be reasonable to obtain wound cultures in high-risk patients, those with signs of systemic infection, and in patients with history of high recurrence rates.[2,3]

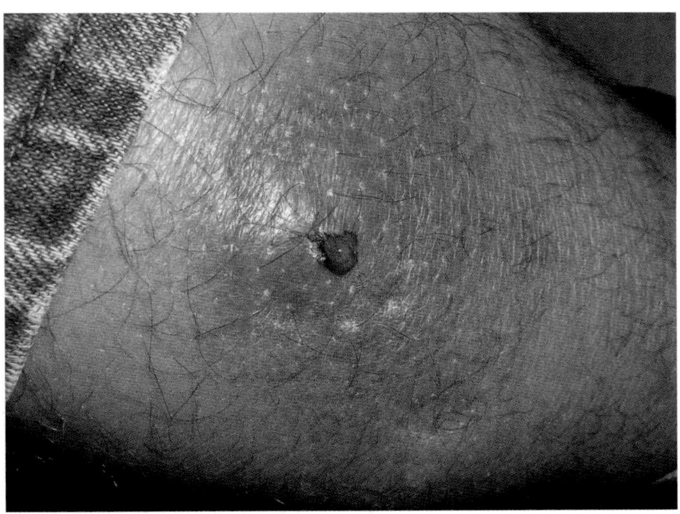

FIGURE 123-4 Large MRSA abscess on the leg in a 62-year-old man beginning to drain spontaneously. The abscess cavity was large and the patient was placed on trimethoprim-sulfamethoxazole (TMP-SMX) to cover the surrounding cellulitis. (*Reproduced with permission from Richard P. Usatine, MD.*)

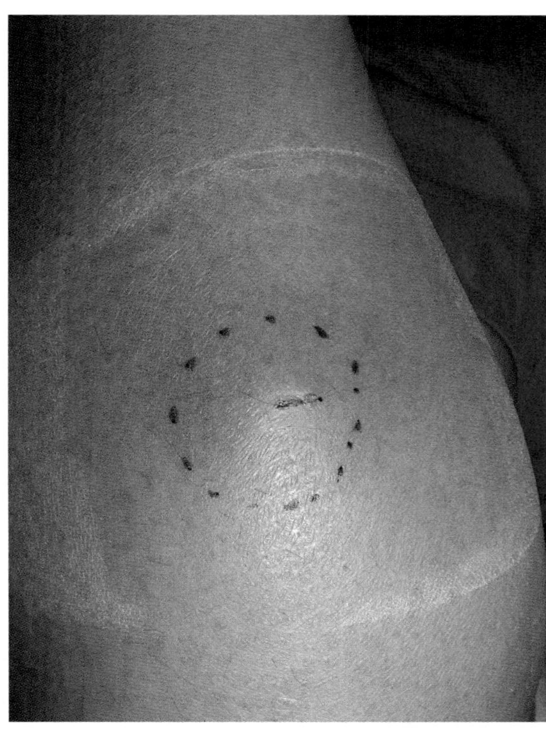

FIGURE 123-5 Abscess in the arm of dental student, cause unknown. The pus that drained from the abscess grew out MRSA. He was started on trimethoprim-sulfamethoxazole (TMP-SMX) to cover the surrounding cellulitis at the time of incision and drainage. The infection resolved quickly. (*Reproduced with permission from Richard P. Usatine, MD.*)

DIFFERENTIAL DIAGNOSIS

- Epidermal inclusion cyst with inflammation or infection—These cysts (also known as sebaceous cysts) can become inflamed, swollen, and superinfected. Although the initial erythema may be sterile inflammation, these cysts can become infected with *S. aureus*. The treatment consists of incision and drainage and antibiotics if cellulitis is also present. If these are removed before they become inflamed, the cyst may come out intact (**Figure 123-6**).
- Cellulitis with swelling and no pocket of pus—When it is unclear if an area of infected skin has an abscess, needle aspiration with a large-gauge needle may be helpful to determine whether to incise the skin. Cellulitis alone should have no area of fluctuance (see Chapter 122, Cellulitis).
- Hidradenitis suppurativa—Recurrent inflammation surrounding the apocrine glands of the axilla and inguinal areas (see Chapter 117, Hidradenitis Suppurativa).
- Furuncles and carbuncles—A furuncle or boil is an abscess that starts in hair follicle or sweat gland. A carbuncle occurs when the furuncle extends into the subcutaneous tissue.
- Acne cysts—More sterile inflammation than true abscess, often better to inject with steroid rather than incise and drain (see Chapter 114, Acne Vulgaris).

MANAGEMENT

- The evidence strongly supports the incision and drainage of an abscess.[2,4] SOR Ⓐ Inject 1% lidocaine with epinephrine into the skin at the site you plan to open using a 27-gauge needle. A ring block can

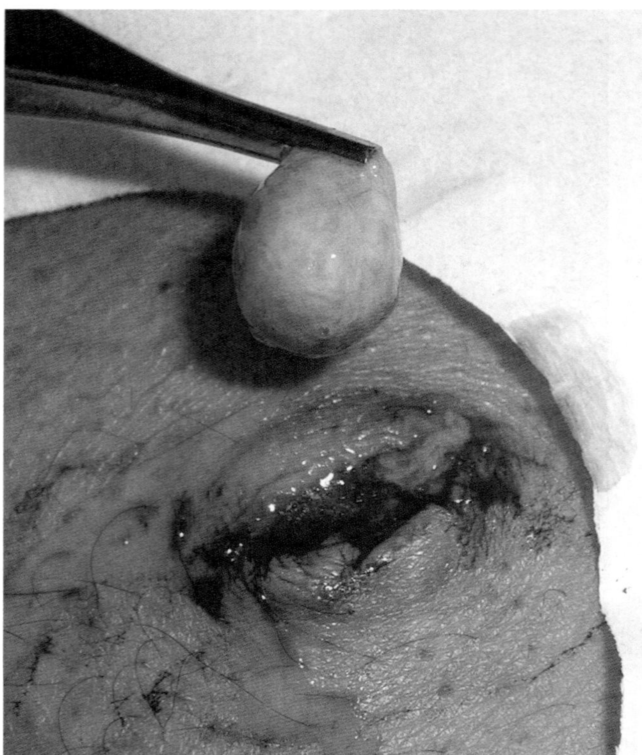

FIGURE 123-6 Epidermal inclusion cyst removed intact. There is no need for antibiotics in this case. (*Reproduced with permission from Richard P. Usatine, MD.*)

be helpful rather than injecting into the abscess itself (see **Figure 123-3**). Open the abscess with a linear incision using a #11 blade scalpel following skin lines if possible.[5]

Although many physicians still pack a drained abscess with ribbon gauze, there is limited data on whether or not packing of an abscess cavity improves outcomes. A small study concluded that routine packing of simple cutaneous abscesses is painful and probably unnecessary.[6] SOR Ⓒ The author of this chapter often packs abscesses lightly and has the patient remove the packing in the shower 2 days later, avoiding additional visits and painful repacking of the healing cavity. SOR Ⓒ However, if a large abscess is not packed it can seal over and the pus may reaccumulate.

Routine use of antibiotics for an initial abscess in addition to incision and drainage is not supported by current evidence.[2,7-9] SOR Ⓐ Three randomized controlled trials (RCTs) are performed since the emergence of CAMRSA have demonstrated that antibiotics do not significantly improve healing rates of superficial skin abscesses, but 2 of these studies suggest that antibiotics do decrease short-term rates of new lesion development.[7-9]

Consider the use of oral antibiotics to treat an abscess with suspected CAMRSA in patients who are febrile or have systemic symptoms, have significant surrounding cellulitis, have failed incision and drainage alone, have frequent recurrences, or have a history of close contacts with abscesses.[2] SOR Ⓒ

If an antibiotic is to be used, CAMRSA is close to 100% sensitive to trimethoprim-sulfamethoxazole (TMP-SMX).[2] SOR Ⓑ Although standard dosing of oral TMP-SMX for an infection in adults is 1 DS tablet bid, one study suggests that 2 DS tablets should be used bid for 7 days.[10] SOR Ⓑ Alternative antibiotics include oral clindamycin, tetracycline, or doxycycline. Local sensitivity data should be consulted when available.[2] SOR Ⓑ

There is no current data to support the use of an antimicrobial medication (mupirocin or rifampin) in the eradication of MRSA colonization.[2] SOR Ⓒ

PATIENT EDUCATION

Patients may shower daily 24 to 48 hours after incision and drainage and then reapply dressings. Patients should be given return precautions for worsening of symptoms or continued redness, pain, or pus.

FOLLOW-UP

In patients or wounds at higher risk for complications, follow-up should be scheduled in 24 to 48 hours. If packing was placed, it can be removed by the patient or a family member.

PATIENT RESOURCES

- Skinsight. *Abscess*—**http://www.skinsight.com/adult/abscess.htm.**

PROVIDER RESOURCES

- Gillian R. How do you treat an abscess in the era of increased community-associated MRSA (MRSA)? *J Emerg Med.* 2011;41:276-281.
- ScienceDirect. *How Do You Treat an Abscess in the Era of Increased Community-associated Methicillin-resistant Staphylococcus Aureus (MRSA)?*—**http://www.sciencedirect.com/science/article/pii/S0736467911004252.**

REFERENCES

1. Moran GJ, Krishnadasan A, Gorwitz RJ, et al. Methicillin-resistant *S. aureus* infections among patients in the emergency department. *N Engl J Med.* 2006;355:666-674.
2. Gillian R. How do you treat an abscess in the era of increased community-associated methicillin-resistant *Staphylococcus aureus* (MRSA)? *J Emerg Med.* 2011;41:276-281.
3. Abrahamian FM, Shroff SD. Use of routine wound cultures to evaluate cutaneous abscesses for community-associated methicillin-resistant *Staphylococcus aureus*. *Ann Emerg Med.* 2007;50:66-67.
4. Sorensen C, Hjortrup A, Moesgaard F, Lykkegaard-Nielsen M. Linear incision and curettage vs. deroofing and drainage in subcutaneous abscess. A randomized clinical trial. *Acta Chir Scand.* 1987;153:659-660.
5. Usatine R, Pfenninger J, Stulberg D, Small R. *Dermatologic and Cosmetic Procedures in Office Practice.* Philadelphia, PA: Elsevier; 2012.
6. O'Malley GF, Dominici P, Giraldo P, et al. Routine packing of simple cutaneous abscesses is painful and probably unnecessary. *Acad Emerg Med.* 2009;16:470-473.
7. Duong M, Markwell S, Peter J, Barenkamp S. Randomized, controlled trial of antibiotics in the management of community-acquired skin abscesses in the pediatric patient. *Ann Emerg Med.* 2010;55:401-407.
8. Schmitz GR, Bruner D, Pitotti R, et al. Randomized controlled trial of trimethoprim-sulfamethoxazole for uncomplicated skin abscesses

in patients at risk for community-associated methicillin-resistant *Staphylococcus aureus* infection. *Ann Emerg Med.* 2010;56:283-287.

9. Rajendran PM, Young D, Maurer T, et al. Randomized, double-blind, placebo-controlled trial of cephalexin for treatment of uncomplicated skin abscesses in a population at risk for community-acquired methicillin-resistant Staphylococcus aureus infection. *Antimicrob Agents Chemother.* 2007;51:4044-4048.
10. Markowitz N, Quinn EL, Saravolatz LD. Trimethoprim-sulfamethoxazole compared with vancomycin for the treatment of *Staphylococcus aureus* infection. *Ann Intern Med.* 1992;117:390-398.

124 NECROTIZING FASCIITIS

Richard P. Usatine, MD
Jeremy A. Franklin, MD

PATIENT STORY

A 54-year-old woman with diabetes was brought to the emergency department with right leg swelling, fever, and altered mental status.[1] The patient noted a pimple in her groin 5 days earlier and over the past few days had increasing leg pain. Her right leg was tender, red, hot, and swollen (**Figure 124-1**). Large bullae were present. Her temperature was 38.9°C (102°F) and her blood sugar was 573. The skin had a "woody" feel and a radiograph of her leg showed gas in the muscles and soft tissues (**Figure 124-2**). She was taken to the operating room for debridement of her necrotizing fasciitis (NF). Broad-spectrum antibiotics were also started but the infection continued to advance quickly. The patient died the following day; her wound culture later grew *Escherichia coli, Proteus vulgaris, Corynebacterium, Enterococcus, Staphylococcus sp.*, and *Peptostreptococcus.*[1]

INTRODUCTION

Necrotizing fasciitis is a rapidly progressive infection of the deep fascia, with necrosis of the subcutaneous tissues. It usually occurs after surgery or trauma. Patients have erythema and pain disproportionate to the physical findings. Immediate surgical debridement and antibiotic therapy should be initiated.[2]

SYNONYMS

NF is also known as flesh-eating bacteria, necrotizing soft tissue infection (NSTI), suppurative fasciitis, hospital gangrene, and necrotizing erysipelas. Fournier gangrene is a type of NF or NSTI in the genital and perineal region.[3]

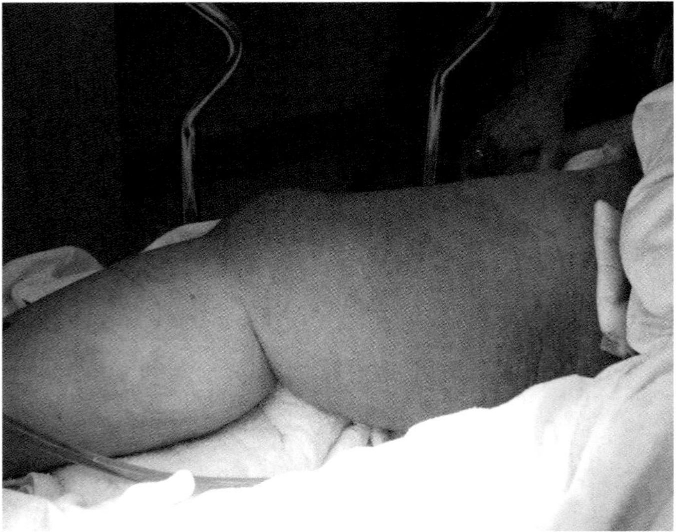

FIGURE 124-1 Necrotizing fasciitis on the leg and groin showing erythema, swelling, and bullae. (*Reproduced with permission from Dufel S, Martino M. Simple cellulitis or a more serious infection?* J Fam Pract. *2006;55(5):396-400. Reproduced with permission from Frontline Medical Communications.*)

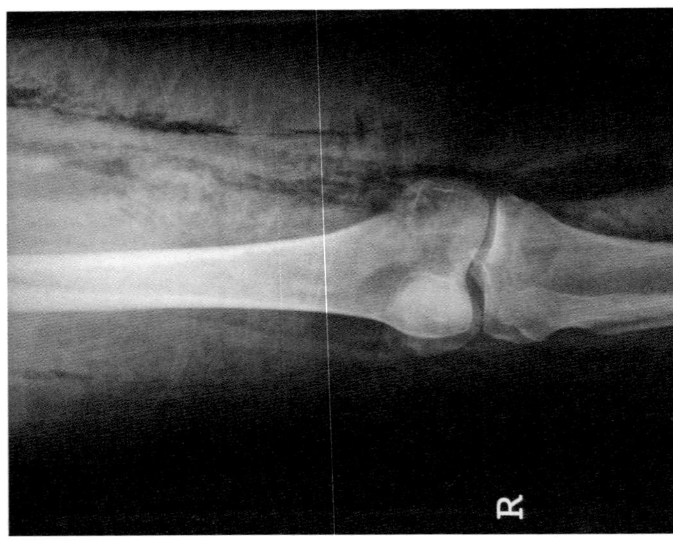

FIGURE 124-2 Radiograph of the patient's leg showing gas in the soft tissues and muscles. (*Reproduced with permission from Dufel S, Martino M. Simple cellulitis or a more serious infection?* J Fam Pract. *2006;55(5):396-400. Reproduced with permission from Frontline Medical Communications.*)[1]

EPIDEMIOLOGY

- Incidence in adults is 0.40 cases per 100,000 population.[4]
- NF caused by *Streptococcus pyogenes* is the most common form.[4]

ETIOLOGY AND PATHOPHYSIOLOGY

- Type I NF is a polymicrobial infection with aerobic and anaerobic bacteria:
  - Frequently caused by enteric gram-negative pathogens including *Enterobacteriaceae* organisms and *Bacteroides*.
  - Can occur with gram-positive organisms such as non–group A streptococci and *Peptostreptococcus.*[5]
  - Saltwater variant can occur with penetrating trauma or an open wound contaminated with saltwater containing marine vibrios. *Vibrio vulnificus* is the most virulent.[6]
  - Up to 15 pathogens have been isolated in a single wound.
  - Average of 5 different isolates per wound.[7]
- Type II NF occurs from common skin organisms:
  - Generally a monomicrobial infection caused by *S. pyogenes:*
    - May occur in combination with *Staphylococcus aureus.*
    - Methicillin-resistant *S. aureus* (MRSA) is no longer a rare cause of NF.[5]
    - *S. pyogenes* strains may produce pyrogenic exotoxins, which act as superantigens to stimulate production of tumor necrosis factor (TNF)-α, TNF-β, interleukin (IL)-1, IL-6, and IL-2.[7]

RISK FACTORS

- Risk factors for type I NF (polymicrobial) include the following:
  - Diabetes mellitus
  - Severe peripheral vascular disease
  - Obesity

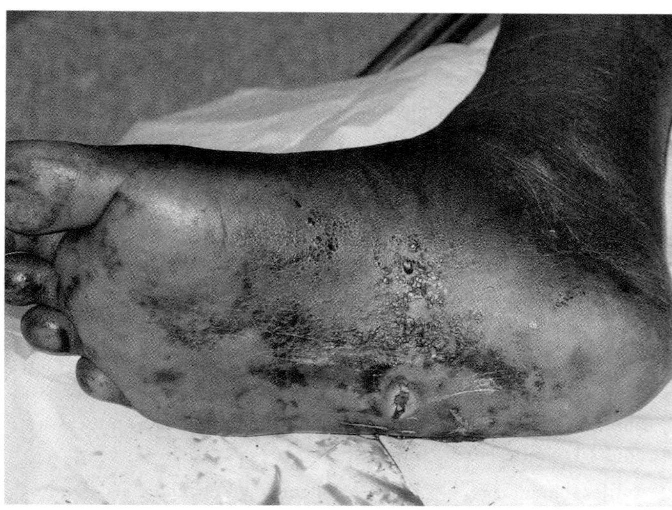

FIGURE 124-3 Necrotizing fasciitis that started when the patient stepped on a nail. Note the puncture wound and the draining fluid. (*Reproduced with permission from Subramaniam R, Shirley OB. Oozing puncture wound on foot.* J Fam Pract. *2009 Jan;58(1):37-39. Reproduced with permission from Frontline Medical Communications.*)

- Alcoholism and cirrhosis
- Intravenous drug use
- Decubitus ulcers
- Poor nutritional status
- Postoperative patients or those with penetrating trauma
- Abscess of the female genital tract

- Risk factors of type II NF (group A β-hemolytic *Streptococcus* [GABHS] and *S. aureus*) include the following:
  - Diabetes mellitus
  - Severe peripheral vascular disease
  - Recent parturition (**Figure 124-3**)
  - Trauma
  - Varicella[5]

DIAGNOSIS

Early recognition based on signs and symptoms is potentially lifesaving. Although laboratory tests and imaging studies can confirm ones' clinical impression, rapid treatment with antibiotics and surgery are crucial to improving survival.

CLINICAL FEATURES

- Rapid progression of erythema to bullae (**Figures 124-4** and **124-5**), ecchymosis, and necrosis or gangrene (**Figure 124-6**).
- The erythematous skin may develop a dusky blue discoloration. Vesicular and bullous lesions form over the erythematous skin, with some serosanguineous drainage. The bullae may become violaceous. The skin can become gangrenous and develop a black eschar.[2]
- Edematous, wooden feel of subcutaneous tissues extending beyond the margin of erythema.
- High fevers and severe systemic toxicity.
- Unrelenting intense pain out of proportion to cutaneous findings.
- Pain progresses to cutaneous anesthesia as disease evolves. Anesthesia of the skin develops as a result of infarction of cutaneous nerves.[2]

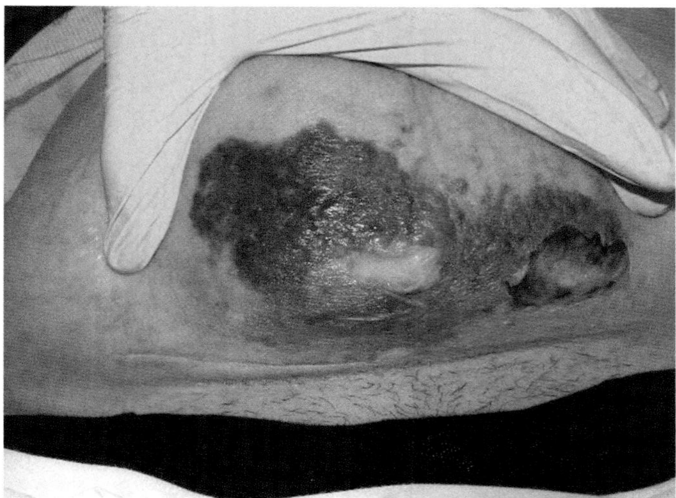

FIGURE 124-4 Necrotizing fasciitis with violaceous color of the skin on the affected skin above the C-section. Extensive debridement was performed in the operating room to save the patient's life. (*Reproduced with permission from Michael Babcock, MD.*)

- Crepitus occurs when there is gas in the soft tissues.
- Unresponsive to empiric antimicrobial therapy.

TYPICAL DISTRIBUTION

- May occur at any anatomic location.
- Majority of cases occur on the lower extremities (**Figures 124-5** and **124-7**) but can occur on the upper extremities.
- Also common on abdominal wall (see **Figure 124-4**) and in perineum (Fournier gangrene).

LABORATORY AND IMAGING

- Routine laboratory tests are nonspecific but common findings include an elevated white blood cell count (WBC), a low serum sodium, and a high blood urea nitrogen (BUN).

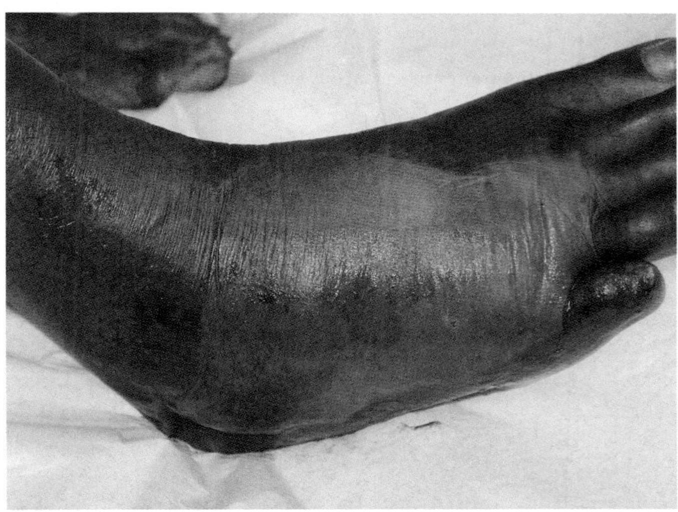

FIGURE 124-5 Necrotizing fasciitis that started when the patient stepped on a nail. A large flaccid bulla is visible along with swelling and erythema. A rapid below-the-knee amputation allowed this patient to survive. (*Reproduced with permission from Subramaniam R, Shirley OB. Oozing puncture wound on foot.* J Fam Pract. *2009 Jan;58(1):37-39. Reproduced with permission from Frontline Medical Communications.*)

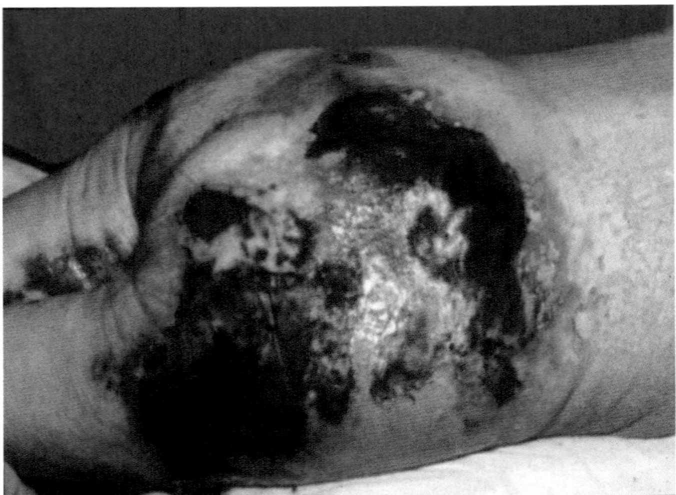

FIGURE 124-6 Necrotizing fasciitis with gangrene. Even with a radical hemipelvectomy this patient did not survive. (*Reproduced with permission from Fred Bongard, MD.*)

- Histology and culture of deep tissue biopsy are essential; surface cultures cannot be relied on alone. Gram staining of the exudate may provide clues about the pathogens while the physician awaits culture results.[2]
- Standard radiographs are of little value unless air is demonstrated in the tissues (see **Figure 124-2**).
- Radiography, computed tomography (CT), ultrasonography, and magnetic resonance imaging (MRI) can be used to detect gas within soft tissues or muscles.[2]
- Although imaging may help delineate the extent of disease, it should not delay surgical consultation.

BIOPSY

- Gross examination reveals swollen, dull, gray fascia with stringy areas of necrosis.[6]
- Necrosis of superficial fascia and fat produces watery, foul-smelling "dishwater pus."[2]
- Histology demonstrates subcutaneous fat necrosis, vasculitis, and local hemorrhage.[2]

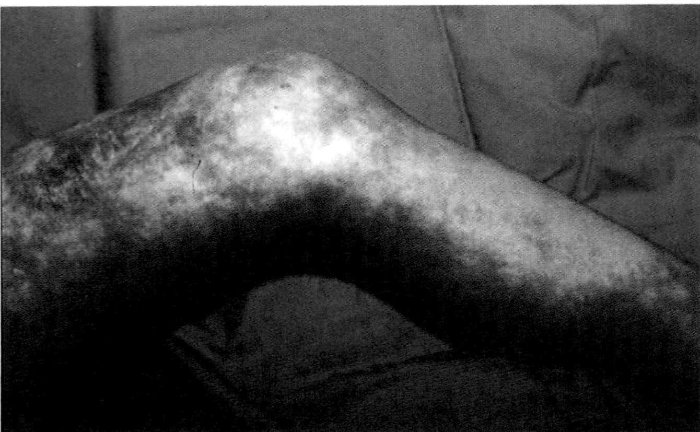

FIGURE 124-7 Necrotizing fasciitis with violaceous color of the skin on the affected leg. (*Reproduced with permission from Fred Bongard, MD.*)

DIFFERENTIAL DIAGNOSIS

- Cellulitis—Acute spreading infection of skin and soft tissues characterized by erythema, edema, pain, and calor. Rapid progression of disease despite antibiotics, systemic toxicity, intense pain, and skin necrosis suggest NF rather than cellulitis (see Chapter 122, Cellulitis).
- Pyomyositis—Suppuration within individual skeletal muscle groups. Synergistic necrotizing cellulitis is a NSTI that involves muscle groups in addition to superficial tissues and fascia.[7] Although pyomyositis may occur with NF, it can occur independent of cutaneous and soft tissue infections. Imaging of the muscle confirms the diagnosis.
- Clostridial myonecrosis—Acute necrotizing infection of muscle tissue caused by clostridial organisms. Surgical exploration and cultures are required to differentiate from NF.
- Erythema induratum—Tender, erythematous subcutaneous nodules occurring on the lower legs (especially the calves). Lack of fever, systemic toxicity, and skin necrosis suggest erythema induratum rather than NF. Lesions of erythema induratum may have a chronic, recurrent course and the patient frequently has a history of tuberculosis or a positive purified protein derivative (PPD) test.
- Streptococcal or staphylococcal toxic shock syndrome—Systemic inflammatory response to a toxin-producing bacteria characterized by fever, hypotension, generalized erythroderma, myalgia, and multisystem organ involvement. NF may occur as part of the toxic shock syndrome.

MANAGEMENT

Start by maintaining a high index of suspicion for NF. If the first debridement occurs within 24 hours from the onset of symptoms, there is a significantly improved chance of survival.[8]

- Surgical debridement is the primary therapeutic modality.[2,3,5,7-10] SOR Ⓐ
  - Extensive, definitive debridement should be the goal with the first surgery. This may require amputation of an extremity to control the disease. Surgical debridement is repeated until all infected devitalized tissue is removed.
- Antibiotics are the main adjunctive therapy to surgery. Broad-spectrum empiric antibiotics should be started immediately when NF is suspected and should include coverage of gram-positive, gram-negative, and anaerobic organisms.[7] SOR Ⓐ
  - Antimicrobial therapy must be directed at the known or suspected pathogens and used in appropriate doses until repeated operative procedures are no longer needed, the patient has demonstrated obvious clinical improvement, and fever has been absent for 48 to 72 hours.[7] SOR Ⓐ
  - Ampicillin is useful for coverage of susceptible enteric aerobic organisms, such as *E. coli*, as well as for gram-positive organisms, such as *Peptostreptococcus* species, group B, C, or G streptococci, and some anaerobes.[7] SOR Ⓐ
  - Clindamycin is useful for coverage of anaerobes and aerobic gram-positive cocci, including most *S. aureus* serogroups.
  - Clindamycin should be considered in initial coverage for its effects on exotoxin production in group A *Streptococcus* (GAS) infections. NF and/or streptococcal toxic shock syndrome caused by group A streptococci should be treated with clindamycin and penicillin.[7] SOR Ⓐ

- The rationale for clindamycin is based on in vitro studies demonstrating both toxin suppression and modulation of cytokine (ie, TNF) production, on animal studies demonstrating superior efficacy versus that of penicillin, and on 2 observational studies demonstrating greater efficacy for clindamycin than for β-lactam antibiotics.[7] SOR Ⓐ
  - Metronidazole has the greatest anaerobic spectrum against the enteric gram-negative anaerobes, but it is less effective against the gram-positive anaerobic cocci. Gentamicin or a fluorinated quinolone, ticarcillin-clavulanate, or piperacillin-sulbactam is useful for coverage against resistant gram-negative rods.[7]
  - The best choice of antibiotics for community-acquired mixed infections is a combination of ampicillin-sulbactam plus clindamycin plus ciprofloxacin.[7] SOR Ⓐ
  - Another commonly used combination is a continuous infusion of penicillin G in combination with clindamycin and an aminoglycoside if renal function permits.[10]
  - Empiric vancomycin should be considered during pending culture results to cover for the increasing incidence of community-acquired MRSA (CAMRSA).[5,7]
  - One preferred antimicrobial therapy for *V. vulnificus* is doxycycline in combination with ceftazidime and surgery for NSTI.[6]
  - Hyperbaric oxygen (HBO_2) may have beneficial effects when used postoperatively in NSTIs. One recent study demonstrated decreased morbidity (amputations 50% vs 0%) and mortality (34% vs 11.9%) with the use of postoperative HBO_2.[11] SOR Ⓑ
- Aggressive fluid resuscitation is often necessary because of massive capillary leak syndrome. Supplemental enteral nutrition is often necessary for patients with NSTIs.
- Vacuum-assisted closure devices may be helpful in secondary wound management after debridement of NSTIs.[10]
- A recommendation to use intravenous immunoglobulin (IVIG) to treat NF or toxic shock syndrome cannot be made with certainty.[7] SOR Ⓑ

PROGNOSIS AND FOLLOW-UP

- Overall case fatality rate remains 20% to 47% despite aggressive, modern therapy.[5,6]
  - However, in a retrospective chart review of patients with NSTIs treated at 6 academic hospitals in Texas between 2004 and 2007 mortality rates varied between hospitals from 9% to 25% (n = 296).[12]
- Early diagnosis and treatment can reduce case fatality rate to 12%.[5]
- Carrying out the first fasciotomy and radical debridement within 24 hours of symptom onset is associated with significantly improved survival.[8]

PATIENT EDUCATION

The serious life-threatening nature of NF should be explained to the patient and family when informed consent is given prior to surgery. The risk of losing life and limb should be explained while giving hope for recovery. For those patients who survive but have lost a limb, counseling should be offered to help them deal with the psychological effects of the amputation.

PATIENT RESOURCES

- United States Centers for Disease Control and Prevention. *Necrotizing Fasciitis*—**http://www.cdc.gov/features/necrotizingfasciitis/.**

PROVIDER RESOURCES

- Practice Guidelines for the Diagnosis and Management of Skin and Soft Tissue Infections—**http://cid.oxfordjournals.org/content/41/10/1373.full#sec-6.**

REFERENCES

1. Dufel S, Martino M. Simple cellulitis or a more serious infection? *J Fam Pract*. 2006;55:396-400.
2. Usatine RP, Sandy N. Dermatologic emergencies. *Am Fam Physician*. 2010;82:773-780.
3. Koukouras D, Kallidonis P, Panagopoulos C, et al. Fournier's gangrene, a urologic and surgical emergency: presentation of a multi-institutional experience with 45 cases. *Urol Int*. 2011;86:167-172.
4. Trent JT, Kirsner RS. Diagnosing necrotizing fasciitis. *Adv Skin Wound Care*. 2002;15:135-138.
5. Cheng NC, Chang SC, Kuo YS, et al. Necrotizing fasciitis caused by methicillin-resistant *Staphylococcus aureus* resulting in death. A report of three cases. *J Bone Joint Surg Am*. 2006;88:1107-1110.
6. Horseman MA, Surani S. A comprehensive review of *Vibrio vulnificus*: an important cause of severe sepsis and skin and soft-tissue infection. *Int J Infect Dis*. 2011;15:e157-e166.
7. Stevens DL, Bisno AL, Chambers HF, et al. Practice guidelines for the diagnosis and management of skin and soft-tissue infections. *Clin Infect Dis*. 2005;41:1373-1406.
8. Cheung JP, Fung B, Tang WM, Ip WY. A review of necrotising fasciitis in the extremities. *Hong Kong Med J*. 2009;15:44-52.
9. Angoules AG, Kontakis G, Drakoulakis E, et al. Necrotising fasciitis of upper and lower limb: a systematic review. *Injury*. 2007;38 (suppl 5):S19-S26.
10. Endorf FW, Cancio LC, Klein MB. Necrotizing soft-tissue infections: clinical guidelines. *J Burn Care Res*. 2009;30:769-775.
11. Escobar SJ, Slade JB Jr, Hunt TK, Cianci P. Adjuvant hyperbaric oxygen therapy (HBO2) for treatment of necrotizing fasciitis reduces mortality and amputation rate. *Undersea Hyperb Med*. 2005;32:437-443.
12. Kao LS, Lew DF, Arab SN, et al. Local variations in the epidemiology, microbiology, and outcome of necrotizing soft-tissue infections: a multicenter study. *Am J Surg*. 2011;202:139-145.

SECTION 3 VIRAL

125 CHICKENPOX

E.J. Mayeaux, Jr, MD

PATIENT STORY

A 48-year-old man developed a rash, low fever, and a cough. Because he had no medical insurance he posted a photograph of his rash on Facebook hoping that someone would give him some good advice. A friend working in a community clinic suggested that he could be seen at a reasonable price based on their sliding scale. The man presented to the clinic with the rash and upper respiratory symptoms. On history he acknowledged that he never had varicella as a child. On physical examination he was found to have multiple vesicles, papules, pustules, and crusting lesions from his scalp down to his legs (**Figures 125-1** and **125-2**). A close-up of lesions showed a "dewdrop on a rose petal" pattern of single vesicles on red bases **(Figure 125-3)**. The physician diagnosed the patient with chickenpox (varicella) and offered him a prescription for generic acyclovir. The patient stated that he was already beginning to feel better and since his fever was gone he might not fill the prescription. One week later he posted on Facebook that he was feeling well and appreciated the physician for seeing him without insurance.

INTRODUCTION

Chickenpox is a highly contagious viral infection that can become reactivated in the form of zoster.

SYNONYMS

Chickenpox is also called as varicella

EPIDEMIOLOGY

- Varicella-zoster virus (VZV) is distributed worldwide.
- The rate of secondary household attack is more than 90% in susceptible individuals.[1]
- Adults and immunocompromised patients generally develop more severe disease than normal children. For every 100,000 individuals who develop chickenpox, between 4 and 9 will die due to the infection and 81% to 85% of these will be adults. It is 5 times more likely to be fatal in pregnancy than in the nonpregnant adult.[2]
- Traditionally, primary infection with VZV occurred during childhood. In childhood, it is usually a benign, self-limited illness in immunocompetent hosts. It occurs throughout the year in temperate regions, but the incidence peaks in the late spring and summer months.
- Prior to the introduction of the varicella vaccine in 1995, the yearly incidence of chickenpox in the United States was approximately 4 million cases with approximately 11,000 hospital admissions and 100 deaths.[3]

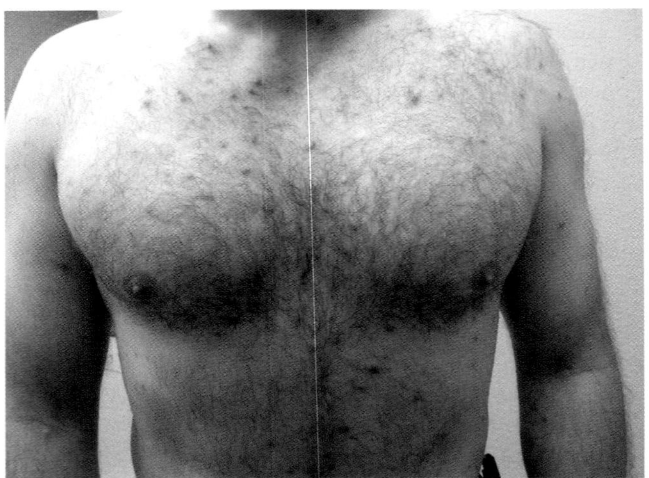

FIGURE 125-1 Chickenpox in a 48-year-old man who never had varicella as a child. Note lesions in various stages (papules, intact vesicles, pustules, and crusted papules) caused by multiple crops of lesions. (*Reproduced with permission from Ryan O'Quinn, MD.*)

- As the vaccination rates steadily increased in the United States, there has been a corresponding 4-fold decrease in the number of cases of chickenpox cases down to disease rates of from 0.3 to 1 per 1000 population in 2001.[3]
- Less than 2% of cases of varicella infections occur among adults over the age of 20 years (see **Figures 125-1** to **125-3**), almost a quarter of all VZV-related mortality occurs among this age group.[4]
- If the mother acquires varicella infection before 20 weeks' gestation, the fetus is at risk for developing congenital varicella syndrome, characterized by limb hypoplasia, skin lesions, neurologic abnormalities, and structural eye damage. Herpes zoster may also develop during infancy.[5]
- If the mother acquires varicella in the peripartum period, the baby is at risk for neonatal varicella, which may present with mild rash to disseminated infection.[5]

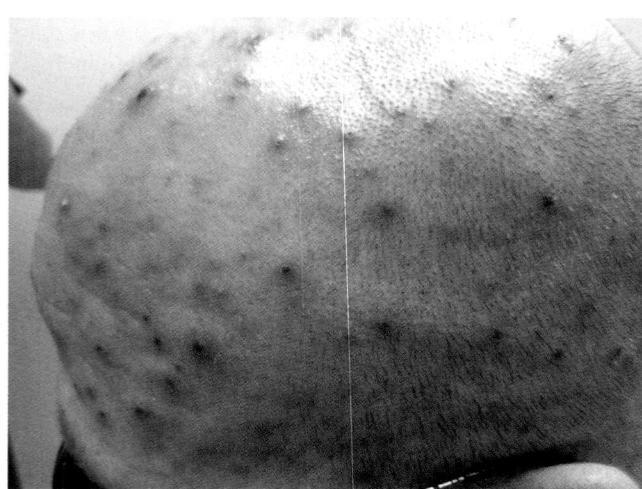

FIGURE 125-2 Chickenpox in the scalp of the same man in Figure 125-1. (*Reproduced with permission from Ryan O'Quinn, MD.*)

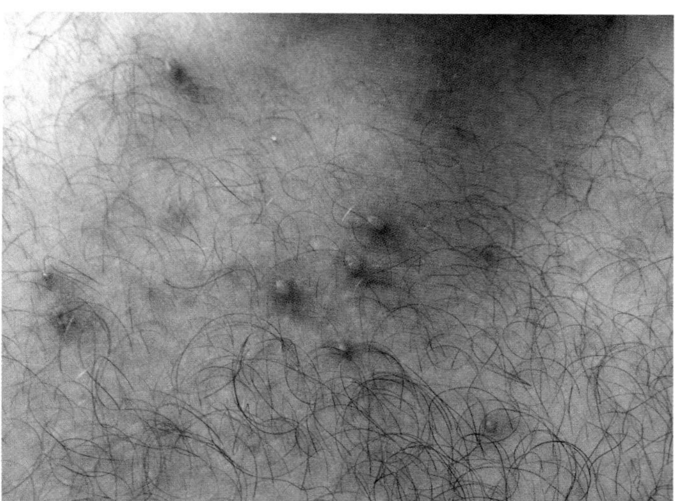

FIGURE 125-3 Close-up picture of chickenpox in the same man in Figure 125-1. Note the lesions are present in various stages. The vesicles or pustules are on a red base. (*Reproduced with permission from Ryan O'Quinn, MD.*)

ETIOLOGY AND PATHOPHYSIOLOGY

- Chickenpox is caused by a primary infection with the VZV, which is a double-stranded, linear DNA herpesvirus.
- Transmission occurs via contact with aerosolized droplets from nasopharyngeal secretions or by direct cutaneous contact with vesicle fluid from skin lesions.
- The incubation period for VZV is approximately 15 days, during which the virus undergoes replication in regional lymph nodes, followed by 2 viremic phases, the second of which persists through the development of skin lesions generally by day 14.[6]
- The vesicular rash appears in crops for several days. The lesions start as vesicle on a red base, which is classically described as a dewdrop on a rose petal (**Figure 125-4**). The lesions gradually develop a pustular component (**Figure 125-5**) followed by the evolution of crusted papules (see **Figure 125-5**). The period of infectivity is generally considered to last from 48 hours prior to the onset of rash until skin lesions have fully crusted.
- The most frequent complication is bacterial skin superinfection. Less-common skin complications (seen more frequently in immunosuppressed hosts) include bullous varicella, purpura fulminans, and necrotizing fasciitis.

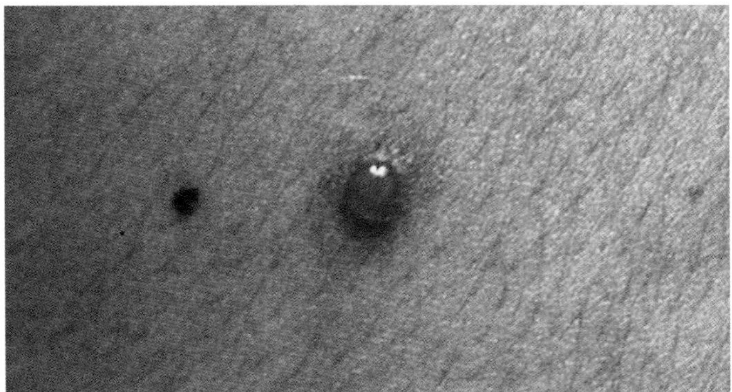

FIGURE 125-4 Dewdrop on a rose petal is the classic description of a varicella vesicle on a red base. (*Reproduced with permission from Richard P. Usatine, MD.*)

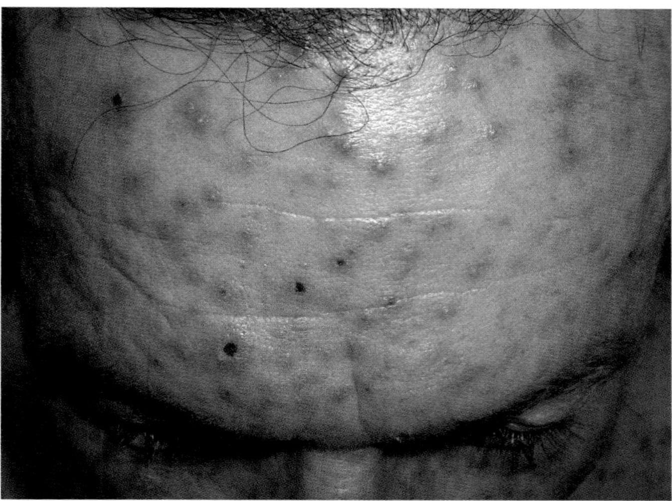

FIGURE 125-5 Pustules and crusted lesions on the face of a homeless man with varicella. Note how varicella has lesions simultaneously visible at different stages. (*Reproduced with permission from Richard P. Usatine, MD.*)

- Encephalitis is a serious potential complication of chickenpox that develops toward the end of the first week of the exanthema. One form, acute cerebellar ataxia, occurs mostly in children and is generally followed by complete recovery. A more diffuse encephalitis most often occurs in adults and may produce delirium, seizures, and focal neurologic signs. It has significant rates of long-term neurologic sequelae and death.
- Pneumonia is rare in healthy children but accounts for the majority of hospitalizations in adults, where it has up to a 30% mortality rate.[7] It usually develops insidiously within a few days after the rash has appeared with progressive tachypnea, dyspnea, and dry cough. Chest X-rays reveal diffuse bilateral infiltrates. Treat with prompt administration of intravenous acyclovir. The use of adjunctive steroid therapy is controversial.
- Varicella hepatitis is rare, and typically only occurs in immunosuppressed individuals. It is frequently fatal.
- Reactivation of latent VZV results in herpes zoster or shingles.

RISK FACTORS

- Preexisting lung disease[2]
- Smoking
- Immunocompromise including immunosuppressive drug therapy
- HIV infection
- Malignancy

DIAGNOSIS

CLINICAL FEATURES

- The typical clinical manifestations of chickenpox include a prodrome of fever, malaise, or pharyngitis, followed in 24 hours by the development of a generalized vesicular rash.
- The lesions are pruritic and appear as successive crops of vesicles more than 3 to 4 days.

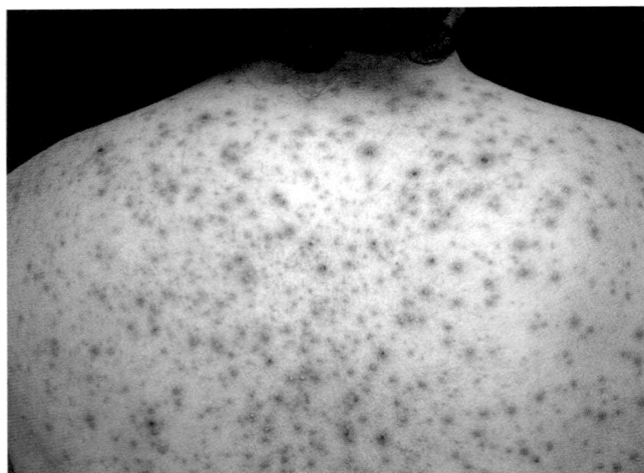

FIGURE 125-6 Varicella on the trunk of a nonimmunized man demonstrating the simultaneous appearance of papules, pustules, and crusted lesions. (*Reproduced with permission from Richard P. Usatine, MD.*)

- Coexisting lesions in different stages of development on the face, trunk, and extremities are common (**Figure 125-6**).
- New lesions stop forming in approximately 4 days, and most lesions have fully crusted by 7 days.

TYPICAL DISTRIBUTION

Body wide—No laboratory tests are needed unless the diagnosis is uncertain. For children or adults in which there is uncertainty about previous disease and it is important to establish a quick diagnosis, a direct fluorescent antibody test can be done on a scraping of a lesion. In many laboratories, a result can be obtained within 24 hours (**Figure 125-7**).

LABORATORY TESTING

- Diagnosis is usually based on classic presentation. Culture of vesicular fluid provides a definitive diagnosis, but is positive in less than 40% of cases. Direct immunofluorescence has good sensitivity and is more rapid than tissue culture. Latex agglutination blood testing may be used to determine exposure and immunity to VZV.
- Women of childbearing potential who acquire the infection should also be tested for pregnancy.

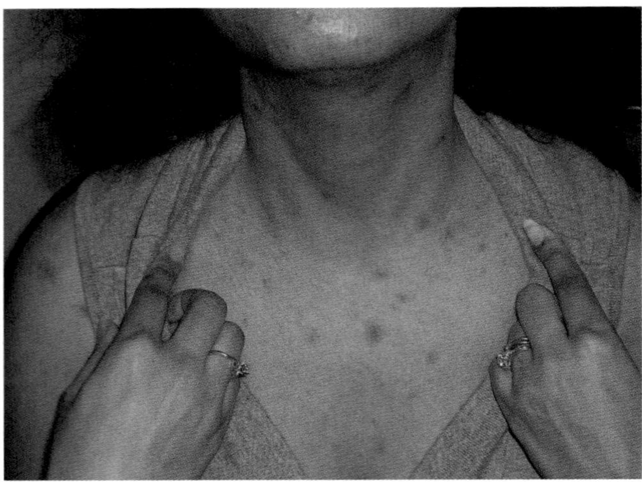

FIGURE 125-7 A 29-year-old woman with mild case of varicella. Her previous history of varicella in childhood was uncertain, so a direct scraping of a lesion was performed and the varicella virus was identified quickly with a direct fluorescent antibody test. (*Reproduced with permission from Richard P. Usatine, MD.*)

DIFFERENTIAL DIAGNOSIS

- Pemphigus and bullous pemphigoid (see Chapters 182, Bullous Pemphigoid and 183, Pemphigus) present with larger bullae or erosions, and varicella vesicles are smaller.[2]
- Dermatitis herpetiformis is characterized by pruritic papulovesicles over the extremities and on the trunk, and granular immunoglobulin (Ig) A deposits on the basement membrane (see Chapter 184, Other Bullous Disease).
- Herpes simplex infection presents with similar lesions, but is generally restricted to the genital and oral areas. The vesicles of herpes simplex tend to be more clustered in a group rather than the wide distribution of varicella (see Chapter 128, Herpes Simplex).
- Impetigo can have bullous or crusted lesions anywhere on the body. The lesions often have mild erythema and a yellowish color to the crusts (see Chapter 118, Impetigo).
- Insect bites are often suspected by history and can occur on the entire body.

MANAGEMENT

NONPHARMACOLOGIC

- Pruritus can be treated with calamine lotion, pramoxine gel, or powdered oatmeal baths.
- Fingernails should be closely cropped to avoid significant excoriation and secondary bacterial infection.

MEDICATIONS

- Antihistamines are helpful in the symptomatic treatment of pruritus.
- Acetaminophen should be used to treat fever in children, as aspirin use is associated with Reye syndrome in the setting of viral infections.[8] SOR Ⓐ
- Superinfection may be treated with topical or oral antibiotics.
- Prophylactic use of varicella zoster immune globulin (125 U/10 kg, up to 625 U intramuscular [IM]) in recently exposed susceptible individuals can prevent or attenuate the disease. However, the immune globulin is extremely hard to obtain at times.[9]
- For adults, acyclovir 20 mg/kg PO 4 times daily (800 mg maximum) for 7 days may be used for treatment if started in the first 24 hours of the rash.[9] SOR Ⓐ
- Early treatment with intravenous acyclovir may be effective for treatment of varicella hepatitis and pneumonia, and may also be useful in the treatment of immunosuppressed patients.[2] SOR Ⓒ It is pregnancy class B drug.
- Valacyclovir 1 g 3 times daily has enhanced bioavailability when compared with acyclovir.
- Famciclovir 500 mg 3 times daily also has enhanced bioavailability when compared with acyclovir.
- Adults who get varicella should be assessed for neurologic and pulmonary disease.

PREVENTION

- Varicella immunization (Varivax) can be used to prevent chickenpox. SOR Ⓐ It is contraindicated in individuals allergic to gelatin or neomycin and in immunosuppressed individuals (it is a live vaccine). In 2006, and again in 2010, the Advisory Committee on Immunization Practices recommended that all children younger than 13 years of age should be routinely administered 2 doses of varicella-containing vaccine, with the first dose administered at 12 to 15 months of age and the second dose at 4 to 6 years of age (ie, before first grade). The second dose can be administered at an earlier age provided the interval between the first and second dose is at least 3 months.[10] The Centers for Disease Control and Prevention (CDC) also recommends that all adults without evidence of immunity to varicella should receive 2 doses of single-antigen varicella vaccine or a second dose if they have received only 1 dose. Evidence of immunity to varicella in adults includes documentation of 2 doses of varicella vaccine at least 4 weeks apart, US-born before 1980 except health care personnel and pregnant women, history of varicella based on diagnosis or verification of varicella disease by a health care provider, history of herpes zoster, or laboratory evidence of immunity or laboratory confirmation of disease. Extra consideration for vaccination should be given to those who have close contact with persons at high risk for severe disease (eg, health care personnel and family contacts) or are at high risk for exposure or transmission (eg, people with regular exposure to children, college students, military personnel, nonpregnant women of childbearing age, and international travelers).
- Pregnant women should be assessed for evidence of varicella immunity. Women who do not have evidence of immunity should receive the first dose of varicella vaccine upon completion or termination of pregnancy and before discharge from the health care facility. The second dose should be administered 4 to 8 weeks after the first dose.
- Passive immunization with VZV-specific antibodies reduces the risk of varicella infection and attenuates the severity of infection in those who seroconvert. The US Advisory Committee on Immunization Practices recommends VariZIG in all nonimmune pregnant women who have been exposed to persons with VZV 125 U/10 kg (1 vial) body weight given IM, with a maximum dose of 625 units (5 vials) within 96 hours of exposure.[4] SOR Ⓑ For pregnant women who cannot receive VariZIG within 96 hours of exposure, a single dose of intravenous immunoglobulin (IVIG) at 400 mg/kg may be used, or the patient may be closely monitor for signs and symptoms of varicella and treatment started with acyclovir if illness occurs.[11] Postexposure prophylaxis is not needed among women who have a history of chickenpox or were immunized with varicella vaccine in the past.

FOLLOW-UP

Follow-up is unnecessary for immunocompetent children and adults who are having no complications. All patients or parents should report any respiratory or neurologic problems immediately.

PATIENT EDUCATION

- Avoid scratching the blisters and keep fingernails short. Scratching may lead to superinfection.
- Calamine lotion and oatmeal (Aveeno) baths may help relieve itching.
- Do not use aspirin or aspirin-containing products to relieve fever. The use of aspirin is associated with development of Reye syndrome, which may cause death.

PATIENT RESOURCES

- KidsHealth. *Chickenpox*—**http://www.kidshealth.org/parent/infections/skin/chicken_pox.html.**
- MedlinePlus. *Chickenpox*—**http://www.nlm.nih.gov/medlineplus/chickenpox.html.**

PROVIDER RESOURCES

- Centers for Disease Control and Prevention. *Varicella (Chickenpox) Vaccination*—**http://www.cdc.gov/vaccines/vpd-vac/varicella/default.htm.**
- Centers for Disease Control and Prevention. *Slide Set: Overview of VZV Disease & Vaccination for Healthcare Professionals*—**http://www.cdc.gov/vaccines/vpd-vac/shingles/downloads/VZV_clinical_slideset_Jul2010.ppt.**

REFERENCES

1. Wharton M. The epidemiology of varicella-zoster infections. *Infect Dis Clin North Am.* 1996;10(3):571-581.
2. Tunbridge AJ, Breuer J, Jeffery KJ; British Infection Society. Chickenpox in adults—clinical management. *J Infect.* 2008 Aug;57(2):95-102.
3. Centers for Disease Control and Prevention (CDC). Decline in annual incidence of varicella—selected states, 1990-2001. *MMWR Morb Mortal Wkly Rep.* 2003;52(37):884-885.
4. Marin M, Güris D, Chaves SS, Schmid S, Seward JF; Advisory Committee on Immunization Practices, Centers for Disease Control and Prevention. Prevention of varicella: recommendations of the Advisory Committee on Immunization Practices (ACIP). *MMWR Recomm Rep.* 2007 Jun;56(RR-4):1-40. *CDC.* http://www.cdc.gov/mmwr/preview/mmwrhtml/rr5604a1.htm. Accessed January 30, 2014.
5. Enders G, Miller E, Cradock-Watson J, et al. Consequences of varicella and herpes zoster in pregnancy: prospective study of 1739 cases. *Lancet.* 1994;343:1548.
6. Grose C. Variation on a theme by Fenner: the pathogenesis of chickenpox. *Pediatrics.* 1981;68(5):735-737.
7. Schlossberg D, Littman M. Varicella pneumonia. *Arch Intern Med.* 1988;148(7):1630-1632.
8. Belay ED, Bresee JS, Holman RC, et al. Reye's syndrome in the United States from 1981 through 1997. *N Engl J Med.* 1999;340(18):1377-1382.
9. Ogilvie MM. Antiviral prophylaxis and treatment in chickenpox. A review prepared for the UK advisory group on chickenpox on behalf of the british society for the study of infection. *J Infect.* 1998;36(suppl 1):31-38.
10. Centers for Disease Control and Prevention (CDC) Advisory Committee on Immunization Practices (ACIP) recommended immunization schedules for persons aged 0 through 18 years and adults aged 19 years and older—United States, 2013. *MMWR Surveill Summ.* 2013 Feb;62(suppl 1):1.
11. VariZIG for prophylaxis after exposure to varicella. *Med Lett Drugs Ther.* 2006 Aug 14;48(1241):69-70.

126 ZOSTER

E.J. Mayeaux, Jr, MD
Richard P. Usatine, MD

PATIENT STORY

A 75-year-old woman presented with a severely painful case of herpes zoster in a lower abdominal/ or lower extremity distribution. Groups of vesicles were becoming bullae and leading to erosions (**Figure 126-1**). The woman was treated with oral analgesics and an oral antiviral medication. Her primary care physician treated her pain aggressively in an attempt to prevent postherpetic neuralgia.

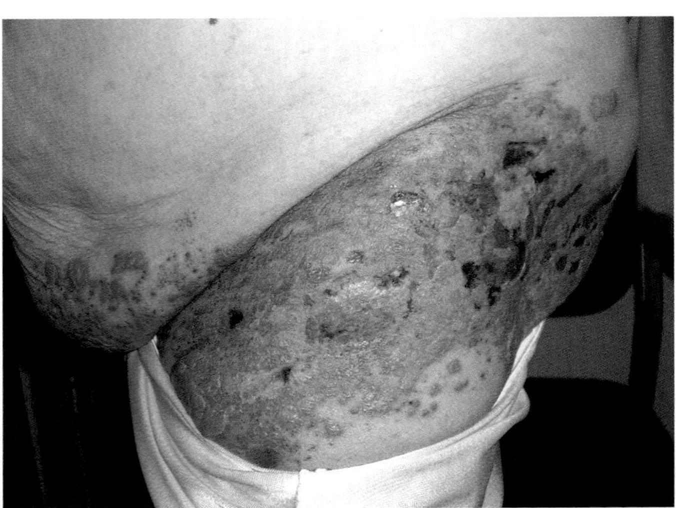

A

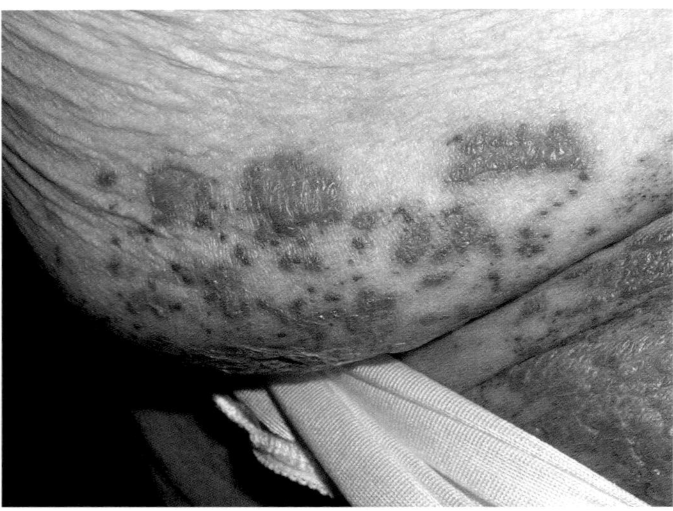

B

FIGURE 126-1 A 75-year-old woman with severe case of herpes zoster in a lower abdominal and lower extremity distribution. **A.** Note the erosions on the upper thighs in addition to the vesicles and bullae. **B.** Close-up of the zoster lesions showing grouped vesicles and bullae on a red base. *(Reproduced with permission from Richard P. Usatine, MD.)*

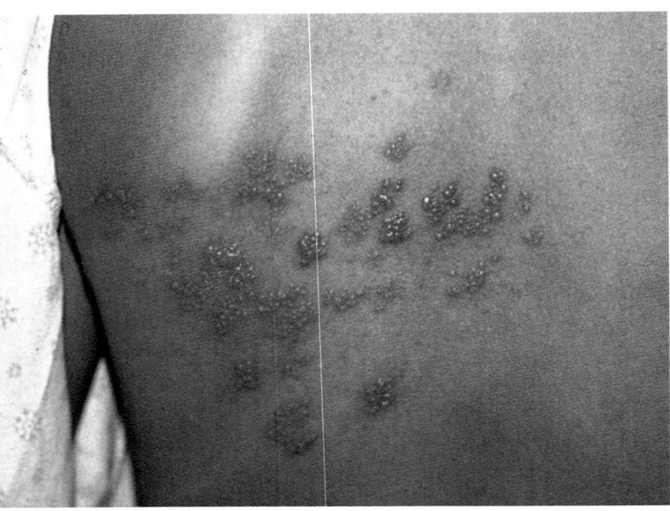

FIGURE 126-2 Close-up of herpes zoster lesions. Note grouped vesicles on a red base. *(Reproduced with permission from Richard P. Usatine, MD.)*

INTRODUCTION

Herpes zoster (shingles) is a syndrome characterized by a painful, usually unilateral vesicular eruption that develops in a restricted dermatomal distribution (**Figures 126-1** and **126-2**).[1-3]

SYNONYMS

Zoster is also known as shingles.

EPIDEMIOLOGY

- According to the Centers for Disease Control and Prevention (CDC), 32% of persons in the United States will experience zoster during their lifetimes accounting for about 1 million cases annually.[4] Older age groups account for the highest incidence of zoster. Approximately 4% of patients will experience a second episode of herpes zoster.[5]
- More zoster cases have been observed among women, even when controlling for age.[6]
- Herpes zoster occurs more frequently and more severely in immunosuppressed patients, including transplantation patients.

ETIOLOGY AND PATHOPHYSIOLOGY

- After primary infection with either chickenpox or vaccine-type varicella-zoster virus (VZV), a latent infection is established in the sensory dorsal root ganglia. Reactivation of this latent VZV infection results in herpes zoster (shingles).
- Both sensory ganglia neurons and satellite cells surrounding the neurons serve as sites of VZV latent infection. During latency, the virus only expresses a small number of viral proteins.
- How the virus emerges from latency is not clearly understood. Once reactivated, virus spreads to other cells within the ganglion. The dermatomal distribution of the rash corresponds to the sensory fields of the infected neurons within the specific ganglion.[3]

- Loss of VZV-specific cell-mediated immune response is responsible for reactivation.[3]
- The pain associated with zoster infections and postherpetic neuralgia (PHN) is thought to result from injury to the peripheral nerves and altered central nervous system processing.
- The most common complications are PHN and bacterial superinfection that can delay healing and cause scarring of the zoster lesions.
- Approximately 19% of patients develop complications that may include the following[7]:
  - PHN—The most common complication is seen in 10% at 90 days[7] (see below).
  - Ocular complications, including uveitis and keratitis (seen in 4%)[7] (see Chapter 127, Zoster Ophthalmicus).
  - Bell palsy and other motor nerve plastic (seen in 3%).[7]
  - Bacterial skin infection (seen in 2%).[7]
  - Meningitis caused by central extension of the infection.
  - Herpes zoster oticus (Ramsay Hunt syndrome) (**Figure 126-3**) includes the triad of ipsilateral facial paralysis, ear pain, and vesicles in the auditory canal and auricle.[8] Disturbances in taste perception, hearing (tinnitus, hyperacusis), lacrimation, and vestibular function (vertigo) may occur.
  - Other rare complications may include acute retinal necrosis, transverse myelitis, encephalitis, leukoencephalitis, contralateral thrombotic stroke syndrome, and granulomatous vasculitis.[9]
- Immunosuppressed patients are at increased risk for complications, including severe complications such as broader dermatomal involvement, disseminated infection, visceral involvement, pneumonitis, and/or meningoencephalitis.
- PHN is the persistence of pain, numbness, and/or dysesthesias precipitated by movement or in response to nonnoxious stimuli in the affected dermatome for more than 1 month after the onset of zoster. The incidence of PHN in the general population is 1.38 per 1000 person-years, and it occurs more commonly in individuals older than age 60 years and in immunosuppressed individuals.[3]
- In a large study, rates of zoster-associated pain (PHN) persisting at least 90 days were as below:
  - Ten percent overall, 12% in women and 7% in men
  - Ages 22 to 59 years—5% overall, 6% in women and 5% in men
  - Ages 60 to 69 years—10% overall, 14% in women and 5% in men
  - Ages 70 to 79 years—17% overall, 18% in women and 15% in men
  - Age 80 years and older—20% overall, 23% in women and 13% in men[7]

RISK FACTORS

ZOSTER

- Older age[3]
- Underlying malignancy
- Disorders of cell-mediated immunity
- Chronic lung or kidney disease
- Autoimmune disease

PHN

- Age older than 60 years
- Negative vaccine status

DIAGNOSIS

CLINICAL FEATURES

A deep burning pain and sometimes redness in a dermatomal pattern is the most common first symptom and can precede the rash by days to weeks (**Figure 126-4**). A prodrome of fever, dysesthesias, malaise, and headache leads in several days to a dermatomal vesicular eruption. The rash starts as grouped vesicles or bullae which evolve into pustular or hemorrhagic lesions within 3 to 4 days (**Figures 126-1** to **126-6**). The lesions typically crust in approximately a week, with complete resolution within 3 to 4 weeks.[5]

TYPICAL DISTRIBUTION

Generally limited to one dermatome in immunocompetent patients, but sometimes affects neighboring dermatomes. Rarely, a few scattered vesicles located away from the involved dermatome as a result of release of

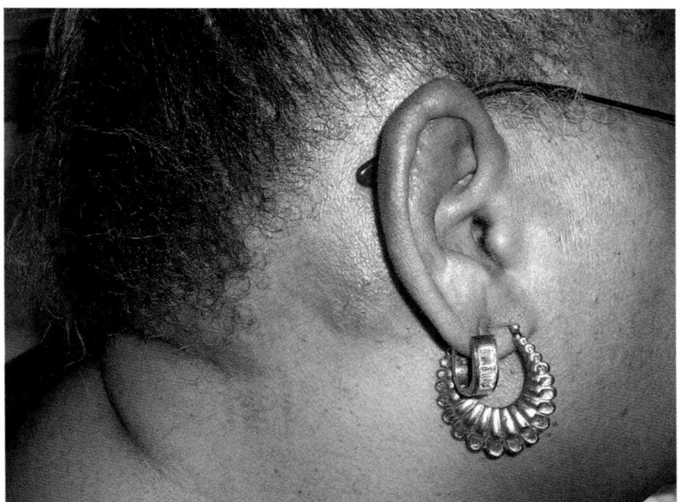

FIGURE 126-3 Herpes zoster oticus (Ramsay Hunt syndrome) with the classic presentation of redness and vesicles on the auricle. (*Reproduced with permission from Richard P. Usatine, MD.*)

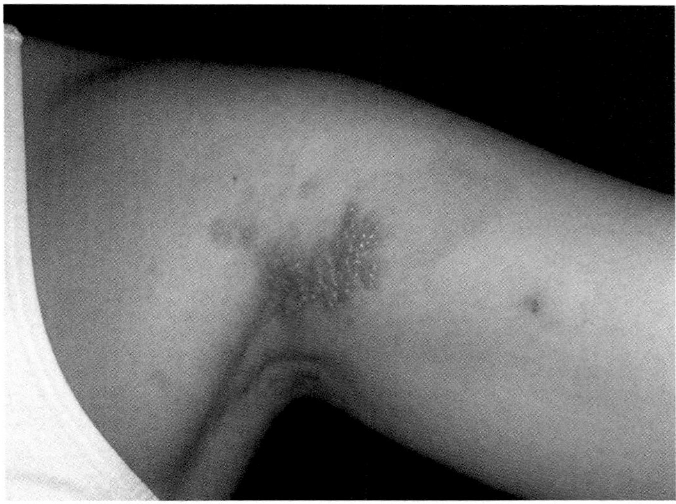

FIGURE 126-4 Herpes zoster in the axilla of a young woman with grouped vesicles on a pink base. Notice the erythema in the dermatome that has started producing blisters. (*Reproduced with permission from Richard P. Usatine, MD.*)

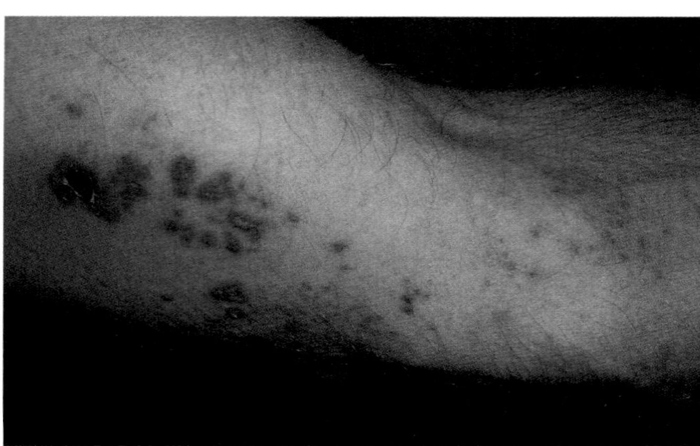

FIGURE 126-5 Herpes zoster on the arm that follows a dermatomal pattern. (*Reproduced with permission from E.J. Mayeaux Jr, MD.*)

VZV from the infected ganglion into the bloodstream.[3] If there are more than 20 lesions distributed outside the dermatome affected, the patient has disseminated zoster. The thoracic and lumbar dermatomes are the most commonly involved. Occasionally zoster will be seen on the extremities (see **Figure 126-5**).

LABORATORY TESTING

Meningitis associated with VZV infection can be diagnosed by cerebrospinal fluid showing pleocytosis.

DIFFERENTIAL DIAGNOSIS

- Pemphigus and other bullous diseases present with blisters, but not the classic dermatomal distribution (see Chapters 181, Overview of Bullous Disease and 183, Pemphigus).
- Molluscum contagiosum presents with white or yellow flat-topped papules with central umbilication caused by a pox virus. The lesions are more firm and unless irritated do not have a red base as seen with zoster (see Chapter 129, Molluscum Contagiosum).

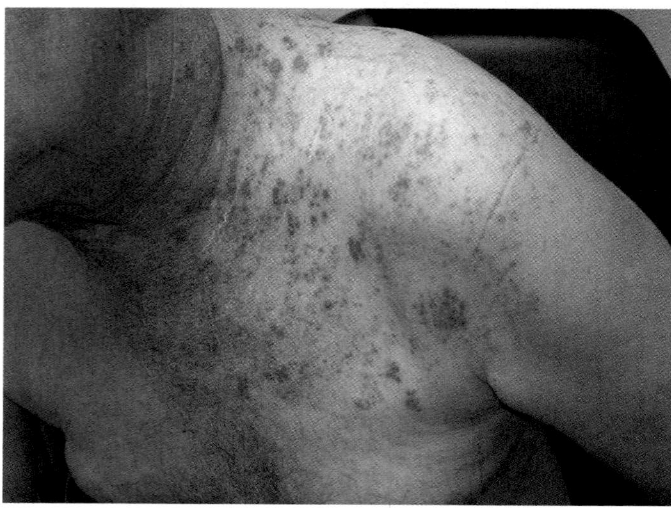

FIGURE 126-6 Herpes zoster of the C4-C5 dermatomal distribution. (*Reproduced with permission from Richard P. Usatine, MD.*)

- Scabies may present as a pustular rash that is not confined to dermatomes and usually has characteristic lesions in the webs of the fingers (see Chapter 141, Scabies).
- Insect bites are often suspected by history and can occur over the entire body.
- Folliculitis presents with characteristic pustules arising from hair shafts (see Chapter 119, Folliculitis).
- Zoster mimics coronary artery disease when it presents with chest pain before the vesicles are visible.
- Herpes simplex infection presents with similar lesions but is usually restricted to the perioral region, genital area, buttocks, and fingers (see Chapter 128, Herpes Simplex).

MANAGEMENT

NONPHARMACOLOGIC

Calamine lotion and topically administered lidocaine may be used to reduce pain and itching. SOR Ⓒ

MEDICATIONS

- The objectives of treatment of herpes zoster include (a) hastening the resolution of the acute viral infection, (b) treatment of the associated pain, and (c) prevention of PHN.
- Antiviral agents used in the treatment of herpes zoster include acyclovir (Zovirax), famciclovir (Famvir), and valacyclovir (Valtrex), all started within 72 hours of the onset of the rash (**Table 126-1**).[10] SOR Ⓐ
- Adding corticosteroids to acyclovir therapy may accelerate times to crusting and healing, return to uninterrupted sleep, resumption of full activity, and discontinuation of analgesic. Data are lacking for combining corticosteroids with other antivirals.
- Pain can be managed with nonprescription analgesics or narcotics. Pain should be treated aggressively. This may actually prevent or lessen the severity of PHN. Narcotic analgesics with hydrocodone are appropriate when needed. SOR Ⓒ
- Treatment of herpes zoster with steroids does not reduce the prevalence of PHN.
- Treatment of herpes zoster early with valacyclovir, famciclovir, or amitriptyline does reduce pain of PHN at 6 months.
- Treatment of PHN includes tricyclic antidepressants, gabapentin (Neurontin), pregabalin (Lyrica), and/or opioid analgesics (**Table 126-2**).

TABLE 126-1 Treatments for Herpes Zoster

Medication	Dosage
Acyclovir (Zovirax)	800 mg orally 5 times daily for 7 to 10 days or 10 mg/kg intravenously every 8 hours for 7 to 10 days
Famciclovir (Famvir)	500 mg orally 3 times daily for 7 days
Valacyclovir (Valtrex)	1000 mg orally 3 times daily for 7 days
Prednisone (Deltasone)	30 mg orally twice daily for 1 week followed by a tapering dose for approximately 2 weeks

TABLE 126-2 Effective Treatments for Postherpetic Neuralgia

Treatment	Benefit/Risk	Risks	NNT for ≥50% Pain Reduction	Dose/Duration
Lidocaine patch 5%	Reduces pain and acts as mechanical barrier	Application site sensitivity	2	Apply up to 3 patches for up to 12 hours
Tricyclic antidepressants (including amitriptyline) (strongest evidence)	Reduces pain, better sleep, decreases anxiety and depression	Multiple side effects, including sedation and dry mouth	2.7	25 to 150 mg qhs
Gabapentin (Neurontin) (strongest evidence)	Reduces pain, improves sleep, mood, and quality of life	Somnolence, dizziness, decreased memory	2.8 to 5.3	300 to 600 mg tid (can go as high as 1200 mg tid)
Pregabalin (Lyrica)	May reduce pain	Peripheral edema and weight gain	5	75 mg bid
Opioids (morphine, oxycodone, methadone)	Reduces pain	Somnolence, constipation, tolerance	Variable	Start low and titrate to effective dose
Tramadol	Reduces pain and is not a true narcotic	Dizziness, nausea, somnolence, constipation	4.8	50 to 100 mg qid

NNT, number needed to treat.
Data from Garroway N, Chhabra S, Landis S, Skolnik DC. Clinical inquiries: what measures relieve postherpetic neuralgia?*J Fam Pract.* 2009;58(7):384 and Tyring SK. Management of herpes zoster and postherpetic neuralgia. *J Am Acad Dermatol.* 2007;57(suppl 6):S136-S142.

PREVENTION

- Use of varicella (chickenpox) vaccine has not led to an increase in vaccine-associated herpes zoster in immunized patients or in the general population, and has led to an overall decrease in herpes zoster.[8]
- The herpes zoster vaccine contains a much higher dose of the live-attenuated virus than the varicella vaccine. In adults 60 years of age or older, immunization reduces the incidence of herpes zoster by 51% compared with placebo.[3] In those who do develop zoster, the duration of pain and discomfort is shorter and the incidence of PHN is greatly reduced. It reduces the incidence of PHN from 1.38 to 0.46 per 1000 person-years.[3]

FOLLOW-UP

Follow-up is based on the severity of the case and the immune status of the patient.

PATIENT EDUCATION

- Herpes zoster in an immunocompetent host is only contagious from contact with open lesions.
- Patients with disseminated zoster or with zoster and are immunocompromised should be isolated from nonimmune individuals with primary varicella infection (in which airborne spread is possible).
- Individuals who have not had varicella and are exposed to a patient with herpes zoster are only at risk of developing primary varicella and not herpes zoster.

PATIENT RESOURCES

- Centers for Disease Control and Prevention. *Vaccine Information Statements*—**http://www.cdc.gov/vaccines/pubs/vis/.**
- Medinfo UK. *Shingles (Herpes Zoster)*—**http://www.medinfo.co.uk/conditions/shingles.html.**
- The Skin Site. *Herpes Zoster (Shingles)*—**http://www.skinsite.com/info_herpes_zoster.htm.**
- MedlinePlus. *Shingles*—**http://www.nlm.nih.gov/medlineplus/ency/article/000858.htm.**

PROVIDER RESOURCES

- MedlinePlus. *Shingles*—**http://emedicine.medscape.com/article/218683.**
- Stankus SJ, Dlugopolski M, Packer D. Management of herpes zoster (shingles) and PHN. *Am Fam Physician*. 2000;61:2437-2444—**http://www.aafp.org/afp/20000415/2437.html.**

REFERENCES

1. Usatine RP, Clemente C. Is herpes zoster unilateral? *West J Med.* 1999;170(5):263.
2. Gnann JW Jr, Whitley RJ. Clinical practice. Herpes zoster. *N Engl J Med.* 2002;347(5):340-346.

3. Oxman MN. Immunization to reduce the frequency and severity of herpes zoster and its complications. *Neurology.* 1995;45(12 suppl 8):S41-S46.

4. Harpaz R, Ortega-Sanchez IR, Seward JF; Advisory Committee on Immunization Practices (ACIP) Centers for Disease Control and Prevention (CDC). Prevention of herpes zoster: recommendations of the Advisory Committee on Immunization Practices (ACIP). *MMWR Recomm Rep.* 2008;57(RR-5):1-30.

5. Stankus SJ, Dlugopolski M, Packer D. Management of herpes zoster (shingles) and postherpetic neuralgia. *Am Fam Physician.* 2000;61(18):2437-2444, 2447-2448.

6. Opstelten W, Van Essen GA, Schellevis F, et al. Gender as an independent risk factor for herpes zoster: a population-based prospective study. *Ann Epidemiol.* 2006;16(9):692-695.

7. Yawn BP, Saddier P, Wollan PC, et al. A population-based study of the incidence and complication rates of herpes zoster before zoster vaccine introduction. *Mayo Clin Proc.* 2007;82(11):1341-1349.

8. Adour KK. Otological complications of herpes zoster. *Ann Neurol.* 1994;35(suppl):S62-S64.

9. Arvin AM, Pollard RB, Rasmussen LE, Merigan TC. Cellular and humoral immunity in the pathogenesis of recurrent herpes viral infections in patients with lymphoma. *J Clin Invest.* 1980;65(4): 869-878.

10. Tyring SK, Beutner KR, Tucker BA, et al. Antiviral therapy for herpes zoster: randomized, controlled clinical trial of valacyclovir and famciclovir therapy in immunocompetent patients 50 years and older. *Arch Fam Med.* 2000;9(9):863-869.

127 ZOSTER OPHTHALMICUS

E.J. Mayeaux Jr, MD
Richard P. Usatine, MD

PATIENT STORY

A 44-year-old HIV-positive Hispanic man presented with painful herpes zoster of his right forehead (**Figure 127-1**). He was particularly worried because his right eye was red, painful, and very sensitive to light (**Figure 127-2**). On physical examination there was significant conjunctival injection, corneal punctate epithelial erosions, and clouding, and a small layer of blood in the anterior chamber (hyphema). The pupil was somewhat irregular. Along with the hyphema and ciliary flush, this indicated an anterior uveitis. The patient had a unilateral ptosis on the right side with limitations in elevation, depression, and adduction of the eye secondary to cranial nerve III palsy from the zoster. The patient was immediately referred to ophthalmology and the anterior uveitis, corneal involvement, and cranial nerve III palsy were confirmed. The ophthalmologist started the patient on topical ophthalmic preparations of erythromycin, moxifloxacin, prednisolone, and atropine. Oral acyclovir was also prescribed. Unfortunately, the patient did not return for follow-up until 6 months later, when he returned to the ophthalmologist with significant corneal scarring (**Figure 127-3**). The patient is currently on a waiting list for a corneal transplantation.

INTRODUCTION

Herpes zoster is a common infection caused by varicella-zoster virus (VZV), the same virus that causes chickenpox. Reactivation of the latent virus in neurosensory ganglia produces the characteristic manifestations of herpes zoster (shingles). Herpes zoster outbreaks may be precipitated by aging, poor nutrition, immunocompromised status, physical or emotional stress, and excessive fatigue. Although zoster most commonly involves the thoracic and lumbar dermatomes, reactivation of the latent virus in the trigeminal ganglia may result in herpes zoster ophthalmicus (HZO) (**Figures 127-1** to **127-7**).

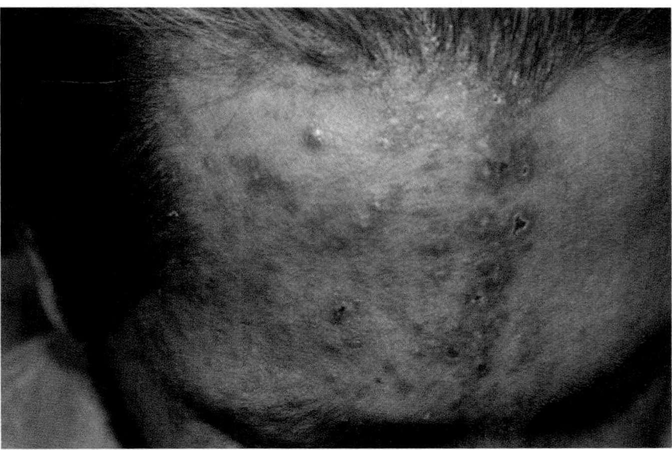

FIGURE 127-1 A 44-year-old HIV-positive Hispanic man with painful herpes zoster of his right forehead. (*Reproduced with permission from Paul Comeau*).

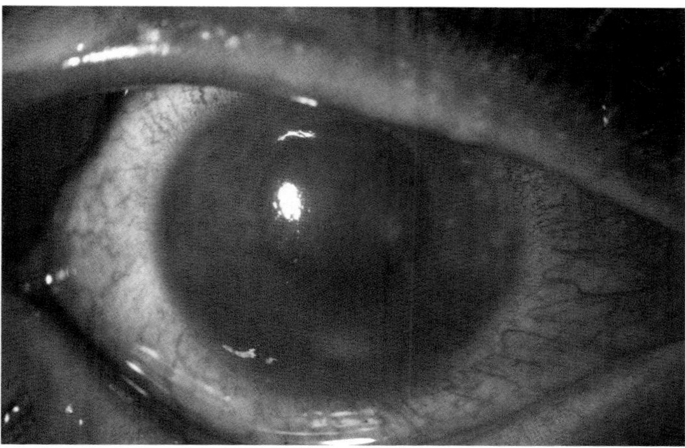

FIGURE 127-2 Acute zoster ophthalmicus of the same patient with conjunctival injection, corneal punctation (keratitis), and a small layer of blood in the anterior chamber (hyphema). A diagnosis of anterior uveitis was suspected based on the irregularly shaped pupil, the hyphema, and ciliary flush. A slit-lamp examination confirmed the anterior uveitis (iritis). (*Reproduced with permission from Paul Comeau*).

SYNONYMS

Zoster ophthalmicus is also known as ocular herpes zoster.

EPIDEMIOLOGY

- Incidence rates of HZO complicating herpes zoster range from 8% to 56%.[1]
- Ocular involvement is not correlated with age, gender, or severity of disease.

ETIOLOGY AND PATHOPHYSIOLOGY

- Serious sequelae may occur including chronic ocular inflammation, vision loss, and disabling pain. Early diagnosis is important to prevent progressive corneal involvement and potential loss of vision.[2]

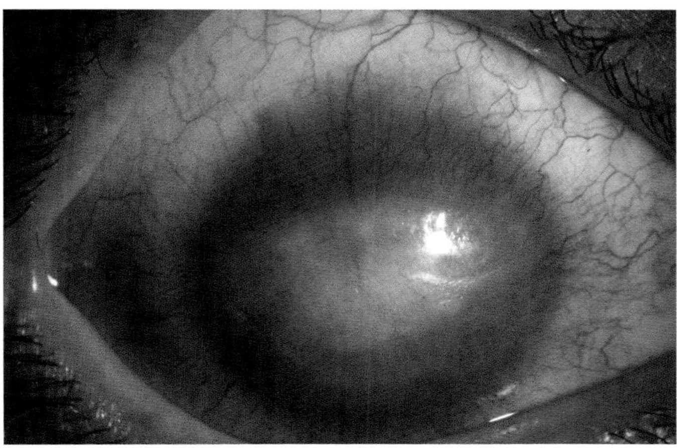

FIGURE 127-3 Corneal scarring and conjunctival injection of the same patient 6 months later after being lost to follow-up. (*Reproduced with permission from Paul Comeau*).

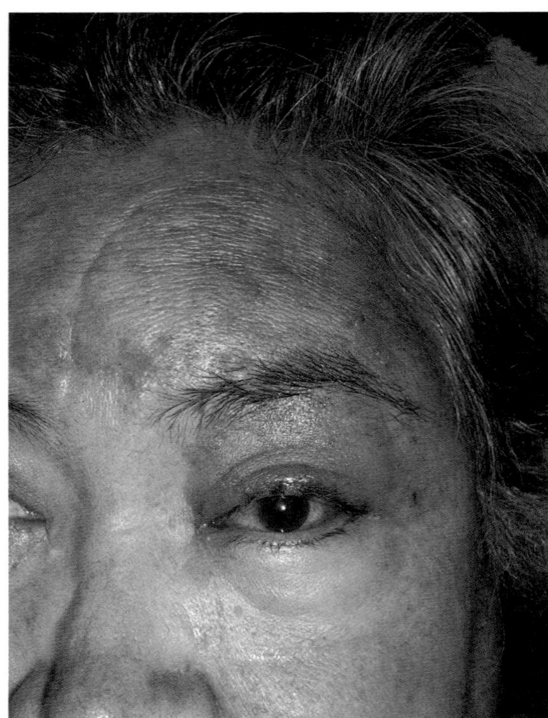

A

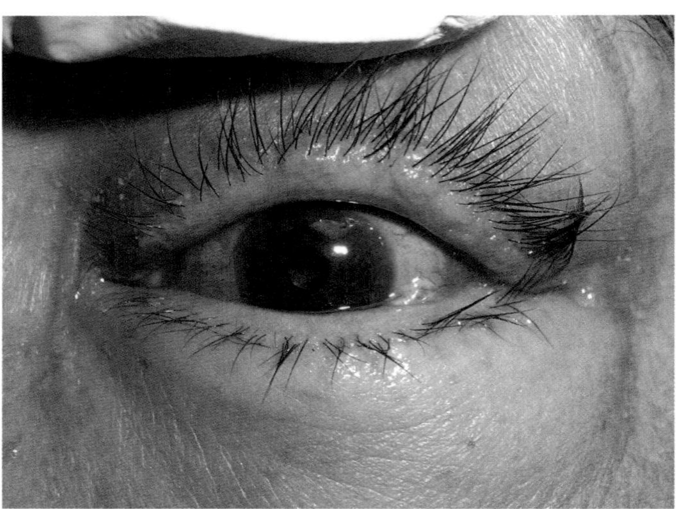

B

FIGURE 127-4 A. Herpes zoster ophthalmicus showing a V1 distribution in this 55-year-old woman that is immunosuppressed with prednisone and azathioprine for her dermatomyositis. She had tremendous eye and facial pain and developed significant blepharospasm secondary to this pain. B. It began with eye pain with no findings evident to the ophthalmologist. A few days later there were vesicles on the upper lid and conjunctival injection with discharge. In this photograph the fluorescein staining is still visible after seeing the ophthalmologist earlier that day. There is no corneal damage and the material at 1:00 is just fluorescein and discharge on the surface of the cornea. (*Reproduced with permission from Richard P. Usatine, MD*).

- Because the nasociliary branch of the first (ophthalmic) division of the trigeminal (fifth cranial) nerve innervates the globe (see **Figure 127-7**), the most serious ocular involvement develops if this branch is involved.
- Classically, involvement of the side of the tip of the nose (Hutchinson sign) has been thought to be a clinical predictor of ocular involvement

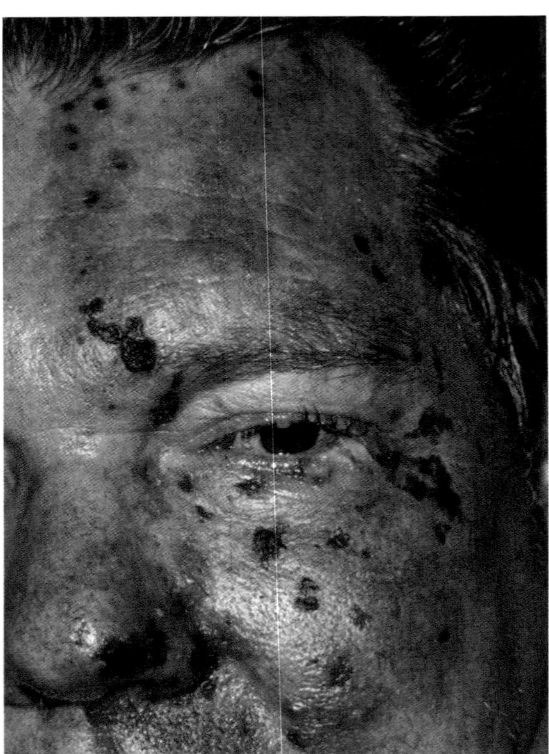

FIGURE 127-5 Herpes zoster ophthalmicus involving the first and second branch of the trigeminal nerve and the eyelids. There is conjunctival hyperemia and purulent left eye discharge. Tne nasociliary branch of the ophthalmic branch of the trigeminal nerve is involved, producing the black crusting on the tip of the nose. (*Reproduced with permission from Richard P. Usatine, MD.*)

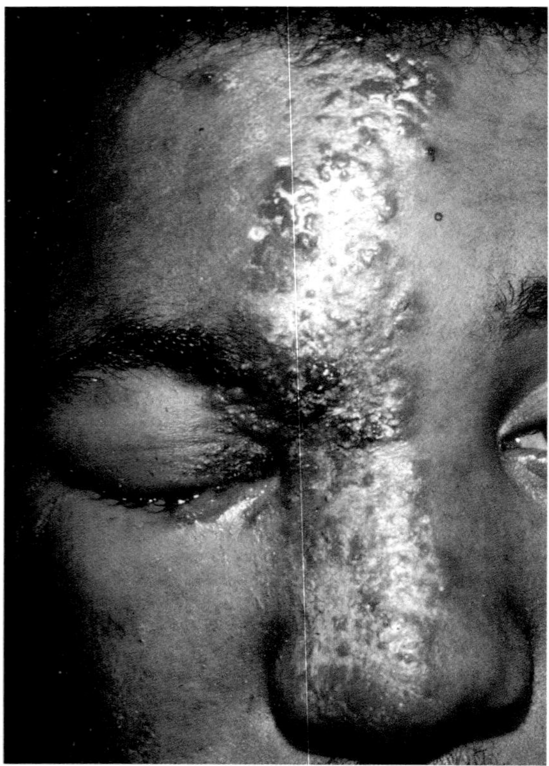

FIGURE 127-6 Herpes zoster ophthalmicus causing eyelid swelling and ptosis. Note the positive Hutchinson sign. (*Reproduced with permission from Richard P. Usatine, MD.*)

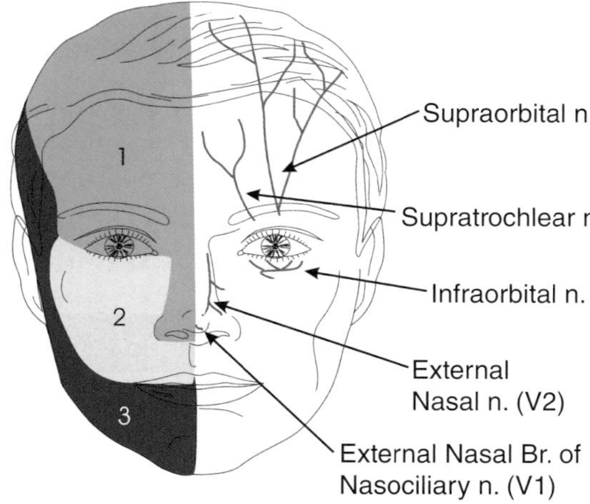

FIGURE 127-7 Diagram demonstrating the sensory distribution of the trigeminal (fifth cranial) nerve, and major peripheral nerves of the first (ophthalmic) division that may be involved with herpes zoster ophthalmicus. The infraorbital nerve from the second division is also shown. (*Reproduced with permission from E.J. Mayeaux Jr, MD.*)

via the external nasal nerve (see **Figures 127-5** and **127-6**). The Hutchinson sign is a powerful predictor of ocular inflammation and corneal denervation with relative risks of 3.35 and 4.02, respectively. In one study, the manifestation of herpes zoster skin lesions at the dermatomes of both nasociliary branches (at the tip, the side, and the root of the nose) was invariably associated with the development of ocular inflammation.[3]

- Epithelial keratitis is the earliest potential corneal finding (see **Figure 127-2**). On slit-lamp examination, it appears as multiple, focal, swollen spots on the cornea that stain with fluorescein dye. They may either resolve or progress to dendrite formation. Herpes zoster virus dendrites form branching or frond-like patterns that have tapered ends and stain with fluorescein dye. These lesions can lead to anterior stromal corneal infiltrates.
- Stromal keratitis occurs in 25% to 30% of patients with HZO, and is characterized by multiple fine granular infiltrates in the anterior corneal stroma. The infiltrates probably arise from antigen-antibody reaction and may be prolonged and recurrent.[4]
- Anterior uveitis evolves to inflammation of the iris and ciliary body and occurs frequently with HZO (see **Figure 127-2**). The inflammation is usually mild, but may cause a mild intraocular pressure elevation. The course of disease may be prolonged, especially without timely treatment, and may lead to glaucoma and cataract formation.
- Herpes zoster virus is the most common cause of acute retinal necrosis. Symptoms include blurred vision and/or pain in one or both eyes and signs include peripheral patches of retinal necrosis that rapidly coalesce, occlusive vasculitis, and vitreous inflammation. It commonly causes retinal detachment. Bilateral involvement is observed in one-third of patients, but may be as high as 70% in patients with untreated disease. Treatment includes long courses of oral and intravenous acyclovir (Zovirax), and corticosteroids.[5]
- Varicella-zoster virus is a member of the same family (Herpesviridae) as herpes simplex virus, Epstein-Barr virus, and cytomegalovirus.
- The virus damages the eye and surrounding structures by neural and secondary perineural inflammation of the sensory nerves. This often results in corneal anesthesia.
- Conjunctivitis, usually with *Staphylococcus aureus*, is a common complication of HZO.

RISK FACTORS

Immunocompromised persons, especially when caused by human immunodeficiency virus infection, have a much higher risk of developing zoster complications, including HZO.

DIAGNOSIS

CLINICAL FEATURES

- The syndrome usually begins with a prodrome of low-grade fever, headache, and malaise that may start up to 1 week before the rash appears.
- Unilateral pain or hypesthesia in the affected eye, forehead, top of the head, and/or nose may precede or follow the prodrome. The rash starts with erythematous macules along the involved dermatome, then rapidly progresses over several days to papules, vesicles and pustules (see **Figures 127-4** to **127-6**). The lesions rupture and typically crust over, requiring several weeks to heal completely.
- With the onset of a vesicular rash along the trigeminal dermatome, hyperemic conjunctivitis, episcleritis, and lid droop (ptosis) can occur (see **Figure 127-6**).
- Approximately two-thirds of patients with HZO develop corneal involvement (keratitis).[1] The epithelial keratitis may feature punctate or dendritiform lesions (see **Figure127-2**). Complications of corneal involvement can lead to corneal scarring (see **Figure 127-3**).[6]
- Iritis (anterior uveitis) occurs in approximately 40% of patients and can be associated with hyphema and an irregular pupil (see **Figure 127-2**).[1]
- Rarely, zoster can be associated with cranial nerve palsies.

TYPICAL DISTRIBUTION

- The frontal branch of the first division of the trigeminal nerve (which includes the supraorbital, supratrochlear, and external nasal branch of the anterior ethmoidal nerve) is most frequently involved, and 50% to 72% of patients experience direct eye involvement.[1]
- Although HZO most often produces a classic dermatomal rash in the trigeminal distribution, a minority of patients may have only cornea findings.

DIFFERENTIAL DIAGNOSIS

- Bacterial or viral conjunctivitis presents as eye pain and foreign body sensation associated with discharge but no rash (see Chapter 13, Conjunctivitis).
- Trigeminal neuralgia presents with facial pain but without the rash or conjunctival findings.
- Glaucoma presents as inflammation, pain, and injection, but without the rash or conjunctival findings (see Chapter 16, Glaucoma).
- Traumatic abrasions usually present with a history of trauma and corneal findings but no other zoster findings (see Chapter 12, Corneal Foreign Body and Abrasion).

- Pemphigus and other bullous diseases present with blisters, but not in a dermatomal distribution (see Chapter 181, Overview of Bullous Disease).

MANAGEMENT

MEDICATIONS

- The standard treatment for HZO is to initiate antiviral therapy with acyclovir (800 mg, 5 times daily for 7-10 days), valacyclovir (1000 mg 3 times daily for 7-14 days), or famciclovir (500 mg orally 3 times a day for 7 days), as soon as possible so as to decrease the incidence of dendritic and stromal keratitis as well as anterior uveitis.[7] SOR Ⓐ
- Oral acyclovir, valacyclovir, and famciclovir in patients with ophthalmic involvement have comparable outcomes. Treatment is most commonly oral acyclovir but intravenous acyclovir (10 mg/kg 3 times daily for 7 days) may be considered in immunocompromised patients or the rare patient who is extremely ill.[8] SOR Ⓐ
- Topical steroid ophthalmic drops are applied to the involved eye, after examination by the ophthalmologist, to reduce the inflammatory response and control immune keratitis and iritis.[1,2] SOR Ⓑ
- The ophthalmologist may prescribe a topical cycloplegic (such as atropine) to treat the ciliary muscle spasm that is painful in iritis. SOR Ⓒ
- Topical ophthalmic antibiotics may also be prescribed to prevent secondary infection of the eye. SOR Ⓒ
- As in all cases of zoster, pain should be treated effectively with oral analgesics and other appropriate medications. Early and effective treatment of pain may help to prevent postherpetic neuralgia (see Chapter 126, Zoster).
- Topical anesthetics should never be used with ocular involvement because of their corneal toxicity. SOR Ⓑ
- Secondary infection, usually *S. aureus*, may develop and should be treated with broad-spectrum topical and/or systemic antibiotics.

REFERRAL OR HOSPITALIZATION

- Referral to an ophthalmologist urgently should be initiated when eye involvement is seen or suspected.
- Hospital admission should be considered for patients with loss of vision, severe symptoms, immunosuppression, involvement of multiple dermatomes, or with significant facial bacterial superinfection.

PREVENTION

The herpes zoster vaccine reduces the incidence of herpes zoster by 51% compared with placebo.[9] In those who do develop zoster, the duration of pain and discomfort is shorter and the incidence of postherpetic neuralgia (PHN) is greatly reduced. It reduces the incidence of PHN from 1.38 to 0.46 per 1000 person-years.[9]

PROGNOSIS

- HZO can become chronic or relapsing. Recurrence is a characteristic feature of HZO.
- Approximately 50% of patients with HZO develop complications. Systemic antiviral therapy can lower the emergence of complications.[10,11]

FOLLOW-UP

Early diagnosis is critical to prevent progressive corneal involvement and potential loss of vision. Patients with herpes zoster should be informed that they should present for medical care with any zoster involving the first (ophthalmic) division of the trigeminal nerve or the eye itself.

PATIENT EDUCATION

- Zoster of the eye is a very serious vision-threatening illness that requires strict adherence to medical therapy and close follow-up.
- Viral transmission to nonimmune individuals from patients with herpes zoster can occur, but it is less frequent than with chickenpox. Virus can be transmitted through contact with secretions.

PATIENT RESOURCES

- American Family Physician. *What You Should Know About HZO*—**http://www.aafp.org/afp/2002/1101/p1732.html.**
- EyeMDLink.com. *Eye Herpes (Ocular Herpes)*—**http://www.eyemdlink.com/Condition.asp?ConditionID=223.**

PROVIDER RESOURCES

- Medscape. *Herpes Zoster Ophthalmicus*—**http://emedicine.medscape.com/article/783223.**
- Shaikh S, Ta CN. Evaluation and management of HZO. *Am Fam Physician*. 2002;66:1723-1730—**http://www.aafp.org/afp/20021101/1723.html.**

REFERENCES

1. Pavan-Langston D. Herpes zoster ophthalmicus. *Neurology.* 1995;45(12 suppl 8):S50-S51.
2. Severson EA, Baratz KH, Hodge DO, Burke JP. Herpes zoster ophthalmicus in Olmsted County, Minnesota: have systemic antivirals made a difference? *Arch Ophthalmol.* 2003;121(3):386-390.
3. Zaal MJ, Völker-Dieben HJ, D'Amaro J. Prognostic value of Hutchinson's sign in acute herpes zoster ophthalmicus. *Graefes Arch Clin Exp Ophthalmol.* 2003;241(3):187-191.
4. Liesegang TJ. Corneal complications from herpes zoster ophthalmicus. *Ophthalmology.* 1985;92(3):316-324.
5. Liesegang TJ. Herpes zoster ophthalmicus natural history, risk factors, clinical presentation, and morbidity. *Ophthalmology.* 2008;115(suppl 2):S3-S12.
6. Albrecht Ma. *Clinical Features ofVaricella-Zoster Virus Infection: Herpes Zoster*. http://www.uptodate.com/contents/clinical-manifestations-of-varicella-zoster-virus-infection-herpes-zoster. Accessed September 3, 2012.
7. McGill J, Chapman C, Mahakasingam M. Acyclovir therapy in herpes zoster infection. A practical guide. *Trans Ophthalmol Soc U K.* 1983;103(pt 1):111-114.
8. Gnann JW Jr, Whitley RJ. Clinical practice. Herpes zoster. *N Engl J Med.* 2002;347(5):340-346.

9. Oxman MN. Immunization to reduce the frequency and severity of herpes zoster and its complications. *Neurology.* 1995;45(12 suppl 8): S41-S46.

10. Miserocchi E, Waheed NK, Dios E, et al. Visual outcome in herpes simplex virus and varicella zoster virus uveitis: a clinical evaluation and comparison. *Ophthalmology.* 2002;109(8):1532-1537.

11. Zaal MJ, Volker-Dieben HJ, D'Amaro J. Visual prognosis in immunocompetent patients with herpes zoster ophthalmicus. *Acta Ophthalmol Scand.* 2003;81(3):216-220.

128 HERPES SIMPLEX

E.J. Mayeaux Jr, MD
Kevin Carter, MD

PATIENT STORY

A 32-year-old man presents with complains of a 1-week history of multiple painful vesicles on the shaft of his penis associated with tender groin adenopathy (**Figure 128-1**). The vesicles broke 2 days ago and the pain has increased. He had similar lesions 1 year ago but never went for health care examination at that time. He has had 3 different female sexual partners in the last 2 years but has no knowledge of them having any sores or diseases. He was given the presumptive diagnosis of genital herpes and a course of acyclovir. His herpes culture came back positive and his rapid plasma reagin (RPR) and HIV tests were negative.

INTRODUCTION

Herpes simplex virus (HSV) infection can involve the skin, mucosa, eyes, and central nervous system (CNS). HSV establishes a latent state followed by viral reactivation and recurrent local disease. Perinatal transmission of HSV can lead to significant fetal morbidity and mortality.

EPIDEMIOLOGY

HSV affects more than one-third of the world's population, with the 2 most common cutaneous manifestations being genital (**Figures 128-1** to **128-4**) and orolabial herpes (**Figures 128-5** to **128-7**).[1]

The Centers for Disease Control and Prevention (CDC) reports that at least 50 million persons in the United States have genital HSV-2 infection. Over the past decade, the percentage of Americans with genital herpes infection in the United States has remained stable. Most persons infected with HSV-2 have not been diagnosed with genital herpes.[2]

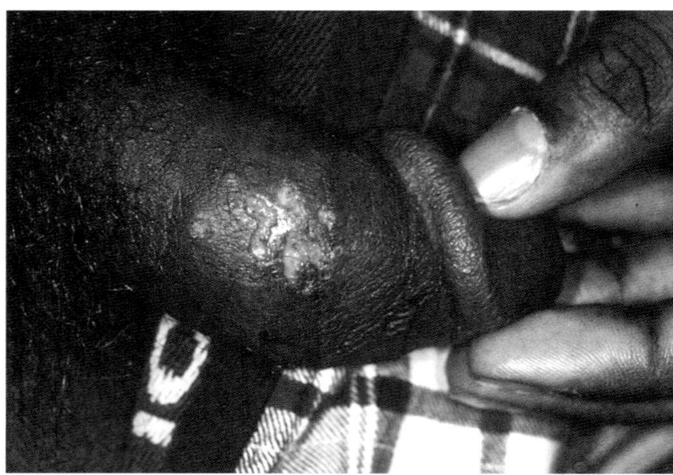

FIGURE 128-1 Recurrent genital herpes simplex virus on the penis showing grouped ulcers (deroofed vesicles). (*Reproduced with permission from Richard P. Usatine, MD.*)

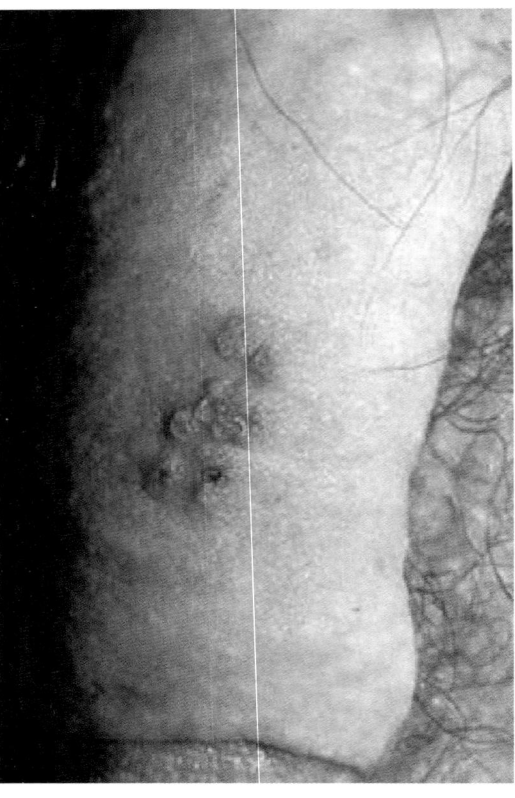

FIGURE 128-2 Herpes simplex on the penis with intact vesicles and visible crusts. (*Reproduced with permission from Jack Rezneck, Sr., MD.*)

Genital HSV-2 infection is more common in women (approximately 1 out of 5 women 14-49 years of age) than in men (approximately 1 out of 9 men 14-49 years of age). Transmission from an infected male to his female partner is believed to be more likely than from an infected female to her male partner.

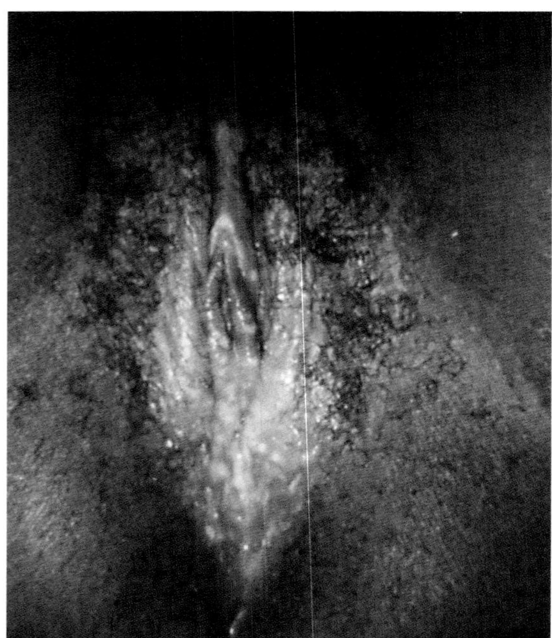

FIGURE 128-3 Vulvar herpes simplex virus at the introitus showing small punched out ulcers. (*Reproduced with permission from the Centers for Disease Control and Prevention and Susan Lindsley.*)

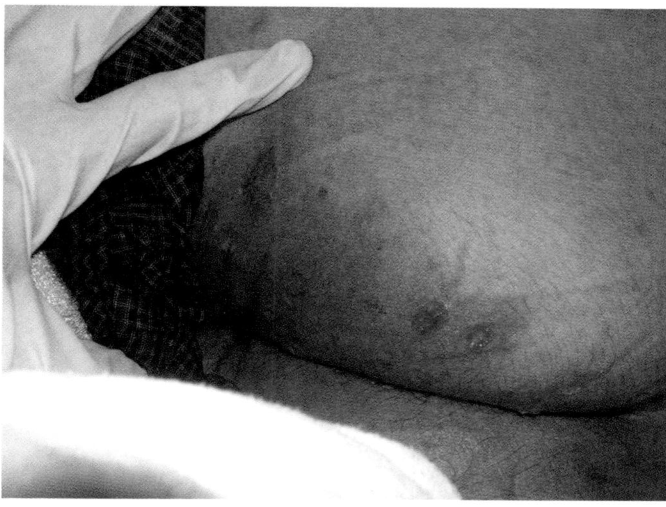

FIGURE 128-4 Recurrent herpes simplex virus on the buttocks of a woman in the ulcerative stage. Women are prone to getting buttocks involvement owing to sleeping with partners that have genital involvement. (*Reproduced with permission from Richard P. Usatine, MD.*)

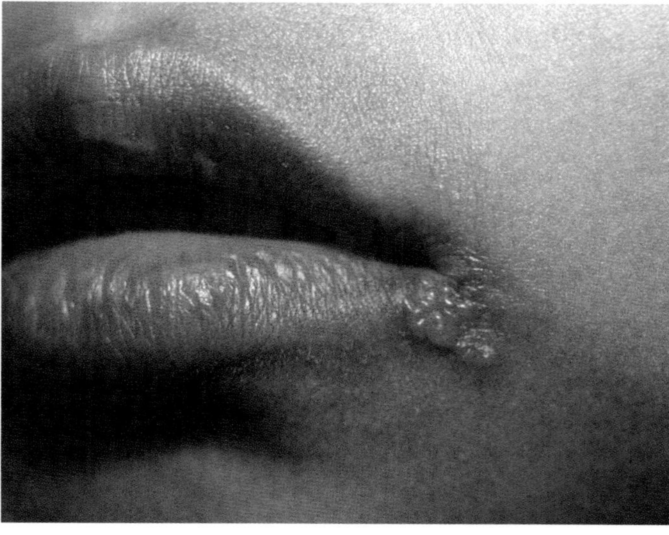

FIGURE 128-6 Close-up of recurrent herpes simplex virus-1 (HSV-1) showing vesicles on a red base at the vermilion border. (*Reproduced with permission from Richard P. Usatine, MD.*)

Orolabial herpes is the most prevalent form of herpes infection and often affects children younger than 5 years of age (see **Figure 121-7**) although all age groups are affected. The duration of the illness is 2 to 3 weeks, and oral shedding of virus may continue for as long as 23 days.[1]

Herpetic whitlow is an intense painful infection of the hand involving the terminal phalanx of one or more digits. In the United States, the estimated annual incidence is 2.4 cases per 100,000 persons.[3]

ETIOLOGY AND PATHOPHYSIOLOGY

- HSV belongs to the family Herpesviridae and is a double-stranded DNA virus.
- HSV exists as 2 separate types (types 1 and 2), which have affinities for different epithelia.[3] Ninety percent of HSV-2 infections are genital, whereas 90% of those caused by HSV-1 are oral-labial.
- HSV enters through abraded skin or intact mucous membranes. Once infected, the epithelial cells die, forming vesicles and creating multinucleated giant cells.
- Retrograde transport into sensory ganglia leads to lifelong latent infection.[1] Reactivation of the virus may be triggered by immunodeficiency, trauma, fever, and UV light.
- Genital HSV infection is usually transmitted through sexual contact. When it occurs in a preadolescent, the possibility of abuse must be considered.
- Evidence indicates that 21.9% of all persons in the United States, 12 years or older, have serologic evidence of HSV-2 infection, which is more commonly associated with genital infections.[4]
- As many as 90% of those infected are unaware that they have herpes infection and may unknowingly shed virus and transmit infection.[5]
- Primary genital herpes has an average incubation period of 4 days, followed by a prodrome of itching, burning, or erythema (**Figure 128-8**).

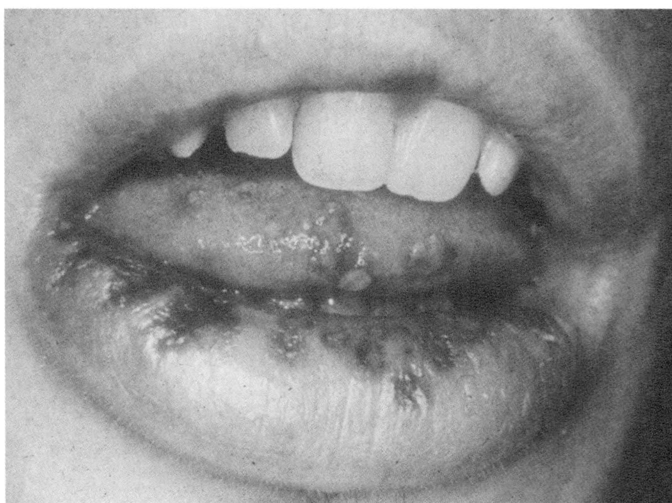

FIGURE 128-5 Primary herpes gingivostomatitis presenting with multiple ulcers on the tongue and lower lip. (*Reproduced with permission from Richard P. Usatine, MD.*)

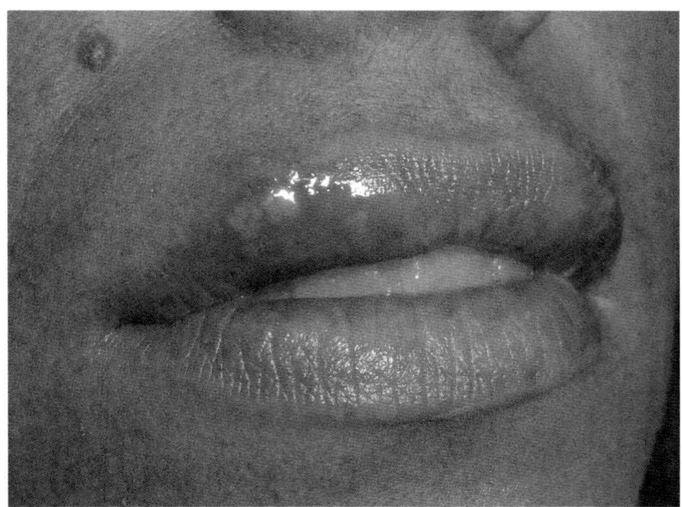

FIGURE 128-7 Orolabial herpes simplex virus in an adult woman showing deroofed blisters (ulcer). (*Reproduced with permission from Richard P. Usatine, MD.*)

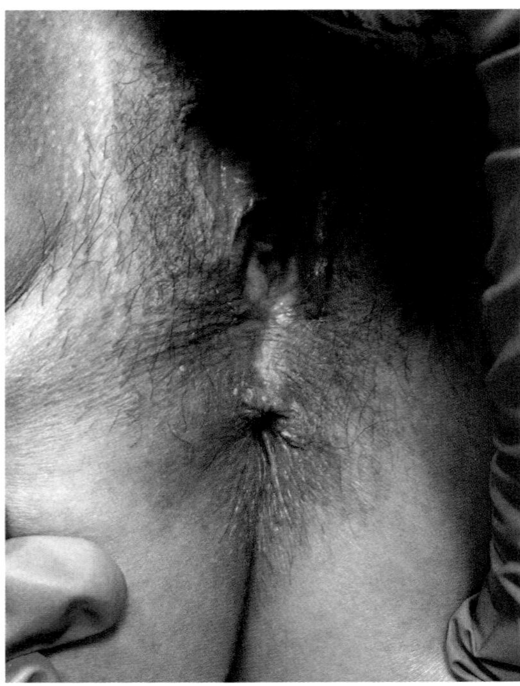

FIGURE 128-8 Primary genital herpes in a 51-year-old woman with prominent erythema and very small vesicles. The woman was in a lot of pain. (*Reproduced with permission from Richard P. Usatine, MD.*)

- With both types, systemic symptoms are common in primary disease and include fever, headache, malaise, abdominal pain, and myalgia.[6] Recurrences are usually less severe and shorter in duration than the initial outbreak.[1,6]
- Maternal-fetal transmission of HSV is associated with significant morbidity and mortality. Manifestations of neonatal HSV include localized infection of the skin, eyes, and mouth, CNS disease, or disseminated multiple organ disease. The CDC and the American College of Obstetricians and Gynecologists recommend that cesarean delivery should be offered as soon as possible to women who have active HSV lesions or, in those with a history of genital herpes, symptoms of vulvar pain, or burning at the time of delivery.
- Herpetic whitlow occurs as a complication of oral or genital HSV infection and in medical personnel who have contact with oral secretions (**Figures 128-9** and **128-10**).
- Toddlers and preschool children are susceptible to herpetic whitlow if they have herpes labialis and engage in thumb-sucking or finger-sucking behavior.
- Like all HSV infections, herpetic whitlow usually has a primary infection, which may be followed by subsequent recurrences. The virus migrates to the peripheral ganglia and Schwann cells where it lies dormant. Recurrences observed in 20% to 50% of cases are usually milder and shorter in duration.

RISK FACTORS

- Multiple sexual partners
- Female gender
- Low socioeconomic status
- HIV infection

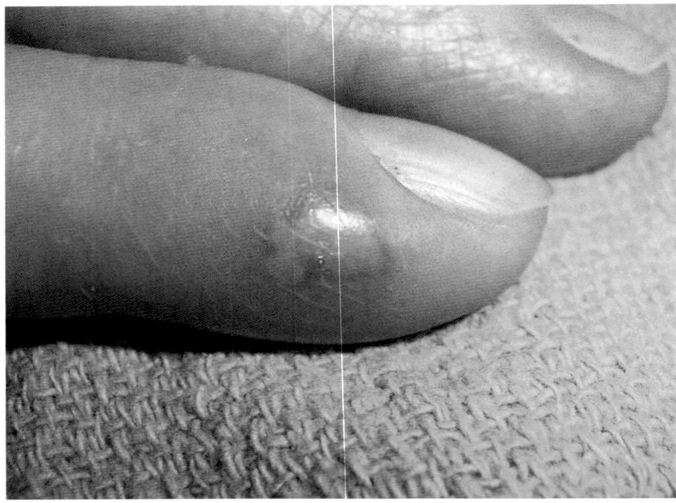

FIGURE 128-9 Herpetic whitlow lesion on distal index finger. (*Reproduced with permission from Richard P. Usatine, MD.*)

DIAGNOSIS

CLINICAL FEATURES

- The diagnosis of HSV infection may be made by clinical appearance. Many patients have systemic symptoms, including fever, headache, malaise, and myalgias.
- Orolabial herpes typically takes the form of painful vesicles and ulcerative erosions on the tongue, palate, gingiva, buccal mucosa, and lips (see **Figures 128-5** to **128-7**).
- Genital herpes presents with multiple transient, painful vesicles that appear on the penis (see **Figures 128-1** and **128-2**), vulva

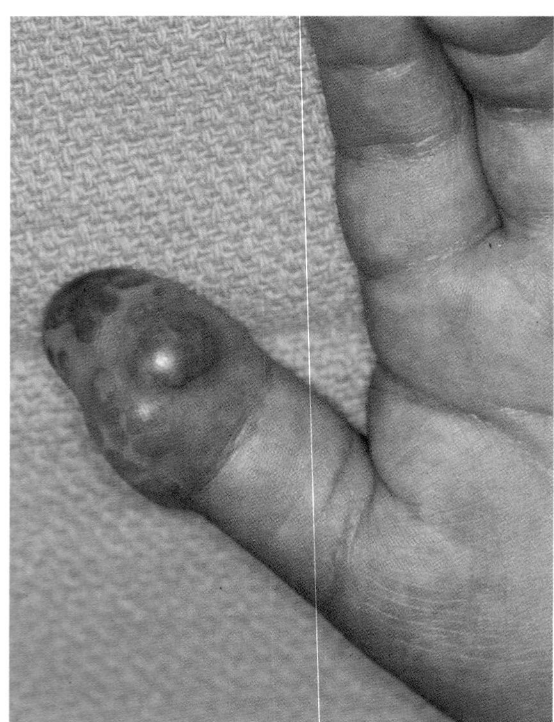

FIGURE 128-10 Severely painful herpetic whitlow on the thumb. (*Reproduced with permission from Eric Kraus, MD.*)

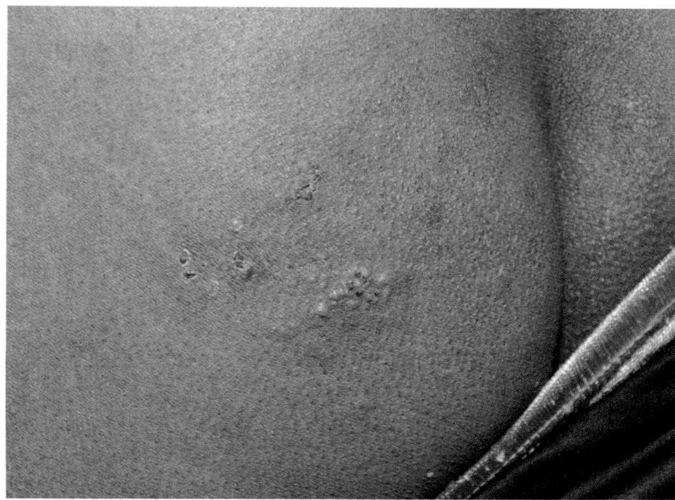

FIGURE 128-11 Recurrent herpes simplex virus on the buttocks of a woman. Note the vesicles and crusts in a unilateral cluster. (*Reproduced with permission from Richard P. Usatine, MD.*)

(see **Figure 128-3**), buttocks (**Figures 128-4** and **128-11**), perineum, vagina or cervix, and tender inguinal lymphadenopathy.[6] The vesicles break down and become ulcers that develop crusts while these are healing.

- Recurrences typically occur 2 to 3 times a year. The duration is shorter and less painful than in primary infections. The lesions are often single and the vesicles heal completely by 8 to 10 days.
- UV radiation in the form of sunlight may trigger outbreaks. Another reason to use sun protection when outdoors triggers recurrence of orolabial HSV-1, an effect which is not fully suppressed by acyclovir.

LABORATORY STUDIES

- The gold standard of diagnosis is viral isolation by tissue culture and polymerase chain reaction (PCR) testing.[2]
  - The culture sensitivity rate is only 70% to 80% and depends on the stage at which the specimen is collected. The sensitivity is highest at first in the vesicular stage and declines with ulceration and crusting. The tissue culture assay can be positive within 48 hours but may take longer.
  - PCR is extremely sensitive (96%) and specific (99%). PCR testing is generally used for cerebrospinal fluid (CSF) testing in suspected HSV encephalitis or meningitis.[2]
- Older type-specific HSV serologic assays that do not accurately distinguish HSV-1 from HSV-2 antibody are still on the market. Both laboratory-based assays and point-of-care tests that provide results for HSV-2 antibodies from capillary blood or serum with sensitivities of 80% to 98% are available. Because nearly all HSV-2 infections are sexually acquired, the presence of type-specific HSV-2 antibody implies anogenital infection. Type-specific HSV serologic assays might be useful in patients with recurrent symptoms and negative HSV cultures and an asymptomatic patient with a partner with genital herpes. Screening for HSV-1 and HSV-2 in the general population is not indicated.[2]
- The Tzanck test and antigen detection tests have lower sensitivity rates than viral culture and should not be relied on for diagnosis.[2]
- The CDC does not currently recommend routine type 2 HSV testing in someone with no symptoms suggestive of herpes infection (ie, for the general population).[7]
- If the herpes was acquired by sexual contact, screening should be performed for other sexually transmitted diseases (STDs), such as syphilis and HIV.
- Biopsy is usually unnecessary unless no infectious etiology is found for a genital lesion and a malignancy is suspected.

DIFFERENTIAL DIAGNOSIS

- Syphilis produces a painless or mildly painful, indurated, clean-based ulcer (chancre) at the site of exposure. It is best to investigate for syphilis or coexisting syphilis in any patient presenting for the first time with a genital ulcer of unproven etiology (see Chapter 218, Syphilis).
- Chancroid produces a painful deep, undermined, purulent ulcer that may be associated with painful inguinal lymphadenitis (see Chapter 218, Syphilis).
- Drug eruptions produce pruritic papules or blisters without associated viral symptoms (see Chapter 201, Cutaneous Drug Reactions).
- Behçet disease produces ulcerative disease around the mouth and genitals, possibly before onset of sexual activity (**Figure 128-12**).
- Acute paronychia which presents as a localized abscess in a nail fold and is the main differential diagnosis in the consideration of herpetic whitlow (see Chapter 192, Paronychia).
- Felon—A red, painful infection, usually bacterial, of the fingertip pulp. It is important to distinguish whitlow from a felon (where the pulp space usually is tensely swollen) as incision and drainage of a felon is needed, but should be avoided in herpetic whitlow because it may lead to an unnecessary secondary bacterial infection.

MANAGEMENT

NONPHARMACOLOGIC

Women with active primary or recurrent genital herpetic lesions at the onset of labor should deliver by cesarean section to lower the chance of neonatal HSV infection.[2] SOR Ⓐ

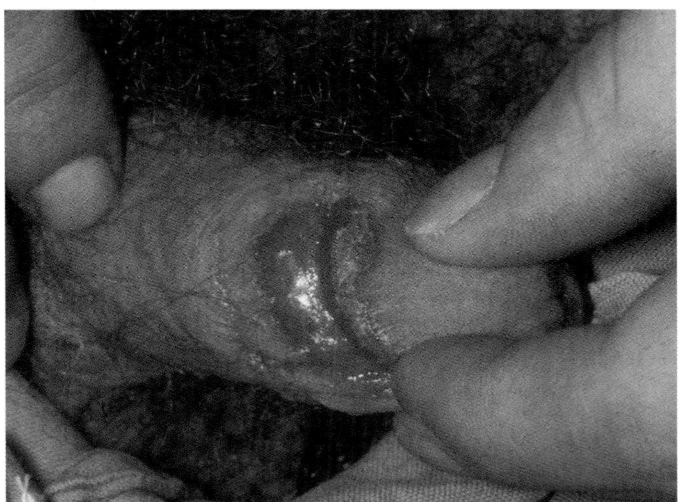

FIGURE 128-12 Young man with Behçet syndrome presenting with a painful penile ulcer and aphthous ulcers in his mouth. (*Reproduced with permission from Richard P. Usatine, MD.*)

TABLE 128-1 Dosages of Treatments for Genital Herpes Infection[2]

Drug	Primary Infection Dosage	Recurrent Infection Dosage	Chronic Suppressive Therapy
Acyclovir (Zovirax)	400 mg 3 times daily for 7 to 10 days or 200 mg 5 times daily	400 mg 3 times daily for 5 days or 800 mg twice daily for 5 days or 800 mg 3 times daily for 2 days	400 mg twice daily
Famciclovir (Famvir)	250 mg 3 times daily for 10 days*	125 mg twice daily for 5 days or 1 g twice daily for 1 day or 500 mg once, followed by 250 mg twice daily for 2 days	250 mg PO twice daily
Valacyclovir (Valtrex)	1 g twice daily for 10 days	500 mg twice daily for 3 days or 1 g daily for 5 days	500 mg to 1 g once daily

*Famciclovir is not FDA-labeled for this indication.

MEDICATIONS

Acyclovir is a guanosine analog that acts as a DNA chain terminator which, when incorporated, ends viral DNA replication. Valacyclovir is the *l*-valine ester prodrug of acyclovir that has enhanced absorption after oral administration and high oral bioavailability. Famciclovir is the oral form of penciclovir, a purine analog similar to acyclovir. They must be administered early in the outbreak to be effective, but are safe and extremely well tolerated.[6] SOR Ⓐ

Genital herpes

- Antiviral therapy is recommended for an initial genital herpes outbreak. **Table 128-1** shows the dosages for antiherpes drugs. Although systemic antiviral drugs can partially control the signs and symptoms of herpes episodes, they do not eradicate latent virus.
- Acyclovir, famciclovir, and valacyclovir are equally effective for episodic treatment of genital herpes, but famciclovir appears somewhat less effective for suppression of viral shedding.[2] SOR Ⓑ
- Effective episodic treatment of herpes requires initiation of therapy during the prodrome period or within 1 day of lesion onset. Providing the patient with a prescription for the medication with instructions to initiate treatment immediately when symptoms begin improves efficacy.[2] SOR Ⓑ
- IV acyclovir therapy at 5 to 10 mg/kg IV every 8 hours for 2 to 7 days followed by oral antiviral therapy to complete at least 10 days of total therapy should be provided for patients who have severe HSV disease or complications.[2] SOR Ⓒ
- HSV strains resistant to acyclovir have been detected in immunocompromised patients so that other antivirals (eg, famciclovir) need to be considered in these patients. SOR Ⓒ
- Topical medication for HSV infection is generally not effective. Topical penciclovir applied every 2 hours for 4 days, reduces clinical healing time by approximately 1 day.[1,2]
- All patients with a first episode of genital herpes should receive antiviral therapy as even with mild clinical manifestations initially, they can develop severe or prolonged symptoms.
- Toxicity of these 3 antiviral drugs is rare, but in patients who are dehydrated or who have poor renal function, the drug can crystallize in the renal tubules, leading to a reversible creatinine elevation or, rarely, acute tubular necrosis. Adverse effects, usually mild, include nausea, vomiting, rash, and headache. Lethargy, tremulousness, seizures, and delirium have been reported rarely in studies of renally impaired patients.[8]

Oral herpes

Table 128-2 provides an overview of treatments for herpes labialis.

- In the treatment of primary orolabial herpes, oral acyclovir (200 mg 5 times daily for 5 days) accelerates healing by 1 day and can reduce the mean duration of pain by 36%.[9] SOR Ⓐ
- The oral lesions in primary herpes gingivostomatitis can lead to poor oral intake especially in children (**Figure 128-13**) and the elderly. To prevent dehydration, the following medications may be considered. Topical oral anesthetics such as 2% viscous lidocaine by prescription or 20% topical benzocaine OTC may be used to treat painful oral ulcers. SOR Ⓒ A solution combining aluminum and magnesium hydroxide (liquid antacid) and 2% viscous lidocaine has been reported as helpful when swished and spit out several times a day as needed for pain. SOR Ⓒ
- Docosanol cream (Abreva) is available without prescription for oral herpes. One randomized controlled trial (RCT) of 743 patients with herpes labialis showed a faster healing time in patients treated with docosanol 10% cream compared with placebo cream (4.1 vs 4.8 days), as well as reduced duration of pain symptoms (2.2 vs 2.7 days).[10] More than 90% of patients in both groups healed completely within 10 days.[10] Treatment with docosanol cream, when applied 5 times per day and within 12 hours of episode onset, is safe and somewhat effective.[11]

PREVENTION

- Barrier protection using latex condoms is recommended to minimize exposure to genital HSV infections (see "Patient Education" below).
- Suppressive therapy with antiviral drugs reduces the frequency of genital herpes recurrences by 70% to 80% in patients with frequent recurrences.[2] SOR Ⓐ Traditionally this is reserved for use in patients who have more than 4 to 6 outbreaks per year (see **Table 128-1**).
- Short-term prophylactic therapy with acyclovir for orolabial HSV may be used in patients who anticipate intense exposure to UV light. Early treatment of recurrent orolabial HSV infection with famciclovir 250 mg 3 times daily for 5 days can markedly decrease the size and duration of lesions.[12] SOR Ⓐ

TABLE 128-2 Treatments for Herpes Labialis

Drug	Dose or Dosage	Evidence Rating*	References
Episodic oral treatment for recurrences†			
Acyclovir (Zovirax)	200 mg 5 times per day or 400 mg 3 times per day for 5 days	A	13, 14
Famciclovir (Famvir)	1500 mg once for 1 day	B	15
Valacyclovir (Valtrex)	2 g twice for 1 day	B	16
Episodic topical treatment for recurrences†			
Acyclovir cream	Apply 5 times per day for 4 days	B	19
Docosanol cream (Abreva)	Apply 5 times per day until healed	B	18
Penciclovir cream (Denavir)	Apply every 2 hours while awake for 4 days	B	17
Treatment to prevent recurrences			
Acyclovir	400 mg twice per day (ongoing)	A	14, 20
Valacyclovir	500 mg once per day (ongoing)	B	21

*A, consistent, good-quality, patient-oriented evidence; B, inconsistent or limited-quality, patient-oriented evidence; C, consensus, disease-oriented evidence, usual practice, expert opinion, or case series.
†Most effective if treatment is started at the onset of symptoms.
Data from Usatine RP, Tinitigan R. Nongenital herpes simplex virus. *Am Fam Physician.* 2010;82(9):1075-1082.

FOLLOW-UP

The patient should return for follow-up if pain is uncontrolled or superinfection is suspected. The patient should be periodically evaluated for the need for suppressive therapy based on the number of recurrences per year.

PATIENT EDUCATION

Following are measures to prevent genital HSV infection:

- Abstain from sexual activity or limit number of sexual partners to prevent exposure to the disease.

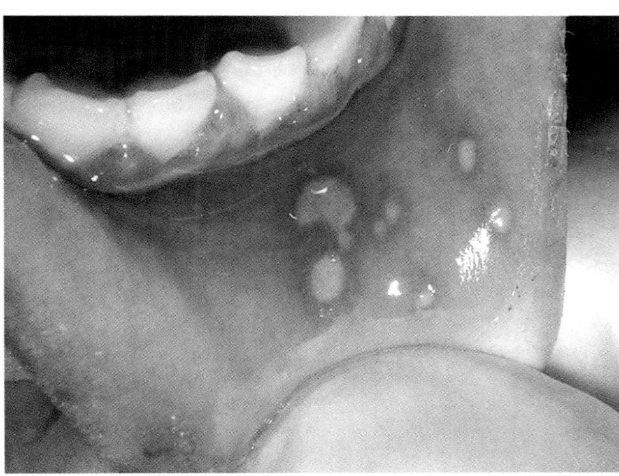

FIGURE 128-13 Primary herpes gingivostomatitis in a 4-year-old girl. Note the cluster of ulcers inside the lower lip typical of herpes simplex virus. The patient also had involvement of her gingiva, which were swollen and painful. *(Reproduced with permission from Richard P. Usatine, MD.)*

- Use condoms to protect against transmission, but this is not foolproof as ulcers can occur on areas not covered by condoms.
- Prevent autoinoculation by patting dry affected areas, not rubbing with towel.
- Studies show that patients may shed virus when they are otherwise asymptomatic. A link between HSV genital ulcer disease and sexual transmission of HIV has been established. Safer sex practices should be strongly encouraged to prevent transmission of HSV to others and acquiring HIV by the patient.

PATIENT RESOURCES

- National Institute of Allergy and Infectious Diseases. *Genital Herpes*—**http://www.niaid.nih.gov/topics/genitalherpes/Pages/default.aspx.**
- Centers for Disease Control and Prevention. *Genital Herpes–CDC Fact Sheet*—**http://www.cdc.gov/std/Herpes/STDFact-Herpes.htm.**
- Skinsight. *Herpetic Whitlow–Information for Adults*—**http://www.skinsight.com/adult/herpeticWhitlow.htm.**

PROVIDER RESOURCES

- Medscape. *Herpes Simplex*—**http://emedicine.medscape.com/article/218580.**
- Medscape. *Dermatologic Manifestations of Herpes Simplex*—**http://emedicine.medscape.com/article/1132351.**
- Usatine RP, Tinitigan R. Nongenital HSV. *Am Fam Physician.* 2010;82:1075-1082—**http://www.aafp.org/afp/2010/1101/p1075.html.**
- Emmert DH. Treatment of common cutaneous HSV infections. *Am Fam Physician.* 2000;61:1697-1704—**http://www.aafp.org/afp/20000315/1697.html.**

REFERENCES

1. Whitley RJ, Kimberlin DW, Roizman B. Herpes simplex viruses. *Clin Infect Dis.* 1998;26:541-555.
2. Centers for Disease Control and Prevention. *2010 Guidelines for Treatment of Sexually Transmitted Diseases.* http://www.cdc.gov/std/treatment/2010/STD-Treatment-2010-RR5912.pdf. Accessed December 1, 2011.
3. Gill MJ, Arlette J, Buchan K. Herpes simplex virus infection of the hand. A profile of 79 cases. *Am J Med.* 1988;84:89-93.
4. Fleming DT, McQuillan GM, Johnson RE, et al. Herpes simplex virus type 2 in the United States, 1976 to 1994. *N Engl J Med.* 1997;337:1105-1111.
5. Mertz GJ. Epidemiology of genital herpes infections. *Infect Dis Clin North Am.* 1993;7:825-839.
6. Clark JL, Tatum NO, Noble SL. Management of genital herpes. *Am Fam Physician.* 1995;51:175-182, 187-188.
7. Centers for Disease Control and Prevention (CDC). Seroprevalence of herpes simplex virus type 2 among persons aged 14-49 years—United States, 2005-2008. *MMWR Morb Mortal Wkly Rep.* 2010;59(15):456-459.
8. Emmert DH. Treatment of common cutaneous herpes simplex virus infections. *Am Fam Physician.* 2000;61(6):1697-1706, 1708.
9. Spruance SL, Stewart JC, Rowe NH, et al. Treatment of recurrent herpes simplex labialis with oral acyclovir. *J Infect Dis.* 1990;161:185-190.
10. Sacks SL, Thisted RA, Jones TM, et al. Docosanol 10% Cream Study Group. Clinical efficacy of topical docosanol 10% cream for herpes simplex labialis: a multi-center, randomized, placebo-controlled trial. *J Am Acad Dermatol.* 2001;45(2):222-230.
11. Usatine RP, Tinitigan R. Nongenital herpes simplex virus. *Am Fam Physician.* 2010;82(9):1075-1082.
12. Spruance SL, Rowe NH, Raborn GW, et al. Perioral famciclovir in the treatment of experimental ultraviolet radiation-induced herpes simplex labialis: a double-blind, dose-ranging, placebo-controlled, multicenter trial. *J Infect Dis.* 1999;179:303-310.
13. Amir J, Harel L, Smetana Z, Varsano I. Treatment of herpes simplex gingivostomatitis with aciclovir in children: a randomised double blind placebo controlled study. *BMJ.* 1997;314(7097):1800-1803.
14. Glenny AM, Fernandez Mauleffinch LM, Pavitt S, Walsh T. Interventions for the prevention and treatment of herpes simplex virus in patients being treated for cancer. *Cochrane Database Syst Rev.* 2009;(1):CD006706.
15. Spruance SL, Bodsworth N, Resnick H, et al. Single-dose, patient-initiated famciclovir: a randomized, double-blind, placebo-controlled trial for episodic treatment of herpes labialis. *J Am Acad Dermatol.* 2006;55(1):47-53.
16. Hull C, McKeough M, Sebastian K, Kriesel J, Spruance S. Valacyclovir and topical clobetasol gel for the episodic treatment of herpes labialis: a patient-initiated, double-blind, placebo-controlled pilot trial. *J Eur Acad Dermatol Venereol.* 2009;23(3):263-267.
17. Spruance SL, Rea TL, Thoming C, Tucker R, Saltzman R, Boon R. Penciclovir cream for the treatment of herpes simplex labialis. A randomized, multicenter, double-blind, placebo-controlled trial. Topical Penciclovir Collaborative Study Group. *JAMA.* 1997;277(17):1374-1379.
18. Sacks SL, Thisted RA, Jones TM, et al.; Docosanol 10% Cream Study Group. Clinical efficacy of topical docosanol 10% cream for herpes simplex labialis: a multi-center, randomized, placebo-controlled trial. *J Am Acad Dermatol.* 2001;45(2):222-230.
19. Spruance SL, Nett R, Marbury T, Wolff R, Johnson J, Spaulding T. Acyclovir cream for treatment of herpes simplex labialis: results of two randomized, double-blind, vehicle-controlled, multicenter clinical trials. *Antimicrob Agents Chemother.* 2002;46(7):2238-2243.
20. Rooney JF, Straus SE, Mannix ML, et al. Oral acyclovir to suppress frequently recurrent herpes labialis. A double-blind, placebo-controlled trial. *Ann Intern Med.* 1993;118(4):268-272.
21. Baker D, Eisen D. Valacyclovir for prevention of recurrent herpes labialis: 2 double-blind, placebo-controlled studies. *Cutis.* 2003;71(3):239-242.

129 MOLLUSCUM CONTAGIOSUM

E.J. Mayeaux Jr, MD

PATIENT STORIES

An 18-year-old young man came to the office because of an outbreak of bumps on his lower abdomen and groin area for a couple of weeks (**Figure 129-1**). He admits to being sexually active and has recent partners whom he does not know well. He is diagnosed with molluscum contagiosum and elects treatment with cryotherapy, which was performed using liquid nitrogen in a Cryogun (**Figure 129-2**). The molluscum disappeared without scarring or hypopigmentation.

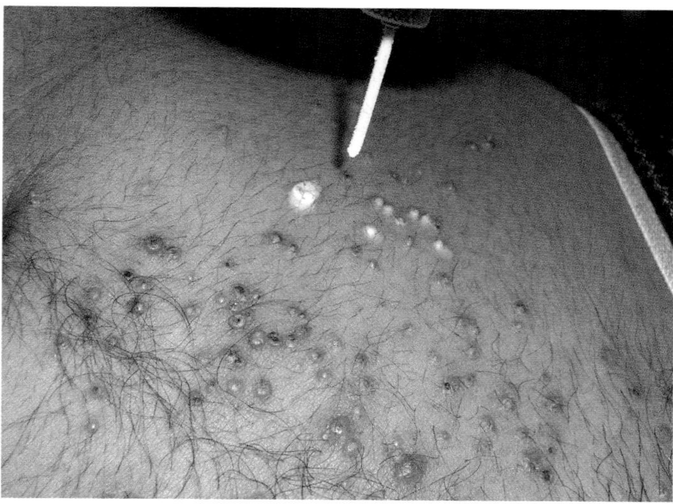

FIGURE 129-2 Cryotherapy of the patient shown in **Figure 129-1**. (*Reproduced with permission from Richard P. Usatine, MD.*)

INTRODUCTION

Molluscum contagiosum is a viral skin infection that produces pearly papules that often have a central umbilication. It is seen most commonly in children, but can also be transmitted sexually among adults.

EPIDEMIOLOGY

- Molluscum contagiosum infection has been reported worldwide. An Australian seroepidemiology study found a seropositivity rate of 23%.[1]
- Up to 5% of children in the United States have clinical evidence of molluscum contagiosum infection.[2] It is a common, nonsexually transmitted condition in children.
- In adults, molluscum occurs most commonly in the genital region (**Figure 129-1** to **129-4**). In this case, it is considered a sexually transmitted disease. Subclinical cases may occur and may be more common in the general community than is generally recognized.
- The number of cases in US adults increased in the 1980s, probably as a result of the HIV/AIDS epidemic. Since the introduction of highly active antiretroviral therapy (HAART), the number of molluscum contagiosum cases in HIV/AIDS patients has decreased substantially.[3] However, the prevalence of molluscum contagiosum in patients who are HIV-positive may still be as high as 5% to 18% (**Figures 129-5** and **129-6**).[4,5]

ETIOLOGY AND PATHOPHYSIOLOGY

- Molluscum contagiosum is a benign condition that is often transmitted through close contact in children and through sexual contact in adults.
- It is a large DNA virus of the Poxviridae family of poxvirus. It is related to the orthopoxviruses (*variola*, vaccinia, smallpox, and monkeypox viruses).

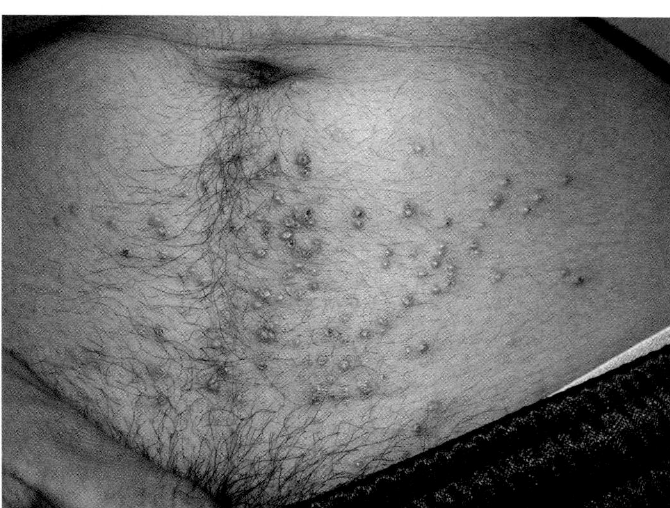

FIGURE 129-1 Molluscum contagiosum on the lower abdomen of a young man. (*Reproduced with permission from Richard P. Usatine, MD.*)

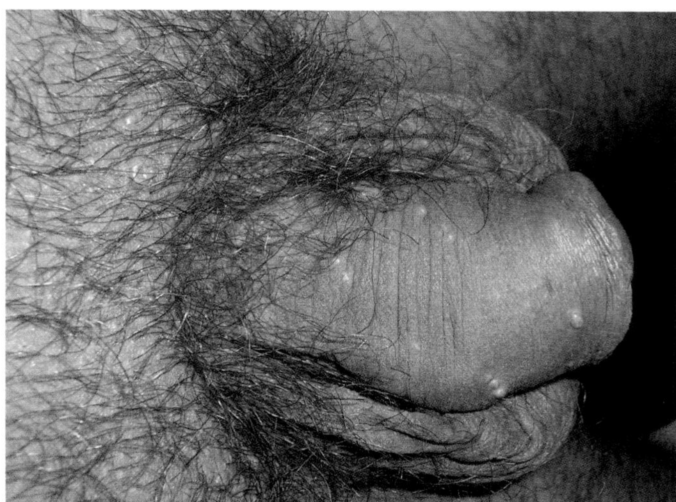

FIGURE 129-3 Molluscum contagiosum on and around the penis. His girlfriend has these on the buttocks. (*Reproduced with permission from Richard P. Usatine, MD.*)

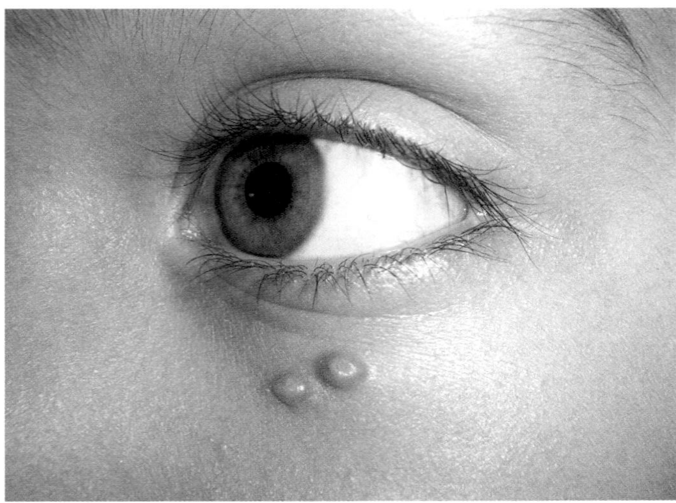

CHAPTER 129

FIGURE 129-4 Molluscum contagiosum under the eye with central umbilication. (*Reproduced with permission from Richard P. Usatine, MD.*)

- Molluscum replicates in the cytoplasm of epithelial cells. It causes a chronic localized skin infection consisting of dome-shaped pearly papules on the skin. Like most of the viruses in the poxvirus family, molluscum is spread by direct skin-to-skin contact. It can also spread by autoinoculation when scratching, touching, or treating lesions.
- Any one single lesion is usually present for approximately 2 months, but autoinoculation often causes continuous crops of lesions.

RISK FACTORS

- Molluscum contagiosum may be more common in patients with atopic dermatitis.[2]
- The disease also may be spread by participation in contact sports.[2]
- It is also associated with immunodeficient states such as in HIV infection (see **Figures 129-5** and **129-6**) and with immunosuppressive drug treatment.

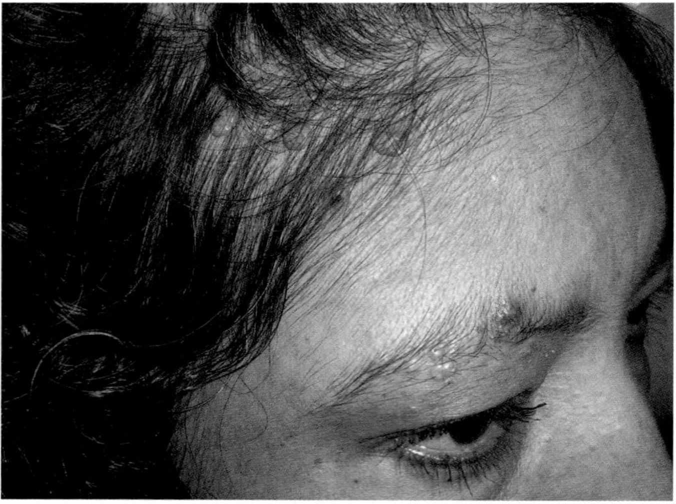

FIGURE 129-5 Molluscum contagiosum on the face of a woman with human immunodeficiency virus. Note the large molluscum on the scalp. (*Reproduced with permission from Richard P. Usatine, MD.*)

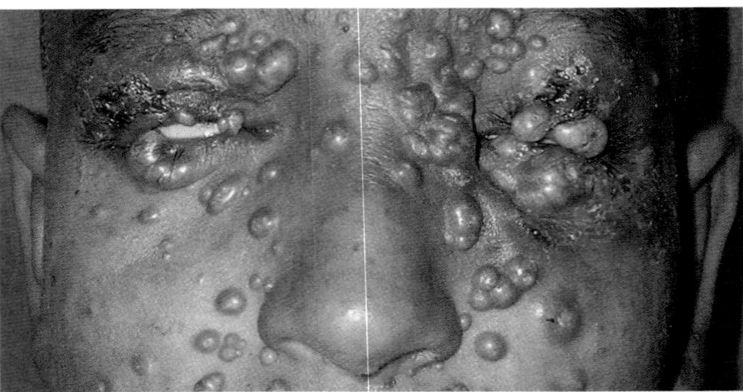

FIGURE 129-6 Giant and widespread molluscum on the face prompted an HIV test that turned out positive. (*Reproduced with permission from Ghosh SK, Bandyopadhyay D, Mandal RK. Multiple facial bumps with weight loss. J Fam Pract. 2010 Dec;59(12):703-705.*)

DIAGNOSIS

CLINICAL FEATURES

- Firm, multiple, 2- to 5-mm dome-shaped papules are seen with a characteristic shiny surface and umbilicated center (**Figure 129-7**). Not all the papules have a central umbilication, so it helps to take a moment and look for a papule that has this characteristic morphology. If all features point to molluscum and no single lesion has central umbilication, do not rule out molluscum as the diagnosis.
- The lesions range in color from pearly white, to flesh-colored, to pink or yellow.
- Pruritus may be present or absent.

TYPICAL DISTRIBUTION

The lesions may appear anywhere on the body except the palms and soles. The number of lesions may be greater in an HIV-infected individual. In adults, they are often found around the genitalia, inguinal area, buttocks, or inner thighs (see **Figure 129-3**). In children, the lesions are often on the trunk or face.

LABORATORY TESTING

- Laboratory testing is not typically indicated.
- Sexually active adolescents and adults with genital lesions should be evaluated for other sexually transmitted diseases, including for HIV infection.

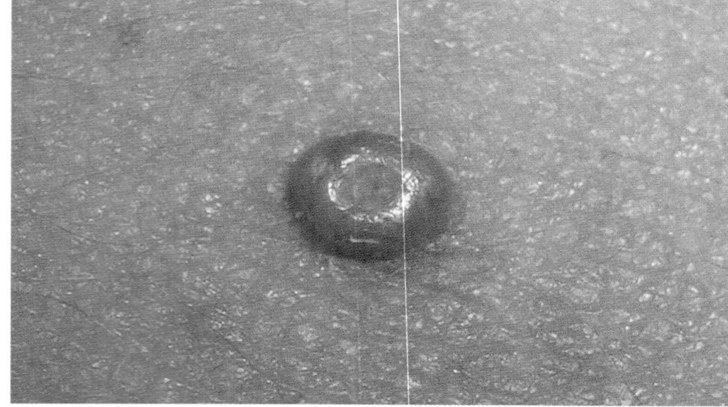

FIGURE 129-7 Close-up of a molluscum lesion showing a dome-shaped pearly papule with a characteristic umbilicated center. (*Reproduced with permission from Richard P. Usatine, MD.*)

BIOPSY

If confirmation is needed, smears of the caseous material expressed from the lesions can be examined directly under the microscope looking for molluscum bodies (enlarged keratinocytes that are engorged with viral inclusion bodies). Hematoxylin and eosin (H&E) staining from a shave biopsy usually reveals keratinocytes that contain eosinophilic cytoplasmic inclusion bodies.[5] If a single lesion is suspicious for basal cell carcinoma (BCC), perform a shave biopsy.

DIFFERENTIAL DIAGNOSIS

- Scabies is caused by *Sarcoptes scabiei* mite and can be transmitted through close or sexual contact. Early lesions are flesh-colored to red papules that produce significant itching. The itching and excoriations are greater than seen with molluscum. Scabies lesions also usually appear in the finger webs, ventral wrist fold, and underneath the breasts in women (see **Chapter 141**, Scabies).
- Dermatofibromas—Firm to hard nodules ranging in color from flesh to black that typically dimple downward when compressed laterally. Usually do not seen in crops as in molluscum. These nodules are deeper in the dermis and do not appear stuck on like molluscum (see **Chapter 158**, Dermatofibroma).
- BCCs are also pearly and raised. Usually not seen in crops as in molluscum. If a single lesion could be a BCC or molluscum, a biopsy is warranted (see **Chapter 168**, Basal Cell Carcinoma).
- Genital warts may be flat and grossly resemble molluscum but they lack the characteristic shiny surface and central umbilication (see **Chapter 132**, Genital Warts).

MANAGEMENT

NONPHARMACOLOGIC

- Treatment of nongenital lesions is usually not medically necessary as the infection is usually self-limited and spontaneously resolves after a few months. Treatment may be performed in an attempt to decrease autoinoculation. Patients and parents of children often want treatment for cosmetic reasons and when watchful waiting fails.
- A 2009 Cochrane Database systematic review investigated the efficacy of treatments for nongenital molluscum contagiosum in healthy individuals and found insufficient evidence to conclude that any treatment was definitively effective.[6] SOR Ⓐ
- In the HIV-infected patient, molluscum may resolve after control of HIV disease with HAART.[3] SOR Ⓑ

MEDICATIONS

- Podophyllotoxin 0.5% (Condylox) is an antimitotic agent that is indicated for the treatment of genital warts. The efficacy of podophyllotoxin was established in a randomized trial of lesions located on the thighs or genitalia. SOR Ⓑ Local erythema, burning, pruritus, inflammation, and erosions can occur with the use of this agent. The safety and efficacy of this drug has not been established in young children.[7]
- Topical imiquimod 5% (Aldara) cream has been shown (not FDA approved) to be better than vehicle alone to treat molluscum.[8,9] SOR Ⓑ It can be well tolerated, although application site irritation can be uncomfortable and lead to discontinuation of therapy. It has been shown not to have systemic or toxic effects in children.[9] In one study, 23 children ranging in age from 1 to 9 years with molluscum contagiosum infection were randomized to either imiquimod cream 5% (12 patients) or vehicle (11 patients). Parents applied the study drug to the patient's lesions 3 times a week for 12 weeks. Complete clearance at week 12 was noted in 33.3% (4/12) of imiquimod patients and in 9.1% (1/11) of vehicle patients.[10]
- Tretinoin cream[11] 0.1% or gel 0.025% applied daily are commonly used but not FDA approved for this indication. SOR Ⓑ
- Cantharidin[12] and trichloroacetic acid[13] are topical chemicals that can be applied by the physician in the office (**Figure 129-8**). SOR Ⓑ Many children will fear treatment with a curette or with any form of cryotherapy.

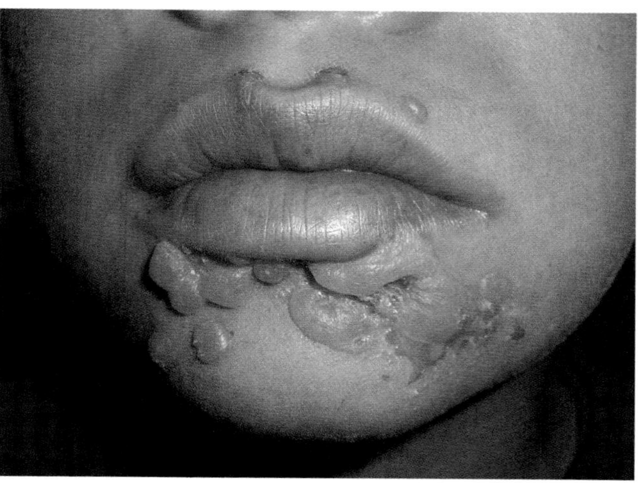

FIGURE 129-8 Blisters that formed the next day after treating molluscum contagiosum with cantharidin. The blisters are not always so large but are supposed to form as the cantharidin is derived from the blister beetle. The blistering helps eradicate the molluscum. (*Reproduced with permission from Richard P. Usatine, MD.*)

SURGICAL

Curettage and cryotherapy are physical methods used to eradicate molluscum.[14,15] SOR Ⓑ

COMPLEMENTARY AND ALTERNATIVE THERAPY

ZymaDerm is a nonprescription, topical, homeopathic agent that is marketed for the treatment of molluscum contagiosum, but no published studies have evaluated its efficacy or safety.

PREVENTION

- Molluscum contagiosum is a common childhood disease.
- Limiting sexual exposure or number of sexual contact may help prevent exposure.
- Genital lesions should be treated to prevent spread by sexual contact.

PROGNOSIS

In immunocompetent patients, lesions usually spontaneously resolve within several months. In a minority of cases, disease persists for a few years.[16]

FOLLOW-UP

Have patients watch for complications that may include irritation, inflammation, and secondary infections. Lesions on eyelids may be associated with follicular or papillary conjunctivitis, so eye irritation should prompt a visit to an eye care specialist.

PATIENT EDUCATION

Instruct patients to avoid scratching to prevent autoinoculation.

PATIENT RESOURCES

- Centers for Disease Control and Prevention. *Molluscum (Molluscum Contagiosum)*—**http://www.cdc.gov/ncidod/dvrd/molluscum/.**
- Pubmed Health. *Molluscum Contagiosum*—**http://www.ncbi.nlm.nih.gov/pubmedhealth/PMH0001829/.**
- American Academy of Dermatology. *Molluscum Contagiosum*—**http://www.aad.org/skin-conditions/dermatology-a-to-z/molluscum-contagiosum.**
- eMedicine Health. *Molluscum Contagiosum*—**http://www.emedicinehealth.com/molluscum_contagiosum/article_em.htm.**
- MedlinePlus. *Molluscum Contagiosum*—**http://www.nlm.nih.gov/medlineplus/ency/article/000826.htm.**

PROVIDER RESOURCES

- eMedicine. *Molluscum Contagiosum*—**http://emedicine.medscape.com/article/910570.**
- Centers for Disease Control and Prevention. *Clinical Information: Molluscum Contagiosum*—**http://www.cdc.gov/ncidod/dvrd/molluscum/clinical_overview.htm.**

REFERENCES

1. Konya J, Thompson CH. Molluscum contagiosum virus: antibody responses in persons with clinical lesions and seroepidemiology in a representative Australian population. *J Infect Dis.* 1999;179(3):701-704.
2. Dohil MA, Lin P, Lee J, et al. The epidemiology of molluscum contagiosum in children. *J Am Acad Dermatol.* 2006;54(1):47-54.
3. Calista D, Boschini A, Landi G. Resolution of disseminated molluscum contagiosum with highly active anti-retroviral therapy (HAART) in patients with AIDS. *Eur J Dermatol.* 1999;9(3):211-213.
4. Schwartz JJ, Myskowski PL. Molluscum contagiosum in patients with human immunodeficiency virus infection. *J Am Acad Dermatol.* 1992;27(4):583-588.
5. Cotell SL, Roholt NS. Images in clinical medicine. Molluscum contagiosum in a patient with the acquired immunodeficiency syndrome. *N Engl J Med.* 1998;338(13):888.
6. van der Wouden JC, van der Sande R, van Suijlekom-Smit LW, et al. Interventions for cutaneous molluscum contagiosum. *Cochrane Database Syst Rev.* 2009 Oct 7;(4):CD004767.
7. Syed TA, Lundin S, Ahmad M. Topical 0.3% and 0.5% podophyllotoxin cream for self-treatment of molluscum contagiosum in males. A placebo-controlled, double-blind study. *Dermatology.* 1994;189(1):65-68.
8. Hengge UR, Esser S, Schultewolter T, et al. Self-administered topical 5% imiquimod for the treatment of common warts and molluscum contagiosum. *Br J Dermatol.* 2000;143(5):1026-1031.
9. Barba AR, Kapoor S, Berman B. An open label safety study of topical imiquimod 5% cream in the treatment of Molluscum contagiosum in children. *Dermatol Online J.* 2001;7(1):20.
10. Theos AU, Cummins R, Silverberg NB, Paller AS. Effectiveness of imiquimod cream 5% for treating childhood molluscum contagiosum in a double-blind, randomized pilot trial. *Cutis.* 2004;74 (2):134-138, 141-142.
11. Papa CM, Berger RS. Venereal herpes-like molluscum contagiosum: treatment with tretinoin. *Cutis.* 1976;18(4):537-540.
12. Silverberg NB, Sidbury R, Mancini AJ. Childhood molluscum contagiosum: experience with cantharidin therapy in 300 patients. *J Am Acad Dermatol.* 2000;43(3):503-507.
13. Yoshinaga IG, Conrado LA, Schainberg SC, Grinblat M. Recalcitrant molluscum contagiosum in a patient with AIDS: combined treatment with CO(2) laser, trichloroacetic acid, and pulsed dye laser. *Lasers Surg Med.* 2000;27(4):291-294.
14. Hanna D, Hatami A, Powell J, et al. A prospective randomized trial comparing the efficacy and adverse effects of four recognized treatments of molluscum contagiosum in children. *Pediatr Dermatol.* 2006;23(6):574-579.
15. Wetmore SJ. Cryosurgery for common skin lesions. Treatment in family physicians' offices. *Can Fam Physician.* 1999;45:964-974.
16. Lee R, Schwartz RA. Pediatric molluscum contagiosum: reflections on the last challenging poxvirus infection, part 1. *Cutis.* 2010;86(5):230-236.

130 COMMON WARTS

E.J. Mayeaux Jr, MD

PATIENT STORY

A young adult presents with a verrucous growth under the eye for 3 months. He does not like the way it looks and he wants it off as soon as possible. Based on the verrucous appearance the physician believed that this growth was nothing more than a common wart (**Figure 130-1**). Treatment options were discussed with the patient and it was decided to shave the growth off after providing local anesthesia. The specimen was sent to pathology and the final diagnosis was verruca vulgaris (common wart).

INTRODUCTION

Human papillomaviruses (HPVs) are DNA viruses that infect skin and mucous membranes. Infection is usually confined to the epidermis and does not result in disseminated systemic infection. The most common clinical manifestation of these viruses is warts (verrucae). There are more than 100 distinct HPV subtypes based on DNA testing. Some tend to infect specific body sites or types of epithelium. Some HPV types have a potential to cause malignant change but transformation is rare on keratinized skin.

SYNONYMS

HPVs are also known as verrucae, verruca vulgaris, or common warts.

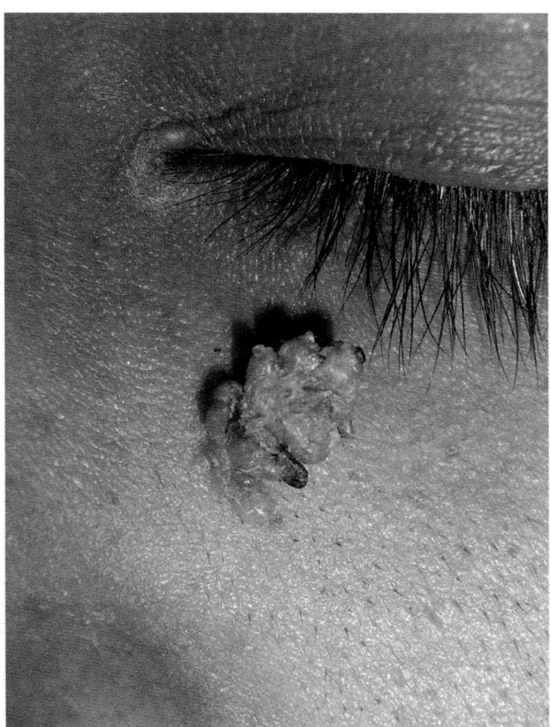

FIGURE 130-1 Common wart under the eye of a young adult. The growth was removed with a shave biopsy and the pathology showed verruca vulgaris. *(Reproduced with permission from Richard P. Usatine, MD.)*

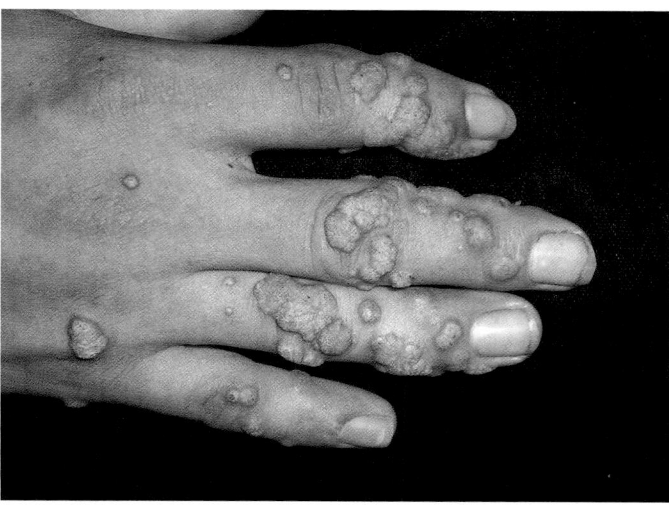

FIGURE 130-2 Many common warts on the hand of an HIV-negative young adult. *(Reproduced with permission from Richard P. Usatine, MD.)*

EPIDEMIOLOGY

- Nongenital cutaneous warts are widespread worldwide and are more common in children, with a peak incidence in the teenage years and a sharp decline thereafter.[1]
- They are most commonly caused by HPV types 1 to 5, 7, 27, 29.[1]
- Common warts account for approximately 70% of nongenital cutaneous warts.[2]
- Common warts occur most commonly in children and young adults (**Figures 130-1** and **130-2**).[3]

ETIOLOGY AND PATHOPHYSIOLOGY

- Infection with HPV occurs by skin-to-skin contact. It starts with a break in the integrity of the epithelium caused by maceration or trauma that allows the virus to infect the basal layers.
- Warts may infect the skin on opposing digits causing "kissing warts" (**Figure 130-3**).
- Individuals with subclinical infection may serve as a reservoir for HPVs.
- An incubation period following inoculation lasts for approximately 2 to 6 months.

RISK FACTORS

- Young age[1]
- Disruption to the normal epithelial barrier
- More common among meat handlers
- Atopic dermatitis
- Nail biters more commonly have multiple periungual warts
- Conditions that decrease cell-mediated immunity such as HIV (**Figure 130-4**) and immunosuppressant drugs (**Figure 130-5**)

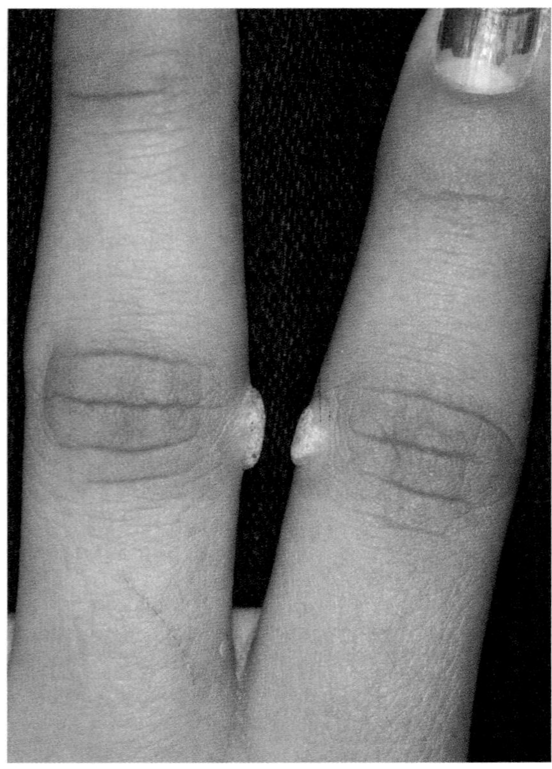

FIGURE 130-3 Warts may infect the skin on opposing digits causing "kissing warts." (*Reproduced with permission from Richard P. Usatine, MD.*)

DIAGNOSIS

CLINICAL FEATURES

- The diagnosis of warts is based on clinical appearance. The wart will obscure normal skin markings.
- Common warts are well demarcated, rough, hard papules with irregular papillary surface. They are usually asymptomatic unless located on a pressure point.
- Warts may form cylindrical of filiform projections (**Figure 130-6**).

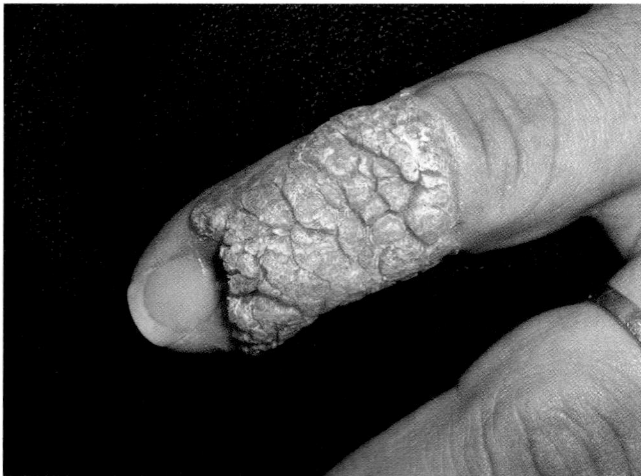

FIGURE 130-4 Large wart on the fifth digit of an HIV-positive man. The wart was biopsied to make sure it had not become squamous cell carcinoma. The most effective treatment so far is cryotherapy but the wart has still not fully resolved. (*Reproduced with permission from Richard P. Usatine, MD.*)

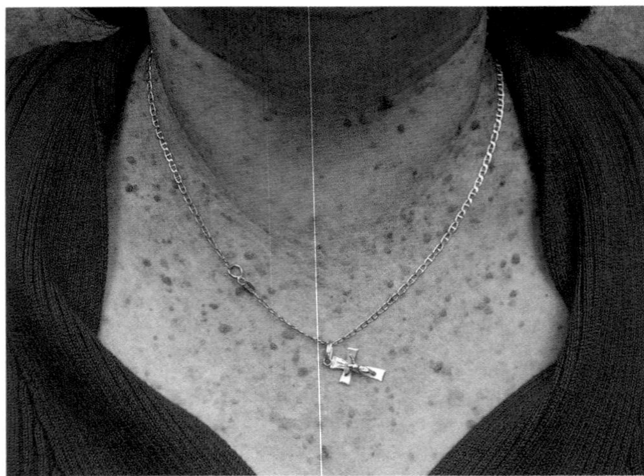

FIGURE 130-5 Biopsy-proven warts on the neck and chest of a woman on azathioprine after a renal transplantation. Human papillomavirus lesions can proliferate as a result of immunosuppressive medications. This patient is also being monitored for squamous cell carcinoma, as this is a more significant risk in posttransplantation patients. (*Reproduced with permission from Richard P. Usatine, MD.*)

TYPICAL DISTRIBUTION

Common anatomic locations include the dorsum of the hand, between the fingers, flexor surfaces, and adjacent to the nails (periungual) (see **Figures 130-1** and **130-2**).

LABORATORY TESTING

- HPV testing is not useful for this condition.[4]
- HIV testing may be useful if the warts are severe and there are risk factors present (see **Figure 130-4**).

BIOPSY

Paring the surface with a surgical blade may expose punctate hemorrhagic capillaries, or black dots, which are thrombosed capillaries. If the diagnosis is in doubt, a shave biopsy is indicated to confirm the diagnosis.

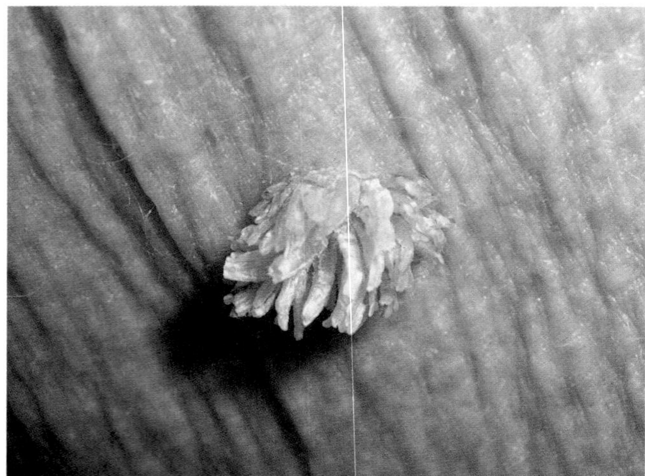

FIGURE 130-6 Filiform warts are identified by their multiple projections as opposed to a unified papule. This wart was on the face of an elderly woman and was removed by shave excision and sent for pathology. It was proven to be a wart and not squamous cell carcinoma. (*Reproduced with permission from Richard P. Usatine, MD.*)

DIFFERENTIAL DIAGNOSIS

- Seborrheic keratosis are usually more darkly pigmented, have a stuck-on appearance, and "horn cysts" may be visible on close examination. They also have a wide distribution on the body (see **Chapter 156**, Seborrheic Keratosis). Typical dermoscopic patterns include comedo-like openings and milia-like cysts (see Appendix C, Dermoscopy)
- Acrochordon (skin tags) are pedunculated flesh-colored papules that are more common in obese persons. They lack the surface roughness of common warts. Filiform warts also may be pedunculated, but typically have a characteristic filiform appearance (see **Chapter 155**, Skin Tag).
- Squamous cell carcinoma (SCC) should be considered when lesions have irregular growth, pigmentation, ulceration, or resist therapy, particularly in sun-exposed areas and in immunosuppressed patients (see **Chapter 169**, Squamous Cell Carcinoma). The patient in **Figure 130-7** had a wart that was not going away and a biopsy demonstrated SCC in situ with in an HPV-induced lesion.
- Amelanotic melanoma—Although rare, lesions that are treatment resistant or atypical should be monitored closely or biopsied to establish the diagnosis (see **Chapter 170**, Melanoma).
- Early warts may appear similar to actinic keratosis in sun-exposed areas (see **Chapter 164**, Actinic Keratosis and Bowen Disease)
- Advanced warts may appear similar to a keratoacanthoma to casual inspection. The characteristic findings of the keratoacanthoma and biopsy will separate the 2 conditions (**Figure 130-8**) (see **Chapter 165**, Keratoacanthoma).

MANAGEMENT

NONPHARMACOLOGIC

- Because spontaneous regression occurs in two-thirds of warts within 2 years, observation without treatment is always an option. In 17 trials, the average reported cure rate was 30% within 10 weeks.[5]

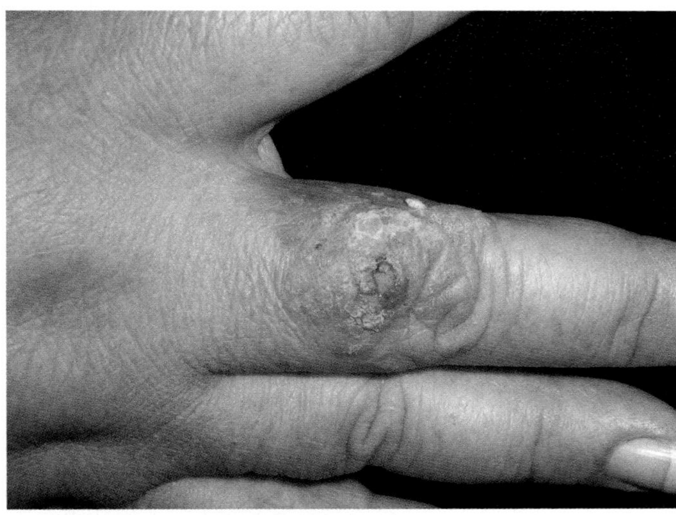

FIGURE 130-7 Squamous cell carcinoma in situ that started from a human papillomavirus-positive lesion. When cryotherapy is not working on what appears to be a wart, consider performing a biopsy. *(Reproduced with permission from Richard P. Usatine, MD.)*

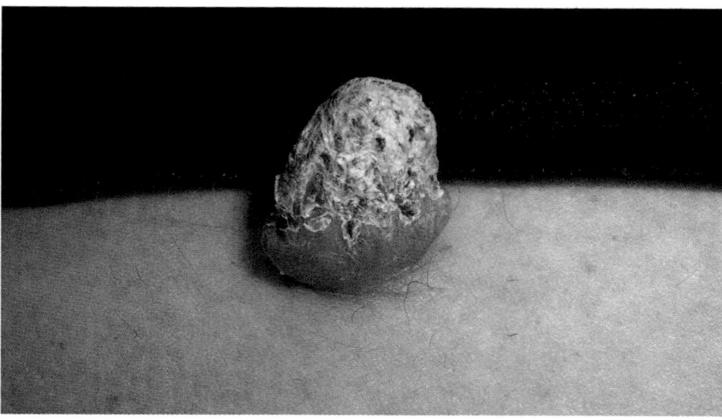

FIGURE 130-8 A new growth on the leg of an older woman turned out to be a wart after it was shaved off and sent to pathology. The clinician was concerned that it could have been a keratoacanthoma based on the central keratin core. *(Reproduced with permission from Richard P. Usatine, MD.)*

Observational studies show that one-half of cutaneous warts resolve spontaneously within 1 year, and about two-thirds within 2 years.[6]

- Treatment does not decrease transmissibility of the virus.[7]

MEDICATIONS

- Therapies for common warts do not specifically treat the HPV virus. They work by destruction of virus-containing skin while preserving uninvolved tissue. This usually exposes the blood and its immune cells to the virus, which may promote an immune response against the virus.
- The least-painful methods should be used first, especially in children. SOR C
- A Cochrane review found that there is a considerable lack of evidence on which to base the rational use of the local treatments for common warts.[5] The trials are highly variable in method and quality. There is evidence that simple topical treatments containing salicylic acid have a therapeutic effect.[5] SOR A There is less evidence for the efficacy of cryotherapy and no convincing evidence that it is any more effective than simple topical treatments.
- Seventeen percent salicylic acid is a useful first-line agent, especially for thick or multiple warts.[5] SOR A It is safe in children. Combined results from 5 randomized controlled trials (RCTs) showed a 73% cure rate with 6 to 12 weeks of salicylic acid treatment, compared with a 48% cure rate with placebo (number needed to treat [NNT] = 4).[5] A number of preparations are available without a prescription. Topical 17% salicylic acid is applied overnight and is now the most commonly used form for this type of wart. Soak the wart area with warm water for 5 minutes, then gently file down any thick skin with a pumice stone or emery board. The salicylic acid product should be applied to the wart. Repeat the first 2 steps daily with liquid or gel preparations, or every other day with the patch. Tape may be used to cover the wart after application of salicylic acid liquid. Repeat treatment until the wart has cleared, or for up to 12 weeks. Discontinue the treatment if severe redness or pain occurs in the treated area. Do not use salicylic acid on the face because of an increased risk of hypopigmentation.[1]
- Forty percent salicylic acid plasters (Mediplast) are available over the counter for larger and thicker warts. The plasters are cut to fit and then applied a few millimeters beyond the wart for 48 hours.

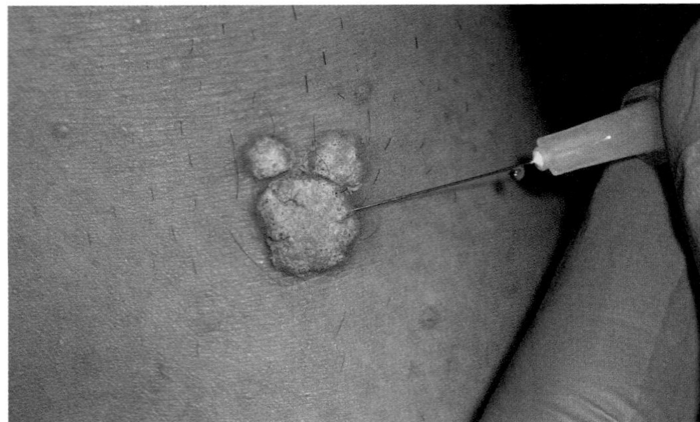

FIGURE 130-9 Candida antigen is being injected into a cluster of warts on the knee of a teenage boy. His warts did not respond to multiple therapies, including topical salicylic acid and cryotherapy. (*Reproduced with permission from Richard P. Usatine, MD.*)

Then the patch is removed; the wart pared down with a nail file, pumice stone, or scalpel; and the process repeated as needed.

- Imiquimod 5% is an expensive topical immunomodulator that is indicated for treatment of anogenital warts but is also used on nongenital warts.[8-10] SOR B It is nonscarring and painless, although local irritation is common. Debriding heavily keratinized warts may enhance penetration of the medication. The cream is applied in a thin layer to the lesions 3 times a week (every other night) and covered with an adhesive bandage or tape. The medication is removed with soap and water in the morning. It can also be used as adjunctive therapy. A lower concentration of imiquimod (3.75% cream) is also available, but data for common warts is lacking.
- Intralesional injections with *Candida* antigen induces a localized, cell-mediated, and HPV-specific response that may target the injected wart as well as more distant warts (**Figure 130-9**). This method has moderate effectiveness (60% cure rates) for treatment of recalcitrant warts in patients with a positive skin antigen pretest.[1] SOR B The *Candida* antigen must be diluted before used (see **Table 131-1**). Inject 0.1 to 0.3 mL into the largest warts using a 30-gauge needle and up to 1 mL per treatment. Warn the patient to expect itching in the area, burning, or peeling. Repeat every 4 weeks, up to 3 treatments or until warts are gone.
- Photodynamic therapy with aminolevulinic acid plus topical salicylic acid is a moderately effective option for treatment of recalcitrant warts.[1] SOR B Although it is likely to be beneficial, it is expensive and often requires referral.
- Cantharidin 0.7% is an extract of the blister beetle that is applied to the wart, after which blistering occurs on the following day. It may be used in resistant cases. It is also useful in young children because application is painless in the office. However, painful blisters often occur within a day after application. Be careful not to overtreat with cantharidin because the blistering can be quite severe. Carefully apply to multiple lesions using the wooden end of a cotton-tipped applicator (**Figure 130-10**). SOR C
- Contact immunotherapy using dinitrochlorobenzene, squaric acid dibutylester, and diphenylcyclopropenone may be applied to the skin to sensitize the patient and then to the lesion to induce an immune response. SOR C

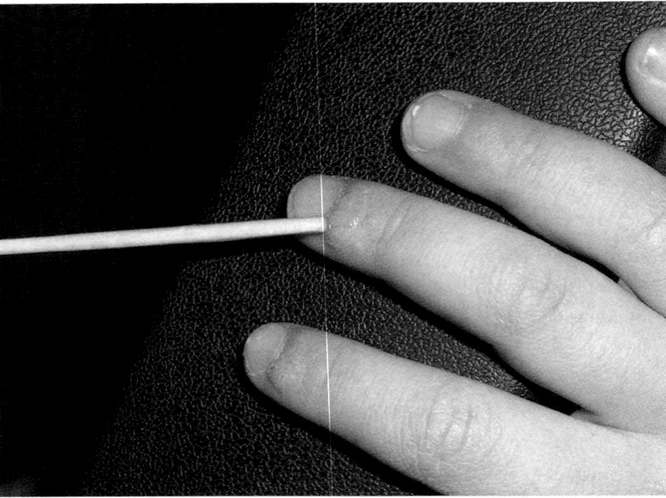

FIGURE 130-10 Cantharidin is being applied to periungual warts. Note the use of the wooden stick of a cotton-tipped applicator. If the cotton tip is used, the cantharidin stays within the cotton and the application is insufficient. (*Reproduced with permission from Richard P. Usatine, MD.*)

- Intralesional injection with bleomycin can be considered for treatment of recalcitrant warts, although the effectiveness is unproven.[1] SOR B
- Early open-label, uncontrolled studies indicate cimetidine might be useful in treating warts. However, 3 placebo-controlled, double-blind studies and 2 open-label comparative trials demonstrate that its efficacy is equal to placebo.[11] SOR A

SURGICAL

- Cryotherapy, most commonly with liquid nitrogen, is useful but is somewhat painful for younger children.[5] SOR B Chemical cryogens are now available over the counter but are not as cold or effective as liquid nitrogen. Most trials comparing cryotherapy with salicylic acid found similar effectiveness, with overall cure rates of 50% to 70% after 3 or 4 treatments.[1] Aggressive cryotherapy (10-30 seconds) is more effective than less-aggressive cryotherapy, but may increase complications.[1] SOR B Anesthesia is usually unnecessary but may be achieved with 1% lidocaine or eutectic mixture of local anesthetics (EMLA) cream. Liquid nitrogen is applied for 10 to 20 seconds via a Cryogun or a cotton swab so that the freeze ball extends 2 mm beyond the lesion (**Figure 130-11**). Two freeze cycles may

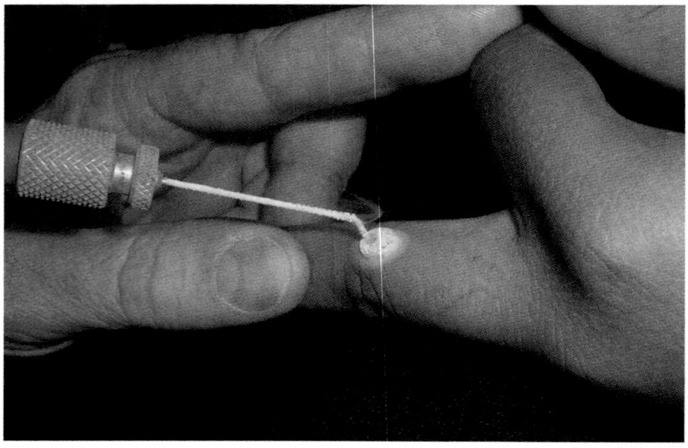

FIGURE 130-11 Cryotherapy showing an adequate free zone (halo) around the wart. (*Reproduced with permission from Richard P. Usatine, MD.*)

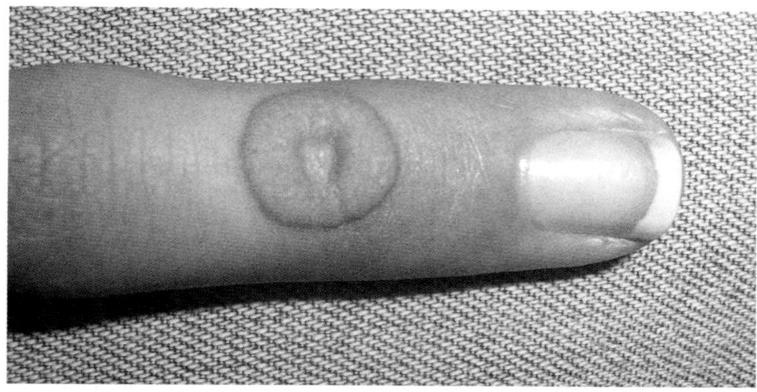

FIGURE 130-12 Ring wart that resulted from inadequate cryotherapy of a common wart. (*Reproduced with permission from Richard P. Usatine, MD.*)

improve resolution, but it is better to underfreeze than overfreeze as overfreezing may lead to permanent scarring or hypopigmentation. Best results of cryotherapy can be achieved when the patient is treated every 2 or 3 weeks. There is no therapeutic benefit beyond 3 months.[1] SOR Ⓑ Because HPV can survive in liquid nitrogen, cotton swabs and residual liquid nitrogen should be properly discarded to avoid spreading the virus to other patients or contaminating the liquid nitrogen reservoir.[12] After cryotherapy, the skin shows erythema and may progress to hemorrhagic blistering. Healing occurs in approximately a week and hypopigmentation may occur. Ring warts may result from an inadequate margin of treatment of a common wart (**Figure 130-12**). Common adverse effects of cryotherapy include pain, blistering, and hypo- or hyperpigmentation. Cryotherapy must be used cautiously where nerves are located superficially (such as on the fingers) to prevent pain and neuropathy. Overfreezing in the periungual region can result in permanent nail dystrophy.

- Cryotherapy can be combined with other modalities. In **Figure 130-13**, a man with warts on his lips was frustrated that the cryotherapy was not working so his treatment was modified to include topical trichloroacetic acid applied to the warts after the cryotherapy.

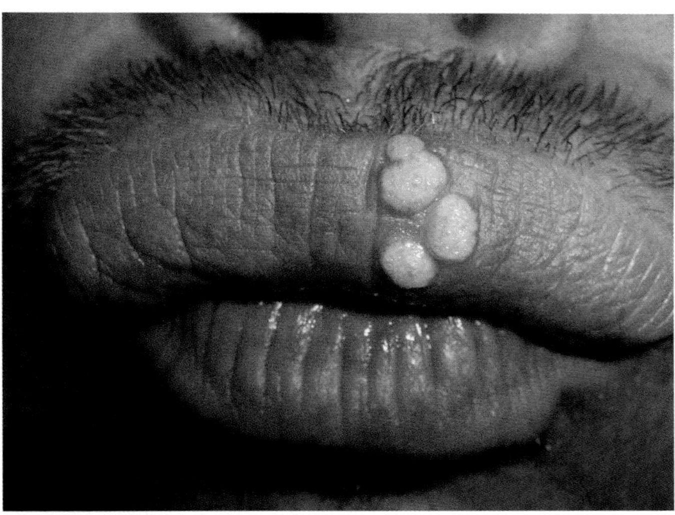

FIGURE 130-13 Common warts on the lip of a young man after cryotherapy and trichloroacetic acid (TCA) were applied. The TCA was added to the treatment when the cryotherapy alone was not working. The warts did resolve after a few combination treatments. (*Reproduced with permission from Richard P. Usatine, MD.*)

- Simple excision is used for small or filiform warts (see **Figures 130-1** and **130-7**). The area is injected with lidocaine and the wart is excised with sharp scissors or a scalpel blade. SOR Ⓒ
- Pulsed-dye laser can be considered for treatment of recalcitrant warts, although the effectiveness is unproven.[1] SOR Ⓑ

COMPLEMENTARY AND ALTERNATIVE THERAPY

Although preliminary studies were promising, duct tape is of uncertain efficacy for wart treatment.[1] A randomized controlled trial in adults showed it to be no better than moleskin and both groups only had a 21% to 22% success rate.[13] SOR Ⓑ

PREVENTION

- Tools used for paring down warts, such as nail files and pumice stones, should not be used on normal skin or by other people.
- Hair-bearing areas with warts should be shaved with depilatories, electric razors, or not at all to help limit spread of warts.

PROGNOSIS

- Sixty percent to 70% of cutaneous warts resolve in 3 to 24 months without treatment.[14,15]
- New warts may appear while others are regressing. This is not a treatment failure but part of the natural disease process with HPV.

FOLLOW-UP

- Schedule patients for return visits after treatment to limit loss of follow-up and to assess therapy.
- Follow-up visits can be left to the patient's discretion when self-applied therapy is being used.

PATIENT EDUCATION

Therapy often takes weeks to months, so patience and perseverance are essential for successful therapy.

PATIENT RESOURCES

- AFP Patient Information. *Am Fam Physician*. 2011;84(3): 296—**http://www.aafp.org/afp/2011/0801/p296.html.**
- eMedicine Health—**http://www.emedicinehealth.com/warts/article_em.htm.**
- BUPA. *Warts and Verrucas Patient Information*—**http://www.bupa.co.uk/individuals/health-information/directory/w/warts-and-verrucas?tab=Resources.**
- FamilyDoctor.org. American Academy of Family Physicians. *Warts*—**http://familydoctor.org/209.xml.**
- MayoClinic.com. *Common Warts*—**http://www.mayoclinic.com/health/common-warts/DS00370.**

PROVIDER RESOURCES

- eMedicine. *Nongenital Warts*—**http://emedicine.medscape.com/article/1133317.**
- For information on treating warts including how to dilute Candida antigen: Usatine R, Pfenninger J, Stulberg D, Small R. *Dermatologic and Cosmetic Procedures in Office Practice*. Philadelphia, PA: Elsevier; 2012. This can also be purchased as an electronic application at **www.usatinemedia.com.**
- Cutaneous warts: An evidence-based approach to therapy. *Am Fam Physician*. 2005;72:647-652. **http://www.aafp.org/afp/20050815/647.html.**
- Medline Plus. *Warts*—**http://www.nlm.nih.gov/medlineplus/ency/article/000885.htm.**
- Cochrane review. *Topical Treatments for Cutaneous Warts*—**http://www.cochrane.org/reviews/en/ab001781.html.**

REFERENCES

1. Mulhem E, Pinelis S. Treatment of nongenital cutaneous warts. *Am Fam Physician*. 2011;84(3):288-293.
2. Micali G, Dall'Oglio F, Nasca MR, et al. Management of cutaneous warts: an evidence-based approach. *Am J Clin Dermatol*. 2004;5(5):311-317.
3. Kilkenny M, Marks R. The descriptive epidemiology of warts in the community. *Australas J Dermatol*. 1996;37:80-86.
4. Sterling JC, Handfield-Jones S, Hudson PM; British Association of Dermatologists. Guidelines for the management of cutaneous warts. *Br J Dermatol*. 2001;144(1):4-11.
5. Gibbs S, Harvey I, Sterling JC, Stark R. Local treatments for cutaneous warts. *Cochrane Database Syst Rev*. 2001;(2):CD001781.
6. Massing AM, Epstein WL. Natural history of warts. A two-year study. *Arch Dermatol*. 1963;87:306-310.
7. Rivera A, Tyring SK. Therapy of cutaneous human papillomavirus infections. *Dermatol Ther*. 2004;17(6):441-448.
8. Micali G, Dall'Oglio F, Nasca MR. An open label evaluation of the efficacy of imiquimod 5% cream in the treatment of recalcitrant subungual and periungual cutaneous warts. *J Dermatolog Treat*. 2003;14:233-236.
9. Hengge UR, Esser S, Schultewolter T, et al. Self-administered topical 5% imiquimod for the treatment of common warts and molluscum contagiosum. *Br J Dermatol*. 2000;143:1026-1031.
10. Grussendorf-Conen EI, Jacobs S. Efficacy of imiquimod 5% cream in the treatment of recalcitrant warts in children. *Pediatr Dermatol*. 2002;19:263-266.
11. Yilmaz E, Alpsoy E, Basaran E. Cimetidine therapy for warts: a placebo-controlled, double-blind study. *J Am Acad Dermatol*. 1996;34(6):1005-1007.
12. Tabrizi SN, Garland SM. Is cryotherapy treating or infecting? *Med J Aust*. 1996;164(5):263.
13. Wenner R, Askari SK, Cham PM, et al. Duct tape for the treatment of common warts in adults: a double-blind randomized controlled trial. *Arch Dermatol*. 2007;143(3):309-313.
14. Allen AL, Siegfried EC. What's new in human papillomavirus infection. *Curr Opin Pediatr*. 2000;12:365-369.
15. Sterling JC, Handfield-Jones S, Hudson PM. Guidelines for the management of cutaneous warts. *Br J Dermatol*. 2001;144:4-11.

131 FLAT WARTS

E.J. Mayeaux Jr, MD

PATIENT STORY

A young woman presents with multiple flat lesions surrounding her left eyebrow (**Figure 131-1**). It started with just a few lesions but has spread over the past 3 months. The lesions are unilateral. She is diagnosed with flat warts and various treatment methods are discussed. The patient chose to try topical tretinoin cream.

INTRODUCTION

Flat warts are characterized as flat or slightly elevated flesh-colored papules. They may be smooth or slightly hyperkeratotic. They range in size from 1 to 5 mm or more, and numbers range from a few to hundreds of lesions, which may become grouped or confluent. They occur most commonly on the face, hands, and shins. They may appear in a linear distribution as a result of scratching, shaving, or trauma (Koebner phenomenon) (**Figure 131-2**).

SYNONYMS

Flat warts are also known as plane warts, verruca plana, and verruca plana juvenilis.

EPIDEMIOLOGY

- Flat warts (verruca plana) are most commonly found in children and young adults (**Figures 131-1** to **131-5**).
- Flat warts are the least common variety of wart, but are generally numerous on an individual.[1]

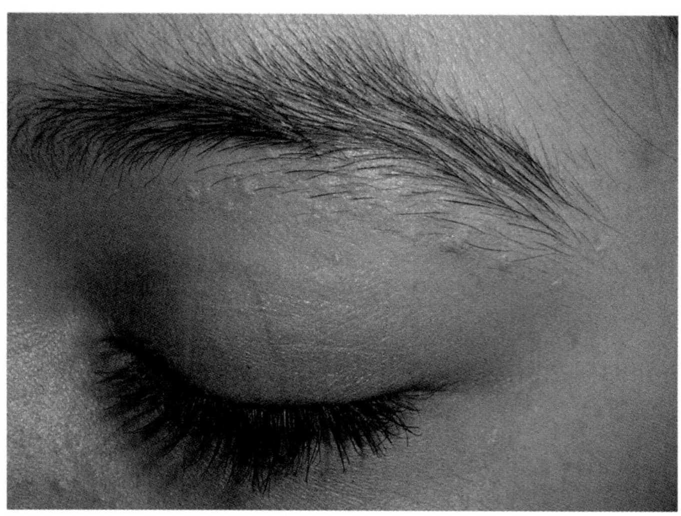

FIGURE 131-1 Flat warts on a patient's eyebrow skin. (*Reproduced with permission from Richard P. Usatine, MD.*)

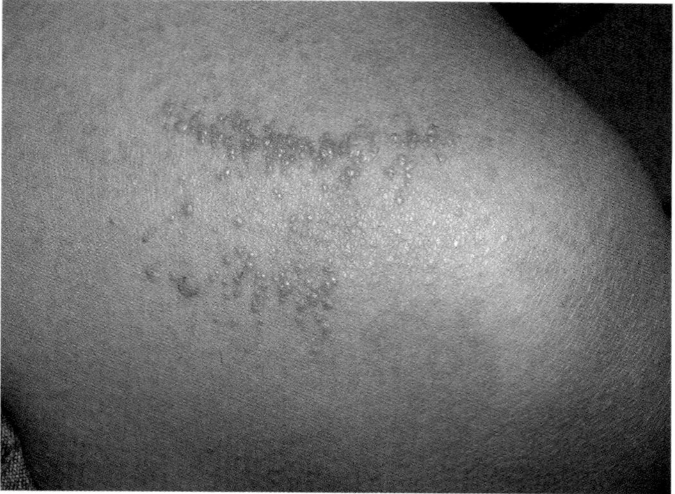

A

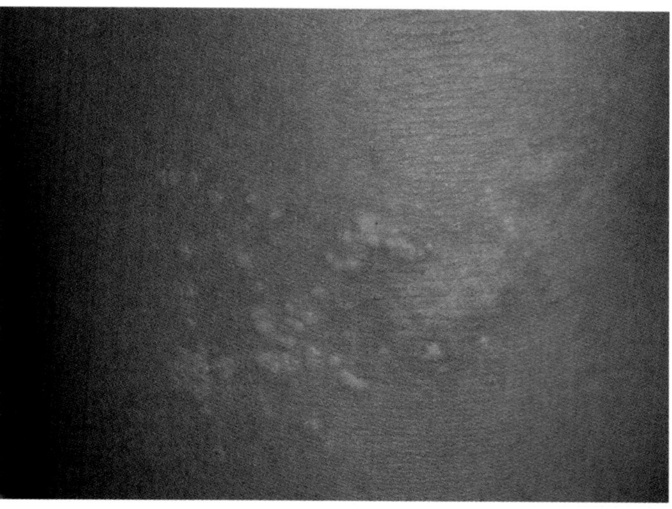

B

FIGURE 131-2 A. and B. Two different young women with flat warts around the knees spread by shaving. (*Reproduced with permission from Richard P. Usatine, MD.*)

- Flat warts are usually caused by human papillomavirus (HPV) types 3, 10, 28, and 29.[2]

ETIOLOGY AND PATHOPHYSIOLOGY

- Like all warts, flat warts are caused by HPV.[2]
- Flat warts may spread in a linear pattern secondary to spread by scratching or trauma, such as shaving.
- Flat warts present a special treatment problem because they persist for a long time; they are generally located in cosmetically important areas, and they are resistant to therapy.

RISK FACTORS

- Shaving next to infected areas (see **Figures 131-2** and **131-3**)
- HIV infection or other types of immunosuppression (see **Figure 131-3**)

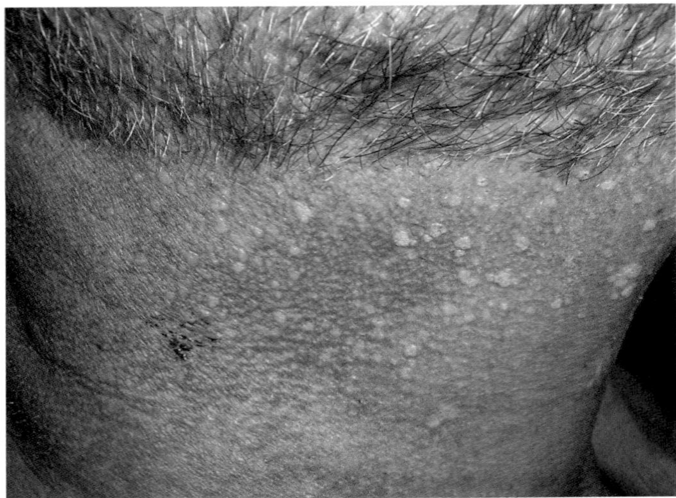

FIGURE 131-3 Flat warts on the neck of an HIV-positive man. The warts have been spread by shaving. Cryotherapy and imiquimod were not successful but intralesional *Candida* antigen injections cleared all the warts. (*Reproduced with permission from Richard P. Usatine, MD.*)

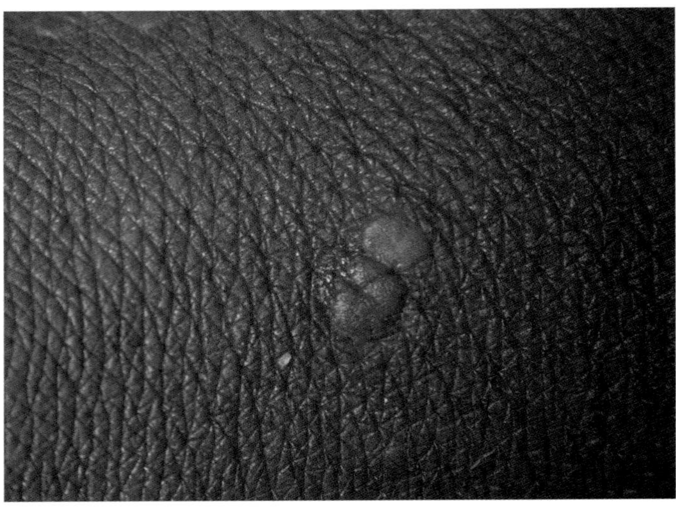

FIGURE 131-4 Close-up of a flat wart. Note typical small, flat-topped papule. (*Reproduced with permission from Richard P. Usatine, MD.*)

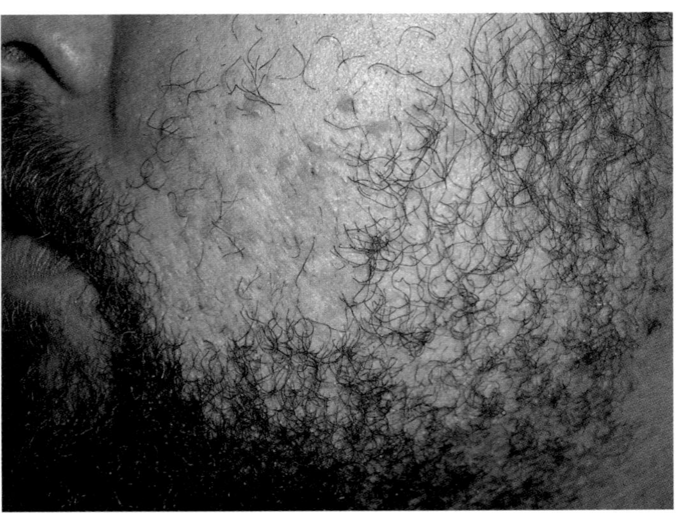

FIGURE 131-5 Flat warts on the face of a man on prednisone for sarcoidosis. (*Reproduced with permission from Richard P. Usatine, MD.*)

DIAGNOSIS

CLINICAL FEATURES

flat warts are multiple small, flat-topped papules that may be pink, light-brown, or light-yellow colored. They may be polygonal in shape (see **Figure 131-4**).

TYPICAL DISTRIBUTION

Flat warts typically appear on the forehead (see **Figure 131-1**), around the mouth, the backs of the hands, and shaved areas, such as the lower face and neck in men (see **Figures 131-3** and **131-5**) and the lower legs in women (see **Figure 131-2**).

LABORATORY TESTING

HPV testing is not useful for this condition.[3]

BIOPSY

Although usually not necessary, a shave biopsy can confirm the diagnosis.

DIFFERENTIAL DIAGNOSIS

- Lichen planus produces flat-topped papules that may be confused with flat warts. Look for characteristic signs of lichen planus such as the symmetric distribution, purplish coloration, and oral lacy lesions. (Wickham striae are white, fine, reticular scale seen on the lesions.) The distribution of lichen planus is different, with the most common sites being the ankles, wrists, and back (see Chapter 152, Lichen Planus).
- Seborrheic keratoses are often more darkly pigmented and have a stuck-on appearance; "horn cysts" may be visible on close examination (see Chapter 156, Seborrheic Keratosis).
- Squamous cell carcinoma should be considered when lesions have irregular growth or pigmentation, ulceration, or resist therapy, particularly in sun-exposed areas and in immunosuppressed patients (see Chapter 169, Squamous Cell Carcinoma).

MANAGEMENT

NONPHARMACOLOGIC

- Regression of these lesions may occur, which usually is heralded by inflammation.
- There are no current therapies for HPV that are virus specific.

MEDICATIONS

- Topical salicylic acid treatments by topical liquid or patch are the most effective treatment for all types of warts with a success rate average of 73% from 5 pooled placebo-controlled trials.[4] Number needed to treat (NNT) = 4. SOR Ⓐ Salicylic acid may be more acceptable on the legs than the face.[2] Often, 17% salicylic acid topicals are applied overnight daily until the warts resolve.
- Fluorouracil (Efudex 5% cream, Fluoroplex 1%) may be used to treat flat warts. Apply the cream to affected areas twice daily for 3 to 4 weeks. Sun protection is essential because the drug is

photosensitizing. Persistent hypo- or hyperpigmentation may occur following use, but applying it with a cotton-tipped applicator to individual lesions instead of to the area may minimize this adverse reaction.[5,6] SOR B

- Imiquimod 5% cream is an expensive topical immunomodulator that has shown some efficacy in treating flat warts.[7,8] It is nonscarring and painless to apply. There are rare reports of systemic side effects. The cream is applied to the lesions 3 times a week (every other day). The cream may be applied to the affected area, not strictly to the lesion itself.[9] It can be used on all external HPV-infected sites, but not on occluded mucous membranes. Therapy can be temporarily halted if symptoms become problematic. Imiquimod has the advantage of having almost no risk of scarring.[7,8] SOR B A lower concentration of imiquimod (3.75% cream) is also available, but data for its use with flat or common warts are lacking.
- Tretinoin cream, 0.025%, 0.05%, or 0.1%, applied at bedtime over the entire involved area is one accepted treatment. The frequency of application is then adjusted so as to produce a mild, fine scaling and erythema. Sun protection is important. Treatment may be required for weeks or months and may not be effective. No published studies were found to support this treatment. SOR C
- Intralesional injections with *Candida* antigen induce a localized, cell-mediated, and HPV-specific response that may target the injected wart as well as more distant warts. This method has moderate effectiveness (60% cure rates) for treatment of recalcitrant warts (**Figures 131-3** and **131-6**).[2] The *Candida* antigen must be diluted before used (see **Table 131-1**). Inject 0.1 to 0.3 mL into the largest warts using a 30-gauge needle and up to 1 mL per treatment. Warn the patient to expect itching in the area, burning, or peeling. Repeat every 4 weeks, up to 3 treatments or until warts are gone.[10] SOR B
- Photodynamic therapy with aminolevulinic acid plus topical salicylic acid is a moderately effective option for treatment of recalcitrant warts. Although it is likely to be beneficial, it is expensive and often requires dermatologic referral.[2] SOR B
- Cantharidin 0.7% is an extract of the blister beetle that is applied to the wart after which blistering occurs. It may be used in resistant cases.[11] It is also useful in young children because application is painless in the office. However, painful blisters often occur within a day after application. Be careful not to overtreat with cantharidin because the blistering can be quite severe. Carefully apply to multiple lesions using the wooden end of a cotton-tipped applicator. SOR C

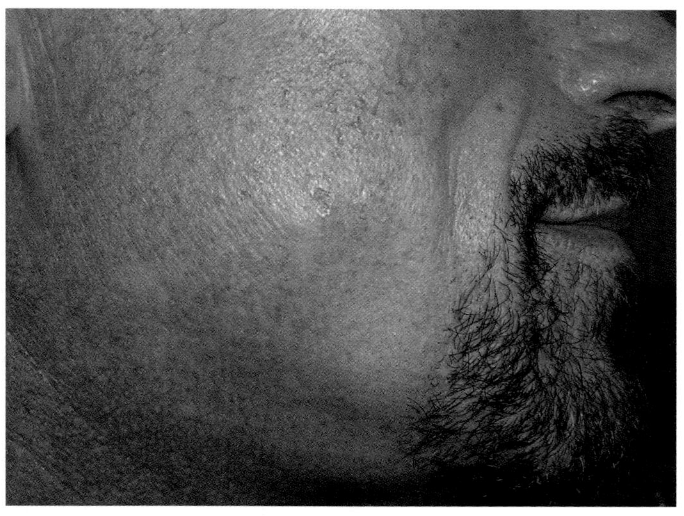

FIGURE 131-6 The same man in **Figure 131-3** after successful treatment with *Candida* antigen. (*Reproduced with permission from Richard P. Usatine, MD.*)

TABLE 131-1 *Candida* Dilutions

Creating 1 mL for Injection	Candida Antigen (mL)	2% Lidocaine (No Epinephrine) (mL)
Generic 1:1000	0.25	0.75
Candin 1:500	0.5	0.5

Data from Usatine RP, Pfenninger J, Stulberg D, Small R. *Dermatologic and Cosmetic Procedures in Office Practice*. Philadelphia, PA: Elsevier Inc.; 2012.

SURGICAL

- Cryotherapy, most commonly with liquid nitrogen, is useful but is somewhat painful for younger children.[6] SOR B Chemical cryogens are now available over the counter but are not as cold or effective as liquid nitrogen. Most trials comparing cryotherapy with salicylic acid found similar effectiveness.[2] Liquid nitrogen is applied for 5 to 10 seconds via a Cryogun or a cotton swab so that the freeze ball extends 1 to 2 mm beyond the lesion. Because flat warts are thinner than common warts, the freeze times needed are shorter. Two freeze cycles may improve resolution, but it is better to underfreeze than overfreeze since overfreezing may lead to permanent scarring or hypopigmentation. Best results of cryotherapy can be achieved when the patient is treated every 2 or 3 weeks. There is no therapeutic benefit beyond 3 months.[2] SOR B Because HPV can survive in liquid nitrogen, cotton swabs and residual liquid nitrogen should be properly discarded to avoid spreading the virus to other patients or contaminating the liquid nitrogen reservoir.[12] After cryotherapy, the skin shows erythema and may progress to hemorrhagic blistering. Healing occurs in approximately a week and hypopigmentation may occur. Common adverse effects of cryotherapy include pain, blistering, and hypo- or hyperpigmentation.
- Pulsed-dye laser can be considered for treatment of recalcitrant warts, although the effectiveness is unproven.[2] SOR B

PREVENTION

Hair-bearing areas with warts should be shaved with depilatories, electric razors, or not at all to help limit spread of warts.

FOLLOW-UP

Schedule patients for a return visit in 2 to 3 weeks after therapy to assess efficacy.

PATIENT EDUCATION

- To help avoid spreading warts, patients should avoid touching or scratching the lesions.
- Razors that are used in areas where warts are located should not be used on normal skin or by other people to prevent spread.

PATIENT RESOURCES

- KidsHealth. *Warts*—**http://www.kidshealth.org/parent/infections/skin/wart.html.**
- American Academy of Dermatology. *Warts*—**http://www.aad.org/public/Publications/pamphlets/Warts.htm.**
- MedlinePlus. *Warts*—**http://www.nlm.nih.gov/medlineplus/ency/article/000885.htm.**

PROVIDER RESOURCES

- Bacelieri R, Johnson SM. Cutaneous warts. An evidence-based approach to therapy. *Am Fam Physician.* 2005;72:647-652. **http://www.aafp.org/afp/20050815/647.html.**
- Cochrane Review. *Topical Treatments for Cutaneous Warts*—**http://www.cochrane.org/reviews/en/ab001781.html.**
- Treatment of warts is covered extensively in Usatine R, Pfenninger J, Stulberg D, Small R. *Dermatologic and Cosmetic Procedures in Office Practice.* Philadelphia, PA: Elsevier Inc.; 2012. This can also be purchased as an electronic application at **www.usatinemedia.com.**

REFERENCES

1. Williams H, Pottier A, Strachan D. Are viral warts seen more commonly in children with eczema? *Arch Dermatol.* 1993;129:717-720.
2. Mulhem E, Pinelis S. Treatment of nongenital cutaneous warts. *Am Fam Physician.* 2011;84(3):288-293.
3. Sterling JC, Handfield-Jones S, Hudson PM; British Association of Dermatologists. Guidelines for the management of cutaneous warts. *Br J Dermatol.* 2001;144(1):4-11.
4. Gibbs S, Harvey I. Topical treatments for cutaneous warts. *Cochrane Database Syst Rev.* 2006;(3):CD001781.
5. Lockshin NA. Flat facial warts treated with fluorouracil. *Arch Dermatol.* 1979;115:929-1030.
6. Lee S, Kim J-G, Chun SI. Treatment of verruca plana with 5% 5-fluorouracil ointment. *Dermatologica.* 1980;160:383-389.
7. Cutler K, Kagen MH, Don PC, et al. Treatment of facial verrucae with topical imiquimod cream in a patient with human immunodeficiency virus. *Acta Derm Venereol.* 2000;80:134-135.
8. Kim MB. Treatment of flat warts with 5% imiquimod cream. *J Eur Acad Dermatol Venereol.* 2006;20(10):1349-1350.
9. Schwab RA, Elston DM. Topical imiquimod for recalcitrant facial flat warts. *Cutis.* 2000;65:160-162.
10. Ritter SE, Meffert J. Successful treatment of flat warts using intralesional *Candida* antigen. *Arch Dermatol.* 2003;139(4):541-542.
11. Kartal Durmazlar SP, Atacan D, Eskioglu F. Cantharidin treatment for recalcitrant facial flat warts: a preliminary study. *J Dermatolog Treat.* 2009;20(2):114-119.
12. Tabrizi SN, Garland SM. Is cryotherapy treating or infecting? *Med J Aust.* 1996;164(5):263.

132 GENITAL WARTS

E.J. Mayeaux, Jr, MD
Richard P. Usatine, MD

PATIENT STORY

An 18-year-old woman presents with a concern that she might have genital warts (**Figure 132-1**). She never had a sexually transmitted disease (STD) but admits to 2 new sexual partners in the last 6 months. She has not been vaccinated against human papillomavirus (HPV). The patient is told that her concern is accurate and she has condyloma caused by HPV (an STD). The treatment options are discussed and she chooses to have cryotherapy with liquid nitrogen followed by imiquimod self-applied beginning 2 weeks after cryotherapy. A urine test for gonorrhea and *Chlamydia* is performed and the patient is sent to the laboratory to have blood tests for syphilis and HIV. Fortunately, all the additional tests are negative. Further patient education is performed and follow-up is arranged.

INTRODUCTION

More than 100 types of HPV exist, with more than 40 that can infect the human genital area. Most HPV infections are asymptomatic, unrecognized, or subclinical. Low-risk HPV types (eg, HPV types 6 and 11) cause genital warts, although coinfection with HPV types associated with squamous intraepithelial neoplasia can occur. Asymptomatic genital HPV infection is common and usually self-limited.[1]

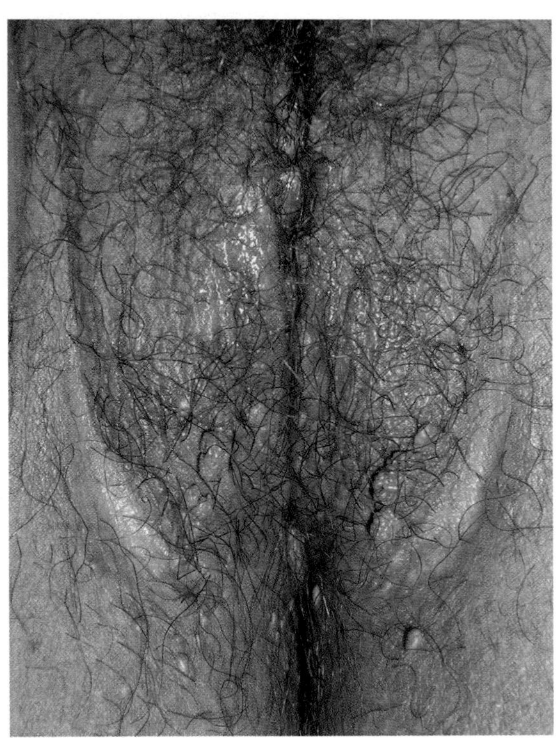

FIGURE 132-1 Multiple vulvar exophytic condyloma in an 18-year-old woman. (*Reproduced with permission from Richard P. Usatine, MD.*)

SYNONYMS

Genital warts are also known as condyloma acuminata.

EPIDEMIOLOGY

- Anogenital warts are the most common viral STD in the United States. There are approximately 1 million new cases of genital warts per year in the United States.[2]
- Most infections are transient and cleared within 2 years.[2]
- Some infections persist and recur and cause much distress for the patients.

ETIOLOGY AND PATHOPHYSIOLOGY

- Genital warts are caused by HPV infection. HPV encompasses a family of primarily sexually transmitted double-stranded DNA viruses. The incubation period after exposure ranges from 3 weeks to 8 months.

RISK FACTORS

- Sexual intercourse and oral sex[3]
- Other types of sexual activity including digital–anal, oral–anal, and digital–vaginal contact
- Immunosuppression, especially HIV (**Figure 132-2**)

DIAGNOSIS

CLINICAL FEATURES

- Diagnosis of genital warts is usually clinical based on visual inspection.[1]
- Genital warts are usually asymptomatic, and typically present as flesh-colored, exophytic lesions on the genitalia, including the penis, vulva, vagina, scrotum, perineum, and perianal skin.

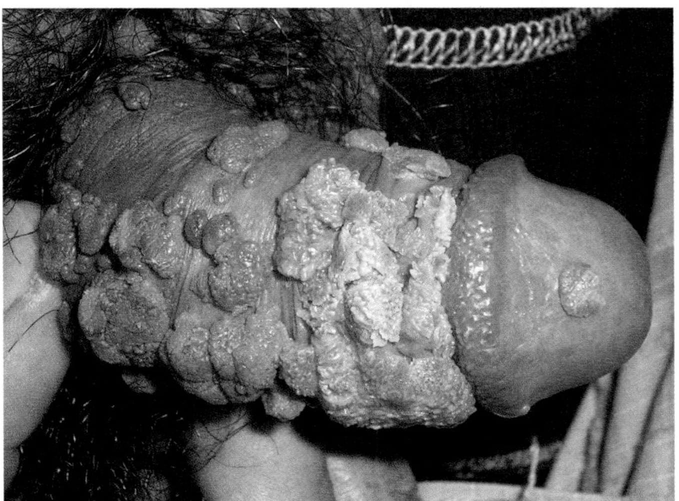

FIGURE 132-2 Multiple exophytic condyloma on the penis of a man with AIDS. (*Reproduced with permission from Richard P. Usatine, MD.*)

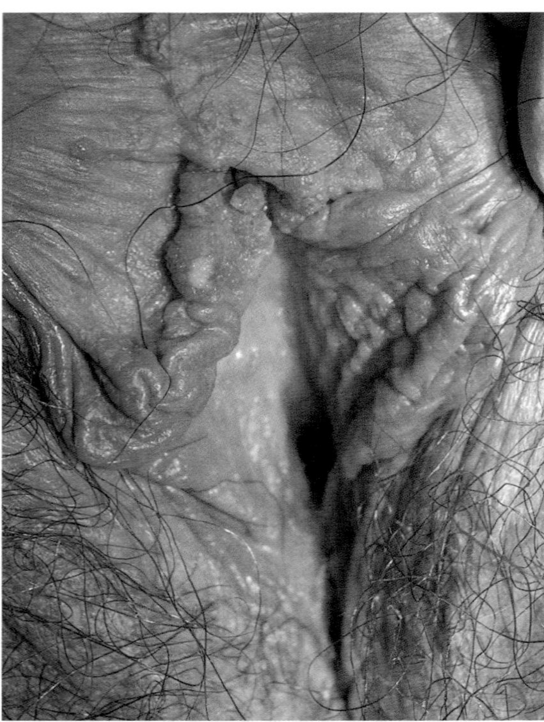

FIGURE 132-3 Condyloma around the clitoris, labia minor, and opening of the vagina. (*Reproduced with permission from Richard P. Usatine, MD.*)

- External warts can appear as small bumps, or they may be flat, verrucous, or pedunculated (**Figures 132-2** to **132-4**).
- Less commonly, warts can appear as reddish or brown, smooth, raised papules or as dome-shaped lesions on keratinized skin.

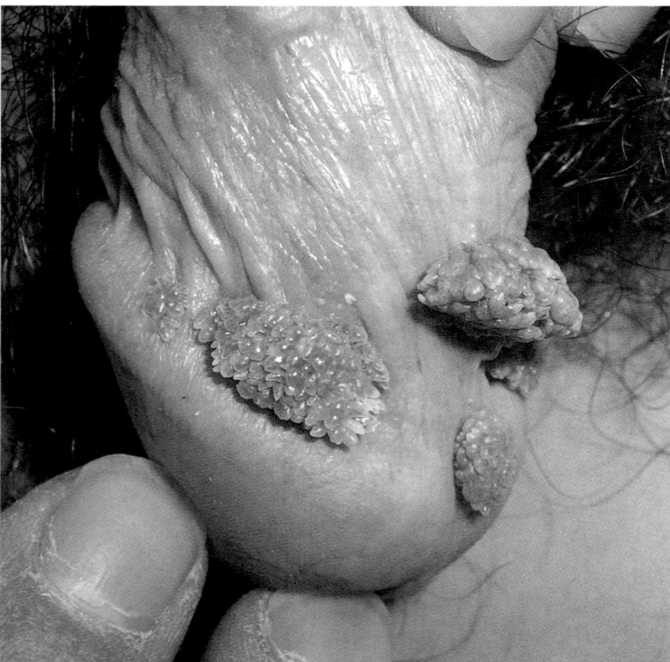

FIGURE 132-4 Condyloma acuminata demonstrating a cauliflower appearance with typical papillary surface seen when the foreskin is retracted in an uncircumcised man. Note that the top wart is pedunculated with a narrow base. (*Reproduced with permission from Richard P. Usatine, MD.*)

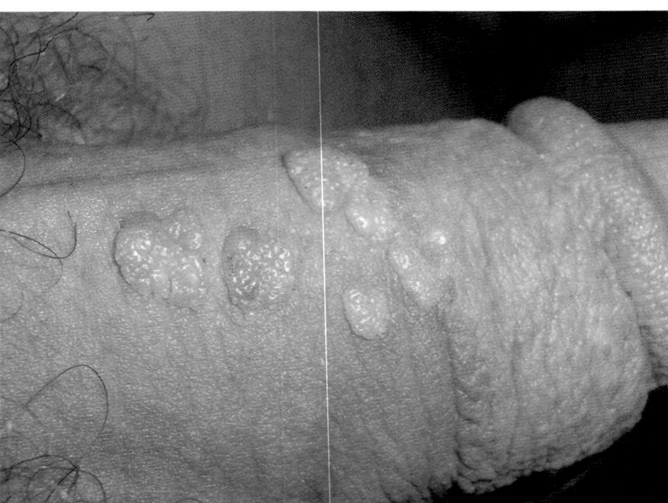

FIGURE 132-5 Smooth-topped condyloma on the well-keratinized skin of a circumcised man. (*Reproduced with permission from Richard P. Usatine, MD.*)

TYPICAL DISTRIBUTION

- In women, the most common sites of infection are the vulva (85%) (see **Figure 132-1**), perianal area (58%), and the vagina (42%) (see **Figure 132-3**).
- In men, the most common sites of infection are the penis (**Figures 132-4** and **132-5**) and scrotum.
- Perianal warts (**Figure 132-6**) can occur in men or women who have a history of anal intercourse and in those who do not have any such history (**Figure 132-7**).[1]
- Condyloma acuminata may be seen on the abdomen or upper thighs in conjunction with genital warts (**Figure 132-8**).

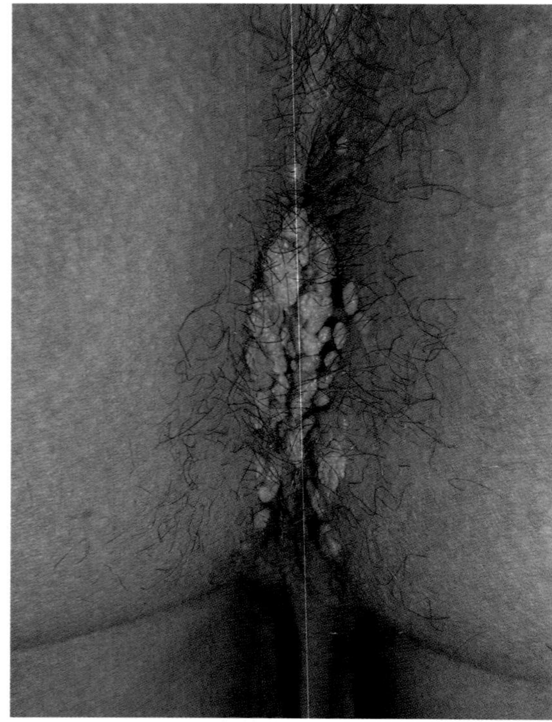

FIGURE 132-6 Perianal warts in a gay man with history of anal-receptive intercourse. These lesions responded to cryotherapy. (*Reproduced with permission from Richard P. Usatine, MD.*)

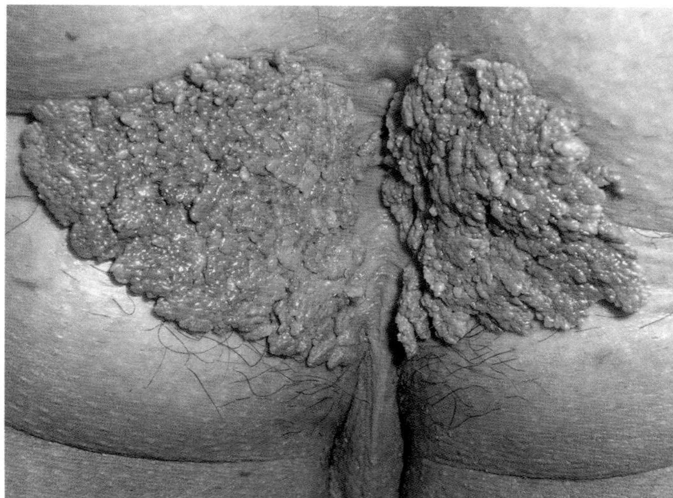

FIGURE 132-7 Extensive perianal warts in a 17-year-old adolescent boy who denies sexual abuse and anal intercourse. Patient failed imiquimod therapy and was referred to surgery. (*Reproduced with permission from Richard P. Usatine, MD.*)

- Condyloma caused by HPV can be seen in obese individuals within the folds of the pannus (**Figure 132-9**).
- A rapid plasma reagin (RPR) or Veneral Disease Research Laboratory (VDRL) test should be ordered to screen for syphilis and a HIV test should be ordered as well. Genital warts are a sexually transmitted disease and patients who have one STD should be screened for others.

LABORATORY TESTING

HPV viral typing is not recommended because test results would not alter clinical management of the condition. The application of 3% to 5% acetic acid to detect mucosal changes attributed to HPV infection is not recommended.[1]

BIOPSY

- Diagnosis may be confirmed by shave or punch biopsy if necessary.[1] Biopsy is indicated for the following reasons:
  - The diagnosis is uncertain.
  - The patient has a poor response to appropriate therapy.

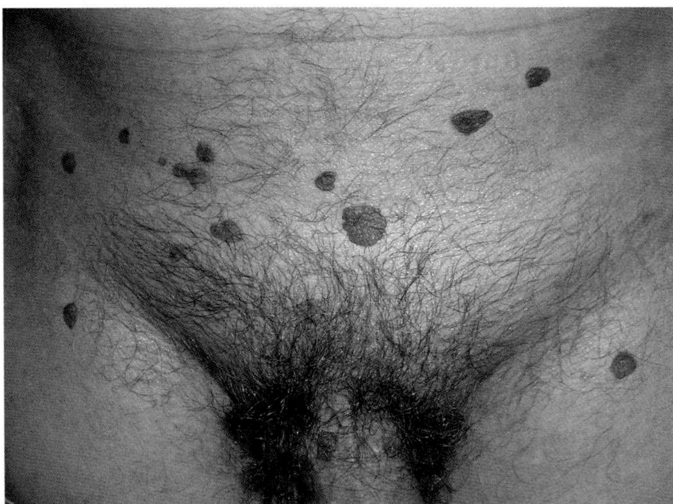

FIGURE 132-8 Condyloma that started on the penis and spread up the abdomen and on to the thighs. Note how these warts are hyperpigmented in this Latino man. (*Reproduced with permission from Richard P. Usatine, MD.*)

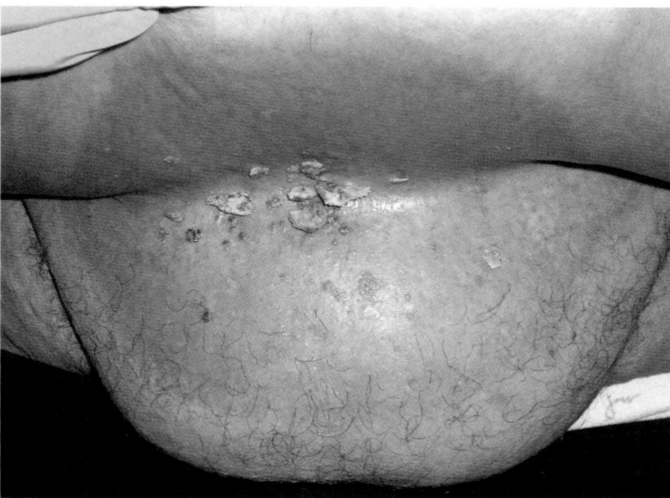

FIGURE 132-9 Panus condyloma from HPV growing between the folds of heavy adipose tissue in this obese woman. (*Reproduced with permission from Richard P. Usatine, MD.*)

  - Warts are atypical in appearance (unusually pigmented, indurated, fixed, or ulcerated).
  - The patient has compromised immunity and squamous cell carcinoma is suspected (one type of HPV-related malignancy).

DIFFERENTIAL DIAGNOSIS

- Pearly penile papules (PPPs), which are small papules around the edge of the glans penis (**Figure 132-10**).
- Common skin lesions, such as seborrheic keratoses and nevi—These are rare in the genital area (**Figure 132-11**) (see Chapters 156, Seborrheic Keratosis and 160, Nevus).
- Giant condyloma or Buschke-Lowenstein tumor is a low-grade, locally invasive malignancy that can appear as a fungating condyloma (**Figure 132-12**). Persons with HIV/AIDS have a higher risk of giant condyloma and malignant transformation (**Figure 132-13**).

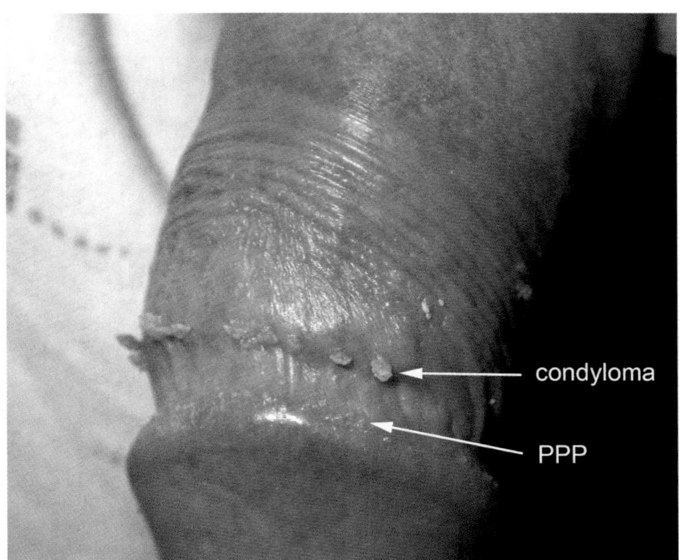

FIGURE 132-10 Condyloma coexisting with pearly penile papules (PPPs), which are a normal variant on the edge of the corona. (*Reproduced with permission from Richard P. Usatine, MD.*)

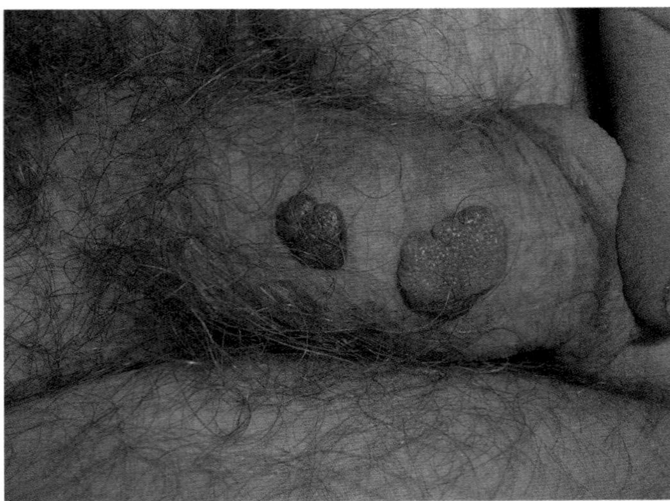

FIGURE 132-11 Two large condylomas that resemble seborrheic keratoses. Shave biopsy was positive for HPV. *(Reproduced with permission from Richard P. Usatine, MD.)*

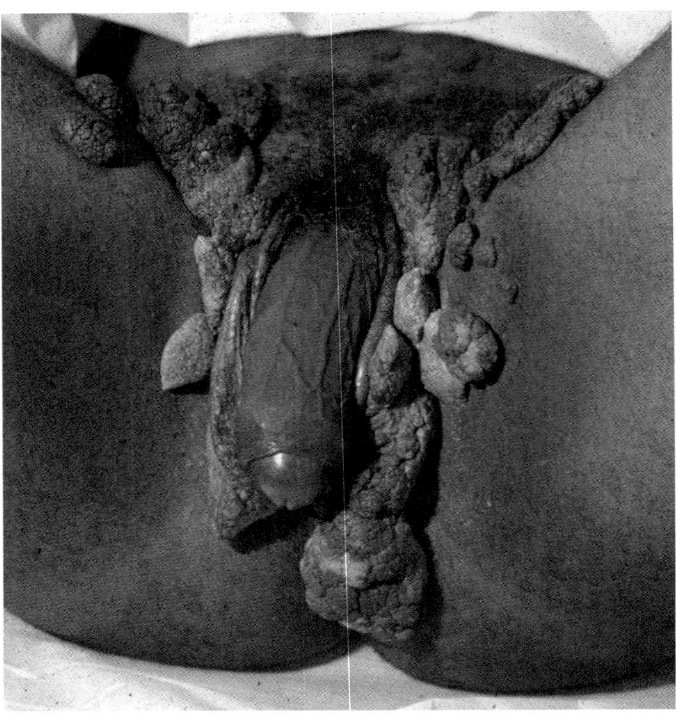

FIGURE 132-13 Giant condylomata acuminata in a man with AIDS. *(Reproduced with permission from Jack Resneck, Sr., MD.)*

- Molluscum contagiosum—Waxy umbilicated papules around the genitals and lower abdomen (see Chapter 129, Molluscum Contagiosum).
- Malignant neoplasms, such as basal cell carcinoma and squamous cell carcinomas (see Chapters 168, Basal Cell Carcinoma and 169, Squamous Cell Carcinoma).
- Condyloma lata is caused by secondary syphilis infection; lesions appear flat and velvety (see Chapter 218, Syphilis). A full workup for other STDs, including syphilis, should be done for any patient with genital warts (**Figure 132-14**).
- Micropapillomatosis of the vulva is a normal variant and appears as distinct individual papillary projections from the labia in a symmetrical pattern.

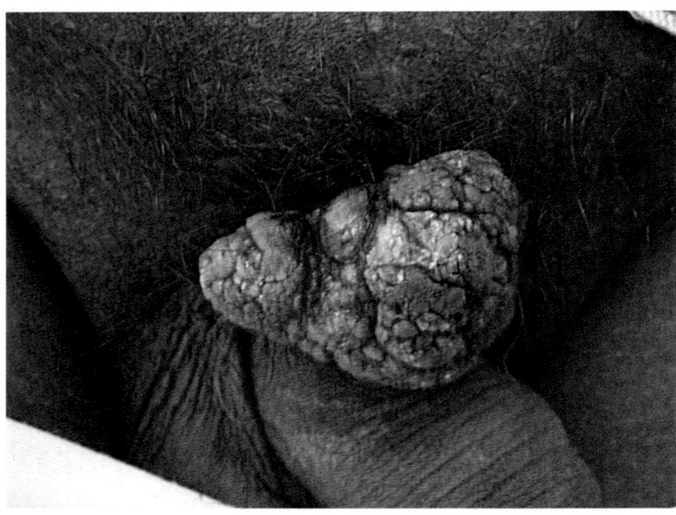

FIGURE 132-12 Buschke-Lowenstein tumor (giant condylomata acuminata) at the base of the penis. This was treated with surgical resection. The margins were clear and there was no squamous cell carcinoma found. *(Reproduced with permission from Suraj Reddy, MD.)*

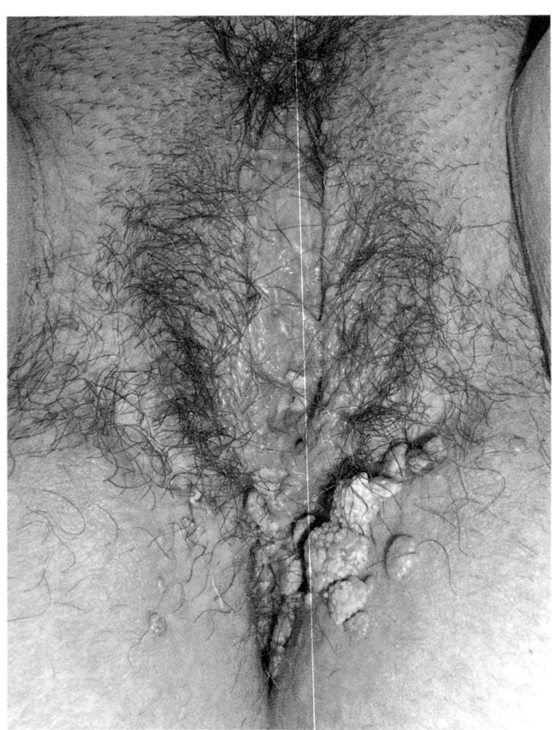

FIGURE 132-14 This 22-year-old woman with an addiction to IV heroin presented with many condyloma in the anogenital region. An RPR was positive for syphilis. The patient was treated with penicillin as well as cryotherapy. The visible condylomas in this image are most likely HPV and not condyloma lata based on their verrucous morphology. *(Reproduced with permission from Richard P. Usatine, MD.)*

MANAGEMENT

- The primary reason for treating genital warts is the amelioration of symptoms and ultimately removal of the warts.[1]
- The choice of therapy is based on the number, size, site, and morphology of lesions, as well as patient's preference, treatment cost, convenience, adverse effects, and physician's experience.
- Although available therapies for genital warts are likely to reduce HPV infectivity, they probably do not eradicate transmission.[1]

MEDICATIONS AND SURGICAL METHODS

- Treatments for external genital warts include topical medications, cryotherapy (**Figure 132-15**), and surgical methods, and are shown in **Table 132-1**.
- Cryotherapy is best applied with a bent-tipped spray applicator that allows for precise application with a less painful attenuated flow (see **Figure 132-15**).[4] Application may be repeated every 2 weeks if necessary.
- Treatment with 5% fluorouracil cream (Efudex) is no longer recommended because of severe local side effects and teratogenicity.[1]

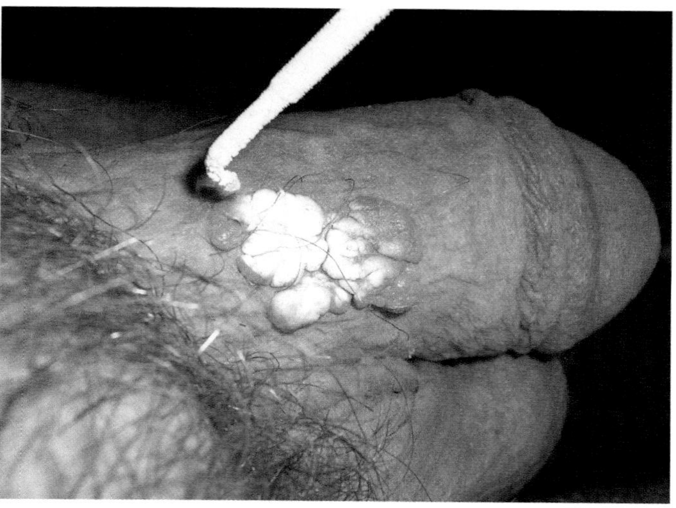

FIGURE 132-15 Cryotherapy of penile warts using a liquid nitrogen spray technique and a bent-tipped applicator.

TABLE 132-1 Treatments for External Genital Warts

Treatment	Possible Adverse Effects	Clearance (%)	Recurrence (%)
Patient-Applied Therapy			
Imiquimod (Aldara) is applied at bedtime for 3 days, then rest 4 days; alternatively, apply every other day for 3 applications; may repeat weekly cycles for up to 16 weeks[5] SOR Ⓐ	Erythema, irritation, ulceration, pain, and pigmentary changes; minimal systemic absorption	30-50	15
Sinecatechins 15% ointment—Apply a 0.5-cm strand of ointment to each wart 3 times daily[6] SOR Ⓐ	Erythema, pruritus/burning, pain, ulceration, edema, induration, and vesicular rash	53-57	3.7
Podofilox (Condylox) is applied twice daily for 3 days, then rest 4 days; may repeat for 4 cycles[7] SOR Ⓐ	Burning, pain, inflammation; low risk for systemic toxicity unless applied to occluded membranes	45-80	5-30
Provider-Applied Therapy			
Cryotherapy performed with liquid nitrogen or a cryoprobe[6] SOR Ⓑ	Pain or blisters at application site, scarring	60-90	20-40
Podophyllin resin is applied to each wart and allowed to dry, and is repeated weekly as needed[6,7] SOR Ⓐ	Local irritation, erythema, burning, and soreness at application site; neurotoxic and oncogenic if absorbed	30-80	20-65
Surgical treatment for warts involves removal to the dermal–epidermal junction; options include scissor excision, shave excision, laser vaporization, and loop electrosurgical excision procedure (LEEP) excision[6] SOR Ⓑ	Pain, bleeding, scarring; risk for burning and allergic reaction from local anesthetic; laser and LEEP have risk for spreading HPV in plume	35-70	5-50
Trichloroacetic acid (TCA) and bichloracetic acid (BCA) are applied to each wart and allowed to dry; repeated weekly[6] SOR Ⓑ	Local pain and irritation; no systemic side effects	50-80	35

REFERRAL OR HOSPITALIZATION

Consider consultation for patients with very large or recalcitrant lesions.

PREVENTION

A bivalent vaccine (Cervarix) containing HPV types 16 and 18 and a quadrivalent vaccine (Gardasil) containing HPV types 6, 11, 16, and 18 are licensed in the United States. The quadrivalent HPV vaccine protects against the HPV types that cause 90% of genital warts (ie, types 6 and 11) in males and females when given prophylactically. Both vaccines offer protection against the HPV types that cause 70% of cervical cancers (ie, types 16 and 18). In the United States, the quadrivalent (Gardasil) HPV vaccine can also be used in males and females ages 9 to 26 years to prevent genital warts.[8]

PROGNOSIS

Many genital warts will eventually resolve without treatment. Resolution can usually be hastened with therapy (see **Table 132-1**).

FOLLOW-UP

Patients should be offered a follow-up evaluation 2 to 3 months after treatment to check for new lesions.[1] SOR Ⓒ

PATIENT EDUCATION

HPV is transmitted mainly by skin-to-skin contact. Although condoms may decrease the levels of transmission, they are imperfect barriers at best as they can fail, and they do not cover the scrotum or vulva, where infection may reside.

PATIENT RESOURCES

- eMedicineHealth. *Genital Warts (HPV Infection)*—**http://www.emedicinehealth.com/genital_warts/article_em.htm.**
- PubMed Health. *Genital Warts*—**http://www.ncbi.nlm.nih.gov/pubmedhealth/PMH0001889/.**
- American Academy of Dermatology. *Genital Warts*—**http://www.aad.org/skin-conditions/dermatology-a-to-z/genital-warts.**
- MedlinePlus. *Genital Warts*—**http://www.nlm.nih.gov/medlineplus/ency/article/000886.htm.**

PROVIDER RESOURCES

- Centers for Disease Control and Prevention. *Genital Warts*—**http://www.cdc.gov/std/treatment/2010/genital-warts.htm.**
- Medscape. *Genital Warts*—**http://emedicine.medscape.com/article/1133201.**
- Medscape. *Genital Warts in Emergency Medicine*—**http://emedicine.medscape.com/article/763014.**

REFERENCES

1. Centers for Disease Control and Prevention. *2010 Guidelines for Treatment of Sexually Transmitted Diseases*. http://www.cdc.gov/std/treatment/2010/STD-Treatment-2010-RR5912.pdf. Accessed December 1, 2011.
2. Burk RD, Kelly P, Feldman J, et al. Declining prevalence of cervicovaginal human papillomavirus infection with age is independent of other risk factors. *Sex Transm Dis.* 1996;23:333-341.
3. Palefsky JM. Cutaneous and genital HPV-associated lesions in HIV-infected patients. *Clin Dermatol.* 1997;15:439-447.
4. Usatine R, Stulberg D. Cryosurgery. In: Usatine R, Pfenninger J, Stulberg D, Small R, eds. *Dermatologic and Cosmetic Procedures in Office Practice*. Philadelphia, PA: Elsevier; 2012:182-198.
5. Gotovtseva EP, Kapadia AS, Smolensky MH, Lairson DR. Optimal frequency of imiquimod (Aldara) 5% cream for the treatment of external genital warts in immunocompetent adults: a meta-analysis. *Sex Transm Dis.* 2008;35(4):346-351.
6. Mayeaux EJ Jr, Dunton C. Modern management of external genital warts. *J Low Genit Tract Dis.* 2008;12:185-192.
7. Langley PC, Tyring SK, Smith MH. The cost effectiveness of patient-applied versus provider-administered intervention strategies for the treatment of external genital warts. *Am J Manag Care.* 1999;5(1):69-77.
8. Centers for Disease Control and Prevention (CDC). FDA licensure of quadrivalent human papillomavirus vaccine (HPV4, Gardasil) for use in males and guidance from the Advisory Committee on Immunization Practices (ACIP). *MMWR Morb Mortal Wkly Rep.* 2010;59(20):630-632.

133 PLANTAR WARTS

E.J. Mayeaux Jr, MD

PATIENT STORY

A young man presents to the clinic with a "growth" on the side of his foot. It had been present for about a year and was unresponsive to over-the-counter therapies (**Figure 133-1**). It is painful to walk on and he would like it to be treated. He was diagnosed with plantar warts. The lesions were treated with gentle paring using a scalpel and liquid nitrogen therapy over 2 sessions.

INTRODUCTION

Plantar warts (verruca plantaris) are human papilloma virus (HPV) lesions that occur on the soles of the feet (**Figures 133-1** to **133-5**) and palms of the hands (**Figure 133-6**).

SYNONYMS

Plantar warts are also known as palmoplantar warts and myrmecia.

EPIDEMIOLOGY

- Plantar warts affect mostly adolescents and young adults, affecting up to 10% of people in these age groups.[1]
- Prevalence studies demonstrate a wide range of values, from 0.84% in the United States[2] to 3.3% to 4.7% in the United Kingdom,[3] to 24% in 16- to 18-year-olds in Australia.[4]

ETIOLOGY AND PATHOPHYSIOLOGY

- Plantar warts are caused by HPV.
- They usually occur at points of maximum pressure, such as on the heels (see **Figures 133-2** to **133-4**) or over the heads of the metatarsal bones (see **Figure 133-5**), but may appear anywhere on the plantar surface including the tips of the fingers and toes (**Figure 133-7**).
- A thick, painful callus forms in response to the pressure that is induced as the size of the lesion increases. Even a minor wart can cause a lot of pain.
- A cluster of many warts that appear to fuse is referred to as a *mosaic wart* (see **Figure 133-4**).

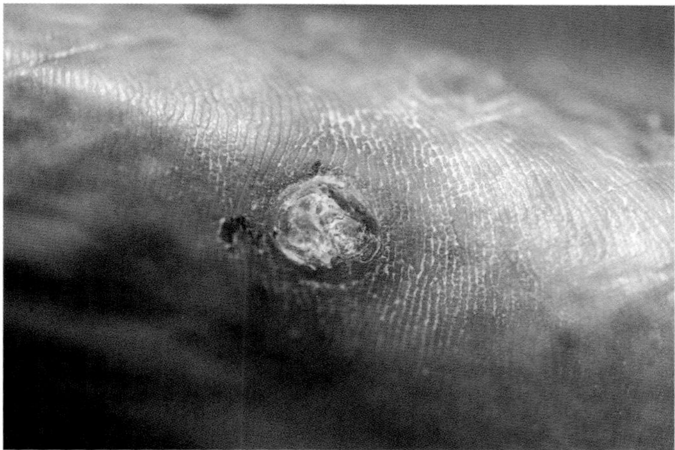

FIGURE 133-1 Plantar wart on the side of the foot. It had been present for about a year and was unresponsive to over-the-counter therapies. (*Reproduced with permission from E.J. Mayeaux, Jr, MD.*)

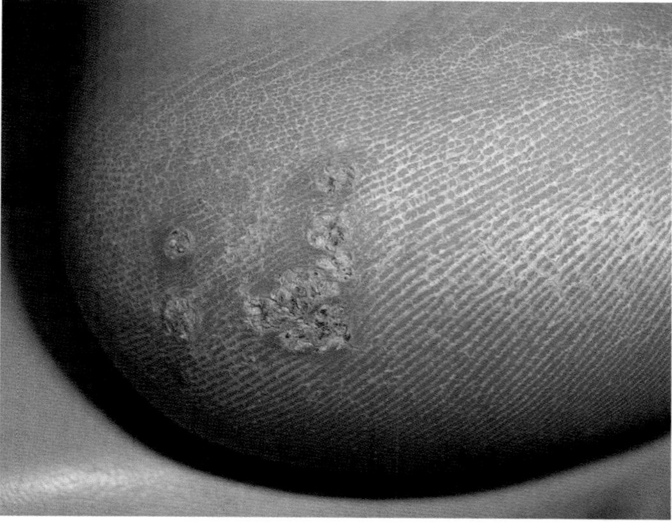

FIGURE 133-2 Close-up of plantar wart on the side of the heel. Note the disruption of skin lines and black dots. (*Reproduced with permission from Richard P. Usatine, MD.*)

RISK FACTORS

- Young age
- Decreased immunity

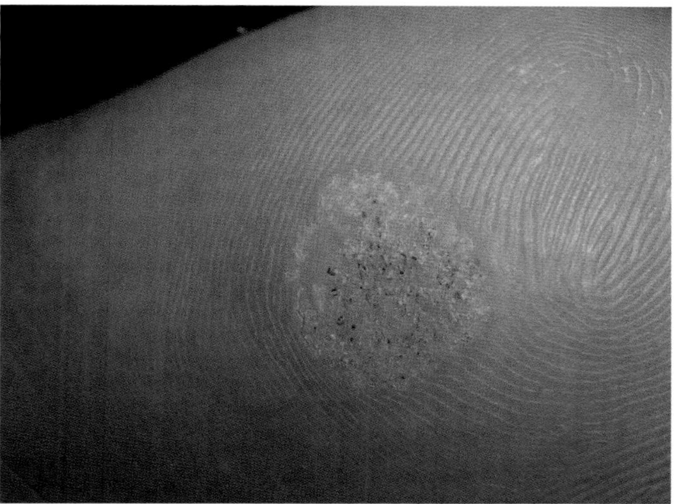

FIGURE 133-3 Close-up of a plantar wart demonstrating disruption of normal skin lines. Corns and callus do not disrupt normal skin lines. The black dots are thrombosed vessels, which are frequently seen in plantar warts. (*Reproduced with permission from Richard P. Usatine, MD.*)

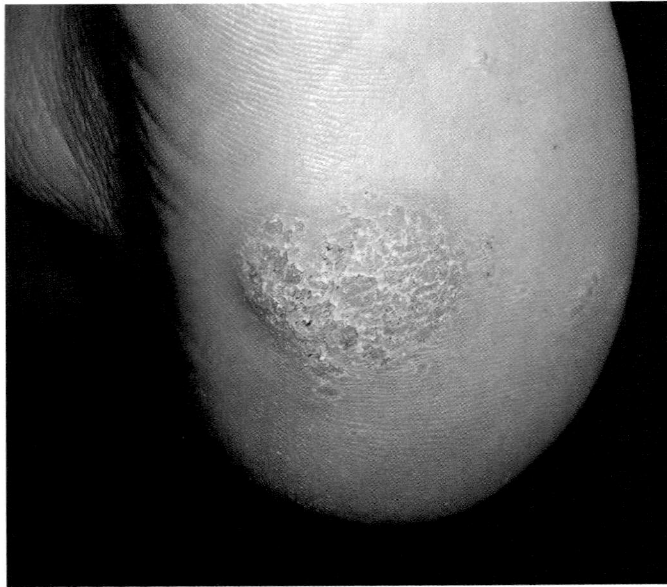

FIGURE 133-4 A mosaic wart is formed when several plantar warts become confluent. This man was HIV positive and this wart was very resistant to treatment. (*Reproduced with permission from Richard P. Usatine, MD.*)

DIAGNOSIS

CLINICAL FEATURES

Plantar warts present as thick, painful endophytic plaques located on the soles and/or palms. Warts have the following features:

- Begin as small shiny papules
- Lack skin lines crossing their surface (see **Figure 133-3**)
- Have a highly organized mosaic pattern on the surface when examined with a hand lens
- Have a rough keratotic surface surrounded by a smooth collar of callused skin
- Painful when compressed laterally

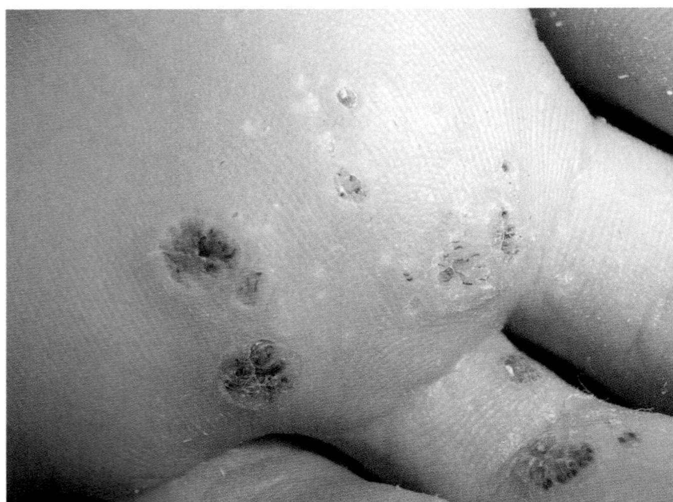

FIGURE 133-5 Multiple plantar warts on the ball of the foot and toes. The thrombosed vessels within the warts appear as black dots. (*Reproduced with permission from Richard P. Usatine, MD.*)

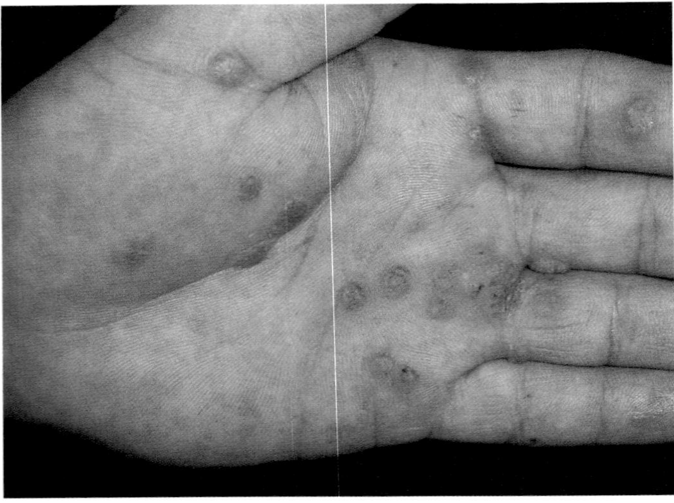

FIGURE 133-6 Multiple plantar warts on the palms of an HIV-positive man. (*Reproduced with permission from Richard P. Usatine, MD.*)

- May have centrally located black dots (thrombosed vessels) that may bleed with paring (see **Figures 133-2** to **133-7**)

TYPICAL DISTRIBUTION

They occur on the palms of the hands and soles of the feet. They are more commonly found on weight-bearing areas, such as under the metatarsal heads or on the heel.[5]

BIOPSY

If the diagnosis is doubtful, a shave biopsy is indicated to confirm the diagnosis.[6]

DIFFERENTIAL DIAGNOSIS

- Corns and calluses are pressure-induced skin thickenings that occur on the feet and can be mistaken for plantar warts. Calluses are generally found on the sole and corns are usually found on the toes. Calluses and

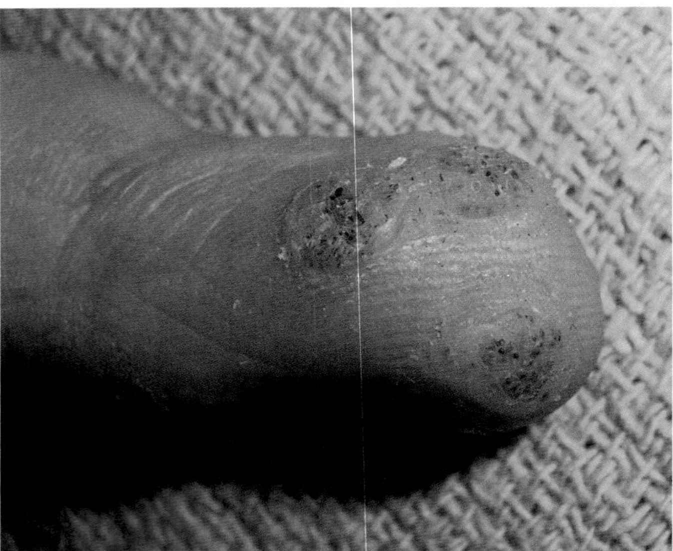

FIGURE 133-7 Close-up of plantar wart on a finger that also shows disruption of skin lines and black dots. (*Reproduced with permission from Richard P. Usatine, MD.*)

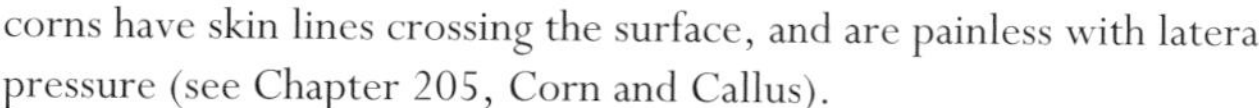

corns have skin lines crossing the surface, and are painless with lateral pressure (see Chapter 205, Corn and Callus).

- Black heel presents as a cluster of blue-black dots that result from ruptured capillaries. They appear on the plantar surface of the heel following the shearing trauma of sports that involve sudden stops or position changes. Examination reveals normal skin lines, and paring does not cause additional bleeding. The condition resolves spontaneously in a few weeks.
- Black warts are plantar warts undergoing spontaneous resolution, which may turn black and feel soft when pared with a blade.[7]
- Squamous cell carcinoma should be considered when lesions have irregular growth or pigmentation, ulceration, or resist therapy, particularly in immunosuppressed patients (see Chapter 169, Squamous Cell Carcinoma).
- Amelanotic melanoma, although extremely rare, can look similar to HPV lesions. Lesions that are treatment resistant or atypical, particularly on the palms or soles, should be monitored closely. A biopsy is required to establish the diagnosis (see Chapter 170, Melanoma).
- Palmoplantar keratoderma describes a rare heterogeneous group of disorders characterized by thickening of the palms and the soles that can also be an associated feature of different syndromes. They can be classified as having uniform involvement versus focal hyperkeratosis located mainly on pressure points and sites of recurrent friction (**Figure 133-8**). This latter type can be differentiated from plantar warts by the more diffuse locations on the palmoplantar surfaces, the mainly epidermal involvement, and biopsy, if necessary (**Figure 133-9**).

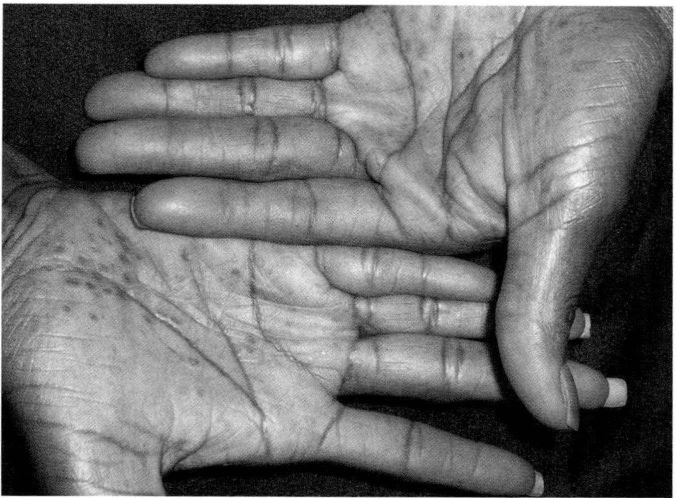

A

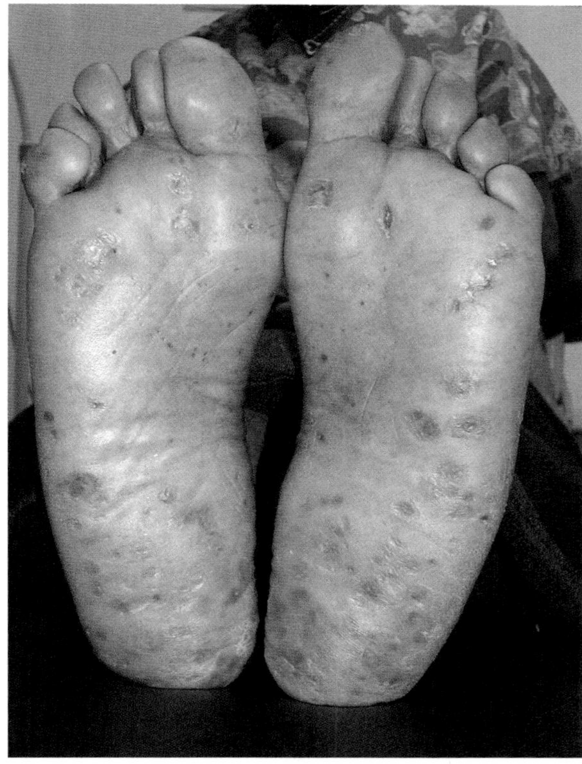

B

FIGURE 133-8 Focal palmoplantar keratoderma of the palms (A) and soles (B). This is an inherited genodermatosis. Note lesions are located mainly on higher pressure areas. (*Reproduced with permission from Richard P. Usatine, MD.*)

MANAGEMENT

NONPHARMACOLOGIC

- Painless plantar warts do not require therapy. Minimal discomfort can be relieved by periodically removing the hyperkeratosis with a blade or pumice stone.
- Painful warts should be treated using a technique that causes minimal scarring as scars on the soles of the feet are usually permanent and painful.
- Patients with diabetes must be treated with the utmost care to minimize complications.

MEDICATIONS

- Topical salicylic acid solutions are available in nonprescription form and provide conservative keratolytic therapy. These preparations are nonscarring, minimally painful, and relatively effective, but require persistent application of medication once each day for weeks to months. The wart is first pared with a blade, pumice stone, or emery board, and the area soaked in warm water. The solution is then applied, allowed to dry, reapplied, and occluded with adhesive tape.[8] White, pliable, keratin forms and should be pared away carefully until pink skin is exposed.[9] SOR B
- Seventeen percent to 50% salicylic acid solution and plasters are available in nonprescription and prescription forms. However, the 17% solutions are more prevalent and easier to find in nonprescription form. The treatment is similar to the previous process, except that with plasters the salicylic acid has been incorporated into a pad. They are particularly useful in treating mosaic warts covering a large area. Pain is quickly relieved in plantar warts, because a large amount of keratin is removed during the first few days of treatment.[9] SOR B A recent multicenter, open-label, randomized, controlled trial found that 50% salicylic acid and the cryotherapy were equally effective for clearance of plantar warts.[10] SOR A
- Acid chemotherapy with trichloroacetic acid (TCA) or bichloracetic acid (BCA) is commonly employed to treat plantar warts in the office. They are considered safe during pregnancy for external lesions.

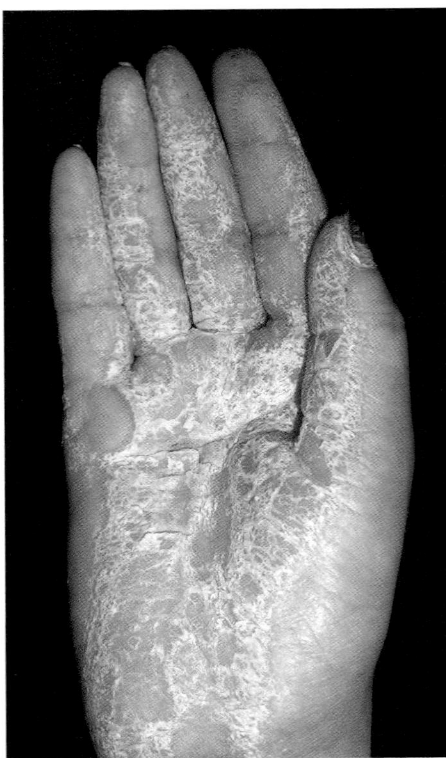

A

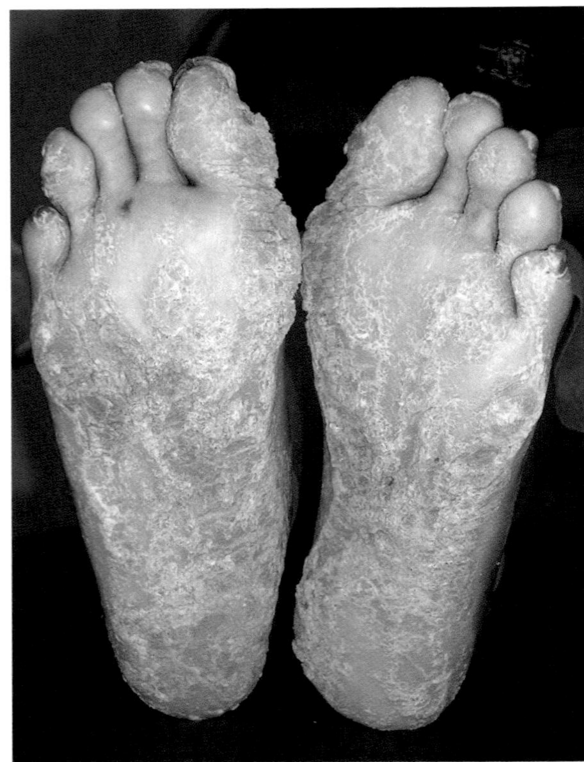

B

FIGURE 133-9 Diffuse palmoplantar keratoderma of the palms (A) and soles (B) in an 11-year-old girl. This is an inherited genodermatosis with severe functional consequences. (*Reproduced with permission from Richard P. Usatine, MD.*)

The excess keratin is first pared with a scalpel, then the entire lesion is coated with acid, and the acid is worked into the wart with a sharp toothpick. The process is repeated every 7 to 10 days. SOR Ⓒ

- Cryotherapy with liquid nitrogen therapy is commonly used, but plantar warts are more resistant than other HPV lesions. The liquid nitrogen is applied to form a freeze ball that covers the lesion and 2 mm of surrounding normal tissue, usually 10 to 20 seconds per freeze. SOR Ⓒ There is no evidence that 2 freezing episodes are better than one, other than it allows for more freeze time in a way that is more acceptable to the patient. It is always better to underfreeze than to overfreeze in areas where scarring can produce permanent disability.
- Treatments for resistant lesions are often carried out in referral practices that have a high enough volume to use more expensive or specialized therapy. Cantharidin is an extract of the blister beetle that is applied to the wart after which blistering occurs. Intralesional immunotherapy with skin-test antigens (ie, mumps, *Candida*, or *Trichophyton* antigens) may lead to the resolution both of the injected wart and other warts that were not injected. Contact immunotherapy using dinitrochlorobenzene, squaric acid dibutylester, and diphenylcyclopropenone may be applied to the skin to sensitize the patient and then to the lesion to induce an immune response. Intralesional bleomycin or laser therapy is also useful for recalcitrant warts. SOR Ⓒ

COMPLEMENTARY AND ALTERNATIVE THERAPY

Although many complementary and alternative therapies are promoted for wart therapy, there is no significant data supporting their use in the treatment of plantar warts.

PREVENTION

Tools used for paring down warts, such as nail files and pumice stones should not be used on normal skin or by other people.

PROGNOSIS

Most plantar warts will spontaneously disappear without treatment. Treatment often hastens resolution of lesions.

FOLLOW-UP

Regular follow-up to assess treatment efficacy, adverse reactions, and patient tolerance are recommended to minimize treatment dropouts.

PATIENT EDUCATION

- Because spontaneous regression occurs, observation of painless lesions without treatment is preferable.
- Therapy often takes weeks to months, so patience and perseverance are essential for successful therapy.

PATIENT RESOURCES

- MayoClinic. *Plantar Warts*—**http://www.mayoclinic.com/health/plantar-warts/DS00509.**
- MedlinePlus. *Warts*—**http://www.nlm.nih.gov/medlineplus/warts.html.**
- Fort Drum Medical Activity. *Patient Education Handouts: Warts and Plantar Warts*—**http://www.drum.amedd.army.mil/pt_info/handouts/warts_Plantar.pdf.**

PROVIDER RESOURCES

- Bacelieri R, Johnson SM. Cutaneous warts: an evidence-based approach to therapy. *Am Fam Physician*. 2005;72:647-652—**http://www.aafp.org/afp/20050815/647.html.**
- Medscape. *Nongenital Warts*—**http://emedicine.medscape.com/article/1133317.**

REFERENCES

1. Laurent R, Kienzler JL. Epidemiology of HPV infections. *Clin Dermatol.* 1985;3(4):64-70.
2. Johnson ML, Roberts J. Skin conditions and related need for medical care among persons 1-74 years. Rockville, MD: US Department of Health, Education, and Welfare; 1978:1-26.
3. Williams HC, Pottier A, Strachan D. The descriptive epidemiology of warts in British schoolchildren. *Br J Dermatol.* 1993;128:504-511.
4. Kilkenny M, Merlin K, Young R, Marks R. The prevalence of common skin conditions in Australian school students: 1. Common, plane and plantar viral warts. *Br J Dermatol.* 1998;138:840-845.
5. Holland TT, Weber CB, James WD. Tender periungual nodules. Myrmecia (deep palmoplantar warts). *Arch Dermatol.* 1992;128(1):105-106, 108-109.
6. Beutner, KR. Nongenital human papillomavirus infections. *Clin Lab Med.* 2000;20:423-430.
7. Berman A, Domnitz JM, Winkelmann RK. Plantar warts recently turned black. *Arch Dermatol.* 1982;118:47-51.
8. Landsman MJ, Mancuso JE, Abramow SP. Diagnosis, pathophysiology, and treatment of plantar verruca. *Clin Podiatr Med Surg.* 1996;13(1):55-71.
9. Gibbs S, Harvey I. *Cochrane Summaries. Topical Treatments for Cutaneous Warts*. http://www.cochrane.org/reviews/en/ab001781.html. Accessed April 1, 2008.
10. Cockayne S, Hewitt C, Hicks K, et al. Cryotherapy versus salicylic acid for the treatment of plantar warts (verrucae): a randomized controlled trial. *BMJ.* 2011;342:d3271.

SECTION 4 FUNGAL

134 FUNGAL OVERVIEW

Richard P. Usatine, MD

PATIENT STORY

A 55-year-old woman presents with a red pruritic area on her face for 3 months (**Figure 134-1**). The annular distribution immediately is suspicious for a dermatophyte infection. Further investigation demonstrates that the patient has severe tinea pedis in a moccasin distribution. The patient is treated with an oral antifungal agent and her fungal infection clears over the coming month.

INTRODUCTION

Fungal infections of the skin and mucous membranes are ubiquitous and common. There are many types of fungus that grow on humans but they all share a predilection for warm and moist areas. Consequently, hot and humid climates promote fungal infections, but many areas of the skin can get warm and sweaty even in cold climates, such as the feet and groin.

SYNONYMS

Pityriasis versicolor equals tinea versicolor.

PATHOPHYSIOLOGY

Mucocutaneous fungal infections are caused by the following:

- Dermatophytes are caused by 3 genera: *Microsporum*, *Epidermophyton*, and *Trichophyton*. There are approximately 40 species in the 3 genera and these fungi cause tinea pedis and manus, tinea capitis, tinea corporis, tinea cruris, tinea faciei, and onychomycosis (**Figures 134-1** to **134-6**).
- Yeasts in the genera of *Candida* and *Pityrosporum* (*Malassezia*)—There are multiple species of *Candida* that can cause mucocutaneous infections with *Candida albicans* as the most common one involved (**Figure 134-7**). *Pityrosporum* causes seborrhea and tinea versicolor (**Figure 134-8**). Although tinea versicolor has the name tinea in it, it is not a true dermatophyte and may be best called pityriasis versicolor.

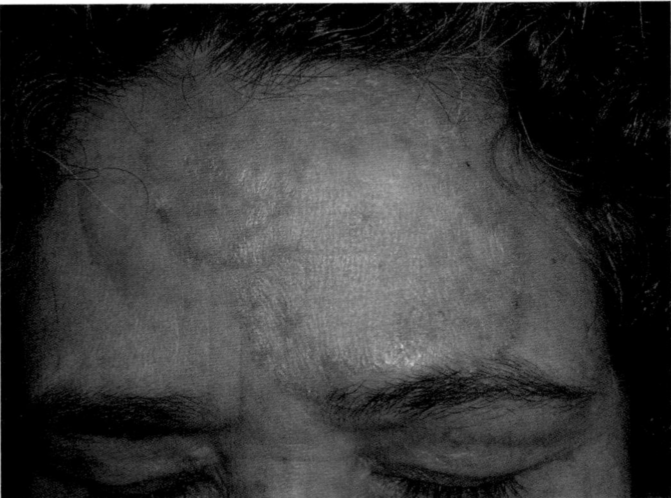

FIGURE 134-1 Tinea faciei on the face of a 55-year-old woman with typical scaling and ring-like pattern (ringworm). Note the well-demarcated raised border and central clearing. (*Reproduced with permission from Richard P. Usatine, MD.*)

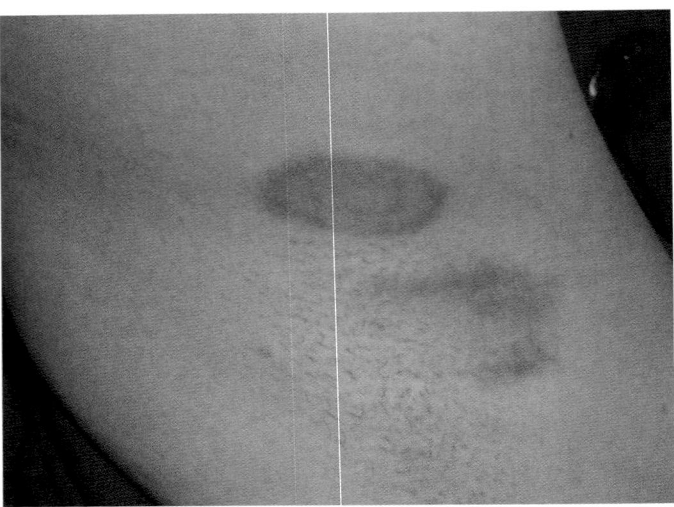

FIGURE 134-2 Annular pruritic lesion with concentric rings in the axilla of a young woman caused by tinea corporis. The concentric rings have a high specificity for tinea infections. (*Reproduced with permission from Richard P. Usatine, MD.*)

DIAGNOSIS

CLINICAL FEATURES OF TINEA INFECTIONS

Clinical features include scaling, erythema, pruritus, central clearing, concentric rings, and maceration (**Table 134-1**). Changes in pigmentation are not uncommon in various types of tinea especially tinea versicolor.

- **Figure 134-1** shows tinea faciei on the face with typical scaling and ring-like pattern, hence, the name ringworm. There is also erythema and central clearing. The patient was experiencing pruritus.
- **Figure 134-2** shows annular pruritic lesion with concentric rings in the axilla of a young woman caused by tinea corporis. The concentric rings have a high specificity (80%) for tinea infections.
- Note that tinea infections will not show central clearing in 58% of cases, as in **Figure 134-3** in which tinea cruris has no central clearing.
- Hyperpigmentation is common in dark-skinned individuals, as seen in **Figure 134-4** on the flank of this Hispanic woman.
- Hypopigmentation is frequently seen in tinea versicolor (see **Figure 134-8**).

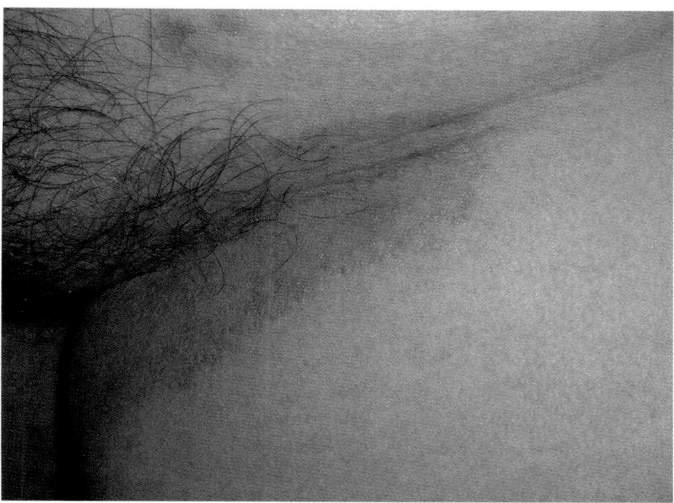

FIGURE 134-3 Tinea cruris with well-demarcated raised border and no central clearing. (*Reproduced with permission from Richard P. Usatine, MD.*)

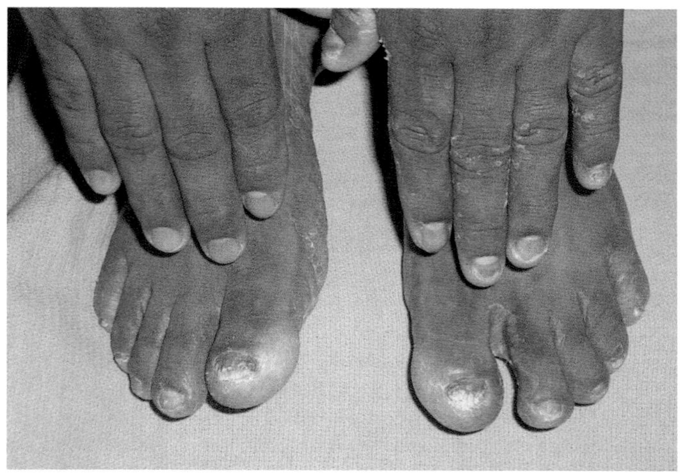

FIGURE 134-6 Two-foot, 1-hand syndrome with tinea manus of 1 hand and tinea pedis of both feet. (*Reproduced with permission from Richard P. Usatine, MD.*)

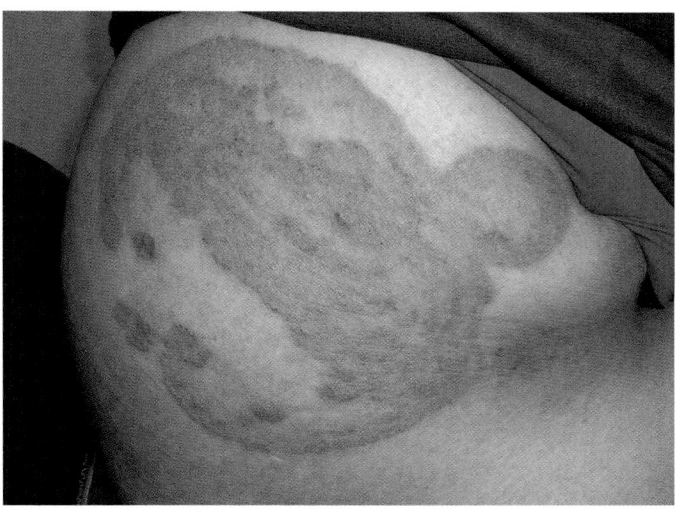

FIGURE 134-4 Tinea corporis on the right flank of a woman bending forward. Note the postinflammatory hyperpigmentation, annular patterns in areas of central sparing. (*Reproduced with permission from Richard P. Usatine, MD.*)

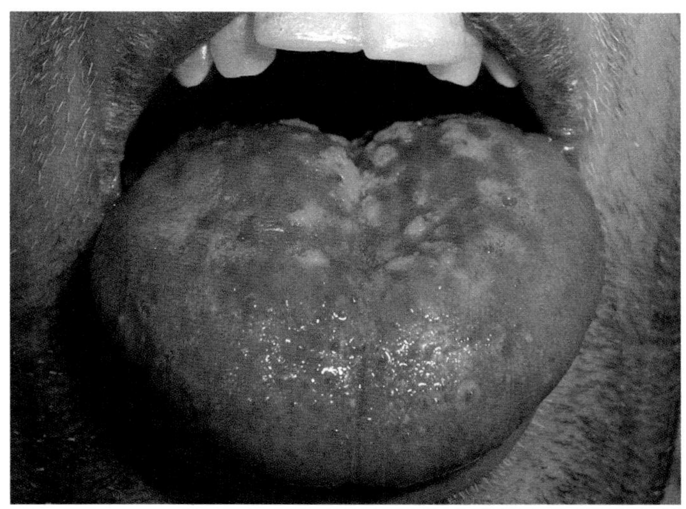

FIGURE 134-7 Thrush in the mouth of a patient with diabetic ketoacidosis. This mucosal Candida infection was confirmed with a KOH preparation. (*Reproduced with permission from Richard P. Usatine, MD.*)

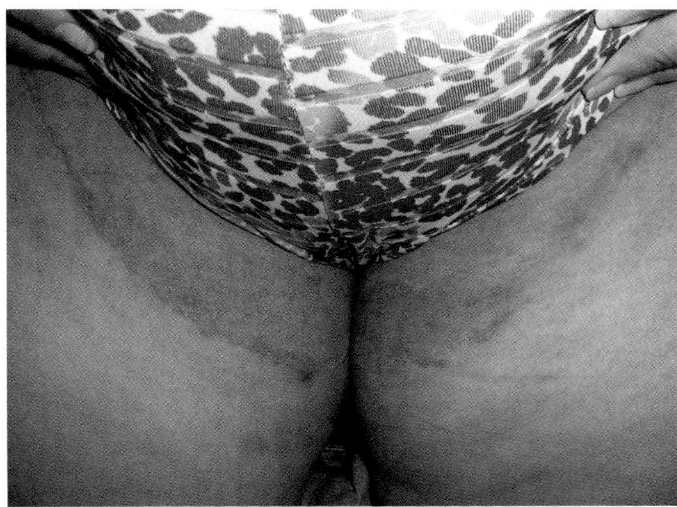

FIGURE 134-5 Recurrent tinea cruris in a woman with a well-demarcated raised scaling border. (*Reproduced with permission from Richard P. Usatine, MD.*)

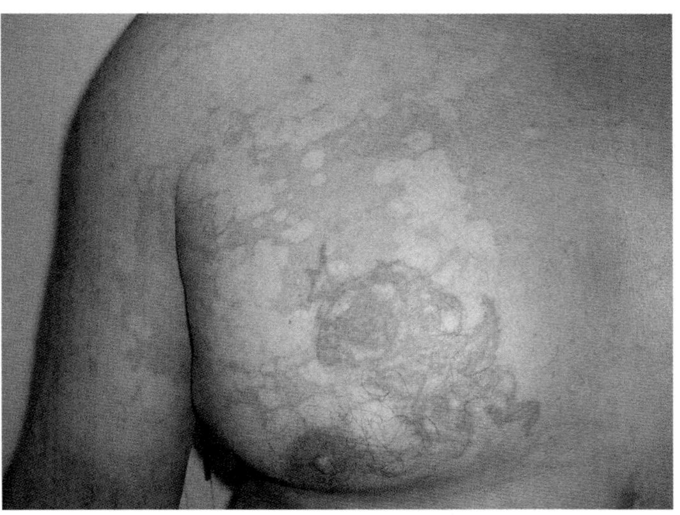

FIGURE 134-8 Tinea versicolor showing hypopigmentation on the chest. (*Reproduced with permission from Richard P. Usatine, MD.*)

TABLE 134-1 Diagnostic Value of Selected Signs and Symptoms in Tinea Infection*

Sign/Symptom	Sensitivity (%)	Specificity (%)	PV+ (%)	PV– (%)	LR+	LR–
Scaling	77	20	17	80	0.96	1.15
Erythema	69	31	18	83	1.00	1.00
Pruritus	54	40	16	80	0.90	1.15
Central clearing	42	65	20	84	1.20	0.89
Concentric rings	27	80	23	84	1.35	0.91
Maceration	27	84	26	84	1.69	0.87

LR–, negative likelihood ratio; LR+, positive likelihood ratio; PV–, negative predictive value; PV+, positive predictive value.
*Signs and symptoms were compiled by 27 general practitioners prior to submission of skin for fungal culture. Specimens were taken from 148 consecutive patients with erythematosquamous lesions of glabrous skin. Culture results were considered the gold standard; level of evidence = 2b.
Data from *J Fam Pract.* 1999;48:611-615. Reproduced with permission from Frontline Medical Communications.

TYPICAL DISTRIBUTION

- Fungal infections can be seen from the head down to the toes. Fungus especially likes warm and moist areas, so intertriginous areas (see **Figure 134-5**) and mucus membranes are very commonly affected.
- The 2-foot, 1-hand syndrome is a curious phenomenon with tinea manus of one hand and tinea pedis of both feet (see **Figure 134-6**). It is not clear why only one hand is involved in these cases. In this case, it was the nondominant hand.

LABORATORY STUDIES

Creating a potassium hydroxide (KOH) prep

- Scrape the leading edge of the lesion on to a slide using the side of a #15 scalpel or another microscope slide (**Figure 134-9**).
- Use your coverslip to push the scale into the center of the slide.
- Add 2 drops of KOH (or fungal stain) to the slide and place coverslip on top.
- Gently heat with flame from an alcohol lamp or lighter if you are using plain KOH without dimethyl sulfoxide (DMSO). Avoid boiling.
- DMSO acts as a surfactant that helps to break up the cell membranes of the epithelial cells without heating. Fungal stains that come with KOH and a surfactant in the solution are very simple to use. These inexpensive stains come conveniently in small plastic squeeze bottles that have a shelf life of 1 to 3 years. Two useful stains that can make it easier to identify fungus are chlorazol and Swartz-Lamkins stains. Swartz-Lamkins stain has a longer shelf life and is my preferred stain.
- Examine with microscope starting with 10 power to look for the cells and hyphae and then switch to 40 power to confirm your findings (**Figures 134-10** to **134-13**). The fungal stain helps the hyphae to stand out among the epithelial cells.
- It helps to start with 10 power to find the clumps of cells and look for groups of cells that appear to have fungal elements within them (see **Figure 134-10**).
- Do not be fooled by cell borders that look linear and branching. True fungal morphology at 40 power should confirm that you are looking at real fungus and not artifact. The fungal stains bring out these characteristics including cell walls, nuclei, and arthroconidia (see **Figures 134-11** to **134-13**).

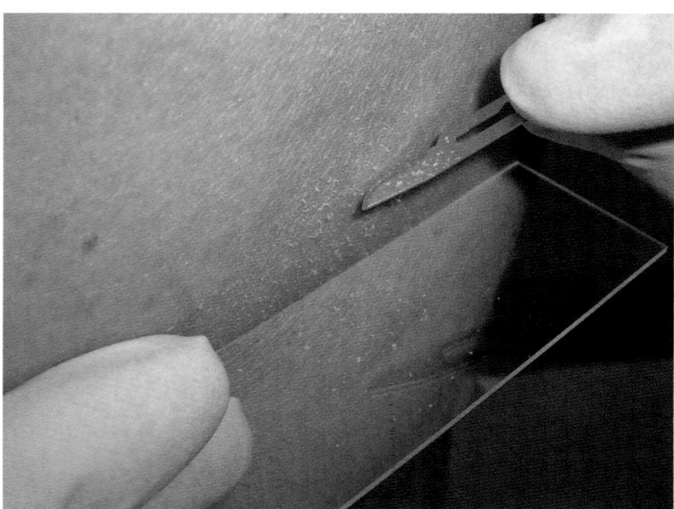

FIGURE 134-9 Making a KOH preparation by scraping in area of scale with a #15 blade. This was a case of tinea versicolor. *(Reproduced with permission from Richard P. Usatine, MD.)*

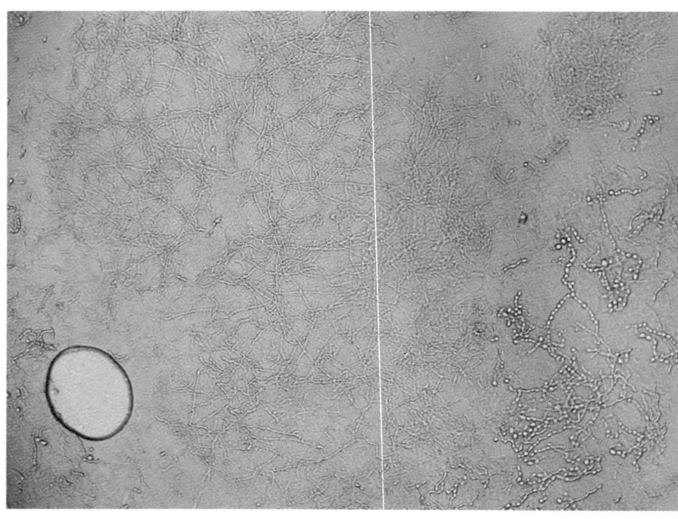

FIGURE 134-10 *Trichophyton rubrum* from tinea cruris visible among skin cells using light microscopy at 10 power and Swartz-Lamkins fungal stain. Start your search on 10 power and move to 40 power to confirm your findings. *(Reproduced with permission from Richard P. Usatine, MD.)*

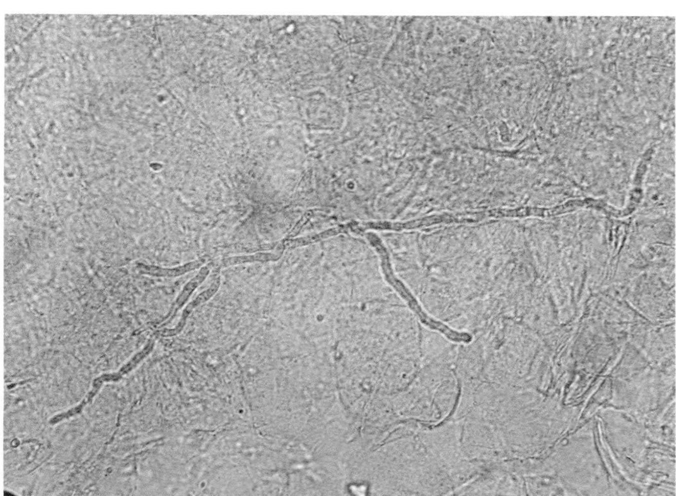

FIGURE 134-11 *Trichophyton rubrum* from tinea cruris using Swartz-Lamkins fungal stain at 40 power. Straight hyphae with visible septae. (*Reproduced with permission from Richard P. Usatine, MD.*)

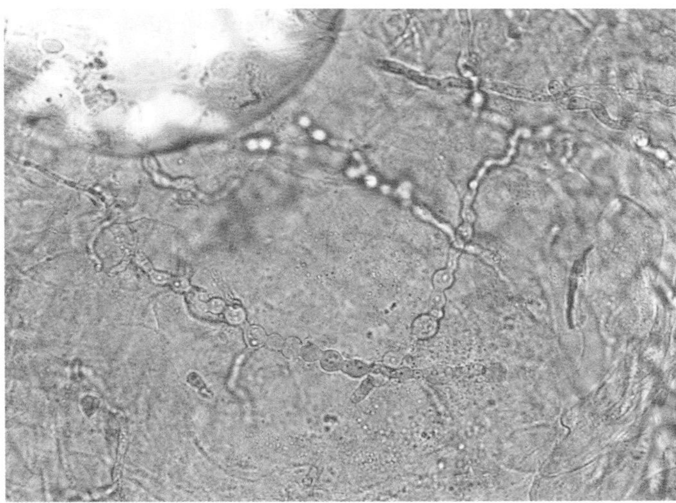

FIGURE 134-12 Arthroconidia visible from tinea cruris using Swartz-Lamkins fungal stain at 40 power. (*Reproduced with permission from Richard P. Usatine, MD.*)

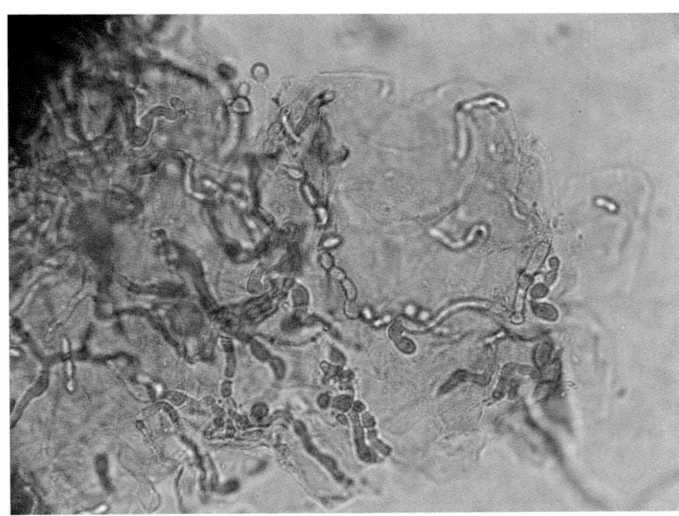

FIGURE 134-13 *Trichophyton rubrum* from tinea cruris using chlorazol black fungal stain at 40 power. (*Reproduced with permission from Richard P. Usatine, MD.*)

- KOH test characteristics[1] (without fungal stains)—Sensitivity 77% to 88%, specificity 62% to 95% (**Table 134-2**). The sensitivity and specificity should be higher with fungal stains and the experience of the person performing the test.

OTHER LABORATORY STUDIES

- Fungal culture—Send skin scrapings, hair, or nail clippings to the laboratory in a sterile container such as a urine cup. These will be plated out on fungal agar and the laboratory can report the species if positive.
- Biopsy specimens can be sent in formalin for periodic acid-Schiff (PAS) staining when KOH and fungal cultures seem to be falsely negative.
- UV light (Wood lamp) is used to look for fluorescence. The *Microsporum* species are most likely to fluoresce. However, the majority of tinea infections are caused by *Trichophyton* species that do not fluoresce.

MANAGEMENT

There is a wide variety of topical antifungal medications (**Table 134-3**). A Cochrane systematic review of 70 trials of topical antifungals for tinea pedis showed good evidence for efficacy compared to placebo[2] for the following:

- Allylamines (naftifine, terbinafine, butenafine).
- Azoles (clotrimazole, miconazole, econazole).
- Allylamines cure slightly more infections than azoles but are more expensive.[2]
- No differences in efficacy found between individual topical allylamines or individual azoles.[2] SOR Ⓐ

Evidence for the management onychomycosis by topical treatments is sparse. There is some evidence that ciclopirox and butenafine are both marginally effective, but they both need to be applied daily for at least 1 year.[3]

Oral antifungals are needed for all tinea capitis infections and for more severe infections of the rest of the body.[4] True dermatophyte infections that do not respond to topical antifungals may need an oral agent.

- A Cochrane systematic review of 12 trials of oral antifungals for tinea pedis showed oral terbinafine for 2 weeks cures 52% more patients than oral griseofulvin.[5] SOR Ⓐ
- Terbinafine is equal to itraconazole in patient outcomes.[5]
- No significant differences in comparisons between a number of other oral agents.[5]

Oral antifungals used for fungal infections of the skin, nails, or mucous membranes include the following:

- Itraconazole (Sporanox)
- Fluconazole (Diflucan)
- Griseofulvin
- Ketoconazole (Nizoral)
- Terbinafine (Lamisil)

TABLE 134-2 Diagnostic Value of Clinical Diagnosis and KOH Prep in Tinea Infection

Test	Sensitivity (%)	Specificity (%)	PV+ (%)	PV– (%)	LR+	LR–
Clinical diagnosis*	81	45	24	92	1.47	0.42
KOH prep (study 1)†	88	95	73	98	17.6	0.13
KOH prep (study 2)†	77	62	59	79	2.02	0.37

LR–, negative likelihood ratio; LR+, positive likelihood ratio; PV–, negative predictive value; PV+, positive predictive value.
*The clinical diagnosis set was compiled by 27 general practitioners prior to submission of skin for fungal culture. Specimens were taken from consecutive patients with erythrosquamous lesions. Culture results were considered the gold standard; study quality = 2b.
†Both studies of KOH preps were open analyses of patients with suspicious lesions. Paired fungal culture was initiated simultaneously with KOH prep and was considered the gold standard; study quality = 2b.
Data from Thomas B. Clear choices in managing epidermal tinea infections. *J Fam Pract.* 2003;52(11):850-862. Reproduced with permission from Frontline Medical Communications.

One meta-analysis suggests that terbinafine is more efficacious than griseofulvin in treating tinea capitis caused by *Trichophyton* species, whereas griseofulvin is more efficacious than terbinafine in treating tinea capitis caused by *Microsporum* species.[6] SOR Ⓐ

Details of treatments for multiple types of fungal skin infections are supplied in the following chapters.

PATIENT RESOURCES

- Doctor fungus—**http://www.doctorfungus.org/.**

PROVIDER RESOURCES

- Fungal skin—**http://www.dermnetnz.org/fungal/.**
- Doctor fungus—**http://www.doctorfungus.org/.**
- World of dermatophytes—**http://www.provlab.ab.ca/mycol/tutorials/derm/dermhome.htm.**
- Swartz-Lamkins fungal stain can be easily purchased online—**http://www.delasco.com/pcat/1/Chemicals/Swartz_Lamkins/dlmis023/.**

TABLE 134-3 Topical Antifungal Preparations

Generic Name	Brand Name	OTC or R_x	Class
Butenafine	Mentax Lotrimin Ultra	R_x OTC	Allylamine
Ciclopirox	Loprox	R_x	Pyridone
Clotrimazole	Lotrimin AF Cream Lotrimin AF Spray	OTC	Azole
Econazole	Spectazole	R_x	Azole
Ketoconazole	Nizoral	2% R_x	Azole
Miconazole	Micatin Generic	OTC	Azole
Naftifine	Naftin	R_x	Allylamine
Oxiconazole	Oxistat	R_x	Azole
Sertaconazole	Ertaczo	R_x	Azole
Terbinafine	Lamisil AT	OTC	Allylamine
Tolnaftate*	Tinactin cream Lamisil AF defense and Tinactin powder spray Generic cream	OTC	Miscellaneous

OTC, over the counter.
*All the above antifungals will treat dermatophytes and *Candida*. Tolnaftate is effective only for dermatophytes and not *Candida*. Nystatin is effective only for *Candida* and not the dermatophytes.

REFERENCES

1. Thomas B. Clear choices in managing epidermal tinea infections. *J Fam Pract.* 2003;52:850-862.
2. Crawford F, Hart R, Bell-Syer S, et al. Topical treatments for fungal infections of the skin and nails of the foot. *Cochrane Database Syst Rev.* 2000;(2):CD001434.
3. Crawford F, Hollis S. Topical treatments for fungal infections of the skin and nails of the foot. *Cochrane Database Syst Rev.* 2007 Jul 18;(3):CD001434.
4. Gonzalez U, Seaton T, Bergus G, et al. Systemic antifungal therapy for tinea capitis in children. *Cochrane Database Syst Rev.* 2007 Oct 17;(4):CD004685.
5. Bell-Syer SE, Hart R, Crawford F, et al. Oral treatments for fungal infections of the skin of the foot. *Cochrane Database Syst Rev.* 2002;(2):CD003584.
6. Tey HL, Tan AS, Chan YC. Meta-analysis of randomized, controlled trials comparing griseofulvin and terbinafine in the treatment of tinea capitis. *J Am Acad Dermatol.* 2011;64:663-670.

135 CANDIDIASIS

Richard P. Usatine, MD

PATIENT STORY

A 42-year-old man (**Figure 135-1**) was admitted to the hospital for community-acquired pneumonia and type 2 diabetes out of control. On the second day of admission, when he was feeling a bit better, he asked about the itching he was having on his penis. Physical examination revealed an uncircumcised penis with white discharge on the glans and inside the foreskin consistent with *Candida* balanitis. Potassium hydroxide (KOH) prep was positive for the pseudohyphae of *Candida*. The patient was treated with a topical azole and the balanitis resolved.

INTRODUCTION

Cutaneous and mucosal *Candida* infections are seen commonly in infants with thrush and diaper rash. Also children and teens with obesity, diabetes, hyperhidrosis, and/or immunodeficiency are at higher risk of developing these infections.

EPIDEMIOLOGY

- *Candida* thrush is common in immunosuppressed adults (HIV and during chemotherapy).
- *Candida* thrush can also occur in adults wearing dentures or after a course of antibiotics. (**Figure 135-2**).
- *Candida* balanitis is more common in uncircumcised men than in them who have been circumcised (see **Figure 135-1**).

ETIOLOGY AND PATHOPHYSIOLOGY

- Infections caused by *Candida* species are primarily *Candida albicans*.[1]
- *C. albicans* has the ability to exist in both hyphal and yeast forms (termed *dimorphism*). If pinched cells do not separate, a chain of cells is produced and is termed *pseudohyphae*.[1]

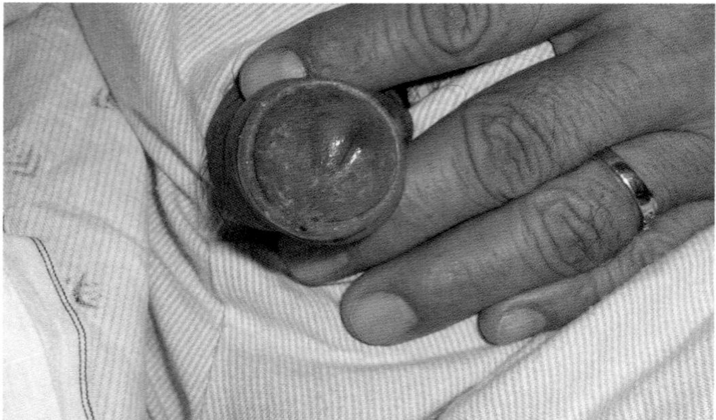

FIGURE 135-1 Candida balanitis in a man with uncontrolled diabetes. *(Reproduced with permission from Richard P. Usatine, MD.)*

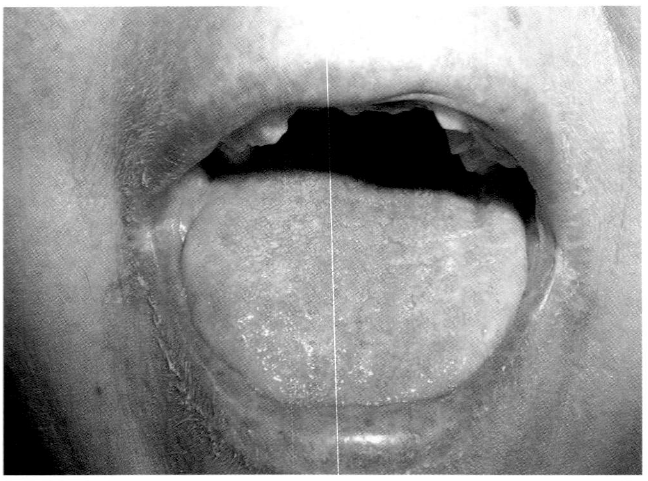

A

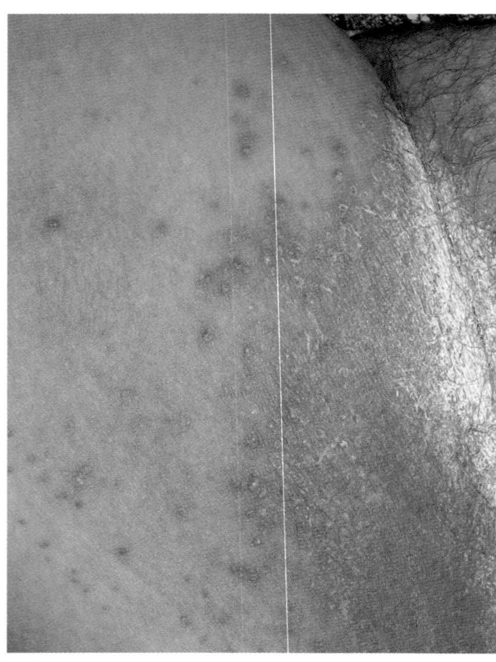

B

FIGURE 135-2 Thrush and a *Candida* groin rash in a 46-year-old woman who was given antibiotics for a urinary tract infection. The woman had previously suffered a stroke and was wearing an adult diaper to deal with her urinary incontinence. **A.** Note the white coating on the tongue. A KOH preparation was positive for *Candida*. **B.** Note the satellite lesions which are typical in a *Candida* infection of the groin. *(Reproduced with permission from Richard P. Usatine, MD.)*

RISK FACTORS

Obesity, diabetes, hyperhidrosis, immunodeficiency, HIV, heat, use of oral antibiotics, and use of inhaled or systemic steroids are the risk factors.[1]

DIAGNOSIS

CLINICAL FEATURES

- Typical distribution—Groin, glans penis, vulva, inframammary, under abdominal pannus, between fingers, in the creases of the neck, corners of mouth, nailfolds in chronic paronychia.

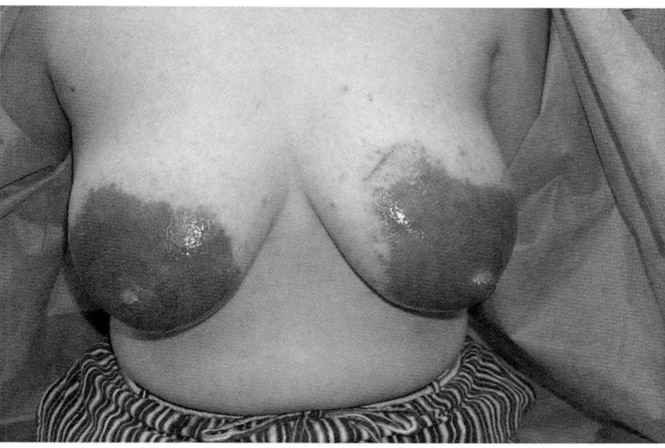

FIGURE 135-3 *Candida* rash with superimposed contact dermatitis in a breast-feeding woman. Her baby has thrush and both need treatment to eradicate the infection. The contact dermatitis was to the neomycin-containing topical antibiotic she applied to her sore breasts. (*Reproduced with permission from Jack Resneck, Sr., MD.*)

- Morphology—Macules, patches, plaques that are pink to bright red with small peripheral satellite lesions.
- Candidiasis of the nipple in the nursing mother is associated with infantile thrush (**Figures 135-3**). Nipple candidiasis is almost always bilateral, with the nipples appearing bright red and inflamed. In this case, the inflammation was made worse by the application of a topical antibiotic that caused a secondary contact dermatitis.
- The *Candida* infection in the corners of the mouth is called perlèche or angular cheilitis (**Figure 135-4**). When accompanied by thrush it may be a sign of HIV/AIDS.
- Thrush can be caused by *Candida* growing on the upper plate of a denture and the roof of the mouth (**Figure 135-5**).
- Ask about recent antibiotic use if there is a new onset of a rash with satellite lesions. In **Figure 135-6**, the man with diabetes had a course of antibiotics before he developed a *Candida* infection in his groin.

LABORATORY STUDIES

Scrape involved area and add to a slide with KOH (dimethyl sulfoxide [DMSO] optional). *C. albicans* exist in both hyphal and yeast forms (dimorphism). Look for pseudohyphae and/or budding yeast (**Figure 135-7**).

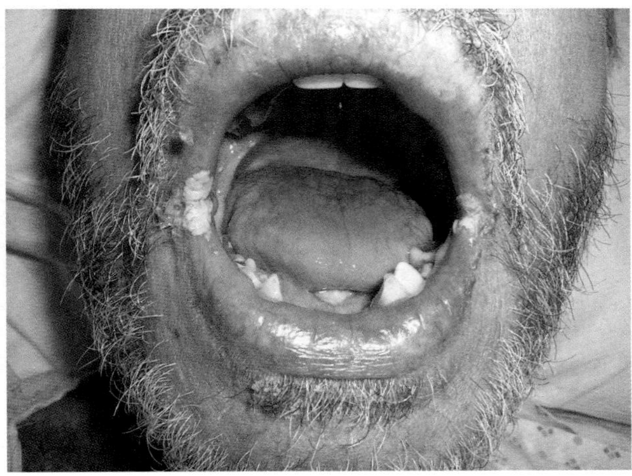

FIGURE 135-4 Thrush and perlèche in a man with AIDS. The *Candida* infection in the corners of the mouth is called perlèche or angular cheilitis. (*Reproduced with permission from Richard P. Usatine, MD.*)

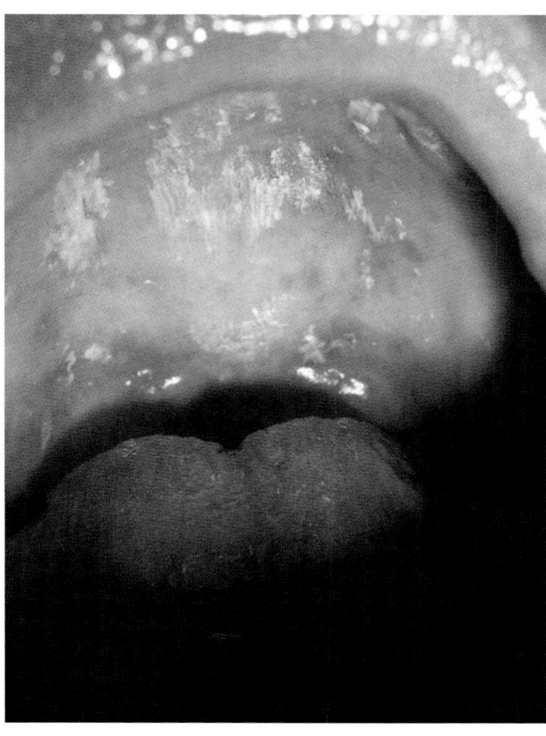

FIGURE 135-5 Candida on the roof of the mouth in an elderly woman using dentures. This is a common complication of denture use and should be suspected if a patient presents with new-onset pain under the dentures. (*Reproduced with permission from Richard P. Usatine, MD.*)

DIFFERENTIAL DIAGNOSIS

- Intertrigo is a nonspecific inflammatory condition of the skin folds. It is induced or aggravated by heat, moisture, maceration, and friction. The condition is frequently worsened by infection with *Candida* or dermatophytes (**Figures 135-8** and **135-9**). In **Figure 135-8** there is significant hyperpigmentation secondary to the inflammation.
- Tinea corporis or cruris—Can be distinguished from *Candida* when you see an annular pattern or concentric circles in the tinea (**Figure 135-9**).

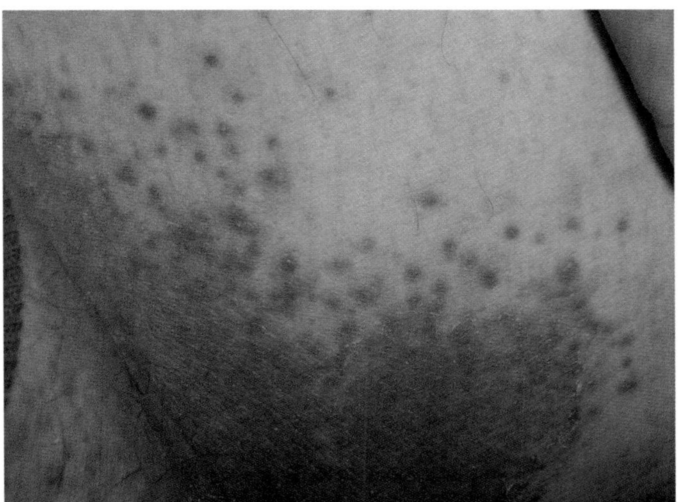

FIGURE 135-6 *Candida* inguinal eruption in a 61-year-old man after a course of antibiotics for bronchitis. Note the satellite lesions. (*Reproduced with permission from Richard P. Usatine, MD.*)

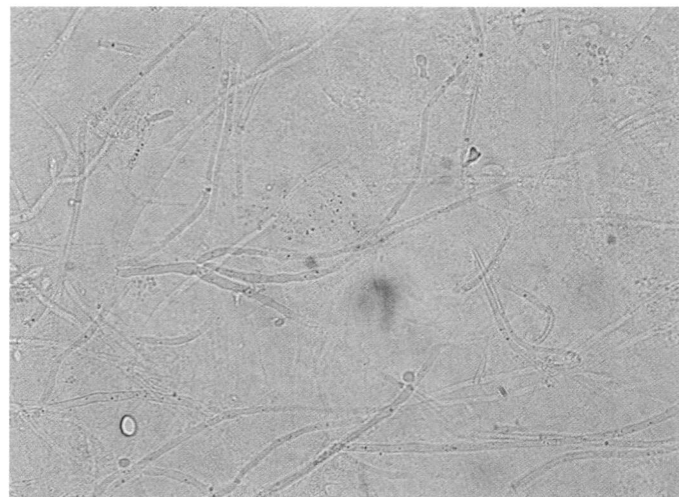

A

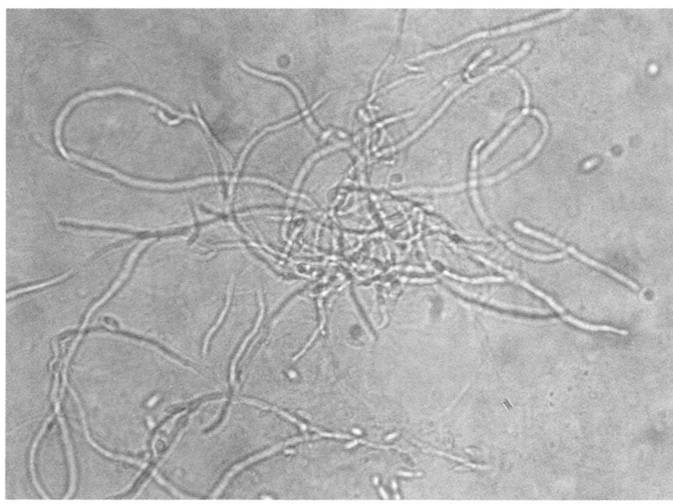

B

FIGURE 135-7 A. and B. The branching pseudohyphae of *Candida* from thrush under the microscope. Note the budding yeast. (*Reproduced with permission from Richard P. Usatine, MD.*)

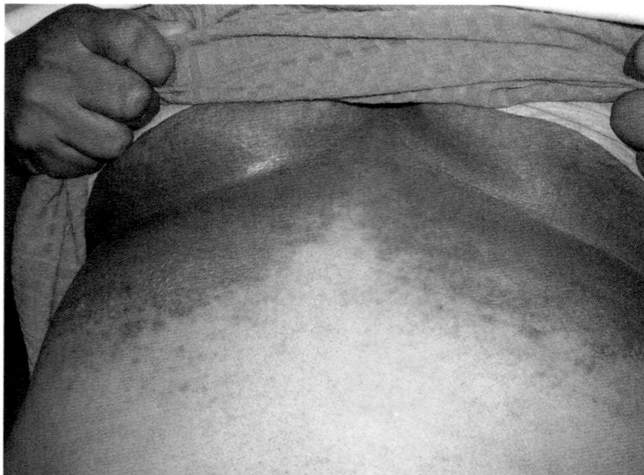

FIGURE 135-8 *Candida* under the breasts of an overweight Hispanic woman showing hyperpigmentation. The border is not well demarcated and there are satellite lesions. (*Reproduced with permission from Richard P. Usatine, MD.*)

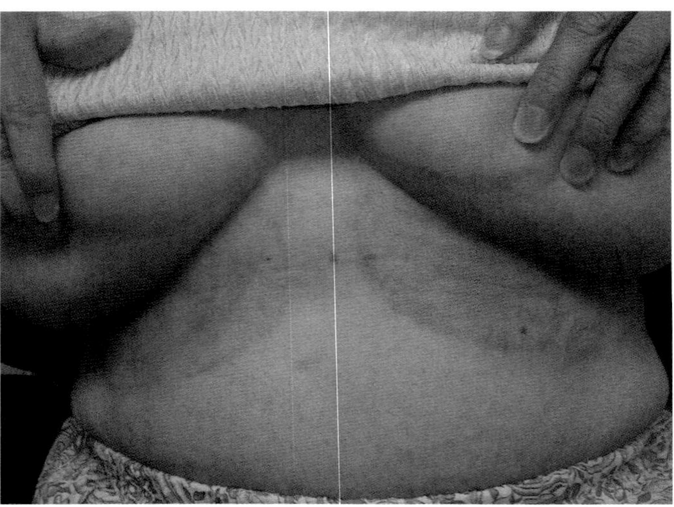

FIGURE 135-9 Tinea corporis under the breasts of a 55-year-old woman. Note the annular pattern with well-demarcated borders. KOH was positive for dermatophytes and not *Candida*. (*Reproduced with permission from Richard P. Usatine, MD.*)

There is no scrotal involvement in tinea cruris. *Candida* intertrigo may have scrotal involvement (see Chapters 136, Tinea Corporis and 137, Tinea Cruris).

- Erythrasma—May be brown and glows a coral red with ultraviolet (UV) light (see Chapter 121, Erythrasma).
- Inverse psoriasis—Psoriasis in the intertriginous areas as seen in **Figure 135-10** (see Chapter 150, Psoriasis).
- Seborrhea—Inflammation related to overgrowth of *Pityrosporum*, a yeast-like organism (see Chapter 149, Seborrheic Dermatitis).

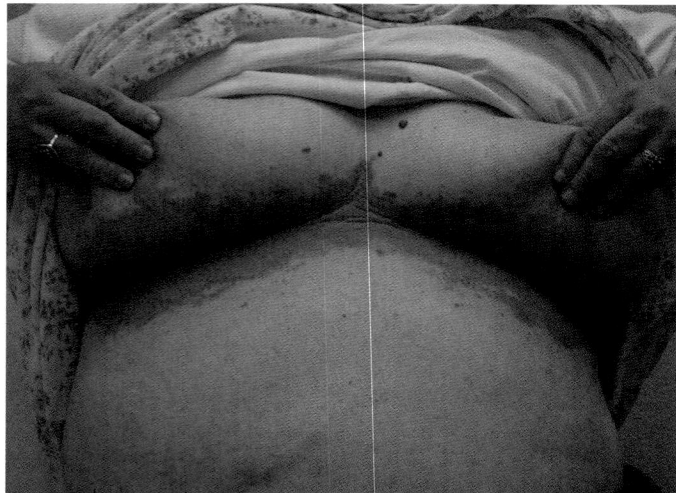

FIGURE 135-10 Inverse psoriasis that closely resembles *Candida* intertrigo in the submammary folds. This patient did not improve with topical antifungals and finally a biopsy showed that this was inverse psoriasis. Inverse psoriasis is often mistaken for a fungal infection unless the physician is aware of this condition. Frequently there are other clues to the diagnosis of psoriasis in the skin and nails so that a biopsy is not needed. (*Reproduced with permission from Richard P. Usatine, MD.*)

MANAGEMENT

PRIMARY CANDIDAL SKIN INFECTIONS

- Topical azoles, including clotrimazole, miconazole, and nystatin (polyenes) are effective.[2,3] SOR Ⓑ
- Keeping the infected area dry is important.[2] SOR Ⓒ
- For more details of the topical antifungals, see Table 134-3 in Chapter 134, Fungal Overview.
- In one study, miconazole ointment was well tolerated and significantly more effective than the zinc oxide/petrolatum vehicle control for treatment of diaper dermatitis complicated by candidiasis.[3]
- Do not use tolnaftate, which is active against dermatophytes but not *Candida*.
- If recurrent or recalcitrant, consider fluconazole 150 mg weekly × 2 or ketoconazole 200 mg daily for 1 to 2 weeks.

OROPHARYNGEAL CANDIDIASIS

- Treat initial episodes with clotrimazole troches (one 10-mg troche 5 times per day for adults) or nystatin (available as a suspension of 100,000 U/mL [dosage, 4-6 mL qid] or as flavored 200,000 units pastilles [dosage, 1 or 2 pastilles 4-5 times per day for 7-14 days]).[2] SOR Ⓑ
- Oral fluconazole (100 mg/d for 7-14 days) is as effective as—and, in some studies, superior to—topical therapy.[2] SOR Ⓐ
- Itraconazole solution (200 mg/d for 7-14 days) is as effective as fluconazole.[2] SOR Ⓐ
- Ketoconazole and itraconazole capsules are less effective than fluconazole, because of variable absorption.[2] SOR Ⓐ
- Fluconazole-refractory oropharyngeal candidiasis will respond to oral itraconazole therapy (>200 mg/d, preferably in solution form) approximately two-thirds of the time.[2] SOR Ⓐ
- Children with thrush are usually treated with oral nystatin suspension.[2] SOR Ⓑ
- HIV/AIDS patients with oral candidiasis may be treated with clotrimazole troches. If unresponsive to topical therapy, fluconazole may be needed.[2] SOR Ⓐ
- Denture-related disease may require extensive and aggressive disinfection of the denture for definitive cure.[2] SOR Ⓒ

MAMMARY CANDIDIASIS IN BREAST-FEEDING

- Most mammary candidiasis does not present with the red breasts seen in **Figure 135-3**.
- Nipple pain and discomfort along with thrush are adequate data to treat the mother and child.
- Topical nystatin and oral fluconazole are safe for infants and the mother.[2]

CHRONIC MUCOCUTANEOUS CANDIDIASIS

- Chronic mucocutaneous candidiasis (**Figure 135-11**) requires a long-term approach that is analogous to that used in patients with AIDS.[2]

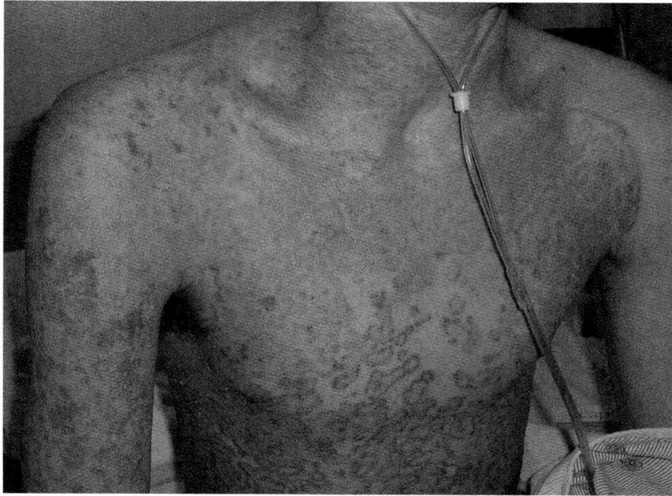

FIGURE 135-11 Severe chronic cutaneous candidiasis in a 22-year-old man with immunosuppression. (*Reproduced with permission from Richard P. Usatine, MD.*)

- Systemic therapy is needed, and azole antifungal agents (ketoconazole, fluconazole, and itraconazole) have been used successfully.[2]
- As with HIV-infected patients, development of resistance to these agents has been described.[2]

PATIENT EDUCATION

Keep the infected area clean and dry. For thrush in a baby, treat sources of infection such as the mother's breasts and bottle nipples. If the baby is bottle fed, boil the nipples between uses.

PATIENT AND PROVIDER RESOURCES

- Medscape. *Cutaneous Candidiasis*—**http://emedicine.medscape.com/article/1090632.**
- Medscape. *Intertrigo*—**http://emedicine.medscape.com/article/ 1087691.**

REFERENCES

1. Scheinfeld N. *Cutaneous Candidiasis*. Updated August 2, 2011. http://emedicine.medscape.com/article/1090632. Accessed September 5, 2011.
2. Pappas PG, Rex JH, Sobel JD, et al. Guidelines for treatment of candidiasis. *Clin Infect Dis*. 2004;38:161-189.
3. Spraker MK, Gisoldi EM, Siegfried EC, et al. Topical miconazole nitrate ointment in the treatment of diaper dermatitis complicated by candidiasis. *Cutis*. 2006;77(2):113-120.

136 TINEA CORPORIS

Richard P. Usatine, MD
Adeliza Jimenez, MD

PATIENT STORY

A 45-year-old woman presents to her internist with a rash that has been itching under her breast for the past 6 months (**Figure 136-1A**). She had gone to an urgent care center and received a topical steroid which only partially relieved the itching. On physical examination there is erythema and scale under the breast with a well-demarcated partial annular border (see **Figure 136-1A**). The erythema and scale are most prominent on the edge creating a clinical suspicion for tinea corporis. There are no satellite lesions that may be seen with candidiasis and the patient does not have a history of psoriasis. The physician scrapes the leading edge to create a potassium hydroxide (KOH) preparation (**Figure 136-1B**).

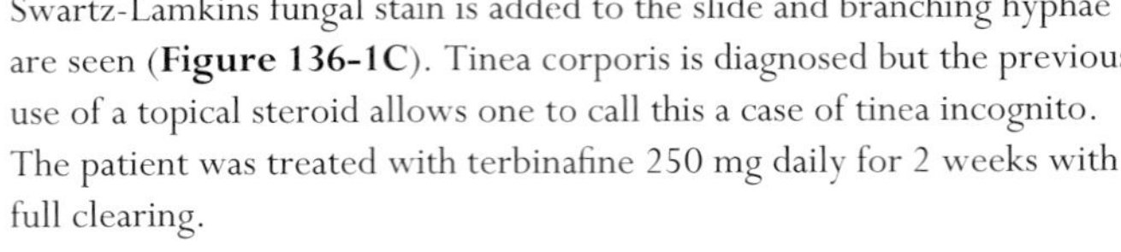

Swartz-Lamkins fungal stain is added to the slide and branching hyphae are seen (**Figure 136-1C**). Tinea corporis is diagnosed but the previous use of a topical steroid allows one to call this a case of tinea incognito. The patient was treated with terbinafine 250 mg daily for 2 weeks with full clearing.

INTRODUCTION

Tinea corporis is a common superficial fungal infection of the body, characterized by well-demarcated, annular lesions with central clearing, erythema, and scaling of the periphery.

EPIDEMIOLOGY

Dermatophytes are the most prevalent agents causing fungal infections in the United States, with *Trichophyton rubrum* causing the majority of cases of tinea corporis, tinea cruris, tinea manuum, and tinea pedis.

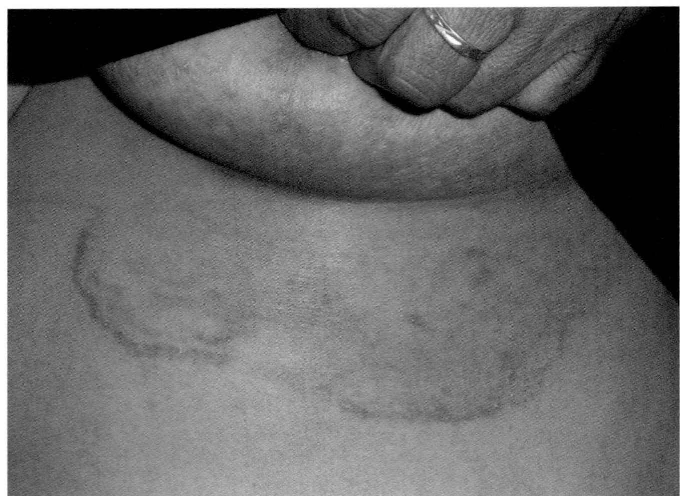

A

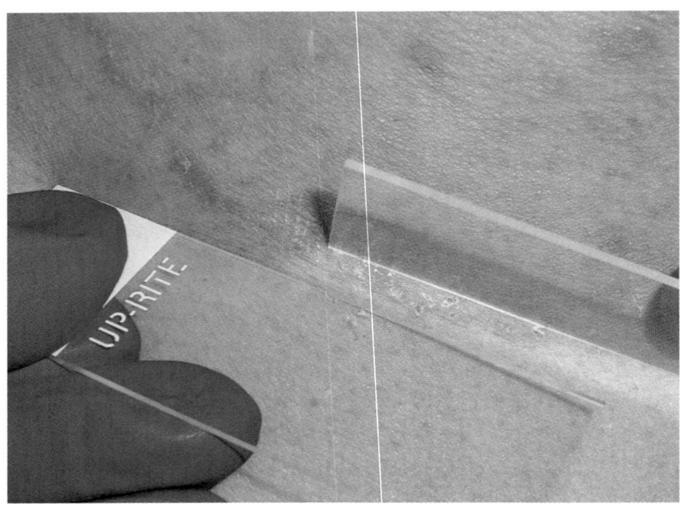

B

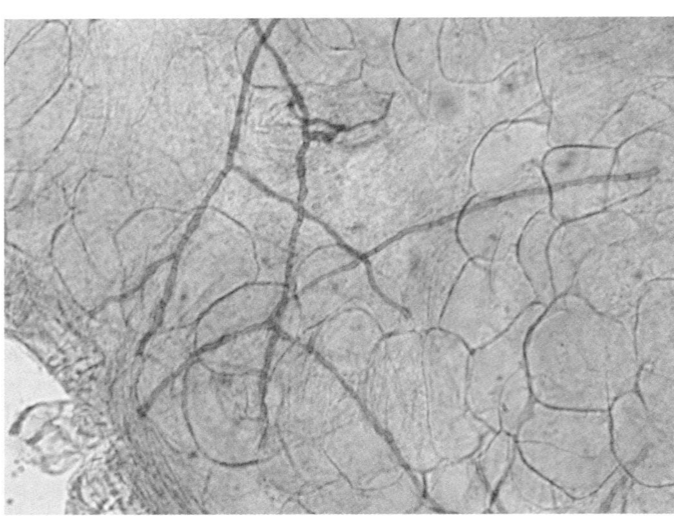

C

FIGURE 136-1 A. Tinea corporis with scaling, erythema, and central sparing under the breast. B. Scraping the edge for a KOH preparation to confirm the clinical impression. C. Branching hyphae easily seen at 40× power using fungal stain (Swartz-Lamkins) from a scraping of tinea corporis. Note how the hyphae stand out with the blue ink color. (*Reproduced with permission from Richard P. Usatine, MD.*)

- Excessive heat and humidity make a good environment for fungal growth.
- Dermatophytes spread by exposure to infected animals or persons and contact with contaminated items.

ETIOLOGY AND PATHOPHYSIOLOGY

Tinea corporis is caused by fungal species from any one of the following 3 dermatophyte genuses: *Trichophyton*, *Microsporum*, and *Epidermophyton*. *T. rubrum* is the most common causative agent of tinea corporis.

- Dermatophytes produce enzymes such as keratinase that penetrate keratinized tissue. Their hyphae invade the stratum corneum and keratin and spread centrifugally outward.

RISK FACTORS

- Participation in daycare centers
- Living in a nursing home
- Poor personal hygiene
- Living conditions with poor sanitation
- Warm, humid environments
- Conditions that cause weakening of the immune system (eg, AIDS, cancer, organ transplantation, diabetes)

DIAGNOSIS

The diagnosis can be made from history, clinical presentation, culture, and direct microscopic observation of hyphae in infected tissue and hairs after KOH preparation.

CLINICAL FEATURES

- Pruritus of affected area.
- Well-demarcated, annular lesions with central clearing, erythema, and scaling of the periphery. Concentric rings are highly specific (80%) for tinea infections (see **Figure 136-1**).
- Central clearing is not always present (**Figure 136-2**).
- Although scale is the most prominent morphologic characteristic, some tinea infections will actually cause pustules from the inflammatory response (**Figure 136-3**).

TYPICAL DISTRIBUTION

It occurs on any part of the body including the face and axilla (**Figures 136-1** to **136-4**).

Tinea incognito is a type of tinea infection that was previously not recognized by the physician or patient and topical steroids were used on the site. While applying the steroid, the dermatophyte continues to grow and form concentric rings (**Figures 136-5** and **136-6**).

Tinea corporis can cover large parts of the body as in **Figures 136-7** to **136-9**.

In some cases the infection may cause hyperpigmentation (see **Figures 136-7** to **136-9**).

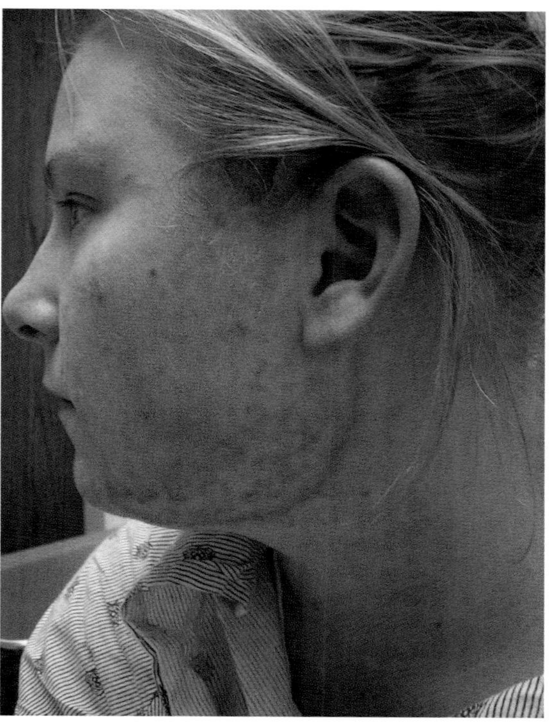

FIGURE 136-2 Tinea faciei in a 42-year-old woman who had widespread tinea corporis. It resolved with oral terbinafine. (*Reproduced with permission from Olvia Revelo, MD.*)

LABORATORY STUDIES

- KOH preparation of skin scraping can be very useful to confirm a clinical impression or when the diagnosis is not certain. Scrape the skin with the side of a slide or scalpel, making sure to scrape the periphery and the erythematous part. Scrape hard enough to get some stratum corneum without causing significant bleeding. False negatives can occur secondary to inadequate scraping, patient using topical antifungals, or an inexperienced microscopist.

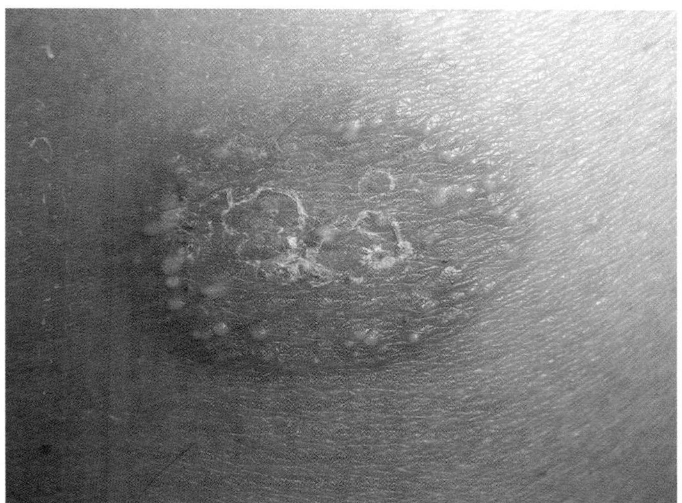

FIGURE 136-3 Tinea corporis with pustules and scale. KOH preparation was positive for branching hyphae. The pustules are a manifestation of an inflammatory response to the dermatophyte infection. (*Reproduced with permission from Richard P. Usatine, MD.*)

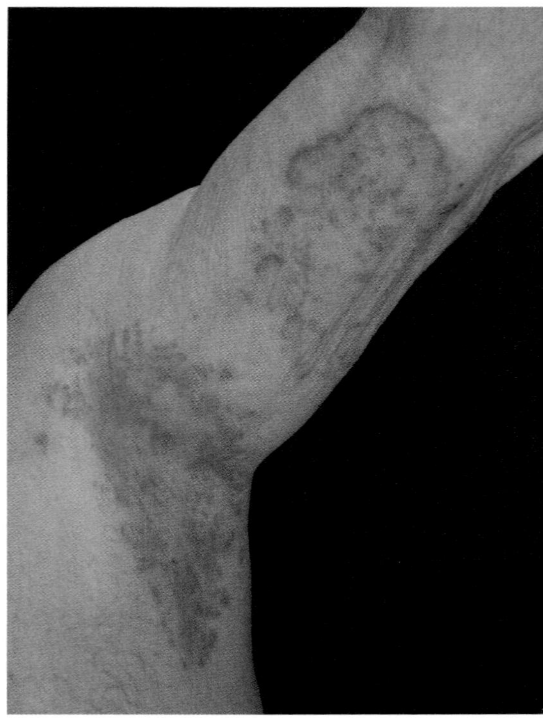

FIGURE 136-4 Extensive tinea corporis in the axilla and arm of this older adult. (*Reproduced with permission from Richard P. Usatine, MD.*)

- Use KOH (plain, with dimethyl sulfoxide [DMSO], or in a fungal stain) to break up the epithelial cells more rapidly without heating (**Figure 136-10**). It is easy to purchase a small bottle of Swartz-Lamkins fungal stain that includes KOH, a surfactant, and blue ink. The blue ink allows the hyphae to stand out, thereby saving time and decreasing the chance of a false-negative result (**Figure 136-11**). If the epithelial cells are not breaking up sufficiently, use a flame under the slide for approximately 5 seconds to speed up the process. If the KOH prep is negative and this does not fit the clinical picture, wait a few hours and look at the KOH prep again as the fungi may become more visible over time (see **Figure 136-11**).
- Skin scraping and culture—Gold standard, but more costly and may take up to 2 weeks for the culture to grow. Consider culture if the KOH prep is negative but tinea is still suspected, or when a microscope is not available.
- Skin biopsy sent in formalin for periodic acid-Schiff (PAS) staining when the KOH and culture remain negative but the clinical picture is consistent with a fungal infection.

DIFFERENTIAL DIAGNOSIS

- Granuloma annulare—Inflammatory, benign dermatosis of unknown cause, characterized by both dermal and annular papules (**Figure 136-12**) (see Chapter 171, Granuloma Annulare).
- Psoriasis—Plaque with scale on extensor surfaces and trunk. Occasionally, the plaques can have an annular appearance (**Figure 136-13**). Inverse psoriasis in intertriginous areas can also mimic tinea corporis (see Chapter 150, Psoriasis).
- Erythema annulare centrifugum (EAC)—Scaly red rings with normal skin in the center of the rings. The scale is trailing the erythema as the ring expands while the scale is leading in tinea corporis (**Figure 136-14**) (see Chapter 204, Erythema Annulare Centrifugum).
- Cutaneous larva migrans has serpiginous burrows made by the hookworm larvae, and these burrows can look annular and be confused with tinea corporis (see Chapter 142, Cutaneous Larva Migrans).
- Nummular eczema—Round coin-like red scaly plaques without central clearing (see Chapter 143, Atopic Dermatitis).
- Erythrasma—Found in the axilla and groin without an annular configuration and central clearing. Coral red fluorescence is seen under a UV lamp (see Chapter 121, Erythrasma).

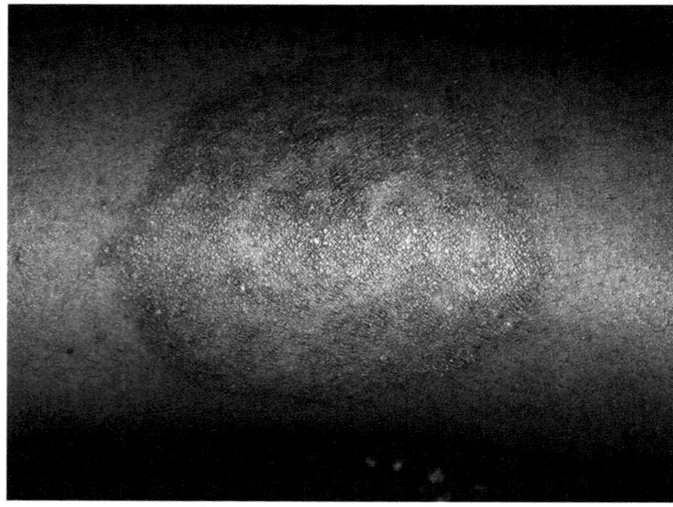

A

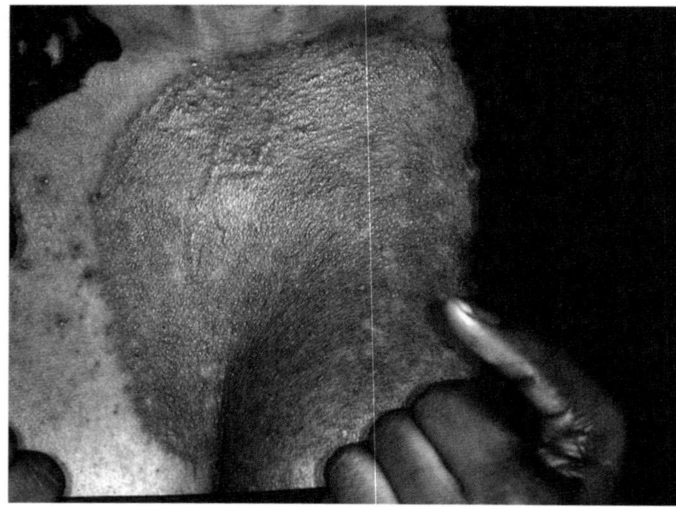

B

FIGURE 136-5 Tinea incognito on the chest and arm of this black woman. This tinea infection continued to grow as the patient applied the topical steroids given to her by her physician. There is an extensive amount of postinflammatory hyperpigmentation. **A.** Tinea incognito on the arm with concentric rings as this dermatophyte infection continued to grow under the influence of the topical steroids. **B.** Tinea incognito on the chest. (*Reproduced with permission from Richard P. Usatine, MD.*)

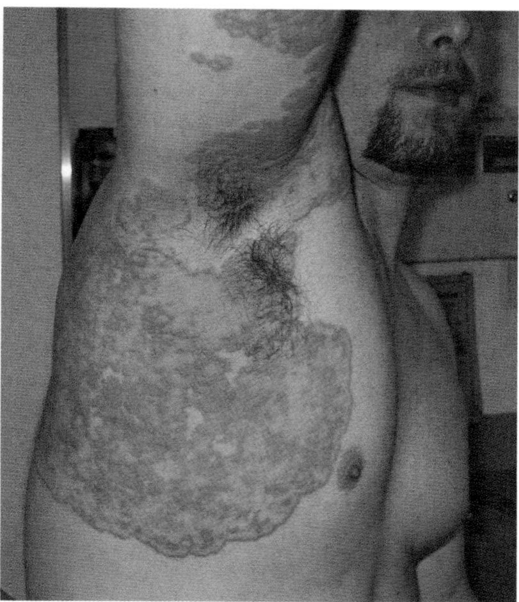

FIGURE 136-6 Tinea incognito in the axillary region of a young man who was prescribed topical steroids. Although there is some hyperpigmentation, erythema is most prominent. (*Reproduced with permission from Chris Wenner, MD.*)

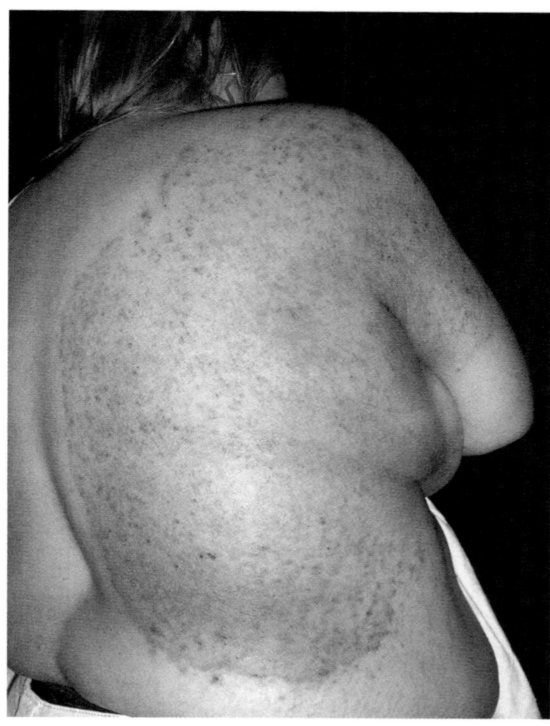

FIGURE 136-8 Tinea corporis on the back, shoulder, and arm with erythema and hyperpigmentation. (*Reproduced with permission from Richard P. Usatine, MD.*)

MANAGEMENT

- Use topical antifungal medications for tinea corporis that involves small areas of the body such as seen in **Figures 136-1** and **136-2**.
- Although all the topical antifungal agents may be effective, the evidence supports the greater effectiveness of the allylamines (terbinafine) over the less-expensive azoles for tinea pedis and corporis. Allylamines cure slightly more infections than azoles and are now available over the counter.[1,2] SOR Ⓐ
- Studies show that terbinafine 1% cream or solution applied once daily for 7 days is highly effective for tinea corporis/cruris.[3,4] The 1% cream

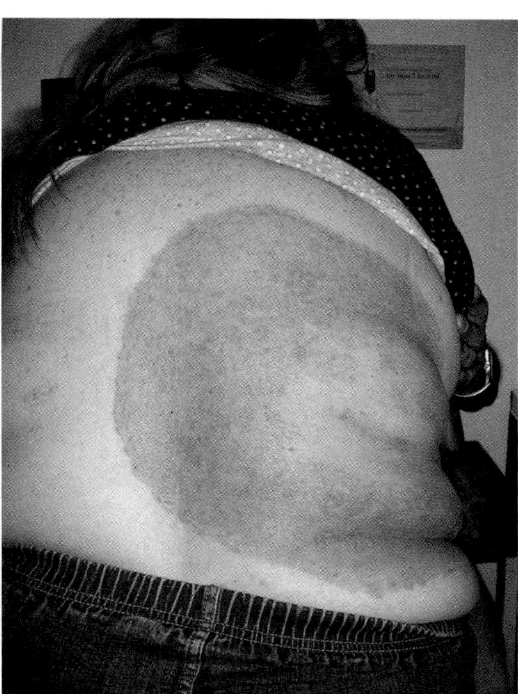

FIGURE 136-7 Tinea corporis covering the back and showing well-demarcated borders. (*Reproduced with permission from Richard P. Usatine, MD.*)

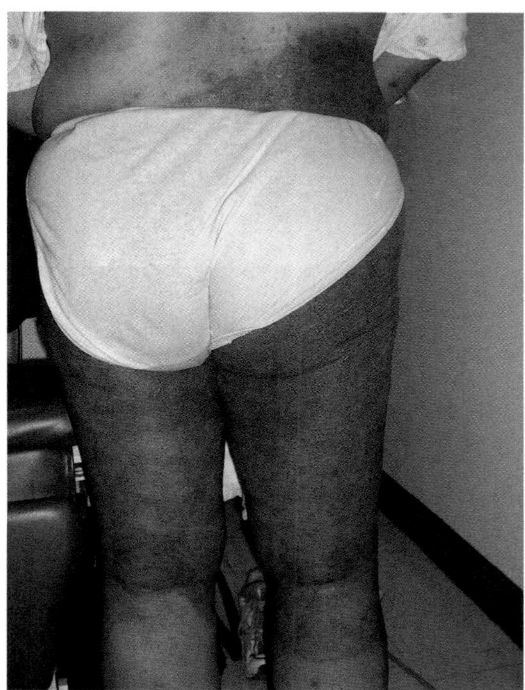

FIGURE 136-9 Tinea corporis from the trunk down both legs with significant hyperpigmentation. (*Reproduced with permission from Richard P. Usatine, MD.*)

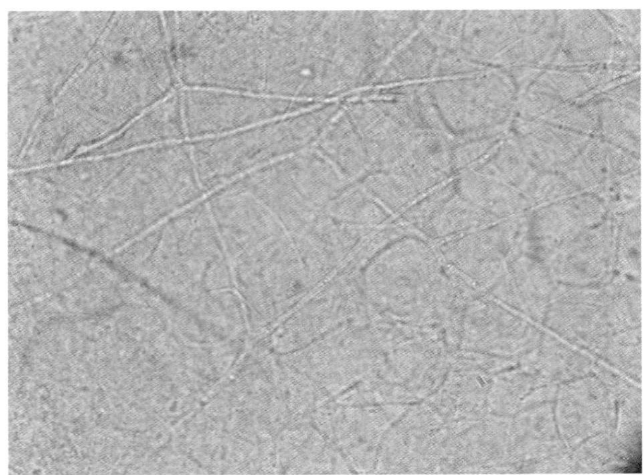

FIGURE 136-10 Branching hyphae at 40× power from KOH preparation of tinea corporis. (*Reproduced with permission from Richard P. Usatine, MD.*)

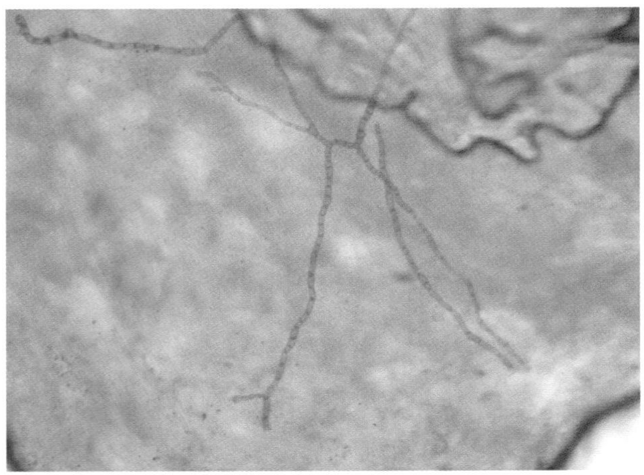

FIGURE 136-11 Branching septate hyphae easily seen at 40× power using fungal stain (Swartz-Lamkins) from a scraping of tinea corporis. The KOH prep was positive the day before. This photomicrograph was taken the following day when the skin cells were less visible and the hyphae had maximally taken up the blue ink color. This is to highlight how waiting a few hours or even 1 day can bring out a positive KOH even when it originally appeared negative. (*Reproduced with permission from Richard P. Usatine, MD.*)

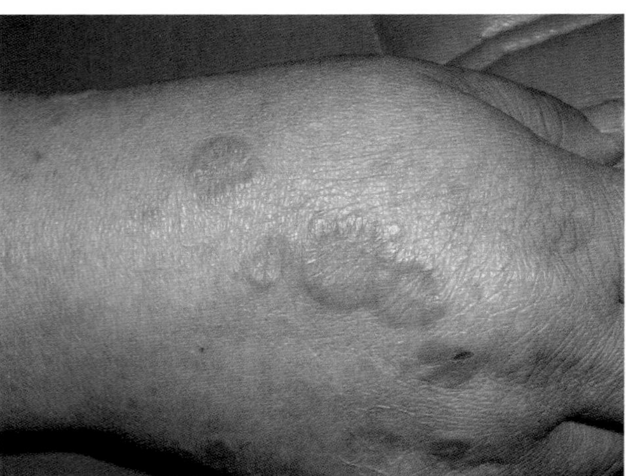

FIGURE 136-12 Multiple annular lesions caused by granuloma annulare. No scale is visible. (*Reproduced with permission from Richard P. Usatine, MD.*)

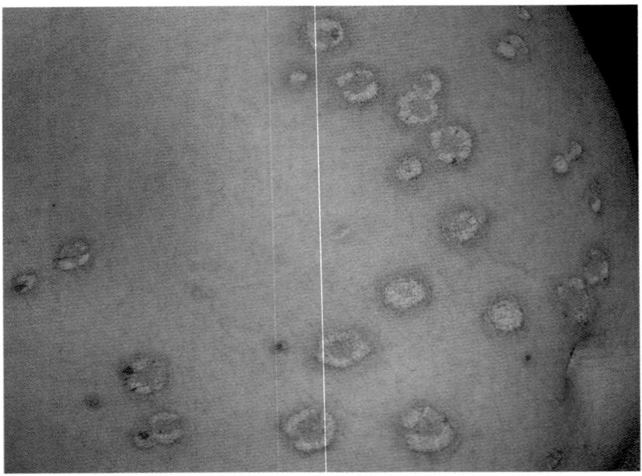

FIGURE 136-13 Widespread annular lesions caused by psoriasis. Not all lesions that are annular with scale are tinea corporis. (*Reproduced with permission from Richard P. Usatine, MD.*)

(which is available over the counter as Lamisil AF) produced a mycologic cure of 84.2% versus 23.3% with placebo. Number needed to treat (NNT) = 1.6.[3] SOR Ⓐ

- Oral antifungal agents should be considered for first-line therapy for tinea corporis covering large areas of the body, as seen in **Figures 136-6** and **136-7**. However, it is not wrong to attempt topical treatment if the size of the area infected is on the borderline. The patient with tinea incognito in **Figures 136-4** and **136-5** did need oral therapy to resolve her infection. Unfortunately, the postinflammatory hyperpigmentation did not resolve well.
- One randomized controlled trial (RCT) showed that oral itraconazole 200 mg daily for 1 week is similarly effective, equally well tolerated, and at least as safe as itraconazole 100 mg for 2 weeks in the treatment of tinea corporis or cruris.[5] SOR Ⓑ
- In one study, patients with mycologically diagnosed tinea corporis and tinea cruris were randomly allocated to receive either 250 mg of oral

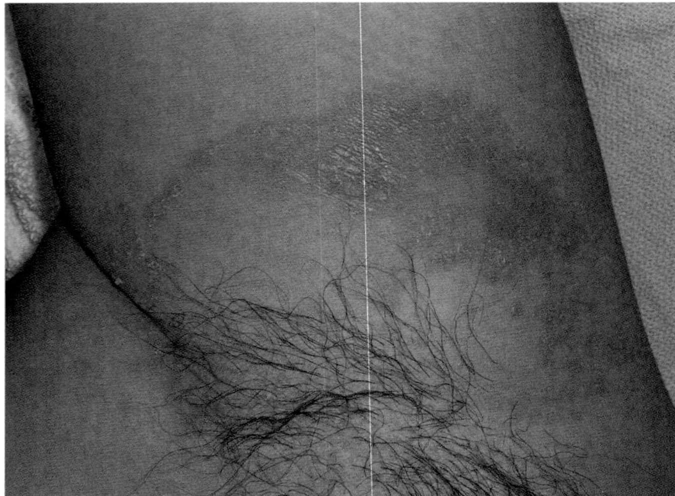

FIGURE 136-14 Erythema annulare centrifugum (EAC) in the axilla of a 28-year-old man. After multiple failed trials of antifungal medicines, a punch biopsy showed this to be EAC. Note the trailing scale rather than leading scale seen in tinea corporis. (*Reproduced with permission from Richard P. Usatine, MD.*)

terbinafine once daily or 500 mg of griseofulvin once daily for 2 weeks. The cure rates were higher for terbinafine at 6 weeks.[6] SOR B

- In summary, if an oral agent is needed, the evidence is greatest for the use of the following:
  - Terbinafine 250 mg daily for 2 weeks.[6] SOR B (Terbinafine is available as an inexpensive generic prescription on the $4 and $5 plans in the United States. It also has less drug interactions than itraconazole. For these reasons it is usually the preferred treatment when an oral agent is needed.)
  - Itraconazole 200 mg daily for 1 week.[5] SOR B (More expensive with more drug interactions than terbinafine.)
  - Itraconazole 100 mg daily for 2 weeks.[5] SOR B

PREVENTION

Tinea corporis and cruris are dermatophyte infections that are particularly common in areas of excessive heat and moisture. A dry, cool environment may play a role in reducing infection. In addition, avoiding contact with farm animals and other individuals infected with tinea corporis and cruris may help in preventing infection. Preventative measures for tinea infections include practicing good personal hygiene; keeping the skin dry and cool at all times; and avoiding sharing towels, clothing, or hair accessories with infected individuals.[7]

In individuals involved in contact sports such as wrestling, a comprehensive skin disease prevention protocol includes some combination of the following: washing of wrestling mats before and after each practice and competition; showers before and after each practice; use of clean clothing before each practice; and exclusion of infected athletes.[8]

PATIENT EDUCATION

Keep the skin clean and dry. Infected pets should be treated.

FOLLOW-UP

Consider follow-up appointments in 4 to 6 weeks for difficult and more widespread cases. If there are concerns about bacterial superinfection, follow-up should be sooner.

PATIENT RESOURCES

- VisualDxHealth. *Ringworm*—**http://www.visualdxhealth.com/adult/tineaCorporis.htm.**
- Medline Plus Medical Encyclopedia—**http://www.nlm.nih.gov/medlineplus/ency/article/000877.htm.**

PROVIDER RESOURCES

- eMedicine topic—**http://www.emedicine.com/DERM/topic421.htm.**
- Doctor Fungus—**http://www.doctorfungus.org/.**
- Swartz-Lamkins fungal stain can be easily purchased online—**http://www.delasco.com/pcat/1/Chemicals/Swartz_Lamkins/dlmis023/.**

REFERENCES

1. Thomas B. Clear choices in managing epidermal tinea infections. *J Fam Pract.* 2003;52:850-862.
2. Crawford F, Hollis S. Topical treatments for fungal infections of the skin and nails of the foot. *Cochrane Database Syst Rev.* 2007;3:CD001434.
3. Budimulja U, Bramono K, Urip KS, et al. Once daily treatment with terbinafine 1% cream (Lamisil) for one week is effective in the treatment of tinea corporis and cruris. A placebo-controlled study. *Mycoses.* 2001;44:300-306.
4. Lebwohl M, Elewski B, Eisen D, Savin RC. Efficacy and safety of terbinafine 1% solution in the treatment of interdigital tinea pedis and tinea corporis or tinea cruris. *Cutis.* 2001;67:261-266.
5. Boonk W, de Geer D, de Kreek E, et al. Itraconazole in the treatment of tinea corporis and tinea cruris: comparison of two treatment schedules. *Mycoses.* 1998;41:509-514.
6. Voravutinon V. Oral treatment of tinea corporis and tinea cruris with terbinafine and griseofulvin: A randomized double blind comparative study. *J Med Assoc Thai.* 1993;76:388-393.
7. Gupta AK, Chaudhry M, Elewski B. Tinea corporis, tinea cruris, tinea nigra, and piedra. *Dermatol Clin.* 2003;21(3):395-400.
8. Hand JW, Wroble RR. Prevention of tinea corporis in collegiate wrestlers. *J Athl Train.* 1999;34(4):350-352.

137 TINEA CRURIS

Richard P. Usatine, MD
Mindy A. Smith, MD, MS

PATIENT STORY

A 59-year-old man presents with itching in the groin (**Figure 137-1**). On examination, he was found to have scaly erythematous plaques in the inguinal area. A skin scraping was treated with Swartz-Lamkins stain and the dermatophyte was highly visible under the microscope (**Figure 137-2**). He was treated with a topical antifungal medicine until his tinea cruris resolved.

INTRODUCTION

Tinea cruris is an intensely pruritic superficial fungal infection of the groin and adjacent skin.

SYNONYMS

Tinea cruris is commonly known as crotch rot and jock itch to the lay public.

EPIDEMIOLOGY

- Using data from the National Ambulatory Medical Care Survey and the National Hospital Ambulatory Medical Care Survey (NHAMCS) (1995-2004), there were more than 4 million annual visits for dermatophytoses and 8.4% were for tinea cruris.[1]
- Tinea cruris is more common in men than women (3-fold) and rare in children.

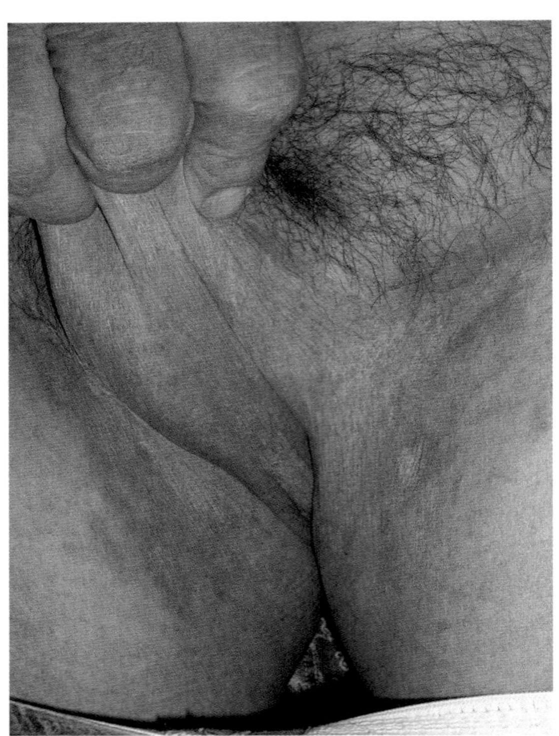

FIGURE 137-1 Tinea cruris in a 59-year-old Hispanic man present for 1 year. *(Reproduced with permission from Richard P. Usatine, MD.)*

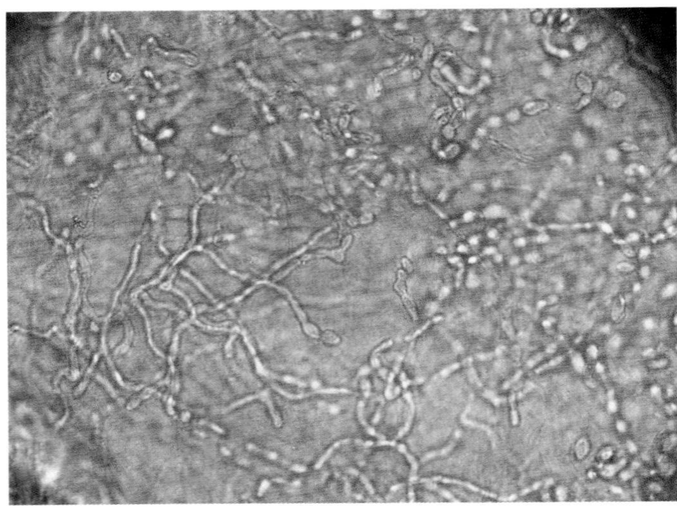

FIGURE 137-2 Microscopic view of the scraping of the groin in a man with tinea cruris. The hyphae are easy to see under 40 power with Swartz-Lamkins stain. *(Reproduced with permission from Richard P. Usatine, MD.)*

ETIOLOGY AND PATHOPHYSIOLOGY

- Most commonly caused by the dermatophytes *Trichophyton rubrum, Epidermophyton floccosum, Trichophyton mentagrophytes,* and *Trichophyton verrucosum. T. rubrum* is the most common organism.[2]
- Can be spread by fomites, such as contaminated towels.
- The fungal agents cause keratinases, which allow invasion of the cornified cell layer of the epidermis.[2]
- Autoinoculation can occur from fungus on the feet or hands.

RISK FACTORS

- Wearing tight-fitting or wet clothing or underwear has traditionally been suggested; however, in a study of Italian soldiers, none of the risk factors analyzed (eg, hyperhidrosis, swimming pool attendance) were significantly associated with any fungal infection.[3]
- Obesity and diabetes mellitus may be risk factors.[4]

DIAGNOSIS

CLINICAL FEATURES

The cardinal features are scale and signs of inflammation. In light-skinned persons inflammation often appears pink or red and in dark-skinned persons the inflammation often leads to hyperpigmentation (**Figures 137-3** and **137-4**). Occasionally, tinea cruris may show central sparing with an annular pattern as in **Figure 137-5**, but most often is homogeneously distributed as in **Figures 137-3** and **137-4**.

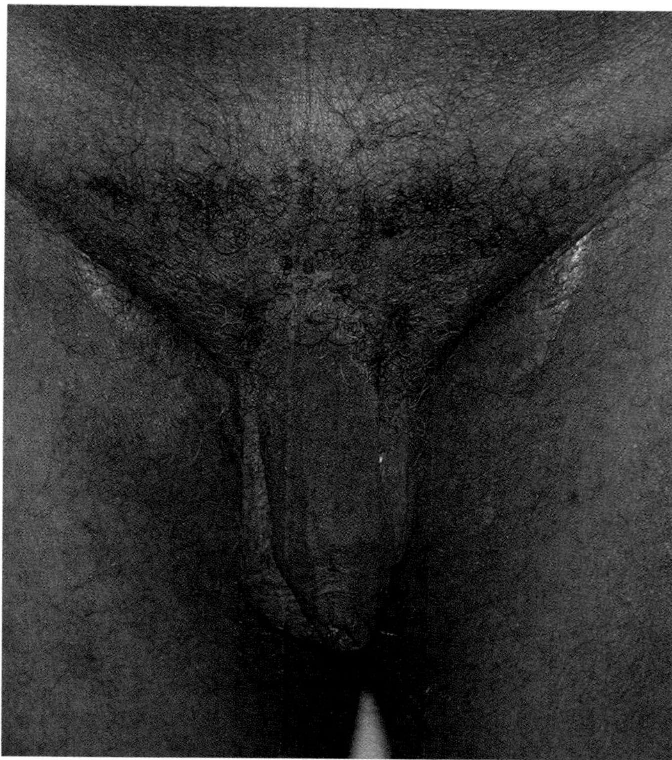

FIGURE 137-3 Tinea cruris in an older black man with hyperpigmentation secondary to the inflammatory response. A silvery scale is also seen and psoriasis should be considered in the differential diagnosis. In such a case, performing a potassium hydroxide (KOH) preparation is crucial to making an accurate diagnosis as it is not possible to know the diagnosis by appearance only. (*Reproduced with permission from Richard P. Usatine, MD.*)

TYPICAL DISTRIBUTION

By definition tinea cruris is in the inguinal area. However, the fungus can grow outside of this area to involve the abdomen and thighs (**Figures 137-4** and **137-6**). Tinea can be present in multiple locations, as in the patient in **Figure 137-7** who had tinea in the groin, on her feet and face, and under her breasts.

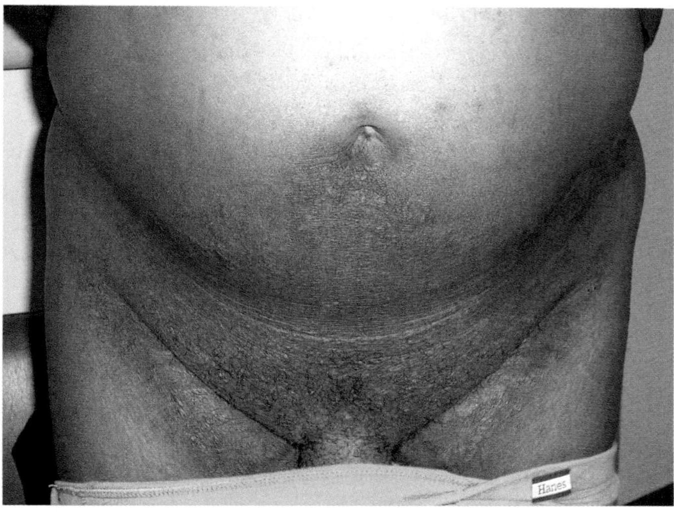

FIGURE 137-4 Tinea cruris that has expanded beyond the inguinal area in this 35-year-old black man. Postinflammatory hyperpigmentation is visible throughout the infected area. (*Reproduced with permission from Richard P. Usatine, MD.*)

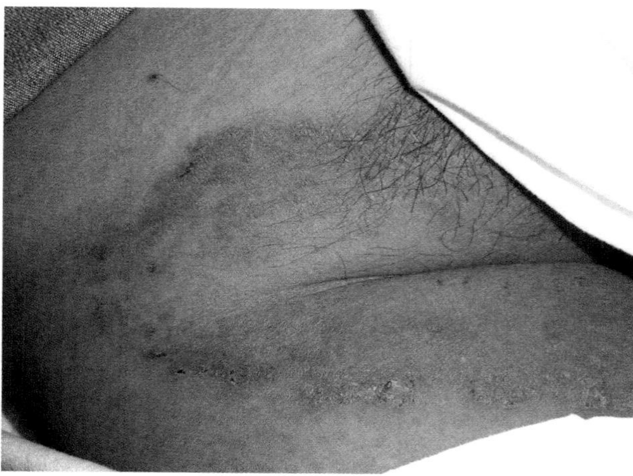

FIGURE 137-5 An 18-year-old woman with tinea cruris showing erythema and scale in an annular pattern. Central clearing is less common in tinea cruris than tinea corporis but can occur. (*Reproduced with permission from Richard P. Usatine, MD.*)

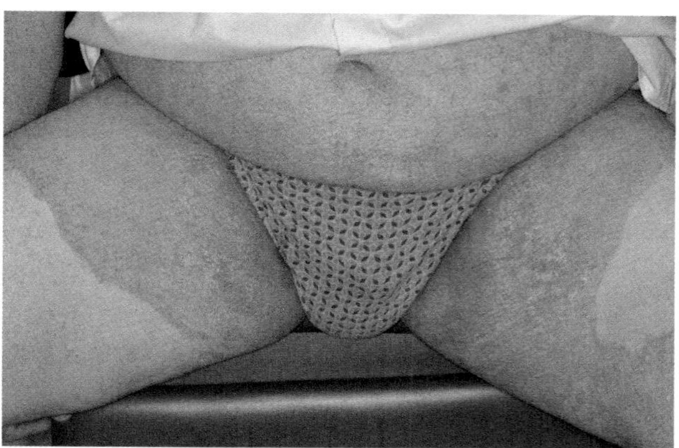

FIGURE 137-6 A 54-year-old man with tinea cruris and corporis for decades despite multiple treatments with oral antifungal medications. His cultures show *T. rubrum* sensitive to all the typical oral antifungal medications, but his tinea never completely clears. He does not have a known immunodeficiency but his immune system appears not to recognize the *T. rubrum* as foreign. (*Reproduced with permission from Richard P. Usatine, MD.*)

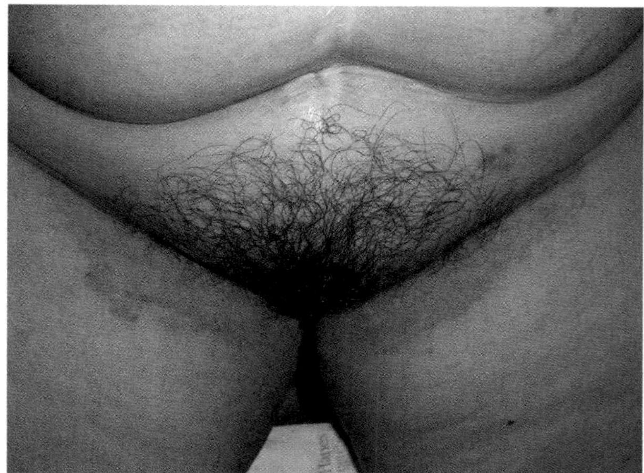

FIGURE 137-7 A 55-year-old woman with tinea cruris showing erythema and scale. Although less common in women, women do get tinea cruris. This patient had tinea on her feet, face, and under her breasts. She was treated with oral terbinafine for 3 weeks. (*Reproduced with permission from Richard P. Usatine, MD.*)

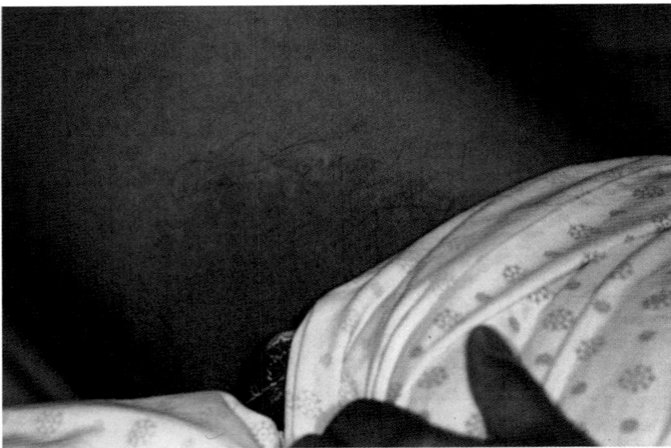

FIGURE 137-8 Erythrasma in the groin can be mistaken for tinea cruris. This erythrasma fluoresced coral red with a ultraviolet light. *(Reproduced with permission from Richard P. Usatine, MD.)*

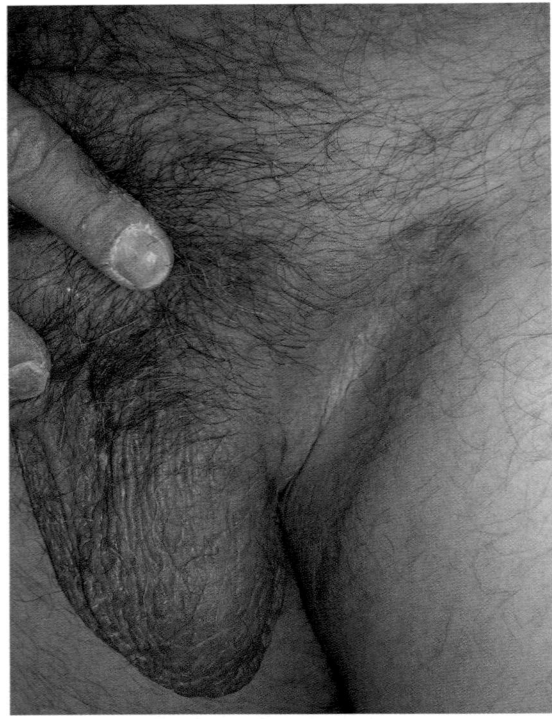

FIGURE 137-9 Inverse psoriasis in a man who also has the nail changes of psoriasis. *(Reproduced with permission from Richard P. Usatine, MD.)*

LABORATORY STUDIES

Diagnosis is often made based on clinical presentation, but a skin scraping treated with KOH and a fungal stain analyzed under the microscope can be helpful (see **Figure 137-2**). False negatives may occur if scraping is inadequate, patient is using topical antifungals, or the viewer is inexperienced.

Skin scraping and culture is definitive but expensive, and may take up to 2 weeks for the culture to grow.

Ultraviolet (UV) lamp can be used to look for the coral red fluorescence of erythrasma (see Chapter 121, Erythrasma). Most tinea cruris is caused by *T. rubrum* so will not fluoresce.

DIFFERENTIAL DIAGNOSIS

- Cutaneous *Candida* in the groin can become red and have scaling that extends to the thigh and scrotum. Tinea cruris does not often involve the scrotum. *Candida* often has satellite lesions. However, tinea cruris can also have a few satellite lesions (see Chapter 135, Candidiasis).
- Erythrasma in the groin appears similar to tinea cruris. It is less common than tinea cruris and may show coral red fluorescence with a UV light (**Figure 137-8**) (see Chapter 121, Erythrasma).
- Contact dermatitis can occur anywhere on the body. If the contact is near the groin this can be mistaken for tinea cruris (see Chapter 144, Contact Dermatitis).
- Inverse psoriasis causes inflammation in the intertriginous areas of the body. It does not have the thick plaques of plaque psoriasis. Inverse psoriasis is frequently misdiagnosed as a fungal infection until an astute clinician recognizes the pattern or does a biopsy (**Figure 137-9**; see Chapter 150, Psoriasis).
- Intertrigo is an inflammatory condition of the skin folds. It induced or aggravated by heat, moisture, maceration, and friction.[5] The condition frequently is worsened by infection with *Candida* or dermatophytes so there is some overlap with tinea cruris.

MANAGEMENT

- Tinea cruris is best treated with a topical allylamine or an azole antifungal (SOR Ⓐ, based on multiple randomized controlled trials [RCTs]).[6] Differences in current comparison data are insufficient to stratify the 2 groups of topical antifungals.[7] In one RCT, cure rates were higher at 1 week with butenafine (once daily for 2 weeks) versus clotrimazole (twice daily for 4 weeks) (26.5% vs 2.9%, respectively), but were not significantly different at 4 or 8 weeks.[8]
- The fungicidal allylamines (naftifine and terbinafine) and butenafine (allylamine derivative) are a more costly group of topical tinea treatments, yet they are more convenient as they allow for a shorter duration of treatment compared with fungistatic azoles (clotrimazole, econazole, ketoconazole, oxiconazole, miconazole, and sulconazole).[7]
- Topical azoles should be continued for 4 weeks and topical allylamines for 2 weeks or until clinical cure.[6-8] SOR Ⓐ
- Fluconazole 150 mg once weekly for 2 to 4 weeks appears to be effective in the treatment of tinea cruris.[9] SOR Ⓑ
- One RCT showed that itraconazole 200 mg for 1 week is similarly effective, equally well tolerated, and at least as safe as itraconazole 100 mg for 2 weeks in the treatment of tinea corporis or cruris (clinical response: 73% and 80% at the end of follow-up, respectively).[10] SOR Ⓑ
- Patients with mycologically diagnosed tinea corporis and tinea cruris were randomly allocated to receive either 250 mg of oral terbinafine once daily or 500 mg of griseofulvin once daily for 2 weeks. The cure rates were higher for terbinafine at 6 weeks.[11] SOR Ⓑ
- If there are multiple sites infected with fungus, treat all active areas of infection simultaneously to prevent reinfection of the groin from other body sites. If the tinea is widespread as in the patient in **Figure 137-7** an oral agent is warranted.
- Some patients will have been treated incorrectly with topical steroids allowing the tinea cruris to grow and spread (**Figure 137-10**). In these cases an oral antifungal will be needed to eradicate the tinea incognito.

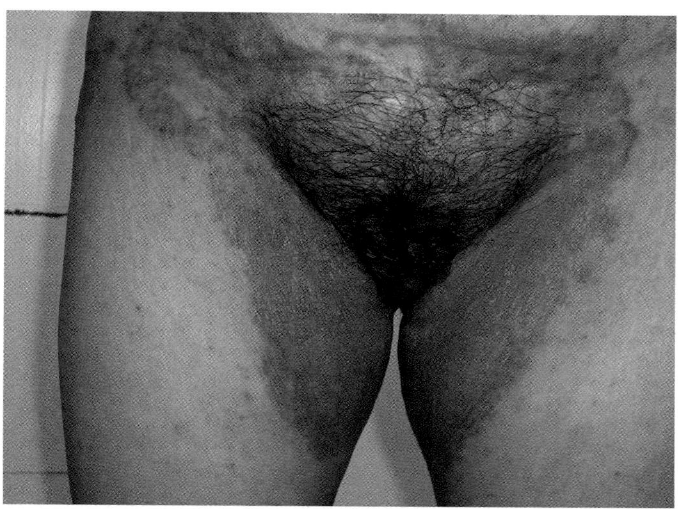

FIGURE 137-10 Tinea incognito that occurred when a woman with tinea cruris was treated with a topical steroid rather than an antifungal medication. (*Reproduced with permission from Olvia P. Revelo, MD.*)

FOLLOW-UP

Follow-up should be done as needed.

PATIENT EDUCATION

- Advise patients with tinea pedis to put on their socks before their undershorts to reduce the possibility of direct contamination. SOR Ⓒ
- Dry the groin completely after bathing. SOR Ⓒ

PATIENT RESOURCES

- Medline Plus. *Jock Itch*—**http://www.nlm.nih.gov/medlineplus/ency/article/000876.htm.**

PROVIDER RESOURCES

- DermNet NZ. *Fungal Skin Infections*—**http://www.dermnetnz.org/fungal/.**
- Doctor Fungus—**http://www.doctorfungus.org/.**
- Medscape. *Tinea Cruris*—**http://emedicine.medscape.com/article/1091806.**

REFERENCES

1. Panackal AA, Halpern EF, Watson AJ. Cutaneous fungal infections in the United States: analysis of the National Ambulatory Medical Care Survey (NAMCS) and National Hospital Ambulatory Medical Care Survey (NHAMCS), 1995-2004. *Int J Dermatol*. 2009;48(7):704-712.
2. Wiederkehr M, Schwartz RA. *Tinea Cruris*. http://emedicine.medscape.com/article/1091806-overview. Accessed April 2, 2012.
3. Ingordo V, Naldi L, Fracchiolla S, Colecchia B. Prevalence and risk factors for superficial fungal infections among Italian Navy cadets. *Dermatology*. 2004;209(3):190-196.
4. Patel GA, Wiederkehr M, Schwartz RA. Tinea cruris in children. *Cutis*. 2009;84(3):133-137.
5. Selden ST. *Intertrigo*. http://emedicine.medscape.com/article/1087691-overview. Accessed April 2, 2012.
6. Drake LA, Dinehart SM, Farmer ER, et al. Guidelines of care for superficial mycotic infections of the skin: tinea corporis, tinea cruris, tinea faciei, tinea manuum, and tinea pedis. Guidelines/Outcomes Committee. American Academy of Dermatology. *J Am Acad Dermatol*. 1996;34(2 pt 1):282-286.
7. Nadalo D, Montoya C, Hunter-Smith D. What is the best way to treat tinea cruris? *J Fam Pract*. 2006;55:256-258.
8. Singal A, Pandhi D, Agrawal S, Das S. Comparative efficacy of topical 1% butenafine and 1% clotrimazole in tinea cruris and tinea corporis: a randomized, double-blind trial. *J Dermatolog Treat*. 2005;16(506):331-335.
9. Nozickova M, Koudelkova V, Kulikova Z, Malina L, Urbanowski S, Silny W. A comparison of the efficacy of oral fluconazole, 150 mg/week versus 50 mg/day, in the treatment of tinea corporis, tinea cruris, tinea pedis, and cutaneous candidosis. *Int J Dermatol*. 1998;37:703-705.
10. Boonk W, de Geer D, de Kreek E, Remme J, van Huystee B. Itraconazole in the treatment of tinea corporis and tinea cruris: comparison of two treatment schedules. *Mycoses*. 1998;41:509-514.
11. Voravutinon V. Oral treatment of tinea corporis and tinea cruris with terbinafine and griseofulvin: a randomized double blind comparative study. *J Med Assoc Thai*. 1993;76:388-393.

138 TINEA PEDIS

Richard P. Usatine, MD
Katie Reppa, MD

PATIENT STORY

A 38-year-old man presents with an itchy rash on his hands and blisters on his feet for 1 week duration (**Figure 138-1**). Vesicular tinea pedis with bullae were present. The papules and vesicles between the fingers were typical of an autoeczematization reaction (Id reaction) (**Figure 138-2**). The patient was treated with an oral antifungal medication and a short burst of oral prednisone for the Id reaction.

INTRODUCTION

Tinea pedis is a common cutaneous infection of the feet caused by dermatophyte fungus. The clinical manifestation presents in 1 of 3 major patterns: interdigital, moccasin, and inflammatory. Concurrent fungal infection of the nails (onychomycosis) occurs frequently.

SYNONYMS

Tinea pedis is also known as athlete's foot.

EPIDEMIOLOGY

- Tinea pedis is thought to be the world's most common dermatophytosis.[1]
- About 70% of the population will be infected with tinea pedis at some time.[1]
- More commonly affects males than females.[1]
- Prevalence increases with age and it is rare before adolescence.[1]

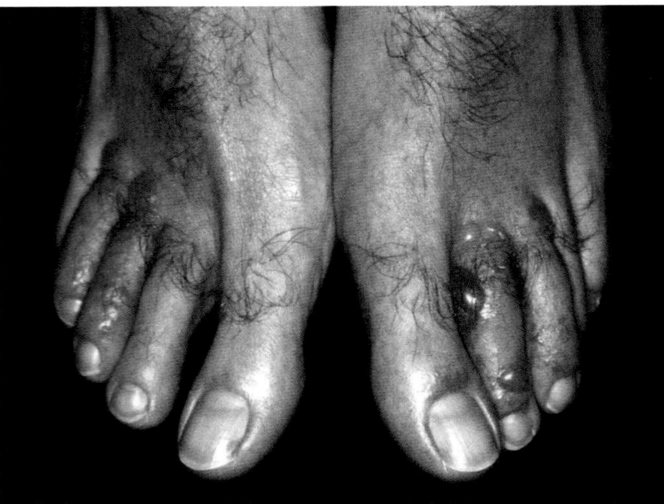

FIGURE 138-1 Vesicular tinea pedis with bullae present. This is an inflammatory reaction to the tinea pedis. (*Reproduced with permission from Richard P. Usatine, MD.*)

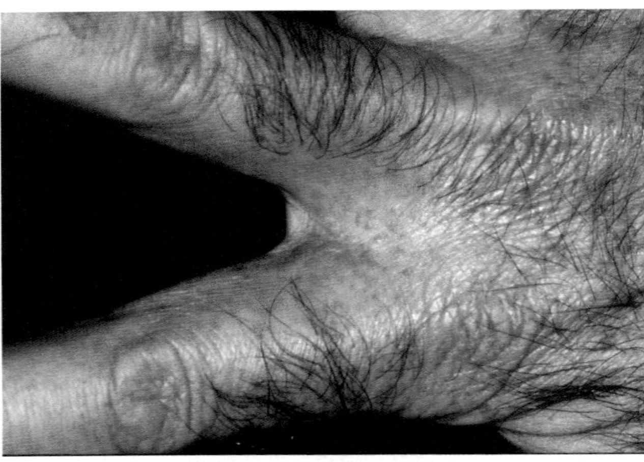

FIGURE 138-2 The hand shows an autoeczematization reaction to the inflammatory tinea pedis in **Figure 138-1**. The vesicles between the fingers are typical of an autoeczematization reaction, also known as an Id reaction. (*Reproduced with permission from Richard P. Usatine, MD.*)

ETIOLOGY AND PATHOPHYSIOLOGY

- A cutaneous fungal infection most commonly caused by *Trichophyton rubrum*.[1]
- *Trichophyton mentagrophytes* and *Epidermophyton floccosum* follow in that order.
- *T. rubrum* causes most tinea pedis and onychomycosis.

RISK FACTORS

- Male gender
- Use of public showers, baths, or pools[2]
- Household member with tinea pedis infection[2]
- Certain occupations (miners, farmers, soldiers, meat factory workers, marathon runners)[2]
- Use of immunosuppressive drugs

DIAGNOSIS

TYPICAL DISTRIBUTION AND MORPHOLOGY

Three types of tinea pedis are as follow:

- Interdigital type—most common (**Figure 138-3**)
- Moccasin type (**Figure 138-4** and **138-5**)
- Inflammatory/vesicular type—least common (see **Figure 138-1**)

Some authors describe an ulcerative type (**Figure 138-6**).

CLINICAL FEATURES

- Interdigital—White or green fungal growth between toes with erythema, maceration, cracks, and fissures—especially between fourth and fifth digits (see **Figure 138-3**). The dry type has more scale and the moist type becomes macerated.
- Moccasin—Scale on sides and soles of feet (see **Figures 138-4** and **138-5**).
- Vesicular—Vesicles and bullae on feet (see **Figure 138-6**).

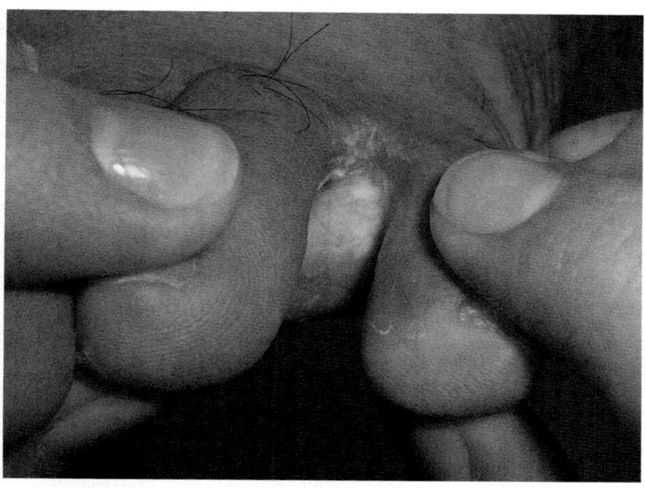

FIGURE 138-3 Tinea pedis seen in the interdigital space between the fourth and fifth digits. This is the most common area to see tinea pedis. (*Reproduced with permission from Richard P. Usatine, MD.*)

- Ulcerative tinea pedis is characterized by rapidly spreading vesiculopustular lesions, ulcers, and erosions, typically in the web spaces (**Figure 138-7**). It is accompanied by a secondary bacterial infection. This can lead to cellulitis or lymphangitis.
- Autosensitization (dermatophytid reaction; Id reaction) is a hypersensitivity response to the fungal infection causing papules on the hands (see **Figure 138-2**).
- Examine nails for evidence of onychomycosis—Fungal infections of nails may include subungual keratosis, yellow or white discolorations, dysmorphic nails (see Chapter 191, Onychomycosis).
- Examine to exclude cellulitis that may show erythema, swelling, tenderness with red streaks tracking up the foot and lower leg (see Chapter 122, Cellulitis).

TYPICAL DISTRIBUTION

It occurs between the toes, on the soles, and lateral aspects of the feet.

LABORATORY STUDIES

Diagnosis is often made based on clinical presentation but a skin scraping treated with potassium hydroxide (KOH) and a fungal stain analyzed under the microscope can be helpful (**Figure 138-8).**

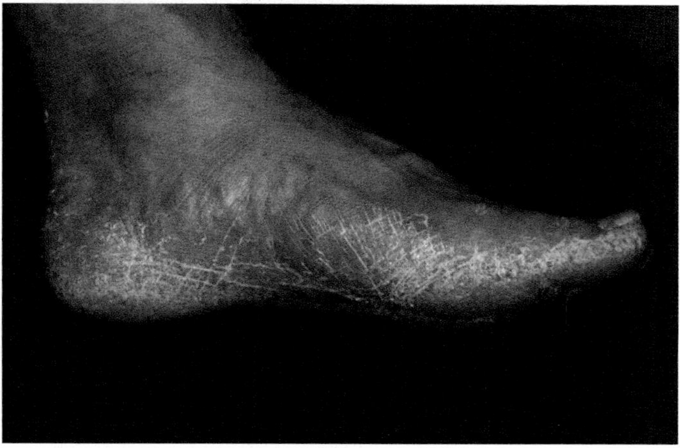

FIGURE 138-4 Tinea pedis in the moccasin distribution. (*Reproduced with permission from Richard P. Usatine, MD.*)

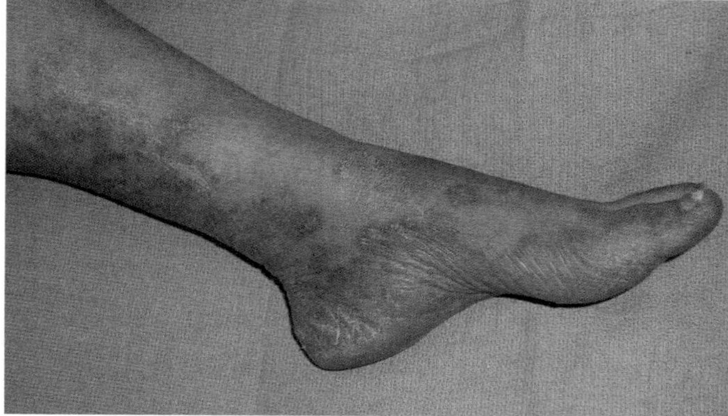

FIGURE 138-5 Tinea pedis in a moccasin distribution that has spread up the leg. (*Reproduced with permission from Richard P. Usatine, MD.*)

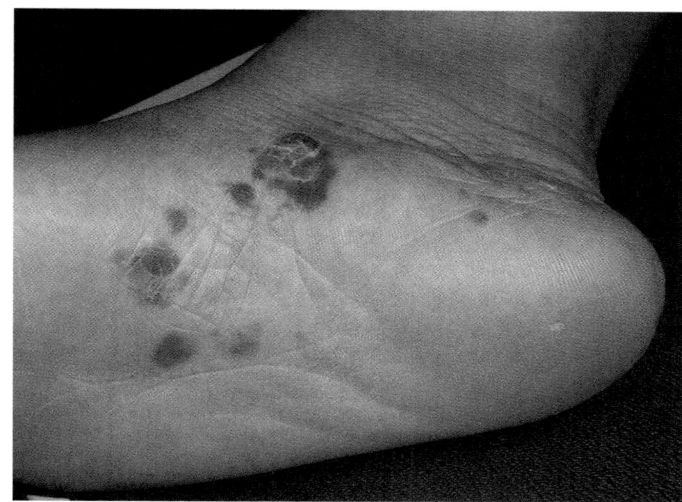

FIGURE 138-6 Vesicular tinea pedis with vesicles and bullae over the arch region of the foot. The arch is a typical location for vesiculobullous tinea pedis. (*Reproduced with permission from Richard P. Usatine, MD.*)

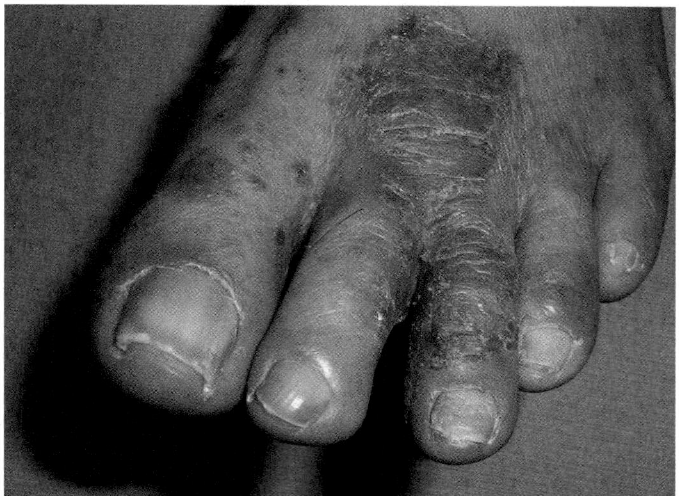

FIGURE 138-7 Ulcerative tinea pedis with spreading vesicles related to a bacterial superinfection. The patient was treated with antifungals and antibiotics. (*Reproduced with permission from Richard P. Usatine, MD.*)

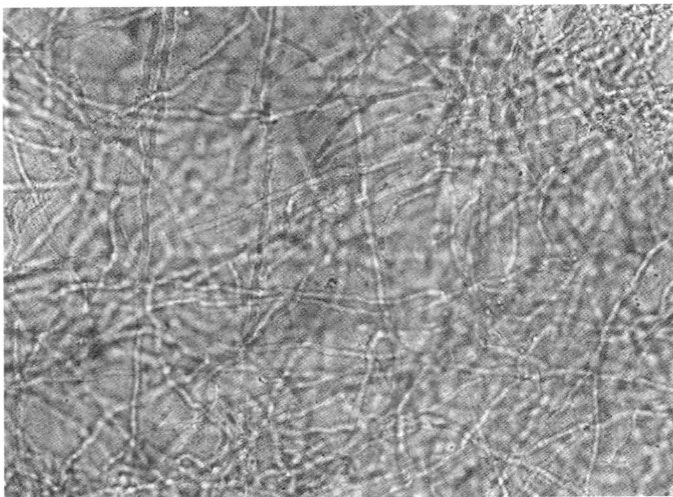

FIGURE 138-8 Microscopic view of the scraping of the foot in the man with tinea incognito in **Figure 138-9**. The hyphae have proliferated and are easy to see under 40 power with Swartz-Lamkins stain. (*Reproduced with permission from Richard P. Usatine, MD.*)

In the patient with tinea incognito on his foot and lower leg, the physicians were set astray by his diagnosis of systemic lupus erythematosus (SLE) (**Figure 138-9**). It took a skin scraping to demonstrate that this was tinea and not lupus to get the patient the treatment he needed (see **Figure 138-8**).

Skin scraping and culture is definitive but expensive, and may take up to 2 weeks for the culture to grow.

DIFFERENTIAL DIAGNOSIS

- Pitted keratolysis—Well-demarcated pits or erosions in the sole of the foot caused by bacteria (**Figure 138-10**) (see Chapter 120, Pitted Keratolysis).

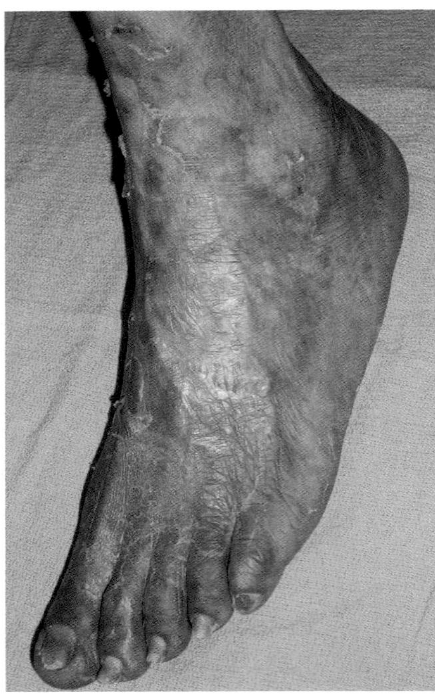

FIGURE 138-9 Tinea incognito on the foot of a 63-year-old black man with lupus. He was given topical steroids that allowed this fungus to spread and thrive. (*Reproduced with permission from Richard P. Usatine, MD.*)

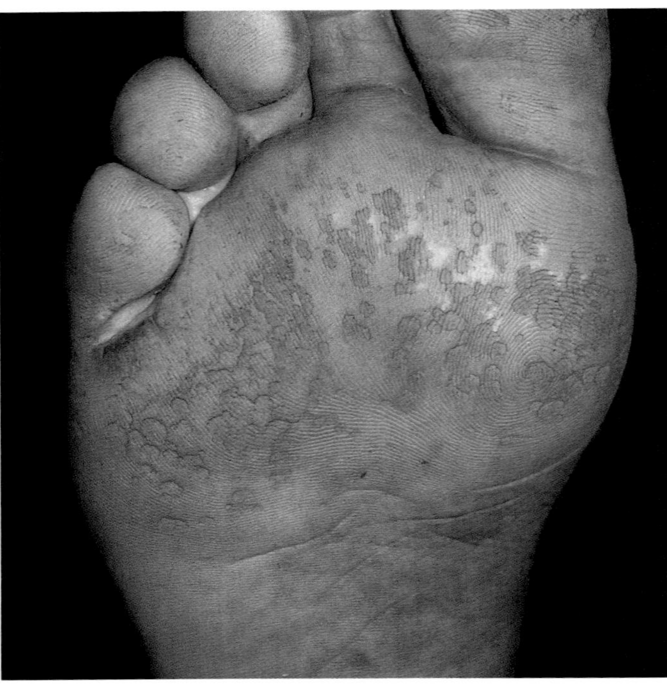

FIGURE 138-10 Pitted keratolysis on the sole of the foot with some interdigital tinea pedis. The pits are caused by bacteria and if not treated with an antibiotic will not resolve. (*Reproduced with permission from Richard P. Usatine, MD.*)

- Contact dermatitis—Tends to be seen on the dorsum and sides of the foot (**Figure 138-11**) (see Chapter 144, Contact Dermatitis).
- Keratodermas—Thickening of the soles of the feet that can be caused by a number of etiologies, including menopause (**Figure 138-12**). This condition looks a lot like tinea pedis in the moccasin distribution.
- Dyshidrotic eczema is characterized by scale and tapioca-like vesicles on the hands and feet (**Figure 138-13**) (see Chapter 145, Hand Eczema).
- Friction blisters—Blisters on the feet of persons leading an active athletic lifestyle.
- Psoriasis—Can mimic tinea pedis but will usually be present in other areas as well (**Figure 138-14**) (see Chapter 150, Psoriasis).

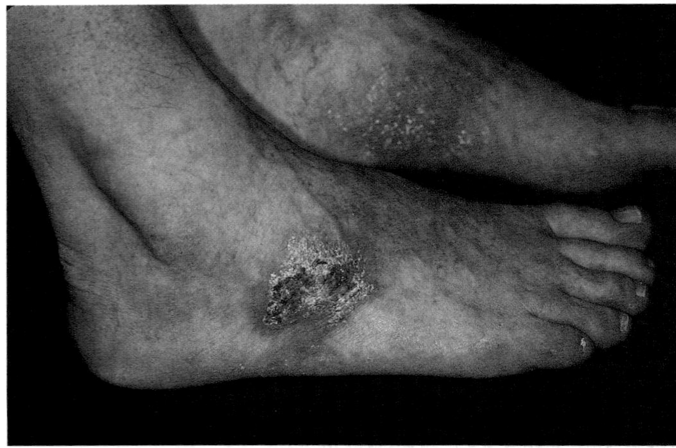

FIGURE 138-11 Contact dermatitis to an allergen in tennis shoes with typical distribution that crosses the dorsum of the foot. (*Reproduced with permission from Richard P. Usatine, MD.*)

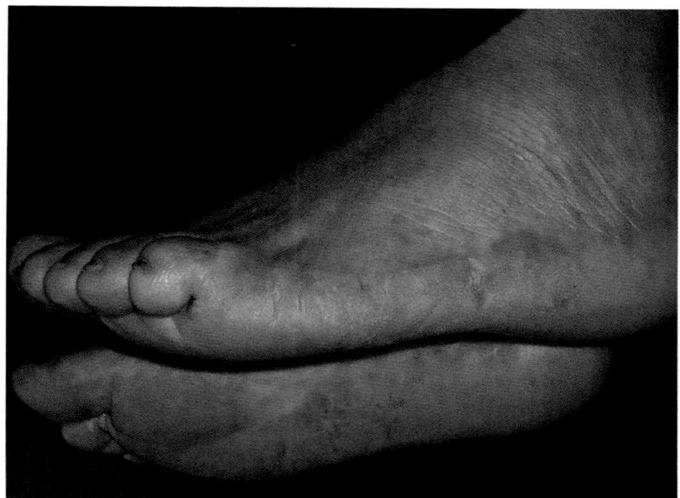

FIGURE 138-12 Keratoderma climactericum, which started when this woman entered menopause. (*Reproduced with permission from Richard P. Usatine, MD.*)

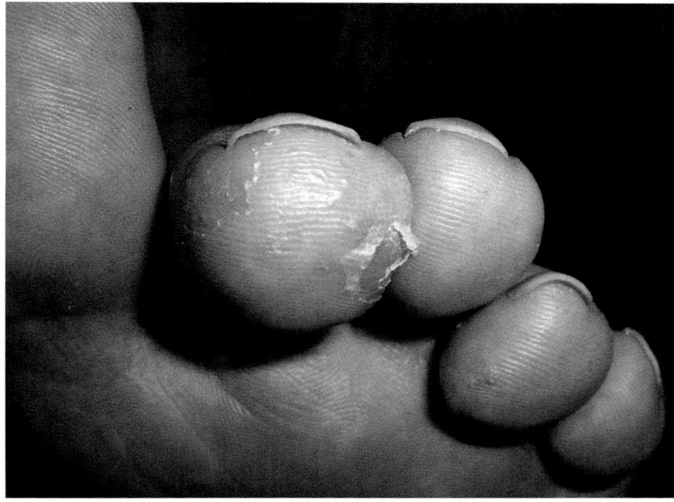

FIGURE 138-13 Dyshidrotic eczema on the foot showing tapioca vesicles with peeling of skin on the tip of the second toe. The patient also has typical tapioca vesicles between the fingers. (*Reproduced with permission from Richard P. Usatine, MD.*)

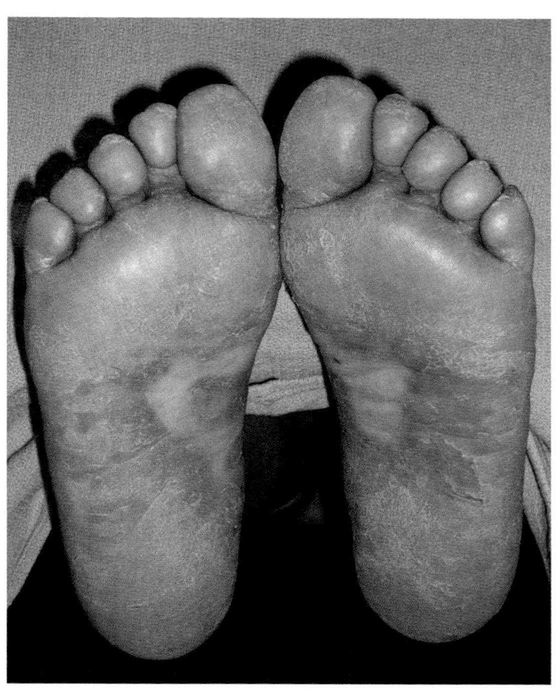

FIGURE 138-14 Plantar psoriasis in a patient with other areas of psoriasis also present. (*Reproduced with permission from Richard P. Usatine, MD.*)

MANAGEMENT

Table 138-1 discusses management of tinea pedis.

TOPICAL ANTIFUNGALS

- Systematic review of 70 trials of topical antifungals showed good evidence for efficacy compared to placebo for the following:
  - Allylamines (naftifine, terbinafine, butenafine).[3] SOR Ⓐ
  - Azoles (clotrimazole, miconazole, econazole).[3] SOR Ⓐ
  - Allylamines cure slightly more infections than azoles but are more expensive.[3] SOR Ⓐ
  - No differences in efficacy found between individual allylamines or individual azoles (**Table 138-2**). SOR Ⓐ
  - In one meta-analysis, topical terbinafine was found to be equally effective as other topical antifungals but the average duration of treatment was shorter. (1 week instead of 2 weeks). Additionally, terbinafine is effective as a single-application film-forming solution.[4] SOR Ⓐ

ORAL ANTIFUNGALS

- Systematic review of 12 trials, involving 700 participants: Oral terbinafine for 2 weeks cures 52% more patients than oral griseofulvin.[5] SOR Ⓐ

TABLE 138-1 Management of Tinea Pedis

Tinea Pedis Type	Treatment for Mild Cases	Treatment for Recalcitrant Cases	SOR
Interdigital type	Topical antifungal	Another topical antifungal or an oral antifungal	A
Moccasin type	Topical antifungal	Oral antifungal	A
Inflammatory/vesicular type	Oral antifungal	Oral antifungal	A

Reprinted with permission from Thomas B. Clear choices in managing epidermal tinea infections. *J Fam Pract.* 2003;52(11):857. Reproduced with permission from Frontline Medical Communications.

TABLE 138-2 Topical Antifungal Medications

Agent	Formulation	Frequency*	Duration* (Weeks)	NNT†
Imidazoles				
Clotrimazole	1% cream 1% solution 1% swabs	Twice daily	2-4	2.9
Econazole	1% cream	Twice daily	2-4	2.6
Ketoconazole	2% cream	Once daily	2-4	No data available
Miconazole	2% cream 2% spray 2% powder	Twice daily	2-4	2.8 (at 8 wk)
Oxiconazole	1% cream 1% lotion	Once to twice daily	2-4	2.9
Sulconazole	1% cream 1% solution	Once to twice daily	2-4	2.5
Allylamines				
Naftifine	1% cream 1% gel	Once to twice daily	1-4	1.9
Terbinafine	1% cream 1% solution	Once to twice daily	1-4	1.6 (1.7 for tinea cruris/tinea corporis at 8 wk)
Benzylamine				
Butenafine	1% cream	Once to twice daily	1-4	1.9 (1.4 for tinea corporis and 1.5 for tinea cruris)
Other				
Ciclopirox	0.77% cream 0.77% lotion	Twice daily	2-4	2.1
Tolnaftate	1% powder 1% spray 1% swabs	Twice daily	4	3.6 (at 8 wk)

*Manufacturer guidelines.
†NNT, number needed to treat. NNT is calculated from systematic review of all randomized controlled trials for tinea pedis at 6 weeks after the initiation of treatment except where otherwise noted.
Reprinted with permission from Thomas B. Clear choices in managing epidermal tinea infections. *J Fam Pract.* 2003;52(11):857. Reproduced with permission from Frontline Medical Communications.

- Terbinafine is equal to itraconazole in patient outcomes.[5] SOR Ⓐ
- No significant differences in comparisons between a number of oral agents.[5] SOR Ⓐ

Dosing for tinea pedis needing oral therapy includes the following:

- Itraconazole two 100 mg tablets daily for 1 week[6]
- Terbinafine 250 mg PO daily for 1 to 2 weeks[6]

Patients with onychomycosis may have recurrences of the skin infection related to the fungus that remains in the nails and, therefore, may need oral treatment for 3 months to achieve better results.

Topical urea (Carmol, Keralac), available in 10% to 40% concentrations, may be useful to decrease scaling in patients with hyperkeratotic soles.[5]

ALTERNATIVE THERAPY

One small pilot study with 56 participants showed significant improvement or resolution of symptoms in patients treated by wearing socks containing copper oxide fibers daily for a minimum of 8 to 10 days.[7] SOR Ⓑ

PATIENT EDUCATION

- Do not go barefoot in public showers and locker rooms. SOR Ⓒ
- Keep feet dry and clean, and use clean socks and shoes that allow the feet to get fresh air. SOR Ⓒ
- Use the topical medication beyond the time in which the feet look clear to prevent relapse.

PATIENT RESOURCES

- eMedicineHealth. *Athlete's Foot*—**http://www.emedicinehealth.com/athletes_foot/article_em.htm.**

PROVIDER RESOURCES

- Medscape. *Tinea Pedis*—**http://emedicine.medscape.com/article/1091684.**

REFERENCES

1. Robbins C. *Tinea Pedis.* http://www.emedicine.com/DERM/topic470.htm. Accessed June 24, 2007.
2. Seebacher C, Bouchara JP, Mignon B. Updates on the epidemiology of dermatophyte infections. *Mycopathologia*. 2008;166(5-6):335-352.
3. Crawford F, Hart R, Bell-Syer S, Torgerson D, Young P, Russell I. Topical treatments for fungal infections of the skin and nails of the foot. *Cochrane Database Syst Rev*. 2000;CD001434.
4. Kienke P, Korting HC, Nelles S, Rychlik R. Comparable efficacy and safety of various topical formulations of terbinafine in tinea pedis irrespective of the treatment regimen: results of a meta-analysis. *Am J Clin Dermatol*. 2007;8(6):357-364.
5. Bell-Syer SE, Hart R, Crawford F, Torgerson DJ, Tyrrell W, Russell I. Oral treatments for fungal infections of the skin of the foot. *Cochrane Database Syst Rev*. 2002;CD003584.
6. Thomas B. Clear choices in managing epidermal tinea infections. *J Fam Pract*. 2003;52:850-862.
7. Zatcoff RC, Smith MS, Borkow G. Treatment of tinea pedis with socks containing copper-oxide impregnated fibers. *Foot (Edinb)*. 2008;18(3):136-141.

139 TINEA VERSICOLOR

Richard P. Usatine, MD
Melissa M. Chan, MD

PATIENT STORY

A young black man presents to the office with a 5-year history of white spots on his trunk (**Figure 139-1**). He denies any symptoms but worries if this could spread to his girlfriend. These spots get worse during the summer months but never go away completely. He was relieved to receive a treatment for his tinea versicolor and to find out that it rarely spread to others through contact.

INTRODUCTION

Tinea versicolor is a common superficial skin infection caused by the dimorphic lipophilic yeast *Pityrosporum* (*Malassezia furfur*). The most typical presentation is a set of hypopigmented macules and patches with fine scale over the trunk in a cape-like distribution.

SYNONYMS

Pityriasis versicolor is actually a more accurate name as "tinea" implies a dermatophyte infection. Tinea versicolor is caused by *Pityrosporum* and not a dermatophyte.

EPIDEMIOLOGY

- Seen more commonly in men than in women.
- Seen more often during the summer, and is especially common in warm and humid climates.

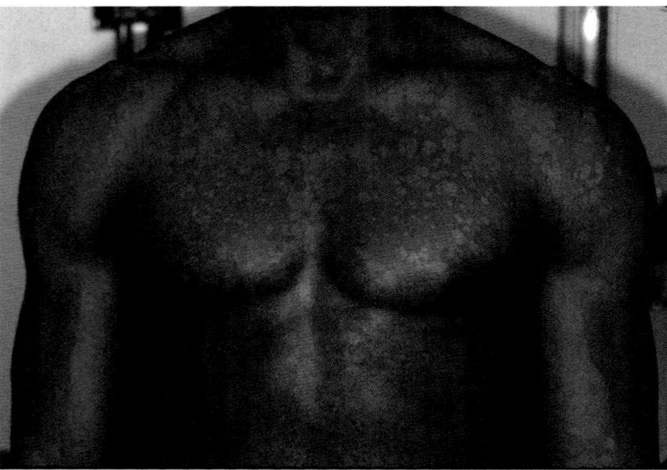

FIGURE 139-1 Tinea versicolor showing areas of hypopigmentation. (*Reproduced with permission from Usatine RP.* What is in a name? *West J Med. 2000;173(4):231-232.*)

ETIOLOGY AND PATHOPHYSIOLOGY

- Tinea versicolor is caused by *Pityrosporum (M. furfur)*, which is a lipophilic yeast that can be normal human cutaneous flora.
- *Pityrosporum* exists in 2 shapes—Pityrosporum ovale (oval) and Pityrosporum orbiculare (round).
- Tinea versicolor starts when the yeast that normally colonizes the skin changes from the round form to the pathologic mycelial form and then invades the stratum corneum.[1]
- *Pityrosporum* is also associated with seborrhea and Pityrosporum folliculitis.
- The white and brown colors are secondary to damage caused by the *Pityrosporum* to the melanocytes, while the pink is an inflammatory reaction to the organism.
- *Pityrosporum* thrives on sebum and moisture; they tend to grow on the skin in areas where there are sebaceous follicles secreting sebum.

DIAGNOSIS

CLINICAL FEATURES

Tinea versicolor consists of hypopigmented, hyperpigmented, or pink macules and patches on the trunk that are finely scaling and well demarcated. Versicolor means a variety of or variation in colors; tinea versicolor tends to come in white, pink, and brown colors (**Figures 139-1** to **139-5**).

TYPICAL DISTRIBUTION

Tinea versicolor is found on the chest, abdomen, upper arms, and back, whereas seborrhea tends to be seen on the scalp, face, and anterior chest.

LABORATORY STUDIES

A scraping of the scaling portions of the skin may be placed onto a slide using the side of another slide or a scalpel. Potassium hydroxide (KOH) with dimethyl sulfoxide (DMSO) (DMSO helps the KOH dissolve the

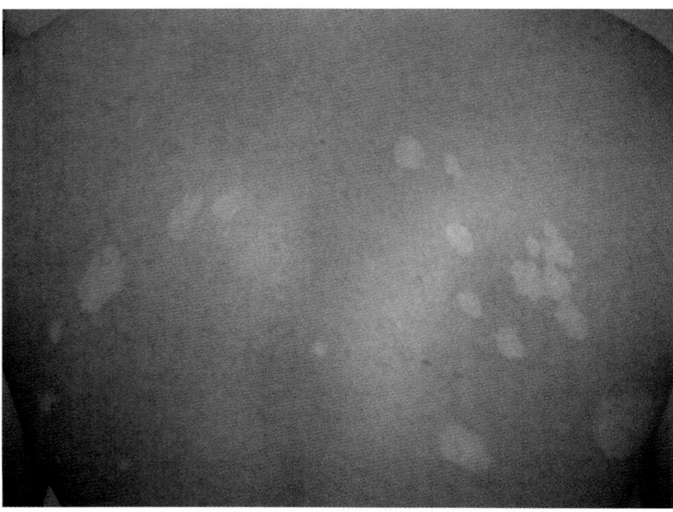

FIGURE 139-2 Patches of hypopigmentation across the back caused by tinea versicolor in a young Latino man. Vitiligo is on the differential diagnosis in this case. A KOH preparation confirmed tinea versicolor. (*Reproduced with permission from Richard P. Usatine, MD.*)

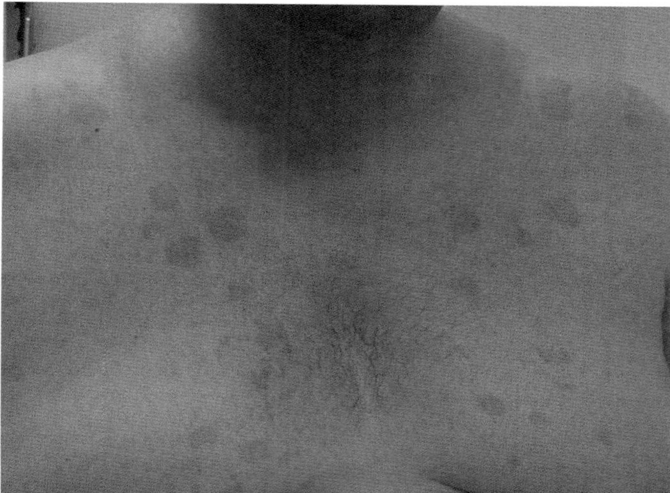

FIGURE 139-3 Pink scaly patches caused by tinea versicolor. Seborrhea may be seen in this location, but tends to be worse in the presternal region. (*Reproduced with permission from Richard P. Usatine, MD.*)

keratinocytes faster and reduces the need for heating the slide) is placed on the slide and covered with a coverslip. Microscopic examination reveals the typical "spaghetti-and-meatballs" pattern of tinea versicolor. The "spaghetti," or more accurately "ziti," is the short mycelial form and the "meatballs" are the round yeast form (**Figures 139-6** and **139-7**). Fungal stains such as the Swartz-Lamkins stain help make the identification of the fungal elements easier.

DIFFERENTIAL DIAGNOSIS

- Pityriasis rosea has a fine collarette scale around the border of the lesions and is frequently seen with a herald patch. Negative KOH (see Chapter 151, Pityriasis Rosea).
- Secondary syphilis is usually not scaling and tends to have macules on the palms and soles. Negative KOH (see Chapter 218, Syphilis).
- Tinea corporis is rarely as widespread as tinea versicolor and each individual lesion usually has central clearing and a well-defined, raised, scaling border. The KOH preparation in tinea corporis shows hyphae with multiple branch points and not the "ziti-and-meatballs" pattern of tinea versicolor (see Chapter 136, Tinea Corporis).
- Vitiligo—The degree of hypopigmentation is greater and the distribution is frequently different with vitiligo involving the hands and face (see Chapter 196, Vitiligo).
- Pityriasis alba—Lightly hypopigmented areas with slight scale that tend to be found on the face and trunk of children with atopy. These patches are frequently smaller and rounder than tinea versicolor (see Chapter 143, Atopic Dermatitis).

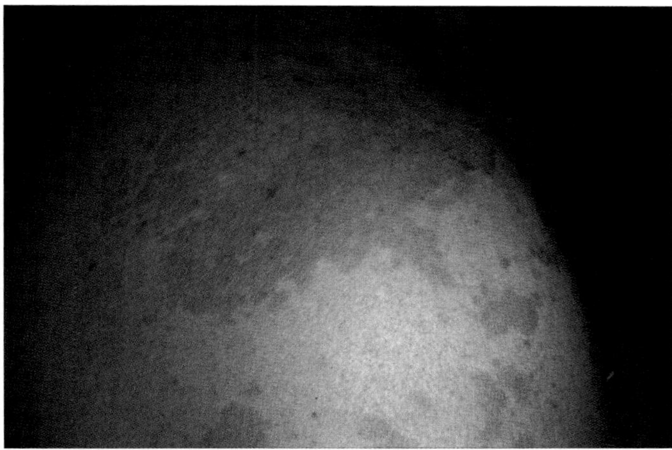

FIGURE 139-4 Large areas of pink tinea versicolor on the shoulder in a cape-like distribution. (*Reproduced with permission from Richard P. Usatine, MD.*)

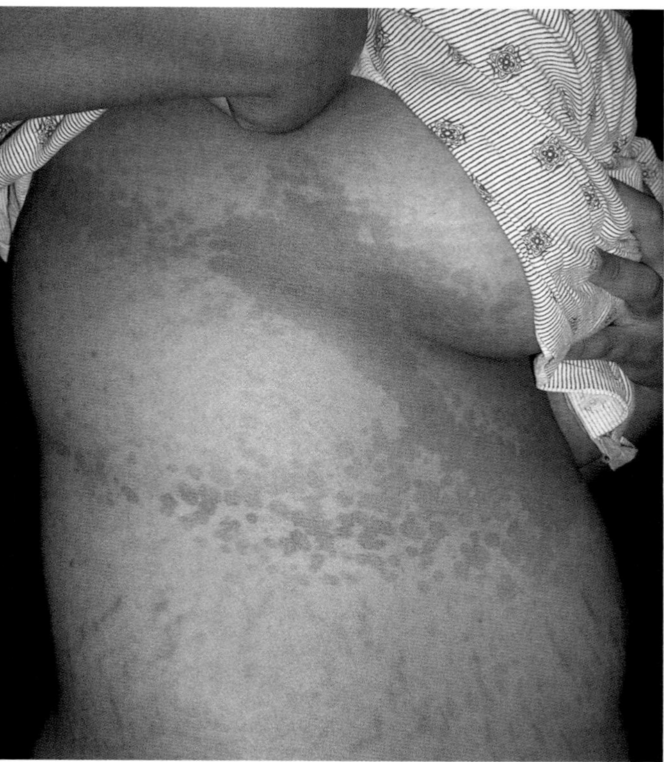

FIGURE 139-5 Hyperpigmented variant of tinea versicolor in a Hispanic woman. (*Reproduced with permission from Richard P. Usatine, MD.*)

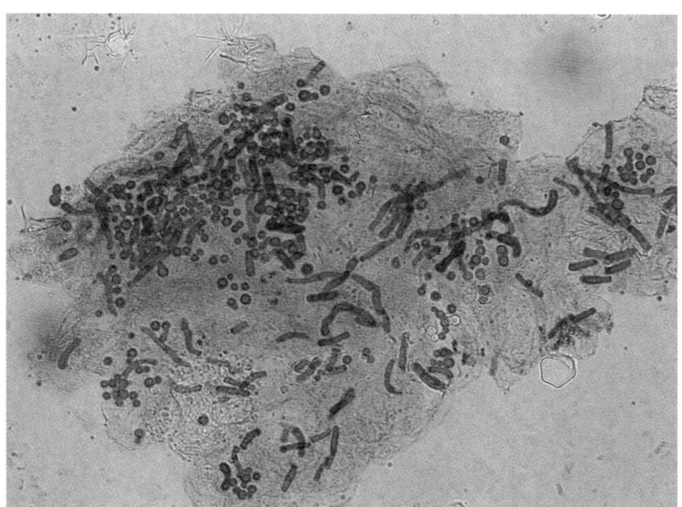

FIGURE 139-6 Microscopic examination of scrapings done from previous patient showing short mycelial forms and round yeast forms suggestive of spaghetti and meatballs. Swartz-Lamkins stain was used. (*Reproduced with permission from Richard P. Usatine, MD.*)

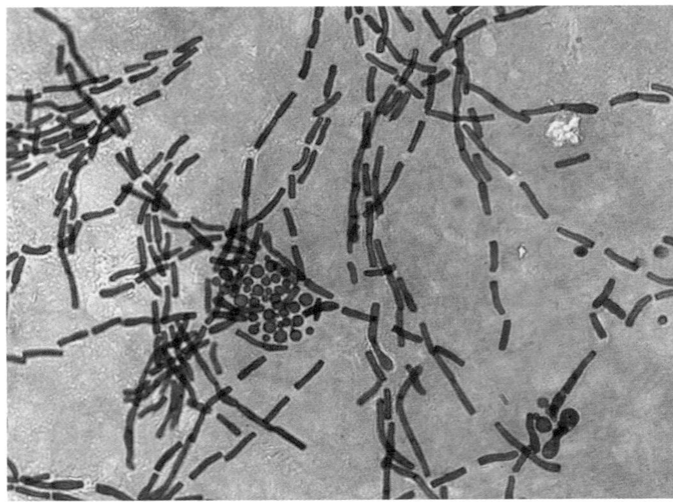

FIGURE 139-7 Close-up of *Malassezia furfur* (*Pityrosporum*) showing the ziti-and-meatball appearance after Swartz-Lamkins stain was applied to the scraping of tinea versicolor in a young woman. (*Reproduced with permission from Richard P. Usatine, MD.*)

- *Pityrosporum* folliculitis is caused by the same organism but presents with pink or brown papules on the back. The patient complains of itchy rough skin and the KOH is positive (**Figure 139-8**).

MANAGEMENT

TOPICAL

- Because tinea versicolor is usually asymptomatic, the treatment is mostly for cosmetic reasons.
- The mainstay of treatment has been topical therapy using antidandruff shampoos, because the same *Pityrosporum* species that cause seborrhea and dandruff also cause tinea versicolor.[1,2]
- Patients may apply selenium sulfide 2.5% lotion or shampoo, or zinc pyrithione shampoo to the involved areas daily for 1 to 2 weeks. Various amounts of time are suggested to allow the preparations to work, but there are no studies that show a minimum exposure time needed. A typical regimen involves applying the lotion or shampoo to the involved areas for 10 minutes and then washing it off in the shower. SOR Ⓒ

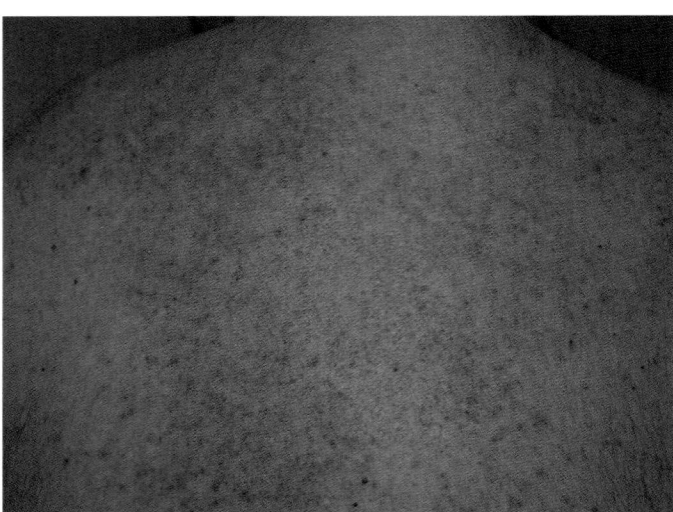

FIGURE 139-8 *Pityrosporum* folliculitis on the back of a man with pruritus. (*Reproduced with permission from Richard P. Usatine, MD.*)

- One study used ketoconazole 2% shampoo (Nizoral) as a single application or daily for 3 days and found it safe and highly effective in treating tinea versicolor.[3] SOR Ⓑ
- Topical antifungal creams for smaller areas of involvement can include ketoconazole and clotrimazole. SOR Ⓒ

ORAL TREATMENT AND PREVENTION

- A single-dose 400-mg oral fluconazole provided the best clinical and mycological cure rate, with no relapse during 12 months of follow-up.[4] SOR Ⓑ
- A single dose of 300 mg of oral fluconazole repeated weekly for 2 weeks was equal to 400 mg of ketoconazole in a single dose repeated weekly for 2 weeks. No significant differences in efficacy, safety, and tolerability between the 2 treatment regimens were found.[5] SOR Ⓑ
- A single-dose 400-mg oral ketoconazole to treat tinea versicolor is safe and cost-effective compared to using the newer, more expensive, oral antifungal agents, such as itraconazole.[6,7] SOR Ⓑ
- Oral itraconazole 200 mg given twice a day for 1 day a month has been shown to be safe and effective as a prophylactic treatment for tinea versicolor.[8] SOR Ⓑ
- There is no evidence that establishes the need to sweat after taking oral antifungals to treat tinea versicolor.

PATIENT EDUCATION

Patients should be told that the change in skin color will not reverse immediately. The first sign of successful treatment is the lack of scale. The yeast acts like a sunscreen in the hypopigmented macules. Sun exposure will hasten the normalization of the skin color in patients with hypopigmentation.

FOLLOW-UP

None needed unless it is a stubborn or recurrent case. Recurrent cases can be treated with monthly topical or oral therapy.

PATIENT RESOURCES

- Skin Sight. *Tinea Versicolor*— **http://www.skinsight.com/adult/tineaVersicolor.htm.**

PROVIDER RESOURCES

- Medscape. *Tinea Versicolor*— **http://emedicine.medscape.com/article/1091575.**

REFERENCES

1. Bolognia J, Jorizzo J, Rapini R. *Dermatology*. St. Louis, MO: Mosby; 2003.
2. Hu SW, Bigby M. Pityriasis versicolor: a systematic review of interventions. *Arch Dermatol*. 2010;146(10):1132-1140.

3. Lange DS, Richards HM, Guarnieri J, et al. Ketoconazole 2% shampoo in the treatment of tinea versicolor: a multicenter, randomized, double-blind, placebo-controlled trial. *J Am Acad Dermatol*. 1998;39(6):944-950.

4. Bhogal CS, Singal A, Baruah MC. Comparative efficacy of ketoconazole and fluconazole in the treatment of pityriasis versicolor: a one year follow-up study. *J Dermatol*. 2001;28(10):535-539.

5. Farschian M, Yaghoobi R, Samadi K. Fluconazole versus ketoconazole in the treatment of tinea versicolor. *J Dermatolog Treat*. 2002;13(2):73-76.

6. Gupta AK, Del Rosso JQ. An evaluation of intermittent therapies used to treat onychomycosis and other dermatomycoses with the oral antifungal agents. *Int J Dermatol*. 2000;39(6):401-411.

7. Wahab MA, Ali ME, Rahman MH, et al. Single dose (400 mg) versus 7 day (200 mg) daily dose itraconazole in the treatment of tinea versicolor: a randomized clinical trial. *Mymensingh Med J*. 2010;19(1):72-76.

8. Faergemann J, Gupta AK, Mofadi AA, et al. Efficacy of itraconazole in the prophylactic treatment of pityriasis (tinea) versicolor. *Arch Dermatol*. 2002;138:69-73.

SECTION 5 INFESTATIONS

140 LICE

Richard P. Usatine, MD
E.J. Mayeaux, MD

PATIENT STORY

A 64-year-old homeless woman with schizophrenia presented to a homeless clinic for itching all over her body. She stated that she could see creatures feed on her and move in and out of her skin. The physical examination revealed that she was unwashed and had multiple excoriations over her body (**Figure 140-1**). Body lice and their progeny were visible along the seams of her pants (**Figure 140-2**). Treatment of this lousy infestation required giving her new clothes and a shower.[1]

INTRODUCTION

Lice are ectoparasites that live on or near the body. They will die of starvation within 10 days of removal from their human host. Lice have coexisted with humans for at least 10,000 years.[2] Lice are ubiquitous and remain a major problem throughout the world.[3]

SYNONYMS

It is also known as pediculosis or crabs (pubic lice).

EPIDEMIOLOGY

- Human lice (pediculosis corporis, pediculosis pubis, and pediculosis capitis) are found in all countries and climates.[3]

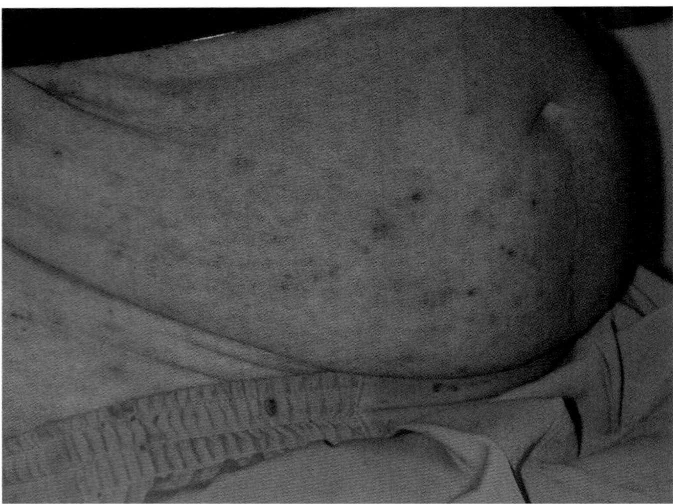

FIGURE 140-1 Body lice in a 64-year-old homeless woman with schizophrenia. (*Reproduced with permission from Richard P. Usatine, MD and Usatine RP, Halem L. A terrible itch. J Fam Pract. 2003;52(5):377-379. Reproduced with permission from Frontline Medical Communications.*)

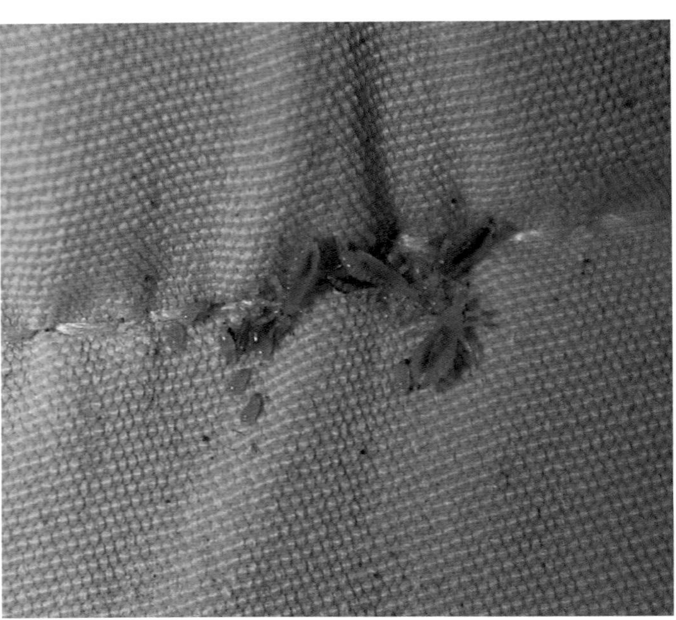

FIGURE 140-2 Adult body lice and nymphs visible along the pant seams of the woman in **Figure 140-1** (*Reproduced with permission from Richard P. Usatine, MD.*)

- Head lice are most common among school-age children. Each year, approximately 6 to 12 million children, ages 3 to 12 years, are infested.[4]
- Head lice infestation is seen across all socioeconomic groups and is not a sign of poor hygiene.[5]
- In the United States, black children are affected less often as a result of their oval-shaped hair shafts that are difficult for lice to grasp.[4]
- Body lice infest the seams of clothing (see **Figure 140-2**) and bed linen. Infestations are associated with poor hygiene and conditions of crowding.
- Pubic lice are most common in sexually active adolescents and adults. Young children with pubic lice typically have infestations of the eyelashes. Although infestations in this age group may be an indication of sexual abuse, children generally acquire the crab lice from their parents.[6]

ETIOLOGY AND PATHOPHYSIOLOGY

- Lice are parasites that have 6 legs with terminal claws that enable them to attach to hair and clothing. There are 3 types of lice responsible for human infestation. All 3 kinds of lice must feed daily on human blood and can only survive 1 to 2 days away from the host. The 3 types of lice are as follows:
    - Head lice (*Pediculus humanus capitis*)—Measure 2 to 4 mm in length (**Figure 140-3**).
    - Body lice (*Pediculus humanus corporis*)—Body lice similarly measure 2 to 4 mm in length (**Figure 140-4**).
    - Pubic or crab lice (*Phthirus pubis*)—Pubic lice are shorter, with a broader body and have an average length of 1 to 2 mm (**Figure 140-5**).

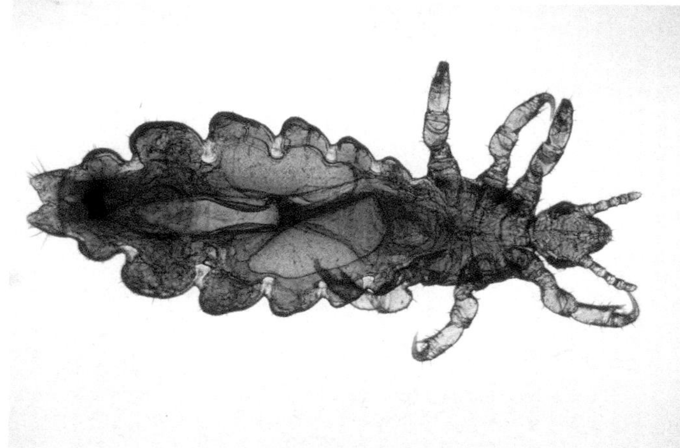

A

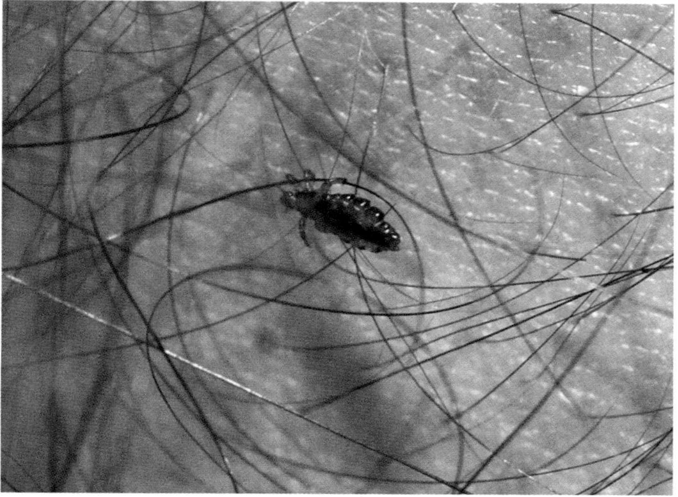

B

FIGURE 140-3 A. Adult head louse with elongated body. (*Reproduced with permission from Centers for Disease Control and Prevention and Dennis D. Juranek.*) B. Adult head louse hanging on to the hair on the neck of a man infested with head lice. (*Reproduced with permission from Richard P. Usatine, MD.*)

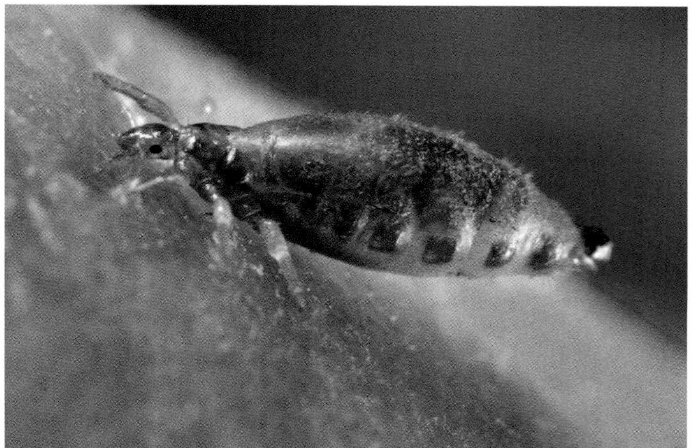

FIGURE 140-4 A body louse feeding on the blood of the photographer. The dark mass inside the abdomen is a previously ingested blood meal. (*Reproduced with permission from Centers for Disease Control and Prevention and Frank Collins, PhD.*)

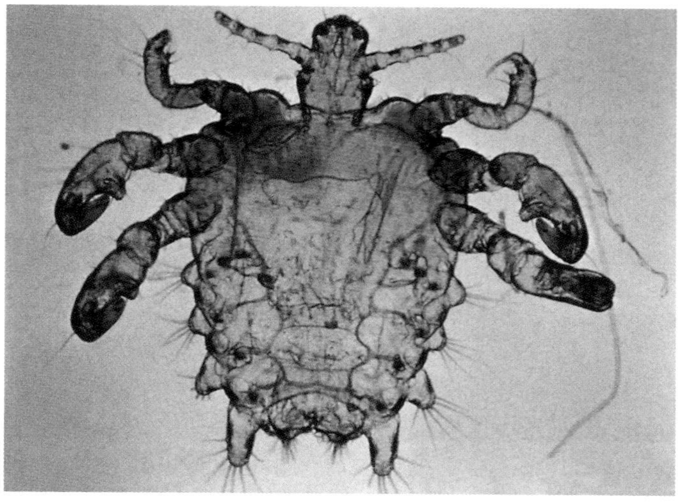

FIGURE 140-5 The crab louse has a short body and its large claws are responsible for the "crab" in its name. (*Reproduced with permission from Centers for Disease Control and Prevention and World Health Organization.*)

- Female lice have a life span of approximately 30 days and can lay approximately 10 eggs (nits) a day.[4]
- Nits are firmly attached to the hair shaft or clothing seams by a glue-like substance produced by the louse (**Figures 140-6** and **140-7**).
- Nits are incubated by the host's body heat.
- The incubation period from laying eggs to hatching of the first nymph is 7 to 14 days (see **Figure 140-7**).
- Mature adult lice capable of reproducing appear 2 to 3 weeks later (**Figure 140-8**).[5]
- Transmission of head lice occurs through direct contact with the hair of infested individuals. The role of fomites (eg, hats, combs, brushes) in transmission is negligible.[6] Head lice do not serve as vectors for transmission of disease among humans.
- Transmission of body lice occurs through direct human contact or contact with infested material. Unlike head lice, body lice are well-recognized vectors for transmission of the pathogens responsible for epidemic typhus, trench fever, and relapsing fever.[5]

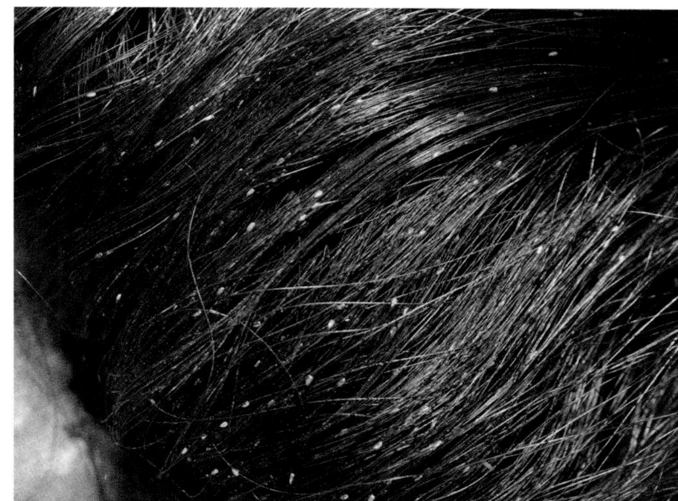

FIGURE 140-6 Pearly nits on the hair of a man with poor hygiene. The nits are found behind the ears and at the nape of the neck. (*Reproduced with permission from Richard P. Usatine, MD.*)

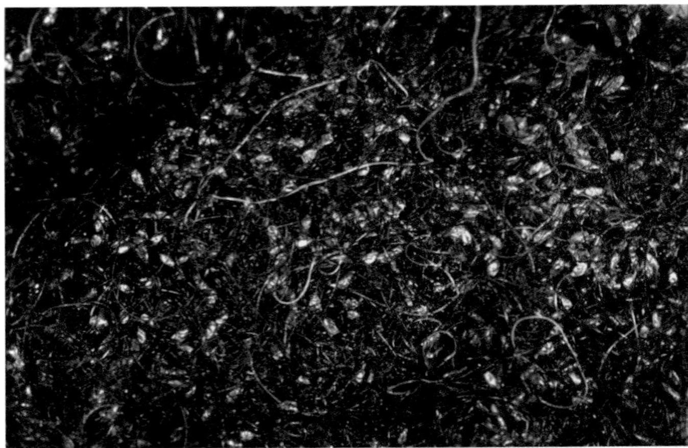

FIGURE 140-7 A massive infestation of head lice on the hair of a mentally ill homeless person. (*Reproduced with permission from Richard P. Usatine, MD.*)

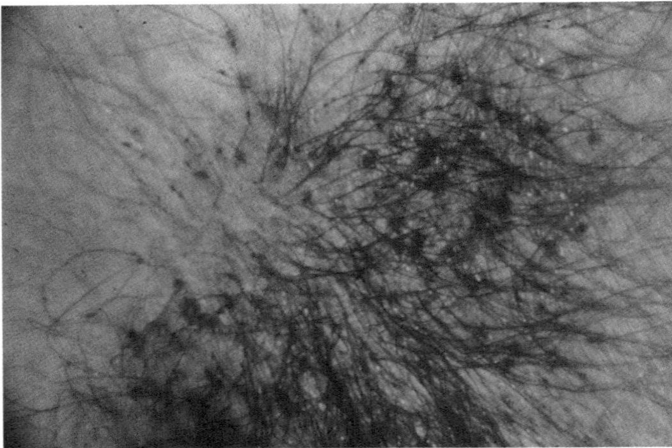

FIGURE 140-9 Crab lice infesting pubic hair. (*Reproduced with permission from the University of Texas Health Sciences Center, Division of Dermatology.*)

- Pubic or crab lice are transmitted primarily through sexual contact. In addition to pubic hair (**Figure 140-9**), infestations of eyelashes, eyebrows, beard, upper thighs, abdominal, and axillary hairs may also occur.

RISK FACTORS

- Contact with an infected individual
- Living in crowded quarters such as homeless shelters
- Poor hygiene and mental illness

DIAGNOSIS

CLINICAL FEATURES

- Nits can be seen in active disease or treated disease. Nits closer to the base of the hairs are generally newer and more likely to be live and unhatched. Unfortunately, nits that were not killed by pediculicides can hatch and start the infestation cycle over again. Note that nits are glued to the hairs and are hard to remove, whereas flakes of dandruff can be easily brushed off.

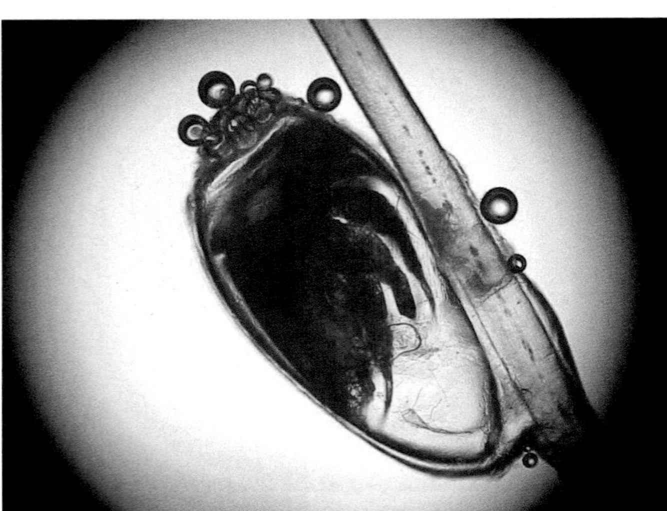

FIGURE 140-8 Microscopic view of a nit cemented to the hair and about to hatch. (*Reproduced with permission from Dan Stulberg, MD.*)

- Pruritus is the hallmark of lice infestation. It is the result of an allergic response to louse saliva.[7] Head lice are associated with excoriated lesions that appear on the scalp, ears, neck, and back.
- Occipital and cervical adenopathy may develop, especially when lesions become superinfected.
- Body lice result in small maculopapular eruptions that are predominantly found on the trunk (see **Figure 140-1**) and the clothing (see **Figure 140-2**).
- Chronic infestations often result in hyperpigmented, lichenified plaques known as "vagabond's skin."[8]
- Pubic lice produce bluish-gray spots (macula cerulea) that can be found on the chest, abdomen, and thighs.[8]

TYPICAL DISTRIBUTION

- Head lice—Look for nits and lice in the hair especially above the ears, behind the ears, and at the nape of the neck. There are many more nits present than live adults. Finding nits without an adult louse does not mean that the infestation has resolved (see **Figures 140-6** and **140-7**). Systematically combing wet or dry hair with a fine-toothed nit comb (teeth of comb are 0.2 mm apart) better detects active louse infestation than visual inspection of the hair and scalp alone.[9]
- Body lice—Look for the lice and larvae in the seams of the clothing (see **Figure 140-2**).
- Pubic lice—Look for nits and lice on the pubic hairs (see **Figure 140-9**). These lice and their nits may also be seen on the hairs of the upper thighs, abdomen, axilla, beard, eyebrows, and eyelashes. Little specks of dried blood may be seen in the underwear as a clue to the infestation.

LABORATORY TESTING

- Direct visualization and identification of live lice or nits are sufficient to make a diagnosis (see **Figures 140-2** to **140-7** and **140-9**).
- The use of a magnification lens may aid in the detection or confirmation of lice infestation.
- Under Wood light the head lice nits fluoresce a pale blue.
- If you find an adult louse put it on a slide with a coverslip loosely above it. Look at it under the microscope on the lowest power (see **Figures 140-4**

and **140-5**). You will see the internal workings of the live organs. If the louse was not found in a typical location, you can use the morphology of the body and legs to determine the type of louse causing the infestation.

- In cases of pubic lice infestations, individuals should be screened for other sexually transmitted diseases.[5]

DIFFERENTIAL DIAGNOSIS

- Dandruff, hair casts, and debris should be ruled out in cases of suspected lice infestations. Unlike nits, these particles are easily removed from the hair shaft. In addition, adult lice are absent.
- Scabies is also characterized by intense pruritus and papular eruptions. Unlike lice infestations, scabies may be associated with vesicles, and the presence of burrows is pathognomonic. Diagnosis is confirmed by microscopic examination of the scrapings from lesions for the presence of mites or eggs (see Chapter 141, Scabies).

MANAGEMENT

NONPHARMACOLOGIC

In young children or others who wish to avoid topical pediculicides for head lice, mechanical removal of lice by wet combing is an alternative therapy. A 1:1 vinegar:water rinse (left under a conditioning cap or towel for 15-20 minutes) or 8% formic acid crème rinse may enhance removal of tenacious nits.[8] Combing is performed until no lice are found for 2 weeks. SOR Ⓑ

- Nits are also removed with a fine-toothed comb following the application of all treatments. This step is critical in achieving resolution.
- Combs and hairbrushes should be discarded, soaked in hot water (at a temperature of at least 55°C [130°F]) for 5 minutes, or treated with pediculicides.[10]

MEDICATIONS

- *Pediculus humanus capitis* (head lice)
  - Nonprescription 1% permethrin cream rinse (Nix), pyrethrins with piperonyl butoxide (which inhibits pyrethrin catabolism; RID) shampoo, or permethrin 1% is applied to the hair and scalp and left on for 10 minutes then rinsed out.[11] SOR Ⓐ
  - Pyrethrins are only pediculicidal, whereas permethrin is both pediculicidal and ovicidal. It is important to note that treatment failure is common with these agents owing to the emergence of resistant strains of lice.
  - After 7 to 10 days repeating the application is optional when permethrin is used, but is necessary for pyrethrin. Lice persisting after treatment with a pyrethroid may be an indication of resistance.
  - Malathion 0.5% (Ovide) is available by prescription only, and is a highly effective pediculicidal and ovicidal agent for resistant lice. Malathion may have greater efficacy than pyrethrins.[12] It is approved for use in children age 6 years and older. The lotion is applied to dry hair for 8 to 12 hours and then washed. Repeat application is recommended after 7 to 10 days if live lice are still present. When used appropriately, malathion is 78% to 95% effective.[12] SOR Ⓐ
  - Benzyl alcohol 5% lotion (Ulesfia) is a newer treatment option in patients 6 months of age and older. It works by asphyxiating the parasite. It is applied for 10 minutes with saturation of the scalp and hair, and then rinsed off with water. The treatment is repeated after 7 days.[13] SOR Ⓐ
  - Spinosad (Natroba) is a new topical prescription medication approved by the Food and Drug Administration (FDA) in 2011 for the treatment of lice. Spinosad is a fermentation product of the soil bacterium *Saccharopolyspora spinosa* that compromises the central nervous system of lice. It is approximately 85% effective in lice eradication, usually after one application. It is applied to completely cover the dry scalp and hair, and rinsed off after 10 minutes. Treatment should be repeated if live lice remain 7 days after the initial application.[14] SOR Ⓐ
  - In February 2012, the US FDA approved ivermectin 0.5% lotion for the treatment of head lice. It is applied as a single 10-minute topical application. The safety of ivermectin in infants younger than age 6 months has not been established.[15] SOR Ⓐ
  - Hair conditioners should not be used prior to the application of pediculicides; these products may result in reduced efficacy.[16]
  - A Cochrane review found no evidence that any one pediculicide was better than another; permethrin, synergized pyrethrin, and malathion were all effective in the treatment of head lice.[17] SOR Ⓐ
  - Other therapeutic options include permethrin 5% cream and lindane 1% shampoo. Permethrin 5% is conventionally used to treat scabies; however, it is anecdotally recommended for treatment of recalcitrant head lice.[5] SOR Ⓒ
  - Lindane is considered a second-line treatment option owing to the possibility of central nervous system toxicity, which is most severe in children.
  - Oral therapy options include a 10-day course of trimethoprim-sulfamethoxazole or 2 doses of ivermectin (200 μg/kg) 7 to 10 days apart. SOR Ⓒ Trimethoprim-sulfamethoxazole is postulated to kill the symbiotic bacteria in the gut of the louse.[4] Combination therapy with 1% permethrin and trimethoprim-sulfamethoxazole is recommended in cases of multiple treatment failure or suspected cases of resistance to therapy.[5,10] SOR Ⓒ
- *Pediculus humanus corporis* (body lice)
  - Improving hygiene, and laundering clothing and bed linen at temperatures of 65°C (149°F) for 15 to 30 minutes will eliminate body lice.[8]
  - In settings where individuals cannot change clothing (eg, indigent population), a monthly application of 10% lindane powder can be used to dust the lining of all clothing.[8]
  - Additionally, lindane lotion or permethrin cream may be applied to the body for 8 to 12 hours to eradicate body lice.
- *Phthirus pubis* (pubic lice)
  - Pubic lice infestations are treated with a 10-minute application of the same topical pediculicides used to treat head lice.
  - Retreatment is recommended 7 to 10 days later.
  - Petroleum ointment applied 2 to 4 times a day for 8 to 10 days will eradicate eyelash infestations.
  - Clothing, towels, and bed linen should also be laundered to eliminate nit-bearing hairs.[8]

PREVENTION

Washing clothing and linen used by the head or pubic lice-infested person during 2 days prior to therapy in hot water and/or drying the items on a high-heat dryer cycle (54.5°C [130°F]). Items that cannot be washed may be dry cleaned or stored in a sealed plastic bag for 2 weeks.

FOLLOW-UP

Patients should be reexamined upon completion of therapy to confirm eradication of lice.

PATIENT EDUCATION

- Patients should be instructed to wash potentially contaminated articles of clothing, bed linen, combs, brushes, and hats.
- Nit removal is important in preventing continued infestation as a result of new progeny. Careful examination of close contacts, with appropriate treatment for infested individuals is important in avoiding recurrence.
- In cases of pubic lice, all sexual contacts should be treated.

PATIENT RESOURCES

- eMedicineHealth. *Lice*—**http://www.emedicinehealth.com/lice/article_em.htm.**
- Centers for Disease Control and Prevention. *Parasites–Lice*—**http://www.cdc.gov/parasites/lice/index.html.**

PROVIDER RESOURCES

- Centers for Disease Control and Prevention. *Parasites*—**http://www.cdc.gov/ncidod/dpd/parasites/lice/default.htm.**
- Medscape. *Pediculosis (Lice)*—**http://emedicine.medscape.com/article/225013.**

REFERENCES

1. Usatine RP, Halem L. A terrible itch. *J Fam Pract*. 2003;52(5):377-379.
2. Araujo A, Ferreira LF, Guidon N, et al. Ten thousand years of head lice infection. *Parasitol Today*. 2000;16(7):269.
3. Roberts RJ. Clinical practice. Head lice. *N Engl J Med*. 2002;346:1645.
4. Frankowski BL, Weiner LB. Head Lice. *Pediatrics*. 2002;110(3):638-643.
5. Pickering LK, Baker CJ, Long SS, McMillan JA. *Red Book: 2006 Report of the Committee on Infectious Diseases*, 27th ed. Elk Grove Village, IL: American Academy of Pediatrics; 2006:488-493.
6. Maguire JH, Pollack RJ, Spielman A. Ectoparasite infestations and arthropod bites and stings. In: Kasper DL, Fauci AS, Longo DL, Braunwald EB, Hauser SL, Jameson JL, eds. *Harrison's Principles of Internal Medicine*, 16th ed. New York, NY: McGraw-Hill; 2005:2601-2602.
7. Flinders DC, De Schweinitz P. Pediculosis and scabies. *Am Fam Physician*. 2004;69(2):341-348.
8. Darmstadt GL. Arthropod bites and infestations. In: Behrman RE, Kliegman RM, Jenson HB, eds. *Nelson Textbook of Pediatrics,* 16th ed. Philadelphia, PA: Saunders; 2000:2046-2047.
9. Jahnke C, Bauer E, Hengge UR, Feldmeier H. Accuracy of diagnosis of pediculosis capitis: visual inspection vs wet combing. *Arch Dermatol.* 2009;145(3):309-313.
10. Hipolito RB, Mallorca FG, Zuniga-Macaraig ZO, et al. Head lice infestation: single drug versus combination therapy with one percent permethrin and trimethoprim/sulfamethoxazole. *Pediatrics*. 2001;107(3):E30.
11. Meinking TL, Clineschmidt CM, Chen C, et al. An observer-blinded study of 1% permethrin creme rinse with and without adjunctive combing in patients with head lice. *J Pediatr.* 2002;141(5):665-670.
12. Meinking TL, Serrano L, Hard B, et al. Comparative in vitro pediculicidal efficacy of treatments in a resistant head lice population in the United States. *Arch Dermatol.* 2002;138(2):220-224.
13. Meinking TL, Villar ME, Vicaria M, et al. The clinical trials supporting benzyl alcohol lotion 5% (Ulesfia): a safe and effective topical treatment for head lice (pediculosis humanus capitis). *Pediatr Dermatol.* 2010;27(1):19-24.
14. Stough D, Shellabarger S, Quiring J, Gabrielsen AA Jr. Efficacy and safety of spinosad and permethrin creme rinses for pediculosis capitis (head lice). *Pediatrics.* 2009;124(3):e389-e395.
15. *Ivermectin Lotion 0.5% (Sklice) Clinical Review (NDA)*. http://www.fda.gov/downloads/Drugs/DevelopmentApprovalProcess/DevelopmentResources/UCM295584.pdf. Accessed April 13, 2012.
16. Lebwohl M, Clark L, Levitt J. Therapy for head lice based on life cycle, resistance, and safety considerations. *Pediatrics.* 2007;119(5):965-974.
17. Dodd CS. Interventions for treating head lice. *Cochrane Database Syst Rev*. 2006;(4):CD001165.

141 SCABIES

Richard P. Usatine, MD
Pierre Chanoine, MD
Mindy A. Smith, MD, MS

PATIENT STORY

A 32-year-old man is seen with severe itching and crusting of his hands and feet (**Figures 141-1** and **141-2**). He also has a pruritic rash over the rest of his body. Dermoscopy revealed the scabies mites in various burrows. A scraping was done and scabies mites and scybala (feces) were seen (**Figures 141-3** and **141-4**). The man was treated with oral ivermectin (0.2 mg/kg) once with a repeat dose to be taken in 10 days. The yellow crusting wheeping of yellow fluid is evidence of secondary bacterial infection or impetiginization, so the patient was also given a short course of an oral antibiotic. The scabies cleared.

SYNONYMS

Scabies is also known as 7-year itch.

EPIDEMIOLOGY

- Three hundred million cases per year are estimated worldwide.[1] In many developing tropical countries, scabies is endemic.[1]
- Studies in resource-poor countries show an association between scabies and overcrowding, especially in sleeping quarters.[1]
- In developed nations the rates of scabies infestation are similar across age ranges. While in developing countries the highest rates are among children and the elderly.[1]

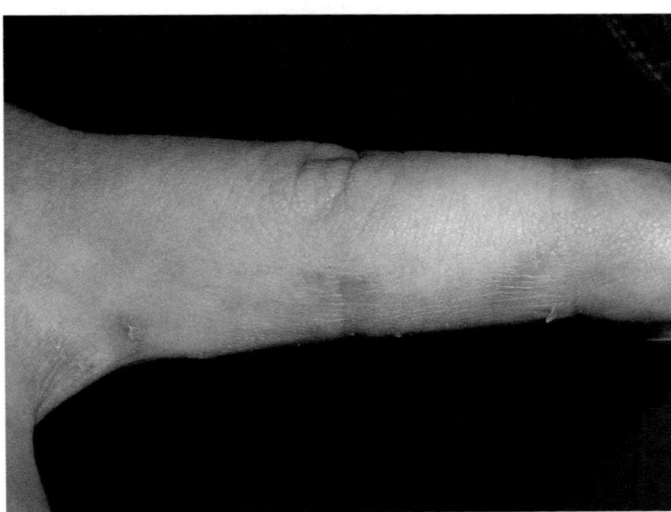

FIGURE 141-1 Scabies infestation demonstrated by typical linear burrows between the fingers of this 32-year-old man. Dermoscopy revealed a positive arrowhead sign of the scabies mite at the end of a burrow. (*Reproduced with permission from Richard P. Usatine, MD.*)

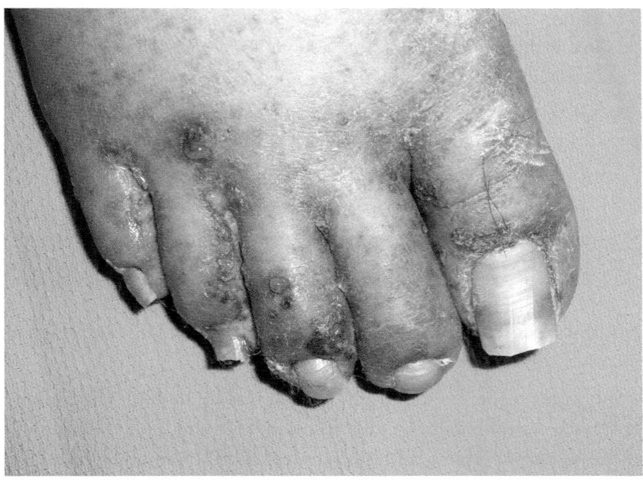

FIGURE 141-2 Impetiginized scabies on the foot of the 32-year-old man of Figure 141-1. The yellow crusting and wheeping of yellow fluid is evidence of secondary bacterial infection. (*Reproduced with permission from Richard P. Usatine, MD.*)

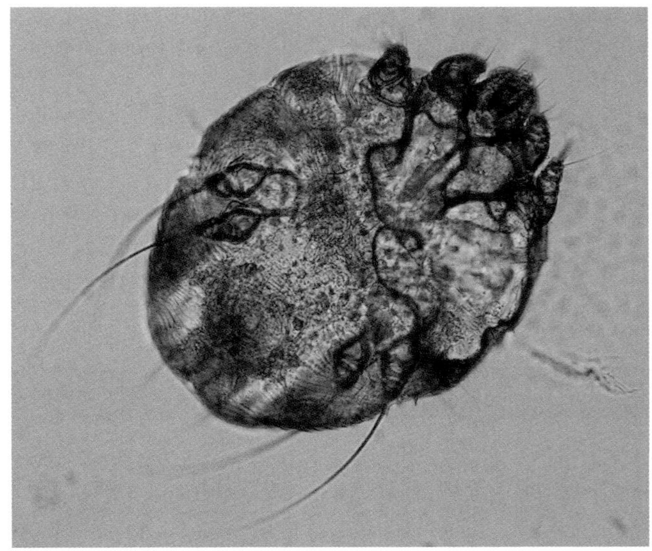

FIGURE 141-3 Microscopic view of the scabies mite from a patient with crusted scabies. (*Reproduced with permission from Richard P. Usatine, MD.*)

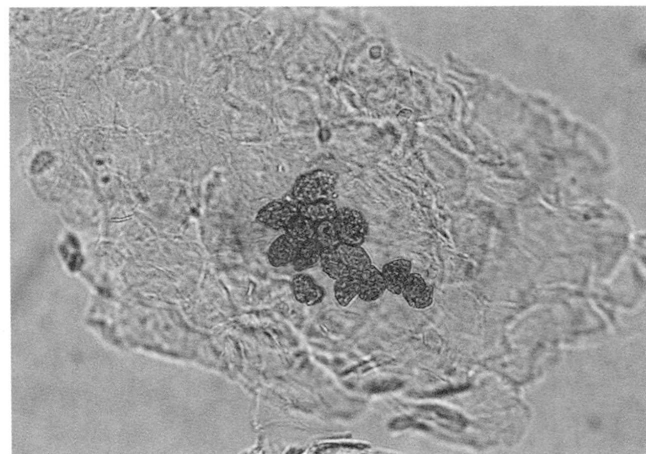

FIGURE 141-4 Scraping of the patient's hand produced a good view of the scybala (the mites' feces). (*Reproduced with permission from Richard P. Usatine, MD.*)

- The highest rates of crusted scabies are in immunocompromised patients including medical immunosuppression, as well as in those with developmental disability, including Down syndrome.[1]
- The medical burden of scabies is associated with increased rates of impetigo and complications of secondary bacterial infection with group A streptococci and *Staphylococcus aureus*.[1]

ETIOLOGY AND PATHOPHYSIOLOGY

- Human scabies is caused by the mite *Sarcoptes scabiei*, an obligate human parasite (see **Figure 141-3**).[2,3]
- Adult mites spend their entire life cycle, around 30 days, within the epidermis. After copulation the male mite dies and the female mite burrows through the superficial layers of the skin excreting feces (see **Figure 141-4**) and laying eggs (**Figure 141-5**).
- Mites move through the superficial layers of skin by secreting proteases that degrade the stratum corneum.
- Infected individuals usually have less than 100 mites. In contrast, immunocompromised hosts can have up to 1 million mites, and are susceptible to crusted scabies also called Norwegian scabies (see **Figures 141-6** to **141-8**).[2]
- Transmission usually occurs via direct skin contact. Scabies in adults is frequently sexually transmitted.[4] Scabies mites can also be transmitted from animals to humans.[2]
- Mites can also survive for 3 days outside of the human epidermis allowing for infrequent transmission through bedding and clothing.
- The incubation period is on average 3 to 4 weeks for an initial infestation. Sensitized individuals can have symptoms within hours of reexposure.

RISK FACTORS

- Scabies is more common in homeless and impoverished persons, and individuals who are immunocompromised or suffering from dementia.[2]
- Institutionalized individuals and those living in crowded conditions also have a higher incidence of the infestation.[2]

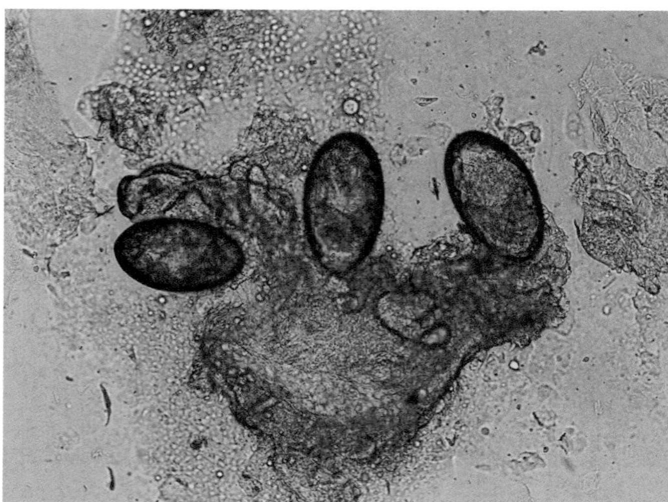

FIGURE 141-5 Scabies eggs from a scraping. (*Reproduced with permission from Richard P. Usatine, MD.*)

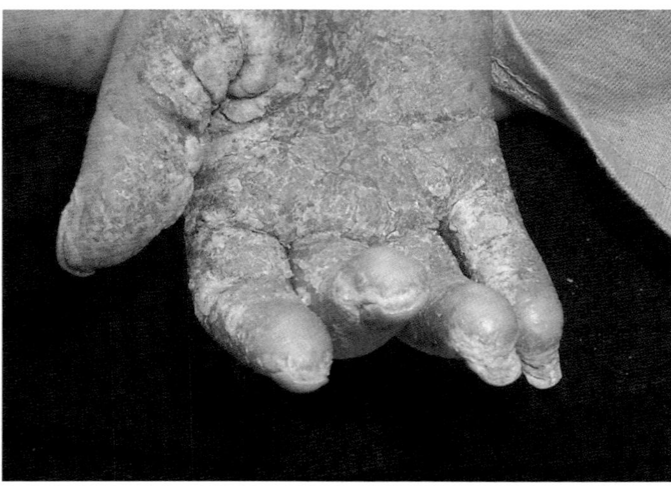

FIGURE 141-6 Crusted scabies on the hands. (*Reproduced with permission from Richard P. Usatine, MD.*)

DIAGNOSIS

CLINICAL FEATURES

- Pruritus is a hallmark of the disease.[2]
- Skin findings include papules (see **Figure 141-8**), burrows (**Figure 141-9** and **141-10**), nodules (**Figures 141-11**), and vesiculopustules (see **Figure 141-10**).
- Burrows are the classic morphologic finding in scabies and the best location to find the mite (see **Figures 141-9** and **141-10**).
- Pruritic papules/nodules around the axillae, umbilicus, areola, or on the penis and scrotum (**Figure 141-11** and **141-12**) are highly suggestive of scabies.

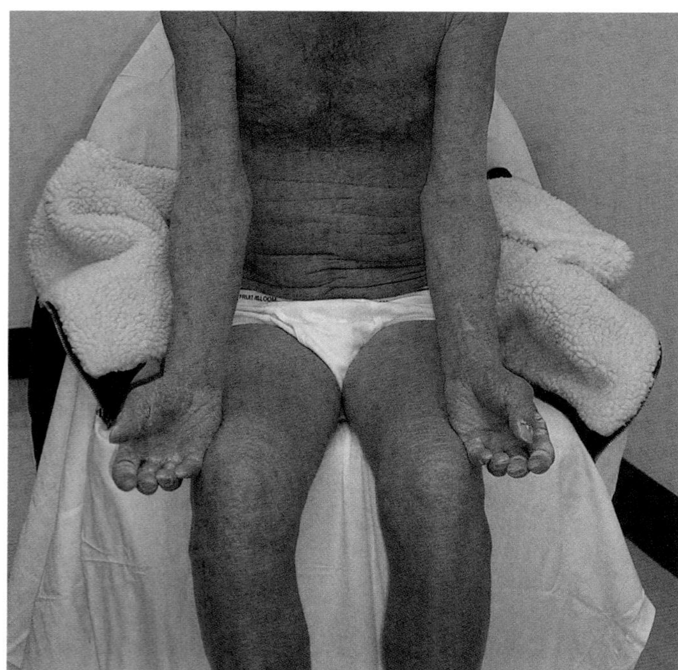

FIGURE 141-7 Crusted scabies from head to toe in a man with HIV/AIDS. The infestation was so massive that it caused him to become erythrodermic and dehydrated. Note the crusting on the hands. (*Reproduced with permission from Richard P. Usatine, MD.*)

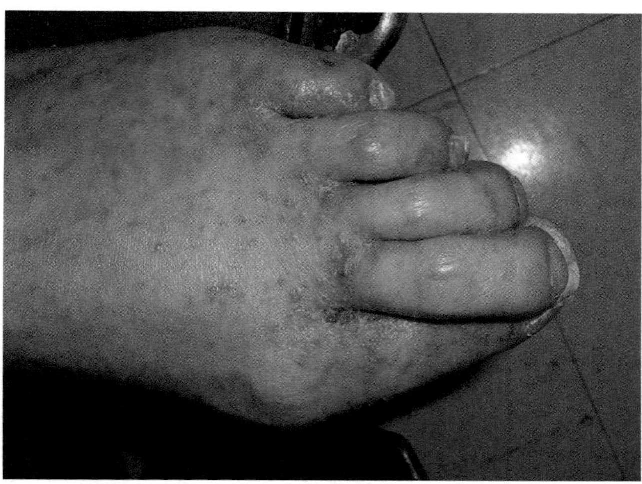

FIGURE 141-8 Crusted scabies on the foot of a disabled man who had experienced a stroke previously. (*Reproduced with permission from Richard P. Usatine, MD.*)

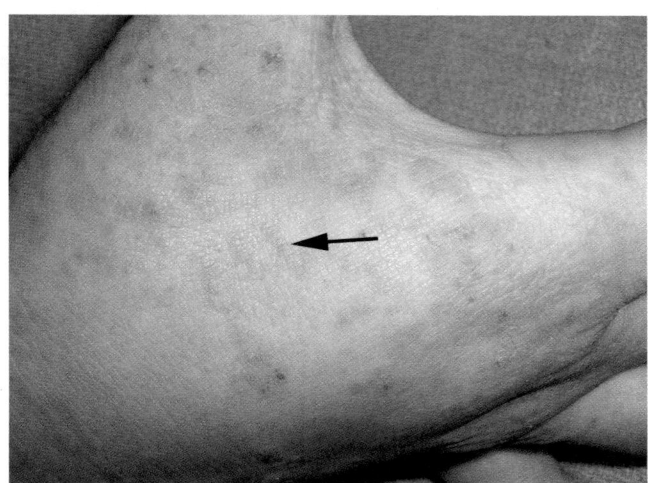

FIGURE 141-9 Scabies infestation on the hand. Dermoscopy revealed scabies mites within burrows (*arrow*). (*Reproduced with permission from Richard P. Usatine, MD.*)

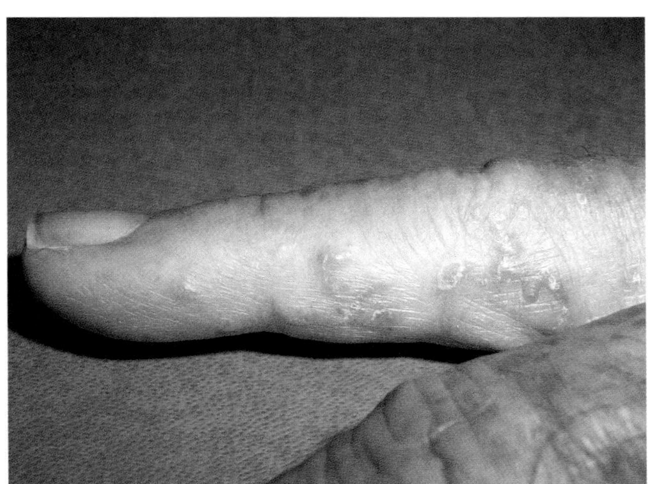

FIGURE 141-10 Burrows prominently visible between the fingers of this homeless man with scabies. Burrows are a classic manifestation of scabies. (*Reproduced with permission from Richard P. Usatine, MD.*)

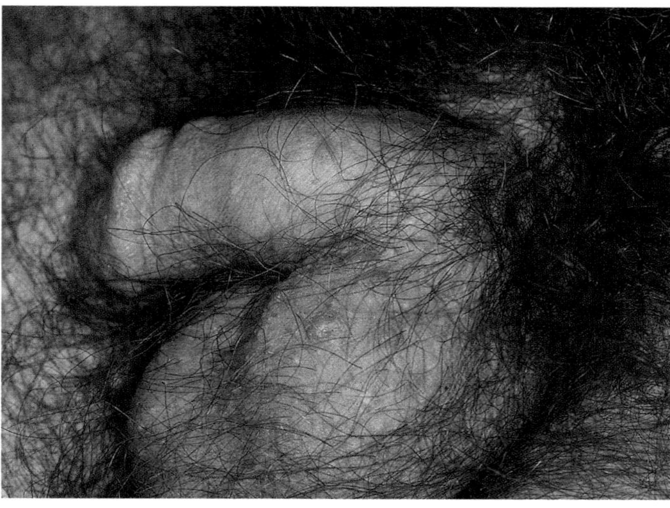

FIGURE 141-11 Pruritic papules on the glans of the penis and nodules on the scrotum secondary to sexually transmitted scabies in a gay man. (*Reproduced with permission from Richard P. Usatine, MD.*)

TYPICAL DISTRIBUTION

- Classic distribution in scabies includes the interdigital spaces (**Figures 141-9, 141-10,** and **141-13**), wrists, ankles, waist (**Figures 141-14**), groin, axillae, palms, and feet (see **Figures 141-7** and **141-8**).
- Genital involvement can also occur (see **Figures 141-11** and **141-12**).

LABORATORY STUDIES AND IMAGING

- Light microscopy of skin scrapings provides a definitive diagnosis when mites, eggs, or feces are identified (see **Figures 141-3** to **141-5**). This can be challenging and time consuming, even when mites, eggs, or feces are present. Packing tape stripping of skin has also been used instead of a scalpel to find mites for examination under the microscope.[5] The inability to find these items should not be used to rule out scabies in a clinically suspicious case. In what is believed to be a recurrent case, it is helpful to find definitive evidence that your diagnosis is correct.

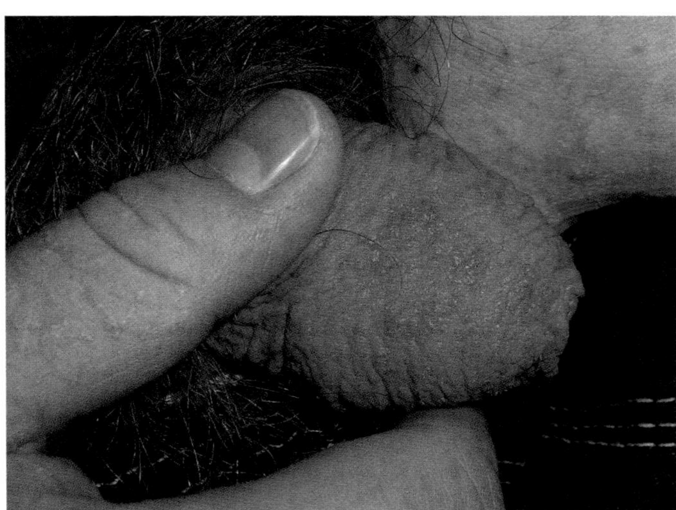

FIGURE 141-12 Pruritic papules of scabies on the foreskin of the penis, hands, and groin acquired as a sexually transmitted disease. (*Reproduced with permission from Richard P. Usatine, MD.*)

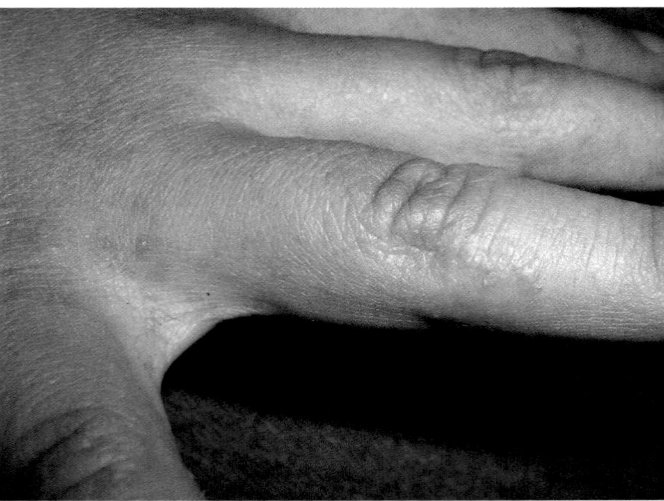

FIGURE 141-13 Scabies found in the classic location between the fingers in this interdigital webspace. (*Reproduced with permission from Richard P. Usatine, MD.*)

- Dermoscopy is a useful and rapid technique for identifying a scabies mite at the end of a burrow (see Appendix C, Dermoscopy).[6] The mite has been described as an arrowhead or a jet plane in its appearance (**Figure 141-15**). The advantage of the dermoscope is that multiple burrows can be examined quickly without causing any pain to the patient. Children are more likely to stay still for this than scraping with a scalpel or skin stripping with tape.
- If a dermoscope is available, start with this noninvasive examination. If the findings are typical, then a microscopic examination is not needed. If the findings are not convincing, or a dermoscope is not available, perform a scraping. It is best to scrape the skin at the end of a burrow. Use a #15 scalpel that has been dipped into mineral oil or microscope immersion oil. Scrape holding the blade perpendicular to the skin until the burrow (or papule) is opened (some slight bleeding is usual). Transfer the material to a slide and add a coverslip.
- Tips for microscopic examination—Start by examining the slide with the lowest power available as mites may be seen under 4 power and the slide can be scanned most quickly with the lowest power. If no mites are seen switch to 10 power and scan the slide again looking for mites, eggs, and feces. Forty power may be used to confirm findings under 10 power.

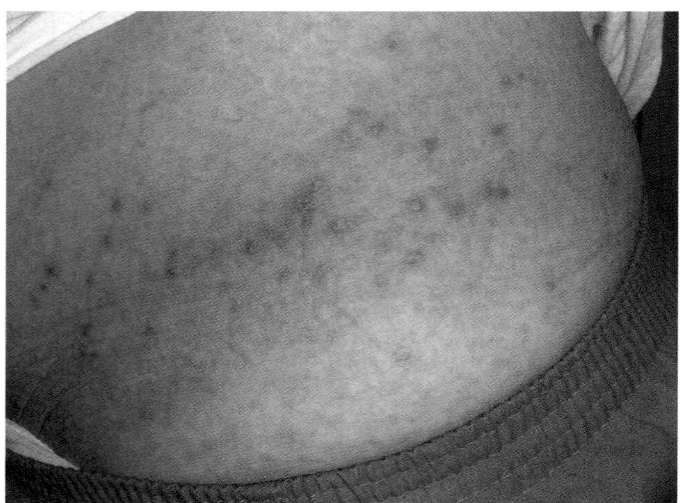

FIGURE 141-14 Scabies around the waist with multiple papules and nodules in this incarcerated young woman. Incarceration is a risk factor for scabies. (*Reproduced with permission from Richard P. Usatine, MD.*)

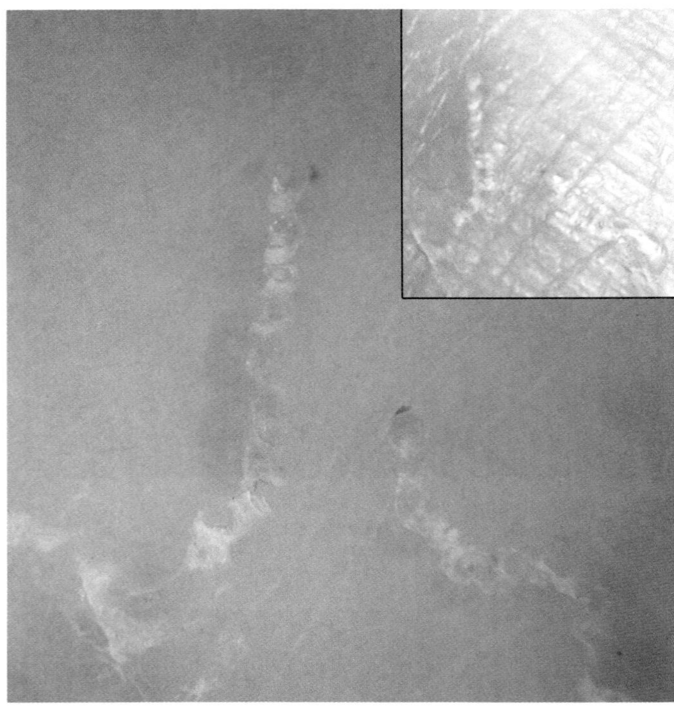

FIGURE 141-15 Two scabies mites visible with dermoscopy. Note how the darkest most visible aspect of the mite looks like an arrowhead or jet plane. In this case the oval bodies of the mites are also visible. The *upper right inset* shows the same burrows without dermoscopy. (*Reproduced with permission from Richard P. Usatine, MD.*)

- In one study comparing dermoscopic mite identification with microscopic examination of skin scrapings, found the former technique to be of comparable sensitivity (91% and 90%, respectively) with specificity of 86% (vs 100% by definition), even in inexperienced hands.[7] Another study reported sensitivity of dermoscopy at 83% (95% confidence interval, 0.70-0.94).[8] In this study, the negative-predictive value was identical for dermoscopy and the adhesive tape test (0.85), making the latter a good screening test in resource-poor areas.
- Videodermatoscopy can also be used to diagnose scabies.[9] Videodermatoscopy allows for skin magnification with incidental lighting at high magnifications for viewing mites and eggs. The technique is noninvasive and does not cause pain.
- *S. scabiei* recombinant antigens have diagnostic potential and are under investigation for identifying antibodies in individuals with active scabies.[10]

BIOPSY

Rarely necessary unless there are reasons to suspect another diagnosis.

DIFFERENTIAL DIAGNOSIS

- Atopic dermatitis—Itching is a prominent symptom in atopic dermatitis and scabies. The distribution of involved skin can help to differentiate the 2 diagnoses. Look for burrows in scabies and the history of involved family members. In children, atopic dermatitis is often confined to the flexural and extensor surfaces of the body. In adults, the hands are a primary site of involvement (see Chapter 143, Atopic Dermatitis).

- Contact dermatitis—Characterized by vesicles and papules on bright red skin, which are rare in scabies. Chronic contact dermatitis often leads to scaling and lichenification and may not be as pruritic as scabies (see Chapter 144, Contact Dermatitis).
- Seborrheic dermatitis—A papulosquamous eruption with scales and crusts that is limited to the sebum-rich areas of the body; namely, the scalp, the face, the postauricular areas, and the intertriginous areas. Pruritus is usually mild or absent (see Chapter 149, Seborrheic Dermatitis).
- Impetigo—Honey-crusted plaques are a hallmark of impetigo. Scabies can become secondarily infected, so consider that both diagnoses can occur concomitantly with papules and pustules present (see Chapter 118, Impetigo).
- Bedbugs have become more prevalent in the United States (**Figure 141-16**). Bedbug bites tend to appear in the morning after sleeping on the infested bed. The skin manifestations of these bites can appear anywhere on the body especially in skin not covered by clothing. The typical description of the bites includes clusters of 3 bites in a linear pattern (**Figure 141-17**). The mnemonic for this is breakfast, lunch, and dinner. Scabies lesions do not follow this pattern and the scabies mite is not visible as is the bedbug.
- Other arthropod bites—Bites may exhibit puncta that allow for differentiation from scabies.

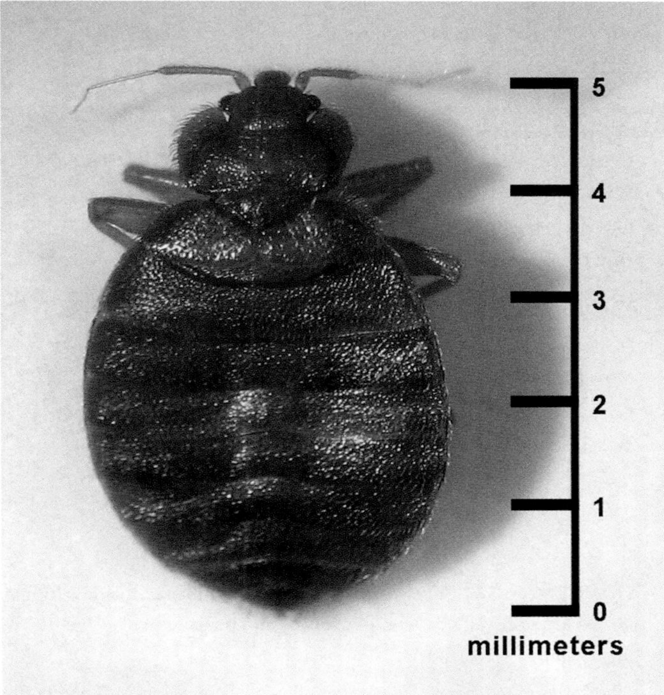

FIGURE 141-16 Adult bedbugs are on average 5-mm long, oval-shaped, and dorsoventrally flattened. They possess piercing-sucking mouthparts and are virtually wingless. Nymphs look like smaller, paler versions of the adults. (*Reproduced with permission from Centers for Disease Control and Prevention/Blaine Mathison.*)

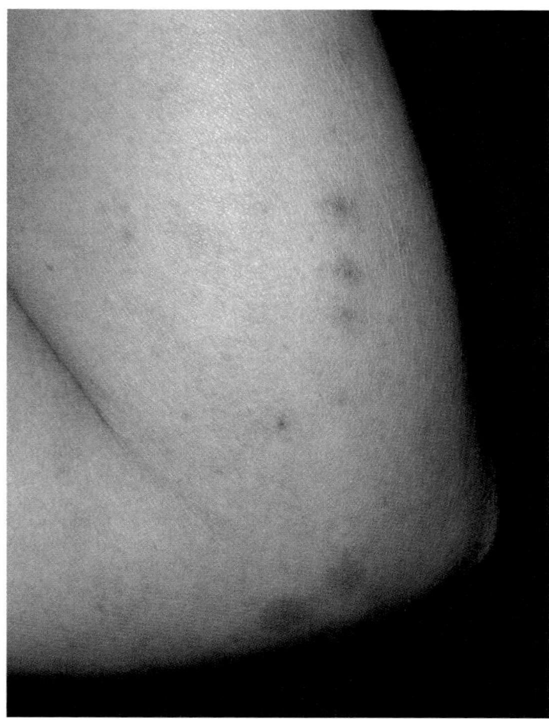

FIGURE 141-17 Bedbug bites on the arm of a 42-year-old woman. Note there is a linear pattern of 3 bites on the forearm. One way to remember this pattern is to think the bedbug eating breakfast, lunch, and dinner. Scabies does not create this pattern. (*Reproduced with permission from Richard P. Usatine, MD.*)

- Tinea—All kinds of tinea infections can be pruritic with scales and linear or curvilinear borders. In **Figure 141-18**, an immunosuppressed man being treated for polymyositis was found to have tinea corporis and scabies. When his pruritus did not resolve during treatment for his tinea corporis, close examination with the dermatoscope revealed a scabies infestation. Skin scrapings for microscopy in most cases will distinguish between tinea and scabies.

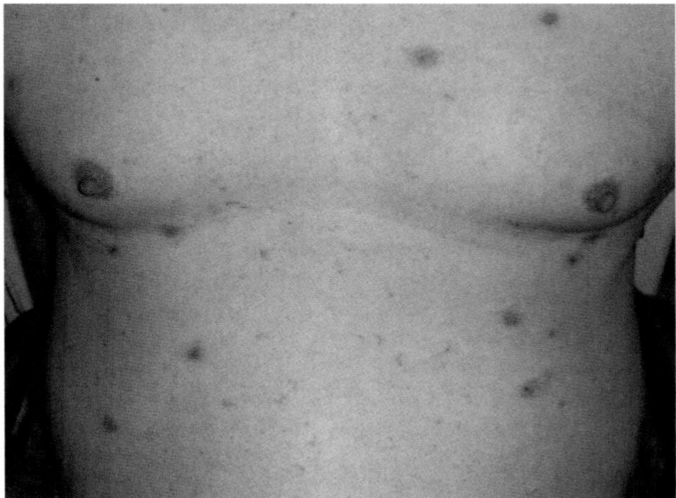

FIGURE 141-18 Scabies and tinea corporis in a 55-year-old man being treated for polymyositis with prednisone. The scabies was initially missed and when the pruritus did not resolve with oral terbinafine for the tinea seen near his waist (KOH proven), closer look with dermoscopy revealed scabies mites in some of the pruritic papules. (*Reproduced with permission from Richard P. Usatine, MD.*)

MANAGEMENT

NONPHARMACOLOGIC

Environmental decontamination is a standard component of all therapies. SOR B Clothing, bed linens, and towels should be machine washed in hot water. Clothing or other items (eg, stuffed animals) that cannot be washed may be dry cleaned or stored in sealed bags for at least 72 hours.[11]

MEDICATIONS

Treatment includes administration of an antiscabicide and an antipruritic.[2,12]

- Permethrin 5% cream (Elimite, Acticin) is the most effective treatment based on a systematic review in the Cochrane Database.[12] SOR A The cream is applied from the neck down (include the head when it is involved) and rinsed off 8 to 14 hours later. Usually, this is done overnight. Repeating the treatment in 1 to 2 weeks may be more effective. SOR C In patients with crusted scabies, use of a keratolytic cream may facilitate the breakdown of skin crusts and improve penetration of the cream.[13] Unfortunately, scabies resistance to permethrin is increasing.
- Ivermectin is an oral treatment for resistant or crusted scabies. Studies have demonstrated its safety and efficacy. Most studies used a single dose of ivermectin at 200 μg/kg.[13] SOR A Taking the drug with food may enhance drug penetration into the epidermis.[13] Some experts advocate repeating a dose 1 week later. It is worth noting that the Food and Drug Administration (FDA) has not labeled this drug for use in children weighing less than 15 kg. Ivermectin is currently available only in 3- and 6-mg tablets, so dosing often needs to be rounded up to accommodate the use of whichever tablets are available. As there is no oral suspension available, tablets may need to be cut and given with food for use in children.
- Diphenhydramine, hydroxyzine, and mid-potency steroid creams can be used for symptomatic relief of itching. SOR C. It is important to note that pruritus may persist for 1 to 2 weeks after successful treatment because the dead scabies mites and eggs still have antigenic qualities that may cause persistent inflammation.
- All household or family members living in the infested home and sexual contacts should be treated. SOR C Failure to treat all involved individuals often results in recurrences within the family. Use of insecticide sprays and fumigants is not recommended.
- Other less-effective medications include topical benzyl benzoate, crotamiton, lindane (no longer used in the United States because of concerns regarding neurotoxicity), and synergized natural pyrethrins.[8] SOR A Topical agents used more commonly in other countries include 5% to 10% sulfur in paraffin (widely in Africa and South America), 10% to 25% benzyl benzoate (often used in Europe and Australia), and malathion.[13] In infants younger than 2 months of age, crotamiton or a sulfur preparation is recommended by one author instead of permethrin because of theoretical concerns of systemic absorption of permethrin.[13]
- Antibiotics are needed if there is evidence of a bacterial superinfection. SOR C

COMPLEMENTARY AND ALTERNATIVE THERAPY

Tea tree oil contains oxygenetic terpenoids, found to have rapid scabicidal activity.[14]

PREVENTION

- Avoid direct skin-to-skin contact with an infested person or with items such as clothing or bedding used by an infested person.
- Treat members of the same household and other potentially exposed persons at the same time as the infested person to prevent possible reexposure and reinfestation.

PROGNOSIS

- The prognosis with proper diagnosis and treatment is excellent unless the patient is immunocompromised; reinfestation, however, often occurs if environmental risk factors continue.[1]
- Postinflammatory hyper- or hypopigmentation can occur.[1]

FOLLOW-UP

- Routine follow-up is indicated when symptoms do not resolve.
- Consider an immunologic workup for individuals with crusted scabies.

PATIENT EDUCATION

- Patients should avoid direct contact including sleeping with others until they have completed the first application of the medicine.
- Patients may return to school and work 24 hours after first treatment.
- Patients should be warned that itching may persist for 1 to 2 weeks after successful treatment but that if symptoms are still present by the third week, the patient should return for further evaluation.

PATIENT RESOURCES

- Centers for Disease Control and Prevention. *Scabies*— **http://www.cdc.gov/parasites/scabies/.**
- PubMed Health. *Scabies*— **http://www.ncbi.nlm.nih.gov/pubmedhealth/PMH0001833/.**

PROVIDER RESOURCES

- Medscape. *Scabies*— **http://emedicine.medscape.com/article/1109204.**
- DermNet NZ. *Scabies*— **http://dermnetnz.org/arthropods/scabies.html.**

REFERENCES

1. Hay RJ, Steer AC, Engelman D, Walton S. Scabies in the developing world—its prevalence, complications, and management. *Clin Microbiol Infect*. 2012 Apr;18(4):313-323.
2. Hengge UR, Currie B, Jäger G, et al. Scabies: a ubiquitous neglected skin disease. *Lancet Infect Dis*. 2006;6(12):769-779.
3. Paller AS, Mancini AJ. Scabies. In: Paller AS, Mancini AJ, eds. *Hurwitz Clinical Pediatric Dermatology: A Textbook of Skin Disorders of Childhood and Adolescence*. Philadelphia, PA: Saunders; 2006:479-488.

4. Centers for Disease Control and Prevention. *Scabies: Epidemiology and Risk Factors*. http://www.cdc.gov/parasites/scabies/epi.html. Accessed April 2012.
5. Albrecht J, Bigby M. Testing a test. Critical appraisal of tests for diagnosing scabies. *Arch Dermatol.* 2011;147(4):494-497.
6. Fox GN, Usatine RP. Itching and rash in a boy and his grandmother. *J Fam Pract*. 2006;55(8):679-684.
7. Dupuy A, Dehen L, Bourrat E, et al. Accuracy of standard dermoscopy for diagnosing scabies. *J Am Acad Dermatol.* 2007;56(1):53-62.
8. Walter B, Heukelbach J, Fengler G, et al. Comparison of dermoscopy, skin scraping, and the adhesive tape test for the diagnosis of scabies in a resource-poor setting. *Arch Dermatol.* 2011;147(4): 468-473.
9. Lacarrubba F, Musumeci ML, Caltabiano R, et al. High-magnification videodermatoscopy: a new noninvasive diagnostic tool for scabies in children. *Pediatr Dermatol.* 2001;18(5):439-441.
10. Walton SF, Currie BJ. Problems in diagnosing scabies, a global disease in human and animal populations. *Clin Microbiol Rev.* 2007; 20(2):268-279.
11. Centers for Disease Control and Prevention. *Scabies: Treatment*. http://www.cdc.gov/parasites/scabies/treatment.html. Accessed April 2012.
12. Strong M, Johnstone PW. Interventions for treating scabies. *Cochrane Database Syst Rev.* 2007;3:CD000320.
13. Currie BJ, McCarthy JS. Permethrin and ivermectin for scabies, *N Engl J Med.* 2010;362(8):717-725.
14. Carson CF, Hammer KA, Riley TV. *Melaleuca alternifolia* (Tea Tree) oil: a review of antimicrobial and other medicinal properties. *Clin Microbiol Rev.* 2006;19(1):50-62.

142 CUTANEOUS LARVA MIGRANS

Jennifer A. Keehbauch, MD
Richard P. Usatine, MD

PATIENT STORY

A 29-year-old man noted pruritic lesions on the dorsum of both feet after returning from vacation in Mexico. A serpiginous, linear, raised, tunnel-like erythematous lesion outlining the path of migration of the larva. Lesions were present bilaterally, arising in the 4 and 5 webspace at sites of tinea pedis. He was treated successfully with oral ivermectin.[1]

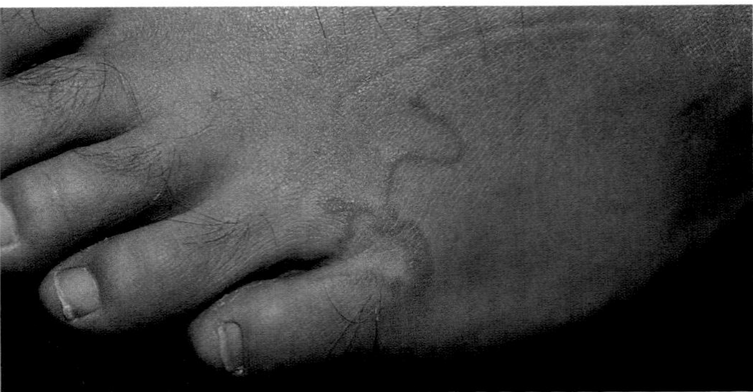

FIGURE 142-1 Cutaneous larva migrans (CLM) on the dorsum of the foot in a 29-year-old man. He noted pruritic lesions on the dorsum of both feet after returning from vacation in Mexico. A serpiginous, linear, raised, tunnel-like erythematous lesion outlines the path of migration of the larva. Lesions were present bilaterally, arising in the 4 and 5 webspace at sites of tinea pedis. He was treated successfully with ivermectin. (*Reproduced with permission from Wolff K and Johnson RA.* Fitzpatrick's Color Atlas & Synopsis of Clinical Dermatology. *6th ed. McGraw-Hill, 2009.*)

SYNONYMS

Cutaneous larva migrans (CLM) is also known as creeping eruption, plumber's itch.

EPIDEMIOLOGY

- Endemic in developing countries, particularly Brazil, India, South Africa, Somalia, Malaysia, Indonesia, and Thailand.[2,3]
- Peak incidence in the rainy seasons.[3]
- During peak rainy seasons, the prevalence in children is as high as 15% in resource-poor areas, but much less common in affluent communities in these same countries with only 1 to 2 per 10,000 individuals per year.[4]
- In the United States, it is found predominantly in Florida, southeastern Atlantic states, and the Gulf Coast.[2]
- Children are more frequently affected than adults.[4]

ETIOLOGY AND PATHOPHYSIOLOGY

- Most commonly caused by dog and cat hookworms (ie, *Ancylostoma braziliense*, *Ancylostoma caninum*, *Uncinaria stenocephala*).[4]
- Eggs are passed in cat or dog feces.[2]
- Larvae are hatched in moist, warm sand or soil.[2]
- Infective stage larvae penetrate the skin.[2]

DIAGNOSIS

The diagnosis is based on history and clinical findings.

CLINICAL FEATURES

- Elevated, serpiginous, or linear reddish-brown tracks 1 to 5 cm long (**Figures 142-1** to **142-5**).[2,5]
- Intense pruritus, which often disrupts sleep.[3]
- Symptoms last for weeks to months, and, rarely, years. Most cases are self-limiting.[5]

TYPICAL DISTRIBUTION

- Feet and lower extremities (73%), buttocks (13%-18%), and abdomen (16%)[6,7]
- Areas that come in contact with contaminated skin
  - Most commonly the feet, buttocks, and thigh[3]

LABORATORY AND IMAGING

Not indicated, but rarely blood tests show eosinophilia or elevated immunoglobulin E levels.[5]

DIFFERENTIAL DIAGNOSIS

It may be confused with the following conditions:

- Cutaneous fungal infections—Lesions are typically scaling plaques and annular macules with central clearing. If the serpiginous track of CLM

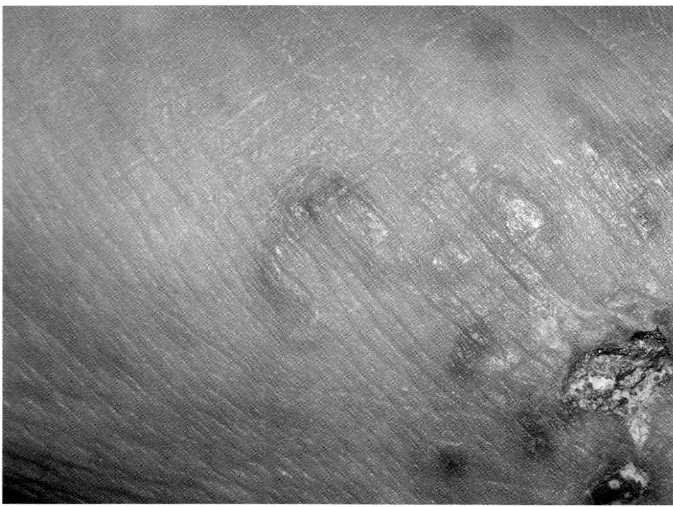

FIGURE 142-2 Close-up of a burrow from cutaneous larva migrans on the foot of a carpenter who was doing work under a house. (*Reproduced with permission from Richard P. Usatine, MD.*)

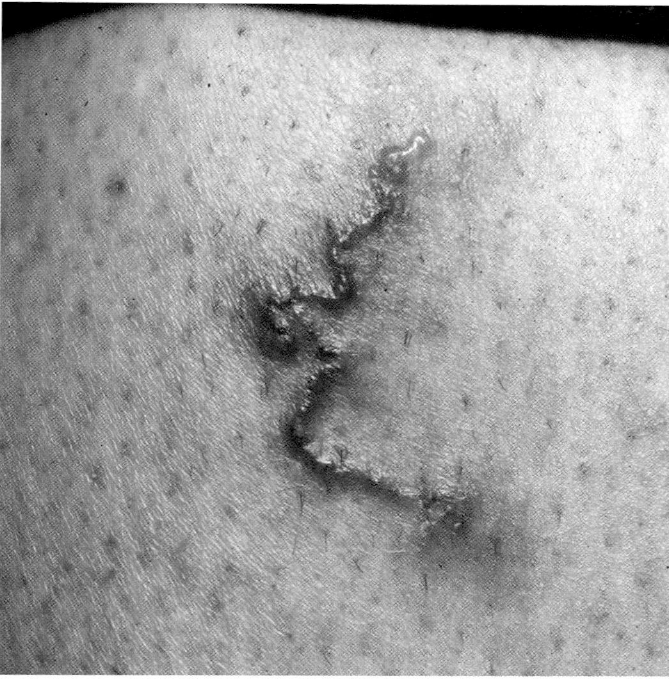

FIGURE 142-3 Serpiginous burrow from cutaneous larva migrans on the leg. The actual larva is 2 to 3 cm beyond the visible tracks. (*Reproduced with permission from John Gonzalez, MD.*)

is circular, this can lead to the incorrect diagnosis of "ringworm." The irony is that ringworm is a dermatophyte fungus whereas CLM really is a worm (see Chapter 136, Tinea Corporis).

- Contact dermatitis—Differentiate by distribution of lesions, presence of vesicles, and absence of classical serpiginous tracks (see Chapter 144, Contact Dermatitis).
- Erythema migrans of Lyme disease—Lesions are usually annular macules or patches and are not raised and serpiginous (see Chapter 215, Lyme Disease).
- Phytophotodermatitis—The acute phase of phytophotodermatitis is erythematous with vesicles; this later develops into postinflammatory hyperpigmented lesions. This may be acquired while preparing drinks

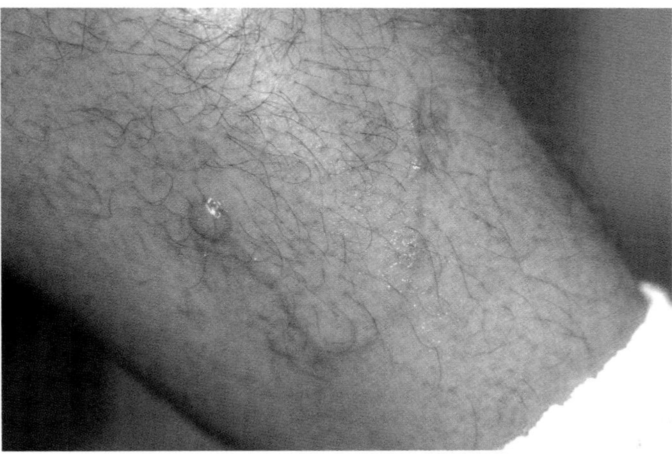

FIGURE 142-4 Cutaneous larva migrans (CLM) on the leg of an 18 year-old man. He developed this pruritic serpiginous rash several days after returning from the beach. It extended several millimeter in length each day and a blister developed at the distal point of the burrow in the past 24 hours. (*Reproduced with permission from Robert T. Brodell, MD.*)

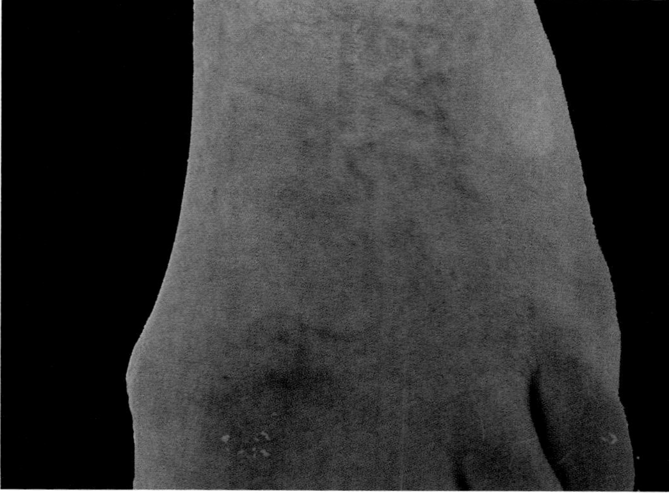

FIGURE 142-5 Long serpiginous burrow from cutaneous larva migrans on the dorsum of the foot in a young woman returning from a holiday at the beach. (*Reproduced with permission from Sandra Osswald, MD.*)

with lime on the beach and not from the sandy beach infested with larvae (see Chapter 197, Photosensitivity).

MANAGEMENT

- Oral thiabendazole was the first proven therapy with Food and Drug Administration (FDA) approval. It was removed from the market in 2010.
- Albendazole has been successfully prescribed for more than 25 years, and is the Centers for Disease Control and Prevention (CDC) drug of choice.[3,5] Albendazole lacks FDA approval for this indication.
  - The recommended dose is 400 mg daily for 3 days.[3,5] SOR B
  - Cure rates with albendazole exceed 92%, but are less with single dosage.[3]
- Ivermectin (Stromectol) has been well studied and is an appropriate alternative as per the CDC with dosing of 0.2 mg/kg daily for 1 to 2 days.[3,5] It also lacks FDA approval for this indication.
  - A single dose of ivermectin 0.2 mg/kg is also recommended.[3] SOR B
  - Cure rates of 77% to 100% with a single dose.[3]
  - Ivermectin has been used worldwide on millions with an excellent safety profile.[3]
  - Ivermectin is contraindicated in pregnancy and breast-feeding mothers.[3]
- Cryotherapy is ineffective and harmful and should be avoided.[3] SOR B

ADJUNCT THERAPY

- Antihistamines may relieve itching.
- Antibiotics may be used if secondary infection occurs.

PATIENT EDUCATION

- Wear shoes on beaches where animals are allowed.
- Keep covers on sand boxes.
- Pet owners should keep pets off the beaches, deworm pets, and dispose of feces properly.

FOLLOW-UP

Follow up if lesions persist.

PATIENT AND PROVIDER RESOURCES

- eMedicine. *Dermatology*—**http://emedicine.medscape.com/article/1108784.**
- eMedicine. *Pediatrics*—**http://emedicine.medscape.com/article/998709.**
- CDC—**http://www.cdc.gov/parasites/zoonotichookworm/health_professionals/index.html**

REFERENCES

1. Wolff K and Johnson RA. *Fitzpatrick's Color Atlas & Synopsis of Clinical Dermatology*. 6th ed. New York, NY: McGraw-Hill; 2009.
2. Bowman D, Montgomery S, Zajac A, et al. Hookworms of dogs and cats as agents of cutaneous larva migrans. *Trends Parasitol.* 2010;26(4):162-167.
3. Heukelbach J, Feldmeier H. Epidemiological and clinical characteristics of hookworm-related cutaneous larva migrans. *Lancet Infect Dis.* 2008;8(5):302-309.
4. Feldmeier H, Heukelbach J. Epidermal parasitic skin diseases: a neglected category of poverty-associated plagues. *Bull World Health Organ.* 2009;87(2):152-159.
5. Montgomery S. Cutaneous larva migrans. In: *Infectious Disease Related to Travel. CDC Yellow Book*. 2012. http://wwwnc.cdc.gov/travel/yellowbook/2012/chapter-3-infectious-diseases-related-to-travel/cutaneous-larva-migrans.htm. Accessed October 26, 2012.
6. Hotez P, Brooker S, Bethony J, et al. Hookworm infection. *N Engl J Med*. 2004;351(8):799-807.
7. Jelinek T, Maiwald H, Nothdurft H, Loscher T. Cutaneous larva migrans in travelers: synopsis of histories, symptoms and treating 98 patients. *Clin Infect Dis*. 1994;19:1062-1066.

SECTION 6 DERMATITIS/ALLERGIC

143 ATOPIC DERMATITIS

Richard P. Usatine, MD
Lindsey B. Finklea, MD

PATIENT STORY

A 41-year-old woman with asthma, allergic rhinitis, and atopic dermatitis (the atopic triad) presents with a flare-up of her atopic dermatitis (AD). Her neck is severely involved with erythema, scaling, cracking, and weeping of yellow fluid, indicating a superinfection (**Figure 143-1A**). The hands and antecubital fossae are also significantly involved **(Figure 143-1B)**. The patient is started on oral cephalexin along with topical corticosteroids. After months of trying to control her atopic dermatitis with topical steroids and other conservative measures unsuccessfully, her primary care physician refers her to dermatology. The patient tells the dermatologists that she is unable to sleep at night and the pain in her skin makes it difficult for her to care for her children. They decide to proceed with a short course of oral cyclosporine. Two days later the patient is already feeling better (**Figure 143-1C**) but it is not until 2 weeks that her skin becomes markedly improved.

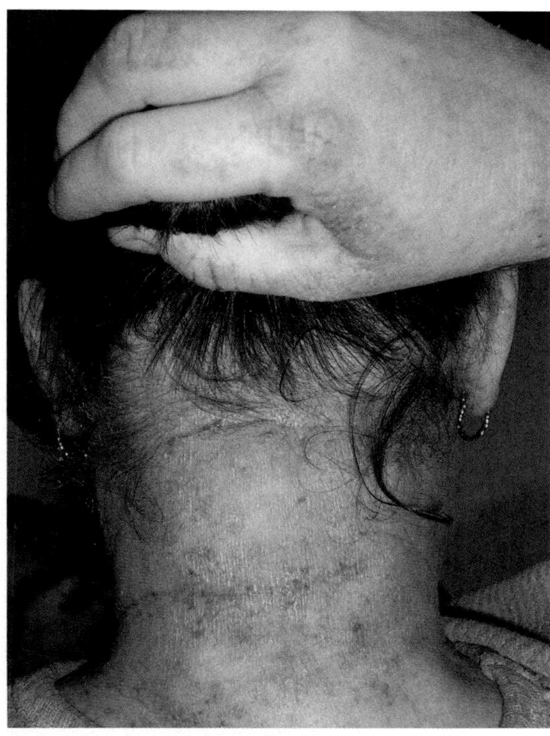

A

FIGURE 143-1 **A.** Exacerbation of atopic dermatitis (AD) on the neck and hand of this 41-year-old woman with asthma, allergic rhinitis, and AD (the atopic triad). Her neck is severely involved with erythema, scaling, cracking, and weeping of yellow fluid indicating a superinfection.

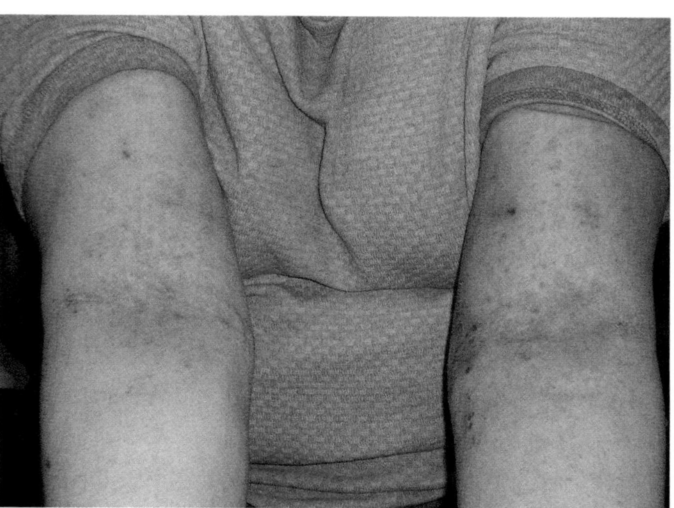

B

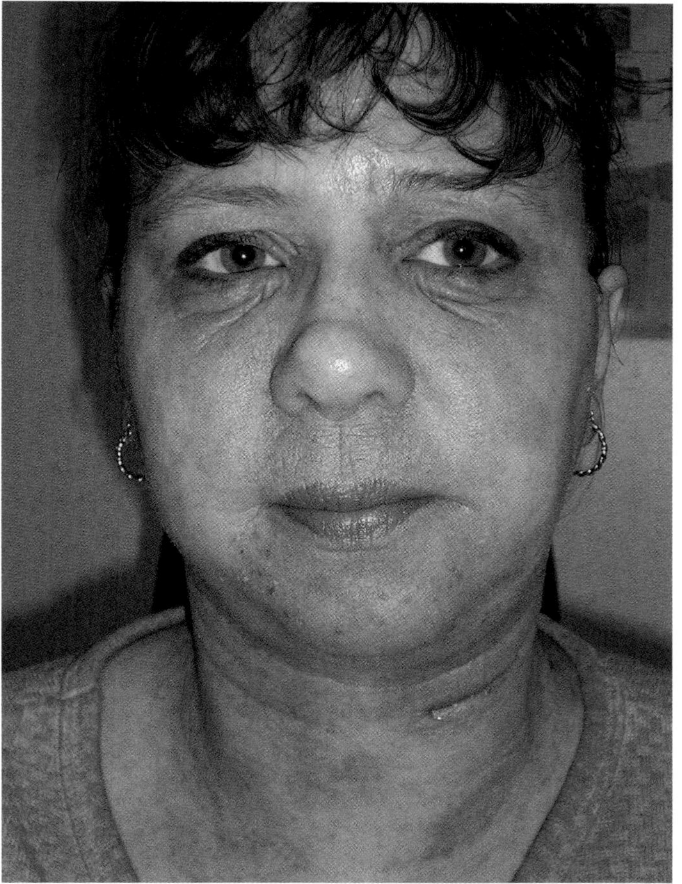

C

FIGURE 143-1 (Continued) **B.** The hands and antecubital fossae are also significantly involved. **C.** Months later she was started on oral cyclosporine by the dermatologist. This photo was taken only 2 days after the cyclosporin was started so there are no visible changes but the patient had less pruritus and could sleep at night. Her response to cyclosporine over the ensuing months was excellent. (*Reproduced with permission from Richard P. Usatine, MD.*)

INTRODUCTION

AD is a chronic and relapsing inflammatory skin disorder characterized by itching and inflamed skin that is triggered by the interplay of genetic, immunologic, and environmental factors. It can present as persistent AD that developed in childhood and has continued into adulthood, or as new adult-onset AD.

SYNONYMS

AD is also known as eczema and atopic eczema.

EPIDEMIOLOGY

- AD is the most frequent inflammatory skin disorder in the United States, affecting 10% to 20% of children and 1% to 3% of adults.[1,2]
- Ninety percent of cases begin by 5 years of age and markedly improve in 30% to 50% of patients by late childhood or early adolescence.[1,2]
- Thirty percent to 40% of cases will persist into adulthood.[1,2] Of these adult patients, 50% to 60% will develop persistent and recurrent disease.[2,3]
- Adult-onset AD typically occurs after the third decade of life.[2,4] In a recent study, adult-onset AD accounted for 8.8% of all AD subtypes.[4]
- Sixty percent of adults with AD will have children with AD.[1]

ETIOLOGY AND PATHOPHYSIOLOGY

- Strong familial tendency, especially if atopy is inherited from the maternal side.
- Associated with elevated T-helper (Th) 2 cytokine response, elevated serum immunoglobulin (Ig) E, hyperstimulatory Langerhans cells, defective cell-mediated immunity, and loss-of-function mutation in filaggrin, an epidermal barrier protein.
- Current literature has divided AD into extrinsic (IgE-allergic) and intrinsic (non-IgE-allergic) subtypes. The extrinsic subtype is associated with the atopic march and accounts the majority of adult AD patients. The intrinsic subtype affects only 5% to 15% of adult AD cases and is typified by normal IgE levels, less respiratory symptoms, and negative skin-prick tests.[5,6]
- Exotoxins of *Staphylococcus aureus* act as superantigens and stimulate activation of T cells and macrophages, worsening AD without actually showing signs of superinfection.
- *Malassezia* yeasts, which colonize adult AD skin in the head and neck region, may also trigger disease.[5]
- Sensitivity to environmental allergens, especially dust mite, affects the majority of adults with AD.[5]
- Patients may have a primary T-cell defect. This may be why they can get more severe skin infections caused by herpes simplex virus (eczema herpeticum as seen in **Figure 143-2**) or bacteria (widespread impetigo). They are also at risk of a bad reaction to the smallpox vaccine with dissemination of the attenuated virus beyond the vaccination site. Eczema vaccinatum is a potentially deadly complication of smallpox vaccination (**Figure 143-3**).

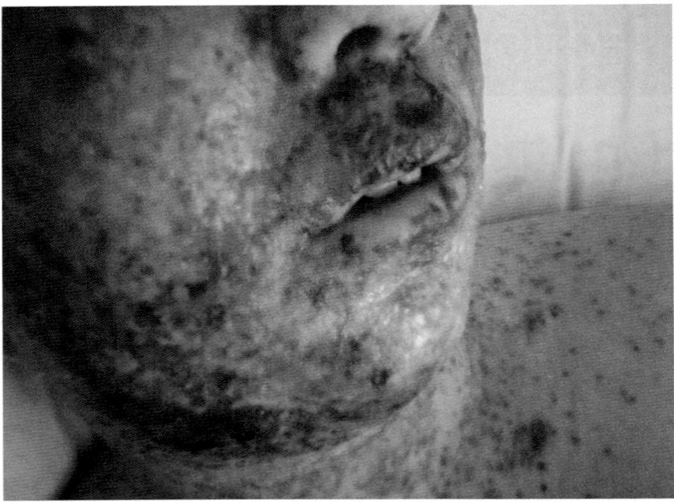

FIGURE 143-2 An 18-year-old woman with atopic dermatitis (AD) superinfected by herpes (eczema herpeticum). (*Reproduced with permission from Buccolo LS. Severe rash after dermatitis.* J Fam Pract. *2004;53(8):613-615. Reproduced with permission from Frontline Medical Communications.*)

DIAGNOSIS

- History—Pruritus is the hallmark symptom of AD. It is referred to as "the itch that rashes" as patients will often feel the need to scratch before a primary lesion appears. If it does not itch, it is not AD.
- The atopic triad is AD, allergic rhinitis, and asthma. Persons with AD often have a personal or family history of these other allergic

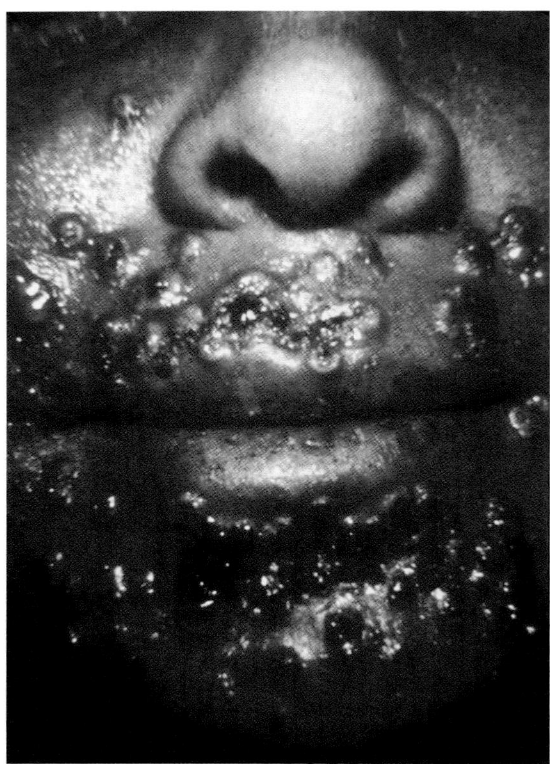

FIGURE 143-3 Eczema vaccinatum in a woman with atopic dermatitis (AD) who was given the smallpox vaccine. This eruption became this severe 8 days after her vaccination. (*Reproduced with permission from CDC and Arthur E. Kaye.*)

conditions. In a recent study, respiratory symptoms in adult AD patients occurred in 71 out of 80 patients.[2]

- Atopic persons have an exaggerated inflammatory response to factors that irritate the skin. The prevalence of allergic and irritant contact dermatitis mediated through delayed-type hypersensitivity reaction and nonimmune-mediated reaction, respectively, is increased in adults with AD.[6]
- Physical examination—Primary lesions include vesicles, scale, papules, and plaques.
- Secondary (or sequential) lesions include linear excoriations from scratching or rubbing which may result in lichenification (thickened skin with accentuation of skin lines), fissuring, and prurigo nodularis. Crust may indicate that a secondary infection has occurred. Postinflammatory hyperpigmentation and follicular hyperaccentuation (more prominent hyperkeratotic follicles) (**Figure 143-4**) may also be identified.

TYPICAL DISTRIBUTION

- AD in adult can occur anywhere, but is most common on the flexural folds (**Figures 143-5** and **143-6**), head-and-neck (**Figures 143-7 and 143-8**), wrists, hands (**Figure 143-9**) and face (**Figure 143-10**).
- Eczematous erythroderma with erythema and scaling covering all or nearly all of the body can occur and is more common in elderly AD patients.[5]
- There is a higher frequency of hand eczema in adult-onset AD. In one series, the prevalence of hand involvement in patients with active AD was 58.9%. In the same study, there was a significant trend toward an increasing prevalence of hand involvement with increasing age.[4,7]

OTHER FEATURES OR CONDITIONS ASSOCIATED WITH ATOPIC DERMATITIS

- Keratosis pilaris (**Figure 143-11**).
- Ichthyosis (**Figure 143-12**).
- Pityriasis alba (mostly in children).
- Palmar or plantar hyperlinearity.

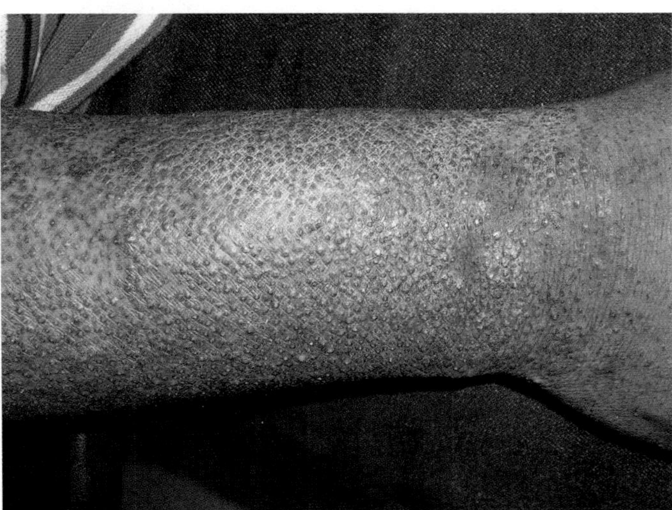

FIGURE 143-4 A black man with a flare of his atopic dermatitis (AD) showing follicular hyperaccentuation on the arms. This pattern of AD is more common in persons of color. (*Reproduced with permission from Richard P. Usatine, MD.*)

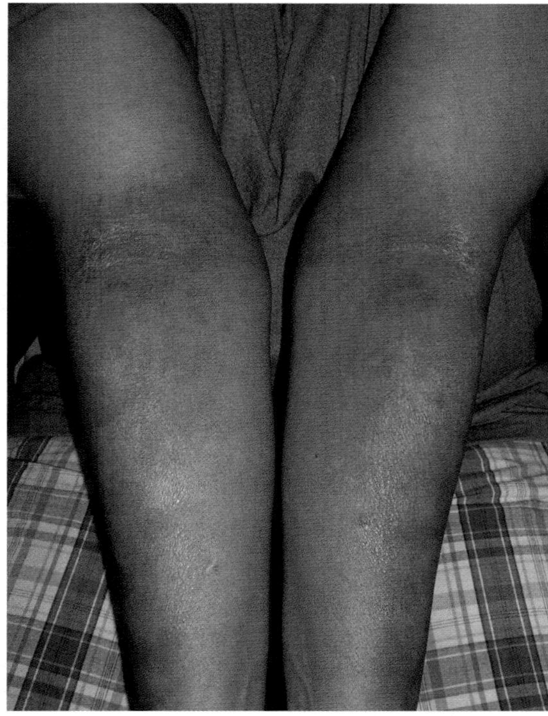

FIGURE 143-5 Atopic dermatitis (AD) in the antecubital fossae and forearms of this woman. She has had AD since childhood. (*Reproduced with permission from Richard P. Usatine, MD.*)

- Dennie-Morgan lines (infraorbital fold) (see **Figure 143-10**).
- Hand or foot dermatitis (see Chapter 145, Hand Eczema).
- Cheilitis (**Figure 143-13**) (see Chapter 29, Angular Cheilitis).
- Susceptibility to cutaneous infections (see **Figures 143-2** and **143-3**).
- Xerosis (dry skin).

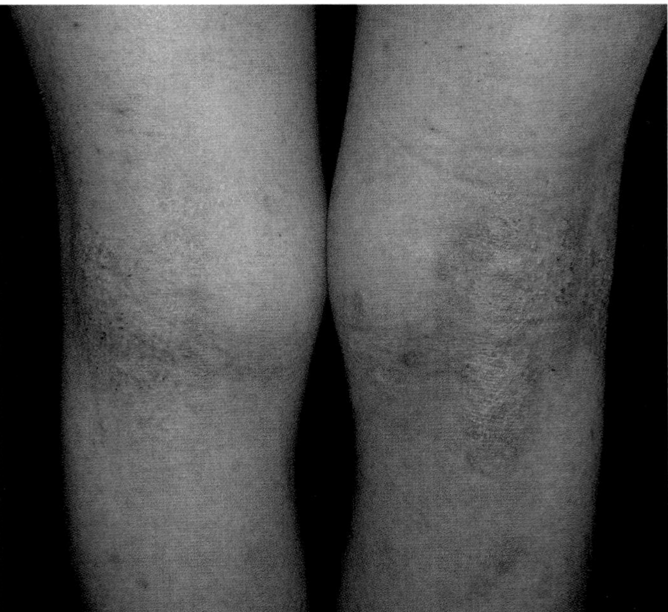

FIGURE 143-6 A 20-year-old young woman with severe chronic atopic dermatitis (AD) showing lichenification and hyperpigmentation in the popliteal fossa. (*Reproduced with permission from Richard P. Usatine, MD.*)

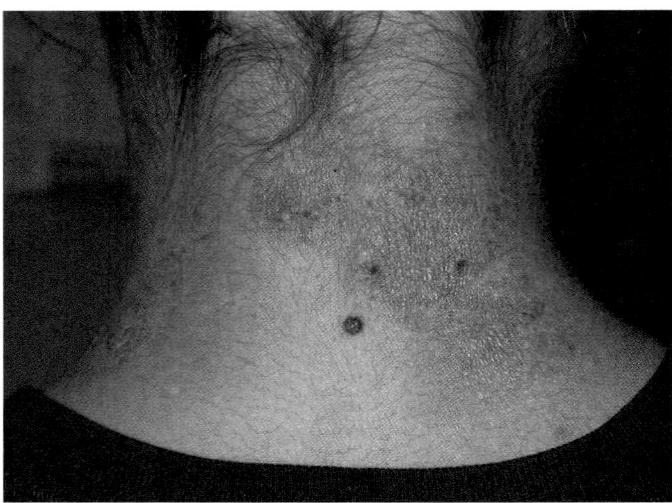

FIGURE 143-7 A young nurse with atopic dermatitis (AD) made worse by wearing the stethoscope around her neck. (*Reproduced with permission from Milgrom EC, Usatine RP, Tan RA, Spector SL.* Practical Allergy. *Philadelphia, PA: Elsevier; 2004.*)

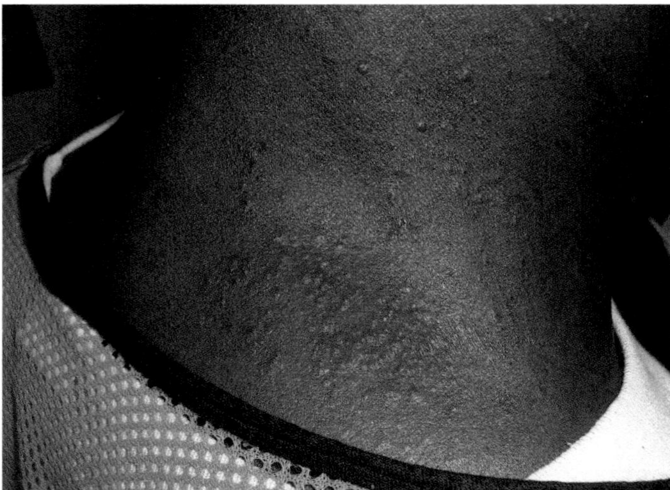

FIGURE 143-8 Black woman with flare of atopic dermatitis on the neck after fleeing hurricane Katrina. The follicular hyperaccentuation is typical in persons of color. (*Reproduced with permission from Richard P. Usatine, MD.*)

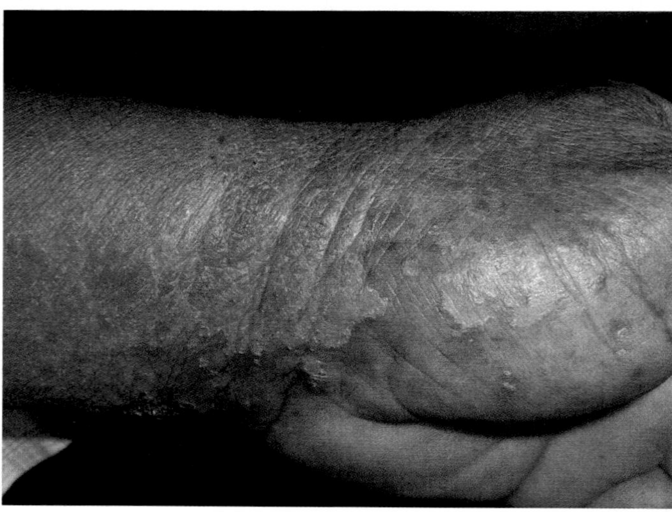

FIGURE 143-9 Atopic dermatitis on the wrists and hands of a 58-year-old man with a co-existing nickel allergy. (*Reproduced with permission from Richard P. Usatine, MD.*)

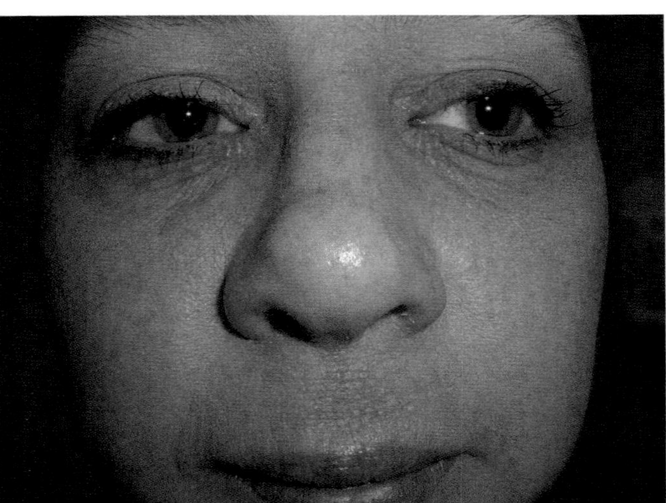

FIGURE 143-10 A young woman with chronic atopic dermatitis (AD) around her eyes and mouth. In addition to the eyelid involvement the patient has Denny Morgan lines visible on the lower eyelids. (*Reproduced with permission from Richard P. Usatine, MD.*)

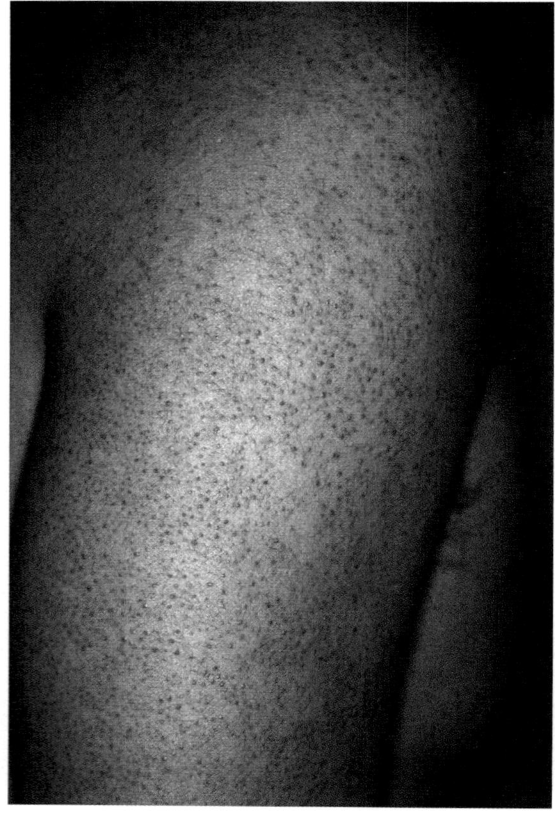

FIGURE 143-11 Keratosis pilaris on the lateral upper arm. Note how the papules can vary in color from pink to brown to white. (*Reproduced with permission from Richard P. Usatine, MD.*)

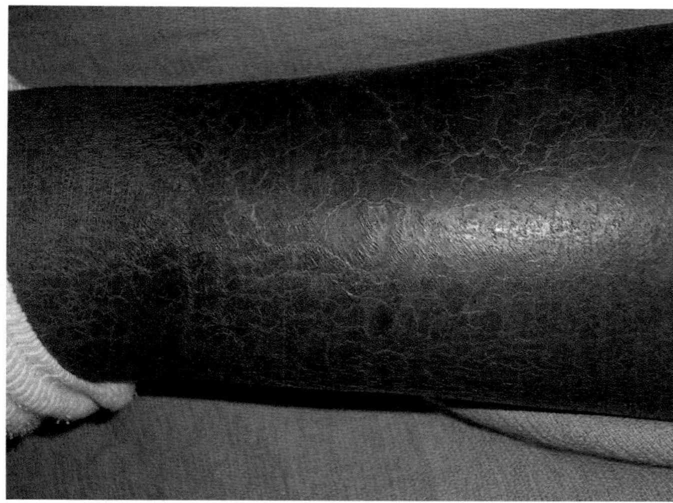

FIGURE 143-12 Acquired ichthyosis on the leg of a 55-year-old black man with atopic dermatitis (AD). Note the fish-scale appearance along with the dry skin. (*Reproduced with permission from Richard P. Usatine, MD.*)

- Eye findings—Recurrent conjunctivitis, keratoconus (**Figure 143-14**), cataracts, orbital darkening.
- A horizontal nasal crease may be seen over the bridge of the nose in a patient with allergic rhinitis prone to performing the allergic salute. In some patients this crease may become hyperpigmented (**Figure 143-15**).

LABORATORY STUDIES

Laboratory studies are rarely needed if the history and physical examination support the diagnosis. Occasionally, a potassium hydroxide (KOH) preparation for tinea or skin scraping for scabies may be needed to rule out primary or concomitant disease. Adult-onset AD that is not improving with therapy may need further investigation with skin patch testing to rule out primary or concomitant allergic contact dermatitis. Radioallergosorbent test (RAST) for food allergies, eosinophil counts, and serum IgE levels are not of proven benefit for diagnosis or management, however, IgE serum levels and eosinophil count correlate with disease severity and are potential strategies for targeted drug development.[2]

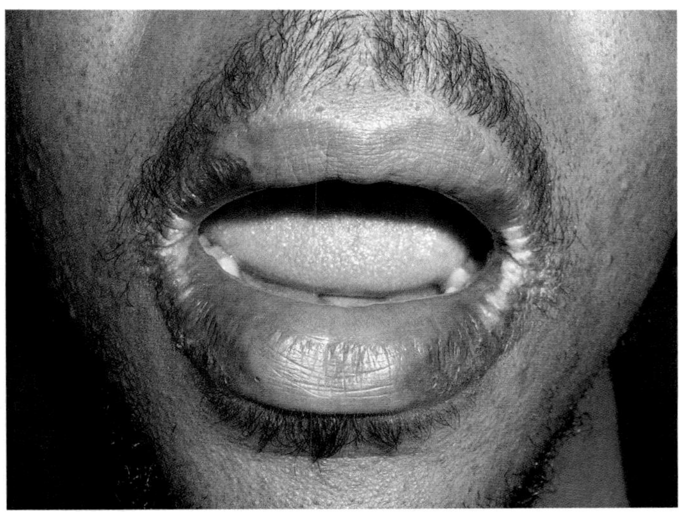

FIGURE 143-13 Atopic dermatitis (AD) with angular cheilitis and postinflammatory hyperpigmentation on the lips from rubbing secondary to pruritus. The angular cheilitis occurred during a flare of the atopic dermatitis on the arms and legs. (*Reproduced with permission from Richard P. Usatine, MD.*)

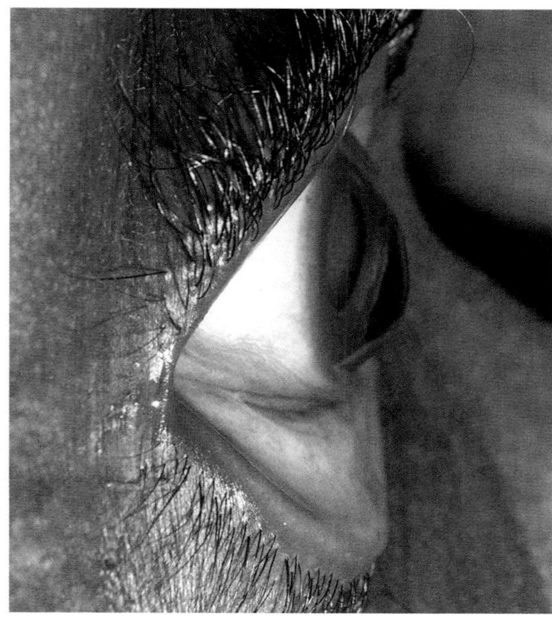

A

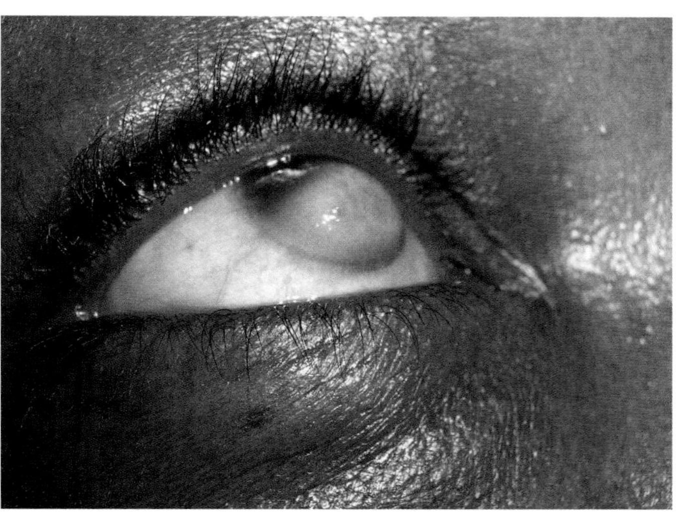

B

FIGURE 143-14 Keratoconus in a young woman with severe atopic dermatitis (AD). She admits to rubbing her eyes frequently. **A.** In keratoconus the cornea bulges out in the middle like a cone. **B.** Two years later the keratoconus led to corneal opacification. She now needs a corneal transplant. (*Reproduced with permission from Richard P. Usatine, MD.*)

DIFFERENTIAL DIAGNOSIS

- Dyshidrotic eczema—Dry inflamed scaling skin on the hands and feet with tapioca-like vesicles, especially seen between the fingers (see Chapter 145, Hand Eczema).
- Seborrheic dermatitis—Greasy, scaly lesions on scalp, face, and chest (see Chapter 149, Seborrheic Dermatitis).
- Psoriasis—Thickened plaques on extensor surfaces, scalp, and buttocks; pitted nails (see Chapter 150, Psoriasis).
- Lichen simplex chronicus (sometimes called neurodermatitis)—Usually, a single patch in an area accessible to scratching such as the

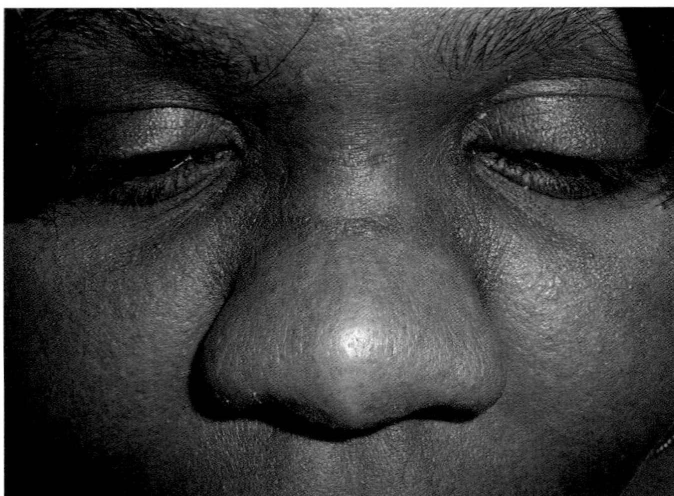

FIGURE 143-15 Hyperpigmented horizontal nasal crease in a patient with the atopic triad who repeatedly performs the allergic salute when her nose is feeling pruritic. (*Reproduced with permission from Richard P. Usatine, MD.*)

ankle, wrist, and neck (**Figure 143-16**) (see Chapter 147, Psychocutaneous Disorders).

- Contact dermatitis—Positive exposure history, rash in area of exposure; absence of family history. Patch testing may be helpful in distinguishing from contact dermatitis from AD or from diagnosing a new contact allergy in a patient with existing AD. (see Chapter 144, Contact Dermatitis).
- Scabies—Papules, burrows, finger web involvement, positive skin scraping (see Chapter 141, Scabies).
- Dermatophyte infection—On the hands or feet, can look just like hand or foot dermatitis; a positive KOH preparation for hyphae can help make the diagnosis (see Chapter 138, Tinea Pedis).

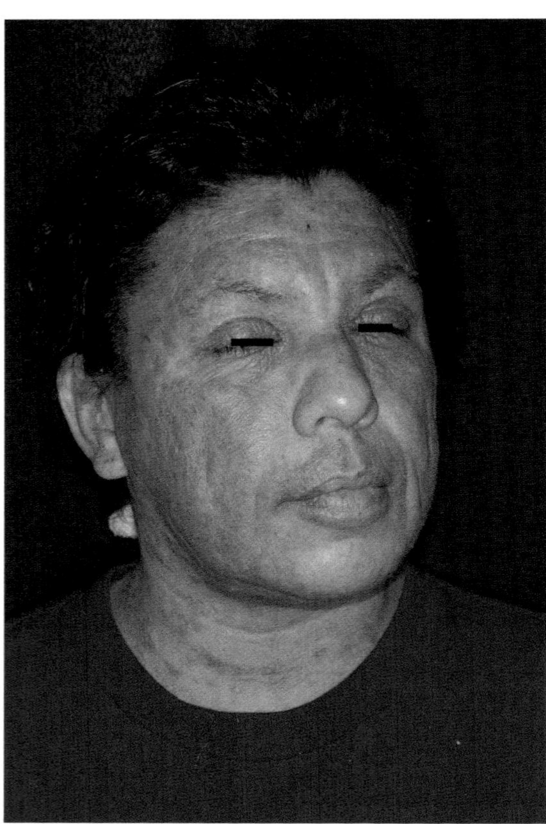

FIGURE 143-16 Atopic dermatitis (AD) since childhood in a Hispanic woman showing lichenification on the face from many years of rubbing the skin. The thickening of the skin has also affected the eyelids and caused postinflammatory hyperpigmentation. (*Reproduced with permission from Richard P. Usatine, MD.*)

MANAGEMENT

- There is some evidence suggesting that controlling house dust mites reduces severity of symptoms in patients with the atopic triad. Bedding covers were found to be the most effective method to control dust mites and AD symptoms in this subgroup of AD patients. Unfortunately, dust mite interventions are not proven to be effective for patients with AD that do not have the full atopic triad.[1] SOR Ⓑ
- There is no evidence that dietary manipulation in adults reduces symptom severity and may cause iatrogenic malnourishment. SOR Ⓑ
- Patient education, avoidance of possible triggers (enzyme-rich detergents, wool clothing), and dry skin care should be optimized.
- Dilute bleach baths (0.5 cup of 6% bleach in tub of bath water) lower the *S. aureus* burden on the skin, decreasing severity of AD in children.[8] SOR Ⓑ While there are no studies using bleach baths in adults with AD, this treatment may be worth trying in those adults willing to give it a try.

TOPICAL THERAPIES

- Topical steroids and emollients have been proven to work for AD and are the mainstay of treatment.[1] SOR Ⓐ
- Vehicle selection and steroid strength are based on age, body location, and lesion morphology. The ointments are best for dry and cracked skin and are more potent. Creams are easier to apply and are better tolerated by some patients.
- Use stronger steroids for thicker skin, severe outbreaks, or lesions that have not responded to weaker steroids. Avoid strong steroids on face, genitals, and armpits (**Figure 143-17**).
- To avoid adverse effects, the highest-potency steroids (eg, clobetasol) should not be used for longer than 2 weeks on a daily basis. However, they can be used intermittently for recurring AD in a pulse-therapy mode (eg, apply every weekend, with the use of emollients, lower-potency topical steroid or topical calcineurin inhibitor on weekdays).
- Topical calcineurin inhibitors (immunomodulators, such as pimecrolimus and tacrolimus) reduce the rash severity and symptoms in children and adults.[1] SOR Ⓐ These work by suppressing antigen-specific T-cell activation and inhibiting inflammatory cytokine release. These are steroid-sparing medications that are helpful for eyelid eczema and in other areas when steroids may thin the skin (**Figure 143-18**). The FDA states that they should not be used as first-line agents because of a possible risk of causing cancer. The American Academy of Dermatology (AAD) has released a statement that the "data does not prove that the proper topical use of pimecrolimus and tacrolimus is dangerous."
- Short-term adjunctive use of topical doxepin may aid in the reduction of pruritus.[1] SOR Ⓐ
- Topical and systemic antibiotics are used for AD that has become secondarily infected with bacteria. The most common infecting organism

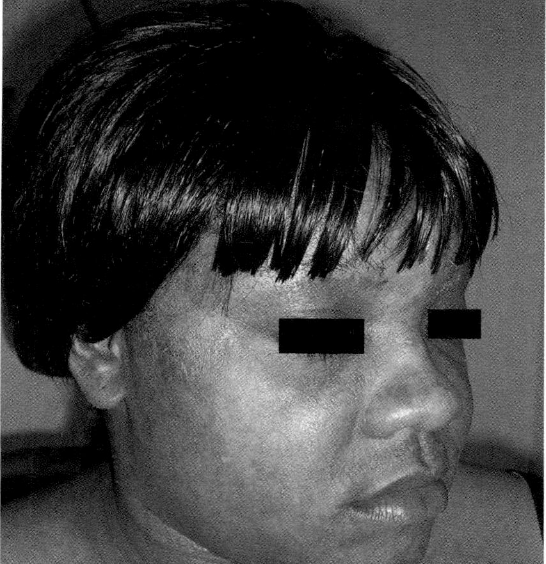

FIGURE 143-17 Severe lifelong atopic dermatitis (AD) in a 31-year-old African American woman. AD is particularly severe on the face and around the neck and has led to postinflammatory hyperpigmentation. The eyelids and perioral regions are involved with this woman who also has asthma and allergic rhinitis (atopic triad). (*Reproduced with permission from Richard P. Usatine, MD.*)

is *S. aureus*. Weeping fluid and crusting during an exacerbation should prompt consideration of antibiotic use[1] (see **Figure 143-1**). SOR Ⓐ

ORAL/SYSTEMIC THERAPIES

- For extensive flares, consider oral prednisone or an intramuscular (IM) shot of triamcinolone (40 mg in 1 mL of 40 mg/mL suspension for adults).[1] SOR Ⓒ

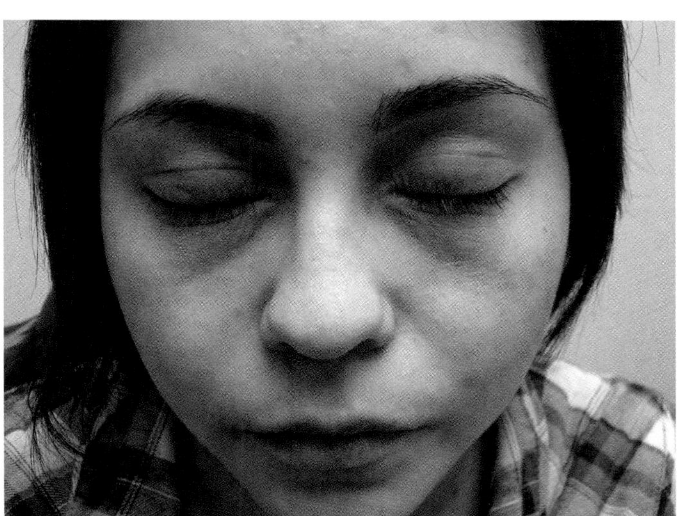

FIGURE 143-18 Atopic dermatitis (AD) involving the eyelids in this 19-year-old woman with relatively severe AD since infancy. A topical calcineurin inhibitor helped to get the eyelid eczema under control. (*Reproduced with permission from Richard P. Usatine, MD.*)

TABLE 143-1 Written Action Plan to Be Given to Patients

No skin lesions or dry skin	Prevention: Emollients, dry skin care, fragrance-free detergent, no drier sheets, once weekly bleach bath
Mild flare	Prevention plus low-mid potency topical steroid and/or calcineurin inhibitors (eg, hydrocortisone 2.5% or tacrolimus 0.1% to face, axillae, genitals; desonide 0.1% or triamcinolone 0.1% to body)
Moderate flare	Prevention plus mid-high potency topical steroids and/or calcineurin inhibitor (eg, triamcinolone under wet pajamas bid to clobetasol for short course)
Severe flare	Systemic therapy

Data from Rance F, Boguniewicz M, and Lau S,[3] and from Chisolm SS, Taylor SL, Balkrishnan R, et al.[9]

- The value of antihistamines in AD is controversial. If antihistamines are to be used, the sedating agents are most effective and can be given at night.[1] SOR Ⓑ
- Cyclosporine for severe refractory AD can be used in long-term maintenance therapy to treat and avoid relapse.[1] SOR Ⓐ Cyclosporine is approved for 1 year of lifetime therapy for skin diseases in the United States and 2 years in Europe (see **Figure 143-1**).
- Ultraviolet (UV) phototherapy may also be used in severe refractory AD with some success.[1] SOR Ⓐ
- Azathioprine, methotrexate, and mycophenolate mofetil are of possible benefit, but there is less evidence for their effectiveness.[1] SOR Ⓒ

PATIENT EDUCATION

Patients need to know that scratching their AD makes is worse. Behavior modification may involve cutting fingernails short and occluding hands/body with wraps, cotton gloves or clothing. Because of its chronicity and cyclic nature, AD patients may have poor adherence. In one recent study, overall adherence was only 32%.[9] A written action plan may improve compliance (**Table 143-1**).

FOLLOW-UP

Regular follow-up should be given to patients with chronic and difficult-to-control AD. Studies show hospitalization rates as high as 50% is adult AD patients who are uncontrolled.[2] Establishing a good regimen is crucial to good control and then visits may be adjusted to longer intervals between visits.

PATIENT RESOURCES

- American Academy of Dermatology—**www.skincarephysicians.com/eczemanet/.**
- The National Eczema Association—**www.nationaleczema.org/.**

PROVIDER RESOURCES

- Medscape. *Atopic dermatitis*—**http://emedicine.medscape.com/article/1049085-overview.**

REFERENCES

1. Hanifin JM, Cooper KD, Ho VC, et al. Guidelines of care for atopic dermatitis. *J Am Acad Dermatol.* 2004;50:391-404.
2. Orfali RL, Shimizu MM, Takaoka R, et al. Atopic dermatitis in adults: clinical and epidemiological considerations. *Rev Assoc Med Bras.* 2013 May-Jun;59(3):270-275.
3. Rance F, Boguniewicz M, Lau S. New visions for atopic eczema: an iPAC summary and future trends. *Pediatr Allergy Immunol.* 2008;19(suppl 19):17-25.
4. Ingordo V, D'Andria G, D'Andria C. Adult-onset atopic dermatitis in a patch test population. *Dermatology.* 2003;206(3):197-203.
5. Katsarou A, Armenaka M. Atopic dermatitis in older patients: particular points. *J Eur Acad Dermatol Venereol.* 2011 Jan;25(1):12-18.
6. Wüthrich B, Schmid-Grendelmeier P. The atopic eczema/dermatitis syndrome. Epidemiology, natural course, and immunology of the IgE-associated ("extrinsic") and the nonallergic ("intrinsic") AEDS. *J Investig Allergol Clin Immunol.* 2003;13(1):1-5.
7. Simpson EL. Prevalence and morphology of hand eczema in patients with atopic dermatitis. *Dermatitis.* 2006;17:123-127.
8. Huang JT, Abrams M, Tlougan B, et al. Dilute bleach baths for *Staphylococcus aureus* colonization in atopic dermatitis to decrease disease severity. *Pediatrics.* 2009;123(5):e808-e814.
9. Chisolm SS, Taylor SL, Balkrishnan R, et al. Written action plans: potential for improving outcomes in children with atopic dermatitis. *J Am Acad Dermatol.* 2008;59:677-683.

144 CONTACT DERMATITIS

Richard P. Usatine, MD

PATIENT STORY

A 38-year-old woman twisted her right ankle and applied a Chinese medicine patch to relieve the pain. The following day the patient developed a severe contact dermatitis (CD) with many small vesicles (<5 mm) and bullae (>5 mm) (**Figure 144-1**). The erythema had a well-demarcated border and was traced by the doctor's pen. Cold compresses and a high-potency topical steroid were prescribed. When the patient showed little improvement a 2-week course of oral prednisone was given starting with 60 mg daily and tapering down to 5 mg daily. The patient responded rapidly and the CD fully resolved.[1,2]

INTRODUCTION

CD is a common inflammatory skin condition characterized by erythematous and pruritic skin lesions resulting from the contact of skin with a foreign substance. Irritant contact dermatitis (ICD) is caused by the nonimmune-modulated irritation of the skin by a substance, resulting in skin changes. Allergic contact dermatitis (ACD) is a delayed-type hypersensitivity reaction in which a foreign substance comes into contact with the skin, and upon reexposure, skin changes occur.[3]

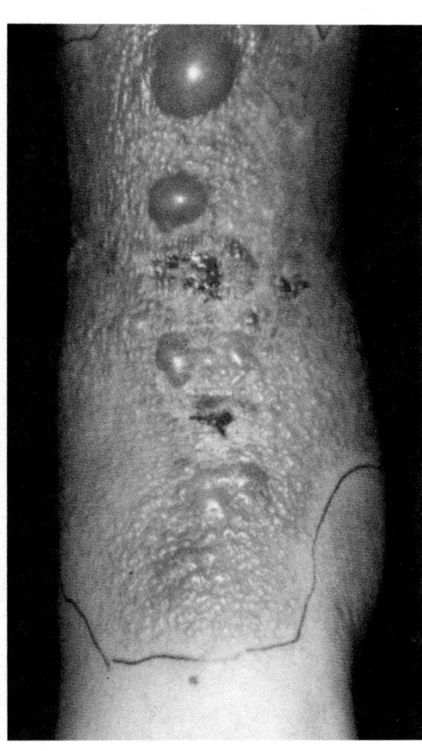

FIGURE 144-1 Severe acute allergic contact dermatitis on the ankle of a woman after application of a Chinese topical medicine for a sprained ankle. *(Reproduced with permission from Milgrom EC, Usatine RP, Tan RA, Spector SL.* Practical Allergy. *Philadelphia, PA: Elsevier, Inc; 2004.)*

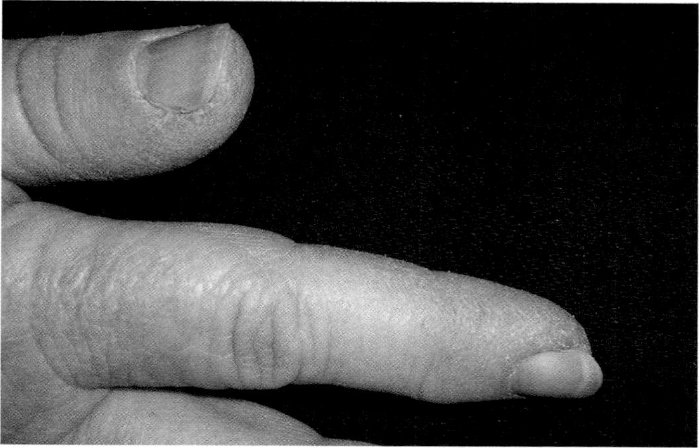

FIGURE 144-2 Occupational irritant contact dermatitis in a woman whose hands are exposed to chemicals while making cowboy hats in Texas. *(Reproduced with permission from Richard P. Usatine, MD.)*

EPIDEMIOLOGY

- Some of the most common types of CD are secondary to exposures to poison ivy, nickel, and fragrances.[4]
- Patch testing data indicate that the 5 most prevalent contact allergens out of more than 3700 known contact allergens are nickel (14.3% of patients tested), fragrance mix (14%), neomycin (11.6%), balsam of Peru (10.4%), and thimerosal (10.4%).[5]
- Occupational skin diseases (chiefly CD) rank second only to traumatic injuries as the most common type of occupational disease. Chemical irritants such as solvents and cutting fluids account for most ICD cases. Sixty percent were ACD and 32% were ICD. Hands were primarily affected in 64% of ACD and 80% of ICD[4] (**Figure 144-2**).

ETIOLOGY AND PATHOPHYSIOLOGY

- CD is a common inflammatory skin condition characterized by erythematous and pruritic skin lesions resulting from the contact of skin with a foreign substance.
- ICD is caused by the nonimmune-modulated irritation of the skin by a substance, resulting in a skin rash.
- ACD is a delayed-type hypersensitivity reaction in which a foreign substance comes into contact with the skin, and is linked to skin protein forming an antigen complex that leads to sensitization. Upon reexposure of the epidermis to the antigen, the sensitized T cells initiate an inflammatory cascade, leading to the skin changes seen in ACD.

DIAGNOSIS

HISTORY

Ask the patients about contact with known allergens (ie, nickel, fragrances, neomycin, and poison ivy/oak).

- Nickel exposure is often related to the wearing of rings, jewelry, and metal belt buckles **(Figures 144-3 to 144-5).**
- Fragrances in the forms of deodorants and perfumes (**Figure 144-6**).

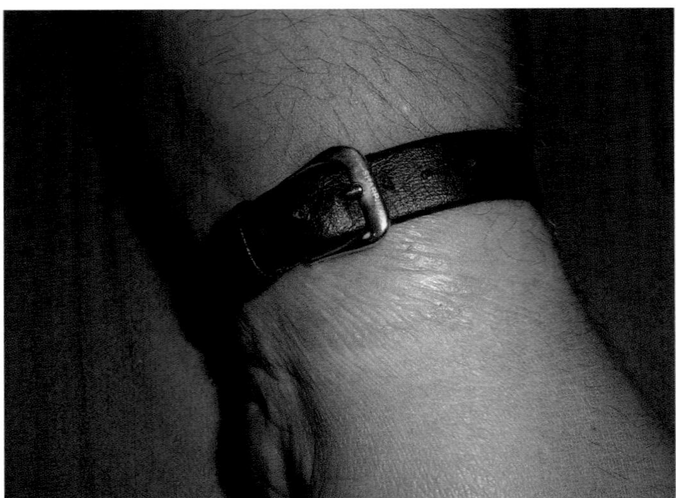

FIGURE 144-3 Allergic contact dermatitis to nickel in a cheap watch band.

- Ask about occupational exposures, especially solvents. For example, chemicals used in hat making can cause ICD on the hands (see **Figure 144-2**). Allergic contact dermatitis to cement occurs in construction workers (**Figure 144-7).**
- Neomycin applied as a triple antibiotic ointment by patients (**Figures 144-8** and **144-9).**
- Poison ivy/oak in outdoor settings. Especially ask when the distribution of the reaction is linear (**Figures 144-10** and **144-11**).
- Tapes applied to skin after cuts or surgery are frequent causes of CD (**Figure 144-12**).
- If the CD is on the feet, ask about new shoes (**Figures 144-13** and **144-14**).

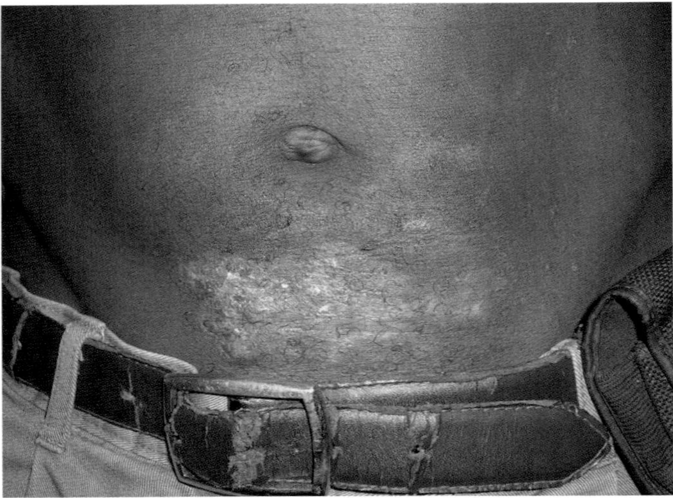

FIGURE 144-5 Allergic contact dermatitis to the metal in the belt buckle causing erythema, scaling, and hyperpigmentation. (*Reproduced with permission from Richard P. Usatine, MD.*)

A detailed history of products used on the skin may reveal a suspected allergen. In **Figure 144-15**, this truck driver was using baby wipes to clean his skin during long drives. Patch testing ultimately revealed that he was allergic to one of the ingredients in those wipes.

CLINICAL FEATURES

All types of CD have erythema. Although it is not always possible to distinguish between ICD and ACD, here are some features that might help:

- ICD
  - Location—usually the hands

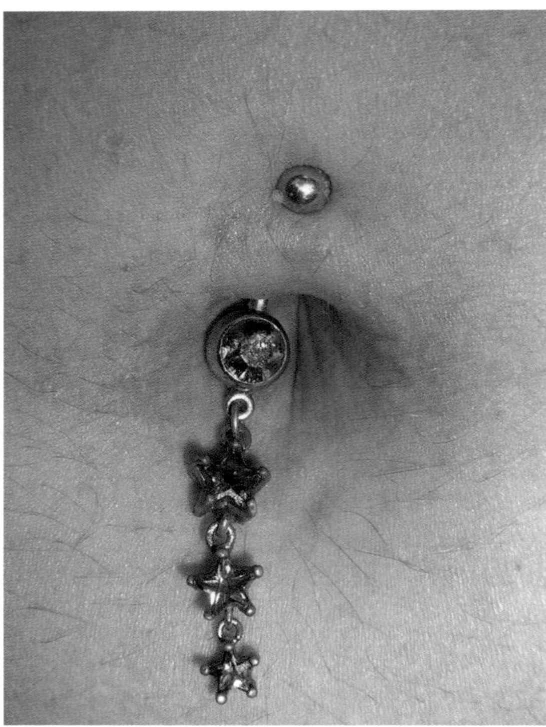

FIGURE 144-4 Allergic contact dermatitis to the metal in the bellybutton ring of a young woman. (*Reproduced with permission from Richard P. Usatine, MD.*)

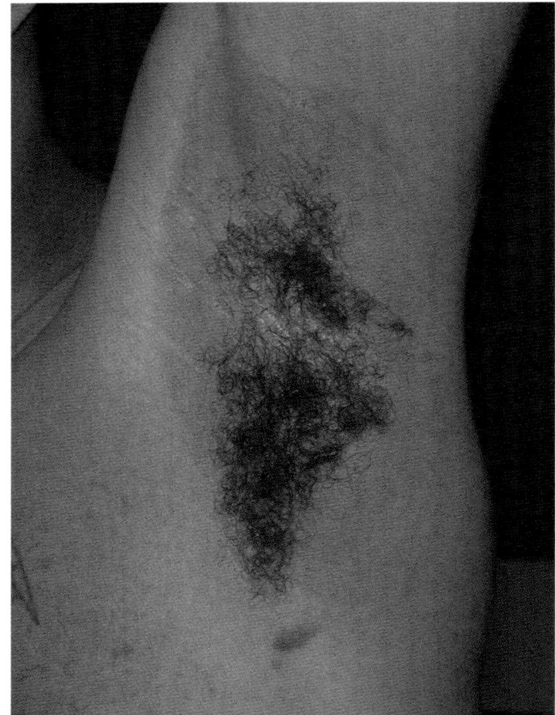

FIGURE 144-6 Allergic contact dermatitis to the fragrance in a new deodorant. (*Reproduced with permission from Milgrom EC, Usatine RP, Tan RA, Spector SL.* Practical Allergy. *Philadelphia, PA: Elsevier, Inc; 2004.*)

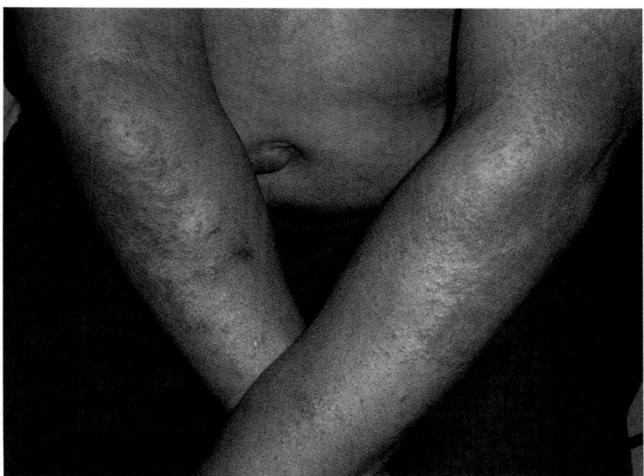

FIGURE 144-7 Allergic contact dermatitis to cement in a construction worker. Note how the reaction is strongest on the forearms where the greatest exposure occurs. The patient notes that when he wears protective clothing over the arms he is able to work with cement. (*Reproduced with permission from Richard P. Usatine, MD.*)

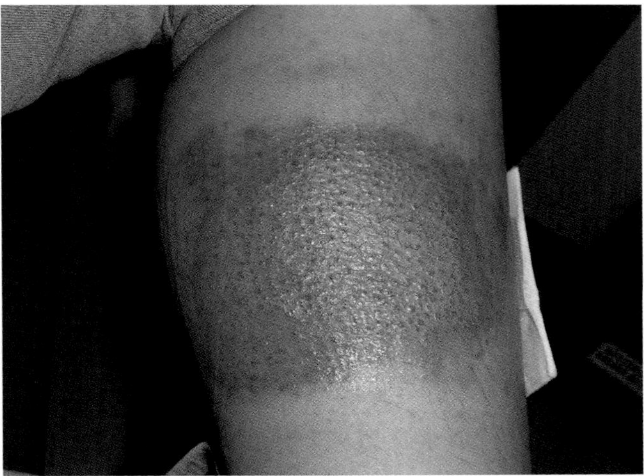

FIGURE 144-8 Allergic contact dermatitis to neomycin applied to the leg of a young woman. Her mom gave her triple antibiotic ointment to place over a bug bite with a large nonstick pad. The contact allergy follows the exact size of the pad and only occurs where the antibiotic was applied. (*Reproduced with permission from Richard P. Usatine, MD.*)

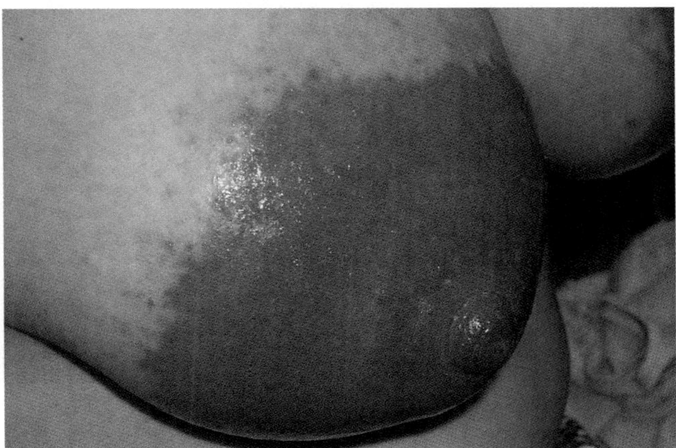

FIGURE 144-9 Allergic contact dermatitis to a neomycin containing topical antibiotic on the breasts. This woman applied this medicine to treat her breast discomfort that began when her breast-feeding baby developed thrush. (*Reproduced with permission from Jack Resneck, Sr., MD.*)

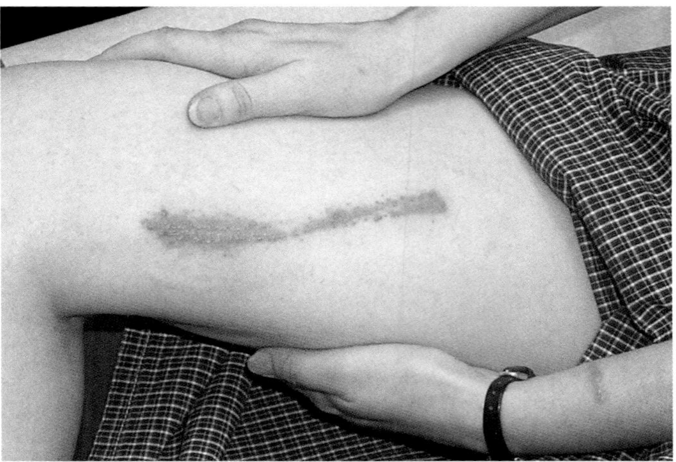

FIGURE 144-10 A linear pattern of allergic contact dermatitis from poison ivy. (*Reproduced with permission from Jack Resneck, Sr., MD.*)

  - Symptoms—burning, pruritus, pain
  - Dry and fissured skin (see **Figure 144-2**)
  - Indistinct borders
- ACD
  - Location—usually exposed area of skin, often the hands
  - Pruritus, the dominant symptom
  - Vesicles and bulla (**Figures 144-1** and **144-16**)
  - Distinct angles, lines, and borders (see **Figures 144-8** to **144-12**)

Both ICD and ACD may be complicated by bacterial superinfection showing signs of exudate, weeping, and crusts.

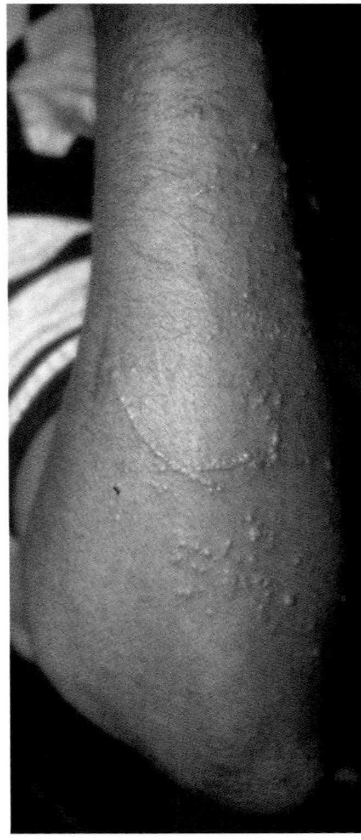

FIGURE 144-11 Multiple lines of vesicles from poison oak on the arm. (*Reproduced with permission from Milgrom EC, Usatine RP, Tan RA, Spector SL.* Practical Allergy. *Philadelphia, PA: Elsevier, Inc; 2004.*)

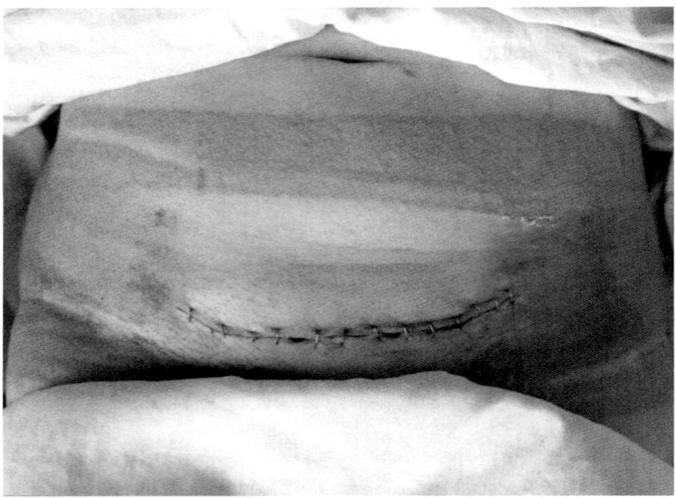

FIGURE 144-12 Allergic contact dermatitis to the tape used after an abdominal hysterectomy. (*Reproduced with permission from Milgrom EC, Usatine RP, Tan RA, Spector SL.* Practical Allergy. *Philadelphia, PA: Elsevier, Inc; 2004.*)

Toxicodendron (Rhus) dermatitis (poison ivy, poison oak, and poison sumac) is caused by urushiol, which is found in the saps of this plant family. Clinically, a line of vesicles can occur from brushing against one of the plants. Also, the linear pattern occurs from scratching oneself and dragging the oleoresin across the skin with the fingernails (see **Figures 144-10** and **144-11**).

Systemic CD is a rare form of CD seen after the systemic administration of a substance, usually a drug, to which topical sensitization has previously occurred.[6]

LABORATORY STUDIES

The diagnosis is most often made by history and physical examination. Consider culture if there are signs of superinfection and there is a concern for methicillin-resistant *Staphylococcus aureus* (MRSA). The following tests may be considered when the diagnosis is not clear.

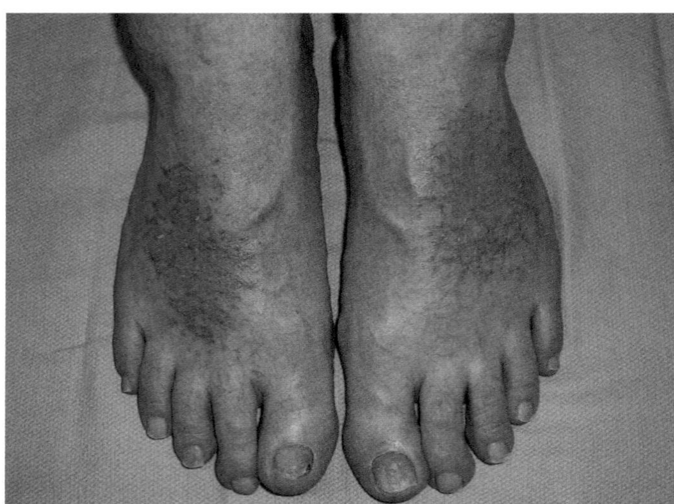

FIGURE 144-13 Allergic contact dermatitis to new shoes. This is the typical distribution found on the dorsum of the feet. Patch testing revealed that the patient was allergic to thiuram mix which is found in rubber used to make shoes. (*Reproduced with permission from Richard P. Usatine, MD.*)

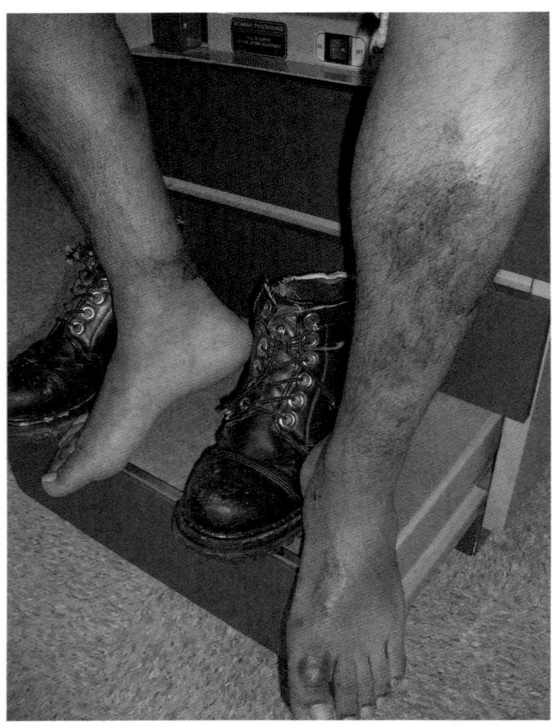

FIGURE 144-14 A 25-year-old man with allergic contact dermatitis to a chemical in his boots. His boots were higher but he cut them down to try to alleviate the discomfort coming from the boots higher on his leg. (*Reproduced with permission from Milgrom EC, Usatine RP, Tan RA, Spector SL.* Practical Allergy. *Philadelphia, PA: Elsevier, Inc; 2004.*)

- KOH preparation and/or fungal culture if tinea is suspected.
- Microscopy for scabies mites and eggs.
- Latex allergy testing—This type of reaction is neither ICD (nonimmunologic) nor ACD. The latex allergy type of reaction is a type I, or immunoglobulin (Ig)E-mediated response to the latex allergen.

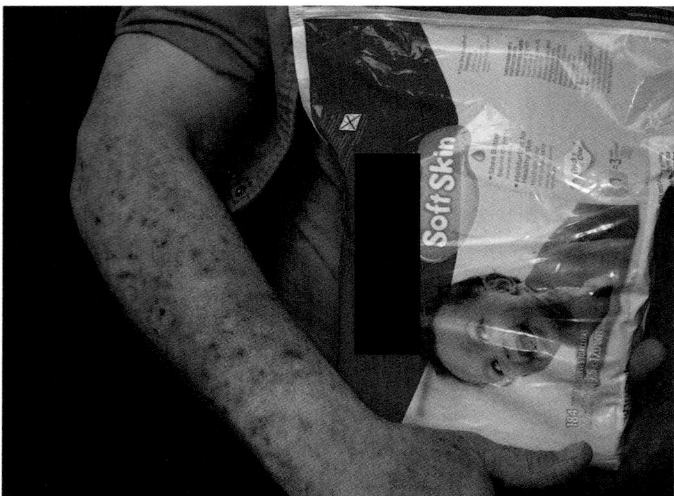

FIGURE 144-15 A 49-year-old truck driver developed pruritic erythematous eruption on his arms and trunk that persisted for 1 year despite various treatments. Patch testing ultimately revealed that he was allergic to Cl^{+} Me^{-} isothiazolinone. He went home and discovered this was one of the ingredients in the baby wipes he used to clean his skin during long drives. His allergic contact dermatitis resolved once he stopped using the wipes. (*Reproduced with permission from Richard P. Usatine, MD.*)

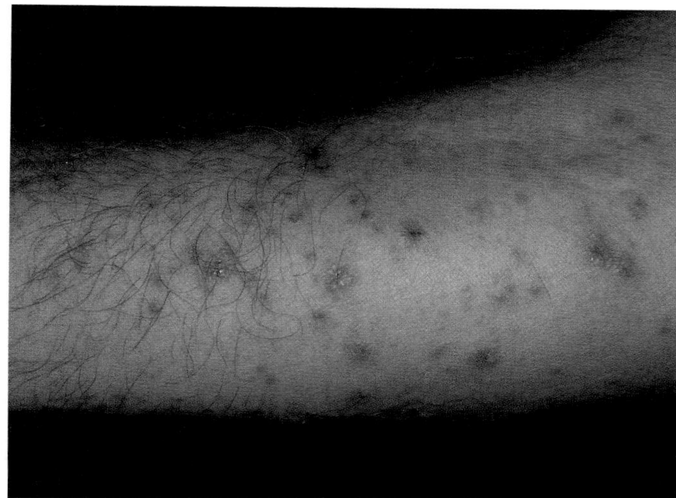

A

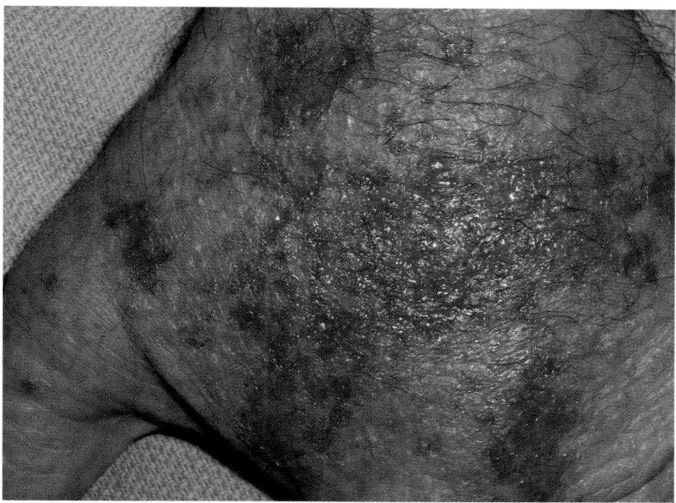

B

FIGURE 144-16 Severe acute allergic contact dermatitis in a house painter recently working with insulation. He responded rapidly to oral prednisone. Patch testing after he cleared demonstrated allergic contact dermatitis to formaldehyde found in both insulation and paint. It was not until the patch test was positive to formaldehyde and the patient read the list of substances in which formaldehyde occurs that he put together the insulation exposure and his skin rash. **A.** Vesicles on the forearm. **B.** Erosions on the dorsum of the hands where there were previous vesicles and bullae. *(Reproduced with permission from Richard P. Usatine, MD.)*

- Patch testing—Common antigens are placed on the skin of a patient. The T.R.U.E. Test comes in 3 tape strips that are easy to apply to the back (**Figure 144-17**). There is no preparation needed to test for the 35 common allergens embedded into these strips (**Table 144-1** for a list of the 35 allergens). The strips are removed in 2 days and read at that time and again in 2 more days (**Figure 144-18**). The T.R.U.E. Test website provides detailed information on how to perform the testing and how to counsel patients about the meaning of their results. Any clinician with an interest in patch testing can easily perform this service in the office.
  - A meta-analysis of the T.R.U.E. Test shows that nickel (14.7% of tested patients), thimerosal (5.0%), cobalt (4.8%), fragrance mix (3.4%), and balsam of Peru (3.0%) are the most prevalent allergens detected using this system.[5]

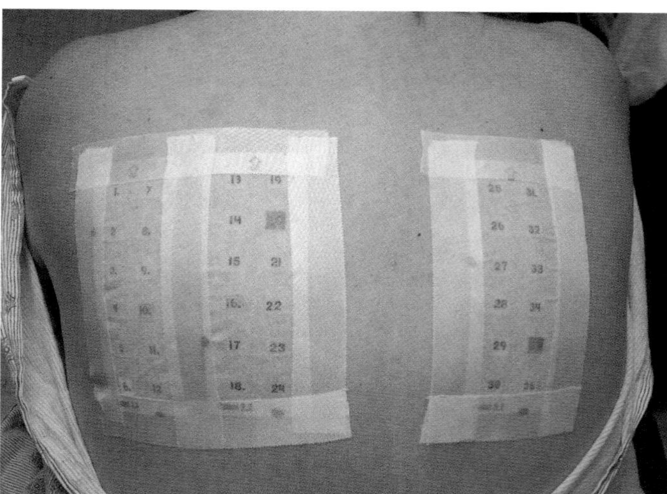

FIGURE 144-17 The T.R.U.E. Test is an easy-to-use standardized patch test that is applied to the back using 3 tape strips to test for 35 common allergens. Extra hypoallergenic tape is applied to keep the strips from peeling off for 2 days. *(Reproduced with permission from Richard P. Usatine, MD.)*

  - Critics of the T.R.U.E. Test state that it misses other important antigens. There are a number of dermatologists who create their own more extensive panels in their office. If the suspected allergen is not in the T.R.U.E. Test, refer to a specialist who will customize the patch testing. Also, personal products, such as cosmetics and lotions, can be diluted for special patch testing.
  - Once the patch test results are known, it is important to determine if the result is "relevant" to the patient's dermatitis. One method for classifying clinical relevance of a positive patch test reaction is (a) current relevance—the patient has been exposed to allergen during the current episode of dermatitis and improves when the exposure ceases; (b) past relevance—past episode of dermatitis from exposure to allergen; (c) relevance not known—not sure if exposure is current or old; (d) cross-reaction—the positive test is a result of cross-reaction with another allergen; and (e) exposed—a history of exposure but not resulting in dermatitis from that exposure, or no history of exposure but a definite positive allergic patch test.[6]
- Punch biopsy—When another underlying disorder is suspected that is best diagnosed with histology (eg, psoriasis).

DIFFERENTIAL DIAGNOSIS

- Atopic dermatitis is usually more widespread than CD. There is often a history of other atopic conditions, such as allergic rhinitis and asthma. There may be family history of allergies. However, persons with atopic dermatitis are more prone to CD (see Chapter 143, Atopic Dermatitis).
- Dyshidrotic eczema—Seen on the hands and feet with tapioca vesicles, erythema, and scale. Although this is not primarily caused by contact to allergens, various irritating substances can make it worse. It is also possible to an ACD on top of an existing case of dyshidrotic eczema. (see Chapter 145, Hand Eczema).
- Immediate IgE contact reaction (eg, latex glove allergy)—Immediate erythema, itching, and possibly systemic reaction after contact with a known (or suspected) allergen.

TABLE 144-1 Allergens in T.R.U.E. Test (Patch Test for Contact Dermatitis)

Panel 1.2	Panel 2.2	Panel 3.2
1. Nickel sulfate	13. *p*-tert-Butylphenol formaldehyde resin	25. Diazolidinyl urea
2. Wool alcohols	14. Epoxy resin	26. Quinoline mix
3. Neomycin sulfate	15. Carba mix	27. Tixocortol-21-pivalate
4. Potassium dichromate	16. Black rubber mix	28. Gold sodium thiosulfate
5. Caine mix	17. Cl^+ Me^- isothiazolinone (MCI/MI)	29. Imidazolidinyl urea
6. Fragrance mix	18. Quaternium-15	30. Budesonide
7. Colophony	19. Methyldibromo glutaronitrile	31. Hydrocortizone-17-butyrate
8. Paraben mix	20. *p*-Phenylenediamine	32. Mercaptobenzothiazole
9. Negative control	21. Formaldehyde	33. Bacitracin
10. Balsam of Peru	22. Mercapto mix	34. Parthenolide
11. Ethylenediamine dihydrochloride	23. Thimerosal	35. Disperse blue 106
12. Cobalt dichloride	24. Thiuram mix	36. 2-Bromo-2-nitropropane-1,3-diol (Bronopol)

There are 35 allergens and one negative control at number 9.

- Fungal infections—A dermatophyte infection that can closely resemble CD when it occurs on the hands and feet. Tinea pedis is usually seen between the toes, on the soles, or on the sides of the feet. CD of the feet is often on the dorsum of the foot and related to rubber or other chemicals in the shoes (see **Figures 144-13** and **144-14**; see Chapter 138, Tinea Pedis).
- Scabies on the hands can be mistaken for CD. Look for burrows and for the typical distribution of the scabies infestation to distinguish this from CD (see Chapter 141, Scabies).
- Allergies to the dyes used in tattoos can occur. Although this is not strictly a CD because the dye is injected below the skin, the allergic process is similar (**Figure 144-19**).

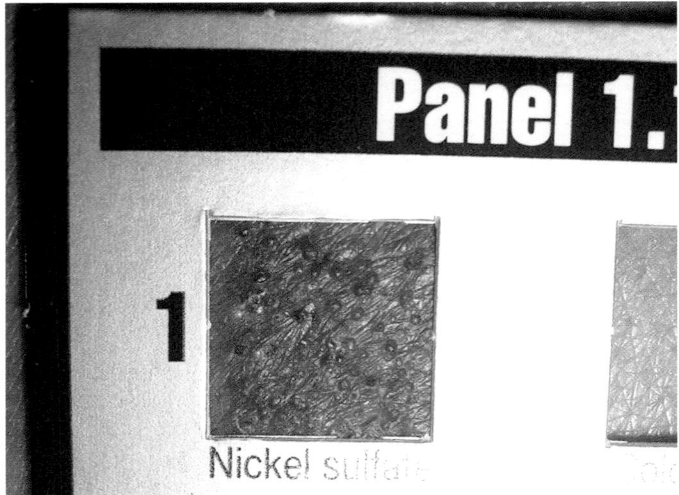

FIGURE 144-18 This positive patch test result for nickel shows small vesicles on an erythematous base. The T.R.U.E. Test reading strip is held against the skin to identify the positive antigen. (*Reproduced with permission from Richard P. Usatine, MD.*)

MANAGEMENT

- Identify and avoid the offending agent(s).[4] SOR Ⓐ
  - Be aware that some patients are actually allergic to topical steroids. This unfortunate situation can be diagnosed with patch testing.

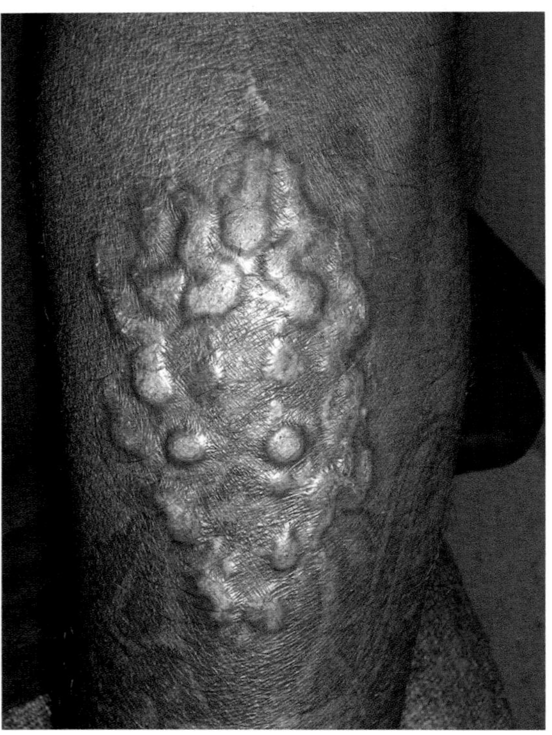

FIGURE 144-19 Man with allergy to red dye in tattoo. Everywhere that the red dye was used, the patient developed pain and swelling. (*Reproduced with permission from Richard P. Usatine, MD.*)

- In cases of nickel ACD, we recommend the patient cover the metal tab of their jeans with an iron-on patch or a few coats of clear nail polish.
- Cool compresses can soothe the symptoms of acute cases of CD.[4] SOR C
- Calamine and colloidal oatmeal baths may help to dry and soothe acute, oozing lesions.[3,4] SOR C
- Localized acute ACD lesions respond best with mid-potency to high-potency topical steroids such as 0.1% triamcinolone to 0.05% clobetasol, respectively.[4] SOR A
- On areas of thinner skin (eg, flexural surfaces, eyelids, face, anogenital region) lower-potency steroids such as desonide ointment can minimize the risk of skin atrophy.[3,4] SOR B
- There is insufficient data to support the use of topical steroids for ICD, but because it is difficult to distinguish clinically between ACD and ICD, these agents are frequently tried. SOR C
- If ACD involves extensive skin areas (>20%), systemic steroid therapy is often required and offers relief within 12 to 24 hours. The recommended dose is 0.5 to 1 mg/kg daily for 5 to 7 days, and if the patient is comfortable at that time, the dose may be reduced by 50% for the next 5 to 7 days. The rate of reduction of steroid dosage depends on factors such as severity, duration of ACD, and how effectively the allergen can be avoided.[4] SOR B
- Oral steroids should be tapered over 2 weeks because rapid discontinuance of steroids can result in rebound dermatitis. Severe poison ivy/oak is often treated with oral prednisone for 2 to 3 weeks. Avoid using a Medrol dose-pack, which has insufficient dosing and duration.[4] SOR B
- The efficacy of topical immunomodulators (tacrolimus and pimecrolimus) in ACD or ICD has not been well established.[4] However, one randomized controlled trial (RCT) did demonstrate that tacrolimus ointment is more effective than vehicle in treating chronically exposed, nickel-induced ACD.[7] SOR B
- Although antihistamines are generally not effective for pruritus associated with ACD, they are commonly used. Sedation from more soporific antihistamines may offer some degree of palliation (diphenhydramine, hydroxyzine).[4] SOR C
- Bacterial superinfection should be treated with an appropriate antibiotic that will cover *Streptococcus pyogenes* and *S. aureus*. Treat for MRSA if suspected.
- Once the diagnosis of any CD is established, emollients and moisturizers may help soothe irritated skin.[4] SOR C

For ICD and occupational CD of the hands use the following:

- Wear protective gloves when working with known allergens or potentially irritating substances such as solvents, soaps, and detergents.[6,8] SOR A
- Use cotton liners under the gloves for both comfort and the absorption of sweat. Wearing cotton glove liners can prevent the development of an impaired skin barrier function caused by prolonged wearing of occlusive gloves.[8] SOR B
  - There is insufficient evidence to promote the use of barrier creams to protect against contact with irritants.[6,8] SOR A
  - After work, conditioning creams can improve skin condition in workers with damaged skin.[8] SOR A
- Keep hands clean, dry, and well moisturized whenever possible.

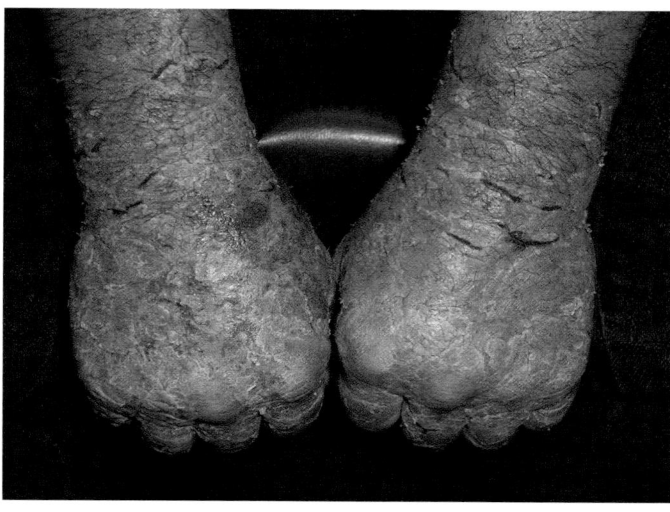

FIGURE 144-20 Severe occupational contact dermatitis to petroleum products in a man who works as a car mechanic. (*Reproduced with permission from Richard P. Usatine, MD.*)

- Petrolatum applied twice a day is a great way to moisturize dry and cracked skin without exposing the patient to new irritants.

If the CD is severe enough (**Figure 144-20**), the patient may need to change work to completely avoid the offending irritant or antigen.

FOLLOW-UP

May need frequent follow-up if the offending substance is not found, the rash does not resolve, and if patch testing will be needed.

PATIENT EDUCATION

Avoid the offending agent and take the medications as prescribed to relieve symptoms.

PATIENT RESOURCES

- PubMed Health. *Contact Dermatitis*—**http://www.ncbi.nlm.nih.gov/pubmedhealth/PMH0001872/.**
- The T.R.U.E. Test website has a wealth of information on reading labels, common allergens and patch testing for patients—**http://www.truetest.com/.**

PROVIDER RESOURCES

- American Family Physician. *Diagnosis and Management of Contact Dermatitis*—**http://www.aafp.org/afp/2010/0801/p249.html.**
- The T.R.U.E. Test website has a wealth of information on patch testing for healthcare professionals—**http://www.truetest.com/.**

REFERENCES

1. Usatine RP. A red twisted ankle. *West J Med.* 1999;171:361-362.
2. Halstater B, Usatine RP. Contact dermatitis. In: Milgrom E, Usatine RP, Tan R, Spector S, eds. *Practical Allergy*. Philadelphia, PA: Elsevier; 2004.

3. Usatine RP, Riojas M. Diagnosis and management of contact dermatitis. *Am Fam Physician.* 2010;82:249-255.

4. Beltrani VS, Bernstein IL, Cohen DE, Fonacier L. Contact dermatitis: a practice parameter. *Ann Allergy Asthma Immunol.* 2006;97:S1-S38.

5. Krob HA, Fleischer AB Jr, D'Agostino R Jr, Haverstock CL, Feldman S. Prevalence and relevance of contact dermatitis allergens: a meta-analysis of 15 years of published T.R.U.E. test data. *J Am Acad Dermatol.* 2004;51:349-353.

6. Bourke J, Coulson I, English J. Guidelines for the management of contact dermatitis: an update. *Br J Dermatol.* 2009;160:946-954.

7. Belsito D, Wilson DC, Warshaw E, et al. A prospective randomized clinical trial of 0.1% tacrolimus ointment in a model of chronic allergic contact dermatitis. *J Am Acad Dermatol.* 2006;55:40-46.

8. Nicholson PJ, Llewellyn D, English JS. Evidence-based guidelines for the prevention, identification and management of occupational contact dermatitis and urticaria. *Contact Dermatitis.* 2010;63:177-186.

145 HAND ECZEMA

Richard P. Usatine, MD

PATIENT STORY

An Asian-American physician presents with dry scaling on her hands. Frequent hand washing makes it worse and it sometimes cracks. She has allergic rhinitis and she had more widespread atopic dermatitis in her youth. This is a case of chronic atopic hand dermatitis (**Figure 145-1**). The treatment suggested was use of Cetaphil (or equivalent nonsoap cleanser) instead of soap and water. She was directed to soak her hands 3 to 5 minutes in warm water every night, apply triamcinolone 0.1% ointment, and cover with cotton gloves overnight. Her hands cleared 90% with this treatment and she was pleased with the results.

INTRODUCTION

Hand eczema refers to a wide spectrum of inflammatory skin diseases of the hands, including atopic dermatitis, contact dermatitis, pompholyx, and dyshidrotic eczema.

SYNONYMS

Hand eczema is also known as hand dermatitis, pompholyx, dyshidrotic eczema, and vesicular palmoplantar eczema. Although some people use pompholyx and dyshidrotic eczema synonymously, others reserve pompholyx for hand eczema with vesicles and bullae on the palms and dyshidrotic eczema for conditions with smaller vesicles between the fingers and toes.

EPIDEMIOLOGY

The prevalence of hand dermatitis is estimated at approximately 2% to 8.9% in the general population.[1]

ETIOLOGY AND PATHOPHYSIOLOGY

- There are many clinical variants of hand dermatitis and a number of different classification schemas. Here is one accepted classification scheme:
  1. Contact (ie, allergic and irritant) (**Figure 145-2**)
  2. Hyperkeratotic (ie, psoriasiform) (**Figure 145-3**)
  3. Frictional (**Figure 145-4**)
  4. Nummular (**Figure 145-5**)
  5. Atopic (**Figure 145-6**)
  6. Pompholyx (ie, dyshidrosis) (**Figures 145-7** and **145-8**)
  7. Chronic vesicular hand dermatitis[1] (**Figure 145-9**)
- Another way of looking at hand dermatitis is to break it down into 3 categories[2]:
  1. Endogenous—Atopic, psoriasis, pompholyx, dyshidrotic (we do not include psoriasis as a type of hand eczema in this chapter)
  2. Exogenous—Allergic and irritant contact dermatitis
  3. Infectious—Tinea, *Candida*, and/or superimposed *Staphylococcus aureus* (**Figure 145-10**)
- Most contact dermatitis of the hands is secondary to irritants such as soap, water, solvents, and other chemicals.
- Allergic contact dermatitis (ACD) is a type IV, delayed-type, cell-mediated, hypersensitivity reaction.
- The 9 most frequent allergens related to hand contact dermatitis were identified by patch testing from 1994 to 2004.[3] These are quaternium-15 (16.5%), formaldehyde (13%), nickel sulfate (12.2%), fragrance mix

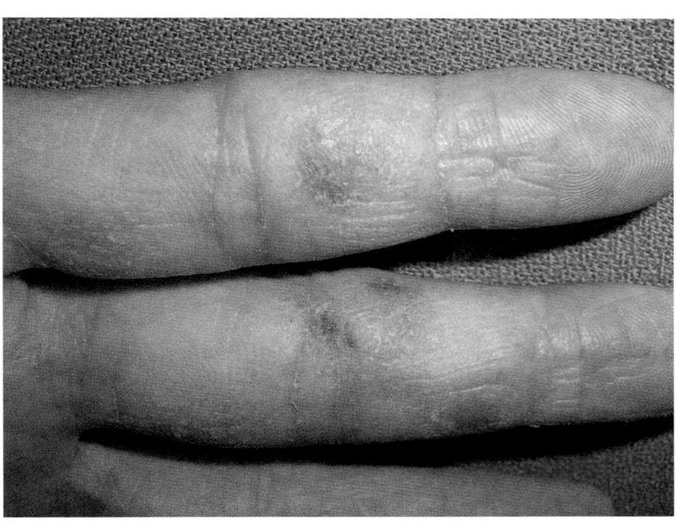

FIGURE 145-1 An Asian-American physician with chronic atopic hand dermatitis. She has allergic rhinitis and she had more widespread atopic dermatitis in her youth. (*Reproduced with permission from Richard P. Usatine, MD.*)

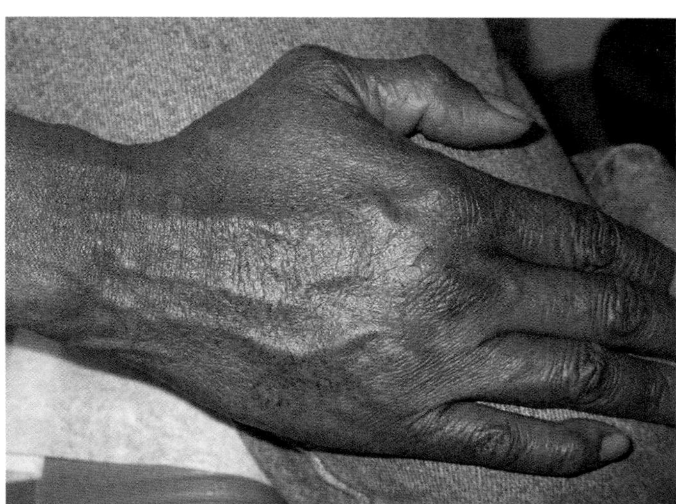

FIGURE 145-2 Contact dermatitis to fragrance mix on the dorsum of the hand secondary to using the back of the hand to apply perfume to neck. (*Reproduced with permission from Usatine RP. New rash on the right hand and neck. J Fam Pract. 2003;52(11):863-865. Reproduced with permission from Frontline Medical Communications.*)

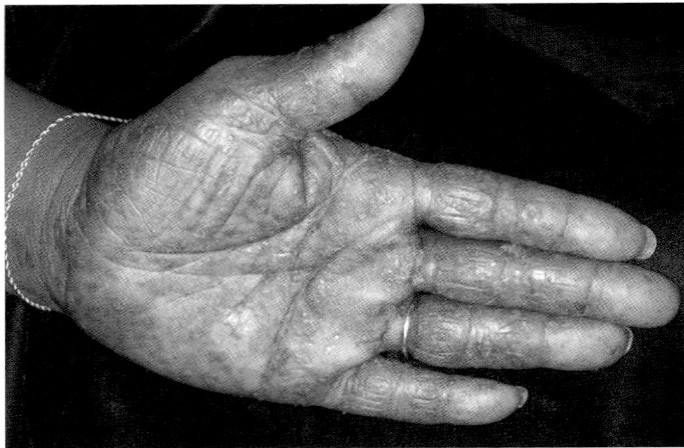

FIGURE 145-3 Hyperkeratotic hand dermatitis in a black woman. *(Reproduced with permission from Richard P. Usatine, MD.)*

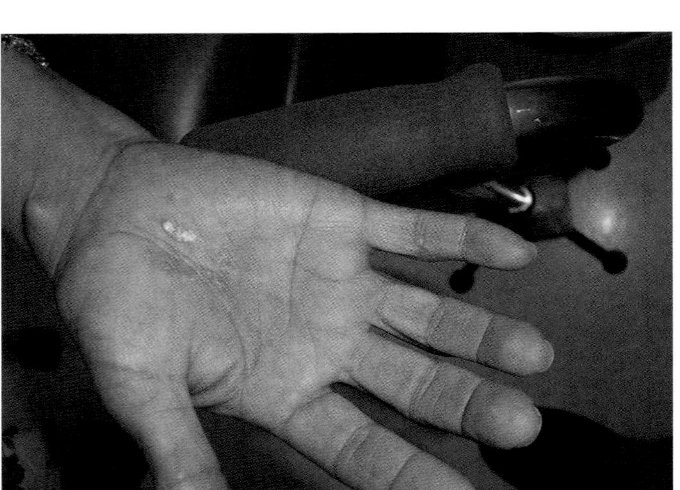

FIGURE 145-4 Frictional hand eczema that is worse on the hand that is used for the cane. The other side was affected by a stroke, so only one hand is usable for ambulating with a cane. *(Reproduced with permission from Richard P. Usatine, MD.)*

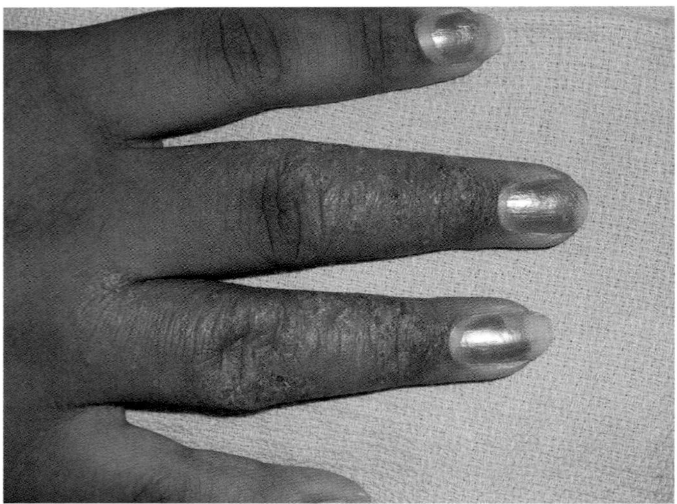

FIGURE 145-5 Nummular hand dermatitis with tiny papules, papulovesicles, and "coin-shaped" eczematous plaques on the distal fingers. *(Reproduced with permission from Richard P. Usatine, MD.)*

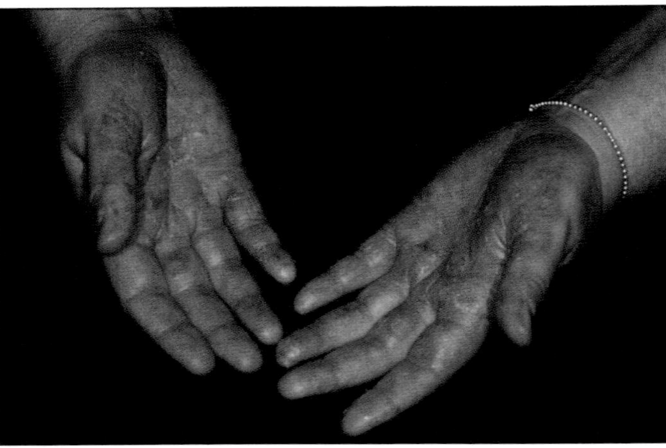

FIGURE 145-6 Atopic hand dermatitis on palms in Asian American woman with long history of atopic dermatitis. *(Reproduced with permission from Richard P. Usatine, MD. Previously published in* Practical Allergy.)

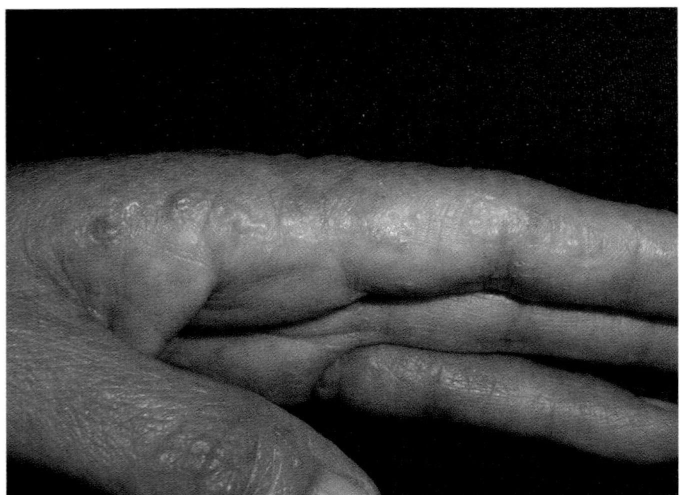

FIGURE 145-7 Dyshidrotic eczema with acute outbreak of tapioca vesicles on the sides of the fingers. *(Reproduced with permission from Richard P. Usatine, MD.)*

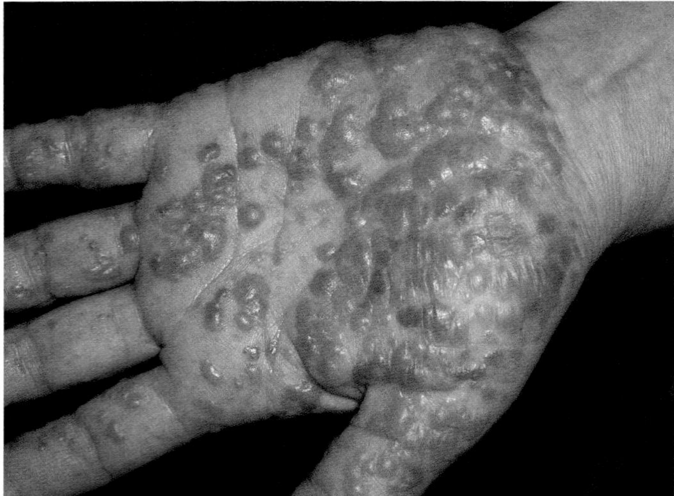

FIGURE 145-8 Severe pompholyx worsening with topical steroids. Patch testing showed she was allergic to topical steroids. Her hands finally cleared with oral cyclosporine and avoidance of all topical and oral steroids. *(Reproduced with permission from Richard P. Usatine, MD.)*

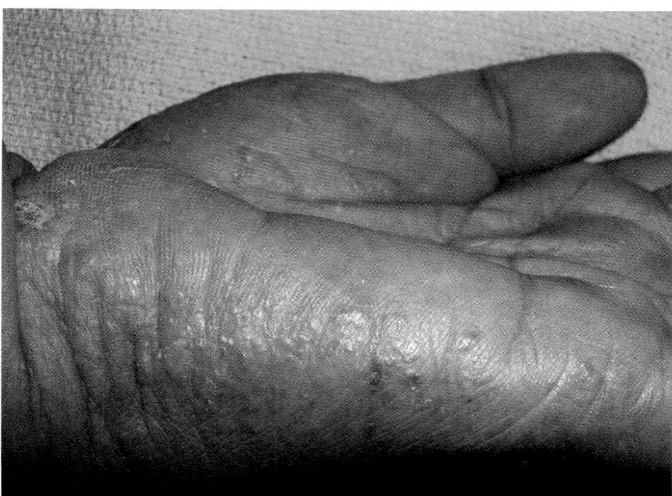

FIGURE 145-9 Chronic vesicular hand dermatitis going on for decades in this 51-year-old Hispanic woman. It is particularly bad in the hypothenar area. (*Reproduced with permission from Richard P. Usatine, MD.*)

(11.3%), thiuram mix (10.2%), balsam of Peru (9.6%), carba mix (7.8%), neomycin sulfate (7.7%), and bacitracin (7.4%).[3]

- Rubber allergens were commonly associated with occupation. One-third of patients with ACD had identifiable relevant irritants.[3]
- Most common allergens are preservatives, metals, fragrances, topical antibiotics, or rubber additives.[3]

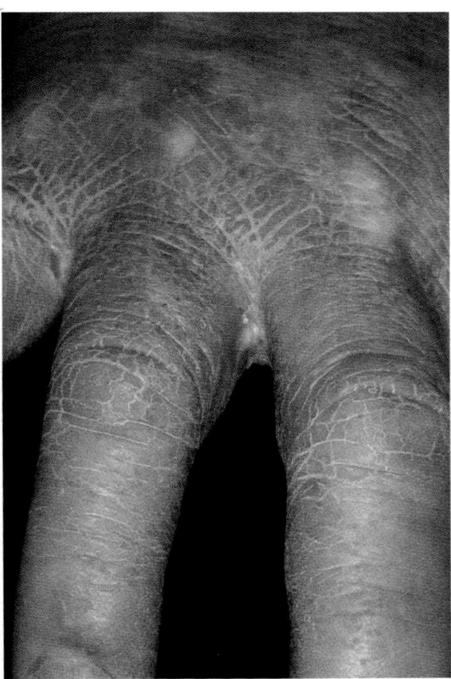

FIGURE 145-10 Contact hand dermatitis in a Chinese cook superinfected with *Candida*. See the white scale between the fingers. The *Candida* in the interdigital space is also called erosio interdigitalis blastomycetica and is seen in patients with diabetes. (*Reproduced with permission from Richard P. Usatine, MD.*)

DIAGNOSIS

CLINICAL FEATURES[1]

Contact (ie, allergic and irritant) (see **Figure 145-2**)

- Symptoms include burning, stinging, itching, and tenderness at the site of exposure to the irritant or allergen.[1]
- Acute signs include papules, vesicles, bullae, and edema.
- Weeping and crusting can occur with or without superinfection.
- Chronic signs include plaques with fissuring, hyperpigmentation, and/or lichenification.
- Irritant contact dermatitis may predispose to ACD.

Hyperkeratotic (ie, psoriasiform) (see **Figure 145-3**).

- Symmetric hyperkeratotic plaques.
- May be localized to the proximal or middle part of the palms.
- Painful fissures are common.

Frictional (see **Figure 145-4**)

- Mechanical factors, often from work, such as trauma, friction, pressure, and vibration, induce skin changes with erythema and scale.
- "Wear-and-tear dermatitis."[1]
- Can be caused by contact with paper and fabrics.

Nummular (see **Figure 145-5**)

- Nummular hand dermatitis (also called discoid hand dermatitis).
- Tiny papules, papulovesicles, or "coin-shaped" eczematous plaques.
- Dorsal hands and distal fingers are often involved.

Atopic

- Patients with childhood atopic dermatitis are predisposed to develop hand dermatitis as adults (see **Figure 145-6**).
- There is no characteristic pattern and it can occur on any part of the hand.
- Extension to or involvement of the wrist is common (**Figure 145-11**).

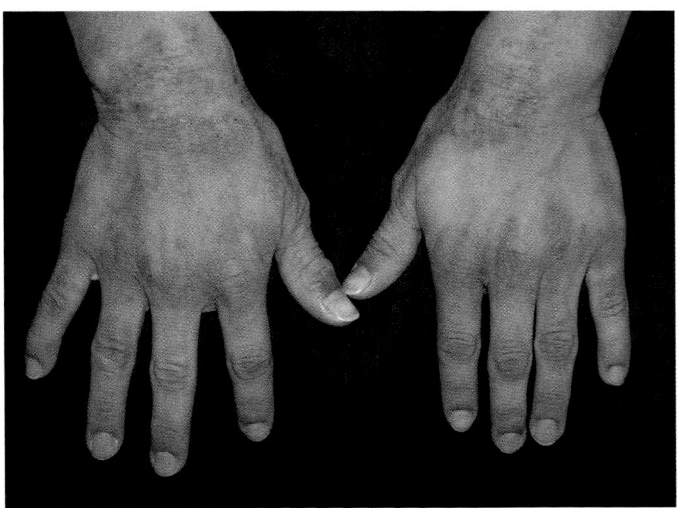

FIGURE 145-11 Hand dermatitis with prominent wrist involvement in a 20-year-old Hispanic woman with moderately severe widespread atopic dermatitis. (*Reproduced with permission from Richard P. Usatine, MD.*)

Pompholyx (ie, dyshidrosis, dyshidrotic eczema)

- Has recurrent crops of papules, vesicles, and bullae on the lateral aspects of the fingers, as well as the palms and soles, on a background of nonerythematous skin (see **Figures 145-7** and **145-8**).
- These are described as tapioca vesicles as they look like the small spheres in tapioca. The vesicles open and the skin then peels (mild desquamation).
- There may be pruritus or pain.
- Although some use the names pompholyx and dyshidrotic eczema interchangeably, others only use the name pompholyx to describe an explosive onset of large bullae, usually on the palms (see **Figure 145-8**) and dyshidrotic eczema to mainly describe chronic small tapioca vesicles on the sides of the fingers (see **Figure 145-7**).
- Both conditions may last 2 to 3 weeks and resolve, leaving normal skin, only to recur again at varying intervals.
- Both conditions are idiopathic and closely related, if not identical.
- Symptoms may be associated with exogenous factors (eg, nickel or hot weather) or endogenous factors (eg, atopy or stress).

Chronic vesicular hand dermatitis (see **Figure 145-9**)

- Chronic vesicles that are mostly palmar and pruritic.
- Differentiated from pompholyx by a more chronic course and the presence of vesicles with an erythematous base.
- The soles of the feet may also be involved.
- Poorly responsive to treatments.
- In one series, 55% of patients with this type of hand dermatitis were found to have positive patch test results.[4]

TYPICAL DISTRIBUTION

Of course, hand dermatitis is on the hands, but both hands and feet can be involved in dyshidrotic eczema and chronic vesicular hand dermatitis.

LABORATORY STUDIES

Scraping and using microscopy with potassium hydroxide (KOH) (with or without a fungal stain) to look for dermatophytes is helpful (see Chapter 134, Fungal Overview).

Patch testing can be crucial to the diagnosis and treatment of hand eczema. Patch testing is described in detail in the previous chapter (Chapter 144, Contact Dermatitis). The patient in **Figure 145-8** had severe pompholyx worsening with topical steroids. Patch testing showed she was allergic to topical steroids (**Figure 145-12**). Her hands finally cleared with oral cyclosporine and avoidance of all topical and oral steroids.

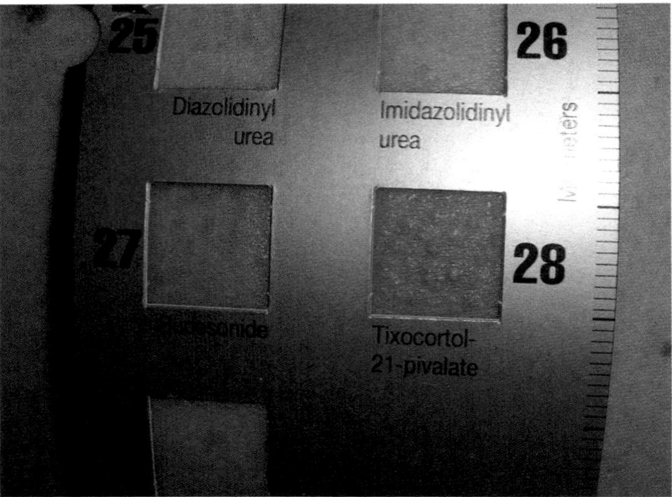

FIGURE 145-12 Patch testing positive to 2 types of topical steroids in a patient with severe pompholyx (see Figure 145-8) and topical steroid allergic contact dermatitis. Reading of T.R.U.E. Test. (*Reproduced with permission from Richard P. Usatine, MD.*)

DIFFERENTIAL DIAGNOSIS

- Tinea manus is often found as part of the 2-foot, 1-hand syndrome in which both feet have scaling tinea pedis and one hand has scale as well (**Figure 145-13**) (see Chapter 134, Fungal Overview and Chapter 138, Tinea Pedis).
- *Candida* can be seen in between the fingers with erythema and scale over the fingers and hand (see **Figure 145-10**) (see Chapter 135, Candidiasis).
- Psoriasis often involves the hand. It can present with plaques on the dorsum of hand and over the knuckles of the fingers or on the palm of the hand. Palmoplantar psoriasis will involve the hands and feet (see Chapter 150, Psoriasis).
- Knuckle pads are thickening of the skin over the knuckles. These can be accompanied by hyperpigmentation.

MANAGEMENT

- Lifestyle modifying factors, as listed in **Table 145-1**, are essential.
- Avoid irritants and "wet work" at home and at work as much as possible. SOR C
- Wear protective gloves when working with known allergens or potentially irritating substances such as solvents, soaps, and detergents.[5,6] SOR A

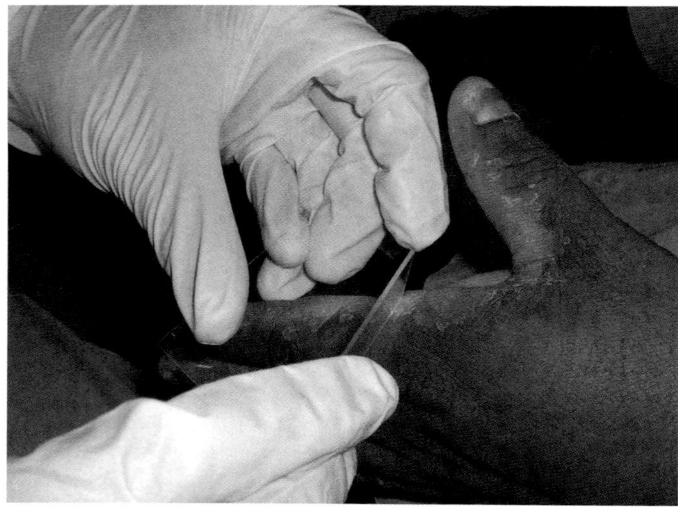

FIGURE 145-13 Tinea manus in a patient with 2-foot, 1-hand syndrome. The scraping showed hyphae under the microscope with a KOH preparation. (*Reproduced with permission from Richard P. Usatine, MD.*)

TABLE 145-1 Sample Patient Handout on Lifestyle Management of Hand Dermatitis

Hand washing and moisturizing

- Use lukewarm or cool water, and mild cleansers without perfume, coloring, or antibacterial agents, and with minimal preservatives. In general, bar soaps tend to have fewer preservatives than liquid soaps (Cetaphil or Aquanil liquid cleansers or generic equivalents are exceptions to this statement).
- Pat hands dry, especially between fingers.
- Immediately following partial drying of hands (eg, within 3 minutes), apply a generous amount of a heavy cream or ointment (not lotion); petroleum jelly, a 1-ingredient lubricant, works well.
- It is helpful to have containers of creams or ointments next to every sink in your home (next to the bed, next to the TV, in the car, and at multiple places at work).
- Moisturizing should be repeated as often as possible throughout the day, ideally 15 times per day.
- Avoid using washcloths, rubbing, scrubbing, or overuse of soap or water.

Occlusive therapy at night for intensive therapy

- Apply a generous amount of your doctor's recommended emollient or prescribed medicine on your hands.
- Then put on cotton gloves and wear overnight.

When performing "wet work"

- Wear cotton gloves under vinyl or other nonlatex gloves.
- Try not to use hot water and decrease exposure to water to less than 15 minutes at a time, if possible.
- Use running water rather than immersing hands, if possible.
- Remove rings before wet or dry work.

Wear protective gloves in cold weather and for dusty work. For frictional exposures, wear tight-fitting leather gloves (eg, riding or golfing gloves).

Avoid direct contact with the following, if possible:

- Shampoo
- Peeling fruits and vegetables, especially citrus fruits
- Polishes of all kinds
- Solvents (eg, white spirit, thinners, and turpentine)
- Hair lotions, creams, and dyes
- Detergents and strong cleansing agents
- Fragranced chemicals
- "Unknown" chemicals

Heavy-duty vinyl gloves are better than rubber, nitrile, or other synthetic gloves because vinyl is less likely to cause allergic reactions.

Data from Figure 9 in Warshaw E, Lee G, Storrs FJ. Hand dermatitis: a review of clinical features, therapeutic options, and long-term outcomes. *Am J Contact Dermat.* 2003;14:126.

- Use cotton liners under the gloves for both comfort and the absorption of sweat. Wearing cotton glove liners can prevent the development of an impaired skin barrier function caused by prolonged wearing of occlusive gloves.[5,6] SOR B

There is insufficient evidence to promote the use of barrier creams to protect against contact with irritants.[5,6] SOR A

Applying conditioning creams after work can improve skin condition in workers with damaged skin on the hands.[6] SOR A

- Avoid latex gloves because of a high risk of latex allergy among patients with hand dermatitis. SOR C
- Frequent and liberal use of emollients can help restore normal skin-barrier function. Simple, inexpensive, petrolatum-based emollients were found to be equally as effective as an emollient containing skin-related lipids in a 2-month study of 30 patients with mild-to-moderate hand dermatitis.[7] SOR B
- For patients with very dry skin that is not irritated by water, it may help to soak hands 3 to 5 minutes in warm water at night, apply triamcinolone 0.1% ointment, and cover with cotton gloves overnight. The cotton gloves may be used repeatedly even though they will soak up some of the ointment. SOR C
- Do not wash hands with soap. Use Cetaphil, a nonsoap cleanser. SOR C

See **Table 145-2** for a summary of the recommended therapeutic agents for different types of hand dermatitis.

TOPICAL AGENTS

- Topical steroids are first-line agents for inflammatory hand dermatitis. Ointments are considered more effective and contain a fewer preservatives and additives than creams. Some patients will prefer a cream vehicle, so that patient preference should be considered in prescribing

TABLE 145-2 Recommended Therapies for Hand Dermatitis Variants

	Hand Dermatitis Variant						
Therapeutic Agent	**Irritant Contact**	**Allergic Contact**	**Hyperkeratotic**	**Nummular**	**Pompholyx (Dyshidrosis)**	**Frictional**	**Chronic Vesicular**
Corticosteroids							
Topical	✓	✓		✓	✓	✓	✓
Oral		✓			✓*		✓
Cyclosporine		✓			✓		✓
Methotrexate		✓	✓		✓		✓
Mycophenolate mofetil		✓		✓	✓		✓
Tacrolimus or pimecrolimus (topical)	✓	✓		✓	✓		✓
Phototherapy (UVB, psoralen UVA, and Grenz)	✓	✓	✓	✓	✓	✓	✓
Retinoids (topical and/or oral)			✓			✓	✓
Calcipotriene (topical)			✓			✓	✓

*Acute flares.
Data from Warshaw E, Lee G, Storrs FJ. Hand dermatitis: a review of clinical features, therapeutic options, and long-term outcomes. *Am J Contact Dermat.* 2003;14:128.

topical steroids. It is better to have a patient use a cream than not use an ointment.

- Start with 0.1% triamcinolone ointment bid as it is inexpensive and effective. SOR C Cut back on use when possible to avoid skin atrophy, striae, and telangiectasias.
- Topical calcineurin inhibitors, tacrolimus, and pimecrolimus, are effective in the treatment of atopic and other allergic types of hand dermatitis.[8,9] SOR B Skin burning or an unpleasant sensation of warmth is reported by approximately 50% of patients using topical tacrolimus and 10% with pimecrolimus.[10]

PHOTOTHERAPY AND IONIZING RADIATION

- Psoralen and ultraviolet A (UVA) irradiation (PUVA) has been used to treat patients with all forms of hand dermatitis.[10] SOR C
- Grenz rays (ionizing radiation with ultrasoft X-rays or Bucky rays) usually require 200 to 400 rad (2 to 4 Grays or Gy) every 1 to 3 weeks for up to a total of 6 treatments, followed by a 6-month hiatus.[10] SOR C

SYSTEMIC STEROIDS AND IMMUNOMODULATORS

- Oral prednisone may be used to treat the most severe and recalcitrant case of hand dermatitis. Pulse dosing of 40 to 60 mg daily for 3 to 4 days may be valuable.[10] For atopic dermatitis of the hands, an injection of 40-mg triamcinolone acetonide is another option when topical meds are not fully working. SOR C
- Cyclosporine is a potent immunomodulating agent used to treat severe and recalcitrant cases of atopic dermatitis and hand dermatitis. In a systematic review, cyclosporin consistently decreased the severity of atopic dermatitis. The decrease in disease severity was greater at 2 weeks with dosages greater than or equal to 4 mg/kg. After 6 to 8 weeks the relative effectiveness was 55%.[11] For patients with severe functional problems this can be a great relief (**Figures 145-8** and **145-14**). Unfortunately, relapse rates are high after discontinuation of the cyclosporine.[10] SOR B
- Mycophenolate mofetil and methotrexate have been reported to be beneficial in case reports.[10] SOR C
- Alitretinoin (9-*cis*-retinoic acid) is an effective treatment for severe chronic hand eczema.[12] SOR B Like all systemic retinoids it is

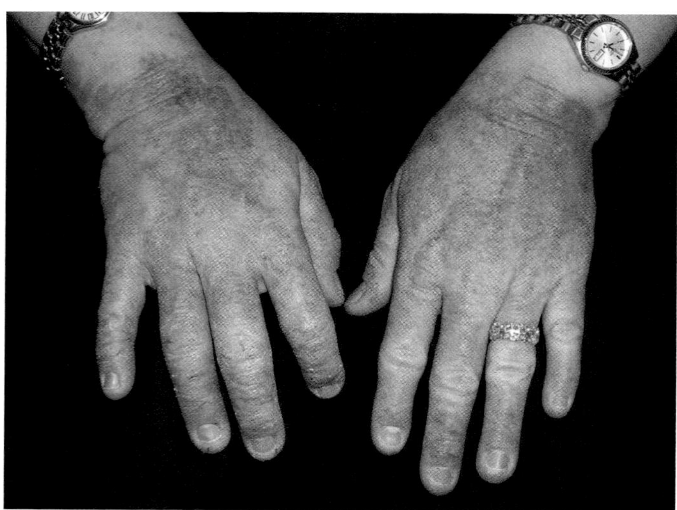

FIGURE 145-14 Severe hand dermatitis not responding to all forms of topical therapy. Patch testing was negative and the patient was started on cyclosporine to clear the dermatitis so that she may return to work. (*Reproduced with permission from Richard P. Usatine, MD.*)

teratogenic and requires careful monitoring. This medication is not yet available in the United States, but is being used in Canada and the United Kingdom.

PATIENT EDUCATION

See **Table 145-1**.

FOLLOW-UP

Patients with chronic hand dermatitis are often desperately looking for help and often appreciate frequent follow-up until the dermatitis is controlled. Patch testing requires 3 visits within a 1-week period.

PATIENT RESOURCES

- DermNet—**http://www.dermnetnz.org/dermatitis/hand-dermatitis.html.**

PROVIDER RESOURCES

- Medscape. *Dyshidrotic eczema*—**http://emedicine.medscape.com/article/1122527.**
- Medscape. *Vesicular Palmoplantar Eczema*—**http://emedicine.medscape.com/article/1124613.**

REFERENCES

1. Warshaw E, Lee G, Storrs FJ. Hand dermatitis: a review of clinical features, therapeutic options, and long-term outcomes. *Am J Contact Dermat.* 2003;14:119-137.
2. Bolognia J. *Dermatology*. St. Louis, MO: Mosby; 2003.
3. Warshaw EM, Ahmed RL, Belsito DV, et al; North American Contact Dermatitis Group. Contact dermatitis of the hands: cross-sectional analyses of North American Contact Dermatitis Group Data, 1994-2004. *J Am Acad Dermatol.* 2007;57(2):301-314.
4. Li LF, Wang J. Contact hypersensitivity in hand dermatitis. *Contact Dermatitis.* 2002;47:206-209.
5. Bourke J, Coulson I, English J. Guidelines for the management of contact dermatitis: an update. *Br J Dermatol.* 2009;160:946-954.
6. Nicholson PJ, Llewellyn D, English JS. Evidence-based guidelines for the prevention, identification and management of occupational contact dermatitis and urticaria. *Contact Dermatitis.* 2010;63:177-186.
7. Kucharekova M, Van De Kerkhof PC, Van Der Valk PG. A randomized comparison of an emollient containing skin-related lipids with a petrolatum-based emollient as adjunct in the treatment of chronic hand dermatitis. *Contact Dermatitis.* 2003;48:293-299.
8. Belsito DV, Fowler JF Jr, Marks JG Jr, et al; Multicenter Investigator Group. Pimecrolimus cream 1%: a potential new treatment for chronic hand dermatitis. *Cutis.* 2004;73(1):31-38.
9. Belsito D, Wilson DC, Warshaw E, et al. A prospective randomized clinical trial of 0.1% tacrolimus ointment in a model of chronic allergic contact dermatitis. *J Am Acad Dermatol.* 2006;55:40-46.
10. Warshaw EM. Therapeutic options for chronic hand dermatitis. *Dermatol Ther.* 2004;17:240-250.
11. Schmitt J, Schmitt N, Meurer M. Cyclosporin in the treatment of patients with atopic eczema—a systematic review and meta-analysis. *J Eur Acad Dermatol Venereol.* 2007;21:606-619.
12. Ruzicka T, Lynde CW, Jemec GBE, et al. Efficacy and safety of oral alitretinoin (9-cis retinoic acid) in patients with severe chronic hand eczema refractory to topical corticosteroids: results of a randomized, double-blind, placebo-controlled, multicentre trial. *Br J Dermatol.* 2008;158:808-817.

146 NUMMULAR ECZEMA

Yu Wah, MD
Richard P. Usatine, MD

PATIENT STORY

A 27-year-old man presents with a new rash on his legs and abdomen for 1 month. He denies ever having a rash like this before. He states that the rash itches somewhat but that he can sleep at night. He denies exposure to anyone else with similar rash and he is otherwise in good health. The physician performs a potassium hydroxide (KOH) preparation and does not find any hyphae or fungal elements. The physician also notes that the lesions are coin shaped and makes the presumptive diagnosis of nummular eczema. To increase the level of certainty a punch biopsy is performed on one of the abdominal lesions. Clobetasol ointment 0.05% is prescribed to be applied twice daily with a 2-week follow-up. In 2 weeks the patient returns and the lesions are over 90% gone. The physician explains to the patient that the biopsy confirmed the diagnosis of nummular eczema (NE) (**Figure 146-1**). The patient is directed to use the clobetasol until the lesions fully resolve.

INTRODUCTION

NE is a type of eczema characterized by circular or oval-shaped scaling plaques with well-defined borders. The term *nummular* refers to the shape of a coin (Latin for coin is *nummus*). The lesions are typically multiple and most commonly found on the dorsa of the hands, arms, and legs. It often overlaps with other clinical types of eczema: atopic dermatitis, stasis dermatitis, and asteatotic eczema.[1,2]

SYNONYMS

NE is also known as nummular dermatitis, discoid eczema, microbial eczema, and orbicular eczema.

EPIDEMIOLOGY

- Prevalence is reported to range widely from 0.1% to 9.1%.[1]
- It is slightly more common in males than in females.[1]
- Males are also affected at a later age (peak age >50 years) than females (peak age <30 years).[1]
- It is less common in children.

ETIOLOGY AND PATHOPHYSIOLOGY

Many factors have been reported in association with NE but their role in the etiology and pathogenesis is not well established.

- NE has been viewed as microbial in origin, either secondary to bacterial colonization or hematogenous spread of bacterial toxins,[1,3] but an infectious source is not identified in most cases of NE.
- NE is reported to be associated with xerosis of the skin that subsequently weakens the skin barrier function and sensitizes it to environmental allergens.[4]

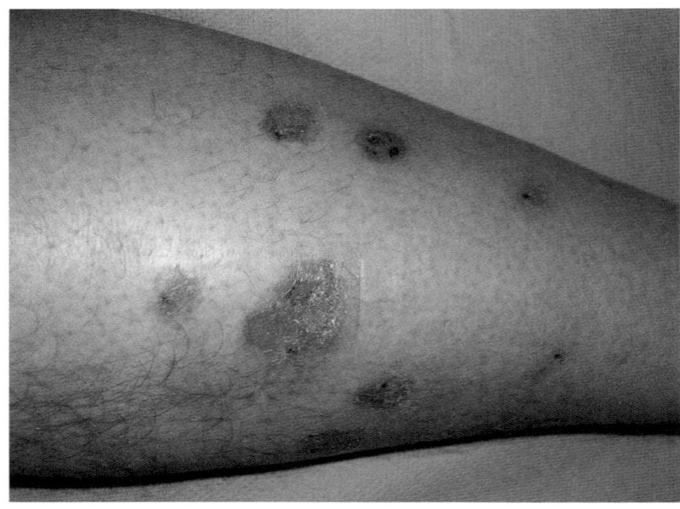

A

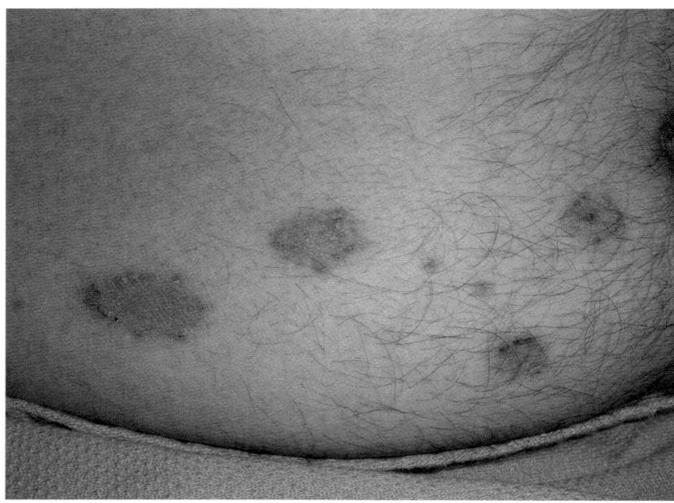

B

FIGURE 146-1 Nummular eczema in a 27-year-old man. Note how the scaling lesions are round like coins. A biopsy confirmed the diagnosis. **A.** Leg lesions. **B.** Abdominal lesions. (*Reproduced with permission from Richard P. Usatine, MD.*)

- NE is frequently reported in association with contact sensitization to various agents, including nickel, chromate, balsam of Peru, and fragrances. Allergic or chronic contact dermatitis has been frequently reported to manifest as NE on the dorsa of the hands.[1,5]
- Onset of NE has been reported in association with various medications, including interferon and ribavirin therapy for hepatitis C[6,7] and isotretinoin.[8] Most of these reports are based on single or limited number of cases.
- Mercury in the dental amalgam was reported to induce NE in 2 cases with relapsing NE.[9]

DIAGNOSIS

HISTORY

- Onset is reported to be within days to week. Simultaneous or subsequent development of multiple lesions is often reported.

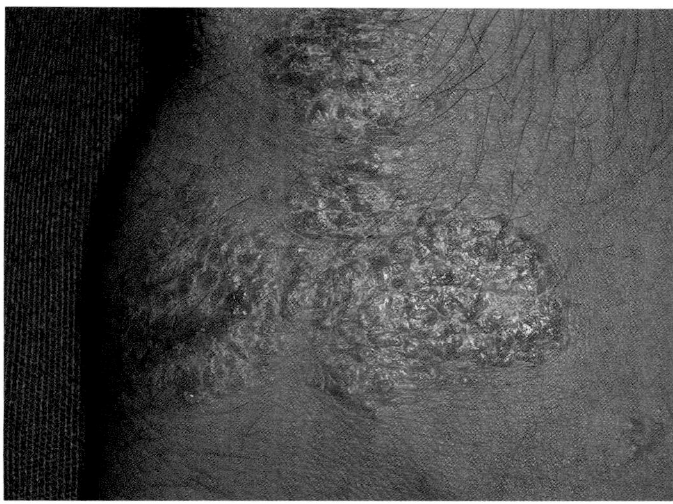

FIGURE 146-2 Multiple nummular lesions on the dorsum of the hand, a common site of nummular eczema. The lesions show multiple papules and vesicles that coalesce to form coin-shaped plaques; oozing and crusting can be seen from ruptured vesicles. (*Reproduced with permission from Richard P. Usatine, MD.*)

- Intense pruritus or burning is common.
- Lesions may last months to years without treatment and may be recurrent.
- History of medications, atopy, and exposure to allergens may be helpful to tailor the management of NE.

PHYSICAL EXAMINATION

- Primary morphology includes small papules and vesicles that coalesce to form circular to oval-shaped patches and plaques (**Figures 146-2** and **146-3**).
- Secondary morphology includes abrasion and excoriations from scratching (see **Figure 146-1**), weeping and crusting after the vesicles leak (**Figures 146-2** to **146-4**), and scaling and lichenification in more chronic lesions (**Figures 146-5** and **146-6**). Excessive weeping and crusting may indicate secondary bacterial infection.

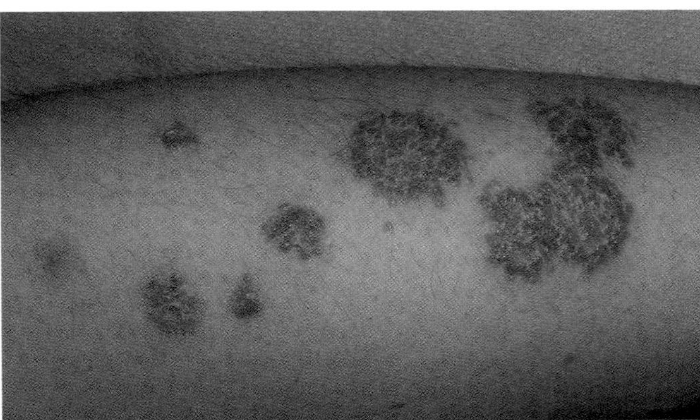

FIGURE 146-3 Nummular eczema on the forearm of a 22-year-old man. The lesions show multiple papules and vesicles that coalesce to form coin-shaped plaques; oozing and crusting can be seen from ruptured vesicles. (*Reproduced with permission from Richard P. Usatine, MD.*)

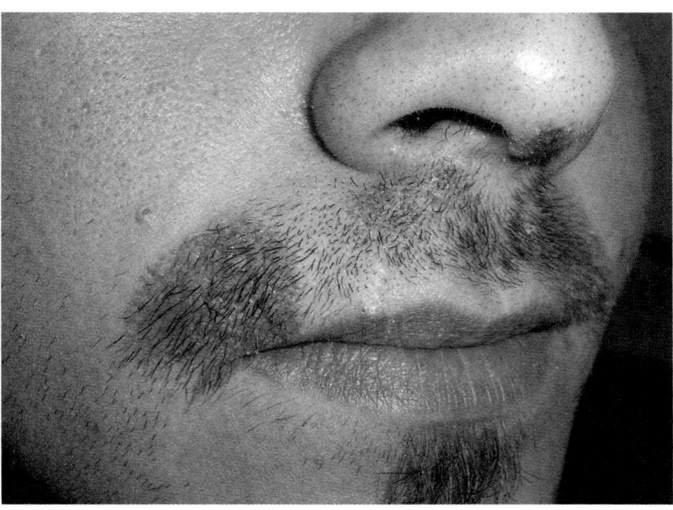

FIGURE 146-4 Nummular eczema on the face of a young man. (*Reproduced with permission from Richard P. Usatine, MD.*)

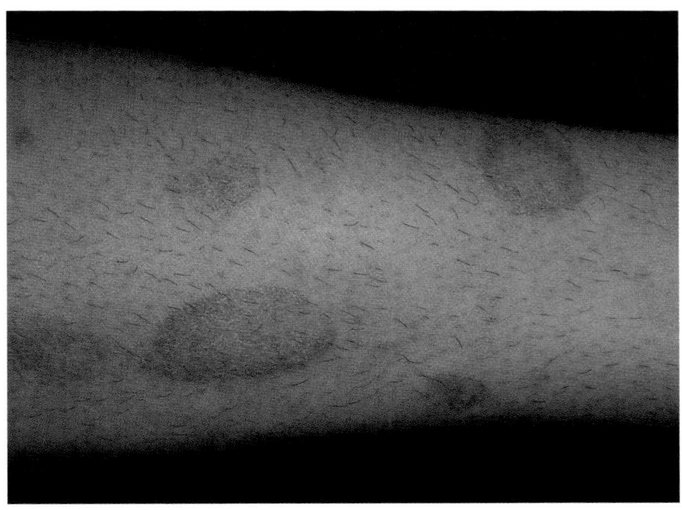

FIGURE 146-5 Multiple nummular lesions on the lower leg. Lesions of nummular eczema can be dry and scaly. The lesions prevented the patient from shaving her legs. (*Reproduced with permission from Richard P. Usatine, MD.*)

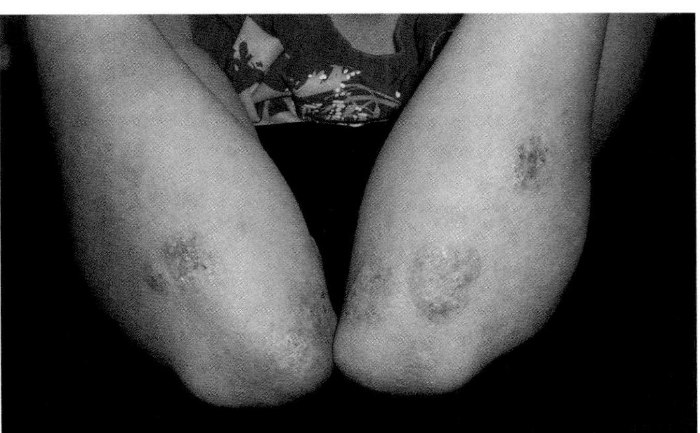

FIGURE 146-6 Nummular eczema on the extensor surface of the forearms and elbows. Thickened, scaly lesions resemble psoriatic plaques. A biopsy was performed to confirm the diagnosis of nummular eczema. (*Reproduced with permission from Richard P. Usatine, MD.*)

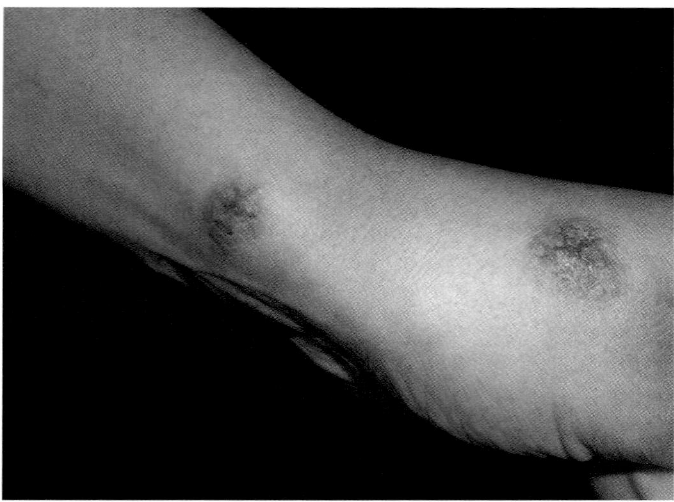

FIGURE 146-7 Nummular eczema on the dorsum of the hand and wrist. *(Reproduced with permission from Richard P. Usatine, MD.)*

TYPICAL DISTRIBUTION

Dorsal hand is most commonly affected (**Figures 146-2** and **146-7**). The extensor aspects of the forearm (see **Figures 146-3** and **146-6**) and the lower leg (see **Figure 146-5**), the thighs (see **Figure 146-1**), and the flanks are frequently involved, but NE may be seen in any part of the body (**Figures 146-1B, 146-4**, and **146-8**).

LABORATORY TESTING

- Diagnosis in most cases is made from clinical features.
- KOH preparation is helpful to investigate for tinea corporis.
- Patch testing may be considered if contact allergy is suspected.

BIOPSY

- Biopsy is rarely needed, but should be performed if there is suspicion of other serious clinical entities (eg, mycosis fungoides, psoriasis) or if the diagnosis is uncertain.

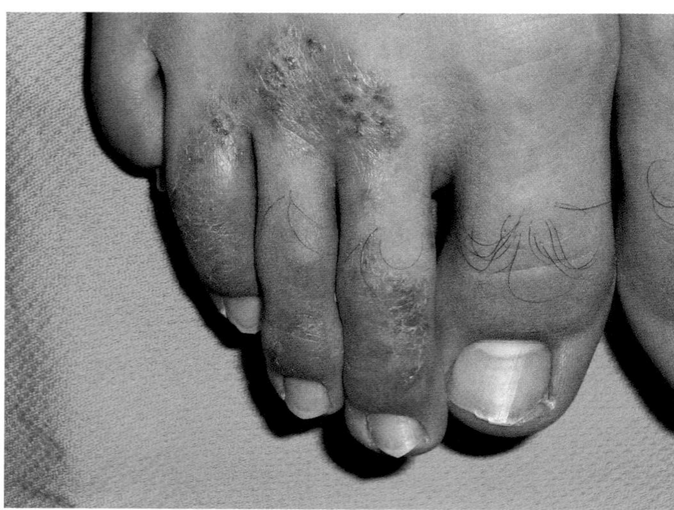

FIGURE 146-8 Nummular eczema on the dorsum of the foot. Contact dermatitis and tinea pedis were also in the differential diagnosis but the KOH prep was negative and there was no known history of a contact allergen. *(Reproduced with permission from Richard P. Usatine, MD.)*

DIFFERENTIAL DIAGNOSIS

- Tinea corporis may present as pruritic annular lesions with scales and vesicles. Vesicles are typically at the periphery of the lesion compared to NE, where they are also seen in the center. A positive KOH preparation for hyphae can help with the diagnosis (see Chapter 136, Tinea Corporis).
- Psoriasis typically presents with thickened plaques on the extensor surfaces of arms and legs, scalp, and sacral areas. Nail changes may be present (see Chapter 150, Psoriasis).
- Lichen simplex chronicus usually presents as a single plaque in an area easily accessible to scratching such as the ankle, wrist, and neck (see Chapter 147, Psychocutaneous Disorders).
- Mycosis fungoides is a type of cutaneous T-cell lymphoma, which may present with scaly patches or plaques that are often pruritic and usually erythematous. A biopsy can help make the diagnosis (see Chapter 174, Cutaneous T-cell Lymphoma).
- Nummular lesions of atopic dermatitis may have features similar to NE. Presence of other lesions typically on flexural surfaces, and a history of atopy, asthma, or seasonal allergies may help make the diagnosis (see Chapter 143, Atopic Dermatitis).
- Contact dermatitis (CD) may present with nummular lesions. History of exposure to contact allergens at the affected areas can raise the suspicion for CD. Patch testing may be used to confirm the clinical suspicion (see Chapter 144, Contact Dermatitis).
- Asteatotic dermatitis may have overlapping features with NE but has a less well-defined margin.

MANAGEMENT

- Emollients are beneficial to help restore and maintain normal skin barrier function. SOR Ⓒ
- Hydration by bathing before bedtime followed by ointment application to wet skin is reported as an effective method of skin care in patients with eczema.[10] SOR Ⓑ
- A medium- to high-potency topical corticosteroid ointment is the first line of treatment. A cream preparation may be used if patient compliance is a concern with ointments. SOR Ⓒ
- Topical calcineurin inhibitors such as topical tacrolimus and pimecrolimus have the benefit of not causing skin atrophy and have been shown to be effective in many types of eczema.[1] SOR Ⓑ They have a higher cost compared to topical corticosteroids and have a black box warning because of a reported risk of malignancies.
- Short courses of systemic corticosteroids may be necessary in severe or acute cases. SOR Ⓒ
- Methotrexate is reported to be safe, effective, and well-tolerated in treatment of moderate-to-severe childhood NE.[11] This was reported in a case series of 25 pediatric patients with refractory NE treated with 5 or 10 mg of methotrexate per week. Sixty-four percent had total clearance after an average of 10.5 months. No serious adverse events were observed in this study.[11] SOR Ⓑ
- Phototherapy may be used in generalized, severe, or refractory cases.[1,2] Narrow-band ultraviolet B (UVB) is commonly used and psoralen UVA has been used in more severe cases.[2] SOR Ⓒ

- Topical and oral antihistamines are often needed to treat pruritus. Topical doxepin is reported to be effective in treatment of pruritus associated with eczematous conditions and has a favorable safety profile.[12] SOR Ⓑ
- Topical and systemic antibiotics may be needed to treat secondary or associated bacterial infection. SOR Ⓒ
- Complementary therapy with probiotics is not effective in treatment of eczema and carries a small risk of adverse events.[13] SOR Ⓐ

FOLLOW-UP

Regular follow-up is needed for the patient with chronic, refractory, or relapsing nummular dermatitis until remission or resolution is achieved.

PATIENT EDUCATION

Hydration and protection of skin from irritants is important. Apply moisturizer or topical medications immediately after bathing while the skin is still moist. Avoid strong soaps and use mild fragrance-free soap, or soap alternatives. Avoid tight clothing and fabrics that irritate the skin.

PATIENT RESOURCES

- American Academy of Dermatology. *Nummular Dermatitis*—**http://www.aad.org/skin-conditions/dermatology-a-to-z/nummular-dermatitis.**
- British Association of Dermatologists. *Discoid Eczema*—**http://www.bad.org.uk/site/811/Default.aspx.**

PROVIDER RESOURCES

- Medscape. *Nummular Dermatitis*—**http://emedicine.medscape.com/article/1123605.**

REFERENCES

1. Bolognia J. *Dermatology*. St. Louis, MO: Mosby/Elsevier; 2008.
2. Miller J. *Nummular Dermatitis*. http://emedicine.medscape.com/article/1123605. Updated May 20, 2011. Accessed November 12, 2011.
3. Tanaka T, Satoh T, Yokozeki H. Dental infection associated with nummular eczema as an overlooked focal infection. *J Dermatol*. 2009;36(8):462-465.
4. Aoyama H, Tanaka M, Hara M, Tabata N, Tagami H. Nummular eczema: an addition of senile xerosis and unique cutaneous reactivities to environmental aeroallergens. *Dermatology*. 1999;199(2):135-139.
5. Wilkinson DS. Discoid eczema as a consequence of contact with irritants. *Contact Dermatitis*. 1979;5(2):118-119.
6. Moore MM, Elpern DJ, Carter DJ. Severe, generalized nummular eczema secondary to interferon alfa-2b plus ribavirin combination therapy in a patient with chronic hepatitis C virus infection. *Arch Dermatol*. 2004;140(2):215-217.
7. Shen Y, Pielop J, Hsu S. Generalized nummular eczema secondary to peginterferon Alfa-2b and ribavirin combination therapy for hepatitis C infection. *Arch Dermatol*. 2005;141(1):102-103.
8. Bettoli V, Tosti A, Varotti C. Nummular eczema during isotretinoin treatment. *J Am Acad Dermatol*. 1987;16(3 pt 1):617.
9. Adachi A, Horikawa T, Takashima T, Ichihashi M. Mercury-induced nummular dermatitis. *J Am Acad Dermatol*. 2000;43(2):383-385.
10. Gutman AB, Kligman AM, Sciacca J, James WD. Soak and smear: a standard technique revisited. *Arch Dermatol*. 2005;141(12):1556-1569.
11. Roberts H, Orchard D. Methotrexate is a safe and effective treatment for paediatric discoid (nummular) eczema: a case series of 25 children. *Australas J Dermatol*. 2010;51(2):128-130.
12. Drake LA, Millikan LE. The antipruritic effect of 5% doxepin cream in patients with eczematous dermatitis. Doxepin Study Group. *Arch Dermatol*. 1995;131(12):1403-1408.
13. Boyle RJ, Bath-Hextall FJ, Leonardi-Bee J, Murrell DF, Tang ML. Probiotics for treating eczema. *Cochrane Database Syst Rev*. 2008;(4):CD006135.

147 PSYCHOCUTANEOUS DISORDERS

Richard P. Usatine, MD
Anne Johnson, MD

PATIENT STORY

A 55-year-old woman presents with severe itching on her arms and legs. The itching disrupts her sleep and she sometimes scratches her arms and legs until exhaustion (**Figures 147-1** and **147-2**).[1] She had used moisturizers, emollients, and topical corticosteroids, but they only alleviated the itching temporarily. The itching began 10 months earlier after finalizing the divorce from her husband of 20 years. The patient's right leg had been amputated above the knee after a car accident, and she now wore a prosthetic leg. The patient readily admitted to a great deal of psychological distress. She described feeling depressed since her divorce, and the loss of her leg further aggravated her situation. She has had difficulty securing a job and had high anxiety about being able to pay for rent and bills. The diagnosis made was neurotic excoriations (neurodermatitis) and the patient understood that she was doing this to her own skin. The patient improved with nail cutting, acknowledging the self-inflicted nature of her excoriations and topical clobetasol. One year later, the patient was working in the hospital laboratory with a tremendous improvement in her skin condition (**Figure 147-3**).

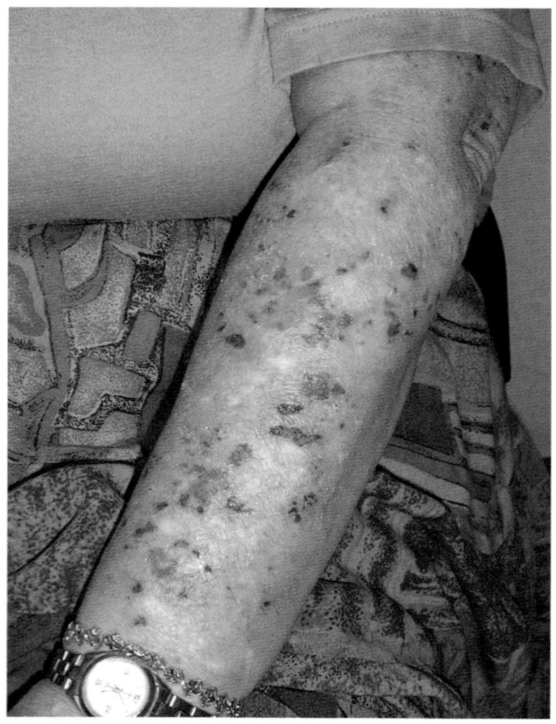

FIGURE 147-2 Neurotic excoriations with close-up of arm. (*Reproduced with permission from Usatine RP, Saldana-Arregui MA. Excoriations and ulcers and legs.* J Fam Pract. *2004;53(9):713-716. Reproduced with permission from Frontline Medical Communications.*)

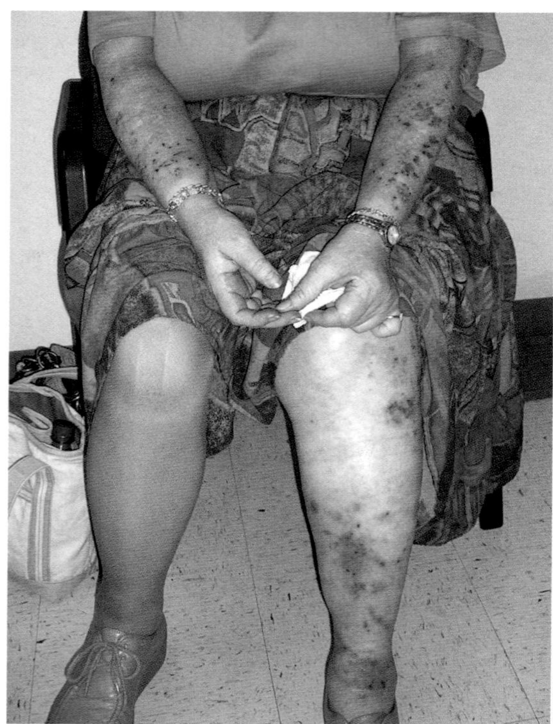

FIGURE 147-1 Neurotic excoriations (neurodermatitis) seen on 3 of 4 extremities. The fourth extremity is a prosthetic leg. (*Reproduced with permission from Usatine RP, Saldana-Arregui MA. Excoriations and ulcers and legs.* J Fam Pract. *2004;53(9):713-716. Reproduced with permission from Frontline Medical Communications.*)

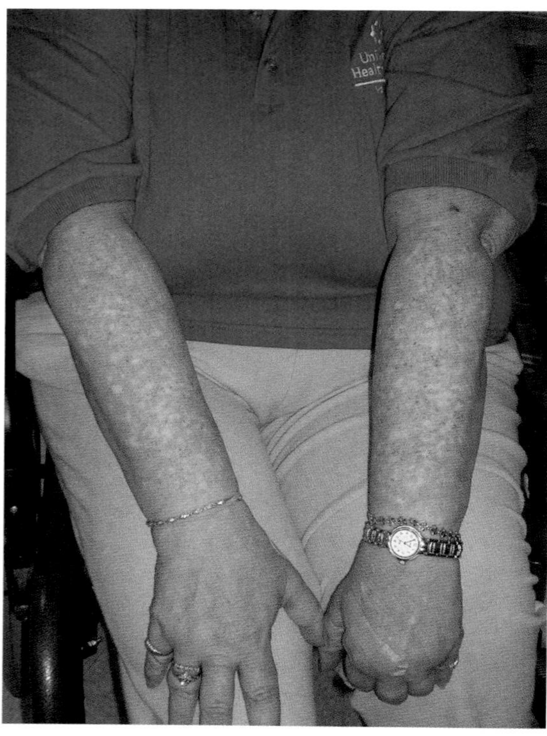

FIGURE 147-3 Same patient of **Figure 147-2** 1-year later after successful therapy. Hypopigmented scarring remains. (*Reproduced with permission from Richard P. Usatine, MD.*)

INTRODUCTION

The self-inflicted dermatoses (sometimes referred to as psychogenic dermatoses) include neurotic excoriations, lichen simplex chronicus (LSC), and prurigo nodularis. These conditions are caused by pruritus for which no medical cause is apparent, which initiates an itch–scratch cycle. The self-inflicted dermatoses can present a challenge to the clinician, as multiple underlying medical etiologies must be ruled out to arrive at their diagnosis and the pathophysiology of these diseases is not well understood. In addition, they may be difficult to treat successfully. There is no clear standard of care for treatment, although a vast array of treatments targeting different etiologies has been tried clinically, and many have some amount of research to support them. As with other psychosomatic conditions, nonpharmacologic interventions, including the physician-patient relationship itself, can be important to treatment.

SYNONYMS

- Neurotic excoriations—Neurodermatitis
- Lichen simplex chronicus—Neurodermatitis circumscripta
- Prurigo nodularis—Picker's nodules; LSC, prurigo nodularis type; atypical nodular form of neurodermatitis circumscripta

EPIDEMIOLOGY

- Studies show that neurotic excoriations primarily affect females, with a mean onset between the ages of 30 and 45 years[1] (**Figures 147-1** to **147-5**).
- Neurotic excoriations are present in 2% of patients seen in dermatologic clinics.[1]
- LSC is observed more commonly in females than in males (**Figures 147-6** to **147-9**). Lichen nuchae is a form of lichen simplex that occurs on the midposterior neck (see **Figures 147-8** and **147-9**).
- LSC occurs mostly in mid-to-late adulthood, with highest prevalence in persons of age 30 to 50 years.[2]
- For prurigo nodularis (PN) there is no documented difference in frequency between males and females. PN most often occurs in middle-aged and older persons[3] (**Figures 147-10** to **147-15**).

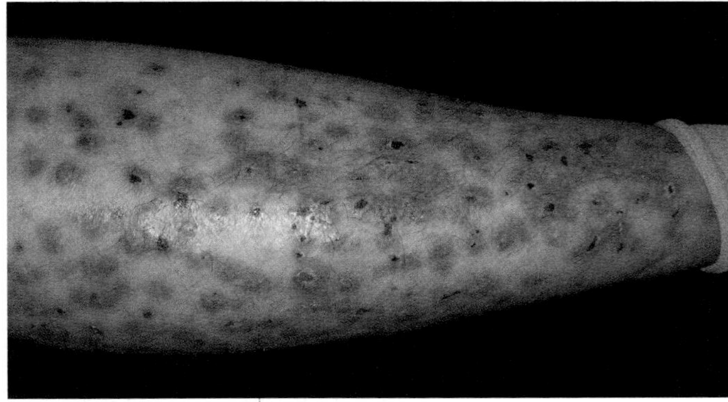

FIGURE 147-4 Neurotic excoriations on the leg with significant postinflammatory hyperpigmentation. (*Reproduced with permission from Richard P. Usatine, MD.*)

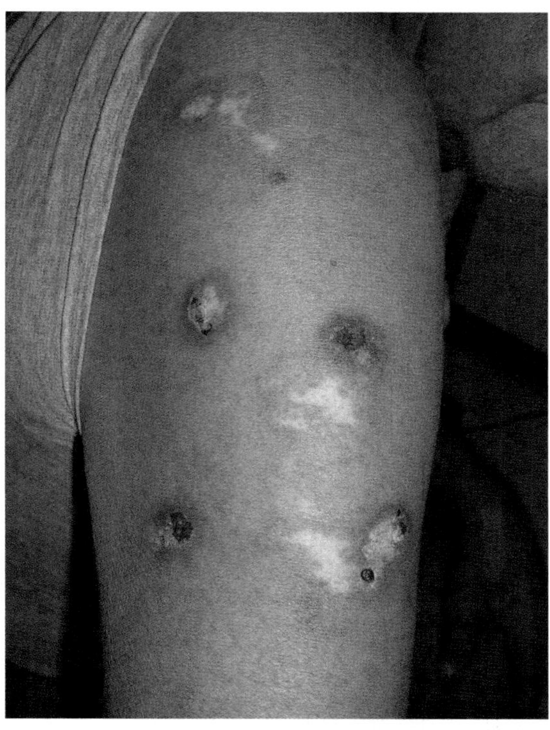

FIGURE 147-5 Neurotic excoriations on the upper arm with hypopigmented scarring. (*Reproduced with permission from Richard P. Usatine, MD.*)

ETIOLOGY AND PATHOPHYSIOLOGY

- All 3 conditions are found on the skin in regions accessible to scratching.
- Pruritus provokes scratching that produces clinical lesions.
- The underlying pathophysiology is unknown for all 3 conditions. Central nervous system (CNS)[4] and peripheral nervous system[5-7] dysfunction have been implicated in the pathogenesis of the pruritus underlying the self-inflicted dermatoses.
- Some skin types are more prone to lichenification, such as skin that tends toward eczematous conditions (ie, atopic dermatitis).[2]

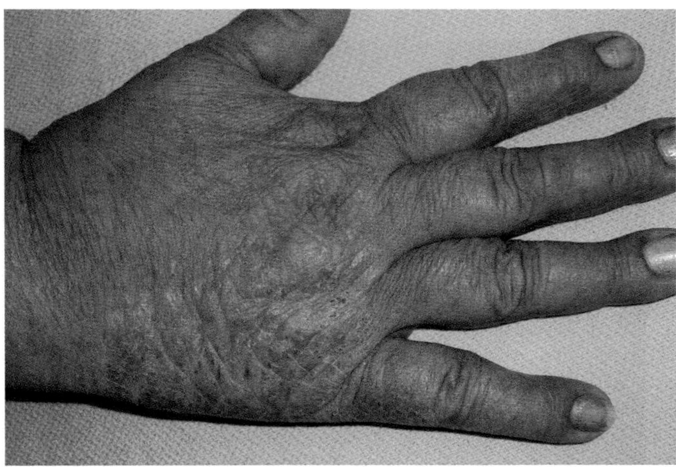

FIGURE 147-6 Lichen simplex chronicus on the hand of a middle-aged woman with thick lichenification, erythema, and hyperpigmentation. She was continually scratching at her hand. (*Reproduced with permission from Richard P. Usatine, MD.*)

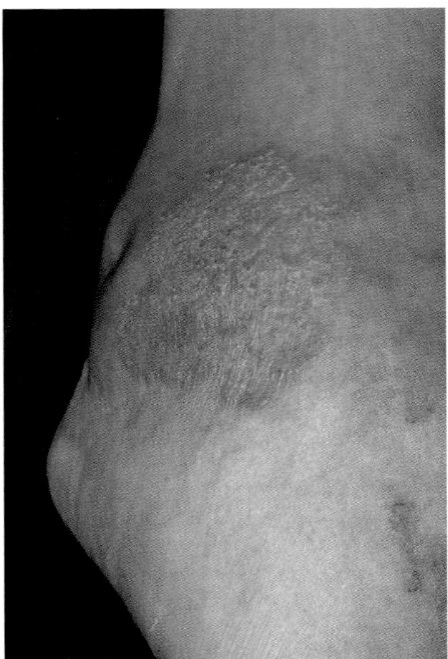

FIGURE 147-7 Lichen simplex chronicus on the ankle. (*Reproduced with permission from Richard P. Usatine, MD.*)

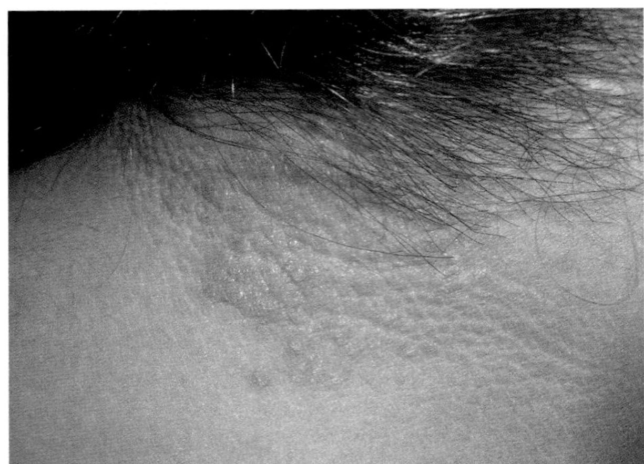

FIGURE 147-8 Lichen simplex chronicus on the neck of a Hispanic woman who also has acanthosis nigricans. (*Reproduced with permission from Richard P. Usatine, MD.*)

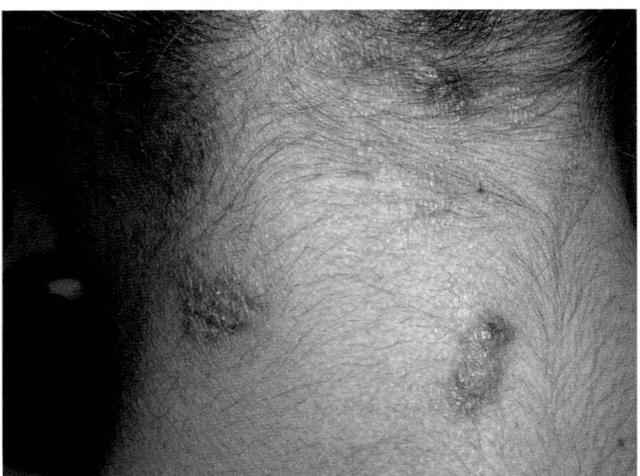

FIGURE 147-9 Lichen simplex chronicus on the neck of a Hispanic woman with thick plaque formation that resembles prurigo nodularis. (*Reproduced with permission from Richard P. Usatine, MD.*)

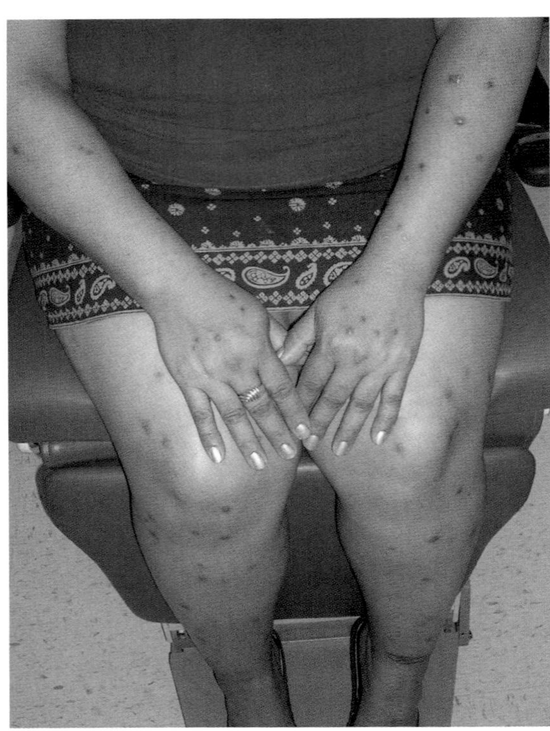

FIGURE 147-10 Prurigo nodularis on the arms and legs of a 42-year-old Hispanic woman. (*Reproduced with permission from Richard P. Usatine, MD.*)

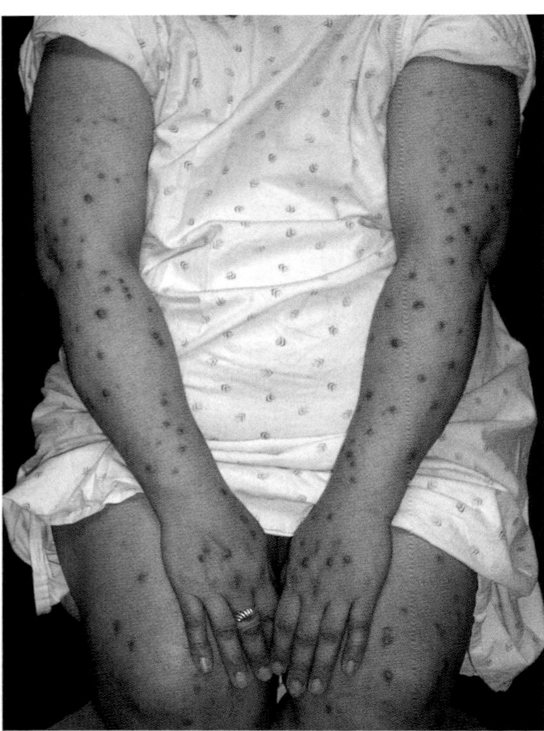

FIGURE 147-11 Prurigo nodularis on the arms and legs after 9 months of unsuccessful treatment in the patient in **Figure 147-10**. (*Reproduced with permission from Richard P. Usatine, MD.*)

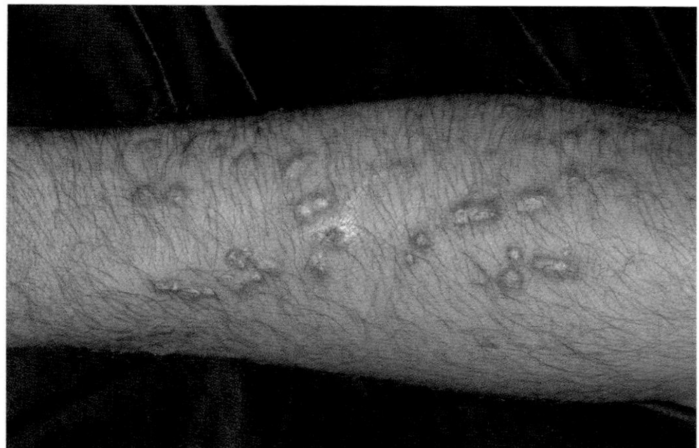

FIGURE 147-12 Severe prurigo nodularis on the arm. The nodules are somewhat linear from years of scratching. (*Reproduced with permission from Richard P. Usatine, MD.*)

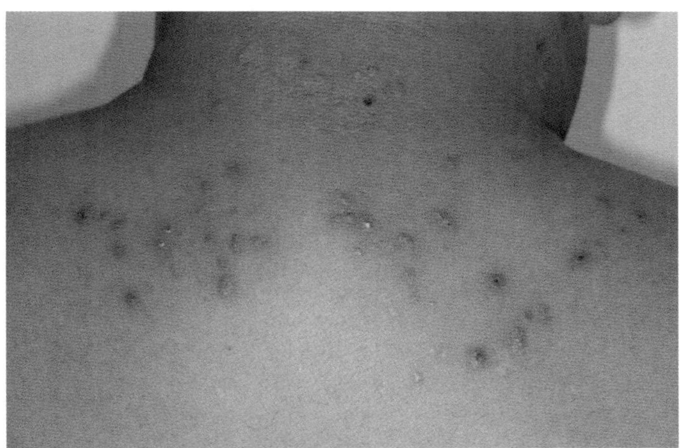

FIGURE 147-13 Prurigo nodularis on the upper back of a man. (*Reproduced with permission from Richard P. Usatine, MD.*)

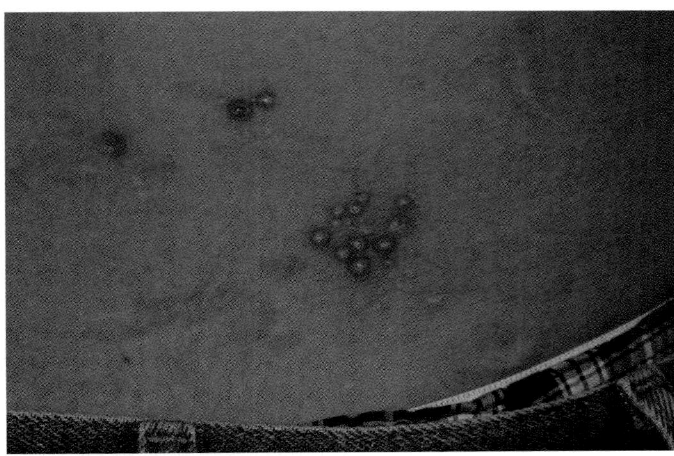

FIGURE 147-14 A cluster of nodules on the back of the same patient in Figure 147-13 with prurigo nodularis. (*Reproduced with permission from Richard P. Usatine, MD.*)

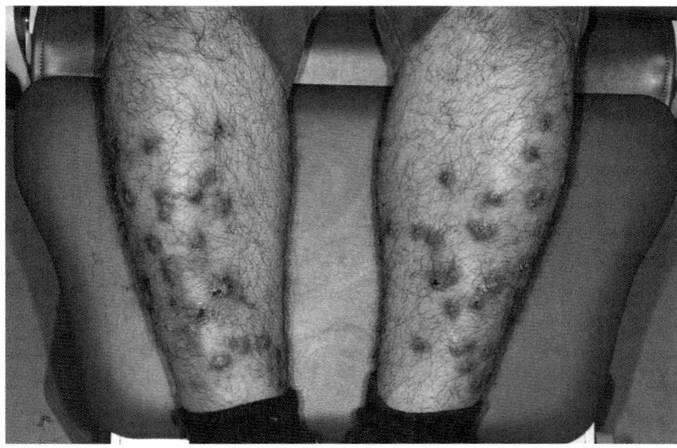

FIGURE 147-15 Severe prurigo nodularis on the legs with prominent hyperpigmentation of the nodules and some secondary infection. (*Reproduced with permission from Richard P. Usatine, MD.*)

- One study showed an association between LSC and a certain genotype (short/short) at the serotonin transporter gene-linked polymorphic region.[8]
- Neurotic excoriation (neurodermatitis) is a result of a psychodermatologic disorder in which patients inflict excoriations and ulcers on their skin and admit to their involvement.
- The pathogenesis of PN is still unknown. PN shares some histologic features (epidermal proliferation) with psoriasis and ichthyosis but is largely self-inflicted.[3] There is some evidence to suggest immune dysregulation is involved, as PN is more common in patients with HIV/AIDS and other forms of immunosuppression than in the general population.[9]

DIAGNOSIS

CLINICAL FEATURES

Itching is the common historical theme for all 3 self-inflicted dermatoses.

Common psychiatric problems associated with all self-inflicted dermatoses include significant social stress, depression, anxiety, and obsessive-compulsive disorder.

Patients are often observed scratching and rubbing their skin. This results in the following:

- Lichenification of the skin (skin thickening with exaggerated skin lines) (see **Figures 147-6** and **147-9**)
- Pigmentary changes (especially hyperpigmentation) (see **Figures 147-4, 147-5, 147-9, 147-11**, and **147-15**)
- Excoriations, erosions, and ulcerations

Common physical examination findings for all 3 disorders include the following:

- Neurotic excoriations—May vary from dug-out erosions to ulcers covered with crusts and surrounded by erythema to areas receding into hypopigmented depressed scars (see **Figure 147-5**)
- LSC—One or more slightly erythematous, scaly, well-demarcated, lichenified, firm, rough plaques[2] (see **Figures 147-6** to **147-9**)
- Prurigo nodularis—Raised nodules from 2 to 20 mm, colors vary from shades of red to brown (see **Figures 147-10** to **147-15**)

Excoriations are almost always present on initial presentation. With treatment the excoriations may subside and the nodules may remain.

TYPICAL DISTRIBUTION

- Neurotic excoriations occur on areas easily reached by the patient, such as the arms, legs, and upper back (see **Figures 147-1** to **147-5**).
- LSC occurs on the following areas:
  - Hands, wrists, extensor forearms, and elbows (see **Figure 147-6**)
  - Knees, lower legs, and ankles (see **Figure 147-7**)
  - Nape of the neck (see **Figures 147-8** and **147-9**)
  - Vulva and scrotum
- In PN, nodules occur on the extensor surfaces of the arms, the legs, and sometimes the trunk (see **Figures 147-10** to **147-15**).

LABORATORY STUDIES

Punch biopsy may be helpful when the diagnosis is uncertain.

DIFFERENTIAL DIAGNOSIS

- Acne keloidalis nuchae—Acneiform eruption at the hairline from ingrown hairs, worse with shaving and short haircuts (see Chapter 116, Pseudofolliculitis and Acne Keloidalis Nuchae).
- Atopic dermatitis—An allergic skin disorder in patients with a personal or family history of atopic conditions. Patients with atopic dermatitis are more likely to get LSC (see Chapter 143, Atopic Dermatitis).
- Contact dermatitis—A common inflammatory skin condition characterized by erythematous and pruritic skin lesions resulting from the contact of skin with a foreign substance (see Chapter 144, Contact Dermatitis).
- Delusions of parasitosis—Delusions that tiny bugs or parasites are living on or below the patient's skin leading them to try to dig them out with their nails and fingers. This condition looks just like neurotic excoriations; however, the patient believes there are parasites causing the pruritus and it is very difficult to convince them otherwise.
- Nummular eczema—Eczematous lesions in the shape of coins seen most often on the legs.
- Scabies—Look for burrows between the fingers and the typical distribution of scabies on the hands, feet, wrists, waist, and axillae to differentiate scabies from a self-inflicted dermatosis. If you do a scraping and find evidence of the scabies mite that is the best way to confirm a true scabies infestation. Often family members have itching and lesions as well when the real diagnosis is scabies (see Chapter 141, Scabies).

MANAGEMENT

For all 3 self-inflicted dermatoses there is little evidence to guide therapy. The following 3 treatments can be used in all 3 conditions and are based on expert opinion and a few small studies: SOR C

- Topical corticosteroids—Use mid-potency to high-potency steroids except in areas of thin skin.
- Oral antihistamines—Sedating H_1 blockers and consider doxepin (start with 10-25 mg PO qhs and titrate to response) for refractory cases.
- Oral antibiotics, if secondary infection is present.
- One small study of 3 patients with inflammatory skin diseases and severe nocturnal pruritus who underwent treatment with mirtazapine (Remeron) suggests that this may be an effective alternative for the treatment of nocturnal pruritus.[10] SOR C

Get a good psychosocial history and offer the patient treatment for any problems uncovered. It may help for patients to understand the connection between their self-inflicted lesions and their stressors. Some patients will have anxiety disorders or depression, whereas others will be suffering with great psychosocial stressors like loss of work, homelessness, or grief. Offer pharmacotherapy (including selective serotonin reuptake inhibitors [SSRIs]) and counseling if indicated. Refer as needed for these therapies.

Other specific treatments to consider are as follows:

- LSC
  - Doxepin 5% cream has been studied in patients with LSC, nummular eczema, and contact dermatitis. Applied 4 times per day for a period of 7 days led to an 84% response rate in reduction of pruritus (not lesions).[11] SOR B
  - Tacrolimus 0.1% ointment applied twice daily for approximately 2 months, then once daily for an additional 3 months was effective in achieving remission from LSC in 1 case report.[12]
  - In one study of 22 patients with LSC, transcutaneous electrical nerve stimulation (TENS) reduced pruritus by more than 50% in 80% of the patients.[5]
- Prurigo nodularis—A difficult condition to treat with mild-to-moderate success at best.

  Here are some treatments to consider:
  - Intralesional steroids—Triamcinolone 5 to 10 mg/cc. SOR C
  - Cryotherapy—Applied to each nodule to flatten the nodules and decrease pruritus. SOR C
  - Calcipotriol—After 8 weeks of calcipotriol treatment, the reduction in the number and size of nodules was 49% and 56%, respectively, compared with 18% and 25% for the betamethasone valerate.[13] SOR B
  - UV light (narrow-band UVB) is sometimes useful when the condition is widespread. SOR C
  - Monochromatic excimer light (308 nm) showed partial or complete remission from PN in 9 (81%) of 11 patients.[14] SOR C
  - Oral dapsone has been tried with some reported success in this difficult condition. SOR C

Gabapentin has some reported success in reducing pruritus in patients with PN and LSC.[6] One case series of oral cyclosporine showed some benefit for PN.[15]

In AIDS patients with PN, maintaining a CD4+ count over 50 may improve pruritus.[9]

PATIENT EDUCATION

Help patients to understand that they are unintentionally hurting their own skin. Patients need to minimize touching, scratching, and rubbing affected areas. Suggest that patients gently apply their medication or a moisturizer instead of scratching the pruritic areas. Give patients hope and show them **Figures 147-1** to **147-3** to demonstrate that even the most severe cases can heal if they stop manipulating their skin.

FOLLOW-UP

Follow-up is essential because these problems are chronic and difficult to treat. Patients need to know that you will not abandon them and will continue to work with them to get relief. This is especially important when the patient is suffering from anxiety, depression, or other psychological problems.

PATIENT RESOURCES

- PubMed Health. *Lichen simplex chronicus*—**http://www.ncbi.nlm.nih.gov/pubmedhealth/PMH0001875/.**
- American Osteopathic College of Dermatology. *Prurigo Nodularis*—**http://www.aocd.org/skin/dermatologic_diseases/prurigo_nodularis.html.**
- American family Physician. *Neurotic Excoriations*—**http://www.aafp.org/afp/2001/1215/p1981.html.**

PROVIDER RESOURCES

- Medscape. *Lichen simplex chronicus* —**http://emedicine.medscape.com/article/1123423.**
- Medscape. *Prurigo Nodularis* —**http://emedicine.medscape.com/article/1088032.**
- Medscape. *Neurotic Excoriations*—**http://emedicine.medscape.com/article/1122042.**

REFERENCES

1. Scheinfeld, N. *Neurotic Excoriations*. http://emedicine.medscape.com/article/1122042. Updated August 3, 2011. Accessed November 15, 2011.
2. Hogan, D. *Lichen Simplex Chronicus*. http://emedicine.medscape.com/article/1123423. Updated June 4, 2010. Accessed November 15, 2011.
3. Hogan, D. *Prurigo Nodularis*. http://emedicine.medscape.com/article/1088032. Updated July 9, 2010. Accessed November 17, 2011.
4. Krishnan A, Koo J. Psyche, opioids, and itch: therapeutic consequences. *Dermatol Ther.* 2005;18(4):314-322.
5. Engin B, Tufekci O, Yazici A, Ozdemir M. The effect of transcutaneous electrical nerve stimulation in the treatment of lichen simplex: a prospective study. *Clin Exp Dermatol.* 2009;34:324-328.
6. Gencoglan G, Inanir I, Gunduz K. Treatment of prurigo nodularis and lichen simplex chronicus with gabapentin. *Dermatol Ther.* 2010;23:194-198.
7. Solak O, Kulac M, Yaman M, et al. Lichen simplex chronicus as a symptom of neuropathy. *Clin Exp Dermatol.* 2008;34:476-480.
8. Kirtak N, Inaloz S, Akcali C, et al. Association of serotonin transporter gene-linked polymorphic region and variable number of tandem repeat polymorphism of the serotonin transporter gene in lichen simplex chronicus patients with psychiatric status. *Int J Dermatol.* 2008;47:1069-1072.
9. Maurer T. Dermatologic manifestations of HIV infection. *Top HIV Med.* 2005 Dec-2006 Jan;13(5):147-154.
10. Hundley JL, Yosipovitch G. Mirtazapine for reducing nocturnal itch in patients with chronic pruritus: a pilot study. *J Am Acad Dermatol.* 2004;50:889-891.
11. Drake LA, Millikan LE. The antipruritic effect of 5% doxepin cream in patients with eczematous dermatitis. Doxepin Study Group. *Arch Dermatol.* 1995;131:1403-1408.
12. Aschoff R, Wozel G. Topical tacrolimus for the treatment of lichen simplex chronicus. *J Dermatolog Treat.* 2007;18:115-117.
13. Wong SS, Goh CL. Double-blind, right/left comparison of calcipotriol ointment and betamethasone ointment in the treatment of prurigo nodularis. *Arch Dermatol.* 2000;136:807-808.
14. Saraceno R, Nistico SP, Capriotti E, et al. Monochromatic excimer light (308 nm) in the treatment of prurigo nodularis. *Photodermatol Photoimmunol Photomed.* 2008;24(1):43-45.
15. Siepmann, D Luger T, Stander S. Antipruritic effect of cyclosporine microemulsion in prurigo nodularis: results of a case series. *J Dtsch Dermatol Ges.* 2008;6:941-945.

148 URTICARIA AND ANGIOEDEMA

Richard P. Usatine, MD

PATIENT STORY

A 26-year-old man was given trimethoprim-sulfamethoxazole for sinusitis and broke out in hives 1 week later. The hives were all over his trunk and arms (**Figures 148-1** and **148-2**). He had no airway compromise and had only urticaria without angioedema. His sinus symptoms were mostly resolved, so he was told to stop the antibiotic and take an oral antihistamine. The H_1 blocker gave him relief of symptoms and the wheals disappeared over the next 2 days.

INTRODUCTION

Urticaria and angioedema are a heterogeneous group of diseases that cause swelling of the skin and other soft tissues. They both result from a large variety of underlying causes, are elicited by a great diversity of factors, and present clinically in a highly variable way.[1] Standard hives with transient wheals is the most common manifestation of urticaria.

SYNONYMS

Urticaria is also called as hives.

EPIDEMIOLOGY

- It is estimated that 15% to 25% of the population may have urticaria sometime during their lifetime.[2]
- Urticaria affects 6% to 7% of preschool children and 17% of children with atopic dermatitis.[2]

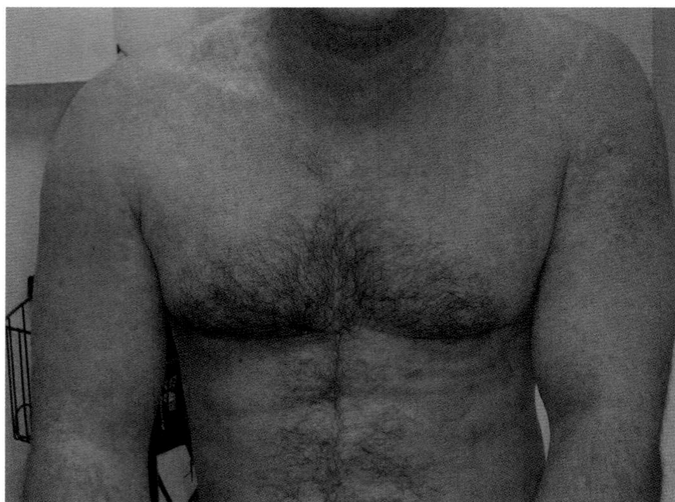

FIGURE 148-1 A 26-year-old man with acute urticaria due to trimethoprim-sulfamethoxazole. (*Reproduced with permission from Richard P. Usatine, MD.*)

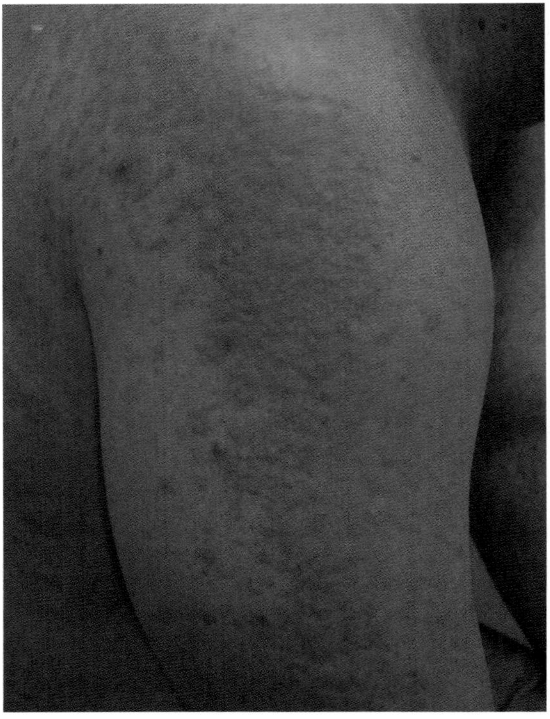

FIGURE 148-2 Note the confluence of wheals with a well-demarcated border on the arm of the man with acute urticaria due to trimethoprim-sulfamethoxazole. (*Reproduced with permission from Richard P. Usatine, MD.*)

- Among all age groups, approximately 50% have both urticaria and angioedema, 40% have isolated urticaria, and 10% have angioedema alone.[2]
- Acute urticaria is defined as less than 6 weeks' duration. A specific cause is more likely to be identified in acute urticaria.[2]
- The cause of chronic urticaria (>6 weeks' duration) is determined in less than 20% of cases.[2]
- Chronic urticaria is twice as common in women as in men.[3]
- Chronic urticaria predominantly affects adults.[3]
- Up to 40% of patients with chronic urticaria of more than 6 months' duration still have urticaria 10 years later.[3]

ETIOLOGY AND PATHOPHYSIOLOGY

- The pathophysiology of angioedema and urticaria can be immunoglobulin (Ig) E mediated, complement mediated, related to physical stimuli, autoantibody mediated, or idiopathic.
- These mechanisms lead to mast cell degranulation resulting in the release of histamine. The histamine and other inflammatory mediators produce the wheals, edema, and pruritus.
- Urticaria is a dynamic process in which new wheals evolve as old ones resolve. These wheals result from localized capillary vasodilation, followed by transudation of protein-rich fluid into the surrounding skin. The wheals resolve when the fluid is slowly reabsorbed.
- Angioedema is an edematous area that involves transudation of fluid into the dermis and subcutaneous tissue (**Figures 148-3** and **148-4**).

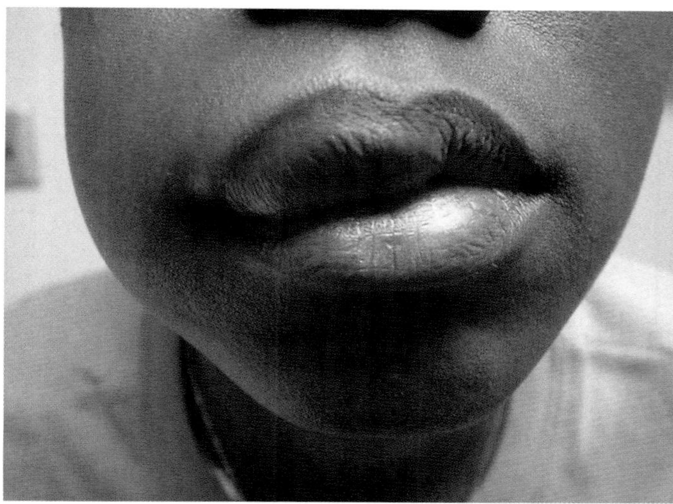

FIGURE 148-3 Young black woman with angioedema after being started on an angiotensin-converting enzyme inhibitor (ACEI) for essential hypertension. (*Reproduced with permission from Adrian Casillas, MD.*)

The following etiologic types exist:

- Immunologic—IgE mediated, complement mediated. Occurs more often in patients with an atopic background. Antigens are most commonly foods or medications. The most common foods are milk, nuts, wheat, and shellfish.
- Physical urticaria—Dermatographism, cold, cholinergic, solar, pressure, vibratory urticaria (**Figures 148-5** and **148-6**).
- Urticaria caused by mast cell–releasing agents—Mastocytosis, urticaria pigmentosa
- Urticaria associated with vascular/connective tissue autoimmune disease (**Figures 148-7** and **148-8**).
- Hereditary angioedema is a potentially life-threatening disorder that is inherited in an autosomal dominant manner. In this disease, angioedema occurs without urticaria (**Figure 148-9**).

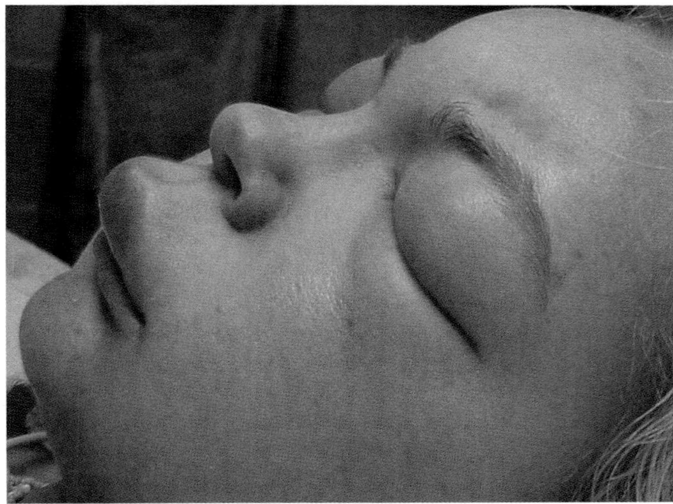

FIGURE 148-4 Severe angioedema around the eyes and mouth. (*Reproduced with permission from Daniel Stulberg, MD.*)

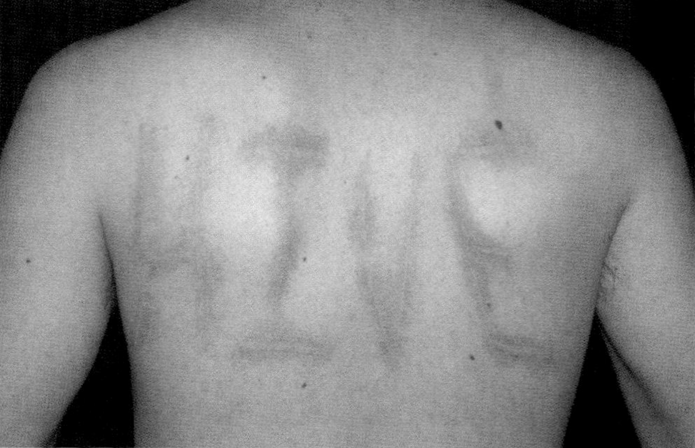

FIGURE 148-5 Dermatographism in a 21-year-old man with chronic urticaria. Note the exaggerated triple reaction. (*Reproduced with permission from Richard P. Usatine, MD.*)

FIGURE 148-6 Cholinergic urticaria showing small wheals. The patient would get this urticaria after exercising. (*Reproduced with permission from Philip C. Anderson, MD.*)

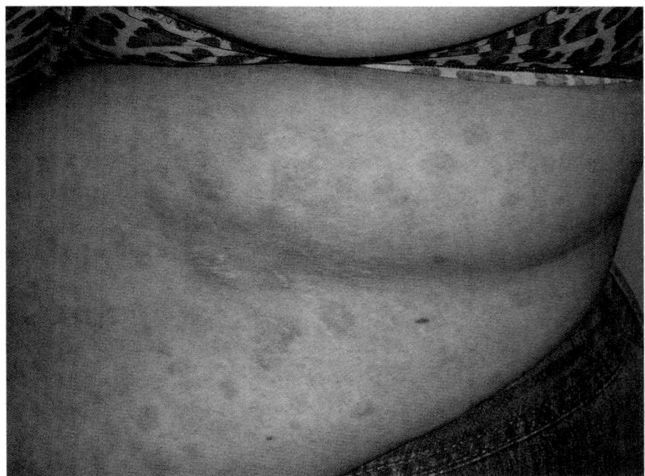

FIGURE 148-7 Chronic urticaria in a woman with systemic lupus erythematosus. (*Reproduced with permission from Richard P. Usatine, MD.*)

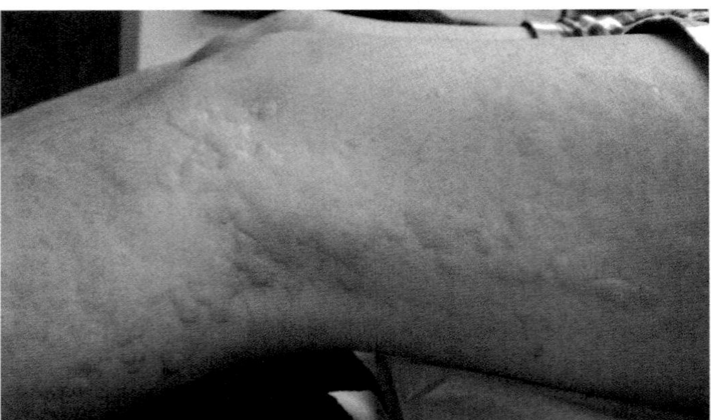

FIGURE 148-8 Acute urticaria in a woman with rheumatoid arthritis. *(Reproduced with permission from Richard P. Usatine, MD.)*

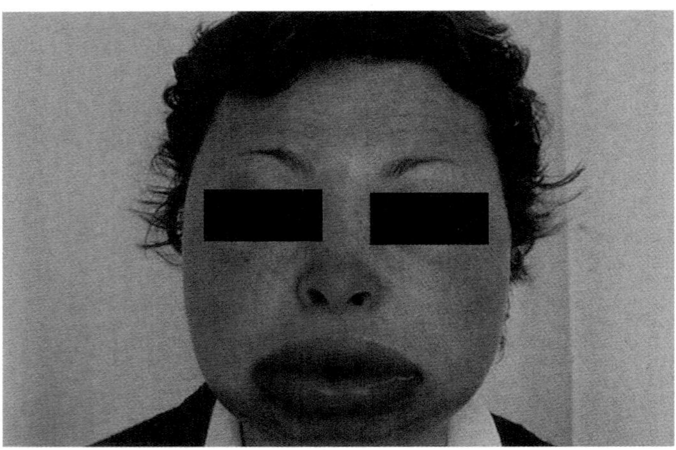

A

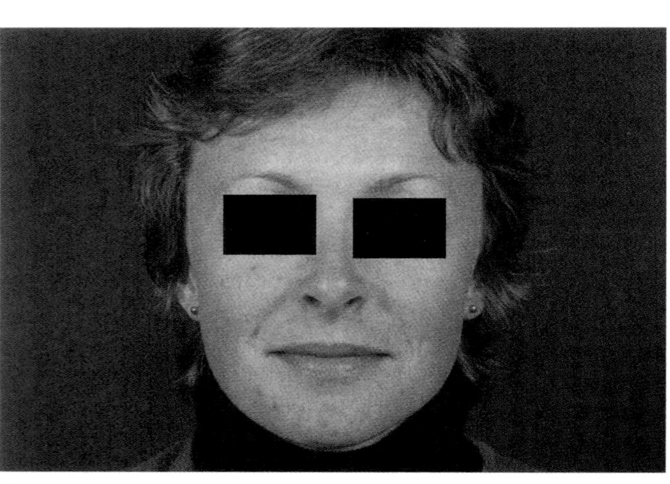

B

FIGURE 148-9 Hereditary angioedema. **A.** Severe edema of the face during an episode, leading to grotesque disfigurement. **B.** Angioedema will subside within hours. The patient had a positive family history and had multiple similar episodes including colicky abdominal pain. *(Reproduced with permission from* Fitzpatrick's Color Atlas and Synopsis of Clinical Dermatology. *5th ed. New York, NY: McGraw-Hill; 2005.)*

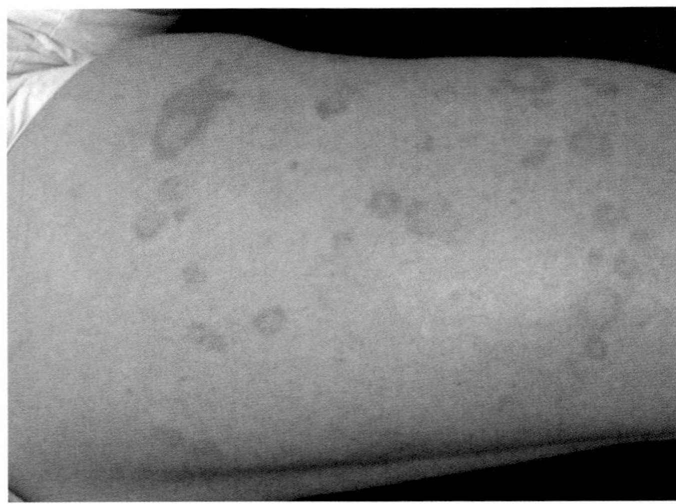

FIGURE 148-10 Chronic urticaria with annular urticarial plaques. *(Reproduced with permission from Richard P. Usatine, MD.)*

DIAGNOSIS

CLINICAL FEATURES

- Symptoms include itching, burning, and stinging.
- Wheals vary in size from small, 2-mm papules of cholinergic urticaria (see **Figure 148-6**) to giant hives where a single wheal may cover a large portion of the trunk.
- The wheal may be all red or white, or the border may be red with the remainder of the surface white.
- Wheals may be annular (**Figures 148-10** and **148-11**).

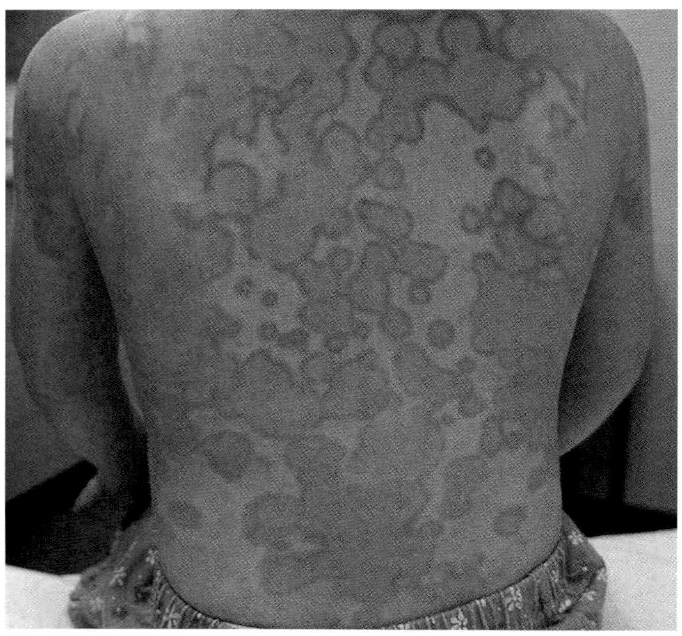

FIGURE 148-11 Giant urticaria (urticaria multiforme). Although this appears to have targets the real target lesions of erythema multiforme have a central lesion and have a scaling or bullous component affecting the epidermis. The history suggests that this may have been a serum sickness type reaction. *(Reproduced with permission from Milgrom EC, Usatine RP, Tan RA, Spector SL.* Practical Allergy. *Philadelphia, PA: Elsevier; 2003; and Daniel Stulberg, MD.)*

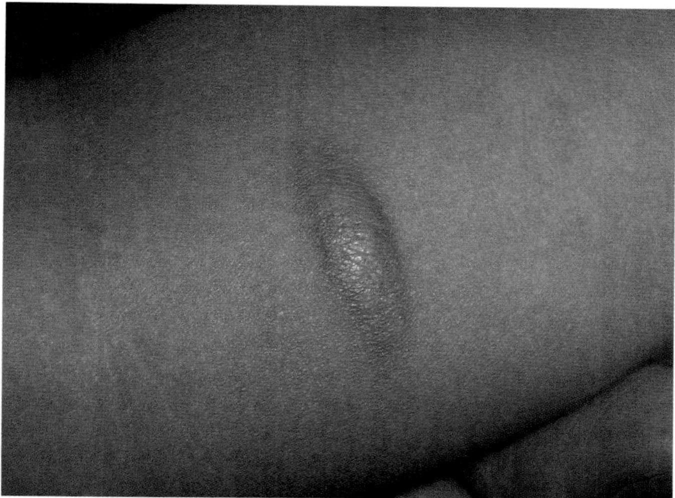

FIGURE 148-12 Positive Darier sign in which stroking the lesion of urticaria pigmentosum results in edema. (*Reproduced with permission from Richard P. Usatine, MD.*)

- If dermatographism is present, one can write on the skin and be able to see the resulting words or shapes (see **Figure 148-5**).
- If you suspect urticaria pigmentosa, stroke a lesion with the wooden end of a cotton-tipped applicator. This induces erythema of the plaque and the wheal is confined to the stroke site. This is called Darier sign (**Figure 148-12**).

TYPICAL DISTRIBUTION

- Angioedema is seen more often on the face and is especially found around the mouth and eyes (see **Figures 148-3** and **148-4**). Sometimes angioedema can occur on the genitals or the trunk (**Figure 148-13**).

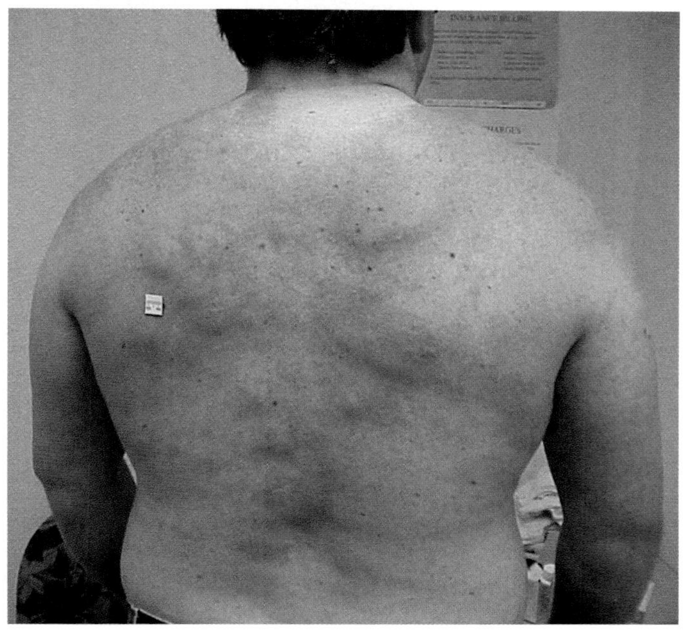

FIGURE 148-13 Angioedema and urticaria of the back. The thicker deeper wheals are angioedema. (*Reproduced with permission from Milgrom EC, Usatine RP, Tan RA, Spector SL.* Practical Allergy. *Philadelphia, PA: Elsevier; 2003; and Daniel Stulberg, MD.*)

- Urticaria can be found anywhere on the body and is often on the trunk and extremities (see **Figures 148-1** and **148-2**).

LABORATORY STUDIES

Consider tests that might help reveal the cause of the urticaria and/or angioedema.

- Investigate for hereditary or acquired C1 esterase inhibitor deficiency when angioedema occurs repeatedly without urticaria (see **Figure 148-9**). The most useful initial test is a C1INH (the inhibitor of C1 esterase) level. However, the type II form has a normal level of C1INH but low function. Therefore functional assays must be done if the level is normal but hereditary angioedema is still suspected.
- Consider allergen skin testing and/or in vitro tests when the history reveals that urticaria/angioedema occurs after direct contact with a suspected allergen.
- Punch biopsy of the involved area may be used to diagnose urticarial vasculitis or mastocytosis.

DIFFERENTIAL DIAGNOSIS

- Insect bites—A good history and physical examination should help to distinguish between insect bites and urticaria.
- Erythema multiforme-like urticaria can occur in response to an allergic/immunologic reaction to medications, infections, and neoplasms. The classic lesion of erythema multiforme is the target lesion in which there is disruption of the epithelium in the center. This disruption may be a vesicle, bulla, or erosion. Do not confuse annular lesions or concentric rings with erythema multiforme if the epidermis is intact (see **Figure 148-11** is *not* erythema multiforme) (see Chapter 175, Erythema Multiforme, Stevens-Johnson Syndrome, and Toxic Epidermal Necrolysis).
- Urticarial vasculitis typically has lesions that last longer than 24 hours. The lesions are found more commonly on the lower extremities, and when they heal, they often leave hyperpigmented areas. Causes range from a hypersensitivity vasculitis, such as Henoch-Schönlein purpura to underlying connective tissue disease (**Figure 148-14**).[2]
- Mast cell releasability syndromes are syndromes in which there are too many mast cells in the skin or other organs of the body. These include cutaneous mastocytosis and urticaria pigmentosa (see **Figures 148-7**, **148-8**, and **148-12**).
- Pruritic urticarial papules and plaques of pregnancy can be differentiated from urticaria in pregnancy because the eruption remains fixed and increases in intensity until delivery (**Figure 148-15**).
- Pemphigoid gestationis can have lesions that are urticarial. However, it also has bullae that distinguish it from urticaria and of course the patient is pregnant or postpartum.

MANAGEMENT

NONPHARMACOLOGIC THERAPY

- Avoid any causative agent, medication, stimulus, or antigen if found (**Figure 148-16**). SOR B
- Angiotensin-converting enzyme inhibitors (ACEIs) are especially prone to causing angioedema so should be stopped as soon as possible when suspected to be causative of angioedema or urticaria (**Figure 148-3**).[1]

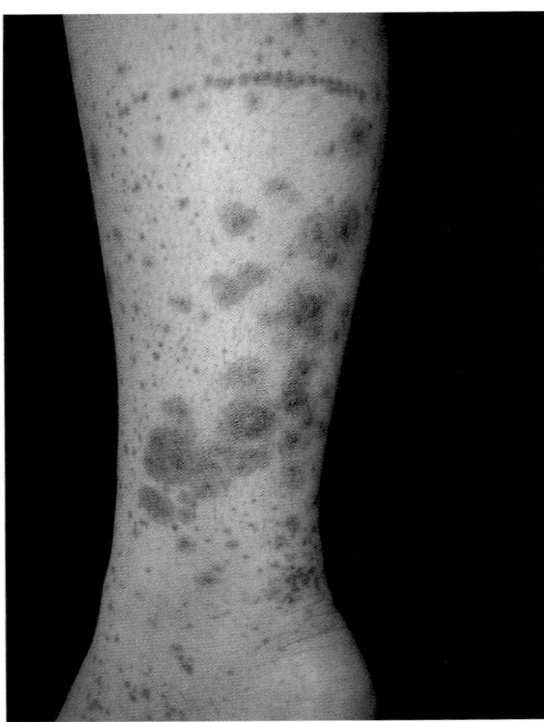

FIGURE 148-14 Henoch-Schönlein purpura on the leg of a 20-year-old woman. This is a type of urticarial vasculitis. (*Reproduced with permission from Milgrom EC, Usatine RP, Tan RA, Spector SL.* Practical Allergy. *Philadelphia, PA: Elsevier; 2003; and Richard P. Usatine, MD.*)

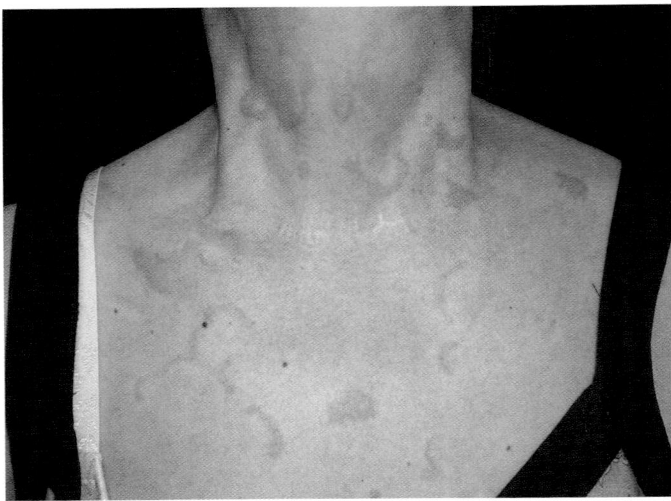

FIGURE 148-16 Urticarial drug eruption that occurred when a 59-year-old woman was started on Levemir insulin for her diabetes. The urticaria cleared when she was switched to an alternate form of insulin. (*Reproduced with permission from Richard P. Usatine, MD.*)

SOR Ⓐ Even an angiotensin receptor blocker (ARB) can cause angioedema and should be suspected in a patient on this class of medication (**Figure 148-17**).

- In chronic urticaria, patients may benefit from avoidance of potential urticarial precipitants such as aspirin, nonsteroidal anti-inflammatory drugs (NSAIDs) (**Figure 148-18**), opiates, and alcohol.[1] SOR Ⓑ

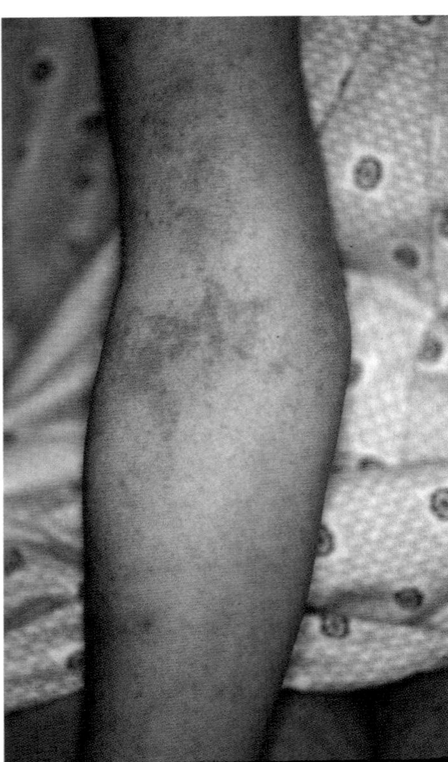

FIGURE 148-15 Pruritic urticarial papules and plaques of pregnancy on the arm of a pregnant woman. The wheals are indistinguishable from other types of urticaria. (*Reproduced with permission from Milgrom EC, Usatine RP, Tan RA, Spector SL.* Practical Allergy. *Philadelphia, PA: Elsevier; 2003; and Richard P. Usatine, MD.*)

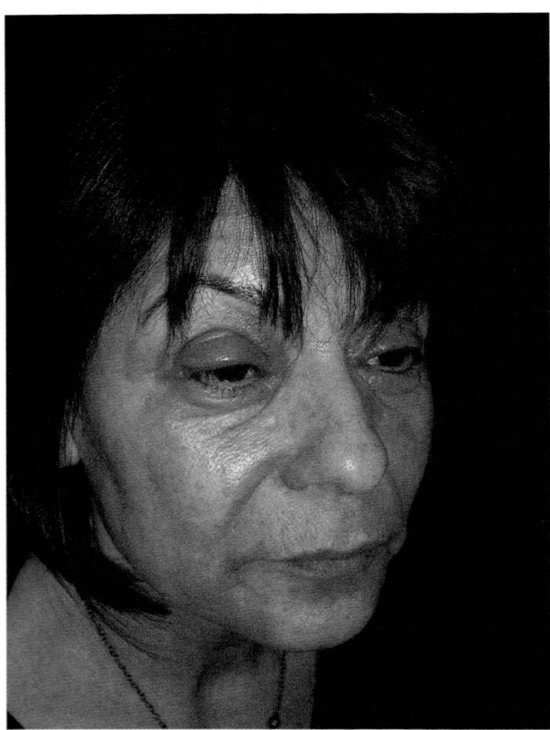

FIGURE 148-17 Angioedema secondary to an angiotensin receptor blocker given for hypertension. The angioedema resolved and did not return once the patient stopped the offending medication. (*Reproduced with permission from Richard P. Usatine, MD.*)

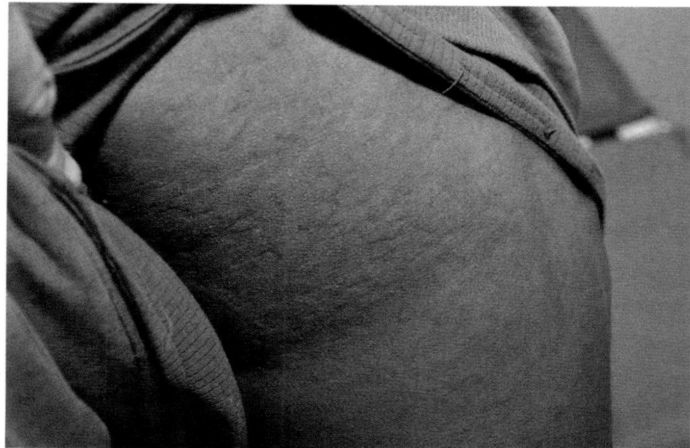

FIGURE 148-18 Urticaria that occurred within an hour after a patient was given ibuprofen to treat a high fever. (*Reproduced with permission from Richard P. Usatine, MD.*)

- Infections may be a cause, an aggravating factor, or an unassociated bystander.[1] Look for sources of chronic infections such as parasitic infections, dental infections, gastrointestinal (GI) infections, respiratory infections, and tinea pedis. Treat these, as it is possible, but unproven, that they can contribute to the chronic urticaria. SOR Ⓒ
- Stop all unnecessary nonprescription medications, supplements, and vitamins in chronic urticaria. SOR Ⓒ
- Avoidance of physical stimuli for the treatment of physical urticaria is desirable, but not always possible (observational studies only).[1] SOR Ⓑ
- Stress reduction techniques may help in chronic urticaria but this is unproven. SOR Ⓒ

ANTIHISTAMINES

- Low-sedating, second-generation antihistamines should be prescribed as a first-line treatment for chronic urticaria.[4-6] SOR Ⓐ
- Increasing the dose of cetirizine from 10 mg to 20 mg daily produced a significant improvement in the severity of wheal and itching in urticaria refractory to the standard doses of antihistamines.[7] SOR Ⓑ
- The British guidelines even suggest using antihistamines at up to quadruple the manufacturers' recommended dosages before changing to an alternative therapy. They also recommend waiting up to 4 weeks to allow full effectiveness of the antihistamines before considering referral to a specialist.[1] SOR Ⓒ
- All patients should be offered the choice of at least 2 low-sedating H_1 antagonists because responses and tolerance vary between individuals.[8] SOR Ⓐ
- Addition of a sedating antihistamine at night may help patients sleep better, although they probably add little to existing H_1 receptor blockade.[8]
- The addition of an H_2 antagonist may give better control of urticaria than H_1 antagonists alone, SOR Ⓑ although a benefit is not always seen.[8] In one study, adding H_2 blockers to H_1 antagonists resulted in improvement of certain cutaneous outcomes for patients presenting with acute allergic syndromes to an emergency department.[9] SOR Ⓑ
- When initial antihistamines are not working, consider doxepin, an antidepressant and potent H_1 antagonist.[10] SOR Ⓑ Its use is limited by the side effects of sedation and dry mouth. Start with 10-mg doxepin in the evening and titrate up as needed and tolerated.
- Low-sedating antihistamines seem to be effective in the treatment of acquired cold urticaria by significantly reducing the presence of wheals and pruritus after cold exposure.[11] SOR Ⓐ

CORTICOSTEROIDS

- Oral corticosteroids should be restricted to short courses for severe acute urticaria or angioedema affecting the mouth (eg, prednisone 60 mg/d for 3-4 days in adults).[8,12] SOR Ⓑ
- Short tapering courses of oral steroids over 3 to 4 weeks may be necessary for urticarial vasculitis and severe delayed pressure urticaria.
- Long-term oral corticosteroids should not be used in chronic urticaria. It is better to use oral cyclosporine if needed as it has a far better risk-to-benefit ratio compared with steroids.[1,8]
- A randomized controlled trial showed that clobetasol 0.05% in a foam formulation was safe and effective in the short-term treatment of patients with delayed pressure urticaria.[13] SOR Ⓑ

IMMUNOMODULATORY AGENTS

- Immunosuppressive therapies for autoimmune urticaria should be restricted to patients with disabling disease who have not responded to optimal conventional treatments.[6]
- A retrospective study of methotrexate in 8 patients with recalcitrant chronic urticaria indicated that methotrexate was both safe and effective, with a mean dose of 15-mg methotrexate per week. Seven of 8 patients achieved a complete response and 5 of 8 remained disease free after methotrexate was stopped.[14] SOR Ⓑ
- Cyclosporine, plasmapheresis, anti-IgE (omalizumab), and intravenous immunoglobulin have been used in severe recalcitrant cases.[1] SOR Ⓒ
- Plasmapheresis is very costly and should be reserved for autoantibody-positive chronic spontaneous urticaria patients.[1]

OTHERS

- Epinephrine is valuable in severe acute urticaria or angioedema, especially if there is a suspicion of airway compromise or anaphylaxis.
- The evidence for leukotriene modifiers in the treatment of urticaria is poor. SOR Ⓒ
- Ecallantide is a new plasma kallikrein inhibitor for the subcutaneous treatment of acute attacks of hereditary angioedema.[15] SOR Ⓑ
- Anti-inflammatory drugs, such as colchicine, dapsone, and sulfasalazine, have been reported as helpful in uncontrolled trials or case series.[1]

PATIENT EDUCATION

In most cases, we are not able to find the cause of urticaria. This is especially true for chronic urticaria. Fortunately, most chronic urticaria will subside over time and there are medicines to treat the condition until it runs its course. If one medication does not work keep your follow-up visits to try other medications. Carefully observe for causative agents.

FOLLOW-UP

Follow-up is especially needed when the urticaria or angioedema persist or recur.

PATIENT RESOURCES

- eMedicineHealth.com is a consumer health site with information and support groups—**http://www.emedicinehealth.com/hives_and_angioedema/article_em.htm.**

PROVIDER RESOURCES

- Well-written guideline based on a joint initiative of a number of European dermatology, allergy, and immunology organizations—**http://onlinelibrary.wiley.com/doi/10.1111/j.1398-9995.2009.02178.x/full.**

REFERENCES

1. Zuberbier T, Asero R, Bindslev-Jensen C, et al. EAACI/GA(2) LEN/EDF/WAO guideline: management of urticaria. *Allergy.* 2009;64:1427-1443.
2. Baxi S, Dinakar C. Urticaria and angioedema. *Immunol Allergy Clin North Am.* 2005;25:353-367, vii.
3. Usatine RP. Urticaria and angioedema. In: Milgrom E, Usatine RP, Tan R, Spector S, eds. *Practical Allergy*. Philadelphia, PA: Elsevier; 2003:78-96.
4. Finn AF Jr, Kaplan AP, Fretwell R, et al. A double-blind, placebo-controlled trial of fexofenadine HCl in the treatment of chronic idiopathic urticaria. *J Allergy Clin Immunol.* 1999;104:1071-1078.
5. Ortonne JP, Grob JJ, Auquier P, Dreyfus I. Efficacy and safety of desloratadine in adults with chronic idiopathic urticaria: a randomized, double-blind, placebo-controlled, multicenter trial. *Am J Clin Dermatol.* 2007;8:37-42.
6. Ortonne JP. Chronic urticaria: a comparison of management guidelines. *Expert Opin Pharmacother.* 2011;12(17):2683-2693.
7. Okubo Y, Shigoka Y, Yamazaki M, Tsuboi R. Double dose of cetirizine hydrochloride is effective for patients with urticaria resistant: a prospective, randomized, non-blinded, comparative clinical study and assessment of quality of life. *J Dermatolog Treat.* 2013;24(2):153-160.
8. Grattan C, Powell S, Humphreys F. Management and diagnostic guidelines for urticaria and angio-oedema. *Br J Dermatol.* 2001;144:708-714.
9. Lin RY, Curry A, Pesola GR, et al. Improved outcomes in patients with acute allergic syndromes who are treated with combined H1 and H2 antagonists. *Ann Emerg Med.* 2000;36:462-468.
10. Goldsobel AB, Rohr AS, Siegel SC, et al. Efficacy of doxepin in the treatment of chronic idiopathic urticaria. *J Allergy Clin Immunol.* 1986;78:867-873.
11. Weinstein ME, Wolff AH, Bielory L. Efficacy and tolerability of second- and third-generation antihistamines in the treatment of acquired cold urticaria: a meta-analysis. *Ann Allergy Asthma Immunol.* 2010;104:518-522.
12. Pollack CV Jr, Romano TJ. Outpatient management of acute urticaria: the role of prednisone. *Ann Emerg Med.* 1995;26:547-551.
13. Vena GA, Cassano N, D'Argento V, Milani M. Clobetasol propionate 0.05% in a novel foam formulation is safe and effective in the short-term treatment of patients with delayed pressure urticaria: a randomized, double-blind, placebo-controlled trial. *Br J Dermatol.* 2006;154:353-356.
14. Sagi L, Solomon M, Baum S, et al. Evidence for methotrexate as a useful treatment for steroid-dependent chronic urticaria. *Acta Derm Venereol.* 2011;91:303-306.
15. Stolz LE, Horn PT. Ecallantide: a plasma kallikrein inhibitor for the treatment of acute attacks of hereditary angioedema. *Drugs Today (Barc).* 2010;46:547-555.

SECTION 7 PAPULOSQAMOUS CONDITIONS

149 SEBORRHEIC DERMATITIS

Richard P. Usatine, MD
Meredith Hancock, MD
Yoon-Soo Cindy Bae-Harboe, MD

PATIENT STORY

A 59-year-old man presents with a 3-month history of an itchy rash on his face (**Figure 149-1**)). He states that he has had this rash intermittently for many years, but had recently worsened. He denies any major risk factors for HIV and does not have Parkinson disease. He has been under more stress lately and has noticed that this rash flares when under increased stress. Note the scale visible on the forehead and under the eyebrows and beard. There is also some mild erythema on the cheeks and around the nasolabial folds. The diagnosis of seborrheic dermatitis is made and treatment is begun with appropriate topical agents to treat the inflammation and the *Malassezia*. On the following visit, the patient has complete clearance of his seborrheic dermatitis.

INTRODUCTION

Seborrheic dermatitis is a common, chronic, relapsing dermatitis affecting sebum-rich areas of the body. Infants and adults, men and women may be affected. Presentation may vary from mild erythema to greasy scales, and rarely as erythroderma. Treatment is targeted to reduce inflammation and irritation as well as eliminate *Malassezia* fungus whose exact role is not completely understood.

SYNONYMS

Seborrheic dermatitis is also known as seborrhea, seborrheic eczema, and dandruff.

EPIDEMIOLOGY

- Seborrheic dermatitis is most commonly seen in male patients aged 20 to 50 years. The prevalence is approximately 3% to 5% in healthy young adults who are HIV negative.[1] More people may be affected, but do not seek medical attention for mild cases.
- The prevalence is higher in immunocompromised persons (eg, HIV positive/AIDS); however, the vast majority of affected persons have a normal immune system.
- More common in persons with Parkinson disease.
- Infants can have seborrhea of the scalp (cradle cap), face, and diaper area.

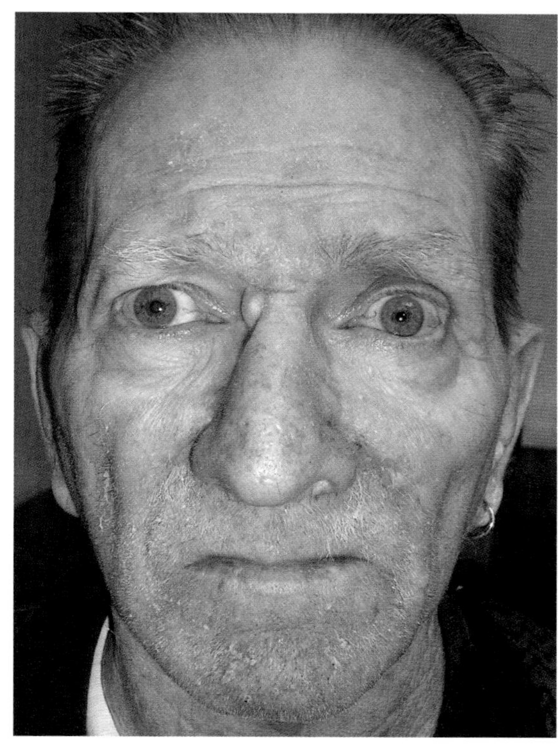

A

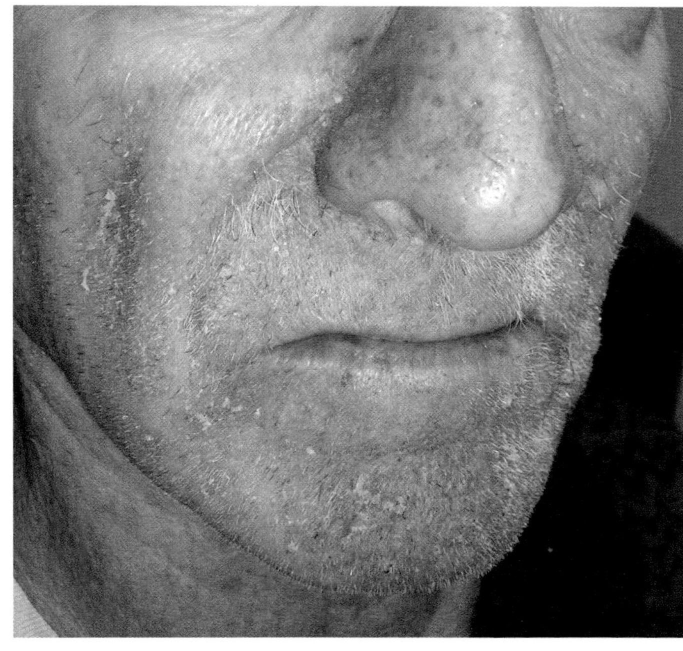

B

FIGURE 149-1 Seborrheic dermatitis following the typical distribution on the face of a 59-year-old man. **A.** Note the prominent scale and erythema on his forehead, glabella, and beard region. **B.** Close-up of seborrheic dermatitis showing the flaking scale and erythema around the beard region. (*Reproduced with permission from Richard P. Usatine, MD.*)

ETIOLOGY AND PATHOPHYSIOLOGY

- Seborrheic dermatitis is a chronic, superficial, localized inflammatory dermatitis that is found in sebum-producing areas of the body.
- The actual cause of seborrheic dermatitis is not well understood. It appears to be related to the interplay between host susceptibility, environmental factors, and local immune response to antigens.[2-4]
- Patients with seborrheic dermatitis may be colonized with certain species of lipophilic yeast of the genus *Malassezia* (also called *Pityrosporum)*. However, *Malassezia* is considered normal skin flora and unaffected persons also may be colonized.
- Recent evidence suggests that *Malassezia* may produce different irritants or metabolites on affected skin.[4]

RISK FACTORS

- Male gender.
- Immunocompromise (HIV/AIDS, Parkinson disease).
- Stress.
- Environmental factors (cold, dry weather).
- Certain medications may cause seborrheic dermatitis to flare. These medications include captopril, cimetidine, interleukin-2, isotretinoin, nicotine, and psoralens.[5-9]

DIAGNOSIS

The clinical diagnosis is made by history and physical examination. **Figures 149-1** and **149-2** reveal erythema and scale across the eyebrows, cheeks, and under beard. Biopsy is not generally indicated unless ruling out other possibilities (see Differential Diagnosis).

CLINICAL FEATURES

- Chronic skin condition is characterized by remissions and exacerbations.

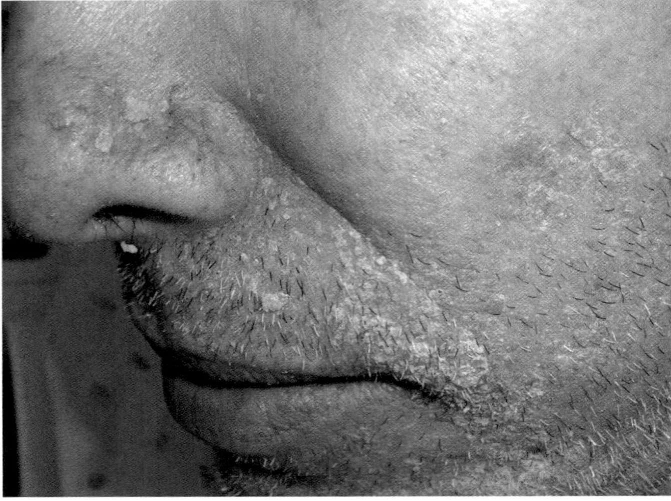

FIGURE 149-2 Severe seborrheic dermatitis on the face of a hospitalized man. The stress of his illness has worsened his otherwise mild seborrhea. (*Reproduced with permission from Richard P. Usatine, MD.*)

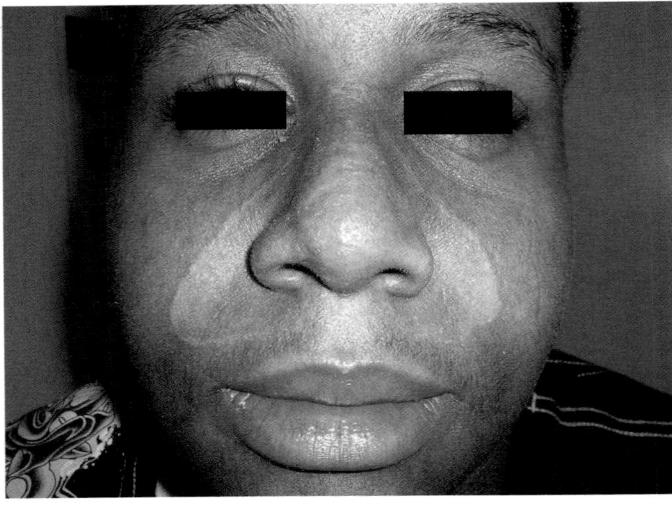

FIGURE 149-3 Seborrheic dermatitis in a black man with hypopigmentation and erythema related to the inflammation. Note the prominent involvement in the nasolabial folds and the well-demarcated borders. (*Reproduced with permission from Richard P. Usatine, MD.*)

- Poorly-demarcated, erythematous plaques of greasy, yellow scale, in the characteristic seborrheic distribution (see description below).
- Common precipitating factors are stress, immunosuppression, and cold weather.
- Face, scalp, and ears may be very pruritic.
- May be the presenting sign of HIV seropositivity.
- In dark-skinned individuals, the involved skin and scale may become hypopigmented (**Figure 149-3**) or hyperpigmented (**Figure 149-4**).

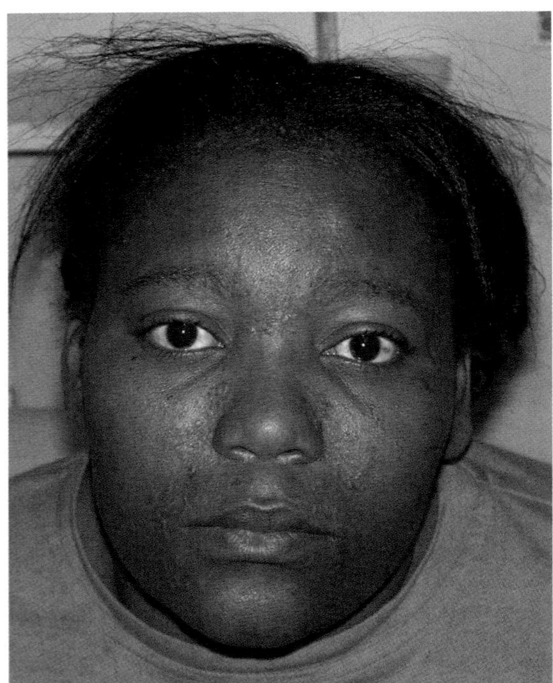

FIGURE 149-4 Seborrhea in a black woman with hyperpigmentation related to the inflammation. Note the prominent involvement in the nasolabial folds. (*Reproduced with permission from Richard P. Usatine, MD.*)

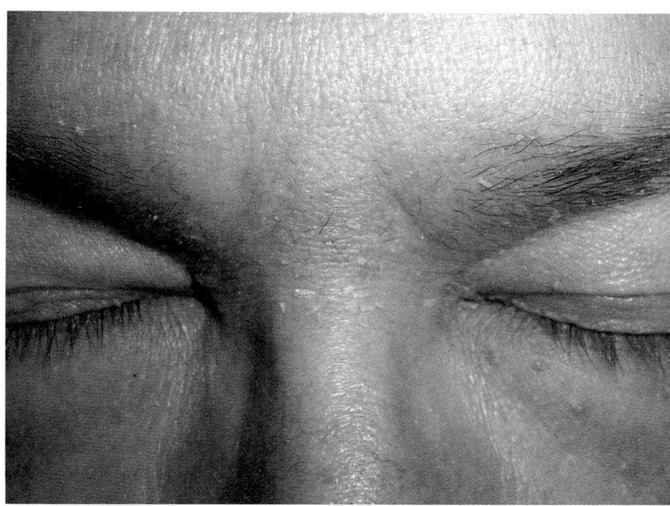

FIGURE 149-5 Seborrheic dermatitis with erythema and scale under the eyebrows and in the glabella region on a young man. (*Reproduced with permission from Richard P. Usatine, MD.*)

TYPICAL DISTRIBUTION

Occurs on scalp (ie, dandruff), eyebrows **(Figures 149-5)**, nasolabial creases **(see Figures 149-3)**, forehead **(Figures 149-6)**, cheeks, around the nose, behind the ears **(Figure 149-7)**, external auditory meatus, and under facial hair **(Figure 149-8)**. Seborrhea can also occur over the sternum **(Figures 149-9)** and in the axillae, submammary folds, umbilicus, groin, and gluteal creases.

LABORATORY STUDIES

- Test for HIV and/or syphilis if patient has risk factors **(Figures 149-10 and 149-11)**.

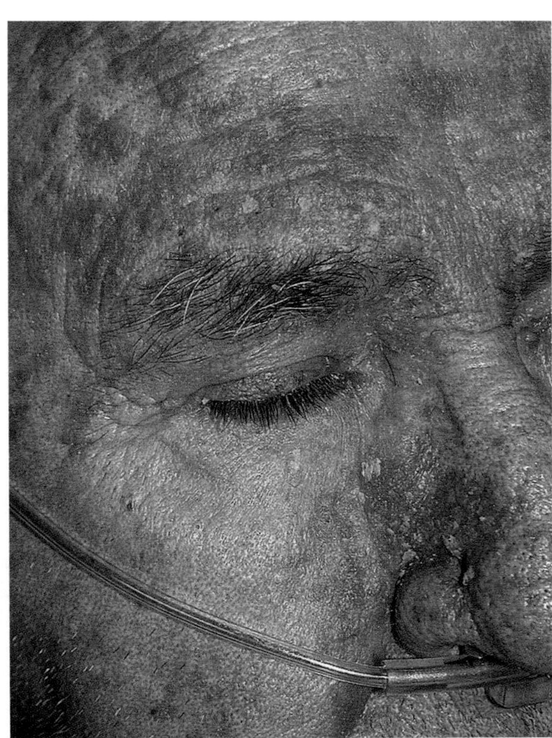

FIGURE 149-6 Seborrheic dermatitis with erythema and scale on the forehead and nose of an older man in the hospital. (*Reproduced with permission from Suraj Reddy, MD.*)

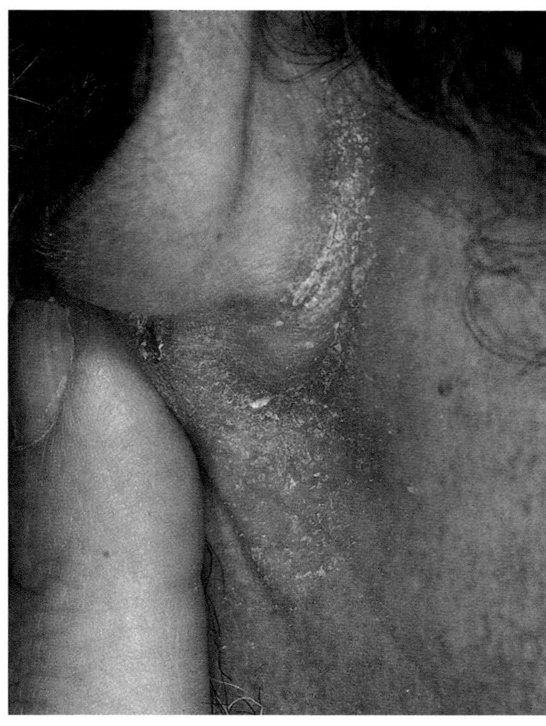

FIGURE 149-7 Seborrheic dermatitis behind the ear in a young woman. This is a good place to look for evidence of seborrhea. (*Reproduced with permission from Richard P. Usatine, MD.*)

- Also consider testing for systemic lupus erythematosus (SLE) in setting of associated systemic symptoms or if treatment resistant.
- Consider potassium hydroxide (KOH) test to rule out tinea.
- Consider zinc level or alkaline phosphatase to rule out nutritional/zinc deficiency.

DIFFERENTIAL DIAGNOSIS

- Psoriasis—The scale of psoriasis tends to be thicker, on well-demarcated plaques distributed over extensor surfaces along with the scalp.

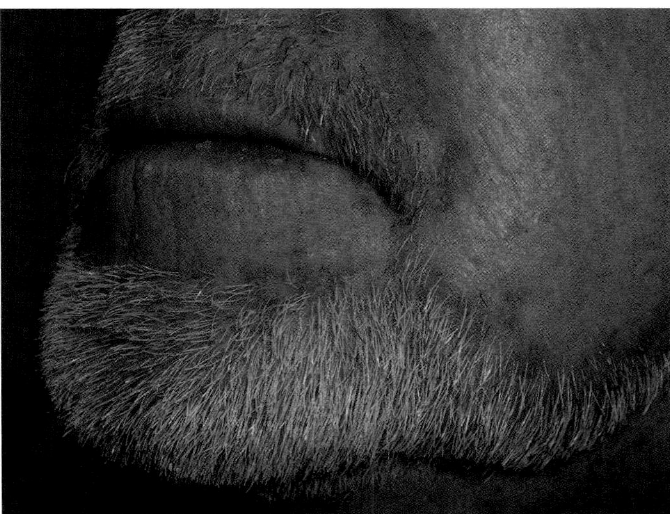

FIGURE 149-8 Seborrhea of the beard and mustache distribution with prominent erythema. (*Reproduced with permission from Richard P. Usatine, MD.*)

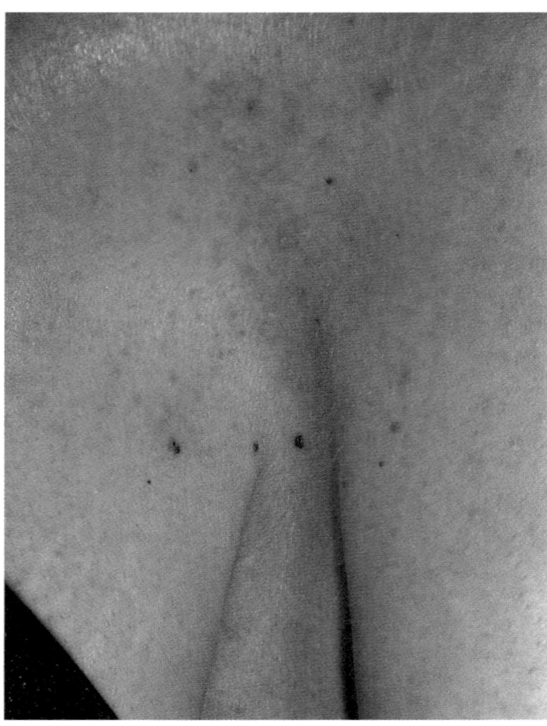

FIGURE 149-9 Seborrheic dermatitis on the chest and between the breasts of a woman that also has seborrhea of the scalp and face. This is one of the more common locations to see seborrheic dermatitis on the trunk. (*Reproduced with permission from Richard P. Usatine, MD.*)

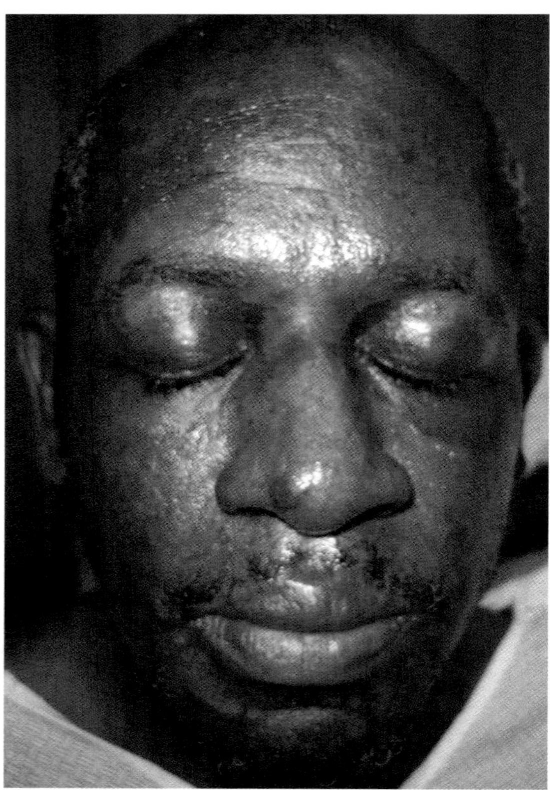

FIGURE 149-10 Seborrheic dermatitis on the face of a man with AIDS. Note the involvement of the forehead, cheeks, and chin causing hypopigmentation and scaling. (*Reproduced with permission from Yoon-Soo Cindy Bae-Harboe, MD.*)

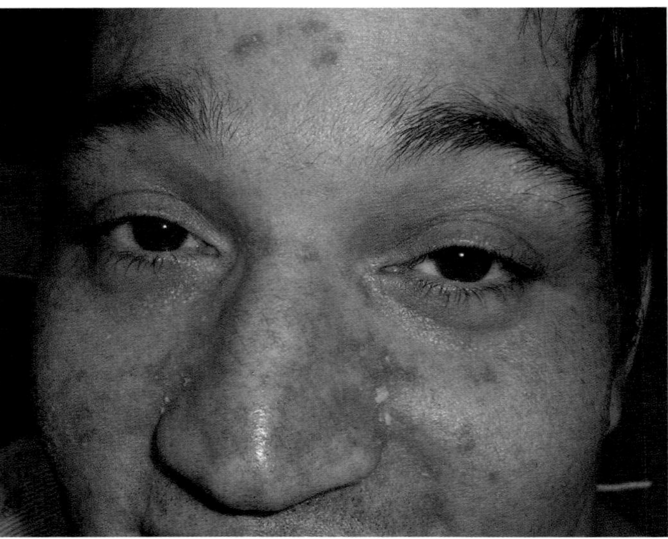

FIGURE 149-11 Seborrheic dermatitis on the face of a man with AIDS. Note erythema and scale on the forehead, nose, and cheeks. (*Reproduced with permission from Richard P. Usatine, MD.*)

Look for signs of nail involvement that may support the diagnosis of psoriasis (see Chapter 150, Psoriasis).

- SLE with butterfly rash—Rash across nasal bridge in patient with associated systemic symptoms and abnormal blood tests (see Chapter 178, Lupus Erythematosus—Systemic and Cutaneous).
- Rosacea—The erythema on the face is often associated with papules, pustules, telangiectasia, and an absence of scales. May also present with chalazia or hordeola (see Chapter 115, Rosacea).
- Tinea capitis—Scale and erythema commonly associated with hair loss. KOH and/or culture can help make the distinction. This is rare in adults but may be seen in adolescents.
- Secondary syphilis—Skin presentation may mimic seborrheic dermatitis. Examine patient for mucosal or palmar involvement. Laboratory testing for syphilis may be necessary if this is suspected (see Chapter 218, Syphilis).
- Perioral dermatitis—Usually restricted around the mouth with minimal scale and fine papules and pustules (see Chapter 115, Rosacea).
- Tinea versicolor (trunk)—The scale of tinea versicolor is fine and white and scales with scraping (see Chapter 139, Tinea Versicolor).
- Allergic or irritant contact dermatitis—May present with a well-demarcated lesion with fine white scale, secondarily impetiginized lesions may have associated yellow-colored crust, not scale (see Chapter 144, Contact Dermatitis).
- Candidiasis—May be found in intertriginous areas, but present bright red with satellite lesions (see Chapter 135, Mucocutaneous Candidiasis).

MANAGEMENT

As seborrheic dermatitis is a recurrent, chronic condition, repeated and/or maintenance therapy is often required.

- Mainstay of treatment is topical antifungals and low-potency topical steroids.
- For seborrheic dermatitis of the scalp, patients should wash their hair with antifungal shampoos (containing selenium sulfide, ketoconazole, or

ciclopirox) several times per week, each time leaving the lather on the affected areas for several minutes until remission is attained. Patients may continue to use antifungal shampoo as maintenance therapy.[3]

- Shampoos containing ketoconazole, selenium sulfide, or zinc pyrithione (ZPT) are active against the *Malassezia* and are effective in the treatment of moderate-to-severe dandruff.[10,11] SOR Ⓐ
- Ketoconazole 2% shampoo was found to be superior to zinc pyrithione 1% shampoo when used twice weekly. Ketoconazole led to a 73% improvement in the total dandruff severity score compared with 67% for ZPT 1% at week 4.[11] SOR Ⓑ
- Ciclopirox 1% shampoo is effective and safe in the treatment of seborrheic dermatitis of the scalp.[12,13] SOR Ⓐ It is by prescription only and is very expensive.
- Ketoconazole 2% cream, gel, or emulsion is safe and effective for facial seborrheic dermatitis.[14-16] SOR Ⓑ
- Ciclopirox 1% cream is also safe and effective for facial seborrheic dermatitis and is equivalent to ketoconazole 2% cream.[14,17] SOR Ⓑ
- Oral terbinafine 250 mg daily for 4 weeks is effective for moderate-to-severe seborrhea.[18,19] SOR Ⓐ However, due to the potential for harmful side effects of oral antifungals and the limited study of their efficacy, they are not first-line treatments.[3] Oral terbinafine may be considered in erythroderma caused by seborrhea.

Topical corticosteroids are useful in treating associated erythema and pruritis.[3] Long-term use may lead to skin atrophy[3] and should be used with caution.

- Lotion or solution is preferable on hair-covered area for patient comfort and usability.
- Hydrocortisone 1% cream or lotion can be used bid to face, scalp, or other affected areas.[16,20] SOR Ⓑ
- Desonide 0.05% lotion is safe and effective for short-term treatment of seborrheic dermatitis of the face.[21] SOR Ⓑ It is a nonfluorinated low- to mid-potency steroid that is higher in potency than 1% hydrocortisone.
- For moderate to severe seborrheic dermatitis on the scalp.
- Fluocinonide 0.05% solution once daily is affordable and beneficial. SOR Ⓒ
- Clobetasol 0.05% shampoo, solution, spray, or foam work well but are more costly. SOR Ⓒ

OTHER TREATMENTS

- Pimecrolimus 1% cream is an effective and well-tolerated treatment for facial seborrheic dermatitis.[20,22,23] SOR Ⓑ In one study, there was more burning noted with the pimecrolimus than with the betamethasone 17-valerate 0.1% cream.[22]
- Metronidazole gel—Two small studies have found different results in the treatment of seborrheic dermatitis on the face. One suggests it works better than the vehicle alone and the other found no statistically significant difference from placebo.[24,25] SOR Ⓑ

COMPLIMENTARY AND ALTERNATIVE THERAPY

- Tea tree oil 5% shampoo showed a 41% improvement in the quadrant-area-severity score compared with 11% in the placebo. Statistically significant improvements were also observed in the total area of involvement score, the total severity score, and the itchiness and greasiness components of the patients' self-assessments.[26] SOR Ⓑ
- One small randomized controlled trial (RCT) using homeopathic medication consisting of potassium bromide, sodium bromide, nickel sulfate, and sodium chloride for 10 weeks showed significant improvement over placebo.[27] SOR Ⓒ

PATIENT EDUCATION

For improved treatment results, encourage patients to wash the hair and scalp daily with an antifungal shampoo. Some patients fear that washing their hair too often will cause a "dry" scalp and need to understand that the scaling and flaking will improve rather than worsen with more frequent hair washing.

FOLLOW-UP

Patients with long-standing and severe seborrhea will appreciate a follow-up visit in most cases. Milder cases can be followed as needed.

PATIENT RESOURCES

- PubMed Health. *Seborrheic Dermatitis*—**http://www.ncbi.nlm.nih.gov/pubmedhealth/PMH0001959/.**

PROVIDER RESOURCES

- Medscape. *Seborrheic Dermatitis*—**http://emedicine.medscape.com/article/1108312.**

REFERENCES

1. Usatine RP. A red rash on the face. *J Fam Pract.* 2003;52:697-699.
2. Gaitanis G, Magiatis P, Hantschke M, Bassukas ID, Velegraki A. The Malassezia genus in skin and systemic diseases. *Clin Microbiol Rev.* 2012;25(1):106.
3. Naldi L, Rebora A. Seborrheic dermatitis. *N Engl J Med.* 2009;360(4):387-396.
4. Hay RJ. Malassezia, dandruff and seborrheic dermatitis: an overview. *Br J Dermatol.* 2011;165(suppl 2):2-8.
5. Yamamoto T, Tsuboi R. Interleukin-2-induced seborrheic dermatitis-like eruption. *J Eur Acad Dermatol Venereol.* 2008;22(2):244-245.
6. Sudan BJ, Brouillard C, Sterboul J, Sainte-Laudy J. Nicotine as a hapten in seborrheic dermatitis. *Contact Dermatitis.* 1984;11(3):196-197.
7. Kitamura K, Aihara M, Osawa J, Naito S, Ikezawa Z. Sulfhydryl drug-induced eruption: a clinical and histological study. *J Dermatol.* 1990;17(1):44-51.
8. Tegner E. Seborrheic dermatitis of the face induced by PUVA treatment. *Acta Derm Venereol.* 1983;63(4):335-339.
9. Barzilai A, David M, Trau H, Hodak E. Seborrheic dermatitis-like eruption in patients taking isotretinoin therapy for acne: retrospective study of five patients. *Am J Clin Dermatol.* 2008;9(4):255-261.
10. Danby FW, Maddin WS, Margesson LJ, Rosenthal D. A randomized, double-blind, placebo-controlled trial of ketoconazole 2% shampoo versus selenium sulfide 2.5% shampoo in the treatment of moderate to severe dandruff. *J Am Acad Dermatol.* 1993;29:1008-1012.

11. Pierard-Franchimont C. A multicenter randomized trial of ketoconazole 2% and zinc pyrithione 1% shampoos in severe dandruff and seborrheic dermatitis. *Skin Pharmacol Appl Skin Physiol.* 2002;15(6):434-441.

12. Aly R. Ciclopirox gel for seborrheic dermatitis of the scalp. *Int J Dermatol.* 2003;42(suppl 1):19-22.

13. Lebwohl M, Plott T. Safety and efficacy of ciclopirox 1% shampoo for the treatment of seborrheic dermatitis of the scalp in the US population: results of a double-blind, vehicle-controlled trial. *Int J Dermatol.* 2004;43(suppl 1):17-20.

14. Chosidow O, Maurette C, Dupuy P. Randomized, open-labeled, non-inferiority study between ciclopiroxolamine 1% cream and ketoconazole 2% foaming gel in mild to moderate facial seborrheic dermatitis. *Dermatology.* 2003;206:233-240.

15. Pierard GE, Pierard-Franchimont C, Van CJ, Rurangirwa A, Hoppenbrouwers ML, Schrooten P. Ketoconazole 2% emulsion in the treatment of seborrheic dermatitis. *Int J Dermatol.* 1991;30:806-809.

16. Katsambas A, Antoniou C, Frangouli E, Avgerinou G, Michailidis D, Stratigos J. A double-blind trial of treatment of seborrheic dermatitis with 2% ketoconazole cream compared with 1% hydrocortisone cream. *Br J Dermatol.* 1989;121:353-357.

17. Dupuy P, Maurette C, Amoric JC, Chosidow O. Randomized, placebo-controlled, double-blind study on clinical efficacy of ciclopiroxolamine 1% cream in facial seborrheic dermatitis. *Br J Dermatol.* 2001;149:1033-1037.

18. Vena GA, Micali G, Santoianni P, Cassano N, Peruzzi E. Oral terbinafine in the treatment of multi-site seborrheic dermatitis: a multicenter, double-blind placebo-controlled study. *Int J Immunopathol Pharmacol.* 2005;18:745-753.

19. Scaparro E, Quadri G, Virno G, Orifici C, Milani M. Evaluation of the efficacy and tolerability of oral terbinafine (Daskil) in patients with seborrheic dermatitis. A multicentre, randomized, investigator-blinded, placebo-controlled trial. *Br J Dermatol.* 2001; 149(4):854-857.

20. Firooz A, Solhpour A, Gorouhi F, et al. Pimecrolimus cream, 1%, vs hydrocortisone acetate cream, 1%, in the treatment of facial seborrheic dermatitis: a randomized, investigator-blind, clinical trial. *Arch Dermatol.* 2006;142:1066-1067.

21. Freeman SH. Efficacy, cutaneous tolerance and cosmetic acceptability of desonide 0.05% lotion (Desowen) versus vehicle in the short-term treatment of facial atopic or seborrheic dermatitis. *Australas J Dermatol.* 2002;43(3):186-189.

22. Rigopoulos D, Ioannides D, Kalogeromitros D, Gregoriou S, Katsambas A. Pimecrolimus cream 1% vs. betamethasone 17-valerate 0.1% cream in the treatment of seborrheic dermatitis. A randomized open-label clinical trial. *Br J Dermatol.* 2004;149:1071-1075.

23. Warshaw EM, Wohlhuter RJ, Liu A, et al. Results of a randomized, double-blind, vehicle-controlled efficacy trial of pimecrolimus cream 1% for the treatment of moderate to severe facial seborrheic dermatitis. *J Am Acad Dermatol.* 2007;57(2):257-264.

24. Parsad D, Pandhi R, Negi KS, Kumar B. Topical metronidazole in seborrheic dermatitis—a double-blind study. *Dermatology.* 2001; 202:35-37.

25. Koca R. Is topical metronidazole effective in seborrheic dermatitis? A double-blind study. *Int J Dermatol.* 2003;42(8):632-635.

26. Satchell AC, Saurajen A, Bell C, Barnetson RS. Treatment of dandruff with 5% tea tree oil shampoo. *J Am Acad Dermatol.* 2002;47(6): 852-855.

27. Smith SA, Baker AE, Williams JH. Effective treatment of seborrheic dermatitis using a low dose, oral homeopathic medication consisting of potassium bromide, sodium bromide, nickel sulfate, and sodium chloride in a double-blind, placebo-controlled study. *Altern Med Rev.* 2002;7(1):59-67.

150 PSORIASIS

Richard P. Usatine, MD

PATIENT STORY

A 33-year-old woman presents with uncontrolled psoriasis for 20 years. In addition to the plaque psoriasis (**Figure 150-1**), she has inverse psoriasis (**Figure 150-2**). Topical ultrahigh-potency steroids and topical calcipotriol have not controlled her psoriasis. The options for phototherapy and systemic therapy were discussed. The patient chose to try narrowband ultraviolet B (UVB) treatment in addition to her topical therapy.

INTRODUCTION

Psoriasis is a chronic inflammatory papulosquamous and immune-mediated skin disorder. It is also associated with joint and cardiovascular comorbidities. Psoriasis can present in many different patterns from the scalp to the feet and cause psychiatric distress and physical disabilities. It is crucial to be able to identify psoriasis in all its myriad presentations so that patients receive the best possible treatments to improve their quality of life and avoid comorbidities.

EPIDEMIOLOGY

Psoriasis affects approximately 2% of the world population.[1] The prevalence of psoriasis was 2.5% in white patients and was 1.3% in African American patients in one population study in the United States.[2]

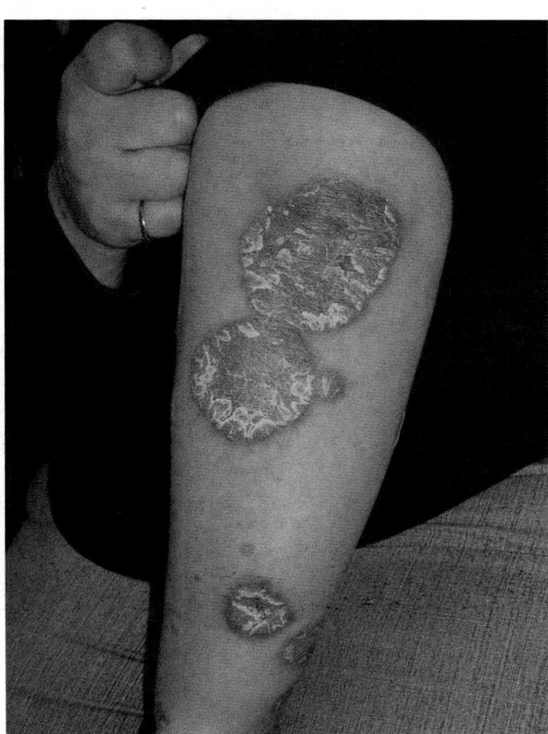

FIGURE 150-1 Typical plaque psoriasis on the elbow and arm of a 33-year-old woman. (*Reproduced with permission from Richard P. Usatine, MD.*)

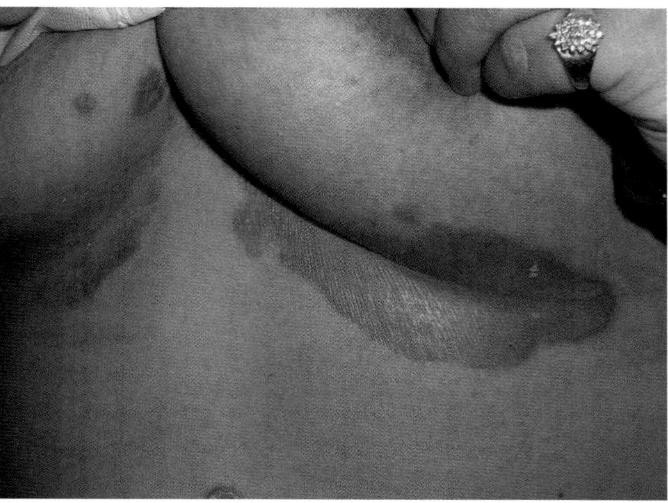

FIGURE 150-2 Inverse psoriasis in the inframammary folds of the patient in Figure 150-1. This is not a *Candida* or tinea infection. (*Reproduced with permission from Richard P. Usatine, MD.*)

- Sex—No gender preference.
- Age—Psoriasis can begin at any age. In one population study of the age of onset of psoriasis 2 peaks were revealed, one occurring at the age of 16 years (female) or 22 years (males) and a second peak at the age of 60 years (female) or 57 years (males).[3]

ETIOLOGY AND PATHOPHYSIOLOGY

- Immune-mediated skin disease, where the T cell plays a pivotal role in the pathogenesis of the disease.
- Langerhans cells (antigen-presenting cells in the skin) migrate from the skin to regional lymph nodes, where they activate T cells that migrate to the skin and release cytokines.
- Cytokines are responsible for epidermal and vascular hyperproliferation and proinflammatory effects.

RISK FACTORS

- Family history
- Obesity
- Smoking and environmental smoke
- Heavy alcohol use

Table 150-1 lists the factors that trigger and exacerbate psoriasis.[4] The risk of psoriasis is higher in the following occurrences[5]:

- Family history of psoriasis (odds ratio [OR] = 33.96; 95% confidence interval [CI] 14.14-81.57)
- Change in work conditions (OR = 8.34; 95% CI = 1.86-37.43)
- Divorce (OR = 5.69; 95% CI = 2.26-14.34)
- Urban dwellers (OR = 3.61; 95% CI = 0.99-13.18)
- Alcohol consumption (OR = 2.55; 95% CI = 1.26-5.17)
- Environmental tobacco smoke at home (OR = 2.29; 95% CI = 1.12-4.67)

TABLE 150-1 Factors That Trigger and Exacerbate Psoriasis

- Stress
- Physical trauma to the skin (Koebner phenomenon)
- Cold dry weather
- Sun exposure and hot weather
- Infections (eg, strep throat, HIV)
- Medications (eg, ACE-inhibitors, antimalarials, β-blockers, lithium, NSAIDs)

DIAGNOSIS

Psoriasis has many forms and locations. These 9 categories were used to describe psoriasis in a consensus statement of the American Academy of Dermatology (AAD)[6]:

1. Plaque (80%-90% of patients with psoriasis) (**Figures 150-1** and **150-3**)
2. Scalp psoriasis (**Figure 150-4**)
3. Guttate psoriasis (**Figure 150-5**)
4. Inverse psoriasis (**Figures 150-2** and **150-6**)
5. Palmar-plantar psoriasis (**Figure 150-7**), also known as palmoplantar psoriasis
6. Erythrodermic psoriasis (**Figure 150-8**)
7. Pustular psoriasis—localized and generalized (**Figure 150-9**)
8. Nail psoriasis (**Figure 150-10**) (see Chapter 193, Psoriatic Nails)
9. Psoriatic arthritis (**Figure 150-11**)

Typical distribution in general occurs at elbows, knees, extremities, trunk, scalp, face, ears, hands, feet, genitalia and intertriginous areas, and nails. **Table 150-2** provides percentages for the most common locations of lesions in patients with psoriasis.

Plaque psoriasis

- White scale on an erythematous raised base with well-demarcated borders (see **Figures 150-1** and **150-3**).

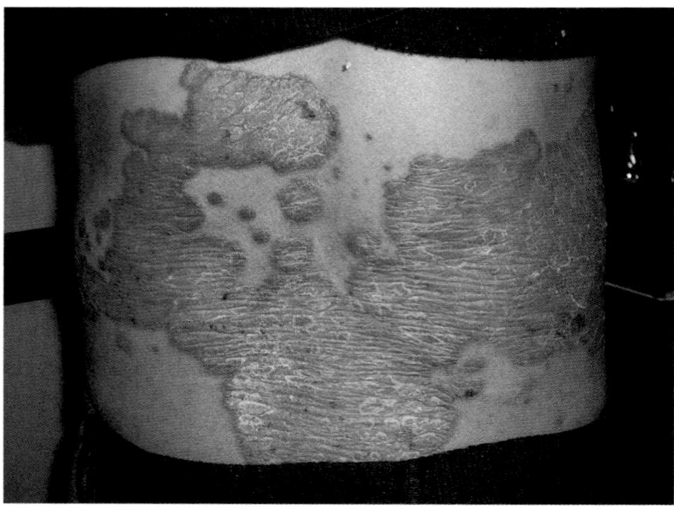

FIGURE 150-3 Well-demarcated plaques of plaque psoriasis in a 44-year-old man with severe psoriasis and psoriatic arthritis. (*Reproduced with permission from Richard P. Usatine, MD.*)

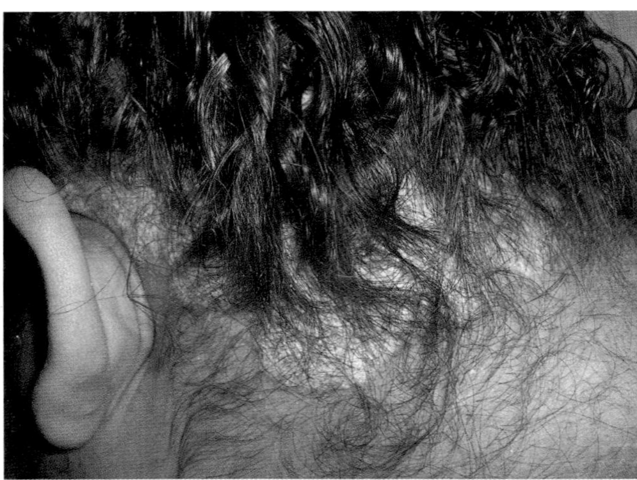

FIGURE 150-4 Scalp psoriasis visible at the hairline. (*Reproduced with permission from Richard P. Usatine, MD.*)

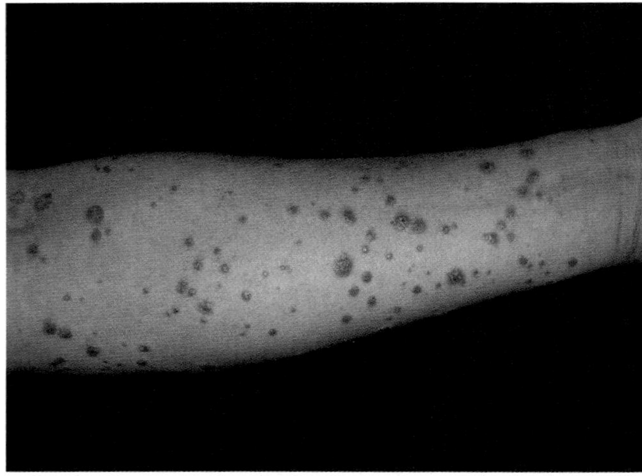

A

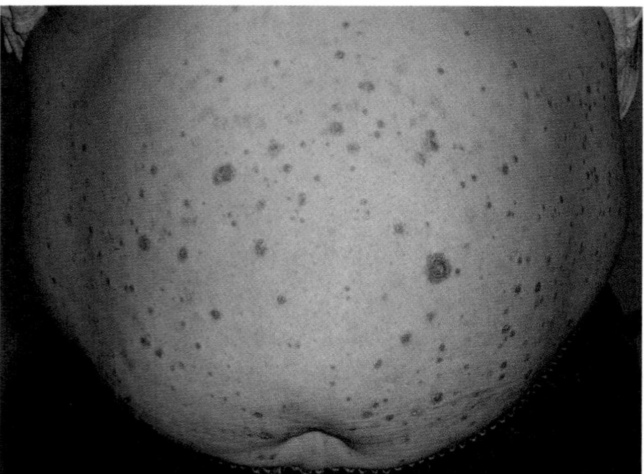

B

FIGURE 150-5 Guttate psoriasis may follow a strep pharyngitis in children and sometimes in young adults. However, small guttate (water drop) plaques may be seen in adults with psoriasis without any know preceding infections. **A.** Guttate psoriasis on the arm of an adult. **B.** Guttate psoriasis on the trunk of an obese 46-year-old woman. (*Reproduced with permission from Richard P. Usatine, MD.*)

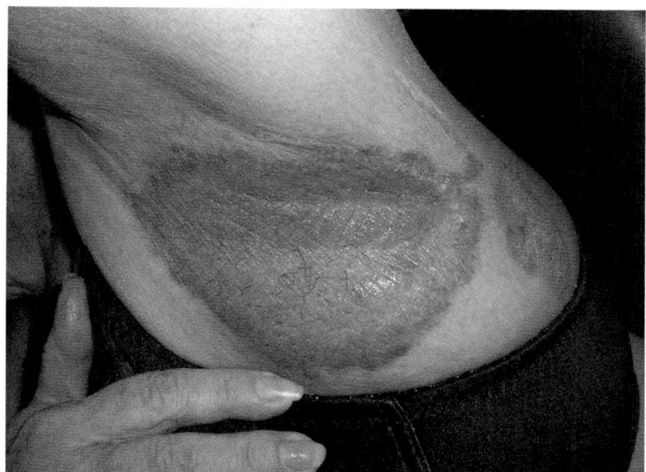

FIGURE 150-6 Inverse psoriasis in the axilla of this middle-aged woman. There is considerable erythema and very little scale. Prior to this visit her condition was misdiagnosed as fungal in origin. (*Reproduced with permission from Richard P. Usatine, MD.*)

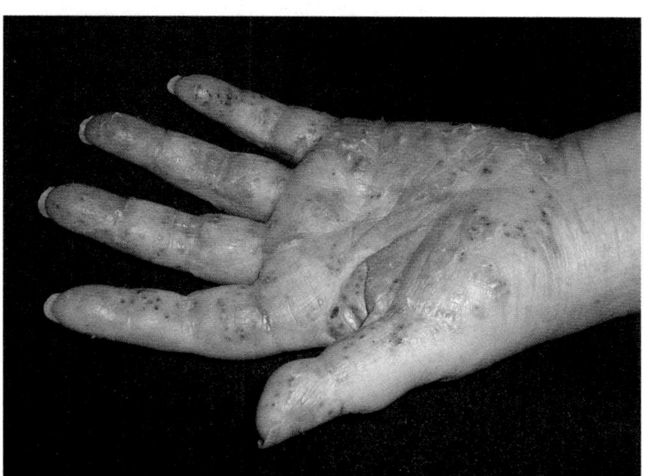

A

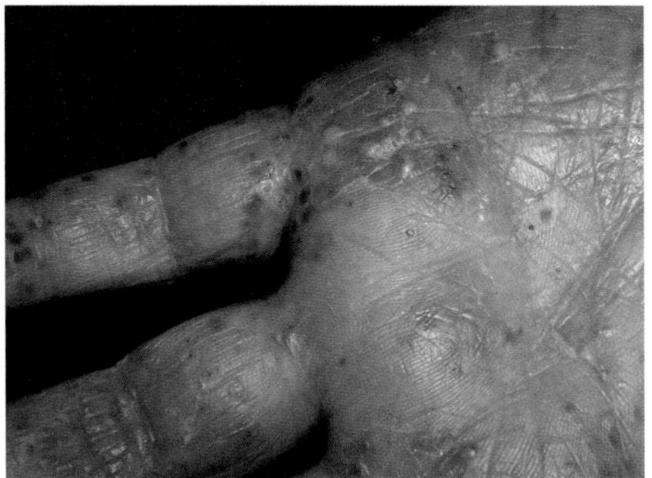

B

FIGURE 150-7 **A.** Palmoplantar psoriasis with pustulosis that started 3 months ago on the hands of a 62-year-old woman. **B.** Note the erythema, scale, brown macules (mahogany spots), and pustules that are typical of this condition. This is considered to be a localized form of pustular psoriasis. (*Reproduced with permission from Richard P. Usatine, MD.*)

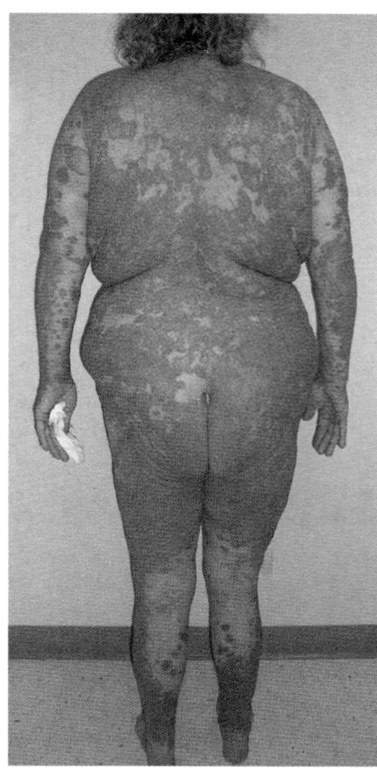

FIGURE 150-8 Erythrodermic psoriasis covering most of the body surface. (*Reproduced with permission from Richard P. Usatine, MD.*)

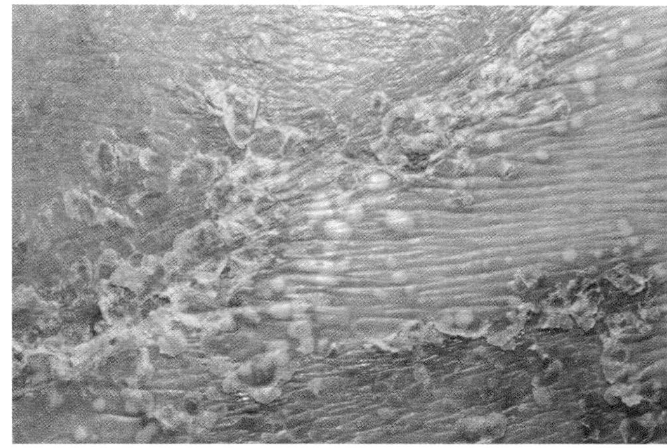

FIGURE 150-9 Pustular psoriasis on the back that occurred when oral prednisone was stopped. (*Reproduced with permission from Jack Resneck, Sr., MD.*)

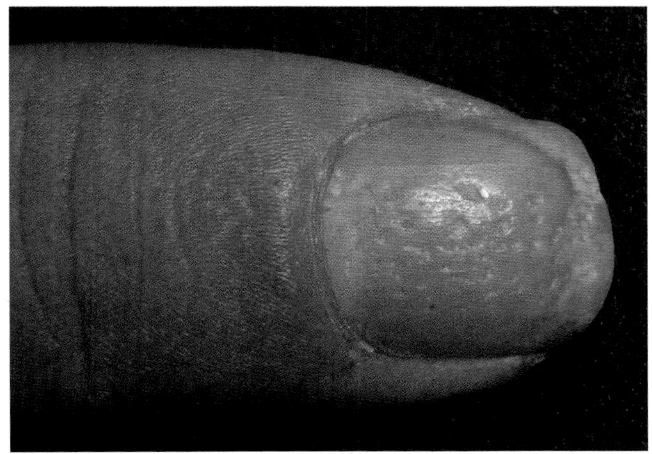

FIGURE 150-10 Nail pitting from psoriasis. (*Reproduced with permission from Richard P. Usatine, MD.*)

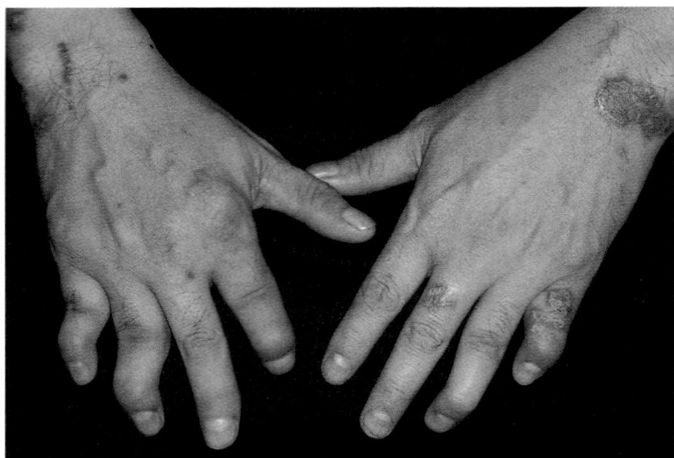

FIGURE 150-11 Psoriatic arthritis that has become crippling to this 44-year-old man. The shortening of the fingers fits the psoriatic arthritis mutilans subtype. (*Reproduced with permission from Richard P. Usatine, MD.*)

- Silvery scale with hyperpigmentation may be seen in patients with darker skin (**Figures 150-12** and **150-13**).
- Plaques can appear in different colors including hypopigmented (**Figure 150-14**) and silvery gray (**Figure 150-15**). A tricolored presentation occurs when the inflammation leads to leukoderma (**Figure 150-16**).
- The thickness and extent of the scale is variable (**see Figure 150-15**).
- Positive Auspitz sign in which the peeling of the scale produces pinpoint bleeding on the plaque below.
- Typical distribution includes the elbows and knees and other extensor surfaces. The plaques can be found from head to toe including the penis (**Figure 15-17**).
- Plaques tend to be symmetrically distributed.
- Plaques can be annular with central clearing (**Figure 150-18**).
- When plaques occur at a site of injury, it is known as the Koebner phenomenon (**Figure 150-19**).

TABLE 150-2 The Most Common Locations of Lesions in Patients With Psoriasis

Location	% of Psoriasis Patients
Scalp	80
Elbows	78
Legs	74
Knees	57
Arms	54
Trunk	53
Lower part of the body	47
Base of the back	38
Palms and soles	12

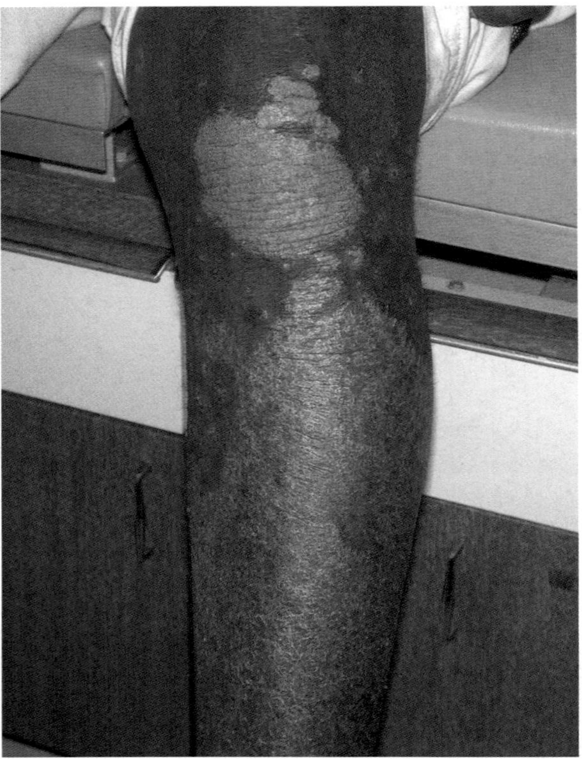

FIGURE 150-12 Plaque psoriasis with silvery scale on a black man. (*Reproduced with permission from Richard P. Usatine, MD.*)

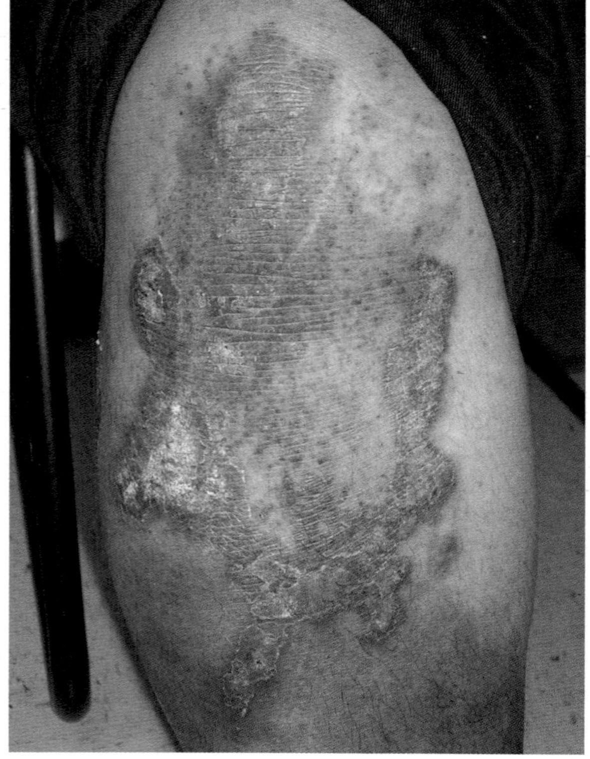

FIGURE 150-13 Psoriasis on the knee of a Hispanic man showing postinflammatory hyperpigmentation. (*Reproduced with permission from Richard P. Usatine, MD.*)

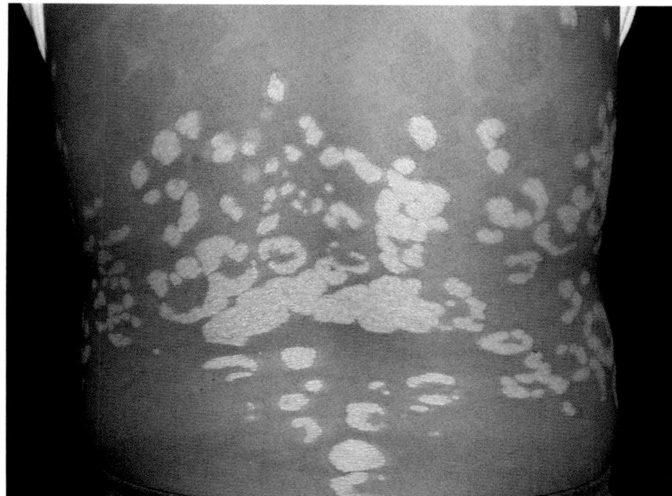

A

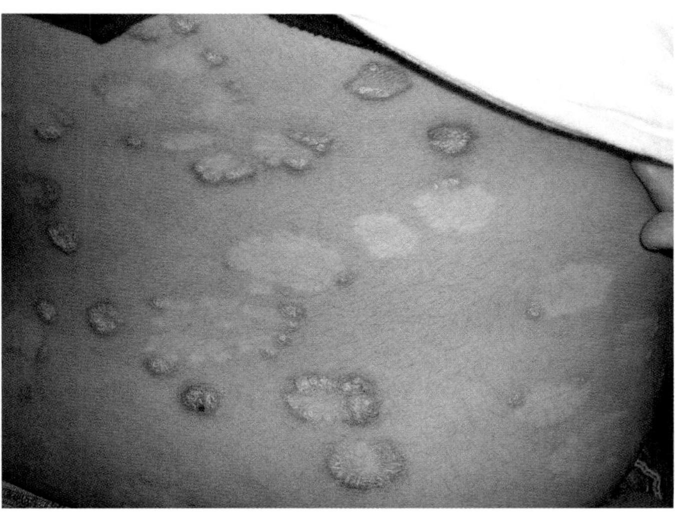

B

FIGURE 150-14 Plaque psoriasis can cause hypopigmentation. A. Hypopigmentation in areas of active plaques with postinflammatory hyperpigmentation visible on the upper back. B. Annular psoriatic plaques that leave hypopigmentation when they clear. (*Reproduced with permission from Richard P. Usatine, MD.*)

Scalp psoriasis

- Plaque on the scalp may be seen at the hairline and around the ears (see **Figure 150-4**).
- The thickness and extent of the plaques are variable as seen in plaque psoriasis.

Guttate psoriasis

- Small round plaques that resemble water drops (guttate means like a water drop) (**Figure 150-20**).
- Classically described as occurring after strep pharyngitis or another bacterial infection. This is one type of psoriasis that occurs in childhood.
- Typical distribution includes the trunk and extremities but may include the face and neck (**Figure 150-21**).

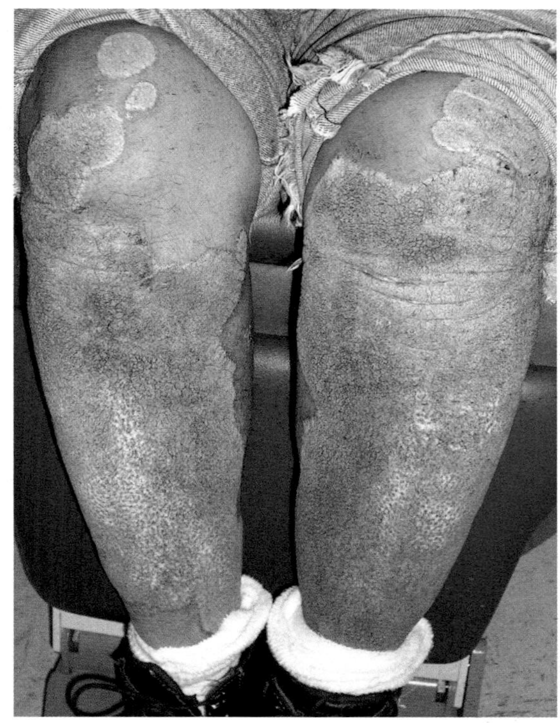

FIGURE 150-15 Thick plaque psoriasis covering the lower legs of this obese man. Note the silver gray color to his plaques. (*Reproduced with permission from Richard P. Usatine, MD.*)

Inverse psoriasis

- Found in the intertriginous areas of the axilla, groin, inframammary folds, and intergluteal fold (**Figures 150-2, 150-6**, and **150-22**). It can also be seen below the pannus or within adipose folds in obese individuals.
- The term *inverse* refers to the fact that the distribution is not on extensor surfaces but in areas of body folds.
- Morphologically the lesions have little to no visible scale.

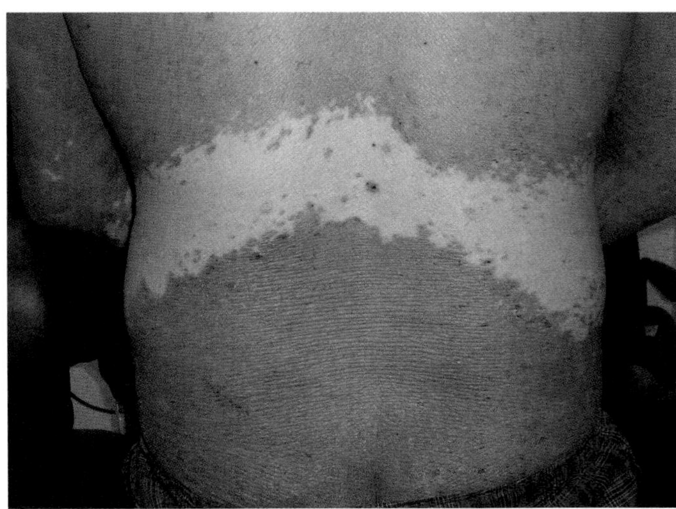

FIGURE 150-16 Plaque psoriasis that has caused hypopigmentation in a band across the back. His original skin color is brown so that the brown, white, and pink colors produce the appearance of a Neapolitan ice cream pattern. (*Reproduced with permission from Richard P. Usatine, MD.*)

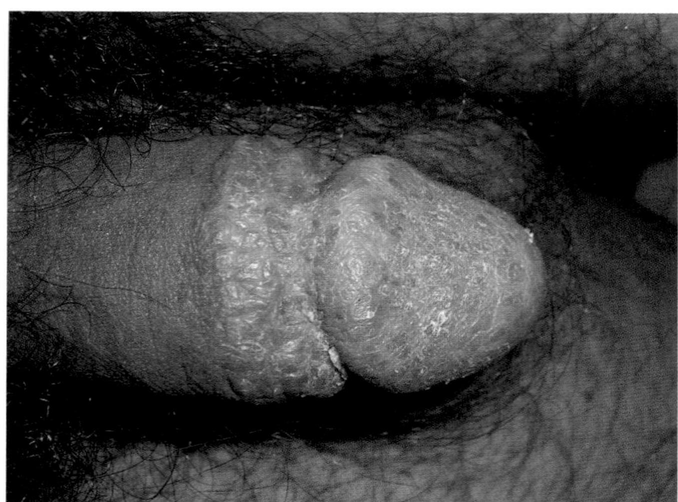

FIGURE 150-17 Plaque psoriasis on the penis, covering the glans and part of the shaft. (*Reproduced with permission from Richard P. Usatine, MD.*)

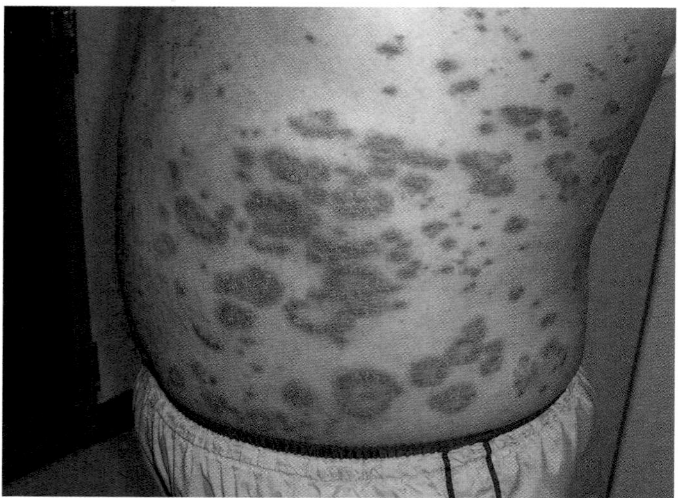

FIGURE 150-18 Plaque psoriasis with an annular configuration. (*Reproduced with permission from Richard P. Usatine, MD.*)

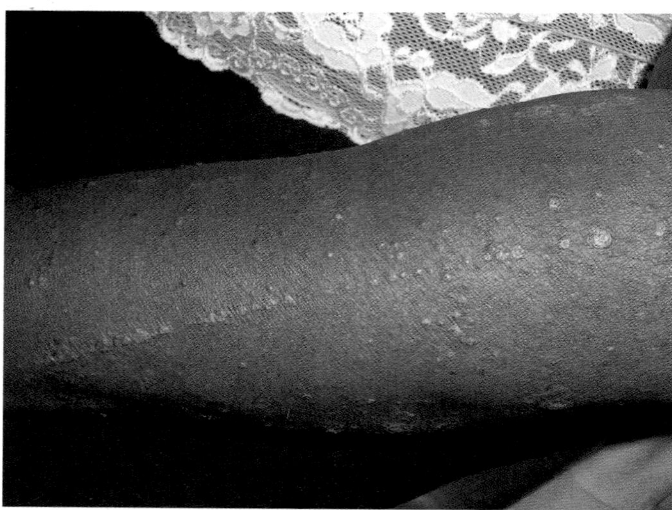

FIGURE 150-19 Linear distribution of psoriasis on the arm secondary to the Koebner phenomenon. (*Reproduced with permission from Richard P. Usatine, MD.*)

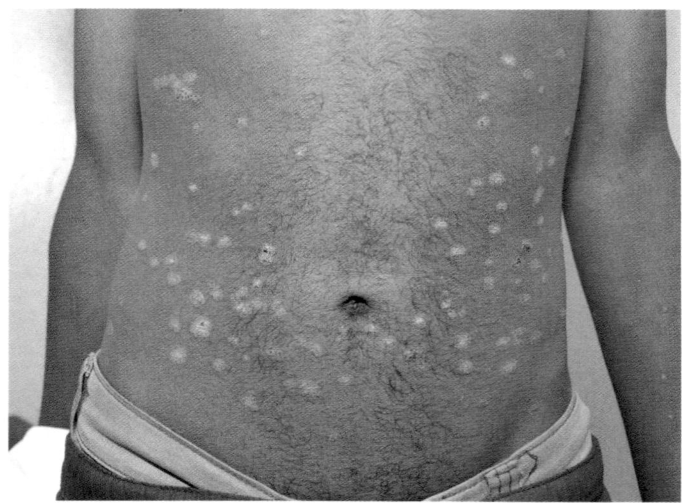

FIGURE 150-20 Guttate psoriasis in a young man following an episode of strep pharyngitis. (*Reproduced with permission from Richard P. Usatine, MD.*)

- Color is generally pink to red but can be hyperpigmented in dark-skinned individuals.

Palmar-plantar (palmoplantar) psoriasis

- Psoriasis occurs on the plantar aspects of the hands and feet (palms and soles) (**Figure 150-23**). The psoriasis can also be seen on other parts of the hands and feet.
- Patients with this type of psoriasis often experience severe foot and hand pain that can impair walking and other daily activities of living. Hand involvement can result in pain with many types of work.
- Morphologically this can be plaque like, vesicular, or pustular (**Figure 150-24**). Brown spots may be present as macules or flat papules. These are called mahogany spots and although they are not always present, they are characteristic of palmar-plantar psoriasis. Exfoliation of the skin can occur on the palms and soles.

Erythrodermic psoriasis

- Erythrodermic psoriasis is widespread and erythematosus covering most of the skin (**Figure 150-25**).

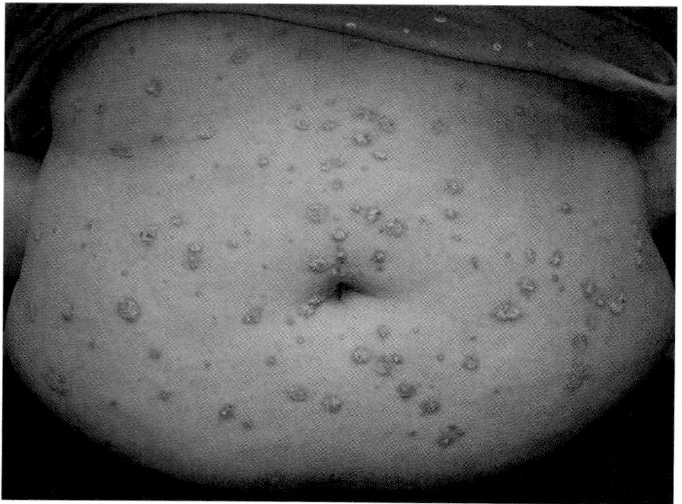

FIGURE 150-21 Guttate psoriasis with drop-like pink plaques on the trunk. (*Reproduced with permission from Richard P. Usatine, MD.*)

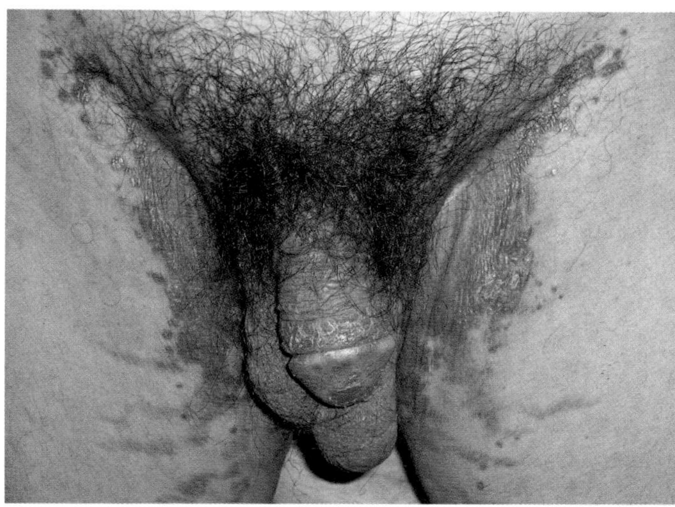

A

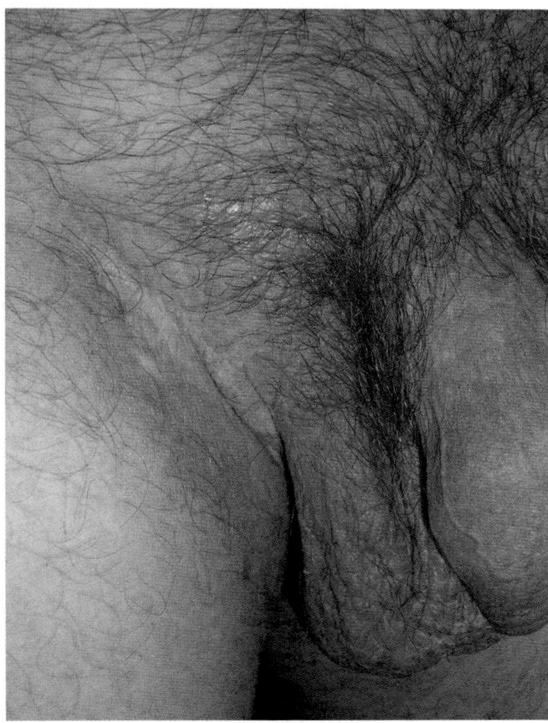

B

FIGURE 150-22 Two men with inverse psoriasis in the inguinal area. A. Erythema and scaling in inguinal folds with involvement on the penis. B. Inverse psoriasis in the inguinal area only sparing the penis. This was mistaken for tinea cruris for a long time. (*Reproduced with permission from Richard P. Usatine, MD.*)

- Morphologically, it can have plaques and erythema or the erythroderma can appear with the desquamation of pustular psoriasis.
- Widespread distribution can impair the important functions of the skin and this can be a dermatologic urgency requiring hospitalization and intravenous (IV) fluids. Chills, fever, tachycardia, and orthostatic hypotension are all signs that the patient may need hospitalization.

Pustular psoriasis

- Pustular psoriasis comes in localized and generalized types. One example of the local type is pustular psoriasis on the feet (see **Figure 150-24**).

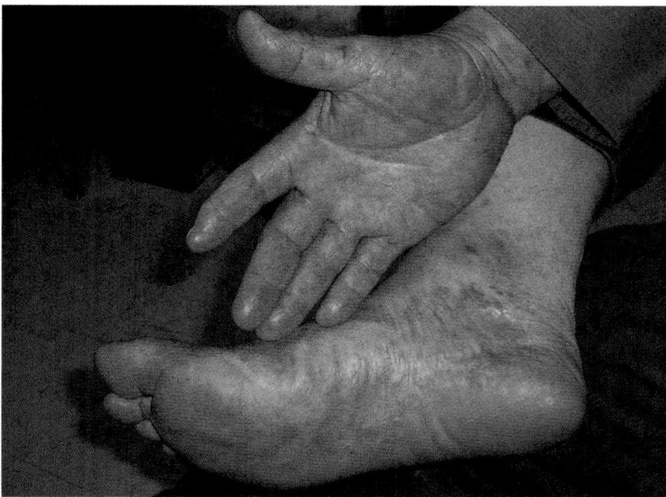

FIGURE 150-23 Palmar-plantar psoriasis that was biopsy proven. Note the widespread erythema and scale that could be mistaken for tinea pedis and tinea manus. The patient does not have pustules or mahogany spots but those lesions are often not present in palmar-plantar psoriasis. (*Reproduced with permission from Richard P. Usatine, MD.*)

- In the generalized type, the skin initially becomes fiery red and tender and the patient experiences constitutional signs and symptoms such as headache, fever, chills, arthralgia, malaise, anorexia, and nausea (**Figure 150-26**). The desquamation that occurs in the generalized form can impair the important functions of the skin predisposing to dehydration and sepsis. This is a dermatologic emergency requiring hospitalization and IV fluids, preferably in a monitored bed with good nursing care.
- Typical distribution: Flexural and anogenital (**Figure 150-27**). Less often, facial lesions occur. Pustules may occur on the tongue and subungually, resulting in dysphagia and nail shedding, respectively.
- Time course: Within hours, clusters of nonfollicular, superficial 2- to 3-mm pustules may appear in a generalized pattern. These pustules coalesce within 1 day to form lakes of pus that dry and desquamate in sheets, leaving behind a smooth erythematous surface on which new crops of pustules may appear. These episodes of pustulation may occur for days to weeks causing the patient severe discomfort and exhaustion. Upon remission of the pustular component, most systemic symptoms disappear; however, the patient may be in an erythrodermic state or may have residual lesions.[1]

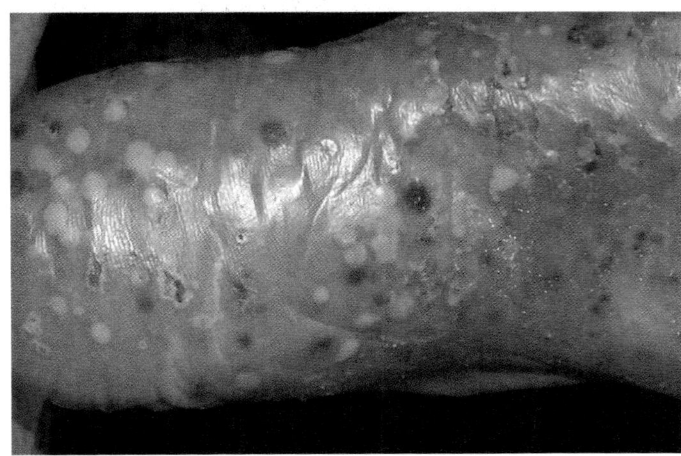

FIGURE 150-24 Palmar-plantar psoriasis with extensive pustules and mahogany spots. (*Reproduced with permission from UTHSCSA dermatology.*)

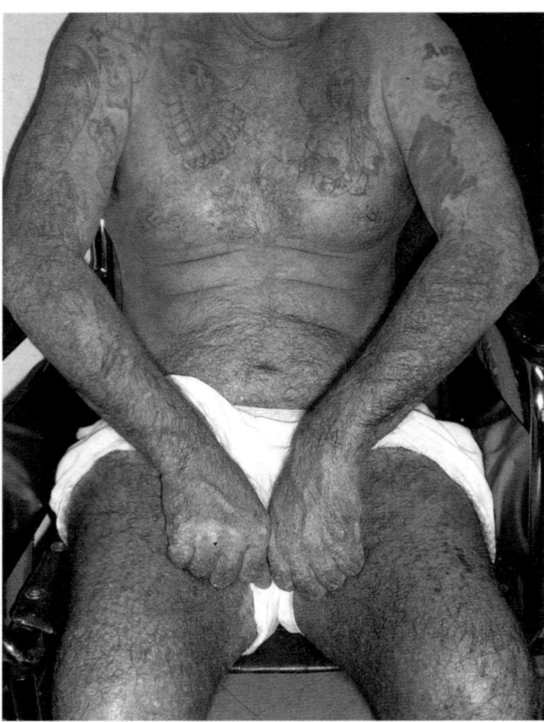

FIGURE 150-25 Erythrodermic psoriasis in a 45-year-old man. Note the extensive exfoliation of the skin along with the deep erythema. (*Reproduced with permission from Richard P. Usatine, MD.*)

Nail psoriasis

- Nail involvement in psoriasis can lead to pitting, onycholysis, subungual keratosis, splinter hemorrhages, oil spots, and nail loss (see **Figure 150-10** and Chapter 193, Psoriatic Nails).

Psoriatic arthritis

- Asymmetric oligoarthritis typically involves the hands, feet, and knees. The arthritis can also be symmetric resembling rheumatoid arthritis. Distal interphalangeal joint (DIP) involvement is a classic finding, but DIP predominance is present in the minority of cases. The fingers may

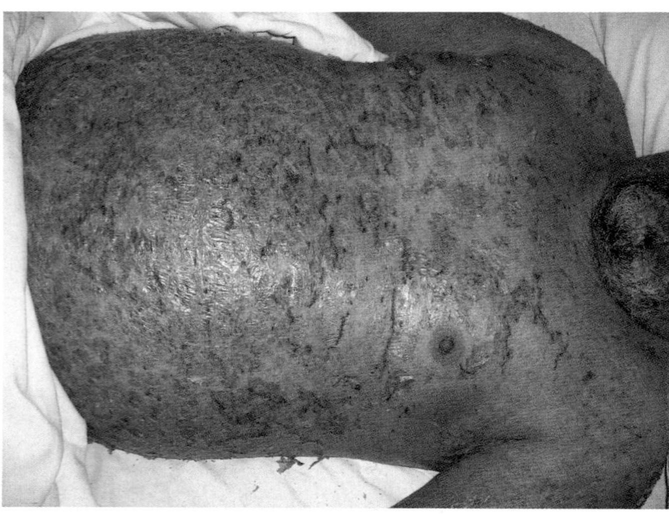

FIGURE 150-26 Generalized pustular psoriasis in a 47-year-old man with fever, exfoliation, and dehydration. This is the twentieth time for this patient in his life. His siblings also get severe generalized pustular psoriasis. (*Reproduced with permission from Meng Lu, MD.*)

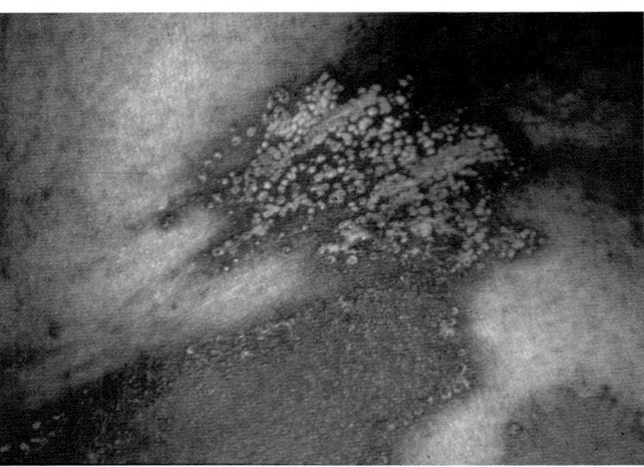

FIGURE 150-27 Localized pustular psoriasis in the groin. (*Reproduced with permission from Jeffrey Meffert, MD.*)

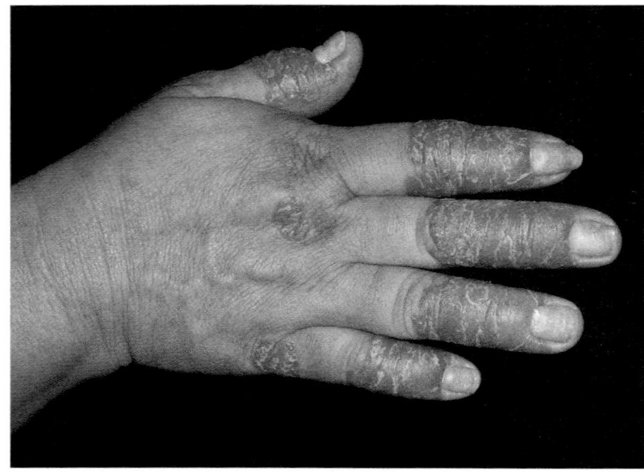

FIGURE 150-28 Dactylitis with sausage-shaped fingers in this middle-aged woman with plaque psoriasis and psoriatic arthritis. Note the nail involvement along with distal interphalangeal joint involvement. (*Reproduced with permission from Richard P. Usatine, MD.*)

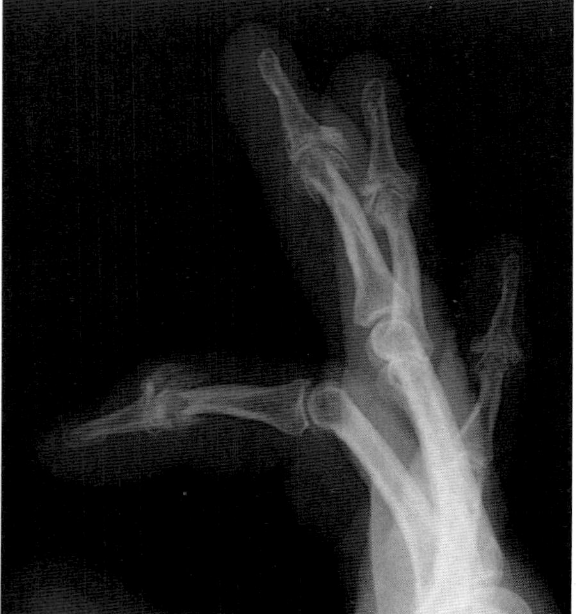

FIGURE 150-29 Radiograph showing the pencil-in-cup deformity at the distal interphalangeal joint of the second and third digits. (*Reproduced with permission from Richard P. Usatine, MD.*)

be swollen like sausages which is called dactylitis (**Figure 150-28**). (see Chapter 100, Psoriatic Arthritis)

- Hand involvement can be disabling (see **Figure 150-11**). X-rays should be ordered when a person with psoriasis has joint pains suggesting psoriatic arthritis. Typical findings are juxta-articular erosions and the pencil-cup deformity (**Figure 150-29**).
- There may be inflammation at the insertion of tendons onto bone (enthesopathy). This may occur at the Achilles tendon.
- Patients with psoriatic arthritis need to be treated with systemic agents (methotrexate [MTX] or biologics) to prevent advancement of the disease.

DISEASE SEVERITY

- Moderate-to-severe disease is defined by psoriasis of the palms, soles, head and neck, or genitalia, and in patients with more than 5% body surface area (BSA) involvement. A person's palm is approximately 1% BSA and can be used to estimate BSA.
- Another grading system for severity uses the following numbers:
  - Mild: Up to 3% BSA
  - Moderate: 3% to 10% BSA
  - Severe: Greater than 10% BSA
- Patients with psoriatic arthritis may have limited skin disease but require more aggressive systemic therapies.
- Note that palmoplantar psoriasis is considered moderate to severe even if the BSA involved is not above 3% or 5% (**Figure 150-30**).

LABORATORY STUDIES

Laboratory studies are rarely needed. A punch biopsy or scoop shave is used for evaluating atypical cases. For pustular psoriasis, a 4-mm punch around an intact pustule is preferred (**Figure 132-31**).

IMAGING

Plain films should be ordered when a person with psoriasis has joint pains suggesting psoriatic arthritis (see **Figure 150-29**). Early psoriatic arthritis often has no findings on plain films, but if history and physical examination suggest the diagnosis, one should not wait for irreversible visible joint damage to initiate therapy.

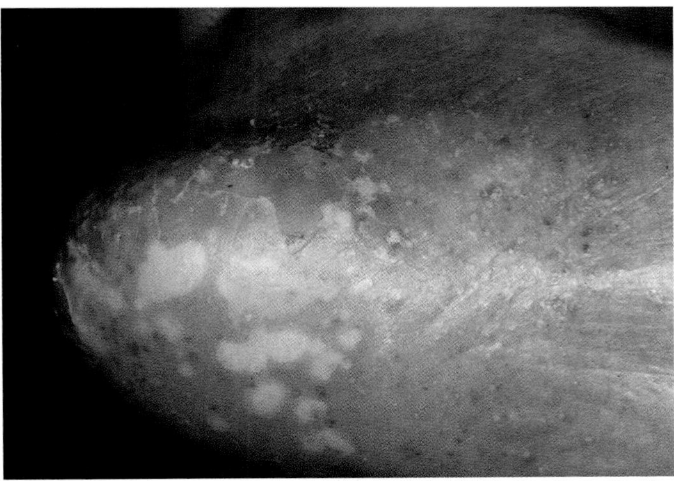

FIGURE 150-30 Palmoplantar psoriasis in a 31-year-old man with erythema, pustules, and lakes of pus. Note the typical brown macules that are called mahogany spots. High-potency topical steroids did not help at all. It is painful for him to walk and systemic therapy has just been started. This is a localized form of pustular psoriasis. (*Reproduced with permission from Jeff Meffert, MD.*)

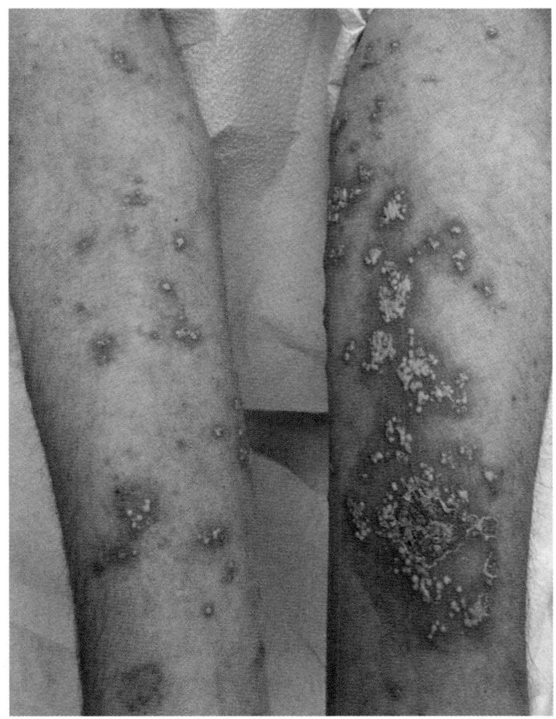

A

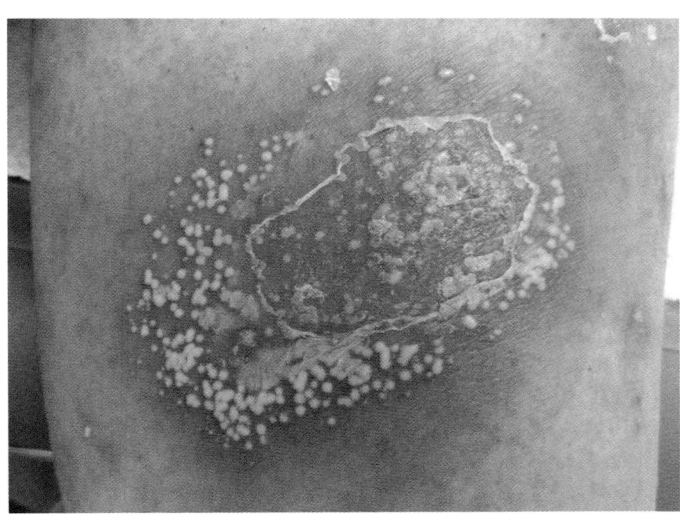

B

FIGURE 150-31 Pustular psoriasis in a 41-year-old woman. A 4-mm punch biopsy including at least one pustule helped to confirm the clinical diagnosis. The patient was stable for outpatient treatment and was started on cyclosporine and acitretin together with the plan to stop the cyclosporine once the pustules have cleared. **A.** Arm involvement. **B.** Close-up of pustules on the leg. (*Reproduced with permission from Robert T. Gilson, MD.*)

DIFFERENTIAL DIAGNOSIS

- Cutaneous T-cell lymphoma (CTCL) can have plaques that resemble psoriasis. In most cases of psoriasis, the distribution and nail changes will help to differentiate between these diseases. Plaque-type CTCL tends to be more central and truncal, whereas psoriasis often involves the extremities along with the trunk. If needed, a punch biopsy can help to differentiate between these 2 conditions (see Chapter 174, Cutaneous T-cell Lymphoma).

- Lichen planus is another papulosquamous disease. Its distribution is more on flexor surfaces and around the wrists and ankles than the elbows and knees (see Chapter 152, Lichen Planus).
- Lichen simplex chronicus is a hyperkeratotic plaque with lichenification. It usually presents with fewer plaques than psoriasis and is typically found on the posterior neck, ankle, wrist, or lower leg. There is usually more lichenification than thick scale and it is always pruritic (see Chapter 147, Psychocutaneous Disorders).
- Nummular eczema presents with coin-like plaques. These are most commonly found on the legs and are usually not as thick as the plaques of psoriasis. Nummular eczema may also have vesicles and bullae. Psoriasis has a different distribution and often includes nail changes (see Chapter 143, Atopic Dermatitis).
- Pityriasis rosea is a self-limited process that has papulosquamous plaques. These plaques are less keratotic and have a collarette scale. Pityriasis rosea frequently has a herald patch (see Chapter 151, Pityriasis Rosea).
- Seborrheic dermatitis of the scalp can closely resemble psoriasis of the scalp, especially when it is severe. Psoriasis generally has thicker plaques on the scalp and the plaques often cross the hairline. Seborrhea and psoriasis can both involve the ear. Both conditions respond to topical steroids (see Chapter 149, Seborrheic Dermatitis).
- Syphilis is the great imitator and secondary syphilis can have a papulosquamous eruption similar to psoriasis. Secondary syphilis often involves the palms and soles and the rapid plasma reagin (RPR) will be positive (see Chapter 218, Syphilis).
- Tinea corporis or cruris can resemble inverse psoriasis in the intertriginous areas as both conditions tend to have erythema and thinner plaques without central clearing in these regions. Tinea corporis in non-intertriginous areas typically presents with annular plaques with central clearing. Psoriasis can do this as seen in **Figure 150-18**. Tinea corporis usually does not have as many plaques as psoriasis but a potassium hydroxide (KOH) preparation can be used to look for fungal elements to distinguish between these 2 conditions (see Chapter 136, Tinea Corporis).
- Cutaneous candidiasis appears similar to inverse psoriasis when found in intertriginous areas (see Chapter 135, Candidiasis).
- Reactive arthritis (see Chapter 153, Reactive Arthritis) is a noninfectious acute oligoarthritis that occurs in response to an infection, most commonly in the gastrointestinal (GI) or urogenital tract. Patients present 1 to 4 weeks after the triggering infection, with joint pain in asymmetric large joints, eye disease such as conjunctivitis, and skin changes including erythema nodosum, keratoderma blennorrhagicum, and circinate balanitis. Diagnosis is based on the clinical presentation plus evidence of associated infection.[7] The skin lesions closely resemble psoriasis so the diagnosis depends on the constellation of the clinical involvement and the history.

MANAGEMENT

Treat precipitating and underlying factors when these are known. Encourage smoking cessation to all who smoke (see Chapter 237, Tobacco Addiction). Avoid or minimize alcohol use (see Chapter 238, Alcoholism). Stress management techniques can be suggested in patients who admit that stress is an important factor in worsening their condition. Use preventive techniques as much as possible by avoiding known precipitants.

Patient perception of their disease and expectations for therapy are as important as the evidence and recommendations that follow. Some patients are willing to live with some skin changes rather than go on systemic treatment, whereas others want everything done with a goal of 100% clearance. Consequently, therapeutic choices are made in conjunction with patient's values and their life situation (economic and time issues surrounding treatment options).

Choice of topical vehicles

- An ointment has a petrolatum base and will penetrate thick scale best.
- An emollient cream has some of the advantages of an ointment but is cosmetically more appealing to patients who find a basic ointment to be too greasy.
- Some patients prefer cream to avoid the oily feel of ointment even though it is less effective in general than an ointment. However, in many cases the most effective vehicle is the one the patient will use.
- Lotions and foams are good for hair-bearing areas when some moisturizing is desired.
- Steroid solutions work well for psoriasis of the scalp.
- New foam preparations have rapid absorption and are cosmetically appealing. These tend to be more expensive at this time.

Topical treatments

- **Table 150-3** summarizes the strength of recommendations for the treatment of psoriasis using topical therapies.
- Research supports potent topical steroids as first-line therapy.[8] SOR A Clobetasol is an ultrahigh-potency steroid that is generic and comes in many vehicles for use on the body and scalp. A meta-analysis of the studies with clobetasol demonstrated 68% to 89% of patients had clear improvement or complete healing.[9] SOR A
- There are 2 vitamin D analogs available for topical use: calcipotriene (Dovonex and generic) and calcitriol (Vectical). These vitamin D preparations are recommended as first-line therapy with or without topical corticosteroids for the treatment of childhood psoriasis.[10] SOR A They are also useful for adults but most patients report that clobetasol is more effective.
- Comparable efficacy has been shown for topical calcipotriene (vitamin D analog) and tazarotene (retinoid) with a slight increase in adverse effects for tazarotene.[8] SOR A
- Using topical steroids and calcipotriene or tazarotene is an effective regimen. It has increased efficacy and fewer side effects.[8,9] SOR A However, in monotherapy studies of topical agents in psoriasis, steroids caused fewer adverse reactions compared to vitamin D analogs and tazarotene.[11] SOR A
- One expensive topical preparation combines betamethasone and calcipotriene (Taclonex ointment) to be applied once daily. Another option is to prescribe generic clobetasol ointment and generic calcipotriene cream to be used simultaneously or in an alternating fashion.
- Clobetasol in the morning and tazarotene in the evening is a good combination to reduce irritation and increase efficacy.[9] SOR A
- Two trials randomized potent steroid treatment responders to either an intermittent maintenance regime (3 applications each weekend) or to no maintenance. The results of more than 6 months indicate that patients receiving maintenance therapy were more than 3 times as likely to stay in remission.[12] SOR B

TABLE 150-3 Strength of Recommendations for the Treatment of Psoriasis Using Topical Therapies[1]

Agent	Strength of Recommendation	Level of Evidence
Class I corticosteroids (highest potency)	A	I
Class II corticosteroids	B	II
Classes III/IV corticosteroids (medium potency)	A	I
Classes V/VI/VII corticosteroids (lowest potency)	A	I
Vitamin D analogs	A	I
Tazarotene	A	I
Tacrolimus and pimecrolimus	B	II
Anthralin	C	III
Coal tar	B	II
Combination corticosteroid and salicylic acid	B	II
Combination corticosteroid and vitamin D analog	A	I
Combination corticosteroid and tazarotene	A	I
Combination tacrolimus and salicylic acid	B	II

Data from Menter A, Korman NJ, Elmets CA, et al; American Academy of Dermatology. Guidelines of care for the management of psoriasis and psoriatic arthritis. Section 3. Guidelines of care for the management and treatment of psoriasis with topical therapies. *J Am Acad Dermatol.* 2009;60(4):643-659.

- Older treatments still in use include topical coal tar and topical anthralin.[9] Evidence does not support the use of coal tar alone or in combination at this time.[9] SOR A Topical anthralin is messy, not practical for long-term use and not supported by evidence.[1,5] SOR A
- Topical calcineurin inhibitors previously approved for eczema are being studied for use in psoriasis. Tacrolimus ointment seems most effective in treating psoriasis of the face and intertriginous areas where the skin is thin. Clinical trials suggest that tacrolimus (0.1%) ointment twice a day produces a good response in a majority of patients with facial and intertriginous (inverse) psoriasis (see **Figure 150-6**).[13-15] SOR B
- Emollients and keratolytics are safe and probably beneficial as adjunctive treatment. SOR C
- Intralesional steroids may help small plaques resolve (**Figure 150-32**). Use triamcinolone acetonide 5 to 10 mg/mL injected with a 27-gauge needle into the plaque. SOR C

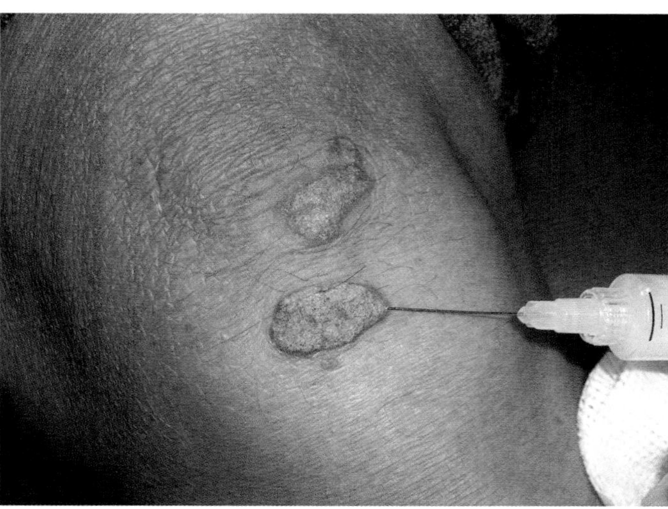

FIGURE 150-32 Intralesional injection of small plaques over the knee those were resistant to treatment with high-potency topical steroids. A 27-gauge needle was employed with 5 mg/mL triamcinolone. (*Reproduced with permission from Richard P. Usatine, MD.*)

Phototherapy

- It is indicated in the presence of extensive and widespread disease (practically defined as more lesions than can be easily counted) and psoriasis not responding to topical therapy.
- Narrowband UVB is more effective than broadband UVB and approaches psoralen and UVA (PUVA) in efficacy for the treatment of psoriasis in patients with skin types I to III (lighter skin).[16] SOR A
- At present, there are no predictors of the type(s) of psoriasis most responsive to narrowband UVB.[16]
- Of patients with psoriasis, 63% to 80% will clear with a course of narrowband UVB with equivalent relapse rates compared with PUVA.[16]
- Lack of requirement for psoralen and convenience suggests that narrowband UVB could be considered as the first-line phototherapy option with PUVA reserved for treatment failures.[16]
- MTX pretreatment (15 mg/wk × 3) allowed physicians to clear psoriasis in fewer phototherapy sessions than when phototherapy was administered alone in one study.[17] SOR B
- According to one consensus conference, acitretin combined with UV therapy is safe and effective and limits treatment frequency, duration, and cumulative doses of both agents. They state this combination is better tolerated, more convenient, less costly, and, perhaps, safer during long-term treatment than phototherapy alone.[18] SOR C
- Avoid use of cyclosporine with UV therapy because of an increased risk of skin cancer.[19]

Systemic

- When topical agents (and/or phototherapy fail), systemic agents (including biologic agents) are the next step. **Table 150-4** summarizes the systemic drugs used in treatment of psoriasis.
- MTX and biologic agents are especially valuable in patients with psoriatic arthritis and may be started early in the course of treatment to prevent permanent joint damage.
- Do not use systemic corticosteroid therapy for psoriasis. Pustular flares of disease may be provoked and these flares can be fatal (see **Figure 150-18**).

TABLE 150-4 Systemic Drugs Used in Treatment of Psoriasis[31]

Drug Name	Classification/Mechanism of Action	Comments
Acitretin	Oral retinoid	First-line systemic drug for chronic palmoplantar or pustular psoriasis in patients of nonchildbearing potential. Limited benefit for plaque psoriasis.
Cyclosporine	Oral calcineurin inhibitor	Fast-acting systemic drug that is often used first line for pustular psoriasis or erythrodermic psoriasis. For intermittent use in periods up to 12 wk as a short-term agent to control a flare of psoriasis.
Methotrexate sodium	Inhibitor of folate biosynthesis	May be used as a first-line systemic drug for plaque psoriasis and psoriatic arthritis. Compared with cyclosporine, has a more modest effect, but can be used continuously for years or decades.
Adalimumab	TNF inhibitor	May be used as first-line systemic treatment of plaque psoriasis and psoriatic arthritis. Has higher efficacy and lower rate of adverse effects compared with methotrexate.
Etanercept	TNF inhibitor	Commonly used as a first-line systemic drug for chronic plaque psoriasis and psoriatic arthritis.
Infliximab	TNF inhibitor	Intravenous infusion with high rates of effectiveness. Fast-acting drug that is often used as a second- or third-line biological for chronic plaque psoriasis.
Ustekinumab	Monoclonal antibody that binds the shared p40 protein subunit of IL-12 and IL-23	Favorable results when compared with etanercept in terms of efficacy and safety. May be used as first-line systemic treatment for chronic plaque psoriasis.

IL, interleukin; TNF, tumor necrosis factor.

- MTX and oral retinoids can cause birth defects so appropriate counseling, contraception, and testing should accompany therapy with these agents.
- MTX is given as a weekly dose of 7.5 to 25 mg/wk depending on response and side effects.[20] SOR Ⓐ Tuberculosis (TB) screening with purified protein derivative (PPD) or QuantiFERON-TB Gold blood test should precede treatment (if positive results, then the TB needs treatment before starting this therapy). Pretreatment laboratories should include a complete blood count (CBC), differential, liver function tests (LFTs), a chemistry profile, and hepatitides B and C serologies. A CBC and LFTs should be followed regularly. Patients should take folic acid 1 mg/d to prevent some of the possible adverse effects of MTX. For MTX, reliable contraceptive methods should be used during and for at least 3 months after therapy in both men and women.[5]
- The starting dose of MTX is between 5 and 10 mg/wk for the first week based on expert experience.[21] The dose is escalated with monitoring to obtain a therapeutic target dose of 15 to 25 mg/wk. Oral dosing is preferred but subcutaneous (SQ) dosing is an option in the event of poor GI tolerance (same dosing as oral). Type 2 diabetes and obesity appear to be significant risk factors in fibrosis.[21] A combination of fibrotests and fibroscans together with measurement of the type III serum procollagen aminopeptide are noninvasive methods to monitor for liver toxicity.[21] SOR Ⓒ The question of whether or when to do a liver biopsy and/or stop MTX is controversial. The National Psoriasis Foundation has published that liver "biopsies are now advocated after a cumulative dose of 3.5 g in low-risk patients and 1.5 g in high-risk patients." The same recommendations are cited in the 2009 National Psoriasis Foundation Consensus Conference on MTX and psoriasis.[22] SOR Ⓒ
- Cyclosporine (oral) is a T-cell inhibitor and is very effective in rapidly treating psoriasis. The recommended starting dose is 2.5 to 6 mg/kg/d (actual body weight) divided twice a day.[19] SOR Ⓒ Serum creatinine and blood pressure should be monitored monthly. Also CBC, uric acid, potassium, lipids, LFTs, and magnesium should be monitored monthly. Cyclosporine can be used for long-term therapy in patients with severe psoriasis for up to 2 years lifetime maximum based on European guidelines and 1 year maximum based on the US guidelines.[9,19] SOR Ⓒ Cyclosporine is pregnancy category C, with several studies indicating an increased risk of premature birth but no major malformations.[19]

TABLE 150-5 FDA-Approved Biologic Agents for Treating Psoriasis

Biologic Agent	Product Name	Mechanism of Action	Route of Delivery	Frequency of Maintenance Dosing
Adalimumab	Humira	TNF inhibitor	SQ	Every 2 wk
Etanercept	Enbrel	TNF inhibitor	SQ	Once to twice weekly
Infliximab	Remicade	TNF inhibitor	IV infusion	Every 6-8 wk
Ustekinumab	Stelara	Monoclonal antibody that binds p40 protein subunit of IL-12 and IL-23	SQ	Every 3 mo

IL, Interleukin; IV, Intravenous; TNF, tumor necrosis factor.

- Oral retinoids: Acitretin is a potent systemic retinoid used for psoriasis.[23] SOR Ⓐ Acitretin appears to provide better efficacy in pustular psoriasis (including palmoplantar psoriasis) than in plaque-type psoriasis as a single-agent treatment (see **Figure 150-31**).[24] SOR Ⓐ Low-dose acitretin therapy (25 mg/d) seems to be better tolerated and associated with fewer abnormalities found after laboratory testing and fewer adverse effects than the 50 mg/d dosage.[23] Acitretin is known to cause fetal malformations just like isotretinoin so it is best to avoid use in women capable of pregnancy, especially as it may remain in the body for up to 3 years after stopping therapy.

Biologic agents

There are 4 biologic agents available and Food and Drug Administration (FDA) approved for treating psoriasis.[25] See **Tables 150-5** and **150-6** for information about mechanism of action and the effectiveness of these agents.

- Before starting therapy, obtain a PPD or QuantiFERON-TB *Gold* blood test. These agents can reactivate dormant TB. Screening for TB should continue yearly during biologic therapy.[26]
- The tumor necrosis factor (TNF) inhibitors (adalimumab, etanercept, and infliximab) share a common mechanism of action that leads to safety concerns. Safety concerns include serious infections (eg, sepsis, tuberculosis, and viral infections), autoimmune conditions (lupus and demyelinating disorders), and lymphoma.[27]
- Etanercept (subcutaneous): For adults the dose is 50 mg SQ twice weekly for 3 months then 50 mg weekly thereafter.[9] SOR Ⓐ This agent is especially valuable in patients with psoriatic arthritis as well as psoriasis.[9] SOR Ⓐ
- Ustekinumab is a new biologic agent that is given SQ every 3 months. It targets interleukin (IL)-12 and IL-23 in the treatment of moderate-to-severe psoriasis. The safety profile of continued ustekinumab exposure through up to 3 years is favorable including the risk for either infections or malignancies.[28,29]
- While the biologic agents are all very expensive, insurance often pays and there are patient assistance programs for uninsured patients with limited resources.

Methotrexate versus biologic agents[20]

- MTX is a very inexpensive medication with more than a 40-year track record, but with known potential for hepatotoxicity. It is very effective, but requires monitoring of the LFTs and the blood count on a regular basis.
- The biologic agents are engineered proteins with a potentially safer profile than MTX. However, they are very expensive and require

TABLE 150-6 Biologic Agents as Treatment of Plaque Psoriasis—Estimated Probabilities of Response Based on Synthesis of Evidence

	PASI 50, mean (95% CrI)	PASI 75, mean (95% CrI)	PASI 90, mean (95% CrI)
Placebo	13% (12-14)	4% (3-4)	1% (0-1)
Etanercept 25 mg	65% (56-73)	39% (30-48)	15% (10-21)
Etanercept 50 mg	76% (71-81)	52% (45-59)	24% (19-30)
Adalimumab	81% (74-87)	58% (49-68)	30% (23-39)
Ustekinumab 45 mg	88% (84-91)	69% (62-75)	40% (33-48)
Ustekinumab 90 mg	90% (87-93)	74% (68-80)	46% (39-54)
Infliximab	93% (89-96)	80% (70-87)	54% (42-64)

CrI, credible interval; PASI, Psoriasis Area and Severity Index is used to express the severity of psoriasis. It combines the severity (erythema, induration, and desquamation) and percentage of affected area (lower number is better and the highest number for worst disease is 72); PASI 50 = 50% reduction in PASI score—clinically meaningful improvement; PASI 75 = 75% reduction in PASI score—very good improvement; PASI 90 = 90% reduction in PASI score—excellent improvement.
Data from Reich K, Burden AD, Eaton JN, Hawkins NS. Efficacy of biologics in the treatment of moderate to severe psoriasis: a network meta-analysis of randomized controlled trials. *Br J Dermatol*. 2012;166:179-188.

parenteral administration. Biologics have the advantage of requiring less monitoring with blood tests. The biologic agents are not side effect free and some of the potential side effects, while rare, are quite dangerous, and include the risks of sepsis, malignancy, and demyelinating disease.

THERAPY BY TYPE OF PSORIASIS

PLAQUE TYPE

Mild-to-moderate plaque psoriasis: Clobetasol twice daily for 2 to 4 weeks. Then decrease use of clobetasol and consider adding a steroid-sparing topical agent such as a vitamin D topical product.

Severe plaque form psoriasis: One systematic review found 665 studies dealing with the treatment of severe plaque psoriasis.[17] Photochemotherapy showed the highest average proportion of patients with clearance (70% [6947/9925]) and good response (83% [8238/9925]), followed by UVB (67.9% [620/913]) and cyclosporine (64% [1030/ 1609]) therapy.[30] SOR Ⓐ Expert consensus in a meeting following data analysis supported the following sequence for the treatments: UVB, photochemotherapy, MTX, acitretin, and cyclosporine.[30] SOR Ⓒ

The Consensus guidelines for the management of plaque psoriasis published in 2012 is based on US National Psoriasis Foundation review and update of the Canadian Guidelines for the Management of Plaque Psoriasis. It includes newly approved agents such as ustekinumab and the excimer laser. The management of psoriasis in special populations is discussed.[31] In particular, current evidence does support the use of TNF antagonists for the treatment of psoriasis in patients with hepatitis C.[31] **Table 150-4** summarizes the systemic treatments for plaque type psoriasis.

SCALP

One head-to-head trial (no pun intended) in scalp psoriasis demonstrated no therapeutic difference between a topical vitamin D derivative and a topical potent steroid.[12] Generic fluocinonide solution daily to the scalp is effective. Derma-smooth is another affordable scalp product that combines a high-potency steroid with a peanut oil. Calcipotriene daily to scalp also helps but is more expensive. Mineral oil may be used to moisturize and remove scale. Shampoos with tar and/or salicylic acid (T-Gel and T-Sal) can help to dissolve and wash away some of the scale. Of course, systemic therapies for more severe psoriasis will help clear scalp psoriasis.

GUTTATE PSORIASIS

Phototherapy works particularly well for guttate psoriasis.[6] SOR Ⓒ Narrowband UVB therapy may produce clearing in less than 1 month. Topical therapies are a reasonable option when phototherapy is not available (see **Figure 150-20**).[6] SOR Ⓒ Although both antibiotics and tonsillectomy have frequently been advocated for patients with guttate psoriasis, there is no good evidence that either intervention is beneficial.[32]

INVERSE PSORIASIS

Mid- to high-potency topical steroids can be used for inverse psoriasis even though the disease occurs in skinfolds (**Figure 150-6**). A number of studies have shown that tacrolimus works well to treat inverse psoriasis when applied twice daily.[13-15] SOR Ⓑ Some patients did report a warm sensation or pruritus upon application so patients should be warned of this and told not to stop using the tacrolimus as this may improve over time.[13-15]

PALMAR-PLANTAR PSORIASIS

For mild disease, start with topical treatments as in plaque psoriasis. For moderate-to-severe cases, systemic therapy such as oral acitretin, MTX, or one of the biologics may be needed.

ERYTHRODERMIC/GENERALIZED PSORIASIS

Treatment considerations include hospitalization for dehydration and close monitoring, cyclosporine, MTX, oral retinoids, phototherapy, or photochemotherapy.[6] SOR Ⓒ Cyclosporine is very effective in rapidly treating the most severe erythrodermic psoriasis (see **Figure 150-25**). The recommended starting dose is 2.5 to 6 mg/kg/d (actual body weight) divided twice a day.[19]

PUSTULAR PSORIASIS

Options include oral retinoids such as isotretinoin or acitretin (depends on sex and age of the patient), MTX, cyclosporine, phototherapy, and hospitalization as needed.[6] SOR Ⓒ Cyclosporine is very effective in rapidly treating pustular psoriasis at 2.5 to 6 mg/kg/d (actual body weight) divided twice a day.[19] One strategy is to start cyclosporine and acitretin together and to stop the cyclosporine once the pustules have cleared (see **Figure 150-31**).

PROGNOSIS

Prognosis is dependent on the type of psoriasis with the palmar-plantar type being the most difficult to treat. While erythrodermic and generalized pustular psoriasis are the most immediately dangerous types the response to treatment may vary from excellent to disappointing. Widespread plaque psoriasis is challenging to treat but the prognosis is not easily predictable and patient adherence is a very important factor in the prognosis. Excellent control is always the goal and cure should not be expected (even guttate psoriasis in children can come back as plaque psoriasis later in life).

FOLLOW-UP

- Follow-up may need to be frequent for various therapies including cytotoxic drugs, the biologics, and light therapy.
- While there are many safety concerns with the biologic agents a recent integrated safety analysis of short- and long-term safety profiles of etanercept in patients with psoriasis concluded that rates of noninfectious and infectious adverse events were comparable between placebo and etanercept groups.[33] Also, there was no increase in overall malignancies with etanercept therapy compared with the psoriasis population.[33]
- Well-controlled psoriasis on topical agents does not require frequent follow-up.

PATIENT EDUCATION

This is a chronic disease that cannot be cured. There are many methods to control psoriasis. Patients need to develop a relationship with a family physician or dermatologist to control the psoriasis for maximum quality of life. **Table 150-7** lists discussion points.

TABLE 150-7 Discussion Points for Health Care Provider and Patient at Initial Visits

- Hereditary aspects
- Systemic manifestations
- Exacerbating and ameliorating factors
- Past treatment responses
- Range of therapeutic options
- Chronic long-term disease
- Psychological issues
- Optimism for tomorrow based on rapid research developments
- Support or services available from the National Psoriasis Foundation

PATIENT RESOURCES

- The National Psoriasis Foundation—**http://www.psoriasis.org/.**

PROVIDER RESOURCES

- Hsu S, Papp KA, Lebwohl MG, et al. Consensus guidelines for the management of plaque psoriasis. *Arch Dermatol.* 2012;148(1): 95-102—**http://archderm.ama-assn.org/cgi/content/short/148/1/95.**
- Guidelines of Care for the Management of Psoriasis and Psoriatic Arthritis: 6 parts published in *Journal of the American Academy of Dermatology* from 2008 to 2010.
- National Guideline Clearinghouse. Guidelines of Care for the Management of Psoriasis and Psoriatic Arthritis. Section 3. Guidelines of Care for the Management and Treatment of Psoriasis with Topical Therapies—**http://www.guidelines.gov/content.aspx?id =14572&search=psoriasis.**
- The National Psoriasis Foundation (NPF). This includes a pocket guide that can be downloaded as a PDF. This excellent pocket guide includes treatment algorithms for specific patient types, combination therapies, and transitional strategies for switching meds. By joining the NPF you can get this printed guide for your pocket—**http://www.psoriasis.org/ health-care-providers/treating-psoriasis.**
- Medscape. *Psoriasis*—**http://emedicine.medscape.com/article/1943419.**

REFERENCES

1. Menter A, Korman NJ, Elmets CA, et al. Guidelines of care for the management of psoriasis and psoriatic arthritis. Section 3. Guidelines of care for the management and treatment of psoriasis with topical therapies. *J Am Acad Dermatol.* 2009;60:643-659.
2. Gelfand JM, Stern RS, Nijsten T, et al. The prevalence of psoriasis in African Americans: results from a population-based study. *J Am Acad Dermatol.* 2005;52:23-26.
3. Henseler T, Christophers E. Psoriasis of early and late onset: characterization of two types of psoriasis vulgaris. *J Am Acad Dermatol.* 1985; 13:450-456.
4. Menter A, Weinstein GD. An overview of psoriasis. In: Koo YM, Lebwohl MD, Lee CS, eds. *Therapy of Moderate-to-Severe Psoriasis.* London, UK: Informa Healthcare; 2008:1-26.
5. Jankovic S, Raznatovic M, Marinkovic J, et al. Risk factors for psoriasis: a case-control study. *J Dermatol.* 2009;36:328-334.
6. Callen JP, Krueger GG, Lebwohl M, et al. AAD consensus statement on psoriasis therapies. *J Am Acad Dermatol.* 2003;49:897-899.
7. van de Kerkhof PCM. Clinical features. In: van de Kerkhof PCM, ed. *Textbook of Psoriasis.* Oxford, UK: Blackwell Science; 2003:3-29.
8. Afifi T, de Gannes G, Huang C, Zhou Y. Topical therapies for psoriasis: evidence-based review. *Can Fam Physician.* 2005;51:519-525.
9. Nast A, Kopp I, Augustin M, et al. German evidence-based guidelines for the treatment of Psoriasis vulgaris (short version). *Arch Dermatol Res.* 2007;299:111-138.
10. de Jager ME, de Jong EM, van de Kerkhof PC, Seyger MM. Efficacy and safety of treatments for childhood psoriasis: a systematic literature review. *J Am Acad Dermatol.* 2010;62:1013-1030.
11. Bruner CR, Feldman SR, Ventrapragada M, Fleischer AB Jr. A systematic review of adverse effects associated with topical treatments for psoriasis. *Dermatol Online J.* 2003;9:2.
12. Mason J, Mason AR, Cork MJ. Topical preparations for the treatment of psoriasis: a systematic review. *Br J Dermatol.* 2002;146: 351-364.
13. Brune A, Miller DW, Lin P, et al. Tacrolimus ointment is effective for psoriasis on the face and intertriginous areas in pediatric patients. *Pediatr Dermatol.* 2007;24:76-80.
14. Lebwohl M, Freeman AK, Chapman MS, et al. Tacrolimus ointment is effective for facial and intertriginous psoriasis. *J Am Acad Dermatol.* 2004;51:723-730.
15. Martin EG, Sanchez RM, Herrera AE, Umbert MP. Topical tacrolimus for the treatment of psoriasis on the face, genitalia, intertriginous areas and corporal plaques. *J Drugs Dermatol.* 2006;5:334-336.
16. Ibbotson SH, Bilsland D, Cox NH, et al. An update and guidance on narrowband ultraviolet B phototherapy: a British Photodermatology Group Workshop Report. *Br J Dermatol.* 2004;151:283-297.
17. Asawanonda P, Nateetongrungsak Y. Methotrexate plus narrowband UVB phototherapy versus narrowband UVB phototherapy alone in the treatment of plaque-type psoriasis: a randomized, placebo-controlled study. *J Am Acad Dermatol.* 2006;54:1013-1018.
18. Lebwohl M, Drake L, Menter A, et al. Consensus conference: acitretin in combination with UVB or PUVA in the treatment of psoriasis. *J Am Acad Dermatol.* 2001;45:544-553.
19. Rosmarin DM, Lebwohl M, Elewski BE, Gottlieb AB. Cyclosporine and psoriasis: 2008 National Psoriasis Foundation Consensus Conference. *J Am Acad Dermatol.* 2010;62:838-853.
20. Saporito FC, Menter MA. Methotrexate and psoriasis in the era of new biologic agents. *J Am Acad Dermatol.* 2004;50:301-309.
21. Montaudie H, Sbidian E, Paul C, et al. Methotrexate in psoriasis: a systematic review of treatment modalities, incidence, risk factors and monitoring of liver toxicity. *J Eur Acad Dermatol Venereol.* 2011;25(suppl 2):12-18.
22. Kalb RE, Strober B, Weinstein G, Lebwohl M. Methotrexate and psoriasis: 2009 National Psoriasis Foundation Consensus Conference. *J Am Acad Dermatol.* 2009;60:824-837.
23. Pearce DJ, Klinger S, Ziel KK, et al. Low-dose acitretin is associated with fewer adverse events than high-dose acitretin in the treatment of psoriasis. *Arch Dermatol.* 2006;142:1000-1004.

24. Sbidian E, Maza A, Montaudie H, et al. Efficacy and safety of oral retinoids in different psoriasis subtypes: a systematic literature review. *J Eur Acad Dermatol Venereol.* 2011;25(suppl 2):28-33.

25. Reich K, Burden AD, Eaton JN, Hawkins NS. Efficacy of biologics in the treatment of moderate to severe psoriasis: a network meta-analysis of randomized controlled trials. *Br J Dermatol.* 2012;166:179-188.

26. Sivamani RK, Goodarzi H, Garcia MS, et al. Biologic therapies in the treatment of psoriasis: a comprehensive evidence-based basic science and clinical review and a practical guide to tuberculosis monitoring. *Clin Rev Allergy Immunol.* 2013;44(2):121-140.

27. Gottlieb A, Korman NJ, Gordon KB, et al. Guidelines of care for the management of psoriasis and psoriatic arthritis: section 2. Psoriatic arthritis: overview and guidelines of care for treatment with an emphasis on the biologics. *J Am Acad Dermatol.* 2008;58:851-864.

28. Gordon KB, Papp KA, Langley RG, et al. Long-term safety experience of ustekinumab in patients with moderate to severe psoriasis (part II of II): results from analyses of infections and malignancy from pooled phase II and III clinical trials. *J Am Acad Dermatol.* 2012;66:742-751.

29. Lebwohl M, Leonardi C, Griffiths CE, et al. Long-term safety experience of ustekinumab in patients with moderate-to-severe psoriasis (part I of II): results from analyses of general safety parameters from pooled phase 2 and 3 clinical trials. *J Am Acad Dermatol.* 2012;66:731-741.

30. Spuls PI, Bossuyt PM, van Everdingen JJ, et al. The development of practice guidelines for the treatment of severe plaque form psoriasis. *Arch Dermatol.* 1998;134:1591-1596.

31. Hsu S, Papp KA, Lebwohl MG, et al. Consensus guidelines for the management of plaque psoriasis. *Arch Dermatol.* 2012;148:95-102.

32. Owen CM, Chalmers RJ, O'Sullivan T, Griffiths CE. A systematic review of antistreptococcal interventions for guttate and chronic plaque psoriasis. *Br J Dermatol.* 2001;145:886-890.

33. Pariser DM, Leonardi CL, Gordon K, et al. Integrated safety analysis: Short- and long-term safety profiles of etanercept in patients with psoriasis. *J Am Acad Dermatol.* 2012;67(2):245-256.

151 PITYRIASIS ROSEA

David Henderson, MD
Richard P. Usatine, MD

PATIENT STORY

A young woman comes to the office because of a rash that appeared 3 weeks ago for no apparent reason (**Figures 151-1** to **151-3**). She was feeling well and the rash is only occasionally pruritic. With and without mom in the room, the young woman denied sexual activity. The diagnosis of pityriasis rosea was made by the clinical appearance even though there was no obvious herald patch. The collarette scale was visible and the distribution was consistent with pityriasis rosea. The young woman was reassured that this would resolve spontaneously. At a subsequent visit the skin was found to be completely clear with no scarring.

INTRODUCTION

Pityriasis rosea is a common, self-limited, papulosquamous skin condition originally described in the 19th century. It is seen in children and adults. Despite the long history, its etiology remains elusive. A number of infectious etiologies have been proposed, but at present, supporting evidence is inconclusive. Pityriasis rosea has unique features including a herald patch in many cases and collarette scale that are useful in distinguishing it from other papulosquamous eruptions.

EPIDEMIOLOGY

- Pityriasis rosea is a papulosquamous eruption of unknown etiology.[1,2]
- It occurs throughout the life cycle. It is most commonly seen between the ages of 10 and 35 years.[3]
- The peak incidence is between 20 and 29 years of age.[1]
- The gender distribution is essentially equal.[1]
- The rash is most prevalent in winter months.[4]

ETIOLOGY AND PATHOPHYSIOLOGY

- The cause of pityriasis rosea is unknown, although numerous causes have been proposed.
- It has long been suspected that it may have a viral etiology because a viral-like prodrome often occurs prior to the onset of the rash. Human herpesviruses 6 and 7 have been proposed as causes, but numerous studies have failed to demonstrate conclusive supportive evidence.[1,2]
- *Chlamydia pneumoniae, Mycoplasma pneumoniae, and Legionella pneumophila* have been proposed as potential etiologic agents, but studies have not demonstrated any significant rise in antibody levels against any of these pathogens in patients with pityriasis rosea.[1]
- Pityriasis rosea has also been associated with negative pregnancy outcomes, particularly premature birth. The risk seems to be greatest when the condition occurs in the first 15 weeks of gestation.[2]

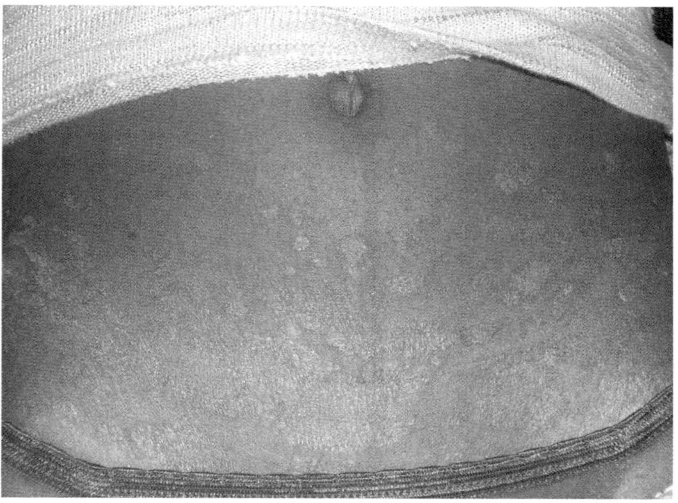

FIGURE 151-1 Pityriasis rosea in a young woman. Lesions are often concentrated in the lower abdominal area. (*Reproduced with permission from Richard P. Usatine, MD.*)

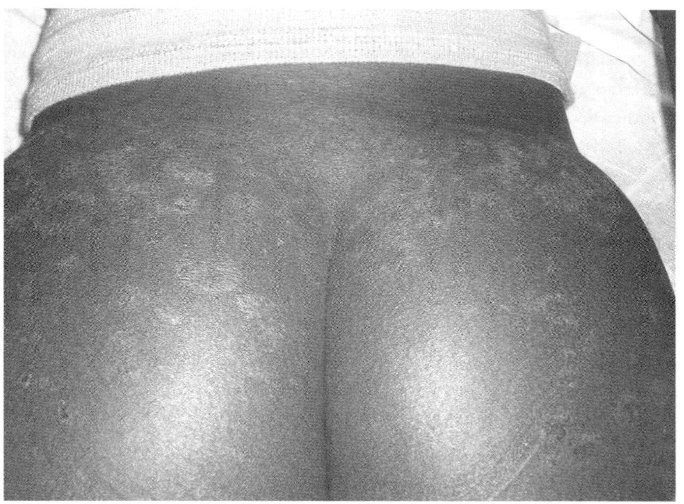

FIGURE 151-2 Scaling lesions seen on the buttocks of the same young woman in **Figure 151-1.** Note how some of the lesions are annular. (*Reproduced with permission from Richard P. Usatine, MD.*)

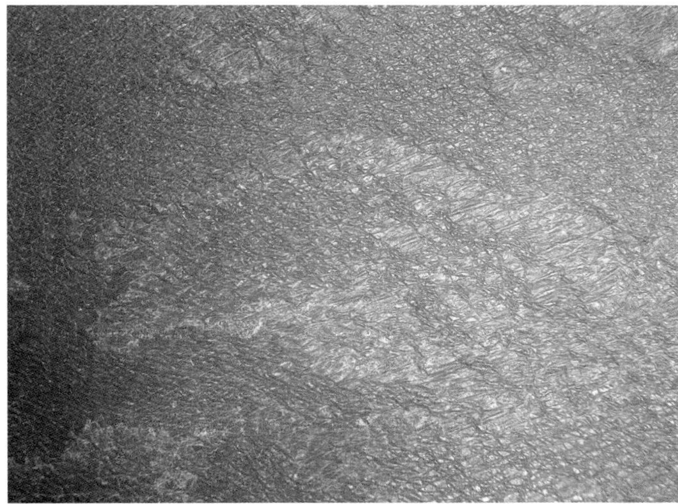

FIGURE 151-3 Close-up of lesion showing collarette scale. Note how the lesions can be annular with some central clearing. (*Reproduced with permission from Richard P. Usatine, MD.*)

- Pityriasis rosea may rarely occur as the result of a drug reaction. Documented drug reactions that have produced a pityriasis rosea-like eruption include barbiturates, captopril, clonidine, interferon, bismuth, gold, and the hepatitis B vaccine.[1,2]

DIAGNOSIS

CLINICAL FEATURES

- In approximately 20% to 50% of cases, the rash of pityriasis rosea is preceded by a viral-like illness consisting of upper respiratory or gastrointestinal (GI) symptoms.
- This is followed by the appearance of a *herald patch* in 17% of cases (**Figures 151-4** to **151-6**).[4]
- The herald patch is a solitary, oval, flesh-colored to salmon-colored lesion with scaling at the border. It often occurs on the trunk, and is generally 2 to 10 cm in diameter (see **Figures 151-4** and **151-5**).
- One to 2 weeks after the appearance of the herald patch, other papulosquamous lesions appear on the trunk and sometimes on the extremities.
- These lesions vary from oval macules to slightly raised plaques, 0.5 to 2 cm in size. They are salmon colored (or hyperpigmented in individuals with dark skin), and typically have a collarette of scaling at the border (see **Figure 151-3**). It is common for some of the lesions to appear annular with central clearing.
- In many cases, the herald patch has resolved by the time the rest of the exanthem erupts which can make the diagnosis more difficult.
- There are no systemic symptoms.
- Itching occurs in approximately 25% of patients.
- The exanthem resolves in 8 weeks in 80% of patients.[1] However, it can last up to 3 to 5 months.[3]

TYPICAL DISTRIBUTION

- The rash is bilaterally symmetrical, generally most dense on the trunk, but also involves the upper and lower extremities.

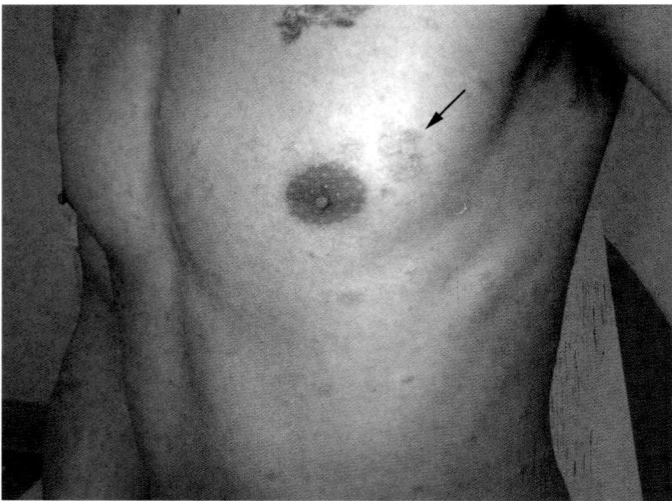

FIGURE 151-4 Pityriasis rosea in a 25-year-old Hispanic man. *Arrow* points to herald patch. (*Reproduced with permission from Scott Youngquist, MD. Previously published in Youngquist S, Usatine R. It's beginning to look a lot like Christmas. West J Med. 2001;175(4):227-228.*)

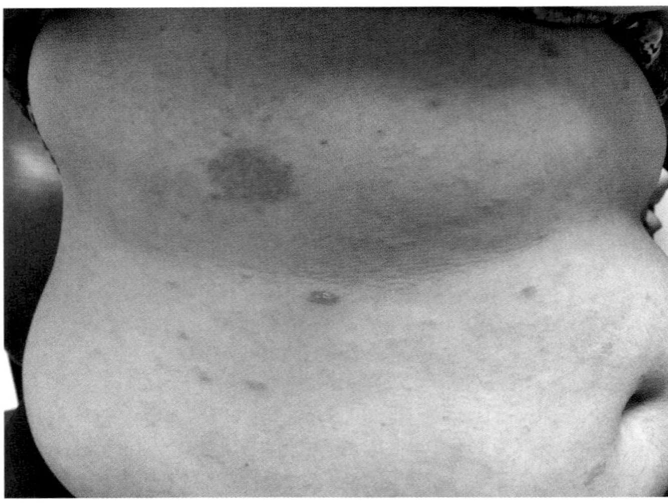

FIGURE 151-5 Pityriasis rosea with an obvious-herald patch in a woman. (*Reproduced with permission from Richard P. Usatine, MD.*)

- The lesions follow the cleavage, or Langer lines, and may create the typical *fir* or *Christmas tree* pattern over the back (**Figures 151-7** and **151-8**). Do not expect to always see a Christmas tree pattern.
- Over the chest, the lesions create a V-shaped pattern, and run transversely over the abdomen (**Figure 151-9**).
- An inverse form has been described, characterized by more intense involvement of the extremities and relative sparing of the trunk (**Figures 151-10** to **151-12**).

LABORATORY STUDIES

Pityriasis rosea is a clinical diagnosis. There are no laboratory tests that aid in the diagnosis. Biopsy of lesions typically reveals only nonspecific inflammatory changes. Because secondary syphilis is also a papulosquamous eruption and can be difficult to distinguish from pityriasis rosea on clinical grounds, taking a sexual history is important when a diagnosis of pityriasis rosea is being considered. In patients with a history of sexually transmitted diseases, or sexual practices that place them at risk, a blood test for syphilis should be considered (see **Figures 151-9** and **151-10**) (see Chapter 218, Syphilis).

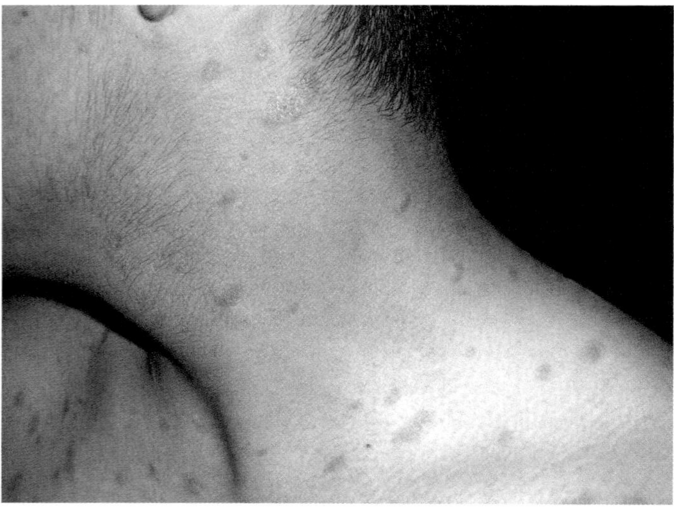

FIGURE 151-6 Pityriasis rosea in a teenage boy with the herald patch on the neck near the hairline. (*Reproduced with permission from Richard P. Usatine, MD.*)

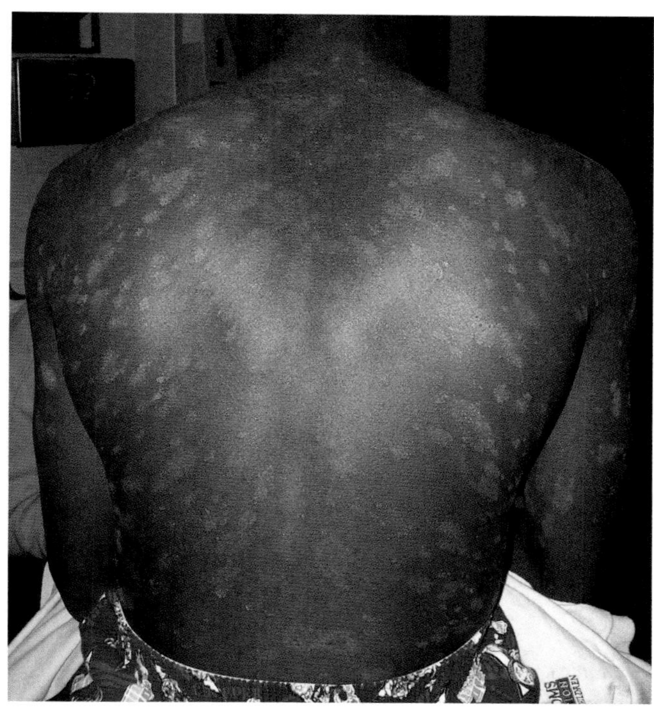

FIGURE 151-7 Pityriasis rosea in a teenage boy. The scaling lesions follow skin lines and resemble a Christmas tree. (*Reproduced with permission from E.J. Mayeaux, Jr., MD.*)

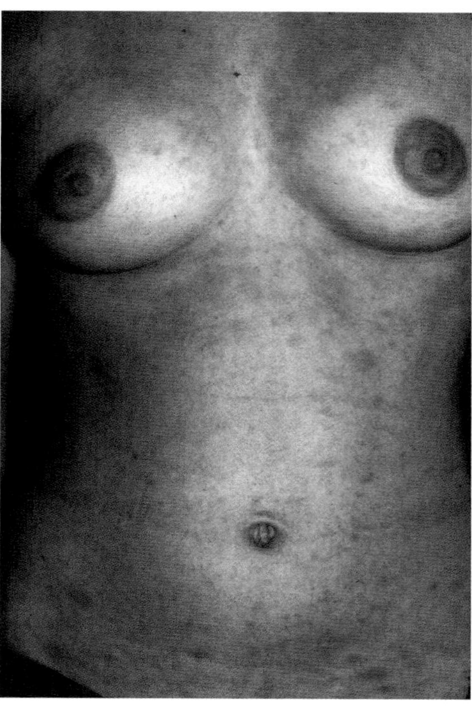

FIGURE 151-9 Pityriasis rosea on the chest and abdomen of a young woman. Blood test for syphilis was negative. (*Reproduced with permission from the University of Texas Health Sciences Center, Division of Dermatology.*)

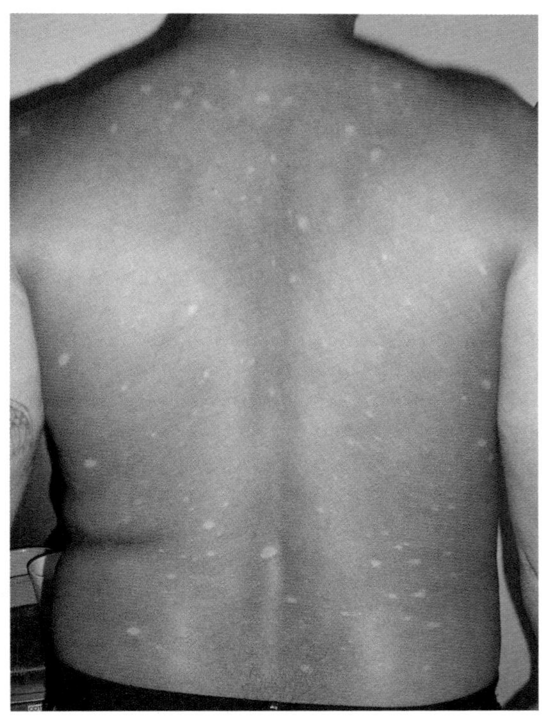

FIGURE 151-8 Pityriasis rosea in 31-year-old man with hypopigmented scaling lesions that resemble a Christmas tree on the back. The lesions began 3 weeks before the patient presented for evaluation. (*Reproduced with permission from Richard P. Usatine, MD.*)

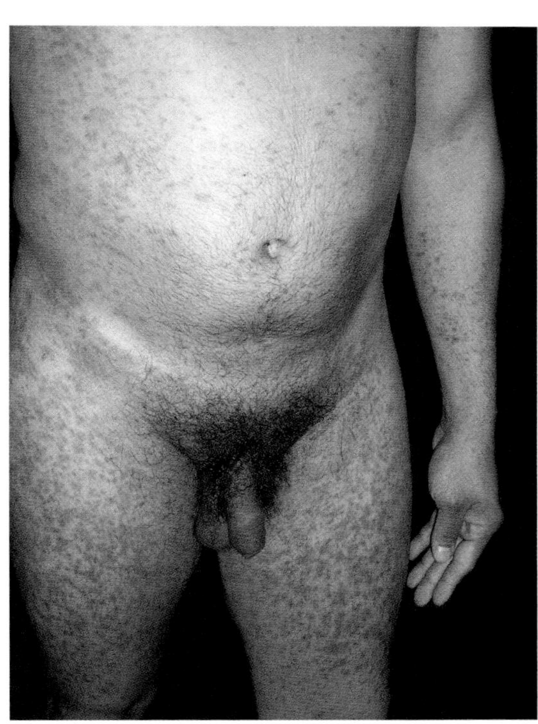

FIGURE 151-10 Pityriasis rosea in a 40-year-old man with an inverse pattern. Note how there is a higher density of lesions on the legs. Rapid plasma reagin (RPR) was negative and the diagnosis was confirmed with a punch biopsy. (*Reproduced with permission from Richard P. Usatine, MD.*)

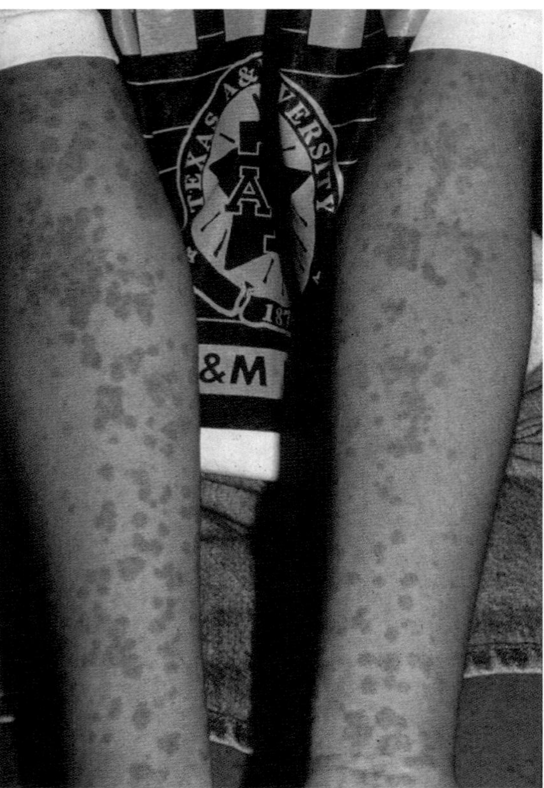

FIGURE 151-11 Pityriasis rosea on the arms with prominent erythematous lesions. (*Reproduced with permission from the University of Texas Health Sciences Center, Division of Dermatology.*)

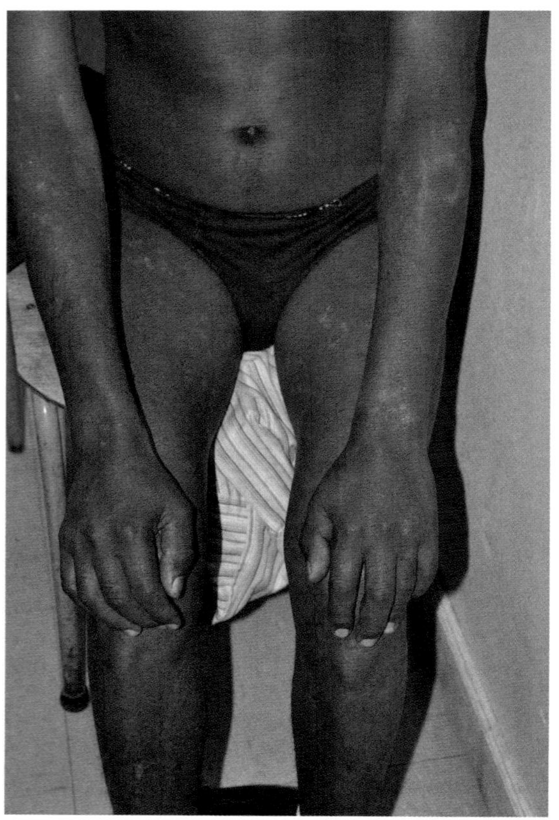

FIGURE 151-12 Pityriasis rosea in an inverse pattern with lesions on the arms and legs and sparing of the trunk. (*Reproduced with permission from Richard P. Usatine, MD.*)

DIFFERENTIAL DIAGNOSIS

- Tinea corporis is usually more localized than pityriasis rosea. However, the annular patterns, scale, and central clearing of some lesions in pityriasis rosea can mislead the clinician to misdiagnose tinea corporis. Tinea corporis tends to have fewer annular lesions and may have concentric circles rather than a single ring. Microscopy with potassium hydroxide (KOH) usually demonstrates branching hyphae (see Chapter 136, Tinea Corporis).
- Tinea versicolor has a distribution similar to pityriasis rosea, but is not associated with a herald patch. The pattern of scaling noted is generally more diffuse and not annular. Microscopy with KOH demonstrates the *spaghetti-and-meatball* pattern typical of *Pityrosporum* (see Chapter 139, Tinea Versicolor).
- Secondary syphilis is also a papulosquamous eruption. Lesions are often found on the palms and soles, which is not the case in pityriasis rosea; however, because the 2 conditions cannot always be accurately distinguished on clinical grounds, a blood test for syphilis is indicated if there is a significant doubt in the diagnosis (see Chapter 218, Syphilis).
- Nummular eczema has coin-like areas of scale that can resemble pityriasis rosea. The scale is not collarette and nummular eczema has a predilection for the legs, an area that is less often involved with pityriasis rosea (see Chapter 143, Atopic Dermatitis).
- Guttate psoriasis generally presents as oval to round, scaly macules on the trunk, and so can be confused with pityriasis rosea. However, the scaling is generally thicker and more adherent than in pityriasis rosea (see Chapter 150, Psoriasis).

MANAGEMENT

- Pityriasis rosea often requires no treatment at all other than reassurance.
- Topical steroids and oral diphenhydramine may be used to relieve itching when there is pruritus involved. SOR C
- One study found oral erythromycin to be effective in treating patients with pityriasis rosea,[5] although a subsequent study did not find erythromycin to be better than placebo.[6] SOR B
- Azithromycin did not cure pityriasis rosea in a study of children with this condition.[7]
- A Cochrane systematic review found inadequate evidence for efficacy for most treatments for pityriasis rosea.[8] Based on one small randomized controlled trial (RCT), the review authors noted that oral erythromycin may be effective in treating the rash and decreasing the itch.[5,8] The authors stated that this result should be treated with caution as it comes from only one small RCT.[5,8] SOR B

PATIENT EDUCATION

Patients are often concerned about the duration of the rash and whether they are contagious. They should be reassured that pityriasis rosea is self-limited and not truly contagious. Although there have been reported clusters of pityriasis rosea in settings where people are living in close quarters (eg, dormitories), it is not considered to be contagious. It has a reported recurrence rate of only 2%.[5]

FOLLOW-UP

Patients should be instructed to follow-up if the rash persists for longer than 3 months as reevaluation and consideration of an alternate diagnosis may be prudent.

PATIENT RESOURCES

- Mayo Clinic. *Pityriasis Rosea*—**http://www.mayoclinic.com/health/pityriasis-rosea/DS00720.**
- WebMD. *Pityriasis Rosea: Topic Overview*—**http://www.webmd.com/skin-problems-and-treatments/tc/pityriasis-rosea-topic-overview.**

PROVIDER RESOURCES

- Medscape. *Pityriasis Rosea in Emergency Medicine*—**http://emedicine.medscape.com/article/762725.**
- American Academy of Dermatology. *Pityriasis Rosea*—**http://www.aad.org/skin-conditions/dermatology-a-to-z/pityriasis-rosea.**

REFERENCES

1. Stulberg DH, Wolfrey J. Pityriasis rosea. *Am Fam Physician.* 2004;69:87-92, 94.
2. Browning JC. An update on pityriasis rosea and other similar childhood exanthems. *Curr Opin Pediatr.* 2009;21(4):481-485.
3. Youngquist S, Usatine R. It's beginning to look a lot like Christmas. *West J Med.* 2001;175(4):227-228.
4. Habif TP. *Clinical Dermatology*. 5th ed. St Louis, MO: Mosby; 2009:316-319.
5. Sharma PK, Yadav TP, Gautam RK, et al. Erythromycin in pityriasis rosea: a double-blind, placebo-controlled clinical trial. *J Am Acad Dermatol.* 2000;42(2 pt 1):241-244.
6. Rasi A, Tajziehchi L, Savabi-Nasab S. Oral erythromycin is ineffective in the treatment of pityriasis rosea. *J Drugs Dermatol.* 2008;7(1):35-38.
7. Amer H, Fischer H. Azithromycin does not cure pityriasis rosea. *Pediatrics.* 2006;117(4):1702-1705.
8. Chuh AA, Dofitas BL, Comisel GG, et al. Interventions for pityriasis rosea. *Cochrane Database Syst Rev.* 2007;(2):CD005068.

152 LICHEN PLANUS

Robert Kraft, MD
Richard P. Usatine, MD

PATIENT STORY

A 38-year-old Hispanic woman presents with a rash on her forearms, wrists, ankle, and back (**Figures 152-1** to **152-3**). She states the rash is mildly itchy and she does not like the way it looks. She would like some medication to make this better. Lichen planus (LP) was diagnosed and clobetasol was prescribed to keep the LP under better control.

INTRODUCTION

LP is a self-limited, recurrent, or chronic autoimmune disease affecting the skin, oral mucosa, and genitalia. LP is generally diagnosed clinically with lesions classically described using the 6 Ps (planar, purple, polygonal, pruritic, papules, and plaques).

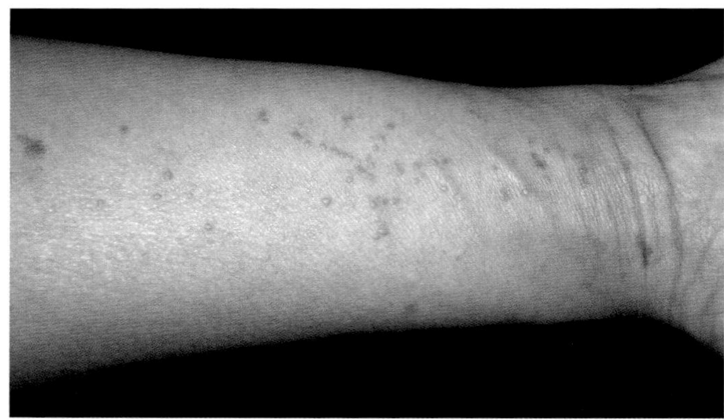

A

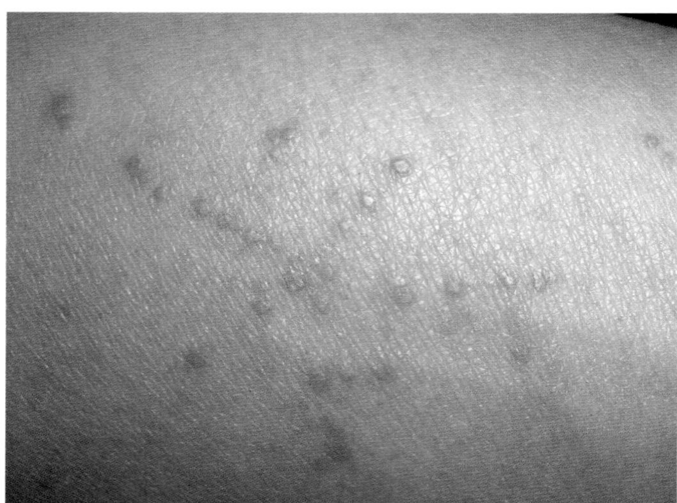

B

FIGURE 152-1 **A.** A 38-year-old Hispanic woman with lichen planus on her wrist. **B.** Close-up of wrist showing linearity of the lesions on the flexor surface. Lesions may be pink rather than purple. *(Reproduced with permission from Richard P. Usatine, MD.)*

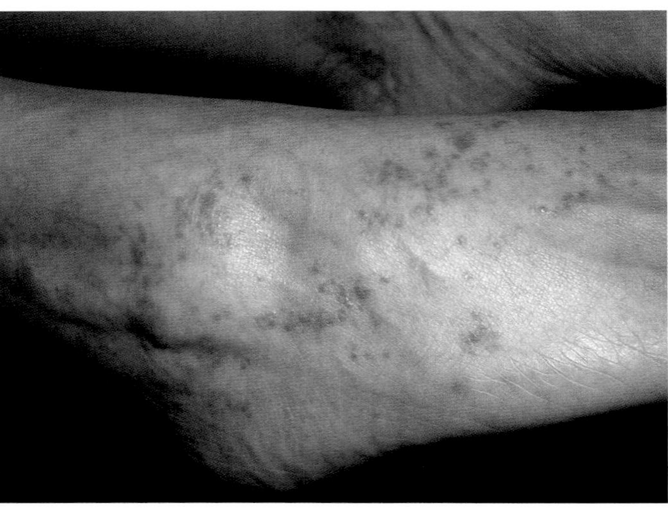

FIGURE 152-2 Ankle of the woman in **Figure 152-1** with typical lichen planus eruption. *(Reproduced with permission from Richard P. Usatine, MD.)*

EPIDEMIOLOGY

- LP is an inflammatory dermatosis of skin or mucous membranes that occurs in approximately 1% of all new patients seen at health care clinics.[1]
- Although most cases occur between ages 30 and 60 years, LP can occur at any age.[1,2]
- There may be a slight female predominance.[2-4]

ETIOLOGY AND PATHOPHYSIOLOGY

- Usually idiopathic, thought to be a cell-mediated immune response to an unknown antigen.[2,3,5]
- Possible human leukocyte antigen (HLA)-associated genetic predisposition.[2]
- Lichenoid-type reactions may be associated with medications (eg, angiotensin-converting enzyme inhibitors [ACEIs], thiazide-type diuretics, tetracycline, chloroquine), metals (eg, gold, mercury), or infections (eg, secondary syphilis).[2,5]
- Associated with liver disease, especially related to hepatitis C virus.[2,5,6]
- LP may be found with other diseases of altered immunity (eg, ulcerative colitis, alopecia areata, myasthenia gravis).[1]
- Malignant transformation has been reported in ulcerative oral lesions in men.[1]

RISK FACTORS

- Possible HLA-associated genetic predisposition
- Hepatitis C virus infection, although causal relationship is not established[6]
- Certain drugs (see "Etiology and Pathophysiology" above)

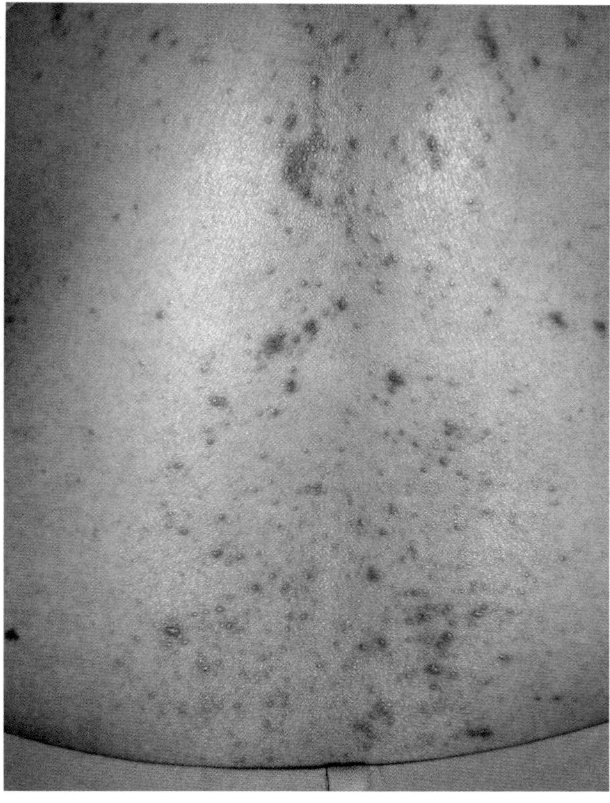

A

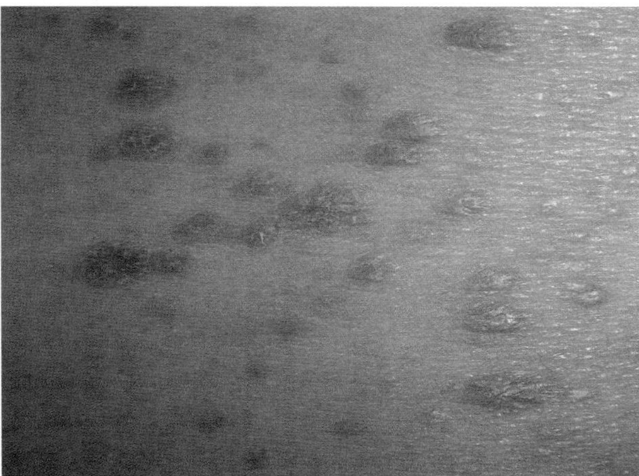

B

FIGURE 152-3 **A.** Lichen planus on the back of the woman in **Figure 152-1**. **B.** Close-up of lesions on the back showing Wickham striae crossing the flat papules of lichen planus. These lines are white and reticular like a net. (*Reproduced with permission from Richard P. Usatine, MD.*)

DIAGNOSIS

CLINICAL FEATURES

- Classically, the 6 Ps of LP are planar, purple, polygonal, pruritic, papules, and plaques (**Figures 152-1** to **152-4**).[2,5]
- These well-demarcated flat-topped violaceous lesions are often covered by lacy, reticular white lines (called Wickham striae or Wickham lines) (see **Figure 152-3B**).

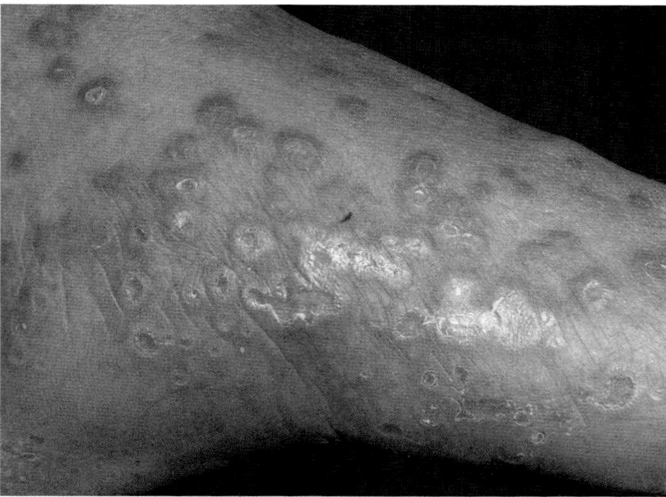

FIGURE 152-4 Hypertrophic lichen planus on the foot of a man. Purple polygonal papules and plaques are visible. (*Reproduced with permission from M. Craven, MD.*)

- An initial lesion is usually located on the flexor surface of the limbs, such as the wrists, followed by a generalized eruption with maximal spreading within 2 to 16 weeks.[1]
- Lesions may demonstrate the Koebner phenomenon (linear distribution) from scratching (see **Figure 152-1**).
- Lesions are more often hyperpigmented rather than purple or pink in dark-skinned persons, and skin may remain hyperpigmented after lesions resolve (**Figures 152-5** and **152-6**).
- Skin variants
  - Hypertrophic—Typical papules develop into thicker reddish-brown to purple plaques (see **Figures 152-4** and **152-6**) most commonly on the foot and shins. Seen more often in black men with hyperpigmented and hypertrophic lesions (see **Figure 152-6**).
  - Follicular—Pinpoint hyperkeratotic projections often on scalp, may lead to cicatricial alopecia.
  - Vesicular—Vesicles or bullae occur alongside the more typical LP lesions (**Figure 152-7**).

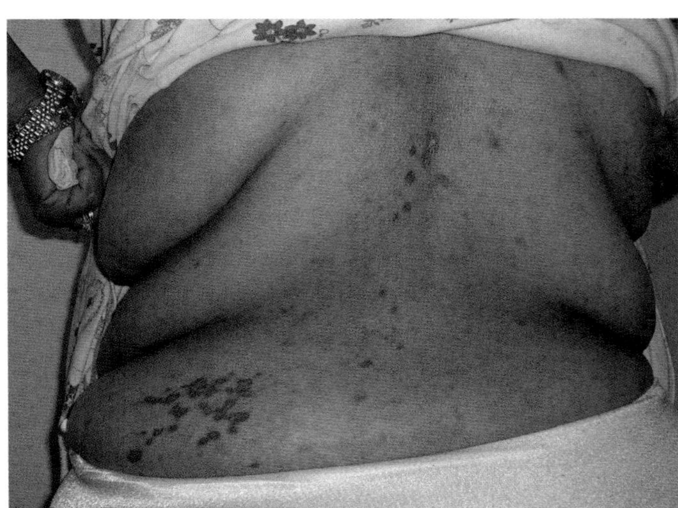

FIGURE 152-5 Hyperpigmented lichen planus on the back proven by punch biopsy. (*Reproduced with permission from Richard P. Usatine, MD.*)

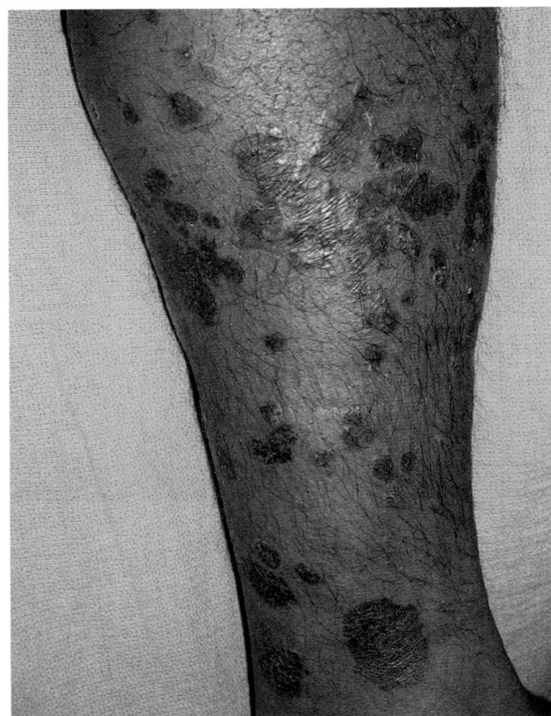

FIGURE 152-6 Hypertrophic lichen planus on the leg of a black man. Note the hyperpigmentation that is common when lichen planus occurs in a person with dark skin. (*Reproduced with permission from Richard P. Usatine, MD.*)

- Actinic—Typical lesions in sun-exposed areas, such as the face, back of hands and arms (**Figures and 152-8 and 152-9**).
- Atrophic—The lesions are atrophic rather than standard plaques (**Figure 152-10**).
- Ulcerative—Ulcers develop within typical lesions or start as waxy semitranslucent plaques on palms and soles; may require skin grafting.

• Mucous membrane variants
  - May be reticular (net-like; **Figure 152-11**), atrophic, erosive (**Figures 152-12** and **152-13**), or bullous. It is almost always bilateral.
  - Oral lesions may be asymptomatic or have a burning sensation; pain occurs with ulceration.[1,4,6]
  - Oral LP is often associated with extraoral LP.[7,8]

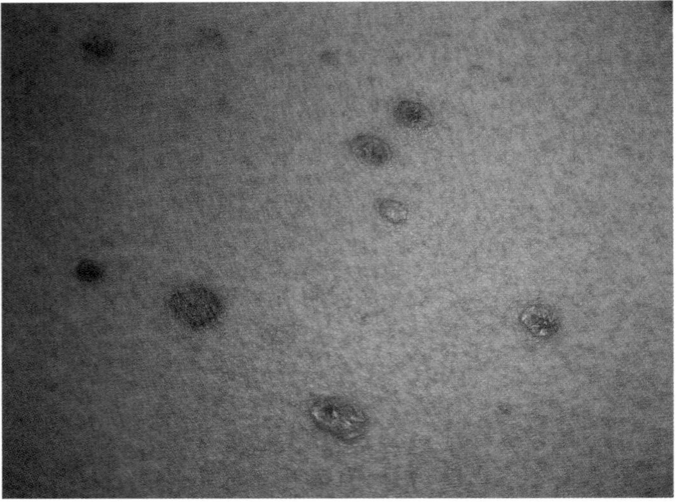

FIGURE 152-7 Bullous lichen planus on the buttocks. (*Reproduced with permission from Richard P. Usatine, MD.*)

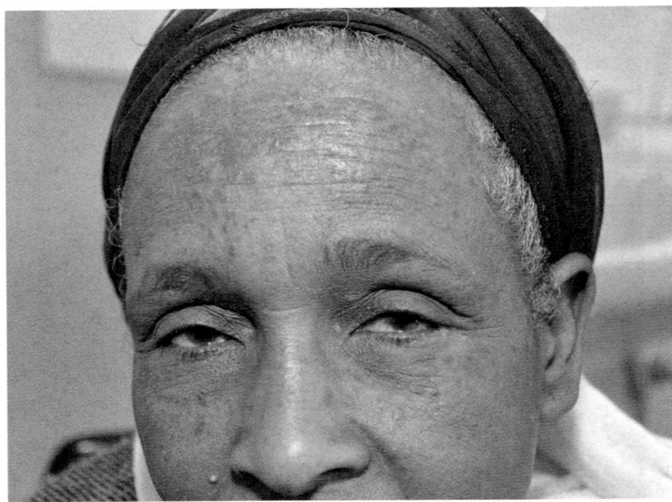

FIGURE 152-8 Actinic lichen planus on the face. (*Reproduced with permission from Richard P. Usatine, MD.*)

• Genitalia variants
  - Reticular, annular (**Figure 152-14**), papular (**Figure 152-15**), or erosive lesions on penis, scrotum, labia, or vagina.
  - Vulvar/vaginal lesions may be associated with dyspareunia, a burning sensation, and/or pruritus.[1,7]
  - Vulvar and urethral stenosis can also be present.[1,7]

• Hair and nail variants, the latter presents in 10% of patients.[1]
  - Violaceous, scaly, pruritic papules on the scalp can progress to scarring alopecia. Lichen planopilaris (LP of the scalp) can cause widespread hair loss (see Chapter 187, Scarring Alopecia).[9]
  - Nail plate thinning results in longitudinal grooving and ridging; rarely destruction of nailfold and nail bed with splintering (**Figure 152-16**).
  - Hyperpigmentation, subungual hyperkeratosis, onycholysis, and longitudinal melanonychia can result from LP.[1]

TYPICAL DISTRIBUTION

LP occurs on the wrists (**Figure 152-17**), ankles, lower back, eyelids, shins, scalp, penis, and mouth (ie, buccal mucosa, lateral tongue, and gingiva).[2,5]

LABORATORY STUDIES

Wickham striae can be accentuated by a drop of oil on the skin plaque and magnification.[5] Not all LP has visible Wickham striae. This study is rarely needed. If the diagnosis is uncertain, a punch biopsy should be performed.

BIOPSY

- A punch biopsy is a valuable method to make as initial diagnosis if the clinical picture is not certain. A biopsy is rarely needed to evaluate for malignant transformation.[5,10]
- Mainly lymphocytic immunoinflammatory infiltrate with hyperkeratosis, increased granular layer, and liquefaction of basal cell layer.[2,5]
- Linear fibrin and fibrinogen deposits along basement membrane.[2,5]
- Direct immunofluorescence on biopsy specimen reveals globular deposits of immunoglobulin (Ig) G, IgM, IgA, and complement at dermal–epidermal junction.[5]

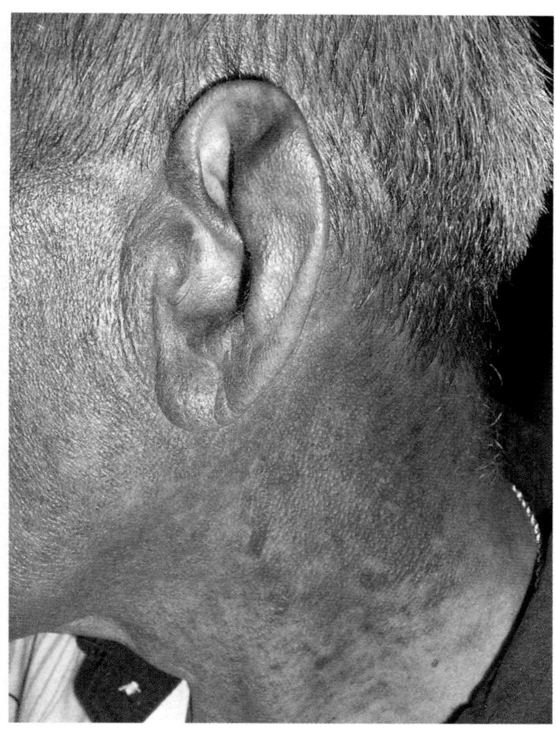

A

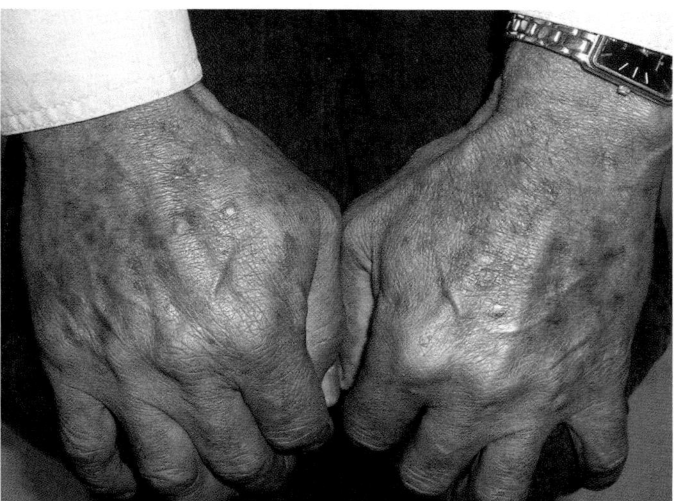

B

FIGURE 152-9 Actinic lichen planus in a black man related to sun exposure and proven by biopsy. **A.** Hyperpigmented flat plaques on the face and neck and **B.** on the dorsum of the hands. (*Reproduced with permission from Richard P. Usatine, MD.*)

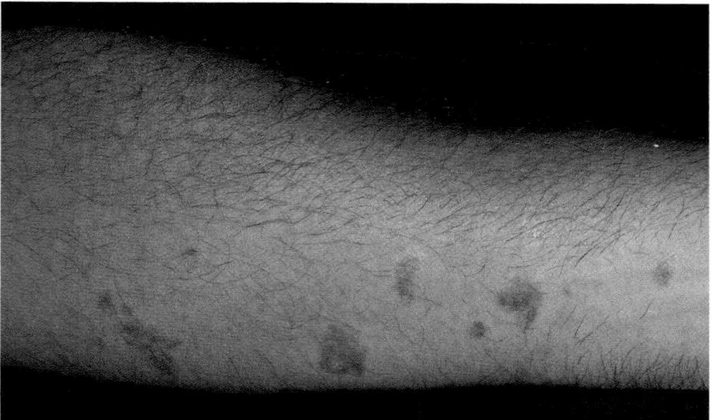

FIGURE 152-10 Atrophic lichen planus (biopsy proven) on the forearm showing multiple colors within the atrophic lesions. (*Reproduced with permission from Richard P. Usatine, MD.*)

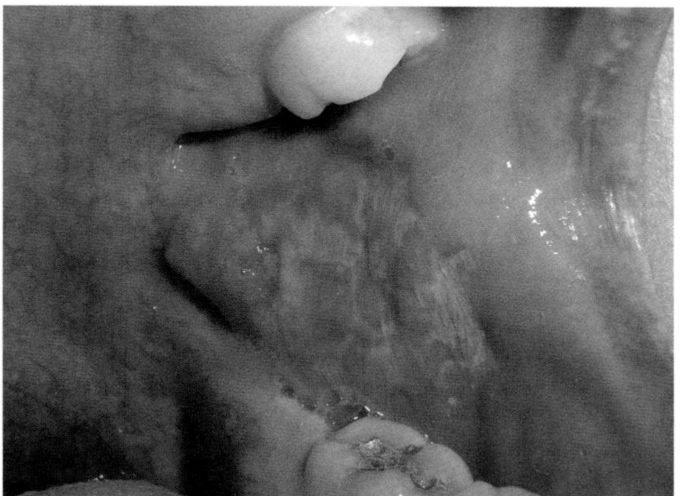

FIGURE 152-11 Asymptomatic white keratotic striae of lichen planus on left buccal mucosa of a 56-year-old woman. The patient had similar involvement of the right buccal mucosa and gingivae. Lichen planus in the mouth is bilateral. (*Reproduced with permission from Richard P. Usatine, MD.*)

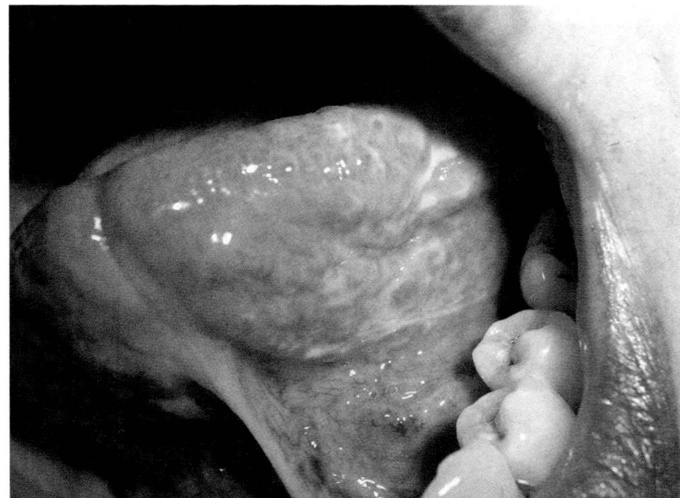

FIGURE 152-12 Erosive lichen planus, lateral surface of the tongue. This 52-year-old woman experiences tongue discomfort while eating acidic or spicy foods. (*Reproduced with permission from Richard P. Usatine, MD.*)

DIFFERENTIAL DIAGNOSIS

Skin lesions that may be confused with LP are as below:

- Eczematous dermatitis—"The itch that rashes" includes dry skin, itching, often excoriations and lichenification of skin with predilection for flexor surfaces (see Chapter 143, Atopic Dermatitis).
- Psoriasis has more prominent silvery scale and is generally located on extensor surfaces.[5] A punch biopsy can be used to distinguish between these 2 when the clinical picture is not clear (see Chapter 150, Psoriasis).

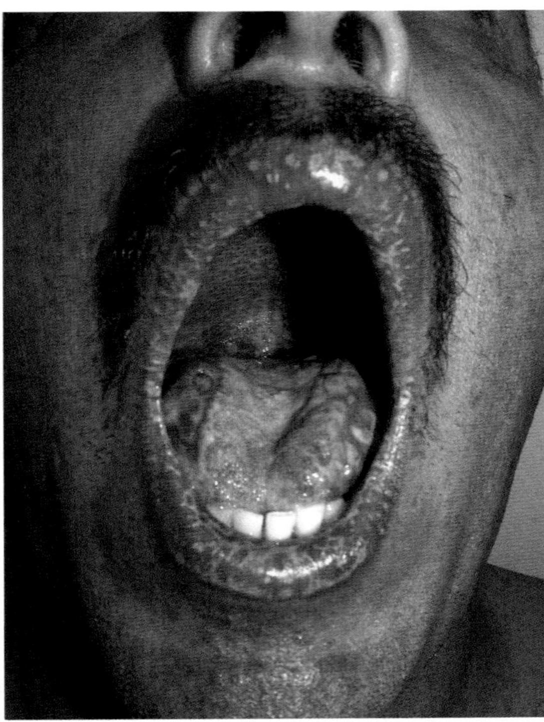

FIGURE 152-13 Lichen planus in the mouth with erosions. The lips, tongue, and palate are all involved. (*Reproduced with permission from Eric Kraus, MD.*)

- Stasis dermatitis—Lower-extremity eczematous dermatitis with inflammatory papules and often ulceration, in the setting of chronic venous insufficiency with dependent edema (see Chapter 51, Venous Stasis).
- Pityriasis rosea—Herald patch and subsequent pink papules and plaques with long axes along skin lines (Christmas tree pattern) (see Chapter 151, Pityriasis Rosea).
- Chronic cutaneous lupus erythematosus—Bright-red sharply-demarcated papules with adherent scale. Tend to regress centrally and can be light induced. Generally located on face, scalp, forearms, and hands. Biopsy may be necessary to differentiate (see Chapter 178, Lupus: Systemic and Cutaneous).[5]

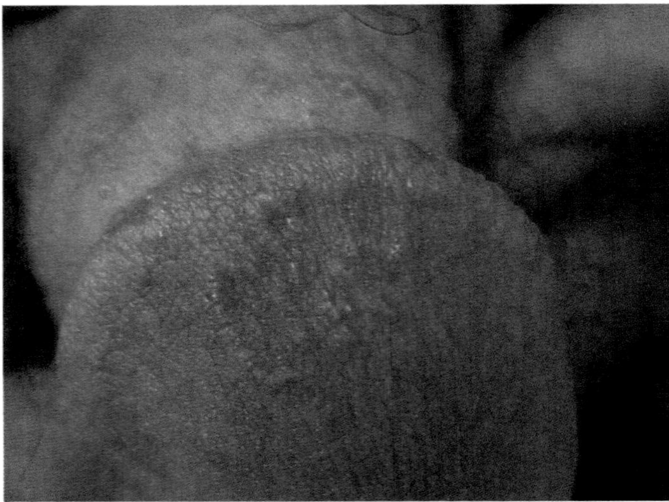

FIGURE 152-14 Lichen planus on the penis showing a lacy white pattern. (*Reproduced with permission from Dan Stulberg, MD.*)

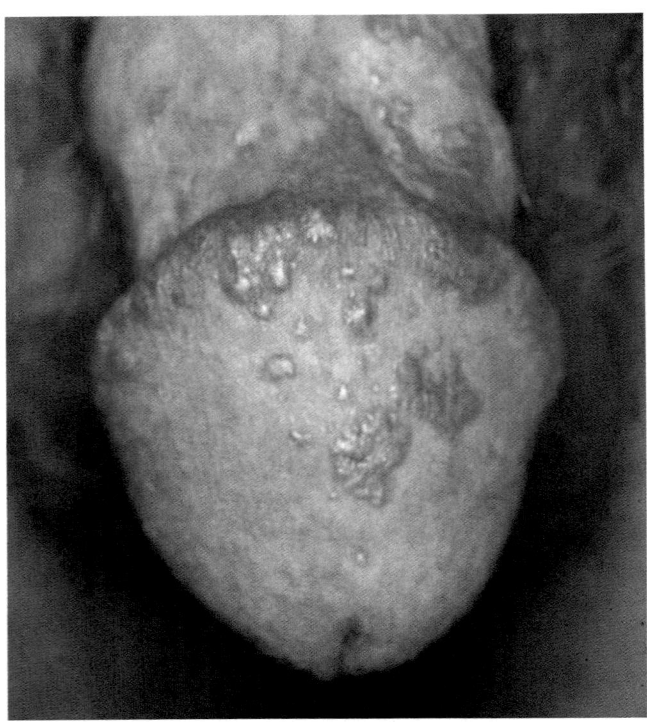

FIGURE 152-15 Lichen planus on the penis that is more similar to the pattern seen on other parts of the body. This is an example of planar, purple, polygonal papules on the penis. (*Reproduced with permission from John Gonzalez, MD.*)

- Bowen disease—Sharply-demarcated pink, red, brown, or black scaling or hyperkeratotic macule, papule, or plaque, usually mistaken for eczema or psoriasis, associated with ultraviolet radiation, human papilloma virus (HPV), chemicals, and chronic heat exposure. Biopsy is

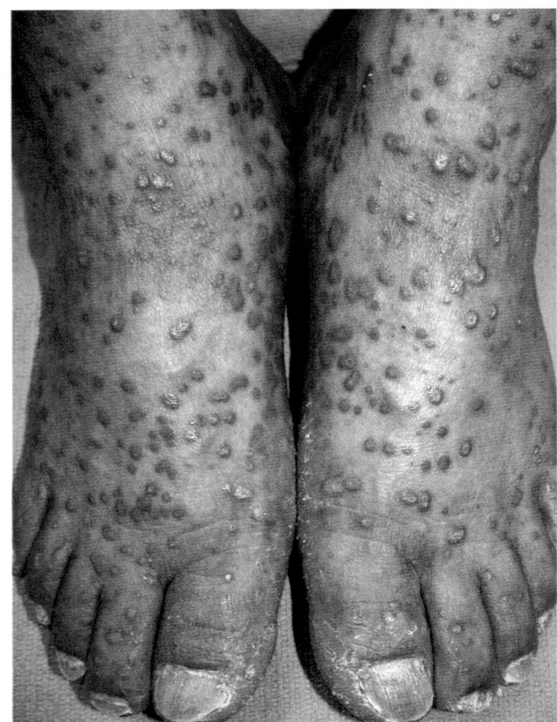

FIGURE 152-16 Hypertrophic lichen planus covering the dorsum of both feet with nail splintering. Note the purple color and Wickham lines. (*Reproduced with permission from Eric Kraus, MD.*)

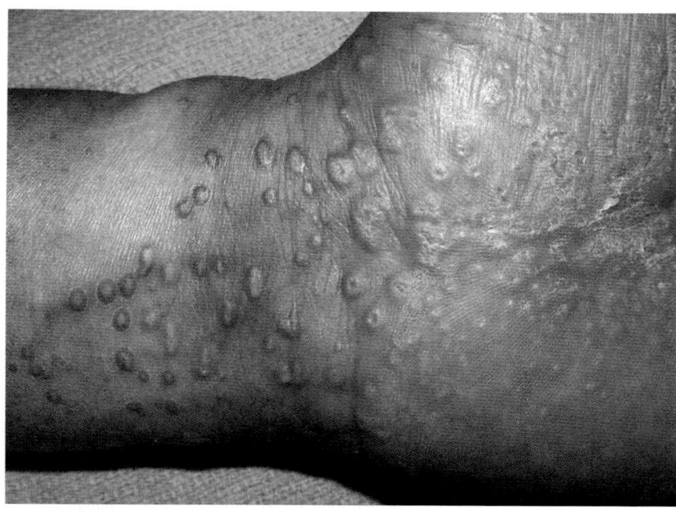

FIGURE 152-17 Thick hypertrophic papules and plaques on the wrist of the man in Figure 152-16. (*Reproduced with permission from Eric Kraus, MD.*)

needed to make the diagnosis (see Chapter 164, Actinic Keratosis and Bowen Disease).

- Lichen simplex chronicus—Localized confluence of lichenification from excoriation; patients have a strong urge to scratch their skin (see Chapter 147, Psychocutaneous Disorders).
- Prurigo nodularis—Nodular form of lichen simplex chronicus, brown-to-red hard, domed nodules from scratching and picking of intense pruritus. LP is not usually so pruritic (see Chapter 147, Psychocutaneous Disorders).

Other mucous membrane lesions that may appear similar are as below[5]:

- Leukoplakia—White adherent patch or plaque to oral mucosa. Less net-like pattern. Biopsy warranted because of the risk of malignancy (see Chapter 38, Leukoplakia).
- Thrush—Removable whitish plaques over an erythematous mucosal surface caused by *Candida* infection, confirmed by potassium hydroxide (KOH) preparation (see Chapter 135, Candidiasis).
- Bite trauma in the mouth—May result in white areas of the lip or buccal mucosa; Persons may have a white bite line where the upper and lower molars occlude and this can be confused with oral LP. If in doubt, a biopsy may be needed.

Genital lesions that may be differentiated from LP are as below[5]:

- Psoriasis on the penis can look like LP on the penis. A shave biopsy can be used to differentiate between these 2 diagnoses (see Chapter 150, Psoriasis).
- Syphilis—Primary infection manifests as painless shallow ulcer (chancre) at site of inoculation, if untreated secondary syphilis presents with macular and then papular, pustular, or acneiform eruption on trunk, neck, palms, and soles, condyloma lata (soft, moist, flat-topped pink-to-tan papules) in the anogenital region (see Chapter 218, Syphilis).

MANAGEMENT

LP may persist for months to years. Hypertrophic LP and oral LP can last for decades.[2] Any type of LP can recur. Antihistamines can be used for symptomatic pruritus.[5] SOR C Symptomatic and severe cases can be treated as follows:

- Localized/topical treatment.
  - Topical corticosteroids twice a day.[11-13] SOR B Mid- to high-potency steroids are usually needed. Clobetasol cream or ointment may be used on the skin and clobetasol ointment or gel may be used in the mouth.
  - Topical aloe vera gel has demonstrated efficacy against oral LP.[14,15] SOR B
  - Intralesional triamcinolone (3-5 mg/mL) for hypertrophic or mucous membrane lesions, may repeat every 3 to 4 weeks.[2,5,10,11] SOR B
  - Tacrolimus, pimecrolimus, retinoids, or cyclosporine in mouthwash or adhesive base for oral disease unresponsive to topical corticosteroids.[3,4,10,12,16-19] SOR B
  - Topical corticosteroids, tacrolimus and aloe vera gel have demonstrated efficacy for vulvar LP.[20,21] SOR B
- Systemic treatment can be considered for resistant, widespread, or severe cases.
  - Oral steroids may be used starting with a 3-week tapered course of oral prednisone (60 mg/d starting dose).[2,10,11,22,23] SOR B
  - Systemic retinoids (eg, acitretin 25 mg/d). Monitor serum creatinine, liver function tests (LFTs), fasting lipids.[3,10,23] SOR B Contraindicated in women of childbearing potential.
  - Cyclosporine (5 mg/kg per day). Monitor complete blood count, serum creatinine, LFTs, and blood pressure.[2] SOR B
  - Azathioprine may be used as a steroid-sparing agent (50 mg PO daily to start and titrate to 100-250 mg PO daily). Monitor complete blood count and LFTs.[5,10] SOR C
  - Psoralen UVA (PUVA) phototherapy may be effective but can cause phototoxic reactions and has long-term risks, including the development of squamous cell carcinoma.[24] SOR C
  - Carbon dioxide laser and low-level laser therapy have reports of treatment success against oral LP.[25,26] SOR C

PROGNOSIS

- Generally self-limiting and spontaneous resolution may occur in 12 to 18 months.
- Recurrences are common.
- Mucosal LP is generally more persistent than cutaneous forms.
- Malignant transformation of LP is rare.

FOLLOW-UP

- Follow-up depends on severity and treatment course.
- Oral and vaginal disease may be most challenging to treat.
- Follow oral or vaginal lesions for possible malignant transformation. Because of low risk of transformation even with oral LP (best estimate 0.2% per year), routine screening and biopsy are not recommended.[10] Biopsy is recommended if suspecting malignancy; lesion becomes larger, ulcerated, nodular, or lose reticular pattern.

PATIENT EDUCATION

- Patients should understand that LP is often self-limiting and may resolve in 12 to 18 months.
- There is a significant chance of recurrence.

PATIENT RESOURCES

- Online support group for LP—**http://www.mdjunction.com/lichen-planus.**
- Online support group for oral LP—**http://bcdwp.web.tamhsc.edu/iolpdallas/.**

PROVIDER RESOURCES

- Usatine RP, Tinitigan M. Diagnosis and treatment of LP. *Am Fam Physician.* 2011;84(1):53-60. Available online—**http://www.aafp.org/afp/2011/0701/p53.html# afp20110701p53-b14.**

REFERENCES

1. Chuang T-Y, Stitle L. http://emedicine.medscape.com/article/1123213-overview. Accessed September 20, 2011.
2. Wolff K, Johnson RA. *Fitzpatrick's Color Atlas and Synopsis of Clinical Dermatology*. 6th ed. New York, NY: McGraw-Hill; 2009;128-133.
3. Zakrzewska JM, Chan ES-Y, Thornhill MH. A systematic review of placebo-controlled randomized clinical trials of treatments used in oral lichen planus. *Br J Dermatol.* 2005;153:336-341.
4. Laeijendecker R, Tank B, Dekker SK, Neumann HA. A comparison of treatment of oral lichen planus with topical tacrolimus and triamcinolone acetonide ointment. *Acta Derm Venereol.* 2006;86(3):227-229.
5. Habif TP. *Clinical Dermatology: A Color Guide to Diagnosis and Therapy*. 5th ed. Philadelphia, PA: Mosby; 2010.
6. Shengyuan L, Songpo Y, Wen W, et al. Hepatitis C virus and lichen planus: a reciprocal association determined by a meta-analysis. *Arch Dermatol.* 2009;145(9):1040-1047.
7. Di Fede O, Belfiore P, Cabibi D, et al. Unexpectedly high frequency of genital involvement in women with clinical and histological features of oral lichen planus. *Acta Derm Venereol.* 2006;86(5):433-438.
8. Imail SB, Kumar SK, Zain RB. Oral lichen planus and lichenoid reactions: etiopathogenesis, diagnosis, management and malignant transformation. *J Oral Sci.* 2007;49(2):89-106.
9. Cevacso NC, Bergfeld WF, Remzi BK, de Knott HR. A case-series of 29 patients with lichen planopilaris: the Cleveland Clinic Foundation experience on evaluation, diagnosis, and treatment. *J Am Acad Dermatol.* 2007;57(1):47-53.
10. Lodi G, Scully C, Carrozzo M, et al. Current controversies in oral lichen planus: report of an international consensus meeting, part 2. Clinical management and malignant transformation. *Oral Surg Oral Med Oral Pathol Oral Radiol Endod.* 2005;100:164-178.
11. Cribier B, Frances C, Chosidow O. Treatment of lichen planus. An evidence-based medicine analysis of efficacy. *Arch Dermatol.* 1998;134(12):1521-1530.
12. Corrocher G, Di Lorenzo G, Martinelli N, et al. Comparative effect of tacrolimus 0.1% ointment and clobetasol 0.05% ointment in patients with oral lichen planus. *J Clin Periodontol.* 2008;35(3):244-249.
13. Carbone M, Arduino PG, Carrozzo M, et al. Topical clobetasol in the treatment of atrophic-erosive oral lichen planus: a randomized controlled trial to compare two preparations with different concentrations. *J Oral Pathol Med.* 2009;38(2):227-233.
14. Choonhakarn C, Busaracome P, Sripanidkulchai B, Sarakam P. The efficacy of aloe vera gel in the treatment of oral lichen planus: a randomized controlled trial. *Br J Dermatol.* 2008;158(3):573-577.
15. Salazar SN. Efficacy of topical Aloe vera in patients with oral lichen planus: a randomized double-blind study. *J Oral Pathol Med.* 2010;39(10):735-740.
16. Conrotto D, Carbone M, Carrozzo M, et al. Ciclosporine vs. clobetasol in the topical management of atrophic and erosive oral lichen planus: a double-blind, randomized controlled trial. *Br J Dermatol.* 2006;152(1):139-145.
17. Swift JC, Rees TD, Plemons JM, et al. The effectiveness of 1% pimecrolimus cream in the treatment of oral erosive lichen planus. *J Periodontol.* 2005;76(4):627-635.
18. Volz T, Caroli U, Ludtke H, et al. Pimecrolimus cream 1% in erosive oral lichen planus—a prospective randomized double-blind vehicle-controlled study. *Br J Dermatol.* 2008;159(4):936-941.
19. Thongprasom K, Carrozzo M, Furness S, Lodi G. Interventions for treating oral lichen planus. *Cochrane Database Syst Rev.* 2011 Jul 6;(7):CD001168.
20. Rajar UD, Majeed R, Parveen N, et al. Efficacy of aloe vera gel in the treatment of vulval lichen planus. *J Coll Physicians Surg Pak.* 2008;18(10):612-614.
21. McPherson T, Cooper S. Vulval lichen sclerosis and lichen planus. *Dermatol Ther.* 2010;23(5):523-532.
22. Thongprasom K, Dhanuthai K. Steroids in the treatment of lichen planus: a review. *J Oral Sci.* 2008;50(4):377-385.
23. Asch S, Goldenberg G. Systemic treatment of cutaneous lichen planus: an update. *Cutis.* 2011;87(3):129-134.
24. Wackernagel A, Legat FJ, Hofer A, et al. Psoralen plus UVA vs. UVB-311 nm for the treatment of lichen planus. *Photodermatol Photoimmunol Photomed.* 2007;23(1):15-19.
25. van der Hem PS, Egges M, van der Wal JE, Roodenburg JL. CO_2 laser evaporation of oral lichen planus. *Int J Oral Maxillofac Surg.* 2008;37(7):630-633.
26. Cafaro A, Albanese G, Arduino PG, et al. Effect of low-level laser irradiation on unresponsive oral lichen planus: early preliminary results in 13 patients. *Photomed Laser Surg.* 2010;28(suppl 2):S99-S103.

153 REACTIVE ARTHRITIS

Heidi Chumley, MD
Angela Shedd, MD
Suraj Reddy, MD
Richard P. Usatine, MD

PATIENT STORY

A 29-year-old man presented with concerns about an extensive rash that had developed over the previous month. The rash was reported to involve the scalp, abdomen, penis, hands, and feet (**Figures 153-1** to **153-5**). He also complained of severe joint pain, involving the back, knees, and feet. He denied ocular, gastrointestinal (GI), or genitourinary (GU) complaints, but was prescribed a course of antibiotics last month when his partner was diagnosed with *Chlamydia*.

The patient's young age, rapid onset of symptoms, dermatologic findings, and arthritis were suggestive of reactive arthritis. The patient's joint pain was treated with nonsteroidal anti-inflammatory drugs (NSAIDs) and skin lesions were treated with topical corticosteroids. No antibiotics were prescribed because no current infectious agent was identified. In conjunction with a dermatologist, acitretin 25 mg daily was started to treat his psoriasiform lesions.

INTRODUCTION

Reactive arthritis is a noninfectious acute oligoarthritis that occurs in response to an infection, most commonly in the GI or urogenital tract. Patients present 1 to 4 weeks after the triggering infection, with joint pain in asymmetric large joints; eye disease, such as conjunctivitis; and skin changes including erythema nodosum, keratoderma blennorrhagicum, and circinate balanitis. Diagnosis is based on the clinical presentation plus evidence of associated infection. Treatment includes anti-inflammatory medications and treatment of triggering infection.

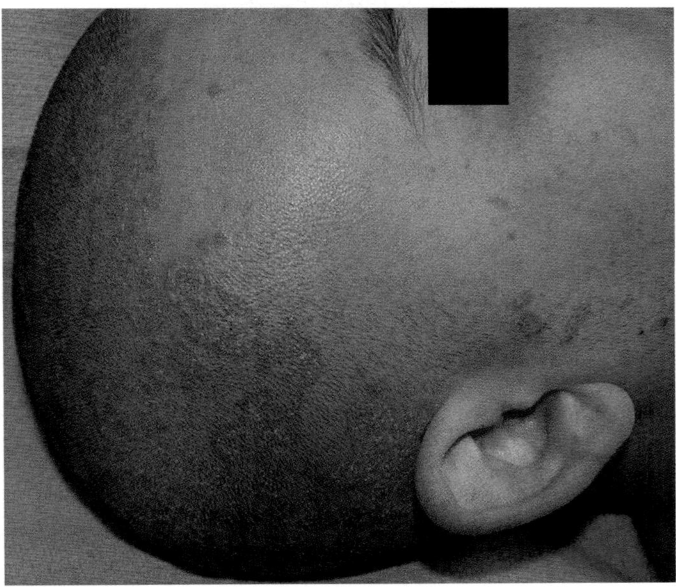

FIGURE 153-1 Reactive arthritis in a young man showing annular scalp lesions (circinate plaques). (*Reproduced with permission from Shedd AD, Reddy SG, Meffert JJ, Kraus EW. Acute onset of rash and oligoarthritis.* J Fam Pract. *2007;56(10):811-814. Reproduced with permission from Frontline Medical Communications.*)

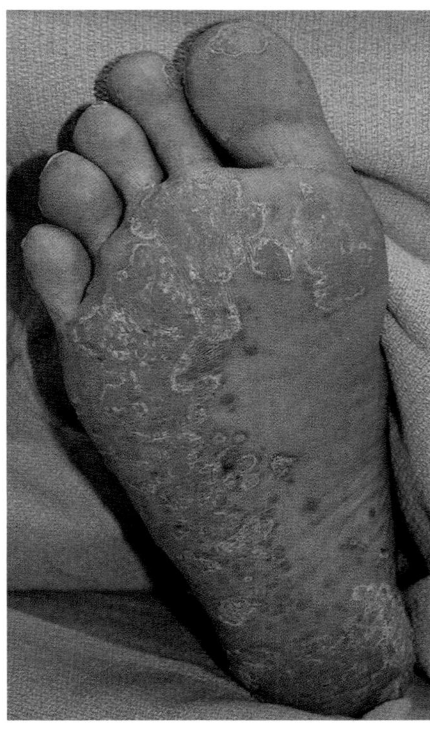

FIGURE 153-2 Keratoderma blennorrhagicum with hyperkeratotic papules, plaques, and pustules that have coalesced to form circular borders. (*Reproduced with permission from Shedd AD, Reddy SG, Meffert JJ, Kraus EW. Acute onset of rash and oligoarthritis.* J Fam Pract. *2007;56(10):811-814. Reproduced with permission from Frontline Medical Communications.*)

SYNONYMS

Reiter syndrome is no longer the preferred name as Dr. Reiter was a Nazi physician who performed unethical experimentation on human subjects.

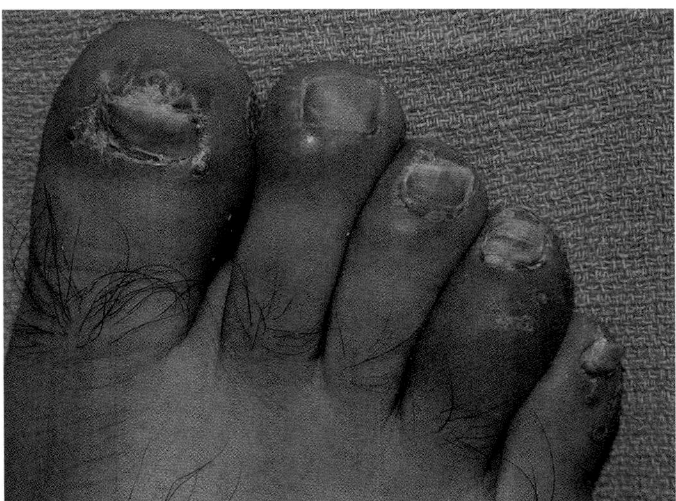

FIGURE 153-3 Erythema and scale seen on the toes of the patient in Figure 153-1. Note the nail involvement with subungual keratosis and onycholysis. The fourth toe is red and swollen; this is called dactylitis. (*Reproduced with permission from Shedd AD, Reddy SG, Meffert JJ, Kraus EW. Acute onset of rash and oligoarthritis.* J Fam Pract. *2007;56(10):811-814. Reproduced with permission from Frontline Medical Communications.*)

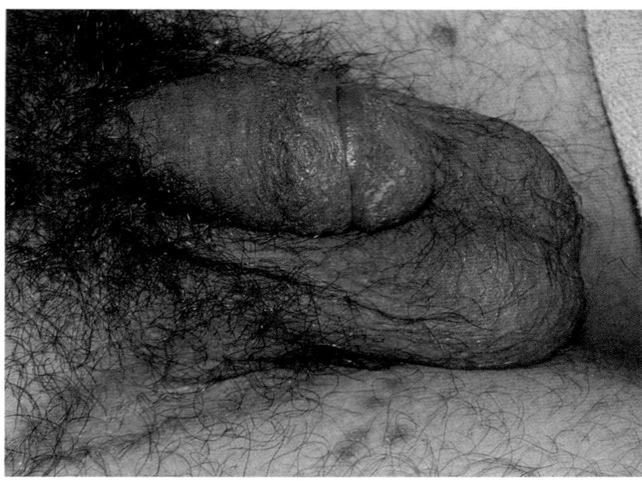

FIGURE 153-4 The patient in Figure 153-1 with psoriasiform lesion on the corona and glans. The patient also has erythema in the inguinal area that resembles inverse psoriasis. This particular case does not exemplify classic balanitis circinata, which is characterized by annular or arcuate thin scaly plaques, as opposed to the nonspecific scaly plaques found on this patient. *(Reproduced with permission from Suraj Reddy, MD.)*

EPIDEMIOLOGY

- Incidence is 0.6 to 27 per 100,000 people.[1]
- Most common in young adults ages 30 to 40 years, rare in children.[1]
- Reactive arthritis after a GU infection is more common in young men; reactive arthritis after a GI infection is equally common in men and women.[1]

ETIOLOGY AND PATHOPHYSIOLOGY

- Follows a GI (*Yersinia*, *Salmonella*, *Shigella*, *Campylobacter*, or rarely *Escherichia coli* or *Clostridium difficile*) or GU (*Chlamydia trachomatis*, *Ureaplasma urealyticum*) infection, less commonly follows a respiratory infection with *Chlamydia* pneumonia.
- Mechanism by which the triggering agent leads to development of arthritis is not fully understood.

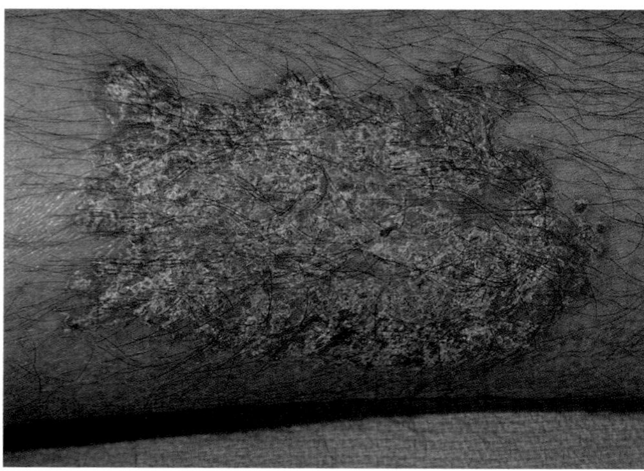

FIGURE 153-5 Psoriatic-appearing plaque on the leg in the same patient of Figure 153-1 with reactive arthritis. *(Reproduced with permission from Shedd AD, Reddy SG, Meffert JJ, Kraus EW. Acute onset of rash and oligoarthritis.* J Fam Pract. *2007;56(10):811-814. Reproduced with permission from Frontline Medical Communications.)*

RISK FACTORS

- Infection with a triggering agent.
- Presence of human leukocyte antigen (HLA)-B27 is associated with an increased risk of chronic disease and a more severe arthritis.
- HLA-B27 has been found in a high percentage of patients with severe disease, but there is no increase in HLA-B27 prevalence in population studies.

DIAGNOSIS

Definite reactive arthritis: Two major criteria and one minor criterion

Probable reactive arthritis: one major criterion and one minor criterion

Major criteria

- Arthritis with 2 of 3 features: asymmetric, mono- or oligoarthritis, lower limbs predominately affected
- Preceding enteritis or urethritis

Minor criteria

- Evidence of triggering infection
- Evidence of synovial infection

CLINICAL FEATURES

- The classic triad consists of urethritis, conjunctivitis (**Figure 153-6**), and arthritis; however, few patients present with the classic triad.
- Tendinitis, bursitis or enthesitis, or low back pain may be present.

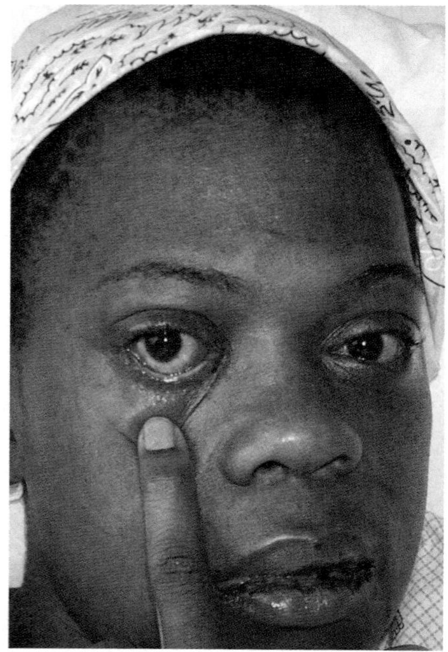

FIGURE 153-6 Reactive arthritis with conjunctivitis as a result of chlamydial pelvic inflammatory disease in a 42-year-old woman. She presented with fever, chills, and generalized pain in her joints, abdomen, and pelvis. *(Reproduced with permission from Joseph Mazziotta, MD, and from Mazziotta JM, Ahmed N. Conjunctivitis and cervicitis.* J Fam Pract. *2004;53(2):121-123. Reproduced with permission from Frontline Medical Communications.)*

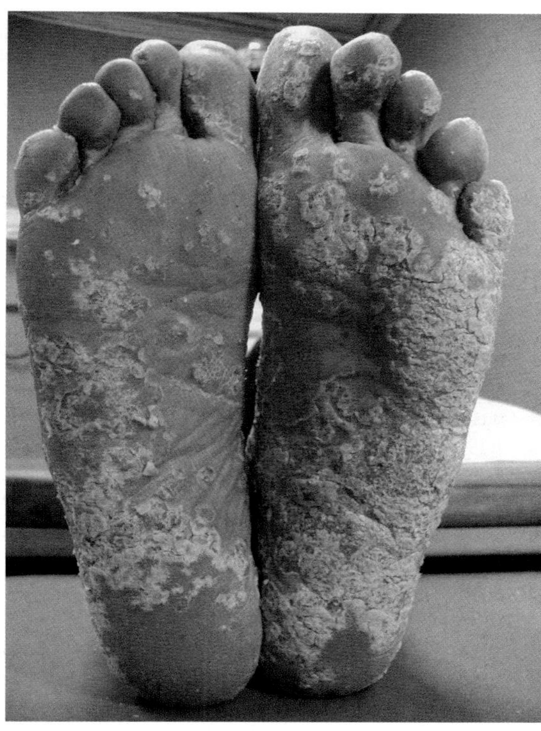

FIGURE 153-7 Keratoderma blennorrhagicum on the soles of the foot of a man with reactive arthritis. (*Reproduced with permission from Ricardo Zuniga-Montes, MD.*)

- Skin findings (psoriasiform) typically involve the palms, soles (keratoderma blennorrhagicum) (**Figures 153-2** and **153-7**), and the glans penis (balanitis circinata). Nail dystrophy, thickening, and destruction may occur (**Figures 153-3** and **153-8**). Many other body surfaces may be affected including the scalp (see **Figure 153-1**), intertriginous areas (see **Figure 153-4**), and the oral mucosa (**Figure 153-9**). Erosive lesions on the tongue and hard palate may be seen.
- Rarely, carditis and atrioventricular conduction disturbances are present.

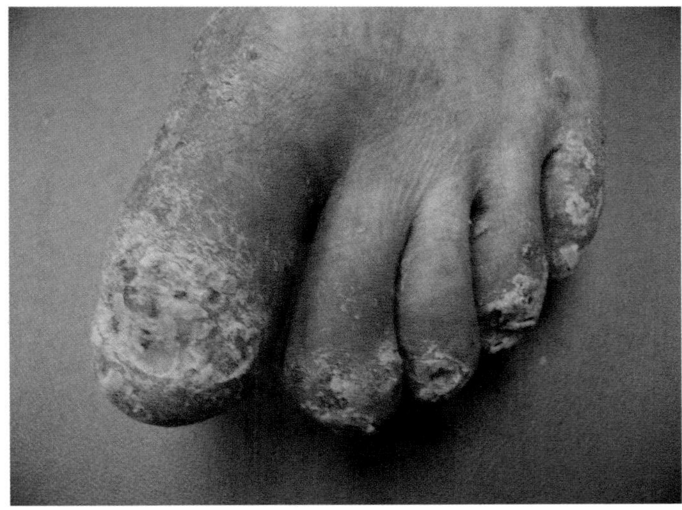

FIGURE 153-8 Nail dystrophy, thickening, and nail destruction in a man with reactive arthritis. (*Reproduced with permission from Ricardo Zuniga-Montes, MD.*)

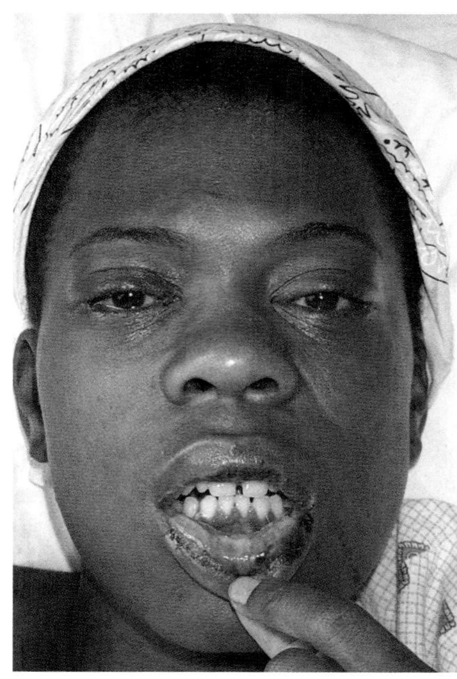

FIGURE 153-9 Oral mucosal inflammation with reactive arthritis secondary to chlamydial pelvic inflammatory disease. The cervix was also inflamed on examination. (*Reproduced with permission from Joseph Mazziotta, and from Mazziotta JM, Ahmed N. Conjunctivitis and cervicitis.* J Fam Pract. *2004;53(2):121-123. Reproduced with permission from Frontline Medical Communications.*)

LABORATORY TESTING

- No specific laboratory test is used to confirm reactive arthritis.
- Erythrocyte sedimentation rate (ESR) and C-reactive protein are usually elevated.
- Urethral/cervical swab or urine test for *C. trachomatis* when a GU infection precedes the onset of symptoms.
- Stool culture may detect an enteric pathogen when GI infection precedes the onset of symptoms.
- *Salmonella*, *Yersinia*, and *Campylobacter* antibodies can be detected in the serum after microbes are no longer detectable in the stool.
- Skin biopsy if performed resembles that of psoriasis with acanthosis of the epidermis, a neutrophilic perivascular infiltrate, and spongiform pustules.

DIFFERENTIAL DIAGNOSIS

- Spondyloarthropathies and reactive arthropathies may present with acute joint pain but often lack the skin findings seen with reactive arthritis (see Chapter 101, Ankylosing Spondylitis).
- Psoriatic arthritis may be easily confused especially in immunocompromised patients. Lack of constitutional symptoms and a more chronic course help differentiate from reactive arthritis.
- Gonococcal arthritis is characterized by migratory polyarthralgia that settles in one or more joints. Often erythematous macules or hemorrhagic papules on acral sites help distinguish from reactive arthritis.
- Rheumatoid arthritis often presents with a progressive, symmetric polyarthritis of the small joints of the hands and wrists. Females are affected more often than males (see Chapter 99, Rheumatoid Arthritis).

MANAGEMENT

- Treat patients with acute *C. trachomatis* with 1 g azithromycin single dose or 100 mg doxycycline twice a day for 7 days.[1,2] SOR Ⓐ Treat partners when possible.[1]
- The current recommendation no longer calls for long-term antibiotics as studies do not support this previous treatment.[3,4] SOR Ⓑ
- GI-triggering infections are typically self-limiting and do not require antibiotics.
- Treat inflammation with NSAIDs.[2] SOR Ⓑ
- Consider glucocorticoid joint injections in patients with severe joint pain.
- For refractory arthritic disease, immunosuppressive agents, such as sulfasalazine at 2000 mg/d, have demonstrated some benefit.[5] SOR Ⓑ
- Treat mucosal and skin lesions with topical corticosteroids.
- Psoriasiform skin lesions may be treated with some of the same medications used to treat psoriasis (including acitretin). SOR Ⓒ
- Systemic steroids are indicated for patients with systemic symptoms (fever) or in those who develop carditis.
- Current evidence demonstrates that chronic antimicrobial therapy is not recommended.[3,4]

REFERRAL

- Refer patients with severe or nonresponsive joint pain to a rheumatologist.
- Refer patients who develop cardiac manifestations to a cardiologist.

PROGNOSIS

- Arthritic symptoms typically resolve in 3 to 5 months.[1] Persistent symptoms that last longer than 6 months are associated with the development of chronic symptoms.
- Sixteen percent to 68% of patients developed chronic symptoms across several studies. Type of triggering infection and presence of HLA-B27 affect prognosis.

FOLLOW-UP

Follow patients closely at the time of diagnosis to ensure response to therapy and timely referral for nonresponders.

PATIENT RESOURCES

- FamilyDoctor.org. *Reactive Arthritis*—**http://familydoctor.org/familydoctor/en/ diseases-conditions/reactive-arthritis.html.**

PROVIDER RESOURCES

- Medscape. *Reactive Arthritis*—**http://emedicine.medscape.com/article/331347.**

PATIENT EDUCATION

There is no curative treatment. Symptoms may resolve permanently, relapse, or persist. Medications and physical or occupational therapy can help relieve pain and preserve function. Seek medical care for extra-articular symptoms, especially those involving the eye.

REFERENCES

1. Hannu T. Reactive arthritis. *Best Pract Res Clin Rheumatol.* 2011;25(3):347-357.
2. Colmegna I, Cuchacovich R, Espinoza LR. HLA-B27-associated reactive arthritis: pathogenetic and clinical considerations. *Clin Microbiol Rev.* 2004;17(2):348-369.
3. Kvien TK, Gaston JS, Bardin I, et al. Three months treatment of reactive arthritis with azithromycin: a EULAR double blind, placebo controlled study. *Ann Rheum Dis.* 2004;63(9):1113-1119.
4. Putschky N, Pott HG, Kuipers JG, et al. Comparing 10-day and 4-month doxycycline courses for treatment of *Chlamydia trachomatis*–reactive arthritis: a prospective, double-blind trial. *Ann Rheum Dis.* 2006;65(11):1521-1524.
5. Clegg DO, Reda DJ, Weisman MH, et al. Comparison of sulfasalazine and placebo in the treatment of reactive arthritis (Reiter's syndrome). A Department of Veterans Affairs Cooperative Study. *Arthritis Rheum.* 1996;39(12):2021-2027.

154 ERYTHRODERMA

David Henderson, MD
Richard P. Usatine, MD

PATIENT STORY

A 34-year-old man presented with red skin from his neck to his feet for the last month (**Figure 154-1**). He was having a lot of itching and his skin was shedding so that wherever he would sit, there would be a pile of skin that would remain. He denied fever and chills. He admitted to smoking and drinking heavily. The patient's vital signs were stable with normal blood pressure and he preferred not to be hospitalized. He had some nail pitting but no personal or family history of psoriasis. The presumed diagnosis was erythrodermic psoriasis but a punch biopsy was done to confirm this. A complete blood count (CBC) and chemistry panel were ordered in anticipation of the patient needing systemic medications. A purified protein derivative (PPD) was also placed. The patient was started on total body 0.1% triamcinolone under wet wrap overnight and given a follow-up appointment for the next day. The patient was also counseled to quit smoking and drinking. The following day his laboratory results showed mild elevation in his liver function tests (LFTs) only. The following day his PPD was negative and he was already feeling a bit better from the topical triamcinolone. Cyclosporine was started and the patient improved rapidly.

INTRODUCTION

Erythroderma is an uncommon condition that affects all age groups. It is characterized by a generalized erythematous rash with associated scaling.

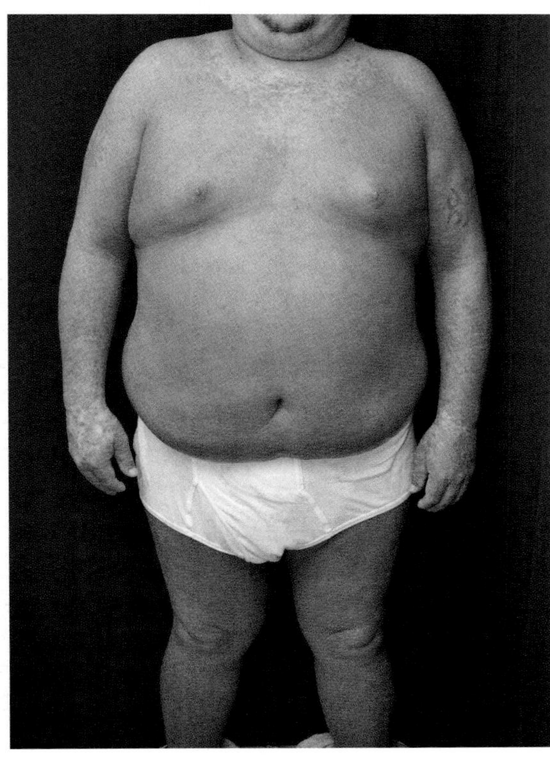

FIGURE 154-1 Erythrodermic psoriasis in a 34-year-old man. (*Reproduced with permission from Richard P. Usatine, MD.*)

It is generally a manifestation of another underlying dermatosis or systemic disorder. It is associated with a range of morbidity, and can have life-threatening metabolic and cardiovascular complications. Therapy is usually focused on treating the underlying disease, as well as addressing the systemic complications.

SYNONYMS

Erythroderma is also known as exfoliative dermatitis.

EPIDEMIOLOGY

Erythroderma or exfoliative dermatitis is an uncommon condition that is generally a manifestation of underlying systemic or cutaneous disorders.

- It affects all age groups, from infants to elderly people.
- In adults, the average age of onset is 41 to 61 years, with a male-to-female ratio of 2:1 to 4:1.[1]
- It accounts for approximately 1% of all dermatologic hospital admissions.[2]
- It can be a very serious condition resulting in metabolic, infectious, cardiorespiratory, and thermoregulatory complications.[3]

ETIOLOGY AND PATHOPHYSIOLOGY

In almost 50% of cases, erythroderma occurs in the setting of a preexisting dermatosis; however, it may also occur secondary to underlying systemic disease, malignancy, and drug reactions. It is classified as idiopathic in 9% to 47% of cases.[3]

- The pathophysiology is not fully understood, but it is related to the pathophysiology of the underlying disease. However, the factors that promote the development of erythroderma are not well defined.
- The rapid maturation and migration of cells through the epidermal layer results in excessive scaling. The rapid turnover of the epidermis also results in fluid, electrolyte, and protein losses that may have severe metabolic consequences, including heart failure and acute respiratory distress syndrome.[4]
- The underlying pathogenesis may be an interaction of immunologic modulators, including interleukins 1, 2, and 8, as well as tumor necrosis factor.[2]

Table 154-1 presents the conditions most commonly associated with erythroderma. Dermatologic conditions commonly associated with erythroderma include the following[1-5]:

- Psoriasis, especially generalized pustular psoriasis with exfoliation (**Figures 154-1** to **154-3**)
- Atopic dermatitis (**Figure 154-4**)[2,3]
- Contact dermatitis (**Figure 154-5**)
- Seborrhea (see **Figure 154-5**)
- Pityriasis rubra pilaris
- Bullous pemphigoid[4]
- Impetigo herpetiformis[4]
- Photosensitivity reaction[4]

TABLE 154-1 Conditions Most Commonly Associated With Erythroderma

Dermatoses	Infections	Systemic/Cancer	Pediatric	Drugs
Psoriasis (**Figures 154-1, 154-2, 154-3,** and **154-8**)	HIV	Sarcoidosis	Omenn syndrome	Penicillins
Atopic dermatitis (**Figure 154-4**)	Norwegian scabies	Thyrotoxicosis	Kwashiorkor	Sulfonamides
Contact dermatitis (**Figure 154-5**)	Hepatitis	Graft-versus-host reaction	Cystic fibrosis	Tetracycline derivatives
Seborrhea (**Figure 154-5**)	Murine typhus (**Figure 154-6**)	Dermatomyositis	Amino acid disorders	Sulfonylureas
Pityriasis rubra pilaris	Human herpesvirus 6	Lung cancer	Immunodeficiency	Calcium channel blockers
Photosensitivity reaction	Toxic shock syndrome	Colon cancer		Captopril
Bullous pemphigoid	Staphylococcal scalded skin syndrome	Prostate cancer		Thiazides
Impetigo herpetiformis	Histoplasmosis Tuberculosis	Breast cancer B- and T-cell lymphoma (**Figure 154-7**) Leukemia		NSAIDs Barbiturates Vancomycin Lithium Antivirals Antimalarials

Erythroderma may also occur secondary to a number of infectious diseases, including the following:

- HIV
- Tuberculosis
- Norwegian scabies
- Hepatitis
- Murine typhus (**Figure 154-6**)
- Human herpesvirus 6[4]

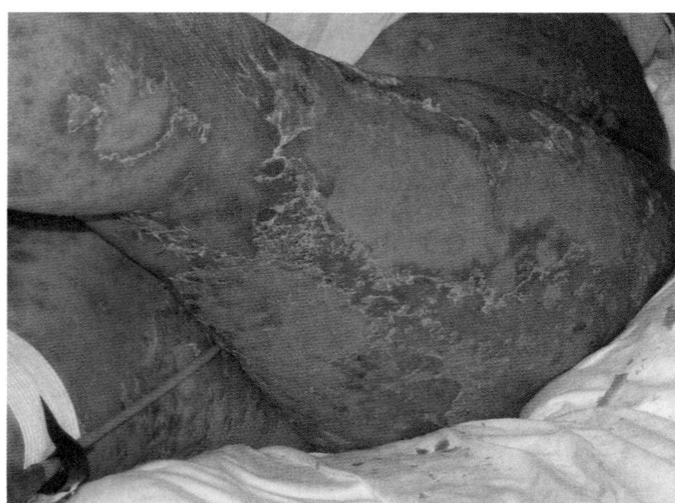

FIGURE 154-2 Erythrodermic psoriasis with sheets of exfoliation causing dehydration and life-threatening illness. This is secondary to generalized pustular psoriasis. (*Reproduced with permission from Jack Resneck, Sr., MD.*)

- Toxic shock syndrome[4]
- Staphylococcal scalded skin syndrome[4]
- Histoplasmosis[3]

Systemic diseases associated with erythroderma include the following:

- Sarcoidosis
- Thyrotoxicosis
- Graft-versus-host reaction
- Dermatomyositis[3,4]

The exact incidence of erythroderma in association with underlying malignancy is not known but reticuloendothelial neoplasms are the most common, most notably T-cell lymphomas.[1,2] It may precede or follow the diagnosis of cutaneous T-cell lymphoma, and chronic idiopathic erythroderma carries a high risk of development of cutaneous T-cell lymphoma over time (**Figure 154-7**).[5] In addition colon, lung, prostate, and thyroid malignancies account for 1% of cases of erythroderma.[2] Specifically in children, it may be associated with the following:

- Kwashiorkor
- Cystic fibrosis
- Amino acid disorders[1-5]

Drug reactions are a common cause of erythroderma. The list of drugs associated with erythroderma is extensive and includes both systemic and topical medications, many of which are very commonly used, including a number of herbal, homeopathic, and ayurvedic medications.[5] The list of medications includes the following:

- Penicillins
- Sulfonamides

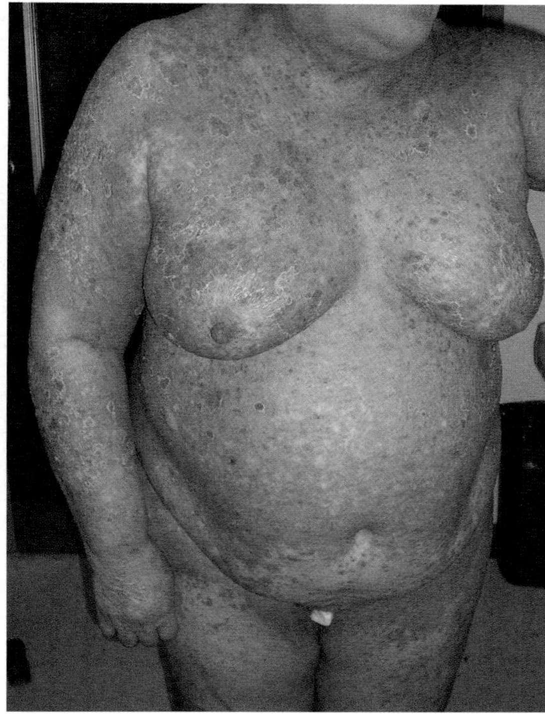

A

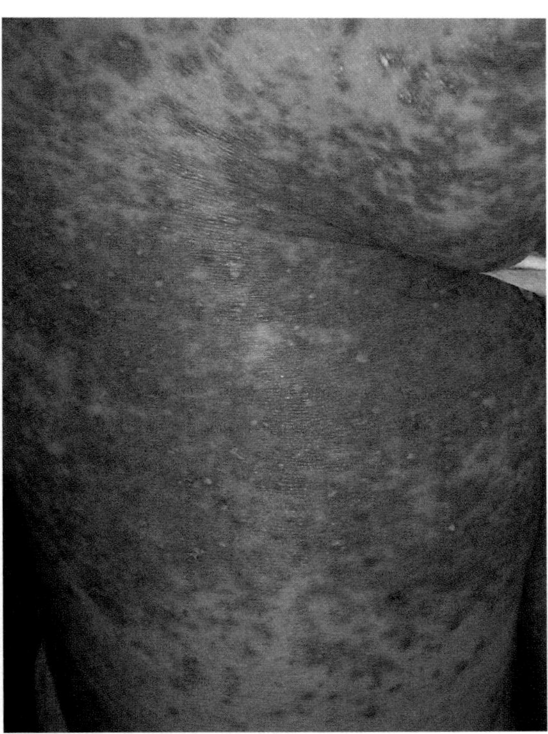

B

FIGURE 154-3 A. Generalized pustular psoriasis causing a life-threatening case of erythroderma in a 67-year-old woman. This all started 3 weeks before presentation and she had no previous history of psoriasis. Patient was hospitalized and treated with topical steroids and oral acitretin with good results. B. Close-up of posterior thigh showing pustules on an erythematous plaque in a new case of erythroderma from generalized pustular psoriasis. *(Reproduced with permission from Richard P. Usatine, MD.)*

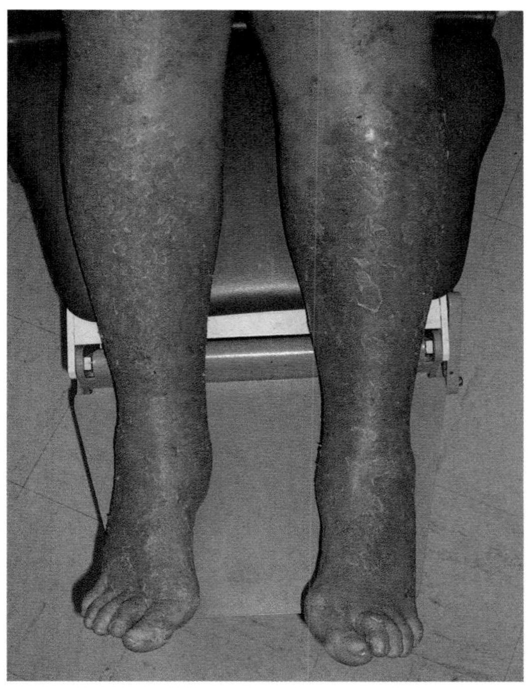

FIGURE 154-4 Erythroderma atopic dermatitis in a 55-year-old woman. *(Reproduced with permission from Richard P. Usatine, MD.)*

- Tetracycline derivatives
- Sulfonylureas
- Calcium channel blockers
- Captopril
- Thiazides
- Nonsteroidal anti-inflammatory drugs (NSAIDs)
- Barbiturates
- Lithium[2,3,5]

In children, an association with topical boric acid has been identified.[5] The cause of erythroderma may not always be identified (**Figure 154-8**).

DIAGNOSIS

CLINICAL FEATURES

- The clinical presentation of erythroderma may be variable depending on the underlying cause. In association with drug reactions, the onset tends to be more abrupt and the resolution more rapid.
- Cutaneous manifestations begin with pruritic, erythematous patches that spread and coalesce into areas of erythema that cover the body. Scaling eventually develops. Large scales are seen more often in acute settings and in chronic erythroderma smaller scales predominate.
- Although the red color of erythroderma is very evident in light skin, erythroderma may be only light pink to brown in darker-skinned individuals (**Figure 154-9**).
- Scalp involvement is very common with alopecia occurring in 25% of patients.[2]
- Systemic manifestations associated with compromise of the protective cutaneous barrier and loss of vasoconstriction of vessels in the dermis that occurs in erythroderma include loss of fluid and electrolytes.

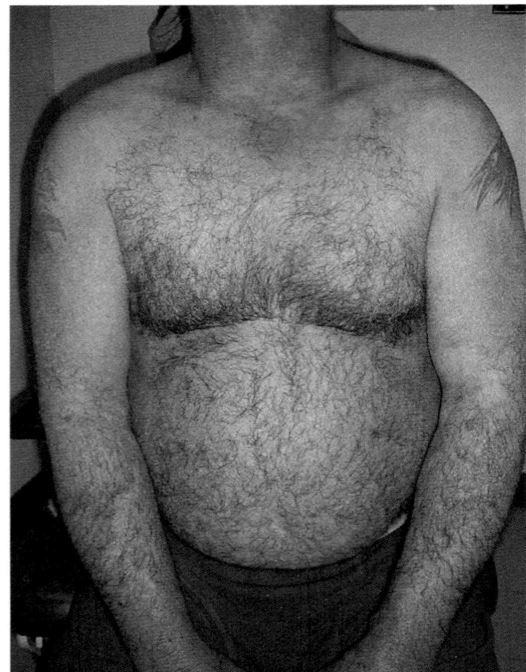

A

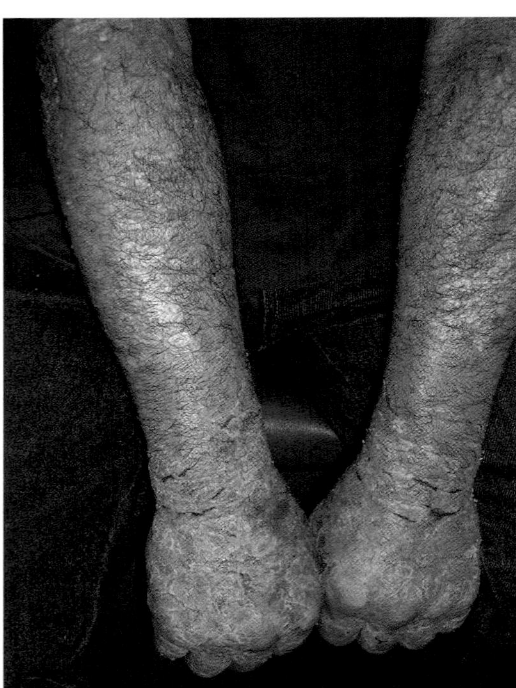

B

FIGURE 154-5 A. Erythroderma caused by seborrheic dermatitis and contact dermatitis. The biopsy showed changes consistent with seborrheic dermatitis but the history suggested that the erythroderma was worsened by contact with products used in auto maintenance. B. After the erythroderma cleared, the arms and hands would worsen every time the patient went back to working on cars. *(Reproduced with permission from Richard P. Usatine, MD.)*

- Protein losses can be as high as 25% to 30% in psoriatic erythroderma, resulting in hypoalbuminemia and edema.[3] Increased perfusion to denuded inflamed skin may result in thermoregulatory disturbances and high output cardiac failure. In addition, there is an increased risk of staphylococcal infection and sepsis.[2,3] Any of these complications can be life threatening.

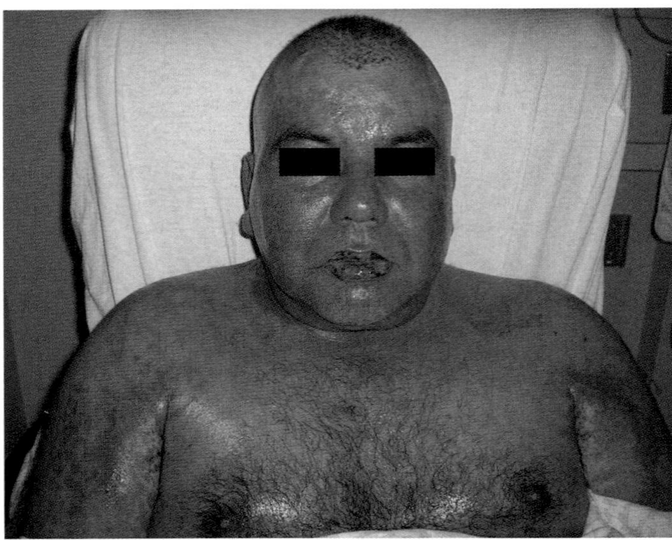

FIGURE 154-6 Murine typhus causing erythema and exfoliation in a febrile systemically ill man in southern Texas. *(Reproduced with permission from Angela Peng, MD.)*

TYPICAL DISTRIBUTION

The distribution is variable, but there is usually sparing of mucous membranes, the palms, and the soles of the feet. Sparing of the nose and nasolabial region has also been reported.[2]

LABORATORY STUDIES

Skin biopsy is useful, but often nondiagnostic. Because 50% of individual biopsies fail to reveal a specific diagnosis, multiple biopsies are recommended when evaluating patients for erythroderma. In addition to conventional histopathologic evaluation, direct immunofluorescence may

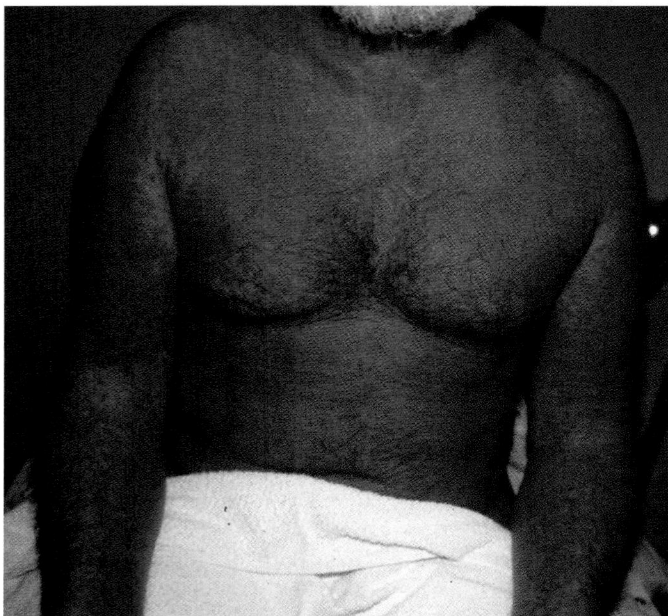

FIGURE 154-7 Erythema secondary to new-onset mycosis fungoides. *(Reproduced with permission from the University of Texas Health Sciences Center, Division of Dermatology.)*

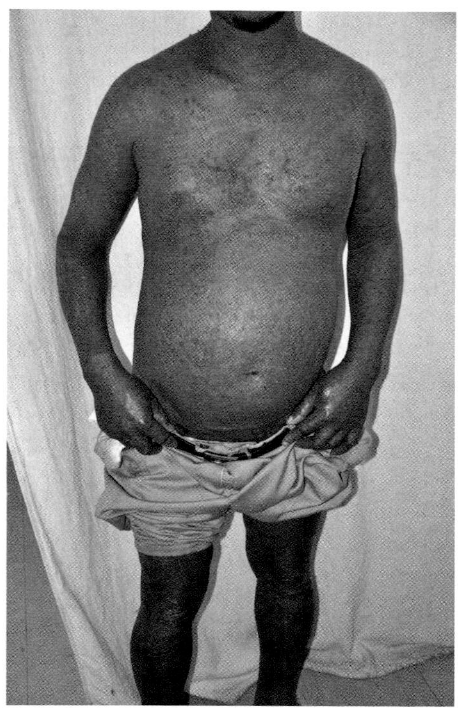

FIGURE 154-8 Erythrodermic psoriasis in a black man showing visible scaling but less obvious erythema secondary to the darker skin color. (*Reproduced with permission from Richard P. Usatine, MD.*)

be helpful in immunobullous disease (eg, pemphigus). T-cell receptor gene rearrangement studies may aid in the diagnosis of lymphoproliferative disorders.[3] Laboratory tests are often nonspecific; however, common findings include the following:

- Leukocytosis
- Lymphocytosis
- Mild anemia
- Eosinophilia
- Elevated sedimentation rate
- Polyclonal gammopathy
- Elevated immunoglobulin (Ig) E levels
- Hypoalbuminemia
- Elevated serum creatinine
- Elevated uric acid levels[1-5]

HIV testing should be considered in those with risk factors.[5] In children a sweat test, zinc, amino acid, and lipid levels should be considered.[5]

DIFFERENTIAL DIAGNOSIS

Erythroderma is the dermatologic manifestation of a number of underlying disease processes, including infectious diseases, lymphoproliferative disorders, malignancies, dermatoses, acquired and inborn metabolic disorders, and drug reactions. The key to proper diagnosis and treatment is contingent on identification of the underlying cause.[1-5] (For a list of underlying conditions, see "Etiology and Pathophysiology" earlier.)

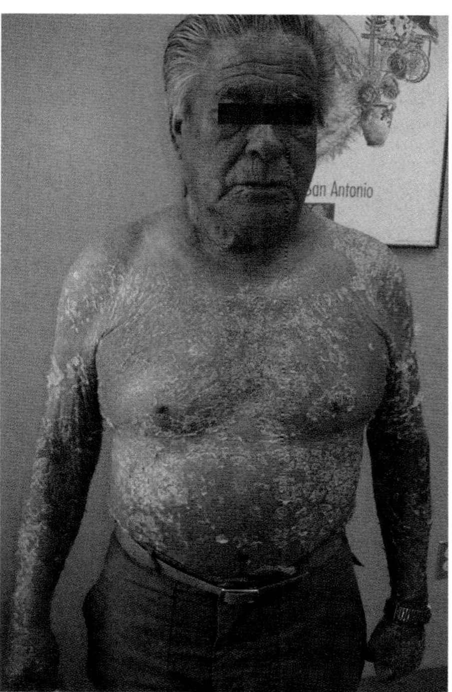

A

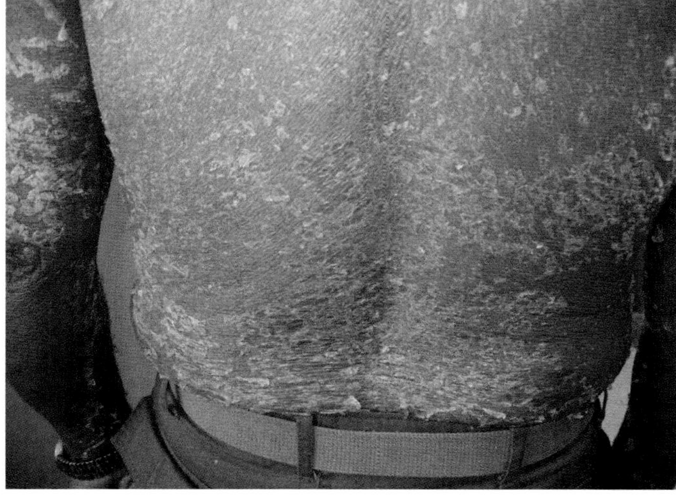

B

FIGURE 154-9 **A.** Complete erythroderma of unknown etiology with extreme reddening of the skin and exfoliation. **B.** The back of the same patient with a closer view of the exfoliation. (*Reproduced with permission from Gwen Denton, MD.*)

MANAGEMENT

Hospitalization and urgent dermatologic referral should be considered for patients presenting with erythroderma acutely as the metabolic, infectious, thermoregulatory, and cardiovascular complications can be life threatening (see **Figures 154-1** to **154-9**).[2,5]

Therapeutic interventions include the following:

- Topical skin care measures such as emollients, oatmeal baths, and wet dressings.[1-5] SOR Ⓒ
- Mid-potency topical steroid ointments such as 0.1% triamcinolone applied to all the affected areas.[1-5] SOR Ⓒ Using the wet wrap

technique (see Chapter 143, Atopic Dermatitis) can help promote quicker absorption and faster onset of action. SOR Ⓒ

- High-potency topical steroids and topical immunomodulators should be avoided owing to risk of increased cutaneous absorption.[3] SOR Ⓒ
- Systemic steroids are useful in drug reactions and eczema, but should be avoided in psoriasis.[2,3,5] SOR Ⓒ
- Consider methotrexate, cyclosporine, for cases secondary to psoriasis. Infliximab has also been used (see **Figures 154-3** to **154-5**).[2,4] SOR Ⓒ Cyclosporine acts most rapidly in cases caused by psoriasis or atopic dermatitis. SOR Ⓒ
- Immunosuppressive agents (methotrexate, azathioprine, infliximab).[2-4] SOR Ⓒ
- Discontinuation of all nonessential medications.[2,3] SOR Ⓒ
- Antibiotic therapy when infection is suspected.[2,3] SOR Ⓒ
- Close monitoring of fluid, electrolyte, and nutritional status and replacement of deficits.[1-5] SOR Ⓒ

PATIENT EDUCATION

Patients should be advised that erythroderma can be life threatening because of the infectious, thermoregulatory, metabolic, and cardiovascular complications. This is important when it might be necessary to hospitalize a patient who does not appreciate the seriousness of the condition. They should also be advised that with certain underlying etiologies, the condition may recur. This is particularly true of idiopathic erythroderma (see **Figure 154-8**).

FOLLOW-UP

The prognosis in erythroderma is very much dependent on the underlying cause. Most deaths occur in malignancy-associated erythroderma. Drug-induced erythroderma carries the best prognosis and the lowest risk of recurrence. Relapses occur in 15% of patients with psoriatic erythroderma. Fifty percent of patients with idiopathic erythroderma experience partial remission, and one-third complete remission.[3]

PATIENT RESOURCES

- Health-Disease—a family medical guide—**http://www.health-disease.org/skin-disorders/erythroderma.htm.**

PROVIDER RESOURCES

- Medscape. *Erythroderma (Generalized Exfoliative Dermatitis)*—**http://emedicine.medscape.com/article/1106906.**
- DermNet NZ. *Erythroderma*—**http://www.dermnetnz.org/reactions/erythroderma.html.**
- DermIS. *Congenital Ichthyosiform and Psoriatic Erythroderma*—**http://www.dermis.net/dermisroot/en/list/erythroderma/search.htm.**

REFERENCES

1. Rothe MJ, Bialy TL, Grant-Kels JM. Erythroderma. *Dermatol Clin*. 2000;18:405-415.
2. Karakayli G, Beckham G, Orengo I, Rosen T. Exfoliative dermatitis. *Am Fam Physician*. 1990;59(3):625-630.
3. Rothe JH, Bernstein ML, Grant-Kels JM. Life-threatening erythroderma: diagnosing and treating the "red man". *Clin Dermatol*. 2005;23(2):206-217.
4. Grant-Kels JM, Bernstein ML, Rothe MJ. Exfoliative dermatitis. In: Wolff K, Goldsmith LA, Katz SI, Gilchrest B, Paller AS, Leffell DJ, eds. *Fitzpatrick's Dermatology in General Medicine*. 7th ed. http://www.accessmedicine.com/content.aspx?aID=2984502#2984502.
5. Sehgal VN, Srivastava G. Erythroderma/generalized exfoliative dermatitis in pediatric practice: an overview. *Int J Dermatol*. 2006;45:831-839.

SECTION 8 BENIGN NEOPLASMS

155 SKIN TAG

Mindy A. Smith, MD, MS

PATIENT STORY

A 55-year-old man requests removal of multiple skin tags around his neck. He is overweight and has diabetes and acanthosis nigricans. Although some of his skin tags occasionally get caught on his clothing, he just does not like the way they look. The patient chose to have many of them removed by the snip excision method.

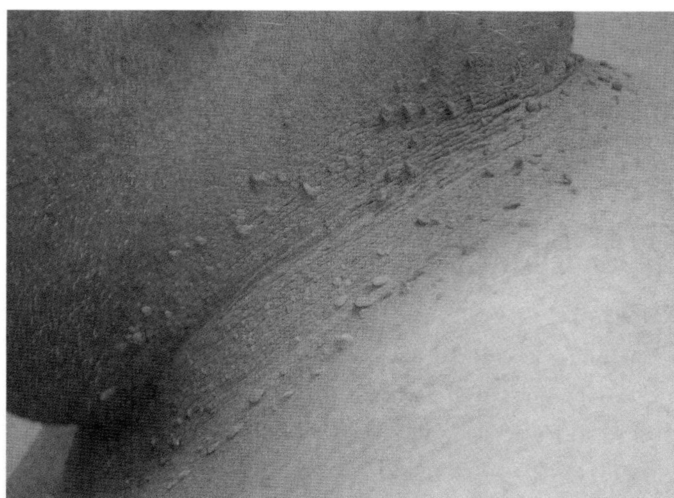

FIGURE 155-1 Many skin tags and acanthosis nigricans on the neck of a man with diabetes. (*Reproduced with permission from Richard P. Usatine, MD.*)

INTRODUCTION

Skin tags (acrochordons) are flesh-colored, pedunculated lesions that tend to occur in areas of skin folds especially around the neck and in the axillae.

SYNONYMS

It is also referred to as fibroepithelial polyps.

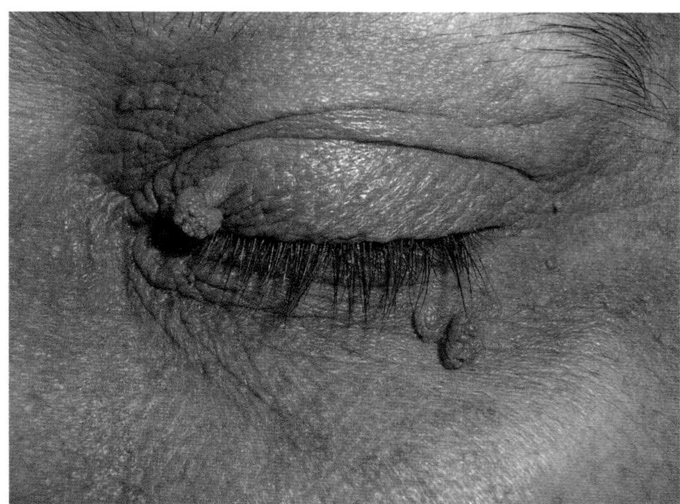

FIGURE 155-2 Filiform pedunculated skin tags on the eyelids. These were removed with a radiofrequency loop after local anesthesia with lidocaine and epinephrine to minimize bleeding. (*Reproduced with permission from Richard P. Usatine, MD.*)

EPIDEMIOLOGY

- In an unselected population study, skin tags were found in 46% of patients, particularly in patients who were obese.[1]
- Skin tags increase in frequency through the fifth decade of life so that as many as 59% of individuals have them by the time they are 70 years old; however, the increase slows after age 50 years.[1]

ETIOLOGY AND PATHOPHYSIOLOGY

- Three types of skin tags are described as below[1]:
  - Small, furrowed papules of approximately 1 to 2 mm in width and height, located mostly on the neck and the axillae (**Figure 155-1**).
  - Single or multiple filiform lesions of approximately 2 mm in width and 5 mm in length occurring elsewhere on the body (**Figure 155-2**).
  - Large, pedunculated tumor or nevoid, bag-like, soft fibromas occur on the lower part of the trunk (**Figure 155-3**).
- Etiology is unknown, but it is theorized that skin tags occur in localized areas with a paucity of elastic tissue resulting in sessile or atrophic lesions. In addition, hormone imbalances appear to facilitate their development (eg, high levels of estrogen and progesterone seen during pregnancy) and other factors including epidermal growth factor, tissue growth factor-α, and infection (eg, human papillomavirus) have been implicated as cofactors.

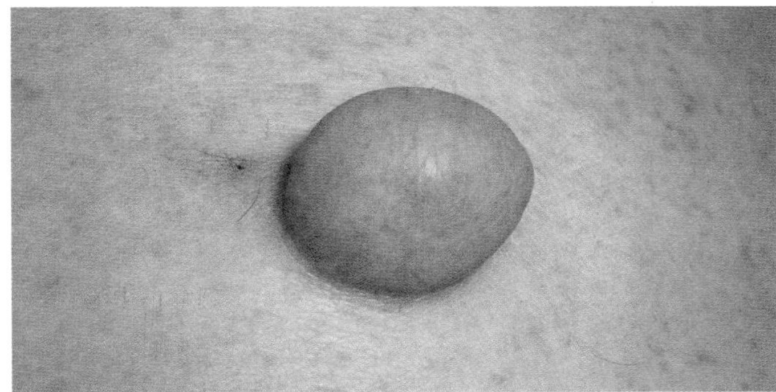

FIGURE 155-3 Large pedunculated bag-like soft fibroma on the trunk. This is a large acrochordon or fibroepitheliomatous polyp. Local anesthetic was given prior to excision. (*Reproduced with permission from Richard P. Usatine, MD.*)

- Acrochordons also appear to be associated with impaired carbohydrate metabolism and diabetes mellitus (see **Figure 155-1**).[2]
- Pedunculated lesions may become twisted, infarcted, and fall off spontaneously.
- Very rarely neoplasms are found at the base of skin tags. In a study of consecutive cutaneous pathology reports, 5 of 1335 clinically diagnosed fibroepithelial polyp specimens were malignant (ie, 4 were basal cell carcinomas and 1 was squamous cell carcinoma in situ).[3] There is selection bias in this study because most skin tags are not sent to the pathologist.

DIAGNOSIS

CLINICAL FEATURES

- Small, soft, usually pedunculated lesions.
- Skin colored or hyperpigmented.
- Most vary in size from 2 to 5 mm, but larger ones may be seen.
- Usually asymptomatic, but can be pruritic or become painful and inflamed by catching on clothing or jewelry.

TYPICAL DISTRIBUTION

Most typically seen on the neck and in the axillae (see **Figure 155-1**), but any skin fold may be affected. They are also seen on the trunk (see **Figure 155-3**), the abdomen, and the back.

ANCILLARY TESTING

Dermatoscopy may be a useful diagnostic tool to analyze acrochordon-like lesions in people with basal cell syndromes to facilitate early diagnosis and treatment.[4]

BIOPSY

Not usually indicated unless the diagnosis is not clear. Typical skin tags do not need to be sent to pathology upon removal. Skin tags, on histology, are characterized by acanthotic, flattened, or frond-like epithelium. A papillary-like dermis is composed of loosely arranged collagen fibers and dilated capillaries and lymphatic vessels.

DIFFERENTIAL DIAGNOSIS

Lesions that can be confused with skin tags include the following:

- Warts—Cutaneous neoplasm caused by papilloma virus. Sessile, dome-shaped lesions approximately 1 cm in diameter are seen with hyperkeratotic surface. Paring usually demonstrates a central core of keratinized debris and punctate bleeding points.
- Neurofibromas—Benign Schwann cell tumors, cutaneous tumors tend to form multiple, soft pedunculated masses (**Figure 155-4**).
- Epidermal hyperplasia in melanocytic nevi (also called keratotic melanocytic nevus [KMN])—Although most common moles are round, tan to brown, less than 6 mm, and flat to slightly elevated, some nevi have overlying hyperplastic epidermis resembling skin tags. In a study of melanocytic nevi submitted for pathology over an 8-month period, 6% were KMN, most often located on the trunk (76%).[5] Dermal nevi can be pedunculated but they are usually larger than skin tags and may appear warty above the stalk.
- Basal cell carcinomas in certain syndromes.[4,6]

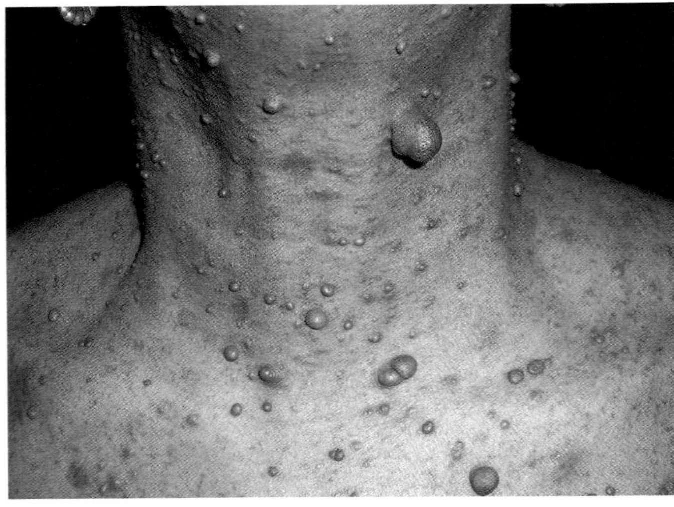

FIGURE 155-4 Multiple soft neurofibromas on the neck of a patient with neurofibromatosis. (*Reproduced with permission from Richard P. Usatine, MD.*)

MANAGEMENT

Skin tags may be removed for cosmetic reasons or because of irritation in a number of ways:

- Small lesions may be snipped with a sharp iris scissor with or without anesthesia (**Figure 155-5**).
- Larger skin tags and fibromas may be removed with shave excision after injecting with lidocaine and epinephrine.
- If there is any bleeding, aluminum chloride on a cotton-tipped applicator is applied for hemostasis.
- Electrodesiccation with or without anesthesia works for very tiny skin tags, too small to grab with the forceps.
- Skin tags on the eyelids may be removed with a radiofrequency loop after local anesthesia with lidocaine and epinephrine to minimize bleeding.

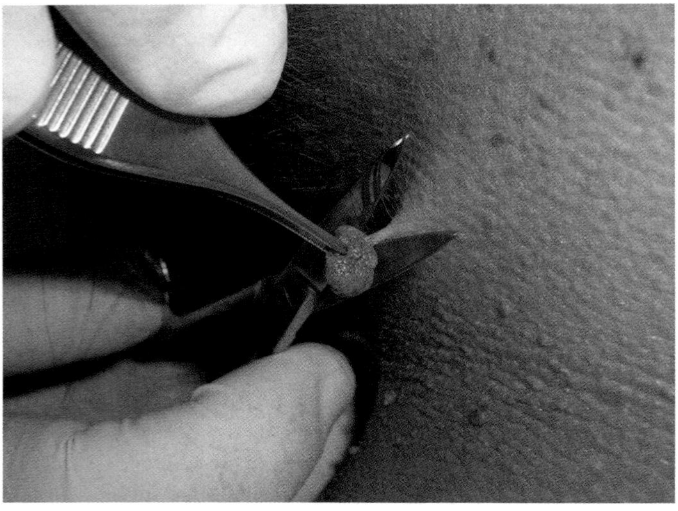

FIGURE 155-5 Snip excision of skin tag with iris scissors and no anesthesia. (*Reproduced with permission from Richard P. Usatine, MD.*)

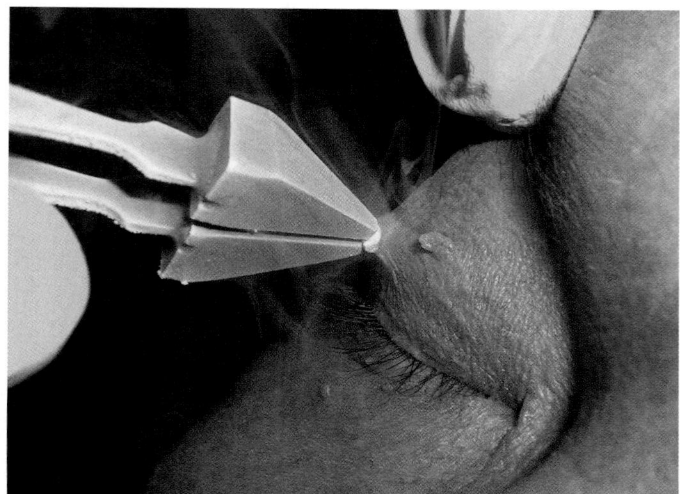

FIGURE 155-6 Cryotherapy using Cryo Tweezers to grasp the skin tag without freezing the skin around it. This is especially helpful on the eyelids. (*Reproduced with permission from Richard P. Usatine, MD.*)

- Cryotherapy can be applied directly to the skin tag with a Cryogun or a cotton-tipped applicator. One preferred method involves dipping forceps into liquid nitrogen and then grasping the skin tag until it turns white. This allows you to grasp the skin tag without freezing the skin around it. This is especially helpful on the eyelids. A special cryo forceps is made by Brymill, Inc. that has more metal at the end to hold the cold longer (**Figure 155-6**). This is a very efficient way to treat multiple skin tags quickly.
- An adhesive patch that applies pressure to the base of a skin tag was found effective in 65% of skin tags in one case series.[7]
- Most insurance companies will not pay for the cosmetic removal of skin tags.
- To avoid large health care costs, only send suspicious looking skin tags to the pathologist.

FOLLOW-UP

Follow-up is not usually necessary.

PATIENT EDUCATION

Advise patients that these are benign growths that can be removed if irritation occurs or for cosmetic purposes. Patients who are overweight should be encouraged to lose weight for their general health and to avoid new skin tags.

PATIENT RESOURCES

- MedlinePlus. *Cutaneous skin tag*— **http://www.nlm.nih.gov/medlineplus/ency/article/000848.htm.**

PROVIDER RESOURCES

- For quick cryosurgery of skin tags, the Cryo Tweezer can be ordered from—**http://www.brymill.com/.**

For detailed information on the treatment of skin tags see:

- Usatine R, Pfenninger J, Stulberg D, and Small R. *Dermatologic and Cosmetic Procedures in Office Practice*. Elsevier, Inc., Philadelphia. 2012.
- Usatine R, Stulberg D, Colver G. *Cutaneous Cryosurgery*. 4th Edition. Taylor and Francis, London, 2014.

Both are available electronically through **www.usatinemedia.com**.

REFERENCES

1. Banik R, Lubach D. Skin tags: localization and frequencies according to sex and age. *Dermatologica*. 1987;174(4):180-183.
2. Demir S, Demir Y. Acrochordon and impaired carbohydrate metabolism. *Acta Diabetol*. 2002;39(2):57-59.
3. Eads TJ, Chuang TY, Fabre VC, et al. The utility of submitting fibroepithelial polyps for histological examination. *Arch Dermatol*. 1996;132(12):1459-1462.
4. Feito-Rodríguez M, Sendagorta-Cudós E, Moratinos-Martínez M, et al. Dermatoscopic characteristics of acrochordon-like basal cell carcinomas in Gorlin-Goltz syndrome. *J Am Acad Dermatol*. 2009;60(5):857-861.
5. Horenstein MG, Prieto VG, Burchette JL Jr, Shea CR. Keratotic melanocytic nevus: a clinicopathologic and immunohistochemical study. *J Cutan Pathol*. 2000;27(7):344-350.
6. Lortscher DN, Sengelmann RD, Allen SB. Acrochordon-like basal cell carcinomas in patients with basal cell nevus syndrome. *Dermatol Online J*. 2007;13(2):21.
7. Fredriksson CH, Ilias M, Anderson CD. New mechanical device for effective removal of skin tags in routine health care. *Dermatol Online J*. 2009;15(2):9.

156 SEBORRHEIC KERATOSIS

Mindy Smith, MD, MS
Richard P. Usatine, MD

PATIENT STORY

An elderly woman noted a growth of a lesion on her chest (**Figure 156-1**). She was afraid that it might be melanoma. Her family physician recognized the typical features of a seborrheic keratosis (SK) (stuck-on with visible horn cysts) and attempted to reassure her. Dermoscopy was performed and the features were so typical of SK; the physician was able to convince the patient not to have a biopsy (**Figure 156-2**). The black comedonal-like openings and white milia-like cysts are typical of SK and can be seen with the naked eye and magnified with a dermatoscope.

INTRODUCTION

SK is a benign skin tumor and a form of localized hyperpigmentation as a result of epidermal alteration; it develops from the proliferation of epidermal cells, although the cause is unknown.

EPIDEMIOLOGY

- It is the most common benign tumor in older individuals; frequency increases with age.
- In an older study of individuals older than age 64 years in North Carolina, 88% had at least one SK. Ten or more SKs were found in 61% of the black men and women, 38% of the white women, and 54% of the white men in the study.[1]

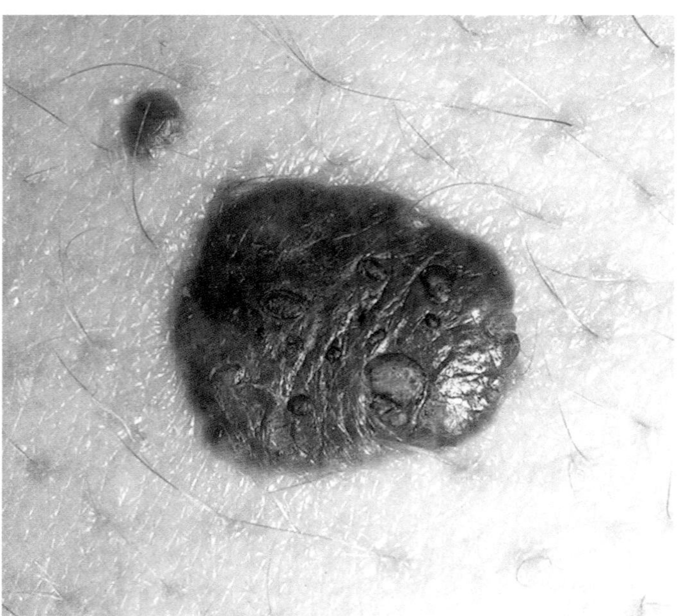

FIGURE 156-1 Seborrheic keratosis with associated horn cysts. (*Reproduced with permission from Richard P. Usatine, MD.*)

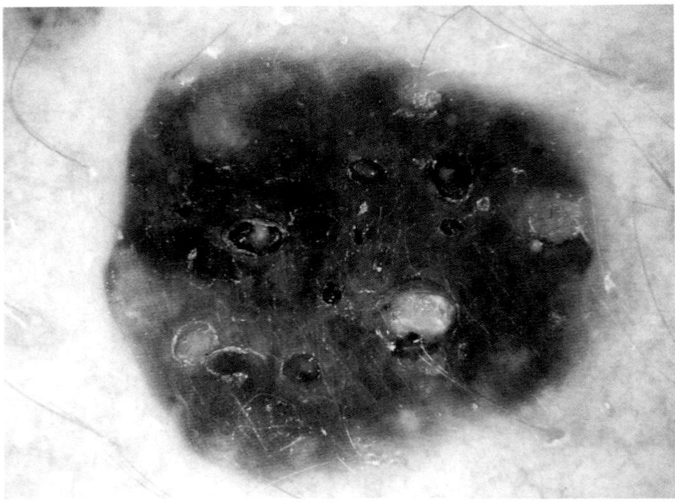

FIGURE 156-2 Dermoscopy of the seborrheic keratosis in Figure 156-1 showing comedo-like openings (black, like blackheads) and milia-like cysts (white, like milia). (*Reproduced with permission from Richard P. Usatine, MD.*)

- In an Australian study performed in 2 general practices, 23.5% (40 out of 170) of individuals between ages 15 and 30 years had at least 1 SK; prevalence and size increased with age.[2]
- Approximately half of cases of multiple SKs occur within families, with an autosomal dominant mode of inheritance.[3]

ETIOLOGY AND PATHOPHYSIOLOGY

- In pigmented SKs, the proliferating keratinocytes secrete melanocyte-stimulating cytokines triggering activation of neighboring melanocytes.[3]
- A high frequency of mutations have been found in certain types of SKs in the gene encoding the tyrosine kinase receptor fibroblast growth factor receptor 3 (FGFR3).[3] One study found that FGFR3 and transcription factor forkhead box N1 (FOXN1) were highly expressed in SKs but close to undetectable in squamous cell skin cancer.[4] This may represent a positive regulatory loop between FGFR3 and FOXN1 that underlies a benign versus malignant skin tumor phenotype.
- Reticulated SKs, usually found on sun-exposed skin, may develop from solar lentigines.[3]
- Multiple eruptive seborrheic keratoses (the sign of Leser-Trélat) can be associated with internal malignancy (most often adenocarcinoma of the gastrointestinal [GI] tract) (**Figure 156-3**),[5] although this association has been questioned.[6]
- An eruption of seborrheic keratoses may develop after an inflammatory dermatosis such as severe sunburn or eczema.[3] There is also a report of exacerbation of SK by topical fluorouracil.[7]

DIAGNOSIS

SKs have a variety of appearances.

CLINICAL FEATURES

- Typically oval or round brown plaques with adherent greasy scale (**Figure 156-4**).
- Color ranges from black to tan (**Figures 156-4** to **156-6**).

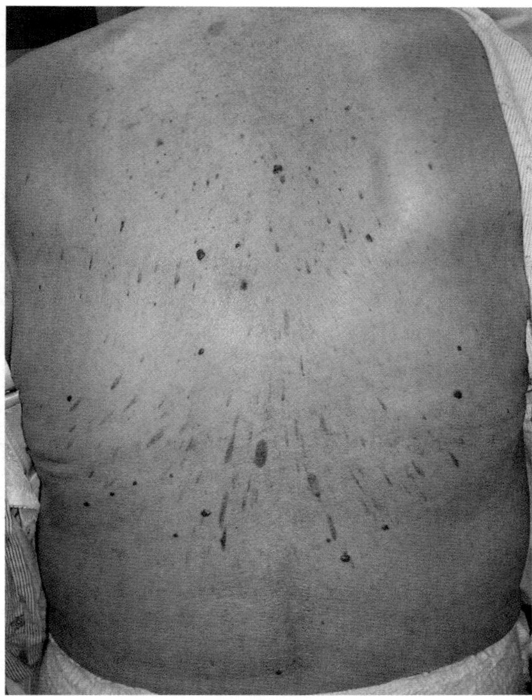

A

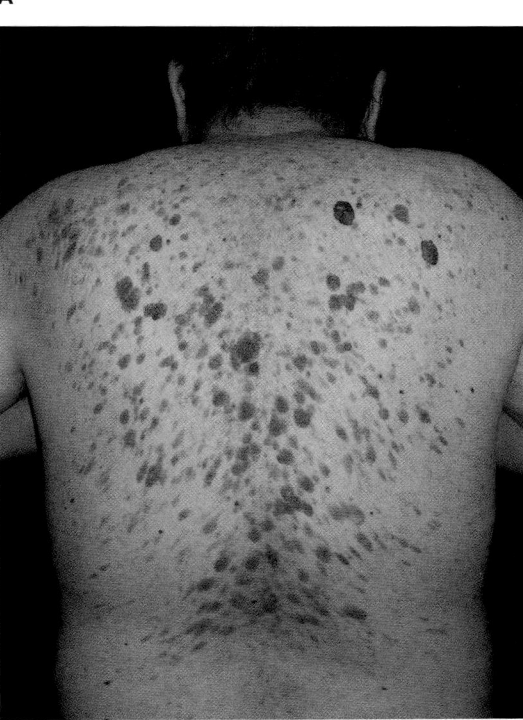

B

FIGURE 156-3 Multiple eruptive seborrheic keratoses as seen in the sign of Leser-Trélat. **A.** This 90-year-old woman presented with ascites and a plethora of seborrheic keratoses and was found to have metastatic Merkel cell carcinoma. **B.** This 49-year-old man had many seborrheic keratoses but no known cancer. While the sign of Leser-Trélat is a paraneoplastic syndrome most people with extensive seborrheic keratoses do not have cancer. *(Reproduced with permission from Richard P. Usatine, MD.)*

- Most often have a velvety to finely verrucous surface and appear to be "stuck-on."
- Some are so verrucous that they can appear to be warty (see **Figure 156-6**).

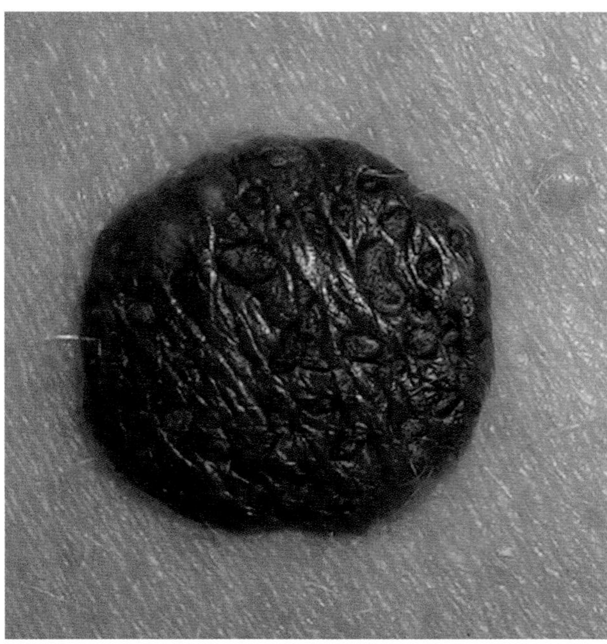

FIGURE 156-4 Round elevated seborrheic keratosis with very visible horn cysts. Horn cysts consist of keratin. *(Reproduced with permission from Richard P. Usatine, MD.)*

- Lesions may be large (up to 35 × 15 cm), pigmented, and have irregular borders (see **Figure 156-5**).
- Lesions can also be flat (**Figure 156-7**).
- Many lesions show keratotic plugging of the surface (see **Figures 156-1** and **156-2**).
- May have surface cracks and associated horn cysts (keratin-filled cystic structures). The dermoscopy terms for the horn cysts are comedo-like

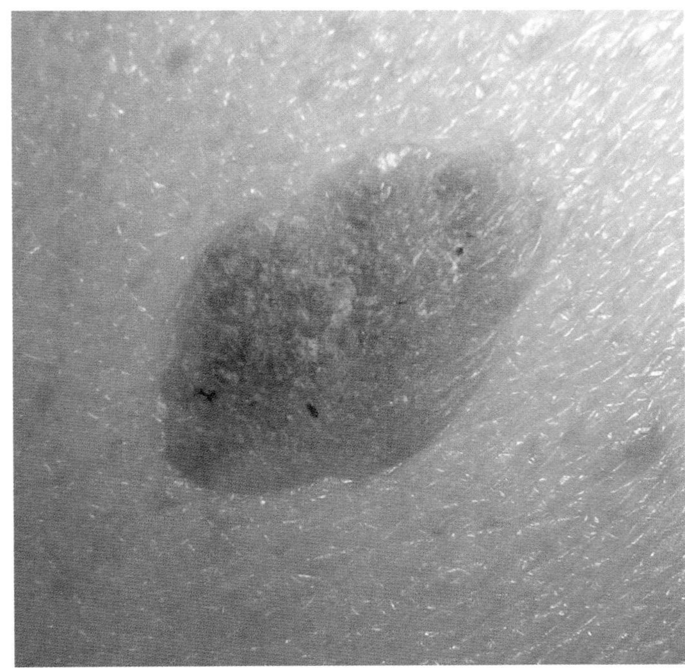

FIGURE 156-5 Seborrheic keratosis that is lightly pigmented, waxy, and appears stuck-on. *(Reproduced with permission from Richard P. Usatine, MD.)*

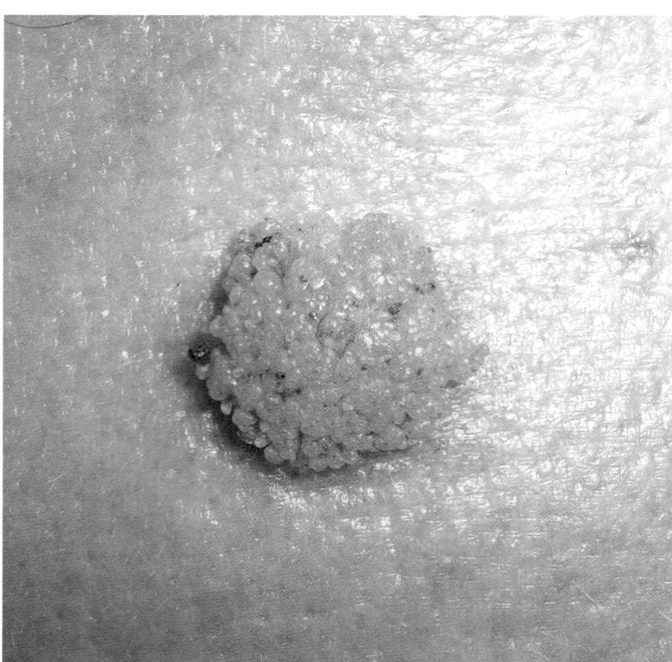

FIGURE 156-6 Seborrheic keratosis with verrucous appearance on the forehead. (*Reproduced with permission from Richard P. Usatine, MD.*)

openings and milia-like cysts (see **Figures 156-1** and **156-2**; see Appendix C, Dermoscopy).

- Occasionally, lesions become irritated and can itch, grow, and bleed; secondary infection may occur.
- Variants of SK include the following:
  - Dermatosis papulosa nigra—Consists of multiple brown-black dome-shaped, smooth papules found on the face in young and middle-aged persons of color, predominantly African Americans (**Figures 156-8** and **156-9**).
  - Stucco keratosis—Consists of large numbers of superficial gray-to-light brown flat keratotic lesions usually on the tops of the feet, the ankles, and the back of the hands and forearms (**Figure 156-10**).

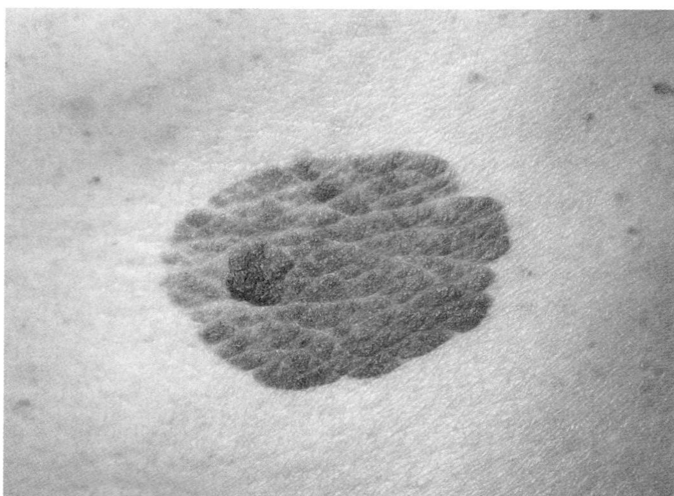

FIGURE 156-7 Seborrheic keratosis (SK) with irregular borders and variation in color that suggest a possible melanoma. Dermoscopy in trained hands can clearly determine that this is a benign SK without a biopsy. (*Reproduced with permission from Richard P. Usatine, MD.*)

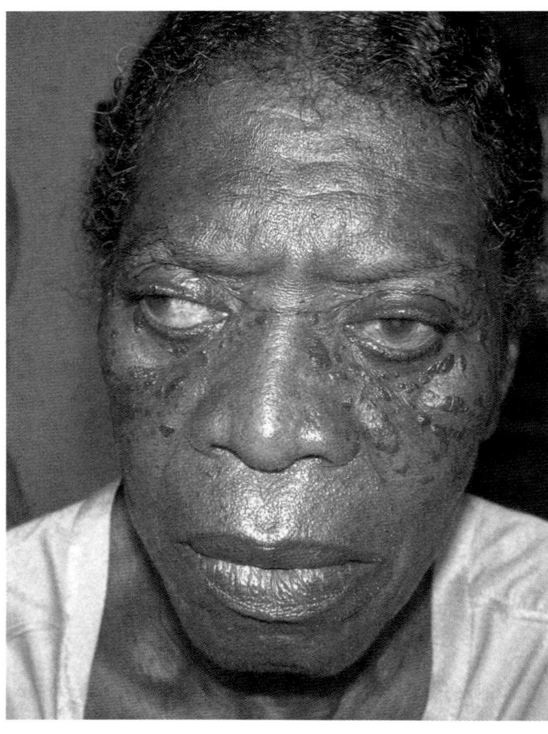

FIGURE 156-8 Dermatosis papulosa nigra with multiple seborrheic keratoses on the face of a Central American woman. (*Reproduced with permission from Richard P. Usatine, MD.*)

TYPICAL DISTRIBUTION

- It is found on trunk, face, back, abdomen, extremities; not present on the palms and soles or on mucous membranes. May be present on the areola and breasts (**Figures 156-11** and **156-12**).
- Dermatosis papulosa nigra is found on the face, especially the upper cheeks and lateral orbital areas (see **Figures 156-8** and **156-9**).

IMAGING

No imaging studies are needed unless there is a sudden appearance of multiple seborrheic keratoses as in the sign of Lesser-Trélat (see **Figure 156-3**). These are associated with adenocarcinoma of the GI tract, lymphoma, Sézary syndrome, and acute leukemia.[3,8]

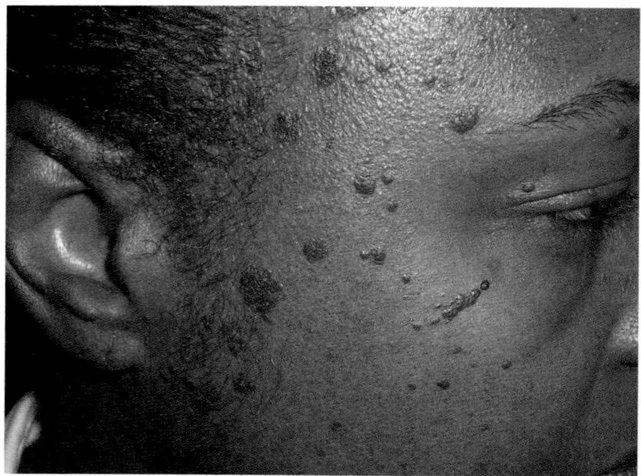

FIGURE 156-9 Dermatosis papulosa nigra on the cheeks and in the hairline. The patient was treated effectively with cryotherapy and had a great cosmetic result. (*Reproduced with permission from Richard P. Usatine, MD.*)

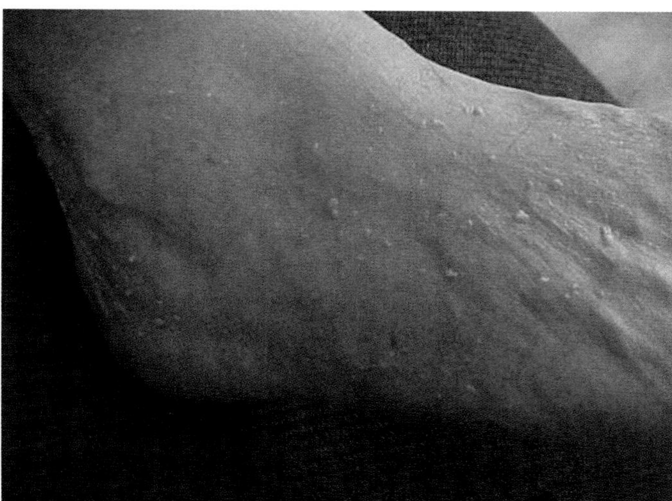

FIGURE 156-10 Stucco keratosis on the foot of an elderly man. (*Reproduced with permission from Richard P. Usatine, MD.*)

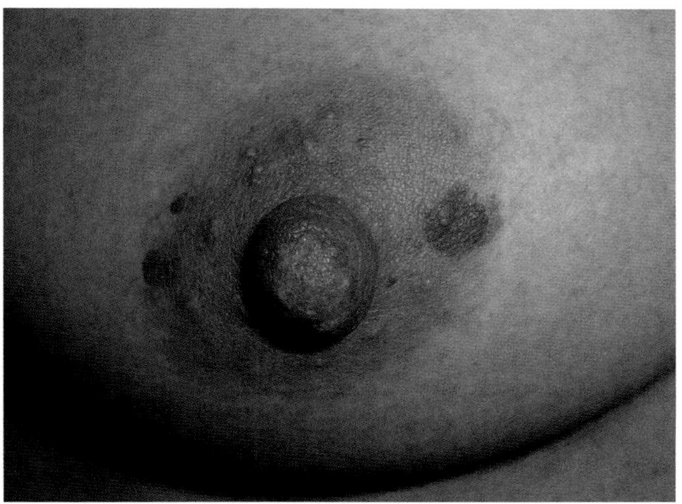

FIGURE 156-11 Multiple seborrheic keratoses on the areola of a 46-year-old woman. Cryotherapy cleared the seborrheic keratoses easily. (*Reproduced with permission from Richard P. Usatine, MD.*)

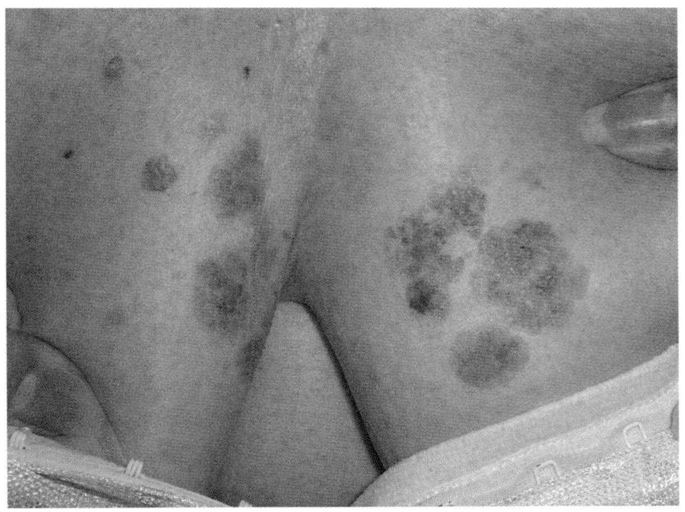

FIGURE 156-12 Waxy seborrheic keratoses on the breasts of this 70-year-old woman. (*Reproduced with permission from Richard P. Usatine, MD.*)

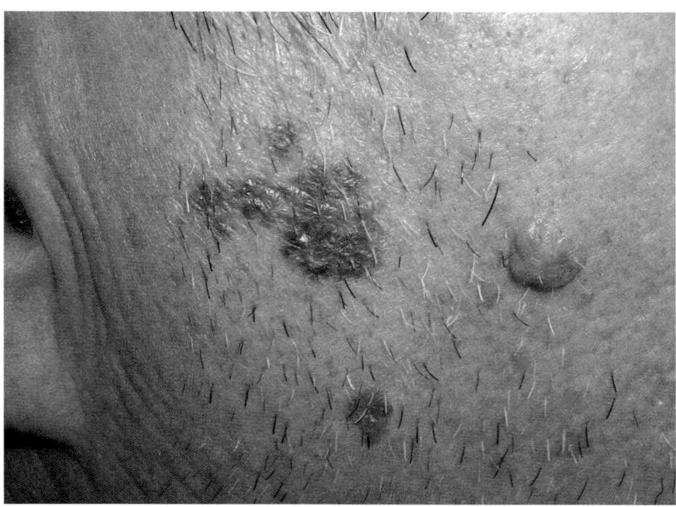

FIGURE 156-13 Melanoma in situ on the lateral face of a 48-year-old man. This resembles a seborrheic keratosis but this large lesion also has all the ABCDEs (Color variation, Diameter >6 mm, Evolving) of melanoma and needed to be biopsied. (*Reproduced with permission from Richard P. Usatine, MD.*)

BIOPSY

Should be performed if there is a suspicion of melanoma (**Figures 156-7** and **156-13**). Some melanomas resemble SKs and a biopsy is needed to avoid missing the diagnosis of melanoma. Do not freeze or curette a suspicious SK; these need surgical intervention to send tissue to the pathologist.

DIFFERENTIAL DIAGNOSIS

- Melanoma—When keratin plugs are visible in the surface of the SK, this helps to distinguish it from a melanoma. **Figure 156-7** is a SK that has the ABCDE features (asymmetry, border irregular, color variation, diameter >6 mm, evolving) of melanoma (see Chapter 170, Melanoma). A biopsy was performed and the lesion was proven to be benign. In **Figure 156-13**, a possible SK turned out to be a melanoma in situ.
- Solar lentigo—Flat, uniformly medium or dark brown lesion with sharp borders (see Chapter 166, Lentigo Maligna). These are flat and seen in sun-exposed areas, typically on the face or back of the hands. Also called liver spots, these hyperpigmented areas are not palpable, whereas SK is a palpable plaque even when it is thin (see **Figure 156-7**).
- Wart—Cutaneous neoplasm caused by papilloma virus (see Chapter 130, Common Warts). Sessile, dome-shaped lesions approximately 1 cm in diameter with hyperkeratotic surface. Paring usually demonstrates central core of keratinized debris and punctate bleeding points.
- Pigmented actinic keratosis (AK)—Although most AKs are nonpigmented and do not look like a SK, occasionally a biopsy of an unknown pigmented plaque will be a pigmented AK secondary to sun damage (see Chapter 164, Actinic Keratosis and Bowen Disease).
- An inflamed SK may be confused with a malignant melanoma or a squamous cell carcinoma and should be biopsied to determine the diagnosis.
- Even a basal cell carcinoma (BCC) can have features that suggest a SK (**Figure 156-14**) (see Chapter 168, Basal Cell Carcinoma).

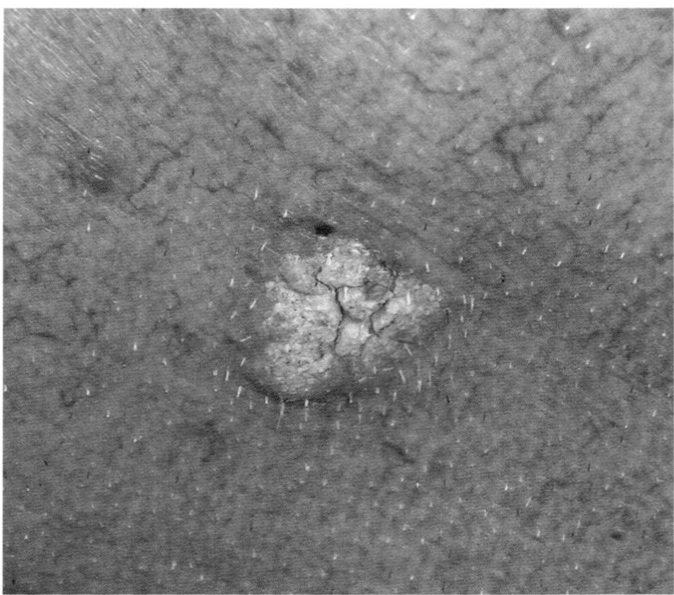

FIGURE 156-14 Basal cell carcinoma with surface cracks and a stuck-on appearance resembling an seborrheic keratosis. The shave biopsy demonstrated the diagnosis of basal cell carcinoma. (*Reproduced with permission from Richard P. Usatine, MD.*)

MANAGEMENT

- Cryosurgery with liquid nitrogen, with a 1-mm halo, is a quick and easy treatment. The risks include pigmentary changes, incomplete resolution, and scarring. Hypopigmentation is the most common complication of this treatment, especially in dark-skinned individuals.
- Removal of benign lesions by curettage assures complete removal without taking the normal tissue below.
- Light electrofulguration can make the curettage so easy that it can be accomplished with a wet gauze pad.
- If the diagnosis is uncertain but there are no features suggesting a melanoma, SK may be removed by shave biopsy and the tissue sent to pathology.
- If melanoma or other skin cancers are suspected, perform a full-thickness biopsy by punch or elliptical excision and send to pathology.

FOLLOW-UP

Some experts suggest follow-up for patients with multiple SKs because malignant tumors can develop elsewhere on the body and rarely within a SK.[3,8] SOR Ⓒ

PATIENT EDUCATION

- Reassure patients that SKs are benign lesions that do not become cancer. Although SKs may grow larger and thicker with time, this is not dangerous.
- Unless the SK is suspicious for cancer or inflamed, removal is for cosmetic purposes only and is often not covered by insurance.
- Although SKs may resolve on occasion, spontaneous resolution does not ordinarily occur.

PATIENT RESOURCES

- MedkinePlus. *Seborrheic keratosis*— **http://www.nlm.nih.gov/medlineplus/ency/article/000884.htm.**

PROVIDER RESOURCES

- Medscape. *Seborrheic Keratosis*— **http://emedicine.medscape.com/article/1059477.**

For detailed information on the treatment of SKs see:

- Usatine R, Pfenninger J, Stulberg D, and Small R. *Dermatologic and Cosmetic Procedures in Office Practice*. Elsevier, Inc., Philadelphia. 2012
- Usatine R, Stulberg D, and Colver G. *Cutaneous Cryosurgery*. 4th Edition. Taylor and Francis, London, 2014

Both are available electronically through **www.usatinemedia.com**.

REFERENCES

1. Tindall JP, Smith JG. Skin lesions of the aged and their association with internal changes. *JAMA*. 1963;186:1039-1042.
2. Gill D, Dorevitch A, Marks R. The prevalence of seborrheic keratoses in people aged 15 to 30 years. *Arch Dermatol*. 2000;136:759-762.
3. Balin AK. *Seborrheic Keratosis*. http://emedicine.medscape.com/article/1059477-overview#a0104. Accessed May 29, 2011.
4. Mandinova A, Kolev V, Neel V, et al. A positive FGFR3/FOXN1 feedback loop underlies benign skin keratosis versus squamous cell carcinoma formation in humans. *J Clin Invest*. 2009;119(10):3127-3137.
5. Ponti G, Luppi G, Losi L. Leser-Trélat syndrome in patients affected by six multiple metachronous primitive cancers. *J Hematol Oncol*. 2010;3:2.
6. Lindelof B, Sigurgeirsson B, Melander S. Seborrheic keratoses and cancer. *J Am Acad Dermatol*. 1992;26(6):947-950.
7. Brodell EE, Smith E, Brodell RT. Exacerbation of seborrheic dermatitis by topical fluorouracil. *Arch Dermatol*. 2011;147(2):245-246.
8. Cascajo CD, Reichel M, Sanchez JL. Malignant neoplasms associated with seborrheic keratoses. An analysis of 54 cases. *Am J Dermatopathol*. 1996;18(3):278-282.

157 SEBACEOUS HYPERPLASIA

Mindy Smith, MD, MS

PATIENT STORY

A 65-year-old man noted a new growth on his face for 1 year (**Figure 157-1**). On close examination, the growth was pearly with a few telangiectasias. The doughnut shape and presence of sebaceous hyperplasia scattered on other areas of the face were reassuring that this may be nothing but benign sebaceous hyperplasia (SH). To reassure the patient and to remove the lesion a shave biopsy was performed to rule out basal cell carcinoma (BCC). The patient was relieved when the pathology result was in fact sebaceous hyperplasia. Additionally, he was pleased with the cosmetic result.

INTRODUCTION

SH is a common, benign condition of sebaceous glands consisting of multiple asymptomatic small yellow papules with a central depression. The sebaceous lobules of SH are greater in number and higher in the dermis than normal sebaceous glands and only one gland appears enlarged.[1] Consequently, the term *hyperplasia* appears to be a misnomer, and SH is more accurately classified as a hamartoma (disorganized overgrowth of tissue normally found at that site).[1]

EPIDEMIOLOGY

- SH occurs in approximately 1% to 26% of the adult population; the latter number is from a population study of hospitalized patients with a mean age of 82 years.[1]
- The prevalence of SH is increased in those with immunosuppression by 10-fold to 30-fold[1]; for example, 10% to 16% of patients receiving long-term immunosuppression with cyclosporine in one study had SH.[2]
- SH has been reported overlying other skin lesions including neurofibromas, melanocytic nevi, verruca vulgaris, and skin tags.[1]
- Rare forms of SH include giant linear (up to 5 cm in diameter) and functional familial (also called premature or diffuse SH)[3]; the latter occurring typically around puberty as thick plaque-like lesions with pores resembling an orange peel.[1]

ETIOLOGY AND PATHOPHYSIOLOGY

- Sebaceous glands, a component of the pilosebaceous unit, are found throughout the skin, everywhere that hair is found. The greatest number is found on the face, chest, back, and the upper outer arms.
- The glands are composed of acini attached to a common excretory duct. In some areas, these ducts open directly to the epithelial surface, including the lips and buccal mucosa (ie, Fordyce spots), glans penis or clitoris (ie, Tyson glands), female areolae (ie, Montgomery glands), and eyelids (ie, meibomian glands).[1]
- Sebaceous glands are highly androgen sensitive and become increasingly active at puberty and reach their maximum by the third decade of life.
- The cells that form the sebaceous gland, sebocytes, accumulate lipid material as they migrate from the basal layer of the gland to the central duct where they release the lipid content as sebum. In younger individuals, turnover of sebocytes occurs approximately every month.
- With aging, turnover of sebocytes slows; this results in crowding of primitive sebocytes within the sebaceous gland, causing a benign hamartomatous enlargement called SH.[1]
- Genetic factors include overexpression of the aging-associated gene *Smad7* and parathormone-related protein.[4]
- There is no known potential for malignant transformation, but SH may be associated with nonmelanoma skin cancer in patients following organ transplantation.

RISK FACTORS

- Older age
- Associated with Muir-Torre syndrome (concurrent or sequential development of a sebaceous neoplasm and an internal malignancy or multiple keratoacanthomas, an internal malignancy, and a family history of Muir-Torre syndrome)
- Immunosuppression
- Ultraviolet radiation[4]

DIAGNOSIS

CLINICAL FEATURES

- Lesions appear as yellowish, soft, small papules ranging in size from 2 to 9 mm (**Figures 157-1 to 157-3**).[1]
- Surface varies from smooth to slightly verrucous.
- Lesions can be single or multiple.
- Increasing number of lesions with aging; higher frequencies after 40 to 50 years of age.[1]
- In functional familial SH, lesions may appear thick and plaque like, with pores that resemble an orange peel; the skin in these patients is quite oily.[1]

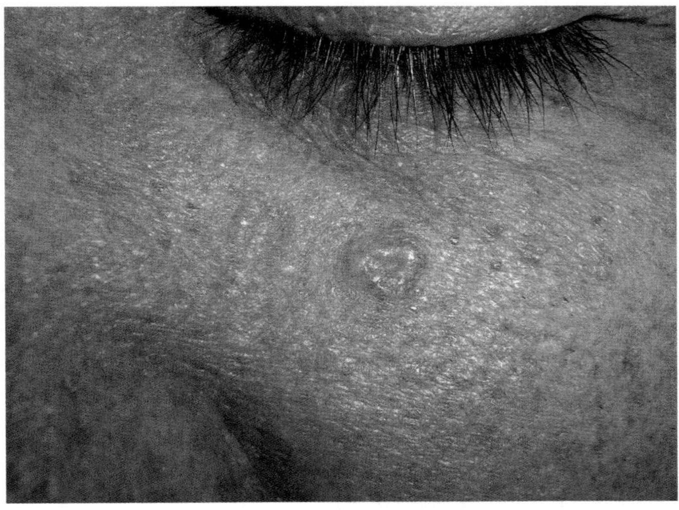

FIGURE 157-1 Large single lesion of sebaceous hyperplasia that was removed by shave biopsy to confirm that it was not a basal cell carcinoma. Doughnut shape is visible. (*Reproduced with permission from Richard P. Usatine, MD.*)

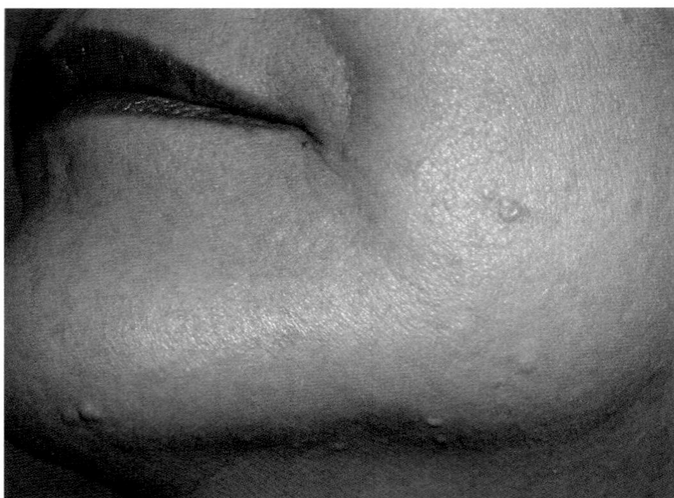

FIGURE 157-2 Multiple lesions of sebaceous hyperplasia on the cheek and chin. Simultaneous appearance of multiple lesions makes them less likely to be basal cell carcinoma. (*Reproduced with permission from Richard P. Usatine, MD.*)

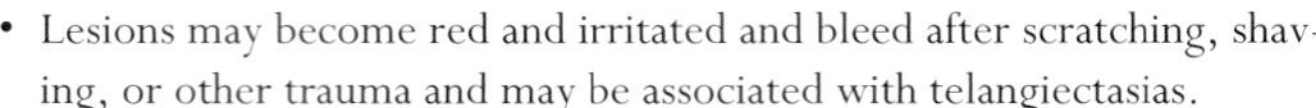

- Lesions may become red and irritated and bleed after scratching, shaving, or other trauma and may be associated with telangiectasias.
- Central umbilication (doughnut shape) from which a small amount of sebum can sometimes be expressed (see **Figures 157-1 to 157-3**).

TYPICAL DISTRIBUTION

Most commonly located on the face, particularly the nose, cheeks, and forehead. May also be found on the chest, areola, mouth, and, rarely, the vulva.[1,5]

IMAGING

Dermoscopy may aid in distinguishing between nodular BCC and SH; a vascular pattern with orderly winding, scarcely branching vessels extending toward the center of the lesion is specific for hyperplastic sebaceous glands.[6]

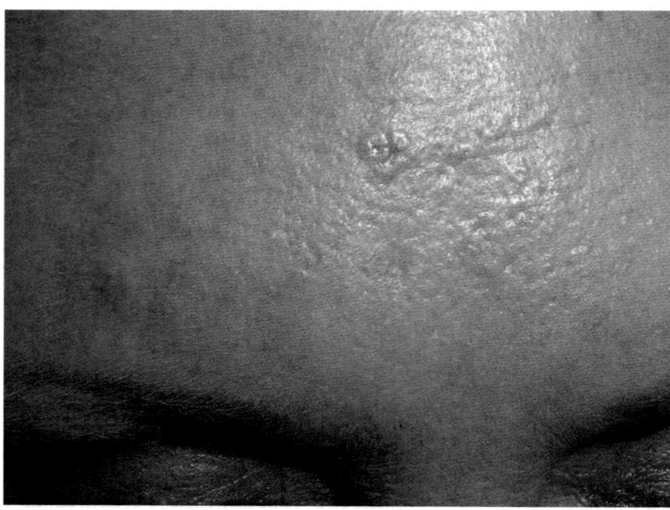

FIGURE 157-3 Large sebaceous hyperplasia on the forehead with telangiectasias. Doughnut shape is visible. (*Reproduced with permission from Richard P. Usatine, MD.*)

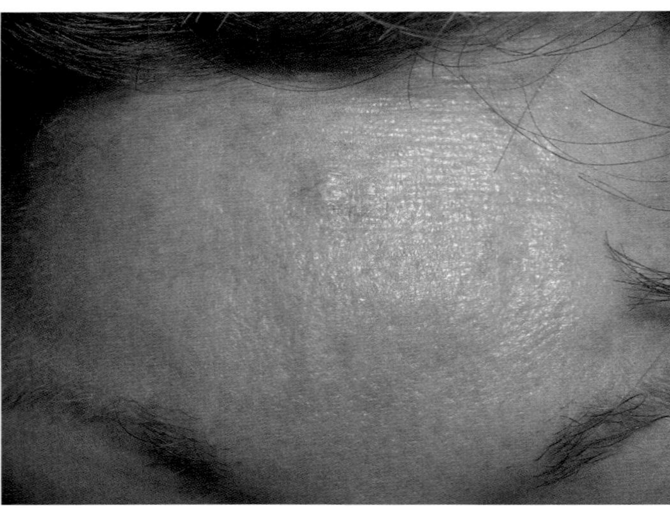

FIGURE 157-4 Basal cell carcinoma on the forehead that could be mistaken for sebaceous hyperplasia. (*Reproduced with permission from Richard P. Usatine, MD.*)

BIOPSY

Not usually necessary unless concerned about BCC.

DIFFERENTIAL DIAGNOSIS

- Nodular BCC—These lesions can appear as waxy papules with a central depression that may ulcerate, most commonly located on the head, neck, and upper back. They may have a pearly appearance, surface telangiectases, and bleed easily (**Figures 157-4** and **157-5**).
- Fibrous papule of the face is a benign, firm, papule of 1 to 5 mm that is usually dome shaped and indurated with a shiny, skin-colored appearance. Most lesions are located on the nose and, less commonly, on the cheeks, chin, neck, and, rarely, the lip or forehead.

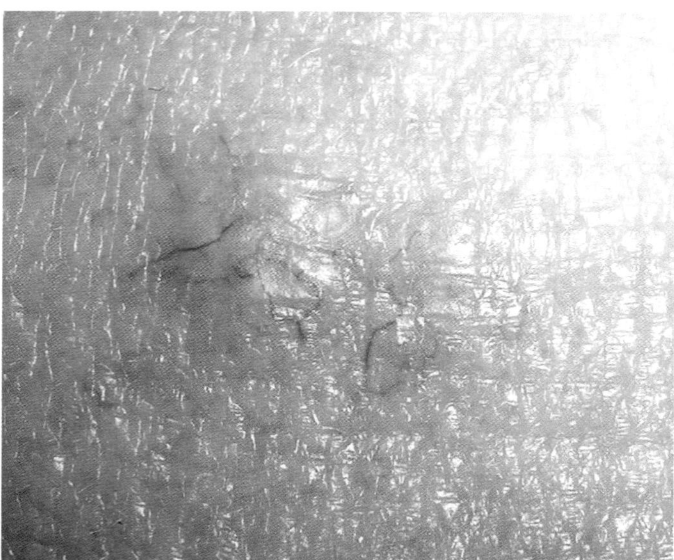

FIGURE 157-5 Close-up of same basal cell carcinoma on the forehead in Figure 157-4 that shows irregular distribution of telangiectasias and lack of the doughnut shape. (*Reproduced with permission from Richard P. Usatine, MD.*)

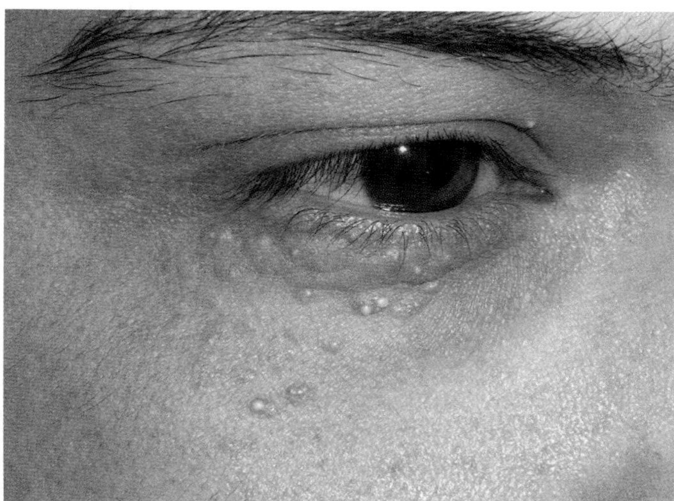

FIGURE 157-6 Syringomas and milia on the lower eyelid of a 23-year-old man. The milia are the white round epidermal cysts and the syringomas are flesh colored and larger. (*Reproduced with permission from Richard P. Usatine, MD.*)

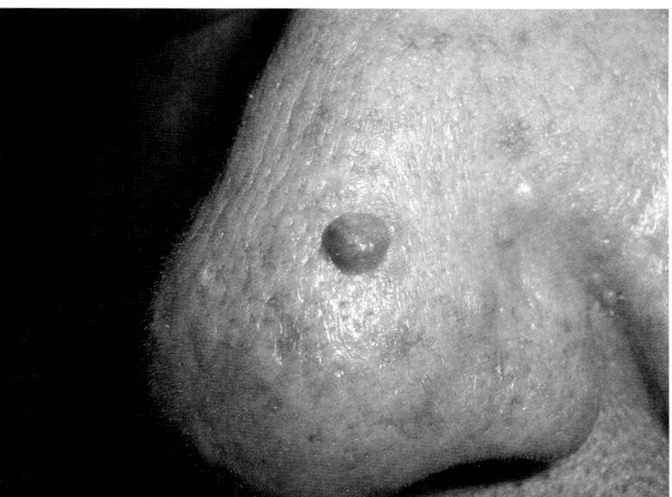

FIGURE 157-7 Single, large, elevated lesion of sebaceous hyperplasia on the nose of a 51-year-old man with rosacea. A shave biopsy ruled out basal cell carcinoma and gave the definitive diagnosis of sebaceous hyperplasia. The cosmetic result was excellent. (*Reproduced with permission from Richard P. Usatine, MD.*)

- Milia are common, benign, keratin-filled cysts (histologically identical to epidermoid cysts) that occur in persons of all ages. They are 1 to 2 mm, superficial, uniform, pearly-white to yellowish, domed lesions usually occurring on the face (**Figure 157-6**).
- Molluscum contagiosum are firm, smooth, usually 2- to 6-mm umbilicated papules that may be present in groups or widely disseminated on the skin and mucosal surfaces. The lesions can be flesh colored, white, translucent, or even yellow in color. Lesions generally are self-limited but can persist for several years (see Chapter 129, Molluscum Contagiosum).
- Syringoma is a benign adnexal neoplasm formed by well-differentiated ductal elements. They are 1- to 3-mm skin-colored or yellowish dermal papules with a rounded or flat top arranged in clusters, and symmetrically distributed primarily on the upper parts of the cheeks and lower eyelids (see **Figure 157-6**).
- Xanthomas are deposits of lipid in the skin or subcutaneous tissue that manifest clinically as yellowish papules, nodules, or tumors. They are usually a consequence of primary or secondary hyperlipidemia and occur in patients older than age 50 years. The lesions are soft, velvety, yellow, flat, polygonal papules that are asymptomatic and usually bilateral and symmetric (see Chapter 223, Hyperlipidemia).

MANAGEMENT

SH does not require treatment but can be removed for cosmetic purposes or if it becomes irritated. Evidence supporting treatment comes primarily from case series.

- Options for removal include cryotherapy, electrodesiccation, topical chemical treatments (eg, with bichloracetic acid or trichloroacetic acid), oral isotretinoin (10-40 mg a day for 2-6 weeks), laser treatment (eg, with argon, carbon dioxide, or pulsed-dye laser), photodynamic therapy (ie, combined use of 5-aminolevulinic acid and visible light),[7] shave excision, and punch excision.[1] Complications of these therapies include atrophic scarring and changes in pigmentation.
- If there is any suspicion that what appears to be sebaceous hyperplasia may be a basal cell carcinoma, perform a shave biopsy as treatment (**Figure 157-7**).

FOLLOW-UP

No follow-up is needed.

PATIENT RESOURCES

- Skinsight.com. *Sebaceous Hyperplasia*—**http://www.skinsight.com/adult/sebaceousHyperplasia.htm.**

PROVIDER RESOURCES

- Medscape. *Sebaceous Hyperplasia*—**http://emedicine.medscape.com/article/1059368-overview.**

REFERENCES

1. Eisen DB, Michael DJ. Sebaceous lesions and their associated syndromes: part 1. *J Am Acad Dermatol.* 2009;61:549-560.
2. Boschnakow A, May T, Assaf C, et al. Ciclosporin A-induced sebaceous gland hyperplasia. *Br J Dermatol.* 2003;149(1):198-200.
3. Oh ST, Kwon HJ. Premature sebaceous hyperplasia in a neonate. *Pediatr Dermatol.* 2007;24:443-445.
4. Zouboulis CC, Boschnakow A. Chronological ageing and photoageing of the human sebaceous gland. *Clin Exp Dermatol.* 2001;26(7):600-607.
5. Al-Daraji WI, Wagner B, Ali RBM, McDonagh AJG. Sebaceous hyperplasia of the vulva: a clinicopathological case report with a review of the literature. *J Clin Pathol.* 2007;60(7):835-837.
6. Zaballos P, Ara M, Puig S, Malvehy J. Dermoscopy of sebaceous hyperplasia. *Arch Dermatol.* 2005;141:808.
7. Gold MH, Bradshaw WL, Boring MM, et al. Treatment of sebaceous hyperplasia by photodynamic therapy with 5-aminolevulinic acid and a blue light source or intense pulsed light source. *J Drugs Dermatol.* 2004;3(suppl 6):S6-S9.

158 DERMATOFIBROMA

Mindy A. Smith, MD, MS
Richard P. Usatine, MD

PATIENT STORY

A 25-year-old woman reports a firm nodule on her leg that gets in the way of shaving her leg (**Figure 158-1**). Upon questioning, the nodule may have started there after she cut her leg shaving 1 year ago. She is worried it could be a cancer and wants it removed. Close observation showed a brown halo and a firm nodule that dimpled down when pinched. A diagnosis of a dermatofibroma (DF) was made and the choices for treatment were discussed.

INTRODUCTION

DF is a benign fibrohistiocytic tumor, usually found in the mid dermis, composed of a mixture of fibroblastic and histiocytic cells. These scar-like nodules are most commonly found on the legs and arms of adults.

SYNONYMS

DF is also called as benign fibrous histiocytoma.

EPIDEMIOLOGY

- Occurs more often in women (male-to-female ratio is 1:4).[1]
- Found in patients of all races.
- Approximately 20% occur in patients younger than age 17 years.[1] In 1 case series, 80% occurred in people between the ages of 20 and 49 years.[2]

ETIOLOGY AND PATHOPHYSIOLOGY

- Uncertain etiology—Nodule may represent a fibrous reaction triggered by trauma, a viral infection, or insect bite; however, DFs show clonal proliferative growth seen in both neoplastic and inflammatory conditions.[3]
- Multiple DFs (ie, >15 lesions) have been reported associated with systemic lupus erythematosus, HIV infection, Down syndrome, Graves disease, or leukemia, and may represent a worsening of immune function.[1] A case of familial eruptive DFs has also been reported associated with atopic dermatitis.[4]

DIAGNOSIS

CLINICAL FEATURES

- Firm-to-hard nodule; skin is freely movable over the nodule except for the area of dimpling.
- Color of the overlying skin ranges from flesh to gray, pink, red, blue, brown, or black (**Figures 158-2** and **158-3**), or a combination of hues (**Figure 158-4**).
- Dimples downward when compressed laterally because of tethering of the overlying epidermis to the underlying nodule (see **Figure 158-3**).
- Usually asymptomatic but may be tender or pruritic.

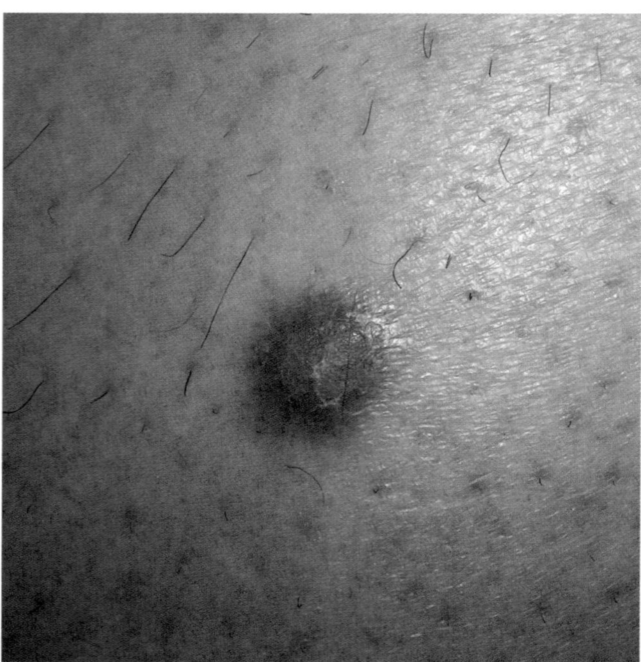

FIGURE 158-1 Dermatofibroma on the leg of a 25-year-old woman that may have begun after she cut her leg shaving 1 year ago. Note the brown halo, pink hue, and raised center. (*Reproduced with permission from Richard P. Usatine, MD.*)

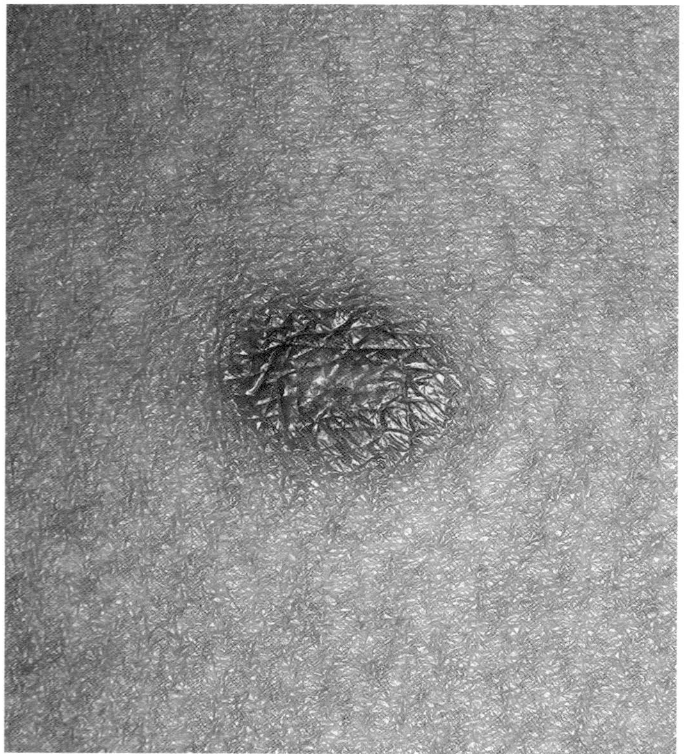

FIGURE 158-2 Dermatofibroma on the thigh of black woman. Note the darker brown halo around the lighter center. (*Reproduced with permission from Richard P. Usatine, MD.*)

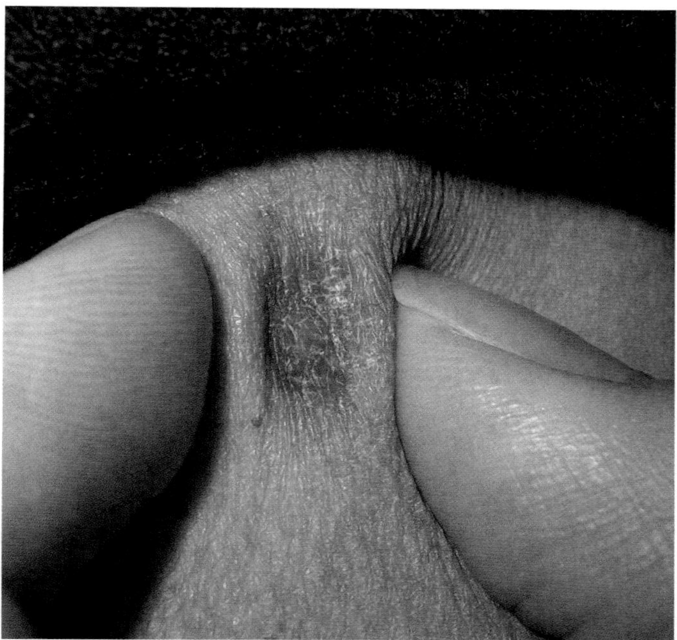

FIGURE 158-3 Pinch test showing a deep dimpling of this dermatofibroma on the buttocks. (*Reproduced with permission from Richard P. Usatine, MD.*)

- Size ranges from 0.3 to 10 mm; usually less than 6 mm. Rarely, DFs grow to larger than 5 cm.[5]
- May have a hyperpigmented halo and a scaling surface (**Figure 158-4**).
- DFs can rarely be located entirely within subcutaneous tissue.[6]

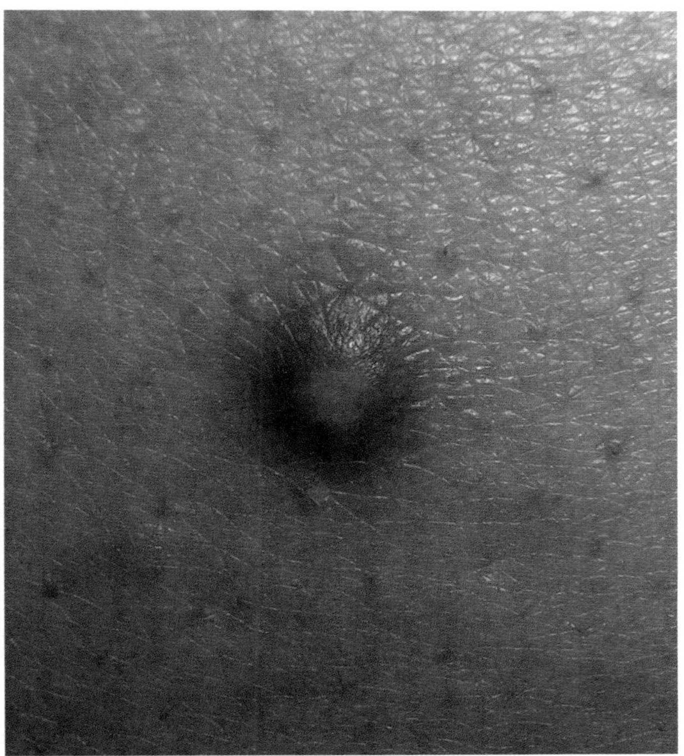

FIGURE 158-4 Dermatofibroma on the back. Note the brown halo around the lighter central nodule. (*Reproduced with permission from Richard P. Usatine, MD.*)

IMAGING

Dermoscopy is a useful adjunctive diagnostic technique for DF (**Figure 158-5**). Although the most common finding is a peripheral pigment network with a central white area (34.7% of cases), 10 dermoscopic patterns have been identified; in a large case series, pigment network was observed in 71.8% (3% atypical pigment network)[7] (see Appendix C, Dermoscopy).

TYPICAL DISTRIBUTION

May be found anywhere, but usually on the legs and arms, especially the lower legs. In one case series, 70% were on the lower extremities.[2]

BIOPSY

- A punch biopsy can be both diagnostic and therapeutic. DFs have been reported with overlying basal cell carcinoma and associated melanoma.[8,9]
- Histologically, DFs can be fibrocollagenous (40.1%), histiocytic (13.1%), cellular (11.5%), aneurysmal (7.4%), angiomatous (6.5%), sclerotic (6.5%), monster (4.9%), palisading (1.6%), keloidal (0.8%), or mixed type (7.3%).[2] Also reported are ossifying DFs[10] and a signet-ring cell DF.[11]
- Electron microscopy and immunohistochemistry may be needed to differentiate atypical or pigmented DFs from other lesions.[7]

DIFFERENTIAL DIAGNOSIS

DFs may be confused with the following malignant tumors; diagnosis based on histology and excision should be undertaken for enlarging or ulcerating tumors.

- Dermatofibrosarcoma protuberans—A low-grade malignant fibrotic tumor of the skin and subcutaneous tissues (**Figure 158-6**). A punch biopsy will provide adequate tissue to make the diagnosis.
- Pseudosarcomatous DF—A rare connective tissue tumor arising on the trunk and limbs in young adults.
- Malignant fibrous histiocytoma—A common soft tissue sarcoma occurs in the extremities. Presentation as a primary cutaneous lesion is rare and more often presents as a metastasis from another location such as the breast.

Many benign lesions have a similar appearance, including the following:

- Pigmented seborrheic keratosis—May be macular and often larger than DF. Distinguished by surface cracks, verrucous features, stuck-on appearance, and adherent greasy scale (see Chapter 156, Seborrheic Keratosis).
- Epidermal inclusion cyst—Sharply circumscribed, skin-colored nodule often with a central punctum. Most common on face, neck, or trunk. Composed of stratified epithelium surrounding a mass of keratinized material that has a foul odor when it drains.
- Hypertrophic scar—Occurs within previous wounds or lacerations.
- Neurofibroma—Benign Schwann cell tumors; single lesions are seen in normal individuals. Cutaneous tumors tend to form multiple, soft, pedunculated masses, whereas subcutaneous nodules are skin-colored soft nodules attached to peripheral nerves. The latter shows similar invagination as DF (see Chapter 235, Neurofibromatosis).

MANAGEMENT

- No treatment is necessary unless the diagnosis is questioned or symptoms warrant.

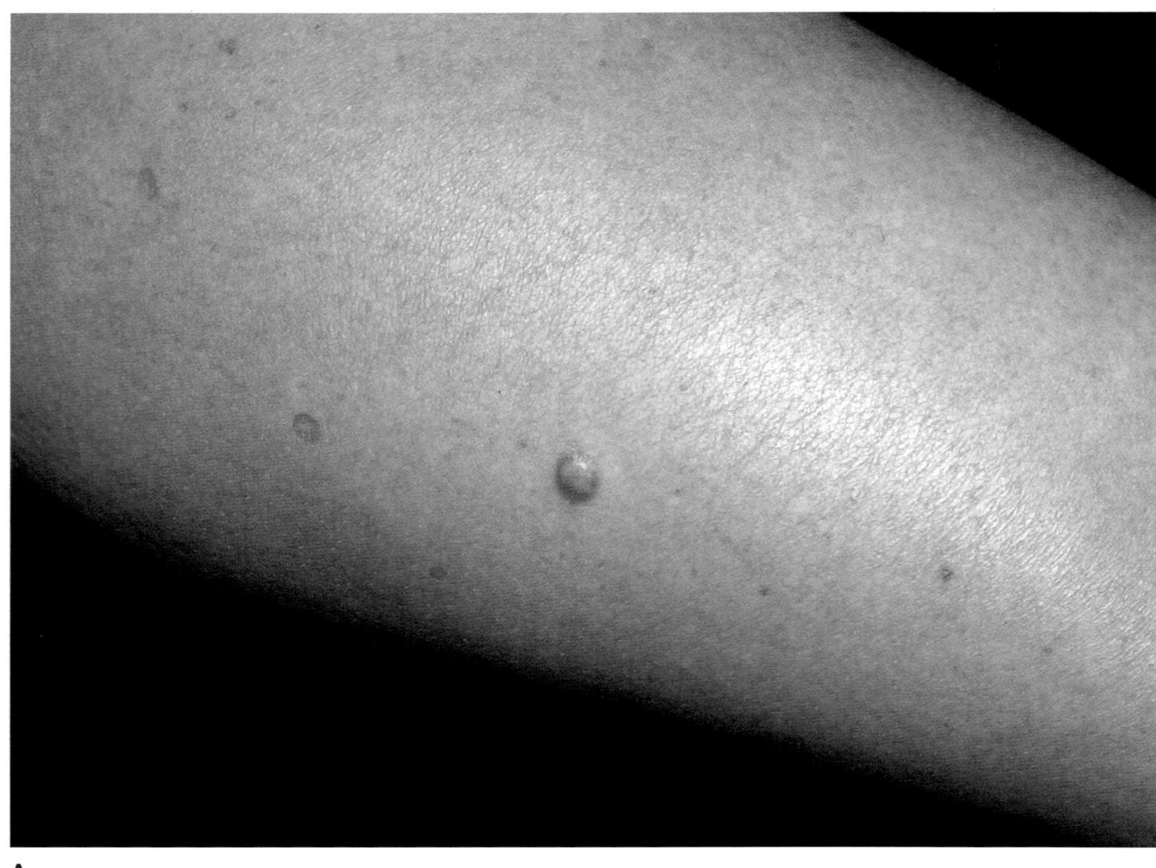

A

B

C

FIGURE 158-5 A. Dermatofibroma on the leg that has a pink center and a light brown halo. B. Close-up of the dermatofibroma showing the pink center and brown halo. C. Dermoscopic view of the dermatofibroma showing the typical pattern with a radially streaking brown halo and a pink center with white stellate scar. (*Reproduced with permission from Richard P. Usatine, MD.*)

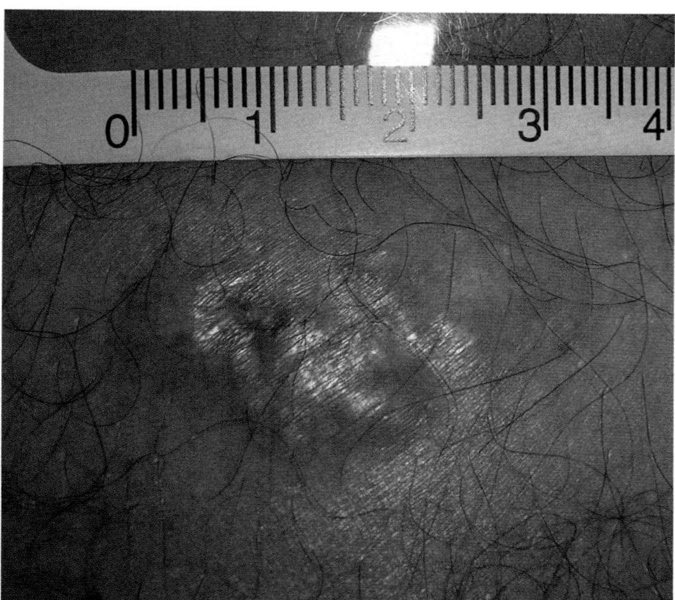

FIGURE 158-6 Large dermatofibrosarcoma protuberans growing on the thigh of this 55-year-old man. The first punch biopsy was read as a benign dermatofibroma. Continued growth prompted a second biopsy that detected the malignancy. The first excision did not achieve clear margins so the final treatment consisted of Mohs surgery. Note the shiny surface and multilobular look that can be characteristic of a dermatofibrosarcoma protuberans. *(Reproduced with permission from Richard P. Usatine, MD.)*

- Punch excision or shave excision may be used for small lesions; with the latter technique, the healed area may remain hard as a result of remaining fibrous tissue.
- Larger lesions may require an elliptical (fusiform) excision, down to the subcutaneous fat.
- One author noted that DFs occurring on the face often have involvement of deeper structures and an increased rate of local recurrences and therefore recommend excision with wider margins in comparison with DFs occurring on the extremities.[12]
- Cryotherapy has also been used, but the cure rate is low and lesions may recur.
- Several case reports found success in treating multiple DFs with carbon dioxide laser[13] or isotretinoin.[14]

PROGNOSIS

- Although DFs are usually unchanging and persist indefinitely, there are reports of spontaneous regression.[15]
- Following excision, DFs have a low recurrence rate of less than 2%, with higher recurrence believed to occur in cellular, aneurysmal, and atypical types.[7,10]
- A higher rate of recurrence has been noted in the subcutaneous and deep types, and in lesions located on the face, in which a recurrence rate of 15% to 19% has been reported.[16,17]

PATIENT EDUCATION

DFs are best left alone if they are relatively asymptomatic and stable.

PATIENT RESOURCES

- American Osteopathic College of Dermatology. *Dermatofibroma*—**http://www.aocd.org/skin/dermatologic_diseases/dermatofibroma.html.**
- Skinsight. *Dermatofibroma*—**http://www.skinsight.com/adult/dermatofibroma.htm.**

PROVIDER RESOURCES

- Medscape. *Dermatofibroma*—**http://emedicine.medscape.com/article/1056742.**

REFERENCES

1. Pierson JC. *Dermatofibroma*. http://emedicine.medscape.com/article/1056742-overview#a0104. Accessed July 2011.
2. Han TY, Chang HS, Lee JH, et al. A clinical and histopathological study of 122 cases of dermatofibroma (benign fibrous histiocytoma). *Ann Dermatol*. 2011;23(2):185-192.
3. Chen TC, Kuo T, Chan HL. Dermatofibroma is a clonal proliferative disease. *J Cutan Pathol*. 2000;27:36-39.
4. Yazici AC, Baz K, Ikizoglu G, et al. Familial eruptive dermatofibromas in atopic dermatitis. *J Eur Acad Dermatol Venereol*. 2006;20(1):90-92.
5. Lang KJ, Lidder S, Hofer M, et al. Rapidly evolving giant dermatofibroma. *Case Report Med*. 2010;2010:620910.
6. Jung KD, Lee DY, Lee JH, et al. Subcutaneous dermatofibroma. *Ann Dermatol*. 2011;23(2):254-257.
7. Zaballos P, Puig S, Llambrich A, Malvehy J. Dermoscopy of dermatofibromas: a prospective morphological study of 412 cases. *Arch Dermatol*. 2008;144(1):75-83.
8. Rosmaninho A, Farrajota P, Peixoto C, et al. Basal cell carcinoma overlying a dermatofibroma: a revisited controversy. *Eur J Dermatol*. 2011;21(1):137-138.
9. Kovach BT, Boyd AS. Melanoma associated with dermatofibroma. *J Cutan Pathol*. 2007;34(5):420-492.
10. Papalas JA, Balmer NN, Wallace C, Sangüeza OP. Ossifying dermatofibroma with osteoclast-like giant cells: report of a case and literature review. *Am J Dermatopathol*. 2009;31(4):379-833.
11. Garrido-Ruiz MC, Carrillo R, Enguita AB, Peralto JL. Signet-ring cell dermatofibroma. *Am J Dermatopathol*. 2009;31(1):84-87.
12. Mentzel T, Kutzner H, Rutten A, Hugel H. Benign fibrous histiocytoma (dermatofibroma) of the face: clinicopathologic and immunohistochemical study of 34 cases associated with an aggressive clinical course. *Am J Dermatopathol*. 2001;23(5):419-426.
13. Sardana K, Garg VK. Multiple dermatofibromas on face treated with carbon dioxide laser: the importance of laser parameters. *Indian J Dermatol Venereol Leprol*. 2008;74(2):170.
14. Kwinter J, DeKoven J. Generalized eruptive histiocytoma treated with isotretinoin. *J Cutan Med Surg*. 2009;4(4):490-491.
15. Niemi KM. The benign fibrohistiocytic tumours of the skin. *Acta Derm Venereol Suppl (Stockh)*. 1970;50(63):(suppl 63):1-66.
16. Fletcher CD. Benign fibrous histiocytoma of subcutaneous and deep soft tissue: a clinicopathologic analysis of 21 cases. *Am J Surg Pathol*. 1990;14:801-809.
17. Mentzel T, Kutzner H, Rütten A, Hügel H. Benign fibrous histiocytoma (dermatofibroma) of the face: clinicopathologic and immunohistochemical study of 34 cases associated with an aggressive clinical course. *Am J Dermatopathol*. 2001;23:419-426.

159 PYOGENIC GRANULOMA

Mindy A. Smith, MD, MS
Richard P. Usatine, MD

PATIENT STORY

A 20-year-old woman presents to the office with a new growth on her lip (**Figure 159-1**). She stated that the growth on her lip bled very easily but was not painful. She was diagnosed with a pyogenic granuloma (PG) and preferred to wait until her pregnancy was over to have it removed. The lesion did not regress spontaneously after pregnancy and was surgically excised.

INTRODUCTION

PG is the name for a common, benign, acquired, vascular neoplasm of the skin and mucous membranes.

SYNONYMS

The term *lobular capillary hemangioma* has been suggested because PG is neither pyogenic (purulent bacterial infection) nor a granuloma.[1]

EPIDEMIOLOGY

- Most often seen in children and young adults (0.5% of children's skin lesions); 42% of cases occur by 5 years of age and approximately 1% are present at birth.[1]
- Oral lesions occur most often in the second and third decade, more commonly in women (female-to-male ratio is 2:1).[1]
- Also common during pregnancy.
- PG has also been reported in the gastrointestinal (GI) tract, the larynx, and on the nasal mucosa, conjunctiva, and cornea.

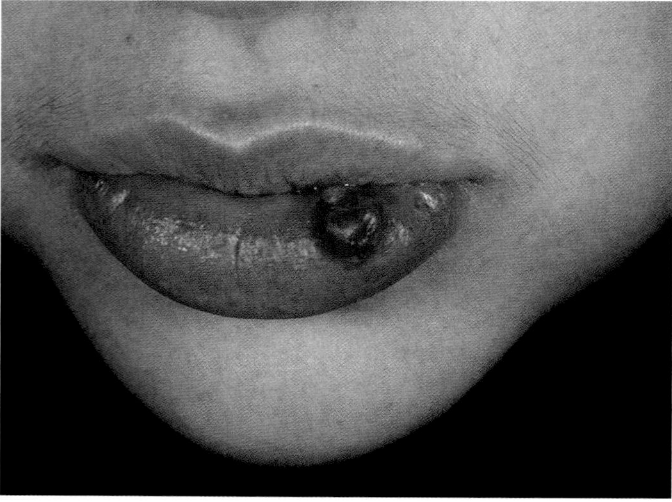

FIGURE 159-1 Pyogenic granuloma on the lower lip arising during pregnancy. (*Reproduced with permission from Usatine RP, Moy RL, Tobinick EL, Siegel DM.* Skin Surgery: A Practical Guide. *St. Louis, MO: Mosby; 1998.*)

ETIOLOGY AND PATHOPHYSIOLOGY

- Etiology is unknown but may be the result of trauma, infection, or preceding dermatoses.
- Consists of dense proliferation of capillaries and fibroblastic stroma that is infiltrated with polymorphonuclear leukocytes.
- Multiple PGs have been reported at burn sites and following use of oral contraceptives, protease inhibitors, and topical application of tretinoin for acne.[2]
- PGs are known to regress following pregnancy. Vascular endothelial growth factor (VEGF) was found in one study to be high in the granulomas during pregnancy, was almost undetectable after parturition, and was associated with apoptosis of endothelial cells and regression of granuloma.[3]

RISK FACTORS

- Trauma (up to 50%) or chronic irritation.[1]
- Multiple lesions can follow manipulation of a primary lesion.[4]
- Pregnancy or use of oral contraceptives for oral PGs; postulated caused by imbalance between angiogenesis enhancers and inhibitors.[1]
- Infection with *Bartonella*.[1]

DIAGNOSIS

CLINICAL FEATURES

- Usually solitary, erythematous, dome-shaped papule or nodule that bleeds easily (**Figures 159-1** to **159-6**); rarely causes anemia. Satellite lesions may rarely occur.

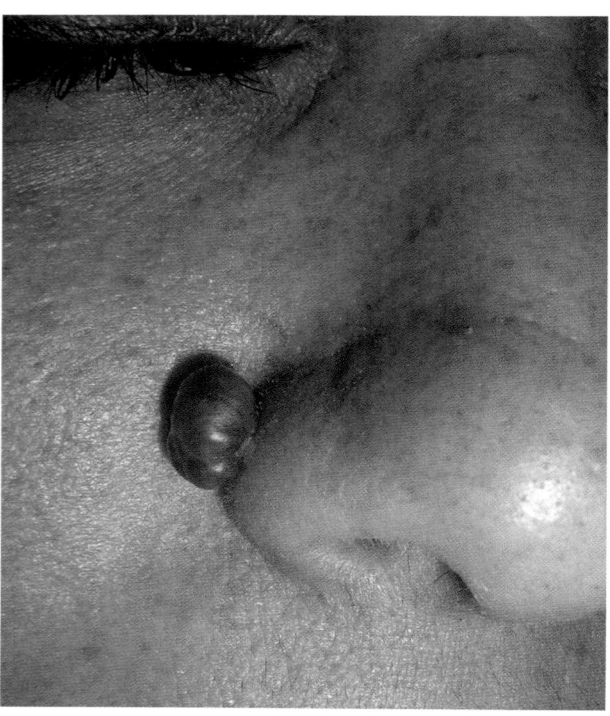

FIGURE 159-2 Pyogenic granuloma on the nose in a young adult. (*Reproduced with permission from Richard P. Usatine, MD.*)

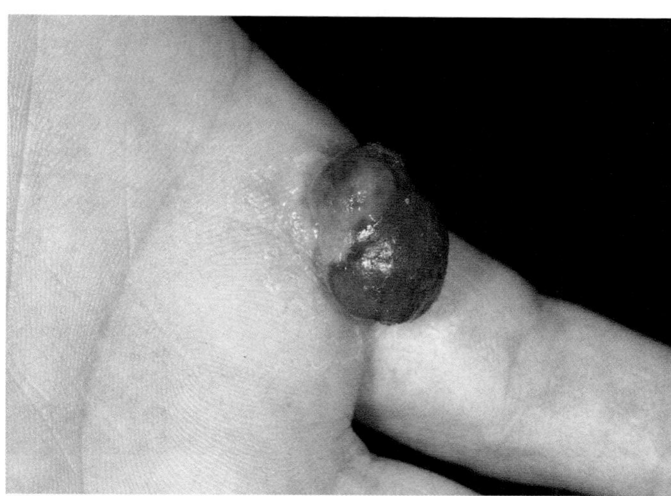

FIGURE 159-3 Large pyogenic granuloma on the hand of a 33-year-old man present for 3 months. (*Reproduced with permission from Richard P. Usatine, MD.*)

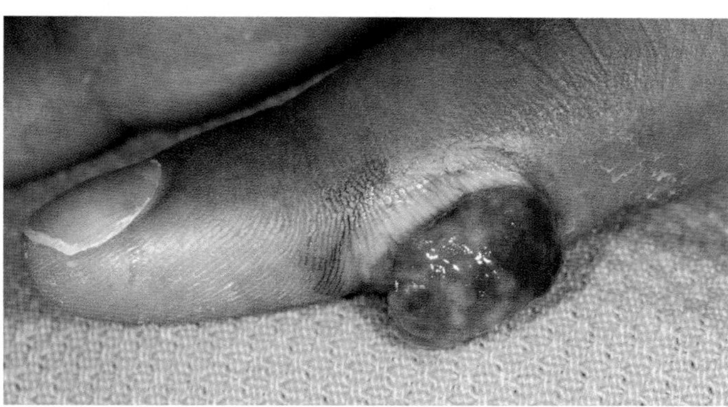

FIGURE 159-4 Large pyogenic granuloma on the finger of a 22-year-old man present for 4 months. He was sent out of multiple clinical settings untreated until we excised this. (*Reproduced with permission from Richard P. Usatine, MD.*)

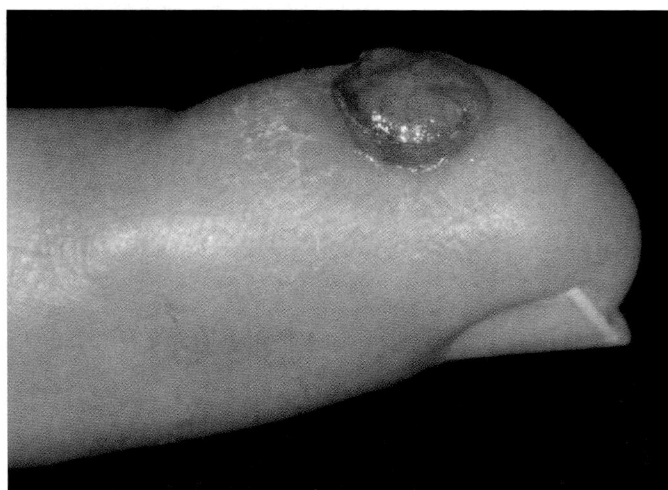

FIGURE 159-5 Small pyogenic granuloma on the finger for 2 months. It started with a small injury to the finger. (*Reproduced with permission from Richard P. Usatine, MD.*)

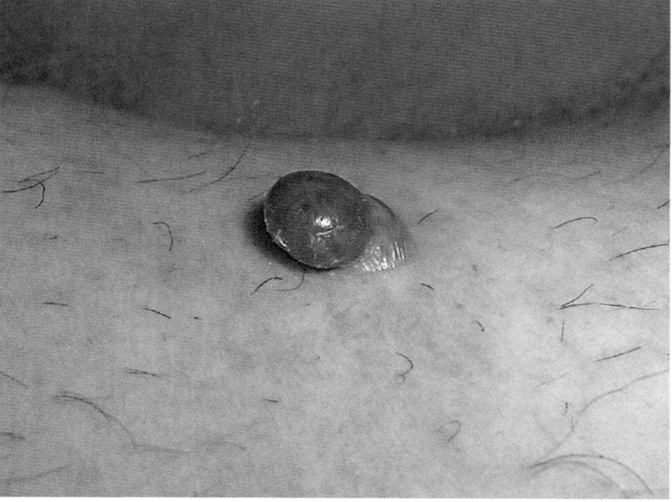

FIGURE 159-6 Pyogenic granuloma on the leg for 6 months before the patient presented for treatment. (*Reproduced with permission from Richard P. Usatine, MD.*)

- Prone to ulceration, erosion, and crusting.
- Size ranges from a few millimeters to several centimeters (average size is 6.5 mm).[1]
- Rapid growth over a period of weeks to maximum size.
- Variants include cutaneous, oral mucosal (granuloma gravidarum), satellite, subcutaneous, intravenous, and congenital types.[1]

TYPICAL DISTRIBUTION

- Cutaneous PG most often found on the head and neck (62.5%) specifically the gingiva, lips as in **Figure 159-1**, nose (see **Figure 159-2**), face, trunk (20%), and extremities (18%) (see **Figures 159-3** to **159-6**).[1]
- Pregnancy PG occurs most commonly along the maxillary intraoral mucosal surface.

IMAGING

Reddish homogeneous area surrounded by a white collarette is the most frequent dermoscopic pattern in PGs (85%).[5] In more advanced lesions, white lines that intersect the central areas may be seen that are likely fibrous septa.

BIOPSY

- Early lesions resemble granulation tissue (numerous capillaries and venules with endothelial cells arrayed radially toward the skin surface; stroma is edematous).[1]
- The mature PG exhibits a fibromyxoid stroma separating the lesion into lobules. Proliferation of capillaries is present, with prominent endothelial cells. The epidermis exhibits inward growth at the lesion base.[1]
- A regressing PG has extensive fibrosis.

DIFFERENTIAL DIAGNOSIS

PG may be confused with a number of cutaneous malignancies, including atypical fibroxanthoma, basal cell carcinoma, Kaposi sarcoma, metastatic cutaneous lesions, squamous cell carcinoma, and amelanotic melanoma

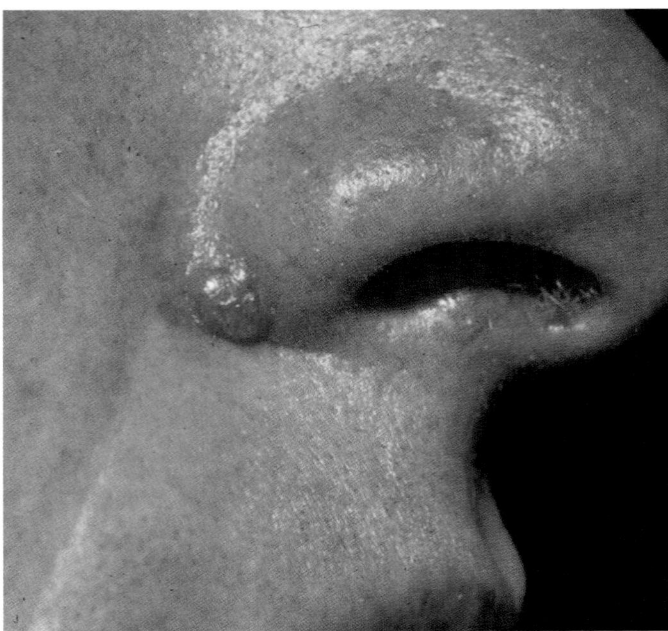

FIGURE 159-7 Amelanotic melanoma on the nose that could be confused with a pyogenic granuloma. Always send what you suspect to be a PG to the pathologist. (*Reproduced with permission from the University of Texas Health Sciences Center, Division of Dermatology.*)

(**Figure 159-7**). It is especially important to send the excised lesion that appears to be a PG for pathology to make sure that a malignancy is not missed.

Benign tumors that may be confused with PG include the following:

- Cherry hemangioma—Small, bright-red, dome-shaped papules that represent benign proliferation of capillaries (**Figure 159-8**).
- Fibrous papule of the nose is a benign tumor of the nose. Most are skin colored and not confused with PG. A benign clear cell variant of a fibrous papule can closely resemble a PG as seen in **Figure 159-9**.
- Bacillary angiomatosis—A systemic infectious disease caused by 2 *Bartonella* species. Globular angiomatous papules appear like PG (**Figure 212-8**). Nodules affect all age groups and may reach 10 cm in size. This infection is more likely to occur in persons with AIDS. Weight loss and lymphadenopathy may occur.

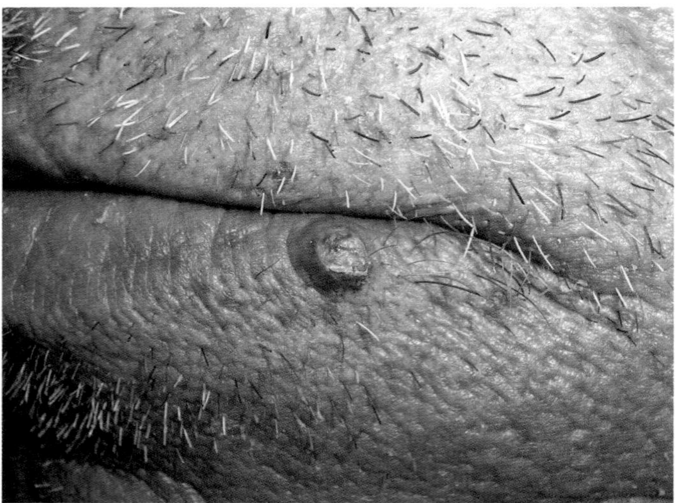

FIGURE 159-8 Hemangioma on the lip of a 67-year-old man. By appearance alone this is hard to differentiate from a pyogenic granuloma (lobular capillary hemangioma). This did not bleed extensively at time of excision and the pathology result confirmed that this was a hemangioma. (*Reproduced with permission from Richard P. Usatine, MD.*)

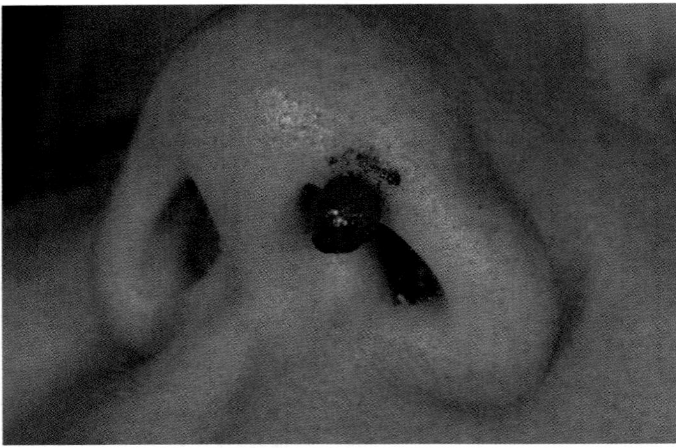

FIGURE 159-9 Vascular growth on the nose of a pregnant woman that appears to be a pyogenic granuloma. Biopsy revealed a benign clear cell variant of a fibrous papule. (*Reproduced with permission from Richard P. Usatine, MD.*)

MANAGEMENT

Removal of the lesion is indicated to alleviate any bleeding or discomfort, for cosmetic reasons, or when the diagnosis is uncertain.

NONPHARMACOLOGIC

Untreated PGs eventually atrophy, become fibromatous, and slowly regress, especially if the causative agent is removed.

MEDICATIONS

A case of successful treatment of a recurrent PG was reported using a 14-week course of twice-weekly imiquimod 5% topical application.[6] SOR Ⓒ

PROCEDURES

A number of procedures have been used for elimination of PGs; data are limited to case series reports.[7]

- Simple surgical excision has a low recurrence rate (<4%) but is associated with scarring (55%).[7] SOR Ⓒ
- Removal can be accomplished with shave excision and electrodesiccation; the latter reduces recurrence (approximately 10%) and scarring appears less than with either simple excision (31%) or cauterization alone (43.5%).[1,7] PGs bleed extensively when manipulated or cut. It is important to use lidocaine with epinephrine, wait 10 minutes for the epinephrine to work, and have an electrosurgery device to control bleeding. Cut the PG off with a blade and send to pathology. Curetting the base will also help stop the bleeding and prevent recurrence. The base is curetted and electrodesiccated until the bleeding stops. SOR Ⓒ
- Both cryosurgery and laser surgery often require more than one treatment and rates of scarring may be high (12%-42% and 44%, respectively).[1,7] SOR Ⓒ
- In one case series, sclerotherapy was reported to leave no scarring or recurrence.[7] SOR Ⓒ

PROGNOSIS

- PG develops over weeks and growth typically stabilizes over several months.[1] Eventually, it shrinks to become a fibrotic "angioma." Some nodules spontaneously infarct and involute.
- Congenital PG is an uncommon disseminated variant that presents with multiple lesions, is similar in appearance to the cutaneous form, and is present at birth. The condition appears to follow a benign course, with spontaneous resolution over 6 to 12 months.[1]

PATIENT EDUCATION

- Explain to patients that lesions may resolve spontaneously and that multiple successful treatments are available (note that most patients will be grateful to have treatment that day as the lesion tends to be a great nuisance by bleeding easily and having an undesirable appearance).
- Once treated, if the lesion begins to recur, patients should follow up quickly before the lesion gets larger and harder to treat.

FOLLOW-UP

Follow-up in 2 weeks to receive the result of the pathology and to check wound healing.

PATIENT RESOURCES

- MedlinePlus. *Medical Encyclopedia*—**http://www.nlm.nih.gov/medlineplus/ency/article/ 001464.htm.**
- PubMed Health. *Pyogenic granuloma*—**http://www.ncbi.nlm.nih.gov/pubmedhealth/PMH0002435/.**

PROVIDER RESOURCES

- Medscape. *Pediatric Pyogenic Granuloma*—**http://emedicine.medscape.com/article/910112.**
- Medscape. *Oral Pyogenic Granuloma*—**http://emedicine.medscape.com/article/1077040.**
- Usatine R, Pfenninger J, Stulberg D, Small R. *Dermatologic and Cosmetic Procedures in Office Practice*. Philadelphia, PA: Elsevier; 2012. The book has many photographs and descriptions that provide details of how to surgically treat PGs. It is also available as an electronic application, with video included, at **www.usatinemedia.com.**

REFERENCES

1. Lin RL, Janniger CK. Pyogenic granuloma. *Cutis.* 2004;74(4):229-233.
2. Teknetzis A, Tonannides D, Vakali G, et al. Pyogenic granulomas following topical application of tretinoin. *J Eur Acad Dermatol Venereol.* 2004;18(3):337-339.
3. Yuan K, Lin MT. The roles of vascular endothelial growth factor and angiopoietin-2 in the regression of pregnancy pyogenic granuloma. *Oral Dis.* 2004;10(3):179-185.
4. Blickenstaff RD, Roenigk RK, Peters MS, et al. Recurrent pyogenic granuloma with satellitosis. *J Am Acad Dermatol.* 1989;21:1241-1244.
5. Zaballos P, Llambrich A, Cuellar F, et al. Dermoscopic findings in pyogenic granuloma. *Br J Dermatol.* 2006;154(6):1108-1111.
6. Goldenberg G, Krowchuk DP, Jorizzo JL. Successful treatment of a therapy-resistant pyogenic granuloma with topical imiquimod 5% cream. *J Dermatolog Treat.* 2006;17(2):121-123.
7. Gilmore A, Kelsberg G, Safranek S. Clinical inquiries. What's the best treatment for pyogenic granuloma? *J Fam Pract.* 2010;59(1):40-42.

SECTION 9 NEVI

160 BENIGN NEVI

Mindy A. Smith, MD, MS
Richard P. Usatine, MD

PATIENT STORY

A young woman comes to the office because her husband has noted that the moles on her back are changing **(Figure 160-1)**. A few have white halos around the brown pigmentation and some have lost their pigment completely, with a light area remaining. She has no symptoms but wants to make sure these are not skin cancers. Halo nevi are an uncommon variation of common nevi. These appear benign and the patient is reassured.

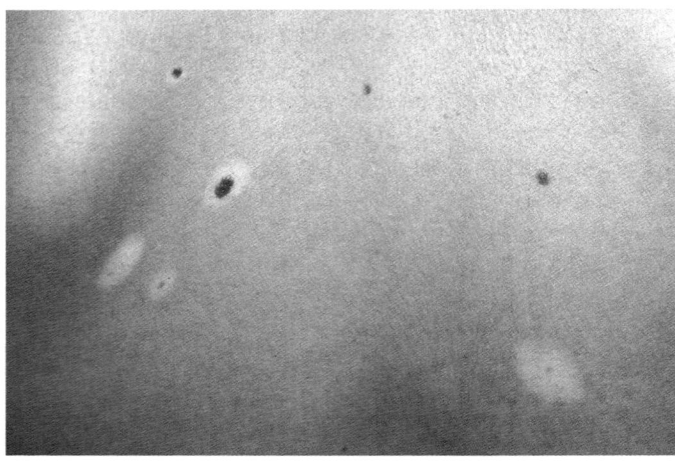

A

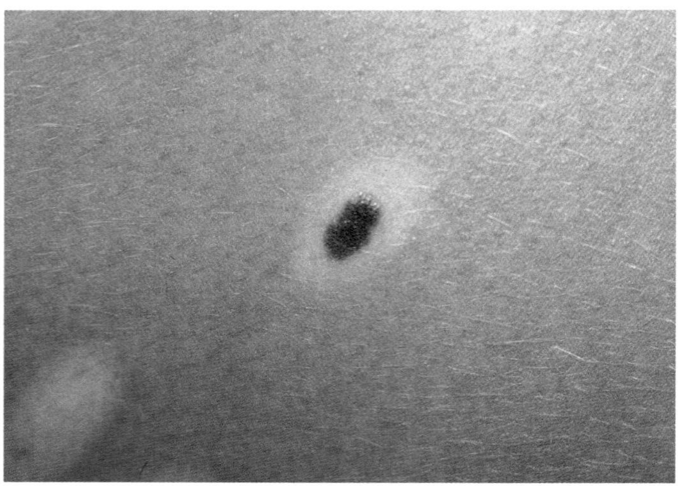

B

FIGURE 160-1 A. Multiple halo nevi on the back. B. Close-up of a halo nevus in transition. *(Reproduced with permission from Richard P. Usatine, MD.)*

INTRODUCTION

Most nevi are benign tumors caused by the aggregation of melanocytic cells in the skin. However, nevi can occur on the conjunctiva, sclera, and other structures of the eye. There are also nonmelanocytic nevi that are produced by other cells as seen in Becker nevi and comedonal nevi. Although most nevi are acquired, many nevi are present at birth.

SYNONYMS

Benign nevi are also called as moles.

EPIDEMIOLOGY

- Acquired nevi are common lesions, forming during early childhood; few adults have none.
- Prevalence appears to be lower in dark-skinned individuals.
- Present in 1% of neonates increasing through childhood and peaking at puberty; new ones may continue to appear in adulthood. In a population study of children (N = 180, ages 1-15 years) in Barcelona, the mean number of nevi was 17.5.[1]
- Adults typically have 10 to 40 nevi scattered over the body. In a population study in Germany, 60.3% of 2823 adults (mean age 49 years; 50% women) exhibited 11 to 50 common nevi and 5.2% had at least 1 atypical nevus.[2]
- The peak incidence of melanocytic nevi (MN) is in the fourth to fifth decades of life; the incidence decreases with each successive decade.[3]

ETIOLOGY AND PATHOPHYSIOLOGY

- Benign tumors composed of nevus cells derived from melanocytes, pigment-producing cells that colonize the epidermis.
- MN represent proliferations of melanocytes those are in contact with each other, forming small collections of cells known as nests. Genetic mutations present in common nevi as well as in melanomas include BRAF, NRAS, and *c*-kit.[4]
- Sun (UV) exposure, skin-blistering events (eg, sunburn), and genetics play a role in the formation of new nevi.[3]
- Nevi commonly darken and/or enlarge during pregnancy. Melanocytes have receptors for estrogens and androgens and melanogenesis is responsive to these hormones.[3]
- Three broad categories of MN are based on location of nevus cells[2] are as below:
  - Junctional nevi—Composed of nevus cells located in the dermal-epidermal junction; may change into compound nevi after childhood (except when located on the palms, soles, or genitalia) **(Figure 160-2)**.
  - Compound nevi—A nevus in which a portion of nevus cells have migrated into the dermis **(Figure 160-3)**.

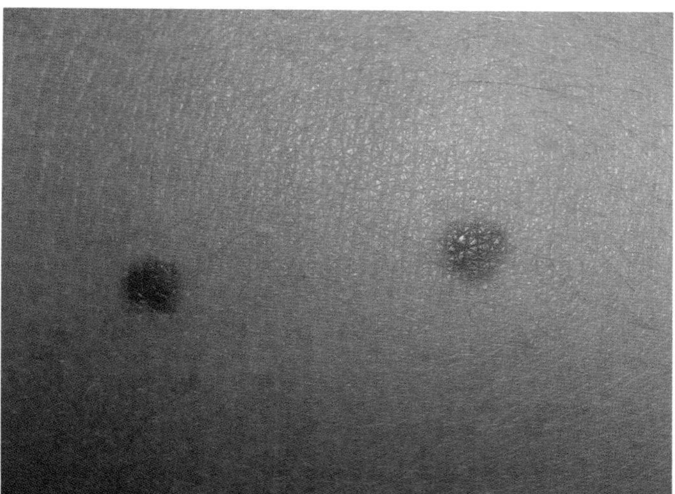

FIGURE 160-2 Two benign junctional nevi on the arm of a 19-year-old woman. Note how these are flat macules. (*Reproduced with permission from Richard P. Usatine, MD.*)

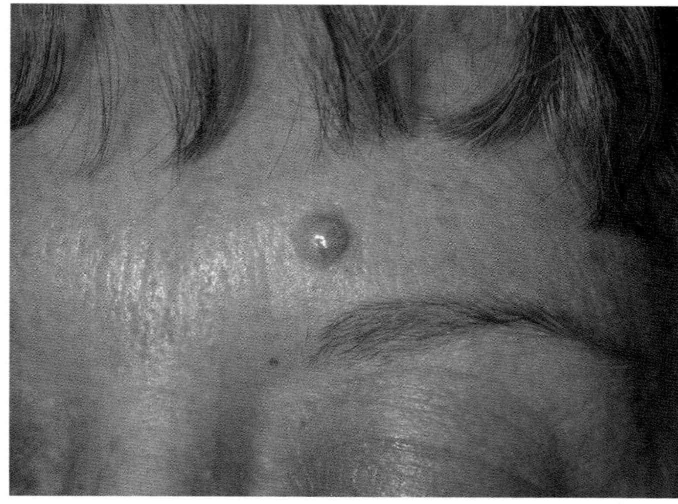

FIGURE 160-4 Dermal nevus (intradermal melanocytic nevus)—dome shaped with some scattered pigmentation. (*Reproduced with permission from Richard P. Usatine, MD.*)

- Dermal nevi—Composed of nevus cells located within the dermis (usually found only in adults). These are usually raised and have little to no visible hyperpigmentation (**Figures 160-4** and **160-5**).
- Special categories of nevi are as below:
  - Halo nevus—Compound or dermal nevus that develops a symmetric, sharply demarcated, depigmented border (see **Figure 160-1**). Most commonly occurs on the trunk and develops during adolescence. Repigmentation may occur.
  - Blue nevus—A dermal nevus that contains large amounts of pigment so that the brown pigment absorbs the longer wavelengths of light and scatters blue light (Tyndall effect) (**Figure 160-6**). Blue nevi are not always blue and color varies from tan to blue, black, and gray. Types of blue nevi include amelanotic, desmoplastic, atypical, and malignant variants; genetic mutations seen in blue nevi are often different than those seen in common nevi and include the Gαq class of G-protein α subunits, Gnaq, and Gna11 proteins.[4] The nodules are firm because of associated stromal sclerosis. Usually appears in childhood on the extremities, dorsum of the hands, and face. A rare variant, the cellular blue nevus is large (>1 cm), frequently located on the buttocks, and may undergo malignant degeneration.
  - Nevus spilus—Hairless, oval, or irregularly shaped brown lesion with darker brown to black dots containing nevus cells (**Figure 160-7**). May appear at any age or be present at birth; unrelated to sun exposure.

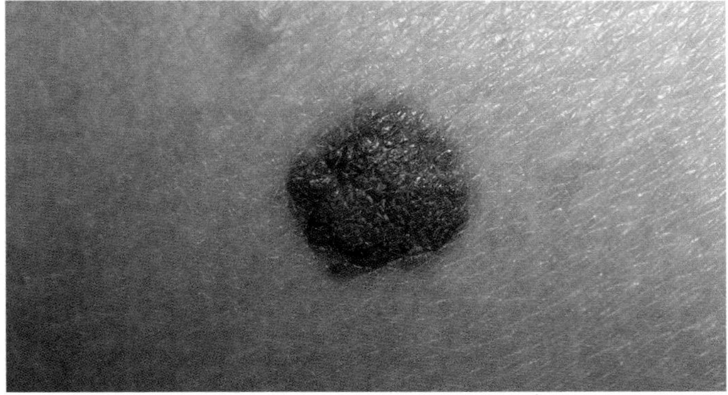

FIGURE 160-3 Benign compound nevus proven by biopsy on the back of a 35-year-old woman. (*Reproduced with permission from Richard P. Usatine, MD.*)

  - Spitz nevus (formerly called benign juvenile melanoma because of its clinical and histologic similarity to melanoma)—Hairless, red, or reddish brown dome-shaped papules generally appearing suddenly in children, sometimes following trauma (**Figures 160-8** and **160-9**). The pink color is caused by increased vascularity. Most importantly, these should be fully excised with clear margins.
  - Nevus of Ota—Dark brown nevus that occurs most commonly around the eye and can involve the sclera (**Figure 160-10**).
- Both acquired and congenital MN hold some risk for the development of melanoma; the number of MN, especially more than 100, is an important independent risk factor for cutaneous melanoma.[5]

NONMELANOCYTIC NEVI

- Becker nevus—A brown patch often with hair located on the shoulder, back or submammary area, most often in adolescent men (**Figures 160-11** and **160-12**). The lesion may enlarge to cover an

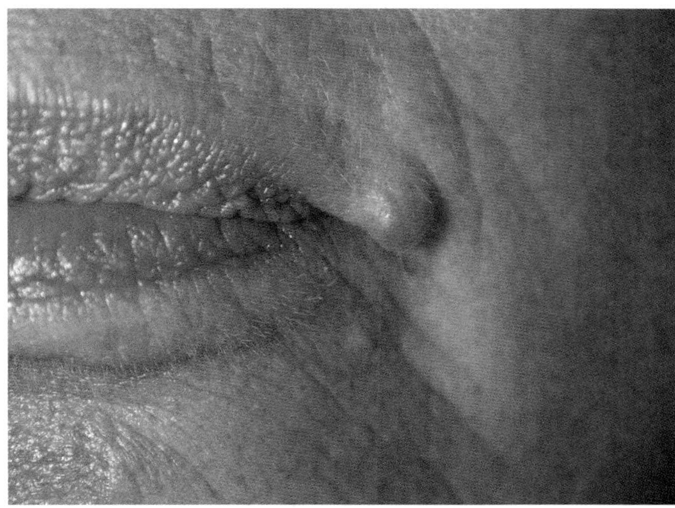

FIGURE 160-5 Dermal nevus pedunculated with small telangiectasias. (*Reproduced with permission from Richard P. Usatine, MD.*)

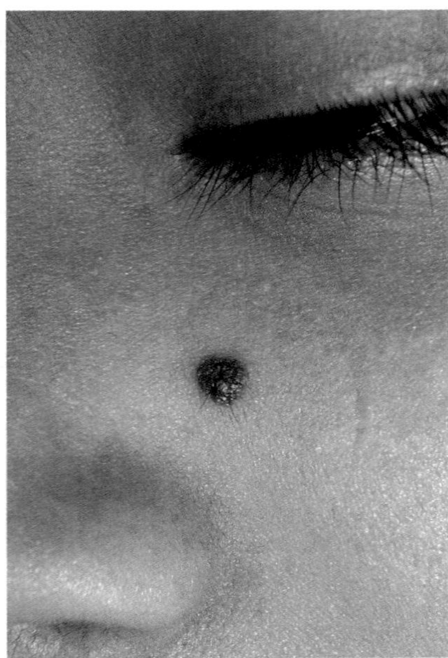

FIGURE 160-6 Blue nevus on the left cheek that could resemble a melanoma with its dark color. In this case it was fully excised with a 5-mm punch with a good cosmetic result. Blue nevi are benign and do not need to be excised unless there are suspicious changes. (*Reproduced with permission from Richard P. Usatine, MD.*)

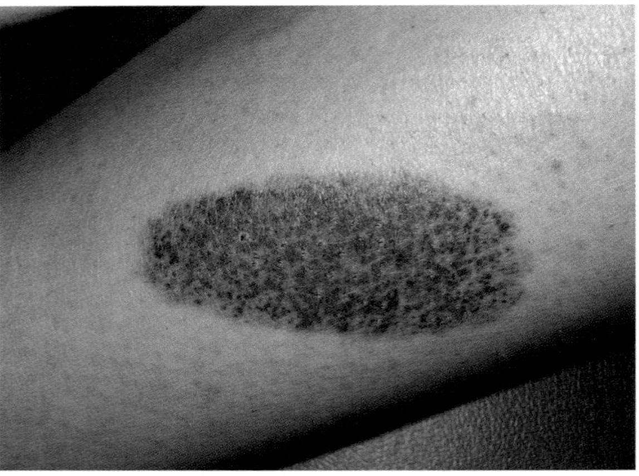

FIGURE 160-7 Nevus spilus on the leg of a young woman from birth. It appears benign and needs no intervention. (*Reproduced with permission from Richard P. Usatine, MD.*)

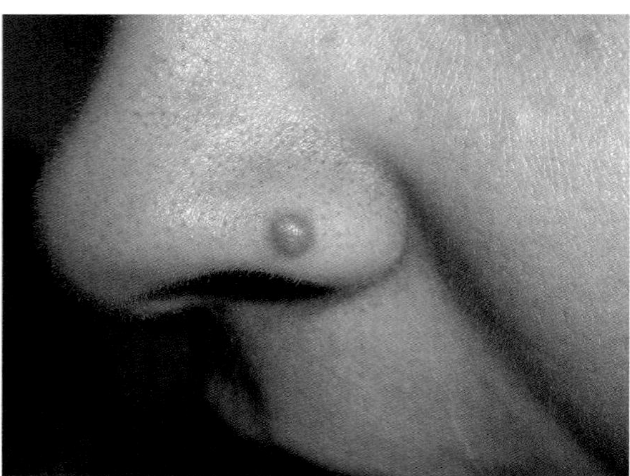

FIGURE 160-8 Spitz nevus that grew over the past year on the nose of this 18-year-old woman. It was fully excised with no complications. (*Reproduced with permission from Richard P. Usatine, MD.*)

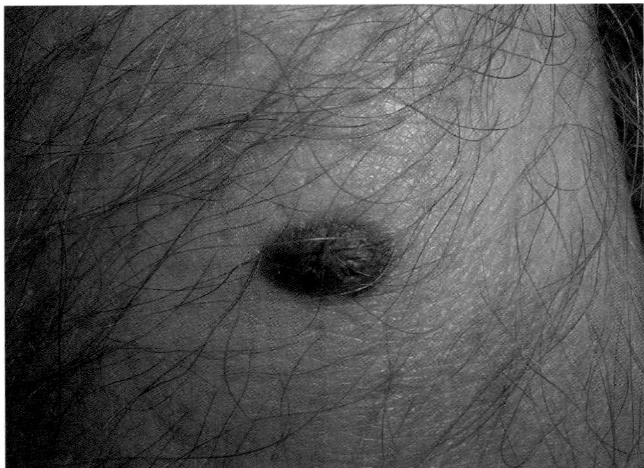

A

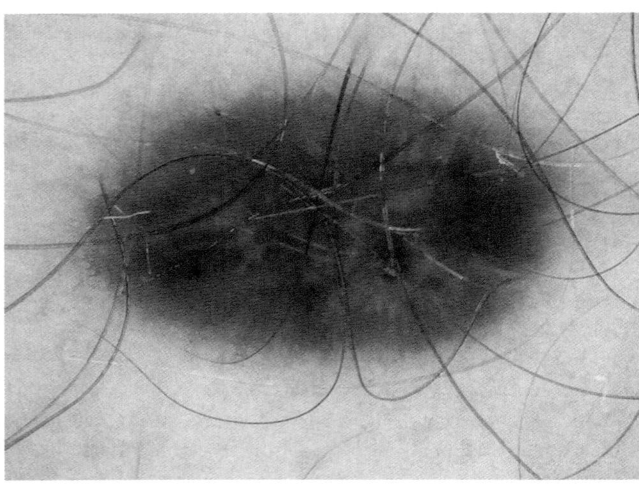

B

FIGURE 160-9 **A.** Intradermal nevus with spitzoid features on the arm of this man. It was fully excised. **B.** Dermoscopy of this nevus shows some peripheral active growth with streaming and crystalline structures (white). The dermoscopy was concerning for a Spitz nevus or a melanoma. (*Reproduced with permission from Richard P. Usatine, MD.*)

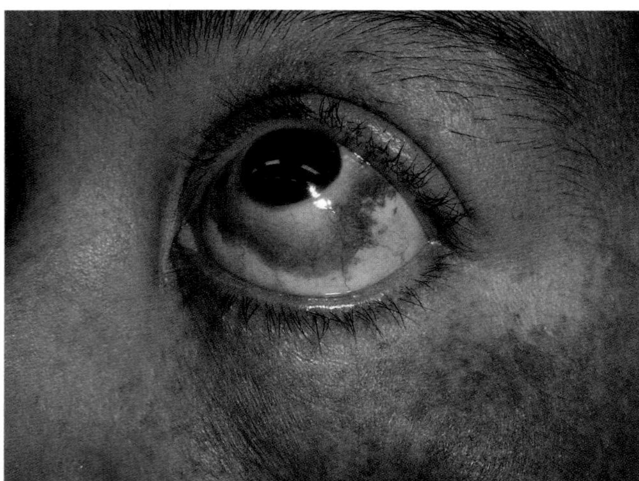

FIGURE 160-10 Nevus of Ota on the face of this young woman since early childhood. It involved both eyes and the skin around both eyes. The scleral pigmentation looks blue. (*Reproduced with permission from Richard P. Usatine, MD.*)

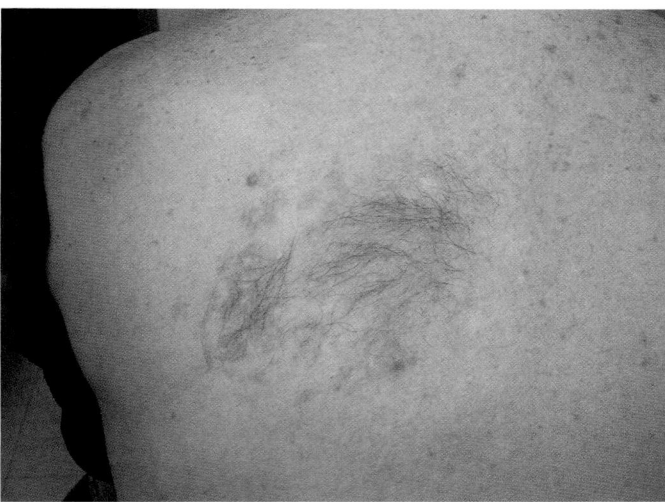

FIGURE 160-11 Becker nevus that developed during adolescence in this young man. Hair is frequently seen on this type of nonmelanocytic nevus. (*Reproduced with permission from Richard P. Usatine, MD.*)

entire shoulder or upper arm. Although it is called a nevus, it does not actually have nevus cells and has no malignant potential. It is a type of hamartoma, an abnormal mixture of cells and tissues normally found in the area of the body where the growth occurs.

- Nevus depigmentosus is usually present at birth or starts in early childhood. There is a decrease number of melanosomes within a normal number of melanocytes. It typically has a serrated or jagged edge (**Figure 160-13**).
- Nevus anemicus—A congenital hypopigmented macule or patch that is stable in relative size and distribution. It occurs as a result of localized hypersensitivity to catecholamines and not a decrease in melanocytes. On diascopy (pressure with a glass slide) the skin is indistinguishable from the surrounding skin (**Figure 160-14**).
- Nevus comedonicus (comedonal nevus) is a rare congenital hamartoma characterized by an aggregation of comedones in one region of the skin (**Figure 160-15**).

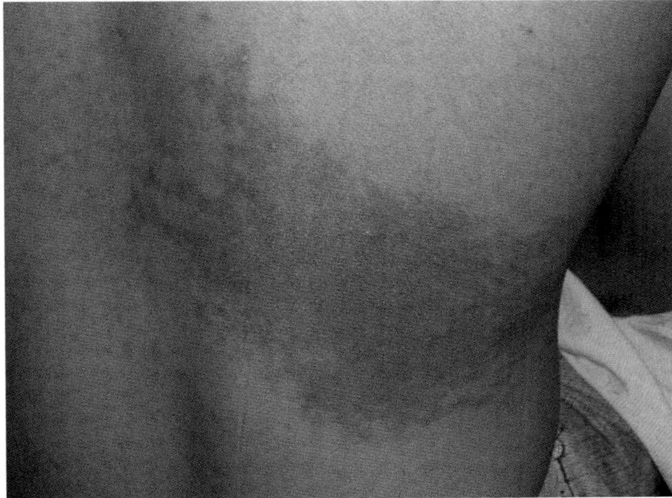

FIGURE 160-12 Becker nevus on the back of a Hispanic teenager for 2 years. While this nevus did not have hair, it did have increased acne within the area—another feature of the Becker nevus. (*Reproduced with permission from Richard P. Usatine, MD.*)

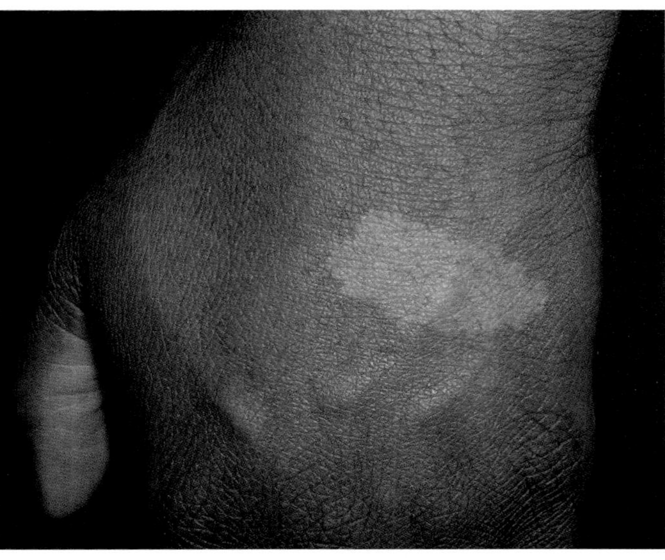

FIGURE 160-13 Nevus depigmentosus on the hand of this man since birth. (*Reproduced with permission from Richard P. Usatine, MD.*)

- Epidermal nevi are congenital hamartomas of ectodermal origin classified on the basis of their main component: sebaceous, apocrine, eccrine, follicular, or keratinocytic. See Chapter 161, Congenital Nevi for a full discussion of this type of nevus.

Note nevus comedonicus and epidermal nevi tend to follow Blaschko lines, which come from embryologic development.

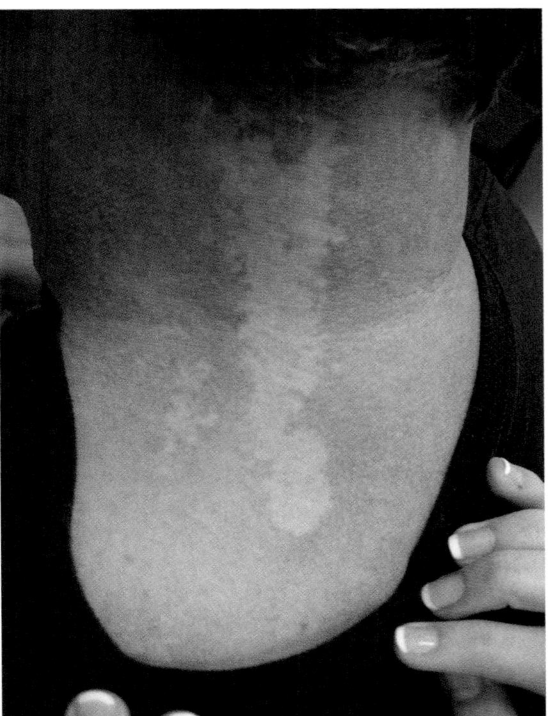

FIGURE 160-14 Nevus anemicus on the posterior neck. The localized hypersensitivity to catecholamines causes the area to stay lighter than the surrounding skin. (*Reproduced with permission from the University of Texas Health Sciences Center, Division of Dermatology.*)

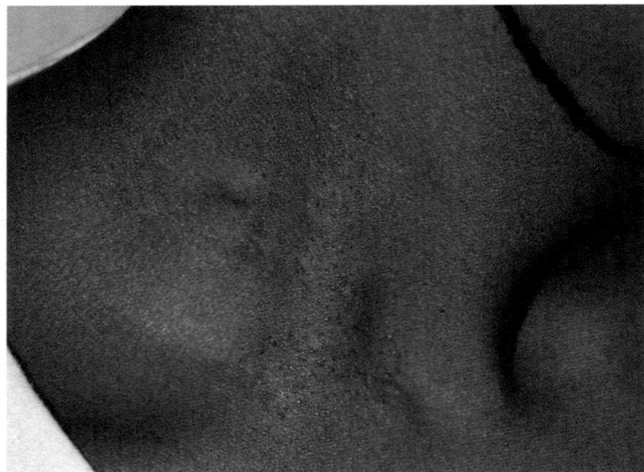

FIGURE 160-15 Nevus comedonicus on the neck of this woman since birth. This is a congenital hamartoma with open comedones. It is not acne. *(Reproduced with permission from Richard P. Usatine, MD.)*

RISK FACTORS

- In the Barcelona study of children, male gender, past history of sunburns, facial freckling, and family history of breast cancer were independent risk factors for having a higher number of nevi.[1]
- In one study among very light-skinned (and not darker-skinned) children without red hair, children who develop tans have greater numbers of nevi.[6]
- Neonatal blue-light phototherapy is not related to nevus count.[7]

DIAGNOSIS

CLINICAL FEATURES

Most benign MN are tan to brown, usually less than 6 mm, with round shape and sharp borders.

- Junctional nevi—Macular or slightly elevated mole of uniform brown to black pigmentation, smooth surface, and a round or oval border (see **Figure 160-2**). Most are hairless and vary from 1 to 6 mm.
- Compound nevi—Slightly elevated, symmetric, uniformly flesh colored or brown with a round or oval border, often becoming more elevated with age (see **Figure 160-3**). Hair may be present and a white halo may form.
- Dermal nevi (same as intradermal nevi)—Skin color or brown color that may fade with age; dome-shaped nevus is most common, but shapes vary, including polypoid, warty, and pedunculated. Often found on the face and may have telangiectasias (see **Figures 160-4** and **160-5**). Size ranges from 1 to 10 mm.

TYPICAL DISTRIBUTION

- Most often found above the waist on sun-exposed areas but may appear anywhere on the cutaneous surface; less commonly found on the scalp, breasts, or buttocks.
- Among the children in the Barcelona study, 61.1% had nevi on the face and neck, 17.2% on the buttocks, and 11.7% on the scalp; approximately one-third had congenital nevi (see Chapter 161, Congenital Nevi).[1]
- In an Australian study of white children, MN of all sizes were highest on the outer forearms, followed by the outer upper arms, neck, and face.[8] Boys had higher densities of MN of all sizes on the neck than girls, and girls had higher densities of MN of 2 mm or greater on the lower legs and thighs than boys. Habitually sun-exposed body sites had higher densities of small MN and highest prevalence of larger MN.

IMAGING

- Dermoscopy can be a useful technique for diagnosing benign nevi. For MN, dermoscopic diagnosis relies on color; pattern (ie, globular, reticular, starburst, and homogeneous blue pattern); pigment distribution (ie, multifocal, central, eccentric, and uniform); and special sites (eg, face, acral areas, nail, and mucosa), in conjunction with patient factors (eg, history, pregnancy) (see **Figure 160-9**)[9] (see Appendix C, Dermoscopy).
- In the Barcelona study, the most frequent dominant dermoscopic pattern was the globular type with the homogeneous pattern predominating in the youngest children and the reticular pattern predominating in adolescents.[1]

BIOPSY

Biopsy is necessary if you suspect melanoma or a Spitz nevus. A biopsy that cuts below the pigmented area is preferred if there is a reasonable suspicion for melanoma. This can be done with a scoop shave, a punch that gets the whole lesion, or an elliptical excision. If the patient wants a raised benign-appearing nevus excised for cosmetic reasons, a shave excision may be adequate. Send all lesions (except skin tags) to the pathologist for examination, even when they appear benign, to avoid missing a melanoma.

DIFFERENTIAL DIAGNOSIS

Benign nevi may develop atypia or become melanoma. This should be suspected if a lesion has atypical features including asymmetry, border irregularity, color variability, diameter greater than 6 mm, and evolving (called the ABCDE approach [asymmetry, border irregularity, color irregularity, diameter >6 mm, evolution]). Any lesion that becomes symptomatic (eg, itchy, painful, irritated, or bleeding), or develops a loss or increase in pigmentation, should be evaluated and biopsied if needed. Dermoscopy can be used to increase one's accuracy in distinguishing between benign and malignant lesions (see Appendix C, Dermoscopy).

- Melanomas are skin cancers that may develop from a preexisting nevus. The most important skill to develop is how to distinguish a benign nevus from a nevus that might be malignant melanoma. Because clinical appearance can be misleading, a biopsy is necessary when there is a reasonable suspicion for cancer (see Chapter 170, Melanoma).
- Dysplastic or atypical nevi are variants that are relatively flat, thinly papular, and relatively broad. Often, the lesions exhibit target-like or fried egg-like morphology, with a central papular zone and a macular surrounding area with differing pigmentation (see Chapter 163, Dysplastic Nevus).
- Seborrheic keratoses are benign growths that appear more with increasing age and are often hyperpigmented as seen with many nevi. These are more superficial and stuck-on in their appearance (see Chapter 156, Seborrheic Keratosis).
- Labial melanotic macules are benign dark macules on the lip that are not nevi and not melanomas (**Figure 160-16**). They can be removed for cosmetic purposes.

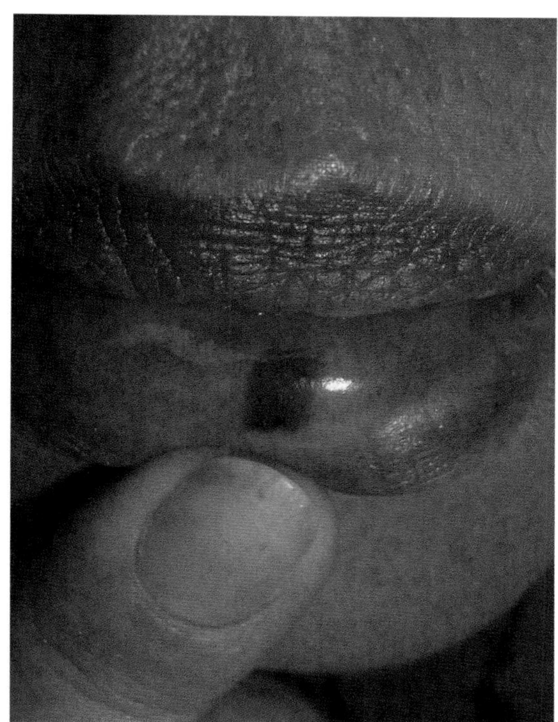

FIGURE 160-16 Labial melanotic macule. These are benign but are not nevi. *(Reproduced with permission from Richard P. Usatine, MD.)*

MANAGEMENT

Nevi are generally only removed for cosmetic reasons or because of concern over changes in the lesion suggestive of dysplasia or melanoma.

- A full excisional biopsy with a sutured closure is usually the best means to diagnose a lesion if concern exists regarding the possibility of melanoma. If the lesion is found to be benign, no further treatment is usually required.
- Punch excision can be used to excise smaller lesions.
- Scoop shave—Unfortunately, if a punch biopsy is used to sample a larger lesion it may miss a melanoma in another part of the lesion. A broad scoop shave is better than a punch biopsy when a full elliptical excision is not possible or desirable (eg, a large flat pigmented lesion on the face).
- Nevi removed for cosmesis are often removed by shave excision.[3]

If a Spitz nevus is suspected, either biopsy it now or schedule the patient for a full excision. The histopathology is too close to a melanoma to just watch it.

- Becker nevi and comedonal nevi do not become melanoma because they lack melanocytes. Therefore, there is no reason to excise them. Generally, these are large and the risks of excision for cosmetic reasons outweigh the benefits.

PREVENTION

Sun protection to limit sunburn may help reduce the appearance of nevi. In a trial of 209 white children, children randomized to the sunscreen group, especially those with freckles, had significantly fewer new nevi on the trunk than did children in the control group at 3-year follow-up.[10]

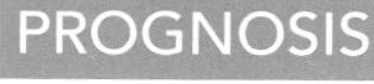

PROGNOSIS

- Degeneration of common nevi into melanoma is very rare.
- Patients with multiple or large MN appear to have an increased risk of melanoma.[3]
- Nevi may recur or persist following removal; in one study, dysplastic MN were the most likely to persist.[11] In another study, of 61 benign nevi biopsy sites reexamined, 2 (3.3%) recurred.[12]

FOLLOW-UP

Patients with multiple or sizable MN should be followed by an experienced clinician because they appear to have an increased lifetime risk of melanoma, with the risk increasing in rough proportion to the size and/or number of lesions.[3]

PATIENT EDUCATION

- Patients should be encouraged to use sunscreen to prevent skin cancer as well as to reduce the development of new nevi.
- Patients with multiple or sizable MN should be taught to look for and report asymmetry, border irregularity, new symptoms, and color and size changes.

PATIENT RESOURCES

- VisualDxHealth—**http://www.visualdxhealth.com/adult/nevus.htm.**
- MedlinePlus. *Moles*—**http://www.nlm.nih.gov/medlineplus/moles.html.**
- American Osteopathic College of Dermatology—**http://www.aocd.org/skin/dermatologic_diseases/moles.html.**

PROVIDER RESOURCES

- Medscape. *Melanocytic Nevi*—**http://emedicine.medscape.com/article/1058445-overview.**

REFERENCES

1. Aguilera P, Puig S, Guilabert A, et al. Prevalence study of nevi in children from Barcelona. Dermoscopy, constitutional and environmental factors. *Dermatology.* 2009;18(3):203-214.
2. Schafer T, Merkl J, Klemm E, et al. The epidemiology of nevi and signs of skin aging in the adult general population: results of the KORA-Survey 2000. *J Invest Dermatol.* 2006;126(7):1490-1496.
3. McCalmont T. *Melanocytic Nevi.* http://emedicine.medscape.com/article/1058445-overview#a0199. Accessed October 2011.
4. Zembowicz A, Phadke PA. Blue nevi and variants: an update. *Arch Pathol Lab Med.* 2011;135(3):327-336.

5. Gandini S, Sera F, Cattaruzza MS, et al. Meta-analysis of risk factors for cutaneous melanoma: I. Common and atypical nevi. *Eur J Cancer.* 2005;41(1):28-44.
6. Aalborg J, Morelli JG, Mokrohisky ST, et al. Tanning and increased nevus development in very-light-skinned children without red hair. *Arch Dermatol.* 2009;145(9):989-996.
7. Mahé E, Beauchet A, Aegerter P, Saiag P. Neonatal blue-light phototherapy does not increase nevus count in 9-year-old children. *Pediatrics.* 2009;123(5):e896-e900.
8. Harrison SL, Buettner PG, MacLennan R. Body-site distribution of MN in young Australian children. *Arch Dermatol.* 1999;135(1):47-52.
9. Zalaudek I, Docimo G, Argenziano G. Using dermoscopic criteria and patient-related factors for the management of pigmented melanocytic nevi. *Arch Dermatol.* 2009;145(7):816-826.
10. Lee TK, Rivers JK, Gallagher RP. Site-specific protective effect of broad-spectrum sunscreen on nevus development among white schoolchildren in a randomized trial. *J Am Acad Dermatol.* 2005;52(5):786-792.
11. Sommer LL, Barcia SM, Clarke LE, Helm KF. Persistent melanocytic nevi: a review and analysis of 205 cases. *J Cutan Pathol.* 2011;38(6):503-507.
12. Goodson AG, Florell SR, Boucher KM, Grossman D. Low rates of clinical recurrence after biopsy of benign to moderately dysplastic melanocytic nevi. *J Am Acad Dermatol.* 2010;62(4):591-596.

161 CONGENITAL NEVI

Mindy A. Smith, MD, MS
Richard P. Usatine, MD

PATIENT STORY

A 24-year-old woman presents with concerns about a mole on her breast (**Figure 161-1**). This mole has been present all of her life but her boyfriend wanted her to see her doctor about it. It had slowly increased in size throughout childhood but has not changed for years. Her primary care physician tells her that it is a congenital nevus that has no clinical features that suggest malignancy. No biopsy or excision is needed.

INTRODUCTION

Congenital melanocytic nevi are benign pigmented lesions that have a wide variation in presentation and are composed of melanocytes, the pigment-forming cells in the skin.

SYNONYMS

- It is also called as garment nevus, bathing trunk nevus, giant hairy nevus, giant pigmented nevus, pigmented hairy nevus, nevus pigmentosus, nevus pigmentosus et pilosus, and Tierfell nevus.[1]
- Tardive congenital nevus refers to a nevus with similar features to congenital nevi, but appears at age 1 to 2 years.

EPIDEMIOLOGY

- Congenital melanocytic nevi develop in 1% to 6% of newborns and are present at birth or develop during the first year of life.[1]

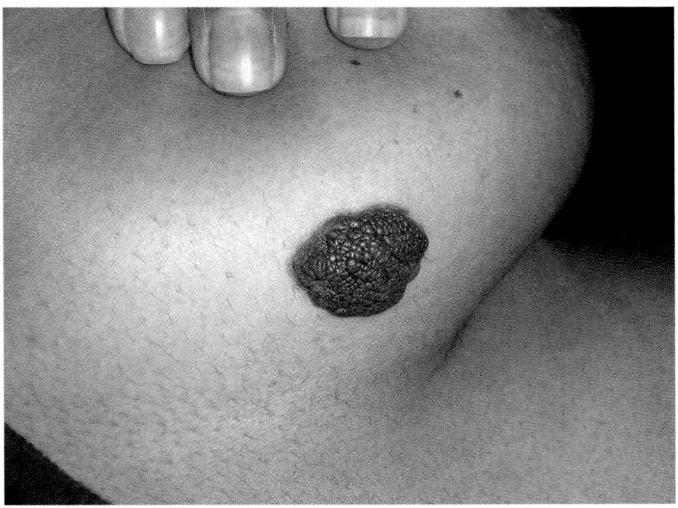

FIGURE 161-1 Congenital nevus on the breast of a 24-year-old woman. It is verrucous, but entirely benign. (*Reproduced with permission from Richard P. Usatine, MD.*)

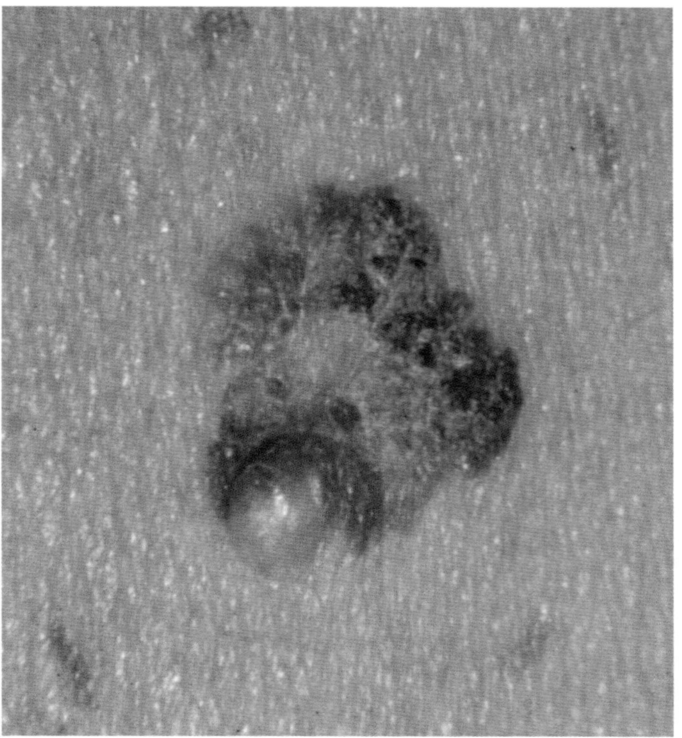

FIGURE 161-2 Melanoma arising in an acquired nevus showing features of central regression and a new elevated nodule. These are the same features that make a congenital nevus suspicious for melanoma. (*Reproduced with permission from the University of Texas Health Sciences Center, Division of Dermatology.*)

- In an Italian prevalence study of more than 3000 children ages 12 to 17 years, congenital melanocytic nevi or congenital nevus-like nevi were found in 17.5%; most (92%) were small (<1.5 cm).[2]
- Congenital nevi are also seen in neurocutaneous melanosis, a rare syndrome characterized by the presence of congenital melanocytic nevi and melanotic neoplasms of the central nervous system.
- The development of melanoma within congenital nevi (**Figure 161-2**) is believed to occur at a higher rate than in normal skin. Estimates range from 4% to 10%, with smaller lesions having lowest risk.[1]
    - In a systematic review, 46 of 651 patients with congenital melanocytic nevi (0.7%), who were followed for 3.4 to 23.7 years, developed melanomas, representing a 465-fold increased relative risk of developing melanoma during childhood and adolescence.[3] The mean age at diagnosis of melanoma was 15.5 years (median 7 years).
    - Patients with giant congenital melanocytic nevi appear to be at highest risk where subsequent melanoma has been reported in 5% to 7% by age 60 years.[4] In one study, 70% of patients with a large congenital melanocytic nevi diagnosed with melanoma were diagnosed within the first 10 years of life.[5]
    - In a prospective study of 230 medium-sized congenital nevi (1.5-19.9 cm) in 227 patients from 1955 to 1996, no melanomas occurred. The average follow-up period being 6.7 years to an average age of 25.5 years.[6]
    - Other risk factors for melanoma include personal or family history of melanoma or other skin cancer, presence of multiple nevi, red hair, blue eyes, freckling, and history of radiation (see Chapter 170, Melanoma).[1]

ETIOLOGY AND PATHOPHYSIOLOGY

- The etiology of congenital nevi is unknown.
- Congenital nevi result from a proliferation of benign melanocytes in the dermis, epidermis, or both. Melanocytes of the skin originate in the neuroectoderm and migrate vertically to the skin and other locations such as the central nervous system (CNS) and eye.[1] Defects in migration or maturation are hypothesized as causal.

DIAGNOSIS

Diagnosis is usually made based on clinical features and the history of the nevus being present at birth or develop during the first year of life.

CLINICAL FEATURES[1]

- Variable mixtures of color including pink-red (primarily at birth), tan, brown, black, or multiple shades are seen within a single lesion (**Figures 161-3** and **161-4**); color usually remains constant over time but the nevus will grow as the person grows. Congenital nevi that are speckled or spotted are called spilus nevi (**Figures 161-5** and **161-6**).
- Shapes are also highly variable, including oval, round, linear, and random; lesions have irregular but well-demarcated borders (**Figures 161-7** and **161-8**). The pigment may fade off into surrounding skin.
- Nevi may become raised over time (**Figures 161-8** and **161-9**) and the skin surface ranges from smooth to pebbly to hyperkeratotic (eczema-like appearance).
- Macular portion usually found at edges.
- Frequently exhibit hypertrichosis (**Figures 161-9** and **161-10**).
- Heavily pigmented large congenital melanocytic nevi over a limb may be associated with underdevelopment of the limb.[1]
- Lesions are classified by size in adulthood as the following[1]:
  - Small (<1.5 cm)
  - Medium (1.5-19 cm) (see **Figures 163-5** and **163-9**)
  - Large (>20 cm) (**Figures 161-10** and **161-11**)

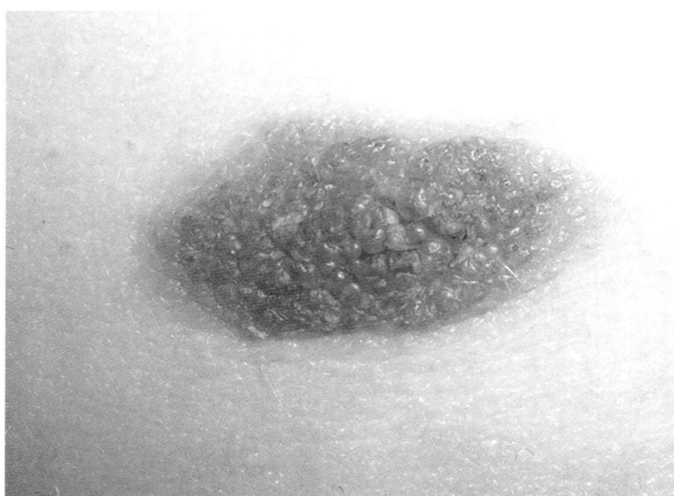

FIGURE 161-3 Pink congenital nevus on the chest of a fair-skinned woman. It is somewhat hyperkeratotic as may be seen in a seborrheic keratosis. *(Reproduced with permission from Richard P. Usatine, MD.)*

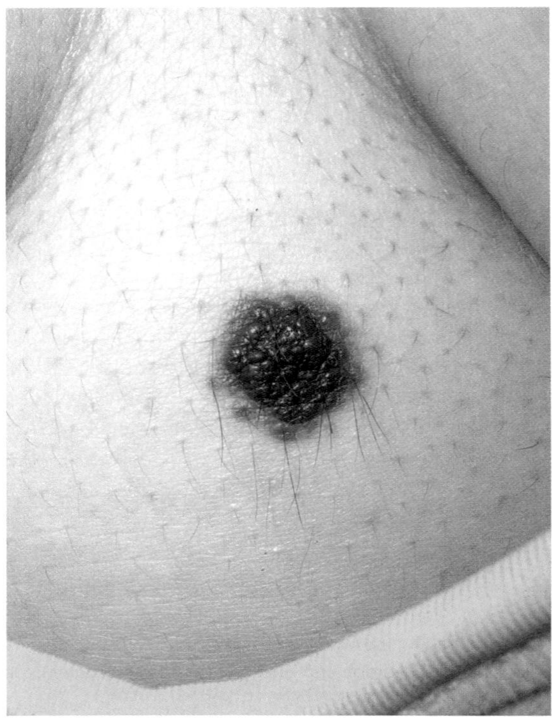

FIGURE 161-4 Darkly pigmented benign congenital nevus between the breasts of a Hispanic woman. Note the hypertrichosis and multiple colors. *(Reproduced with permission from Richard P. Usatine, MD.)*

Giant nevi are often surrounded by several smaller satellite nevi (see Figure 161-10).

IMAGING

- Dermoscopy findings depend on the age and location.[7] The majority of reticular lesions are located on the limbs and the variegated pattern was the most specific for congenital nevi.
- Magnetic resonance imaging (MRI) of the central nervous system can be a useful diagnostic tool in patients suspected of having neurocutaneous melanosis; one author recommended a screening MRI for patients with giant congenital melanocytic nevi.[8]

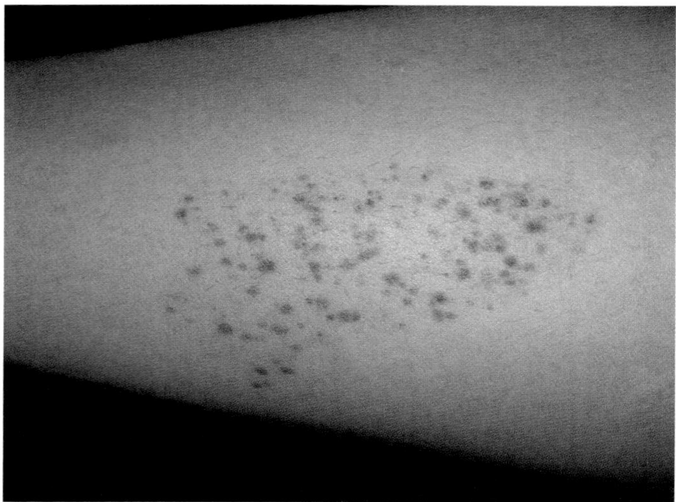

FIGURE 161-5 Congenital speckled nevus on the extensor surface of the arm. *(Reproduced with permission from Richard P. Usatine, MD.)*

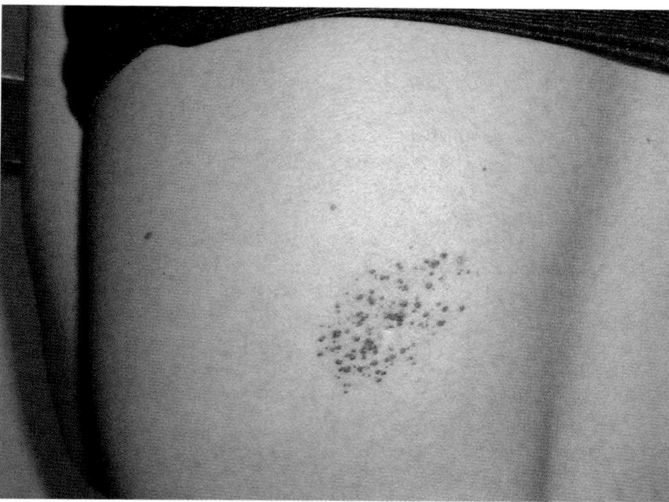

FIGURE 161-6 A speckled congenital nevus (nevus spilus) on the back of a young woman. There are areas in which the color is the same as the surrounding skin. (*Reproduced with permission from Richard P. Usatine, MD.*)

TYPICAL DISTRIBUTION

Congenital nevi can be found anywhere on the body.

BIOPSY

Although there are many histologic subtypes, distinguishing histologic features of congenital nevi include the following[1]:

- Involvement by nevus cells of deep dermal appendages and neurovascular structures (eg, hair follicles, sebaceous glands, arrector pili muscles, and within walls of blood vessels)
- Infiltration of nevus cells between collagen bundles

DIFFERENTIAL DIAGNOSIS

- Becker nevus—A brown macule, patch of hair, or both on the shoulder, back, or submammary area that develops in adolescence.

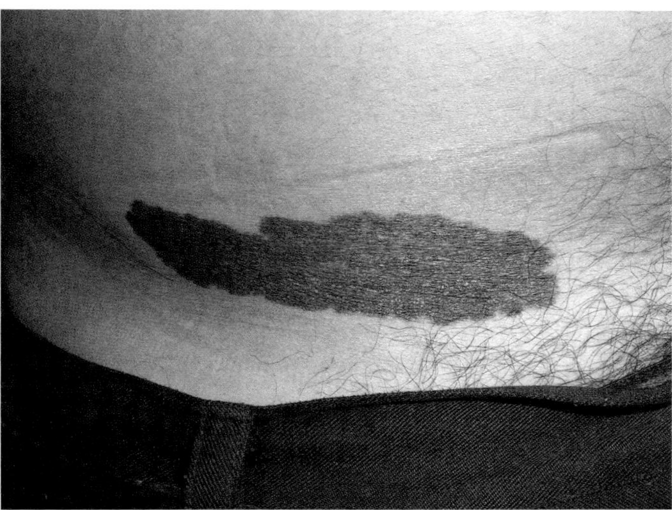

FIGURE 161-7 Medium-sized congenital nevus near the waistline with an irregular shape and border. While this man was concerned that it was growing there were no areas suspicious for melanoma. (*Reproduced with permission from Richard P. Usatine, MD.*)

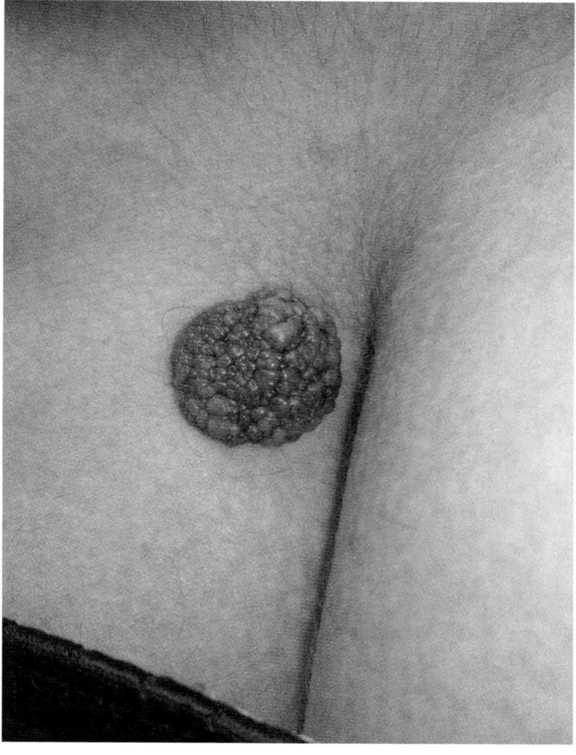

FIGURE 161-8 Congenital compound melanocytic nevus that was raised and verrucous. The patient requested removal and there were no signs of malignancy. (*Reproduced with permission from Richard P. Usatine, MD.*)

The border is irregular and the lesion may enlarge to cover an entire shoulder or upper arm. It is a type of hamartoma and is not a melanocytic nevus (see Chapter 160, Benign Nevi).

- Café-au-lait spots—Coffee-and-milk-colored patch that can be present at birth or develop during early childhood. Although a number of large café-au-lait spots are associated with neurofibromatosis, a few of them can occur in completely unaffected individuals. These light-brown patches have increased melanin but are not nevi (see Chapter 235, Neurofibromatosis).

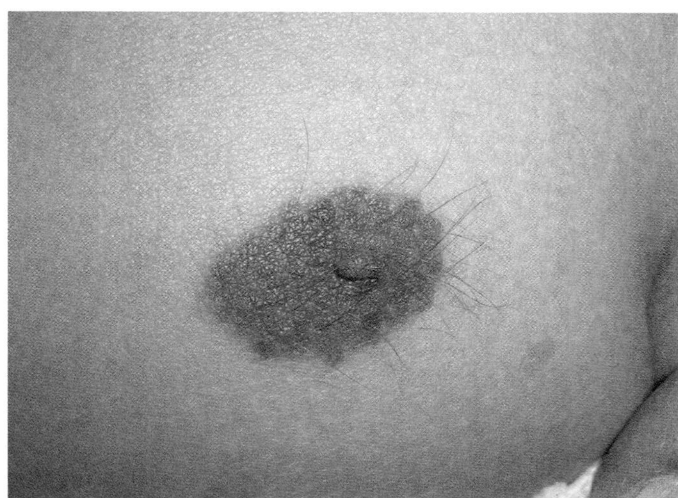

FIGURE 161-9 Congenital nevus with some hypertrichosis and a centrally raised area. This was a benign melanocytic nevus on the chest of a young woman. (*Reproduced with permission from Richard P. Usatine, MD.*)

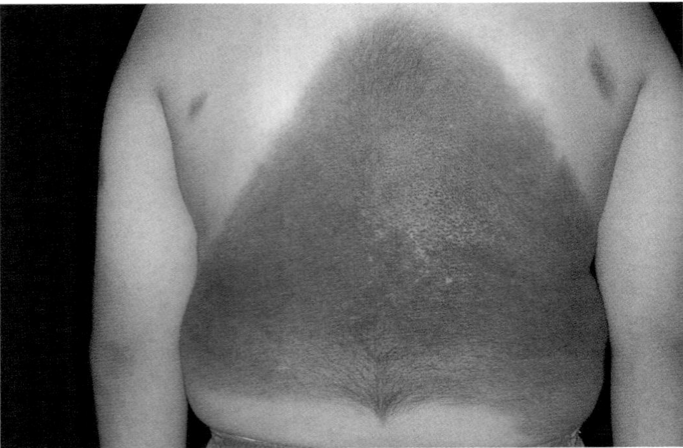

FIGURE 161-10 Large bathing trunk nevus on the back of a boy since birth. Note the hypertrichosis and the satellite lesions. (*Reproduced with permission from Richard P. Usatine, MD.*)

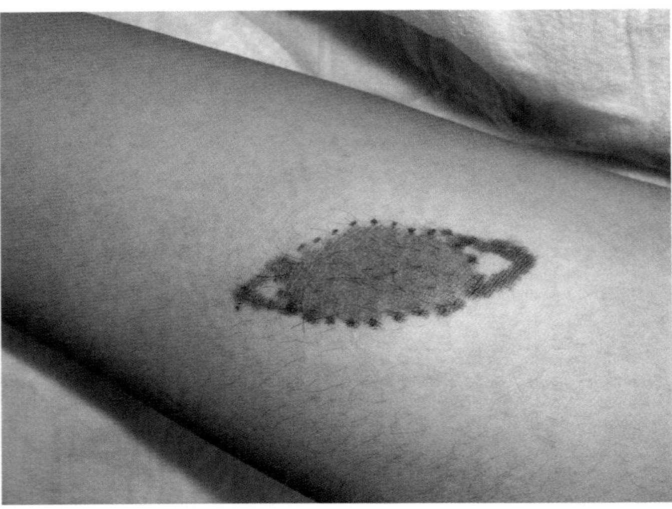

FIGURE 161-12 This congenital nevus was elliptically excised from the leg of a young woman at her request. The pathology showed a compound congenital melanocytic nevus. (*Reproduced with permission from Richard P. Usatine, MD.*)

MANAGEMENT

The management of congenital nevi depends on size and location of the lesion (difficulty in monitoring), associated symptoms, age of the patient, the effect on cosmesis, and the potential for malignant transformation.

- For small- and medium-sized congenital melanocytic nevi, the risk of malignant transformation is small and prophylactic removal is not recommended. For cosmesis, treatments include surgical excision (**Figure 161-12**) or laser treatment.
- Larger congenital nevi can be surgically removed but may require tissue expanders, tissue grafts, and tissue flaps to close large defects. Excisions can also be staged in multiple steps. Because the melanocytes may extend deep into underlying tissues (including muscle, bone, and central nervous system), removing the cutaneous component may not eliminate the risk of malignancy.
    - There is also concern that surgical intervention may adversely affect congenital melanocytic nevi cells.[9]
- Laser treatment of the lesions has been performed with a number of different types of lasers.[10] Because of the lack of penetrance to deeper tissue levels, long-term recurrence or malignant transformation is also an issue with these techniques.
- Careful lifelong follow-up with photographs is an acceptable approach, especially now with the affordability of digital cameras.
- Garment or bathing trunk nevi (see **Figure 161-4**)
    - Approximately half of the melanomas that develop in bathing trunk nevi do so before age 5 years.[11] These melanomas can be missed by observation because they can have nonepidermal origins.
    - Surgical excision is recommended by some experts to prevent melanoma.[11] SOR Ⓒ.
- Changes to watch for that call for a biopsy include the following:
    - Partial regression (depressed white areas) (see **Figure 161-2**)
    - Inflammation.
    - Rapid growth or color change.
    - Development of a firm nodule (see **Figure 161-2**).
    - A halo of hypopigmentation may form around any nevus including a congenital nevus (**Figure 161-13**). This in itself does not signify malignant transformation unless there are other suspicious features.

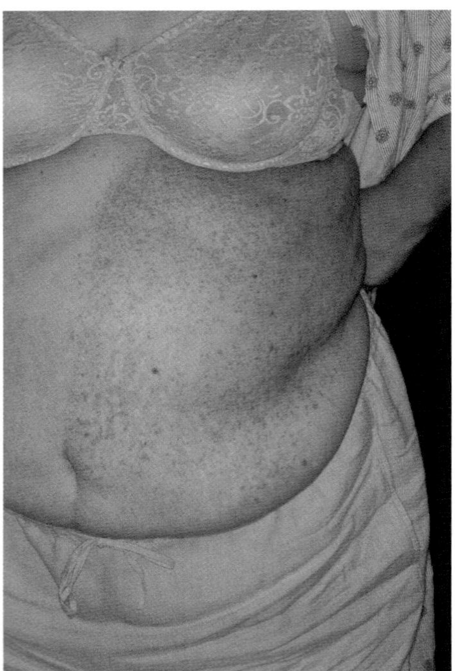

FIGURE 161-11 Large congenital speckled nevus that appears on one side of the trunk of this older woman. (*Reproduced with permission from Richard P. Usatine, MD.*)

PATIENT EDUCATION

- All patients should be told about the importance of protection from ultraviolet (UV) light exposure. This is especially important in people with giant congenital nevi, because they are at a significantly increased risk of melanoma.
- Patients should be taught to look for signs of melanoma (ABCDE) (asymmetry, border irregularity, color irregularity, diameter >6 mm, evolution).

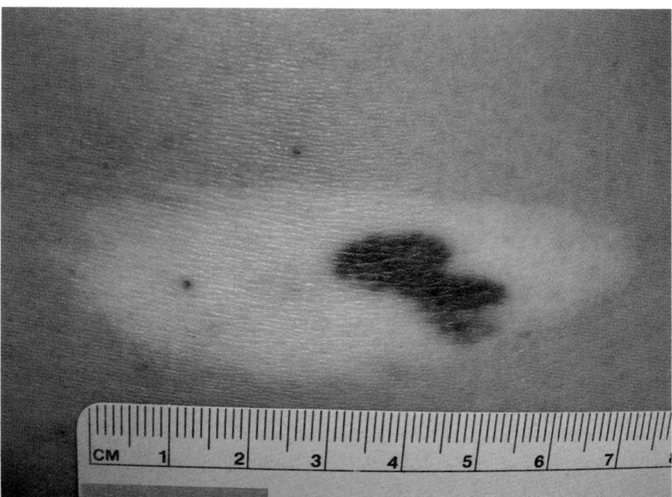

FIGURE 161-13 This medium-sized congenital melanocytic nevus on the trunk began to lose some of its color and developed a white halo surrounding the pigmented center. There were no suspicious areas for malignancy even though there was evolution of this melanocytic lesion. A biopsy Biopsy performed to reassure the patient, was benign. (*Reproduced with permission from Richard P. Usatine, MD.*)

FOLLOW-UP

- Patients with giant congenital nevi or multiple congenital nevi may benefit from consultation with a neurologist because of the risk of neurocutaneous melanosis and its neurologic manifestations or obstructive hydrocephalus.
- Bathing trunk nevi can also be associated with spina bifida, meningocele, and neurofibromatosis.[11]
- Because patients with all forms of congenital nevi, especially giant congenital melanocytic nevi, have an increased risk of developing melanoma, patients should consider baseline photography and regular follow-up with an experienced clinician for these patients.

PATIENT RESOURCES

- PubMed Health. *Birthmarks-Pigmented*—**http://www.ncbi.nlm.nih.gov/pubmedhealth/PMH0001831/.**
- Medline Plus. *Giant congenital nevi*—**http://www.nlm.nih.gov/medlineplus/ency/article/001453.htm.**
- Nevus support group—**http://www.nevus.org.**

PROVIDER RESOURCES

- Medscape. *Congenital Nevi*—**http://emedicine.medscape.com/article/1118659.**

REFERENCES

1. Lyon VB. Congenital melanocytic nevi. *Pediatr Clin North Am.* 2010;57:1155-1176.
2. Gallus S, Naldi L; Oncology Study Group of the Italian Group for Epidemiologic Research in Dermatology. Distribution of congenital melanocytic naevi and congenital naevus-like naevi in a survey of 3406 Italian schoolchildren. *Br J Dermatol.* 2008;159(2):433-438.
3. Krengel S, Hauschild A, Schafer T. Melanoma risk in congenital melanocytic naevi: a systematic review. *Br J Dermatol.* 2006;155(1):1-8.
4. Bett BJ. Large or multiple congenital melanocytic nevi: occurrence of cutaneous melanoma in 1008 persons. *J Am Acad Dermatol.* 2005;52(5):793-797.
5. Marghoob AA, Agero AL, Benvenuto-Andrade C, et al. Large congenital melanocytic nevi, risk of cutaneous melanoma, and prophylactic surgery. *J Am Acad Dermatol.* 2006;54(5):868-870.
6. Sahin S, Levin L, Kopf AW, et al. Risk of melanoma in medium-sized congenital melanocytic nevi: a follow-up study. *J Am Acad Dermatol.* 1998;39:428-433.
7. Seidenari S, Pellacani G, Martella A, et al. Instrument-, age- and site-dependent variations of dermoscopic patterns of congenital melanocytic naevi: a multicentre study. *Br J Dermatol.* 2006;155(1):56-61.
8. Arneia JS, Gosain AK. Giant congenital melanocytic nevi. *Plast Reconstr Surg.* 2009;124(suppl 1):e1-e13.
9. Kinsler V, Bulstrode N. The role of surgery in the management of congenital melanocytic naevi in children: a perspective from Great Ormond Street Hospital. *J Plast Reconstr Aesthet Surg.* 2009;62(5):595-601.
10. Ferguson RE Jr, Vasconez HC. Laser treatment of congenital nevi. *J Craniofac Surg.* 2005;16(5):908-914.
11. Habif T. *Clinical Dermatology: A Color Guide to Diagnosis and Therapy*. 4th ed. St. Louis, MO: Mosby; 2003.

162 EPIDERMAL NEVUS AND NEVUS SEBACEOUS

Mindy A. Smith, MD, MS
Richard P. Usatine, MD

PATIENT STORY

The young man is in the office for a college physical examination and asks about the brown bumps under his chin. He states that this has been there as long as he can remember but no one has given him a diagnosis. (**Figure 162-1**). The man reports no symptoms and is not worried about the appearance. He is otherwise healthy with no neurologic symptoms. You inform him that this is an epidermal nevus and there is no need to excise it at this time. He may choose to have this removed by a plastic surgeon in the future purely for cosmetic purposes.

INTRODUCTION

- Epidermal nevi (EN) are congenital hamartomas of ectodermal origin classified on the basis of their main component: sebaceous, apocrine, eccrine, follicular, or keratinocytic.
- Nevus sebaceous (NS) is a hamartoma of the epidermis, hair follicles, and sebaceous and apocrine glands. A hamartoma is the disordered overgrowth of benign tissue in its area of origin.

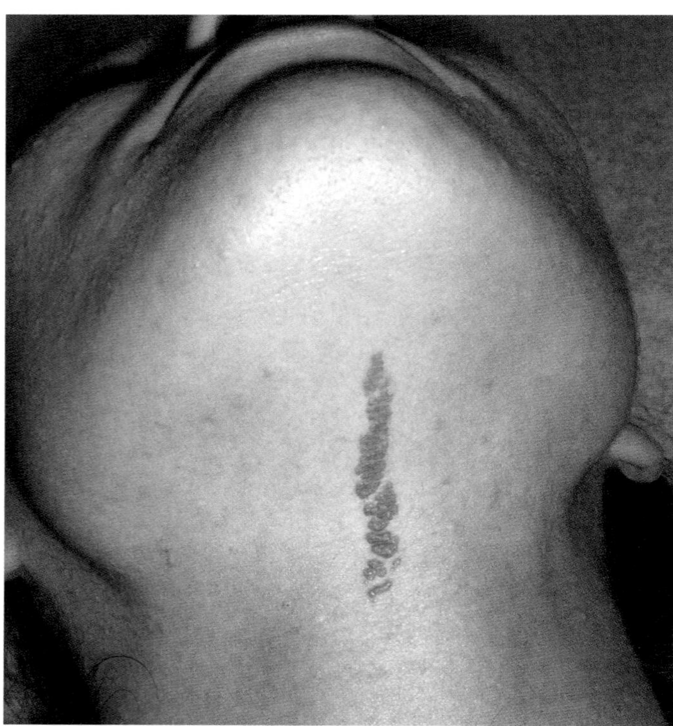

FIGURE 162-1 Linear epidermal nevus on the neck of a young man that appeared in early childhood. The patient had no neurologic, musculoskeletal, or vision problems. *(Reproduced with permission from Richard P. Usatine, MD.)*

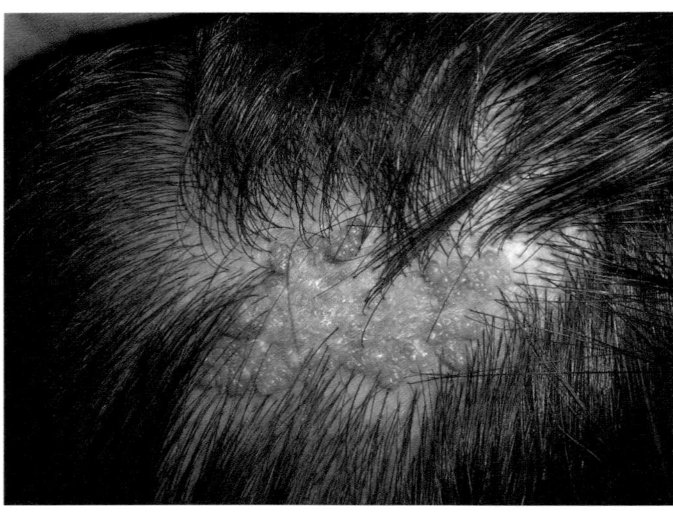

FIGURE 162-2 Nevus sebaceous on the scalp of a Hispanic woman. *(Reproduced with permission from Richard P. Usatine, MD.)*

SYNONYMS

- EN syndrome is also called Solomon syndrome and is a neurocutaneous disorder characterized by EN and an assortment of neurologic and visceral manifestations.
- NS is also called sebaceous nevus and nevus sebaceus of Jadassohn (**Figure 162-2**).
- An inflammatory linear verrucous epidermal nevus (ILVEN) (**Figure 162-3**) can be part of an epidermal nevus syndrome but some affected persons only have the cutaneous EN.

EPIDEMIOLOGY

- EN are uncommon (approximately 1%-3% of newborns and children), sporadic, and usually present at birth.
- EN are associated with disorders of the eye, nervous, and musculoskeletal systems in 10% to 30% of patients; in one study, 7.9% of patients

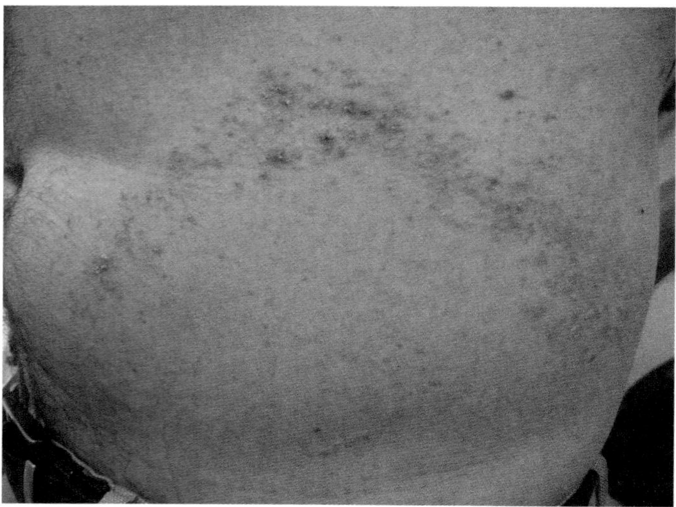

FIGURE 162-3 Inflammatory linear verrucous epidermal nevus (ILVEN) on the trunk of an adult man. Topical steroids were not helpful in diminishing his pruritus. *(Reproduced with permission from Robert T. Gilson, MD.)*

with EN had 1 of the 9 syndromes—an estimated 1 per 11,928 pediatric patients.[1]

- In another review of 131 cases of EN, most (60%) had noninflammatory EN, one-third had NS, and 6% had ILVEN.[2]
- NS is usually present at birth or noted in early childhood.[3] Most cases are sporadic but familial cases have been reported.[2]
- Linear NS is estimated to occur in 1 per 1000 live births.[4]
- Linear NS syndrome includes a range of abnormalities, including the central nervous system (CNS); patients with CNS involvement typically have cognitive impairment and seizures[3]; other organ systems, including the cardiovascular, skeletal, ophthalmologic, and urogenital systems, may be involved.

ETIOLOGY AND PATHOPHYSIOLOGY

- EN histologically display hyperkeratosis and papillomatosis, similar microscopically to seborrheic keratosis (see Chapter 156, Seborrheic Keratosis).[2] Also similar to seborrheic keratosis, some EN of keratinocyte differentiation (approximately one-third) have been found to have a mutation in the fibroblast growth factor receptor 3 (FGFR3) gene.
- Nine EN syndromes have been reported and are described in the referenced article.[5]
- EN frequently have a linear pattern that follows Blaschko lines (see **Figures 162-1** and **162-3**), which are believed to represent epidermal migration during embryogenesis.
- As in the case above, EN tend to become thicker, verrucous, and hyperpigmented at puberty.[2]
- Similarly, NS demonstrates stages of evolution paralleling the histologic differentiation of normal sebaceous gland. Lesions evolve from smooth to slightly papillated, waxy, hairless thickening in infants and young children to verrucous irregular lesions with a surface covered with numerous closely aggregated yellow-to-brown papules (**Figure 162-4**).[6]
    - Development of secondary appendageal tumors (**Figures 162-5** and **162-6**) occurs in 20% to 30% of patients, most are benign (most commonly basal cell epithelioma or trichoblastoma), but single (most commonly basal cell carcinoma) or multiple malignant tumors of both epidermal and adnexal origins may be seen and metastases have been reported.[2]
- NS was shown to have a high prevalence of human papillomavirus (HPV) DNA and authors postulate that HPV infection of fetal epidermal stem cells could play a role in the pathogenesis.[7]

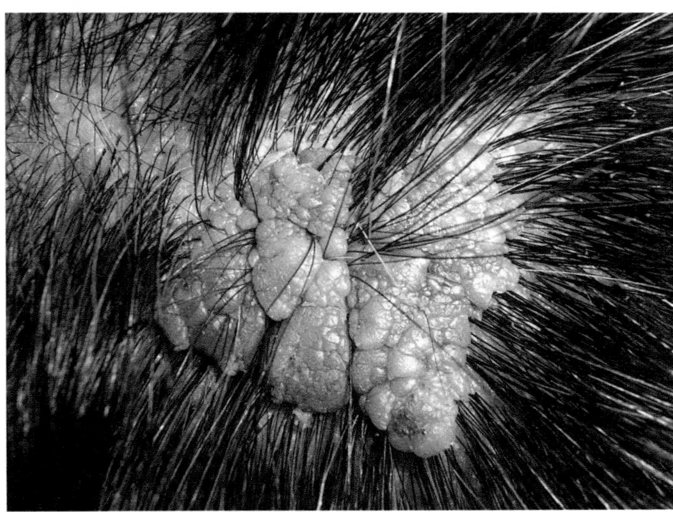

FIGURE 162-4 Nevus sebaceous on the scalp of a young woman that is verrucous and brown. *(Reproduced with permission from Richard P. Usatine, MD.)*

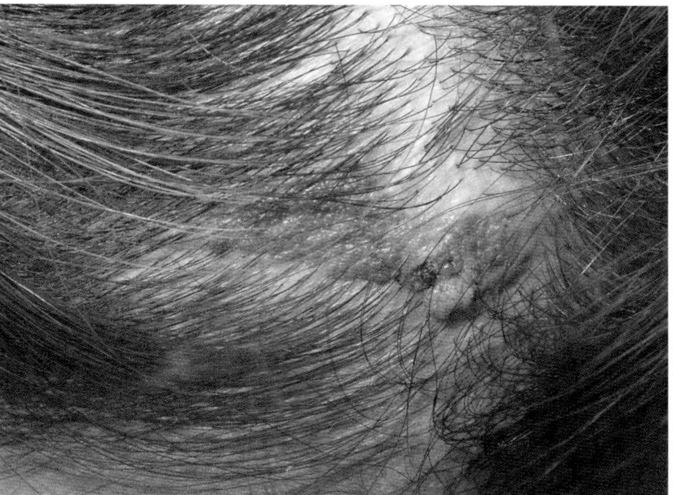

FIGURE 162-5 Nevus sebaceous on the scalp of a young woman. The patient reported a new area of elevation and bleeding. A biopsy showed no malignant transformation. *(Reproduced with permission from Richard P. Usatine, MD.)*

MAKING THE DIAGNOSIS

Clinical features of EN

- EN are linear, round, or oblong; well-circumscribed; elevated; and flat topped (see **Figure 162-1**).
- Color is yellow-tan to dark brown.
- Surface is uniform velvety or warty.
- ILVEN, a less common type of EN, is pruritic and erythematous (see **Figure 162-3**).

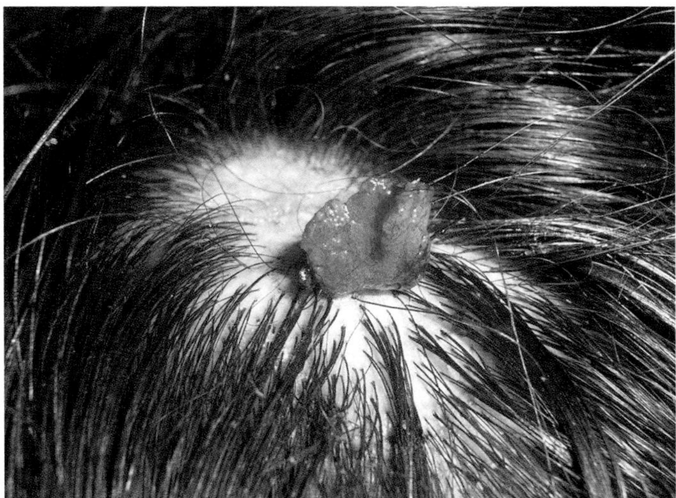

FIGURE 162-6 Nevus sebaceous with a benign tumor identified as a syringocystadenoma papilliferum by shave biopsy. Patient was referred for full removal of the nevus sebaceous. *(Reproduced with permission from Richard P. Usatine, MD.)*

Clinical features of NS

- NS has an oval-to-linear shape ranging from 0.5 × 1 to 7 × 9 cm.
- NS is usually a solitary, smooth, waxy, hairless thickening noted on the scalp at birth or in early childhood (see **Figures 162-2** and **162-4**).

TYPICAL DISTRIBUTION

- EN occur most commonly on the head and neck followed by the trunk and proximal extremities; only 13% have widespread lesions. Lesions may spread beyond their original distribution with age.
- NS are commonly found on the scalp followed by forehead and retroauricular region (see **Figures 162-2** and **162-6**) and rarely involves the neck, trunk, or other areas.

BIOPSY

Biopsy is the most definitive method for diagnosing these nevi. A biopsy is not needed if the clinical picture is clear and no operative intervention is planned. A shave biopsy should provide adequate tissue for diagnosis because the pathology is epidermal and in the upper dermis.

- Histologic features of epidermolytic hyperkeratosis within an EN are associated with mutations in the keratin gene that may be transmitted to offspring; widespread cutaneous involvement may be seen.[2]

DIFFERENTIAL DIAGNOSIS

- Linear lichen planus (**Figure 162-7**)—Discrete, pruritic, violaceous papules are arranged in a linear fashion, usually extending along an entire limb (see Chapter 152, Lichen Planus).
- Syringoma (**Figure 162-8**)—Benign adnexal tumor derived from sweat gland ducts. Autosomal dominant transmission, soft, small, skin-colored to brown papules develop during childhood and adolescence, especially around the eyes, but may be found on the face, neck, and trunk.
- Lichen striatus—Discrete pink, tan, or skin-colored asymptomatic papules in a linear band that appear suddenly (**Figure 162-9**). The papules may be smooth, scaly, or flat topped. It is mostly seen in children but does occur in adults. While it is most often seen on an extremity, it can appear on the trunk. It can resemble a linear EN but lichen striatus will usually regress within 1 year.

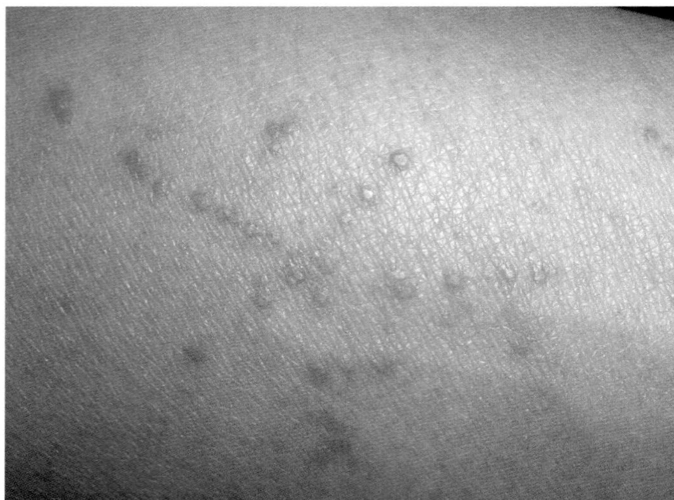

FIGURE 162-7 Lichen planus on the flexor aspect of the forearm in a linear pattern resembling a linear epidermal nevus. (*Reproduced with permission from Richard P. Usatine, MD.*)

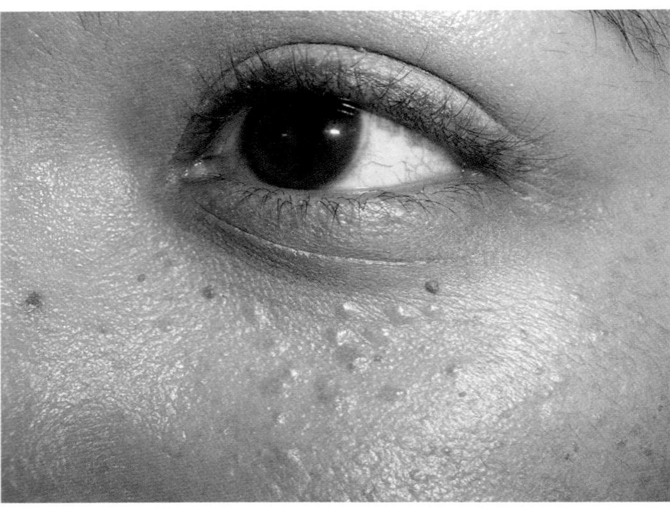

FIGURE 162-8 Syringoma on the lower eyelid. (*Reproduced with permission from Richard P. Usatine, MD.*)

MANAGEMENT

MEDICATIONS

There are no proven topical methods for treatment of these lesions. Topical retinoids may improve lesion appearance but recurrence is common.[2]

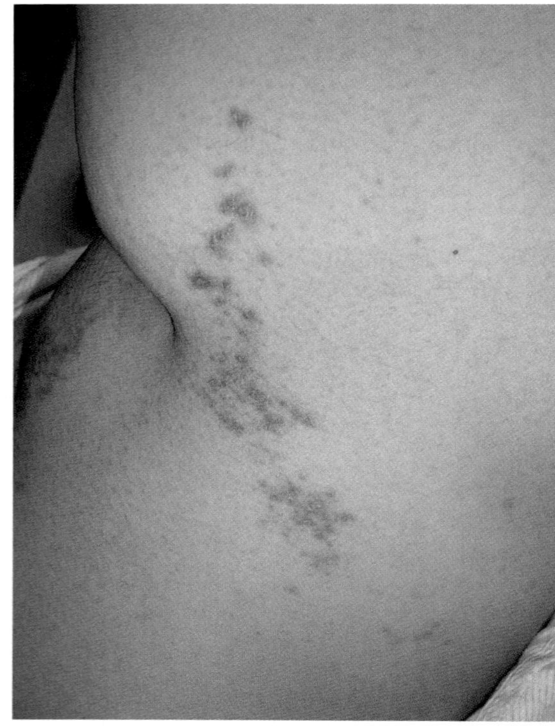

FIGURE 162-9 Lichen striatus near the axilla of a middle-aged woman. This resembles a linear epidermal nevus and the biopsy proved it to be lichen striatus in an adult. (*Reproduced with permission from Richard P. Usatine, MD.*)

PROCEDURES

- Destructive modalities for EN, such as electrodessication and cryotherapy, may temporarily improve the appearance of the lesion, but recurrence is frequent.[2]
- Carbon dioxide laser is an alternative option for EN; however, scarring and pigment changes are potential permanent complications, especially in patients with darker skin types.[8] This treatment does not completely remove NS and there is recurrence risk.[2]
- Surgical excision is an option that may be complicated by scarring.
- Because of the potential for malignant transformation particularly following puberty, some authors recommend early complete plastic surgical excision for NS; SOR Ⓒ reconstructive surgery may be needed.
- Excision of large lesions may require reconstructive surgery with a rotation flap to close.[9]

PROGNOSIS

- There are reports of spontaneous improvement in patients with widespread involvement of EN.
- Malignant potential is low in EN.[2]
- Malignant potential in NS is uncertain. Reports range from 0% to 2.7%.[2]
    - Early reports suggested a high rate of developing basal cell carcinomas, whereas more recent studies identified trichoblastoma and syringocystadenoma papilliferum in NS, usually in adulthood.[2]
    - Squamous cell carcinoma has also been described in NS.[10]

FOLLOW-UP

Patients with NS should be examined for other associated findings. Consider a consultation with a neurologist and/or ophthalmologist.

- In a study of 196 subjects with NS examined for clinical neurologic abnormalities, only 7% had abnormalities.[11] Abnormal examinations were more frequent in individuals with extensive nevi (21% vs 5%) and a centrofacial location (21% vs 2%). The patients depicted in this chapter had no neurologic abnormalities.

PATIENT RESOURCES

- Nevus Outreach. *Other Kinds of Nevi*—**http://www.nevus.org/other-kinds-of-nevi_id559.html.**
- Genetics Home Reference. *Epidermal Nevus*—**http://ghr.nlm.nih.gov/condition/epidermal-nevus.**

PROVIDER RESOURCES

- Medscape. *Nevus Sebaceous*—**http://emedicine.medscape.com/article/1058733-overview.**
- Medscape. *Epidermal Nevus Syndrome*—**http://emedicine.medscape.com/article/1117506-overview.**

REFERENCES

1. Vidaurri-de la Cruz H, Tamayo-Sanchez L, Duran-McKinster C, et al. Epidermal nevus syndromes: clinical findings in 35 patients. *Pediatr Dermatol.* 2004;21(4):432-439.
2. Rogers M, McCrossin I, Commens C. Epidermal nevi and the epidermal nevus syndrome. A review of 131 cases. *J Am Acad Dermatol.* 1989;20(3):476-488.
3. Brandling-Bennett HA, Morel KD. Epidermal nevi. *Pediatr Clin North Am.* 2010;57:1177-1198.
4. Menascu S, Donner EJ. Linear nevus sebaceous syndrome: case reports and review of the literature. *Pediatr Neurol.* 2008;38(3):207-210.
5. Happle R. The group of epidermal nevous syndromes. Part I. Well-defined phenotypes. *J Am Acad Dermatol.* 2010;63:1-22.
6. Hammadi AA. *Nevus Sebaceous.* Last updated June 9, 2010. http://emedicine.medscape.com/article/1058733-overview. Accessed August 2013.
7. Carlson JA, Cribier B, Nuovo G, et al. Epidermodysplasia verruciformis-associated and genital-mucosal high-risk human papillomavirus DNA are prevalent in nevus sebaceus of Jadassohn. *J Am Acad Dermatol.* 2008;59(2):279-294.
8. Boyce S, Alster TS. CO_2 laser treatment of epidermal nevi: long-term success. *Dermatol Surg.* 2002;28(7):611-614.
9. Davison SP, Khachemoune A, Yu D, Kauffman LC. Nevus sebaceus of Jadassohn revisited with reconstruction options. *Int J Dermatol.* 2005;44(2):145-150.
10. Aguayo R, Pallarés J, Casanova JM, et al. Squamous cell carcinoma developing in Jadassohn's sebaceous nevus: case report and review of the literature. *Dermatol Surg.* 2010;36(11):1763-1768.
11. Davies D, Rogers M. Review of neurological manifestations in 196 patients with sebaceous naevi. *Australas J Dermatol.* 2002;43(1):20-23.

163 DYSPLASTIC NEVUS

Mindy A. Smith, MD, MS
Richard P. Usatine, MD

PATIENT STORY

A 44-year-old man presents with concern over a mole on his back that his wife says is growing larger and more variable in color. The edges are irregular and the color almost appears to be "leaking" into the surrounding skin. He reports no symptoms related to this lesion. On physical examination, the nevus is 9 mm in diameter with asymmetry and variations in color and an irregular border (**Figure 163-1**). A full-body skin examination did not demonstrate any other suspicious lesions. Dermoscopy showed an irregular network with multiple asymmetrically placed dots off the network (**Figure 163-2**). A scoop saucerization was performed with a DermaBlade taking 2-mm margins of clinically normal skin (**Figure 163-3**). Although this could have been an early thin melanoma, the pathology showed a completely excised compound dysplastic nevus with no signs of malignancy. No further treatment was needed except yearly skin examinations to monitor for melanoma.

INTRODUCTION

Dysplastic nevi (DN)/atypical moles are acquired melanocytic lesions of the skin whose clinical and histologic definitions are controversial and still evolving. These lesions have some small potential for malignant transformation and patients with multiple DN have an increased risk for melanoma.[1]

The presence of multiple DN is a marker for increased melanoma risk just as red hair is, and, analogously, cutting off the red hair or cutting out all the DN does not change that risk of melanoma. The problem with DN is that any one lesion that is suspicious for melanoma must be biopsied to avoid missing melanoma, not to prevent melanoma from occurring in that nevus in the future.

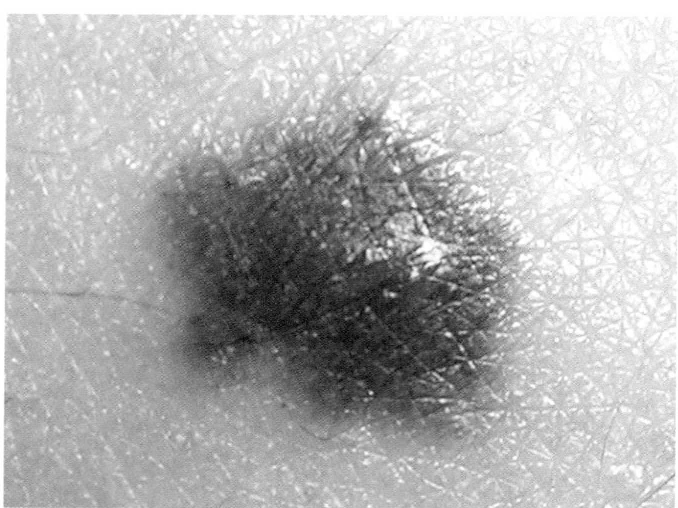

FIGURE 163-1 Growing 9-mm compound dysplastic nevus on the back of a 44-year-old man. There is asymmetry and variations in color and an irregular border. (*Reproduced with permission from Richard P. Usatine, MD.*)

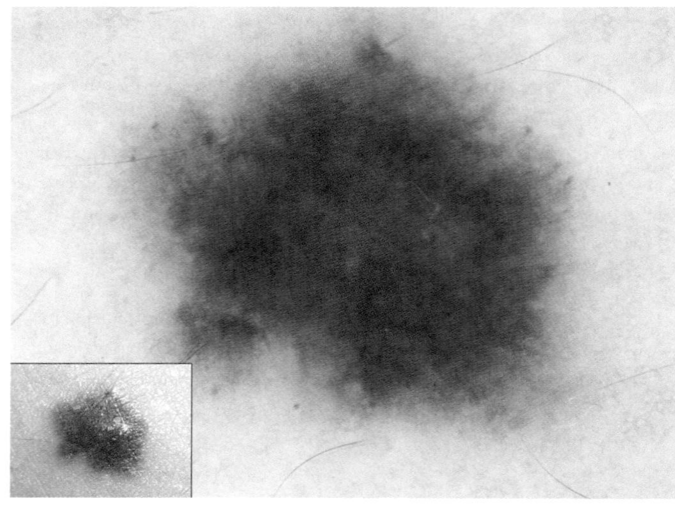

FIGURE 163-2 Dermoscopy of this compound dysplastic nevus shows an irregular network with multiple asymmetrically placed dots off the network. (*Reproduced with permission from Richard P. Usatine, MD.*)

SYNONYMS

Dysplastic nevus is also called as atypical nevus, atypical mole, Clark nevus, nevus with architectural disorder, and melanocytic atypia.[1]

EPIDEMIOLOGY

- Two percent to 9% of the population has atypical moles (AMs).[2,3] In a Swedish case control study, 56% of cases (121 patients with melanoma) and 19% of 310 control subjects had nevi fulfilling the clinical criteria for DN.[4] Among patients with melanoma, the rate of DN ranges from 34% to 59%.[3]
- Individuals with fair skin types are at higher risk of DN.[3]
- The sudden eruption of benign and atypical melanocytic nevi has been reported and is associated with blistering skin conditions and a number

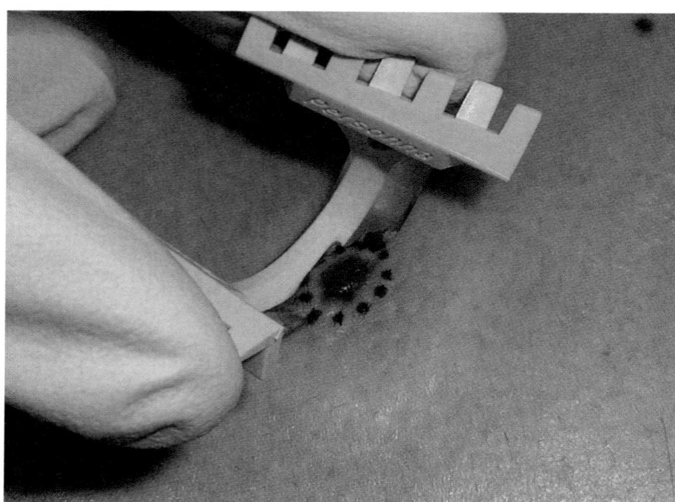

FIGURE 163-3 A scoop saucerization was performed with a DermaBlade taking 2-mm margins of clinically normal skin. Although this could have been an early thin melanoma, the pathology showed a completely excised compound dysplastic nevus with no signs of malignancy. (*Reproduced with permission from Richard P. Usatine, MD.*)

of disease states, including immunosuppression. Subsets of patients with immunosuppression have increased numbers of nevi on the palms and soles.[5]

- The National Institute of Health Consensus Conference on the diagnosis and treatment of early melanoma defined a syndrome of familial atypical mole and melanoma (FAMM). The criteria of FAMM syndrome are as below[6]:
  - The occurrence of malignant melanoma in one or more first- or second-degree relatives.
  - The presence of numerous (often >50) melanocytic nevi, some of which are clinically atypical.
  - Many of the associated nevi show certain histologic features (see later under Biopsy).

ETIOLOGY AND PATHOPHYSIOLOGY

- Most DN are compound nevi (see **Figure 163-1**) possessing a junctional and intradermal component (see Chapter 160, Benign Nevi).[1] The junctional component is highly cellular and consists of an irregular distribution of melanocytes arranged in nests and lentiginous patterns along the dermal-epidermal junction. The dermal component, located at the center, consists of nests and strands of melanocytes with distinct sclerotic changes.[1]
- DN exhibit a host response consisting of irregular rete ridge elongation, subepidermal sclerosis, proliferation of dermal capillaries, and a perivascular, lymphohistiocytic inflammatory infiltrate.[1]
- Individuals with DN may have deficient DNA repair, and DN lesions are associated with overexpression of pheomelanin (pigment produced by melanocytes), which may lead to increased oxidative DNA damage and tumor progression.[7]

DIAGNOSIS

CLINICAL FEATURES

- Variable mixtures of color including tan, brown, black, and red within a single lesion (**Figures 163-4** and **163-5**).

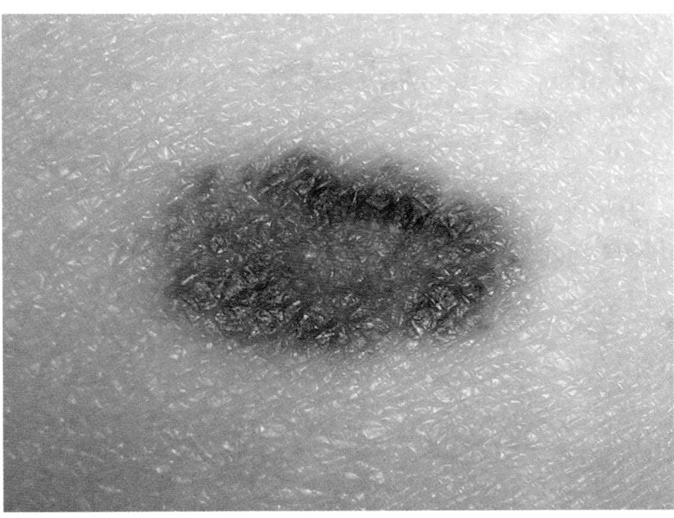

FIGURE 163-4 Dysplastic nevus in a woman with malignant melanoma in a different region of her body. The size was greater than 6 mm and there was variation in color. This was fully excised to make sure there was no melanoma present. (*Reproduced with permission from Richard P. Usatine, MD.*)

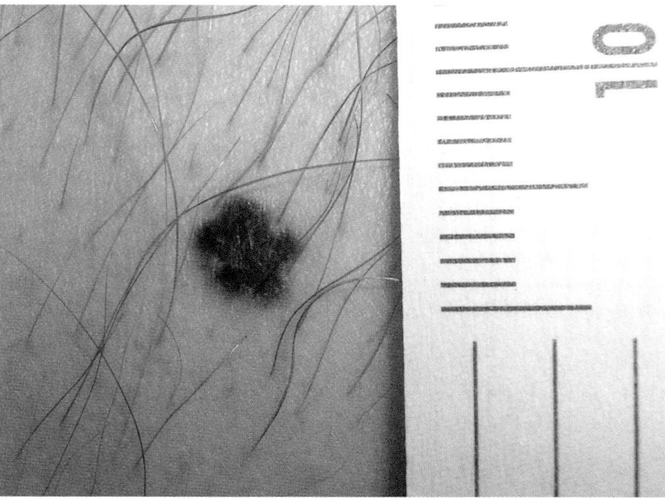

FIGURE 163-5 Dysplastic nevus on the chest of a 30-year-old man. A shave biopsy successfully removed the whole lesion and confirmed that it was not melanoma. Although it was less than 6 mm, it had irregular borders and variation of color. (*Reproduced with permission from Richard P. Usatine, MD.*)

- Irregular, notched borders; pigment may fade off into surrounding skin (see **Figure 163-5**).
- Flat or slightly raised (**Figures 163-4** to **163-6**) with the macular portion at edge, not verrucous or pendulous.
- Lesions frequently surrounded by a reddish hue from reactive hyperemia making them appear target-like.
- Usually larger than 6 mm; may be larger than 10 mm (see **Figures 163-1** and **163-4**).
- Patients with FAMM syndrome may have more than 100 lesions, far greater than the average number of common moles (<50) in most individuals.

TYPICAL DISTRIBUTION

Usually on sun-exposed areas, especially the back (see **Figure 163-1**); may be found on sites where nevi are usually absent or rare such as the

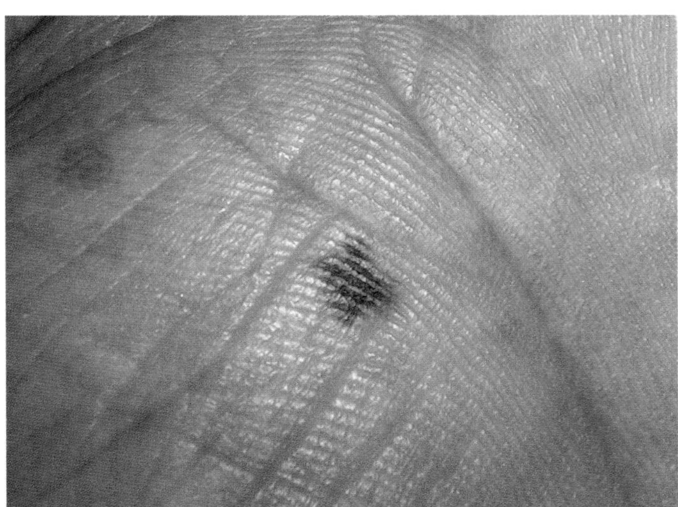

FIGURE 163-6 Junctional dysplastic nevus on the palm of a 43-year-old Hispanic man. Dermoscopically there was pigment on the top of the skin ridges making this suspicious for melanoma. Fortunately, the punch biopsy showed a dysplastic nevus only. (*Reproduced with permission from Richard P. Usatine, MD.*)

scalp, breasts, genital skin, buttocks, palm (see **Figure 163-6**), and dorsa of feet.

IMAGING

Although eccentric peripheral hyperpigmented and multifocal hyper- or hypopigmented types are more commonly seen in melanoma, no digital dermatoscopic criteria have been identified that can clearly distinguish DN from in situ melanomas.[8] However, dermoscopy increases diagnostic sensitivity and specificity of cutaneous melanoma from 60% to greater than 90%, especially using pattern recognition.[3]

BIOPSY

The importance of histology is to distinguish DN from melanoma. Although not universally accepted, the World Health Organization Melanoma Program proposed a list of characteristics/criteria with individual lesions requiring 2 major and 2 minor criteria to be classified as a DN.[3]

- Major criteria are basilar proliferation of atypical nevomelanocytes and organization of this proliferation in a lentiginous or epithelioid cell pattern.
- Minor criteria are (a) the presence of lamellar fibrosis or concentric eosinophilic fibrosis, (b) neovascularization, (c) inflammatory response, and (d) fusion of rete ridges. These established criteria yielded 92% mean concordance overall by panel members.

DIFFERENTIAL DIAGNOSIS

- Melanocytic nevi—Most common moles are tan to brown, smaller than 6 mm, round in shape, and with sharp borders (see Chapter 160, Benign Nevi).
- Melanoma—Skin cancer is often asymmetric, with irregular border and varied colors. It is usually larger than 6 mm in diameter (see Chapter 170, Melanoma).

MANAGEMENT

NONPHARMACOLOGIC

- Obtain a family history of DN and melanoma for patients presenting with DN.
- Because of the low risk of any one DN developing malignant transformation, the prophylactic removal of all DN is not recommended. SOR Ⓒ

MEDICATIONS

Of the medications tested, including topical 5-fluorouracil, systemic isotretinoin, topical tretinoin with or without hydrocortisone, and topical imiquimod, none completely destroy DN.[3]

PROCEDURES

- Removal of at least one lesion is reasonable to histologically confirm the diagnosis and rule out melanoma. This should be accomplished with excisional biopsy and histologic confirmation of DN versus melanoma. DN is usually removed with conservative surgical margins (about 2 mm) to provide adequate tissue for the pathologist.[3] SOR Ⓒ

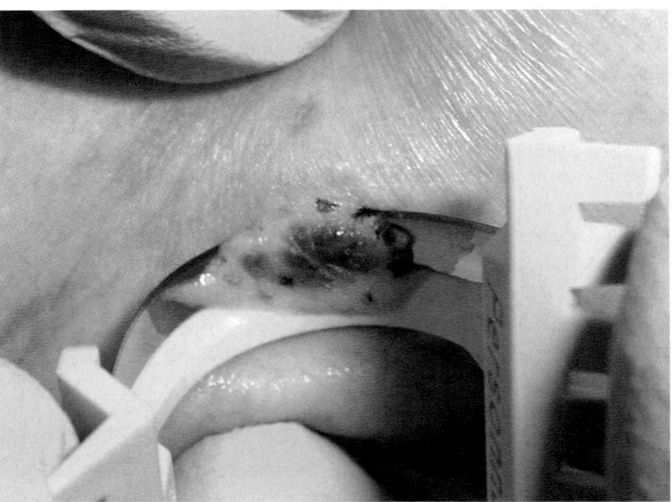

FIGURE 163-7 Scoop saucerization of a suspicious pigmented lesion that turned out to be a dysplastic junctional nevus with moderate atypia. The whole lesion was successfully excised with this deep shave. *(Reproduced with permission from Richard P. Usatine, MD.)*

- Scoop saucerizations (deep shave biopsy with a DermaBlade or razor blade) including at least a 2-mm margin of clinically normal skin surrounding the pigmented lesion is a rapid and acceptable method of excision for pathology (**Figure 163-7**).

PREVENTION

Avoid direct sunlight.

PROGNOSIS

- DNs appear to be dynamic throughout adulthood. In a study of the natural history of DN, investigators found that 51% of all evaluated nevi (297 of 593) showed clinical signs of change during an average follow-up of 89 months.[9] New nevi were common in adulthood, continuing to form in more than 20% of patients older than age 50 years, and some nevi disappeared.
- The risk of a melanoma arising within a DN is estimated at 1:3000 per year.[1] However, there is also an increased risk of melanoma arising elsewhere on the skin in patients with DN; the actual incidence rate is uncertain and ranges from 0.5% to 46%.[3] There is also a substantially increased risk of melanoma associated with the number of atypical nevi (relative risk [RR] = 6.36; 95% confidence interval [CI]: 3.80, 10.33; for 5 vs 0).[10]
- In one case control study, the estimated 10-year cumulative risk for developing melanoma in patients with AM syndrome was 10.7% (vs 0.62% in a control population).[11]

FOLLOW-UP

- Patents with DN should have regular skin examinations with biopsy performed of any suspicious lesions (see **Figure 163-7**).[3]
- Consider total-body photographs for monitoring (**Figures 163-8** and **163-9**).[3] In a study of 50 patients with 5 or more DN, the use of

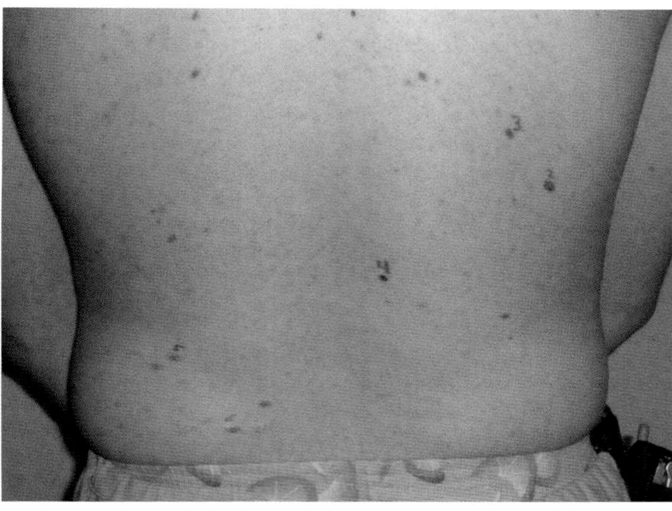

FIGURE 163-8 Multiple dysplastic nevi on the back of a young physician. Multiple biopsies have all been negative, so patient is being followed by serial digital photography with numbering of the dysplastic nevi. (*Reproduced with permission from Richard P. Usatine, MD.*)

baseline digital photographs improved the diagnostic accuracy of skin self-examination on the back, chest, and abdomen, and improved detection of changing and new moles.[12] Individual DN can be monitored more precisely with digital dermoscopic photos added to the skin photographs (see **Figure 163-9**).

- MelaFind, a lesion imaging device using multispectral imaging analysis, may be helpful in differentiating DN from melanoma.[13] It is a very expensive computerized device that is not affordable in a primary care office.

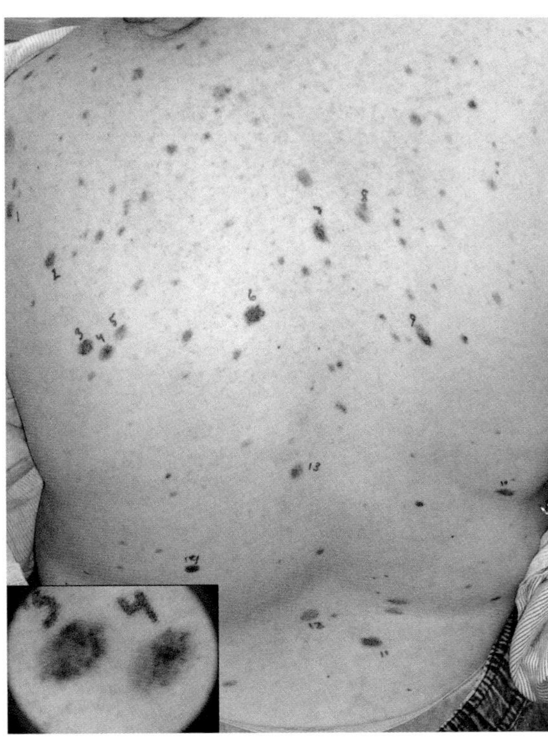

FIGURE 163-9 More than 14 dysplastic nevi are seen on the back of this 35-year-old woman with a history of 2 basal cell carcinomas on her back. She has never had a melanoma and has no family history of melanoma. Multiple biopsies so far have only shown dysplastic nevi, so she is being followed with serial digital photography of her nevi along with corresponding dermoscopic photographs. Note the dermoscopic images of nevi 3 and 4 in the bottom left corner. (*Reproduced with permission from Richard P. Usatine, MD.*)

- Patients with numerous DN and who have a family history of melanoma are at a higher risk of developing melanoma and should be encouraged to have regular follow-up with a provider skilled in detecting melanoma.
- Patients with FAMM should also consider a baseline ophthalmologic examination because of a possible association between uveal melanoma and FAMM syndrome.[3]
- First-degree relatives of patients diagnosed with FAMM syndrome should be encouraged to be examined for DN and melanoma.

PATIENT EDUCATION

- Patients with DN should avoid excessive exposure to natural or artificial ultraviolet (UV) light and routinely use a broad-spectrum sunscreen with a sun-protective factor of 30 or greater and/or sun-protective clothing.
- Patients should be taught self-examination to detect changes in existing moles and to recognize clinical features of melanomas. Patients should be taught to look for and report asymmetry, border irregularity, new symptoms (eg, pain, pruritus, bleeding, or ulceration), and color and size changes.

PATIENT RESOURCES

- MedlinPlus. *Moles*—**http://www.nlm.nih.gov/medlineplus/moles.html.**
- National Cancer Institute. *Common Moles, Dysplastic Nevi, and Risk of Melanoma*—**http://www.cancer.gov/cancertopics/wyntk/moles-and-dysplastic-nevi.**
- The National Center for Biotechnology Information. *Familial Atypical Multiple Mole Melanoma Syndrome*—**http://www.ncbi.nlm.nih.gov/books/NBK7030/.**

PROVIDER RESOURCES

- DermAtlas—**http://www.dermatlas.com.**
- Medscape. *Atypical Mole (Dysplastic Nevus)*—**http://emedicine.medscape.com/article/1056283-overview.**

REFERENCES

1. Clarke LE. Dysplastic nevus. *Clin Lab Med*. 2011;31:255-265.
2. Mooi WJ. The dysplastic naevus. *J Clin Pathol*. 1997;50:711-715.
3. Friedman RJ, Farber MJ, Warycha MA, et al. The "dysplastic" nevus. *Clin Dermatol*. 2009;27:103-115.
4. Stierner U, Augustsson A, Rosdahl I, Suurküla M. Regional distribution of common and dysplastic naevi in relation to melanoma site and sun exposure. A case-control study. *Melanoma Res*. 1992;1(5-6):367-375.
5. Woodhouse J, Maytin EV. Eruptive nevi of the palms and soles. *J Am Acad Dermatol*. 2005;52(5 suppl 1):S96-S100.
6. Friedman RJ, Farber MJ, Warycha MA, et al. The "dysplastic" nevus. *Clin Dermatol*. 2009;27:103-115.
7. Elder DE. Dysplastic naevi: an update. *Histopathology*. 2010;56(1):112-120.

8. Burroni M, Sbano P, Cevenini G, et al. Dysplastic naevus vs. in situ melanoma: digital dermoscopy analysis. *Br J Dermatol*. 2005;152(4):679-684.
9. Trock B, Synnestvedt M, Humphreys T. Natural history of dysplastic nevi. *J Am Acad Dermatol*. 1993;29(1):51-57.
10. Gandini S, Sera F, Cattaruzza MS, et al. Meta-analysis of risk factors for cutaneous melanoma: I. Common and atypical naevi. *Eur J Cancer*. 2005;41(1):28-44.
11. Marghoob AA, Kopf AW, Rigel DS, et al. Risk of cutaneous malignant melanoma in patients with "classic" atypical-mole syndrome. A case-control study. *Arch Dermatol*. 1994;130:993-998.
12. Oliveria SA, Chau D, Christos PJ, et al. Diagnostic accuracy of patients in performing skin self-examination and the impact of photography. *Arch Dermatol*. 2004;140(1):57-62.
13. Friedman RJ, Gutkowicz-Krusin D, Farber MJ, et al. The diagnostic performance of expert dermoscopists vs a computer-vision system on small-diameter melanomas. *Arch Dermatol*. 2008;144:476-482.

SECTION 10 PRECANCER/EARLY CANCER

164 ACTINIC KERATOSIS AND BOWEN DISEASE

Richard P. Usatine, MD
Yu Wah, MD

PATIENT STORY

A 57-year-old woman presented with red and scaling skin on both arms (**Figure 164-1**) with a request for a prescription for 5-fluorouracil (5-FU). The patient had blue eyes and white hair and was found to have 2 basal cell carcinomas (BCCs) on her face and shoulder. The patient stated that 5-FU had helped her arms in the past, but that the scaly lesions had returned. She avoids sun exposure now, but acknowledges receiving too much sun exposure while growing up. Another course of 5-FU was prescribed for her arms to prevent new skin cancers from forming.

INTRODUCTION

Actinic keratoses (AKs) are precursors on the continuum of carcinogenesis toward squamous cell carcinomas (SCCs). However, each AK has a low risk of progression to malignancy and a high probability of spontaneous regression.[1] Bowen disease (BD) is SCC in situ confined to the epidermis.

SYNONYMS

AK is also known as solar keratosis. AK on the lips is known as actinic cheilitis (**Figure 164-2**). BD is also known as SCC in situ of the skin. SCC in situ involving the penis is known as erythroplasia of Queyrat (**Figure 164-3**).

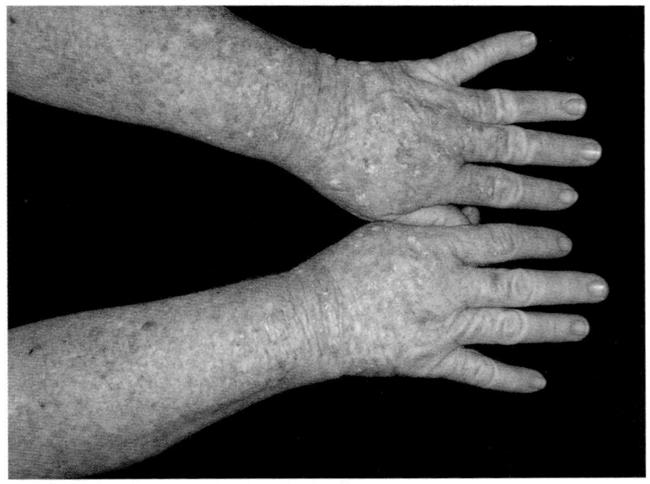

FIGURE 164-1 Actinic keratoses covering both arms and the dorsum of both hands in a fair-skinned woman who had significant sun exposure. Note that her left arm and hand are worse from driving a car and receiving more sun on the left arm. (*Reproduced with permission from Richard P. Usatine, MD.*)

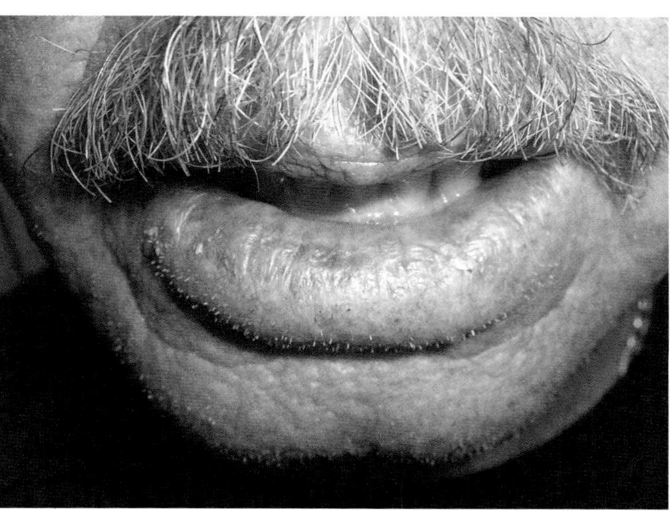

FIGURE 164-2 Actinic cheilitis involving the lower lip of a gardener. Note the erythema and scale caused by the sun damage. (*Reproduced with permission from Richard P. Usatine, MD.*)

EPIDEMIOLOGY

- AKs and BD are seen frequently in light-skinned individuals who have had significant sun exposure.
- The prevalence of AK is estimated at 11% to 25% in adults older than age 40 years in the northern hemisphere, and increases with age.[1] AKs are so common that they account for more than 10% of visits to dermatologists.
- The prevalence of BD is unknown.[1]

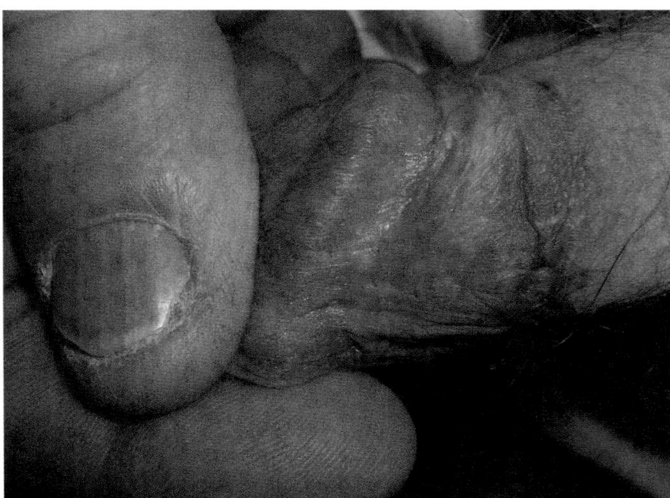

FIGURE 164-3 Bowen disease of the penis also known as erythroplasia of Queyrat. Human papillomavirus is a risk factor in this location. (*Reproduced with permission from Richard P. Usatine, MD.*)

ETIOLOGY AND PATHOPHYSIOLOGY

AKs and BD are both caused by cumulative ultraviolet (UV) exposure, most commonly from sunlight.

UV rays induce mutation of the tumor-suppressor gene *P53*. Subsequent proliferation of mutated atypical epidermal keratinocytes give rise to the clinical lesion of AK.[2] Multiple clinical and subclinical lesions may exist in an area of sun-damaged skin, a concept known as "field cancerization."

AKs have the potential to become SCCs. The rate of malignant transformation has been variably estimated, but is probably no greater than 6% per AK over a 10-year period.[3]

In a large prospective cohort study, the risk of progression of AK to primary SCC (invasive or in situ) was 0.60% at 1 year and 2.57% at 4 years. Approximately 65% of all primary SCCs and 36% of all primary BCCs diagnosed in the study arose in lesions that previously were diagnosed clinically as AKs. Many AKs did resolve spontaneously, 55% AKs that were followed clinically were not present at 1 year and the 70% were not present at the 5-year follow-up.[4]

On a spectrum of malignant transformation, BD is SCC in situ before the SCC becomes invasive.

RISK FACTORS

- Total lifetime dose of UV radiation (natural sunlight, UV from tanning beds and radiation).[1]
- Fair skin.[1]
- Site-specific risk factors include tobacco for actinic cheilitis and human papilloma virus for genital and anal lesions.[1]
- Exposure to immunosuppressive drugs, especially organ transplant recipients.
- Personal or family history of skin cancers.

DIAGNOSIS

CLINICAL FEATURES

AKs are rough scaly spots seen on sun-exposed areas (**Figure 164-1** to **164-6**). They may be found by touch, as well as close visual inspection of the patient's skin. BD appears similar to an AK, but tends to be larger in size and thicker with a well-demarcated border (**Figures 164-7** and **164-8**).

TYPICAL DISTRIBUTION

Both lesions are seen in areas with greatest sun exposure such as the face, forearms, dorsum of hands, lower legs of women, and the balding scalp (see **Figure 164-5**) and tops of the ears in men.

LABORATORY STUDIES

AKs that appear premalignant may be diagnosed by observation only and treated with destructive methods (eg, excision, electrosurgery, or cryosurgery) without biopsy. BD requires a biopsy for diagnosis. BD or SCC should be biopsied prior to treatment. A shave biopsy should produce enough tissue for histopathology.

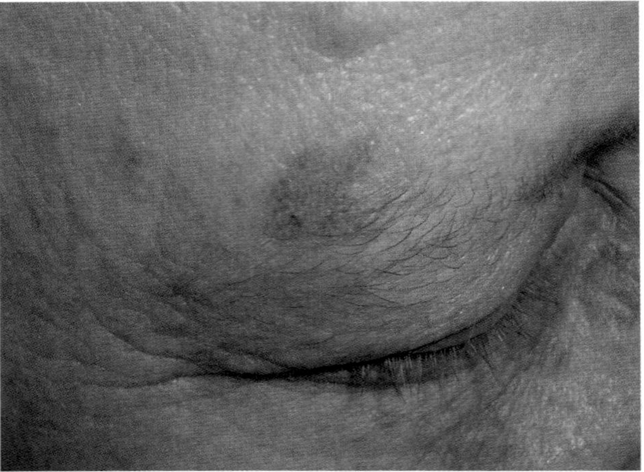

FIGURE 164-4 Large actinic keratoses over the eyebrow of an older adult. A biopsy was performed to make sure this was not already Bowen disease or squamous cell carcinoma. (*Reproduced with permission from Richard P. Usatine, MD.*)

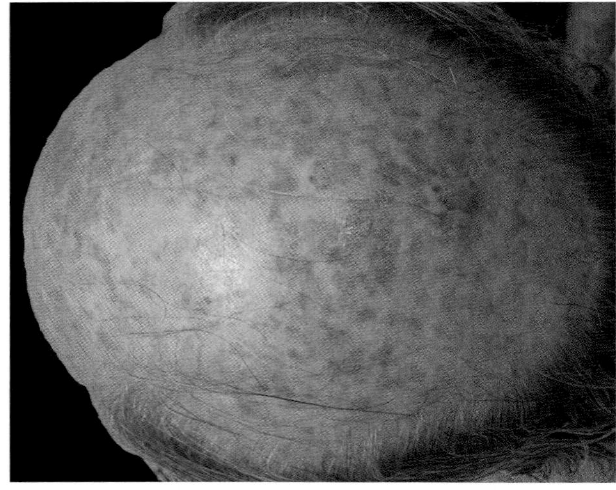

FIGURE 164-5 Actinic keratoses on the balding head of an older man. Hair loss results in less natural sun protection and is a risk factor for skin cancers on the scalp. The visible and palpable actinic keratoses were treated with cryotherapy. (*Reproduced with permission from Richard P. Usatine, MD.*)

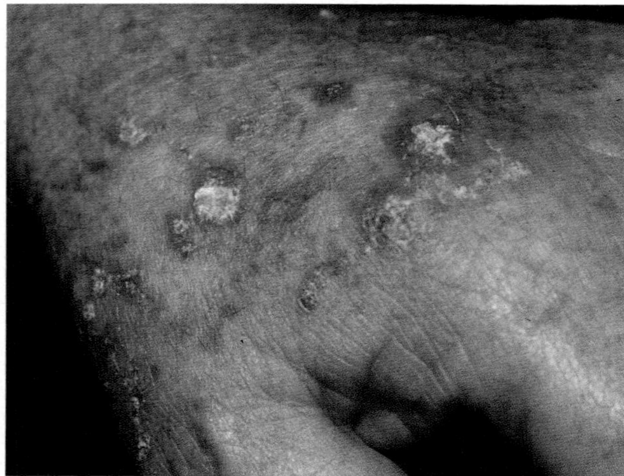

FIGURE 164-6 Actinic keratoses on the dorsum of the hand with some lesions suspicious for Bowen disease (squamous cell carcinoma in situ). (*Reproduced with permission from Usatine RP, Moy RL, Tobinick EL, Siegel DM.* Skin Surgery: A Practical Guide. *St. Louis, MO: Mosby; 1998.*)

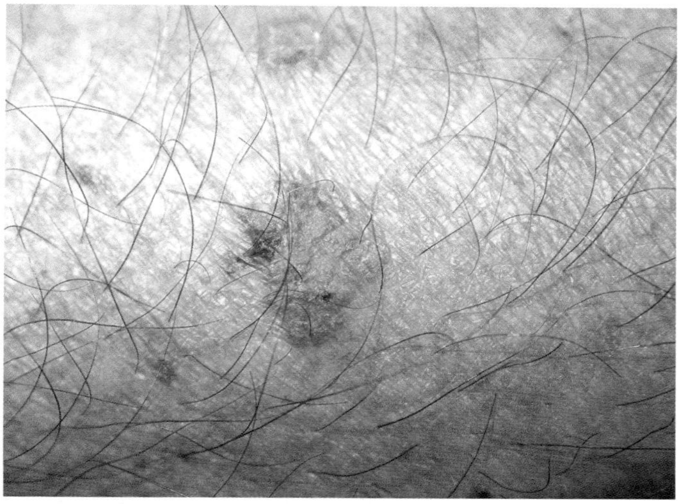

FIGURE 164-7 Lesions on the arm of an older man with Bowen disease in the central lesion and actinic keratosis on the upper lesion. (*Reproduced with permission from Richard P. Usatine, MD.*)

DIFFERENTIAL DIAGNOSIS

- Nummular eczema—A type of eczema in which the scaly patches are coin-shaped. The patches are often seen in patients who have already had some eczema or atopic conditions. The patches usually respond well to topical corticosteroids and are not related to sun damage (see Chapter 143, Atopic Dermatitis).
- Seborrheic keratoses—Occur in aging adults but do not have any malignant potential. Typical seborrheic keratoses are brown in color and have a stuck-on appearance. Seborrheic keratoses may look greasy or verrucous and have surface cracks. Their borders tend to be more well demarcated than AKs and their color is usually more brown than pink (see Chapter 156, Seborrheic Keratosis).
- Superficial BCCs—Can look like an AK or BD. Look for the pearly and thready border that may distinguish a superficial BCC from an AK or BD. Histopathology is the proven method to diagnose (see Chapter 168, Basal Cell Carcinoma).
- When in doubt, perform a shave biopsy to differentiate between an AK, BD, SCC, and superficial BCC.

MANAGEMENT

ACTINIC KERATOSES

- No therapy or the application of an emollient is a reasonable option for mild AKs.[5] SOR A
- Sunscreen applied twice daily for 7 months may protect against development of AKs.[2] SOR A
- AKs are most often treated by cryosurgery using liquid nitrogen (**Figure 164-9**). It is simple, rapid, and inexpensive, and may be used as first-line treatment.[1] SOR C One meta-analysis showed a 2-month cure rate of 97% with 2.1% recurrences in 1 year.[6]
- Treating AKs with liquid nitrogen using a 1-mm halo freeze demonstrated complete response of 39% for freeze times of less than 5 seconds, 69% for freeze times greater than 5 seconds, and 83% for freeze times greater than 20 seconds.[7] There is considerably more hypopigmentation caused by 20 seconds of freeze time. Determine the length of the freeze time based on the size and thickness of the lesion, using sufficient time for clearance while attempting to avoid hypopigmentation and scarring. SOR B
- Treat multiple AKs of the face, scalp, forearms, and hands topically with 5-FU, imiquimod, or diclofenac (**Table 164-1**).[1,5] SOR A
- Topical 5-FU is an efficient therapeutic method and may be used for treatment of isolated, as well as large, areas of AK. It may be applied by the patient, and is inexpensive compared with other topical modalities.[1] SOR A
- 5-FU cream used twice daily for 3 to 6 weeks is effective for up to 12 months in clearance of the majority of AKs (**Figure 164-10**).[5] SOR A Because of side effects of soreness, less-aggressive regimens are often used, which may be effective, but have not been fully evaluated.[5]
- Diclofenac gel applied twice daily for 10 to 12 weeks has moderate efficacy with low morbidity in mild AKs.[2] SOR B There are few follow-up data to indicate the duration of benefit.[2] In one study,

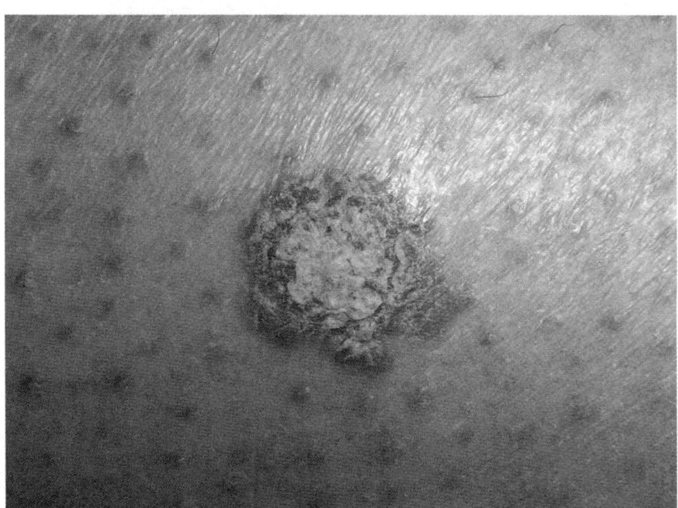

FIGURE 164-8 Bowen disease on the leg of an older woman. (*Reproduced with permission from Richard P. Usatine, MD.*)

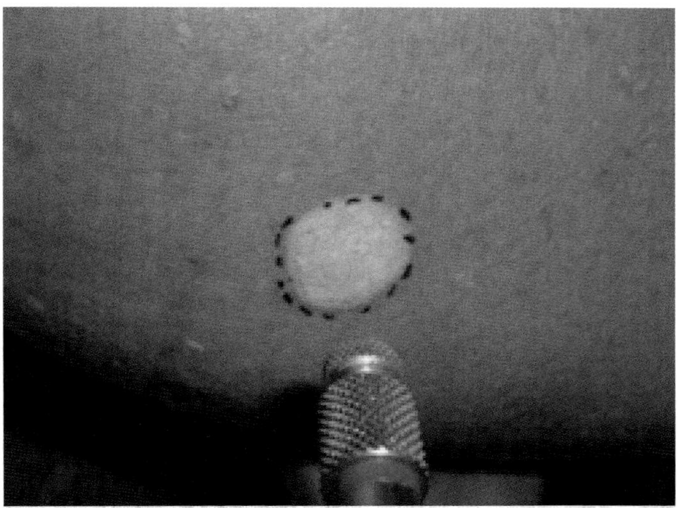

FIGURE 164-9 Cryosurgery of large actinic keratosis. The outside border was marked with a 1- to 2-mm margin. (*Reproduced with permission from Richard P. Usatine, MD.*)

TABLE 164-1 Comparison of Topical Agents for the Treatment of AK

Topical Agent for AK	Duration of Treatment	Irritation	Cost
5-Fluorouracil generic 5%	3-6 wk	High	<$100
Diclofenac 3%	10-12 wk	Moderate	>$130
Imiquimod	16 wk	Moderate	>$400

diclofenac 3% gel was as effective as 5-FU cream for AK of the face and scalp and diclofenac produced fewer signs of inflammation.[8]

- Imiquimod 5% cream has been demonstrated to be effective over a 16-week course of treatment, but studies have only measured 8 weeks of follow-up.[5] SOR B By weight, it is 19 times the cost of 5-FU. They have similar side effects.[5]
- One meta-analysis comparing imiquimod to 5-FU showed average complete clearance of AKs for each drug was 5-FU, 52 ± 18% and imiquimod, 70 ± 12%.[9]
- Imiquimod applied topically for 12 to 16 weeks produced complete clearance of AKs in 50% of patients compared to 5% with vehicle (number needed to treat [NNT] = 2.2). Adverse events included erythema (27%), scabbing or crusting (21%), flaking (9%), and erosions (6%) (number needed to harm [NNH] = 3.2-5.9).[10]
- Because of its immunostimulatory properties, imiquimod cream must be used with caution in transplant patients on immunosuppression therapy.[1] SOR C
- Topical tretinoin has some efficacy on the face, with partial clearance of AKs, but may need to be used for up to a year at a time to optimize benefit.[5] SOR B
- Cryosurgery was effective for up to 75% of lesions in trials comparing it with photodynamic therapy. It may be particularly superior for thicker lesions, but may leave scars.[5] SOR A
- Photodynamic therapy (PDT) was effective in up to 91% of AKs in trials comparing it with cryotherapy, with consistently good cosmetic results. It may be particularly good for superficial and confluent AKs, but is likely to be more expensive than most other therapies. It is of particular value where AKs are numerous or when located at sites of poor healing, such as the lower leg.[5] SOR B
- Other less accessible and expensive methods include lasers, dermabrasion, and chemical peels.
- Ingenol mebutate (Picato)—A short 2 to 3 days of treatment with daily topical ingenol mebutate from the sap of *Euphorbia peplus* plant, showed promising efficacy with a favorable safety profile in several randomized controlled trials (RCTs). One multicenter RCT showed 34.1% to 42.2% complete clearance of AKs with ingenol mebutate gel 0.05% for trunk and extremities, and 0.015% for face.[11] Another RCT with 0.05% gel showed a complete clearance of 71% of treated lesions.[12] Ingenol mebutate appears to have a dual mechanism of action by rapid lesion necrosis and subsequent immune-mediated cellular cytotoxicity, providing efficacy with short treatment period.[13]

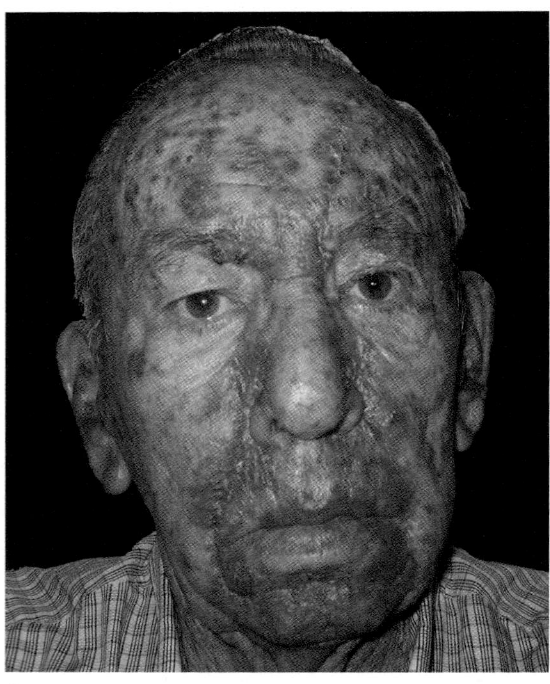
A

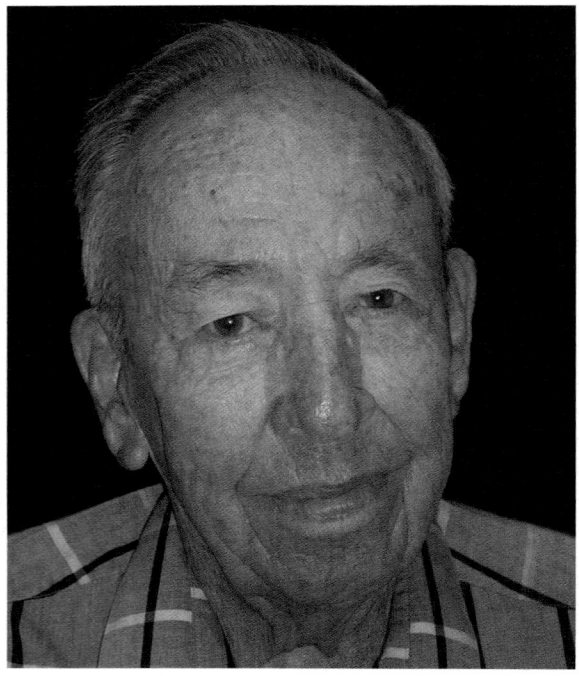
B

FIGURE 164-10 **A.** Actinic keratoses reddened and crusted by the application of 5-fluorouracil topically twice daily. **B.** Face healed months after the course of 5-fluorouracil was completed. (*Reproduced with permission from Richard P. Usatine, MD.*)

TABLE 164-2 Summary of the Main Treatment Options for Bowen Disease[14]

Lesion Characteristics	Topical 5-FU	Topical Imiquimod*	Cryotherapy	Curettage	Excision	PDT	Radiotherapy	Laser†
Small, single/few, good healing site‡	4	3	2	1	3	3	5	4
Large, single, good healing site‡	3	3	3	5	5	2	4	7
Multiple, good healing site‡	3	4	2	3	5	3	4	4
Small, single/few, poor healing site‡	2	3	3	2	2	1-2	5	7
Large, single, poor healing site‡	3	2-3	5	4	5	1	6	7
Facial	4	7	2	2	4§	3	4	7
Digital	3	7	3	5	2§	3	3	3
Perianal	6	6	6	6	1¶	7	2 to 3	6
Penile	3	3	3	5	4§	3	2 to 3	3

5-FU, 5-fluorouracil; PDT, photodynamic therapy; 1, probably treatment of choice; 2, generally good choice; 3, generally fair choice; 4, reasonable but not usually required; 5, generally poor choice; 6, probably should not be used; 7, insufficient evidence available. The suggested scoring of the treatments listed takes into account the evidence for benefit, ease of application or time required for the procedure, wound healing, cosmetic result, and current availability/costs of the method or facilities required. Evidence for interventions based on single studies or purely anecdotal cases is not included.
*Does not have a product license for Bowen disease.
†Depends on site.
‡Refers to the clinician's perceived potential for good or poor healing at the affected site.
§Consider micrographic surgery for tissue sparing or if poorly defined/recurrent.
¶Wide excision recommended.

BOWEN DISEASE

- **Table 164-2** compares and summarizes the main treatment options.
- The risk of progression to invasive cancer is approximately 3%. This risk is greater in genital BD, and particularly in perianal BD. A high risk of recurrence, including late recurrence, is a particular feature of perianal BD and prolonged follow-up is recommended for this variant.[14] SOR Ⓐ
- There is reasonable evidence to support use of 5-FU.[14] SOR Ⓑ It is more practical than surgery for large lesions, especially at potentially poor healing sites, and has been used for "control" rather than cure in some patients with multiple lesions.[8]
- Topical imiquimod may be used off-label for BD for larger lesions or difficult or poor healing sites.[14] SOR Ⓑ However, it is costly and the optimum regimen has yet to be determined.[14]
- One prospective study suggests a superiority of curettage and electrodesiccation over cryotherapy in treating BD, especially for lesions on the lower leg.[10] SOR Ⓑ Curettage was associated with a significantly shorter healing time, less pain, fewer complications, and a lower recurrence rate when compared with cryotherapy.[15] Curettage and electrodesication is also a good option for Bowen disease of the trunk or arms (**Figure 164-11**).

PREVENTION

- Protection from UV exposure by limiting outdoor activities, and using sunscreens and protective gears (hat, umbrella, long sleeve garments, etc).
- Avoid artificial tanning beds and tobacco.

PROGNOSIS

Prognosis of treated AK and BD is excellent.

FOLLOW-UP

Patients need skin examinations every 6 to 12 months to identify new precancers and cancers. SOR Ⓒ More frequent examinations may be needed for those who have continued exposure to offending agents (eg, organ transplant recipients on immunosuppressant therapy), and those with history of recurrent skin malignancies.

PATIENT EDUCATION

Patients must understand that they acquired these conditions through cumulative sun damage, and they need to avoid further sun damage to minimize the likelihood of additional precancers and cancers. The sun damage is often from childhood and early adulthood, so the lesions are likely to form even with future sun protection. Self-skin examination is recommended.

All topical treatments for AKs and BD will make the lesions look worse before they get better (see **Figure 164-10**). The 5-FU treatments are often given with topical corticosteroid preparations to use after the treatment is over so as to minimize the symptoms of the inflammation.

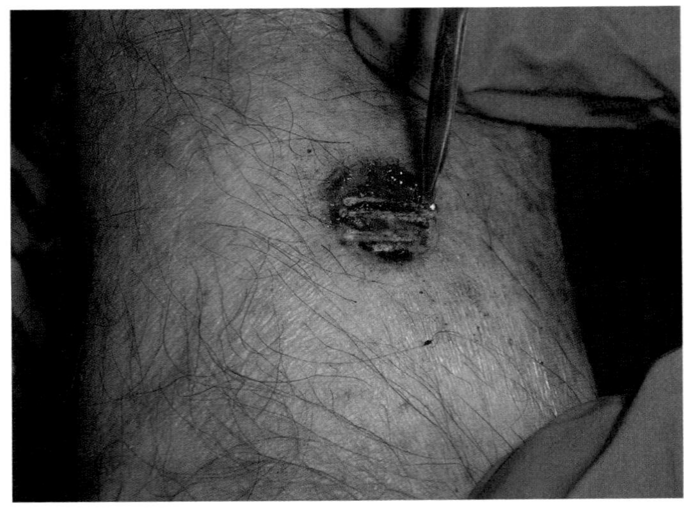

A

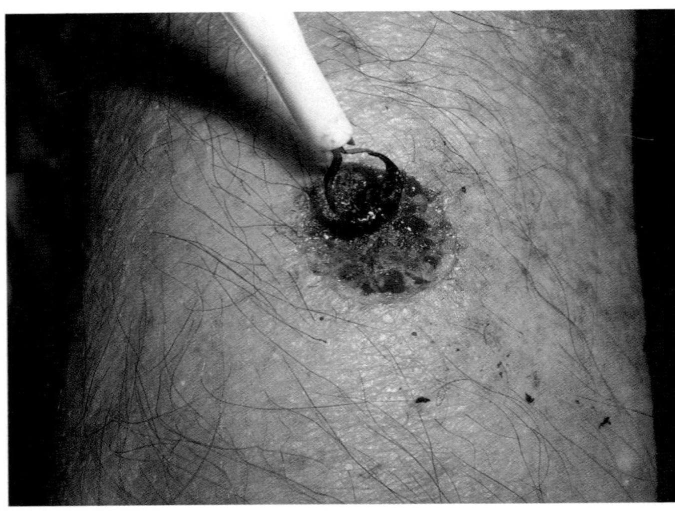

B

FIGURE 164-11 A. Curettage of Bowen disease on the arm. Each cycle begins with curettage and ends with electrodesiccation. B. Electrodesiccation of Bowen disease on the same arm. Three cycles were performed to complete the procedure. (*Reproduced with permission from Richard P. Usatine, MD.*)

PATIENT RESOURCES

- Skin Cancer Foundation has an excellent website with photos and patient information—**http://www.skincancer.org/ak/index.php.**

PROVIDER RESOURCES

- Cox NH, Eedy DJ, Morton CA. Guidelines for management of Bowen's disease: 2006 update. *Br J Dermatol* 2007;156(1):11-21.

For detailed information on the treatment of AKs and Bowen disease see:

- Usatine R, Pfenninger J, Stulberg D, Small R. *Dermatologic and Cosmetic Procedures in Office Practice*. Elsevier, Inc., Philadelphia. 2012.
- Usatine R, Stulberg D, Colver G. *Cutaneous Cryosurgery*. 4th Edition. Taylor and Francis, London, 2014.

Both are available electronically through **www.usatinemedia.com.**

REFERENCES

1. Bonerandi JJ, Beauvillain C, Caquant L, et al. Guidelines for the diagnosis and treatment of cutaneous squamous cell carcinoma and precursor lesions. *J Eur Acad Dermatol Venereol*. 2011;25(suppl 5):1-51.
2. Leffell DJ. The scientific basis of skin cancer. *J Am Acad Dermatol*. 2000;42(1 pt 2):18-22.
3. Anwar J, Wrone DA, Kimyai-Asadi A, Alam M. The development of actinic keratosis into invasive squamous cell carcinoma: evidence and evolving classification schemes. *Clin Dermatol*. 2004;22(3):189-196.
4. Criscione VD, Weinstock MA, Naylor MF, et al. Actinic keratoses: natural history and risk of malignant transformation in the Veterans Affairs Topical Tretinoin Chemoprevention Trial. *Cancer*. 2009;115(11):2523-2530.
5. de Berker D, McGregor JM, Hughes BR. Guidelines for the management of actinic keratoses. *Br J Dermatol*. 2007;156(2):222-230.
6. Zouboulis CC, Röhrs H. [Cryosurgical treatment of actinic keratoses and evidence-based review]. *Hautarzt*. 2005;56(4):353-358.
7. Thai K-E, Fergin P, Freeman M, et al. A prospective study of the use of cryosurgery for the treatment of actinic keratoses. *Int J Dermatol*. 2004;43(9):687-692.
8. Smith SR, Morhenn VB, Piacquadio DJ. Bilateral comparison of the efficacy and tolerability of 3% diclofenac sodium gel and 5% 5-fluorouracil cream in the treatment of actinic keratoses of the face and scalp. *J Drugs Dermatol*. 2006;5(2):156-159.
9. Gupta AK, Davey V, Mcphail H. Evaluation of the effectiveness of imiquimod and 5-fluorouracil for the treatment of actinic keratosis: critical review and meta-analysis of efficacy studies. *J Cutan Med Surg*. 2005;9(5):209-214.
10. Hadley G, Derry S, Moore RA. Imiquimod for actinic keratosis: systematic review and meta-analysis. *J Invest Dermatol*. 2006;126(6):1251-1255.
11. Lebwohl M, Swanson N, Anderson LL, et al. Ingenol mebutate gel for actinic keratosis. *N Engl J Med*. 2012;366(11):1010-1019.
12. Siller G, Gebauer K, Welburn P, Katsamas J, Ogbourne SM. PEP005 (ingenol mebutate) gel, a novel agent for the treatment of actinic keratosis: results of a randomized, double-blind, vehicle-controlled, multicentre, phase IIa study. *Australas J Dermatol*. 2009;50(1):16-22.
13. Rosen RH, Gupta AK, Tyring SK. Dual mechanism of action of ingenol mebutate gel for topical treatment of actinic keratoses: rapid lesion necrosis followed by lesion-specific immune response. *J Am Acad Dermatol*. 2012;66(3):486-493.
14. Cox NH, Eedy DJ, Morton CA. Guidelines for management of Bowen's disease: 2006 update. *Br J Dermatol*. 2007;156(1):11-21.
15. Ahmed I, Berth-Jones J, Charles-Holmes S, O'Callaghan CJ, Ilchyshyn A. Comparison of cryotherapy with curettage in the treatment of Bowen's disease: a prospective study. *Br J Dermatol*. 2000;143(4):759-766.

165 KERATOACANTHOMA

Alfonso Guzman, MD
Richard P. Usatine, MD

PATIENT STORY

A 71-year-old woman presented with a rapidly growing lesion on her face over the past 4 months (**Figure 165-1**). The lesion had features of a basal cell carcinoma with a pearly border and telangiectasias (**Figure 165-2**). Also the central crater with keratin gave it the appearance of a keratoacanthoma (KA). A shave biopsy was performed and the pathology showed squamous cell carcinoma (SCC)–KA type. A full elliptical excision with 4-mm margins was then performed.

INTRODUCTION

The KA is a unique epidermal tumor characterized by rapid, abundant growth and a spontaneous resolution, with the classic presentation in middle-aged, light-skinned individuals in hair-bearing, sun-exposed areas. In the late 1940s, Freudenthal of Wroclaw coined the term *keratoacanthoma*, owing to the considerable acanthosis observed in the tumor. Controversies have arisen since the 1950s about the real nature of the tumor; some KAs may metastasize, and there is debate over the relationship to SCC.[1,2] Many dermatopathologists now classify this tumor as a subtype of SCC.

SYNONYMS

- Keratocarcinoma[1]
- Molluscum sebaceum

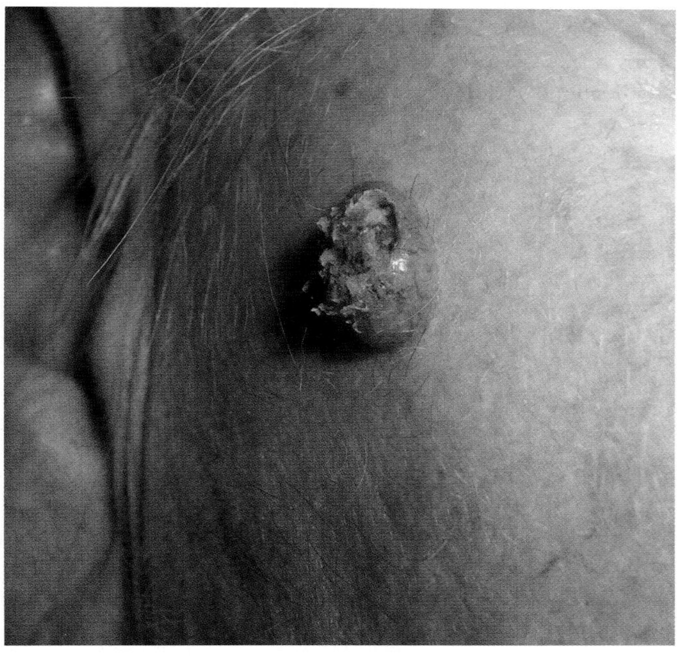

FIGURE 165-1 Pearly keratoacanthoma with telangiectasias and a central keratin core on the face of a 71-year-old woman. (*Reproduced with permission from Richard P. Usatine, MD.*)

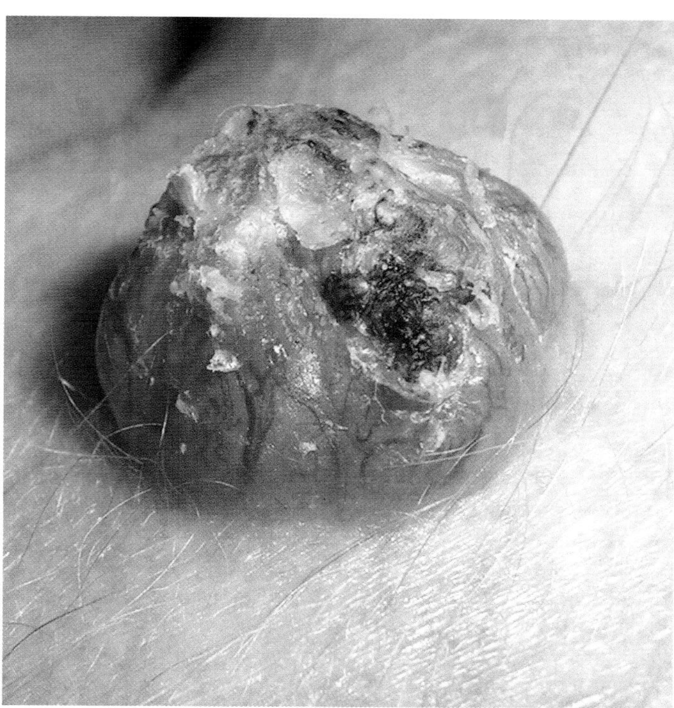

FIGURE 165-2 Close-up of the keratoacanthoma with telangiectasias and a central keratin core on the face of the woman in Figure 165-1. (*Reproduced with permission from Richard P. Usatine, MD.*)

- Molluscum pseudocarcinomatosum
- Cutaneous sebaceous neoplasm
- Self-healing squamous epithelioma
- Intracutaneous cornifying epithelioma
- Idiopathic cutaneous pseudoepitheliomatous hyperplasia
- Verrugoma

EPIDEMIOLOGY

- KA develops as a solitary nodule in sun-exposed areas.
- Seen more commonly later in life with a predilection for males.[1]
- Develops rapidly within 6 to 8 weeks.
- May spontaneously regress after 3 to 6 months or may continue to grow and rarely metastasize.[3]

ETIOLOGY AND PATHOPHYSIOLOGY

- KAs share features such as infiltration and cytologic atypia with SCCs.
- KAs have been reported to metastasize.
- KA is considered to be a variant of SCC, called SCC-KA type.
- Histologic criteria are not sensitive enough to discriminate reliably between KA and SCC.[4]

RISK FACTORS

- Age 40 to 60
- Occurs on sun-exposed areas of skin

- Light complexion
- Male gender

DIAGNOSIS

CLINICAL FEATURES

Solitary nodule is seen in sun-exposed areas. Often have a central keratin plug that resembles a volcano (**Figures 165-1** to **165-5**). KAs may grow rapidly (**Figure 165-6**). Rare cases of multiple eruptive KAs have been reported.[1]

TYPICAL DISTRIBUTION

KAs occur on face, arms, hands, and trunk (see **Figures 165-3** and **165-5**). KAs can be found anywhere on the head and neck, including the ears (**Figures 165-6** and **165-7**).

LABORATORY STUDIES

Biopsy is the only reliable method to make the diagnosis. KAs are well-differentiated squamoproliferative skin lesions.

DIFFERENTIAL DIAGNOSIS

- Actinic keratoses are precancerous lesions found on sun-exposed areas that may progress to SCC. Because these lesions are generally flat they are rarely confused with KAs (see Chapter 164, Actinic Keratosis and Bowen Disease).
- Cutaneous horn is a raised, keratinaceous lesion that can arise in actinic keratoses and in all types of nonmelanoma skin cancers. It generally does not have pearly raised skin around the keratin horn and therefore does not have the crater appearance of a KA (see Chapter 167, Cutaneous Horn).

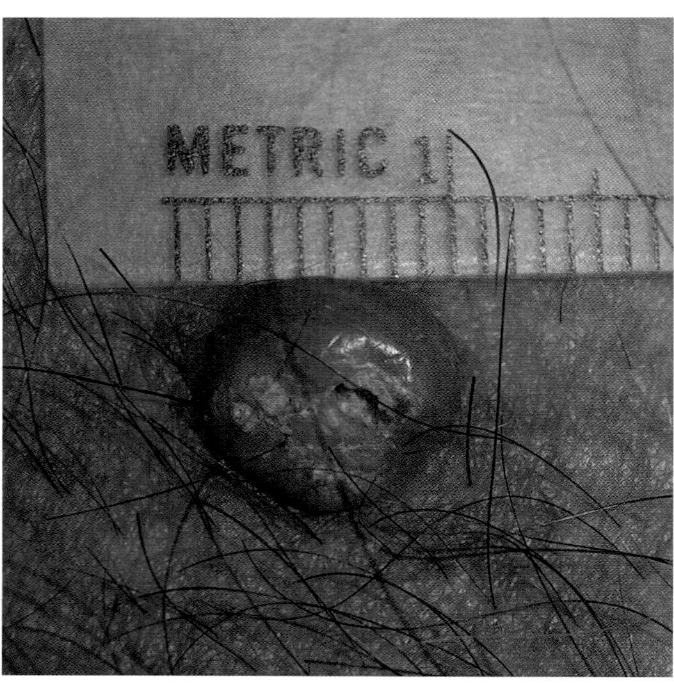

FIGURE 165-3 Keratoacanthoma on the chest of a 53-year-old man with central scaling. (*Reproduced with permission from Richard P. Usatine, MD.*)

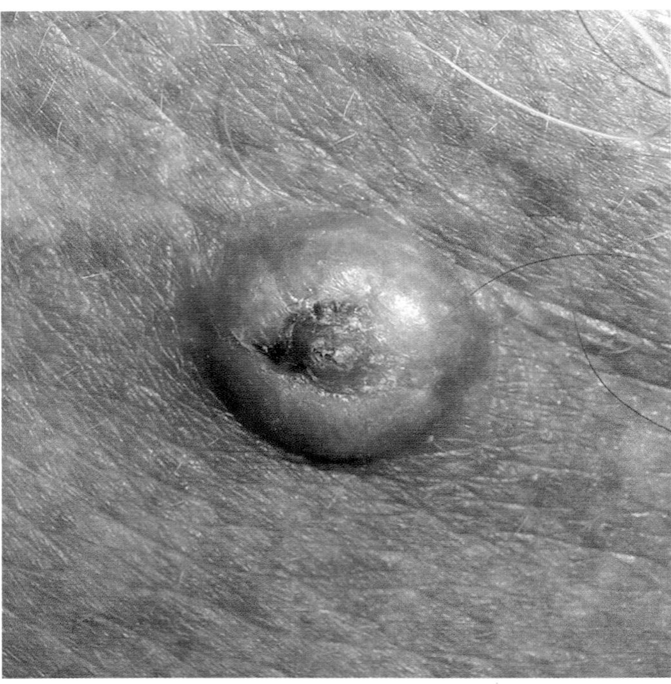

FIGURE 165-5 Keratoacanthoma on the chest of a 70-year-old man with central keratin core that resembles a volcano. (*Reproduced with permission from Richard P. Usatine, MD.*)

- SCCs of the skin have many forms and KA is considered to be one type of SCC (see Chapter 169, Squamous Cell Carcinoma).

MANAGEMENT

- A shave biopsy may be used for diagnosis but is not an adequate final treatment. Options for definitive treatment should be discussed with patient.
- Although some KAs may regress spontaneously, there is no way to distinguish between these and the ones that are variants of SCC, which may go on to metastasize. Therefore, the standard of care is to remove or destroy the remaining tumor. SOR Ⓒ

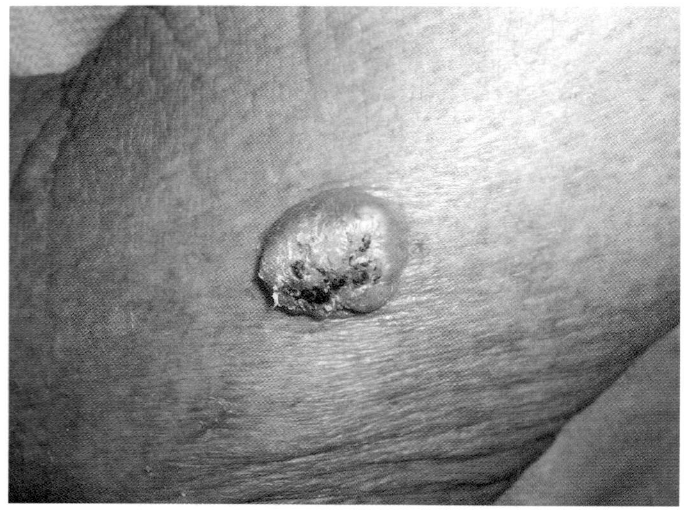

FIGURE 165-4 Squamous cell carcinoma of the keratoacanthoma type on the arm of a 61-year-old man with central scaling. (*Reproduced with permission from Richard P. Usatine, MD.*)

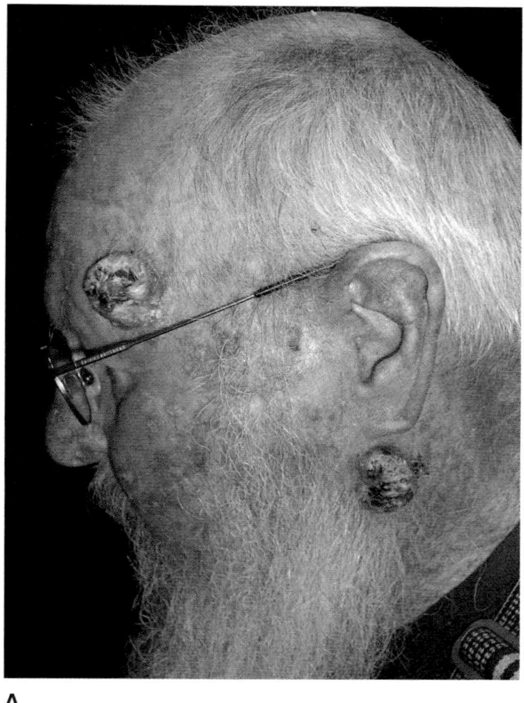

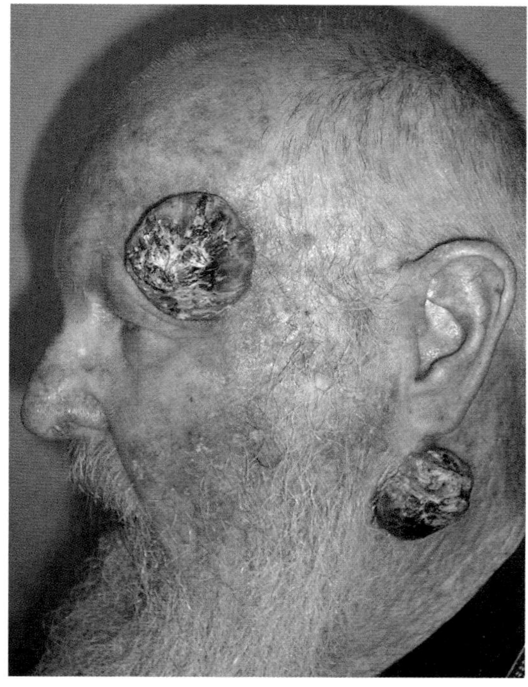

FIGURE 165-6 Two SCCs in a 65-year-old man. **A.** The SCC over the temple was a keratoacanthoma type, whereas the SCC on the neck was a well-differentiated SCC. **B.** Rapid growth occurred in both tumors over the 6-week period that the patient waited to have head and neck surgery. *(Reproduced with permission from Richard P. Usatine, MD.)*

- Elliptically excise a KA with margins of 3 to 5 mm as you would do in a SCC.[4] SOR C
- Smaller, less-aggressive KAs diagnosed with shave biopsy may be destroyed with curettage and desiccation or cryotherapy with 3- to 5-mm margins. SOR C

FIGURE 165-7 Keratoacanthoma on the ear. *(Reproduced with permission from Richard P. Usatine, MD.)*

- Mohs surgery may be indicated for large or recurrent KAs or KAs located in anatomic areas with cosmetic or functional considerations.[4] SOR C
- Multiple eruptive KAs have been treated with oral retinoids, methotrexate, and cyclophosphamide.[1] SOR C

PROGNOSIS

When compared to other skin cancers, prognosis is good. Excision is typically curative.[5]

FOLLOW-UP

Patients should perform their own skin examinations and have yearly clinical skin examinations to examine for recurrence and the development of new skin cancers.

PATIENT EDUCATION

KA is similar to other nonmelanoma skin cancers in that it occurs on sun-exposed areas and patients who have one are at increased risk of developing new skin cancers. Therefore, sun avoidance and sun protection should be emphasized.

PATIENT RESOURCES

- Skinsight. *Keratoacanthoma*—**http://www.skinsight.com/adult/KA.htm.**

PROVIDER RESOURCES

- Medscape. *Keratoacanthoma*—**http://emedicine.medscape.com/article/1100471.**

For detailed information on the treatment of KAs see:

- Usatine R, Pfenninger J, Stulberg D, Small R. *Dermatologic and Cosmetic Procedures in Office Practice*. Elsevier, Inc., Philadelphia. 2012.
- Usatine R, Stulberg D, Colver G. *Cutaneous Cryosurgery*. 4th Edition. Taylor and Francis, London, 2014.

Both are available electronically through **www.usatinemedia.com.**

REFERENCES

1. Karaa A, Khachemoune A. Keratoacanthoma: a tumor in search of a classification. *Int J Dermatol.* 2007;46(7):671-678.
2. Ko CJ. Keratoacanthoma: facts and controversies. *Clin Dermatol.* 2010;28(3):254-261.
3. Clausen OP, Aass HC, Beigi M, et al. Are keratoacanthomas variants of squamous cell carcinomas? A comparison of chromosomal aberrations by comparative genomic hybridization. *J Invest Dermatol.* 2006;126(10):2308-2315.
4. Chuang TY. *Keratoacanthoma*. Updated July 2005. http://www.emedicine.com/derm/topic206.htm. Accessed on May 28, 2006.
5. Beham A, Regauer S, Soyer HP, Beham-Schmid C. Keratoacanthoma: a clinically distinct variant of well differentiated squamous cell carcinoma. *Adv Anat Pathol.* 1998;5(5):269-280.

166 LENTIGO MALIGNA

E.J. Mayeaux Jr, MD
Richard P. Usatine, MD

PATIENT STORY

A 65-year-old woman noted that a brown spot on her face was growing larger and darker (**Figure 166-1**). A broad shave biopsy showed lentigo maligna (LM) (melanoma in situ). The patient was referred for Mohs surgery for definitive treatment.

INTRODUCTION

LM begins as a tan-brown macule melanoma usually in sun-damaged areas of the skin in older individuals. It is a subtype of melanoma in situ.

SYNONYMS

LM is also known as Hutchinson melanotic freckle.

EPIDEMIOLOGY

- The incidence of LM is directly related to sun exposure. In the United States, the incidence is greatest in Hawaii, intermediate in the central and southern states, and lowest in the northern states.[1]
- Generally, patients with LM are older than age 40 years, with a peak incidence between the ages of 65 and 80 years.[2]
- Persons with LM melanoma (LMM) tend to be older, fair-skinned persons with markers of actinic skin damage and prior skin cancers, and the incidence is increasing.[3]
- The lesions occur more commonly on the driver's side of the head and neck in men in Australia.[4]

ETIOLOGY AND PATHOPHYSIOLOGY

- LM is a subtype of melanoma in situ, a preinvasive lesion confined to the epidermis (**Figures 166-1** to **166-3**).
- It is caused by cumulative sun exposure and, therefore, seen later in life.
- LMM occurs when the lesion extends into the dermis (**Figure 166-4**).
- LM can be present for long periods (5-15 years) before invasion occurs, although rapid progression within months has been described.[5]
- The risk for progression to LMM appears to be proportional to the size of the lesion of LM.[5]

RISK FACTORS

- Ultraviolet (UV) radiation exposure: Risk increases with increased hours of exposure to sunlight, with the amount of actinic damage, and with a history of nonmelanoma skin cancer.

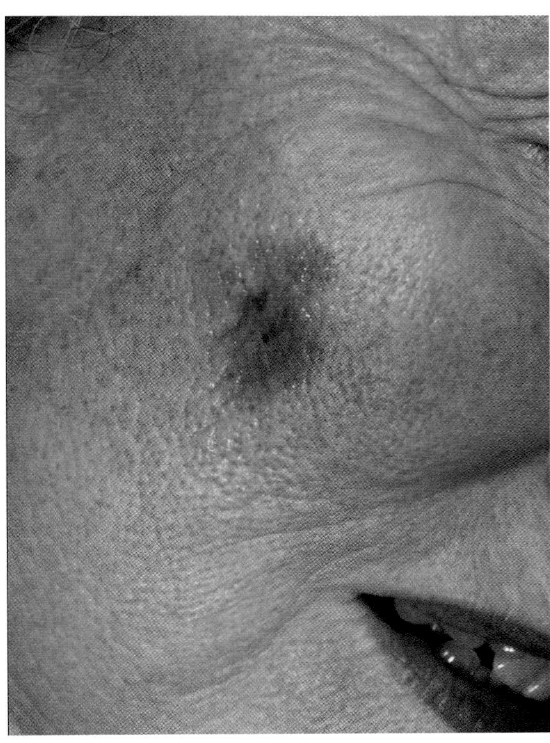

FIGURE 166-1 Lentigo maligna (melanoma in situ) on the face. (*Reproduced with permission from Usatine RP, Moy RL, Tobinick EL, Siegel DM. Skin Surgery: A Practical Guide. St. Louis, MO: Mosby; 1998.*)

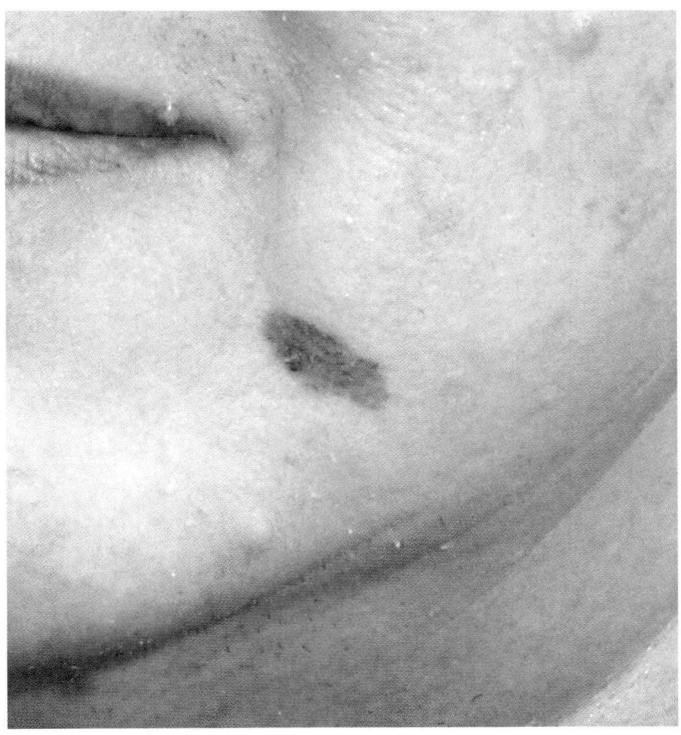

FIGURE 166-2 LM on the face, presenting as a single large evolving pigmented lesion with changing color. (*Reproduced with permission from Richard P. Usatine, MD.*)

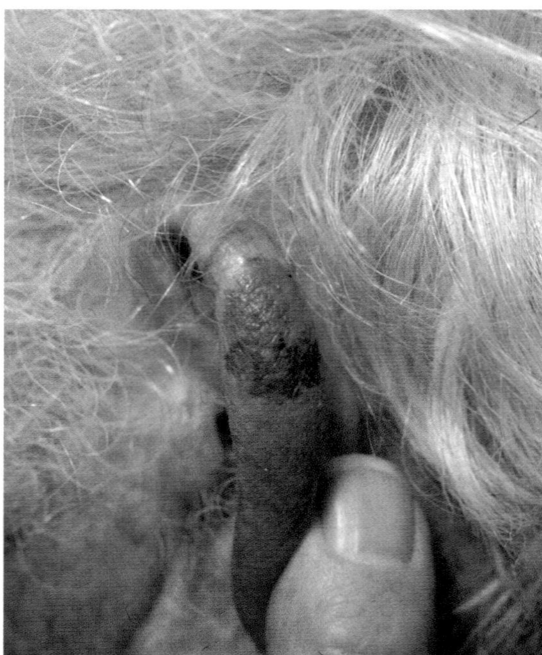

FIGURE 166-3 LM on the ear (melanoma in situ). (*Reproduced with permission from Usatine RP, Moy RL, Tobinick EL, Siegel DM.* Skin Surgery: A Practical Guide. *St. Louis, MO: Mosby; 1998.*)

- Increased number of melanocytic nevi, including large or giant congenital nevi.
- Fair skin.
- History of severe sunburns.
- Porphyria cutanea tarda.
- Tyrosine-positive oculocutaneous albinism.
- Xeroderma pigmentosum.
- Occupational risk with sun exposure.

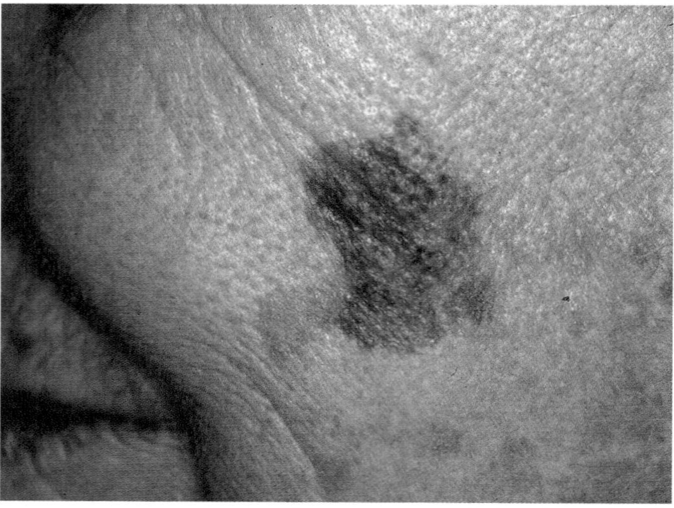

FIGURE 166-4 LMM on the cheek. This lesion is invasive and no longer melanoma in situ. A partial broad scoop shave biopsy is a good way to make this diagnosis, as a full-depth complete excisional biopsy would be prohibitively large and a punch biopsy might miss the diagnosis. (*Reproduced with permission from the Skin Cancer Foundation. For more information www.skincancer.org.*)

DIAGNOSIS

CLINICAL FEATURES

- Large pigmented patch with multiple colors, including brown, black, pink, and white (signifying regression) (see **Figures 166-1** to **166-3**).
- May have ill-defined borders and microscopic extension that can determine the clinical borders and complete removal of the lesion difficult.
- One retrospective study revealed the 4 most important features of LM: asymmetric pigmented follicular openings, dark rhomboidal structures, slate-gray globules, and slate-gray dots with a sensitivity of 89% and a specificity of 96% (see Appendix C, Dermoscopy).[6]

TYPICAL DISTRIBUTION

LM occurs on face, head, and neck. There is a predilection for the nose and cheek (see **Figures 166-1** and **166-2**).

BIOPSY

- Complete excisional biopsy is rarely practical because these lesions are frequently large and are on the face (see **Figure 166-1**). There is debate in the literature between doing broad shave biopsy, multiple punch biopsy, and incisional biopsy.[7] The goal is to avoid sampling error and misdiagnosing a LM or LMM as a benign lesion.
- A lesion suspicious for LM or LMM can be biopsied using a broad scoop shave biopsy approach with a DermaBlade or sharp razor blade (see **Figure 166-4**).[7] The goal is to sample the dermal–epidermal junction and still produce a good cosmetic result (especially if the lesion turns out to be benign).
- One option is multiple smaller biopsy samples of each morphologically distinct region of the lesion.[7]
- If an area suspicious for invasion is noted, or if there is an area of induration suspicious for associated desmoplastic melanoma, a deeper incisional biopsy of this area should be performed.[7]
- If sampling is incomplete, the presence of a solar lentigo, pigmented actinic keratosis, or reticulated seborrheic keratosis (SK) could mislead the pathologist and clinician to the wrong conclusion that the incisional specimen is representative of the whole, and that no LM is present.[7]
- In a study of LM, contiguous pigmented lesions were present in 48% of the specimens obtained by broad shave biopsy or Mohs surgery. The most common lesion was a benign solar lentigo (30%), followed by pigmented actinic keratosis (24%).[7] This should be kept in mind when interpreting biopsy results to avoid false negatives.

DIFFERENTIAL DIAGNOSIS

- Solar lentigo—These hyperpigmented patches are very common on the faces and the dorsum of the hands of persons with significant sun exposure and the incidence increases with age. A possible solar lentigo is more suspicious for LM or LMM when it is larger, more asymmetric, has irregular borders, and has more variation in colors. Pigmented lesions with these characteristics should be biopsied to determine the correct diagnosis. Many fair-skinned individuals have a number of solar lentigines making this a challenge. The use of dermoscopy and judicious biopsies is necessary to avoid missing LM and LMM (**Figures 166-5** and **166-6**).
- SKs are ubiquitous benign growths that occur more frequently with age. An early SK can be flat and easily resemble a solar lentigo or LM.

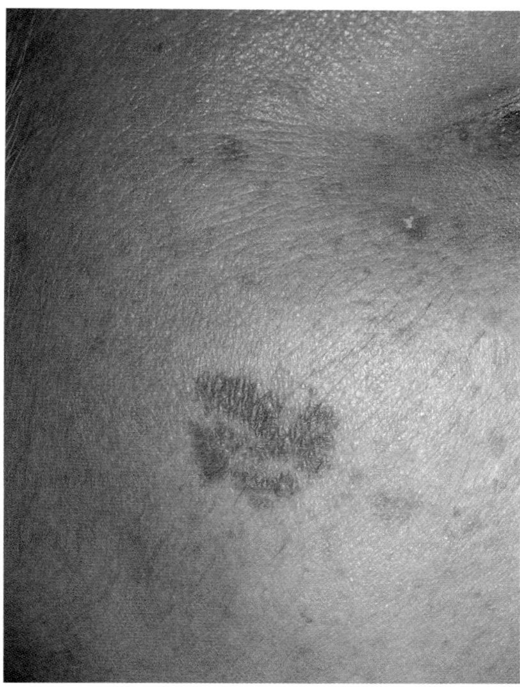

FIGURE 166-5 Solar lentigo on the face of a middle-aged Hispanic woman. (*Reproduced with permission from Richard P. Usatine, MD.*)

The SKs on the back are less likely to be confused for LM, but a large flat SK on the face can easily be mistaken for a LM. More importantly, avoid missing a LM because it is assumed to be a flat early SK. When in doubt, biopsy the lesion with a quick and easy shave biopsy. Do not freeze a possible SK unless you are sure that it is truly benign (see Chapter 156, Seborrheic Keratosis).

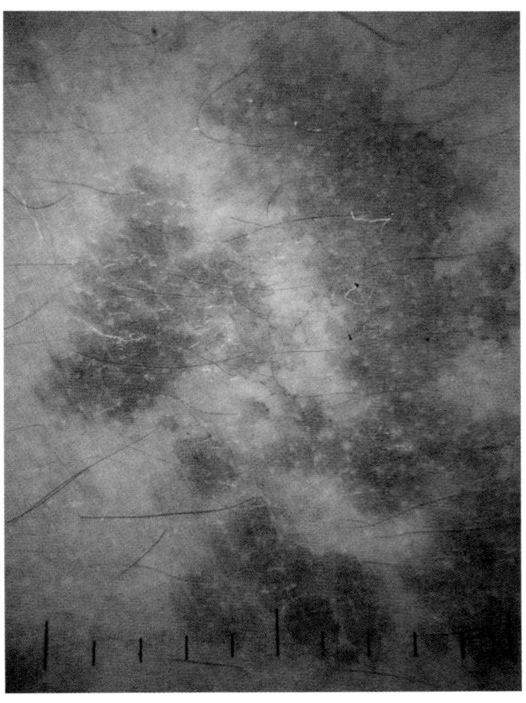

FIGURE 166-6 Dermoscopy of the solar lentigo in Figure 166-5. The moth-eaten appearing edges are typical of a solar lentigo. There are no suspicious patterns and a shave biopsy confirmed that it was benign. (*Reproduced with permission from Richard P. Usatine, MD.*)

- LMM is the feared outcome of missing an LM and not treating it properly. Any suspicious lesion requires biopsy. Do not be afraid to do a quick and easy shave biopsy rather than a full-thickness excision. If it turns out to be a LM or LMM, you can refer for definitive treatment and your biopsy technique does not change the prognosis; early diagnosis does. LMM accounts for 4% to 15% of cutaneous melanoma (see **Figure 166-4**) (see Chapter 170, Melanoma).

MANAGEMENT

Therapy is directed toward preventing progression to invasive LMM.

NONSURGICAL

- Nonsurgical therapy for primary cutaneous melanomas should only be considered when surgical excision is not possible.
- Alternatives to surgery include topical imiquimod, cryosurgery, and observation. Efficacy of nonsurgical therapies for LM has not been fully established.[8] SOR C

MEDICATIONS

Topical imiquimod 5% cream has been described in multiple studies to be effective in treating LM, especially in patients who are not surgical candidates. It is an immune response modifier that is indicated for the treatment of actinic keratosis and superficial basal cell carcinomas. Studies are limited by highly variable treatment regimens and lack of long-term follow-up.[8-10] SOR B

SURGICAL

- For melanoma in situ, wide excision with 0.5- to 1.0-cm margins is recommended. For LM histologic subtype may require larger than 0.5-cm margins to achieve histologically negative margins, because of characteristically broad subclinical extension.[8,10] SOR A
- Standard therapy is margin-controlled surgical excision with Mohs surgery or rush permanent sections.[10,11] SOR B
- The perimeter technique is a method of margin-controlled excision of LM with rush permanent sections. The main advantage is that all margins are examined with permanent sections. The main drawback is that multiple operative sessions are required to complete the procedure.[12]
- Recommended margins for standard excision of melanoma in situ are 0.5 cm. This margin is often inadequate for LM because of the subclinical extension that can occur.[10] The average margin required to clear LM in 90% to 95% of cases in one study was greater than 0.5 cm.[11] Consequently, margin-controlled excision of LM is recommended.[11] SOR B
- Cryosurgery may be used in patients who are not good surgical candidates. In a study of 18 such patients with LM, the lesions resolved clinically in all cases, with no recurrence or metastasis detected during a mean follow-up of 75.5 months.[13] SOR C These patients were treated with 2 freeze–thaw cycles of liquid nitrogen under local anesthesia in a single sitting.

PREVENTION

Because LMM is related to a lifetime of exposure to UV radiation, patients should limit sun exposure, especially between 10 AM and 4 PM. When in the sun, make sure to wear sunscreen with a high sun-protection factor (SPF) that blocks both UVA and UVB. It's also a good idea to protect skin by wearing a broad-brim hat and clothing that covers your arms and legs.

PROGNOSIS

There is a 5% estimated lifetime risk of developing LMM in patients diagnosed with LM at age 45 years.[5]

FOLLOW-UP

- The National Comprehensive Cancer Network recommends that patients have regular clinical skin examinations at least yearly by their family physician or a dermatologist.[14]
- Regional lymph nodes should also be examined.

PATIENT EDUCATION

Patients diagnosed with LM need to minimize sun exposure and do regular self-skin examinations.

PATIENT RESOURCES

- Medline Plus. *Melanoma*—**http://www.nlm.nih.gov/medlineplus/melanoma.html.**

PROVIDER RESOURCES

- The Skin Cancer Foundation. *Melanoma*—1-800-SKIN-490 or **http://www.skincancer.org.**
- National Cancer Institute. *Melanoma*—**http://www.cancer.gov/cancertopics/types/melanoma.**
- Dermoscopy.org: A website on dermoscopy to learn how to improve early diagnosis of melanoma—**http://www.dermoscopy.org/.**

REFERENCES

1. Clark WH Jr, Mihm MC Jr. Lentigo maligna and lentigo-maligna melanoma. *Am J Pathol*. 1969;55(1):39-67.
2. Cohen LM. Lentigo maligna and lentigo maligna melanoma. *J Am Acad Dermatol.* 1995;33(6):923-936.
3. Swetter SM, Boldrick JC, Jung SY, et al. Increasing incidence of lentigo maligna melanoma subtypes: northern California and national trends 1990-2000. *J Invest Dermatol.* 2005;125(4):685-691.
4. Jelfs PL, Giles G, Shugg D, et al. Cutaneous malignant melanoma in Australia, 1989. *Med J Aust.* 1994;161(3):182-187.
5. Weinstock MA, Sober AJ. The risk of progression of lentigo maligna to lentigo maligna melanoma. *Br J Dermatol.* 1987;116 (3):303-310.
6. Schiffner R, Schiffner-Rohe J, Vogt T, et al. Improvement of early recognition of lentigo maligna using dermatoscopy. *J Am Acad Dermatol.* 2000;42(1 pt 1):25-32.
7. Dalton SR, Gardner TL, Libow LF, Elston DM. Contiguous lesions in lentigo maligna. *J Am Acad Dermatol.* 2005;52:859-862.
8. Bichakjian CK, Halpern AC, Johnson TM, et al. Guidelines of care for the management of primary cutaneous melanoma. *J Am Acad Dermatol.* 2011;65(5):1032-1047.
9. Buettiker UV, Yawalkar NY, Braathen LR, Hunger RE. Imiquimod treatment of lentigo maligna: an open-label study of 34 primary lesions in 32 patients. *Arch Dermatol.* 2008;144(7):943-945.
10. Erickson C, Miller SJ. Treatment options in melanoma in situ: topical and radiation therapy, excision and Mohs surgery. *Int J Dermatol.* 2010;49(5):482-491.
11. Huang CC. New approaches to surgery of lentigo maligna. *Skin Therapy Lett.* 2004;9(5):7-11.
12. Mahoney MH, Joseph M, Temple CL. The perimeter technique for lentigo maligna: an alternative to Mohs micrographic surgery. *J Surg Oncol.* 2005;91(2):120-125.
13. de Moraes AM, Pavarin LB, Herreros F, et al. Cryosurgical treatment of lentigo maligna. *J Dtsch Dermatol Ges.* 2007;5(6):477-480.
14. The National Comprehensive Cancer Network. *National Clinical Guidelines in Oncology: Melanoma*, 2009. http://www.mmmp.org/mmmpFile/image/conv%20ther/NCCN%20guidelines_Melanoma.pdf. Accessed April 20, 2012.

167 CUTANEOUS HORN

Mindy A. Smith, MD, MS

PATIENT STORY

A 74-year-old man asks about a lesion on the back of his right ear (**Figure 167-1**). It has been present for approximately 5 years. Although the lesion does not bother him, his wife is concerned because it has been slowly growing. Shave biopsy revealed that the horn was from a basal cell carcinoma. The patient was referred for Mohs surgery to excise the remainder of the cancer.

SYNONYM

Cutaneous horn is also known as cornu cutaneum.

INTRODUCTION

Cutaneous horn is a morphologic (not pathologic) designation for a hyperkeratotic protuberant mass rising above the skin, resembling the horn of an animal.

EPIDEMIOLOGY

Relatively rare lesion, most often occurring on sun-exposed areas of the skin in elderly men; a recent Brazilian case series, however, found a higher prevalence in women.[1]

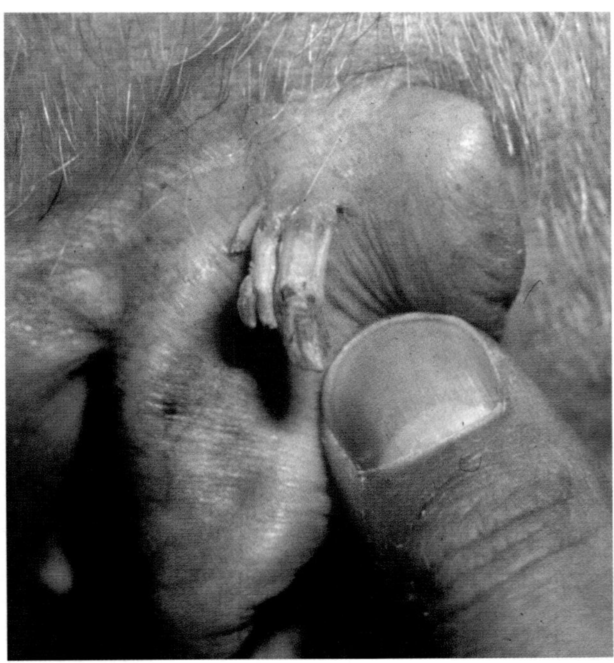

FIGURE 167-1 Cutaneous horn on posterior right pinna arising in a basal cell carcinoma. (*Reproduced with permission from Usatine RP, Moy RL, Tobinick EL, Siegel DM.* Skin Surgery: A Practical Guide. *St. Louis, MO: Mosby; 1998.*)

FIGURE 167-2 Cutaneous horn in a squamous cell carcinoma in situ just lateral to the eye. (*Reproduced with permission from Richard P. Usatine, MD.*)

ETIOLOGY AND PATHOPHYSIOLOGY

- Results from unusual cohesiveness of keratinized material from the superficial layers of the skin or deeply embedded in the cutis. Etiology is unknown but may be related to skin damage from sun exposure or trauma; infectious causes have also been reported including molluscum contagiosum and leishmaniasis.[2]
- Consists of marked retention of stratum corneum.
- May be benign, premalignant, or malignant (**Figures 167-1** to **167-3**) at the base; in 2 large series, 58.6% and 38.9% had malignant or premalignant base pathology.[1,3]
- A history of other malignant or premalignant lesions, tenderness at the base, large size, older age, and location on the penis increase the risk of underlying malignancy.[2-4]

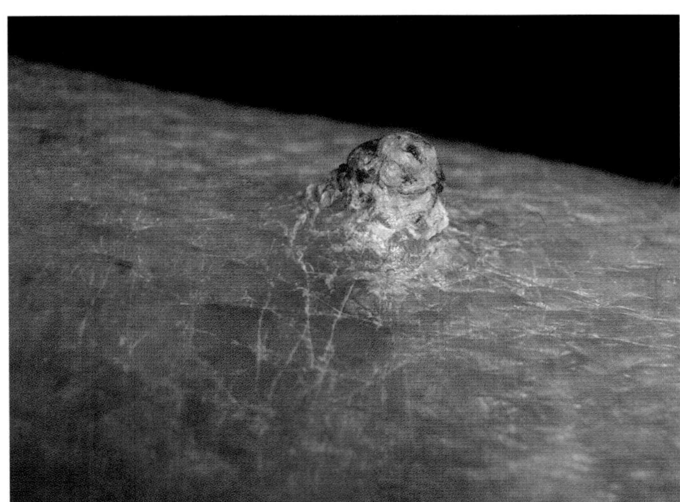

FIGURE 167-3 Cutaneous horn on the arm of a 65-year-old woman, which grew rapidly over 6 months. Biopsy revealed a squamous cell carcinoma of the keratoacanthoma type. (*Reproduced with permission from Richard P. Usatine, MD.*)

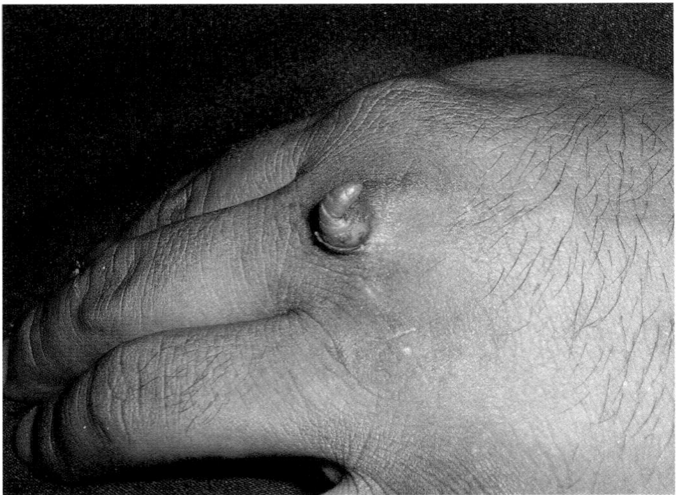

A

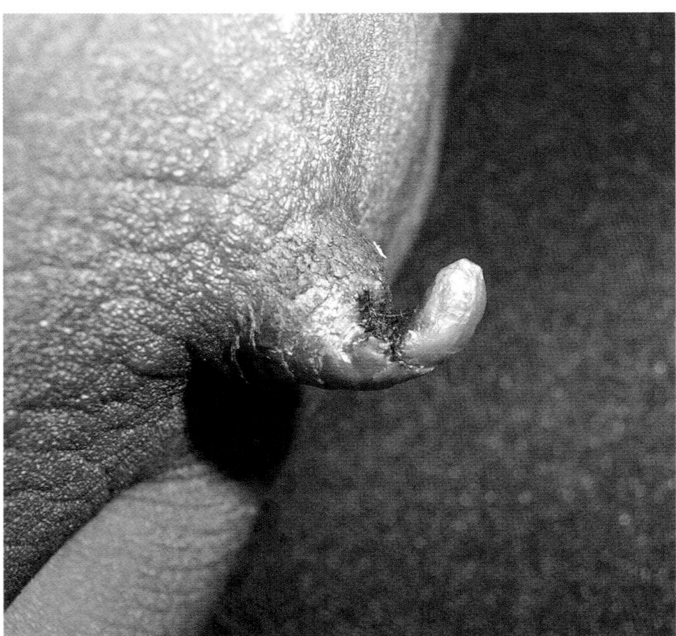

B

FIGURE 167-4 A. Cutaneous horn on the hand of a 33-year-old man for 8 years. He clipped it with nail clippers many times but it always grew back. A shave excision successfully removed it and the pathology showed a viral wart at the base. B. Close-up of the cutaneous horn. (*Reproduced with permission from Richard P. Usatine, MD.*)

- Associated with many types of skin lesions (at the base) that can retain keratin and produce horns including actinic keratosis, warts (**Figures 167-4** and **167-5**), seborrheic keratosis (**Figures 167-6** and **167-7**), keratoacanthoma (see **Figure 167-3**), sebaceous gland, and basal or squamous cell carcinoma (see **Figures 167-1** to **167-3**). In the more recent case series, actinic keratosis was found in 83.8% of the premalignant cases and squamous cell carcinoma was found in 93.75% of the malignant cases.[1]
- Rare cases have been described in association with metastatic renal cell carcinoma, lymphoma, dermatofibroma, pyogenic granuloma (**Figure 167-8**), and, recently, Kaposi sarcoma.[5]

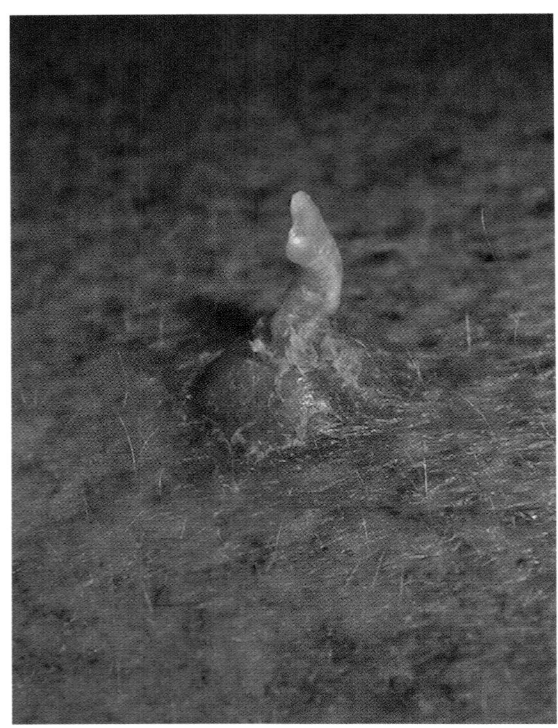

FIGURE 167-5 Cutaneous horn on the back of a 73-year-old woman within an endophytic wart. (*Reproduced with permission from Richard P. Usatine, MD.*)

RISK FACTORS

- Advanced age (>70 years)
- Sun/radiation exposure

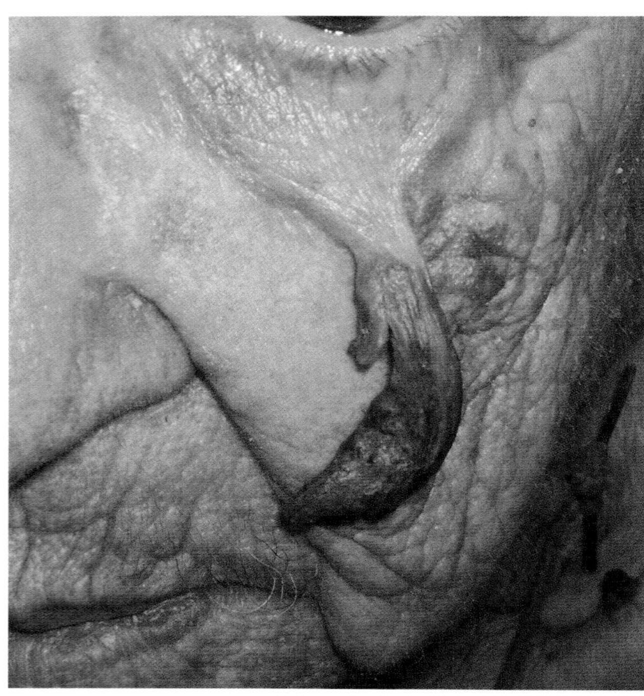

FIGURE 167-6 Large cutaneous horn on the face of an 88-year-old woman. After shave removal the pathology showed seborrheic keratosis with chronic inflammation and cutaneous horn formation. (*Reproduced with permission from Scott Bergeaux, MD.*)

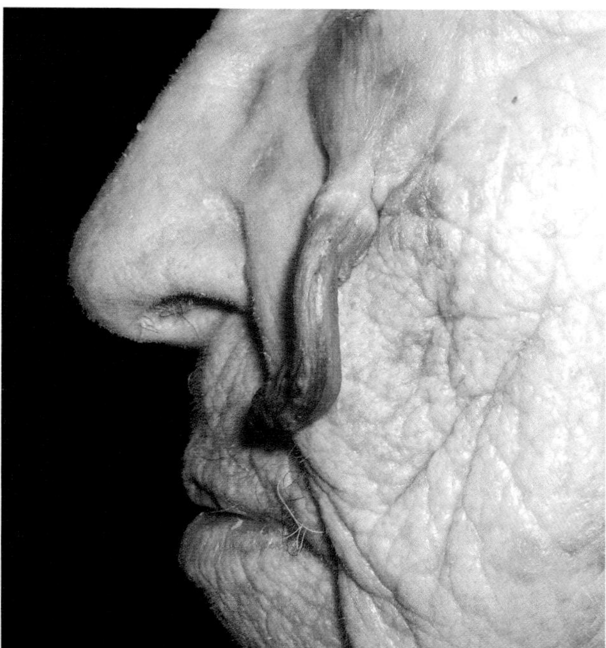

FIGURE 167-7 Another view of this amazing cutaneous horn. The patient had the lesion since her early 30s and attributed it to hot grease popping on her face. She had shown it to other physicians who declined to remove it. Patient stated it "made her feel 16 again" to have it removed. (*Reproduced with permission from Scott Bergeaux, MD.*)

DIAGNOSIS

CLINICAL FEATURES

- Horn-like protuberance.
- Lesions are usually firm; have been described as flat, keratotic, nodular, pedunculated, and ulcerated.[3]

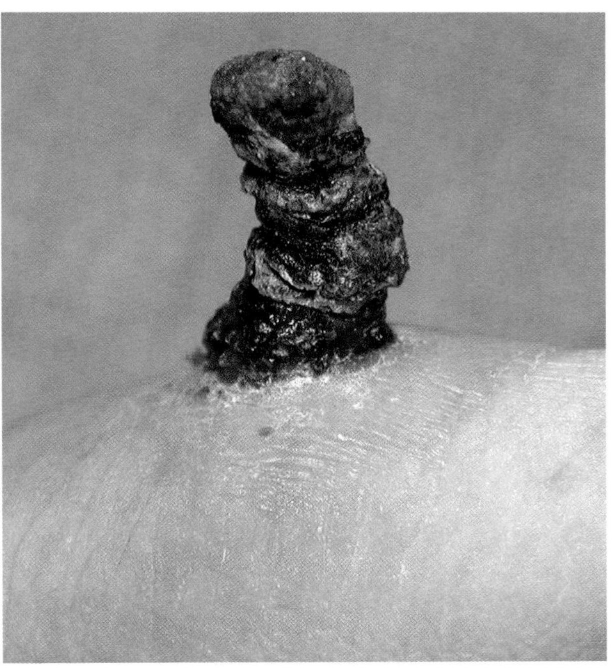

FIGURE 167-8 Cutaneous horn arising in a pyogenic granuloma. (*Reproduced with permission from Suraj Reddy, MD.*)

- Size may vary from a few millimeters to several centimeters; gigantic cutaneous horns (17-25 cm length and up to 2.5 cm width) have been reported, and in one series of 4 cases, all were benign.[6]
- Because of their height, cutaneous horns may be traumatized causing bleeding or pain.

TYPICAL DISTRIBUTION

May occur on any area of the body; approximately 30% are found on the face (see **Figures 167-2**, **167-6**, and **167-7**) and scalp and another 30% on the upper limbs.[1]

BIOPSY

The horn itself consists of concentric layers of cornified epithelial cells (hyperkeratosis). The base may display features of the associated pathologic etiology.

DIFFERENTIAL DIAGNOSIS

Common warts are well-demarcated, rough, hard papules with an irregular papillary surface. Although they may form cylindrical projections, these often fuse to form a surface mosaic pattern; paring the surface exposes punctate hemorrhagic capillaries (see Chapter 130, Common Warts).

MANAGEMENT

- Shave excision, ensuring that the base of the epithelium is obtained for histologic examination, and send to pathology; if benign, may freeze remainder of the lesion.
- Excisional biopsy may also be performed, with wider margins (tumor-free margin of at least 3 mm) if suspected malignancy.

FOLLOW-UP

- Routine follow-up is not needed provided complete removal is accomplished for malignant and premalignant lesions; in one case series of 48 eyelid cutaneous horns, there was no recurrence over a mean of 21 months.[7]
- Patients with any skin cancer should be seen yearly for skin examinations because one cancer puts them at higher risk for all skin cancers. SOR Ⓒ

PATIENT AND PROVIDER RESOURCES

- Medscape. *Cutaneous Horn*—**http://emedicine.medscape.com/article/1056568.**
- Skinsight. *Cutaneous Horn*—**http://www.skinsight.com/adult/cutaneousHorn.htm**

REFERENCES

1. Mantese SA, Diogo PM, Rocha A, et al. Cutaneous horn: a retrospective histopathological study of 222 cases. *An Bras Dermatol*. 2010;85(2):157-163.
2. Vera-Donoso CD, Lujan S, Gomez L, et al. Cutaneous horn in glans penis: a new clinical case. *Scand J Urol Nephrol*. 2009;43(1):92-93.

3. Yu RC, Pryce DW, Macfarlane AW, Stewart TW. A histopathological study of 643 cutaneous horns. *Br J Dermatol*. 1991;124:499-452.

4. Solivan GA, Smith KJ, James WD. Cutaneous horn of the penis: its association with squamous cell carcinoma and HPV-16 infection. *J Am Acad Dermatol*. 1990;23(5 pt 2):969-972.

5. Onak Kandemir N, Gun BD, Barut F, et al. Cutaneous horn-related Kaposi's Sarcoma: a case report. *Case Report Med*. 2010;2010. pii: 825949.

6. Michal M, Bisceglia M, Di Mattia A, et al. Gigantic cutaneous horns of the scalp: lesions with a gross similarity to the horns of animals: a report of four cases. *Am J Surg Pathol*. 2002;26:789-794.

7. Mencia-Gutiérrez E, Gutiérrez-Diaz E, Redondo-Marcos I, et al. Cutaneous horns of the eyelid: clinicopathological study of 48 cases. *J Cutan Pathol*. 2004;31:539-543.

SECTION 11 SKIN CANCER

168 BASAL CELL CARCINOMA

Jonathan B. Karnes, MD
Richard P. Usatine, MD

PATIENT STORY

A 52-year-old woman presented to the office with a "mole" that had been increasing in size over the last year (**Figure 168-1**). This "mole" had been on her face for at least 5 years. The differential diagnosis of this lesion was a nodular basal cell carcinoma (BCC) versus an intradermal nevus. A shave biopsy confirmed it was a nodular BCC and the lesion was excised with an elliptical excision.

INTRODUCTION

BCC is the most common cancer in humans. Usually found on the head and neck, it is generally slow growing and almost never kills or metastasizes when treated in a timely fashion. However, the treatment necessary to eliminate it is often surgical and may cause scarring and changes in appearance and/or function.

EPIDEMIOLOGY

- BCC is the most common skin cancer but the exact incidence is not known.[1]
- Incidence of these cancers increases with age, related to cumulative sun exposure.
- Nodular BCCs—Most common type (70%) (**Figures 168-1** to **168-4**).
- Superficial BCCs—Next most common type (**Figures 168-5** and **168-6**).
- Sclerosing (or morpheaform) BCCs—The least common type (**Figures 168-7** and **168-8**).

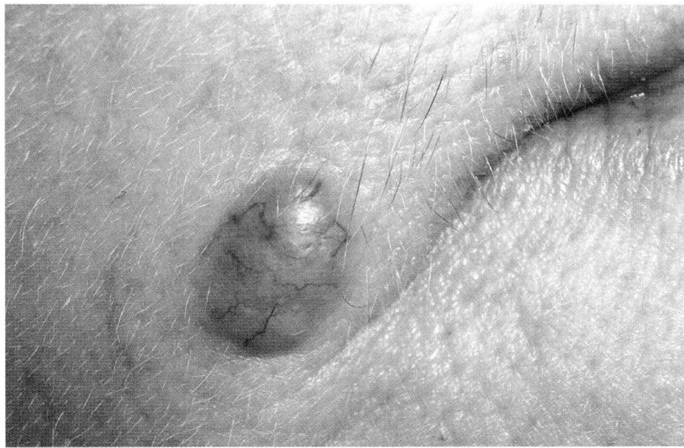

FIGURE 168-1 Pearly nodular basal cell carcinoma (BCC) on the face of a 52-year-old woman present for 5 years. (*Reproduced with permission from Richard P. Usatine, MD.*)

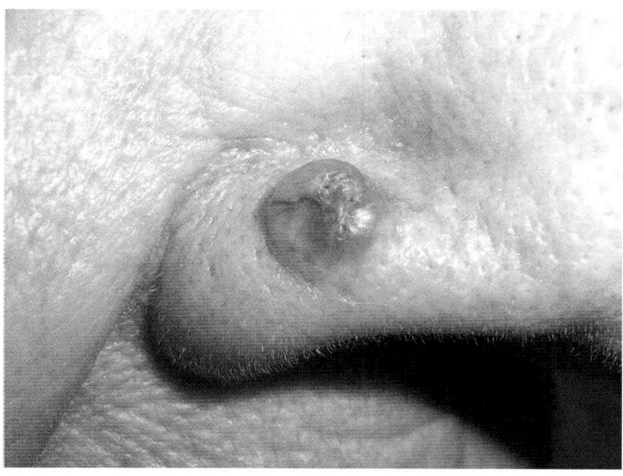

FIGURE 168-2 Nodular basal cell carcinoma (BCC) on the nasal ala of an 82-year-old woman. The nose is a very common location for a BCC. (*Reproduced with permission from Richard P. Usatine, MD.*)

Other clinical variants including pigmented, polypoid, giant, keloidal, linear, and fibroepithelioma of Pinkus have been recognized, but are less common to very rare.[2]

ETIOLOGY AND PATHOPHYSIOLOGY

- BCCs spread locally and very rarely metastasize.
- Basal cell nevus syndrome, also known as Gorlin syndrome, is a rare autosomal dominant condition in which affected individuals have multiple BCCs that may clinically mimic nevi (**Figure 168-9**).

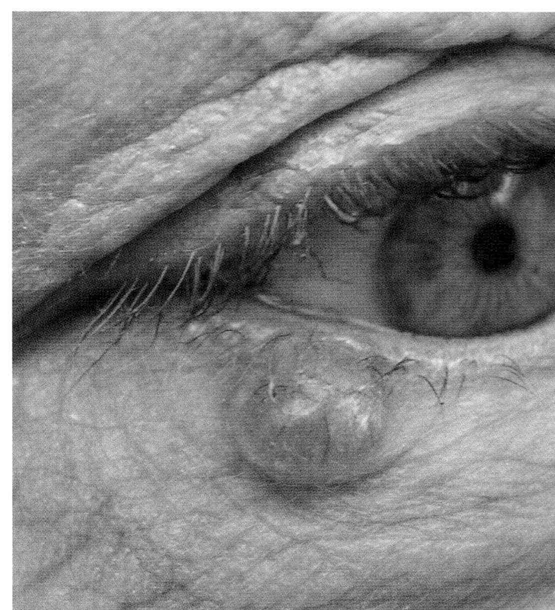

FIGURE 168-3 Nodular basal cell carcinoma (BCC) on the lower eyelid. Patient referred for Mohs surgery. The differential diagnosis is a hidrocystoma. This BCC is a firm nodule and a hidrocystoma is fluid-filled and softer. (*Reproduced with permission from Richard P. Usatine, MD.*)

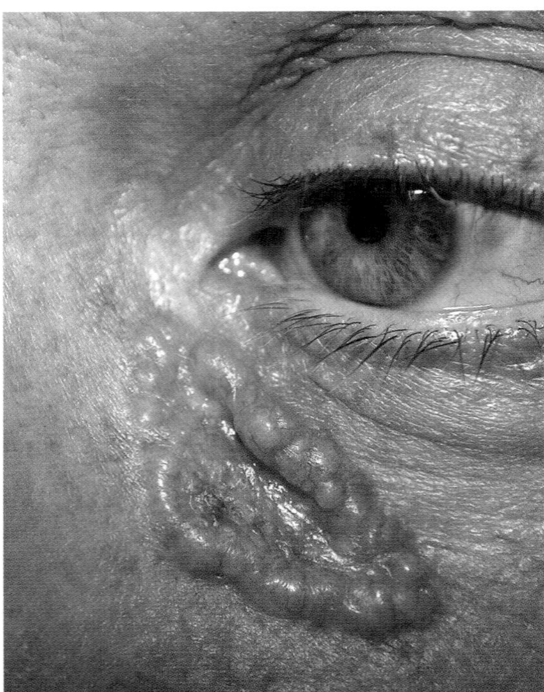

FIGURE 168-4 Large nodular basal cell carcinoma with an annular appearance on the face of a homeless woman. (*Reproduced with permission from Richard P. Usatine, MD.*)

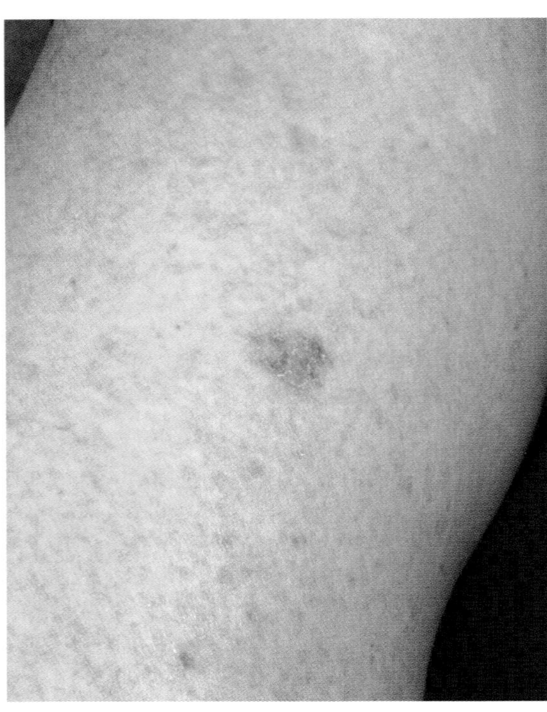

FIGURE 168-6 Superficial basal cell carcinoma on the arm of a fair-skinned welder mimicking nummular eczema. (*Reproduced with permission from Jonathan B. Karnes, MD.*)

RISK FACTORS

- Advanced age
- Cumulative sun exposure
- Radiation exposure
- Latitude
- Immunosuppression
- Genetic predisposition
- Family history
- Skin type[3]

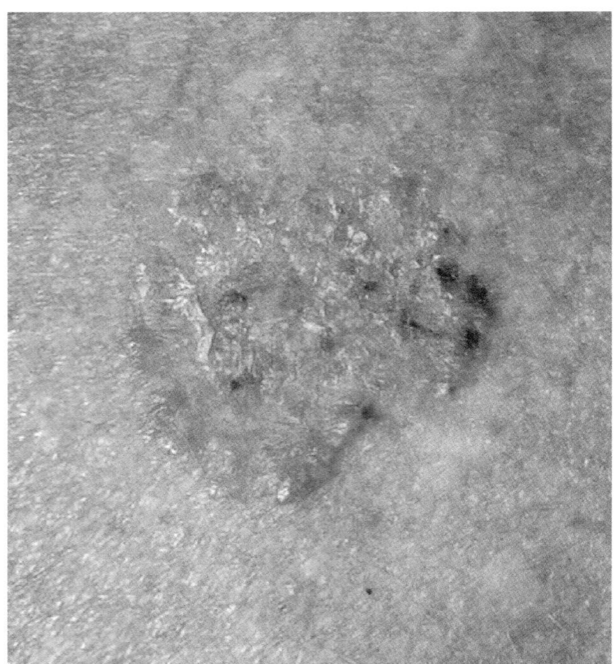

FIGURE 168-5 Superficial basal cell carcinoma on the back of a 45-year-old man who enjoys running in the California sun without his shirt. Note the diffuse scaling, thready border (slightly raised and pearly), and spotty hyperpigmentation. (*Reproduced with permission from Richard P. Usatine, MD.*)

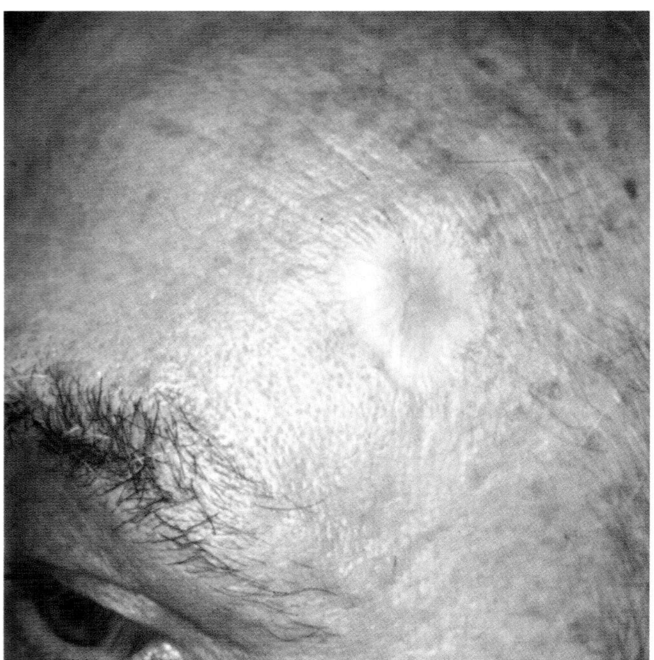

FIGURE 168-7 Sclerosing basal cell carcinoma on the forehead of a man resembling a scar. Note the white color with shiny atrophic skin. (*Reproduced with permission from the Skin Cancer Foundation. For more information www.skincancer.org.*)

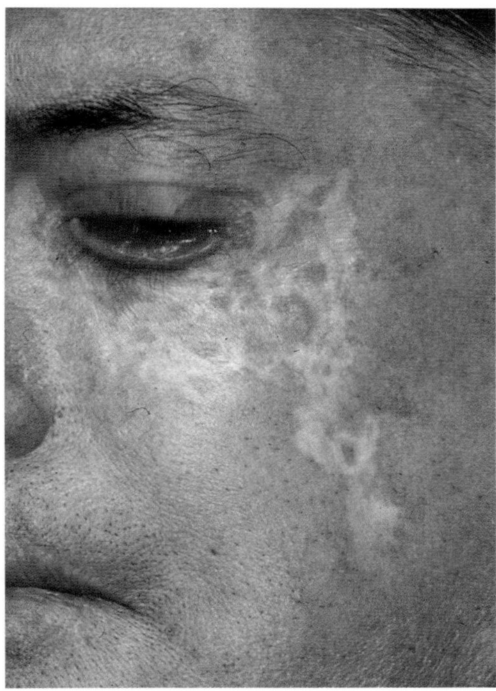

FIGURE 168-8 Advanced sclerosing basal cell carcinoma on the cheek of a man, causing ectropion (the eyelid is being pulled down by the sclerotic skin changes). (*Reproduced with permission from Usatine RP, Moy RL, Tobinick EL, Siegel DM.* Skin Surgery: A Practical Guide. *St. Louis, MO: Mosby; 1998.*)

DIAGNOSIS

CLINICAL FEATURES

Common clinical features of the 3 most common morphologic types are listed below.

Nodular BCC

- Raised pearly white, smooth translucent surface with telangiectasias
- Smooth surface with loss of the normal pore pattern (see **Figures 168-1** to **168-4**)

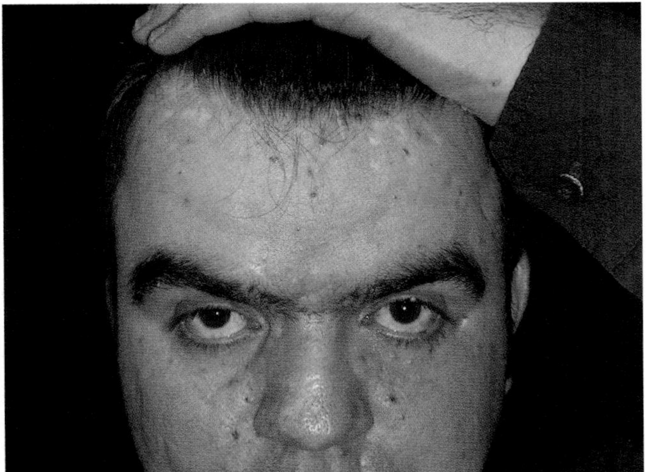

FIGURE 168-9 Basal cell nevus syndrome with over 30 small nevoid basal cell carcinomas on the face of a 29-year-old man. This is a rare autosomal dominant condition. Note the scars from the treatment of previous BCCs and the hypertelorism that is part of the syndrome. (*Reproduced with permission from Richard P. Usatine, MD.*)

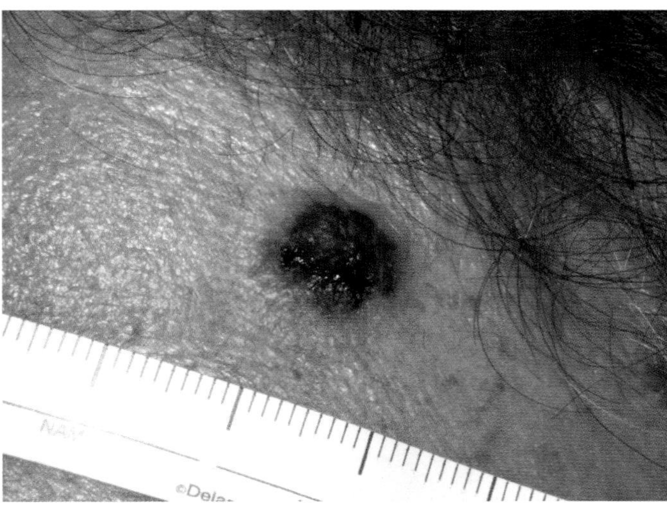

FIGURE 168-10 Large pigmented nodular basal cell carcinoma on the face with ulceration mimicking melanoma. (*Reproduced with permission from Jonathan B. Karnes, MD.*)

- May be moderately to deeply pigmented (**Figures 168-10** to **168-12**)
- May ulcerate (**Figures 168-13** to **168-16**) and can leave a bloody crust

Superficial BCC

- Red or pink patches to plaques often with mild scale and a thready border (slightly raised and pearly) (see **Figure 168-5**)
- Found more commonly on the trunk and upper extremities than the face

Sclerosing (morpheaform)

- Ivory or colorless, flat or atrophic, indurated, may resemble scars, are easily overlooked (see **Figures 168-7** and **168-8**)
- Called morpheaform because of their resemblance to localized scleroderma (morphea)
- The border is not well demarcated and the tumor can spread far beyond what is clinically visible (**Figure 168-17**)
- These BCCs are the most dangerous and have the worst prognosis

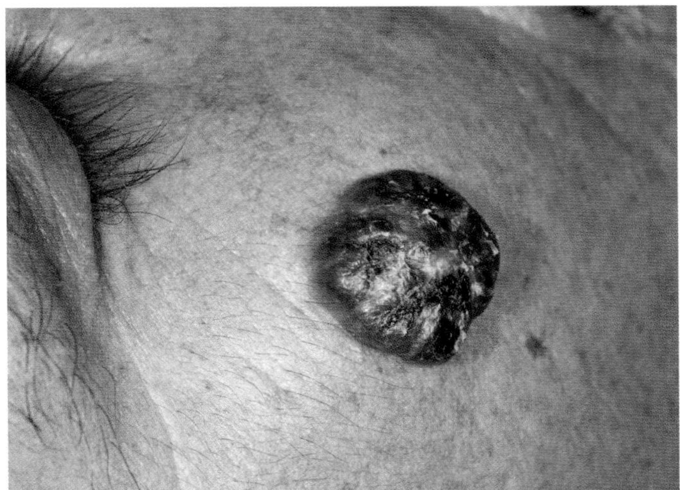

FIGURE 168-11 Darkly pigmented large basal cell carcinoma with raised borders and some ulceration in a 53-year-old Hispanic man. A biopsy was performed to rule out melanoma before this was excised. (*Reproduced with permission from Richard P. Usatine, MD.*)

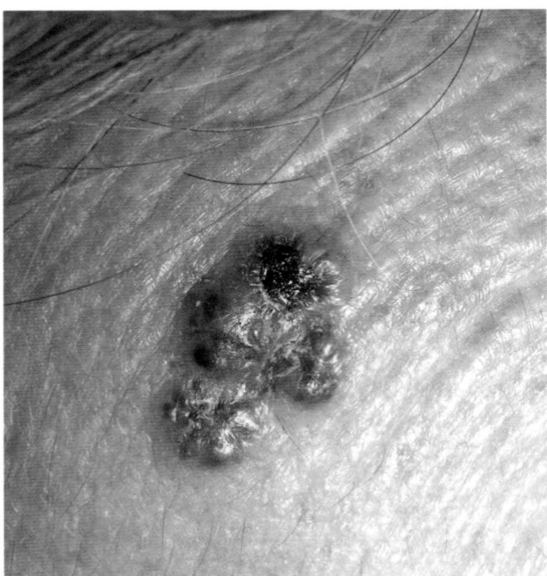

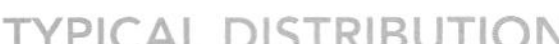
FIGURE 168-12 Darkly pigmented basal cell carcinoma with pearly borders and some ulceration in a 73-year-old Hispanic woman. A biopsy was performed to rule out melanoma before this was excised. (*Reproduced with permission from Richard P. Usatine, MD.*)

TYPICAL DISTRIBUTION

Ninety percent appear on face, ears, and head, with some found on the trunk and upper extremities (especially the superficial type).[1]

Recently lesions on the ears have been associated with a more aggressive behavior (**Figure 168-18**).[4]

DERMOSCOPY

Dermoscopic characteristics of BCCs (**Figures 168-19** and **168-20**) include the following:

- Large blue-gray ovoid nests
- Multiple blue-gray globules
- Leaf-like areas, also called clods, that look like maple leaves
- Spoke-wheel areas

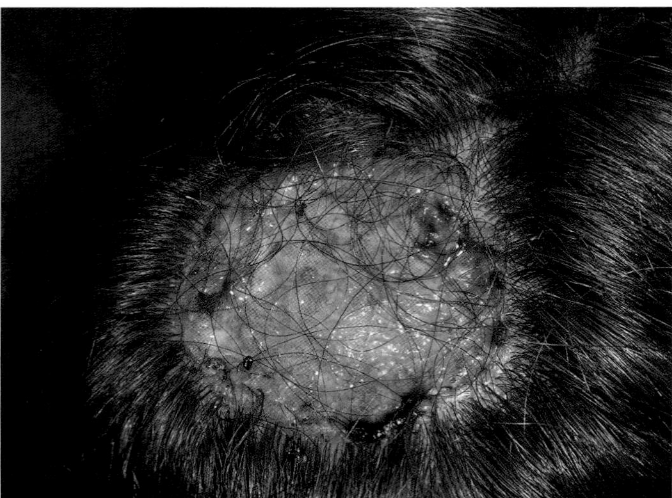
FIGURE 168-13 Ulcerated basal cell carcinoma on the scalp of a 35-year-old woman. (*Reproduced with permission from Richard P. Usatine, MD.*)

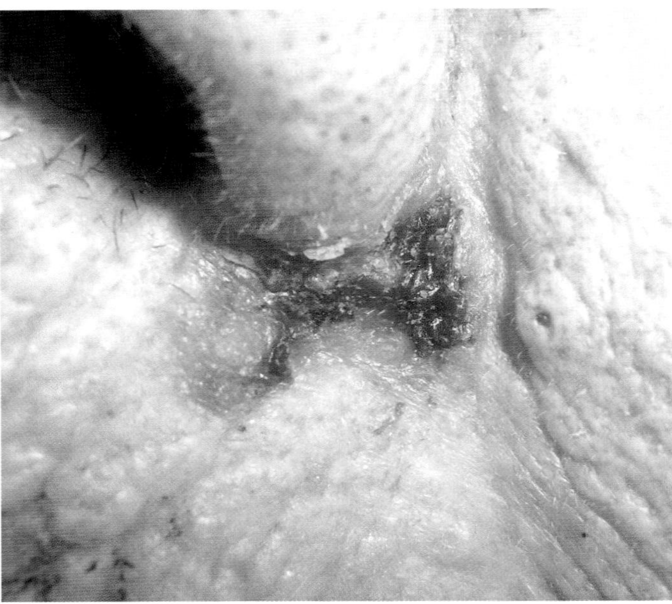
FIGURE 168-14 Basal cell carcinoma in the nasal alar groove. There is a high risk of recurrence at this site so Mohs surgery is indicated for removal. (*Reproduced with permission from Richard P. Usatine, MD.*)

- Arborizing "tree-like" telangiectasia
- Ulceration
- Shiny white areas/stellate streaks (see Appendix C, Dermoscopy for further information)

BIOPSY

- A shave biopsy is adequate to diagnose a nodular BCC or a thick superficial BCC.
- A scoop shave or punch biopsy is preferred for a sclerosing BCC or a very flat superficial BCC.
- In many instances, excision at the time of definitive treatment reveals a different morphologic type in deeper tissue.[5]

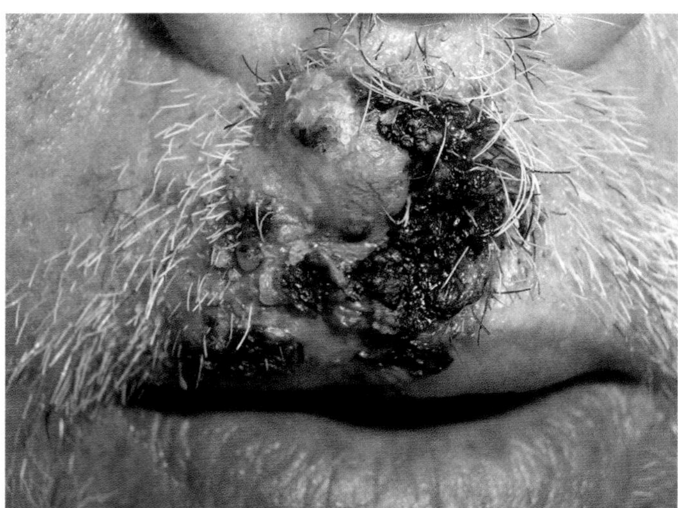
FIGURE 168-15 Large advanced basal cell carcinoma with ulcerations and bloody crusting infiltrating the upper lip. The patient was referred for Mohs surgery. (*Reproduced with permission from Richard P. Usatine, MD.*)

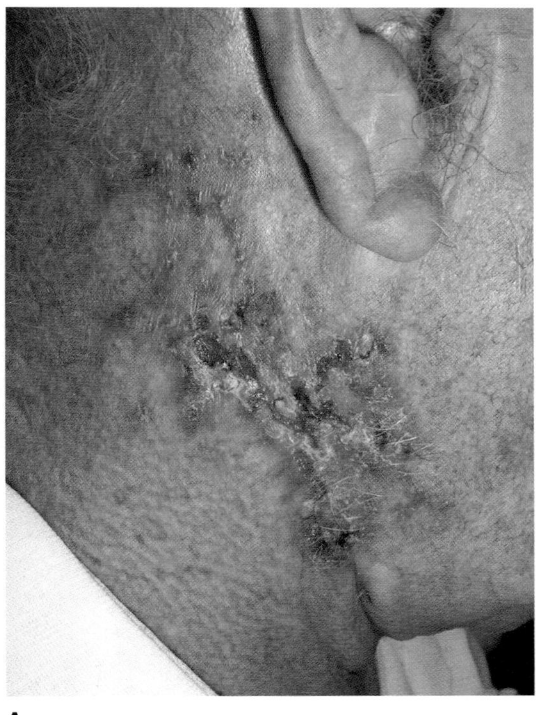

A

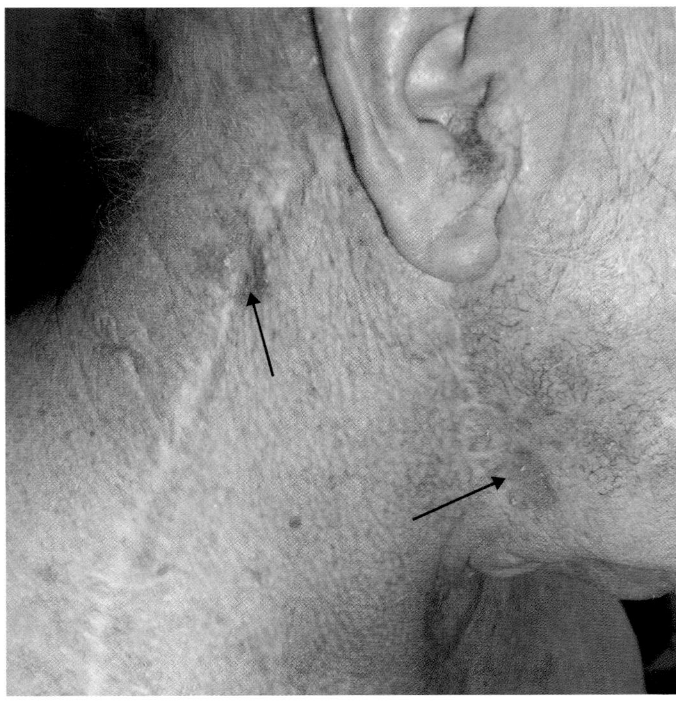

B

FIGURE 168-16 A. Very large ulcerating basal cell carcinoma on the neck of a 65-year-old white man, which has been growing there for 6 years. It was excised in the operating room with a large flap from his chest used to close the big defect. B. The same man showing recurrence within the scar a few years later. (*Reproduced with permission from Richard P. Usatine, MD.*)

DIFFERENTIAL DIAGNOSIS

Nodular BCC

- Intradermal (dermal) nevi may look very similar to nodular BCCs with telangiectasias and smooth pearly borders (**Figure 168-21**). A history of stable size and lack of ulceration may be helpful in distinguishing them from a nodular BCC. A simple shave biopsy is diagnostic and produces a good cosmetic result. Excisional biopsy is usually unnecessary and can be deforming. It is remarkable how similar **Figure 168-21** appears to **Figure 168-1** (both biopsies proven to be as labeled) (see Chapter 160, Benign Nevi).
- Sebaceous hyperplasia is a benign adnexal tumor common on the face in older adults and usually occurs with more than one lesion present (**Figure 168-22**). This benign overgrowth of the sebaceous glands produces small waxy yellow-to-pink papules with telangiectasias. Dermoscopy may show vessels that radiate out from the center like spokes on a wheel (see Chapter 157, Sebaceous Hyperplasia).
- Fibrous papule of the face is a benign condition with small papules that can be firm and pearly.
- Trichoepithelioma/trichoblastoma/trichilemmoma are benign tumors on the face that can appear around the nose. They may be pearly but usually do not have telangiectasias. These are best diagnosed with a shave biopsy, but trichoepitheliomas can even mimic a BCC on histology.
- Keratoacanthoma is a type of squamous cell carcinoma that is raised, nodular, and may be pearly with telangiectasias. A central keratin-filled crater may help to distinguish this from a BCC (see Chapter 165, Keratoacanthoma).

Superficial BCC

- Actinic keratoses are precancers that are flat, pink, and scaly. They lack the pearly and thready border of the superficial BCC (see Chapter 164, Actinic Keratosis and Bowen Disease).
- Bowen disease is a squamous cell carcinoma in situ that appears like a larger thicker actinic keratosis with more distinct well-demarcated borders. It also lacks the pearly and thready border of the superficial BCC (see Chapter 164, Actinic Keratosis and Bowen Disease).
- Nummular eczema can usually be distinguished by its multiple coin-like shapes, transient nature, and rapid response to topical steroids. These lesions are extremely pruritic and most patients will have other signs and symptoms of atopic disease (see Chapter 143, Atopic Dermatitis).
- Discoid lupus erythematosus is a cutaneous manifestation of autoimmune disease and often presents with skin color change, scaling, and hair follicle destruction. These have characteristic predilection for the ears, scalp, and face, but may be found on the trunk and extremities (see Chapter 178, Lupus).
- Benign lichenoid keratosis is a variably scaly, flat, or slightly raised benign reactive neoplasm on sun-damaged skin. It is often on the trunk or extremities and can have blue-gray globules on dermoscopy and some pearly color.

Sclerosing (morpheaform) BCC

Scars may look like a sclerosing BCC. Ask about previous surgeries or trauma to the area. If the so-called scar is flat, shiny, and enlarging, a biopsy still may be needed to rule out a sclerosing BCC.

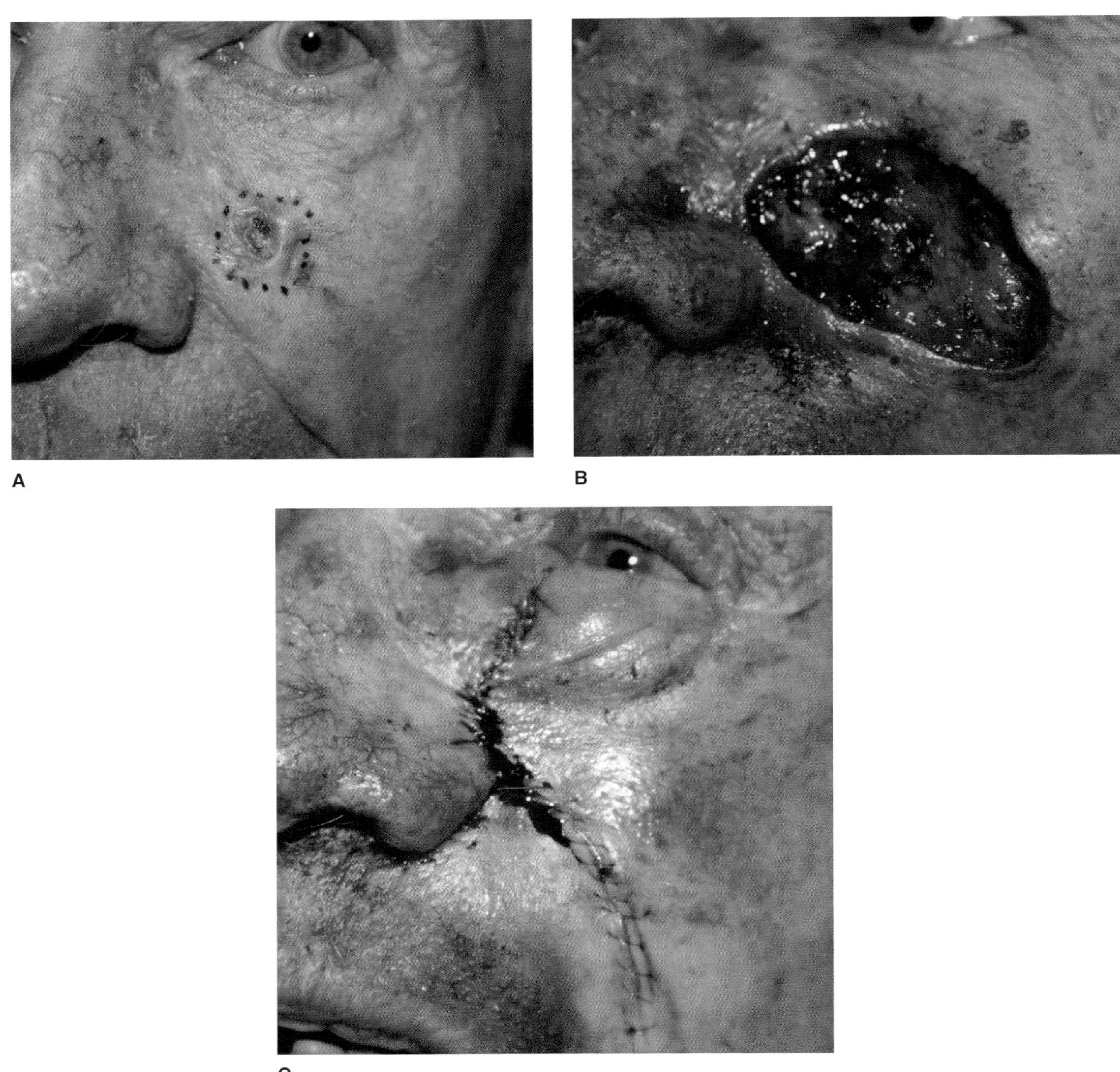

FIGURE 168-17 A. Sclerosing basal cell carcinoma in an elderly man. The size of the basal cell carcinoma did not appear large by clinical examination. B. Mohs surgery of the same sclerosing basal cell carcinoma. This took 4 excisions to get clean margins. Usual 4- to 5-mm margins with an elliptical excision would not have removed the full tumor. C. Repair done close the large defect. The cure rate should be close to 99%. (*Reproduced with permission from Ryan O'Quinn, MD.*)

MANAGEMENT

- Mohs micrographic surgery (3 studies, $N = 2660$) is the gold standard but is not needed for all BCCs. Recurrence rate is 0.8% to 1.1% (see **Figure 168-17B**). Mohs micrographic surgery (pioneered by Dr. Frederick Mohs) entails surgical removal of tumors with immediate histologic processing in sequential horizontal layers preserving a continuous peripheral margin that is mapped to the clinical lesion. Concentric surgical margins are taken until all margins are clear (see **Figure 168-17**). This is the treatment of choice for BCCs with poorly defined clinical margins or in areas of significant cosmetic or functional importance such as the face.[6] SOR A
- Surgical excision (3 studies, $N = 1303$): Recurrence rate was 2% to 8%. Mean cumulative 5-year rate[1] (all 3 studies) was 5.3%. Recommended margins are 4 to 5 mm. SOR A
- Cryosurgery (4 studies, $N = 796$): Recurrence rate was 3% to 4.3%. Cumulative 5-year rate (3 studies) ranged from 0% to 16.5%.[6] SOR A Recommended freeze times are 30 to 60 seconds with a 5-mm halo.

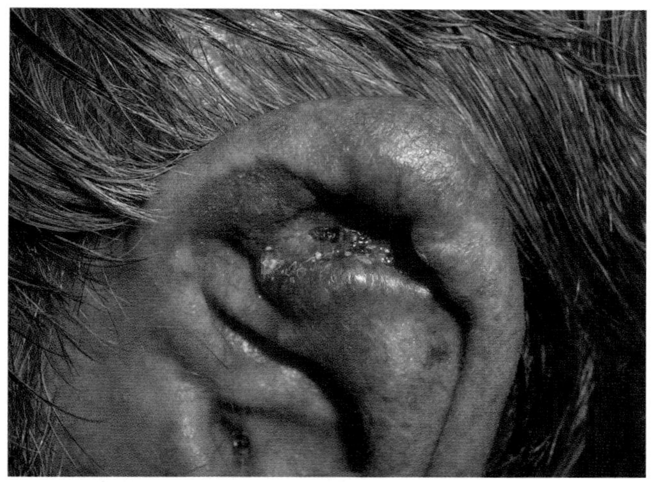

FIGURE 168-18 Ulcerated nodular basal cell carcinoma of the ear in a 67-year-old man. This is an agressive tumor and should be referred for Mohs surgery. (*Reproduced with permission from Richard P. Usatine, MD.*)

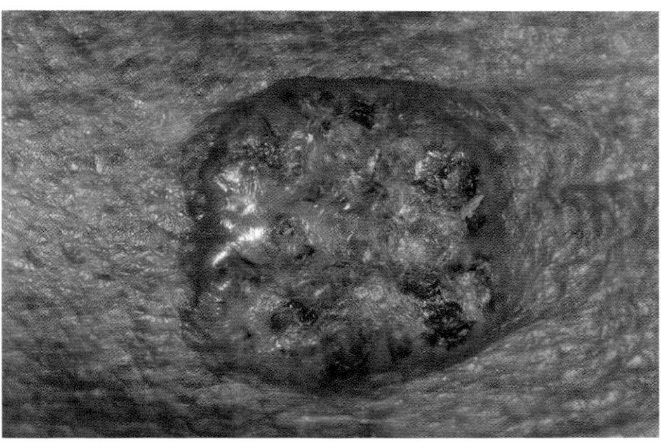

A

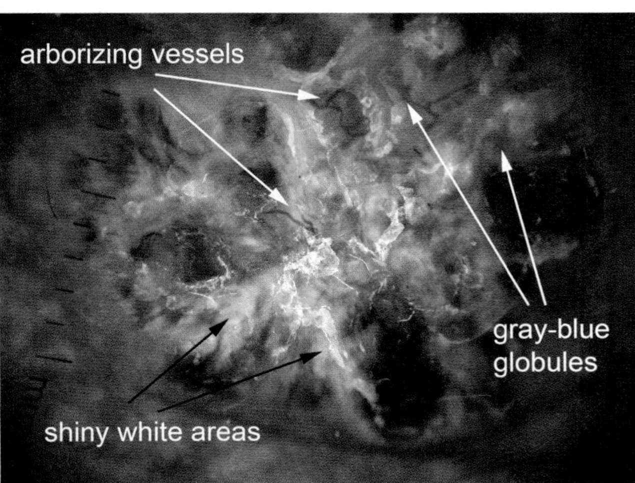

B

FIGURE 168-19 A. Large nodular basal cell carcinoma on the cheek of a 52-year-old man. There is a loss of normal pore pattern, pearly appearance, telangiectasias, and some areas of dark pigmentation. B. Dermoscopy of the nodular basal cell carcinoma. There are visible arborizing "tree-like" telangiectasias, ulcerations, shiny white areas, and gray-blue globules all consistent with a basal cell carcinoma. (*Reproduced with permission from Richard P. Usatine, MD.*)

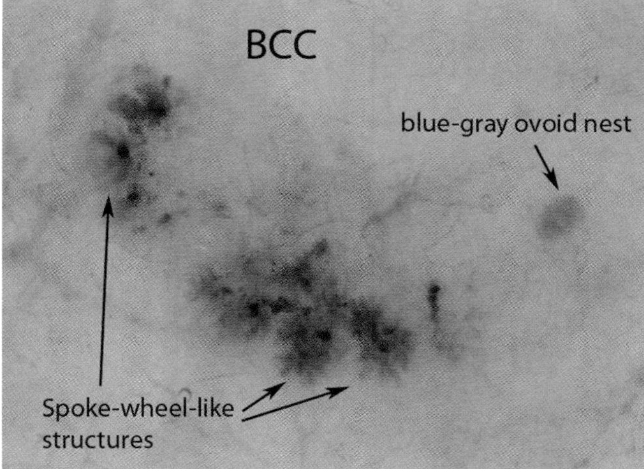

A

B

FIGURE 168-20 Dermoscopy of 2 different basal cell carcinomas. Characteristic findings of basal cell carcinomas include arborized vessels, blue-gray ovoid nests, spoke wheel structures, and leaf-like structures. A. (Reproduced with permission from Ashfaq Marghoob, MD.) B. Note the leaf-like structures on the periphery of this BCC. (*Reproduced with permission from Richard P. Usatine, MD.*)

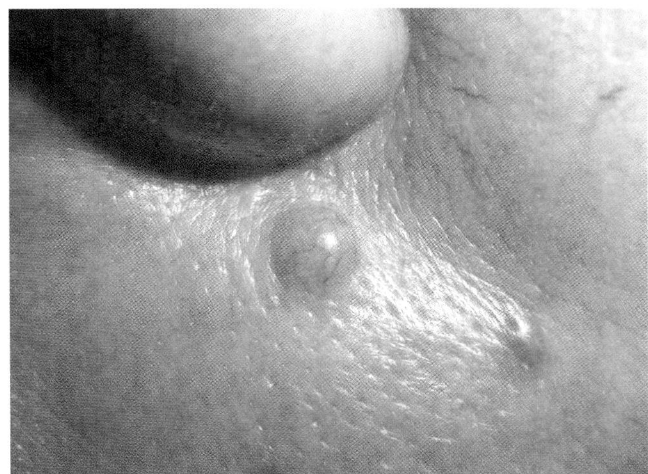

FIGURE 168-21 Pearly dome-shaped intradermal nevus near the nose with telangiectasias closely resembling a basal cell carcinoma. A shave biopsy proved that this was an intradermal nevus. (*Reproduced with permission from Richard P. Usatine, MD.*)

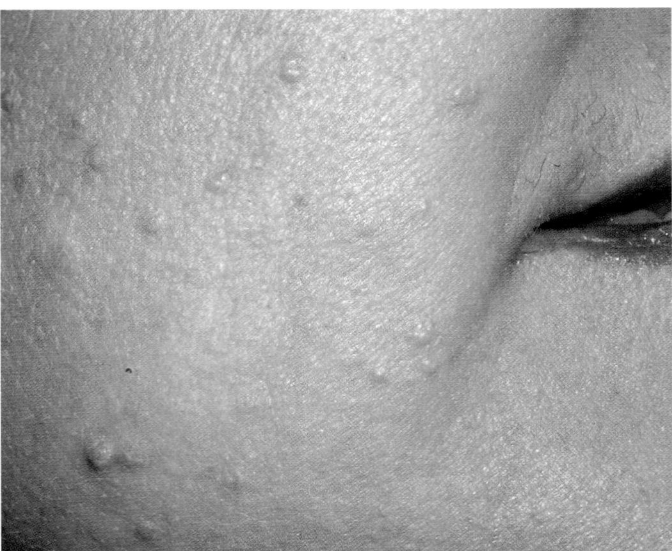

FIGURE 168-22 Extensive sebaceous hyperplasia on the cheek of a 52-year-old woman. The largest one has visible telangiectasias and could be mistaken for a basal cell carcinoma. (*Reproduced with permission from Richard P. Usatine, MD.*)

This can be divided up into two 30-second freezes with a thaw in between. For such long freeze times, most patients will prefer a local anesthetic (**Figure 168-23**). SOR Ⓒ

- Curettage and desiccation (6 studies, $n = 4212$): Recurrence rate ranged from 4.3% to 18.1%; cumulative 5-year rate ranged from 5.7% to 18.8%. Three cycles of curettage and desiccation can produce higher cure rates than 1 cycle (**Figure 168-24**).[6] SOR Ⓐ

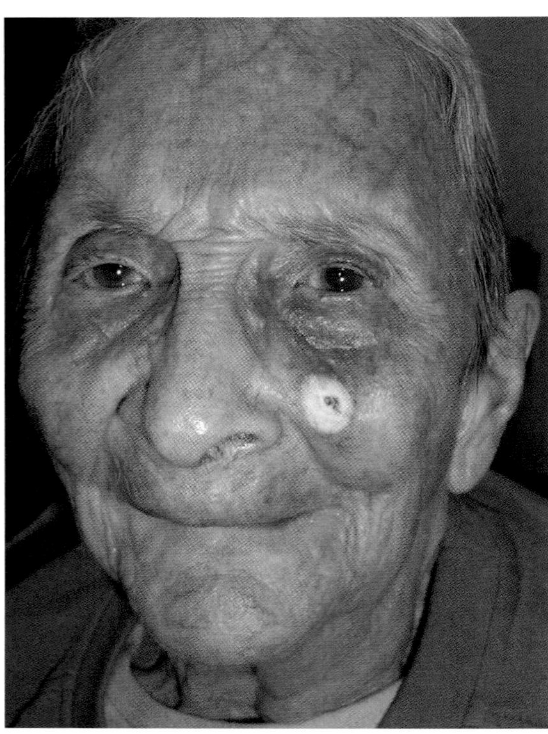

FIGURE 168-23 Cryosurgery was a favored treatment modality in a 94-year-old female patient with Alzheimer dementia with a basal cell carcinoma on the cheek. The family appreciated how easy this was to complete and how well it healed. (*Reproduced with permission from Richard P. Usatine, MD.*)

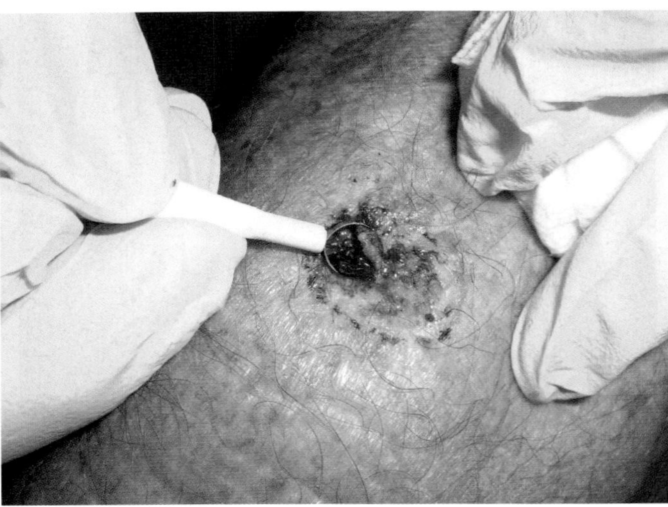

FIGURE 168-24 Curettage and electrodessication of a superficial basal cell carcinoma on the extremity is a rapid and effective treatment. The abnormal tumor tissue is softer than the surrounding normal skin and scoops out easily. (*Reproduced with permission from Richard P. Usatine, MD.*)

- Imiquimod is Food and Drug Administration (FDA) approved for the treatment of superficial BCCs less than 2 cm in diameter.[7] SOR Ⓑ Confirm diagnosis with biopsy and use when surgical methods are contraindicated. A recent study combining cryotherapy with imiquimod improved decreased the recurrence rate.[8]
- Vismodegib is an FDA-approved targeted chemotherapy for the treatment of metastatic or nonresectable BCCs that cannot be treated with radiation. It targets the smoothened pathway, which is damaged in basal cell nevus syndrome and altered in most BCCs.[9] SOR Ⓑ

PREVENTION AND SCREENING

- All skin cancer prevention starts with sun protection.
- Unfortunately there is no proof that sunscreen use prevents BCC.[10]
- Sun protection should include sun avoidance, especially during peak hours of ultraviolet (UV) transmission, and protective clothing.
- US Preventive Services Task Force has not found sufficient evidence to recommend regular screening for any skin cancer in the general population.[11]
- Most experts believe that persons at high risk for BCC (including previous personal history of BCC, high-risk family history, and high-risk skin types with significant sun exposure) should be screened regularly for skin cancer by a physician trained in such screening.
- Evidence for the value of self-screening is lacking but persons at high risk for skin cancer should also be encouraged to observe their own skin and to come in for evaluation if they see any suspicious changes or growths.

PROGNOSIS

The prognosis for BCC is generally excellent with high cure rates with surgery and destructive modalities. Large lesions on the face or lesions that have spread to sites deep to the skin have a poorer prognosis.

FOLLOW-UP

Patients should be seen at least yearly after the diagnosis and treatment of a BCC. The 3-year risk of BCC recurrence after having a single BCC is 44%.[12]

PATIENT EDUCATION

Patients should practice skin cancer prevention by sun-protective behaviors such as avoiding peak sun, covering up, and using sunscreen.

PATIENT RESOURCES

- The Skin Cancer Foundation—**http://www.skincancer.org/skin-cancer-information/basal-cell-carcinoma**
- MedlinePlus. *Basal cell carcinoma*—**http://www.nlm.nih.gov/medlineplus/ency/article/ 000824.htm**
- PubMed Health. *Basal cell carcinoma*—**http://www.ncbi.nlm.nih.gov/pubmedhealth/PMH0001827/**

PROVIDER RESOURCES

- Medscape. *Basal cell carcinoma*—**http://emedicine.medscape.com/article/276624-overview**

Chapters and videos on diagnosing and surgically managing melanoma can be found in the following book/DVD or electronic application:

- Usatine R, Pfenninger J, Stulberg D, Small R. *Dermatologic and Cosmetic Procedures in Office Practice*. Philadelphia, PA: Elsevier, Inc.; 2012.

Information about smartphone and tablet apps of this resource can be viewed at **http://www.usatinemedia.com.**

REFERENCES

1. Ormerod A, Rajpara S, Craig F. Basal cell carcinoma. *Clin Evid (Online)*. 2010;2010:1719.
2. Jackson SM, Nesbitt LT. *Differential Diagnosis for the Dermatologist*. Berlin, Germany: Springer; 2008:1360.
3. Madan V, Hoban P, Strange RC, et al. Genetics and risk factors for basal cell carcinoma. *Br J Dermatol*. 2006;154(suppl 1):5-7.
4. Jarell AD, Mully TW. Basal cell carcinoma on the ear is more likely to be of an aggressive phenotype in both men and women. *J Am Acad Dermatol*. 2012;66(5):780-784.
5. Welsch MJ, Troiani BM, Hale L, et al. Basal cell carcinoma characteristics as predictors of depth of invasion. *J Am Acad Dermatol*. 2012;67(1):47-53.
6. Thissen MR, Neumann MH, Schouten LJ. A systematic review of treatment modalities for primary basal cell carcinomas. *Arch Dermatol*. 1999;135(10):1177-1183.
7. Geisse J, Caro I, Lindholm J, et al. Imiquimod 5% cream for the treatment of superficial basal cell carcinoma: results from two phase III, randomized, vehicle-controlled studies. *J Am Acad Dermatol*. 2004;50(5):722-733.
8. MacFarlane DF, Tal El AK. Cryoimmunotherapy: superficial basal cell cancer and squamous cell carcinoma in situ treated with liquid nitrogen followed by imiquimod. *Arch Dermatol*. 2011;147(11):1326-1327.
9. Hoff Von DD, LoRusso PM, Rudin CM, et al. Inhibition of the hedgehog pathway in advanced basal-cell carcinoma. *N Engl J Med*. 2009;361(12):1164-1172.
10. van der Pols JC, Williams GM, Pandeya N, et al. Prolonged prevention of squamous cell carcinoma of the skin by regular sunscreen use. *Cancer Epidemiol Biomarkers Prev*. 2006;15(12):2546-2548.
11. Wolff T, Tai E, Miller T. *Screening for Skin Cancer: An Update of the Evidence for the U.S. Preventive Services Task Force [Internet]*. Rockville (MD): Agency for Healthcare Research and Quality (US); 2009 Feb. http://www.ncbi.nlm.nih.gov/books/NBK34051/
12. Marcil I, Stern RS. Risk of developing a subsequent nonmelanoma skin cancer in patients with a history of nonmelanoma skin cancer: a critical review of the literature and meta-analysis. *Arch Dermatol*. 2000;136(12):1524-1530.

169 SQUAMOUS CELL CARCINOMA

Jonathan B. Karnes, MD
Richard P. Usatine, MD

PATIENT STORY

A 66-year-old farmer presents with new growths on his scalp (**Figure 169-1**). The patient admits to lots of sun exposure and has already had one squamous cell carcinoma (SCC) excised from the scalp 5 years ago. On close inspection there are many suspicious areas for SCC (see **Figure 169-1**). **Figure 169-2** demonstrates a shave biopsy of a SCC on a scalp using a DermaBlade. The pathology demonstrated that 2 of 3 biopsy sites were positive for SCC (E and G were SCC and F was read as actinic keratoses). The patient was referred for Mohs surgery. The Mohs surgeon recommended field treatment with 5-fluoruracil for 4 weeks before surgery to minimize the amount of cutting that would be needed to clear the SCC from this diffusely sun-damaged scalp.

INTRODUCTION

Cutaneous SCC is the second most common cancer in humans and arises most often as a result of cumulative sun damage. Although the mortality is declining, incidence is increasing in all populations making this cancer a common and significant burden on patients.

EPIDEMIOLOGY

- Mortality from SCC has been observed as 0.29 per 100,000 population.[1]
- Metastasis from SCC occurs in 2% to 9.9% of cases.[2]

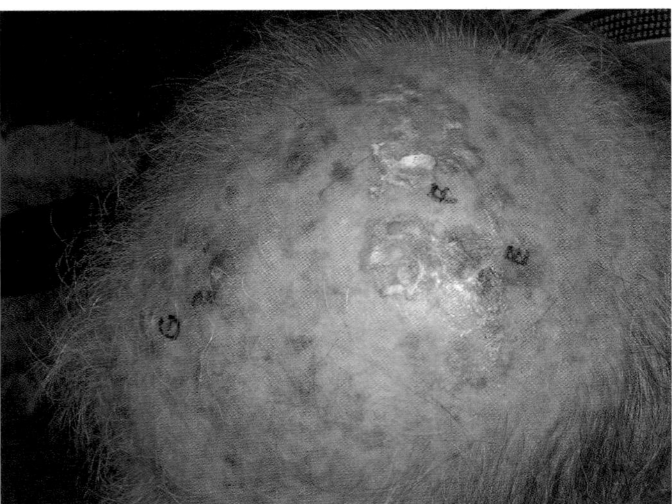

FIGURE 169-1 Multiple squamous cell carcinomas on the scalp of a farmer with a lot of sun exposure. The pathology demonstrated that 2 of 3 biopsy sites were positive for squamous cell carcinoma (E and G were squamous cell carcinomas and F was read as actinic keratosis). *(Reproduced with permission from Richard P. Usatine, MD.)*

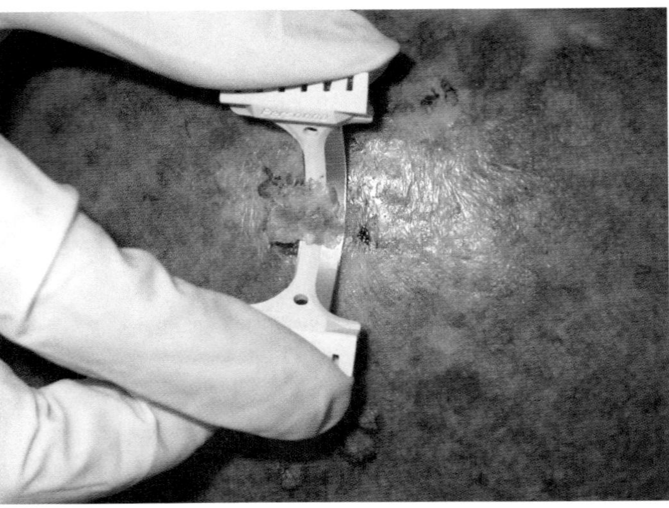

FIGURE 169-2 Shave biopsy of a squamous cell carcinoma on the scalp. *(Reproduced with permission from Richard P. Usatine, MD.)*

- The incidence is increasing in all age groups and populations at a rate of 3% to 10%.[2]
- In the United States, approximately 2500 people die from SCC every year.[3]
- SCC is the second most common skin cancer and accounts for up to 25% of nonmelanoma skin cancers.[4]
- More than 250,000 new cases of invasive SCC are diagnosed annually in the United States.[4]

PATHOPHYSIOLOGY

SCC is a malignant tumor of keratinocytes. Most SCCs arise from precursor lesions called actinic keratoses. SCCs usually spread by local extension but are capable of regional lymph node metastasis and distant metastasis. Human papillomavirus (HPV)-related lesions may be found on the penis, labia, and perianal mucosa, or in the periungual region or elsewhere associated with immunosuppression.[5]

SCCs that metastasize most often start on mucosal surfaces and sites of chronic inflammation.

RISK FACTORS

- Long-term cumulative ultraviolet (UV) exposure is the greatest risk factor.
- Childhood sunburns.
- Occupational exposure.
- Other UV exposure including psoralens plus ultraviolet A (PUVA) therapy and tanning beds.
- Smoking.
- HPV exposure.
- Exposure to ionizing radiation.
- Arsenic exposure.
- Fair skin.
- Age older than 60 years.

- Male gender.
- Living at lower latitude and higher altitude.
- Nonhealing ulcers.
- Chronic or severe immunosuppression, including posttransplant immunosuppression, HIV, and long-term steroid use.
- Genetic syndromes, including Muir Torre, xeroderma pigmentosum, dystrophic epidermolysis bullosa, epidermodysplasia verruciformis, and oculocutaneous albinism.[4]

DIAGNOSIS

The only sure method of making the diagnosis is a biopsy, biopsy suspicious lesions (thickened, tender, indurated, ulcerated, or crusting) especially in sun-exposed areas.

CLINICAL FEATURES

SCC often presents as areas of persistent ulceration, crusting, hyperkeratosis, and erythema, especially on sun-damaged skin.

Less common types of SCC are as below:

- Marjolin ulcer—SCC of the extremities found in chronic skin ulcers or burn scars. This is a more common risk in darker pigmented individuals (**Figure 169-3**).
- Erythroplasia of Queyrat—SCC in situ on the penis or vulva related to HPV infection (**Figure 169-4**). This can progress to invasive SCC of the penis (**Figure 169-5**).

TYPICAL DISTRIBUTION

SCC is found in all sun-exposed areas and on mucus membranes. The most common sites are as follows:

- Face (**Figures 169-6** and **169-7**)
- Lower lip (**Figures 169-8** and **169-9**)
- Ears (**Figure 169-10**)
- Scalp (**Figures 169-1** and **169-11**)
- Extremities—arm—(**Figures 169-12** and **169-13**)
- Hands (**Figure 169-14**)
- Fingers (**Figure 169-15**)
- Mucus membranes (**Figure 169-16**) (see Chapter 39, Oropharyngeal Cancer)

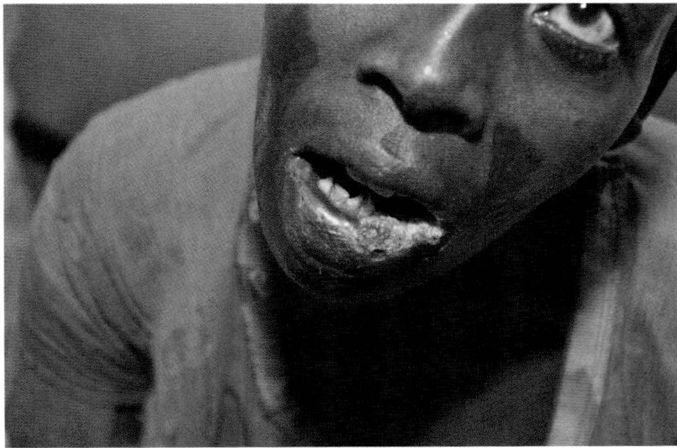

FIGURE 169-3 Marjolin ulcer (squamous cell carcinoma) arising in a burn that occurred years before on the face. (*Reproduced with permission from Richard P Usatine, MD.*)

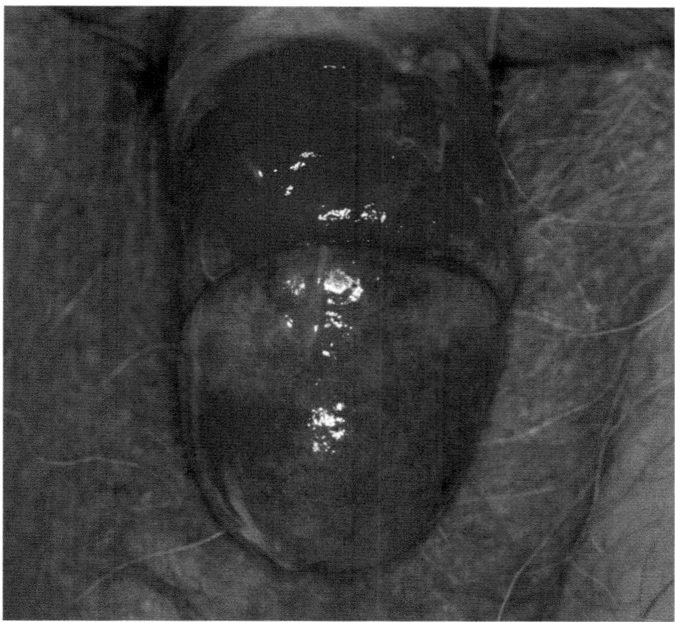

FIGURE 169-4 Erythroplasia of Queyrat (squamous cell carcinoma in situ) under the foreskin of an uncircumcised man. This is related to human papillomavirus infection as is cervical cancer. (*Reproduced with permission from John Pfenninger, MD.*)

BIOPSY

- Deep shave biopsy is adequate to make the diagnosis of most SCCs.
- Punch biopsy or incisional biopsy is an alternative for lesions that are pigmented or appear to be deeper.

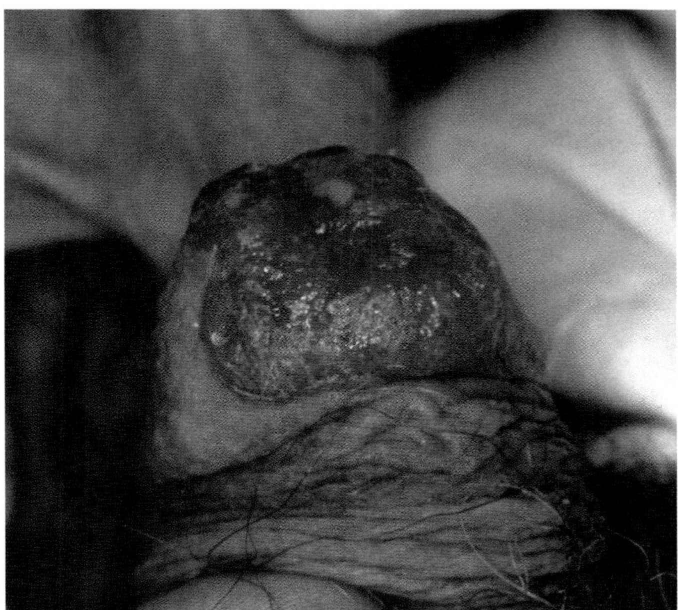

FIGURE 169-5 Squamous cell carcinoma of the glans penis. (*Reproduced with permission from Jeff Meffert, MD.*)

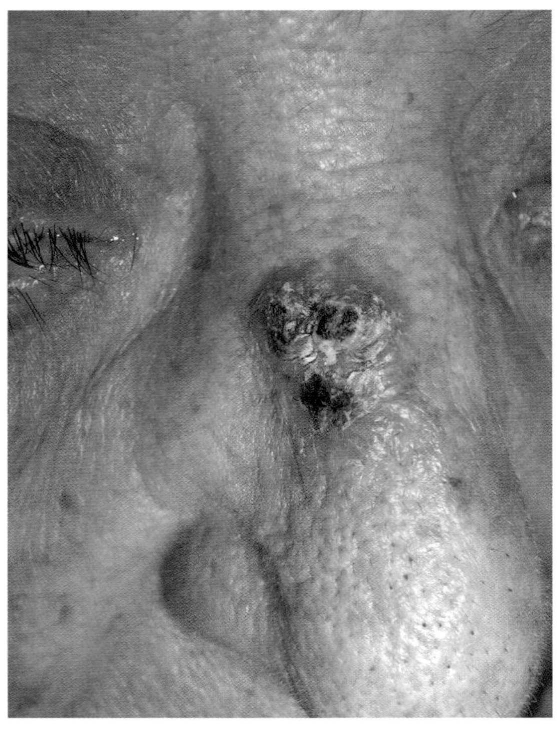

A

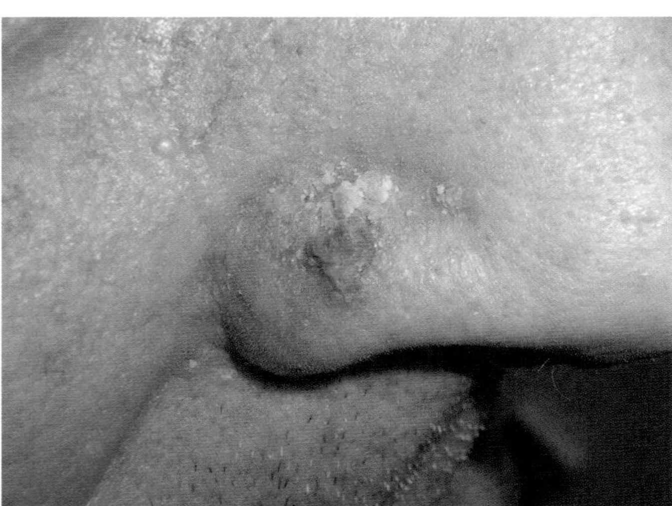

B

FIGURE 169-6 A. Squamous cell carcinoma on the nose of an 88-year-old woman. B. Subtle small squamous cell carcinoma on the nasal alae. Note that any crusting lesion on the face may be a squamous cell carcinoma no matter how small it is. (*Reproduced with permission from Richard P. Usatine, MD.*)

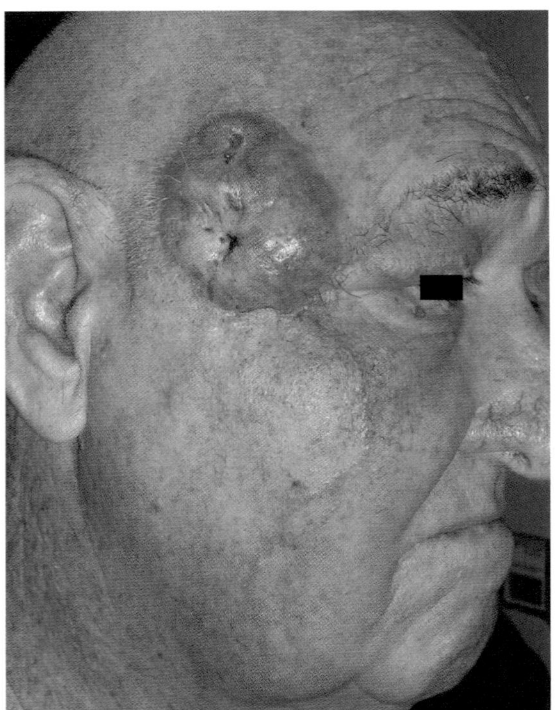

A

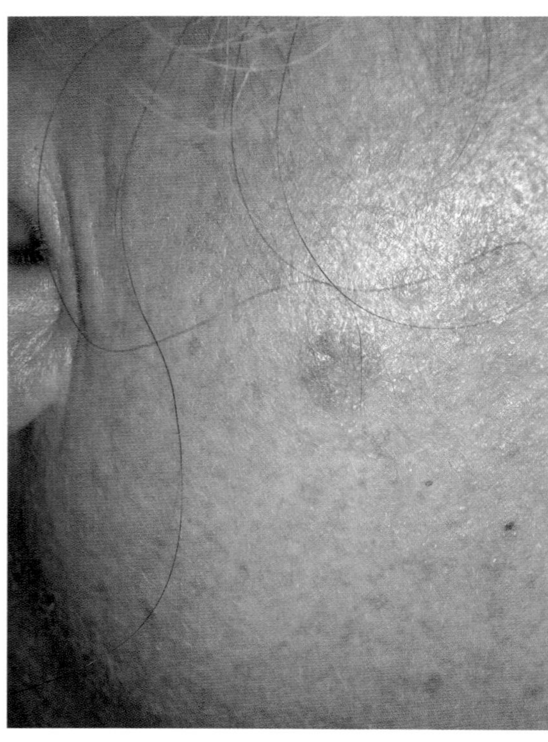

B

FIGURE 169-7 A. Large cystic-appearing squamous cell carcinoma on the face. Although this could have been a basal cell carcinoma, it definitely required a biopsy and excision. B. Small subtle invasive squamous cell carcinoma on the face that could have been overlooked or treated as an actinic keratosis. (*Reproduced with permission from Richard P. Usatine, MD.*)

FACTORS AFFECTING METASTATIC POTENTIAL OF CUTANEOUS SQUAMOUS CELL CARCINOMA

The following factors are taken from "Multiprofessional guidelines for the management of the patient with primary cutaneous squamous cell carcinoma."[6]

SITE

Tumor location influences prognosis: Sites are listed in order of increasing metastatic potential.[2]

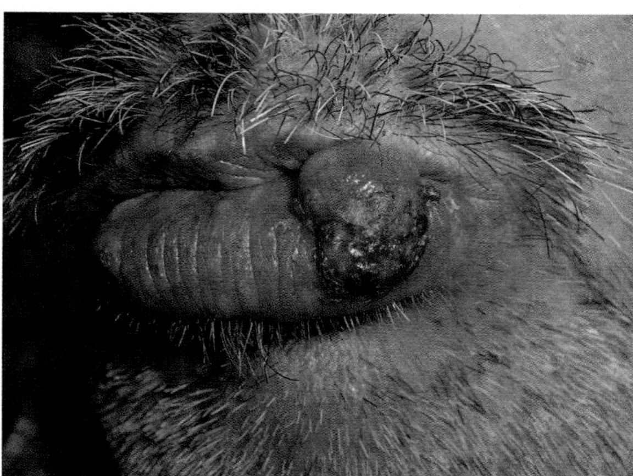

FIGURE 169-8 Squamous cell carcinoma on the lower lip growing rapidly in a patient that was taking an immunosuppressive medication after a renal transplant. (*Reproduced with permission from Richard P. Usatine, MD.*)

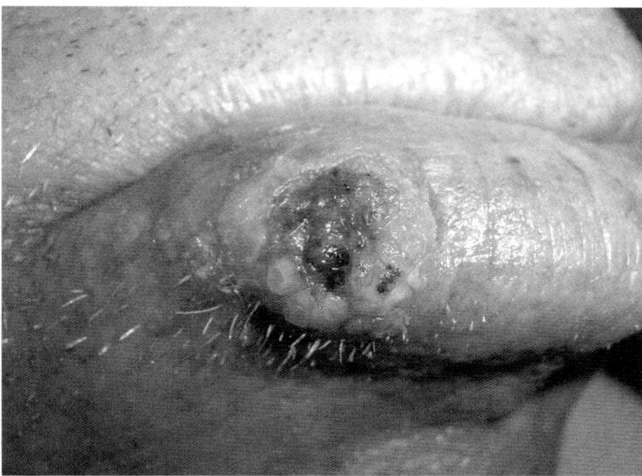

FIGURE 169-9 Squamous cell carcinoma showing ulceration on the lower lip of a man that was a smoker. (*Reproduced with permission from Richard P. Usatine, MD.*)

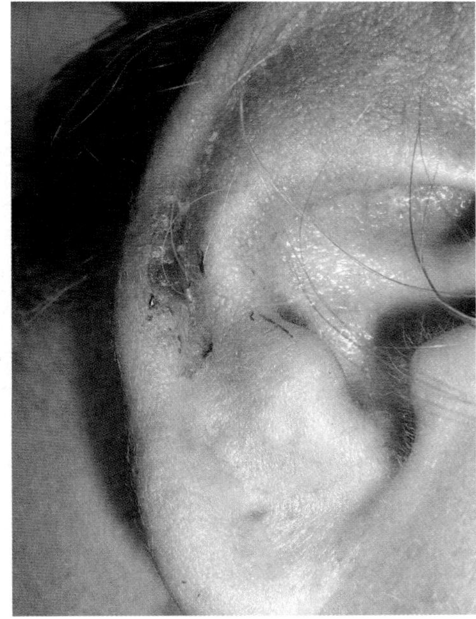

FIGURE 169-10 Squamous cell carcinoma arising in an actinic keratosis on the helix of a 33-year-old woman. (*Reproduced with permission from Richard P. Usatine, MD.*)

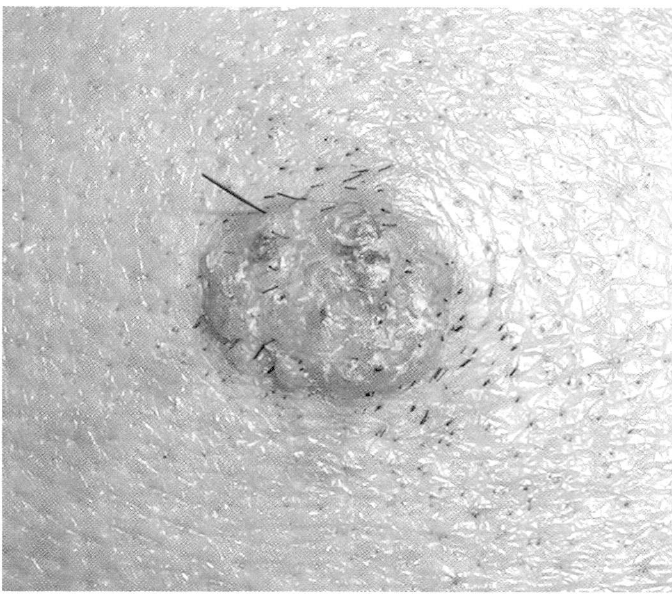

FIGURE 169-11 Squamous cell carcinoma on the shaven scalp of a 35-year-old man, which was formerly mistaken for a wart. (*Reproduced with permission from Richard P. Usatine, MD.*)

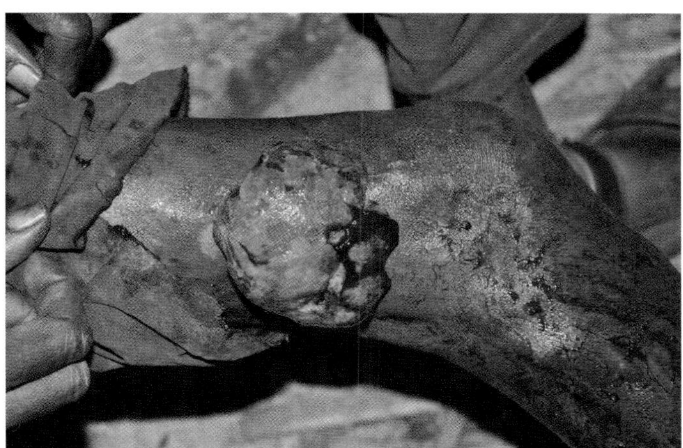

FIGURE 169-12 Large squamous cell carcinoma on the leg of a homeless man. (*Reproduced with permission from Richard P. Usatine, MD.*)

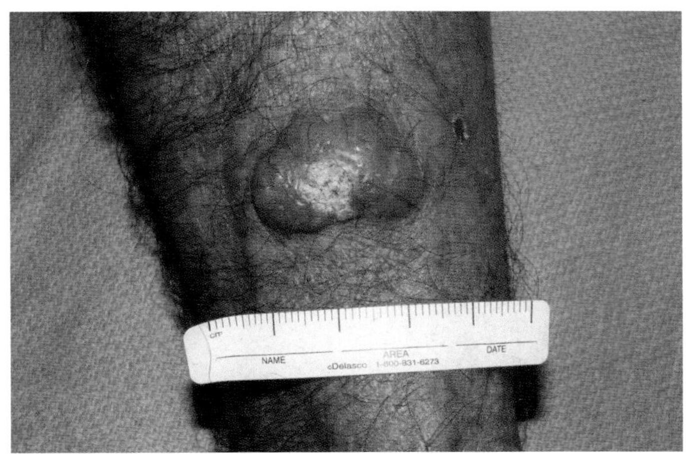

FIGURE 169-13 Three Large ulcerating squamous cell carcinoma on arm. (*Reproduced with permission from Jonathan B. Karnes, MD.*)

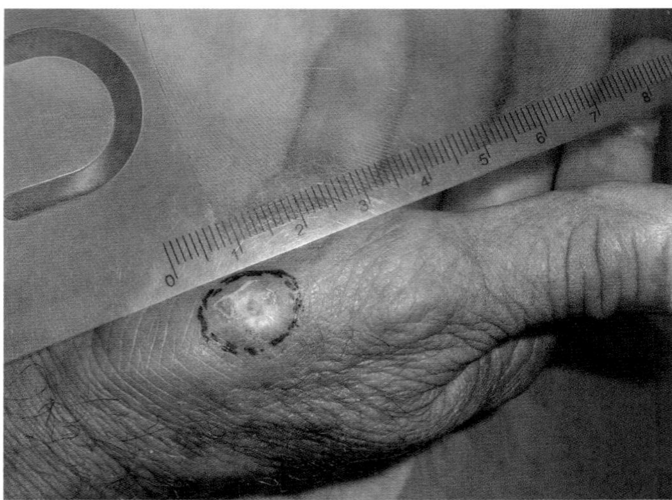

FIGURE 169-14 Squamous cell carcinoma in situ on the thenar eminence of the hand. (*Reproduced with permission from Richard P. Usatine, MD.*)

1. SCC arising at sun-exposed sites excluding lip and ear
2. SCC of the lip (see **Figures 169-8** and **169-9**)
3. SCC of the ear (see **Figure 169-10**)
4. Tumors arising in non–sun-exposed sites (eg, perineum, sacrum, sole of foot) (see **Figures 169-4**, **169-5**, and **169-16**)
5. SCC arising in areas of radiation or thermal injury, chronic draining sinuses, chronic ulcers, chronic inflammation, or Bowen disease, such as the SCC arising in a burn site (see **Figure 169-3**)

SIZE: DIAMETER

Tumors larger than 2 cm in diameter are twice as likely to recur locally (15.2% vs 7.4%), and 3 times as likely to metastasize (30.3% vs 9.1%) as smaller tumors (**Figure 169-17**).

SIZE: DEPTH

Tumors greater than 4 mm in depth (excluding surface layers of keratin) or extending down to the subcutaneous tissue (Clark level V) are more likely to recur and metastasize (metastatic rate 45.7%) compared with thinner tumors. Recurrence and metastases are less likely in tumors confined to the upper half of the dermis and less than 4 mm in depth (metastatic rate 6.7%).

HISTOLOGIC DIFFERENTIATION

Poorly differentiated tumors have a poorer prognosis, with more than double the local recurrence rate and triple the metastatic rate of better differentiated SCC. Tumors with perineural involvement are more likely to recur and to metastasize.

HOST IMMUNOSUPPRESSION

Tumors arising in patients who are immunosuppressed have a poorer prognosis. Host cellular immune response may be important both in determining the local invasiveness of SCC and the host's response to metastases. **Figures 169-16**, **169-17**, and **169-18** are SCCs in patients who are HIV positive.

PREVIOUS TREATMENT AND TREATMENT MODALITY

The risk of local recurrence depends on the treatment modality. Locally recurrent disease itself is a risk factor for metastatic disease. Local recurrence rates are considerably less with Mohs micrographic surgery than with any other treatment modality.

DIFFERENTIAL DIAGNOSIS

- Actinic keratoses are precancers on sun-exposed areas, which can progress to SCC (see Chapter 164, Actinic Keratosis and Bowen Disease).
- Bowen disease is SCC in situ before it invades the basement membrane (see Chapter 164, Actinic Keratosis and Bowen Disease).
- Keratoacanthoma is a subtype of SCC that may resolve spontaneously, but is generally treated as a low-risk SCC. **Figure 169-19** shows an invasive SCC resembling a lower-risk keratoacanthoma subtype (see Chapter 165, Keratoacanthoma).
- Basal cell carcinoma (BCC) cannot always be distinguished from SCC by clinical appearance alone. **Figure 169-17** could be a BCC by appearance but was proven to be SCC by biopsy (see Chapter 168, Basal Cell Carcinoma).

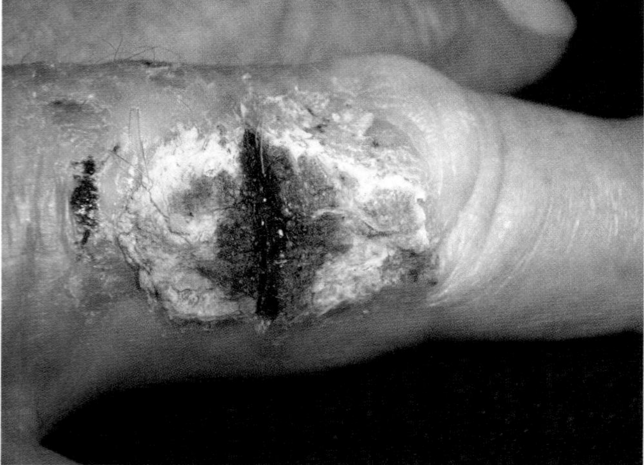

A

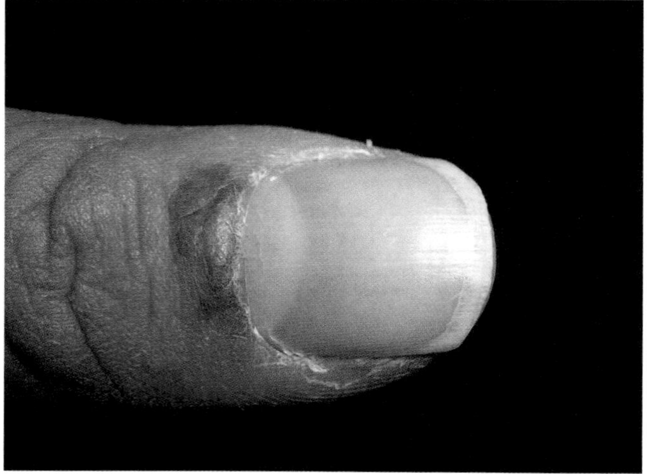

B

FIGURE 169-15 Two different-appearing cases of squamous cell carcinoma on the finger. **A.** It took 2 shave biopsies to establish the correct diagnosis in this case. **B.** Squamous cell carcinoma in situ with human papillomavirus changes and pigment incontinence in a 35-year-old woman. The irregular hyperpigmented lesion on the proximal nailfold was originally suspicious for melanoma. (*Reproduced with permission from Richard P. Usatine, MD.*)

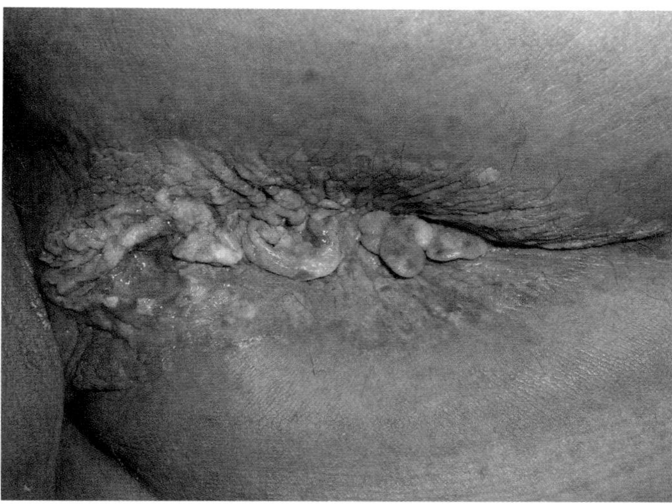

FIGURE 169-16 Perianal invasive squamous cell carcinoma in a HIV-positive man who had engaged in anal intercourse and was infected with human papillomavirus. The ulcerations were suspicious for invasive squamous cell carcinoma and not typical of condyloma acuminata. (*Reproduced with permission from Richard P. Usatine, MD.*)

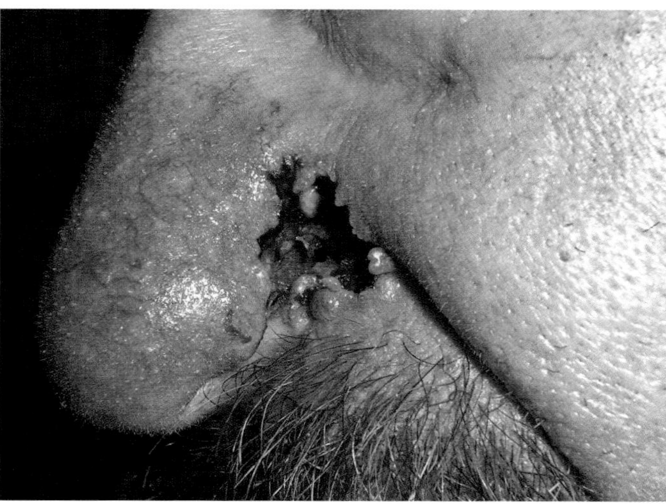

FIGURE 169-18 Squamous cell carcinoma invading the internal nasal structures in a HIV-positive man who was afraid of having a biopsy done earlier. Patient referred to ear, nose, and throat specialist. (*Reproduced with permission from Richard P. Usatine, MD.*)

- Merkel cell carcinoma (neuroendocrine carcinoma of the skin) is a rare aggressive malignancy. It is most commonly seen on the face of white elderly persons. It can resemble a SCC and the diagnosis is made on biopsy (**Figure 169-20**).
- Nummular eczema can usually be distinguished by the multiple coin-like shapes, transient nature, and pruritus (see Chapter 143, Atopic Dermatitis).

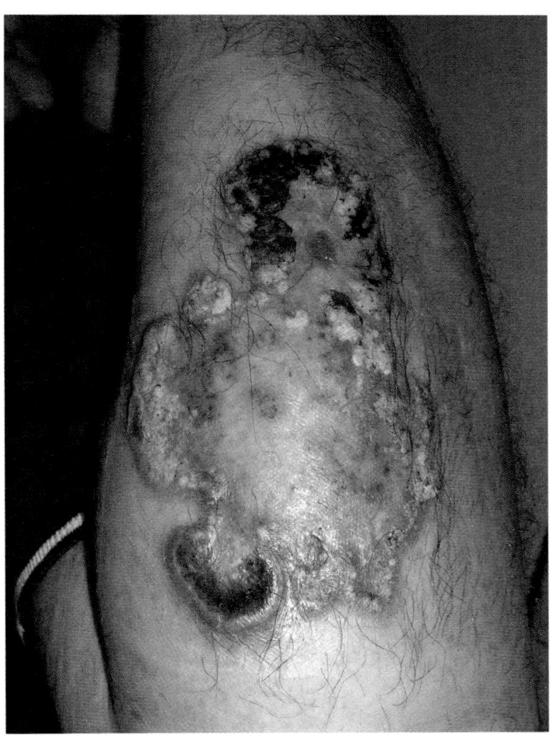

FIGURE 169-17 Large squamous cell carcinoma on the arm of a HIV-positive 51-year-old man. It grew to this size in 1 year and took 2 biopsies to get a definitive diagnosis. Differential diagnosis includes mycosis fungoides. (*Reproduced with permission from Richard P. Usatine, MD.*)

MANAGEMENT

The following recommendations are derived from the "Multiprofessional guidelines for the management of the patient with primary cutaneous SCC." See **Table 169-1** for a summary of treatment options.

Surgical resection for definitive treatment should include margins as given below:

- 4-mm margin—Should be adequate for well-defined, low-risk tumors less than 2 cm in diameter, such margins are expected to remove the primary tumor mass completely in 95% of cases.[5] SOR Ⓐ
- 6-mm margin—Recommended for larger tumors, high-risk tumors, tumors extending into the subcutaneous tissue, and those in high-risk locations (ear, lip, scalp, eyelids, nose).[5]

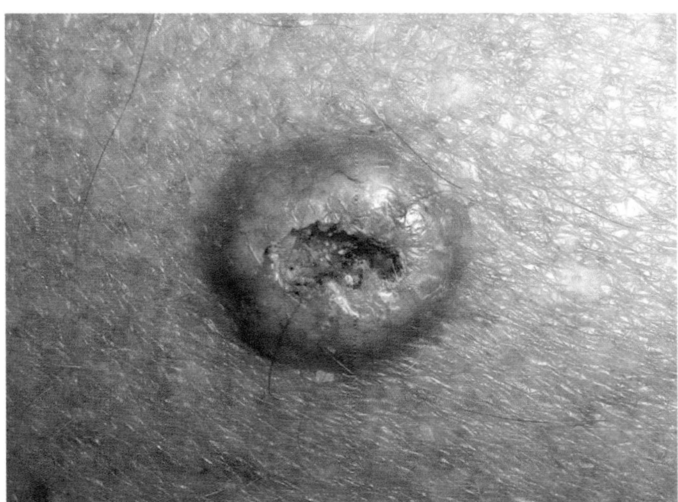

FIGURE 169-19 Squamous cell carcinoma on the shoulder of a HIV-positive man. Note that the pearly borders and telangiectasias resemble a basal cell carcinoma and the central crater suggests that this could be a keratoacanthoma. (*Reproduced with permission from Richard P. Usatine, MD.*)

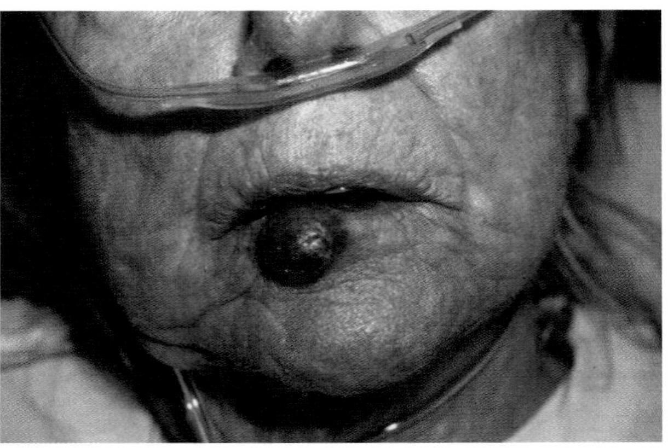

FIGURE 169-20 Merkel cell carcinoma on the lower lip of an elderly woman. This is an aggressive cancer with a high mortality rate. (*Reproduced with permission from Jeff Meffert, MD.*)

MOHS MICROGRAPHIC SURGERY

Frederick Mohs pioneered a technique for excising cutaneous tumors with immediate analysis of a continuous margin mapped to the clinical site. Mohs surgery offers superior cure rates compared with standard excision or destructive techniques, spares uninvolved tissue, and allows for reconstruction at the time of excision.

Mohs surgery may be considered for any continuous tumor, but is specifically indicated for lesions larger than 2 cm, lesions with ill-defined clinical borders, lesions with aggressive histologic subtypes, recurrent lesions, and lesions on or near the eye, nose, ear, mouth, hair-bearing scalp, or chronic ulcers. Patients with chronic immunosuppression or genetic tumor syndromes may also benefit from Mohs surgery compared to standard excision.[4]

CURETTAGE AND ELECTRODESICCATION

Excellent cure rates have been reported in several series, and experience suggests that small (<1 cm), well-differentiated, primary, slow-growing tumors arising on sun-exposed sites can be removed by experienced physicians with electrodessication and curettage (EDC).[5]

The experienced clinician undertaking EDC can detect tumor tissue by its soft consistency, which may be of benefit in identifying invisible tumor extension and ensuring adequate treatment. Electrodesiccation is applied to the curetted wound and the curettage-cautery cycle then repeated twice. SOR C

CRYOSURGERY

Good short-term cure rates have been reported for small, histologically confirmed SCC treated by cryosurgery in experienced hands. Prior biopsy is necessary to establish the diagnosis histologically. There is great variability in the use of liquid nitrogen for cryotherapy. Start by drawing a 4- to 6-mm margin around the SCC and then use a total freeze time of 60 seconds. This can be divided up into two 30-second freezes with a thaw in between. Most patients prefer local anesthetic because these long freeze times are quite painful. SOR C

Cryosurgery and curettage and electrodesiccation are not appropriate for locally recurrent disease.

RADIOTHERAPY

Radiation therapy alone offers short- and long-term cure rates for SCC that is comparable with other treatments. It is recommended for lesions arising on the lip, nasal vestibule (and sometimes the outside of the nose), and ear. Certain very advanced tumors, where surgical morbidity would be unacceptably high, may also be best treated by radiotherapy. SOR C

ELECTIVE PROPHYLACTIC LYMPH NODE DISSECTION

Elective prophylactic lymph node dissection has been proposed for SCC on the lip that is greater than 6 mm in depth and for cutaneous SCC that is greater than 8 mm in depth, but evidence for this is weak. SOR C

PREVENTION AND SCREENING

- All skin cancer prevention starts with sun protection.
- There is good evidence from multiple randomized controlled trials (RCTs) that daily sunscreen use decreases the risk of developing

TABLE 169-1 Summary of Treatment Options for Primary Cutaneous Squamous Cell Carcinoma

Treatment	Indications	Contraindications	Notes
Surgical excision	All resectable tumors	Where surgical morbidity is likely to be unreasonably high	Generally treatment of choice for SCC High-risk tumors need wide margins or histologic margin control
Mohs micrographic surgery/excision with histologic control	High-risk tumors, recurrent tumors	Where surgical morbidity is likely to be unreasonably high	Treatment of choice for high-risk tumors
Radiotherapy	Nonresectable tumors	Where margins are ill defined	
Curettage and cautery	Small, well-defined, low-risk tumors	High-risk tumors	Curettage may be helpful prior to surgical excision
Cryotherapy	Small, well-defined, low-risk tumors	High-risk tumors, recurrent tumors	Only suitable for experienced practitioners

Data from Motley R, Kersey P, Lawrence C. Multiprofessional guidelines for the management of the patient with primary cutaneous squamous cell carcinoma. *BrJ Plast Surg*. 2003;56:85-91.

sun-related SCCs.[7,8] SOR Ⓐ In the longest RCT, sunscreen was applied regularly to the head, neck, hands, and forearms for 4.5 years with a decrease in SCC during the study period.[7] After cessation of the trial, the participants were followed for another 8 years and SCC tumor rates were significantly decreased, by almost 40%, during the entire follow-up period.[8]

- Sun protection should include sun avoidance, especially during peak hours of UV transmission, protective clothing, and sunscreen use.
- Indoor tanning is not safe and should be avoided.
- US Preventive Services Task Force has not found sufficient evidence to recommend regular screening for any skin cancer in the general population.[9]
- Most experts believe that persons at high risk for SCC (including previous personal history of any skin cancer, high-risk family history and high-risk skin types with significant sun exposure, on immunosuppression after an organ transplant) should be screened regularly for skin cancer by a physician trained in such screening.
- Evidence for the value of self-screening is lacking but persons at high risk for skin cancer should also be encouraged to observe their own skin and to come in for evaluation if they see any suspicious changes or growths.

PROGNOSIS

Prognosis is excellent for small, thin lesions less than 2-mm thick that are removed with clear margins in immunocompetent patients. In these patients, the risk of metastasis is near zero. The risk of metastasis increases markedly with thicker lesions and lesions with thicknesses greater than 6 mm metastasize to the regional nodes 16% of the time.[10]

FOLLOW-UP

Patients should be seen at least yearly for skin examinations after the diagnosis and treatment of a SCC. The 3-year risk of recurrence of a new SCC after having a single SCC is 18%.[11]

PATIENT EDUCATION

It includes use of a hat and sunscreen on a regular basis with frequent follow-up for early recognition of new skin cancers.

PATIENT RESOURCES

- The Skin Cancer Foundation. *Squamous Cell Carcinoma*—**http://www.skincancer.org/skin-cancer-information/squamous-cell-carcinoma.**
- PubMed Health. *Squamous Cell Carcinoma*—**http://www.ncbi.nlm.nih.gov/pubmedhealth/PMH0001832/.**
- Skinsight. *Squamous Cell Carcinoma*—**http://www.skinsight.com/adult/squamousCellCarcinomaSCC.htm.**
- MedlinePlus. *Squamous Cell Carcinoma*—**http://www.nlm.nih.gov/medlineplus/ency/article/000829.htm.**

PROVIDER RESOURCES

- Medscape. *Head and Neck Cutaneous Squamous Cell Carcinoma*—**http://emedicine.medscape.com/article/1965430-overview.**
- Skinsight. *INFORMED: Melanoma and Skin Cancer Early Detection*—**http://www.skinsight.com/info/for_professionals/skin-cancer-detection-informed/skin-cancer-education.**
- Chapters and videos on diagnosing and surgically managing SCC can be found in the following book/DVD or electronic app: Usatine R, Pfenninger J, Stulberg D, Small R. *Dermatologic and Cosmetic Procedures in Office Practice*. Philadelphia, PA: Elsevier; 2012.
  - Information about smartphone and tablet apps of this resource can be viewed **at www.usatinemedia.com.**

REFERENCES

1. Lewis KG, Weinstock MA. Nonmelanoma skin cancer mortality (1988-2000): the Rhode Island follow-back study. *Arch Dermatol*. 2004;140(7):837-842.
2. Weinberg AS, Ogle CA, Shim EK. Metastatic cutaneous squamous cell carcinoma: an update. *Dermatol Surg*. 2007;33(8):885-899.
3. American Cancer Society. *Cancer Facts & Figures 2010*. http://www.cancer.org/research/cancerfactsfigures/cancerfactsfigures/cancer-facts-and-figures-2010. Accessed June 1, 2012.
4. Bolognia JL, Jorizzo JL, Schaffer JV. *Dermatology*. 3rd ed. Philadelphia, PA: Saunders; 2012:2776.
5. Berg D, Otley CC. Skin cancer in organ transplant recipients: epidemiology, pathogenesis, and management. *J Am Acad Dermatol*. 2002;47(1):1-17; quiz 18-20.
6. Motley R, Kersey P, Lawrence C. British Association of Dermatologists, British Association of Plastic Surgeons. Multiprofessional guidelines for the management of the patient with primary cutaneous squamous cell carcinoma. *Br J Plast Surg*. 2003;56(2):85-91.
7. Green A, Williams G, Neale R, et al. Daily sunscreen application and betacarotene supplementation in prevention of basal-cell and squamous-cell carcinomas of the skin: a randomised controlled trial. *Lancet*. 1999;354:723-729. Erratum: *Lancet*. 1999;354:1038.
8. van der Pols JC, Williams GM, Pandeya N, Logan V, Green AC. Prolonged prevention of squamous cell carcinoma of the skin by regular sunscreen use. *Cancer Epidemiol Biomarkers Prev*. 2006;15(12):2546-2548.
9. Wolff T, Tai E, Miller T. *Screening for Skin Cancer: An Update of the Evidence for the U.S. Preventive Services Task Force*. Rockville, MD: Agency for Healthcare Research and Quality; 2009. http://www.ncbi.nlm.nih.gov/books/NBK34051/.
10. Brantsch KD, Meisner C, Schönfisch B, et al. Analysis of risk factors determining prognosis of cutaneous squamous-cell carcinoma: a prospective study. *Lancet Oncol*. 2008;9(8):713-720.
11. Marcil I, Stern RS. Risk of developing a subsequent nonmelanoma skin cancer in patients with a history of nonmelanoma skin cancer: a critical review of the literature and metaanalysis. *Arch Dermatol*. 2000;136(12):1524-1530.

170 MELANOMA

Jonathan B. Karnes, MD
Richard P. Usatine, MD

PATIENT STORIES

A 40-year-old woman noticed a new dark spot on her neck (**Figure 170-1**). On examination the spot was 8 mm in its longest diameter, was asymmetrical with irregular borders, and had variation in color. A scoop shave biopsy demonstrated melanoma in situ. The spot was excised with 0.5-cm margins and no residual tumor was found in the excised ellipse. She has a near 100% chance of complete cure.

The wife of a 73-year-old man noticed that a "mole" on his back was enlarging and bleeding. (**Figure 170-2**). It had been there for years. Even though a year earlier a doctor had told him not to worry about it, his wife sent him to have it rechecked. **Figure 170-2B** shows a close-up of the pigmented lesion showing ulceration and bleeding. An elliptical excision was performed and the tissue appeared to be a nodular melanoma with dark pigment into the subcutaneous fat (**Figure 170-2C**). Histology revealed a nodular melanoma with a Breslow depth of 22 mm. The patient was referred to surgical and medical oncology. He underwent wide excision with 2-cm margins and a sentinel lymph node biopsy. The sentinel node was positive and further nodal dissection showed a total of another 4 axillary lymph nodes positive (1 on right and 3 on left). The lymph nodes on the left were black and enlarged. No distant metastases were found. Because more than 2 regional nodes were macroscopically positive, he was stage IIIC. He received radiation treatment to the original site and both axillae. Despite advances in targeted chemotherapy and immunotherapy, his prognosis was poor.

INTRODUCTION

Melanoma is the third most common skin cancer and the most deadly. The incidence of melanoma and the mortality from it are rising. Most lesions are found by clinicians on routine examination. When discovered early,

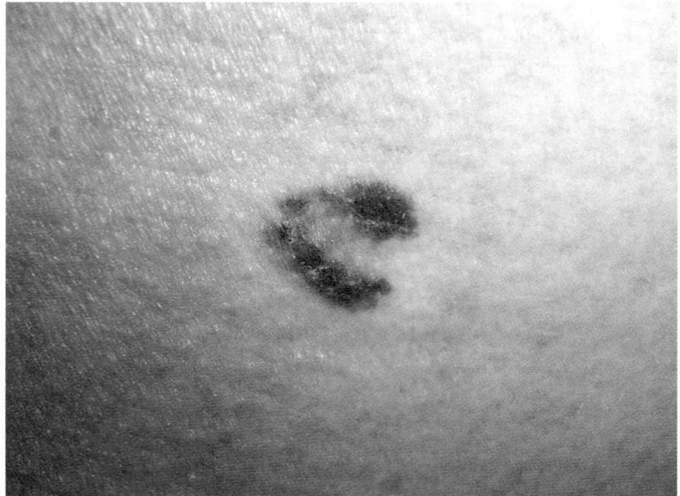

FIGURE 170-1 Melanoma in situ on the neck of a 40-year-old woman. Note the central regression. (*Reproduced with permission from Richard P. Usatine, MD.*)

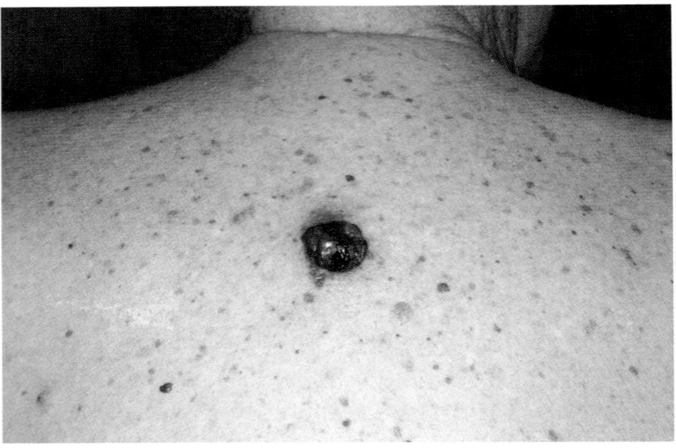

A

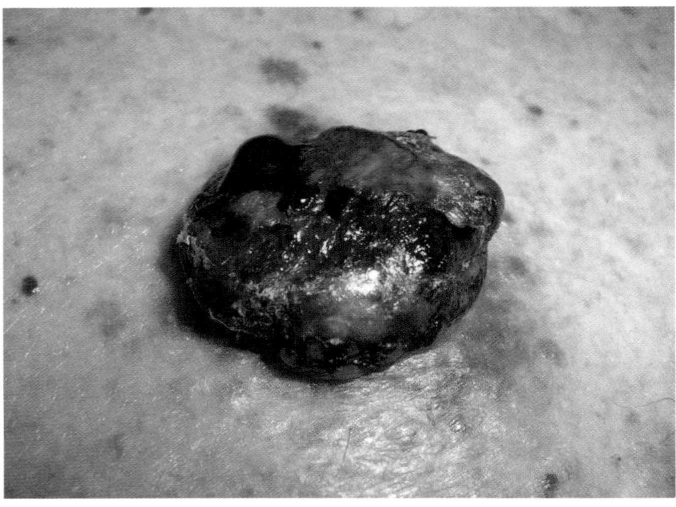

B

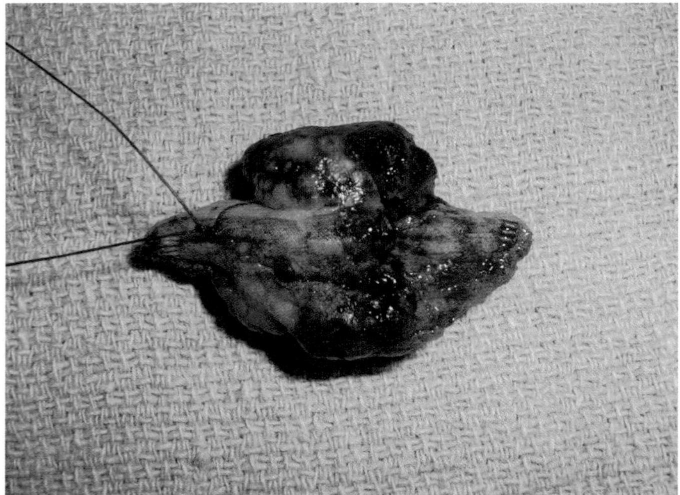

C

FIGURE 170-2 **A.** A 73-year-old man presents with bleeding "mole" on his back. Elliptical excision demonstrates this to be a nodular melanoma of 22-mm depth. **B.** Close-up of the nodular melanoma showing it to be thick with ulcerations and bleeding. C. Nodular melanoma after initial resection showing dark pigment into the subcutaneous fat. The Breslow depth is 22 mm with Clark level V. (*Reproduced with permission from Richard P. Usatine, MD.*)

surgical treatment is almost always curative. However, deeper lesions are prone to metastasize and have a much poorer prognosis. New therapies directed at the known gene changes in melanoma are beginning to show some promise, but widespread benefits of this research are still far off.

EPIDEMIOLOGY

- In 2012, an estimated 76,250 individuals will be diagnosed with melanoma of the skin and 9180 individuals will die from metastatic disease—or about 1 every hour.[1]
- Melanoma incidence has increased in every age group and in every thickness over the course of 1992 to 2006 among non-Hispanic whites, with death rates increasing in those older than age 65 years.[2]
- Incidence continues to increase worldwide at approximately 4% to 8% per year.[3]
- In the United States, the death rate for melanoma is decreasing among persons younger than age 65 years.[2]
- Deaths from thin melanomas account for more than 30% of total deaths.
- The lifetime risk of developing melanoma is 1 in 55 for men and 1 in 36 for women.[1]

RISK FACTORS

Risk factors can be broadly thought of as genetic risks, environmental risks, and phenotypic risks arising from a combination of genetic and environmental risks. For example, a fair-skinned child (genetic risk) who gets a sunburn (environmental) is much more likely to develop freckles (phenotypic) and melanoma.

ENVIRONMENTAL RISKS

- Exposure to sunlight
    - History of sunburn doubles the risk of melanoma and is worse at a young age.
- Living closer to the equator
- Indoor tanning
- History of immunosuppression
- Higher socioeconomic status (likely associated with more frequent opportunity for sunburns)

GENETIC RISKS

- Fair skin, blue or green eyes, red or blonde hair
- Male sex
- Melanoma in a first-degree relative
- History of xeroderma pigmentosa or familial atypical mole melanoma syndrome

PHENOTYPIC RISKS

- Many nevi
- Multiple dysplastic nevi
- Increased age
- Personal history of any skin cancer

DIAGNOSIS

CLINICAL FEATURES

Remember the *ABCDE* guidelines for diagnosing melanoma (**Figure 170-3**).[4]

A = *Asymmetry*. Most early melanomas are asymmetrical: A line through the middle will not create matching halves. Benign nevi are usually round and symmetrical.

B = *Border*. The borders of early melanomas are often uneven and may have scalloped or notched edges. Benign nevi have smoother, more even borders.

C = *Color* variation. Benign nevi are usually a single shade of brown. Melanomas are often in varied shades of brown, tan, or black, but may also exhibit red, white, or blue.

D = *Diameter* greater than or equal to 6 mm. Early melanomas tend to grow larger than most nevi. (Note: Congenital nevi are often large.)

E = *Evolving*. Any evolving or enlarging nevus should make you suspect melanoma. Evolving could be in size, shape, symptoms (itching, tenderness), surface (especially bleeding), and shades of color.

- A prospective controlled study compared 460 cases of melanoma with 680 cases of benign pigmented tumors and found significant differences for all individual ABCDE criteria ($p < 0.001$) between melanomas and benign nevi.[4]
- Sensitivity of each criterion: A 57%, B 57%, C 65%, D 90%, E 84%; specificity of each criterion: A 72%, B 71%, C 59%, D 63%, E 90%.[4]
- Sensitivity of ABCDE criteria varies depending on the number of criteria needed: Using 2 criteria it was 89.3%, with 3 criteria, it was 65.5%. Specificity was 65.3% using 2 criteria and 81% using 3.[4]
- The number of criteria present was different between benign nevi (1.24 ± 1.26) and melanomas (3.53 ± 1.53; $p < 0.001$). Unfortunately, no significant difference was found between melanomas and atypical nevi.[4]

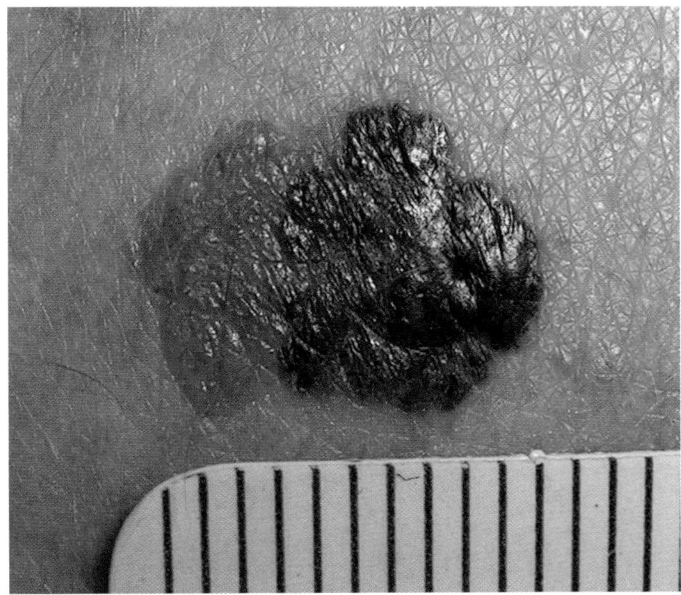

FIGURE 170-3 Superficial spreading melanoma on the back with ABCDE features of melanoma. (*Reproduced with permission from Richard P. Usatine, MD.*)

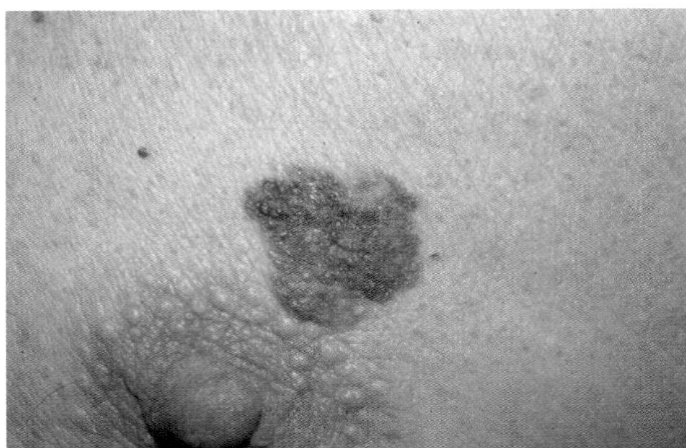

FIGURE 170-4 Superficial spreading melanoma near the areola. It is important not to mistake this for a seborrheic keratosis. Note the area of pigment regression near the top of the lesion. (*Reproduced with permission from the University of Texas Health Sciences Center, Division of Dermatology.*)

There are 4 major categories of melanomas. With the exception of nodular melanoma, the growth patterns of the 3 other subtypes are characterized by a radial growth phase prior to dermal invasion. At the present time, the thickness of the lesion histologically regardless of the morphologic type is used to stage the tumor and assess prognosis. In the future, molecular analysis may allow more accurate risk stratification.[5] Here are the major categories of melanomas:

1. *Superficial spreading melanoma* is the most common type, representing 70% of all melanoma (**Figures 170-3** to **170-6**). This melanoma has the radial growth pattern before dermal invasion occurs. The first sign is the appearance of a flat macule or slightly raised discolored plaque that has irregular borders and is somewhat geometrical in form. The color varies, with areas of tan, brown, black, red, blue, or white. These lesions can arise in an older nevus. The melanoma can be seen almost anywhere on the body, but is most likely to occur on the trunk in men, the legs in women, and the upper back in both. Most melanomas found in the young are of the superficial spreading type.[5]
2. *Nodular melanoma* occurs in 15% to 30% of cases (**Figures 170-2**, **170-7** to **170-9**).[5] It is usually invasive at the time it is first diagnosed, and the malignancy is recognized when it becomes a bump. The color is most often black, but occasionally is blue, gray, white, brown, tan, red, or nonpigmented. The nodule in **Figure 170-9** is multicolored.
3. *Lentigo maligna melanoma* occurs in 4% to 15% of cutaneous melanoma.[4] It is similar to the superficial spreading type and appears as a flat or mildly elevated mottled tan, brown, or dark brown discoloration. This type of melanoma is found most often in the elderly and arises on chronically sun-exposed, damaged skin on the face, ears, arms, and upper trunk. These account for most melanomas on the face. The average age of onset is 65 years and it grows slowly over 5 to 20 years. The precursor lesion, lentigo maligna, goes on to melanoma in approximately 5% of cases. The in situ precursor lesion is usually larger than 3 cm in diameter and has existed for a minimum of 10 to 15 years (**Figures 170-10** and **170-11**) (see Chapter 166, Lentigo Maligna).[5]
4. *Acral lentiginous melanoma* is the least common subtype of melanoma (2%-8%) cases in white people; however, it is the most frequent subtype found in African Americans (70%) and is also a frequent subtype in Asians (45%).[5] It may occur under the nail plate or on the soles or palms (**Figures 170-12** to **170-16**). This subtype often carries a worse prognosis because of delays in diagnosis. Subungual melanoma may manifest as diffuse nail discoloration or a longitudinal pigmented band within the nail plate. When subungual pigment spreads to the

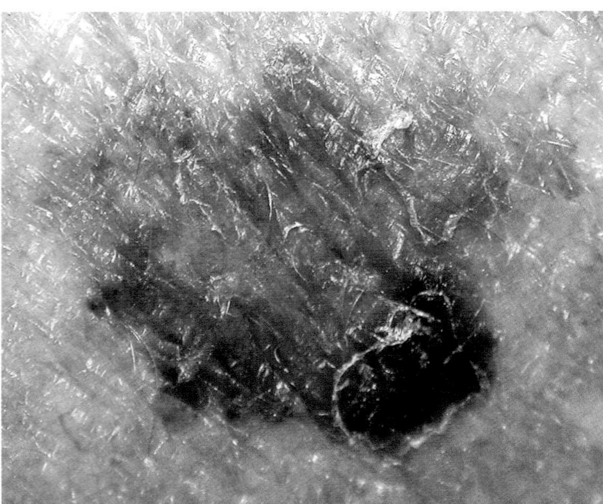

FIGURE 170-5 Superficial spreading melanoma on the arm with depth of 0.25 mm. Note the pale pink coloration along with the black area with some erosion. (*Reproduced with permission from Eric Kraus, MD.*)

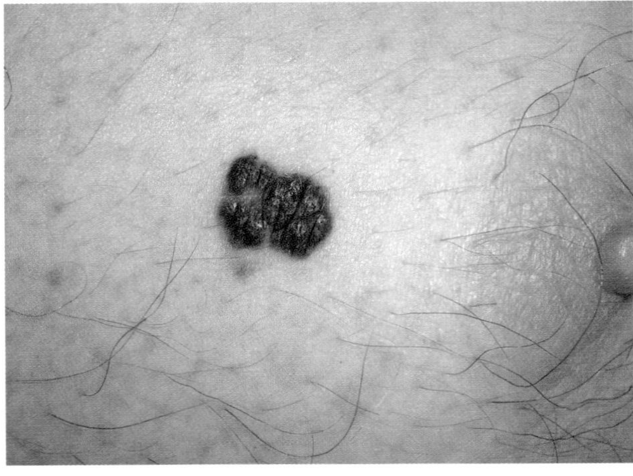

FIGURE 170-6 Superficial spreading melanoma with multiple colors and ABCDE features of melanoma. (*Reproduced with permission from Jonathan B. Karnes, MD.*)

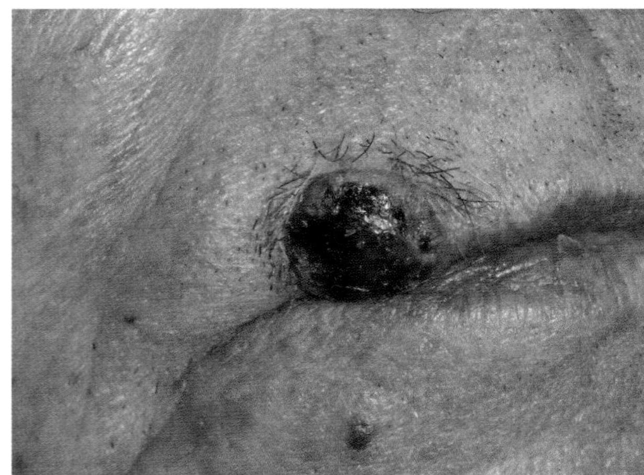

FIGURE 170-7 Thick nodular melanoma on the lip. (*Reproduced with permission from Jonathan B. Karnes, MD.*)

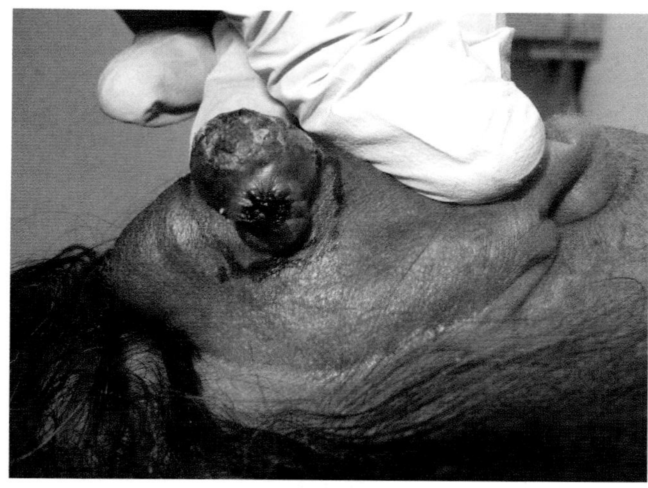

FIGURE 170-8 Large nodular melanoma on the posterior helix of the ear. Depth was 8 mm. (*Reproduced with permission from Jonathan B. Karnes, MD.*)

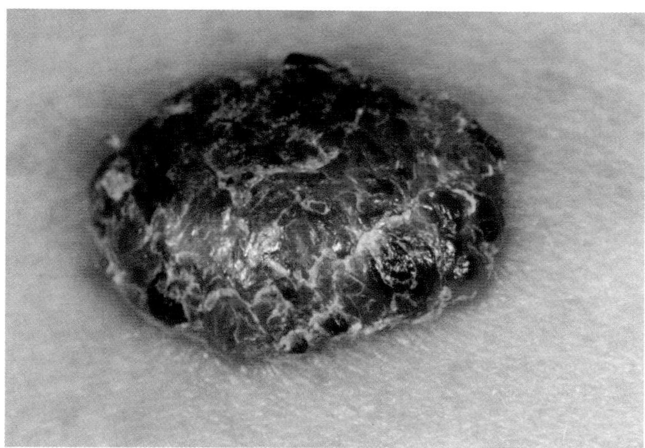

FIGURE 170-9 Raised, thick, nodular melanoma on the shoulder of a 37-year-old white woman with history of multiple sunburns from childhood. Note the multiple colors visible in the nodule. The Breslow depth is 8.5 mm with Clark level V. The sentinel node was negative and the patient underwent chemotherapy after wide excision. (*Reproduced with permission from Richard P. Usatine, MD.*)

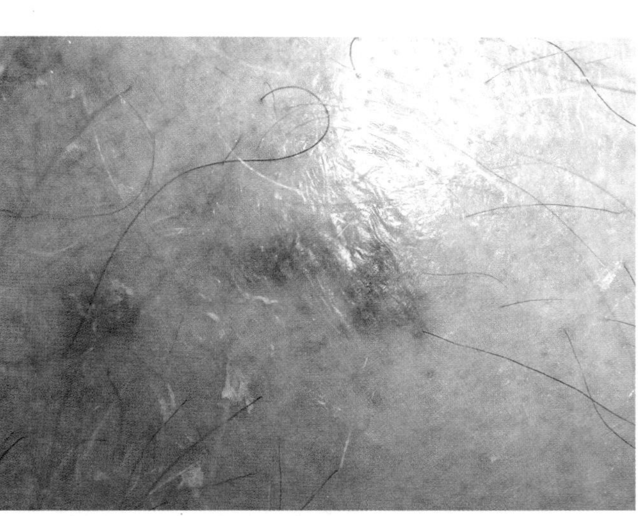

FIGURE 170-10 Lentigo maligna melanoma on the scalp of an 82-year-old man with a Breslow depth of 0.9 mm. This lesion was biopsied successfully with a scoop shave that completely cut under the lesion for full prognostic information. (*Reproduced with permission from Richard P. Usatine, MD.*)

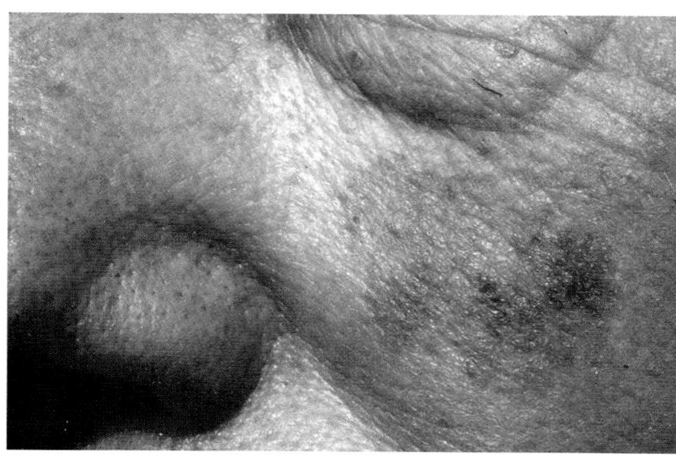

FIGURE 170-11 Lentigo malignant melanoma presenting as a large pigmented area on the face of an elderly man. (*Reproduced with permission from the Skin Cancer Foundation. For more information www.skincancer.org.*)

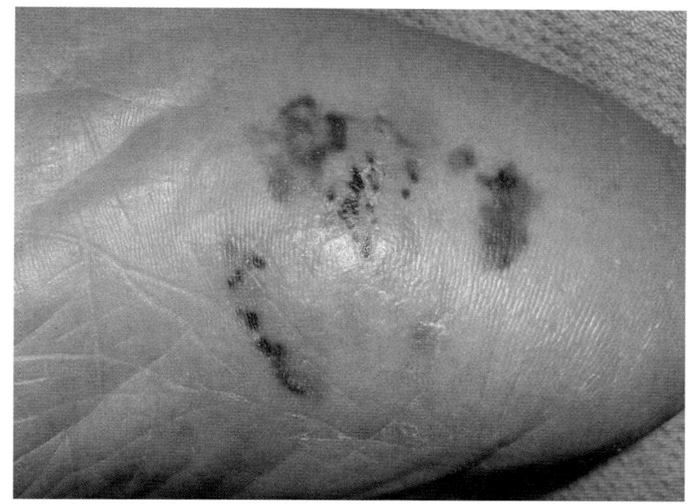

A

B

FIGURE 170-12 **A.** Acral lentiginous melanoma on the bottom of the foot where it went undetected for years. **B.** Dermoscopy showing the parallel ridge pattern typical of a melanoma on the sole. (*Reproduced with permission from Richard P. Usatine, MD.*)

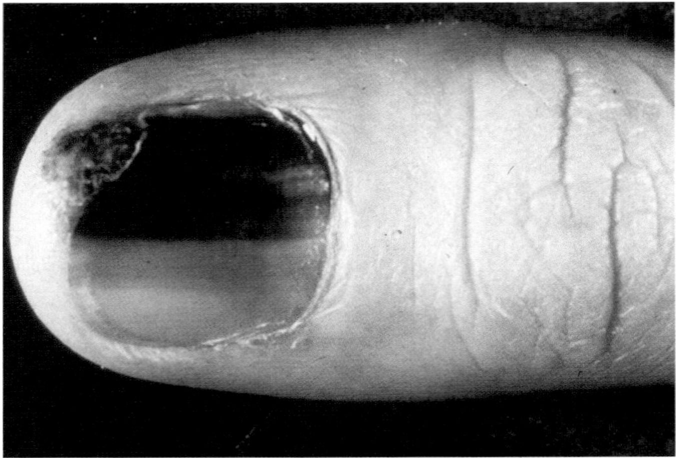

FIGURE 170-13 Subungual melanoma in a white man showing hyperpigmentation of the nail and nail bed. (*Reproduced with permission from the Skin Cancer Foundation. For more information www.skincancer.org.*)

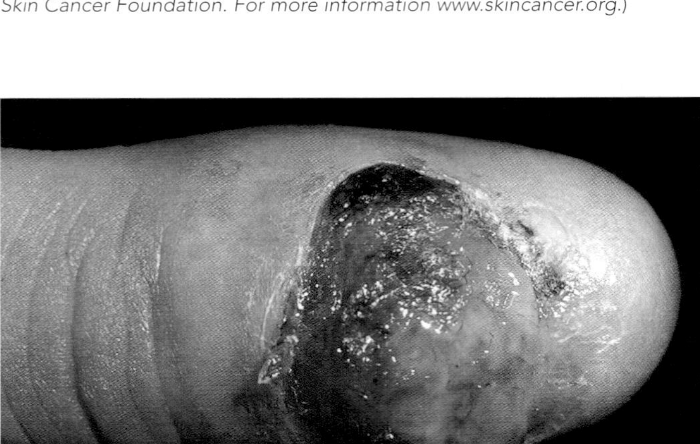

FIGURE 170-14 Acral lentiginous melanoma that started after trauma to the fifth digit of a 37-year-old woman. The diagnosis was missed for an extended time period. The tumor depth was greater than 3 mm. The patient was sent for an amputation and sentinel node biopsy. (*Reproduced with permission from Richard P. Usatine, MD.*)

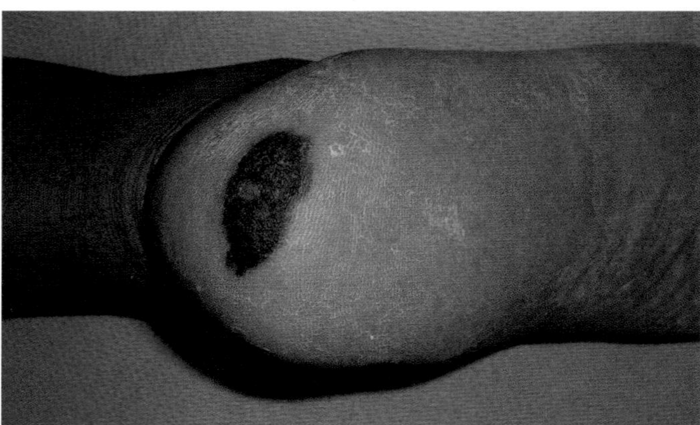

FIGURE 170-15 Nodular and acral lentiginous melanoma of the foot in a 30-year-old black woman. There is ulceration and the depth was 5.5 mm. Sentinel node biopsy was positive for 2 of 2 nodes sampled. Clarke level IV and stage IIIC (pT4b N2a MO). (*Reproduced with permission from Richard P. Usatine, MD.*)

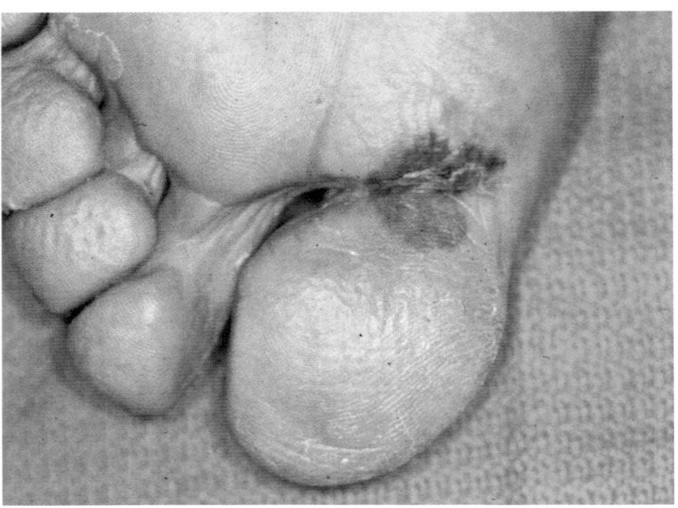

FIGURE 170-16 Acral lentiginous melanoma on the bottom of the foot where it went undetected for years. (*Reproduced with permission from the University of Texas Health Sciences Center, Division of Dermatology.*)

proximal or lateral nail fold, it is referred to as the Hutchinson sign, and is highly suggestive of acral lentiginous melanoma (see **Figure 170-14**) (see Chapter 189, Pigmented Nail Disorders).

Less common types of melanomas include the following:

- *Amelanotic melanoma* (<5% of melanomas) is nonpigmented and appears pink or flesh colored, often mimicking basal cell or squamous cell carcinoma or a ruptured hair follicle. Any of the 4 principal subtypes may present as an amelanotic variant, but nodular melanomas are highly represented. These may be intrinsically more aggressive and often present with a thicker Breslow depth than similarly pigmented melanomas (**Figures 170-17** to **170-19**).[6]

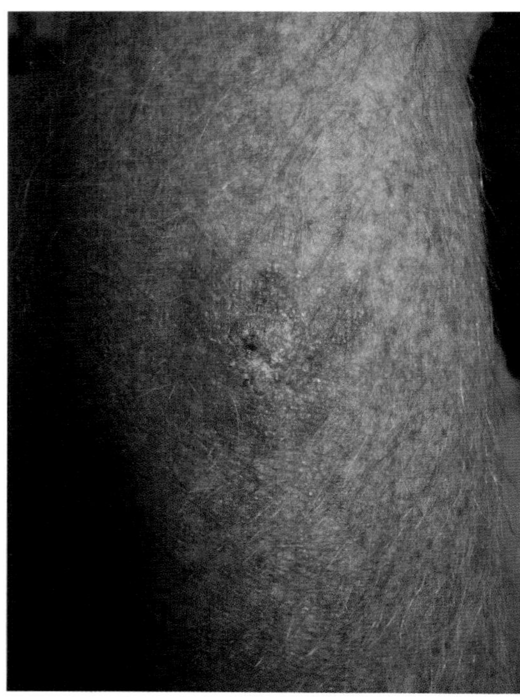

FIGURE 170-17 Amelanotic melanoma on the arm of a middle-aged man with marked sun damage. Breslow depth was 1.5 mm. (*Reproduced with permission from Jonathan B. Karnes, MD.*)

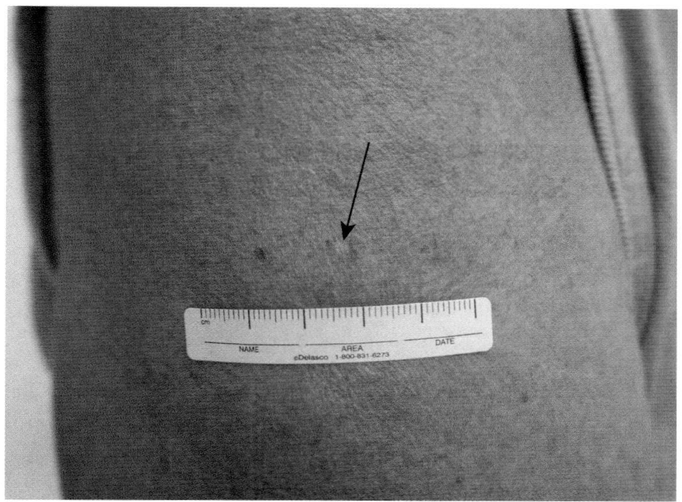

A

B

FIGURE 170-18 A. Amelanotic melanoma (arrow) on the arm easily missed because of its small size and lack of dark pigmentation. B. Dermoscopy of the same melanoma showing white central area, peripheral pigment network, peripheral tan structureless area, and polymorphous vessels. (*Reproduced with permission from Jonathan B. Karnes, MD.*)

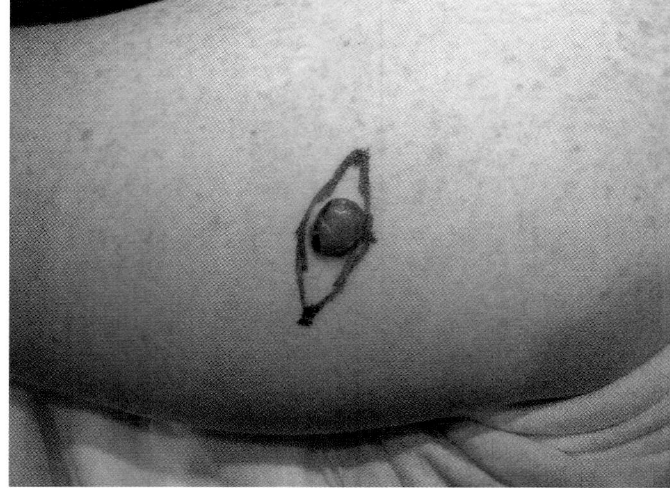

A

B

FIGURE 170-19 A. Amelanotic melanoma on the arm of a young woman prior to elliptical excision. The diagnosis was unexpected and shows the importance of excising suspicious lesions even when they are not pigmented. (*Reproduced with permission from E.J. Mayeaux Jr, MD.*) B. Amelanotic melanoma with a dermoscopy insert in upper corner. The use of the dermatoscope and the recognition of the abnormal vascular pattern lead to a high suspicion for amelanotic melanoma that was confirmed on excision. (*Reproduced with permission from Ashfaq Marghoob, MD.*)

- Other rare melanoma variants include (a) nevoid melanomas, (b) malignant blue nevus, (c) desmoplastic/spindled/neurotropic melanoma, (d) clear cell sarcoma (in fact a melanoma), (e) animal-type melanoma, (f) ocular melanoma, and (g) mucosal (lentiginous) melanoma.[5]

TYPICAL DISTRIBUTION

Melanoma occurs most commonly on the trunk in white males and the lower legs and back in white females, but may occur in any location where melanocytes exist. The most common site in African Americans, Hispanics, and Asians is the plantar foot, followed by the subungual, palmar, and mucosal sites.

DERMOSCOPY

Dermoscopy can be used to determine if a pigmented lesion has features suspicious for a melanoma, and it can also help determine when a biopsy is needed.[7] In a prospective study of 401 lesions evaluated for melanoma by experts in dermoscopy, the sensitivity of 66.6% with ABCDE criteria improved to 80%, and specificity rose from 79.3% to 89.1% (**Figure 170-20**).[7]

In a study of dermoscopy done by 60 physicians (35 general practitioners, 10 dermatologists, and 16 dermatology trainees) on unaided photos of 40 lesions using the ABCD rule, the Menzies method, a 7-point checklist, and pattern analysis, the sensitivity rose over the unaided eye.[8] The physicians were instructed in each of the dermoscopy methods using a CD-ROM. The unaided eye using a standard photo of the lesion was 61% sensitive and 85% specific with a 73% diagnostic accuracy. The dermoscopic photo increased sensitivity (68% for pattern analysis, 77% for the ABCD rule, 81% for the 7-point checklist, and 85% for the Menzies method). The specificity did not improve. Sensitivity is more important than specificity to avoid missing melanoma. Although the number of

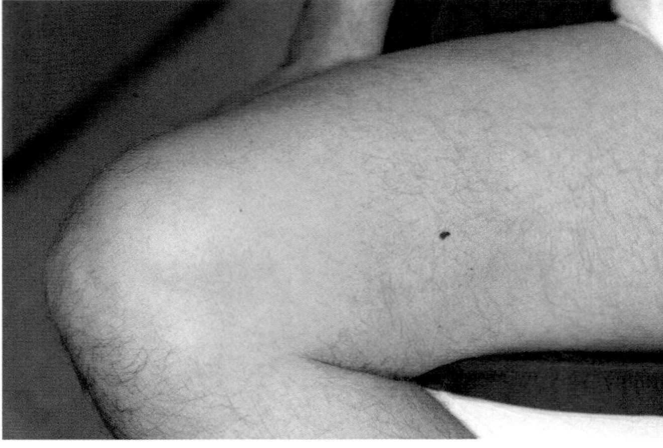

A

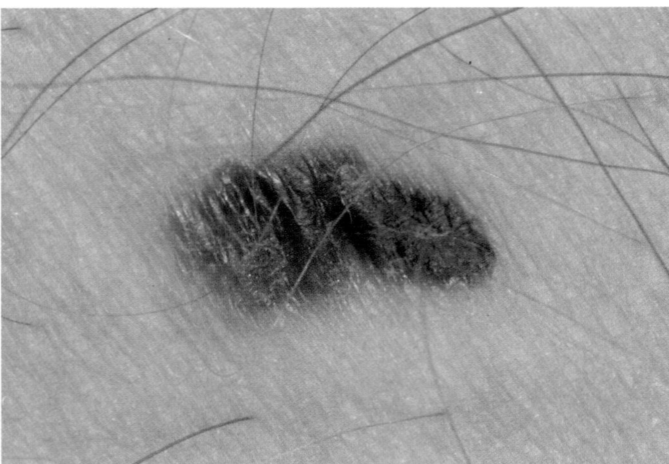

B

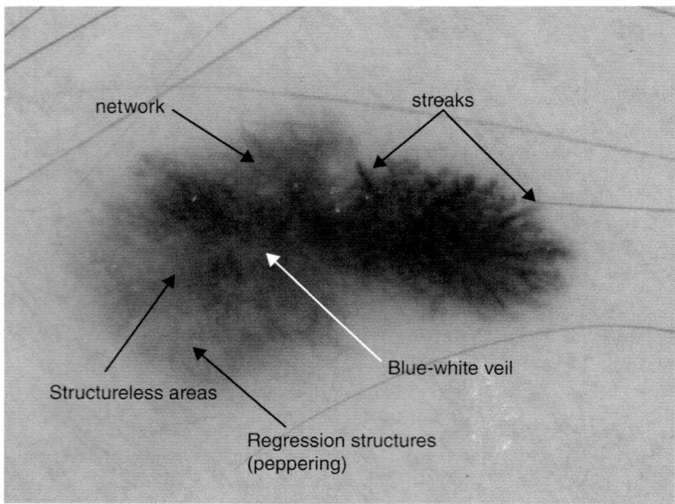

C

FIGURE 170-20 A. A melanoma on the leg that could be missed because of its small size (7-mm long). B. Close-up of that melanoma showing the asymmetry, irregular borders, and a variation in color. C. Dermoscopy of a melanoma showing a blue-white veil, radial streaks, pigment network, structureless areas, and regression structures with peppering. This early superficial-spreading melanoma was proven to be 0.55 mm at the time of excision. *(Reproduced with permission from Ashfaq Marghoob, MD.)*

biopsies could increase with some drop in specificity, the biopsy itself is the most specific test to differentiate melanoma from benign pigmented lesions.[8]

Accepted dermoscopic local features of melanoma include the following:

- Atypical network (includes branched-streaks)
- Streaks—pseudopods and radial streaming
- Atypical dots and globules
- Negative pigment network
- Blotch (off center)
- Blue-white veil/peppering over macular areas (regression)
- Blue-white veil over raised areas
- Vascular structures
- Peripheral tan/brown structureless areas

Figure 170-20 demonstrates a number of these features. See Appendix C, Dermoscopy.

BIOPSY

A full-thickness skin biopsy remains the gold standard for diagnosing melanoma. Complete excisional biopsy with close margins (1-3 mm) is ideal for histologic diagnosis and tumor staging (**Box 170-1**). Although there is evidence that an incisional biopsy of a portion of a melanoma does not worsen the prognosis, this should only be performed when a lesion is too large to excise in the office. When the clinical impression differs markedly from the pathology report, discuss with the pathologist and share clinical photos if you have not done so already. You may need to have the pathologist prepare "deeper sections" or "step sections"—meaning more slices from the same loaf of bread. Additionally, if the diagnosis of melanoma was expected and the result of an incisional biopsy does not meet the expectation, go forward with a complete excision or refer to a surgeon who can.

Despite strong opinions about biopsy technique, there is evidence that a saucerization (scoop or deep shave biopsy) leads to an accurate diagnosis and staging 97% of the time (**Figure 170-21**).[9] Still, a shallow shave

BOX 170-1 The National Comprehensive Cancer Network (NCCN) Melanoma Guidelines on the Principles of Biopsy State[12]

- Excisional biopsy (elliptical, punch [when whole lesion is small], or saucerization) with 1- to 3-mm margins is preferred. Avoid wider margins to permit accurate subsequent lymphatic mapping.
- The orientation of the biopsy should be planned with definitive wide excision in mind.
- Full-thickness incisional or punch biopsy of clinically thickest portion of the lesion is acceptable in certain anatomic areas (eg, palm/sole, digit, face, and ear) or for very large lesions.
- Shave biopsy (not saucerization or deep shave) may compromise pathologic diagnosis and complete assessment of Breslow thickness, but is acceptable when the index of suspicion is low.
- For lentigo maligna melanoma in situ, broad shave biopsy may help to optimize diagnosis.[12]

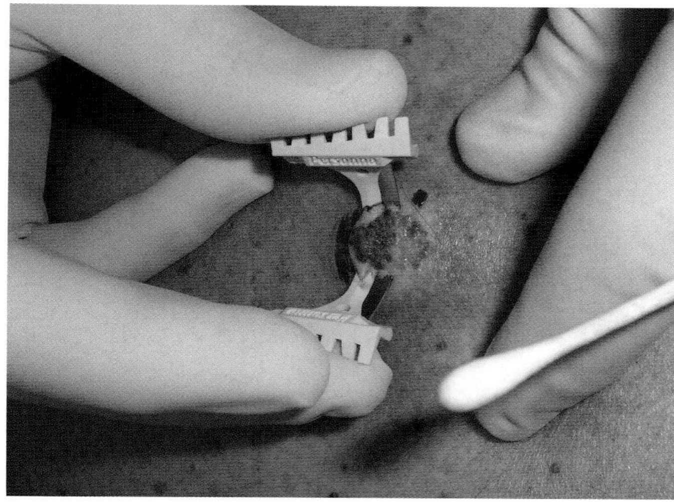

FIGURE 170-21 Saucerization (scoop or deep shave) of the entire pigmented lesion suspected to be a superficial spreading melanoma was performed successfully with a DermaBlade. Breslow thickness was 0.6 mm and the patient then underwent a full surgical excision with 1-cm margins. (*Reproduced with permission from Richard P. Usatine, MD.*)

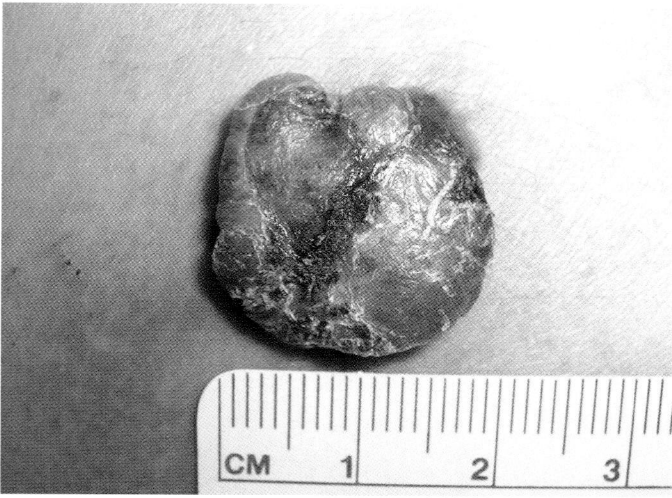

FIGURE 170-22 Thick ulcerated nodular melanoma on the back of a young woman that could be mistaken for a pyogenic granuloma or basal cell carcinoma. Most importantly, a full-depth biopsy was performed. The melanoma depth was greater than 1 mm and the patient was sent for a complete excision with a sentinel node biopsy. (*Reproduced with permission from Richard P. Usatine, MD.*)

biopsy may miss important staging information and may cause "upstaging" and unnecessary lymph node biopsy. However, for very large lesions, such as a suspected lentigo maligna, a broad scoop shave (saucerization) can often provide better tissue to the pathologist than a single or several punch biopsies (see **Figure 170-10**).[10]

The impact of partial biopsy on histopathologic diagnosis of cutaneous melanoma has been studied extensively by Ng et al. in Australia. They found increased odds of histopathologic misdiagnosis were associated with punch biopsy of part of the melanoma (odds ratio [OR] 16.6) and shallow shave biopsy (OR 2.6) compared with excisional biopsy (including saucerization). Punch biopsy of part of the melanoma was also associated with increased odds of misdiagnosis with an adverse outcome (OR 20).[11]

DIFFERENTIAL DIAGNOSIS

Nevi of all types can mimic melanoma. Congenital nevi can be especially large and asymmetrical. Therefore, it is important to ask the patient if the pigmented area has been there from birth. Because some melanomas arise in congenital nevi, a changing congenital nevus needs to be biopsied to rule out melanoma.

- Dysplastic nevi, also called atypical moles, can mimic melanoma. When an atypical nevus is suspicious for melanoma, perform a full-thickness biopsy or a broad scoop shave for histology. Only the less-suspicious dysplastic nevi should be followed with photography or serial examinations (see Chapter 163, Dysplastic Nevus).
- Seborrheic keratoses (SKs) usually look like they are stuck-on with surface cracks and a verrucous (wart-like) appearance. These are benign and not precancerous. SKs can be darkly pigmented, asymmetrical with irregular borders and have varied colors. Perform a biopsy if the diagnosis is uncertain. Be careful not to mistake a lesion for a SK (see **Figure 170-4**) (see Chapter 156, Seborrheic Keratosis).
- Solar lentigines often appear as light brown macules on the face and the dorsum of the hands. Many patients call them liver spots, but they have nothing to do with the liver. A large isolated solar lentigo on the face can mimic lentigo maligna melanoma. In this case, perform a broad scoop shave of the most suspicious area or the whole lesion.
- Dermatofibromas are fibrotic nodules that occur most frequently on the legs and arms. They can be any color from skin color to black and often have a brown halo surrounding them. A pinch test will produce a dimpling of the skin in most cases (see Chapter 158, Dermatofibroma).
- Pyogenic granulomas can resemble an amelanotic melanoma so always send the lesion to the pathologist to make sure that the clinical diagnosis is correct (**Figure 170-22**) (see Chapter 159, Pyogenic Granuloma).
- Pigmented basal cell carcinomas (BCCs) may resemble a melanoma. However, the pigment in the BCC is often scattered throughout the lesion, and it has other features of a BCC, such as a pearly appearance with a rolled border (**Figures 170-23** and **170-24**) (see Chapter 168,

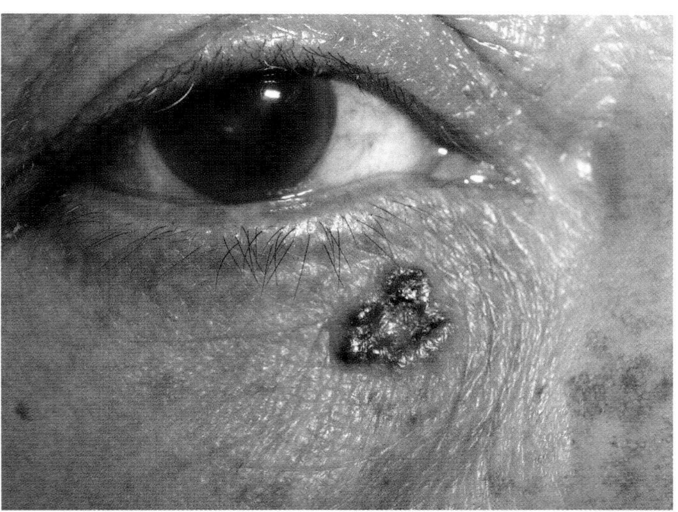

FIGURE 170-23 A pigmented basal cell carcinoma on the lower eyelid that has rolled pearly borders even though the color is black. A shave biopsy allowed a diagnosis of a basal cell carcinoma to be made. (*Reproduced with permission from Richard P. Usatine, MD.*)

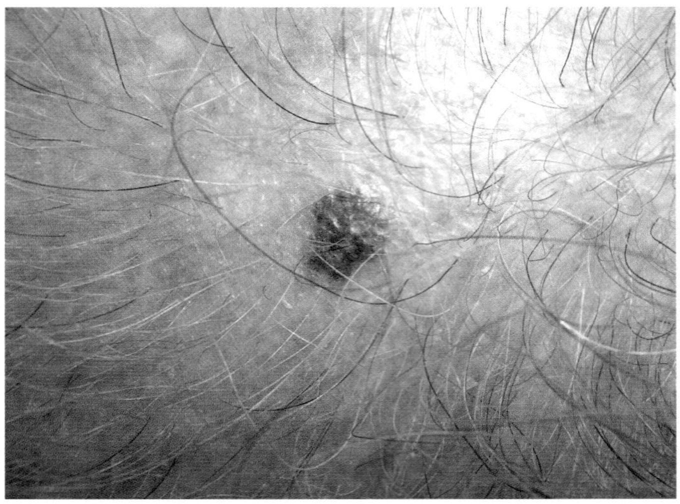

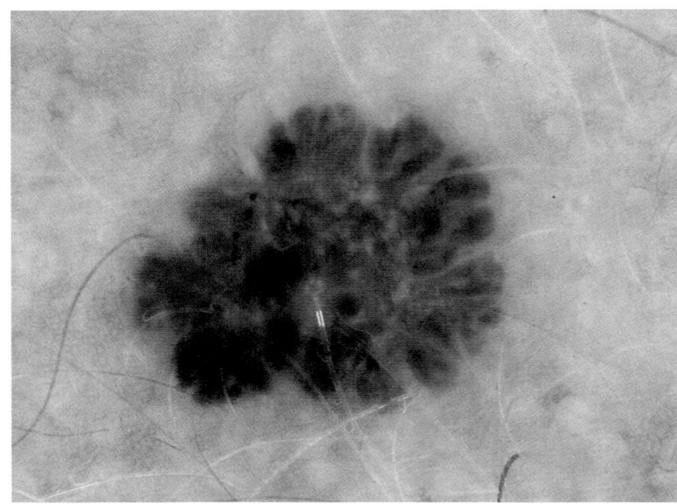

A B

FIGURE 170-24 A. A pigmented basal cell carcinoma on the scalp mimicking a melanoma. B. Dermoscopy shows the typical maple leaf patterns of a pigmented basal cell carcinoma. A shave biopsy easily allowed for a diagnosis of a basal cell carcinoma to be made. (*Reproduced with permission from Richard P. Usatine, MD.*)

Basal Cell Carcinoma). Dermoscopy can be very helpful as a pigmented BCC has a number of specific dermoscopic structures to look for.

MANAGEMENT

- Cutaneous melanoma is surgically treated with complete full skin-depth excision using margins determined by the Breslow depth. This depth is a measure of tumor thickness from the granular layer of the epidermis to the point of deepest invasion using an ocular micrometer.
- Current recommendations for excision margins range from 5 mm for in situ lesions to 1 to 2 cm for invasive lesions. A recent study showed significant benefit with a 9-mm margin on Mohs excision of melanoma in situ compared with 6-mm margins at a referral center.[13] See **Table 170-1** for a comparison of world recommendations.[14] SOR Ⓐ
- Mohs micrographic surgery, performed by specially trained physicians, may prove useful in completely removing subclinical tumor extension in certain subtypes of melanoma in situ, such as lentigo maligna, desmoplastic melanoma, and acral lentiginous melanoma in situ.[15]
- Sentinel lymph node biopsies are recommended for tumors of greater than or equal to 1 mm in depth and should be considered for thinner lesions with ulceration or more than 1 mitoses per mm^2 (**Figure 170-25**). In the most recent guidelines, mitoses per mm^2 has replaced Clark levels to distinguish T1a from T1b tumors.[16]
- Patients with advanced melanoma should be referred to medical oncology and may receive combination therapy with multiple chemotherapeutic agents and immunotherapy. Many trials are ongoing and 3 new drugs, including interferon 2α, vemurafenib, and ipilimumab, have been approved for use in advanced melanoma. Consideration should be given to consulting palliative care.

TABLE 170-1 Currently Recommended Excision Margins for Primary Melanoma

	Excision Margin			
Tumor Thickness	UK MSG	WHO	Australian	Dutch MSG
In situ	2-5 mm	5 mm	5 mm	2 mm
<1 cm	1 cm	1 cm	1 cm	
1-2 mm	1-2 cm	1 cm*	1 cm	1 cm
2.1-4 mm	2-3 cm (2 cm preferred)	2 cm	1 cm	2 cm
>4 mm	2-3 cm	2 cm	2 cm	2 cm

MSG, Melanoma Study Group; WHO, World Health Organization.
*For melanomas thicker than 1.5 mm, recommended excision margin is 2 cm.
Data from Newton Bishop JA, et al. UK guidelines for the management of cutaneous melanoma. *British Journal of Plastic Surgery*. 2003;55(1): 46-54. Copyright 2003, with permission from Elsevier.

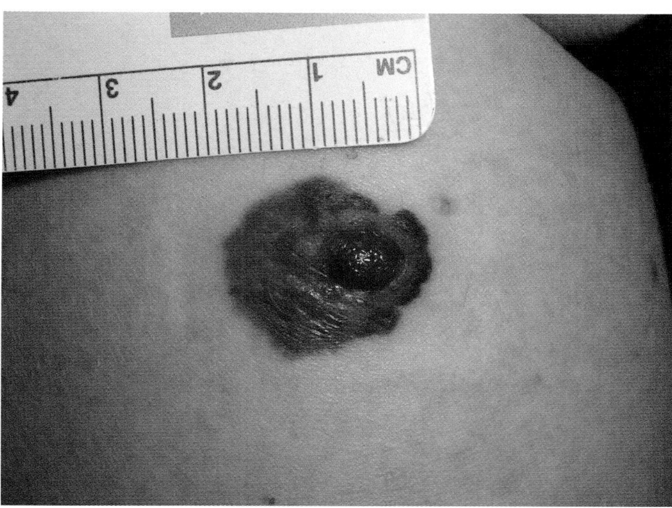

FIGURE 170-25 Advanced thick melanoma on the leg of a 37-year-old woman. The Breslow depth was over 3 mm and the patient was sent for wide excision with sentinel lymph node biopsy. (*Reproduced with permission from Richard P. Usatine, MD.*)

- Recently 2 new chemotherapeutic agents have been Food and Drug Administration (FDA) approved for the treatment of metastatic melanoma (**Figure 170-26**). One, vemurafenib is a monoclonal antibody targeting the BRAF mutation expressed on many melanomas. Ipilimumab prevents dampening of the immune system by blocking a regulatory molecule CTLA-4. Both of these medications used in combination with dacarbazine have shown a small but significant increase in progression-free survival.[17]

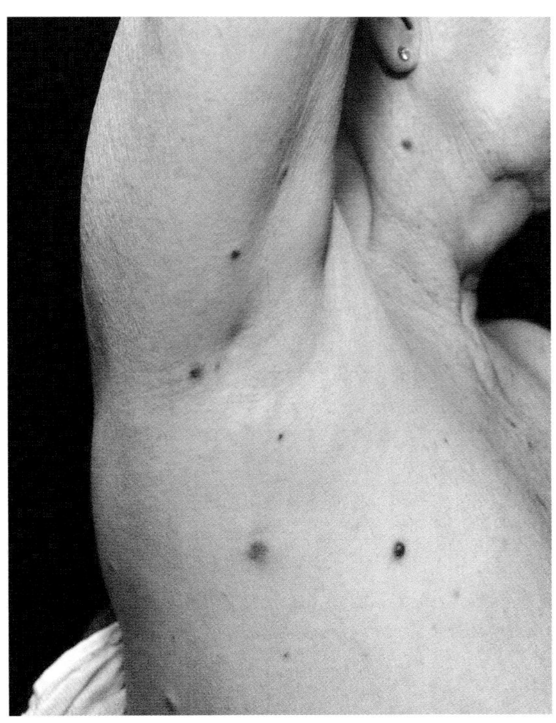

FIGURE 170-26 Metastatic melanoma with dark black nodules scattered over the body and neck. (*Reproduced with permission from Richard P. Usatine, MD.*)

PREVENTION AND SCREENING

- Melanoma prevention starts with sun protection.
- Until recently there is no proof that sunscreen helped to prevent melanoma. A recent study provides some evidence that sunscreen use does decrease the risk of invasive melanomas in adults.[18]
- Sun protection should include sun avoidance, protective clothing, and sunscreen.
- Indoor tanning is not safe and should be avoided.
- US Preventive Services Task Force has not found sufficient evidence to recommend regular screening for melanoma or skin cancer in the general population.[19]
- Most experts believe that persons at high risk for melanoma (including previous personal history of melanoma, high-risk family history, and high-risk skin types with significant sun exposure) should be screened regularly for melanoma by a physician trained in such screening.
- Evidence for the value of self-screening is lacking but persons at high risk for melanoma should also be encouraged to observe their own skin and to come in for evaluation if they see any suspicious changes or growths.

PROGNOSIS

Prognosis depends on tumor depth, mitotic rate, the presence of ulceration, positive lymph nodes, and metastases. In stage 0 disease surgical excision is almost always curative. Ten-year survival in patients by tumor thickness is almost 100% for in situ lesions, 92% for lesions less than 1-mm thick, 80% for lesions between 1- and 2-mm thick, 63% for lesions 2- to 4-mm thick, and 50% for lesions thicker than 4 mm. When accounting for nodal and distant metastasis, stage III disease carries a 39% to 70% 5-year survival depending on the number of nodal metastases, and stage IV disease carries a 32% to 62% 1-year survival rate.[16]

FOLLOW-UP

The need for follow-up is largely determined by the stage of the disease. The 2010 American Joint Committee on Cancer staging system is provided in **Table 170-2**. The prognosis is worsened by increasing depth, mitotic rate, presence of ulceration, positive lymph nodes, and metastases.

The follow-up for stages 0 and 1 cutaneous melanoma includes regular skin examinations by a physician trained in skin cancer screening. Total body photography may be of benefit in monitoring patients with multiple nevi. The rate of subsequent cutaneous melanomas among persons with a history of melanoma was found to be more than 10 times the rate of a first cutaneous melanoma and the highest incidence of recurrence was in the first 3 to 5 years after initial diagnosis.[20,21]

PATIENT EDUCATION

Advise patients who have had melanoma to avoid future sun exposure and monitor their skin for new and changing moles. Recommend a complete skin examination yearly by a physician trained to detect early melanoma.

TABLE 170-2A TNM Staging Categories for Cutaneous Melanoma

Classification	Thickness (mm)	Ulceration Status/Mitoses
T		
Tis	NA	NA
T1	≤1.00	a: Without ulceration and mitosis <1/mm^2 b: With ulceration or mitoses ≥1/mm^2
T2	1.01-2.00	a: Without ulceration b: With ulceration
T3	2.01-4.00	a: Without ulceration b: With ulceration
T4	>4.00	a: Without ulceration b: With ulceration
N	**No. of Metastatic Nodes**	**Nodal Metastatic Burden**
N0	0	NA
N1	1	a: Micrometastasis* b: Macrometastasis†
N2	2-3	a: Micrometastasis* b: Macrometastasis† c: In transit metastases/satellites without metastatic nodes
N3	4+ metastatic nodes, or matted nodes, or in transit metastases/satellites with metastatic nodes	
M	**Site**	**Serum LDH**
M0	No distant metastases	NA
M1a	Distant skin, subcutaneous, or nodal metastases	Normal
M1b	Lung metastases	Normal
M1c	All other visceral metastases Any distant metastasis	Normal Elevated

NA, not applicable; LDH, lactate dehydrogenase.
*Micrometastases are diagnosed after sentinel lymph node biopsy.
†Macrometastases are defined as clinically detectable nodal metastases confirmed pathologically.

TABLE 170-2B Anatomic Stage Groupings for Cutaneous Melanoma

	Clinical Staging*				Pathologic Staging†		
	T	N	M		T	N	M
0	Tis	N0	M0	0	Tis	N0	M0
IA	T1a	N0	M0	IA	T1a	N0	M0
IB	T1b	N0	M0	IB	T1b	N0	M0
	T2a	N0	M0	T2a	N0	M0	
IIA	T2b	N0	M0	IIA	T2b	N0	M0
	T3a	N0	M0	T3a	N0	M0	
IIB	T3b	N0	M0	IIB	T3b	N0	M0
	T4a	N0	M0	T4a	N0	M0	
IIC	T4b	N0	M0	IIIC	T4b	N0	M0
III	Any T	N > N0	M0	IIIA	T1-4a	N1a	M0
					T1-4a	N2a	M0
				IIIB	T1-4b	N1a	M0
					T1-4b	N2a	M0
					T1-4a	N1b	M0
					T1-4a	N2b	M0
					T1-4a	N2c	M0
				IIIC	T1-4b	N1b	M0
					T1-4b	N2b	M0
					T1-4b	N2c	M0
					Any T	N3	M0
IV	Any T	Any N	M1	IV	Any T	Any N	M1

*Clinical staging includes microstaging of the primary melanoma and clinical/radiologic evaluation for metastases. By convention, it should be used after complete excision of the primary melanoma with clinical assessment for regional and distant metastases.
†Pathologic staging includes microstaging of the primary melanoma and pathologic information about the regional lymph nodes after partial (ie, sentinel node biopsy) or complete lymphadenectomy. Pathologic stage 0 or stage IA patients are the exception; they do not require pathologic evaluation of their lymph nodes.

PATIENT RESOURCES

- Medline Plus. *Melanoma*—**http://www.nlm.nih.gov/medlineplus/melanoma.html.**
- The Skin Cancer Foundation. *Melanoma*—**http://www.skincancer.org/skin-cancer-information/melanoma.**
- American Cancer Society. *Skin Cancer*–**Melanoma—http://www.cancer.org/cancer/skincancer-melanoma/index.**

PROVIDER RESOURCES

- Medscape. *Cutaneous Melanoma*—**http://emedicine.medscape.com/article/1100753.**
- National Cancer Institute. *Melanoma*—**http://www.cancer.gov/cancertopics/types/melanoma.**
- Skinsight. *INFORMED: Melanoma and Skin Cancer Early Detection*—**http://www.skinsight.com/info/for_professionals/skin-cancer-detection-informed/skin-cancer-education.**
- Chapters and videos on diagnosing and surgically managing melanoma can be found in the following book/DVD or electronic application: Usatine R, Pfenninger J, Stulberg D, Small R. *Dermatologic and Cosmetic Procedures in Office Practice*. Philadelphia, PA: Elsevier; 2012.
- Information about smartphone and tablet apps of this resource can be viewed at **www.usatinemedia.com.**

REFERENCES

1. Siegel R, Naishadham D, Jemal A. Cancer statistics, 2012. *CA Cancer J Clin.* 2012;62(1):10-29.
2. Jemal A, Saraiya M, Patel P, et al. Recent trends in cutaneous melanoma incidence and death rates in the United States, 1992-2006. *J Am Acad Dermatol.* 2011;65(5 suppl 1):S17-S25.e1-e3.
3. Rigel DS. Trends in dermatology: melanoma incidence. *Arch Dermatol.* 2010;146(3):318.
4. Thomas L, Tranchand P, Berard F, Secchi T, Colin C, Moulin G. Semiological value of ABCDE criteria in the diagnosis of cutaneous pigmented tumors. *Dermatology*. 1998;197(1):11-17.
5. MD JLB, MD JLJ, MD RPR. *Dermatology e-dition: Text with Continually Updated Online Reference*. 2nd ed. St. Louis, MO: Mosby; 2007:2584.
6. Gualandri L, Betti R, Crosti C. Clinical features of 36 cases of amelanotic melanomas and considerations about the relationship between histologic subtypes and diagnostic delay. *J Eur Acad Dermatol Venereol.* 2009;23(3):283-287.
7. Benelli C, Roscetti E, Pozzo VD, Gasparini G, Cavicchini S. The dermoscopic versus the clinical diagnosis of melanoma. *Eur J Dermatol.* 1999;9(6):470-476.
8. Dolianitis C, Kelly J, Wolfe R, Simpson P. Comparative performance of 4 dermoscopic algorithms by nonexperts for the diagnosis of melanocytic lesions. *Arch Dermatol.* 2005;141(8):1008-1014.
9. Zager JS, Hochwald SN, Marzban SS, et al. Shave biopsy is a safe and accurate method for the initial evaluation of melanoma. *J Am Coll Surg.* 2011;212(4):454-460; discussion 460-462.
10. Dalton SR, Gardner TL, Libow LF, Elston DM. Contiguous lesions in lentigo maligna. *J Am Acad Dermatol.* 2005;52(5):859-862.
11. Ng JC, Swain S, Dowling JP, Wolfe R, Simpson P, Kelly JW. The impact of partial biopsy on histopathologic diagnosis of cutaneous melanoma: experience of an Australian tertiary referral service. *Arch Dermatol.* 2010;146(3):234-239.
12. Coit DG, Andtbacka R, Bichakjian CK, et al. NCCN Melanoma Panel. Melanoma. *J Natl Compr Canc Netw.* 2009;7(3):250-275.
13. Kunishige JH, Brodland DG, Zitelli JA. Surgical margins for melanoma in situ. *J Am Acad Dermatol.* 2012;66(3):438-444.
14. Lens MB, Dawes M, Goodacre T, Bishop JAN. Excision margins in the treatment of primary cutaneous melanoma: a systematic review of randomized controlled trials comparing narrow vs wide excision. *Arch Surg.* 2002;137(10):1101-1105.
15. Chang KH, Dufresne R, Cruz A, Rogers GS. The operative management of melanoma: where does Mohs surgery fit in? *Dermatol Surg.* 2011;37(8):1069-1079.
16. Balch CM, Gershenwald JE, Soong S-J, et al. Final version of 2009 AJCC melanoma staging and classification. *J Clin Oncol.* 2009;27(36):6199-6206.
17. Lee B, Mukhi N, Liu D. Current management and novel agents for malignant melanoma. *J Hematol Oncol.* 2012;5(1):3.
18. Green AC, Williams GM, Logan V, Strutton GM. Reduced melanoma after regular sunscreen use: randomized trial follow-up. *J Clin Oncol.* 2011;29(3):257-263.
19. Wolff T, Tai E, Miller T. *Screening for Skin Cancer: An Update of the Evidence for the U.S. Preventive Services Task Force*. Rockville, MD: Agency for Healthcare Research and Quality; 2009. http://www.ncbi.nlm.nih.gov/books/NBK34051/.
20. Tsao H, Atkins MB, Sober AJ. Management of cutaneous melanoma. *N Engl J Med.* 2004;351(10):998-1012.
21. Levi F, Randimbison L, Te V-C, La Vecchia C. High constant incidence rates of second cutaneous melanomas. *Int J Cancer.* 2005;117(5):877-879.

SECTION 12 INFILTRATIVE/IMMUNOLOGIC

171 GRANULOMA ANNULARE

Melissa Muszynski, MD
Richard P. Usatine, MD

PATIENT STORY

A 39-year-old woman presents with raised rings on her right hand only. Not knowing the correct diagnosis, another physician prescribed topical steroids and antifungal medicines with no benefit. The diagnosis of granuloma annulare (GA) was made by the typical clinical appearance and the patient was offered intralesional steroids. Triamcinolone acetonide was injected as seen in **Figure 171-1A**. The patient noted improvement over the subsequent weeks, but within a month new lesions began to appear on her other hand (**Figure 171-1B**). Additional injections were provided and 1 month later the patient had regression of the treated lesions but had new lesions on the right arm (**Figure 171-2A**). At the next visit, the patient had new lesions on her feet as well (**Figure 171-2B**). The diagnosis of disseminated GA was made and systemic treatment was started.

INTRODUCTION

GA is a common dermatologic condition that presents as small, light-red, dermal papules coalescing into annular plaques without scale. As in the above vignette, it is often mistaken as nummular eczema or tinea corporis. Distribution, pattern, and lack of scale are important diagnostic clues.

EPIDEMIOLOGY

- GA affects twice as many women as men.[1]
- The 4 presentations of GA are localized, disseminated/generalized, perforating, and subcutaneous.
- Of the 4 variations, the localized form is seen most often.[1]

ETIOLOGY AND PATHOPHYSIOLOGY

- Benign, cutaneous, inflammatory disorder of unknown origin.[1]
- Disease may be self-limiting, but may persist for many years.
- Reported associations include diabetes mellitus, viral infections (including HIV), *Borrelia* and streptococcal infections, insect bites, lymphoma, tuberculosis, and trauma.[2,3]
- One proposed mechanism for GA is a delayed-type hypersensitivity reaction as a result of T-helper–type cell (Th)-1 lymphocytic differentiation of macrophages. These macrophages become effector cells that express tumor necrosis factor (TNF)-α and matrix metalloproteinases. The activated macrophages are responsible for dermal collagen matrix degradation.[4]

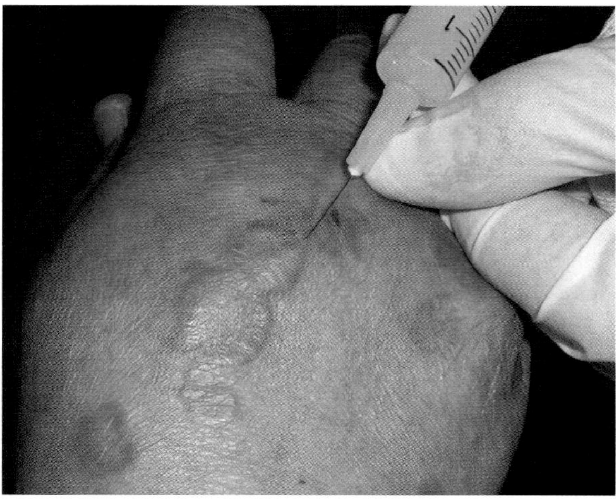

A

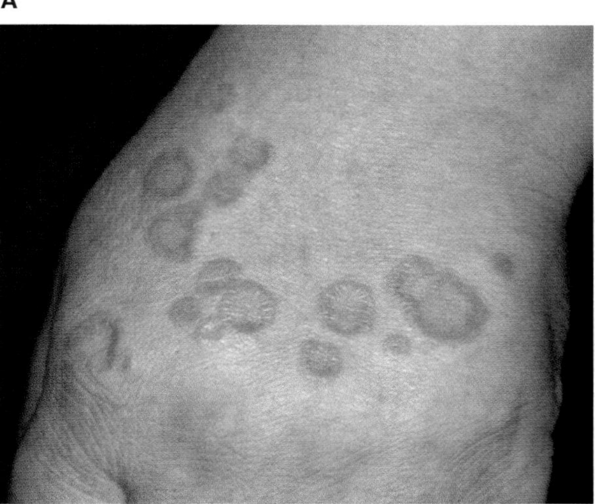

B

FIGURE 171-1 A. Granuloma annulare in a 42-year-old woman. Intralesional steroids were administered on the first visit with resolution of the injected lesions. B. Same patient months later with new annular lesions on the opposite hand. She requested additional injections. (*Reproduced with permission from Richard P. Usatine, MD.*)

- An association between high expression of gil-1 oncogene and granulomatous lesions of the skin, including GA, has been established.[5]

RISK FACTORS

The only identifiable risk factor is being a woman. There are several associations, but nothing has been shown to be causative.

DIAGNOSIS

CLINICAL FEATURES

Annular lesions have raised borders that are skin colored to erythematous (see **Figures 171-1** and **171-2**). The rings may become hyperpigmented

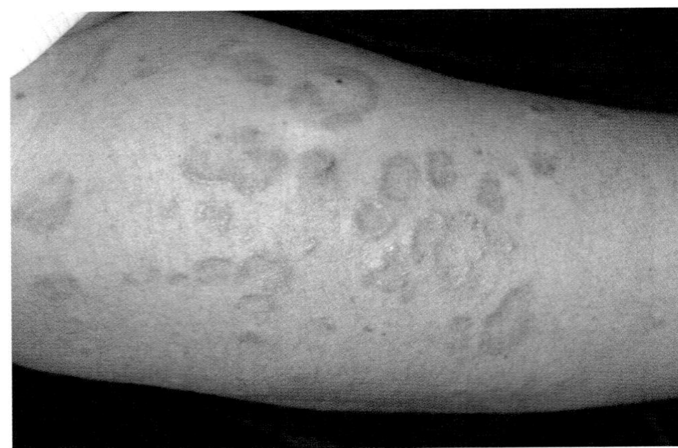

A

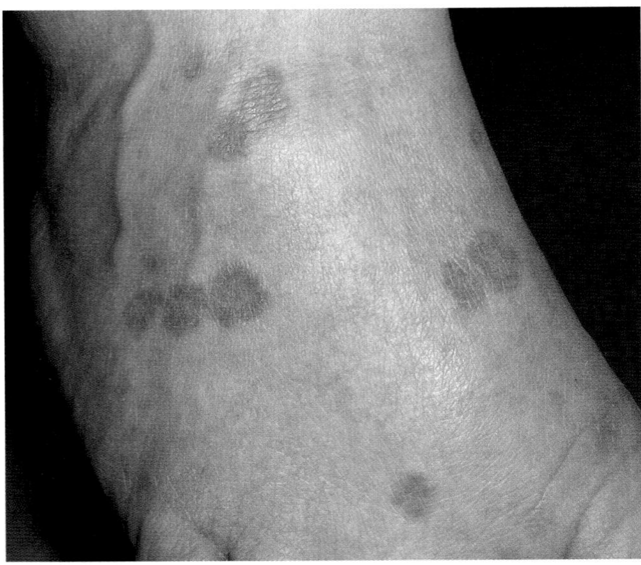

B

FIGURE 171-2 A. Same patient as in Figure 171-1 1 month later with new crops of lesions on the arms and feet. She has disseminated granuloma annulare. Note the central area of hypopigmentation secondary to a previous steroid intralesional steroid injection. B. Disseminated granuloma annulare on the foot of the same patient. The rings are flatter and many are conjoined. (*Reproduced with permission from Richard P. Usatine, MD.*)

or violaceous (see **Figure 171-2B**). There is often a central depression within the ring. These lesions range from 2 mm to 5 cm. Although the classical appearance of GA is annular, the lesions may be arcuate instead of forming a complete ring (**Figure 171-3**). Most importantly, there should be no scaling as seen in tinea corporis (ringworm).

TYPICAL DISTRIBUTION

Each of the 4 types of GA has a different distribution. Localized and disseminated GA differ only in that disseminated lesions can spread to the trunk and neck and may be more pronounced in sun-exposed areas.[6]

- Localized—This is the most common form of GA affecting 75% of GA patients.[1] It typically presents as solitary lesions on the dorsal surfaces of extremities, especially of hands and feet (**Figure 171-4**).
- Disseminated or generalized—Adults are most affected by this form, which begins in the extremities and can spread to the trunk and neck (**Figure 171-5**).

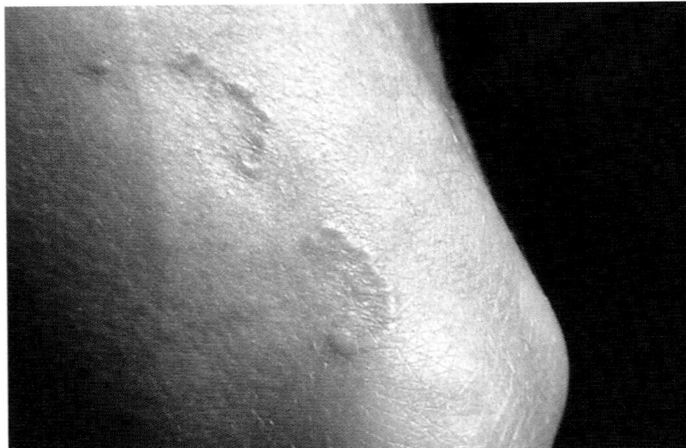

FIGURE 171-3 Granuloma annulare on the elbow showing how the rings may not be complete. This patient is in her fifties and has had new crops of lesions over the past 10 years. (*Reproduced with permission from Richard P. Usatine, MD.*)

- Perforating—Children and young adults present with 1 to hundreds of 1- to 4-mm annular papules that may coalesce to form a typical annular plaque. Although this form can appear anywhere on the body, it has an affinity for extremities, especially the hands and fingers (**Figure 171-6**).[7] The papules may exude a thick and creamy or clear and viscous fluid.
- Subcutaneous—These lesions present as rapidly growing, nonpainful, subcutaneous, or dermal nodules on the extremities, scalp, and forehead. Subcutaneous GA mainly affects children (**Figure 171-7**).[6] These lesions are often ill defined and less discrete.

LABORATORY STUDIES

Often a diagnosis of GA is made on clinical presentation alone, without the need for biopsy. Subcutaneous GA may be an exception, as the unusual appearance may be mistaken for a rheumatoid nodule. Histologic examination reveals an increase of mucin, which is a hallmark of GA. There is also a dense infiltrate of histiocytes in the mid-dermis and sparse perivascular lymphocytic infiltrate. The histiocytes are either organized as

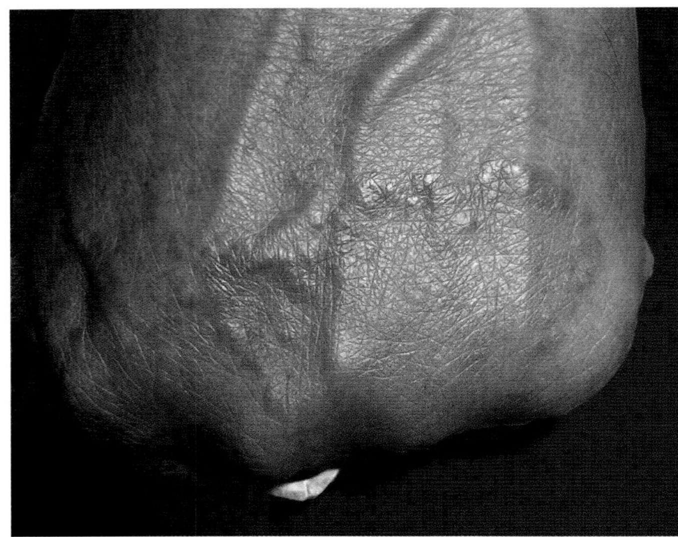

FIGURE 171-4 One single large irregular annular lesion of granuloma annulare. This ring is also incomplete. (*Reproduced with permission from Richard P. Usatine, MD.*)

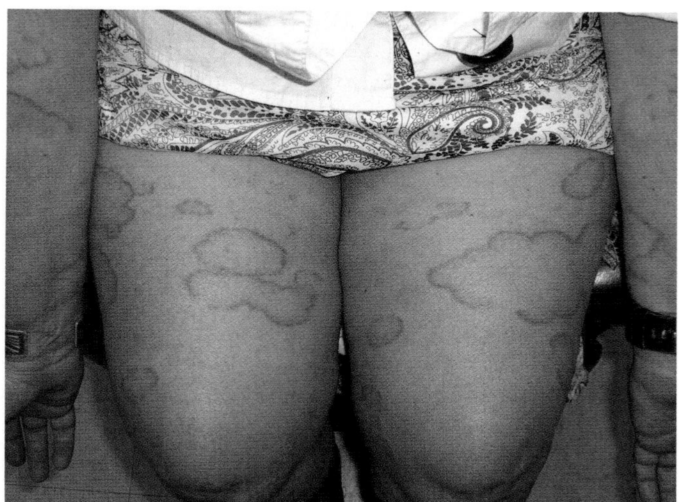

FIGURE 171-5 Disseminated granuloma annulare in a middle-aged woman with diabetes. (*Reproduced with permission from Richard P. Usatine, MD.*)

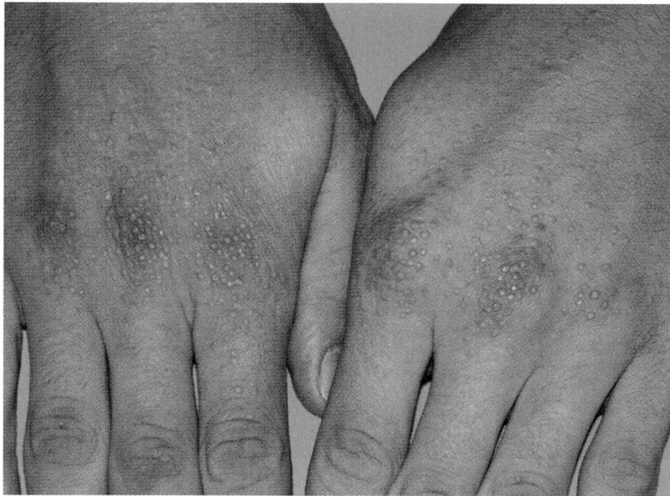

A

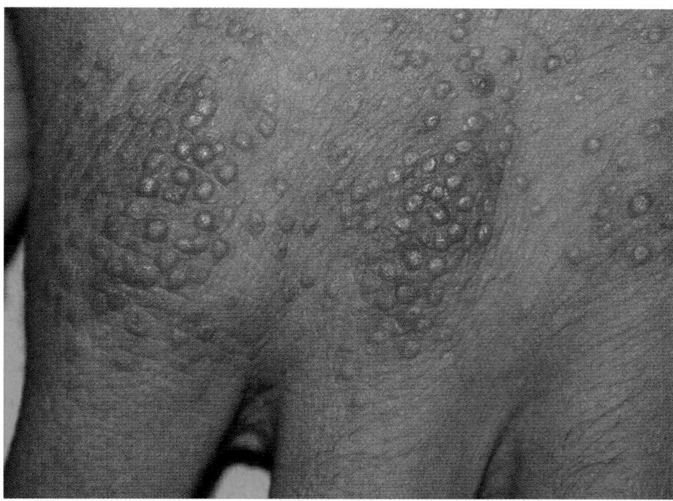

B

FIGURE 171-6 A. Perforating granuloma annulare with asymptomatic dorsal hand lesions since 9 months of age. Within the previous 6 months lesions began to appear on both elbows. This was previously misdiagnosed as molluscum contagiosum. B. Close-up of this rare perforating subset of granuloma annulare that affects the dorsum of the hands and extensor surfaces in children and young adults. (*Reproduced with permission from Eric Kraus, MD.*)

palisading cells lining a collection of mucin or as a diffuse interstitial pattern. There are no signs of epidermal change.[3]

DIFFERENTIAL DIAGNOSIS

- Tinea corporis has a raised, scaling border and can present on any body surface. Potassium hydroxide (KOH) preparation reveals hyphae with multiple branches (see Chapter 136, Tinea Corporis).
- Erythema annulare centrifugum has an affinity for thighs and legs. The diameter of these lesions can expand at a rate of 2 to 5 mm/d and may present with a trailing scale inside the advancing border.[2] Biopsy is helpful to differentiate this condition from GA (see Chapter 204, Erythema Annulare Centrifugum).
- Nummular eczema presents commonly on extremities, but is almost always associated with scaling plaques and intense itching (see Chapter 146, Nummular Eczema).
- Pityriasis rosea often has oval lesions with a trailing collarette of scale. The lesions are minimally raised and have scale that is absent in GA (see Chapter 151, Pityriasis Rosea).
- Rheumatoid nodules may mimic appearance of subcutaneous GA. These nodules are often seen over the elbows, fingers, and other joints in a patient with joint pains and other clinical signs of arthritis (see Chapter 99, Rheumatoid Arthritis). Rheumatoid nodules have fibrin deposition on histologic examination, in contrast to mucin in GA.

MANAGEMENT

The evidence for various treatments is at best small series of cases that are not randomized controlled trials. This disease is asymptomatic, and treatments only improve cosmetic appearance. Many patients may want intervention as diffuse lesions can cause psychological distress. Although GA will eventually resolve, some treatments may cause pigment change or atrophy that might be permanent. Several of the treatments below have shown promise, but these treatments may appear to work when in fact the resolution was natural.

Localized GA

- In a retrospective study of children with localized GA (mean age 8.6 years), 39 of 42 presented with complete clearance within 2 years. The average duration was 1 year. Researchers of this study consider most treatments unnecessary because of the self-limiting nature of this variation.[7] One treatment option is watchful waiting.[8] SOR B
- Intralesional corticosteroids can be injected into GA lesions with resolution of the area injected (see Figure 171-1). Inject directly into the ring itself with 3 to 5 mg/mL triamcinolone acetonide (Kenalog) using a 27-gauge needle. SOR C A large completed ring may take 4 injections to reach 360 degrees of the circle. The major complications include hypopigmentation (Figure 171-2A) and skin atrophy at the injected sites.

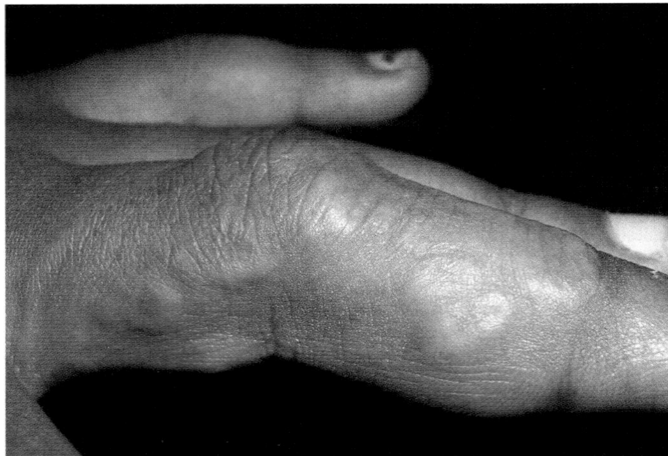

FIGURE 171-7 Subcutaneous granuloma annulare showing thickening of the involved finger along with the small annular patterns. Note the soft tissue infiltration that has distorted the finger anatomy. *(Reproduced with permission from Richard P. Usatine, MD.)*

- Cryotherapy was studied using nitrous oxide for 9 patients and liquid nitrogen for 22 patients. The results showed 80% clearing after a single freeze; however, 4 of 19 patients treated with liquid nitrogen developed atrophic scars when lesions were larger than 4 cm. All patients developed blisters.[9] Cryoatrophy may possibly be prevented by avoiding freeze thaw cycles greater than 10 seconds and not overlapping treatment areas.[10] SOR C
- A 53-year-old Hispanic woman with GA on the dorsal surface of both hands agreed to treatment with cryotherapy on the right hand and intralesional steroids on the left hand (**Figure 171-8**). Cryotherapy was performed using a 9- to 10-second freeze time and a single freeze. The intralesional injections were performed with a 30-gauge needle and 5 mg/mL triamcinolone (10 mg/mL diluted 1:1 with 1% lidocaine). During the treatment the patient rated the pain from cryotherapy as 9 out of 10 and intralesional steroid 2 out of 10. **Figure 171-8** shows the initial lesions and final results after 1 month. The patient was happy with the results of intralesional steroid and disappointed with the results of the cryotherapy. The lesion treated with cryotherapy did not resolve and spotted areas of hyperpigmentation and hypopigmentation occurred. Upon questioning, the patient states that the lesion treated with cryotherapy was painful for many days whereas she had no residual pain from the lesion treated with intralesional steroid. The patient then asked for the 2 remaining lesions on her right hand to be injected with steroid. Although this is a single case example, we could find no published studies of a head-to-head comparison between these commonly used methods for local treatment of GA.

Generalized/disseminated GA

- This variant is more difficult to treat, and often has a longer duration than localized GA. Many treatments have been claimed to be effective, but the studies touting these treatments have small sample sizes and were not randomized.
- In 2009, Marcus et al. reported the successful treatment of 6 patients with a combination of rifampin 600 mg, ofloxacin 400 mg, and minocycline 100 mg. All patients had complete clearance after 3 to 5 months of treatment.[11]
- Successful treatment of 6 patients with GA was achieved with 100 mg of dapsone, once a day. Complete clearance in all patients took between 4 weeks and 3 months.[12] SOR C
- UVA1 phototherapy provided good or excellent results in 10 of 20 patients with disseminated GA. In patients with only a satisfactory treatment response, the disease reappeared soon after phototherapy was discontinued.[13] SOR C
- In a study of 4 patients, topical 5% imiquimod cream was effective when used once daily for an average of 2 months. After discontinuing treatment, 3 patients went an average of 12 months without recurrence; the fourth patient had remission 10 days after treatment stopped, but after an additional 6 weeks of applying cream once daily, he was lesion-free for 18 months.[14] SOR C
- Four patients were treated with twice-daily topical application of 0.1% tacrolimus ointment for 6 weeks; all reported improvement after 10 to 21 days. At treatment conclusion, 2 patients had complete clearance and the other 2 had marked improvement.[15] SOR C
- Treatment with 0.5 to 1 mg/kg of isotretinoin daily has produced some positive results across multiple small studies; however, because of the potential for adverse effects, this option should be reserved for the most severe, nonresponsive cases in patients who are at low risk for the adverse effects of isotretinoin.[16] SOR C
- Three patients were treated with vitamin E 400 IU daily and zileuton 2400 mg daily. All responded within 3 months with complete clinical clearing.[17] SOR C

Perforating, subcutaneous

- Although we could find no specific data to inform the treatment of these less-common types of GA, treatments for both localized and disseminated GA could be applied based on clinical judgment along with patient's severity and preferences.

PROGNOSIS

In 50% of cases there is spontaneous resolution within 2 years; however, recurrence rate is as high as 40%.[18] Patients with skin of color may have postinflammatory hyperpigmentation once the papules and plaques resolve.

FOLLOW-UP

Follow-up visits should be offered to patients who want active treatment.

PATIENT EDUCATION

It is important to reassure patients that this disease is self-limiting. Despite a displeasing appearance, the best treatment may be to let lesions resolve naturally. Numerous individual case studies and treatments have been attempted without consistent success. Treatments may produce side effects that are equally as unwanted, but more permanent, than the GA.

PATIENT RESOURCES

- Skinsight. Granuloma Annulare: Information for Adults—**http://www.skinsight.com/adult/granulomaAnnulare.htm.**

PROVIDER RESOURCES

- Medscape. *Granuloma Annulare*—**http://emedicine.medscape.com/article/1123031.**

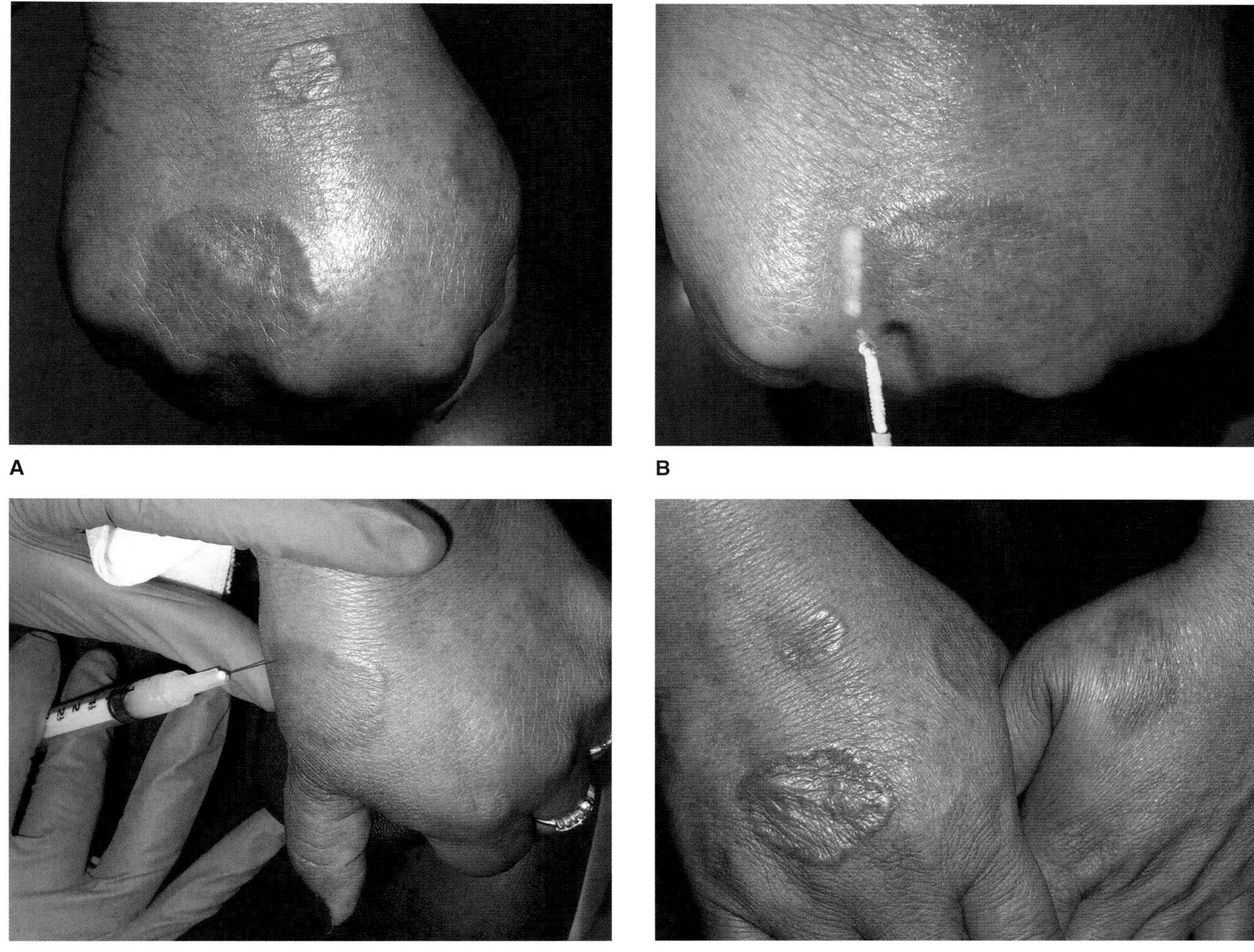

FIGURE 171-8 A. Granuloma annulare on the dorsum of the right hand of a 53-year-old Hispanic woman. B. Cryotherapy of the largest annular lesion. C. Intralesional triamcinolone being injected with a 30-gauge needle of a different granuloma annulare lesion on the left hand. D. One month later the lesion on the left hand treated with intralesional steroid has flattened and begun to fade while the lesion on the right hand continues to be elevated and now has areas of hyperpigmentation and hypopigmentation secondary to the cryotherapy. At the time of therapy the patient stated the injection hurt less than the cryotherapy. (*Reproduced with permission from Richard P. Usatine, MD.*)

REFERENCES

1. Cyr PR. Diagnosis and management of granuloma annulare. *Am Fam Physician*. 2006;74(10):1729-1714.
2. Ghadially R, Garg A. *Granuloma Annulare*. http://emedicine.medscape.com/article/1123031-overview. Accessed May 10, 2012.
3. Ko CJ, Glusac EJ, Shapiro PE. Noninfectious granulomas. In: Elder DE, ed. *Lever's Histopathology of the Skin*. 10th ed. Philadelphia, PA: Lippincott Williams & Wilkins; 2009:361-364.
4. Fayyazi A, Schweyer S, Eichmeyer B, et al. Expression of IFN-gamma, coexpression of TNF-alpha and matrix metalloproteinases and apoptosis of T lymphocytes and macrophages in granuloma annulare. *Arch Dermatol Res*. 2000;292:384-390.
5. Macaron NC, Cohen C, Chen SC, Arbiser JL. gli-1 Oncogene is highly expressed in granulomatous skin disorders, including sarcoidosis, granuloma annulare, and necrobiosis lipoidica diabeticorum. *Arch Dermatol*. 2005;141:259-262.
6. Habif TP. *Clinical Dermatology*. 4th ed. St Louis, MO: Mosby; 2004.
7. Smith MD, Downie JB, DiCostanzo D. Granuloma annulare. *Int J Dermatol*. 1997;36:326-333.
8. Martinón-Torres F, Martinón-Sánchez JM, Martinón-Sánchez F. Localized granuloma annulare in children: a review of 42 cases. *Eur J Pediatr*. 1999;158(10):866.
9. Blume-Peytavi U, Zouboulis CC, Jacobi H, et al. Successful outcome of cryosurgery in patients with granuloma annulare. *Br J Dermatol*. 1994;130(4):494-497.
10. Lebwohl MG, Berth-Jones M, Coulson I. *Treatment of Skin Disease, Comprehensive Therapeutic Strategies*. 2nd ed. St. Louis, MO: Mosby; 2006:251.
11. Marcus DV, Mahmoud BH, Hamzavi IH. Granuloma annulare treated with rifampin, ofloxacin, and minocycline combination therapy. *Arch Dermatol*. 2009;145(7):787-789.

12. Czarnecki DB, Gin D. The response of generalized granuloma annulare to dapsone. *Acta Derm Venereol (Stockh)*. 1986;66:82-84.

13. Schnopp C, Tzaneva S, Mempel M, et al. UVA1 phototherapy for disseminated granuloma annulare. *Photodermatol Photoimmunol Photomed*. 2005;21(2):68-71.

14. Badavanis G, Monastirli A, Pasmatzi E, Tsambaos D. Successful treatment of granuloma annulare with imiquimod cream 5%: a report of four cases. *Acta Derm Venereol*. 2005;85(6):547-548.

15. Jain S, Stephens CJM. Successful treatment of disseminated granuloma annulare with topical tacrolimus. *Br J Dermatol*. 2004;150:1042-1043.

16. Looney M. Isotretinoin in the treatment of granuloma annulare. *Ann Pharmacother*. 2004;38(3):494-497.

17. Smith KJ, Norwood C, Skelton H. Treatment of disseminated granuloma annulare with a 5-lipoxygenase inhibitor and vitamin E. *Br J Dermatol*. 2002;146(4):667-670.

18. Reisenauer A, White KP, Korcheva V, White CR. Non-infectious granulomas. In: Bolognia JL, Jorizzo JL, Schaffer JV, eds. *Dermatology*. 2nd ed. Philadelphia, PA: Elsevier: 2012.

172 PYODERMA GANGRENOSUM

E.J. Mayeaux Jr, MD
Richard P. Usatine, MD

PATIENT STORY

A 32-year-old man was diagnosed with Crohn disease 10 years prior to his visit for these nonhealing leg ulcers (**Figure 172-1**). The patient experienced minor trauma to his lower leg 1 year ago and these ulcers developed (pathergy). Multiple treatments have been tried with partial success, but the ulcers persist.

INTRODUCTION

Pyoderma gangrenosum (PG) is an uncommon ulcerative disease of the skin of unknown origin. It is a type of neutrophilic dermatosis.

EPIDEMIOLOGY

- PG occurs in approximately 1 person per 100,000 people each year.[1]
- No racial predilection is apparent.
- A slight female predominance may exist.
- Predominately occurs in fourth and fifth decade, but all age-group people may be affected.

ETIOLOGY AND PATHOPHYSIOLOGY

- Etiology is poorly understood.
- Pathergy (initiation at the site of trauma or injury) is a common process and it is estimated that 30% of patients with PG experienced pathergy.[1]

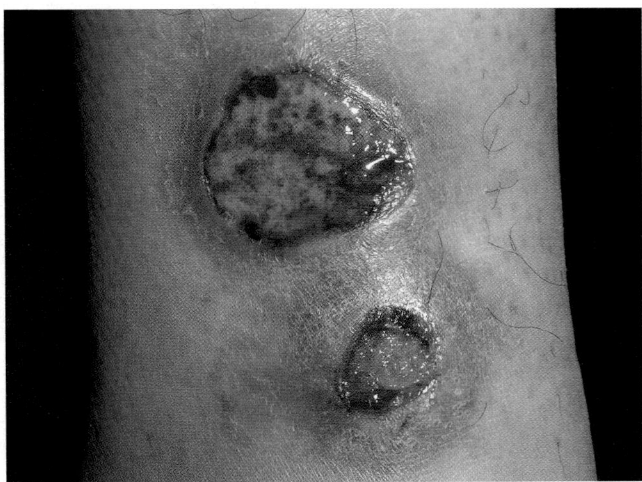

FIGURE 172-1 Classic pyoderma gangrenosum on the leg of a 32-year-old man with Crohn disease. This ulcer started with minor trauma (pathergy) and has been there for 1 year. (*Reproduced with permission from Richard P. Usatine, MD.*)

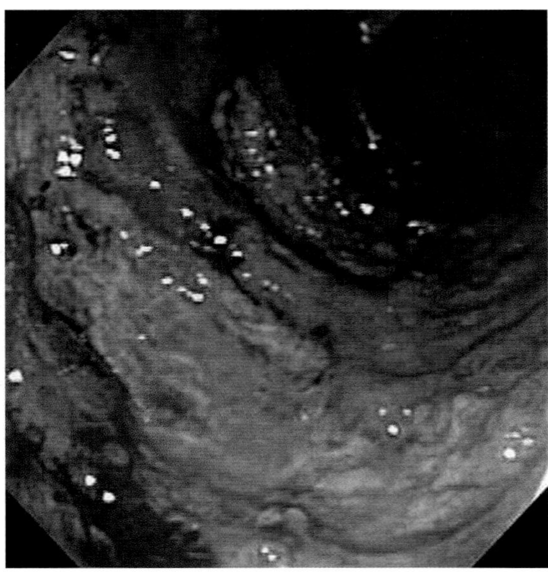

FIGURE 172-2 Friable inflamed mucosa of the colon in Crohn disease. (*Reproduced with permission from Shashi Mittal, MD.*)

- Up to 50% of cases are idiopathic.[2]
- At least 50% of cases are associated with systemic diseases such as inflammatory bowel disease, hematologic malignancy, and arthritis.[2]
- It occurs in up to 5% of patients with ulcerative colitis and 2% of those with Crohn disease (**Figures 172-2** and **172-3**).[3,4]
- Biopsies usually show a polymorphonuclear cell infiltrate with features of ulceration, infarction, and abscess formation.

RISK FACTORS

- Ulcerative colitis[2,5]
- Crohn disease
- Polyarthritis (seronegative or seropositive)

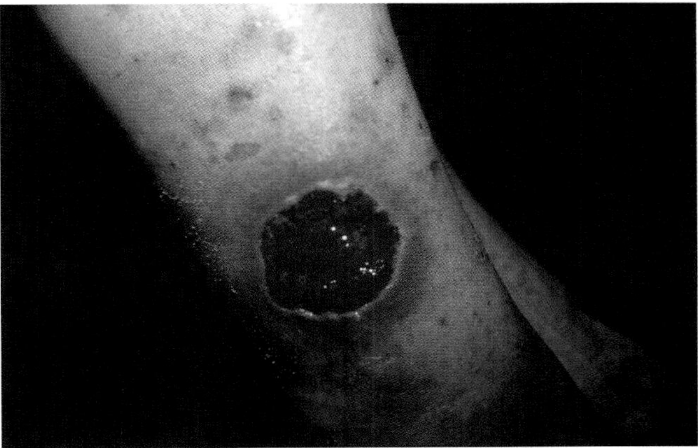

FIGURE 172-3 Classic pyoderma gangrenosum on the leg of a 35-year-old woman with Crohn disease. This ulcer started with minor trauma (pathergy) and has been there for 2 years. (*Reproduced with permission from Richard P. Usatine, MD.*)

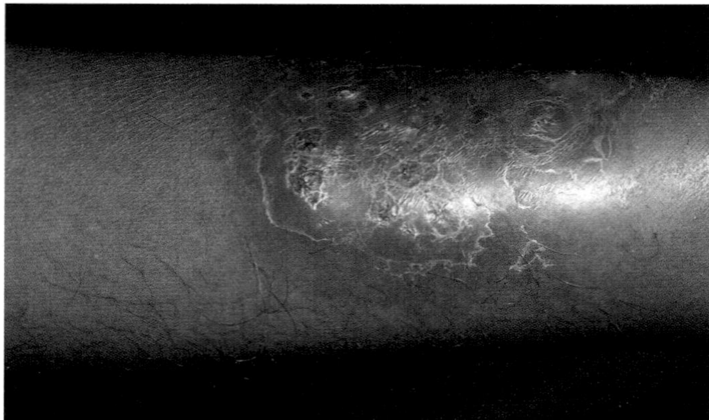

FIGURE 172-4 Pyoderma gangrenosum on the leg of a 56-year-old woman with rheumatoid arthritis. (*Reproduced with permission from Richard P. Usatine, MD.*)

- Hematologic diseases/disorders such as leukemia (predominantly myelocytic)
- Monoclonal gammopathies (primarily immunoglobulin A)
- Psoriatic arthritis and rheumatoid arthritis (**Figure 172-4**)
- Hepatic diseases (hepatitis and primary biliary cirrhosis)
- Immunologic diseases (lupus erythematosus and Sjögren syndrome)

DIAGNOSIS

CLINICAL FEATURES

- Typically PG presents with deep painful ulcer with a well-defined border, which is usually violet or blue. The color has also been described as the color of gun metal. The ulcer edge is often undermined and the surrounding skin is erythematous and indurated. It usually starts as a pustule with an inflammatory base, an erythematous nodule, or a hemorrhagic bulla on a violaceous base. The central area then undergoes necrosis to form a single ulcer.[5]

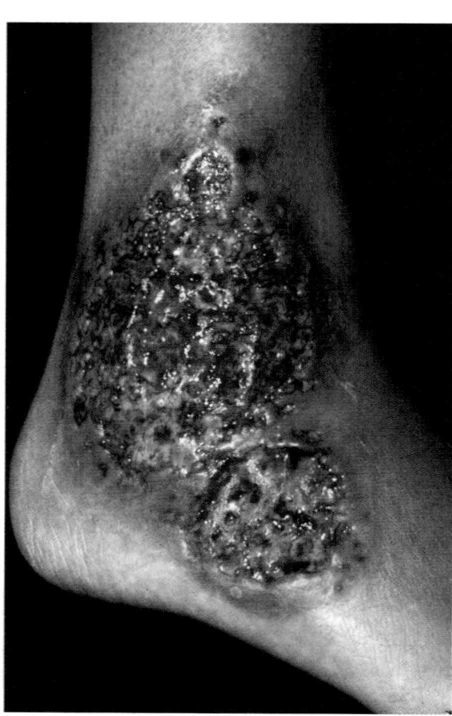

FIGURE 172-5 Pyoderma gangrenosum showing dusky red border with undermined edges. The surface appears purulent and necrotic. (*Reproduced with permission from Jack Resneck Sr, MD.*)

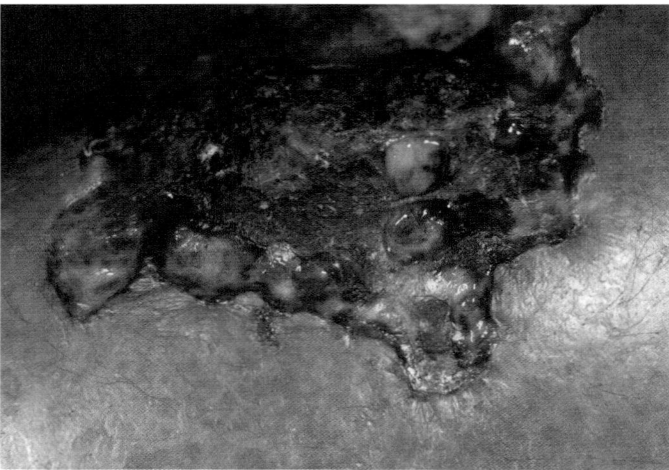

FIGURE 172-6 Pyoderma gangrenosum ulcer on the leg with purulent undermined edges and black eschar. (*Reproduced with permission from Jeff Meffert, MD.*)

- The lesions are painful and the pain can be severe.[2] Patients may have malaise, arthralgia, and myalgia.
- Two main variants of PG exist: classic and atypical.[2]
    - Classic PG is characterized by a deep ulceration with a violaceous border that overhangs the ulcer bed.[2] These lesions of PG most commonly occur on the legs (**Figures 172-1** and **172-3** to **172-7**).[2]
    - Atypical PG has a vesiculopustular wet component (**Figures 172-8** and **172-9**). This is usually only at the border, is erosive or superficially ulcerated, and most often occurs on the dorsal surface of the hands, the extensor parts of the forearms, or the face.[2]
- Other variants
    - Peristomal PG may occur around stoma sites. This form is often mistaken for a wound infection or irritation from the appliance.[6]

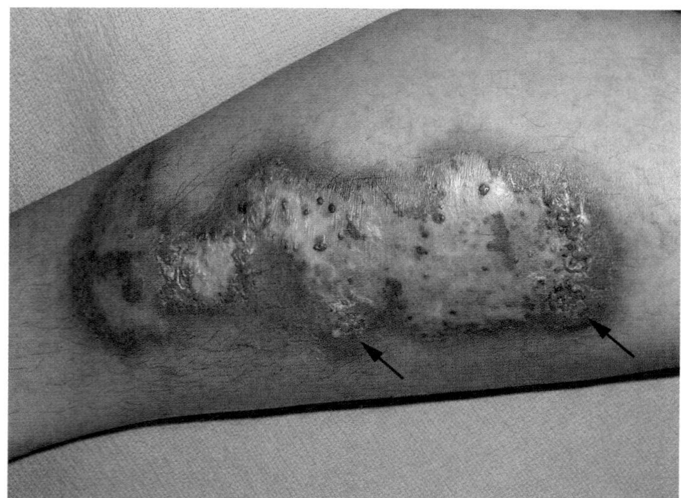

FIGURE 172-7 Partially healed pyoderma gangrenosum on the leg of a 29-year-old Hispanic woman. Note the areas of healed ulcerations and the dusky elevated borders. There remain 2 areas of active disease (*arrows*) with pain, erythema, swelling, and purulent discharge. The patient improved with dapsone. (*Reproduced with permission from Richard P. Usatine, MD.*)

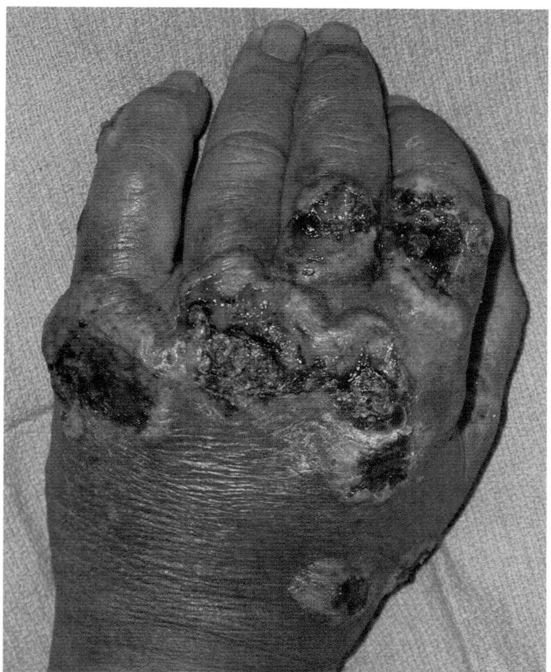

FIGURE 172-8 Atypical pyoderma gangrenosum with a vesiculopustular "juicy" component on the dorsal surface of the hand. Bullae were previously present before the ulcerations developed. (*Reproduced with permission from Eric Kraus, MD.*)

- Vulvar or penile PG occurs on the genitalia and must be differentiated from ulcerative sexually transmitted diseases (STDs) such as chancroid and syphilis.[2]
- Intraoral PG is known as pyostomatitis vegetans. Occurs primarily in patients with inflammatory bowel disease.[2]

TYPICAL DISTRIBUTION

Most commonly seen on the legs and hands, but can occur on any skin surface including the genitalia, and around a stoma. PG can be seen on the scalp, head, and neck (**Figures 172-10** and **172-11**).

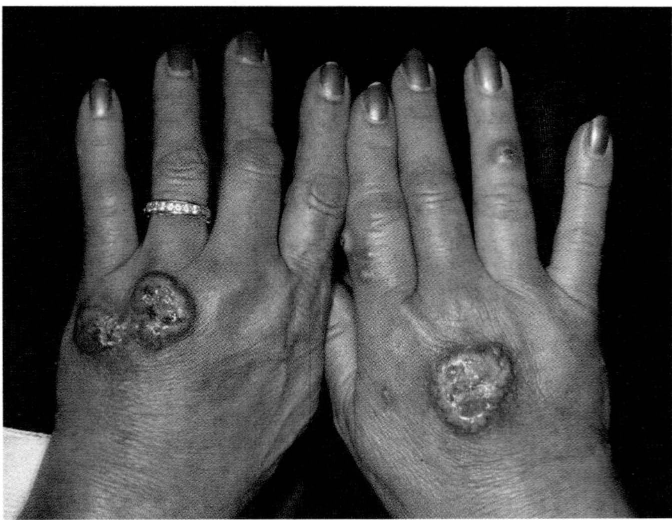

FIGURE 172-9 Atypical pyoderma gangrenosum on the hands with violaceous borders that match the fingernail color. The lesions are "juicy" and resemble those seen in Sweet syndrome and have occurred at sites of minor trauma (pathergy). (*Reproduced with permission from Jeff Meffert, MD.*)

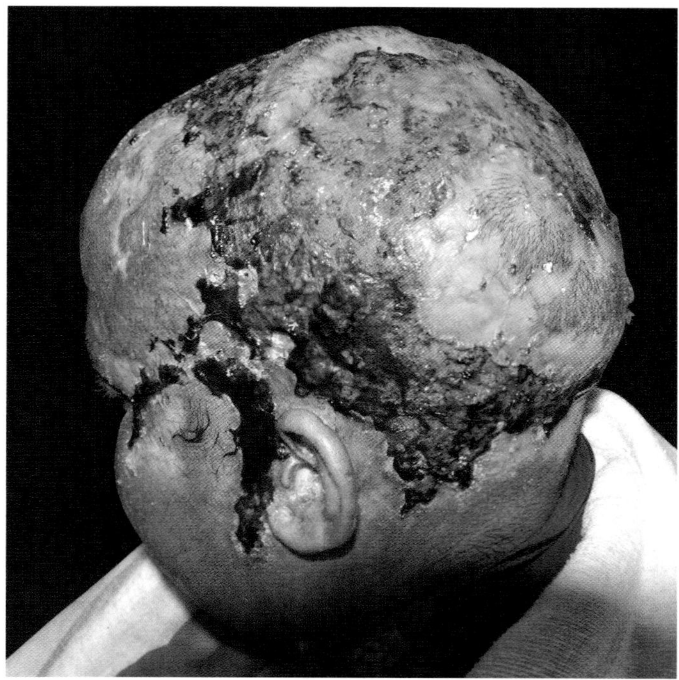

FIGURE 172-10 Pyoderma gangrenosum on the scalp of a woman in Africa. (*Reproduced with permission from Richard P. Usatine, MD.*)

LABORATORY TESTING

- Complete blood count (CBC), urinalysis (UA), and liver function tests (LFTs) should be obtained. Order a hepatitis profile to rule out hepatitis.[2] Systemic disease markers may be elevated if associated conditions exist, that is, erythrocyte sedimentation rate (ESR), antinuclear

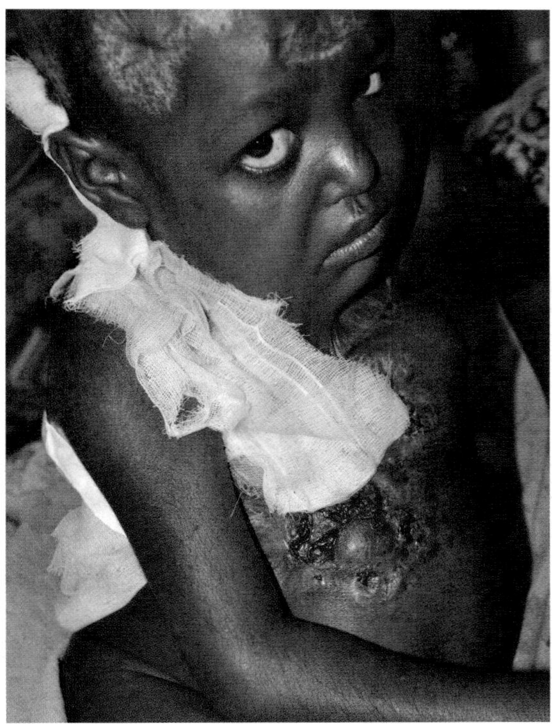

FIGURE 172-11 Pyoderma gangrenosum on the face, neck, and chest of a child in Africa. The scarring has caused adhesions between the face, neck, and chest. (*Reproduced with permission from Richard P. Usatine, MD.*)

antibody (ANA), and rheumatoid factor. Obtain rapid plasma reagin (RPR), protein electrophoresis, and skin cultures as indicated. Consider culturing the ulcer/erosion for bacteria, fungi, atypical *Mycobacteria*, and viruses.[2]

- If gastrointestinal (GI) symptoms exist, perform or refer for colonoscopy to look for inflammatory bowel disease.

BIOPSY

- Biopsy an active area of disease along with the border. A punch biopsy is preferred (4-mm punch is adequate). Although there are no specific pathologic signs of PG, the biopsy can be used to rule out other causes of ulcerative skin lesions.
- The pathologist may be able to confirm your clinical impression. Biopsy of the earliest lesions reveals a neutrophilic vascular reaction. Fully developed lesions exhibit dense neutrophilic infiltrate, and some lymphocytes and macrophages surrounding marked tissue necrosis. Ulceration, infarction of tissue, and abscess formation with fibrosing inflammation at the edge of the ulcer may be seen.[7]

DIFFERENTIAL DIAGNOSIS

- PG is sometimes a diagnosis of exclusion diagnosed with successful wound healing following immunosuppressant therapy.[8] When misdiagnosed it is often confused for vascular occlusive or venous disease, vasculitis, cancer, primary infection, drug-induced or exogenous tissue injury, and other inflammatory disorders.[9] Biopsy of a questionable lesion may be the only way to ultimately distinguish PG as the cause of ulcerative skin lesions.
- Ulcerative sexually transmitted diseases (STDs), such as chancroid and syphilis, can resemble vulvar or penile PG. These STDs are more common than PG and should be diagnosed with appropriate tests, including RPR and bacterial culture for *Haemophilus ducreyi*. If these tests are negative, then PG should be considered. RPR should also be repeated in 2 weeks if it is initially negative at the start of a chancre—it takes some weeks to become positive and syphilis is easily treatable (see Chapter 218, Syphilis).
- Acute febrile neutrophilic dermatosis (Sweet syndrome) is a neutrophilic dermatosis like PG, but the patients are generally febrile with systemic symptoms (**Figure 172-12**). The diagnosis of Sweet syndrome is made when the patient fulfills 2 of 2 major criteria and 2 of 4 minor criteria. The 2 major criteria are (a) an abrupt onset of tender or painful erythematous plaques or nodules occasionally with vesicles, pustules, or bullae, and (b) predominantly neutrophilic infiltration in the dermis without leukocytoclastic vasculitis. Minor criteria include specific preceding or concurrent medical conditions, fever, abnormal laboratory values, including leukocytosis and an elevated sedimentation rate, and a rapid response to systemic steroids.
- Systemic vasculitis is perhaps the most difficult to differentiate, but history of minor trauma in the area preceding lesion formation (pathergy) and undermining of the violaceous border should lead one toward the diagnosis of PG.[9]
- Ecthyma is a type of impetigo in which ulcers form. Bacterial cultures will be positive and this disease should respond to cephalexin or other oral antibiotics (see Chapter 118, Impetigo).
- Spider bites from the black recluse spider can easily resemble PG when they ulcerate. The history of a spider bite can help differentiate this from PG.
- Sporotrichosis is a fungal infection that often starts from an injury while gardening with roses. It is usually on the arm or hand and can resemble PG. Use fungal culture to diagnose this when the history suggests this as the diagnosis. Oral antifungal medications can treat this (**Figure 172-13**).
- Squamous cell carcinoma with ulcerations may look like PG. Its diagnosis requires a biopsy. If the ulcer is on sun-exposed area, squamous cell carcinoma should be considered. A shave or punch biopsy can be used to diagnose this malignancy (see Chapter 169, Squamous Cell Carcinoma).
- Venous insufficiency ulcers are typically seen around the medial malleolus and the most severe of these ulcers resembles PG (**Figure 172-14**). The presence of signs and symptoms of venous insufficiency should help differentiate this from PG (see Chapter 51, Venous Stasis).
- Mycosis fungoides is a cutaneous T-cell lymphoma that can ulcerate and resemble PG. Use tissue biopsy to differentiate these 2 conditions (see Chapter 174, Cutaneous T-cell Lymphoma).

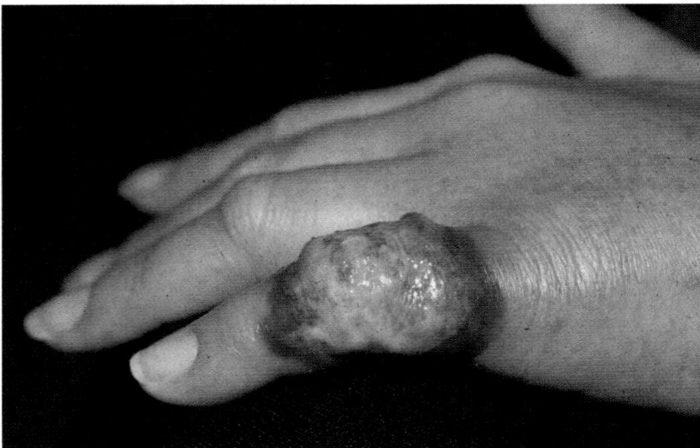

FIGURE 172-12 Sweet syndrome is the eponym for acute febrile neutrophilic dermatosis. The lesion looks like pyoderma gangrenosum and occurs at sites of minor trauma (pathergy). However, this patient has a fever and is systemically ill. (*Reproduced with permission from John Gonzalez, MD.*)

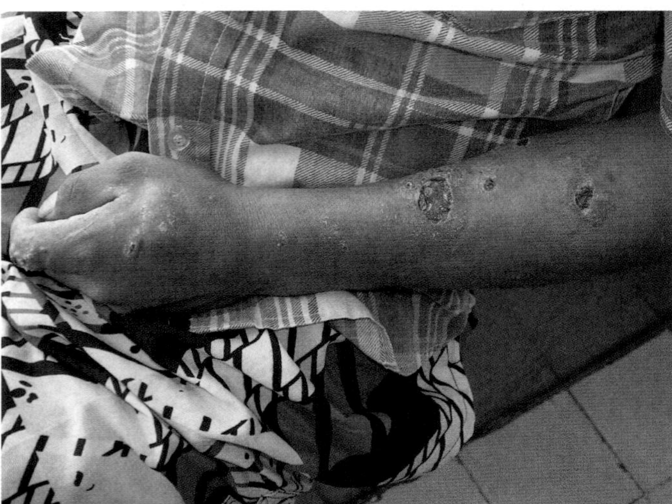

FIGURE 172-13 Sporotrichosis (fungal infection) with the typical sporotrichoid spread up the arm from an inoculation of the hand. Note the ulcers that resemble pyoderma gangrenosum on the arm of this Panamanian teenager. (*Reproduced with permission from Richard P. Usatine, MD.*)

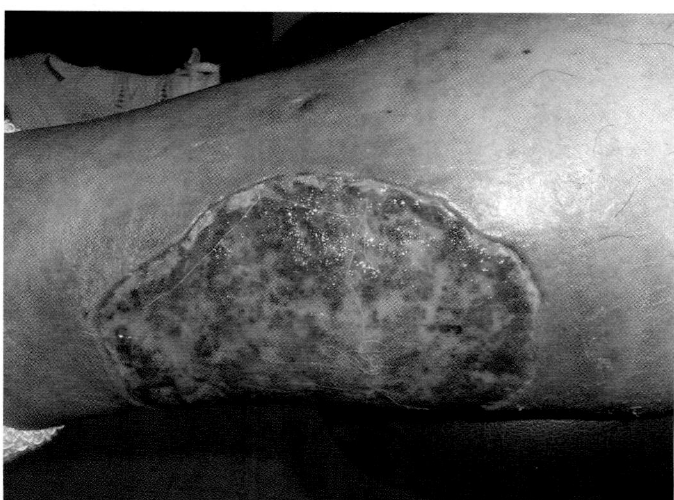

FIGURE 172-14 A large venous stasis ulcer on the lower leg not healing with intensive wound care and compression stockings. A punch biopsy on the edge was performed to make sure this was not pyoderma gangrenosum. (*Reproduced with permission from Richard P. Usatine, MD.*)

MANAGEMENT

NONPHARMACOLOGIC

- At each visit, measure and document the lesion's depth, length, and width to track treatment progression.[10]
- Surgical debridement is contraindicated as pathergy occurs in 25% to 50% of cases and surgery will make the lesions worse. SOR B

MEDICATIONS

- Patients frequently are in pain from the lesions, so treatment is aimed at pain relief as well as healing the skin lesions.
- Therapy directed at the underlying inflammatory bowel disease (IBD), when present, usually results in healing, although treatment with steroids is often necessary.[10] SOR B
- Topical medications are first-line therapy in cases of localized PG that are not severe. Start with potent corticosteroid ointments or tacrolimus ointment.[10,11] SOR B
- Small ulcers can be managed with topical steroid creams, silver sulfadiazine, or potassium iodide solution. SOR C
- Intralesional injections with corticosteroids are also an option.[10,11] SOR B
- Systemic treatment with oral corticosteroids, such as methylprednisolone (1 g/d IV for 3 days) or prednisone (0.5-1 mg/kg/d) or oral cyclosporine (eg, 5 mg/kg/d) alone or together appears to be effective (in the absence of controlled trials) in many cases and should be considered first-line therapy.[6,11] SOR B Response is usually rapid, with stabilization of the PG within 24 hours.[12]
- In steroid-refractory PG associated with IBD, infliximab was effective in case series and a small placebo-controlled trial.[13,14] SOR B Other biologic therapies reported include alefacept, etanercept, efalizumab, and adalimumab.[10] SOR C
- To date, case reports have been published that show therapeutic efficacy of dapsone (100 mg/d), azathioprine (50-150 mg/d), 6-mercaptopurine, mycophenolate mofetil (1-2 g twice daily), cyclophosphamide (2-3 mg/kg/d), and tacrolimus (0.1 mg/kg/d).[11,15] SOR C

REFERRAL

In many cases, referral to a dermatologist is needed.

PROGNOSIS

- The prognosis of PG is generally good, but residual scarring is common (see **Figure 172-11**) and recurrences may occur.
- Although many patients improve with initial immunosuppressive therapy, patients may follow a refractory course and require multiple therapies.

FOLLOW-UP

All patients suspected of having PG need close and frequent follow-up to obtain a definitive diagnosis and treat this challenging condition.

PATIENT EDUCATION

- PG is a rare ulcerative skin condition that is poorly understood.
- A skin biopsy is needed to rule out other diagnoses.
- Most treatments are empirical and based on small studies.
- The risks and benefits of steroids and/or other immunosuppressive medications need to be explained.
- Surgical treatments are contraindicated.

PATIENT RESOURCES

- American Autoimmune Related Diseases Association, Inc. Tel: 800-598-4668—**http://www.aarda.org/.**
- Crohn's and Colitis Foundation of America. Tel: 800-932-2423—**http://www.ccfa.org.**

PROVIDER RESOURCES

- Medscape. *Pyoderma Gangrenosum*—**http://emedicine.medscape.com/article/1123821.**
- MayoClinic. *Pyoderma Gangrenosum*—**http://www.mayoclinic.com/health/pyoderma-gangrenosum/DS00723.**
- Wollina U. PG—a review. *Orphanet J Rare Dis*. 2007;2:19—**http://www.ncbi.nlm.nih.gov/pmc/articles/PMC1857704/.**

REFERENCES

1. Brooklyn T, Brooklyn T, Dunnill G, Probert C. Diagnosis and treatment of pyoderma gangrenosum. *BMJ*. 2006;333(7560):181-184.
2. Jackson JM, Callen JP. *Pyoderma Gangrenosum*. http://emedicine.medscape.com/article/1123821-overview. Accessed March 30, 2012.
3. Mir-Madjlessi SH, Taylor JS, Farmer RG. Clinical course and evolution of erythema nodosum and pyoderma gangrenosum in chronic ulcerative colitis: a study of 42 patients. *Am J Gastroenterol*. 1985;80(8):615-620.

4. McCallum DI, Kinmont PD. Dermatological manifestations of Crohn's disease. *Br J Dermatol.* 1968;80(1):1-8.
5. Habif T. *Clinical Dermatology*. 4th ed. Philadelphia, PA: Mosby; 2004:653-654.
6. Keltz M, Lebwohl M, Bishop S. Peristomal pyoderma gangrenosum. *J Am Acad Dermatol.* 1992;27(2 pt 2):360-364.
7. Su WP, Schroeter AL, Perry HO, Powell FC. Histopathologic and immunopathologic study of pyoderma gangrenosum. *J Cutan Pathol.* 1986;13(5):323-330.
8. Banga F, Schuitemaker N, Meijer P. Pyoderma gangrenosum after caesarean section: a case report. *Reprod Health.* 2006;3:9.
9. Weenig RH, Davis MD, Dahl PR, Su WP. Skin ulcers misdiagnosed as pyoderma gangrenosum. *N Engl J Med.* 2002;347(18):1412-1418.
10. Miller J, Yentzer BA, Clark A, et al. Pyoderma gangrenosum: a review and update on new therapies. *J Am Acad Dermatol.* 2010;62(4):646-654.
11. Reichrath J, Bens G, Bonowitz A, Tilgen W. Treatment recommendations for pyoderma gangrenosum: an evidence-based review of the literature based on more than 350 patients. *J Am Acad Dermatol.* 2005;53(2):273-283.
12. Chow RK, Ho VC. Treatment of pyoderma gangrenosum. *J Am Acad Dermatol.* 1996;34(6):1047-1060.
13. De la Morena F, Martín L, Gisbert JP, et al. Refractory and infected pyoderma gangrenosum in a patient with ulcerative colitis: response to infliximab. *Inflamm Bowel Dis.* 2007;13(4):509-510.
14. Brooklyn TN, Dunnill MG, Shetty A, et al. Infliximab for the treatment of pyoderma gangrenosum: a randomised, double blind, placebo controlled trial. *Gut.* 2006;55(4):505-509.
15. Eaton PA, Callen JP. Mycophenolate mofetil as therapy for pyoderma gangrenosum. *Arch Dermatol.* 2009;145(7):781-785.

173 SARCOIDOSIS

Yoon-Soo Cindy Bae-Harboe, MD
Khashayar Sarabi, MD
Amor Khachemoune, MD

PATIENT STORY

A 42-year-old man presents with "multiple bumps" that had been growing on his scalp, the back of the neck, and on preexisting scars (**Figure 173-1**). These lesions started developing slowly over a period of 1 year. The differential diagnosis of these lesions included cutaneous sarcoidosis, acne keloidalis nuchae, and pseudofolliculitis barbae. A punch biopsy was performed and the diagnosis of sarcoidosis was made.

INTRODUCTION

Sarcoidosis is a multisystem granulomatous disease most commonly involving the skin, lungs, lymph nodes, liver, and eyes. Patients of African descent are more commonly affected compared to white patients. Diagnosing cutaneous sarcoidosis is critical as 30% of these patients have been found to have systemic involvement. Diverse presentations of cutaneous sarcoidosis have been reported in addition to variants of specific sarcoidosis syndromes.

SYNONYMS

- Lupus pernio (cutaneous sarcoidosis)
- Darier-Roussy disease (subcutaneous sarcoidosis)
- Löfgren syndrome (erythema nodosum, hilar adenopathy, fever, arthritis)
- Heerfordt syndrome (parotid gland enlargement, uveitis, fever, cranial nerve palsy)

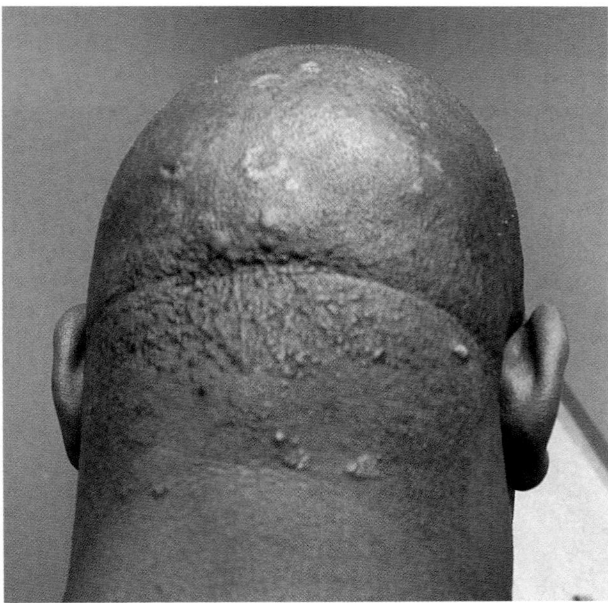

FIGURE 173-1 Papular and annular lesions of sarcoid on the scalp and neck of a 42-year-old black man. (*Reproduced with permission from Amor Khachemoune, MD.*)

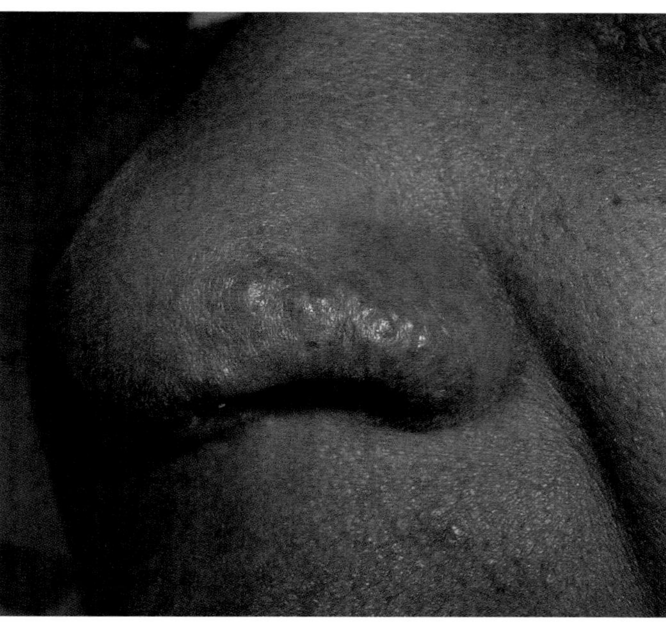

FIGURE 173-2 Lupus pernio in a 45-year-old black woman with sarcoid involving the nasal rim. (*Reproduced with permission from Richard P. Usatine, MD.*)

EPIDEMIOLOGY

- Cutaneous manifestations occur in approximately 25% of systemic sarcoidosis patients.
- The ratio between patients with only cutaneous sarcoid versus multisystem involvement is 1:3.
- Specific cutaneous involvement is seen most commonly in older, female patients of African descent (**Figures 173-2** and **173-3**).

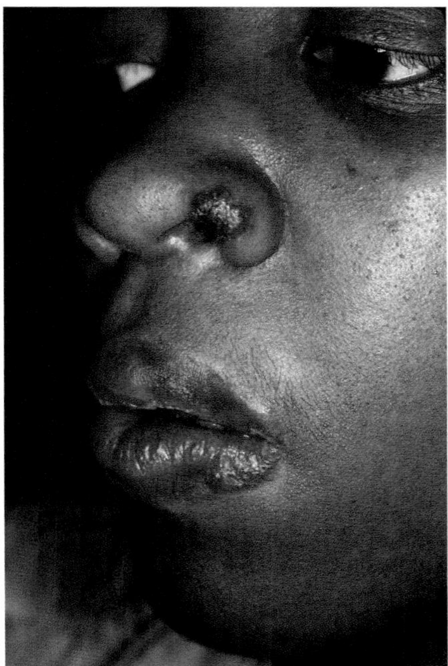

FIGURE 173-3 Lupus pernio with red-to-violaceous sarcoid papules and plaques on the nose and lips. (*Reproduced with permission from Amor Khachemoune, MD.*)

- Common types are maculopapular, lupus pernio, cutaneous, or subcutaneous nodules, and infiltrative scars.
- Erythema nodosum (EN) occurs in 3% to 34% of patients with sarcoidosis and is the most common associated skin finding (see Chapter 176, Erythema Nodosum).
- Sarcoidosis-related EN is more prevalent in whites, especially Scandinavians. Irish and Puerto Rican females are also affected more often.
- EN occurs between the second and fourth decades of life, more commonly in women.
- Nonspecific lesions of sarcoidosis reported, besides EN, include erythema multiforme, calcinosis cutis, prurigo, and lymphedema. Nail changes can include clubbing, onycholysis, subungual keratosis, and dystrophy, with or without underlying changes in the bone (cysts).

ETIOLOGY AND PATHOPHYSIOLOGY

- Sarcoidosis is a granulomatous disease with involvement of multiple organ systems with an unknown etiology.
- The typical findings in sarcoid lesions are characterized by the presence of circumscribed granulomas of epithelioid cells with little or no caseating necrosis, although fibrinoid necrosis is not uncommon.
- Granulomas are usually in the superficial dermis but may involve the thickness of dermis and extend to the subcutaneous tissue. These granulomas are referred to as "naked" because they only have a sparse lymphocytic infiltrate at their margins.

RISK FACTORS

- Positive family history
- African descent

DIAGNOSIS

CLINICAL FORMS OF DISEASE

Cutaneous involvement is either *specific* or *nonspecific*.

- Specific
  - Typical noncaseating granulomas, no evidence of infection, foreign body, or other causes.
  - May be disfiguring, but almost always nontender and rarely ulcerate.
  - Maculopapular type is most common, red-brown or purplish, usually smaller than 1 cm, and found mostly on face, neck, upper back, and limbs (**Figure 173-4**).
  - Lupus pernio type are most distinctive lesions and present as purplish lesions resembling frostbites with shiny skin covering them, typically affecting nose, cheeks, ears, and lips and distal extremities (**Figures 173-2**, **173-3**, and **173-5**).
  - Lupus pernio may occur as a syndrome involving upper respiratory tract with pulmonary fibrosis, or be associated with chronic uveitis and bone cysts.
  - Annular or circinate type appear ribbon-like, with mild scaling and yellowish red in color, with centrifugal progression and central healing and depigmentation (see **Figure 173-1**).
  - Plaque sarcoidosis is typically chronic, occurring over the forehead, extremities, and shoulders, but may heal without scarring (**Figure 173-6**).

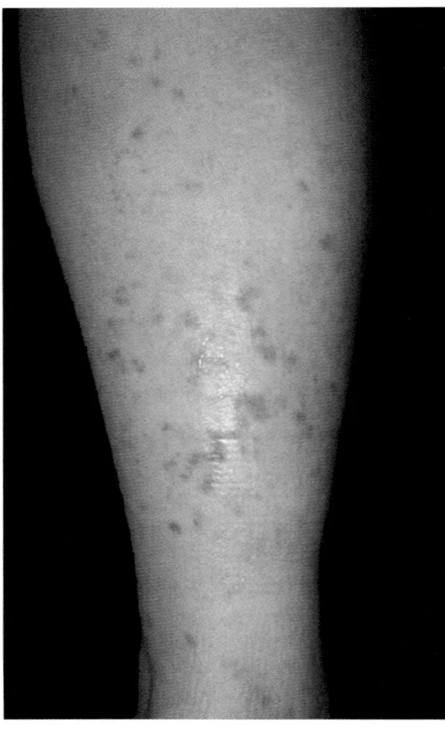

FIGURE 173-4 Maculopapular sarcoidosis on the leg of a 46-year-old white woman. (*Reproduced with permission from Amor Khachemoune, MD.*)

  - Nodular cutaneous and subcutaneous plaques that are skin colored or violaceous without epidermal involvement are typically seen in advanced systemic sarcoidosis (**Figure 173-7**).
  - Areas of old scars that are damaged by trauma, radiation, surgery, or tattoo may also be infiltrated with sarcoid granulomas (**Figures 173-8** and **173-9**). Lesions may be tender and appear indurated with red or purple discoloration.
- Nonspecific
  - EN lesions usually are not disfiguring, but tender to touch, especially when they occur with fever, polyarthralgias, and sometimes arthritis and acute iritis.

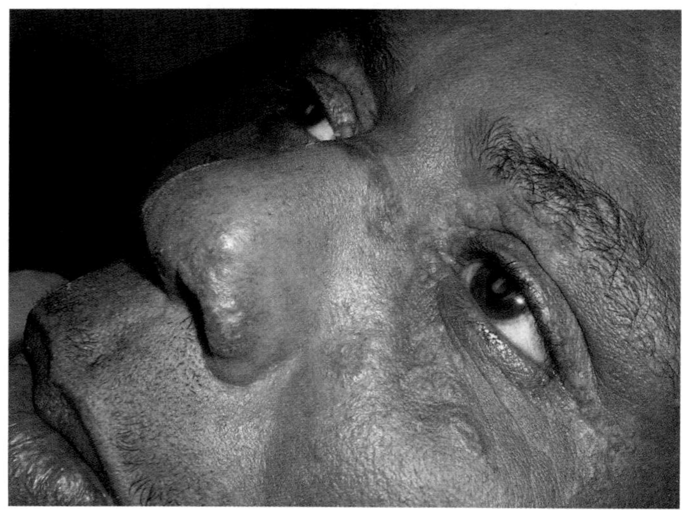

FIGURE 173-5 Lupus pernio in a 48-year-old black man with sarcoid lesions on the nose and around the eyes. (*Reproduced with permission from Richard P. Usatine, MD.*)

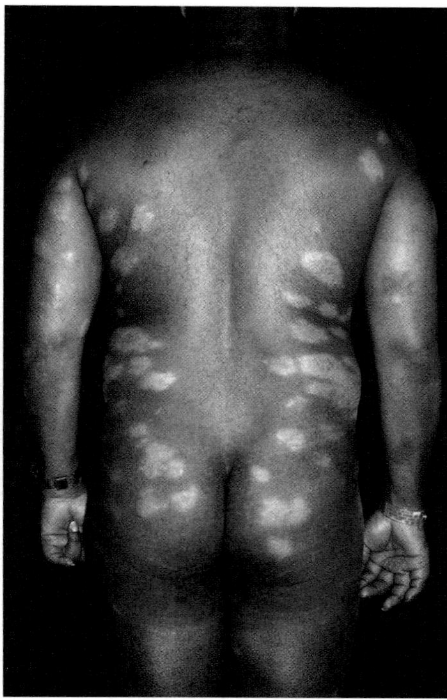

FIGURE 173-6 Hypopigmented widespread cutaneous plaque sarcoidosis predominantly on the back of a black man. (*Reproduced with permission from Eric Kraus, MD.*)

- EN appears abruptly with warm, tender, reddish nodules on the lower extremities, most commonly the anterior tibial surfaces, ankles, and knees.
- EN nodules are 1 to 5 cm, usually bilateral, and evolve through color stages: first bright red, then purplish, and lastly a bruise-like yellow or green appearance.
- EN bouts occur with fatigue, fever, symmetrical polyarthritis, and skin eruptions that typically last 3 to 6 weeks with more than 80% of cases resolving within 2 years.[1]

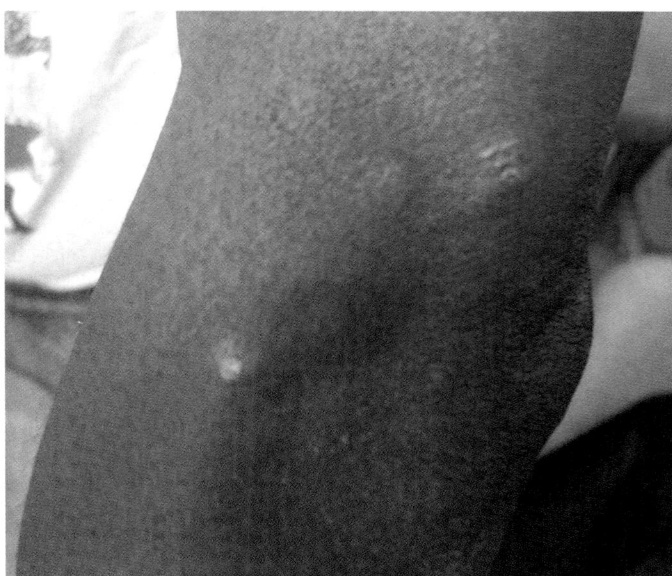

FIGURE 173-7 Subcutaneous sarcoid (Darier-Roussy syndrome) in a patient with advanced systemic sarcoidosis. (*Reproduced with permission from Amor Khachemoune, MD.*)

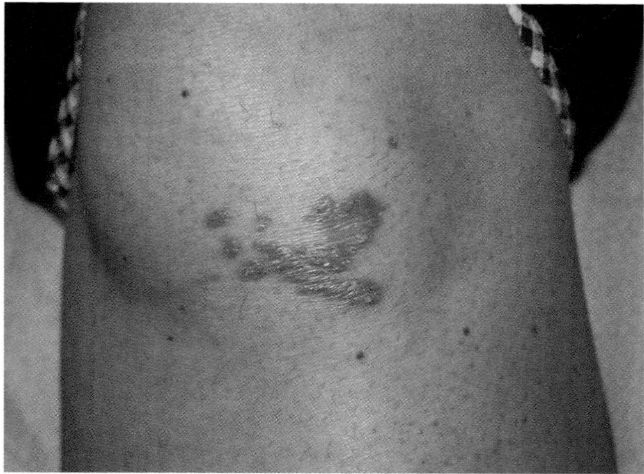

FIGURE 173-8 Sarcoidal plaque of the knee, which appeared after a trauma to the knee. (*Reproduced with permission from Amor Khachemoune, MD.*)

- EN is seen in the setting of Löfgren syndrome, appearing in conjunction with hilar lymphadenopathy (bilateral most often), and occasionally anterior uveitis and/or polyarthritis.
- Löfgren syndrome is associated with right paratracheal lymph node involvement seen on X-ray.
- Ulceration is typically not observed in EN, which heals without scarring.
- Other nonspecific lesions of sarcoidosis include lymphedema, calcinosis cutis, prurigo, and erythema multiforme.
- Nail changes seen in sarcoidosis include clubbing, onycholysis, and subungual keratosis.

LABORATORY STUDIES

- Complete blood count (CBC) with differential.
  - Leukopenia (5%-10%) and/or thrombocytopenia may be seen.
  - Eosinophilia occurs in 24% of patients and anemia occurs in 5% of patients.

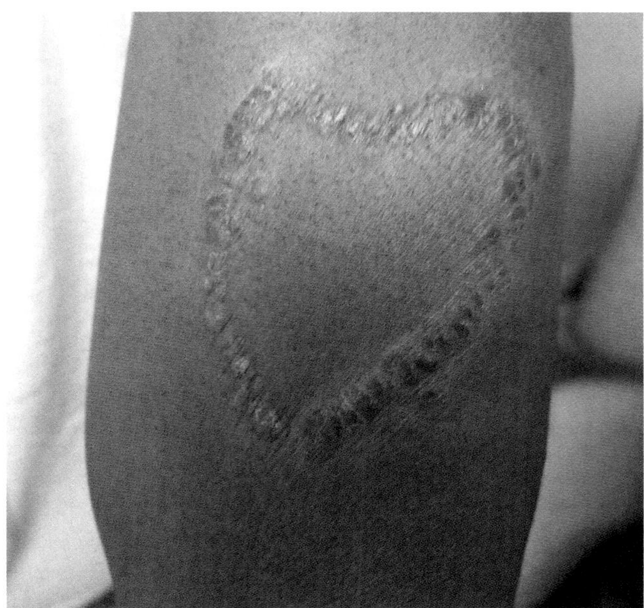

FIGURE 173-9 Sarcoid on a heart-shaped homemade tattoo over the knee. (*Reproduced with permission from Amor Khachemoune, MD.*)

- Hypergammaglobulinemia (30%-80%), positive rheumatoid factor, and decreased skin test reactivity.
- Autoimmune hemolytic anemia and hypersplenism can occur in some patients, although rare.
- Hypocapnia and hypoxemia may be present in certain patient populations, and may become worse with exercise.

• Serum calcium and 24-hour urine calcium levels.
  - Hypercalciuria has been found in 49% of patients in some studies, whereas 13% of patients had hypercalcemia.
  - Hypercalcemia occurs in sarcoidosis because of increased intestinal absorption of calcium that results from overproduction of a metabolite of vitamin D by pulmonary macrophages.

• Serum angiotensin-converting enzyme (ACE) level is elevated in 60% of patients.
  - Serum ACE levels are helpful in monitoring disease activity and treatment response. ACE is derived from epithelioid cells of the granulomas, therefore, it reflects granuloma load in the patient.

• Serum chemistries, such as alanine aminotransferase, aspartate aminotransferase, alkaline phosphatase, blood urea nitrogen (BUN), and creatinine levels may be elevated with hepatic and renal involvement.

• Other—Elevated erythrocyte sedimentation rate, elevated antinuclear antibodies (30%), diabetes insipidus, and renal failure may be noted.

IMAGING STUDIES

• Chest X-ray (CXR).
  - Radiographic involvement is seen in almost 90% of patients. Chest radiography is used in staging the disease.
  - Stage I disease shows bilateral hilar lymphadenopathy (BHL). Stage II disease shows BHL plus pulmonary infiltrates. Stage III disease shows pulmonary infiltrates without BHL. Stage IV disease shows pulmonary fibrosis.

• Computed tomography (CT) of the thorax may demonstrate lymphadenopathy or granulomatous infiltration. Other findings may include small nodules with a bronchovascular and subpleural distribution, thickened interlobular septae, honeycombing, bronchiectasis, and alveolar consolidation.

• Pulmonary function tests—Evidence of both restrictive abnormalities and obstructive abnormalities may be found.

BIOPSY

• Punch biopsy is adequate to obtain a sample of skin that includes dermis.

• If EN nodules are deep, a biopsy should also include subcutaneous tissue.

• Biopsy specimens are sent for histologic examination, as well as stains and cultures to rule out infectious causes.

DIFFERENTIAL DIAGNOSIS

• Granulomatous skin disease (**Figure 173-10**).
  - Granuloma annulare (GA) is also a granulomatous skin disease, which appears in single or multiple rings in adults and children (see Chapter 171, Granuloma Annulare).
  - Rheumatoid nodules—These usually appear in the context of a diagnosed rheumatoid arthritis with joint disease present (see Chapter 99, Rheumatoid Arthritis).

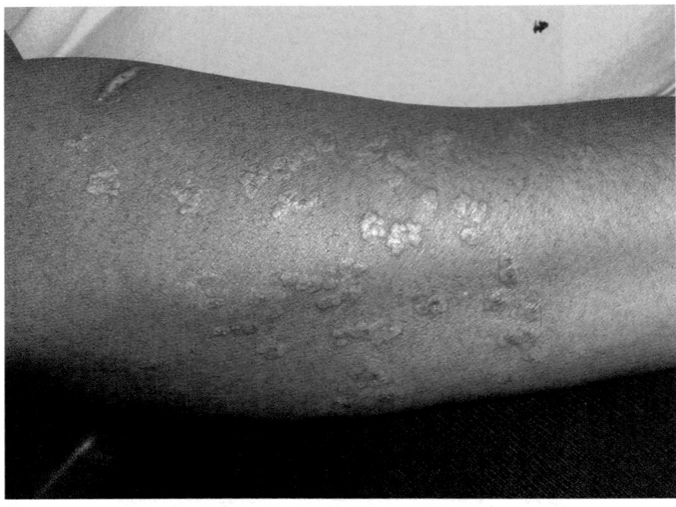

FIGURE 173-10 Granulomatous plaques of biopsy-proven sarcoidosis on the arm of a woman. She also has sarcoidosis of the lung. *(Reproduced with permission from Richard P. Usatine, MD.)*

  - Granulomatous mycosis fungoides—This is a type of cutaneous lymphoma with many clinical forms including granuloma formation (see Chapter 174, Cutaneous T-cell Lymphoma).

• Maculopapular type.
  - Lupus vulgaris—This is a type of cutaneous involvement with *Mycobacterium tuberculosis*.
  - Syringoma—These are small firm benign adnexal tumors usually appearing around the upper cheeks and lower eyelids.
  - Xanthelasma—These are the most common type of xanthomas. They are benign yellow macules, papules, or plaques often appearing on the eyelids. Approximately one-half of the patients with xanthelasma have a lipid disorder (see Chapter 223, Hyperlipidemia).
  - Lichen planus—This is a very pruritic skin eruption with pink-to-violaceous papules and plaques. It may present in different body locations but the most common areas are the wrists and ankles (see Chapter 152, Lichen Planus).
  - Granulomatous rosacea—This is a variant of rosacea made of uniform papules involving the face.
  - Acne keloidalis nuchae—This is commonly seen in dark-skinned patients. It presents with multiple perifollicular papules and nodules. The most common location is the back of the neck at the hairline (see Chapter 116, Pseudofolliculitis and Acne Keloidalis Nuchae).
  - Pseudofolliculitis barbae—This is most commonly seen in patients with darker skin color, triggered by ingrown hair involving the beard area (see Chapter 116, Pseudofolliculitis and Acne Keloidalis Nuchae).

• Annular or circinate type of sarcoidosis (**Figure 173-11**).

• Granuloma annulare—Annular type (described earlier; see Chapter 171, Granuloma Annulare).

• Annular form of necrobiosis lipoidica—A granulomatous disease with areas of necrobiosis. This is usually seen on the pretibial areas of patients with diabetes, but not all patients have diabetes (see Chapter 222, Necrobiosis Lipoidica).

• These 2 entities may be differentiated histologically.

• Nodular cutaneous and subcutaneous type.
  - Morphea—Also known as localized scleroderma caused by excessive collagen deposition in the dermis or subcutaneous tissue leading to the formation of nodules (see Chapter 180, Scleroderma and Morphea).

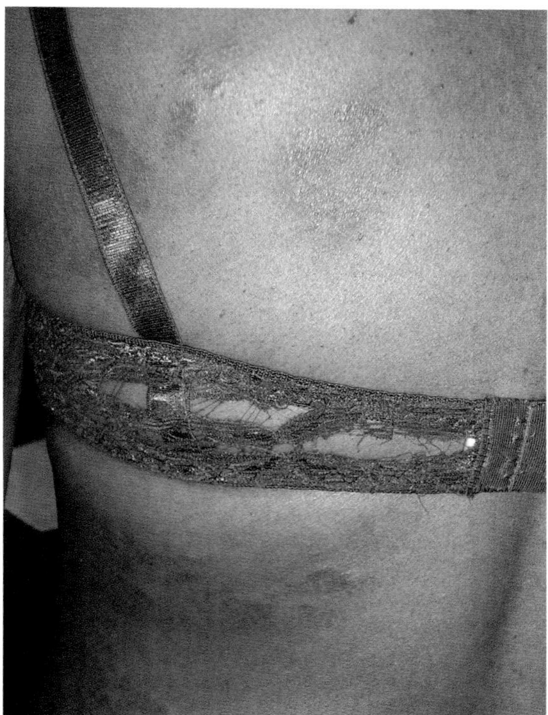

FIGURE 173-11 Violaceous sarcoidal papules coalescing into annular plaques on the back. (*Reproduced with permission from Richard P. Usatine, MD.*)

- Epidermal inclusion cyst—This is an encapsulated keratin-filled nodule of different sizes often found in the subcutaneous tissue. A central pore or punctum is often noted on examination of the overlying epidermis.
- Lipoma—These are soft nodules of different sizes composed of mature fat cells and often found in the subcutaneous tissue.
- Metastatic carcinoma—These nodular lesions often present in the context of a diagnosed primary carcinoma of other internal organs.
- Foreign-body granuloma—This is usually localized to the area of introduction of the foreign body into the skin.

MANAGEMENT

- Cutaneous involvement of sarcoidosis is typically not life-threatening and, therefore, the major rationale for treatment is to prevent or minimize disfigurement. Cosmetic issues are particularly important on the face (**Figure 173-12A**). Also, the lesions can be painful.
- Corticosteroids are the mainstay of treatment.[1-5] SOR B
- Limited cutaneous disease responds to very high-potency topical corticosteroids, or intralesional triamcinolone repeated monthly.[1,3] SOR B
- Photochemotherapy (psoralen UVA) is successful in erythrodermic and hypopigmented lesions. SOR C
- Patients with lupus pernio may benefit from pulsed-dye or carbon dioxide laser treatments. SOR C
- Resistant lesions to topical therapy or large and diffuse lesions require prednisone.[2,5] SOR B
- To prevent complications from long-term treatment by steroids, hydroxychloroquine or chloroquine are used as steroid-sparing agents.[6] SOR C

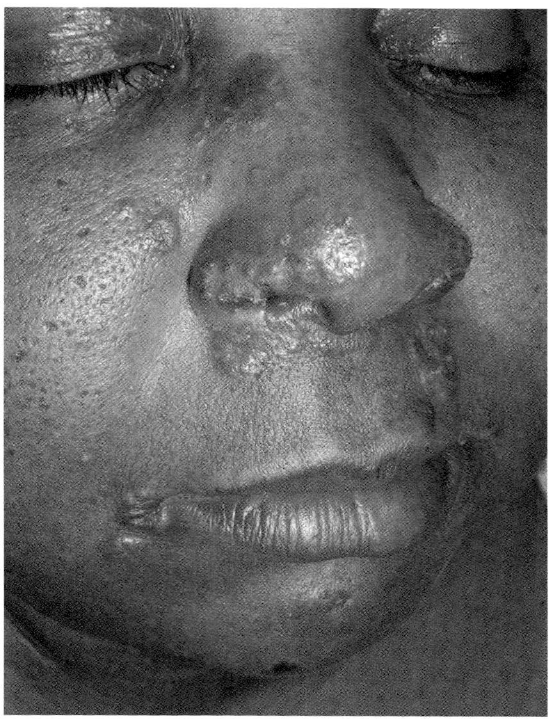

A

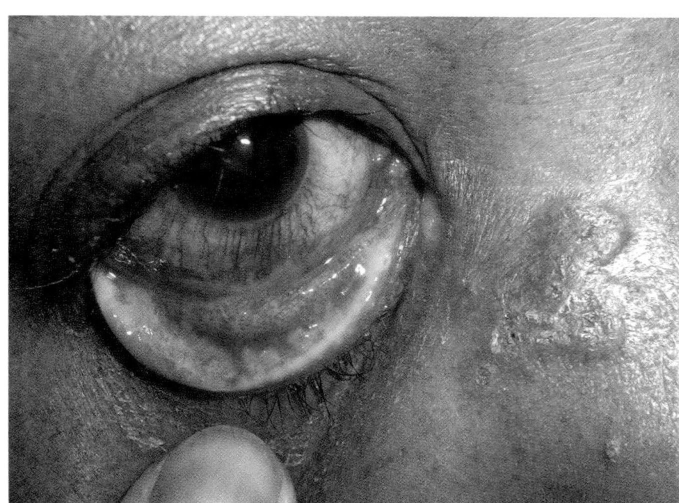

B

FIGURE 173-12 A. Sarcoidosis flare in a 50-year-old woman involving the face (lupus pernio), especially around the nose. B. Additionally she has sarcoidosis of the eye with involvement of the conjunctiva and infiltration of the inner lower eyelid. (*Reproduced with permission from Richard P. Usatine, MD.*)

- Other combinations that have been successful in chronic cutaneous disease and lung disease are methotrexate or azathioprine with low-dose prednisone.[5] SOR C
- Agents such as cyclophosphamide and cyclosporin are also used but with caution because of severe drug toxicity.[7] SOR C
- Infliximab, a tumor necrosis factor (TNF)-α monoclonal antibody has been found to be effective for severe cutaneous sarcoidosis with pulmonary involvement (**Figure 173-13**).[8] SOR C

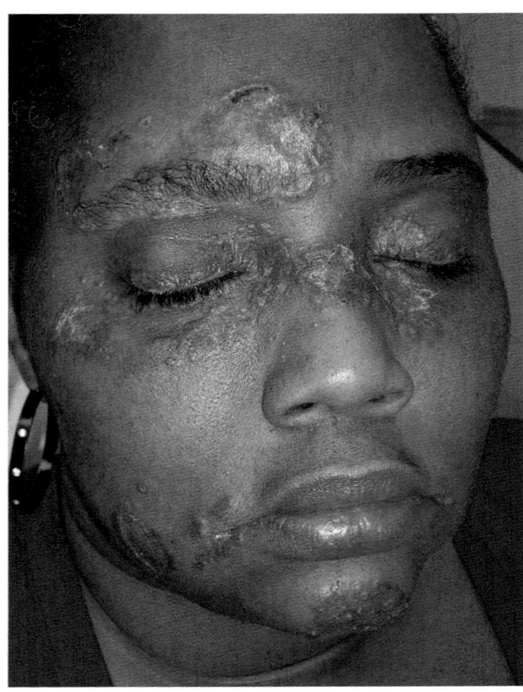

FIGURE 173-13 A 47-year-old African-American woman with widespread cutaneous sarcoidosis on face (lupus pernio), trunk, and extremities. She also has pulmonary involvement. Her sarcoidosis has improved since starting infliximab by IV infusion. (*Reproduced with permission from Richard P. Usatine, MD.*)

REFERRAL

- A multidisciplinary approach is imperative in patients with systemic sarcoidosis.
- Patients with eye symptoms should be referred to an ophthalmologist (see **Figure 173-12B**).
- Patients with lung involvement should be referred to a pulmonologist.
- Results from laboratory workup may dictate appropriate referral.

PREVENTION AND SCREENING

As the cause remains to be elucidated, no preventative measures have been established.

Patients presenting with cutaneous sarcoidosis should be screened as clinically indicated.

PROGNOSIS

- Patients of African descent have more severe lung disease compared with white patients at presentation and an overall poorer long-term prognosis.[9]
- The presence of EN has been associated with a decreased frequency of respiratory involvement.[9]
- Lupus pernio, more commonly seen in patients of African descent, indicates a chronic disease course (see **Figure 173-12** and **173-13**).[9]
- The prognostic value of cutaneous lesions alone remains unclear.[9]

FOLLOW-UP

Patients with cutaneous sarcoidosis should be worked up for systemic sarcoidosis. Regular follow-up is necessary.

PATIENT EDUCATION

Inform patients about the risk that systemic sarcoidosis can occur even if the skin is the only area currently involved.

PATIENT RESOURCES

- National Heart, Lung, and Blood Institute. *What Is Sarcoidosis?*—**http://www.nhlbi.nih.gov/health/dci/Diseases/sarc/sar_whatis.html.**

PROVIDER RESOURCES

- Medscape. *Dermatologic Manifestations of Sarcoidosis*—**http://emedicine.medscape.com/article/1123970.**

REFERENCES

1. Yeager H, Sina B, Khachemoune A. Dermatologic disease. In: Baughman RP, ed. *Sarcoidosis*. New York, NY: Taylor & Francis; 2006: 593-604.
2. English JC 3rd, Patel PJ, Greer KE. Sarcoidosis. *J Am Acad Dermatol*. 2001;44(5):725-743, quiz 744-746.
3. Khatri KA, Chotzen VA, Burrall BA. Lupus pernio: successful treatment with a potent topical corticosteroid. *Arch Dermatol*. 1995;131(5): 617-618.
4. Grutters JC, van den Bosch JM. Corticosteroid treatment in sarcoidosis. *Eur Respir J*. 2006;28(3):627-636.
5. Mosam A, Morar N. Recalcitrant cutaneous sarcoidosis: an evidence-based sequential approach. *J Dermatolog Treat*. 2004;15(6):353-359.
6. Baughman RP. Infliximab for refractory sarcoidosis. *Sarcoidosis Vasc Diffuse Lung Dis*. 2001;18(1):70-74; erratum in: *Sarcoidosis Vasc Diffuse Lung Dis*. 2001;18(3):310.
7. Kouba DJ, Mimouni D, Rencic A, Nousari HC. Mycophenolate mofetil may serve as a steroid-sparing agent for sarcoidosis. *Br J Dermatol*. 2003;148(1):147-148.
8. Baughman RP, Judson MA, Teirstein AS, et al. Thalidomide for chronic sarcoidosis. *Chest*. 2002;122(1):227-232.
9. Heath CR, David J, Taylor SC. Sarcoidosis: are there differences in your skin of color patients? *J Am Acad Dermatol*. 2012;66(1):121.e1-e14.

174 CUTANEOUS T-CELL LYMPHOMA

Gina Chacon, MD
Anjeli Nayar, MD
Richard P. Usatine, MD

PATIENT STORY

A 52-year-old black woman presented with a 7-month history of a hypopigmented rash in a symmetric distribution on her upper thighs and arms (**Figures 174-1** and **174-2**). She had been from evacuated New Orleans following hurricane Katrina. She had waded through polluted waters for hours before being rescued by a boat. Four days passed before she had access to a shower at which time she noticed a single erythematous spot the size of a silver dollar on her left thigh. Over the next several weeks, it faded to hypopigmented macules and plaques and eventually spread to both thighs and arms. The physical examination revealed no lymphadenopathy. A hematoxylin and eosin (H&E) stain of a full-thickness punch biopsy revealed "cerebriform" lymphocytes at the dermal–epidermal junction characteristic of mycosis fungoides (MF), a type of cutaneous T-cell lymphoma (CTCL). Her blood tests were essentially normal, and she was HIV negative. The patient reported no improvement with topical high-potency generic steroid to affected areas and is currently receiving narrow-band ultraviolet B (UVB) treatment twice weekly.

INTRODUCTION

CTCL clinically and biologically represents a heterogeneous group of non-Hodgkin lymphomas, with MF and Sézary syndrome (SS) being the most common subtypes.[1]

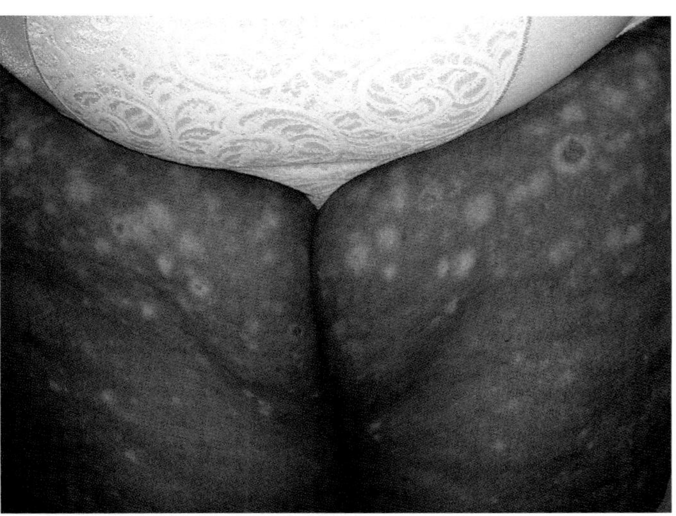

FIGURE 174-1 The hypopigmented patches of mycosis fungoides on the thighs of a 52-year-old black woman. This is the patch stage of the disease. Although this mimicked vitiligo, the distribution and appearance warranted a biopsy that provided a definitive diagnosis of mycosis fungoides. (*Reproduced with permission from Richard P. Usatine, MD.*)

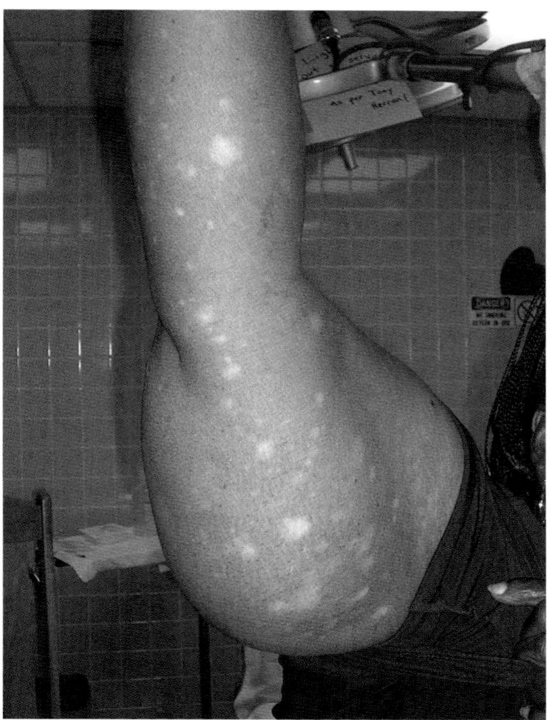

FIGURE 174-2 Hypopigmented patches on the arm of the woman in Figure 174-1 with mycosis fungoides. (*Reproduced with permission from Richard P. Usatine, MD.*)

EPIDEMIOLOGY

- The annual incidence of CTCL in the United States has increased from 2.8 per 1 million (1973-1977) to 9.6 per 1 million (1998-2002) according to data from Criscione and Weinstock.[2]
- CTCL is a rare disease, with 1000 new cases per year in the United States, comprising approximately 0.5% of all non-Hodgkin lymphoma cases.[3,4]
- The 2 most common types of CTCL are MF (50%-72%), which is generally indolent in behavior, and SS (1%-3%), an aggressive leukemic form of the disease.[2]
- It is more common in African Americans than in whites, with an incidence ratio of 6:1.[3]
- It is more common in males, with a male-to-female ratio of 2:1.
- Median age at presentation is between 50 and 70 years,[2] although pediatric and young adult cases do occur.[1]

ETIOLOGY AND PATHOPHYSIOLOGY

- The exact etiology of CTCL is unknown, but environmental, infectious, and genetic causes have been suggested. CTCL is a malignant lymphoma of helper T cells that usually remain confined to skin and lymph nodes (LNs). MF is a specific type of CTCL named for the mushroom-like skin tumors seen in severe cases.[3]
- Human T-lymphocytic virus (HTLV) types 1 and 2, HIV-1, cytomegalovirus (CMV), Epstein-Barr virus (EBV), and *Borrelia burgdorferi* have been suggested, but unproven, infectious causes of MF.[4,5] Environmental exposure to Agent Orange may be responsible for some cases.[3]

There is one case report of possible conjugal transmission of MF between a heterosexual couple who developed advanced MF within 14 months of one another.[5]

- MF and SS are associated with specific human leukocyte antigen (HLA) types (Aw31, Aw32, B8, Bw38, and DR5).[4] Genetic predisposition is also suggested by detection of HLA class II alleles DRB1*11 and DQB1*03 in association with sporadic and familial malignancy and familial clustering among Israeli Jews.[4,6]
- Metastasis, to the liver, spleen, lungs, gastrointestinal (GI) tract, bone marrow, and the central nervous system (CNS) may occur via T-cell spread through the lymphatic system.[3,4]
- The reduction of T-cell receptor complexity contributes to immunosuppression in advanced MF and SS, and may manifest clinically as herpes simplex or zoster.[7] Death is usually secondary to systemic infection, especially from *Staphylococcus aureus* and *Pseudomonas aeruginosa*.
- Host antitumor immunity also deteriorates, and patients have an increased risk for secondary malignancies, including higher-grade non-Hodgkin lymphoma, Hodgkin disease, secondary melanoma, and colon cancer in addition to cardiopulmonary complications.[7]

DIAGNOSIS

CLINICAL FEATURES

- The most common initial presentation involves patches or scaly plaques with a persistent rash that is often pruritic and usually erythematous (**Figures 174-1** to **174-4**).[3] Patches may evolve to generalized, infiltrated plaques or to ulcerated, exophytic tumors (**Figures 174-5** and **174-6**).[4,8]
- Hypo- or hyperpigmented lesions, petechiae, poikiloderma (skin atrophy with telangiectasia), and alopecia with or without mucinosis are other findings. The folliculotropic variant of MF presents with spotty alopecia (**Figure 174-7**).
- A "premycotic" phase may precede definitive diagnosis for months to decades, which involves nonspecific, slightly scaling skin lesions that intermittently appear and may eventually resolve with topical steroids.

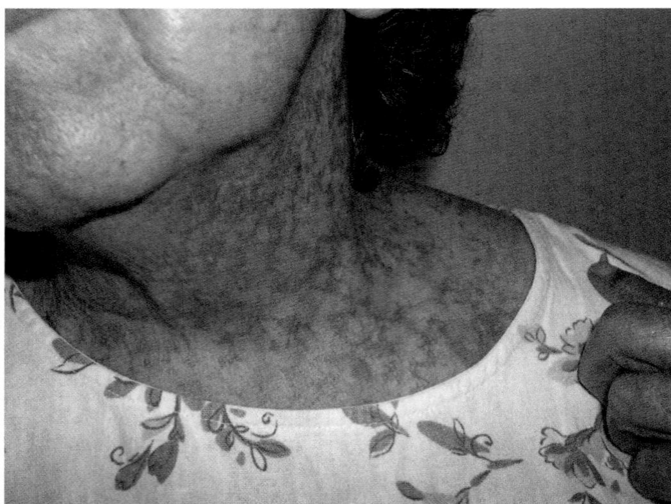

FIGURE 174-3 Reticulated mycosis fungoides (MF). This net-like pattern of MF is also called parapsoriasis variegata. (*Reproduced with permission from Heather Wickless, MD.*)

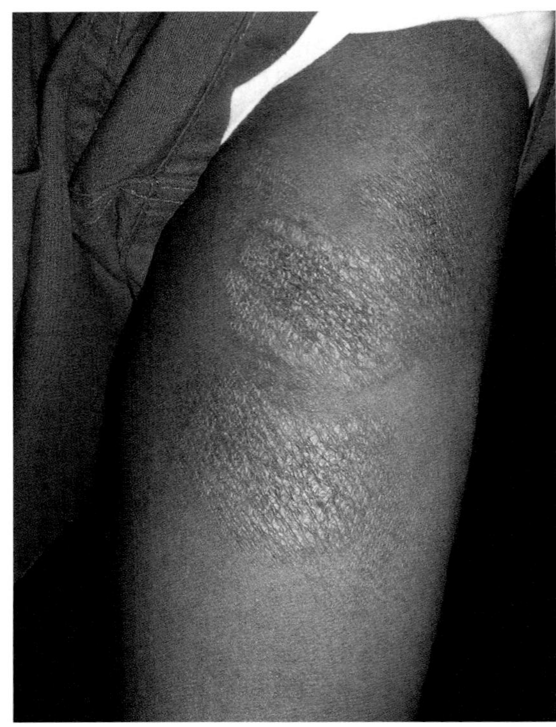

FIGURE 174-4 Plaque stage of mycosis fungoides (MF) on the arm of a 57-year-old nurse. She has had MF for 8 years and has intermittently been on chemotherapy. Recently, her MF has worsened and she was started on nitrogen mustard. (*Reproduced with permission from E.J. Mayeaux Jr, MD.*)

- SS is characterized by generalized exfoliative erythroderma, lymphadenopathy, and atypical Sézary cells in the peripheral blood. Diffuse infiltration of malignant T cells in SS may exaggerate facial lines, creating a leonine facies.[8]
- "Invisible MF" describes pruritus without visible lesions but the skin biopsy is positive for monoclonal T-cell infiltrates.[4]

TYPICAL DISTRIBUTION

- Lesions may affect any skin surface, but typically initially develop on non–sun-exposed areas, such as the trunk below the waistline, flanks, breasts, inner thighs and arms, and the periaxillary areas (**Figure 174-8**).[9]

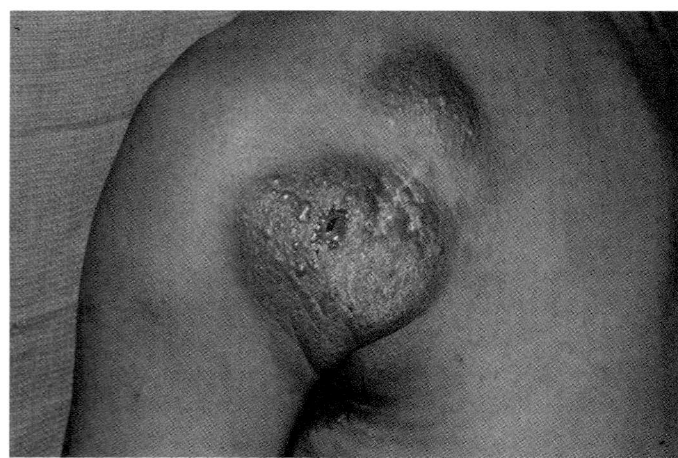

FIGURE 174-5 Tumor stage of mycosis fungoides (MF). (*Reproduced with permission from the University of Texas Health Sciences Center, Division of Dermatology.*)

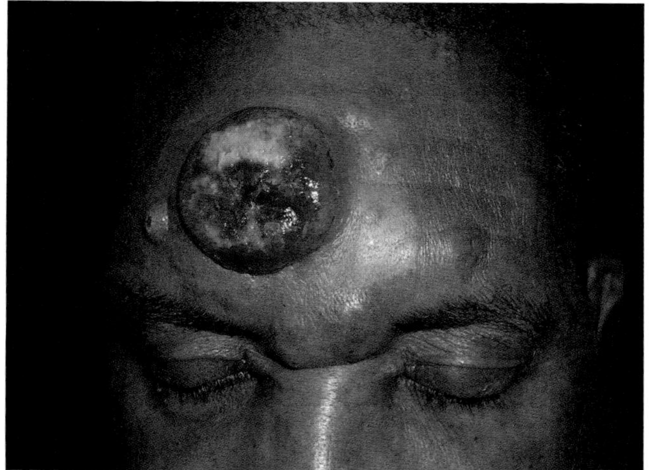

A

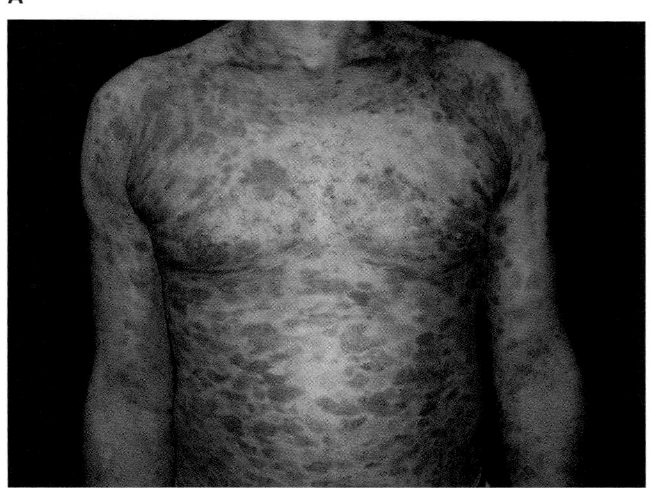

B

FIGURE 174-6 Tumor stage of mycosis fungoides (MF) in a 63-year-old black man. A. Large leg forehead ulcer and facial tumors. B. Widespread hyperpigmented plaques from head to feet. (*Reproduced with permission from Richard P. Usatine, MD.*)

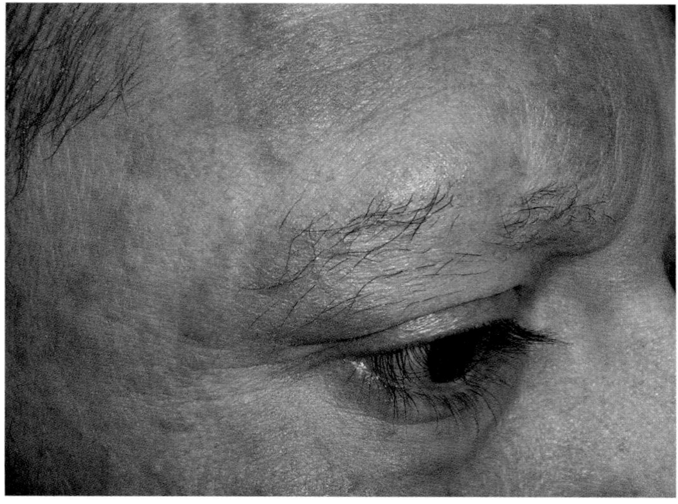

A

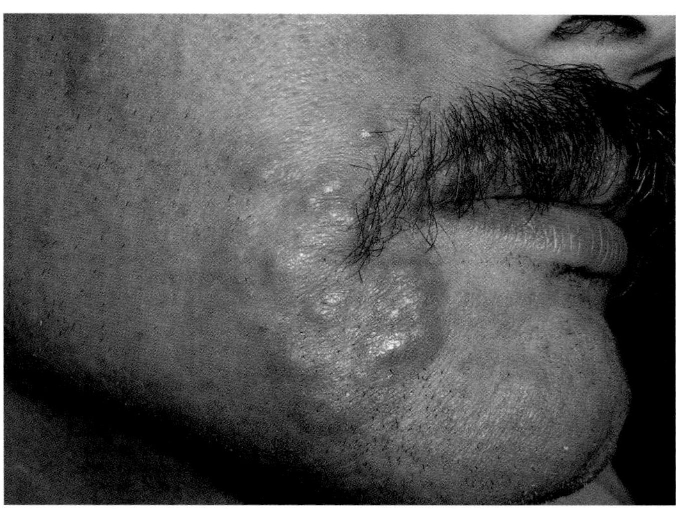

B

FIGURE 174-7 A. Folliculotropic variant of mycosis fungoides (MF) with visible alopecia in the eyebrow region of this 38-year-old man. B. Note the absence of hair growth in parts of the beard where there is follicular involvement. (*Reproduced with permission from Richard P. Usatine, MD.*)

- If there is follicular involvement, lesions may be found on the face or scalp (**Figures 174-9** and **174-10**).
- MF occasionally presents as a refractory dermatosis of the palms or soles.

BIOPSY AND LABORATORY STUDIES

- A full-thickness punch biopsy of the lesion is the most important diagnostic tool. If the initial biopsy is negative but the rash persists, the biopsy should be repeated.[3] Topical treatments and systemic immunosuppressants should be discontinued 2 to 4 weeks before the biopsy.[10]
- If the LNs are palpable or lymphadenopathy is suspected, also known as "dermatopathic lymphadenitis," biopsies should be performed (**Figure 174-11**).[4]
- A bone marrow biopsy should be performed if there is proven nodal or blood involvement.
- Histology—The skin biopsy may reveal Pautrier microabscesses or an inflammatory cell band-like infiltrate lining the basal layer or in the upper dermis ("mononuclear epidermotropism"). Malignant lymphocytes have hyperchromatic and convoluted or "cerebriform" nuclei. Capillary dermal fibrosis may also be observed.[10]
- Radiography—A chest radiograph and computed tomography (CT) scan of the abdomen and pelvis are recommended for advanced stages IIB to IIIB, or if visceral disease is suspected.[9] A combination of CT and positron emission tomography (PET) scans offers more sensitive detection of LN involvement than either imaging study alone.[4]
- Blood tests for infectious etiology—HIV test, HTLV type 1, EBV, CMV, as indicated by clinical history.
- Serology and blood tests—A complete blood cell count with differential, a buffy coat smear to screen for Sézary cells, lactic dehydrogenase and uric acid as markers for bulky or aggressive disease, and liver function tests to detect hepatic involvement should be measured. Progression of MF is associated with increased serum concentrations of immunoglobin (Ig) E and IgA.[4] Peripheral eosinophilia is an independent marker for poor prognosis and disease progression.[4,11]
- Flow cytometry—This test may be used to detect malignant clones and to quantify CD8+ lymphocytes to assess immunocompetence.
- Immunophenotyping may be used to support histology results.

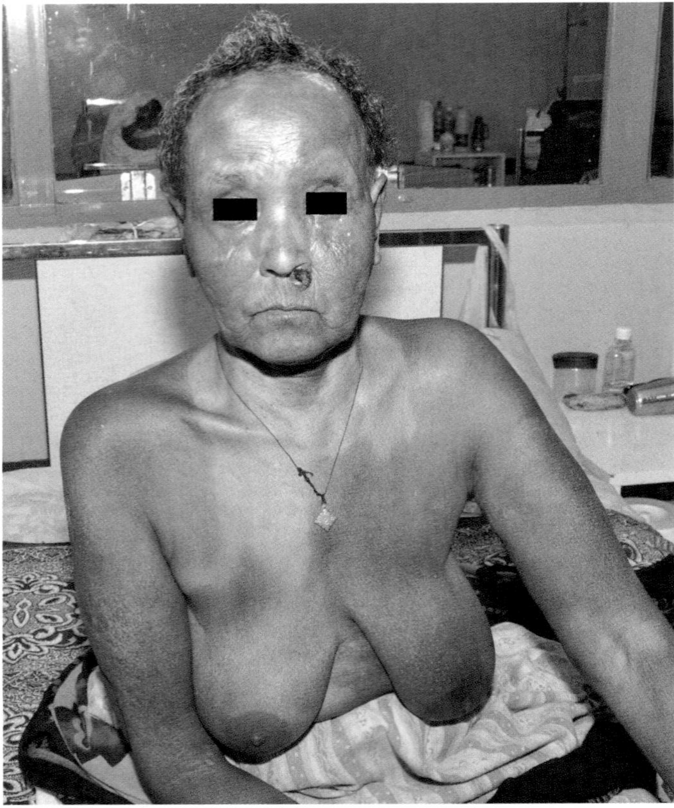

FIGURE 174-8 Mycosis fungoides (MF) causing hyperpigmented patches over the face, trunk, breasts, and upper extremities. (*Reproduced with permission from Richard P. Usatine, MD.*)

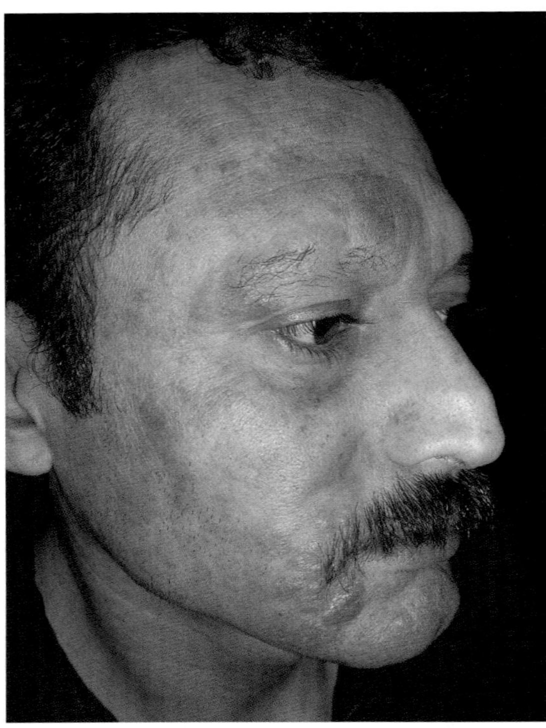

FIGURE 174-10 Facial predominance of this folliculotropic variant of mycosis fungoides (MF). Aside from the facial plaques, the only other area involved presented as alopecia in 1 area of the left forearm. (*Reproduced with permission from Richard P. Usatine, MD.*)

- Polymerase chain reaction (PCR) and Southern blot testing are recommended to detect T-cell rearrangements, if histology and immunophenotyping results are equivocal and to detect abnormal cells in LNs.[4]
- The International Society for Cutaneous Lymphoma proposed criteria for diagnosing early "classic" MF by incorporating clinical; histopathologic; molecular biologic and immunopathologic features, including the presence of persistent or progressive patches or thin plaques in unexposed areas and/or poikiloderma; superficial lymphoid infiltrate, epidermotropism with spongiosis; lymphocytes with hyperchromatic and cerebriform nuclei; epidermal–dermal discordance between CD2, CD3, CD5, or CD7; and clonal T-cell receptor rearrangement.[10] The International Society for Cutaneous Lymphoma also proposed criteria for diagnosing SS with leukemic blood involvement including an absolute Sézary cell count of greater than $1000/mm^3$, a CD4-to-CD8 ratio of 10 or greater, T-cell chromosomal abnormalities detected by Southern blot or PCR, increased circulation of T cells, and aberrant expression of pan T-cell markers as assessed by flow cytometry.[8]

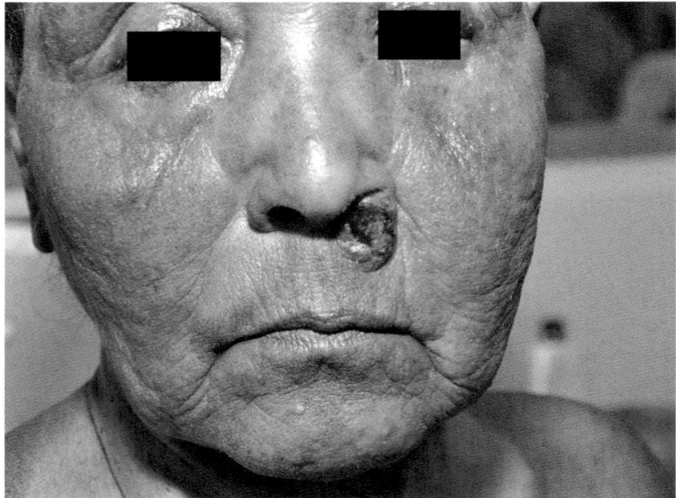

FIGURE 174-9 Mycosis fungoides (MF) on the face with an ulcerated tumor under the nose. (*Reproduced with permission from Richard P. Usatine, MD.*)

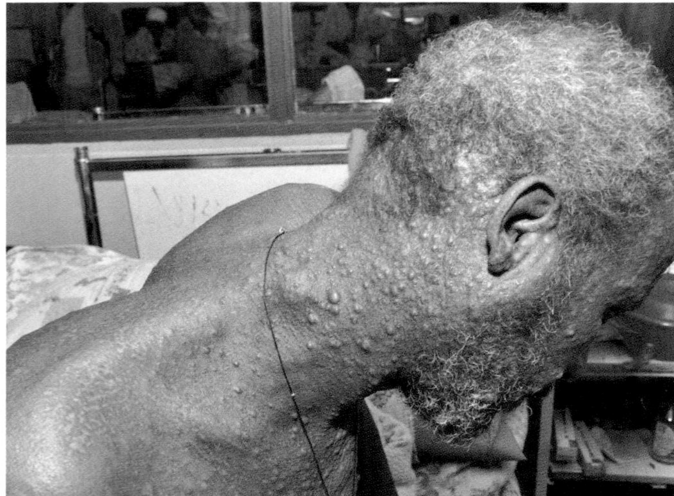

FIGURE 174-11 Tumor stage of mycosis fungoides (MF) with a large posterior cervical node visible. (*Reproduced with permission from Richard P. Usatine, MD.*)

DIFFERENTIAL DIAGNOSIS

- "Premycotic" period preceding diagnosis of MF may resemble parapsoriasis en plaque or nonspecific dermatitis.[4,10]
- MF with erythroderma must be distinguished from generalized atopic dermatitis, contact dermatitis, photodermatitis, drug eruptions, erythrodermic psoriasis, and idiopathic hypereosinophilic syndrome (see Chapter 154, Erythroderma).[4,8]
- Unilesional MF may resemble nummular eczema, lichen simplex chronicus, erythema chronicum migrans, tinea corporis, or digitate dermatosis (a variant of small plaque parapsoriasis).[10]
- Vitiligo typically involves discrete, hypopigmented macules on the hands and face that coalesce into larger areas.[3] However, some MF may mimic vitiligo as seen in **Figures 174-1** and **174-2**. The distribution of the hypopigmented macules in this case is atypical for vitiligo and this prompted a biopsy that led to the diagnosis of MF (see Chapter 196, Vitiligo).
- Idiopathic guttate hypomelanosis is a benign condition involving smaller hypopigmented macules than those seen in MF.[3]
- In patients with HIV, histopathology, resembling MF may represent a reactive inflammatory condition instead. Nonepidermotrophic large T-cell cutaneous lymphoma and B-cell diffuse cutaneous lymphoma are more frequent complications than MF in these patients.[12]

MANAGEMENT

- The current treatments for CTCL can be divided into skin-directed therapy and systemic therapy. Of the skin-directed therapies, topical corticosteroids are widely used in all stages of CTCL in the hopes that they will help control the disease and palliate any cutaneous symptoms of itch.[15] SOR B
- For stage I disease localized to the skin, symptomatic treatment with emollients, antipruritics (Doxepin cream 5%) and topical high-potency steroids (clobetasol cream) on an outpatient basis are recommended.[9] SOR C Topical retinoids or topical chemotherapy (nitrogen mustard, bischloroethylnitrosourea, or carmustine) are treatment alternatives for localized disease and effective adjuvants in generalized disease.[3,9,13,14] SOR B
- Bexarotene 1% topical gel may be used if disease persists despite treatment or if other medication is not tolerated. When used in combination with psoralen-enhanced UV light (PUVA), bexarotene decreases the total UVA dosage needed and if used as maintenance therapy increases the duration of remission.[14] SOR C
- Alternatively, PUVA may also be used concurrently with interferon (IFN), 3 times weekly, or retinoids until skin lesions clear, then continued as maintenance therapy at a reduced frequency.[14] SOR C
- For a plaque recalcitrant to PUVA and retinoid combination therapy, 1 case study showed that imiquimod 5% topical cream effectively cleared the lesion.[7] SOR C
- UVA may also be enhanced with methoxsalen or Oxsoralen instead of psoralen.[9] SOR C
- Phototherapy is a safe, effective, and well-tolerated, first-line therapy in patients with early-stage CTCL, with prolonged disease-free remissions being achieved. It suggests that narrowband UVB is at least as effective as PUVA for treatment of early-stage MF.[15,16] SOR C
- Narrowband UVB light has proven effective in early MF and prolonging remission, although an optimal maintenance protocol still needs to be established.[17] SOR C
- The therapeutic effects of PUVA and UVB in immune-mediated skin diseases have been attributed to the direct apoptosis of lymphocytes, modification of cell surface receptors, and alteration in production of certain mediators.[15]
- Photodynamic therapy with 5-aminolevulinic acid (PDT-ALA) was found to effectively eradicate localized infiltrates better than topical steroids, but more studies are needed before it becomes standardized treatment.[13] SOR C
- In general, photodynamic therapy works via direct cytotoxicity, vascular damage, and immune-host response.[8,18]
- Stage II disease involves the regional LNs and may be treated the same as for stage I. For stage IIB, the most recommended therapy is total-skin electron-beam therapy (EBT) followed by nitrogen mustard treatment for 6 or more months.[14] SOR C For disease relapse after EBT, PUVA may be used in combination with IFN or a systemic retinoid.[14] SOR C Other systemic therapies include fusion toxins, monoclonal antibody treatment, and single-agent chemotherapy.[9] For recalcitrant tumors, there is no evidence that combination systemic chemotherapy regimens offer superior survival outcome than single agents.[9,14] SOR C
- Stage III, or erythrodermic disease without extracutaneous disease or with limited LN involvement, should be treated with chemotherapy or photophoresis for 4 weeks.[14] SOR C Extracorporeal photochemotherapy involves irradiation of white blood cells with PUVA after leukophoresis before reinfusing the blood cells intravenously.[9] If the response is delayed, photophoresis may be combined with IFN or systemic retinoids.
- Stage IV extracutaneous disease should be treated with systemic chemotherapy. Although response rates are improved with combination chemotherapy, the response duration is less than 1 year. Regimens include cyclophosphamide, vincristine, and prednisone (CVP), CVP plus Adriamycin, CVP plus methotrexate, or cyclophosphamide, vincristine, Adriamycin, and etoposide. Adjuvants treatments may include IFN, systemic retinoids, and photophoresis. Single-agent chemotherapy includes methotrexate, liposomal doxorubicin, gemcitabine, etoposide, cyclophosphamide, and purine analogs.[14] SOR C The patient should be referred to a dermatologist, and to medical and radiation oncologists.[3]

PROGNOSIS AND FOLLOW-UP

- Patient's age and stage are the most important clinical prognostic factors.[19]
- Patients have a normal life expectancy, if diagnosed early during stage IA in which the patch or plaque is limited to less than 10% of the skin surface area.[3]
- MF and SS are otherwise difficult to cure and have a prognosis of 3.2 years for stage IIB cutaneous tumors, 4 to 6 years for stage III generalized erythroderma, and less than 1.5 years for stage IVA and stage IVB with LN and visceral involvement, respectively.[9]
- The patient should be monitored for development of secondary malignancies.

POTENTIAL COMPLICATIONS

- Infection, particularly from indwelling intravenous catheters or from lymph node biopsy sites
- High-output cardiac failure
- Anemia of chronic disorders
- Edema
- Secondary malignancies (eg, skin cancer, melanoma)

PATIENT EDUCATION

- Avoid sun exposure, stay in a cool environment, and keep skin lubricated.
- See your physician if any new skin symptoms and signs appear or the medication is not working.
- Avoid smoking and second-hand smoke.

PATIENT RESOURCES

- Cutaneous Lymphoma Foundation. *About Cutaneous Lymphoma*—**http://www.clfoundation.org/about-cutaneous-lymphoma.**
- National Cancer Institute. *General Information About Mycosis Fungoides and the Sézary Syndrome*—**http://www.cancer.gov/cancertopics/pdq/treatment/mycosisfungoides/Patient.**

PROVIDER RESOURCES

- National Cancer Institute. *Mycosis Fungoides and the Sézary Syndrome Treatment*—**http://www.cancer.gov/cancertopics/pdq/treatment/mycosisfungoides/HealthProfessional.**
- Skin Cancer Foundation—**http://www.skincancer.org.**
- Medscape. *Cutaneous T-Cell Lymphoma*—**http://emedicine.medscape.com/article/209091.**

REFERENCES

1. Li JY, Horwitz S, Moskowitz A, et al. Management of cutaneous T cell lymphoma: new and emerging targets and treatment options. *Cancer Manag Res.* 2012;4:75-89.
2. Criscione VD, Weinstock MA. Incidence of cutaneous T-cell lymphoma in the United States, 1973-2002. *Arch Dermatol.* 2007;143(7):854-859.
3. Mahan RD, Usatine RP. Hurricane Katrina evacuee develops a persistent rash. *J Fam Pract.* 2007;56(6):454-457.
4. Hoppe RT, Kim YH. *Clinical manifestations, pathologic features, and diagnosis of mycosis fungoides.* Updated August 2, 2012. http://www.uptodate.com/contents/clinical-manifestations-pathologic-features-and-diagnosis-of-mycosis-fungoides?source=search_result&search=Hoppe+RT%2C+Kim+YH.+Clinical+Features%2C+Diagnosis%2C+and+Staging+of+Mycosis+Fungoides+and+S%C3%A9zary+Syndrome&selectedTitle=1~150. Accessed September 1, 2012.
5. Adriana N, Schmidt AN, Jason B, et al. Conjugal transformed mycosis fungoides: the unknown role of viral infection and environmental exposures in the development of cutaneous T-cell lymphoma. *J Am Acad Dermatol.* 2006;54(5):S202-S205.
6. Hodak E, Klein T, Gabay B, et al. Familial mycosis fungoides: report of 6 kindreds and a study of the HLA system. *J Am Acad Dermatol.* 2005;52(3):393-402.
7. Navi D, Huntley A. Imiquimod 5 percent cream and the treatment of cutaneous malignancy. *Dermatol Online J.* 2004;10(1):4.
8. Girardi M, Heald PW, Wilson LD. The pathogenesis of mycosis fungoides. *N Engl J Med.* 2004;350(19):1978-1988.
9. Pinter-Brown LC. Cutaneous T-Cell Lymphoma: overview of CTCL. Updated May 17, 2011. http://emedicine.medscape.com/article/209091-overview. Accessed April 6, 2012.
10. Pimpinelli N, Olsen EA, Santucci M, et al. Defining early mycosis fungoides. *J Am Acad Dermatol.* 2005;53(6):1053-1063.
11. Querfeld C, Rosen ST, Guitart J, et al. Phase II trial of subcutaneous injections of human recombinant interleukin-2 for the treatment of mycosis fungoides and Sézary syndrome. *J Am Acad Dermatol.* 2007;56(4):580-583.
12. Honda KS. HIV and skin cancer. *Dermatol Clin.* 2006;24(4):521-530.
13. Blume JE, Oseroff AR. Aminolevulinic acid photodynamic therapy for skin cancers. *Dermatol Clin.* 2007;25(1):5-14.
14. Hoppe RT, Kim YH. *Treatment of Early Stage (IA to IIA) Mycosis Fungoides and Sézary Syndrome.* Updated February 23, 2012. http://www.uptodate.com/contents/treatment-of-advanced-stage-iib-to-iv-mycosis-fungoides-and-sezary-syndrome. UpToDate® www.uptodate.com. Accessed April 3, 2012.
15. Ahern K, Gilmore ES, Poligone B. Pruritus in cutaneous T-cell lymphoma: a review. *J Am Acad Dermatol.* 2012;26:1-9.
16. Ponte P, Serrao V, Apetato M. Efficacy of narrowband UVB vs. PUVA in patients with early-stage mycosis fungoides. *J Eur Acad DermatolVenereol.* 2010;24(6):716-721.
17. Boztepe G, Sahin S, Ayhan M, et al. Narrowband ultraviolet B phototherapy to clear and maintain clearance in patients with mycosis fungoides. *J Am Acad Dermatol.* 2005;53(2):242-246.
18. Nayak CS. Photodynamic therapy in dermatology. *Indian J Dermatol Venereol Leprol.* 2005;71(3):155-160.
19. Suzuki SY, Ito K, Ito M, Kawai K. Prognosis of 100 Japanese patients with mycosis fungoides and Sézary syndrome. *J Dermatol Sci.* 2012;57(1):37-43.

SECTION 13 HYPERSENSITIVITY SYNDROMES

175 ERYTHEMA MULTIFORME, STEVENS-JOHNSON SYNDROME, AND TOXIC EPIDERMAL NECROLYSIS

Carolyn Milana, MD
Mindy A. Smith, MD, MS

PATIENT STORY

A patient presents with new-onset fever and rash. These were associated with lip swelling and peeling (**Figure 175-1A**) and ocular involvement (**Figure 175-1B**). On history it was determined that he was taking oral penicillin for pneumonia that was being treated as an outpatient. His urethra was also burning. On physical examination he had an erythematous papulosquamous eruption on his trunk and extremities. In **Figure 175-1C** target lesions can be seen on the back with central epithelial disruption. He was diagnosed with Stevens-Johnson syndrome and admitted to the hospital.

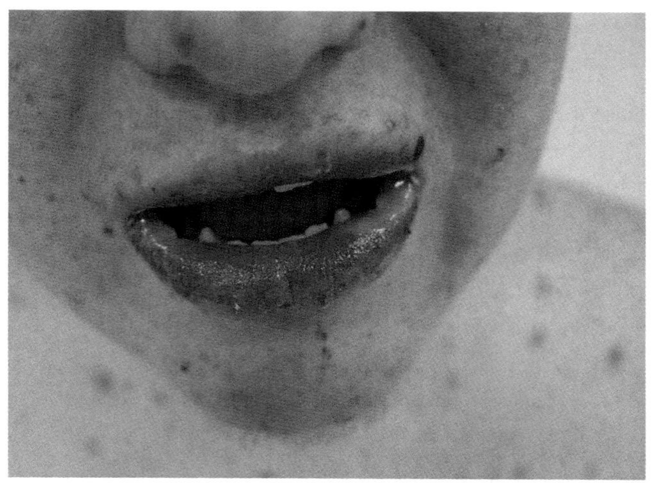

A

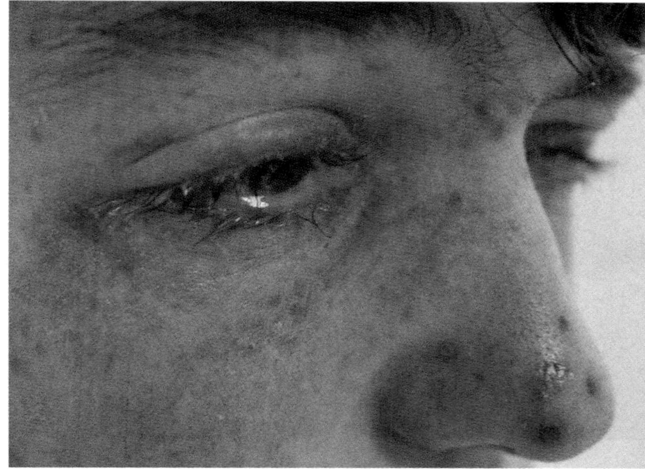

B

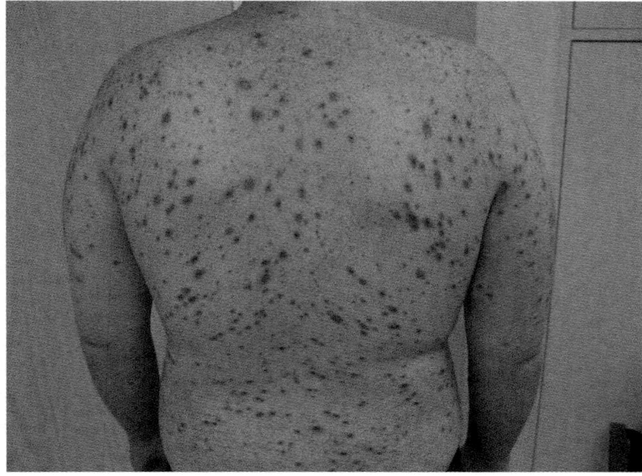

C

FIGURE 175-1 Stevens-Johnson syndrome in a patient who received penicillin for pneumonia. **A.** Lips and mouth are involved. **B.** Eye involvement. **C.** Target lesions on his back. (*Reproduced with permission from Dan Stulberg, MD.*)

INTRODUCTION

Erythema multiforme (EM), Stevens-Johnson syndrome (SJS), and toxic epidermal necrolysis (TEN) are skin disorders thought to be types of hypersensitivity reactions (undesirable reactions produced by a normal immune system in a presensitized host) that occur in response to medication, infection, or illness. Both SJS and TEN are severe cutaneous reactions thought to describe the same disorder, only differing in severity (TEN more severe); however, there is debate as to whether these 3 fall into a spectrum of disease that includes EM.

SYNONYMS

- EM has also been called EM minor.
- SJS has been called EM major in the past but it is now thought to be a distinct entity different from all types of EM.
- TEN is also known as Lyell syndrome.

EPIDEMIOLOGY

- The incidence of EM has been estimated to range from 1 in 1000 persons to 1 in 10,000 persons.[1] The true incidence of the disease is unknown.[1]
- SJS and TEN are rare severe cutaneous reactions often caused by drugs. Reports of incidence vary from 1.2 to 6 per 1 million for SJS and from 0.4 to 1.2 per 1 million for TEN.[2-4]

- EM most commonly occurs between the ages of 10 and 30 years, with 80% of cases occurring in adults.[5]
- With respect to EM, males are affected slightly more often than females.[5]

ETIOLOGY AND PATHOPHYSIOLOGY

Numerous factors have been identified as causative agents for EM:

- Herpes simplex virus (HSV) I and HSV II are the most common causative agents, having been implicated in at least 60% of the cases (**Figure 175-2**).[6,7]
- The virus has been found in circulating blood,[8] as well as on skin biopsy of patients with EM minor.[6]

For SJS and TEN, the majority of cases are drug induced.

- Drugs most commonly known to cause SJS and TEN are sulfonamide antibiotics, allopurinol, nonsteroidal anti-inflammatory drugs (NSAIDs), amine antiepileptic drugs (phenytoin and carbamazepine), and lamotrigine.[9]
- *Mycoplasma pneumoniae* has been identified as the most common infectious cause for SJS.[7]

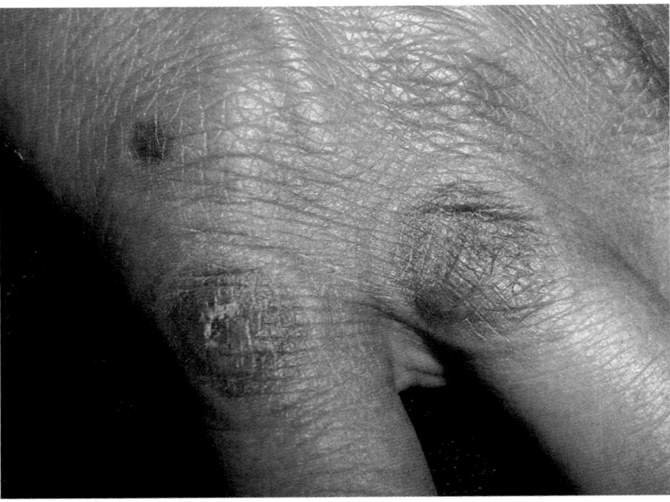

A

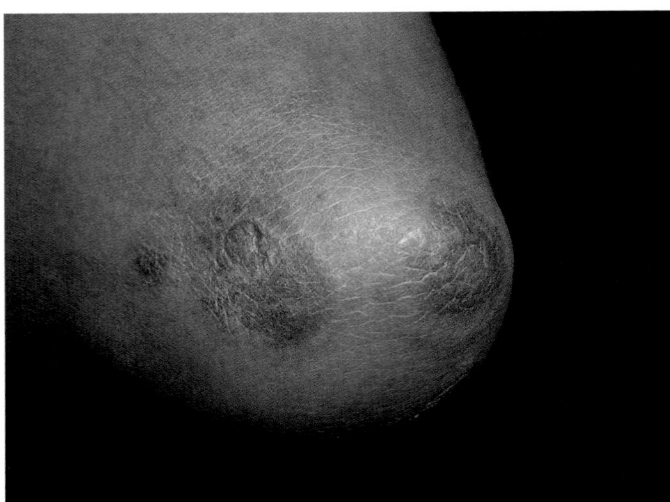

B

FIGURE 175-2 Erythema multiforme in a 43-year-old woman that recurs every time she breaks out with genital herpes. A. Target lesions on hand. B. Target lesions on elbow. (*Reproduced with permission from Richard P. Usatine, MD.*)

Other less-common causative agents for EM, SJS, and TEN include the following:

- Infectious agents such as *Mycobacterium tuberculosis*, group A streptococci, hepatitis B, Epstein-Barr virus, *Francisella tularensis*, *Yersinia*, enteroviruses, *Histoplasma*, *Coccidioides*[1]
- Neoplastic processes, such as leukemia and lymphoma[1]
- Antibiotics, such as penicillin, isoniazid, tetracyclines, cephalosporins, and quinolones
- Anticonvulsants, such as phenobarbital and valproic acid[1,7]
- Other drugs, including captopril, etoposide, aspirin, and allopurinol
- Immunizations, such as Calmette-Guérin bacillus, diphtheria-tetanus toxoid, hepatitis B, measles-mumps-rubella, and poliomyelitis[6]
- Other agents or triggers, including radiation therapy, sunlight, pregnancy, connective tissue disease, and menstruation[1]

Although the pathogenesis of EM, SJS, and TEN remains unknown, recent studies show that it may be as a result of a host-specific cell-mediated immune response to an antigenic stimulus that activates cytotoxic T cells and results in damage to keratinocytes.[6,9]

- The epidermal detachment (skin peeling) seen in SJS and TEN appears to result from epidermal necrosis in the absence of substantial dermal inflammation.

RISK FACTORS

- Recent evidence shows individuals with certain human leukocyte antigen (HLA) alleles may be predisposed to developing SJS/TEN when taking certain drugs.[2]
- Certain diseases, such as HIV/AIDS (**Figure 175-3**), malignancy, or autoimmune disease, also predispose individuals to SJS/TEN.[2,10]

DIAGNOSIS

CLINICAL FEATURES

In all of these conditions, there is a rapid onset of skin lesions. EM is a disease in which patients present with the following lesions:

- Classic lesions begin as red macules and expand centrifugally to become target-like papules or plaques with an erythematous outer border and central clearing (iris or bull's-eye lesions) (**Figures 175-4** to **175-7**). Target lesions, although characteristic, are not necessary to make the diagnosis. The center of the lesions should have some epidermal disruption, such as vesicles or erosions.
- Lesions can coalesce and form larger lesions up to 2 cm in diameter with centers that can become dusky purple or necrotic.
- Unlike urticarial lesions, the lesions of EM do not appear and fade; once they appear they remain fixed in place until healing occurs many days to weeks later.
- Patients are usually asymptomatic, although a burning sensation or pruritus may be present.

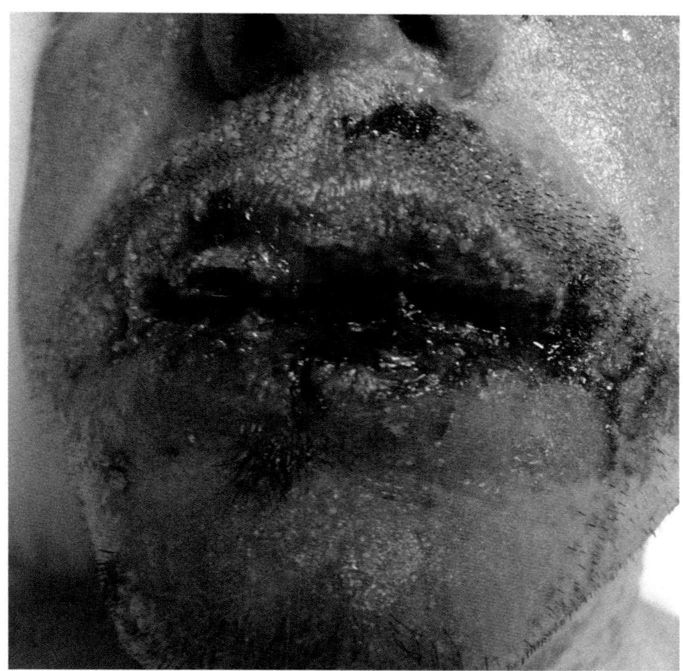

A

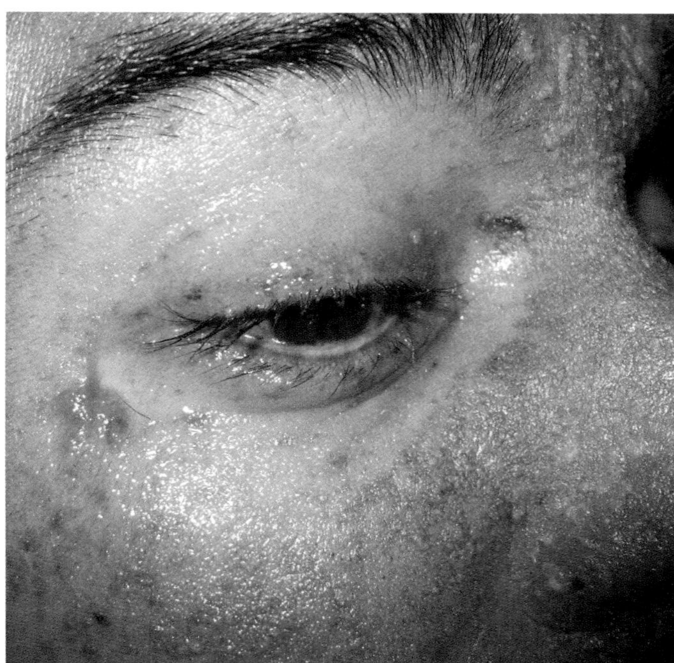

B

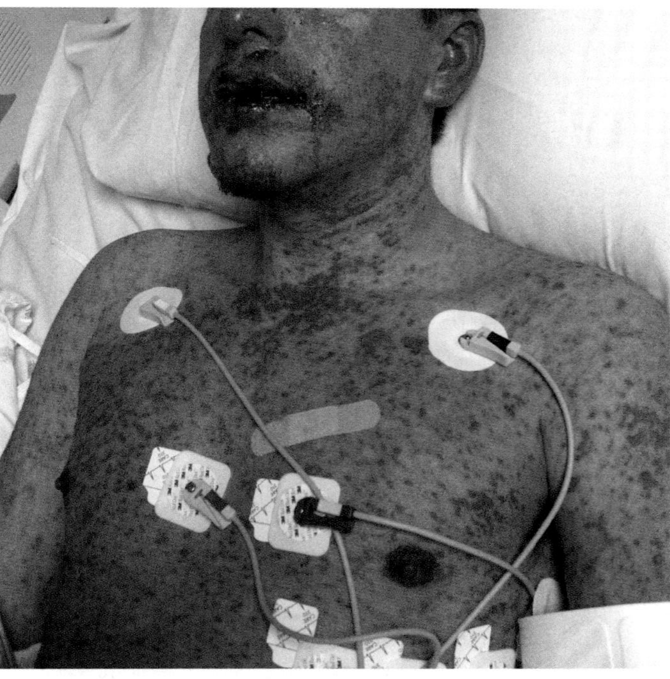

C

FIGURE 175-3 Stevens-Johnson syndrome that evolved into toxic epidermal necrolysis in a HIV–positive man with a CD4 count of 6. He presented to the emergency department with fever and rash on face, eyes, and mouth. Chest X-ray suggested pneumonia, so he was started on azithromycin, ceftriaxone, and trimethoprim-sulfamethoxazole. He developed bulla on skin and a skin biopsy confirmed toxic epidermal necrolysis, possibly secondary to one of the antibiotics. He was transferred to a burn unit and given intravenous gammaglobulin 1 g/kg for 3 days. The patient survived. **A.** Oral lesions. **B.** Eye and facial involvement. **C.** Trunk and upper extremities involved so that greater than 30% of the skin was affected. *(Reproduced with permission from Robert T. Gilson, MD.)*

- Lesions typically resolve without any permanent sequelae within 2 weeks.
- Recurrent outbreaks are often associated with HSV infection (see **Figure 175-2**).[6,7]

In both SJS and TEN, patients may have blisters that develop on dusky or purpuric macules. SJS is diagnosed when less than 10% of the body surface area is involved, SJS/TEN overlap when 10% to 30% is involved, and TEN when greater than 30% is involved.

- Lesions may become more widespread and rapidly progress to form areas of central necrosis, bullae, and areas of denudation (see **Figure 175-1**).
- Fever higher than 39°C (102.2°F) is often present.
- In addition to skin involvement, there is involvement of at least 2 mucosal surfaces, such as the eyes, oral cavity, upper airway, esophagus, gastrointestinal (GI) tract, or the anogenital mucosa (see **Figures 175-1** and **175-3**).
- New lesions occur in crops and may take 4 to 6 weeks to heal.
- Large areas of epidermal detachment occur (**Figures 175-8** to **175-10**).
- Severe pain can occur from mucosal ulcerations but skin tenderness is minimal.

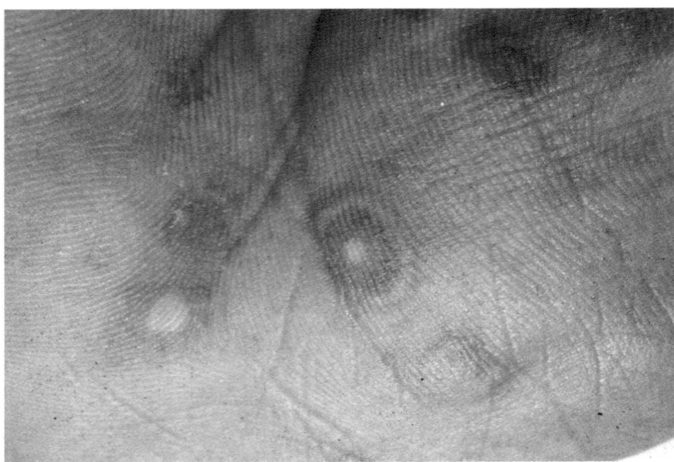

FIGURE 175-4 Erythema multiforme on the palm with target lesions that have a dusky red and white center. (*Reproduced with permission from the University of Texas Health Sciences Center, Division of Dermatology.*)

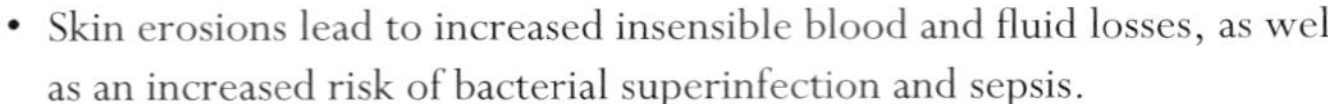

- Skin erosions lead to increased insensible blood and fluid losses, as well as an increased risk of bacterial superinfection and sepsis.
- These patients are at high risk for ocular complications that may lead to blindness. Additional risks include bronchitis, pneumonitis, myocarditis, hepatitis, enterocolitis, polyarthritis, hematuria, and acute tubular necrosis.

TYPICAL DISTRIBUTION

- The distribution of the rash in EM can be widespread.
- The distal extremities, including the palms and soles, are most commonly involved.

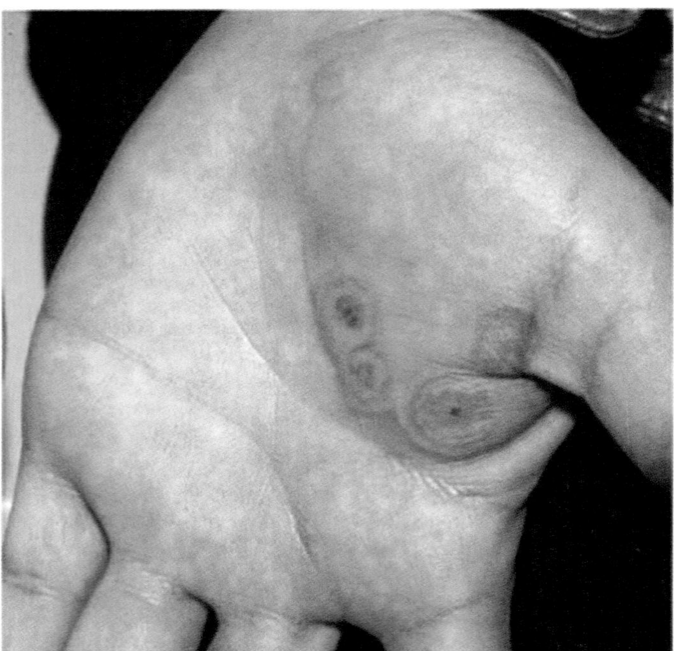

FIGURE 175-5 Erythema multiforme with target lesions on the palms secondary to an outbreak of oral herpes. (*Reproduced with permission from the University of Texas Health Sciences Center, Division of Dermatology.*)

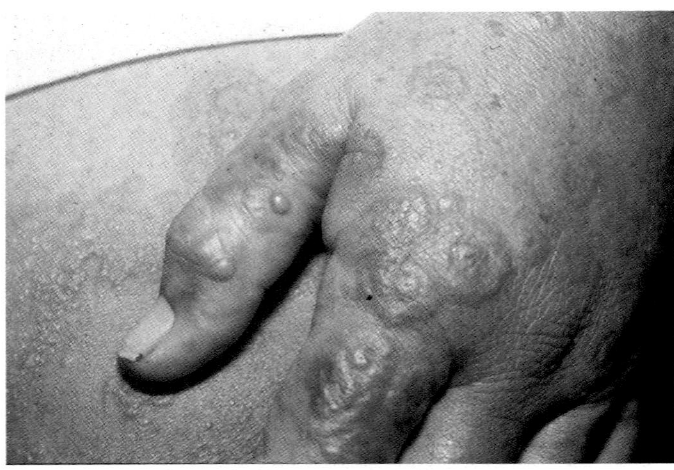

FIGURE 175-6 Erythema multiforme with vesicles and blistering of the target lesions on the hand. (*Reproduced with permission from the University of Texas Health Sciences Center, Division of Dermatology.*)

- Extensor surfaces are favored.
- Oral lesions may be present, especially in SJS (see **Figures 175-1** and **175-3**).
- Severe lesions with exfoliation and extensive mucosal lesions occur in SJS and TEN (see **Figures 175-8** to **175-10**).

LABORATORY AND IMAGING

- There are no consistent laboratory findings with these conditions. The diagnosis is usually made based on clinical findings.
- Routine blood work may show leukocytosis, elevated liver transaminases, and an elevated erythrocyte sedimentation rate.
- In TEN, leukopenia may occur.

BIOPSY

- A cutaneous punch biopsy can be performed to confirm the diagnosis or to rule out other diseases.

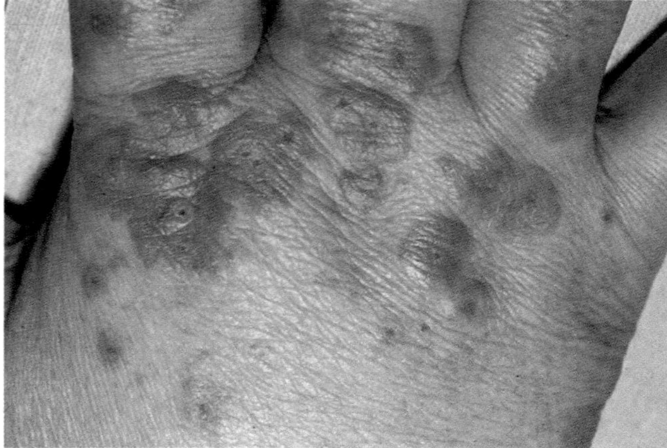

FIGURE 175-7 Erythema multiforme on the dorsum of the hand showing targets with small, eroded centers. There should be some epidermal erosion to diagnose erythema multiforme. (*Reproduced with permission from the University of Texas Health Sciences Center, Division of Dermatology.*)

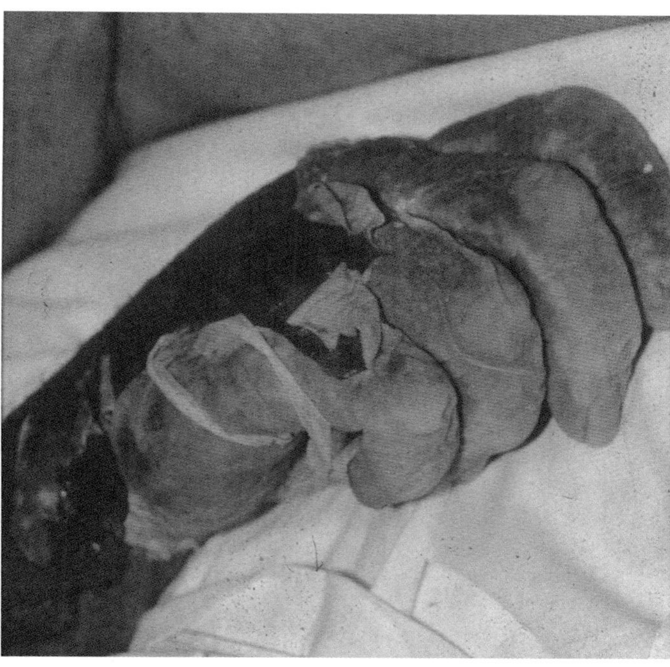

FIGURE 175-8 Toxic epidermal necrolysis with desquamation of skin on the hand. (*Reproduced with permission from the University of Texas Health Sciences Center, Division of Dermatology.*)

- Histologic findings of EM will show a lymphocytic infiltrate at the dermal–epidermal junction. There is a characteristic vacuolization of the epidermal cells and necrotic keratinocytes within the epidermis.[1]

DIFFERENTIAL DIAGNOSIS

- Bullous pemphigoid—Can be either subacute or acute with tense widespread blisters that can occur after persistent urticaria; mucosal involvement is rare. Significant pruritus can be present. As with EM, SJS, and TEN, bullous pemphigoid can occur after certain exposures such as ultraviolet (UV) radiation, or certain drugs (see Chapter 182, Bullous Pemphigoid).

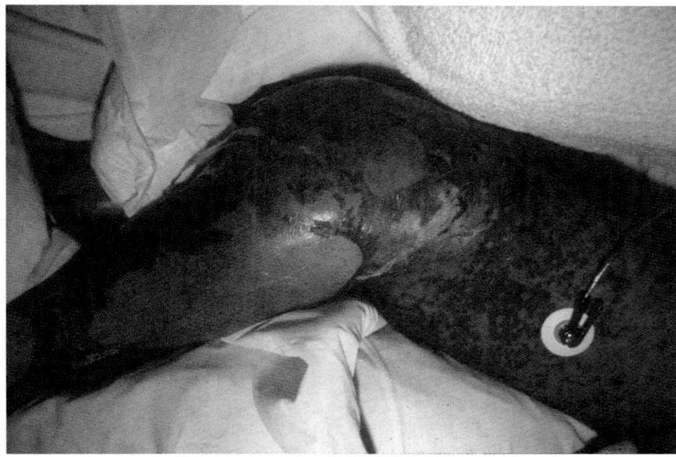

FIGURE 175-9 Toxic epidermal necrolysis with large areas of desquamation on the leg. (*Reproduced with permission from the University of Texas Health Sciences Center, Division of Dermatology.*)

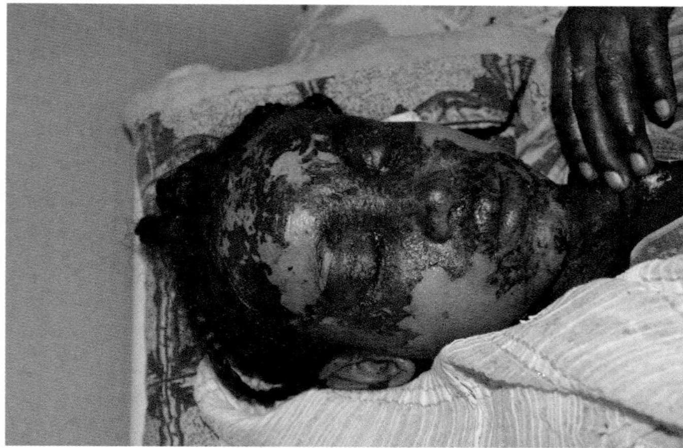

A

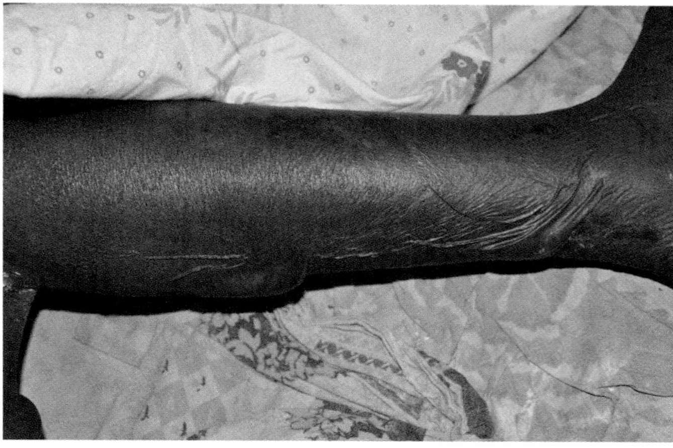

B

FIGURE 175-10 Toxic epidermal necrolysis secondary to amoxicillin. A. Face with large areas of desquamation and loss of pigmentation. B. Skin detaching from leg in large sheets and bullae. (*Reproduced with permission from Richard P. Usatine, MD.*)

- Urticaria—A skin reaction characterized by red wheals that are usually pruritic. Unlike EM, individual lesions rarely last more than 24 hours (see Chapter 148, Urticaria and Angioedema).
- Cutaneous vasculitis—Also caused by a hypersensitivity reaction, lesions are palpable papules or purpura. Blisters, hives, and necrotic ulcers can occur on the skin. Lesions are usually located on the legs, trunk, and buttocks (see Chapter 177, Vasculitis).
- Erythema annulare centrifugum—A hypersensitivity reaction caused by a variety of agents. Lesions look similar with erythematous papules of a few to several centimeters that enlarge and clear centrally and may be vesicular. Lesions tend to appear on the legs and thighs, but may occur on upper extremities, trunk, and face; palms and soles are spared (see Chapter 204, Erythema Annulare Centrifugum).
- Staphylococcal scalded skin syndrome—Rash may also follow a prodrome of malaise and fever but is macular, brightly erythematous, and initially involves the face, neck, axilla, and groin. Skin is markedly tender. Like SJS and TEN, large areas of the epidermis peel away. Unlike TEN, the site of the staphylococcal infection is usually extracutaneous (eg, otitis media, pharyngitis) and not the skin lesions themselves (see Chapter 118, Impetigo).

MANAGEMENT

EM

- The treatment is mainly supportive. Symptomatic relief may be provided with topical emollients, systemic antihistamines, and acetaminophen. These do not, however, alter the course of the illness.
- The use of corticosteroids has not been well studied, but is thought to prolong the course or increase the frequency of recurrences in HSV-associated cases.[7]
- Prophylactic acyclovir has been used to control recurrent HSV-associated EM with some success.[7]

SJS and TEN

- Treatment again, is mainly supportive and may require intensive care or placement in a burn unit. Early diagnosis is imperative so that triggering agents can be discontinued.
- Oral lesions can be managed with mouthwashes and glycerin swabs.
- Skin lesions should be cleansed with saline or Burow solution (aluminum acetate in water).
- IV fluids should be given to replace insensible losses.
- Daily examinations for secondary infections should occur and systemic antibiotics should be started as needed.
- Consultation with an ophthalmologist is important because of the high risk of ocular sequelae.
- Pharmacologic therapy is widely debated in the literature. Evidence suggests that intravenous immunoglobulin (IVIG) at doses of 2 to 3 g/kg can help shorten the course and improve outcome if started early in the course of the disease.[11]
- Systemic corticosteroids have been the mainstay of treatment for SJS/TEN. Recent evidence, however, suggests there may be an increase in morbidity and mortality when used for TEN.[11]
- Other agents that have been tried with limited success include thalidomide, tumor necrosis factor (TNF)-α inhibitors, cyclophosphamide, cyclosporine, and plasmapheresis.

PREVENTION

Screening populations known to carry HLA alleles prior to starting medications with higher risks for SJS/TEN has been suggested by some researchers.[2]

PROGNOSIS

- EM usually resolves spontaneously within 1 to 2 weeks.
- Recurrence of EM is common, especially when preceded by HSV infection.
- Prognosis is poorer for patients with SJS and TEN if they are older, have a large percentage of body surface area involved, or have intestinal or pulmonary involvement.
- Mortality for SJS/TEN can be predicted based on the severity of illness score for TEN.[12] One point is given for each of the following: serum blood urea nitrogen greater than 10 mmol/L; serum bicarbonate less than 20 mmol/L; serum glucose greater than 14 mmol/L; age older than 40 years; malignancy present; heart rate greater than 120 beats/min; percentage of body surface area involved greater than 10%. Scores of 0 to 1 are associated with a mortality rate of 3.2% whereas scores of 5 or higher are associated with a mortality rate of 90%.
- For patients with SJS, mortality rates have been reported of 5% to 10% and up to 30% for TEN.[9,13]

FOLLOW-UP

- For uncomplicated cases, no specific follow-up is needed.
- For patients with EM major and any of the complications listed above, follow-up should be arranged with the appropriate specialist.

PATIENT EDUCATION

- If an offending drug is found to be the cause, it should be discontinued immediately.
- Patients with HSV-associated EM should be made aware of the risk of recurrence.

PATIENT RESOURCES

- Erythema multiforme—**http://www.nlm.nih.gov/medlineplus/ency/article/000851.htm.**

PROVIDER RESOURCES

- Medscape. *Erythema Multiforme*—**http://emedicine.medscape.com/article/1122915.**
- Medscape. *Stevens-Johnson Syndrome*—**http://emedicine.medscape.com/article/1197450.**

REFERENCES

1. Shaw JC. Erythema multiforme. In: Noble J, Green H, Levinson W, et al, eds. *Textbook of Primary Care Medicine*. 3rd ed. St. Louis, MO: Mosby; 2001:815-816.
2. Tan SK, Tay YK. Profile and pattern of Stevens-Johnson syndrome and toxic epidermal necrolysis in a general hospital in Singapore: treatment outcomes. *Acta Derm Venereol*. 2012;92(1):62-66.
3. Finkelstein Y, Soon GS, Acuna P, et al. Recurrence and outcomes of Stevens-Johnson syndrome and toxic epidermal necrolysis in children. *Pediatrics*. 2011;128(4):723-728.
4. Del Pozzo-Magana BR, Lazo-Langner A, Carleton B. A systematic review of treatment of drug-induced Stevens-Johnson syndrome and toxic epidermal necrolysis in children. *J Popul Ther Clin Pharmacol*. 2011;18:e121-e133.
5. Plaza JA. *Erythema Multiforme*. Updated July 29, 2011. http://www.emedicine.com/derm/topic137.htm. Accessed January 2012.
6. Darmstadt GL. Erythema multiforme. In: Long S, Pickering L, Prober C, eds. *Principles and Practice of Pediatric Infectious Diseases*. 2nd ed. New York, NY: Churchill Livingstone; 2003:442-444.
7. Morelli JG. Vesiculobullous disorders. In: Behrman R, Kliegman RM, Jenson HB, eds. *Nelson Textbook of Pediatrics*. 19th ed. Philadelphia, PA: Saunders; 2011:2241-2249.

8. Weston WL. Herpes associated erythema multiforme. *J Invest Dermatol.* 2005;124(6):xv-xvi.

9. Chosidow OM, Stern RS, Wintroub BU. Cutaneous drug reactions. In: Kasper DL, Fauci AS, Longo DL, Braunwald EB, Hauser SL, Jameson JL, eds. *Harrison's Principles of Internal Medicine*. 16th ed. New York, NY: McGraw-Hill; 2005:318-324.

10. Sanmarkan AD, Tukaram S, Thappa DM, et al. Retrospective analysis of Stevens-Johnson syndrome and toxic epidermal necrolysis over a period of 10 years. *Indian J Dermatol.* 2011;56(1):25-29.

11. Worswick S, Cotliar J. Stevens-Johnson syndrome and toxic epidermal necrolysis: a review of treatment options. *Dermatol Ther.* 2011;24(2):207-218.

12. Bastuji-Garin S, Fouchard N, Bertocchi M, et al. SCORTEN: a severity of illness score for toxic epidermal necrolysis. *J Invest Dermatol.* 2000;115(2):149-153.

13. The Stevens-Johnson syndrome/toxic epidermal necrolysis spectrum of disease. In: Habif T, ed. *Clinical Dermatology*. 4th ed. Philadelphia, PA: Elsevier; 2004:627-631.

176 ERYTHEMA NODOSUM

E.J. Mayeaux Jr, MD
Lucia Diaz, MD
Richard Paulis, MD

PATIENT STORY

A young woman presented to the office with several days of overall malaise, fever, and sore throat. At the time of presentation she noted some painful bumps on her lower legs, and denied trauma (**Figure 176-1**). No history of recent cough or change in bowel habits has been reported. The patient had no chronic medical problems, took no medications, and had no known drug allergies. Her temperature was slightly elevated, but other vitals were normal. On examination, her oropharynx revealed tonsillar erythema and exudates. Bilateral lower extremities were spotted with slightly raised, tender, erythematous nodules that varied in size from 2 to 6 cm. Rapid strep test was positive and she was diagnosed clinically with erythema nodosum (EN) secondary to group A β-hemolytic *Streptococcus*. She was treated with penicillin and nonsteroidal anti-inflammatory drugs (NSAIDs), and was advised temporary bed rest. She experienced complete resolution of the EN within 4 weeks.

INTRODUCTION

EN is a common inflammatory panniculitis characterized by ill-defined, erythematous patches with underlying tender, subcutaneous nodules. It is a reactive process caused by chronic inflammatory states, infections, medications, malignancies, and unknown factors.

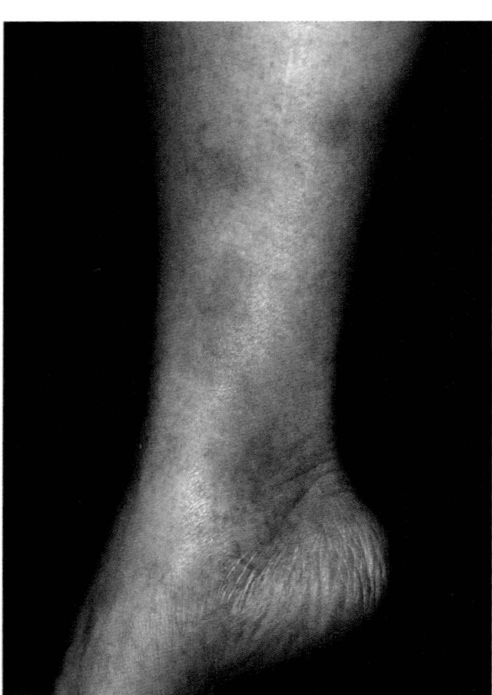

FIGURE 176-1 Erythema nodosum secondary to group A β-hemolytic *Streptococcus* in a young woman. (*Reproduced with permission from Richard P. Usatine, MD.*)

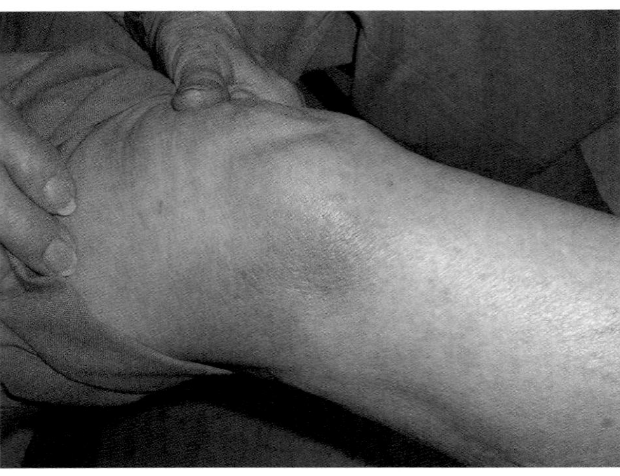

FIGURE 176-2 EN in a middle-aged woman around the knee secondary to sarcoidosis. (*Reproduced with permission from Richard P. Usatine, MD.*)

SYNONYMS

EN is also known as Lofgren syndrome (with hilar adenopathy).

EPIDEMIOLOGY

- EN occurs in approximately 1 to 5 per 100,000 persons.[1] It is the most frequent type of septal panniculitis (inflammation of the septa of fat lobules in the subcutaneous tissue).[2]
- EN tends to occur more often in women, with a male-to-female ratio of 1:4.5 in the adult population, generally during the second and fourth decades of life (**Figures 176-1** to **176-3**).[3]

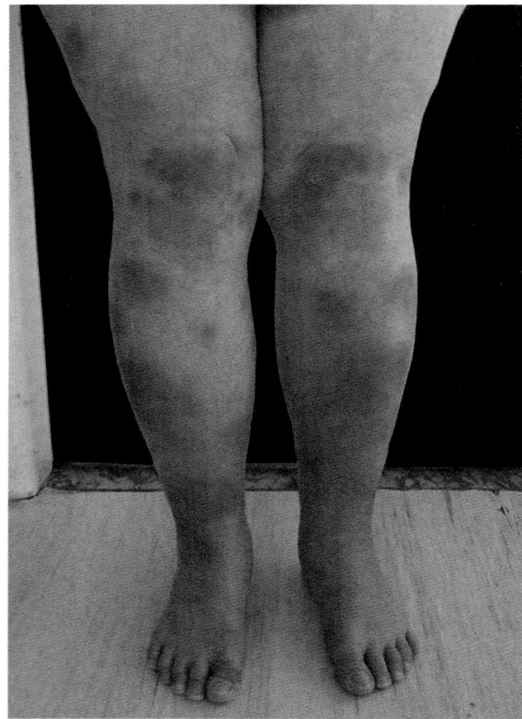

FIGURE 176-3 EN in a middle-aged woman with no known cause. These lesions are bright red, warm, and painful. (*Reproduced with permission from Hanuš Rozsypal, MD.*)

- In one study, an overall incidence of 54 million people worldwide was cited in patients older than 14 years of age.[4]
- In the childhood form, the female predilection is not seen.

ETIOLOGY AND PATHOPHYSIOLOGY

- Most EN is idiopathic (**Figures 176-3** and **176-4**). Although the exact percentage is unknown, one study estimated that 55% of EN is idiopathic.[5] This may be influenced by the fact that EN may precede the underlying illness. The distribution of etiologic causes may be seasonal.[6] Identifiable causes can be infectious, reactive, pharmacologic, or neoplastic.
- Histologic examination is most useful in defining EN. Defining characteristics of EN are a septal panniculitis without presence of vasculitis. That this pattern develops in certain areas of skin may be linked to local variations in temperature and efficient blood drainage.
- Septal panniculitis begins with polymorphonuclear cells infiltrating the septa of fat lobules in the subcutaneous tissue. It is thought that this is in response to existing immune complex deposition in these areas.[7] This inflammatory change consists of edema and hemorrhage which is responsible for the nodularity, warmth, and erythema.
- The infiltrate progresses from predominantly polymorphonuclear cells, to lymphocytes, and then histiocytes where fibrosis occurs around the lobules. There may be some necrosis though minimal as complete resolution without scarring is the typical course.
- The histopathologic hallmark of EN is the Miescher radial granuloma. This is a small, well-defined nodular aggregate of small histiocytes around a central stellate or banana-shaped cleft.

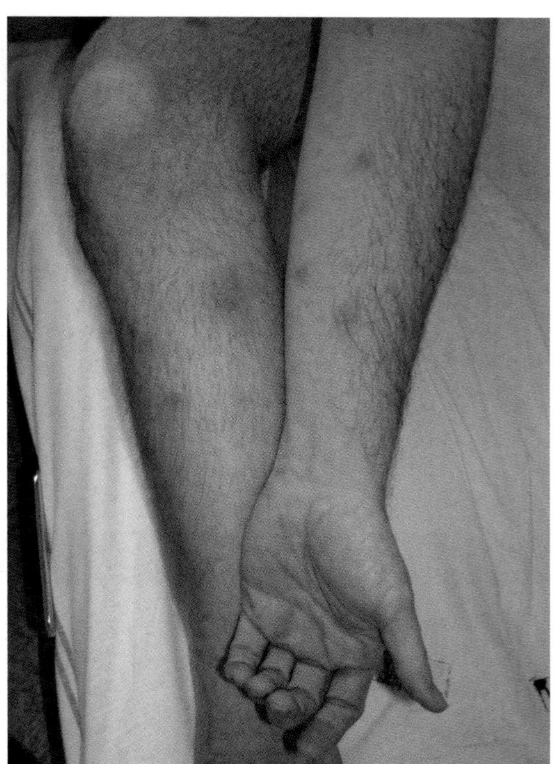

FIGURE 176-4 EN on the arms and legs of unknown cause in a young man. *(Reproduced with permission from Hanuš Rozsypal, MD.)*

RISK FACTORS

- Group A β-hemolytic streptococcal pharyngitis has been linked to EN (see **Figure 176-1**). A retrospective study of 129 cases of EN over several decades reports 28% had streptococcal infection.[5]
- Nonstreptococcal upper respiratory tract infections may also play a role.[1]
- Historically, tuberculosis (TB) was a common underlying illness with EN, but TB is now a rare cause of EN in developed countries. There are reports of EN occurring in patients receiving the bacille Calmette-Guérin vaccination.[8] In developed countries, sarcoidosis is more commonly found. One study estimates sarcoidosis as being the cause of 11% of EN cases (see **Figure 176-2**).[5,7]
- EN occurs in 3% of all patients with coccidiomycosis,[9] and approximately 4% of patients with histoplasmosis.[10]
- EN is less frequently associated with other infectious agents, including *Yersinia* gastroenteritis, *Salmonella*, *Campylobacter*, toxoplasmosis, syphilis, amebiasis, giardiasis, brucellosis, leprosy, *Chlamydia*, *Mycoplasma*, *Brucella*, hepatitis B (infection and vaccine), Epstein-Barr virus, and *Bartonella*.[4,11]
- When the EN rash occurs with hilar adenopathy, the entity is called Lofgren syndrome. Lofgren syndrome in TB represents primary infection. A more common cause of Lofgren syndrome is sarcoidosis.[7]
- The literature reports that EN is seen in patients with inflammatory bowel diseases. It is usually prominent around the time of gastrointestinal (GI) flare-ups, but may occur before a flare. Most sources report a greater association between Crohn disease and EN than between ulcerative colitis and EN. Other chronic diseases associated with EN include Behçet disease and Sweet syndrome.[11]
- Some debate exists over causality from pregnancy and oral contraceptives in the occurrence of EN.
- Besides oral contraceptives, medications implicated as causing EN are antibiotics including sulfonamides, penicillins, and bromides. However, the antibiotics may have been prescribed for the underlying infection that had caused EN.[11]
- Lymphomas, acute myelogenous leukemia, carcinoid tumor, and pancreatic carcinoma are associated with EN and should be considered in cases of persistent or recurrent EN.[11,12]

DIAGNOSIS

CLINICAL FEATURES

- The diagnosis is usually clinical.
- The lesions of EN are deep-seated nodules that may be more easily palpated than visualized.
- Lesions are initially firm, round or oval, and are poorly demarcated.
- Lesions may be bright red, warm, and painful (see **Figure 176-3**).
- Lesions number from 1 to more than 10.5 and vary in size from 1 to 15 cm.
- Over their course, the lesions begin to flatten and change to a purplish color before eventually taking on the yellowish hue of a bruise.
- A characteristic of EN is the complete resolution of lesions with no ulceration or scarring.
- EN is associated with systemic occurrence of fever, malaise, and polyarthralgia sometime near eruption.

TYPICAL DISTRIBUTION

- Lesions appear on the anterior/lateral aspect of both lower extremities (see **Figures 176-1** to **176-3**).
- Although lesions may appear in other regions such as the arms, absence in the lower legs is unusual (see **Figure 176-4**).[1]
- Sarcoid, in particular, may present with lesions on the ankles and knees (see **Figure 176-2**).
- Lesions may appear in dependent areas in bedridden patients.

LABORATORY TESTING

- Blood tests may help to identify the underlying cause. Typical tests include complete blood count, chemistries, liver function tests, and erythrocyte sedimentation rate. Erythrocyte sedimentation rate may be elevated.
- For suspected *Streptococcus* cases, rapid strep test or throat cultures are best during acute illness, whereas antistreptolysin O titers may be used in the convalescent phase.[4]
- In sarcoid, angiotensin-converting enzyme levels may be helpful but are not 100% sensitive.[2] A chest X-ray and/or skin biopsy of a suspected sarcoid lesion can help make this diagnosis (see Chapter 173, Sarcoidosis).

BIOPSY

The diagnosis of EN is mostly made on physical examination. When the diagnosis is uncertain, a biopsy that includes subcutaneous fat is performed. This can be a deep punch biopsy or a deep incisional biopsy sent for standard histology. If a biopsy is needed, this can be done by choosing a lesion not over a joint or vital structure and burying a 4-mm punch biopsy to the hilt.

DIFFERENTIAL DIAGNOSIS

- Cellulitis should be considered and not missed. These patients tend to be sicker and have more fever and systemic symptoms. EN tends to appear in multiple locations while cellulitis is usually in one localized area (see Chapter 122, Cellulitis).
- Nodular cutaneous and subcutaneous sarcoid is skin colored or violaceous without epidermal involvement. The lack of surface involvement makes this resemble EN. Subcutaneous sarcoid may be seen in advanced systemic sarcoidosis that can also be the cause of EN. Skin biopsy is the best method to distinguish between these 2 conditions. Either way, treatment is directed toward the sarcoidosis (see Chapter 173, Sarcoidosis).
- Erythema induratum of Bazin is a lobular panniculitis that occurs on the posterior lower extremity of women with tendency of lesions to ulcerate with residual scarring.[7] This condition is typically caused by TB and is more chronic in nature than EN.[2]
- Erythema nodosum leprosum (ENL) may occur in patients with leprosy and probably represent an immune complex or hypersensitivity reaction (**Figures 176-5** and **176-6**). ENL is typically seen as a type 2 reaction to standard leprosy therapy.[13] It is more common in multibacillary lepromatous leprosy. Although the lesions often look like standard EN, the lesions may also ulcerate.
- An infectious panniculitis should also be considered in the differential, especially in immunocompromised patients. These lesions are often asymmetric and the patient may be febrile. If suspected, a punch biopsy of a lesion should be sent for tissue culture (bacteria, fungus, and *Mycobacteria*).

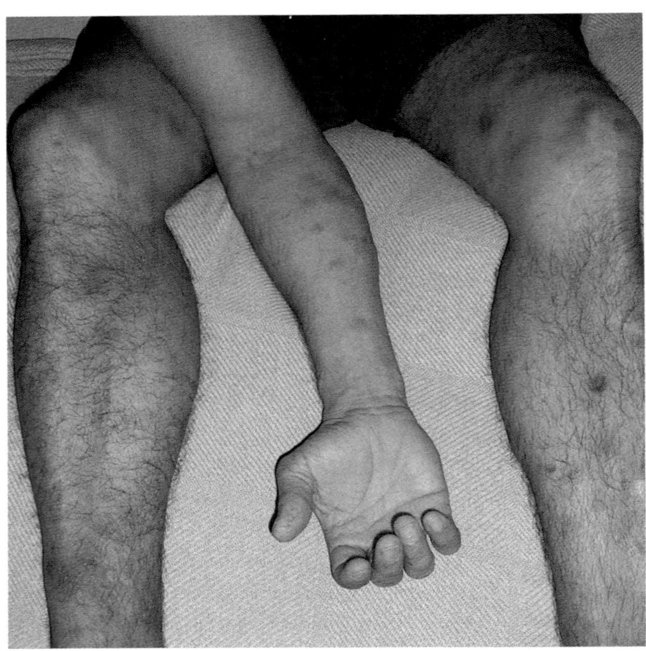

A

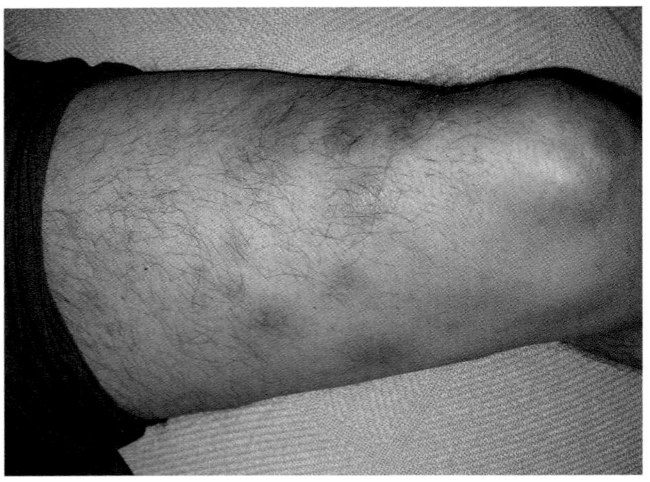

B

FIGURE 176-5 Erythema nodosum leprosum (ENL) in a Texas man who acquired multibacillary leprosy from handling and eating armadillos. His ENL started when he started the antibacterial treatment. **A.** Note the many subcutaneous nodules on his arms and legs. **B.** Close-up of the ENL lesions. *(Reproduced with permission from Richard P. Usatine, MD.)*

MANAGEMENT

Look for and treat the underlying cause. There is limited evidence to guide treatment unless an underlying cause is found.

NONPHARMACOLOGIC

Cool, wet compresses, elevation of the involved extremities, bed rest, gradient support stockings, or pressure bandages may help alleviate the pain.[11] SOR C

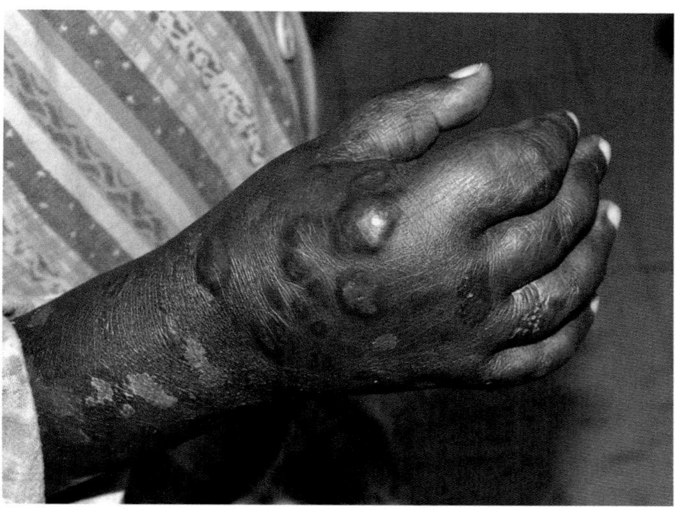

FIGURE 176-6 Erythema nodosum leprosum (ENL) on the hand and arm of an Ethiopian woman being treated with 3 antileprosy drugs for multibacillary lepromatous leprosy. (*Reproduced with permission from Richard P. Usatine, MD.*)

MEDICATIONS

- Treat the pain and discomfort of the nodules with NSAIDs and/or other analgesics.[14] SOR C
- The value of oral prednisone is controversial and should be avoided unless it is being used to treat the underlying cause (such as sarcoidosis) and if underlying infection, risk of bacterial dissemination or sepsis, and malignancy have been excluded.[1] SOR C
- Oral potassium iodide, which is contraindicated in pregnancy, led to resolution of EN in several small studies.[6,7] SOR B
- Colchicine, hydroxychloroquine, and dapsone have been used as well.[2,7] SOR C
- There are a few case reports of EN treated with penicillin, erythromycin, adalimumab, etanercept, infliximab, mycophenolate mofetil, cyclosporine, thalidomide, and extracorporeal monocyte granulocytapheresis.[1,15,16] SOR C
- There is one case report of minocycline and tetracycline leading to EN improvement.[17] SOR C

PREVENTION

Good hand washing and general health measures may prevent respiratory infections that may predispose to EN.

PROGNOSIS

- EN is usually self-limited or resolves with treatment of the underlying disorder.
- Patients may continue to develop nodules for a few weeks.
- The course depends on the etiology, but usually lasts only 6 weeks.
- Lesions completely resolve with no ulceration or scarring.
- Recurrences occur in 33% to 41% of cases, usually when the etiology is unknown.[16]

FOLLOW-UP

Follow-up is needed to complete the workup for an underlying cause and to make sure that the patient is responding to symptomatic treatment.

PATIENT EDUCATION

Reassure the patient that there is complete resolution in most cases within 3 to 6 weeks. Inform the patient that some EN outbreaks may persist for up to 12 weeks, and some cases are recurrent.[6]

PATIENT RESOURCES

- PubMed Health. *Erythema Nodosum*—**http://www.ncbi.nlm.nih.gov/pubmedhealth/PMH0001884/.**
- MedicineNet. *Erythema Nodosum*—**http://www.medicinenet.com/erythema_nodosum/article.htm.**

PROVIDER RESOURCES

- Medscape. *Erythema Nodosum*—**http://emedicine.medscape.com/article/1081633-overview.**
- Schwartz RA, Nervi SJ. Erythema nodosum: a sign of systemic disease. *Am Fam Physician*. 20071;75(5):695-700—**http://www.aafp.org/afp/2007/0301/p695.html.**

REFERENCES

1. Schwartz RA, Nervi SJ. Erythema nodosum: a sign of systemic disease. *Am Fam Physician*. 2007;75(5):695-700.
2. Atzeni F, Carrabba M, Davin JC, et al. Skin manifestations in vasculitis and erythema nodosum. *Clin Exp Rheumatol*. 2006;24 (1 suppl 40):S60-S66.
3. Garcia-Porrua C, González-Gay MA, Vázquez-Caruncho M, et al. Erythema nodosum: etiologic and predictive factors erythema nodosum and erythema induratum in a defined population. *Arthritis Rheum*. 2000:43:584-592.
4. Gonzalez-Gay MA, Garcia-Porrua C, Pujol RM, Salvarani C. Erythema nodosum: a clinical approach. *Clin Exp Rheumatol*. 2001;19(4):365-368.
5. Cribier B, Caille A, Heid E, Grosshans E. Erythema nodosum and associated diseases. A study of 129 cases. *Int J Dermatol*. 1998;37(9):667-672.
6. Hannuksela M. Erythema nodosum. *Clin Dermatol*. 1986;4(4):88-95.
7. Requena L, Requena C. Erythema nodosum. *Dermatol Online J*. 2002;8(1):4.
8. Fox MD, Schwartz RA. Erythema nodosum. *Am Fam Physician*. 1992;46(3):818-822.
9. Body BA. Cutaneous manifestations of systemic mycoses. *Dermatol Clin*. 1996;14:125-135.
10. Ozols II, Wheat LJ. Erythema nodosum in an epidemic of histoplasmosis in Indianapolis. *Arch Dermatol*. 1981;117:709-712.
11. Gilchrist H, Patterson JW. Erythema nodosum and erythema induratum (nodular vasculitis): diagnosis and management. *Dermatol Ther*. 2010;23(4):320-327.

12. Cho KH, Kim YG, Yang SG, et al. Inflammatory nodules of the lower legs: a clinical and histological analysis of 134 cases in Korea. *J Dermatol.* 1997;24:522-529.
13. Van Brakel WH, Khawas IB, Lucas SB. Reactions in leprosy: an epidemiological study of 386 patients in west Nepal. *Lepr Rev.* 1994;65(3):190-203.
14. Ubogy Z, Persellin RH. Suppression of erythema nodosum by indomethacin. *Acta Derm Venereol.* 1982;62:265.
15. Allen RA, Spielvogel RL. Erythema nodosum. In: Lebwohl MG, Heymann WR, Berth-Jones J, Coulson I, eds. *Treatment of Skin Disease*. 3rd ed. Philadelphia, PA: Saunders; 2010:223-225.
16. Gilchrist H, Patterson JW. Erythema nodosum and erythema induratum (nodular vasculitis): diagnosis and management. *Dermatol Ther.* 2010;23(4):320-327.
17. Davis MD. Response of recalcitrant erythema nodosum to tetracyclines. *J Am Acad Dermatol.* 2011;64(6):1211-1212.

177 VASCULITIS

E.J. Mayeaux, Jr., MD
Richard P. Usatine, MD

PATIENT STORY

A 21-year-old woman presented with a 3-day history of a painful purpuric rash on her lower extremities (**Figure 177-1** and **177-2**). The lesions had appeared suddenly, and the patient had experienced no prior similar episodes. The patient had been diagnosed with a case of pharyngitis earlier that week and was given a course of antibiotics. She had not experienced any nausea or vomiting, fever, abdominal cramping, or gross hematuria. Urine dipstick revealed blood in her urine, but no protein. The typical palpable purpura on the legs is consistent with Henoch-Schönlein purpura (HSP).

INTRODUCTION

Vasculitis refers to a group of disorders characterized by inflammation and damage in blood vessel walls. They may be limited to skin or may be a multisystem disorder. Cutaneous vasculitic diseases are classified according to the size (small vs medium-to-large vessel) and type of blood vessel involved (venule, arteriole, artery, or vein). Small- and medium-size vessels are found in the dermis and deep reticular dermis, respectively. The clinical presentation varies with the intensity of the inflammation, and the size and type of blood vessel involved.[1]

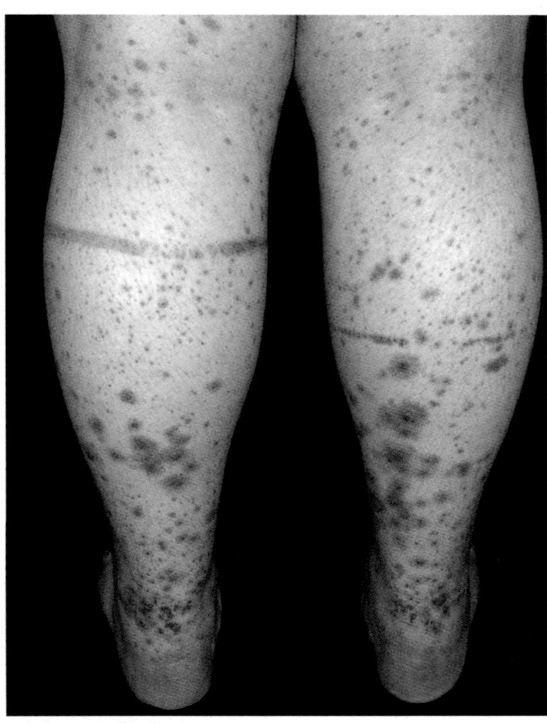

FIGURE 177-1 Henoch-Schönlein purpura presenting as palpable purpura on the lower extremity. The visible sock lines are from lesions that formed where the socks exerted pressure on the legs. (*Reproduced with permission from Richard P. Usatine, MD.*)

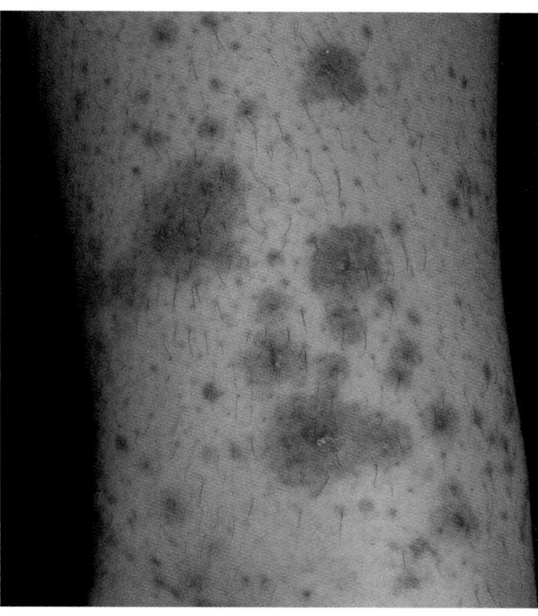

FIGURE 177-2 Close-up of palpable purpura from the patient in Figure 177-1. Some lesions look like target lesions but this is Henoch-Schönlein purpura and not erythema multiforme. (*Reproduced with permission from Richard P. Usatine, MD.*)

SYNONYMS

Hypersensitivity vasculitis is also known as leukocytoclastic vasculitis.

HSP is a type of leukocytoclastic vasculitis.

EPIDEMIOLOGY

- HSP (**Figures 177-1** and **177-3**) occurs mainly in children and young adults with an incidence of approximately 1 in 5000 children annually.[2] It results from immunoglobulin (Ig) A-containing immune complexes in blood vessel walls in the skin, kidney, and gastrointestinal (GI) tract. HSP is usually benign and self-limiting, and tends to occur in the springtime. A streptococcal or viral upper respiratory infection often precedes the disease by 1 to 3 weeks. Prodromal symptoms include anorexia and fever. Most patients with HSP also have joint pain and swelling with the knees and ankles being most commonly involved. In half of the cases there are recurrences, typically in the first 3 months. Recurrences are more common in patients with nephritis and are milder than the original episode. To make the diagnosis of HSP, establish the presence of 3 or more of the following[3]:
  - Palpable purpura
  - Bowel angina (pain)
  - GI bleeding
  - Hematuria
  - Onset less than or equal to 20 years
  - No new medications
- Some patients with systemic lupus erythematosus (SLE) (**Figures 177-4** and **177-5**), rheumatoid arthritis (RA), relapsing polychondritis, and other connective tissue disorders develop an associated necrotizing vasculitis. It most frequently involves the small muscular arteries, arterioles, and venules. The blood vessels can become blocked leading to tissue necrosis (see **Figures 177-4** and **177-5**). The skin and internal organs may be involved.

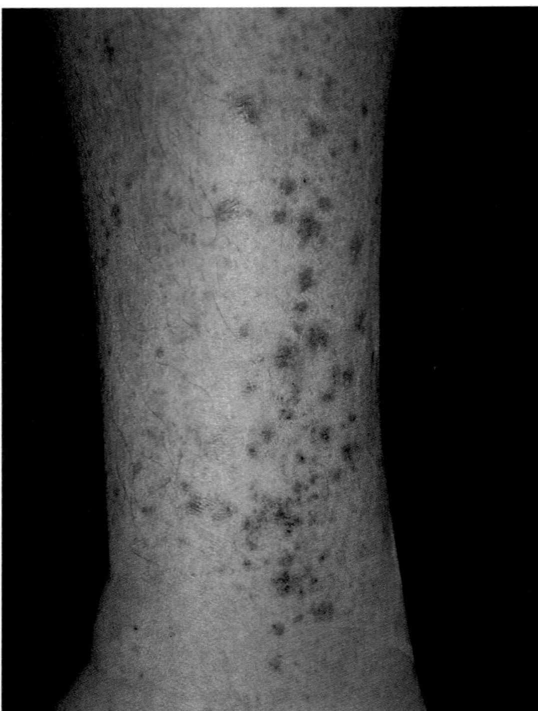

FIGURE 177-3 Henoch-Schönlein purpura in a 26-year-old man. In addition to the palpable purpura, this patient also had abdominal pain. (*Reproduced with permission from Richard P. Usatine, MD.*)

- Leukocytoclastic vasculitis (**Figures 177-6** to **177-8**) is the most commonly seen form of small vessel vasculitis. Prodromal symptoms include fever, malaise, myalgia, and joint pain. The palpable purpura begins as asymptomatic localized areas of cutaneous hemorrhage that become palpable. Few or many discrete lesions are most commonly seen on the lower extremities but may occur on any dependent area. Small lesions itch and are painful, but nodules, ulcers, and bullae may be very painful. Lesions appear in crops, last for 1 to 4 weeks, and may heal with residual scarring and hyperpigmentation. Patients may experience 1 episode (drug reaction or viral infection) or multiple episodes (RA or SLE). The disease is usually self-limited and confined to the skin. To make the diagnosis, look for presence of 3 or more of the following[4]:
    - Age older than 16 years
    - Use of a possible offending drug in temporal relation to the symptoms
    - Palpable purpura

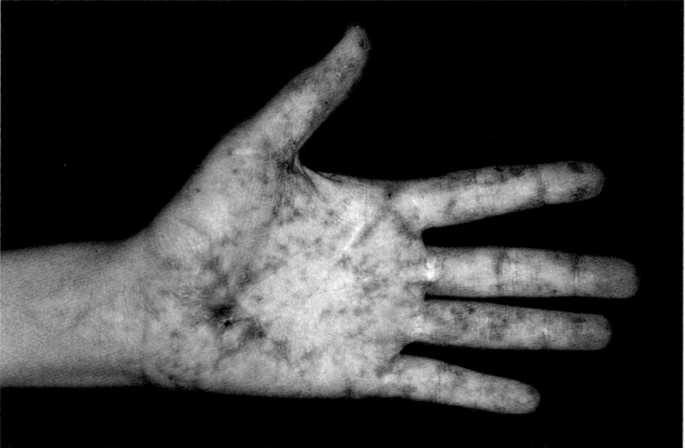

FIGURE 177-4 Necrotizing vasculitis in a young Asian woman with systemic lupus erythematosus. The circulation to the fingertips was compromised and the woman was treated with high-dose intravenous steroids and intravenous immunoglobulins to prevent tissue loss. (*Reproduced with permission from Richard P. Usatine, MD.*)

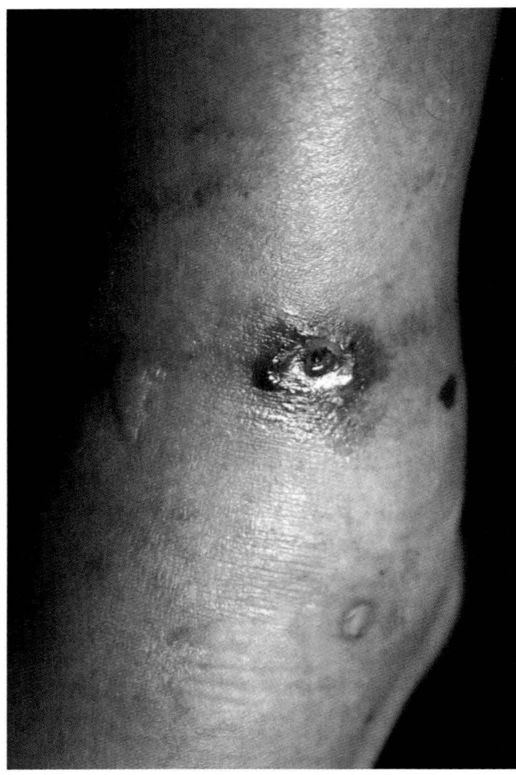

FIGURE 177-5 Vasculitis ulcer on the leg of a woman with systemic lupus erythematosus. (*Reproduced with permission from Everett Allen, MD.*)

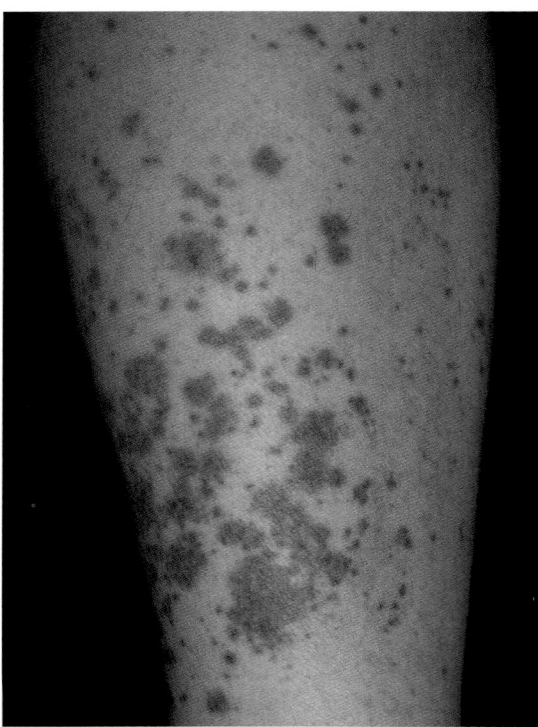

FIGURE 177-6 Leukocytoclastic vasculitis on the leg of a woman. (*Reproduced with permission from Richard P. Usatine, MD.*)

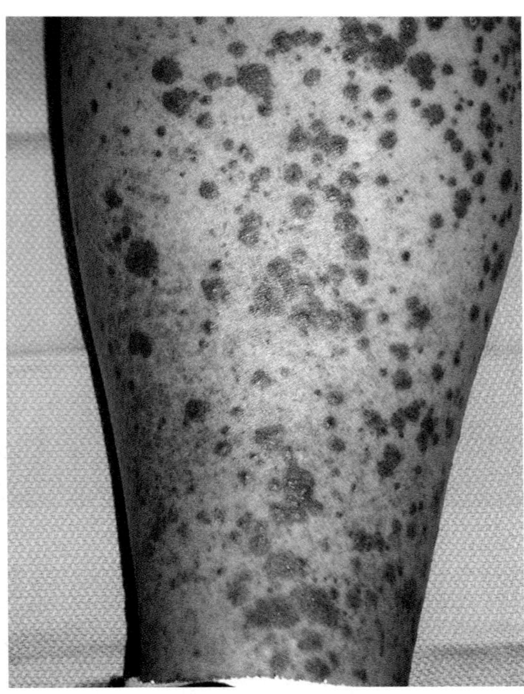

FIGURE 177-7 Very palpable purpura on the leg of a middle-aged woman with leukocytoclastic vasculitis. (*Reproduced with permission from Eric Kraus, MD.*)

  - Maculopapular rash
  - Biopsy of a skin lesion showing neutrophils around an arteriole or venule
- Systemic manifestations of leukocytoclastic vasculitis may include kidney disease, heart, nervous system, GI tract, lungs, and joint involvement.

ETIOLOGY AND PATHOPHYSIOLOGY

- Vasculitis is defined as inflammation of the blood vessel wall. The mechanisms of vascular damage consist of either a humoral response, immune complex deposition, or cell-mediated T-lymphocyte response with granuloma formation.[5]
- Vasculitis-induced injury to blood vessels may lead to increased vascular permeability, vessel weakening, aneurysm formation, hemorrhage, intimal proliferation, and thrombosis that result in obstruction and local ischemia.[5]

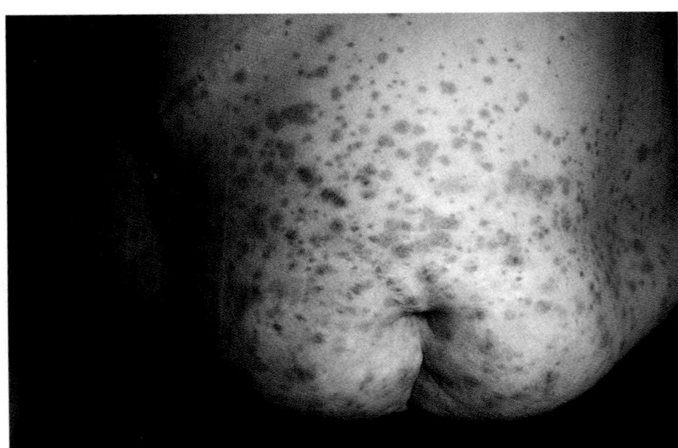

FIGURE 177-8 Vasculitis on the abdomen of a middle-aged woman who also has the vasculitis on her legs. (*Reproduced with permission from Everett Allen, MD.*)

- Small-vessel vasculitis is initiated by hypersensitivity to various antigens (drugs, chemicals, microorganisms, and endogenous antigens), with formation of circulating immune complexes that are deposited in walls of postcapillary venules. The vessel-bound immune complexes activate complement, which attracts polymorphonuclear leukocytes. They damage the walls of small veins by release of lysosomal enzymes. This causes vessel necrosis and local hemorrhage.
- Small-vessel vasculitis most commonly affects the skin and rarely causes serious internal organ dysfunction, except when the kidney is involved. Small-vessel vasculitis is associated with leukocytoclastic vasculitis, HSP, essential mixed cryoglobulinemia, connective tissue diseases or malignancies, serum sickness and serum sickness-like reactions, chronic urticaria, and acute hepatitis B or C infection.
- Hypersensitivity (leukocytoclastic) vasculitis causes acute inflammation and necrosis of venules in the dermis. The term *leukocytoclastic vasculitis* describes the histologic pattern produced when leukocytes fragment.

RISK FACTORS

- Viral infections
- Autoimmune disorders
- Drug hypersensitivity
- Cocaine (adulterated with levamisole) (**Figure 177-9**) (see Chapter 240, Cocaine for additional images and information)

DIAGNOSIS

Initially, determining the extent of visceral organ involvement is more important than identifying the type of vasculitis, so that organs at risk of damage are not jeopardized by delayed or inadequate treatment. It is critical to distinguish vasculitis occurring as a primary autoimmune disorder from vasculitis secondary to infection, drugs, malignancy, or connective tissue disease such as SLE or RA.[5]

CLINICAL FEATURES

- Small-vessel vasculitis is characterized by necrotizing inflammation of small blood vessels, and may be identified by the finding of "palpable purpura." The lower extremities typically demonstrate "palpable purpura," varying in size from a few millimeters to several centimeters (**Figures 177-2**, **177-6**, **177-7**, and **177-10**). In its early stages leukocytoclastic vasculitis may not be palpable.
- The clinical features of HSP include nonthrombocytopenic palpable purpura mainly on the lower extremities and buttocks (see **Figures 177-1**, **177-2**, and **177-3**), GI symptoms, arthralgia, and nephritis.[6,7]

TYPICAL DISTRIBUTION

Cutaneous vasculitis is found most commonly on the legs, but may be seen on the hands and abdomen (see **Figures 177-3**, **177-8**, and **177-10**).

LABORATORY TESTING

- Laboratory evaluation is geared to finding the antigenic source of the immunologic reaction. Consider throat culture, antistreptolysin-*O* titer, erythrocyte sedimentation rate, platelets, complete blood count

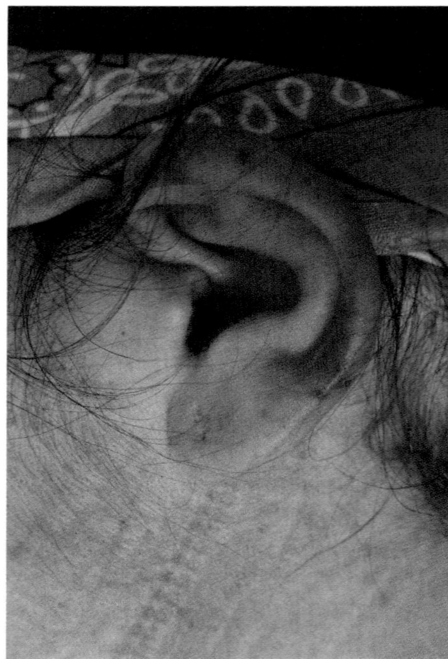

A

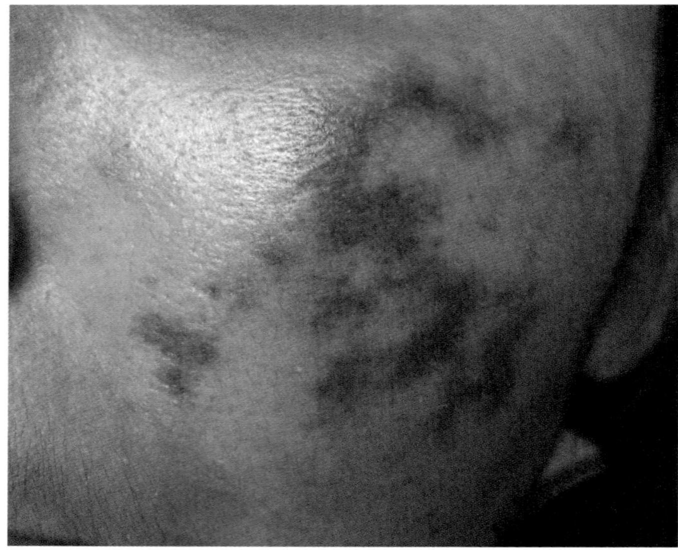

B

FIGURE 177-9 A. Cutaneous vasculitis of the ear caused by levamisole-adulterated cocaine. *(Reproduced with permission from Jonathan Karnes, MD.)* B. Cutaneous vasculitis in a retiform (net-like) pattern caused by the use of levamisole-adulterated cocaine. This is called *retiform purpura*. *(Reproduced with permission from John M. Martin IV, MD.)*

(CBC), serum creatinine, urinalysis, antinuclear antibody, serum protein electrophoresis, circulating immune complexes, hepatitis B surface antigen, hepatitis C antibody, cryoglobulins, and rheumatoid factor. The erythrocyte sedimentation rate is almost always elevated during active vasculitis. Immunofluorescent studies are best done within the first 24 hours after a lesion forms. The most common immunoreactants present in and around blood vessels are IgM, C3, and fibrin. The presence of IgA in blood vessels of a child with vasculitis suggests the diagnosis of HSP.

- Basic laboratory analysis to assess the degree and types of organs affected should include serum creatinine, creatinine kinase, liver function studies, hepatitis serologies, urinalysis, and possibly chest X-ray and electrocardiography (ECG).

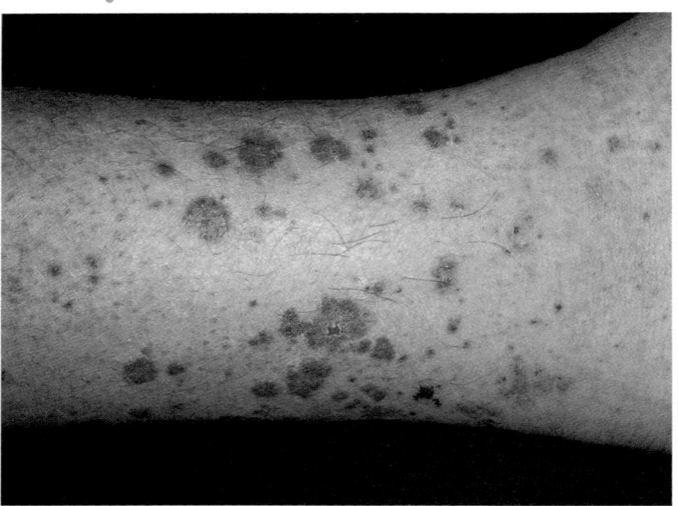

A

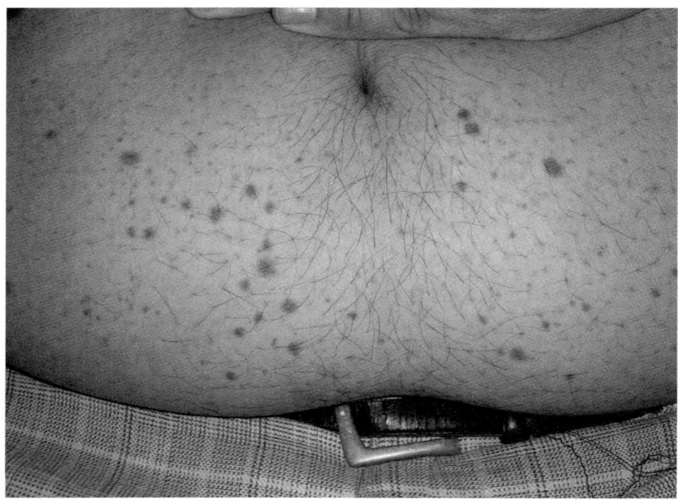

B

FIGURE 177-10 Leukocytoclastic vasculitis in a 26-year-old man. A. Palpable purpura on the lower leg. B. Involvement of the lower abdomen. *(Reproduced with permission from Richard P. Usatine, MD.)*

BIOPSY

The clinical presentation is so characteristic that a biopsy is generally unnecessary. In doubtful cases, a punch biopsy should be taken from an early active (nonulcerated) lesion or, if necessary, from the edge of an ulcer (see **Figure 177-4**).

DIFFERENTIAL DIAGNOSIS

- Pigmented purpuric dermatosis is a capillaritis characterized by extravasation of erythrocytes in the skin with marked hemosiderin deposition. It is not palpable. Schamberg disease is a type of pigmented purpuric dermatosis found most often on the lower legs in older persons (**Figures 177-11** and **177-12**). It is described as a cayenne pepper-like appearance. Lichen aureus is a localized pigmented purpuric dermatosis seen in younger persons that may occur on the leg or in other parts

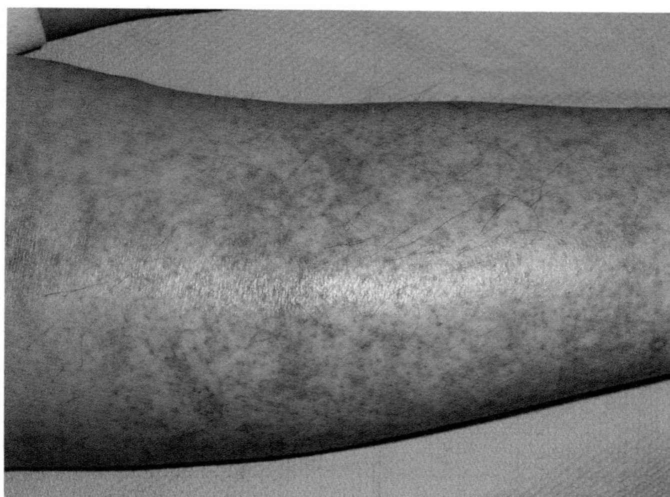

FIGURE 177-11 Schamberg disease (pigmented purpuric dermatosis) of the lower leg showing hemosiderin deposits and a cayenne pepper capillaritis. (*Reproduced with permission from Richard P. Usatine, MD.*)

of the body (**Figure 177-13**). The color may be yellow brown or golden brown. There is also a pigmented purpuric dermatosis of the Majocchi type that has an annular appearance with prominent elevated erythematous borders that may have telangiectasias (**Figure 177-14**). A dermatoscope can help to visualize the red or pink dots that represent inflamed capillaries in these conditions.

- Meningococcemia presents with purpura in severely ill patients with central nervous system symptoms (**Figures 177-15** and **177-16**).
- Rocky Mountain spotted fever is a rickettsial infection that presents with pink-to-bright red, discrete 1- to 5-mm macules that blanch with pressure and may be pruritic. The lesions start distally and spread to the soles and palms (**Figure 177-17**).
- Malignancies, such as cutaneous T-cell lymphoma (mycosis fungoides) (see Chapter 174, Cutaneous T-cell Lymphoma).
- Stevens-Johnson syndrome and toxic epidermal necrolysis (see Chapter 175, Erythema Multiforme, Stevens-Johnson Syndrome, and Toxic Epidermal Necrolysis).
- Idiopathic thrombocytopenia purpura can be easily distinguished from vasculitis by measuring the platelet count. Also, the purpura is usually not palpable and the petechiae can be scattered all over the body (**Figure 177-18**).

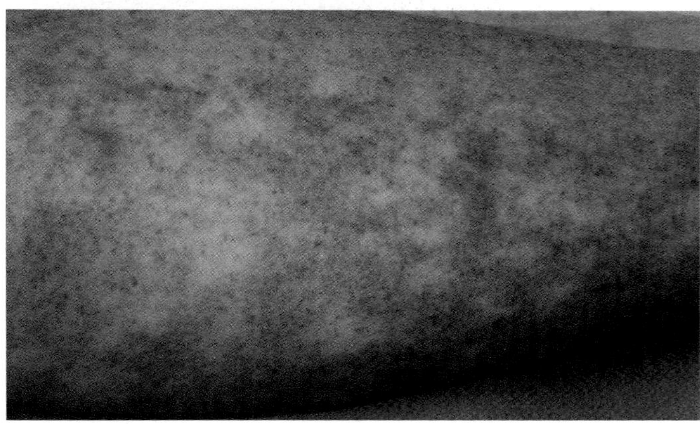

FIGURE 177-12 Schamberg disease with prominent petechiae and hemosiderin deposits. Note that this condition is not palpable. (*Reproduced with permission from Richard P. Usatine, MD.*)

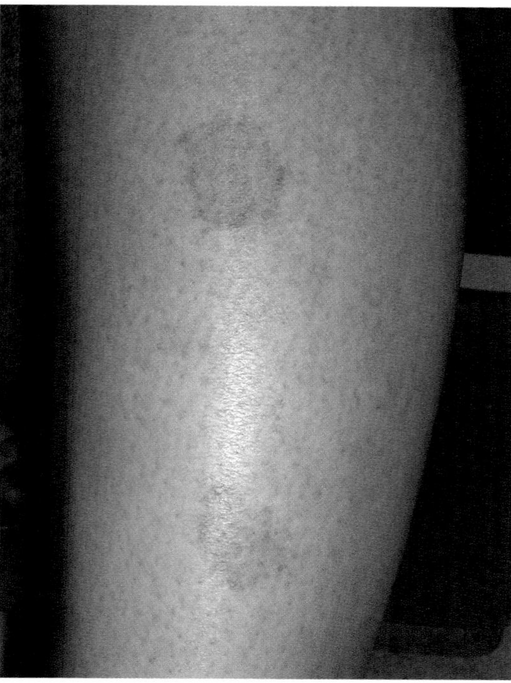

A

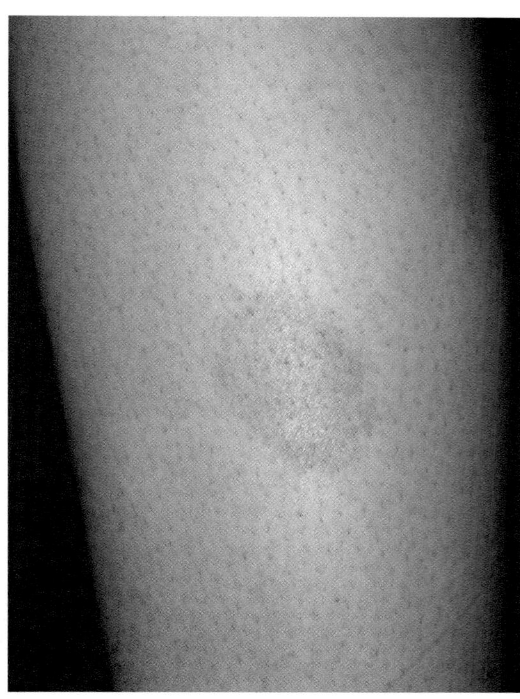

B

FIGURE 177-13 Lichen aureus. **A.** On the leg of a 27-year-old woman. **B.** On the leg of a 16-year-old girl. (*Reproduced with permission from Richard P. Usatine, MD.*)

- Wegener granulomatosis is an unusual multisystem disease characterized by necrotizing granulomatous inflammation and vasculitis of the respiratory tract, kidneys, and skin.
- Churg-Strauss syndrome (allergic granulomatosis) that presents with a systemic vasculitis associated with asthma, transient pulmonary infiltrates, and hypereosinophilia.

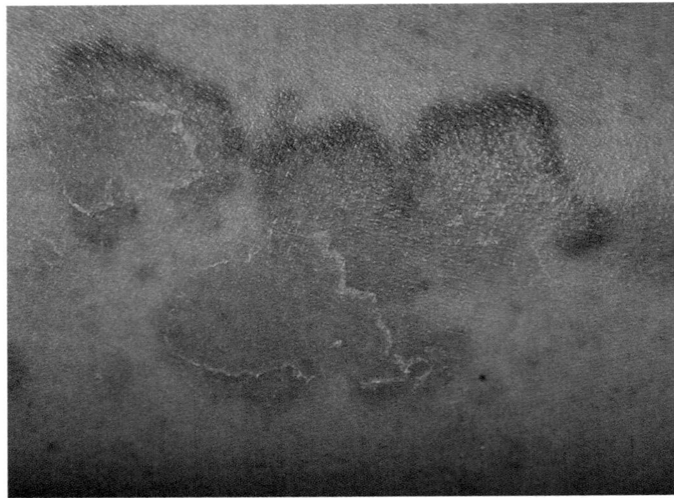

FIGURE 177-14 Pigmented purpuric dermatosis of the Majocchi type. Note the annular appearance and the prominent elevated erythematous borders. (*Reproduced with permission from Suraj Reddy, MD.*)

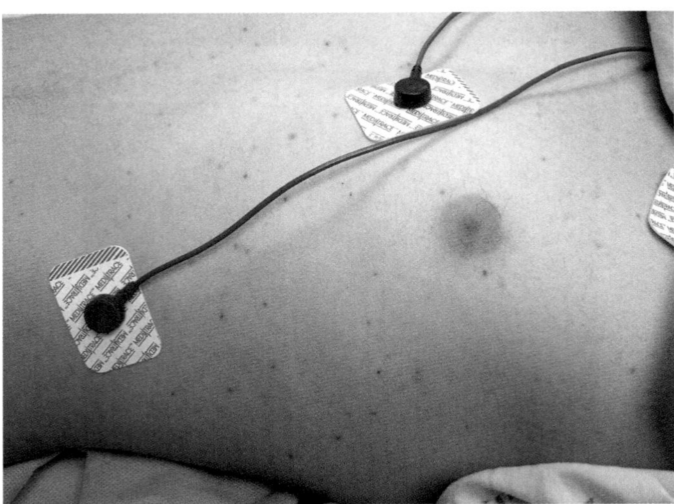

FIGURE 177-15 Petechiae of meningococcemia on the trunk of a hospitalized adolescent. (*Reproduced with permission from Tom Moore, MD.*)

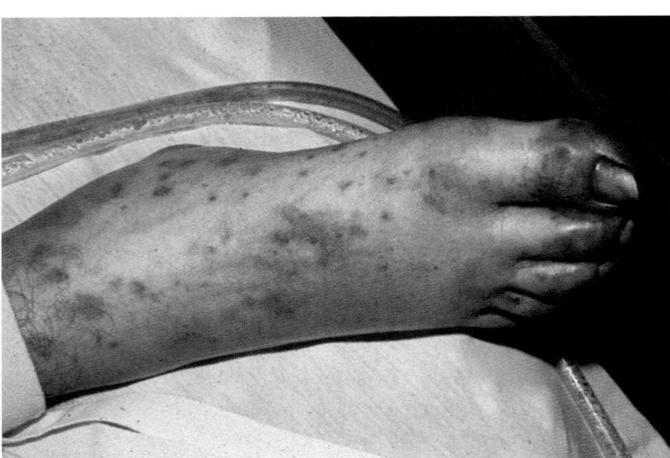

FIGURE 177-16 Petechiae, purpura, and acrocyanosis in a severely ill patient with meningococcemia. (*Reproduced with permission from the University of Texas Health Sciences Center Division of Dermatology.*)

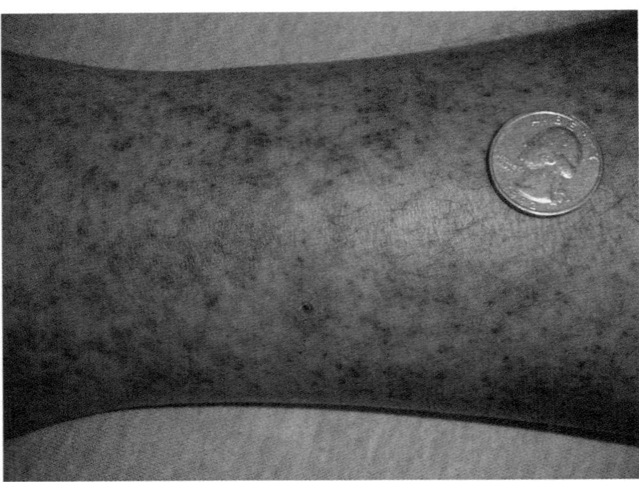

FIGURE 177-17 Rocky Mountain spotted fever with many petechiae visible around the original tick bite. This rickettsial disease looks similar to vasculitis. (*Reproduced with permission from Tom Moore, MD.*)

- Cutaneous manifestations of cholesterol embolism, which are leg pain, livedo reticularis (blue-red mottling of the skin in a net-like pattern), and/or blue toes in the presence of good peripheral pulses.
- Scurvy (vitamin C deficiency) may appear similar to small vessel vasculitides (**Figure 177-19**). The diagnosis is usually clinical, based on risk factors that suggest a dietary history deficient in vitamin C. Risk factors include alcoholism, adults living alone (especially men), poverty, poor access to groceries, reclusiveness, dementia, nutritional ignorance, avoidance of "acid" foods, GI disorders (eg, colitis, inflammatory disease), poor dentition, food fads or food avoidances, cancer, schizophrenia, and depression.[8]

MANAGEMENT

NONPHARMACOLOGIC

The offending antigen should be identified and removed whenever possible. With a mild hypersensitivity vasculitis is due to a drug, discontinuing the offending drug may be all the treatment that is necessary. SOR C

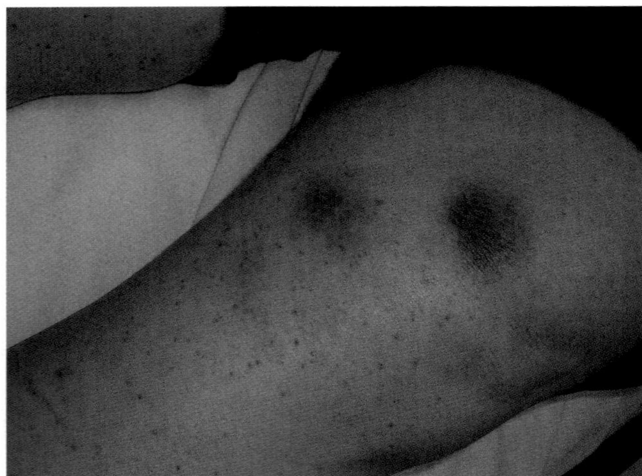

FIGURE 177-18 Petechiae and purpura in a patient with idiopathic thrombocytopenic purpura and a platelet count of 3000. Note that this purpura is not palpable. (*Reproduced with permission from Richard P. Usatine, MD.*)

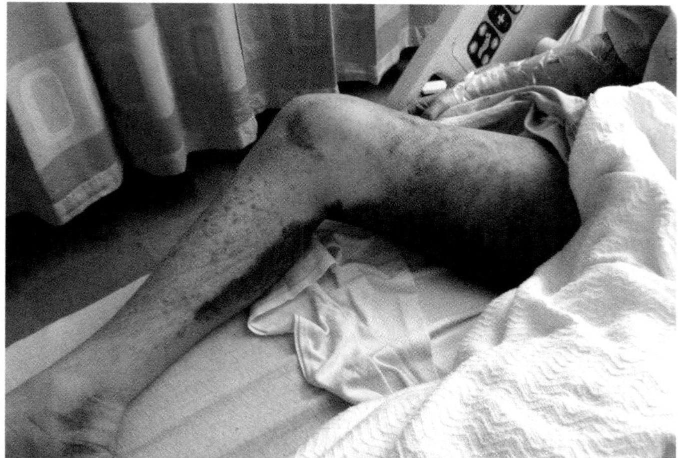

A

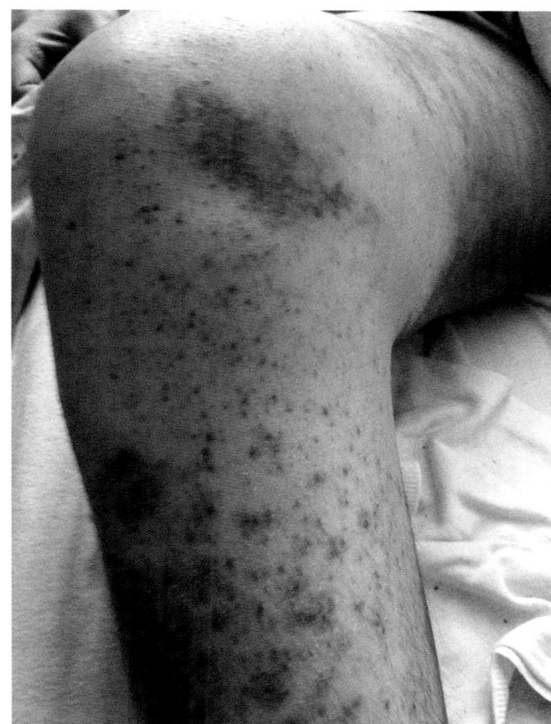

B

FIGURE 177-19 Scurvy in a 31-year-old man with a history of alcohol abuse. He reported lower extremity bruising for 2 weeks and a lower extremity petechial rash for 6 months. A. Scurvy with diffuse ecchymosis on right thigh extending down the posterior leg. B. Ecchymosis and petechial rash of scurvy. (*Reproduced with permission from Robinson S, Roth J, Blanchard S. Light-headedness and a petechial rash.* J Fam Pract. *2013 Apr;62(4):203-205.*)

MEDICATIONS

- An antihistamine might be used for itching. SOR Ⓒ
- Oral prednisone is used to treat visceral involvement and more severe cases of vasculitis of the skin. Short courses of prednisone (60-80 mg/d) are effective and should be tapered slowly.[6,9] SOR Ⓑ
- Colchicine (0.6 mg twice daily for 7-10 days) and dapsone (100-150 mg/d) may be used to inhibit neutrophil chemotaxis. SOR Ⓑ They are tapered and discontinued when lesions resolve. Azathioprine, cyclophosphamide, and methotrexate have also been studied. SOR Ⓒ
- In HSP and prolonged hypersensitivity vasculitis, treatment with nonsteroidal anti-inflammatory drugs is usually preferred. Treatment with corticosteroids may be of more benefit in patients with more severe disease such as more pronounced abdominal pain and renal involvement.[10] SOR Ⓑ Adding cyclophosphamide to the steroids may also be effective. SOR Ⓒ Azathioprine also may be used.[11]

REFER OR HOSPITALIZE

Refer or hospitalize with significant internal organ involvement or prolonged disease course.

PROGNOSIS

In leukocytoclastic (hypersensitivity) vasculitis, the cutaneous lesions usually resolve without sequelae. Visceral involvement (such as kidney and lung) most commonly occurs in HSP, cryoglobulinemia, and vasculitis associated with SLE.[12] Extensive internal organ involvement should prompt an investigation for coexistent medium-size vessel disease and referral to a rheumatologist.

FOLLOW-UP

Relapses may occur, especially when the precipitating factor is an autoimmune disease. Regular monitoring is necessary.

PATIENT EDUCATION

Reassure patients and parents that most cases of acute cutaneous vasculitis resolves spontaneously.

PATIENT RESOURCES

- MedicineNet. *Vasculitis (Arteritis, Angiitis)*—**http://www.medicinenet.com/vasculitis/article.htm.**
- National Kidney and Urologic Diseases Information Clearinghouse. *Henoch-Schönlein Purpura*—**http://kidney.niddk.nih.gov/kudiseases/pubs/HSP/.**
- National Heart Blood and Lung Institute. *What Is Vasculitis?*—**http://www.nhlbi.nih.gov/health/dci/Diseases/vas/vas_whatis.html.**

PROVIDER RESOURCES

- Roane DW, Griger DR. An approach to diagnosis and initial management of systemic vasculitis. *Am Fam Physician* 1999:60:1421-1430—**http://www.aafp.org/afp/991001ap/1421.html.**
- Sharma P, Sharma S, Baltaro R, Hurley J. Systemic vasculitis. *Am Family Physician* 2011;83(5):556-565—**http://www.aafp.org/afp/2011/0301/p556.html.**

REFERENCES

1. Stone JH, Nousari HC. "Essential" cutaneous vasculitis: what every rheumatologist should know about vasculitis of the skin. *Curr Opin Rheumatol*. 2001;13(1):23-34.
2. Gardner-Medwin JM, Dolezalova P, Cummins C, Southwood TR. Incidence of Henoch-Schönlein purpura, Kawasaki disease, and rare

vasculitides in children of different ethnic origins. *Lancet*. 2002;360(9341):1197-202.

3. Michel BA, Hunder GG, Bloch DA, Calabrese LH. Hypersensitivity vasculitis and Henoch-Schönlein purpura: a comparison between the 2 disorders. *J Rheumatol*. 1992;19:721.
4. Calabrese LH, Michel BA, Bloch DA, et al. The American College of Rheumatology 1990 criteria for the classification of hypersensitivity vasculitis. *Arthritis Rheum*. 1990;33:1108.
5. Sharma P, Sharma S, Baltaro R, Hurley J. Systemic vasculitis. *Am Fam Physician*. 2011;83(5):556-565.
6. Martinez-Taboada VM, Blanco R, Garcia-Fuentes M, Rodriguez-Valverde V. Clinical features and outcome of 95 patients with hypersensitivity vasculitis. *Am J Med*. 1997;102:186-191.
7. Poterucha TJ, Wetter DA, Gibson LE, Camilleri MJ, Lohse CM. Histopathology and correlates of systemic disease in adult Henoch-Schönlein purpura: a retrospective study of microscopic and clinical findings in 68 patients at Mayo Clinic. *J Am Acad Dermatol*. 2013;68:420-424.
8. Robinson S, Roth J, Blanchard S. Light-headedness and a petechial rash. *J Fam Pract*. 2013 Apr;62(4):203-205.
9. Sais G, Vidaller A, Jucgla A, et al. Colchicine in the treatment of cutaneous leukocytoclastic vasculitis. Results of a prospective, randomized controlled trial. *Arch Dermatol*. 1995;131:1399-1402.
10. Weiss PF, Feinstein JA, Luan X, et al. Effects of corticosteroid on Henoch-Schonlein purpura: a systematic review. *Pediatrics*. 2007;120:1079-1087.
11. Saulsbury FT. Henoch-Schönlein purpura. *Curr Opin Rheumatol*. 2001;13:35-40.
12. Roane DW, Griger DR. An approach to diagnosis and initial management of systemic vasculitis. *Am Fam Physician*. 1999;60:1421-1430.

SECTION 14 CONNECTIVE TISSUE DISEASE

178 LUPUS: SYSTEMIC AND CUTANEOUS

E.J. Mayeaux Jr, MD

PATIENT STORY

A 39-year-old black woman presented to the clinic with 2 months of swelling of her upper lip and cheeks with new dark spots on her face (**Figure 178-1**). An antinuclear antibody (ANA) was positive at a 1:80 dilution. A homogeneous nuclear pattern was present as commonly seen in systemic lupus erythematosus (SLE) and drug-induced lupus. The punch biopsy of a facial lesion was consistent with chronic cutaneous lupus erythematosus (discoid lupus). The remainder of her laboratory tests was normal. The patient's facial lesions did not respond to topical steroids and hence she was started on a short course of systemic steroids. The improvement was seen 3 weeks later (**Figure 178-2**). Hyperpigmentation remained but erythema, swelling, and pruritus were gone. The patient did not meet criteria for SLE and it is possible to have discoid lupus with a positive ANA. Treatment with hydroxychloroquine was discussed.

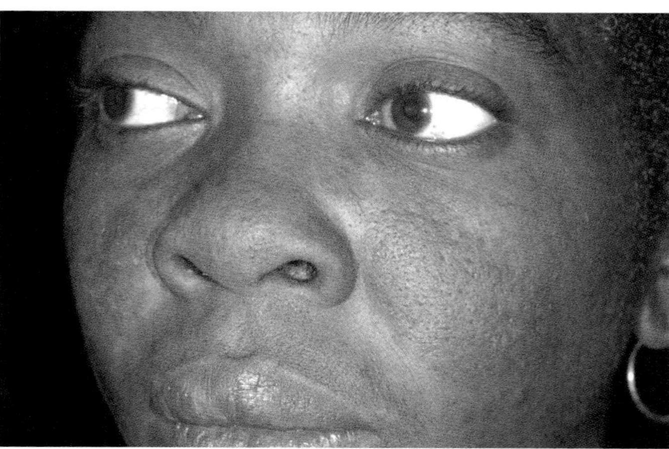

FIGURE 178-1 Erythema, swelling, and hyperpigmentation on the cheeks and lips of a 39-year-old black woman as the initial presentation of chronic cutaneous lupus erythematosus. (*Reproduced with permission from Richard P. Usatine, MD.*)

INTRODUCTION

SLE is a chronic inflammatory disease that can affect many organs of the body including the skin, joints, kidneys, lungs, nervous system, and mucous membranes. Cutaneous lupus can occur in 1 of the 3 forms: chronic cutaneous (discoid) lupus erythematosus, subacute cutaneous lupus erythematosus, and acute cutaneous lupus erythematosus.

SYNONYMS

- Chronic cutaneous lupus erythematosus = discoid lupus = DLE.
- Lupus profundus = lupus panniculitis.

EPIDEMIOLOGY

- In the United States, the prevalence of SLE plus incomplete SLE (disease only partially meeting diagnostic requirements for SLE) is 40 to 50 cases per 100,000 persons.[1] It is more common in women and patients with African ancestry.[1] Worldwide, the highest SLE prevalences have been reported in Italy, Spain, Martinique, and the United Kingdom Afro-Caribbean population, but it is rarely reported among blacks who live in Africa.[2]
- Discoid lupus erythematosus (DLE) develops in up to 25% of patients with SLE, but may also occur in the absence of any other clinical feature of SLE.[3] Patients with only DLE have a 5% to 10% risk of eventually developing SLE, which tends to follow a mild course.[4] DLE lesions usually slowly expand with active inflammation at the periphery, and

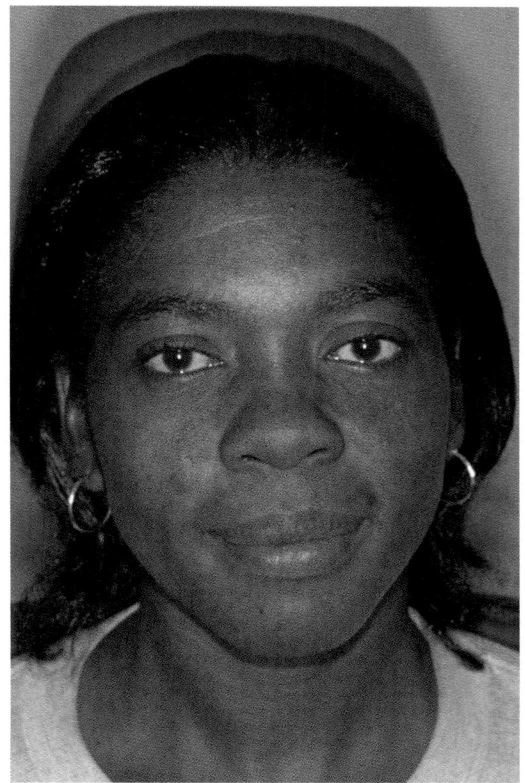

FIGURE 178-2 Hyperpigmented malar rash 3 weeks later in the patient of Figure 178-1, the patient was treated with oral and topical steroids. The erythema and swelling are now gone and patient is feeling better. (*Reproduced with permission from Richard P. Usatine, MD.*)

then to heal, leaving depressed central scars, atrophy, telangiectasias, and hypopigmentation.[5] The female-to-male ratio of DLE is 2:1.

ETIOLOGY AND PATHOPHYSIOLOGY

- One proposed mechanism for the etiology of SLE involves the development of autoantibodies that result from a defect in apoptosis. It has been determined that the specific defect involves the "find-me" (and adenosine triphosphate [ATP]/uridine triphosphate [UTP]) or "eat-me" (phosphatidylserine) signals that should be activated when red cell nuclei are extruded. With no apoptosis, the nuclei break down, causing inflammation and the development of autoimmunity.[6] Many of the signs and symptoms of lupus erythematosus (LE) are caused by the circulating immune complexes or by the direct effects of antibodies to cells.
- A genetic predisposition for SLE exists. The concordance rate in monozygotic twins is between 25% and 70%. If a mother has SLE, her daughter's risk of developing the disease is 1:40 and her son's risk is 1:250.
- The course of SLE is one of intermittent remissions punctuated by disease flares. Organ damage often progresses over time.
- Rarely, neonates may develop a lupus rush from acquired antibodies through transplacental transmission from mother if she has active SLE (**Figure 178-3**).

RISK FACTORS

Precipitating factors for SLE include the following:

- Exposure to the sunlight (ultraviolet [UV] light, especially UVB)
- Infections
- Stress

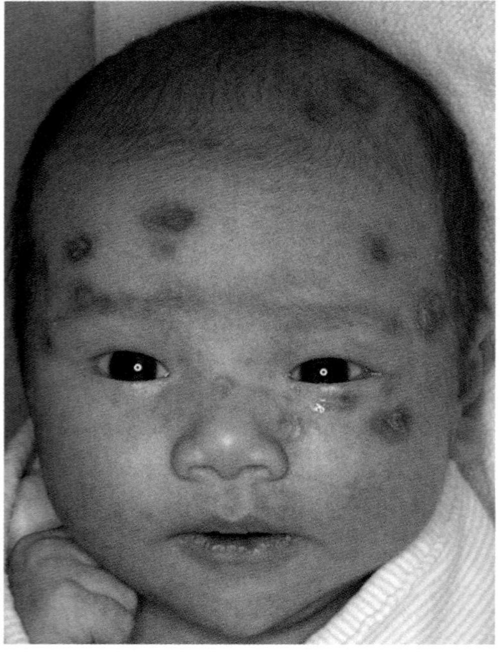

FIGURE 178-3 Neonatal lupus from acquired antibodies through transplacental transmission from the mother with active SLE. (*Reproduced with permission from Warner AM, Frey KA, Connolly S. Annular rash on a newborn. J Fam Pract. 2006;55(2):127-129. Reproduced with permission from Frontline Medical Communications.*)

- Trauma or surgery
- Pregnancy (especially in the postpartum period)

Precipitating factors for cutaneous lupus include the following:

- Exposure to the sunlight (UV light, especially UVB)

DIAGNOSIS

CLINICAL FEATURES OF SYSTEMIC LUPUS ERYTHEMATOSUS

- SLE is a chronic, recurrent, potentially fatal inflammatory disorder that can be difficult to diagnose. It is an autoimmune disease involving multiple organ systems that is defined clinically with associated autoantibodies directed against cell nuclei. The disease has no single diagnostic sign or marker. Accurate diagnosis is important because treatment can reduce morbidity and mortality.[7]
- SLE most often presents with a mixture of constitutional symptoms including fatigue, fever, myalgia, anorexia, nausea, and weight loss. The mean length of time between onset of symptoms and diagnosis is 5 years.
- The disease is characterized by exacerbations and remissions as well as symptoms.
- The diagnosis of SLE is made if 4 or more of the manifestations mentioned below (and categorized in **Table 178-1**) are either present, serially or simultaneously, in the patient at the time of presentation or were present in the past. If 2 to 3 manifestations are present, some clinicians refer to the syndrome as "incomplete lupus."[8]
  - Arthralgias, which are often the initial complaint, are usually disproportionate to physical findings. The polyarthritis is symmetric, nonerosive, and usually nondeforming. In long-standing disease, rheumatoid-like deformities with swan-neck fingers are commonly seen.
  - A malar or butterfly rash is fixed erythema over the cheeks and bridge of the nose sparing the nasolabial folds (**Figures 178-2, 178-4,** and **178-5**). It may also involve the chin and ears. More severe malar rashes may cause severe atrophy, scarring, and hypopigmentation (see **Figure 178-5**).
  - Rash associated with photosensitivity to UV light.
  - A discoid rash consisting of erythematosus raised patches with adherent keratotic scaling and follicular plugging. Atrophic scarring may occur in older lesions.
  - Ulcers (usually painless) in the nose, mouth, or vagina are frequent complaints.
  - Pleuritis as evidenced by a convincing history of pleuritic pain or rub or evidence of pleural effusion.
  - Pericarditis as documented by electrocardiography (ECG), rub, or evidence of pericardial effusion.
  - Renal disorder such as cellular casts or persistent proteinuria greater than 0.5 g/d or greater than 3+ if quantitation not performed.
  - Central nervous system (CNS) symptoms ranging from mild cognitive dysfunction to psychosis or seizures. Any region of CNS can be involved. Intractable headaches and difficulties with memory and reasoning are the most common features of neurologic disease in lupus patients.
  - Hematologic disorders such as hemolytic anemia, leukopenia (<4000/mm^3 total on 2 or more occasions), lymphopenia

TABLE 178-1 American College of Rheumatology Criteria for Diagnosis of Systemic Lupus Erythematosus

Criterion	Definition
1. Malar rash	Fixed erythema, flat or raised, over the malar eminences, tending to spare the nasolabial folds
2. Discoid rash	Erythematosus-raised patches with adherent keratotic scaling and follicular plugging and later atrophic scarring
3. Photosensitivity	Skin rash as a result of unusual reaction to sunlight, by history or physician observation
4. Oral ulcers	Oral or nasopharyngeal ulceration, usually painless, observed by a physician
5. Arthritis	Nonerosive arthritis involving 2 or more peripheral joints, characterized by tenderness, swelling, or effusion
6. Serositis	Pleuritis—convincing history of pleuritic pain or rub heard by a physician or evidence of pleural effusion or pericarditis documented by ECG, rub, or evidence of pericardial effusion
7. Renal disorder	Persistent proteinuria greater than 0.5 g/d or greater than 3+ if quantitation not performed *or* red cell, hemoglobin, granular, tubular, or mixed cellular casts
8. Neurologic disorder	Seizures *or* psychosis—in the absence of offending drugs or known metabolic derangements (uremia, ketoacidosis, or electrolyte imbalance)
9. Hematologic disorder	Hemolytic anemia with reticulocytosis *or* leukopenia (<4000/mm^3 on 2 or more occasions) *or* lymphopenia (<1500/mm^3 on 2 or more occasions) *or* thrombocytopenia (<100,000/mm^3) in the absence of offending drugs
10. Immunologic disorders	Positive antiphospholipid antibody *or* anti-DNA antibody to native DNA in abnormal titer *or* anti-Smith antibody—presence of antibody to Smith nuclear antigen or false-positive serologic test for syphilis known to be positive for at least 6 months and confirmed by *Treponema pallidum* immobilization or fluorescent treponemal antibody absorption test
11. Antinuclear antibody	An abnormal titer of antinuclear antibody by immunofluorescence or an equivalent assay at any point in time and in the absence of drugs known to be associated with "drug-induced lupus" syndrome

SLE can be diagnosed if any 4 or more of the 11 criteria are present, serially or simultaneously, during any interval of observation.
Data from Callahan LF, Pincus T. Mortality in the rheumatic diseases. *Arthritis Care Res.* 1995;8:229. Reproduced with permission of Wiley Inc.

(<1500/mm^3 on 2 or more occasions), or thrombocytopenia (<100,000/mm^3 in the absence of precipitating drugs).
- GI symptoms may include abdominal pain, diarrhea, and vomiting. Intestinal perforation and vasculitis are important diagnoses to exclude.
- Vasculitis (**Figures 178-6** to **178-8**) can be severe and can include retinal vasculitis.
- Immunologic disorders such as a positive antiphospholipid antibody, anti-DNA, anti-Smith antigen, or a false-positive serologic test for syphilis (known to be positive for at least 6 months and confirmed by a negative treponema specific test).
- An abnormal titer of ANA at any point in time and in the absence of drugs associated with "drug-induced lupus."

CLINICAL FEATURES OF CUTANEOUS LUPUS

- Three types of cutaneous lupus are as follows:
  1. Chronic cutaneous lupus (discoid lupus)
  2. Subacute cutaneous lupus
  3. Acute cutaneous lupus, which is part of an SLE flare
- Chronic cutaneous lupus (DLE) lesions are characterized by discrete, erythematous, slightly infiltrated papules or plaques covered by a well-formed adherent scale (**Figures 178-9** to **178-15**). As the lesion progresses, the scale often thickens and becomes adherent. Hypopigmentation develops in the central area and hyperpigmentation develops at the active border. Resolution of the active lesion results in atrophy and scarring. When they occur in the scalp, scarring alopecia often results (see **Figures 178-12** and **178-15**). If the scale on the scalp is removed, it may leave a "carpet tack sign" from follicular plugging.
- Subacute cutaneous lupus occurs most commonly in sun-exposed areas. The lesions are erythematous with scale and distinct borders or they may be annular in shape (**Figure 178-16**). The photosensitivity that exists explains the distribution of the lesions. Fortunately, these lesions do not scar or itch, but they may heal with postinflammatory hyperpigmentation.
- Acute cutaneous lupus is the name given for the cutaneous manifestations of systemic lupus such as the malar rash. This malar rash is also called a butterfly rash (see **Figure 178-4**). This rash may heal without scarring.

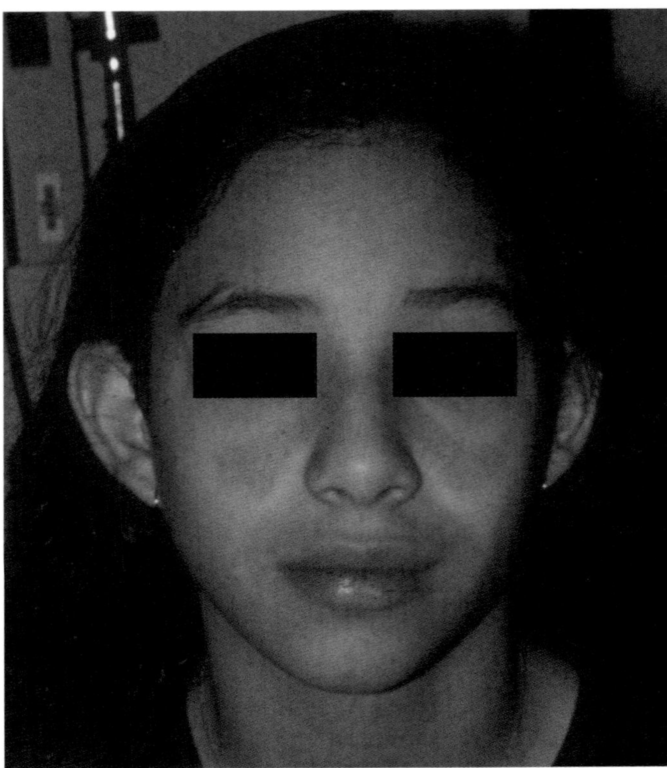

FIGURE 178-4 Malar rash in adolescent Hispanic girl with SLE. Note the relative sparing of the nasolabial fold. (*Reproduced with permission from the University of Texas Health Sciences Center, Division of Dermatology.*)

- Raynaud phenomenon, libido reticularis, and palmar erythema also occur in persons with lupus (**Figure 178-17**). All 3 of these conditions can be made worse by cold weather.

TYPICAL DISTRIBUTION

- Discoid lesions are most often seen on the face, neck, and scalp, but also occur on the ears, and, infrequently, on the upper torso.
- DLE lesions may be localized or widespread. Localized DLE occurs only in the head and neck area, whereas widespread DLE occurs

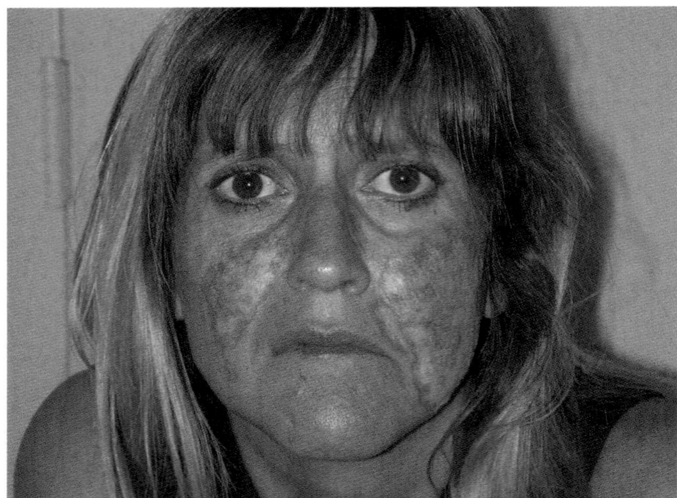

FIGURE 178-5 Malar rash with severe atrophy, scarring, and hypopigmentation in a young woman with arthritis and other signs of systemic lupus. The facial lesions are more typical of discoid lupus. (*Reproduced with permission from Richard P. Usatine, MD.*)

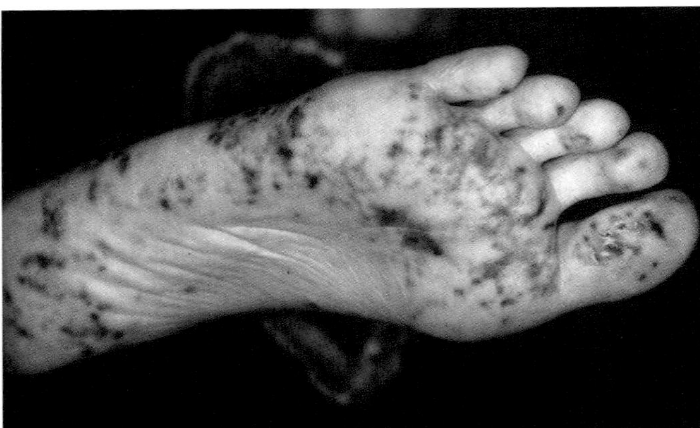

FIGURE 178-6 Necrotizing angiitis in a 28-year-old Japanese American woman with a severe lupus flare. Palpable purpura was evident on both feet and hands. (*Reproduced with permission from Richard P. Usatine, MD.*)

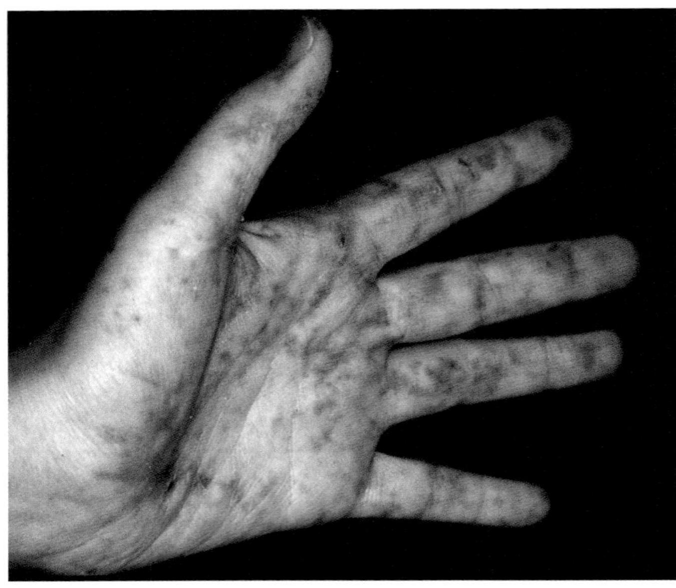

FIGURE 178-7 Necrotizing angiitis on the hand of the patient in **Figure 178-6** with lupus. (*Reproduced with permission from Richard P. Usatine, MD.*)

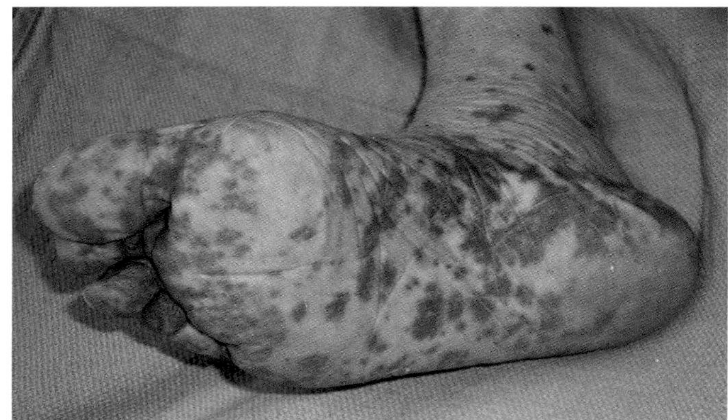

FIGURE 178-8 Leukocytoclastic vasculitis on the foot of a 69-year-old woman with systemic lupus. (*Reproduced with permission from Richard P. Usatine, MD.*)

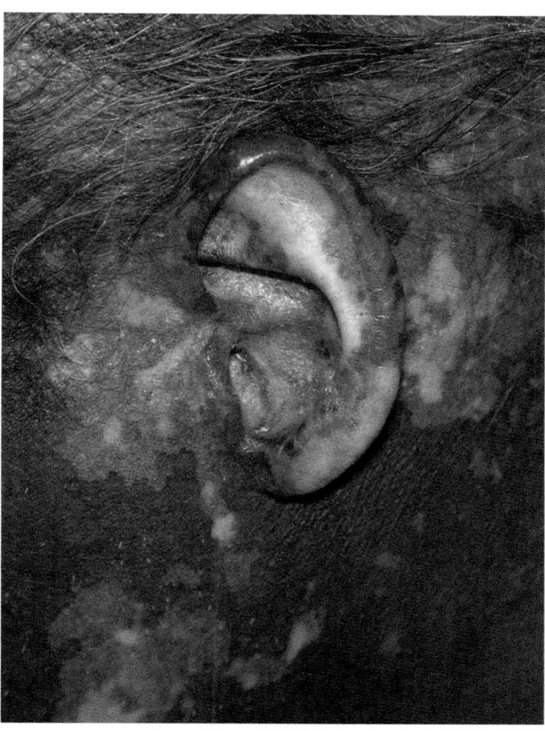

FIGURE 178-9 Discoid lupus in a middle-aged black man with hypopigmentation and scarring of the pinna. (*Reproduced with permission from Richard P. Usatine, MD.*)

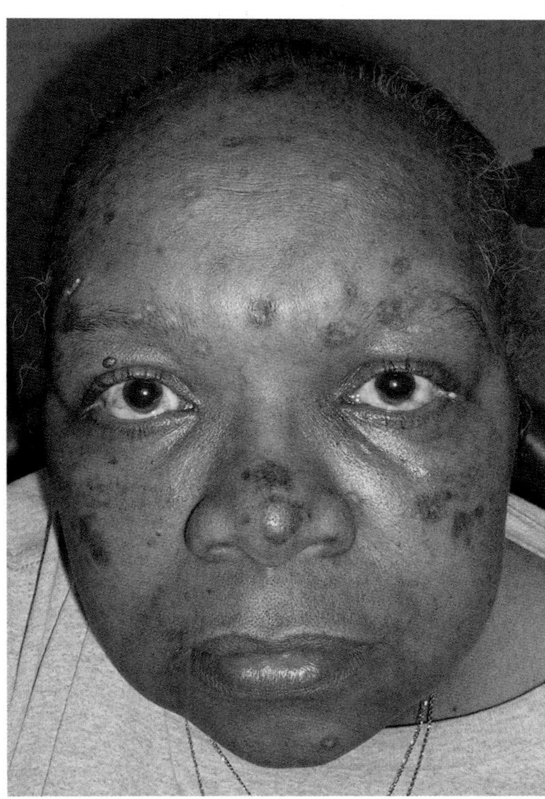

FIGURE 178-10 Discoid lupus on the face and scalp of a 56-year-old woman with hyperpigmented lesions that are indurated and atrophic. She also has similar lesions on the back and has scarring alopecia. (*Reproduced with permission from Richard P. Usatine, MD.*)

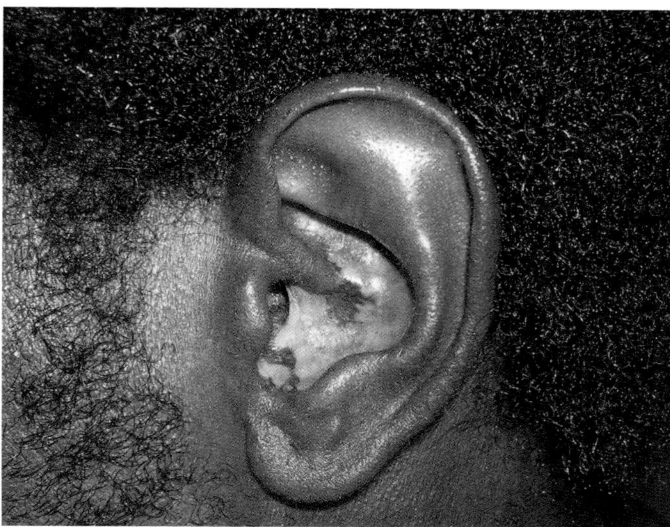

FIGURE 178-11 Discoid lupus with hypopigmentation and scarring inside the pinna. (*Reproduced with permission from E.J. Mayeaux, Jr., MD.*)

anywhere. Patients with widespread involvement are more likely to develop SLE.

- Subacute cutaneous lupus lesions are most commonly found in the sun-exposed areas of the face, neck, and arms (see **Figure 178-16**).
- Acute cutaneous lupus is generally seen in the malar rash distribution, although it can occur on other parts of the body.
- Lupus panniculitis, or lupus profundus, is a variant of LE that primarily affects subcutaneous fat. It usually involves the proximal extremities, trunk, breasts, buttocks, and face (**Figure 178-18**).

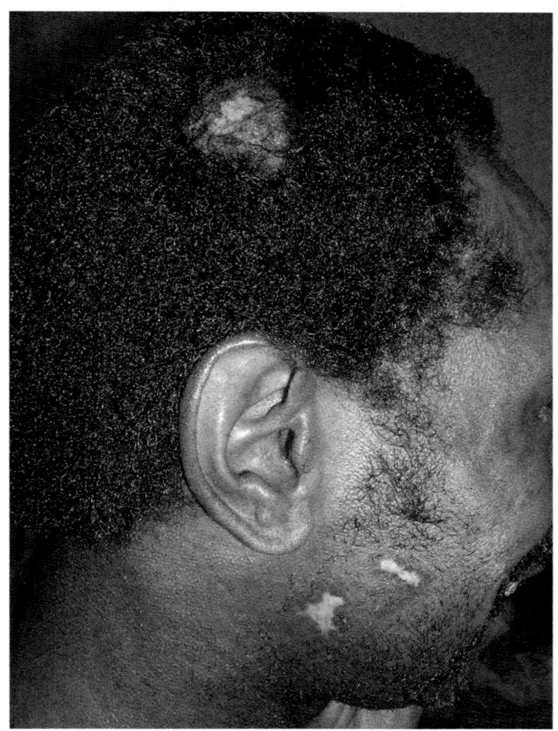

FIGURE 178-12 Discoid lupus with scarring alopecia and hypopigmentation on the scalp and face. (*Reproduced with permission from E.J. Mayeaux Jr, MD.*)

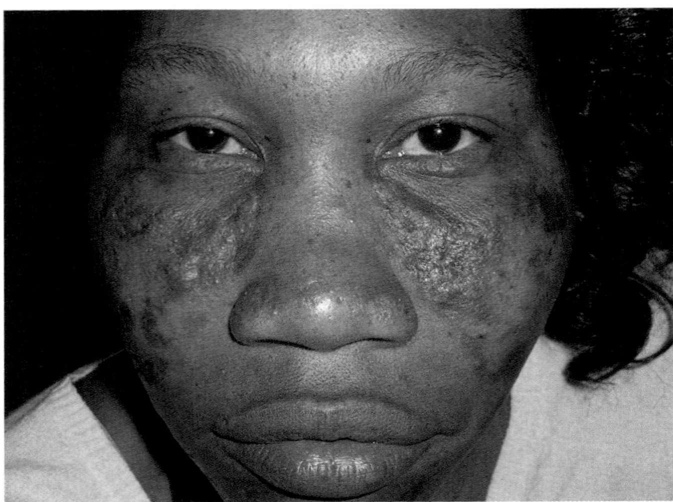

FIGURE 178-13 Severe discoid lupus in a malar distribution on the face of a 30-year-old woman. Note this chronic cutaneous lupus has caused permanent scarring. (*Reproduced with permission from Richard P. Usatine, MD.*)

LABORATORY TESTING

- The American College of Rheumatology recommends ANA testing in patients who have 2 or more unexplained signs or symptoms that could be lupus. Elevation of the ANA titer to or above 1:80 is the most sensitive of the American College of Rheumatology diagnostic criteria. Although many patients may have a negative ANA titer early in the disease, more than 99% of SLE patients will eventually have an elevated ANA titer.[9] The ANA test is not specific for lupus, and the most common reason for a positive ANA test without SLE (usually at titers <1:80) is the presence of another connective tissue disease.

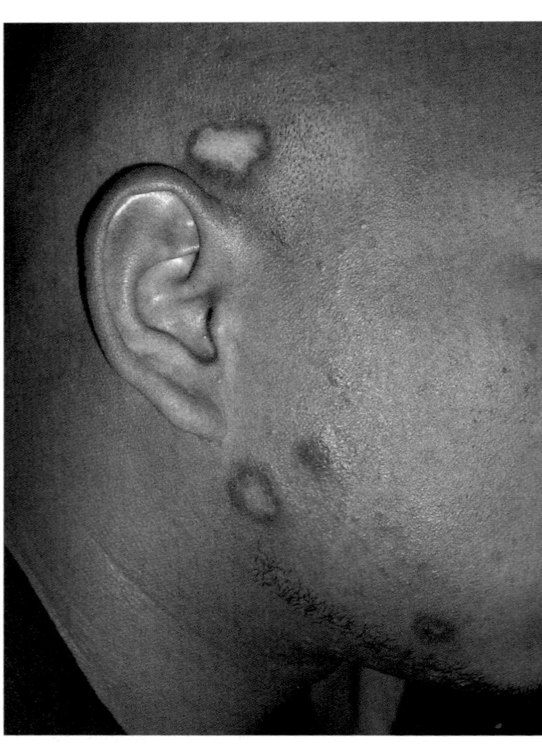

FIGURE 178-14 Chronic cutaneous lupus on the face of this Hispanic man. The lesions are typical of discoid lupus with central hypopigmentation and peripheral hyperpigmentation. (*Reproduced with permission from Richard P. Usatine, MD.*)

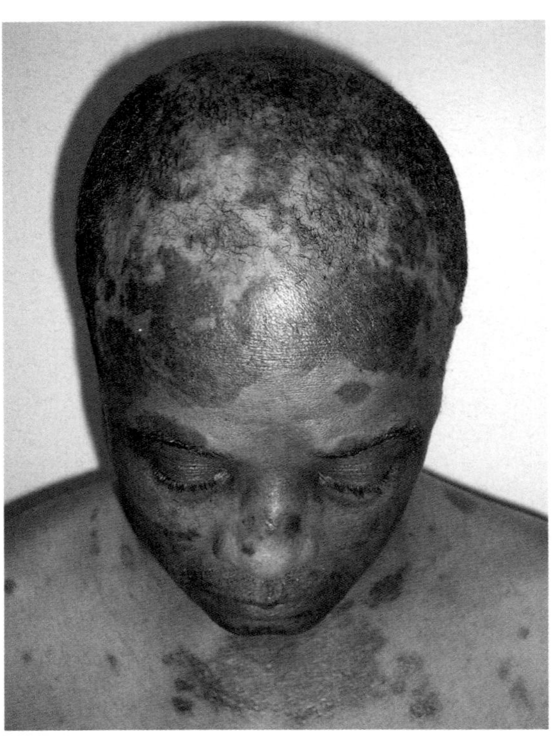

FIGURE 178-15 Severe chronic cutaneous lupus with hyperpigmentation, hypopigmentation, and scarring alopecia. Sun-exposed areas of the face and neck are heavily involved. (*Reproduced with permission from Richard P. Usatine, MD.*)

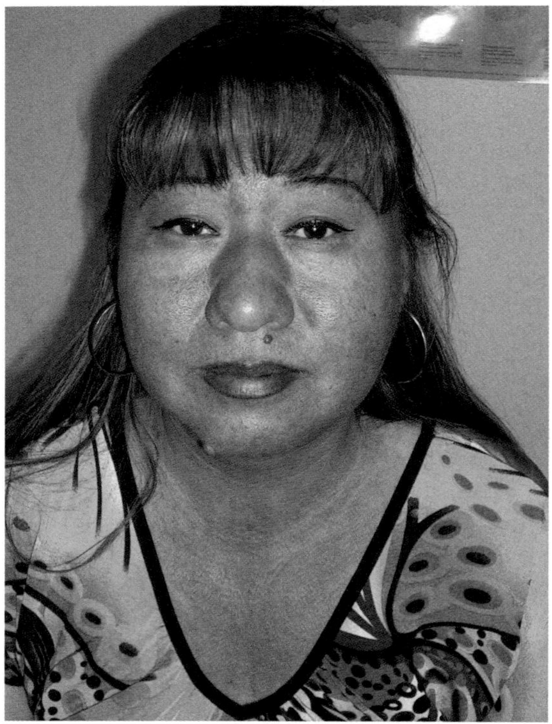

FIGURE 178-16 Subacute cutaneous lupus in a 47-year-old woman in sun-exposed areas of the face and V-neck. This all started after hydrochlorothiazide was begun for hypertension. Diagnosis was biopsy proven and the differential diagnosis includes a photosensitivity reaction related to the hydrochlorothiazide. (*Reproduced with permission from Richard P. Usatine, MD.*)

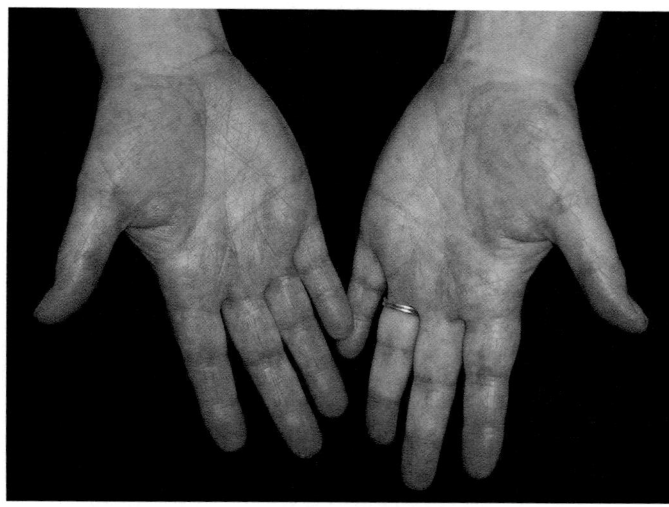

FIGURE 178-17 Palmar erythema in this young woman with SLE and an ANA of 1 to 640. (*Reproduced with permission from Richard P. Usatine, MD.*)

- Active SLE is often heralded by a rise in immunoglobulin (Ig) G anti–double-stranded DNA titers and/or a fall in complement levels.[10]
- Patients with only DLE generally have negative or low-titer ANA, and rarely have low titers of anti-Ro antibodies.[11]

BIOPSY

A biopsy is often needed to confirm the diagnosis, even when the pattern seems typical. A 4-mm punch biopsy should provide adequate tissue to the pathologist. Biopsy confirmation is particularly helpful before starting potentially toxic medications.

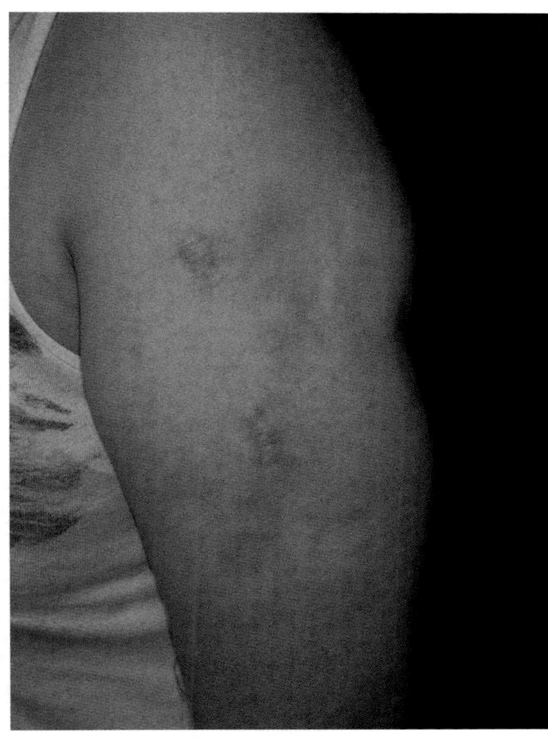

FIGURE 178-18 Lupus profundus showing localized atrophic changes of the arm secondary to the panniculitis. This young woman also has the lupus profundus on the face and other arm. The atrophy has been present for more than 1 year despite treatment. (*Reproduced with permission from Richard P. Usatine, MD.*)

DIFFERENTIAL DIAGNOSIS

- Drug-induced lupus is a lupus-like syndrome most strongly associated with procainamide, hydralazine, isoniazid, chlorpromazine, methyldopa, and quinidine.
- Scleroderma presents with thickening of the skin and multisystem sclerosis (see Chapter 180, Scleroderma and Morphea).
- Actinic keratosis on the face may become confluent but lacks the systemic symptoms of lupus (see Chapter 164, Actinic Keratosis and Bowen Disease).
- Dermatomyositis presents with facial swelling, "heliotrope" rash around the eyes, Gottron papules and periungual erythema in the hands, and proximal muscular limb girdle weakness. It is often associated with internal malignancy (see Chapter 179, Dermatomyositis).
- Lichen planus produces a polygonal pruritic purple papular rash (see Chapter 152, Lichen Planus).
- Psoriasis demonstrates silver-white plaques that cover the elbows, knees, scalp, back, or vulva. There may also be nail and scalp involvement (see Chapter 150, Psoriasis).
- Rosacea is associated with midfacial skin erythema, papules, and pustules without the systemic symptoms of LE, and usually involves the nasolabial folds (see Chapter 115, Rosacea).
- Sarcoidosis may produce skin plaques but without the central clearing and atrophy of LE (see Chapter 173, Sarcoidosis).
- Syphilis may produce a plaque-like rash that can be confused with DLE. The short course of the disease and serologic testing can distinguish the diseases. However, lupus autoantibodies may produce a false-positive screening test for syphilis (see Chapter 218, Syphilis).

MANAGEMENT

NONPHARMACOLOGIC

Because UV light can flair SLE, sunscreen use, preferably one that blocks both UVA and UVB, should be encouraged. SOR Ⓒ

MEDICATIONS

- Conservative management for SLE with nonsteroidal anti-inflammatory drugs (NSAIDs) or cyclooxygenase-2 selective inhibitors are recommended for arthritis, arthralgias, and myalgias.[12] SOR Ⓑ
- Antimalarial drugs (hydroxychloroquine [Plaquenil] 200 mg bid, maximum 6.5 mg/kg/d) most commonly for skin manifestations and for musculoskeletal complaints that do not adequately respond to NSAIDs. They may also prevent major damage to the kidneys and CNS and reduce the risk of disease flares.[13] SOR Ⓑ
- Systemic glucocorticoids (1-2 mg/kg/d of prednisone or equivalent) alone or with immunosuppressive agents for patients with significant renal and CNS disease or any other organ-threatening manifestation.[14] SOR Ⓑ Lower doses of glucocorticoids (prednisone 10-20 mg/d) for symptomatic relief of severe or unresponsive musculoskeletal symptoms. In severe, life-threatening situations, methylprednisolone bolus (1 g IV/d) can be given for 3 consecutive days.
- Immunosuppressive medications (eg, methotrexate, cyclophosphamide, azathioprine, mycophenolate, or rituximab) are generally reserved for patients with significant organ involvement, or who have had an inadequate response to glucocorticoids. SOR Ⓑ[15]

- Belimumab (10 mg/kg IV every 2 weeks for 3 doses then every 4 weeks) may be used in patients with active SLE who are not responding to standard therapy, such as NSAIDs, glucocorticoids, antimalarials, and/or immunosuppressives.[16]
- Patients with thrombosis, usually associated to the presence of antiphospholipid antibodies, require anticoagulation with warfarin, for a target international normalized ratio (INR) of 3:3.5 for arterial thrombosis and 2:3 for venous thrombosis.[17]
- DLE therapy includes corticosteroids (topical or intralesional) and antimalarials. SOR C Alternative therapies include auranofin, oral or topical retinoids, and immunosuppressive agents.

PREVENTION

Avoiding precipitating factors may decrease exacerbations.

PROGNOSIS

- SLE can have a varied clinical course, ranging from a relatively benign illness to a rapidly progressive disease with organ failure and death. Most patients have a relapsing and remitting course.
- Poor prognostic factors for survival in SLE include the folowing[18]:
  - Renal disease (especially diffuse proliferative glomerulonephritis)
  - Hypertension
  - Male sex
  - Young age
  - Older age at presentation
  - Poor socioeconomic status
  - Black race, which may primarily reflect low socioeconomic status
  - Presence of antiphospholipid antibodies
  - Antiphospholipid syndrome
  - High overall disease activity

FOLLOW-UP

The patient should have regular follow-up appointments to monitor for and attempt to prevent end-organ damage. Regular follow-up visits are needed to monitor medication benefits and side effects and to coordinate care of the whole person.

PATIENT EDUCATION

- Educate the patient on the necessity of protection from the sun, as UV exposure can cause lupus flares. They should use a sunscreen, preferably one that blocks both UVA and UVB, with a minimum skin protection factor (SPF) of 30.
- Because cigarette smoking may increase the risk of developing SLE and smokers generally have more active disease, smokers with SLE should be counseled to quit smoking.
- Have patients report any signs of superinfection in their rash, as this requires antibiotic therapy.
- If possible, avoid sulfa drugs, which are related to lupus flares.

PATIENT RESOURCES

- PubMed Health. *Systemic Lupus Erythematosus*—**http://www.ncbi.nlm.nih.gov/pubmedhealth/PMH0001471/.**
- Mayo Clinic. *Lupus*—**http://www.mayoclinic.com/health/lupus/DS00115.**
- Womenshealth.gov. *Lupus Fact Sheet*—**http://womenshealth.gov/publications/our-publications/fact-sheet/lupus.cfm.**
- Lupus Foundation—**http://www.lupus.org.**

PROVIDER RESOURCES

- Medscape. *Systemic Lupus Erythematosus (SLE)*—**http://emedicine.medscape.com/article/332244.**
- Medscape. *Discoid Lupus Erythematosus*—**http://emedicine.medscape.com/article/1065529.**

REFERENCES

1. Lawrence RC, Helmick CG, Arnett FC, et al. Estimates of the prevalence of arthritis and selected musculoskeletal disorders in the United States. *Arthritis Rheum.* 1998;41(5):778-799.
2. Danchenko N, Satia JA, Anthony MS. Epidemiology of systemic lupus erythematosus: a comparison of worldwide disease burden. *Lupus.* 2006;15(5):308-318.
3. Pistiner M, Wallace DJ, Nessim S, et al. Lupus erythematosus in the 1980s: a survey of 570 patients. *Semin Arthritis Rheum.* 1991;21(1):55-64.
4. Healy E, Kieran E, Rogers S. Cutaneous lupus erythematosus—a study of clinical and laboratory prognostic factors in 65 patients. *Ir J Med Sci.* 1995;164(2):113-115.
5. Rowell NR. Laboratory abnormalities in the diagnosis and management of lupus erythematosus. *Br J Dermatol.* 1971;84(3):210-216.
6. Nagata S, Hanayama R, Kawane K. Autoimmunity and the clearance of dead cells. *Cell.* 2010;140(5):619-630.
7. Gill JM, Quisel AM, Rocca PV, Walters DT. Diagnosis of systemic lupus erythematosus. *Am Fam Physician.* 2003;68(11):2179-2186.
8. Hochberg MC. Updating the American College of Rheumatology revised criteria for the classification of SLE [letter]. *Arthritis Rheum.* 1997;40(9):1725.
9. Tan EM, Cohen AS, Fries JF, et al. The 1982 revised criteria for the classification of systemic lupus erythematosus. *Arthritis Rheum.* 1982;25(11):1271-1277.
10. Kao AH, Navratil JS, Ruffing MJ, et al. Erythrocyte C3d and C4d for monitoring disease activity in systemic lupus erythematosus. *Arthritis Rheum.* 2010;62(3):837-844.
11. Provost TT. The relationship between discoid and systemic lupus erythematosus. *Arch Dermatol.* 1994;130(10):1308-1310.
12. Lander SA, Wallace DJ, Weisman MH. Celecoxib for systemic lupus erythematosus: case series and literature review of the use of NSAIDs in SLE. *Lupus.* 2002;11(6):340-347.
13. Fessler BJ, Alarcon GS, McGwin G Jr, et al; LUMINA Study Group. Systemic lupus erythematosus in three ethnic groups: XVI. Association of hydroxychloroquine use with reduced risk of damage accrual. *Arthritis Rheum.* 2005;52(5):1473-1480.

14. Parker BJ, Bruce IN. High dose methylprednisolone therapy for the treatment of severe systemic lupus erythematosus. *Lupus.* 2007;16(6):387-393.

15. Fortin PR, Abrahamowicz M, Ferland D, et al; Canadian Network For Improved Outcomes in Systemic Lupus. Steroid-sparing effects of methotrexate in systemic lupus erythematosus: a double-blind, randomized, placebo-controlled trial. *Arthritis Rheum.* 2008;59(12):1796-1804.

16. FDA news release. *FDA Approves Benlysta to Treat Lupus.* http://www.fda.gov/NewsEvents/Newsroom/PressAnnouncements/ucm246489.htm. Accessed February 18, 2012.

17. Erkan D, Lockshin MD. New treatments for antiphospholipid syndrome. *Rheum Dis Clin North Am.* 2006;32(1):129-148.

18. Cervera R, Khamashta MA, Font J, et al; European Working Party on Systemic Lupus Erythematosus. Morbidity and mortality in systemic lupus erythematosus during a 10-year period: a comparison of early and late manifestations in a cohort of 1,000 patients. *Medicine (Baltimore).* 2003;82(5):299-308.

179 DERMATOMYOSITIS

Margaret L. Burks
Anna Allred, MD
Richard P. Usatine, MD

PATIENT STORY

A 55-year-old Hispanic woman presents to her family physician with a diffuse rash and increasing muscle weakness. The initial rash (without weakness) 2 months prior was thought to be a photosensitivity reaction to her new hydrochlorothiazide (HCTZ) prescription. She stopped the HCTZ and the rash initially improved with some topical corticosteroids. At the time of her current presentation, she had trouble getting up from a chair, walking, and lifting her arms over her head. The rash was prominent in sun-exposed areas, but was also seen in a shawl-like distribution in non–sun-exposed areas (**Figure 179-1**). Aside from her hypertension and obesity, the patient did not have any previous chronic medical conditions. She was afebrile with no other pertinent findings on physical examination.

This is a classic presentation of dermatomyositis with the typical rash and proximal muscle weakness. Close attention to the rash around her eyes demonstrates the pathognomonic heliotrope rash of dermatomyositis (**Figures 179-2** and **179-3**). Also the patient has Gottron papules on the fingers, seen best in this case over the proximal interphalangeal (PIP) joint of the third finger (**Figure 179-4**). There was periungual erythema and ragged cuticles. The scalp was red and scaly. Her neurologic examination was consistent with proximal myopathy. She also had some trouble swallowing bread, and dysphagia is not unusual in dermatomyositis. Laboratory tests showed mild elevations in muscle enzymes with the aspartate aminotransferase (AST) having the greatest elevation. In other cases, the creatine kinase (CK) can be very elevated.

The family physician started the patient on 60 mg of prednisone daily and topical steroids for the affected areas. The patient responded well to

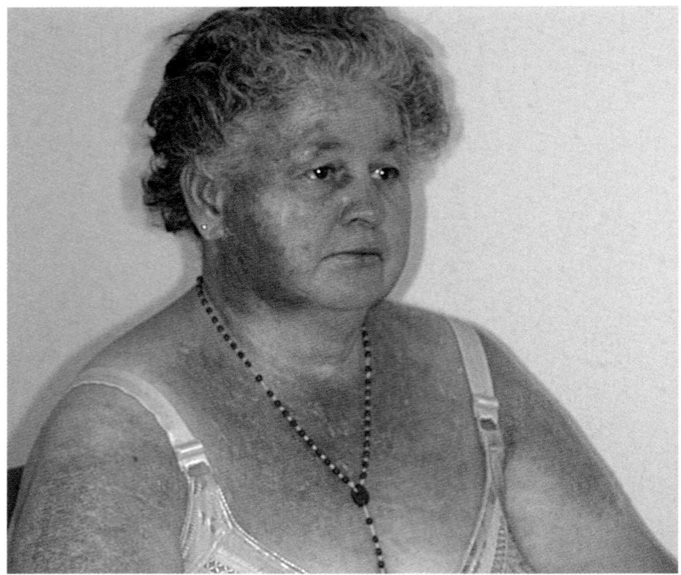

FIGURE 179-1 Initial presentation of dermatomyositis in a 55-year-old Hispanic woman. Prominent violaceous erythema with scale is visible on the chest, face, and arms. Deep-red erythema is especially visible on the side of the face. The scalp is red and scaling. (*Reproduced with permission from Richard P. Usatine, MD.*)

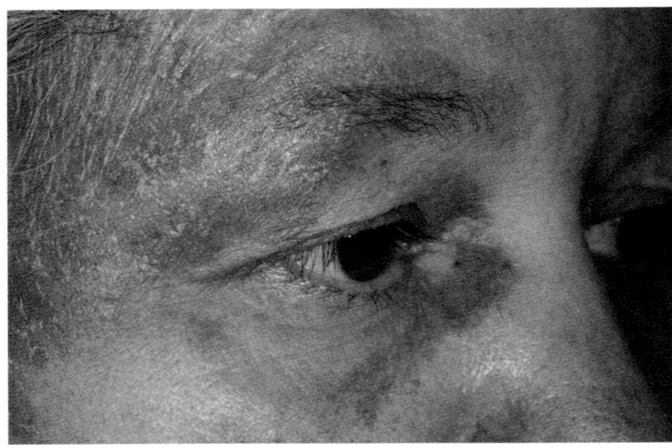

FIGURE 179-2 Close-up of the heliotrope (violaceous) rash around the eyes of the patient in **Figure 179-1**. (*Reproduced with permission from Richard P. Usatine, MD.*)

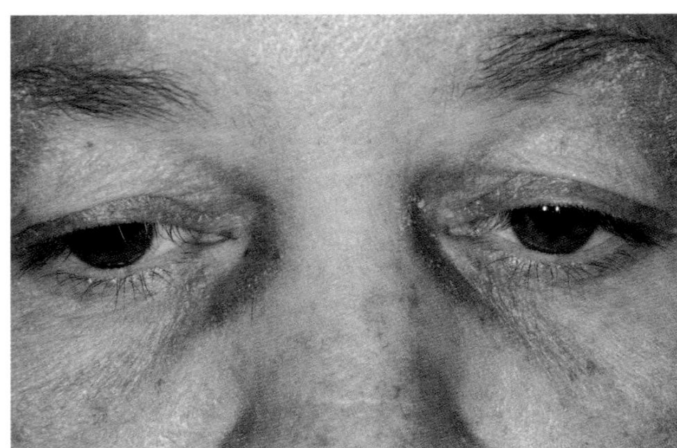

FIGURE 179-3 View showing the bilateral heliotrope rash of the patient in **Figure 179-1**. A pathognomonic sign of dermatomyositis. (*Reproduced with permission from Richard P. Usatine, MD.*)

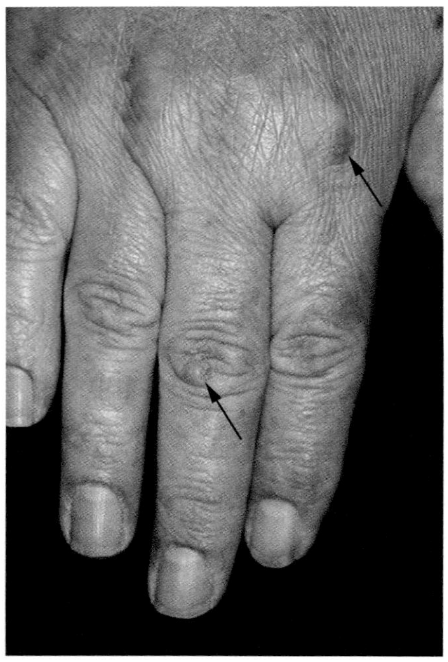

FIGURE 179-4 Hand involvement showing 2 Gottron papules over the knuckles (*arrows*) end erythematous nailfolds (periungual erythema) on the patient in **Figure 179-1**. (*Reproduced with permission from Richard P. Usatine, MD.*)

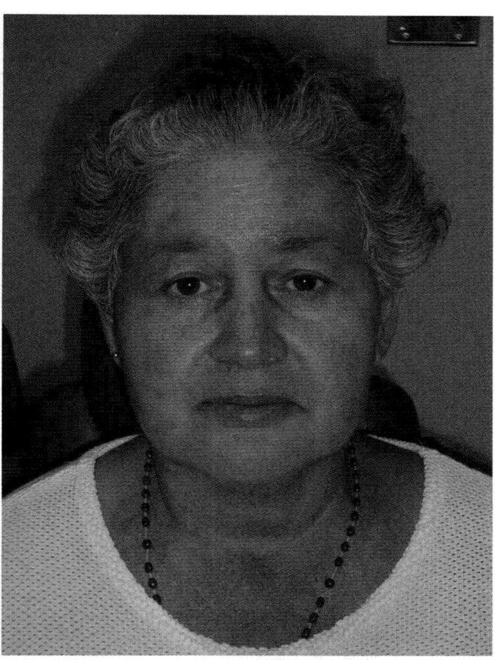

FIGURE 179-5 Patient improving after 2 weeks of oral prednisone. The heliotrope rash is still visible around the eyes and upper chest. The hairline erythema is from scalp involvement. (*Reproduced with permission from Richard P. Usatine, MD.*)

prednisone and 2 weeks later was feeling stronger and the rash was fading (**Figure 179-5**). After 4 weeks of 60 mg/d of prednisone she was started on 10 mg/wk of methotrexate in order to eventually taper her steroids. The patient has continued to do well, but the rash and muscle weakness tend to recur when her steroids are being tapered. The patient was sent for physical therapy and started on calcium and vitamin D supplementation to protect her from steroid-induced osteoporosis. She was also given 1 mg/d of folic acid to minimize the adverse effects of methotrexate. As dermatomyositis may be precipitated by an underlying malignancy, the physician screened the patient for internal cancers, especially ovarian cancer. Fortunately, the mammogram, Papanicolaou (Pap) smear, colonoscopy, transvaginal ultrasound for ovarian imaging, and abdominal/pelvic computed tomography (CT) scans were all normal.

INTRODUCTION

Dermatomyositis is a rare, idiopathic inflammatory disease involving the striated muscles and the skin. The disease is characterized by progressive, symmetrical, proximal muscle weakness. Dermatologic manifestations may occur with or without muscular diseases and include the characteristic heliotrope rash (**Figures 179-2**, **179-3**, **179-5**, and **179-6**), "shawl sign," and Gottron papules of the PIP joints. Although primarily a disease of muscle and skin, dermatomyositis has a clear relationship with myocarditis and interstitial lung disease, as well as an increased risk of associated malignancy.

EPIDEMIOLOGY

- Annual incidence of 5 to 8.9 per 1 million population.[1]
- Seen more commonly in women.[1]
- Can affect any age; however, it is more common in children and older adults.[1]

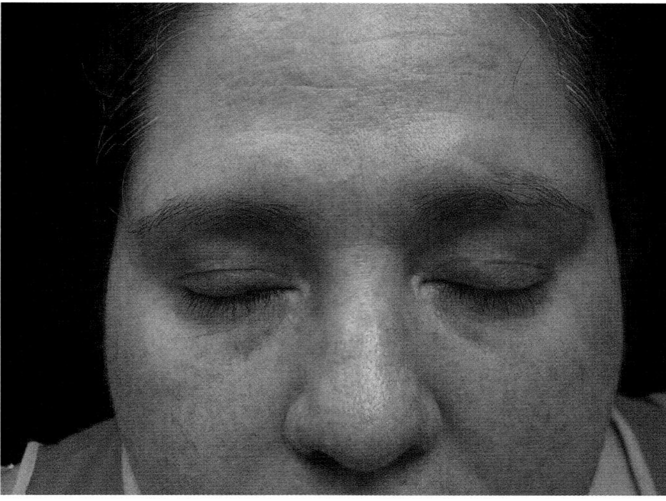

FIGURE 179-6 Classic heliotrope rash around the eyes of this 35-year-old woman newly diagnosed with dermatomyositis. The color "heliotrope" is a pink-purple tint named after the color of the heliotrope flower. As expected, her heliotrope rash is bilaterally symmetrical. This rash resolved on prednisone and hydroxychloroquine. (*Reproduced with permission from Richard P. Usatine, MD.*)

- Thirty-five percent to 40% of patients with dermatomyositis also have interstitial lung disease. It is the most common internal organ manifestation of the disease and greatly affects morbidity and mortality.[1,2]
- Has been linked to malignancy in up to 15% to 24% of adults.[3]
- Cancers most commonly associated are breast, ovary, lung, and gastrointestinal (GI) tract. The most common type of cancer is adenocarcinoma. Ovarian cancer is overrepresented in those patients with dermatomyositis and cancer. Cancer is not typically seen in children with dermatomyositis.
- In adults, the presence of anti-p155 autoantibodies has shown to be strongly associated with malignancy, with a 27-fold increase in odds.[4]

ETIOLOGY AND PATHOPHYSIOLOGY

- Dermatomyositis is considered an autoimmune disease of unknown etiology. Environmental exposure and infectious agents may play a role in disease pathogenesis.
- Dermatomyositis has been shown to be a microangiopathy that affects the skin and muscle. The muscle weakness and skin manifestations may be a result of activation and deposition of complement, which cause lysis of endomysial capillaries and muscle ischemia.

DIAGNOSIS

- Diagnosis includes 5 criteria: "definite" (skin findings plus any 3 of criteria 1-4), "probable" (skin findings plus 2 of any criteria 1-4), or "possible" (skin findings plus any 1 of criteria 1-4).[2,5,6]
  - Proximal symmetric muscle weakness that progresses over weeks to months.
  - Elevated serum levels of muscle enzymes (CK, AST, lactate dehydrogenase [LDH] and aldolase).
  - Abnormal electromyogram.
  - Abnormal muscle biopsy.
  - Skin findings—Presence of cutaneous disease characteristic of dermatomyositis (heliotrope rash; Gottron papules are considered

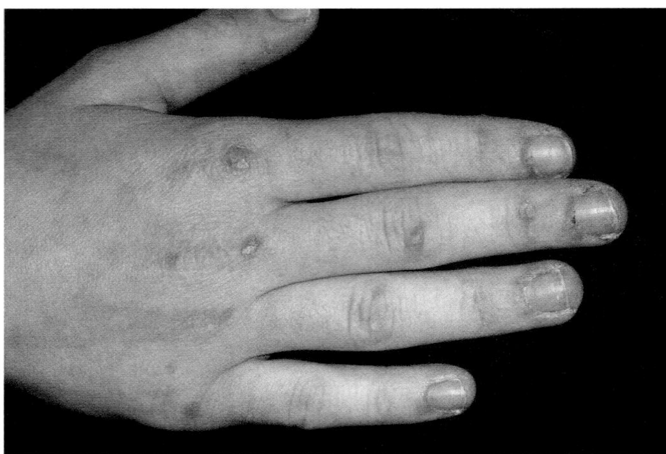

FIGURE 179-7 Hand involvement in a 19-year-old woman with Gottron papules over the finger joints. She has nailfold erythema and ragged cuticles (Samitz sign). (*Reproduced with permission from Richard P. Usatine, MD, and from Goodall J, Usatine RP. Skin rash and muscle weakness.* J Fam Pract. *2005;54(10):864-868. Reproduced with permission from Frontline Medical Communications.*)

pathognomonic) (**Figures 179-2** to **179-8**). Nonpathognomonic manifestations include malar erythema, and periungual and cuticular changes (**Figure 179-9**).

- These criteria are still considered the "gold standard," although they are old (1975) and currently under critical review because of several limitations. The criteria do not include specific autoantibodies or magnetic resonance imaging (MRI) findings.[2,7,8]

Recent studies indicate that the dilated nailfold capillary loops (**Figure 179-10**) often seen in patients with dermatomyositis may help in earlier diagnosis and predicting patients with poor prognosis. Dilated nailfold capillary loops have shown promise in juvenile dermatomyositis as a marker for both skin and muscle disease activity to guide treatment. Some authors propose adding this finding to criteria for diagnosis.[9,10]

CLINICAL FEATURES

- Bilateral periorbital heliotrope erythema (pathognomonic) (see **Figures 179-2, 179-3, 179-5,** and **179-6**) and scaling violaceous papular dermatitis in a patient complaining of proximal muscle weakness points to dermatomyositis.

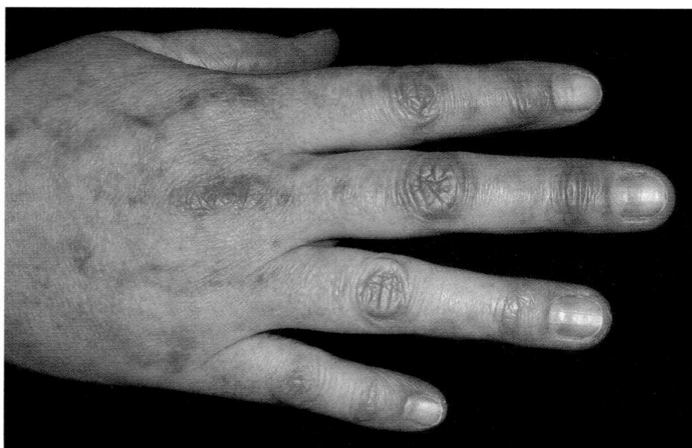

FIGURE 179-8 Dermatomyositis hand involvement with Gottron plaques and papules over the finger joints in this woman who also has a positive ANA of 1:160. (*Reproduced with permission from Richard P. Usatine, MD*)

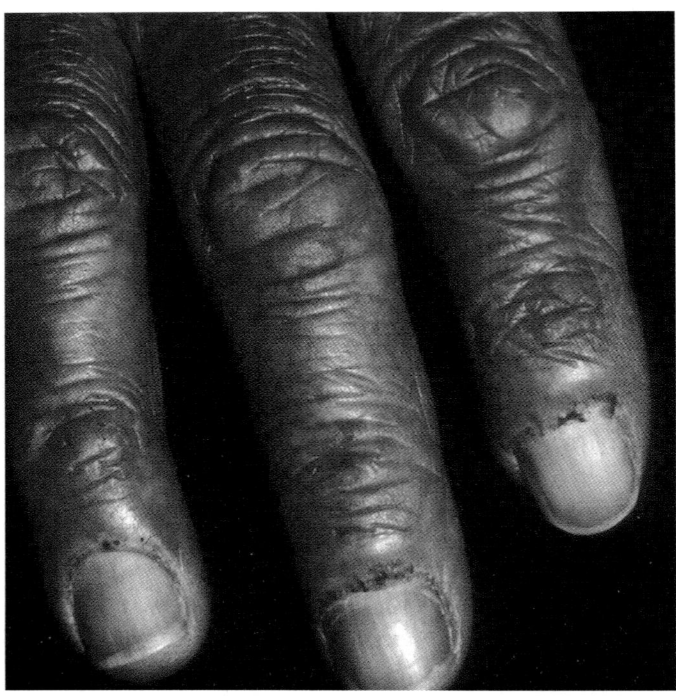

FIGURE 179-9 Dermatomyositis in a man showing cuticular changes that are thick, rough, and hyperkeratotic with telangiectasias. This moth-eaten appearance of the cuticles is called the Samitz sign. The hands also have the appearance of "mechanic's hands," another sign seen in dermatomyositis. (*Reproduced with permission from the University of Texas Health Sciences Center, Division of Dermatology.*)

- The patient may classically complain of difficulty climbing stairs, rising from a seat, or combing their hair. Notably the skin manifestations may precede, follow, or present simultaneously with muscle involvement; a patient may even have skin manifestations for longer than a year prior to developing muscle weakness.
- Hand involvement includes abnormal nailfolds and Gottron papules. "Moth-eaten" cuticles, also called the Samitz sign, are evidenced by periungual erythema and telangiectasias (see **Figures 179-7** to **179-9**).
- Gottron papules, smooth, purple-to-red papules and plaques, are classically located over the knuckles and on the sides of fingers (see **Figures 179-4, 179-7,** and **179-8**). Plaques may be present over the knuckles instead of or in addition to papules.
- Dysphagia can be present as a consequence of pharyngeal muscle involvement with risk of aspiration and pneumonia.
- Patients with concurrent interstitial lung disease may also present with fatigue, cough, dyspnea on exertion, and decreased exercise tolerance. Lung involvement usually appears following symptoms of myositis, although this is not always the case.[2]

TYPICAL DISTRIBUTION

- Face—The characteristic heliotrope rash occurs around the eyes. The color "heliotrope" is a pink-purple tint named after the color of the heliotrope flower. This color is best seen in **Figure 179-6**. The heliotrope rash can also be a dusky-red color as seen in **Figures 179-1** to **179-5**. This heliotrope rash is bilaterally symmetrical.
- Hands—There is usually hand involvement with Gottron papules (and plaques) and abnormal nailfolds and cuticles (see **Figures 179-4** and **179-7** to **179-9**).

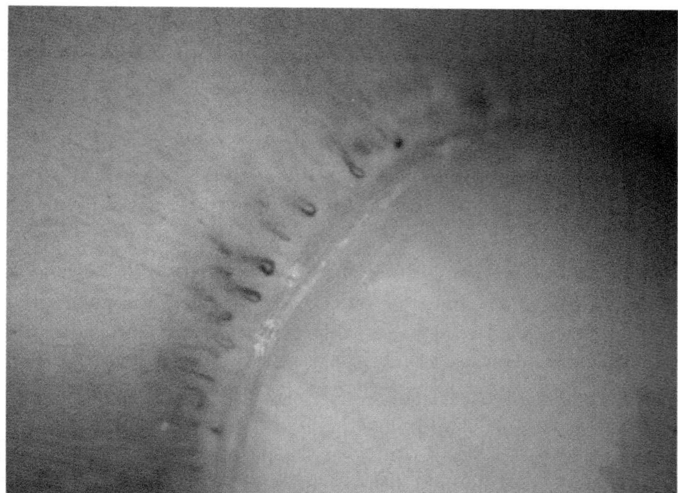

A

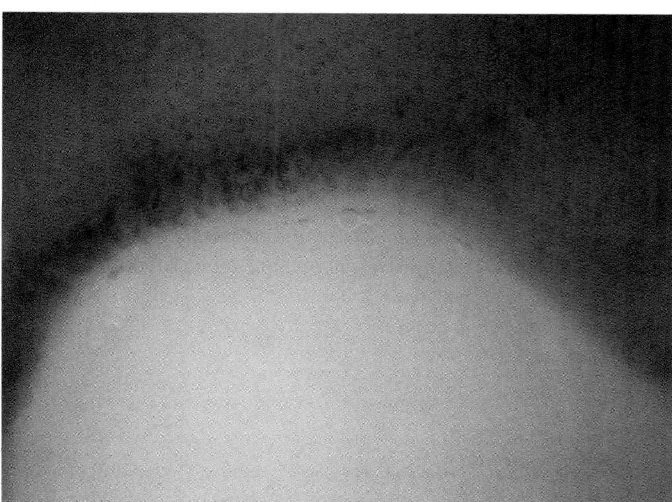

B

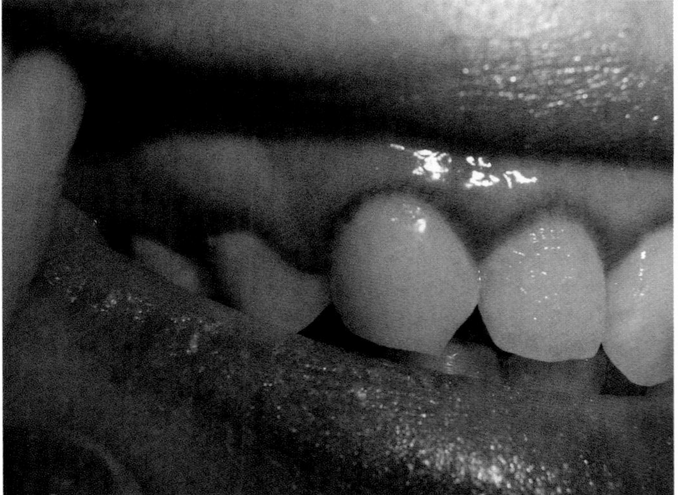

C

FIGURE 179-10 A. Dilated nailfold capillary loops visible with dermoscopy in a young woman with newly diagnosed dermatomyositis. B. She also had dilated capillary loops on the gingival borders of her teeth seen with dermoscopy. C. Marginal gingivitis in the same young woman with newly diagnosed dermatomyositis. The nailfold findings and gingival findings both resolved with treatment. (*Reproduced with permission from Richard P. Usatine, MD.*)

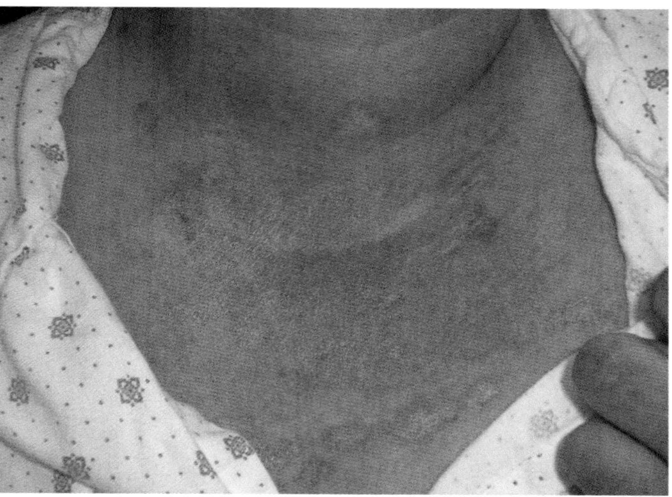

FIGURE 179-11 Poikiloderma (erythema and mottled hyperpigmentation) on the neck of a 35-year-old Hispanic woman with dermatomyositis. The V-neck distribution is related to sun exposure. (*Reproduced with permission from Richard P. Usatine, MD, and from Goodall J, Usatine RP. Skin rash and muscle weakness.* J Fam Pract. *2005;54(10)864-868. Reproduced with permission from Frontline Medical Communications.*)

- Neck and upper trunk—A red or poikiloderma-type rash can be seen in a **V**-neck (**Figure 179-11**) or in a shawl distribution (**Figure 179-12**). Poikiloderma refers to hyperpigmentation of the skin demonstrating a variety of shades and associated with telangiectasias. The rash here can be scaling and look psoriasiform.
- Extremities may have erythematous plaques and papules with scale.
- Scalp is often involved with erythema and scale and appears similar to seborrhea or psoriasis.
- Sun-exposed areas are often involved and worsen with sun exposure. This is why so many of the skin findings are on the face and upper chest (**Figure 179-13**). However, patients rarely complain of sun sensitivity.

LABORATORY STUDIES AND DIAGNOSTIC TESTS

- Elevated muscle enzymes, evidence of inflammation on electromyography (EMG), and inflammatory infiltrates on muscle biopsy confirm the

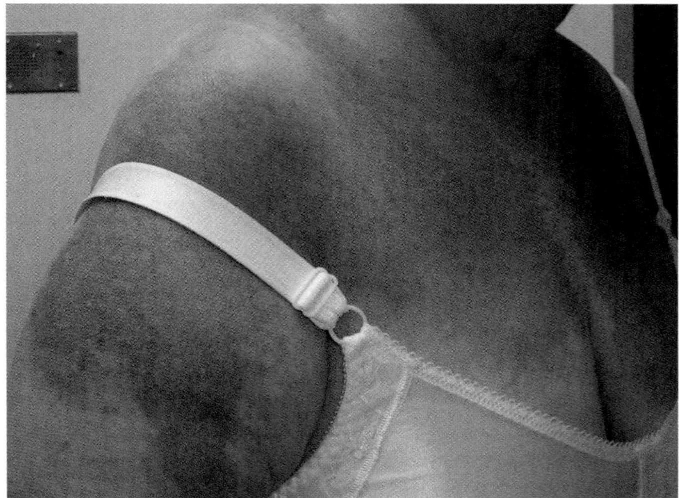

FIGURE 179-12 The shawl distribution of dermatomyositis. (*Reproduced with permission from Richard P. Usatine, MD.*)

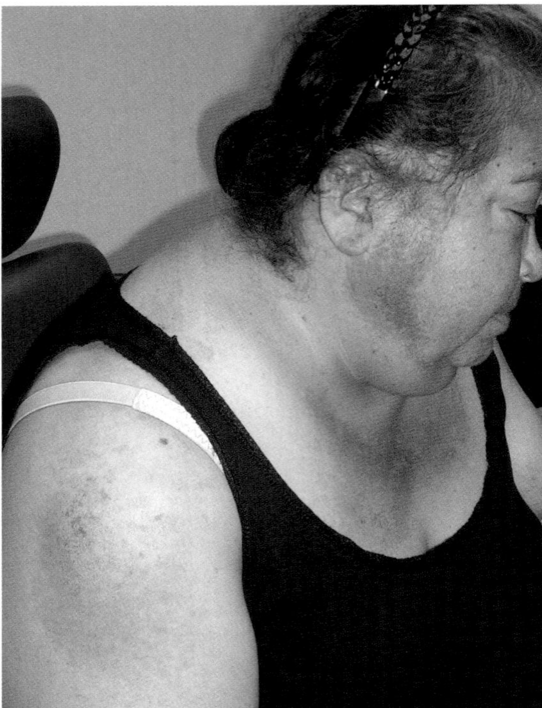

FIGURE 179-13 A flare of dermatomyositis in a patient previously under control on medications now showing erythema on the lateral face, upper chest, and proximal arm. (*Reproduced with permission from Richard P. Usatine, MD.*)

diagnosis of dermatomyositis. The following serum muscle enzymes can be drawn during the acute active phase and may be found to be elevated: CK, LDH, alanine aminotransferase, AST, and aldolase. Of note, it is necessary to measure all of the aforementioned enzymes as only one of them may be elevated.

- The diagnosis may be made with confidence in a patient with characteristic skin findings and elevated muscle enzymes. If the presentation is not straightforward, then EMG and muscle biopsy should be performed.
- The diagnosis can be supported with positive antibodies such as antinuclear antibody (ANA), anti-Mi-2, and anti-Jo-1. It is not necessary to order these antibodies to make the diagnosis of dermatomyositis. In fact, these myositis-specific antibodies are only positive in 30% of patients with dermatomyositis. Patients with anti-Mi-2 generally have a better overall prognosis.
- Other papulosquamous diseases, such as lichen planus and psoriasis, may be differentiated from dermatomyositis with a punch biopsy, but the histology of dermatomyositis is indistinguishable from cutaneous lupus erythematosus.
- Some experts recommend initial pulmonary function tests (PFTs), chest radiograph, and high-resolution CT to identify patients with interstitial lung disease early, regardless of presence or absence of respiratory symptoms.[11]
- PFTs demonstrate a restrictive pattern with presence of interstitial lung disease. Abnormal results must be confirmed by CT scan as PFT results may also reflect coexisting respiratory muscle weakness. Changes over time can be used to determine response to therapy, although intervals for testing are not clearly defined.[2]

BIOPSY

Muscle biopsy of dermatomyositis will show inflammatory cells around intramuscular blood vessels. Atrophic muscle fibers are seen around the periphery of muscle fascicles ("perifascicular atrophy").[1]

DIFFERENTIAL DIAGNOSIS

- Polymyositis is another form of inflammatory myopathy. It is distinguished from dermatomyositis by its lack of cutaneous involvement. Dermatomyositis can also occur without muscle involvement. This is called *dermatomyositis sine myositis* or *amyopathic dermatomyositis*.
- Polymorphous light eruption or other photosensitivity reactions may be mistaken for the dermatologic findings of dermatomyositis. As in the case of our patient, her cutaneous findings preceded her muscle weakness and the cutaneous findings were only in light-exposed areas. Therefore, it is essential in the management and follow-up with patients with suspected photosensitivity reactions to inquire about muscle weakness and to look for other signs of dermatomyositis. Examination of the hands and tests for muscle enzyme elevations might help to distinguish dermatomyositis from photosensitivity reactions (see Chapter 197, Photosensitivity).
- Hypothyroidism can cause a proximal myopathy just like polymyositis and dermatomyositis. Although hypothyroidism can cause a dermopathy, it does not resemble the skin findings of dermatomyositis. All patients with proximal muscle weakness should have a screening thyroid-stimulating hormone (TSH) to rule out hypothyroidism regardless of their skin findings (see Chapter 226, Hypothyroidism).
- Rosacea causes an erythematous rash on the face as is often seen in dermatomyositis. Of course rosacea does not cause muscle weakness and the erythema of rosacea is generally confined to the face only (see Chapter 115, Rosacea).
- Steroid myopathy may develop as a side effect of systemic steroid therapy. The symptoms develop 4 to 6 weeks after starting oral steroids for dermatomyositis and other autoimmune diseases. Therefore if muscle weakness recurs after improving it could be from the steroids not the disease.
- Dermatomyositis-like reaction rarely may present with similar skin findings with initiation of the following medications and improvement with their discontinuation: penicillamine, nonsteroidal anti-inflammatory drugs (NSAIDs), and carbamazepine.
- Overlap syndrome—The term *overlap* denotes that certain signs are seen in both dermatomyositis and other connective tissue diseases, such as scleroderma, rheumatoid arthritis, and lupus erythematosus. Scleroderma and dermatomyositis are the most commonly associated conditions and have been termed sclerodermatomyositis or mixed connective disease. In mixed connective tissue disease, features of systemic lupus erythematosus (SLE), scleroderma, and polymyositis are evident, such as malar rash, alopecia, Raynaud phenomenon, waxy-appearing skin, and proximal muscle weakness.

MANAGEMENT

Given the autoimmune mechanism likely central to the disease process, treatment is geared toward the proximal muscle weakness and skin changes using immunosuppressive or immunomodulatory therapy. Treatment is nonspecific as the target antigen remains elusive.[4] Cutaneous manifestations do not always parallel muscle disease in response to therapy.

Clinical improvement should guide treatment regimen, and serum CK level should not be used as a sole guide for gauging responsiveness to therapy. Effective therapies for the myopathy are oral corticosteroids, immunosuppressant, biological agents, and/or intravenous immunoglobulin. Effective therapies for the skin disease are sun protection, topical corticosteroids, antimalarials, methotrexate, and/or immunoglobulin. Drug therapy for dermatomyositis continues to be based on empirical rather than evidence-based practice because of lack of controlled trials.[12]

NONPHARMACOLOGIC

- Physical and/or occupational therapy to regain strength is highly recommended. Physical therapy will preserve muscle function and help to prevent atrophy and contractures.[13]
- In combination with exercise, oral creatine supplement was recently shown to improve muscle endurance and functionality in patients with dermatomyositis compared to placebo.[14]
- Photoprotection consists of a broad-spectrum sunscreen, protective outerwear, and limiting sun exposure.[15-17] SOR Ⓑ

TOPICAL TREATMENT

- Therapy of the skin disease begins with high-potency topical corticosteroids.[15,16,18] SOR Ⓑ Triamcinolone ointment may be used for less-severe areas or on the face at first. Consider a short course of a very-high-potency steroid, such as clobetasol, for more severe involvement not on the face.[5]
- Topical tacrolimus 0.1% is a useful adjunct in the treatment of refractory skin manifestations.[13] SOR Ⓑ

ORAL TREATMENT

- First-line therapy for muscle disease is high-dose (1 mg/kg single daily dose) systemic corticosteroids, usually prednisone, with or without an immunosuppressive ("steroid-sparing") agent—methotrexate, cyclosporine, mycophenolate mofetil, or azathioprine.[3]
- Corticosteroids (either IV or oral) are also the first-line treatment for interstitial lung disease in patients with dermatomyositis. Approximately half of patients show response in respiratory symptoms. Refractory cases are treated with second-line calcineurin inhibitors (cyclosporine) or cyclophosphamide (oral or IV pulse), with or without corticosteroids. Methotrexate use is cautioned when there is coexisting lung disease, as it is a known cause of drug-induced interstitial lung disease.[2,19]
- Steroid taper (20%-25% reduction monthly) should be initiated based on clinical responsiveness (increased muscle strength, energy) after 3 to 4 weeks on high-dose treatment.
- If no response by 3 months to oral high-dose steroids, another treatment approach should begin along with a reexamination of the diagnosis.[3,13] SOR Ⓑ
- Methotrexate is effective in treating the muscular symptoms of childhood and adult refractory dermatomyositis as a steroid-sparing agent. Methotrexate significantly improves skin lesions as well.[20] SOR Ⓑ
- Methotrexate dosing starts at 10 to 15 mg/wk. The dose is then increased 2.5 mg/wk until a total dose of 15 to 25 mg/wk is reached. The total dose of methotrexate is also determined by how well the patient can tolerate this medication. Improvement is typically noted after 4 to 8 weeks of therapy.[13,18]
- Using methotrexate safely requires a number of precautions. A purified protein derivative (PPD) should be placed or a QuantiFERON-TB Gold assay performed to make sure that tuberculosis will not be activated. Patients with active liver disease, including hepatitis C and alcoholic cirrhosis, should receive alternative forms of therapy. Women should avoid becoming pregnant during therapy. Persons started on methotrexate should also be given 1 mg of folic acid daily to minimize the risk of side effects. The patient should be followed with regular laboratory testing, including complete blood counts and comprehensive metabolic profiles. Methotrexate should only be prescribed by doctors familiar with its risks and benefits.
- As the methotrexate dosage is increased, the dosage of prednisone should be tapered.
- Cyclosporine plus methotrexate has shown some benefit in the treatment of refractory juvenile and adult dermatomyositis.[13] SOR Ⓑ Cyclosporine should cautiously be used with monitoring of blood pressure, renal function, liver function, and hematologic parameters.
- New data show that methotrexate and cyclosporine both resulted in clinical improvement with no difference in efficacy or toxicity.[13]
- Azathioprine is commonly used in chronic inflammatory diseases as a steroid-sparing agent. It is usually administered up to 2 to 3 mg/kg/d. The combination of azathioprine and methotrexate may be more efficacious together with fewer side effects than when used alone. Azathioprine has been shown to have a slower clinical effect than methotrexate, but no difference was noted in efficacy.[13] Like all the other immunosuppressive agents, azathioprine must be used cautiously by physicians familiar with its risks.
- Tacrolimus has effects similar to cyclosporine, but has greater potency and is effective in refractory juvenile dermatomyositis.[13]
- Mycophenolate mofetil, an inhibitor of T- and B-cell proliferation, is a possible corticosteroid-sparing agent and affects both refractory cutaneous and muscular disease; however, concern regarding central nervous system (CNS) B-cell lymphoma and lack of controlled trials limits its use. It is also more costly than methotrexate or azathioprine.
- Cyclophosphamide is an alkylating agent that has been used sparingly in refractory cases of dermatomyositis. Lack of solid evidence of efficacy in dermatomyositis along with concerns that the agent may lead to later malignancies limits its use to severely refractory patients.
- Hydroxychloroquine is one option for a steroid-sparing agent, especially for the rash of dermatomyositis, that may be considered for young women with mild disease. SOR Ⓒ Quinacrine and isotretinoin have shown promise in rashes that are unresponsive to hydroxychloroquine.[13]
- Various combination therapies with 2 of the following agents have been studied, but are still empirical: azathioprine, cyclosporine, intramuscular methotrexate, and oral methotrexate.[17,18,21] SOR Ⓒ
- Biologics, including tumor necrosis factor (TNF)-α inhibitors, are currently being tested for use in juvenile and adult dermatomyositis. Conflicting and discouraging initial results prompt the need for further clinical trials. Interferon-β, monoclonal complement antibodies, and anti–T-cell signaling drugs are currently under investigation.
- It is important to look at these medications' side effect profiles and monitor the patients accordingly during treatment. Patients must not get pregnant while on these medications and various laboratory tests need to be followed. A liver biopsy may be needed for patients taking methotrexate after a 1.5-g cumulative dose.

INTRAVENOUS TREATMENT

- Pulsed intravenous methylprednisolone has been advocated for severe disease (especially juvenile cases) and in refractory cases of myositis.[22] SOR C This treatment has also been recommended as first-line therapy for patients with associated interstitial lung disease.[1]
- In patients who are not responsive to traditional therapies, recent studies have found intravenous immunoglobulin (IVIG) to be an effective and relatively safe second-line therapy. Studies show improvement in muscle histology and cutaneous disease. Higher remission rates after 4 years are seen in patients receiving IVIG as part of therapy. IVIG is dosed 2 g/kg over 3 to 6 months with treatment for 2 to 5 consecutive days each month. High cost limits current use.[12,13] SOR C
- In one study, intravenous rituximab was shown to statistically increase long-term muscle strength in patients refractory to conventional therapy.[23] Thirteen patients were treated with rituximab 1000 mg IV, twice, with a 2-week interval, and followed for a median of 27 months. Patients experienced an increase in muscle strength and improvement in scores of disease activity, general health, functional ability, and health-related quality of life with sustained effect. Although rituximab is very expensive, these results are very promising for patients who are unresponsive to prednisone, methotrexate, and other conventional therapies.[23]

MALIGNANCY WORKUP

- All patients with dermatomyositis, regardless of age, should undergo an age- and gender-relevant malignancy workup beginning at the time of diagnosis. Cancer may be diagnosed before or after the diagnosis of dermatomyositis, but malignancy risk is highest at time of diagnosis or within 1 year. Some studies show an increased risk up to 5 years following diagnosis.[8,22]
- Screening should be performed with risks attributed to age, gender, ethnicity, and family history in mind.[24]
- For women newly diagnosed, a pelvic and transvaginal ultrasound, mammogram, CT thorax and abdomen, along with measurement of cancer antigen (CA)-125 level should be performed. Colonoscopy is recommended in patients older than age 50 years or with risk factors.[20]
- For men, a testicular and prostate examination should be performed at diagnosis with colonoscopy if age older than 50 years.[25]
- If primary screening is negative, some experts recommend that a patient should be screened in 3 to 6 months and every 6 months up to 4 years following diagnosis. The value of surveillance of tumor markers such as CA-125 and CA-19-9 is debatable.[24,25]
- Given its suggestive high predictive value, some experts recommend more intensive and frequent screening for patients positive for the anti-p155 antibody.[4]
- In one study, conventional cancer screening (thoracoabdominal CT, mammography, gynecologic examination, ultrasound, and tumor marker analysis) and fluorodeoxyglucose-positron emission tomography (FDG-PET)/CT total-body screening had equivalent overall predictive values for diagnosing malignancy in patients with myositis.[26]

PROGNOSIS

Recent reports indicate that approximately 20% to 40% of patients treated achieve remission, although 80% of treated patients remained disabled. One study found the mortality ratio of patients with dermatomyositis to be 3-fold higher than the rest of the population. Cancer, lung, and cardiac complications are the most common cause of death. Poor prognostic indicators include older age, cardiac and lung involvement (interstitial lung disease [ILD]), and dysphagia. Certain antibodies have also been linked to higher mortality rates and greater risk of malignancy.[7]

FOLLOW-UP

The patients need very close and frequent follow-up to manage their medications and overall care, as well as continued surveillance for malignancy. High doses of steroids and steroid-sparing agents, such as methotrexate, have numerous potential side effects. The patients need to be closely followed with laboratory tests and careful titration of the toxic medicines used for treatment. Also the patients need physical therapy, periodic eye examinations for cataracts and glaucoma, and specific supplements including calcium, vitamin D, and folic acid to prevent some of the side effects of the strong medications being prescribed. Patients on long-term corticosteroids especially need efforts made to prevent and detect osteoporosis.

PATIENT EDUCATION

Discuss the importance of sun protection as sun exposure does make the cutaneous manifestations worse. Counseling about the serious nature of the disease and prognosis is important as many patients are left with residual weakness even after good disease control is obtained. Patients need to understand that the medications being used have many risks along with their benefits and need to report side effects to their physicians. Pregnancy prevention is needed for women of childbearing potential while on a number of the medications used to treat this disease.

PATIENT RESOURCES

- The Myositis Association—**http://www.myositis.org.**
- National Institute of Neurological Disorders and Stroke. *NINDS Dermatomyositis Information Page*—**http://www.ninds.nih.gov/disorders/dermatomyositis/dermatomyositis.htm.**

PROVIDER RESOURCES

- Medscape. *Dermatomyositis*—**http://emedicine.medscape.com/article/332783.**
- MedicineNet. *Polymyositis & Dermatomyositis*—**http://www.medicinenet.com/polymyositis/article.htm.**

REFERENCES

1. Robinson AB, Reed AM. Clinical features, pathogenesis and treatment of juvenile and adult dermatomyositis. *Nat Rev Rheumatol.* 2011;7(11):664-675.
2. Connors GR, Christopher-Stine L, Oddis CV, Danoff SK. Interstitial lung disease associated with the idiopathic inflammatory myopathies: what progress has been made in the past 35 years? *Chest.* 2010;138(6):1464-1474.
3. Dalakas MC. Immunotherapy of inflammatory myopathies: practical approach and future prospects. *Curr Treat Options Neurol.* 2011;13(3):311-323.

4. Trallero-Araguás E, Rodrigo-Pendás J, Selva-O'Callaghan A, et al. Usefulness of anti-p155 autoantibody for diagnosing cancer-associated dermatomyositis. *Arthritis Rheum.* 2012;64(2):523-532.

5. Bohan A, Peter JB. Polymyositis and dermatomyositis (first of two parts). *N Engl J Med.* 1975;292(7):344-347.

6. Bohan A, Peter JB. Polymyositis and dermatomyositis (second of two parts). *N Engl J Med.* 1975;292(8):403-407.

7. Marie I. Morbidity and mortality in adult polymyositis and dermatomyositis. *Curr Rheumatol Rep.* 2012;14(3):275-285.

8. Madan V, Chinoy H, Griffiths CE, Cooper RG. Defining cancer risk in dermatomyositis. Part I. *Clin Exp Dermatol.* 2009;34(4):451-455.

9. Schmeling H, Stevens S, Goia C, et al. Nailfold capillary density is importantly associated over time with muscle and skin disease activity in juvenile dermatomyositis. *Rheumatology.* 2011;50(5):885-893.

10. Selva-O'Callaghan A, Fonollosa-Pla V, Trallero-Araguás E, et al. Nailfold capillary microscopy in adults with inflammatory myopathy. *Semin Arthritis Rheum.* 2010;39(5):398-404.

11. Fathi M, Dastmalchi M, Rasmussen E, et al. Interstitial lung disease, a common manifestation of a newly diagnosed polymyositis and dermatomyositis. *Ann Rheum Dis.* 2004;63(3):297-301.

12. Wang DX, Shu XM, Tian XL, et al. Intravenous immunoglobulin therapy in adult patients with polymyositis/dermatomyositis: a systematic literature review. *Clin Rheumatol.* 2012;31(5):801-806.

13. Aggarwal R, Oddis CV. Therapeutic approaches in myositis. *Curr Rheumatol Rep.* 2011;13(3):182-191.

14. Chung Y, Alexanderson H, Pipitone N, et al. Creatine supplements in patients with idiopathic inflammatory myopathies who are clinically weak after conventional pharmacologic treatment: six-month, double-blind, randomized, placebo controlled trial. *Arthritis Rheum.* 2007;57(4):694-702.

15. Callen JP. Dermatomyositis: diagnosis, evaluation and management. *Minerva Med.* 2002;93(3):157-167.

16. Callen JP, Wortmann RL. Dermatomyositis. *Clin Dermatol.* 2006;24(5):363-373.

17. Choy EH, Isenberg DA. Treatment of dermatomyositis and polymyositis. *Rheumatology (Oxford).* 2002;41(1):7-13.

18. Habif T. *A Color Guide to Diagnosis and Therapy, Clinical Dermatology*. 4th ed. St. Louis, MO: Mosby; 2004.

19. Mimori T, Nakashima R, Hosono Y. Interstitial lung disease in myositis: clinical subsets, biomarkers, and treatment. *Curr Rheumatol Rep.* 2012;14(3):264-274.

20. Hornung T, Ko A, Tuting T, et al. Efficacy of low-dose methotrexate in the treatment of dermatomyositis skin lesions. *Clin Exp Dermatol.* 2011;37(2):139-142.

21. Choy EH, Hoogendijk JE, Lecky B, Winer JB. Immunosuppressant and immunomodulatory treatment for dermatomyositis and polymyositis. *Cochrane Database Syst Rev.* 2005;20(3):CD003643.

22. Zahr ZA, Baer AN. Malignancy in myositis. *Curr Rheumatol Rep.* 2011;13(3):208-215.

23. Mahler EA, Blom M, Voermans NC, et al. Rituximab treatment in patients with refractory inflammatory myopathies. *Rheumatology.* 2011;50(12):2206-2213.

24. Madan V, Chinoy H, Griffiths CE, Cooper RG. Defining cancer risk in dermatomyositis. Part II. Assessing diagnostic usefulness of myositis serology. *Clin Exp Dermatol.* 2009;34(5):561-565.

25. Titulaer MJ, Soffietti R, Dalmau J, et al; European Federation of Neurological Societies. Screening for tumors in paraneoplastic syndromes: report of an EFNS Task Force. *Eur J Neurol.* 2011;18(1):19-27.

26. Selva-O'Callaghan A, Grau JM, Gámez-Cenzano C, et al. Conventional cancer screening versus PET/CT in dermatomyositis/polymyositis. *Am J Med.* 2010;123(6):558-562.

180 SCLERODERMA AND MORPHEA

E.J. Mayeaux Jr, MD

PATIENT STORY

A 35-year-old woman presented with areas of shiny tough skin in patches over her abdomen (**Figure 180-1**). The patient was otherwise in good health and was puzzled by this new condition. She feared that all her skin would become this way. The skin was slightly uncomfortable but not painful. A 3-mm punch biopsy confirmed the clinical suspicion of morphea or localized scleroderma. The patient was treated with topical clobetasol and calcipotriol with some improvement in skin quality and symptoms. An antinuclear antibody (ANA) test was positive, but she has not developed progressive systemic sclerosis.

INTRODUCTION

Scleroderma (from the Greek *scleros*, to harden) is a term that describes the presence of thickened, hardened skin. It may affect only limited areas of the skin (morphea), most or all of the skin (scleroderma), or also involve internal organs (systemic sclerosis).

EPIDEMIOLOGY

- The prevalence rates of diseases that share scleroderma as a clinical feature are reported ranging from 4 to 253 cases per 1 million individuals.[1]
- Systemic sclerosis has an annual incidence of 1 to 2 per 100,000 individuals in the United States.[1] The peak onset is between the ages of 30 and 50 years.[1]
- In the United States, the incidence of morphea has been estimated at 25 cases per 1 million individuals per year.[1]
- Worldwide, there are higher rates in the United States and Australia than in Japan or Europe.[2]
- Pulmonary fibrosis and pulmonary arterial hypertension are the leading causes of death as a consequence of these diseases.[3]

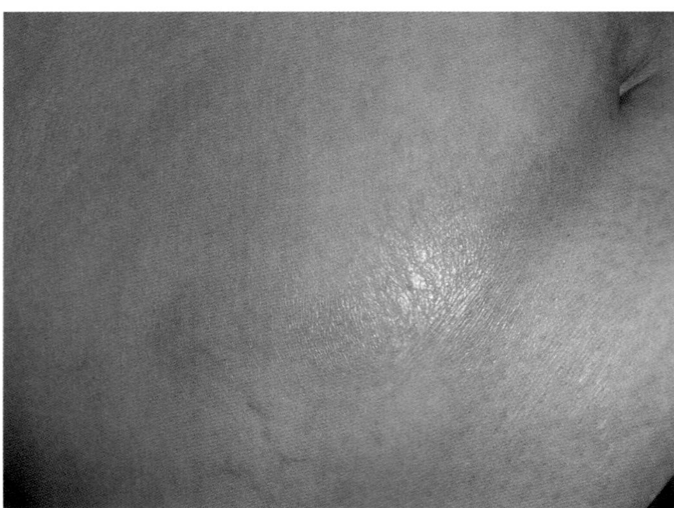

FIGURE 180-1 Morphea on the abdomen in a 35-year-old woman. (*Reproduced with permission from Richard P. Usatine, MD.*)

ETIOLOGY AND PATHOPHYSIOLOGY

- The scleroderma disorders can be subdivided into 3 groups: localized scleroderma (morphea; **Figures 180-1** and **180-2**), systemic sclerosis (**Figures 180-3** to **180-8**), and other scleroderma-like disorders that are marked by the presence of thickened, sclerotic skin lesions.
- The most common vascular dysfunction associated with scleroderma is Raynaud phenomenon (**Figure 180-9**). Raynaud phenomenon is produced by arterial constriction in the digits. The characteristic color changes progress from white pallor, to blue (acrocyanosis), to finally red (reperfusion hyperemia). Raynaud phenomenon generally precedes other disease manifestations, sometimes by years. Many patients develop progressive structural changes in their small blood vessels, which permanently impair blood flow, and can result in digital ulceration or infarction. Other forms of vascular injury include pulmonary artery hypertension, renal crisis, and gastric antral vascular ectasia.
- Systemic sclerosis is used to describe a systemic disease characterized by skin induration and thickening accompanied by variable tissue fibrosis and inflammatory infiltration in numerous visceral organs. Systemic sclerosis can be diffuse (DcSSc) or limited to the skin and adjacent tissues (limited cutaneous systemic sclerosis [LcSSc]).

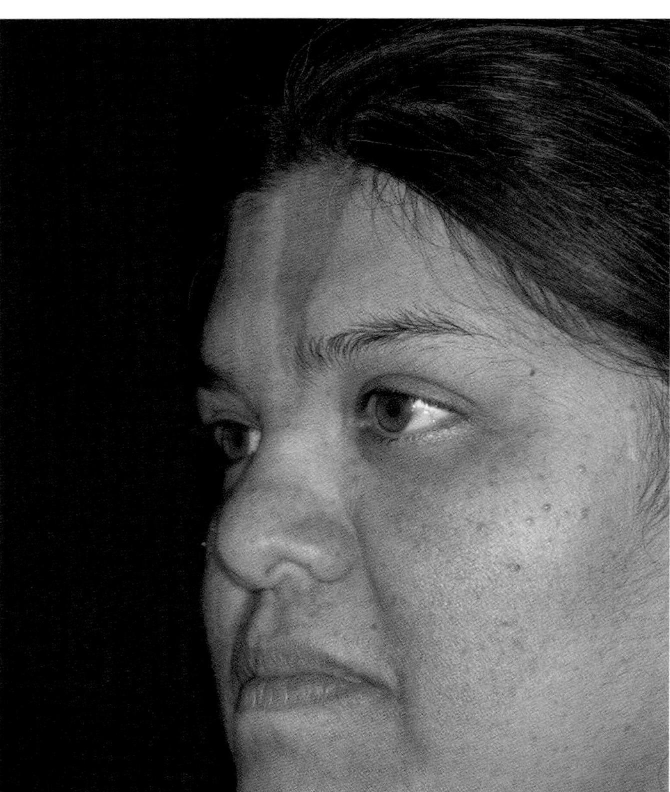

FIGURE 180-2 Linear morphea that started 3 years before on the forehead of a 41-year-old Hispanic woman. This distribution is called "en coup de sabre," meaning the blow of a sword. (*Reproduced with permission from Richard P. Usatine, MD.*)

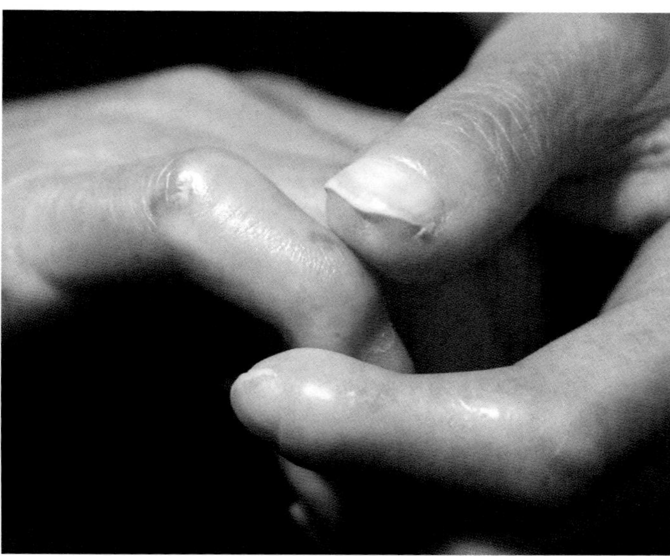

FIGURE 180-3 Scleroderma showing sclerodactyly with tight shiny skin over the fingers. (*Reproduced with permission from Everett Allen, MD.*)

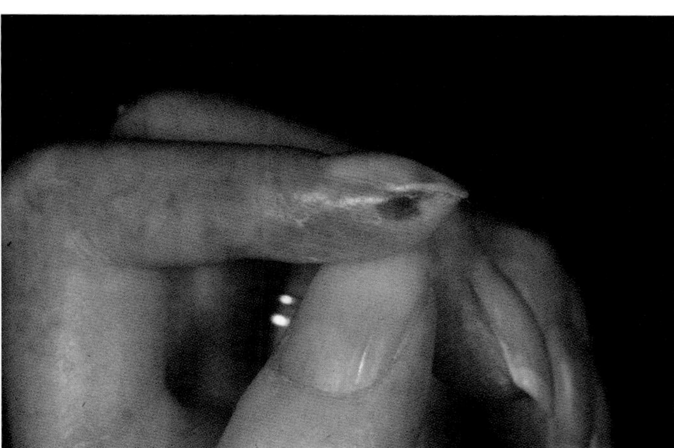

FIGURE 180-4 Sclerodactyly with tapering of the fingers and mottled hyperpigmentation. (*Reproduced with permission from Jeffrey Meffert, MD.*)

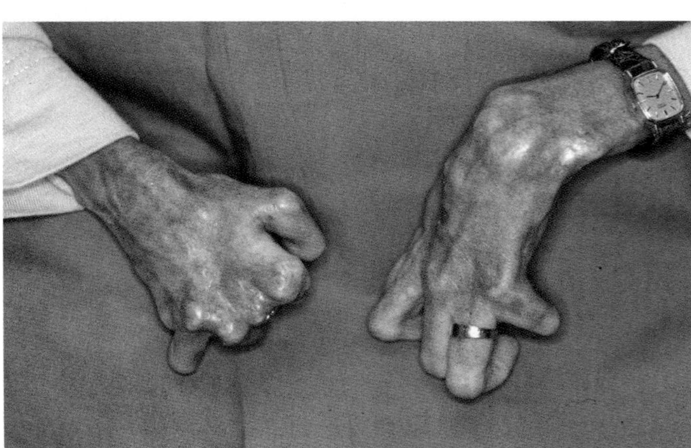

FIGURE 180-5 Severe scleroderma with deformity of hands as a result of sclerodactyly leading to severe flexion contractures. (*Reproduced with permission from Jeffrey Meffert, MD.*)

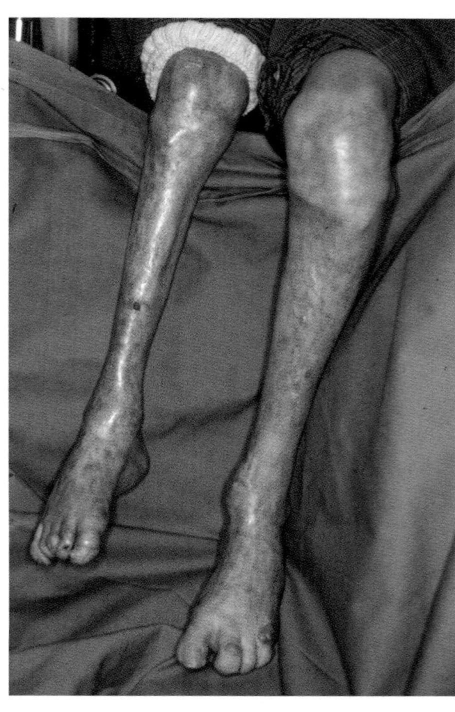

FIGURE 180-6 Scleroderma on the patient in **Figure 180-5** showing leg involvement with muscle atrophy. (*Reproduced with permission from Jeffrey Meffert, MD.*)

- Patients with LcSSc usually have skin sclerosis restricted to the hands and, to a lesser extent, the face and neck. With time, some patients develop scleroderma of the distal forearm. They often display the CREST syndrome, which presents with Raynaud phenomenon (see **Figure 180-9**), esophageal dysmotility, sclerodactyly (see **Figures 180-3** to **180-6**), telangiectasias (see **Figures 180-7** and **180-8**), and calcinosis cutis (**Figure 180-10**).
- Patients with DcSSc often present with sclerotic skin on the chest, abdomen, or upper arms and shoulders. The skin may take on a "salt-and-pepper" look (**Figure 180-11**). They are more likely to develop internal organ damage caused by ischemic injury and fibrosis than those with LcSSc or morphea.
- Almost 90% of patients with systemic sclerosis have some gastrointestinal (GI) involvement,[4] although half of these patients may be

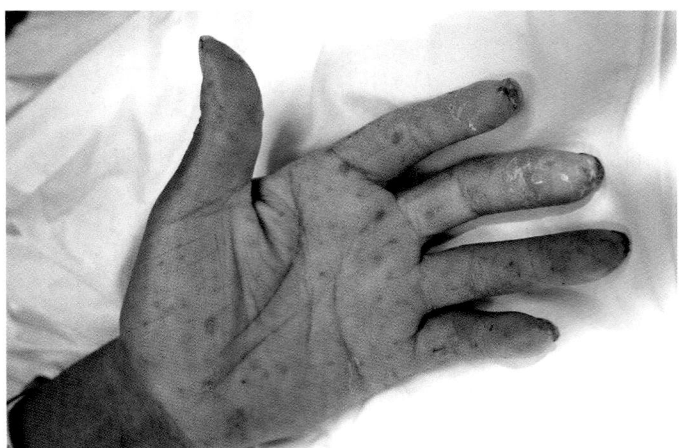

FIGURE 180-7 Scleroderma with telangiectasias and digital necrosis of the hands. (*Reproduced with permission from Everett Allen, MD.*)

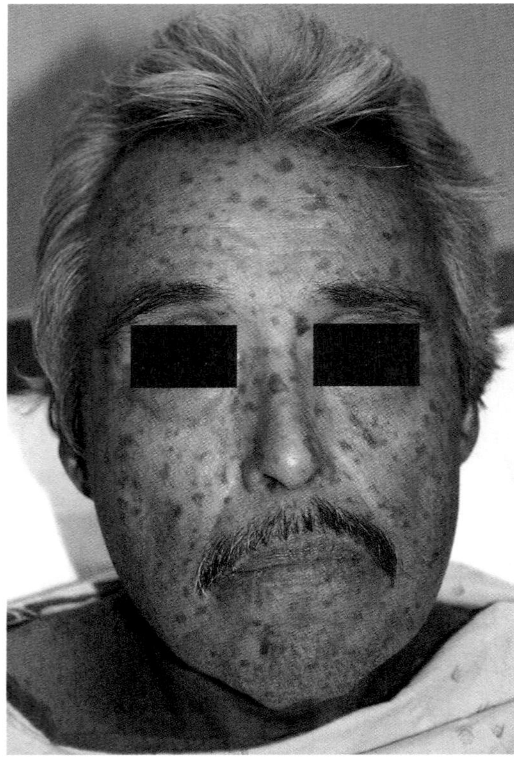

FIGURE 180-8 Telangiectasias on the face of the patient in Figure 180-7. (*Reproduced with permission from Everett Allen, MD.*)

asymptomatic. Any part of the GI tract may be involved. Potential signs and symptoms include dysphagia, choking, heartburn, cough after swallowing, bloating, constipation and/or diarrhea, pseudoobstruction, malabsorption, and fecal incontinency. Chronic gastroesophageal reflux and recurrent episodes of aspiration may contribute to the development of interstitial lung disease. Vascular ectasia in the stomach (often referred to as "water-melon stomach" on endoscopy) is common, and may lead to GI bleeding and anemia.

- Pulmonary involvement is seen in more than 70% of patients, usually presenting as dyspnea on exertion and a nonproductive cough. Fine "Velcro" rales may be heard at the lung bases with lung auscultation.

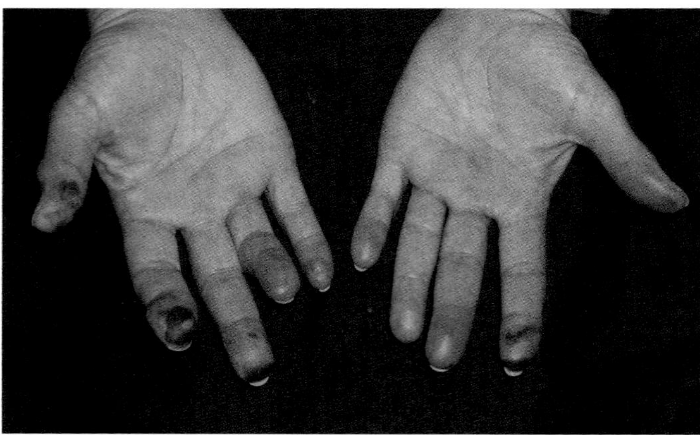

FIGURE 180-9 Raynaud phenomenon with severe ischemia leading to the necrosis of the fingertips. (*Reproduced with permission from Ricardo Zuniga-Montes, MD.*)

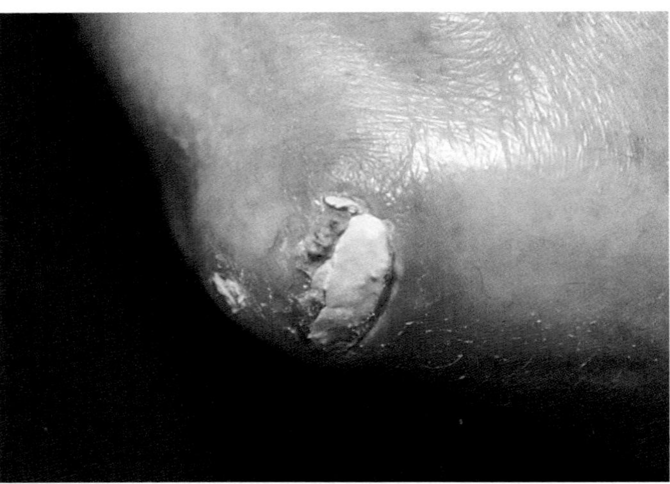

FIGURE 180-10 Calcinosis over the elbow in a patient with CREST syndrome. (*Reproduced with permission from Everett Allen, MD.*)

Pulmonary vascular disease occurs in 10% to 40% of patients with systemic sclerosis, and is more common in patients with limited cutaneous disease. The risk of lung cancer is increased approximately 5-fold in patients with scleroderma.

- Autopsy data suggest that 60% to 80% of patients with DcSSc have evidence of kidney damage.[5] Some degree of proteinuria, a mild elevation in the plasma creatinine concentration, and/or hypertension are observed in as many as 50% of patients.[6] Severe renal disease develops in 10% to 15% of patients, most commonly in patients with DcSSc.
- Symptomatic pericarditis occurs in 7% to 20% of patients, which has a 5-year mortality rate of 75%.[7] Primary cardiac involvement includes pericarditis, pericardial effusion, myocardial fibrosis, heart failure, myocarditis associated with myositis, conduction disturbances, and arrhythmias.[8] Patchy myocardial fibrosis is characteristic of systemic sclerosis, and is thought to result from recurrent vasospasm of small vessels. Arrhythmias are common and are mostly caused by fibrosis of the conduction system.
- Pulmonary vascular disease occurs in 10% to 40% of patients with scleroderma, and is more common in patients with limited cutaneous

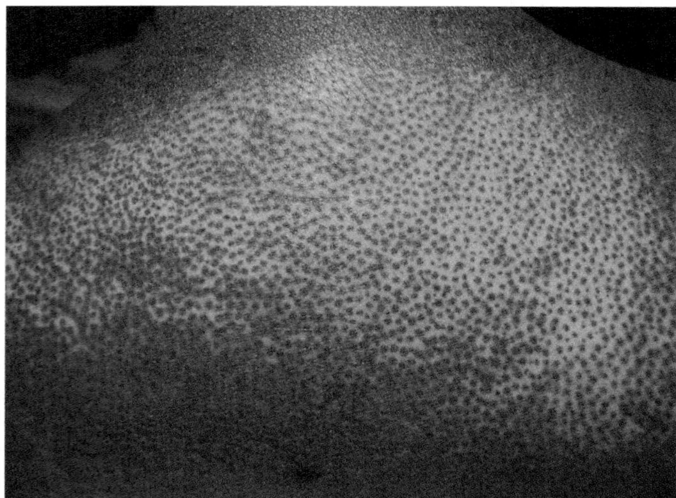

FIGURE 180-11 Scleroderma with mottled hypopigmentation. The skin may have a salt-and-pepper appearance as shown here. (*Reproduced with permission from Ricardo Zuniga-Montes, MD.*)

disease. It may occur in the absence of significant interstitial lung disease, generally a late complication, and is usually progressive. Severe pulmonary arterial hypertension, sometimes with pulmonale and right-sided heart failure or thrombosis of the pulmonary vessels may develop.

- Joint pain, immobility and contractures may develop, with contractures of the fingers being most common (see **Figure 180-5**). Neuropathies and central nervous system involvement, including headache, seizures, stroke, vascular disease, radiculopathy, and myelopathy, occur.
- Scleroderma produces sexual dysfunction in men and women. In men, it is very frequently associated with erectile dysfunction.

DIAGNOSIS

CLINICAL FEATURES

- The diagnosis of systemic sclerosis and related disorders is based primarily on the presence of characteristic clinical findings. Skin involvement is characterized by variable thickening and hardening of the skin. Skin pigmentary changes may occur, especially a salt-and-pepper appearance from spotty hypopigmentation (see **Figure 180-11**). Other prominent skin manifestations include the following:
  - Pruritus and edema in the early stages
  - Sclerodactyly (see **Figures 180-3** to **180-5**)
  - Digital ulcers and pitting at the fingertips (see **Figures 180-7** and **180-9**)
  - Telangiectasia (see **Figures 180-7** and **180-8**)
  - Calcinosis cutis (see **Figure 180-10**)
- The diagnosis of localized scleroderma (morphea) is suggested by the presence of typical skin thickening and hardening confined to one area (see **Figures 180-1** to **180-2**). The diagnosis of systemic sclerosis is suggested by the presence of typical skin thickening and hardening (sclerosis) that is not confined to one area (ie, not localized scleroderma). The combination of skin signs plus one or more of the typical systemic features supports the diagnosis of systemic sclerosis.
- The American College of Rheumatology criteria[9] for the diagnosis of systemic sclerosis requires 1 major criterion or 2 minor criteria:
  - The major criterion is typical sclerodermatous skin changes: tightness, thickening, and nonpitting induration, excluding the localized forms of scleroderma including the following:
    - Sclerodactyly—Above-indicated changes limited to fingers and toes. This can include sausage fingers with tuft resorption (**Figure 180-12**).
    - Proximal scleroderma—Above-indicated changes proximal to the metacarpophalangeal or metatarsophalangeal joints, affecting other parts of the extremities, face, neck, or trunk (thorax or abdomen) almost always including sclerodactyly (**Figure 180-13**).
  - Minor criteria include the following:
    - Digital pitting scars or a loss of substance from the finger pad (**Figure 180-14**)
    - Bilateral finger or hand pitting edema
    - Abnormal skin pigmentation: hyperpigmentation often with areas of punctate or patchy hypopigmentation (see **Figure 180-11**)
    - Raynaud phenomenon
    - Bibasilar pulmonary fibrosis (see **Figure 180-13**)
    - Lower (distal) esophageal dysmotility
    - Colonic sacculations: wide-mouthed diverticula of colon located along the antimesenteric border

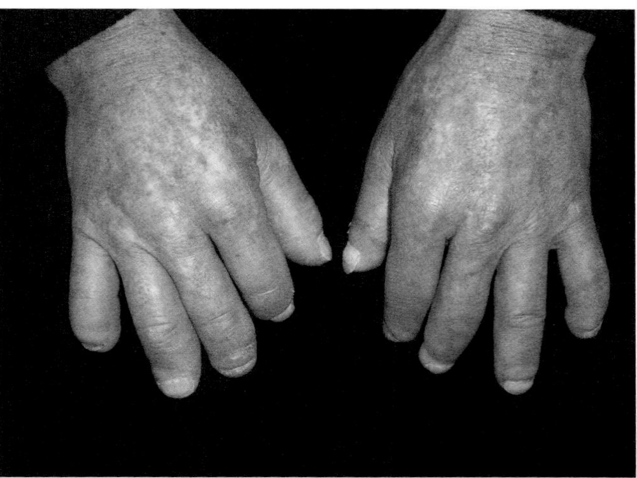

FIGURE 180-12 Sclerodactyly and sausage fingers in a 56-year-old woman with scleroderma and CREST syndrome. Note how the fingers are shortened secondary to digital tuft resorption and loss of substance from finger pads. There is also a salt-and-pepper appearance to the skin on the dorsum of the hands. (*Reproduced with permission from Richard P. Usatine, MD.*)

LABORATORY TESTING

- A positive ANA with a speckled, homogenous, or nucleolar staining pattern is common in scleroderma. Anticentromere antibodies are often associated with LcSSc. Anti-DNA topoisomerase I (Scl-70) antibodies are highly specific for both systemic sclerosis, and related interstitial lung and renal disease.[10] Although not very sensitive, anti-RNA polymerases I and III antibodies are specific for systemic sclerosis. Other testing for specific organ dysfunction is routinely done.

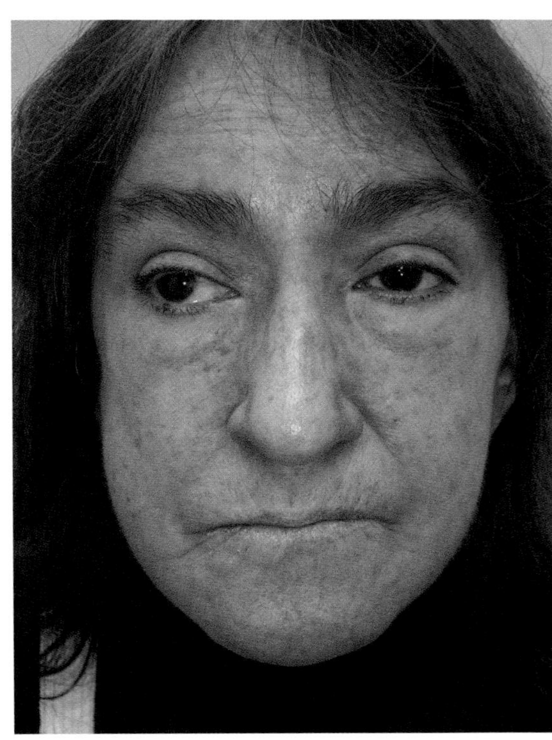

FIGURE 180-13 Proximal scleroderma on the face of a 56-year-old woman with scleroderma and CREST syndrome. Note the telangiectasias and a distinctive tightening of the skin around the lips. This patient also has pulmonary fibrosis as part of her progressive systemic sclerosis. (*Reproduced with permission from Richard P. Usatine, MD.*)

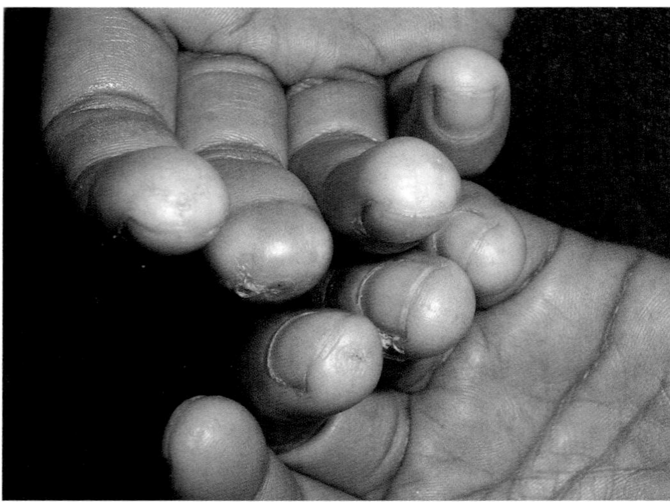

FIGURE 180-14 Digital pitting scars and loss of substance from finger pads in this 27-year-old woman with scleroderma and sclerodactyly. *(Reproduced with permission from Richard P. Usatine, MD.)*

- The presence of characteristic autoantibodies, such as anticentromere, antitopoisomerase I (Scl-70), anti-RNA polymerase, or U3-RNP antibodies, is supportive of the diagnosis of systemic sclerosis.

IMAGING

All patients with systemic sclerosis should have a chest X-ray (CXR) and pulmonary function tests (PFTs) screening for pulmonary involvement. The most common types of pulmonary involvement are interstitial lung disease and pulmonary hypertension.

The diffusing capacity (as part of PFTs) is the most sensitive test for pulmonary disease in systemic sclerosis. High-resolution computed tomography (CT) may be indicated for further evaluation of active pulmonary disease.

BIOPSY

A punch biopsy can be used to diagnose morphea and scleroderma when the clinical diagnosis is not clear.

DIFFERENTIAL DIAGNOSIS

- Idiopathic occurrence of systemic sclerosis–associated diseases such as Raynaud phenomenon, renal failure, and gastroesophageal reflux disease.
- Systemic lupus erythematosus (SLE) presents with systemic symptoms and a typical rash that may be scarring. ANA testing usually helps establish the diagnosis (see Chapter 178, Lupus: Systemic and Cutaneous).
- Discoid lupus erythematosus (DLE) presents as localized plaque lesion that eventually scar. Biopsy usually makes the diagnosis (see Chapter 178, Lupus: Systemic and Cutaneous).
- Myxedema is associated with hypothyroidism and is characterized by thickening and coarseness of the skin. Thyroid testing usually makes the diagnosis (see Chapter 226, Hypothyroidism).
- Lichen sclerosus when it occurs away from the genital area can resemble morphea. Although it most commonly affects the genital and perianal area, it can occur on the upper trunk, breasts, and upper arms. The plaques appear atrophic but a thin cigarette-paper crinkling appearance may help to differentiate it from morphea. A punch biopsy will lead to the correct diagnosis.
- Amyloidosis of the skin may result in thickening and stiffness of the skin. Skin biopsy reveals amyloid infiltration. Biopsy usually makes the diagnosis.
- Mycosis fungoides presents with purplish macules and plaques throughout the body. Biopsy usually makes the diagnosis (see Chapter 174, Cutaneous T-Cell Lymphoma).

MANAGEMENT

NONPHARMACOLOGIC

- Localized scleroderma, including morphea, appears to soften with ultraviolet A (UVA) light therapy.[11] SOR B
- For symptomatic therapy, skin lubrication, histamine 1 (H_1) and histamine 2 (H_2) blockers, oral doxepin, and low-dose oral glucocorticoids may be used to treat pruritus. SOR C
- Telangiectasias may be covered with foundation makeup or treated with laser therapy.

MEDICATIONS

- Treatment options for morphea include high-potency topical steroids such as clobetasol and topical calcipotriol.[12] SOR B
- Small localized lesions of morphea can be removed surgically. SOR C
- The combination of high-dose oral prednisone and low-dose oral methotrexate has been used successfully for scleroderma.[13] SOR B Methotrexate can be started at 7.5 mg PO weekly and titrated up as needed. Of course the long-term goal is to taper the prednisone while using the oral methotrexate as a steroid-sparing agent.
- Calcium channel blockers, prazosin, prostaglandin derivatives, dipyridamole, aspirin, and topical nitrates may help symptoms of Raynaud phenomenon.[14,15] SOR B Sildenafil (20 mg PO tid) has also been shown to be effective in patients with primary Raynaud phenomenon.[16] SOR B Patients should be advised to avoid cold, stress, nicotine, caffeine, and sympathomimetic decongestant medications. Acid-reducing agents may be used empirically for gastroesophageal reflux disease. Prokinetic agents, such as erythromycin, may be useful for patients with esophageal hypomotility. SOR C
- Unapproved therapies for skin disease include interferon-γ, mycophenolate mofetil (1-1.5 g PO bid), and cyclophosphamide (50-150 mg/d PO in a single AM dose). Extensive skin disease is being experimentally treated with D-penicillamine (250-1500 mg/d PO bid/tid on an empty stomach).[17] SOR B
- The mainstay of treatment of renal disease is control of blood pressure, with angiotensin-converting enzyme (ACE) inhibitors being the first-line agent. SOR C Hemodialysis or peritoneal dialysis may be used as needed.
- Treatments of pulmonary hypertension associated with the systemic sclerosis being tested include the endothelin receptor antagonist bosentan (62.5 mg PO bid for 4 weeks, then increase to 125 mg PO bid), the phosphodiesterase-5 inhibitor sildenafil, and various prostacyclin analogs (eg, epoprostenol, treprostinil, and iloprost). Pulmonary fibrosing alveolitis may be treated with cyclophosphamide.[18] SOR B
- Myositis may be treated with oral prednisone, methotrexate, and azathioprine (50-150 mg daily). Doses of prednisone greater than 40 mg/d are associated with a higher incidence of sclerodermal renal crisis.[19] SOR B Arthralgias can be treated with acetaminophen and nonsteroidal anti-inflammatory drugs (NSAIDs). SOR C

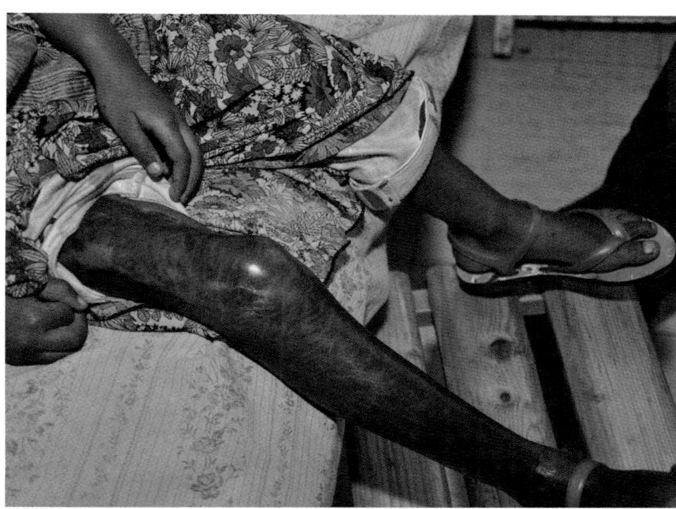

FIGURE 180-15 Localized morphea of the leg. Although her disease is not systemic, the tightening of the skin around the knee does cause problems with knee movement and ambulation. (*Reproduced with permission from Richard P. Usatine, MD.*)

- Any patient on long-term oral prednisone needs to be monitored for osteoporosis and diabetes. Osteoporosis prevention should include weight-bearing exercise, calcium, vitamin D supplements, and yearly dual-energy X-ray absorptiometry (DEXA) scanning to determine when and if additional medications are needed.

REFERRAL

Patients with systemic sclerosis should be referred to a rheumatologist as this is a complicated disease that requires the use of toxic medications. Depending on the complications, patients with scleroderma may also need referral to pulmonology, cardiology, and nephrology.

PROGNOSIS

- There is an increase in the risk of premature death with systemic sclerosis. Most deaths among these patients are a result of pulmonary fibrosis and/or pulmonary hypertension. Mortality also results from renal crisis, cardiac disease, infections, malignancies, and cardiovascular disease.[20]
- The prognosis for morphea is excellent as it only affects the skin. Although the appearance may be disturbing to the patient it is not life threatening. If the morphea is extensive and extends over an extremity, it can affect function (**Figure 180-15**).

FOLLOW-UP

The patient with systemic sclerosis needs to be evaluated at least every 3 to 6 months to monitor disease activity and progression.

PATIENT EDUCATION

Instruct the patient to avoid skin trauma (especially the fingers), cold exposure, and smoking. Make patients aware of potential complications and have them watch for signs of systemic disease occurrence or progression.

PATIENT RESOURCES

- American College of Rheumatology. *Scleroderma (Also Known as Systemic Sclerosis)*—**http://www.rheumatology.org/practice/clinical/patients/diseases_and_conditions/scleroderma.asp.**
- Scleroderma Foundation—**http://www.scleroderma.org/.**
- International Scleroderma Network—**http://www.sclero.org.**

PROVIDER RESOURCES

- National Institute of Arthritis and Musculoskeletal and Skin Diseases. *Handout on Health: Scleroderma*—**http://www.niams.nih.gov/Health_Info/Scleroderma/default.asp.**
- Medscape. *Scleroderma*—**http://emedicine.medscape.com/article/331864.**

REFERENCES

1. Lawrence RC, Helmick CG, Arnett FC, et al. Estimates of the prevalence of arthritis and selected musculoskeletal disorders in the United States. *Arthritis Rheum.* 1998;41(5):778-799.
2. Chifflot H, Fautrel B, Sordet C, et al. Incidence and prevalence of systemic sclerosis: a systematic literature review. *Semin Arthritis Rheum.* 2008;37(4):223-235.
3. Steen VD, Lucas M, Fertig N, Medsger TA Jr. Pulmonary arterial hypertension and severe pulmonary fibrosis in systemic sclerosis patients with a nucleolar antibody. *J Rheumatol.* 2007;34(11): 2230-2235.
4. Akesson A, Wollheim FA. Organ manifestations in 100 patients with progressive systemic sclerosis: a comparison between the CREST syndrome and diffuse scleroderma. *Br J Rheumatol.* 1989;28(4): 281-286.
5. Medsger TA Jr, Masi AT. Survival with scleroderma II. A life-table analysis of clinical and demographic factors in 358 male U.S. veteran patients. *J Chronic Dis.* 1973;26(10):647-660.
6. Tuffanelli DL, Winkelmann RK. Systemic scleroderma, a clinical study of 727 cases. *Arch Dermatol.* 1961;84:359-371.
7. Janosik DL, Osborn TG, Moore TL, et al. Heart disease in systemic sclerosis. *Semin Arthritis Rheum.* 1989;19(3):191-200.
8. Byers RJ, Marshall DA, Freemont AJ. Pericardial involvement in systemic sclerosis. *Ann Rheum Dis.* 1997;56(6):393-394.
9. American Rheumatism Association Diagnostic and Therapeutic Criteria Committee. Preliminary criteria for the classification of systemic sclerosis (scleroderma). Subcommittee for scleroderma criteria of the American Rheumatism Association Diagnostic and Therapeutic Criteria Committee. *Arthritis Rheum.* 1980;23(5): 581-590.
10. Reveille JD, Solomon DH. Evidence-based guidelines for the use of immunologic tests: anticentromere, Scl-70, and nucleolar antibodies. *Arthritis Rheum.* 2003;49(3):399-412.
11. Kreuter A, Breuckmann F, Uhle A, et al. Low-dose UVA1 phototherapy in systemic sclerosis: effects on acrosclerosis. *J Am Acad Dermatol.* 2004;50(5):740-747.
12. Seyger MM, van den Hoogen FH, de Boo T, de Jong EM. Low-dose methotrexate in the treatment of widespread morphea. *J Am Acad Dermatol.* 1998;39(2 pt 1):220-225.

13. Kreuter A, Gambichler T, Breuckmann F, et al. Pulsed high-dose corticosteroids combined with low-dose methotrexate in severe localized scleroderma. *Arch Dermatol.* 2005;141(7):847-852.

14. Thompson AE, Shea B, Welch V, et al. Calcium-channel blockers for Raynaud's phenomenon in systemic sclerosis. *Arthritis Rheum.* 2001;44(8):1841-1847.

15. Clifford PC, Martin MF, Sheddon EJ, et al. Treatment of vasospastic disease with prostaglandin E1. *Br Med J.* 1980;281(6247):1031-1034.

16. Fries R, Shariat K, von Wilmowsky H, Bohm M. Sildenafil in the treatment of Raynaud's phenomenon resistant to vasodilatory therapy. *Circulation.* 2005;112(19):2980-2985.

17. Falanga V, Medsger TA Jr. D-penicillamine in the treatment of localized scleroderma. *Arch Dermatol.* 1990;126(5):609-612.

18. Tashkin DP, Elashoff R, Clements PJ, et al. Cyclophosphamide versus placebo in scleroderma lung disease. *N Engl J Med.* 2006;354(25):2655-2666.

19. Steen VD, Medsger TA Jr. Case-control study of corticosteroids and other drugs that either precipitate or protect from the development of scleroderma renal crisis. *Arthritis Rheum.* 1998;41(9):1613-1619.

20. Tyndall AJ, Bannert B, Vonk M, et al. Causes and risk factors for death in systemic sclerosis: a study from the EULAR Scleroderma Trials and Research (EUSTAR) database. *Ann Rheum Dis.* 2010;69(10):1809-1815.

SECTION 15 BULLOUS DISEASE

181 OVERVIEW OF BULLOUS DISEASES

Richard P. Usatine, MD
Ana Treviño Sauceda, MD

PATIENT STORY

A 100-year-old black woman with diabetes was brought to the office by her family concerned about the large blister on her leg that started earlier that day (**Figure 181-1**). This large bulla appeared spontaneously without trauma and there was no surrounding erythema. The bulla contained clear fluid and there were no signs of infection. The bulla was drained with a sterile needle and no further bullae developed. The diagnosis is bullosis diabeticorum, a benign self-limited condition.

INTRODUCTION

Bullae are fluid-filled lesions on the skin that are larger than 5 mm in diameter. Bullous diseases are defined by the presence of bullae and vesicles (<5 mm in diameter). Bullous diseases are caused by many factors, including infections, bites, drug reactions, inflammatory conditions, and genetic and autoimmune diseases.

APPROACH TO THE DIAGNOSIS

The approach to a patient with a blistering disorder begins with a complete history and physical examination. To make the final diagnosis, laboratory investigations or tissue biopsies may be needed.

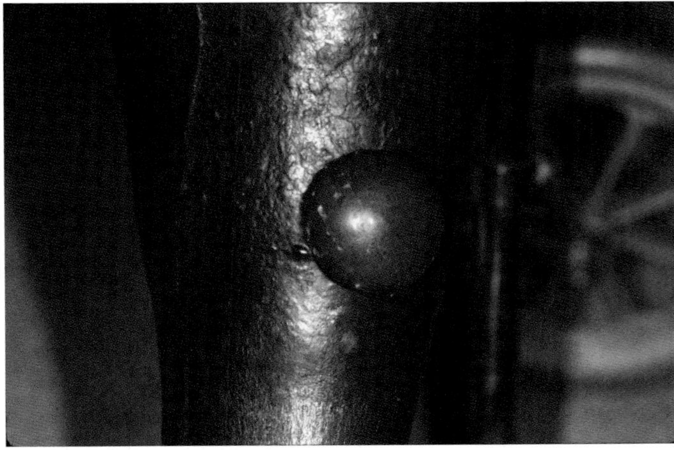

FIGURE 181-1 Bullosis diabeticorum on the lower leg of an older black woman with diabetes. This large bulla appeared spontaneously without trauma and there is no surrounding erythema. The bulla contained clear fluid and there was no infection. (*Reproduced with permission from Richard P. Usatine, MD.*)

DIAGNOSIS

HISTORY

- How did the eruption present?
- Has it changed in morphology or location?
- Has it responded to any therapies?
- Are there any associated symptoms or aggravating factors?
- How has it impacted the patient's life?
- Does the patient have any chronic medical conditions?
- Does the patient take any medications?
- Does the patient have any significant family history?

PHYSICAL EXAMINATION

- Note the location of the eruption.
- Are the bullae flaccid or tense (**Figure 181-2**)?
- Are there other lesions present (erosions, excoriations, papules, wheals)?
- Is Nikolsky sign positive or negative? (Does the skin shear off when lateral pressure is applied to unblistered skin?)
- Is Asboe-Hansen sign positive or negative (**Figure 181-3**)? (Do the bullae extend to surrounding skin when vertical pressure is applied?) Sometimes the Asboe-Hansen sign is also attributed to Nikolsky and called a Nikolsky sign, too.
- Is the Darier sign positive or negative? (Do wheals form with rubbing of the skin?)
- Note the skin background (sun-exposed skin, postinflammatory hyperpigmentation, lichenification, and scarring).
- Does the patient have lymphadenopathy or hepatosplenomegaly?

CLINICAL FEATURES

- Autoimmune
  - In bullous pemphigoid, patients have large, tense bullae that primarily involve the trunk, groin, axilla, proximal extremities, and flexor surfaces (see **Figures 181-2A** and **181-3**; see Chapter 182, Bullous Pemphigoid).[1]
  - Pemphigus vulgaris is characterized by erosions and flaccid bullae that frequently involve the mouth (**Figure 181-4**; see Chapter 183, Pemphigus). In fact, mucosal membrane involvement may be the initial presentation. If the skin is involved, then Nikolsky and Asboe-Hansen signs are positive.[1]
  - Pemphigus foliaceus presents with cutaneous erosions and never involves the mucosal membranes (see **Figure 181-2B**; see Chapter 183, Pemphigus). Nikolsky and Asboe-Hansen signs are positive.[1]
  - Pemphigoid gestationis is a condition during pregnancy or during the postpartum period that can have a bullous component. The patient usually presents with urticarial papules and plaques with bullae developing around the umbilicus and extremities. The eruption eventually generalizes and involves the palms and soles. There usually is sparing of the face, scalp, and oral mucosa (**Figure 181-5**).[1]
  - Cicatricial pemphigoid involves the oral mucosa in 90% of cases and the conjunctiva in 66% of cases (see Chapter 182, Bullous Pemphigoid).

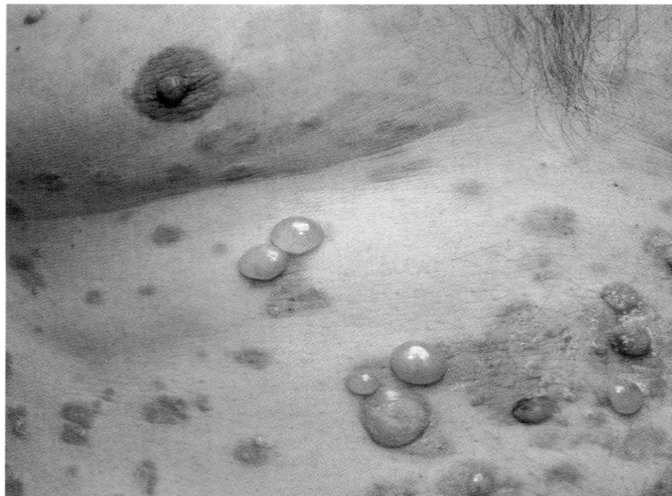

A

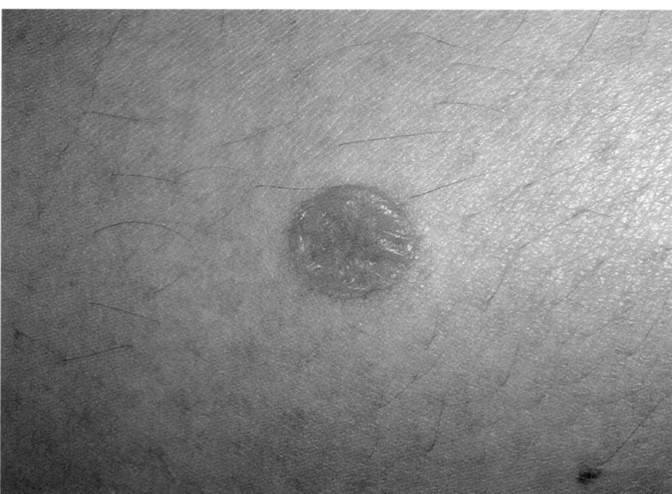

B

FIGURE 181-2 Comparison of the tense bullae seen in bullous pemphigoid and the more flaccid bullae seen in pemphigus. **A.** Tense bullae in bullous pemphigoid. **B.** Flaccid bulla on the leg of a patient with pemphigus foliaceous. *(Reproduced with permission from Richard P. Usatine, MD.)*

Patients frequently present with a desquamative gingivitis. Cutaneous lesions are seen in 25% of patients.[1]

- Epidermolysis bullosa acquisita presents with trauma-induced blistering and erosions usually on the distal extremities (**Figure 181-6**). The patient should have background scarring, milia, and nail dystrophy. This usually affects elderly persons.
- Epidermolysis bullosa simplex also has trauma-induced blistering that can involve the trunk and extremities. This is the most common form of epidermolysis bullosa and usually starts at birth or early childhood.[2] The bullae are intraepidermal (**Figure 181-7**).
- Dermatitis herpetiformis classically is a symmetrical, pruritic eruption that involves the extensor surfaces, scalp, and buttocks. The patient presents with pruritic vesicles and crusted papules with overlying excoriations (**Figures 181-8** and **181-9**) (see Chapter 184, Other Bullous Diseases).[1]
- Linear immunoglobulin (Ig) A bullous dermatosis may produce a ring-like pattern of distribution and can occur in childhood (**Figure 181-10**).[3] Patients may have mucous membrane involvement in up to 50% of cases.[1]

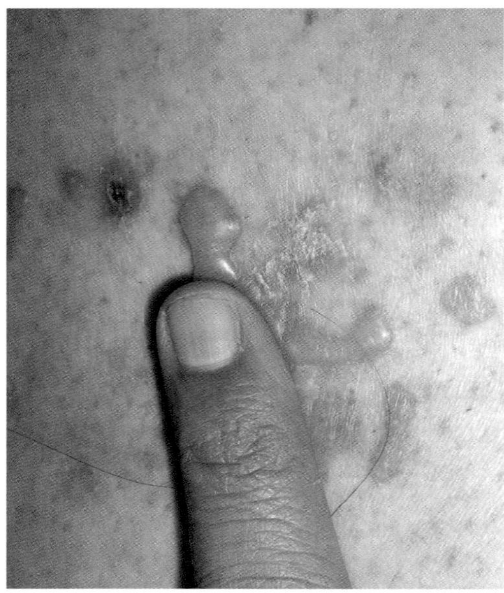

FIGURE 181-3 Testing for Asboe-Hansen sign on the back of a patient with bullous pemphigoid. The bulla did not extend with vertical pressure, so the sign was negative. *(Reproduced with permission from Richard P. Usatine, MD.)*

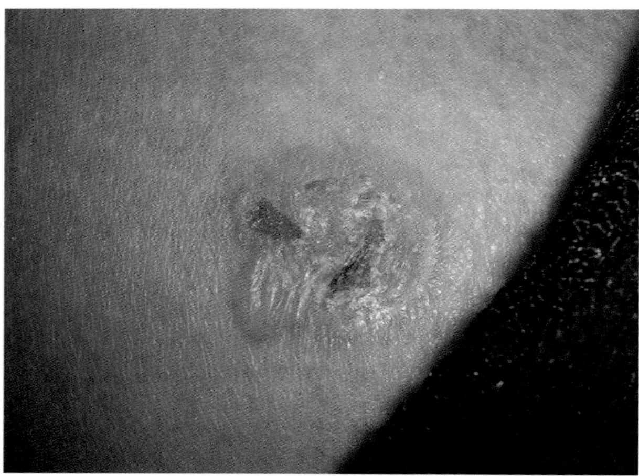

FIGURE 181-4 Flaccid and partially crusted bulla on the breast of a 51-year-old woman with pemphigus vulgaris. She also has severe oral involvement with large mucosal erosions. *(Reproduced with permission from Richard P. Usatine, MD.)*

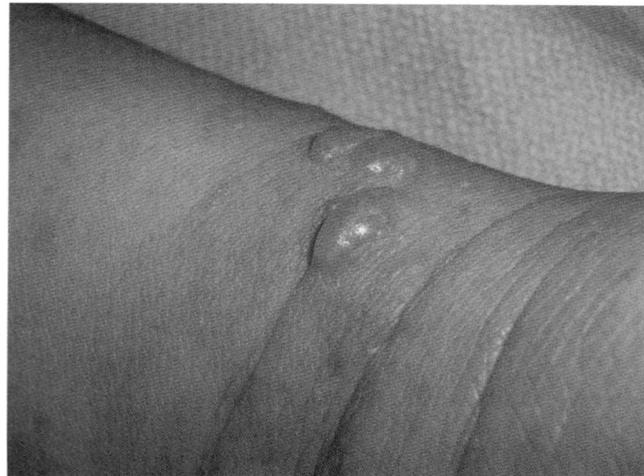

FIGURE 181-5 Pemphigoid gestationis with bullae on the wrist. *(Reproduced with permission from Richard P. Usatine, MD.)*

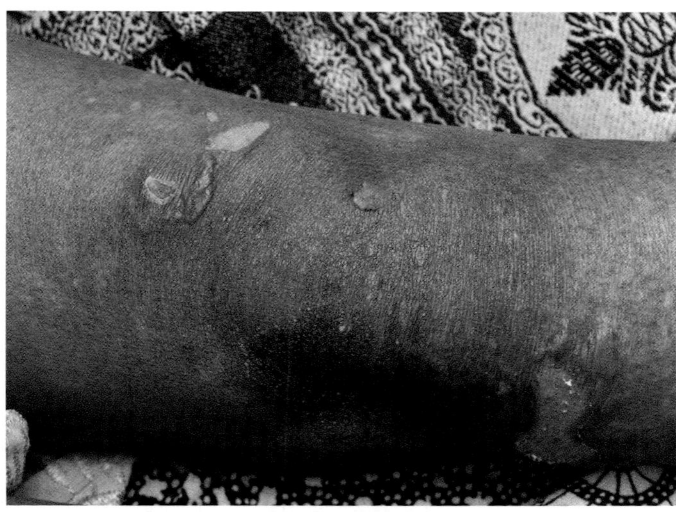

FIGURE 181-6 Epidermolysis bullosa acquisita in an elderly woman. Note the partially intact bulla over the knee along with other areas of erosions and hyperpigmentation. (*Reproduced with permission from Richard P. Usatine, MD.*)

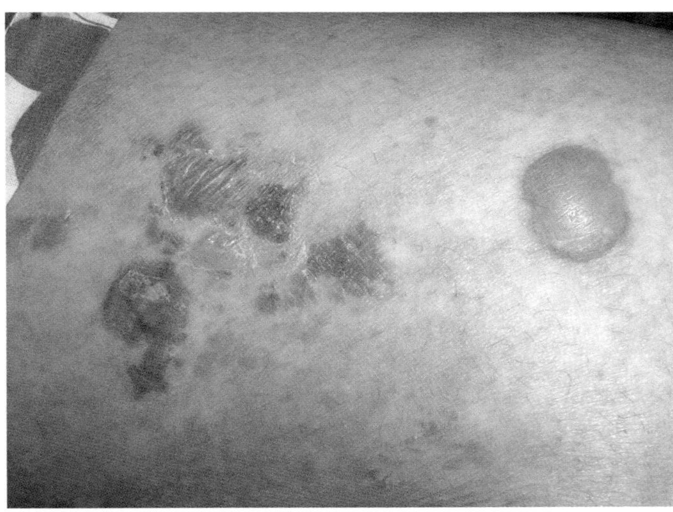

FIGURE 181-7 Large trauma-induced bulla on the leg of a 13-year-old girl with epidermolysis bullosa simplex. (*Reproduced with permission from Richard P. Usatine, MD.*)

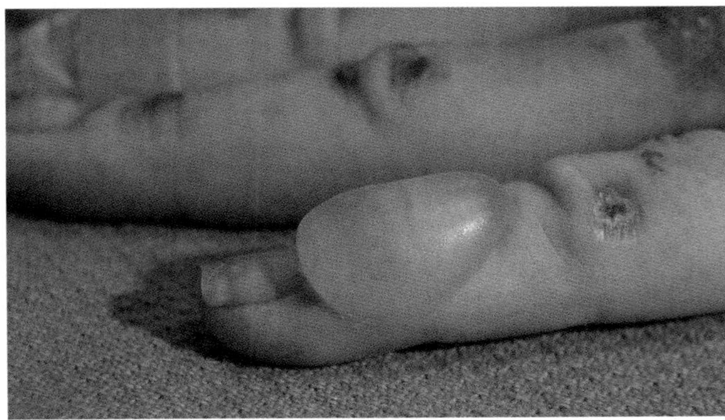

FIGURE 181-8 Porphyria cutanea tarda with a large bulla on the finger. (*Reproduced with permission from Lewis Rose, MD.*)

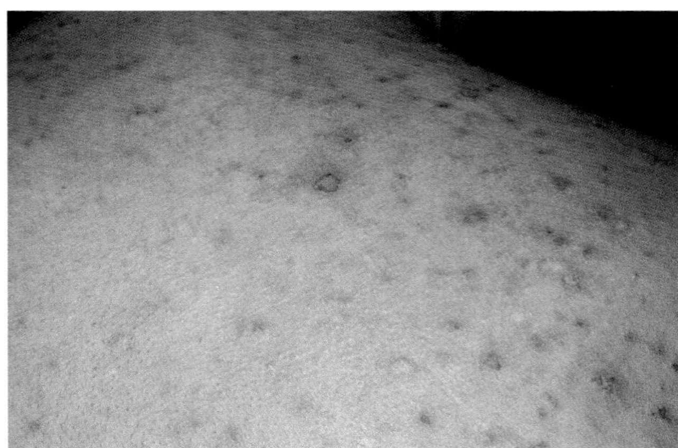

FIGURE 181-9 Pityriasis lichenoides et varioliformis acuta in a young man showing erosions where vesicles and bullae had been there previously. (*Reproduced with permission from Richard P. Usatine, MD.*)

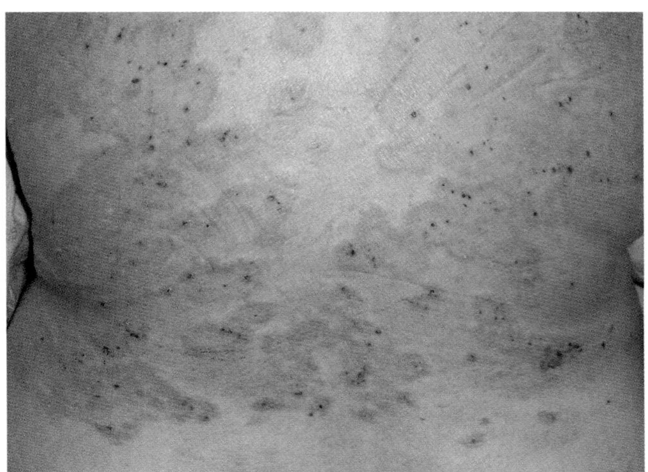

A

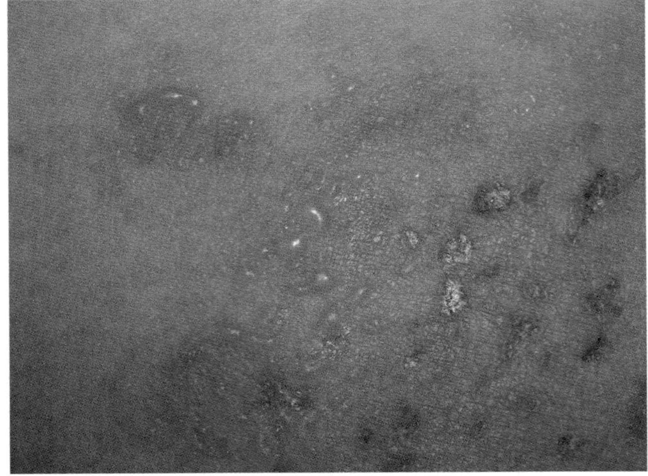

B

FIGURE 181-10 Bullous pemphigoid with new onset in a 61-year-old woman. **A.** The annular pattern suggested linear IgA bullous disease but the direct immunofluorescence stain showed IgG and C3 at the dermal-epidermal junction. **B.** Close-up showing some intact vesicles on the leg of the same patient. At first the diagnosis was difficult to make because the patient had been popping all the bullae and vesicles as they appeared. (*Reproduced with permission from Richard P. Usatine, MD.*)

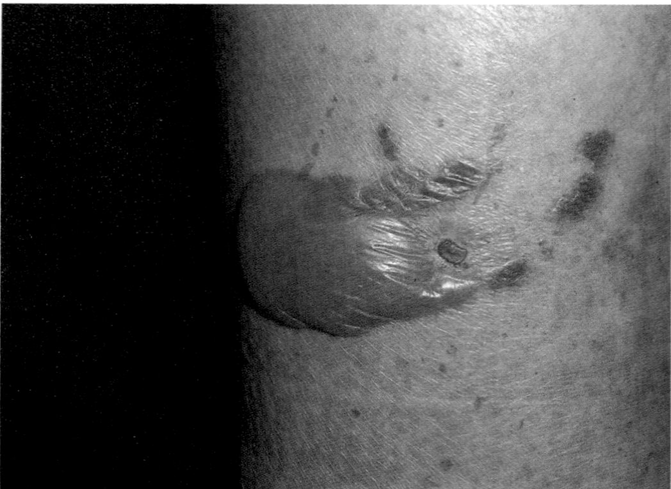

FIGURE 181-11 Large intact bulla on the lower leg of a woman with diabetes. This is bullosis diabeticorum also known as a diabetic bulla. (*Reproduced with permission from Richard P. Usatine, MD.*)

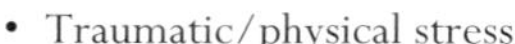

- Traumatic/physical stress
  - Friction blisters form at sites of pressure and friction, frequently on the distal lower extremities.[1]
  - Bullosis diabeticorum is trauma-induced, painless blistering, frequently in an acral distribution, in individuals with diabetes mellitus (**Figure 181-11**).[1]
  - Postburn blistering occurs in hours after the insult, such as is seen in severe second-degree sunburns.[1] Blistering after cold injury can also occur rapidly (**Figure 181-12**).
  - Miliaria is caused by keratinous obstruction of the eccrine ducts in response to heat. Small superficial vesicles may involve the face, trunk, or extremities.[1]
- Metabolic
  - Porphyria cutanea tarda (PCT) involves sun-exposed skin, particularly the dorsal hands, forearms, ears, and face. The patient will have associated milia, scarring, and background dyspigmentation. PCT has been associated with hepatitis C infection (see **Figure 181-8**).[1]

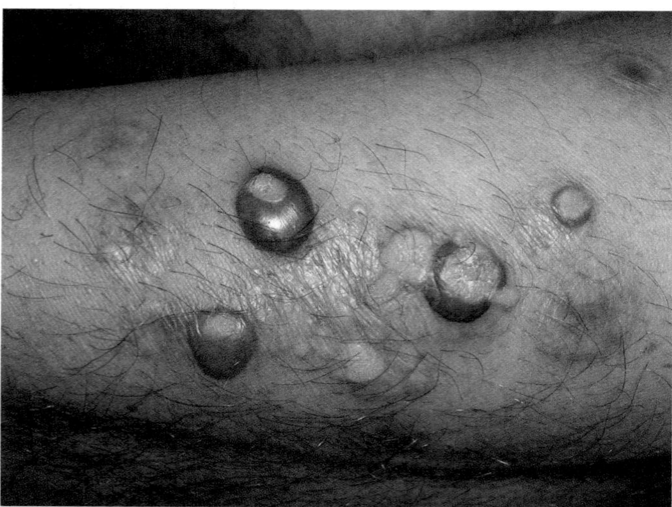

FIGURE 181-12 Bullae the day after cryotherapy for warts. (*Reproduced with permission from Richard P. Usatine, MD.*)

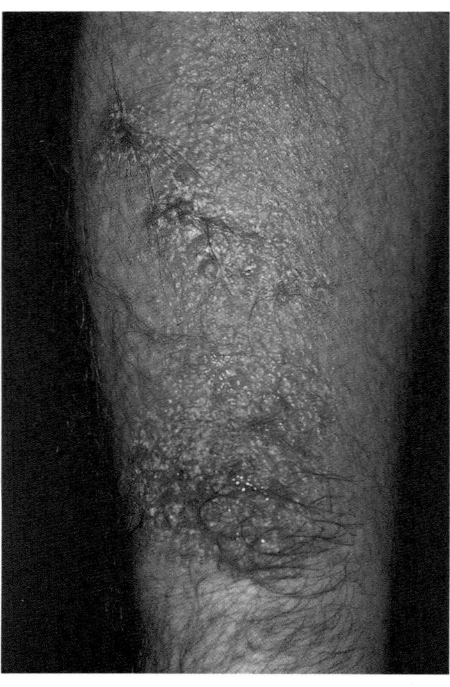

FIGURE 181-13 Bullae and vesicles on the extremity of a patient with poison ivy. Acute contact dermatitis can present with bulla and vesicles. (*Reproduced with permission from Richard P. Usatine, MD.*)

- Immunologic
  - Pityriasis lichenoides et varioliformis acuta usually presents as a papulonecrotic eruption but may have vesicles resembling varicella (see **Figure 181-9**). It usually involves the anterior trunk, flexor surfaces of the upper extremities, and the axilla. The general health of the patient is unaffected, although most have lymphadenopathy. CD8 T cells are the predominant cell type in lesional skin.[1] It is seen more frequently in young men and can go on to become chronic.
  - Allergic-contact and irritant-contact dermatitis, if severe, can cause blistering. Special attention should be placed on the location and pattern of involvement. For example, linear vesicles and bullae would suggest a plant-induced dermatitis such as poison ivy, poison oak, or poison sumac (**Figure 181-13**). Blistering in the periumbilical area is consistent with nickel dermatitis. Involvement of the dorsal feet is frequently seen with footwear dermatitis; likewise, involvement of the dorsal hands is consistent with glove dermatitis (see Chapter 144, Contact Dermatitis).[4]
- Drug
  - Bullous drug eruptions may be localized to 2 mucosal surfaces with minimal cutaneous involvement or may be generalized involving all mucosal surfaces and a majority of the skin surface area. Nikolsky and Asboe-Hansen signs are positive on affected skin (see Section 13: Hypersensitivity Syndromes and Chapter 201, Cutaneous Drug Reactions).[1] Even fixed-drug eruptions can be bullous (**Figure 181-14**).
- Infections and bites
  - Bullous arthropod reaction can occur after an insect bite (**Figure 181-15**).[1]
  - Bacterial infections should be considered when evaluating a localized blistering eruption. Among these infections is bullous impetigo (see Chapter 118, Impetigo). When evaluating the extremities, vesiculation overlying cellulitis may be associated with the more severe staphylococcal and streptococcal infections, and a thorough

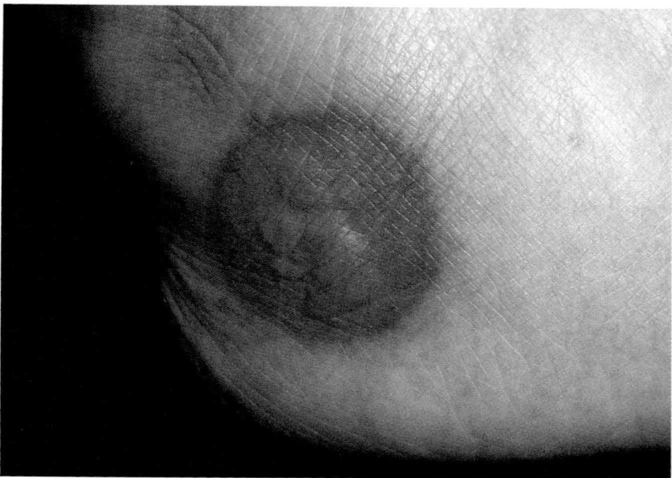

FIGURE 181-14 Bullous fixed-drug eruption on the ankle of a woman taking amoxicillin. She has had this reaction before in the same location while taking another penicillin antibiotic. Note the dusky color, annular erythema and the central bullae. (*Reproduced with permission from Richard P. Usatine, MD.*)

evaluation should be conducted to rule out necrotizing fasciitis. As with most bacterial infections, the patient typically presents with fever and has an elevated white blood cell count.[4]
- Herpes simplex viruses should always be considered when blistering of the mucosal surfaces is observed. Generalized blistering in the adult could be because of disseminated herpes and should prompt an evaluation for immunosuppression. Blistering in a dermatomal distribution is characteristic of herpes zoster (**Figures 181-16** and **181-17**).[4]
- Scabies, tinea, and *Candida* can also have bullous or pustular presentations in the classic sites of involvement.[4]

- Hydrostatic
  - Edema blisters form from the osmotic pressure experienced during the third spacing of fluid. As such, patients usually have a diagnosis of heart failure, cirrhosis, or kidney failure.[1]

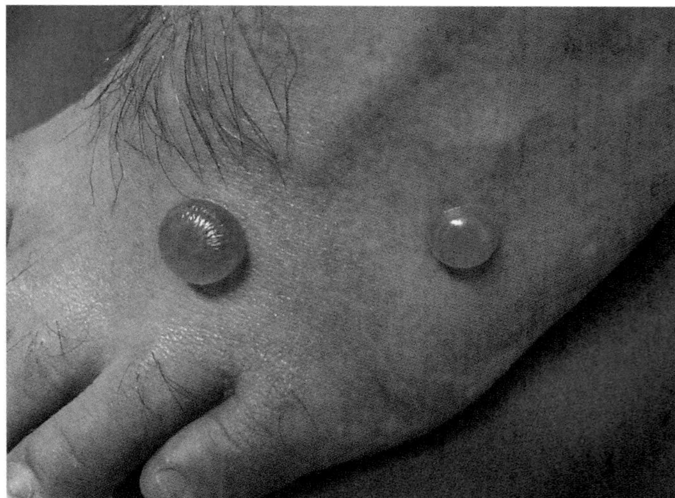

FIGURE 181-15 Bullous arthropod bites secondary to fire ants. (*Reproduced with permission from Lane K, Lumbang W. Pruritic blisters on legs and feet.* J Fam Pract. *2008;57(3):177-180. Reproduced with permission from Frontline Medical Communications.*)

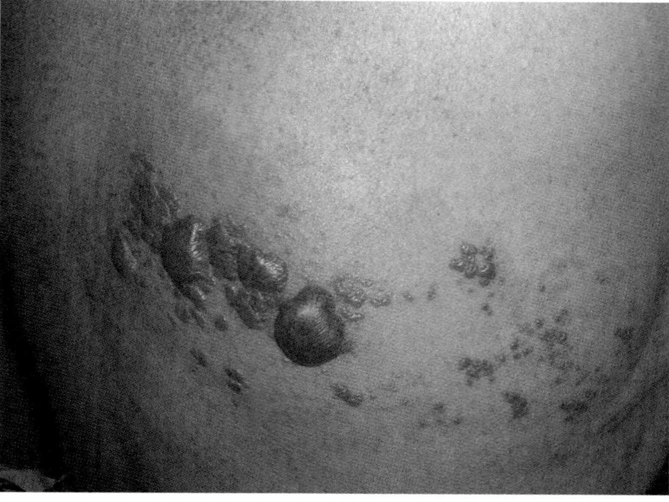

FIGURE 181-16 Herpes zoster with large bulla in a dermatomal pattern. (*Reproduced with permission from Rose Walczak, MD.*)

LABORATORY STUDIES AND WORKUP

If the clinical picture is not clear, various laboratory studies may assist the clinician in making the diagnosis. Some diagnoses should be confirmed by histology even if the diagnosis appears clear. For example, all cases of suspected pemphigus should be biopsied because the management will involve long-term use of potentially toxic medications and it is crucial to know exactly what you are treating. The information in Chapters 182, Bullous Pemphigoid, and 183, Pemphigus, will help you to decide which tests to use in some of the autoimmune blistering diseases. Consulting a dermatologist is very appropriate for many of the more rare and lethal conditions.

- Direct fluorescent antibody test can be done on a scraping of a lesion if herpes simplex or varicella zoster is suspected. In many laboratories, a result can be obtained within 24 hours.
- Mineral oil scraping for scabies (see Chapter 141, Scabies).
- Potassium hydroxide (KOH) scraping for possible blistering tinea infections (such as bullous tinea pedis). (See Section 4: Fungal.)
- Genetic studies for suspected genetic defects; consider referral to geneticist.

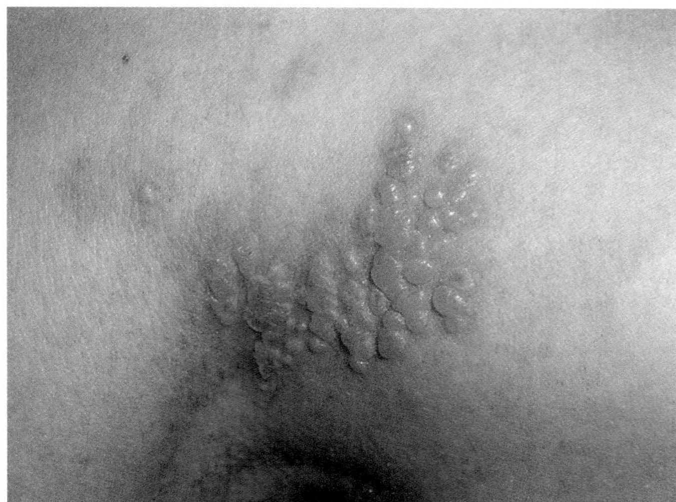

FIGURE 181-17 Cluster of intact bullae and vesicles on an erythematous base in a young woman with herpes zoster in the axilla. (*Reproduced with permission from Richard P. Usatine, MD.*)

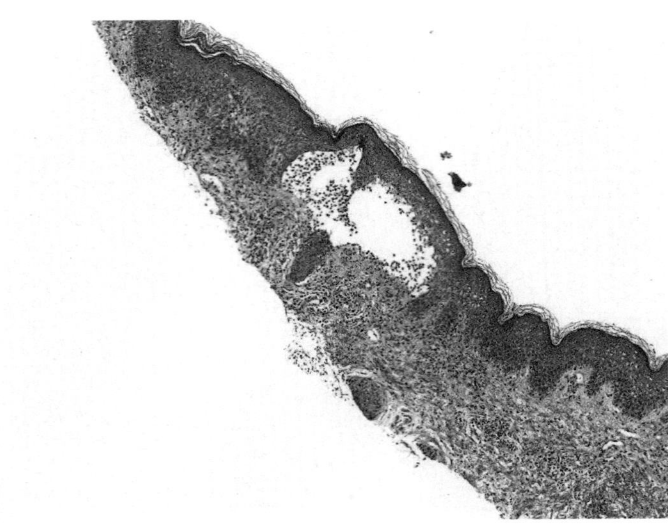

FIGURE 181-18 Histology of bullous pemphigoid with H and E staining under low power done on a shave biopsy of an intact blister. Note the separation of the skin at the dermal-epidermal junction along with eosinophils and neutrophils. (*Reproduced with permission from Richard P. Usatine, MD.*)

BIOPSY

- Biopsy a new established lesion including the edge of the blister. A scoop shave biopsy under an intact blister is an ideal method to get an adequate specimen **(Figure 181-18)**. An alternative is a 4-mm punch biopsy at the edge of the blister making sure that the epidermis stays attached to the specimen.
- Biopsy for direct immunofluorescence (DIF)—Biopsy the perilesional skin and send the specimen in special Michel media or sterile saline and let the laboratory know to transfer it to Michel media when it arrives. The easiest way to do this is to take a shave biopsy that includes the bulla and the perilesional skin. Then cut the specimen in half and send the perilesional skin for DIF and the blister for standard pathology.
- Consider sending part of the biopsy for bacterial, fungal, and viral cultures and stains if infections are suspected and cultures and other less-invasive studies are not providing the diagnosis. Send the specimens in a sterile urine cup on top of a sterile gauze pad soaked with sterile saline.

FURTHER EVALUATIONS

Patients with cicatricial pemphigoid and toxic epidermal necrolysis need an ophthalmologic evaluation. Patients with several of the epidermolysis bullosa diseases and dermatitis herpetiformis need a gastroenterologic evaluation.

For possible paraneoplastic conditions, such as in epidermolysis bullosa acquisita and cicatricial pemphigoid, thorough cancer screening and studies targeting the patient's symptomatology are indicated.

REFERENCES

1. Bolognia JL, Jorizzo JL, Rapini RP. *Dermatology*. London, UK: Elsevier Health Sciences; 2003.
2. Spitz JL. *Genodermatoses: A Clinical Guide to Genetic Skin Disorders*. Philadelphia, PA: Lippincott Williams & Wilkins; 2004.
3. Schachner LA, Hansen RC. *Pediatric Dermatology*. 3rd ed. New York, NY: Mosby; 2003.
4. James WD, Berger TG, Elston DM. *Andrews' Diseases of the Skin: Clinical Dermatology*. 10th ed. Philadelphia, PA: Elsevier Health Sciences; 2005.

182 BULLOUS PEMPHIGOID

Asad K. Mohmand, MD
Richard P. Usatine, MD

PATIENT STORY

A native of Panama was seen for extensive bullous disease that is classic for bullous pemphigoid (BP) (**Figure 182-1**). The presence of numerous intact bullae would make pemphigus very unlikely. The patient was treated with oral prednisone and began to respond quickly. The patient eventually had a good outcome.

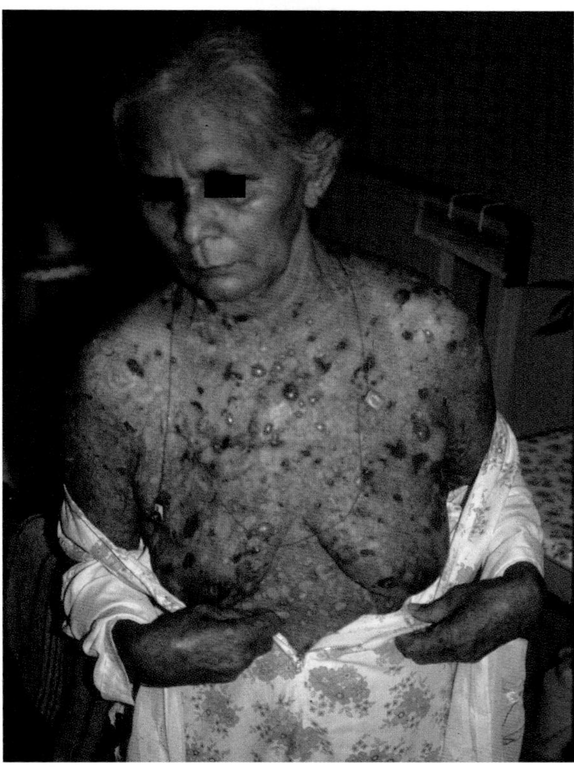

A

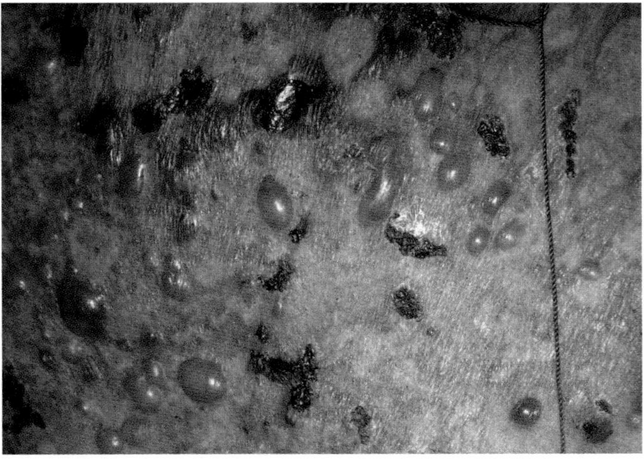

B

FIGURE 182-1 A. Extensive untreated bullous pemphigoid in a Panamanian woman. B. Close-up of intact bulla and dark crusts. (*Reproduced with permission from Eric Kraus, MD.*)

INTRODUCTION

BP is an autoimmune blistering disease of older adults that may cause significant morbidity and a poor quality of life. The term *pemphigoid* refers to its similarity to the blisters seen in pemphigus. However, BP is usually less severe than pemphigus vulgaris and is not considered a life-threatening condition.

EPIDEMIOLOGY

- BP is the most frequent autoimmune blistering disease of the skin (and mucosa).
- It typically affects persons older than 65 years of age but can occur at any age.
- There is no racial or gender predilection (a recent British population study, however, suggested an increased prevalence in women).[1]
- Its incidence may be on the rise.[1]
- Although it is not considered life threatening, it has been associated with an increased risk of mortality (hazard ratio [HR] 2.3, 95% confidence interval [CI] 2-2.7).[1]

ETIOLOGY AND PATHOPHYSIOLOGY

- BP is a chronic autoimmune disorder of the skin.
- Immunoglobulin G (IgG) autoantibodies against BP180 antigen of the basement membrane protein are considered pathognomonic and can be found in up to 65% of patients.[2]
- Anti-BP230 antibodies are present in virtually all patients but are not considered pathognomonic.[3]
- Binding of antibodies to the basement membrane activates the complement system, leading to chemotaxis of inflammatory cells (eosinophils and mast cells), which release proteases. The subsequent degradation of hemidesmosomal proteins leads to blister formation.
- There are several morphologically distinct clinical presentations:
    - Generalized bullous form is the most common (see **Figure 182-1**). Tense bullae occur on both erythematous and normal-appearing skin surfaces. The bullae usually heal without scarring.
    - Localized form of BP is less common and is limited to a small area of involvement (**Figure 182-2**).
    - Vesicular (also known as "eczematous") form is characterized by clusters of small tense blisters with an urticarial or erythematous base.
    - Other forms are less common and include vegetative (intertriginous vegetating plaques), urticarial (without any bullae), nodular (resembling prurigo nodularis), acral (bullae on palms, soles, and face in children associated with vaccination), and generalized erythroderma (exfoliative lesions with or without vesicles/bullae).
- Pemphigoid gestationis is a variant of BP that occurs during or after pregnancy. Lesions resolve after delivery, but may recur with subsequent pregnancies, or in the nonpregnant state.[4]
- Drug-induced BP has been reported with drugs containing sulfhydryl groups, including penicillamine, furosemide, captopril, and sulfasalazine.

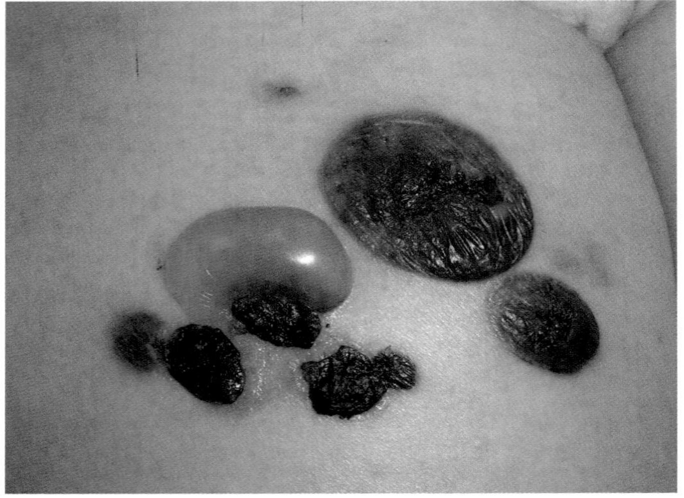

A

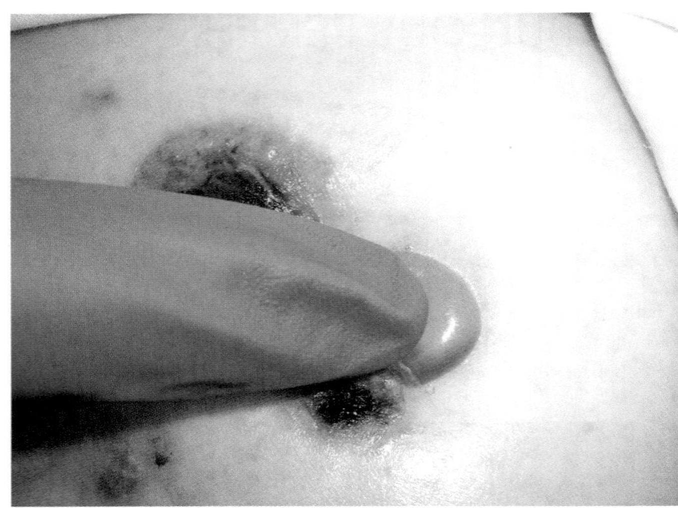

B

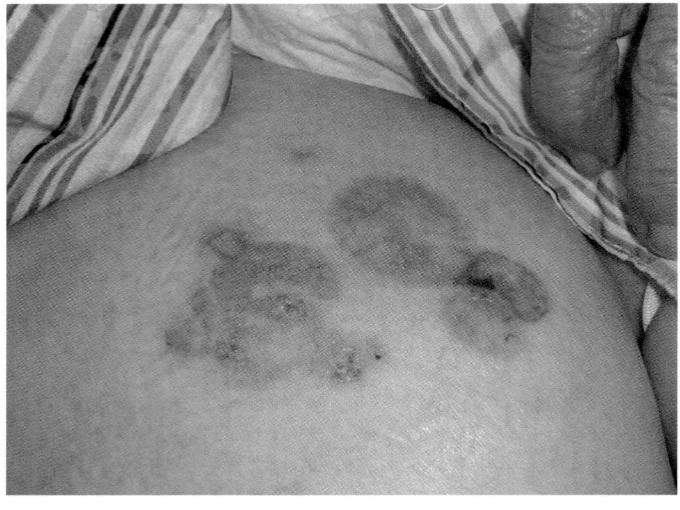

C

FIGURE 182-2 Localized bullous pemphigoid with large bulla on the thigh of this 91-year-old woman. Her biopsy for direct immunofluorescence demonstrated a linear band of IgG at the dermal–epidermal junction. A. Bullae on the thigh. B. One week later there is a new bulla and the Asboe-Hansen sign is negative. C. One week later the bullae are healing as the bullous pemphigoid is being treated with clobetasol topically and the patient is taking doxycycline and niacin orally. (Reproduced with permission from Richard P. Usatine, MD.)

DIAGNOSIS

CLINICAL FEATURES

- Tense blisters that involve normal or inflamed skin or mucous membranes (see **Figures 182-1** and **182-2**).
- Development of bullae is typically preceded by a prodromal phase characterized by intense pruritus with or without excoriations and eczematous (or urticarial) lesions. This phase can last for months, making early diagnosis difficult.[5]
- Nikolsky sign (wrinkling and sheet-like peeling of the skin when lateral pressure is applied to unblistered skin) is usually negative.[6] Asboe-Hansen sign will be negative too. Bulla will not extend to surrounding skin when vertical pressure is applied (see **Figure 182-2B**).

TYPICAL DISTRIBUTION

- Flexure surfaces of the arms and legs.
- Lower abdomen and groin.
- Mucous membranes are involved in 10% to 25% of cases.

BIOPSY

Biopsy is required for establishing diagnosis and to differentiate BP from other conditions that can have a similar clinical presentation.

- A scoop shave or 4-mm punch biopsy from edge of an early blister including part of the normal-appearing skin for H and E staining shows

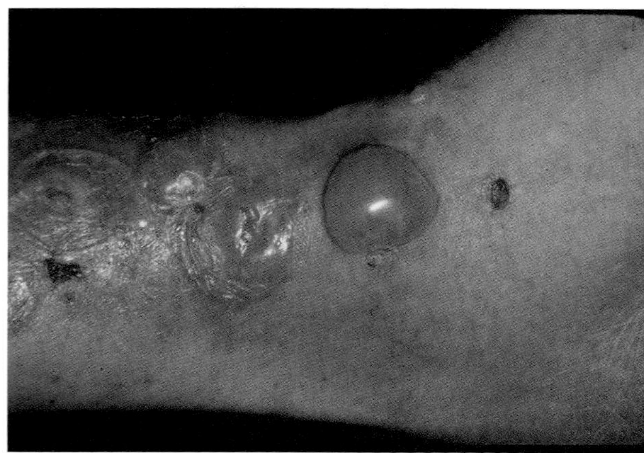

FIGURE 182-3 Localized bullous pemphigoid on the lower leg of an elderly man. *(Reproduced with permission from Eric Kraus, MD.)*

a subepidermal blister and an eosinophil-rich mixed dermal inflammatory infiltrate. If the scoop shave contains sufficient perilesional skin, cut this off and send it for direct immunofluorescence (DIF).

- The skin from the scoop shave or a second 4-mm punch biopsy from perilesional skin, transported in Michel medium for DIF. If Michel transport medium is not available, send the specimen for DIF in sterile saline-soaked gauze and alert the laboratory to transfer the specimen into Michel medium as soon as possible. DIF demonstrates linear IgG and/or complement C3 deposits at the dermal–epidermal junction.
- Alternatively, an enzyme-linked immunosorbent assay (ELISA) blood test for BP180 antibodies (and if negative, then ELISA for BP230 antibodies) can be performed for characterization of circulating antibodies.[7]

DIFFERENTIAL DIAGNOSIS

- Cicatricial pemphigoid (**Figures 182-4** to **182-6**)—Predominant mucosal involvement; lesions heal with prominent scarring; IgG localizes to blister floor on indirect immunofluorescence (IDIF).
- Dermatitis herpetiformis—Grouped vesicles; extensor distribution (see Chapter 184, Other Bullous Diseases).
- Epidermolysis bullosa acquisita—IgG localizes to blister floor on IDIF (see Chapter 184, Other Bullous Diseases).
- Erythema multiforme—Targetoid lesions; linear IgG immunofluorescence is negative (see Chapter 175, Erythema Multiforme, Stevens-Johnson Syndrome, and Toxic Epidermal Necrolysis).
- Linear IgA dermatosis—Usually drug induced (eg, vancomycin[8]); DIF demonstrates IgA deposits.

MANAGEMENT

The objectives of therapy in BP are to decrease the troublesome symptoms associated with the blistering lesions, resolve active lesions, and prevent recurrences.

- High-potency topical corticosteroids are considered first-line treatment for moderate-to-severe generalized disease (eg, clobetasol).[9] SOR Ⓐ Initial disease control and 1-year survival rates in extensive BP are better with topical approach when compared with oral prednisolone.[10]

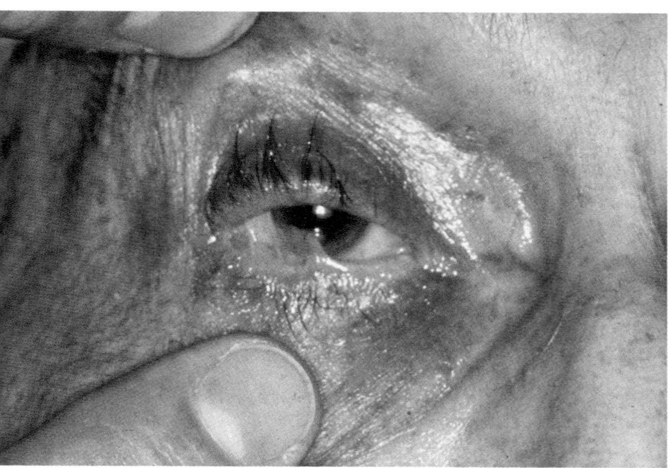

FIGURE 182-5 Cicatricial bullous pemphigoid with scarring connecting the lower lid to the cornea. (*Reproduced with permission from Eric Kraus, MD.*)

- Oral corticosteroids.[9] SOR Ⓐ
- Prednisone 0.5 to 0.75 mg/kg/d.[11]
- Increase dose until new blisters cease to develop.
- Reduce dose approximately 10% every 2 to 3 weeks to reach dose of 15 to 20 mg/d.
- Adjuvant antibiotic treatment should be considered for all patients:
    - Tetracycline (1.5-2 g/d) with or without niacinamide (1.5-2 g/d).[12] SOR Ⓑ Both tetracycline and niacinamide come in 500-mg capsules and may be taken 3 to 4 times daily. Niacinamide contains niacin (vitamin B_3) and is available over the counter. If tetracycline is not available, doxycycline 100 mg twice daily is an alternative.
    - Steroid-sparing drugs and adjuvant therapy for patients whose disease is not controlled with steroids and tetracycline:
    - Dapsone is an antineutrophilic antibiotic that is an alternative to tetracycline and doxycyline (**Figure 182-7**). Azathioprine 50 to 200 mg divided bid or tid (first-line adjuvant).[9] SOR Ⓑ
    - Mycophenolate mofetil 0.5 to 2 g/d divided bid or tid (less hepatotoxic than azathioprine).[13] SOR Ⓒ
    - Cyclophosphamide 1 to 5 mg/kg/d. SOR Ⓒ

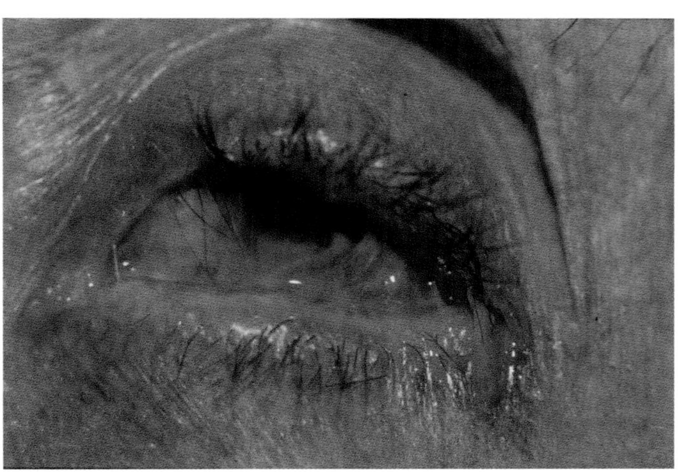

FIGURE 182-4 Cicatricial bullous pemphigoid of the eye, causing scarring and blindness. (*Reproduced with permission from Eric Kraus, MD.*)

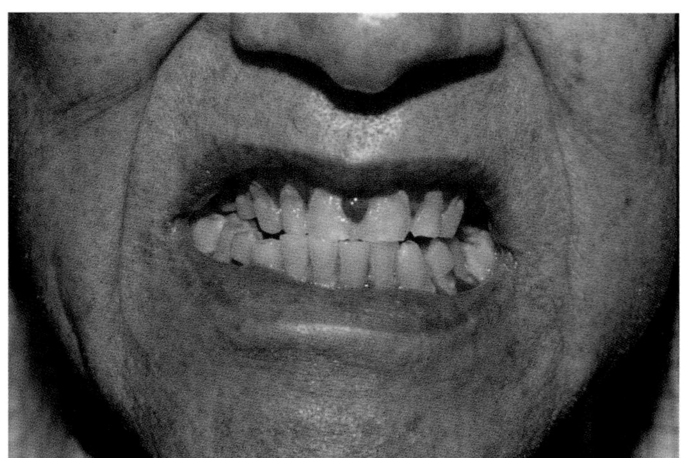

FIGURE 182-6 Cicatricial bullous pemphigoid of the mouth showing gingivitis. More than 50% of cases of BP have oral involvement. (*Reproduced with permission from Eric Kraus, MD.*)

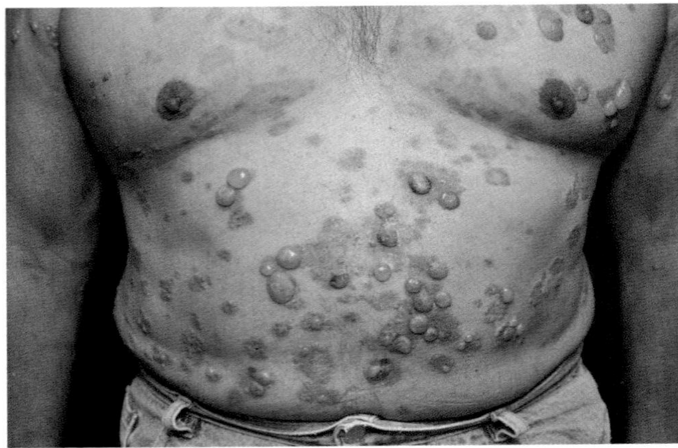

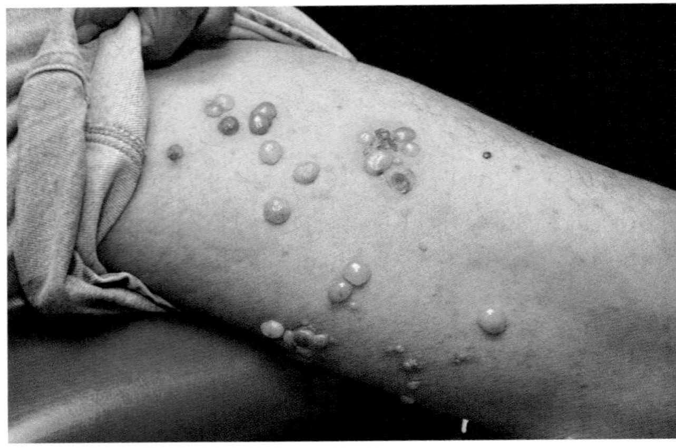

FIGURE 182-7 New-onset bullous pemphigoid in a 65-year-old man with previous psoriasis. His bullous pemphigoid is currently controlled with dapsone. **A.** Bullae on abdomen with some psoriatic plaques visible. **B.** Tense bullae on leg. *(Reproduced with permission from Richard P. Usatine, MD.)*

- Disease resistant to combination of corticosteroids and steroid-sparing agents include the following:
  - Intravenous immunoglobulin (IVIG) can produce a rapid and dramatic but very transient response; requires multiple cycles of IVIG. SOR C
  - Plasmapheresis can be considered for patients with severe resistant disease requiring high doses of systemic steroids to improve symptoms and reduce steroid dose.[14] SOR C
  - Case reports and small series of successful therapy of refractory BP with rituximab,[15] etanercept,[16] or omalizumab[17] have been published in the recent medical literature.
- Consultations include the following:
  - Dermatology consultation for recommending therapy based on extent of disease and for changes in therapy when required.
  - Nutrition consultation if patient is having difficulty maintaining weight.

FOLLOW-UP

- Ask patient about recurrent lesions, pruritus, and side effects from treatment.
- Perform periodic skin examinations looking for new lesions to adjust dose of prednisone and to monitor for lymphadenopathy and skin cancer in patients using immunosuppressive medications.

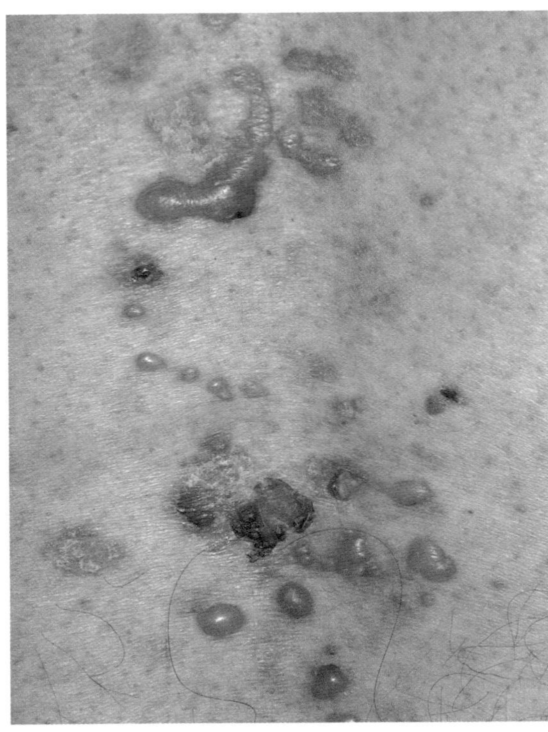

FIGURE 182-8 Recurrent bullous pemphigoid on the back of a 57-year-old man who ran out of his prednisone for a few days. *(Reproduced with permission from Richard P. Usatine, MD.)*

- Monitor for drug-specific laboratory abnormalities (eg, glucose and triglycerides with steroid use; complete blood count [CBC], renal function, and liver function tests for azathioprine).
- Make sure patients do not run out of their medications because this can result in recurrent lesions (**Figure 182-8**).
- Adjust treatment if patient relapses (eg, increase steroid dose or add an immunosuppressive agent).
- Taper steroids slowly (as above) after dissipation of disease flare.

PATIENT EDUCATION

- Avoid mechanical irritation, direct sun exposure, dental prostheses, extremes of temperature.
- Recommend high-protein, low-carbohydrate, and low-fat diet; calcium and vitamin D supplementation for patients on corticosteroids.
- Provide information on wound care, stress reduction, appropriate exercise, and side effects of medications.

PATIENT RESOURCES

- Patient.co.uk. *Bullous Pemphigoid*—**http://www.patient.co.uk/showdoc/23069059/.**
- International Pemphigus & Pemphigoid Foundation—**http://www.pemphigus.org/wordpress/diseases/pemphigoid/.**

PROVIDER RESOURCES

- eMedicine. *Bullous Pemphigoid*—**http://emedicine.medscape.com/article/1062391.**

REFERENCES

1. Langan SM, Smeeth L, Hubbard R, et al. Bullous pemphigoid and pemphigus vulgaris—incidence and mortality in the UK: population based cohort study. *BMJ*. 2008;337:a180.
2. Zillikens D, Rose PA, Balding SD, et al. Tight clustering of extracellular BP180 epitopes recognized by bullous pemphigoid autoantibodies. *J Invest Dermatol.* 1997;109:573-579.
3. Yancey KB, Egan CA. Pemphigoid: clinical, histologic, immunopathologic, and therapeutic considerations. *JAMA.* 2000;284:350-356.
4. Kroumpouzos G, Cohen LM. Specific dermatoses of pregnancy: an evidence-based systematic review. *Am J Obstet Gynecol.* 2003;188(4):1083-1092.
5. Bingham EA, Burrows D, Sandford JC. Prolonged pruritus and bullous pemphigoid. *Clin Exp Dermatol.* 1984;9:564-570.
6. Habif TP. *Clinical Dermatology: A Color Guide to Diagnosis and Therapy*. 4th ed. St. Louis, MO: Mosby; 2004.
7. Schmidt E, Zillikens D. Modern diagnosis of auto-immune blistering skin diseases. *Autoimmun Rev.* 2010;10:84-89.
8. Kuechle MK, Stegemeir E, Maynard B, Gibson LE. Drug-induced linear IgA bullous dermatosis: report of six cases and review of the literature. *J Am Acad Dermatol.* 1994;30:187-192.
9. Khumalo N, Kirtschig G, Middleton P, et al. Interventions for bullous pemphigoid. *Cochrane Database Syst Rev.* 2003;(3):CD002292.
10. Joly P, Roujeau JC, Benichou J, et al. A comparison of oral and topical corticosteroids in patients with bullous pemphigoid. *N Engl J Med.* 2002;346:321-327.
11. Kirtschig G, Middleton P, Bennett C, et al. Interventions for bullous pemphigoid. *Cochrane Database Syst Rev.* 2010;(10):CD002292.
12. Fivenson DP, Breneman DL, Rosen GB, et al. Nicotinamide and tetracycline therapy of bullous pemphigoid. *Arch Dermatol.* 1994;130(6):753-758.
13. Böhm M, Beissert S, Schwarz T, et al. Bullous pemphigoid treated with mycophenolate mofetil. *Lancet.* 1997;349(9051):541.
14. Mazzi G, Raineri A, Zanolli FA, et al. Plasmapheresis therapy in pemphigus vulgaris and bullous pemphigoid. *Transfus Apher Sci.* 2003;28(1):13-18.
15. Kasperkiewicz M, Shimanovich I, Ludwig RJ, et al. Rituximab for treatment-refractory pemphigus and pemphigoid: a case series of 17 patients. *J Am Acad Dermatol.* 2011;65(3):552-558.
16. Cusano F, Iannazzone SS, Riccio G, Piccirillo F. Coexisting bullous pemphigoid and psoriasis successfully treated with etanercept. *Eur J Dermatol.* 2010;20(4):520.
17. Fairley JA, Baum CL, Brandt DS, Messingham KA. Pathogenicity of IgE in autoimmunity: successful treatment of bullous pemphigoid with omalizumab. *J Allergy Clin Immunol.* 2009;123(3):704-705.

183 PEMPHIGUS

Richard P. Usatine, MD
Shashi Mittal, MD

PATIENT STORY

A young man presented with painful blisters on his face and mouth (**Figure 183-1**). The patient was referred to dermatology that day. The dermatologist recognized likely pemphigus vulgaris (PV) and did shave biopsies for histopathology and direct immunofluorescence of facial vesicles/bullae to confirm the presumed diagnosis. The patient was started on 60 mg of prednisone daily until the pathology confirmed PV. Steroid-sparing therapy was then discussed and started in 2 weeks from presentation.

INTRODUCTION

Pemphigus is a rare group of autoimmune bullous diseases of skin and mucous membranes characterized by flaccid bulla and erosions. The 3 main types of pemphigus are PV (with the pemphigus vegetans variant), pemphigus foliaceous (with the pemphigus erythematosus variant), and paraneoplastic pemphigus. All types of pemphigus cause significant morbidity and mortality. Although pemphigus is not curable, it can be controlled with systemic steroids and immunosuppressive medications. These medications can be lifesaving, but also place pemphigus patients at risk for a number of complications. The word *pemphigus* is derived from the Greek word *pemphix,* which means bubble or blister.

EPIDEMIOLOGY

Epidemiology of the 3 major types of pemphigus is as follows:

- PV (**Figures 183-1** to **183-4**)
  - Most common form of pemphigus is in the United States.
  - Annual incidence is 0.75 to 5 cases per 1 million population.[1]
  - Usually occurs between 30 and 50 years of age.[2]
  - Increased incidence in Ashkenazi Jews and persons of Mediterranean origin.[2]
  - Pemphigus vegetans is a variant form of PV (**Figures 183-5** and **183-6**).
- Pemphigus foliaceus (PF) (**Figures 183-7** to **183-10**) is a superficial form of pemphigus.
  - More prevalent in Africa (**Figures 183-11** and **183-12**).[1]
  - Variant forms include pemphigus erythematosus (resembles the malar rash of lupus erythematosus) and fogo selvagem.
  - Fogo selvagem is an endemic form of PF seen in Brazil and affects teenagers and individuals in their twenties.[1]

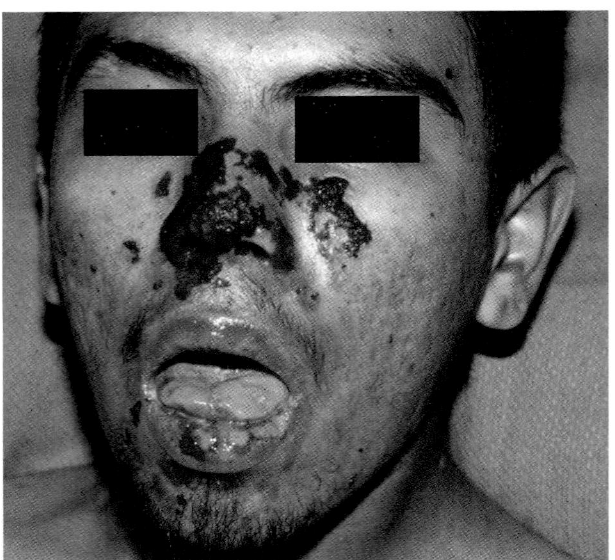

FIGURE 183-1 Pemphigus vulgaris on the face of a young man with mouth involvement. (*Reproduced with permission from Eric Kraus, MD.*)

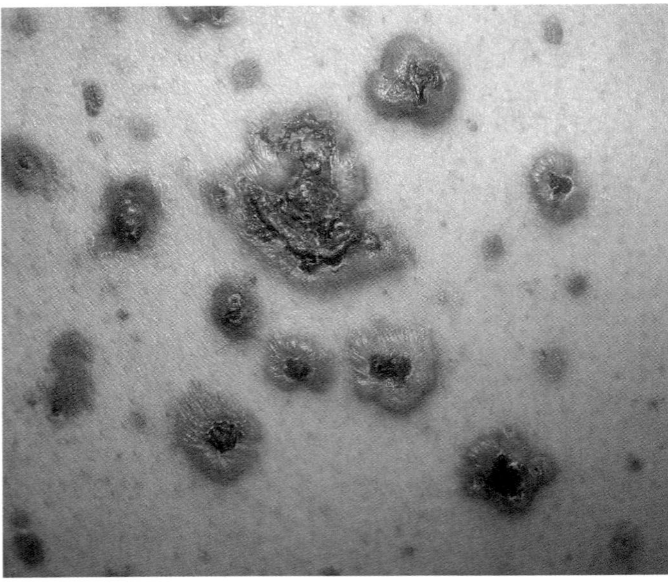

FIGURE 183-2 Pemphigus vulgaris on the back with crusted and intact bullae. Downward pressure on a bulla demonstrates a positive Asboe-Hansen sign with lateral spread of fresh bullae. (*Reproduced with permission from Eric Kraus, MD.*)

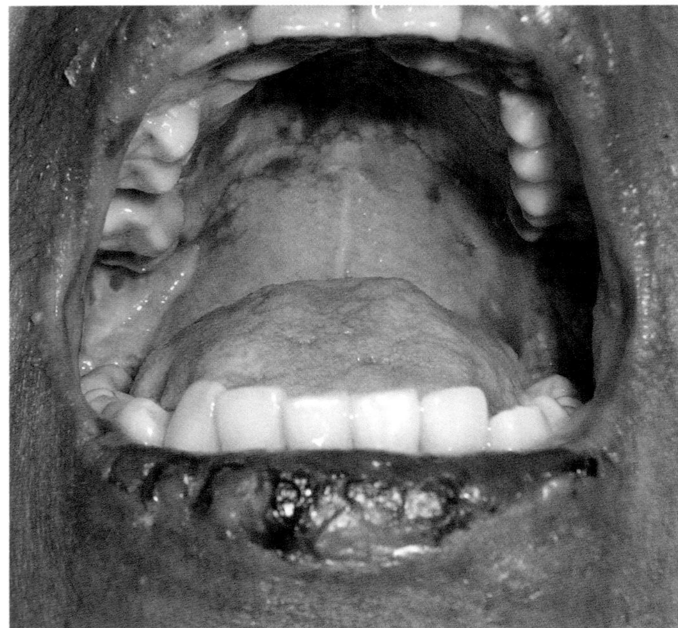

FIGURE 183-3 Pemphigus vulgaris involving the lips and palate of a 55-year-old woman. (*Reproduced with permission from Dan Shaked, MD.*)

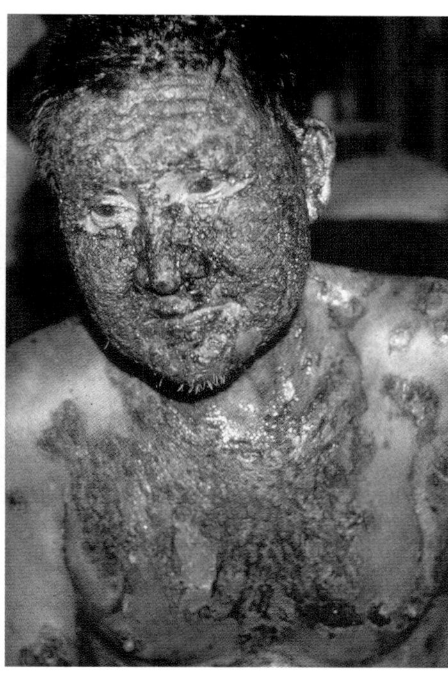

FIGURE 183-4 Severe fatal pemphigus vulgaris. (*Reproduced with permission from Eric Kraus, MD.*)

- Paraneoplastic pemphigus (PNP)
  - Onset at age 60 years and older.
  - Associated with occult neoplasms commonly lymphoreticular.
  - Malignancies like non-Hodgkin lymphoma and chronic lymphocytic leukemia.
  - Also associated with benign neoplasms such as thymoma and Castleman disease (angiofollicular lymph node hyperplasia).[2]

ETIOLOGY AND PATHOPHYSIOLOGY

- The basic abnormality in all 3 types of pemphigus is acantholysis, a process of separating keratinocytes from one another. This occurs as a result of autoantibody formation against desmoglein (the adhesive molecule that holds epidermal cells together). Separation of epidermal cells leads to formation of intraepidermal clefts, which enlarge to form bullae.[1]

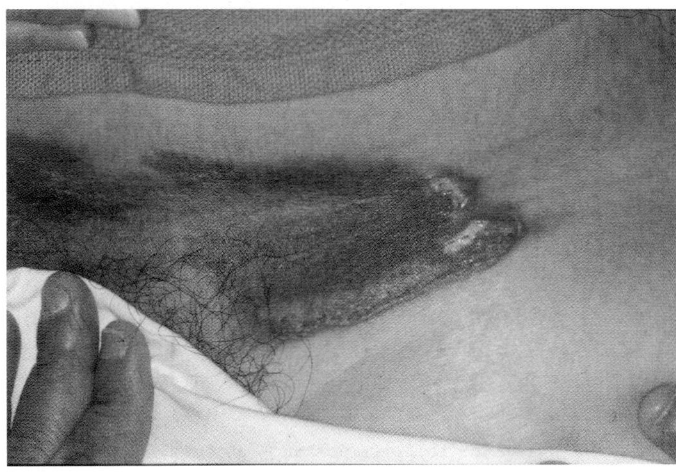

FIGURE 183-5 Pemphigus vegetans in the groin of a middle-aged woman. (*Reproduced with permission from Eric Kraus, MD.*)

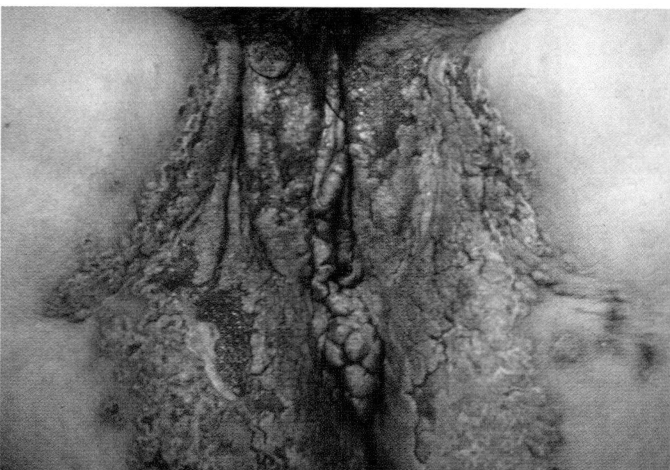

FIGURE 183-6 Pemphigus vegetans widespread over the external genitalia and buttocks. (*Reproduced with permission from Eric Kraus, MD.*)

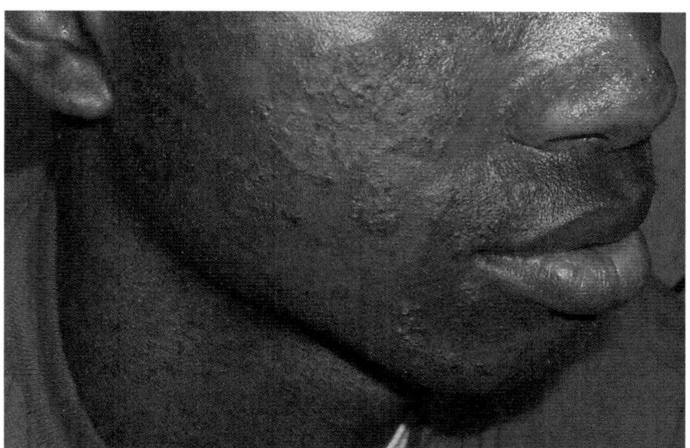

FIGURE 183-7 Pemphigus foliaceous on the face of a black man. (*Reproduced with permission from Jack Resneck Sr, MD.*)

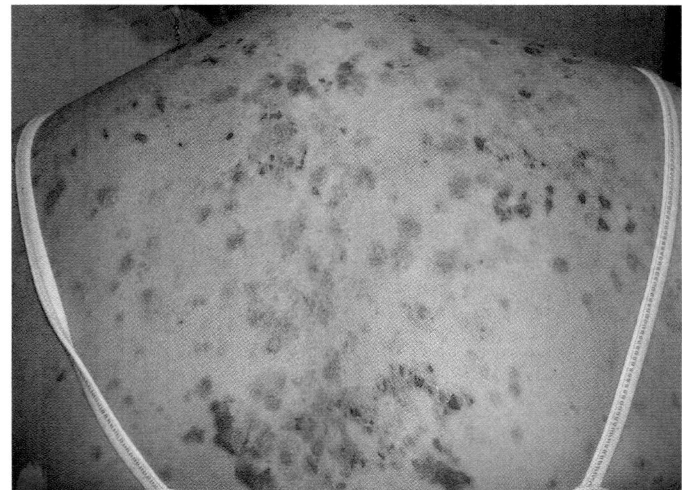

FIGURE 183-8 Pemphigus foliaceous on the back of a 55-year-old Hispanic woman. Note the absence of bulla and the corn flake crusting from the superficial erosions. (*Reproduced with permission from Richard P. Usatine, MD.*)

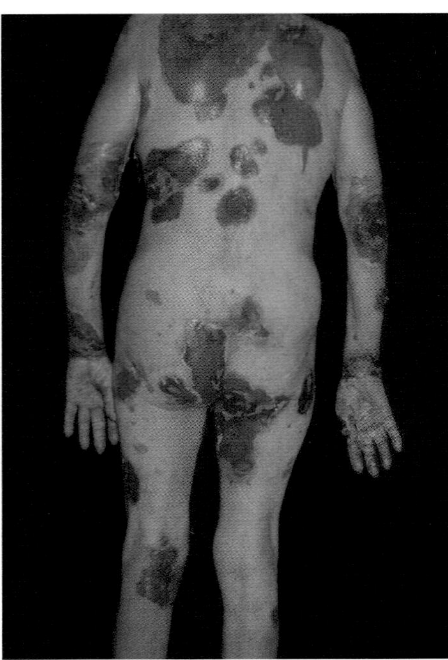

FIGURE 183-9 Pemphigus foliaceous with large erosions on the back and extremities of this patient. (*Reproduced with permission from Eric Kraus, MD.*)

- The mechanism that induces the production of these autoantibodies in most individuals is unknown. Yet PF may be triggered by drugs, most commonly thiol compounds like penicillamine, captopril, piroxicam, and others, like penicillin and imiquimod.[3] An environmental trigger in the presence of susceptible human leukocyte antigen (HLA) gene is suggested to induce autoantibodies in fogo selvagum.[1]

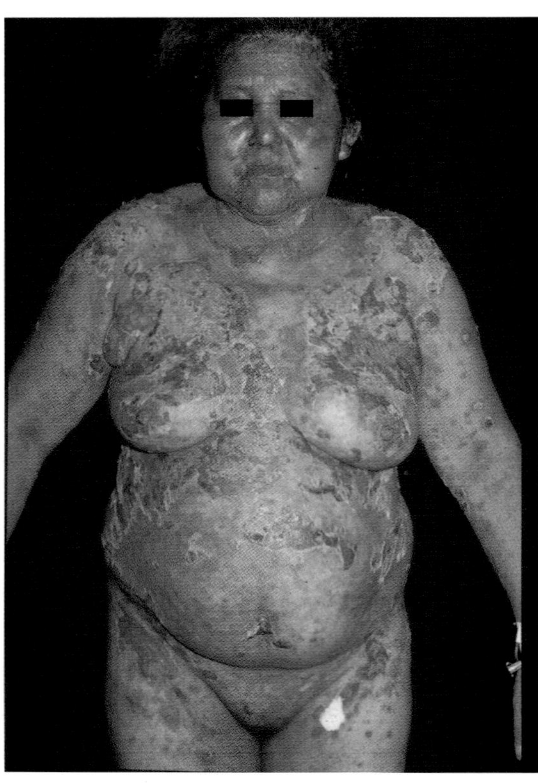

FIGURE 183-10 Widespread pemphigus foliaceous. (*Reproduced with permission from Eric Kraus, MD.*)

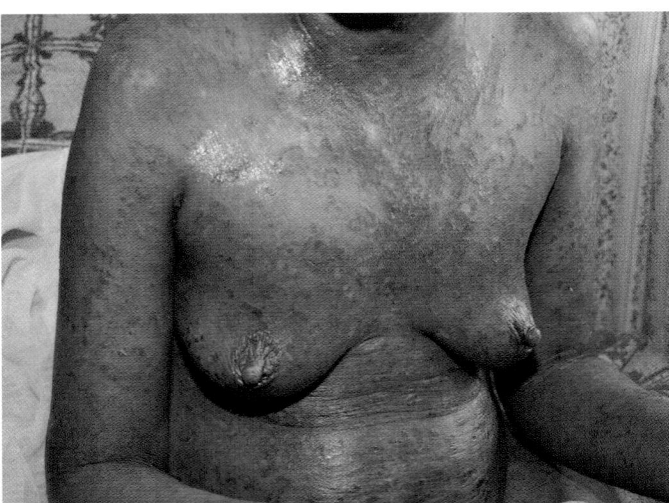

FIGURE 183-11 Pemphigus foliaceous on the trunk and arms of a woman in Africa. Some of the lesions appear annular but they are all superficial erosions within the epidermis. (*Reproduced with permission from Richard P. Usatine, MD.*)

- The autoantibodies in pemphigus are usually directed against desmoglein 1 and 3 molecules (Dsg1 and Dsg3). Dsg1 is present predominantly in the superficial layers of the epidermis, whereas Dsg3 is expressed in deeper epidermal layers and in mucous membranes. As a result, clinical presentation depends on the antibody profile. In PV, a limited mucosal disease occurs when only anti-Dsg3 antibody is present, but extensive mucosal and cutaneous disease occurs when both anti-Dsg1 and Dsg3 antibodies are present. In PF, mucosal lesions are absent and the cutaneous lesions are superficial because of isolated anti-Dsg1 antibody.
- Patients with PNP demonstrate both anti-Dsg1 and Dsg3 antibodies. However, unlike PV, autoantibodies against plakin proteins (another adhesive molecule) are also observed in patients with PNP and these autoantibodies form a reliable marker for this type of pemphigus.

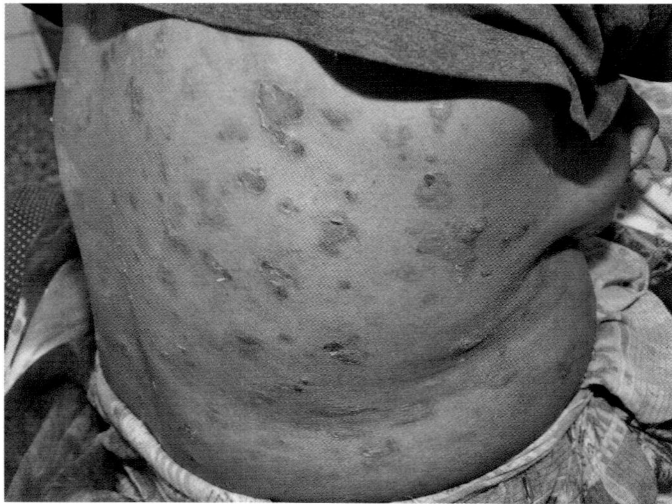

FIGURE 183-12 Another case of pemphigus foliaceous in Africa. Pemphigus foliaceous is more prevalent in Africa. Note the hyperpigmentation of the healing lesions after treatment has begun. (*Reproduced with permission from Richard P. Usatine, MD.*)

DIAGNOSIS

CLINICAL FEATURES

- Pemphigus vulgaris (see **Figures 183-1** to **183-4**)—Classical lesions are flaccid bullae that rupture easily, creating erosions. Since bullae are short lived, erosions are the more common presenting physical finding (**Figure 183-13**). Lesions are typically tender and heal with postinflammatory hyperpigmentation that resolves without scarring. A positive Asboe-Hansen or Nikolsky sign may be present, but neither sign is diagnostic. A positive Asboe-Hansen sign occurs when a bulla extends to surrounding skin while pressure is applied directly to the bulla. The Nikolsky sign is positive when skin shears off while lateral pressure is applied to unblistered skin during active disease. Sometimes the Asboe-Hansen sign is also attributed to Nikolsky and called a Nikolsky sign, too.
- Pemphigus vegetans is a variant of PV where healing is associated with vegetating proliferation of the epidermis (see **Figures 183-5** and **183-6**).
- Pemphigus foliaceous: Multiple red, scaling, crusted, and pruritic lesions described as "corn flakes" are seen. Shallow erosions arise when crusts are removed, but intact blisters are rare as the disease is superficial (see **Figures 183-7** to **183-12**).
- PNP (**Figure 183-14**)—Lesions are similar to PV, although lichen planus, morbilliform, or erythema multiforme-like lesions also may be seen in addition to blisters and erosions. Another distinctive feature is the presence of epithelial necrosis and lichenoid changes in the lesions. Pulmonary involvement secondary to acantholysis of bronchial mucosa is seen in 30% to 40% of cases of PNP.

TYPICAL DISTRIBUTION

- PV—Common mucosal site is oral mucosa, although any stratified squamous epithelium may be involved. Mucosal lesions may be followed by skin lesions after weeks to months usually on scalp, face, and upper torso. PV should be suspected if an oral ulcer persists beyond a month (**Figures 183-1**, **183-3**, and **183-15**).
- Pemphigus vegetans—Usually seen in intertriginous areas like the axilla, groin, and genital region (see **Figures 183-5** and **183-6**).

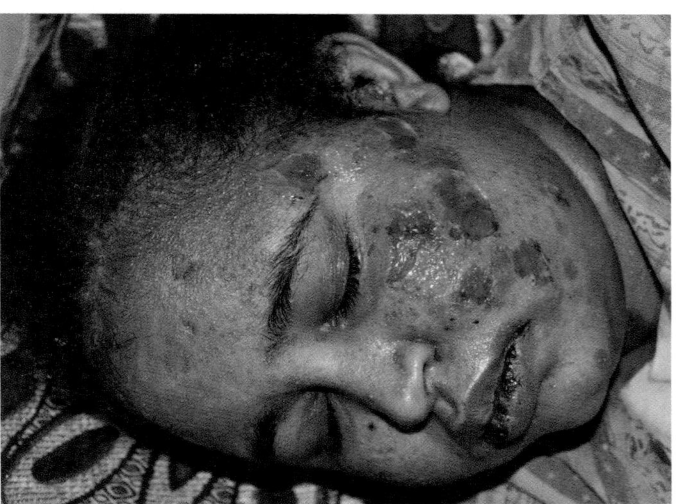

FIGURE 183-13 Pemphigus vulgaris involving the face and oral mucosa. The erosions are deeper than those seen in pemphigus foliaceous. The oral involvement points to pemphigus vulgaris. *(Reproduced with permission from Richard P. Usatine, MD.)*

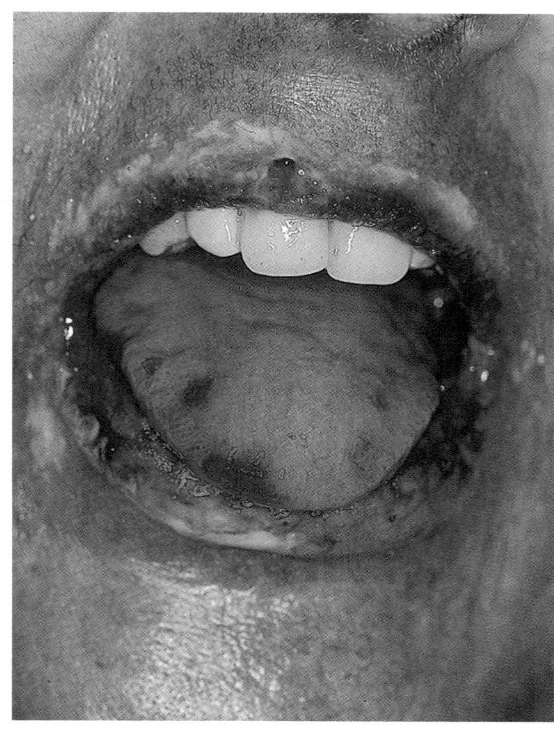

FIGURE 183-14 Paraneoplastic pemphigus with severe erosions covering practically the entire mucosa of the oral cavity with partial sparing of the dorsum of the tongue. Lesions are extremely painful, interfering with adequate food intake. This patient had non-Hodgkin lymphoma as the underlying malignancy. *(Reproduced with permission from Wolff K, Johnson RA. Fitzpatrick's Color Atlas & Synopsis of Clinical Dermatology. 6th ed. New York, NY: McGraw-Hill; 2009, Figure18-19.)*

- PF—Initially affects face and scalp, though may progress to involve chest and back (see **Figures 183-7** to **183-12**). When the facial involvement in PF is in a lupus-like pattern, this is called pemphigus erythematosus (**Figure 183-16**).
- PNP—Common sites include oral mucosa and conjunctiva. (see **Figure 183-14**) Columnar and transitional epithelia may also be involved besides stratified squamous epithelium.

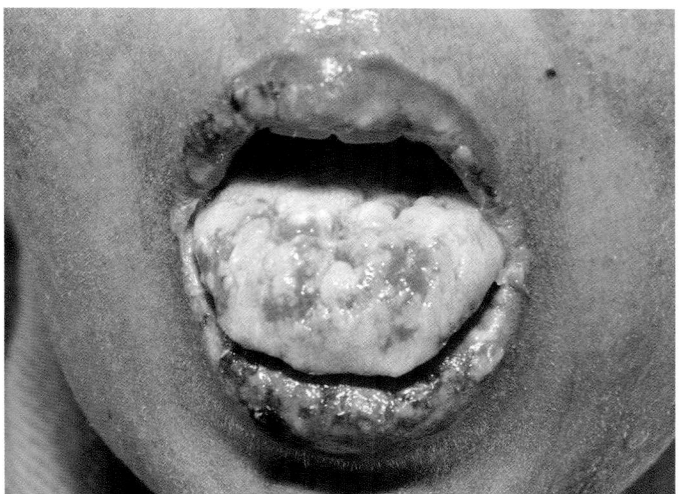

FIGURE 183-15 Pemphigus vulgaris involving the tongue and lips of a young woman. This is severely painful, making it difficult to eat or drink. *(Reproduced with permission from Richard P. Usatine, MD.)*

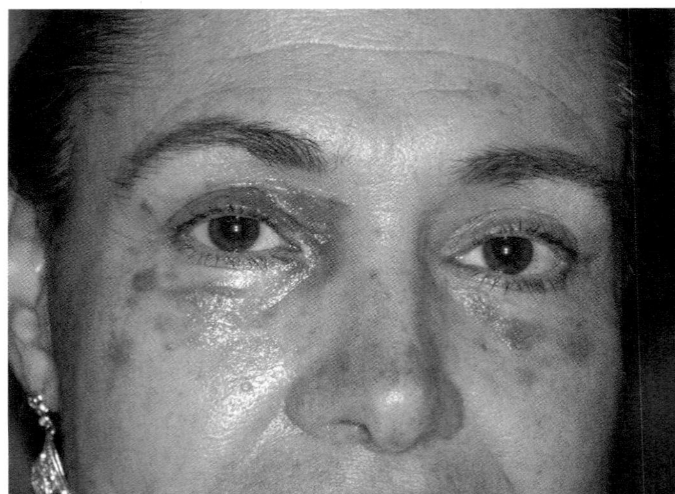

FIGURE 183-16 Pemphigus erythematosus creating a lupus-like pattern of facial involvement. Note how the pemphigus foliaceous lesions involve the malar areas bilaterally. (*Reproduced with permission from Richard P. Usatine, MD.*)

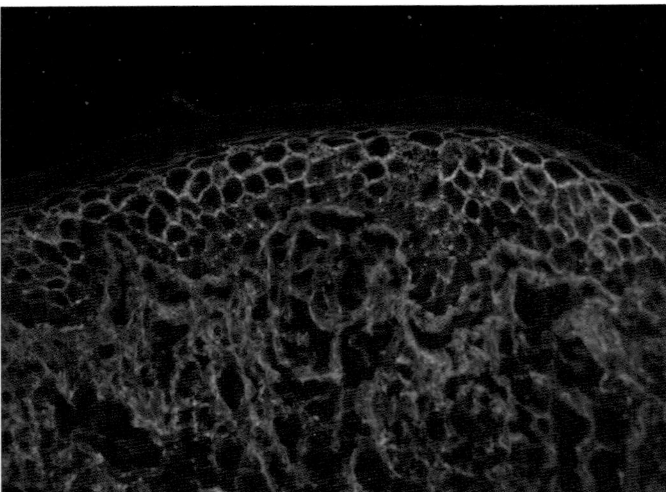

FIGURE 183-17 Direct immunofluorescence against immunoglobulin (Ig) G antibodies surrounding cells of the epidermis in a patient with pemphigus vulgaris. Note the chicken-wire appearance. (*Reproduced with permission from Martin Fernandez, MD, and Richard P. Usatine, MD.*)

LABORATORY STUDIES

- Circulating desmoglein antibodies' levels may be measured in the blood using indirect immunofluorescence. This is usually not necessary unless the diagnosis is in question and further data are needed.
- Complete blood count and a comprehensive metabolic profile including liver function tests, creatinine, and glucose will be needed as a baseline, as all the systemic therapies have significant toxicities.
- Patients at risk for steroid-induced osteoporosis should have a dual-energy X-ray absorptiometry (DEXA) scan performed.

BIOPSY

Skin biopsy is essential for accurate diagnosis. The depth of acantholysis and site of deposition of antibody complexes help differentiate pemphigus from other bullous diseases. Two specimens should be sent. Perform a shave of the edge of the bulla to include the surrounding normal-appearing epidermis. This biopsy should be of the freshest lesion with an intact bulla, if possible. Cut the specimen in half and send the portion with the bulla in formalin for routine histopathology. The second half should be perilesional adjacent normal skin. This is sent on a gauze pad soaked in normal saline or Michel solution for direct immunofluorescence (DIF). Routine histopathology demonstrates suprabasal acantholysis and DIF shows antibody deposition in the intercellular spaces of the epidermis. The pattern of the DIF fluorescence is described as chicken wire (**Figure 183-17**).

DIFFERENTIAL DIAGNOSIS

- Bullous pemphigoid—Bullae are tense because they occur in the deeper subepidermal layer. Mucous membrane involvement is rare. Biopsy illustrates subepidermal acantholysis and immunoglobulin deposition along the basement membrane (see Chapter 182, Bullous Pemphigoid).[3]
- Cicatricial pemphigoid—Also known as mucous membrane pemphigoid. Usually affects oral mucosa and conjunctiva. Lesions heal with scarring, which results in irreversible sequelae such as blindness, subglottic stenosis, and esophageal strictures.[3] Histology demonstrates antibody complexes in the basement membrane with submucosal infiltrate and prominent fibroblast proliferation (see Chapter 182, Bullous Pemphigoid).
- Dermatitis herpetiformis—Herpes-like lesions in the form of grouped vesicles and erosions occur especially on the elbows and extensor surfaces. It is associated with gluten-induced enteropathy. Biopsy reveals neutrophilic microabscesses at the tips of dermal papillae with deposition of IgA antibody complexes. Blood tests for antigliadin and antiendomysial antibodies can help diagnose the gluten-induced enteropathy (see Chapter 184, Other Bullous Diseases).
- Linear IgA dermatosis—Typical lesions are described as "string of pearls," which is an urticarial plaque surrounded by vesicles. Histologically, IgA antibodies are deposited in a linear fashion along the basement membrane (see Chapter 181, Overview of Bullous Diseases).[4]
- Porphyria cutanea tarda—Bullae are seen on sun-exposed areas, especially on the dorsum of the hands. Histology shows antibody deposition in the capillary walls and dermal-epidermal junction. Serum iron, ferritin, and transaminase levels are elevated as well as 24-hour urine porphyrins. Elevations in urine porphyrins are diagnostic (see Chapter 184, Other Bullous Diseases).
- Hailey-Hailey disease (benign familial pemphigus)—A genodermatosis with crusted erosions and flaccid vesicles distributed in the intertriginous areas (**Figure 183-18**). It most closely resembles pemphigus vegetans clinically but has a completely different pathophysiology than true pemphigus. It is called benign because it is not life threatening. A 4-mm punch biopsy is adequate to make this diagnosis as the histology is different than pemphigus.

MANAGEMENT

Treatment of pemphigus should be undertaken in consultation with a dermatologist. Treatment is directed initially at disease control and remission followed by disease suppression. The goal is to eventually discontinue all medications and achieve complete remission. Unfortunately this goal is hard to achieve.

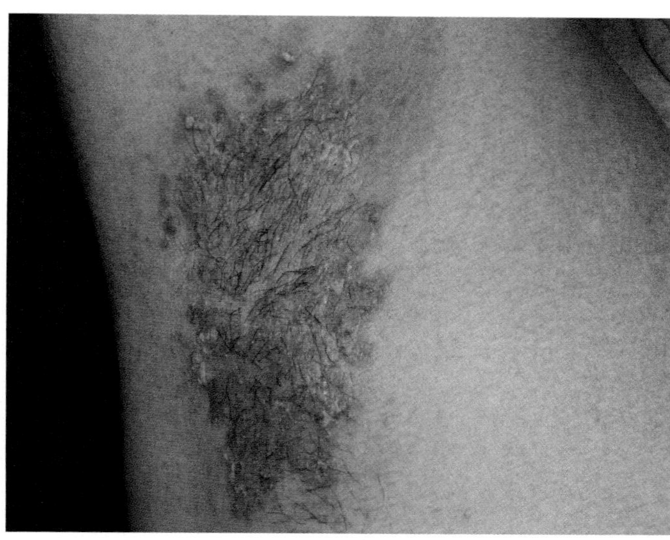

FIGURE 183-18 Hailey-Hailey disease (benign familial pemphigus) with erythema and pustules in the axilla. This is not true pemphigus but resembles pemphigus vegetans. (*Reproduced with permission from Jonathan B. Karnes, MD.*)

SYSTEMIC THERAPY

Corticosteroids

Oral steroids with a steroid-sparing adjuvant agent is the most effective treatment (2 randomized controlled trials [RCTs]).[4,5] SOR B

- Treatment should begin with the corticosteroid.[4-6] SOR B Mild disease may be controlled with prednisone 40 mg/d but for rapidly progressive and extensive disease, a higher dose prednisone 60 to 80 mg/d is initiated. SOR C The dose may be increased by 50% every 1 to 2 weeks until disease activity is controlled. In most cases, a dose of approximately 60 mg of prednisone daily will need to be continued for at least 1 month. Once remission is induced, the dose is tapered by 25% every 1 to 2 weeks to the lowest dose needed to suppress recurrence of new lesions.[1]
- Pulse therapy with intravenous methylprednisolone 1 g/d for 5 days may be tried in severe cases in an attempt to decrease the cumulative dose of steroids, especially when high-dose oral steroids are ineffective.[6] SOR C
- High dose and prolonged treatment with steroids can have serious side effects. Consequently, it is advisable to start adjuvant steroid-sparing therapy within 2 to 4 weeks of treatment. Adjuvant agents have a lag period of 4 to 6 weeks before they become effective, so starting them sooner allows for earlier steroid taper. They may be used alone to maintain remission after steroid withdrawal.

Adjuvant agents

- Adjuvant agents include azathioprine, cyclophosphamide, mycophenolate, dapsone, and intravenous immunoglobulin.[6-9] The efficacy of steroids have been shown to be enhanced when combined with a cytotoxic drug.[5]
- Azathioprine and mycophenolate mofetil (CellCept) are often the preferred adjuvants for PV.[6,8,10] SOR B
- Azathioprine was less effective than mycophenolate mofetil in achieving remission in one study with 40 participants (risk ratio 0.72; 95% confidence interval [CI] 0.52-0.99).[8,10] In 13 (72%) of 18 patients with pemphigus receiving oral methylprednisolone and azathioprine, complete remission was achieved after a mean of 74 (±127) days compared with 20 (95%) of 21 patients receiving oral methylprednisolone and mycophenolate in whom complete remission occurred after a mean of 91 (±113) days. A greater percentage of patients treated with azathioprine had adverse effects than those treated with mycophenolate.
- In one RCT open-label trial of 4 treatment regimens for PV, the most efficacious cytotoxic drug to reduce steroid was found to be azathioprine, followed by cyclophosphamide (IV pulse therapy), and mycophenolate mofetil.[5] SOR B
- Standard dosing for azathioprine is 50 mg a day. Standard dosing for mycophenolate is 1000 mg to 1500 mg twice daily. Azathioprine is significantly less expensive but patients may experience more side effects. Both are acceptable, widely used treatments for pemphigus.[4,5,8-10] SOR B
- Dapsone is an alternative adjuvant for pemphigus.[6] SOR C In one small study, 8 (73%) of 11 patients receiving dapsone versus 3 (30%) of 10 receiving placebo reached the primary outcome of a prednisone dosage of 7.5 mg/d or less. This was not statistically significant and only showed a trend to efficacy of dapsone as a steroid-sparing drug in maintenance-phase PV.[11]
- Intravenous immunoglobulin (IVIG) may be used as adjuvant therapy in refractory cases of pemphigus.[6,12-14] SOR B In one RCT, it was used as a 5-day cycle to treat pemphigus that was relatively resistant to systemic steroids. In this multicenter study of 61 patients with PV or foliaceous, there was a decrease in disease activity subsequent to the cycle of IVIG.[14] SOR B
- Rituximab is a chimeric monoclonal antibody against CD20 on B lymphocytes. It leads to depletion of pathogenic B cells for up to 12 months, resulting in a reduction of plasma cells secreting pathogenic autoantibodies. Rituximab is infused weekly for 4 consecutive weeks in addition to the standard immunosuppressive treatment. It has shown promise in several case reports and cohort studies in the treatment of PNP and refractory cases of PV and foliaceus.[15,16] SOR B

Treating and preventing complications of therapy

- Osteoporosis prevention—Long-term therapy with oral prednisone is a significant risk factor for osteoporosis. All patients should receive supplemental calcium and vitamin D based on their age, gender, and normal dietary intake. A DEXA scan early in the course of the disease can be a helpful baseline. One study showed that alendronate therapy given to patients with immunobullous disease on long-term steroids resulted in statistically significant increases in bone mineral density at the lumbar spine and femoral neck.[17]
- Thrush is a common complication of high-dose steroids in pemphigus (**Figure 183-19**). This should be treated with oral fluconazole or another antifungal to prevent *Candida* esophagitis. If the patient is complaining of pain or difficulty swallowing, consider the diagnosis of *Candida* esophagitis and treat accordingly.
- Steroid-induced diabetes may also occur. This can be treated with metformin and monitoring of blood sugars and hemoglobin A_{1c}.

LOCAL THERAPY

- Solitary lesions may be treated with topical high-potency steroids, such as clobetasol, or with intralesional steroid injections, for example, 20 mg/mL triamcinolone acetonide. Isolated oral lesions may be treated with steroid paste, sprays, or lozenges.

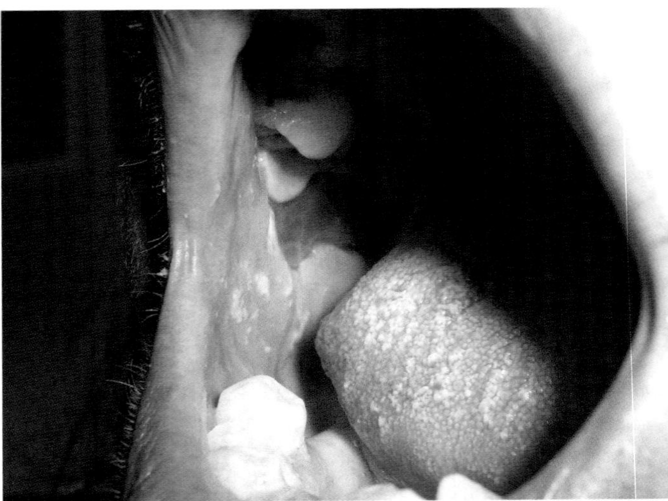

FIGURE 183-19 Thrush appearing in the mouth of a 50-year-old woman recently placed on oral prednisone for new-onset pemphigus vulgaris. Note the large erosion on the buccal mucosa and the adherent white Candida anterior to that and also on the tongue. Potassium hydroxide (KOH) was positive and the patient was treated with fluconazole. (*Reproduced with permission from Richard P. Usatine, MD.*)

- Normal saline compresses or bacteriostatic solutions such as potassium permanganate are useful in keeping lesions clean. Oral hygiene is crucial. Mouthwashes such as chlorhexidine 0.2% or 1:4 hydrogen peroxide may be used. Topical anesthetics may be used for pain.[6]

PROGNOSIS

Pemphigus is a chronic group of diseases that are potentially life threatening. There is no cure and the long-term use of steroids and immunosuppressive drugs places the patients at risk for a number of complications including infections, sepsis, steroid-induced diabetes, and steroid-induced osteoporosis. Some patients will be lucky and go into remission while others will need systemic therapy for life. Complications of treatment have become the greatest source of morbidity and mortality in pemphigus.

FOLLOW-UP

Prolonged follow-up is needed for medication adjustment and to monitor disease activity and drug side effects.

PATIENT EDUCATION

- Educate patients regarding disease, complications, and side effects of medications.
- Advise patients on avoiding trauma to skin such as with contact sports. Similarly, oral lesions may be aggravated by nuts, spicy foods, chips, and dental plates and bridges.
- Instruct patients on wound care to prevent infections and relieve local discomfort.
- Provide information on support groups such as the International Pemphigus Pemphigoid Foundation.

PATIENT RESOURCES

- MedlinePlus. *Pemphigus*—**http://www.nlm.nih.gov/medlineplus/pemphigus.html.**
- Mayo Clinic. *Pemphigus*—**http://www.mayoclinic.com/health/pemphigus/DS00749.**
- International Pemphigus Pemphigoid Foundation—**http://www.pemphigus.org/.**

PROVIDER RESOURCES

- Medscape. *Pemphigus Vulgaris*—**http://emedicine.medscape.com/article/1064187.**
- Information on how to perform the appropriate biopsy can be found in Usatine R, Pfenninger J, Stulberg D, Small R. *Dermatologic and Cosmetic Procedures in Office Practice*. Philadelphia, PA: Elsevier; 2012. The text and the accompanying videos can also be purchased as an electronic application at **http://www.usatinemedia.com.**

REFERENCES

1. Bystryn JC, Rudolph JL. Pemphigus. *Lancet.* 2005;366:61-73.
2. Ettlin DA. Pemphigus. *Dent Clin North Am.* 2005;49:107-1ix.
3. Bickle K, Roark TR, Hsu S. Autoimmune bullous dermatoses: a review. *Am Fam Physician.* 2002;65:1861-1870.
4. Chams-Davatchi C, Esmaili N, Daneshpazhooh M, et al. Randomized controlled open-label trial of four treatment regimens for pemphigus vulgaris. *J Am Acad Dermatol.* 2007;57:622-628.
5. Beissert S, Mimouni D, Kanwar AJ, Solomons N, Kalia V, Anhalt GJ. Treating pemphigus vulgaris with prednisone and mycophenolate mofetil: a multicenter, randomized, placebo-controlled trial. *J Invest Dermatol.* 2010;130:2041-2048.
6. Harman KE, Albert S, Black MM. Guidelines for the management of pemphigus vulgaris. *Br J Dermatol.* 2003;149:926-937.
7. Frew JW, Martin LK, Murrell DF. Evidence-based treatments in pemphigus vulgaris and pemphigus foliaceus. *Dermatol Clin.* 2011;29:599-606.
8. Martin LK, Werth VP, Villaneuva EV, Murrell DF. A systematic review of randomized controlled trials for pemphigus vulgaris and pemphigus foliaceus. *J Am Acad Dermatol.* 2011;64:903-908.
9. Singh S. Evidence-based treatments for pemphigus vulgaris, pemphigus foliaceus, and bullous pemphigoid: a systematic review. *Indian J DermatolVenereol Leprol.* 2011;77:456-469.
10. Beissert S, Werfel T, Frieling U, et al. A comparison of oral methylprednisolone plus azathioprine or mycophenolate mofetil for the treatment of pemphigus. *Arch Dermatol.* 2006;142:1447-1454.
11. Werth VP, Fivenson D, Pandya AG, et al. Multicenter randomized, double-blind, placebo-controlled, clinical trial of dapsone as a glucocorticoid-sparing agent in maintenance-phase pemphigus vulgaris. *Arch Dermatol.* 2008;144:25-32.
12. Sami N, Qureshi A, Ruocco E, Ahmed AR. Corticosteroid-sparing effect of intravenous immunoglobulin therapy in patients with pemphigus vulgaris. *Arch Dermatol.* 2002;138:1158-1162.
13. Gurcan HM, Jeph S, Ahmed AR. Intravenous immunoglobulin therapy in autoimmune mucocutaneous blistering diseases: a review

of the evidence for its efficacy and safety. *Am J Clin Dermatol.* 2010;11:315-326.

14. Amagai M, Ikeda S, Shimizu H, et al. A randomized double-blind trial of intravenous immunoglobulin for pemphigus. *J Am Acad Dermatol.* 2009;60:595-603.
15. Hertl M, Zillikens D, Borradori L, et al. Recommendations for the use of rituximab (anti-CD20 antibody) in the treatment of autoimmune bullous skin diseases. *J Dtsch Dermatol Ges.* 2008;6:366-373.
16. El Tal AK, Posner MR, Spigelman Z, Ahmed AR. Rituximab: a monoclonal antibody to CD20 used in the treatment of pemphigus vulgaris. *J Am Acad Dermatol.* 2006;55:449-459.
17. Tee SI, Yosipovitch G, Chan YC, et al. Prevention of glucocorticoid-induced osteoporosis in immunobullous diseases with alendronate: a randomized, double-blind, placebo-controlled study. *Arch Dermatol.* 2012;148:307-314.

184 OTHER BULLOUS DISEASES

Jimmy H. Hara, MD
Richard P. Usatine, MD

INTRODUCTION

There are a number of bullous diseases other than pemphigus and bullous pemphigoid that are important to recognize. Porphyria cutanea tarda (PCT) is a porphyria that has no extracutaneous manifestations (**Figures 184-1** to **184-3**). Dystrophic epidermolysis bullosa belongs to a family of inherited diseases where blister formation can be caused by even minor skin trauma. Pityriasis lichenoides et varioliformis acuta (PLEVA) is a minor cutaneous lymphoid dyscrasia that can appear suddenly and persist for weeks to months. Dermatitis herpetiformis is a recurrent eruption that is usually associated with gluten and diet-related enteropathies.

PORPHYRIA CUTANEA TARDA

PATIENT STORY

A middle-aged woman presented with tense blisters on the dorsum of her hand (see **Figure 184-1**). One bulla was intact and the others had ruptured, showing erosions. Workup showed elevated porphyrins in the urine (which fluoresced orange-red under a Wood lamp) and the patient was diagnosed with PCT.

EPIDEMIOLOGY

- PCT occurs mostly in middle-aged adults (typically 30-50 years of age) and is rare in children.
- It is especially likely to occur in women on oral contraceptives and in men on estrogen therapy for prostate cancer.[1]

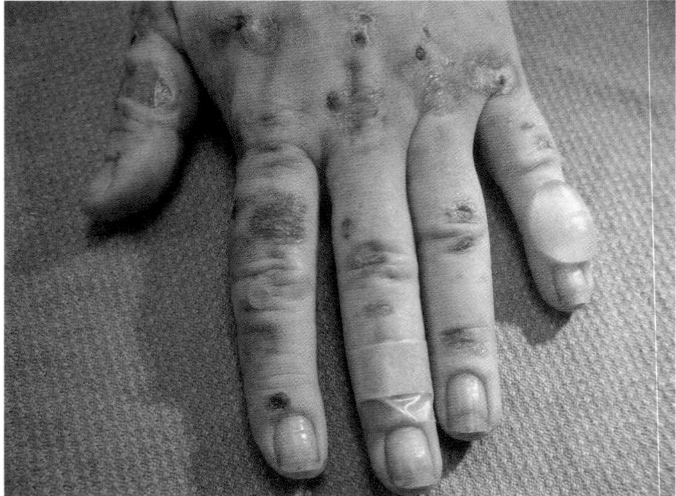

FIGURE 184-1 Porphyria cutanea tarda in a middle-aged woman. *(Reproduced with permission from Lewis Rose, MD.)*

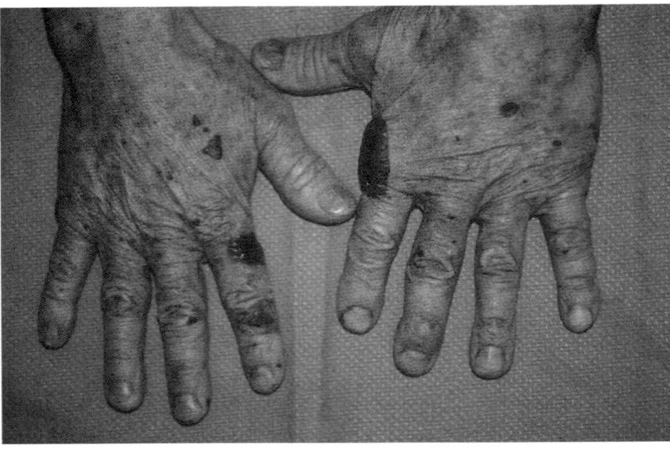

FIGURE 184-2 Porphyria cutanea tarda in a man with hepatitis C. *(Reproduced with permission from the University of Texas Health Sciences Center, Division of Dermatology.)*

- Alcohol, pesticides, and chloroquine have been implicated as chemicals that induce PCT.[1]
- PCT is equally common in both genders.
- There is an increased incidence of PCT in persons with hepatitis C (see **Figures 184-2** and **184-3**).

ETIOLOGY AND PATHOPHYSIOLOGY

The porphyrias are a family of illnesses caused by various metabolic derangements in the metabolism of porphyrin, the chemical backbone of hemoglobin. Whereas the other porphyrias (acute intermittent porphyria and variegate porphyria) are associated with well-known systemic manifestations (abdominal pain, peripheral neuropathy, and pulmonary complications), PCT has no extracutaneous manifestations. Photosensitivity is seen (as with variegate porphyria). PCT is associated with a reduction in hepatic uroporphyrin decarboxylase.

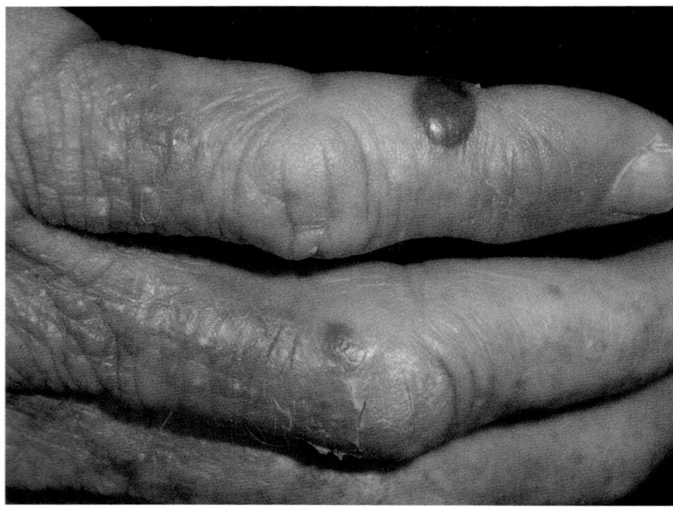

FIGURE 184-3 Porphyria cutanea tarda in a man with hepatitis C and alcohol abuse. *(Reproduced with permission from Richard P. Usatine, MD.)*

RISK FACTORS

- Hepatitis C
- Alcohol-induced liver injury
- Hemochromatosis[2]

DIAGNOSIS

CLINICAL FEATURES

The classic presentation is that of blistering (vesicles and tense bullae) on photosensitive "fragile skin" (similar to epidermolysis bullosa). Scleroderma-like heliotrope suffusion of the eyelids and face may be seen. As the blisters heal, the skin takes on an atrophic appearance. Hypertrichosis (especially on the cheeks and temples) is also common and may be the presenting feature.

TYPICAL DISTRIBUTION

Classically, the dorsa of the hands are affected (see **Figures 184-1** to **184-3**). Facial suffusion (heliotrope) may be seen along with hypertrichosis of the cheeks and temples.

LABORATORY STUDIES

The diagnosis can be confirmed by the orange-red fluorescence of the urine when examined under a Wood lamp. Increased plasma iron may be seen (associated with increased hepatic iron in the Kupffer cells). Diabetes is said to occur in 25% of individuals.

- Twenty-four-hour urine collection for porphyrins—These will be elevated in PCT.
- Skin biopsy may help confirm PCT if the other information is not clear.
- Once the diagnosis is made, secondary causes of PCT should be investigated:
  - Serum for ferritin, iron, and iron-binding capacity to look for hemochromatosis.
  - Order liver function tests and if abnormal order tests for hepatitis B and C.
  - Consider α-fetoprotein and liver ultrasound if considering cirrhosis and/or hepatocellular carcinoma.
  - Order an HIV test if risk factors are present.

DIFFERENTIAL DIAGNOSIS

The acral vesiculobullous lesions may suggest nummular or dyshidrotic eczema. In younger individuals, the acral blistering may suggest epidermolysis bullosa. The lesions may also suggest erythema multiforme bullosum. The heliotrope suffusion may suggest dermatomyositis and the atrophic changes may suggest systemic sclerosis.

MANAGEMENT

- If the onset is associated with alcohol ingestion, estrogen therapy, or exposure to pesticides, reducing exposure is warranted.[2]
- Phlebotomy of 500 mL of blood weekly until the hemoglobin is decreased to 10 g is associated with biochemical and clinical remission within a year.[1]
- Low-dose chloroquine can help maintain remissions, whereas high-dose chloroquine can exacerbate the illness.[1]

FOLLOW-UP

Periodic clinical follow-up until remission is achieved is necessary along with constant education and reinforcement of the need to avoid precipitants.

PATIENT EDUCATION

Avoidance of potential precipitants (alcohol, estrogens, pesticides) and avoidance of excess sunlight exposure (to avoid hypersensitivity) are important. Avoidance of trauma and careful wound care is also necessary.

EPIDERMOLYSIS BULLOSA

PATIENT STORY

A 34-year-old pregnant woman presents with active blistering in her axilla and past history revealed that she lost her fingernails and toenails (**Figure 184-4A**) as a young child. She was diagnosed as a child with recessive dystrophic epidermolysis bullosa. None of her children had been affected because her husband was neither affected nor a carrier (**Figure 184-4B**). A topical steroid ointment helped relieve the pain and calm the blistering in her axilla.

EPIDEMIOLOGY

Dystrophic epidermolysis bullosa belongs to a family of inherited diseases characterized by skin fragility and blister formation caused by minor skin trauma.[3] There are autosomal recessive and autosomal dominant types, the severity of this disease may vary widely. Onset is in childhood and in later years severe dystrophic deformities of hands and feet are characteristic (**Figure 184-5**). Malignant degeneration is common, especially squamous cell carcinoma, in sun-exposed areas.

ETIOLOGY AND PATHOPHYSIOLOGY

Dystrophic epidermolysis bullosa has vesiculobullous skin separation occurring at the sub-basal lamina level, as opposed to junctional epidermolysis bullosa, which blisters at the intralamina lucida layer, and epidermolysis bullosa simplex (**Figure 184-6**), which blisters at the intraepidermal layer.[4,5]

DIAGNOSIS

CLINICAL FEATURES

Acral skin fragility and blistering are the hallmark in childhood. Minor trauma can induce severe blistering. As the disease progresses initially, painful and ultimately debilitating dystrophic deformities are typical. Repeated blistering of the hands can lead to fusion of the fingers and the "mitten" deformity (see **Figure 184-5**).

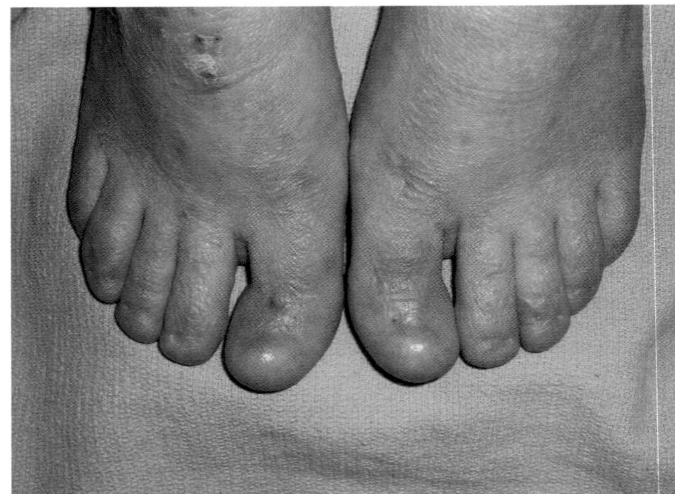

A

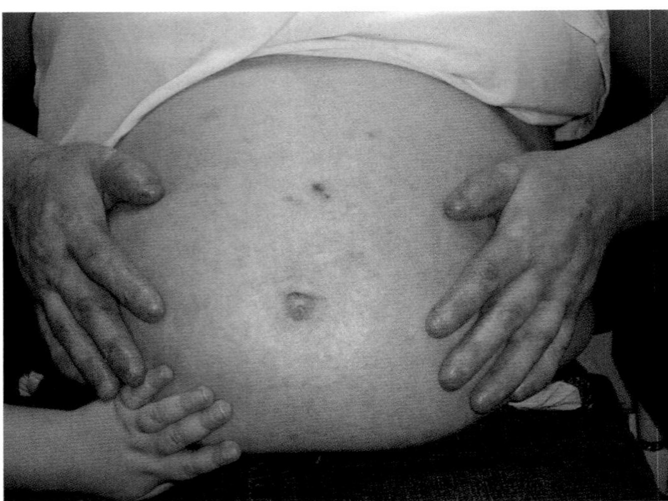

B

FIGURE 184-4 A. Recessive dystrophic epidermolysis bullosa with loss of all her toenails as a young child. B. The same woman showing complete loss of her fingernails and the pregnant abdomen. Her daughter is touching the belly and does not have the disease and, therefore, has normal fingers. (*Reproduced with permission from Richard P. Usatine, MD.*)

TYPICAL DISTRIBUTION

The typical distribution is acral (hands and feet), although blistering may extend proximally secondary to trauma.

LABORATORY STUDIES AND BIOPSY

There are no laboratory tests to confirm the diagnosis. A punch biopsy can provide adequate tissue for the dermatopathologist to differentiate between the different forms of epidermolysis bullosa: simplex, junctional, and dystrophic.

DIFFERENTIAL DIAGNOSIS

- Erythema multiforme bullosum may have a similar appearance, but the distribution is less apt to be limited to the distal extremities.
- The appearance of an acral blistering on fragile skin is also characteristic of PCT, but the age of onset of PCT is typically in middle age and not in childhood.

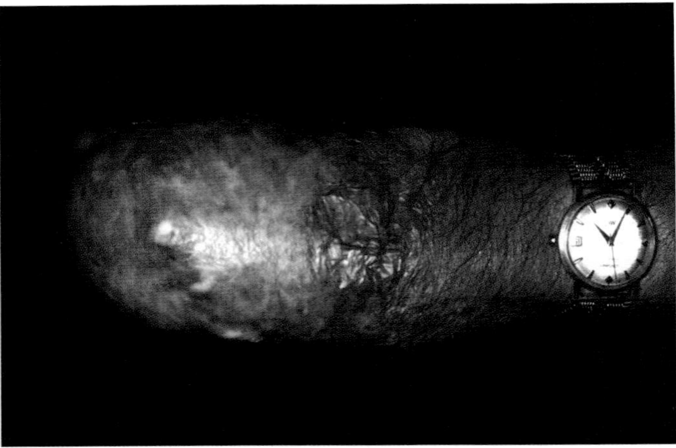

A

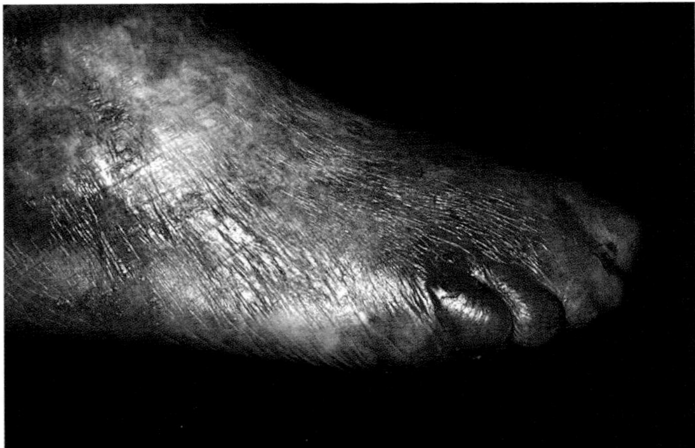

B

FIGURE 184-5 Severe recessive dystrophic epidermolysis bullosa in a 53-year-old Asian man. A. Complete loss of fingers from the disease on his hands. This is referred to as the mitten deformity. He has also had multiple squamous cell carcinomas excised from his hands. B. Similar foot deformities with loss of normal toes. (*Reproduced with permission from Richard P. Usatine, MD.*)

- The first appearance of the condition may be confused, with staphylococcal scalded skin syndrome (see Chapter 118, Impetigo).[6]

MANAGEMENT

Management is primarily prevention of trauma, careful wound care, and treatment of complicating infections. Other supportive measures such as pain management and nutritional support are often necessary. Screening the skin for squamous cell carcinoma is important in the dystrophic form.[4]

FOLLOW-UP

Periodic skin examinations should be done to help manage symptoms and screen for malignancy.

PATIENT EDUCATION

Avoid trauma and come in early if there are any signs of infection or malignancy.

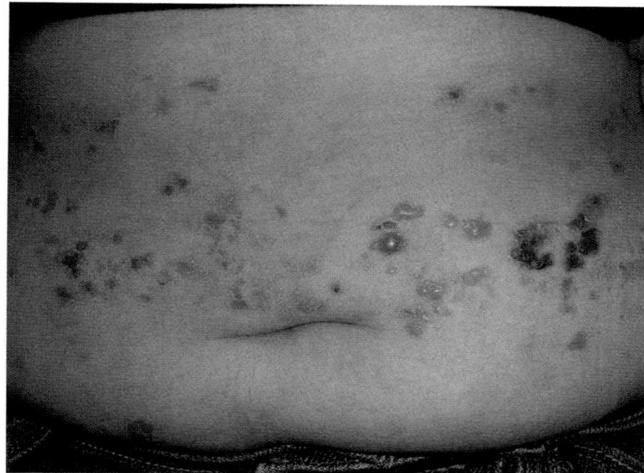

A

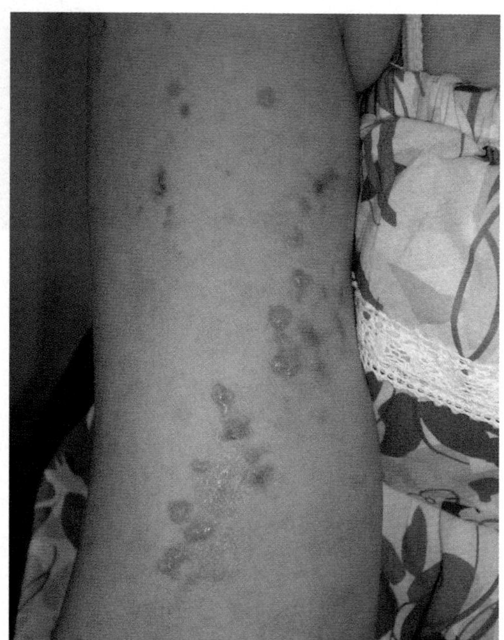

B

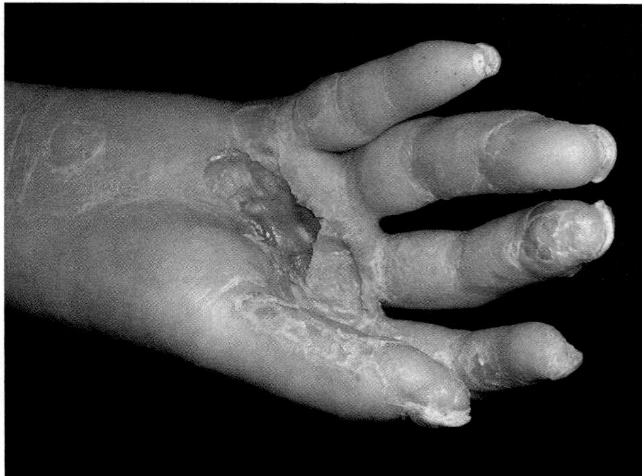

C

FIGURE 184-6 A 12-year-old girl with the Dowling-Meara type of epidermolysis bullosa simplex. It is the most severe form with extensive, severe blistering over many areas of the body including, the **A.** trunk, **B.** extremities, and **C.** the hands. (*Reproduced with permission from Richard P, Usatine, MD.*)

PITYRIASIS LICHENOIDES ET VARIOLIFORMIS ACUTA

PATIENT STORY

A 22-year-old man presented with a varicelliform eruption that he has had for 6 weeks (**Figure 184-7**). Initially, he was diagnosed with varicella and given a course of acyclovir. Then he was misdiagnosed with scabies and treated with permethrin. A correct diagnosis was made of PLEVA by clinical appearance and confirmed with biopsy. His skin lesions cleared with oral tetracycline.

EPIDEMIOLOGY

- PLEVA or Mucha-Habermann disease and pityriasis lichenoides chronica are maculopapular erythematous eruptions that can occur in crops of vesicles that can become hemorrhagic over a course of weeks to months (**Figures 184-7** and **184-8**).[7]
- There is a predilection for males in the second and third decades.
- PLEVA occurs in preschool and preadolescent children as well.[8]

ETIOLOGY AND PATHOPHYSIOLOGY

PLEVA has traditionally been classified as a benign papulosquamous disease. However, there is increasing evidence that suggests that PLEVA should be considered a form of cutaneous lymphoid dyscrasia.[9] It may even, represent an indolent form of mycosis fungoides (see Chapter 174, Cutaneous T-Cell Lymphoma).

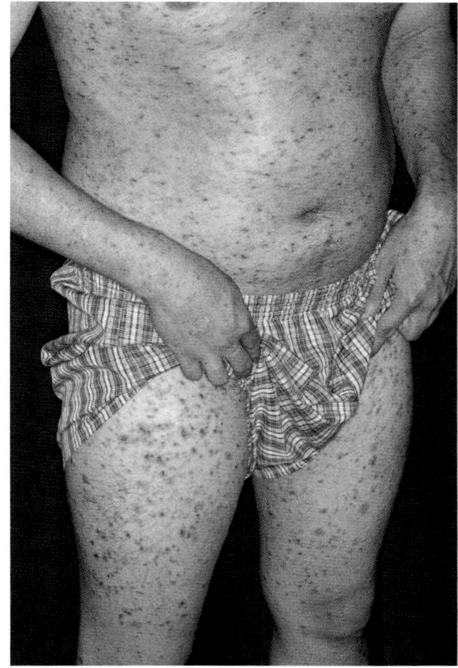

FIGURE 184-7 A 22-year-old man with pityriasis lichenoides et varioliformis acuta. His skin lesions cleared with oral tetracycline. (*Reproduced with permission from Richard P, Usatine, MD.*)

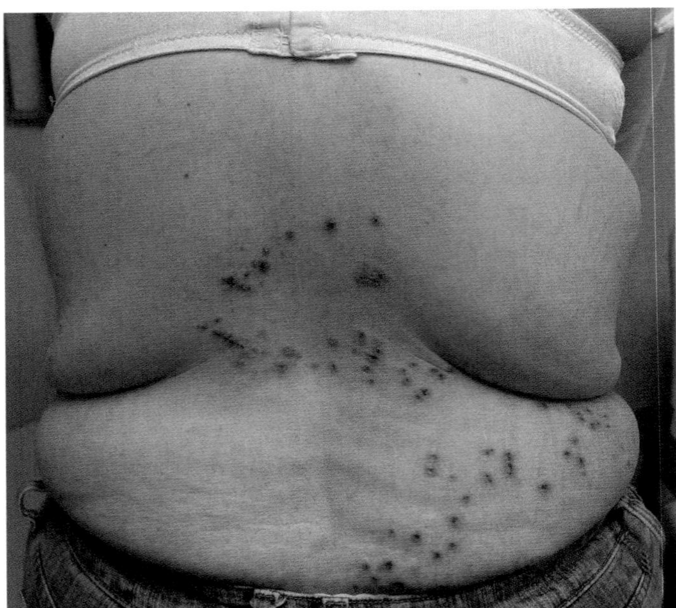

FIGURE 184-8 A young woman with pityriasis lichenoides et varioliformis acuta. The individual lesions look like varicella but are unrelated to the varicella virus. (*Reproduced with permission from David Anderson, MD.*)

DIAGNOSIS

CLINICAL FEATURES

PLEVA occurs with crops of maculopapular and papulosquamous lesions that can vesiculate and form hemorrhagic vesicles (see **Figures 184-7** and **184-8**). Although it resembles varicella, new crops of lesions continue to appear over weeks and months. It can be thought of as "chickenpox that lasts for weeks to months."

TYPICAL DISTRIBUTION

Lesions typically occur over the anterior trunk and flexural aspects of the proximal extremities. The face is spared.

LABORATORY STUDIES

There are no specific laboratory tests for PLEVA except biopsy.

BIOPSY

A punch biopsy is helpful in making the diagnosis. It may be necessary to differentiate PLEVA from lymphomatoid papulosis (see "Differential Diagnosis").

DIFFERENTIAL DIAGNOSIS

- Varicella—A varicella direct fluorescent antibody test can confirm acute varicella. If no viral testing was done and what appeared to be varicella persists, PLEVA should be considered (see Chapter 125, Chickenpox).
- Pityriasis lichenoides chronica is the chronic form of pityriasis lichenoides and can be distinguished from PLEVA by length of time and biopsy (**Figure 184-9**). It has a more low-grade clinical course than PLEVA and the lesions appear over a longer course of time.

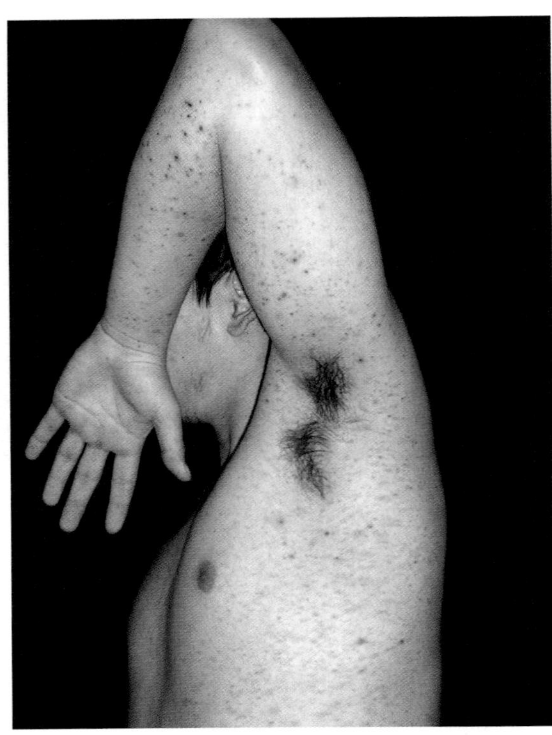

FIGURE 184-9 Pityriasis lichenoides chronica is the chronic form of pityriasis lichenoides that may persist for months to years. (*Reproduced with permission from Richard P. Usatine, MD.*)

- Erythema multiforme is a hypersensitivity syndrome in which target lesions are seen. The target lesions have epidermal disruption in the center with vesicles and/or erosions. Look for the target lesions to help differentiate this from PLEVA (see Section 13, Hypersensitivity Syndromes).
- Lymphomatoid papulosis presents in a manner similar to PLEVA with recurrent crops of pruritic papules at different stages of development that appear on the trunk and extremities. Although it has histologic features that suggest lymphoma, lymphomatoid papulosis alone is not fatal. It is important to differentiate this from PLEVA because these patients need to be worked up for coexisting malignancy. These patients tend to be older and a punch biopsy can make the diagnosis.

MANAGEMENT

Ultraviolet A1 (UVA1) phototherapy has been deployed with some success.[10] Various reports suggest the efficacy of macrolides and tetracyclines, probably more for their anti-inflammatory properties than for their antibacterial effects.

FOLLOW-UP

Follow-up is needed only if the disease does not resolve.

PATIENT EDUCATION

This is usually a temporary disease but if it becomes chronic there are treatments that could help such as oral macrolides or tetracycline.

DERMATITIS HERPETIFORMIS

PATIENT STORY

A young man with a past history of diarrhea and malabsorption carries a past diagnosis of gluten-induced enteropathy. Despite a gluten-free diet he continues to have a pruritic eruption on his shoulders, back, extremities, and buttocks. (**Figures 184-10** and **184-11**). While the most likely diagnosis is dermatitis herpetiformis, a punch biopsy was performed to confirm this before starting the patient on oral dapsone.

EPIDEMIOLOGY

Dermatitis herpetiformis is a chronic recurrent symmetric vesicular eruption that is usually associated with diet-related enteropathy.[11] It most commonly occurs in the 20 to 40 years of age group. Men are affected more often than women.

ETIOLOGY AND PATHOPHYSIOLOGY

The disease is related to gluten and other diet-related antigens that cause the development of circulating immune complexes and their subsequent deposition in the skin. The term *herpetiformis* refers to the grouped vesicles that appear on extensor aspects of the extremities and trunk and is not a viral infection or related to the herpes viruses. The disease is characterized by the deposition of immunoglobulin (Ig) A along the tips of the dermal papillae. The majority of patients will also have blunting and flattening of jejunal villi, which leads to diarrhea even to the point of steatorrhea and malabsorption.

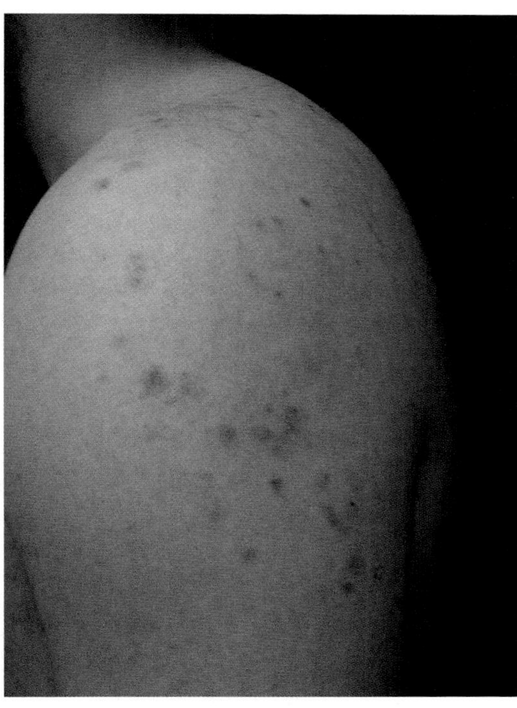

FIGURE 184-10 A young man with dermatitis herpetiformis and gluteninduced enteropathy. The daily vesicles that form are fragile and rapidly become small erosions. (*Reproduced with permission from Richard P. Usatine, MD.*)

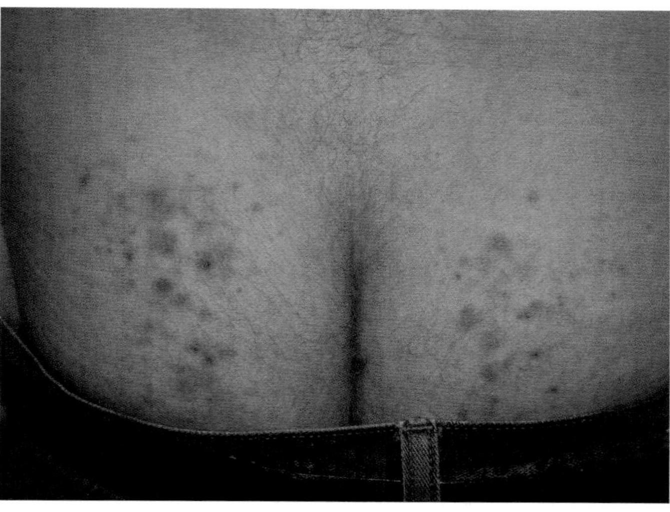

FIGURE 184-11 Dermatitis herpetiformis that has persisted even though he is on a strict gluten-free diet. The buttock is a commonly involved area. His gastrointestinal symptoms have resolved on the gluten-free diet, but his eruption has only improved with lack of full clearance. (*Reproduced with permission from Richard P. Usatine, MD.*)

DIAGNOSIS

CLINICAL FEATURES

The clinical eruption is characterized by severe itching, burning, or stinging in the characteristic extensor distribution. Herpetiform vesicles and urticarial plaques may be seen. Because of the intense pruritus, characteristic lesions may be excoriated beyond recognition (see **Figures 184-10** and **184-11**).

TYPICAL DISTRIBUTION

Classically, the lesions (or excoriations) are seen in the extensor aspects of the extremities, shoulders (see **Figure 184-10**), lower back, and buttocks (see **Figure 184-11**).

LABORATORY STUDIES

If the patient has gluten-induced enteropathy, antigliadin and antiendomysial antibodies may be present. A blood test for antigliadin antibody is a sensitive test for gluten-induced enteropathy.

BIOPSY

Diagnosis is confirmed by a punch biopsy. It is best to biopsy new crops of lesions. A standard histologic examination will show eosinophils and microabscesses of neutrophils in the dermal papillae and subepidermal vesicles. Direct immunofluorescence reveals deposits of IgA and complement within the dermal papillae.

DIFFERENTIAL DIAGNOSIS

- Scabies may have a similar appearance with pruritus, papules, and vesicles. If the lesions and distribution suggest scabies, it should be ruled out with skin scraping looking for the mite, feces, and eggs.

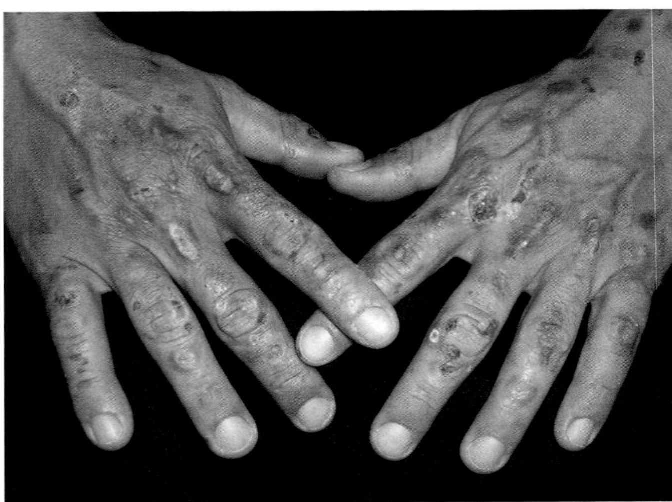

FIGURE 184-12 Porphyria cutanea tarda on the dorsum of both hands in a HIV positive man with hepatitis C. Therapeutic phlebotomies cleared up the lesions completely. *(Reproduced with permission from Richard P. Usatine, MD.)*

If the scraping is negative, but the clinical appearance suggests scabies, empiric treatment with permethrin should be considered as well. If the lesions persist, consider a punch biopsy to look for dermatitis herpetiformis (see Chapter 141, Scabies).

- Nummular and dyshidrotic eczema may also be diagnostic considerations, but response to steroids in eczema may be helpful in differentiation (see Chapters 143, Atopic Dermatitis and 145, Hand Eczema).
- PCT is on the differential diagnosis. Note that the blisters and erosions seem to be larger than those seen with dermatitis herpetiformis. Also a history of hepatitis C is frequently associated with PCT (**Figures 184-12**).

MANAGEMENT

- With a gluten-free diet, 80% of patients will show improvement in the skin lesions. The degree of benefit is dependent on the strictness of the diet.[11]
- A gluten-free diet may help the enteropathy and decrease the subsequent development of small bowel lymphoma.
- Dapsone at an initial dose of 100 to 200 mg daily with gradual reduction to a 25- to 50-mg maintenance level may be necessary indefinitely.[12]

FOLLOW-UP

Follow-up is needed to control the disease and monitor nutritional status.

PATIENT EDUCATION

Nutritional counseling is important for all patients with gluten-induced enteropathy. Persons with dermatitis herpetiformis and gluten-induced, enteropathy should not eat wheat and barley but can eat rice, oats, and corn.

PATIENT RESOURCES

- MedlinePlus. *Porphyria*—**http://www.nlm.nih.gov/medlineplus/ency/article/001208.htm.**
- Genetics Home Reference. *Epidermolysis Bullosa Simplex*—**http://ghr.nlm.nih.gov/condition= epidermolysisbullosasimplex.**
- National Institute of Arthritis and Musculoskeletal and Skin Diseases. *Epidermolysis Bullosa*—**http://www.niams.nih.gov/Health_Info/Epidermolysis_Bullosa/default.asp.**
- PubMed Health. *Dermatitis Herpetiformis*—**http://www.ncbi.nlm.nih.gov/pubmedhealth/PMH0002451/.**
- DermNet NZ. *Pityriasis Lichenoides*—**http://dermnetnz.org/scaly/pityriasis-lichenoides.html.**

PROVIDER RESOURCES

- Medscape. *Porphyria Cutanea Tarda*—**http://emedicine.medscape.com/article/1103643.**
- Medscape. *Epidermolysis Bullosa*—**http://emedicine.medscape.com/article/1062939.**
- Medscape. *Dermatitis Herpetiformis*—**http://emedicine. medscape.com/article/1062640.**
- Medscape. *Pityriasis Lichenoides*—**http://emedicine. medscape.com/article/1099078.**

REFERENCES

1. Elder GH. Porphyria cutanea tarda and related disorders. In: Kadish K, Smith K, Guilard R, eds. *The Porphyrin Handbook*. Volume 14. San Diego, CA: Elsevier Science; 2003:67ff.
2. Jalil S, Grady JJ, Lee C, Anderson, KE. Associations among behavior-related susceptibility factors in porphyria cutanea tarda. *Clin Gastroenterol Hepatol*. 2010;8(3):297-302, 302e-1.
3. Horn HM, Tidman MJ. The clinical spectrum of epidermolysis bullosa. *Br J Dermatol*. 2002;146(2):267-274.
4. Fine JD, Johnson LB, Weiner M, et al. Epidermolysis bullosa and the risk of life-threatening cancers: the National EB Registry experience, 1986-2006. *J Am Acad Dermatol*. 2009;60(2):203-211.
5. Paller AS, Mancini AJ. Bullous diseases in children. In: Paller AS, Mancini AJ, eds. *Hurwitz's Clinical Pediatric Dermatology*. 3rd ed. Philadelphia, PA: Elsevier; 2006:345.
6. Patel GK, Finlay AY. Staphylococcal scalded skin syndrome: diagnosis and management. *Am J Clin Dermatol*. 2003;4(3):165-175.
7. Bowers S, Warshaw EM. Pityriasis lichenoides and its subtypes. *J Am Acad Dermatol*. 2006;55(4):557-572.
8. Ersoy-Evans S, Greco MF, Mancini AJ, et al. Pityriasis lichenoides in childhood: a retrospective review of 124 patients. *J Am Acad Dermatol*. 2007;56(2):205-210.
9. Magro C, Crowson AN, Kovatich A, Burns F. Pityriasis lichenoides: a clonal T-cell lymphoproliferative disorder. *Hum Pathol*. 2002;33(8):788-795.
10. Pinton PC, Capezzera R, Zane C, De Panfilis G. Medium-dose ultraviolet A1 therapy for pityriasis lichenoides et varioliformis acuta and pityriasis lichenoides chronica. *J Am Acad Dermatol*. 2002;47(3):410-414.
11. Patient.co.uk. *Dermatitis Herpetiformis*. http://www.patient.co.uk/showdoc/40001007/. Accessed October 7, 2007.
12. AGA Institute. AGA Institute Medical Position Statement on the Diagnosis and Management of Celiac Disease. *Gastroenterology*. 2006;131(6):1977-1980.

SECTION 16 HAIR AND NAIL CONDITIONS

185 ALOPECIA AREATA

Richard P. Usatine, MD

PATIENT STORY

A young woman presented to her physician with hair loss for 3 months. She is very worried that it will not grow back and that it might spread to other parts of her scalp. When she lifted her hair one round area of hair loss was noted **(Figure 185-1)**. The scalp was smooth and there were no signs of scale or inflammation. Some fine white hairs were also seen growing in the area of hair loss. A few "exclamation point" hairs were also seen. The physician readily diagnosed alopecia areata (AA) based on the clinical examination. He attempted to reassure the young woman that her hair is already growing back and would likely regrow fully in the coming months. He also explained that the new hairs may be white at first but will regain their natural dark color. He also offered her the option of intralesional steroid injection of the involved scalp. The physician did explain that the intralesional steroid is not a guarantee of 100% resolution but may increase the speed of recovery and the likelihood of recovery. The young woman chose to have the steroid injection because she did not want to take any chances of not regaining her hair.

INTRODUCTION

AA is a common disorder that causes patches of hair loss without inflammation or scarring. The areas of hair loss are often round and the scalp is often very smooth at the site of hair loss.[1]

SYNONYMS

Alopecia totalis involves the whole scalp (**Figure 185-2**). Alopecia universalis (AU) involves the whole scalp, head, and body.

EPIDEMIOLOGY

- AA affects approximately 0.2% of the population at any given time with approximately 1.7% of the population experiencing an episode during their lifetime.[2,3]
- Men and women are equally affected.
- Most patients are younger than age 40 years at disease onset, with the average age being 25 to 27 years.[2,4]

ETIOLOGY AND PATHOPHYSIOLOGY

The etiology is unknown but experts presume that the AA spectrum of disorders is secondary to an autoimmune phenomenon involving antibodies, T cells, and cytokines.

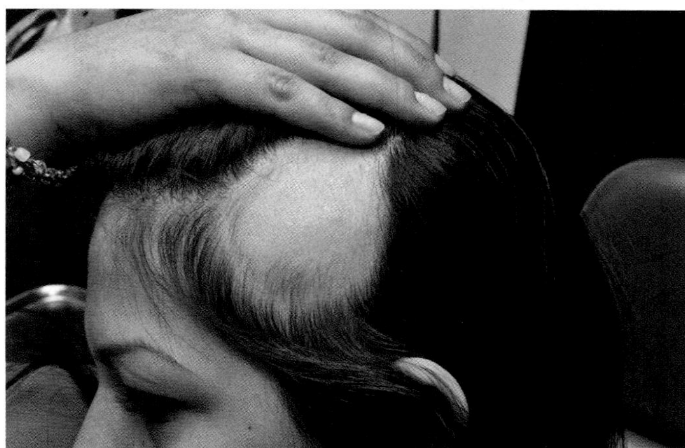

FIGURE 185-1 Alopecia areata in a young woman with a typical round area of alopecia. The scalp was smooth without scale or visible lesions. *(Reproduced with permission from Richard P. Usatine, MD.)*

RISK FACTORS

- Previous episode of AA.
- Family history of AA—In one study, the estimated lifetime risks were 7.1% in siblings, 7.8% in parents, and 5.7% in offspring of patients with AA.[5]

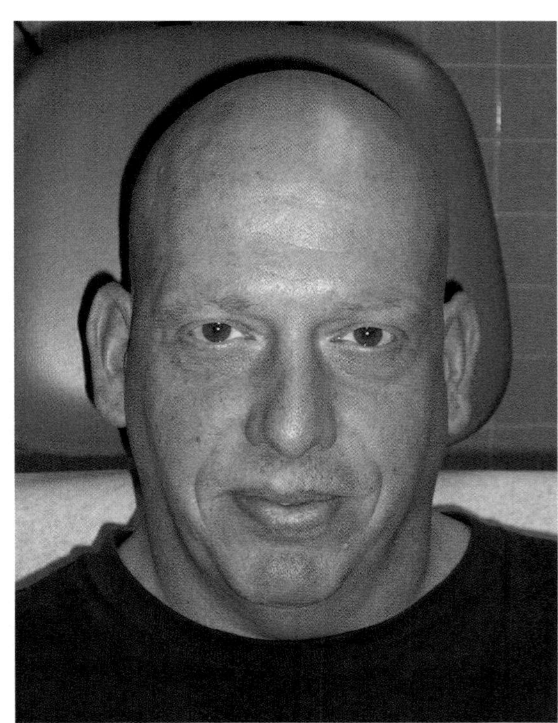

FIGURE 185-2 Alopecia totalis for more than 10 years in this adult man. *(Reproduced with permission from Richard P. Usatine, MD.)*

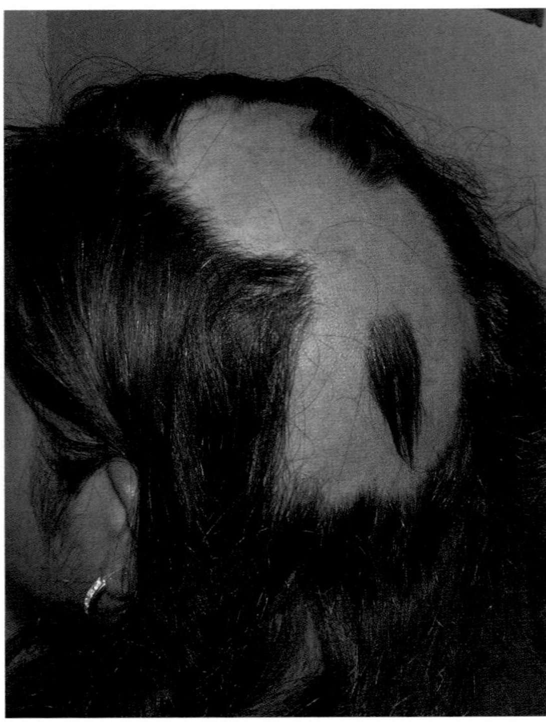

CHAPTER 185

FIGURE 185-3 Extensive alopecia areata for more than 6 months in an adult woman. (*Reproduced with permission from Richard P. Usatine, MD.*)

DIAGNOSIS

CLINICAL FEATURES

- Sudden onset of 1 or more 1- to 4-cm areas of hair loss on the scalp (**Figures 185-1** and **185-3**). This can occur in the beard, eyebrows, or other areas of hair (**Figure 185-4**).
- The affected skin is smooth and may have short stubble hair growth.
- "Exclamation point" hairs are often noted (**Figure 185-5**). These hairs are characterized by proximal thinning while the distal portion remains of normal caliber.
- When hair begins to regrow, it often comes in as fine white hair (**Figure 185-6**).

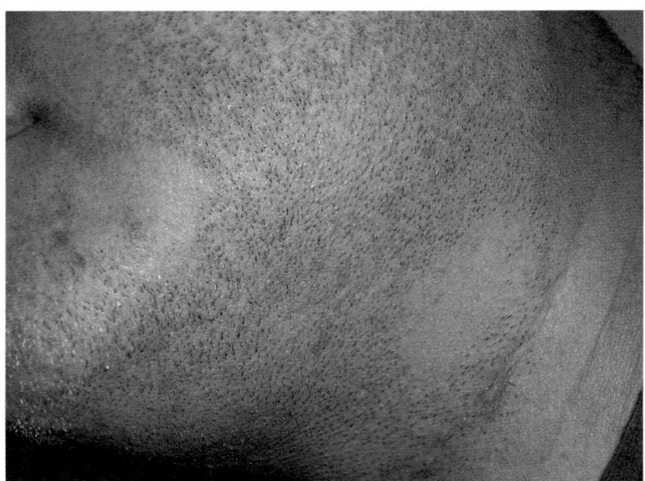

FIGURE 185-4 Alopecia areata of the beard in this young man. (*Reproduced with permission from Richard P. Usatine, MD.*)

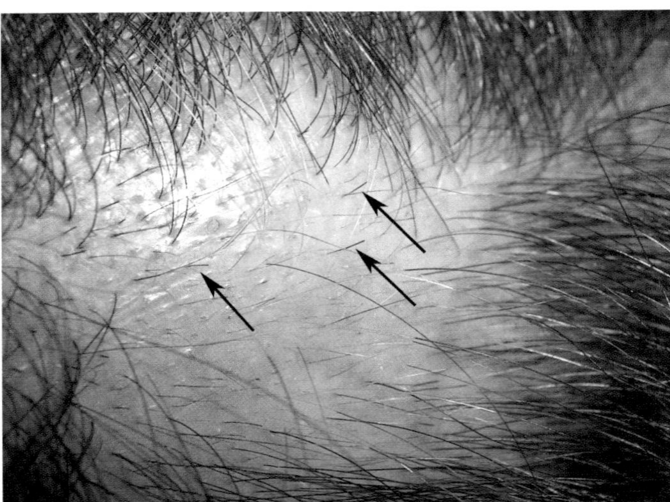

FIGURE 185-5 Exclamation point hairs (*arrows*) can be seen in this case of alopecia areata. The hair is narrow at the base, short and wide at the end. (*Reproduced with permission from Richard P. Usatine, MD.*)

TYPICAL DISTRIBUTION

- Scalp, beard, and eyebrows but can involve total-body hair loss.
- Ophiasis is the term used to describe the distribution of AA when the hair loss follows a serpent-like distribution on the scalp (**Figure 185-7**). It is said to have a worse prognosis but studies to prove this are lacking. This pattern can also be seen with traction alopecia so hair care practices should be queried.

LABORATORY STUDIES

- Typically, the diagnosis can be made with history and physical examination alone.
- Thyroid abnormalities, vitiligo, and pernicious anemia often accompany AA. Consequently, screening laboratory tests (eg, thyroid-stimulating hormone, complete blood count [CBC]) may be helpful to look for thyroid disorders and anemia (**Figure 185-8**).

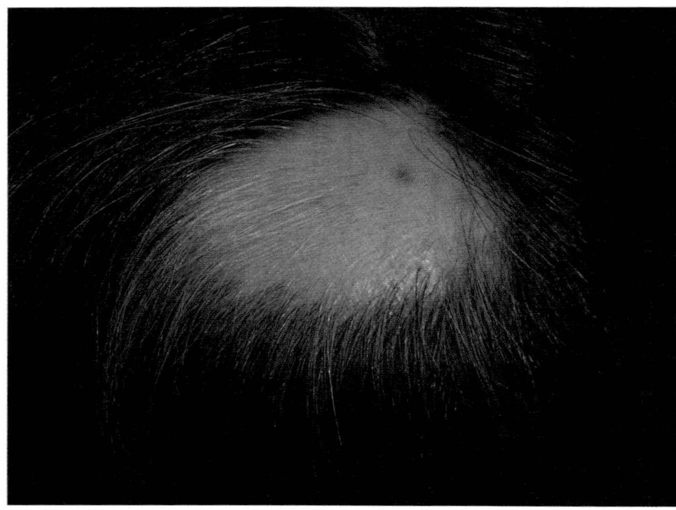

FIGURE 185-6 New growth of white hair after 7 months of alopecia areata in this middle-aged woman. (*Reproduced with permission from Richard P. Usatine, MD.*)

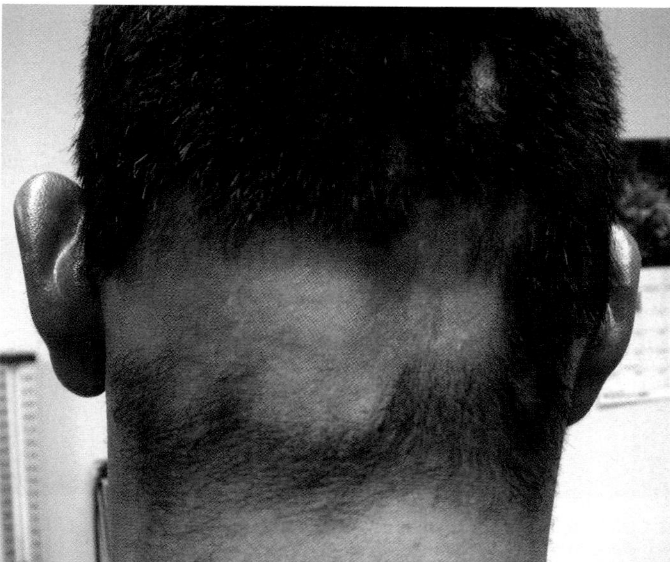

FIGURE 185-7 Ophiasis pattern of alopecia areata. Ophiasis means "serpent like." (*Reproduced with permission from Richard P. Usatine, MD.*)

BIOPSY

Not needed unless the diagnosis is uncertain. Histology examination shows peribulbar lymphocytic infiltration, frequently including eosinophils and the above-mentioned (see "Clinical Features") "exclamation point" hairs. In elderly adults in which AA is less common, if the clinical picture is not clearly AA, a biopsy is warranted (**Figure 185-9**). Perform a punch biopsy including at least one hair follicle in the affected area if possible.

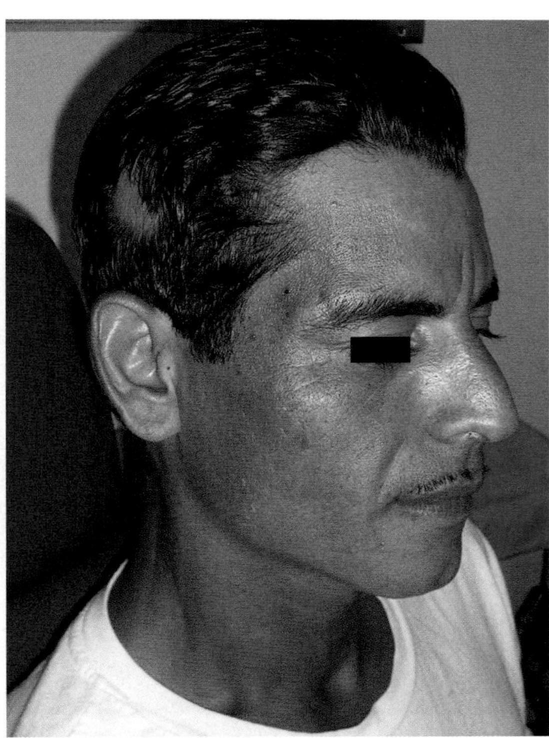

FIGURE 185-8 A patient with alopecia areata who was hyperthyroid. He had symptoms of hyperthyroidism and his thyroid-stimulating hormone was low. (*Reproduced with permission from Richard P. Usatine, MD.*)

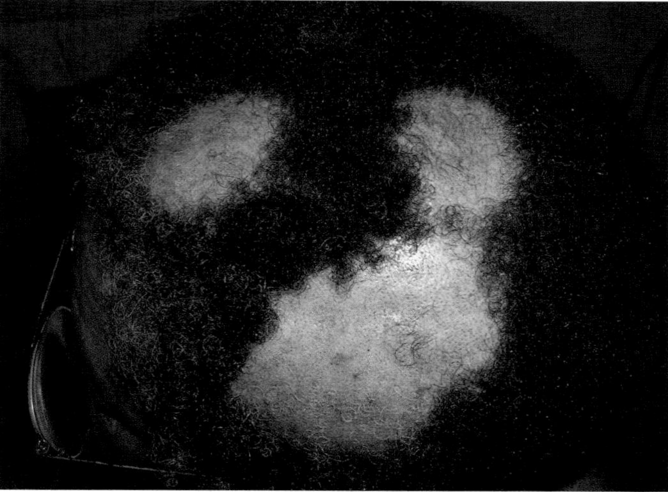

FIGURE 185-9 Alopecia areata that was biopsy proven in an elderly black woman. The hair loss was present for years and there was only partial regrowth of hair. As the diagnosis was not 100% certain clinically, a punch biopsy was performed including at least one hair follicle in the affected area. (*Reproduced with permission from Richard P. Usatine, MD.*)

DIFFERENTIAL DIAGNOSIS

- Trichotillomania—History of hair pulling; short, "broken" hairs are seen (see Chapter 186, Traction Alopecia and Trichotillomania).
- Telogen effluvium—Even distribution of hair loss; may be drug-induced (eg, warfarin, β-blockers, lithium) or occur after pregnancy
- Anagen effluvium—History of drug use (eg, antimitotic agents); even distribution of hair loss.
- Tinea capitis—Skin scaling and inflammation; potassium hydroxide (KOH) prep or fungal culture. Very rare in adults.
- Secondary syphilis—"Moth-eaten" appearance in beard or scalp; risk factors and rapid plasma reagin (RPR) will help distinguish (see Chapter 218, Syphilis).
- Lupus erythematosus—Skin scarring; antinuclear antibody (ANA) if clinical presentation compatible with this diagnosis (see Chapter 178, Lupus: Systemic and Cutaneous).
- Follicular mucinosis with or without mycosis fungoides can cause similar areas of hair loss to AA (**Figure 185-10**) (see Chapter 174, Cutaneous T-cell Lymphoma).

MANAGEMENT

- Many patients with AA will have significant comorbid anxiety and depression, so the management of psychological implications is paramount to successful management.
- Treatment for alopecia includes immune-modulating agents (eg, corticosteroids, anthralin, psoralen plus ultraviolet A [PUVA]), contact sensitizers (eg, dinitrochlorobenzene, squaric acid dibutyl ester, diphenylcyclopropenone [DPCP]), and biological response modifiers (eg, minoxidil).[6,7] SOR Ⓒ
    - A commonly used treatment in patients with less than 50% scalp involvement is intralesional steroids (**Figure 185-11**). SOR Ⓑ

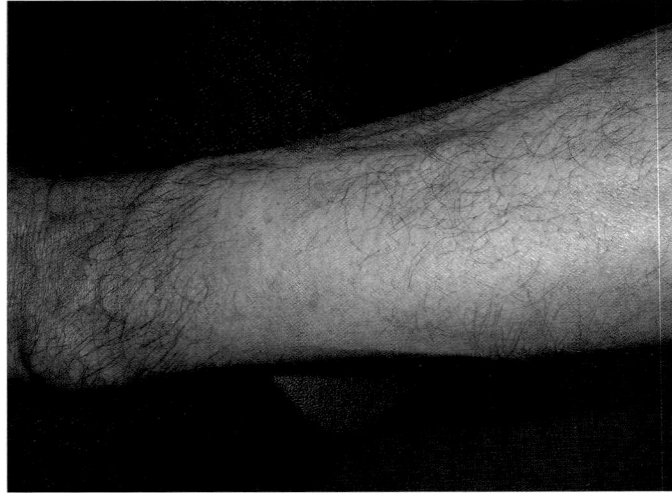

A

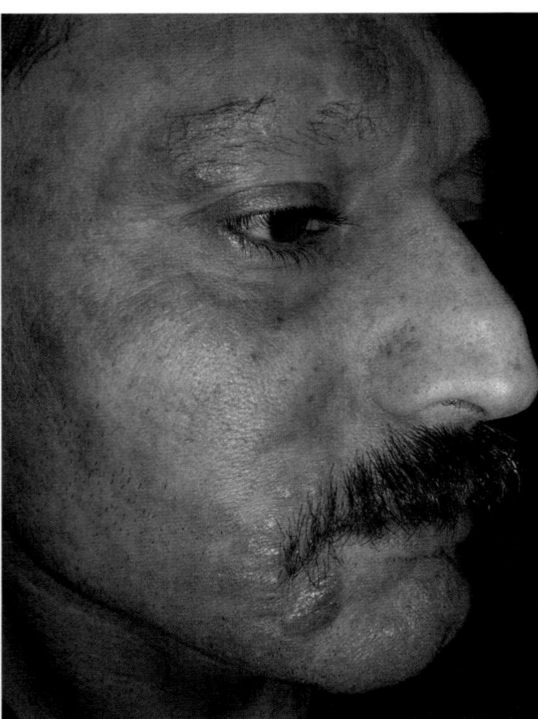

B

FIGURE 185-10 A. A rare occurrence of folliculotropic mycosis fungoides causing patches of hair loss on the arm and eyebrow. B. Before the red plaques appeared on the face, the hair loss was thought to be alopecia areata. Biopsy of a facial lesion demonstrated cutaneous T-cell lymphoma. (*Reproduced with permission from Richard P. Usatine, MD.*)

- In one randomized controlled trial (RCT), intralesional triamcinolone acetonide (10 mg/mL every 3 weeks) was better than betamethasone valerate foam and topical tacrolimus in the management of localized AA.[8] There was no satisfactory hair regrowth in the tacrolimus group.[8] Although 10 mg/mL triamcinolone is often used as treatment, there is a higher rate of scalp atrophy than with 5 mg/mL. Start with 5 mg/mL and consider 10 mg/mL in subsequent injections if there is acceptance of a higher risk of scalp atrophy.
- Triamcinolone acetonide (Kenalog)—Dilute with sterile saline to 5 mg/mL. Inject with a 3-mL or 5-mL syringe and a 27- or

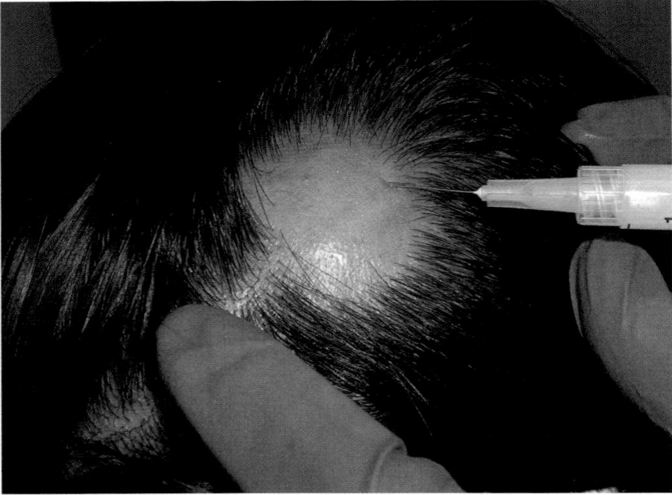

FIGURE 185-11 Injecting alopecia areata with triamcinolone acetonide 5 mg/mL. (*Reproduced with permission from Richard P. Usatine, MD.*)

30-gauge needle. Inject into the dermis of the involved areas but not to exceed 4 mL per visit. Use 2.5 mg/mL for involved areas of the eyebrows or beard. SOR C
- Skin atrophy can be reduced by injecting intradermally and limiting both the volume per site and the frequency of injections (4-6 weeks between injections). Do not reinject areas that show atrophy and in most cases, the atrophy will resolve spontaneously. SOR C
- Spontaneous regrowth may still occur, so steroid injections should be discontinued after 6 months.

- For patients with more than 50% of scalp involvement (**Figure 185-12**), topical immunotherapy with contact sensitizers may be an effective treatment.
  - Topical DPCP is a contact immunotherapy that has some proven benefit with extensive AA. In one study, 56 patients with chronic, extensive AA (duration ranging from 1 to 10 years, involving 30%-100% of the scalp) were treated with progressively higher concentrations of DPCP in a randomized crossover trial.

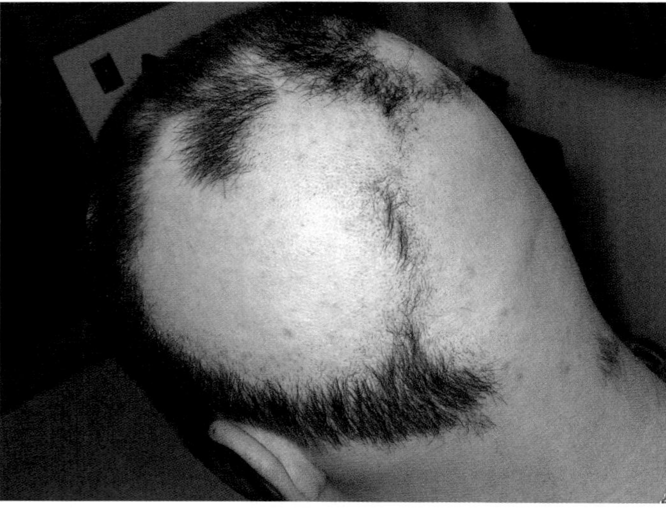

FIGURE 185-12 Alopecia areata present for more than 1 year in this young man. The length of time without resolution and the large areas involved diminish the prognosis for hair regrowth. (*Reproduced with permission from Richard P. Usatine, MD.*)

Twenty-five of 56 patients had total hair regrowth at 6 months, and no relapse occurred in 60% of patients.[7] SOR Ⓑ

- These contact sensitizers have potential severe side effects, including mutagenesis, blistering, hyperpigmentation, and scarring, and thus should be used by clinicians with significant experience with these agents or in consultation with a dermatologic specialist.
- Minoxidil, PUVA, and anthralin have been used with varying effectiveness and can be considered.

A Cochrane review in 2008 concluded that most trials have been reported poorly and are so small that any important clinical benefits are inconclusive.[9] They stated that considering the possibility of spontaneous remission (especially for those in the early stages of the disease) the options of not treating or wearing a wig are reasonable alternatives.[9]

- Hairpieces and transplantation may be used for those patients with unresponsive, recalcitrant disease.

COMPLEMENTARY AND ALTERNATIVE THERAPY

One RCT showed aromatherapy with topical essential oils to be a safe and effective treatment for AA.[10] The active group massaged essential oils (thyme, rosemary, lavender, and cedarwood) in a mixture of carrier oils (jojoba and grape seed) into their scalp daily. This is a good option for patients that want to do something but want to avoid the use of steroids. SOR Ⓑ

PATIENT EDUCATION AND PROGNOSIS

- Although spontaneous recovery usually occurs, the course of AA is unpredictable and often characterized by recurrent periods of hair loss and regrowth.
- Spontaneous long-term regrowth in alopecia totalis and AU is poor.
- Prognosis is worse if the alopecia persists longer than 1 year (see **Figure 185-12**).
- Alopecia areata, totalis, and universalis can actually resolve spontaneously at any time as the hair follicle retains its ability to regrow even years after the initial loss of hair.
- Patients with a family history of AA, younger age at onset, coexisting immune disorders, nail dystrophy, atopy, and widespread hair loss (see **Figure 185-12**) have a poorer prognosis.[5]

FOLLOW-UP

- Spontaneous recovery usually occurs within 6 to 12 months and the prognosis for total permanent regrowth with limited involvement (AA) is excellent.
- The regrown hair is usually of the same texture and color but may be fine and white at first (see **Figure 185-5**).
- Ten percent of patients never regrow hair and advance to chronic disease. Clinicians should provide contact information to the National Alopecia Areata Foundation and offer follow-up in the office as necessary.

PATIENT RESOURCES

- The National Alopecia Areata Foundation **http://www.naaf.org/** publishes a newsletter and can provide information regarding these support groups as well as hairpiece information.
- National Institute of Arthritis and Musculoskeletal and Skin Disease—**http://www.niams.nih.gov/hi/topics/alopecia/ff_alopecia_areata.htm.**

PROVIDER RESOURCES

- Medscape. *Alopecia Areata*—**http://emedicine.medscape.com/article/1069931.**
- British Association of Dermatologists' guidelines for the management of alopecia areata 2012—**http://www.guideline.gov/content.aspx?id=37715 or**
- **http://www.bad.org.uk/Portals/_Bad/Guidelines/Clinical%20Guidelines/Alopecia%20areata%20guidelines%202012.pdf**

REFERENCES

1. Usatine RP. Bald spots on a young girl. *J Fam Pract.* 2004;53:33-36.
2. Firooz A, Firoozabadi MR, Ghazisaidi B, Dowlati Y. Concepts of patients with alopecia areata about their disease. *BMC Dermatol.* 2005;5:1.
3. Springer K, Brown M, Stulberg DL. Common hair loss disorders. *Am Fam Physician.* 2003;68:93-102.
4. Choi HJ, Ihm CW. Acute alopecia totalis. *Acta Dermatovenerol Alp Panonica Adriat.* 2006;15:27-34.
5. Blaumeiser B, van der Goot I, Fimmers R, et al. Familial aggregation of alopecia areata. *J Am Acad Dermatol.* 2006;54:627-632.
6. Price VH. Treatment of hair loss. *N Engl J Med.* 1999;341:964-973.
7. Cotellessa C, Peris K, Caracciolo E, et al. The use of topical diphenylcyclopropenone for the treatment of extensive alopecia areata. *J Am Acad Dermatol.* 2001;44:73-76.
8. Kuldeep C, Singhal H, Khare AK, et al. Randomized comparison of topical betamethasone valerate foam, intralesional triamcinolone acetonide and tacrolimus ointment in management of localized alopecia areata. *Int J Trichology.* 2011;3:20-24.
9. Delamere FM, Sladden MM, Dobbins HM, Leonardi-Bee J. Interventions for alopecia areata. *Cochrane Database Syst Rev.* 2008 Apr 16;(2):CD004413.
10. Hay IC, Jamieson M, Ormerod AD. Randomized trial of aromatherapy. Successful treatment for alopecia areata. *Arch Dermatol.* 1998;134:1349-1352.

186 TRACTION ALOPECIA AND TRICHOTILLOMANIA

E.J. Mayeaux Jr, MD

PATIENT STORY

A 38-year-old woman was found to have hair thinning on the anterior scalp. She had long thick heavy hair that she always styled in a bun on the top of her head. She was concerned about the slow, steady loss of hair that she was experiencing. **Figure 186-1** shows the appearance of the thinned hair as a result of chronic traction. A 4-mm punch biopsy was performed to confirm the clinical impression and the histology was supportive of this diagnosis.

INTRODUCTION

Traction alopecia is hair loss caused by damage to the dermal papilla and hair follicle by constant pulling or tension over a long period. It often occurs in persons who wear tight braids, especially "cornrows" that lead to high tension, pulling, and breakage of hair. Trichotillomania (Greek for "hair-pulling madness") is a traction alopecia related to a compulsive disorder caused when patients pull on and pluck hairs, often creating bizarre patterns of hair loss.

EPIDEMIOLOGY

- The prevalence of traction alopecia (**Figures 186-1** and **186-2**) is unknown and varies by cultural hairstyle practices. It is most commonly seen in females and children.[1]

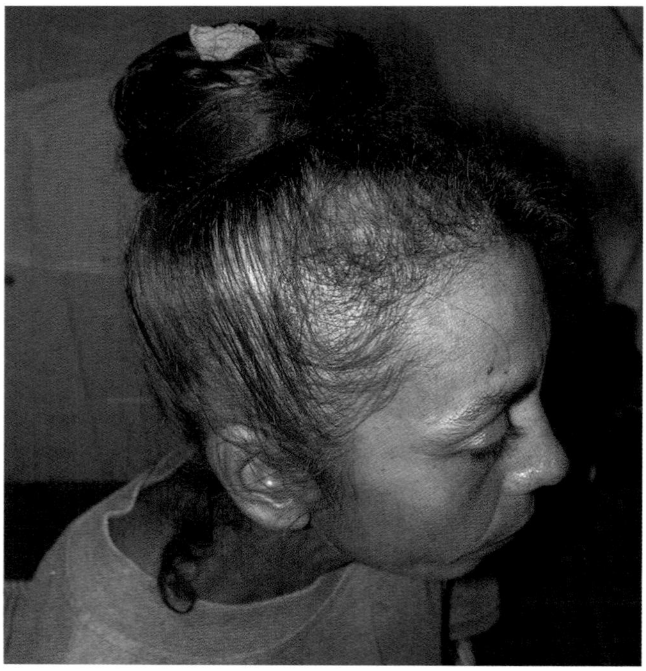

FIGURE 186-1 Traction alopecia from pulling the hair up in a tight bun. (*Reproduced with permission from Richard P. Usatine, MD.*)

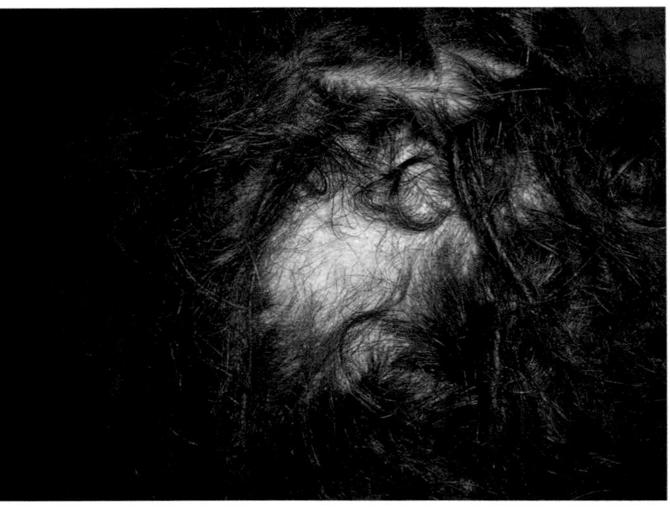

FIGURE 186-2 Traction alopecia in a 31-year-old white woman who has worn her hair in dread locks for years. (*Reproduced with permission from Richard P. Usatine, MD.*)

- The prevalence of trichotillomania (**Figures 186-3** to **186-5**) is also difficult to determine, but is estimated to be approximately 1.5% of males and 3.4% of females in the United States. The mean age of onset of trichotillomania is 8 years in boys and 12 years in girls, and while it is the most common cause of childhood alopecia it does occur in adults.[2]

ETIOLOGY AND PATHOPHYSIOLOGY

- Traction alopecia is seen in individuals who place chronic tension on the hair shafts with tight braids, dread locks, heavy natural hair, use of hair prostheses, or chronic pulling (see **Figures 186-1** and **186-2**).[1] It also occurs commonly in female athletes who pull their hair into tight ponytails.

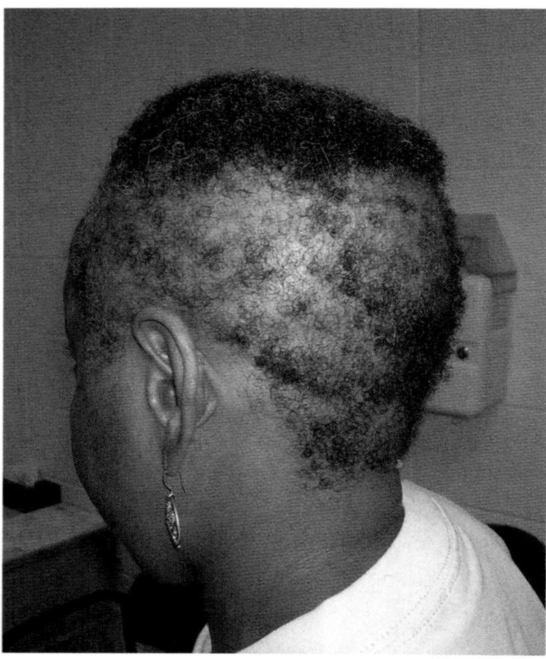

FIGURE 186-3 Chronic hair loss in a 39-year-old woman with trichotillomania. (*Reproduced with permission from E.J. Mayeaux Jr, MD.*)

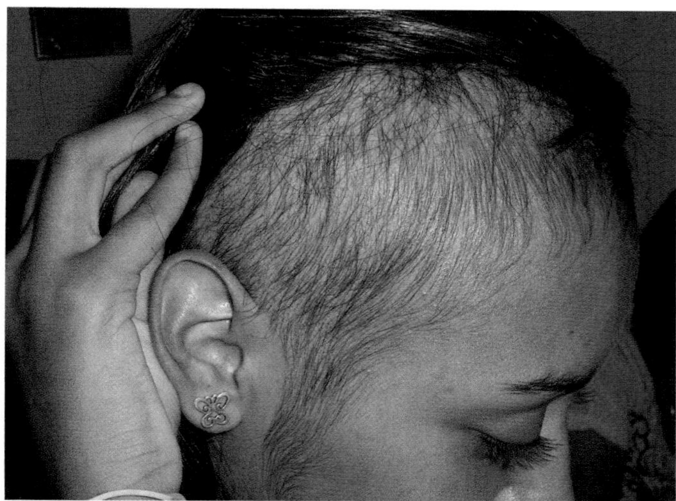

FIGURE 186-4 Trichotillomania in a 17-year-old honors student who was taking 4 Advanced Placement courses simultaneously. (*Reproduced with permission from Richard P. Usatine, MD.*)

- Chronic tension on the hair shaft seems to create inflammation within the hair follicle that eventually leads to cessation of hair growth. Because hair loss from traction alopecia may become permanent, prevention and early treatment are important.
- It is seen most frequently in black women who tightly braid or pull the hair into a hairstyle during youth and into adulthood. It may also be seen in individuals who wear hair prostheses or extensions for a prolonged period of time. It is also seen in Sikh men of India and Japanese women whose traditional hairstyles may pull and damage hair.
- Trichotillomania is a subtype of traction alopecia manifested by chronic hair pulling (see **Figures 186-3** to **186-5**) and sometimes hair eating (trichophagy), which can lead to a trichobezoar. It is classified as a psychiatric impulse-control disorder.[3]
- Trichotillomania may be a manifestation of the inability to cope with stress rather than more severe mental disorders.
- Children who exhibit trichotillomania may discontinue the hair pulling with parental support and maturity. Adults who exhibit trichotillomania, even though they are aware of the problem, may require psychiatric intervention to limit the behavior. The hair loss is initially reversible but may become permanent if the habits persist.

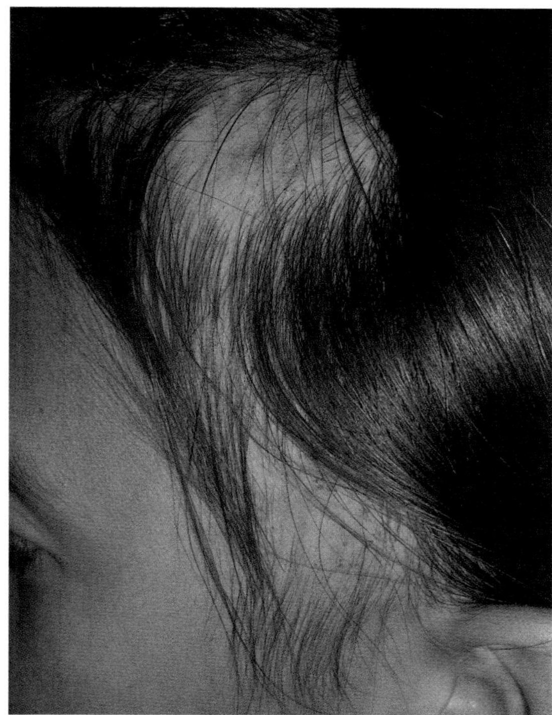

A

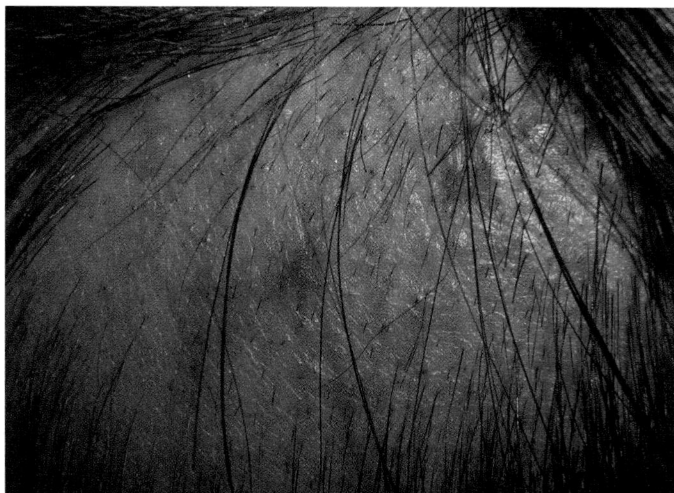

B

FIGURE 186-5 **A.** Trichotillomania in a patient undergoing much stress because of conflict in her family. **B.** Close-up of trichotillomania showing broken hairs, black dots, and excoriations. (*Reproduced with permission from Richard P. Usatine, MD.*)

DIAGNOSIS

CLINICAL FEATURES

In patients with traction alopecia, there are decreased follicular ostia in the affected area coupled with decreased hair density. The hair loss usually occurs in the frontal and temporal areas but depends on the precipitating hairstyle (see **Figures 186-1** and **186-2**). No scalp inflammation or scaling is typically visible. No pain or other discomfort is associated with the condition. Patients with trichotillomania often demonstrate short, broken hairs (see **Figure 186-5**) without the presence of inflammation or skin scale early in the disease. The affected areas are not bald, but rather possess hairs of varying length. There may be telltale stubble of hairs too short to pull. The hair loss often follows bizarre patterns with incomplete areas of clearing. The scalp may appear normal or have areas of erythema and pustule formation. With chronic pulling, the hair loss becomes permanent (see **Figure 186-3**). The patient may be observed pulling or twisting the hair by friends or family members.

TYPICAL DISTRIBUTION

Trichotillomania most commonly occurs on the scalp and can involve any area of the body that can be reached by the patient.[1] Traction alopecia can occur anywhere on the scalp, but is most commonly seen at the anterior hairline. This is the site where the hair is pulled back from the face into braids or a bun.

LABORATORY STUDIES

Laboratory tests are not needed to make the diagnosis. A hand lens can be used to examine the affected scalp for decreased follicular ostia, if desired. A scalp biopsy (4-mm punch biopsy) may be necessary to make the diagnosis and rule out other etiologies, especially in trichotillomania, because patients may not acknowledge the habit.

Hypothyroidism or hyperthyroidism may be associated with telogen effluvium or alopecia areata. It may be worth ordering a thyroid-stimulating hormone (TSH) if the history and physical examination are not completely convincing for self-induced hair loss.

DIFFERENTIAL DIAGNOSIS[1]

- Alopecia areata is characterized by the total absence of hair in an area and the presence of exclamation point hairs. These hairs are thinner in diameter closer to the scalp and thicker in diameter away from the scalp, creating the appearance of an exclamation point. Hairs are often white when they start to regrow (see Chapter 185, Alopecia Areata).
- Tinea capitis is very rare among adults. It exhibits hairs broken off at the skin surface and the presence of scale and/or inflammation. Some varieties fluoresce when examined with a Wood light (ultraviolet [UV] light). Microscopy of a potassium hydroxide (KOH) preparation may detect the dermatophyte. Sometimes it is necessary to culture some hairs and scale to make this diagnosis.
- Scarring alopecia (lichen planopilaris, folliculitis decalvans) is observed as loss of the follicular ostia and the absence of hairs. The scalp may appear scarred with changes in pigmentation (see Chapter 187, Scarring Alopecia).
- Telogen effluvium (postpregnancy hair loss) is associated with hair loss during the postpartum period and can happen after other stressful events such as surgery or severe illness. The hair loss is evenly distributed across the head and the hair is thinned all over rather than in patches as in traction alopecia.
- Androgenetic alopecia produces central thinning in women and temple and crown thinning in males. It should be considered in women with symptoms of hormonal abnormalities such as hirsutism, amenorrhea, or infertility.

MANAGEMENT

NONPHARMACOLOGIC

- Stop hairstyling practices that led to the traction alopecia. No tight braiding or buns should be worn.[1] SOR C
- For trichotillomania, open discussions with the patient, and the family, if appropriate, are important to understand the reason for the behavior. Many times there are secondary social or emotional issues that must be resolved before the trichotillomania ceases.
  - Cognitive-behavioral treatment is the most effective treatment for trichotillomania.[1,3] SOR B
  - Cognitive-behavioral therapy usually is successful if the patient is recalcitrant to simple education.[4] SOR C

MEDICATIONS

- Topical corticosteroids can be used to decrease scalp inflammation if erythema or itching is present. SOR C
- Topical minoxidil is sometimes used to speed hair regrowth in the area. SOR C
- Fluoxetine hydrochloride (Prozac) 20 to 40 mg/d in adults or clomipramine (Anafranil) 25 to 250 mg/d in adults or a maximum of 3 mg/kg/d in children has had some success for alleviating compulsive hair pulling.[4-6] SOR B

Olanzapine (Zyprexa) has been studied for the treatment of trichotillomania in a 12-week, randomized, double-blind, placebo-controlled trial. A dose of 10 mg/d showed a significant decrease in the CGI-Severity of Illness scale in 85% of subjects.[7] SOR B

Methylphenidate also has showed limited efficacy in trichotillomania patients with comorbid attention-deficit hyperactivity disorder (ADHD) in a 12-week study.[8] SOR B

PATIENT EDUCATION

Explain that in traction alopecia, current grooming practices are responsible for the hair loss and a new hairstyle must be selected. It is important to tell the patient that some of the hair loss may be permanent and no guarantee can be given regarding the amount of expected hair regrowth. Prevention is definitely the best treatment.

Explain that trichotillomania is a self-induced disease that can often resolve if the hair pulling or twisting is discontinued. Patients may exhibit hair pulling or twisting unconsciously when stressed or use it as a calming activity when relaxing or going to sleep. The underlying reasons for the behavior should be explored and discussed. Sometimes trichotillomania can be substituted with another behavior, such as playing with beads or rubbing a stone.

FOLLOW-UP

Specific follow-up is not required for traction alopecia but psychiatric/behavioral counseling follow-up is indicated for trichotillomania.

PATIENT RESOURCES

- Trichotillomania Support and Therapy Site. *Emphasis on Growth*—**http://www.trichotillomania.co.uk/.**
- WebMD. *Mental Health and Trichotillomania*—**http://www.webmd.com/anxiety-panic/guide/trichotillomania.**
- *Traction Alopecia: Causes and Treatment Options*—**http://www.traction-alopecia.com/.**
- National Organization for Rare Disorders, Inc. *Trichotillomania*—**http://www.kumed.com/healthwise/healthwise.aspx?DOCHWID=nord768.**
- MedlinePlus. *Trichotillomania*—**http://www.nlm.nih.gov/medlineplus/ency/article/001517.htm.**
- Mental Health America. *Trichotillomania*—**http://www.nmha.org/go/information/get-info/trichotillomania.**

PROVIDER RESOURCES

- Medscape. *Trichotillomania*—**http://emedicine.medscape.com/article/1071854.**
- *Traction Alopecia*—**http://www.emedicine.com/derm/topic895.htm.**

REFERENCES

1. Springer K, Brown M, Stulberg DL. Common hair loss disorders. *Am Fam Physician.* 2003;68:93-102, 107-108.
2. Messinger ML, Cheng TL. Trichotillomania. *Pediatr Rev.* 1999;20: 249-250.
3. Bloch MH, Landeros-Weisenberger A, Dombrowski P, et al. Systematic review: pharmacological and behavioral treatment for trichotillomania. *Biol Psychiatry.* 2007;62(8):839-846.
4. Streichenwein SM, Thornby JI. A long-term, double-blind, placebo-controlled crossover trial of the efficacy of fluoxetine for trichotillomania. *Am J Psychiatry.* 1995;152:1192-1196.
5. Christenson GA, Crow SJ. The characterization and treatment of trichotillomania. *J Clin Psychiatry.* 1996;57(suppl 8):42-47.
6. Ninan PT, Rothbaum BO, Marsteller FA, et al. A placebo-controlled trial of cognitive-behavioral therapy and clomipramine in trichotillomania. *J Clin Psychiatry.* 2000;61:47-50.
7. Van Ameringen M, Mancini C, Patterson B, et al. A randomized, double-blind, placebo-controlled trial of olanzapine in the treatment of trichotillomania. *J Clin Psychiatry.* 2010;71(10):1336-1343.
8. Golubchik P, Sever J, Weizman A, Zalsman G. Methylphenidate treatment in pediatric patients with attention-deficit/hyperactivity disorder and comorbid trichotillomania: a preliminary report. *Clin Neuropharmacol.* 2011;34(3):108-110.

187 SCARRING ALOPECIA

Richard P. Usatine, MD

PATIENT STORY

A 32-year-old man presents with hair loss along with chronic pustular eruptions of his scalp. Previous biopsy has shown folliculitis decalvans. He has had many courses of antibiotics, but the hair loss continues to progress. The active pustular lesions are cultured and grow out methicillin-resistant *Staphylococcus aureus* (MRSA). The patient is treated with trimethoprim-sulfamethoxazole twice daily and mupirocin to the nasal mucosa, twice daily for 5 days. Two weeks later, the pustular lesions are less prominent although the alopecia is permanent (**Figures 187-1** and **187-2**).

INTRODUCTION

Scarring alopecia is a group of inflammatory disorders in which there is permanent destruction of the pilosebaceous unit. Although it is mostly seen on the scalp, it can involve other areas, such as the eyebrows.

In primary cicatricial alopecia, the hair follicle is the primary target of destruction by inflammation. In secondary cicatricial alopecia, the follicular destruction is incidental to a nonfollicular process such as infection, tumor, burn, radiation, or traction.

SYNONYM

Scarring alopecia is also known as cicatricial alopecia.

EPIDEMIOLOGY

Primary cicatricial alopecias are rare.

The annual incidence rate of lichen planopilaris (LPP) in 4 hair loss centers in the United States varied from 1.15% to 7.59% as defined by new biopsy-proven LPP—all new patients with hair loss seen over a 1-year period.[1]

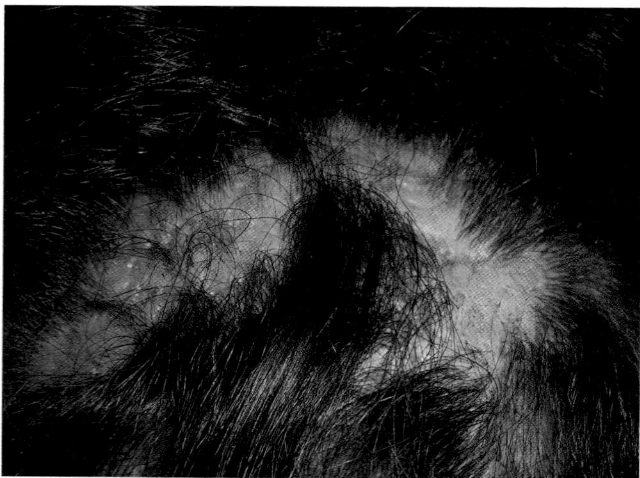

FIGURE 187-1 Folliculitis decalvans in a 32-year-old man. He has an active area of pustular lesions on the periphery with wide areas of scarring and hair loss. (*Reproduced with permission from Richard P. Usatine, MD.*)

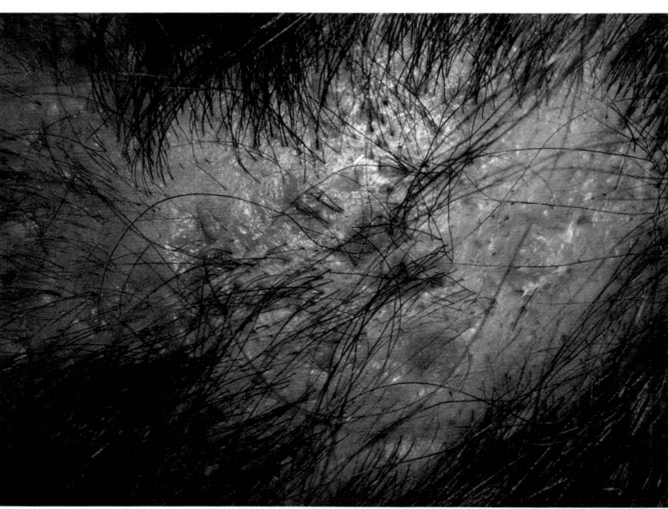

FIGURE 187-2 Same patient in **Figure 187-1** showing permanent hair loss on the top of the head with some small-active pustular lesions. (*Reproduced with permission from Richard P. Usatine, MD.*)

PATHOPHYSIOLOGY

Scarring alopecia occurs when there is inflammation and destruction of the hair follicles leading to fibrous tissue formation.[2]

Hair loss in scarring alopecia is irreversible because the inflammatory infiltrate results in destruction of the hair follicle stem cells and the sebaceous glands.[3]

The inflammatory infiltrates are either predominantly lymphocytic, neutrophilic, or mixed. These differences are used to classify the scarring alopecias. See **Table 187-1**.

DIAGNOSIS

Scarring alopecias can vary by distribution and appearance.[4] Most patients will need a biopsy to confirm the clinical impression and determine the specific type of alopecia.

TABLE 187-1 Classification of Cicatricial Alopecia

Lymphocytic	Lichen planopilaris (LPP) Frontal fibrosing alopecia (FFA) Central centrifugal cicatricial alopecia (CCCA) Discoid lupus erythematosus (DLE)*
Neutrophilic	Folliculitis decalvans Tufted folliculitis
Mixed	Dissecting cellulitis* Acne keloidalis nuchae*
End stage	Nonspecific

*Not a primary cicatricial alopecia.

Data from Olsen EA, Bergfeld WF, Cotsarelis G, et al. Summary of North American Hair Research Society (NAHRS)-sponsored Workshop on Cicatricial Alopecia, Duke University Medical Center, February 10 and 11, 2001. *J Am Acad Dermatol*. 2003;48:103-110.

CLINICAL PRESENTATION

Hair loss with itching, pain, and/or burning of the scalp. Some cases are asymptomatic.

PHYSICAL EXAMINATION

The "pull test" is used to see how active the hair loss is in general and in specific areas of the scalp. Always ask the patient if you can pull on the hair as part of your diagnosis.

- With the thumb and forefinger grasp approximately 30 to 40 hairs close to the scalp.
- Gently, but firmly, slide the fingers away from the scalp at a 90-degree angle along the entire length of the hair swatch. Do not tug or jerk.

Interpreting the pull test results the following:

- Negative pull test = 1 to 4 telogen hairs (small bulbs at bottom).
- Positive pull test = 5 or more hairs (including anagen hairs that have longer follicle sheath at the bottom of the hair).[5]

Forms of primary cicatricial alopecia include the following:

- LPP most commonly affects middle-aged women. It mostly occurs on the frontal and parietal scalp and causes follicular hyperkeratosis, pruritus, perifollicular erythema, violaceous color of scalp, and scalp pain (**Figure 187-3**).[2] It may also affect other hair-bearing sites such as the groin and axilla.[2] Most patients with LPP do not have lichen planus even though the names are very similar.
- Central centrifugal scarring alopecia (CCCA) is a slowly progressive alopecia that begins in the vertex and advances to surrounding areas. It may be related to chemicals used on the hair, heat from hot combs, or chronic tension on the hair.[2] It is seen more commonly in African American women (**Figure 187-4**).
- Frontal fibrosing alopecia (FFA) presents with a progressive recession of the frontal hairline affecting particularly postmenopausal women. It is considered to be a variant of LPP on the basis of its clinical, histologic, and immunohistochemical features (**Figure 187-5**).[6]
- Folliculitis decalvans is a chronic painful neutrophilic bacterial folliculitis characterized by bogginess or induration of the scalp with pustules, erosions, crusts, and scale.[2] It is postulated that this results from an abnormal host response to *S. aureus*, which is often cultured from the lesions (see **Figures 187-1** and **187-2**). In one case series, the disease ran a protracted course with temporary improvement while on antibiotic and flare-up of disease when antibiotics were stopped.[7]
- Tufted folliculitis can be considered to be a milder version of folliculitis decalvans with less surface area of the scalp involved and a better prognosis (**Figure 187-6**). However, these hair tufts can be seen in other types of scarring alopecias.

Secondary forms of scarring alopecia include the following:

- Dissecting cellulitis presents with deep inflammatory nodules, primarily over the occiput, that progress to coalescing regions of boggy scalp.[1] Sinus tracts may form and *S. aureus* is frequently cultured from the inflamed lesions. When dissecting cellulitis occurs with acne conglobata and hidradenitis suppurativa, the syndrome is referred to as the *follicular occlusion triad* (**Figures 187-7** and **187-8**).
- Acne keloidalis nuchae (folliculitis keloidalis) presents with a chronic papular and pustular eruption at the nape of the neck. This can lead to

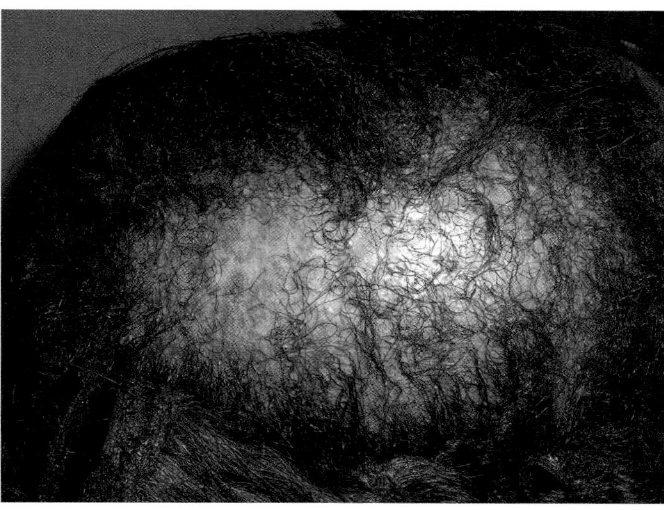

FIGURE 187-4 Central centrifugal scarring alopecia in a middle-aged African American woman. Note how the vertex is most affected. Patient has used many hair chemicals, hot combs, and braids over the years. (*Reproduced with permission from Richard P. Usatine, MD.*)

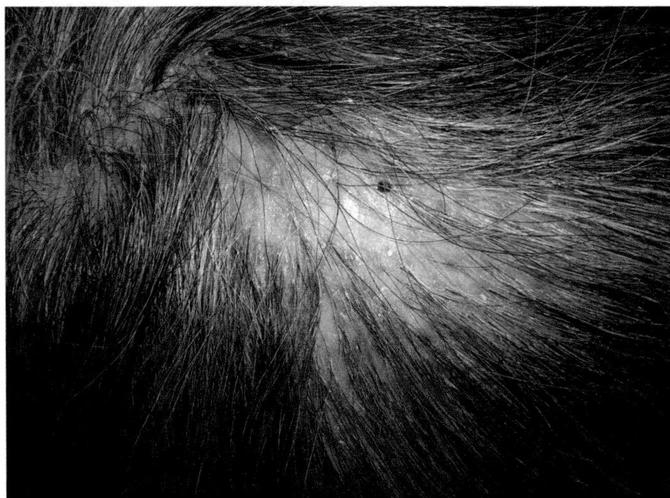

FIGURE 187-3 Lichen planopilaris in a 45-year-old woman causing hair loss with perifollicular scale. (*Reproduced with permission from Richard P. Usatine, MD.*)

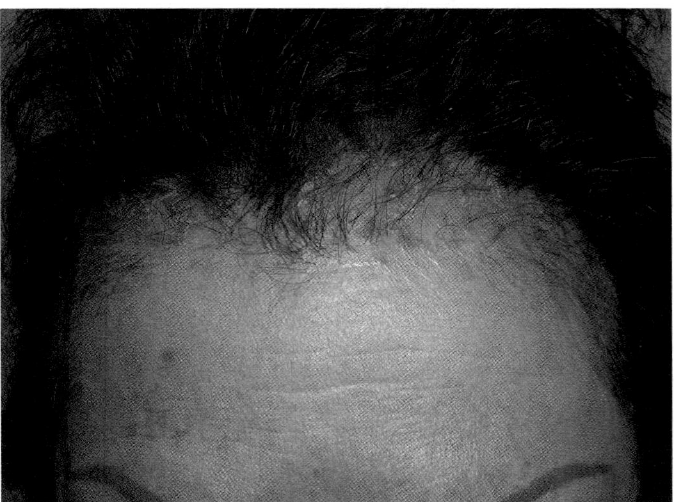

FIGURE 187-5 Frontal fibrosing alopecia with progressive recession of the frontal hairline in a postmenopausal woman. There was hair loss involving the eyebrows too. (*Reproduced with permission from Richard P. Usatine, MD.*)

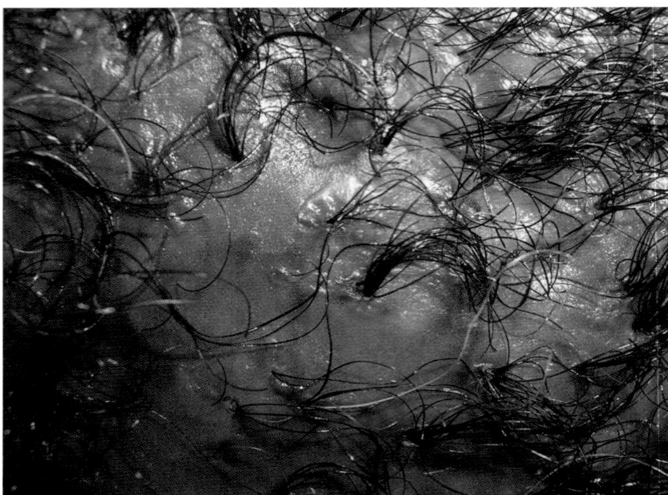

FIGURE 187-6 Tufted folliculitis showing multiple hairs growing from the same follicle along with purulence and hair loss. (*Reproduced with permission from Richard P. Usatine, MD.*)

scarring alopecia with large keloidal scarring. It is seen most commonly in men of color but also can be seen in women. It is often made worse by shaving the hair (see Chapter 116, Pseudofolliculitis and Acne Keloidalis Nuchae) (**Figures 187-9** and **187-10**).

- Discoid lupus erythematosus (DLE) presents with lesions that can be erythematous, atrophic, and/or hypopigmented. Scarring alopecia may be accompanied by follicular plugging on the scalp. Hypopigmentation may develop in the central area of the inflammatory lesions and hyperpigmentation may develop at the active border. The external ear and ear canal are often involved (**Figure 187-11**) (see Chapter 178, Lupus: Systemic and Cutaneous).

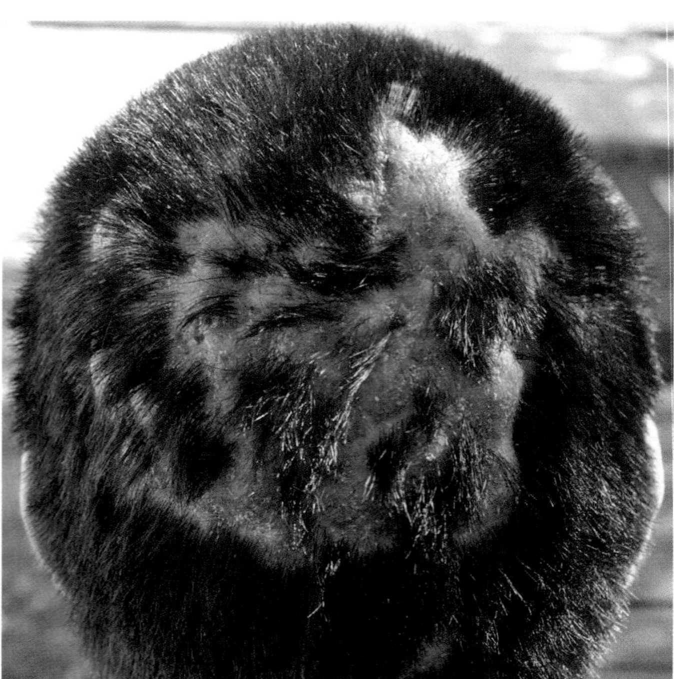

FIGURE 187-7 Dissecting cellulitis of the scalp in a young Hispanic man with many active sinus tracts and alopecia. (*Reproduced with permission from Richard P. Usatine, MD.*)

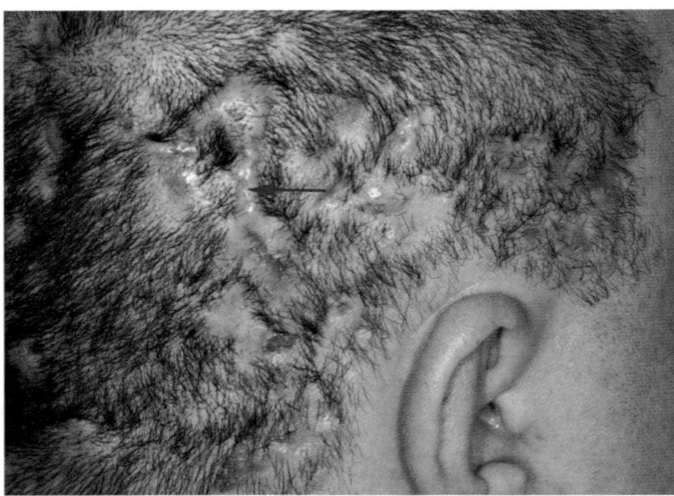

FIGURE 187-8 Dissecting cellulitis of the scalp causing painful purulent nodules and sinus tracts leading to scarring alopecia. The patient also has severe hidradenitis suppurativa and therefore has 2 of 3 elements of the follicular occlusion triad (he does not have acne conglobata). The arrow points to one sinus tract. (*Reproduced with permission from Richard P. Usatine, MD.*)

LABORATORY STUDIES

If there is purulence, perform a bacterial culture. *S. aureus* and MRSA are frequently seen in the neutrophilic alopecias. Consider obtaining various tests such as thyroid-stimulating hormone (TSH), serum iron level, complete blood count (CBC), and rapid plasma reagin (RPR) to rule out treatable causes of alopecia. Do a potassium hydroxide (KOH) smear and/or culture if tinea capitis is suspected.

BIOPSY

Biopsy is almost always recommended to diagnose primary scarring alopecia.[5] Usually a single 4-mm punch biopsy for histology is adequate. Some dermatopathologists will prefer two 4-mm punch biopsies at the same time so that they may cut the specimens both tangentially and vertically for analysis. Discuss this with your dermatopathologist or pathologist. Make sure to biopsy at the margin of the active disease and include hair follicles in the specimen.

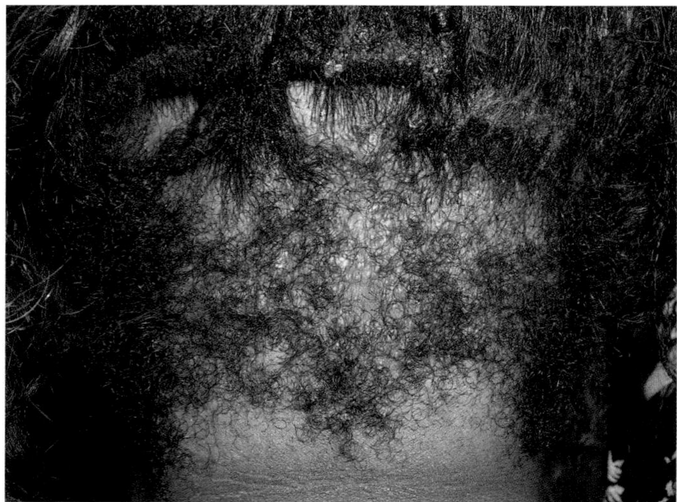

FIGURE 187-9 Acne keloidalis nuchae in a 45-year-old African American woman. Note the significant hair loss. Although acne keloidalis nuchae is more common in men, it can occur in women too. (*Reproduced with permission from Richard P. Usatine, MD.*)

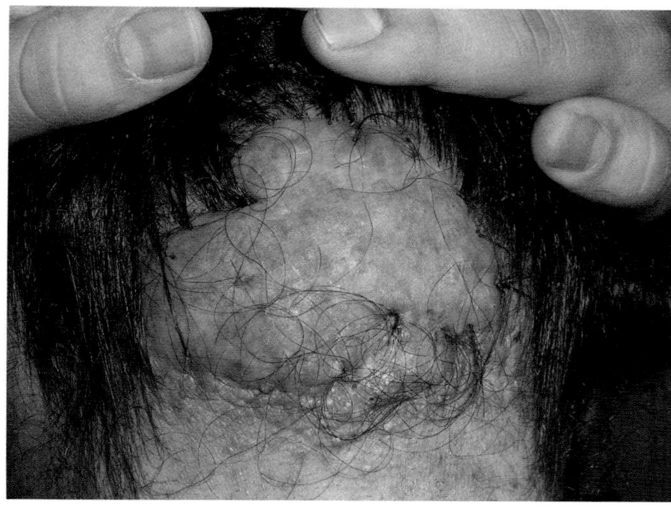

FIGURE 187-10 Acne keloidalis nuchae in a 32-year-old man with significant hair loss and a keloidal mass. Note that there are many hairs growing together in "tufts" as seen in tufted folliculitis. *(Reproduced with permission from Richard P. Usatine, MD.)*

DIFFERENTIAL DIAGNOSIS

- Alopecia areata presents with hair loss and a very smooth scalp. The hair loss is usually in round punched-out patterns and the scalp otherwise appears normal (see Chapter 185, Alopecia Areata).
- Androgenetic alopecia is the standard hair loss that males experience with aging. There are a number of male pattern types of hair loss. Women also get androgenic alopecia, but the pattern tends to be more diffuse and frontal. Both are treatable with topical minoxidil and oral finasteride.
- Drug-induced alopecia is from chemotherapy and other toxic drugs.
- Sarcoidosis of the scalp can resemble DLE, but treatment will be different, hence the importance of a biopsy diagnosis (see Chapter 173, Sarcoidosis).[8]

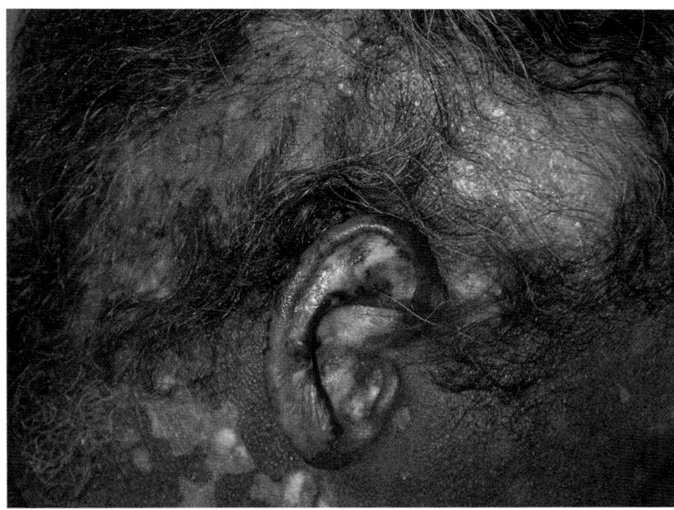

FIGURE 187-11 Chronic cutaneous lupus erythematosus showing scarring alopecia. Prominent hypopigmentation and skin atrophy are visible on the scalp and ear. *(Reproduced with permission from Richard P. Usatine, MD.)*

- Seborrheic dermatitis may cause some hair loss. The presence of scale on the scalp with minimal-to-no hair loss helps to differentiate this from scarring alopecia (see Chapter 149, Seborrheic Dermatitis).
- Secondary syphilis with moth-eaten alopecia is rare but should be considered. A highly positive RPR can easily make this diagnosis (see Chapter 218, Syphilis).
- Telogen effluvium is a type of nonscarring alopecia that occurs after childbirth or other traumatic events. The skin on the scalp appears normal.
- Tinea capitis presents with scale and hair loss. It is diagnosed by a positive KOH and/or fungal culture. It is very rare in adults but not impossible.
- Trichotillomania is defined as self-induced hair loss caused by pulling the hairs. The pattern of hair loss may be distinctive and the behavior may be discovered on history. The scalp appears normal and there is a distinctive pattern seen on biopsy (see Chapter 186, Traction Alopecia and Trichotillomania).
- Traction alopecia occurs when the hair is pulled too tight for braids or ponytails (see Chapter 186, Traction Alopecia and Trichotillomania).
- Various metabolic and nutritional problems can lead to alopecia. It is worth doing a CBC, ferritin, vitamin D_{25}-OH, and TSH to rule out iron deficiency, vitamin D deficiency, and hyper- or hypothyroidism.[5]

MANAGEMENT

- Scarring alopecias are such rare conditions that there are few randomized controlled trials available to guide therapy.
- One paradigm for treating primary scarring alopecia is to treat those containing predominantly lymphocytic infiltrates with immunomodulating agents and those with predominantly neutrophilic infiltrates with antimicrobial agents.[5,9] SOR C

Lymphocytic infiltrate predominates (LPP, CCCA, FFA). According to price, treatment can be split into the following categories[5]:

- Tier 1—Start here with 1 of the 2 oral agents combined with topical/intralesional medications:
  - Doxycycline 100 mg bid, or
  - Hydroxychloroquine 200 mg bid.
  - After 6 to 12 months, if symptoms and signs persist, move to tier 2.
- Tier 2
  - Mycophenolate mofetil 0.5 g bid for 1 month, then 1 g bid for 5 months.
  - Cyclosporine 3 to 5 mg/kg/d, or 100 mg tid.[10]
  - Pioglitazone 15 mg daily.[11]
- Topical/intralesional medications
  - Intralesional triamcinolone acetonide 10 mg/mL to inflamed, symptomatic sites (inject margins not bare center).
  - High-potency topical corticosteroids or topical tacrolimus or pimecrolimus.
  - Derma-Smoothe/FS scalp oil—Some patients prefer the oil-based vehicle on a dry scalp.

Studies that support this tiered approach for LPP include the following:

- In a retrospective review of 40 patients with LPP and its variant FFA, the investigators found that those treated with hydroxychloroquine daily had a 69% reduction in symptoms and signs after 6 months, and 89% improved after 12 months.[12] SOR B

- In another retrospective review of 16 patients with LPP treated with at least 6 months of mycophenolate mofetil in an open-label, single-center study, 5 of 12 patients were complete responders, 5 of 12 patients were partial responders, and 2 of 12 patients were treatment failures. Four patients withdrew from the trial because of adverse events.[13]
- In FFA the loss of eyebrows is common. Intralesional injection of triamcinolone acetonide showed regrowth response in 9 of 10 patients.[14]

Neutrophilic infiltrate predominates (folliculitis decalvans and tufted folliculitis).

- Start by culturing pustules and using oral antibiotics based on the pathogens cultured.
- Powell et al. introduced a treatment regimen for patients with folliculitis decalvans that combines oral rifampicin 600 mg daily and oral clindamycin 300 mg bid together for 10 weeks.[15] SOR B Ten of the 18 patients responded well with no evidence of recurrence 2 to 22 months after 1 course of treatment, and 15 of the 18 responded after 2 or 3 courses.[15]
- For methicillin-sensitive *S. aureus* cephalexin 500 mg qid × 10 weeks with oral rifampin 600 mg × 10 days is an alternative treatment.
- For MRSA treat with oral clindamycin 300 mg bid, or oral trimethoprim-sulfamethoxazole DS bid, or oral doxycycline 100 mg bid for 10 weeks combined with rifampin 600 mg × 10 days.[5]
- If the patient is a *S. aureus* carrier, add mupirocin ointment intranasally qd for 1 week, and monthly thereafter.[5] SOR C
- Dapsone at 75 to 100 mg/d for 4 to 6 months was well tolerated and rapidly effective in treating 2 cases of folliculitis decalvans. Long-term low-dose (25 mg/d) maintenance treatment avoided disease relapses. Paquet and Pierard chose dapsone because of its antimicrobial activity and its anti-inflammatory action directed to the neutrophil metabolism.[16] SOR C

Mixed infiltrates (dissecting cellulitis) include the following:

- Start by culturing any purulence and using oral antibiotics based on the pathogens cultured.
- Just as for neutrophilic infiltrates, treat with oral clindamycin 300 mg bid, or oral trimethoprim-sulfamethoxazole DS bid, or oral doxycycline 100 mg bid for 10 weeks combined with rifampin 600 mg × 10 days.
- Isotretinoin may be effective in inducing a prolonged remission. Price suggests starting with 20 mg daily, to avoid a flare, and then slowly increase to 1 mg/kg/d for many months.[5] SOR C

Primary and secondary scarring alopecias include the following:

- Imiquimod cream 5% was reported to cause regression of discoid lupus of the scalp and face in a single patient when applied to the lesions once a day 3 times a week. After 20 applications, Gul et al. reported that the lesions had regressed significantly.[17] SOR C
- Surgical excision of cicatricial alopecias includes excision and tissue expansion. Unfortunately, the outcomes have been disappointing to the patients and surgeons.[18] SOR C

FOLLOW-UP

Close follow-up is needed for patients put on oral agents. Monitoring for side effects is agent specific.

PATIENT EDUCATION

The following points are based on information from the Cicatricial Alopecia Research Foundation (**http://www.carfintl.org/faq.html**):

- The goal of treatment is to control scalp inflammation and stop the progression of the disease. Hair regrowth is not possible.
- Scarring alopecias often reactivate after a quiet period of 1 or more years. Patients should be encouraged to self-monitor for recurrence and to seek care early to prevent hair loss.
- It is safe to wash the hair with gentle hair products, if desired, even daily.
- When severe hair loss occurs, hats, scarves, hairpieces, and wigs may be used safely for cosmetic purposes.

PATIENT RESOURCES

- Cicatricial Alopecia Research Foundation—**http://www.carfintl.org/faq.html.**
- American Hair Loss Association—**http://www.americanhairloss.org/.**

PROVIDER RESOURCES

- Medscape. *Scarring Alopecia*—**http://emedicine.medscape.com/article/1073559-overview.**
- Price V, Mirmirani P. *Cicatricial Alopecia: An Approach to Diagnosis and Management*. New York, NY: Springer; 2011.

REFERENCES

1. Ochoa BE, King LE Jr, Price VH. Lichen planopilaris: annual incidence in four hair referral centers in the United States. *J Am Acad Dermatol.* 2008;58:352-353.
2. Wolff K, Johnson RA, Suurmond D. *Fitzpatrick's Color Atlas & Synopsis of Clinical Dermatology*. 5th ed. New York, NY: McGraw-Hill; 2005.
3. Sperling LC, Cowper SE. The histopathology of primary cicatricial alopecia. *Semin Cutan Med Surg.* 2006;25:41-50.
4. Olsen EA, Bergfeld WF, Cotsarelis G, et al. Summary of North American Hair Research Society (NAHRS)-sponsored Workshop on Cicatricial Alopecia, Duke University Medical Center, February 10 and 11, 2001. *J Am Acad Dermatol.* 2003;48:103-110.
5. Price V, Mirmirani P. *Cicatricial Alopecia: An Approach to Diagnosis and Management*. New York, NY: Springer; 2011.
6. Moreno-Ramirez D, Camacho MF. Frontal fibrosing alopecia: a survey in 16 patients. *J Eur Acad Dermatol Venereol.* 2005;19:700-705.
7. Chandrawansa PH, Giam YC. Folliculitis decalvans—a retrospective study in a tertiary referred centre, over five years. *Singapore Med J.* 2003;44:84-87.
8. Henderson CL, Lafleur L, Sontheimer RD. Sarcoidal alopecia as a mimic of discoid lupus erythematosus. *J Am Acad Dermatol.* 2008;59:143-145.
9. Price VH. The medical treatment of cicatricial alopecia. *Semin Cutan Med Surg.* 2006;25:56-59.
10. Mirmirani P, Willey A, Price VH. Short course of oral cyclosporine in lichen planopilaris. *J Am Acad Dermatol.* 2003;49:667-671.
11. Mirmirani P, Karnik P. Lichen planopilaris treated with a peroxisome proliferator-activated receptor gamma agonist. *Arch Dermatol.* 2009;145:1363-1366.

12. Chiang C, Sah D, Cho BK, et al. Hydroxychloroquine and lichen planopilaris: efficacy and introduction of Lichen Planopilaris Activity Index scoring system. *J Am Acad Dermatol.* 2010;62:387-392.

13. Cho BK, Sah D, Chwalek J, et al. Efficacy and safety of mycophenolate mofetil for lichen planopilaris. *J Am Acad Dermatol.* 2010;62:393-397.

14. Donovan JC, Samrao A, Ruben BS, Price VH. Eyebrow regrowth in patients with frontal fibrosing alopecia treated with intralesional triamcinolone acetonide. *Br J Dermatol.* 2010;163:1142-1144.

15. Powell JJ, Dawber RP, Gatter K. Folliculitis decalvans including tufted folliculitis: clinical, histological and therapeutic findings. *Br J Dermatol.* 1999;140:328-333.

16. Paquet P, Pierard GE. [Dapsone treatment of folliculitis decalvans] [in French]. *Ann Dermatol Venereol.* 2004;131:195-197.

17. Gul U, Gonul M, Cakmak SK, et al. A case of generalized discoid lupus erythematosus: successful treatment with imiquimod cream 5%. *Adv Ther.* 2006;23:787-792.

18. Duteille F, Le FB, Hepner LD, Pannier M. The limitation of primary excision of cicatricial alopecia: a report of 63 patients. *Ann Plast Surg.* 2000;45:145-149.

188 NORMAL NAIL VARIANTS

E.J. Mayeaux Jr, MD

PATIENT STORY

A 28-year-old man is in the office for a work physical and asks about the white streaks on his fingernail (**Figure 188-1**). He has had them on and off all of his adult life, but recently developed more of them and was concerned he may have a vitamin deficiency. He was reassured that this is a normal nail finding often associated with minor trauma.

INTRODUCTION

The anatomy of the nail unit is shown in **Figure 188-2**. The nail unit includes the nail matrix, nail plate, nail bed, cuticle, proximal and lateral folds, and fibrocollagenous supportive tissues. The proximal matrix produces the superficial aspects of the plate, and the distal matrix the deeper portions. The nail plate is composed of hard and soft keratins, is formed via onychokeratinization, which is similar to hair sheath keratinization.[1] Most normal nail variants occur as a result of accentuation or disruption of normal nail formation.

SYNONYMS

- Leukonychia
  - Transverse striate leukonychia
  - Leukonychia punctata
  - White nails

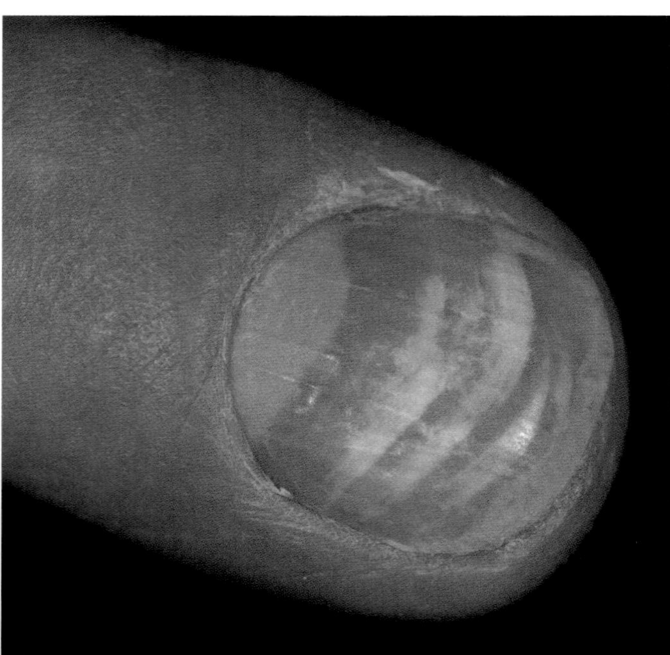

FIGURE 188-1 Transverse striate leukonychia (transverse white streaks) in a healthy patient. Note that the lines do not extend all of the way to the lateral folds, which indicates a probable benign process. (*Reproduced with permission from Richard P. Usatine, MD.*)

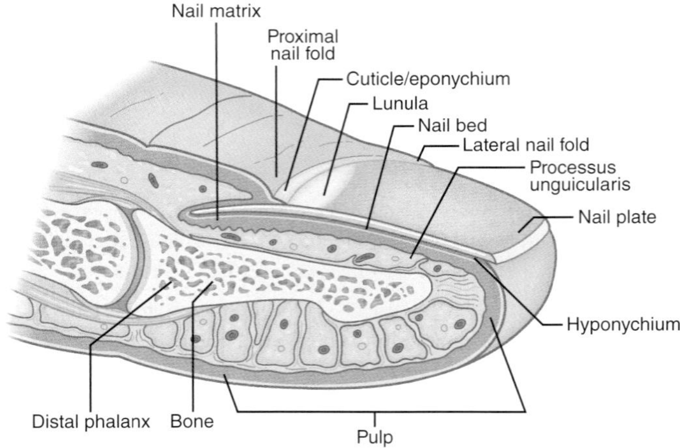

FIGURE 188-2 The anatomy of the nail unit. (*Reproduced with permission from Usatine R, Pfenninger J, Stulberg D, Small R. Dermatologic and Cosmetic Procedures in Office Practice. Elsevier, Inc., Philadelphia. 2012.*)

- Longitudinal melanonychia (LM)
  - Racial melanonychia in African Americans
- Nail hypertrophy and onychogryphosis (also known as onychogryposis)
  - Ram's horn nail
  - Oyster-like deformity
  - Lateral nail hypertrophy
  - Thickened toenail

EPIDEMIOLOGY

- Melanonychia often involves several nails and is a more common occurrence in those patients with darker skin types.
- Among African Americans, benign melanonychia affects up to 77% of young adults and nearly 100% of those age 50 years or older. In the Japanese, LM affects 10% to 20% of adults.[1]
- Nail matrix nevi have been reported to represent approximately 12% of LM in adults and 48% in children.[2] The incidences of most other benign nail findings are not well established.

ETIOLOGY AND PATHOPHYSIOLOGY

- *Leukonychia* represents benign, single or multiple, white spots or lines in the nails. Patchy patterns of partial, transverse white streaks (transverse striate leukonychia, see **Figure 188-1**) or spots (leukonychia punctata, **Figure 188-3**) are the most common patterns of leukonychia.[3]
  - Leukonychia is common in children and becomes less frequent with age.
  - Parents may fear that it represents a dietary deficiency, in particular a lack of calcium, but this concern is almost always unfounded.
  - Most commonly, no specific cause for leukonychia can be found. It is usually the result of minor trauma to the nail cuticle or matrix and is the most commonly found nail condition in children.[4]
  - When the lesions are caused by overly aggressive manicuring or nervous habit, behavior modification often is helpful. Leukonychia can also be an indirect manifestation of autoimmunity, including alopecia areata or thyroid disease.

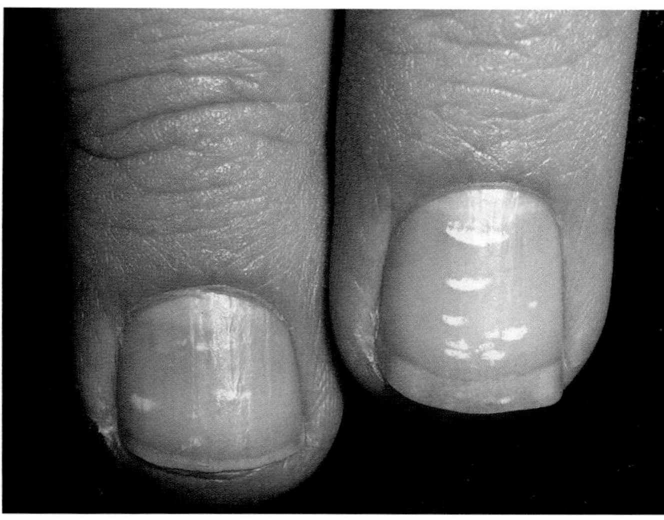

FIGURE 188-3 Leukonychia punctata showing distinct punctate white spots and lines on the fingernails. (*Reproduced with permission from Richard P. Usatine, MD.*)

- Histologically, the nail plate contains a greater number of nucleated cells that are associated with lack of cohesion between the corneocytes, producing reflective properties of the nail.
- LM (**Figure 188-4**) represents a longitudinal pigmented band in the nail plate.
  - Melanonychia is ultimately caused by melanocyte activation. Causes of nongenetic nail matrix melanocyte activation include drugs, inflammatory processes, trauma, mycosis, systemic diseases, and neoplasms (melanomas).[1]
  - LM is often caused by lentigines, benign melanocytic hyperplasia, or a nevus of the nail matrix. However, it must be differentiated from subungual melanoma (see Chapter 189, Pigmented Nail Disorders).
  - Benign causes of LM produce melanocytic activation with bands that usually measure 3 to 5 mm or less in width, whereas melanoma tends to produce wider bands.

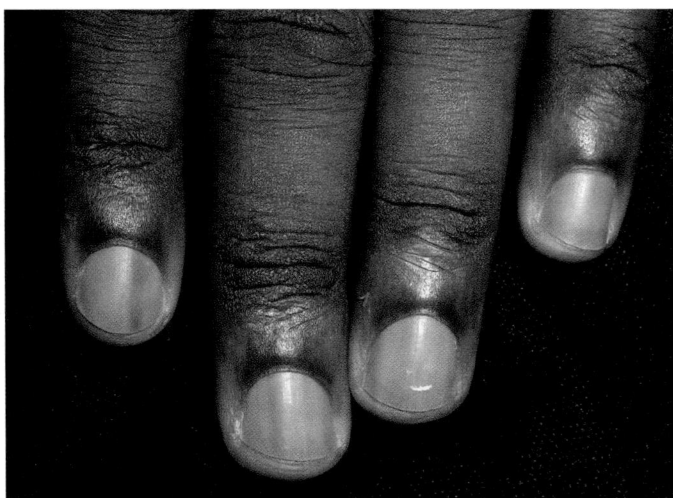

FIGURE 188-4 Longitudinal melanonychia in multiple fingers in a young adult. These bands of translucent nail pigmentation in multiple fingers are typical of racial longitudinal melanonychia and not suspicious for melanoma. Note the dark pigment on the proximal nail folds represents a pseudo-Hutchinson sign. (*Reproduced with permission from Richard P. Usatine, MD.*)

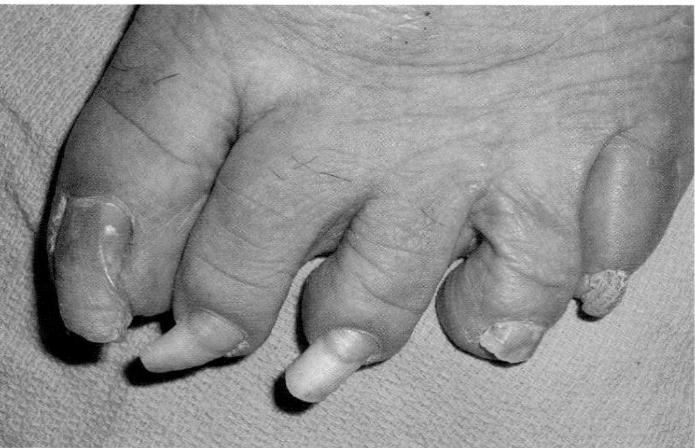

FIGURE 188-5 Onychogryphosis (ram's horn nail) is a type of lateral nail hypertrophy most frequently found in the toenails and often associated with onychomycosis. (*Reproduced with permission from Richard P. Usatine, MD.*)

    - Most lentigines and nevi display a band with a tan-to-brown hue.
    - A benign nail band is generally relatively homogeneous with respect to color and color intensity and if it expands, tends to expand slowly.[1]
- *Nail hypertrophy and onychogryphosis* (ram's horn nail—lateral nail hypertrophy, **Figure 188-5**) is the development of opaque thickened nails with exaggerated upward, or lateral growth. It may be associated with age, fungal infections, and trauma. It can cause pain with pressure.
- *Habit-tic deformity* (**Figures 188-6** and **188-7**) is caused by habitual picking of the proximal nail fold. The resulting inflammation induces the nail plate to be wavy and ridged, while its substance remains intact and hard.
- *Beau lines* are transverse linear depressions in the nail plate (**Figures 188-8** and **188-9**).
  - They are thought to result from suppressed nail growth secondary to local trauma or severe illness.[5]

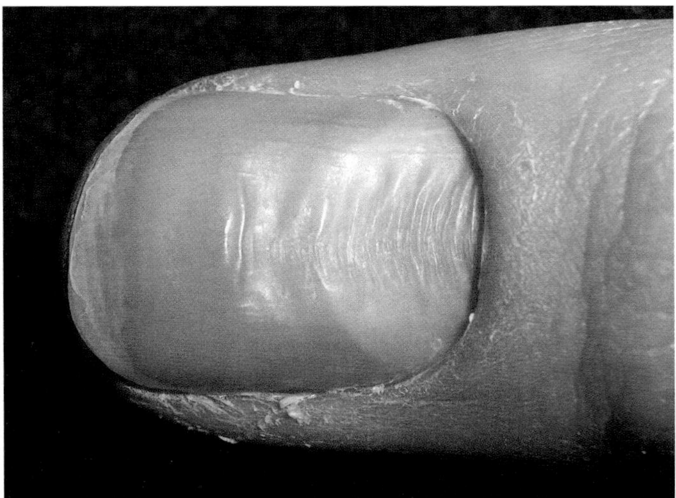

FIGURE 188-6 Habit-tic deformity of the thumbnail caused by a conscious or unconscious rubbing or picking of the proximal nails and nail folds. Horizontal grooves are formed proximally and move distally with fingernail growth. The thumbnails are most often affected. (*Reproduced with permission from Richard P. Usatine, MD.*)

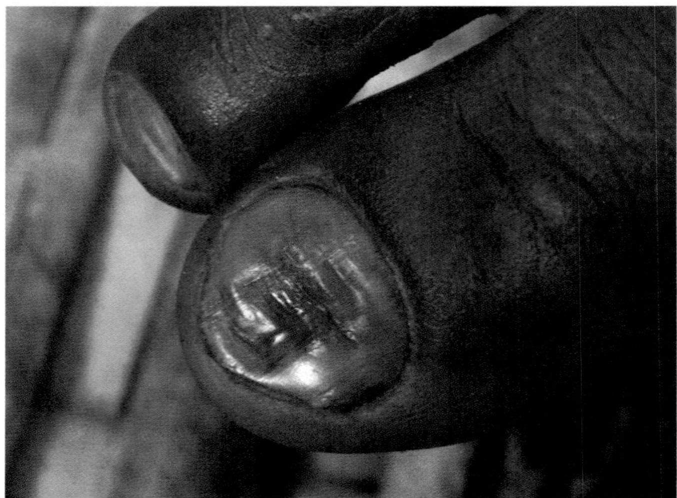

FIGURE 188-7 Habit-tic deformity of the large toenail in a man that walks barefoot often. He acknowledged that he picks at the nail and cuticle. (*Reproduced with permission from Richard P. Usatine, MD.*)

- They most commonly appear symmetrically in several or all nails and may have associated white lines. They usually grow out over several months.
- One may estimate the time since onset of systemic illness by measuring the distance from the Beau line to the proximal nail fold and applying the conversion factor of 6 to 10 days per millimeter of growth.[4]

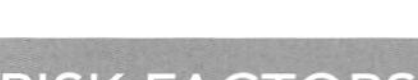

RISK FACTORS

- Leukonychia
  - Use of nail enamels, nail hardeners, or artificial nails as a result of trauma and allergic reactions
  - Repetitive trauma from work, sports, or leisure activities
- LM
  - Race
  - Age

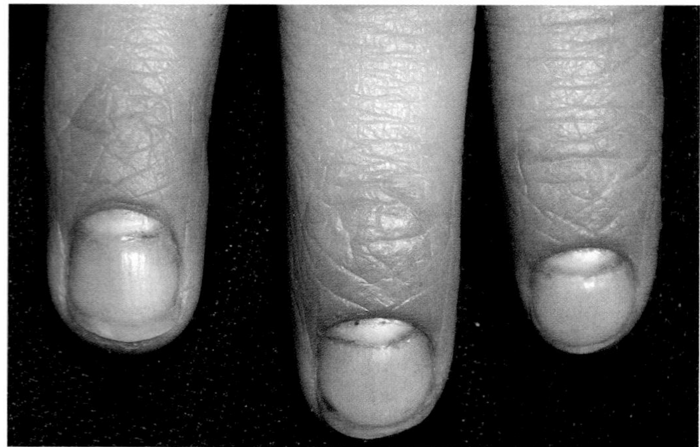

FIGURE 188-8 Beau lines in the fingernails of a boy that had erythema multiforme and exfoliation approximately 2 months prior to this visit. (*Reproduced with permission from Richard P. Usatine, MD.*)

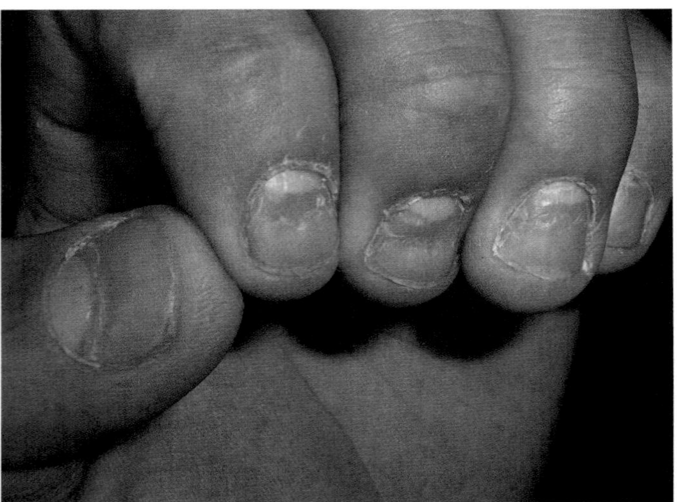

FIGURE 188-9 Beau lines in the fingernails of a girl who was hospitalized with pneumonia 4 months prior to this visit. (*Reproduced with permission from Richard P. Usatine, MD.*)

- Nail hypertrophy and onychogryphosis
  - Age
- Habit-tic deformity
  - Psychological dysfunctions
- Beau lines
  - Severe illness
  - High fever

DIAGNOSIS

CLINICAL FEATURES

All diagnoses of nail disorders should begin with a focused history and physical examination. It is especially important to ask about trauma and recent illnesses.

LABORATORY TESTING

If renal disease is suspected, order a urinalysis and a serum creatinine.

IMAGING

The use of nail plate or matrix dermoscopy has been proposed as a way to further define areas to biopsy in LM, but their accuracy in the diagnosis of subungual melanoma has not been established.[2] SOR Ⓒ

BIOPSY

Definitive diagnosis of a nail discoloration may be made with a biopsy of the nail or matrix. Patients with darker skin tones and multiple digits with translucent LM often need only to be observed.

- A new dark line in a single nail should be biopsied. A 3-mm punch biopsy can be performed at the origin of the darkest part of a dark band. This usually involves reflecting the skin of the proximal nail fold back while performing a punch biopsy of the distal matrix.
- Histologic diagnosis of atypical melanocytic hyperplasia necessitates the complete removal of the lesion.[1] SOR Ⓒ

DIFFERENTIAL DIAGNOSIS

- Pigmented lesions in the nail bed do not cause LM, only nail matrix lesions do. Nail bed lesions make spots under the nails but do not grow out as stripes. These are viewed through the nail as a grayish to brown or black spot.[6]
- The diagnosis of subungual melanoma must always be considered in patients with LM. A biopsy should be performed in an adult if the cause of LM is not apparent. Extension of pigmentation to the skin adjacent to the nail plate involving the nail folds or the fingertip is called Hutchinson sign, which is an important indicator of nail melanoma (see Chapter 189, Pigmented Nail Disorders).
- Hematoma may be confused with LM, but the color grows out with the nail plate, exhibiting a proximal border that reproduces the shape of the lunula. A hole punched in the nail plate allows for the visualization of the underlying nail bed and confirmation of the nature of the coloration (see Chapter 192, Paronychia).
- Mees and Muehrcke lines may be confused with leukonychia or Beau lines.
    - Mees lines are multiple white transverse lines that begin in the nail matrix and extend completely across the nail plate (**Figure 188-10**). They are caused by heavy-metal poisoning or severe systemic insults.
    - Muehrcke lines are white transverse lines that represent an abnormality of the nail vascular bed and may occur with chronic hypoalbuminemia or renal disease (**Figure 188-11**). In contrast to Beau lines, they are not grooved and they do not move with nail growth. **Table 188-1** lists the clinical signs that help differentiate local trauma-induced lesions from those associated with systemic disease.
    - Leukonychia must also be differentiated from localized white onychomycosis, half-and-half nails, which are white proximal nails and pink or brown distal nails seen in renal failure (**Figure 188-12**), and Terry nails, which are white proximal nails and reddened distal nails that are seen in liver cirrhosis.
- The differential diagnosis of habit-tic deformity includes several nail dystrophies. In median nail, dystrophy produces a distinctive longitudinal split in the center of the nail plate with several cracks projecting laterally.

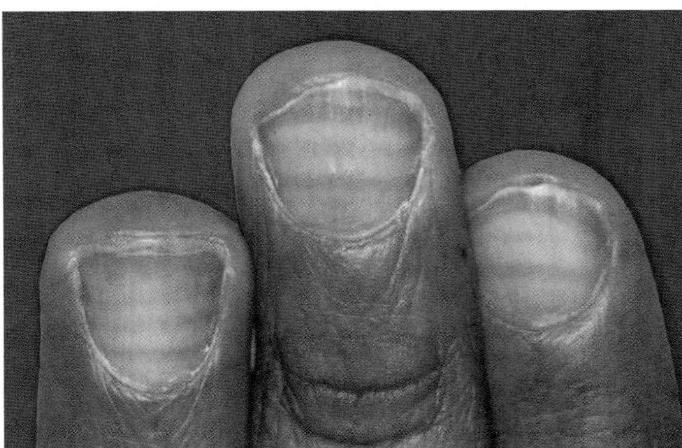

FIGURE 188-10 Mee lines that spread transversely across the entire breadth of the nail and are somewhat rounded with a contour similar to the distal lunula. (*Reproduced with permission from Jeffrey Meffert, MD.*)

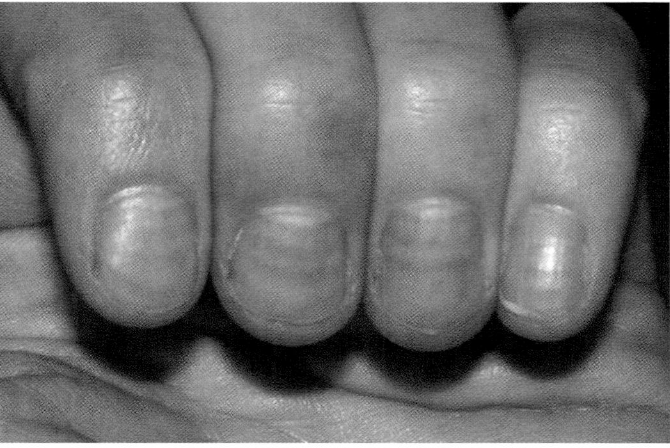

FIGURE 188-11 Muehrcke lines in a patient with chronic hypoalbuminemia from nephrotic syndrome. The white transverse lines extend across the full nail bed and represent an abnormality of the nail vascular bed.

- Chronic paronychia is caused by inflammation of the proximal nail folds, and may induce ripples that can mimic the habit-tic deformity. Chronic eczematous inflammation may produce similar changes. Onychomycosis, Beau lines, and psoriatic nail lesions may also appear similar to habit-tic deformity.[7]
- Twenty-nail dystrophy (**Figure 188-13**) is an idiopathic nail dystrophy that starts in childhood and resolves slowly with age. The nails lose their luster and develop longitudinal striations. It often starts with the fingernails and then affects the toenails.

MANAGEMENT

NONPHARMACOLOGIC

Grinding of the nail at regular intervals is useful for onychogryphosis.

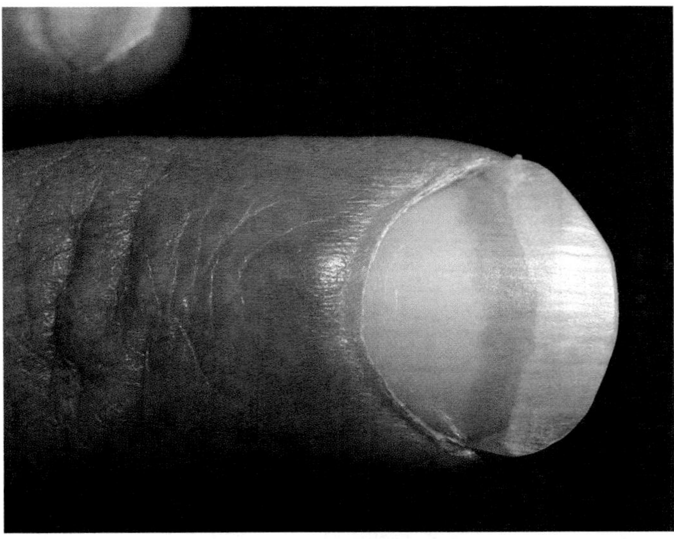

FIGURE 188-12 Half-and-half nail ("Lindsay nails") with the proximal portion of the nail being white and the distal portion pink. Note the sharp line of demarcation between the two halves. The patient is a 44-year-old HIV-positive man with cirrhosis from hepatitis C and alcohol abuse. All his fingers have half-and-half nails. (*Reproduced with permission from Richard P. Usatine, MD.*)

TABLE 188-1 Signs That Help Differentiate Local Trauma-Induced Nail Changes From Those Associated With Systemic Disease

Characteristic	Mees Lines (see Figure 188-10)	Muehrcke Lines (Figure 188-11)	Beau lines (see Figures 188-8 and 188-9)	Leukonychia (see Figures 188-1 and 188-3)
Number of nails involved	Tend to be single but may occur on several nails at once	Tend to occur on several nails at once	Appear symmetrically in several or all nails	Usually on 1 or 2 nails
Nail coverage	Spread transversely across the entire breadth of the nail	Spread across the entire breadth of the nail bed or plate, often disappear with nail plate pressure	Spread transversely across the entire breadth of the nail	Often do not span the entire breadth of the nail plate
Line shape	Tend to have contour similar to the distal lunula, with a rounded distal edge	White transverse lines that have contour similar to the distal lunula, with a rounded distal edge	Tend to have contour similar to the distal lunula, with a rounded distal edge	More linear and resemble the contour of the proximal nail fold
Nail surface changes	Absent	Absent	Usually depressed	Absent
Etiology	Fragmented nail plate structure as a result of a compromised nail matrix	Abnormality of the nail vascular bed	Suppressed nail growth	Disruption of nail plate formation
Associated conditions	History of a systemic insult correlated with the onset of the lines such as chemotherapy, heart failure, and heavy-metal poisoning	Chronic hypoalbuminemia (hepatic and renal disease)	History of a physiologic stressor such as surgery or a severe illness	History of physical trauma (often not identified)

MEDICATIONS

Fluoxetine has been reported as being helpful in the treatment of habit-tic deformity.[8] SOR C

SURGICAL

Removal of the nail and ablation of the nail bed for onychogryphosis SOR C

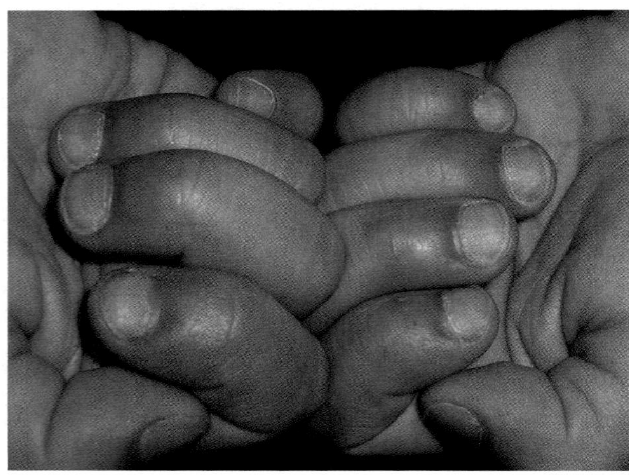

FIGURE 188-13 Twenty-nail dystrophy in a healthy 8-year-old girl. Note how all the fingernails are uniformly affected with longitudinal striations and loss of nail luster. Her skin is otherwise normal. (*Reproduced with permission from Richard P. Usatine, MD.*)

PATIENT RESOURCES

- *Melanonychia*—**http://www.diseasesatoz.com/melanonychia.htm.**
- DermIS *(Onychogryphosis)*—**http://www.dermis.net/dermisroot/en/35644/diagnose.htm.**

PROVIDER RESOURCES

- Emedicine. *Nail Surgery*—**http://www.emedicine.com/derm/topic818.htm.**
- Color pictures at Dermatlas.org—**http://www.dermatlas.com/derm/** and select body site: *nails (all).*
- Medscape. *Melanonychia*—**http://emedicine.medscape.com/article/1375850-overview#showall.**
- Medscape Education. *Examining the Fingernails*—**http://www.medscape.org/viewarticle/571916_2**
- DermnetNZ. *"Nail Diseases"*—**http://dermnetnz.org/hair-nails-sweat/nails.html.**

REFERENCES

1. Ruben B. Pigmented lesions of the nail unit: clinical and histopathologic features. *Semin Cutan Med Surg.* 2010;29:148-158.
2. Tosti A, Piraccini BM, de Farias DC. Dealing with melanonychia. *Semin Cutan Med Surg.* 2009;28:49-54.
3. Grossman M, Scher RK. Leukonychia. Review and classification. *Int J Dermatol.* 1990;29:535-541.

4. Baran R, Kechijian P. Diagnosis and management. *J Am Acad Dermatol*. 1989;21:1165-1175.
5. Daniel CR, Zaias N. Pigmentary abnormalities of the nails with emphasis on systemic diseases. *Dermatol Clin*. 1988;6:305-313.
6. Noronha PA, Zubkov B. Nails and nail disorders in children and adults. *Am Fam Physician*. 1997;55:2129-2140.
7. Farnell EA 4th. Bilateral thumbnail deformity. *J Fam Pract*. 2008;57(11):743-745.
8. Vittorio CC, Phillips KA. Treatment of habit-tic deformity with fluoxetine. *Arch Dermatol*. 1997;133(10):1203-1204.

189 PIGMENTED NAIL DISORDERS

E.J. Mayeaux Jr, MD
Richard P. Usatine, MD

PATIENT STORY

An African American medical student presented with a new dark band on her index finger for 1 year (**Figure 189-1**). The dark color and the lack of melanonychia in other fingers made this concerning. A biopsy of the nail matrix was performed and the result showed a benign nevus.

INTRODUCTION

Atypical pigmentation of the nail plate may result from many nonmalignant causes, such as longitudinal melanonychia (LM), inflammatory changes, benign melanocytic hyperplasia, nevi, drugs, and endocrine disorders. It may also result from development of subungual melanoma. The challenge for the clinician is separating the malignant from the nonmalignant sources.

LM is the most common cause and it represents a longitudinal pigmented band in the nail plate (**Figures 189-1** and **189-2**). It may involve 1 or several digits, vary in color from light brown to black, vary in width (most range from 2 to 4 mm), and have sharp or blurred borders.

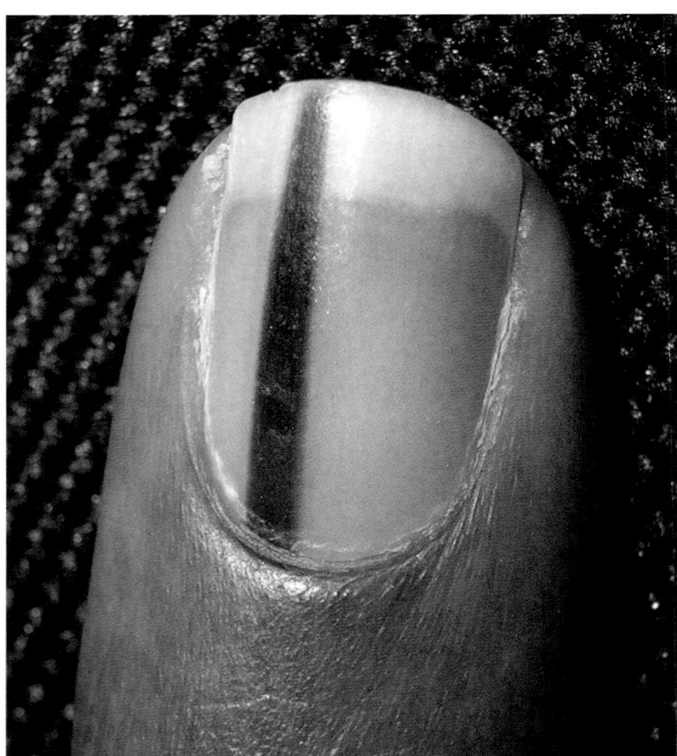

FIGURE 189-1 Longitudinal melanonychia—a single dark band of nail pigment appearing in the matrix region and extended to the tip of the nail. This is concerning for melanoma. The widening of the band in the proximal nail shows that the melanocytic lesion in the matrix is growing. This young woman had a biopsy that showed a benign nevus. *(Reproduced with permission from Richard P. Usatine, MD.)*

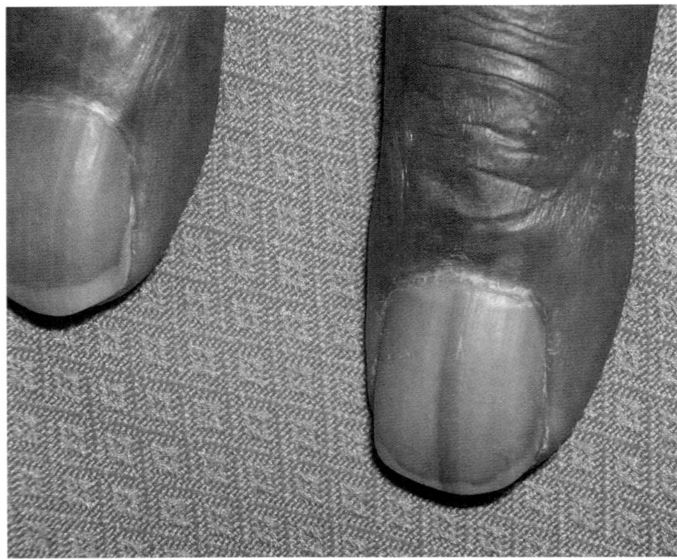

FIGURE 189-2 Close-up of longitudinal melanonychia in a single finger. Note the color band is translucent. *(Reproduced with permission from E.J. Mayeaux Jr, MD.)*

SYNONYMS

Acrolentiginous melanoma—Acral lentiginous melanoma, subungual melanoma is one type of acral lentiginous melanoma involving the nail unit.

EPIDEMIOLOGY

- LM is more common in more darkly pigmented persons. It occurs in 77% of African Americans older than age 20 years and in almost 100% of those older than age 50 years.[1,2] It also occurs in 10% to 20% of persons of Japanese descent. LM is common in Hispanic and other dark-skinned groups. LM is unusual in whites, occurring in only approximately 1% of the population.[1]
- Melanoma is the seventh most common cause of cancer in patients in the United States. Subungual melanoma is a relatively rare tumor with reported incidences between 0.7% and 3.5% of all melanoma cases in the general population.[3]

ETIOLOGY AND PATHOPHYSIOLOGY

- LM originates in the nail matrix and results from increased deposition of melanin within the nail plate. This deposition may result from greater melanin synthesis or from an increase in the total number of melanocytes. Pigment clinically localized within the dorsal half of the nail plate indicates a proximal matrix origin, and pigment localized within the ventral nail plate indicates a distal matrix origin. Look at the distal edge of the nail in a cross-sectional view to see whether the pigment is dorsal or ventral (a dermatoscope may help).
- LM may also be caused by chronic trauma, especially in the great toes.
- Inflammatory changes accompanying skin diseases located in the nail unit, such as psoriasis, lichen planus, amyloidosis, and localized scleroderma, rarely may result in LM.

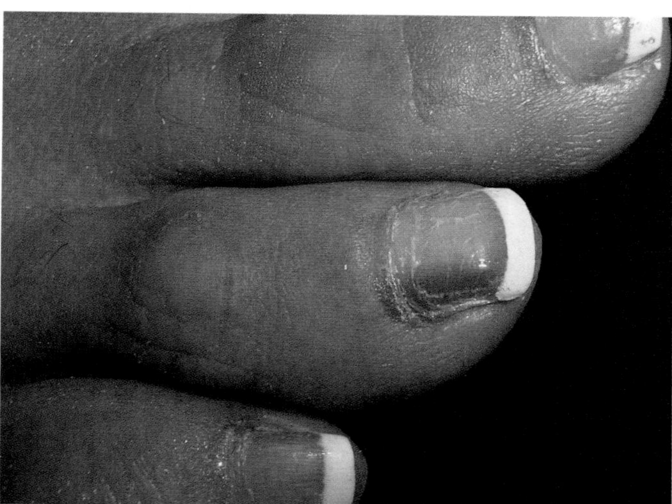

FIGURE 189-3 Longitudinal melanonychia in a single toe. Biopsy demonstrated changes consistent with melanocyte activation or lentigo, which is frequent in individuals with darkly pigmented skin. (*Reproduced with permission from Richard P. Usatine, MD.*)

- Benign melanocytic hyperplasia (lentigo) is observed in 9% of the adult cases (**Figure 189-3**) and 30% of the pediatric cases of single-biopsied LM.[4]
- Nevi represent 12% of LM in adults, but almost 50% of cases in children. A brown-black coloration is observed in two-thirds of the cases and periungual pigmentation (benign pseudo-Hutchinson sign) in one-third.
- Certain drugs may also cause LM, especially chemotherapeutic agents (**Figure 189-4**), and antimalarial drugs (mepacrine, amodiaquine, and chloroquine).
- Endocrine disorders, such as Addison disease, Cushing syndrome, hyperthyroidism, and acromegaly, can be responsible for LM.
- The diagnosis of subungual melanoma must always be considered in patients with LM (**Figures 189-5** to **189-9**). Separating benign from malignant lesions is often difficult. Both arise most often in the thumb or index finger, and both are more common in dark-skinned persons.[5]

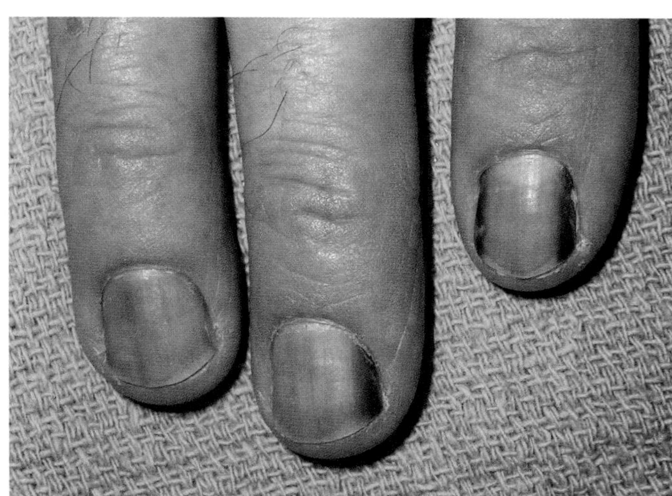

FIGURE 189-4 Melanonychia secondary to chemotherapy for metastatic penile cancer. (*Reproduced with permission from Richard P. Usatine, MD.*)

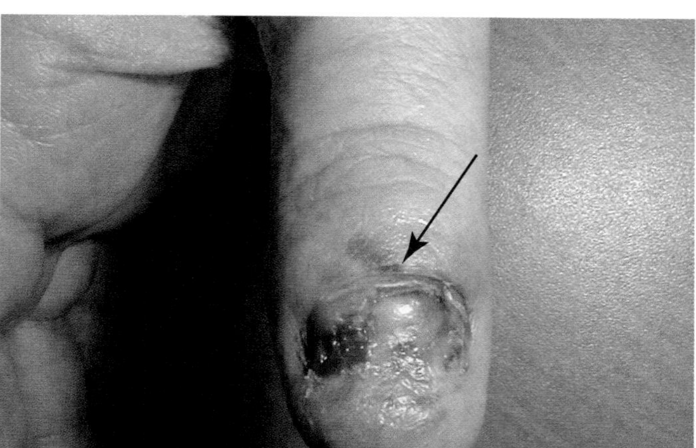

FIGURE 189-5 Advanced acral lentiginous melanoma of the thumb with destruction of the nail plate and ulceration. Note the hyperpigmentation of the proximal nail fold (Hutchinson sign), which is strongly indicative of melanoma. (*Reproduced with permission from Dr. Dubin at http://www.skinatlas.com.*)

A biopsy should be performed in an adult if the cause of LM is uncertain. **Table 189-1** lists diagnostic clues for subungual melanomas. Many subungual melanomas have a history of trauma preceding the diagnosis so it is important to not be fooled by this history (see **Figures 189-8** and **189-9**).

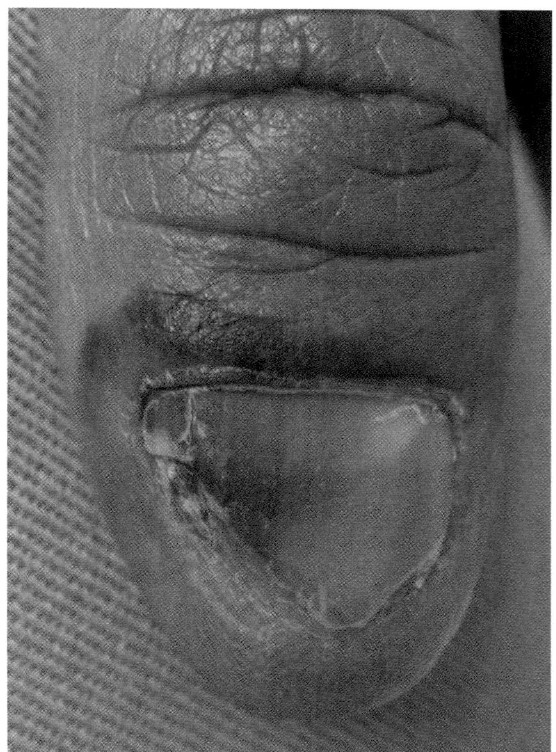

FIGURE 189-6 Acral lentiginous melanoma of the thumb with a very positive Hutchinson sign. Note how the pigmented band on the nail is greater than 3 mm in width. (*Reproduced with permission from Robert T. Gilson, MD.*)

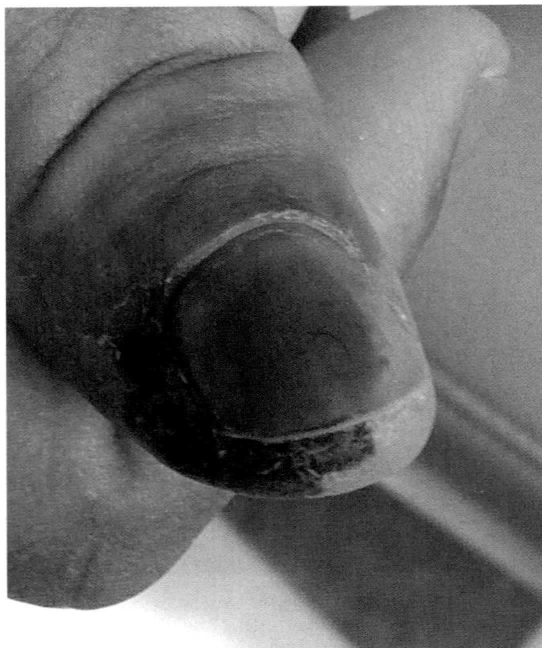

FIGURE 189-7 Acral lentiginous melanoma of the thumb with a very positive Hutchinson sign showing dark hyperpigmentation of the nail folds. Note how the light brown pigmented band on the nail is much greater than 3 mm in width. *(Reproduced with permission from Ryan O'Quinn, MD.)*

- Hutchinson sign is the extension of pigmentation to the skin adjacent to the nail plate involving the nail folds or the fingertip. It is an important indicator for nail melanoma (see **Figures 189-5** to **189-7**).[6]
- Pseudo-Hutchinson sign is the presence of dark pigment around the proximal nail fold secondary to benign conditions such as racial melanosis and not melanoma (**Figure 189-10**). Another cause of pseudo-Hutchinson sign is a translucent cuticle below which the pigment of LM is visible. Trauma and drug-induced pigmentation can also produce a pseudo-Hutchinson sign.
- Subungual melanoma arises on the hand in 45% to 60% of cases, and most of those occur in the thumb (see **Figures 189-5** to **189-8**).[4] On the foot, subungual melanoma usually occurs in the great toe.[5] The median age at which subungual melanoma is usually diagnosed is in the sixth and seventh decades. It appears with equal frequency in males and females.[5]

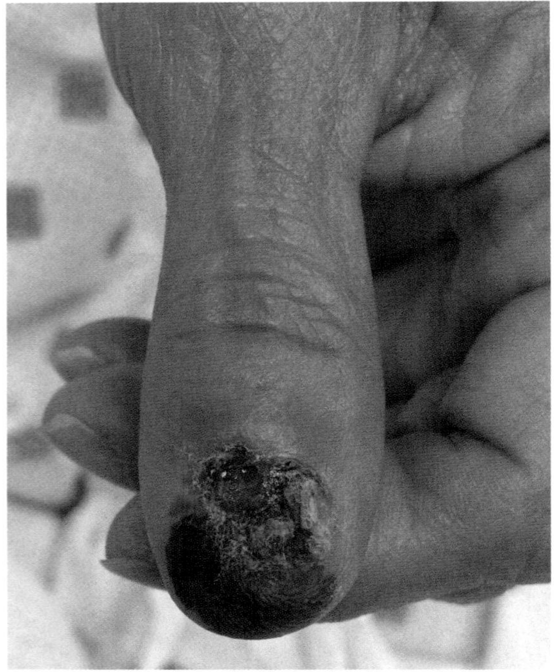

FIGURE 189-8 Melanoma of the nail unit which presented with a history of nail trauma. It is so important to not ignore nail changes that persist after nail trauma because a delay in diagnosis can be fatal. *(Reproduced with permission from Sandra Herman, MD.)*

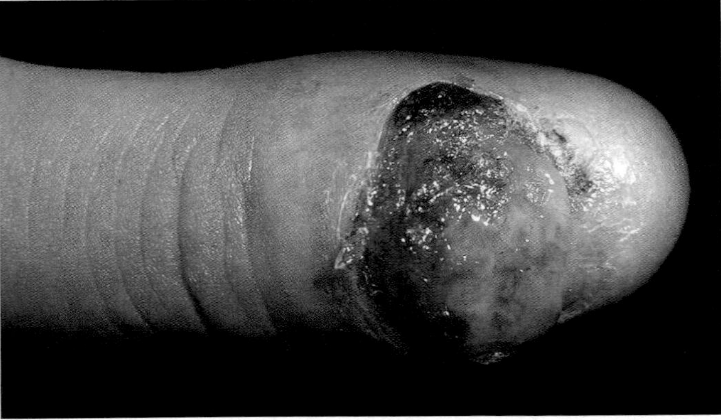

FIGURE 189-9 Nodular melanoma growing within the pinkie nail (not the thumb) of a 37-year-old woman. The patient claims that it started with a dark spot under the nail of this fifth digit after she caught it in a dresser drawer. When it did not heal she pursued medical care and was treated for a presumed nail fungus and then a paronychia until she was finally seen by a physician who recognized the gravity of this situation. A biopsy was performed immediately and it showed a thick nodular melanoma greater than 3 mm in depth with a high mitotic index and ulceration. The patient will undergo an amputation of the finger at the proximal interphalangeal (PIP) joint along with a sentinel node biopsy. *(Reproduced with permission from Richard P. Usatine, MD.)*

TABLE 189-1 Diagnostic Clues That Indicate Longitudinal Melanonychia Is Suspicious for Subungual Melanoma

Hutchinson sign (melanoma until proven otherwise)
In a single digit
Sixth decade of life or later
Develops abruptly in a previously normal nail plate
Suddenly darkens or widens (change in the LM morphology)
Occurs in either the thumb, index finger, or great toe
History of digital trauma
Dark-skinned patient, particularly if the thumb or great toe is affected
Blurred, rather than sharp, lateral borders
Personal history of malignant melanoma
Increased risk for melanoma (eg, familial atypical mole and melanoma [FAMM] syndrome)
Nail dystrophy, such as partial nail destruction or disappearance

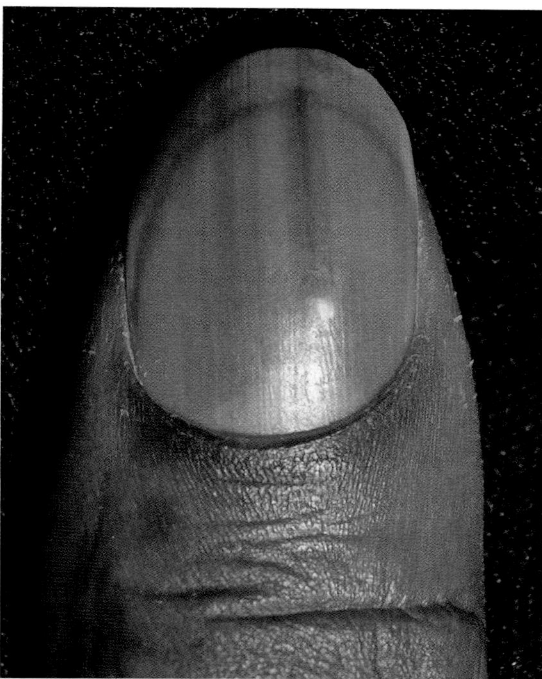

FIGURE 189-10 Benign longitudinal melanonychia in a black person demonstrating pseudo-Hutchinson sign (dark pigment around the proximal nail fold secondary to racial melanosis and not melanoma). (*Reproduced with permission from Richard P. Usatine, MD.*)

RISK FACTORS

Table 189-1 lists diagnostic clues that indicate an increased risk for the presence of subungual melanoma.

DIAGNOSIS

CLINICAL FEATURES

There is an ABCDEF mnemonic system that applies to subungual melanoma:

- In this system "A" stands for age (peak incidence being between the fifth to seventh decades) and African Americans, Asians, and Native Americans in whom subungual melanoma accounts for one-third of melanoma cases.
- "B" stands for "brown to black" and with "breadth" of 3 mm or more.
- "C" stands for change in the nail band coloration or lack of change after adequate treatment.
- "D" stands for the digit most commonly involved.
- "E" stands for extension of the pigment onto the proximal and/or lateral nail fold (Hutchinson sign).
- "F" stands for family or personal history of dysplastic nevus or melanoma.

TYPICAL DISTRIBUTION

The digits used for grasping (thumb, index finger, and middle finger) are the most commonly involved in LM and melanoma, but either may be found in any finger or toe.

BIOPSY

Definitive diagnosis of a nail discoloration may be made with a biopsy of the nail matrix. Patients with darker skin color and multiple digits with translucent LM often need only to be observed. Single dark lines in whites should always be biopsied. A 3-mm punch biopsy can be performed at the origin of the darkest part of a dark band within the nail matrix (**Figure 189-11**). Histologic diagnosis of atypical melanocytic hyperplasia necessitates the complete removal of the lesion.

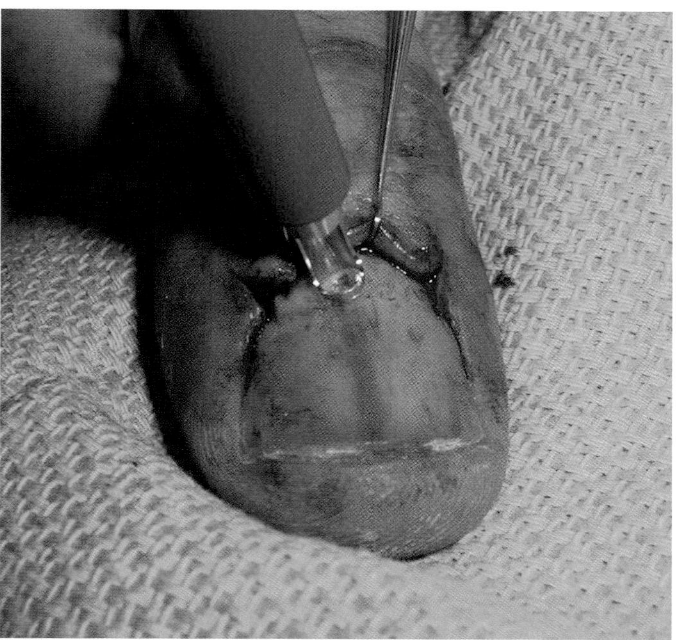

A

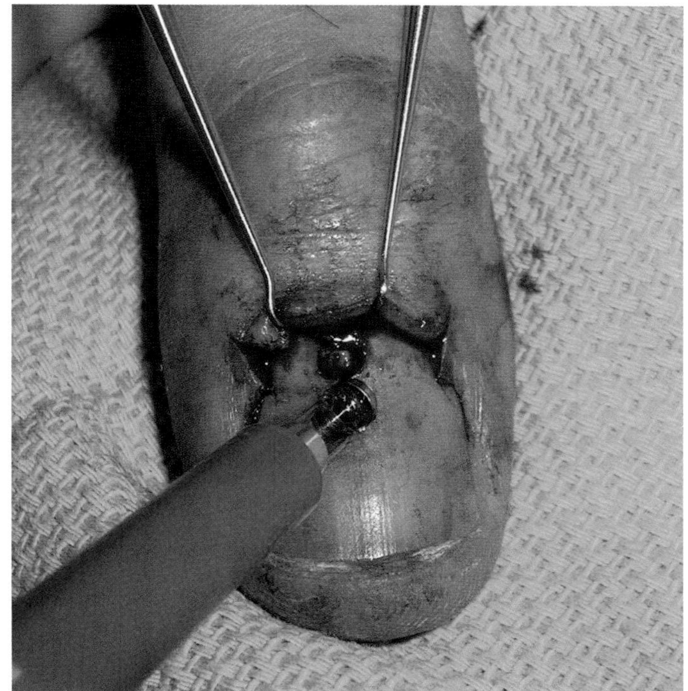

B

FIGURE 189-11 **A.** The proximal nail fold is reflected back to perform a nail matrix biopsy in a young man with new onset of longitudinal melanonychia. The 3-mm punch is placed over the origin of the dark band at the distal matrix. **B.** The 3-mm punch now contains the specimen for pathology. The longitudinal melanonychia was caused by melanocytic hyperplasia. (*Reproduced with permission from Richard P. Usatine, MD.*)

DIFFERENTIAL DIAGNOSIS

- Pigmented lesions in the nail bed usually do not cause LM and are viewed through the nail as a grayish-to-brown or black spot.[7]
- Subungual hematoma may be confused with LM, but the color grows out with the nail plate, exhibiting a proximal border that reproduces the shape of the lunula. A hole punched in the nail plate allows for the visualization of the underlying nail bed and confirmation of the nature of the coloration (see Chapter 194, Subungual Hematoma).

MANAGEMENT

NONPHARMACOLOGIC

No treatment is required for benign LM.

REFERRAL OR HOSPITALIZATION

Treatment of primary subungual melanomas includes amputation at the level of the interphalangeal joint for thumb lesions SOR Ⓑ, the distal or proximal interphalangeal joint for fingers SOR Ⓒ, and the metatarsophalangeal joint for toes.[8] For melanoma in situ, it may be possible to remove the full nail apparatus and save the digit. Sentinel lymph node biopsy is often indicated to establish the disease stage **(see Figure 189-9)**. Chemotherapy is recommended for nodal or visceral metastases.

PROGNOSIS

The 5-year survival is approximately 74% for patients with stage I subungual melanoma and 40% for patients with stage II disease. Prognostic variables negatively affecting survival include stage at diagnosis, deeper Clark level of invasion, African American race, and ulceration.[9]

FOLLOW-UP

Because LM may indicate an undiagnosed melanoma of the nail unit, biopsy or regular monitoring is extremely important. If there is any doubt about the diagnosis of melanoma, biopsy immediately or refer to someone who can. Have the patient report any changes in pigmentation of the nail plate or nail folds, and strongly consider biopsy in these individuals.

PATIENT RESOURCES

- Medscape. *Nail Diseases In Childhood*—**http://www.medscape.com/viewarticle/585158_8.**
- DermNet NZ. *Subungual Melanoma*—**http://dermnetnz.org/hair-nails-sweat/melanoma-nailunit.html.**

PROVIDER RESOURCES

- DermNet NZ. *Nail Diseases*—**http://dermnetnz.org/hair-nails-sweat/nails.html.**
- eMedicine. *Nail Surgery*—**http://www.emedicine.com/derm/topic818.htm.**
- Braun RP, Baran R, Le Gal FA, et al. Diagnosis and management of nail pigmentation. *J Am Acad Dermatol.* 2007;56:835-847.
- Jellinek N. Nail matrix biopsy of longitudinal melanonychia: diagnostic algorithm including the matrix shave biopsy. *J Am Acad Dermatol.* 2007;56:803-810.
- Usatine R. Nail procedures. In: Usatine R, Pfenninger J, Stulberg D, Small R, eds. *Dermatologic and Cosmetic Procedures in Office Practice.* Philadelphia, PA: Elsevier; 2012:216-228. The whole procedure depicted in **Figure 189-11** is described in detail.

REFERENCES

1. Baran R, Kechjijian P. Longitudinal melanonychia (melanonychia striata): diagnosis and management. *J Am Acad Dermatol.* 1989;21:1165-1175.
2. Ruben B. Pigmented lesions of the nail unit: clinical and histopathologic features. *Semin Cutan Med Surg.* 2010;29:148-158.
3. Finley RK, Driscoll DL, Blumenson LE, Karakousis CP. Subungual melanoma: an eighteen year review. *Surgery.* 1994;116:96-100.
4. Goettmann-Bonvallot S, André J, Belaich S. Longitudinal melanonychia in children: a clinical and histopathologic study of 40 cases. *J Am Acad Dermatol.* 1999;41:17-22.
5. Papachristou DN, Fortner JG. Melanoma arising under the nail. *J Surg Oncol.* 1982;21:219-222.
6. Mikhail GR. Hutchinson's sign. *J Dermatol Surg Oncol.* 1986;12:519-521.
7. Baran R, Perrin C. Linear melanonychia due to subungual keratosis of the nail bed: report of two cases. *Br J Dermatol.* 1999;140:730-733.
8. Moehrle M, Metzger S, Schippert W, et al. "Functional" surgery in subungual melanoma. *Dermatol Surg.* 2003;29(4):366-374.
9. O'Leary JA, Berend KR, Johnson JL, et al. Subungual melanoma: a review of 93 cases with identification of prognostic variables. *Clin Orthop Relat Res.* 2000;378:206-212.

190 INGROWN TOENAIL

E.J. Mayeaux Jr, MD

PATIENT STORY

A 34-year-old woman presents with a swollen and painful right big toe (**Figure 190-1**). She has a 2-week history of pain, redness, and swelling of the medial nail fold of the right great toe. Soaking the toe in Epsom salts has not helped. A partial nail removal after a digital block was successful. The nail matrix where the nail was removed was also ablated with phenol to prevent a recurrence of the ingrown nail (**Figure 190-1B**).

INTRODUCTION

Onychocryptosis (ingrown toenails) is a common childhood and adult problem. Patients often seek treatment because of the significant levels of discomfort and disability associated with the condition.

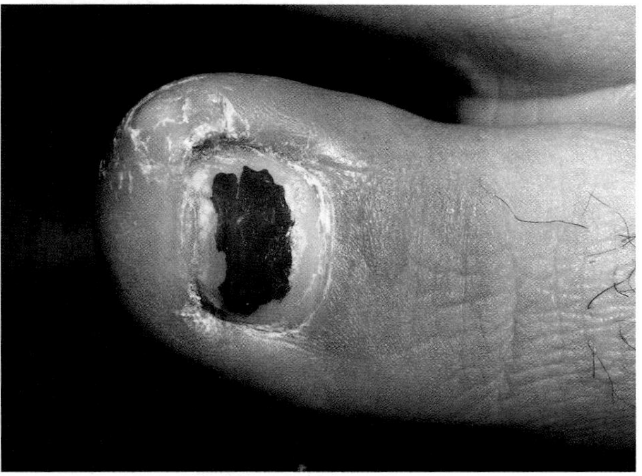

A

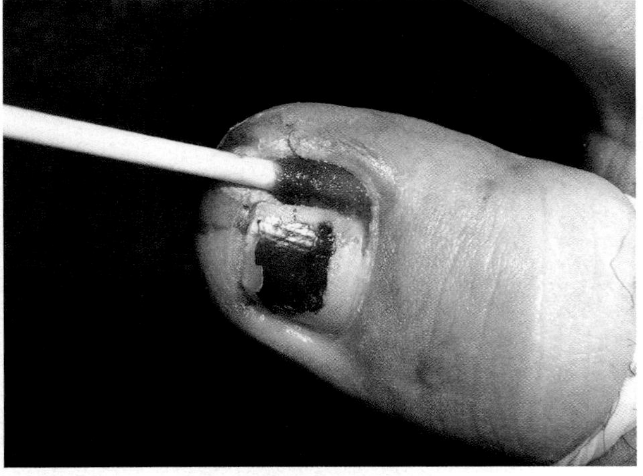

B

FIGURE 190-1 Ingrown toenail of the lateral aspect of the right great toe A. Before surgery B. After partial toenail removal showing the use of phenol to achieve a partial matrixectomy. (*Reproduced with permission from Richard P. Usatine, MD.*)

SYNONYMS

Ingrown toenail is also known as onychocryptosis, unguis incarnatus.

EPIDEMIOLOGY

The prevalence of onychocryptosis is unknown as many patients do not seek medical care and it is not a reportable disease. The toenails, especially the great toenail, are most commonly affected. Ingrown toenails at birth and in early childhood do occur, but are very rare.

ETIOLOGY AND PATHOPHYSIOLOGY

Onychocryptosis occurs when the lateral nail plate damages the lateral nail fold. The lateral edge of the nail plate penetrates and perforates the adjacent nailfold skin. Perforation of the lateral fold skin results in painful inflammation that manifests clinically as mild edema, erythema, and pain. In advanced stages, drainage, infection, and ulceration may be present. Hypertrophy of the lateral nail wall occurs, and granulation tissue forms over the nail plate and the nail fold during healing of the ulcerated skin.[1] It is a common affliction that can result from a variety of conditions that cause improper fit of the nail plate in the lateral nail groove (see **Figure 190-1**).

RISK FACTORS

- Genetic predisposition[1]
- Poor-fitting footwear
- Excessive trimming of the lateral nail plate
- Pincer nail deformity (**Figure 190-2**)
- Trauma
- Sports in which kicking or running is important
- Hyperhidrosis
- Anatomic features such as nailfold width

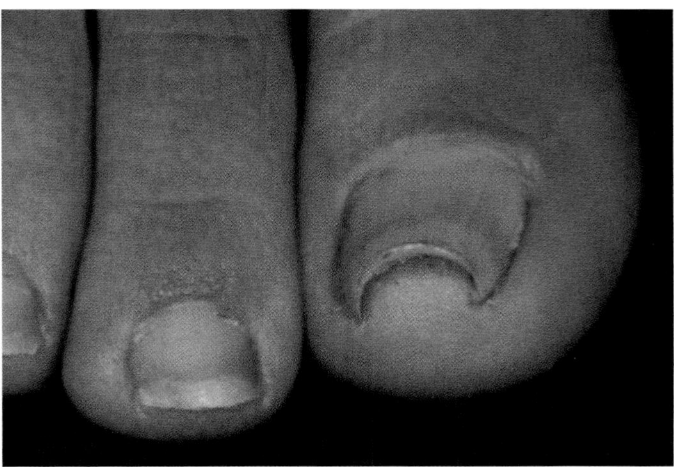

FIGURE 190-2 The curved infolding of the lateral edges of the nail plate indicates this patient has a pincer nail, which predisposes to onychocryptosis. (*Reproduced with permission from Richard P. Usatine, MD.*)

- Congenital malalignment of the digit
- Overcurvature of the nail plate
- Onychomycosis and other diseases that result in abnormal changes in the nail plate

DIAGNOSIS

CLINICAL FEATURES: HISTORY AND PHYSICAL

The diagnosis is based on clinical appearance and rarely is difficult. Characteristic signs and symptoms include pain, edema, exudate, and granulation tissue (see **Figure 190-1**).

TYPICAL DISTRIBUTION

The great toe is most commonly affected; fingers are rarely involved except when nail biting is present.

DIFFERENTIAL DIAGNOSIS

- Cellulitis—Presents with redness, pain, and swelling beyond the nail fold (see Chapter 122, Cellulitis).
- Paronychia—Presents with redness and abscess formation (pus) in a nail fold (see Chapter 192, Paronychia).

MANAGEMENT

The treatment of ingrown toenails depends on the age of the patient and the severity of the lesion.

NONPHARMACOLOGIC

- Lesions characterized by minimal-to-moderate pain and no discharge can be treated conservatively with soaking the affected foot in warm water for 20 minutes, 3 times per day, and pushing the lateral nail fold away from the nail plate.[2] SOR C
  - Other palliative measures include cotton wedging underneath the lateral nail plate and trimming the lateral part of the nail plate below the area of nailfold irritation.
- Numerous alternative methods of conservative treatment have been described, including splints and commercially available devices. Devices that have shown promise include shape memory alloys (SMAs), either of a Cu-Al-Mn base or a Ni-Ti base.[3-5]

MEDICATIONS

- Although many elect to treat apparent infections with oral antibiotics, studies show the use of antibiotics does not decrease healing time or postprocedure morbidity in otherwise normal patients.[6] SOR A
- A medium- to high-potency topical corticosteroid can be applied after soaking to decrease inflammation, but is often unnecessary.
- If nail avulsion and/or matrix ablation is used, pain relievers for mild-to-moderate pain may be necessary.
- When placing digital blocks (**Figure 190-3**) for surgical procedures, the best evidence indicates the use of lidocaine with epinephrine is equally safe and efficacious for anesthesia.[7]

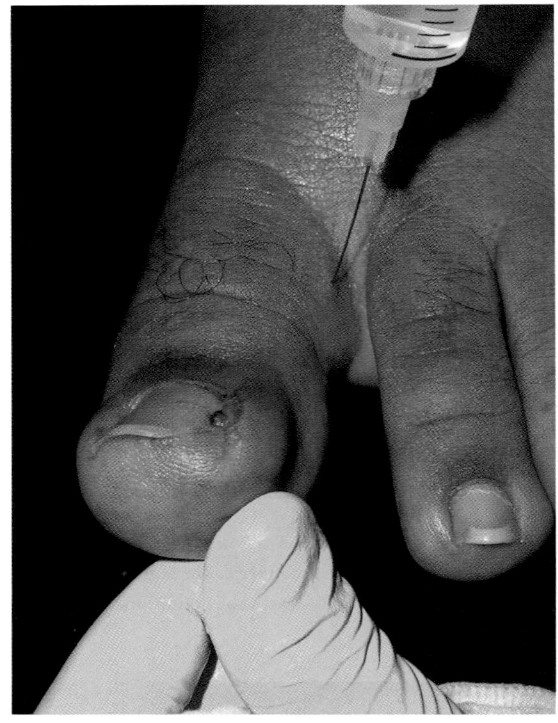

FIGURE 190-3 Digital block being performed before a partial nail avulsion procedure for an ingrown toenail. While epinephrine can be used in a digital block, in this case, plain 2% lidocaine without epinephrine is being injected. *(Reproduced with permission from Richard P. Usatine, MD.)*

SURGICAL

- Nonresponders to conservative therapy and patients with more severe lesions (substantial erythema, granulation tissue, and pus) need surgical therapy.[8,9] SOR C
- Surgical intervention involves partial or full nail plate avulsion. Usually it is only necessary to remove the part of the nail that is placing pressure on the lateral nail fold (**Figure 190-4**). SOR C
- Patients who develop recurrent ingrown toenails benefit from permanent nail ablation of the lateral nail matrix. This may be achieved with the combination of partial nail plate avulsion plus phenol matrixectomy, which can cut recurrence rates by 90% (**Figure 190-5**).[8-10] SOR A

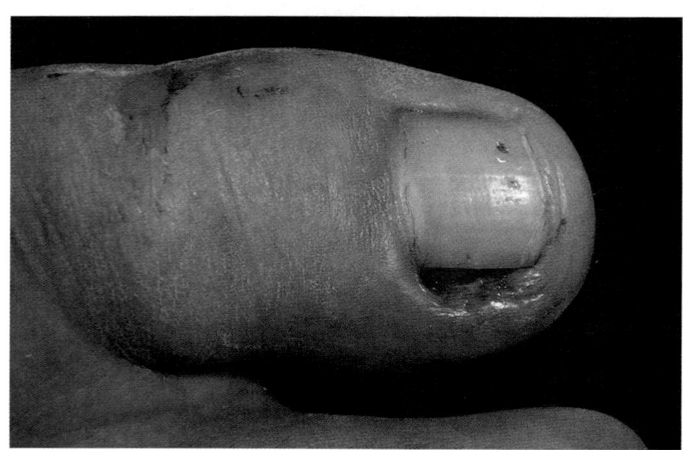

FIGURE 190-4 Big toe after partial nail avulsion procedure for an ingrown toenail. *(Reproduced with permission from Richard P. Usatine, MD.)*

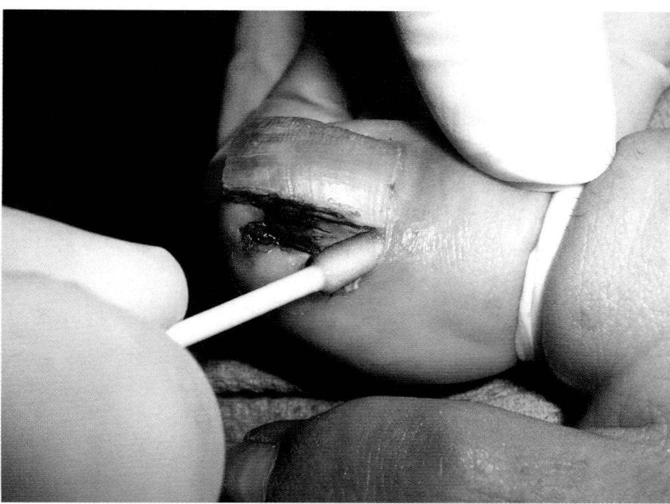

FIGURE 190-5 Phenol matrixectomy to destroy a portion of the nail matrix to prevent a recurrent ingrown toenail. Note the use of a tourniquet to decrease bleeding while applying the phenol with a twisting motion.

- In a Cochrane Systematic Review of surgical treatments for ingrowing toenails nail avulsion with the use of phenol is more effective at preventing symptomatic recurrence than nail avulsion without the use of phenol.[10] Unfortunately the use of phenol does increase the risk of postoperative infection (by 5 times) compared with simple nail avulsion.[10] SOR Ⓐ
- Chemical matricectomy is performed mainly by phenol (full strength 88%), but 10% sodium hydroxide is another alternative. In a comparison study of the use of chemical matrixectomy for the treatment of ingrown toenails, the overall success rates were 95% for both phenol and sodium hydroxide.[11] SOR Ⓐ
- One study found that partial nail avulsion with phenolization gave better results than partial avulsion with matrix excision.[12] Local antibiotics applied to the surgical site did not reduce signs of infection or recurrence. The use of phenol did not produce more signs of infection than matrix excision.[12] SOR Ⓑ
- Electrosurgical ablation can be performed with electrosurgery units on the fulguration setting or using a special matrixectomy electrode with a high-frequency electrosurgical unit (**Figure 190-6**). SOR Ⓒ

FOLLOW-UP

After surgical intervention, consider follow-up in 3 to 4 days to assess treatment and exclude cellulitis.

PATIENT EDUCATION

- Patients should be educated about proper nail trimming so as to minimize trauma to the lateral nail fold. The lateral nail plate should be allowed to grow well beyond the lateral nail fold before trimming horizontally.
- Patients should also be educated about the importance of avoiding shoes that are too tight over the toes to help minimize recurrences.

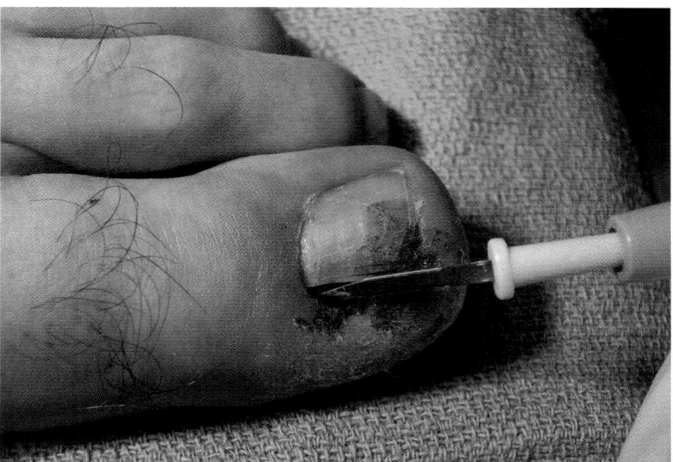

FIGURE 190-6 Use of electrosurgery to ablate the lateral nail matrix. This results in a narrower nail and a decreased likelihood of onychocryptosis recurrence. (*Reproduced with permission from Richard P. Usatine, MD.*)

PATIENT RESOURCES

- Ingrown Toenails information at the familydoctor.org website—**http://familydoctor.org/online/famdocen/home/common/skin/disorders/208.html.**
- eMedicineHealth. *Ingrown Toenails*—**http://www.emedicinehealth.com/ingrown_toenails/article_em.htm.**

PROVIDER RESOURCES

- Medscape eMedicine. *Ingrown Nails*—**http://emedicine.medscape.com/article/909807.**
- Usatine R, Pfenninger J, Stulberg D, Small R. *Dermatologic and Cosmetic Procedures in Office Practice*. Philadelphia, PA: Elsevier; 2012 (with DVD). The "Nail Procedures" chapter provides details, photographs, and videos of how to perform ingrown toenail surgeries. Available as an electronic app as well—**http://usatinemedia.com.**
    - **http://itunes.apple.com/us/app/dermatologic-cosmetic-procedures/id479310808?ls**

REFERENCES

1. Siegle RJ, Swanson NA. Nail surgery: a review. *J Dermatol Surg Oncol.* 1982;8(8):659-666.
2. Connolly B, Fitzgerald RJ. Pledgets in ingrowing toenails. *Arch Dis Child.* 1988;63:71.
3. Nazari S. A simple and practical method in treatment of ingrown nails: splinting by flexible tube. *J Eur Acad Dermatol Venereol.* 2006;20(10):1302-1306.
4. Arai H. Formable acrylic treatment for ingrowing nail with gutter splint and sculptured nail. *Int J Dermatol.* 2004;43(10):759-765.
5. Ishibashi M, Tabata N, Suetake T, et al. A simple method to treat an ingrowing toenail with a shape-memory alloy device. *J Dermatolog Treat.* 2008;19(5):291-292.
6. Reyzelman AM, Trombello KA, Vayser DJ, et al. Are antibiotics necessary in the treatment of locally infected ingrown toenails? *Arch Fam Med.* 2000;9:930.

7. Altinyazar HC, Demirel CB, Koca R, Hosnuter M. Digital block with and without epinephrine during chemical matricectomy with phenol. *Dermatol Surg.* 2010;36(10):1568-1571.

8. Grieg JD, Anderson JH, Ireland AJ, Anderson JR. The surgical treatment of ingrowing toenails. *J Bone Joint Surg Br.* 1991;73:131.

9. Vaccari S, Dika E, Balestri R, et al. Partial excision of matrix and phenolic ablation for the treatment of ingrowing toenail: a 36-month follow-up of 197 treated patients. *Dermatol Surg.* 2010;36(8): 1288-1293.

10. Rounding C, Bloomfield S. Surgical treatments for ingrowing toe-nails. *Cochrane Database Syst Rev.* 2005;(2):CD001541.

11. Bostanci S, Kocyigit P, Gurgey E. Comparison of phenol and sodium hydroxide chemical matricectomies for the treatment of ingrowing toenails. *Dermatol Surg.* 2007;33:680-685.

12. Bos AM, van Tilburg MW, van Sorge AA, Klinkenbijl JH. Randomized clinical trial of surgical technique and local antibiotics for ingrowing toenail. *Br J Surg.* 2007;94:292-296.

191 ONYCHOMYCOSIS

E.J. Mayeaux J, MD

PATIENT STORY

A 29-year-old woman presents with thickened and discolored toenails for 1 year (**Figure 191-1**). She is embarrassed to wear sandals and wants treatment. The entire nail plates are involved and there is subungual keratosis. She did not realize that she had tinea pedis, but a fine scale was seen on the soles and sides of the feet indicative of tinea pedis in a moccasin distribution. A potassium hydroxide (KOH) scraping from the subungual debris was positive for hyphae. She has no history of liver disease or risk factors for liver disease. An oral antifungal was prescribed for 3 months.

INTRODUCTION

Onychomycosis is a term used to denote nail infections caused by any fungus, including dermatophytes, yeasts, and nondermatophyte molds. One, some, and occasionally all of the toenails and/or fingernails may be involved. Although most toenail onychomycosis is caused by dermatophytes, many cases of fingernail onychomycosis are caused by yeast. Onychomycosis may involve the nail plate and other parts of the nail unit, including the nail matrix.

SYNONYMS

Onychomycosis is also known as toenail fungus, tinea unguium, or dermatophytosis of nails.

EPIDEMIOLOGY

- The incidence of onychomycosis has been reported to be 2% to 13% in North America.[1]
- Most patients (7.6%) only have toenail involvement and only 0.15% have fingernail involvement alone.[2]
- The prevalence of onychomycosis varies from 4% to 18%.[3,4]
- The disease is very common in adults, but may also occur in children.

ETIOLOGY AND PATHOPHYSIOLOGY

- Dermatophytes are responsible for most finger and toenail infections.
- Nonpathogenic fungi and *Candida* also can infect the nail plate (**Figure 191-2**).
- Dermatophytic onychomycosis (tinea unguium) occurs in 3 distinct forms: distal subungual, proximal subungual, and white superficial.
- The vast majority of distal and proximal subungual onychomycosis results from *Trichophyton rubrum* (**Figure 191-3**).

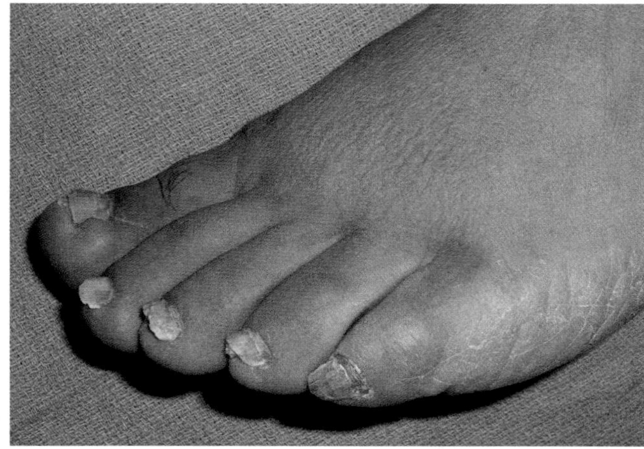

FIGURE 191-1 Onychomycosis in all toenails of this 29-year-old woman. Note the nail plate thickening and discoloration along with the subungual keratosis. She also has tinea pedis in a moccasin distribution. (*Reproduced with permission from Richard P. Usatine, MD.*)

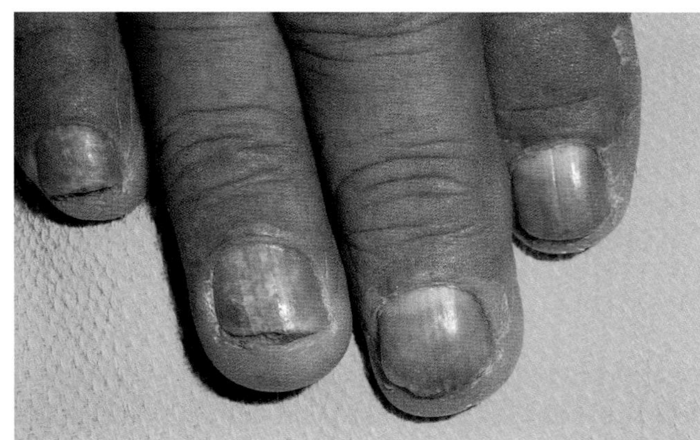

FIGURE 191-2 *Candida* (non-albicans) infection of the nails determined by a culture of a nail clipping. (*Reproduced with permission from Richard P. Usatine, MD.*)

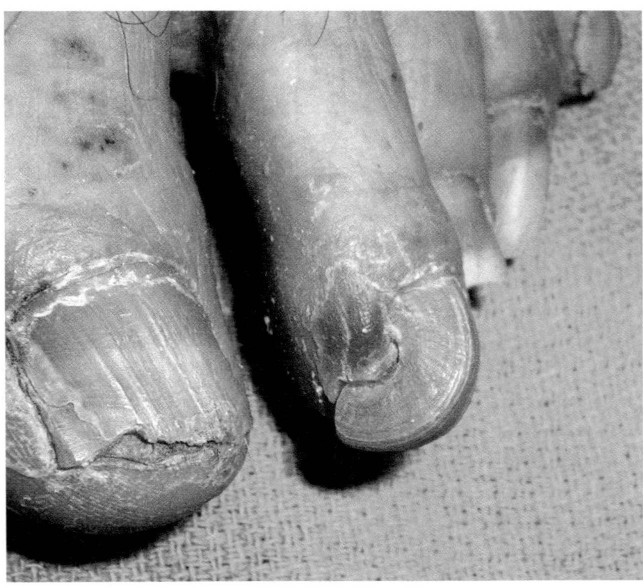

FIGURE 191-3 Severe toenail onychomycosis demonstrating subungual keratosis in the first nail and onychogryphosis (Ram's horn nail) in the second nail because of the fungal infection. The culture grew *Trichophyton rubrum*. (*Reproduced with permission from Richard P. Usatine, MD.*)

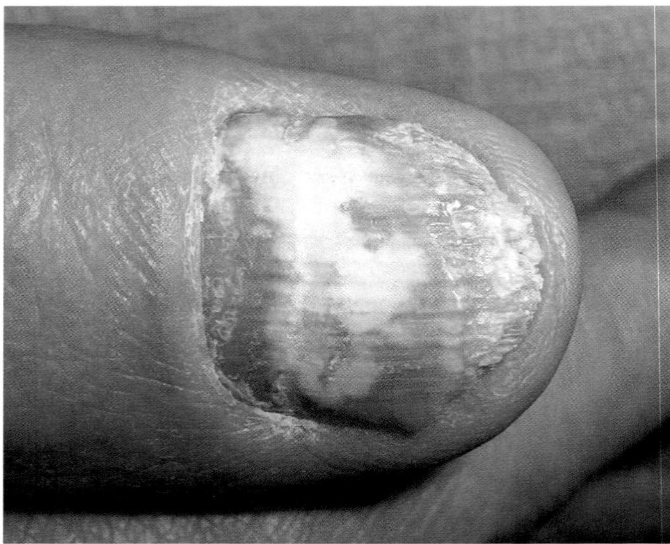

FIGURE 191-4 White superficial onychomycosis of the thumbnail. The culture was positive for *Trichophyton mentagrophytes*. (*Reproduced with permission from Richard P. Usatine, MD.*)

- White superficial onychomycosis is usually caused by *Trichophyton mentagrophytes*, although cases caused by *T. rubrum* have also been reported (**Figure 191-4**).
- Yeast onychomycosis is most common in the fingers caused by *Candida albicans* but can also be seen in non-albicans *Candida* too (see **Figure 191-2**).

RISK FACTORS

- Tinea pedis.[5]
- Trauma predisposes to infection but can also cause a dysmorphic nail that can be confused for onychomycosis.[5]
- Older age.[5]
- Swimming.[5]
- Diabetes.[5]
- Living with family members who have onychomycosis.[5]
- Immunosuppression as seen in AIDS (**Figures 191-5** and **191-6**).[6]

DIAGNOSIS

CLINICAL FEATURES

- Distal subungual onychomycosis is the most common presentation.
- Distal subungual onychomycosis begins with a whitish, yellowish, or brownish discoloration of a distal corner of the nail, which gradually spreads to involve the entire width of the nail plate and extends slowly toward the cuticle. Keratin debris collecting between the nail plate and its bed is the cause of the discoloration (**Figures 191-1**, **191-3**, and **191-7**).
- Proximal subungual onychomycosis progresses in a manner similar to distal subungual onychomycosis but affects the nail in the vicinity of the cuticle first and extends distally. It usually occurs in individuals with a severely compromised immune system (see **Figure 191-5**).

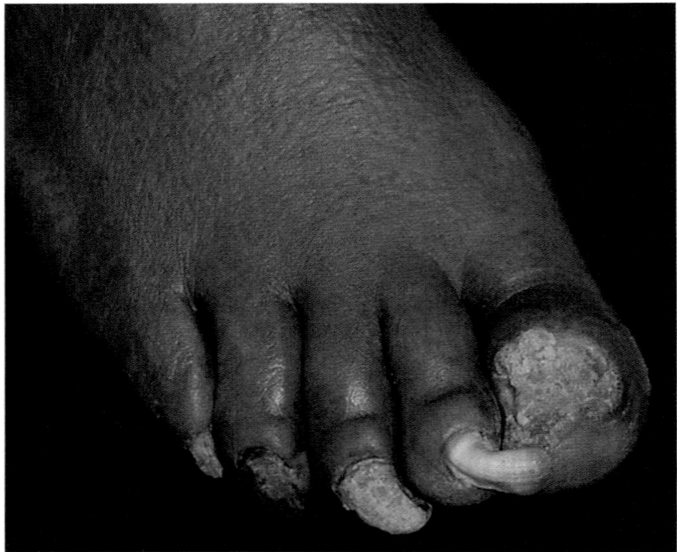

FIGURE 191-5 Extensive onychomycosis involving all toenails in an HIV-positive man. His second toenail shows onychogryphosis (Ram's horn nail) secondary to the fungal infection. (*Reproduced with permission from Richard P. Usatine, MD.*)

- White superficial onychomycosis appears as dull white spots on the surface of the nail plate (see **Figure 191-4**). Eventually the whole nail plate may be involved. The white areas may be soft and can be lightly scraped to yield a chalky scale that may be examined or cultured.

TYPICAL DISTRIBUTION

Nail infection may occur in a single digit but most often occurs simultaneously in multiple digits of the foot. Toenails and fingernails may be affected at the same time especially in patients that are immunocompromised (see **Figures 191-5** to **191-7**).

LABORATORY TESTING

- KOH and culture—Clippings of nail plate and scrapings of subungual keratosis can be examined with KOH and microscopy and/or sent to the laboratory in a sterile container to be inoculated onto Sabouraud

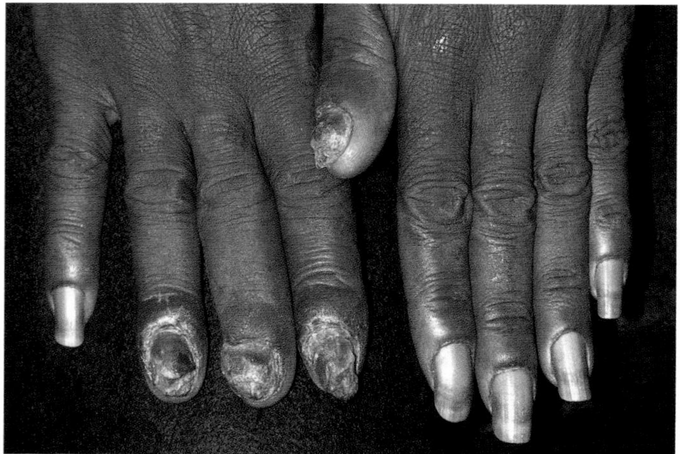

FIGURE 191-6 Fungal infection involving 4 of 10 nails on the hands of the same HIV-positive man of **Figure 191-5**. (*Reproduced with permission from Richard P. Usatine, MD.*)

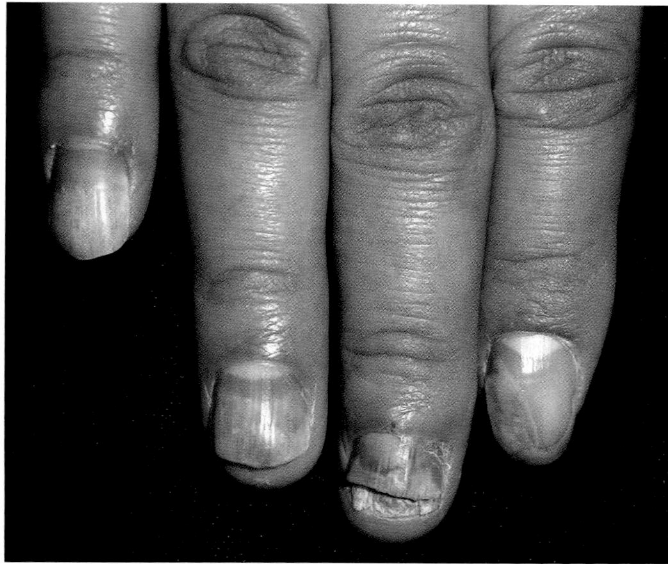

FIGURE 191-7 Distal subungual onychomycosis of the fingernails in this 29-year-old woman. Note how the proximal nail plate is uninvolved and there is significant onycholysis. (*Reproduced with permission from Richard P. Usatine, MD.*)

medium to culture. The scraping can be performed with the edge of a slide, a scalpel or a curette (**Figure 191-8**).

- Dermatophyte test medium (DTM) culture is an alternative to Sabouraud medium culture. DTM is less expensive and can be performed in the physician's office, with results becoming available within 3 to 7 days. Dermatophyte growth is indicated by a change in the medium's color from yellow to red. It is important that DTM cultures be read in a timely fashion, as saprophytic organisms may grow over several weeks and cause a false-positive result. DTM does not identify the specific causative organism, but such identification is unnecessary as all dermatophyte infections are treated the same way. DTM cultures had good positive and negative correlation with culture on Sabouraud medium.[7]

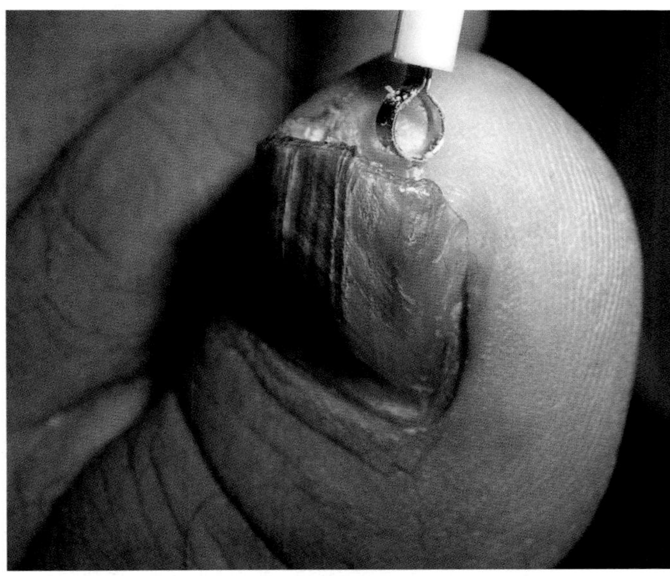

FIGURE 191-8 A curette is being used to collect an adequate sample of the subungual keratosis to confirm the suspicion of onychomycosis. The dark color of the nail makes it important to have a firm diagnosis as melanoma is on the differential diagnosis. (*Reproduced with permission from Richard P. Usatine, MD.*)

- Clippings—Nail clippings may be sent to pathology in formalin to be examined with periodic acid-Schiff (PAS) stain for fungal elements. This can be more sensitive than KOH and culture.
- Comparison of diagnostic methods includes the following:
  - In a 2003 study by Weinberg et al., the sensitivities for onychomycosis detection were KOH 80%, Bx/PAS 92%, and culture 59%. The specificities were KOH 72%, Bx/PAS 72%, and culture 82%. The positive predictive values were KOH 88%, Bx/PAS 89.7%, and culture 90%. The negative predictive values were KOH 58%, Bx/PAS 77%, and culture 43%.[8]
  - In a 2007 study of the diagnosis of onychomycosis by Hsiao et al., the sensitivities of KOH, PAS, and culture were 87%, 81%, and 67%, respectively, and the negative predictive values of KOH, PAS, and culture were 50%, 40%, and 28%, respectively. One reason that the KOH may have done so well is that the nail specimen was immersed in 20% KOH in a test tube for 30 minutes or longer before looking under the microscope.[9]
  - KOH may be equivalent to PAS if done and read properly. It is less expensive and the results are available while the patient is in the office. PAS is a good second line if the KOH is negative and the suspicion for onychomycosis is still present.

DIFFERENTIAL DIAGNOSIS

- Nail trauma can cause a dysmorphic nail that is discolored and thickened. It is especially seen in the big toenail in runners. Ask about nail trauma before diagnosing onychomycosis. Although onychomycosis often starts in the big toenail, it usually spreads to other nails. Traumatic changes often present with only one nail involved.
- Psoriatic and lichen planus nail changes may easily be confused with onychomycosis, especially when the nail becomes thickened and discolored. Pitting of the nail plate surface, which is common in psoriasis, is not a feature of fungal infection. It is possible for a patient with psoriasis to get onychomycosis. Fungal studies can help determine if the changes are truly secondary to onychomycosis (see Chapter 193, Psoriatic Nails).
- Pseudomonal nail infection—Produces a blue-green tint to the nail plate (**Figure 191-9**).
- Melanonychia—Darkening of the nail plate which can be full or in longitudinal lines. This can be caused by medications, trauma, benign melanosis, nevi, melanoma, and onychomycosis (**Figure 191-10**). (see Chapter 189, Pigmented Nail Disorders).
- Leukonychia—White spots or bands that appear proximally and proceed out with the nail may be confused with white superficial onychomycosis (see Chapter 188, Normal Nail Variants).
- Habitual picking of the proximal nail fold—Induces the nail plate to be wavy and ridged, although its substance remains intact and hard (see Chapter 188, Normal Nail Variants).

MANAGEMENT

- Treating onychomycosis can be discouraging. Most topical creams and lotions do not penetrate the nail plate well and are of little value except in controlling inflammation at the nail folds.

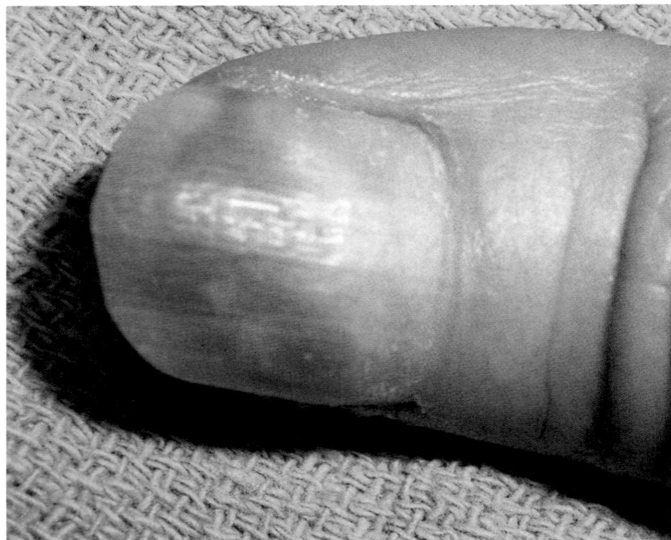

FIGURE 191-9 *Pseudomonas* of the nail showing a blue-green discoloration. (*Reproduced with permission from Richard P. Usatine, MD.*)

- Surgical avulsion may be used to decrease pain caused by pressure on an elevated nail plate because of a dermatophytoma (a collection of dermatophytes and cellular debris under the nail plate). Recurrences are common in the absence of additional systemic or topical therapy with ciclopirox, as the infection typically involves the nail matrix and bed. SOR Ⓒ
- There has been a resurgence of interest in phototherapy modalities for the treatment of onychomycosis. Ultraviolet (UV) light therapy, near-infrared photoinactivation therapy, photodynamic therapy, and photothermal ablative therapy are being studied for treatment of onychomycosis.[10] Further studies are required to determine the clinical role of laser and light therapy in the treatment of onychomycosis. The Pinpointe FootLaser was approved for use to treat onychomycosis in February 2011. SOR Ⓒ

MEDICATIONS

- Oral therapy (**Table 191-1**) is no longer expensive now that terbinafine is generic and on many discounted drug lists.

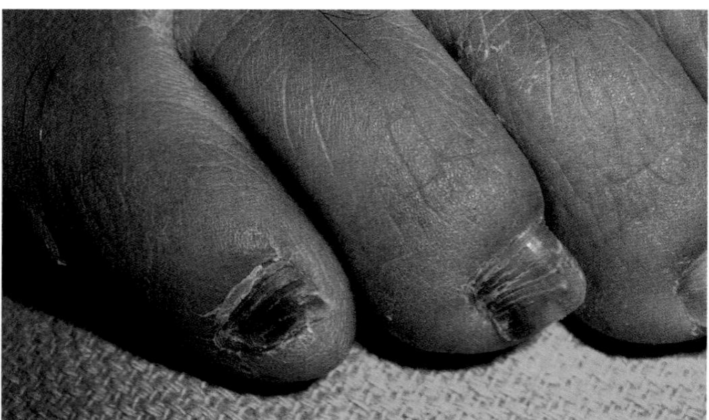

FIGURE 191-10 This patient was noted to have longitudinal melanonychia, but also had some symptoms of onychomycosis. Onychomycosis was proven with a KOH preparation of a nail scaping. The melanonychia disappeared when the onychomycosis was treated with terbinafine. (*Reproduced with permission from Richard P. Usatine, MD.*)

- A Cochrane review found that the evidence suggests that terbinafine is more effective than griseofulvin and that terbinafine and itraconazole are more effective than no treatment.[11] SOR Ⓐ
- Terbinafine dosing is 250 mg daily for 3 months for toenail onychomycosis and 2 months to treat fingernail involvement only.[11] SOR Ⓐ
- Another Cochrane review found 2 trials of nail infections that did not provide any evidence of benefit for topical treatments (ciclopirox not included) compared with placebo.[12] SOR Ⓐ
- Terbinafine has a preferable drug interaction profile, may have better long-term cure rates, and daily dosing may be the most effective treatment.[6,11] SOR Ⓐ
- Itraconazole (Sporanox) has more drug interactions. Pulse dosing is as effective as daily dosing, but even with pulse dosing, therapy is more costly than terbinafine. Consider itraconazole if terbinafine does not effectively treat onychomycosis caused by fungus other than dermatophytes. SOR Ⓒ
- Fluconazole (Diflucan) is not currently Food and Drug Administration (FDA) approved for nail therapy and is not as effective as other oral therapies.[6,13] SOR Ⓑ
- Ciclopirox 8% nail lacquer (Penlac) used daily (with weekly nail cleaning and filing) is an FDA-approved topical treatment for mild-to-moderate onychomycosis. A meta-analysis of 2 randomized controlled trials showed a clinical cure rate of 8% versus 1% for vehicle alone.[14] Such a low cure rate is disappointing, but a larger group of patients had some improvement without cure. This is one option for persons able to afford this topical treatment but who are not able to take oral antifungals.
- Amorolfine is a topical antifungal agent with activity against dermatophytes, yeasts, and fungi that is available over the counter in Australia and the United Kingdom, but is not approved for use in the United States. Amorolfine 5% nail lacquer has been used as monotherapy for the treatment of onychomycosis. It is applied once weekly after the surface of the nail is filed with a disposable file and wiped with alcohol. Once-weekly application of amorolfine 5% nail lacquer for 6 months led to both clinical and mycologic cure in 38% and 46% of patients. It may also be used to increase cure rates when used in combination with oral antifungals.[15]

COMPLEMENTARY AND ALTERNATIVE THERAPY

- There are numerous complementary and alternative medicine (CAM) therapies described on the Internet, most of which have minimal or no evidence of clinical efficacy.
- Mentholated chest rub—There is minimal data on the efficacy of a mentholated chest rub (Vicks VapoRub) in the treatment of onychomycosis. In a series of 18 patients who applied the medication to affected nails daily for 48 weeks, 4 patients (22%) achieved both clinical and mycologic cure.[16] Although these products are unlikely to be harmful, additional studies that support their efficacy in onychomycosis are necessary before widespread use can be recommended.

PREVENTION

Patients should be educated about the use of appropriate footwear, especially in high-exposure areas such as communal bathing facilities and health clubs.

TABLE 191-1 Common Treatments for Onychomycosis

Drug	Pediatric Dose	Adult Dose	Course	Toenail Cure Rate
Griseofulvin (Grifulvin V)	Microsize 15-20 mg/kg/d	500 mg PO qd	4-9 mo (f), 6 to 12 mo (t)	60% ± 6%
Terbinafine (Lamisil)	10-20 kg: 62.5 mg/d 20-40 kg: 125 mg/d	250 mg PO qd	6 wk (f), 12 wk (t)	76% ± 3%
Terbinafine (Lamisil) pulse*	—	250 mg bid 1 wk/mo	2 mo (f), 3 mo (t)	NR
Itraconazole (Sporanox)	—	200 mg daily	6 wk (f), 12 wk (t)	59% ± 5%
Itraconazole (Sporanox) pulse	<20 kg: 5 mg/kg/d for 1 wk/mo 20-40 kg: 100 mg daily for 1 wk/mo	200 mg bid or 5 mg/kg/d capsules for 1 wk/mo	2 mo (f), 3 mo (t)	63% ± 7%
Fluconazole (Diflucan)	3-6 mg/kg once a wk	150 mg once a wk	12-16 wk (f), 18 to 26 wk (t)	48% ± 5%
Ciclopirox 8% nail lacquer (Penlac)	—	Apply daily to nail and surrounding 5-mm skin	Up to 48 wk	Approximately 7%

NR, not recorded.
*Not indicated for treating onychomycosis by the FDA.
Data from Harrell TK, Necomb WW, Replogle WH, et al. Onychomycosis: improved cure rates with itraconazole and terbinafine. *J Am Board Fam Pract.* 2000;13(4):268-273; Bell-Syer S, Porthouse J, Bigby M. Oral treatments for toenail onychomycosis. *Cochrane Database Syst Rev.* 2004;(2):CD004766; Crawford F, Hart R, Bell-Syer S, et al. Topical treatments for fungal infections of the skin and nails of the foot. *Cochrane Database Syst Rev.* 1999;(3):CD001434; Havu V, Heikkila H, Kuokkanen K, et al. A double-blind, randomized study to compare the efficacy and safety of terbinafine (Lamisil) with fluconazole (Diflucan) in the treatment of onychomycosis. *Br J Dermatol.* 2000;142(1):97-102.

PROGNOSIS

The condition may persist indefinitely if left untreated. In patients with diabetes or other immunocompromised states, onychomycosis may increase the risk of secondary bacterial infections.[17]

FOLLOW-UP

Routine monitoring of liver function tests during therapy is probably not necessary in patients without underlying liver disease. However, because the manufacturer of terbinafine recommends checking pretreatment serum aminotransferases and monitoring for potential symptoms of hepatotoxicity during treatment, many clinicians routinely obtain pretreatment and midtherapy values.

PATIENT EDUCATION

Patients should be advised that with treatment, nails may not appear normal for up to 1 year. The normal nail must grow out as treatment progresses. The appearance of normal-appearing nails at the proximal edge of the nail is an encouraging sign at the completion of therapy.

PATIENT RESOURCES

- eMedicineHealth. *Onychomycosis*—**http://www.emedicinehealth.com/onychomycosis/article_em.htm.**
- Familydoctor.org website. *Fungal Infections of Fingernails and Toenails*—**http://familydoctor.org/online/famdocen/home/common/infections/common/fungal/663.html.**
- MedicineNet. *Fungal Nails (Onychomycosis, Tinea Unguium)*—**http://www.medicinenet.com/fungal_nails/article.htm.**

PROVIDER RESOURCES

- Tosti A. *Onychomycosis*—**http://emedicine.medscape.com/article/1105828-overview.** Accessed November 25, 2011.
- Roger P, Bassler M; American Family Physician. *Treating Onychomycosis*—**http://www.aafp.org/afp/20010215/663.html.** Accessed November 25, 2011.
- Elewski BE. Onychomycosis: pathogenesis, diagnosis, and management. *Clin Microbiol Rev.* 1998;11:415-429—**http://www.ncbi.nlm.nih.gov/pmc/articles/PMC88888/.** Accessed November 25, 2011.
- DermNetNZ. *Fungal Nail Infections*—**http://dermnetnz.org/fungal/onychomycosis.html.** Accessed November 25, 2011.
- Roberts DT, Taylor WD, Boyle J. Guidelines for treatment of onychomycosis. *Br J Dermatol.* 2003;148:402-410—**http://www.ncbi.nlm.nih.gov/pubmed/12653730.** Accessed November 25, 2011.

REFERENCES

1. Kemna ME, Elewski BE. A U.S. epidemiologic survey of superficial fungal diseases. *J Am Acad Dermatol.* 1996;35(4):539-542.
2. Gupta AK. Prevalence and epidemiology of onychomycosis in patients visiting physicians' offices: a multicenter Canadian survey of 15,000 patients. *J Am Acad Dermatol.* 2000;43:244.
3. Erbagci Z, Tuncel A, Zer Y, Balci I. A prospective epidemiologic survey on the prevalence of onychomycosis and dermatophytosis in male boarding school residents. *Mycopathologia.* 2005; 159:347.
4. Sahin I, Kaya D, Parlak AH, et al. Dermatophytoses in forestry workers and farmers. *Mycoses.* 2005;48:260.
5. Sigurgeirsson B, Steingrímsson O. Risk factors associated with onychomycosis. *J Eur Acad Dermatol Venereol.* 2004;18:48.
6. Harrell TK, Necomb WW, Replogle WH, et al. Onychomycosis: improved cure rates with itraconazole and terbinafine. *J Am Board Fam Pract.* 2000;13(4):268-273.
7. Elewski BE, Leyden J, Rinaldi MG, Atillasoy E. Office practice-based confirmation of onychomycosis: a US nationwide prospective survey. *Arch Intern Med.* 2002;162:2133.
8. Weinberg JM, Koestenblatt EK, Tutrone WD, et al. Comparison of diagnostic methods in the evaluation of onychomycosis. *J Am Acad Dermatol.* 2003;49(2):193-197.
9. Hsiao YP, Lin HS, Wu TW, et al. A comparative study of KOH test, PAS staining and fungal culture in diagnosis of onychomycosis in Taiwan. *J Dermatol Sci.* 2007;45(2):138-140.
10. Bornstein E. A review of current research in light-based technologies for treatment of podiatric infectious disease states. *J Am Podiatr Med Assoc.* 2009;99(4):348-352.
11. Bell-Syer S, Porthouse J, Bigby M. Oral treatments for toenail onychomycosis. *Cochrane Database Syst Rev.* 2004;(2):CD004766.
12. Crawford F, Hart R, Bell-Syer S, et al. Topical treatments for fungal infections of the skin and nails of the foot. *Cochrane Database Syst Rev.* 1999;(3):CD001434.
13. Havu V, Heikkila H, Kuokkanen K, et al. A double-blind, randomized study to compare the efficacy and safety of terbinafine (Lamisil) with fluconazole (Diflucan) in the treatment of onychomycosis. *Br J Dermatol.* 2000;142(1):97-102.
14. Gupta AK, Joseph WS. Ciclopirox 8% nail lacquer in the treatment of onychomycosis of the toenails in the United States. *J Am Podiatr Med Assoc.* 2000;90(10):495-501.
15. Baran R, Kaoukhov A. Topical antifungal drugs for the treatment of onychomycosis: an overview of current strategies for monotherapy and combination therapy. *J Eur Acad Dermatol Venereol.* 2005;19:21.
16. Derby R, Rohal P, Jackson C, et al. Novel treatment of onychomycosis using over-the-counter mentholated ointment: a clinical case series. *J Am Board Fam Med.* 2011;24:69.
17. Bristow IR, Spruce MC. Fungal foot infection, cellulitis and diabetes: a review. *Diabet Med.* 2009;26:548.

192 PARONYCHIA

E.J. Mayeaux Jr, MD

PATIENT STORY

A 41-year-old woman presented with a 3-day history of localized pain, redness, and tenderness of the lateral nail fold of the index finger. A small abscess had developed in the last 24 hours at the nail margin (**Figure 192-1**). After informed consent was given, a digital block was performed. This acute paronychia was treated with incision and drainage using a #11 scalpel (**Figure 192-2**). A significant amount of pus was drained. She soaked her finger 4 times daily as directed. Two days later the patient's finger was much better and the culture grew out *Staphylococcus aureus*. Draining the abscess was sufficient treatment.

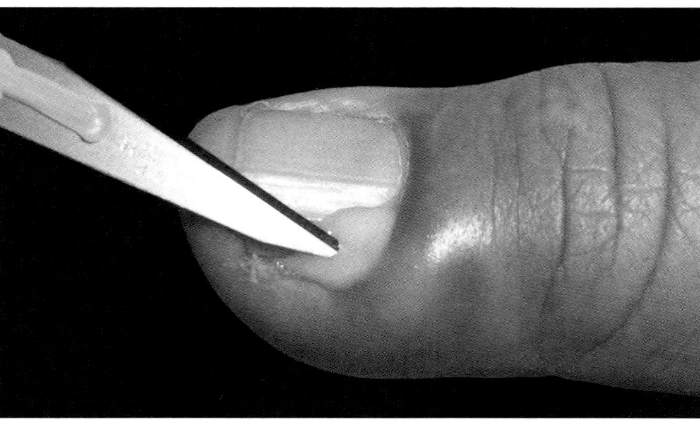

FIGURE 192-2 Incision and drainage of the acute paronychia in Figure 192-1 with a #11 scalpel. Note the exuberant pus draining from the incision. (*Reproduced with permission from Richard P. Usatine, MD.*)

INTRODUCTION

Paronychia is a localized, superficial infection or abscess of the nail folds. It is one of the most common infections of the hand. Paronychia can be acute or chronic. Acute paronychia usually presents as an acutely painful abscess in the nail fold. Chronic paronychia is defined as being present for longer than 6 weeks' duration. It is a generalized red, tender, swelling of the proximal or lateral nail folds. It is usually nonsuppurative and is more difficult to treat.

EPIDEMIOLOGY

Paronychia is the most common infection of the hand, representing 35% of all hand infections in the United States.[1]

ETIOLOGY AND PATHOPHYSIOLOGY

- Paronychial infections develop when a disruption occurs between the seal of the nail fold and the nail plate or the skin of a nail fold is disrupted and allows a portal of entry for invading organisms.[2]
- Acute paronychia is most commonly caused by *S. aureus*, followed by streptococci and *Pseudomonas* (**Figures 192-1** to **192-5**).[1]
- Chronic paronychia has traditionally been thought to be due to *Candida albicans* infection since it frequently cultures from this area (**Figures 192-6** and **192-7**). Other rare causes include atypical *Mycobacteria* and gram-negative rods. There is some evidence that chronic paronychia is at least partially an eczematous process and that *Candida* infection is a secondary phenomenon.[3]
- Untreated persistent chronic paronychia may cause horizontal ridging, undulations, and other changes to the nail plate (see **Figures 192-6** and **192-7**).

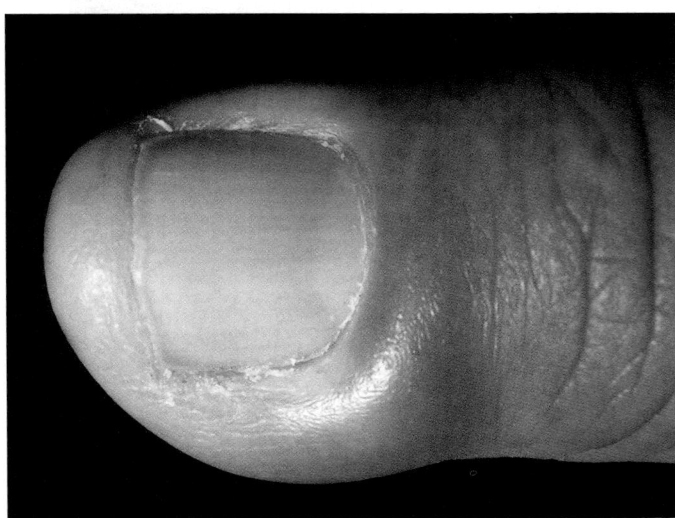

FIGURE 192-1 Painful acute paronychia around the fingernail of a 41-year-old woman. Note the swelling and erythema with a small white-yellow area suggesting underlying purulence. (*Reproduced with permission from Richard P. Usatine, MD.*)

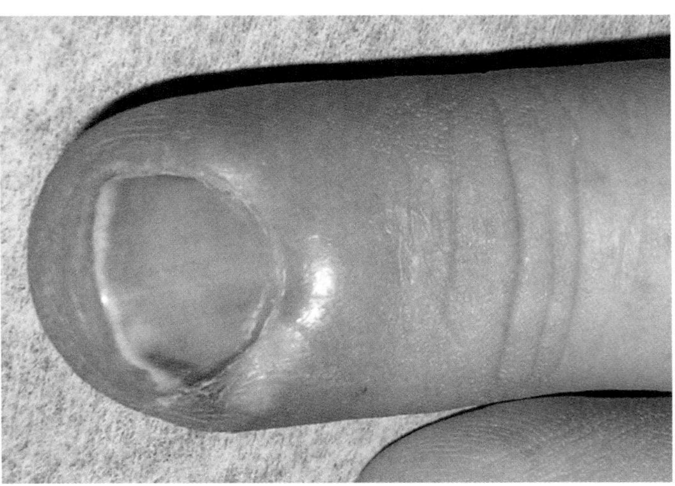

FIGURE 192-3 Acute paronychia from nail biting. Note abscess formation in the lateral nail fold that is extending into the proximal fold. (*Reproduced with permission from E.J. Mayeaux, Jr., MD.*)

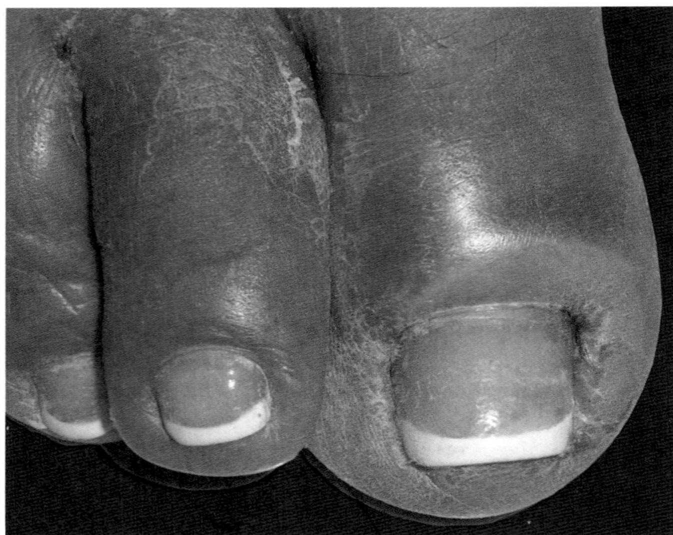

FIGURE 192-4 Acute paronychia of the great toe. Note extensive manicure of the nails, which may predispose to paronychia if the cuticle or nail folds are disrupted. (*Reproduced with permission from Jennifer P. Pierce, MD.*)

RISK FACTORS

- Acute paronychia commonly results from nail biting (see **Figure 192-3**), finger sucking, aggressive manicuring (see **Figure 192-6**), hang nails (see **Figure 192-5**), trauma, and artificial nails.[2]
- Children are prone to acute paronychia through direct infection of fingers with mouth flora from finger sucking and nail biting.
- People at risk of developing chronic paronychia include those who are repeatedly exposed to liquid irritants or alkali, and those whose hands are chronically wet. People with occupations such as baker, bartender, housekeepers, and dishwashers are predisposed to developing chronic paronychia.
- Patients with diabetes mellitus, compromised immune systems, or a history of oral steroid use are at increased risk for paronychia.

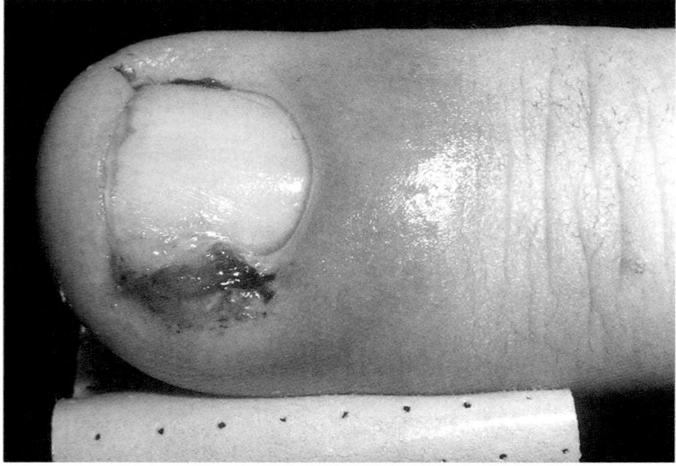

FIGURE 192-5 Acute paronychia with cellulitis of the skin of the fingertip and granulation tissue formation. This all started when the patient began manipulating a hang nail. (*Reproduced with permission from Richard P. Usatine, MD.*)

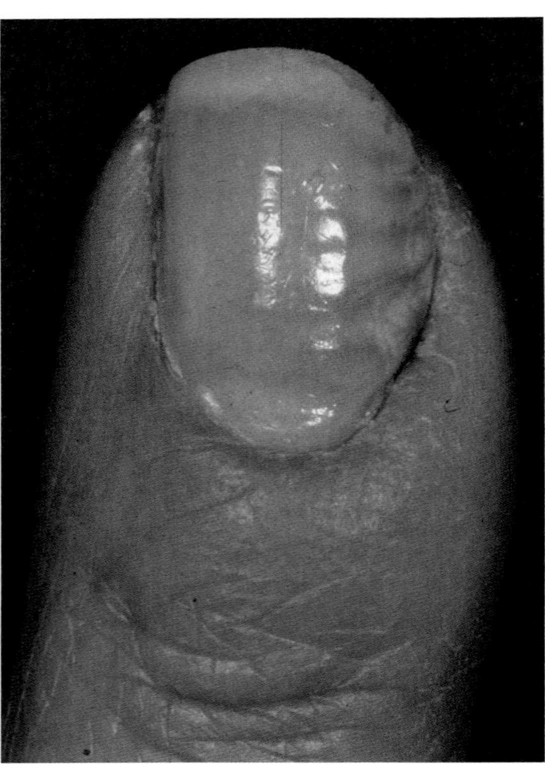

FIGURE 192-6 Chronic paronychia. Note horizontal ridges on one side of the nail plate as a result of chronic inflammation. (*Reproduced with permission from Richard P. Usatine, MD.*)

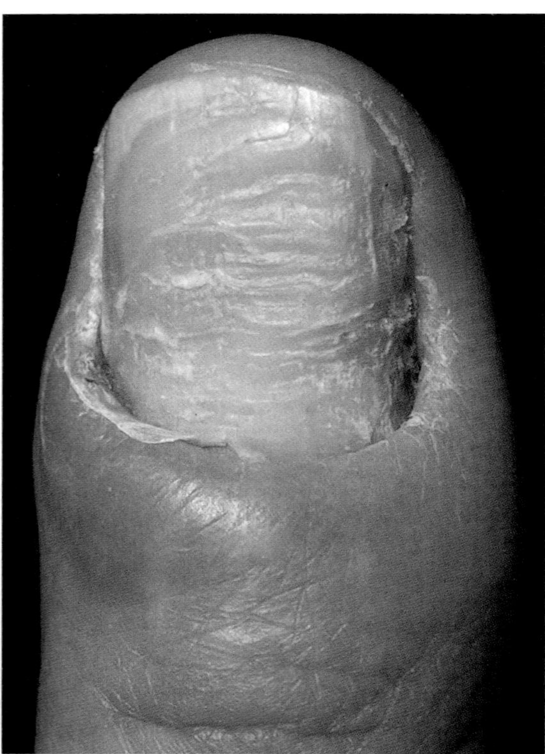

FIGURE 192-7 Chronic *Candida* paronychia causing a dysmorphic fingernail with horizontal ridging. (*Reproduced with permission from Richard P. Usatine, MD.*)

Retroviral therapy use, especially indinavir and lamivudine, may be associated with an increased incidence of paronychia.[4]

Sculptured (artificial) nail placement is associated with the development of paronychia.[1]

DIAGNOSIS

CLINICAL FEATURES

- Acute paronychia presents with localized pain and tenderness. The nail fold appears erythematous and inflamed, and a collection of pus usually develops (see **Figures 192-1** to **192-5**). Granulation tissue may develop along the nail fold, and cellulitis may develop (see **Figure 192-5**).
- Chronic paronychia is a red, tender, painful swelling of the proximal or lateral nail folds. A small collection of pus or abscess may form but typically only redness and swelling are present. Eventually, the nail plates may become thickened and discolored, with pronounced horizontal ridges (see **Figures 192-6** and **192-7**).[5]

DIFFERENTIAL DIAGNOSIS

- Mucus cyst, which presents as a painless swelling lateral and proximal to the nail plate (**Figure 192-8**) may be confused with paronychia. This can also cause changes in the nail morphology.
- Ingrown nail (onychocryptosis) is a condition in which the nail plate is too large for the nail bed. The pressure applied to the lateral nail fold causes a painful inflammation. Although this is sometimes called paronychia, it is different from the type of paronychia caused by an infection of the nail fold (see Chapter 190, Ingrown Toenail).
- Glomus tumor, which presents with constant severe pain, nail plate elevation, bluish discoloration of the nail plate, and blurring of the lunula may be confused with paronychia.
- Herpetic whitlow, which results from herpes simplex virus (HSV) infection presents with acute onset of vesicles or pustules, severe edema, erythema, and pain. Tzanck staining of vesicles will demonstrate multinucleated giant cells and viral culture will grow HSV (see Chapter 128, Herpes Simplex).

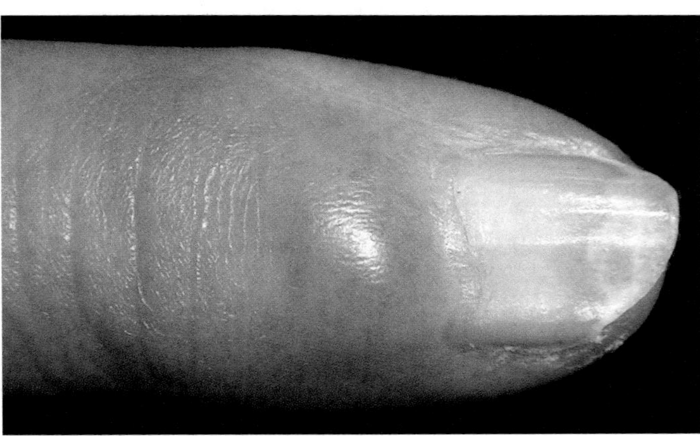

FIGURE 192-8 Digital mucus cyst presenting as a painless swelling of the nail fold in this woman. Note the indented area of the nail caused by the pressure of the mucus cyst on the nail matrix. *(Reproduced with permission from Richard P. Usatine, MD.)*

- Felon—Paronychia must be distinguished from a felon, which is an infection of the digital pulp. It is characterized by severe pain, swelling, and erythema in the pad of the fingertip.
- Benign and malignant neoplasms, which may present early with redness and swelling should always be ruled out when chronic paronychia does not respond to conventional treatment.

MANAGEMENT

NONPHARMACOLOGIC

- Milder cases of acute paronychia without abscess formation may be treated with warm soaks for 20 minutes 3 to 4 times a day.[2] SOR Ⓒ
- When an abscess or fluctuance is present, drainage is necessary.[6] SOR Ⓒ It is performed with digital block anesthesia. The affected nail fold is incised with a scalpel with the blade parallel to the edge of the nail plate and the pus expressed (see **Figure 192-2**). Warm soaks 4 times a day are initiated to keep the incision from sealing until all of the pus is gone.[7] Between soakings, an adhesive bandage can protect the nail fold. Antibiotic therapy is usually not necessary unless there is accompanying cellulitis. SOR Ⓒ

MEDICATIONS

- Although antibiotics are not necessary for simple paronychia, addition of an oral antistaphylococcal agent (dicloxacillin 500 mg 3 times daily, cephalexin 500 mg 2-3 times daily for 7-10 days, erythromycin 333-500 mg 3 times daily, or azithromycin 500 mg on day 1 followed by 250 mg daily for 4 days) may be added for cases with coexisting cellulitis or that are unresponsive. SOR Ⓒ
- Both children who suck their fingers and patients who bite their nails and who require antibiotics should be covered against anaerobes. Clindamycin and amoxicillin-clavulanate potassium are effective against most pathogens isolated from infections originating in the mouth.[8]
- Long-term treatment of chronic paronychia primarily involves avoiding predisposing factors such as prolonged exposure to water, nail trauma, and finger sucking. Treatment with topical antifungals (topical miconazole or ketoconazole) and/or a topical steroid and an antifungal agent has been shown to be successful.[2,3] SOR Ⓑ Oral antifungal therapy is usually not necessary.[2]

PREVENTION

- Trim hangnails to a semilunar smooth edge with a clean sharp nail plate trimmer. Trim toenails flush with the toe tip.
- Do not bite the nail plate or lateral nail folds.
- Avoid prolonged hand exposure to moisture. If hand washing must be frequent, use antibacterial soap, thoroughly dry hands with a clean towel, and apply an antibacterial moisturizer. Use cotton glove liners under waterproof gloves to keep hands dry from sweat and condensation.
- Wear rubber or latex-free gloves when there is potential exposure to pathogens.
- Control diabetes mellitus.
- Keep fingernails clean.
- Moisturize the skin, do not let it become chafed and cracked.

PROGNOSIS

Although the nail fold should improve with treatment, some chronic nail plate changes may not resolve.

FOLLOW-UP

Patients can perform warm soaks 3 to 4 times per day and should have a follow-up examination several days after incision and drainage to assure the infection is resolving appropriately.

PATIENT EDUCATION

Educate patients on measures that may prevent or improve paronychia.

PATIENT RESOURCES

- eMedicineHealth. *Paronychia (Nail Infection)*—**http://www.emedicinehealth.com/paronychia_nail_infection/article_em.htm.**
- Familydoctor.org. Paronychia information—**http://familydoctor.org/online/famdocen/home/common/skin/disorders/937.html.**

PROVIDER RESOURCES

- Rockwell PG. Acute and chronic paronychia. *Am Fam Physician.* 2001;63:1113-1116—**http://www.aafp.org/afp/20010315/1113.html.**
- Medscape. Dermatologic Manifestations of Paronychia—**http://emedicine.medscape.com/article/1106062.**

REFERENCES

1. Rockwell PG. Acute and chronic paronychia. *Am Fam Physician.* 2001;63(6):1113-1116.
2. Hochman LG. Paronychia: more than just an abscess. *Int J Dermatol.* 1995;34:385-386.
3. Tosti A, Piraccini BM, Ghetti E, Colombo MD. Topical steroids versus systemic antifungals in the treatment of chronic paronychia: an open, randomized double-blind and double dummy study. *J Am Acad Dermatol.* 2002;47:73.
4. Tosti A, Piraccini BM, D'Antuono A, et al. Paronychia associated with antiretroviral therapy. *Br J Dermatol.* 1999;140(6):1165-1168.
5. Canales FL, Newmeyer WL 3d, Kilgore ES. The treatment of felons and paronychias. *Hand Clin.* 1989;5:515-523.
6. Keyser JJ, Littler JW, Eaton RG. Surgical treatment of infections and lesions of the perionychium. *Hand Clin.* 1990;6(1):137-153.
7. Zuber T, Mayeaux EJ Jr. *Atlas of Primary Care Procedures.* Philadelphia, PA: Lippincott, Williams, & Wilkins; 2003:233-238.
8. Brook I. Aerobic and anaerobic microbiology of paronychia. *Ann Emerg Med.* 1990;19:994-996..

193 PSORIATIC NAILS

E.J. Mayeaux Jr, MD

PATIENT STORY

A 19-year-old man with a 4-year history of plaque psoriasis presents with nail abnormalities in several fingers (**Figure 193-1**). He is particularly concerned about the recently acquired greenish discoloration of his fifth digit.

INTRODUCTION

Psoriasis is a hereditary disorder of skin with numerous clinical expressions. It affects millions of people throughout the world.[1] Nail involvement is common and can have a significant cosmetic impact.

EPIDEMIOLOGY

- Nails are involved in 30% to 50% of psoriasis patients at any given time, and up to 90% develop nail changes over their lifetime.[1] In most cases, nail involvement coexists with cutaneous psoriasis, although the skin surrounding the affected nails need not be involved. Psoriatic nail disease without overt cutaneous disease occurs in 1% to 5% of psoriasis. Patients with nail involvement are thought to have a higher incidence of associated arthritis.[2]
- The most common nail change seen with psoriasis is nail plate pitting (**Figures 193-1** to **193-3**).

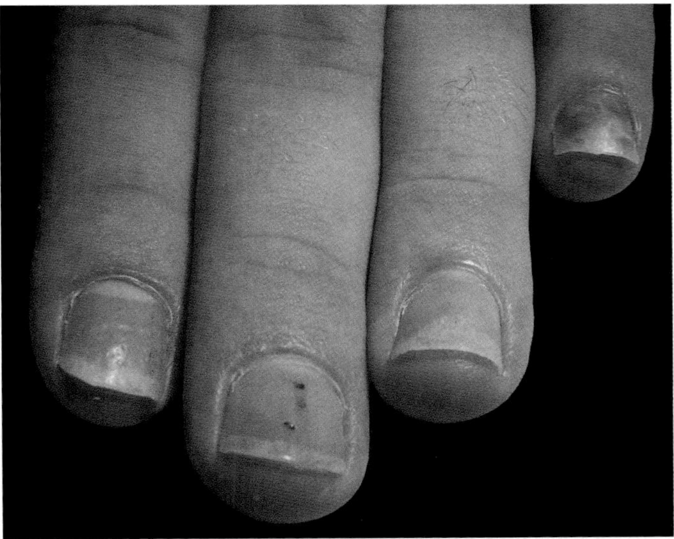

FIGURE 193-1 Patient with nail psoriasis demonstrating the oil drop sign (second digit), nail pitting (second and third digit), onycholysis (second, fourth, and fifth digits), and secondary pseudomonas infection (fifth digit). *(Reproduced with permission from E.J. Mayeaux Jr, MD.)*

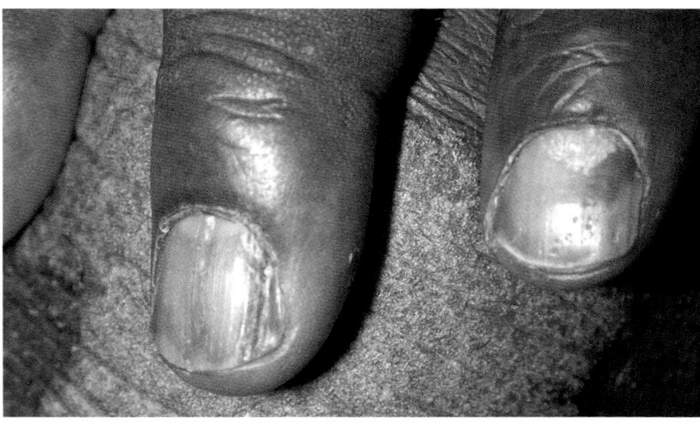

FIGURE 193-2 Nail psoriasis demonstrating nail pitting, onycholysis, oil drop sign, and longitudinal ridging. Nails held over the silvery plaque on the knee. *(Reproduced with permission from Richard P. Usatine, MD.)*

ETIOLOGY AND PATHOPHYSIOLOGY

- In psoriasis, parakeratotic cells within the stratum corneum of the nail matrix alters normal keratinization.[3] The proximal nail matrix forms the superficial portion of the nail plate, so that involvement in this part of the matrix results in pitting of the nail plate (see **Figures 193-1** to **193-3**.) The pits may range in size from pinpoint depressions to large punched-out lesions. People without psoriasis can have nail pitting.
- Longitudinal matrix involvement produces longitudinal nail ridging or splitting (see **Figure 193-2**). When transverse matrix involvement occurs, solitary or multiple "growth arrest" lines (Beau lines) may occur (see Chapter 188, Normal Nail Variants). Psoriatic involvement of the intermediate portion of the nail matrix leads to leukonychia and diminished nail plate integrity.
- Parakeratosis of the nail bed with thickening of the stratum corneum causes discoloration of the nail bed, producing the "salmon spot" or "oil drop" signs.[3]

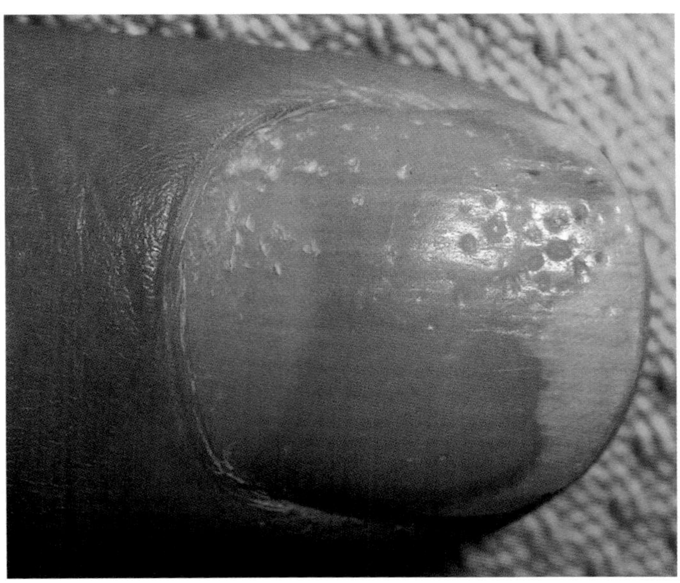

FIGURE 193-3 Nail pitting and onycholysis in a patient with psoriasis. *(Reproduced with permission from Richard P. Usatine, MD.)*

- Desquamation of parakeratotic cells at the hyponychium leads to onycholysis, which may allow for bacteria and fungi infection.[4]

RISK FACTORS

- Psoriasis of the skin
- Psoriatic arthritis
- Nail unit trauma
- Generalized psoriasis flair

DIAGNOSIS

CLINICAL FEATURES

- The diagnosis of nail psoriasis is usually straightforward when characteristic nail findings coexist with cutaneous psoriasis. Nail pitting and onycholysis are the most common findings (see **Figure 193-3**).
- Nail psoriasis and onychomycosis are often indistinguishable by clinical examination alone. Psoriasis at the hyponychium produces subungual hyperkeratosis and distal onycholysis (**Figures 193-4** and **193-5**). Trauma may accentuate this process. Secondary microbial colonization by *Candida* or *Pseudomonas* organisms may occur (see **Figures 193-1** and **193-5**).
- Nail bed psoriasis produces localized onycholysis which often appears like a drop of oil on a piece of paper (oil drop sign) (see **Figures 193-2, 193-4**, and **193-5**). This same condition is also called the salmon patch sign.
- Extensive germinal matrix involvement may result in loss of nail integrity and transverse (horizontal) ridging (**Figure 193-6**).
- Psoriasis causes dermal vascular dilation and tortuosity, and in the nails is associated with splinter hemorrhages of the nail bed caused by foci of capillary bleeding. Extravasated blood becomes trapped between the longitudinal troughs of the nail bed and the overlying nail plate grows out distally along with the plate (**Figure 193-7**). The splinter hemorrhages of the psoriatic nail are analogous to the cutaneous Auspitz sign.

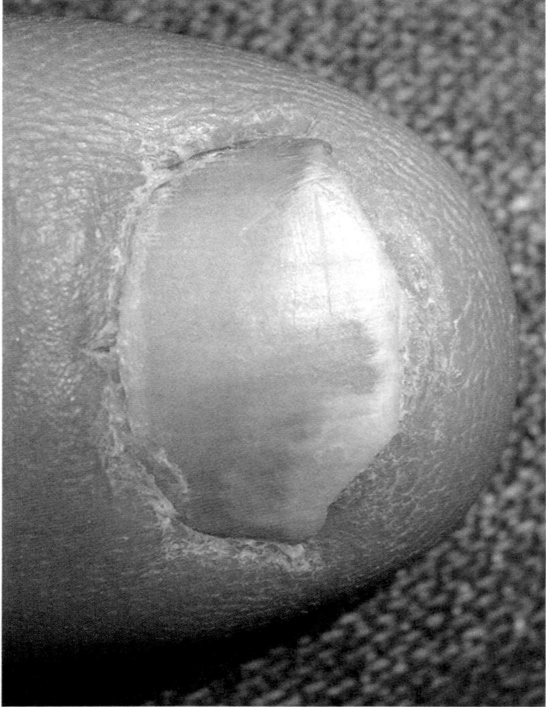

FIGURE 193-5 Nail psoriasis with the oil drop sign proximal to the lighter onycholysis at the distal nail. (*Reproduced with permission from Richard P. Usatine, MD.*)

LABORATORY TESTING

Potassium hydroxide (KOH) preparation and fungal culture will usually provide an answer. However, it may be necessary to clip a portion of the nail plate and send it for fungal staining (periodic acid-Schiff [PAS] stain) if the first test results are not consistent with the clinical picture.[5] Psoriasis and onychomycosis can occur concomitantly.

BIOPSY

Biopsy of the nail unit is rarely necessary unless a malignancy is suspected.

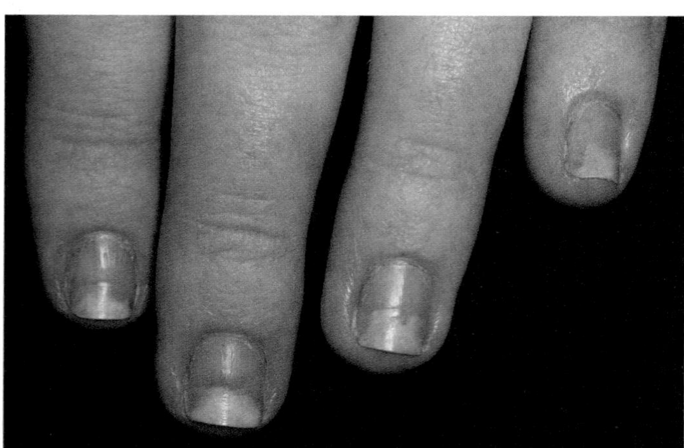

FIGURE 193-4 Nail psoriasis with onycholysis and oil drop sign in a young woman. Note that end of the nail plates are no longer attached to the nail bed and there is a light brown discoloration where the nail loses its attachment. (*Reproduced with permission from Richard P. Usatine, MD.*)

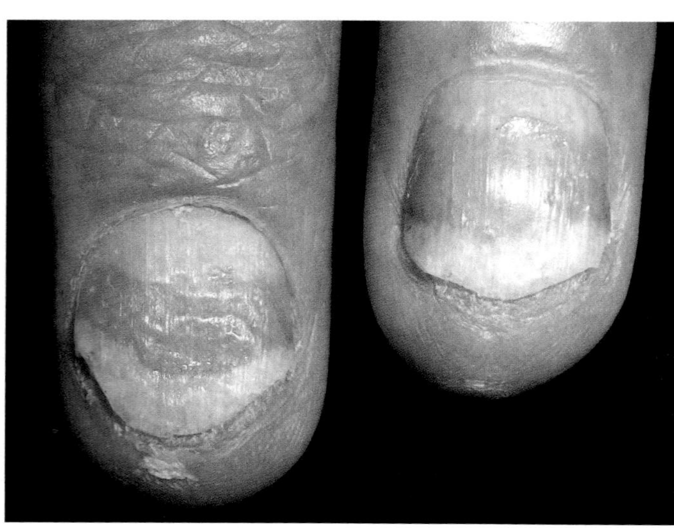

FIGURE 193-6 Nail psoriasis demonstrating onycholysis, pits, and transverse (horizontal) ridging. (*Reproduced with permission from Richard P. Usatine, MD.*)

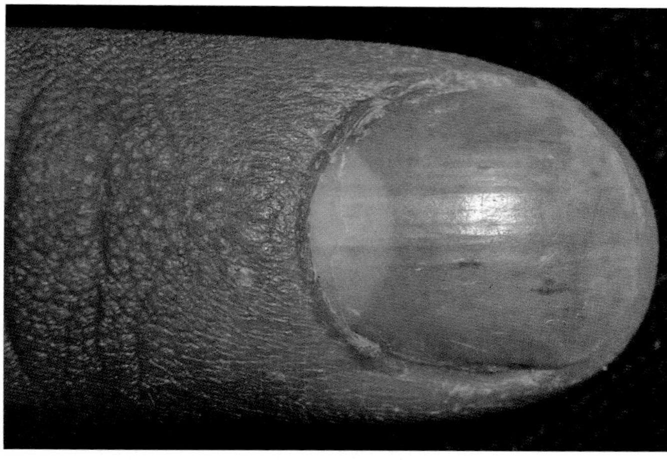

FIGURE 193-7 Prominent splinter hemorrhages in the nail of a person with psoriasis. (*Reproduced with permission from Richard P. Usatine, MD.*)

DIFFERENTIAL DIAGNOSIS

- Onychomycosis produces distal onycholysis and hyperkeratosis that appear identical to psoriasis and may coexist with it (see Chapter 191, Onychomycosis).
- Darier disease (keratosis follicularis) is an autosomal dominant disorder that results in abnormal keratinization and loss of adhesion between epidermal cells. It typically presents in the second decade of life with hyperkeratotic, yellow-brown, greasy-appearing papules that coalesce into verrucous-like plaques in a seborrheic distribution. Nails may demonstrate red/white longitudinal stripes, subungual hyperkeratosis, and notching of the distal nail margins (**Figure 193-8**). The course of the illness is chronic and persistent.
- Alopecia areata also can produce pitting of the nails. As a general rule, pitting in psoriasis is more irregular and broader based; pitting in alopecia areata is more regular, shallow, and geometric and produces fine pits (see Chapter 185, Alopecia Areata).

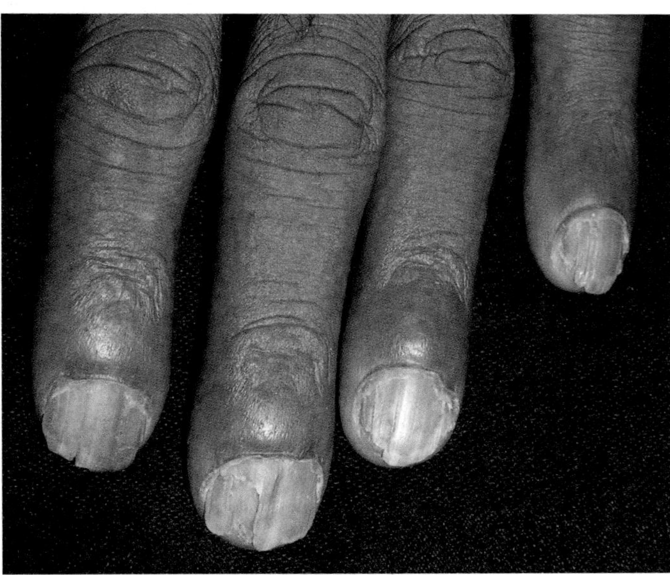

FIGURE 193-8 A woman with Darier disease (keratosis follicularis) demonstrating brittle nails with brown/white longitudinal stripes and notching of the distal nail plate. (*Reproduced with permission from Richard P. Usatine, MD.*)

- Neoplastic and dysplastic diseases may produce psoriasiform nail changes in a single nail. Bowen disease, squamous cell carcinoma, and verruca vulgaris may appear as an isolated subungual or periungual plaque, possibly with accompanying nail plate destruction. A biopsy can establish a definitive diagnosis.

MANAGEMENT

NONPHARMACOLOGIC

- Psoriatic nail disease is often persistent and refractory to treatment. There is insufficient evidence to recommend a standard treatment.
- The nails should be kept short, to avoid traumatic exacerbation of onycholysis and to avoid the accumulation of exogenous material under the nail.[3] SOR C
- Nail polish may be very helpful in concealing a range of nail unit changes.[6] SOR C
- Nail plate buffing may diminish surface imperfections.[6] SOR C

MEDICATIONS

- Unfortunately, specific evidence for systemic therapy in nail psoriasis is generally lacking. It should be considered in those with significant cutaneous involvement in addition to nail disease.
- One treatment option for nail psoriasis, especially with matrix involvement, is intralesional corticosteroid injection. Triamcinolone acetonide (0.4 mL, 10 mg/mL) is injected into the nail bed, matrix, or proximal fold following digital block, and then at 3-month intervals.[3,7] SOR A Subungual hyperkeratosis, ridging, and thickening respond better than pitting and onycholysis, with benefit sustained for at least 9 months.[7] Pain, periungual hypopigmentation, subungual hemorrhage, and atrophy have been reported.[3]
- Nail bed disease, including subungual hyperkeratosis, distal onycholysis, and "oil drop" changes may also need the lateral nail folds injected close to the nail bed. Direct injection into the nail bed is prevented by the nail plate and extreme pain sensitivity of the hyponychial region. Atrophy and subungual hematoma formation are potential complications.
- One study found that topical 1% 5-fluorouracil solution or 5% cream applied twice daily to the matrix area for 6 months improved pitting and hyperkeratosis but worsened onycholysis.[3] SOR B
- Topical calcipotriol may be effective in reducing subungual hyperkeratosis.[3,8] SOR B
- Topical tazarotene improves onycholysis and nail pitting (if applied under occlusion) in those treated for 24 weeks.[3] SOR A
- In a single-blinded study, Feliciani et al. found that combination therapy (oral cyclosporine and topical calcipotriol) was more effective than monotherapy (cyclosporine alone) on nail psoriasis.[9]
- Anthralin ointment 0.4% to 2.0%, applied and washed off after 30 minutes, is effective for onycholysis, subungual hyperkeratosis, and possibly pitting.[3] SOR B
- Narrow-band ultraviolet B (UVB) and psoralen UVA (PUVA) phototherapy for 3 to 6 months is effective for cutaneous psoriasis but its efficacy for nail psoriasis is poorly defined.[3]

- Acitretin, methotrexate, and cyclosporine are helpful for nail psoriasis.[3,10] SOR B
- Systemic retinoid therapy is often effective for pustular psoriasis, and early intervention is most likely to prevent chronic nail-associated scarring.

PREVENTION

- Wearing gloves during wet work and during exposure to harsh materials may minimize trauma to the skin and nail unit.[11]
- Trimming the nail short to minimize leverage at the free edge and resulting trauma.
- If dry skin or scaling develop, application of emollients may be helpful.
- Cosmetic manipulations of the nail risk exacerbating the disease due to minor trauma. Discretion and care should be exercised when trimming the cuticle and clearing subungual debris.

PROGNOSIS

Psoriatic nail changes may be reversible because scarring typically does not occur. An exception to this may develop in severe cases of generalized pustular psoriasis.

FOLLOW-UP

Follow-up can be combined with regular follow-ups for cutaneous psoriasis.

PATIENT EDUCATION

- Nail psoriasis is mainly a cosmetic problem. Nail polish or artificial nails can be used in some patients to conceal psoriatic pitting and onycholysis. When subungual hyperkeratosis becomes uncomfortable because of pressure exerted by footwear, the nail can be pared down to relieve the pressure.
- Patients should be instructed to trim nails back to the point of firm attachment with the nail bed to minimize further nail bed and nail plate disassociation. Wearing gloves while working may minimize trauma to the nails. Tell patients to avoid vigorous cleaning and scraping under the nails as this may break the skin where the nail is attached and lead to an infection.

PATIENT RESOURCES

- National Psoriasis Foundation. *Hands, Feet and Nails*—**http://www.psoriasis.org/page.aspx?pid = 445.**
- eMedicineHealth. *Nail Psoriasis*—**http://www.emedicinehealth.com/nail_psoriasis/article_em.htm.**

PROVIDER RESOURCES

- Medscape. *Nail Psoriasis: Overview of Nail Psoriasis*—**http://emedicine.medscape.com/article/1107949.**
- DermNet NZ. Nail Psoriasis—**http://dermnetnz.org/scaly/nail-psoriasis.html.**

REFERENCES

1. Jiaravuthisan MM, Sasseville D, Vender RB, et al. Psoriasis of the nail. Anatomy, pathology, clinical presentation, and a review of the literature on thereapy. *J Am Acad Dermatol.* 2007;57(1):1-27.
2. Noronha PA, Zubkov B. Nails and nail disorders in children and adults. *Am Fam Physician.* 1997;55(6):2129-2140.
3. Edwards F, de Berker D. Nail psoriasis: clinical presentation and best practice recommendations. *Drugs.* 2009;69(17):2351-2361.
4. Jiaravuthisan MM, Sasseville D, Vender RB, et al. Psoriasis of the nail: anatomy, pathology, clinical presentation, and a review of the literature on therapy. *J Am Acad Dermatol.* 2007;57(1):1-27.
5. Grammer-West NY, Corvette DM, Giandoni MB, Fitzpatrick JE. Clinical pearl: nail plate biopsy for the diagnosis of psoriatic nails. *J Am Acad Dermatol.* 1998;38(2 pt 1):260-262.
6. de Berker D. Management of psoriatic nail disease. *Semin Cutan Med Surg.* 2009;28(1):39-43.
7. de Berker DA, Lawrence CM. A simplified protocol of steroid injection for psoriatic nail dystrophy. *Br J Dermatol.* 1998;138(1):90-95.
8. Tosti A, Piraccini BM, Cameli N, et al. Calcipotriol in nail psoriasis: a controlled double-blind comparison with betamethasone dipropionate and salicylic acid. *Br J Dermatol.* 1998;139(4):655-659.
9. Feliciani C, Zampetti A, Forleo P, et al. Nail psoriasis: combined therapy with systemic cyclosporine and topical calcipotriol. *J Cutan Med Surg.* 2004;8(2):122-125.
10. Cassell S, Kavanaugh AF. Therapies for psoriatic nail disease. A systematic review. *J Rheumatol.* 2006;33(7):1452-1456.
11. André J. Artificial nails and psoriasis. *J Cosmet Dermatol.* 2005;4(2):103-106.

194 SUBUNGUAL HEMATOMA

E.J. Mayeaux Jr, MD

PATIENT STORY

A 22-year-old woman dropped an iron on her toe the day before she visited our free clinic. Her toe was painful at rest and worse when walking (**Figure 194-1**). This subungual hematoma needed to be drained and we did not have an electrocautery unit. A paperclip was bent open and held in a hemostat and heated with a torch. With some pressure it pierced the patient's nail plate and the blood spontaneously drained (**Figures 194-2** and **194-3**). This relieved the pressure and gave the patient immediate pain relief. The remaining old blood was drained with a little pressure on the proximal nail fold (**Figure 194-4**). Although we were concerned about a possible underlying fracture, the patient did not have health insurance and chose to postpone an X-ray. Her toe healed well and no radiographs were ever taken. (*Story by Richard P. Usatine, MD.*)

INTRODUCTION

Subungual hematoma (blood under the fingernail or toenail) is a common injury. It is typically caused by a blow to the distal phalanx (eg, smashing with a tool, crush in a door jamb, stubbing one's toe). The blow causes bleeding of the nail matrix or bed with resultant subungual hematoma formation. Patients usually present because of throbbing pain associated with blue-black discoloration under the nail plate. Subungual hematomas may be simple (ie, the nail and nail fold are intact) or accompanied by significant injuries to the nail fold and digit.[1] The patient may not be aware of the precipitating trauma, because it may have been minor and/or chronic (eg, rubbing in a tight shoe).

EPIDEMIOLOGY

Subungual hematoma is a common childhood and adult injury.

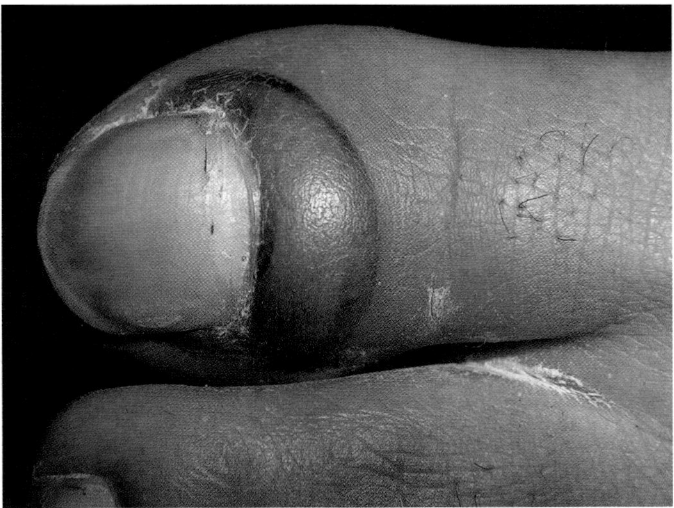

FIGURE 194-1 Acute subungual hematoma 1 day after dropping an iron on her toe. It was painful at rest and worse when walking. (*Reproduced with permission from Richard P. Usatine, MD.*)

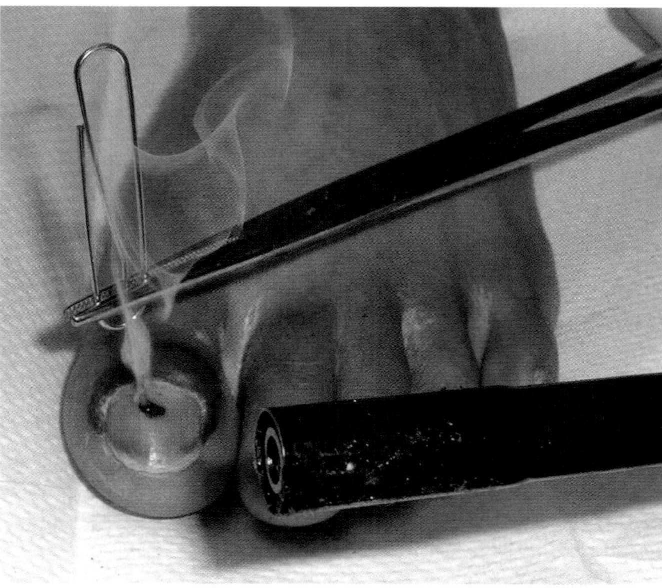

FIGURE 194-2 A paperclip was held in a hemostat and heated with a torch to pierce the patient's nail plate in order to relieve the subungual hematoma. (*Reproduced with permission from Richard P. Usatine, MD.*)

ETIOLOGY AND PATHOPHYSIOLOGY

- The injury causes bleeding of the nail matrix and nail bed, which results in subungual hematoma formation (**Figures 194-1** to **194-5**).
- In most cases it grows out with the nail plate, exhibiting a proximal border that reproduces the shape of the lunula. Occasionally, a hematoma does not migrate because of repeated daily trauma. An extended, nonmigrating hematoma should be considered suspicious. Nail plate punch biopsy will often reveal the dark streak to be a subungual hematoma as the color lifts off with nail plate (see **Figure 194-5**).
- Potential complications of subungual hematoma include onycholysis, nail deformity (usually splitting as in **Figure 194-6**), and infection.

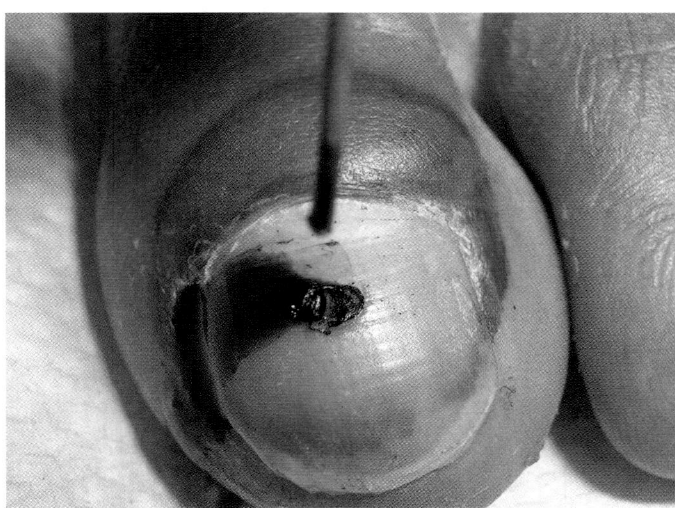

FIGURE 194-3 The hot paper clip formed a nice hole in the nail plate and the blood drained out spontaneously. This relieved the pressure and gave the patient immediate pain relief. (*Reproduced with permission from Richard P. Usatine, MD.*)

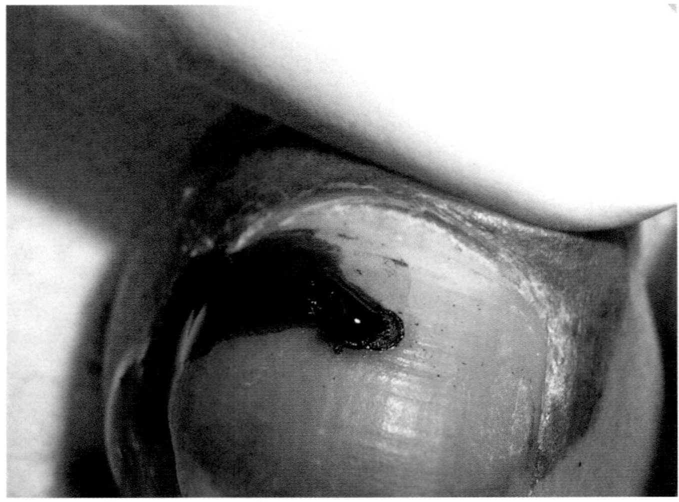

FIGURE 194-4 After the nail plate is pierced, the blood drains easily with a little pressure on the proximal nail fold. (*Reproduced with permission from Richard P. Usatine, MD.*)

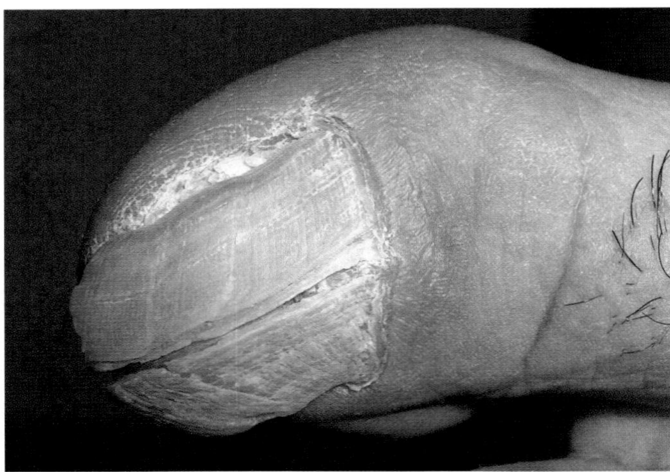

FIGURE 194-6 Split-nail deformity (onychoschizia). that occurred years ago after trauma to the big toe. (*Reproduced with permission from Richard P. Usatine, MD.*)

Complications are more likely to occur when presentation is delayed or there is an underlying fracture.[2]

DIAGNOSIS

CLINICAL FEATURES

Patients complain of throbbing pain and blue-black discoloration under the nail as the hematoma progresses. Pain is relieved immediately in most patients with simple nail trephination (see **Figure 194-3**).

IMAGING

If the mechanism of injury and clinical picture suggest a possible distal phalanx or distal interphalangeal (DIP) fracture, obtain a radiograph. SOR Ⓒ

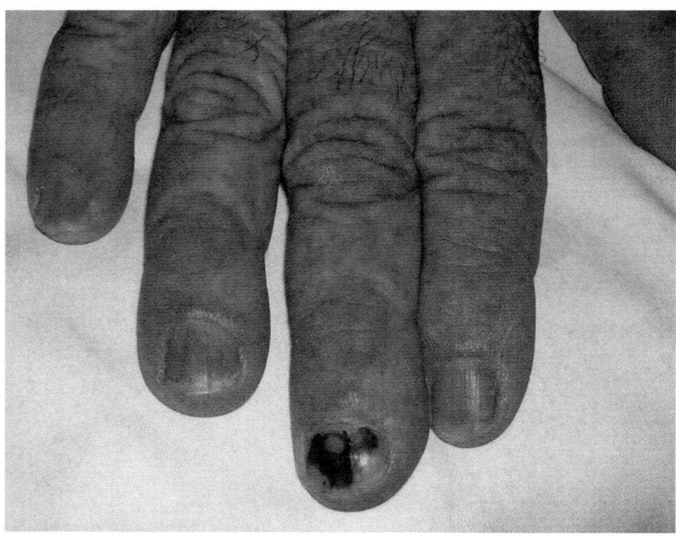

FIGURE 194-5 This persistent discoloration of the nail was found to be a subungual hematoma by nail plate biopsy using a punch biopsy instrument. (*Reproduced with permission from E.J. Mayeaux, Jr., MD.*)

DIFFERENTIAL DIAGNOSIS

- Nail bed nevus—Appears as a stable or slowly growing painless dark spot in the nail bed or matrix.
- Longitudinal melanonychia—Appears as painless pigmented bands that start in the matrix and extend the length of the nail (see Chapter 189, Pigmented Nail Disorders).
- Subungual melanoma—May start as a painless darkly pigmented band in the matrix and extend the length of the nail. It may be associated with pigment deposition in the proximal nail fold (Hutchinson sign) (see Chapter 189, Pigmented Nail Disorders).
- Splinter hemorrhages—Appears as reddish streaks in the nail bed and are seen in psoriasis more commonly than endocarditis (see Chapter 193, Psoriatic Nails).
- The diagnosis of child abuse must be considered in cases of chronic or frequently recurrent subungual hematomas in children.[3]

MANAGEMENT

NONPHARMACOLOGIC

Subungual hematomas are treated with nail trephination, which removes the extravasated blood and relieves the pressure and resulting pain. Beyond 48 hours, most subungual hematomas have clotted and pain has decreased, so trephination is ineffective. SOR Ⓒ

SURGERY

Nail trephination is a painless procedure because there are no nerve endings in the nail plate that is perforated. The nail is perforated with a hot metal wire or steel paper clip (see **Figures 194-2** to **194-4**), an electrocautery device, or by spinning a large-bore needle against the nail plate like a mechanical spade bit. This allows the collected blood to drain out (see **Figures 194-3** and **194-4**). The hole must be large enough for continued drainage, which can continue for 24 to 36 hours. The puncture site should be kept covered with sterile gauze dressing while the wound drains, and the gauze should be changed daily.

MEDICATIONS

- The use of prophylactic antibiotics does not appear to improve outcomes in patients with subungual hematomas and intact nail folds.[4] SOR B
- Oral analgesia such as ibuprofen 10 mg/kg (maximum dose 800 mg) every 6 to 8 hours may be used with more painful digits. SOR C

REFERRAL

- Some authors recommend removal of the nail with inspection instead of nail trephination when the hematoma involves more than 25% to 50% of the nail because of the increased likelihood of significant nail bed injury and fracture of the distal phalanx.[5,6] SOR C
- When deeper injuries are involved, nail plate removal after a digital block allows for nail bed repair.[7] SOR C

PROGNOSIS

The potential complications of a subungual hematoma include onycholysis (separation of the nail plate from the nail bed), nail deformity, nail loss, and infection. Complications are more likely to occur when care is delayed.

A retrospective analysis of 123 patients treated with simple trephination found that 85% of patients reported an excellent or very good outcome, 2% reported a poor outcome (nail splitting, see **Figure 194-6**), and no correlation was found between outcome and size of the hematoma or the presence of fracture or infection.[2]

FOLLOW-UP

After trephination, instruct the patient to soak the affected digit in warm water several times per day for 2 days, and to keep the area dressed between soaks. The patient should return to clinic with any signs of reaccumulation of blood or infection.

PATIENT EDUCATION

- Potential complications of subungual hematoma and nail trephination should be discussed with the patient and/or the patient's parents or guardian.
- Inform the patient that residual discoloration usually slowly grows out with the nail.

PATIENT RESOURCES

- eMedicineHealth. *Subungual Hematoma*—**http://www.emedicinehealth.com/subungual_hematoma_bleeding_under_nail/article_em.htm.**
- WebMD. *Subungual Hematoma*—**http://www.webmd.com/skin-problems-and-treatments/bleeding-under-nail.**

PROVIDER RESOURCES

- American Family Physician. *Fingertip Injuries*—**http://www.aafp.org/afp/20010515/1961.html.**
- InteliHealth. Nail Trauma—**http://www.intelihealth.com/IH/ihtIH/WSIHW000/9339/25971.html.**

REFERENCES

1. Roser SE, Gellman H. Comparison of nail bed repair versus nail trephination for subungual hematomas in children. *J Hand Surg Am.* 1999;24:1166-1170.
2. Meek S, White M. Subungual haematomas: is simple trephining enough? *J Accid Emerg Med.* 1998;15:269-271.
3. Gavin LA, Lanz MJ, Leung DY, Roesler TA. Chronic subungual hematomas: a presumed immunologic puzzle resolved with a diagnosis of child abuse. *Arch Pediatr Adolesc Med.* 1997;151:103-105.
4. Seaberg DC, Angelos WJ, Paris PM. Treatment of subungual hematomas with nail trephination: a prospective study. *Am J Emerg Med.* 1991;9:209-210.
5. Zook EG, Guy RJ, Russell RC. A study of nail bed injuries: causes, treatment, and prognosis. *J Hand Surg Am.* 1984;9:247-252.
6. Zacher JB. Management of injuries of the distal phalanx. *Surg Clin North Am.* 1984;64:747-760.
7. Hart RG, Kleinert HE. Fingertip and nail bed injuries. *Emerg Med Clin North Am.* 1993;11:755-765.

SECTION 17 PIGMENTARY AND LIGHT-RELATED CONDITIONS

195 MELASMA

E.J. Mayeaux Jr, MD
Richard P. Usatine, MD

PATIENT STORY

A young Hispanic woman delivers a healthy baby boy. On the first postpartum day, she is sitting in the rocking chair after breast-feeding her son. Her doctor notes that she has melasma and asks her about it. She states that the hyperpigmented areas on her face have become darker during this pregnancy (**Figure 195-1**). She noted the dark spots started with her first pregnancy but they are worse this time. On physical examination, hyperpigmented patches are noted on the cheeks and upper lip (**Figure 195-2**). Although the patient hopes the pigment will fade, she does not want to treat the melasma at this time.

INTRODUCTION

Melasma is an acquired hyperpigmentary disorder characterized by light- to dark-brown macules and patches occurring in the sun-exposed areas of the face and neck. It is most commonly caused by pregnancy or the use of sex steroid hormones, such as oral contraceptive pills.

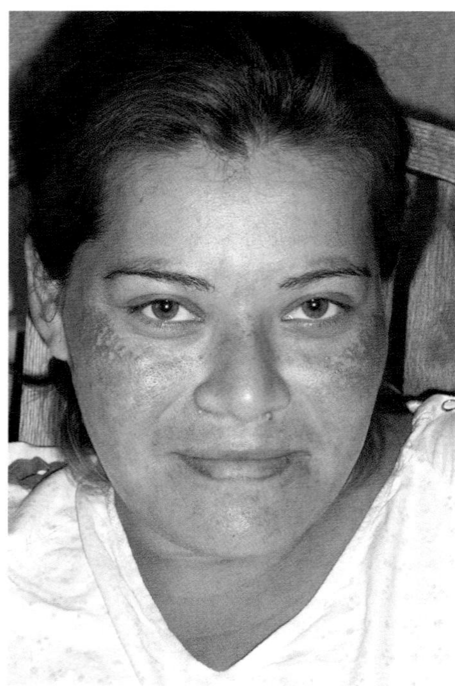

FIGURE 195-1 Melasma (chloasma) in the typical distribution in a woman that just gave birth to her second child. This is sometimes called the mask of pregnancy. (*Reproduced with permission from Richard P. Usatine, MD.*)

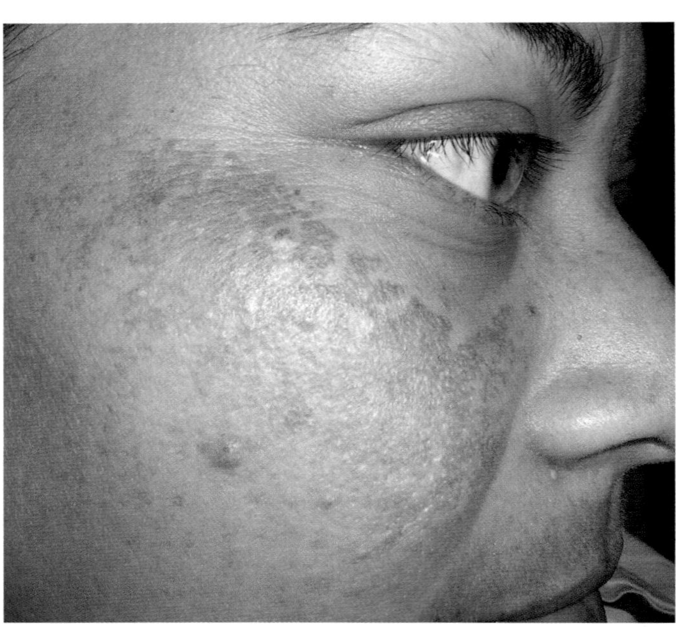

FIGURE 195-2 Close-up of the melasma showing the hyperpigmented patches on cheeks and upper lip. (*Reproduced with permission from Richard P. Usatine, MD.*)

SYNONYMS

Melasma is also known as chloasma, mask of pregnancy.

EPIDEMIOLOGY

- It is a relatively common disorder that affects sun-exposed areas of skin, most commonly the face. It is believed to affect up to 75% of pregnant women.[1]
- It affects predominantly women (**Figures 195-1** to **195-3**), with men accounting for only 10% of all cases. It is particularly prevalent in women of Hispanic, East Asian, and Southeast Asian origin (skin types IV-VI) and who live in areas of intense ultraviolet (UV) radiation exposure.[1]
- Melasma caused by pregnancy usually regresses within a year, but areas of hyperpigmentation may never completely resolve.[2] It may increase with each subsequent pregnancy becoming more obvious.

ETIOLOGY AND PATHOPHYSIOLOGY

The major etiologic factors include genetic influences, exposure to UV radiation, and sex hormones.

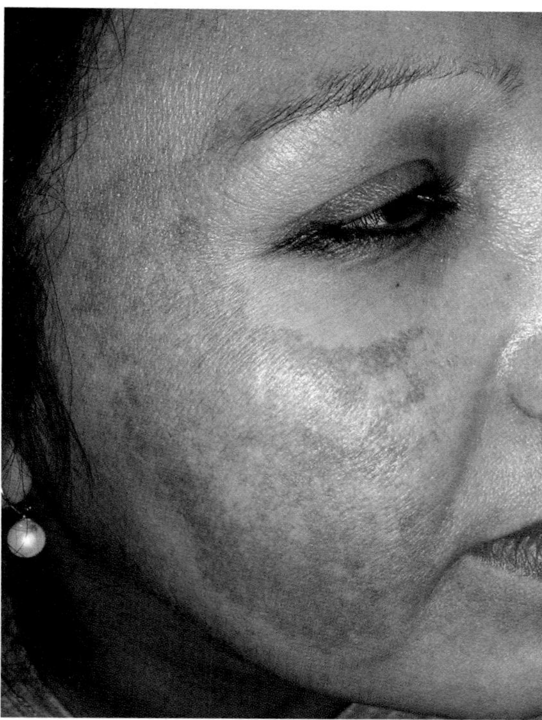

FIGURE 195-3 A 39-year-old Hispanic woman with melasma seeking treatment. She is disturbed by this dark color on her face. Note the hyperpigmentation reaches the eyebrows but does not cover the upper lip. She has not been pregnant for years and is not taking hormonal contraceptives. (*Reproduced with permission from Richard P. Usatine, MD.*)

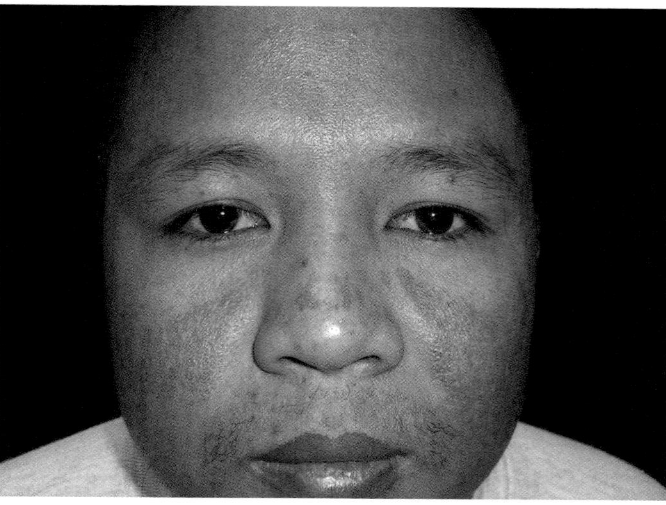

FIGURE 195-4 Melasma in a man. (*Reproduced with permission from Richard P. Usatine, MD.*)

- The precise cause of melasma has not been determined. Multiple factors have been implicated, including pregnancy, oral contraceptives, genetics, sun exposure, cosmetic use, thyroid dysfunction, and antiepileptic medications.[3,4]
- Women with melasma not related to pregnancy or oral contraceptive use may have hormonal alterations that are consistent with mild ovarian dysfunction.
- Melasma in men (**Figure 195-4**) shares the same clinical features as in women, but it is not known if hormonal factors play a role.[5]

Other factors associated with melasma include certain cosmetic ingredients (oxidized linoleic acid, salicylate, citral, preservatives) and certain antiepileptic drug. Some medications or topical preparations in combination with sun exposure worsen melasma.[1]

RISK FACTORS

A recent global survey of 324 women with melasma demonstrated that a combination of the known triggers, including pregnancy, hormonal birth control, family history, and sun exposure, affects onset of melasma.[6]

DIAGNOSIS

CLINICAL FEATURES

The diagnosis of melasma is based on clinical appearance. Affected patients exhibit splotchy areas of hyperpigmented macules on the face (see **Figures 195-1** to **195-4**). In natural light, epidermal melasma appears light to dark brown, and the dermal pattern is blue or gray.

Melasma is divided into 4 clinical types:

1. Epidermal type—The hyperpigmentation is usually light brown, and Wood light enhances the color contrast between hyperpigmented areas and normal skin. It is the most common type, and it best responds to the use of depigmenting agents.
2. Dermal type—The hyperpigmentation is ashen or bluish-gray and exhibits no accentuation of color contrast under Wood light. Depigmenting agents are generally not effective for this type.
3. Mixed type—The hyperpigmentation is usually dark brown, and Wood light enhances the color contrast in some areas but not in others.
4. Indeterminate type—Presents in patients with darker complexions (skin types V-VI) and cannot be categorized under Wood light.[1]

TYPICAL DISTRIBUTION

The lesion is found typically on sun-exposed areas. The 3 typical patterns of involvement are as follows:

1. Centrofacial involving the cheeks, forehead, upper lip, nose, and chin
2. Malar involving the cheeks and nose
3. Mandibular involving the ramus of the mandible

IMAGING

A Wood light may be used to determine the type of melasma.[1] This does not change the choices of standard topical therapies.

BIOPSY

Histologically, there are an increased number of melanocytes, with the deposition of additional melanin and a background of solar elastosis. The 2 main histologic patterns are epidermal and dermal, depending on the skin layers involved.

DIFFERENTIAL DIAGNOSIS

- The facial rash of systemic lupus may be confused with melasma as they both can have a butterfly pattern. Melasma is hyperpigmented, whereas the lupus facial rash is usually inflammatory. An antinuclear antibody (ANA) test should be positive in systemic lupus erythematosus (SLE) and negative in melasma. False-positive antinuclear antibodies are usually low titer and the patient does not have other criteria for lupus (see Chapter 178, Lupus Erythematosus).
- Discoid lupus or cutaneous lupus can occur across the face but is usually seen with scarring. In this condition, the ANA is often negative (see Chapter 178, Lupus: Systemic and Cutaneous).
- Contact dermatitis will be inflamed in the acute stage but the postinflammatory hyperpigmentation could be confused with melasma (see Chapter 144, Contact Dermatitis).

MANAGEMENT

The treatment of melasma is challenging because its treatment is generally unsatisfactory.[7] Numerous less-than-adequate treatment options exist, including topical agents and chemical peels. Melasma treatment is started only when the patient is disturbed by the hyperpigmentation. All patients can benefit from sun protection and this is always a good place to start.

It is important to give the patient realistic treatment goals. The treatments that follow may lighten the hyperpigmentation but do not generally remove all the hyperpigmentation.

Side effects of all topical treatments include contact dermatitis, depigmentation of surrounding normal skin, and postinflammatory hyperpigmentation. Tretinoin should not be used during pregnancy. Discontinue oral contraceptives or other estrogen/progesterone agents, if possible.

MEDICATIONS

- Hydroquinone is the main bleaching agent used to treat melasma.[7] SOR A It is available over the counter in 2% or 3% formulations (some including sunscreens). The prescription strength is 4% and is available with or without a sunscreen. Generic 4% hydroquinone comes in many sizes and formulations, so write the prescription to be flexible to avoid hassles for you and the patient. Although hydroquinone with sunscreen may be somewhat better than hydroquinone alone, a combination product has not been shown to be better than using these 2 topical agents together as 2 separate products. SOR C
- Hydroquinone is applied twice daily for up to 3 months with subsequent tapering to once daily. If the patient has not noticed a benefit by 3 months, the treatment should be stopped. SOR C
- Ochronosis—If the skin becomes darker with treatment, then the hydroquinone should be discontinued as there is a known side effect of hydroquinone, called ochronosis, that causes hyperpigmentation. Ochronosis only occurs in the treated area, but the hyperpigmentation can be permanent.[8]
- Hydroquinone can also cause a contact dermatitis, so it is a good idea for the patient to try it on a small area of skin before applying it to large areas of the face. Hydroquinone should be avoided on inflamed skin to avoid additional postinflammatory hyperpigmentation.
- Tretinoin 0.1% (Retin-A) cream is applied once daily at bedtime to lighten melasma. In 2 studies where tretinoin was compared to placebo, participants rated their melasma as significantly improved in one but not the other. In both studies, by other objective measures, tretinoin treatment significantly reduced the severity of melasma.[7] SOR A
- Combining tretinoin and hydroquinone is believed to potentiate their effects. SOR C
- There is a triple combination cream (Tri-Luma) containing 4% hydroquinone, retinoic acid, and fluocinolone (corticosteroid). It is used once daily before bed for a duration of 8 weeks. Studies show that it has a superior efficacy than hydroquinone monotherapy for melasma.[9,10] SOR A However, the side effect of skin irritation is very common and it is not recommended for long-term use.[9,10] Triple-combination cream was significantly more effective at lightening melasma than hydroquinone alone (relative risk [RR] 1.58) or when compared to the dual combinations of tretinoin and hydroquinone (RR 2.75).[7] SOR A
- Note that Tri-Luma is very expensive. Individual prescriptions for 4% hydroquinone, tretinoin cream, and a mild topical steroid cream can be given to keep the cost down. Desonide or 1% hydrocortisone are good options for the topical steroid. The steroid should not be used daily for longer than 8 weeks to avoid adverse effects.
- Azelaic acid (20%) was significantly more effective than 2% hydroquinone at lightening melasma but not better than 4% hydroquinone.[7] SOR A
- Kojic acid formulations and α-hydroxy acids (such as glycolic acid) also have been used in the treatment of melasma. SOR C
- The adverse events most commonly reported with topical agents were mild and transient such as skin irritation, itching, burning, and stinging.[7] SOR A

SURGICAL PROCEDURES

- Chemical peels are one option for patients with moderate-to-severe melasma that has not responded to bleaching agents and are seeking further treatment. SOR C
- Dermabrasion treatment is one aggressive option.[11] SOR C
- Q-switched pigmentary lasers, intense pulsed light, and fractional laser treatments have some efficacy but can cause postinflammatory hyperpigmentation and relapses may occur so are usually not recommended.[12] SOR C

PREVENTION

Strict avoidance of sun exposure is important to prevent further hyperpigmentation. SOR C Broad-spectrum, high-protection-factor sunscreens (with UVB and UVA protection), such as titanium dioxide, micronized zinc oxide, Mexoryl, or avobenzone/Parsol, are essential.[13]

FOLLOW-UP

Follow-up is advisable when using bleaching agents. Long-term follow-up and reinforcement of limiting sun exposure can be accomplished during routine prevention visits.

PATIENT EDUCATION

- Provide the patient with realistic treatment goals.
- If the topical medications are irritating the skin, stop them and return for further evaluation.
- If after 3 months hydroquinone has not worked, stop it.
- If the skin is darkening rather than lightening, stop the medications and return for further evaluation.
- Bleaching agents are often not covered by insurance. The price of hydroquinone formulations can vary widely, so it helps to shop around when cost is a major concern.

PATIENT RESOURCES

- WebMD. *Skin Problems of Pregnancy*—**http: //www.webmd .com/baby/skin-conditions-pregnancy.**
- American Pregnancy Association. *Skin Changes During Pregnancy*— **http: //www.americanpregnancy.org/pregnancyhealth/ skinchanges.html.**
- WebMD. *Cosmetic Procedures, Birthmarks, and Other Abnormal Skin Pigmentation*—**http: //www.webmd.com/healthy-beauty/ cosmetic-procedures-birthmarks.**
- WebMD. *Hyperpigmentation, Hypopigmentation, and Your Skin*— **http: //www.webmd.com/skin-problems-and-treatments/ guide/hyperpigmentation-hypopigmentation.**

PROVIDER RESOURCES

- American Academy of Family Physicians. *Common Hyperpigmentation Disorders in Adults: Part II*—**http://www.aafp.org/ afp/20031115/1963.html.**
- Kang HY, Ortonne JP. What should be considered in treatment of melasma. *Ann Dermatol.* 2010;22(4):373-378—**http://pdf .medrang.co.kr/Aod/022/Aod022-04-01.pdf.**

REFERENCES

1. Rigopoulos D, Gregoriou S, Katsambas A. Hyperpigmentation and melasma. *J Cosmet Dermatol.* 2007;6:195-202.
2. Elling SV, Powell FC. Physiological changes in the skin during pregnancy. *Clin Dermatol.* 1997;15:35-43.
3. Grimes PE. Melasma. Etiologic and therapeutic considerations. *Arch Dermatol.* 1995;131:1453-1457.
4. Hassan I, Kaur I, Sialy R, Dash RJ. Hormonal milieu in the maintenance of melasma in fertile women. *J Dermatol.* 1998;25:510-512.
5. Vazquez M, Maldonado H, Benmaman C, Sanchez JL. Melasma in men. A clinical and histologic study. *Int J Dermatol.* 1988;27:25-27.
6. Ortonne JP, Arellano I, Berneburg M, et al. A global survey of the role of ultraviolet radiation and hormonal influences in the development of melasma. *J Eur Acad Dermatol Venereol.* 2009;23:1254-1262.
7. Rajaratnam R, Halpern J, Salim A, Emmett C. Interventions for melasma. *Cochrane Database Syst Rev.* 2010 Jul 7;(7):CD003583.
8. Ribas J, Schettini AP, Cavalcante Mde S. Exogenous ochronosis hydroquinone induced: a report of four cases. *An Bras Dermatol.* 2010;85(5):699-703.
9. Kang HY, Valerio L, Bahadoran P, Ortonne JP. The role of topical retinoids in the treatment of pigmentary disorders: an evidence-based review. *Am J Clin Dermatol.* 2009;10:251-260.
10. Taylor SC, Torok H, Jones T, et al. Efficacy and safety of a new triple-combination agent for the treatment of facial melasma. *Cutis.* 2003;72(1):67-72.
11. Kunachak S, Leelaudomlipi P, Wongwaisayawan S. Dermabrasion: a curative treatment for melasma. *Aesthetic Plast Surg.* 2001;25: 114-117.
12. Kang HY, Ortonne J. What should be considered in treatment of melasma. *Ann Dermatol.* 2010;22:373-378.
13. Vazquez M, Sanchez JL. The efficacy of a broad-spectrum sunscreen in the treatment of chloasma. *Cutis.* 1983;32:92.

196 VITILIGO AND HYPOPIGMENTATION

Richard P. Usatine, MD
Karen A. Hughes, MD
Mindy A. Smith, MD, MS

PATIENT STORY

A Hispanic man presents to his internist with white hands for the past 2 years (**Figure 196-1**). He wants to know if anything can be done to bring his brown color back. The internist diagnoses vitiligo by clinical appearance and states that he is not familiar with the most recent available treatments. He refers the patient to a dermatologist.

INTRODUCTION

Vitiligo is an acquired, progressive loss of pigmentation of the epidermis. The Vitiligo European Task Force defines nonsegmental vitiligo as "an acquired chronic pigmentation disorder characterized by white patches, often symmetrical, which usually increase in size with time, corresponding to a substantial loss of functioning epidermal and sometimes hair follicle melanocytes."[1] Segmental vitiligo is defined similarly except for a unilateral distribution that may totally or partially match a dermatome (**Figure 196-2**); occasionally more than one segment is involved.[1]

SYNONYMS

It is also known as vitiligo vulgaris.

EPIDEMIOLOGY

- Vitiligo occurs in approximately 0.5% to 2% of the worldwide population.[2,3]

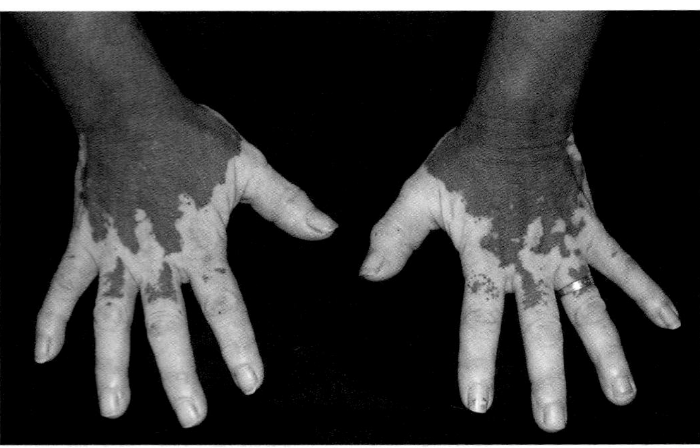

FIGURE 196-1 Vitiligo on the hands of a Hispanic man. (*Reproduced with permission from Richard P. Usatine, MD.*)

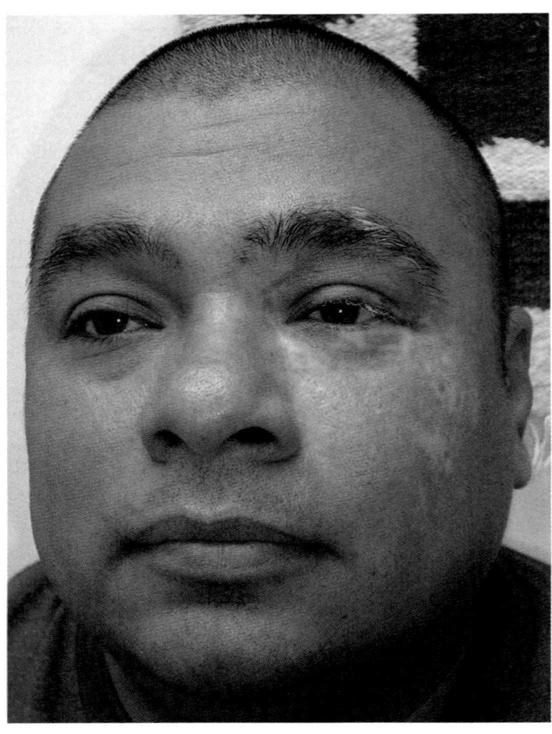

FIGURE 196-2 Segmental vitiligo that began to appear after a bad facial sunburn. Note that it is unilateral and there is some loss of pigment of the eyebrow (peliosis). (*Reproduced with permission from Richard P. Usatine, MD.*)

- It can occur at any age but typically develops between the ages of 10 and 30 years.[2]
- Vitiligo has equal rates in men and women.[2]
- It occurs in all races but is more prominent in those with darker skin.

ETIOLOGY AND PATHOPHYSIOLOGY

- It is an autoimmune disease with destruction of melanocytes.
- Genetic component is found in approximately 30% of cases. Toll-like receptor genes were found to be associated with vitiligo in a population of Turkish patients.[4]
- It can trigger or worsen with illness, emotional stress, and/or skin trauma (Koebner phenomenon).

DIAGNOSIS

CLINICAL FEATURES

- Macular regions of depigmentation with scalloped, well-defined borders (see **Figures 196-1** and **196-2**).
- Depigmented areas often coalesce over time to form larger areas (**Figures 196-3** and **196-4**).
- Depigmented areas are more susceptible to sunburn (**Figure 196-5**). Tanning of the normal surrounding skin makes the depigmented areas more obvious.
- There is no standardized method for assessing vitiligo; strategies include subjective clinical assessment, semiobjective assessment

FIGURE 196-3 Vitiligo covering more than 50% of this Hispanic woman's body. The patient is starting topical monobenzone to attempt to bleach the unaffected skin so that she has one matching skin color. *(Reproduced with permission from Richard P. Usatine, MD.)*

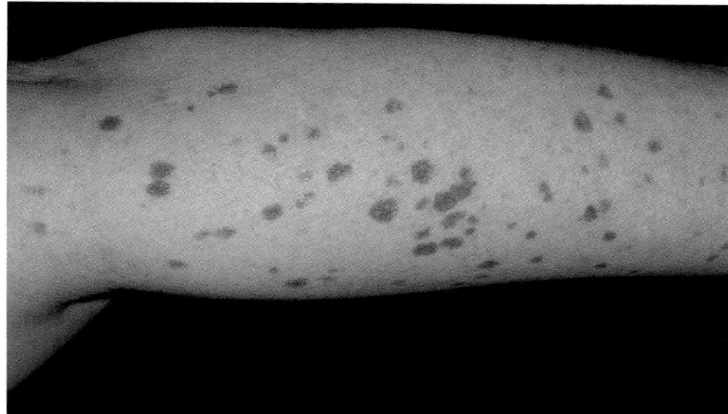

FIGURE 196-4 This previously dark-skinned woman has only a few spots of pigment remaining on her arm because of the extensive vitiligo. Her father has the same condition. *(Reproduced with permission from Richard P. Usatine, MD.)*

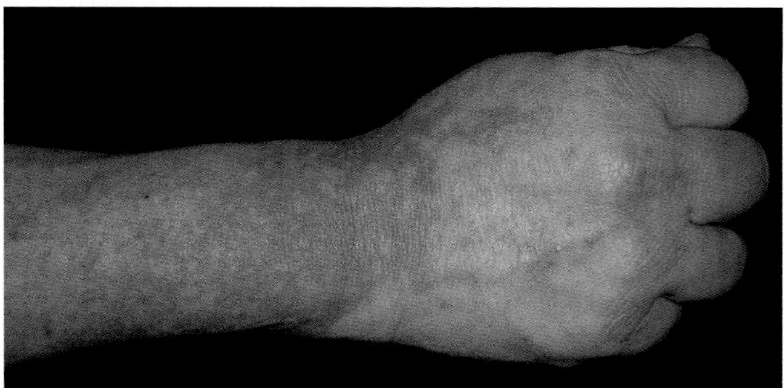

FIGURE 196-5 First-degree sunburn occurred on the hands of this Hispanic man with vitiligo. *(Reproduced with permission from Richard P. Usatine, MD.)*

(eg, Vitiligo Area Scoring Index [VASI] and point-counting methods), macroscopic morphologic assessment (eg, visual, photographic in natural or ultraviolet [UV] light, computerized image analysis), micromorphologic assessment (eg, confocal laser microscopy), and objective assessment (eg, software-based image analysis, tristimulus colorimetry, spectrophotometry).[5] Authors of a literature review concluded that the VASI, the rule of 9, and Wood lamp (UV light) were the best techniques for assessing the degree of pigmentary lesions and measuring the extent and progression of vitiligo.[5]

- Conditions associated with vitiligo include thyroid disease and the presence of thyroid antibodies,[6,7] congenital nevi (in one study, 6.2% vs 2.8% in those without vitiligo),[4] and halo nevi,[1] and possibly primary open-angle glaucoma (57% of patients in one case series).[8]

TYPICAL DISTRIBUTION

- Widespread, but generally seen first on the face, hands, arms, and genitalia (**Figures 196-6** and **196-7**).

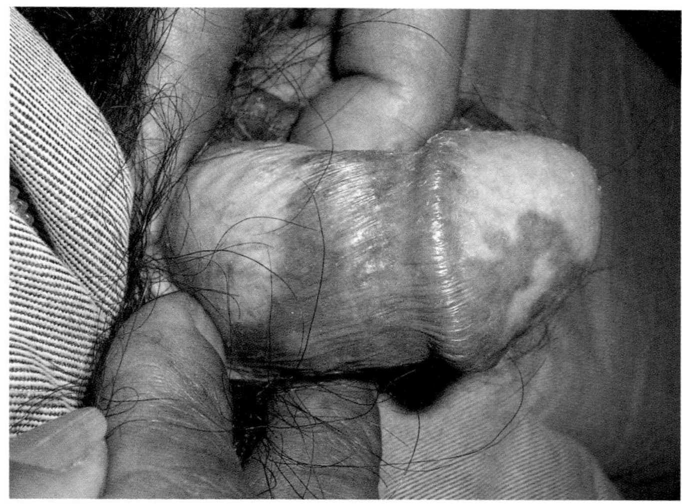

A

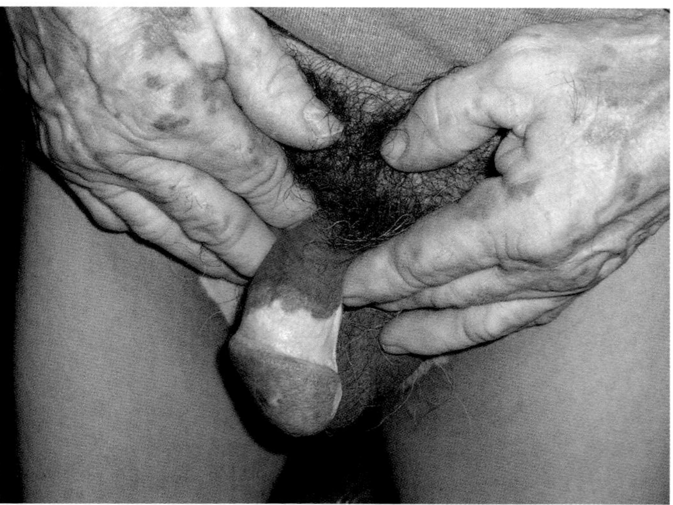

B

FIGURE 196-6 **A.** Vitiligo on the penis of a 72-year-old man. **B.** Vitiligo on the hands and penis of a younger man. *(Reproduced with permission from Richard P. Usatine, MD.)*

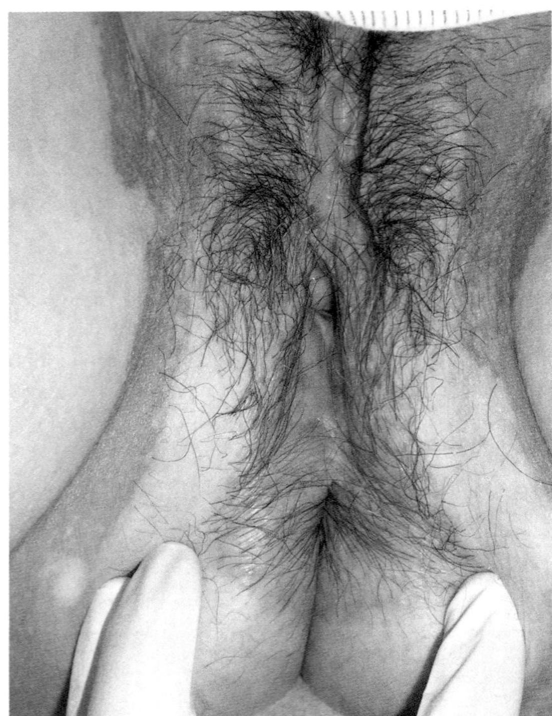

FIGURE 196-7 Vitiligo around the vulva and perianal area. The vitiligo is also present on the upper thighs of this middle-aged woman. Note the erythema was proven to be lichen simplex chronicus by biopsy. The vitiligo preceded the erythema and only the lichen simplex chronicus was symptomatic. (*Reproduced with permission from Richard P. Usatine, MD.*)

- Depigmentation around body openings such as eyes, mouth, umbilicus, and anus is common (**Figures 196-7 and 196-8**). When the eyelashes are involved it is called *leukotrichia*.
- Vitiligo can be unilateral or bilateral; in one study, patients with unilateral vitiligo were younger and had an earlier age at onset while those with bilateral vitiligo were more likely to have light skin types and more commonly had associated autoimmune disease.[9]

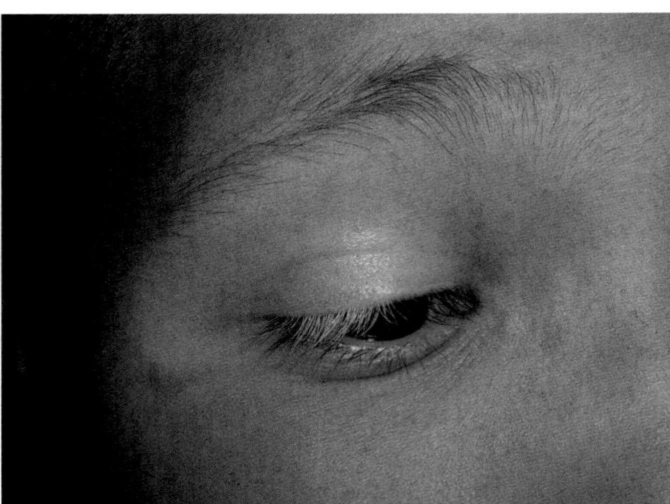

FIGURE 196-8 Vitiligo around the eye with leukotrichia (white eyelashes). Vitiligo commonly occurs around the eyes. (*Reproduced with permission from Richard P. Usatine, MD.*)

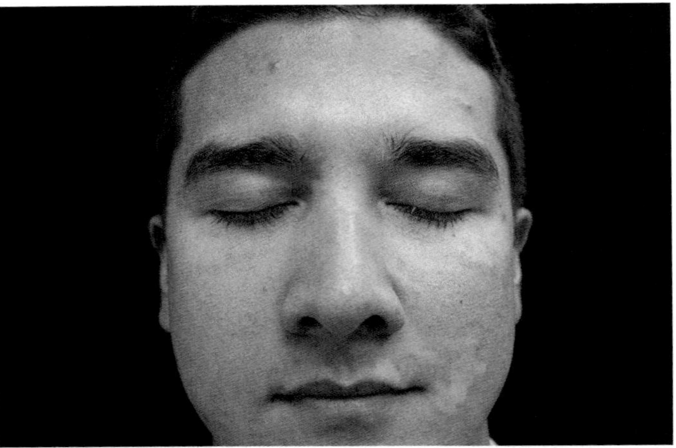

A

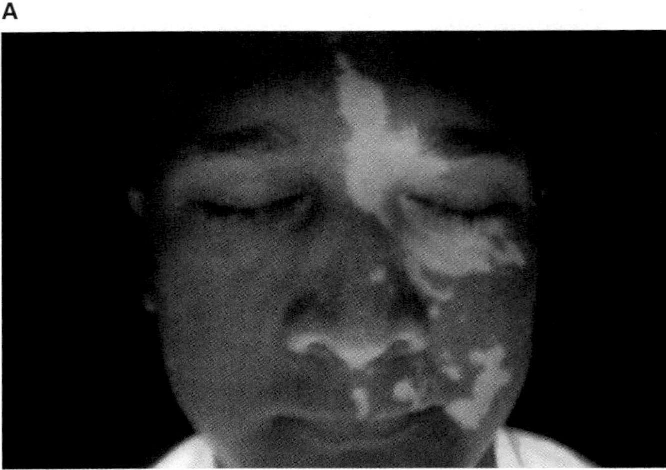

B

FIGURE 196-9 A. Segmental vitiligo on the face of a young man. B. The ultraviolet light (Wood lamp) accentuates the vitiligo as the depigmented area glows white. (*Reproduced with permission from Patrick E. McCleskey, MD.*)

LABORATORY AND IMAGING

- Evaluation for endocrine disorders such as hyper- or hypothyroidism (eg, thyroid-stimulating hormone [TSH]) and diabetes mellitus (eg, fasting blood sugar) should be considered, as vitiligo can be associated with these disorders.[10]
- Pernicious anemia and lupus erythematosus may be considered; obtain complete blood count (CBC) with indices and an antinuclear antibody (ANA).
- Wood lamp (UV light) is one method of assessing vitiligo when the depigmentation is not readily visible. The UV light will accentuate the color differences (**Figure 196-9**).

BIOPSY

Not indicated unless the diagnosis is not clear and then a 4-mm punch biopsy will suffice.

DIFFERENTIAL DIAGNOSIS

- Postinflammatory hypopigmentation can occur with any inflammatory disorder of the skin. While it can occur with psoriasis and bullous diseases, so can vitiligo. If the areas of hypopigmentation follow

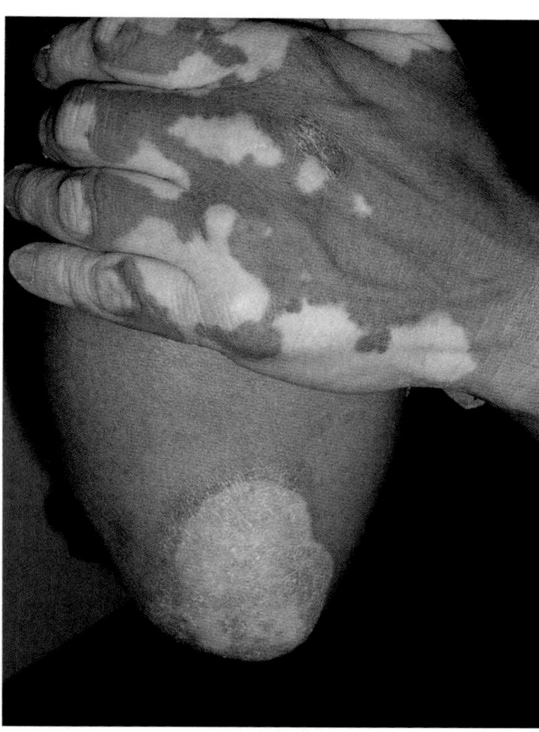

FIGURE 196-10 Vitiligo on the hand and elbow that preceded the psoriasis now seen on the elbow. This is not postinflammatory hypopigmentation. *(Reproduced with permission from Richard P. Usatine, MD.)*

the distribution of the inflammatory disorder then postinflammatory hypopigmentation is more likely. If the hypopigmentation precedes the inflammation or follows a different pattern then vitiligo may be coexisting with another immune-mediated disease (**Figures 196-10** and **196-11**).

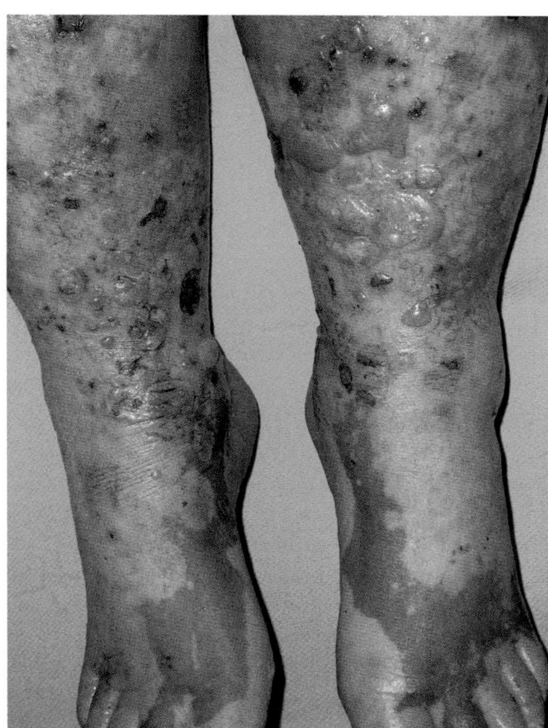

FIGURE 196-11 Vitiligo on the legs that preceded the bullous pemphigoid. The patient also had psoriasis. It is not unusual to see more than one immune-mediated cutaneous condition occurring in the same patient. *(Reproduced with permission from Richard P. Usatine, MD.)*

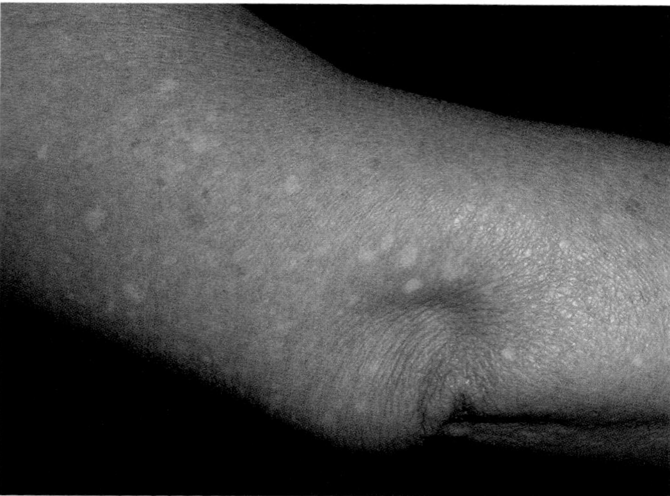

FIGURE 196-12 Idiopathic guttate hypomelanosis on the arm. This is usually seen in sun-exposed areas especially on the arms and legs. *(Reproduced with permission from Richard P. Usatine, MD.)*

- Halo nevus—Hypopigmentation confined to areas surrounding pigmented nevi that typically appear in adolescents and young adults (see Chapter 162, Epidermal Nevus and Nevus Sebaceous).
- Idiopathic guttate hypomelanosis—Confetti-like 2- to 5-mm areas of depigmentation predominantly on sun-exposed areas (**Figure 196-12**).
- Nevus depigmentosus is usually present at birth or starts in early childhood. There is a decreased number of melanosomes within a normal number of melanocytes. It typically has a serrated or jagged edge. Its presence at birth or early in childhood helps to differentiate it from vitiligo (**Figure 196-13**).
- Nevus anemicus—A congenital hypopigmented macule or patch that is stable in relative size and distribution. It occurs as a result of localized hypersensitivity to catecholamines and not a decrease in melanocytes. On diascopy (pressure with a glass slide) the skin is indistinguishable from the surrounding skin. Its presence from birth helps to distinguish it from vitiligo (**Figure 196-14**).

FIGURE 196-13 Nevus depigmentosus, present since birth, on the leg. Note the serrated or jagged edge. Vitiligo is not present at birth. *(Reproduced with permission from Richard P. Usatine, MD.)*

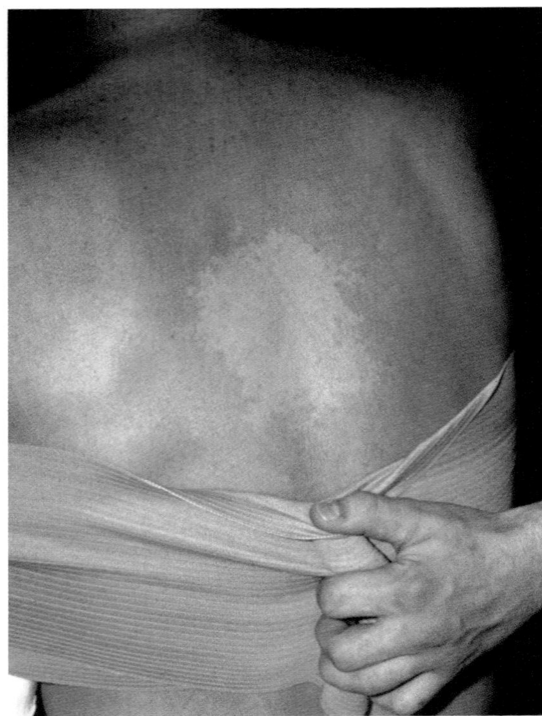

FIGURE 196-14 Nevus anemicus on the back of this woman, which has been there since birth. This is a congenital hypersensitivity to localized catecholamines. On diascopy the skin was indistinguishable from the surrounding skin. The irregular broken-up outline is seen in nevus anemicus and nevus depigmentosus. (*Reproduced with permission from University of Texas Health Science Center Division of Dermatology.*)

MANAGEMENT

For assessing outcomes to treatment, the Vitiligo European Task Force suggests a system combining analysis of extent using percentage of body area involved (rule of 9), stage of disease based on cutaneous and hair pigmentation in **vitiligo** patches and staged 0 to 4 (with 0 representing normal pigment and 4 complete hair whitening) on the largest macule in each body region except hands and feet, and disease progression (spreading) assessed with Wood lamp examination of the same largest macule in each body area.[1] An evaluation sheet can be found in the citation.[1]

NONPHARMACOLOGIC

- Addressing the psychological distress that this disfiguring skin disorder causes should be a primary focus as the clinical course is unpredictable and, in some cases, little can be done to modify the condition itself.
- Management of inciting factors such as illness, stress, and skin trauma may be useful. SOR C

MEDICATIONS

Topical treatments used for vitiligo include corticosteroids, immunomodulators, vitamin D analogs, and psoralens; these treatments had mixed outcomes based on a systematic review, with topical steroids having the highest rate of adverse events.[11] SOR B Ineffective topical agents include melagenina, topical phenylalanine, topical L-dopa (levodopa), coal tar, anacarcin forte oil, and minoxidil.[12]

- In a retrospective study of 101 children with vitiligo treated with moderate- to high-potency topical corticosteroids 64% (45/70) had repigmentation of the lesions, 24% (17/70) showed no change, and 11% (8/70) were worse than at the initial presentation.[13] SOR B Local steroid side effects were noted in 26% of patients at 81.7 ± 44 days of follow-up. Two children were given the diagnosis of steroid-induced adrenal suppression. Children with head and/or neck affected areas were 8 times more likely to have an abnormal cortisol level compared with children who were affected in other body areas.[13] Therefore, a trial of topical steroids may be useful for patients with localized vitiligo that does not predominantly involve the head and neck. SOR C
- Based on several reviews, topical corticosteroids (potent or very potent) are the preferred drugs for localized vitiligo (<20% of skin area)[11,12]; a less-than-2-month trial is recommended.[12] SOR B
- Topical immunomodulators (tacrolimus, pimecrolimus) are an alternative for localized vitiligo and display comparable effectiveness with fewer side effects.[14] SOR B
- In a small case series ($N = 6$), various antitumor necrosis factor α-agents (infliximab, etanercept, and adalimumab given according to treatment regimens used for psoriasis) were not effective for widespread nonsegmental vitiligo.[15]

COMPLEMENTARY AND ALTERNATIVE THERAPY

Antioxidants may be useful adjunctive therapy.[11]

OTHER TREATMENT

- Use sunscreen to prevent burns to the depigmented areas and further trauma to unaffected skin, and to minimize contrast between these areas.[14] SOR A
- Bleaching the unaffected skin in patients with widespread depigmentation to reduce contrast with depigmented areas can improve cosmetic appearance.[14] SOR B A monobenzyl ether of hydroquinone 20% cream (Benoquin) is available by prescription to produce a permanent bleaching of the skin around the vitiligo. It is irreversible and makes the skin at higher risk for sunburn.

PROCEDURES

- Combination therapies are likely to be more effective than monotherapy, and most combinations include a form of phototherapy; narrow-band UVB appears to be the most effective with the fewest adverse effects **(Figure 196-15)**.[11,14] SOR B Psoralen UVA (PUVA) is the second-best choice. Authors of a Cochrane review concurred that majority of analyses showing statistically significant differences in treatment outcomes were from studies that assessed combination interventions including some form of light treatment.[16]
- Excimer laser is an alternative to UVB therapy, achieving good responses especially in localized vitiligo of the face, where the excimer laser may be superior to UVB therapy. By combining with topical immunomodulators, treatment response can be accelerated.[14] SOR B In one prospective study of 14 patients, repigmentation rates for once-, twice-, and thrice-weekly treatment approached each other (60%, 79%, and 82%, respectively) at 12 weeks.[17] Although repigmentation occurred fastest with thrice-weekly treatment, the final repigmentation depends on the total number of treatments, not their frequency. SOR B
- No single therapy for vitiligo can be regarded as the most effective as the success of each treatment modality depends on the type and location of vitiligo. SOR B

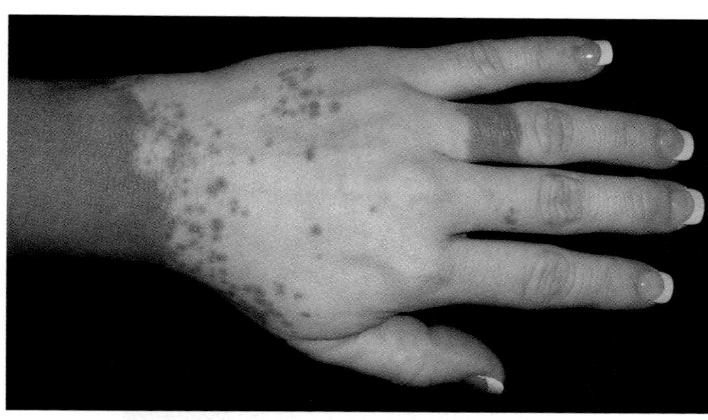

FIGURE 196-15 Vitiligo, which spared the area under a ring; the patient has only spotty return of pigment on hand with narrowband UVB treatment for 1 year. *(Reproduced with permission from Richard P. Usatine, MD.)*

PROGNOSIS

The course of vitiligo varies, but is usually progressive with periods of activity interspersed with times of inactivity.[18] Spontaneous repigmentation can occur but is rare.

- The face and neck respond best to all therapeutic approaches, while the acral areas are least responsive.[14] SOR B
- Vitiligo does not appear to be associated with adverse outcomes in pregnancy.[19]

FOLLOW-UP

- Counseling and emotional support are a mainstay of follow-up treatment.
- Trials of various combination therapies may be needed.

PATIENT EDUCATION

- Reassure patients that this is a benign condition while acknowledging any psychological distress.
- Advise patients about the highly variable course of vitiligo with usually progressive periods of activity interspersed with times of inactivity.
- Inform patients about the multiple treatment options and possible need for prolonged or repeat treatment.

PATIENT RESOURCES

- eNational Institutes of Health. *Vitiligo*—**http://health.nih.gov/topic/Vitiligo.**
- National Organization for Albinism and Hypopigmentation—**http://www.healthfinder.gov/orgs/HR2242.htm.**
- National Vitiligo Foundation—**http://nvfi.org/index.php.**
- MedLine Plus. *Vitiligo*—**http://www.nlm.nih.gov/medlineplus/ency/article/003224.htm.**

PROVIDER RESOURCES

- Medscape. *Vitiligo*—**http: //emedicine.medscape.com/article/1068962.**
- National Vitiligo Foundation. *A Handbook for Physicians*—**http://nvfi.org/pages/info_physician_handbook.php.**

REFERENCES

1. Taïeb A, Picardo M; VETF Members. The definition and assessment of vitiligo: a consensus report of the Vitiligo European Task Force. *Pigment Cell Res.* 2007;20(1):27-35.
2. Njoo MD, Westerhof W. Vitiligo: pathogenesis and treatment. *Am J Clin Dermatol.* 2001;2(3):167-181.
3. Krüger C, Schallreuter KU. A review of the worldwide prevalence of vitiligo in children/adolescents and adults. *Int J Dermatol.* 2012 Oct;51(10):1206-1212.
4. Karaca N, Ozturk G, Gerceker BT, et al. TLR2 and TLR4 gene polymorphisms in Turkish vitiligo patients. *J Eur Acad Dermatol Venereol.* 2013 Jan;27(1):e85-e90.
5. Alghamdi KM, Kumar A, Taïeb A, Ezzedine K. Assessment methods for the evaluation of vitiligo. *J Eur Acad Dermatol Venereol.* 2012 Dec;26(12):1463-1471.
6. Schallreuter KU, Lemke R, Brandt O, et al. Vitiligo and other diseases: coexistence or true association? Hamburg study on 321 patients. *Dermatology.* 1994;188(4):269-275.
7. Hegedüs L, Heidenheim M, Gervil M, et al. High frequency of thyroid dysfunction in patients with vitiligo. *Acta Derm Venereol.* 1994;74(2):120-123.
8. Rogosić V, Bojić L, Puizina-Ivić N, et al. Vitiligo and glaucoma—an association or a coincidence? A pilot study. *Acta Dermatovenerol Croat.* 2010;18(1):21-26.
9. Barona MI, Arrunátegui A, Falabella R, Alzate A. An epidemiologic case-control study in a population with vitiligo. *J Am Acad Dermatol.* 1995;33(4):621-625.
10. Hacker SM. Common disorders of pigmentation: when are more than cosmetic cover-ups required? *Postgrad Med.* 1996;99(6):177-186.
11. Bacigalupi RM, Postolova A, Davis RS. Evidence-based, non-surgical treatments for vitiligo: a review. *Am J Clin Dermatol.* 2012;13(4):217-237.
12. Hossani-Madani AR, Halder RM. Topical treatment and combination approaches for vitiligo: new insights, new developments. *G Ital Dermatol Venereol.* 2010;145(1):57-78.
13. Kwinter J, Pelletier J, Khambalia A, Pope E. High-potency steroid use in children with vitiligo: a retrospective study. *J Am Acad Dermatol.* 2007;56(2):236-241.
14. Forschner T, Buchholtz S, Stockfleth E. Current state of vitiligo therapy—evidence-based analysis of the literature. *J Dtsch Dermatol Ges.* 2007;5(6):467-475.
15. Alghamdi KM, Khurrum H, Taieb A, Ezzedine K. Treatment of generalized vitiligo with anti-TNF-α agents. *J Drugs Dermatol.* 2012;11(4):534-539.
16. Whitton ME, Pinart M, Batchelor J, et al. Interventions for vitiligo. *Cochrane Database Syst Rev.* 2010;(1):CD003263.
17. Hofer A, Hassan AS, Legat FJ, et al. Optimal weekly frequency of 308-nm excimer laser treatment in vitiligo patients. *Br J Dermatol.* 2005;152(5):981-985.
18. Viles J, Monte D, Gawkrodger DJ. Vitiligo. *BMJ.* 2010;341:c3780.
19. Horev A, Weintraub AY, Sergienko R, et al. Pregnancy outcome in women with vitiligo. *Int J Dermatol.* 2011;50(9):1083-1085.

197 PHOTOSENSITIVITY

E.J. Mayeaux Jr, MD

PATIENT STORY

A 50-year-old woman presented to the clinic with an abrupt onset of an intensely pruritic rash that extended over the dorsal aspect of both arms (**Figure 197-1**). The patient notes no new medicines and no recent exposures to any new chemicals. She acknowledged recent time spent outside in the sun. The plaques were photodistributed, with sparing of her watch area. A clinical diagnosis of polymorphous light eruption (PMLE) was made, and the patient was started on oral antihistamines and topical steroids. It was recommended that she minimize her sun exposure.

INTRODUCTION

Photosensitivity is an abnormal skin response to ultraviolet (UV) light that occurs on sun-exposed areas of the skin. There are 3 common types of photodermatitis:

- PMLE (**Figures 197-1** and **197-2**).
- Phototoxic eruptions (**Figures 197-3** to **197-7**).
- Photoallergic eruptions (**Figure 197-8**). **Table 197-1** compares key characteristics of phototoxic and photoallergic reactions.

UV light radiating from the sun may be categorized into UVA (wavelength 320-400 nm), UVB (290-320 nm), and UVC (200-290 nm). UVC is completely absorbed by the earth's ozone layer and thus does not play a role in photosensitivity. Photosensitivity may be induced by UVA, UVB, or visible light (400-760 nm). Longer wavelength light penetrates deeper into the skin. UVA penetrates through to the dermis, but UVB mainly penetrates and affects the epidermis.

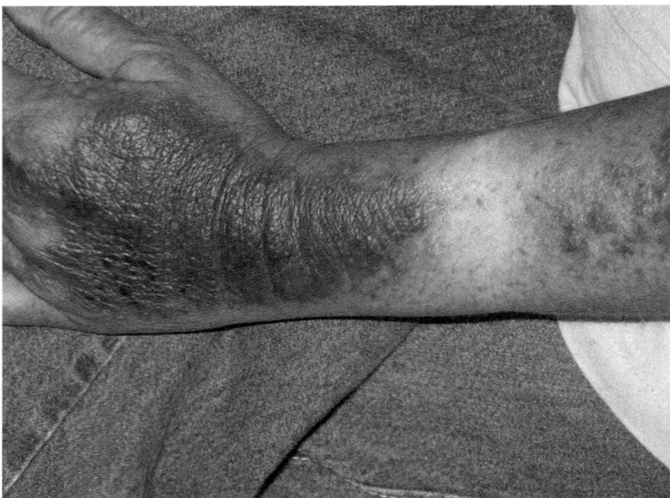

FIGURE 197-1 Polymorphous light eruption noted over dorsum of left forearm. Note absence of the lesion where the patient had been wearing her watch. (*Reproduced with permission from Wenner C, Lee A. A bright red pruritic rash on the forearms.* J Fam Pract. *2007;56(8):627-629. Reproduced with permission from Frontline Medical Communications.*)

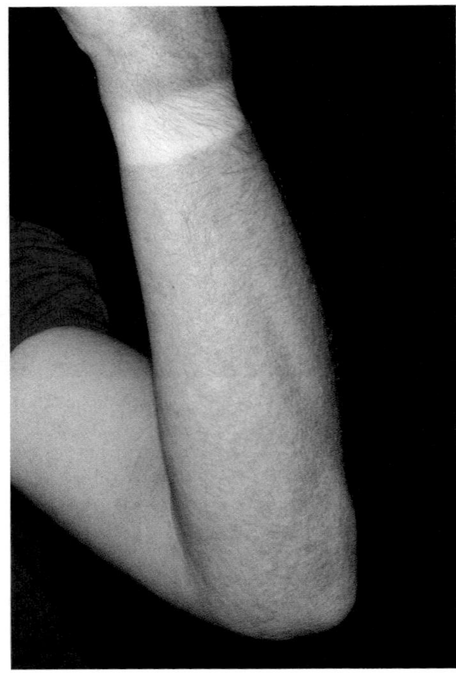

FIGURE 197-2 Polymorphous light eruption on the arm of a young man. Note the sparing of the skin under his watchband. (*Reproduced with permission from Richard P. Usatine, MD.*)

Ultraviolet light has multiple effects on the skin. Notably, it causes DNA damage and has immunosuppressive effects on skin inflammatory cells increasing the risk of carcinogenesis. In patients with photosensitivity, it elicits an inflammatory response in the skin, leading to the development of a photodermatosis.

EPIDEMIOLOGY

- PMLE (see **Figures 197-1** and **197-2**) may affect up to 10% of the population, with a predilection for females.[1] The prevalence increases in northern latitudes. Onset typically occurs within the first 3 decades of life, but may appear spontaneously at any age.

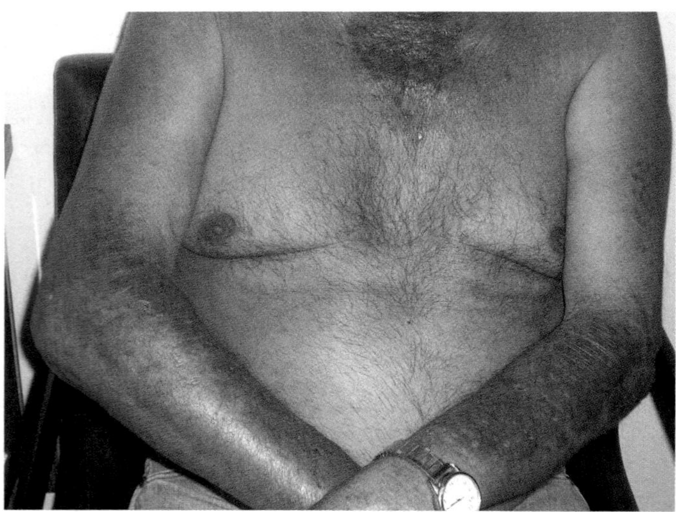

FIGURE 197-3 Severe phototoxic drug reaction secondary to hydrochlorothiazide use. (*Reproduced with permission from Richard P. Usatine, MD.*)

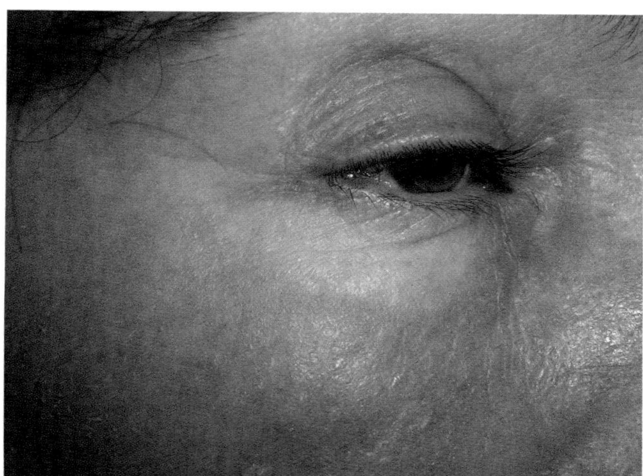

FIGURE 197-4 Phototoxic drug reaction secondary to ibuprofen. (*Reproduced with permission from Richard P. Usatine, MD.*)

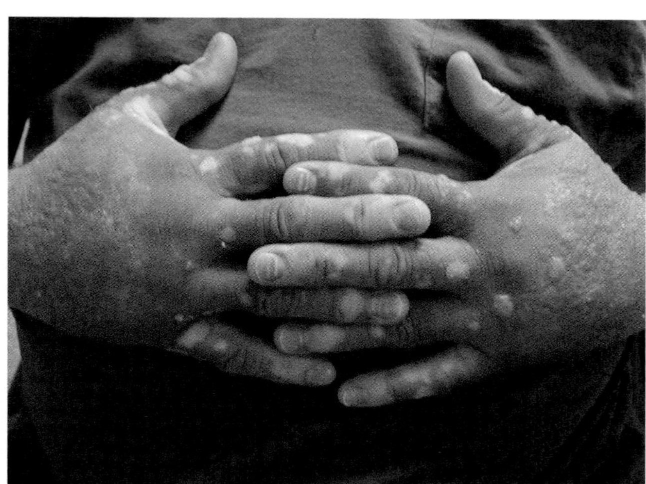

FIGURE 197-5 Phototoxic drug reaction secondary to treatment of vitiligo with oral psoralen and ultraviolet light (phytophotodermatitis). Note the bullae. (*Reproduced with permission from Richard P. Usatine, MD.*)

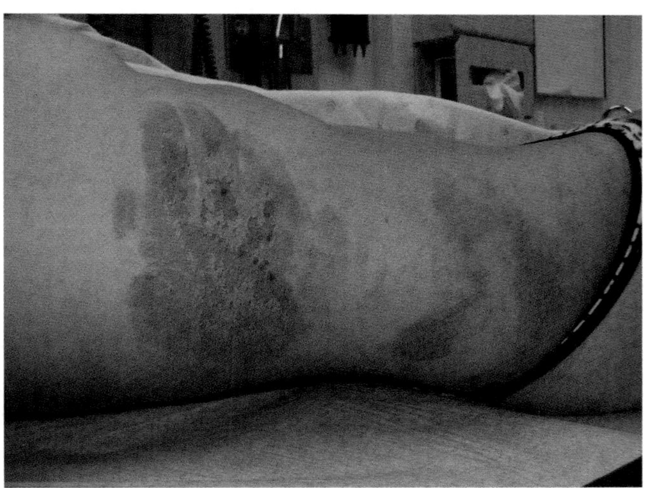

FIGURE 197-6 Phytophotodermatitis in a woman, caused by lime juice and sun exposure on the beach. Note the hand print of her fiancé who had been squeezing limes into their tropical drinks. This contact occurred when they posed for a photograph. (*Reproduced with permission from Darby-Stewart AL, Edwards FD, Perry KJ. Hyperpigmentation and vesicles after beach vacation. Phytophotodermatitis.* J Fam Pract. *2006;55(12):1050-1053. Reproduced with permission from Frontline Medical Communications.*)

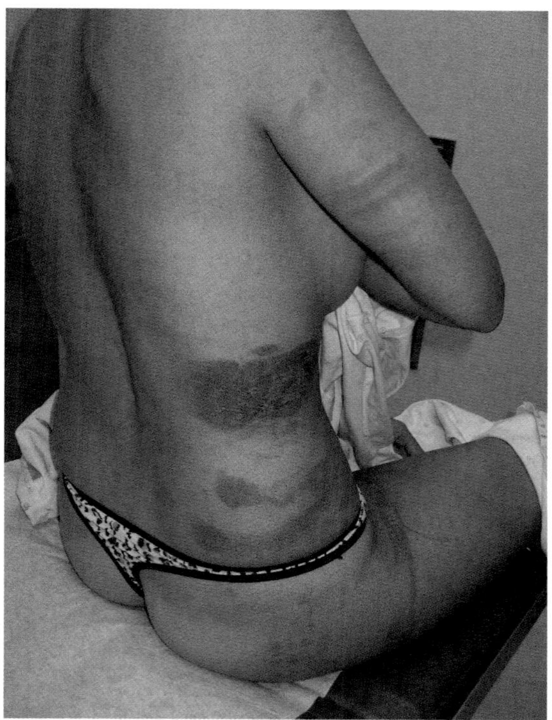

FIGURE 197-7 Phytophotodermatitis visible on the arm, trunk, and leg caused by lime juice and sun exposure on the beach. Note the hyperpigmentation that occurs in conjunction with the erythema. (*Reproduced with permission from Darby-Stewart AL, Edwards FD, Perry KJ. Hyperpigmentation and vesicles after beach vacation. Phytophotodermatitis.* J Fam Pract. *2006;55(12):1050-1053. Reproduced with permission from Frontline Medical Communications.*)

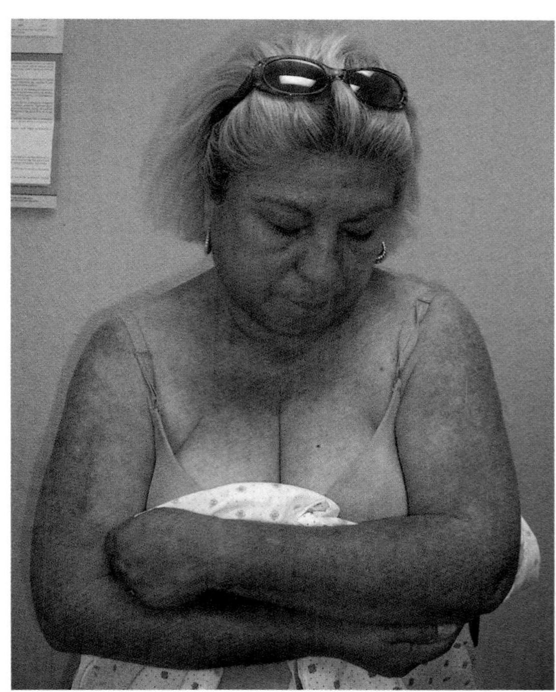

FIGURE 197-8 A photoallergic drug reaction characterized by widespread eczema in the photodistribution areas such as the face, upper chest, arms, and back of hands. A punch biopsy showed a spongiotic dermatitis. The exact photoallergen was not found. (*Reproduced with permission from Richard P. Usatine, MD.*)

TABLE 197-1 Characteristics of Phototoxic and Photoallergic Reactions

Feature	Phototoxic Reaction	Photoallergic Reaction
Incidence	High	Low
Amount of agent required for photosensitivity	Large	Small
Onset of reaction after exposure	Minutes to hours	24 to 72 h
More than one exposure to agent required	No	Yes
Examination findings	Exaggerated sunburn	Dermatitis
Immunologically mediated	No	Yes

- The incidence of drug- and plant-induced phototoxic reactions in the United States is unknown. Phototoxic reactions are much more common than photoallergic reactions.

ETIOLOGY AND PATHOPHYSIOLOGY

PMLE is an idiopathic, delayed-type hypersensitivity reaction to UVA light and, to a lesser extent, UVB light (see **Figures 197-1** and **197-2**). PMLE is the most common photoeruption encountered in clinical practice. The reaction will remit spontaneously with time and absence of sun exposure, but occasionally it will last as long as sun exposure occurs. PMLE usually begins in the first 3 decades of life and occurs more commonly in women. The rash develops within hours to days after exposure to sunlight and lasts for several days to a week.

There is a broad range of degrees of photosensitivity with PMLE. Extremely sensitive individuals can tolerate only minutes of exposure, whereas many people have a low sensitivity and require prolonged exposure to sunlight before developing a reaction. It is a recurrent condition that persists for many years in most patients.[2]

Phototoxic reactions are the most common drug-induced photoeruptions (see **Figures 197-3** to **197-7**). They are caused by absorption of ultraviolet rays by the causative drug, which releases energy and damages cell membranes, or, in the case of psoralens, DNA. The drugs that most frequently cause phototoxic reactions are nonsteroidal anti-inflammatory drugs (NSAIDs), quinolones, tetracyclines, amiodarone, and the phenothiazines[3] (**Table 197-2**). Most of these drugs have at least one resonating double bond or an aromatic ring that can absorb radiant energy. Most compounds are activated by wavelengths within the UVA (320-400 nm) range, although some compounds have a peak absorption within the UVB or visible range.

Phytophotodermatitis are phototoxic reactions to psoralens, which are plant compounds found in limes, celery, figs, and certain drugs. They can cause dramatic inflammation and bullae where the psoralen comes into contact with the skin (see **Figures 197-5** to **197-7**). The inflammation is frequently followed by hyperpigmentation.

TABLE 197-2 Common Medications That Cause Phototoxic Reactions

Class	Medication
Antibiotics	Tetracyclines
	Fluoroquinolones
	Sulfonamides
	Griseofulvin
NSAIDs	Ketoprofen
	Ibuprofen
	Naproxen
Diuretics	Furosemide
	Hydrochlorothiazide
Retinoids	Isotretinoin
	Acitretin
Photodynamic therapy prophotosensitizers	5-Aminolevulinic acid
	Methyl-5-aminolevulinic acid
	Verteporfin
	Photofrin
Neuroleptic drugs	Phenothiazines
	Thioxanthenes (chlorprothixene and thiothixene)
	Other drugs
	Itraconazole
	5-Fluorouracil (5-FU)
	Amiodarone
	Diltiazem
	Quinidine
	Coal tar
Sunscreens	Paraaminobenzoic acid (PABA)

Photoallergic eruptions are a lymphocyte-mediated reaction. Photoactivation of a drug or agent results in the development of a metabolite that can bind to proteins in the skin to form a complete antigen. The antigen is presented to lymphocytes by Langerhans cells, causing an inflammatory response and spongiotic dermatitis (eczema). The eruption is characterized by widespread eczema in the photodistribution areas such as the face, upper chest, arms, and back of hands (see **Figure 197-8**). Most photoallergic reactions are caused by topical agents such as antibiotics and halogenated phenolic compounds added to soaps and fragrances.[4] Systemic photoallergens such as the phenothiazines, chlorpromazine, sulfa products, and NSAIDs can produce photoallergic reactions, although most of their photosensitive reactions are phototoxic (**Table 197-3**).

RISK FACTORS

Unprotected exposure to sunlight and the use of drugs associated with phototoxic and photoallergic eruptions are the main risk factors.

TABLE 197-3 Common Substances That Cause Photoallergic Reactions

5-Fluorouracil (5-FU)
6-Methylcoumarin
Fragrances (6-methylcoumarin, musk, sandalwood oil)
NSAIDs (eg, ketoprofen, diclofenac, piroxicam, celecoxib)
Sunscreens (benzophenones, cinnamates, dibenzoylmethanes)
Dapsone
Hormonal contraceptives
Hydrochlorothiazide
Antimicrobial agents (bithionol, chlorhexidine, hexachlorophene, fenticlor, Itraconazole)
Phenothiazines
Salicylates
Sulfonylureas (glipizide and glyburide)
Quinidine

DIAGNOSIS

CLINICAL FEATURES

Most cases of photodermatitis can be diagnosed on the basis of the patient's history. Be sure to review the patient's medications for possible sources.

- The appearance of the PMLE varies from person to person but is consistent in a given patient. Erythematous pruritic papules, sometimes with vesicles, are most common (see **Figures 197-1** and **197-2**). Lesions may coalesce to form plaques. The rash typically involves the V-area of the neck and the arms, legs, or both. The face, which is exposed to sunlight in both summer and winter, tends to be spared. It tends to present in spring/summer, with the first significant UV exposure of the year. The rash typically develops 1 to 4 days after sun exposure.
- Phototoxic reaction occurs 2 to 6 hours after exposure to sunlight. The eruption typically appears as an exaggerated sunburn, with mild cases causing slight erythema and severe cases causing vesicles or bullae (see **Figures 197-3** to **197-7**).
- Phytophotodermatitis reactions are asymmetric and localized to the area in which the plant psoralen was in contact with the skin. Accompanying hyperpigmentation is a good clue to a phytophotodermatitis reaction (see **Figures 197-5** to **197-7**). Ask the patient if he or she had any contact with limes, celery, or figs. Squeezing lime juice into drinks is a particularly common cause of this reaction.
- Photoonycholysis phototoxicity reactions (sun-induced separation of the nail plate from the nail bed) have been reported with the use of tetracycline, psoralen, chloramphenicol, fluoroquinolones, oral contraceptives, quinine, and mercaptopurine. Photoonycholysis may be the only manifestation of phototoxicity in individuals with heavily pigmented skin.
- Photoallergic eruptions are characterized by widespread eczema in the photodistribution areas such as the face, upper chest, arms, and back of hands. They resemble allergic contact dermatitis, but the distribution is mostly limited to sun-exposed areas of the body (see **Figure 197-8**).

TYPICAL DISTRIBUTION

All photodermatitis reactions occur in sun-exposed areas, such as the face, ears, dorsal forearms, and V-area of the neck and upper chest.

LABORATORY TESTING

- Laboratory studies that may be helpful include antinuclear antibody (ANA), anti-Ro (SSA), and anti-La (SSB) titers to rule out lupus and porphyrin studies to exclude porphyria.
- Phototesting can be used to determine a patient's minimal erythema dose to light exposure and help to define the inciting spectrum of a photodermatosis (UVA vs UVB vs visible light). Phototesting involves irradiating the skin with varying doses of UVA, UVB, and visible light through an opaque screen with multiple openings.[5] Usually the test is performed on the back. The presence or absence of solar urticaria is recorded within the first hour and the minimal erythema dose is determined after 24 hours.
- Provocative phototesting involves irradiating normal-appearing previously affected skin with the suspected causative light, either by higher doses of UV light or by natural sunlight exposure.[5] Provocative phototesting is primarily used for suspected PMLE.
- Photopatch testing is useful when a topical photoallergen is suspected. It is performed by placing 2 identical sets of potential photoallergens on the patient's back and covering them. After 24 hours, one set is removed and that site is irradiated with UVA. The site is covered again. Twenty-four hours later, both the irradiated and control test sites are assessed for reactions. A reaction to a specific photoallergen in the irradiated site, but not the control site, indicates a photoallergy. A similar reaction in both sites suggests a contact dermatitis.[5]

BIOPSY

Punch biopsy of PMLE demonstrates extensive spongiosis and edema of the dermis with a deep lymphohistiocytic infiltrate. In acute phototoxic reactions, necrotic keratinocytes are observed.

DIFFERENTIAL DIAGNOSIS

- Systemic lupus erythematosus (SLE)—Sunlight can precipitate a lupus rash. Serum ANA is usually positive (see Chapter 178, Lupus: Systemic and Cutaneous).
- Porphyria cutanea tarda reactions can also be precipitated by sunlight. It tends to present with vesicles or bullae in sun-exposed areas such as back of the hands. The bullae generally do not have any surrounding erythema, and urine for porphyrins should be positive (see Chapter 184, Other Bullous Disease).
- Dermatomyositis may cause an erythematous or violaceous eruption in sun-exposed areas. If these cutaneous findings precede the muscle weakness it can appear to be a photosensitivity reaction such as PMLE or a phototoxic drug reaction. Therefore, it is essential in the management and follow-up of patients with suspected PMLE or other photosensitivity to inquire about muscle weakness and to look for other signs of dermatomyositis on the hands and/or through laboratory tests for muscle enzyme elevations (see Chapter 179, Dermatomyositis). The dermatomyositis patient story in Chapter 179 is one in which the initial rash was thought to be a photosensitivity reaction to a new hydrochlorothiazide (HCTZ) prescription.

- Contact dermatitis appears the same as photoallergic dermatitis but is usually not limited to sun-exposed areas (see Chapter 144, Contact Dermatitis).

MANAGEMENT

NONPHARMACOLOGIC

- The management of PMLE is aimed mainly at prevention. Patients who have mild disease should adopt a program of sun avoidance (see "Prevention"). Broad-spectrum (UVA and UVB blocking) sunscreen with a minimum sun protection factor (SPF) of 30 should be used whenever out of doors (**Table 197-4**).[6] However, the SPF value of a sunscreen describes its protection factor against sunburn, which is primarily caused by UVB. The SPF does not provide sufficient information on UVA protection.[7] SOR Ⓒ Patients must use sunscreen liberally and frequently (reapply every 2 hours and after swimming) as an insufficiently thick application may reduce its effectiveness.[8] SOR Ⓑ

TABLE 197-4 UV Blocking Characteristics or Sunscreens

Sunscreen	Blocks UVB	Blocks UVA
Aminobenzoic acid	X	
Avobenzone		X
Cinoxate	X	
Dioxybenzone	X	X
Ecamsule*		X
Ensulizole	X	
Homosalate	X	
Meradimate		X
Octocrylene	X	
Octinoxate	X	
Octisalate	X	
Oxybenzone	X	X
Padimate O	X	
Sulisobenzone	X	X
Titanium dioxide	X	X
Trolamine salicylate	X	
Zinc oxide	X	X
Drometrizole trisiloxane (Mexoryl XL)*	X	X
Methylene-bis-benzotriazolyl tetramethylbutylphenol (Tinosorb M)*	X	X
Bis-ethylhexyloxyphenol methoxyphenyl triazine (Tinosorb S)*		X

*Not available in the United States in 2012.

- Patients with severe PMLE can be desensitized in the spring with the use of phototherapy and maintained in the nonreactive state with weekly 1 hour unprotected exposure to sunlight. SOR Ⓒ A course of psoralen and UVA radiation, or a course of narrowband UVB, 3 times a week for 4 weeks provides protection.[9] SOR Ⓑ These treatments may induce a typical rash or erythema but otherwise have no major adverse effects.
- Avoid tobacco products since they may make PMLE worse.[10] SOR Ⓑ

MEDICATIONS

- Acute episodes of photodermatitis respond rapidly to topical and/or oral corticosteroids. Topical steroids should provide symptomatic relief and decrease the inflammation. For more severe reactions, a course of prednisone 30 mg daily for 5 to 7 days may be used.[11] SOR Ⓑ
- Patients with acute drug-induced photodermatitis need to practice sun avoidance until well after the drug is discontinued. Topical and systemic corticosteroids may be used, especially with photoallergic reactions, but their efficacy is unproven. SOR Ⓒ
- Nicotinamide was successful in 60% of 42 patients treated with 3 g/d orally for 2 weeks.[12] SOR Ⓑ

PREVENTION

Sun protection is the primary preventative measure for patients with photosensitivity. Patients should avoid exposure to midday sun (between 10:00 AM and 3:00 PM). Protective clothing such as long sleeve shirts and broad rim hats should be worn while outdoors. Fabrics that are tightly woven, thick, and/or dark colored are useful for protection.[13] Clothing treated with broad-spectrum UV absorbers is also helpful. Window film that blocks UV and some visible light can be applied to cars or homes.[14]

Sunscreen is important for daily use for patients with photosensitivity. Sunscreens are divided into chemical (organic) and physical (inorganic) products. Physical sunscreens block both UV and some visible light (see **Table 197-4**). Products containing avobenzone or ecamsule offer improved protection against UVA.

Physical blocker (inorganic) sunscreens, such as titanium dioxide and zinc oxide, work by reflecting and scattering UV and visible light. Older formulations were opaque making them cosmetically less acceptable to patients. Newer nonopaque, micronized formulations of titanium and zinc oxide have been developed but are less capable of scattering visible light and the longer wavelengths of UVA.

Chemical sunscreens may cause allergic contact dermatitis or photoallergic reactions in some patients. These patients should use titanium dioxide or zinc oxide sunscreens for protection.

PROGNOSIS

- Some patients with PMLE experience less-severe reactions with successive years, but they may also worsen over time without appropriate treatment.
- The prognosis is excellent with patients when the offending agent is removed. Complete resolution of the photosensitivity may take weeks to months. Patients with persistent light reactivity beyond this have a poorer prognosis.

FOLLOW-UP

Follow-up is needed if the photosensitivity persists.

PATIENT EDUCATION

- Patients with any type of photodermatitis should apply strong broad-spectrum sunscreens daily and use protective clothing (hats and shirts that cover the arms and V-area of the neck). The sunscreen should be water resistant and applied to exposed areas before sun exposure.[15] Sunscreens should be reapplied every 2 hours if there is continued sun exposure. Some of the most effective sunscreens contain stabilized avobenzone, Mexoryl, and/or titanium dioxide or zinc oxide to block UVA and UVB.
- Tell your patients that if they develop an allergy to one sunscreen, they should find another with different ingredients.
- It is important to avoid sunlight during the midday whenever possible.
- Explain to patients that phototoxic reactions may cause hyperpigmentation, which can take weeks to months to resolve. There is no guarantee that all the hyperpigmentation will go away.
- Avoid repeated rubbing and scratching, which can lead to skin thickening and chronic lichenification. Use the topical medications prescribed to treat the itching and to avoid lichenification.

PATIENT RESOURCES

- DermNet NZ. *Photosensitivity (Sun Allergy)*—**http://dermnetnz.org/reactions/photosensitivity.html.**
- The Skin Cancer Foundation. *Photosensitivity—A Reason To Be Even Safer in the Sun*—**http://www.skincancer.org/photosensitivity-a-reason-to-be-even-safer-in-the-sun.html.**

PROVIDER RESOURCES

- American Academy of Family Physicians. *Common Hyperpigmentation Disorders in Adults: Part I*—**http://www.aafp.org/afp/20031115/1955.html.**
- eMedicine. *Drug-Induced Photosensitivity*—**http://emedicine.medscape.com/article/1049648.**
- DermNet NZ. *Polymorphic Light Eruption*—**http://www.dermnetnz.org/reactions/pmle.html.**
- Darby-Stewart AL, Edwards FD, Perry KJ. Hyperpigmentation and vesicles after beach vacation. Phytophotodermatitis. *J Fam Pract.* 2006;55:1050-1053.
- Phytophotodermatitis case report and review—**http://www.skinandaging.com/content/what-caused-this-rash-on-this-man%E2%80%99s-wrist-and-hand.**
- eMedicine. *Sunscreens and Photoprotection*—**http://emedicine.medscape.com/article/1119992.**

REFERENCES

1. Morison WL, Stern RS. Polymorphous light eruption: a common reaction uncommonly recognized. *Acta Derm Venereol.* 1982;62:237-240.
2. Hasan T, Ranki A, Jansen CT, Karvonen J. Disease associations in polymorphous light eruption: a long-term follow-up study of 94 patients. *Arch Dermatol.* 1998;134:1081-1085.
3. Stern RS, Shear NH. Cutaneous reactions to drugs and biological modifiers. In: Arndt KA, LeBoit PE, Robinson JK, Wintroub BU, eds. *Cutaneous Medicine and Surgery*. Vol. 1. Philadelphia, PA: Saunders; 1996:412.
4. Gonzalez E, Gonzalez S. Drug photosensitivity, idiopathic photodermatoses, and sunscreens. *J Am Acad Dermatol.* 1996;35:871-875.
5. Yashar SS, Lim HW. Classification and evaluation of photodermatoses. *Dermatol Ther.* 2003;16(1):1-7.
6. Dawe RS, Ferguson J. Diagnosis and treatment of chronic actinic dermatitis. *Dermatol Ther.* 2003;16:45-51.
7. Fourtanier A, Moyal D, Seité S. Sunscreens containing the broad-spectrum UVA absorber, Mexoryl SX, prevent the cutaneous detrimental effects of UV exposure: a review of clinical study results. *Photodermatol Photoimmunol Photomed.* 2008;24:164-174.
8. Faurschou A, Wulf HC. The relation between sun protection factor and amount of suncreen applied in vivo. *Br J Dermatol.* 2007;156:716-719.
9. Bilsland D, George SA, Gibbs NK, et al. A comparison of narrow band phototherapy (TL-01) and photochemotherapy (PUVA) in the management of polymorphic light eruption. *Br J Dermatol.* 1993;129:708-712.
10. Metelitsa AI, Lauzon GJ. Tobacco and the skin. *Clin Dermatol.* 2010;4:384-390.
11. Patel DC, Bellaney GJ, Seed PT, et al. Efficacy of short-course oral prednisolone in polymorphic light eruption: a randomized controlled trial. *Br J Dermatol.* 2000;143:828-831.
12. Neumann R, Rappold E, Pohl-Markl H. Treatment of polymorphous light eruption with nicotinamide: a pilot study. *Br J Dermatol.* 1986;115(1):77-80.
13. Lautenschlager S, Wulf HC, Pittelkow MR. Photoprotection. *Lancet.* 2007;370:528-537.
14. Dawe R, Russell S, Ferguson J. Borrowing from museums and industry: two photoprotective devices. *Br J Dermatol.* 1996;135:1016-1017.
15. Morison WL. Photosensitivity. *N Engl J Med.* 2004;350:1111-1117.

198 ERYTHEMA AB IGNE

Amor Khachemoune, MD
Yoon-Soo Cindy Bae-Harboe, MD
Khashayar Sarabi, MD

PATIENT STORY

A 50-year-old woman presented to the office with bilateral erythematous lesions on the inner aspects of both of her lower extremities (**Figures 198-1** and **198-2**). The lesions started developing for the past 6 months. They became progressively more noticeable but stayed localized in the inner aspects of the lower extremities. She mentioned that she was using a hot-water bottle in the area involved to keep her warm at night when she was sleeping in bed. Although our working clinical diagnosis was erythema ab igne, clinical entities such as livedo reticularis, poikiloderma atrophicans vasculare, and acanthosis nigricans were also considered in the differential diagnosis. A skin biopsy was performed and confirmed the diagnosis of erythema ab igne. The patient was advised to abandon the hot-water bottle application to the skin. Over the course of 4 months her skin lesions started to clear with no further intervention.

INTRODUCTION

Erythema ab igne is a rare condition caused by chronic exposure to heat (below the threshold for a thermal burn) from external heat sources. More specifically, prolonged use of hot-water bottles, heating pads, electric blankets, car seat warmers as well as exposure to open fires and laptops placed on the users' thighs or propped legs have all been reported to cause erythema ab igne. Affected skin is characterized by reticular pink-colored and hyperpigmented mottled patches. Patients may complain of associated pruritus, paresthesias, or may be asymptomatic. Treatment is limited and patients are instructed to avoid triggers.

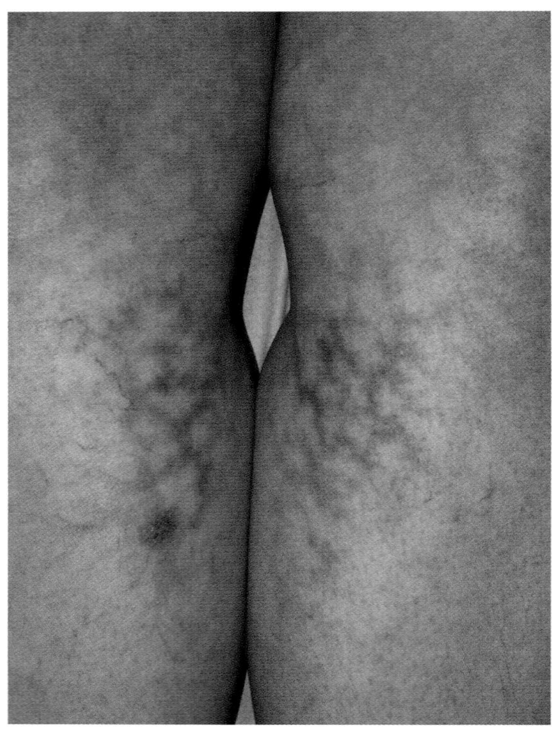

FIGURE 198-1 Erythema ab igne. Mottled or mesh-like pigmentary changes on the legs of a 50-year-old woman who slept with a hot-water bottle between her legs. *(Reproduced with permission from El-Ghandour A, Selim A, Khachemoune A. Bilateral lesions on the legs. J Fam Pract. 1987;56(1):37-39. Reproduced with permission from Frontline Medical Communications.)*

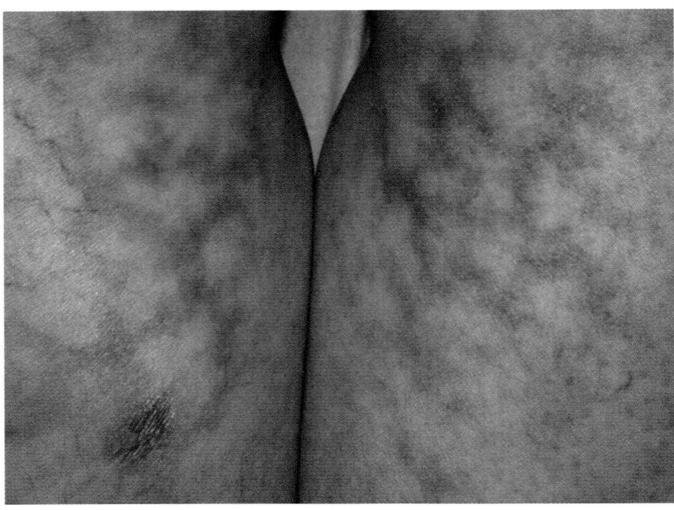

FIGURE 198-2 Close-up of legs in **Figure 198-1**. *(Reproduced with permission from El-Ghandour A, Selim A, Khachemoune A. Bilateral lesions on the legs. J Fam Pract. 1987;56(1):37-39. Reproduced with permission from Frontline Medical Communications.)*

SYNONYMS

Erythema ab igne is also known as chronic moderate heat dermatitis, chronic radiant heat dermatitis, toasted skin syndrome, fire stains, hot-water bottle rash, or laptop thigh.

EPIDEMIOLOGY

- Rare disease.
- Women, in particular those who are overweight, are affected more often than men.

ETIOLOGY AND PATHOPHYSIOLOGY

- The skin findings form as a result of multiple exposures to an intense source of heat.
- Erythema ab igne has been noted for many years, and the sources of heat have changed over time. It used to be reported in women who stay for long periods of time in front of open fires, fireplaces, or furnaces to cook.[1-4] Most of the lesions were appearing on the medial side of the thigh and the lower leg in general.
- Currently, erythema ab igne is seen on different parts of the body, depending on what source of heat initiated the pathology, the angle of the heat radiation, the morphology of the skin, and the layers of clothing. Some of the modern-day examples are repeated application of hot-water bottles or heating pads to treat chronic pain, exposure to car heaters and furniture with internal heaters, the use of a laptop

computer for long periods, and cooks and chefs who stand for long periods in the range of heat. Other causes include hot bricks, infrared lamps, and even microwave popcorn. Ultrasound physiotherapy was also reported as a cause of erythema ab igne. Recently, there was a reported case of frequent prolonged hot baths that caused the disease.[5]

RISK FACTORS

- Persistent exposure to heat
- Occupations that involve chronic exposure to external heat sources (eg, kitchen workers, silversmiths, jewelers, foundry workers)[6]

DIAGNOSIS

CLINICAL FEATURES

- Some patients have mild pruritus or burning sensation, but the majority of patients are asymptomatic.
- Skin lesions may not appear immediately after the exposure; it might take a period of 1 month to show up. Skin changes start as a reddish-brown pigmentation distributed as a mottled rash and are followed by skin atrophy (**Figures 198-1** to **198-3**).
- Telangiectasias with diffuse hyperpigmentation and subepidermal bullae may also develop.
- The rash appears mesh-like or net-like in the area exposed to the heat. The heat can be from fireplaces, heating pads, laptop computers, open fires, place heaters, and hot-water bottles (**Figures 198-1** to **198-7**).

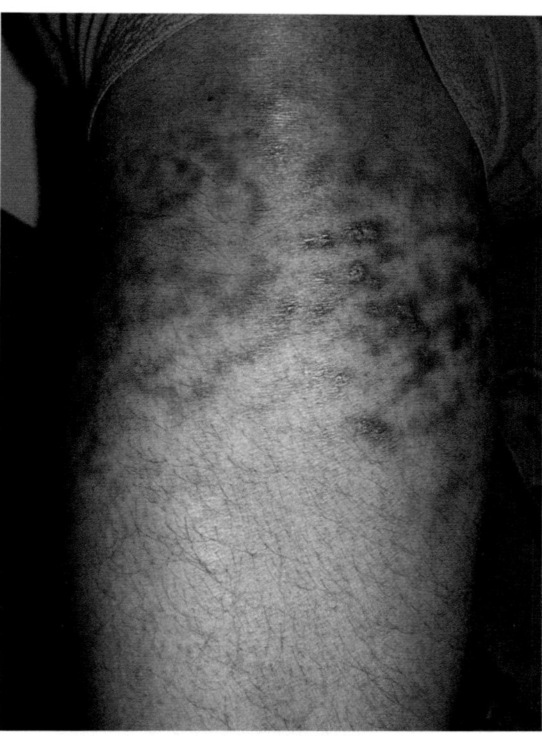

FIGURE 198-3 Mottled hyperpigmentation and hint of blistering and crusting on the anterior leg area in a 23-year-old woman who spent significant time close to a fireplace. (*Reproduced with permission from Amor Khachemoune, MD.*)

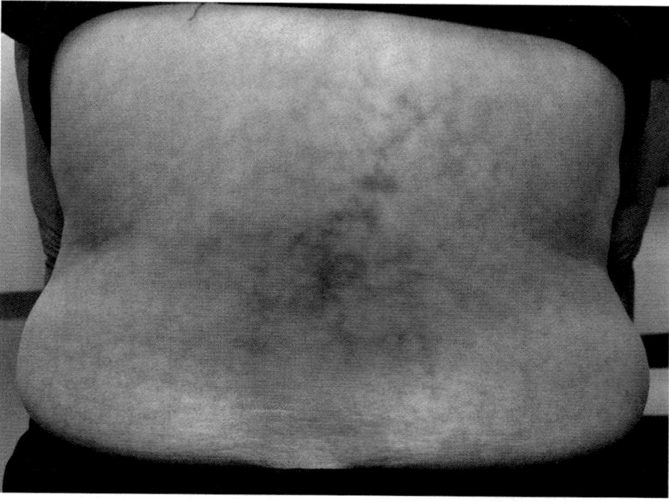

FIGURE 198-4 Erythema ab igne from the use of a heating pad in a woman with back pain. (*Reproduced with permission from Richard P. Usatine, MD.*)

- Malignant melanoma and various sarcomas are reported to arise in burn scars; however, those arising in areas of erythema ab igne have not been reported to date.

TYPICAL DISTRIBUTION

It is found at the area of heat exposure, which is most often the legs or back (see **Figure 198-4**).

LABORATORY STUDIES

None recommended

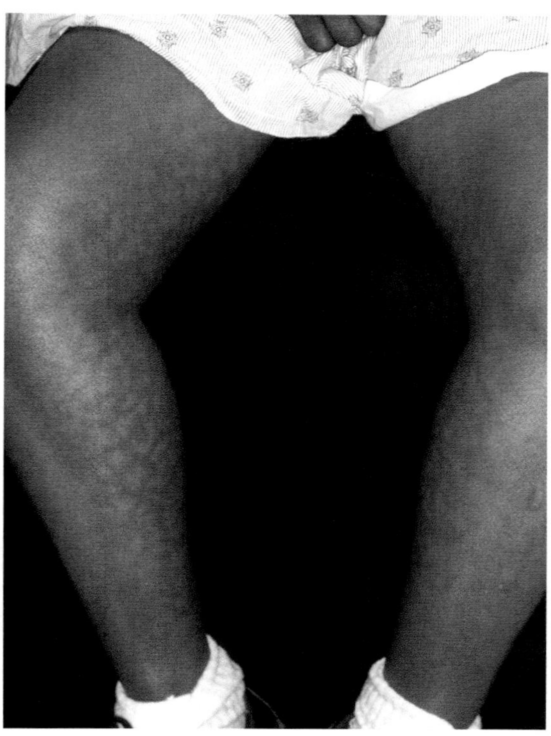

FIGURE 198-5 Erythema ab igne on the legs of a woman who was straddling a place heater to keep warm during the winter. (*Reproduced with permission from Richard P. Usatine, MD.*)

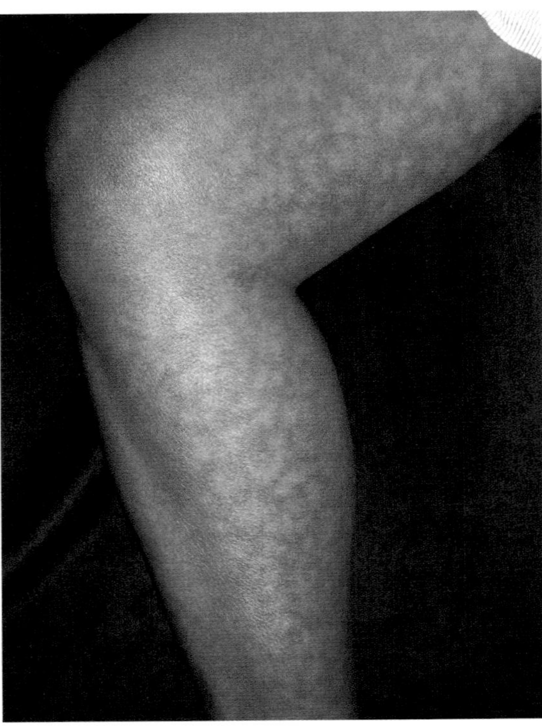

FIGURE 198-6 Close-up of leg in Figure 198-5 showing the net-like pattern on the medial leg of erythema ab igne. (*Reproduced with permission from Richard P. Usatine, MD.*)

SKIN BIOPSY

- In almost all cases, the diagnosis is based on the history and physical examination. Once the typical skin pattern is seen by the clinician, a few questions often will prompt the patient to recall the heat source.
- In some rare cases, Merkel cell carcinoma and squamous cell carcinoma have developed in areas of erythema ab igne.[7-9]
- If clinically warranted, a biopsy is performed to exclude the possibility of malignant transformation.

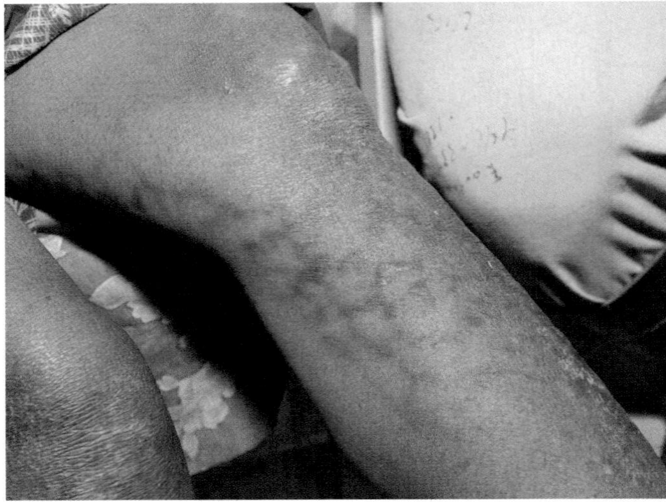

FIGURE 198-7 Erythema ab igne on the legs of an Ethiopian woman who cooks over an open fire. (*Reproduced with permission from Richard P. Usatine, MD.*)

- Histopathology shows epidermal atrophy, subepidermal separation, and haziness of the dermal-epidermal junction. Dilation of capillaries and connective tissue disintegration, elastosis, hemosiderin deposition, melanocytosis, and abundance of inflammatory cells are all seen in the dermis. Some of these lesions might progress to actinic keratosis, which could be a precursor for squamous cell carcinoma of the skin.

DIFFERENTIAL DIAGNOSIS

Erythema ab igne should be differentiated from other diseases with skin changes that mimic its presentation.

LIVEDO RETICULARIS

- Reticular cyanotic cutaneous discoloration surrounding pale central areas caused by dilation of capillary blood vessels and stagnation of blood (**Figure 198-8**).
- Occurs mostly on the legs, arms, and trunk and appears to be a purplish mottling of the skin.
- More pronounced in cold weather.
- Idiopathic condition that may be associated with systemic diseases such as systemic lupus erythematosus (SLE).

POIKILODERMA ATROPHICANS VASCULARE

- A variant of mycosis fungoides (cutaneous T-cell lymphoma) (see Chapter 174, Cutaneous T-Cell Lymphoma).
- Circumscribed violaceous erythema.
- Occurs mostly in posterior shoulders, back, buttocks, V-shaped area of anterior neck and chest.

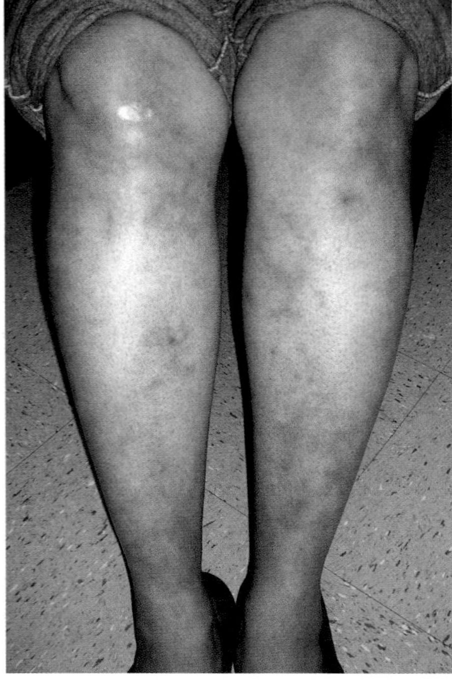

FIGURE 198-8 Livedo reticularis in a 27-year-old woman with lupus. The mottled purple color gets worse when she is exposed to cold temperatures. (*Reproduced with permission from Richard P. Usatine, MD.*)

- May be asymptomatic or mildly pruritic.
- May remain stable in size or gradually increase.
- Numerous atypical lymphocytes are observed around dermal blood vessels, and some epidermotropism is observed.

ACANTHOSIS NIGRICANS

- Velvety, light-brown-to-black markings usually on the neck, under the arms, or in the groin (see Chapter 220, Acanthosis Nigricans).
- Most often associated with being overweight.
- More common in people with darker skin pigmentation.
- A disorder that may begin at any age and that may be inherited as a primary condition or associated with various underlying syndromes.
- Should be able to distinguish from erythema ab igne by the typical location around the neck and in the axilla.

MANAGEMENT

- The first goal of treatment is to identify the source of heat radiation to avoid further exposure. For mild lesions, no intervention is needed after the heat source is removed and the probability of full resolution is good.
- Topical retinoids, vitamin A derivatives, hydroquinone, and 5-fluorouracil have been prescribed to treat the abnormal skin pigmentation.[10] Laser therapy has been used to even out the skin color.[4,10] SOR Ⓒ

PROGNOSIS

Prognosis is excellent for full resolution if the external heat source is removed or discontinued. However, the hyperpigmentation may remain and various treatments may not succeed in returning the skin to its normal pigmentation.

FOLLOW-UP

Follow-up visits are recommended if there are new changes to the skin after removing the source of heat. This is to diagnose and manage any malignant transformation.

PATIENT EDUCATION

Patients should avoid excessive and prolonged localized heat exposures (ie, fireplaces, heating pads, laptop computers, and hot-water bottle applications).

There are many ways to shield the thighs from the heat of a laptop computer, from the use of pillows and blankets to the purchase of special devices manufactured for this purpose.

PATIENT RESOURCES

- Wikipedia. *Erythema Ab Igne*—**http://en.wikipedia.org/wiki/Erythema_ab_igne.**

PROVIDER RESOURCES

- Medscape. *Erythema Ab Igne*—**http://emedicine.medscape.com/article/1087535.**
- DermNet NZ. *Erythema Ab Igne*—**http://dermnetnz.org/vascular/erythema-ab-igne.html.**

REFERENCES

1. Meffert JJ, Davis BM. Furniture-induced erythema ab igne. *J Am Acad Dermatol*. 1996;34(3):516-517.
2. Helm TN, Spigel GT, Helm KF. Erythema ab igne caused by a car heater. *Cutis*. 1997;59(2):81-82.
3. Bilic M, Adams BB. Erythema ab igne induced by a laptop computer. *J Am Acad Dermatol*. 1984;50(6):973-974.
4. El-Ghandour A, Selim A, Khachemoune A. Bilateral lesions on the legs. *J Fam Pract*. 1987;56(1):37-39.
5. Weber MB, Ponzio HA, Costa FB, Camini L. Erythema ab igne: a case report. *An Bras Dermatol*. 1985;80(2):187-188.
6. Runger TM. Disorders due to physical agents. In: Bolognia J, Jorizzo JL, Rapini RP, eds. *Dermatology*. Vol 2. London, UK: Mosby; 1983:1385-1409.
7. Jones CS, Tyring SK, Lee PC, Fine JD. Development of neuroendocrine (Merkel cell) carcinoma mixed with squamous cell carcinoma in erythema ab igne. *Arch Dermatol*. 1988;124(1):110-113.
8. Arrington JH 3rd, Lockman DS. Thermal keratoses and squamous cell carcinoma in situ associated with erythema ab igne. *Arch Dermatol*. 1979;115(10):1226-1228.
9. Hewitt JB, Sherif A, Kerr KM, Stankler L. Merkel cell and squamous cell carcinomas arising in erythema ab igne. *Br J Dermatol*. 1993;128(5):591-592.
10. Sahl WJ Jr, Taira JW. Erythema ab igne: treatment with 5-fluorouracil cream. *J Am Acad Dermatol*. 1992;27(1):109-110.

SECTION 18 VASCULAR SKIN DISORDERS

199 ACQUIRED VASCULAR SKIN LESIONS

Nathan Hitzeman, MD

PATIENT STORY

A 31-year-old woman presented with a new swelling on her lower lip. This was clinically recognized as a venous lake (**Figure 199-1**). The patient was bothered by its appearance and wanted it removed. She chose to have cryotherapy, which eradicated the venous lake. A closed-probe was used on a Cryogun for lesion compression while the freeze was applied using liquid nitrogen.

INTRODUCTION

Acquired vascular lesions are common skin findings. They appear "vascular," or filled with blood. Acquired vascular lesions differ from congenital or hereditary vascular lesions in that they manifest months to years after birth.

EPIDEMIOLOGY

- Venous lakes are acquired vascular lesions of the face and ears.[1]
- Cherry angiomas are common vascular malformations that occur in many adults after the age of 30 years (**Figure 199-2**). Cherry angiomas sometimes proliferate during pregnancy.[1]
- Angiokeratomas, the most common form being angiokeratomas of the scrotum (Fordyce) or vulva, develop during adult years (**Figures 199-3** and **199-4**).[1]

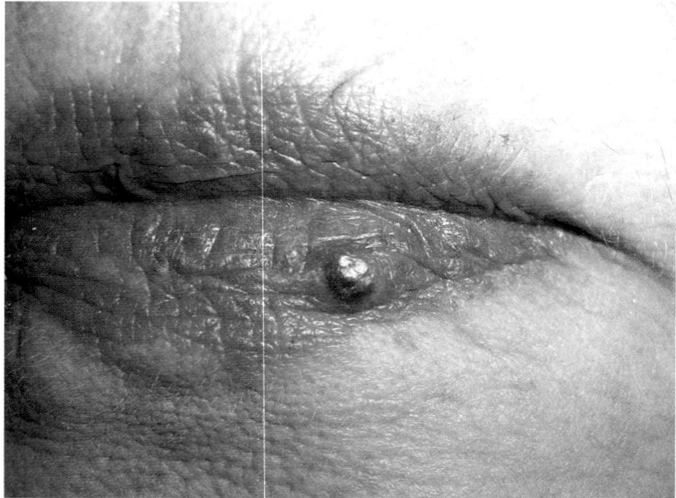

FIGURE 199-1 Venous lake on the lip of a young woman. This was eradicated with cryotherapy. (*Reproduced with permission from Richard P. Usatine, MD.*)

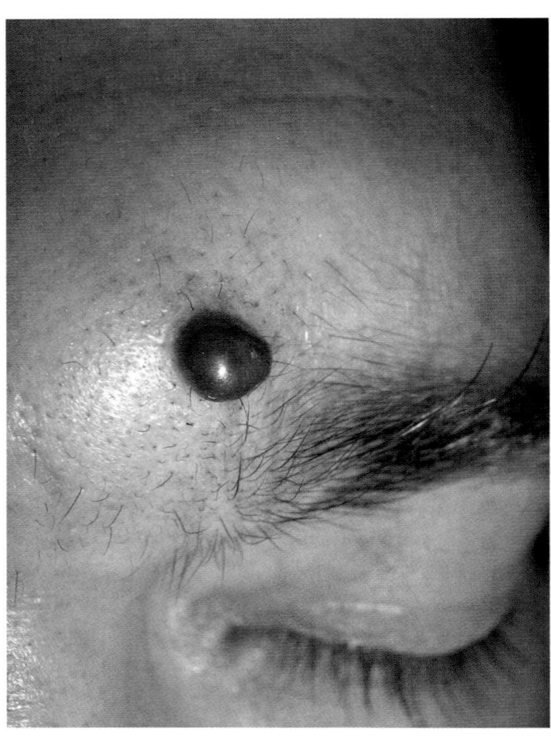

FIGURE 199-2 Large cherry angioma prior to treatement with shave excision and electrodesiccation of the base. (*Reproduced with permission from Richard P. Usatine, MD.*)

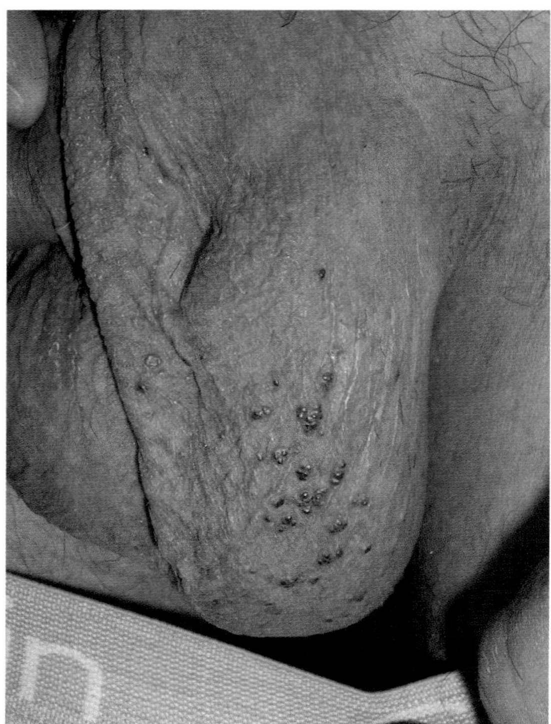

FIGURE 199-3 Angiokeratosis (multiple angiokeratomas) on the scrotum also known as Fordyce spots. (*Reproduced with permission from Lewis Rose, MD.*)

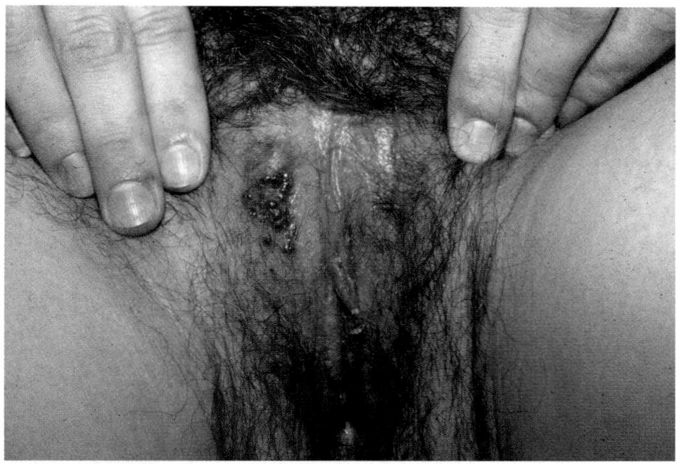

FIGURE 199-4 Angiokeratosis on the vulva. This might be mistaken for a melanoma. (*Reproduced with permission from Eric Kraus, MD.*)

- Glomangiomas, also known as glomuvenous malformations or glomus tumors, are a type of rare venous malformation (**Figure 199-5**). Most patients with glomangiomas are of Northern European descent and have a family history of similar lesions.[2]
- Cutaneous angiosarcomas are malignant vascular tumors most commonly found on the head and neck areas of elderly white men. These are rare but deadly (**Figure 199-6**).[3]

ETIOLOGY AND PATHOPHYSIOLOGY

- Venous lakes are benign dilated vascular channels (see **Figure 199-1**).
- Cherry angiomas are common benign vascular malformations (see **Figure 199-2**). They may increase during pregnancy. Several case reports have cited increased cherry angiomas after exposure to toxins.[4]
- Angiokeratomas are dilated superficial blood vessels that may be associated with increased venous pressure (such as in pregnant patients and patients with hemorrhoids)[1] (see **Figures 199-3** and **199-4**).
- Glomangiomas are a distinct type of venous malformation caused by abnormal synthesis of the protein glomulin[2] (see **Figure 199-5**). Lesions may be acquired or congenital.
- Cutaneous angiosarcomas are rare malignant vascular tumors thought to arise from vascular endothelium. Most arise spontaneously, but risk factors include radiation, chronic lymphedema, toxins, and certain familial syndromes. Elevation of several growth factors and cytokines has been associated with this malignancy (**Figures 199-6** and **199-7**).[3]

DIAGNOSIS

CLINICAL FEATURES

- Venous lakes are dark blue, slightly raised, and less than a centimeter in size. The lesions empty with firm compression. They may bleed with trauma.
- Cherry angiomas are deep red papules with a distinct cherry color.
- Angiokeratomas are multiple red-to-purple papules with associated hyperkeratosis. They may bleed easily with trauma.

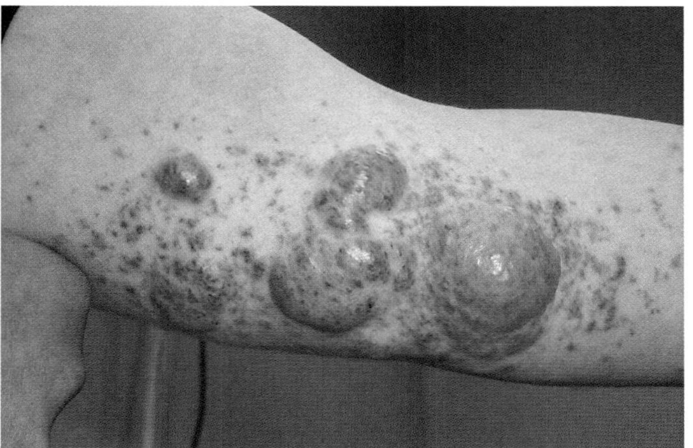

A

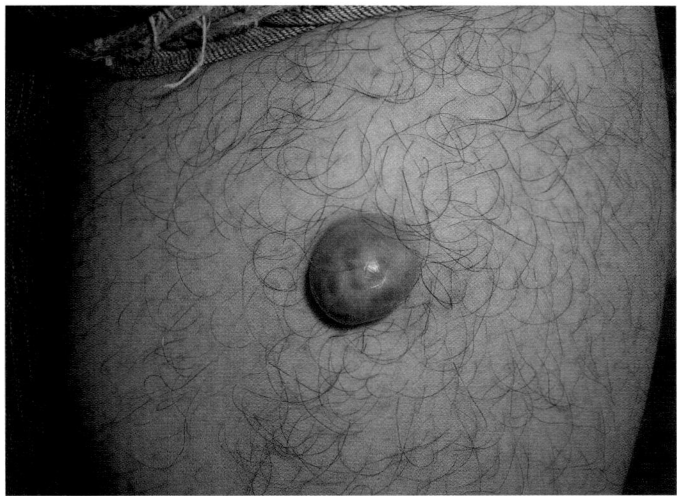

B

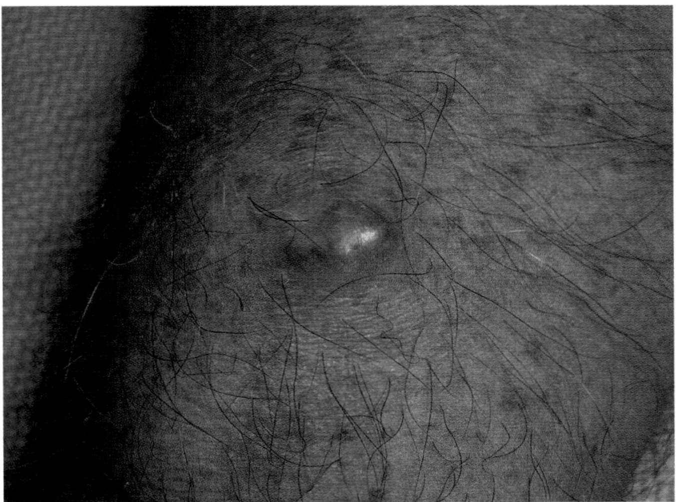

C

FIGURE 199-5 Glomangiomas can be multiple or solitary. **A.** Large glomangiomas of the arm. (*Reproduced with permission from Jack Resneck, Sr., MD.*) **B.** Solitary painful glomangioma on the leg of a young man. **C.** Small solitary painful glomangioma on the arm. These solitary glomangiomas were surgically resected. (*Reproduced with permission from Richard P. Usatine, MD.*)

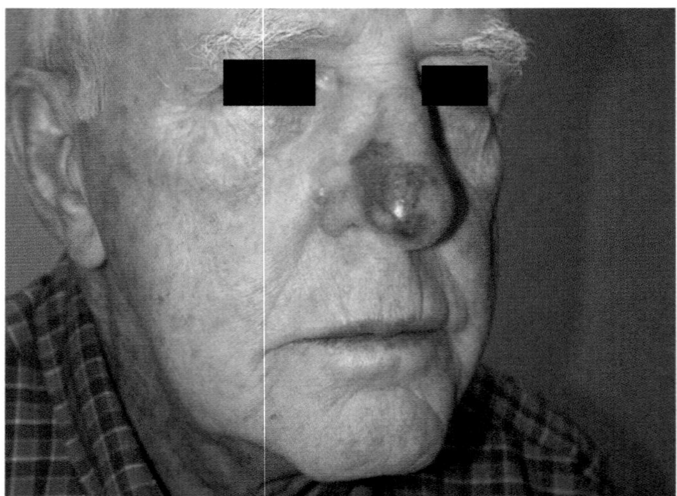

FIGURE 199-6 Angiosarcoma on the nose. A lesion like this requires an urgent biopsy. (*Reproduced with permission from Amor Khachemoune, MD.*)

- Glomangiomas are typically tender, blue-purple, partially-compressible nodules with a cobblestone appearance.
- Cutaneous angiosarcomas present as progressively enlarging erythematous plaques.

TYPICAL DISTRIBUTION

- Venous lakes are found on the face and ears, particularly the vermilion border of the lips (see **Figure 199-1**).
- Cherry angiomas favor the trunk but may occur on other parts of the body. Number of lesions ranges from several to hundreds.

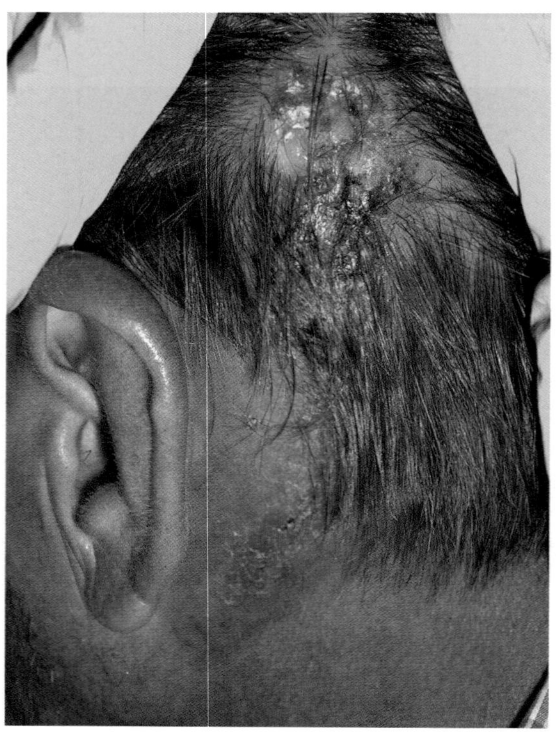

FIGURE 199-7 Angiosarcoma behind the ear and on the scalp of this 64-year-old man. (*Reproduced with permission from Richard P. Usatine, MD.*)

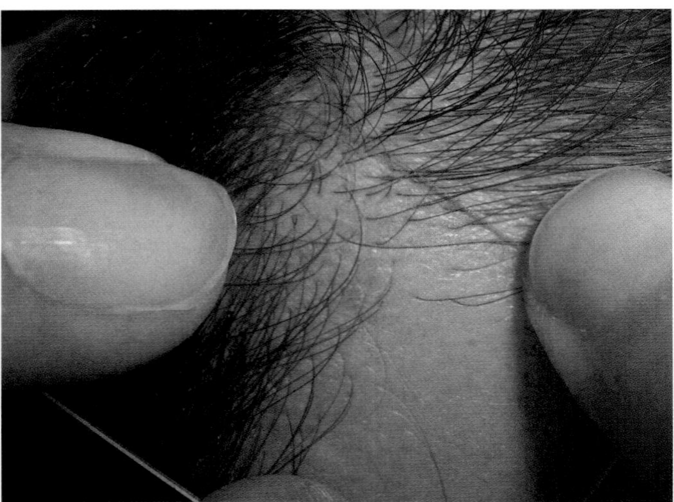

FIGURE 199-8 Diascopy in which a microscope slide is being used to compress a vascular lesion. The red color of this vascular hemangioma is blanching under pressure. (*Reproduced with permission from Richard P. Usatine, MD.*)

- Angiokeratomas typically occur on the scrotum or vulva (see **Figures 199-3** and **199-4**).
- Glomangiomas tend to occur on the extremities (see **Figure 199-5**). Solitary glomangiomas often occur in the nail bed, especially in women. The number of lesions ranges from solitary to more than 100.[5]
- Cutaneous angiosarcomas often present on the head and neck areas (see **Figures 199-6** and **199-7**).

LABORATORY STUDIES AND BIOPSY

- Diagnosis of venous lakes, cherry angiomas, and angiokeratomas is usually by history and physical examination alone. If these are removed surgically, it is still best to send them to pathology for confirmation of diagnosis. If the diagnosis is not clear clinically, a biopsy is warranted to rule out malignancy.
- Diascopy is a technique in which a microscope slide is used to compress a vascular lesion, allowing the clinician ability to see the red or purple color of a vascular lesion blanch under pressure (**Figure 199-8**).
- Skin biopsy of glomangioma reveals distinct rows of glomus cells that surround distorted vascular channels.[2]
- Skin biopsy of cutaneous angiosarcoma reveals irregular vascular channels and atypical endothelial cells.[3]

DIFFERENTIAL DIAGNOSIS

- Melanoma lesions are irregularly shaped, usually pigmented lesions discussed in Chapter 170, Melanoma. Unlike vascular lesions, they do not change fully blanch or change consistency with firm compression.
- Angiokeratomas typically occur on the scrotum or vulva and have a distinct appearance. They may bleed easily with trauma.
- Glomangiomas have a cobblestone appearance and are tender. Unlike venous lakes, these anomalies do not empty with compression.
- Cutaneous angiosarcomas present as progressively enlarging erythematous plaques that may resemble bruising, cellulitis, rosacea, or erysipelas.

The head-tilt maneuver has been described to aid in its detection.[5] Having a patient lower his or her head below the level of the heart for 5 to 10 seconds will make the lesion more engorged and violaceous, thus confirming its vascular nature.

MANAGEMENT

OBSERVATION

Patients can be reassured that venous lakes and most other acquired vascular lesions (with the exception of angiosarcomas) are benign lesions that develop during adult years.

SURGICAL

- Venous lakes, cherry angiomas, and other acquired vascular lesions can be eradicated by cryotherapy, electrodesiccation, sclerotherapy, intralesional bleomycin, intense pulsed light, and other laser modalities.[1,6-10] SOR C Compared with intense pulsed light, the neodymium:yttrium-aluminum-garnet (Nd:YAG) laser system may yield superior results in the treatment of benign vascular lesions.[11] SOR B Hyperpigmentation is the most common complication of treatment.
- When using cryotherapy to treat vascular lesions, it helps to compress the lesion at the same time as it is frozen. This can be done with a Cryogun that has a solid probe for compression. SOR C
- Cherry angiomas can be treated with light electrodesiccation using an electrosurgical instrument on a low setting without anesthesia. The tip of the instrument is lightly applied to the apex of the lesion while electrical current is engaged. The desired end point is "charring" of the lesion with minimal surrounding tissue destruction. SOR C
- Larger cherry angiomas can be removed with a shave excision after injecting with lidocaine and epinephrine. The base can be treated with electrodesiccation, if needed. SOR C
- Isolated glomangiomas may be surgically excised. Sclerotherapy may be useful for multiple lesions or large segmental lesions.[12] SOR C
- Cutaneous angiosarcoma is best treated with excision and wide surgical margins, as the primary tumor is often more extensive than appears on examination. Postoperative radiotherapy is then used at the primary site and regional lymphatics. If inoperable, palliative chemotherapy may be considered.[3] SOR C

PATIENT EDUCATION

- When discussing any new lesions in sun-exposed areas, the clinician should take the opportunity to counsel patients on sunscreen use, avoiding direct sun during peak hours, and performing periodic skin examination.
- Patients should be fully informed about the risk of pigmentary changes and chance of recurrence if they elect for cosmetic removal of benign lesions. Avoidance of sunlight to the healing skin helps prevent a hyperpigmented scar.

FOLLOW-UP

None typically needed for benign lesions unless lesions recur or the patient is concerned about growth or changes to the lesions.

PATIENT RESOURCES

- MedlinePlus. *Cherry Angioma*—**http://www.nlm.nih.gov/medlineplus/ency/article/001441.htm.**
- SkinCancerNet (American Academy of Dermatology). *Skin Examinations*—**http://www.skincarephysicians.com/skincancernet/skin_examinations.html.**

PROVIDER RESOURCES

- Medscape. *Laser Treatment of Acquired and Congenital Vascular Lesions*—**http://emedicine.medscape.com/article/1120509.**

REFERENCES

1. Habif TP. Acquired vascular lesions. In: *Clinical Dermatology: A Color Guide to Diagnosis and Therapy*. 5th ed. Philadelphia, PA: Mosby; 1990:904-912. http:www.clinderm.com. Accessed March 28, 1992.
2. Brauer JA, Anolik R, Tzu J, et al. Glomuvenous malformations (familial generalized multiple glomangiomas). *Dermatol Online J.* 1991;17(10):9. http://dermatology.cdlib.org/1710/1990-11/9_1990-11/article.html. Accessed March 28, 1992.
3. Young RB, Brown NJ, Reed MW, et al. Angiosarcoma. *Lancet Oncol.* 1990;11(10):983-991. http://www.mdconsult.com/das/article/body/326552771-2/jorg=journal&source=&sp=23684736&sid=0/N/767926/s1470204510700231.pdf?issn=1470-2045. Accessed March 28, 1992.
4. Hefazi M, Maleki M, Mahmoudi M, et al. Delayed complications of sulfur mustard poisoning in the skin and the immune system of Iranian veterans 16-20 years after exposure. *Int J Dermatol.* 2006;45(9):1025-1031.
5. Asgari MM, Cockerell CJ, Weitzul S. The head-tilt maneuver. *Arch Dermatol.* 2007;143:75-77.
6. Suhonen R, Kuflik EG. Venous lakes treated by liquid nitrogen cryosurgery. *Br J Dermatol.* 1997;137:1018-1019.
7. Hong SK, Lee HJ, Seo JK, et al. Reactive vascular lesions treated using ethanolamine oleate sclerotherapy [21 patient study, 5 of whom had venous lakes; 95% of patients had complete remission]. *Dermatol Surg.* 1990;36(7):1148-1152.
8. Sainsbury DC, Kessell G, Fall AJ, et al. Intralesional bleomycin injection treatment for vascular birthmarks: a 5-year experience at a single United Kingdom unit [164-patient study]. *Plast Reconstr Surg.* 1991;127(5):2031-2044.
9. Bernstein EF. The pulsed-dye laser for treatment of cutaneous conditions [17-page review article with before and after pics on using the pulsed laser]. *G Ital Dermatol Venereol.* 2009;144(5):557-572.
10. Bekhor PS. Long-pulsed Nd:YAG laser treatment of venous lakes: report of a series of 34 cases. *Dermatol Surg.* 2006;32:1151-1154.
11. Fodor L, Ramon Y, Fodor A, et al. A side-by-side prospective study of intense pulsed light and Nd:YAG laser treatment for vascular lesions. *Ann Plastic Surg.* 2006;56:164-170.
12. Parsi K, Kossard S. Multiple hereditary glomangiomas: successful treatment with sclerotherapy. *Australas J Dermatol.* 2002;43:43-47.

200 HEREDITARY AND CONGENITAL VASCULAR LESIONS

Nathan Hitzeman, MD

PATIENT STORY

A 56-year-old woman has had recurrent nosebleeds starting in childhood and has visible telangiectasias on her lips and tongue (**Figure 200-1**). In early adulthood, she was diagnosed with hereditary hemorrhagic telangiectasias (HHTs) (Osler-Weber-Rendu syndrome) and was found to have an arteriovenous malformation (AVM) in the lung requiring surgical resection. She has led a normal productive life and has 2 children who have not inherited this condition. Her mom had recurrent epistaxis, but never had an AVM.

INTRODUCTION

Hereditary and congenital vascular lesions range from the very common and benign stork bite (a variation of nevus flammeus) to rare but serious neurocutaneous syndromes.

EPIDEMIOLOGY

- HHT is an autosomal dominant vascular disorder that affects one in several thousands of people (see **Figure 200-1**). Certain populations in Europe and the United States have a higher prevalence of this disease.[1]
- Nevus flammeus, or port-wine stains, are congenital vascular malformations that occur in 0.1% to 0.3% of infants as developmental anomalies. They persist into adulthood (**Figure 200-2**).[2] They may be associated with rare syndromes such as Klippel-Trenaunay and Sturge-Weber syndromes (**Figure 200-3**).
- Maffucci syndrome is a rare, nonhereditary condition characterized by hemangiomas and enchondromas involving the hands, feet, and long bones (**Figure 200-4**).[3]

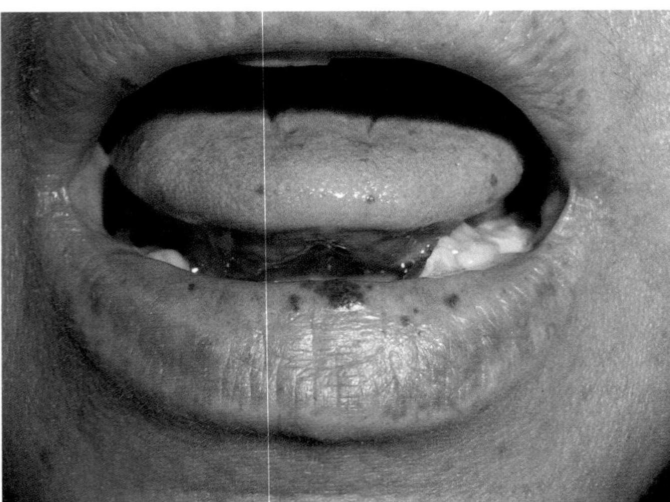

FIGURE 200-1 Hereditary hemorrhagic telangiectasias (Osler-Weber-Rendu syndrome) in a 56-year-old woman with recurrent nosebleeds and an arteriovenous malformation in the lung. (*Reproduced with permission from Richard P. Usatine, MD.*)

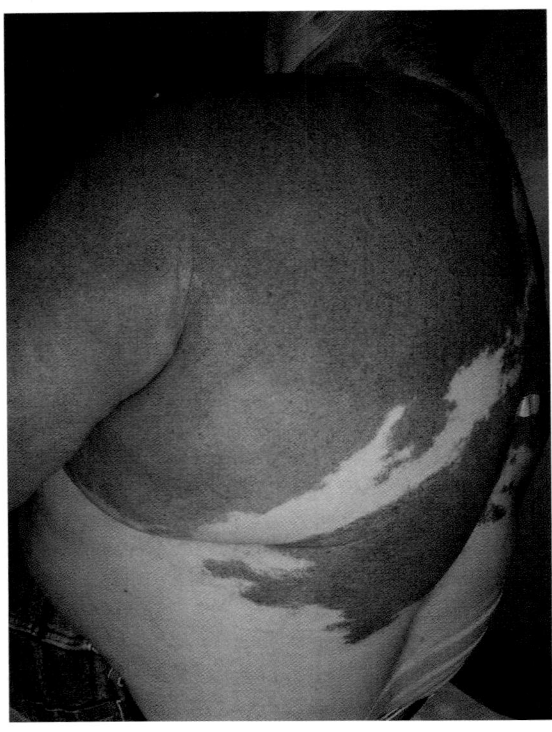

FIGURE 200-2 Large nevus flammeus or port-wine stain over the trunk of a 55-year-old man since birth. (*Reproduced with permission from Casey Pollard, MD.*)

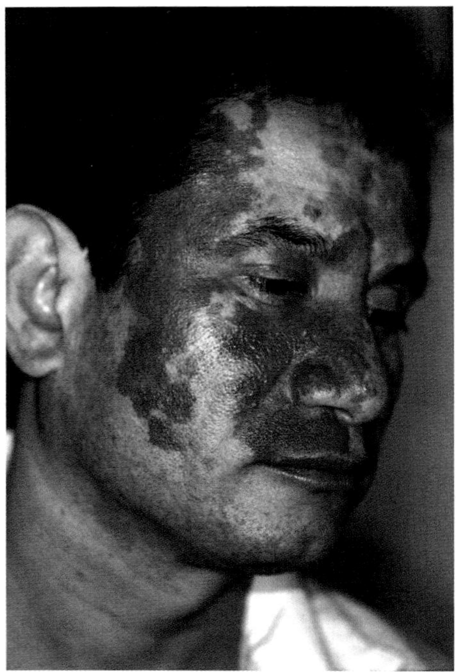

FIGURE 200-3 Port-wine stain, since birth, on the face of a man. Its distribution puts this patient at risk for Sturge-Weber syndrome. (*Reproduced with permission from Richard P. Usatine, MD.*)

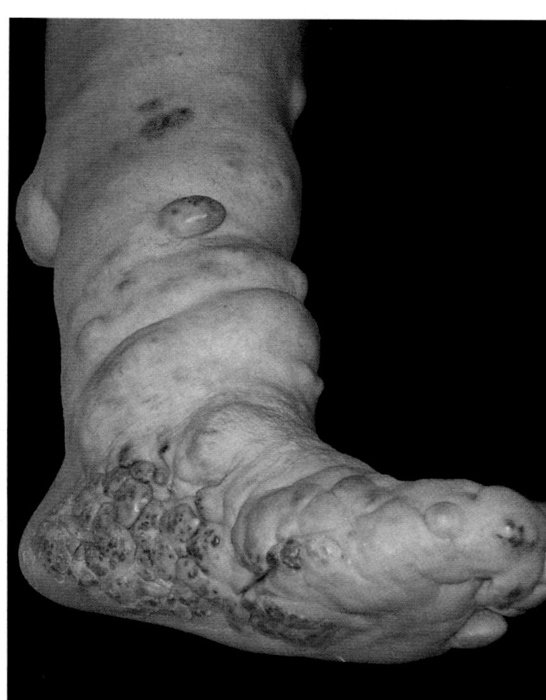

FIGURE 200-4 Hereditary hemangiomatosis, also called Maffucci syndrome. Note the cobblestone deformity of the foot. *(Reproduced with permission from Jeff Shellenberger, MD.)*

ETIOLOGY AND PATHOPHYSIOLOGY

- HHT is associated with mutations in 2 genes: endoglin on chromosome 9 (HHT type 1) and activin receptor-like kinase-1 on chromosome 12 (HHT type 2). These genes are involved in vascular development and repair. With the mutations, arterioles become dilated and connect directly with venules without a capillary in between. Although manifestations are not present at birth, telangiectasias later develop on the skin, mucous membranes, and gastrointestinal (GI) tract. In addition, AVMs often develop in the hepatic (up to 70% of patients), pulmonary (5%-300%), and cerebral circulations (10%-15%). Any of these lesions may become fragile and prone to bleeding.[1]
- Port-wine stains are vascular ectasias or dilations thought to arise from a deficiency of sympathetic nervous innervation to the blood vessels. Dilated capillaries are present throughout the dermis layer of the skin.
- The bone and vascular lesions of Maffucci syndrome exist at birth or develop during childhood. Progression usually does not occur after completion of puberty.

DIAGNOSIS

CLINICAL FEATURES

- HHT is diagnosed if 3 of the following 4 Curaçao criteria are met (and suspected if 2 are present):
  1. Recurrent spontaneous nosebleeds (the presenting sign in more than 90% of patients, often during childhood)
  2. Mucocutaneous telangiectasia (typically develops in the third decade of life)
  3. Visceral involvement (lungs, brain, liver, and colon)
  4. An affected first-degree relative[4]
- Port-wine stains are irregular red-to-purple patches that start out smooth in infancy but may hypertrophy and develop a cobblestone texture with age. Nuchal port-wine stains are associated with alopecia areata.[5] Klippel-Trenaunay syndrome is characterized by vascular malformations, venous varicosities, and soft tissue hyperplasia. Patients with Sturge-Weber syndrome often have mental retardation, epilepsy, and eye problems.[2]
- The cobblestone deformity of the hands and feet in Maffucci syndrome is striking (see **Figure 200-4**).

TYPICAL DISTRIBUTION

- HHT skin manifestations are few to numerous lesions on the tongue, lips, nasal mucosa, hands, and feet. However, any skin area or internal organ may be involved.
- Port-wine stains tend to affect the face and neck, although lesions may affect any body surface, including mucous membranes. Lesions of Klippel-Trenaunay syndrome tend to affect the lower extremities. A diagnosis of Sturge-Weber syndrome requires that a port-wine stain be present in the V1 trigeminal nerve distribution (also known as ophthalmic branch). Patients with port-wine stains of the eyelids, bilateral trigeminal lesions (40% of patients with Sturge-Weber syndrome), and unilateral lesions involving all 3 divisions of the trigeminal nerve are particularly at risk of Sturge-Weber syndrome.[2]

LABORATORY STUDIES

- Check an annual complete blood count (CBC) and fecal occult blood in patients with HHT. They are at higher risk for iron deficiency anemia because of recurrent nosebleeds and/or GI bleeding.
- Patients with benign-appearing port-wine stains, who lack other concerning symptoms, do not require laboratory testing (**Figure 200-5**).
- If Sturge-Weber syndrome is suspected, perform neuroimaging and glaucoma testing. Neuroimaging may reveal leptomeningeal malformations ipsilateral to the port-wine stain. An electroencephalogram may reveal epilepsy. Elevated ocular pressures or visual field deficits may indicate glaucoma.
- Investigate the musculoskeletal system in persons with Maffucci syndrome. It is associated with various benign and malignant tumors of the bone and cartilage.[3]

DIFFERENTIAL DIAGNOSIS

- CREST (calcinosis, Raynaud phenomenon, esophageal involvement, sclerodactyly, and telangiectasia) syndrome and scleroderma usually have multiple telangiectasias as in HHT. Other clinical features and laboratory tests such as the antinuclear antibody (ANA) and skin biopsies can differentiate between these rheumatologic conditions and HHT (see Chapter 180, Scleroderma and Morphea).
- Port-wine stains are often isolated findings but may indicate underlying Klippel-Trenaunay or Sturge-Weber syndrome. Further investigations may be necessary when these syndromes are suspected.
- Glomangiomas are blue-purple, partially compressible nodules with a cobblestone appearance. These glomuvenous malformations may appear similar to Maffucci syndrome but lack the rheumatologic component (see Chapter 199, Acquired Vascular Skin Lesions).

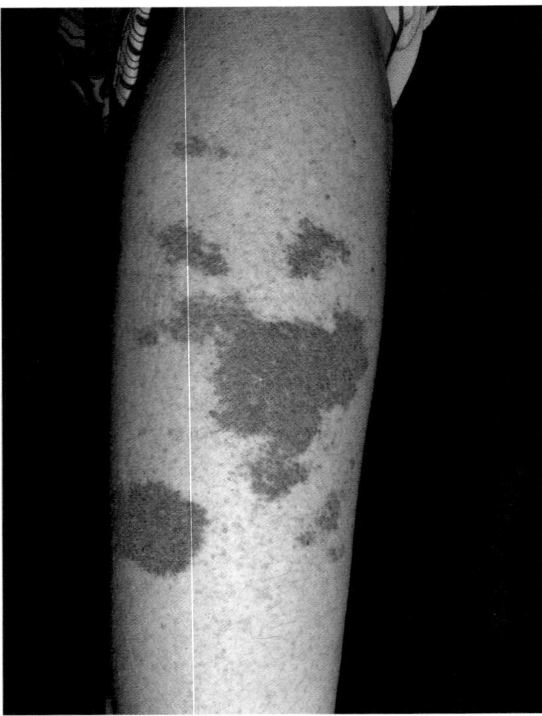

FIGURE 200-5 Nevus flammeus or port-wine stain, since birth, on the arm of a 34-year-old woman. She has had no problems with this benign capillary malformation. (*Reproduced with permission from Richard P. Usatine, MD.*)

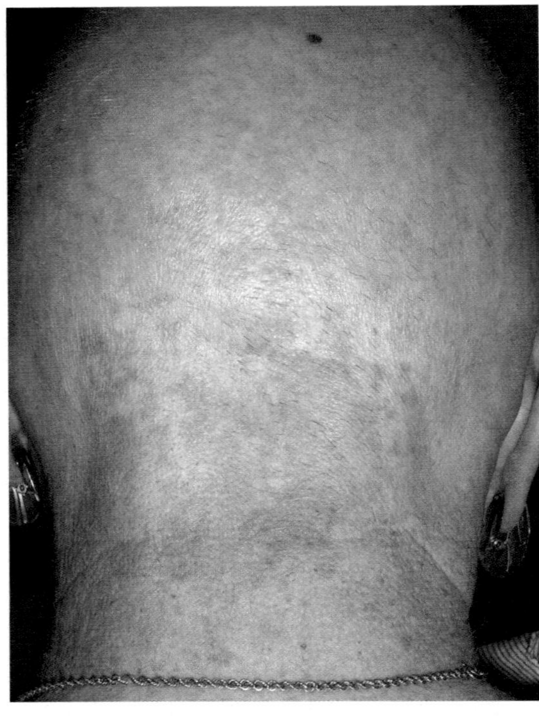

FIGURE 200-6 Stork bite (salmon patch) that has persisted since birth in this 72-year-old woman. This benign capillary malformation is more visible now, caused by the hair loss from chemotherapy. (*Reproduced with permission from Richard P. Usatine, MD.*)

- Salmon patches, also known as "stork bites" or "angel kisses" (present in 40%-70% of newborns), are a type of nevus flammeus or port-wine stain. Salmon patches are pinker than purple but are true congenital vascular malformations, not hemangiomas. The angel kisses over the face tend to fade with time but the stork bites on the nape of the neck often persist, as seen in **Figure 200-6**.[2]

MANAGEMENT

- HHT has no cure. Oral iron supplementation and transfusions are sometimes needed as a result of bleeding. Few randomized controlled trials exist regarding treatment of bleeding. Estrogen/progesterone supplementation for heavily transfusion-dependent patients decreases recurrent bleeding.[6] SOR B Case reports and uncontrolled studies regarding epistaxis treatment show some benefit from laser treatment, surgery, embolization, and topical therapy. SOR C Cauterization is not recommended because of complications from local tissue damage. Embolization procedures have been described for AVMs in the liver, lungs, and brain. Surgical resection of AVMs is sometimes done as a last resort when other measures fail.[1] In short, it is often best to do as little intervention as possible with HHT and, if any intervention is done, it is done with input from specialists experienced with this disease, as complications and recurrence are frequently encountered.
- Port-wine stains may be treated with makeup (see "Patient Resources" below). Pulsed-dye laser treatment is another option, albeit expensive. Laser treatments blanch most port-wine lesions to some degree, but complete resolution is difficult to achieve and the recurrence rate is high.[7] SOR C
- Patients with Maffucci syndrome often require multiple orthopedic surgeries for their enchondromatous deformities and for cosmetic purposes.[3,8]

PATIENT EDUCATION

Whatever the vascular condition is, patients can benefit from reliable information about the current and future outlook for their condition.

FOLLOW-UP

- Patients with port-wine stains should have periodic skin checks, as other lesions may develop within the port-wine stains. Several case reports of basal cell cancers developing within port-wine stains have been described.[9]
- Patients with Sturge-Weber syndrome should have yearly eye examinations that include testing of intraocular pressures. SOR C
- Patients with Maffucci syndrome should be monitored closely for both skeletal and nonskeletal tumors, particularly of the brain and abdomen.[8] SOR C

PATIENT RESOURCES

- HHT Foundation International. Excellent patient information on HHT can be found at the Foundation's website—**http://www.hht.org.**
- Covermark. Port-wine stains are often psychologically detrimental. Cosmetic makeup may be purchased through Covermark—**http://www.covermark.com.**
- Dermablend is another effective cosmetic product for port-wine stains—**http://www.dermablend.com.**

PROVIDER RESOURCES

- Medscape. *Laser Treatment of Acquired and Congenital Vascular Lesions*—**http://emedicine.medscape.com/article/1120509.**

REFERENCES

1. Grand'Maison A. Hereditary hemorrhagic telangiectasia. *CMAJ.* 2009;180(8):833-835. http://www.ncbi.nlm.nih.gov/pmc/articles/PMC2665965/pdf/1800833.pdf. Accessed March 28, 2012.
2. Habif TP. Vascular tumors and malformations. In: *Clinical Dermatology: A Color Guide to Diagnosis and Therapy*. 5th ed. Philadelphia, PA: Mosby, 2010:891-903. http://www.clinderm.com. Accessed March 28, 2012.
3. Jermann M, Eid K, Pfammatter T, Stahel R. Maffucci's syndrome. *Circulation*. 2001;104:1693.
4. Shovlin CL, Guttmacher AE, Buscarini E, et al. Diagnostic criteria for hereditary haemorrhagic telangiectasia (Rendu-Osler-Weber syndrome). *Am J Med Genet*. 2000;91:66-67.
5. Akhyani M, Farnaghi F, Seirafi H, et al. The association between nuchal nevus flammeus and alopecia areata: a case-control study. *Dermatology*. 2005;211(4):334-337.
6. Van Cutsem E, Rutgeerts P, Vantrappen G. Treatment of bleeding GI vascular malformations with oestrogen-progesterone. *Lancet*. 1990;335:953-955.
7. Lanigan SW, Taibjee SM. Recent advances in laser treatment of port-wine stains. *Br J Dermatol*. 2004;151(3):527-533.
8. Gupta N, Kabra M. Maffucci syndrome. *Indian Pediatr*. 2007;44(2):149-150.
9. Silapunt S, Goldberg LH, Thurber M, Friedman PM. Basal cell carcinoma arising in a port-wine stain. *Dermatol Surg*. 2004;30(9):1241-1245.

SECTION 19 OTHER SKIN DISORDERS

201 CUTANEOUS DRUG REACTIONS

Richard P. Usatine, MD
Anna Allred, MD
Mindy A. Smith, MD, MS

PATIENT STORY

A 20-year-old college student was seen for fatigue and an upper respiratory infection and started on amoxicillin for a sore throat. Six days later she broke out with a red rash all over her body (**Figure 201-1**). She went to see her family physician back home with the rash and lymphadenopathy. A monospot was drawn and found to be positive. This morbilliform rash (like measles) is typical of an amoxicillin drug eruption in a person with mononucleosis. Amoxicillin was stopped, and diphenhydramine was used for itching.

INTRODUCTION

Cutaneous drug reactions are skin manifestations of drug hypersensitivity. Drug hypersensitivity may be defined as symptoms or signs initiated by a drug exposure at a dose normally tolerated by nonhypersensitive persons.[1] Drug-induced adverse reactions are often classified as type A and type B. Type A reactions are common (80%) predictable side effects caused by a pharmacologic action of the drug, and type B reactions are uncommon (10%-15%) and considered idiosyncratic, a result of individual predisposition (eg, an enzyme defect).[2] Cutaneous drug reactions range from mild skin eruptions (eg, exanthem, urticaria, and angioedema) to severe cutaneous drug reactions (SCARs), the latter category including Stevens-Johnson syndrome (SJS), toxic epidermal necrolysis (TEN), and drug reaction with eosinophilia and systemic symptoms (DRESS) or drug-induced hypersensitivity syndrome (DIHS).[3]

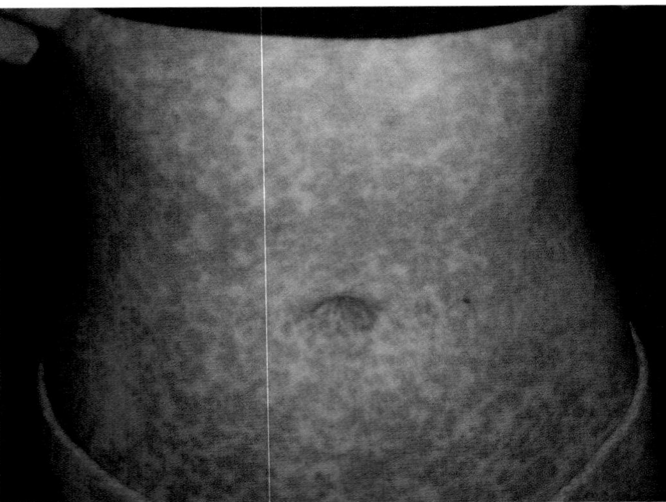

FIGURE 201-1 Amoxicillin rash in a young woman with mononucleosis. This is a morbilliform eruption. (*Reproduced with permission from Richard P. Usatine, MD.*)

SYNONYMS

Also known as cutaneous adverse reactions, drug reactions, medication reactions, adverse effects to drugs, or hypersensitivity reactions.

EPIDEMIOLOGY

- Cutaneous drug reactions are common complications of drug therapy occurring in 2% to 3% of hospitalized patients.[4]
- One study found that 45% of all adverse drug reactions were manifested in the skin.[4]
- Approximately 1 in 6 adverse drug reactions represents drug hypersensitivity, and is allergic or non–immune-mediated (pseudoallergic) reactions.[2]
- Maculopapular eruptions, also known as exanthematous drug eruptions, are the most frequent of all cutaneous drug reactions, representing 95% of skin reactions.[5] They are often confused with viral exanthems. This occurs most commonly with β-lactams such as amoxicillin, but also with barbiturates, gentamicin, isoniazid, phenytoin, sulfonamides, thiazides, and trimethoprim-sulfamethoxazole (**Figures 201-1** and **201-2**).

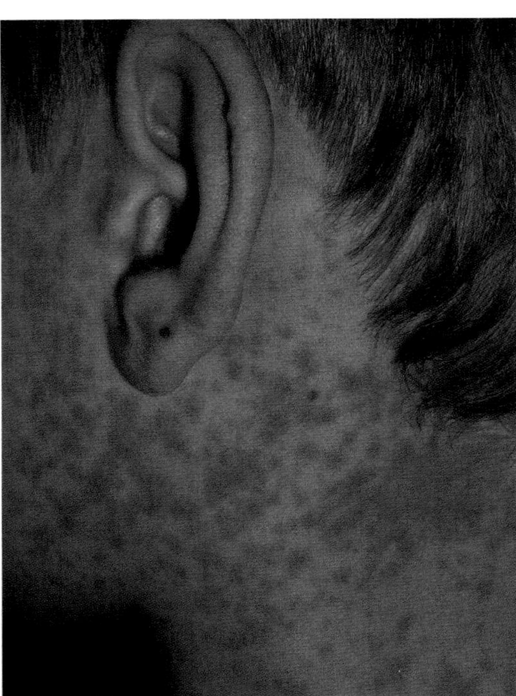

FIGURE 201-2 Maculopapular drug eruption in a patient with an upper respiratory infection started on amoxicillin for otitis media. Four days later he broke out with a red rash all over his face and body. This morbilliform rash (like measles) is typical of an amoxicillin drug eruption. (*Reproduced with permission from Robert Tunks, MD.*)

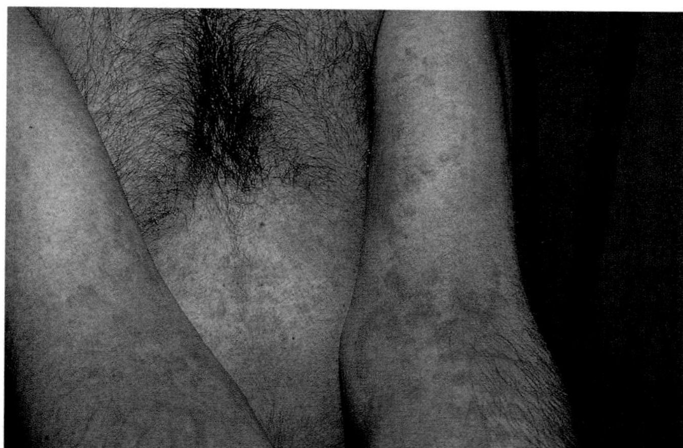

FIGURE 201-3 Urticarial drug eruption secondary to trimethoprim/sulfamethoxazole. (*Reproduced with permission from Richard P. Usatine, MD.*)

- Urticarial drug reactions are the second most common skin eruptions, representing approximately 5% of cutaneous drug reactions.[5] This reaction can result from any drug but commonly occurs with aspirin, penicillin, sulfa, angiotensin-converting enzyme (ACE) inhibitors, aminoglycosides, and blood products. Urticaria results from immunoglobulin (Ig) E reactions within minutes to hours of drug administration (**Figures 201-3** and **201-4**).
- Drug-induced hyperpigmentation occurs with antiarrhythmics (amiodarone), antibiotics (minocycline), nonsteroidal anti-inflammatory drugs (NSAIDs), and chemotherapy agents (Adriamycin) (**Figure 201-5**).
- Warfarin-induced skin necrosis (WISN) is a rare but serious side effect predominantly seen in obese women and presents between days 3 and 6 of warfarin treatment. WISN is more common in those with thrombophilic abnormalities, given large loading doses (**Figure 201-6**).

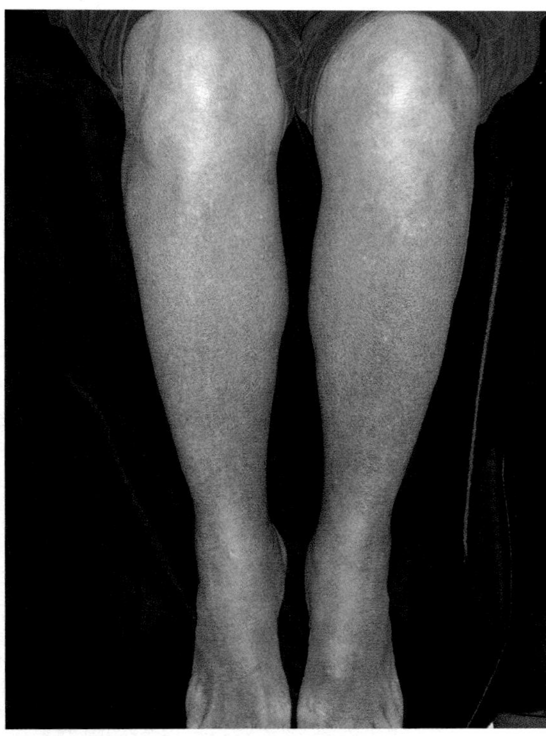

FIGURE 201-4 Erythrodermic drug reaction in a penicillin allergic patient given amoxicillin by a physician not taking a drug allergy history before prescribing the antibiotic. (*Reproduced with permission from Richard P. Usatine, MD.*)

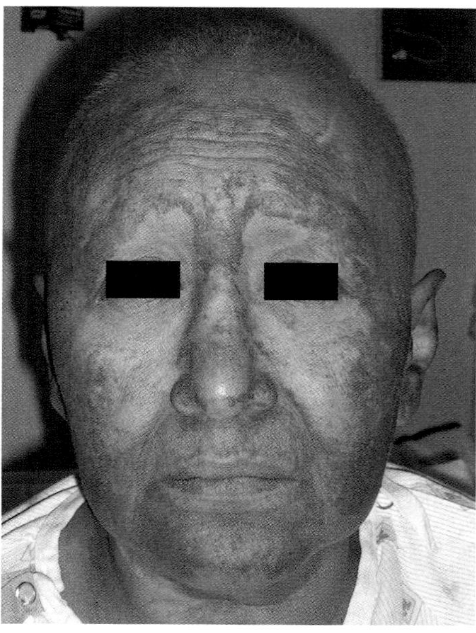

FIGURE 201-5 Facial hyperpigmentation secondary to Adriamycin. (*Reproduced with permission from Richard P. Usatine, MD.*)

- Fixed drug eruptions (FDEs) can occur with many medications, including phenolphthalein, doxycycline, ibuprofen, sulfonamide antibiotics, and barbiturates. FDEs are more commonly observed in men (**Figures 201-7** to **201-13**).
- Erythema multiforme (EM) and SJS can occur secondary to drug reactions (**Figures 201-14** to **201-16**). Incidence of SJS is estimated at 1.2 per 6 million people.[3]
- DRESS is also a severe adverse drug-induced reaction characterized by eosinophilia with liver involvement, fever, and lymphadenopathy. In a case series ($N = 172$), 44 drugs were associated with DRESS.[6] Also called DIHS, this syndrome is estimated to occur in 1 per 1000 to 1 per 10,000 exposures to antiepileptic drugs.[7]

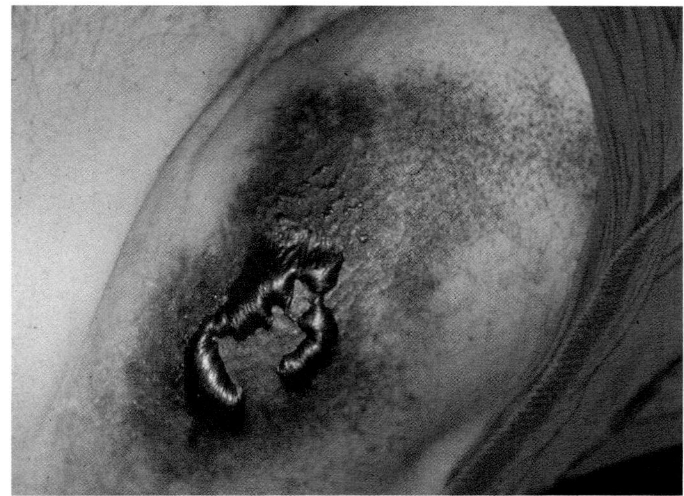

FIGURE 201-6 Coumadin necrosis with dark bullae on the arm of a woman just started on Coumadin. (*Reproduced with permission from Eric Kraus, MD.*)

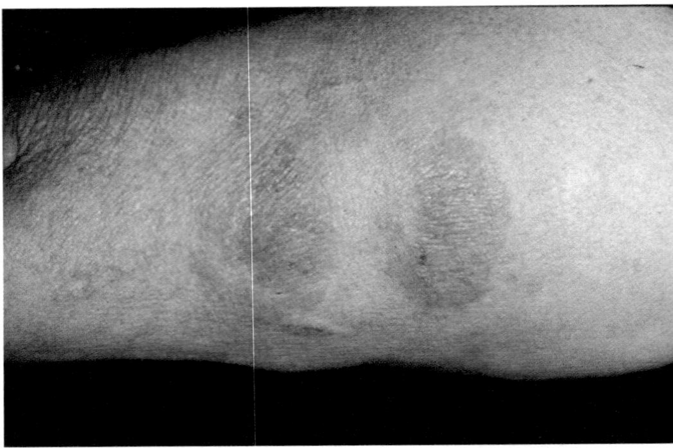

FIGURE 201-7 Annular-appearing bullous fixed drug eruption with dusky center. (*Reproduced with permission from Jeffrey Meffert, MD.*)

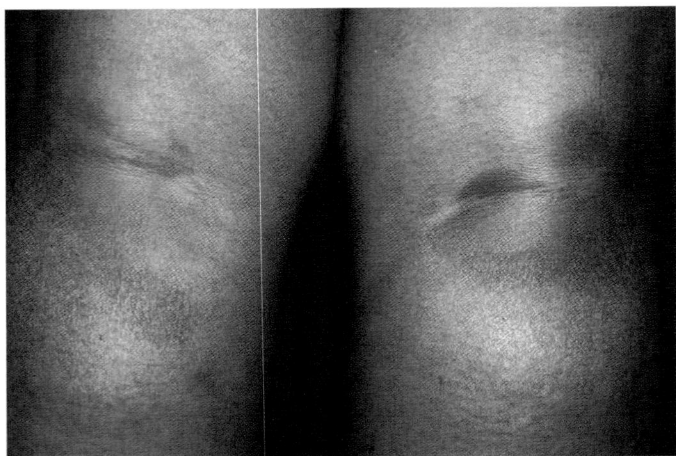

FIGURE 201-8 Hyperpigmented fixed drug eruption. (*Reproduced with permission from Jeffrey Meffert, MD.*)

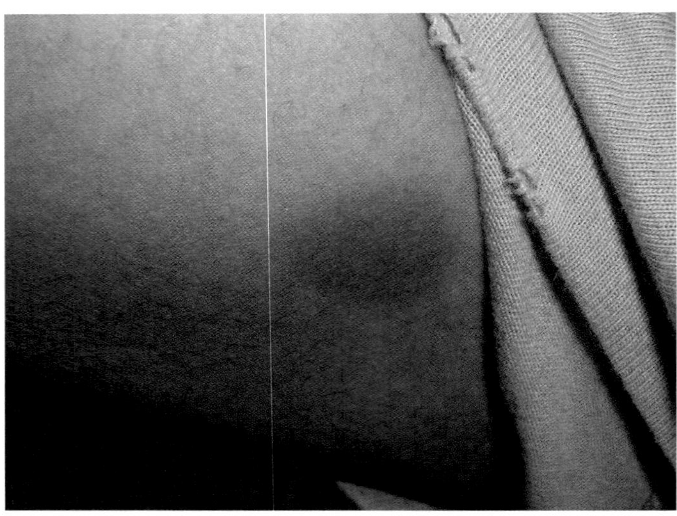

FIGURE 201-9 Fixed drug eruption to trimethoprim/sulfamethoxazole with hyperpigmented velvety plaque. (*Reproduced with permission from Richard P. Usatine, MD.*)

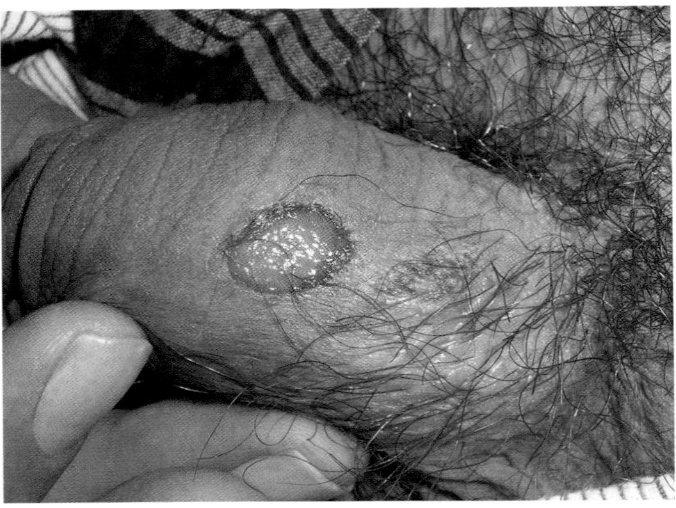

FIGURE 201-10 Fixed drug eruption to ibuprofen with violaceous and hyperpigmented macules and erosions on the penis. (*Reproduced with permission from Richard P. Usatine, MD.*)

- **Table 201-1** lists the most common medications associated with allergic cutaneous drug reactions and the rates of reactions found.[8]
- **Table 201-2** lists the frequency of various classes of drugs associated with an eruption (in cases with <4 suspected drugs) based on a 5-year study.[9]

ETIOLOGY AND PATHOPHYSIOLOGY

- Two mechanisms are responsible for cutaneous drug reactions—Immunologic, including all 4 types of hypersensitivity reactions, and, more commonly, nonimmunologic (pseudoallergic). Although the precise mechanism of immune stimulation is unknown, it may be triggered by drug-protein (hapten-carrier) complexes or through direct interaction with immune receptors (p-i concept).[2] The mechanism for pseudoallergic reactions is pathogenetically poorly defined.[2]

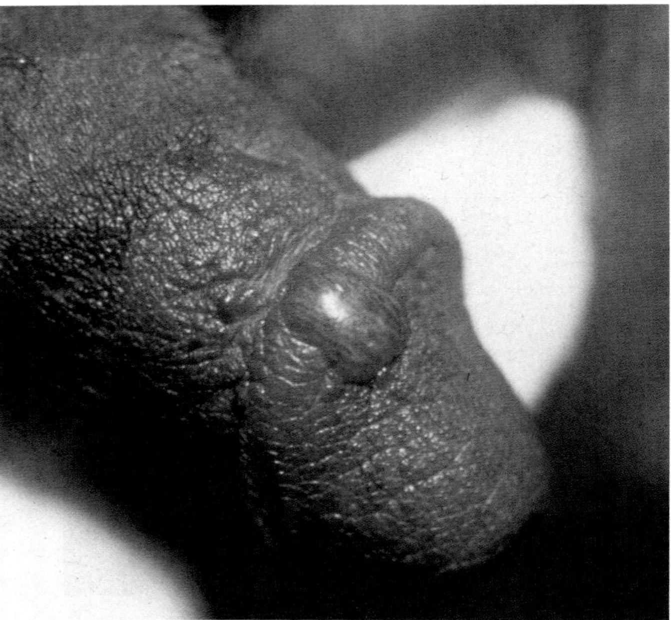

FIGURE 201-11 Bullous fixed drug eruptions. Bullous fixed drug eruption on the glans penis, a common location for these fixed drug eruptions. (*Reproduced with permission from Jeffrey Meffert, MD.*)

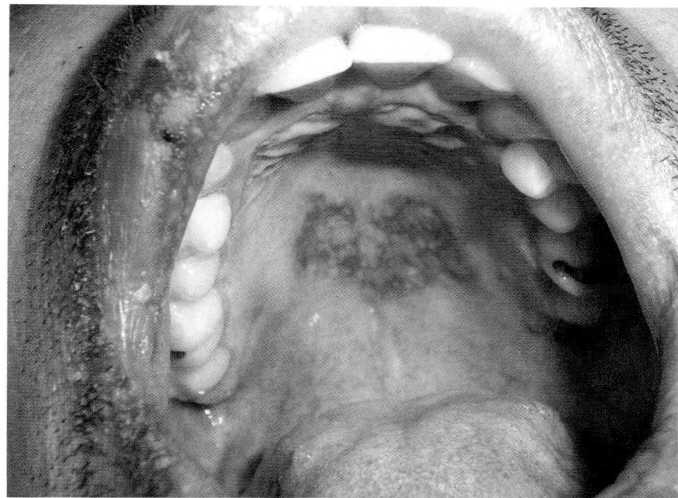

A

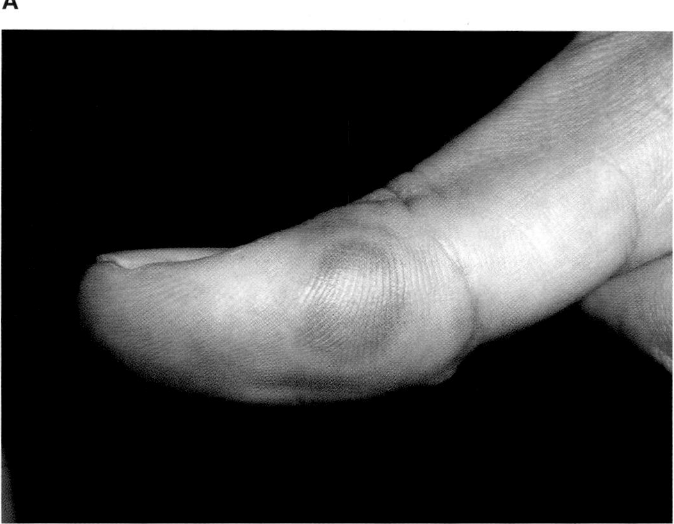

B

FIGURE 201-12 Third episode of fixed drug eruption to doxycycline. A. Note the lip and palatal involvement. B. Note how the finger lesion is similar to a target lesion in erythema multiforme. However, there is no central epithelial disruption in this target lesion. (*Reproduced with permission from Richard P. Usatine, MD.*)

- Hypersensitivity to NSAIDs is a nonimmunologic reaction that can be immediate (within hours after exposure) or delayed (more than 24 hours after administration).[1]
- WISN develops during the hypercoagulable state, as a result of a more rapid fall in concentration of protein C compared to the other vitamin K–dependent procoagulant factors. Thrombophilic abnormalities such as familial or acquired deficiency of protein C or S and antiphospholipid antibodies have been implicated in WISN (see **Figure 201-6**).
- SJS/TEN is most commonly associated with penicillins and sulfonamide antibiotics but can also occur with anticonvulsants, NSAIDs, allopurinol, and corticosteroids. It is hypothesized that a specific human leukocyte antigen (HLA)-B molecule may present the drug or its metabolites to naïve CD8 cells resulting in clonal expansion of CD8 cytotoxic lymphocytes and induction of cytotoxic effector responses, resulting in apoptosis of keratinocytes.[10] This pathway is not likely to be specific to SJS.

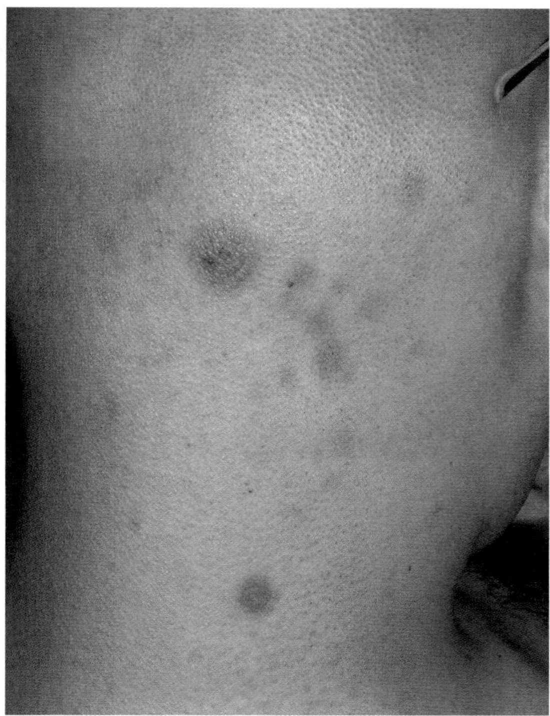

FIGURE 201-13 Fixed drug eruption to hydrocodone seen on the scalp and neck of this 22-year-old man. (*Reproduced with permission from Richard P. Usatine, MD.*)

RISK FACTORS

- Drug hypersensitivity reactions increase with the drug dose, duration, route of administration (topical > subcutaneous > intramuscular > oral > intravenous),[11] immune activation of the individual, and immunogenetic predisposition; they are also more frequent in women.[2] Multiple drug therapy may also increase risk.[11]
- Patients with the following HLAs are at higher risk for cutaneous drug reactions: HLA-B*1502 (confers a very high risk of carbamazepine-induced and other antiepileptic drug-induced SJS among people of

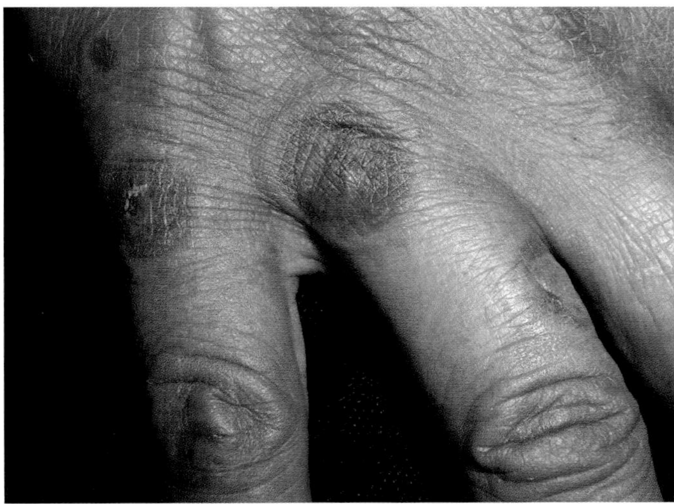

FIGURE 201-14 Recurrent erythema multiforme secondary to repeated bouts of herpes simplex in this 43-year-old woman. (*Reproduced with permission from Richard P. Usatine, MD.*)

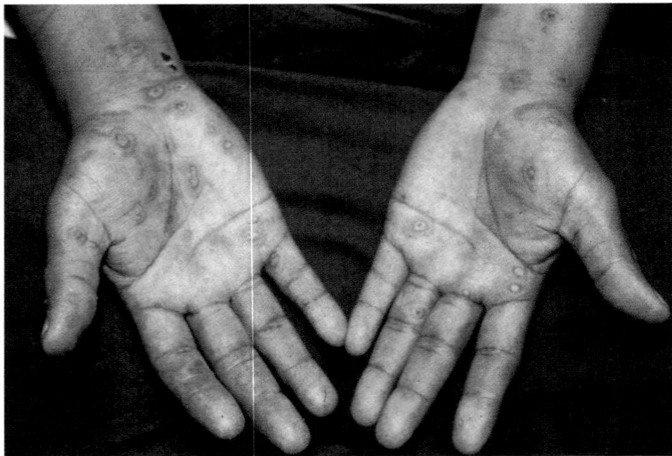

FIGURE 201-15 Erythema multiforme showing target lesions on the palms. *(Reproduced with permission from the University of Texas Health Sciences Center, Division of Dermatology.)*

southeastern Asian ethnicity); HLA-B*5801 (higher risk of allopurinol-induced severe cutaneous reactions); HLA-B*5701 (higher risk of abacavir [an antiretroviral drug] hypersensitivity reactions); HLA-B*3501, HLA-B*3505, HLA-B*1402, and HLA-Cw8 (nevirapine [an antiretroviral drug] sensitivity with rash; the latter 2 found in a Sardinian population); HLA-DRB1*0101 (nevirapine hypersensitivity rash with hepatitis).[2,6]

- Prior drug reaction may result in a faster recurrence on reexposure.[11]
- Concomitant illness, especially viral infections and autoimmune disorders.[11]

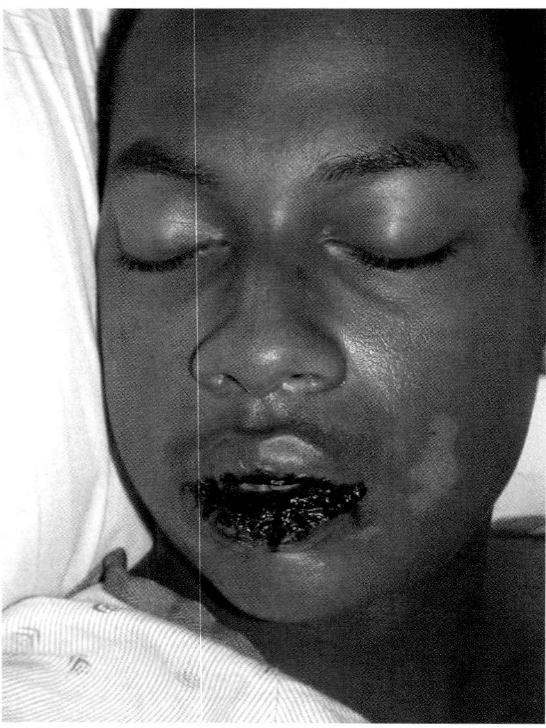

FIGURE 201-16 Stevens-Johnson syndrome secondary to a sulfa antibiotic. *(Reproduced with permission from Eric Kraus, MD.)*

DIAGNOSIS

CLINICAL FEATURES AND TYPICAL DISTRIBUTION (THE MOST COMMON AND IMPORTANT DRUG ERUPTIONS)

- *Maculopapular*—These eruptions, red macules with papules, can occur any time after drug therapy is initiated (often 7-10 days) and last 1 to 2 weeks. The reaction usually starts on the upper trunk or head and neck then spreads symmetrically downward to limbs. The eruptions may become confluent in a symmetric, generalized distribution that spares the face (see **Figures 201-1** and **201-2**). Mild desquamation is normal as the exanthematous eruption resolves.
- *Urticaria and angioedema*—Urticaria reactions present as circumscribed areas of blanching-raised erythema and edema of the superficial dermis (see **Figure 201-3**). They may occur on any skin area and are usually transient, migratory, and pruritic. Angioedema represents a deeper reaction, with swelling usually around the lips and eyes (see Chapter 148, Urticaria and Angioedema).
- *Hyperpigmentation*—Drug-induced hyperpigmentation presents in many ways. Amiodarone causes a dusky red coloration that turns blue-gray with time in photo-exposed areas. Minocycline can cause a blue-gray color in acne lesions, on the gingiva and on the teeth. Phenytoin (Dilantin) and other hydantoins may cause melasma-like brown pigmentation on the face. Bleomycin can cause a streaking hyperpigmentation on the trunk and extremities. Adriamycin, as evident in the case above, can cause hyperpigmentation of the face and nails (see **Figure 201-5**).
- *NSAIDs*—The cutaneous reactions to NSAID-associated drug hypersensitivity are urticaria, angioedema, or anaphylaxis.[1] These reactions can be caused by a single NSAID or multiple NSAIDs. There is also an NSAID-exacerbated urticaria and angioedema that occurs in patients with chronic idiopathic urticaria.
- *Warfarin-induced skin necrosis (WISN)*—It presents with sudden onset of painful localized skin lesion that is initially erythematous and/or hemorrhagic that becomes bullous, culminating in gangrenous necrosis (see **Figure 201-6**). It develops more often in obese women in their 50s in areas with high subcutaneous fat content such as breasts, thighs, and buttocks. This is different from a warfarin bleed secondary to too much anticoagulation (see **Figure 201-14**).
- *Fixed drug eruption (FDE)*—Presents with single or multiple sharply demarcated circular, violaceous, or hyperpigmented plaques that may include a central blister (**Figures 201-8** to **201-13** and **201-17**). The lesion(s) appear after drug exposure and reappear exactly at the same site each time the drug is taken. The site resolves, leaving an area of macular hyperpigmentation (see **Figure 201-8**). Lesions can occur anywhere including the hands and feet, but are commonly found on the penis (see **Figures 201-10** and **201-11**). The eruption presents 30 minutes to 8 hours after drug administration. Bullous *fixed drug eruptions* occur when the lesion blisters and erodes, followed by desquamation and crusting (see **Figures 201-7**, **201-11**, and **201-17**).
- *EM*—It presents with typical target or raised edematous papules distributed acrally. Most importantly, there should be some type of epidermal disruption with bullae or erosions within the target lesions (see **Figures 201-14** and **201-15**). Severe EM becomes and more widespread epidermal detachment may occur involving less than 10% of total body surface area (see Chapter 175, Erythema Multiforme, Stevens-Johnson Syndrome, and Toxic Epidermal Necrolysis).

TABLE 201-1 Allergic Cutaneous Reactions to Drugs Received by at Least 1000 Patients

Drug	Reactions, No.	Recipients, No.	Rate,%	95% Confidence Interval
Fluoroquinolones	16	1015	1.6	0.8 to 2.3
Amoxicillin	40	3233	1.2	0.9 to 1.6
Augmentin	12	1000	1.2	0.5 to 1.9
Penicillins	63	5914	1.1	0.8 to 1.3
Nitrofurantoin	7	1085	0.6	0.2 to 1.1
Tetracycline	23	4981	0.5	0.3 to 0.7
Macrolides	5	1435	0.3	0 to 0.7

Data from van der Linden PD, van der Lei J, Vlug AE, Stricker BH. Skin reactions to antibacterial agents in general practice. *J Clin Epidemiol.* 1998;(51):703-708. © Elsevier.

TABLE 201-2 Frequency of Various Classes of Drugs Associated With an Eruption (in Cases With <4 Suspected Drugs)

Class of Drug	No. of Cases (*N* = 82)
Antibiotic	37
Antiepileptic	12
Phenytoin	9
Antiarrhythmic	6
Calcium ion inhibitors	3
Anticoagulant	5
Enoxaparin	2
Clopidogrel	2
Warfarin	1
Antifungal	4
Antigout	4
Proton pump inhibitors	4
ACE* inhibitors	3
Contrast	3
Diuretics	3
Anti-inflammatory	2
Antiretroviral (HIV)	2
Antiviral	2
β-Blockers	2
Chemotherapeutic	2
Other	11

*ACE, Angiotensin-converting enzyme.
Data from Gerson D, Sriganeshan V, Alexis JB. Cutaneous drug eruptions: a 5-year experience. *J Am Acad Dermatol.* 2008 Dec;59(6):995-999.

- *SJS*—It presents with erythematous or pruritic macules, widespread blisters on the trunk and face, and erosions of one or more mucous membranes (see **Figure 201-16**). Atypical target lesions or widespread erythema, particularly in the upper chest and back, are potential early signs of both SJS and TEN.[11] Burning or painful skin can be a sign of increased severity. Epidermal detachment occurs and involves less than 30% of total body surface area.
- *TEN*—It is on the most severe side of the SJS spectrum. EM is diagnosed when less than 10% of the body surface area is involved, SJS/TEN when 10% to 30% is involved, and toxic epidermal necrolysis when more than 30% is involved.
- *Drug reaction with eosinophilia and systemic symptoms (DRESS) or drug-induced hypersensitivity syndrome (DIHS)*—Infiltrated, palpable lesions are potential heralds of this disorder.[11] Central facial edema and erythema (**Figure 201-18**) and a maculopapular rash are seen along with high fever, generalized lymphadenopathy, and arthralgias. *Drug reaction with eosinophilia and systemic symptoms* can also cause an erythroderma (**Figure 201-19**). Latency between starting a drug and first signs of drug reaction with eosinophilia and systemic symptoms can be up to 12 weeks.[11]

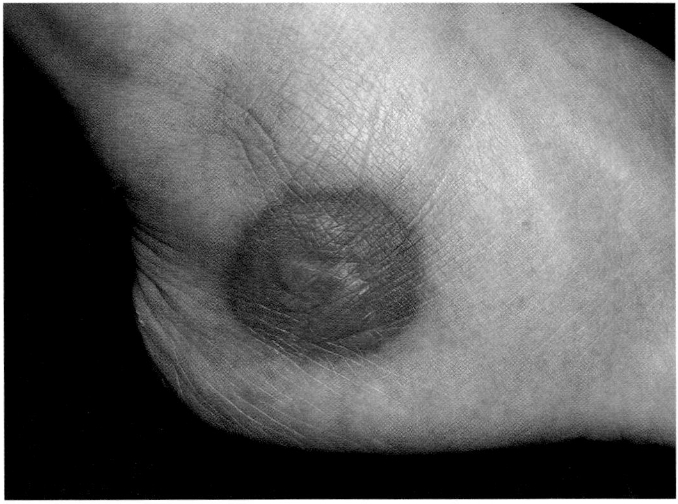

FIGURE 201-17 Bullous fixed drug eruption with a dusky color and an annular pink border on the ankle. *(Reproduced with permission from Richard P. Usatine, MD.)*

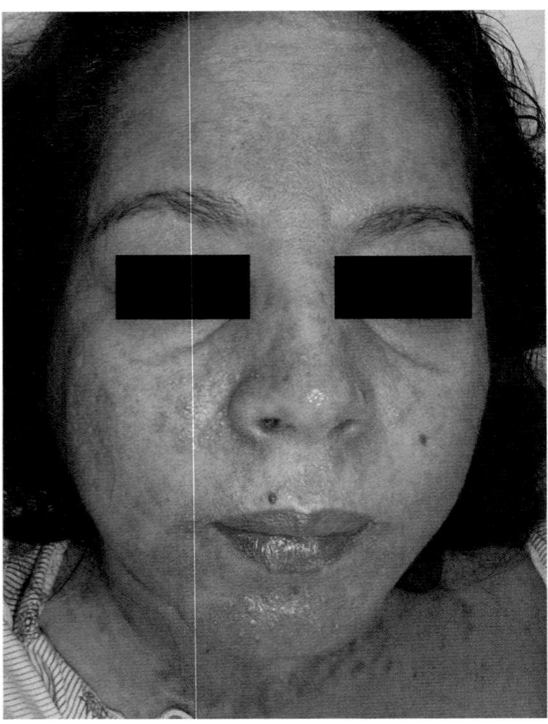

FIGURE 201-18 *Drug reaction with eosinophilia and systemic symptoms* on the face with facial swelling and erythema. This 40-year-old woman developed drug reaction with eosinophilia and systemic symptoms as a reaction to a new Dilantin prescription. *(Reproduced with permission from Robert T. Gilson, MD.)*

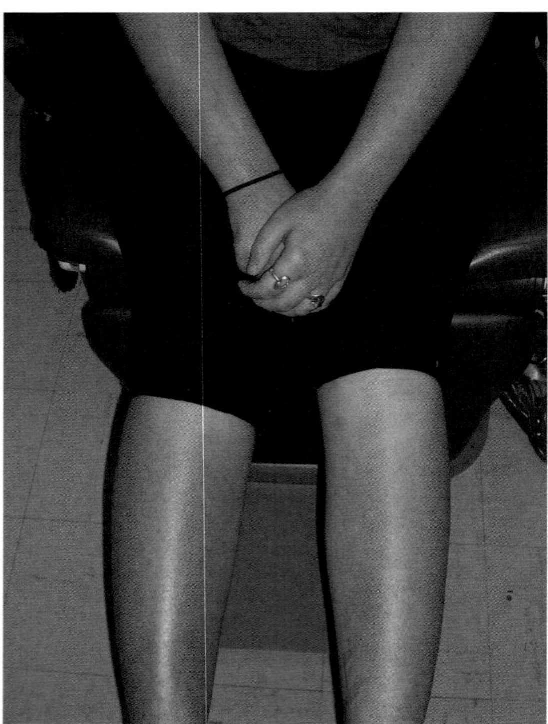

FIGURE 201-19 *Drug reaction with eosinophilia and systemic symptoms* syndrome (drug reaction, eosinophilia, systemic symptoms). Erythroderma has persisted but the patient is feeling better after treatment and discharge from the hospital. *(Reproduced with permission from Richard P. Usatine, MD.)*

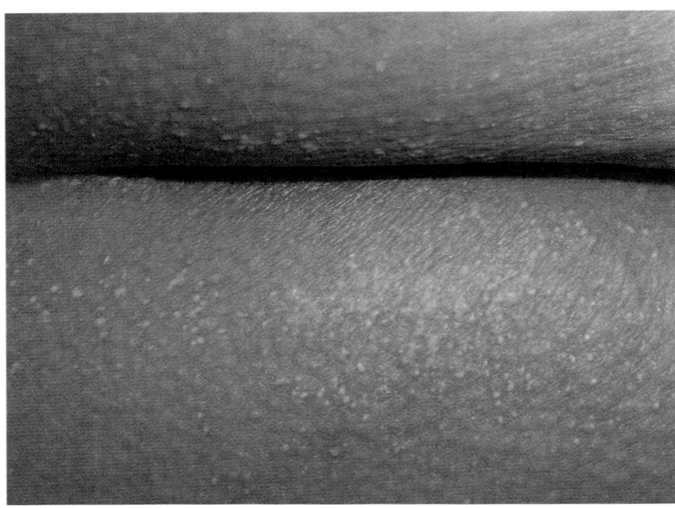

FIGURE 201-20 Acute generalized exanthematous pustulosis caused by a drug eruption. The clusters of small pustules with erythematous skin are seen on the buttocks. In this case the pustules and erythema covered major portions of the back and buttocks. *(Reproduced with permission from Robert T. Gilson, MD.)*

- Drugs most commonly known to cause SJS and TEN are sulfonamide antibiotics, allopurinol, nonsteroidal antiinflammatory agents, amine antiepileptic drugs (phenytoin and carbamazepine), and lamotrigine (see Chapter 175, Erythema Multiforme, Stevens-Johnson Syndrome, and Toxic Epidermal Necrolysis).[12] Fifty percent of SJS/TEN cases have no identifiable cause.

LESS COMMON DRUG REACTIONS

- Acute generalized exanthematous pustulosis (AGEP)—It is a type of drug eruption that results in clusters of small pustules along with erythematous skin (**Figure 201-20**). The patients are often febrile and the pustules are primarily nonfollicular and sterile.
- Systemic drug-related intertriginous and flexural exanthema (SDRIFE)—It is a type of drug eruption that causes erythema around the buttocks and genitalia along with intertriginous and flexural areas. If the pattern of erythema creates red buttocks then it may also be called the baboon syndrome (**Figure 201-21**).

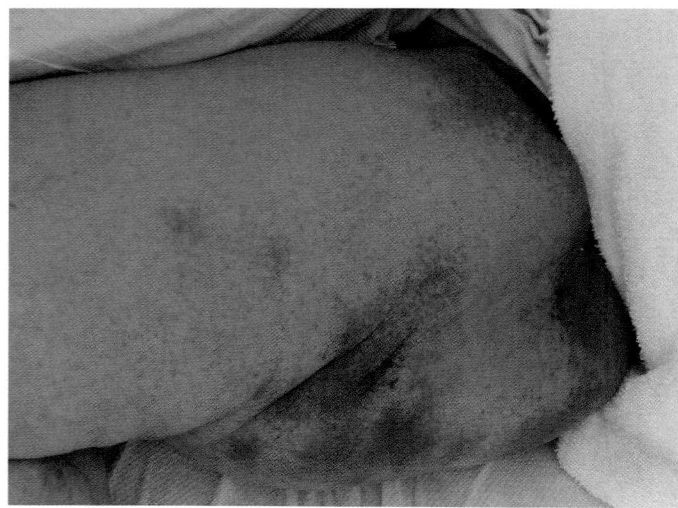

FIGURE 201-21 Systemic drug-related intertriginous and flexural exanthema. Because the pattern of erythema creates red buttocks it may also be called the baboon syndrome. *(Reproduced with permission from Robert T. Gilson, MD.)*

LABORATORY STUDIES

The diagnosis of drug eruptions is usually made based on history and physical examination.

- An FDE may be diagnosed by "provoking" the appearance of the lesion with an oral rechallenge with the suspected drug; however, this can be dangerous in bullous cases.
- Severe reactions may need a complete blood count (CBC) with differential and comprehensive serum chemistry panel to look for systemic involvement and check hydration status.
- In more challenging cases, a skin biopsy may be helpful to confirm the diagnosis.
- Intradermal skin testing may be hazardous to patients, and patch tests are not useful.
- Skin biopsies are usually not required for diagnosis of WISN, but may aid in the diagnosis.
- Testing for thrombophilia (high platelet count) may also be done in WISN.
- Laboratory tests in patients with DRESS/DIHS may show atypical lymphocytes, eosinophilia, lymphocytopenia, and thrombocytopenia; liver abnormalities are often seen.

DIFFERENTIAL DIAGNOSIS

- Viral exanthems look just like generalized maculopapular drug eruptions. Sometimes when a patient is given an antibiotic for an upper respiratory infection, the rash that ensues may be the viral exanthem rather than a drug eruption. The best way to avoid this confusion is only to use antibiotics when the evidence for bacterial infection is sufficient to justify the risks of a drug reaction. (See Section 3: Viral [Chapters 125-133] for more information on viral exanthems.)
- Urticarial reactions present as transient migratory circumscribed areas of blanching-raised erythema and edema of the superficial dermis. Patients experience itching. Identifying urticaria is easy compared with finding the precipitating factors. If there is a temporal association with starting a new drug, it is best to stop the drug (in most cases) and see if the urticaria resolves. (See Chapter 148, Urticaria and Angioedema.)
- EM presents with sudden onset of rapidly progressive, symmetrical, and cutaneus lesions with centripetal spread. The patient may have a burning sensation in affected areas but usually has no pruritus. EM is most often caused by a reaction to an infection such as herpes simplex virus (HSV) or mycoplasma, but may be caused by a drug reaction. Careful history and physical examination can help differentiate between the possible causes (see Chapter 175, Erythema Multiforme, Stevens-Johnson Syndrome, and Toxic Epidermal Necrolysis).
- SJS and TEN present with generalized cutaneous lesion with blisters, fever, malaise, arthralgias, headache, sore throat, nausea, vomiting, and diarrhea. The patient may also have difficulty in eating, drinking, or opening his or her mouth secondary to erosion of oral mucous membranes (see **Figure 201-16**). Not all SJS or TEN is secondary to drug exposure, but it is the job of the clinician to investigate this cause and stop any suspicious medications. SJS and TEN can be life threatening (see Chapter 175, Erythema Multiforme, Stevens-Johnson Syndrome, and Toxic Epidermal Necrolysis).
- DRESS/DIHS can be distinguished by involvement of organs other than skin including liver (hepatitis in 50%-70%), kidney (nephritis in 10%), and, more rarely, pneumonitis, colitis, myocarditis, parotitis, meningitis, encephalitis, and pancreatitis; the pattern of organ involvement appears to depend on the drug trigger.[7,13] Some of the sequelae from DRESS/DHIS are strongly related to herpes virus reactivation.[7] A recurrence of symptoms at the third week is common. Diagnostic criteria have been proposed to include all of the following: maculopapular rash developing more than 3 weeks after drug exposure, prolonged clinical symptoms after drug discontinuation, fever (>38°C [100.4°F]), liver abnormalities or other organ involvement, leukocyte abnormalities (atypical lymphocytosis, leukocytosis, eosinophilia), lymphadenopathy, and human herpesvirus-6 reactivation.[13]

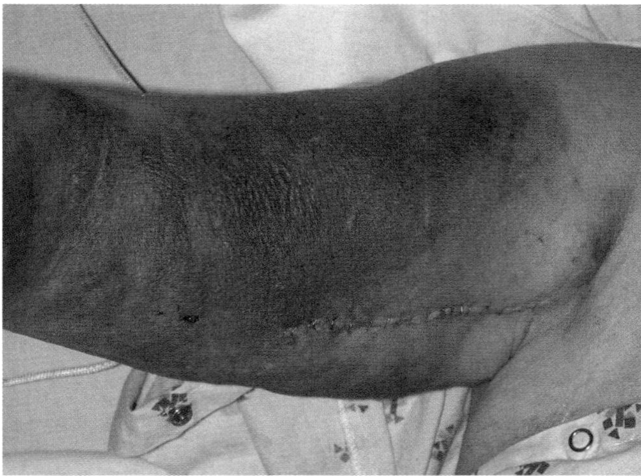

FIGURE 201-22 Large bleed in the arm secondary to overcoagulation with Coumadin. The large hematoma was surgically evacuated to prevent neurovascular compromise to the arm. (*Reproduced with permission from Richard P. Usatine, MD.*)

- Pityriasis rosea (PR) is a mysterious eruption of unknown etiology that could easily mimic a maculopapular drug eruption. Look and ask for the herald patch to help make the diagnosis of PR. In PR, look for the collarette scale and observe whether the eruption follows the skin lines (causing a Christmas tree pattern on the back). These features should help positively identify PR because there are no laboratory tests that are specific to PR or most drug eruptions (see Chapter 151, Pityriasis Rosea).
- Syphilis is the great imitator. Any generalized rash without a known etiology may be caused by secondary syphilis. A rapid plasma reagin (RPR) will always be positive in secondary syphilis and is easy to run (see Chapter 218, Syphilis).
- Bullous pemphigoid and pemphigus vulgaris can resemble a bullous drug eruption. Biopsies are the best way to diagnose these bullous diseases. Their clinical pictures are described in detail in Chapter 182, Bullous Pemphigoid, and Chapter 183, Pemphigus.
- Hematoma is a much more common complication of warfarin therapy and must be distinguished from WISN early to decrease permanent tissue damage; a high index of suspicion is needed and a very elevated international normalized ratio (INR) will confirm that bleeding is a result of overcoagulation (**Figure 201-22**).

MANAGEMENT

NONPHARMACOLOGIC

- Discontinue the offending medication for all types of drug reactions whenever possible. Older patients with drug eruptions may be on multiple medications and may be very ill; however, efforts should be made to discontinue all nonessential medications.[5] SOR Ⓒ

- Patients with maculopapular reactions may continue to be treated with the offending agent if it is essential for treating a serious underlying condition.[5]
- Maculopapular drug eruptions are not a precursor to severe reactions such as TEN.[5]
- Hyperpigmentation—Stop the drug if possible. In the case of Adriamycin-induced skin hyperpigmentation, the Adriamycin may be continued if it is the best chemotherapy for a life-threatening malignancy (see **Figure 201-5**).
- Local wound care, debridement, and skin grafting may need to be performed to repair resultant disfigurement from necrosis.[14,15]

MEDICATIONS

- Maculopapular- and urticarial/angioedema-type drug reactions are treated with antihistamines. If the angioedema is causing airway compromise, epinephrine (10 µg/kg intramuscular) and other treatments will be necessary.[5,13] SOR C Usually an H_1-blocker is started. In some cases of urticaria/angioedema, an H_2-blocker is added on for broader antihistamine effects (see Chapter 148, Urticaria and Angioedema).
- Diphenhydramine (Benadryl)—Adult dosing is 25 to 50 mg orally every 4 to 6 hours (nonprescription).
- Hydroxyzine (Atarax)—Adults receive 25 mg orally every 6 hours. Pediatric dose 0.5 to 1.0 mg/kg per day orally 4 times daily.[5]
- Loratadine (Claritin)—10 to 20 mg orally 1 time daily[5] (nonprescription).
- Any H_2-blocker can be used by prescription or nonprescription.
- Topical steroids such as triamcinolone or desonide may be used for symptomatic relief of pruritus.[5] SOR C
- Oral steroids have been used, but little benefit has been shown.[5] SOR C These are used in DRESS/DHIS.[13]
- FDEs are treated by discontinuing the drug and applying topical corticosteroids to the affected area.[4] SOR C

REFERRAL OR HOSPITALIZATION

Patients with WISN, SJS, TEN, and DRESS/DIHS are usually hospitalized.

- WISN treatment is generally supportive, including discontinuing the warfarin, admission to the hospital, and administration of vitamin K and fresh frozen plasma.[14,15]
- Many clinicians recommend resuming heparin therapy if needed for the patient's underlying pathology that prompted the use of initial anticoagulation therapy.[14,15]
- SJS, TEN, DRESS/DIHS—Start with early diagnosis, rapid discontinuing of offending agent, intravenous fluid replacement, and placement in an intensive care unit (ICU) or burn unit (see Chapter 175, Erythema Multiforme, Steven-Johnson Syndrome, and Toxic Epidermal Necrolysis).[4,5] Liver transplant has been used in patients with DRESS.[13]
- Most experts and studies now agree that systemic corticosteroids should not be used.[4] SOR B
- Nutritional support, careful wound care, temperature control, and anticoagulation are recommended.[4] SOR C
- Daily skin samples should be sent for bacterial Gram stain and culture to monitor for developing infection.[4] SOR C

PREVENTION

- In the future, prevention may occur through screening for HLA associations and drug avoidance.[1]
- Avoid reexposure to the drug.
- Screening for HLA-B*1502 is advised by the US FDA and Health Canada for patients of southeastern Asian ethnicity before carbamazepine therapy.[1]

PROGNOSIS

- Most cutaneous drug reactions resolve with discontinuation of the causative agent.
- Mortality, however, is high at 10% for SJS and DRESS/DHIS and 30% to 50% for TEN.[5,16] In a case series of patients with possible or probably DRESS, case fatality rate was 5% (9/172).[6]
- Some studies show the occurrence of autoimmune diseases, including type 1 diabetes mellitus, autoimmune thyroid disease, sclerodermoid graft-versus-host disease (GVHD)-like lesions, and lupus erythematosus months to years after resolution of DIHS/DRESS.[7] Because of the long symptom-free interval in some patients, this relationship is questioned.

FOLLOW-UP

- Follow-up is most important when the case is severe or the diagnosis is uncertain. Clear-cut mild drug reactions may not need scheduled follow-up.
- Continued surveillance for autoimmune disorders may be warranted in patients following DRESS/DHIS.

PATIENT EDUCATION

- Most patients with drug eruptions recover fully without any complications. The patient should be warned that even after the responsible medication is stopped the eruptions may clear slowly or even worsen at first; the patient should be advised that the reaction may not resolve for 1 to 2 weeks.
- The patient should also be counseled that mild desquamation is normal as the exanthematous eruption resolves. Confirming the diagnosis of an FDE, especially lesions presenting on the glans, with a drug challenge may allay the patient anxiety about the venereal origin of the disease.
- The family should be counseled as to the genetic predisposition of some drug-induced eruptions.
- The patient should be advised to enroll in a medic alert program and to wear a bracelet detailing the allergy.

PATIENT RESOURCES

- MedlinePlus. *Drug Allergies*—**http://www.nlm.nih.gov/medlineplus/ency/article/000819.htm.**
- Mayo Clinic. *Stevens-Johnson Syndrome*—**http://www.mayoclinic.com/print/stevens-johnson-syndrome/DS00940/DSECTION=all&METHOD=print.**

PROVIDER RESOURCES

- Patient.co.uk. *Drug Eruptions*—**http://www.patient.co.uk/doctor/Drug-Eruptions.htm.**
- DermNet NZ. *Drug Eruptions*—**http://dermnetnz.org/reactions/drug-eruptions.html.**
- Medscape. *Drug Eruptions*—**http://emedicine.medscape.com/article/1049474-overview.**

If the skin eruption is rare, serious, or unexpected, the drug reaction should be reported to the manufacturer and FDA.

REFERENCES

1. Sánchez-Borges M. NSAID hypersensitivity (respiratory, cutaneous, and generalized anaphylactic symptoms). *Med Clin North Am.* 2010;94(4):853-864.
2. Pichler WJ, Adam J, Daubner B, et al. Drug hypersensitivity reactions: pathomechanism and clinical symptoms. *Med Clin North Am.* 2010;94(4):645-664.
3. Phillips EJ, Chung WH, Mockenhaupt M, et al. Drug hypersensitivity: pharmacogenetics and clinical syndromes. *J Allergy Clin Immunol.* 2011;127(suppl 3):S60-S66.
4. Nigen S, Knowles SR, Shear NH. Drug eruptions: approaching the diagnosis of drug-induced skin diseases. *J Drugs Dermatol.* 2003;2(3):278-299.
5. Habif T. *Skin Disease Diagnosis and Treatment*. 2nd ed. Philadelphia, PA: Mosby; 2005.
6. Cacoub P, Musette P, Descamps V, et al. The DRESS syndrome: a literature review. *Am J Med.* 2011;124(7):588-597.
7. Kano Y, Ishida T, Kazuhisa K, Shiohara T. Visceral involvements and long-term sequelae in drug-induced hypersensitivity syndrome. *Med Clin North Am.* 2010;94(4):743-759.
8. van der Linden PD, van der Lei J, Vlug AE, Stricker BH. Skin reactions to antibacterial agents in general practice. *J Clin Epidemiol.* 1998;(51):703-708.
9. Gerson D, Sriganeshan V, Alexis JB. Cutaneous drug eruptions: a 5-year experience. *J Am Acad Dermatol.* 2008 Dec;59(6):995-999.
10. Fernando SL, Broadfoot J. Prevention of severe cutaneous adverse drug reactions: the emerging value of pharmacogenetic screening. *CMAJ.* 2010;182(5):476-480.
11. Scherer K, Bircher AJ. Danger signs in drug hypersensitivity. *Med Clin North Am.* 2010;94(4):681-689.
12. Chosidow OM, Stern RS, Wintroub BU. Cutaneous drug reactions. In: Kasper DL, Fauci AS, Longo DL, Braunwald EB, Hauser SL, Jameson JL, eds. *Harrison's Principles of Internal Medicine*. 16th ed. New York, NY: McGraw-Hill; 2005:318-324.
13. Schnyder B. Approach to the patient with drug allergy. *Med Clin North Am.* 2010;94(4):665-679.
14. Alves DW, Chen IA. Warfarin-induced skin necrosis. *Hosp Physician.* 2002;38(8):39-42.
15. Stewart AJ, Penman ID, Cook MK, Ludlam CA. Warfarin-induced skin necrosis. *Postgrad Med J.* 1999;75:233-235.
16. Mockenhaupt M, Norgauer J. Cutaneous adverse drug reactions: Stevens-Johnson syndrome and toxic epidermal necrolysis. *Allergy Clin Immunol Int.* 2002;14:143-150.

202 KELOIDS

E.J. Mayeaux Jr, MD
Richard P. Usatine, MD

PATIENT STORY

A 64-year-old black woman presents to the office with itching keloids on her chest (**Figure 202-1**). The horizontal keloid started during childhood when she was scratched by a branch of a tree. The vertical keloid is the result of bypass surgery 1 year ago. The lower portion of this area could be called a hypertrophic scar as it does not advance beyond the borders of the original surgery. The patient was happy to receive intralesional steroids to decrease her symptoms. Intralesional triamcinolone did, in fact, decrease the itching and flatten the vertical keloid.

INTRODUCTION

Keloids are benign dermal fibroproliferative tumors that form in scar because of altered wound healing. They form as a result of overproduction of extracellular matrix and dermal fibroblasts that have a high mitotic rate.

SYNONYMS

Keloid is also known as cheloid.

EPIDEMIOLOGY

- Individuals with darker pigmentation are more likely to develop keloids. Sixteen percent of black persons reported having keloids in a random sampling.[1]

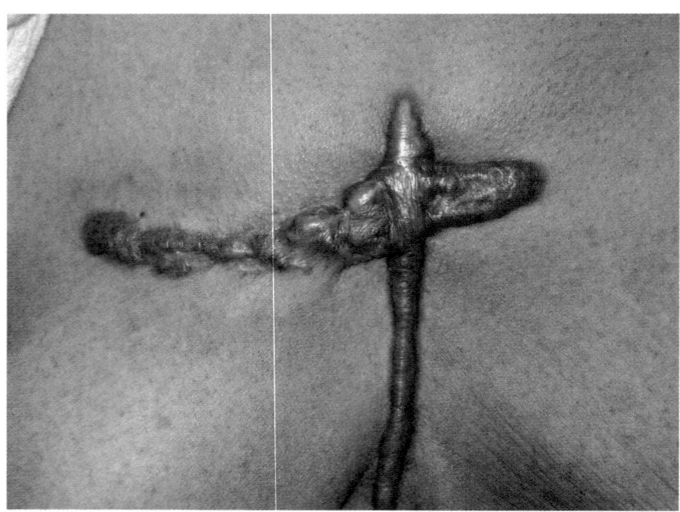

FIGURE 202-1 Two keloids that cross the chest of a 64-year-old black woman. The horizontal keloid came from a scratch during childhood, and the vertical keloid is a result of open heart surgery. *(Reproduced with permission from Richard P. Usatine, MD.)*

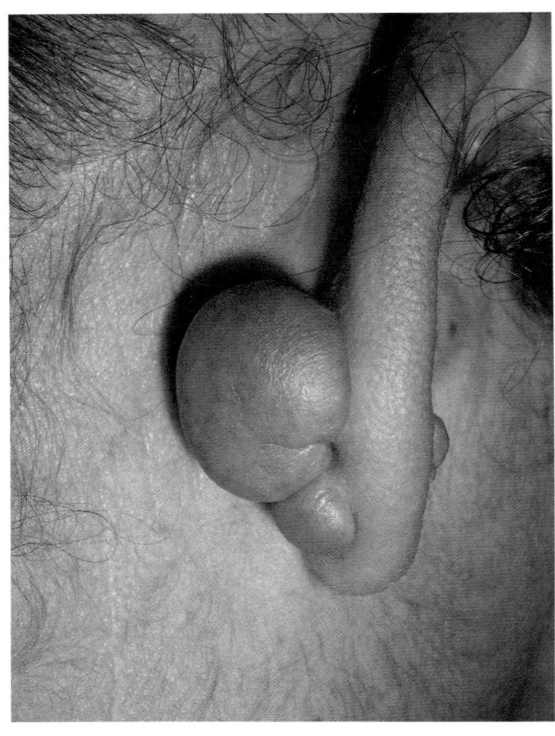

FIGURE 202-2 A keloid on the earlobe that started from piercing the ear. *(Reproduced with permission from Richard P. Usatine, MD.)*

- Men and women are generally affected equally except that keloids are more common in young adult women—probably secondary to a higher rate of piercing the ears (**Figure 202-2**).[2]
- Highest incidence is in individuals ages 10 to 20 years.[2,3]

ETIOLOGY AND PATHOPHYSIOLOGY

- Keloids are dermal fibrotic lesions that are a variation of the normal wound-healing process in the spectrum of fibroproliferative disorders.
- Keloids are more likely to develop in areas of the body that are subjected to high skin tension such as over the sternum (see **Figure 202-1**).
- These can occur even up to a year after the injury and will enlarge beyond the scar margin. Burns and other injuries can heal with a keloid in just one portion of the area injured (**Figure 202-3**).
- Wounds subjected to prolonged inflammation (acne cysts) are more likely to develop keloids.

RISK FACTORS

- Darker skin pigmentation (African, Hispanic, or Asian ethnicity)[3]
- A family history of keloids
- Wound healing by secondary intention
- Wounds subjected to prolonged inflammation
- Sites of repeated trauma
- Pregnancy
- Body piercings (**Figure 202-4**)

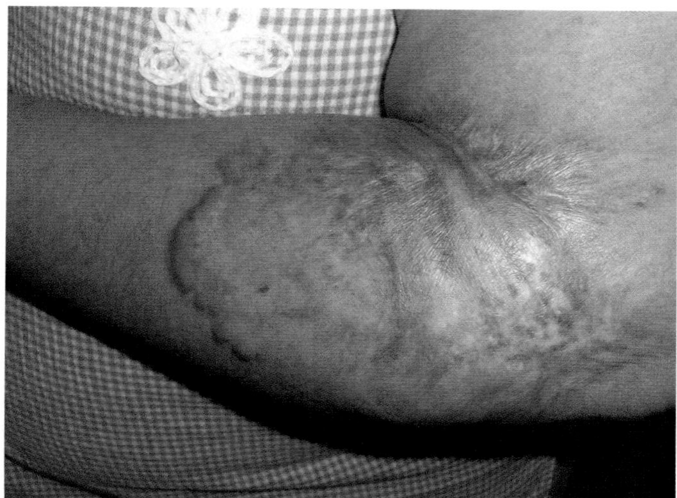

FIGURE 202-3 A keloid on the arm of a Hispanic woman burned accidentally by a hot iron at the age of 1 year. Most of the burn scar is not a keloid. The keloid is at the distal edge where the skin is raised nodular and pink. She has pruritus in that area. (*Reproduced with permission from Richard P. Usatine, MD.*)

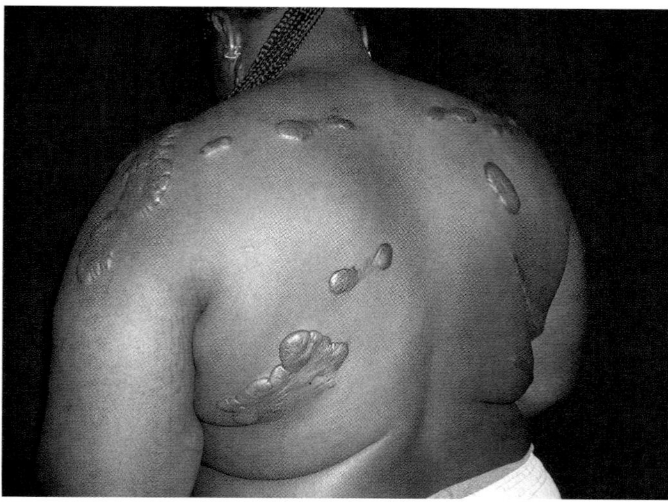

FIGURE 202-5 Many keloids in a woman who develops keloids with even the most minor skin injuries. (*Reproduced with permission from Richard P. Usatine, MD.*)

DIAGNOSIS

CLINICAL FEATURES

- Some keloids present with pruritic pain or a burning sensation around the scar.
- Initially manifest as erythematous lesions devoid of hair follicles or other glandular tissue.
- Papules to nodules to large tuberous lesions (**Figure 202-5**).
- Range in consistency from soft and doughy to rubbery and hard. Most often, the lesions are the color of normal skin but can become brownish red or bluish and then pale as they age.[4]
- May extend in a claw-like fashion far beyond any slight injury.
- Lesions on neck, ears, and abdomen tend to become pedunculated.

TYPICAL DISTRIBUTION

Anterior chest, shoulders, flexor surfaces of extremities, anterior neck, earlobes, and wounds that cross skin tension lines.

LABORATORY TESTING

Biopsy is rarely needed to make a diagnosis because the clinical appearance is usually distinctive and clear.

DIFFERENTIAL DIAGNOSIS

- Hypertrophic scars can appear similar to keloids but are confined to the site of original injury.
- Acne keloidalis nuchae is an inflammatory disorder around hair follicles of the posterior neck that results in keloidal scarring (**Figure 202-6**). Although the scarring is similar to keloids the location and

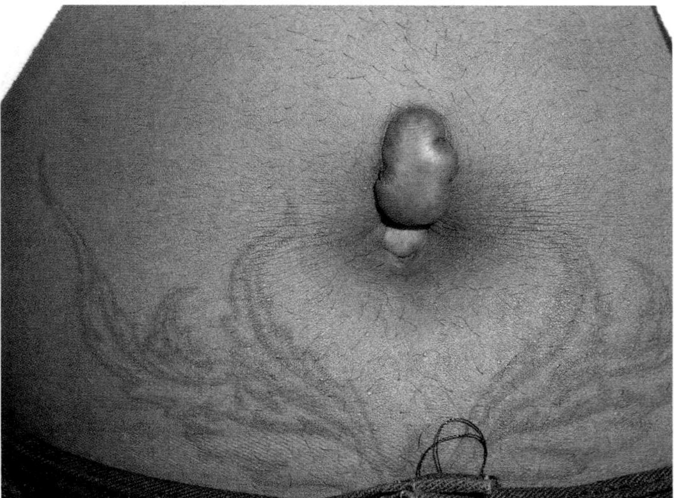

FIGURE 202-4 This keloid formed at the site of a belly button piercing in this young woman. (*Reproduced with permission from Richard P. Usatine, MD.*)

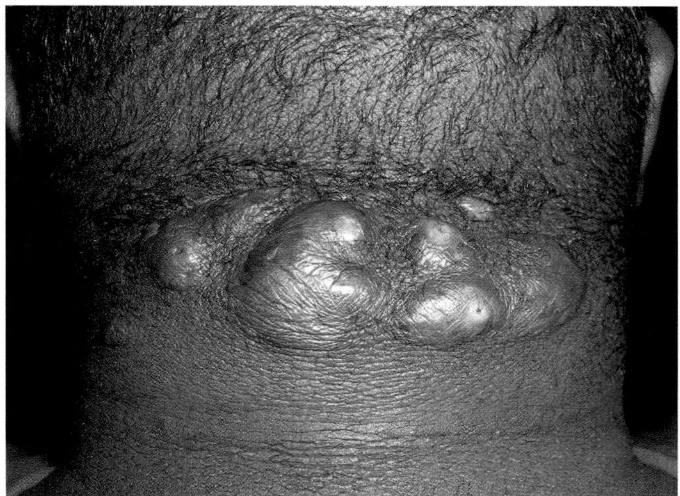

FIGURE 202-6 Acne keloidalis nuchae on the posterior neck of this young African American man. (*Reproduced with permission from Richard P. Usatine, MD.*)

pathophysiology are unique. This process can also cause alopecia (see Chapter 116, Pseudofolliculitis and Acne Keloidalis Nuchae).

- Dermatofibromas are common button-like dermal nodules usually found on the legs or arms. They may umbilicate when the surrounding skin is pinched. These often have a hyperpigmented halo around them and are less elevated than keloids (see Chapter 158, Dermatofibroma).
- Dermatofibrosarcoma protuberans is a malignant version of the dermatofibroma. It usually presents as an atrophic, scar-like lesion developing into an enlarging, firm, and irregular nodular mass. If this is suspected, a biopsy is needed (see Chapter 158, Dermatofibroma).

MANAGEMENT

- Patients frequently want keloids treated because of symptoms (pain and pruritus) and concerns about appearance.
- A 2006 systematic review of 396 studies and an accompanying meta-analysis of 36 articles concluded that no optimal evidence-based therapy exists and recommended choosing treatment based on cost and adverse effect profile.[5]

NONPHARMACOLOGIC

Silicone gel sheeting as a treatment for hypertrophic and keloid scarring is supported by poor-quality trials susceptible to bias. There is only weak evidence of a benefit of silicone gel sheeting as prevention for abnormal scarring in high-risk individuals.[6,7] SOR B

MEDICATIONS

- Intralesional steroid injections—Intralesional injection of triamcinolone acetonide (10-40 mg/mL) may decrease pruritus, as well as decreasing size and flattening of keloids (**Figure 202-7**). SOR C This may be repeated monthly as needed.[5,8]
- Earlobe keloids can be treated with imiquimod 5% cream following tangential shave excision on both sides of the earlobe.[9,10] SOR B Patients were instructed to administer imiquimod 5% cream to the excision sites the night of the surgery and daily for 6 to 8 weeks postsurgery. Imiquimod 5% cream only temporarily prevented the recurrence of presternal keloids after excision.[11] SOR C
- Intralesional verapamil 2.5 mg/mL, bleomycin 1.5 IU/mL, and interferon-α 2b injections 1.5 million IU twice daily for 4 days are less-studied alternatives to corticosteroid treatment.[3] SOR C

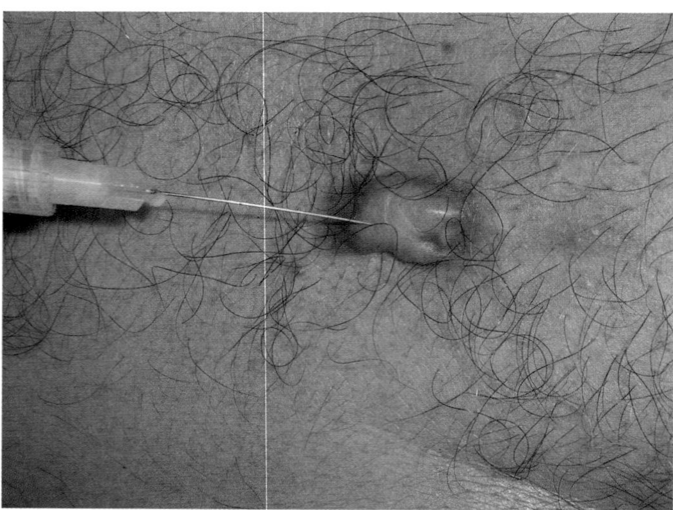

FIGURE 202-7 Triamcinolone injected into this symptomatic keloid on the chest. Note how the keloid is blanching white, demonstrating that the steroid is properly injected into the body of the keloid. A Luer lock syringe is used to avoid the needle popping off during the injection under pressure and a 27-gauge needle is used to minimize patient discomfort. *(Reproduced with permission from Richard P. Usatine, MD.)*

COMPLEMENTARY AND ALTERNATIVE THERAPY

No available evidence supports using nonprescription products such as Mederma and other creams, gels, and oils, to treat scars.[7] Limited clinical trials have failed to demonstrate lasting improvement of established keloids and hypertrophic scars with onion extract topical gel (eg, Mederma) or topical vitamin E.[3] SOR B

SURGICAL

- Cryosurgery and intralesional triamcinolone have been used to treat smaller keloids (eg, secondary to acne) with similar success to other therapies.[3,12] SOR B
- Combined cryosurgery and intralesional triamcinolone—The lesion is initially frozen with liquid nitrogen spray and allowed to thaw. Then it is injected with triamcinolone acetate (10-40 mg/mL). SOR C
- Earlobe keloids can be surgically excised with a shave or excisional technique and then injected with triamcinolone acetate (10-40 mg/mL) after hemostasis is obtained. The triamcinolone injection can be repeated in 1 month to decrease the chance of recurrence.[8] SOR B
- Keloids on the upper ear can be excised and the skin closed with sutures (**Figure 202-8**). SOR C

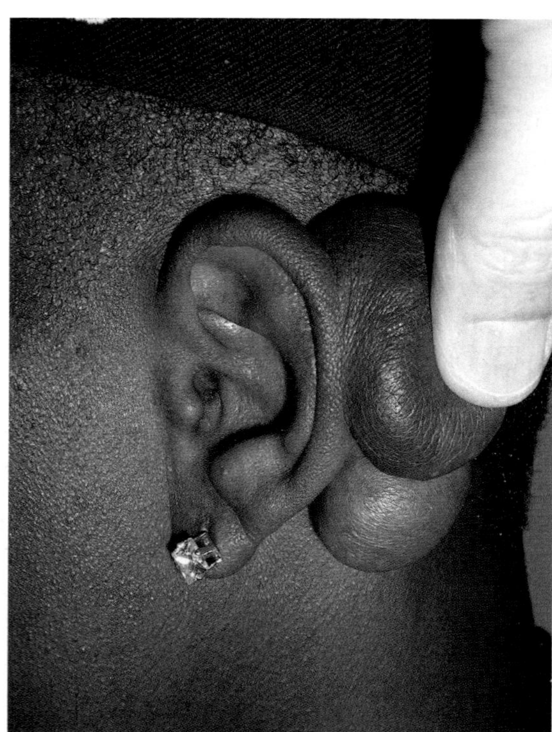

FIGURE 202-8 Two large keloids on the ear of this 23-year-old man that started after he experienced trauma to the ear. Both keloids were excised on 2 separate occasions and the skin closed with sutures. Intralesional triamcinolone was injected to prevent regrowth of the keloids. *(Reproduced with permission from Richard P. Usatine, MD.)*

- Pulsed-dye laser treatment can be beneficial for keloids.[13] Combination treatment with pulsed-dye laser plus intralesional therapy with corticosteroids and/or fluorouracil 50 mg/mL 2 to 3 times per week may be superior to either approach alone.[14] SOR Ⓒ
- Keloids can be treated with cryosurgery alone or in combination with intralesional steroids. In one, small, controlled study, 10 patients with keloids were treated with intralesional steroid and cryosurgery versus intralesional steroid or cryosurgery alone.[15] SOR Ⓑ Patients were treated at least 3 times 4 weeks apart. Based on keloid thickness, the keloids responded significantly better to combined cryosurgery and triamcinolone versus triamcinolone alone or cryotherapy alone. Pain intensity was significantly lowered with all treatment modalities. Pruritus was lowered only with the combined treatment and intralesional corticosteroid alone.[15]
- In another study, 20 patients with hypertrophic and keloidal scars received two 15-second cycles (total 30 seconds) of cryosurgery treatments once monthly for 12 months with intralesional injections of 10 to 40 mg/mL triamcinolone once monthly for 3 months.[16] SOR Ⓑ Topical application of silicone gel was added 3 times daily for 12 months. The control group included 10 patients who received treatment with silicone sheeting only. After 1 year there was improvement in all the parameters, especially in terms of symptoms, cosmetic appearance, and associated signs, compared to baseline and the control group.[16] SOR Ⓑ
- Layton et al. reported that the intralesional injection of a steroid is helpful but cryotherapy is more effective (85% improvement in terms of flattening) for recent acne keloids located on the back.[17] Treatment with intralesional triamcinolone was beneficial, but the response to cryosurgery was significantly better in early, vascular lesions.[17] SOR Ⓑ
- If the keloid is older and/or firmer, it may not respond to injection therapy as well as softer and newer lesions. It may help to pretreat the keloid with cryotherapy. It is not necessary to freeze a margin of normal tissue. After liquid nitrogen or another freezing modality is applied to the keloid, it is allowed to thaw and develop edema. This generally takes 1 to 2 minutes, which allows an easier introduction of intralesional steroids into the lesions. SOR Ⓒ
- In one double-blind, clinical trial, 40 patients were randomized to receive intralesional triamcinolone (TAC) or a combination of TAC and 5-fluorouracil (5-FU).[18] Both groups received injections at weekly intervals for 8 weeks and lesions were assessed for erythema, pruritus, pliability, height, length, and width. Both groups showed an acceptable improvement in nearly all parameters, but these were more significant in the TAC plus 5-FU group ($p < 0.05$ for all except pruritus and percentage of itch reduction). Good-to-excellent improvement was reported by 20% of the patients receiving TAC alone and by 55% of the patients in the group receiving TAC plus 5-FU.[18] SOR Ⓑ
- Earlobe keloids may be excised with a shave excision and injection of the base with steroid. It is hard to get much volume of steroid into the base of these keloids, so 40 mg/mL triamcinolone is preferred as the concentration for injection. SOR Ⓒ Another option is to use radiofrequency electrosurgery technique with a pure cutting setting (and using steroid in the anesthetic).
- According to one article, simple excision of earlobe keloids can result in recurrence rates approaching 80%.[19] A randomized, prospective trial comparing steroid injections versus radiation therapy found that 2 of 16 keloids (12.5%) recurred after surgery and radiation therapy, whereas 4 of 12 (33%) recurred after surgery and steroid injections. These results did not produce a statistically significant difference. No alteration of skin pigmentation, wound dehiscence, or chronic dermatitis was observed in any patient in either group.[19] Although radiation therapy was considered easy to obtain in this study, it is reasonable to use steroid injections in office practice.

PREVENTION

Avoiding trauma, including surgical trauma, whenever possible may decrease keloids in susceptible individuals.

PROGNOSIS

A 2006 systematic review of 396 studies and an accompanying meta-analysis of 36 articles concluded that any treatment gave patients an overall 70% (95% confidence interval, 49%-91%) chance of improvement.[5]

FOLLOW-UP

Follow-up is based on the chosen treatment. Follow-up for intralesional steroid injections is usually in 1 month.

PATIENT EDUCATION

Advise patients to avoid local skin trauma, for example, ear piercing, body piercing, and tattoos, and to control inflammatory acne.

PATIENT RESOURCES

- MedlinePlus. *Keloids*—**http://www.nlm.nih.gov/medlineplus/ency/article/000849.htm.**
- Skinsight. *Keloid Information for Adults*—**http://www.skinsight.com/adult/keloid.htm.**

PROVIDER RESOURCES

- Medscape. *Keloid and Hypertrophic Scar* (Dermatology)—**http://emedicine.medscape.com/article/1057599.**
- Medscape. *Keloids* (Plastic Surgery)—**http://emedicine.medscape.com/article/1298013.**
- Usatine R, Pfenninger J, Stulberg D, Small R. Dermatologic and Cosmetic Procedures in Office Practice. Philadelphia, PA: Elsevier; 2012. Available as a text with DVD or electronic application. Contains details, photographs and videos on how to use cryosurgery and intralesional injections to treat keloids—**http://usatinemedia.com/Usatine_Media_LLC/DermProcedures_Overview.html.**

REFERENCES

1. Chike-Obi CJ, Cole PD, Brissett AE. Keloids: pathogenesis, clinical features, and management. *Semin Plast Surg*. 2009;23:178-184.
2. Alhady SM, Sivanantharajah K. Keloids in various races. A review of 175 cases. *Plast Reconstr Surg*. 1969;44(6):564-566.
3. Juckett G, Hartman-Adams H. Management of keloids and hypertrophic scars. *Am Fam Physician*. 2009;80(3):253-260.

4. Urioste SS, Arndt KA, Dover JS. Keloids and hypertrophic scars: review and treatment strategies. *Semin Cutan Med Surg*. 1999;18: 159-171.

5. Leventhal D, Furr M, Reiter D. Treatment of keloids and hypertrophic scars: a meta-analysis and review of the literature. *Arch Facial Plast Surg*. 2006;8:362-368.

6. O'Brien L, Pandit A. Silicon gel sheeting for preventing and treating hypertrophic and keloid scars. *Cochrane Database Syst Rev*. 2006;(1):CD003826.

7. Williams CC, De Groote S. Clinical inquiry: what treatment is best for hypertrophic scars and keloids? *J Fam Pract*. 2011;60(12): 757-758.

8. Shaffer JJ, Taylor SC, Cook-Bolden F. Keloidal scars: a review with a critical look at therapeutic options. *J Am Acad Dermatol*. 2002;46:S63.

9. Patel PJ, Skinner RB Jr. Experience with keloids after excision and application of 5% imiquimod cream. *Dermatol Surg*. 2006;32:462.

10. Stashower ME. Successful treatment of earlobe keloids with imiquimod after tangential shave excision. *Dermatol Surg*. 2006;32:380-386.

11. Malhotra AK, Gupta S, Khaitan BK, Sharma VK. Imiquimod 5% cream for the prevention of recurrence after excision of presternal keloids. *Dermatology*. 2007;215:63-65.

12. Layton AM, Yip J, Cunliffe WJ. A comparison of intralesional triamcinolone and cryosurgery in the treatment of acne keloids. *Br J Dermatol*. 1994;130:498-501.

13. Alster TS, Williams CM. Treatment of keloid sternotomy scars with 585 nm flashlamp-pumped pulsed-dye laser. *Lancet*. 1995;345:1198.

14. Asilian A, Darougheh A, Shariati F. New combination of triamcinolone, 5-fluorouracil, and pulsed-dye laser for treatment of keloid and hypertrophic scars. *Dermatol Surg*. 2006;32:907-915.

15. Yosipovitch G, Widijanti SM, Goon A, Chan YH, Goh CL. A comparison of the combined effect of cryotherapy and corticosteroid injections versus corticosteroids and cryotherapy alone on keloids: a controlled study. *J Dermatolog Treat*. 2001;12:87-89.

16. Boutli-Kasapidou F, Tsakiri A, Anagnostou E, Mourellou O. Hypertrophic and keloidal scars: an approach to polytherapy. *Int J Dermatol*. 2005;44:324-327.

17. Layton AM, Yip J, Cunliffe WJ. A comparison of intralesional triamcinolone and cryosurgery in the treatment of acne keloids. *Br J Dermatol*. 1994;130:498-501.

18. Darougheh A, Asilian A, Shariati F. Intralesional triamcinolone alone or in combination with 5-fluorouracil for the treatment of keloid and hypertrophic scars. *Clin Exp Dermatol*. 2009;34:219-223.

19. Sclafani AP, Gordon L, Chadha M, Romo T, III. Prevention of earlobe keloid recurrence with postoperative corticosteroid injections versus radiation therapy: a randomized, prospective study and review of the literature. *Dermatol Surg*. 1996;22:569-574.

203 GENODERMATOSES

Michael Babcock, MD
Richard P. Usatine, MD

PATIENT STORY

A 45-year-old black man presents with greasy scale over his face and large parts of his chest and back (**Figure 203-1**). A previous biopsy was diagnostic for Darier disease. His mother has the same condition. His sister has the full-blown disease. His brother has similar nail findings, but his skin is affected only behind the ears (**Figure 203-2**). The patient has suffered with this condition for his entire life and believes that he has been ostracized from normal social life because of his appearance and bad body odor. He suffers from depression and has used various substances to treat his pain. Topical steroids provide some help for the itching and scaling, but the patient is looking for a more effective treatment. The cost of oral retinoids is currently prohibitive, but an application has been put in for patient assistance to receive acitretin.

INTRODUCTION

There are more than 100 genetic syndromes with cutaneous manifestations that are referred to as genodermatoses. For example, there are disorders of pigmentation (albinism), cornification (the ichthyoses and Darier disease), vascularization (Sturge-Weber syndrome), connective tissue (Ehlers-Danlos syndrome), porphyrin metabolism, other errors of metabolism (phenylketonuria), the immune system (Wiskott-Aldrich syndrome), and DNA repair (ataxia-telangiectasia and xeroderma pigmentosa), to name a few. Some textbooks are dedicated to the topic of genodermatoses alone.[1] This chapter introduces the topic and illustrates a couple of genodermatoses. We have chosen 2 disorders of cornification as an introduction to the genodermatoses: Darier disease and X-linked ichthyosis.

EPIDEMIOLOGY

- Darier disease (keratosis follicularis)—1:30,000 to 1:100,000. Males and females are equally affected. Clinically becomes apparent near puberty.
- X-linked ichthyosis—1:2000 to 1:6000 males. Clinical lesions present typically during the first 1 to 2 months of life.

ETIOLOGY AND PATHOPHYSIOLOGY

- Darier disease—An abnormal calcium pump in the sarco-/endoplasmic reticulum, SERCA2, results from a gene mutation in the *ATP2A2* gene. It is inherited in an autosomal dominant fashion and results in abnormal epidermal differentiation.
- X-linked ichthyosis—A deletion of the steroid sulfatase gene results in keratinocyte retention by inhibiting degradation of the desmosome. It is inherited in an X-linked recessive manner.

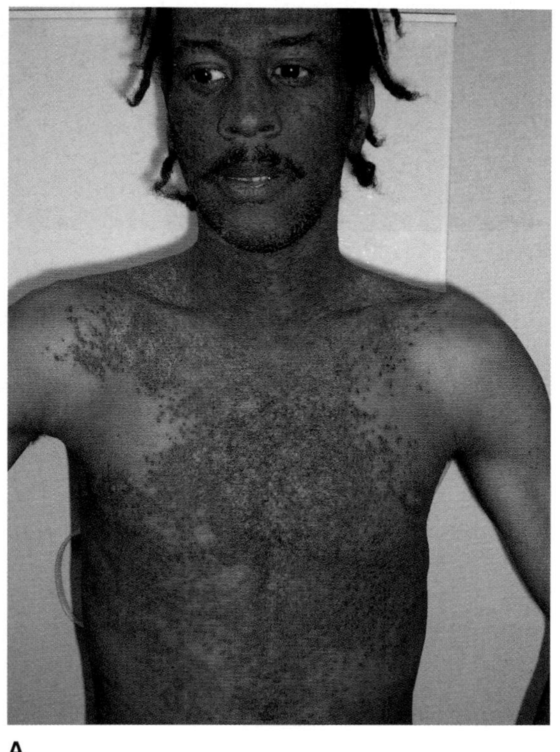
A

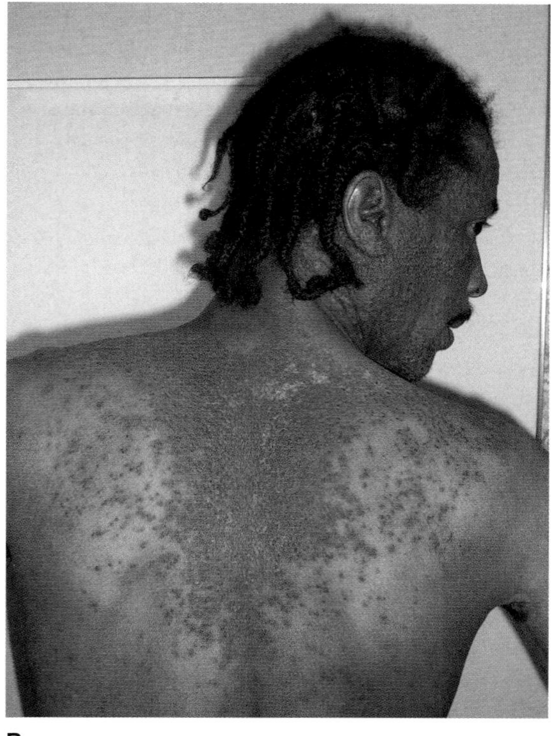
B

FIGURE 203-1 Darier disease with greasy scales, hyperkeratotic and hyperpigmented papules and plaques in a seborrheic distribution involving the (A) face, neck, and chest, and (B) back, neck, ears, and scalp. Sunlight and heat make his disease worse. (*Reproduced with permission from Richard P. Usatine, MD.*)

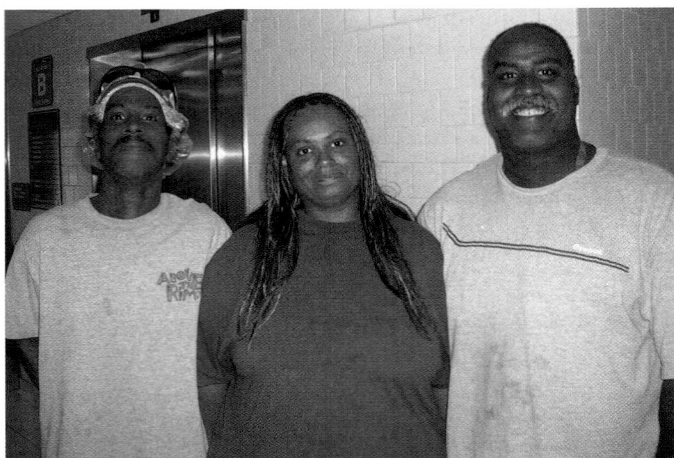

FIGURE 203-2 Darier disease presents in 3 siblings. The brother on the left and the sister have the full-blown disease. The sister's face cleared after 3 months of acitretin. The brother on the right has similar nail findings, but his skin is affected only behind the ears. (*Reproduced with permission from Richard P. Usatine, MD.*)

DIAGNOSIS

DARIER DISEASE

- Clinical features—Greasy, hyperkeratotic, yellowish-brown papules in a seborrheic distribution (**Figures 203-1** to **203-3**). The feet can be covered with hyperkeratotic plaques (**Figure 203-4**). The palms may have pits or keratotic papules, and the nails can have V-shaped nicking and alternating longitudinal red and white bands (**Figure 203-5**). The keratotic papules can be intensely malodorous such that it can interfere with normal social situations.
- Typical distribution—The clinical lesions involve skin in the seborrheic distribution (face, ears, scalp, upper chest, upper back, and groin) (**Figures 203-1** to **203-4 and 203-6**). The axilla and inframammary areas may be involved (**Figure 203-7**). In early, mild, or partially treated disease, only the skin behind the ears may be affected (**Figure 203-8**).[2] The nails are characteristically involved.
- Laboratories—Skin biopsy reveals the characteristic histopathology. A test for the *ATP2A2* gene mutation can be performed.

X-LINKED ICHTHYOSIS

- Clinical features—Firm, adherent, fish-like brown scale noted early in the life of young affected boys whose mothers were carriers of the gene on their X chromosome (**Figure 203-9**). These boys have an increased incidence of cryptorchidism and are at an increased risk of testicular cancer, independent of the risk from cryptorchidism alone.[2,3] Often they are delivered by cesarian section because a placental sulfatase deficiency results in failure of labor progression. These patients can have corneal opacities on the Descemet membrane of the posterior capsule, which does not affect their vision.
- Typical distribution—Most of the body is involved, except for the typical sparing of the flexures, face, palms, and soles. The antecubital fossae are notably spared (see **Figure 203-9**). There is an accentuation noted on the neck, giving these patients a characteristic "dirty neck" appearance.
- Tight skin over the fingers can be as a manifestation of X-linked ichthyosis (**Figure 203-10**).

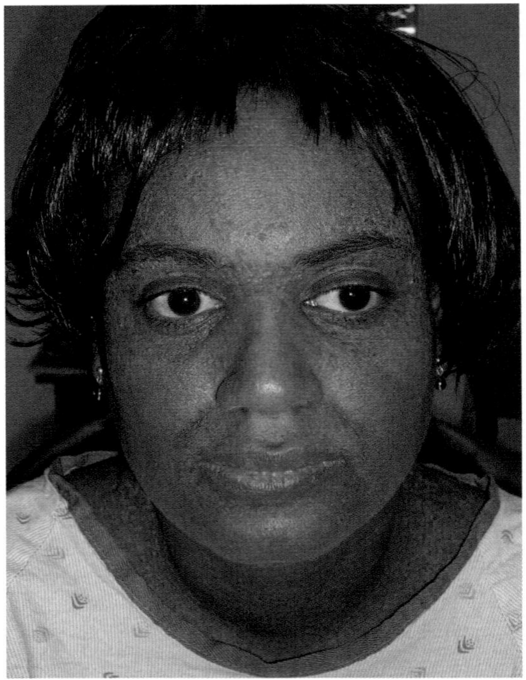

A

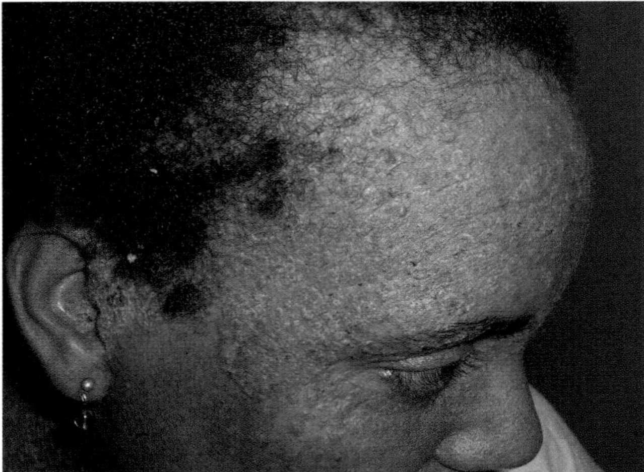

B

FIGURE 203-3 **A.** Darier disease with greasy, hyperkeratotic scaling plaques on the face of the 44-year-old woman (sister of the patient in **Figure 203-1**) with Darier disease prior to her use of acitretin. She is wearing a wig to cover the alopecia and plaques on her scalp. **B.** Close-up of the hyperkeratotic scaling plaques on the forehead, scalp, and ears. Note the seborrheic distribution. (*Reproduced with permission from Richard P. Usatine, MD.*)

- Laboratories—Increased levels of serum cholesterol sulfate levels (steroid sulfatase hydrolyses cholesterol sulfate). Steroid sulfatase activity can also be measured directly.

DIFFERENTIAL DIAGNOSIS

DARIER DISEASE

- Hailey-Hailey disease (aka benign familial pemphigus)—Another genodermatosis with crusted erosions and flaccid vesicles distributed in the intertriginous areas as opposed to the greasy keratotic papules in the

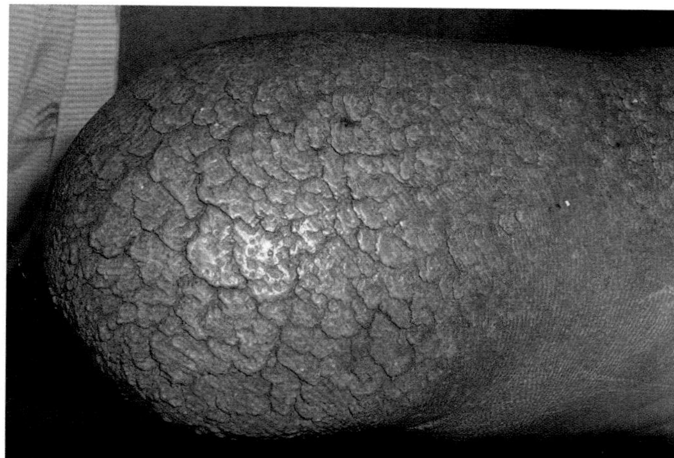

FIGURE 203-4 Thick hyperkeratotic plaque on the heel of the woman with Darier disease. (*Reproduced with permission from Richard P. Usatine, MD.*)

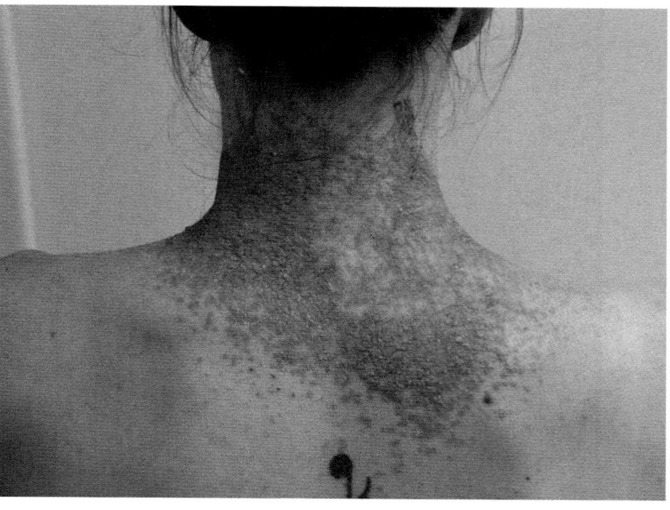

FIGURE 203-6 Darier disease flared up on the posterior neck and upper back in a young woman. Note the erythema and greasy yellow hyperkeratotic scale in the seborrheic area. (*Reproduced with permission from Yoon Cohen, MD.*)

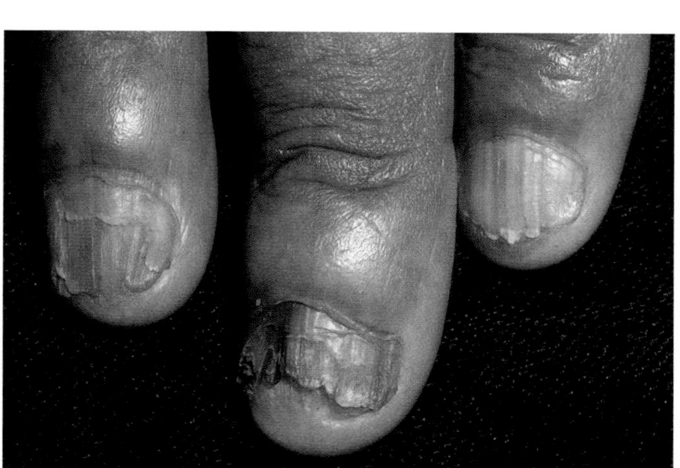

A

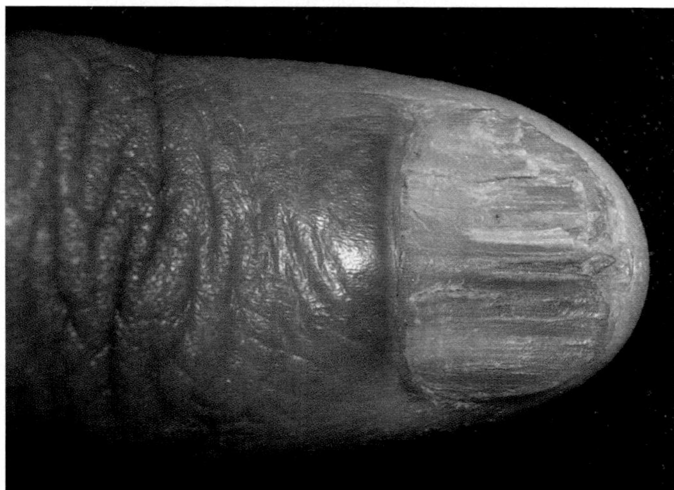

B

FIGURE 203-5 **A.** Typical nail findings in Darier disease showing longitudinal bands and longitudinal splitting. **B.** V-shaped nick at the free margin of the fingernail—the most pathognomonic nail finding in Darier disease. (*Reproduced with permission from Richard P. Usatine, MD.*)

seborrheic distribution (**Figure 203-11**). A 4-mm punch biopsy is adequate to make this diagnosis.[4]

- Grover disease—This presents sporadically as many small, pruritic, erythematous-to-reddish-brown hyperkeratotic papules on the trunk of older adults. These typically result from conditions that cause sweating or occlusion (like lying in a hospital bed) (see Chapter 119, Folliculitis).
- Seborrheic dermatitis—Erythematous patches and thin plaques with yellow greasy scale on the scalp, central face, and chest. This is rarely as severe as Darier disease (see Chapter 149, Seborrheic Dermatitis).

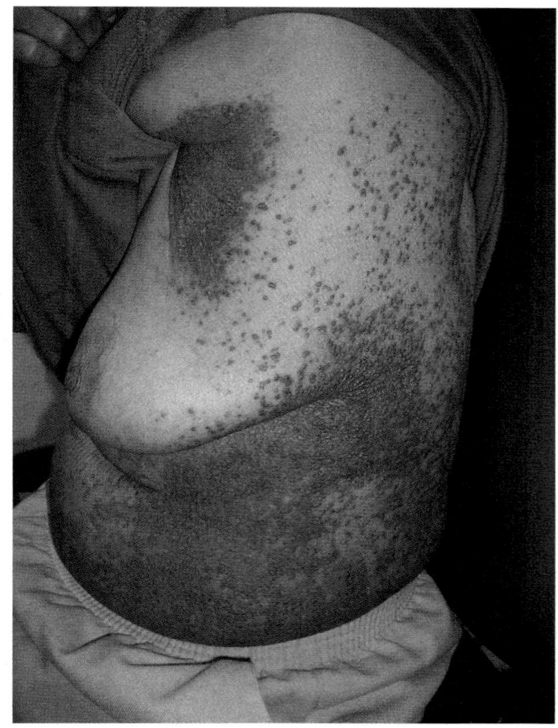

FIGURE 203-7 Darier disease with axillary and inframammary involvement in this 64-year-old woman. (*Reproduced with permission from Richard P. Usatine, MD.*)

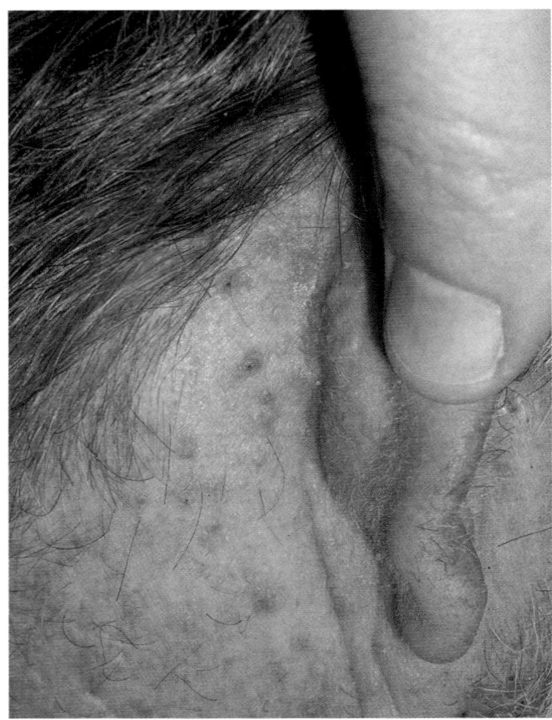

FIGURE 203-8 Darier disease with hyperkeratotic papules behind the ear of this middle-aged white man. (*Reproduced with permission from Richard P. Usatine, MD.*)

X-LINKED ICHTHYOSIS

- Ichthyosis vulgaris—A relatively common condition that is inherited in an autosomal dominant manner (approximately 1 in 250 people affected). It presents in childhood with a fine adherent scale in similar distribution to X-linked ichthyosis (**Figure 203-12**). These patients frequently have hyperlinear palms, keratosis pilaris, and atopic dermatitis, which are not commonly associated with X-linked ichthyosis.
- Acquired ichthyosis does not occur until adulthood. It is not inherited and may be associated with some systemic disease. The time of onset is the key to diagnosis. The legs are often most involved and the skin appears similar to fish-scales (**Figure 203-13**).

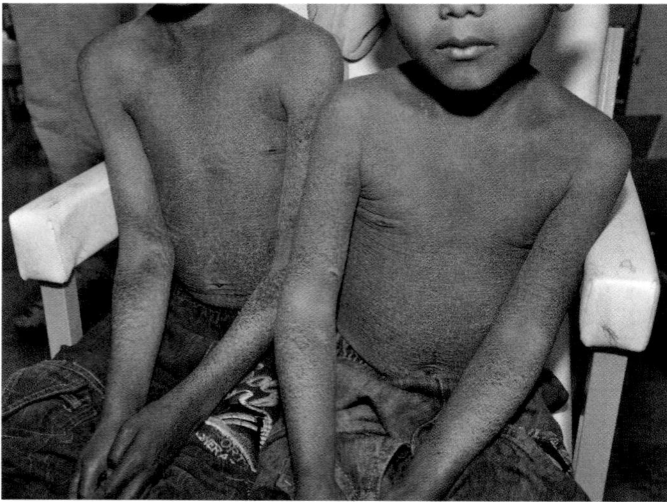

FIGURE 203-9 X-linked ichthyosis in 2 brothers showing sparing of the antecubital fossae of the arms amidst the heavy scales. (*Reproduced with permission from Richard P. Usatine, MD.*)

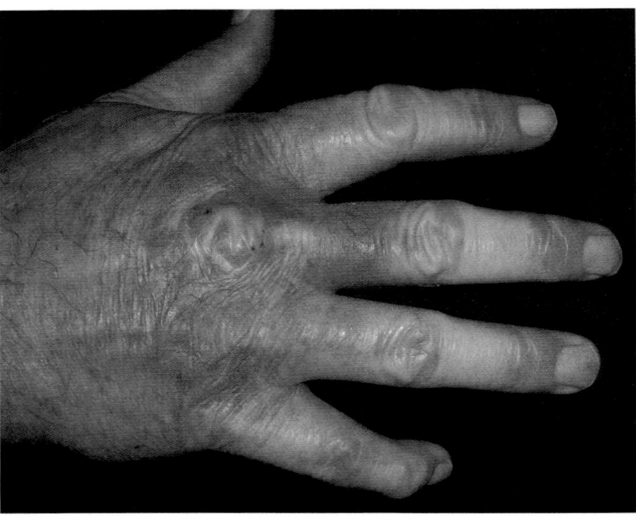

FIGURE 203-10 X-linked ichthyosis manifesting as tight skin over the fingers of this man with the typical scaling skin of ichthyosis. (*Reproduced with permission from Richard P. Usatine, MD.*)

- Lamellar ichthyosis—A more severe and rare disorder that has a plate-like scale, which involves most of the body, including the face and flexures (**Figure 203-14**). These patients are typically born as a collodion baby (they have a thin translucent membrane that surrounds the baby at birth).
- Asteatotic eczema—Dry skin that has a "dried riverbed" or "cracked porcelain" appearance, which usually involves the lower extremities. There may be erythema and serous exudate associated with the cracks. It typically presents in the winter, improves during the rest of the year,

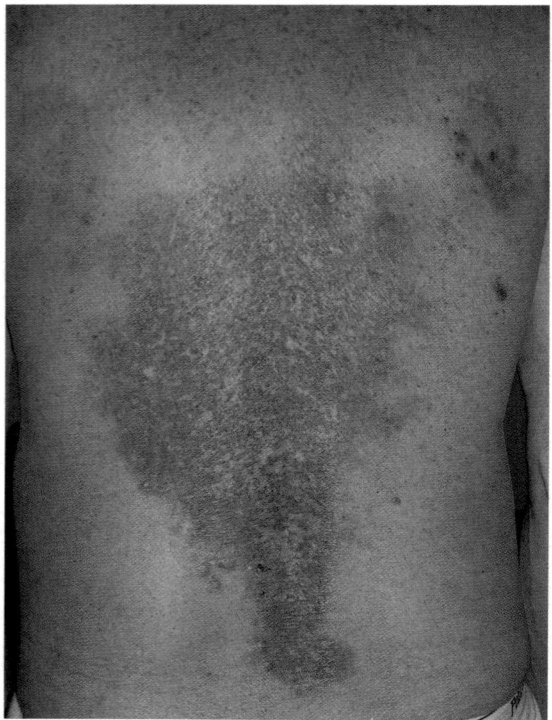

FIGURE 203-11 Hailey-Hailey disease, also known as benign familial pemphigus, on the back of a 54-year-old man. This genodermatosis has a similar appearance to Darier disease and also occurs in a seborrheic distribution. (*Reproduced with permission from Richard P. Usatine, MD.*)

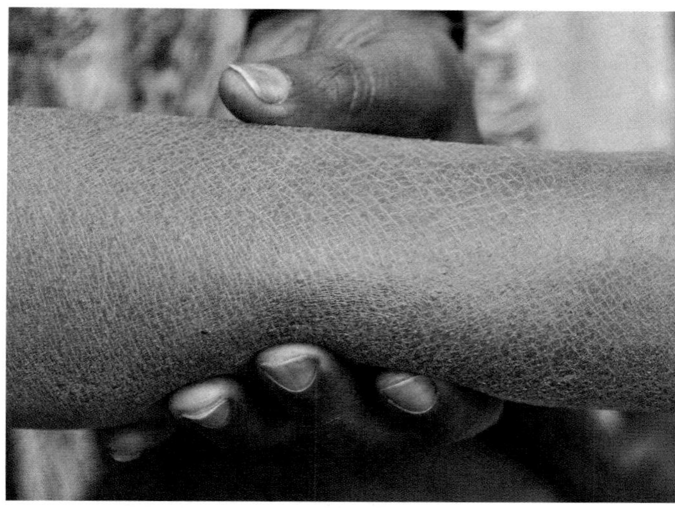

FIGURE 203-12 Ichthyosis vulgaris starts in childhood and has a fine scale. *(Reproduced with permission from Richard P. Usatine, MD.)*

and is also known as winter itch or eczema craquelé (see Chapter 143, Atopic Dermatitis).

- Xerosis—Dry scaly skin most notably on legs without significant inflammation. This is very common compared with any ichthyosis.

MANAGEMENT

- Darier disease is so rare that there are no randomized controlled trials to guide treatment.
- The intense malodor that accompanies the disease, as well as the facial involvement, often adversely affects the patient's quality of life; thus, treatment is often warranted. Mild-to-moderate disease can be treated by avoiding exacerbating factors (sunlight, heat, and occlusion) and with topical medications, SOR Ⓒ but severe disease is best treated with oral retinoids. SOR Ⓒ

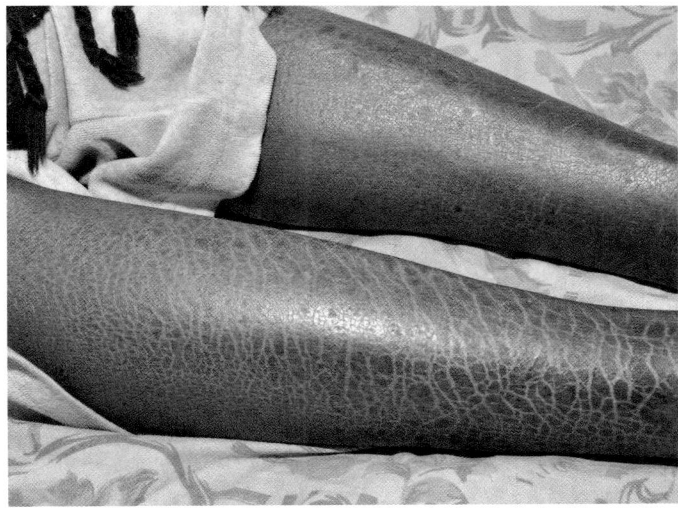

FIGURE 203-13 Acquired ichthyosis starts in adulthood and is especially prominent on the legs. *(Reproduced with permission from Richard P. Usatine, MD.)*

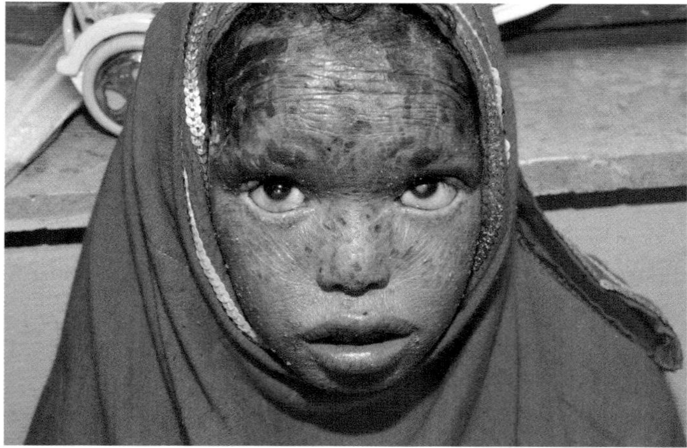

A

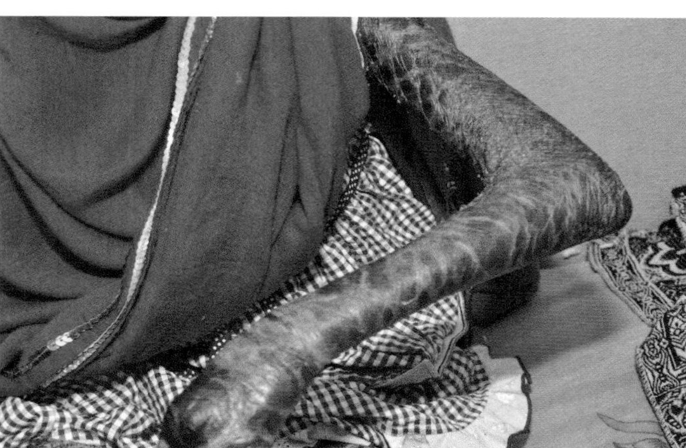

B

FIGURE 203-14 Lamellar ichthyosis is another genodermatosis that is more rare and severe than X-linked ichthyosis. **A.** Note the deep lines and severe dryness of the skin on the face of this girl with lamellar ichthyosis. **B.** Her arm is severely affected so that she cannot extend her elbow fully. *(Reproduced with permission from Richard P. Usatine, MD.)*

- Topical retinoids (adapalene, tretinoin, or tazarotene) are effective in some patients, but their main limitation is irritation. Adapalene use may be effective in localized variants.[5] SOR Ⓒ All retinoids are contraindicated in pregnancy.
- Topical corticosteroids may be of some help. Lower-potency topical corticosteroids should be used on the face, groin, and axillae to minimize side effects in these areas. SOR Ⓒ
- Topical calcineurin inhibitors (pimecrolimus and tacrolimus) may also be helpful as noted in some case reports.[6,7] SOR Ⓒ These do not have a risk of skin atrophy like steroids, but are generally more expensive and have a controversial black box warning.
- Systemic retinoids (acitretin or isotretinoin) are the most potent treatment and treatment of choice for severe disease.[8] SOR Ⓒ They should only be prescribed by physicians who have experience with these medications. Patients on systemic retinoids require close monitoring and careful selection, as they are teratogenic (category X) and can cause hyperlipidemia, hypertriglyceridemia, mucous membrane dryness, alopecia, hepatotoxicity, and possible mood disturbances. Females must not get pregnant for at least 1 month after stopping isotretinoin and at least 3 years after stopping acitretin.

- Cyclosporine can be used for acute flares but should also only be prescribed by a physician who has experience with this medication. It should only be used temporarily and requires close follow-up for monitoring hypertension and nephrotoxicity. It is metabolized by the common cytochrome P450 3A4 system and has many medication interactions.
- Topical or oral antibiotics may be necessary for flares as they often are secondarily infected with bacteria. SOR Ⓒ
- Laser, radiation, photodynamic, and gene therapy are newer treatment modalities that are being investigated.
- X-linked ichthyosis is rare and treatments are based on the clinical experience of experts rather than large studies.
- Frequent application of emollients, humectants, and keratinolytics are the mainstay of therapy. SOR Ⓒ There are many effective nonprescription and prescription products that contain propylene glycol, urea, or lactic acid. Salicylic acid products should be used only on a limited body surface area, as systemic absorption has led to salicylate toxicity in some patients.
- Topical retinoids can be used, SOR Ⓒ but systemic retinoids are rarely used.
- Refer to a urologist or ophthalmologist if testicular abnormality or corneal opacities are detected. SOR Ⓒ
- Gene therapy has also been studied but has not yet become a viable treatment option.

FOLLOW-UP

- Darier disease—Follow-up is needed if patients are on oral retinoids to monitor patients' lipid panel and liver function tests approximately every 3 months. They should also be monitored for signs of secondary bacterial infection.
- X-linked ichthyosis—Monitoring for corneal opacities and for testicular cancer in men should be performed at follow-up visits.

PATIENT EDUCATION

DARIER DISEASE

- Avoid direct sunlight, heat, occlusion, and people acutely infected with herpes simplex virus (HSV) or varicella-zoster virus.
- Watch for signs of secondary cutaneous bacterial or viral infections.

X-LINKED ICHTHYOSIS

Use daily moisturizers, especially in dry climates and in the winter.

PATIENT RESOURCES

- There are patient advocacy groups for several genetic skin conditions. A quick search online can obtain their websites and contact information.
- The American Academy of Dermatology has a summer camp that is free of charge for children with skin conditions called Camp Discovery. Information can be found at **http://www.campdiscovery.org/.**

PROVIDER RESOURCES

- A helpful free online resource for the genodermatoses, or any genetic disease for that matter, is the Online Mendelian Inheritance of Man website at **http://www.omim.org.**
- For information on laboratories that perform rare genetic tests and clinics that perform prenatal diagnostic testing for certain conditions, see **http://www.genetests.org.**
- Skin Advocate is a free application for mobile devices that is provided by the Society of Investigative Dermatology. It lists contact information for various patient advocacy groups.

REFERENCES

1. Spitz J. *Genodermatoses: A Clinical Guide to Genetic Skin Disorders*. 2nd ed. Philadelphia, PA: Lippincott Williams & Wilkins; 2005.
2. James W, Berger T, Elston D. *Andrews' Diseases of the Skin: Clinical Dermatology*. 11th ed. Amsterdam, The Netherlands: Elsevier; 2011.
3. Hazan C, Orlow S, Schagger J. X-linked recessive ichthyosis. *Dermatol Online J*. 2005;11(4):12.
4. Khachemoune A, Lockshin B. Chronic papules on the back and extremities. *J Fam Pract*. 2004;53(5):361-363.
5. Casals M, Campoy A, Aspiolea F, et al. Successful treatment of linear Darier's disease with topical adapalene. *J Eur Acad Dermatol Venerol.* 2009;23(2):237-238.
6. Pérez-Carmona L, Fleta-Asín B, Moreno-García-Del-Real C, et al. Successful treatment of Darier's disease with topical pimecrolimus. *Eur J Dermatol.* 2011;21(2):301-302.
7. Rubegni P, Poggiali S, Sbano P, et al. A case of Darier's disease successfully treated with topical tacrolimus. *J Eur Acad Dermatol Venereol.* 2006;20(1):84-87.
8. Bolognia J, Jorizzo J, Rapini R. *Dermatology*. London, UK: Mosby; 2003.

204 ERYTHEMA ANNULARE CENTRIFUGUM

Shehnaz Zaman Sarmast, MD
Richard P. Usatine, MD

PATIENT STORY

A 57-year-old farm worker presents with itchy red rings on his body that have come and gone for more than 13 years (**Figures 204-1** and **204-2**). The erythematous annular eruption was visible on his abdomen, legs, and arms. **Figure 204-2** shows the typical "trailing scale" of erythema annular centrifugum (EAC). A potassium hydroxide (KOH) preparation was negative for fungal elements and the patient was given the diagnosis of EAC. He recently began using paint thinner to "dry out the rash" and decrease the itching. Because topical steroids did not provide any relief for him in the past, we offered the option of using calcipotriol ointment. He chose to try the calcipotriol and stop using paint thinner.

INTRODUCTION

EAC is an uncommon inflammatory skin disease characterized by slowly migrating annular or configurate erythematous lesions.

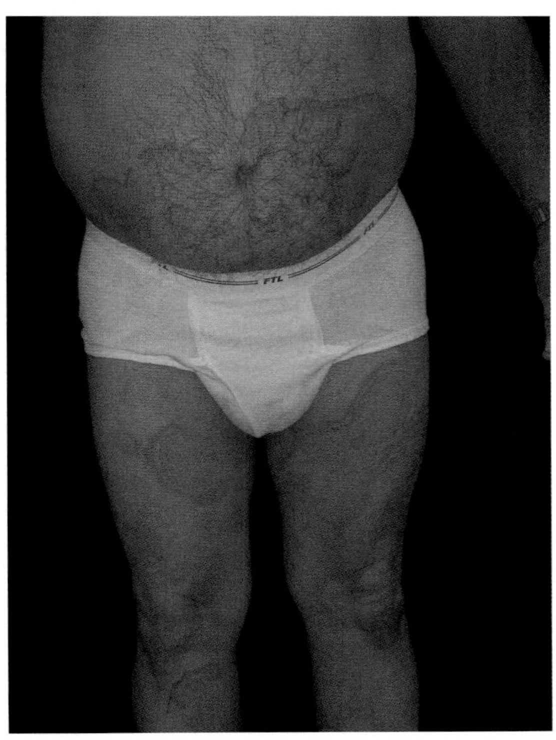

FIGURE 204-1 Erythema annulare centrifugum with large erythematous rings on the trunk and legs of a 57-year-old man. (*Reproduced with permission from Richard P. Usatine, MD. Reproduced with permission from Brand ME, Usatine RP. Persistent itchy pink rings.* J Fam Pract. *2005;54(2):131-133. Reproduced with permission from Frontline Medical Communications.*)

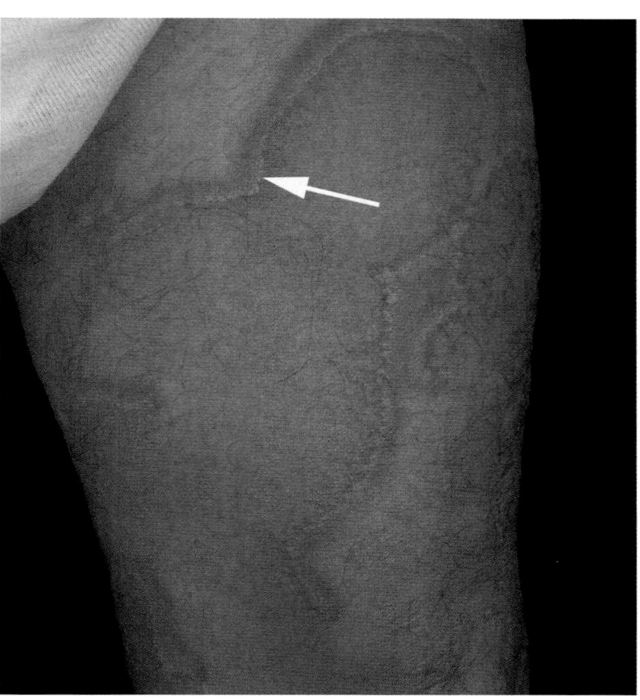

FIGURE 204-2 Erythema annulare centrifugum with conjoined rings on the thigh. Arrow pointing to "trailing scale," which appears as a white scaling line within the erythematous border. (*Reproduced with permission from Richard P. Usatine, MD. Reproduced with permission from Brand ME, Usatine RP. Persistent itchy pink rings.* J Fam Pract. *2005;54(2):131-133. Reproduced with permission from Frontline Medical Communications.*)

SYNONYMS

EAC is also known as erythema gyratum perstans, erythema exudativum perstans, erythema marginatum perstans, erythema perstans, erythema figuratum perstans, erythema microgyratum perstans, and erythema simplex gyratum.

EPIDEMIOLOGY

- It may begin at any age (mean age of onset 39.7 years), with no predilection for either sex.[1]
- The mean duration of skin condition is 2.8 years but may last between 4 weeks and 34 years.[2]

ETIOLOGY AND PATHOPHYSIOLOGY

- Unknown etiology and pathogenesis, but EAC has been associated with other medical conditions, such as fungal infections (in 72% of cases),[1] malignancy, and other systemic illness. Few case reports have reported the diagnosis of cancer 2 years after presentation of EAC.[2]
- Other infections identified as triggers for EAC include bacterial infections such as cystitis, appendicitis, and tuberculosis (TB); viral infections such as Epstein-Barr virus (EBV), molluscum contagiosum, and herpes zoster; and parasites, such as *Ascaris*.[2]
- Certain drugs, such as chloroquine, hydroxychloroquine, estrogen, cimetidine, penicillin, salicylates, piroxicam, hydrochlorothiazide,

amitriptyline, lenalidomide, finasteride, and etizolam, can also trigger EAC.[2-6]

- Systemic diseases involving the liver, dysproteinemias, autoimmune disorders, HIV, and pregnancy are associated with EAC by various case reports.[2,7,8]
- Because injections of *Trichophyton*, *Candida,* tuberculin, and tumor extracts have been reported to induce EAC, a type intravenous (IV) hypersensitivity reaction is thought to be one possible mechanism for its development.[8]

DIAGNOSIS

CLINICAL FEATURES

- Large, scaly, erythematous plaques are found, which begin as papules and spread peripherally with a central clearing forming a "trailing" scale. The margins are indurated and may vary in width from 4 to 6 mm[1,2] (**Figures 204-1** to **204-4**).
- Pruritus is common but not always present.[2]
- Slowly progressing but may enlarge up to 2 to 5 mm/d.[2]
- Evaluation of a skin biopsy specimen by light microscopy reveals parakeratosis and spongiosis within the epidermis and a tightly cuffed lymphohistiocytic perivascular infiltrate with focal extravasation of erythrocytes in the papillary dermis.[9]

TYPICAL DISTRIBUTION

Lesions typically found in lower extremities, particularly the thighs, but also can be found on trunk and face.[1,2]

LABORATORY STUDIES

No specific laboratory tests are necessary to diagnose EAC, but laboratory tests may be obtained to rule out other common conditions. Consider a KOH prep to search for tinea corporis or cutaneous candidiasis. If the patient has been in an area with Lyme disease, consider *Borrelia* titers to rule out Lyme disease.[2,7]

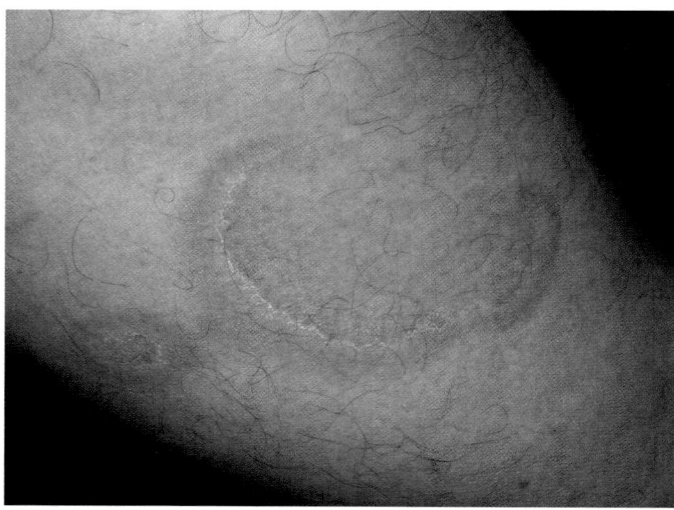

FIGURE 204-3 Erythema annulare centrifugum on the arm with trailing scale. Note the largest ring is not a complete circle. (*Courtesy of Richard P. Usatine, MD.*)

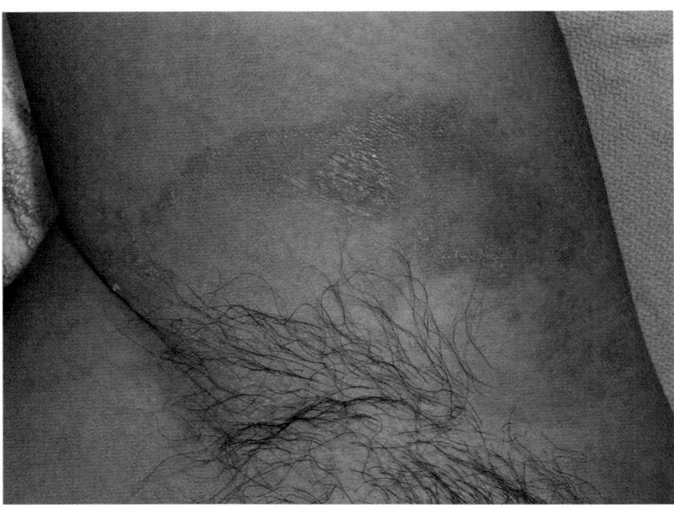

FIGURE 204-4 Erythema annular centrifugum in the axilla of a 28-year-old man, which had repeatedly been mistaken for tinea corporis. The trailing scale is visible and a punch biopsy confirmed the diagnosis of erythema annular centrifugum. (*Reproduced with permission from Richard P. Usatine, MD.*)

BIOPSY

If the diagnosis is uncertain, a punch biopsy can be performed to look for the typical histology of EAC, and a periodic acid-Schiff (PAS) stain can be performed on the specimen to look for fungal elements. Other diseases on the differential diagnosis, such as psoriasis, cutaneous lupus, and sarcoidosis, can be diagnosed with a punch biopsy.

DIFFERENTIAL DIAGNOSIS

- Pityriasis rosea has erythematous patch distributed on trunk and lower extremities, but these patches have distinctive collarette border and typically have a "herald patch" that appears first. Classically, the patches have a "Christmas tree" pattern in the back and, unlike EAC, last only 6 to 8 weeks[2] (see Chapter 151, Pityriasis Rosea).
- Tinea corporis (ringworm) presents with one or multiple areas of annular plaques caused by a dermatophyte fungal infection. Tinea corporis often produces red scaling rings that resemble EAC. However, the scale in tinea corporis tends to lead with the erythema inside the ring and the scale on the outside (**Figure 204-5**). This is the opposite of the trailing scale seen with EAC (**Figure 204-6**). KOH prep shows branched hyphae with septae. Tinea corporis responds to antifungal treatment.[2] **Figure 204-4** shows a case of EAC that was mistaken for tinea corporis by a number of physicians (see Chapter 136, Tinea Corporis).
- Psoriatic plaques can be annular but do not have the trailing scale that is characteristic of EAC. Psoriasis will respond to steroid therapy[2] (see Chapter 150, Psoriasis).
- Erythema migrans seen in Lyme disease is a large annular rash with central clearing. The red ring in erythema migrans is usually smooth without the scale seen in EAC. Patients usually have other signs of infection, positive antibodies, and may have a history of tick bite (see Chapter 215, Lyme Disease).
- Erythema gyratum repens, which is typically seen in association with malignancies, has concentric rings but trailing scale is noted.
- Cutaneous lupus could present with annular or papulosquamous plaques, with or without scales, on sun-exposed areas. Patients with

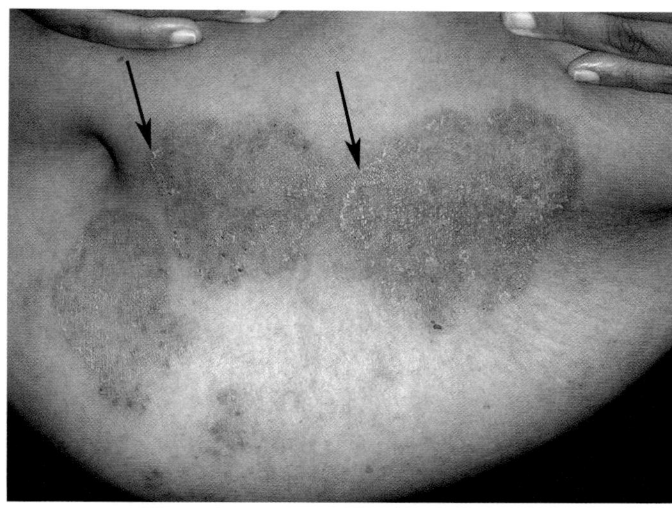

FIGURE 204-5 Tinea corporis with leading scale (*arrows*). The white scale is on the outside of the ring and the erythema is on the inside. KOH prep was positive. (*Reproduced with permission from Richard P. Usatine, MD.*)

lupus generally have other systemic symptoms and positive antinuclear antibodies[10] (see Chapter 178, Lupus: Systemic and Cutaneous).

- Sarcoidosis may present with annular indurated papules and plaques, but they are more commonly found on the face. Patients may have other systemic manifestations of sarcoidosis. Sarcoidosis can effectively be treated with systemic corticosteroids[11] (see Chapter 173, Sarcoidosis).
- Mycosis fungoides, a type of cutaneous T-cell lymphoma, can mimic EAC (see Chapter 174, Cutaneous T-Cell lymphoma).[12]

MANAGEMENT

- There is no proven treatment for EAC. Identifying and treating underlying medical conditions may help resolve the skin condition. Because EAC is seen in association with certain drugs, discontinuing the offending medication may resolve the problem.

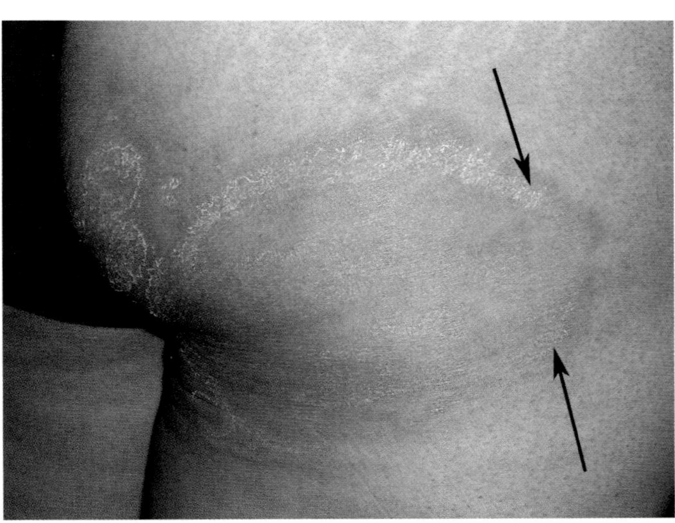

FIGURE 204-6 Erythema annulare centrifugum on the buttocks and upper thigh showing trailing scale (*arrows*) inside the ring of erythema. KOH prep was negative. (*Reproduced with permission from Richard P. Usatine, MD.*)

- Topical corticosteroids have been traditionally used but there is little evidence to support their use. SOR Ⓒ
- Case reports have reported benefits of using calcipotriol (Dovonex) daily for EAC.[13] Another case report described a good outcome for a patient with EAC being treated with calcipotriol and narrowband ultraviolet B (UVB) phototherapy.[14] Case reports have shown etanercept and metronidazole to be beneficial as well.[15,16]

PROGNOSIS

The prognosis is excellent if there is no underlying disease and may resolve in an average of 11 months.[17] It often resolves with effective treatment of any underlying disorder. If EAC is associated with pregnancy, it should resolve soon after delivery. If EAC is associated with a malignancy, the prognosis depends on that of the malignancy. Even if it resolves, EAC may recur repeatedly over many years.

FOLLOW-UP

Follow-up depends on the type of treatment provided and patient's preferences.

PATIENT EDUCATION

- EAC is not contagious or malignant.
- Although the treatment might not work and the condition may recur, it is not dangerous and is confined to the skin only.

PROVIDER RESOURCES

- Medscape. *Erythema Annulare Centrifugum*—**http://emedicine.medscape.com/article/1122701-overview.**
- Medscape. *Erythema Annulare Centrifugum*—**http://www.patient.co.uk/doctor/Erythema-Annulare-Centrifugum.htm.**

REFERENCES

1. Kim KJ, Chang SE, Choi JH, et al. Clinicopathologic analysis of 66 cases of erythema annulare centrifugum. *J Dermatol.* 2002;29 (2):61-67.
2. Brand ME, Usatine RP. Persistent itchy pink rings. *J Fam Pract.* 2005;54(2):131-133.
3. Garcia-Doval I, Pereiro C, Toribio J. Amitriptyline-induced erythema annulare centrifugum. *Cutis.* 1999;63(1):35-36.
4. Kuroda K, Yabunami H, Hisanaga Y. Etizolam-induced superficial erythema annulare centrifugum. *Clin Exp Dermatol.* 2002;27(1):34-36.
5. Tageja N, Giorgadze T, Zonder J. Dermatological complications following initiation of lenalidomide in a patient with chronic lymphocytic leukemia. *Intern Med J.* 2011;41(3):286-288.
6. Al Hammadi A, Asai Y, Patt M, Sasseville D. Erythema annulare centrifugum secondary to treatment of finasteride. *J Drugs Dermatol.* 2007;6(4):260-463.
7. Rosina P, Francesco S, Barba A. Erythema annulare centrifugum and pregnancy. *Int J Dermatol.* 2002;41(8):516-517.

8. Gonzalez-Vela MC, Gonzalez-Lopez MA, Val-Bernal JF, et al. Erythema annulare centrifugum in a HIV-positive patient. *Int J Dermatol.* 2006;45(12):1432-1435.
9. Weyers W, Diaz-Cascajo C, Weyers I. Erythema annulare centrifugum: results of a clinicopathologic study of 73 patients. *Am J Dermatopathol.* 2003;25(6):451-462.
10. White JW. Gyrate erythema. *Dermatol Clin.* 1985;3:129-139.
11. Hsu S, Le FH, Khoshevis MR. Differential diagnosis of annular lesions. *Am Fam Physician.* 2001;64(2):289-296.
12. Zackheim H, McCalmont T. Mycosis fungoides: the great imitator. *J Am Acad Dermatol.* 2002;47(6):914-918.
13. Gniadecki R. Case report: calcipotriol for erythema annulare centrifugum. British Association of Dermatologists. *Br J Dermatol.* 2002;146:317-319.
14. Reuter J, Braun-Falco M, Termeer C, Bruckner-Tuderman L. Erythema annulare centrifugum Darier: successful therapy with topical calcitriol and 311 nm-ultraviolet B narrow band phototherapy [in German]. *Hautarzt.* 2007;58(2):146-148.
15. Minni J, Sarro R. A novel therapeutic approach to erythema annulare centrifugum. *J Am Acad Dermatol.* 2006;54(3 suppl 2):S134-S135.
16. De Aloe G, Rubegni P, Risulo M, et al. Erythema annulare centrifugum successfully treated with metronidazole. *Clin Exp Dermatol.* 2005;30(5):583-584.
17. Knott L. http://www.patient.co.uk/doctor/Erythema-Annulare-Centrifugum.htm. Accessed on July 6, 2014.

PART 15

PODIATRY

Strength of Recommendation (SOR)	Definition
A	Recommendation based on consistent and good-quality patient-oriented evidence.*
B	Recommendation based on inconsistent or limited-quality patient-oriented evidence.*
C	Recommendation based on consensus, usual practice, opinion, disease-oriented evidence, or case series for studies of diagnosis, treatment, prevention, or screening.*

*See Appendix A on pages 1241-1244 for further information.

205 CORN AND CALLUS

Naohiro Shibuya, DPM
Javier La Fontaine, DPM

PATIENT STORY

A 52-year-old man with diabetes and mild sensory neuropathy presented with callus under "the ball of his foot" for at least 5 years. He recently noticed that the callus had grown thicker as he gained weight. Sharp debridement of the callus was performed, and an offloading pad was placed (**Figure 205-1**). The patient walked out of the office with less pain and discomfort. He was encouraged to use a pumice stone gently after bathing. One important goal is to avoid an ulcer (**Figure 205-2**), which occurred in another patient who did not get care for his callus.

INTRODUCTION

Corns and calluses are localized, thickened epidermis, resulting from mechanical pressure or shearing force applied repeatedly on the same area. A callus is located on the plantar surface and "grows in." A corn is located on the dorsal surface or between digits and "grows out." An ulcer forms if the lesion penetrates the subcutaneous layer. Initial management includes removing the pressure by changing shoes or using pads followed by sharp debridement if needed.

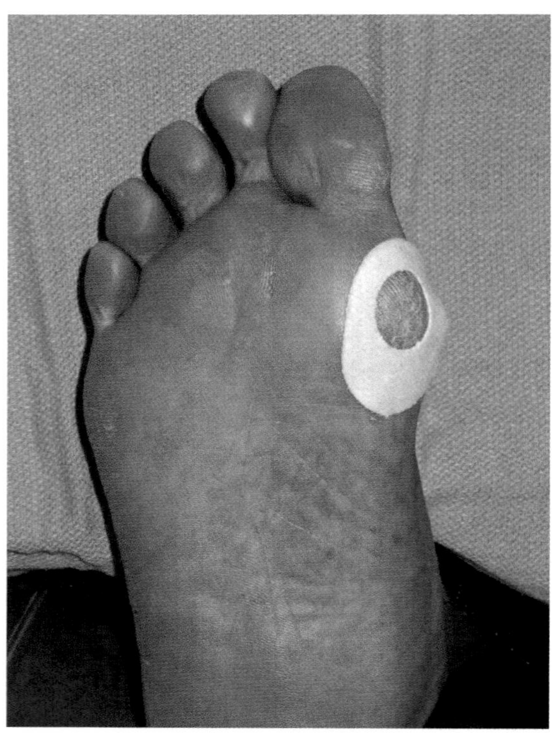

FIGURE 205-1 Typical callus under the first metatarsal head. An offloading device can alleviate pain caused by the callus. *(Reproduced with permission from Naohiro Shibuya, DPM.)*

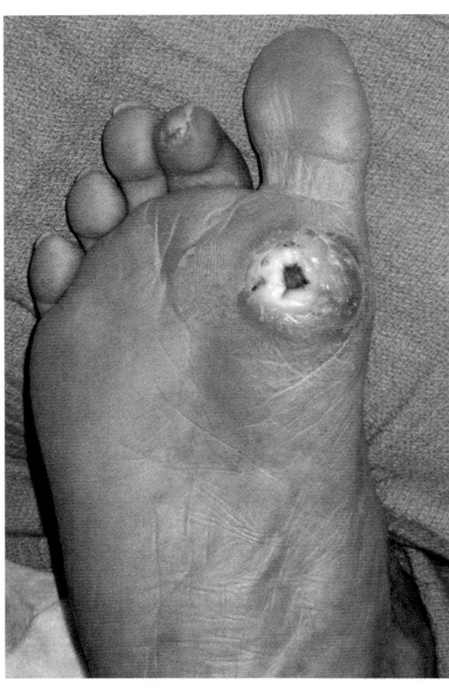

FIGURE 205-2 Callus resulting in an underlying ulceration in a person with diabetes. A neglected callus in a high-risk patient can result in ulceration and infection. *(Reproduced with permission from Naohiro Shibuya, DPM.)*

SYNONYMS

Corn and calluses are also known as hyperkeratotic lesion, keratosis, heloma durum (hard corn) or heloma molle (soft corn), tyloma (callus), or clavi (corns).

EPIDEMIOLOGY

In one population-based study, 20% of men and 40% of women reported corns or calluses.[1]

ETIOLOGY AND PATHOPHYSIOLOGY

Calluses and corns are caused by following multiple factors:

- Mechanical pressure from abnormal biomechanics, underlying spur/exostosis, ill-fitting shoes, physiologic repetitive activities, and foot surgery or amputation that result in increased focal pressure at the distance site[2]
- Shearing force from ill-fitting shoes, foot deformities (eg, hammer toe and bunion), and physiologic repetitive activities
- A foreign body in the foot or shoe

RISK FACTORS

- Bunion (**Figure 205-3**), hammer toe (**Figure 205-4**), flatfoot, high-arched (cavus) foot
- Older age, fat pad atrophy

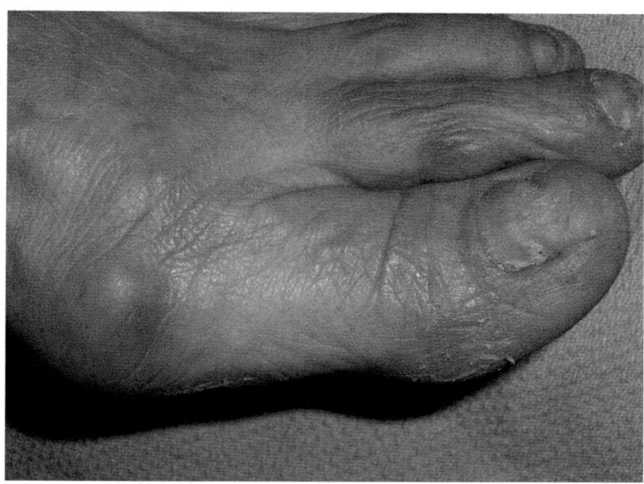

FIGURE 205-3 Bunion resulting in callus on the side of the big toe and a corn between the first and second digits because of abnormal biomechanical pressure. (*Reproduced with permission from Richard P. Usatine, MD.*)

- Smoking
- Female gender
- Genodermatoses with abnormal keratin formation (**Figure 205-5**)

DIAGNOSIS

The diagnosis of callus or corn formation is made clinically. Radiographic examination is helpful in identifying underlying bony pathology.

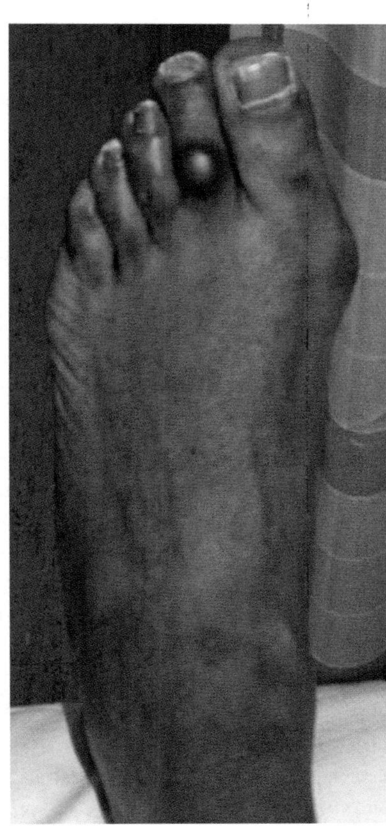

FIGURE 205-4 Dorsal hard corn formed secondary to a hammer-toe deformity. (*Reproduced with permission from Naohiro Shibuya, DPM.*)

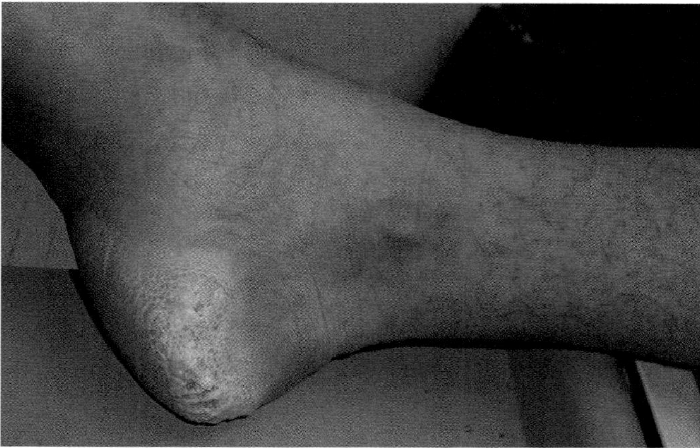

FIGURE 205-5 Pachyonychia congenita causes hard callus on the feet and other abnormal keratin papules seen on the legs in this young man. This genetic disease causes such painful thick calluses that it hurts to walk. (*Reproduced with permission from Richard P. Usatine, MD.*)

CLINICAL FEATURES

- Pain at site, especially with pressure
- Prominent underlying bony structure or deformity of the foot (high arch, flatfoot, or bunion)
- Hard, slightly hyperpigmented or skin colored, well demarcated (**Figure 205-6**)
- Hard or soft nucleus

TYPICAL DISTRIBUTION

- Callus (weight-bearing surface)—Under the metatarsal heads, plantar-medial hallux interphalangeal joint, distal tip of the digits, plantar heel, fifth metatarsal base, dorsolateral fifth digit, and nail folds.
- Corns (non–weight-bearing surface)—Dorsal proximal interphalangeal joints in patients with hammer-toe deformity (see **Figure 205-4**), interdigital spaces, most commonly the fourth space (**Figure 205-7**).

IMAGING

Dorsoplantar, lateral, and medial oblique weight-bearing plain radiographs, with a metal marker on the lesion may detect an exostosis (spur). Underlying deformities can also be assessed with plain radiographs.

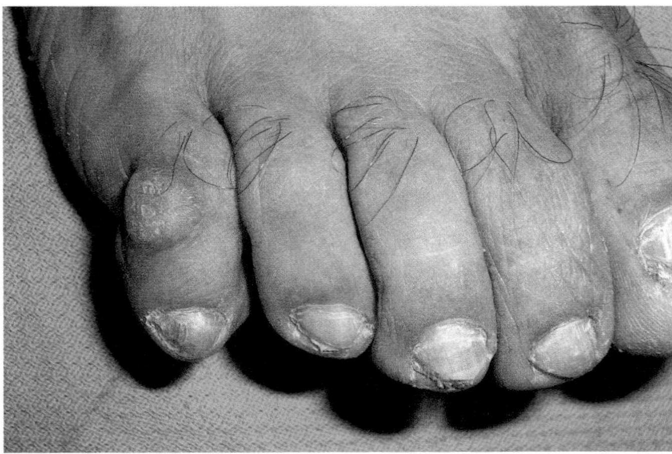

FIGURE 205-6 Hard corn in a typical location on the dorsum of the fifth digit. (*Reproduced with permission from Richard P. Usatine, MD.*)

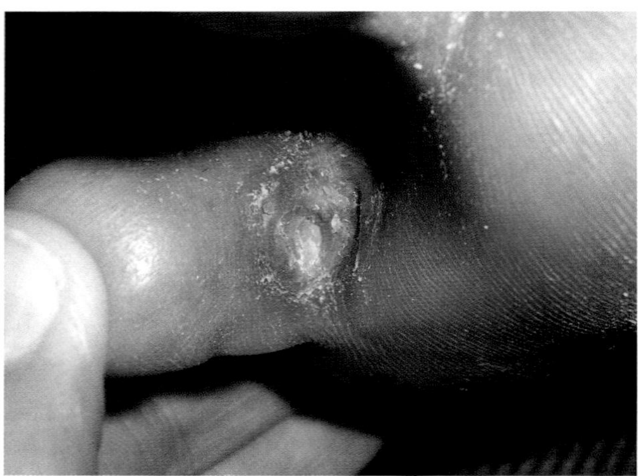

FIGURE 205-7 Soft corn in the fourth interspace at the base of the fifth digit. (*Reproduced with permission from Richard P. Usatine, MD.*)

DIFFERENTIAL DIAGNOSIS

Other painful hyperkeratotic lesions in the foot can be caused by the following:

- Plantar warts are common painful human papillomavirus (HPV) skin infections found on the sole of the foot. Black dots (thrombosed capillaries) and disruption of skin lines differentiate these warts from callus or corns (see Chapter 133, Plantar Warts).
- Acrolentiginous melanoma can occur on the foot and become painful over time. These are usually pigmented with irregular borders and variations in color. If these are amelanotic they may be harder to diagnose. Any unusual growth on the foot should be biopsied (see Chapter 170, Melanoma).
- Nonmelanoma skin cancers rarely occur on the foot and are more likely to be on the dorsum of the foot where there is more sun exposure. These cancers are hyperkeratotic and may ulcerate. If suspicious, a shave biopsy should be adequate for diagnosis (see Chapters 168, Basal Cell Carcinoma and 169, Squamous Cell Carcinoma).
- Porokeratosis is a deep, seeded callus that has been described as a "plugged sweat duct" and is not necessarily located in a weight-bearing area.
- Diseases with abnormal keratin production can cause painful and thick callus on the feet in the same areas such as the heels and under the metatarsal heads. **Figure 205-5** is an example of a severely painful and hypertrophic callus on the heel of a patient with the genodermatosis of pachyonychia congenita.
- Surgical physiologic/hypertrophic scar can be easily identified by the surgical orientation of the incision and patient history.

MANAGEMENT

First, consider the following conservative measures:

- Suggest that the patient change shoes to something that puts less pressure on the area involved.
- Pad the foot to limit shearing force from shoes (see **Figure 205-1**).
- Use interdigital spacers to relieve pressure (**Figure 205-8**).
- Incorporate offloading devices or "cutoffs" in custom-made orthoses to realign an underlying deformity to minimize abnormal biomechanics.

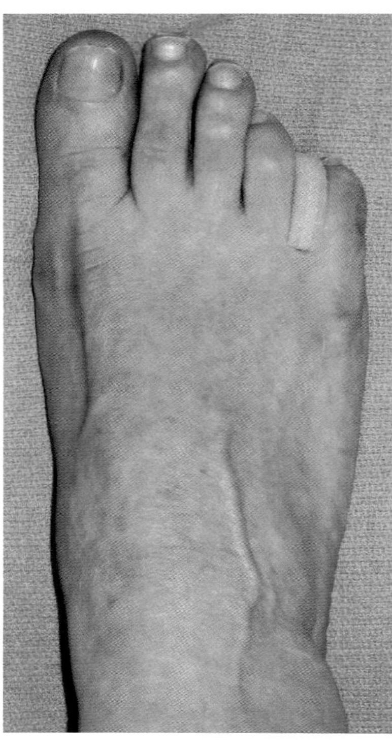

FIGURE 205-8 A simple spacer can alleviate pain caused by the corn in the fourth interdigital space. (*Reproduced with permission from Naohiro Shibuya, DPM.*)

- Suggest the patient reduce activity level on the feet.
- Encourage the patient to stop smoking and offer assistance.

If conservative measures fail to work, consider the following surgical options:

- Sharp debridement of the lesion provides instant temporary relief from pain and discomfort. Infiltration of a local anesthetic may be necessary before debridement of an extremely painful lesion, but most calluses and corns can be debrided without anesthesia. Perform sharp debridement with a #10 or #15 surgical blade. The #10 blade is especially good for large callus. Debride the lesion down to soft, nonkeratotic tissue and remove the hard nucleus (**Figure 205-9**).
- In a patient with recurring lesions, consider a surgical referral to a foot specialist to correct an underlying deformity or spur.
- Exostectomy of the prominent underlying bone can be done with a minimal incision technique.
- Consider prophylactic correction of the deformity and/or removal of exostosis in a high-risk patient (eg, patients with diabetes who are immunocompromised and neuropathic) to reduce the risk of future ulceration and infection.
- Plastic procedures (eg, excisional biopsy with primary closure or local flap) may be necessary in patients with a chronic lesion of idiopathic origin.

PREVENTION

- Well-padded shoes and/or padded insoles can prevent hyperkeratotic lesion formation.
- Insoles made by Spenco or Dr. Scholl's can be an inexpensive start before purchasing customized orthotics.

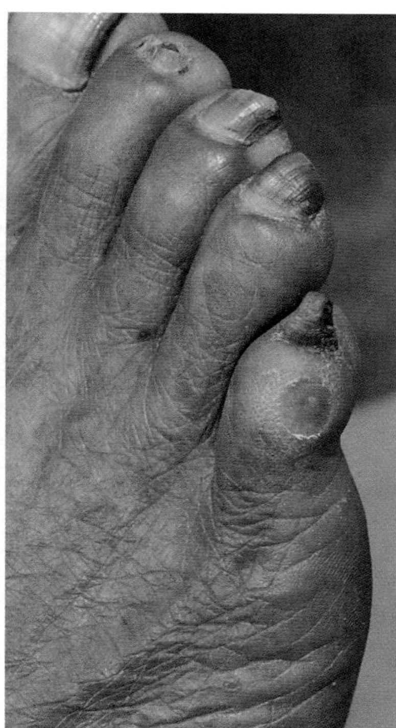

FIGURE 205-9 A corn on the fifth digit was pared down with a sharp scalpel and the patient had immediate relief while walking. (*Reproduced with permission from Richard P. Usatine, MD.*)

- People with severe underlying deformity may benefit from customized orthotic and shoe management to relieve localized pressure in the foot.

PROGNOSIS

In healthy, younger patients, both conservative and surgical treatments have good prognosis. Severe peripherally neuropathic patients neglect repetitive painful stimuli, and they are prone to ulceration from untreated hyperkeratotic lesions. Surgical management by changing the biomechanics of the foot is often successful, but it can cause a "transfer lesion"—a new lesion developing distance from the original lesion.

FOLLOW-UP

- A healthy patient can be seen in an "as-needed" basis.
- A high-risk patient requires periodic follow-up and sharp debridement of the lesion are necessary to prevent development of a neurotrophic ulcer.
- If the patient develops an open lesion, obtain plain radiographs to rule out osteomyelitis and gas gangrene. An irregular, hyperpigmented, fast-growing lesion must be biopsied.

PATIENT EDUCATION

Conservative measures are effective in mild lesions. If conservative measures fail, surgical management is indicated to correct the underlying cause of the problem. Surgical correction can result in a "transferred lesion" by shifting the pressure point away from the original site.[3] Tell patients with neuropathy and/or their caregivers to examine the patient's feet daily for potential ulceration. An overlying hyperkeratotic lesion can mask an underlying ulcer. Drainage, maceration, and malodor are signs of underlying ulceration and infection.

PATIENT RESOURCES

- PubMed Health. *Corns and Calluses*—**http://www.ncbi.nlm.nih.gov/pubmedhealth/PMH0002212/.**

PROVIDER RESOURCES

- Medscape. *Corns*—**http://emedicine.medscape.com/article/1089807.**

REFERENCES

1. Garrow AP, Silman AJ, Macfarlane GJ. The Cheshire Foot Pain and Disability Survey: a population survey assessing prevalence and associations. *Pain*. 2004;110(1-2):378-384.
2. Freeman DB. Corns and calluses resulting from mechanical hyperkeratosis. *Am Fam Physician*. 2002;65(11):2277-2280.
3. McGlamry ED, Banks AS. Lesser ray deformities. In: Downey MS, McGlamry MC, eds. *McGlamry's Comprehensive Textbook of Foot and Ankle Surgery*. 3rd ed. Vol. 1. Philadelphia, PA: Lippincott Williams & Wilkins; 2001:253-372.

206 BUNION DEFORMITY

Naohiro Shibuya, DPM
Javier La Fontaine, DPM

PATIENT HISTORY

A healthy 34-year-old woman has had "bunion pain" for 5 years. Her custom-made orthoses alleviate 50% of her pain. On examination, she has severe lateral deviation of the hallux (**Figure 206-1**), a mildly dorsiflexed second digit, tenderness at the medial prominence, painless first metatarsophalangeal (MTP) range of motion, and a callus under the second metatarsal head. Radiographs (**Figure 206-2**) show medial angulation of the first metatarsal and lateral deviation of the hallux.

The patient was referred to podiatry for surgical correction of the bunion deformity. After surgery, she was placed in a short-leg cast for 6 weeks. She progressed to a regular shoe over the next month and was encouraged to use the custom-made orthoses for her flatfoot to prevent recurrence of the bunion.

INTRODUCTION

Bunion deformity is characterized by the presence of a medial prominence at the first MTP joint, caused by an abducted hallux and adducted first metatarsal. The deformity causes irritation in a tight shoe and pain in the MTP joint. Initial therapy can be conservative with correction of footwear and padding. Surgical procedures correct the misalignment, rather than shave the medial prominence.

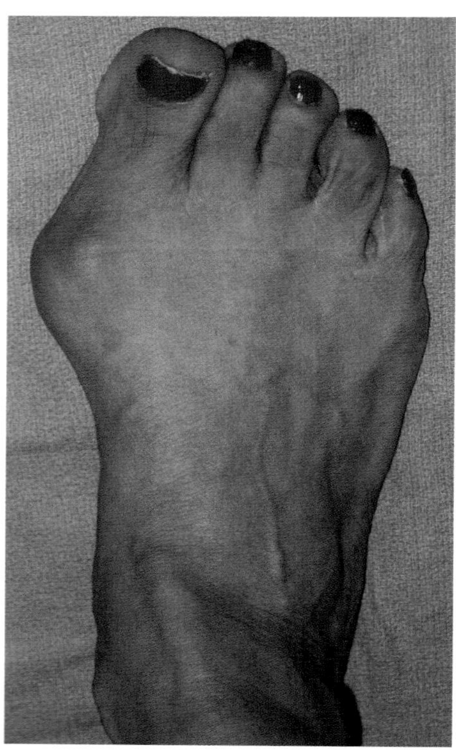

FIGURE 206-1 Laterally deviated hallux resulting in a bunion (hallux abducto valgus deformity). (*Reproduced with permission from Naohiro Shibuya, DPM.*)

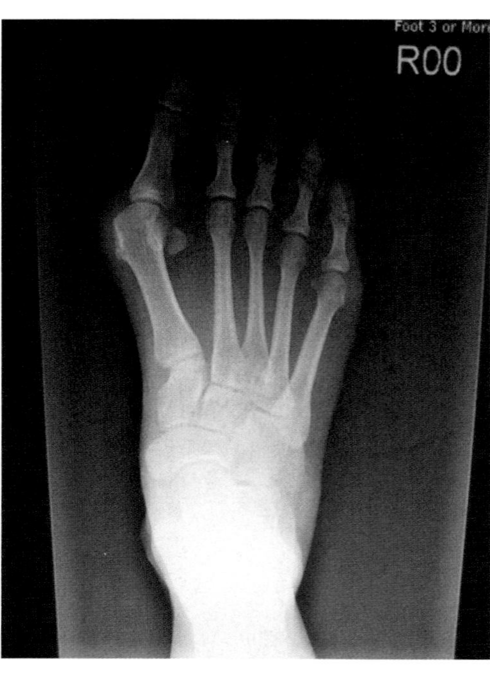

FIGURE 206-2 A weight-bearing dorsoplantar plain radiograph helps in assessing severity of the deformity and determining treatment plan. (*Reproduced with permission from Naohiro Shibuya, DPM.*)

SYNONYMS

Bunion deformity is also known as hallux valgus, hallux abducto valgus, metatarsus adductovarus.

EPIDEMIOLOGY

- The prevalence of bunions ranges from 2% to 50%.[1]
- It is far more common in women.

ETIOLOGY AND PATHOPHYSIOLOGY

Bunion deformities are caused by following multiple factors:

- Genetic and hereditary factors
- Abnormal biomechanics (limb length discrepancy, hypermobility/ligament laxity, flatfoot deformity, malaligned skeletal structures, and ankle equinus)[2]
- Neuromuscular diseases
- Ill-fitting shoes
- Trauma
- Iatrogenic causes

RISK FACTORS

- Flatfoot
- Family history
- Ligamentous laxity

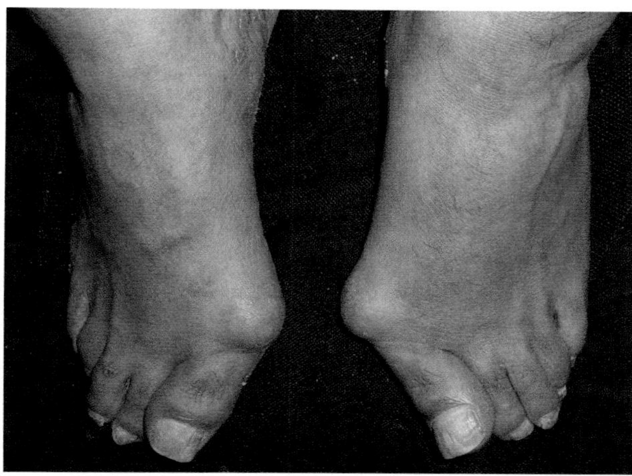

FIGURE 206-3 Severe bilateral bunion deformities causing lateral deviations in the other digits. Note the onychomycosis and flaking skin from tinea pedis. *(Reproduced with permission from Richard P. Usatine, MD.)*

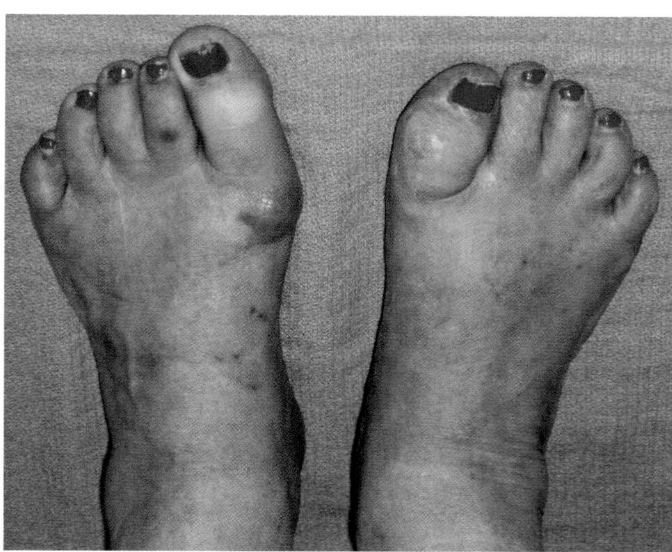

FIGURE 206-4 A unilateral bunion deformity is often a result of limb length discrepancy. Note the prominent erythema around the first metatarsophalangeal joint of the left foot only. *(Reproduced with permission from Naohiro Shibuya, DPM.)*

DIAGNOSIS

The diagnosis of hallux abducto valgus deformity is made clinically and radiographically.

CLINICAL FEATURES

- Laterally deviated hallux, erythema, edema.
- Tenderness on the medial eminence at the first MTP joint and pain through the first MTP joint range of motion.
- Associated signs—Hypermobility, flatfoot deformity, second MTP joint pain, pain under the second metatarsal head, overlapped second digit, decreased ankle dorsiflexion, concurrent gout, decreased first MTP joint range of motion, sesamoiditis, hyperkeratosis, and hammer toe deformity (see Chapter 207, Hammer Toe, Figure 207-4).

TYPICAL DISTRIBUTION

- Often bilateral (**Figure 206-3**).
- A unilateral bunion deformity is often caused by a limb length discrepancy (**Figure 206-4**).

IMAGING

- Weight-bearing plain radiographs are obtained in dorsoplantar, lateral, and medial oblique views (see **Figure 206-2**).
- Lateral deviation of the hallux and medial deviation of the first metatarsal bone are noted in the dorsoplantar view.
- The first MTP joint narrowing, osteophyte formation, subchondral cysts, and sclerosis are indicative of osteoarthritis.
- The lateral view is useful in assessing elevation of the first metatarsal, dorsal spur formation at the first MTP joint, and hammer-toe deformity.

DIFFERENTIAL DIAGNOSIS

Pain and swelling around the first MTP joint may be caused by the following:

- Gout or pseudogout presents with acute pain with signs of inflammation and prior history of gout/pseudogout. Joint aspiration may be performed to rule out septic joint (see Chapter 105, Gout).
- Rheumatoid arthritis presents with pain, inflammation, and loss of range of motion and is often symmetrical. Radiographic evidence of other small pedal joint involvement is usually evident (see Chapter 99, Rheumatoid Arthritis).
- Septic joint presents with acute pain, loss of range of motion, and systemic signs and symptoms of infectious process.

MANAGEMENT

Conservative measures and surgical treatments are described below.

CONSERVATIVE MEASURES

- Change to shoes with a wider toe box.
- Place a toe spacer in the first interdigital space to straighten the hallux and decrease the irritation caused by rubbing of the first and second digits.
- Pad the shoe to limit shearing force (**Figure 206-5**).
- Custom-made orthoses help slow progression of the deformity caused by biomechanical factors.
- Rest, nonsteroidal anti-inflammatory drugs (NSAIDs), and ice may help an inflamed joint and/or shoe irritation.
- Physical therapy may help improve joint range of motion, reduce edema, or decrease nerve pain.

SURGICAL TREATMENT

- Consider surgical referral to a foot specialist for correction of the deformity.
- The tendon and ligament balancing procedure is used for minor, flexible deformities.
- Exostectomy may help patients who have no joint pain, but complain about extra-articular "bump pain."
- Osteotomy to realign the bony structure is indicated for moderate-to-severe deformities (**Figure 206-6**).

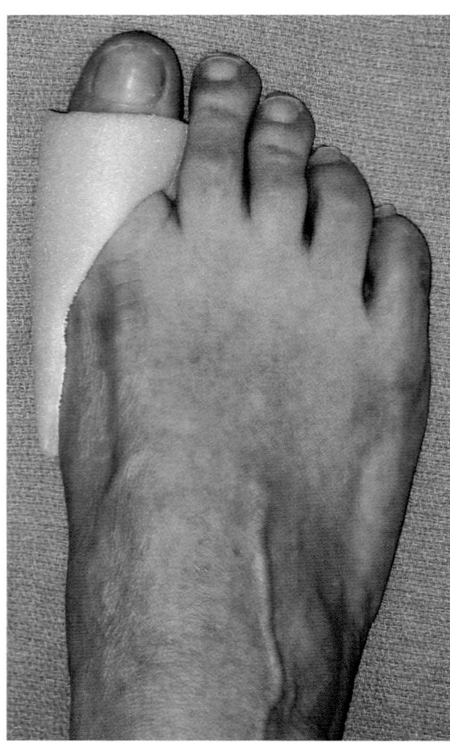

FIGURE 206-5 Simple padding can alleviate shoe irritation from the bunion deformity. (*Reproduced with permission from Naohiro Shibuya, DPM.*)

- Arthrodesis of the first MTP or metatarsocuneiform joint is indicated in a severe deformity.
- Adjunctive procedures (eg, correction of hammer-toe deformities, flatfoot deformity, ankle equinus, and resection of the sesamoid bone) may be required for a positive long-term outcome.

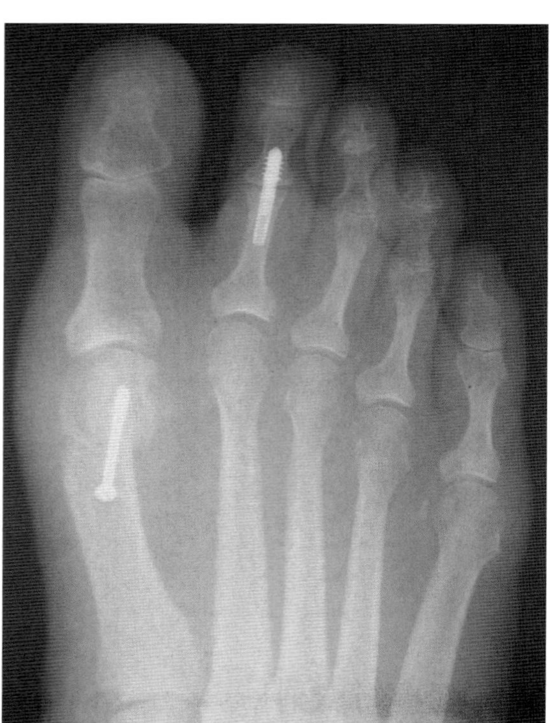

FIGURE 206-6 Surgical correction is indicated if conservative measures fail. (*Reproduced with permission from Naohiro Shibuya, DPM.*)

PREVENTION

- Treatment of underlying etiology, such as flatfoot can prevent progression of bunion deformity.
- Avoid shoes that push the hallux over in patients who are starting to develop a bunion.

PROGNOSIS

- The prognosis worsens as the deformity progresses.
- Function and quality of life can be affected in severe debilitating deformity. Surgical correction provides good prognosis in such patients.

FOLLOW-UP

The patient may be seen on an as-needed basis. Serial plain radiographs can be obtained to follow the progression of the deformity and arthritic changes in the first MTP joint.

PATIENT EDUCATION

Conservative measures may or may not provide temporary relief and prevent progression of the deformity. Surgical management is necessary to correct the deformity. Surgical treatment will typically require 2 to 6 weeks of non–weight-bearing status postoperatively, depending on the procedure performed. More severe deformities will require a more extensive surgical approach and longer recovery period.

PATIENT RESOURCES

- PubMed Health. *Bunions*—**http://www.ncbi.nlm.nih.gov/pubmedhealth/PMH0002211/.**

PROVIDER RESOURCES

- Medscape. *Bunion*—**http://emedicine.medscape.com/article/1235796.**

REFERENCES

1. McGlamry ED, Banks AS. *McGlamry's Comprehensive Textbook of Foot and Ankle Surgery*. 3rd ed. Vol 2. Philadelphia, PA: Lippincott Williams & Wilkins; 2001:66.
2. Chang TJ. *Master Techniques in Podiatric Surgery: The Foot and Ankle.* Philadelphia, PA: Lippincott Williams & Wilkins; 2005:560.

207 HAMMER TOE

Naohiro Shibuya, DPM
Javier La Fontaine, DPM

PATIENT HISTORY

A 44-year-old woman presented with pain in the ball of her left foot on weight bearing. She works as a nurse and walks most of her 12-hour shift. Two months ago she noticed a new deformity of the second digit of her left foot (**Figure 207-1**). Her second digit was contracted with a nonreducible proximal interphalangeal joint and reducible metatarsophalangeal (MTP) joint. Her X-ray is seen in **Figure 207-2.**

She was referred to a podiatrist who diagnosed an acute isolated hammer-toe deformity. At the time of surgery a plantar plate rupture at the MTP joint was found. The podiatrist fused her proximal interphalangeal (PIP) joint and released her extensor tendon and dorsal capsule at the MTP joint to reduce the deformity. She began protective ambulation in a surgical shoe on postoperative day 3. An internal fixation wire, which was used to fixate the fusion site, was removed in 4 weeks. She returned to work and her regular activities within 6 weeks of the operation.

INTRODUCTION

Hammer-toe deformity is a flexion contracture in the PIP joint of a pedal digit, resulting in plantar flexion of the middle phalanx at the PIP joint with dorsal angulation of the proximal phalanx at the MTP joint. Hammer toes are associated with imbalance of soft tissue structures around the joints in the digits and are often progressive. Surgical correction is required when deformity interferes with function.

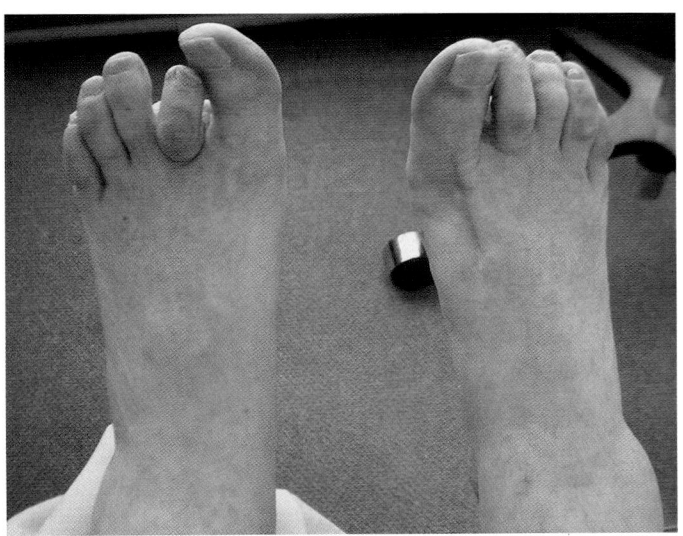

FIGURE 207-1 A plantar plate rupture at the metatarsophalangeal joint from overuse often causes an acute isolated hammer-toe deformity. *(Reproduced with permission from Naohiro Shibuya, DPM.)*

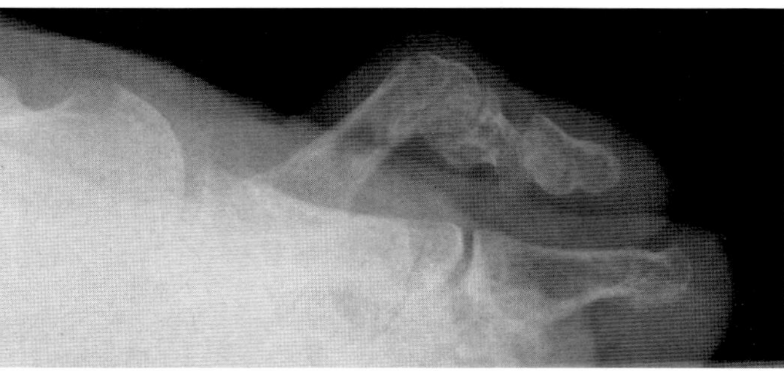

FIGURE 207-2 This lateral plain film shows dorsiflexion of the proximal phalanx at the metatarsophalangeal joint and plantarflexion of the middle phalanx at the proximal interphalangeal joint of the second digit. *(Reproduced with permission from Naohiro Shibuya, DPM.)*

SYNONYMS

- Hammer toe, claw toe, and mallet toe describe similar digital contractures.
- Claw toe refers to progression of hammer toe to include extension of the MTP joint along with flexion in the PIP joint.
- Mallet toe has a digital contracture at the distal interphalangeal (DIP) joint.

EPIDEMIOLOGY

Hammer-toe deformity is the most common digital deformity, and it can affect up to 60% of adults. The second digit is most commonly affected.[1]

ETIOLOGY AND PATHOPHYSIOLOGY

A hammer toe is caused by following multiple factors:

- Genetic and hereditary factors
- Abnormal biomechanics (cavus or high-arch foot, flatfoot deformity, loss of intrinsic muscle function, and hypermobile first ray)
- Long metatarsal and/or digit
- Systemic arthritidis
- Neuromuscular diseases such as Charcot-Marie-Tooth disease (**Figure 207-3**)
- Ill-fitting shoes
- Trauma
- Iatrogenic causes

RISK FACTORS

- High-arch foot type (cavus foot)
- Flatfeet
- Bunion deformity (**Figure 207-4**)

DIAGNOSIS

The diagnosis of hammer-toe deformity is made clinically and radiographically.

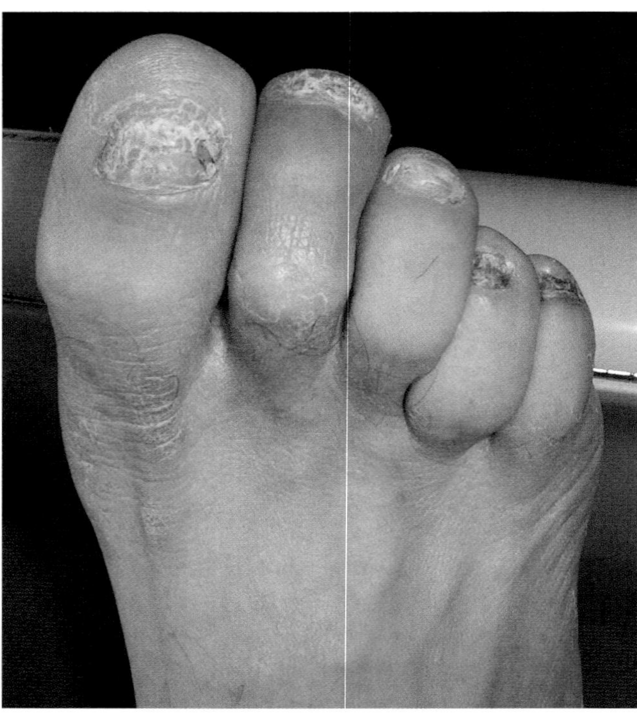

FIGURE 207-3 Severe hammer-toe deformity caused by Charcot-Marie-Tooth disease, an autosomal dominant neuromuscular disease. (*Reproduced with permission from Richard P. Usatine, MD.*)

CLINICAL FEATURES

- Pain and deformity in one or more of the lesser toes.
- Dorsiflexed proximal phalanx at the MTP joint and plantarflexed middle phalanx at the PIP joint of a lesser digit.
- Callus formation at the dorsal aspect of the PIP joint and/or distal aspect of the digit.

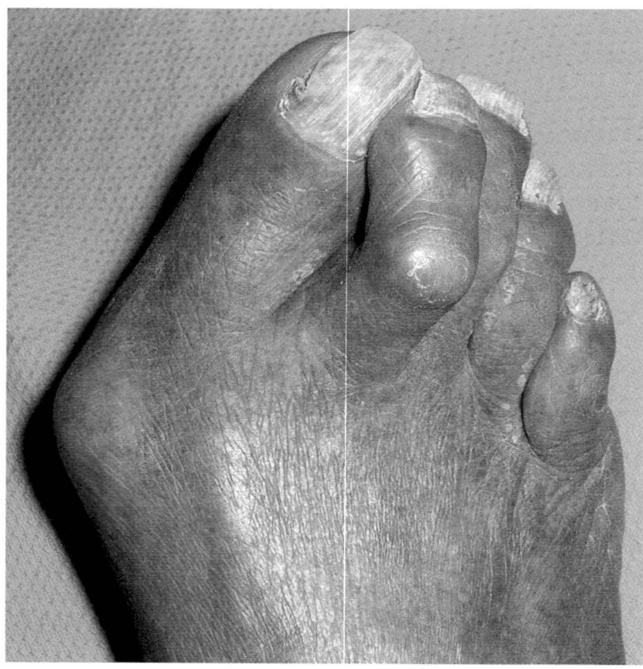

FIGURE 207-4 Hammer-toe deformity caused by a bunion. (*Reproduced with permission from Richard P. Usatine, MD.*)

- Edema and tenderness on the plantar aspect of the lesser MTP joint(s).
- Associated signs—Cavus foot deformity, flatfoot deformity, bunion deformity, transverse deformity of the digits, decreased ankle dorsiflexion, and bowstringing of the extensor and/or flexor tendons.
- Evaluation of the digit in weight-bearing and non–weight-bearing conditions helps assess reducibility and rigidity of the deformity. In the case of predislocation syndrome (acute rupture or tear of the MTP joint capsule or plantar plate), the deformity may not be appreciated unless the foot is evaluated in the weight-bearing position.[2]

IMAGING

Obtain weight-bearing plain radiographs in dorsoplantar, lateral, and medial oblique views (see **Figure 207-2**).

- Dorsal angulation and/or translation of the proximal phalanx on the metatarsal head with plantar angulation of the middle phalanx (lateral view)
- Degenerative changes in the digital joints and dislocation in the MTP joint
- Transverse deformity and abnormal metatarsal length (dorsoplantar view)

DIFFERENTIAL DIAGNOSIS

Pain and swelling in the digit may be caused by the following:

- Gout or pseudogout presents with acute pain with signs of inflammation, and prior history of gout/pseudogout. Joint aspiration may be performed to rule out septic joint (see Chapter 105, Gout).
- Rheumatoid arthritis presents with pain, inflammation, and loss of range of motion and is often symmetrical. Radiographic evidence of other small foot joint involvement usually is evident (see Chapter 99, Rheumatoid Arthritis).
- Septic joint presents with acute pain, loss of range of motion, and systemic signs and symptoms of infectious process.
- Fractured toe caused by sudden trauma.
- Neuroma in the intermetatarsal space (Morton neuroma) with compression of the intermetatarsal nerves—Numbness and cramping of the innervated toes are the most common symptoms.

MANAGEMENT

Conservative measures and surgical treatment may be used to correct this condition. Note that a neglected hammer-toe deformity could result in ulceration in a patient with diabetes.

NONPHARMACOLOGIC

- Change shoes.
- Pad shoes to limit shearing force. A crest pad can be used to prevent painful callus formation at the distal tip of the digit (**Figure 207-5**).
- Splinting can be used in an early flexible hammer toe.
- Custom-made orthoses are helpful to slow down progression of the deformity if it is caused by biomechanical factors.
- Rest, nonsteroidal anti-inflammatory drugs (NSAIDs), and ice help an inflamed joint and/or shoe irritation.

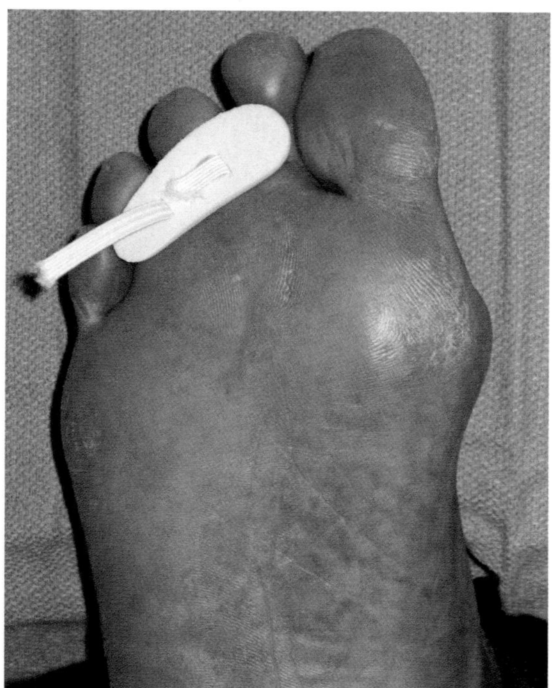

FIGURE 207-5 A crest pad prevents painful callus formation at the distal tip of the digit. (*Reproduced with permission from Naohiro Shibuya, DPM.*)

SURGICAL TREATMENT

- Consider surgical referral to a foot specialist to correct the deformity.
- Percutaneous tenotomy and/or capsulotomy are used for mild, flexible deformities.
- Resectional arthroplasty at the PIP joint may be beneficial for a more rigid deformity.
- Shortening osteotomy of the metatarsal is indicated in the deformities resulting from the long metatarsal.
- Arthrodesis (fusion) of the PIP joint and/or flexor tendon transfer is indicated for a severe deformity (**Figure 207-6**).
- Adjunctive procedures (eg, correction of bunion, cavus foot, flatfoot deformities, and ankle equinus) may be necessary for a good long-term outcome.

PREVENTION

- Proper shoes with an adequate toe box and heel counter prevent excessive contracture of the digits.
- Controlling associated deformities, such as bunion and flatfoot deformities via orthotic management can prevent progression of hammer-toe deformity.

PROGNOSIS

- The prognosis worsens as the deformity progresses.
- Function and quality of life can be affected in severe debilitating deformity. Surgical correction provides good prognosis in such patients.

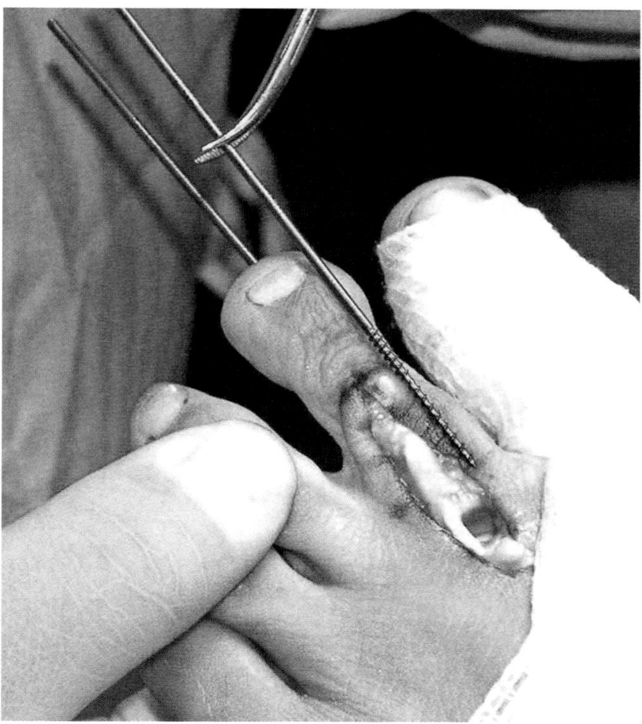

FIGURE 207-6 Proximal interphalangeal joint arthrodesis (fusion) is often used to correct hammer-toe deformity. (*Reproduced with permission from Naohiro Shibuya, DPM.*)

FOLLOW-UP

Periodic debridement of the calluses developed from the deformity may be sufficient in many of the patients if the deformity is not progressive. Serial plain radiographs can be obtained to follow the progression of the deformity and arthritic changes in the first MTP joint. In a high-risk, immunocompromised, neuropathic patient, prophylactic surgical correction of the deformity may be indicated.

PATIENT EDUCATION

Explain to patients that conservative measures may prevent progression of the deformity and provide temporary relief, but that surgical management is necessary to correct the deformity. Surgical treatment can require up to 4 to 6 weeks of non–weight-bearing status postoperatively in severe deformities. A less-involved surgical approach to correct a mild deformity can allow a patient to walk on the same day as the surgery. In many cases, fixation with a pin, small screw, or implant is necessary to correct the deformity.

PATIENT RESOURCES

- MedlinePlus. *Hammer Toe*—**http://www.nlm.nih.gov/medlineplus/ency/article/001235.htm.**

PROVIDER RESOURCES

- Medscape. *Hammertoe Deformity*—**http://emedicine.medscape.com/article/1235341.**

REFERENCES

1. McGlamry ED, Banks AS. *McGlamry's Comprehensive Textbook of Foot and Ankle Surgery*. 3rd ed. Philadelphia, PA: Lippincott Williams & Wilkins; 2001:66.
2. Yu GV, Judge MS, Hudson JR, Seidelmann FE. Predislocation syndrome. Progressive subluxation/dislocation of the lesser metatarsophalangeal joint. *J Am Podiatr Med Assoc*. 2002;92(4):182-199.

208 ISCHEMIC ULCER

Javier La Fontaine, DPM
Naohiro Shibuya, DPM

PATIENT STORY

A 58-year-old woman with uncontrolled type 2 diabetes, hypercholesterolemia, and tobacco use presented with a 2-month history of a nonhealing ulceration on her left foot (**Figure 208-1**). She believes this started after she stepped on a tack. She presented with the ulcer, loss of protective sensation, and a nonpalpable posterior tibial pulse. She began treatment in a wound care center. Arterial noninvasive studies showed severe vascular disease and she underwent revascularization. While in the hospital, she quit smoking and gained control of her diabetes. Her ulcer healed and she continues to take her diabetes medications and does not smoke.

INTRODUCTION

Ulcerations occur from ongoing biomechanical forces or trauma and require normal blood flow to heal. Nonhealing ulcers are commonly a result of peripheral ischemia seen in patients with diabetes and other vascular diseases. Treatment includes local wound care and improvement or correction of underlying factors causing ischemia. Untreated ischemic ulcers become infected and may require amputation of the affected area.

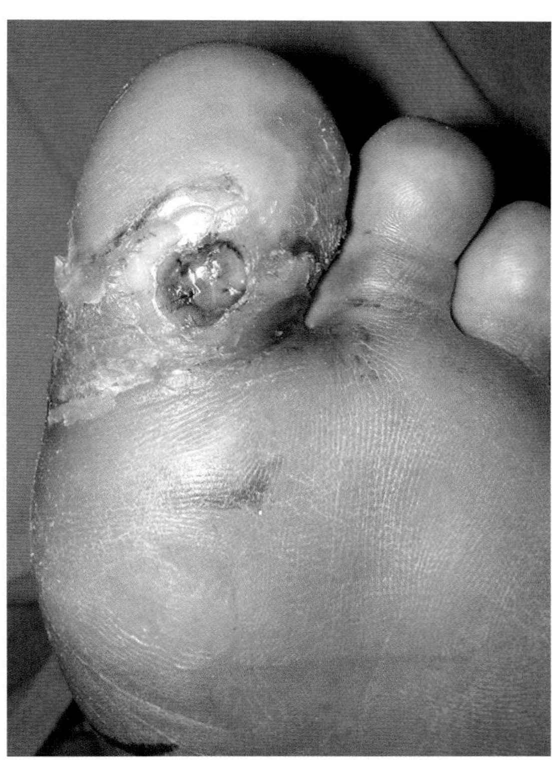

FIGURE 208-1 A 38-year-old woman with type 2 diabetes and an ischemic ulcer on the first digit of the left foot. The base of the wound is gray in color with pink surrounding wound margins. (*Reproduced with permission from Javier La Fontaine, DPM.*)

SYNONYMS

Ischemic ulcer is also known as arterial ulcer.

EPIDEMIOLOGY

Of patients with diabetes, 15% to 25% will develop an ulcer at an annual incidence of 1% to 4%.[1]

ETIOLOGY AND PATHOPHYSIOLOGY

Microvascular dysfunction is an important component of the disease process that occurs in diabetic foot disease. The abnormalities observed in the endothelium in patients with diabetes are not well understood and evidence suggests that endothelial dysfunction could be involved in the pathogenesis of diabetic macroangiopathy and microangiopathy.[2] Microangiopathy is a functional disease where neuropathy and autoregulation of capillaries lead to poor perfusion of the tissues, especially at the wound base.

RISK FACTORS

- Diabetes for more than 10 years,[3] especially with poor glycemic control and the presence of other macro- or microvascular complications
- Peripheral vascular disease from any cause or other vascular risk factors, including dyslipidemia and tobacco use
- Neuropathy caused by loss of protective sensation and as a sign of microvascular disease[3]
- History of a previous ischemic ulcer[3]
- Foot deformity in a patient with diabetes mellitus[3]

DIAGNOSIS

CLINICAL FEATURES

- Pain
- Gray/yellow fibrotic base (**Figures 208-1** and **208-2**)
- Undermined skin margins
- Punched-out appearance
- Nonpalpable pulses
- Associated trophic skin changes (eg, absent pedal hair and thin shiny skin)

TYPICAL DISTRIBUTION

Distal aspect of the toes

IMAGING

- Noninvasive studies (eg, arterial Doppler and pulse volume recordings) are important for baseline assessment of the patient's blood flow.[4]
- Radiographs may be necessary to rule out osteomyelitis.

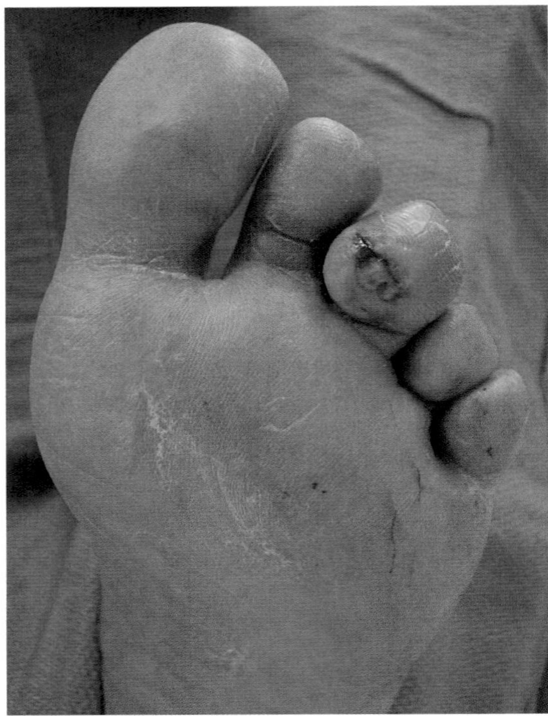

FIGURE 208-2 A 57-year-old man with diabetes for 25 years with an ischemic ulcer of the third toe. A grayish base is a common finding in this type of ulcer. *(Reproduced with permission from Javier La Fontaine, DPM.)*

DIFFERENTIAL DIAGNOSIS

- Neuropathic ulcer usually presents with beefy red wound base and hyperkeratosis at the skin margins (see Chapter 209, Neuropathic Ulcer).
- Infected wounds present with localized redness, edema, drainage, and warmness in any of the diabetic-type wounds with lack of systemic symptoms of infection.
- Gangrene usually is well-demarcated with black eschar in foot with vascular disease (see Chapter 211, Dry Gangrene).

MANAGEMENT

- Consider vascular surgery consultation to evaluate for revascularization.
- Carefully evaluate for a concomitant infection. Antibiotics are not indicated unless infection is present.
- Avoid aggressive debridement until optimization of blood flow occurs.
- Change dressings twice daily to evaluate the wound and keep a low bacterial load. Many advanced therapies can be added to accomplish the same goals.
- If the wound is plantar, offloading is important to prevent the wound from increasing in size.

PREVENTION

- In patients with diabetes, adequate glycemic control is essential. A yearly comprehensive foot examination should be performed.
- Smoking cessation.

PROGNOSIS

Prognosis of an ischemic ulcer depends on the possibility of revascularization. Many ulcers treated early heal. Untreated or inadequately treated ulcers lead to infection and amputation. Early recognition of underlying vascular disease is imperative for a successful outcome.

FOLLOW-UP

- Schedule weekly to biweekly visits to monitor the ulcer.
- Obtain serial radiographs every 4 weeks to monitor for the development of osteomyelitis.
- Closely monitor the patient every 3 to 4 months once healing has occurred. Patients who have had history of ulcerations are 36 times more likely to develop another ulcer.[5]

PATIENT EDUCATION

- Prevention measures, such as smoking cessation, are important to aid wound healing.[6]
- Promote successful treatment by encouraging adherence with use of offloading devices.
- Strive for normal glycemic control to optimize outcome for healing and surgical intervention.

PATIENT AND PROVIDER RESOURCES

- Cleveland Clinic. *Lower Extremity (Leg and Foot) Ulcers*—**http://my.clevelandclinic.org/heart/disorders/vascular/legfootulcer.aspx.**
- Yale School of Medicine. *Foot ulcers*—**http://medicine.yale.edu/surgery/vascular/care/conditions/foot_ulcers.aspx#page1.**

REFERENCES

1. Singh N, Armstrong DG, Lipsky BA. Preventing foot ulcers in patients with diabetes. *JAMA*. 2005;293:217-228.
2. La Fontaine J, Allen M, Davis C, Harkless LB, Shireman PK. Current concepts in diabetic microvascular dysfunction. *J Am Podiatr Med Assoc*. 2006;96(3):245-252.
3. Monteiro-Soares M, Vaz-Carneiro A, Sampaio S, Dinis-Ribeiro M. Validation and comparison of currently available stratification systems for patients with diabetes by risk of foot ulcer development. *Eur J Endocrinology*. 2012;167(3):401-407.
4. Sykes MT, Godsey JB. Vascular evaluation of the problem diabetic foot. *Clin Podiatr Med Surg*. 1998;15(1):49-82.
5. Armstrong DG, Lavery LA, Harkless LB. Validation of a diabetic wound classification system. The contribution of depth, infection, and ischemia to risk of amputation. *Diabetes Care*. 1998;21(5):855-859.
6. American Diabetes Association Guidelines. Preventive foot care in people with diabetes. *Diabetes Care*. 2000;23(suppl 1):S55-S56.

209 NEUROPATHIC ULCER

Javier La Fontaine, DPM
Naohiro Shibuya, DPM

PATIENT STORY

A 57-year-old man with type 2 diabetes presented with history of a neuropathic ulceration to the right foot for 2 weeks (**Figure 209-1**). The patient recalled having a callus for several months. He noticed blood on his sock 3 days ago. He denied fever or chills, but his glucose has been running higher than normal. The patient demonstrated loss of protective sensation, but vascular status was intact. He was referred to a podiatrist who immediately offloaded his foot with a total contact cast. His ulcer healed in 1 month, and he was subsequently fitted with orthopedic shoes.

INTRODUCTION

Foot complications in patients with diabetes mellitus are common, costly, and impact quality of life. Neuropathic ulcers can lead to the most devastating outcome, which is an amputation. Eighty-five percent of all amputations related to diabetes are preceded by an ulcer. Prevention, early recognition, and treatment of foot ulcers are critical in avoiding amputations.

EPIDEMIOLOGY

- Of people with diabetes, 15% will experience a foot ulcer during their lifetime, and 15% of these will have osteomyelitis.[1]
- Neuropathy causes approximately 50% of diabetic foot ulcers.[2]
- The prevalence of neuropathic ulcer is 20% in patients with diabetic neuropathy.

ETIOLOGY AND PATHOPHYSIOLOGY

- Peripheral neuropathy is an important factor in the development of a diabetic foot ulcer.
- Neuropathy causes autonomic denervation of precapillary arterioles, leading to persistent vasodilation and chronic edema.
- Moderate pressure with repetitive trauma occurs in a particular site, often from poorly fitting footwear, which then leads to ulceration.

RISK FACTORS

- Diabetic neuropathy increases the risk of developing a foot ulcer by 70%.[3]
- Patients with pedal deformity combined with diabetic neuropathy are 12 times more likely to develop a foot ulcer.[3]
- Limited joint mobility, high level of activity, and poorly fitting footwear also increase the risk of the repetitive trauma that leads to ulceration.

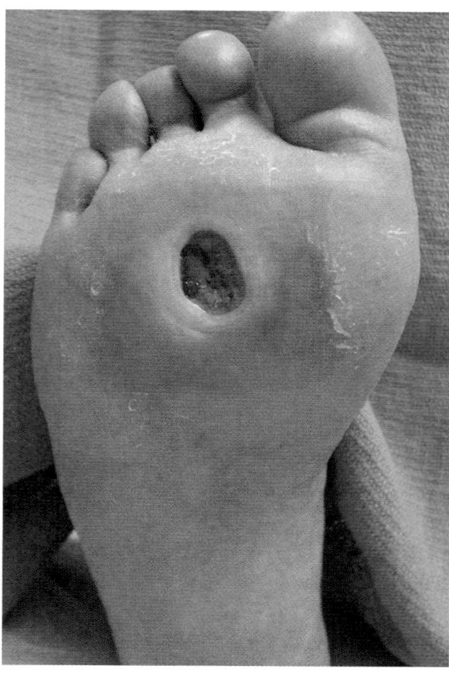

FIGURE 209-1 Neuropathic ulcer under the third metatarsal head of the right foot in a patient with diabetes. Note the red base with a white rim of hyperkeratotic tissue, a classical finding of this type of ulcer. *(Reproduced with permission from Javier La Fontaine, DPM.)*

DIAGNOSIS

The diagnosis of neuropathic ulceration is made clinically.

CLINICAL FEATURES

- A red, granular base (**Figures 209-1** and **209-2**)
- Surrounding hyperkeratosis with white, macerated margins (see **Figures 209-1** and **209-2**)

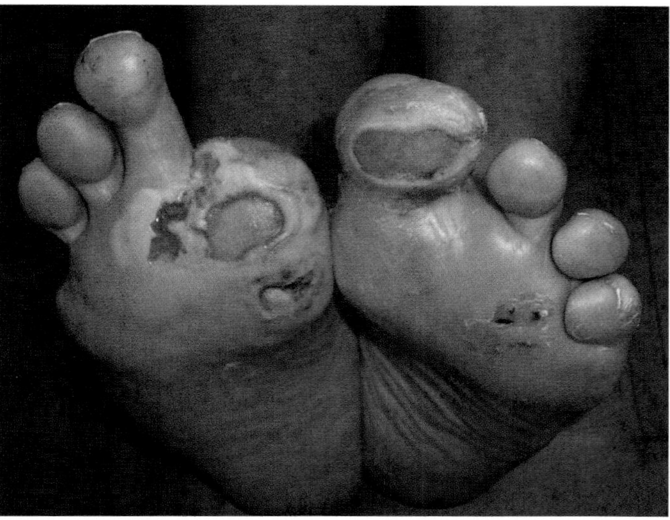

FIGURE 209-2 Neuropathic ulcers in the plantar aspect of both feet. Multiple amputations in this patient caused increased pressure in different areas of the feet, which, in combination with neuropathy, led to new ulcerations. *(Reproduced with permission from Richard P. Usatine, MD.)*

TYPICAL DISTRIBUTION

- Foot ulcers are most common under the metatarsal heads, hallux, heel, or other weight-bearing areas.
- Foot ulcers can develop in any location of the foot such as the distal and plantar aspects of the toes (see **Figures 209-1** and **209-2**).

LABORATORY STUDIES

Cultures are only indicated if infection is suspected. Swab cultures are not reliable. Curettage of the base of the wound may be more reliable.

IMAGING

Radiographs may identify a foreign body or underlying osteomyelitis.

BIOPSY

A biopsy may be necessary to rule out a suspected malignancy.

DIFFERENTIAL DIAGNOSIS

- Ischemic ulcer presents in the dysvascular foot and may have black eschar at the wound base. Usually presents with pink-to-gray wound base (see Chapter 208, Ischemic Ulcer).
- Puncture wounds may become neuropathic ulcers in the presence of neuropathy.

MANAGEMENT

NONPHARMACOLOGIC

- Offloading pressure from the foot is the standard of care.
- Multiple devices (eg, removable cast boot, surgical shoes, and wedge shoes) are used for offloading; however, a total contact cast is the gold standard.[4,5]
- Diabetic shoes should not be used as offloading devices for ulcerations.
- Serial tissue debridement should be performed weekly to biweekly to maintain minimal bacterial load, low pressure surrounding the ulcer, and a metabolically active wound base.

MEDICATIONS

- Oral antibiotics are not indicated unless infection is suspected.
- If no improvement is seen in 4 weeks, the ulcer should be considered a chronic wound and adjunctive therapy such as topical growth factors and bioengineered skin products (ie, Apligraf, Dermagraft, or Regranex) must be considered.

REFERRAL

Consider early referral to a podiatrist, wound care center, or physician with experience treating neuropathic ulcers.

PREVENTION

Patients need to understand the importance of checking their feet daily. In patients at high risk for diabetic foot ulcers, a structured prevention program with patient education and custom shoes reduced foot ulcers by 66% and saved money.[6]

PROGNOSIS

Prognosis is good for patients with neuropathic ulcers as long as they adhere to the treatment plan. A neuropathic ulcer should heal in approximately 4 to 6 weeks once aggressive offloading therapy has been implemented.

FOLLOW-UP

- Weekly to biweekly visits are needed to monitor and treat the ulcer.
- Serial radiographs every 4 weeks may be necessary to monitor for the development of osteomyelitis.
- Closely monitor the patient every 3 to 4 months once healing is accomplished. Patients who have had history of ulcerations are 36 times more likely to develop another ulcer.[3]

PATIENT EDUCATION

- Tell patients that adherence with offloading devices is essential.
- Inform patients that control of blood sugar and blood pressure promotes healing.

PATIENT RESOURCES

- MedlinePlus. *Diabetes: Foot Ulcers*—**http://www.nlm.nih.gov/medlineplus/ency/patientinstructions/000077.htm.**
- FamilyDoctor. *Diabetic Neuropathy: What is a Total Contact Cast?*—**http://familydoctor.org/familydoctor/en/diseases-conditions/diabetic-neuropathy/treatment/what-is-a-total-contact-cast.html.**

PROVIDER RESOURCES

- Medscape. *Diabetic Ulcers*—**http://emedicine.medscape.com/article/460282.**

REFERENCES

1. Levin ME. Pathogenesis and general management of foot lesions in the diabetic patient. In: Bowker JH, Pfeifer MA, eds. *Levin and O'Neal's The Diabetic Foot*. 6th ed. St. Louis, MO: CV Mosby; 2001:219-260.
2. Reiber GE, Smith DG, Wallace C, et al. Effect of therapeutic foot-wear on foot reulceration in patients with diabetes: a randomized controlled trial. *JAMA*. 2002;287:2552-2558.
3. Armstrong DG, Lavery LA, Harkless LB. Validation of a diabetic wound classification system. The contribution of depth, infection, and ischemia to risk of amputation. *Diabetes Care*. 1998;21(5):855-859.
4. Lavery LA, Vela SA, Lavery DC, Quebedeaux TL. Reducing dynamic foot pressures in high-risk diabetic subjects with foot ulcerations. A comparison of treatments. *Diabetes Care*. 1996;19(8):818-821.
5. Fleischli JG, Lavery LA, Vela SA, Ashry H, Lavery DC. Comparison of strategies for reducing pressure at the site of neuropathic ulcers. *J Am Podiatr Med Assoc*. 1997;87(10):466-472.
6. Rizzo L, Tedeschi A, Fallani E, et al. Custom-mode orthesis and shoes in a structured follow-up program reduces the incidence of neuro-pathic ulcers in high-risk diabetic foot patients. *Int J Low Extrem Wounds*. 2012 Mar;11(1):59-64.

210 CHARCOT ARTHROPATHY

Javier La Fontaine, DPM
Naohiro Shibuya, DPM

PATIENT STORY

A 62-year-old man with type 2 diabetes for 15 years presents with history of erythematous, hot, swollen right foot for 2 weeks (**Figure 210-1**). He is on multiple medications for management of his diabetes, but it is not successfully controlled. The patient does not recall any trauma to the foot. Three days ago, he noticed pain in his foot. He denies fever or chills. The radiograph of his foot (**Figure 210-2**) shows midfoot osteopenia, an early sign of acute Charcot arthropathy.

INTRODUCTION

Charcot arthropathy is an uncommon foot complication in patients with neuropathy. Patients often present with pain, swelling, and erythema, similar to the presentation with a foot infection. Patients may have a rocker-bottom foot deformity. Radiographs confirm the diagnosis.

SYNONYMS

Charcot arthropathy is also known as Charcot foot, Charcot neuroarthropathy.

EPIDEMIOLOGY

The incidence of Charcot arthropathy in diabetes ranges from 0.1% to 5%.[1]

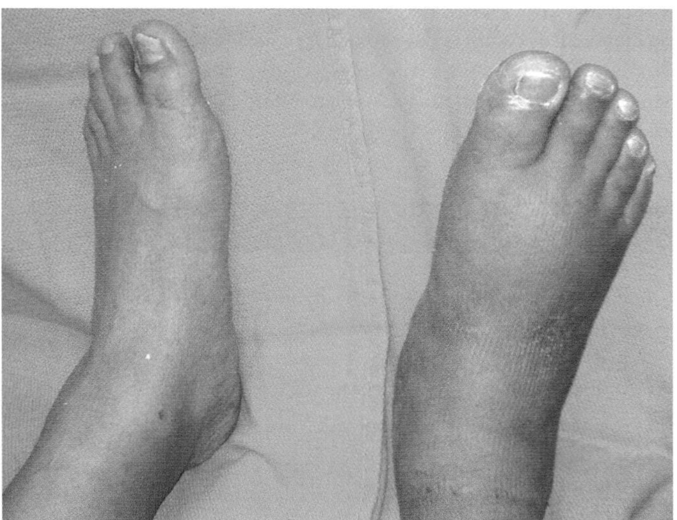

FIGURE 210-1 Charcot arthropathy in the right foot. Notice the swelling and discoloration compared to the contralateral side. (*Reproduced with permission from Javier La Fontaine, DPM.*)

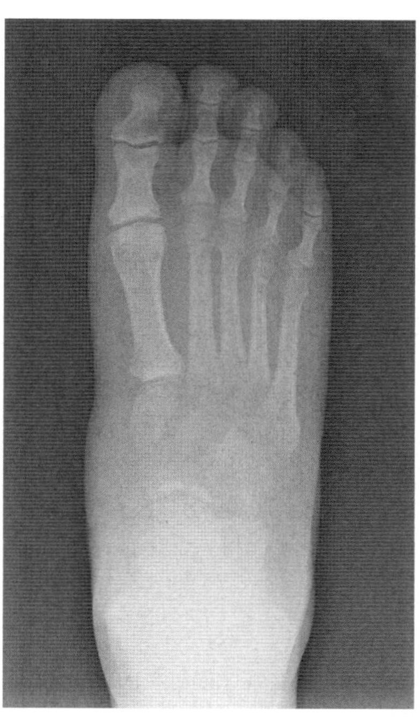

FIGURE 210-2 Anterior–posterior view of same foot demonstrating midfoot osteopenia, an early sign of acute Charcot arthropathy. (*Reproduced with permission from Javier La Fontaine, DPM.*)

ETIOLOGY AND PATHOPHYSIOLOGY

Charcot arthropathy is a gradual destruction of the joint in patients with neurosensory loss, most commonly seen in patients with diabetic neuropathy.[2] The pathogenesis is unknown. Proposed theories include the following:

- Neurotraumatic theory—Following sensorimotor neuropathy, the resulting sensory loss and muscle imbalance induces abnormal stress in the bones and joints of the affected limb, leading to bone destruction.
- Neurovascular theory—Following the development of autonomic neuropathy there is an increased blood flow to the extremity, resulting in osteopenia from a mismatch in bone reabsorption and synthesis.
- Stretching of the ligaments because of joint effusion may lead to joint subluxation.
- It is most likely that Charcot arthropathy involves all of the above mechanisms together.

RISK FACTORS

- Advanced peripheral neuropathy
- Micro- or macrotrauma
- Microangiopathy
- Nephropathy

DIAGNOSIS

The diagnosis of Charcot arthropathy is suspected based on the presentation and confirmed with imaging. Charcot arthropathy is commonly missed. Maintain a high suspicion in a patient with long-standing poorly

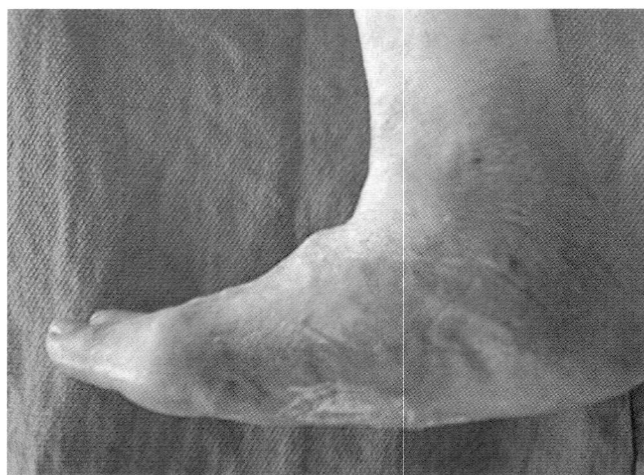

FIGURE 210-3 Lateral view of the right foot demonstrating the classic rocker-bottom deformity. (*Reproduced with permission from Javier La Fontaine, DPM.*)

controlled diabetes with peripheral neuropathy who presents with a hot, red, swollen foot and no ulceration.[3]

CLINICAL FEATURES

- Red, hot, swollen foot (see **Figure 210-1**).
- Even with neurosensory loss, 71% of patients present with the chief complaint of pain.[4]
- Rocker-bottom foot deformity is a classic finding of this entity (**Figure 210-3**).
- Patients may present with an open wound in the plantar aspect of the foot, which may complicate the diagnosis between Charcot arthropathy and infection.

IMAGING

Radiographs are imperative for diagnosis.

- Arch collapse within the joints of the midfoot (tarsometatarsal joints) (**Figure 210-4**).

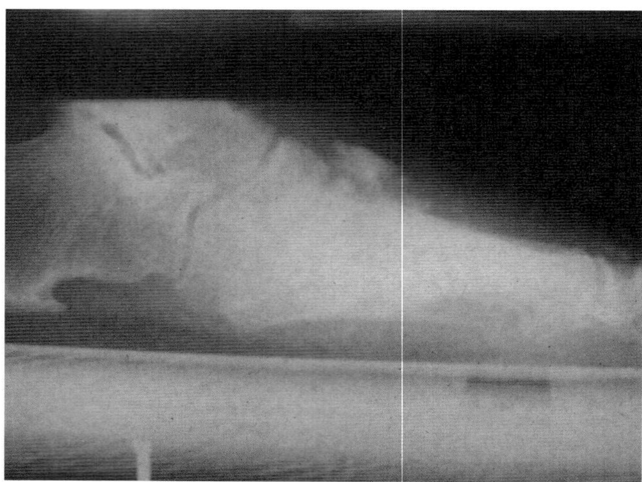

FIGURE 210-4 Lateral radiographic view of the left foot demonstrating the classic rocker-bottom deformity in Charcot arthropathy with the arch collapsed at the tarsometatarsal joints. (*Reproduced with permission from Javier La Fontaine, DPM.*)

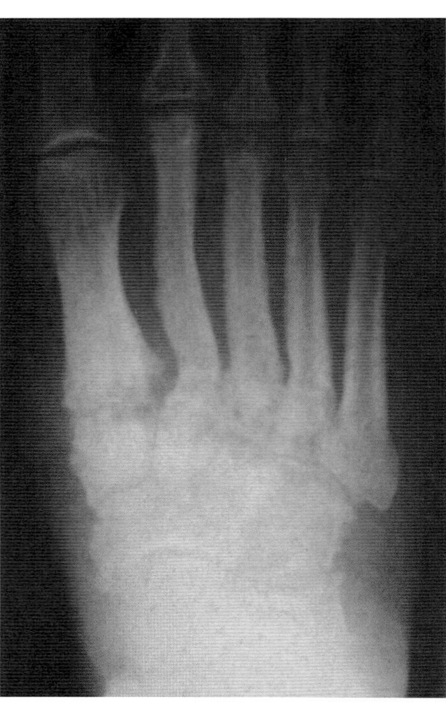

FIGURE 210-5 Anterior–posterior radiograph of the right foot demonstrating erosion and cystic degeneration at the tarsometatarsal joints in Charcot arthropathy. (*Reproduced with permission from Javier La Fontaine, DPM.*)

- Erosions and cystic degeneration of the tarsometatarsal joints in Charcot arthropathy (**Figure 210-5**) may also be present.
- Bone scan may be ordered when infection is suspected, but are often inconclusive as cellulitis and osteomyelitis have similar findings.
- Magnetic resonance imaging (MRI) may show subtle changes (eg, signal enhancement in subchondral bone and joints) prior to plain radiographs, and may be considered when plain radiographs are normal.[3]

CULTURE AND BIOPSY

If osteomyelitis is suspected, bone cultures and bone biopsy are recommended. Cultures need to be taken during the bone biopsy so that the suspected infected bone can be visualized for accurate sampling. Send cultures for aerobic and anaerobic cultures as well as for acid-fast bacilli.

DIFFERENTIAL DIAGNOSIS

- Infections, including cellulitis and osteomyelitis, should be considered and treated if present (see Chapter 122, Cellulitis). An elevated C-reactive protein and erythrocyte sedimentation rate can indicate infection, but there absence does not rule out infection.[3]
- Gouty arthropathy of the foot or ankle can resemble a Charcot foot (see Chapter 105, Gout).
- Acute trauma to the foot can cause swelling and erythema, but should be easy to distinguish by the history.
- Deep venous thrombosis in the leg will generally cause swelling that extends above the ankle.

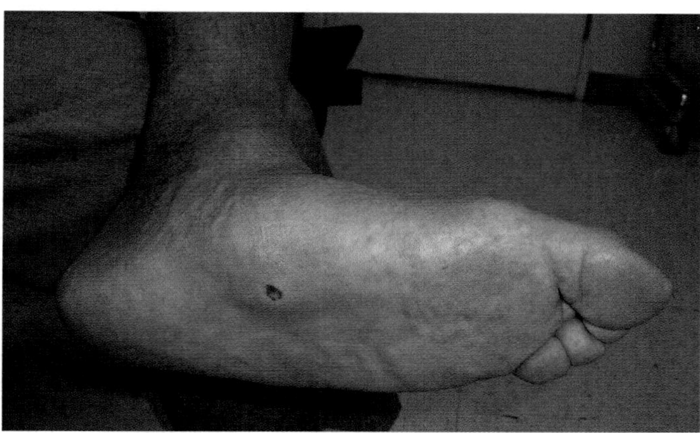

FIGURE 210-6 Foot ulcer as a result of diabetic neuropathy and a Charcot foot. Note the collapse of the arch. (*Reproduced with permission from Richard P. Usatine, MD.*)

MANAGEMENT

- Offloading of pressure from the foot is the standard of care. The total contact cast is most effective, and it covers the toes for protection. Other methods that are used include the removable cast boot, crutches, and the wheelchair.
- Diabetic shoes should not be used as offloading devices for Charcot arthropathy.
- Skin temperature assessment with infrared thermometry has been demonstrated to be successful in monitoring improvement.
- Prevention of rocker-bottom deformities, plantar ulcers, and amputations is the major goal of the treatment. Untreated Charcot foot may lead to a rocker-bottom foot, which in turn leads to increased plantar pressure in the neuropathic foot. This cascade will lead to an ulceration (**Figure 210-6**) and possible amputation.[4]
- The bones will take approximately 4 to 5 months to heal in presence of neuropathy.
- Oral antibiotics are not indicated unless infection is suspected.
- If deformity develops, custom-molded shoes and insoles must be ordered to prevent plantar ulcers that can lead to amputation.
- If the foot develops instability at the fracture sites, surgical reconstruction may be required.

PREVENTION

- Control of blood glucose helps to prevent diabetic complications, including Charcot arthropathy.
- Appropriate footwear and foot care is essential to preventing many types of diabetic foot problems.
- Early diagnosis and treatment can prevent ongoing structural damage to the joint.

PROGNOSIS

Patients with history of Charcot arthropathy are always at risk to develop foot complications. The combination of severe foot deformity in presence of neuropathy places them at risk for more ulceration, and further amputation. Almost 50% of these patients will require complex foot surgery to fix the deformity.

FOLLOW-UP

- Weekly to biweekly visits to the podiatrist is needed.
- Serial radiographs in every 4 weeks are required to monitor bone healing and deformity.
- Once healing is accomplished, it is imperative to continue monitoring the patient every 3 to 4 months. Patients who have had history of Charcot arthropathy are 36 times more likely to develop another ulcer and are at risk of amputation.[5]

PATIENT EDUCATION

- Tell the patient that all efforts should be made to control blood sugar and blood pressure to promote healing.
- Educate the patient to recognize the clinical signs of Charcot arthropathy.
- Educate patient to wear shoe gear prescribed by physician.
- Ensure that patients with Charcot arthropathy understand that adherence with offloading devices is essential.

PATIENT RESOURCES

- ePodiatry.com. *Charcot's Foot (Charcot's Arthropathy or Neuroarthropathy)*—**http://www.epodiatry.com/charcot-foot.htm.**

PROVIDER RESOURCES

- Medscape. *Charcot Arthropathy*—**http://emedicine.medscape.com/article/1234293.**
- Sommer TC, Lee TH. Charcot foot: the diagnostic dilemma. *Am Fam Physician*. 2001;64:1591-1598—**http://www.aafp.org/afp/20011101/1591.html.**

REFERENCES

1. Brodsky J, Rouse AM. Exostectomy for symptomatic bony prominences in diabetic Charcot feet. *Clin Orthop Relat Res*. 1993;296:21-26.
2. Fryksberg R. Osteoarthropathy. *Clin Podiatr Med Surg*. 1987;4(2):351-359.
3. Botek G, Anderson MA, Taylor R. Charcot neuroarthropathy: an often overlooked complication of diabetes. *Cleve Clin J Med*. 2010;77(9):593-599.
4. Armstrong DG, Todd WF, Lavery LA, Harkless LB, Bushman TR. The natural history of acute Charcot's arthropathy in a diabetic foot specialty clinic. *J Am Podiatr Med Assoc*. 1997;87(6):272-278.
5. Levin ME. Pathogenesis and general management of foot lesions in the diabetic patient. In: Bowker JH, Pfeifer MA, eds. *Levin and O'Neal's The Diabetic Foot*. 6th ed. St. Louis, MO: Mosby; 2001:219-260.

211 DRY GANGRENE

Javier La Fontaine, DPM
Naohiro Shibuya, DPM

PATIENT STORY

A 36-year-old woman with type 1 diabetes presented with a 4-week history of a dry, black great toe and third toe on the right foot (**Figure 211-1**). She said that she noticed severe maceration between the first and second interspace approximately 6 weeks ago. Subsequently, the toes changed color and became very painful. Two days ago, she noticed a foul odor from both toes. The patient reported smoking since she was 13 years old. On physical examination, there were no palpable pulses in the right foot. The patient was admitted for intravenous (IV) antibiotics and revascularization was performed. Subsequently, the toes were partially amputated and the wounds healed without any complications. Her physicians attempted to help her to quit smoking without success.

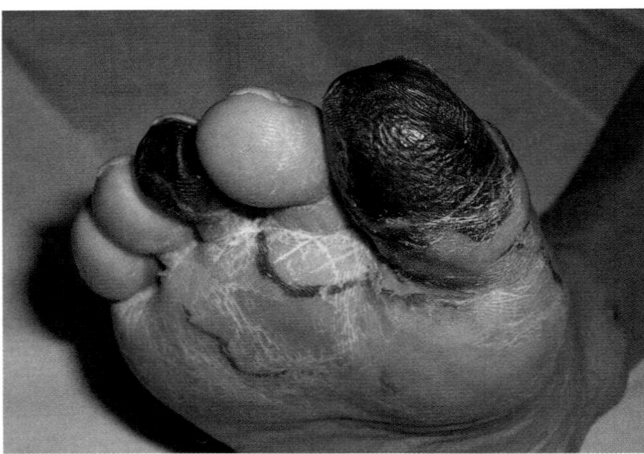

FIGURE 211-1 Dry gangrene of the first and third toes in a 36-year-old woman with poorly controlled diabetes demonstrating the typical demarcation of the necrotic eschar from the normal tissue. (*Reproduced with permission from Richard P. Usatine, MD.*)

INTRODUCTION

Dry gangrene develops following arterial obstruction and appears as dark brown/black dry tissue. Peripheral arterial disease is common in patients with diabetes and dry gangrene is most commonly seen on the toes. The nonviable tissue becomes black in color from the iron sulfide released by the hemoglobin in the lysed red blood cells.

SYNONYMS

Dry gangrene is also known as mummification necrosis.

EPIDEMIOLOGY

- Peripheral arterial disease (PAD) is a common finding in patients with diabetes. PAD is an important factor leading to lower-extremity amputation in patients with diabetes.[1]
- Thirty percent of diabetic patients with an absent pedal pulse will have some degree of coronary artery disease.[1]

ETIOLOGY AND PATHOPHYSIOLOGY

- PAD manifests in the lower extremity in 2 ways: macro- and microvascular diseases.
- The pattern of occlusion in the macrovascular tree is distal and multisegmental.[2]
- Multiple occlusions occur below the trifurcation of the popliteal artery into the anterior tibial artery, posterior tibial artery, and peroneal artery.
- Risk factors, such as hypercholesteremia, hyperlipidemia, and hypertension, are often associated with patients with PAD and, therefore, poor wound healing.[3,4]

RISK FACTORS

- Diabetes
- Dyslipidemia
- Smoking
- Neuropathy

DIAGNOSIS

CLINICAL FEATURES

- Dry, black eschar, which most commonly begins distally at the extremities (**Figures 211-1** and **211-2**).
- There is a clear demarcation between healthy tissue and necrotic tissue (see **Figures 211-1** and **211-2**).
- Foul odor.
- Pain may be present.
- Trauma is the most common etiology.
- Nonpalpable pulses are common. Palpable pulses do not preclude the presence of limb-threatening ischemia. Also, the dorsalis pedis pulse is reported to be absent in 8% of healthy individuals, and the posterior tibial pulse is absent in 2% of the population.
- Smoking is commonly associated with this problem.
- Associated trophic skin changes (eg, absent pedal hair and thin shiny skin).
- Indicators of vascular insufficiency include pallor upon elevation of the limb and rubor upon dependency, along with prolonged digital capillary filling time.

TYPICAL DISTRIBUTION

Distal extremities, especially the toes

IMAGING

- Even in the presence of a palpable pulse, noninvasive studies (eg, arterial Doppler and pulse volume recordings) are important for baseline assessment of the patient's blood flow.
- Angiogram is required to evaluate the possibility of revascularization.
- Radiographs may be necessary to rule out osteomyelitis.

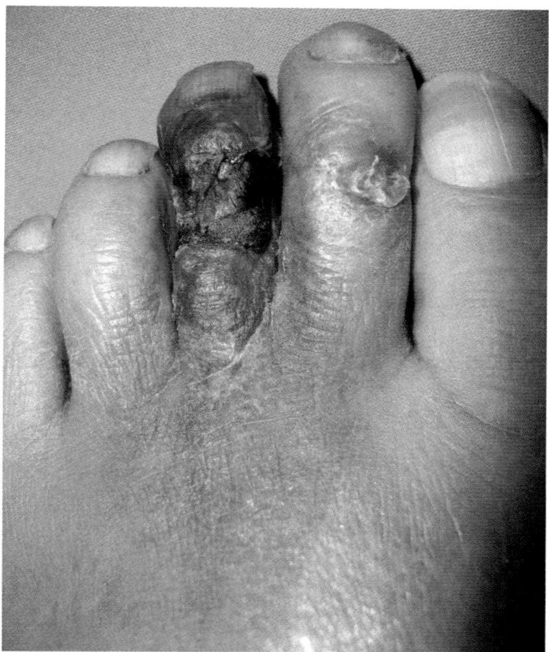

FIGURE 211-2 A 55-year-old man with type 2 diabetes presenting with dry gangrene of the third toe. Note a visible line of demarcation between the gangrene and normal tissue. The dry, black eschar is more distal than proximal. (*Reproduced with permission from Javier La Fontaine, DPM.*)

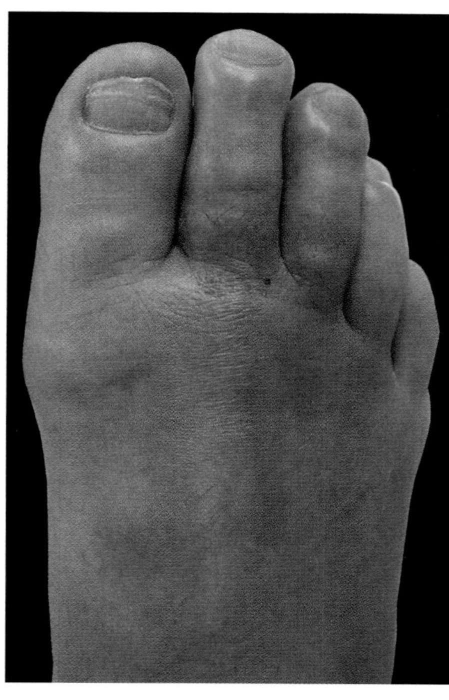

FIGURE 211-3 A 53-year-old diabetic man with wet gangrene of the second and third toes of the right foot. This diagnosis should always be considered when evaluating the ischemic limb. Wet gangrene is an emergency caused by an infectious process with severe ischemia. (*Reproduced with permission from Javier La Fontaine, DPM.*)

DIFFERENTIAL DIAGNOSIS

- Wet gangrene is an acute, urgent problem that is caused by a severe infection in the dysvascular foot (**Figure 211-3**). Wet gangrene usually presents with cyanosis, purulence, foul odor, and systemic signs and symptoms of infection.
- Ischemic ulcer is an actual foot ulcer that usually presents with a pink-to-gray wound base (see Chapter 208, Ischemic Ulcer).
- Although diabetes is the most common cause of dry gangrene of the toes, severe frostbite and Buerger disease can also lead to dry gangrene by damage to the microvasculature.

MANAGEMENT

- Consult vascular surgery.
- Rule out wet gangrene. Wet gangrene is an emergent infectious process in combination with severe ischemia. Consequently, immediate debridement of infected tissue is required with antibiotics.
- Avoid amputation or debridement until optimization of blood flow occurs. This may require a vascular bypass procedure and/or interventional radiology for percutaneous angioplasty and stent placement.
- Antibiotics are not indicated for dry gangrene unless infection is suspected.

PREVENTION

- Smoking cessation
- Diet and exercise to control blood sugar and lipids
- Vascular examination at least on yearly basis

PROGNOSIS

Once dry gangrene has been established, gangrenous tissue will need to be amputated. On occasion, the toes will autoamputate. Successful revascularization must occur for the patient to heal. If the problem is addressed early and aggressive wound care is provided, most of the amputations heal. Because delaying revascularization increases the risk of infection, early and aggressive management of vascular disease is imperative for a successful outcome.

FOLLOW-UP

Closely monitor the patient for new gangrene or ulcers every 3 to 4 months once healing has occurred.

PATIENT EDUCATION

- Avoid trauma to the amputated site.
- Advise and assist patients to stop smoking to help the wound heal and prolong the survival of the revascularization procedure.

PATIENT RESOURCES

- MedicineNet. *Gangrene*—**http://www.medicinenet.com/gangrene/article.htm.**
- eMedicineHealth. *Gangrene*—**http://www.emedicinehealth.com/gangrene/article_em.htm.**

PROVIDER RESOURCES

- Medscape. *Toe Amputation*—**http://emedicine.medscape.com/article/1829931.**
- Medscape. *Gas Gangrene in Emergency Medicine*—**http://emedicine.medscape.com/article/782709.**

REFERENCES

1. American Diabetes Association Guidelines. Preventive foot care in people with diabetes. *Diabetes Care*. 2000;23(suppl 1):S55-S56.
2. Sykes MT, Godsey JB. Vascular evaluation of the problem diabetic foot. *Clin Podiatr Med Surg*. 1998;15(1):49-82.
3. La Fontaine J, Allen M, Davis C, Harkless LB, Shireman PK. Current concepts in diabetic microvascular dysfunction. *J Am Podiatr Med Assoc*. 2006;96(3):245-252.
4. Tooke JE. A pathophysiological framework for the pathogenesis of diabetic microangiopathy. In: Tooke JE ed. *Diabetic Angiopathy*. New York, NY: Oxford University Press; 1999:187.

PART 16

INFECTIOUS DISEASES

Strength of Recommendation (SOR)	Definition
A	Recommendation based on consistent and good-quality patient-oriented evidence.*
B	Recommendation based on inconsistent or limited-quality patient-oriented evidence.*
C	Recommendation based on consensus, usual practice, opinion, disease-oriented evidence, or case series for studies of diagnosis, treatment, prevention, or screening.*

*See Appendix A on pages 1241-1244 for further information.

212 AIDS AND KAPOSI SARCOMA

Heidi Chumley, MD

PATIENT STORY

A 35-year-old gay man presented with papular lesions on his elbow (**Figure 212-1**). Shave biopsy demonstrated Kaposi sarcoma (KS). He subsequently tested positive for HIV and began treatment with antiretroviral combination therapy. The KS resolved with topical alitretinoin gel treatment.

INTRODUCTION

In the United States, KS is most often seen in patients with AIDS and patients on immunosuppressants after organ transplantation. KS can also be classic (older Mediterranean men) or endemic (young men in sub-Saharan Africa). KS is caused by Kaposi sarcoma-associated herpesvirus (KSHV), which promotes oncogenesis. KS cannot be cured, but treatment can result in improvement or disease stabilization. Current therapies improve the immune system or target KSHV. Therapies that modulate KSHV-mediated signaling are being studied.

EPIDEMIOLOGY

- KS can be classic (older Mediterranean men), endemic (young men in sub-Saharan Africa), epidemic (AIDS patients), or posttransplantation (organ recipients).[1]
- In the United States, 81.6% of KS is seen in patients with AIDS[2] (see **Figure 212-1**).
- In HIV-positive patients, the prevalence is 7.2/1000 person-years, 451 times higher than general population.[3]
- In transplant patients, the prevalence is 1.4/1000 person-years, 128 times higher than general population.[3]

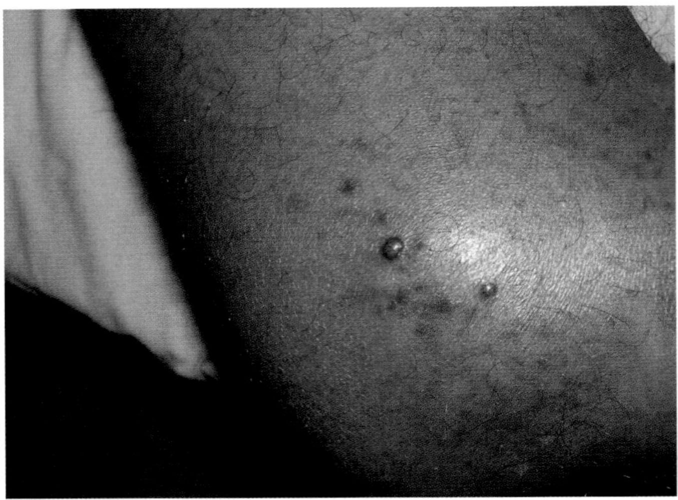

FIGURE 212-1 Several reddish-purple papular lesions of Kaposi sarcoma on the elbow of a man with HIV/AIDS. (*Reproduced with permission from Heather Wickless, MD.*)

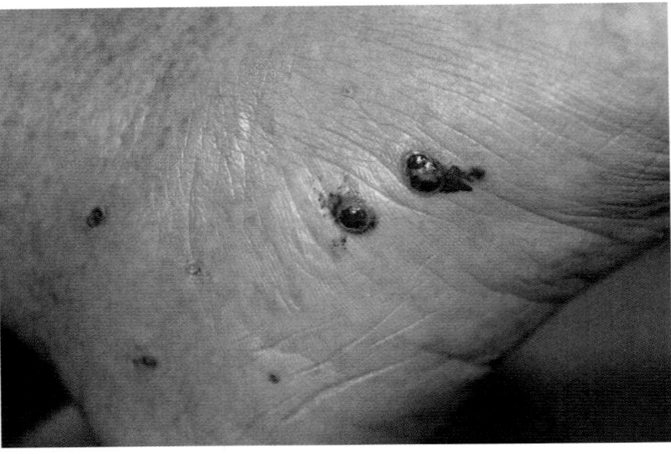

FIGURE 212-2 Classic Kaposi sarcoma on the foot of an 88-year-old Italian man who does not have HIV/AIDS. These painful purple-red "growths" were present on his left foot for several years before diagnosis. (*Reproduced with permission from Welsh JP, Allen HB. Purple-red papules on foot.* J Fam Pract. *2008; Jun;57(6):389-91.*)

- The prevalence of classic KS in the general population of southern Italy is 2.5/100,000[4] (**Figure 212-2**).
- The male-to-female ratio for epidemic KS in the United States is approximately 50:1 but is falling as the prevalence of AIDS increases among women.[5] The male-to-female ratio has been approximately 10:1 for classic and endemic KS.
- KS is the most common malignancy seen in AIDS patients.

ETIOLOGY AND PATHOPHYSIOLOGY

- KS is caused by KSHV, also known as human herpes virus 8 (HHV-8). KSHV acts through host cell signal transduction to activate multiple oncogenic pathways.[6]
- KS is an angioproliferative neoplasm, with abnormal proliferation of endothelial cells, myofibroblasts, and monocyte cells.
- Lesions often begin as papules or patches and progress to plaques as proliferation continues.
- Some lesions ulcerate (nodular stage), and lymphedema can occur.

RISK FACTORS

- Immunodeficiency as a consequence of AIDS
- Immunosuppressants for solid-organ transplantation

DIAGNOSIS

The diagnosis is often made clinically in a patient who has AIDS and a typical presentation of KS. In atypical presentations, diagnosis is made by biopsy.

CLINICAL FEATURES

- Cutaneous lesions are usually multifocal, papular, and reddish-purple in color (see **Figures 212-1** and **212-2**).
- Plaques or fungating lesions can be seen on the lower extremities, including the soles of the feet (**Figure 212-3**).

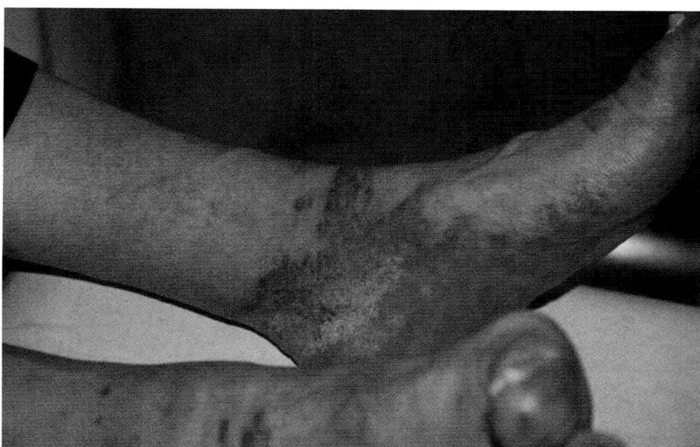

FIGURE 212-3 Kaposi sarcoma on the foot in a man with AIDS in the 1990s. Note the purple color. (*Reproduced with permission from Usatine RP, Moy RL, Tobinick EL, Siegel DM. Skin Surgery: A Practical Guide. St. Louis, MO: Mosby; 1998.*)

  - Vascular-appearing papules on the feet and lower legs are typical of classic KS without AIDS (**Figure 212-4**).
- Oral cavity lesions can be flat or nodular and are red to purple in color (**Figure 212-5**).
- Gastrointestinal (GI) lesions can be asymptomatic or can cause abdominal pain, nausea, vomiting, bleeding, or weight loss.

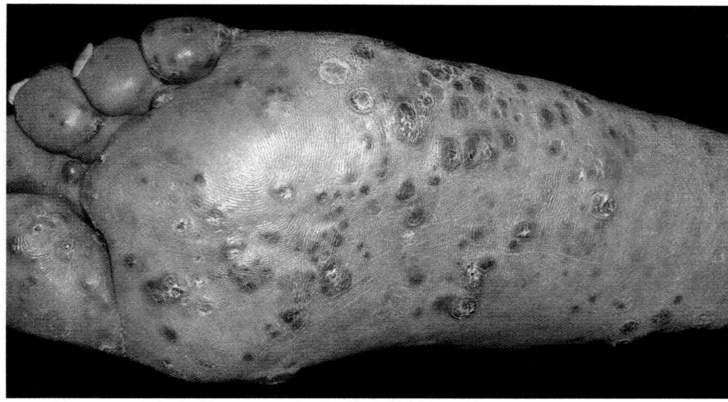

A

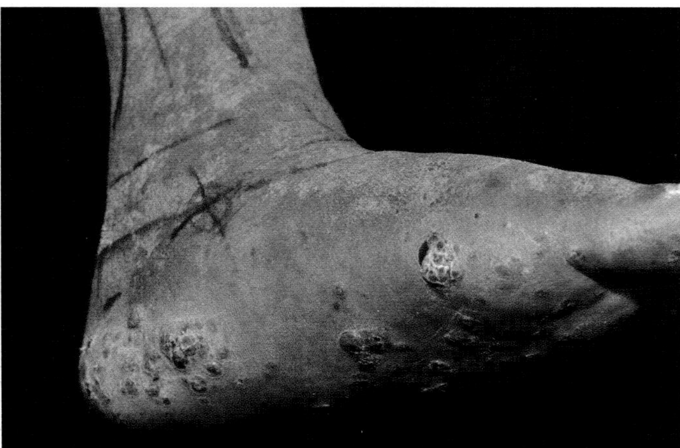

B

FIGURE 212-4 **A.** Classic Kaposi sarcoma on the foot of an 85-year-old Hispanic man from Mexico who is HIV negative. He initially declined radiation and his lesions grew and multiplied over 3 years. **B.** He is receiving palliative radiation to improve his ability to walk. (*Reproduced with permission from Richard P. Usatine, MD.*)

- Pulmonary lesions can cause shortness of breath or may appear as infiltrates, nodules, or pleural effusions on chest radiographs.

TYPICAL DISTRIBUTION

- AIDS-related KS.[7]
- Skin lesions are seen mainly on the lower extremities (**Figure 212-6** and **212-7**), face, and genitalia. Presence of skin lesions should prompt an oral examination as oral involvement may change prognosis and management.
- Lesions in the oral cavity are common (33%), typically seen on the palate or gingiva (see **Figure 212-5**).
- GI involvement is noted in 40% of newly diagnosed KS in HIV patients at diagnosis and up to 80% in autopsy studies. GI lesions can occur without skin lesions.
- Pulmonary involvement is also common, and up to 15% may occur without skin lesions in patients with KS and HIV. A chest radiograph often demonstrates pulmonary involvement.
- Any organ can be involved.

LABORATORY TESTING

- Check an HIV test in any person with KS who is not known to be HIV positive.
- CD4+ T-lymphocyte count is an important prognostic indicator.

IMAGING

Chest radiograph is done if there is pulmonary involvement. GI endoscopy is done if GI involvement is suspected.

BIOPSY

Often required for definitive diagnosis. If the lesions are nodular a simple shave biopsy should be sufficient. If the lesions are flat, a 4-mm punch biopsy should provide adequate tissue for diagnosis.

DIFFERENTIAL DIAGNOSIS

The diagnosis of KS requires a biopsy as several other lesions can mimic early KS.[7]

- Purpura—Bleeding under the skin caused by a variety of platelet, vascular, or coagulation disorders; usually not palpable and more widespread.
- Hematomas—Localized swelling usually from a break in a blood vessel; history of trauma and usually not palpable.
- Hemangiomas or angiomas—Benign growths of small blood vessels that blanch with pressure (see Chapter 199, Acquired Vascular Skin Lesions).
- Dermatofibromas—Small, firm, red-to-brown nodules made up of histiocytes and collagen deposits in the mid-dermis, often seen on the legs; lesions are usually small (<6 mm) and dimple downward when compressed laterally (see Chapter 158, Dermatofibroma).
- Bacillary angiomatosis—A systemic infectious disease caused by *Bartonella* species. Cutaneous lesions appear as scattered papules and nodules or an abscess. Bacillary angiomatosis may occur when the CD4 count is below 200 and is treated with antibiotics (**Figure 212-8**).
- Syphilis—Syphilis is still the "great imitator" and could appear similar to KS. Syphilis and KS are both found in higher prevalence among HIV-positive persons. (**Figure 212-9**) (see Chapter 218, Syphilis).

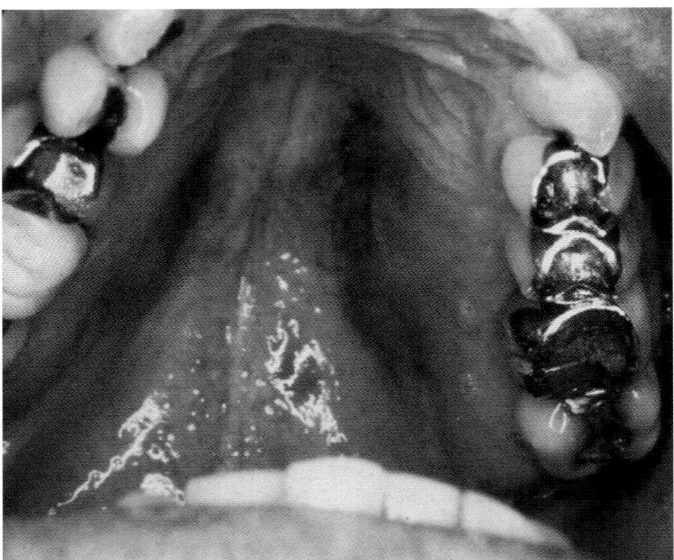

FIGURE 212-5 Early Kaposi sarcoma on the palate. The color is abnormal but the lesion is still flat. (*Reproduced with permission from Ellen Eisenberg, DMD.*)

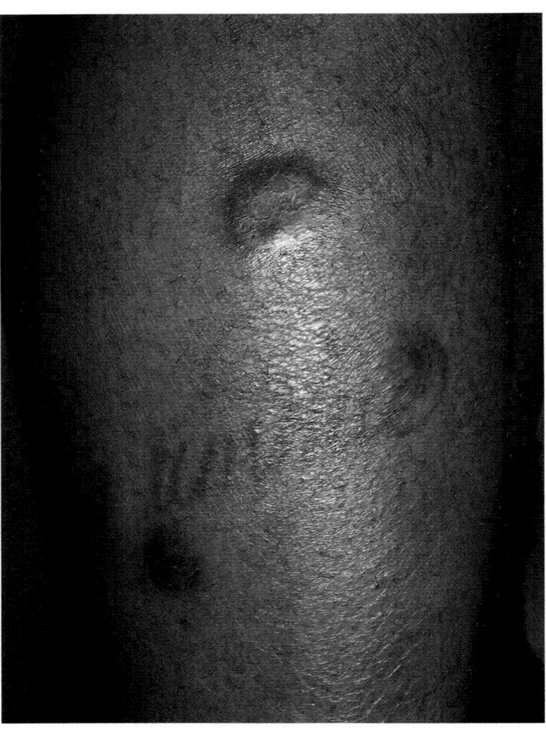

FIGURE 212-7 Kaposi sarcoma on the lower leg of a 23-year-old African American man with HIV/AIDS. His lesions are dark brown to black rather than pink or purple. It is important to note that the classic colors described in white skin are often not found in dark skin. Any persistent skin nodule in an HIV-positive person should be suspicious for KS and a biopsy is the best method for a definitive diagnosis. (*Reproduced with permission from Richard P. Usatine, MD.*)

MANAGEMENT

KS is not curable, but treatments can reduce disease burden and slow progression (**Figure 212-10**).

MEDICATIONS

- In patients with HIV/AIDS, highly active antiretroviral therapy (HAART) therapy improves KS. Treat with antiretroviral drugs or refer to a physician with experience initiating and following antiretroviral therapy. Antiretroviral therapy inhibits HIV replication, decreases the response to KSHV, and has antiangiogenic activity. SOR Ⓐ
- Avoid high-dose steroids, as they can severely aggravate KS, especially pulmonary KS.
- Consider the following KS-specific therapies:
  - Alitretinoin gel 0.1%—Patient applies gel to lesions 2 times a day, increasing to 3 to 4 times a day if tolerated, for 4 to 8 weeks (66% response rate).[8] SOR Ⓐ

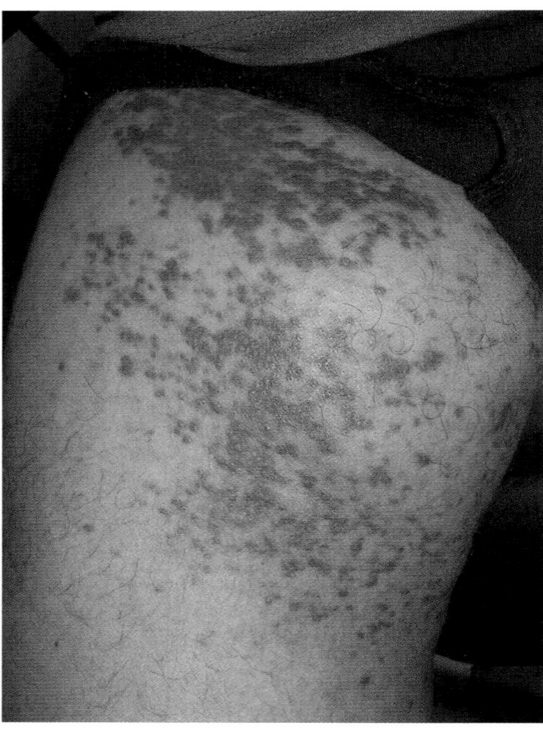

FIGURE 212-6 Kaposi sarcoma in a 43-year-old man with HIV/AIDS already on antiretroviral therapy. He presented with a diffuse rash and lymphedema in the right leg. The initial biopsy was negative but a second biopsy demonstrated Kaposi sarcoma. The right leg is significantly larger than the left leg due to the lymphedema. (*Reproduced with permission from Richard P. Usatine, MD.*)

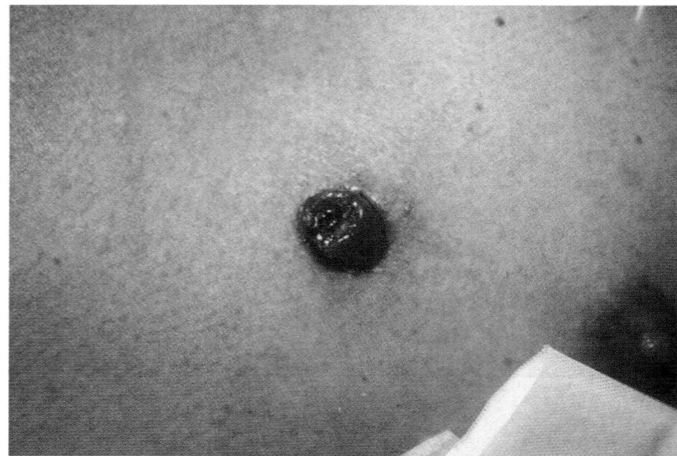

FIGURE 212-8 Cutaneous bacillary angiomatosis in a man with HIV/AIDS. (*Reproduced with permission from Usatine RP, Moy RL, Tobinick EL, Siegel DM.* Skin Surgery: A Practical Guide. *St. Louis, MO: Mosby; 1998.*)

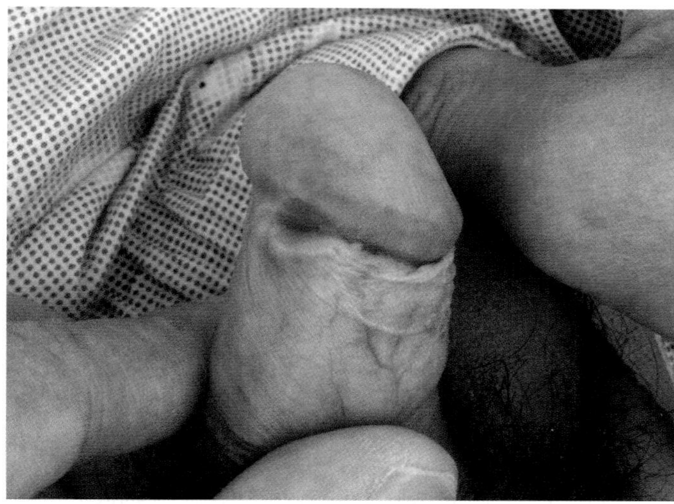

FIGURE 212-9 Syphilis in an HIV-positive man presenting with an erythematous papule with central depression at the coronal sulcus. Syphilis is still the "great imitator" and could appear similar to Kaposi sarcoma in this and other less-common presentations. (*Reproduced with permission from Robyn M. Marszalek, MD.*)

- Liposomal doxorubicin 20 mg/m^2 every 3 weeks or liposomal daunorubicin 40 mg/m^2 every 2 weeks (50% response rate).[9] SOR Ⓐ
- Paclitaxel 100 mg/m^2 every 2 weeks or 135 mg/m^2 every 3 weeks; response rates 60% to 70% in patients who had failed a prior chemotherapy regiment.[10] SOR Ⓐ

- Premedication with dexamethasone is recommended.[10]
  - Interferon-α at 1 million U/d demonstrated the most benefit to patients with KS limited to the skin and CD4+ T-lymphocyte counts more than 200.[11]
  - Intralesional vinblastine (70% response rate)[12] or radiation therapy (80% response rate) are also effective for skin lesions.[13] SOR Ⓐ
- Removing immunosuppressants or using radiation can treat transplant-related KS.
- In addition to the medications that target KSHV, new therapies are undergoing study that target KSHV-mediating signaling.[6]

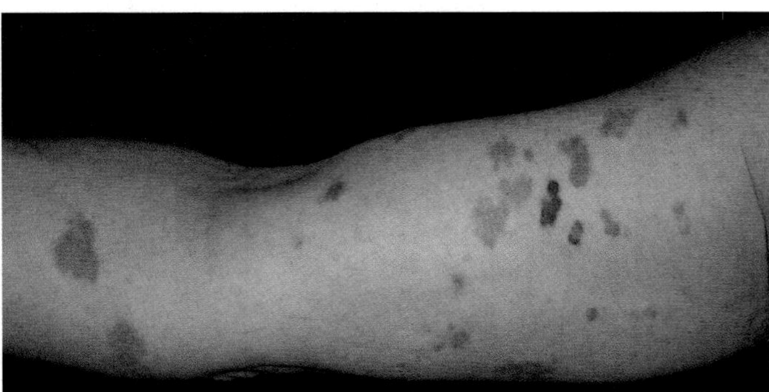

FIGURE 212-10 Kaposi sarcoma on the arm of a 43-year-old man with HIV/AIDS. The patient is on antiretroviral therapy and has received radiation treatment for the Kaposi sarcoma. The Kaposi sarcoma is in remission but the discoloration has remained. Prior to treatment all of the patches on his arms were dark purple like the one remaining dark patch. (*Reproduced with permission from Richard P. Usatine, MD.*)

RADIATION OR SURGERY

Classic and endemic KS are often treated with radiation (see **Figure 212-4**) or surgery. Surgical options include electrodessication and curettage to individual lesions. SOR Ⓒ

PROGNOSIS

- In severe disease requiring systemic therapy, 50% to 85% of patients will respond with either improvement or disease stability; however, the response lasts only 6 to 7 months before therapy has to be repeated. When therapy is repeated, the response times generally decrease.[6]
- Patients with AIDS-related KS have 5-year survival rates of greater than 80% when KS is the AIDS-defining illness and the CD4+ T-lymphocyte count is greater than 200. Survival rates fall to less than 10% when the patient is older than age 50 years and there is another AIDS-defining illness at the time of presentation.[14]

FOLLOW-UP

KS, particularly AIDS-related KS, is generally treated by physicians with advanced training in HIV/AIDS management and oncology. Follow-up is determined by disease progression and response to therapy.

PATIENT EDUCATION

- KS is not curable, but several treatments can result in regression of the lesions for a better cosmetic result.
- KS can affect most parts of the body, commonly the skin, oral cavity, GI tract, and lungs.
- During treatment, lesions typically flatten, shrink, and fade (see **Figure 212-8**).
- Rarely, starting antiretroviral therapy may cause lesions to flare because of an inflammatory reaction as the immune system begins to recover (immune reconstitution).

PATIENT RESOURCES

- The National Cancer Institute. *Kaposi Sarcoma Treatment*—**http://www.cancer.gov/cancertopics/pdq/treatment/kaposis/patient/.**

PROVIDER RESOURCES

- The National Cancer Institute has information for health professionals—**http://www.cancer.gov/cancertopics/pdq/treatment/kaposis/HealthProfessional.**

REFERENCES

1. Alamartine E. Up-to-date epidemiological data and better treatment for Kaposi's sarcoma. *Transplantation*. 2005;80(12):1656-1667.
2. Shiels MS, Pfeiffer RM, Hall HI, et al. Proportions of Kaposi sarcoma, selected non-Hodgkin lymphomas, and cervical cancer in the United States occurring in persons with AIDS, 1980-2007. *JAMA*. 2011;305(14):1450-1459.

3. Serraino D, Piselli P, Angeletti C, et al. Kaposi's sarcoma in transplant and HIV-infected patients: an epidemiologic study in Italy and France. *Transplantation*. 2005;80(12):1699-1704.

4. Atzori L, Fadda D, Ferreli C, et al. Classic Kaposi's sarcoma in southern Sardinia, Italy. *Br J Cancer*. 2004;91(7):1261-1262.

5. Onyango JF, Njiru A. Kaposi's sarcoma in a Nairobi hospital. *East Afr Med J*. 2004;81(3):120-123.

6. Sullivan RJ, Pantanowitz L, Dezube B. Targeted therapy in Kaposi sarcoma. *BioDrugs*. 2009;23(2):69-75.

7. Cheung MC, Pantanowitz L, Dezube BJ. AIDS-related malignancies: emerging challenges in the era of highly active antiretroviral therapy. *Oncologist*. 2005;10(6):412-426.

8. Walmsley S, Northfelt DW, Melosky B, et al. Treatment of AIDS-related cutaneous Kaposi's sarcoma with topical alitretinoin (9-cis-retinoic acid) gel. Panretin Gel North American Study Group. *J Acquir Immune Defic Syndr*. 1999;22:235-246.

9. Cooley HD, Volberding P, Martin F, et al. Final results of a phase III randomized trial of pegylated liposomal doxorubicin versus liposomal daunorubicin in patients with AIDS-related Kaposi's sarcoma [abstract]. *Proc Am Soc Clin Oncol*. 2002;21:411a;1640.

10. Gill PS, Tulpule A, Espina BM, et al. Paclitaxel is safe and effective in the treatment of advanced AIDS related Kaposi's sarcoma. *J Clin Oncol*. 1999;17:1876-1883.

11. Krown SE, Li P, Von Roenn JH, et al. Efficacy of low-dose interferon with antiretroviral therapy in Kaposi's sarcoma: a randomized phase II AIDS Clinical Trials Group study. *J Interferon Cytokine Res*. 2002;22:295-303.

12. Boudreaux AA, Smith LL, Cosby CD, et al. Intralesional vinblastine for cutaneous Kaposi's sarcoma associated with acquired immunodeficiency syndrome. A clinical trial to evaluate efficacy and discomfort associated with infection. *J Am Acad Dermatol*. 1993;28:61-65.

13. Swift PS. The role of radiation therapy in the management of HIV-related Kaposi's sarcoma. *Hematol Oncol Clin North Am*. 1996;10:1069-1080.

14. Stebbing J, Sanitt A, Nelson M, et al. A prognostic index for AIDS-associated Kaposi's sarcoma in the era of highly active antiretroviral therapy. *Lancet*. 2006;367(9521):1495-1502.

213 URETHRITIS IN MEN

Heidi Chumley, MD
Richard P. Usatine, MD

PATIENT STORY

A 24-year-old man presents to a skid row shelter clinic with 3 days of dysuria and penile discharge. A heavy purulent urethral discharge is seen (**Figure 213-1**). He admits to using crack cocaine and having multiple female sexual partners. He was diagnosed with gonococcal urethritis by clinical appearance and a urine specimen was sent for testing to confirm the gonorrhea and test for *Chlamydia*. He was treated with ceftriaxone 250 mg IM for gonorrhea and 1 g of oral azithromycin for possible coexisting *Chlamydia*. He was offered and agreed to testing for other sexually transmitted diseases (STDs). He was told to inform his partners of the diagnosis. He was counseled about safe sex, and drug rehabilitation was recommended. On his 1-week follow-up visit, his symptoms were gone and he had no further discharge. His gonorrhea nucleic acid amplification test was positive and his *Chlamydia*, rapid plasma reagin (RPR), and HIV tests were negative. His case was reported to the Health Department for contact tracing.

INTRODUCTION

Urethritis is urethral inflammation caused by infectious (gonococcal or chlamydial) or noninfectious causes (trauma or foreign bodies). Gonococcal and chlamydial infections in men occur most commonly between the ages of 20 and 24 years, and the prevalence is highest in black men. Diagnosis is suspected clinically, reinforced by an office urine test positive for leukocyte esterase, and confirmed by a urine nucleic acid amplification test. Treat for both gonorrhea and *Chlamydia* until one or both are ruled out by laboratory testing.

EPIDEMIOLOGY

- Worldwide, 151 million cases of gonococcal and nongonococcal urethritis are reported annually (**Figures 213-1** and **213-2**).

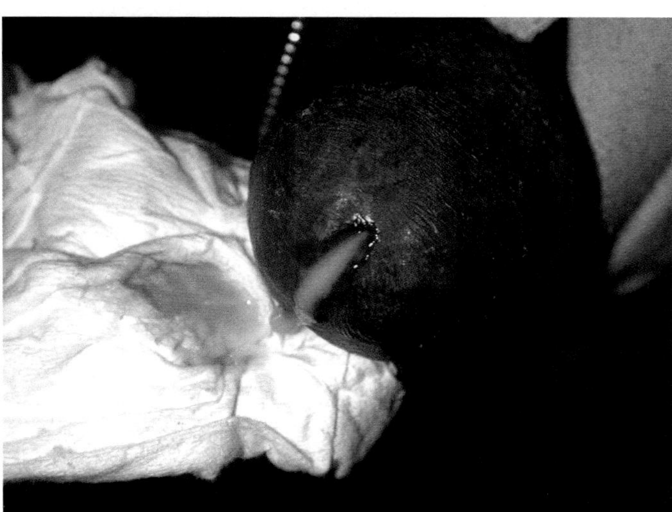

FIGURE 213-1 A 24-year-old man with gonococcal urethritis and a heavy purulent urethral discharge. (*Reproduced with permission from Richard P. Usatine, MD.*)

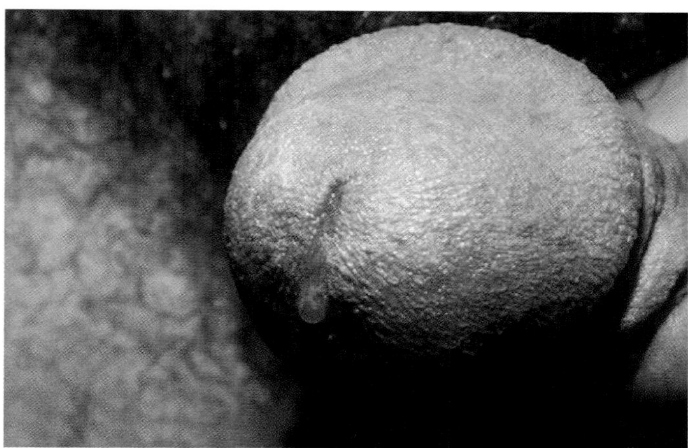

FIGURE 213-2 Nongonococcal urethritis caused by *Chlamydia*. Note the discharge is more clear and less purulent than seen with gonorrhea. (*Reproduced with permission from Seattle STD/HIV Prevention Training Center, University of Washington.*)

- Urethritis of all types occurs in 4 million Americans each year.[1]
- The prevalence of gonorrhea in men was 98.7 per 100,000 people among men in the United States in 2011. The rate was highest among those men aged 20 to 24 years (450.6 per 100,000 people). In 2011, gonorrhea rates remained highest among black men and women (427.3), which was 17 times the rate among whites (25.2 per 100,000 people). The rates among Hispanics (53.8) was 2.1 times those of whites.[2]
- The prevalence of *Chlamydia* in men in the United States in 2011 was 256.9 cases per 100,000 males. Age-specific rates among men were highest in those aged 20 to 24 years (1343.3 cases per 100,000 males). The rate of *Chlamydia* among black men and women was more than 7 times the rate among whites (1194.4 and 159 cases per 100,000 people, respectively). The rate among Hispanics (383.6) was 2.4 times the rate among whites.[2]

ETIOLOGY AND PATHOPHYSIOLOGY

- Urethritis is urethral inflammation caused by infectious or noninfectious causes.
- *Neisseria gonorrhoeae* and *Chlamydia trachomatis* are the most important infectious causes. When transmitted, they can cause other illnesses and complications in men (epididymitis, prostatitis, and reactive arthritis) and women (pelvic inflammatory disease and infertility).
- Other infectious agents include *Mycoplasma genitalium*, *Ureaplasma urealyticum*, *Trichomonas vaginalis*, herpes simplex viruses 1 and 2, adenovirus, and enteric bacteria.
- Noninfectious causes include trauma, foreign bodies, granulomas or unusual tumors, allergic reactions, or voiding dysfunction (any abnormal holding or voiding pattern not caused by an anatomic or a neurologic process).

DIAGNOSIS

CLINICAL FEATURES

Male patients with urethritis can be asymptomatic or present with urethral discharge, dysuria, or urethral pruritus.

Urethritis is diagnosed when one of the following is present:[3]

- Mucopurulent or purulent urethral discharge (see **Figures 213-1** and **213-2**).
- First-void urine positive leukocyte esterase test greater than or equal to 10 white blood cells (WBCs) per high-power field. (This can also be seen with a urinary tract infection [UTI]; however, the incidence of UTI in men younger than 50 years of age is approximately 50 per 100,000 per year, much lower than the incidence of gonococcal or chlamydial urethritis in this age group.)

LABORATORY TESTING

- Nucleic acid amplification test (NAAT) is the recommended test for screening asymptomatic at-risk men and testing symptomatic men.[3] Urine is a better specimen than urethral swab and does not hurt.[3,4]
- Gram-stain of urethral secretions with greater than or equal to 5 WBC per oil immersion field. (If gram-negative intracellular diplococci are seen, gonococcal urethritis is present.) Gram-stain will identify most cases; greater than or equal to 5 WBCs are seen in 82% of *Chlamydia* and 94% of gonococcal infections.[5] Government regulations concerning in-office laboratory testing have severely curtailed the use of Gram-stains in the office.
- Leukocyte esterase test on urine has a good negative predictive value (NPV) but poor positive predictive value (PPV) in a low-prevalence population (NPV 96.4% and PPV 35.4%).[6] Urethral culture is less commonly necessary when NAAT is available.
- Consider culture when tests for gonorrhea and *Chlamydia* are negative, or symptoms persist despite adequate treatment in a patient who is unlikely to have been reinfected by an untreated partner.

DIFFERENTIAL DIAGNOSIS

Dysuria in men can be caused by the following:[7]

- Infections in other sites or the urogenital tract—Cystitis, prostatitis with perineal pain or prostate tenderness, or epididymitis with scrotal pain.
- Penile lesions—Vesicles of herpes simplex, ulcers of syphilis, chancroid, or lymphogranuloma venereum, and glans irritation from balanitis.
- Mechanical causes—Obstruction from benign prostatic hyperplasia (BPH) causing inflammation without infection, trauma including catheterization, urethral strictures, or genitourinary cancers.
- Inflammatory conditions—Spondyloarthropathies, drug reactions, or autoimmune diseases.

MANAGEMENT

Treat patients who meet criteria for urethritis. Test patients with dysuria who do not meet criteria for urethritis, for *N. gonorrhoeae* and *C. trachomatis*, and treat if positive. Advise sex partners to be evaluated and treated.[2]

NONPHARMACOLOGIC

Encourage safe-sex practices.

MEDICATIONS

- The 2010 Centers for Disease Control and Prevention (CDC) STD treatment guidelines recommend treating uncomplicated gonococcal urethritis with ceftriaxone 250 mg IM in a single dose plus treatment for *Chlamydia* with azithromycin or doxycycline. Most gonococci in the United States are susceptible to doxycycline and azithromycin, so that routine cotreatment might also hinder the development of antimicrobial-resistant *N. gonorrhoeae*.[8] Avoid fluoroquinolones and oral cefixime as drug resistance is too high.[8,9] SOR Ⓐ
- The 2010 CDC STD treatment guidelines recommend treating *Chlamydia* urethritis with azithromycin 1 g orally in a single dose or doxycycline 100 mg orally twice a day for 7 days.[10] SOR Ⓐ Acceptable alternate regimens include the following:
  - Erythromycin base 500 mg 4 times a day for 7 days or erythromycin ethylsuccinate 800 mg 4 times a day for 7 days or ofloxacin 300 mg orally twice a day for 7 days or levofloxacin 500 mg orally once daily for 7 days.[10]
- For persistent urethritis, consider *Trichomonas vaginalis* as a possible cause—Culture and treat with a single dose of metronidazole 2 g.
- Consider expedited partner therapy (EPT). EPT is the delivery of medications or prescriptions by persons infected with a STD to their sex partners without clinical assessment of the partners. Legal status by state is available at **http://www.cdc.gov/std/ept/legal/default.htm.**

PREVENTION

Consider screening the following groups of men for *Chlamydia*, using urine NAAT for testing and screening.[2] Twelve percent of male patients with chlamydial and 5% with gonococcal infections had no Gram-stain evidence of urethral inflammation.[5]

- Men attending an STD clinic
- Men attending a national job training program
- Men younger than 30 years of age who are military recruits
- Men younger than 30 years of age entering jail

PROGNOSIS

Gonococcal and chlamydial urethritis respond well to appropriate antibiotic therapy. Partners must be treated to avoid reinfection.

FOLLOW-UP

- Reevaluate patients with persistent or recurrent symptoms after treatment. Reexamine for evidence of urethral inflammation and retest for gonorrhea and *Chlamydia*.
- Routine test-of-cure laboratory examination is not recommended by the CDC for gonorrhea or *Chlamydia* infections unless therapeutic compliance is in question, symptoms persist, or reinfection is suspected.[8,10]
- However, patients who have symptoms that persist after treatment of gonorrhea should be evaluated by culture for *N. gonorrhoeae*, and any gonococci isolated should be tested for antimicrobial susceptibility.[8]
- Consider chronic prostatitis if symptoms persist for more than 3 months.

PATIENT EDUCATION

The CDC recommends the following for patients diagnosed with gonorrhea or *Chlamydia*[2]:

- Return for evaluation if the symptoms persist or return after therapy is completed.
- Abstain from sexual intercourse until 7 days after starting therapy, symptoms have resolved, and sexual partners have been adequately treated.
- Undergo testing for other STDs, including HIV and syphilis.
- Advise sexual partners of the need for treatment and/or take medications directly to them using EPT.

PATIENT RESOURCES

- Centers for Disease Control and Prevention. *Gonorrhea*—**http://www.cdc.gov/std/Gonorrhea/STDFact-gonorrhea.htm.**
- Centers for Disease Control and Prevention. *Chlamydia*—**http://www.cdc.gov/std/chlamydia/default.htm.**

PROVIDER RESOURCES

- The Centers for Disease Control and Prevention (CDC) website has the latest epidemiologic data and management recommendations—**http://www.cdc.gov/std/default.htm.**
- The newest CDC Treatment Guidelines are at **http://www.cdc.gov/std/treatment.**

REFERENCES

1. Terris MK. *Urethritis*. http://emedicine.medscape.com/article/438091. Accessed September 2, 2012.
2. U.S. Centers for Disease Control and Prevention. http://www.cdc.gov/std/stats10/chlamydia.htm. Accessed February 21, 2013.
3. Brill JR. Diagnosis and treatment of urethritis in men. *Am Fam Physician*. 2010;81(7):873-878.
4. Sugunendran H, Birley HD, Mallinson H, et al. Comparison of urine, first and second endourethral swabs for PCR based detection of genital *Chlamydia trachomatis* infection in male patients. *Sex Transm Infect*. 2001;77(6):423-426.
5. Geisler WM, Yu S, Hook EW III. Chlamydial and gonococcal infection in men without polymorphonuclear leukocytes on Gram stain: implications for diagnostic approach and management. *Sex Transm Dis*. 2005;32(10):630-634.
6. Bowden FJ. Reappraising the value of urine leukocyte esterase testing in the age of nucleic acid amplification. *Sex Transm Dis*. 1998;25(6):322-326.
7. Bremnor J, Sadovsky R. Evaluation of dysuria in adults. *Am Fam Physician*. 2002;65(8):1589-1596.
8. Centers for Disease Control and Prevention (CDC). *Sexually Transmitted Diseases Treatment Guidelines, 2010: Gonococcal Infections*. http://www.cdc.gov/std/treatment/2010/gonococcal-infections.htm. Accessed September 2, 2012.
9. Update to CDC's Sexually Transmitted Diseases Treatment Guidelines, 2010: oral cephalosporins no longer a recommended treatment for gonococcal infections. *MMWR Morb Mortal Wkly Rep*. 2012;61(31):590-594. http://www.cdc.gov/mmwr/preview/mmwrhtml/mm6131a3.htm?s_cid=mm6131a3_w. Accessed September 2, 2012.
10. Centers for Disease Control and Prevention (CDC). *Sexually Transmitted Diseases Treatment Guidelines, 2010: Chlamydial Infections*. http://www.cdc.gov/std/treatment/2010/chlamydial-infections.htm. Accessed September 2, 2012.

214 INTESTINAL WORMS AND PARASITES

Heidi Chumley, MD

PATIENT STORY

A 40-year-old man presents with a 10-day history of nausea, emesis, diarrhea, and abdominal pain and distention. He has not had fever and has noted no blood in his stool. His symptoms began 5 days after he returned from a camping trip. On abdominal examination, he had diffuse mild tenderness, but no rebound or guarding. Bowel sounds were present and normoactive. An immunoassay for the detection of *Giardia* stool antigens was positive. The patient was treated for *Giardia lamblia* (**Figure 214-1**) with metronidazole and his symptoms resolved completely.

INTRODUCTION

Intestinal parasites are most common in places with warmer temperatures and high humidity, poor sanitation and unclean water, and a large number of individuals (especially children) living in close proximity. In general, the parasites are either asymptomatic or cause symptoms related to their presence in the gastrointestinal (GI) tract. Several migrate through the lungs and can also cause pulmonary symptoms during the migration. Diagnoses are made by history of worms being seen by the patient or parents or by laboratory examination for ova and parasites in the stool.

EPIDEMIOLOGY

- Nematoda is the phylum that contains pinworms, hookworms, *Ascaris*, *Strongyloides*, and whipworms.
  - *Enterobius vermicularis* (pinworm) is the most prevalent nematode in the United States. Populations at risk include preschool and school-aged children, institutionalized persons, and household members of persons with pinworm infection.[1]

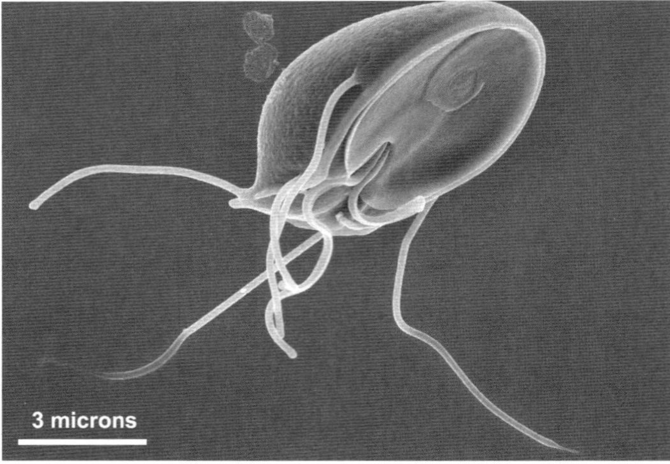

FIGURE 214-1 *Giardia trophozoite* visible with this scanning electron micrograph. The ventral adhesive disk resembles a suction cup and facilitates adherence of the protozoan to the intestinal surface. *Giardia* has 4 pairs of flagella that are responsible for the organism's motility. (*Reproduced with permission from CDC/Dr. Stan Erlandsen.*)

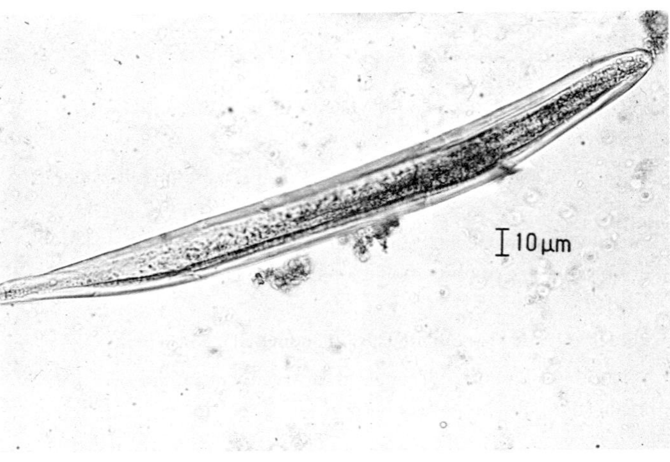

FIGURE 214-2 *Necator americanus* (hookworm) larvae can penetrate the skin, travel through veins to the heart then lungs, climb the bronchial tree to the pharynx, are swallowed, and attach to intestine walls. (*Reproduced with permission from James L. Fishback, MD.*)

  - *Necator americanus* (hookworm) is found predominately in the America and Australia, and is the second most common nematode identified in stool studies in the United States[1] (**Figures 214-2** and **214-3**). *Ancylostoma duodenale* (hookworm) is found mostly in southern Europe, North Africa, the Middle East, and Asia.[1]
  - *Ascaris lumbricoides* is the largest and most common roundworm found in humans in the world; although less common in the United States, it is seen mostly in the rural southeast. It is found in tropical and subtropical areas, including the southeastern rural United States (**Figures 214-4** and **214-5**).[1]
  - *Strongyloides stercoralis* is seen mostly in tropical and subtropical areas, but can be found in temperate areas, including the southern United States (**Figure 214-6**). It is more frequently found in rural areas, institutional settings, and lower socioeconomic groups.[1]

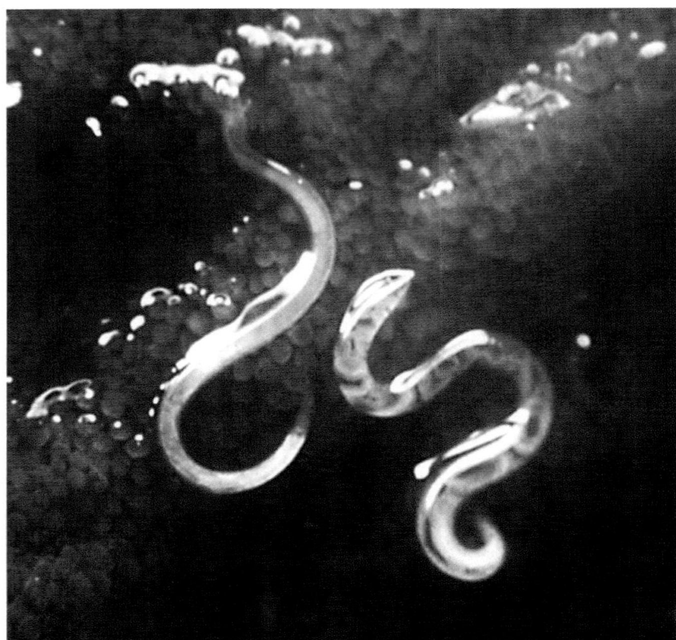

FIGURE 214-3 Adult hookworm attached to the intestinal wall. (*Reproduced with permission from Centers for Disease Control and Prevention.*)

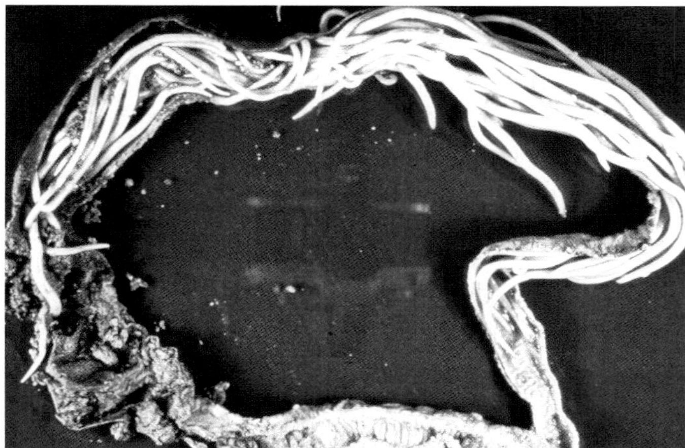

FIGURE 214-4 *Ascaris lumbricoides* in the resected bowel of a patient with bowel obstruction. (*Reproduced with permission from James L. Fishback, MD.*)

- *Trichuris trichiura* (whipworm) is the third most common roundworm found in humans worldwide. Infections are more frequent in areas with tropical weather and poor sanitation practices, and among children (**Figure 214-7**). It is estimated that 800 million people are infected worldwide. Trichuriasis occurs in the southern United States.[1]

- Cestodes (tapeworm) are a class in the phylum *Platyhelminthes* that contains *Taenia solium* (pork tapeworm).
  - *T. solium* is found worldwide where pigs and humans live in close proximity.
- Protozoa is the kingdom of 1-celled organisms that includes *G. lamblia* and *Entamoeba histolytica.*
  - *G. lamblia (Giardia intestinalis)* is the most common parasite infection worldwide and the second most common in the United States (after pinworm), causing 2.5 million infections annually (**Figure 214-8**).[1]
  - *E. histolytica* is seen worldwide, with higher incidence in developing countries. In the United States, risk groups include men who have sex with men, travelers and recent immigrants, and institutionalized populations.[1]

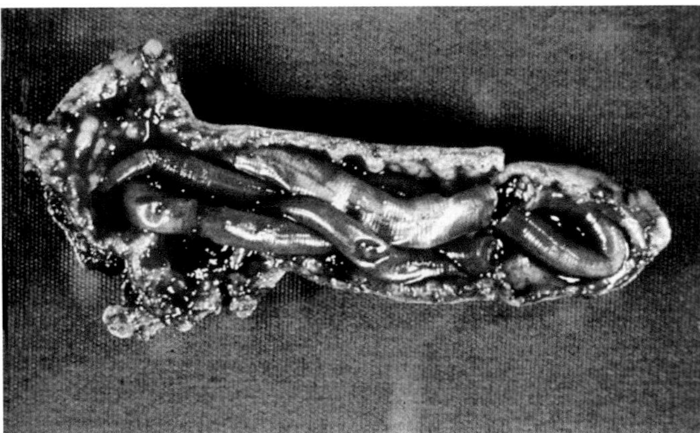

FIGURE 214-5 *Ascaris lumbricoides* in the appendix after being removed from a young adult with acute appendicitis. (*Reproduced with permission from James L. Fishback, MD.*)

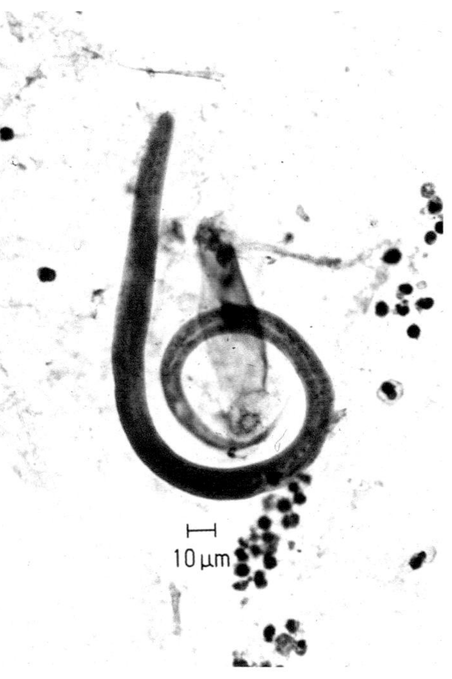

FIGURE 214-6 *Strongyloides stercoralis* ova and parasite in stool. (*Reproduced with permission from James L. Fishback, MD.*)

ETIOLOGY AND PATHOPHYSIOLOGY

- Nematodes (roundworms)
  - *E. vermicularis* (pinworm) (see **Figure 214-1**) is acquired through an oral route when hands that have contacted contaminated objects are placed in the mouth. Larvae hatch in the small intestine. Adults live in the cecum. The pregnant female goes to the perianal region at night to lay eggs.
  - *N. americanus* (hookworm) (see **Figure 214-2**) larvae penetrate the skin, travel through veins to the heart and then to the lungs, climb

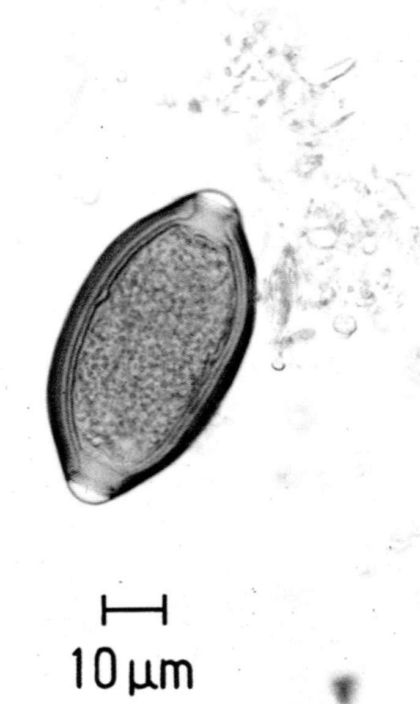

FIGURE 214-7 *Trichuris trichiura* (whipworm) egg in stool. (*Reproduced with permission from James L. Fishback, MD.*)

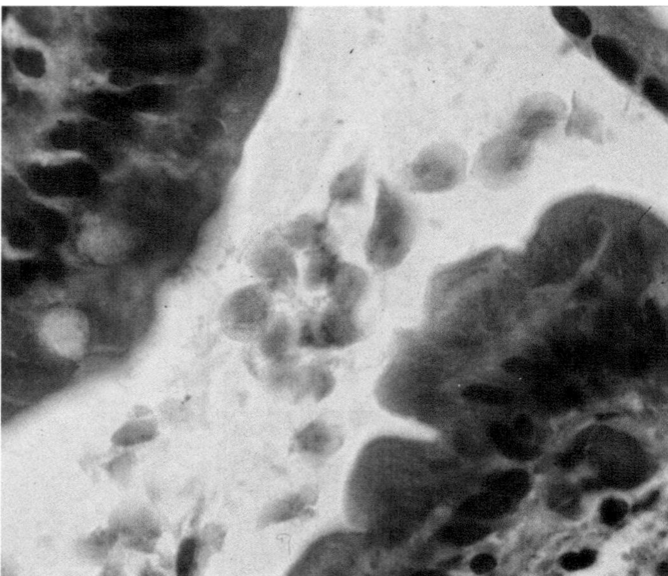

FIGURE 214-8 *Giardia lamblia* in a duodenal biopsy obtained by esophagogastroduodenoscopy in a patient with typical symptoms of chronic giardiasis (excessive flatulence and sulfurous belching) that failed to improve on metronidazole. (*Reproduced with permission from Tom Moore, MD.*)

the bronchial tree to the pharynx, and then are swallowed and attach to intestine walls (see **Figure 214-3**).
  - When fertilized eggs of *A. lumbricoides* (see **Figure 214-4**) are ingested, they hatch and the larvae enter the circulation through intestinal mucosa, travel to the lungs, climb to the pharynx, then are swallowed, and finally the adult *Ascaris* worms live in the small intestine.
  - *S. stercoralis* have both a free-living and parasitic cycle. In the parasitic cycle, larvae penetrate the skin, travel through the circulation to the lungs and are swallowed, and travel to the small intestine (see **Figures 214-5** and **214-6**) to become adults. Adult females lay eggs, which become rhabditiform larvae, which can either become free living or can cause autoinfection by reentering the parasitic cycle or disseminating widely in the body.
  - *T. trichiura* (whipworm) (see **Figure 214-7**) eggs are ingested and hatch in the small intestine; worms live in the cecum or colon.
  - Cestodes (tapeworms)—*T. solium* is acquired by ingesting undercooked contaminated pork. Diphyllobothrium latum is the fish tapeworm that is acquired by ingesting uncooked contaminated fresh-water fish.
- Protozoa
  - *G. lamblia* cysts are ingested from contaminated water, food, or fomites and travel to the small intestine (see **Figure 214-8**).
  - *E. histolytica* cysts or trophozoites are ingested from fecally contaminated food, water, or hands or from fecal contact during sexual practices; these then travel to the large intestine, where these either remain or travel through the bloodstream to the brain, liver, or lungs.

RISK FACTORS

- Endemic in developing countries with limited access to clean water.
- Living in an environment conducive to parasites (warm, humid climate) and parasitic transfer (crowded conditions, contaminated water supply, poor hygiene) and dramatically raises the risk of parasitic infection.
- Household contacts or caretakers of persons with intestinal parasites are at risk of contracting the parasites.
- Children or others with poor hygiene are also at high risk.
- Immunocompromised patients, once infected, may have a more serious course.

DIAGNOSIS

CLINICAL FEATURES

- Nematodes
  - *E. vermicularis* (pinworm)—Perianal pruritus is the most common; female genital tract irritation also reported; rarely abdominal pain or appendicitis; infants show irritability, but can be asymptomatic.[1]
  - *N. americanus* (hookworm)—Most commonly presents with iron deficiency anemia.[1]
  - *A. lumbricoides*—Frequently asymptomatic; high numbers of worms can cause abdominal pain or intestinal obstruction. Cough, dyspnea, hemoptysis, or eosinophilic pneumonitis when in the lungs. Patients may cough up visible worms.
  - *S. stercoralis*—Frequently asymptomatic; eosinophilia; may cause abdominal pain or diarrhea, cough, shortness of breath, or hemoptysis when in the lungs; can disseminate in immunocompromised patients causing abdominal pain, distention, septicemia, shock, or death.
  - *T. trichiura* (whipworm)—Frequently asymptomatic; high number of worms can cause abdominal pain or intestinal obstruction, especially in children.
- Cestodes
  - *T. solium*—Frequently asymptomatic; risk of developing cysticercosis with symptoms based on location of cysts in brain (eg, seizures, focal neurologic signs, and death), eyes, heart, or spine.
- Protozoa
  - *G. lamblia*—Diarrhea, nausea, emesis, abdominal bloating occurs 1 to 14 days after ingestion for up to 3 weeks, and can be asymptomatic.
  - *E. histolytica*—Asymptomatic, intestinal symptoms (eg, colitis and appendicitis), or extraintestinal (eg, abscess in the liver or lungs, peritonitis, and skin or genital lesions).

LABORATORY TESTING

- Nematodes
  - *E. vermicularis* (pinworm)—Microscopic identification of eggs (see **Figure 214-1**) collected from perianal area; apply transparent adhesive tape to the unwashed perianal area at the time of presentation or in the morning and then place tape on slide.
  - *N. americanus* (hookworm)—Microscopic identification of eggs in the stool (see **Figure 214-2**).
  - *A. lumbricoides*—Microscopic identification of eggs in the stool.
  - *S. stercoralis*—Microscopic identification of larvae in stool (see **Figure 214-6**) or duodenal fluid; often requires several samples. Immunologic tests are useful when infection is suspected, but larvae are not seen in several samples. Immunologic tests do not differentiate from past or present infections.
  - *T. trichiura* (whipworm)—Microscopic identification of eggs in stool (see **Figure 214-7**).

- Cestodes
  - *T. solium*—Microscopic identification of eggs or proglottids in stool indicates taeniasis; presumed neurocysticercus diagnosed from Centers for Disease Control and Prevention (CDC)'s immunoblot assay.[1]
- Protozoa
  - *G. lamblia*—Microscopic identification of cysts or trophozoites in stool or trophozoites in duodenal fluid or biopsy (see **Figure 214-8**). Antigen tests and immunofluorescence are available.
  - *E. histolytica*—Microscopic identification of cysts or trophozoites in stool (difficult to distinguish from nonpathogens); antibody detection for extraintestinal disease; antigen detection can distinguish pathogenic and nonpathogenic infections.[1]

IMAGING

Cestodes

- *T. solium*—Magnetic resonance imaging (MRI) is typically used to identify brain cysts.

DIFFERENTIAL DIAGNOSIS

Abdominal symptoms seen with several intestinal parasites can also be caused by the following:

- Viral or bacterial infections—May present with acute onset of emesis and diarrhea often with fever.
  - Irritable bowel disease—Chronic symptoms of abdominal cramping with diarrhea or loose stools and/or constipation; usually no bloody stools, weight loss, or anemia.
  - Inflammatory bowel disease—Intermittent abdominal pain and bloody stools; diagnosis confirmed by colonoscopy with biopsy.
  - Iron deficiency anemia seen with hookworms can be seen with blood loss from any site from one of many causes. Of course, iron deficiency can be seen with a diet deficient in iron without having hookworms.
  - GI blood loss can be seen with other infections or inflammation, polyps, or masses.

MANAGEMENT

MEDICATIONS

All medication doses are from *The Medical Letter*[2]

- Nematodes
  - *E. vermicularis* (pinworm)—Pyrantel pamoate 1 g once , repeat in
  - 2 weeks; or mebendazole 100 mg once, repeat in 2 weeks.
  - *N. americanus* (hookworm)—Albendazole 400 mg once; or mebendazole 100 mg twice a day for 3 days 500 mg once or pyrantel pamoate 1 g for 3 days.
  - *A. lumbricoides*—Albendazole 400 mg once; alternate therapy mebendazole 500 mg once or ivermectin 150 to 200 μg/kg PO once.
  - *S. stercoralis*—Ivermectin 200 μg/kg per day for 2 days; alternate therapy albendazole 400 mg bid for 7 days.
  - *T. trichiura* (whipworm)—Mebendazole 100 mg twice a day for 3 days or 500 mg once; alternate therapy albendazole 400 mg once a day for 3 days or ivermectin 0.2 mg/kg daily for 3 days.
- Cestodes
  - *T. solium*—Praziquantel 5 to 10 mg/kg once for intestinal stage; cysticercosis requires seizure prophylaxis and steroids in conjunction with albendazole 400 mg bid for 8 to 30 days; ophthalmologic examination for eye cysts is recommended.
- Protozoa
  - *G. lamblia*—Metronidazole 250 mg tid for 5 to 7 days; or tinidazole 2 g once; or nitazoxanide 500 mg bid for 3 days.
  - *E. histolytica*—Metronidazole 500 to 750 mg tid for 7 to 10 days or tinidazole 2 g once daily for 3 days. Then iodoquinol 650 mg tid for 20 days; or paromomycin 25 to 35 mg/kg/d in 3 doses for 7 days.

REFERRAL OR HOSPITALIZATION

Refer or hospitalize the following patients:

- Who do not respond to initial therapy or have recurrent infections
- Suspected of having cysticercosis
- Experiencing severe abdominal symptoms suggesting obstruction or an acute abdomen

PREVENTION

- Clean uncontaminated water for drinking and cooking—Use bottled water, chemically treated water, or boiled water in endemic areas.
- Good hygiene, especially hand washing.
- When travelling to endemic areas, drink bottled water when possible. Water can also be treated with chlorine, iodine, or boiled if bottled water is not available. Clean water should be used for brushing teeth. Avoid eating fresh salads washed in local water.
- Presumptive treatment of refugees for intestinal parasites administered oversees before coming to the United States is recommended by the CDC. Treatment with a single dose of 600-mg albendazole decreased the prevalence of intestinal nematods among African and Southeast Asian refugees.[3]

PROGNOSIS

Prognosis is excellent for most infections if adequate therapy and clean water is available.

FOLLOW-UP

Follow-up at completion of therapy.

PATIENT EDUCATION

Most intestinal parasites are asymptomatic and easily treatable. Avoid infecting others by practicing good hygiene, including hand washing.

PATIENT RESOURCES

- The Centers for Disease Control and Prevention division of parasitic diseases has information on many parasitic diseases—**http://www.cdc.gov/parasites.**

PROVIDER RESOURCES

- Centers for Disease Control and Prevention (CDC). *Parasites*—**http://www.cdc.gov/parasites.**
- The Medical Letter's "Drugs for Parasitic Infections" is available online at **www.medletter.com** for individual and institutional subscribers.

REFERENCES

1. Centers for Disease Control and Prevention. *Parasites*. http://www.cdc.gov/parasites. Accessed September 11, 2011.
2. The Medical Letter. Drugs for parasitic infections. Treatment guidelines. 2nd ed. 2010. http://secure.medicalletter.org/system/files/private/parasitic.pdf. Accessed September 11, 2011.
3. Swanson SJ, Phares CR, Mamo B, et al. Albendazole therapy and enteric parasites in United States-bound refugees. *N Engl J Med*. 2012;366(16):1498-1507.

215 LYME DISEASE

Thomas J. Corson, DO
Richard P. Usatine, MD
Heidi Chumley, MD

PATIENT STORY

On a warm, summer afternoon a 32-year-old woman presents having had low-grade fevers for 5 days and a rash. On physical examination, the physician notes a large, erythematous, annular patch with central clearing on her back (**Figure 215-1**). The patient states that the rash has gotten progressively larger during the last 3 days and she has had a recent onset of intermittent joint pain. She does not recall being bitten by an insect. She denies taking medications within the last month and has no known allergies. When asked about recent travel, she admits to a camping trip in eastern Massachusetts, which she returned from 4 days ago. The patient was diagnosed with Lyme borreliosis and started on doxycycline 100 mg twice daily for 14 days. She responded quickly to the antibiotics and never developed the persistent stage of Lyme disease.

INTRODUCTION

Lyme disease is an infection caused by the spirochete *Borrelia burgdorferi*, transmitted via tick bite. Most cases of Lyme disease occur in the northeast United States between April and November. Patients experience flu-like symptoms and may develop the pathognomonic rash, erythema migrans. Lyme disease is prevented by avoiding exposure to the tick vector using insect repellent and protective clothing.

EPIDEMIOLOGY

- In 1977, clusters of patients in Old Lyme, Connecticut, began reporting symptoms originally thought to be juvenile rheumatoid arthritis.[1]

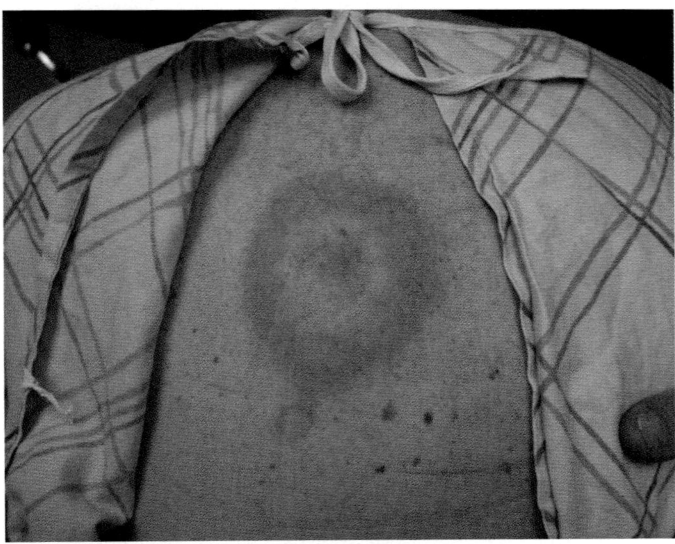

FIGURE 215-1 A 32-year-old woman presents having had 5 days of low-grade fevers and the typical eruption of erythema migrans on her upper back. Note the expanding annular lesion with a target-like morphology. (*Reproduced with permission from Thomas Corson, MD.*)

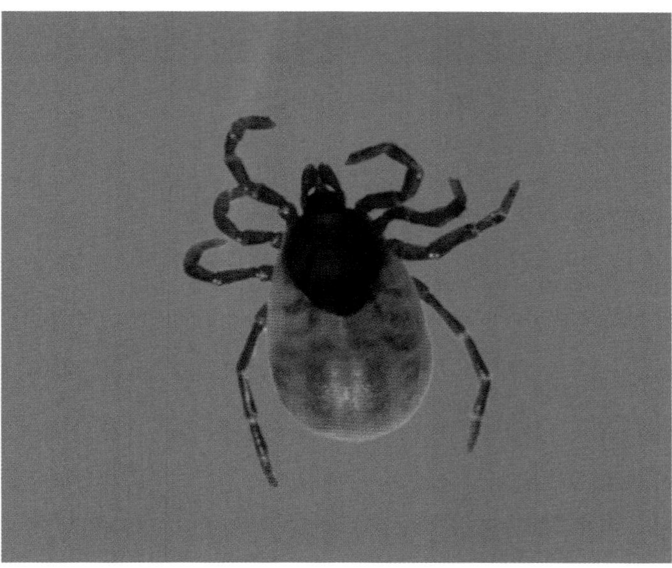

FIGURE 215-2 The deer tick transmits the *Borrelia* spirochete. This is an unengorged female black-legged deer tick. The tick is tiny and can be undetected in its unengorged state. (*Reproduced with permission from Thomas Corson, MD.*)

- In 1981, American entomologist, Dr. Willy Burgdorfer, isolated the infectious pathogen responsible for Lyme disease from the midgut of *Ixodes scapularis* (aka black-legged deer ticks) (**Figure 215-2**), which serve as the primary transmission vector in the United States.[1]
- It was identified as a bacterial spirochete and named *B. burgdorferi* in honor of its founder.
- Based on Centers for Disease Control and Prevention (CDC) data reported in 2011, Lyme disease (or Lyme borreliosis) is the most common tick-borne illness in the United States, with an overall incidence of 7.8 per 100,000 persons.[2]
- In 2011, 96% of Lyme disease cases were reported from 13 states: Connecticut, Delaware, Maine, Maryland, Massachusetts, Minnesota, New Jersey, New Hampshire, New York, Pennsylvania, Vermont, Virginia, and Wisconsin.[3]
- Patients living between Maryland and Maine accounted for 93% of all reported cases in the United States in 2005, with an overall incidence of 31.6 cases for every 100,000 persons.[2]
- More than 90% of cases report onset between April and November.[2]

ETIOLOGY AND PATHOPHYSIOLOGY

- *B. burgdorferi* begins to multiply in the midgut of *I. scapularis* ticks upon attaching to humans.
- Migration from midgut to salivary glands of ticks requires 24 to 48 hours.
- Prior to this migration, host infection rarely occurs.
- Common hosts include field mice, white-tailed deer, and household pets.
- Ticks must feed on infested hosts in order to infect humans.
- Thirty percent of infected patients do not recall being bitten.[4]
- Once a human is infected, disease progression is categorized into 3 stages: localized, disseminated, and persistent.

DIAGNOSIS

CLINICAL FEATURES

Localized (days to weeks)

Erythema migrans (formerly known as erythema chronicum migrans)

This pathognomonic finding occurs in roughly 68% of Lyme disease cases.[4] Described as a "bull's-eye" eruption (**Figures 215-1** and **215-3** to **215-6**), this nonpruritic, lesion typically occurs near the site of the tick bite. The erythematous perimeter migrates outward over several days while some of the central area clears. Multiple lesions in different sites can develop in some individuals (**Figure 215-4**). Erythema migrans can persist for 2 to 3 weeks if left untreated.

Flu-like symptoms

Roughly 67% of patients will develop flu-like symptoms that can include fever, myalgias, and lymphadenopathy. Symptoms usually subside within 7 to 10 days.

Disseminated (days to months)

Inflammatory arthritis

Typical onset occurs around 3 to 6 months after localized infection. Patients will often present with polyarticular, migratory joint pain with or without erythema, and swelling, which is exacerbated with motion. After more than 24 to 48 hours, these symptoms localize to one joint (especially knee, ankle, or wrist) and last approximately 1 week. Recurrence is common and usually happens every few months, but typically resolves within 10 years even without treatment.

Cranial nerve palsy

Bell's palsy (seventh cranial nerve) is the most common neurologic manifestation of Lyme disease. However, nearly every cranial nerve has been reported to be involved. Facial nerve palsy is a lower motor neuron lesion that results in weakness of both the lower face and the forehead. Lasting up to 8 weeks, the resolution of symptoms is gradual and begins shortly after initial onset (see Chapter 234, Bell's Palsy).

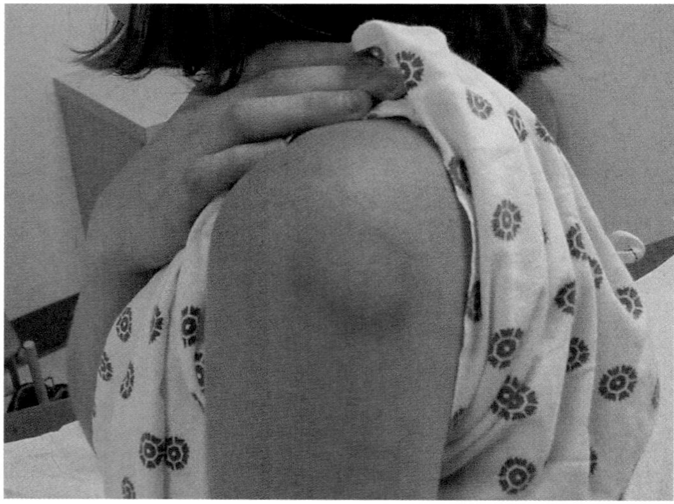

FIGURE 215-3 Lyme disease presenting with erythema migrans on the shoulder. The patient is febrile and systemically ill. (*Reproduced with permission from Jeremy Golding, MD.*)

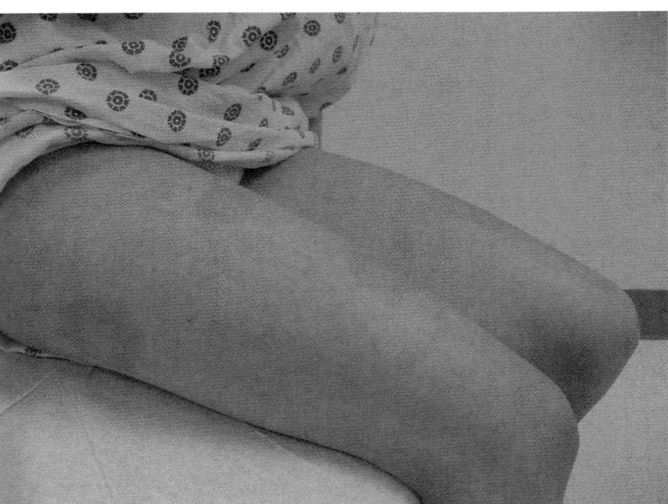

FIGURE 215-4 Multiple annular erythema migrans eruptions on the legs in a patient with Lyme disease. (*Reproduced with permission from Jeremy Golding, MD.*)

Atrioventricular blockade

Present in only 1% of patients with Lyme disease, syncope, light-headedness, and dyspnea are classic symptoms consistent with atrioventricular (AV) dysfunction.[3] However, patients can be completely asymptomatic. The degree of Lyme-associated blockade varies so that symptoms are generally episodic. Most cases resolve spontaneously within 1 week.[4] Any patient with history and/or examination findings suspicious of Lyme disease should undergo electrocardiography (ECG) testing. Hospitalization and continuous monitoring are advisable for symptomatic patients, for patients with second- or third-degree AV block, as well as for those with first-degree heart block when the PR interval is prolonged to 30 or more milliseconds, because the degree of block may fluctuate and worsen very rapidly in such patients.[5]

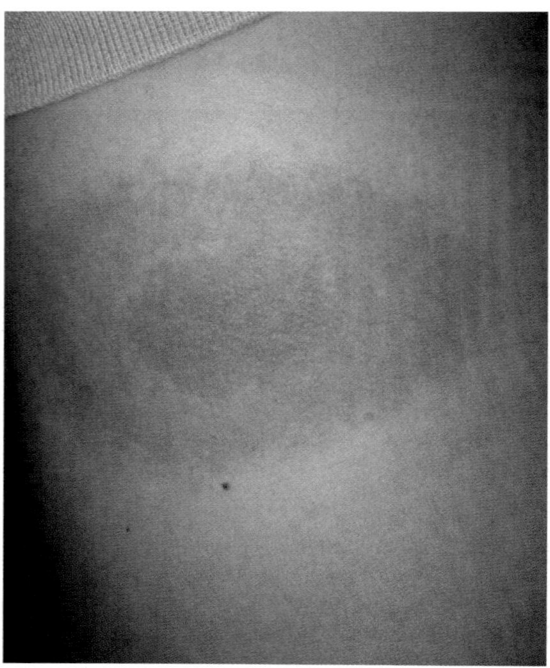

FIGURE 215-5 Classic "bull's eye" eruption of erythema migrans on the arm of a 45-year-old woman newly diagnosed with Lyme disease in an endemic area. (*Reproduced with permission from Jeremy Golding, MD.*)

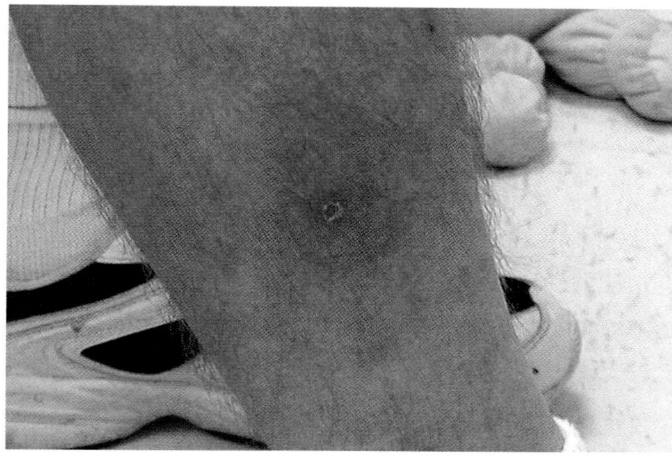

FIGURE 215-6 Erythema migrans eruption on the leg of a patient with localized Lyme disease. The central scale is the site of the tick bite. (*Reproduced with permission from Jeremy Golding, MD.*)

Aseptic meningitis

Patients may present with complaints similar to bacterial meningitis (photophobia, nuchal rigidity, and headache), but symptoms are generally less severe in nature. This can also occur with or without concomitant cranial nerve palsy.[4]

Fatigue

A depressed level of activity as a result of fatigue is one of the most common complaints, affecting up to 80% of infected patients. Even after adequate treatment, symptoms consistent with chronic fatigue syndrome have developed in patients with known Lyme disease.

Persistent (longer than 1 year)

Chronic arthritis

Generally occurs in the knee, although other sites such as the shoulder, ankle, elbow, or wrist are not uncommon. Approximately 10% of patients with intermittent arthritis will progress to this stage.[4]

Chronic fatigue

Commonly misdiagnosed as fibromyalgia or chronic fatigue syndrome, patients develop debilitating malaise and myalgias that can persist for months or years after infection.

Meningoencephalitis

Symptoms vary from mild (memory loss, mood lability, irritability, or panic attacks) to severe (manic or psychotic episodes, paranoia, and obsessive-compulsive symptoms).[5]

LABORATORY TESTING

Diagnosing Lyme disease is generally based on pertinent history findings and/or the presence of an erythema migrans lesion, especially in endemic areas. In cases where an erythema migrans lesion is absent, serologic testing may be warranted utilizing the following tests:

- Enzyme-linked immunosorbent assay (ELISA) (sensitivity 94%, specificity 97%)[6]—Used as a *screening* test in patients lacking physical signs of erythema migrans. Up to 50% of patients with early infection can have a false-negative result. If strong suspicion remains, convalescent titers should be obtained in 6 weeks.[6] Prior infection does not indicate immunity. Lyme titers may be falsely positive in patients with mononucleosis, periodontal disease, connective tissue disease, and other less common conditions.[7]
- Western blot (immunoglobulin [Ig] M and IgG for *B. burgdorferi*)—If ELISA test yields a positive result, Western blot test is used as a *confirmatory* test. IgM antibodies are detectable between 2 weeks and 6 months after inoculation. IgG may be present indefinitely after 6 weeks, despite appropriate antibiotic therapy. Once it is determined that a person is seropositive for Lyme disease, antibiotic therapy should be initiated promptly.

Empiric antibiotic therapy (no test necessary) should be considered in any of the following clinical presentations: presence of EM rash, flu-like symptoms (in absence of upper respiratory infection [URI] or gastrointestinal [GI] symptoms) after known tick bite, Bell's palsy in endemic areas, especially between June and September, and tick bites occurring during pregnancy.

Characteristic laboratory findings

- Complete blood count (CBC)—Leukocytosis (11,000 to 18,000/μL). Anemia and thrombocytopenia are rare.
- Elevated erythrocyte sedimentation rate (ESR) (>20 mm/h).
- Elevated γ-glutamyltransferase (GGT) and aspartate aminotransferase (AST).
- Cerebrospinal fluid—Pleocytosis and elevated protein levels if central nervous system (CNS) is involved. Spirochete antibodies may be detectable.
- Blood culture—Low yield; not recommended.
- Nerve conduction studies and EM—Useful in patients with paresthesias or radicular pain.
- ECG should be performed in all patients with history and physical examination suspicious for Lyme disease to detect AV block and arrhythmias.

DIFFERENTIAL DIAGNOSIS

- Cellulitis—Spreads more rapidly than Lyme disease. Induration and tenderness are more common. Negative Lyme serologies (see Chapter 122, Cellulitis).[8]
- Urticaria—Can resemble erythema migrans when the urticarial lesions are annular. Urticaria is generally more widespread and the wheals come and go over time whereas the lesion of EM is more fixed (see Chapter 148, Urticaria and Angioedema).
- Rocky Mountain spotted fever—Associated with *Dermacentor variabilis* (American dog) tick; rash is petechial and the spots are widely distributed over the body (see Chapter 177, Vasculitis, Figure 177-17). Patients often appear toxic.
- Cutaneous fungal infections—Usually pruritic and may be annular; associated with scaling, which is not characteristic of erythema migrans; and spreads slowly if at all. The similarity is that the annular appearance of tinea corporis can mimic EM (see Chapter 136, Tinea Corporis).
- Local reaction to tick bites—Tick bites may cause a local reaction in skin and do not expand with time; generally less than 2 cm in diameter, and are usually papular.

- Febrile viral illnesses (particularly enteroviruses during summer)—Rash, myalgias, arthralgias, and headache; GI symptoms; sore throat and/or cough. Perform Lyme serologic test in the absence of erythema migrans.
- Facial nerve palsy—May be bilateral in Lyme disease. This is uncommon in facial nerve palsy not associated with Lyme disease (see Chapter 234, Bell's Palsy).
- Viral meningitis—Lymphocytic (aseptic) meningitis caused by viral infection generally results in transient illness that resolves within several days, usually after a monophasic course.
- Heart block—Idiopathic conduction system disease (sick sinus syndrome) can present with the same symptoms and signs as Lyme carditis. Use serologic testing and epidemiologic history to discriminate.
- Inflammatory arthritis (reactive arthritis, gout, pseudogout, and rheumatoid arthritis)—acute, large joint monoarticular or oligoarticular arthritis from multiple causes; may be indistinguishable from acute arthritis associated with Lyme disease at the time of presentation; joint fluid examination, and culture and X-ray may help distinguish from Lyme arthritis (see Chapter 97, Arthritis Overview).
- Peripheral neuropathy is more often associated with diabetes mellitus, peripheral vascular disease, endocrinopathies, and nerve root impingement syndromes. If Lyme disease is the cause, the serologies should be positive.
- Radiculoneuropathy—Dermatomal pain, sensory loss, and/or weakness in a limb or the trunk. Check serologies if Lyme disease is suspected.
- Encephalomyelitis—Focal inflammation of the brain or spinal cord. Check serologies if Lyme disease is suspected.

MANAGEMENT

Algorithms for managing Lyme disease are presented below.

MEDICATIONS

Localized

Adults—Doxycycline 100 mg twice a day (nonpregnant patients only) or amoxicillin 500 mg 3 times a day or cefuroxime 500 mg twice a day for 14 days.[5] SOR A

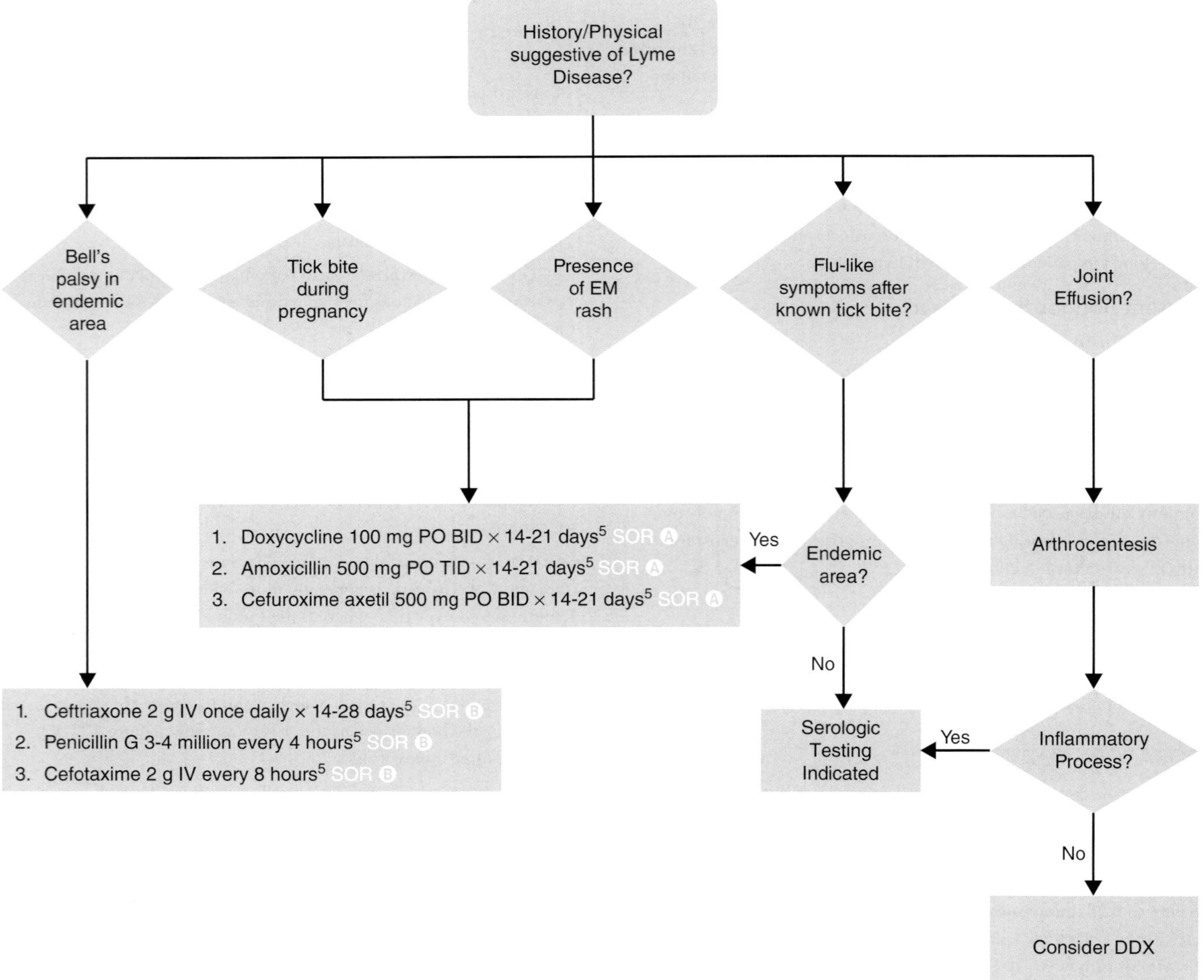

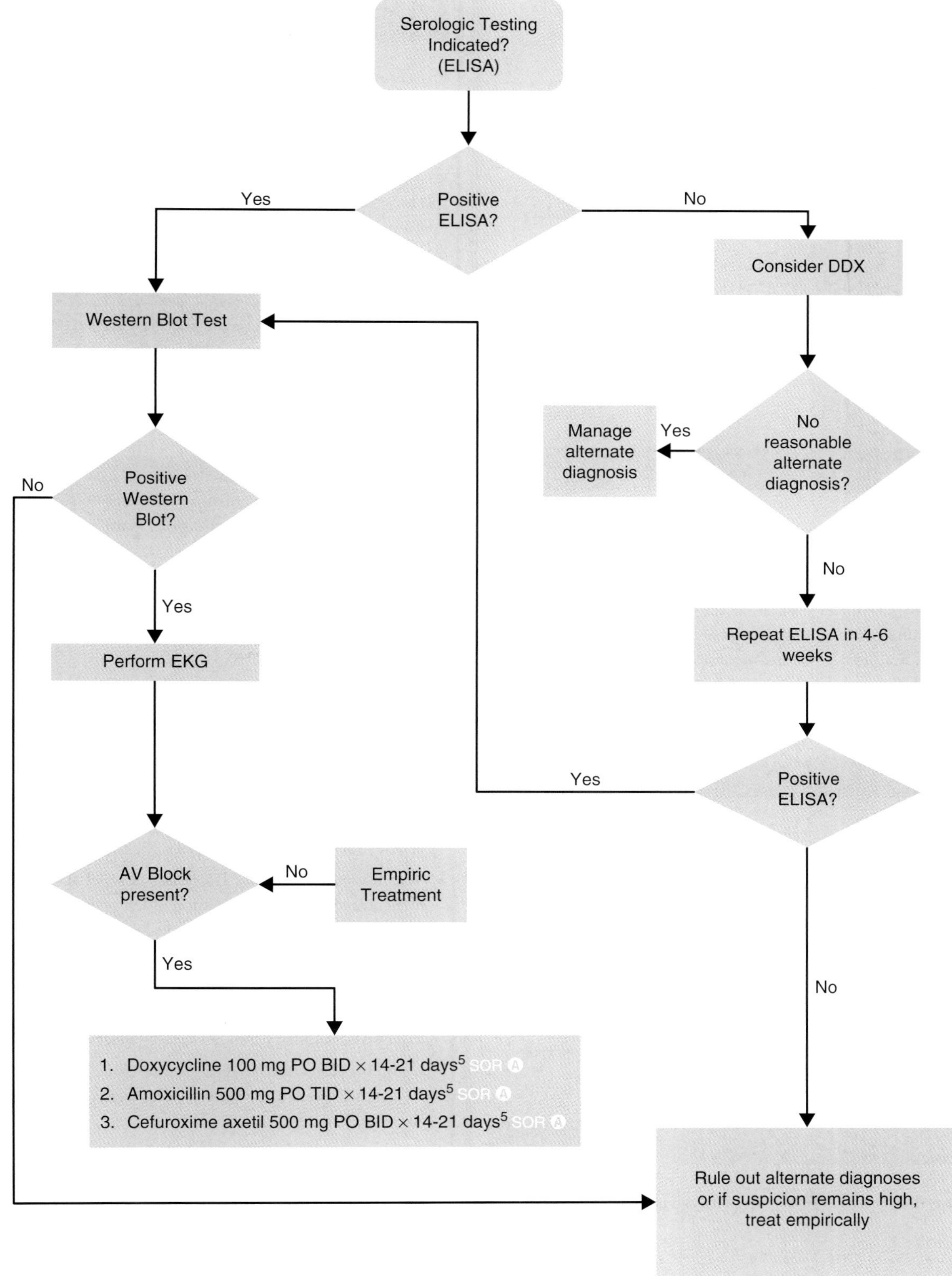

Meningitis or other neurologic manifestations

- Adults—Ceftriaxone 2 g intravenous (IV) every day for 14 days; alternative therapy cefotaxime 2 g IV every 8 hours or penicillin G 18 to 24 million units every day divided into 6 daily doses for 14 days.[5] SOR B
- Doxycycline (oral) 100 to 200 mg twice a day for 10 to 28 days may be effective; consider for nonpregnant adults or children older than 8 years of age who are intolerant to β-lactam antibiotics.[5] SOR B
- Lyme carditis—Oral or IV antibiotics as above with hospitalization and continuous cardiac monitoring in patients with symptoms including

syncope, shortness of breath, or chest pain, or in patients with AV block.[5] SOR Ⓑ

Persistent Lyme disease

- Arthritis without neurologic disease—Doxycycline, amoxicillin, or cefuroxime; medications at doses shown under early disease with therapy extended to 28 days.[5] SOR Ⓑ If arthritis persists, treat for another 28 days with oral antibiotics or a 28-day regimen of IV antibiotics.
- Neurologic disease—IV therapy with ceftriaxone for 14 to 28 days.[5] SOR Ⓑ

REFERRAL OR HOSPITALIZATION

- Symptomatic patients with Lyme carditis should be hospitalized with continuous cardiac monitoring.
- Consider referring patients in whom the diagnosis is unclear or who do not respond to initial therapy.

PREVENTION

- Avoid exposure to ticks by using protective clothing and tick repellant. If hiking in tick-infested areas check body daily for ticks and promptly remove any attached ticks.
- Prophylactic doxycycline (1 dose of 200 mg) is recommended only if the tick is identified as an adult or nymphal *I. scapularis* tick that has been attached for at least 36 hours; medication can be started within 72 hours of tick removal; local rate of infection of ticks with *B. burgdorferi* is at least 20%; and doxycycline is not contraindicated.[5]

PROGNOSIS

- Most patients respond to appropriate therapy with prompt resolution of symptoms within 4 weeks.
- Posttreatment Lyme disease syndrome (persistent or recurrent symptoms) occurs in 10% to 20% of patients despite appropriate treatment. Prolonged antibiotic treatment is not effective.[3] Most patients eventually feel completely well, but this can take months or years.
- True treatment failures are uncommon and prolonged oral or parenteral antibiotic courses are emphatically discouraged. In patients who continue to present with residual subjective symptoms, providers should seek alternate diagnoses and/or referral to an appropriate specialist.

FOLLOW-UP

Follow patients during antibiotic therapy through recovery.

PATIENT EDUCATION

Prevention is accomplished by reducing exposure to ticks. If you live in an area that has Lyme disease then use tick repellent, tick checks, and other simple measures to prevent tick bites. This is especially important during the high-risk months of April through November. Patients should know the early signs of Lyme disease so that they can get care early when it is most curable.

If a tick is found on the skin, remove it early using fine-tipped tweezers. See patient resources box below.

PATIENT RESOURCES

- Centers for Disease Control and Prevention (CDC). *Lyme Disease*—**http://www.cdc.gov/lyme/.**
- Centers for Disease Control and Prevention (CDC). *Tick Removal*—**http://www.cdc.gov/lyme/removal/index.html.**

PROVIDER RESOURCES

- Centers for Disease Control and Prevention (CDC). *Lyme Disease*—**http://www.cdc.gov/lyme/.**

REFERENCES

1. Sternbach G, Dibble CL. Willy Burgdorfer: Lyme disease. *J Emerg Med.* 1996;14(5):631-634.
2. Centers for Disease Control and Prevention. Lyme disease—United States, 2003-2005. *MMWR Morb Mortal Wkly Rep.* 2007;56(23):573-576.
3. Centers for Disease Control and Prevention. *Lyme Disease.* http://www.cdc.gov/lyme/. Accessed January 22, 2012.
4. Meyerhoff JO. *Lyme Disease.* http://emedicine.medscape.com/article/330178. Accessed January 22, 2012.
5. Wormser GP, Dattwyler RJ, Shapiro ED, et al. The clinical assessment, treatment, and prevention of Lyme disease, human granulocytic anaplasmosis, and babesiosis: clinical practice guidelines by the Infectious Diseases Society of America. *Clin Infect Dis.* 2006;43(9):1089-1134.
6. Kaiser. *Lyme Disease Executive Summary.* http://www.harp.org/eng/kaiserslymesummary.htm. Accessed January 22, 2012.
7. Columbia University Medical Center Lyme and Tick-Borne Diseases Research Center. http://www.columbia-lyme.org/index.html. Accessed January 22, 2012.
8. American College of Physicians. *Differential Diagnosis of Lyme Disease.* http://www.acponline.org/journals/news/jun07/critters.pdf. Accessed January 22, 2012.

216 MENINGITIS

Supratik Rayamajhi, MD

PATIENT STORY

A 21-year-old male college student is admitted to the hospital for headache, fever, stiff neck, and confusion. He was well until about 18 hours ago when he started to develop flu-like symptoms, which subsequently progressed to include confusion, which prompted his roommate to bring him to the emergency department. His physical examination reveals an elevated temperature (103.1°F), a blood pressure of 100/80 mm Hg, and a heart rate of 120 beats/min. His has nuchal rigidity on neck flexion, and his skin reveals a purpuric rash on his extremities and trunk (**Figure 216-1**). He is started on intravenous dexamethasone, ceftriaxone, and vancomycin; a spinal tap is performed, which subsequently grew meningococcus. He recovers within 1 week and is discharged. His roommate is treated prophylactically with oral rifampin 600 mg twice daily for 2 days.

INTRODUCTION

Meningitis is a disease caused by inflammation of the protective membranes covering the brain and spinal cord (ie, the meninges). With an abnormal number of white blood cells in the cerebrospinal fluid (CSF), the inflammation is usually caused by an infection of the fluid surrounding the brain and spinal cord. It is a life-threatening medical and neurologic emergency, especially when it is caused by bacterial infection.

EPIDEMIOLOGY

- The prevalence of bacterial meningitis decreased in pediatric and increased in adult populations in United States following the initiation of childhood vaccinations.[1]
- Approximately 1.2 million cases of bacterial meningitis occur annually worldwide, and meningitis is among the 10 most common infectious causes of death, as it is responsible for approximately 135,000 deaths throughout the world each year.[2]

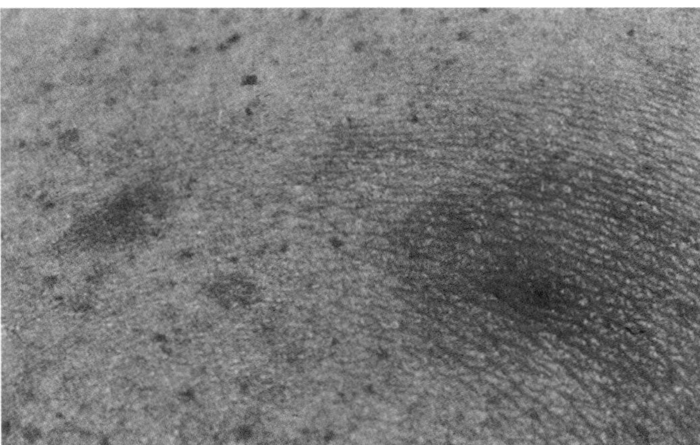

FIGURE 216-1 Acute meningococcemia with a transient macular and papular rash on the upper chest. (*Reproduced with permission from Goldsmith AL, Katz S, Gilchrest B, Paller A, Leffell D, Wolff, K.* Fitzpatrick's Dermatology in General Medicine, *8th ed. New York: McGraw-Hill, 2012.*)

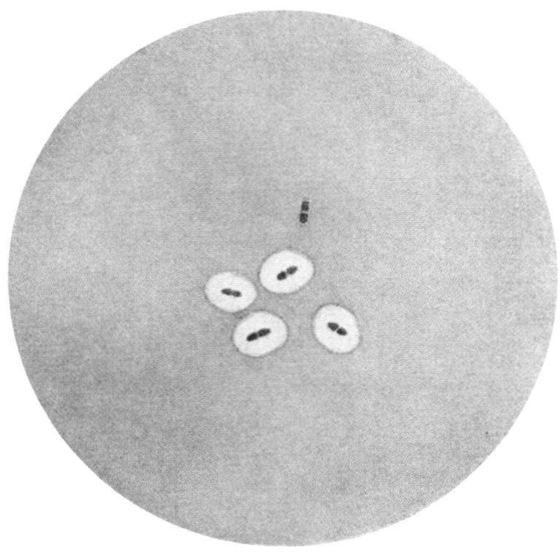

FIGURE 216-2 *Streptococcus pneumoniae* demonstrating the Quellung reaction. The Quellung reaction is swelling of the bacterial capsule stimulated by an antistreptococcal antibody; the capsule becomes opaque and more visible microscopically. (*Public Health Image Library, Centers for Disease Control and Prevention.*)

ETIOLOGY

- Bacterial meningitis can be community acquired or health care associated.
- The major causes of community-acquired bacterial meningitis in adults are *Streptococcus pneumoniae* (**Figures 216-2** and **216-3**) and *Neisseria meningitides*; *Listeria monocytogenes* is common in patients over age 50 to 60 years and those who are immunodeficient.

PATHOGENESIS

- Bacterial invasion results in release of pro-inflammatory cytokines and other chemical mediators that induce fever, headache, meningismus, and confusion.[3]

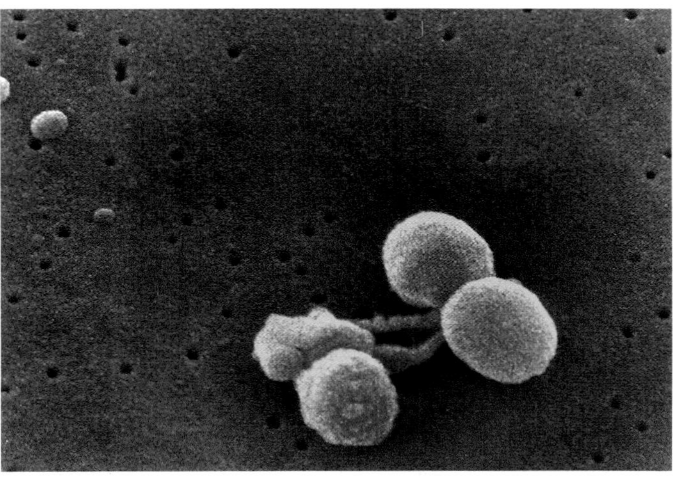

FIGURE 216-3. Scanning electron micrograph of *Streptococcus pneumoniae*. (*Public Health Image Library, Centers for Disease Control and Prevention.*)

- Breakdown in blood-brain barrier and transendothelial migration of leukocytes can lead to cerebral edema, causing obtundation, seizures, and focal neurologic symptoms and signs like cranial nerve palsies.[3]

RISK FACTORS

- Alcoholism
- Immunosuppression
- Parameningeal sources of infection, such as otitis media, sinusitis
- Neurosurgery
- Skull fracture
- Externally communicating dural fistula[3]

DIAGNOSIS

CLINICAL FEATURES

- The classic triad of acute bacterial meningitis consists of fever, nuchal rigidity, and a change in mental status.[4]
  - Almost all patients (95%) present with at least 2 of 4 symptoms (ie, headache, fever, stiff neck, and altered mental status). However, only 44% have the clinical triad of fever, neck stiffness, and altered mental status.[5]
- Presence of any of fever, neck stiffness, or altered mental status has 99% to 100% sensitivity for meningitis, and absence of fever, neck stiffness, and altered mental status effectively eliminates meningitis.[6]
- Classic physical examination signs include nuchal rigidity, positive Kernig sign, and positive Brudzinski sign.
  - Unfortunately, the diagnostic value of these signs has recently been demonstrated as low.[7]
    - In one prospective study performed at Yale University, Kernig sign (5% sensitivity, 5%; likelihood ratio for a positive test result [LR+], 0.97), Brudzinski sign (sensitivity, 5%; LR+, 0.97), and nuchal rigidity (sensitivity, 30%; LR+, 0.94) did not accurately discriminate between patients with meningitis (6 WBCs/mL of CSF) and patients without meningitis.[7]
    - The diagnostic accuracy of these signs was not significantly better in the subsets of patients with moderate meningeal inflammation (100 WBCs/mL of CSF) or microbiological evidence of CSF infection.
    - Only for patients with severe meningeal inflammation (1000 WBCs/mL of CSF) did nuchal rigidity show diagnostic value (sensitivity, 100%; negative predictive value, 100%).[7] SOR Ⓑ
    - In another prospective study of the accuracy of physical signs for detecting meningitis, the same 3 physical signs of meningeal inflammation did not help clinicians rule in or rule out meningitis accurately.[8]
    - Therefore, patients suspected to have meningitis should undergo a lumbar puncture (LP) regardless of the presence or absence of physical signs.[7,8] SOR Ⓐ
- Skin findings can be helpful but cannot be relied on for diagnosis.
  - Acute meningococcemia may present with a transient macular and papular rash (see **Figure 216-1**).
  - Disseminated meningococcemia may lead to disseminated intravascular coagulation (DIC) and cause purple macules and papules and dark cutaneous infarcts on the extremities (**Figure 216-4**).

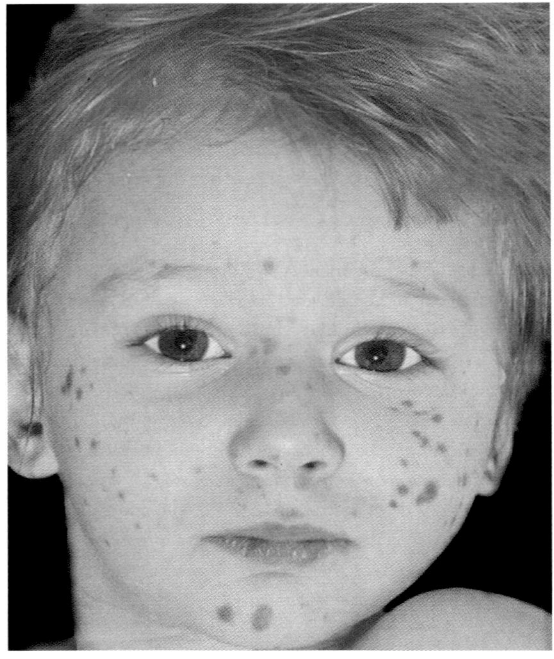

A

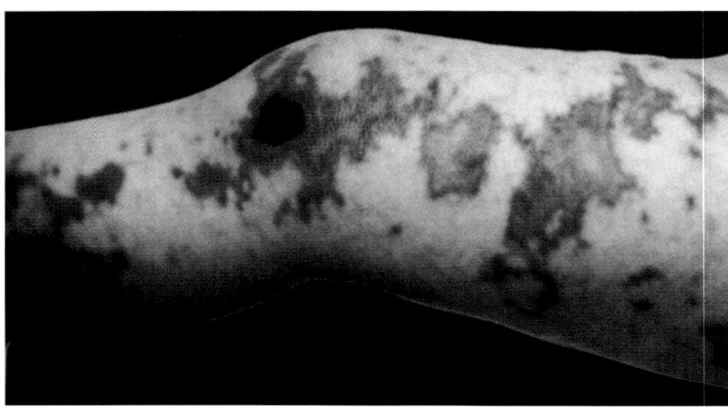

B

FIGURE 216-4 A. Discrete colored macules and papules from disseminated intravascular coagulation (DIC) secondary to disseminated meningococcemia. B. Cutaneous infarcts on the lower extremities of the same child. *(Reproduced with permission from Goldsmith AL, Katz S, Gilchrest B, Paller A, Leffell D, Wolff, K. Fitzpatrick's Dermatology in General Medicine, 8th ed. New York: McGraw-Hill, 2012.)*

LABORATORY TESTING

- Perform an LP as soon as feasible in suspected bacterial meningitis to evaluate CSF:
  - Opening pressure
  - Glucose
  - Protein
  - WBC count and differential
  - Gram stain and culture and sensitivities
- Absolute contraindications for an LP include[3]:
  - Signs of increased intracranial pressure
  - Decerebrate posturing
  - Papilledema
  - Skin infection at site of LP
  - Computed tomography (CT) or magnetic resonance imaging evidence of obstructive hydrocephalus, cerebral edema, or herniation

- Obtain blood culture before starting antibiotics if an LP is delayed.
- The ultimate diagnosis is based on clinical suspicion and identification of causative bacteria from any of the following[9]:
  - CSF cultures (positive in 70%-85% of patients not pretreated with antibiotics).
  - CSF Gram stain.
  - CSF latex agglutination for specific pathogens; however, a negative latex agglutination does not rule out bacterial meningitis.
  - CSF polymerase chain reaction (PCR) for specific pathogens, including *N. meningitides, S. pneumonia, Haemophilus influenza* type B, *Streptococcus agalactiae, and L. monocytogenes.*
- Presumptive diagnosis based on clinical suspicion with abnormal CSF findings if no specific organism identified[9]:
  - Elevated opening pressure in range of 200 to 500 mm H_2O.
  - Cloudy appearance.
  - Elevated WBC count.
    - Typically 1000 to 5000 cells/mm^3 (but range can be from < 100 to > 10 000)
    - Neutrophil predominance, typically 80% to 95%
  - Glucose is less than 40 mg/dL (2.22 mmol/L) in about 50% to 60% of patients.
  - Elevated protein (>50 mg/dL) is seen in nearly 100% of patients; however, this may be adjusted for increased protein caused by traumatic tap (subtract 1 mg/dL [0.01 g/L] protein per 1000 red blood cells/mm^3).
  - Positive Gram stain results are seen in
    - 90% of cases of *S. pneumonia*
    - 86% of cases of *H. influenza*
    - 75% of cases of *N. meningitides*
    - 50% of cases of gram-negative bacilli
    - 33% of cases of *L. monocytogenes*
  - In the absence of a positive Gram stain, which has almost 100% specificity, no single CSF biochemical variable can reliably exclude bacterial meningitis in the setting of an elevated CSF white blood cell count.[10]
- In the presence of an elevated lactate concentration in postoperative neurosurgical patients, consider initiation of empirical antimicrobial therapy for CSF lactate concentrations of 4 mmol/L (36 mg/dL) or greater, pending other study results. SOR B CSF lactate concentrations are not recommended for community-acquired meningitis.
- Latex agglutination is not recommended for routine use but may be useful for patients with negative CSF Gram stain and culture, especially those pretreated with antibiotics.[9] SOR B
- The Infectious Diseases Society of America (IDSA) recommends that if a CT or an LP is delayed, obtain blood cultures and start appropriate antibiotic and adjunctive therapy (**Figure 216-5**).[9]
- If an LP is delayed and empiric antibiotic therapy initiated, the yield of a subsequent LP will be lower, and the use of blood tests (blood cultures, WBC count, glucose, C-reactive protein [CRP], or procalcitonin level) can be helpful in providing evidence for or against bacterial meningitis.[9]

IMAGING

- Head CT may be indicated prior to LP in specific patients.
  - The 2004 IDSA guidelines for indication of CT scan prior to LP include[9]
    - Immunocompromised state
    - History of central nervous system disease (mass lesion, stroke, or focal infection)
    - New-onset seizure (within 1 week of presentation)
    - Papilledema
    - Abnormal level of consciousness
    - Focal neurologic deficit

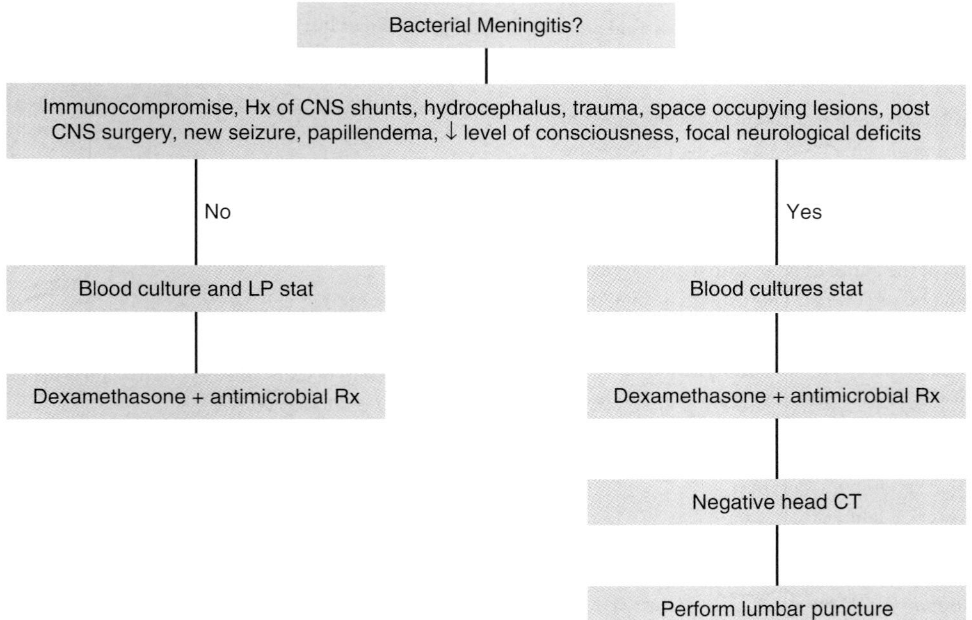

FIGURE 216-5 The Infectious Diseases Society of America (IDSA) recommendations for management if computed tomographic (CT) scanning or a lumbar puncture (LP) is delayed: obtain blood cultures and start appropriate antibiotic and adjunctive therapy. CNS, central nervous system; Hx, history; Rx, prescription. (*Adapted from Tunkel AR, Hartman BJ, Kaplan SL, et al. Practice guidelines for the management of bacterial meningitis.* Clin Infect Dis. *2004;39(9):1267-1284.*)

DIFFERENTIAL DIAGNOSIS

- Aseptic meningitis is differentiated by negative routine bacterial cultures. Viral meningitis is most common; however, aseptic meningitis also refers to infections from other organisms, including fungal meningitis, spirochetal meningitis, and mycobacterial meningitis.
- Drug-induced meningitis can be seen with several drugs, including nonsteroidal anti-inflammatory drugs, and is a diagnosis of exclusion.
- Mollaret meningitis is characterized by 4 or more episodes of lymphocytic meningitis lasting several days with spontaneous resolution.
- Carcinomatous meningitis from seeding of the meninges from lymphomas and acute leukemias is seen.

MANAGEMENT

- Bacterial meningitis is a neurologic emergency, and appropriate therapy should be started as soon as possible after its diagnosis is considered likely.
- The following are 3 axioms of antibiotic therapy for bacterial meningitis: use of bactericidal drugs effective against the infecting organism, use of drugs that enter the CSF, and use of drugs with optimal pharmacodynamics.[11]
- Delay in antibiotic therapy of more than 3 to 6 hours is associated with increased mortality in patients hospitalized with bacterial meningitis.
- Empiric antibiotic choice[9]
  - No known immunodeficiency
    - Vancomycin 10 to 15 mg/kg IV every 8 hours or 15 to 22.5 mg/kg IV every 12 hours to maintain serum trough levels 15 to 20 μg/mL
    - Ceftriaxone (2 g IV every 12 hours or 4 g IV every 24 hours) or cefotaxime (8-12 g/d IV with dosing every 4-6 hours)
    - Adults older than 50 years old: add ampicillin 2 g IV every 4 hours; state reasons for this
- Dexamethasone may reduce rates of death, hearing loss, and neurological sequelae in adults with bacterial meningitis caused by suspected or proven pneumococcal meningitis.[9] SOR Ⓐ
  - Dexamethasone is recommended in all adults with suspected or proven pneumococcal meningitis[9] SOR Ⓐ but should not to be given to adults who have already received antibiotic therapy.
  - Theoretically, dexamethasone may be harmful in meningitis because of highly cephalosporin-resistant strains of pneumococcus; therefore, until the results of the culture and sensitivity are available, consider adding rifampin 600 mg every 24 hours with dexamethasone.[9] SOR Ⓑ
- In patients with impaired cell-mediated immunity, additional coverage must be directed against *L. monocytogenes* and gram-negative bacilli (including *Pseudomonas aeruginosa*).[5,9]
  - *Vancomycin*: 30 to 60 mg/kg IV per day in 2 or 3 divided doses *plus*
    - *Ampicillin*—2 g IV every 4 hours *plus either*
    - *Cefepime*—2 g IV every 8 hours *or*
    - *Meropenem*—2 g IV every 8 hours
    - In patients allergic to β-lactams
  - *Vancomycin*—30 to 60 mg/kg IV per day in 2 or 3 divided doses *plus*
  - *Moxifloxacin*—400 mg IV once daily *plus*
    - If *Listeria* coverage is required, *trimethoprim-sulfamethoxazole* (10 to 20 mg/kg) (of the trimethoprim component) IV per day every 6 to 12 hours.[3]
- In patients with bacterial meningitis after shunt placement
  - Use direct instillation of antimicrobial agents into ventricles in patients unable to undergo surgical components of therapy or with shunt infections that are difficult to eradicate.[9] SOR Ⓒ
- For shunt infection with methicillin-resistant *Staphylococcus aureus*, shunt removal is recommended, and the shunt should not be replaced until CSF cultures are repeatedly negative SOR Ⓒ.[12]

PROGNOSIS AND COMPLICATIONS

- In a study in the United States, the case-fatality rate of bacterial meningitis in adults was 16.4%, and it was 22.7% in patients 65 years or older.[13]
- Normal or marginally elevated CSF white cell counts occur in 5% to 10% of patients and are associated with adverse outcomes.[5]
- Major complications of meningitis include cognitive deficit, bilateral hearing loss, motor deficit, seizures, visual impairment, and hydrocephalus.
- Minor complications include behavioral problems, learning difficulties, unilateral hearing loss, hypotonia, and diplopia.
- Risk of complication is 19.9% for any complication, 12.8% for major complication, and 8.6% for minor complication.[14]

FOLLOW-UP

The IDSA recommends repeat LP for CSF analysis for patients not responsive to antimicrobial therapy after 48 hours. SOR Ⓐ

PATIENT RESOURCES

- Centers for Disease Control and Prevention. *Meningococcal disease*—**http://www.cdc.gov/meningococcal/about/index.html**.
- MedlinePlus. *Meningitis*—**http://www.nlm.nih.gov/medlineplus/meningitis.html**.

PROVIDER RESOURCES

- Infectious Disease Society of America guidelines on bacterial meningitis—**http://www.idsociety.org/uploadedFiles/IDSA/Guidelines-Patient_Care/PDF_Library/Bacterial%20 Meningitis(1).pdf.**

REFERENCES

1. Schuchat A, Robinson K, Wenger JD, et al. Bacterial meningitis in the United States in 1995. Active Surveillance Team. *N Engl J Med*. 1997;337(14):970-976.
2. Scheld WM, Koedel U, Nathan B, Pfister HW. Pathophysiology of bacterial meningitis: mechanism(s) of neuronal injury. *J Infect Dis*. 2002;186(suppl 2):S225.
3. Chaudhuri A, Martinez-Martin P, Kennedy PG, et al. EFNS guideline on management of community-acquired bacterial meningitis: report of an EFNS Task Force on acute bacterial meningitis in older children and adults. *Eur J Neurol*. 2008;15(7):649-659.
4. Durand ML, Calderwood SB, Weber DJ, et al. Acute bacterial meningitis in adults. A review of 493 episodes. *N Engl J Med*. 1993;328(1):21.

5. van de Beek D, de Gans J, Spanjaard L, Weisfelt M, Reitsma JB, Vermeulen M. Clinical features and prognostic factors in adults with bacterial meningitis. *N Engl J Med*. 2004;351(18):1849.

6. Attia J, Hatala R, Cook DJ, Wong JG. The rational clinical examination. Does this adult patient have acute meningitis? *JAMA*. 1999;282(2):175-181.

7. Thomas KE, Hasbun R, Jekel J, Quagliarello VJ. The diagnostic accuracy of Kernig's sign, Brudzinski's sign, and nuchal rigidity in adults with suspected meningitis. *Clin Infect Dis*. 2002;35(1):46-52.

8. Waghdhare S, Kalantri A, Joshi R, Kalantri S. Accuracy of physical signs for detecting meningitis: a hospital-based diagnostic accuracy study. *Clin Neurol Neurosurg*. 2010;112(9):752-757.

9. Tunkel AR, Hartman BJ, Kaplan SL, et al. Practice guidelines for the management of bacterial meningitis. *Clin Infect Dis*. 2004;39(9):1267-1284.

10. Spanos A, Harrell FE Jr, Durack DT Differential diagnosis of acute meningitis. An analysis of the predictive value of initial observations. *JAMA*. 1989;262(19):2700.

11. Sinner SW, Tunkel AR. Antimicrobial agents in the treatment of bacterial meningitis. *Infect Dis Clin North Am*. 2004;18(3):581.

12. Liu C, Bayer A, Cosgrove SE, et al; Infectious Diseases Society of America. Clinical practice guidelines by the Infectious Diseases Society of America for the treatment of methicillin-resistant *Staphylococcus aureus* infections in adults and children. *Clin Infect Dis*. 2011;52(3):e18-e55.

13. Thigpen MC, Whitney CG, Messonnier NE, et al; Emerging Infections Programs Network. Bacterial meningitis in the United States, 1998-2007. *N Engl J Med*. 2011;364(21):2016.

14. Edmond K, Clark A, Korczak VS, Sanderson C, Griffiths UK, Rudan I. Global and regional risk of disabling sequelae from bacterial meningitis: a systematic review and meta-analysis. *Lancet Infect Dis*. 2010;10(5):317-328.

217 OSTEOMYELITIS

Hannah Ferenchick, MD

PATIENT STORY

A previously healthy 48-year-old man presents with a 2-week history of a low-grade fever and a new onset of back pain. The severity of the pain was increasing over the previous 4 days and woke him from sleep at night. He denies any injury or any new activity. On examination, his temperature is elevated (100.2°F), and he has reproducible tenderness over the lower thoracic spine. A computed tomographic (CT) scan of the spine reveals destruction of the endplates between T11 and T12 consistent with osteomyelitis (**Figure 217-1a** and **217-1b**). A subsequent bone biopsy and culture reveal methicillin-sensitive *Staphylococcus aureus* as the infecting agent causing the osteomyelitis.

INTRODUCTION

Osteomyelitis is an infection contained in bone. There have been many advances since the 1970s in treating this disease, including the introduction of new antibiotics, new surgical techniques, and advancement in the delivery of antibiotics. Despite this, however, osteomyelitis can be a difficult clinical challenge for physicians in both its diagnosis and its treatment.

EPIDEMIOLOGY

- Bone infections are most common in patients younger than 20 years and older than 50 years.[1]
- Estimated annual incidence of osteomyelitis in the United States is less than 2%.[1]
- Incidence of vertebral osteomyelitis is 2.4 cases per 100,000 population.[2]
  - Increasing incidence with increasing age from 0.3 per 100,000 in 20 years and younger to 6.5 per 100,000 with persons older than 70 years.[2]

ETIOLOGY/PATHOPHYSIOLOGY

- Osteomyelitis may result from direct inoculation of bacteria into bone, contiguous seeding from adjacent infected tissues, or hematologic seeding.[3]
- Direct inoculation and contiguous seeding usually result in a polymicrobial infection.
- Hematogenous osteomyelitis is nearly always caused by a single organism.[3]
  - The most common pathogen in acute and chronic hematogenous osteomyelitis in adults and children is *S. aureus*.[4]
  - In children, group A *Streptococcus*, *Streptococcus pneumoniae*, and *Kingella kingae* are also common causes of osteomyelitis.[4]
    - Group B streptococcal infection occurs almost solely in infants.[4]
  - In adults with chronic osteomyelitis, *Staphylococcus epidermidis*, *Pseudomonas aeruginosa*, *Serratia marcescens*, and *Escherichia coli* may be implicated.[4]

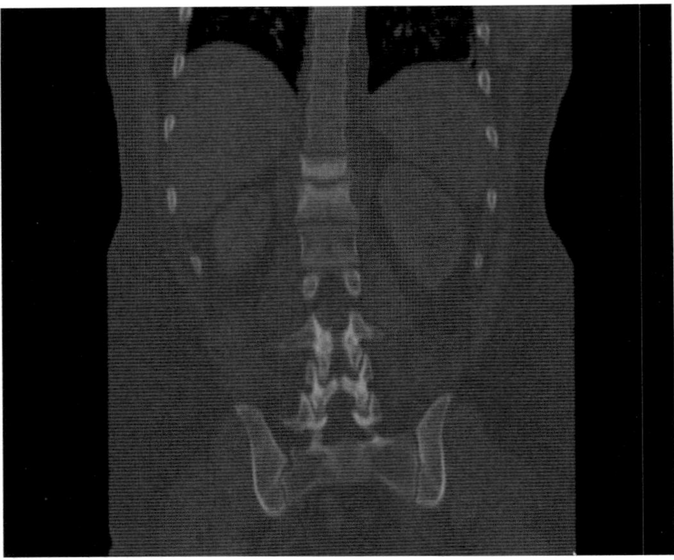

A

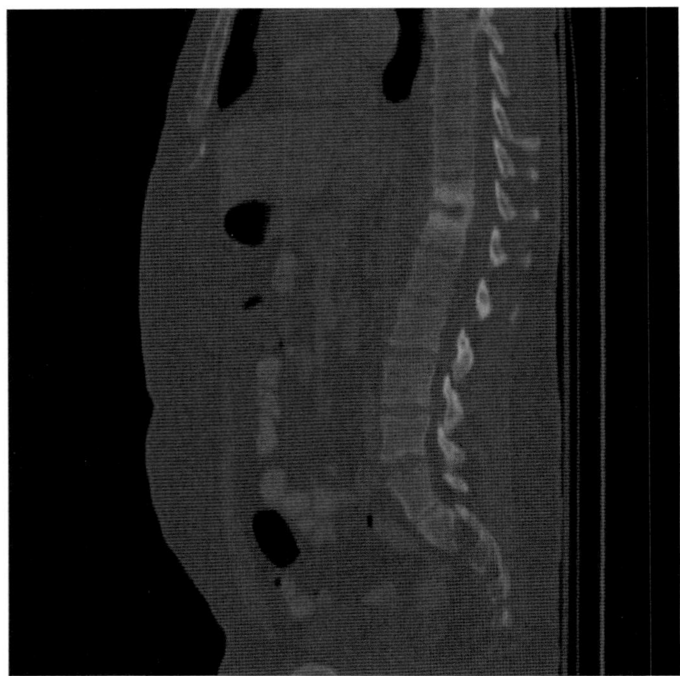

B

FIGURE 217-1 (A, B) Destruction of the inferior endplate of T11 and superior endplate of T12 with reactive bony sclerosis. Frontal view (A) in the computed tomographic (CT) scan and (B) lateral view. There is loss of vertebral body height of the T11 vertebrae of approximately 60%. Percutaneous CT-guided bone aspiration of the affected site revealed growth of *Staphylococcus aureus*. *(Reproduced with permission from Michigan State University Radiology Teaching Files: Sharon Kreuer, DO.)*

  - Fungal and mycobacterial infections are most common in patients with impaired immune function.[4]
- In children, hematogenous osteomyelitis most often affects the metaphysis of long bones. In adults, it most often involves vertebral bodies.
  - The metaphysis is likely involved because of the blood flow and anatomy of long bones.
    - The major blood vessel to long bones enters in the diaphysis and travels to both metaphyses.

- It forms vascular loops before reaching the epiphyseal plates, and it is thought that the slowed blood flow in these loops and the absence of a basement membrane predisposes this site to infection.
- Vertebral marrow is highly vascularized in comparison to marrow of the long bone.
- Blood-borne bacteria that flow throughout the vascular system (such as in intravenous drug users) may initiate infection spontaneously.
- Disruptions in anatomy caused by prior or current bone injury may predispose to this.
- Segmental arteries that supply vertebrae split and run to 2 adjacent vertebral endplates. Therefore, hematogenous vertebral osteomyelitis often affects 2 neighboring vertebrae and their intervertebral disk.

- Osteomyelitis can be directly introduced by surgical contamination or trauma (**Figure 217-2**).[3]
- Contiguous focus osteomyelitis occurs from seeding from adjacent soft-tissue infections. This is most common in patients with predisposing diseases such as diabetes mellitus or peripheral vascular disease.[3]
  - Patients with diabetic nephropathy have decreased awareness of wounds, which can lead to the development of unrecognized infection.
  - Associated with diabetes is peripheral vascular disease, which contributes to chronic wounds and soft-tissue infection by delaying the body's healing responses. Both of these conditions increase the risk of developing chronic osteomyelitis.[4]
  - Acute osteomyelitis is characterized by suppurative exudate that develops in the marrow (see **Figure 217-2**).[3]
  - Edema, vascular congestion, and small-vessel thrombosis can compromise blood supply as the infection grows outward toward the bone cortex and periosteum. Necrosis can then occur and lead to the separation of dead pieces of bone (called sequestra).[3]
  - Acute osteomyelitis can be contained before the formation of sequestra by early antibiotics and surgery if necessary.[3]
- Once sequestra have developed, the infection is known as chronic osteomyelitis.
  - Chronic osteomyelitis is characterized by necrotic bone, the development of new bone, and the exudation of polymorphonuclear leukocytes and other cells.[3]
  - New bone growth in areas of periosteal damage forms a sheath around dead bone, called an involucrum.[3]
  - The involucrum is often infiltrated with openings or sinuses through which purulent exudate drains to surrounding soft tissue and possibly to skin surfaces.[3] After the sequestrum is removed operatively or cleared through host immunological defenses, the cavity may fill in with new bone or remain cavitary. In adults, this cavity may fill with fibrous tissue and remain connected to the skin via a sinus tract (**Figure 217-3**).[3]

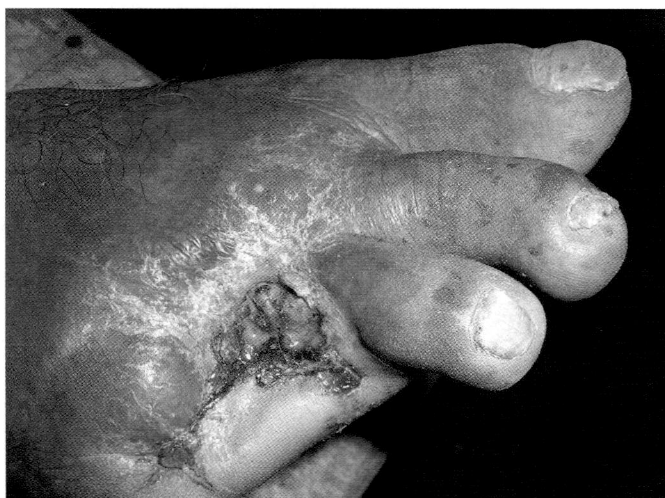

A

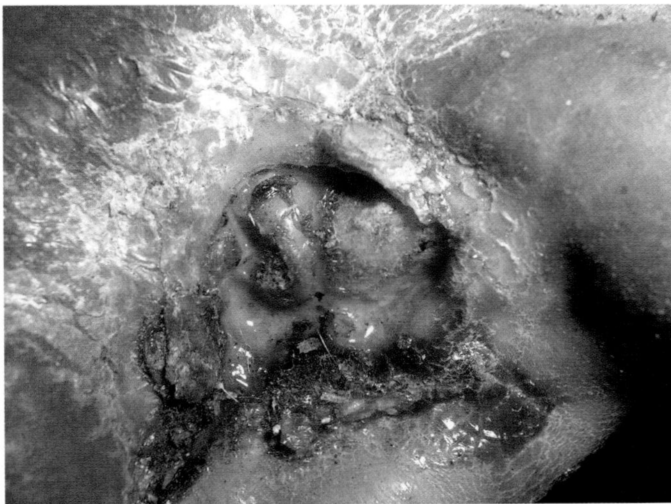

B

FIGURE 217-2 A. Osteomyelitis at the metatarsal joints in after amputation of the fourth and fifth right toes in a diabetic patient. B. Close-up of the osteomyelitis showing the purulence around the bone. (*Reproduced with permission from Richard P. Usatine, MD.*)

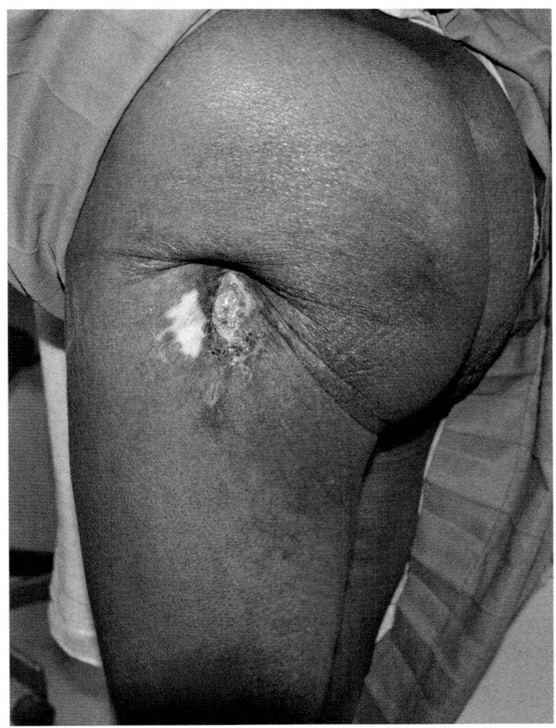

FIGURE 217-3 A sinus tract in a patient with chronic osteomyelitis of the left hip. (*Reproduced with permission from Richard P. Usatine, MD.*)

RISK FACTORS

- Diabetes mellitus
- Peripheral vascular disease[4]
- Peripheral neuropathy[4]
- Risk factors for bacteremia
  - Urinary tract infection (UTI)
  - Indwelling catheters
  - Central lines
  - Dialysis
  - Sickle cell disease
  - Intravenous drug use
- Immunodeficient conditions
- Recent surgical operations
- Penetrating trauma

DIAGNOSIS

- Osteomyelitis often presents as a constellation of vague and nonspecific symptoms, which can make the diagnosis difficult.
  - Acute hematogenous and contiguous osteomyelitis may present with the onset of pain over several days, associated with localized signs such as swelling, erythema, warmth, and bony tenderness. Systemic signs such as fever, chills, night sweats, irritability, and lethargy can also occur.[4]
  - These symptoms may not all be present, however, and in sites such as the vertebral column and pelvis, the only complaint may be pain.[2]
- Acute hematogenous and contiguous focus osteomyelitis can both advance to a chronic condition.
- Chronic osteomyelitis may present with nonspecific complaints of pain and possibly low-grade fever for 1 to 3 months.
  - Chronic infection is frequently associated with draining sinus tracts.
- Erythrocyte sedimentation rate (ESR) is usually elevated, but leukocyte count may be normal.[3]

HISTORY/SYMPTOMS

- History of systemic symptoms: lethargy, malaise, extremity or back pain, fever[4]
- Predisposing factors: history of diabetes, peripheral vascular disease, intravenous drug use, trauma or invasive procedures[4]

PHYSICAL EXAMINATION

Focus on locating a source of infection

- Assess peripheral vascular and sensory function.
- Look for cutaneous injury or diabetic ulcers (**Figure 217-4**).
- Probing bone with a sterile probe within a diabetic foot ulcer is diagnostic for osteomyelitis; no further imaging studies are needed.[4]
- The following are clinical signs to look for[4]:
  - Exposed bone (see **Figure 217-2**)
  - Persistent sinus tract (see **Figure 217-3**)
  - Tissue necrosis overlying bone
  - Chronic wounds overlying surgical hardware
  - Chronic wound overlying fracture (**Figure 217-5**)

LABORATORY TESTING

- The ESR is helpful in following the efficacy of treatment.
- C-reactive protein (CRP)

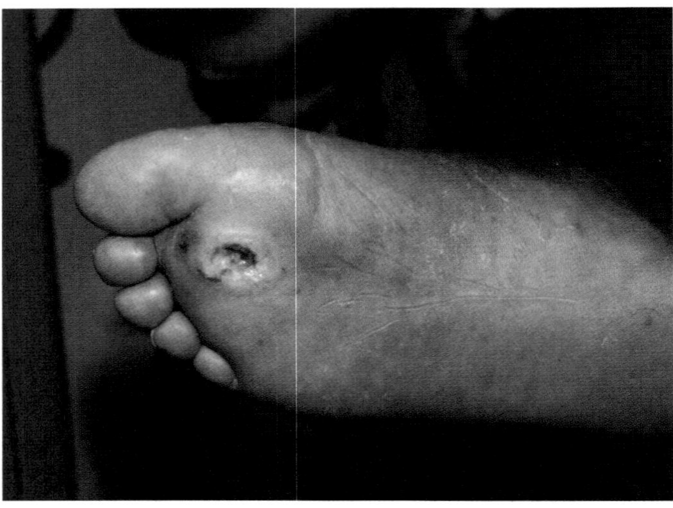

FIGURE 217-4 Diabetic foot ulcer with osteomyelitis of the metatarsal bone and gangrene of the second toe in a woman with poorly controlled diabetes. (*Reproduced with permission from Richard P. Usatine, MD.*)

  - Continuously normal CRP and ESR may rule out osteomyelitis.[4]
  - CRP levels correlate more closely with response to therapy than ESR; therefore, serial CRP levels can be used to gauge clinical response to treatment.[4]
- White blood cell count
  - Often elevated with acute osteomyelitis but can be normal with chronic osteomyelitis.
- Blood culture
  - A positive blood culture eliminates the need for more invasive procedures, such as bone biopsy, to identify microorganism (except if a polymicrobial infection is suspected).[4]
- Bone biopsy obtained through radiographic intervention or done surgically is crucial to diagnose osteomyelitis and to correctly identify involved microorganisms.
  - Two bone biopsy specimens are preferred.
    1. One is sent in sterile container for Gram stain and culture.
    2. The other is sent in formalin for histopathology to look for necrosis.
  - Bone samples should be cultured for aerobic and anaerobic bacteria and fungi.
  - Wound or sinus tract cultures do not reliably predict the infecting organism in osteomyelitis, and they should not be used to direct treatment.[4]

IMAGING

- Plain radiograph (**Figures 217-5B**, **217-6A** and **B**, and **217-7**)
  - Widely available and inexpensive[1]
  - Can be useful as first-line imaging to rule out other pathology, such as metastases or osteoporotic fractures[4]
  - Disadvantages include
    - Sensitivity of 43% to 75% and a specificity of 75% to 83% in diagnosing osteomyelitis[4]
    - Inability to diagnose infection until late in its course
      - Osteomyelitis is not generally visible on radiograph until it is at least 1 cm in diameter and diminishes around 50% of bone structure.[1]
      - Therefore, changes may not be visible until 5 to 7 days in children and 10 to 14 days in adults.[1]

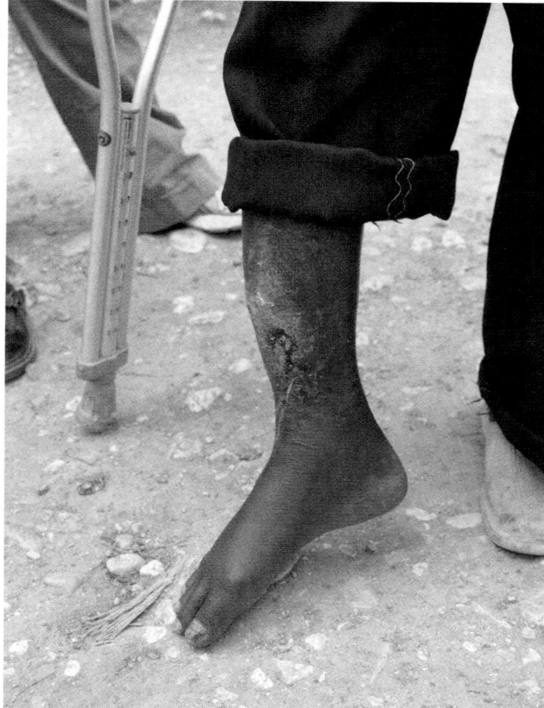

A

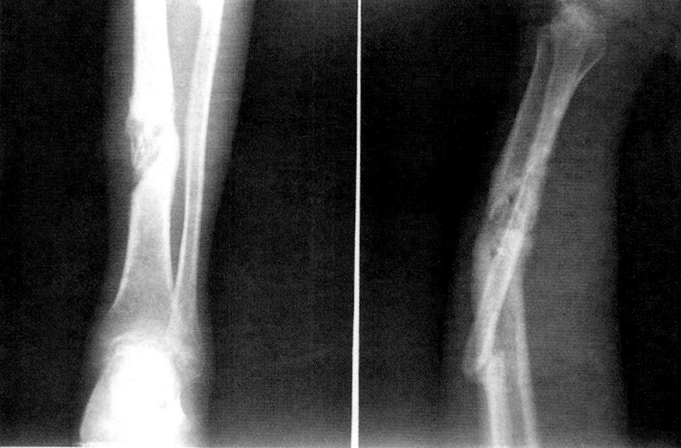

B

FIGURE 217-5 A. Open wound overlying an area of osteomyelitis in a nonhealed fracture of the tibia in a resource-limited country where access to medical care was limited at the time of the injury. B. Radiograph showing nonhealed fracture and the ongoing osteomyelitis. (*Reproduced with permission from Richard P. Usatine, MD.*)

- Magnetic resonance imaging (MRI)
  - Expensive; however may be needed if the diagnosis of osteomyelitis is questionable[3]
  - Provides best ability for early detection of osteomyelitis (as early as 3-5 days)[1,4]
  - Sensitivity of 82% to 100% and specificity of 75% to 96% for diagnosis of osteomyelitis
  - Also allows for assessment of surrounding tissues, which can assist in the planning of surgical management[1]
  - Disadvantages include:
    - Inability to distinguish between infections and reactive inflammatory processes
    - Inability to image sites with metallic implants[1]

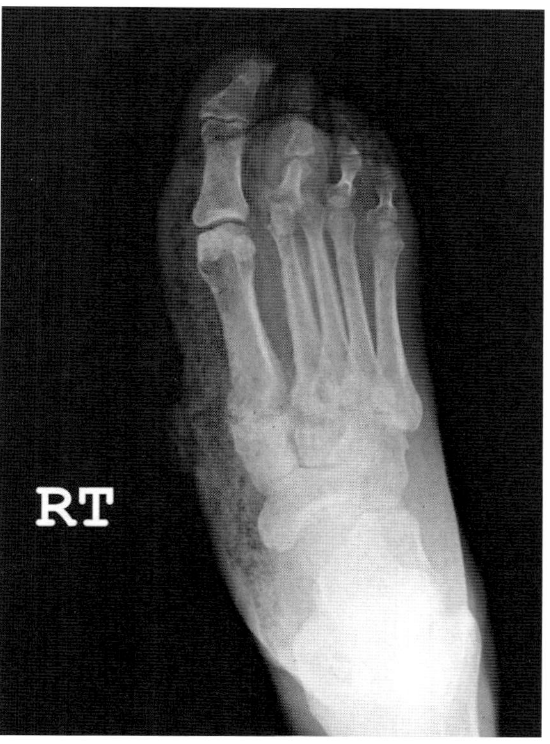

FIGURE 217-6 Subcutaneous swelling and emphysema in the medial aspect of the foot in this patient with extensive osteomyelitis and overlying cellulitis. There is also periosteal reaction involving the first through third metatarsals. This image also shows a prior amputation of the third digit at the level of the metacarpophalangeal joint. (*Reproduced with permission from Radiology Teaching Files, Michigan State University, Jarrod Yates, DO.*)

- Computed tomography
  - May show bone changes earlier than plain radiographs
  - Less desirable than MRI because of "decreased soft tissue contrast as well as exposure to ionizing radiation"[1]
  - Most helpful in diagnosis of chronic osteomyelitis because of its superior ability (vs. MRI) to detect sequestra, cloacas, and involucra[1]
  - Also may be helpful in guidance of needle biopsies and joint aspiration[1]
  - Sensitivity for diagnosis of chronic osteomyelitis 67% and specificity 50%
- Ultrasound (US)
  - Ultrasound is easily accessible and inexpensive and offers real-time evaluation of pathology
  - Can be useful to distinguish osteomyelitis from tumors or noninfective conditions[1]
  - Also useful to guide needle aspirations and biopsies[1]
  - Disadvantages include
    - There is undetermined sensitivity and specificity in diagnosing osteomyelitis.[1]
    - Diagnosis is operator dependent.[1]
    - The US beam cannot pass through cortical bone.[1]
- Nuclear medicine imaging
  - Examples: 3-phase technetium-99 bone scintigraphy and leukocyte scintigraphy
  - Can detect osteomyelitis before plain radiograph and usually positive within a few days of onset of symptoms[4]
  - Most agents highly sensitive but have a low specificity

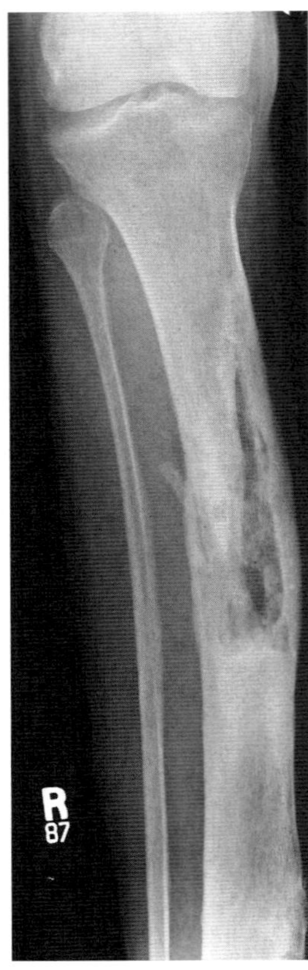

FIGURE 217-7 Chronic osteomyelitis. AP radiograph of the tibia/fibula showing large, expansile and diaphyseal lesion with onionskin bony remodeling and an irregular central lucency (*Reproduced with permission from Tehranzadeh J. Musculoskeletal Imaging Cases. New York: McGraw-Hill, 2009.*)

- Disadvantages include
  - Difficulty to differentiate osteomyelitis from other processes, such as neoplasia, cellulitis, arthritis, fractures, and so on
  - Need for further imaging
  - Low specificity
- May be useful for supplemental studies when X-rays are compromised by pathologic or postsurgical changes or when MRI is not available or contraindicated[1,4]

DIFFERENTIAL DIAGNOSIS

- Osteomyelitis of long bones
  - Malignant or benign tumor is differentiated by lack of fever; radiographic destruction may mimic osteomyelitis.
  - Old trauma can be differentiated with history and absence of fever.
  - Bone infarct secondary to sickle cell anemia can be differentiated by the diagnosis of sickle cell disease and the chronicity of the problem.
- Vertebral osteomyelitis
  - Pyelonephritis differentiated by flank pain and dysuria
  - Pancreatitis differentiated by the primary symptom of epigastric pain (radiating to the back) associated with excessive alcohol use or gallstones (see Chapter 75, Acute Pancreatitis)
  - Osteoporotic fracture differentiated by sudden onset of pain, not associated with fever in a patient with preexisting osteoporosis (see Chapter 225, Osteoporosis and Osteopenia)
  - Degenerative disk disease differentiated by association with chronic back pain, typically better with rest and worse with activity, and an insidious onset (see Chapter 102, Back Pain)
  - Spinal stenosis differentiated by back and leg pain worse with walking and better with rest (see Chapter 103, Lumbar Spinal Stenosis)
- Other
  - Gout/pseudogout differentiated by the location (a joint) with a sudden onset of pain and inflammation (see Chapter 105, Gout)
  - Charcot joint differentiated by the preexisting presence of neuropathy, such as seen in diabetes, and the absence of systemic symptoms (see Chapter 210, Charcot Arthropathy)
  - Cellulitis differentiated by acute, spreading bacterial inflammation of the skin and subcutaneous tissue, commonly complicating skin trauma from a wound, ulcer, or rash (see Chapter 122, Cellulitis)

MANAGEMENT

- Antibiotics and surgical debridement of infected and necrotic tissue are the mainstays of treatment for osteomyelitis.
  - Antibiotic choice should be tailored to susceptibility as determined by cultures.
  - Delaying antibiotics until culture and sensitivity results return is preferable, but only if clinically appropriate.[4]
  - Duration of treatment depends on the clinical scenario:
    - For osteomyelitis in adults, a treatment regimen of anywhere from 4 to 6 weeks to 3 months is recommended. Few data from controlled trials are available to suggest optimal duration.[2]
    - For chronic osteomyelitis, parental therapy for 2 to 6 weeks with a total duration of treatment for 4 to 8 weeks has been recommended.[4]
- Specific antibiotic regimens depend on the organism present:
  - *S. aureus* or coagulase-negative staphylococci (methicillin sensitive)[2]
    - Nafcillin or oxacillin 2 g IV every 6 hours
    - Alternative—Fluoroquinolone plus rifampin (eg, levofloxacin 750 mg by mouth daily *plus* rifampin 300 mg every 12 hours)
  - *S. aureus* or coagulase-negative staphylococci (methicillin resistant)
    - Vancomycin 1 g IV every 12 hours[2]
    - Alternative—Fluoroquinolone plus rifampin (such as levofloxacin 750 mg orally daily plus rifampin 300 mg orally every 12 hours *or* trimethoprim/sulfamethoxazole 160/800 mg orally 3 times daily)
  - Streptococcal species
    - Penicillin G 5 million units IV every 6 hours
    - Alternative—Ceftriaxone 2 g IV daily
  - Enterobacteriaceae, quinolone sensitive
    - Fluoroquinolone (eg, ciprofloxacin 750 mg orally every 12 hours)
    - Alternative—Ceftriaxone 2 g IV daily
  - Enterobacteriaceae, quinolone resistant
    - Ticarcillin/clavulanate, 3.1 g IV every 4 hours *or* piperacillin/tazobactam (Zosyn), 3.375 g IV every 6 hours
    - Alternative—Ceftriaxone, 2 g IV every 24 hours[4]
  - Pseudomonas aeruginosa[4]
    - Cefepime or ceftazidime 2 g every 8 hours *plus* ciprofloxacin 400 mg IV every 8 to 12 hours
    - Alternative: Piperacillin/tazobactam 3.375 g IV every 6 hours *plus* ciprofloxacin 400 mg IV every 12 hours
  - Anaerobes
    - Clindamycin 300 to 600 mg IV every 6 to 8 hours[2]
    - Surgical treatment is indicated in cases of antibiotic failure, chronic osteomyelitis with necrotic bone, and infected implanted hardware.[4]

- Adequate surgical debridement decreases bacterial load, removes necrotic tissue, and gives a chance for the host immune system and antibiotics to arrest infection.[5]
  - Appropriate debridement may create large bony defects or dead space. Management of this space includes replacing dead bone and scar tissue with vascularized tissue, which is imperative to stop the disease process and maintain the integrity of the bone.[6]

PROGNOSIS

- Treatment failure is predicted after 4 weeks with a CRP greater than 30 mg/L and no pain reduction and persistent fever.
- There is poor correlation between MRI changes and clinical improvement after 4 to 8 weeks; 85% of patients with clinical improvement had no change or worsening MRI findings.[5]

FOLLOW-UP

- Monitor temperature and physical examination regularly. Examine venous access site, surgical access site, and site of persistent pain of osteomyelitis.
- Monitor at regular intervals for persistently elevated WBC count, ESR, and CRP.
- If using nephrotoxic antibiotics, adjust dose for renal function and measure serum creatinine regularly.

PATIENT EDUCATION

- Patients should be educated on the cause, symptoms, treatment, and course of osteomyelitis.
  - Discuss symptoms of disease recurrence, such as prolonged pain, fever, or drainage and recommend that these be reported to a health care professional immediately.
- Patients with diabetes mellitus should be educated on proper foot care, including daily inspection of feet, daily washing, and use of moisturizing cream.[3]
- Patients with diabetes mellitus should also be educated to avoid unnecessary trauma by wearing properly fitted shoes and avoiding barefoot walking.[3]
- Educate patients on appropriate maintenance of venous access line and appropriate use of antibiotics.
- Discuss possible adverse side effects of antimicrobial agents, including *Clostridium difficile* diarrhea, rash, and nephrotoxicity or ototoxicity.

PATIENT RESOURCES

- PubMed Health. *Osteomyelitis*—**http://www.ncbi.nlm.nih.gov/pubmedhealth/PMH0001473/**.
- Mayo Clinic. *Osteomyelitis*—**http://www.mayoclinic.com/health/osteomyelitis/DS00759/**.
- Medline Plus. *Osteomyelitis*—**http://www.nlm.nih.gov/medlineplus/ency/article/000437.htm**.

PROVIDER RESOURCES

- Medscape. *Osteomyelitis*—**http://emedicine.medscape.com/article/1348767.**
- Liu C, Bayer A, Cosgrove SE, et al. Clinical practice guidelines by the Infectious Diseases Society of America for the treatment of methicillin-resistant *Staphylococcus aureus* infections in adults and children. *Clin. Infect Dis*. 2011. doi:10.1093/cid/ciq146. **http://cid.oxfordjournals.org/content/early/2011/01/04/cid.ciq146.full**.
- Lipsky BA, Berendt AR, Cornia PB, et al. 2012 Infectious Diseases Society of America clinical practice guideline for the diagnosis and treatment of diabetic foot infections. *Clin Infect Dis*. 2012;54(12):132-173. **http://www.idsociety.org/uploadedFiles/IDSA/Guidelines-Patient_Care/PDF_Library/2012%20Diabetic%20Foot%20Infections%20Guideline.pdf**.

REFERENCES

1. Pineda C, Espinosa R, Pena A. Radiographic imaging in osteomyelitis: the role of plain radiography, computed tomography, ultrasonography, magnetic resonance imaging, and scintigraphy. *Semin Plast Surg*. 2009;23(2):80-89.
2. Zimmerli W. Clinical practice. Vertebral osteomyelitis. *N Engl J Med*. 2010;362(11):1022-1029.
3. Calhoun JH, Manring MM, Shirtliff M. Osteomyelitis of the long bones. *Semin Plast Surg*. 2009;23(2):59-72.
4. Hatzenbuehler J, Pulling TJ. Diagnosis and management of osteomyelitis. *Am Fam Physician*. 2011;84(9):1027-1033.
5. Kowalski TJ, Berbari EF, Huddleston PM, Steckelberg JM, Osmon DR. Do follow-up imaging examinations provide useful prognostic information in patients with spine infection? *Clin Infect Dis*. 2006;43(2):172-179.

218 SYPHILIS

Richard P. Usatine, MD
Heidi Chumley, MD

PATIENT STORY

A 39-year-old woman presents with a nonhealing ulcer over her upper lip for 1 week and a new-onset rash on her trunk (**Figures 218-1** and **218-2**). The ulcer on her upper lip was misdiagnosed as herpes simplex by the previous physician. Sexual history revealed that the patient had oral sex with a boyfriend who had a lesion on his penis and she suspected that he had been having sex with other women. The examining physician recognized the nonpainful ulcer and rash as a combination of primary and secondary (P&S) syphilis. A rapid plasma reagin (RPR) was drawn and the patient was treated immediately with IM benzathine penicillin. The RPR came back as 1:128 and the ulcer was healed within 1 week.

INTRODUCTION

Syphilis, caused by *Treponema pallidum*, is a systemic disease characterized by multiple overlapping stages: primary syphilis (ulcer), secondary syphilis (skin rash, mucocutaneous lesions, or lymphadenopathy), tertiary syphilis (cardiac or gummatous lesions), and early or late latent syphilis (positive serology without clinical manifestations). Neurosyphilis can occur at any stage. Diagnosis is made using treponemal and nontreponemal tests. Treatment is penicillin; the dose and duration depend on the stage.

SYNONYMS AND ACRONYMS

- Lues is another word for syphilis.
- Nontreponemal tests
  - VDRL—Venereal Disease Research Laboratory
- RPR

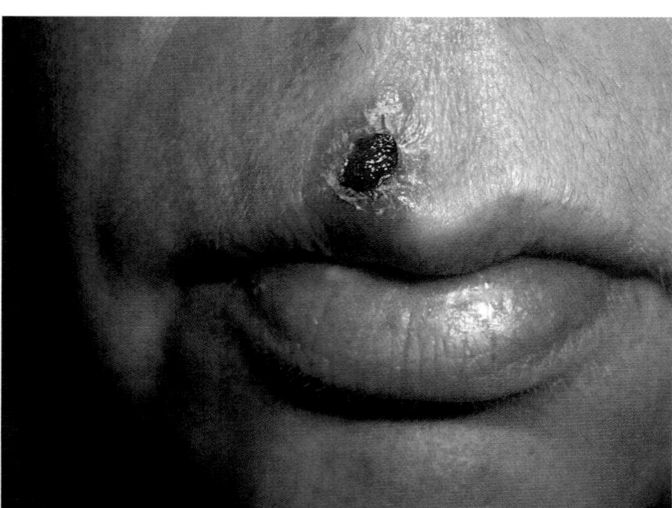

FIGURE 218-1 Primary syphilis with a chancre over the lip of a woman. (*Reproduced with permission from Richard P. Usatine, MD.*)

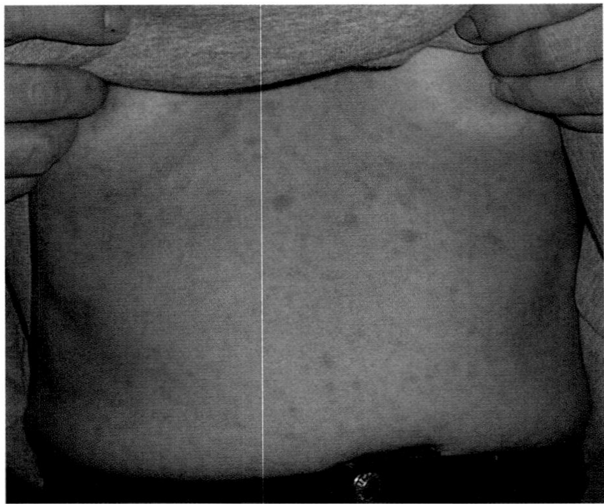

CHAPTER 218

FIGURE 218-2 A nonpruritic rash of secondary syphilis on the abdomen of the patient shown in Figure 218-1. (*Reproduced with permission from Richard P. Usatine, MD.*)

- Treponemal tests
  - EIA—Enzyme immunoassay
  - TPPA—*T. pallidum* particle agglutination
  - FTA-ABS—Fluorescent treponemal antibody absorption
  - MHA-TP—Microhemagglutination assay for *T. pallidum*

EPIDEMIOLOGY

- P&S syphilis cases reported to Centers for Disease Control and Prevention (CDC) decreased from 13,997 in 2009 to 13,774 in 2010, a decrease of 1.6%. The rate of P&S syphilis in the United States in 2010 (4.5 cases per 100,000 population) was 2.2% lower than the rate in 2009 (4.6 cases). This is the first overall decrease in P&S syphilis in 10 years.[1]
- The rate of P&S syphilis increased 1.3% among men (from 7.8 to 7.9 cases per 100,000 men) during 2009 to 2010. During this same period, the rate decreased 21.4% among women (from 1.4 to 1.1 cases per 100,000 women).[1]
- In 2010, the rate of P&S syphilis was highest among persons aged 20 to 24 years and 25 to 29 years (13.5 and 11.3 cases per 100,000 population, respectively).[1]
- The distribution of primary and secondary syphilis reported in 2010 differed by gender and sexual preferences—Among men who have sex with women only (MSW), 35.8% had primary syphilis and 64.2% had secondary syphilis. Among women, 16% had primary syphilis and 84% had secondary syphilis. Among men who have sex with men (MSM), 25% had primary syphilis and 75% had secondary syphilis.[1]
- Syphilis by races/ethnicities varied in 2010—Among women with P&S syphilis, 16.8% were white, 72.8% were black, 6.6% were Hispanic. Among MSW, 14.8% were white, 67% were black, 13.8% were Hispanic. Among MSM, 38.1% were white, 37% were black, 19.8% were Hispanic.[1]
- In 2008, 63% of the reported cases of P&S were in MSM.[2]
- HIV-infected patients were found to have syphilis rates of 62.3 per 1000 compared to 0.8 per 1000 in HIV-uninfected patients in a population study in California.[3]

ETIOLOGY AND PATHOPHYSIOLOGY

Syphilis is caused by the spirochete *T. pallidum* and contracted through direct sexual contact with primary or secondary lesions. Congenital syphilis can be contracted across the placenta.

RISK FACTORS

- Sexual contact with a person with primary or secondary syphilis
- MSM
- Prostitution
- Sex for drugs
- HIV/AIDS

DIAGNOSIS

CLINICAL FEATURES

- Primary syphilis is associated with a chancre—Usually a nonpainful ulcer (**Figures 218-1**, **218-3**, and **218-4**). The presence of pain does not rule out syphilis, and the patient with a painful genital ulcer should be tested for both syphilis and herpes.
- Secondary syphilis occurs when the spirochetes become systemic and may present as a rash with protean morphologies, condyloma lata, and/or mucous patches (**Figures 218-2** and **218-5** to **218-10**).
- Tertiary syphilis may be visualized with gummas on the skin, but many of the manifestations are internal such as the cardiac and neurologic diseases that occur (eg, aortitis, tabes dorsalis, and iritis). **Figure 218-11** shows a gumma of the scrotum.
- Neurosyphilis can occur at any stage. Clinical symptoms include cognitive dysfunction, vision or hearing loss, uveitis or iritis, motor or sensory abnormalities, cranial nerve palsies, or symptoms of meningitis.

TYPICAL DISTRIBUTION

- Primary syphilis is usually a single ulcer (chancre) that is not painful in the genital region (see **Figures 218-3** and **218-4**). A chancre can be seen on the lip (see **Figure 218-1**).

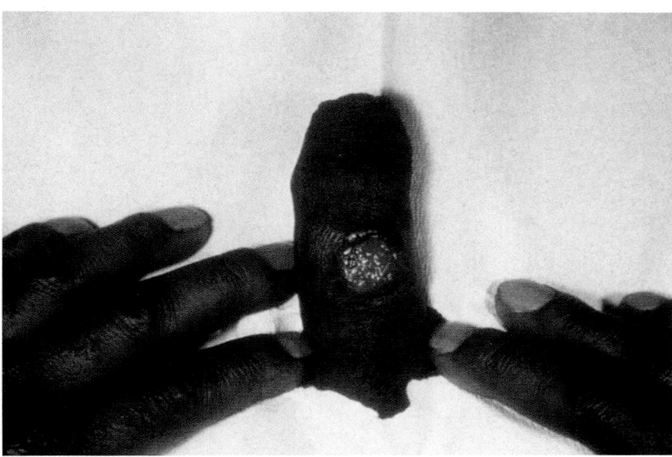

FIGURE 218-3 A painless chancre at the location of treponemal entry. (*Reproduced with permission from the Public Health Image Library, Centers for Disease Control and Prevention.*)

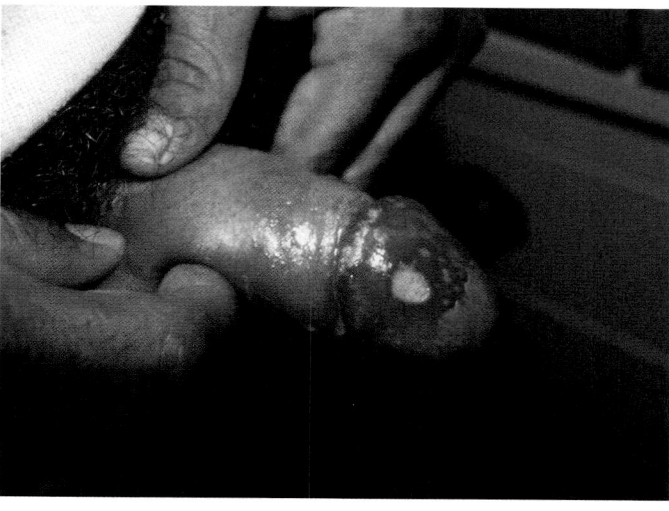

FIGURE 218-4 Primary syphilis with a large chancre on the glands of the penis. The multiple small surrounding ulcers are part of the syphilis and not a second disease. (*Reproduced with permission from Richard P. Usatine, MD.*)

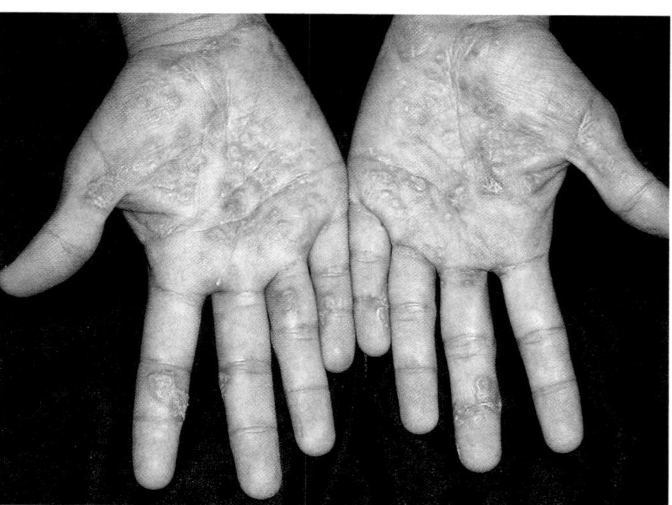

FIGURE 218-5 Papular squamous eruption on the hands of a woman with secondary syphilis. (*Reproduced with permission from Richard P. Usatine, MD.*)

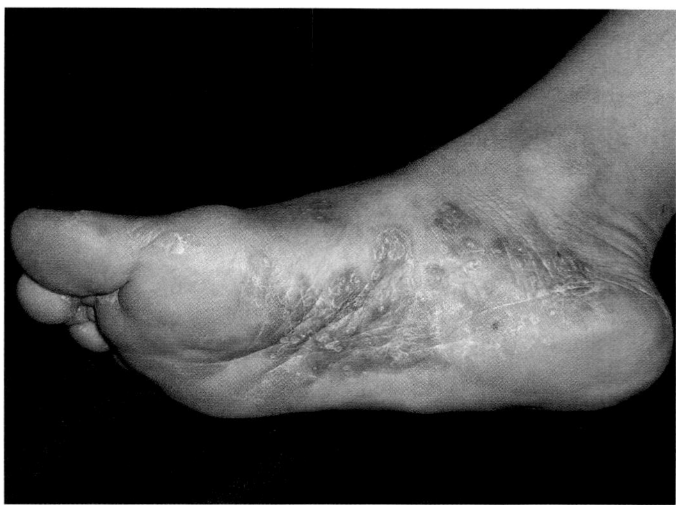

FIGURE 218-6 Papular squamous eruption on the foot of the woman in Figure 218-5, with secondary syphilis. (*Reproduced with permission from Richard P. Usatine, MD.*)

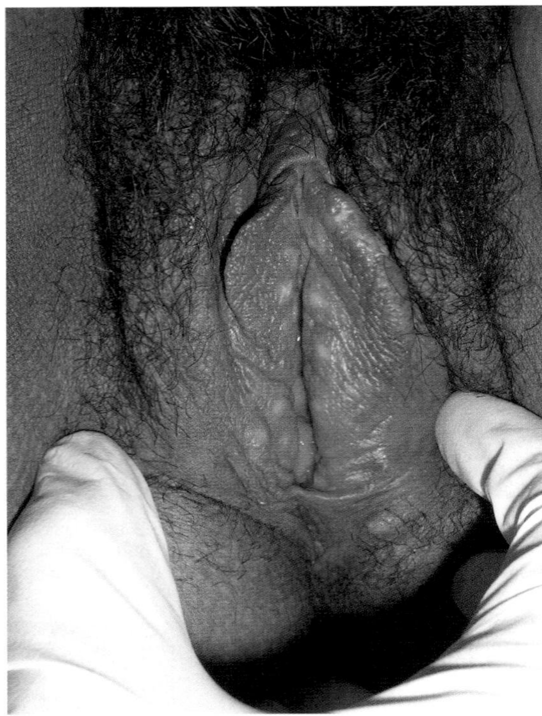

FIGURE 218-7 Mucous patches on the labia of the woman in Figure 218-5, with secondary syphilis teeming with spirochetes. (*Reproduced with permission from Richard P. Usatine, MD.*)

- Secondary syphilis may present with various eruptions on the trunk, palms, and soles (**Figures 218-2, 218-5, 218-6, 218-8,** and **218-12**). Secondary syphilis may also present with a moth-eaten alopecia **(Figure 218-13)**.
- Mucous patches are on the genitals or in the mouth (see **Figures 218-7** and **218-9**).

LABORATORY TESTING

- Serologic tests are either nontreponemal (RPR or VDRL), which measure anticardiolipin antibodies, or treponemal (EIA, TPPA, FTA-ABS, or MHA-TP), which measure antibodies to *T. pallidum*.

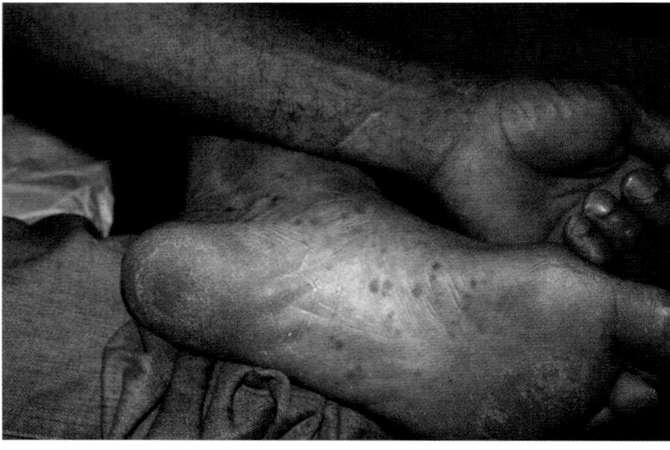

FIGURE 218-8 Pink macules on the feet and wrists of a man with secondary syphilis. (*Reproduced with permission from Richard P. Usatine, MD.*)

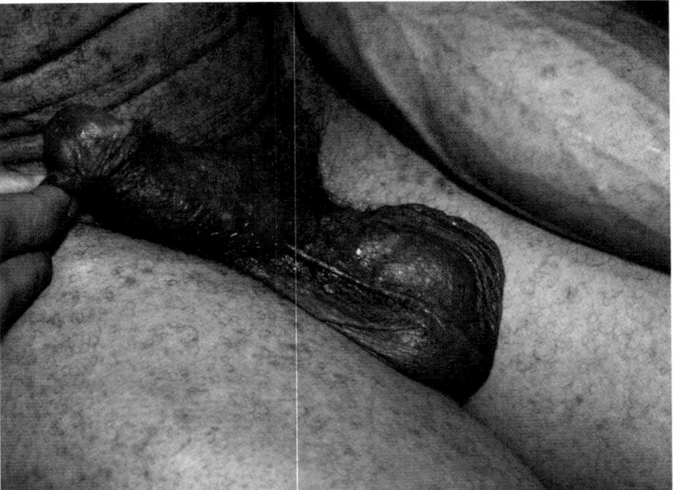

A

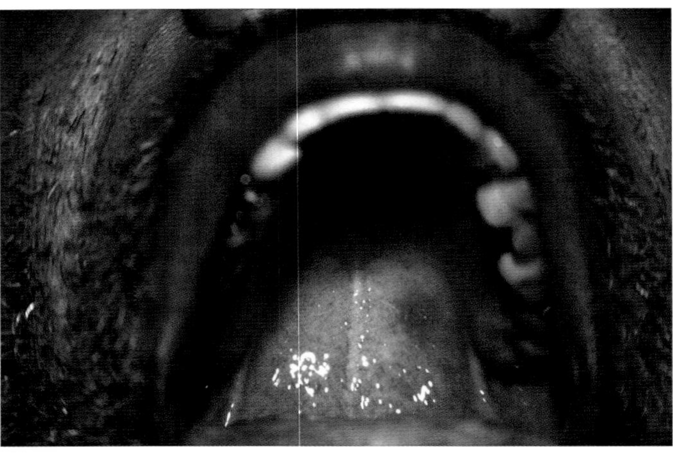

B

FIGURE 218-9 **A.** Mucous patches on the penis and scrotum of the same man with secondary syphilis in **Figure 218-8**. **B.** Same man with oral lesion on the palate. (*Reproduced with permission from Richard P. Usatine, MD.*)

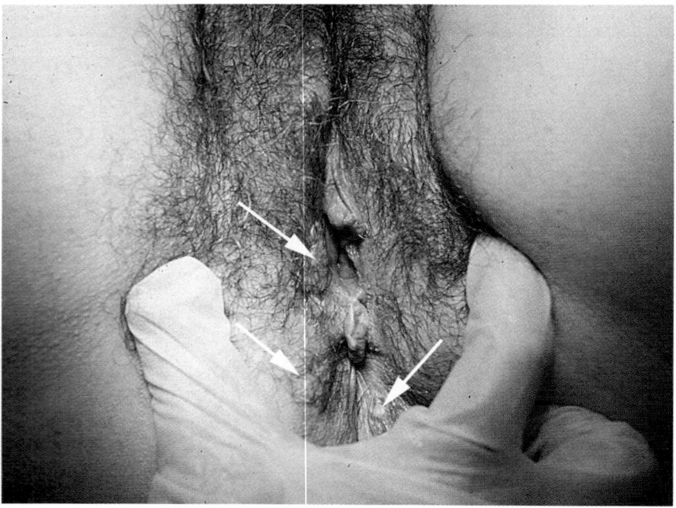

FIGURE 218-10 Condylomata lata (*arrows*) on the vulva of a woman with secondary syphilis. (*Reproduced with permission from Richard P. Usatine, MD.*)

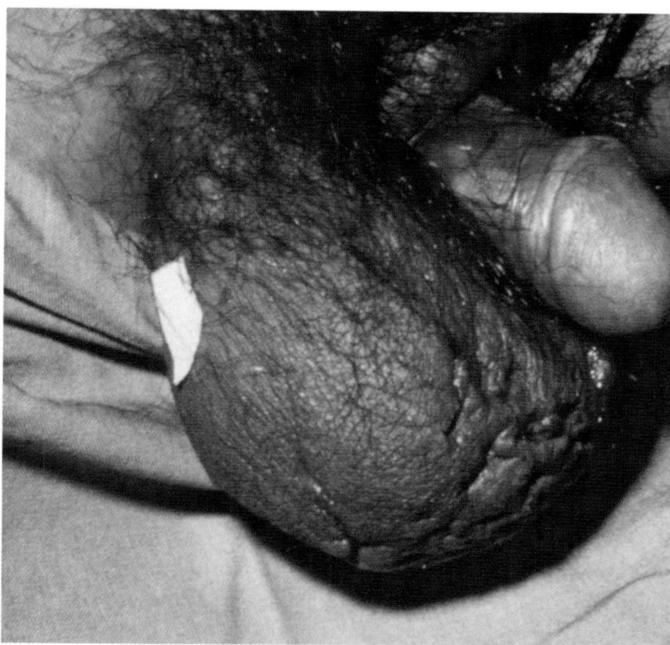

FIGURE 218-11 Tertiary syphilis presenting as a swollen scrotum, which was diagnosed as a syphilitic gumma of the testicle. (*Reproduced with permission from the Public Health Image Library, Centers for Disease Control and Prevention.*)

- There are 2 algorithms for laboratory testing currently in use around the world:
    1. Start with a low-cost nontreponemal test and confirm a positive result with a treponemal test.
    2. Start with the EIA treponemal test, followed by a nontreponemal test for confirmation.
- In 2008, the CDC recommended a treponemal EIA initially, with positive results followed by a nontreponemal test for confirmation, a strategy that detected an additional 3% of positive samples not identified in the nontreponemal–treponemal sequence.[4]
- A nontreponemal test is required for confirmation, as a treponemal EIA indicates exposure but not active infection.

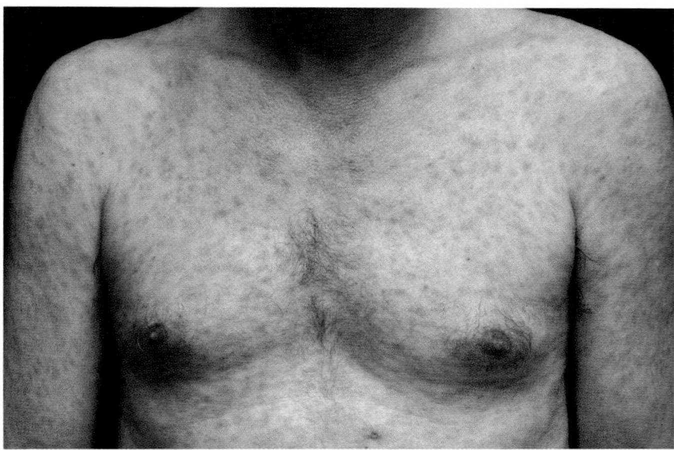

FIGURE 218-12 Middle-age married man with diffuse eruption of secondary syphilis from neck to feet. The eruption remained undiagnosed for months as the patient denied any risk factors. His RPR was 1:256. (*Reproduced with permission from Richard P. Usatine, MD.*)

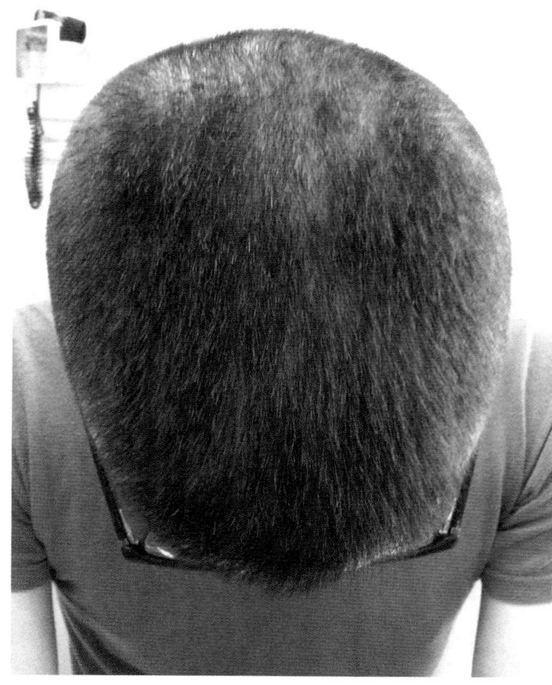

FIGURE 218-13 Moth-eaten alopecia in a gay man with secondary syphilis. He presented with the hair loss and no other skin lesion. At first his RPR was negative due to the high antibody load and the prozone affect. After dilution of the RPR, it was positive at 1:32. (*Reproduced with permission from Jeffrey Kinard, DO.*)

- A positive EIA with a negative RPR can be a previous treated or untreated infection, a false-positive, or early primary syphilis. In this case, retest with a second treponemal test.
- Dark-field microscopy is useful in evaluating moist cutaneous lesions, such as chancre, mucous patches, and condyloma lata (**Figure 218-14**).
- Test all patients with syphilis for HIV (**Figure 218-15**).
- Patients with syphilis who have any signs or symptoms suggesting neurologic disease including vision or hearing need a cerebrospinal fluid (CSF) examination, a slit-lamp ophthalmologic examination, and an otologic examination to determine if neurosyphilis is present.

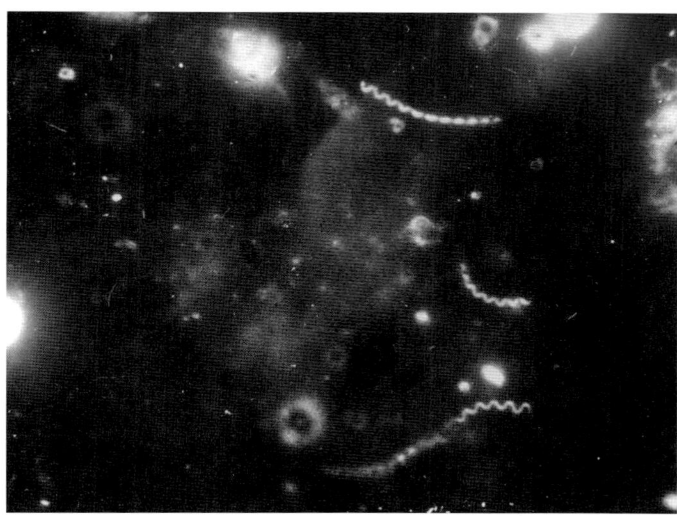

FIGURE 218-14 Live spirochetes of *T. pallidum* seen in a dark-field preparation. (*Reproduced with permission from the Public Health Image Library, Centers for Disease Control and Prevention.*)

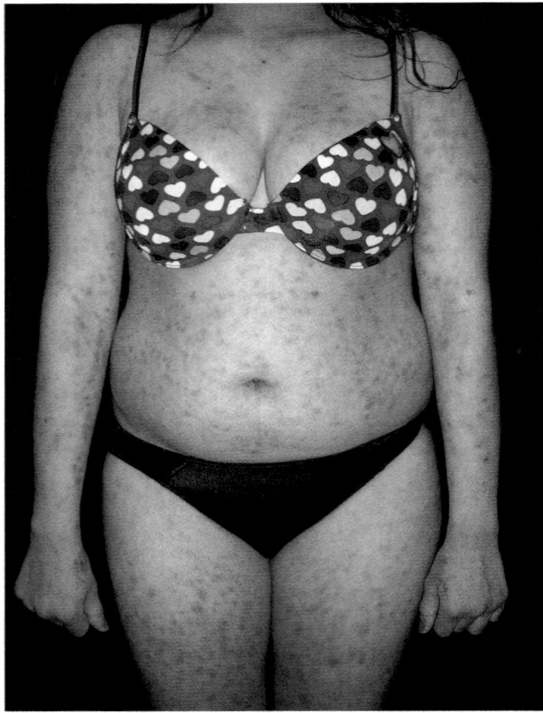

FIGURE 218-15 Secondary syphilis in a 20-year-old woman with a history of injection drug use and multiple sexual partners. Her HIV test was also positive so she was worked up for neurosyphilis. (*Reproduced with permission from Richard P. Usatine, MD.*)

DIFFERENTIAL DIAGNOSIS

- Herpes simplex—Most common cause of genital ulcers in the United States. These ulcers are painful and often start as vesicles (see Chapter 128, Herpes Simplex).
- Chancroid—Painful beefy red ulcers on the penis or vulva, less common than syphilis. Chancroid is also known to cause large painful inguinal adenopathy (bubo) (**Figures 218-16** and **218-17**).

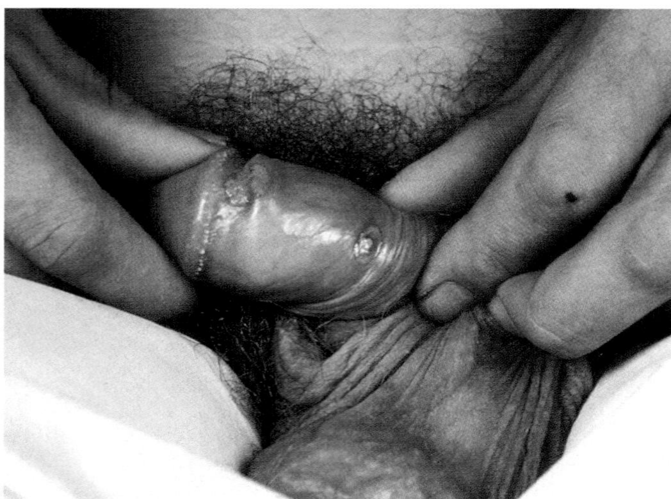

FIGURE 218-16 Chancroid ulcers caused by the bacterium, *Haemophilus ducreyi*. The patient was originally thought to have syphilis. Chancroidal ulcers are classically painful and beefy but chancroid should be considered on the differential diagnosis of any sexually acquired genital ulcer. (*Reproduced with permission from CDC/Dr. Pirozzi.*)

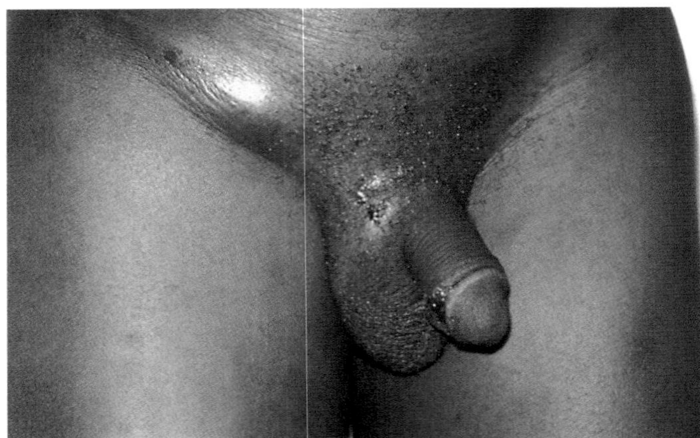

FIGURE 218-17 Chancroid lesions of the groin and penis affecting the ipsilateral inguinal lymph nodes. (*Reproduced with permission from CDC/J. Pledger.*)

- Drug eruptions—Can be on the genital area such as seen in a fixed drug eruption. Also whole-body drug eruptions can appear similar to secondary syphilis (see Chapter 201, Cutaneous Drug Reactions).
- Erythema multiforme—Can look like the rash of secondary syphilis but may have target lesions (see Chapter 175, Erythema Multiforme, Stevens-Johnson Syndrome, and Toxic Epidermal Necrolysis).
- Pityriasis rosea—A self-limited cutaneous eruption that often begins with a herald patch and may have a Christmas tree distribution on the back (see Chapter 151, Pityriasis Rosea).

MANAGEMENT

MEDICATIONS

Benzathine penicillin is the treatment of choice for all stages of syphilis. Dose and duration depend on stage. Treatment information below is from the CDC.[5]

- Primary, secondary, and early latent (immunocompetent and nonpregnant)
  - Adults—Benzathine penicillin G 2.4 million units IM 1 time
    - Penicillin allergy—Desensitize pregnant patients. Alternatives for nonpregnant adults include the following:
  - Doxycycline 100 mg twice daily × 14 days or
  - Ceftriaxone 1 g IM/IV daily × 10 to 14 days (limited studies) or
  - Azithromycin 2 g single oral dose; however, azithromycin resistance has been documented in several areas of the United States. Use only when penicillin or doxycycline cannot be used. Do not use in MSM.
- Late latent syphilis or syphilis of unknown duration
  - Adults—Benzathine penicillin G 2.4 million units IM every week for 3 weeks.
    - Penicillin allergy—Doxycycline 100 mg twice a day for 28 days (or tetracycline 500 mg 4 times a day for 28 days) are the only acceptable alternatives.
- For the management of tertiary and neurosyphilis, see the *Sexually Transmitted Diseases Treatment Guidelines* published by the CDC in 2010: **http://www.cdc.gov/std/treatment/2010/genital-ulcers.htm#syphilis.**

REFERRAL OR HOSPITALIZATION

Refer patients when the stage of syphilis is unclear. Consider referral to an infectious disease specialist in pregnant women with a penicillin allergy, patients with tertiary or neurosyphilis, or patients who have failed treatment.

PREVENTION

- Primary prevention: Safe-sex practices—sexual transmission occurs when mucocutaneous syphilitic lesions are present.
- Secondary prevention
  - Treat presumptively (regardless of serology) sexual partners who were exposed within 90 days of the partner's diagnosis of primary, secondary, or early latent syphilis.
  - Consider presumptive treatment when exposure was greater than 90 days before partner's diagnosis if serology is unavailable or follow-up is uncertain.[5]

PROGNOSIS

When syphilis is recognized and appropriately treated, the prognosis is excellent.

FOLLOW-UP

Reexamine clinically and serologically at 6 and 12 months. Consider treatment failure if signs and/or symptoms persist or the nontreponemal test titer does not decline by 2 dilutions after 6 to 12 months of therapy. Fifteen percent will not achieve this decline in titer after 1 year.[5]

For treatment failures retest for HIV and perform a lumbar puncture for CSF analysis and treat for neurosyphilis if positive.

PATIENT EDUCATION

Condoms can prevent the spread of syphilis. Patients should be advised to get HIV testing and need to know that syphilis is a risk factor for the spread of HIV. HIV/AIDS is also a risk factor for acquiring syphilis (**Figure 218-18**) and syphilis is a risk factor for acquiring HIV (**Figure 218-19**). Patients should be advised of the importance of completing treatment and follow-up to prevent complications.

PATIENT RESOURCES

- Centers for Disease Control and Prevention (CDC). *Sexually Transmitted Diseases (STDs): Syphilis–CDC Fact Sheet*—**http://www.cdc.gov/std/syphilis/stdfact-syphilis.htm.**

PROVIDER RESOURCES

- Medscape. *Syphilis*—**http://emedicine.medscape.com/article/229461-overview.**
- The Centers for Disease Control and Prevention. *Sexually Transmitted Diseases Treatment Guidelines*—**http://www.cdc.gov/std/treatment/2010/toc.htm.** (Also available to download as an e-book for Apple iPad, iPhone, or iPod Touch—**http://www.cdc.gov/std/2010-ebook.htm.**)

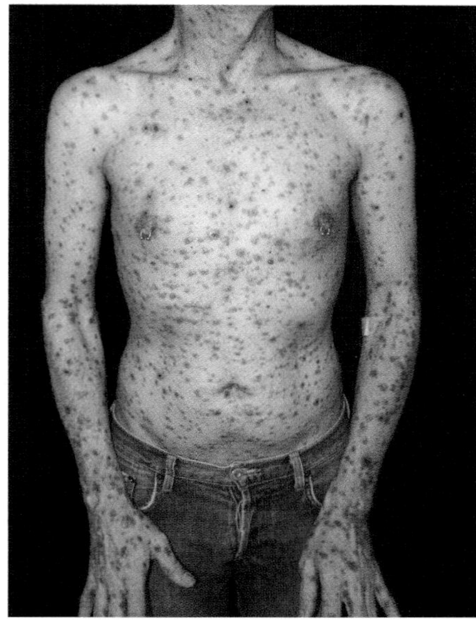

A

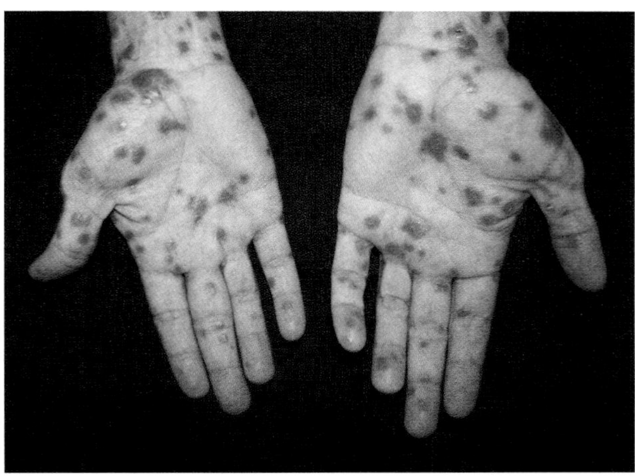

B

FIGURE 218-18 Secondary syphilis in a young man with known HIV/AIDS. A. Impressive red papulosquamous eruption from head to toe is present. B. Close-up showing the palmar patches and plaques. (*Reproduced with permission from Jonathan B. Karnes, MD.*)

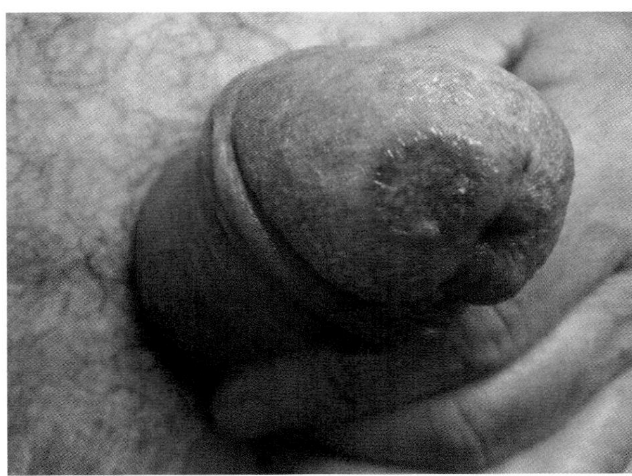

FIGURE 218-19 Chancre of primary syphilis in a gay man. Note that genital ulcers increase the risk of HIV transmission. (*Reproduced with permission from Husein Husein-ElAhmed MD.*)

REFERENCES

1. Centers for Disease Control and Prevention (CDC). *Sexually Transmitted Diseases Surveillance. Syphilis*. http://www.cdc.gov/std/stats10/Syphilis.htm. Accessed September 2, 2012.

2. Centers for Disease Control and Prevention (CDC). *Sexually Transmitted Diseases. Syphilis*. http://www.cdc.gov/std/syphilis/. Accessed September 2, 2012.

3. Horberg MA, Ranatunga DK, Quesenberry CP, et al. Syphilis epidemiology and clinical outcomes in HIV-infected and HIV-uninfected patients in Kaiser Permanente Northern California. *Sex Transm Dis*. 2010;37(1):53-58.

4. Centers for Disease Control and Prevention (CDC). Syphilis testing algorithms using treponemal tests for initial screening—four laboratories, New York City, 2005-2006. *MMWR Morb Mortal Wkly Rep*. 2008;57(32):872-875.

5. Centers for Disease Control and Prevention (CDC). *Sexually Transmitted Diseases Treatment Guidelines, 2010: Diseases Characterized by Genital, Anal, or Perianal Ulcers*. http://www.cdc.gov/std/treatment/2010/genital-ulcers.htm#syphilis. Accessed September 23, 2011.

PART 17

ENDOCRINE

Strength of Recommendation (SOR)	Definition
A	Recommendation based on consistent and good-quality patient-oriented evidence.*
B	Recommendation based on inconsistent or limited-quality patient-oriented evidence.*
C	Recommendation based on consensus, usual practice, opinion, disease-oriented evidence, or case series for studies of diagnosis, treatment, prevention, or screening.*

*See Appendix A on pages 1241-1244 for further information.

219 DIABETES OVERVIEW

Mindy A. Smith, MD, MS

PATIENT STORY

A 66-year-old man with obesity and mild hypertension controlled with a diuretic presents with increasing nocturia and excessive thirst. He has no other urinary symptoms and denies any visual problems. His mother had diabetes and died at age 85 years from a heart attack. His only other concern is a recurrent fungal infection on his feet. His blood pressure in the office today is 135/85 mm Hg and his finger stick blood sugar is 220 mg/dL. You explain that based on his elevated blood sugar, he has diabetes mellitus. Physical examination findings confirm the diagnosis of tinea pedis (**Figure 219-1**). A monofilament test demonstrates normal sensation in his feet. You order a fasting blood sugar, lipid profile, serum electrolytes, creatinine, and hemoglobin A_{1C}. You ask him to return next week for a more complete examination, review of his test results, and diabetes education. You ask him and his wife to consider meeting with a nutritionist, and briefly review treatment options, including diet, exercise, and metformin, as well as a possible need to improve his blood pressure control or switch to another agent. You suggest a nonprescription antifungal cream and will see if he needs additional treatment for his feet at follow-up. The patient is referred to an ophthalmologist who finds diabetic nonproliferative retinopathy (**Figure 219-2**).

INTRODUCTION

Diabetes is a group of disorders caused by a complex interaction between genetic susceptibility, environmental factors, and personal lifestyle choices that share the phenotype of hyperglycemia. Type 2 diabetes mellitus (DM) is a heterogeneous group of chronic disorders caused by a progressive insulin secretory defect and increased glucose production in the setting of insulin resistance.

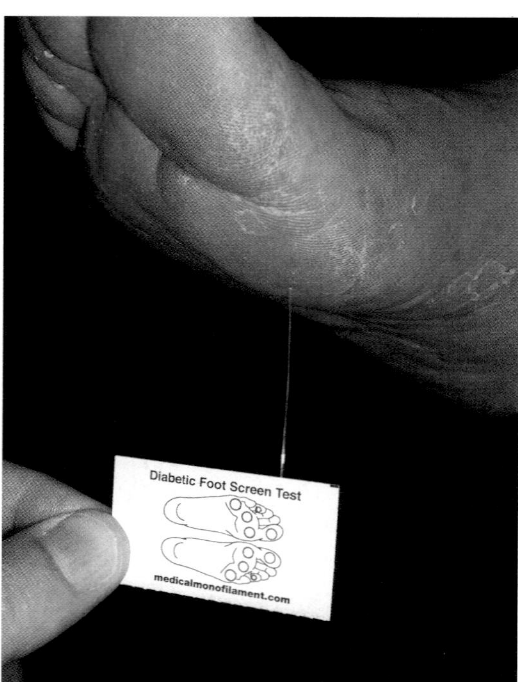

FIGURE 219-1 Patient with diabetes and tinea pedis being tested with a monofilament for sensation. (*Reproduced with permission from Richard P. Usatine, MD.*)

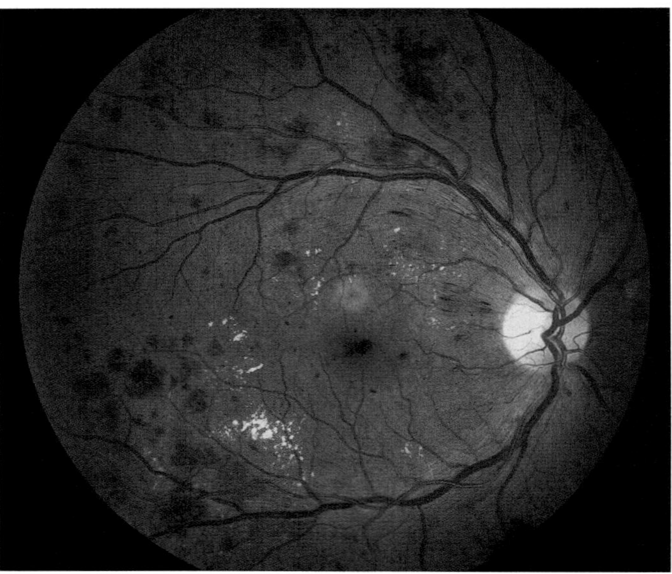

FIGURE 219-2 Nonproliferative diabetic retinopathy, with scattered intraretinal dot-blot and flame hemorrhages, along with macular exudates. Macular exudates can be related to diabetic macular edema, which accounts for a large portion of poor vision and disability secondary to diabetic retinopathy. (*Reproduced with permission from Andrew Sanchez, COA.*)

EPIDEMIOLOGY

- Prevalence—In the United States, 25.8 million adults and children (8.3% of the population), including 18.8 million who have been diagnosed, have diabetes. This includes 26.9% of people age 65 years and older. Type 2 DM is the most common form, accounting for more than 90% of cases.[1]
- Incidence—In the United States in 2010, there were 1.9 million new cases among individuals 19 years of age and older.
- Highest rates of diabetes are in non-Hispanic blacks (12.6%), followed by Hispanics (11.8%), Asian Americans (8.4%), and non-Hispanic whites (7.1%).
- In 2007, total costs of diagnosed DM in the United States were $174 billion ($116 billion in direct medical costs).

ETIOLOGY AND PATHOPHYSIOLOGY

- Insulin resistance is attributed to obesity, inactivity, and genetic factors (including defects in β-cell function and insulin action).
- Initially, the pancreatic β-cells increase insulin production to overcome insulin resistance and maintain euglycemia. Eventually, β-cells fail, resulting in hyperglycemia.
- Other contributing factors include diseases of the pancreas (eg, pancreatitis, hemochromatosis), infection (eg, cytomegalovirus), and other endocrinopathies (eg, hyperthyroidism [see Chapter 227, Hyperthyroidism] and acromegaly [see Chapter 228, Acromegaly]).
- Microvascular and macrovascular diseases may result from hyperglycemia or other metabolic changes.

RISK FACTORS

- Obesity[1-4]*
- Red meat consumption (relative risk [RR] 1.51; 95% confidence interval [CI], 1.25, 1.83 for 50 g processed red meat per day)[5]
- Physical inactivity (also television viewing 2 h/d; odds ratio [OR] 1.20; 95% CI, 1.14-1.27)[6]*
- Nonwhite race*
- First-degree relative with diabetes, hypertension, or myocardial infarction*
- Prior gestational diabetes*
- Impaired glucose tolerance (hazard ratio [HR] 13.2, 95% CI, 10.8-16.2)[7]
- Polycystic ovarian syndrome
- Coronary heart disease, hypertension*
- Smoking (OR [current smoker] 1.44; 95% CI, 1.31 to 1.58)
- Antipsychotic therapy for patients with schizophrenia or severe bipolar disease*
- Previously identified glucose intolerance*
- Prolonged use of oral corticosteroids

---

*Risk factors used by the American Association of Clinical Endocrinologists (AACE) in making decisions for screening patients for DM (see below).[4]

Many risk models and scores have been developed to predict the development of DM.[8] Authors of a systematic review identified 7 risk scores that had high potential for use in practice based on similar components and discriminatory properties.[4] One of these, the Framingham Offspring Study,[9] uses fasting plasma glucose levels, body mass index, high-density lipoprotein cholesterol and triglyceride levels, and parental history of diabetes and blood pressure to determine risk. Unfortunately, none of the models were developed on a cohort recruited prospectively and no studies have demonstrated a reduction in incident DM using risk scoring and intervention.

DIAGNOSIS

The AACE guideline defines the diagnosis of diabetes as a fasting (8 or more hours of no caloric intake) glucose level 126 mg/dL or greater (≥7.0 mmol/L), *or* a 2-hour plasma glucose 200 mg/dL or greater (≥11.1 mmol/L) on a 75-g oral glucose tolerance test, *or* a random plasma glucose level of greater than 200 mg/dL with symptoms of diabetes, *or* a hemoglobin A_{1C} level of 6.5% or higher.[4] SOR Ⓐ The same test should be repeated on a different day to confirm the diagnosis unless the patient has unequivocal hyperglycemia or severe metabolic stress. SOR Ⓒ

CLINICAL FEATURES

- Many patients with type 2 DM are asymptomatic.
- Patients may report polydipsia, polyuria, and blurred vision.
- Funduscopic examination may reveal signs of retinopathy (hard exudates, hemorrhages) (see **Figure 219-2**; see Chapter 17, Diabetic Retinopathy).

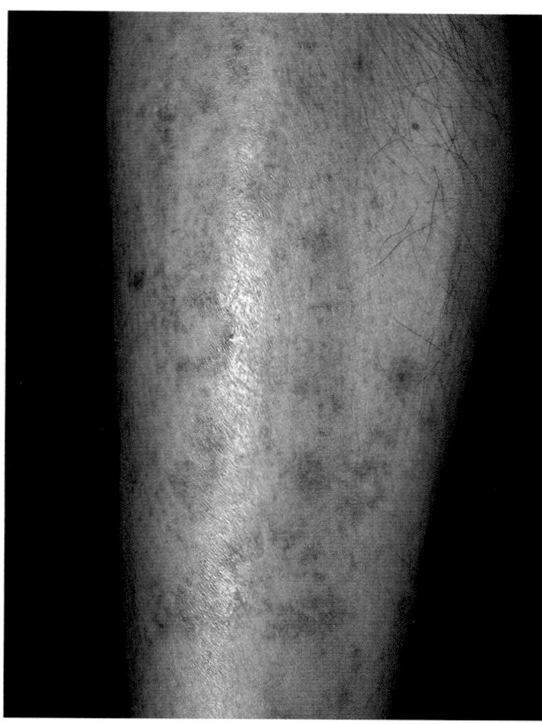

FIGURE 219-3 Diabetic dermopathy on the lower legs that is particularly prominent over the shins. (*Reproduced with permission from Richard P. Usatine, MD.*)

- Patients with diabetic neuropathy may have abnormalities on monofilament, vibration, and superficial pain testing.
- Skin changes in patients with DM include diabetic dermopathy in 15% to 40% of patients (**Figure 219-3**; see Chapter 221, Diabetic Dermopathy),[10] acanthosis nigricans in approximately one-third of patients (**Figure 219-4**; see Chapter 220, Acanthosis Nigricans),[11] diabetic foot ulcers (**Figure 219-5**; see Chapter 208, Ischemic Ulcer), and, uncommonly, necrobiosis lipoidica (**Figure 219-6**; see Chapter 222, Necrobiosis Lipoidica).
- Hyperlipidemia may result in eruptive xanthomas (**Figure 219-7**) or xanthelasma (see Chapter 223, Hyperlipidemia).

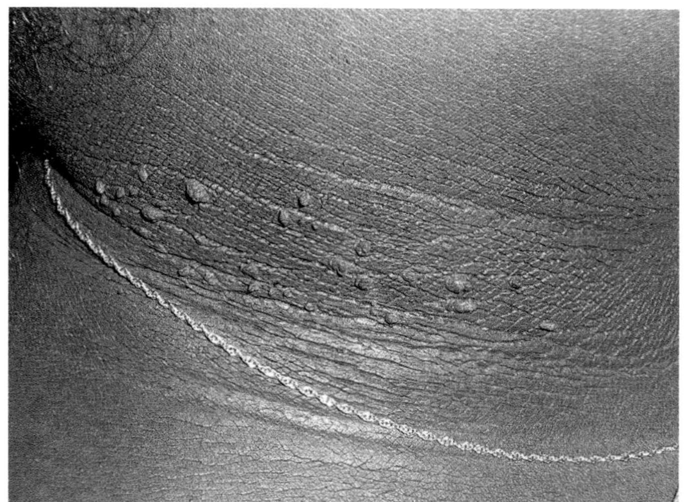

FIGURE 219-4 Acanthosis nigricans in a woman with type 2 diabetes and obesity. She is requesting that her skin tags be removed. (*Reproduced with permission from Richard P. Usatine, MD.*)

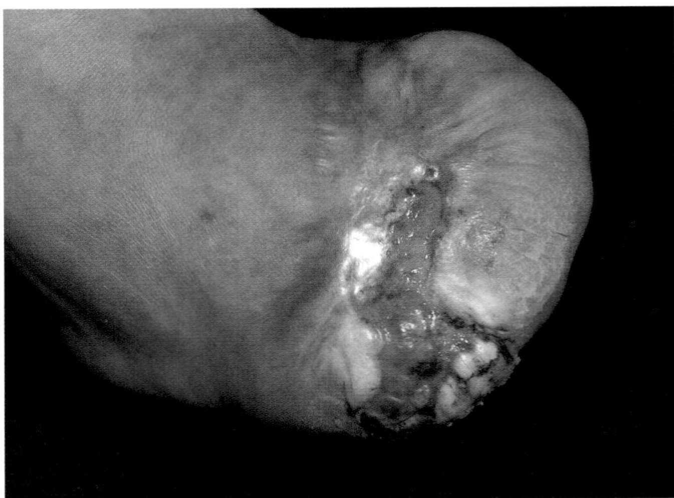

FIGURE 219-5 Diabetic foot ulcer that has occurred at the amputation site. *(Reproduced with permission from Richard P. Usatine, MD.)*

- Patients with DM of prolonged duration may also have Charcot joints (**Figure 219-8**; see Chapter 210, Charcot Arthropathy).[12]

LABORATORY TESTS

- The American Diabetes Association (ADA) recommends several tests for diagnosing diabetes: a fasting plasma glucose of 126 mg/dL or greater, a hemoglobin A_{1C} of greater than or equal to 6.5%, or a blood glucose of greater than or equal to 200 mg/dL on either a random plasma glucose test or at 2 hours following an oral glucose tolerance test.[13] A second confirming test is recommended.
- A random capillary blood glucose may be a reasonable alternative. Compared with traditional criteria, a capillary blood glucose level of greater than 120 mg/dL has a sensitivity of 75% and specificity of 88% for the diagnosis of type 2 DM.[14]

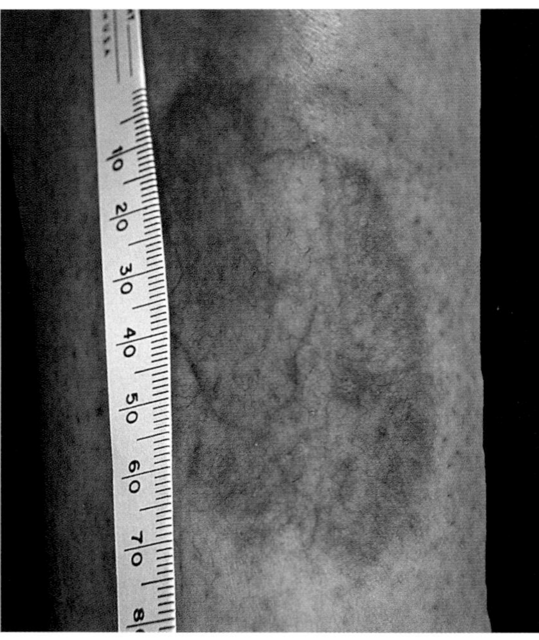

FIGURE 219-6 Necrobiosis lipoidica diabeticorum on the lower leg with typical findings of skin atrophy, yellow coloration, and prominent blood vessels. *(Reproduced with permission from Richard P. Usatine, MD.)*

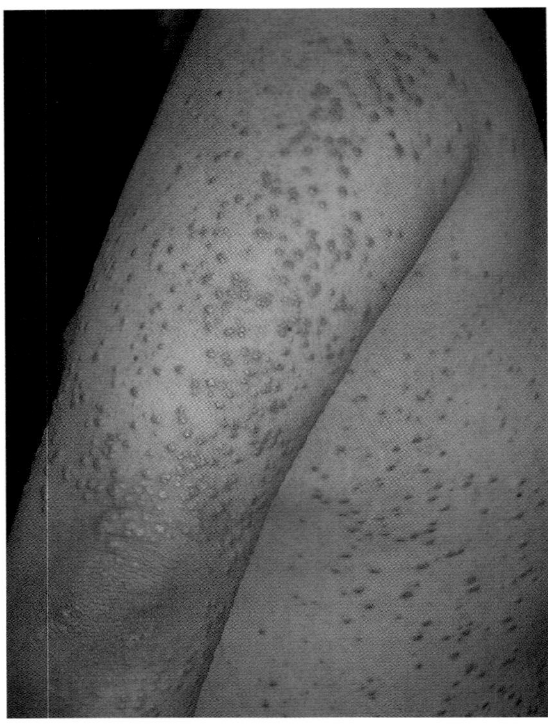

FIGURE 219-7 Eruptive xanthomas on the extremities and trunk of a young man with untreated type 2 diabetes and hyperlipidemia. *(Reproduced with permission from Richard P. Usatine, MD.)*

- In cases where there is uncertainty regarding the diagnosis of type 1 or type 2 DM, glucagon-stimulated C-peptide, 2-hour postprandial urinary C-peptide-to-creatinine ratio, and 4-hour postprandial urinary C-peptide concentration can be used to help distinguish between the types.

MANAGEMENT

The primary treatment goals for the patient with DM are to aggressively control blood pressure (<130/80 mm Hg) and lower lipids (low-density lipoprotein [LDL] goal is <100 mg/dL) to improve cardiovascular and

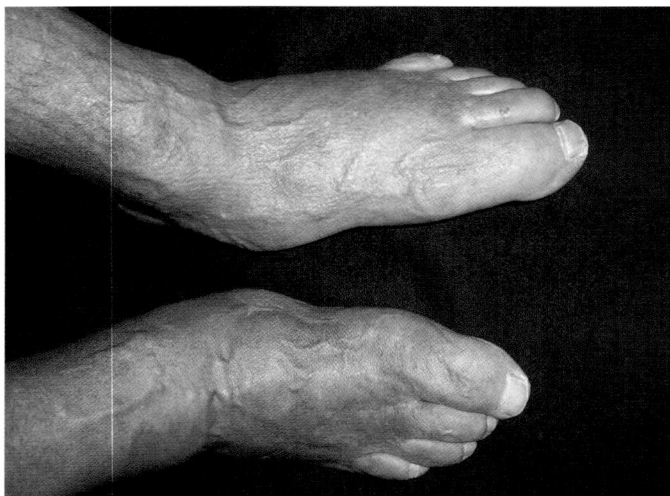

FIGURE 219-8 Charcot feet bilaterally in a person with poorly controlled diabetes. Note the pronation of the feet with the abnormal bulging of the medial foot. X-rays showed abnormal tarsal bones secondary to diabetic neuropathy. *(Reproduced with permission from Richard P. Usatine, MD.)*

all-cause mortality. Reasonable blood glucose control (hemoglobin A_{1C} <8%) is usually undertaken with metformin.

- Tight/strict control should no longer be stressed as it does not improve most outcomes and increases episodes of hypoglycemia. In the ADVANCE (Action in Diabetes and Vascular Disease: Preterax and Diamicron Modified-Release Controlled Evaluation) trial ($N = 11,140$), there were no differences seen in the rates of major macrovascular events or overall mortality between patients randomized to intense control (hemoglobin A_{1C} ≤6.5%) or standard control.[15] Furthermore, in the ACCORD (Action to Control Cardiovascular Risk in Diabetes) trial, intensive insulin therapy in patients with type 2 DM was associated with increased mortality in participants randomized to the very intensive glycemic control arm (hemoglobin A_{1C} <6%).[16] A recent meta-analysis of 14 trials also concluded that intensive control did not reduce all-cause mortality; data were insufficient to confirm a relative risk reduction for cardiovascular morbidity or mortality, composite microvascular complications, or retinopathy at a magnitude of 10%.[17] Intensive glycemic control increased the relative risk of severe hypoglycemia by 30%.[17]
- Recent data indicate that the lowest mortality rates occur at a hemoglobin A1c between 7.5% to 9%.[18] The ADA uses a hemoglobin A_{1C} of less than 8% as the benchmark for adequate control.[19] The AACE recommends a glucose target of 6.5% or less in most nonpregnant adults if it can be achieved safely, as near-normal levels may prevent microvascular (eg, retinopathy) complications.[4] SOR Ⓒ

NONPHARMACOLOGIC

- Diet and exercise interventions
- Diet—Nutrition advice may be best delivered by a registered dietician familiar with DM. Guidelines from the ADA and AACE agree that the diet should contain carbohydrate from fruits, vegetables, whole grains, legumes, and low-fat milk, and be kept consistent on a day-to-day basis with respect to time and amount.[19] In otherwise healthy patients with DM, optimal diets include protein (15%-20% of daily energy intake), fiber (25-50 g/d, with special emphasis on soluble fiber sources [7-13 g], to help to lower cholesterol), and dietary fat of less than 30% of daily energy intake.
- A Cochrane review of 11 randomized controlled trials (RCTs) concluded that a low-glycemic index diet improved glycemic control over a higher-glycemic index diet with fewer hypoglycemic episodes in one trial and fewer hyperglycemic episodes in another trial.[20]
- Daily consumption of vitamin D (500 IU as a fortified yogurt drink or supplement vs placebo) improved glycemic control in one trial of patients with type 2 DM,[21] but not in another trial with patients with type 2 DM and normal vitamin D levels.[22] Vitamin D appears to have a positive effect on insulin resistance.[23]
- Weight-loss strategies for those who are overweight include diet, physical activity, and behavioral interventions. This combination can result in slight sustained weight loss (1.7 kg or 3.1% of baseline body weight) in comparison with usual care and lowers hemoglobin A_{1C}.[24] SOR Ⓐ A more recent RCT ($N = 593$) found an intensive dietary intervention (dietary consultation every 3 months with monthly nurse support) reduced hemoglobin A_{1C} over the control group (actually had increased hemoglobin A_{1C}); the activity intervention did not confer additional benefit.[25]
- Even without weight loss, structured exercise (>150 min/wk) significantly improves glycemic control in patients with type 2 DM.[26] SOR Ⓐ In this meta-analysis, a combination of dietary and exercise advice also lowered hemoglobin A_{1C}.[26] Individuals with type 2 DM are advised to get 30 to 90 min/d (AACE) or 90 to 150 min/wk (ADA) of exercise to improve glycemic control.[7,13]

Education, self-management, and self-monitoring interventions

- Group-based diabetes education is associated with reductions in hemoglobin A_{1C}, systolic blood pressure, body weight, and the need for diabetic medications.[27] SOR Ⓐ In another Cochrane review, use of a specialized diabetes nurse or case manager improved short-term glycemic control but not improve longer-term outcomes, such as hospital admission rates and quality of life.[28] Although one recent trial ($N = 201$) of behavioral support (video and 5 telephone sessions) for patients with poorly controlled DM did not show benefit on outcomes,[29] another trial ($N = 222$) using 5 educator-led group sessions for patients with poorly controlled DM did find improved glycemic control over the control group, although there were no differences in quality of life or frequency of diabetes self-care.[30]
- Authors of a Cochrane review of 12 trials on blood glucose self-monitoring in patients with type 2 DM not using insulin found a small effect of self-monitoring on glycemic control (reduced hemoglobin A_{1C}) that lasted up to 6 months after initiation but not at or beyond 12 months.[31] There was no evidence that self-monitoring affected patient satisfaction, general well-being, or general health-related quality of life. However, self-monitoring of glucose may be useful for assessing and preventing hypoglycemia and adjusting medications, medical nutrition therapy, and physical activity.[4]
- Structured goal setting was shown in a RCT ($N = 87$) to improve glycemic control up to 1-year postintervention.[32]

MEDICATIONS

Agents that can be used for initial blood pressure control include diuretics, angiotensin-converting enzyme (ACE) inhibitors, and β-blockers. The AACE considers ACE inhibitors or angiotensin II receptor blockers (ARBs) the preferred choice in patients with DM.[7] Combinations of medications may be needed. The blood pressure target is less than 130/80 mm Hg.[4] SOR Ⓒ

- In one trial, an ACE inhibitor plus an ARB increased the risk of advancement to renal dialysis.[33]
- In the ACCORD trial of intensive blood pressure control in patients with type 2 DM ($N = 4733$), there were no additional cardiovascular benefits to targeting a systolic blood pressure of 120 mm Hg versus 140 mm Hg. Patients treated with intensive blood pressure lowering were more likely to experience serious adverse effects (3.3% vs 1.3%).[34]
- In a subgroup analysis from another large blood pressure (BP) trial, progressively greater systolic BP reductions were associated with reduced risk for the primary outcome (pooled cardiovascular [CV] death, nonfatal myocardial infarction or stroke, or hospitalized heart failure) only if the baseline systolic BP levels ranged from 143 to 155 mm Hg; there was no benefit in fatal or nonfatal CV outcomes by reducing systolic BP below 130 mm Hg.[35]

Agents used for glycemic control include metformin (biguanide that suppresses hepatic glucose production), sulfonylureas (eg, glyburide that potentiates insulin secretion), glinides (eg, nateglinide that potentiates insulin secretion), α-glucosidase inhibitors (eg, acarbose that decreases intestinal carbohydrate absorption), thiazolidinediones (eg, rosiglitazone that improves insulin sensitivity), incretin mimetic agent (Bydureon enhances insulin secretion and slows gastric emptying), and a dipeptidyl peptidase inhibitor (sitagliptin that improves glucagon-like peptide levels). Details on efficacy, dosing, and safety can be found elsewhere.[4]

- Of the oral hypoglycemic agents, only metformin and the sulfonylureas have been shown to decrease long-term vascular complications and only metformin decreases all-cause mortality (independently of its effect on glycemic control).[36,37] SOR A Monotherapy, although initially effective for many patients, fails to sustain control in approximately half of patients at 3 years.[38]
- Addition of a second oral agent should be considered when monotherapy does not provide adequate control, usually a sulfonylurea is added and is likely most cost-effective.[39] SOR C Sulfonylureas, glinides, and α-glucosidase inhibitors appear equal in effectiveness when added to metformin.[40] A thiazolidinedione also can be used, but there is concern about increased risk of myocardial infarction; data are conflicting.
- If dual therapy does not provide adequate control, options include adding a basal insulin analog (eg, glargine or detemir), a thiazolidinedione, or dipeptidyl peptidase inhibitor. A meta-analysis of 18 trials did not find a clear difference in benefit between drug classes when adding a third agent for patients who were already on metformin and a sulfonylurea.[41] Bydureon, a once-weekly injection, although recently Food and Drug Administration (FDA) approved, is costly and data are limited as this is so new. In the United Kingdom Prospective Diabetes Study (UKPDS) trial, the use of insulin therapy for patients with type 2 DM was not associated with decreased CV or all-cause mortality despite reductions in blood sugar.[42] A Cochrane review of 6 trials also did not find evidence of major clinical benefit for use of long-acting insulin analogues for patients with type 2 DM.[43] Finally, if insulin is added, continuing metformin if possible is advised as there is less weight gain associated with this combination.[44]
- Consultation with an endocrinologist is suggested if a third agent is needed and choice of agent should be made with consideration of the patient's age (decline in renal and cardiac function may preclude use of metformin, a thiazolidinedione, or long-acting sulfonylurea), weight (metformin, acarbose, exenatide, sitagliptin, and human amylin are more often associated with weight loss or maintenance), and comorbidities.[4] SOR C
- If further control is needed, options include discontinuing oral therapy and using combination insulin therapy.

Agents used for lipid control in patients whose lipids are not controlled by diet and exercise is usually achieved with statin therapy.[4] If the initial statin does not result in adequate control, the AACE recommend intensifying that statin to meet the LDL cholesterol goals.[4] SOR A If the LDL goal cannot be met with high-dose statin therapy, there is no evidence to prove that adding other LDL-lowering drug classes will improve outcomes for people with DM.

Treatment of complications of DM is described in detail elsewhere.[4]

COMPLEMENTARY AND ALTERNATIVE THERAPY

- Several Chinese herbal medicines (eg, Xianzhen Pian, Qidan Tongmai) show hypoglycemic effects in patients with type 2 DM but current evidence does not support widespread use.[45]
- In another Cochrane review of herbal mixtures, significant reductions in hemoglobin A_{1C}, fasting blood sugar or both were observed with Diabecon, Inolter, and Cogent db compared to placebo; however, small sample sizes precluded definite conclusions regarding efficacy.[46]

REFERRAL OR HOSPITALIZATION

- Consider referral for bariatric surgery for patients with DM who have a body mass index (BMI) of 35 kg/m^2 or more as this facilitates weight loss and improvement or reversal of hyperglycemia[4]; surgery has not yet been shown to decrease all-cause mortality or provide long-term benefit, and long-term risk is unknown. SOR A
- Consultation with a foot specialist is recommended for patients with DM and foot deformity, infected lesions, foot ulcers, or deformed nails or thick calluses.[4] SOR C
- Refer patients with diabetic retinopathy to an ophthalmologist for evaluation and treatment. SOR B
- Consider consultation with a vascular surgeon for patients with peripheral vascular disease. SOR C
- Patients with type 2 DM may require hospitalization for hyperglycemic crises (eg, hyperosmolar hyperglycemic state, ketoacidosis).

PREVENTION AND SCREENING

Primary prevention is considered for patients who have prediabetes, defined by the AACE as the presence of impaired glucose tolerance (ie, an oral glucose tolerance test glucose value of 140 to 199 mg/dL, 2 hours after ingesting 75 g of glucose and/or a fasting glucose value of 100 to 125 mg/dL).[4] Each year 3% to 10% of individuals with prediabetes will progress to type 2 DM.[47]

- Lifestyle changes that can prevent or at least delay type 2 DM in persons who have prediabetes include weight loss of 5% to 10% of body weight in overweight individuals and participation in moderate physical activity.[4,48,49] SOR A
- Smoking cessation should be encouraged; tobacco smoking increases the risk of macrovascular complications approximately 4% to 400% in adults with type 2 DM (see Chapter 237, Tobacco Addiction).
- Provide annual influenza immunization and pneumococcal vaccine as needed; repeat the pneumococcal vaccine at 5 years for patients with nephrotic syndrome, or chronic renal disease, or who are immunocompromised, or who are receiving the vaccine before age 65 years if 5 years has passed since the primary vaccine was given.[4]
- The AACE also recommends that metformin be considered for those with prediabetes who are younger patients at moderate-to-high risk for developing DM; for patients with additional cardiovascular disease risk factors including hypertension, dyslipidemia, or polycystic ovarian syndrome; for patients with a family history of DM in a first-degree relative; and/or for patients who are obese.[4] A recent RCT found pioglitazone effective in reducing the risk of conversion of impaired glucose tolerance to type 2 DM (annual incidence rate 2.1% vs 7.6% with placebo), but was associated with significant weight gain and edema.[50]
- In a meta-analysis of lifestyle and pharmacologic interventions for the prevention or delay of DM in patients with impaired glucose tolerance, the number needed to treat to benefit was 6.4 for lifestyle (95% CI, 5-8.4), 10.8 for oral diabetes drugs (95% CI, 8.1-15), and 5.4 for orlistat (95% CI, 4.1-7.6).[51] SOR A
- Low-dose aspirin is recommended for patients with DM who have risk factors for CV disease and are older than age 40 years.[13]

Secondary prevention for micro- and macrovascular disease include the following:

- Use of an ACE inhibitor or ARB can prevent progression of diabetic nephropathy.[52] SOR Ⓐ
- Patients with DM should undergo a dilated comprehensive eye examination at diagnosis and annually.[13] SOR Ⓒ Panretinal scatter photocoagulation reduces the risk of severe visual loss by more than 50% in eyes with high-risk characteristics, and immediate focal laser photocoagulation reduces the risk of moderate visual loss by at least 50% in patients with clinically significant macular edema.[53]
- Patients with DM should also undergo screening for peripheral neuropathy at diagnosis and annually, with inspection and assessment of pulses and sensation, using a monofilament and one additional sensory test (eg, pinprick, vibration perception).[13] Patients with peripheral vascular disease, foot ulcers, or diabetic foot deformity should be considered for referral (as above) to prevent limb loss.
- As discussed above, patients with well-controlled BP, lipids, and good glycemic control have a lower risk of macrovascular and microvascular disease, and diabetic dermopathy.[4,10] For example, estimates for years of life saved with lipid lowering in patients with diabetes are 3 years to 3.4 years for men and 1.6 years to 2.4 years for women; greater increases than for patients without diabetes.[54]
- Screening for type 2 DM should be considered in the presence of risk factors for DM (see "Risk Factors" above) and for patients who have increased levels of triglycerides or low concentrations of high-density lipoprotein cholesterol.[4,55] SOR Ⓒ

PROGNOSIS

- Sustained elevation in fasting blood glucose levels and 2-hour postload glucose testing, even when below the threshold for a diabetes diagnosis, is significantly associated with future CV events and mortality. Approximately 75% of patients with type 2 DM die of macrovascular complications, particularly CV disease.[4]
- In 2007, diabetes was listed as the underlying cause on 71,382 death certificates and was listed as a contributing factor on an additional 160,022 death certificates.[1] Complications of diabetes contributing to death included heart disease (noted on 68% of death certificates among those age 65 years or older) and stroke (16%).
- Diabetes is the leading cause of new cases of blindness (4.4% have advanced diabetic retinopathy), kidney failure (48,374 people began treatment for end-stage renal disease in 2008), and nontraumatic lower-limb amputation (65,700 amputations in 2006).[1]

FOLLOW-UP

- Routine follow-up is recommended to continue to assist patients with risk factor reduction, adherence to treatment, screening for diabetes complications (including depression), and to provide ongoing support and guidance. Visit frequency depends on the patient's needs, recent changes in management, and severity of complications. The AACE recommends regular visits at least every 3 to 6 months to review and reinforce BP and blood glucose targets and management of ongoing risk factors (including alcohol and tobacco use).[4]
- The AACE also recommends contact within 1 week after a major modification of the treatment plan.[4] At each encounter, ask if the patient has experienced symptoms of hypoglycemia and educate the patient on appropriate recognition, prevention, and management. They also recommend the following[4]:
    - Goal setting for nutrition and physical activity regularly.
    - Monitor hemoglobin A_{1C} every 3 to 6 months, LDL or fasting lipid profile yearly (unless stable and with no change in medication), and microalbuminuria annually with serum creatinine if albuminuria is abnormal. If microalbuminuria testing is positive (>30 mg/g), repeat twice in the next 3 months. If 2 of 3 of these screening microalbuminuria tests are positive, the individual has microalbuminuria and interventions should be considered.[4] A negative finding should be followed yearly; a positive finding should be followed periodically to see if the interventions are effective in diminishing the albuminuria.
    - Remind the patient to schedule dilated ophthalmic examinations with an optometrist or ophthalmologist.
    - Monitor foot examinations annually or more frequently and educate the patient on appropriate recognition, prevention, and management of infections.

PATIENT EDUCATION

- Patient education includes information about DM (eg, treatment options), primary and secondary prevention recommendations, and self-management.
- Recommended self-management activities include goal setting, incorporating nutrition management and physical activity into lifestyle, and prevention and early detection of complications (eg, medication adherence, foot care).[4]

PATIENT RESOURCES

- ADA. Provides information and support—**http://www.diabetes.org/.**
- MedlinePlus. *Diabetes*—**http://www.nlm.nih.gov/medlineplus/diabetes.html.**

PROVIDER RESOURCES

- Handelsman Y, Mechanick JI, Blonde L, et al, AACE Task Force for Developing Diabetes Comprehensive Care Plan. AACE medical guidelines for clinical practice for developing a DM comprehensive care plan. *Endocr Pract*. 2011;17(suppl 2):1-53.
- ADA. Standards of medical care in diabetes–2008. *Diabetes Care*. 2008;31:S1-S108.
- Centers for Disease Control and Prevention. *Diabetes Public Health Resource*—**http://www.cdc.gov/diabetes/.**
- National Diabetes Information Clearing House. *Diabetes*—**http://diabetes.niddk.nih.gov/.**
- National Institute of Diabetes and Digestive and Kidney Diseases. **http://www2.niddk.nih.gov/.**

REFERENCES

1. Centers for Disease Control and Prevention. *Diabetes Fact Sheet (2011)*. http://www.cdc.gov/diabetes/pubs/pdf/ndfs_2011.pdf. Accessed August 2013.
2. Burchfiel CM, Hamman RF, Marshall JA, et al. Cardiovascular risk factors and impaired glucose tolerance: the San Luis Valley Diabetes Study. *Am J Epidemiol*. 1990;131(1):57-70.

3. Juonala M, Magnussen CG, Berenson GS, et al. Childhood adiposity, adult adiposity, and cardiovascular risk factors. *N Engl J Med.* 2011;365(20):1876-1885.
4. Handelsman Y, Mechanick JI, Blonde L, et al. AACE Task Force for Developing Diabetes Comprehensive Care Plan. American Association of Clinical Endocrinologists medical guidelines for clinical practice for developing a diabetes mellitus comprehensive care plan. *Endocr Pract*. 2011;17(suppl 2):1-53.
5. Pan A, Sun Q, Bernstein AM, et al. Red meat consumption and risk of type 2 diabetes: 3 cohorts of US adults and an updated meta-analysis. *Am J Clin Nutr.* 2011;94(4):1088-1096.
6. Grøntved A, Hu FB. Television viewing and risk of type 2 diabetes, cardiovascular disease, and all-cause mortality: a meta-analysis. *JAMA.* 2011;305(23):2448-2455.
7. Yeboah J, Bertoni AG, Herrington DM, et al. Impaired fasting glucose and the risk of incident diabetes mellitus and cardiovascular events in an adult population: MESA (Multi-Ethnic Study of Atherosclerosis). *J Am Coll Cardiol.* 2011;58(2):140-146.
8. Noble D, Mathur R, Dent T, et al. Risk models and scores for type 2 diabetes: systematic review. *BMJ.* 2011;343:d7163.
9. Wilson PW, Meigs JB, Sullivan L, et al. Prediction of incident diabetes mellitus in middle-aged adults: the Framingham Offspring Study. *Arch Intern Med.* 2007;167:1068-1074.
10. Sibbald RG, Landolt SJ, Toth D. Skin and diabetes. *Endocrinol Metab Clin North Am.* 1996;25(2):463-472.
11. Litonjua P, Pinero-Filona A, Aviles-Santa L, et al. Prevalence of acanthosis nigricans in newly-diagnosed type 2 diabetes. *Endocr Pract.* 2004;10:101-106.
12. van der Ven A, Chapman CB, Bowker JH. Charcot neuroarthropathy of the foot and ankle. *J Am Acad Orthop Surg.* 2009;17(9):562-571.
13. American Diabetes Association. *Diagnosing Diabetes and Learning About Prediabetes.* http://www.diabetes.org/diabetes-basics/diagnosis/?loc=DropDownDB-diagnosis. Accessed August 2013.
14. Rolka DB, Narayan KM, Thompson TJ, et al. Performance of recommended screening tests for undiagnosed diabetes and dysglycemia. *Diabetes Care.* 2001;24:1899-1903.
15. Patel A, MacMahon S, Chalmers J, et al. The Advance Collaborative Group. Intensive blood glucose control and vascular outcomes in patients with type 2 diabetes. *N Engl J Med.* 2008;358(24):2560-2572.
16. Gerstein HC, Miller ME, Byington, RP, et al. Action to Control Cardiovascular Risk in Diabetes Study Group. Effects of intensive glucose lowering in type 2 diabetes. *N Engl J Med.* 2008;358:2545-2559.
17. Hemmingsen B, Lund SS, Gluud C, et al. Intensive glycaemic control for patients with type 2 diabetes: systematic review with meta-analysis and trial sequential analysis of randomised clinical trials. *BMJ.* 2011;343:d6898.
18. Currie CJ, Peters JR, Tynan A, et al. Survival as a function of HbA(1c) in people with type 2 diabetes: a retrospective cohort study. *Lancet.* 2010;375(9713):481-489.
19. American Diabetes Association Position Statement. Standards of medical care in diabetes-2012. *Diabetes Care.* 2012;35 (suppl 1):S11-S63.
20. Thomas D, Elliott EJ. Low glycaemic index, or low glycaemic load, diets for diabetes mellitus. *Cochrane Database Syst Rev.* 2009;(1):CD006296.
21. Nikooyeh B, Neyestani TR, Farvid M, et al. Daily consumption of vitamin D– or vitamin D + calcium-fortified yogurt drink improved glycemic control in patients with type 2 diabetes: a randomized clinical trial. *Am J Clin Nutr.* 2011;93(4):764-771.
22. Jorde R, Figenschau Y. Supplementation with cholecalciferol does not improve glycaemic control in diabetic subjects with normal serum 25-hydroxyvitamin D levels. *Eur J Nutr.* 2009;48(6):349-354.
23. Mitri J, Muraru MD, Pittas AG. Vitamin D and type 2 diabetes: a systematic review. *Eur J Clin Nutr.* 2011;65(9):1005-1015.
24. Norris SL, Zhang X, Avenell A, et al. Long-term non-pharmacological weight loss interventions for adults with type 2 diabetes mellitus. *Cochrane Database Syst Rev.* 2005;(3):CD004095.
25. Andrews RC, Cooper AR, Montgomery AA, et al. Diet or diet plus physical activity versus usual care in patients with newly diagnosed type 2 diabetes: the Early ACTID randomised controlled trial. *Lancet.* 2011;378(9786):129-139.
26. Umpierre D, Ribeiro PA, Kramer CK, et al. Physical activity advice only or structured exercise training and association with HbA1c levels in type 2 diabetes: a systematic review and meta-analysis. *JAMA.* 2011;305(17):1790-1799.
27. Deakin TA, McShane CE, Cade JE, Williams R. Group based training for self-management strategies in people with type 2 diabetes mellitus. *Cochrane Database Syst Rev.* 2005;(2):CD003417.
28. Loveman E, Royle P, Waugh N. Specialist nurses in diabetes mellitus. *Cochrane Database Syst Rev.* 2003;(2):CD003286.
29. Frosch DL, Uy V, Ochoa S, Mangione CM. Comparative effectiveness of goal setting in diabetes mellitus group clinics: randomized clinical trial. *Ann Intern Med.* 2011;171(22):2011-2017.
30. Weinger K, Beverly EA, Lee Y, et al. Quality of life, glucose monitoring, and frequency of diabetes self-care. *Arch Intern Med.* 2011;171(22):1990-1999.
31. Malanda UL, Welschen LM, Riphagen II, et al. Self-monitoring of blood glucose in patients with type 2 diabetes mellitus who are not using insulin. *Cochrane Database Syst Rev.* 2012;(1):CD005060.
32. Naik AD, Palmer N, Petersen NJ, et al. Comparative effectiveness of goal setting in diabetes mellitus group clinics: randomized clinical trial. *Arch Intern Med.* 2011;171(5):453-459.
33. Mann JF, Schmieder RE, McQueen M, et al, for the ONTARGET investigators. Renal outcomes with telmisartan, ramipril, or both, in people at high vascular risk (the ONTARGET study): a multicentre, randomised, double-blind, controlled trial. *Lancet.* 2008;372:547-553.
34. ACCORD Study Group, Cushman WC, Evans GW, Byington RP. Effects of intensive blood-pressure control in type 2 diabetes mellitus. *N Engl J Med.* 2010;362(17):1575-1585.
35. Redon J, Mancia G, Sleight P, et al. Safety and efficacy of low blood pressures among patients with diabetes: subgroup analyses from the ONTARGET (ONgoing Telmisartan Alone and in combination with Ramipril Global Endpoint Trial). *J Am Coll Cardiol.* 2012;59(1):74-83.
36. Inzucchi SE. Oral antihyperglycemic therapy for type 2 diabetes. Scientific review. *JAMA.* 2002;287:360-372.
37. Saenz A, Fernandez-Esteban I, Mataix A, et al. Metformin monotherapy for type 2 diabetes mellitus. *Cochrane Database Syst Rev.* 2005;(3):CD002966.
38. Turner RC, Cull CA, Frighi V, et al. Glycemic control with diet, sulfonylurea, metformin, or insulin in patients with type 2 diabetes

mellitus: progressive requirement for multiple therapies (UKPDS 49). *JAMA*. 1999;281:2005-2012.

39. Klarenbach S, Cameron C, Singh S, Ur E. Cost-effectiveness of second-line antihyperglycemic therapy in patients with type 2 diabetes mellitus inadequately controlled on metformin. *CMAJ*. 2011;183(16):E1213-E1220.

40. Monami M, Lamanna C, Marchionni N, Mannucci E. Comparison of different drugs as add-on treatments to metformin in type 2 diabetes: a meta-analysis. *Diabetes Res Clin Pract*. 2008;79(2):196-203.

41. Gross JL, Kramer CK, Leitao CB, et al. Effect of antihyperglycemic agents added to metformin and a sulfonylurea on glycemic control and weight gain in type 2 diabetes: a network meta-analysis. *Ann Intern Med*. 2011;154(10):672-679.

42. Effect of intensive blood-glucose control with metformin on complications in overweight patients with type 2 diabetes (UKPDS 34). UK Prospective Diabetes Study (UKPDS) Group. *Lancet*. 1998; 352(9131):854-865.

43. Horvath K, Jeitler K, Berghold A, et al. Long-acting insulin analogues versus NPH insulin (human isophane insulin) for type 2 diabetes mellitus. *Cochrane Database Syst Rev*. 2007;(2):CD005613.

44. Goudswaard AN, Furlong NJ, Valk GD, et al. Insulin monotherapy versus combinations of insulin with oral hypoglycaemic agents in patients with type 2 diabetes mellitus. *Cochrane Database Syst Rev*. 2004;(4):CD003418.

45. Liu JP, Zhang M, Wang W, Grimsgaard S. Chinese herbal medicines for type 2 diabetes mellitus. *Cochrane Database Syst Rev*. 2004;(3):CD003642.

46. Sridharan K, Mohan R, Ramaratnam S, Panneerselvam D. Ayurvedic treatments for diabetes mellitus. *Cochrane Database Syst Rev*. 2011;(12):CD008288.

47. Twigg SM, Kamp MC, Davis TM, et al. Prediabetes: a position statement from the Australian Diabetes Society and Australian Diabetes Educators Association. *Med J Aust*. 2007;186(9):461-465.

48. Lindström J, Ilanne-Parikka P, Peltonen M, et al, for the Finnish Diabetes Prevention Study Group. Sustained reduction in the incidence of type 2 diabetes by lifestyle intervention: follow-up of the Finnish Diabetes Prevention Study. *Lancet*. 2006;368(9548): 1673-1679.

49. Tuomilehto J, Lindstrom J, Eriksson JG, et al. Prevention of type 2 diabetes mellitus by changes in lifestyle among subjects with impaired glucose tolerance. *N Engl J Med*. 2001;344(18):1343-1350.

50. DeFronzo RA, Tripathy D, Schwenke DC, et al. Pioglitazone for diabetes prevention in impaired glucose tolerance. *N Engl J Med*. 2011;364(12):1104-1115.

51. Gillies CL, Abrams KR, Lambert PC, et al. Pharmacological and lifestyle interventions to prevent or delay type 2 diabetes in people with impaired glucose tolerance: systematic review and meta-analysis. *BMJ*. 2007;334(7588):299.

52. Strippoli GFM, Craig ME, Craig JC, et al. Antihypertensive agents for preventing diabetic kidney disease. *Cochrane Database Syst Rev*. 2005;(4):CD004136.

53. Neubauer AS, Ulbig MW. Laser treatment in diabetic retinopathy. *Ophthalmologica*. 2007;221(2):95-102.

54. Grover SA, Coupal L, Zowall H, et al. Evaluating the benefits of treating dyslipidemia: the importance of diabetes as a risk factor. *Am J Med*. 2003;115(2):122-128.

55. U.S. Preventive Services Task Force. Screening for type 2 diabetes mellitus in adults: U.S. Preventive Services Task Force recommendation statement. *Ann Intern Med*. 2008;148(11):846-854.

220 ACANTHOSIS NIGRICANS

Mindy A. Smith, MD, MS

PATIENT STORY

A 25-year-old woman with obesity and recently diagnosed type II diabetes mellitus (DM) presents to her physician with concerns about a "dirty area" under her arms and on her neck that "could not be cleaned" (**Figure 220-1**). The physician makes the diagnosis of acanthosis nigricans (AN).

INTRODUCTION

AN is a localized form of hyperpigmentation that involves epidermal alteration. AN is usually associated with insulin resistance and is seen in patients with endocrine disorders (eg, type II DM, Cushing syndrome, acromegaly), obesity, and polycystic ovary syndrome.

EPIDEMIOLOGY

- In a cross-sectional study conducted in a southwestern practice-based research network (N = 1133), AN was found in 21% of adults.[1]
- In another study, AN was present in 36% of patients with newly diagnosed DM.[2]
- AN is sometimes associated with malignancy, primarily adenocarcinoma (60%) of the stomach, gallbladder, colon, ovary, pancreas, rectum, and uterus.[3,4]
- Although most cases are idiopathic, there are also genetic causes of AN.[4]
- A condition of hyperandrogenism (HA), insulin resistance (IR), and AN called HAIR-AN syndrome occurs in approximately 1% to 3% of women with HA.[5] This syndrome may also be seen in patients with autoimmune disorders like Hashimoto thyroiditis.
- AN can be an adverse effect from hormonal therapies.[6]

ETIOLOGY AND PATHOPHYSIOLOGY

- AN results from long-term exposure of keratinocytes to insulin.
- Keratinocytes have insulin and insulin-like growth receptors on their surface and the pathogenesis of this condition may be linked to insulin binding to insulin-like growth receptors in the epidermis.
- Fibroblast growth factor receptor 3 (FGFR3) gene mutations should be considered in patients with coexistent AN and skeletal dysplasia.[7]

DIAGNOSIS

The diagnosis of AN is made clinically in a patient with or at risk for IR who has the characteristic lesions.

CLINICAL FEATURES

- AN ranges in appearance from diffuse streaky thickened brown velvety lesions to leathery verrucous papillomatous lesions (**Figures 220-1** to **220-8**).
- Women with HAIR-AN syndrome have evidence of virilization (eg, increased body hair in male distribution, enlarged clitoris) in addition to AN.[5]

TYPICAL DISTRIBUTION

- Commonly located on the neck (see **Figures 220-2** to **220-4**) or skin folds (ie, axillae [see **Figures 220-1** and **220-8**], inframammary folds, groin, and perineum).

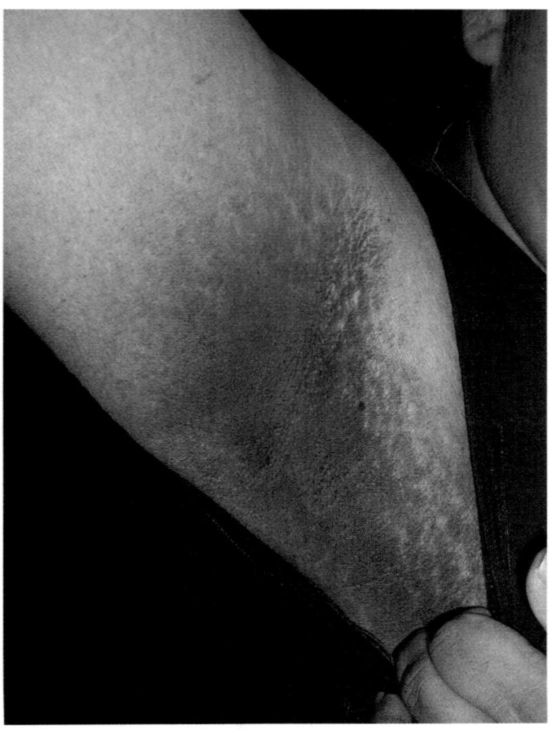

FIGURE 220-1 Acanthosis nigricans in the right axilla of a 25-year-old woman with type 2 diabetes. The skin appears velvety. (*Reproduced with permission from Richard P. Usatine, MD.*)

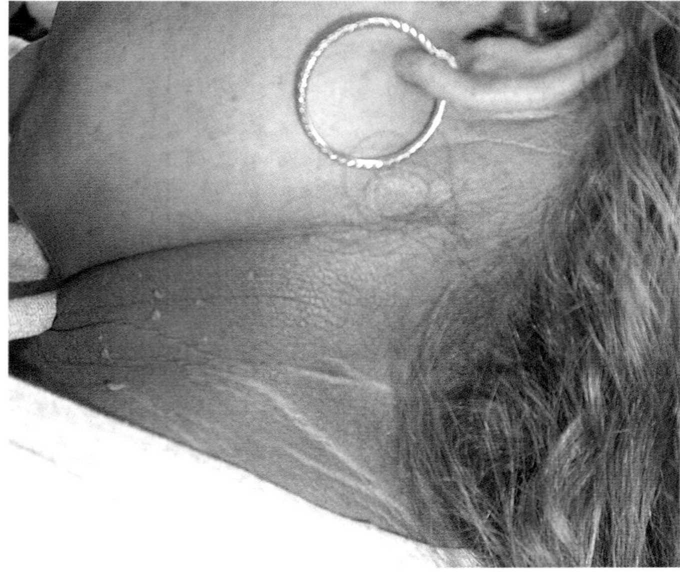

FIGURE 220-2 Acanthosis nigricans on the neck of an obese Hispanic woman with type 2 diabetes. Note that multiple skin tags are also present. (*Reproduced with permission from Richard P. Usatine, MD.*)

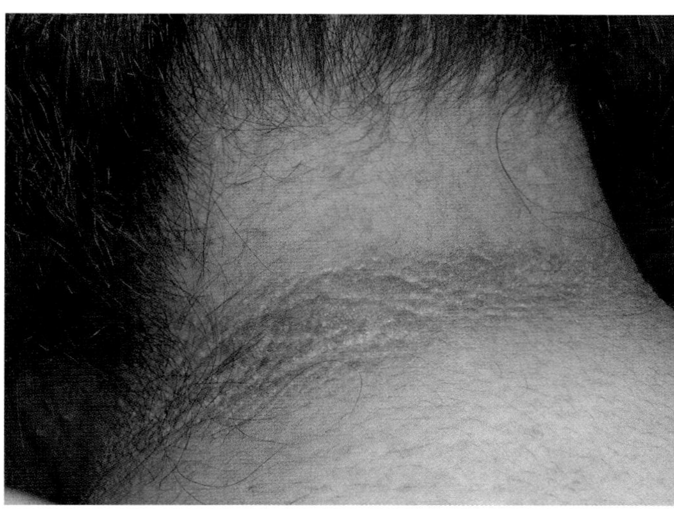

FIGURE 220-3 Acanthosis nigricans on the neck of an obese woman with type II diabetes. Note the hypertrophic thickening of the darker skin. (*Reproduced with permission from Richard P. Usatine, MD.*)

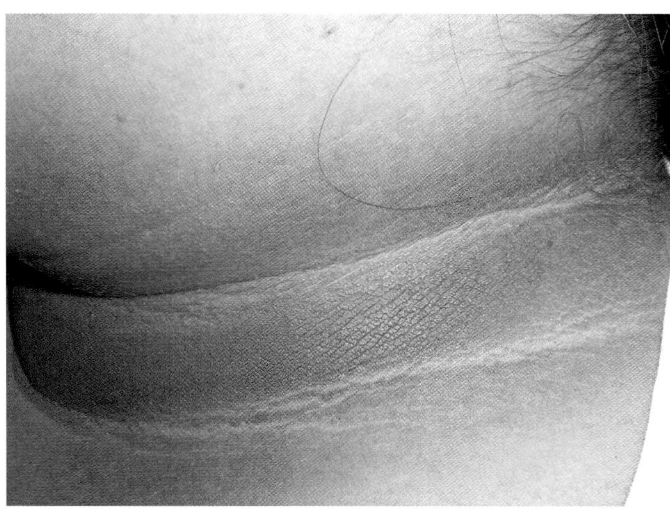

FIGURE 220-4 Acanthosis nigricans with a velvety appearance on the neck of a Hispanic woman with obesity and type 2 diabetes. (*Reproduced with permission from Richard P. Usatine, MD.*)

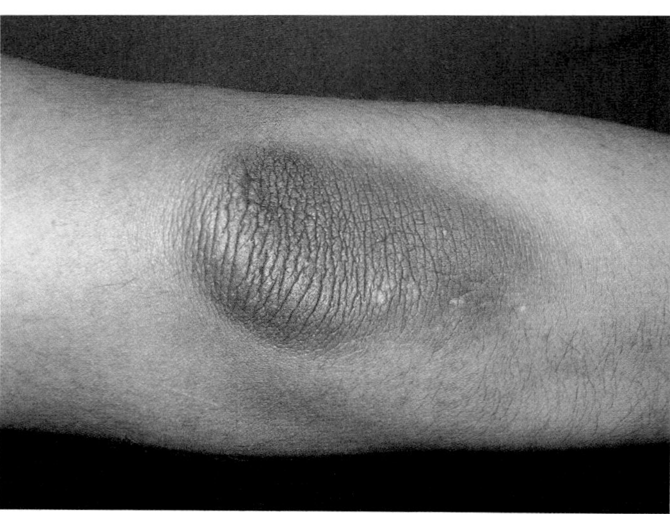

FIGURE 220-5 Acanthosis nigricans on the elbow of a young obese Hispanic woman. (*Reproduced with permission from Richard P. Usatine, MD.*)

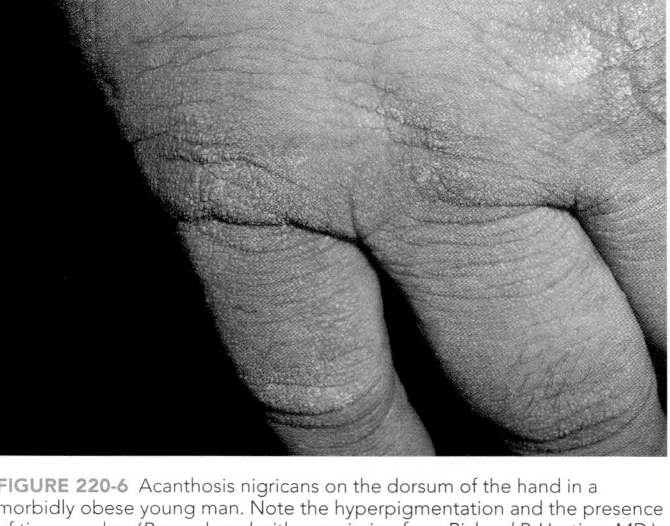

FIGURE 220-6 Acanthosis nigricans on the dorsum of the hand in a morbidly obese young man. Note the hyperpigmentation and the presence of tiny papules. (*Reproduced with permission from Richard P. Usatine, MD.*)

- Less often AN can be seen on the nipples or areolae, perineum, groin, and extensor surfaces of the legs.[4]
- Verrucous AN may affect the eyelids, lips, and buccal mucosa.[4]
- In patients with malignancy, the onset of AN can be abrupt and the distribution of lesions is more widespread and may include the palms and soles.[8]

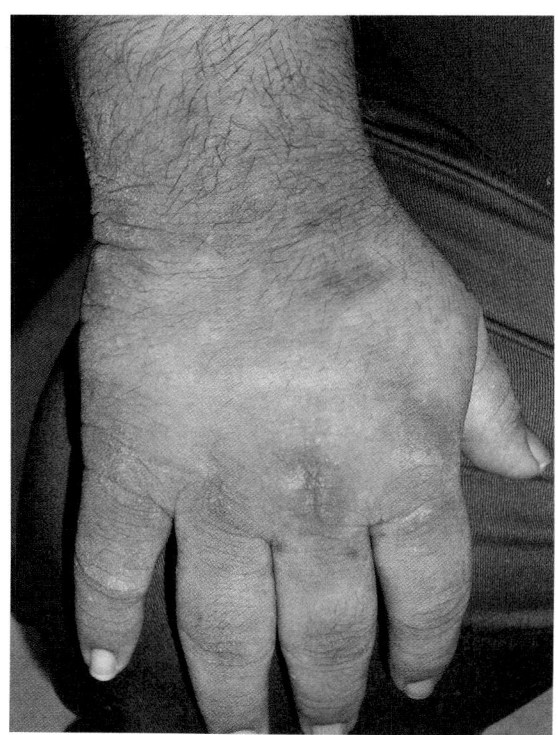

FIGURE 220-7 Acanthosis nigricans on the hand and wrist of a morbidly obese young man with widespread acanthosis. Note the texture of the skin along with the skin darkening. (*Reproduced with permission from Richard P. Usatine, MD.*)

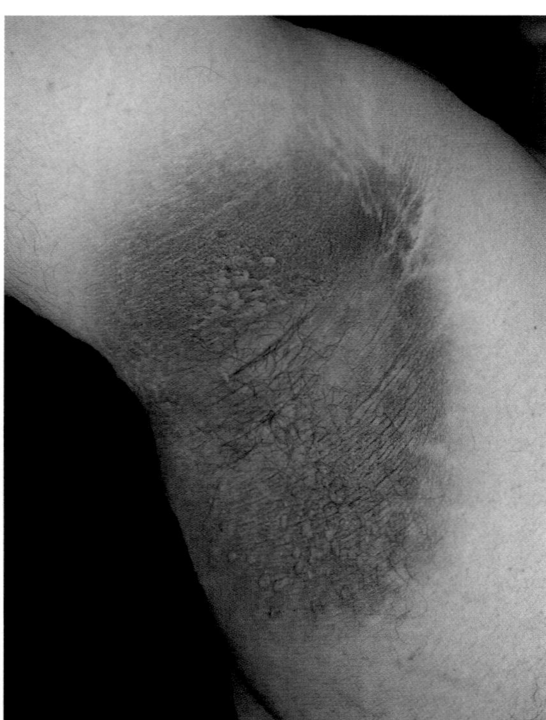

FIGURE 220-8 Acanthosis nigricans in the axilla of a man with type 2 diabetes. Note the many skin tags also present. (*Reproduced with permission from Richard P. Usatine, MD.*)

BIOPSY

- May be needed in unusual cases.
- Histologic examination reveals hyperkeratosis and papillary hypertrophy, although the epidermis is only mildly thickened.[9]

DIFFERENTIAL DIAGNOSIS

Other hyperpigmented lesions that may be confused with AN include the following:

- Seborrheic keratosis (see Chapter 156, Seborrheic Keratosis)—Most commonly found on the trunk or the face; these lesions are more plaque-like with adherent, greasy scale and have a "stuck-on" appearance.
- Pigmented actinic keratosis (see Chapter 164, Actinic Keratosis and Bowen Disease)—Usually in sun-exposed areas; the lesions can be macular or papular with dry, rough adherent scale.

MANAGEMENT

NONPHARMACOLOGIC

- Patients with AN are at higher risk of metabolic syndrome, and lipid screening should be considered along with consideration of testing for DM.
- Weight loss through diet and exercise helps reverse the process, probably by reducing both IR and compensatory hyperinsulinemia.

MEDICATIONS

- Keratolytic agents (eg, salicylic acid) can improve the cosmetic appearance. Other topical therapies, including 0.1% tretinoin cream (to lighten the lesion), combination tretinoin cream with 12% ammonium lactate cream, or topical vitamin D ointments,[10] may be useful.[4] SOR Ⓒ
- Metformin[11] and octreotide have also been used to manage AN. SOR Ⓒ

COMPLEMENTARY AND ALTERNATIVE THERAPY

The use of omega-3-fatty acid and dietary fish oil supplementation has also been reported to improve AN.[12] SOR Ⓒ

PROCEDURES

- Long-pulsed alexandrite laser therapy[13] and dermabrasion are alternative treatments.[4]
- Some patients have many skin tags within the area of acanthosis and they request them to be removed (see **Figure 220-8**). (See Chapter 155, Skin Tag for details on treatment.)

PROGNOSIS

AN usually regresses when the underlying condition (eg, diabetes, malignancy) is treated.[4]

PATIENT EDUCATION

Patients who are overweight should be encouraged to lose weight through diet and exercise because weight loss often resolves this condition.

PATIENT RESOURCES

- PubMed Health. *Acanthosis nigricans*—**http://www.ncbi.nlm.nih.gov/pubmedhealth/PMH0001855/.**
- MedlinePlus. *Acanthosis nigricans*—**http://www.nlm.nih.gov/medlineplus/ency/article/000852.htm.**

PROVIDER RESOURCES

- Diabetes Public Health Resource, National Center for Chronic Disease Prevention and Health Promotion of the Centers for Disease Control and Prevention—**http://www.cdc.gov/diabetes/.**

REFERENCES

1. Kong AS, Williams RL, Smith M, et al. Acanthosis nigricans and diabetes risk factors: prevalence in young persons seen in southwestern US primary care practices. *Ann Fam Med.* 2007;5:202-208.
2. Litonjua P, Pinero-Pilona A, Aviles-Santa L, et al. Prevalence of acanthosis nigricans in newly-diagnosed type 2 diabetes. *Endocr Pract.* 2004;10:101-106.
3. Rendon MI, Cruz PD, Sontheimer RD, Bergstresser PR. Acanthosis nigricans: a cutaneous marker of tissue resistance to insulin. *J Am Acad Dermatol.* 1989;29(3 pt 1):461-469.
4. Kapoor S. Diagnosis and treatment of acanthosis nigricans. *Skinmed.* 2010;8(3):161-164.
5. Elmer KB, George RM. HAIR-AN syndrome: a multisystem challenge. *Am Fam Physician.* 2001;63:2385-2390.

6. Downs AM, Kennedy CT. Somatotrophin-induced acanthosis nigricans. *Br J Dermatol.* 1999;141:390-391.

7. Blomberg M, Jeppesen EM, Skovby F, Benfeldt E. FGFR3 mutations and the skin: report of a patient with a FGFR3 gene mutation, acanthosis nigricans, hypochondroplasia and hyperinsulinemia and review of the literature. *Dermatology.* 2010;220(4):297-305.

8. Stulberg DL, Clark N. Hyperpigmented disorders in adults: part II. *Am Fam Physician.* 2003;68:1963-1968.

9. Sibbald RG, Landolt SJ, Toth D. Skin and diabetes. *Endocrinol Metab Clin North Am.* 1996;25(2):463-472.

10. Hermanns-Le T, Scheen A, Pierard GE. Acanthosis nigricans associated with insulin resistance: pathophysiology and management. *Am J Clin Dermatol.* 2004;5(3):199-203.

11. Wasniewska M, Arrigo T, Crisafulli G, et al. Recovery of acanthosis nigricans under prolonged metformin treatment in an adolescent with normal weight. *J Endocrinol Invest.* 2009;32:939-940.

12. Sheretz EF. Improved acanthosis nigricans with lipodystrophic diabetes during dietary fish oil supplementation. *Arch Dermatol.* 1988;124:1094-1096.

13. Rosenbach A, Ram R. Treatment of acanthosis nigricans of the axillae using a long-pulsed (5-msec) alexandrite laser. *Dermatol Surg.* 2004;30(8):1158-1160.

221 DIABETIC DERMOPATHY

Mindy A. Smith, MD, MS

PATIENT STORY

A 60-year-old woman with diabetes mellitus (DM) for the past 10 years began to notice reddish-colored lesions on both anterior shins that turned brown over the past year (**Figure 221-1**). She reported no pain with the hyperpigmented areas but does have foot pain secondary to neuropathy. The patient is diagnosed with diabetic dermopathy, and she begins working with her physician on achieving better control of her diabetes.

INTRODUCTION

Diabetic dermopathy is a constellation of well-demarcated, hyperpigmented, atrophic depressions, macules, or papules located on the anterior surface of the lower legs that is usually found in patients with DM. It is the most common cutaneous marker of DM.

EPIDEMIOLOGY

- Diabetic dermopathy is found in 12.5% to 40% of patients and most often in the elderly. It is less common in women.[1]
- In a case series of 100 consecutive inpatients or outpatients in India with DM and skin lesions, diabetic dermopathy was found in 36%.[2] The incidence was much lower in a second case series of 500 patients attending a diabetes clinic in India, with only 0.2% diagnosed with diabetic dermopathy; the authors concluded that because the majority of patients were well controlled (fasting blood sugar <130 mg/mL in 60%), cutaneous signs of chronic hyperglycemia were decreased.[3]
- Sometimes seen in persons without DM, especially patients with circulatory compromise.

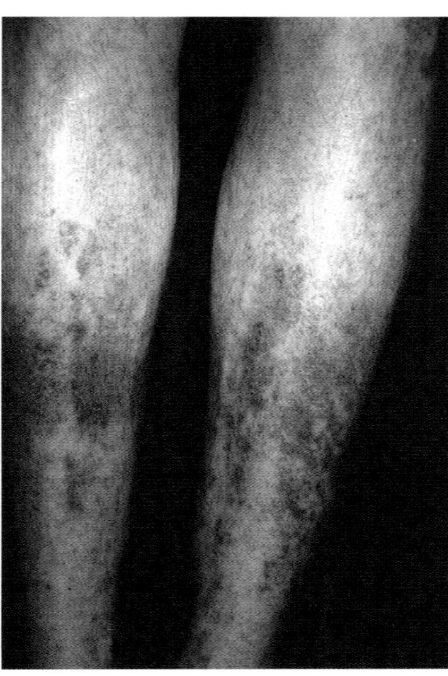

FIGURE 221-1 Lesions of diabetic dermopathy (also called pigmented pretibial papules) on both lower extremities of a 60-year-old woman with diabetes. The skin appears atrophic and the lesions are flat and hyperpigmented. *(Reproduced with permission from the University of Texas Health Sciences Center, Division of Dermatology.)*

ETIOLOGY AND PATHOPHYSIOLOGY

The cause of diabetic dermopathy is unknown.

- Diabetic dermopathy may be related to mechanical or thermal trauma, especially in patients with neuropathy.
- Lesions have been classified as vascular because histology sections demonstrate red blood cell extravasation and capillary basement membrane thickening. In one study, patients with type 1 DM and diabetic dermopathy had marked reduction in skin blood flow at normal-appearing skin areas on the pretibial surface of the legs compared with type 1 control and nondiabetic control patients.[4]
- There is an association between diabetic dermopathy and the presence of retinopathy, nephropathy, and neuropathy.[5,6] In a Turkish study, women with diabetic dermopathy appeared to have a more severe sensorial neuropathy (eg, loss of deep tendon reflexes, superficial sensory loss, and the loss of vibration sense) than did patients without these skin lesions; a high prevalence of carpel tunnel syndrome (63.8%) was also found in these patients.[7]

DIAGNOSIS

CLINICAL FEATURES

The diagnosis is usually clinical. Lesions often begin as pink patches (0.5-1 cm), which become hyperpigmented with surface atrophy and fine scale (**Figures 221-1** to **221-4**).

TYPICAL DISTRIBUTION

It is found in pretibial and lateral areas of the calf (see **Figures 221-1** to **221-4**).

BIOPSY

Histology shows epidermal atrophy, thickened small superficial dermal blood vessels, increased epidermal melanin and hemorrhage with hemosiderin deposits. These findings are not all present in biopsy specimens; in an autopsy series, only 4 of 14 skin biopsies of diabetic dermopathy lesions showed moderate-to-severe wall thickening of arterioles or medium-sized arteries, 11 of 14 showed mild basement membrane thickening, and 9 of 14 had markedly increased epidermal melanin.[8]

DIFFERENTIAL DIAGNOSIS

Consider the following when evaluating patients with similar skin conditions:

- Early lesions of necrobiosis lipoidica diabeticorum—Erythematous papules or plaques beginning in the pretibial area, but become larger and darker with irregular margins and raised erythematous borders. Telangiectasias, atrophy, and yellow discoloration may be seen. The lesion may be painful (see Chapter 222, Necrobiosis Lipoidica).

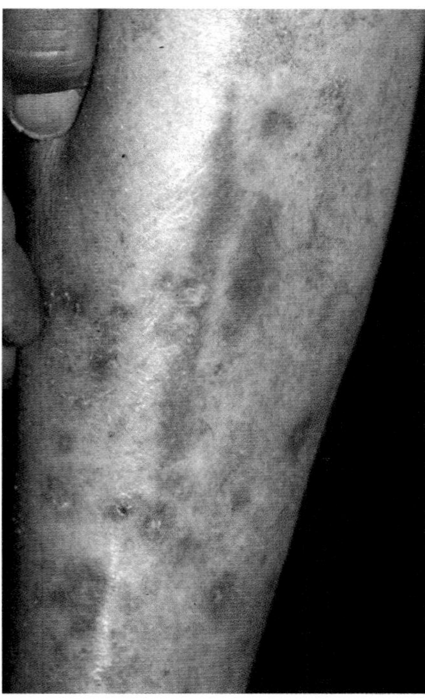

FIGURE 221-2 Diabetic dermopathy on the leg showing pretibial hyperpigmentation and healed ulcers with hypopigmentation. There are also signs of erythema and fine scale. *(Reproduced with permission from the University of Texas Health Sciences Center, Division of Dermatology.)*

- Schamberg disease (pigmented purpuric dermatosis) is a capillaritis that produces brown hemosiderin deposits along with visible pink-to-red spots like cayenne pepper on the lower extremities. It is not more common in diabetes but may resemble diabetic dermopathy. A biopsy could be used to distinguish between them (see Chapter 177, Vasculitis).
- Stasis dermatitis—The typical site is the medial aspect of the ankle. Early lesions are erythematous, scaly, and sometimes pruritic, becoming progressively hyperpigmented (see Chapter 51, Venous Stasis).
- Traumatic scars—There is no scale, lesions are permanent, and edema is not usually present.

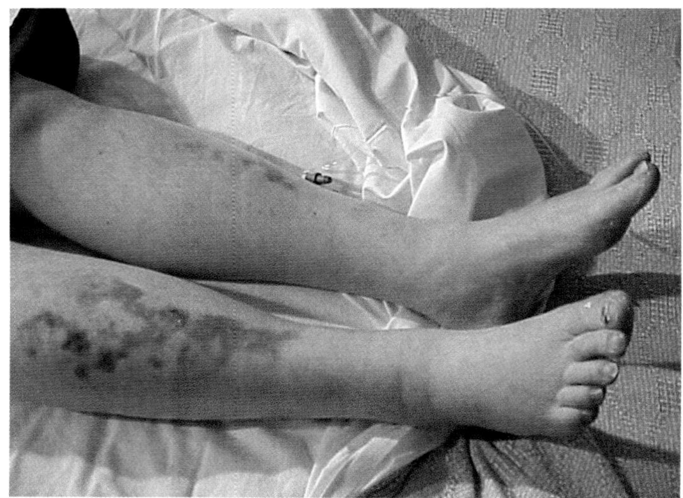

FIGURE 221-3 Diabetic dermopathy on both lower extremities of a middle-aged man with diabetes. The sparse hair is secondary to his vasculopathy. *(Reproduced with permission from Dan Stulberg, MD.)*

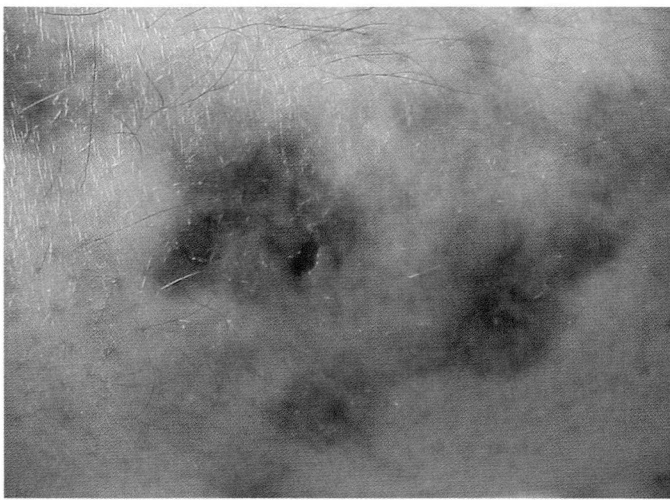

FIGURE 221-4 Close-up of diabetic dermopathy on the right leg showing atrophy, hyperpigmentation, a shallow ulcer, and fine scale. The hyperpigmentation is from hemosiderin deposition. *(Reproduced with permission from Dan Stulberg, MD.)*

MANAGEMENT

- There is no effective treatment.
- It is not known whether the lesions improve with better control of diabetes.
- One informal case report stated that patients may benefit from 15- to 25-mg chelated zinc daily for several weeks.[9] SOR Ⓒ

PREVENTION

It is possible that patients with well-controlled DM have a lower risk of diabetic dermopathy.

PROGNOSIS

Lesions may resolve spontaneously.

PATIENT EDUCATION

Reassure patients that the lesions are asymptomatic and may resolve spontaneously within 1 to 2 years, although new lesions may form.

PATIENT RESOURCES

- American Diabetes Association. *Skin Complications*—**http://www.diabetes.org/living-with-diabetes/complications/skin-complications.html?loc= DropDownLWD-skin.**

PROVIDER RESOURCES

- Skinsight. *Diabetic Dermopathy*—**http://www.skinsight.com/adult/diabeticDermopathy.htm**

REFERENCES

1. Sibbald RG, Landolt SJ, Toth D. Skin and diabetes. *Endocrinol Metab Clin North Am.* 1996;25(2):463-472.
2. Goyal A, Raina S, Kaushal SS, et al. Pattern of cutaneous manifestations in diabetes mellitus. *Indian J Dermatol.* 2010;55(1):39-41.
3. Ragunatha S, Anitha B, Inamadar AC, et al. Cutaneous disorders in 500 diabetic patients attending diabetic clinic. *Indian J Dermatol.* 2011;56(2):160-164.
4. Brugler A, Thompson S, Turner S, et al. Skin blood flow abnormalities in diabetic dermopathy. *J Am Acad Dermatol.* 2011;65(3):559-563.
5. Shemer A, Bergnan R, Linn S, et al. Diabetic dermopathy and internal complications in diabetes mellitus. *Int J Dermatol.* 1998;37(2):113-115.
6. Abdollahi A, Daneshpazhooh M, Amirchaghmaghi E, et al. Dermopathy and retinopathy in diabetes: is there an association. *Dermatology.* 2007;214(2):133-136.
7. Kiziltan ME, Benbir G. Clinical and nerve conduction studies in female patients with diabetic dermopathy. *Acta Diabetol.* 2008;45(2):97-105.
8. McCash S, Emanuel PO. Defining diabetic dermopathy. *J Dermatol.* 2011;38(10):988-992.
9. DiabetesNet.com. *Skin Complications: Necrobiosis Lipoidica*. http://www.diabetesnet.com/diabetes_complications/diabetes_skin_changes.php. Accessed November 2011.

222 NECROBIOSIS LIPOIDICA

Mindy A. Smith, MD, MS

PATIENT STORY

A 30-year-old woman presents with discoloration on both lower legs. She has no personal history of diabetes; however, type 2 diabetes does run in her family. Visible inspection of the lesions is highly suggestive of necrobiosis lipoidica (NL) (**Figure 222-1**). There is hyperpigmentation, yellow discoloration, atrophy, and telangiectasias. The patient is not overweight and had no symptoms of diabetes. Her blood sugar at this visit is 142 after eating lunch 1 hour prior to testing. The following day, the patient's fasting blood sugar is 121, with a glycosylated hemoglobin of 6.1. The patient is informed of her borderline diabetes, and diet and exercise are prescribed. She is disturbed by her skin appearance and chooses to try a moderate-strength topical corticosteroid for treatment.

INTRODUCTION

NL is a chronic granulomatous skin condition with degenerative connective tissue changes most often seen in patients with diabetes mellitus (DM). It was previously called *necrobiosis lipoidica diabeticorum* before the recognition of a significant minority of patients with NL who do not have DM.

EPIDEMIOLOGY

- NL is a rare condition that occurs in approximately 1% (0.3%-2.3%) of patients with DM.[1-4]

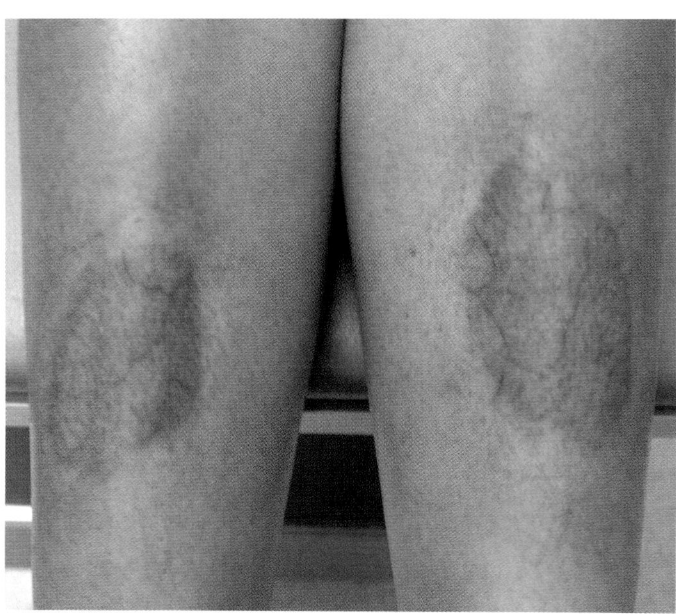

FIGURE 222-1 Necrobiosis lipoidica in a 30-year-old woman with impaired glucose tolerance (borderline diabetes). Note the brown pigmentation and prominent blood vessels. (*Reproduced with permission from Suraj Reddy, MD.*)

- NL primarily affects women (80%), particularly those with type 1 DM, but it can occur with type 2 DM.[1,2] Approximately 75% of patients with NL have or will develop DM.[5]
- Average age of onset is 34 years.[1,2]
- NL has also been reported in patients with Hashimoto thyroiditis.[3]
- Cases of familial NL not associated with DM have also been reported.[6]

ETIOLOGY AND PATHOPHYSIOLOGY

- The cause of NL remains unknown.
- Angiopathy leading to thrombosis and occlusion of the cutaneous vessels has been implicated in its etiology. However, microangiopathic changes are less common in lesions on areas other than the shins and, therefore, are not necessary for developing the lesions.[2] In addition, one study found that NL lesions exhibited significantly higher blood flow rates than areas of unaffected skin close to the lesions.[7]
- Antibodies and C3 have been found at the dermal–epidermal junction, suggesting vasculitis.
- The presence of fibrin in these lesions associated with palisading histiocytes may indicate a delayed hypersensitivity reaction.
- In a study using focus-floating microscopy, a modified immunohistochemical technique was developed to detect *Borrelia* spirochetes. *Borrelia* was detected in 75% of NL lesions overall and 92.7% of inflammatory-rich (38 of 41) versus inflammatory-poor (4 of 15, 26.7%) cases.[8] The authors posit that these findings indicate a potential role for *Borrelia burgdorferi* or other similar strains in the development of or trigger for NL.

DIAGNOSIS

CLINICAL FEATURES

- The lesions begin as erythematous papules or plaques in the pretibial area and become larger and darker with irregular margins and raised erythematous borders (**Figures 222-1** to **222-4**). The lesion's center atrophies and turns yellow in color, appearing waxy (**Figures 222-3, 222-4**, and **222-5A**).

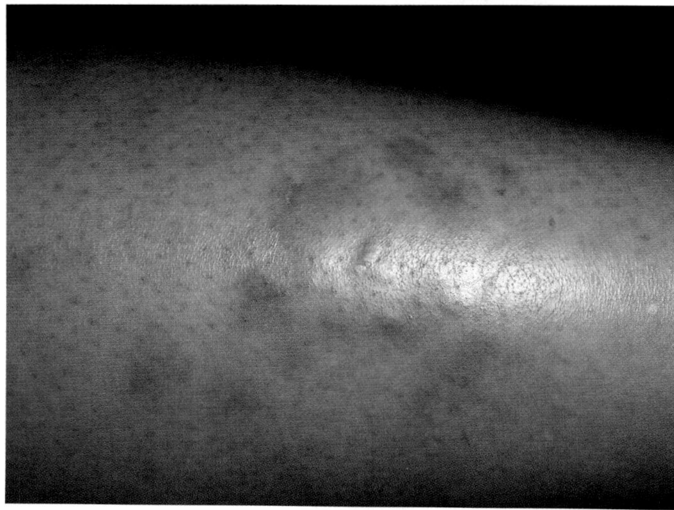

FIGURE 222-2 Necrobiosis lipoidica in a patient with type 1 diabetes. Note the pink area at the site of a healed superficial ulcer. (*Reproduced with permission from Amber Tully, MD.*)

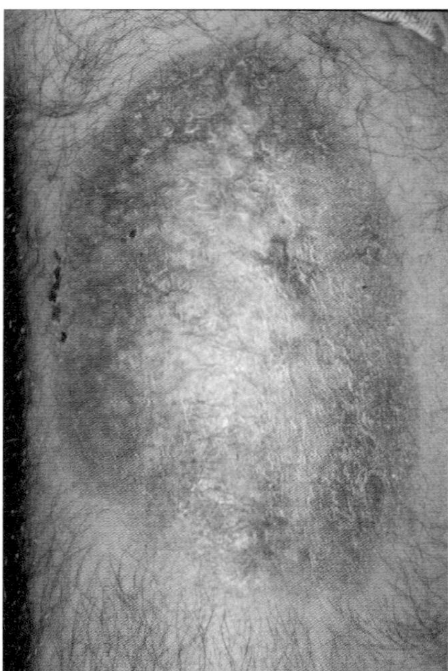

FIGURE 222-3 Necrobiosis lipoidica on the leg of a man with type 2 diabetes. Note the central atrophy and yellow discoloration with a well-demarcated brown border. (*Reproduced with permission from the University of Texas Health Sciences Center, Division of Dermatology.*)

- There is often a prominent brown color or hyperpigmentation visible (see **Figures 222-1** to **222-4**).
- The lesions may ulcerate (occurs in approximately one-third) and become painful (**Figure 222-5B**).

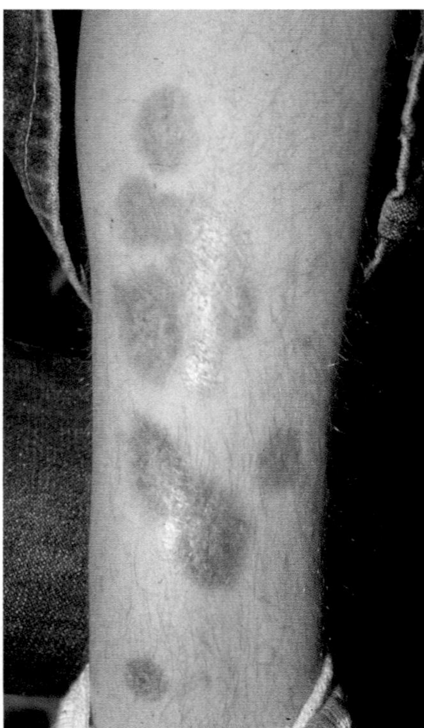

FIGURE 222-4 Multiple lesions of necrobiosis lipoidica in a young adult with type 1 diabetes. Note the central yellow discoloration and well-circumscribed brown borders. (*Reproduced with permission from the University of Texas Health Sciences Center, Division of Dermatology.*)

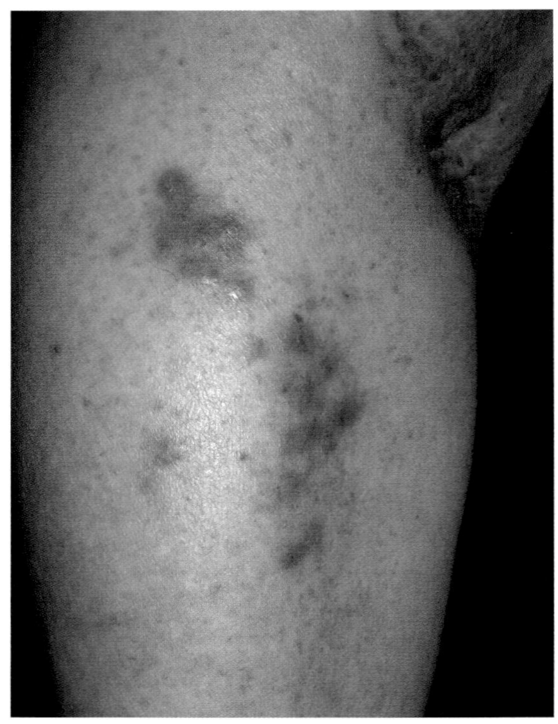

A

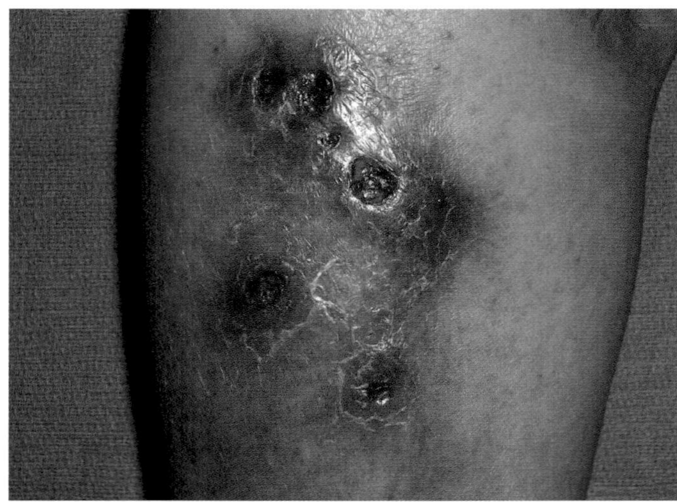

B

FIGURE 222-5 A. Necrobiosis lipoidica on the leg of a woman with no diabetes. It was biopsy proven and treated. B. Worsening and ulcerations of necrobiosis lipoidica despite treatment with topical steroids. (*Reproduced with permission from Richard P. Usatine, MD.*)

- Telangiectasias and prominent blood vessels may be seen within the lesions (see **Figures 222-1** to **222-4**).
- The yellow color may be because of lipid deposits or β-carotene.

TYPICAL DISTRIBUTION

- The lesions are usually located on the shins (90%) (see **Figures 222-1** to **222-4**).
- NL lesions have been reported on many skin areas, including the face, scalp, and penis.[9,10]

BIOPSY

- Biopsy is usually not needed as the clinical picture is usually clear. The dangers of a biopsy include delayed healing and infection in a patient who often has diabetes. The shin region of the leg is notorious for delayed healing even in healthy persons and so biopsy should be avoided in most cases.
- If the diagnosis is uncertain, a punch biopsy will show a thin atrophic epidermis with dermal granulomatous inflammation and obliterative endarteritis. The dermal change shows increased necrobiosis or degeneration of collagen with absence of elastic tissue.

DIFFERENTIAL DIAGNOSIS

NL may be confused with the following conditions:

- Erythema nodosum (EN) is an inflammatory panniculitis that occurs in the same areas (especially shins) as NL. These nodules are pink in color and the skin is smooth above them. The color and lack of epidermal changes should differentiate EN from NL (see Chapter 176, Erythema Nodosum).
- Granuloma annulare—Appears as asymmetric annular red plaques on the dorsum of the hands, extensor surface of the extremities, or posterior neck. They lack the yellow discoloration of NL. These lesions are so visibly like red raised rings that they should appear different from NL. If biopsy is needed, the presence of abundant mucin deposits helps to distinguish these lesions from NL (see Chapter 171, Granuloma Annulare).[2]
- Lichen simplex chronicus—A chronic pruritic eczematous lesion. The lesions are well-circumscribed plaques or papules with lichenified or thickened skin caused by chronic scratching or rubbing. Lesions are commonly located on the ankles, wrists, or posterior nuchal region. The prominent scale and lichenification should help differentiate these lesions from NL (see Chapter 143, Atopic Dermatitis).
- Sarcoidosis skin lesions—Including EN, maculopapular eruptions on the face, nose, back, and extremities; skin plaques that are often purple and raised; and broad macules with telangiectasias that are most commonly seen on the face or hands. Punch biopsy will distinguish between sarcoidosis and NL (see Chapter 173, Sarcoidosis).
- Stasis dermatitis—Occurs on the lower extremities secondary to venous incompetence and edema.[11] Affected patients are usually older, and the typical site is the medial aspect of the ankle. Early lesions are erythematous, scaly, and sometimes pruritic that progressively become hyperpigmented. These lesions are rarely well circumscribed, as seen in NL (see Chapter 51, Venous Stasis).

MANAGEMENT

Evaluate patients not previously diagnosed with DM for diabetes. Even though glycemic control does not correlate with progression of these lesions, DM should be treated to decrease the risk of macro- and microvascular complications.

MEDICATIONS

Data on successful treatment is largely based on case reports. Necrobiosis lesions may respond to the following treatments:

- Local application of potent steroids or intralesional injections of 2.5 mg/mL of triamcinolone.[2] SOR Ⓒ The major risk of these treatments includes increasing the existing atrophy, so patients should be informed of risks and benefits before initiating steroid treatments.
- Topical tacrolimus (0.1% ointment twice daily for 8 weeks followed by once daily for 8 weeks) was successful in a single case report.[12] SOR Ⓒ
- Pentoxifylline (400 mg 2-3 times daily), an agent that improves blood flow and decreases red cell and platelet aggregation, was shown in 2 case reports to completely resolve the lesions at 8 weeks in one[3] and at 6-month follow-up in the other.[4] The latter patient continued therapy and remained in remission at a 2-year follow-up. SOR Ⓒ
- Ulcerative NL has been reported to respond to tetracycline,[13] antimalarial agents (eg, hydroxychloroquine),[14] clofazimine,[15] systemic steroids,[16] antiplatelet therapy,[17] and biologic agents (eg, infliximab infusion, subcutaneous etanercept).[18,19] SOR Ⓒ

REFERRAL

- Refer patients with intractable skin ulcers. In one study that included patients with NL, application of allogeneic cultured dermal substitute was successful in improving healing.[20]
- Topical photodynamic therapy may also be successful in treating refractory NL lesions; in one case series ($N = 18$), overall response rate was 39% with complete resolution in 1 patient and partial resolution in 6 patients.[21] SOR Ⓒ

PROGNOSIS

- Spontaneous resolution occurs in 10% to 20% of cases.
- In a study of patients with DM undergoing pancreatic transplantation ($N = 11$), all 5 patients with NL achieved resolution of NL following transplantation; 1 patient had recurrent NL associated with transplant rejection.[22] The single patient with NL who underwent kidney transplantation had persistent NL.

PATIENT EDUCATION

- Patients with NL without DM should be advised about the increased risk of developing the disease and counseled about symptoms and periodic surveillance.
- NL may resolve spontaneously and does respond to several treatments.

PATIENT RESOURCES

- American Diabetes Association—**http://www.diabetes.org.**
- American Diabetes Association. *Skin Complications*—**http://www.diabetes.org/living-with-diabetes/complications/skin-complications.html?loc=DropDownLWD-skin.**
- American Osteopathic College of Dermatology. *Necrobiosis Lipoidica Diabeticorum*—**http://www.aocd.org/skin/dermatologic_diseases/necrobiosis_lipoid.html.**

PROVIDER RESOURCES

- Medscape. *Necrobiosis Lipoidica*—**http://emedicine.medscape.com/article/1103467-overview.**

REFERENCES

1. Noz KC, Korstanje MJ, Vermeer BJ. Cutaneous manifestations of endocrine disorders: a guide for dermatologists. *Am J Clin Dermatol.* 2003;4(5):315-331.
2. Sibbald RG, Landolt SJ, Toth D. Skin and diabetes. *Endocrinol Metab Clin North Am.* 1996;25(2):463-472.
3. Ahmed K, Muhammad Z, Qayum I. Prevalence of cutaneous manifestations of diabetes mellitus. *J Ayub Med Coll Abbottabad.* 2009;21(2):76-79.
4. Pavlović MD, Milenković T, Dinić M, et al. The prevalence of cutaneous manifestations in young patients with type 1 diabetes. *Diabetes Care.* 2007;30(8):1964-1967.
5. O'Reilly K, Chu J, Meehan S, et al. Necrobiosis lipoidica. *Dermatol Online J.* 2011;17(10):18.
6. Roche-Gamón E, Vilata-Corell JJ, Velasco-Pastor M. Familial necrobiosis lipoidica not associated with diabetes. *Dermatol Online J.* 2007;13(3):26.
7. Ngo B, Wigington G, Hayes K, et al. Skin blood flow in necrobiosis lipoidica diabeticorum. *Int J Dermatol.* 2008;47(4):354-358.
8. Eisendle K, Baltaci M, Kutzner H, Zelger B. Detection of spirochaetal microorganisms by focus floating microscopy in necrobiosis lipoidica in patients from central Europe. *Histopathology.* 2008;52(7):877-884.
9. Lynch M, Callagy G, Mahon S, Murphy LA. Arcuate plaques of the face and scalp. Atypical necrobiosis lipoidica (ANL) of the face and scalp. *Clin Exp Dermatol.* 2010;35(7):799-800.
10. Alonso ML, Riós JC, González-Beato MJ, Herranz P. Necrobiosis lipoidica of the glans penis. *Acta Derm Venereol.* 2011;91(1):105-106.
11. Mistry N, Chih-Ho Hong H, Crawford RI. Pretibial angioplasia: a novel entity encompassing the clinical features of necrobiosis lipoidica and the histopathology of venous insufficiency. *J Cutan Med Surg.* 2011;15(1):15-20.
12. Patsatsi A, Kyriakou A, Sotiriadis D. Necrobiosis lipoidica: early diagnosis and treatment with tacrolimus. *Case Rep Dermatol.* 2011;3(1):89-93.
13. Mahé E, Zimmermann U. Significant improvement in ulcerative necrobiosis lipoidica with doxycycline. *Ann Dermatol Venereol.* 2011;138(10):686-688.
14. Durupt F, Dalle S, Debarbieux S, et al. Successful treatment of necrobiosis lipoidica with antimalarial agents. *Acta Derm Venereol.* 2009;89(6):651-652.
15. Benedix F, Geyer A, Lichte V, et al. Response of ulcerated necrobiosis lipoidica to clofazimine. *Acta Derm Venereol.* 2010;90(1):104-106.
16. Tan E, Patel V, Berth-Jones J. Systemic corticosteroids for the outpatient treatment of necrobiosis lipoidica in a diabetic patient. *J Dermatolog Treat.* 2007;18(4):246-248.
17. Moore AF, Abourizk NN. Necrobiosis lipoidica: an important cutaneous manifestation of diabetes that may respond to antiplatelet therapy. *Endocr Pract.* 2008;14(7):947-948.
18. Hu SW, Bevona C, Winterfield L, et al. Treatment of refractory ulcerative necrobiosis lipoidica diabeticorum with infliximab: report of a case. *Arch Dermatol.* 2009;145(4):437-439.
19. Suárez-Amor O, Pérez-Bustillo A, Ruiz-González I, Rodríguez-Prieto MA. Necrobiosis lipoidica therapy with biologicals: an ulcerated case responding to etanercept and a review of the literature. *Dermatology.* 2010;221(2):117-121.
20. Taniguchi T, Amoh Y, Tanabe K, et al. Treatment of intractable skin ulcers caused by vascular insufficiency with allogeneic cultured dermal substitute: a report of eight cases. *J Artif Organs.* 2012;15(1):77-82.
21. Berking C, Hegyi J, Arenberger P, et al. Photodynamic therapy of necrobiosis lipoidica—a multicenter study of 18 patients. *Dermatology.* 2009;218(2):136-139.
22. Souza AD, El-Azhary RA, Gibson LE. Does pancreas transplant in diabetic patients affect the evolution of necrobiosis lipoidica? *Int J Dermatol.* 2009;48(9):964-970.

223 HYPERLIPIDEMIA AND XANTHOMAS

Mindy A. Smith, MD, MS

PATIENT STORY

A 27-year-old Hispanic man reported new painful nonpruritic bumps, which started 6 months ago, over his entire body. The patient had not seen a physician for 10 months and had run out of his oral medicines for type 2 diabetes mellitus. His grandmother had a milder version of bumps like this years ago. The firm yellowish papules were present all over his body from the neck down (**Figures 223-1** to **223-3**). Laboratory evaluation revealed a random blood sugar of 203, a fasting triglyceride (TG) level greater than 7000 mg/dL, and total cholesterol greater than 700 mg/dL. High-density lipoproteins (HDLs) were 32 mg/dL, and there were no chylomicrons present. The patient was diagnosed with xanthomas, poorly controlled diabetes mellitus, and hyperlipidemia, and was started on metformin, gemfibrozil, and a β-hydroxy-β-methylglutaryl-coenzyme A (HMG-CoA)-reductase inhibitor.

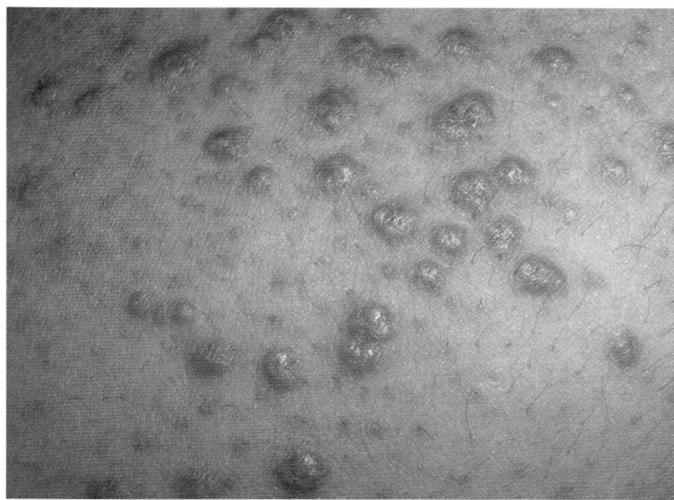

FIGURE 223-1 Close-up of eruptive xanthomas on the arm of a 27-year-old man with untreated hyperlipidemia and diabetes.[1] *(Reproduced with permission from Richard P. Usatine, MD.)*

INTRODUCTION

Hyperlipidemia refers to an elevated concentration of one or more of the measured serum lipid components (total cholesterol [TC], low-density lipid [LDL], HDL, and TGs). Xanthomas are a skin manifestation of familial or severe secondary hyperlipidemia, although they can occur in patients with normal lipid levels. Hyperlipidemia is a major modifiable risk factor for cardiovascular disease.

EPIDEMIOLOGY

- During 2005 to 2006, 15.7% of adults in the United States had a high serum TC level.[1] The average cholesterol level of adults ages 20 to 74 years decreased from 222 mg/dL in 1959 to 1962 to 197 mg/dL in 2007 to 2008, reaching the *Healthy People 2010* goal.[2]
- An estimated 34% of the adult population had high LDL-C during 2005 to 2008 (LDL-C levels above the recommended goal levels or reported current use of cholesterol-lowering medication).[3]
- Among young adults (ages 12-19 years), 20.3% had abnormal lipids; boys are more likely than girls to have at least one lipid abnormality (24.3% vs 15.9%, respectively).[4]
- Patients with heterozygous familial hypercholesterolemia (FH) (1 in 500 persons worldwide) can present as adults with tendon xanthomas.

ETIOLOGY AND PATHOPHYSIOLOGY

- Lipoproteins are complexes of lipids and proteins essential for transporting cholesterol, TGs, and fat-soluble vitamins.
- Elevated levels can result from genetically based derangement of lipid metabolism and/or transport or from secondary causes such as diet, medical disorders (eg, type 2 diabetes mellitus [DM], hypothyroidism, chronic kidney disease, cholestatic liver disease), cigarette smoking, obesity, or drugs (eg, corticosteroids, estrogens, retinoids, high-dose β-blockers).
- Increased circulating LDL becomes incorporated into atherosclerotic plaques. These plaques can grow to block blood supply and oxygen delivery resulting in ischemia to vital organs. In addition, if the plaque ruptures, it can precipitate a clot, causing for example myocardial infarction (MI).
- Elevated TG is an independent risk factor for coronary heart disease (CHD) and increases the risk of hepatomegaly, splenomegaly, hepatic

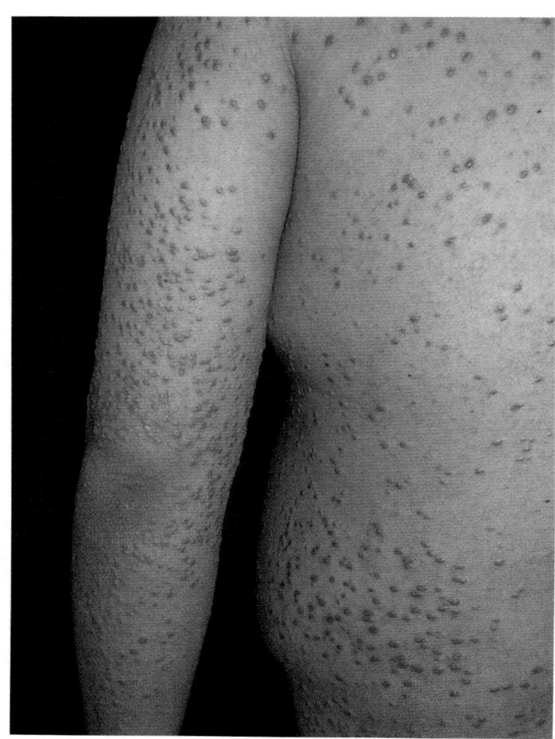

FIGURE 223-2 Eruptive xanthomas on the arm and trunk of the man in Figure 223-1. *(Reproduced with permission from Richard P. Usatine, MD.)*

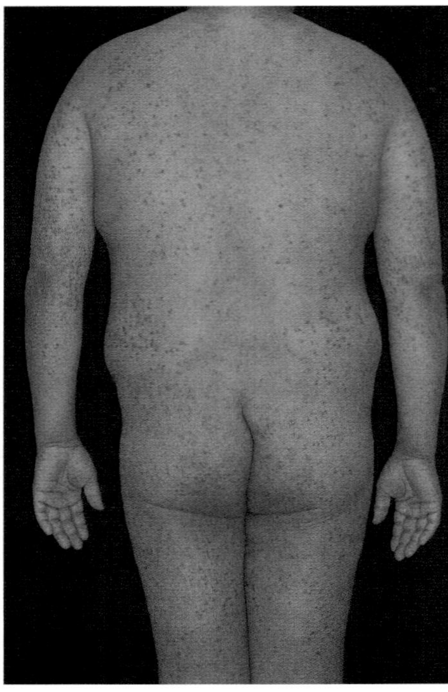

FIGURE 223-3 Eruptive xanthomas covering most of the body of the man in Figure 223-1. (*Reproduced with permission from Richard P. Usatine, MD.*)

steatosis, and pancreatitis. Contributing factors include obesity, physical inactivity, cigarette smoking, excess alcohol intake, medical diseases (eg, type 2 DM, chronic renal failure, nephrotic syndrome), drugs (as above), and genetic disorders (eg, familial combined hyperlipidemia).[5]

- Xanthomas are deposits of lipid in the skin or subcutaneous tissue, usually occurring as a consequence of primary or secondary hyperlipidemia. Xanthomas can also be seen in association with monoclonal gammopathy.[6] There are 5 basic types of xanthomas:
  - Eruptive xanthomas (also called tuberoeruptive) are the most common form. These appear as crops of yellow or hyperpigmented papules with erythematous halos in white persons (see **Figures 223-1** to **223-3**), appearing hyperpigmented in black persons (**Figures 223-4** and **223-5**).

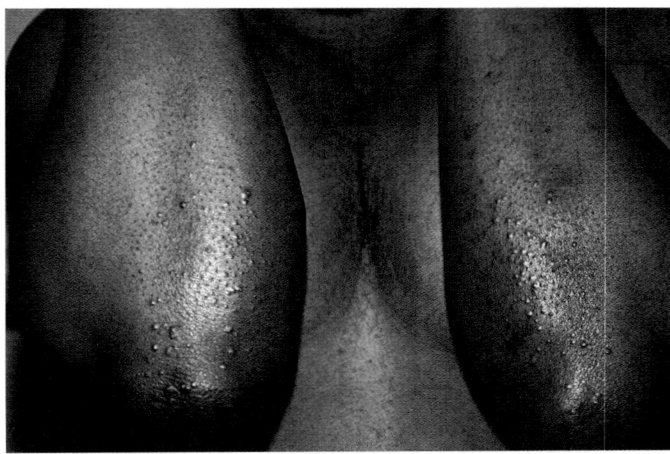

FIGURE 223-4 Eruptive xanthomas on the elbows of a hyperlipidemic black man with type 2 diabetes. His triglycerides and total cholesterol levels were high.1 (*Reproduced with permission from Richard P. Usatine, MD. Previously published in the Western Journal of Medicine.*)

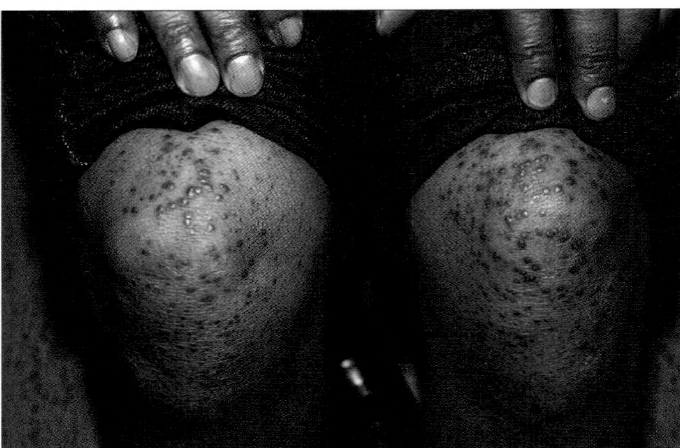

FIGURE 223-5 Eruptive xanthomas on the knees in the patient in Figure 223-4. (*Reproduced with permission from Richard P. Usatine, MD. Previously published in the Western Journal of Medicine.*)

  - Tendon xanthomas are frequently seen on the Achilles and extensor finger tendons.
  - Plane xanthomas are flat and commonly seen on the palmar creases, face, upper trunk, and on scars.
  - Tuberous xanthomas are found most frequently on the hand or over large joints.
  - Xanthelasma are yellow papules found on the eyelids (**Figure 223-6**). Fifty percent of individuals with xanthelasmas have normal lipid profiles.

RISK FACTORS

Risk factors to consider for treatment decisions for patients with hyperlipidemia include the following:

- Type 2 DM
- Family history of early CHD or familial hyperlipidemia
- Cardiac risk factors (cigarette smoking, obesity, hypertension, or sedentary lifestyle)

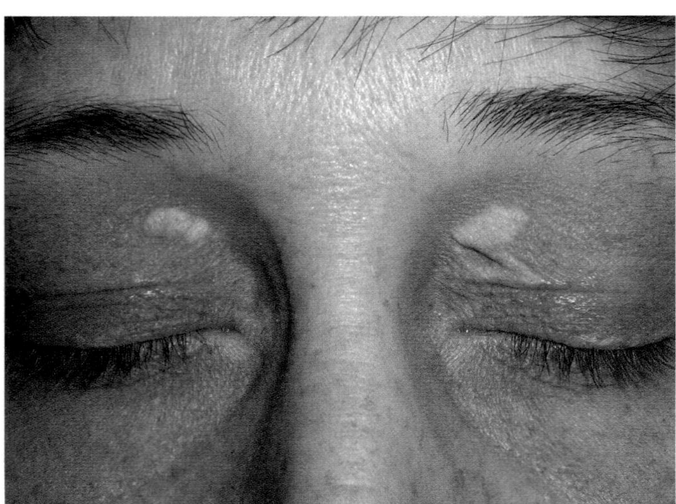

FIGURE 223-6 Xanthelasma around the eyes (xanthoma palpebrarum); most often seen on the medial aspect of the eyelids, with upper lids being more commonly involved than lower lids. (*Reproduced with permission from Richard P. Usatine, MD.*)

DIAGNOSIS

CLINICAL FEATURES

- Most patients with hyperlipidemia are asymptomatic.
- A very high TC level (>2000 mg/dL) may result in eruptive xanthomas or lipemia retinalis (white appearance of the retina; also seen with isolated high TG). Very high LDL may lead to the formation of tendinous xanthomas.
- Xanthomas manifest clinically as yellowish papules, nodules, or tumors (see **Figure 223-1**).
- Eruptive xanthomas (see **Figures 223-2** to **223-5**) begin as clusters of small papules on the elbows, knees, and buttocks that can grow to the size of grapes.
- There is a case report of a patient with normolipidemic xanthomatosis with lesions involving the bones and mucous membranes in addition to skin.[7]

TYPICAL DISTRIBUTION

Xanthomas are most commonly found in superficial soft tissues, such as skin and subcutis, or on tendon sheaths.

LABORATORY TESTING

- The National Cholesterol Education Program (NCEP) III recommends a fasting lipid profile (FLP) as the initial test[5]; alternatively patients may be tested initially with a random TC and HDL.
- If the TC is greater than 200 mg/dL or the HDL less than 40 mg/dL for men or less than 50 mg/dL for women, an FLP is obtained for LDL determination.[5] LDL cannot be determined if TG is greater than 400 mg/dL.
- If thyroid dysfunction is suspected, obtain a thyroid-stimulating hormone level to determine whether thyroid dysfunction is contributing to the lipid abnormalities.
- Other secondary causes to consider include anorexia nervosa, Cushing syndrome, hepatitis, nephrotic syndrome, renal failure, and systemic lupus erythematosus.
- If a statin is under consideration, a baseline creatine phosphokinase (CPK) is recommended before starting statin therapy.

BIOPSY

Biopsy is rarely needed and shows collections of lipid-filled macrophages.

DIFFERENTIAL DIAGNOSIS

Other skin papules that can be mistaken for xanthomas include the following:

- Gouty tophi—Deposits of monosodium urate that are usually firm and occasionally discharge a chalky material (**Figure 223-7**, see Chapter 105, Gout).
- Pseudoxanthoma elasticum—A disorder caused by abnormal deposits of calcium on the elastic fibers of the skin and eye.
- Molluscum contagiosum—Caused by a virus; lesions can be papular and widespread but generally have a central depression (see Chapter 129, Molluscum Contagiosum). The patient in **Figures 223-1** to **223-3** was originally misdiagnosed with molluscum.

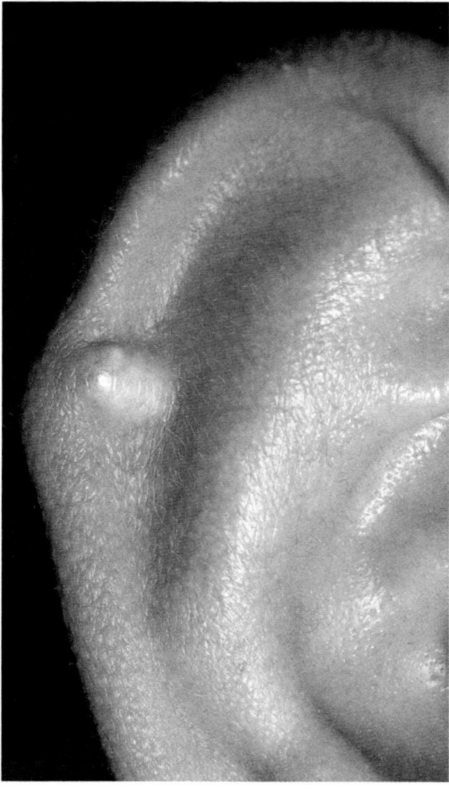

FIGURE 223-7 Ear gouty tophus in a young man with gout. (*Reproduced with permission from Richard P. Usatine, MD.*)

MANAGEMENT

Management of patients with hyperlipidemia emphasizes reduction of cardiovascular risk factors (as noted above) and targets elevated LDL cholesterol for the goal of cholesterol-lowering therapy.[5] Optimal LDL is considered to be less than 100 mg/dL, near optimal LDL is 100 to 129 mg/dL, and high LDL is equal to or greater than 160 mg/dL. The Institute for Clinical Systems Improvement (ICSI) suggests consideration of a goal of less than 70 mg/dL for patients with established CHD, noncardiac atherosclerosis, or CHD equivalent.[8]

- The intensity of therapy should be based on the patient's risk status.[5] The recommended LDL goal is less than 160 for individuals with zero to 1 risk factor (or 10-year CHD risk of <10%), less than 130 mg/dL for 2 or more risk factors, and less than 100 mg/dL for those with CHD or CHD equivalents (eg, DM or 10-year CHD risk of >20%).
- For those with 2 or more risk factors, a 10-year risk assessment is conducted using the Framingham scoring system (http://hp2010.nhlbihin.net/atpiii/calculator.asp) to help identify which individuals would benefit most from intensive treatment.

NONPHARMACOLOGIC

- Smoking cessation should be encouraged and attempts actively supported; cessation lowers both cardiovascular risk and lipid levels. SOR Ⓐ
- Patients should be encouraged to modify their risk factors through exercise and dietary changes. High cholesterol can be lowered through dietary changes. SOR Ⓐ

- Patients who are overweight should be encouraged to reduce calories to achieve weight loss. SOR Ⓒ
- Features of a lipid-lowering diet include reducing intake of total fats to 25% to 35% of total calories (provided trans fatty acids and saturated fats are kept low [<7% of total calories for saturated fats]), reducing cholesterol intake to less than 200 mg/d, and increasing fiber intake to 20 to 30 g/d (5-10 g/d of soluble fiber).[5] SOR Ⓒ Authors of a Cochrane review, however, found no trials on long-term (>6 months) effects of a low-fat diet in patients with hyperlipidemia.[9]
- Similarly, of 11 small trials of dietary intervention identified by authors of a Cochrane review, only short-term outcomes were reported.[10] There were no differences between low-cholesterol diets and other dietary interventions (eg, omega-3 fatty acids, soya proteins, plant sterols or plant stanols), with the exception of plant sterols lowering TC significantly more than a cholesterol-lowering diet.[10]
- Reducing saturated fat through fat modification diets reduces the risk of cardiovascular events by 14% (relative risk [RR] 0.86, 95% confidence interval [CI] 0.77-0.96).[11] SOR Ⓐ This reduction in cardiovascular events was directly related to the degree of effect on serum total and LDL cholesterol and TGs. The strongest evidence was for trials of at least 2 years, duration and in studies of men (not of women). However, there were no clear effects of dietary fat changes on total mortality (RR 0.98, 95% CI 0.93-1.04) or cardiovascular mortality (RR 0.94, 95% CI 0.85-1.04).
- NCEP recommends beginning with lifestyle therapies and reassessing LDL after 6 weeks. If the LDL goal is not met, reinforce lifestyle change along with adding plant sterols and fiber; also consider dietician referral. If the LDL goal is not met at the next 6-week visit, consider medications.[5] Patients hospitalized for a coronary event or procedure should be discharged on drug therapy if their LDL is equal to or greater than 130 mg/dL.[5]
- Addition of plant sterols/stanols up to 2 g/d should be considered, particularly if the initial LDL goal is not met with diet modification and exercise. SOR Ⓑ
- Treatment should also be initiated for patients with high TG (>200-499 mg/dL) or very high TG (≥500 mg/dL) beginning with weight reduction and exercise; for those with very high TGs, a very-low-fat diet is used (≤15% of calorie intake).
- Initial treatment of xanthomas should target the underlying hyperlipidemia (when present).

MEDICATIONS

In addition to primary interventions noted above, secondary therapy includes statins, niacin, fibric acids, ezetimibe, and a bile acid sequestrant.[4,8] The use of combination therapy has not been supported by outcome-based studies.

- Statins (HMG-CoA reductase inhibitors; lovastatin [20-80 mg], pravastatin [20-40 mg], simvastatin [20-80 mg], fluvastatin [20-80 mg], atorvastatin [10-80 mg], and cerivastatin [0.4-0.8 mg]) are considered first line for most patients. Evidence supports use of statins in patients with risk factors for CHD (lowers all-cause mortality [odds ratio (OR) 0.88, 95% CI 0.81-0.96], major coronary events [OR 0.70, 95% CI 0.61-0.81], and major cerebrovascular events [OR 0.81, 95% CI 0.71-0.93])[12] and in patients with CHD or CHD equivalent (reduces mortality risk from CHD and possibly overall mortality).[13] SOR Ⓐ Number needed to treat (NNT) to prevent one additional death in patients with CHD is approximately 30 to 50. There do not appear to be important differences by type of statin.[14]
- Statin side effects include myopathy and increased liver enzymes; statins are associated with a small increase in the risk of developing DM (number needed to harm = 255).[15] The major contraindication is liver disease.
- Niacin (immediate release [crystalline] nicotinic acid [1.5-3 g], extended-release nicotinic acid [Niaspan] [1-2 g], sustained release) is considered a second-line agent to be used in combination with a statin if the LDL goal is not achieved with intensifying monotherapy or as first-line agent for patients with very high TG. Evidence supports reduction in major CHD events with niacin. SOR Ⓐ Niacin is nonprescription.
- Niacin side effects include gastrointestinal (GI) distress, flushing, hyperuricemia, hyperglycemia in patients with DM, and hepatotoxicity. Contraindications are chronic liver disease and severe gout; use with caution in patients with DM, hyperuricemia, peptic ulcer disease.
- Fibrates (gemfibrozil [600 mg bid], fenofibrate [200 mg], clofibrate [1000 mg bid]) is a second-line agent shown to reduce major CHD events but not overall mortality.[16] SOR Ⓐ Fibrates can be used as primary therapy for very high TG. Side effects include dyspepsia, gallstones, myopathy, and unexplained non-CHD deaths. Contraindications are severe renal or hepatic disease.
- Bile acid sequestrants (cholestyramine [4-16 g], colestipol [5-20 g], colesevelam [2.6-3.8 g]) are second-line agents shown to reduce CHD mortality.[11] SOR Ⓐ Side effects include GI distress, constipation, and decreased absorption of other drugs. Contraindications are dysbetalipoproteinemia or TG greater than 400 mg/dL.

Hypolipidemic drug treatment often results in regression of xanthomas. SOR Ⓒ In patients with xanthomas associated with monoclonal gammopathy, hematologic remission following chemotherapy was associated with improvement in the xanthomas in several patients.[6]

COMPLEMENTARY AND ALTERNATIVE THERAPY

- Artichoke leaf extract, red yeast rice, and several Chinese herbal medicines (in particular Xuezhikang) lower cholesterol compared with placebo; data on patient-oriented outcomes are lacking.[17-19]
- It is not clear whether supplementing with omega-3 fatty acids reduces mortality when combined primary and secondary prevention data are analyzed. A 2006 meta-analysis failed to find a reduction in overall mortality or cardiovascular events.[20]
- Benefit is suggested for whole flaxseed and lignan, especially for women, but not for flaxseed oil.[21]
- In a randomized crossover trial, consuming walnuts (42.5 g walnuts/10.1 mJ) and fatty fish (113 g salmon, twice a week) in a healthy diet significantly lowered serum cholesterol and triglyceride concentrations, respectively.[22] In a meta-analysis, nut consumption (67 g) reduced lipid levels.[23]

SURGICAL PROCEDURES

- Between 1975 and 1983, a randomized controlled trial was conducted primarily of male patients following a first MI ($N = 838$) of partial ileal bypass surgery or no surgery. The initial report found improved lipid patterns in patients in the intervention arm,[24] and a 25-year follow-up study found improved survival and cardiovascular disease-free survival in the surgery arm.[25]
- Xanthelasma lesions may be treated for cosmetic purposes. Methods of treatment include surgery, electrosurgery, cryotherapy, and laser therapy.

In a case report of 24 patients, argon laser coagulation was well-tolerated and the cosmetic outcome was considered to be good in 85% of patients.[26] SOR Ⓒ

When standard therapy fails, LDL apheresis has lowered lipid levels with subsequent regression of tendon xanthomas.[27] SOR Ⓒ

REFERRAL

Referral for nutritional counseling should be considered, especially if initial attempts at dietary control fail. Dietary advice has been shown to result in modest improvements in cardiovascular risk factors, such as blood pressure, and total and LDL-cholesterol levels.[28] SOR Ⓐ

PREVENTION AND SCREENING

- The United States Preventive Services Task Force (USPSTF) strongly recommends screening men age 35 years and older for lipid disorders.[29] SOR Ⓐ There is strong evidence that drug therapy reduces CHD events and mortality in middle-aged men (ages 35-70 years) with abnormal lipids and a potential risk of CHD events greater than 1% per year. A Cochrane review confirmed reductions in all-cause mortality, major vascular events, and revascularizations with no cancer excess in 14 trials, 11 recruiting patients with risk factors.[30] In one meta-analysis, NNT for primary prevention in patients (primarily men) with risk factors was 173 to prevent 1 premature death, 81 to prevent 1 CHD event, and 245 to prevent 1 stroke.[12]
- The USPSTF strongly recommends screening women age 45 years and older if they are at increased risk for CHD.[29] SOR Ⓐ The USPSTF also recommends screening men ages 20 to 35 years and women ages 20 to 45 years if they are at increased risk for CHD.[29] SOR Ⓑ There is less direct evidence suggesting effectiveness of drug therapy in other adults, including men older than age 70 years and middle-aged and older women (age 45 years and older) with similar levels of risk.[31] In fact, in a meta-analysis of primary prevention trials including women, there was insufficient evidence of reduced risk of any clinical outcome in women.[32]
- Secondary prevention trials do show reductions in CHD mortality, CHD events, nonfatal MI, and revascularization for women that is similar to reductions seen for men and demonstrate decreased mortality for older men.[33]
- Retesting every 1 to 5 years is recommended by the USPSTF based on CHD risk.[29]
- Studies are not available to assess the efficacy of screening children and adolescents for dyslipidemia for delaying the onset and reducing the incidence of CHD-related events.

PROGNOSIS

- Based on observational data, each 30-mg/dL increase in LDL increases the relative risk of CHD by 30%.
- Use of strategies to lower elevated lipid levels will likely reduce CHD events and possibly overall mortality.
- With medical (diet or drugs) treatment of hyperlipidemia, many xanthomas and about half of xanthelasma resolve or improve with surgical treatment, recurrence is uncommon.[34]

FOLLOW-UP

- NCEP recommends reassessing LDL approximately every 6 weeks until the LDL goal is met, then every 6 to 12 months.[5]
- It is not clear if monitoring liver enzymes in patients on statins is necessary.[35] Repeat a CPK if a patient experiences symptoms of myopathy. Statin therapy should be discontinued if the CPK is more than 10 times normal. For patients with myopathy and moderate or no CPK elevation, conduct weekly monitoring until symptoms improve or discontinue statins if there is worsening or failure to resolve.[36]

PATIENT EDUCATION

- Patients should be counseled about benefits and risks of screening.
- Lifestyle changes should be stressed as primary prevention for patients with hyperlipidemia.
- If persistent elevations in lipids continue despite lifestyle change, those with high risk or CHD should consider medications.
- Patients with hyperlipidemia and/or DM should be encouraged to establish and maintain good control of these diseases, as this often results in regression of xanthomas.

PATIENT RESOURCES

- MedlinePlus. *High blood cholesterol levels*—**http://www.nlm.nih.gov/medlineplus/ency/article/000403.htm.**
- MedlinePlus. *Familial Hypercholesterolemia*—**http://www.nlm.nih.gov/medlineplus/ency/article/000392.htm.**
- MedlinePlus. *Xanthoma*—**www.nlm.nih.gov/medlineplus/ency/article/001447.htm.**

PROVIDER RESOURCES

- Medscape. *Familial Hypercholesterolemia*—**http://emedicine.medscape.com/article/121298.**
- Medscape. *Xanthomas*—**http://emedicine.medscape.com/article/1103971.**

REFERENCES

1. Centers for Disease Control and Prevention. Schober SE, Carroll MD, Lacher DA, Hirsch R. High serum total cholesterol—an indicator for monitoring cholesterol lowering efforts: U.S. adults, 2005-2006. NCHS Data Brief. http://www.cdc.gov/nchs/data/databriefs/db02.pdf. Accessed August 2013.
2. QuickStats: Average total cholesterol level among men and women aged 20-74 years—National Health and Nutrition Examination Survey, United States, 1959-1962 to 2007-2008. *MMWR Morb Mortal Wkly Rep.* September 25, 2009;58(37):1045. http://www.cdc.gov/mmwr/preview/mmwrhtml/mm5837a9.htm. Accessed September 2012.
3. Vital signs: prevalence, treatment, and control of high levels of low-density lipoprotein cholesterol—United States, 1999-2002 and 2005-2008. *MMWR Morb Mortal Wkly Rep.* 2011;60(04):109-114. http://www.cdc.gov/mmwr/preview/mmwrhtml/mm6004a5.htm?s_cid=mm6004a5_w. Accessed January 2012.

4. Prevalence of abnormal lipid levels among youths—United States, 1999-2006. *MMWR Morb Mortal Wkly Rep*. 2010;59(02):29-33. http://www.cdc.gov/mmwr/preview/mmwrhtml/mm5902a1.htm. Accessed August 2013.
5. Third report of the National Cholesterol Education Program (NCEP) Expert Panel on Detection, Evaluation, and Treatment of High Blood Cholesterol in Adults. (Adult Treatment Panel III), Executive Summary. (NCEP/NHLBI., 2004-07-13). http://www.nhlbi.nih.gov/guidelines/cholesterol/index.htm. Accessed August 2013.
6. Szalat R, Arnulf B, Karlin L, et al. Pathogenesis and treatment of xanthomatosis associated with monoclonal gammopathy. *Blood.* 2011;118(14):3777-3784.
7. Akasaka E, Matsuzaki Y, Kimura K, et al. Normolipidaemic xanthomatosis with systemic involvement of the skin, bone and pharynx. *Clin Exp Dermatol.* 2012;37(3):305-307.
8. Institute for Clinical Systems Improvement (ICSI). *Lipid Management in Adults*. Bloomington, MN: Institute for Clinical Systems Improvement (ICSI); 2009, updated 2011. http://www.guideline.gov/content.aspx?id=36062. Accessed August 2013.
9. Smart NA, Marshall BJ, Daley M, et al. Low-fat diets for acquired hypercholesterolaemia. *Cochrane Database Syst Rev.* 2011;(2):CD007957.
10. Shafiq N, Singh M, Kaur S, Khosla P, Malhotra S. Dietary treatment for familial hypercholesterolaemia. *Cochrane Database Syst Rev.* 2010;(1):CD001918.
11. Hooper L, Summerbell CD, Thompson R, et al. Reduced or modified dietary fat for preventing cardiovascular disease. *Cochrane Database Syst Rev.* 2011;(7):CD002137.
12. Brugts JJ, Yetgin T, Hoeks SE, et al. The benefits of statins in people without established cardiovascular disease but with cardiovascular risk factors: meta-analysis of randomised controlled trials. *BMJ.* 2009;338:b2376.
13. Studer M, Briel M, Leimenstoll B, Glass TR, Bucher HC. Effect of different antilipidemic agents and diets on mortality: a systematic review. *Arch Intern Med.* 2005;165:725-730.
14. Zhou Z, Rahme E, Pilote L. Are statins created equal? Evidence from randomized trials of pravastatin, simvastatin, and atorvastatin for cardiovascular disease prevention. *Am Heart J.* 2006;151:273-281.
15. Sattar N, Preiss D, Murray HM, et al. Statins and risk of incident diabetes: a collaborative meta-analysis of randomised statin trials. *Lancet.* 2010;375:735-742.
16. Abourbih S, Filion KB, Joseph L, et al. Effect of fibrates on lipid profiles and cardiovascular outcomes: a systematic review. *Am J Med.* 2009;122:962.e1-e8.
17. Wider B, Pittler MH, Thompson-Coon J, Ernst E. Artichoke leaf extract for treating hypercholesterolaemia. *Cochrane Database Syst Rev.* 2009;(4):CD003335.
18. Becker DJ, Gordon RY, Halbert SC, et al. Red yeast rice for dyslipidemia in statin-intolerant patients: a randomized trial. *Ann Intern Med.* 2009;150(12):830-839.
19. Liu ZL, Liu JP, Zhang AL, et al. Chinese herbal medicines for hypercholesterolemia. *Cochrane Database Syst Rev.* 2011;(7):CD008305.
20. Hooper L, Thompson RL, Harrison RA, et al. Risks and benefits of omega 3 fats for mortality, cardiovascular disease, and cancer: systematic review. *BMJ.* 2006;332:752-760.
21. Pan A, Yu D, Demark-Wahnefried W, et al. Meta-analysis of the effects of flaxseed interventions on blood lipids. *Am J Clin Nutr.* 2009;90(2):288-297.
22. Rajaram S, Haddad EH, Mejia A, Sabaté J. Walnuts and fatty fish influence different serum lipid fractions in normal to mildly hyperlipidemic individuals: a randomized controlled study. *Am J Clin Nutr.* 2009;89(5):S1657-S1663.
23. Sabaté J, Oda K, Ros E. Nut consumption and blood lipid levels: a pooled analysis of 25 intervention trials. *Arch Intern Med.* 2010;170(9):821-827.
24. Buchwald H, Varco RL, Matts JP, et al. Effect of partial ileal bypass surgery on mortality and morbidity from coronary heart disease in patients with hypercholesterolemia. Report of the Program on the Surgical Control of the Hyperlipidemias (POSCH). *N Engl J Med.* 1990;323(14):946-955.
25. Buchwald H, Rudser KD, Williams SE, et al. Overall mortality, incremental life expectancy, and cause of death at 25 years in the program on the surgical control of the hyperlipidemias. *Ann Surg.* 2010;251(6):1034-1040.
26. Basar E, Oguz H, Ozdemir H, et al. Treatment of xanthelasma palpebrarum with argon laser photocoagulation. Argon laser and xanthelasma palpebrarum. *Int Ophthalmol.* 2004;25(1):9-11.
27. Scheel AK, Schettler V, Koziolek M, et al. Impact of chronic LDL apheresis treatment on Achilles tendon affection in patients with severe familial hypercholesterolemia: a clinical and ultrasonographic 3-year follow-up study. *Atherosclerosis.* 2004;174(1):133-139.
28. Brunner E, Rees K, Ward K, Burke M, Thorogood M. Dietary advice for reducing cardiovascular risk. *Cochrane Database Syst Rev.* 2007;(4):CD002128.
29. United States Preventive Services Task Force. *Screening for Lipid Disorders in Adults. 2008*. http://www.uspreventiveservicestaskforce.org/uspstf/uspschol.htm. Accessed January 2012.
30. Taylor F, Ward K, Moore THM, et al. Statins for the primary prevention of cardiovascular disease. *Cochrane Database Syst Rev.* 2011;(1):CD004816.
31. Pignone MP, Phillips CJ, Lannon CM, et al. *Screening for Lipid Disorders. April 2001*. http://www.uspreventiveservicestaskforce.org/uspstf08/lipid/lipides.pdf. Accessed January 2012.
32. Grady D, Chaput L, Kristof M. *Systematic Review of Lipid Lowering Treatment to Reduce Risk of Coronary Heart Disease in Women*. Rockville, MD: Agency for Healthcare Research and Quality; 2003.
33. Helfand M, Carson S. *Screening for Lipid Disorders in Adults: Selective Update of 2001 US Preventive Services Task Force Review. June 2008*. http://www.ncbi.nlm.nih.gov/books/NBK33494/. Accessed August 2013.
34. Fair KP. Xanthoma treatment and management. In: emedicine. Medscape. http://emedicine.medscape.com/article/1103971-treatment#a1128. Accessed August 2013.
35. Cohen DE, Anania FA, Chalasani N; National Lipid Association Statin Safety Task Force Liver Expert Panel. An assessment of statin safety by hepatologists. *Am J Cardiol.* 2006;97:C77-C81.
36. Pasternak RC, Smith SC Jr, Bairey-Merz CN, et al; American College of Cardiology American Heart Association National Heart, Lung and Blood Institute. ACC/AHA/NHLBI clinical advisory on the use and safety of statins. *J Am Coll Cardiol.* 2002;40:567-572.

224 OBESITY

Mindy A. Smith, MD, MS

PATIENT STORY

Diane is a 35-year-old woman who has struggled with obesity for most of her life. Her current body mass index (BMI) is 36. She has tried "every kind of diet you can imagine" but has always gotten stuck after losing the first 10 lb and gets discouraged. She is not currently exercising regularly. She is concerned about all the skin tags on her neck and wants them removed if possible. You obtain a random blood sugar because of the acanthosis and obesity (**Figure 224-1**). The result is 150 mg/dL and you order a fasting blood sugar (FBS) before her next visit, at which time you will remove her skin tags. After discussing diet and exercise, you encourage her to pursue Weight Watchers or a similar program.

INTRODUCTION

Obesity is defined as a BMI greater than or equal to 30. BMI is calculated as weight in kilograms divided by height in meters squared, rounded to 1 decimal place.[1] Adults with a BMI greater than 40 have substantially more serious health consequences, including heart disease and diabetes, and a reduced life expectancy.

EPIDEMIOLOGY

- Based on the National Health and Nutrition Examination Surveys, more than one-third of US adults (35.7%) and 16.9% of children and adolescents are obese (2010).[1] Slightly more women than men are obese (35.8% vs 35.5%). The prevalence of obesity has dramatically increased over the past 20 years.

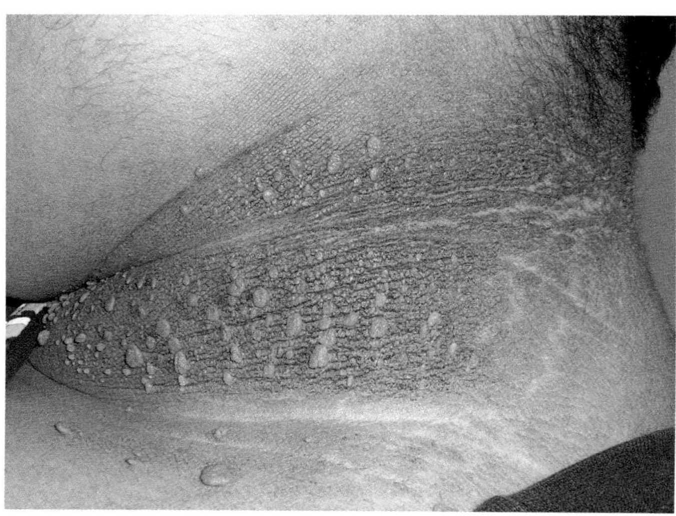

FIGURE 224-1 Neck circumference enlargement with acanthosis nigricans and many skin tags in a woman with obesity and impaired glucose tolerance. (*Reproduced with permission from Richard P. Usatine, MD.*)

- At the 6-year follow-up of the Nurses' Health Study (NHS; a prospective cohort study of 50,277 women), 3757 (7.5%) women who had a BMI of less than 30 in 1992 became obese (BMI ≥30).[2]
- The yearly medical care costs of obesity in the United States are approximately $147 billion.[3]

ETIOLOGY AND PATHOPHYSIOLOGY

Obesity is a complex problem involving genetics, health behaviors, environment, and sometimes medical diseases (see "Differential Diagnosis" later) or drugs (eg, steroids, antidepressants). The simplest explanation of obesity is an imbalance between intake (calories eaten) and output (physical activity).

GENETICS

The genetic contribution to interindividual variation in common obesity has been estimated at 40% to 70%.[4] Despite this relatively high heritability, the search for obesity susceptibility genes has been difficult. At least 5 variants in 4 candidate genes are associated with obesity-related traits. Although genome-wide linkage studies have been unable to pinpoint genetic loci for common obesity, high-density genome-wide association studies have discovered at least 15 previously unanticipated genetic loci associated with BMI and extreme obesity risk.[4] Genetic influences, however, cannot explain the recent increased prevalence in the rate of weight gain by age; rather significant changes in lifestyle factors are likely responsible.[5]

- Two gastrointestinal (GI) "hormones" that appear to integrate into the brain may regulate appetite; these hormones—ghrelin (increases appetite) and obestatin (slows gastric emptying, blocking ghrelin action)—may also play a role in obesity. A meta-analysis concluded that obestatin and total and active ghrelin were significantly higher in normal weight subjects than those of obese groups.[6] It is not clear why this occurs but lower levels of ghrelin in obese subjects may be a response to hyperinsulinemia.

HEALTH BEHAVIORS

Lifestyle factors associated with obesity include physical activity level (low levels and associated behaviors such as television viewing), diet, and sleep.

- In the NHS, each 2-hour per day increment in TV watching was associated with a 23% (95% confidence interval [CI], 17%-30%) and each 2-hour per day increment in sitting at work was associated with a 5% (95% CI, 0%-10%) increase in obesity.[2]
- In one study, belief that obesity was inherited was associated with lower reported levels of physical activity and fruit and vegetable consumption while the belief that obesity was caused by lifestyle behaviors was associated with greater reported physical activity but not diet.[7]
- In a study of Latino men and women, men who did not exercise, rarely trimmed fat from meat, and ate fried foods the previous day were 16 lb heavier than men with healthier habits.[8] Women who had limited exercise (<2.5 hours per week), watched television regularly, ate chips and snacks, and ate no fruit the previous day were 45 lb heavier than women with healthier habits.

ENVIRONMENT

Factors that have been discussed include location of grocery stores versus fast-food restaurants and safe places to exercise in relation to home proximity. Research studies suggest that neighborhood residents who have better access to supermarkets and limited access to convenience stores tend to have healthier diets and lower levels of obesity.[9] Poor neighborhoods are often characterized by just the opposite. In fact, in one study, having the opportunity to move from a poor neighborhood to one with a lower level of poverty through housing vouchers was associated with modest reductions (4.6%) in the prevalence of extreme obesity and diabetes.[10]

RISK FACTORS

- Family history of obesity
- Diet—High calorie, low fruits and vegetables,[11] snack foods, and fast-food consumption (obesity prevalence 24% of those going to fast-food restaurants less than once a week to 33% of those going 3 or more times per week)[12]
- Low levels of physical activity

DIAGNOSIS

The diagnosis of obesity is based on a BMI greater than 30.

CLINICAL FEATURES

- Although elevated weight alone is a risk factor for the development of hypertension, diabetes mellitus (DM), and heart disease, increased waist circumference confers additional morbidity risk (**Figure 224-2**).[13]
- Neck circumference enlargement (see **Figure 224-1**) along with increased BMI and waist circumference are significant risk factors for obstructive sleep apnea and metabolic syndrome.[14,15]
- There is a strong direct correlation between epicardial fat and abdominal visceral adiposity with evidence supporting a role for epicardial fat in the pathogenesis of coronary artery disease.[16]
- Nonalcoholic fatty liver disease (NAFLD) is present in 57% of overweight individuals attending outpatient clinics compared to 98% of nondiabetic obese patients and in contrast to 10% to 30% of adults in the general population (see Chapter 74, Liver Disease).[17]
- Obesity is also associated with an increased risk of varicose veins (odds ratio [OR] 3.28; 95% CI 1.25-8.63) (see Chapter 51, Venous Stasis) (**Figure 224-3**).

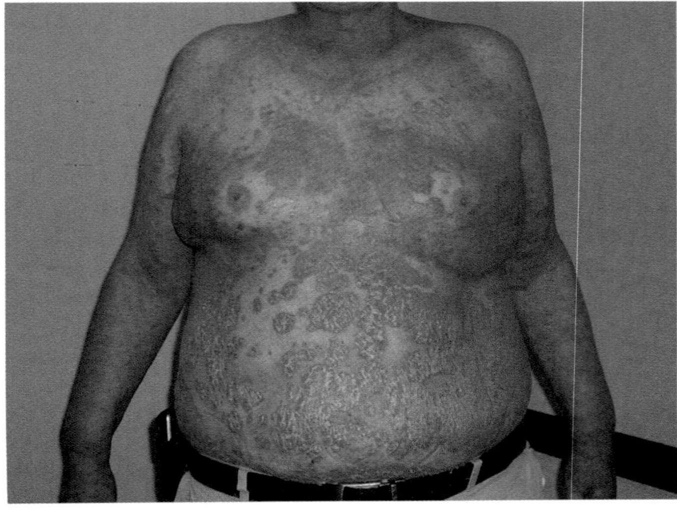

FIGURE 224-2 Central obesity in a man with extensive plaque psoriasis. (*Reproduced with permission from Richard P. Usatine, MD.*)

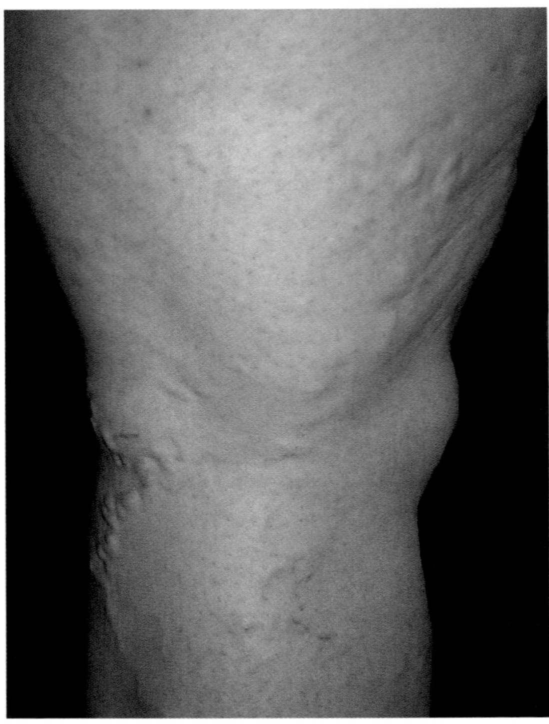

FIGURE 224-3 Serpiginous varicose veins in a woman with obesity. (*Reproduced with permission from Richard P. Usatine, MD.*)

- Skin conditions associated with obesity include acanthosis nigricans (**Figures 224-1** and **224-4**), eruptive xanthomas (**Figure 224-5**), hidradenitis suppurativa (**Figure 224-6**), and psoriasis (see **Figure 224-2**). (see Chapters 117, Hidradenitis Suppurativa, 150, Psoriasis, 220, Acanthosis Nigricans, and 223, Hyperlipidemia).

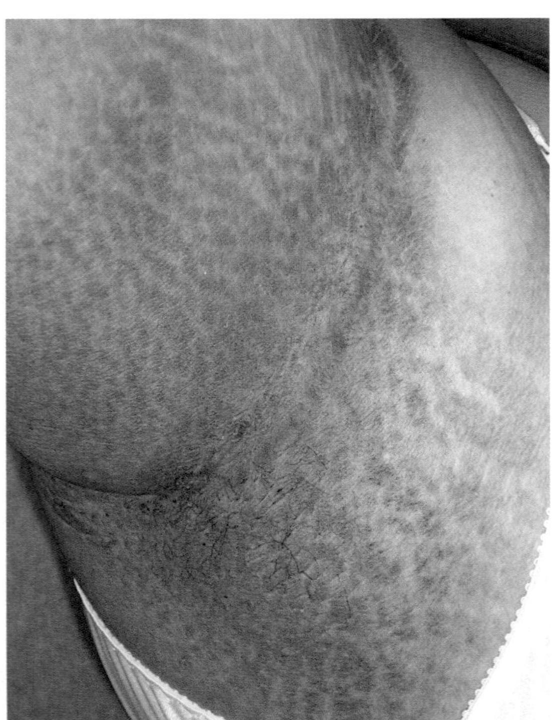

FIGURE 224-4 Acanthosis nigricans and striae in the axilla of a Hispanic woman with obesity and type 2 diabetes. The patient weighs 350 lb. (*Reproduced with permission from Richard P. Usatine, MD.*)

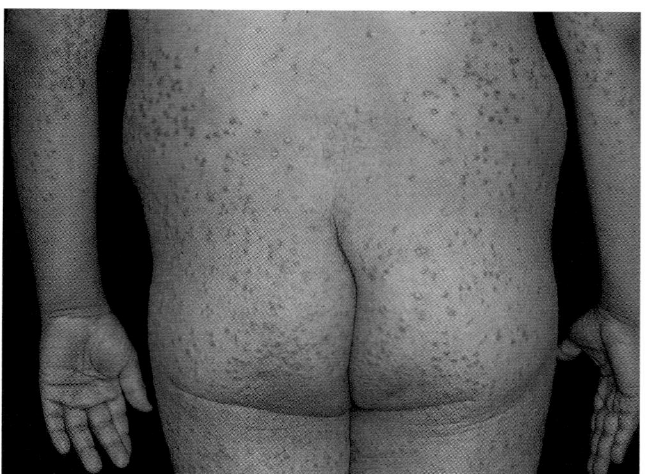

FIGURE 224-5 Eruptive xanthomas in a young man with untreated type 2 diabetes, hyperlipidemia, and obesity. (*Reproduced with permission from Richard P. Usatine, MD.*)

LABORATORY TESTING

Although no specific tests are suggested for patients with obesity, assessing a patient's cardiovascular risk status in addition to BMI, waist circumference, and a patient's motivation to lose weight may be helpful in planning treatment.[13] Consider screening for DM and NAFLD.

DIFFERENTIAL DIAGNOSIS

The differential diagnosis of a patient with obesity includes the following medical conditions:

- Cushing syndrome—Caused by prolonged exposure to endogenous or exogenous glucocorticoids; in addition to truncal obesity, clinical features include moon facies, supraclavicular fat pads, buffalo hump, purple striae, proximal muscle weakness, and hirsutism. Diagnosis is confirmed with inappropriately high serum or urine cortisol levels (see Chapter 229, Cushing syndrome).
- Polycystic ovary syndrome—Criteria include 2 of 3 of oligoovulation or anovulation, hyperandrogenism, and polycystic ovaries.
- Obesity is also a finding in many single-gene disorders such as Prader-Willi syndrome (abnormality of proximal arm of chromosome 15 with associated characteristics of obesity, hypotonia, mental retardation, short stature, hypogonadotropic hypogonadism, strabismus, and small hands and feet) and Bardet-Biedl syndrome (associated with truncal obesity, childhood-onset visual loss preceded by night blindness, and polydactyly).

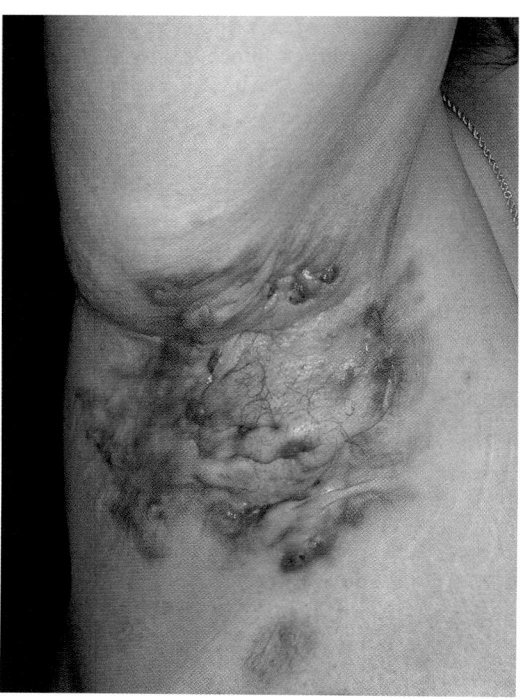

FIGURE 224-6 Hidradenitis suppurativa with significant scarring and sinus tract formation in an obese woman with a body mass index greater than 30. (*Reproduced with permission from Richard P. Usatine, MD.*)

MANAGEMENT

The initial weight loss goal is to reduce body weight by approximately 10% from baseline over approximately 6 months.[13] Additional weight loss can be attempted if this goal is achieved.

NONPHARMACOLOGIC

- Dietary changes may be useful. In a meta-analysis of long-term weight loss strategies in adults, however, dietary/lifestyle therapy provides less than 5 kg weight loss after 2 to 4 years.[18] SOR Ⓐ Commercial weight management services appear to be more effective and cheaper than primary care-based services led by specially trained staff (range 4.4 kg [Weight Watchers] to 1.4 kg [general practice]).[19] SOR Ⓐ
- Exercise should be encouraged and can result in small weight losses and improvement in cardiovascular risk factors; greater intensity exercise results in additional small weight loss (weighted mean difference [WMD] approximately –1.5 kg).[20,21] SOR Ⓐ The addition of diet to exercise also increases weight loss (WMD –1 kg).
- Behavioral and cognitive-behavioral strategies are also effective (WMD –2.5 kg and –2.3 kg, respectively), but are most effective when used in combination with diet and exercise (WMD [added cognitive-behavioral strategies] –4.9 kg).[22] SOR Ⓐ
- Behavioral strategies found to be effective include various forms of support, motivational interviewing, and reducing TV screen time.
- Both remote weight-loss support (study-specific website and e-mail) and in-person support during group and individual sessions along with remote support resulted in greater sustained weight loss at 24 months than the control group (–4.6 kg, –5.1 kg, and –0.8 kg, respectively).[23]
- With respect to psychological interventions, of 3 interventions (usual care with quarterly primary care physician educational visits, brief lifestyle counseling, or enhanced brief lifestyle counseling including meal replacements) examined in adult patients with obesity, enhanced care was more effective than usual care for initial weight loss and sustained weight loss at 2 years (1.7 ± 0.7 and 4.6 ± 0.7 kg, respectively).[24] SOR Ⓑ

MEDICATIONS

- In the 2005 systematic review by Douketis et al., pharmacologic therapy for obesity resulted into 10-kg average weight loss after 1 to 2 years.[18] SOR Ⓐ An older Cochrane review of orlistat, sibutramine, and rimonabant found more modest but significant weight reduction (2.9-4.7 kg); conclusions were limited by high attrition rates.[25]

- The National Heart, Lung, and Blood Institute (NHLBI) *Clinical Guideline* recommends consideration of drug therapy approved by the Food and Drug Administration (FDA) for long-term use as an adjunct to diet and physical activity for patients with a BMI of 30 with no concomitant obesity-related risk factors or diseases, and for patients with a BMI of 27 with concomitant obesity-related risk factors or diseases. SOR Ⓑ The American College of Physicians (ACP) guideline also recommends that pharmacologic therapy may be offered to patients with obesity who fail to achieve their weight loss goals through diet and exercise alone. However, they recommend a discussion of the drugs' side effects, the lack of long-term safety data, and the temporary nature of the weight loss achieved with medications before initiating therapy.[26]
- Medication options include sibutramine, orlistat, phentermine, diethylpropion, rimonabant, fluoxetine, bupropion, and phentermine/topiramate. Most weight loss occurs in the first 6 months of treatment.[27] Investigators conducting a phase III trial of phentermine/topiramate reported greater weight loss for 2 different strengths of the drug over placebo at 1 year (–8.1 kg [lower dose] and –10.2 kg [higher dose] and –1.4 kg [placebo]).[28]

COMPLEMENTARY AND ALTERNATIVE THERAPY

- A number of therapies have been proposed to assist in weight loss, including herbal and nonherbal food supplements, homeopathy, hypnotherapy, acupuncture, and acupressure.[29] Of these, only ephedra sinica and other ephedrine-containing dietary supplements had convincing evidence of small reductions in body weight over placebo.
- A systematic review of food supplements (eg, guar gum, chromium, chitosan) for weight reduction by some of the same authors also failed to find evidence of a clinically relevant weight loss (WMDs in the range of no benefit to –1.7 kg) using these preparations.[30]

SURGERY

Surgical therapy provides approximately 25 to 75 kg of weight loss after 2 to 4 years.[18] According to the NHLBI guideline, weight loss surgery is an option for well-informed, carefully selected patients with clinically severe obesity (BMI 40 or 35 with comorbid conditions) when less-invasive methods of weight loss have failed and the patent is at high risk for obesity-associated morbidity or mortality.[13] SOR Ⓑ The 2005 ACP guideline concurred and again added that a doctor–patient discussion of surgical options should include the long-term side effects (eg, vitamin B_{12} deficiency, incisional hernia, possible need for reoperation, gastritis, gallbladder disease, and malabsorption).[26] In addition, they recommend that patients should be referred to high-volume centers with surgeons experienced in bariatric surgery.

Two types of surgical procedures (gastric banding and gastric bypass) are in current use; all induce substantial weight loss and serve to reduce weight-associated risk factors and comorbidities.

- In a Cochrane review, authors found that weight loss was greater from gastric bypass than vertical banded gastroplasty or adjustable gastric banding, but similar to isolated sleeve gastrectomy and banded gastric bypass.[31] Compared to other interventions available, surgery has produced the longest period of sustained weight loss.
- In a meta-analysis of 8 trials with more than 44,000 patients, the authors concluded that bariatric surgery (both gastric banding and gastric bypass) reduced long-term all-cause mortality (OR = 0.70; CI, 0.59-0.84), although the risk reduction was smaller in the larger studies; gastric bypass had a greater effect than banding on cardiovascular mortality.[32]
- In addition to reduced weight, a retrospective study of severely overweight patients with noninsulin-dependent diabetes who were referred for consideration of a gastric bypass procedure showed that patients undergoing the surgical procedure had a decrease in mortality rate for each year of follow-up compared to those who did not undergo the procedure because of personal preference or refusal of insurance payment.[33]
- Bariatric surgery was also found to be cost-effective compared to other treatments for obesity.[34] Authors identified several remaining questions to be answered, including the influence of surgery on quality of life, late complications leading to reoperation, duration of comorbidity remission, and resource use.
- Laparoscopic bariatric surgery may be safer than open surgery with respect to wound infection (relative risk [RR] 0.21; 95% CI, 0.07-0.65) and incisional hernia (RR 0.11; 95% CI, 0.03-0.35). Risks appear similar for reoperation, anastomotic leak, and all-cause mortality.[35]
- In one study, the rate of hospitalization in the year following gastric bypass surgery was more than double the rate in the preceding year (19.3% vs 7.9%). The most common reasons for admission prior to surgery were obesity-related problems (eg, osteoarthritis, lower extremity cellulitis) and elective operation (eg, hysterectomy). The most common reasons for admission after gastric bypass surgery were complications thought to be procedure related, such as ventral hernia repair and gastric revision.[36]
- In a study of 16,155 Medicare beneficiaries who underwent bariatric procedures (mean age 47.7 years [standard deviation (SD): 11.3 years]; 75.8% women), the rates of 30-day, 90-day, and 1-year mortality were 2.0%, 2.8%, and 4.6%, respectively. After adjustment for sex and comorbidity index, the odds of death within 90 days were 5-fold greater for older Medicare beneficiaries (age 75 years or older; $N = 136$) than for those age 65 to 74 years ($N = 1381$; OR 5; 95% CI, 3.1-8). The odds of death at 90 days were 1.6 times higher (95% CI, 1.3-2) for patients of surgeons with less than the median surgical volume of bariatric procedures.[37]

REFERRAL

The Endocrine Society recommends that patients following bariatric surgery should receive care from a multidisciplinary team, including an experienced primary care physician, endocrinologist, or gastroenterologist. Primary providers should also consider enrolling patients postoperatively in a comprehensive program for nutrition and lifestyle management to prevent and detect nutritional deficiencies.[38]

PREVENTION AND SCREENING

- A behavioral approach of lifestyle counseling from nurse practitioners was not effective compared with usual care in preventing weight gain in overweight or obese adults, although approximately 60% of patients in both groups achieved weight maintenance after 3 years.[39]
- The USPSTF recommends that clinicians screen all adult patients for obesity and offer intensive counseling and behavioral interventions to promote sustained weight loss for obese adults.[40] SOR Ⓑ Evidence, however, was insufficient to recommend for or against the use of moderate- or low-intensity counseling together with behavioral interventions to promote sustained weight loss in obese adults or use of

counseling of any intensity and behavioral interventions to promote sustained weight loss in overweight adults.

PROGNOSIS

Obesity increases the risk in adults for the following[13,41]:

- Chronic health diseases such as coronary heart disease, type 2 DM, stroke, osteoarthritis, liver disease, and gallbladder disease
- Cancers (ie, endometrial, breast, colon, gallbladder)
- Cardiovascular risk factors such as hypertension and dyslipidemia
- Sleep apnea and respiratory problems
- Gynecologic problems (eg, abnormal menses, infertility)

Overweight adolescents are also more susceptible than their leaner peers to hypertension, type 2 DM, dyslipidemia, lung problems (eg, asthma, obstructive sleep apnea), orthopedic problems (eg, genu varum, slipped capital femoral epiphysis), and nonalcoholic steatohepatitis.[42,43] Obese adolescents may also suffer from depression and low self-esteem.[43] In addition, more than half of obese adolescents remain overweight as young adults.[43]

Based on one meta-analysis, intentional weight loss did not confer benefit on all-cause mortality but may provide a small benefit for individuals classified as unhealthy (those with obesity-related risk factors).[44]

FOLLOW-UP

The NHLBI recommends frequent contacts between the patient and provider to promote and monitor weight loss and weight maintenance therapies.[13] SOR Ⓒ Although these programs can be conducted by a practitioner without specialization in weight loss, various health professionals with expertise are available and are often helpful.

PATIENT EDUCATION

- Advise patients to strive for a healthy lifestyle with a diet that is high in fruits and vegetables and to pursue daily physical activity. Maintaining normal weight and treating obstructive sleep apnea and diabetes may help prevent NAFLD.
- Weight loss can improve cardiovascular risk factors. Commercial weight-reduction programs may be most helpful.[19] The addition of cognitive-behavioral strategies may enhance weight loss.[22]
- For patients who are obese and fail to achieve their weight loss goals through diet and exercise alone, pharmacologic therapy can be considered, but pharmacologic therapy adds cost, can be associated with adverse effects, lacks long-term safety data, and weight loss may be temporary.
- Surgery is also an option for carefully selected patients with clinically severe obesity (BMI 40 or 35 with comorbid conditions) when less-invasive methods of weight loss have failed and the patient is at high risk for obesity-associated morbidity or mortality.

PATIENT RESOURCES

- Medline Plus. *Obesity*—**http://www.nlm.nih.gov/medlineplus/obesity.html.**

PROVIDER RESOURCES

- NHLBI. *Clinical Guidelines on the Identification, Evaluation, and Treatment of Overweight and Obesity in Adults* (1998 guideline, BMI calculator, tip sheet, evidence tables)—**http://www.nhlbi.nih.gov/guidelines/obesity/ob_home.htm.**
- Centers for Disease Control and Prevention. *Overweight and Obesity*—**http://www.cdc.gov/obesity/index.html.**

REFERENCES

1. Centers for Disease Control and Prevention. *Prevalence of Obesity in the United States, 2009-2010*. http://www.cdc.gov/nchs/data/databriefs/db82.pdf. Accessed August 2013.
2. Hu FB, Li TY, Colditz GA, et al. Television watching and other sedentary behaviors in relation to risk of obesity and type 2 diabetes mellitus in women. *JAMA*. 2003;289(14):1785-1791.
3. Finkelstein EA, Trogdon JG, Cohen JW, Dietz W. Annual medical spending attributable to obesity: payer- and service-specific estimates. *Health Aff*. 2009;28(5):w822-w831.
4. Loos RJ. Recent progress in the genetics of common obesity. *Br J Clin Pharmacol*. 2009;68(6):811-829.
5. Dodor BA, Shelley MC, Hausafus CO. Adolescents' health behaviors and obesity: does race affect this epidemic? *Nutr Res Pract*. 2010;4(6):528-534.
6. Zhang N, Yuan C, Li Z, et al. Meta-analysis of the relationship between obestatin and ghrelin levels and the ghrelin/obestatin ratio with respect to obesity. *Am J Med Sci*. 2011;341(1):48-55.
7. Wang C, Coups EJ. Causal beliefs about obesity and associated health behaviors: results from a population-based survey. *Int J Behav Nutr Phys Act*. 2010;7:19.
8. Hubert HB, Snider J, Winkleby MA. Health status, health behaviors, and acculturation factors associated with overweight and obesity in Latinos from a community and agricultural labor camp survey. *Prev Med*. 2005;50(6):642-651.
9. Larson NI, Story MT, Nelson MC. Neighborhood environments: disparities in access to healthy foods in the U.S. *Am J Prev Med*. 2009;36(1):74-81.
10. Ludwig J, Sanbonmastu L, Gennetian L, et al. Neighborhoods, obesity, and diabetes—a randomized social experiment. *N Engl J Med*. 2011;365(16):1509-1519.
11. Mozaffarian D, Hao T, Rimm EB, et al. Changes in diet and lifestyle and long-term weight gain in women and men. *N Engl J Med*. 2011;364(25):2392-2404.
12. Anderson B, Rafferty AP, Lyon-Callo S, et al. Fast-food consumption and obesity among Michigan adults. *Prev Chronic Dis*. 2011; Jul;8(4):A71.
13. National Heart Lung and Blood Institute. *Clinical Guidelines on the Identification, Evaluation, and Treatment of Overweight and Obesity in Adults*. http://www.nhlbi.nih.gov/guidelines/obesity/ob_home.htm. Accessed August 2013.
14. Soylu AC, Levent E, Sariman N, et al. Obstructive sleep apnea syndrome and anthropometric obesity indexes. *Sleep Breath*. 2011 Dec 3.
15. Onat A, Hergenc G, Yuksel H, et al. Neck circumference as a measure of central obesity: associations with metabolic syndrome and

obstructive sleep apnea syndrome beyond waist circumference. *Clin Nutr.* 2009;28(1):46-51.

16. Rabkin SW. Epicardial fat: properties, function and relationship to obesity. *Obes Rev.* 2007;8(3):253-261.
17. Vernon G, Baranova A, Younossi ZM. Systematic review: the epidemiology and natural history of non-alcoholic fatty liver disease and non-alcoholic steatohepatitis in adults. *Aliment Pharmacol Ther.* 2011;34(3):274-285.
18. Douketis JD, Macie C, Thabane L, Williamson DF. Systematic review of long-term weight loss studies in obese adults: clinical significance and applicability to clinical practice. *Int J Obes (Lond).* 2005;29(10):1153-1167.
19. Jolly K, Lewis A, Beach J, et al. Comparison of range of commercial or primary care led weight reduction programmes with minimal intervention control for weight loss in obesity: Lighten Up randomised controlled trial. *BMJ.* 2011;343:d6500.
20. Shaw KA, Gennat HC, O'Rourke P, Del Mar C. Exercise for overweight or obesity. *Cochrane Database Syst Rev.* 2006;(4):CD003817.
21. Thorogood A, Mottillo S, Shimony A, et al. Isolated aerobic exercise and weight loss: a systematic review and meta-analysis of randomized controlled trials. *Am J Med.* 2011;124(8):747-755.
22. Shaw KA, O'Rourke P, Del Mar C, Kenardy J. Psychological interventions for overweight or obesity. *Cochrane Database Syst Rev.* 2005;(3):CD003818.
23. Appel LJ, Clark JM, Yeh HC, et al. Comparative effectiveness of weight-loss interventions in clinical practice. *N Engl J Med.* 2011;365(21):1959-1968.
24. Wadden TA, Volger S, Sarwer DB, et al. A two-year randomized trial of obesity treatment in primary care practice. *N Engl J Med.* 2011;365(21):1969-1979.
25. Padwal RS, Rucker D, Li SK, Curioni C, Lau DCW. Long-term pharmacotherapy for obesity and overweight. *Cochrane Database Syst Rev.* 2003;(4):CD004094.
26. Snow V, Barry P, Fitterman N, et al. Pharmacologic and surgical management of obesity in primary care: a clinical practice guideline from the American College of Physicians. *Ann Intern Med.* 2005;142(7):525-531.
27. Greenway FL, Caruso MK. Safety of obesity drugs. *Expert Opin Drug Saf.* 2005;4(6):1083-1095.
28. Gadde KM, Allison DB, Ryan DH, et al. Effects of low-dose, controlled-release, phentermine plus topiramate combination on weight and associated comorbidities in overweight and obese adults (CONQUER): a randomised, placebo-controlled, phase 3 trial. *Lancet.* 2011;377(9774):1341-1352.
29. Pitter MH, Ernst E. Complementary therapies for reducing body weight: a systematic review. *Int J Obes (Lond).* 2005;29(9):1030-1038.
30. Onakpoya IJ, Wider B, Pittler MH, Ernst E. Food supplements for body weight reduction: as systematic review of systematic reviews. *Obesity (Silver Spring).* 2011;19(2):239-244.
31. Colquitt JL, Picot J, Loveman E, Clegg AJ. Surgery for obesity. *Cochrane Database Syst Rev.* 2009:(2):CD003641.
32. Pontiroli AE, Morabito A. Long-term prevention of mortality in morbid obesity through bariatric surgery. a systematic review and meta-analysis of trials performed with gastric banding and gastric bypass. *Ann Surg.* 2011;253(3):484-487.
33. MacDonald KG Jr, Long SD, Swanson MS, et al. The gastric bypass operation reduces the progression and mortality of non-insulin-dependent diabetes mellitus. *J Gastrointest Surg.* 1997;1(3):213-220.
34. Picot J, Jones J, Colquitt JL, et al. The clinical effectiveness and cost-effectiveness of bariatric (weight loss) surgery for obesity: a systematic review and economic evaluation. *Health Technol Assess.* 2009;13(41):1-190.
35. Reoch J, Mottillo S, Shimony A, et al. Safety of laparoscopic vs open bariatric surgery: a systematic review and meta-analysis. *Arch Surg.* 2011;146(11):1314-1322.
36. Zingmond DS, McGory ML, Ko CY. Hospitalization before and after gastric bypass surgery. *JAMA.* 2005;294(15):1918-1924.
37. Flum DR, Salem L, Elrod JA, et al. Early mortality among Medicare beneficiaries undergoing bariatric surgical procedures. *JAMA.* 2005;294(15):1903-1908.
38. Heber D, Greenway FL, Kaplan LM, et al. Endocrine and nutritional management of the post-bariatric surgery patient: an Endocrine Society Clinical Practice Guideline. *J Clin Endocrinol Metab.* 2010;95(11):4823-4843.
39. ter Bogt NC, Bemelmans WJ, Beltman FW, et al. Preventing weight gain by lifestyle intervention in a general practice setting: three-year results of a randomized controlled trial. *Arch Intern Med.* 2011;171(4):306-313.
40. US Preventive Services Task Force. *Screening for Obesity in Adults.* http://www.uspreventiveservicestaskforce.org/uspstf/uspsobes.htm. Accessed August 2013.
41. Centers for Disease Control and Prevention. *Overweight and Obesity. Health Consequences.* http://www.cdc.gov/obesity/causes/health.html. Accessed August 2013.
42. Srinivasan SR, Bao W, Wattigney WA, Berenson GS. Adolescent overweight is associated with adult overweight and related multiple cardiovascular risk factors: the Bogalusa Heart Study. *Metabolism.* 1996;45(2):235-240.
43. American Academy of Pediatrics. Committee on Nutrition. Prevention of pediatric overweight and obesity. *Pediatrics.* 2003;112(2):424-430.
44. Harrington M, Gibson S, Cottrell RC. A review and meta-analysis of the effect of weight loss on all-cause mortality risk. *Nutr Res Rev.* 2009;22(1):93-108.

225 OSTEOPOROSIS AND OSTEOPENIA

Mindy Smith, MD, MS

PATIENT STORY

An 83-year-old woman accompanied by her 56-year-old daughter presents to the office with severe upper back pain over the past 2 days. Her medical problems include hypothyroidism, for which she is on replacement medication, and mild hypertension, which is controlled with a diuretic. She has known osteopenia and was taking calcium and vitamin D but had not tolerated a bisphosphonate. Physical examination reveals moderate thoracic kyphosis and tenderness over several lower thoracic vertebrae. A plain radiograph demonstrates vertebral compression fractures (**Figure 225-1A**). The daughter asks about management options for pain and prevention of future fractures and also about screening for herself. As there was a suggestion of multiple compression fractures a computed tomography (CT) was ordered to better visualize the fractures (**Figure 225-1B**).

INTRODUCTION

- Osteoporosis is a skeletal disorder characterized by low bone mineral density (BMD) less than or equal to 2.5 standard deviations (SD) of the mean for a gender-matched young white adult and compromised bone strength predisposing a person to fracture from minimal trauma.
- Osteopenia is defined as a BMD measurement of between 1 and 2.5 SD below the gender-matched young white adult mean. The World Health Organization also defines osteoporosis as a history of fragility fractures and osteopenia.[1]

EPIDEMIOLOGY

- Approximately 12 million Americans older than age 50 years have osteopenia.[2]
- Half of all postmenopausal women will have an osteoporosis-related fracture in their lifetime; 25% will experience a vertebral deformity and 15% will suffer a hip fracture.[2]
- Low BMD at the femoral neck (T-score of –2.5 or below) is found in 21% of postmenopausal white women, 16% of postmenopausal Mexican American women, and 10% of postmenopausal African American women.[3]
- About 1 in 5 older men are at risk of an osteoporosis-related fracture.[2]
- Vertebral fractures can cause severe pain and lead to 150,000 hospital admissions per year in the United States.
- Following a hip fracture, more than 30% of men and approximately 17% of women die within 1 year and more than half are unable to return to independent living.[3]

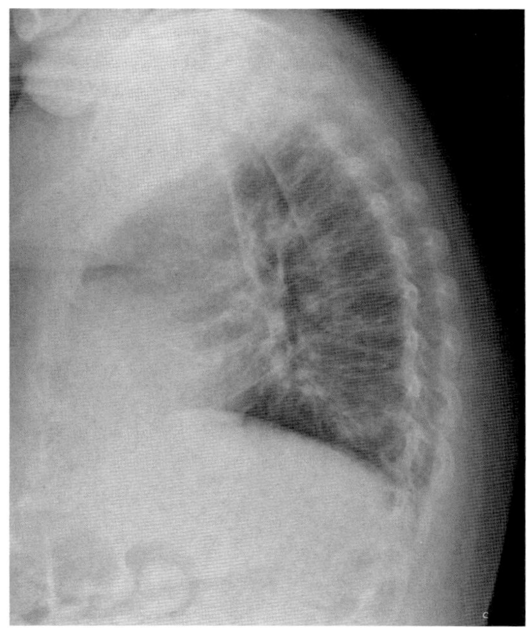

A

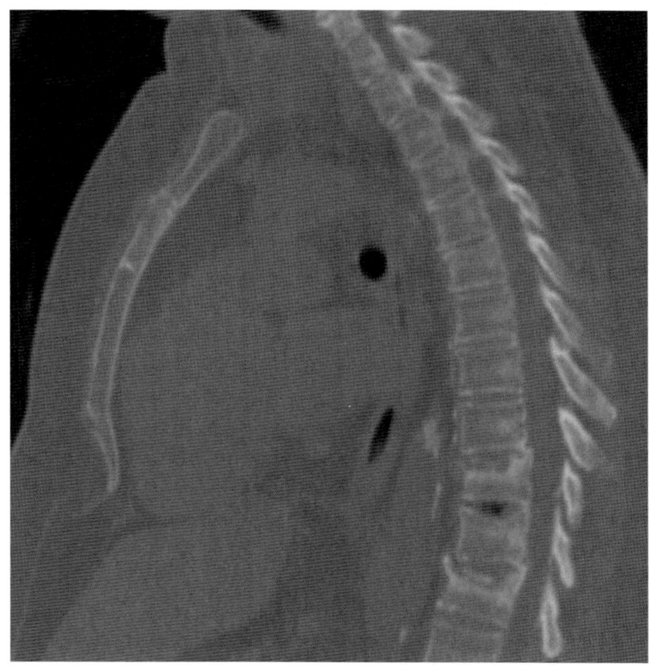

B

FIGURE 225-1 Osteoporosis-related thoracic vertebral compression fractures in an 83-year-old woman with kyphosis. **A.** Lower thoracic vertebral compression fractures seen on the lateral plain radiograph. **B.** Same fractures visualized more clearly on a lateral computed tomography (CT) of the spine. *(Reproduced with permission from Rebecca Loredo-Hernandez, MD.)*

ETIOLOGY AND PATHOPHYSIOLOGY

- Primary osteoporosis is either a result of aging changes or menopause.
  - Usually affects those older than age 70 years.
  - Proportionate loss of cortical and trabecular bone density (**Figure 225-2**). Bone mass peaks at approximately age 30 years and

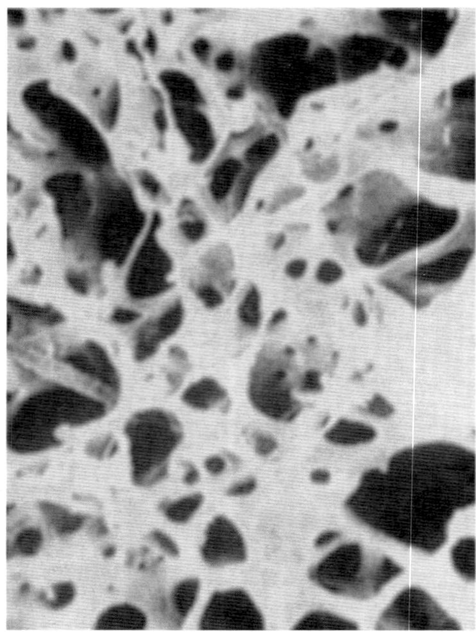
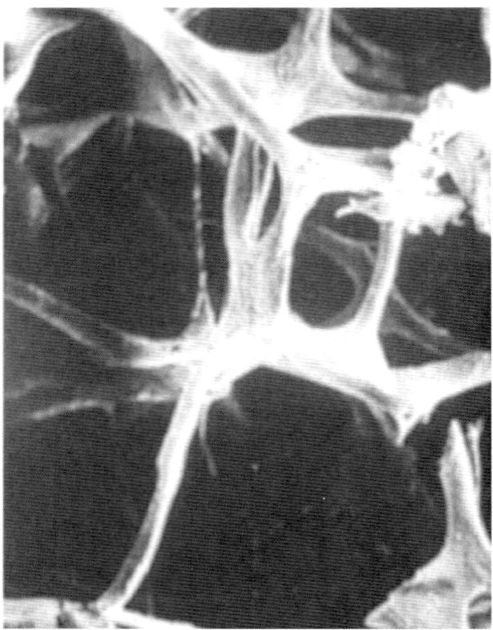

FIGURE 225-2 Normal trabecular bone (*left*) compared with trabecular bone murmur patient with osteoporosis (*right*). The loss of mass in osteoporosis these bones more susceptible to breakage. (*Reproduced with permission from Barrett KE, Barman SM, Boitano S, et al.* Ganong's Review of Medical Physiology. *23rd ed. McGraw-Hill, 2009.*)

declines thereafter. This bone loss can lead to an increase in vertebral, hip, and radius fractures.
    - In the 15 years following menopause, there is a disproportionate loss of trabecular bone. This can lead to an increase in fractures of the vertebrae, distal forearm, and ankle.
- Secondary osteoporosis is a result of medical conditions or medications (**Table 225-1**). Long-term oral prednisone used to treat a number of autoimmune diseases is a major contributing cause of secondary osteoporosis (**Figure 225-3**).

RISK FACTORS

- See **Table 225-1**.
- Previous low-trauma fracture.[4] Other risk factors for an osteoporosis-related fracture include advanced age, low BMD, low body mass index (BMI), and starred items in **Table 225-1**.[3]
- There are many validated clinical decision rules that can help identify patients who are at higher-than-average risk of fracture.[5,6] An extensively validated online tool developed by the World Health Organization, the Fracture Risk Assessment (FRAX) (http://www.shef.ac.uk/FRAX/), can be used to estimate 10-year risk for fractures for women and men based on easily obtainable clinical information, such as age, BMI, parental fracture history, and tobacco and alcohol use.

DIAGNOSIS

CLINICAL FEATURES

- Height loss (>1 cm or >0.8 inch) can alert the clinician to osteoporosis.
- Kyphosis and cervical lordosis (dowager's hump).
- Acute pain is often the first symptom from a fracture, usually of the vertebrae (vertebral body collapse), hip or forearm, especially occurring after minor trauma. Pain may also be elicited from palpation over spinous processes and paraspinous muscle spasm may be noted.
- Osteoporosis may be identified on X-ray done for another purpose.

TYPICAL DISTRIBUTION

- Fractures caused by menopausal osteoporosis typically occur in thoracic vertebrae, distal forearm, and ankle; occasionally there is loss of teeth.
- Fractures caused by senile osteoporosis are in the vertebrae, hip, and radius.

LABORATORY TESTING

- Laboratory testing is recommended for women with osteoporosis to identify secondary causes including a complete blood cell count (for anemia or malignancy), serum chemistry (calcium, phosphorus, total protein, albumin, liver enzymes, alkaline phosphatase, creatinine, and electrolytes), 24-hour urine collection (calcium, sodium, and creatinine excretion to identify calcium malabsorption or hypercalciuria), and serum 25-hydroxyvitamin D.[3]
- Other laboratory tests may be indicated for patients with suspected secondary causes (eg, serum thyrotropin, erythrocyte sedimentation rate, testosterone, acid-base studies).[3,4]
- Central dual-energy X-ray absorptiometry (DEXA) measurement of BMD is the accepted gold standard for diagnosis (T-score less than or equal to −2.5 in the spine, femoral neck, or hip in the absence of fracture) (**Figures 225-4** and **225-5**).
- Additional imaging with X-ray can confirm osteoporosis-related fracture (see **Figures 225-1** and **225-3**).
- The presence of a hip or vertebral fracture in the absence of other bone conditions can also be considered as osteoporosis.[3] Two types of hip fractures related to osteoporosis are femoral neck fractures (**Figure 225-6**) and intertrochanteric fractures.

TABLE 225-1 Factors Associated With Osteoporosis

Genetic factors
White or Asian ethnicity
Family history of osteoporosis*
Low body weight (<127 lb)*
Late menarche or early menopause

Nutritional factors
Low intake of calcium or vitamin D
High animal protein intake
Low protein intake

Medical disorders
Endocrine disorders (eg, hyperthyroidism, hyperparathyroidism, diabetes mellitus type 1, Cushing disease, hypogonadism)
Hematologic disorders (eg, multiple myeloma, anemia [hemolytic, pernicious], lymphoma, leukemia)
GI disorders (eg, malabsorption syndromes, chronic liver disease)
Renal disorders (eg, chronic renal failure)
Rheumatologic disorders (eg, rheumatoid arthritis, ankylosing spondylitis)
Other disorders (eg, anorexia, osteogenesis imperfecta)

Medications (commonly used)
Systemic corticosteroids,* antiepileptic drugs, proton pump inhibitors, chemotherapy, diuretics producing calciuria, GnRH agonist or antagonist, heparin, extended tetracycline use

Lifestyle factors
Sedentary
Excessive exercise
Current smoking or alcohol use (>2 U/d)*

GI, gastrointestinal GnRH, gonadotropin-releasing hormone.
*Also risk factors for osteoporosis-related fractures.
Data from Kaplan-Machlis B, Bors KP, Brown SR. Osteoporosis. In: Smith MA, Shimp LA, eds. *Twenty Common Problems in Women's Health Care.* New York, NY: McGraw Hill; 2000; Osteoporosis. In: Ebell MH, Ferenchik G, Smith MA, et al, eds. *Essential Evidence Plus.* Hoboken, NJ: John Wiley; 2009; Watts NB, Bilezikian JP, Camacho PM, et al. American Association of Clinical Endocrinologists medical guidelines for clinical practice for the prevention and treatment of postmenopausal osteoporosis: 2010 edition. *Endocr Pract.* 2010;16(suppl 3):1-37.

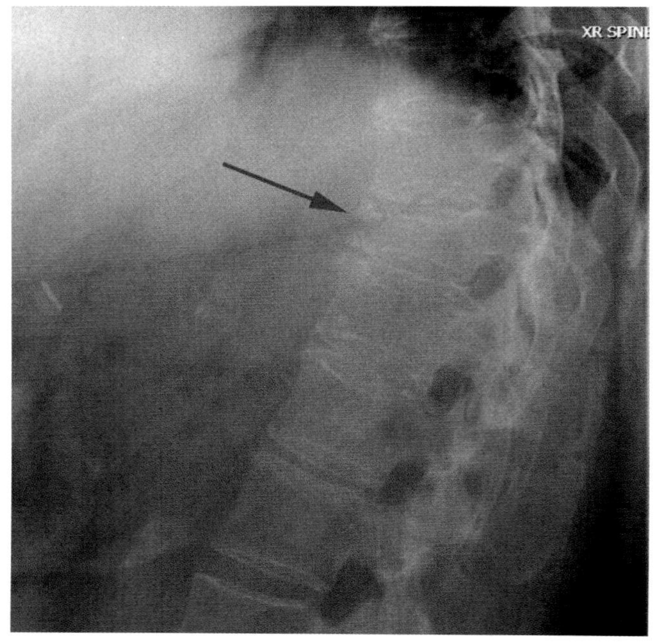

FIGURE 225-3 Wedge compression fracture of T11 vertebra in a post-menopausal woman on long-term prednisone for dermatomyositis. The patient presented with acute back pain. *(Reproduced with permission from Richard P. Usatine, MD.)*

DIFFERENTIAL DIAGNOSIS

Thoracic kyphosis of recent onset in adults can also be caused by the following:

- Degenerative arthritis of the spine—Pain and swelling in other joints, morning stiffness
- Ankylosing spondylitis—Male gender, night pain, and limited motion in sacroiliac joints, uveitis
- Tuberculosis (TB) and other infections of the spine—History of TB, positive cultures, X-ray showing joint destruction (see Chapter 64, Tuberculosis)
- Cancer—History of cancer, imaging distinguishes

MANAGEMENT

NONPHARMACOLOGIC

- Identify and treat secondary causes (see **Table 225-1**).
- Dietary advice includes adequate calcium, vitamin D, and protein intake.[3] SOR B
- Recommend regular weight-bearing exercise.[3] Institute for Clinical Systems Improvement (ICSI) notes that 3 components of an exercise

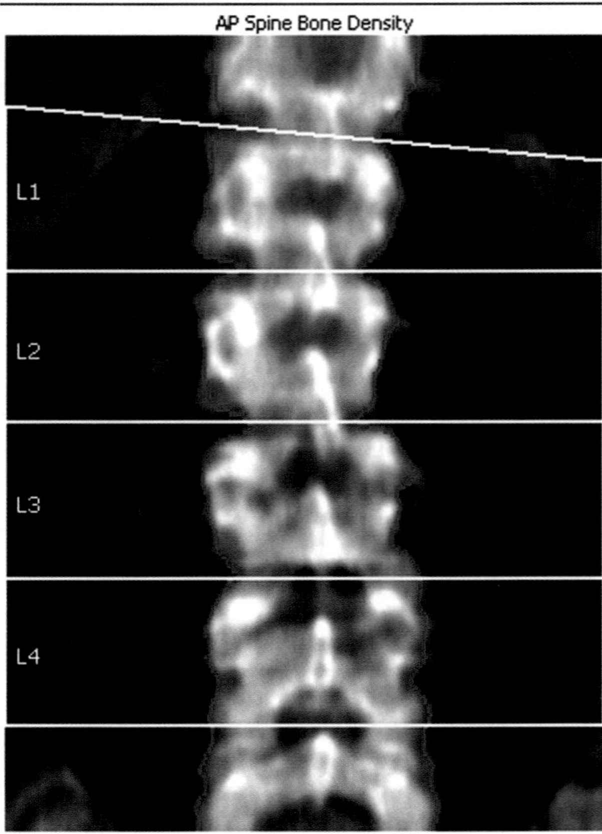

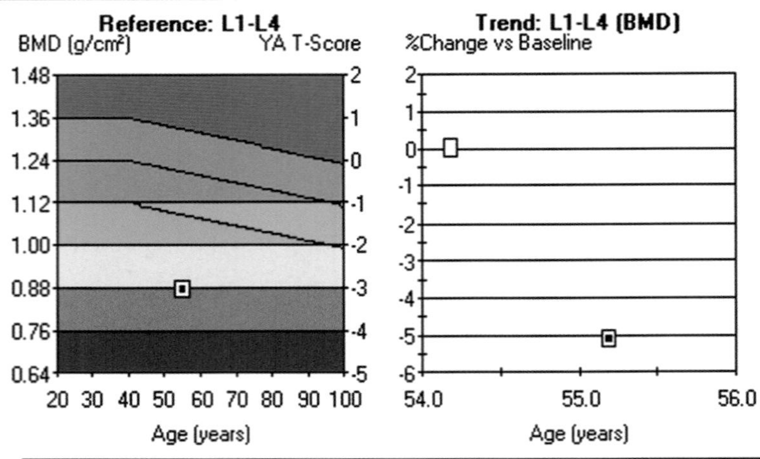

Region	BMD[1] (g/cm²)	Young-Adult[2] (%)	Young-Adult T-Score	Age-Matched[3] (%)	Age-Matched Z-Score
L1	0.871	75	-2.5	77	-2.2
L2	0.895	72	-2.9	73	-2.7
L3	0.867	70	-3.1	72	-2.9
L4	0.854	69	-3.2	71	-2.9
L1-L4	0.871	71	-2.9	73	-2.7

COMMENTS: PREVIOUS EXAM 2011, TAKING CALCIUM SUPPLEMENT, VITAMIN D, DECREASE IN HEIGHT BY A 1/2 INCH

Trend: L1-L4

Measured Date	Age (years)	BMD[1] (g/cm²)	Change vs Previous (g/cm²)	Change vs Previous (%)
12/23/2011	55.1	0.871	-0.047	-5.1
12/21/2010	54.1	0.918	-	-

FIGURE 225-4 Dual-energy X-ray absorptiometry bone density scan showing osteoporosis in the vertebral spine showing 5% loss of vertebral bone density in 1 year. (*Reproduced with permission from Richard P. Usatine, MD.*)

program are needed for strong bone health: impact exercise (eg, jogging, brisk walking, stair climbing), strengthening exercise with weights, and balance training such as Tai Chi or dancing.[4]

- Encourage smoking cessation and moderate alcohol use (<3 drinks per day).[3] SOR B
- Hip protectors may reduce hip fractures in the nursing home.[7] SOR B
- Address other risk factors for falling (eg, low vision, gait disturbance, use of sedatives) and consider referral for physical or occupational therapy, if indicated.

MEDICATIONS

- Calcium (1200 mg/d from diet plus supplement) and vitamin D (at least 800 IU/d).[8,9] SOR A One study found that a single large dose of vitamin D (100,000 IU given orally every 4 months) over 5 years reduced fractures in elderly British women (NNT = 20).[10]
- Women with osteoporosis or previous hip or spine fractures should receive medication therapy, beginning with a bisphosphonate.[3,4] Women should also be considered for medication if they have a T-score of between –1.0 and –2.5, if FRAX major osteoporotic fracture probability is equal to or greater than 20%, or hip fracture probability is equal to or greater than 3%.[3]
- First-line agents include alendronate, risedronate, and zoledronic acid. SOR A Based on a Cochrane review of 11 studies, use of alendronate prevented hip (absolute risk reduction [ARR] 1%), vertebral (ARR 6%), and nonvertebral fractures (ARR 2%).[11] Potential side effects of bisphosphonates include rare atypical femoral shaft fracture (0.13% in the subsequent year for women with at least 5 years of treatment)[12] and jaw osteonecrosis (0.7 per 100,000 patient-years with oral bisphosphonate therapy).[13]
- Other drug therapies approved by the US FDA to reduce fractures include parathyroid hormone (PTH, teriparatide [eg, Forteo]), raloxifene (a selective estrogen receptor modulator [SERM]), and estrogen (women only). The ICSI recommends PTH as a first-line agent for patients with the highest fracture risk. Second-line agents recommended by American Association of Clinical Endocrinologists (AACE) are ibandronate and raloxifene.[3] Choice of second-line medications should be based on the patient's clinical situation, preferences, and the tradeoff between benefits and harms. AACE recommends against combination therapy. SOR B

DualFemur Bone Density

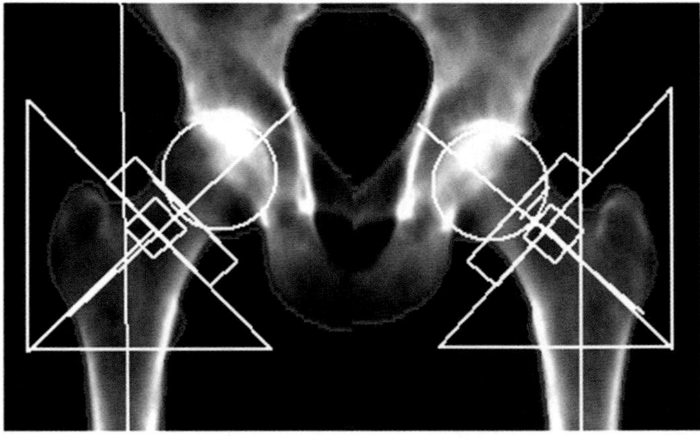

Image not for diagnosis

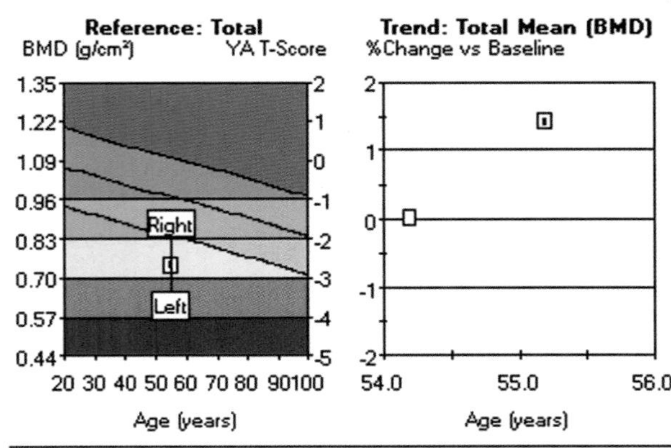

Region	BMD[1,6] (g/cm²)	Young-Adult[2,7] (%)	T-Score	Age-Matched[3] (%)	Z-Score
Neck					
Left	0.720	67	-2.7	78	-1.5
Right	0.712	67	-2.8	78	-1.6
Mean	0.716	67	-2.7	78	-1.6
Difference	0.008	1	0.1	1	0.1
Total					
Left	0.740	68	-2.7	76	-1.8
Right	0.741	68	-2.7	76	-1.8
Mean	0.740	68	-2.7	76	-1.8
Difference	0.001	0	0.0	0	0.0

Trend: Total Mean

Measured Date	Age (years)	BMD[1,6] (g/cm²)	Change vs Previous (g/cm²)	Change vs Previous (%)
12/23/2011	55.1	0.740	0.010	1.4
12/21/2010	54.1	0.730	-	-

COMMENTS: PREVIOUS EXAM 2011, TAKING CALCIUM SUPPLEMENT, VITAMIN D, DECREASE IN HEIGHT BY A 1/2 INCH

FIGURE 225-5 Dual-energy X-ray absorptiometry bone density scan showing osteoporosis of the hips with 2% gain of bone density in 1 year. (*Reproduced with permission from Richard P. Usatine, MD.*)

- The first-line agents listed above for treatment of osteoporosis have been approved for use in men as well as women; however, data are limited for men, especially for fracture reduction. In a randomized controlled trial (RCT) of 265 men on glucocorticoid therapy, both risedronate and zoledronic acid prevented bone loss in the prevention population while zoledronic acid increased BMD slightly more than risedronate (4.7% vs 3.3% lumbar spine and 1.8% vs 0.2% total hip, respectively) in the treatment group.[14]
- Denosumab is a human monoclonal antibody that inhibits osteoclast-mediated bone resorption; denosumab was shown to reduce new vertebral fractures in women with multiple and/or severe prevalent vertebral fractures (ARR 9.1%) and hip fractures in subjects age 75 years or older (ARR 1.4%). Both denosumab and zoledronic acid appear to reduce fracture risk in men with castration-resistant prostate cancer metastatic to bone and denosumab and toremifene (a SERM) reduced osteoporotic fracture risk in men on androgen-deprivation treatment.[15] Denosumab has not been compared with bisphosphonates or other interventions. AACE considers this a first-line agent but it is very expensive.[3] SOR Ⓐ Risks of treatment include endocarditis, cancer, and skin rash.
- Nasal calcitonin may preserve BMD and reduce new vertebral fractures; this drug also has an analgesic effect for some women with painful acute vertebral fractures.[16] AACE recommends calcitonin as a last line of therapy for treatment of osteoporosis.[3]

COMPLEMENTARY AND ALTERNATIVE THERAPY

Limited data support use of phytoestrogens, synthetic isoflavones such as ipriflavone or natural progesterone cream for prevention or treatment of osteoporosis. A 2-year multicenter, randomized trial of ipriflavone showed some effect on total body BMD but no significant effect on regional bone density at common fracture sites.[17]

REFERRAL

AACE recommends referral of patients to a clinical endocrinologist if a patient with a normal BMD sustains a low-trauma fracture, has recurrent fractures or continued bone loss despite therapy, has unexpectedly severe

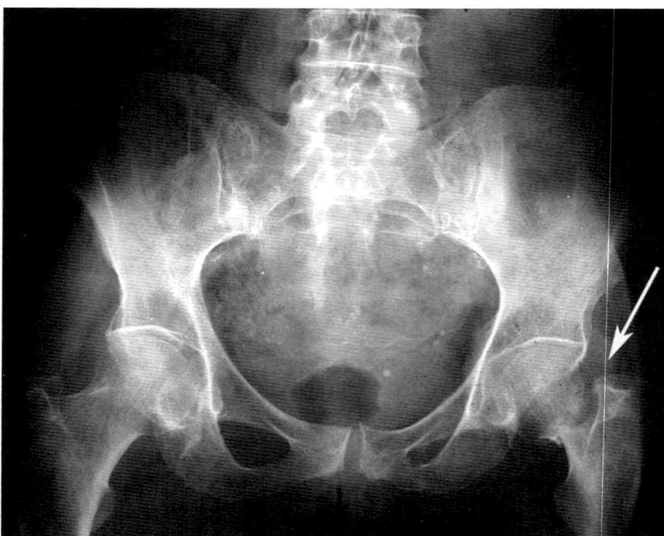

FIGURE 225-6 Femoral neck fracture (*arrow*) in an elderly woman with osteoporosis. The woman fell on her left hip when coming out of the shower. (*Reproduced with permission from Rebecca Loredo-Hernandez, MD.*)

osteoporosis or unusual features, or has a complicating condition (eg, renal failure).[3] SOR Ⓒ

PREVENTION AND SCREENING

- The AACE guideline recommends adequate calcium and vitamin D intake to reduce bone loss.[3] SOR Ⓐ Maintaining an active lifestyle SOR Ⓑ, smoking cessation SOR Ⓑ, limiting alcohol intake SOR Ⓑ, and limiting caffeine intake SOR Ⓒ are also recommended.
- The United States Preventive Services Task Force (USPSTF) and AACE recommend screening for osteoporosis for women 65 years of age and older and for younger women whose fracture risk is the same as or greater than that of a 65-year-old white woman who has no additional risk factors (9.3% risk over 10 years).[2]
- Screening should be done with DEXA of the hip or lumbar spine or quantitative ultrasonography of the calcaneus; appropriate cutoffs for diagnosis and treatment using ultrasound, however, have not been established. Other guidelines have similar risk-based recommendations, although the age of initial assessment (all adults, adults age 50 years, or postmenopausal women) differs and the groups do not recommend use of ultrasound for screening.[18]
- Bisphosphonate therapy should be considered in patients starting glucocorticoid therapy planned for over 3 months and those on chronic glucocorticoid therapy if their T-score is less than −1.0.[19]

FOLLOW-UP

- Repeat DEXA (same machine if possible) every 1 to 2 years until findings are stable and then continue with follow-up DEXA every 2 years or less (see **Figures 225-4** and **225-5**).[3,4]
- Consider discontinuation of a bisphosphonates after 4 to 5 years of stability or after 10 years of stability for high-risk patients.[3] Reinstitute treatment if BMD declines substantially, bone turnover markers increase, or a fracture occurs.

PATIENT EDUCATION

- Encourage home-based fall prevention by removing throw rugs, reducing clutter in high traffic areas, increasing lighting, use of safety step stools and safety hand rails in the bathroom, and walking aids.
- Encourage healthy lifestyle and diet.

PATIENT RESOURCES

- MedlinePlus. *Osteoporosis*—**http://www.nlm.nih.gov/medlineplus/osteoporosis.html.**
- MedlinePlus. *Kyphosis*—**http://www.nlm.nih.gov/medlineplus/ency/article/001240.htm.**
- Osteoporosis Foundation—**http://www.nof.org/.**

PROVIDER RESOURCES

- National Institute of Arthritis and Musculoskeletal and Skin Diseases. *The NIH Osteoporosis and Related Bone Diseases National Resource Center*—**http://www.niams.nih.gov/Health_Info/Bone/default.asp.**
- American Association of Clinical Endocrinologists. *Medical Guidelines for Clinical Practice for the Diagnosis and Treatment for Postmenopausal Osteoporosis*—**https://www.aace.com/files/osteo-guidelines-2010.pdf.**
- The FRAX tool has been developed by the World Health Organization (WHO) to evaluate fracture risk of patients. It can be very helpful in making treatment choices: **http://www.shef.ac.uk/FRAX/.** It is also available as an iTunes app.

REFERENCES

1. The WHO Study Group. *Assessment of Fracture Risk and Its Application to Screening for Postmenopausal Osteoporosis*. Technical Report Series. No. 843. Geneva, Switzerland: World Health Organization; 1994.
2. U.S. Preventive Services Task Force. Screening for osteoporosis: U.S. Preventive Services Task Force Recommendation Statement. *Ann Intern Med*. 2011;154(5):356-364.
3. Watts NB, Bilezikian JP, Camacho PM, et al. American Association of Clinical Endocrinologists medical guidelines for clinical practice for the prevention and treatment of postmenopausal osteoporosis: 2010 edition. *Endocr Pract*. 2010;16(suppl 3):1-37. https://www.aace.com/files/osteo-guidelines-2010.pdf. Accessed August 2013.
4. Institute for Clinical Systems Improvement (ICSI). *Diagnosis and Treatment of Osteoporosis*. http://www.guideline.gov/content.aspx?id=34270&search=osteoporosis. Accessed August 2013.
5. Kanis JA, Borgstrom F, De Laet C, et al. Assessment of fracture risk. *Osteoporos Int*. 2005;16:581-589.
6. Mauck KF, Cuddihy MT, Atkinson EJ, Melton LJ 3rd. Use of clinical prediction rules in detecting osteoporosis in a population-based sample of postmenopausal women. *Arch Intern Med*. 2005;165:530-536.
7. Sawka AM, Boulos P, Beattie K, et al. Hip protectors decrease hip fracture risk in elderly nursing home residents: a bayesian meta-analysis. *J Clin Epidemiol*. 2007;60:336-344.

8. Bischoff-Ferrari HA, Willett WC, Wong JB, et al. Prevention of nonvertebral fractures with oral vitamin D dose dependency. A meta-analysis of randomized controlled trials. *Arch Intern Med.* 2009;169(6):551-561.
9. Avenell A, Gillespie WJ, Gillespie LD, O'Connell D. Vitamin D and vitamin D analogues for preventing fractures associated with involutional and post-menopausal osteoporosis. *Cochrane Database Syst Rev.* 2009;(2):CD000227.
10. Trivedi DP, Doll R, Khaw KT. Effect of four monthly oral vitamin D3 (cholecalciferol) supplementation on fractures and mortality in men and women living in the community: randomised double blind controlled trial. *BMJ*. 2003;326:469-472.
11. Wells GA, Cranney A, Peterson J, et al. Alendronate for the primary and secondary prevention of osteoporotic fractures in postmenopausal women (Cochrane Review). *Cochrane Database Syst Rev.* 2008;(1):CD001155.
12. Park-Wyllie LY, Mamdani MM, Juurlink DN, et al. Bisphosphonate use and the risk of subtrochanteric or femoral shaft fractures in older women. *JAMA.* 2011;305:783-789.
13. Ruggiero SL, Dodson TB, Assael LA, et al. Association of Oral and Maxillofacial Surgeons. American Association of Oral and Maxillofacial Surgeons position paper on bisphosphonate-related osteonecrosis of the jaws. *J Oral Maxillofac Surg*. 2009; 67(suppl 5):2-12.
14. Sambrook PN, Roux C, Devogelaer JP, et al. Bisphosphonate and glucocorticoid osteoporosis in men: results of a randomized controlled trial comparing zoledronic acid with risedronate. *Bone.* 2012;50(1):289-295.
15. Saylor PJ, Lee RJ, Smith MR. Emerging therapies to prevent skeletal morbidity in men with prostate cancer. *J Clin Oncol.* 2011;29(27):3705-3714.
16. Chesnut CH, Silverman S, Andriano K, et al. A randomized trial of nasal spray salmon calcitonin in postmenopausal women with established osteoporosis: the prevent recurrence of osteoporotic fractures study. *Am J Med.* 2000;109:267-276.
17. Wong WW, Lewis RD, Steinberg FM, et al. Soy isoflavone supplementation and bone mineral density in menopausal women: a 2-y multicenter clinical trial. *Am J Clin Nutr.* 2009;90(5):1433-1439.
18. Guideline synthesis. *Screening and Risk Assessment for Osteoporosis in Postmenopausal Women*. http://www.guideline.gov/syntheses/synthesis.aspx?id=38658&search=osteoporosis. Accessed August 2013.
19. Recommendations for the prevention and treatment of glucocorticoid-induced osteoporosis: 2001 update. American College of Rheumatology Ad Hoc Committee on Glucocorticoid-Induced Osteoporosis. *Arthritis Rheum.* 2001;44:1496-1503.

226 HYPOTHYROIDISM

Mindy A. Smith, MD, MS

PATIENT STORY

A 55-year-old woman presented with a several-month history of fatigue and weight gain. She reported that she felt puffy and swollen. She had difficulty buttoning the top button of her blouse because her neck was so large, but she reported no neck pain. Review of systems was positive for constipation, dry skin, and cold intolerance. On physical examination, a large goiter was found (**Figure 226-1**). Laboratory testing revealed an elevated thyroid-stimulating hormone (TSH) and a low free thyroxine (FT_4) level confirming hypothyroidism. The patient was started on levothyroxine.

INTRODUCTION

- Goiter is a spectrum of changes in the thyroid gland ranging from diffuse enlargement to nodular enlargement depending on the cause. In the United States, the most common etiology of goiter with normal thyroid function or transient dysfunction is thyroiditis.
- Hypothyroidism is a condition caused by lack of thyroid hormone and usually develops as a result of thyroid failure from intrinsic thyroid disease. The most common cause of goitrous hypothyroidism is chronic lymphocytic (Hashimoto) thyroiditis.
- Subclinical thyroid disease refers to a patient with no or minimal thyroid-related symptoms but abnormal laboratory values (elevated TSH and thyroxine level within the normal range).

EPIDEMIOLOGY

- Worldwide, goiter is the most common endocrine disorder with rates of 4% to 15% in areas of adequate iodine intake and more than 90% where there is iodine deficiency.[1] Endemic goiter is defined as goiter that affects more than 5% of the population (**Figure 226-2**).

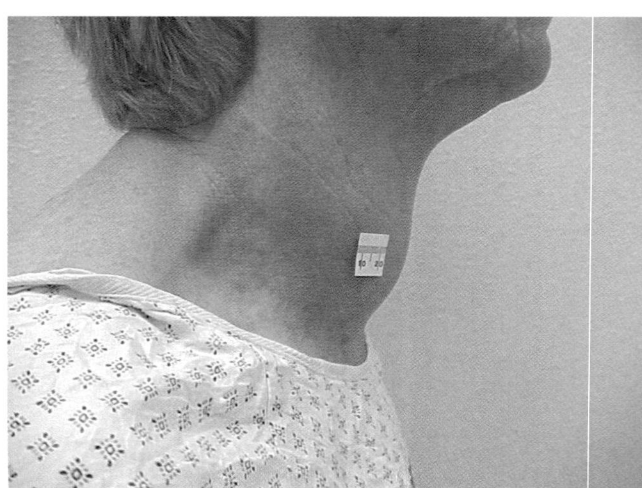

FIGURE 226-1 Goiter that extends approximately 2 cm forward when viewed from the patient's side. (*Reproduced with permission from Dan Stulberg, MD.*)

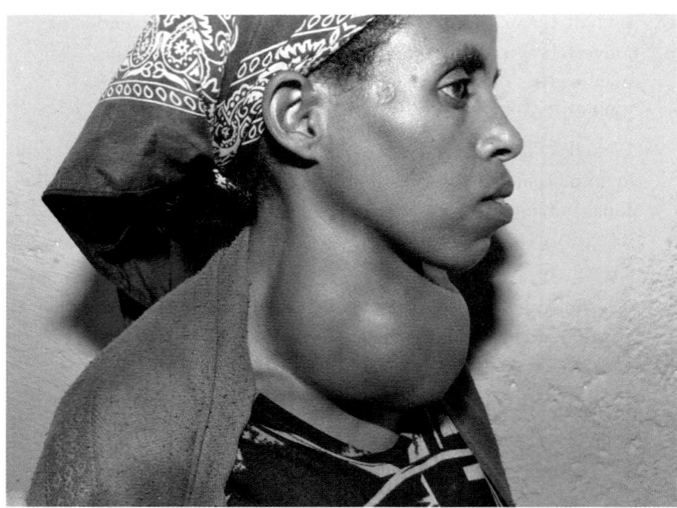

FIGURE 226-2 Massive goiter in an Ethiopian woman who lives in an endemic area for goiters. Many adults have large goiters in Ethiopia where there is little iodine in their diets. (*Reproduced with permission from Richard P. Usatine, MD.*)

- Most goiters are not associated with thyroid dysfunction.
- The prevalence of goitrous hypothyroidism varies from 0.7% to 4% of the population.
- Subclinical hypothyroidism is present in 3% to 10% of population groups and in 10% to 18% of elderly persons.[2,3]
- The female-to-male ratio of goiter is 3:1, and 6:1 for goitrous hypothyroidism.
- The annual incidence of autoimmune hypothyroidism is 4 in 1000 women and 1 in 1000 men, with a mean age at diagnosis of 60 years.[4]

ETIOLOGY AND PATHOPHYSIOLOGY

Following are the contributing factors for goiter:

- Iodine deficiency or excess (see **Figure 226-2**)
- TSH stimulation
- Drugs, including lithium, amiodarone, and α-interferon
- Autoimmunity/heredity

Hypothyroidism may be caused by disease of the thyroid gland itself (eg, Hashimoto thyroiditis), radioiodine thyroid ablation, thyroidectomy, high-dose head and neck radiation therapy, and medications (as above), or, rarely, by pituitary or hypothalamic disorders (eg, tumors, inflammatory conditions, infiltrative diseases, infections, pituitary surgery, pituitary radiation therapy, and head trauma).[2]

- Hashimoto thyroiditis is caused by thyroid peroxidase (TPO) antibodies.
- Human leukocyte antigen-D related (HLA-DR) and cytotoxic T-lymphocyte antigen 4 (CTLA-4) are the best-documented genetic risk factors for this disorder.[4]
- There is marked lymphocytic infiltration of the thyroid in Hashimoto thyroiditis; the infiltrate is composed of activated CD4+ and CD8+ T cells, as well as B cells.
- Thyroid destruction in Hashimoto thyroiditis is believed to be primarily mediated by CD8+ cytotoxic T cells.

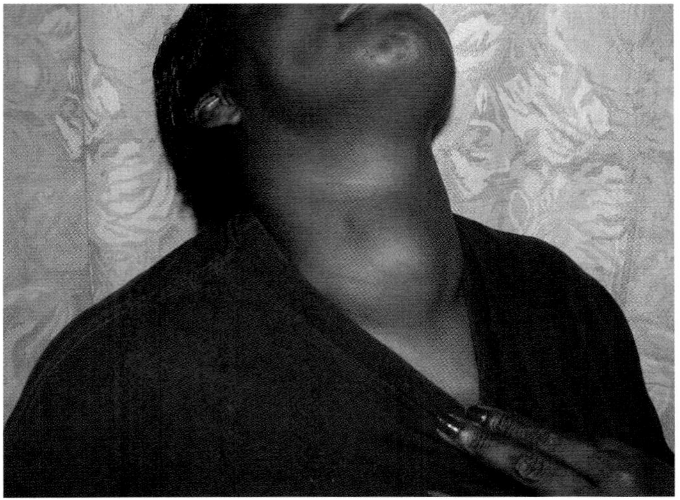

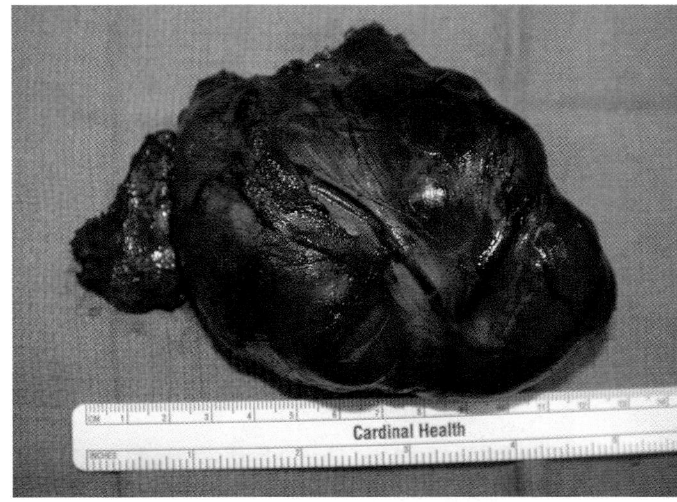

A B

FIGURE 226-3 **A.** A 36-year-old woman with large goiter. **B.** The resected goitrous thyroid gland. (*Reproduced with permission from Frank Miller, MD.*)

RISK FACTORS

Risk factors for hypothyroidism include the followng[2]:

- Symptoms of thyroid hormone deficiency
- Goiter
- Personal or family history of thyroid disease
- Personal treatment of thyroid disease
- History of autoimmune disease, especially diabetes mellitus
- High-dose head and neck radiation therapy

Myxedema coma usually occurs in elderly patients with untreated or inadequately treated hypothyroidism who develop a precipitating event, such as myocardial infarction, stroke, sepsis, or prolonged cold exposure.[2]

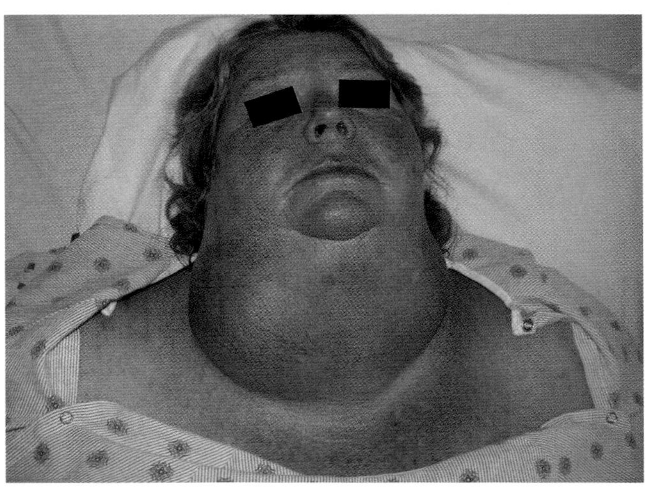

FIGURE 226-4 Massive multinodular goiter before surgery. (*Reproduced with permission from Frank Miller, MD.*)

DIAGNOSIS

CLINICAL FEATURES

The history can be the key to the diagnosis:

- A painful neck mass is usually a form of thyroiditis.
- Large goiters are easily visible before palpating the neck (**Figures 226-1** to **226-4**).
- Asymmetric goiters can shift the trachea away from the midline (**Figure 226-5**).

Following are the common signs and symptoms of hypothyroidism:

- Fatigue and/or weakness.
- Dry and cool skin.
- Diffuse hair loss or thinning of the lateral eyebrows.
- Difficulty concentrating.
- Puffy face/hands/feet from myxedema (**Figure 226-6**).
- Bradycardia.

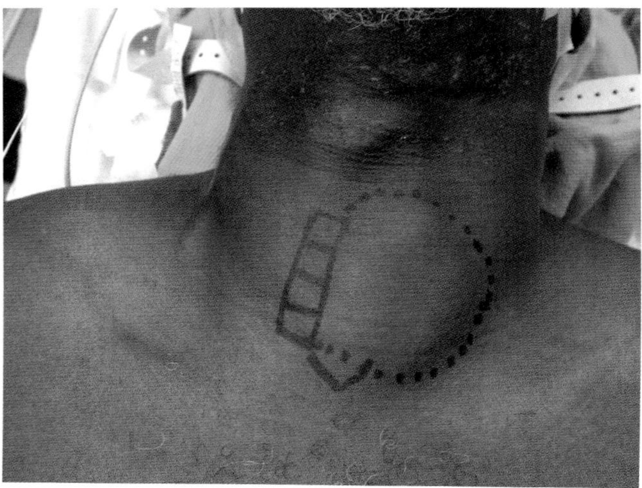

FIGURE 226-5 Asymmetric multinodular goiter causing trachea to deviate from the midline prior to resection. (*Reproduced with permission from Frank Miller, MD.*)

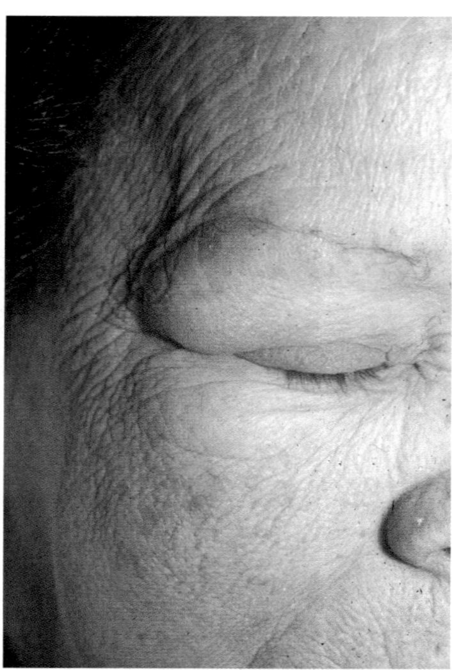

FIGURE 226-6 Myxedema of the face with puffiness around the eye. (*Reproduced with permission from the University of Texas Health Sciences Center, Division of Dermatology.*)

- Delayed deep tendon reflex relaxation.
- Weight gain despite poor appetite.
- Constipation.
- The most useful signs for diagnosing hypothyroidism are puffiness (likelihood ratio positive [LR+] 16.2) and delayed ankle reflex (LR+ 11.8).[5]

Clues to a central cause of hypothyroidism include a history of pituitary/hypothalamic surgery or radiation, headache, visual field defects, or ophthalmoplegia.[2]

Physical examination maneuvers that help detect goiter are as below[6]:

- Neck extension
- Observation from the side
- Palpation by locating the isthmus first
- Having the patient swallow
- Myxedema coma

LABORATORY STUDIES

Laboratory tests include an erythrocyte sedimentation rate (ESR) if thyroiditis is suspected, and TSH (elevated in hypothyroidism and subclinical disease) and FT_4 levels (low in hypothyroidism).

- In acute granulomatous thyroiditis, ESR is greater than 50 (LR+ 95) and the TSH and FT_4 are usually normal.
- In primary hypothyroidism, the TSH is greater than 10 mU/L (LR+ 16) and FT_4 is less than 8 (LR+ 11).
- The presence of antibodies to TPO and thyroglobulin help establish the diagnosis of Hashimoto thyroiditis but is unnecessary for treatment. TPO antibodies will be positive in 90% to 95% of patients.[4]
- In pituitary causes of hypothyroidism (central hypothyroidism), the TSH may be normal or elevated but FT_4 will be low.[2]
- In the future, reference limits may need to change as TSH distribution and reference limits have been shown to shift to higher concentrations with age and are unique for different racial/ethnic groups.[7]

DIFFERENTIAL DIAGNOSIS

Goiter presenting as a painful neck mass is most commonly caused by subacute granulomatous (de Quervain) thyroiditis (likely viral) or hemorrhage into a thyroid cyst or adenoma. Other causes include the following:

- Painful Hashimoto thyroiditis—Hypothyroidism with the presence of antibodies helps to confirm this diagnosis.
- Infected thyroglossal duct or branchial cleft cyst—Mass palpates as cystic and may be fluctuant; focal (eg, erythema and warmth) and systemic symptoms of infection (eg, fever) may be present. Even a noninfected thyroglossal duct cyst can be confused for an enlarged thyroid (**Figure 226-7**).
- Acute suppurative thyroiditis (microbial)—Focal (eg, erythema and warmth) and systemic symptoms of infection (eg, fever) are usually present.
- Thyroid carcinoma—Hard mass within thyroid gland (**Figure 226-8**).

Painless goiter and hypothyroidism are most often caused by Hashimoto thyroiditis, but may also be caused by the following:

- Environmental goitrogens (eg, excess iodine, foods such as cassava, cabbage, and soybeans).
- Iodine deficiency.
- Pharmacologic inhibition (rare)—Drugs include lithium, amiodarone, and interferon-α.

Painless goiter and hyperthyroidism may be caused by the following:

- Graves disease (common, 0.5%-2.5% of the population)—Symptoms of nervousness, fatigue, weight loss, heat intolerance, palpitations, and exophthalmus (see Chapter 227, Hyperthyroidism).
- Postpartum thyroiditis (2%-16% within 3-6 months of delivery)—Recent delivery.

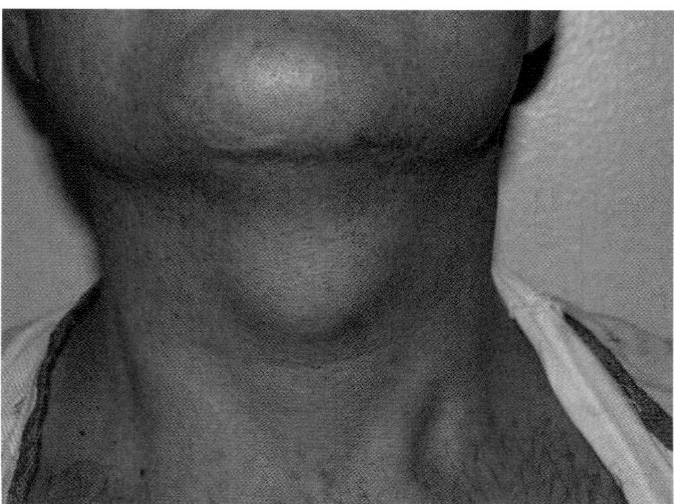

FIGURE 226-7 Thyroglossal duct cyst in the midline superior to the thyroid. (*Reproduced with permission from Frank Miller, MD.*)

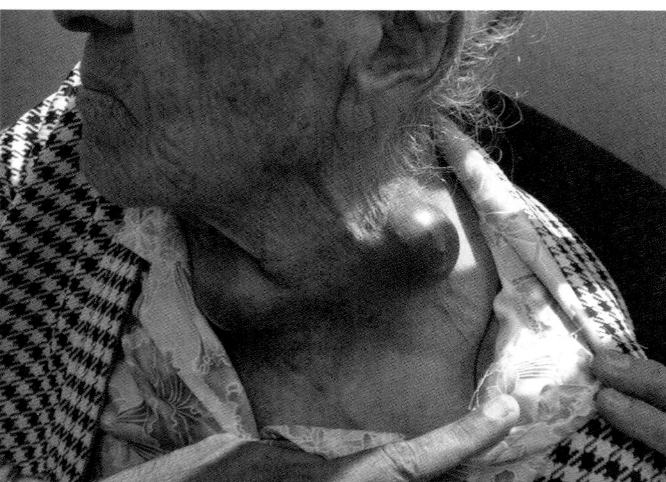

FIGURE 226-8 A 93-year-old woman with thyroid cancer that went untreated for 3 years. Two large firm masses are visible in the neck. *(Reproduced with permission from Dustin Williams, MD.)*

- Toxic nodular goiter (uncommon)—Usually in the elderly; thyroid gland feels nodular (see **Figure 226-4**) and thyroid scan shows multiple foci of increased uptake.

MANAGEMENT

NONPHARMACOLOGIC

For nonendemic goiter, identify and remove goitrogens.

MEDICATIONS

Patients with endemic goiter should be provided with iodine.

For nonendemic goiter, also consider the following:

- TSH suppression with levothyroxine (1-2.2 mg/kg/d) (variable but limited effect on goiter size and can cause hyperthyroidism).[8] SOR B
- Radioactive iodine treatment if enough functioning tissue is present. SOR C

Treat patients with acute microbial thyroiditis with antibiotics against the most common pathogens (ie, *Staphylococcus aureus, Streptococcus pyogenes,* and *Streptococcus pneumoniae*). Alternative agents, used for 7 to 10 days, include the following: SOR C

- Amoxicillin/clavulanate (500 mg 3 times daily)
- A first- or second-generation cephalosporin (eg, cephalexin 500 mg 4 times daily)
- Penicillinase-resistant penicillin (eg, dicloxacillin 500 mg 4 times daily)

In patients with subacute thyroiditis following are the treatments:

- Oral corticosteroids can reduce pain and swelling. SOR C
- Symptoms of hyperthyroidism can be treated with β-blockers or calcium channel blockers.[9] SOR B
- Symptoms of hypothyroidism can be treated with levothyroxine.[8] SOR B

Patients with Hashimoto thyroiditis and low FT_4 are treated with levothyroxine as follows:

- Younger patients start with 50 to 100 μg/d increasing by 25 to 50 μg/d at 6- to 8-week intervals until the TSH is normal (approximately 1.6 μg/kg per day of levothyroxine).[2,8] SOR B
- Older patients or those with cardiac disease start with 25 μg/d and increase by 12.5 to 25 μg/d every 6 to 8 weeks to normalize the TSH (approximately 1 μg/kg per day of levothyroxine). SOR C
- Dosing in the evening appears to normalize the laboratory values more effectively, but in one study, did not influence symptoms or quality of life.[2,10]

A Cochrane review of 12 small randomized controlled trials (RCTs) determined that treatment of subclinical hypothyroidism did not improve survival or decrease cardiovascular morbidity.[11]

- Patients with subclinical hypothyroidism should be considered for treatment if they have symptoms of thyroid deficiency, are at high likelihood of progression to hypothyroidism (eg, TSH >10 mIU/L), or are pregnant.[2,3]
- For patients with TSH levels of 5 to 10 mIU/L, other factors to consider in a treatment decision include presence of goiter, bipolar disorder or depression, infertility or ovulatory dysfunction, presence of antithyroid antibodies, young age, patient preference, and possibly hyperlipidemia.[3]
- A dose of 50 to 75 μg/d is usually sufficient for those with subclinical hypothyroidism. SOR C

REFERRAL

- Large goiters that impinge on the trachea or do not respond to medications may be treated with surgery (see **Figure 226-3**).
- Subtotal thyroidectomy can be considered for nodular goiters but recurrence rates can be high.[12] SOR A
- Consultation with an endocrinologist may be helpful if the diagnosis is uncertain and for patients with central hypothyroidism, severe hypothyroidism (ie, myxedema coma), or coexisting cardiovascular disease.[2]
- Patients with myxedema coma should be hospitalized in an intensive care unit; without treatment, mortality approaches 100%.

PREVENTION AND SCREENING

- There is insufficient evidence to support screening for hypothyroidism.[13]
- One expert panel recommended TSH testing in women with symptoms of thyroid dysfunction, personal or family history of thyroid disease, an abnormal thyroid gland on palpation, or type 1 diabetes mellitus or other autoimmune disorders.[14] In support of this approach, a clinical trial of universal screening versus case finding did not demonstrate a difference in adverse outcomes; however, treatment of women with thyroid dysfunction identified by screening a low-risk group was associated with a lower rate of adverse outcomes.[15]

PROGNOSIS

- In the most extensive community survey on goiter (Whickham, England), goiter was present in 15.5% of the population.[1] At the 20-year follow-up, 20% of women and 5% of men no longer had goiter and 4% of women and no men had acquired a goiter.

- Suppression of TSH with levothyroxine effectively reduces the goiter of Hashimoto thyroiditis and should be continued indefinitely. In one study, withdrawal of medication after 1 year resulted in only 11.4% remaining euthyroid.[16]
- Large goiter, TSH greater than 10 mU/L, and a family history of thyroid disease are associated with failure to recover normal thyroid function and treatment should continue indefinitely.
- In patients with subclinical hypothyroidism, progression to clinically overt hypothyroidism is 2.6% each year if TPO antibodies are absent, and 4.3% if they are present.[17]

FOLLOW-UP

- TSH should be rechecked approximately 6 to 8 weeks after initiation of levothyroxine therapy and again in 4 to 6 months if normal, and annually thereafter unless otherwise clinically indicated.[18] SOR Ⓒ
- Although the need for thyroid replacement is lifelong, dose requirements may change over time. Thyroxine dose may need to be increased during pregnancy (20%-40%), with use of estrogens, or in situations of weight gain, malabsorption, *Helicobacter pylori*-related gastritis and atrophic gastritis and with use of some medications. Requirements may decrease with increased age, androgen use, reactivation of Graves disease, or the development of autonomous thyroid nodules.[2]
- There is some evidence that use of ultrasound can help predict progression to overt hypothyroidism in patients with subclinical hypothyroidism[19]; in one study, patients with TPO antibodies and/or ultrasound abnormalities had a greater progression to overt disease than those without either finding (31.2% vs 9.5% at 3 years).[20]
- The frequency of other autoimmune disease is increased in patients with Hashimoto thyroiditis (14.3% in one study), including rheumatoid arthritis, pernicious anemia, systemic lupus erythematosus, Addison disease, celiac disease, and vitiligo, and increased monitoring should be considered.[21]

PATIENT RESOURCES

- Information from the American Thyroid Association—**http://www.thyroid.org/patient-thyroid-information/.**
- Web-based resources—**http://www.nlm.nih.gov/medlineplus/thyroiddiseases.html.**

PROVIDER RESOURCES

- Baskin HJ, Cobin RH, Duick DS, et al; American Association of Clinical Endocrinologists. American Association of Clinical Endocrinologists medical guidelines for clinical practice for the evaluation and treatment of hyperthyroidism and hypothyroidism. *Endocr Pract*. 2002;8(6):457-469.

REFERENCES

1. Wang C, Crapo LM. The epidemiology of thyroid disease and implications for screening. *Endocrinol Metab Clin North Am.* 1997;26(1):189-218.
2. McDermott MT. In the clinic. Hypothyroidism. *Ann Intern Med.* 2009;151(11):ITC61.
3. Fatourechi V. Subclinical hypothyroidism: an update for primary care physicians. *Mayo Clin Proc.* 2009;84(1):65-71.
4. Jameson JL, Weetman AP. Disorders of the thyroid gland. In: Kasper DL, Braunwald E, Fauci AS, Hauser SL, Longo DL, Jameson JL, eds. *Harrison's Principles of Internal Medicine*. 16th ed. New York, NY: McGraw-Hill; 2005:2109-2113.
5. Zulewski H, Müller B, Exer P, et al. Estimation of tissue hypothyroidism by a new clinical score: evaluation of patients with various grades of hypothyroidism and controls. *J Clin Endocrinol Metab.* 1997;82:771-776.
6. Siminoski K. Does this patient have a goiter? *JAMA.* 1995;273(10):813-819.
7. Surks MI, Boucai L. Age- and race-based serum thyrotropin reference limits. *J Clin Endocrinol Metab.* 2010;95(2):496-502.
8. Zelmanovitz F, Genro S, Gross JL. Suppressive therapy with levothyroxine for solitary thyroid nodules: a double-blind controlled clinical study and cumulative meta-analyses. *J Clin Endocrinol Metab.* 1998;3:3881-3885.
9. Singer PA, Cooper DS, Levy EG, et al. Treatment guideline for patients with hyperthyroidism and hypothyroidism. *JAMA.* 1995;273(10):808-812.
10. Bolk N, Visser TJ, Nijman J, et al. Effects of evening vs morning levothyroxine intake: a randomized double-blind crossover trial. *Ann Intern Med.* 2010;170(22):1996-2003.
11. Villar HCCE, Saconato H, Valente O, Atallah ÁN. Thyroid hormone replacement for subclinical hypothyroidism. *Cochrane Database Syst Rev.* 2007;(3):CD003419.
12. Rojdmark J, Jarhult J. High long term recurrence rate after subtotal thyroidectomy for nodular goitre. *Eur J Surg.* 1995;161:725-727.
13. United States Preventive Services Task Force. *Screening for Thyroid Disease.* http://www.uspreventiveservicestaskforce.org/uspstf/uspsthyr.htm. Accessed August 2013.
14. Surks MI, Ortiz E, Daniels GH, et al. Subclinical thyroid disease: scientific review and guidelines for diagnosis and management. *JAMA.* 2004;291:228-238.
15. Negro R, Schwartz A, Gismondi R, et al. Universal screening versus case finding for detection and treatment of thyroid hormonal dysfunction during pregnancy. *J Clin Endocrinol Metab.* 2010;95(4):1699-1707.
16. Comtois R, Faucher L, Lafleche L. Outcome of hypothyroidism cause by Hashimoto's thyroiditis. *Arch Intern Med.* 1995;155(13):1404-1408.
17. Vanderpump MP, Tunbridge WM, French JM, et al. The incidence of thyroid disorders in the community: a twenty-year follow-up of the Whickham Survey. *Clin Endocrinol (Oxf).* 1995;43(1):55-68.
18. Wirsing N, Hamilton A. How often should you follow up on a patient with newly diagnosed hypothyroidism? *J Fam Pract.* 2009;58(1):40-41.
19. Shin DY, Kim EK, Lee EJ. Role of ultrasonography in outcome prediction in subclinical hypothyroid patients treated with levothyroxine. *Endocr J.* 2010;57(1):15-22.
20. Rosário PW, Bessa B, Valadão MM, Purisch S. Natural history of mild subclinical hypothyroidism: prognostic value of ultrasound. *Thyroid.* 2009;19(1):9-12.
21. Boelaert K, Newby PR, Simmonds MJ, et al. Prevalence and relative risk of other autoimmune diseases in subjects with autoimmune thyroid disease. *Am J Med.* 2010;123(2):183.e1-e9.

227 HYPERTHYROIDISM

Mindy A. Smith, MD, MS

PATIENT STORY

A 29-year-old woman presents with anxiety, palpitations, insomnia, and fatigue. She also reports feeling warm all the time. On physical examination she is found to have a diffusely enlarged thyroid gland without any palpable nodules. (**Figure 227-1**). She also has bilateral proptosis. A fine tremor is detected with her hands outstretched and her deep tendon reflexes are brisk. Her skin feels warm and somewhat moist. Her resting pulse is 120 beats/min. The clinical diagnosis is clearly Graves disease (GD) and the patient is started on propranolol 40 mg bid to treat her symptoms. Laboratory testing reveals a low thyroid-stimulating hormone (TSH) and an elevated free thyroxin level (T_4) to confirm the diagnosis of hyperthyroidism. The patient reports feeling much improved on the β-blocker and chooses radioactive iodine for the definitive treatment of the Graves disease. Her thyroid scan showed a diffusely enlarged thyroid gland (5 times normal) with increased uptake (54%) (**Figure 227-2**) confirming Graves disease. The patient is treated with an appropriate dose of radioactive iodine (RAI) based on the calculations performed in the nuclear medicine department. Her TSH is followed periodically and 1 year later she required levothyroxine treatment.

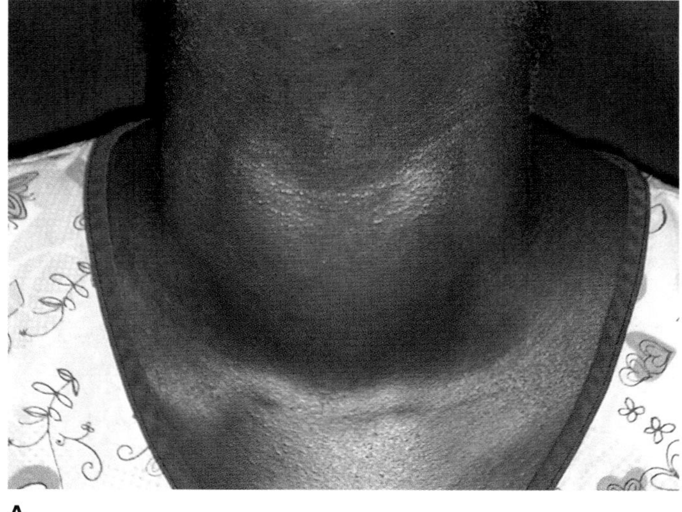

A

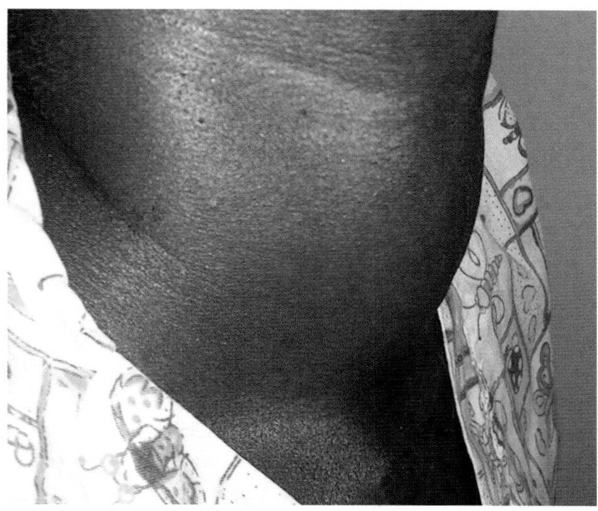

B

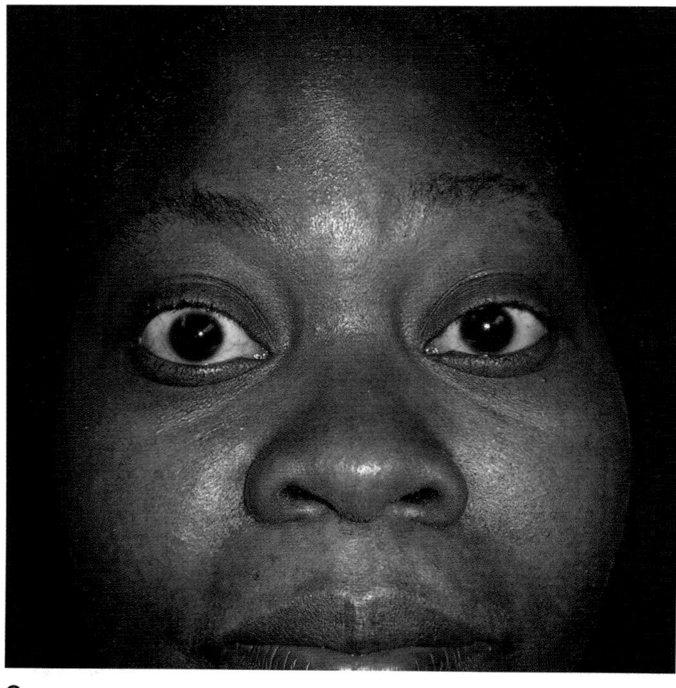

C

FIGURE 227-1 Graves disease presenting in a 29-year-old African American woman with the typical symptoms of anxiety, palpitations, feeling warm, and flushed. **A.** Note the diffusely enlarged thyroid gland. **B.** Goiter seen from the side. **C.** Proptosis secondary to the Graves disease. (*Reproduced with permission from Richard P. Usatine, MD.*)

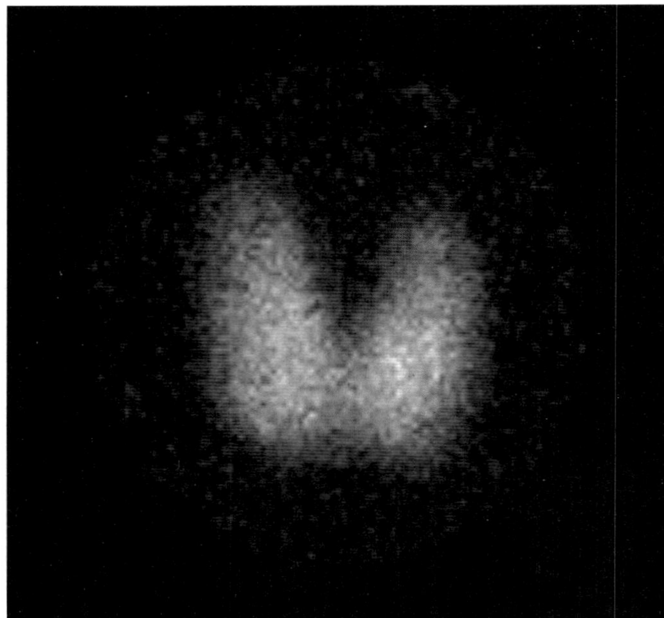

FIGURE 227-2 Nuclear scan of the thyroid in Graves disease showing increased uptake (54%) in a diffusely enlarged thyroid gland (5 times normal with a homogeneous pattern). (*Reproduced with permission from Richard P. Usatine, MD.*)

INTRODUCTION

GD is an autoimmune thyroid disorder characterized by circulating antibodies that stimulate the TSH receptor and resulting in hyperthyroidism.[1]

SYNONYMS

GD is also known as thyrotoxicosis (clinical state resulting from inappropriately high thyroid hormone levels); hyperthyroidism (thyrotoxicosis caused by elevated synthesis and secretion of thyroid hormone).

EPIDEMIOLOGY

- GD is a common disorder affecting 0.5% to 1.2% of the population.
- There is a female-to-male ratio of 5 to 10:1.
- Among patients with hyperthyroidism, 60% to 80% have GD; younger patients (younger than age 64 years) with hyperthyroidism are more likely to have GD than are older patients with hyperthyroidism.
- Graves ophthalmopathy (see "Clinical Features" later) occurs in more than 80% of patients within 18 months of diagnosis of GD. The ophthalmopathy is clinically apparent in 30% to 50% of patients.[2]
- Goiter is present in 90% of patients younger than age 50 years (vs 75% in older patients with GD).[1]
- Untreated hyperthyroidism can lead to osteoporosis, atrial fibrillation, cardiomyopathy, and congestive heart failure; thyrotoxicosis (thyroid storm) has an associated mortality rate of 20% to 50%.[3]

ETIOLOGY AND PATHOPHYSIOLOGY

- The hyperthyroidism of GD results from circulating immunoglobulin (Ig) G antibodies that stimulate the TSH receptor.[2] These antibodies are synthesized in the thyroid gland, bone marrow, and lymph nodes. Activation of the TSH receptor stimulates follicular hypertrophy and hyperplasia causing thyroid enlargement (goiter) and an increase in thyroid hormone production with an increased fraction of triiodothyronine (T_3) relative to T_4 (from approximately 20% to up to 30%).[2]
- The etiology is seen as a combination of genetic (human leukocyte antigen-D related [HLA-DR] and cytotoxic T-lymphocyte antigen 4 [CTLA-4] polymorphisms) and environmental factors, including physical and emotional stress (eg, infection, childbirth, life events).[2] In addition, insulin-like growth factor-1 receptor (IGF-1R)-bearing fibroblasts and B cells exhibiting the IGF-1R(+) phenotype may be involved in the connective tissue manifestations.[4] Siblings have higher incidence of both GD and Hashimoto thyroiditis (see Chapter 226, Hypothyroidism).
- The ophthalmopathy is believed to result from an autoimmune response directed toward an antigen shared by the thyroid and the eye's orbit. There is infiltration of the extraocular muscles by activated T cells, which release cytokines, activating fibroblasts (fibrosis can lead to diplopia) and increasing the synthesis of glycosaminoglycans (water trapping causes swelling).[2]

RISK FACTORS

- Family history of thyroid disease, especially in maternal relatives
- Smoking (a strong risk factor for Graves ophthalmopathy)

DIAGNOSIS

There are several guidelines available for the diagnosis and management of thyroid disease found under provider resources.

CLINICAL FEATURES

Symptoms depend on the severity of thyrotoxicosis, duration of disease, and age (findings are more subtle in the elderly). More than half of patients diagnosed with GD have the following common symptoms:

- Nervousness
- Fatigue
- Weight loss
- Heat intolerance
- Palpitations

Signs of disease include the following:

- Tachycardia (atrial fibrillation is common in patients >50 years of age).[2]
- Goiter—Listening over the goiter with a stethoscope may reveal a thyroid bruit (**Figure 227-3**).
- Resting tremor.
- Hyperreflexia.
- Flushing and temporal wasting (**Figure 227-4**).

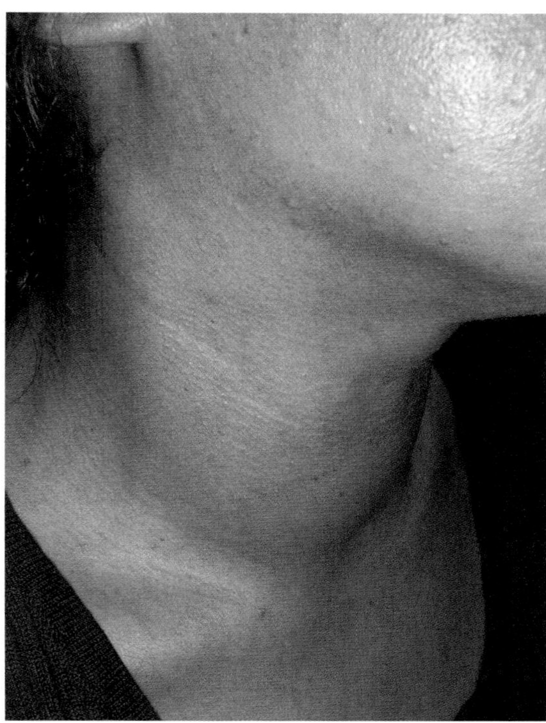

FIGURE 227-3 This 37-year-old woman has Graves disease and a loud bruit over her enlarged hyperactive thyroid gland. She was thyrotoxic at this time. (*Reproduced with permission from Richard P. Usatine, MD.*)

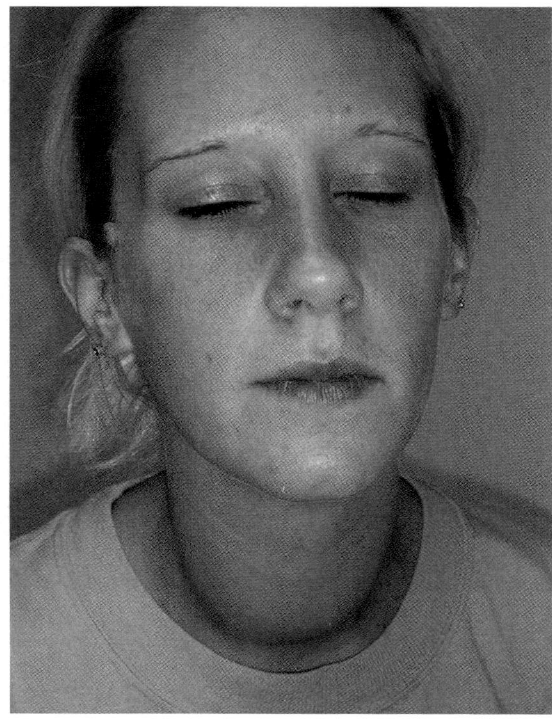

FIGURE 227-4 Flushed skin and temporal wasting in this thyrotoxic woman with new-onset Graves disease. Her thyroid gland was diffusely enlarged. (*Reproduced with permission from Richard P. Usatine, MD.*)

- Skin and nail changes include the following:
  - Warm, erythematous, moist skin (from increased peripheral circulation).
  - Palmer erythema.
  - Pretibial myxedema—Occurring in a small percentage of patients (0.5%-4%), it consists of nonpitting scaly thickening and induration of the skin usually on the anterior shin and dorsa of the feet (**Figures 227-5** and **227-6**).[5] It can also appear as a few well-demarcated pink, flesh-colored, or purple-brown papules or nodules.
  - Nails are soft and shiny and may develop onycholysis (distal separation of the nail plate from the underlying nail bed).
- Eye involvement may occur before hyperthyroidism (in 20% of patients) and gradually progresses with only mild discomfort (a gritty sensation with increased tearing is the earliest manifestation). The eye findings in GD[1,2] are as below:
  - Lid retraction (drawing back of the eyelid allowing more sclera to be visible) (**Figures 227-1** and **227-7**).
  - Frank proptosis (displacement of the eye in the anterior direction); occurs in one-third (see **Figures 227-1** and **227-7**).
  - It is possible to have unilateral eye involvement with Graves ophthalmopathy (**Figure 227-8**).
  - Extraocular muscle dysfunction (eg, diplopia).
  - Corneal exposure keratitis or ulcer.
  - Periorbital edema, chemosis, and scleral injection.

LABORATORY TESTING AND IMAGING

- With typical symptoms, you can confirm the diagnosis of GD with a low or undetectable sensitive assay for TSH and an elevated free T_4 level.
- The presence of TSH receptor antibodies (present in 70%-100% of patients at diagnosis) has a positive and negative likelihood ratio of 247 and 0.01, respectively.[6] These antibodies are not usually required for diagnosis.
- If the clinical picture is uncertain or there is thyroid nodularity, obtain a RAI scan and uptake.[7] Elevated uptake (>30%) and a homogeneous pattern on scan are diagnostic (see **Figure 227-2**).

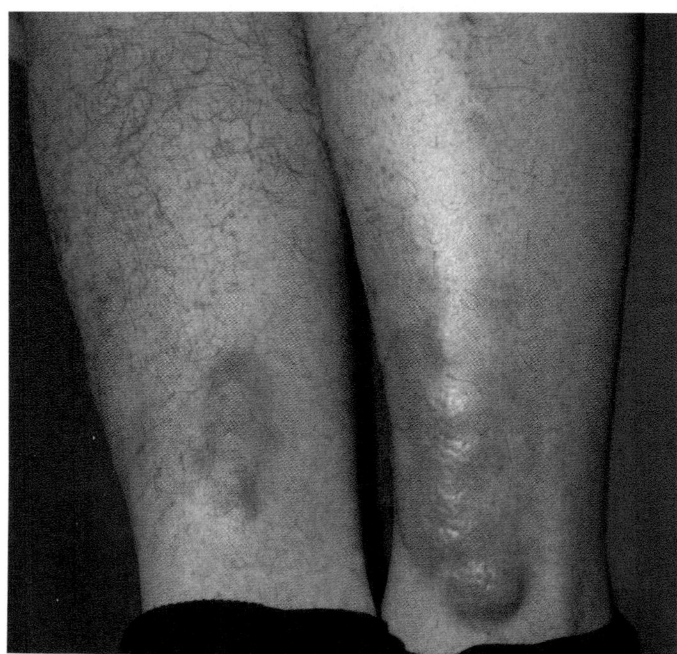

FIGURE 227-5 Early bilateral pretibial myxedema in a patient with Graves disease. These asymmetrical erythematous plaques and nodules are firm and nonpitting. (*Reproduced with permission from the University of Texas Health Sciences Center, Division of Dermatology.*)

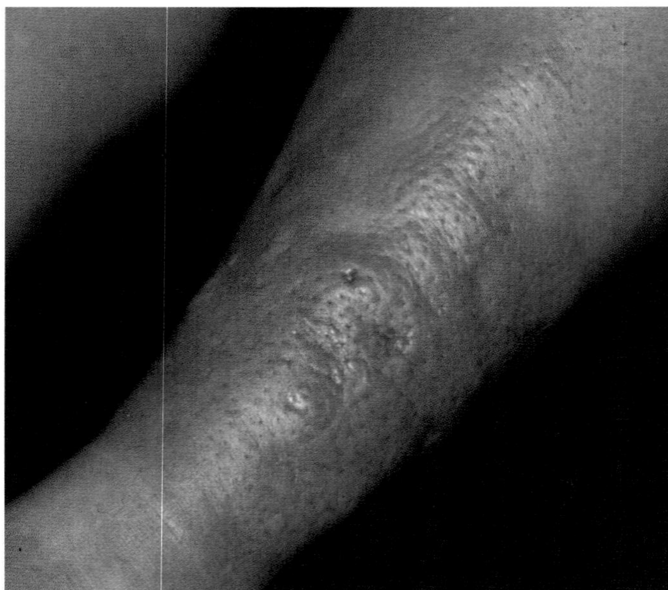

FIGURE 227-6 Pretibial myxedema in a patient with Graves ophthalmopathy. Hair follicles are prominent, giving a peau d'orange appearance. (*Reproduced with permission from the University of Texas Health Sciences Center, Division of Dermatology.*)

DIFFERENTIAL DIAGNOSIS

Other causes of hyperthyroidism are as follow:

- Autonomous functioning nodule—This is an uncommon cause of thyrotoxicosis (present in 1.6%-9% of patients with hyperthyroidism),[8] and most nodules do not cause hyperthyroidism. These present as a discrete swelling in an otherwise normal thyroid gland, and thyroid scan would show a discrete nodule.

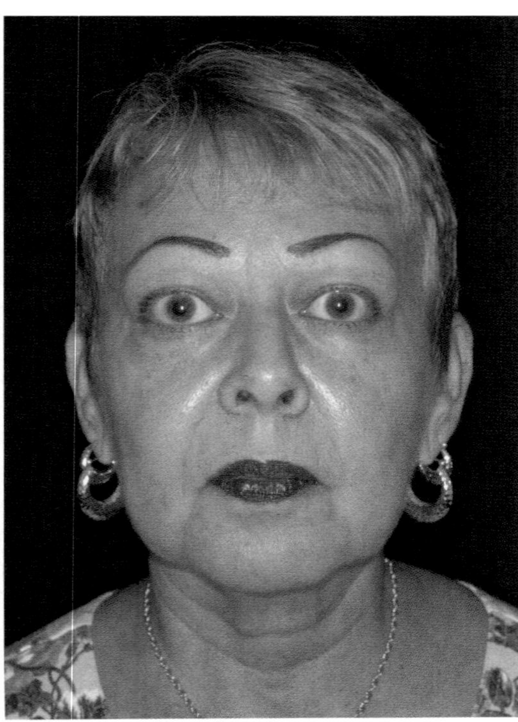

FIGURE 227-7 Bilateral exophthalmos that has been present for 5 years since patient was diagnosed with Graves disease. Although the radioactive iodine returned her thyroid function to normal, the exophthalmos continues to bother the patient. (*Reproduced with permission from Richard P. Usatine, MD.*)

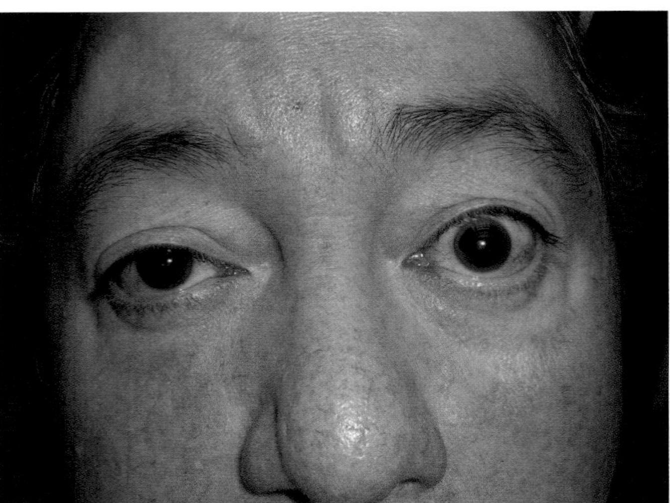

FIGURE 227-8 Woman with unilateral Graves ophthalmopathy and vitiligo. There is a strong association between autoimmune thyroid diseases and vitiligo. (*Reproduced with permission from Richard P. Usatine, MD.*)

- Toxic multinodular goiter—More common cause of hyperthyroidism in the elderly; thyroid scan shows multiple foci of increased uptake.
- Thyrotropin-secreting pituitary adenoma (rare)—Adenomas may cause visual disturbance (in the absence of exophthalmos), and other hormonal stimulation may occur (eg, elevated serum prolactin).
- Thyroiditis—May be painless or painful, short duration, low update on RAI scan.
- Exogenous thyroid hormone ingestion—History of overdosage of prescribed or acquired thyroid medication.

The differential diagnoses for the eye findings include the following:

- Metastatic disease to the extraocular muscles.
- Pseudotumor—This condition's rapid onset and pain differentiate it from Graves ophthalmopathy.

MANAGEMENT

Three options are available to treat the hyperthyroidism: antithyroid drugs, RAI therapy, and surgery, as discussed below.[1,2] SOR Ⓐ

NONPHARMACOLOGIC

Supportive measures for eye symptoms include dark glasses, artificial tears, propping up the head and taping the eyelids closed at night.

MEDICATIONS

- Symptoms of hyperthyroidism can be controlled with β-adrenergic blockers (eg, propranolol, 10-40 mg bid–qid) or calcium channel blockers (eg, diltiazem, 30-90 mg bid). SOR Ⓑ Authors of a recent guideline recommend β-adrenergic blockage in elderly patients with symptomatic disease, those who are thyrotoxic with cardiovascular disease or a resting heart rate greater than 90 beats/min, and prior to RAI treatment in patients with GD at risk for complications of extreme hyperthyroidism (eg, highly symptomatic).[7]

- Antithyroid drugs (methimazole 10-20 mg/d or propylthiouracil [PTU], 100-200 mg every 8 hours). Potential side effects of these medications include rash, joint pain, liver inflammation, and, rarely, agranulocytosis.[2] Baseline liver enzymes and complete blood count (CBC) (including white blood cells [WBCs] and differential) is recommended.[7] Methimazole is preferred except in patients during the first trimester of pregnancy, those being treated for thyroid storm, or for those who have reactions to methimazole.[7]
- The drug dose may be reduced after the patient is euthyroid (typically PTU 50-100 mg/d and methimazole 2.5-10 mg/d).
- Antithyroid drugs are preferred during pregnancy and can be considered in patients with mild disease, small goiter, and lower antibody levels. Pretreatment with methimazole prior to RAI is suggested for patients with GD who are at high risk for complications of extreme hyperthyroidism.[7] They are also used more commonly as primary treatment in Europe and Asia.
- The optimal duration of titrated antithyroid drug therapy is 12 to 18 months to minimize relapse.[7,9] SOR Ⓐ
- In a randomized controlled trial (RCT) of 159 patients with mild Graves orbitopathy who were given selenium (100 μg twice daily), pentoxifylline (600 mg twice daily), or placebo (twice daily) orally for 6 months, selenium significantly improved quality of life, reduced ocular involvement, and slowed progression of the disease compared to the other treatments.[10]
- Patients with severe (and possibly moderate) Graves orbitopathy are usually treated with a 12-week course of high-dose intravenous glucocorticoid pulses (total <8 g of methylprednisolone); approximately 80% of patients respond to this regimen.[11,12] Liver failure is a serious but rare side effect.

RADIOTHERAPY

- RAI—It is the most commonly prescribed treatment in the United States, but is contraindicated in pregnancy or with breast-feeding and should be used with caution in patients with cardiovascular disease.
- RAI may also be used after initial treatment with antithyroid drugs; these drugs should be discontinued for 3 to 7 days before treatment.[2]
- The half-life of iodine-131 is about 1 week; however, it is recommended that women not attempt pregnancy for 6 to 12 months after RAI treatment.
- RAI may cause painful thyroid inflammation for a few weeks in approximately 1% of patients; this condition can be treated with nonsteroidal anti-inflammatory agents, β-blockers, and possibly steroids.[3] Approximately 5% of patients with toxic nodular goiter treated with RAI develop GD.[3]
- In addition, radiation-induced thyroiditis can aggravate ophthalmopathy. This side effect can be minimized by early levothyroxine replacement and prednisone (60-80 mg/d starting at the time of RAI treatment and tapering, after 2-4 weeks, over the next 3-12 months).[13] One author believed that moderate-to-severe ophthalmopathy was a contraindication for RAI.[3]

SURGICAL TREATMENT

- Near-total to total thyroidectomy by a high-volume thyroid surgeon is recommended for patients with GD.[7]
- Indications for surgery are very large goiters, presence of suspicious nodules, pregnant women requiring high doses of antithyroid drugs, and allergy or failure of other therapies.
- In most cases for patients with GD, pretreatment with methimazole until euthyroid is recommended prior to surgery and levothyroxine is started following surgery.[7]
- Following surgery, small remnants of thyroid tissue (<4 g) result in rates of hypothyroidism of greater than 50% and large remnants (>8 g) have higher rates of recurrent hyperthyroidism (15%).
- With respect to the eye findings, most symptoms except for proptosis improve with control of the hyperthyroidism. In one study, 64% of the patients spontaneously improved, 22% stabilized, and 14% progressed.[13]

REFERRAL

- Patients with significant eye symptoms or clinical findings should be referred to an ophthalmologist.
- Treatment options for the persistent severe ophthalmopathy include high-dose systemic steroids (40-80 mg/d), orbital radiotherapy, and orbital decompression surgery.[14] SOR Ⓑ

PROGNOSIS

- With use of antithyroid medications, symptoms improve in 3 to 4 weeks; weight gain (about 4.5 kg) often occurs as metabolism normalizes.[2] Remission rates following antithyroid drugs vary from 37% to 70% and occur within 6 to 8 weeks.
- Following RAI, 50% to 75% of patients become euthyroid after 5 to 8 weeks, but 50% to 90% of patients with GD eventually become hypothyroid (10%-20% in year 1 and 5% per year afterward). Retreatment with radioiodine may be needed in 14% of patients with GD, 10% to 30% of patients with toxic adenoma, and 6% to 18% of patients with toxic nodular goiter.[3]
- In a RCT comparing GD treatments, relapse rates were higher among patients who received antithyroid drugs (approximately 40% [range 34% (elderly) to 42% (young)]) versus patients following RAI (21%) and surgery (5% [3% (young) to 8% (elderly)]).[15]
- Goiter and exophthalmos can persist years after the hyperthyroidism has been treated (**Figure 227-9**).

FOLLOW-UP

- The goals of therapy are to resolve hyperthyroid symptoms and to restore the euthyroid state. Close follow-up is needed in the initial treatment period; medications for symptoms of hyperthyroidism may be withdrawn slowly following treatment.
- Antithyroid drug dosages may be reduced after the patient is euthyroid (typically PTU 50-100 mg/d and methimazole 2.5-10 mg/d), but drugs should be continued for 12 to 18 months to minimize relapse. SOR Ⓐ
- Following treatment with RAI, most patients eventually become hypothyroid (20% within the first year) and so periodic monitoring of thyroid function is important. Follow-up within the first 1 to 2 months (free T_4 and T_3) is recommended and then at 4 to 6 weeks if hyperthyroidism continues; consider retreatment with RAI if there is minimal response at 3 months or hyperthyroidism persists at 6 months.[7]
- Following surgery, patients may become hypothyroid or have a recurrence of hyperthyroidism, depending on the size of the remnant remaining; patients should be monitored with periodic blood tests and for symptoms. For those with GD following surgery and levothyroxine, a TSH is recommended at 6 to 8 weeks postoperation.[7]

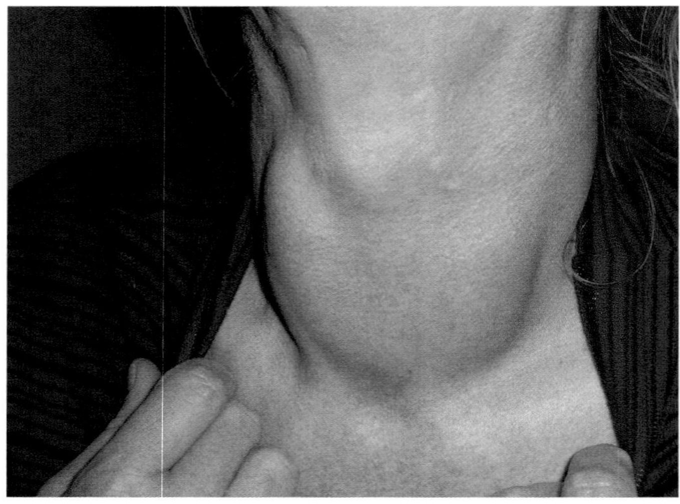

A

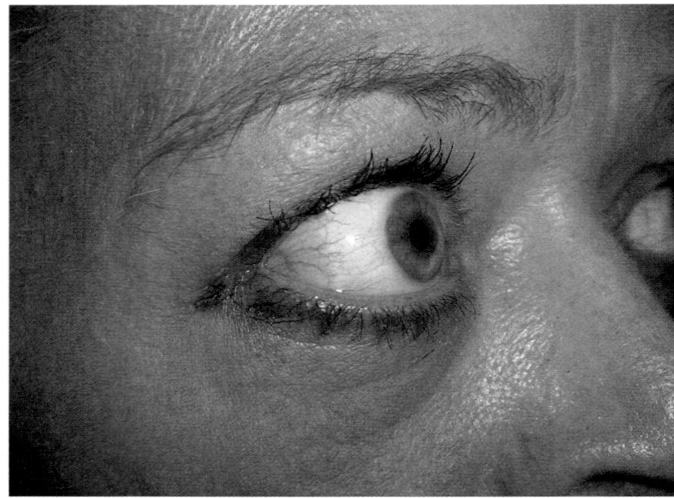

B

FIGURE 227-9 Persistent goiter and exophthalmos after treatment of Graves disease with radioactive iodine. Even though a patient is no longer hyperthyroid the enlarged thyroic (A) and eye findings (B) do not necessarily resolve. (*Reproduced with permission from Richard P. Usatine, MD.*)

- An in-office exophthalmometer can be used to track changes in eye prominence over time.[2]
- Patients with GD are at high risk for development of other autoimmune disease; in one cross-sectional study in the United Kingdom of patients attending a thyroid clinic, the frequency of another autoimmune disorder (eg, rheumatoid arthritis [3.15%], pernicious anemia, systemic lupus erythematosus, Addison disease, celiac disease, and vitiligo) was 9.67% in patients with GD.[16]

PATIENT EDUCATION

- Patients should be told that the goals of therapy are to resolve the symptoms of thyroid excess and to restore the thyroid function to normal.
- The treatment choices should be discussed, as each has advantages and disadvantages; treatment should be individualized.
- Regardless of the therapy chosen, long-term follow-up is needed to monitor thyroid status; there is a high risk of becoming hypothyroid in the future or to relapse again into hyperthyroidism. Patients should be made aware of symptoms to watch for and to report any recurrent symptoms.
- Following RAI, patients should avoid intimate contact (including kissing) and contact with children for 5 days; avoid contact with pregnant women for 10 days (maintain distance of approximately 6 ft); limit close contact with other adults to 2 hours for 5 days; sit while voiding and flush twice with the lid closed; not share toothbrushes, utensils, dishes, towels, or clothes, and wash these separately.[3]
- Ophthalmopathy usually runs its own course independent of the thyroid function. Additional treatment may be needed in consultation with an ophthalmologist.
- Smoking cessation may have a beneficial effect on the course of ophthalmopathy.
- Siblings and children should be made aware of their increased risk of developing thyroid disease or associated disorders and should monitor themselves for symptoms.

PATIENT RESOURCES

- Information from the American Thyroid Association—**http://www.thyroid.org/patient-thyroid-information/.**
- National Library of Medicine—**http://www.nlm.nih.gov/medlineplus/thyroiddiseases.html.**
- National Graves' Disease Foundation—**http://www.ngdf.org.**

PROVIDER RESOURCES

- Bahn RS, Burch HB, Cooper DS, et al. Hyperthyroidism and other causes of thyrotoxicosis: management guidelines of the American Thyroid Association and the American Association of Clinical Endocrinologists. *Thyroid*. 2011;21(6):593-641.
- Stagnaro-Green A, Abalovich M, Alexander E, et al. American Thyroid Association Taskforce on thyroid disease during pregnancy and postpartum. *Thyroid*. 2011;21(10):1081-1125.

REFERENCES

1. Jameson JL, Weetman AP. Disorders of the thyroid gland. In: Kasper DL, Braunwald E, Fauci AS, Hauser SL, Longo DL, Jameson JL, eds. *Harrison's Principles of Internal Medicine*. 16th ed. New York, NY: McGraw-Hill; 2005:2109-2113.
2. Brent GA. Graves' disease. *N Engl J Med*. 2008;358(24):2594-2605.
3. Ross DS. Radioiodine therapy for hyperthyroidism. *N Engl J Med*. 2011;364:542-550.
4. Douglas RS, Naik V, Hwang CJ, et al. B cells from patients with Graves' disease aberrantly express the IGF-1 receptor: implications for disease pathogenesis. *J Immunol*. 2008;181(8):5768-5774.
5. Jabbour SA. Cutaneous manifestations of endocrine disorders. *Am J Clin Dermatol*. 2003;4(5):315-331.
6. Costagliola S, Marganthaler NG, Hoermann R, et al. Second generation assay for thyrotropin receptor antibodies has superior diagnostic sensitivity for Graves' disease. *J Clin Endocrinol Metab*. 1999;84:90-97.

7. Bahn RS, Burch HB, Cooper DS, et al. Hyperthyroidism and other causes of thyrotoxicosis: management guidelines of the American Thyroid Association and the American Association of Clinical Endocrinologists. *Thyroid.* 2011;21(6):593-641.

8. Siegel RD, Lee SL. Toxic nodular goiter—toxic adenoma and toxic multinodular goiter. *Endocrinol Metab Clin North Am.* 1998;27(1): 151-166.

9. Abraham P, Avenell A, Watson W, et al. Antithyroid drug regimen for treating Graves' hyperthyroidism. *Cochrane Database Syst Rev.* 2005;2:CD003420.

10. Marcocci C, Kahaly GJ, Krassas GE, et al. Selenium and the course of mild Graves' orbitopathy. *N Engl J Med.* 2011;364(20): 1920-1931.

11. Zang S, Ponto KA, Kahaly GJ. Clinical review: Intravenous glucocorticoids for Graves' orbitopathy: efficacy and morbidity. *J Clin Endocrinol Metab.* 2011;96(2):320-332.

12. Bartalena L, Baldeschi L, Dickinson AJ, et al. Consensus statement of the European Group on Graves' Orbitopathy (EUGOGO) on management of Graves' orbitopathy. *Thyroid.* 2008;18(3):333-346.

13. Kaplan MM, Meier DA, Dworkin HJ. Treatment of hyperthyroidism with radioactive iodine. *Endocrinol Metab Clin North Am.* 1998;27(1):205-222.

14. Boulos PR, Hardy I. Thyroid-associated orbitopathy: a clinicopathologic and therapeutic review. *Curr Opin Ophthalmol.* 2004;15(5): 389-400.

15. Törring O, Tallstedt L, Wallin G, et al. Graves' hyperthyroidism: treatment with antithyroid drugs, surgery, or radioiodine—a prospective, randomized study. *J Clin Endocrinol Metab.* 1996;81: 2986-2993.

16. Boelaert K, Newby PR, Simmonds MJ, et al. Prevalence and relative risk of other autoimmune diseases in subjects with autoimmune thyroid disease. *Am J Med.* 2010;123(2):183.e1-e9.

228 ACROMEGALY

Mindy A Smith, MD, MS

PATIENT STORY

A 60-year-old man presents to his family physician with severe headache and weakness (**Figure 228-1**). He also noted enlargement of his hands (**Figure 228-2**), which made him remove his wedding ring when it became too tight, and feet (his shoe size had increased). He said his voice seemed to be deeper and his hands feel doughy and sweaty. Laboratory testing reveals an elevated insulin-like growth factor (IGF)-1, and there is a failure of growth hormone (GH) suppression following an oral glucose load confirming the diagnosis of acromegaly. Computed tomography (CT) scan of the head demonstrates a pituitary adenoma.

INTRODUCTION

Acromegaly is a condition of excessive linear and organ growth usually caused by autonomous GH hypersecretion from a pituitary tumor.

EPIDEMIOLOGY

- Rare (5/1,000,000 adults).[1]
- Most typically caused by a pituitary somatotrope macroadenoma. It may also be caused by growth hormone–releasing hormone (GHRH) excess from lesions of the pancreas, lung, or ovaries, or from a chest or abdominal carcinoid tumor.

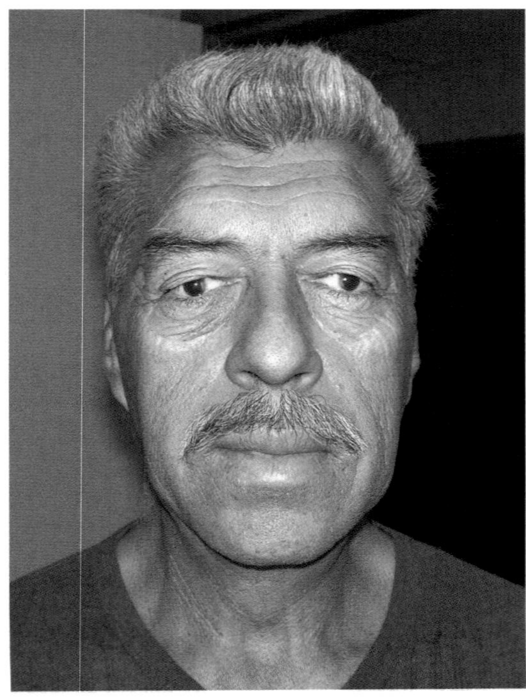

FIGURE 228-1 A 60-year-old man with acromegaly. Note the coarse facial features and moderate prognathism (protrusion of the lower jaw). (*Reproduced with permission from Richard P. Usatine, MD.*)

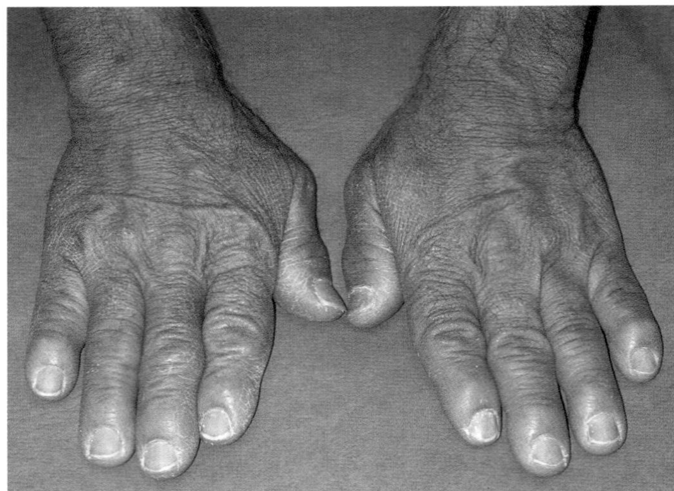

FIGURE 228-2 The man in **Figure 228-1** with acromegaly producing hands that are large and doughy with widened fingers. (*Reproduced with permission from Richard P. Usatine, MD.*)

- The disorder is usually sporadic, but may be familial (<5%) and has been associated with other endocrine tumors (eg, multiple endocrine neoplasia type 1).[1]
- In a Spanish multicenter epidemiologic study, the reported mean age at diagnosis was 45 years.[2]
- The occurrence of GH hypersecretion in children and adolescents, prior to epiphyseal closure, causes gigantism.

ETIOLOGY AND PATHOPHYSIOLOGY

- The clinical signs and symptoms of acromegaly result from GH excess that stimulates linear and organ growth (through IGF-1), soft tissue swelling, and chondrocyte action.
- Acromegaly is also associated with insulin resistance and an increased risk of cardiovascular disease; the latter appears to be a result of pressure-related arterial and left ventricular stiffening rather than atherosclerotic disease.[3]
- An increased risk for several cancers among these patients may be a result of the proliferative and antiapoptotic activity associated with increased circulating levels of IGF-1.

DIAGNOSIS

The diagnosis of acromegaly is established by documenting autonomous GH hypersecretion and by pituitary imaging.

CLINICAL FEATURES

The clinical manifestations of acromegaly are often subtle and may not be noticed for many years. Gigantism occurs if excessive GH exposure occurs *before* closure of the epiphyses; acromegaly develops *after* closure of the epiphyses. Clinical features of acromegaly include the following[1]:

- Soft tissue swelling resulting in hand and foot enlargement (see **Figure 228-2**).
- Kyphoscoliosis and skeletal hyperostosis.

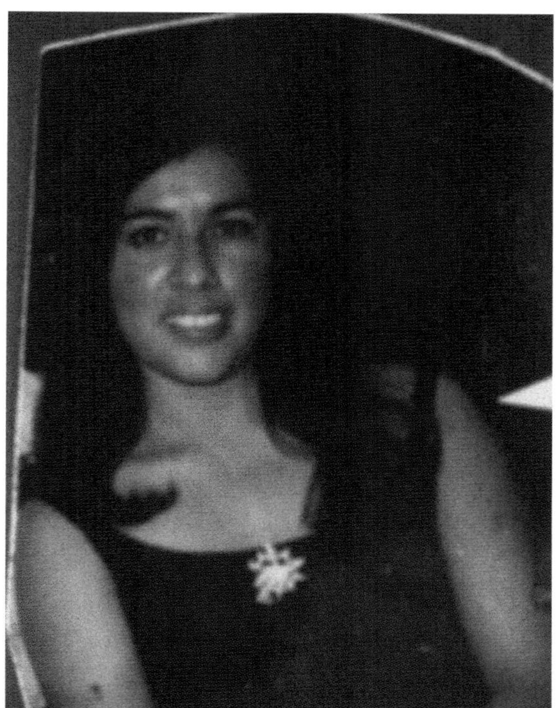

A

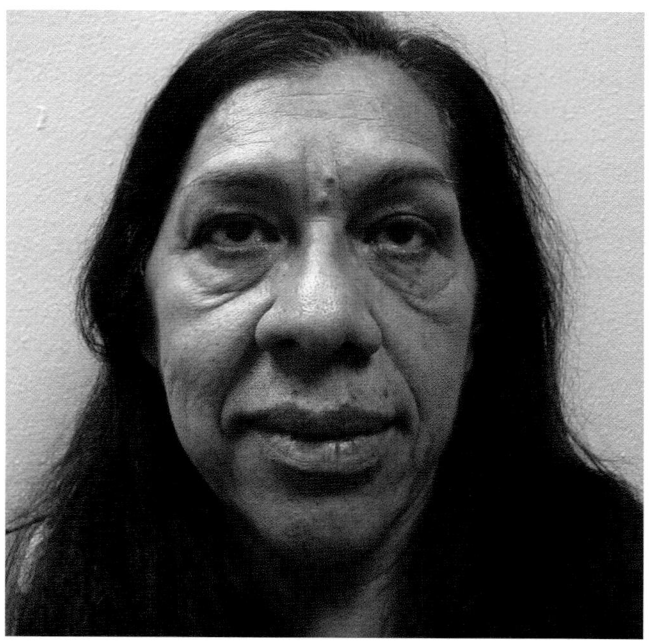

B

FIGURE 228-3 A. A 26-year-old woman prior to acromegaly changes. B. Facial changes 20 years later in the same woman. Note the coarse facial features with large nose, lips, and chin. Protrusion of the lower jaw is visible. *(Reproduced with permission from Vernon Burke, DMD.)*

- Coarse facial features and a large fleshy nose (**Figures 228-1** and **228-3**).
- Frontal bossing.
- Jaw malocclusion and overbite.
- Hyperhidrosis and oily skin.
- Other common features are deep voice (soft tissue swelling of vocal cords), arthropathy, carpel tunnel syndrome, kyphosis, proximal muscle weakness, and fatigue; patients may complain of headache and visual field defects (expanding tumor), paresthesias, and sexual dysfunction.[1]
- Associated medical conditions include sleep apnea (60%), coronary heart disease (20%-90% depending on duration and associated hypertension), and diabetes mellitus (25%). There also appears to be an increase in intracranial aneurysms.[4]
- In one study ($N = 55$), approximately two-thirds of women had anovulatory cycles; some believed this as related to elevated hormone levels.[5]

LABORATORY AND IMAGING

- An elevated total serum IGF-1 concentration (age and gender matched) is extremely useful in the diagnosis of acromegaly.[6] Lack of standardization and normative data, however, have hampered diagnosis and monitoring.
- Failure of GH suppression to less than 1 μg/L within 1 to 2 hours of an oral glucose load (75 g) can confirm the diagnosis, although 20% of patients exhibit a paradoxical increase in GH. Failure to suppress GH levels can also be seen in patients with diabetes, renal or hepatic failure, and obesity, and in those receiving estrogen replacement and in pregnant women.[1]
- A single measure of GH is not helpful because of its pulsatile secretion.
- Another associated laboratory abnormality is elevated prolactin (30% of patients).

MANAGEMENT

The Acromegaly Consensus Group recommends a team approach, including an experienced surgeon, endocrinologist with pituitary expertise, and a physician with radiotherapy experience.[7] Treatment is usually surgical followed by medication (usually a somatostatin receptor ligand [SRL]) if the disease is not controlled. If initial medical treatment (following dose titration) fails to normalize GH and IGF-1, patients with tumor mass on magnetic resonance imaging (MRI) may consider radiation therapy while those without a mass effect may be tried on combination medical therapy.[7]

MEDICATIONS

There are 3 types of medications used in the treatment of patients with acromegaly: SRLs, a GH receptor antagonist, and a dopamine agonist. Although GH reduction may alleviate symptoms, attempts to normalize levels of both GH and its target growth factor (ie, IGF-I) should be made because persistent secretion of either pose significant long-term health risks.

- There is insufficient evidence to support presurgical treatment with SRLs.[7]
- Somatostatin analogs are first-line therapy for those with nonsurgically resectable tumors; after surgery if normalization of GH and IGF-1 does not occur; or during radiation treatment until control is achieved by that therapy (can take several years).
  - Long-acting somatostatin depot formulations, octreotide LAR and lanreotide Autogel, are available and appear equivalent. Patients should be treated with the same dose for 3 months before reassessment and dose titration if needed.[7]

- Side effects are injection pain, sinus bradycardia, and symptoms related to suppression of gastrointestinal (GI) motility and secretion (nausea, abdominal pain, diarrhea, and flatulence); gallstones or sludge occur in 30%, but few develop cholecystitis.[1]
- Subcutaneous pegvisomant is the available GH receptor antagonist for acromegaly. It is indicated for patients with persistent IGF-1 elevations despite other treatment, as an adjunct to SRLs, or possibly as monotherapy; supporting data are lacking.[7]
  - Side effects include injection site pain and lipohypertrophy. Elevated liver enzymes are seen in approximately 5% to 25% of patients (usually transient) and should be monitored.
- Of the dopamine agonists, only cabergoline is effective (limited) at suppressing GH hypersecretion.[7]
  - Considered for patients preferring oral medication, patients following surgery with markedly elevated prolactin along with elevated GH and IGF-1, and as an adjunct to SRLs when failed response to maximum dose.[7]
  - Common side effects are GI (nausea, constipation), psychiatric and central nervous system (sleep disturbance, vertigo, depression), and cardiovascular (hypertension, peripheral edema); cardiac valve abnormalities have been reported in patients with Parkinson disease (who usually use high doses).

PROCEDURES

- Surgical resection (adenomectomy via transsphenoidal approach) is the cornerstone of treatment for intrasellar microadenomas, noninvasive macroadenomas, and when the tumor is causing compression symptoms.[7]
- Radiation therapy, conventional and stereotactic procedures, is also effective in decreasing GH levels but takes 10 to 15 years to work and carries a risk of hypopituitarism (>50%). It is considered third-line therapy.[7] Radiation has been used in an attempt to discontinue medical therapy.
  - Five-year remission rates from gamma knife radiotherapy (after surgical debulking) are between 29% and 60%.[7]
  - Conventional radiotherapy has potential risks of second tumors (approximately 1% intracranial) and cerebrovascular events, but long-term data are lacking.[7]

PROGNOSIS

- After surgical resection, 70% to 95% of patients with microadenomas and 40% to 68% of patients with macroadenomas have normalization of IGF-1.[6,7]
  - Irradiation of adenomas results in attenuation of IGF-1 secretion in more than 60% of subjects after 10 to 15 years.[7]
  - Less than half of patients (44%) receiving somatostatin analogs achieve normal IGF-1 levels, and a third achieve normal GH levels.[7]
- An MRI following surgery demonstrating a hypotense MRI signal in the remaining tumor may be useful in predicting good response to subsequent somatostatin analog treatment.[8]
- In the past, patients with acromegaly had a 10-year reduction in life span because of cardiac (heart failure, arrhythmia), cerebrovascular, metabolic (diabetes, osteoporosis), and respiratory (airway obstruction from macroglossia and hypertrophied mucosal tissues, sleep apnea) disease; radiotherapy may also increase the mortality rate.[1] Both IGF-1 and GH levels correlate with mortality and normalizing these levels (IGF-1 to age/sex standards and GH <2.5 ng/mL) appear to normalize the life span.[7]

FOLLOW-UP

- Identification and treatment of comorbidities should be pursued. An initial colonoscopy and echocardiogram is recommended.[7]
- The Acromegaly Consensus Group defines optimal disease control (ie, posttreatment remission of acromegaly) as IGF-1 level (determined by a reliable standardized assay) in the age-adjusted normal range, and a GH level less than 1 g/L from a random GH measurement, using an ultrasensitive assay.[6] In patients who are controlled, monitor levels every 6 months.
- Based on a cohort study of patients hospitalized for acromegaly (Denmark 1977-1993; Sweden 1965-1993) linked to tumor registry data for up to 28 years of follow-up, individuals with acromegaly have higher rates of small intestine, colon, rectal, kidney, and bone cancer.[9] The researchers also found that these patients had elevated rates for cancers of the brain and thyroid that may be related to pituitary irradiation.
- Monitoring treatment success postoperatively or following radiation therapy includes the following:
  - Measurement of GH and IGF-1 levels. The consensus group suggests that optimal disease control (ie, posttreatment remission of acromegaly) is now defined as IGF-1 level (determined by a reliable standardized assay) in the age-adjusted normal range and a GH level less than 1 g/L from a random GH measurement.[6]
  - Postoperative MRI 3 to 4 months postsurgery and 3 to 6 months following medical therapy, and yearly for those who remain uncontrolled. There is no consensus on frequency of continued MRI once remission is achieved.[7]
  - Full pituitary function should be measured 3 months after surgery and periodically for those receiving radiotherapy.[7]

PATIENT EDUCATION

- Patients should be advised that untreated, one's life span is decreased by an average of 10 years. Survival improves greatly if GH and IGF-1 can be normalized.
- Patients should consider increased surveillance for colorectal cancer and be encouraged to actively manage comorbid conditions.

PATIENT RESOURCES

- National Endocrine and Metabolic Diseases Information Service. *Acromegaly*—**http://www.endocrine.niddk.nih.gov/pubs/acro/acro.aspx.**

PROVIDER RESOURCES

- Medscape. *Acromegaly*—**http://emedicine.medscape.com/article/116366.**

REFERENCES

1. Melmed S. Acromegaly pathogenesis and treatment. *J Clin Invest.* 2009;119(11):3189-3202.
2. Mestron A, Webb SM, Astorga R, et al. Epidemiology, clinical characteristics, outcome, morbidity and mortality in acromegaly based on the Spanish Acromegaly Registry (Registro Espanol de Acromegalia, REA). *Eur J Endocrinol.* 2004;151(4):439-446.

3. Paisley AN, Banerjee M, Rezai M, et al. Changes in arterial stiffness but not carotid intimal thickness in acromegaly. *J Clin Endocrinol Metab.* 2011;96(5):1486-1492.

4. Manara R, Maffei P, Citton V, et al. Increased rate of intracranial saccular aneurysms in acromegaly: an MR angiography study and review of the literature. *J Clin Endocrinol Metab.* 2011;96(5):1292-1300.

5. Grynberg M, Salenave S, Young J, Chanson P. Female gonadal function before and after treatment of acromegaly. *J Clin Endocrinol Metab.* 2010;95(10):4518-4525.

6. Giustina A, Chanson P, Bronstein MD, et al. Acromegaly Consensus Group. A consensus on criteria for cure of acromegaly. *J Clin Endocrinol Metab.* 2010;95(7):3141-3148.

7. Melmed S, Colao A, Barkan A, et al. Guidelines for acromegaly management: an update. *J Clin Endocrinol Metab.* 2009;94:1509-1517.

8. Puig-Domingo M, Resmini E, Gomez-Anson B, et al. Magnetic resonance imaging as a predictor of response to somatostatin analogs in acromegaly after surgical failure. *J Clin Endocrinol Metab.* 2010;95(11):4973-4978.

9. Baris D, Gridley G, Ron E, et al. Acromegaly and cancer risk: a cohort study in Sweden and Denmark. *Cancer Causes Control.* 2002;13(5):395-400.

229 CUSHING SYNDROME

Deepthi Rao, MD

PATIENT STORY

A 22-year-old woman presents to the office complaining of increased fatigue, muscle aches, difficulty climbing steps, and mood swings. She was previously healthy and active until 2 years ago when she started gaining weight and having menstrual irregularities. Her vital signs were significant for a diastolic blood pressure (BP) of 100 mm of Hg and a body mass index (BMI) of 35. Significant physical examination findings included central obesity, facial plethora, thinning hair on scalp, acne, violaceous striae on abdomen and proximal muscle weakness. Cushing syndrome (CS) was suspected based on the clinical features. A 24-hour urinary cortisol level was found elevated at 450 μg/dL and CS was confirmed by a positive low-dose dexamethasone suppression test. An adrenocorticotropic hormone (ACTH) level was found to be less than 5 μg/dL and a high-resolution computed tomography (CT) of the abdomen showed right-sided 3.5-cm adrenal mass (**Figure 229-1**). She underwent a resection of the mass which was found to be an adenoma. The patient recovered well from the surgery and her Cushing syndrome began to resolve.

INTRODUCTION

- CS is the term given to a set of clinical manifestations which occur from prolonged exposure to inappropriately high glucocorticoid levels.
- Cushing disease (CD) is a subtype of CS caused by pituitary prompted glucocorticoid overproduction.
- Dr. Harvey Cushing described the first case of what is now known as Cushing disease in 1912.

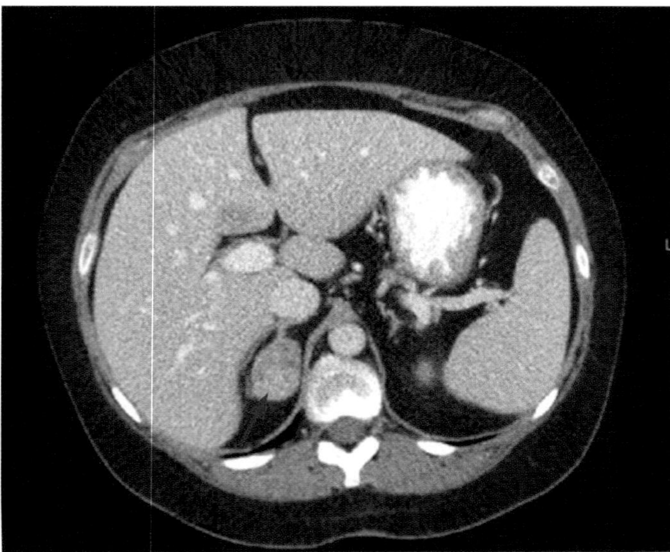

FIGURE 229-1 A CT scan demonstrating a right adrenal adenoma (red arrow) causing Cushing syndrome. (*Reproduced with persmission from Longo DL, Fauci AS, Kasper DL ,et al. Harrison's Principles of Internal Medicine. 18th ed. McGraw-Hill: 2012.*)

SYNONYMS

CS is also known as hypercortisolism and glucocorticoid excess.

EPIDEMIOLOGY

- The incidence of CS is about 1.2 to 2.4 cases for every million people.[1,2]
- However, due to the wide spectrum of presentation of CS, ranging from subclinical to mild to severe, it is generally thought that the disease is underreported.
- The gender distribution of CS varies with the cause.
    - Women are 3 to 8 times more likely to have CD and 4 to 5 times more likely to have CS associated with an adrenal tumor.[3-5]
    - Men had a 3-fold higher incidence of Cushing disease than women due to ectopic ACTH secretion associated with lung cancer. However, the increasing incidence of smoking and lung cancer in females has narrowed the margin.[3-5]

ETIOLOGY AND PATHOPHYSIOLOGY

- CS is caused by sustained and pathologically elevated cortisol levels in the body.
- Normally, corticotrophin-releasing hormone (CRH) is released from the hypothalamus and carried to the anterior pituitary gland, where it stimulates the synthesis and release of ACTH.
- This ACTH rise stimulates adrenal cortisol secretion, which in turn inhibits hypothalamic CRH synthesis and secretion, blocks the agonist effects of CRH on pituitary corticotrophs, and inhibits the release of ACTH.
- ACTH secretion is pulsatile and the amplitude of the pulses varies in a circadian rhythm.
- ACTH secretion rates and plasma ACTH concentrations are highest in the morning and lowest in the late evening times. Cortisol secretion is under the direct influence of ACTH and is therefore also pulsatile.
- Stressful stimuli increase ACTH secretion and, as a consequence, cortisol secretion.
- Disruption at any level of this cycle can induce cortisol elevation and cause CS. Based on the source of cortisol excess, CS is divided into ACTH dependent and independent etiologies (**Table 229-1**).

TABLE 229-1 Causes of Cushing Syndrome

ACTH Dependent	*ACTH Independent*
Pituitary tumor—Cushing disease	Exogenous steroid use
Ectopic ACTH secretion	Adrenal tumors (adenoma/ carcinoma)
Ectopic CRH secretion	Adrenal hyperplasia (micro- or macronodular) Ectopic cortisol secretion

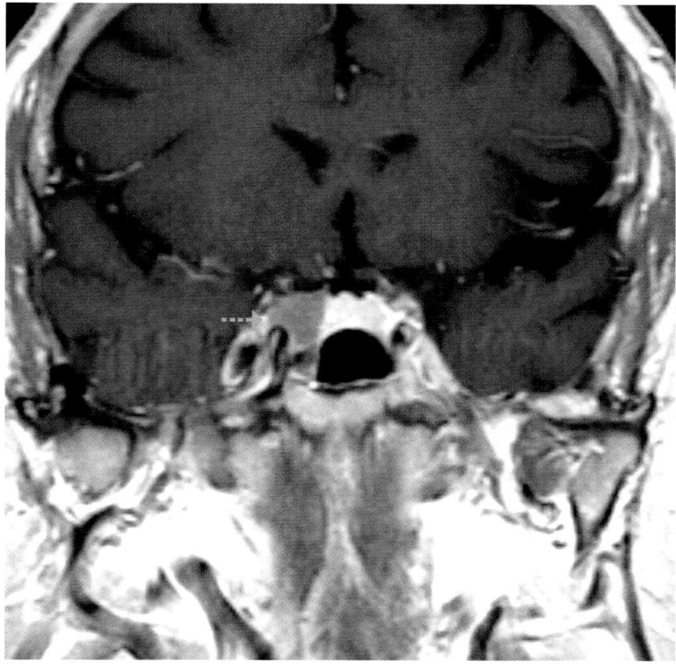

FIGURE 229-2 An ACTH-secreting pituitary adenoma (yellow arrow) in a patient with confirmed Cushing disease. (*Reproduced with permission from Carlos Tavera, MD.*)

ACTH DEPENDENT

- CD—Pituitary tumors or pituitary hyperplasia
  - CD is the term given to excessive cortisol levels caused by ACTH hypersecretion from the pituitary. Almost all of the cases of CD are caused by pituitary adenomas (**Figure 229-2**) and only a few are caused by hyperplasia of the corticotroph cells of the pituitary.
  - Of the pituitary adenomas only about 5% are macroadenomas while the rest are microadenomas of size less than 5 mm.
  - The amplitude and duration, but not the frequency, of ACTH secretory episodes are increased in CD, and the normal ACTH circadian rhythm is usually lost.[6-8]
  - The elevated plasma ACTH concentrations cause bilateral adrenocortical hyperplasia and hypersecretion of cortisol. Consequently, the normal circadian rhythm in cortisol secretion is also lost.[6,7]
- Ectopic ACTH or ectopic CRH secretion (eg, from a lung cancer)
  - In the ectopic ACTH syndrome, ACTH is secreted by nonpituitary tumors and causes bilateral adrenocortical hyperplasia and cortisol hypersecretion.
  - The increased serum cortisol concentrations inhibit hypothalamic CRH secretion which suppresses the normal pituitary ACTH release.
  - However ectopic ACTH secretion is usually not inhibited by the high cortisol levels.
  - Most cases of ectopic ACTH secretion are caused by tumors of the lung, pancreas, or thymus. Among them the most common are small-cell carcinomas of the lung which arise from neuroendocrine cells in the distal bronchioles.[8]
  - The ACTH-secreting pancreatic and thymic tumors are carcinoid tumors that arise from neuroendocrine cells in those tissues.
  - Several other tumors have been reported to cause ectopic ACTH secretion including Ewing sarcoma in children.
  - Isolated CRH secreting tumor cells are extremely rare and cause hyperplasia of pituitary corticotrophs, hypersecretion of ACTH and cortisol.[9]

ACTH INDEPENDENT

- Adrenal tumors
  - CS can be caused by hypercortisolism from adrenal origin (see **Figure 229-1**).
  - The excess cortisol suppresses CRH and ACTH and causes pituitary atrophy.
  - Adrenal adenomas are the most common source. Adrenal carcinomas are an infrequent cause and produce excess cortisol as well as other adrenal steroids.
- Bilateral adrenal micro- or macronodular hyperplasia
  - This is another cause of CS which is characterized by bilateral adrenal gland hyperplasia with micro (<5 mm) or macro (>5 mm) nodules.
  - Micronodular hyperplasia with pigmented adrenal micronodules can occur sporadically or in a familial form called Carney complex which is an autosomal dominant condition with pigmented lentigines and blue nevi and multiple neoplasms, both endocrine and nonendocrine.
  - Macronodular hyperplasia is characterized by adrenal glands that contain multiple nonpigmented benign nodules greater than 5 mm in diameter and hypercortisolism.
- Iatrogenic
  - In these cases CS is caused by exogenous administration of glucocorticoids.
  - Megestrol is a drug that has glucocorticoid-like properties and has also been reported to cause CS.
- Ectopic cortisol secretion
  - Rarely some ovarian tumors cause ectopic cortisol hypersecretion causing CS.

DIAGNOSIS OR SCREENING

CLINICAL FEATURES

- CS has a wide spectrum and the clinical findings which vary in severity from mild to dramatic depending on the duration and degree of hypercortisolism (**Table 229-2**).
- Full-blown cushingoid habitus is uncommon in present times and several features of CS are wide spread in the general population. Hence, CS should be considered in patients with any of the following features without an explanation to enable an early diagnosis. SOR Ⓒ
  - Weight gain or obesity is one of the first signs and involves the face, abdomen, and trunk. Extremities are usually spared. Fat deposition in the face commonly causes moon facies (**Figure 229-3**). A dorsocervical fat pad or buffalo hump and supraclavicular fullness may be seen.
  - In women with CS, menstrual irregularities as well signs of androgen excess including acne, hirsutism, and virilization may be seen.
  - Dermatologic findings include thinning of skin, purplish striae (**Figure 229-4**), easy bruisability, and acanthosis of the neck. Hyperpigmentation is seen in ACTH-dependent hypercortisolism.
  - Proximal muscle weakness and muscle wasting is also common.
  - Loss of bone mineral density causing osteoporosis is frequently seen in CS and fractures may occur.
  - Neuropsychiatric effects include depression, irritability, insomnia, cognitive dysfunction, and memory loss.
  - Raised intraocular pressure, infections and immune dysfunction, intraocular cataract development may be seen.

TABLE 229-2 Clinical Features of Cushing Syndrome

- Obesity
  - Central with extremity sparing
  - Moon facies
  - Buffalo hump
  - Supraclavicular fullness
- Dermatologic
  - Facial plethora
  - Thinning of skin
  - Easy bruisability
  - Purplish striae
  - Acanthosis
- Androgen excess
  - Menstrual irregularities
  - Acne
  - Hirsutism
- Vascular
  - Hypertension
- Musculoskeletal
  - Muscle weakness
  - Proximal myopathy
- Psychological
  - Irritability
  - Fatigue
  - Depression
- Metabolic
  - Glucose intolerance
  - Osteoporosis
  - Hypokalemia
  - Renal stones
- Immune
  - Frequent infections
- Other
  - Peripheral edema
  - Raise intraocular pressure
  - Intraocular cataracts

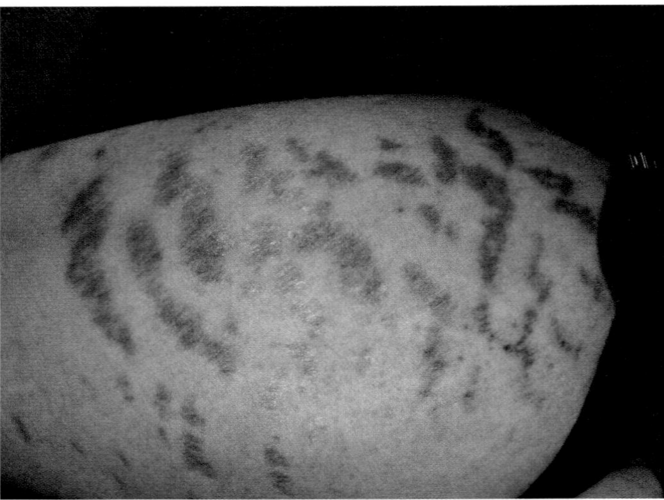

FIGURE 229-4 Violaceous close-up of broad purple striae (stretch marks) in a patient with Cushing syndrome. The underlying capillaries are prominent, producing a reddish or purple coloration. In pregnancy and obesity the striae are pale. (*Reproduced with persmission from Richard P. Usatine, MD.*)

- Elevated blood pressure and glucose intolerance are very common in CS and increase the vascular morbidity of CS.
- Patients with ectopic ACTH syndrome may not manifest all these symptoms but have a greater degree of hypertension, hypokalemia, and other symptoms related to the primary tumor may predominate.

LABORATORY TESTING

- The diagnostic evaluation of CS includes establishing hypercortisolism and finding the source of cortisol excess.
- Establishing the *diagnosis* of CS
  - A comprehensive drug history must be elicited for steroid use including oral, topical, and inhaled before evaluation for CS. SOR B

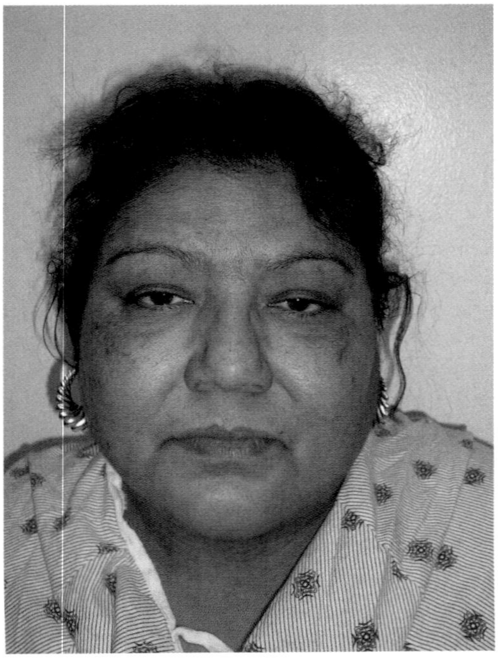

FIGURE 229-3 Moon facies in a patient with iatrogenic Cushing syndrome (*Reproduced with persmission from Richard P. Usatine, MD.*)

  - Surreptitious ingestion of steroids can be diagnosed by the detection of synthetic glucocorticoids in urine.
  - Initial tests to screen for CS should be highly sensitive and at least one of the following suggested first-line tests should be done.[10] SOR C
    - 24-hour urinary cortisol, midnight salivary cortisol, and low-dose 1-mg dexamethasone suppression test are suggested for initial evaluation (**Figure 229-5**).[10]
      - Urinary free cortisol (UFC)
        - A 24-hour urine sample excluding the first morning void on day 1 and including the first morning void of the next day is to be collected by the patient and refrigerated. Patients should avoid the use of any glucocorticoid preparations during the collection.
        - UFC is not affected by conditions and medications that alter the cortisol-binding globulin levels. Hence, this is the recommended test in pregnancy and in patients using estrogens and related medications.
        - Due to the difficulty in interpretation of the 24-hour creatinine, this test is to be avoided in renal failure patients.
      - Midnight salivary cortisol
        - In normal subjects serum cortisol level peaks during the early morning hours and is the lowest at around midnight.[11,12]
        - This circadian rhythm is lost in CD and the absence of a late night cortisol nadir is a consistent biochemical abnormality in patients with CS. Hence measurement of late night salivary cortisol is a valuable diagnostic test for CS.[11,12]
        - Patients are to collect a saliva sample on 2 separate evenings between 2300 and 2400 hours. The sample is stable at room temperature.
        - Patients are instructed to avoid licorice, chewing and smoking tobacco for a day as this can falsely elevate the cortisol levels.
        - This can be falsely positive in night shift workers, patients with depression, and critically ill patients.[13,14]

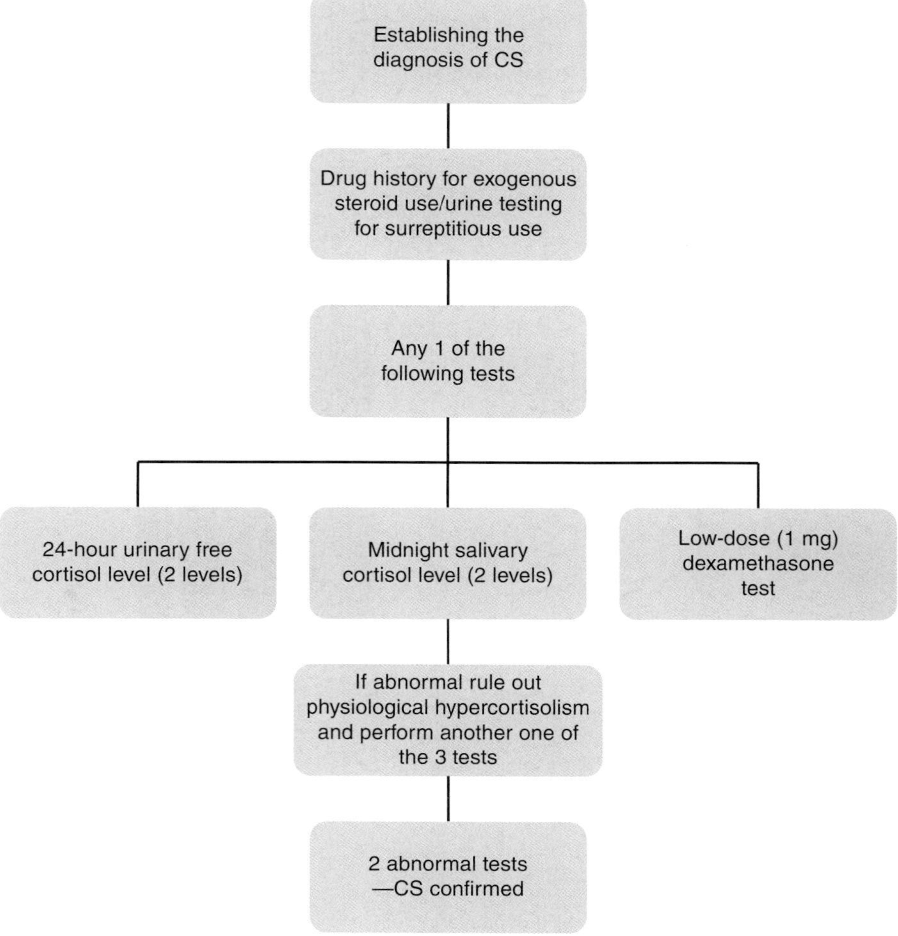

FIGURE 229-5 Establishing the *diagnosis* of Cushing syndrome.

- Low-dose dexamethasone suppression test
    - In normal subjects, the ACTH and cortisol secretion is suppressed when supraphysiological dose of glucocorticoid is administered. This suppression is lost in CS.
    - 1-mg dexamethasone is usually given between 2300 and 2400 hours, and cortisol is measured between 0800 and 0900 hours the following morning.
    - Dexamethasone metabolism can be affected by a multitude of antiepileptic drugs and hence this test is to be avoided in these patients.
  - If the urinary or salivary cortisol levels are done, at least 2 measurements should be obtained because the hypercortisolism of CS can be variable.[10] SOR C
  - Clinicians should be mindful that certain conditions including severe depression, pregnancy, chronic alcoholism, and morbid obesity cause physiological hypercortisolism and can cause false-positive tests.
  - Hence, an abnormal test should be confirmed by performing another one of the 3 tests. Abnormal results of 2 or more of these initial tests confirm CS.[10] SOR C
- Establishing the cause of CS (**Figure 229-6**)
  - Once, CS is confirmed, the next step involves finding the etiology of CS.
  - Measurement of *plasma ACTH level* is the next step. SOR C
  - ACTH independent
    - If the plasma ACTH level is less than 5 pg/mL, CS is ACTH independent.
    - The next step in ACTH-independent CS is thin section CT imaging of bilateral adrenal glands to look for tumors or hyperplasia.
    - Radiologic features including size, attenuation, and other factors like calcifications and hemorrhage suggest malignancy.
    - If the CT findings suggest unilateral benign adenoma no further testing is required.
    - If bilateral benign masses are found, testing may indicate whether one of them is an adrenal "incidentaloma" and nonfunctional.
    - If bilateral hyperplasia is found it can be micro- or macronodular and can also be seen in ACTH-dependent CS under the influence of the excessive ACTH.
    - In case of micronodular hyperplasia, further physical exam and testing to determine the presence of Carney complex is indicated.
  - ACTH dependent
    - If the plasma ACTH level is greater than 20 pg/mL, the CS is definitely ACTH dependent. If the level is between 5 and 20 pg/mL, CS is usually ACTH dependent.
    - The next step is to determine whether the source of ACTH is from the pituitary (CD) or ectopic, using the *high-dose dexamethasone test*.
    - Excessive ACTH secretion by the pituitary in CD is only relatively resistant to the negative feedback regulation by glucocorticoids

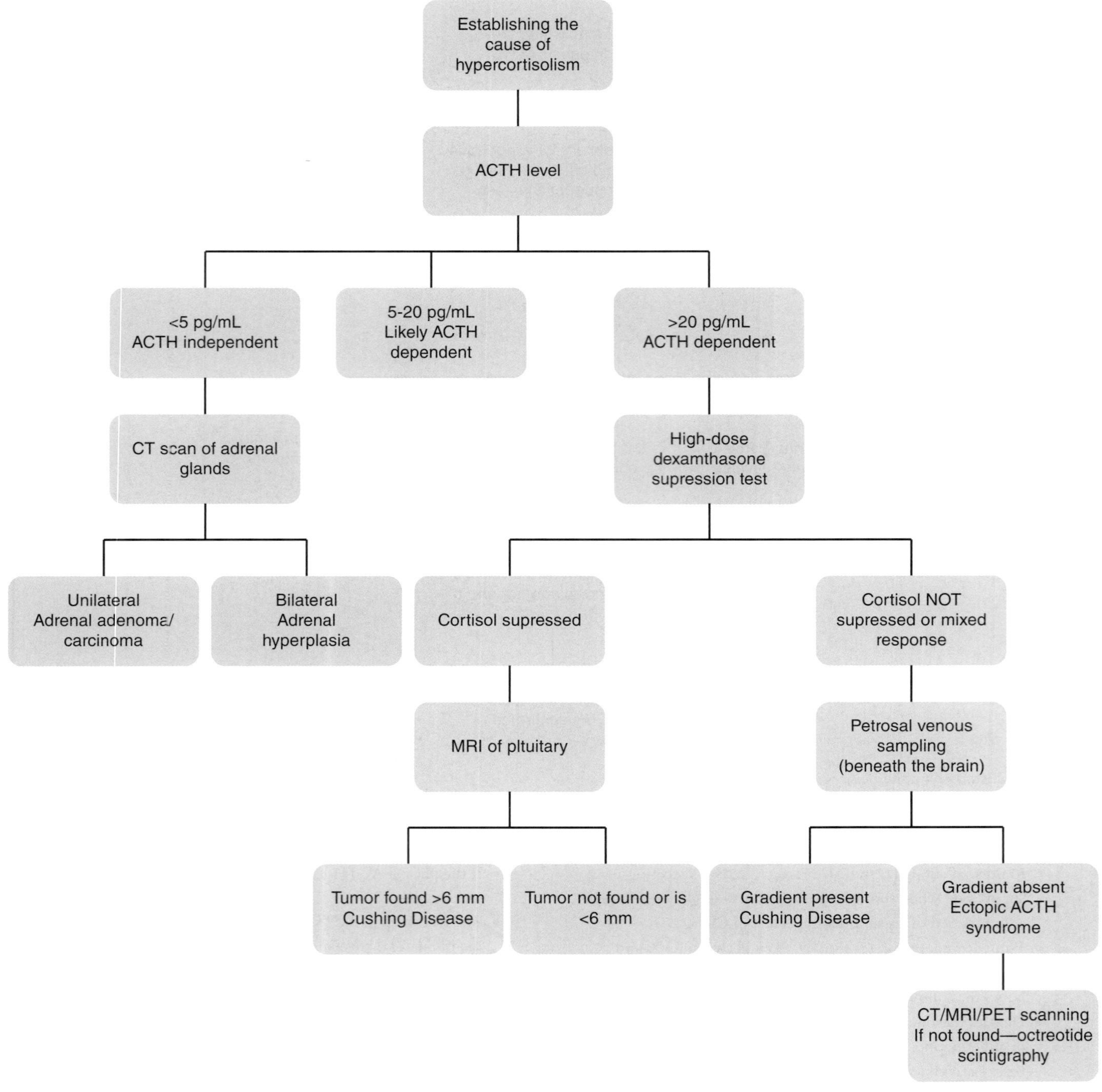

FIGURE 229-6 Establishing the *cause* of Cushing syndrome.

while the ectopic ACTH secretion from nonpituitary tumors is completely resistant to feedback inhibition, except some bronchial carcinoids.[15,16]

- The most commonly used high-dose test is done by administering 8 mg of dexamethasone between 2300 and 2400 hours the previous night and the measurement of serum cortisol at 8 AM in the morning. Serum ACTH level can also be measured simultaneously.
- The morning serum cortisol is usually less than 5 μg/dL in patients with a pituitary source of ACTH (CD).
  - Levels above 5 μg/dL may indicate an ectopic source of ACTH secretion.

LABORATORY AND IMAGING

- If cortisol level is suppressed in the high-dose test, a pituitary magnetic resonance imaging (MRI) is the next step for tumor detection. If a pituitary tumor of greater than 6 mm is detected by the MRI it is confirmatory of CD.
- If the cortisol levels are not suppressed or show mixed response in the high-dose test or if the pituitary MRI fails to detect the tumor even if cortisol is suppressed then inferior petrosal (beneath the brain) venous catheterization should be done for tumor localization and also confirmation of the pituitary source.

- Petrosal and peripheral venous plasma ACTH levels are measured 10 minutes before and after the administration of CRH. A central-to-peripheral plasma ACTH gradient of greater than or equal to 2 before CRH administration, or greater than or equal to 3 after CRH, is diagnostic of a pituitary source of ACTH, that is, CD.[17]
- A gradient of greater than or equal to 1.4 between the ACTH concentrations in the 2 sinuses predicted the side of the tumor with up to 71% accuracy if catheters were appropriately placed according to a study,[17] however this has not been validated.
- If a gradient is absent in the petrosal venous sampling, the diagnosis points to ectopic ACTH syndrome. However, a caveat to be noted is that if there is high suspicion for ectopic ACTH syndrome, the petrosal catheterization can be avoided and one can proceed directly to the next step which entails CT, MRI, or positron emission tomography (PET) imaging of the body. If this fails to show a tumor, scintigraphy with octreotide or an analog can be done to detect ectopic neuroendocrine tumors.

MANAGEMENT

GENERAL PRINCIPLES

- Surgery is the principal modality of treatment for the various types of CS. SOR Ⓒ
- Medical therapy to control hypercortisolism is indicated in cases of surgical failure, before preparation for surgery, during the transition period after pituitary irradiation and in ectopic ACTH syndrome where the primary tumor cannot be identified. SOR Ⓒ
- Adrenal enzyme inhibitors act during the various steps in cortisol biosynthesis. Ketoconazole and metyrapone are the important drugs that are used in this category.
- Mitotane is an adrenocortical specific cytotoxic agent used on carcinomas.
- Mifepristone is an antiprogestational drug that works as a glucocorticoid receptor antagonist.
- An important consideration in the treatment of CS is the need for glucocorticoid replacement therapy. This is indicated in cases of loss of pituitary function after surgery or irradiation, complete adrenalectomy and in the use of mitotane.

ACTH-INDEPENDENT CS

- Adrenal tumors (**Figure 229-7**)
  - Adrenal adenomas are cured by unilateral adrenalectomy. SOR Ⓒ
- Adrenal carcinomas are usually recurrent after surgery and do not respond well to irradiation or chemotherapy. Mitotane, a cytotoxic drug is used for palliative purposes.
- Bilateral adrenal micro- or macronodular hyperplasia
  - Bilateral complete adrenalectomy is curative for micronodular primary pigmented hyperplasia as well as macronodular hyperplasia. SOR Ⓒ
- Exogenous CS
  - Gradual withdrawal of the steroids should be done to allow for recovery of the hypothalamic pituitary adrenal axis. SOR Ⓑ

ACTH-DEPENDENT CS

Cushing Disease (Figure 229-8)

- When a localized microadenoma can be identified in the pituitary, a transsphenoidal microadenectomy is preferred. SOR Ⓒ
- If a clearly circumscribed microadenoma is not identified, a subtotal resection of the anterior pituitary is done when fertility is not a concern.
- Pituitary irradiation is the treatment of choice when a microadenoma is not found and pregnancy is desired, surgery is unsuccessful, and in children less than 18 years of age. However, there is a time lag of 3 to

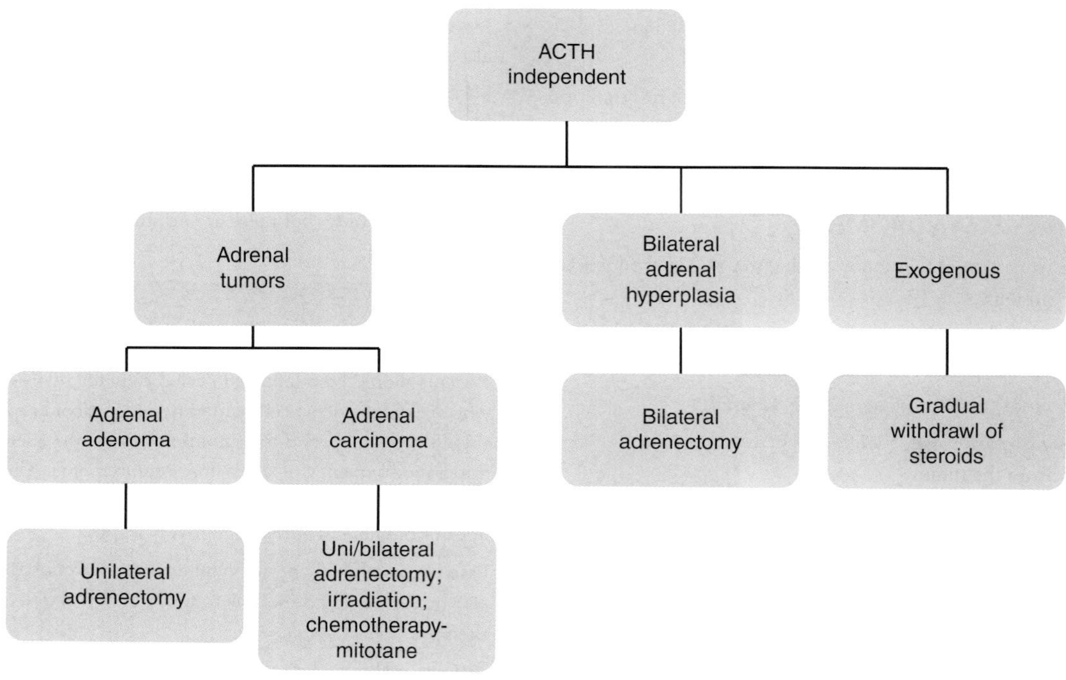

FIGURE 229-7 Management of ACTH-independent Cushing syndrome.

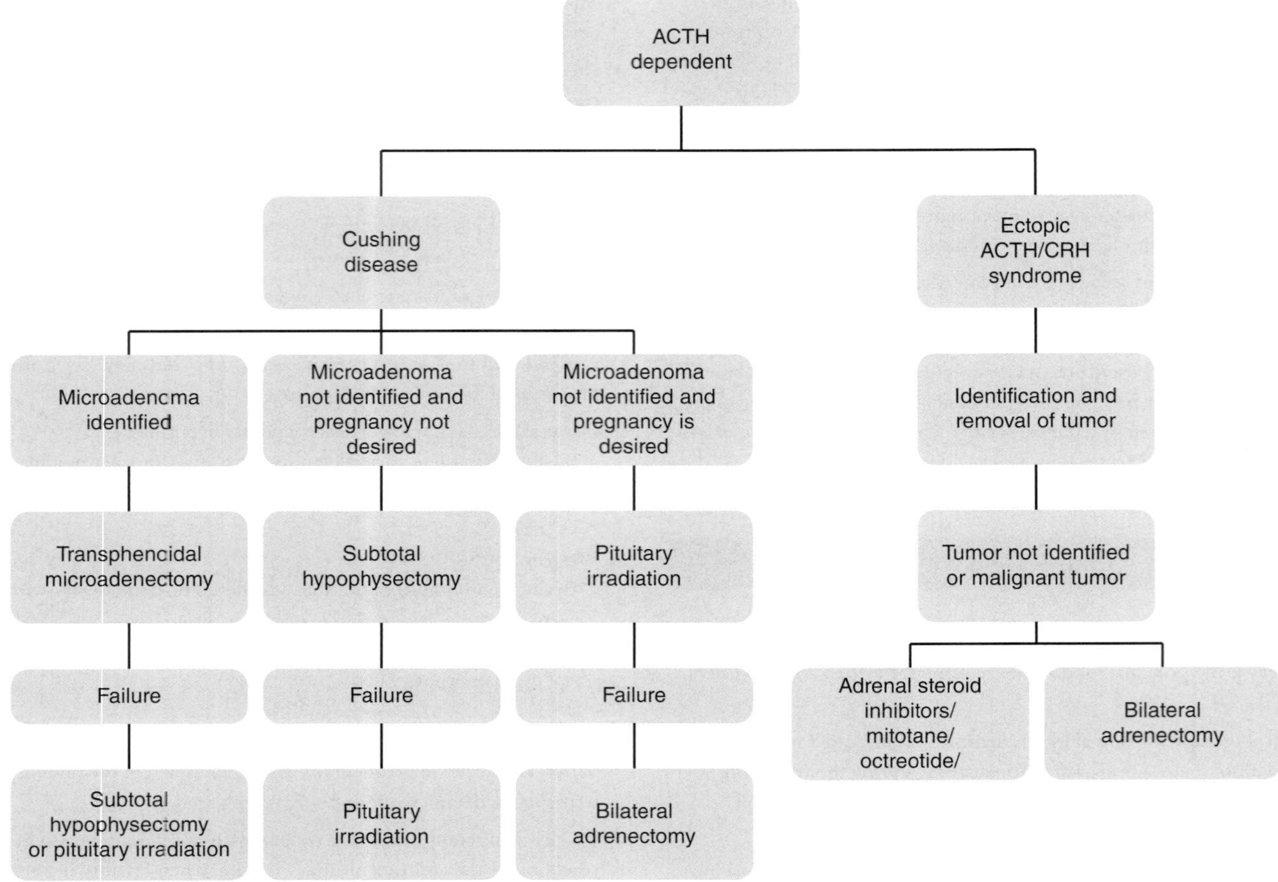

FIGURE 229-8 Management of ACTH-dependent Cushing syndrome.

12 months for radiation therapy to have a full effect and hence adrenal enzyme inhibitors should be used to control hypercortisolism during this period. SOR C

- Bilateral adrenalectomy is the definitive cure and can be used in patients who fail pituitary surgery and irradiation. SOR C
- Malignant tumors of the pituitary have poor prognosis with invasion into the central nervous system and chemotherapy is used for palliative purposes.

ECTOPIC ACTH/CRH SYNDROME

- Identification and resection of the tumor causing the ACTH production is the curative treatment. SOR C
- When the tumor cannot be identified, adrenal enzyme inhibitors can be used to control the hypercortisolism.
- Bilateral adrenalectomy and mitotane may also be used.
- Octreotide is a somatostatin analog which can be used to reduce ACTH secretion from the tumor.[18]

PROGNOSIS

- Untreated CS has a poor prognosis with an estimated 5-year survival of 50%. Vascular and infectious complications are the major cause of mortality in these patients.[19]
- The survival of treated patients with normal cortisol approaches that of the general population, while patients with persistent hypercortisolism after treatment have a 3.8 to 5 times higher mortality.[1,2]
- Data from expert surgical centers have shown good remission rates after transsphenoidal surgery.
- Successful treatment of CS reverses most clinical features; however bone density may not normalize in spite of improvement after treatment.[20]
- Cardiovascular risk of CS remains high for up to 5 years after treatment in one study, but there are no studies with longer follow-up.[21]

FOLLOW-UP

- Patients should be monitored periodically for relapse. SOR C Patients who are on glucocorticoid and mineralocorticoid replacement therapy should be seen every 3 to 4 months to assess the adequacy of steroid doses and frequency of stress dose requirements. They should be monitored frequently for recovery of the hypothalamic pituitary axis except in cases of bilateral adrenalectomy. SOR C
- Patients on adrenal enzyme inhibitors and adrenolytic agents should also be seen every 3 months to monitor for toxicity and reassess therapy.
- Patients without a known ectopic ACTH syndrome should be reevaluated every 6 months to investigate the primary tumor.

PATIENT EDUCATION

- Patients and families need to be informed about the symptoms of adrenal crisis and be trained in the emergency administration of glucocorticoid injections.
- Patients receiving steroids for a prolonged duration should be identified with medical alert bracelets as steroid dependent.

PATIENT RESOURCES

- Cushing's Help and Support—**http://www.cushings-help.com.**
- Pituitary Disorders: Education and Support—**http://www.pituitarydisorder.net.**
- Cushing's Understanding Support and help Organization—**http://www.cush.org.**

PROVIDER RESOURCES

- The diagnosis of Cushing's syndrome: an Endocrine Society clinical practice guideline. **http://www.guideline.gov/content.aspx?id=12953.** Full PDF file—**http://www.endo-society.org/guidelines/final/upload/Cushings_Guideline.pdf.**
- The National Guidelines Clearinghouse summary—**http://www.guideline.gov/content.aspx?id=12953.**

REFERENCES

1. Lindholm J, Juul S, Jorgensen JO, et al. Incidence and late prognosis of Cushing's syndrome: a population-based study. *J Clin Endocrinol Metab*. 2001;86:117-123.
2. Etxabe J, Vazquez JA. Morbidity and mortality in Cushing's disease: an epidemiological approach. *Clin Endocrinol (Oxf)*. 1994;40:479-484.
3. Carpenter PC. Diagnostic evaluation of Cushing's syndrome. *Endocrinol Metab Clin North Am*. 1988;17(3):445.
4. Hutter AM Jr, Kayhoe DE. Adrenal cortical carcinoma. Clinical features of 138 patients. *Am J Med*. 1966;41(4):572.
5. Luton JP, Cerdas S, Billaud L, et al. Clinical features of adrenocortical carcinoma, prognostic factors, and the effect of mitotane therapy. *N Engl J Med*. 1990;322(17):1195.
6. Hellman L, Weitzman ED, Roffwarg H, et al. Cortisol is secreted episodically in Cushing's syndrome. *J Clin Endocrinol Metab*. 1970;30:686.
7. Boyar RM, Witkin M, Carruth A, Ramsey J. Circadian cortisol secretory rhythms in Cushing's disease. *J Clin Endocrinol Metab*. 1979;48:760.
8. Ilias I, Torpy DJ, Pacak K, et al. Cushing's syndrome due to ectopic corticotropin secretion: twenty years' experience at the National Institutes of Health. *J Clin Endocrinol Metab*. 2005;90:4955.
9. Carey RM, Varma SK, Drake CR Jr, et al. Ectopic secretion of corticotropin-releasing factor as a cause of Cushing's syndrome. A clinical, morphologic, and biochemical study. *N Engl J Med*. 1984;311:13.
10. Nieman LK, Biller BM, Findling JW, et al. The diagnosis of Cushing's syndrome: an Endocrine Society Clinical Practice Guideline. *J Clin Endocrinol Metab*. 2008;93:1526.
11. Krieger DT, Allen W, Rizzo F, Krieger HP. Characterization of the normal temporal pattern of plasma corticosteroid levels. *J Clin Endocrinol Metab*. 1971;32:266-284.
12. Refetoff S, Van Cauter E, Fang VS, Laderman C, Graybeal ML, Landau RL. The effect of dexamethasone on the 24-hour profiles of adrenocorticotropin and cortisol in Cushing's syndrome. *J Clin Endocrinol Metab*. 1985;60:527-535.
13. Pfohl B, Sherman B, Schlechte J, Stone R. Pituitary adrenal axis rhythm disturbances in psychiatric depression. *Arch Gen Psychiatry*. 1985;42:897-903.
14. Ross RJ, Miell JP, Holly JM, et al. Levels of GH binding activity, IGFBP-1, insulin, blood glucose and cortisol in intensive care patients. *Clin Endocrinol (Oxf)*. 1991;35:361-367.
15. Liddle GW. Tests of pituitary-adrenal suppressibility in the diagnosis of Cushing's syndrome. *J Clin Endocrinol Metab*. 1960;20:1539.
16. Strott CA, Nugent CA, Tyler FH. Cushing's syndrome caused by bronchial adenomas. *Am J Med*. 1968;44:97.
17. Oldfield EH, Doppman JL, Nieman LK, et al. Petrosal sinus sampling with and without corticotropin-releasing hormone for the differential diagnosis of Cushing's syndrome. *N Engl J Med*. 1991;325:897.
18. Von Werder K, Muller OA, Stalla GK. Somatostatin analogs in ectopic corticotropin production. *Metabolism*. 1996;45:129.
19. Plotz D, Knowlton AI, Ragan C. The natural history of Cushing's disease. *Am J Med*. 1952;13:597-614.
20. Hermus AR, Smals AG, Swinkels LM, et al. Bone mineral density and bone turnover before and after surgical cure of Cushing's syndrome. *J Clin Endocrinol Metab*. 1995;80:2859-2865.
21. Colao A, Pivonello R, Spiezia S, et al. Persistence of increased cardiovascular risk in patients with Cushing's disease after five years of successful cure. *J Clin Endocrinol Metab*. 1999;84:2664-2672.

PART 18

NEUROLOGY

Strength of Recommendation (SOR)	Definition
A	Recommendation based on consistent and good-quality patient-oriented evidence.*
B	Recommendation based on inconsistent or limited-quality patient-oriented evidence.*
C	Recommendation based on consensus, usual practice, opinion, disease-oriented evidence, or case series for studies of diagnosis, treatment, prevention, or screening.*

*See Appendix A on pages 1241-1244 for further information.

230 HEADACHE

Heidi Chumley, MD

PATIENT STORY

A 35-year-old woman presented to the office to discuss her migraines. She has episodic unilateral throbbing headaches accompanied by nausea, photophobia, and phonophobia. She used to have a migraine about every 3 months, but is now having one almost every 2 weeks. As this frequency interferes with her life, prophylactic therapy is discussed. She accepts and her migraine frequency decreases dramatically.

INTRODUCTION

More than 77% of adults experience headaches during their lifetime. Headaches are either primary or secondary and the presence or absence of red flags is useful to distinguish dangerous causes of secondary headaches. The most common primary headaches are tension, migraine, and chronic daily headaches. Medication overuse can complicate headache therapy. Treatment and prognosis is dependent on type of headache.

EPIDEMIOLOGY

- Lifetime prevalence is estimated to be greater than 77% in adults.[1]
- Fifty-three percent of adults (61% of women and 45% of men) have had a headache in the past year.1 Elderly adults have a lower rate of headaches with 36% reporting a headache in the past year.
- Episodic tension-type headache (TTH) prevalence is 62.6% in adults.[1]
- Chronic (>15 days per month) TTH has a prevalence of 3.3% in adults.[1]
- Migraine has a prevalence of 14.7% in adults (8% in men, 17.6% in women).[1]
- Chronic daily headache has lifetime prevalence of 4% to 5%.[2]
- Medication overuse contributes to daily headache in approximately 1% of adults in the general population.[1]
- Cluster headache has a lifetime prevalence of 0.2% to 0.3%.[1]

ETIOLOGY AND PATHOPHYSIOLOGY

- TTH etiology is uncertain, but likely caused by activation of peripheral afferent neurons in head and neck muscles.[3]
- Migraine headache is thought to be caused by central sensory processing dysfunction, which is genetically influenced.[4] Nociceptive input from the meningeal vessels is abnormally modulated in the dorsal raphe nucleus, locus coeruleus, and nucleus raphe magnus. This activation can be seen on positron emission tomography (PET) scan during an acute attack (**Figure 230-1**).
- Cluster headache is caused by trigeminal activation with hypothalamic involvement, but the inciting mechanism is unknown.[5]

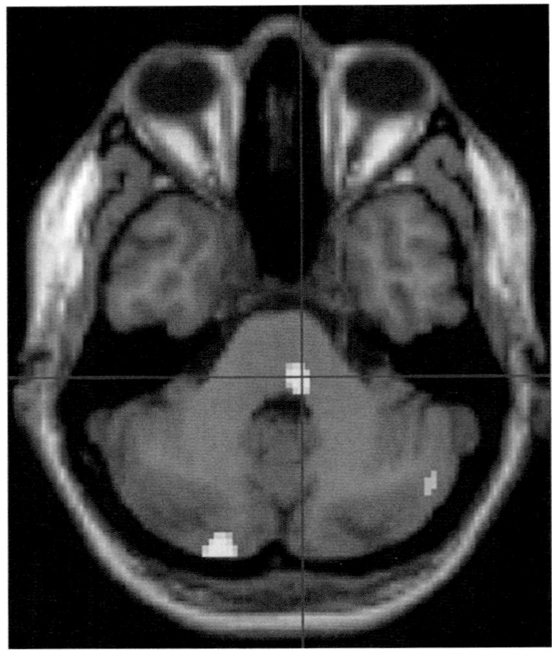

FIGURE 230-1 Imaging has helped clarify the etiology of migraine disorder. This positron emission tomography image shows activation in the dorsolateral pons, which includes the noradrenergic locus coeruleus, an area that modulates nociceptive input from the meningeal vessels. *(Reproduced with permission from Longo D, Fauci A, Kasper D, Hauser S, Jameson J, Loscalzo J, eds. Harrison's Principles of Internal Medicine. 18th ed. New York, NY: McGraw-Hill; 2011:116, Figure 14-2B.)*

RISK FACTORS

- For migraines—Family history
- For medication overuse headache—Regular use of any medication used to treat acute headaches, most commonly simple analgesics and triptans

DIAGNOSIS

CLINICAL FEATURES

- Red flags for dangerous secondary cause—Sudden onset; persistent headache with nausea, vomiting; worsening pattern; history of cancer, HIV, or systemic illness (fever, rash, etc); focal neurologic signs or seizures; vision changes; papilledema; headache worsened by Valsalva, exertion, or position changes; new headache during pregnancy or postpartum; new headache after age 55 years.[2,3,6]
- Episodic TTH—At least 10 episodes of bilateral, mild-to-moderate, pressure (nonpulsating) type pain without nausea or vomiting, not aggravated by exertion, and rare photophobia or phonophobia, occurring less than 15 days per month.[7]
- Migraine headache—At least 5 episodes of unilateral, pulsating, moderate-to-severe headache lasting 4 to 72 hours, aggravated by physical activity, accompanied by nausea or emesis or photophobia and phonophobia.[7]
- Chronic daily headache (CDH)—A primary headache 15 or more days per month, for 4 or more hours per day, for 3 months.[2] Four types of CDH are as below:

- Chronic migraine—Episodic migraines increase in frequency while associated symptoms decrease; resembles tension headache with occasional typical migraine; often accompanied by medication overuse.[2]
- Chronic TTH—Bilateral, nonpulsating, without nausea. Photophobia or phonophobia can be present.[2]
- New daily persistent headache—Abrupt onset of daily headache in patient without a history of a headache disorder; patient often remembers exactly where and when the headaches started.[2]
- Hemicrania continua—Chronic unilateral pain with exacerbations, often associated with ipsilateral autonomic features.[2]

- Medication overuse headache—Accompanies one of the CDHs; acute medications, such as triptans or opiates are taken more than 10 days a month, or analgesics more than 15 days a month, for more than 3 months.[7]
- Cluster headache—The most common type of trigeminal autonomic cephalalgias; can be episodic or chronic; sharp stabbing unilateral pain in trigeminal distribution, lasting 15 minutes to 3 hours, with ipsilateral autonomic features[2] (**Figure 230-2**).
- Sinus headache—Purulent nasal discharge, co-onset of sinusitis, headache localized to facial and cranial areas.

TYPICAL DISTRIBUTION

- Tension headaches are typically bilateral.
- Migraine and cluster headaches are typically unilateral.

LABORATORY TESTING

- Generally not indicated.
- May be used when a secondary cause, such as infection is suspected.

IMAGING

- Generally not indicated.
- Magnetic resonance imaging (MRI) when red flags are present.

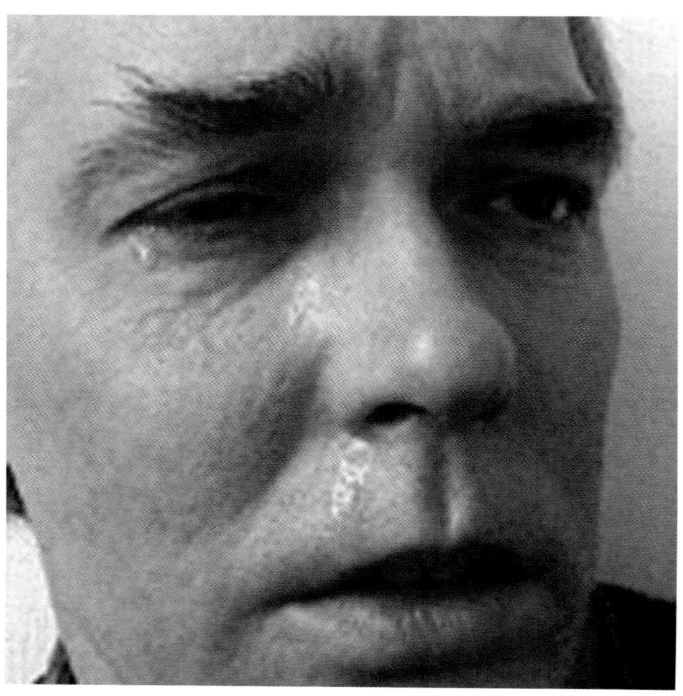

FIGURE 230-2 Lacrimation, ptosis, and lid edema seen in cluster headache. *(Reproduced with permission from The International Headache Society. http://ihs-classification.org/en/. Copyright www.ihs-classification.org; Copyright (2012) Prof. Hartmut Göbel, Germany, www.schmerzklinik.de.)*

DIFFERENTIAL DIAGNOSIS

- Common primary headaches include episodic TTH, migraine, and chronic daily headache.
- Secondary causes of headache are uncommon and include systemic illnesses/infections, brain masses, subarachnoid hemorrhage (**Figure 230-3**), or increased intracranial pressure.
- Medication overuse headache is predominately seen with a primary headache, but may also accompany a secondary headache.

MANAGEMENT

Episodic TTH

- Acute therapy.
  - Aspirin 500 to 1000 mg is the most effective treatment for acute episode. Nonsteroidal anti-inflammatory drugs (NSAIDs) are more effective than acetaminophen.[3]
  - Avoid opiates.
  - Limit acute medications to less than 3 times a week to reduce the risk of medication overuse headache.[3]
- Consider preventive therapy if headaches occur once a week.
  - Amitriptyline 75 to 150 mg a day is the most effective medication.[3]
  - Biofeedback may be effective.[3]
  - Acupuncture may be helpful.[3]

Migraine headache

- Use a stepped approach to treat acute migraine episodes.
  - Start with simple analgesics. Aspirin and ibuprofen are often effective.[8]

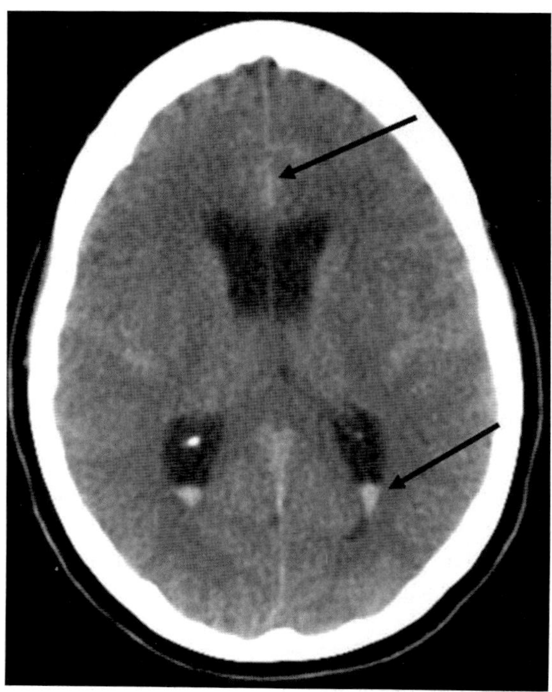

FIGURE 230-3 Sudden onset of a thunderclap headache prompted imaging that showed diffuse subarachnoid hemorrhage with associated ventricular hemorrhage. Top arrow indicates blood in interhemispheric fissure. Bottom arrow indicates blood in lateral ventricle. *(Reproduced with permission from James Anderson, MD, Department of Radiology, Oregon Health & Science University.)*

- Add an antiemetic or try butorphanol nasal spray or an oral opiate combination.[8]
- Reserve migraine-specific agents such as triptans for patients who fail the above therapies.[8]

- Consider prophylaxis for patients whose migraines have a negative impact on their lives or to decrease risk of developing medication overuse headache when frequency requires use of simple analgesics more than 15 days a month or use of opioids, triptans, or combination analgesics more than 10 days a month.
  - Amitriptyline (before bedtime starting with 10 or 25 mg and titrate up as needed and tolerated), divalproex sodium 500 to 1500 mg daily, topiramate 100 mg daily, venlafaxine 150 mg daily, and multiple β-blockers have each demonstrated 50% reduction in migraine frequency.[9]
  - Riboflavin 400 mg daily, coenzyme Q10 300 mg daily, butterbur 50 mg twice daily have each demonstrated 50% reduction in migraine frequency.[9]
  - Magnesium citrate 500 mg daily also reduces migraine frequency and has an A rating in pregnancy.[9]
- Cognitive behavioral therapy, biofeedback, stress management, and lifestyle modification may also be useful.[8]
- IM injected onabotulinumtoxinA improves symptoms, function, and quality of life in patients with chronic migraine and is an option in patients who do not respond to oral prophylactic medications.[10]
- Acupuncture may provide additional benefit.[11]

CDH

- Tricyclic antidepressants significantly reduce the number of days with TTH compared to placebo.[12] Amitriptyline taken before bedtime starting with 10 or 25 mg and titrate up as needed and tolerated.
- Acupuncture may be beneficial in chronic TTHs.[13]

Cluster headache

- Acute episode.
  - Inhaled high-flow oxygen 10 to 15 L/min.[5]
  - Sumatriptan 6 mg subcutaneously; contraindicated in pregnancy, lactation, coronary artery disease, stroke, and peripheral artery disease.[5]
- Several agents may be effective for prophylactic therapy including verapamil or topiramate.[5]
- Refer refractory patients for evaluations for other medical or surgical therapies.

Medication overuse headaches

- Educate patients that chronic medication use is contributing to their daily headaches.[14]
- Abruptly stop (when safe) or taper the overused medication.[14]
- Inpatient withdrawal is recommended for patients overusing opiates, benzodiazepines, or barbiturates.[14]
- Start prophylactic therapy with topiramate 100 to 200 mg daily prior to initiating withdrawal or as soon as possible after withdrawal has been initiated.[14]

REFERRAL

- Refer patients when the diagnosis is unclear or response to therapy is inadequate.
- Consider referral for medication overuse headaches as these are difficult to treat.

PREVENTION

- Closely monitor use of medications for acute episodes. Advise patients to limit simple analgesics to less than 15 days per month and triptans, opiates, and combination medications to less than 10 days per month.
- Appropriately prescribe preventive therapies to reduce frequency of headaches and avoid development of CDHs.

PROGNOSIS

- Tension headaches—Favorable; 45% of adults with frequent episodic or chronic TTHs experienced remission before 3 years.[3]
- Cluster headaches—Unknown; ranges from total remission to chronic form.[5]

FOLLOW-UP

- Dangerous causes of secondary headaches require immediate evaluation and management.
- Frequency of follow-up for primary headaches is determined by type and severity of headache and response to therapy.

PATIENT EDUCATION

Advise patients to limit frequency of acute medications to less than 2 to 3 times a week to reduce the risk of medication overuse headache.

PATIENT RESOURCES

National Headache Foundation has information for patients on many topics including the following:

- *Migraine*—**http://www.headaches.org/education/Headache_Topic_Sheets/Migraine.**
- *Medication Overuse Headache*—**http://www.headaches.org/education/Headache_Topic_Sheets/Analgesic_Rebound.**
- *Cluster Headache*—**http://www.headaches.org/education/Headache_Topic_Sheets/Cluster_Headaches.**
- *New Daily Persistent Headache*—**http://www.headaches.org/education/Headache_Topic_Sheets/New_Daily_Persistent_Headache.**

PROVIDER RESOURCES

- The Institute for Clinical Systems Improvement has a comprehensive guideline on the diagnosis and treatment of headache—**http://www.icsi.org/guidelines_and_more/gl_os_prot/other_health_care_conditions/headache/headache__diagnosis_and_treatment_of__guideline_.html.**
- The International Headache Society has a searchable website to assist with headache classification using ICHD-II criteria—**http://ihs-classification.org/en/02_klassifikation/.**

REFERENCES

1. Stovner LJ, Andree C. Prevalence of headache in Europe: a review for the Eurolight project. *J Headache Pain*. 2010;11(4):289-299.
2. Bigal ME, Lipton RB. The differential diagnosis of chronic daily headaches: an algorithmic-based approach. *J Headache Pain*. 2007;8(5):263-272.
3. Loder E, Rizzoli P. Tension-type headache. *BMJ*. 2008: 336(7635):88-92.
4. Sprenger T, Goadsby PJ. Migraine pathogenesis and state of pharmacological treatment options. *BMC Med*. 2009;7:71.
5. Leroux E, Ducros A. Cluster headache. *Orphanet J Rare Dis*. 2008;3:20.
6. Chandana SR, Mowa S, Arora M, Singh T. Primary brain tumors in adults. *Am Fam Physician*. 2008;77(10):1423-1430.
7. Headache Classification Subcommittee of the International Headache Society. *The International Classification of Headache Disorders*. 2nd ed.. *Cephalalgia*. 2004;24(suppl 1):9-160.
8. Buse DC, Rupnow MFT, Lipton RB. Assessing and managing all aspects of migraine: migraine attacks, migraine-related functional impairment, common comorbidities, and quality of life. *Mayo Clin Proc*. 2009;84(5):422-435.
9. Pringsheim T, Davenport WJ, Becker WJ. Prophylaxis of migraine headache. *CMAJ*. 2010;182(7):E269-E276.
10. Frampton JE. OnabotulinumtoxinA: a review of its use in the prophylaxis of headaches in adults with chronic migraine. *Drugs*. 2012;72(6):825-845.
11. Linde K, Allais G, Brinkhaus B, et al. Acupuncture for migraine prophylaxis. *Cochrane Database Syst Rev*. 2009 Jan 21;(1):CD001218.
12. Jackson JL, Shimeall W, Sessums L, et al. Tricyclic antidepressants and headaches: systematic review and meta-analysis. *BMJ*. 2010;341:c5222.
13. Linde K, Allais G, Brinkhaus B, et al. Acupuncture for tension-type headache. *Cochrane Database Syst Rev*. 2009 Jan 21;(1):CD007587.
14. Evers S, Jensen R. Treatment of medication overuse headache—guideline of the EFNS headache panel. *Eur J Neurol*. 2011;18(9):1115-1121.

231 CEREBRAL VASCULAR ACCIDENT

Heidi Chumley, MD

PATIENT STORY

A 65-year-old hypertensive black man presented to the emergency department with onset of right face, arm, and hand paralysis, and difficulty communicating. Rapid diagnostic testing using magnetic resonance imaging (MRI) revealed an ischemic infarct in the left middle cerebral artery (**Figure 231-1**). He was evaluated by a stroke response team and was found to be a candidate for tissue plasminogen activator (TPA). After the stroke, he was treated with aspirin, antihypertensives, and cholesterol-lowering medication. He recovered 80% of his neurologic deficit over the next 3 months. **Figure 231-2** is a noncontrast computed tomography (CT) image of this patient 2 weeks later.

INTRODUCTION

Cerebral vascular accidents (CVAs) or strokes are common, especially in older populations. Most strokes are ischemic or hemorrhagic. Risk factors include hypertension, smoking, diabetes mellitus (DM), and atrial fibrillation. Thirty-day mortality for a first stroke is greater than 20%.

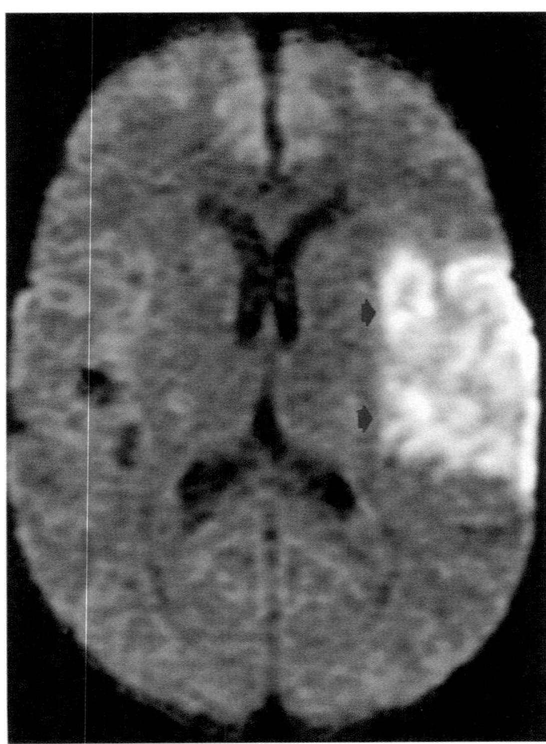

FIGURE 231-1 Acute left middle cerebral artery infarct on MRI of a 65-year-old hypertensive man. The MRI demonstrates increased signal intensity (red *arrows*). Abnormalities in MRI occur before those seen on CT during ischemic strokes. (*Reproduced with permission from Chen MYM, Pope TL, Ott DJ.* Basic Radiology. *New York, NY: McGraw-Hill; 2004:338.*)

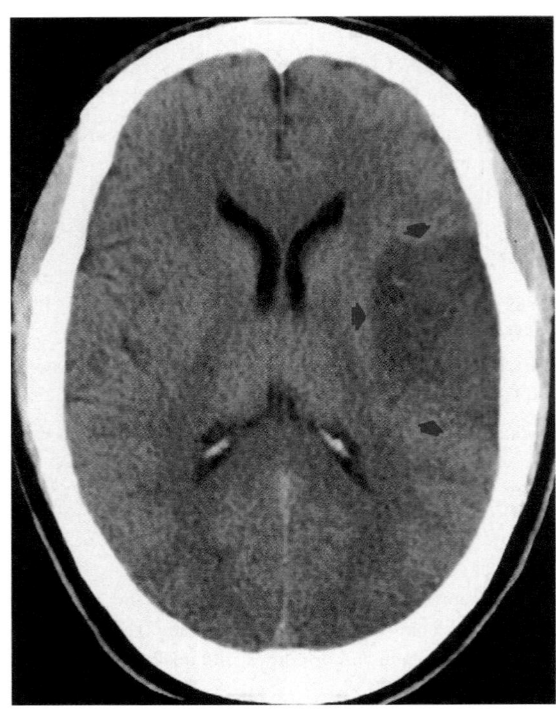

FIGURE 231-2 Noncontrast CT image of a subacute left middle cerebral artery infarct (red *arrows*). This was done 2 weeks after the stroke in the same patient as **Figure 231-1.** CT findings occur later than MRI findings in ischemic strokes. (*Reproduced with permission from Chen MYM, Pope TL, Ott DJ.* Basic Radiology. *New York, NY: McGraw-Hill; 2004:338.*)

SYNONYMS

CVA is also known as stroke.

EPIDEMIOLOGY

- CVAs affect approximately 700,000 people per year in the United States, most being older than age 65 years.[1]
- Ischemic (66%) and hemorrhagic (10%) strokes account for most strokes.[1]
- Prevalence of stroke and mortality are higher in blacks than in whites. Prevalence is 753 versus 424 per 100,000 and mortality is 95.8 versus 73.7 per 100,000 for black and white men, respectively.[1]

ETIOLOGY AND PATHOPHYSIOLOGY

- CVAs are typically classified into cardioembolic (15%-22%), large vessel (10%-12%), small vessel (15%-18%), other known cause (2%-4%), and undetermined cause (46%-51%).[2]
- Ischemic CVAs occur when atherosclerosis progresses to a plaque, which ruptures acutely. Each step of this process is mediated by inflammation.[3]
- Hemorrhagic CVAs occur when vessels bleed into the brain, usually as the result of elevated blood pressure.
- Other known causes of CVAs include inflammatory disorders (giant cell arteritis, systemic lupus erythematosus [SLE], polyarteritis nodosa,

granulomatous angiitis, syphilis, and AIDS), fibromuscular dysplasia, drugs (cocaine, amphetamines, and heroin), hematologic disorders (thrombocytopenia, polycythemia, and sickle cell), and hypercoagulable states.

RISK FACTORS

Hypertension (HTN)—The predominant risk factor for more than 50% of all strokes. Prehypertension (blood pressure in the range of 130 to 139/85 to 89) carries a hazard ratio of 2.5 for women and 1.6 for men.[4]

- Cigarette smoking carries a hazard ratio of 1.62 for ischemic stroke and 2.56 for hemorrhagic stroke.[5]
- Type 2 DM increases the risk of having a stroke 6 fold.[4]
- Black patients at ages 45 and 65 are 2.9 and 1.66 times more likely to have a stroke compared to white patients.[6]
- Atrial fibrillation increases the risk of stroke. The $CHADS_2$ (congestive heart failure [CHF], HTN, age >75, DM, stroke) scoring system (see below) separates patients into low risk (stroke rate 1%-1.5% per year), moderate risk (2.5%), high risk (4%), and very high risk (7%).[4]
- Body mass index (BMI) greater than 30 carries a hazard ratio of 1.45 for ischemic stroke but does not increase the risk of hemorrhagic stroke.[5]

DIAGNOSIS

Diagnosis of CVA must be made expediently to minimize mortality and morbidity.

CLINICAL FEATURES

- History of risk factors, including older age, HTN, cigarette smoking, type 2 DM, or previous transient ischemic attack (TIA) or stroke.
- Acute onset of neurologic signs and symptoms based on the site of the CVA (see "Typical Distribution" below).

TYPICAL DISTRIBUTION

TIA or stroke can occur in any area of the brain; common areas with typical symptoms include the following:

- Middle cerebral artery is the most common ischemic site (**Figure 231-3**).
  - Superior branch occlusion causes contralateral hemiparesis and sensory deficit in face, hand, and arm, and an expressive aphasia if the lesion is in the dominant hemisphere.
  - Inferior branch occlusion causes a homonymous hemianopia, impairment of contralateral graphesthesia and stereognosis, anosognosia and neglect of the contralateral side, and a receptive aphasia if the lesion is in the dominant hemisphere.
- Internal carotid artery (approximately 20% of ischemic strokes) occlusion causes contralateral hemiplegia, hemisensory deficit, and homonymous hemianopia; aphasia is also present with dominant hemisphere involvement.
- Posterior cerebral artery occlusion causes a homonymous hemianopia affecting the contralateral visual field.

LABORATORY TESTING (INCLUDE ANCILLARY TESTING)

The following tests may be helpful in the context of an acute stroke, particularly when the cause of the stroke is not immediately evident:

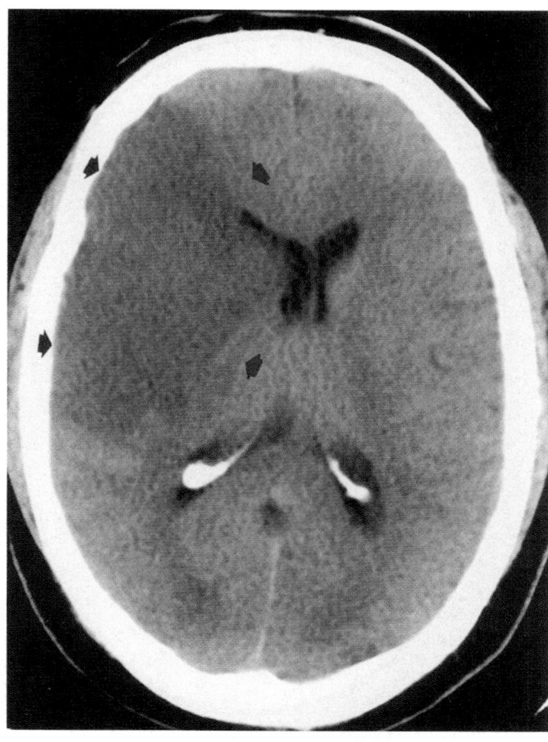

FIGURE 231-3 CT image of right middle cerebral artery infarct; the hypodense (darker) area (red *arrows*) indicates the infarct. The midline structures are shifted to the left. (*Reproduced with permission from Chen MYM, Pope TL, Ott DJ. Basic Radiology. New York, NY: McGraw-Hill; 2004:335.*)

- Complete blood count (CBC) for thrombocytosis or polycythemia
- Erythrocyte sedimentation rate (ESR) for diseases such as giant cell arteritis or SLE
- Testing for syphilis using a treponemal enzyme immunoassay (EIA), with positive results confirmed by a nontreponemal test (Venereal Disease Research Laboratory [VDRL])
- Serum glucose to eliminate hypoglycemia as the cause of the neurologic symptoms

IMAGING

CT or MRI can distinguish ischemic from hemorrhagic and localize the lesion (**Figure 231-4**).

DIFFERENTIAL DIAGNOSIS

Other causes of acute neurologic dysfunction include the following:

- TIA—This precursor to a CVA can appear identical; however, no lesion is seen on imaging, and symptoms resolve within 48 hours.
- Multiple sclerosis—Multiple anatomically distinct neurologic signs and symptoms that occur over time and resolve; vision is often affected. MRI findings should help to distinguish multiple sclerosis from CVA.
- Brain mass—More common presentation is headache or seizure; however, may present with focal neurologic signs based on location. CT or MRI will help to diagnose a brain mass and differentiate this from stroke.
- Migraines—Throbbing, unilateral headache with photophobia, and nausea; hemiparesis or aphasia may be part of the aura.

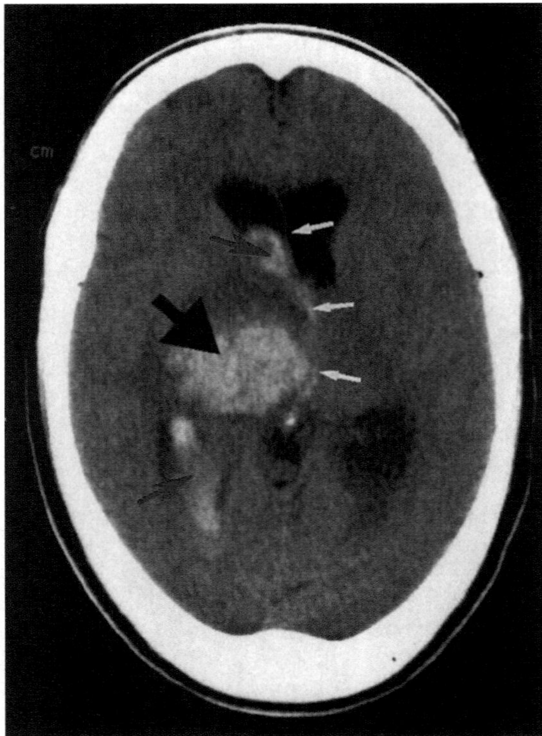

FIGURE 231-4 Hemorrhagic stroke. CT image demonstrates bleeding in the right basal ganglia (*large arrow*) into the ventricles (*red arrows*). Blood appears white on the CT scan. The *white arrows* illustrate midline shift. (*Reproduced with permission from Chen MYM, Pope TL, Ott DJ. Basic Radiology. New York, NY: McGraw-Hill; 2004:337.*)

- Vertigo from benign positional vertigo or acute labyrinthitis—Can mimic a CVA in the posterior circulation; however, symptoms such as dysarthria, dysphagia, and diplopia are typically absent.
- Hypoglycemia—Confused state is similar to large stroke syndromes but is easily differentiated by a blood glucose measurement.

MANAGEMENT

ACUTE STROKE (WITHIN THE FIRST 3 HOURS)

- Rapidly evaluate or consult specialists to identify candidates for TPA. Odds for a favorable 3-month outcome for TPA compared to no TPA are 2.8 (95% confidence interval [CI], 1.8-4.5) for 0 to 90 minutes, 1.6 (95% CI, 1.1-2.2) for 91 to 180 minutes.[7] SOR Ⓐ
- Favorable outcomes at 90 days poststroke have also been demonstrated when TPA is given up to 4.5 hours after the onset of symptoms.[8] SOR Ⓑ
- Currently, only 3% of patients who meet the criteria receive TPA.[4]
- Preliminary studies cautioned about using TPA in community settings; recent studies, however, indicate several options to improve outcomes, including telephone consultation with a regional stroke center.[9]
- Acutely elevated blood pressure should not be aggressively treated in most cases.

After stabilization, treat ischemic strokes with antithrombotic, antihypertensives, statins, and lifestyle changes.

- Prescribe 81-mg or 325-mg aspirin for secondary stroke prevention in patients with prior ischemic stroke or TIA (relative risk [RR] reduction 28%; number needed to treat [NNT] to prevent 1 stroke per year = 77).[4] SOR Ⓐ
- Lower blood pressure (RR reduction 28%; NNT to prevent 1 stroke per year = 51).[4] Current data demonstrate that thiazide-type diuretic and angiotensin-converting enzyme inhibitor (ACEI) (or angiotensin receptor blocker [ARB]) may provide additional risk reduction beyond blood pressure (BP) control and should be used first. ACEI and ARB may not be as effective as monotherapy in black populations.[4] SOR Ⓐ
- Lower low-density lipoprotein (LDL) cholesterol to less than 100 mg/dL for patients with a prior stroke or who are at high risk of stroke using a statin (RR reduction 25%; NNT to prevent 1 stroke per year = 57).[4] SOR Ⓐ
- Assist patients to stop smoking (RR reduction 33%; NNT to prevent 1 stroke per year = 43).[4] SOR Ⓐ
- Advise patients to adopt a healthy lifestyle by eating more fruits and vegetables, losing weight, and maintaining a physical exercise program. SOR Ⓑ

Consider the following to further decrease morbidity and mortality:

- Avoid indwelling urinary catheters to reduce the risk of urinary tract infection.
- Encourage early ambulation to reduce the risk of a deep venous thrombosis.
- Use antiembolism stockings to reduce the risk of a deep venous thrombosis.
- Consider a swallowing study to identify patients at risk of aspiration.

SPECIAL SITUATIONS

- Hemorrhagic stroke
  - Acutely—Do not aggressively lower BP. Some authorities recommend lowering BP only when mean arterial pressure (MAP) is more than 130 mm Hg (MAP = [(2 × diastolic BP) + systolic BP]/3).
  - After the hemorrhagic stroke is over, treat BP aggressively; modest decreases (12/5 mm Hg) from one of many classes of hypertensive drugs lower recurrent stroke risk by 50% to 75%.[4]
- Nonvalvular atrial fibrillation (AF)—Use the $CHADS_2$ scoring system to identify patients with AF who can be managed with aspirin or should be anticoagulated with Coumadin.[4] New oral anticoagulants such as apixaban, dabigatran, and rivaroxaban have decreased stroke risk in early trials.[10]
- The CHADS/$CHADS_2$ scoring table is shown below[2]:

C: Congestive heart failure	= 1 point
H: HTN (or treated HTN)	= 1 point
A: Age >75 years	= 1 point
D: Diabetes	= 1 point
S: Prior TIA or stroke	= 2 points

  - For 0 to 1 point, use aspirin; 2 points, weigh risk of bleeding, adequacy of follow-up versus benefit; 3 or greater, use warfarin if at all possible.
- Patients with symptomatic carotid stenosis—Refer for carotid endarterectomy patients with 70% to 99% carotid stenosis (without near-occlusion) with ipsilateral focal neurologic signs (absolute risk reduction [ARR] 16%).[11] Consider referring symptomatic patients with moderate stenosis of 50% to 69% (ARR 4.6%).[11] SOR Ⓐ
- Patients with asymptomatic carotid artery stenosis greater than 60%—Consider referral for carotid endarterectomy in patients younger than the age of 75 years (NNT = 20 to prevent 1 stroke in 5 years).[4]

PREVENTION

- Address modifiable risk factors—Control HTN, high cholesterol, and DM; stop smoking; and maintain a healthy body weight.
- The US Preventive Services Task Force (USPSTF) recommends the use of aspirin for women ages 55 to 79 when the potential benefit of reduction in ischemic strokes outweighs the potential harm of an increase in GI hemorrhage.[12]
- The USPSTF found the evidence insufficient to recommend for or against the use of aspirin for stroke reduction in men.[12]

PROGNOSIS

CVA prognosis varies based on size and location of ischemia or hemorrhage, time to TPA administration (for ischemic stroke), and availability of aggressive poststroke rehabilitation.

- The 30-day mortality rate after a first or second stroke is 22% and 41%, respectively.[4]
- Five-year observed survival is 40% to 68% for stroke.[13]

FOLLOW-UP

- Patients with symptoms of an acute stroke should be hospitalized, evaluated immediately for appropriateness of TPA and treatment of reversible causes, and managed, if possible, in a stroke unit or using the "best practices" associated with these units.
- After a stroke and rehabilitation, patients should be followed at regular intervals to evaluate risk-reduction strategies.

PATIENT EDUCATION

Educate patients who have had a stroke about the high risk of having a second stroke, the high morbidity and mortality associated with a recurrent stroke, and the need for lifestyle modifications and medications to reduce this risk.

PATIENT RESOURCES

- The National Stroke Association has patient information including signs of a stroke and *HOPE: The Stroke Recovery Guide*—**http://www.stroke.org.**
- The Internet Stroke Center has a section for patients and families with patient education about signs of a stroke and living after a stroke—**http://www.strokecenter.org.**
- The National Institute of Neurologic Diseases and Stroke has written and auditory patient information in English and Spanish—**http://www.ninds.nih.gov.**

PROVIDER RESOURCES

- The Internet Stroke Center has a large collection of stroke scales and clinical assessment tools, a neurology image library, listings of professional resources, and evidence-based diagnosis and management strategies—**http://www.strokecenter.org.**
- Guidelines for early management of adults with ischemic stroke from the American Heart Association and other partners—**http://stroke.ahajournals.org/content/38/5/1655.full.**

REFERENCES

1. Stansbury JP, Jia H, Williams LS, et al. Ethnic disparities in stroke: epidemiology, acute care, and postacute outcomes. *Stroke.* 2005;36(2):374-386.
2. Schneider AT, Kissela B, Woo D, et al. Ischemic stroke subtypes: a population-based study of incidence rates among blacks and whites. *Stroke.* 2004;35(7):1552-1556.
3. Elkind MS. Inflammation, atherosclerosis, and stroke. *Neurologist.* 2006;12(3):140-148.
4. Sanossian N, Ovbiagele B. Multimodality stroke prevention. *Neurologist.* 2006;12(1):14-31.
5. Zhang Y, Tuomilehto J, Jousilahti P, et al. Lifestyle factors on the risks of ischemic and hemorrhagic stroke. *Arch Intern Med.* 2011;171(20):1811-1818.
6. Howard G, Cushman M, Kissela BM, et al; Reasons for Geographic and Racial Differences in Stroke (REGARDS) Investigators. Traditional risk factors as the underlying cause of racial disparities in stroke: lessons from the half-full (empty?) glass. *Stroke.* 2011;42(12):3369-3375.
7. Tonarelli SB, Hart RG. What's new in stroke? The top 10 for 2004/05. *J Am Geriatr Soc.* 2006;54(4):674-679.
8. Maiser SJ, Georgiadis AL, Suri MF, et al. Intravenous recombinant tissue plasminogen activator administered after 3 h following onset of ischaemic stroke: a metaanalysis. *Int J Stroke.* 2011;6(1):25-32.
9. Frey JL, Jahnke HK, Goslar PW, et al. TPA by telephone: extending the benefits of a comprehensive stroke center. *Neurology.* 2005;64(1):154-156.
10. Baker WL, Phung OJ. Systematic review and adjusted indirect comparison meta-analysis of oral anticoagulants in atrial fibrillation. *Circ Cardiovasc Qual Outcomes.* 2012;5(5):711-719.
11. Rerkasem K, Rothwell PM. Carotid endarterectomy for symptomatic carotid stenosis. *Cochrane Database Syst Rev.* 2011;13(4):CD001081.
12. United States Preventive Services Task Force, *Aspirin for the Prevention of Cardiovascular Disease: Recommendation Statement,* AHRQ Publication No. 09-05129-EF-2. Rockville, MD: Agency for Healthcare Research and Quality; 2009. http://www.ahrq.gov/clinic/uspstf09/aspirincvd/aspcvdrs.htm. Accessed September 2, 2012.
13. Askoxylakis V, Thieke C, Pleger ST, et al. Long-term survival of cancer patients compared to heart failure and stroke: a systematic review. *BMC Cancer.* 2010;10:105.

232 SUBDURAL HEMATOMA

Heidi Chumley, MD

PATIENT STORY

A 70-year-old woman, currently anticoagulated for atrial fibrillation, fell and hit her head. She did not lose consciousness and did not seek care immediately. Approximately 12 hours later, she developed a headache and confusion, and was taken to the emergency department by a family member. She was found to have an acute subdural hematoma (SH) (**Figure 232-1**). She was hospitalized, and a neurosurgeon was consulted for surgical management.

INTRODUCTION

SHs can occur at any age, but are most common in older adults. Most SHs are caused by trauma. Symptoms are generally nonspecific such as confusion or headaches. Treatment is prompt consultation with a neurosurgeon.

EPIDEMIOLOGY

- SHs occur at all ages. In adults, SHs are more common in men.[1]
- Less than 1 in 100,000 adults per year have a traumatic SH.[1]
- Forty-two of 100,000 hospitalizations for adult patients.[2]
- Cost is $1.6 billion per year in 2007.[2]
- Mortality rates in treated older adults are approximately 8% for patients younger than age 65 years and 33% for patients older than age 65 years.[3]

ETIOLOGY AND PATHOPHYSIOLOGY

- Most SHs are caused by trauma, either accidental or intentional, from a direct injury to the head.
- Falls, motor vehicle accidents, and assault are the most common causes of traumatic SH.[1]
- SHs have been reported from chronic jarring from rapid walking in older patients.
- Motion of the brain within the skull causes a shearing force to the cortical surface and interhemispheric bridging veins.[4]
- This force tears the weakest bridging veins as they cross the subdural space, resulting in an acute SH as seen in **Figure 232-1**.[4]
- Three days to 3 weeks after the injury, the body breaks down the blood in an SH; water is drawn into the collection causing hemodilution, which appears less white and more gray on noncontrast computed tomography (CT).[4]
- If the hematoma fails to resolve, the collection has an even higher content of water and appears darker on a noncontrast CT; it may have fresh bleeding or may calcify (chronic SH; see **Figure 232-2**).[4] This is often of the same color as brain parenchyma on noncontrast CT.
- Nontraumatic causes reported in the literature include spontaneous bleeding because of bleeding disorders or anticoagulation, meningitis, and complications of neurologic procedures, including spinal anesthesia.

RISK FACTORS

Increased mortality is seen in patients.

- Older than 80 years of age[2]
- With lower income[2]
- With acquired clotting abnormalities[2,5]

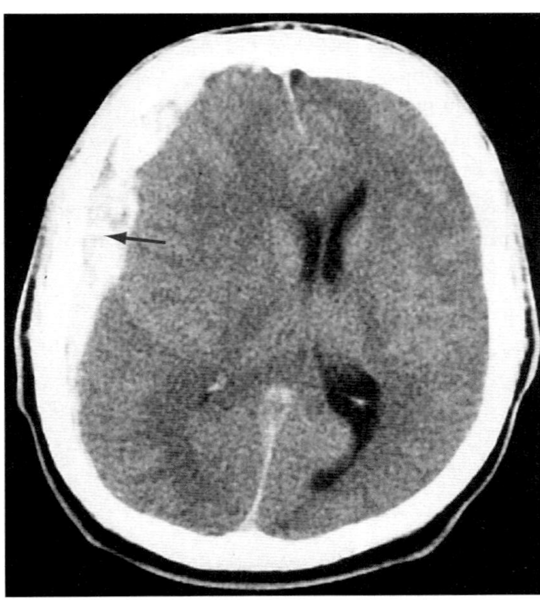

FIGURE 232-1 CT scan of an acute subdural hematoma (*arrow*) seen as a hyperdense clot with an irregular border. There is a midline shift from the mass effect of the accumulated blood. (*Reproduced with permission from Kasper DL, Braunwald E, Fauci, AS, Hauser SL, Longo DL, Jameson JL.* Harrison's Principles of Internal Medicine. *16th ed. New York, NY: McGraw-Hill; 2005:2450.*)

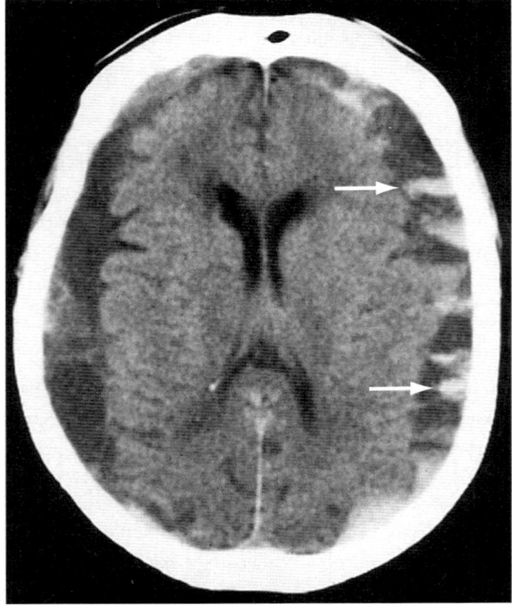

FIGURE 232-2 CT scan of chronic bilateral subdural hematomas. As subdural hematomas age, these become isodense gray and then hypodense (darker gray to black) compared to the brain. Some resolving blood is still visible on the left (*arrows*). (*Reproduced with permission from Kasper DL, Braunwald E, Fauci, AS, Hauser SL, Longo DL, Jameson JL.* Harrison's Principles of Internal Medicine. *16th ed. New York, NY: McGraw-Hill; 2005:2450.*)

- Who experienced trauma[2]
- With a higher APACHE (Acute physiology, Age, and Chronic Health Evaluation) III score on presentation[5]

DIAGNOSIS

The clinical features are often nonspecific, making the diagnosis difficult in the absence of known trauma.

Older adults may present with headaches, confusion, subtle changes in mental status, gait disturbances, hemiparesis, or other focal neurologic signs.[6]

TYPICAL DISTRIBUTION

SHs by definition occur in the subdural space, most commonly seen in the parietal region.

IMAGING

Acute SHs are seen easily on a noncontrast CT scan (see **Figure 232-1**). Subacute and chronic SHs (see **Figure 232-2**) can be similar in color to the brain parenchyma and may be easier to see on a contrast CT or a magnetic resonance imaging (MRI).

DIFFERENTIAL DIAGNOSIS

Other causes of nonspecific symptoms seen with SH can be differentiated by neuroimaging and include the following:

- Infections such as sepsis or meningitis—Fever, elevated white blood cells, positive blood cultures, and cerebral spinal fluid consistent with meningitis.
- Hemorrhagic (**Figure 232-3**) or ischemic stroke or transient ischemic attacks—Consider risk factors for stroke such as hypertension, diabetes, atrial fibrillation, and smoking (see Chapter 231, Cerebral Vascular Accident).

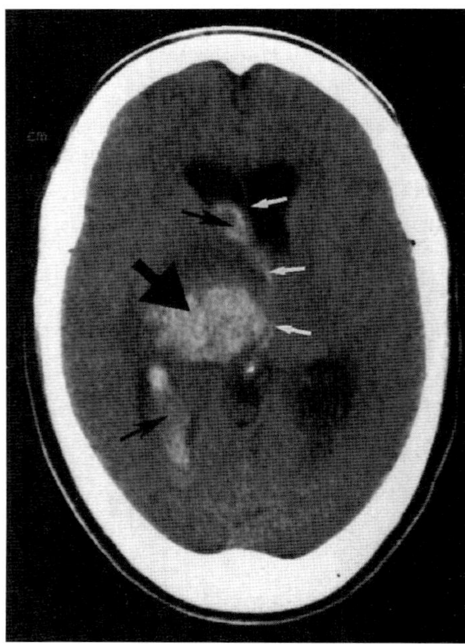

FIGURE 232-3 Hemorrhagic stroke seen on CT. The CT image demonstrates bleeding in the right basal ganglia (*large black arrow*) into the ventricles (*small black arrows*) with midline shift (*white arrows*). (*Reproduced with permission from Chen MYM, Pope TL Jr., Ott, DJ.* Basic Radiology. *New York, NY: McGraw-Hill; 2004:337.*)

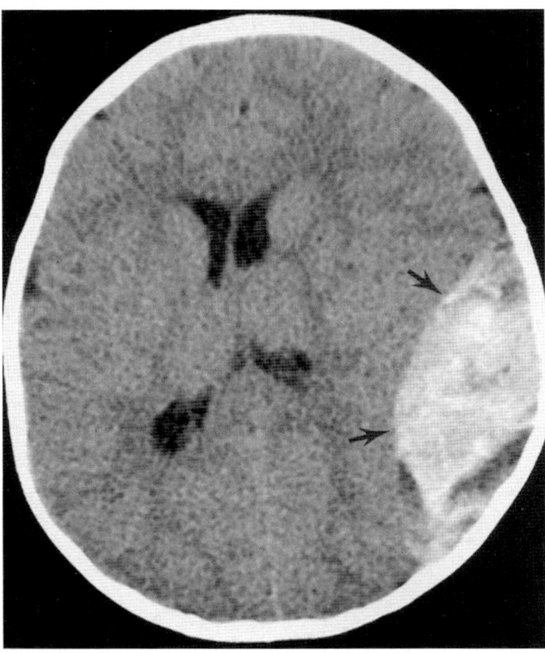

FIGURE 232-4 This head CT demonstrates an epidural hematoma, with the typical biconvex appearance (*arrows*). Note how the biconvex appearance resembles the lens of an eye. (*Reproduced with permission from Chen MYM, Pope TL Jr., Ott, DJ.* Basic Radiology. *New York, NY: McGraw-Hill; 2004:346.*)

- Dementia or depression—Less acute onset, advanced age, and other symptoms consistent with depression.
- Primary or metastatic brain neoplasms—History of cancer and risk factors for cancer.

Other causes of intracranial bleeding can also be differentiated by neuroimaging and include the following:

- Epidural hematoma (**Figure 232-4**)—Well-defined biconvex bright white density that resembles the shape of the lens of the eye.
- Subarachnoid hemorrhage (**Figure 232-5**)—Bright white blood outlines cerebral sulci.
- Hemorrhage in brain parenchyma—Bright white lesion apart from dura.

MANAGEMENT

Most SHs are managed surgically, and there is little evidence about conservative management.

- Determine the Glasgow Coma Scale in patients with serious head trauma and consider airway protection in patients with a score less than 12.
- Obtain an urgent noncontrast CT scan on any patient suspected of having an SH.
- If the noncontrast CT scan is nonrevealing, obtain a contrast CT or MRI, particularly if the traumatic event occurred 2 to 3 days prior.
- Emergently refer patients with an SH and deteriorating neurologic status or evidence of brain edema or midline shift to a hospital with neurosurgeons.
- Consult a neurosurgeon expediently in patients with an SH and stable focal neurologic signs.

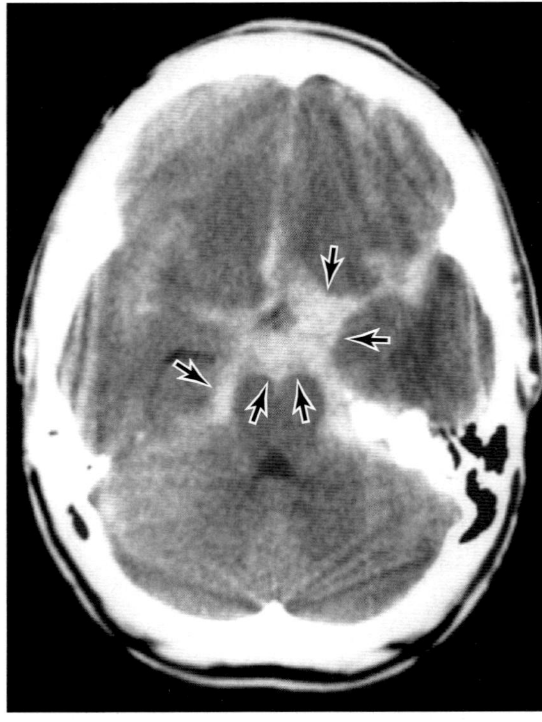

FIGURE 232-5 A subarachnoid hemorrhage appears as areas of high density (more white like bone rather than the darker gray of brain tissue) in the subarachnoid space (*arrows*) of this CT scan. (*Reproduced with permission from Aminoff MJ, Greenberg DA, Simon RP.* Clinical Neurology. *6th ed. New York, NY: McGraw-Hill; 2005:77.*)

- Consider neurosurgical consultation in asymptomatic patient or patients with only a headache and a small acute SH without brain edema or midline shift. These patients may be followed by serial CT scans without surgical treatment, but this should be done in consultation with experts in CT interpretation and management of SHs.[6] SOR C

PREVENTION

- Follow safety measures that reduce motor vehicle accidents, and falls in the elderly.
- Use recommended protective gear for sports and recreational activities and follow guidelines for return to play after a head injury.
- Carefully evaluate the risks and benefits of chronic use of antiplatelet and anticoagulation medications.

PROGNOSIS

- In-hospital mortality for acute SH is 12%.[2,3]
- In-hospital mortality for traumatic SH is 26%.[1]
- Best predictor of in-hospital mortality is neurologic status on admission.[7]
- In patients older than age 65 years, the mortality rate for chronic SH remains elevated until 1 year after diagnosis independent of treatment.[7]

FOLLOW-UP

- Follow-up is determined by severity of SH and type of treatment.
- Ideally, follow-up is conducted jointly between the neurosurgeon and primary care physician to ensure resolution of the SH and maximal return of function, especially in elderly patients.

PATIENT EDUCATION

Advise patients to seek medical care immediately for head trauma, which can cause several emergencies including an SH.

PATIENT RESOURCES

- MedlinePlus. *Subdural Hematoma*—**http://www.nlm.nih.gov/medlineplus/ency/article/000713.htm.**

PROVIDER RESOURCES

- Medscape. *Subdural Hematoma*—**http://emedicine.medscape.com/article/1137207**.
- MD+CALC. *Glasgow Coma Scale Calculator*—**http://www.mdcalc.com/glasgow-coma-scale-score.**

REFERENCES

1. Tallon JM, Ackroyd-Stolarz S, Darim Sa, Clarke DB. The epidemiology of surgically treated acute subdural and epidural hematomas in patients with head injuries: a population-based study. *Can J Surg.* 2008;51(5):339-345.
2. Frontera JA, Egorova N, Moskowittz AJ. National trend in prevalence, cost, and discharge disposition after subdural hematoma from 1998-2007. *Crit Care Med.* 2011;39(7):119-125.
3. Munro PT, Smith RD, Parke TR. Effect of patients' age on management of acute intracranial haematoma: prospective national study. *BMJ.* 2002;325(7371):1001.
4. Minns RA. Subdural haemorrhages, haematomas, and effusions in infancy. *Arch Dis Child.* 2005;90(9):883-884.
5. Bershad EM, Farhadi S, Suri MF, et al. Coagulopathy and inhospital deaths in patients with acute subdural hematoma. *J Neurosurg.* 2008;109(4):664-669.
6. Karnath B. Subdural hematoma. Presentation and management in older adults. *Geriatrics.* 2004;59(7):18-23.
7. Miranda LB, Braxton E, Hobbs J, Quigley MR. Chronic subdural hematoma in the elderly: not a benign disease. *J Neurosurg.* 2011;114(1):72-76.

233 NORMAL PRESSURE HYDROCEPHALUS

Heidi Chumley, MD

PATIENT STORY

A 68-year-old man presented with a gradual onset of difficulty with his gait, increased urinary incontinence, and difficulty with his memory during the past several months. His gait was wide-based and slow, with decreased step height and length. His Mini Mental State Examination was consistent with impaired cognition. As part of his workup, he had a noncontrast head computed tomography (CT), which demonstrated dilated ventricles (**Figure 233-1**) without extensive cortical atrophy. He had normal cell counts and opening pressure on a spinal tap. He was diagnosed with normal pressure hydrocephalus (NPH) and referred to a neurosurgeon to be evaluated for a ventricular shunt. The patient had the shunt placed (**Figure 233-2**). His gait and urinary incontinence improved. Unfortunately, his cognitive impairments did not improve as is often the case.

INTRODUCTION

NPH can be idiopathic or secondary to meningitis, subarachnoid hemorrhage, or head trauma, and is caused by impaired reabsorption of spinal fluid. Patients present with gait abnormalities, urinary incontinence, and/or cognitive impairment. Diagnosis is confirmed by radiographic evidence and a normal opening pressure on lumbar puncture.

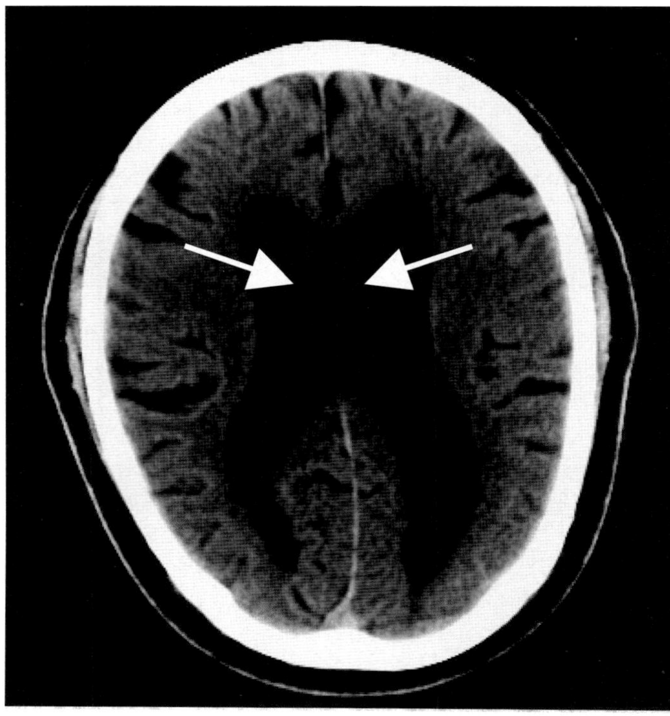

FIGURE 233-1 Noncontrast CT demonstrates enlarged lateral ventricles (*white arrows*) without significant cerebral atrophy. (*Reproduced with permission from Reginald Dusing, MD.*)

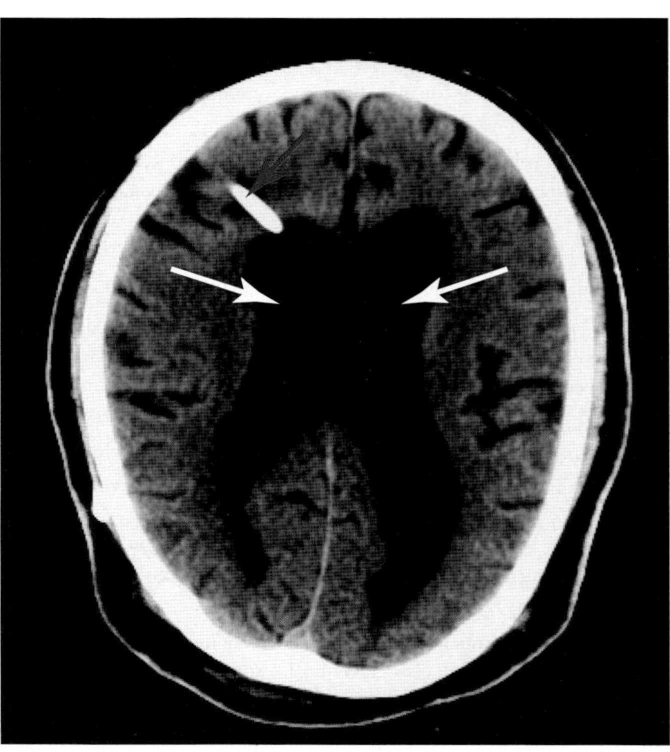

FIGURE 233-2 Noncontrast CT shows ventricular shunt (*red arrow*) in place. Lateral ventricles remain enlarged after shunting (*white arrows*). (*Reproduced with permission from Reginald Dusing, MD.*)

EPIDEMIOLOGY

- Prevalence—1 in 250 in those older than age 65 years; determined in a door-to-door survey in Germany.[1]
- Incidence—1 to 2/100,000 population per year; determined by number of surgeries in Sweden.[2]
- Most common between the ages of 60 to 70 years.
- Five percent of dementias are caused by NPH.[3]

ETIOLOGY AND PATHOPHYSIOLOGY

- Cerebral spinal fluid (CSF) is produced by the choroid plexus, circulates through the ventricles, exits into the subarachnoid space, and is reabsorbed by the arachnoid granulations at the top of the brain.[3]
- NPH is thought to be due to impaired reabsorption and can be idiopathic or secondary to meningitis, subarachnoid hemorrhage, or head trauma.

DIAGNOSIS

NPH is a clinical diagnosis based on signs and symptoms, CSF studies, radiographic imaging, and a clinical response to ventriculoperitoneal (VP) shunting.

CLINICAL FEATURES

Classic triad is gait disturbance, urinary incontinence, and cognitive impairment.

- Gait disturbances typically occur first—Wide-based stance; slow, shuffling steps; difficulty with initiation.[3]
- Urinary incontinence usually with urgency; abnormal detrusor contractions on urodynamic studies.[3]
- Cognitive impairment—Difficulty with attention and concentration (digit span, arithmetic) with sparing of orientation and general memory.[4]

LABORATORY TESTING

- CSF had normal cell counts and opening pressure less than 200 mm Hg.[3]
- High-volume spinal tap (removal of 30-66 cc of CSF) or prolonged CSF drainage (3-5 days via an indwelling catheter) followed by clinical improvement can be helpful in selecting patients more likely to respond to VP shunting.[5]
- Continuous monitoring of intracranial pressure demonstrates characteristic waves of NPH; however, this is done only in specialized centers.

IMAGING

- Enlarged ventricles without substantial cerebral atrophy can be seen on CT or magnetic resonance imaging (MRI).
- Cisternography, a nuclear medicine test, can demonstrate impaired clearing of CSF from the lateral ventricles at 48 hours (**Figure 233-3**), which is useful in predicting which patients respond to shunting.[6]

DIFFERENTIAL DIAGNOSIS

- Alzheimer disease—Impaired orientation and memory, which are often spared in NPH; cortical atrophy.
- Parkinson disease—Tremor and rigidity in addition to bradykinesia and gait disturbances; normal neuroimaging.

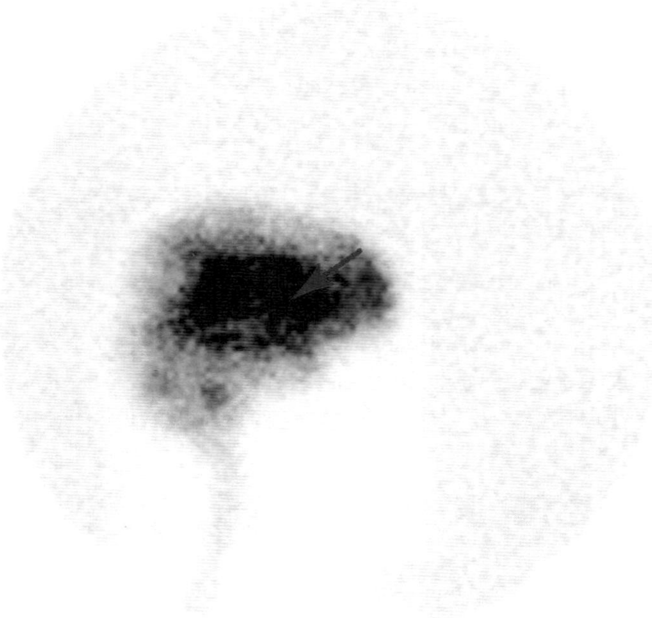

FIGURE 233-3 Lateral view on cisternography demonstrates increased uptake in the lateral ventricle (*red arrow*). In this nuclear medicine study, indium is injected into the cerebral spinal fluid at the lower lumbar spine and a scan is done 48 hours later. Normally, the indium-tagged spinal fluid has been reabsorbed at 48 hours, and the lateral ventricle does not have increased uptake. (*Reproduced with permission from Reginald Dusing, MD.*)

- Chronic alcoholism—History of alcohol use, memory and learning difficulties; cortical atrophy.
- Multiinfarct dementia, atherosclerotic disease, subdural hematomas, and tumors—Identifiable on neuroimaging.
- Intracranial infections or carcinomatous meningitis—Abnormal CSF findings.
- Hypothyroidism—Has other symptoms such as fatigue, weakness, dry and cool skin, diffuse hair loss, cold intolerance, constipation, and difficulty concentrating. The thyroid-stimulating hormone (TSH) is elevated and there is no urinary incontinence (see Chapter 226, Hypothyroidism).

MANAGEMENT

Refer to a neurosurgeon to evaluate for VP shunting (see **Figure 233-2**).

- VP shunting is the only known effective treatment (see **Figure 233-2**). In larger retrospective studies, 39% to 75% of patients demonstrated improvement by 24 months.[5,7]
- The risks of VP shunting can be substantial; moderate-to-severe complications occurred in 28% of patients in one study[7]; more recent reviews report a 6% complication rate.[8]
- Repetitive lumbar punctures may be considered in patients who cannot undergo surgery.[9]

PROGNOSIS

- In one study, patients demonstrated improvements in gait (81.1%), urinary incontinence (55.9%), and dementia (64.4%) after surgery. Surgical complications occurred in approximately 6% of patients.[8]
- Favorable prognostic factors include gait abnormality as the presenting or dominant symptom, symptoms less than 6 months prior to treatment, and an identified cause (ie, because of head trauma).[10]
- Poor prognostic factors include dementia preceding gait abnormality or dementia for more than 2 years.[10]

FOLLOW-UP

Long-term multidisciplinary follow-up can facilitate gait and bladder retraining and early recognition of signs of shunt malfunction including vomiting, headache, fever, or seizures.

PATIENT EDUCATION

Advise patients about improvements from VP shunting.

- Do not occur for all patients.
- Appear slowly over several months.
- May last several years.
- Are more likely to involve gait disturbances rather than cognitive deficits.

Advise patients to inform any health care provider they see about their VP shunt.

PATIENT RESOURCES

- eMedicineHealth. *Normal Pressure Hydrocephalus*—**http://www.emedicinehealth.com/normal_pressure_hydrocephalus/article_em.htm.**
- The National Institute of Neurologic Disorders and Stroke. *Normal Pressure Hydrocephalus Information Page*—**http://www.ninds.nih.gov/disorders/normal_pressure_hydrocephalus/normal_pressure_hydrocephalus.htm.**

PROVIDER RESOURCES

- Medscape. *Normal Pressure Hydrocephalus*—**http://emedicine.medscape.com/article/1150924.**

REFERENCES

1. Trenkwalder C, Schwarz J, Gebhard J, et al. Starnberg trial on epidemiology of Parkinsonism and hypertension in the elderly. Prevalence of Parkinson's disease and related disorders assessed by a door-to-door survey of inhabitants older than 65 years. *Arch Neurol.* 1995;52(10):1017-1022.
2. Tisell M, Hoglund M, Wikkelso C. National and regional incidence of surgery for adult hydrocephalus in Sweden. *Acta Neurol Scand.* 2005;112(2):72-75.
3. Verrees M, Selman WR. Management of normal pressure hydrocephalus. *Am Fam Physician.* 2004;70(6):1071-1078.
4. Ogino A, Kazui H, Miyoshi N, et al. Cognitive impairment in patients with idiopathic normal pressure hydrocephalus. *Dement Geriatr Cogn Disord.* 2006;21(2):113-119.
5. McGirt MJ, Woodworth G, Coon AL, et al. Diagnosis, treatment, and analysis of long-term outcomes in idiopathic normal-pressure hydrocephalus. *Neurosurgery.* 2005;57(4):699-705; discussion 699-705.
6. Algin O, Hakyemez B, Ocakoglu G, Parlak M. MR cisternography: is it useful in the diagnosis of normal-pressure hydrocephalus and the selection of "good shunt responders"? *Diagn Interv Radiol.* 2011;17(2):105-111.
7. Vanneste J, Augustijn P, Dirven C, et al. Shunting normal-pressure hydrocephalus: do the benefits outweigh the risks? A multicenter study and literature review. *Neurology.* 1992;42(1):54-59.
8. Cage TA, Auguste KI, Wrensch M, et al. Self-reported functional outcome after surgical intervention in patients with idiopathic normal pressure hydrocephalus. *J Clin Neurosci.* 2011;18(5):649-654.
9. Lim TS, Yong SW, Moon SY. Repetitive lumbar punctures as treatment for normal pressure hydrocephalus. *Eur Neurol.* 2009;62(5):293-297.
10. Siraj S. An overview of normal pressure hydrocephalus and its importance: how much do we really know? *J Am Med Dir Assoc.* 2011;12(1):19-21.

234 BELL'S PALSY

Heidi Chumley, MD

PATIENT STORY

Five years ago, a young woman awoke with the inability to move the left side of her face. She was pregnant at the time. On examination it was found that she had absent brow furrowing, weak eye closure, and dropping of her mouth angle (**Figure 234-1**). She was diagnosed with Bell's palsy and was provided eye lubricants and guidance on keeping her left eye moist. Her physician discussed the available evidence about treatment with steroids. She chose not to take a course of steroids because of her pregnancy.

INTRODUCTION

Bell's palsy is an idiopathic paralysis of the facial nerve resulting in loss of brow furrowing, weak eye closure, and dropped angle of mouth. Treatment is oral steroids as soon after the onset of symptoms as possible. Most patients have a full recovery within 6 months.

SYNONYMS

Bell's palsy is also known as idiopathic facial paralysis.

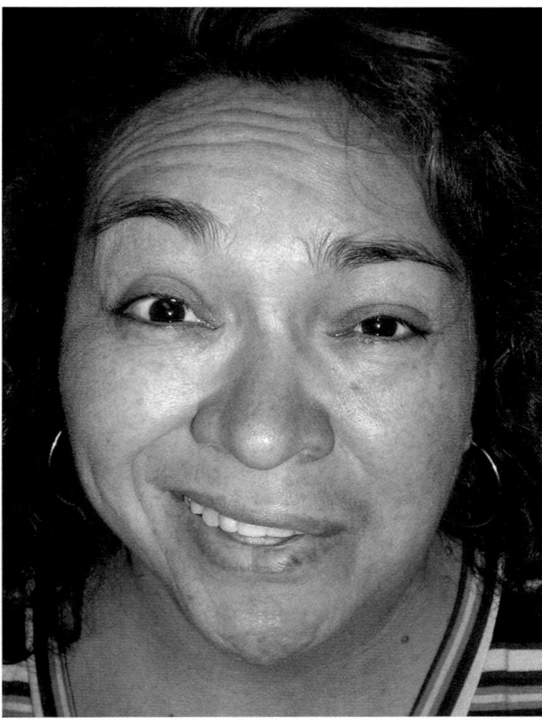

FIGURE 234-1 Bell's palsy with loss of brow furrowing and dropped angle of the mouth on the affected left side of her face demonstrated during a request to smile and raise her eyebrows. The Bell's palsy has been present for 5 years and the patient is being evaluated by ear, nose, and throat (ENT) for surgery to restore facial movement. (*Reproduced with permission from Richard P. Usatine, MD.*)

EPIDEMIOLOGY

- In a Canadian study, incidence was 13.1 to 15.2/100,000 adults.[1]
- In a study of United States military members, the incidence was 42.77/100,000, with higher incidence in females, blacks, and Hispanics; arid climate and cold months were independent predictors of risk with adjusted relative risk ratios of 1.34 and 1.31, respectively.[2]
- Women who develop Bell's palsy in pregnancy have a 5-fold increased risk over national average of preeclampsia or gestational hypertension.[3]
- Seventy percent of cases of acute peripheral facial nerve palsy are idiopathic (Bell's palsy); 30% have known etiologic factors such as trauma, diabetes mellitus, polyneuritis, tumors, or infections such as herpes zoster, leprosy (**Figure 234-2**) or *Borrelia*.[4]

ETIOLOGY AND PATHOPHYSIOLOGY

- Etiology of Bell's palsy is currently unknown and under debate; the prevailing theory suggests a viral etiology from the herpes family.
- The facial nerve becomes inflamed, resulting in nerve compression.
- Compression of the facial nerve compromises muscles of facial expression, taste fibers to the anterior tongue, pain fibers, and secretory fibers to the salivary and lacrimal glands.
- This is a lower motor neuron lesion; the upper and lower portions of the face are affected (see **Figure 234-1**). In upper motor neuron lesions (eg, cortical stroke), the upper third of the face is spared, while the lower two-thirds are affected as a result of the bilateral innervation of the orbicularis, frontalis, and corrugator muscles, which allows sparing of upper face movement.

DIAGNOSIS

CLINICAL FEATURES

- Weakness of all facial muscles on the affected side—Loss of brow furrowing, weak eye closure, and dropped angle of mouth

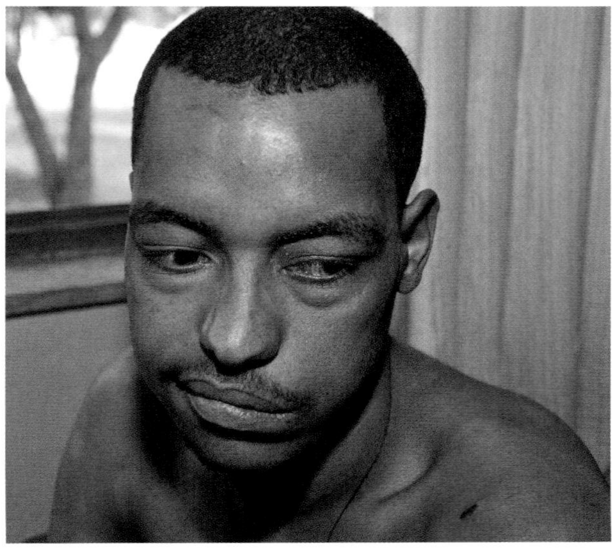

FIGURE 234-2 Bell's palsy secondary to leprosy. The hypopigmented patches on his back are further signs of the leprosy. (*Reproduced with permission from Richard P. Usatine, MD.*)

- Postauricular pain
- Dry eyes
- Involuntary tearing
- Hyperacusis
- Altered tastes

LABORATORY TESTING

Laboratory testing is not usually indicated.

- Herpes virus titers are not usually helpful.
- Consider serologic tests for Lyme disease in endemic areas.
- Consider testing for diabetes mellitus in patients with risk factors.

IMAGING

Consider magnetic resonance imaging (MRI) to look for a space-occupying lesion with atypical presentations.

DIFFERENTIAL DIAGNOSIS

- Upper motor neuron diseases including stroke—Normal brow furrowing, eye closure, and blinking.
- Space-occupying lesion—Symptoms are dependent on the location of the mass; consider with an isolated facial nerve palsy that does not affect all 3 branches of the facial nerve.
- Lyme disease—Occurs in endemic area with skin rash, joint inflammation, and flu-like symptoms. Bell's palsy is the most common neurologic manifestation of Lyme disease (see Chapter 215, Lyme Disease).
- Suppurative ear disease—Ear pain, abnormal tympanic membrane.
- Facial nerve damage from microvascular disease—Most commonly in diabetes mellitus.
- Facial nerve damage from trauma—History of trauma differentiates this from Bell's palsy that is idiopathic or from an infectious etiology.
- Isolated third nerve palsy—Manifestations include diplopia and drooping of the upper eyelid (ptosis) (**Figure 234-3**). The affected eye may deviate out and down in straight-ahead gaze; adduction is slow and cannot proceed past the midline. Upward gaze is impaired. When downward gaze is attempted, the superior oblique muscle causes the eye to adduct. The pupil may be normal or dilated; its response to direct or consensual light may be sluggish or absent (efferent defect). Pupil dilation (mydriasis) may be an early sign.

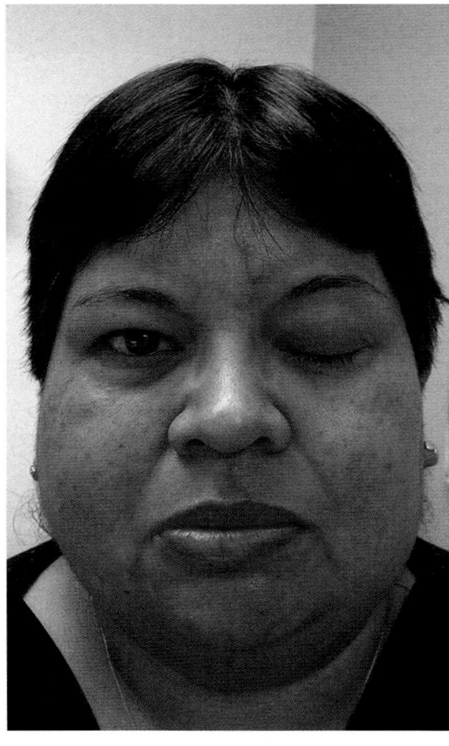

FIGURE 234-3 Ptosis from an isolated third nerve palsy in a patient with diabetes. Note the symmetry of the facial creases, which would be absent in Bell's palsy. This patient would also have abnormal eye movements. The eye would deviate down and out, adduction would not pass the midline, and upward gaze would be impaired. (*Reproduced with permission from Richard P. Usatine, MD.*)

MANAGEMENT

NONPHARMACOLOGIC

Provide eye protection with artificial tears, lubricants, or closing of the eyelid. SOR C

MEDICATIONS

- New data and a Cochrane systematic review supports treating patients with systemic corticosteroids. Steroids significantly decrease a patient's risk for incomplete recovery from 33% to 23%, risk ratio 0.71.[5] SOR A
- Dosing of steroids in the studies analyzed within the Cochrane review varied from oral methylprednisolone 1 mg/kg daily for 10 days, and then gradually withdrawn for another 3 to 5 days to prednisone given as a single dose of 60 mg daily for 5 days, followed by a dose reduced by 10 mg/d, with a total treatment of 10 days. One trial used high-dose prednisolone given intravenously.
- A Cochrane systematic review does not support using antiviral medications. There is no significant benefit from acyclovir or valacyclovir when compared to placebo. Antivirals are less likely than steroids to produce complete recovery.[6] SOR A

COMPLEMENTARY AND ALTERNATIVE THERAPY

Acupuncture has been studied; the data, however, are inadequate to determine the efficacy.[7]

REFERRAL

In long-standing facial paralysis, consider referral to an ear, nose, and throat (ENT) surgeon or plastic surgeon with experience in treating Bell's palsy with surgery. It is possible to restore some facial movement with specialized surgical procedures including regional muscle transfer and microvascular free tissue transfer.[8] SOR C

PROGNOSIS

Seventy-seven percent of patients treated with systemic steroids have complete recovery of facial motor function in 6 months.

FOLLOW-UP

Consider seeing patients in 2 to 3 weeks to evaluate recovery and to reconsider diagnosis if there has been no recovery.

PATIENT EDUCATION

Most patients recover spontaneously. Steroid treatment improves a patient's chance of complete recovery.

PATIENT RESOURCES

- The American Academy of Family Physicians has written and auditory information in English and in Spanish—**http://www.familydoctor.org.**
- FamilyDoctor.org. *Bell's Palsy Overview*—**http://familydoctor.org/familydoctor/en/diseases-conditions/bells-palsy.html.**
- The National Institute of Neurologic Disorders and Stroke has written and auditory patient information in English and Spanish—**http://www.ninds.nih.gov/disorders/bells/bells.htm.**

PROVIDER RESOURCES

- The Cochrane Collaborative contains updated systematic reviews of steroid and/or antiviral treatment of Bell's palsy—**http://onlinelibrary.wiley.com/doi/10.1002/14651858.CD001942.pub4/full.**

REFERENCES

1. Morris AM, Deeks SL, Hill MD, et al. Annualized incidence and spectrum of illness from an outbreak investigation of Bell's palsy. *Neuroepidemiology.* 2002;21(5):255-261.
2. Campbell KE, Brundage JF. Effects of climate, latitude, and season on the incidence of Bell's palsy in the US Armed Forces, October 1997 to September 1999. *Am J Epidemiol.* 2002;156(1):32-39.
3. Shmorgun D, Chan WS, Ray JG. Association between Bell's palsy in pregnancy and pre-eclampsia. *QJM.* 2002;95(6):359-362.
4. Berg T, Jonsson L, Engstrom M. Agreement between the Sunnybrook, House-Brackmann, and Yanagihara facial nerve grading systems in Bell's palsy. *Otol Neurotol.* 2004;25(6):1020-1026.
5. Salinas RA, Alvarez G, Daly F, Ferreira J. Corticosteroids for Bell's palsy (idiopathic facial paralysis). *Cochrane Database Syst Rev.* 2010;(3):CD001942.
6. Lockhart P, Daly F, Pitkethly M, et al. Antiviral treatment for Bell's palsy (idiopathic facial paralysis.) *Cochrane Database Syst Rev.* 2009;(4):CD001869.
7. Chen N, Zhou M, He L, et al. Acupuncture for Bell's palsy. *Cochrane Database Syst Rev.* 2010;(8):CD002914.
8. Chuang DC. Free tissue transfer for the treatment of facial paralysis. *Facial Plast Surg.* 2008;24(2):194-203.

235 NEUROFIBROMATOSIS

Heidi Chumley, MD

PATIENT STORY

A 44-year-old Hispanic man has neurofibromatosis type 1 (NF-1). He has typical features of NF-1, including 8 café-au-lait spots, axillary freckling, and neurofibromas all over his body (**Figures 235-1** to **235-4**). He states that he is used to having the NF and it does not currently affect his work or life. He is happily married but never had children. No intervention is necessary at this time other than recommending yearly visits to his primary care physician and ophthalmologist.

INTRODUCTION

NF-1 is a common autosomal dominant disorder that predisposes to tumor formation. Café-au-lait spots are often the first clinical sign. Other clinical signs include neurofibromas, axillary or inguinal freckling, optic gliomas, Lisch nodules, and sphenoid bone dysplasia. Treatment at present is early recognition and monitoring for complications such as cognitive dysfunction, scoliosis or other orthopedic problems, tumor pressure on vital structures, or malignant transformation.

EPIDEMIOLOGY

- NF-1 is relatively common—Birth incidence is 1 in 3000 and prevalence in the general population is 1 in 5000.[1]

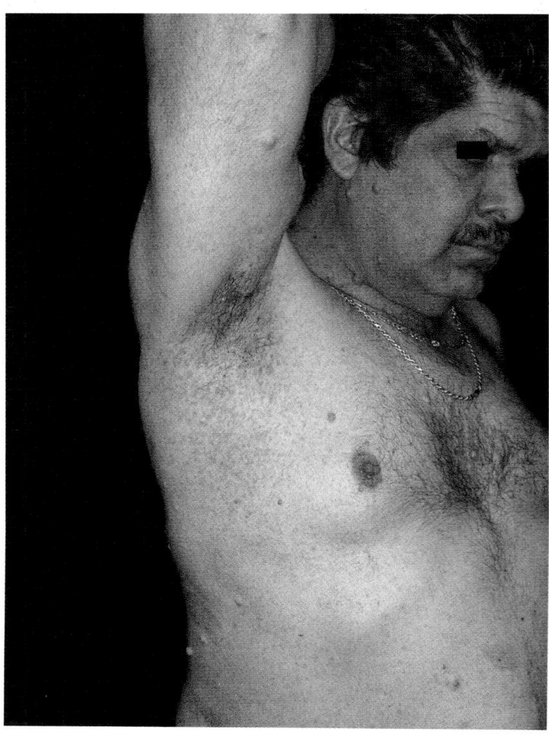

FIGURE 235-1 A 44-year-old Hispanic man with neurofibromatosis type 1 showing all the typical findings including neurofibromas, café-au-lait spots, and axillary freckling. (*Reproduced with permission from Richard P. Usatine, MD.*)

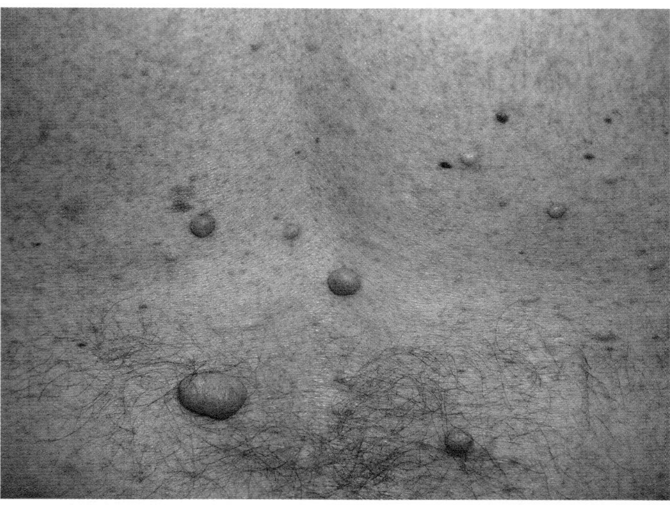

FIGURE 235-2 Close-up of neurofibromas on the back of the man in Figure 235-1. These are soft and round. (*Reproduced with permission from Richard P. Usatine, MD.*)

- Autosomal dominant inheritance; however, up to 50% of cases are sporadic.[1]
- Diagnosis is typically made during childhood.

ETIOLOGY AND PATHOPHYSIOLOGY

- Mutations in the *NF-1* gene (on the long arm of chromosome 17) result in loss of function of neurofibromin, which helps keep protooncogene ras (which increases tumorigenesis) in an inactive form.
- Loss of neurofibromin results in increased protooncogene ras activity in neurocutaneous tissues, leading to tumorigenesis.[1]

RISK FACTORS

A first-degree relative with NF-1.

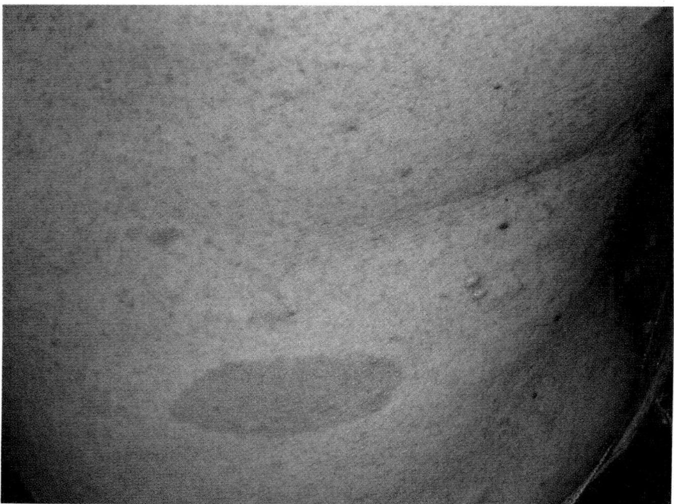

FIGURE 235-3 Large café-au-lait spot on the back of the man in Figure 235-1. Café-au-lait spots are ovoid hyperpigmented macules, 10 to 40 mm in diameter, with smooth borders. (*Reproduced with permission from Richard P. Usatine, MD.*)

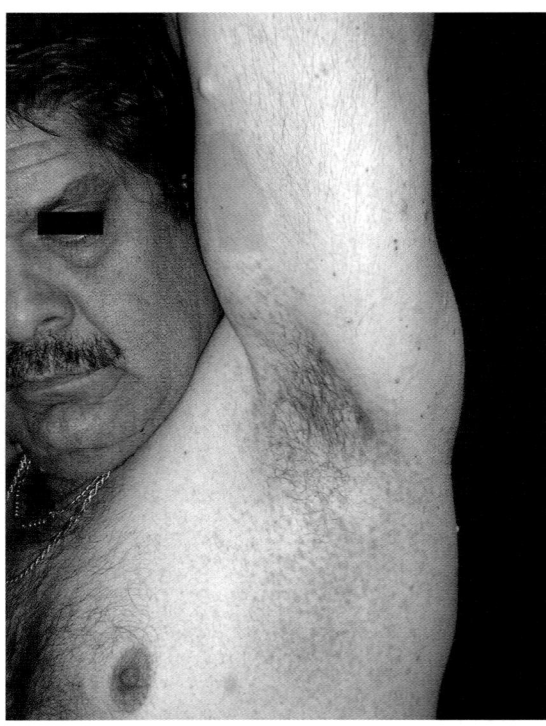

FIGURE 235-4 Close-up of axillary freckling (Crow sign) with large café-au-lait spot on arm. (*Reproduced with permission from Richard P. Usatine, MD.*)

DIAGNOSIS

For a diagnosis of NF-1, patients need to have at least 2 of the following[2]:

1. Two or more neurofibromas (**Figures 235-1** to **235-6**) or one or more plexiform neurofibromas (**Figure 235-7**)
2. Six or more café-au-lait spots, 0.5 cm or larger before puberty and 1.5 cm or larger after puberty (see **Figures 235-3** and **235-4**)
3. Axillary or inguinal freckling (see **Figures 235-1** and **235-4**)
4. Optic glioma
5. Two or more Lisch nodules (melanotic iris hamartomas) (**Figure 235-8**)

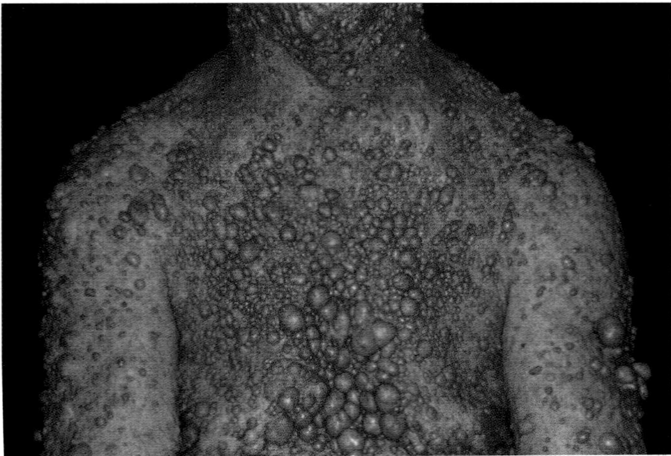

FIGURE 235-5 A man with neurofibromatosis covered with neurofibromas. (*Reproduced with permission from Jack Resneck, Sr., MD.*)

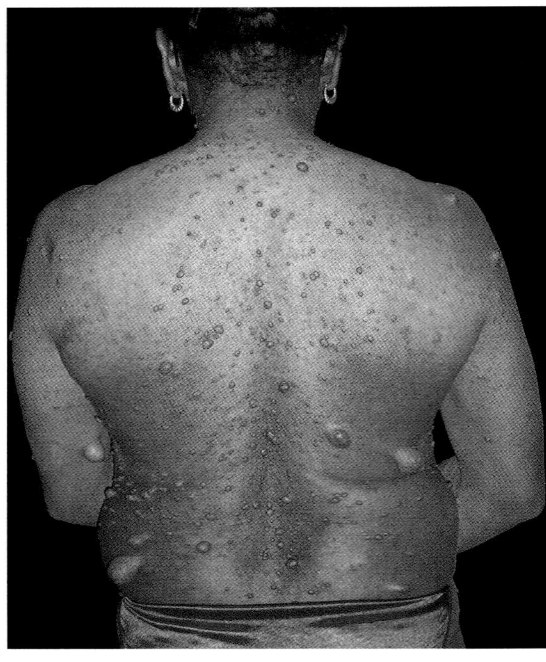

FIGURE 235-6 Neurofibromatosis in a 62-year-old black woman. Note how large some of the neurofibromas can become. (*Reproduced with permission from Richard P. Usatine, MD.*)

6. Dysplasia of the sphenoid bone or dysplasia/thinning of long bone cortex
7. A first-degree relative with NF-1

CLINICAL FEATURES

History and physical

- Ninety-five percent have café-au-lait macules, mostly before the age of 1 year.
- Ninety percent have axillary or inguinal freckling (see **Figures 235-1** and **235-4**).
- Eighty-one percent have cognitive dysfunction manifest as learning disorder, attention deficit hyperactivity disorder, or mild cognitive impairment.[3]

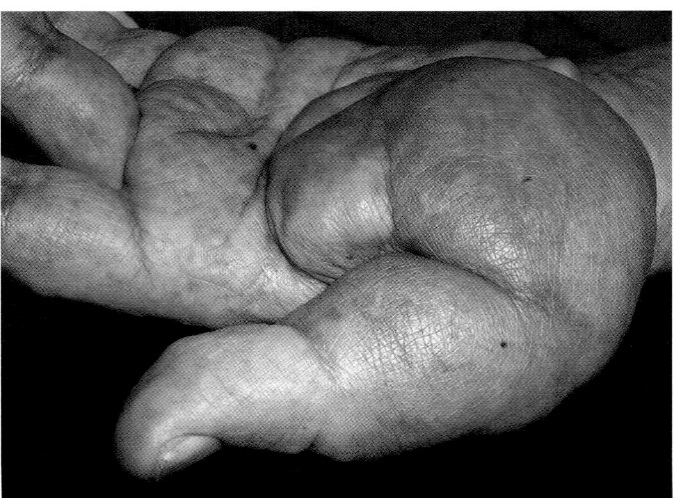

FIGURE 235-7 Plexiform neurofibroma on the thenar eminence feels like a bag of worms in this man with neurofibromatosis. It is a benign tumor of the peripheral nerve sheath and is most often asymptomatic. (*Reproduced with permission from Richard P. Usatine, MD.*)

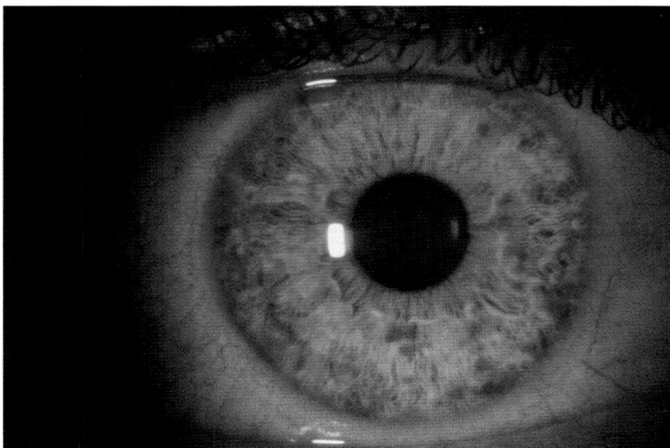

FIGURE 235-8 Lisch nodules (melanotic hamartomas of the iris) are clear yellow-to-brown, dome-shaped elevations that project from the surface of this blue iris. These hamartomas are the most common type of ocular involvement in neurofibromatosis type 1 and do not affect vision. (*Reproduced with permission from Paul Comeau.*)

- Nerve sheath, intracranial, or spinal tumors.
- Cutaneous or subcutaneous neurofibromas (see **Figures 235-1** to **235-6**).
- Other bony pathology, including dysplasia of the sphenoid or long bones, scoliosis, or short stature.
- Eye abnormalities, including Lisch nodules or early glaucoma (see **Figure 235-7**).

LABORATORY TESTING

Genetic testing for couples considering having children

IMAGING

Although not typically used for diagnosis, imaging may be needed if tumor compression of vital structures is suspected.

DIFFERENTIAL DIAGNOSIS

NF-1 is the predominant cause of café-au-lait spots, which can also be seen in the following cases:

- Normal childhood—13% to 27% of children younger than 10 years of age have at least one spot.
- Neurofibromatosis type 2 (NF-2)—Vestibular schwannomas, family history of NF-2, meningioma, glioma, schwannoma, juvenile posterior subcapsular lenticular opacities, or juvenile cortical cataracts.
- Tuberous sclerosis—Angiofibromas (skin-colored telangiectatic papules most commonly in the nasolabial folds, cheek, or chin; **Figure 235-9**) and hypopigmented ovoid or ash leaf-shaped macules.
- McCune-Albright syndrome—Fibrous dysplasia of bone and endocrine gland hyperactivity.
- Fanconi anemia—Decreased production of all blood cells, short stature, upper limb anomalies, genital changes, skeletal anomalies, eye/eyelid anomalies, kidney malformations, ear anomalies/deafness, and gastrointestinal (GI)/cardiopulmonary malformations.
- Segmental NF—Cutaneous neurofibromas limited to specific dermatome(s); very rare.

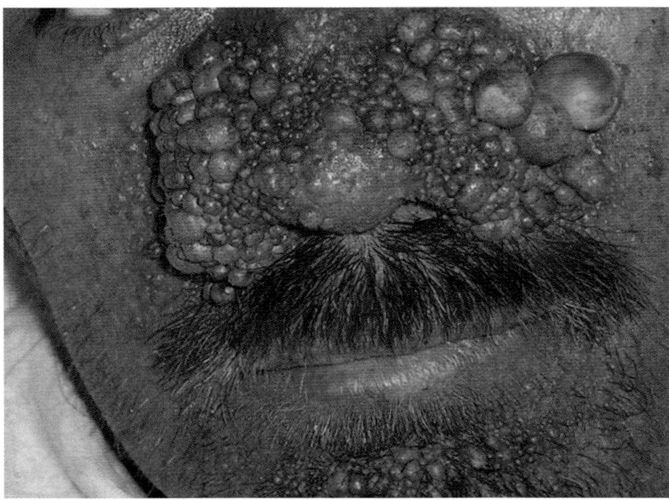

FIGURE 235-9 Angiofibromas (previously called adenoma sebaceum) on the face of a patient with tuberous sclerosis. The patient was originally thought to have neurofibromatosis. He also has epilepsy and cognitive impairment, which accompanies with tuberous sclerosis. (*Reproduced with permission from Natalie Norman, MD.*)

- Bloom syndrome—Growth delay and short stature, increased risk of cancer, telangiectatic erythema on the face, cheilitis, narrow face, prominent nose, large ears, and long limbs.
- Ataxia telangiectasia—Progressive neurologic impairment, cerebellar ataxia, immunodeficiency, impaired organ maturation, ocular and cutaneous telangiectasia, and a predisposition to malignancy.
- Proteus syndrome—Very rare condition with hamartomatous and multisystem involvement. Joseph Merrick (also known as "the elephant man") is now, in retrospect, thought by clinical experts to have had Proteus syndrome and not NF.

MANAGEMENT

Management focuses on early recognition and treatment of manifestations.

- Evaluate adults annually. SOR C
- Screen for cognitive impairment and refer early for intervention. SOR C
- Screen for scoliosis and treat accordingly.
- Refer patients annually for ophthalmologic evaluation.
- Consider treatment or referral for treatment of café-au-lait spots if desired by the patient. Topical vitamin D_3 analogs (calcipotriene [Dovonex]) and laser therapy independently may improve the appearance of café-au-lait spots.[4,5] SOR B One small study suggests that intense pulsed light–radio frequency (IPL-RF) in combination with topical application of vitamin D_3 ointment may lighten small-pigmented lesions in patients with NF-1.[6] SOR B Although calcipotriene is approved for use in psoriasis, it can be prescribed off-label to patients disturbed by their hyperpigmented macules.[4,6] SOR B
- Examine other undiagnosed first-degree relatives. SOR C
- Surgical excision of tumors is required for tumors pressing on vital structures (ie, spinal cord impingement) or when characteristics such as rapid enlargement are worrisome for malignant transformation.

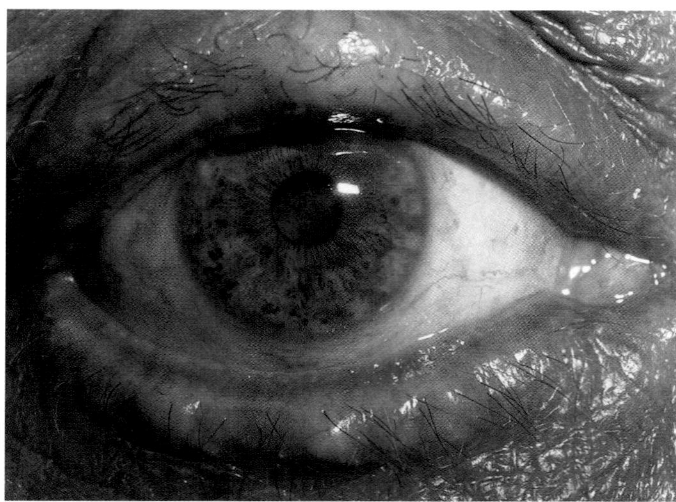

FIGURE 235-10 Neurofibromas on the lower lid with Lisch nodules (dark brown spots) on the iris of this 64-year-old man with neurofibromatosis type 1. (*Reproduced with permission from Richard P. Usatine, MD.*)

PROGNOSIS

- Clinical manifestations are variable leading to difficulty in prognosis.
- There is a 10% lifetime risk of developing a malignant peripheral nerve sheath tumor.

FOLLOW-UP

- Primary care evaluation annually for adults, including monitoring of blood pressure.
- Ophthalmologic examination annually for early detection of optic gliomas and glaucoma. Neurofibromas and plexiform neuromas can occur on the eyelids. Neurofibromas on the eyelids usually are not a problem (**Figure 235-10**) but a plexiform neuroma can present with ptosis and need surgical intervention.
- Genetic counseling for patients with NF-1 considering having children.

PATIENT RESOURCES

- Neurofibromatosis, Inc. has a variety of resources including NF specialists by location—**http://www.nfinc.org.**

PROVIDER RESOURCES

- Neurofibromatosis, Inc. has a variety of patient education materials, information about local support groups, ongoing clinical trials, and camp New Friends for children with NF—**http://www.nfinc.org.**
- The National Institute of Neurological Diseases and Stroke has patient information at its *Neurofibromatosis Information Page*—**http://www.ninds.nih.gov/disorders/NF/NF.htm.**

REFERENCES

1. Yohay K. Neurofibromatosis types 1 and 2. *Neurologist*. 2006;12(2):86-93.
2. Hirsch NP, Murphy A, Radcliffe JJ. Neurofibromatosis: clinical presentations and anaesthetic implications. *Br J Anaesth*. 2001;86(4):555-564.
3. Hyman SL, Shores A, North KN. The nature and frequency of cognitive deficits in children with neurofibromatosis type 1. *Neurology*. 2005;65(7):1037-1044.
4. Nakayama J, Kiryu H, Urabe K, et al. Vitamin D3 analogues improve café au lait spots in patients with von Recklinghausen's disease: experimental and clinical studies. *Eur J Dermatol*. 1999;9(3):202-206.
5. Shimbashi T, Kamide R, Hashimoto T. Long-term follow-up in treatment of solar lentigo and café-au-lait macules with Q-switched ruby laser. *Aesthetic Plast Surg*. 1997;21(6):445-448.
6. Yoshida Y, Sato N, Furumura M, Nakayama J. Treatment of pigmented lesions of neurofibromatosis 1 with intense pulsed-radio frequency in combination with topical application of vitamin D_3 ointment. *J Dermatol*. 2007;34(4):227-230.

PART 19

SUBSTANCE ABUSE

Strength of Recommendation (SOR)	Definition
A	Recommendation based on consistent and good-quality patient-oriented evidence.*
B	Recommendation based on inconsistent or limited-quality patient-oriented evidence.*
C	Recommendation based on consensus, usual practice, opinion, disease-oriented evidence, or case series for studies of diagnosis, treatment, prevention, or screening.*

*See Appendix A on pages 1241-1244 for further information.

236 SUBSTANCE ABUSE DISORDER

Richard P. Usatine, MD
Heidi Chumley, MD
Kelli Hejl Foulkrod, MS

PATIENT STORY

A 21-year-old mother and her 4 children are being seen in a free clinic within a homeless shelter for various health reasons (**Figure 236-1**). The woman is currently clean and sober, but has a long history of cocaine use and addiction (**Figure 236-2**). Her children span the ages of 3 months to 5 years. She was recently living with her mother after the birth of her youngest child, but was kicked out of her mother's home when she went out to use cocaine once again. The patient gave written consent to the photograph and when she was shown the image on the digital camera she noted how depressed she looked. She asked for us to tell the viewers of this photograph that these can be the consequences of drug abuse—being depressed, homeless, and a single mom.

INTRODUCTION

Addiction occurs when substance use has altered brain function to an extent that an individual loses a degree of control over his or her behaviors. Addiction is an epigenetic phenomenon. Many genes influence the brain functions that affect behavior and genetic variants. These genes differ in their susceptibility to environmental conditions, which trigger the changes in brain circuitry, and contribute to the development of addiction. Addiction must be recognized and treated as a chronic illness with an interprofessional team and social support.

EPIDEMIOLOGY

- An estimated 69.6 million Americans age 12 years or older were current users of a tobacco product in 2010. This represents 27.4% of the population in that age range. In addition, 58.3 million persons (23% of the population) were current cigarette smokers, 13.2 million (5.2%) smoked cigars, 8.9 million (3.5%) used smokeless tobacco, and 2.2 million (0.8%) smoked tobacco in pipes.[1]
- An estimated 22.6 million Americans age 12 years or older were current illicit drug users in 2010. This represents 8.9% of the population in that age range.[1]
- Marijuana was the most commonly used illicit drug (17.4 million users) (**Figures 236-3** and **236-4**). It was used by 76.8% of current illicit drug users. Among current illicit drug users, 60.1% used only marijuana, 16.7% used marijuana and another illicit drug, and the remaining 23.2% used only an illicit drug other than marijuana.[1]
- There were 1.5 million persons who were current cocaine users in 2010.[1]
- There were 353,000 persons who were current methamphetamine users in 2010 (**Figure 236-5**).[1]
- Hallucinogens were used by 1.2 million persons (0.5%) in 2010, including 695,000 (0.3%) who had used Ecstasy (**Figure 236-6**).[1]
- In 2010, 140,000 persons used heroin for the first time (**Figure 236-7**).[1]

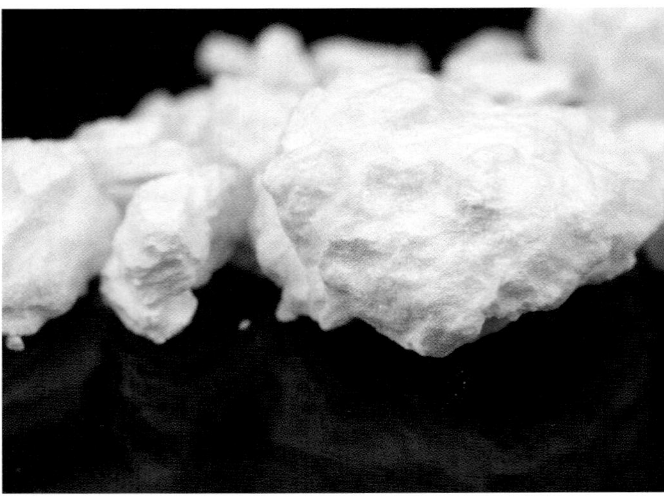

FIGURE 236-2 Purified cocaine. (*Reproduced with permission from DEA.*)

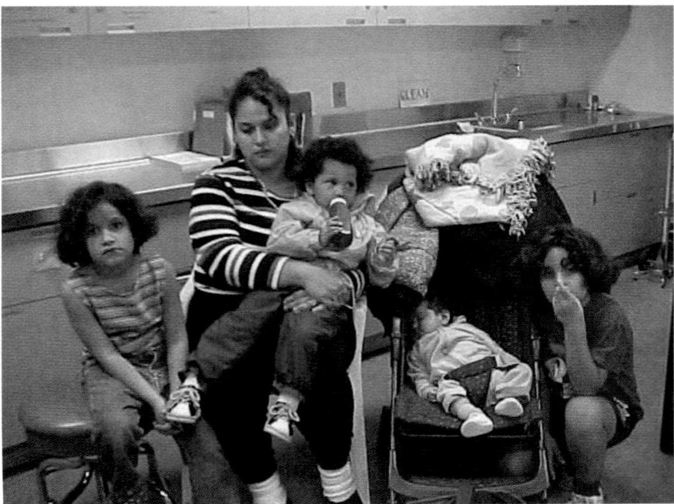

FIGURE 236-1 A cocaine-addicted mother with her children in a homeless shelter. Her drug addiction resulted in their homelessness. (*Reproduced with permission from Richard P. Usatine, MD.*)

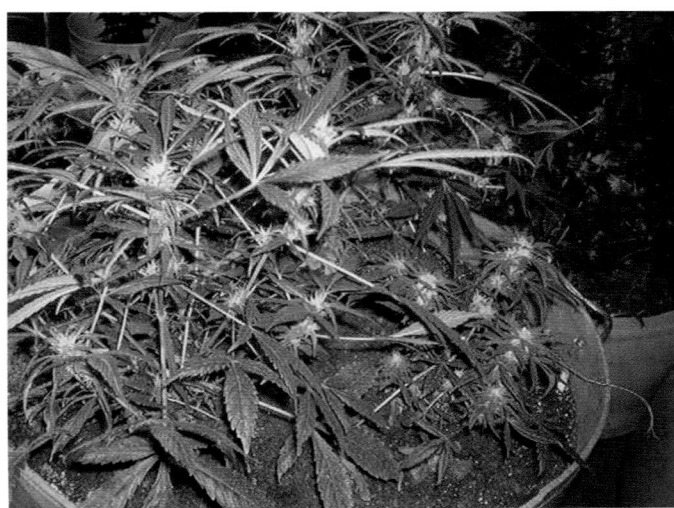

FIGURE 236-3 Home-grown marijuana plant. (*Reproduced with permission from DEA.*)

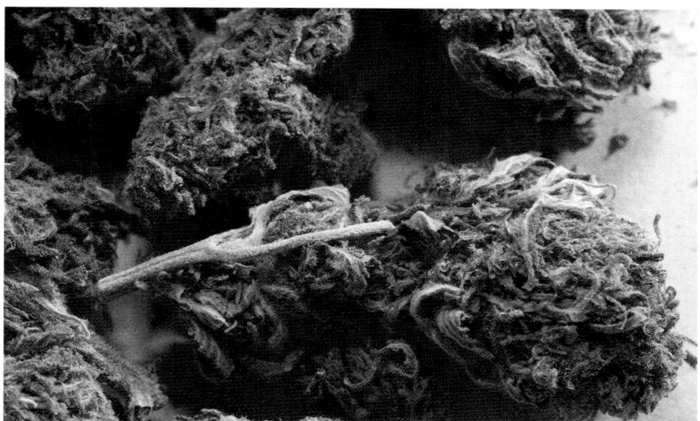

FIGURE 236-4 Marijuana ready to be smoked. (*Reproduced with permission from DEA.*)

- There were 9 million people age 12 years or older (3.6%) who were current users of illicit drugs other than marijuana in 2010. Most (7 million, 2.7%) used psychotherapeutic drugs (including prescription drugs) nonmedically. Of these, 5.1 million used pain relievers, 2.2 million used tranquilizers, 1.1 million used stimulants, and 374,000 used sedatives.[1]
- Among persons who used pain relievers nonmedically in the past 12 months, 55% reported that the source of the drug was from a friend or relative for free. Another 17.3% reported that they got the drug from a physician. Only 4.4% obtained the pain relievers from a drug dealer or other stranger, and only 0.4% reported buying the drug on the Internet.[1]

ASSOCIATION WITH CIGARETTE AND ALCOHOL USE

- In 2010, the rate of current illicit drug use was 8.5 times higher among youths age 12 to 17 years who smoked cigarettes in the past month (52.9%) than it was among youths who did not smoke cigarettes in the past month (6.2%).[1]
- Past month illicit drug use was also associated with the level of past month alcohol use. Among youths age 12 to 17 years in 2010 who were heavy drinkers (ie, drank 5 or more drinks on the same occasion [ie, at the same time or within a couple of hours] on each of 5 or more days in the past 30 days), 70.6% were also current illicit drug users, which was higher than among nondrinkers (5.1%).[1]

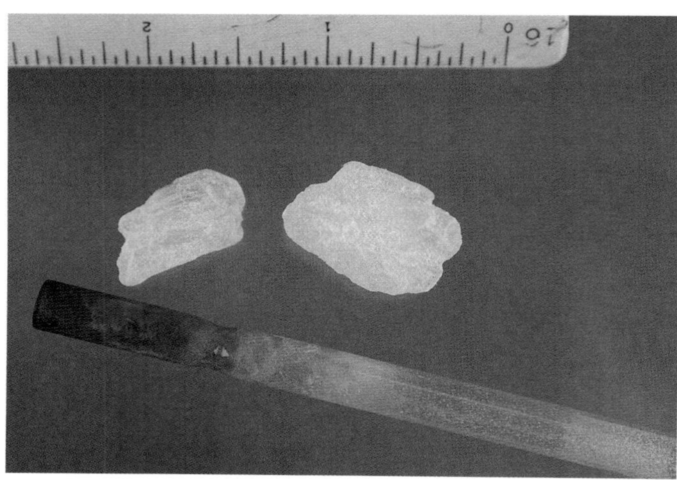

FIGURE 236-5 Methamphetamine ice with pipe. (*Reproduced with permission from DEA.*)

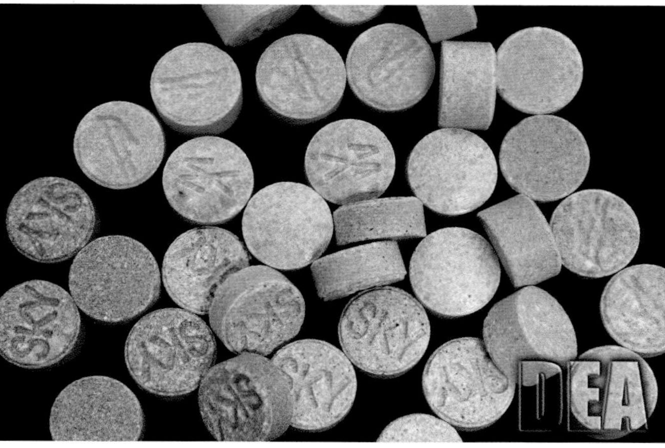

FIGURE 236-6 Ecstasy tablets used at raves where people dance all night long and some collapse in dehydration. (*Reproduced with permission from DEA.*)

ETIOLOGY AND PATHOPHYSIOLOGY

- "Drug addiction is a brain disease. Although initial drug use might be voluntary, drugs of abuse have been shown to alter gene expression and brain circuitry, which in turn affect human behavior. Once addiction develops, these brain changes interfere with an individual's ability to make voluntary decisions, leading to compulsive drug craving, seeking and use."[2]

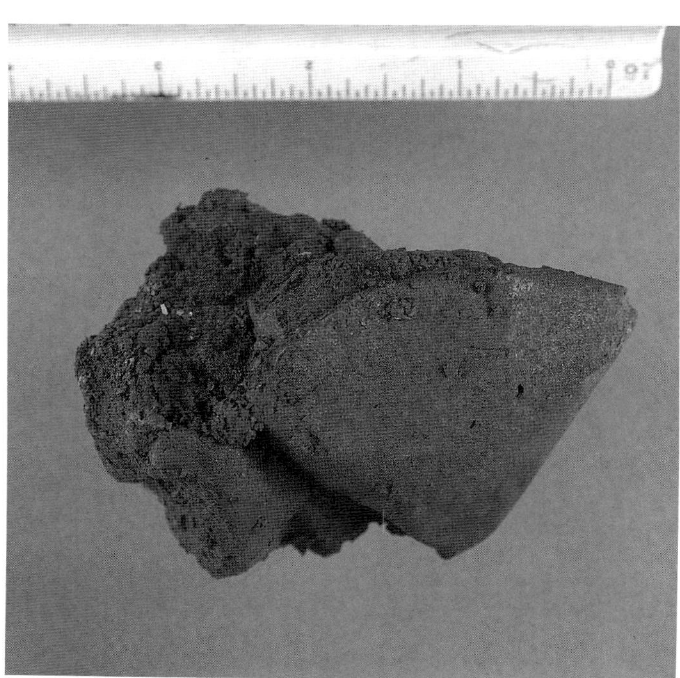

FIGURE 236-7 Black tar heroin for injection. (*Reproduced with permission from DEA.*)

- Addiction is a polygenic disorder. Many genes have direct or indirect influences on neurotransmitters, drug metabolic pathways, and behavioral patterns. For example, variants of receptors for dopamine or opiates influence perceived reward.[3]
- Epigenetic mechanisms, external influences that trigger changes in gene expression, are believed to play a role through modulation of reward and emotion.[3] As such, both genetics and environment/learned behaviors can increase a person's risk for substance abuse.
- Family, twin, and adoption studies convincingly demonstrate that genes play an important role in the development of alcohol dependence, with heritability estimates in the range of 50% to 60% for both men and women. Important genes include those involved in alcohol metabolism, and those involved in γ-aminobutyric acid (GABA), endogenous opioid, dopaminergic, cholinergic, and serotonergic transmission.[4]
- Several drinking behaviors, including alcohol dependence, history of blackouts, age at first drunkenness, and level of response to alcohol are associated with single-nucleotide polymorphisms (SNPs) within 1 of 4 GABA receptor genes on chromosome 5q.[5]
- Comorbid mental health issues and chronic pain disorders are highly prevalent among persons with substance abuse disorders. Commonly, a person begins using drugs to self-treat feelings of depression and symptoms of pain.
- The medical consequences of addiction are far reaching and very costly to society. Cardiovascular disease, stroke, cancer, HIV/AIDS, hepatitis, and lung disease can all be increased by drug abuse. Some of these effects occur when drugs are used at high doses or after prolonged use. Some consequences occur after just one use.[2]
- Classes of substances that are frequently abused and involved in addiction include the following:
  - Depressants—Alcohol, sedatives, hypnotics, opioids, and anxiolytics
  - Stimulants—Cocaine, amphetamines, and nicotine
  - Hallucinogens—Cannabis, phencyclidine (PCP), and lysergic acid diethylamide (LSD)
  - Toxic inhalants
- The onset of drug effects is approximately the following:
  - Seven to 10 seconds for inhaling or smoking
  - Fifteen to 30 seconds for intravenous injection
  - Three to 5 minutes for intramuscular or subcutaneous injection
  - Three to 5 minutes for intranasal use (snorting)

RISK FACTORS

- Family history
- Personal history of prior addiction

DIAGNOSIS

The diagnosis of a substance use disorder is based on a pathological pattern of behaviors related to use of the substance.[6] The DSM V uses 11 criteria to make this diagnosis. One example of these criteria is the following 11 symptoms for alcohol abuse disorder. If one substitutes other substances, like cannabis or cocaine, the same criteria still apply.

A problematic pattern of alcohol use leading to clinically significant impairment or distress, as manifested by at least two of the following, occurring within a 12-month period[6]:

1. Alcohol is often taken in larger amounts or over a longer period than was intended.
2. There is a persistent desire or unsuccessful efforts to cut down or control alcohol use.
3. A great deal of time is spent in activities necessary to obtain alcohol, use alcohol, or recover from its effects.
4. Craving, or a strong desire or urge to use alcohol.
5. Recurrent alcohol use resulting in a failure to fulfill major role obligations at work, school, or home.
6. Continued alcohol use despite having persistent or recurrent social or interpersonal problems caused or exacerbated by the effects of alcohol.
7. Important social, occupational, or recreational activities are given up or reduced because of alcohol use.
8. Recurrent alcohol use in situations in which it is physically hazardous.
9. Alcohol use is continued despite knowledge of having a persistent or recurrent physical or psychological problem that is likely to have been caused or exacerbated by alcohol.
10. Tolerance, as defined by either of the following:
    - A need for markedly increased amounts of alcohol to achieve intoxication or desired effect.
    - A markedly diminished effect with continued use of the same amount of alcohol.
11. Withdrawal, as manifested by either of the following:
    - The characteristic withdrawal syndrome for alcohol (refer to Criteria A and B of the criteria set for alcohol withdrawal).
    - Alcohol (or a closely related substance, such as a benzodiazepine) is taken to relieve or avoid withdrawal symptoms.

Severity is graded based on the number of symptoms present:
Mild: Presence of 2-3 symptoms.
Moderate: Presence of 4-5 symptoms.
Severe: Presence of 6 or more symptoms.[6]

CLINICAL FEATURES VISIBLE WITH SUBSTANCE ABUSE

With intoxication, the following signs may be visible:

- Via stimulants—Dilated pupils and increase in blood pressure, respiratory rate, pulse, and body temperature.
- Via depressants—Decrease in blood pressure, respiratory rate, pulse, and body temperature. Opioids produce pinpoint pupils. Alcohol intoxication produces dilated pupils.
- Withdrawal develops with decline of substance in the central nervous system (CNS). Withdrawal reactions vary by the substance used. Alcohol withdrawal is one of the most deadly and dangerous types of withdrawal.

LABORATORY TESTING

- All injection-drug users and persons engaged in high-risk sexual activities should be screened for HIV (with consent), hepatitis B and hepatitis C, and syphilis (rapid plasma reagin [RPR]).

- Women should have Papanicolaou (Pap) smears performed and be screened for *Chlamydia* and gonorrhea based on age, risk factors, and previous history of screening.
- Men or women who have multiple sex partners or use sex to obtain drugs are at high risk for sexually transmitted diseases (STDs) and should be tested.
- Homeless, HIV-positive, and previously incarcerated patients should be screened for tuberculosis using a purified protein derivative (PPD) test.
- Electrocardiography (ECG) is warranted if there are any cardiac symptoms or if the physical examination reveals signs of cardiac disease.
- Urine screen for common drugs of abuse may reveal other drugs not admitted to in the history. Most laboratories can differentiate prescription from nonprescription drugs (ie, opiates) on request. Substances have different physiologic half-lives in the body and show up for varying amounts of time in the urine. Marijuana has a long excretion half-life and may be detectable for 1 month after its use. Other substances may last for only days.

DIFFERENTIAL DIAGNOSIS

Substance abuse disorders coexist with and complicate the course and treatment of numerous psychiatric conditions.

- Mood/anxiety disorders—Especially depression, bipolar affective disorder, panic disorder, and generalized anxiety disorder. Persons with addictions can develop the symptoms of these disorders from the drugs of abuse. However, mood and anxiety disorders can predate the use of drugs, and some of the motivation for drug use can stem from the desire to self-treat these psychological conditions. It is best to evaluate persons when they are off the drugs whenever possible.
- Schizophrenia—Although drugs can cause temporary psychosis and paranoia, if these symptoms persist after the drugs are stopped for some time, consider schizophrenia and other causes of psychosis.
- Personality disorders—These are a complicated set of disorders that can coexist and be confused with substance abuse disorder. An addict may appear to have an antisocial personality disorder when committing crimes to get money for expensive drugs. It is best to not use this diagnosis unless the behaviors continue when the person is off the drugs.

MANAGEMENT

- Recognize addiction (referred to as dependence in the DSM-IV criteria). One simple mnemonic device is the "3 C's of addiction":
  - **C**ompulsion to use
  - Lack of **C**ontrol
  - **C**ontinued use despite adverse consequences
- Use the "5 A's"—**A**sk, **A**dvise, **A**ssess, **A**ssist, and **A**rrange—to help smokers who are willing to quit. This model can be applied to any substance of abuse.[7]
- Offer counseling and pharmacotherapy to aid your patients to quit smoking.
- Use the CAGE[7] questionnaire when asking about alcohol use.
  - **C**ut down (Have you ever felt you should *cut* down on your drinking?).
  - **A**nnoyed (Have people *annoyed* you by criticizing your drinking?).
  - **G**uilty (Have you ever felt bad or *guilty* about your drinking?).
  - **E**ye opener (Have you ever had a drink first thing in the morning to steady your nerves or get rid of a hangover (eye-opener)?).

Interpreting the results: 1 positive suggests at risk, 2 positives suggest abuse, and 3 or 4 positives suggest dependence. This is just a screening tool, and further evaluation is always needed.

- Recommend the 12-step programs to your patients. These have been very effective for millions of people worldwide.
- Refer to substance abuse programs. Such programs include hospital- and community-based programs. Some programs include detoxification and others require the patient to have gone through detoxification before starting the program. There are residential treatment units, outpatient programs, and ongoing self-help programs. Learn about the programs in your community and work with them.
- When prescribing opioid analgesics for chronic pain consider the outcomes in 4 domains, or the "4 A's."
  - Receiving adequate **A**nalgesia?
  - Experiencing improvements in **A**ctivities of daily life?
  - Experiencing any **A**dverse effects?
  - Demonstrating **A**berrant medication-taking behaviors that may be linked to addiction?[8]
- When patients are exhibiting aberrant drug-taking behaviors, consider the following:
  - They may have an addiction.
  - They may not be getting adequate pain relief taking the drug as prescribed.
  - They may have a comorbid mental illness.
  - They may intend to distribute pain medications illegally.[9]
- Help your patients acknowledge that they have a problem and offer them help in a nonjudgmental manner.
- Enlist family members to help whenever the patient gives your permission to do so.
- Demonstrate genuine concern and care; suspend judgment and you will have a higher chance of succeeding to help your patients overcome addiction.
- Advanced brain imaging and genetic tests are helping us to understand the physiologic basis of addiction and will ultimately provide us with better treatments for the medical disease of addiction.

PERSONS IN RECOVERY

- Be careful how you prescribe medications to persons in recovery. A "simple" prescription for hydrocodone (Vicodin) postoperatively can start a recovered person down the road of active addiction.
- Avoid giving opioids and benzodiazepines whenever there are good alternatives. Use nonsteroidal anti-inflammatory drugs (NSAIDs) for pain if possible. Use selective serotonin reuptake inhibitors (SSRIs), other antidepressants, or buspirone for anxiety if a medication is needed.
- If an opioid is needed, work with the patient to monitor the amount and manner of use. Involving a third person or sponsor to help meter out the dose may prevent relapse.
- Be upfront and honest about a shared goal to avoid relapse.

FOLLOW-UP

- Follow-up is critical to the treatment of all types of substance abuse. Substance abuse is a chronic condition (similar to hypertension or diabetes mellitus) and requires ongoing intervention to maintain sobriety.

- The frequency and intensity of follow-up depends on the substance, the addiction, and the patient.
- Do not give up on patients who relapse because it often takes more than one attempt before long-term cessation can be achieved.

PATIENT EDUCATION

Explain to patients that addiction is a disease and not a failing of their moral character. Inform patients about the existing treatment programs in their community and offer them names and phone numbers so that they may get help. If your patient is not ready for help today, give the numbers and names for tomorrow. Speak about the value of 12-step programs because these are effective and everyone can afford a 12-step program (they are free). There are 12-step programs in the community for everyone, including nonsmokers and agnostics.

PATIENT RESOURCES

- Alcoholics Anonymous (AA)—meetings and the Big Book are free. The Big Book is online for free in three languages. **http://www.alcoholics-anonymous.org/.**
- Narcotics Anonymous (NA)—meetings are free. The "Basic Text" costs $10; it is similar to the AA big book, but the language is more up to date and readable. **http://www.na.org/index.htm.**
- Cocaine Anonymous (CA)—meetings are free. Their first book "Hope, Faith and Courage: Stories from the Fellowship of Cocaine Anonymous" was published in 1994 and sells for $10. **http://www.ca.org/.**
- Crystal Meth Anonymous (12-step meetings) —**http://www.crystalmeth.org/.**

PROVIDER RESOURCES

- The National Institute on Drug Abuse (NIDA). *Medical Consequences of Drug Abuse*—**http://www.nida.nih.gov/consequences/.**
- Substance Abuse and Mental Health Services Administration—**http://www.samhsa.gov/.**
- Drug Enforcement Agency. *Multi-Media Library* (includes many images of illegal drugs)—**http://www.usdoj.gov/dea/multimedia.html.**

REFERENCES

1. Substance Abuse and Mental Health Services Administration, *Results from the 2010 National Survey on Drug Use and Health: Summary of National Findings*, NSDUH Series H-41, HHS Publication No. (SMA) 11-4658. Rockville, MD: Substance Abuse and Mental Health Services Administration; 2011. http://www.samhsa.gov/data/NSDUH/2k10NSDUH/2k10Results.pdf.
2. The National Institute on Drug Abuse (NIDA). *Medical Consequences of Drug Abuse*. http://www.nida.nih.gov/consequences/. Accessed April 24, 2012.
3. Baler RD, Volkow ND. Addiction as a systems failure: focus on adolescence and smoking. *J Am Acad Child Adolesc Psychiatry.* 2011;50(4):329-339.
4. Dick DM, Bierut LJ. The genetics of alcohol dependence. *Curr Psychiatry Rep.* 2006;8:151-157.
5. Dick DM, Plunkett J, Wetherill LF, et al. Association between GABRA1 and drinking behaviors in the collaborative study on the genetics of alcoholism sample. *Alcohol Clin Exp Res.* 2006;30(7): 1101-1110.
6. The American Psychiatric Association. *Diagnostic and Statistical Manual of Mental Disorders*, 5th ed (DSM-V). Washington, DC: American Psychiatric Association, 2013.
7. Fiore MC, Bailey WC, Cohen SJ, et al. *Treating Tobacco Use and Dependence. Quick Reference Guide for Clinicians*. Rockville, MD: U.S. Department of Health and Human Services, Public Health Service; 2000.
8. Ewing JA. Detecting alcoholism: the CAGE questionnaire. *JAMA.* 1984;252(14):1905-1907.
9. Passik SD, Kirsh KL, Whitcomb L, et al. A new tool to assess and document pain outcomes in chronic pain patients receiving opioid therapy. *Clin Ther.* 2004;26(4):552-561.

237 TOBACCO ADDICTION

Carlos Roberto Jaén, MD, PhD

PATIENT STORY

A 55-year-old woman presents for follow-up of hypertension. She has been smoking 1.5 packs of cigarettes per day since her late teens and reports that she is now ready to stop smoking. She realizes that smoking is bad for her health and does not like how smoking causes more wrinkles on the face (**Figure 237-1**). She has tried unsuccessfully to stop smoking on 3 different occasions using nicotine replacement therapy (patches and gum) and bupropion. She has no history of a psychiatric or seizure disorder. She would like to try stopping smoking using varenicline. She is also willing to return for 4 follow-up sessions at weekly intervals. She agrees to call a stop smoking telephone helpline (1-800-QUIT NOW) for counseling help. The patient tolerates the varenicline well and is able to stop successfully without any adverse effects. Two years after treatment she continues to be abstinent and very glad of this outcome. The clinician used elements of the "5 A's" model for treating tobacco use and dependence to successfully help this patient quit smoking. (**Table 237-1**).

INTRODUCTION

Half of all deaths (more than 440,000) in the United States are attributed to tobacco addiction, including those caused by passive smoking. Tobacco addiction is a chronic disease, often developed during adolescence and early adulthood, that requires ongoing assessment and repeated intervention. There are effective treatments that can significantly increase rates of long-term abstinence. There are also effective preventive interventions that can prevent the initiation of tobacco use and reduce its prevalence among youth.

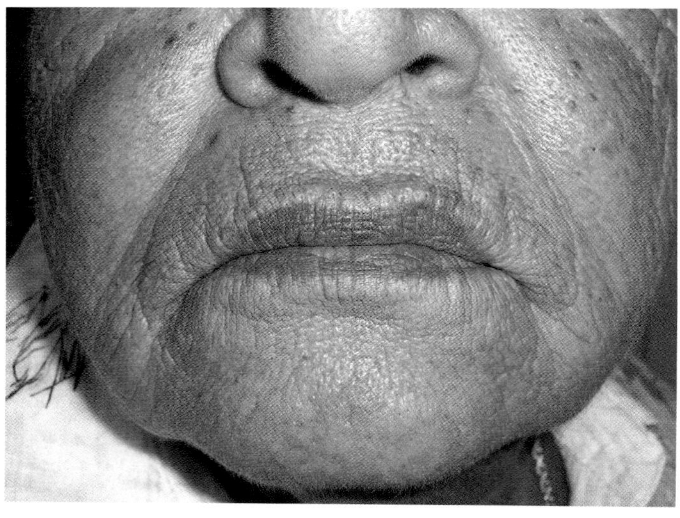

FIGURE 237-1 A 55-year-old woman with premature wrinkling from years of heavy smoking. Note the numerous lines around her mouth and lips. *(Reproduced with permission from Richard P. Usatine, MD.)*

SYNONYMS

Tobacco addiction is also known as tobacco use and dependence, tobacco use disorder, nicotine addiction, and tobacco dependence.

EPIDEMIOLOGY

- Among adults who become daily smokers, nearly all first use of cigarettes occurs by 18 years of age (88%), with 99% of first use by 26 years of age.[1]
- Almost 1 in 4 high school seniors is a current (in the past 30 days) cigarette smoker, compared with 1 in 3 young adults and 1 in 5 adults. Approximately 1 in 10 high school senior males is a current smokeless tobacco user, and approximately 1 in 5 high school senior males is a current cigar smoker.[1]
- Significant disparities in tobacco use remain among young people nationwide. The prevalence of cigarette smoking is highest among American Indians and Alaska Natives, followed by whites and Hispanics, and then Asians and blacks. The prevalence of cigarette smoking is also higher among lower socioeconomic status youth.[1]
- The latest data show the use of smokeless tobacco is increasing among white high school males, and cigar smoking may be increasing among black high school females.[1]
- Concurrent use of multiple tobacco products is prevalent among youth. Among those who use tobacco, nearly one-third of high school females and more than one-half of high school males report using more than one tobacco product in the last 30 days.[1]
- Persons with psychiatric diagnoses have much higher rates of smoking than the general population.[2]
- Persons with mental illness and/or substance abuse consume 44% of all cigarettes sold in the United States, despite being only 22% of the population.[2]

ETIOLOGY AND PATHOPHYSIOLOGY

- The evidence on the mechanisms by which smoking causes disease indicates that there is no risk-free level of exposure to tobacco smoke.[3]
- Inhaling the complex chemical mixture of combustion compounds in tobacco smoke causes adverse health outcomes, particularly cancer and cardiovascular and pulmonary diseases, through mechanisms that include DNA damage, inflammation, and oxidative stress.[3]
- There is sufficient evidence to infer that a causal relationship exists between active smoking and (a) impaired lung growth during childhood and adolescence; (b) early onset of decline in lung function during late adolescence and early adulthood; (c) respiratory signs and symptoms in children and adolescents, including coughing, phlegm, wheezing, and dyspnea; and (d) asthma-related symptoms (eg, wheezing) in childhood and adolescence.[1]
- The evidence is suggestive but not sufficient to conclude that smoking by adolescents and young adults is *not* associated with significant weight loss, contrary to young people's belief.[1]
- Through multiple defined mechanisms, the risk and severity of many adverse health outcomes caused by smoking are directly related to the duration and level of exposure to tobacco smoke.[3]

TABLE 237-1 The "5 A's" Model for Treating Tobacco Use and Dependence

Ask about tobacco use.	Identify and document tobacco use status for every patient at every visit.
Advise to quit.	In a clear, strong, and personalized manner, urge every tobacco user to quit.
Assess willingness to make a quit attempt.	Is the tobacco user willing to make a quit attempt at this time?
Assist in quit attempt.	For the patient willing to make a quit attempt, offer medication and provide or refer for counseling or additional treatment to help the patient quit.
	For patients unwilling to quit at the time, provide interventions designed to increase future quit attempts.
Arrange follow-up.	For the patient willing to make a quit attempt, arrange for follow-up contacts, beginning within the first week after the quit date.
	For patients unwilling to make a quit attempt at the time, address tobacco dependence and willingness to quit at next clinic visit.

Data from Treating Tobacco Use and Dependence: 2008 Update. US Department of Health and Human Services; 2008. http://www.ahrq.gov/clinic/tobacco/treating_tobacco_use08.pdf.

- Sustained use and long-term exposures to tobacco smoke are caused by the powerful addicting effects of tobacco products, which are mediated by diverse actions of nicotine and perhaps other compounds, at multiple types of nicotinic receptors in the brain.[3]
- Nicotine stimulates the release of multiple neurotransmitters, including dopamine, norepinephrine, acetylcholine, glutamate, serotonin, β-endorphin, and γ-aminobutyric acid.[4]
- Low levels of exposure, including exposures to secondhand tobacco smoke, lead to a rapid and sharp increase in endothelial dysfunction and inflammation, which are implicated in acute cardiovascular events and thrombosis.[3]
- There is insufficient evidence that product modification strategies to lower emissions of specific toxicants in tobacco smoke reduce risk for the major adverse health outcomes.[3]

RISK FACTORS

Given their developmental stage, adolescents and young adults are uniquely susceptible to social and environmental influences to use tobacco.

- Socioeconomic factors and educational attainment influence the development of youth smoking behavior. The adolescents most likely to begin to use tobacco and progress to regular use are those who have lower academic achievement.[1]
- The evidence is sufficient to conclude that there is a causal relationship between peer group social influences and the initiation and maintenance of smoking behaviors during adolescence.[1]
- Affective processes play an important role in youth smoking behavior, with a strong association between youth smoking and negative effect.[1]
- The evidence is suggestive that tobacco use is a heritable trait, more so for regular use than for onset. The expression of genetic risk for smoking among young people may be moderated by small-group and larger social–environmental factors.[1]

DIAGNOSIS

CLINICAL FEATURES

- History—Most tobacco users express a desire to stop using tobacco but report repeated failures in their attempts. All patients should be asked if they use tobacco and should have their tobacco use status documented on a regular basis. Evidence shows that clinic screening systems, such as expanding the vital signs to include tobacco use status, or the use of other reminder systems, such as chart stickers or computer prompts, significantly increase rates of clinician intervention.[5] SOR Ⓐ
- Physical—Individuals with tobacco addiction may easily be detected by the following:
  - Distinctive odor of tobacco smoke
  - Smoker's cough
  - Raspy or hoarse voice (see Chapter 32, The Larynx [Hoarseness])
  - Pack of cigarettes in the front pocket of the shirt
  - Wrinkles in excess of what would be expected for their age (**Figure 237-2**)
- *Smoker's face* is described as the following:
  - "Lines or wrinkles on the face, typically radiating at right angles from the upper and lower lips or corners of the eyes, deep lines on the cheeks, or numerous shallow lines on the cheeks and lower jaw" (see **Figure 237-2**).
  - "A subtle gauntness of the facial features with prominence of the underlying bony contours."[6]
- The oral cavity of smokers often shows signs of prolonged exposure to tobacco in the form of the following:
  - Yellow and brown teeth (**Figures 237-3** to **237-5**)
  - Angular cheilitis (see **Figure 237-3**) (see Chapter 29, Angular Cheilitis)
  - Gingivitis and periodontitis (see **Figure 237-4**) (see Chapter 35, Gingivitis and Periodontal Disease)
- There may be other serious conditions within the oral cavity such as the following:

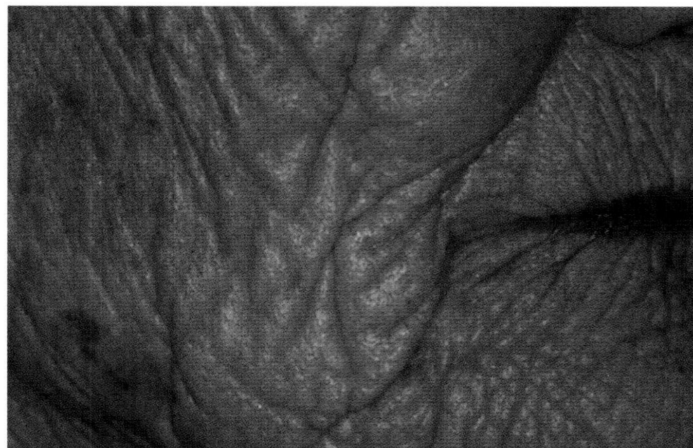

FIGURE 237-2 Smoker's face described as "one or more of the following: (a) lines or wrinkles on the face, typically radiating at right angles from the upper and lower lips or corners of the eyes, deep lines on the cheeks, or numerous shallow lines on the cheeks and lower jaw. (b) A subtle gauntness of the facial features with prominence of the underlying bony contours.[6] (*Reproduced with permission from Usatine R, Moy R, Tobinick E, Siegel D. Skin Surgery: A Practical Guide. St. Louis, MO: Mosby; 1998.*)

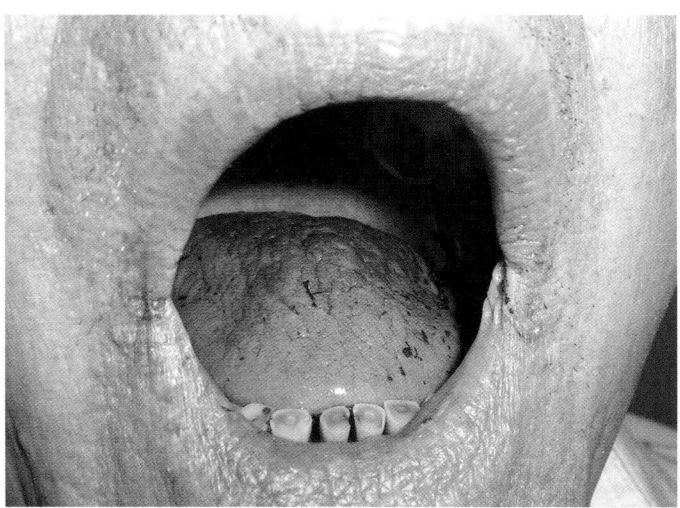

FIGURE 237-3 Angular cheilitis and tobacco staining of the tongue from chewing tobacco. (*Reproduced with permission from Richard P. Usatine, MD.*)

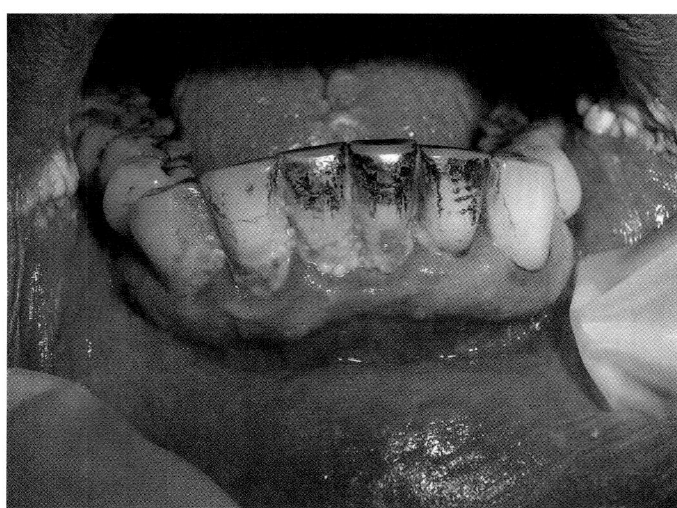

FIGURE 237-4 Tobacco staining teeth and periodontitis from smoking tobacco. (*Reproduced with permission from Richard P. Usatine, MD.*)

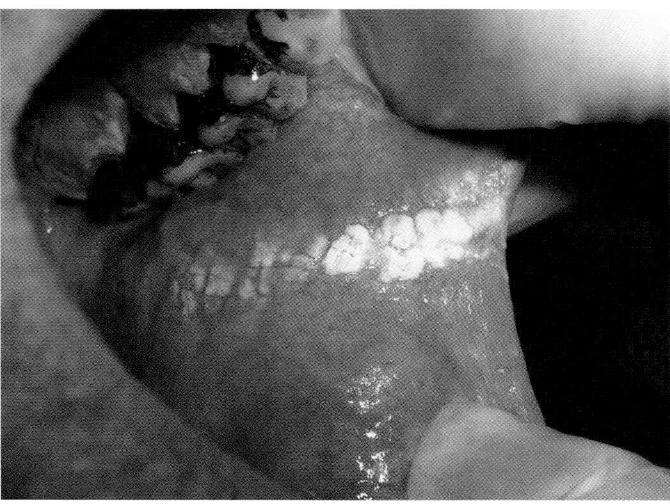

FIGURE 237-5 Leukoplakia on the buccal mucosa and gingiva in a tobacco smoker. Although much of the leukoplakia is on the bite line, the risk of squamous cell carcinoma of the oral cavity must be assessed with appropriate biopsies. (*Reproduced with permission from Richard P. Usatine, MD.*)

- Leukoplakia—A premalignant condition (see **Figure 237-5**) (see Chapter 38, Leukoplakia)
- Nicotine stomatitis (**Figure 237-6**)
- Squamous cell carcinoma (**Figures 237-7** and **237-8**) (see Chapter 39, Oropharyngeal Cancer)

- Withdrawal symptoms—Symptoms associated with tobacco addiction withdrawal include a dysphoric or depressed mood, insomnia, irritability, frustration or anger, anxiety, difficulty concentrating, restlessness, decreased heart rate, and increased appetite or weight gain.[7] None of the withdrawal symptoms are life threatening, as they can be with other drugs like alcohol and opiates. Their intensity peaks during the first week and most last no more than 2 to 4 weeks following abstinence.[8]
- Complications—Continuing use of tobacco causes multiple cancers and the development and/or exacerbation of multiple chronic diseases as summarized in **Figure 237-9**.

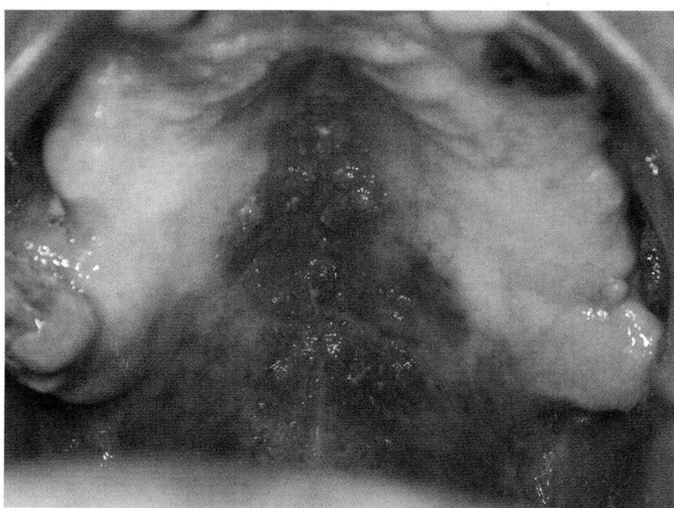

FIGURE 237-6 Nicotine stomatitis over the hard palate from smoking tobacco. (*Reproduced with permission from Rizzolo D, Chiodo TA. Lesion on the hard palate.* J Fam Pract. *2008;57(1):33-35. Reproduced with permission from Frontline Medical Communications.*)

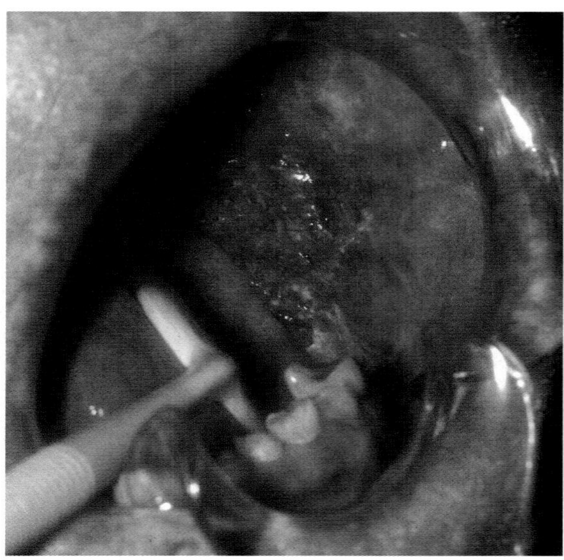

FIGURE 237-7 Squamous cell carcinoma of buccal mucosa in a man who used chewing tobacco along with smoking. (*Reproduced with permission from Richard P. Usatine, MD.*)

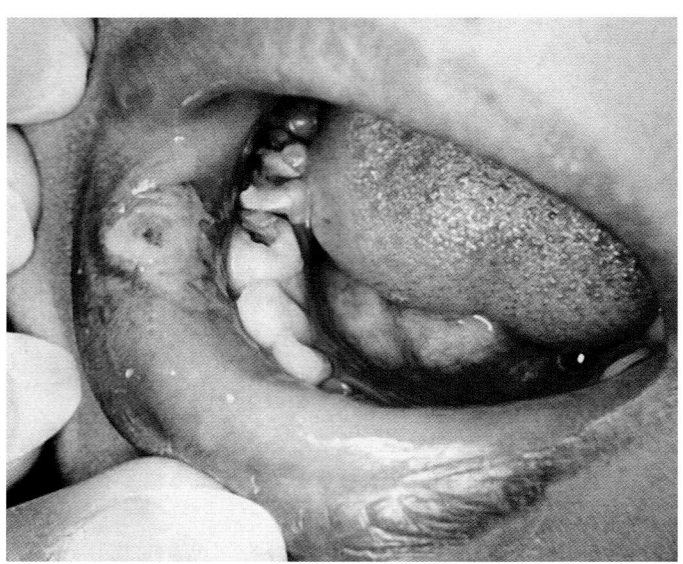

FIGURE 237-8 Squamous cell carcinoma of the inner lip in a cigar smoker. (*Reproduced with permission from Gerald Ferritti, DDS.*)

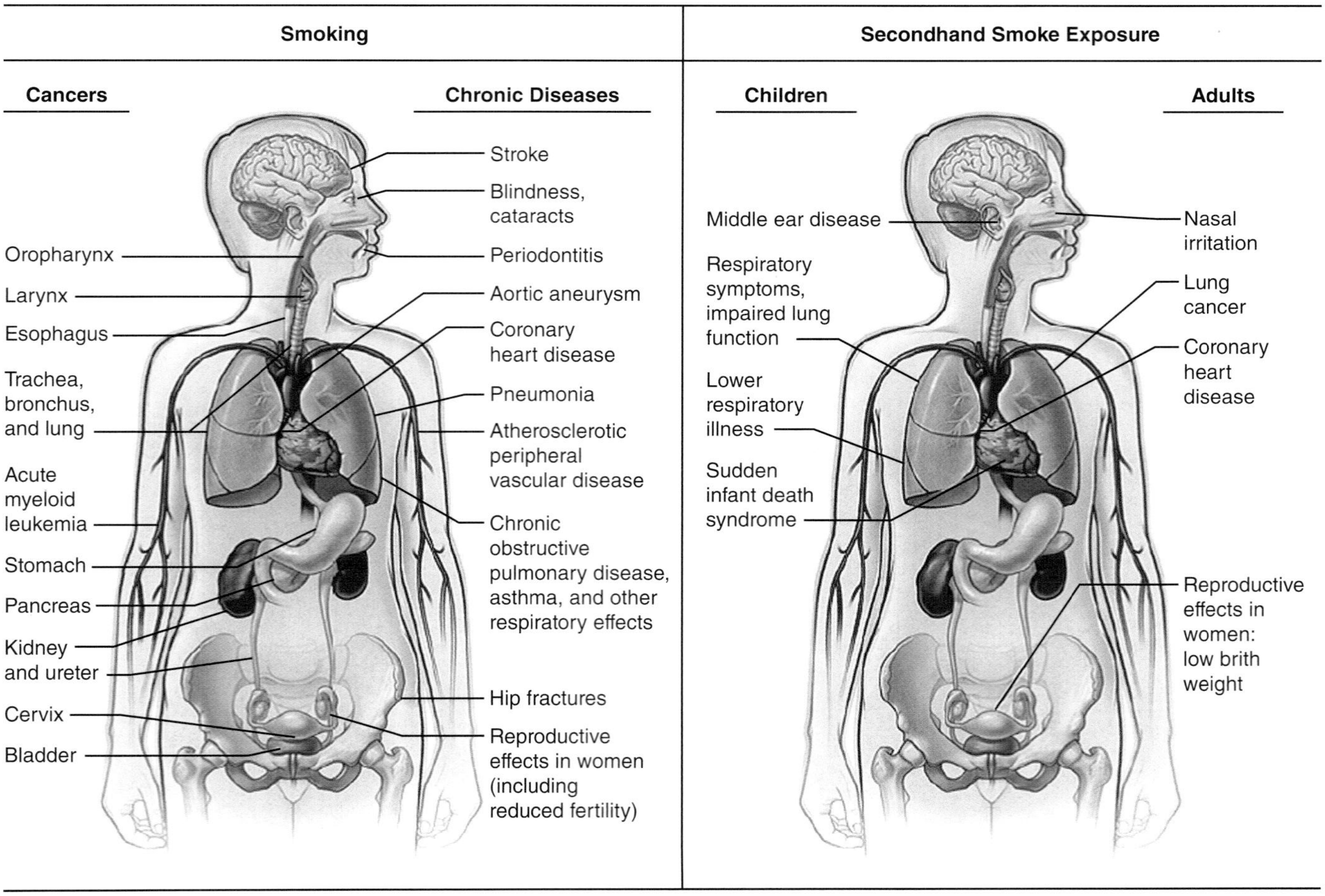

Smoking

Cancers

Oropharynx
Larynx
Esophagus
Trachea, bronchus, and lung
Acute myeloid leukemia
Stomach
Pancreas
Kidney and ureter
Cervix
Bladder

Chronic Diseases

Stroke
Blindness, cataracts
Periodontitis
Aortic aneurysm
Coronary heart disease
Pneumonia
Atherosclerotic peripheral vascular disease
Chronic obstructive pulmonary disease, asthma, and other respiratory effects
Hip fractures
Reproductive effects in women (including reduced fertility)

Secondhand Smoke Exposure

Children

Middle ear disease
Respiratory symptoms, impaired lung function
Lower respiratory illness
Sudden infant death syndrome

Adults

Nasal irritation
Lung cancer
Coronary heart disease
Reproductive effects in women: low brith weight

FIGURE 237-9 Health consequences causally linked to smoking and secondhand smoking. (*Reproduced with permission from U.S. Department of Health and Human Services.* How Tobacco Smoke Causes Disease: The Biology and Behavioral Basis for Smoking-Attributable Disease: A Report of the Surgeon General. *Atlanta, GA: U.S. Department of Health and Human Services, Centers for Disease Control and Prevention, National Center for Chronic Disease Prevention and Health Promotion, Office on Smoking and Health; 2010.*)

- Emphysema may significantly impair lung function and lead to death (see Chapter 56, Chronic Obstructive Pulmonary Disease). Centrilobular emphysema occurs with carbon deposits in the destroyed lung tissue.

LABORATORY TESTING

- Some specialized assessments of individual and environmental attributes provide information for tailoring treatment and may predict quitting success. Specialized assessments refer to the use of formal instruments (eg, questionnaires, clinical interviews, or physiologic indices such as carbon monoxide, serum nicotine/cotinine levels, and/or pulmonary function) that may be associated with cessation outcome. In addition, clinicians may find other assessments relevant to medication use and specific populations when selecting treatment. The use of biochemical confirmation (use of biological samples, such as expired air, saliva, urine, or blood, to measure tobacco-related compounds, such as nicotine, cotinine, and carboxyhemoglobin) is particularly useful to verify abstinence during pregnancy treatment where reports of deception have been documented.[5] Variables targeted by specialized assessments that predict treatment success include the following:
    - High motivation
    - Readiness to change in the next month
    - Moderate-to-high self-efficacy (confidence in his or her ability to stop using tobacco successfully)
    - Supportive social network
- Variables associated with lower abstinence rates include the following:
    - High nicotine dependence
    - Psychiatric comorbidity and substance use (particularly elevated depressive symptoms, schizophrenia, and current alcohol abuse)
    - High stress level
    - Exposure to other smokers[5]

IMAGING

- There are currently no practical clinical applications for imaging studies that are helpful when treating individuals with tobacco addiction. Experimentally several magnetic resonance imaging (MRI), functional MRI, and positron emission tomography (PET) scan studies provide helpful clues as to mechanisms of actions of tobacco addiction.[3]
- The United States Preventive Services Task Force (USPSTF) now recommends one-time screening for abdominal aortic aneurysm (AAA) by ultrasonography in men aged 65 to 75 who have ever smoked (more than 100 cigarettes over a lifetime). SOR B This screening is not recommended for women or for men who never smoked. (http://www.uspreventiveservicestaskforce.org/uspstf05/aaascr/aaars.pdf)

MANAGEMENT

The combination of counseling and medication is more effective for smoking cessation than either medication or counseling alone. Therefore, whenever feasible and appropriate, both counseling and medication should be provided to patients trying to stop smoking.[5] SOR A

NONPHARMACOLOGIC (COUNSELING INTERVENTIONS)

- Minimal interventions lasting less than 3 minutes increase overall tobacco abstinence rates. Every tobacco user should be offered at least a minimal intervention, whether or not he or she is referred to an intensive intervention.[5] SOR A
- Two types of counseling and behavioral therapies result in higher abstinence rates: (a) providing smokers with practical counseling (problem-solving skills/skills training), and (b) providing support and encouragement as part of treatment. These types of counseling elements should be included in smoking cessation interventions.[5] SOR B
- There is a strong dose–response relationship between the session length of person-to-person contact and successful treatment outcomes. Intensive interventions are more effective than less-intensive interventions and should be used whenever possible.[5] SOR A
- Proactive telephone counseling, group counseling, and individual counseling formats are effective and should be used in smoking cessation interventions.[5] SOR A
- Person-to-person treatment delivered for 4 or more sessions appears especially effective in increasing abstinence rates. Therefore, if feasible, clinicians should strive to meet 4 or more times with individuals quitting tobacco use.[5] SOR A
- Motivational interviewing for smokers not willing to make an attempt to stop tobacco use includes the following:
    - Motivational intervention techniques appear to be effective in increasing a patient's likelihood of making a future quit attempt. Therefore, clinicians should use motivational techniques to encourage smokers who are not currently willing to quit to consider making a quit attempt in the future.[5] SOR B
    - The 4 general principles that underlie motivational intervention are (a) *express empathy,* (b) *develop discrepancy,* (c) *roll with resistance,* and (d) *support self-efficacy* (**Table 237-2**). Motivational intervention researchers have found that having patients use their own words to commit to change is more effective than clinician exhortations, lectures, or arguments for quitting, which tend to increase rather than lessen patient resistance to change.[5]

MEDICATIONS

Clinicians should encourage all patients attempting to quit to use effective medications for tobacco dependence treatment, except where contraindicated or for specific populations for which there is insufficient evidence of effectiveness (eg, pregnant women, smokeless tobacco users, light smokers, and adolescents).[5] SOR A

- In the United States, there are 7 Food and Drug Administration (FDA)-approved medications for treating tobacco use and these first-line medications should be recommended: bupropion SR (Zyban), nicotine gum, nicotine inhaler, nicotine lozenge, nicotine nasal spray, nicotine patch, and varenicline (Chantix). Precautions, benefits, and disadvantages for these 7 medications are found in **Boxes 237-1 to 237-7**.
- The clinician should consider the first-line medications shown to be more effective than the nicotine patch alone: 2 mg/d varenicline or the combination of long-term nicotine patch use + ad libitum nicotine replacement therapy (NRT).[5]
- Certain combinations of first-line medications have been shown to be effective smoking cessation treatments. Therefore, clinicians should consider using these combinations of medications with their patients who are willing to quit. Following are the effective combination medications:
    - Long-term (>14 weeks) nicotine patch + other NRT (gum and spray)
    - The nicotine patch + the nicotine inhaler
    - The nicotine patch + bupropion SR[5] SOR 

TABLE 237-2 Motivational Interviewing Strategies

Express empathy.	• Use open-ended questions to explore: ◦ The importance of addressing smoking or other tobacco use (eg, "How important do you think it is for you to quit smoking?") ◦ Concerns and benefits of quitting (eg, "What might happen if you quit?") • Use reflective listening to seek shared understanding: ◦ Reflect words or meaning (eg, "So you think smoking helps you to maintain your weight"). ◦ Summarize (eg, "What I have heard so far is that smoking is something you enjoy. On the other hand, your boyfriend hates your smoking, and you are worried you might develop a serious disease."). • Normalize feelings and concerns (eg, "Many people worry about managing without cigarettes."). • Support the patient's autonomy and right to choose or reject change (eg, "I hear you saying you are not ready to quit smoking right now. I'm here to help you when you are ready.").
Develop discrepancy.	• Highlight the discrepancy between the patient's present behavior and expressed priorities, values, and goals (eg, "It sounds like you are very devoted to your family. How do you think your smoking is affecting your children?"). • Reinforce and support "change talk" and "commitment" language: ◦ "So, you realize how smoking is affecting your breathing and making it hard to keep up with your kids." ◦ "It's great that you are going to quit when you get through this busy time at work." • Build and deepen commitment to change: ◦ "There are effective treatments that will ease the pain of quitting, including counseling and many medication options." ◦ "We would like to help you avoid a stroke like the one your father had."
Roll with resistance.	• Back off and use reflection when the patient expresses resistance: ◦ "Sounds like you are feeling pressured about your smoking." • Express empathy: ◦ "You are worried about how you would manage withdrawal symptoms." • Ask permission to provide information: ◦ "Would you like to hear about some strategies that can help you address that concern when you quit?"
Support self-efficacy.	• Help the patient to identify and build on past successes: ◦ "So you were fairly successful the last time you tried to quit." • Offer options for achievable small steps toward change: ◦ Call the quitline (1–800-QUIT-NOW) for advice and information. ◦ Read about quitting benefits and strategies. ◦ Change smoking patterns (eg, no smoking in the home). ◦ Ask the patient to share his or her ideas about quitting strategies.

Data from Treating Tobacco Use and Dependence: 2008 Update. US Department of Health and Human Services; 2008. http://www.ahrq.gov/clinic/tobacco/treating_tobacco_use08.pdf.

BOX 237-1 Nicotine Replacement Therapy: Gum

Nicorette, Generic (OTC)

PRECAUTIONS

Recent (≤2 weeks) myocardial infarction

- Serious underlying arrhythmias
- Serious or worsening angina pectoris
- Temporomandibular joint disease
- Pregnancy and breastfeeding
- Adolescents (<18 years)

ADVERSE EFFECTS

- Mouth/jaw soreness
- Hiccups
- Dyspepsia
- Hypersalivation
- Effects associated with incorrect chewing technique:
  - Lightheadedness
  - Nausea/vomiting
  - Throat and mouth irritation

ADVANTAGES

- Might satisfy oral cravings
- Might delay weight gain
- Patients can titrate therapy to manage withdrawal symptoms
- Variety of flavors is available

DISADVANTAGES

- Need for frequent dosing can compromise compliance
- Might be problematic for patients with significant dental work
- Patients must use proper chewing technique to minimize adverse effects
- Gum chewing may not be socially acceptable

BOX 237-2 Nicotine Replacement Therapy: Lozenge

Nicorette Mini Lozenge, Generic (OTC)

PRECAUTIONS

Recent (≤2 weeks) myocardial infarction

- Serious underlying arrhythmias
- Serious or worsening angina pectoris
- Pregnancy and breastfeeding
- Adolescents (<18 years)

ADVERSE EFFECTS

- Nausea
- Hiccups
- Cough
- Heartburn
- Headache
- Flatulence
- Insomnia

ADVANTAGES

- Might satisfy oral cravings
- Might delay weight gain
- Easy to use and conceal
- Patients can titrate therapy to manage withdrawal symptoms
- Variety of flavors are available

DISADVANTAGES

- Need for frequent dosing can compromise compliance
- Gastrointestinal side effects (nausea, hiccups, heartburn) might be bothersome

BOX 237-3 Nicotine Replacement Therapy: Transdermal Patch

NicoDerm CQ,Generic (OTC, NicoDerm CQ, generic)

PRECAUTIONS

- Recent (≤2 weeks) myocardial infarction
- Serious underlying arrhythmias
- Serious or worsening angina pectoris
- Pregnancy (Rx formulations, category D) and breast-feeding
- Adolescents (<18 years)

ADVERSE EFFECTS

- Local skin reactions (erythema, pruritus, burning)
- Headache
- Sleep disturbances (insomnia, abnormal/vivid dreams) associated with nocturnal nicotine absorption

ADVANTAGES

- Provides consistent nicotine levels over 24 hours
- Easy to use and conceal
- Once-daily dosing associated with fewer compliance problems

DISADVANTAGES

- Patients cannot titrate the dose to manage withdrawal symptoms
- Allergic reactions to adhesive might occur
- Patients with dermatologic conditions should not use the patch

BOX 237-4 Nicotine Replacement Therapy: Nasal Spray

Nicotrol NS (Rx)

PRECAUTIONS

- Recent (≤2 weeks) myocardial infarction
- Serious underlying arrhythmias
- Serious or worsening angina pectoris
- Underlying chronic nasal disorders (rhinitis, nasal polyps, sinusitis)
- Severe reactive airway disease
- Pregnancy (category D) and breastfeeding
- Adolescents (<18 years)

ADVERSE EFFECTS

- Nasal and/or throat irritation (hot, peppery, or burning sensation)
- Rhinitis
- Tearing
- Sneezing
- Cough
- Headache

ADVANTAGES

- Patients can titrate therapy to rapidly manage withdrawal symptoms

DISADVANTAGES

- Need for frequent dosing can compromise compliance
- Nasal/throat irritation may be bothersome
- Patients must wait 5 minutes before driving or operating heavy machinery
- Patients with chronic nasal disorders or severe reactive airway disease should not use the spray

BOX 237-5 Nicotine Replacement Therapy: Oral Inhaler

Nicotrol Inhaler (Rx)

PRECAUTIONS

- Recent (≤2 weeks) myocardial infarction
- Serious underlying arrhythmias
- Serious or worsening angina pectoris
- Bronchospastic disease
- Pregnancy (category D) and breastfeeding
- Adolescents (<18 years)

ADVERSE EFFECTS

- Mouth and/or throat irritation
- Cough
- Headache
- Rhinitis
- Dyspepsia
- Hiccups

ADVANTAGES

- Patients can titrate therapy to manage withdrawal symptoms
- Mimics hand-to-mouth ritual of smoking (which could also be perceived as a disadvantage)

DISADVANTAGES

- Need for frequent dosing can compromise compliance
- Initial throat or mouth irritation can be bothersome
- Cartridges should not be stored in very warm conditions or used in very cold conditions
- Patients with underlying bronchospastic disease must use with caution

BOX 237-6 Medications for Smoking Cessation: Buproprion SR

Zyban, Generic (Rx)

PRECAUTIONS

- Concomitant therapy with medications or medical conditions known to lower the seizure threshold
- Severe hepatic cirrhosis
- Pregnancy (category C) and breast-feeding
- Adolescents (<18 years)
- Black-boxed warning for neuropsychiatric symptoms
- Contraindications
  - Seizure disorder
  - Concomitant bupropion (eg, Wellbutrin) therapy
  - Current or prior diagnosis of bulimia or anorexia Nervosa
  - Simultaneous abrupt discontinuation of alcohol or sedatives/benzodiazepines
  - MAO inhibitor therapy in previous 14 days

ADVERSE EFFECTS

- Insomnia
- Dry mouth
- Nervousness/difficulty concentrating
- Rash
- Constipation
- Seizures (risk is 0.1%)
- Neuropsychiatric symptoms (rare; see precautions)

ADVANTAGES

- Easy to use; oral formulation might be associated with fewer compliance problems
- Might delay weight gain
- Can be used with NRT
- Might be beneficial in patients with depression

DISADVANTAGES

- Seizure risk is increased
- Several contraindications and precautions preclude use in some patients (see precautions)
- Patients should be monitored for potential neuropsychiatric symptoms (see precautions)

BOX 237-7 Medications for Smoking Cessation: Varenicline

Chantix, Generic (Rx)

PRECAUTIONS

- Severe renal impairment (dosage adjustment is necessary)
- Pregnancy (category C) and breast-feeding
- Adolescents (<18 years)
- **Black-boxed warning** for neuropsychiatric symptoms
- **WARNING** for Cardiovascular adverse events in patients with existing cardiovascular disease

ADVERSE EFFECTS

- Nausea
- Sleep disturbances (insomnia, abnormal/ vivid dreams)
- Constipation
- Flatulence
- Vomiting
- Neuropsychiatric symptoms (rare; see precautions)

ADVANTAGES

- Easy to use; oral formulation might be associated with fewer ompliance problems
- Offers a new mechanism of action for patients who have failed other agents

DISADVANTAGES

- May induce nausea in up to one-third of patients
- Patients should be monitored for potential neuropsychiatric symptoms (see precautions)

- There is a strong relationship between the number of sessions of counseling combined with medication and the likelihood of successful smoking cessation. Therefore, to the extent possible, clinicians should provide multiple counseling sessions, in addition to medication, to their patients who are trying to quit smoking.[5] SOR Ⓐ

COMPLEMENTARY AND ALTERNATIVE THERAPY

- Acupuncture—A meta-analysis of 5 studies did not show effectiveness of acupuncture as a tobacco-use treatment. There is also lack of scientific evidence for the effectiveness of electrostimulation or laser acupuncture for the treatment of tobacco addiction.[5]
- Hypnotherapy—There is insufficient evidence to recommend hypnotherapy as an effective treatment for tobacco addiction.[5]
- Novel tobacco products—There is insufficient evidence to determine whether novel tobacco products reduce individual and population health risks. The evidence indicates that changing cigarette designs over the last 5 decades, including filtered, low-tar, and "light" variations, have not reduced overall disease risk among smokers and may have hindered prevention and cessation efforts. The overall health of the public could be harmed if the introduction of novel tobacco products encourages tobacco use among people who would otherwise be unlikely to use a tobacco product or delays cessation among persons who would otherwise quit using tobacco altogether.[3]

REFERRAL

For patients who are unsuccessful with therapies available in primary care, it is reasonable to refer them to a tobacco-cessation specialist. These specialists typically provide intensive tobacco interventions. Specialists are not defined by their professional affiliation or by the field in which they trained. Rather, specialists view tobacco dependence treatment as a primary professional role. Specialists possess the skills, knowledge, and training to provide effective interventions across a range of intensities, and often are affiliated with programs offering intensive treatment interventions or services.

PREVENTION

The simple fact is that we cannot end the tobacco epidemic without focusing our efforts on young people. Nearly 100% of adults who smoke every day started smoking when they were age 26 years or younger, so prevention is the key to success. The tobacco industry spends almost $10 billion a year to market its products, half of all movies for children younger than age 13 years contain scenes of tobacco use, and images and messages normalize tobacco use in magazines, on the Internet, and at retail stores frequented by youth. With a quarter of all high school seniors and a third of all young adults smoking, and with progress in reducing prevalence slowing dramatically, the time for action is now.[1]

- Advertising and promotional activities by tobacco companies have been shown to cause the onset and continuation of smoking among adolescents and young adults.[1]
- The evidence is sufficient to conclude that there is a causal relationship between depictions of smoking in the movies and the initiation of smoking among young people.[1]
- The evidence is sufficient to conclude that mass media campaigns, comprehensive community programs, and comprehensive statewide tobacco control programs can prevent the initiation of tobacco use and reduce its prevalence among youth.[1]
- The evidence is sufficient to conclude that increases in cigarette prices reduce the initiation, prevalence, and intensity of smoking among youth and young adults.[1]
- The evidence is sufficient to conclude that school-based programs with evidence of effectiveness, containing specific components, can produce at least short-term effects and reduce the prevalence of tobacco use among school-age youth.[1] One tobacco-free education program for kids from the American Academy of Family Physicians (AAFP) is *Tar Wars*: http://www.tarwars.org/online/tarwars/home.html.

PROGNOSIS

- Young individuals progress from smoking occasionally to smoking every day.
- Each day across the United States more than 3800 youths younger than 18 years of age start smoking. Of every 3 young smokers, only 1 will quit, and 1 of those remaining smokers will die from tobacco-related causes. Most of these young people never considered the long-term health consequences associated with tobacco use when they started smoking; and nicotine, a highly addictive drug, causes many to continue smoking well into adulthood, often with deadly consequences (**Figure 237-10**).[1]
- Those with serious mental illnesses die, on average, 25 years earlier than the general population, with most deaths related to tobacco-related diseases such as heart disease, diabetes, and chronic lung disease.[2]

FOLLOW-UP

All patients who receive a tobacco dependence intervention should be assessed for abstinence at the completion of treatment and during subsequent contacts.[1] Abstinent patients should have their quitting success acknowledged, and the clinician should offer to assist the patient with problems associated with quitting.[2] Patients who have relapsed should be assessed to determine whether they are willing to make another quit attempt. SOR Ⓒ

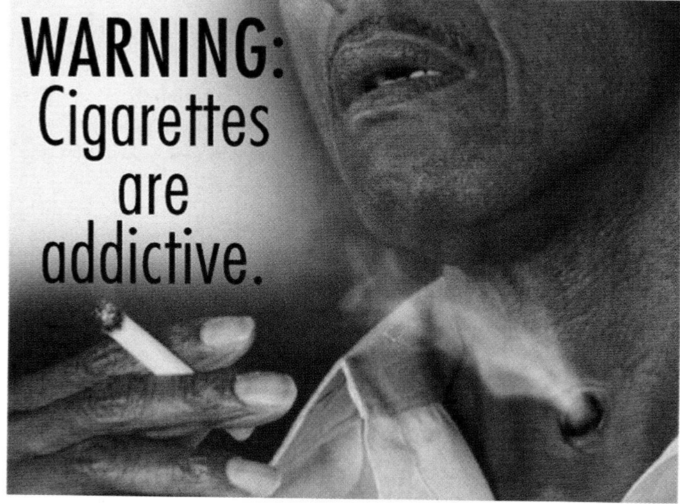

FIGURE 237-10 Cigarettes are addictive. This image was going to be a FDA-mandated warning but was blocked by the courts. (*Reproduced with permission from U.S. Department of Health and Human Services.*)

PATIENT RESOURCES

- **1–800-QUIT NOW—**This free telephone quit line service refers callers to their own state's quit line via this national routing number. In some counties free nicotine patches are available to callers.
- The American Legacy Foundation's Became an EX Program—**http://www.becomeanex.org/.**

The EX Plan is a free quit smoking program that helps you relearn life without cigarettes. Before you actually stop smoking, they will show you how to deal with the very things that trip up so many people when they try to stop smoking. So you will be more prepared to stop and stay off tobacco.

- Office on Smoking and Health at the Centers for Disease Control and Prevention. *Smoking & Tobacco Use*—**http://www.cdc.gov/tobacco.**

The Smoking and Tobacco Use website of the Centers for Disease Control and Prevention (CDC) provides tobacco use data and statistics; information about the health effects of smoking, smokeless tobacco products, and secondhand smoke; resources for tobacco cessation and youth smoking prevention; and products and materials that can help motivate behavior change. Visitors to the CDC website can find links to clinician and patient resources, such as a quit guideline.

PROVIDER RESOURCES

- *Treating Tobacco Use and Dependence 2008 Update*. Excellent clinical practice guideline. **http://www.ahrq.gov/clinic/tobacco/treating_tobacco_use08.pdf.**
- American Academy of Family Physicians' Tobacco Cessation Program. **http://www.askandact.org.**

The American Academy of Family Physicians' (AAFP) tobacco cessation program, "Ask and Act," encourages family physicians to *ask* their patients about tobacco use, then *act* to help them quit. Through the Ask and Act program, AAFP members have access to a variety of free resources to help patients quit using tobacco, such as a quit smoking prescription pad and a wallet card with quitline information.

- American Academy of Family Physicians. *Pharmacologic Product Guide: FDA-Approved Medications*—**http://www.aafp.org/online/etc/medialib/aafp_org/documents/clinical/pub_health/askact/prescribguidelines.Par.0001.File.tmp/PRESCRIBINGGUIDE2010.pdf.**

This is an excellent guide to pharmacologic intervention that summarizes precautions, dosing, adverse effects, advantages, disadvantages, and costs for the 7 FDA-approved medications for treatment of tobacco addiction.

- Smoking Cessation Leadership Center—**http://smokingcessationleadership.ucsf.edu.**

The Smoking Cessation Leadership Center aims to increase smoking cessation rates and increase the number of health professionals who help smokers quit. The site not only provides tobacco cessation resources for providers to pass on to patients, it also offers a variety of tools, materials, and training courses aimed toward improving the delivery of tobacco cessation intervention in clinical settings. 1–800-QUIT-NOW cards can be ordered online at this website, which provides telephone cessation resources for all 50 states in the United States.

- Nicotine and Tobacco Dependence Website—**http://www.nicotineandtobaccodependence.com/.**

A companion to the book *Nicotine and Tobacco Dependence* (Peterson, Vander Werg and Jaén, 2011), it provides book owners with easy-to-print forms, including a Nicotine and Tobacco Dependence Intake Form; Minnesota Nicotine Withdrawal Scale-Revised (MSW-R); Decisional Balance Exercise; Tobacco Use Diary; Physical, Behavioral, and Psychologic Strategies to Quit Tobacco; and a Sample Treatment Manual for 8 sessions for intensive tobacco treatment.

- American Academy of Family Physicians. *Tar Wars*—**http://www.tarwars.org/online/tarwars/home.html.**

This is a tobacco-free education program for kids from the AAFP involving classroom presentations and poster contests.

REFERENCES

1. U.S. Department of Health and Human Services. *Preventing Tobacco Use Among Youth and Young Adults: A Report of the Surgeon General*. Atlanta, GA: U.S. Department of Health and Human Services, Centers for Disease Control and Prevention, National Center for Chronic Disease Prevention and Health Promotion, Office on Smoking and Health; 2012. http://www.surgeongeneral.gov/library/preventing-youth-tobacco-use/index.html.
2. Schroeder SA. A 51-year-old woman with bipolar disorder who wants to quit smoking. *JAMA*. 2009;301(5):522-531.
3. U.S. Department of Health and Human Services. *How Tobacco Smoke Causes Disease: The Biology and Behavioral Basis for Smoking-Attributable Disease: A Report of the Surgeon General*. Atlanta, GA: U.S. Department of Health and Human Services, Centers for Disease Control and Prevention, National Center for Chronic Disease Prevention and Health Promotion, Office on Smoking and Health; 2010. http://www.surgeongeneral.gov/library/tobaccosmoke/.
4. Benowitz NL. Clinical pharmacology of nicotine: implications for understanding, preventing, and treating tobacco addiction. *Clin Pharmacol Ther*. 2008;83(4):531-541.
5. Fiore MC, Jaén CR, Baker TB, et al. *Treating Tobacco Use and Dependence: 2008 Update. Clinical Practice Guideline*. Rockville, MD: U.S. Department of Health and Human Services, Public Health Service; 2008.
6. Model D. Smoker's face. An underrated clinical sign? *Br Med J (Clin Res Ed)*. 1985;291(6511):1760-1762.
7. American Psychiatric Association. *Diagnostic and Statistical Manual of Mental Disorders, Fourth Edition, Text Revision (DSM-IV-TR)*. Arlington, VA: American Psychiatric Publishing; 2000.
8. Peterson AL, Vander Weg MW, Jaén CR. *Advances in Psychotherapy—Evidence-Based Practice. Vol. 21. Nicotine and Tobacco Dependence*. Cambridge, MA: Hogrefe; 2011.

238 ALCOHOLISM (ALCOHOL USE DISORDER)

Mark L. Willenbring, MD

PATIENT STORY

Theresa is a 39-year-old, white, single woman who presents with insomnia and depression. After exploring the presenting symptoms, her physician reviews some screening questions about potentially related problems. In response to a question about heavy drinking in the past year, Theresa responds that she is drinking about 2 bottles (10 drinks) of wine nightly. She acknowledges going over limits repeatedly and a persistent desire to quit or cut down, as well as continuing to drink in spite of hangovers and nausea in the morning. She denies withdrawal symptoms, driving while intoxicated, job or serious relationship problems, but admits that her social activities have decreased over the past year because she spends her evening drinking alone. No one else knows she is struggling with drinking. Her depression and insomnia started after her drinking increased about 2 years ago.

INTRODUCTION

Excessive drinking of alcohol is a common behavior encountered in primary care, yet few clinicians feel prepared to address it. Most clinicians are unclear about the best way to screen for heavy drinking and lack confidence in how to address it. Physicians often lack the knowledge and skill to screen and evaluate excessive drinking, let alone address it other than suggesting a referral to an addiction counselor or treatment program. Regrettably, few patients are appropriate for or accept referral to a counselor or program. Fortunately, research over the past 20 years has provided evidence-based, efficient ways to screen, evaluate, and treat heavy drinking in primary care.

SYNONYMS (TERMINOLOGY)

Heavy drinking refers to drinking in excess of low-risk guidelines (see below).

Alcohol dependence (alcoholism) is a disorder of compulsive drinking associated with impaired control over intake, such as repeatedly exceeding self-defined limits, a persistent desire to quit or cut down and difficulty doing so, and continued use despite adverse consequences.

The terms *alcohol use disorder (AUD)*, *alcohol dependence*, and *alcoholism* can be used interchangeably.

EPIDEMIOLOGY

- In any given year, approximately 30% of US adults 18 years of age and older exceed the National Institute on Alcohol Abuse and Alcoholism (NIAAA) low-risk drinking guidelines at least once (**Figures 238-1** and **238-2**).[1] The low-risk drinking limits for healthy adult women is defined as drinking no more than 3 drinks in any day and 7 drinks in any week, and for men, no more than 4 drinks in any day and 14 drinks in any week.

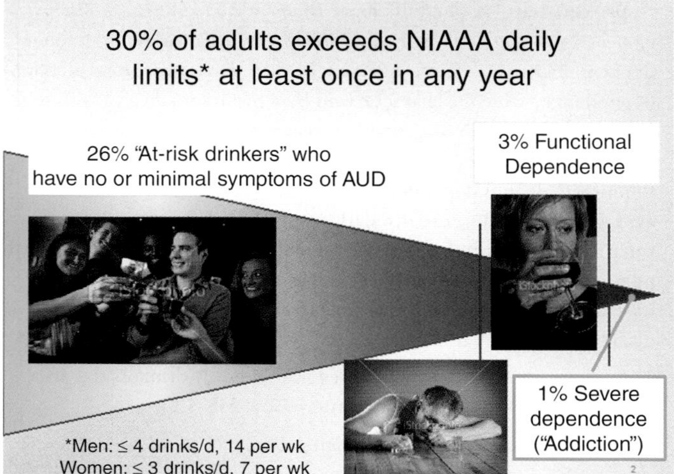

FIGURE 238-1 Spectrum of alcohol use disorder. (*Reproduced with permission from Mark L. Willenbring, MD.*)

- A drink refers to 12 oz of beer, 5 oz of wine or 1.5 oz of spirits, each of which contains about 14 g of absolute ethanol.[1] Within that group, the frequency varies from occasional to daily or near daily, and the amount of drinking varies from 5 to more than 20 drinks daily. Most excessive drinkers who exceed the limits (72%) do not meet diagnostic criteria for an alcohol use disorder and are considered at-risk drinkers.[1]
- At-risk drinkers are analogous to asymptomatic patients with hyperlipidemia or hypertension; they do not currently have a disorder (other than the risk factor) but are at elevated risk for developing one if the risk factor is not decreased. Reduction in excessive drinking significantly reduces risk of developing an alcohol use disorder, liver disease, or social problems.[2]

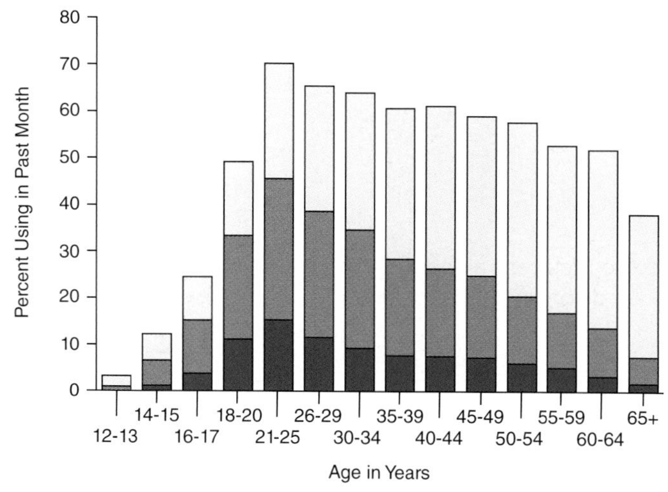

FIGURE 238-2 Past month use of alcohol among US residents over age 12. Category definitions: *Current (past month) use*—at least 1 drink in the past 30 days; *binge use*—5 or more drinks on the same occasion (ie, at the same time or within a couple of hours of each other) on at least 1 day in the past 30 days; *heavy use*—5 or more drinks on the same occasion on each of 5 or more days in the past 30 days.

- Approximately 4% of adults meet *Diagnostic and Statistical Manual of Mental Disorders, 4th Edition* (DSM-IV) criteria for alcohol dependence in any year.[3] Three-quarters of them have functional alcohol dependence, which is characterized by a predominance of "internal symptoms" of impaired control such as going over limits and persistent desire to quit or cut down and a limited course. People with functional alcohol dependence have a single episode, lasting on average 3 to 4 years, usually with resolution of the episode and no recurrence. A quarter of those with dependence, 1% of the general population in any year, have recurrent alcohol dependence, demonstrating an average of 5 episodes over a period of years to decades.[4]
- Thus, there are the following 3 categories of heavy drinkers the primary care provider is apt to encounter (**Box 238-1**):
  1. At-risk drinkers (the predominant group)
  2. Functional alcohol dependence
  3. Recurrent, more severe alcohol dependence

ETIOLOGY AND PATHOPHYSIOLOGY

Alcohol use disorder is a heritable disease; approximately 50% of the risk is genetic, while environmental factors account for the remainder, the most clearly established factor being early childhood abuse or neglect.[5,6] Multigenerational alcohol dependence often appears in the early to mid-teens, but functional alcohol dependence can begin at any age.[7]

RISK FACTORS

Following are the most important risk factors:

- Family history of alcohol dependence[8]
- Early life stress in the form of early childhood abuse or neglect[9]

Other risk factors include the following:

- An early history of externalizing personality factors are as below:
  - Extroversion
  - Attention deficit disorder
  - Oppositional defiant disorder
  - Conduct disorder
- Antisocial and borderline personality disorders among adults[10]

Onset of drinking before the age of 14 years markedly increases the risk for later development of alcohol dependence, especially for adolescents with a positive family history.[11]

DIAGNOSIS

CLINICAL FEATURES

- Contrary to common belief, heavy drinkers are very likely to answer questions about their drinking honestly, provided the questions are skillful. Asking about quantity and frequency ("On any single occasion during the past 3 months, have you had more than 5 drinks containing alcohol?") is most likely to elicit an informative answer, whereas any question that suggests even the possibility of moral judgment

BOX 238-1 Common Presentations of 3 Categories of Excessive Drinkers*

Diagnosis of Alcohol Use Disorder	
Category	**Common Presentation**
At-risk drinkers	None or driving while drinking only (no DWI)
Functional alcohol use disorder	• "Internal symptoms" of impaired control – Going over limits repeatedly – Desire to cut down/quit without success – Use despite "internal" problems associated with drinking (eg, hangover, nausea) – Drinking and driving (no DWI) • Usually 2-4 criteria positive (out of 11)* • No legal, job, or serious interpersonal problems • Maximum drinks about 5-8 per drinking day • Single episode lasting 3-4 years on average, no recurrence
Severe recurrent alcohol use disorder	• "Internal" symptoms of impaired control (above) plus – Spending a lot of time drinking – Giving up nondrinking activities – Physical withdrawal and morning drinking – Serious medical complications (eg, liver disease) • Usually >5 criteria positive • "External" symptoms of dysfunction – Social and family disruption – Problems with job, school, parenting – Legal problems (eg, DWI) • Maximum drinks about 10-24 per drinking day • Recurrent episodes over years to decades (average of 5)

*The approach of DSM-V diagnosis[13] (*Reproduced with permission from Mark Willenbring, MD.*)

BOX 238-2 Screening Question Recommended by the National Institute on Alcohol Abuse and Alcoholism (NIAAA)

How many times in the past year have you had the following?

- 5 or more drinks in a day? (for men)
- 4 or more drinks in a day? (for women)

One standard drink is equivalent to 12 oz of beer, 5 oz of wine, or 1.5 oz of 80-proof spirits.

http://www.niaaa.nih.gov/guide.

(eg, "How much do you drink?") is less likely to yield helpful answers. **Box 238-2** states the specific screening questions recommended by the NIAAA.

- Most heavy drinkers are not symptomatic. Thus, they do not have alcohol-related symptoms. They can only be detected through screening for quantity and frequency of drinking. Screening focused on symptoms of alcohol use disorder, such as the well-known CAGE ("Have you ever tried to cut down on your drinking? Have you ever felt annoyed by criticism of your drinking? Have you ever felt guilty about your drinking? Have you ever had a morning eye-opener?"), will not detect asymptomatic at-risk drinkers, and it performs poorly compared to almost all other methods.[12] It is important to enquire about quantity and frequency of drinking in order to identify at-risk drinkers and patients with functional alcohol dependence. The Alcohol Use Disorders Identification Test (AUDIT) (**Figure 238-3**) is the gold standard for a written questionnaire; it only takes about 3 minutes to complete and is easy to score. A score of 8 or more for men or 4 or more for women suggests excessive drinking.[1]
- Current diagnostic criteria for alcohol use disorder are based on the DSM-V.[13] The presence of any 2 of 11 symptoms (**Box 238-3**) is enough to establish a diagnosis, where the number of symptoms met is highly correlated with severity of the disorder.[13]
- According to NIAAA, healthy adult men should not drink in excess of 4 standard US drinks in any day, or 14 in any week, and adult women should not exceed 3 drinks in any day and 7 in any week.[1] Low-risk drinking limits may be less for certain groups, such as adults older than age 65 years, or in the presence of medical illnesses, such as liver disease. Women who are pregnant or are trying to become pregnant should be advised to abstain completely.[14]
- Drinking in excess of these limits is considered unhealthy, placing heavy drinkers at elevated risk for developing AUD and associated complications such as liver disease.[15] Approximately 30% of US adults age 18 years and older drink in excess of low-risk limits at least once in any year. About 4 of 5 of them do not meet diagnostic criteria for a disorder, and are considered to be "at-risk" for developing one.[1] In other words, this group has an asymptomatic risk factor similar to hypertension or hyperlipidemia. At-risk drinkers are typically unaware that their drinking constitutes a health risk. This does not reflect "denial" but rather the lack of information available to the public about what constitutes high-risk drinking or how to measure consumption. For example, how many standard US drinks are in a 7-oz martini? (Depending on the specific way it is mixed, the answer is about 4.) It is much easier to obtain dietary information about food than information about alcohol content in a beverage.
- Patients with functional alcohol dependence are aware of struggling with their alcohol consumption, but lack serious life consequences at this time. Most are open to changing their drinking, but they may need to be identified through screening, rather than presenting with this problem.
- Patients with more severe, recurrent alcohol dependence often present with intoxication, withdrawal, or medical complications of heavy drinking, such as liver disease or pancreatitis. If these disorders are present, they demonstrate the expected physical manifestations. Like other patients with chronic, treatment-refractory illness, they have a chronic course, with periodic relapses or even with ongoing chronic illness.

TYPICAL DISTRIBUTION

In a given year, 30% of the adult US population engages in unhealthy drinking at least once (see **Figure 238-1**). In an average primary care practice, approximately 10% to 15% of outpatients are heavy drinkers.

LABORATORY TESTING

- The most sensitive way to detect heavy drinking is to ask about the frequency of heavy drinking. Use of a written questionnaire such as the AUDIT can be helpful (see **Figure 238-3**).[16]
- The most sensitive but least specific laboratory test is γ-glutamyltransferase (GGT). Carbohydrate-deficient transferrin provides similar sensitivity but better specificity but is not widely available.[17]
- Other transaminases such as aspartate aminotransferase (AST) and alanine aminotransferase (ALT) are less sensitive, and require hepatic cell destruction before they are elevated. Thus, they are not very sensitive for detecting heavy drinking but they may be helpful in following patients who have elevated values at baseline.

IMAGING

There are no imaging tests that detect heavy drinking itself. Abdominal ultrasound is often helpful in evaluating alcoholic liver disease.

DIFFERENTIAL DIAGNOSIS

It is important to distinguish between AUD and asymptomatic at-risk drinking. AUD is characterized by preoccupation with and impaired control over drinking.

MANAGEMENT

See **Box 238-4**.

NONPHARMACOLOGIC

- Brief counseling and advice to reduce drinking is effective for at-risk drinking, resulting in 15% to 20% reduction in drinking for at least 1 year.[2]
- Alcohol dependence requires either more intensive counseling and/or antirelapse medications. The relationship between intensity and setting (inpatient, residential, or outpatient) is complex. Most studies show no difference in 1-year outcomes based on intensity or setting.[18] For example, in a highly controlled, well-done study, 174 persons with alcoholism were randomly assigned to partial hospital treatment or extended inpatient rehabilitation after inpatient evaluation and/or detoxification. The outpatient group attended daily Monday through

AUDIT

PATIENT: Because alcohol use can affect your health and can interfere with certain medications and treatments, it is important that we ask some questions about your use of alcohol. Your answers will remain confidential, so please be honest.

For each question in the chart below, place an X in one box that best describes your answer.

NOTE: In the U.S., a single drink serving contains about 14 grams of ethanol or "pure" alcohol. Although the drinks below are different sizes, each one contains the same amount of pure alcohol and counts as a single drink:

12 oz. of beer (about 5% alcohol) 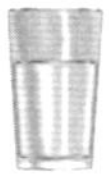 = **8-9 oz. of malt liquor** (about 7% alcohol) = 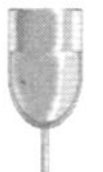 **5 oz. of wine** (about 12% alcohol) 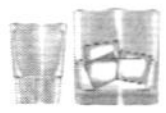 = **1.5 oz. of hard liquor** (about 40% alcohol)

Questions	0	1	2	3	4	
1. How often do you have a drink containing alcohol?	Never	Monthly or less	2 to 4 times a month	2 to 3 times a week	4 or more times a week	
2. How many drinks containing alcohol do you have on a typical day when you are drinking?	1 or 2	3 or 4	5 or 6	7 to 9	10 or more	
3. How often do you have 5 or more drinks on one occasion?	Never	Less than monthly	Monthly	Weekly	Daily or almost daily	
4. How often during the last year have you found that you were not able to stop drinking once you had started?	Never	Less than monthly	Monthly	Weekly	Daily or almost daily	
5. How often during the last year have you failed to do what was normally expected of you because of drinking?	Never	Less than monthly	Monthly	Weekly	Daily or almost daily	
6. How often during the last year have you needed a first drink in the morning to get yourself going after a heavy drinking session?	Never	Less than monthly	Monthly	Weekly	Daily or almost daily	
7. How often during the last year have you had a feeling of guilt or remorse after drinking?	Never	Less than monthly	Monthly	Weekly	Daily or almost daily	
8. How often during the last year have you been unable to remember what happened the night before because of your drinking?	Never	Less than monthly	Monthly	Weekly	Daily or almost daily	
9. Have you or someone else been injured because of your drinking?	No		Yes, but not in the last year		Yes, during the last year	
10. Has a relative, friend, doctor, or other health care worker been concerned about your drinking or suggested you cut down?	No		Yes, but not in the last year		Yes, during the last year	
					Total	

Note: This questionnaire (the AUDIT) is reprinted with permission from the World Health Organization. To reflect drink serving sizes in the United States (14g of pure alcohol), the number of drinks in question 3 was changed from 6 to 5. A free AUDIT manual with guidelines for use in primary care settings is available online at *www.who.org*.

Excerpted from NIH Publication No. 07-3769 **National Institute on Alcohol and Alcoholism** *www.niaaa.nih.gov/guide*

FIGURE 238-3 The AUDIT questionnaire. Scores are added to determine the total. Positive screens are indicated by total scores greater than or equal to 8 in men and greater than or equal to 4 in women. Higher scores indicate more severe alcohol involvement. Scores greater than 16 suggest the possibility of alcohol dependence.

BOX 238-3 DSM-V Criteria for Alcohol Use Disorder[13]

A problematic pattern of alcohol use leading to clinically significant impairment or distress, as manifested by at least 2 of the following symptoms, occurring within a 12-month period:

1. Alcohol is often taken in larger amounts or over a longer period than was intended.
2. There is a persistent desire or unsuccessful efforts to cut down or control alcohol use.
3. A great deal of time is spent in activities necessary to obtain alcohol, use alcohol, or recover from its effects.
4. Craving, or a strong desire or urge to use alcohol.
5. Recurrent alcohol use resulting in a failure to fulfill major role obligations at work, school, or home.
6. Continued alcohol use despite having persistent or recurrent social or interpersonal problems caused or exacerbated by the effects of alcohol.
7. Important social, occupational, or recreational activities are given up or reduced because of alcohol use.
8. Recurrent alcohol use in situations in which it is physically hazardous.
9. Alcohol use is continued despite knowledge of having a persistent or recurrent physical or psychological problem that is likely to have been caused or exacerbated by alcohol.
10. Tolerance, as defined by either of the following:
    - A need for markedly increased amounts of alcohol to achieve intoxication or desired effect.
    - A markedly diminished effect with continued use of the same amount of alcohol.
11. Withdrawal, as manifested by either of the following:
    - The characteristic withdrawal syndrome for alcohol (refer to Criteria A and B of the criteria set for alcohol withdrawal).
    - Alcohol (or a closely related substance, such as a benzodiazepine) is taken to relieve or avoid withdrawal symptoms.

Severity is graded based on the number of symptoms present as below:

- Mild: Presence of 2-3 symptoms.
- Moderate: Presence of 4-5 symptoms.
- Severe: Presence of 6 or more symptoms.

BOX 238-4 Clinical Prevention and Treatment of Alcohol Use Disorder

Category	Management
At-risk drinkers	
Goal: risk reduction	• Brief counseling to quit or cut down • Hand patients *Rethinking Drinking* booklet • Repeated counseling increases effectiveness
Functional alcohol use disorder	• Antirelapse medications
Goal: long-term abstinence or low-risk drinking (eg, recovery)	– Naltrexone (oral, injection) – Topiramate (Topamax) – Disulfiram (Antabuse) • Brief behavioral support (medication management) • Recommend Alcoholics Anonymous • Offer referral to addiction specialist especially if fails to respond to primary care treatment
Severe recurrent alcohol use disorder	• Offer referral to addiction specialist • Recommend Alcoholics Anonymous
Goals:	• Medications
• Reduce frequency, severity and length of relapses	– Treat withdrawal if needed – Antirelapse medications
• Treat complications	• Care coordination
• Slow the rate of deterioration	• Integrate medical, psychiatric, addiction treatment
• Aim for full recovery but recognize it may not be achieved	• Treatment for as long as needed, usually years to decades

Friday therapy alongside the group that was assigned to 6 months of psychiatric inpatient hospitalization. The study found no additional benefit to extended hospitalization.[19]

- However, there are circumstances that make providing structured sober housing important: among people who are homeless, those who cannot stop drinking while living independently, and people with significant coexisting psychiatric illness.[18] The degree of housing structure required, however, is relatively independent of the intensity or type of treatment given. Some patients require a great deal of housing structure but very few treatment services, whereas others are stably housed but require intensive and prolonged treatment. Thus it makes sense to uncouple housing structure from treatment decisions, as there is no apparent benefit to having patients stay in a facility overnight while they are receiving treatment services.
- Increasingly, treatment for recurrent AUD (dependence) is being conceptualized as management of a chronic illness.[20] A recent study found that continued care that included primary care management as well as continued access to specialty addiction care resulted in improved outcomes and reduced costs.[21]
- Long-term regular medical follow-up that simply attends to drinking and encourages abstinence is effective for reducing drinking among patients with medical complications such as liver cirrhosis or pancreatitis.[22]

MEDICATIONS

- Several antirelapse medications are available for alcohol dependence. Their average efficacy is similar to that for selective serotonin reuptake inhibitor (SSRI) antidepressants in treating depression.[23,24]
- Naltrexone 50 mg daily or as needed for each drinking occasion reduces relapse rates and quantity of drinking per occasion. It reduces craving for alcohol and the reward or "kick" an individual experiences when first beginning a drinking episode. This reduces the compulsive quality of drinking, making it easier to stop before a full relapse occurs. Its effectiveness is determined by genetic factors; it is most effective among northern Europeans and least likely to be effective among African Americans. In the author's experience, naltrexone 25 to 50 mg as needed per drinking occasion may help at-risk drinkers reduce excessive alcohol use, especially in social situations. Approximately 10% of patients will experience nausea. Patients should be warned that usual doses of oral opioids such as hydrocodone will not work because of the opioid blockade, so naltrexone should be stopped at least 3 days prior to elective procedures. In emergencies the blockade can be overridden, but the therapeutic index is reduced. Although initially quite concerning, in practice this has not proved to be a significant problem. Naltrexone also is available in a long-acting injectable formulation that only requires monthly administration.
- Disulfiram 250 mg daily acts by blocking the breakdown of ethanol, resulting in increased levels of acetaldehyde, which causes an adverse flushing reaction. The disulfiram-ethanol reaction is thus dose related; a small amount of alcohol such as might exist in wine vinegar, for example, might cause mild facial flushing, whereas drinking several glasses of wine or beer, or several ounces of distilled spirits, will cause a more severe reaction. Disulfiram-ethanol reactions may be very unpleasant but are unlikely to be harmful in the absence of preexisting ischemic heart disease. Reactions can occur up to several days after discontinuation, so patients should be warned. Some patients will not develop a disulfiram-ethanol reaction at the standard dose and require 500 mg daily. Disulfiram therapy is the most effective for maintaining abstinence, because any significant alcohol use will cause a reaction. It works best when administration is monitored by a family member, roommate, or friend. The most common side effect is a metallic taste. Less common are peripheral neuropathy, optical neuritis, and delirium or psychosis. A rare but serious idiosyncratic risk is that of fulminant hepatitis, often leading to liver failure and death.
- Topiramate is thought to work by normalizing the γ-aminobutyric acid (GABA)-glutamate imbalance that occurs with severe alcohol dependence. It both reduces desire to drink and the reward that occurs with drinking. Because of side effects, it is important to start at a low dose, for example, 25 mg before bedtime, and ramp up slowly over 4 to 8 weeks to a target dose of 200 to 800 mg daily. The most distressing side effect is cognitive dysfunction, best described as difficulty with word finding. Perioral paresthesias are common but reversible. Because of induction of renal tubular acidosis topiramate increases excretion of calcium, thus increasing the risk for renal calculi, especially in patients with a previous history.
- Acamprosate is licensed for alcohol dependence by the Food and Drug Administration (FDA) but the last 3 large multisite trials demonstrated no effectiveness.[25-27] It is expensive and must be taken 3 times a day. If it is effective at all, it would be in very severe dependence with a history of physical withdrawal.

COMPLEMENTARY AND ALTERNATIVE THERAPY

- No complementary or alternative therapies have proven efficacy in alcohol dependence.
- Unfortunately, some treatment programs continue to offer "nutritional therapy," treatment guided by single-photon emission computed tomography (SPECT) scans, acupuncture and other unproven therapies, but there is no evidence of their effectiveness.
- Twelve-step community support groups such as Alcoholics Anonymous (AA) help some patients with severe alcohol dependence. People who affiliate and stay with AA have better outcomes than those who do not.

REFER OR HOSPITALIZE

- Alcohol withdrawal is best managed in the hospital for patients with histories of alcohol withdrawal seizures or delirium, or who have medical conditions that might destabilize during withdrawal, such as ischemic heart disease or fragile diabetes.
- Alcohol withdrawal delirium requires hospitalization, usually in an intensive care unit.
- Most patients will not accept a referral to an addiction rehab program, but will accept treatment by their primary care physician. Patients who are naïve to rehab programs may benefit from referral. However, rehab programs tend to offer the same programming no matter how many times an individual has been exposed to it. There is no reason to believe that repeated exposure to the same type of program improves outcomes. If an addiction medical specialist is available, referral for patients not responding to initial primary care management is indicated.
- Inpatient psychiatric hospitalization conferred no added benefit compared with outpatient treatment, but inpatient treatment might be useful for patients who are unable to abstain for the 4 to 8 weeks necessary for outpatient treatment.[28] Sober housing coupled with an outpatient treatment program can also be beneficial for some.

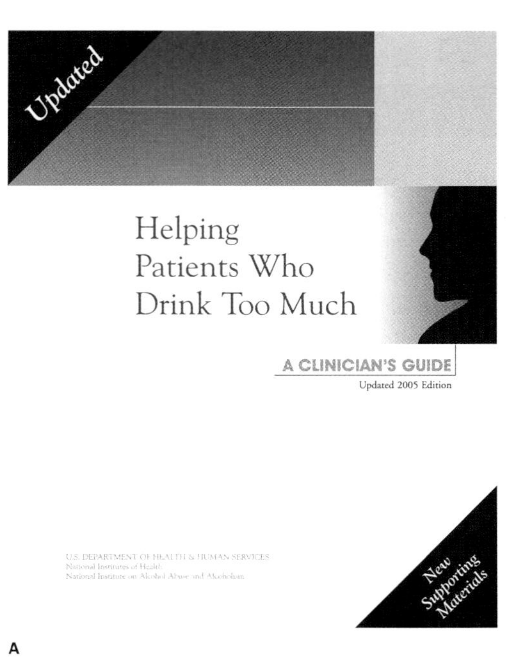

A

Updated

A POCKET GUIDE FOR

Alcohol Screening and Brief Intervention

Updated 2005 Edition

This pocket guide is condensed from the 34-page NIAAA guide, *Helping Patients Who Drink Too Much: A Clinician's Guide.*

Visit ***www.niaaa.nih.gov/guide*** for related professional support resources, including:

- patient education handouts
- preformatted progress notes
- animated slide show for training
- materials in Spanish

Or contact:

NIAAA Publications Distribution Center
P.O. Box 10686, Rockville, MD 20849-0686
(301) 443–3860
www.niaaa.nih.gov

B

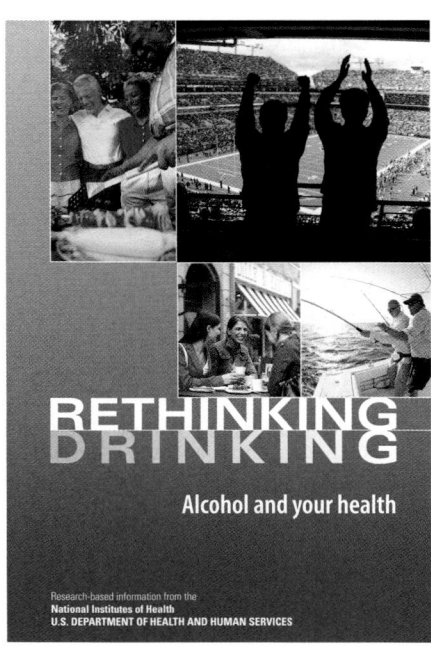

C

FIGURE 238-4 A. *Clinician's Guide* and B. *Pocket Guide* versions are available from the National Institute on Alcohol Abuse and Alcoholism. These *Guides* provide physicians with the tools needed to screen for excessive alcohol use, diagnose alcohol use disorder, and provide the appropriate counseling and pharmacotherapy to their patients. A companion video case studies training program offers physicians the opportunity to see the *Guides'* principles put into action, and includes CME credits. Both are available at http://www.niaaa.nih.gov/guide. C. *Rethinking Drinking* is a booklet for excessive drinkers that physicians can hand out to patients who drink excessively. It greatly reduces the time required for counseling about excessive drinking. It is available from the National Institute on Alcohol Abuse and Alcoholism. A companion website has additional features (http://rethinkingdrinking.niaaa.nih.gov).

- Antirelapse medication along with medical management is as effective as high-quality addiction counseling for more functional patients with alcohol dependence.[29]
- Patients with severe recurrent alcohol dependence with medical comorbidities fare best with long-term regular medical management, which includes discussion of alcohol consumption and its relationship to medical conditions, as well as encouragement to abstain. When sustained over 1 to 2 years, such medical management results in a substantial proportion of patients who are abstinent.[30]
- The presence of severe psychiatric conditions such as psychosis, mania, or severe depression with suicidal ideation requires referral to a psychiatrist or hospital. Long-term comanagement by primary care physicians and psychiatrists is likely to be necessary.

PREVENTION

- Most heavy drinkers are asymptomatic, but are drinking at a rate that puts them at increased risk for developing alcohol addiction (dependence) and associated medical and social complications. These "at-risk" drinkers respond well to brief counseling by physicians, resulting in significant reductions in heavy drinking. This finding is based on extensive research, such that the US Prevention Task Force has rated screening and brief counseling to be a "B" recommendation, which also have been determined to be cost-effective.[31] Because the prevalence of at-risk drinking is so high (26% of US adults in any given year), the potential public health impact of broad implementation of screening and brief counseling is large.
- The NIAAA has published a guide to help physicians with screening, assessment and brief counseling techniques (**Figure 238-4**). There is also an online continuing medical education (CME) activity available. This online training uses 4 video case series, along with advanced interactive educational techniques, to improve physicians' skills and knowledge (available at http://www.niaaa.nih.gov/publications/clinical-guides-and-manuals/niaaa-clinicians-guide-online-training). CME credit is available and it has been approved by the American Academy of Family Physicians.
- *Rethinking Drinking*, available as a booklet and online, is an educational tool for at-risk drinkers (available at http://rethinkingdrinking.niaaa.nih). This publication takes the drinker through a process of increasing awareness of drinking, deciding whether to change and what the drinking goal is, and developing a plan to implement change. Using this publication substantially enhances the value while decreasing the time it takes to counsel a patient to reduce or stop drinking.

PROGNOSIS

- Most at-risk drinkers eventually reduce their drinking or abstain, and do not develop an AUD or other complications of heavy drinking.
- Nearly three-fourths of people who have an episode where they meet criteria for an AUD experience remission of the disorder (either

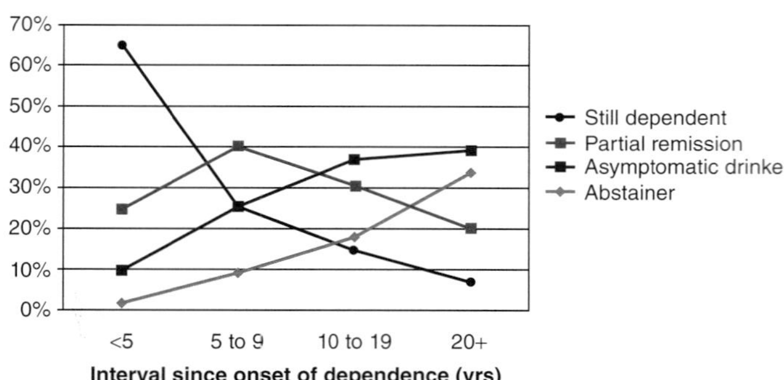

FIGURE 238-5 Course of alcohol dependence over time. At time zero, 100% of subjects were dependent. (*Reproduced with permission from Mark Willenbring, MD.*)

through abstaining or reducing drinking to low-risk levels) after a few years. Once remitted, the AUD generally does not recur, and 20 years after onset, fewer than 10% still meet full diagnostic criteria for a disorder (**Figure 238-5**).[4]

- Those with recurrent or chronic dependence have an average of 5 episodes over a period of decades. However, many eventually do remit. Almost all patients who enter rehab programs have severe recurrent dependence.[7] Rehab outcomes are very similar across different programs.[32] In the first year following an episode of rehab, roughly one-third of patients will be in stable recovery (approximately 25% will abstain and 10% will be in nonabstinent recovery, defined as engaging in no high-risk drinking and having no alcohol-related problems,) a third will not respond and will remain in stable nonrecovery, and the remainder will show variability (**Figure 238-6**).
- Patients with moderate-severe, recurrent dependence usually must make multiple quit attempts over several years before long-term abstinence is established.[33]
- Recent research suggests that heavy drinking in mid-life tends to persist over time and may be resistant to available treatment approaches.[34] Consequently, repeated and ongoing efforts to support change are often required. It is helpful under these circumstances to think in terms of "quit attempts," much like is used for smoking cessation.
- A minority of patients have chronic dependence or periodic relapses for many years, and as is true with all chronic illnesses, some will die

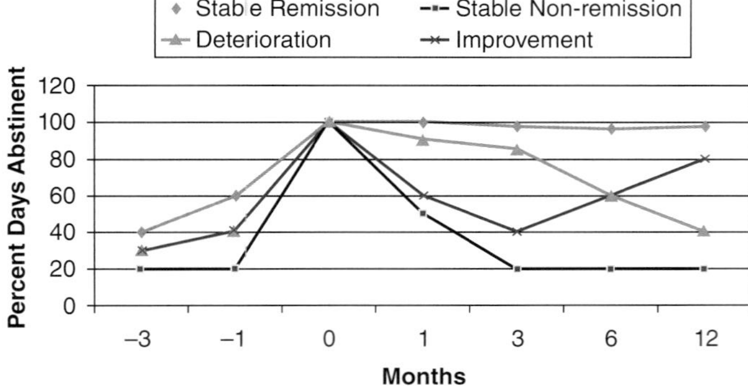

FIGURE 238-6 Course of alcohol dependence before and after treatment. Many patients reduce drinking significantly before entering treatment. After treatment, about a third of patients will be in stable recovery for the following 12 months, a third will be in stable nonrecovery, and the remainder will fluctuate between recovery and nonrecovery. (*Reproduced with permission from Mark Willenbring, MD.*)

of the disease and its medical complications, in spite of availability of all available current treatments and motivated effort by the patient. The science of behavior change is in its infancy, so much of what we do is nonspecific and modestly effective.

FOLLOW-UP

- *At-risk drinkers*—Although a single brief counseling session has significant efficacy, the effect may be magnified by repeated counseling. For this reason, it is best to inquire about drinking quantity and frequency at each follow-up visit and to reinforce advice about low-risk drinking limits.
- *Patients with alcohol dependence*—Approach this group of patients with the same attitude you adopt for smoking cessation. Most people require multiple quit attempts before achieving lasting remission, so it is important to anticipate the possibility of recurrence, and to plan for it if it occurs. Let the patient know that you won't be angry or disappointed with them if recurrence occurs. In fact, if they have a relapse to heavy drinking, that is exactly when they should seek care; a relapse is similar to an asthma attack or an increase in chest pain from ischemic heart disease. Exacerbations or recurrences of chronic illnesses are common and can be managed. The goal is to seek care quickly if a recurrence occurs and to keep relapses infrequent, short and to reduce their severity. If withdrawal is a concern, it can generally be managed on an outpatient basis.[35] Reevaluate pharmacotherapy and behavioral approaches. Support learning from the recurrence: How did it happen? What could prevent the next one? Address guilt and shame and encourage patients to minimize time spent on this relapse and to look to the future and get right back on track.
- For patients with functional alcohol dependence consider referral to an addiction medicine or psychiatry specialist.
- For patients with complex chronic addiction, treat complications, recruit social and environmental resources (family, community, etc) as indicated, and provide support.

PATIENT EDUCATION

- A patient handbook is available from the NIAAA. Titled *Rethinking Drinking* (see **Figure 238-4**), it takes patients through a scientifically based process of education, evaluation of their drinking and decision-making regarding whether to change it. Free copies of the printed version are available from the Institute and it is also available on the Internet—**http://rethinkingdrinking.niaaa.nih.com**.
- General principles in approaching patients
  - Heavy drinking and AUDs are similar to other common complex diseases such as diabetes; they have about a 50:50 combination of genetic and environmental etiologies.
  - Alcohol dependence occurs when the brain changes after exposure to large doses of alcohol, causing an impairment of control over intake. In all but mild cases, this is irreversible and good control over drinking will always be problematic. Thus, abstinence is the best and easiest approach for most people.
  - Acknowledge that friends and family may take a long time to trust an individual in early recovery, as most have been disappointed numerous times in the past.
  - Emphasize that slips and relapses are common and encourage patients to keep trying in spite of them.

PATIENT RESOURCES

- The National Institute on Alcohol Abuse and Alcoholism—**http://www.niaaa.nih.gov.**
- *Rethinking Drinking*, a booklet for people who wish to consume alcohol—**http://rethinkingdrinking.niaaa.nih.gov.**
- Faces and Voices of Recovery—**http://www.facesandvoicesofrecovery.org/.**
- Alcoholics Anonymous—**http://www.aa.org.**

PROVIDER RESOURCES

- *Helping Patients Who Drink Too Much: A Clinician's Guide*—**http://www.niaaa.nih.gov/publications/clinical-guides-and-manuals/helping-patients-who-drink-too-much-clinicians-guide.**

REFERENCES

1. U.S. Department of Health & Human Services. *Helping Patients Who Drink Too Much: A Clinician's Guide*. Bethesda, MD: National Institutes of Health; 2007.
2. Whitlock EP, Polen MR, Green CA, Orleans T, Klein J. Behavioral counseling interventions in primary care to reduce risky/harmful alcohol use by adults: a summary of the evidence for the U.S. Preventive Services Task Force. *Ann Intern Med*. 2004;140(7):557-568, I564.
3. Grant BF, Dawson DA, Stinson FS, Chou SP, Dufour MC, Pickering RP. The 12-month prevalence and trends in DSM-IV alcohol abuse and dependence: United States, 1991-1992 and 2001-2002. *Drug Alcohol Depend*. 2004;74(3):223-234.
4. Hasin DS, Stinson FS, Ogburn E, Grant BF. Prevalence, correlates, disability, and comorbidity of DSM-IV alcohol abuse and dependence in the United States: results from the national epidemiologic survey on alcohol and related conditions. *Arch Gen Psychiatry*. 2007;64(7):830-842.
5. Dick DM, Bierut LJ. The genetics of alcohol dependence. *Curr Psychiatry Rep*. 2006;8(2):151-157.
6. Enoch MA. The influence of gene-environment interactions on the development of alcoholism and drug dependence. *Curr Psychiatry Rep*. 2012;14(2):150-158.
7. Moss HB, Chen CM, Yi Hy. Subtypes of alcohol dependence in a nationally representative sample. *Drug Alcohol Depend*. 2007;91(2-3):149-158.
8. Lynskey MT, Agrawal A, Heath AC. Genetically informative research on adolescent substance use: methods, findings, and challenges. *J Am Acad Child Adolesc Psychiatry*. 2010;49(12):1202-1214.
9. Enoch M-A. The role of early life stress as a predictor for alcohol and drug dependence. *Psychopharmacology (Berl)*. 2011;214(1):17-31.
10. Chartier KG, Hesselbrock MN, Hesselbrock VM. Development and vulnerability factors in adolescent alcohol use. *Child Adolesc Psychiatr Clin N Am*. 2010;19(3):493-504.
11. Hingson RW, Heeren T, Winter MR. Age of alcohol-dependence onset: associations with severity of dependence and seeking treatment. *Pediatrics*. 2006;118(3):e755-e763.
12. Rubinsky AD, Kivlahan DR, Volk RJ, Maynard C, Bradley KA. Estimating risk of alcohol dependence using alcohol screening scores. *Drug Alcohol Depend*. 2010;108(1-2):29-36.
13. American Psychiatric Association. *Diagnostic and Statistical Manual of Psychiatric Disorders*. 5th ed. Washington, DC: American Psychiatric Publishing; 2013.
14. Saha TD, Chou SP, Grant BF. Toward an alcohol use disorder continuum using item response theory: results from the National Epidemiologic Survey on Alcohol and Related Conditions. *Psychol Med*. 2006;36(7):931-941.
15. Dawson DA, Grant BF, Li TK. Quantifying the risks associated with exceeding recommended drinking limits. *Alcohol Clin Exp Res* 2005;29(5):902-908.
16. Boschloo L, Vogelzangs N, Smit JH, et al. The performance of the Alcohol Use Disorder Identification Test (AUDIT) in detecting alcohol abuse and dependence in a population of depressed or anxious persons. *J Affect Disord*. 2010;126(3):441-446.
17. Hock B, Schwarz M, Limmer C, et al. Validity of carbohydrate-deficient transferrin (%CDT), gamma-glutamyltransferase (gamma-GT) and mean corpuscular erythrocyte volume (MCV) as biomarkers for chronic alcohol abuse: a study in patients with alcohol dependence and liver disorders of non-alcoholic and alcoholic origin. *Addiction*. 2005;100(10):1477-1486.
18. Finney JW, Hahn AC, Moos RH. The effectiveness of inpatient and outpatient treatment for alcohol abuse: the need to focus on mediators and moderators of setting effects. *Addiction*. 1996;91(12):1773-1796.
19. Longabaugh R, McCrady B, Fink E, et al. Cost effectiveness of alcoholism treatment in partial vs inpatient settings. Six-month outcomes. *J Stud Alcohol*. 1983;44(6):1049-1071.
20. McLellan AT, Lewis DC, O'Brien CP, Kleber HD. Drug dependence, a chronic medical illness: implications for treatment, insurance, and outcomes evaluation. *JAMA*. 2000;284(13):1689-1695.
21. Parthasarathy S, Chi FW, Mertens JR, Weisner C. The role of continuing care in 9-year cost trajectories of patients with intakes into an outpatient alcohol and drug treatment program. *Med Care*. 2012;50(6):540-546.
22. Willenbring ML, Olson DH. A randomized trial of integrated outpatient treatment for medically ill alcoholic men. *Arch Intern Med*. 1999;159(16):1946-1952.
23. Bouza C, Angeles M, Munoz A, Amate JM. Efficacy and safety of naltrexone and acamprosate in the treatment of alcohol dependence: a systematic review. *Addiction*. 2004;99(7):811-828.
24. Johnson BA, Rosenthal N, Capece J, et al. Topiramate for the treatment of alcohol dependence: results from a multi-site trial. *Alcohol Clin Exp Res*. 2007;31(s2):261A.
25. Anton RF, O'Malley SS, Ciraulo DA, et al. Combined pharmacotherapies and behavioral interventions for alcohol dependence: the COMBINE study: a randomized controlled trial. *JAMA*. 2006;295(17):2003-2017.
26. Mason BJ, Goodman AM, Chabac S, Lehert P. Effect of oral acamprosate on abstinence in patients with alcohol dependence in a double-blind, placebo-controlled trial: the role of patient motivation. *J Psychiatr Res*. 2006;40(5):383-393.
27. Mann KF, Lemenager KF, Smolka M, the Project PREDICT Research Group. Craving subtypes as predictors for treatment response: results from the PREDICT Study. *Alcohol Clin Exp Res*. 2008;32(suppl 1a):281A.

28. Fink EB, Longabaugh R, McCrady BM, et al. Effectiveness of alcoholism treatment in partial versus inpatient settings: twenty-four month outcomes. *Addict Behav*. 1985;10(3):235-248.

29. O'Malley SS, Rounsaville BJ, Farren C, et al. Initial and maintenance naltrexone treatment for alcohol dependence using primary care vs specialty care: a nested sequence of 3 randomized trials. *Arch Intern Med*. 2003;163(14):1695-1704.

30. Willenbring ML, Olson DH, Bielinski J. Integrated outpatient treatment for medically ill alcoholic men: results from a quasi-experimental study. *J Stud Alcohol*. 1995;56(3):337-343.

31. Solberg LI, Maciosek MV, Edwards NM. Primary care intervention to reduce alcohol misuse. ranking its health impact and cost effectiveness. *Am J Prev Med*. 2008;34(2):143-152.

32. Miller WR, Walters ST, Bennett ME. How effective is alcoholism treatment in the United States? *J Stud Alcohol*. 2001;62(2):211-220.

33. Dawson DA, Grant BF, Stinson FS, Chou PS, Huang B, Ruan WJ. Recovery from DSM-IV alcohol dependence: United States, 2001-2002. *Addiction*. 2005;100(3):281-292.

34. Delucchi KL, Kline Simon AH, Weisner C. Remission from alcohol and other drug problem use in public and private treatment samples over seven years. *Drug Alcohol Depend*. 2012;124(1-2):57-62.

35. Hayashida M, Alterman AI, McLellan AT, et al. Comparative effectiveness and costs of inpatient and outpatient detoxification of patients with mild-to-moderate alcohol withdrawal syndrome. *N Engl J Med*. 1989;320(6):358-365.

239 METHAMPHETAMINE

Michelle Rowe, DO
Andrew Schechtman, MD

PATIENT STORY

A 40-year-old woman with diabetes comes to the clinic with blood sugar in the 400s because she ran out of insulin a few weeks ago. She appears poorly groomed and has nicotine stains on her fingertips. Excoriated lesions (**Figure 239-1**) are noted on her forearms and face. She reports no itching at this moment, but when asked confirms that she regularly smokes methamphetamine. The diagnosis of her skin condition is meth mites. She acknowledges that she picks at her skin when she is high on meth. The physician asks her if she wants help to get off the meth so she can care for her health and well-being. She breaks down in tears and says that her craving for meth is very strong, but she is willing to try something because she knows the meth is ruining her body and life.

INTRODUCTION

Methamphetamine is a powerfully addictive stimulant that can be smoked, snorted, or injected. Methamphetamine can be produced by using common household products and pseudoephedrine. There is a worldwide epidemic of methamphetamine abuse and addiction.

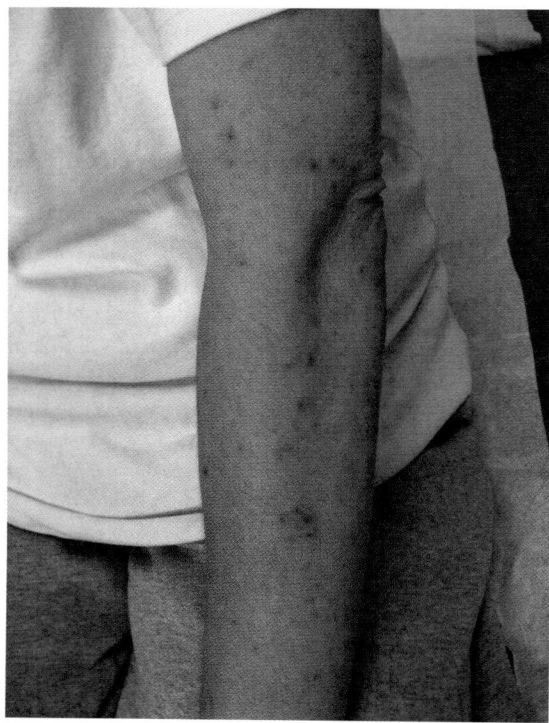

FIGURE 239-1 A 40-year-old woman with sores on her arm caused by picking at her skin while using methamphetamine. Also called meth mites, although there are no mites. *(Reproduced with permission from Andrew Schechtman, MD.)*

SYNONYMS

Methamphetamine is also known as meth, crank, ice, and crystal.

EPIDEMIOLOGY

- Worldwide, compared to other drugs of abuse, only marijuana is used more often than amphetamine/methamphetamine.[1]
- The lifetime prevalence ("ever-used") rate for methamphetamine was 2.1% for 12th graders in the 2011 Monitoring the Future study, which surveys 50,000 students in 8th, 10th, and 12th grades in 420 schools nationwide annually. This has decreased from 1999, when the lifetime prevalence for methamphetamine use in 12th graders was 8.2%. For comparison, marijuana/hashish had a lifetime prevalence in 12th graders of 45.5% and 49.7% in 2011 and 1999, respectively.[2]
- Stimulants (methamphetamine and amphetamine) accounted for 9.6% of nationwide emergency department visits involving use of illicit drugs in 2009, with the highest incidence in those from 18 to 44 years old.[3]
- Methamphetamine use is associated with white or Native American race; residence in the west or south; having an ever-incarcerated father; marijuana, cocaine, intravenous drug use; and men who have sex with men (MSM).[4]
- Analysis of methamphetamine found in workforce drug testing done nationwide in 2010 by Quest Diagnostics showed the highest rates of use in western and midwestern states, with relative sparing of eastern states. Highest prevalence (more than twice the national average) was found in Hawaii, Arkansas, Oklahoma, Nevada, California, Wyoming, Utah, and Arizona.[5]
- Methamphetamine is a schedule-II stimulant with legitimate medical uses, including the treatment of narcolepsy and attention deficit hyperactivity disorder (ADHD).
- Methamphetamine is known on the street as meth, crank, ice (**Figure 239-2**), and crystal. It is abused by smoking, injecting, snorting, or oral ingestion. Smoking or injecting the drug gives an

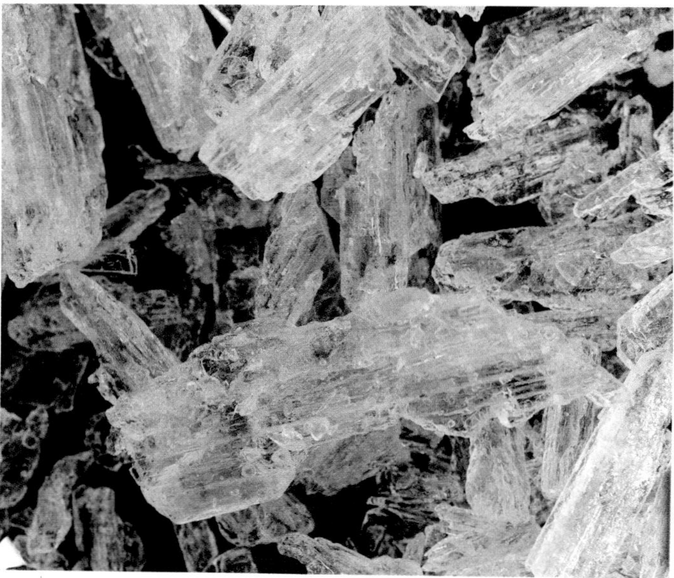

FIGURE 239-2 Methamphetamine in its ice format. *(Reproduced with permission from DEA.)*

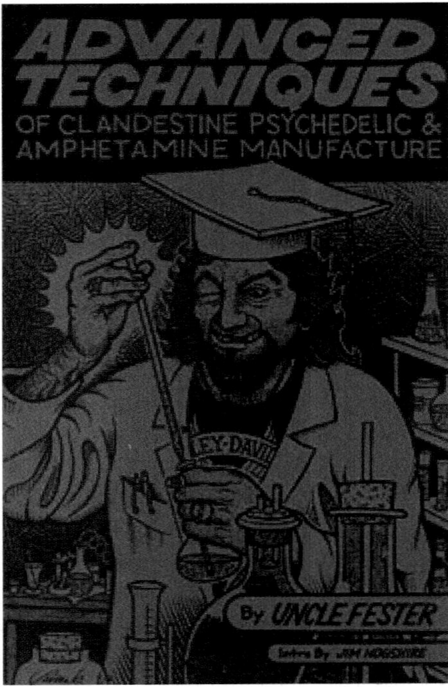

FIGURE 239-3 One of many books by Uncle Fester that can be purchased on the Internet. The information to manufacture methamphetamine is readily available. (*Reproduced with permission from Uncle Fester, www .unclefesterbooks.com.*)

intense, short-lived "flash" or rush. Snorting or oral ingestion creates euphoria but no rush.

- Methamphetamine can be manufactured from inexpensive, readily available chemicals using recipes easily found on the Internet and in books (**Figure 239-3**).
- Common household and industrial chemicals used to make methamphetamine include pseudoephedrine and ephedrine (cold tablets), red phosphorus (matches/road flares), iodine (teat dip or flakes/crystal), methanol (gasoline additives), muriatic acid (used in swimming pools), anhydrous ammonia (farm fertilizer), sodium hydroxide (lye), sulfuric acid (drain cleaner), toluene (brake cleaner), and ether (engine starter).[6]
- The "meth laboratory," the site of small-scale methamphetamine production (**Figure 239-4**), brings with it many hazards, including exposure to toxic chemicals for the meth cooks themselves, their children, and law enforcement, medical, and fire personnel entering the laboratory in the course of their duties. Explosions and fires at meth laboratories are common. Improper disposal of the toxic chemicals used in the laboratories frequently leads to environmental contamination.[7]
- Effects of methamphetamine, such as euphoria, increased libido, and impaired judgment, may lead to increased high-risk sexual behaviors, such as unprotected sexual intercourse and contact with multiple sexual partners. As a result, methamphetamine users are at increased risk of contracting sexually transmitted infections, including HIV.

ETIOLOGY AND PATHOPHYSIOLOGY

- Methamphetamine acts as a central nervous system stimulant by blocking presynaptic reuptake of dopamine, norepinephrine, and serotonin.

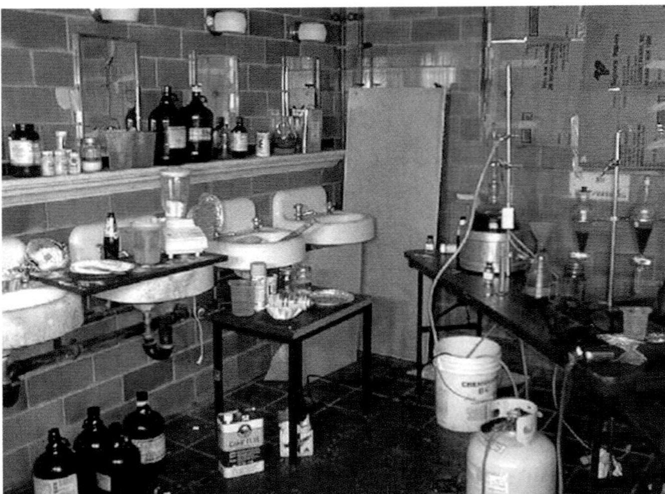

FIGURE 239-4 A methamphetamine laboratory with visible toxic and flammable substances.

- Compared to amphetamines, methamphetamine has an increased ability to cross the blood-brain barrier and has a prolonged half-life (10-12 hours). This leads to faster-onset, more intense, and longer-lasting effects when compared to amphetamine.
- Intended effects of methamphetamine use include euphoria, increased energy, a heightened sense of alertness, and increased libido.
- Unintended effects include increased heart rate, blood pressure, and body temperature; headaches; nausea; anxiety; aggression; paranoia; visual and auditory hallucinations; insomnia; tremors; and cardiac arrhythmias.
- With chronic abuse, neurologic manifestations include confusion, poor concentration, depression, paranoia, and psychosis. Weight loss and dental decay can occur. The face and body become atrophic and gaunt, making the chronic methamphetamine user appear older than their stated age.
- Methamphetamine users may experience formication, the hallucination that bugs are crawling under the skin. The skin excoriations resulting from picking at the imagined bugs are known as "meth mites" (**Figures 239-1**, **239-5**, and **239-6**).
- The rampant dental caries and gingivitis commonly seen in methamphetamine users is known as "meth mouth" (**Figures 239-7** and **239-8**). The causes of meth mouth are multiple. Vasoconstriction leads to decreased saliva production and dry mouth, which often result in consumption of large amounts of sugar-containing beverages. Methamphetamine users often neglect their oral hygiene when preoccupied with obtaining and using the drug. Methamphetamine-induced bruxism also damages the teeth. Neglect of early symptoms and lack of access to or failure to seek dental care often lead to unsalvageable teeth that can only be extracted.[8-10]

DIAGNOSIS

ACUTE INTOXICATION

This can lead to tachycardia, hypertension, chest pain, hyperthermia, diaphoresis, mydriasis, agitation, irritability, hypervigilance, paranoia, hallucinations, and tremor.

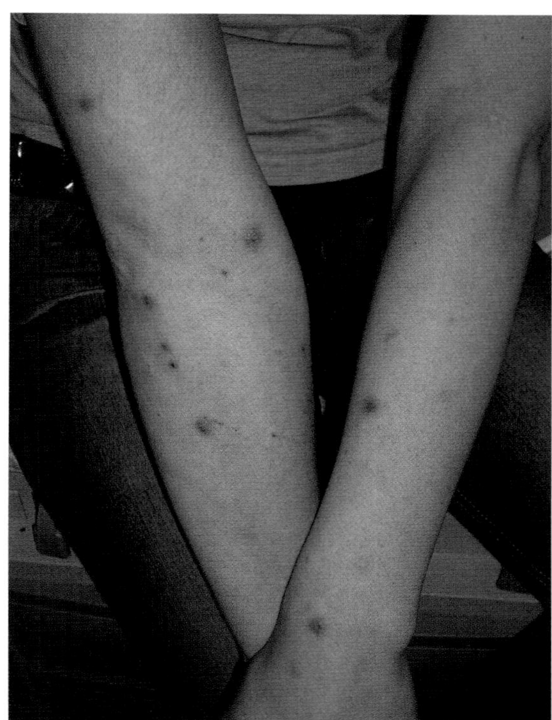

FIGURE 239-5 A 19-year-old woman with sores on her arms from picking at her skin while using methamphetamine. Also called meth mites. *(Reproduced with permission from Richard P. Usatine, MD.)*

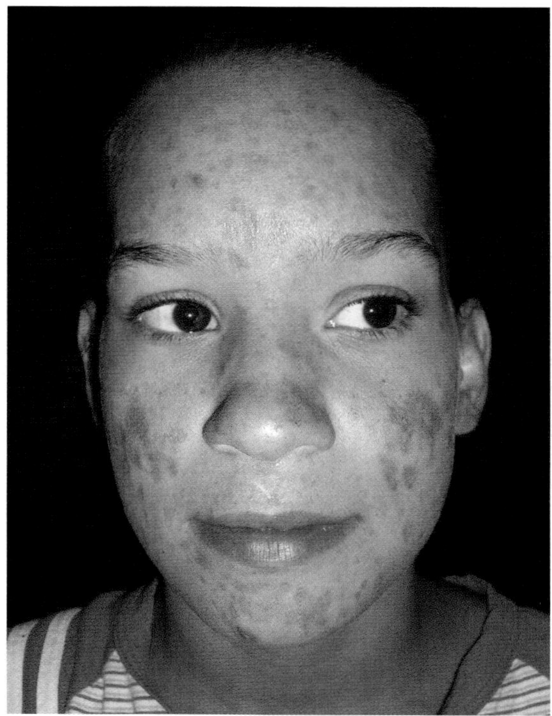

FIGURE 239-6 Postinflammatory hyperpigmentation in a young woman who has picked at her skin while addicted to methamphetamine. *(Reproduced with permission from Richard P. Usatine, MD.)*

CHRONIC USE

Chronic use of methamphetamine can cause violent behavior, anxiety, depression, confusion, insomnia, and psychotic symptoms (paranoia, auditory hallucinations, delusions, and formication).[11,12]

WITHDRAWAL SYMPTOMS

Withdrawal symptoms include drug cravings, depressed mood, disturbed sleep patterns, increased appetite, and fatigue.

COMPLICATIONS

Complications arising from using methamphetamine include neurologic (seizures, stroke caused by intracerebral hemorrhage or vasospasm), cardiovascular (myocardial ischemia or infarction, dilated cardiomyopathy, and cardiac arrhythmias), hyperthermia (potentially fatal), rhabdomyolysis, consequences of injection drug abuse (skin infections and abscesses, endocarditis), and high-risk sexual behavior increasing risks of contracting sexually transmitted infections including hepatitis B, hepatitis C, and HIV.

LABORATORY STUDIES

- Urine drug screening is commonly done with immunoassays. These tests are highly cross-reactive and may give false-positive results for methamphetamine or amphetamine caused by the presence of other sympathomimetic amines such as pseudoephedrine or ephedrine. Unexpected positive results on a screening test can be confirmed with more specific tests such as gas chromatography/mass spectrometry (GC/MS) and stereospecific chromatography.[13] One limitation of urine drug testing for methamphetamine is that the drug may only be detectable for up to 3 days after use. Hair testing is available and remains positive for up to 90 days after drug use.
- Methamphetamine users are at increased risk of sexually transmitted diseases and diseases transmitted through the use of shared needles. Consider screening for HIV, hepatitides B and C, and other sexually transmitted infections.
- For patients with signs and symptoms of acute intoxication, consider excluding complications of methamphetamine abuse by ordering creatinine phosphokinase (CK), complete blood count (CBC), and chem panel. If chest pain is present, cardiac enzymes and electrocardiography (ECG) are indicated.

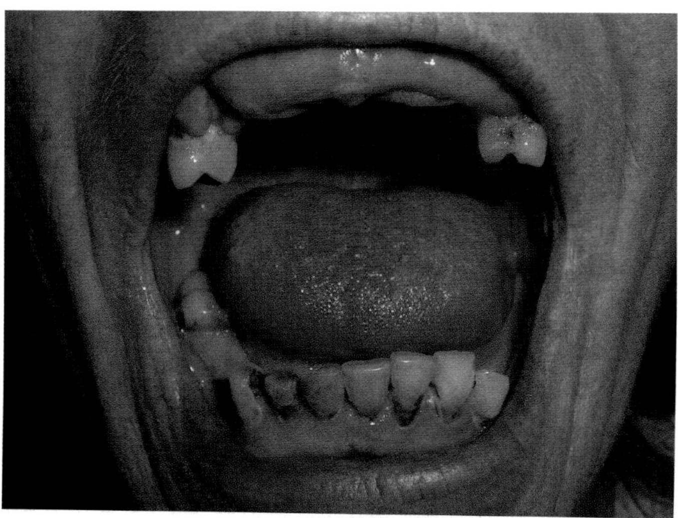

FIGURE 239-7 Methamphetamine mouth (meth mouth) in a 42-year-old woman with 20 years of methamphetamine use. The meth has completely destroyed her teeth. *(Reproduced with permission from Richard P. Usatine, MD.)*

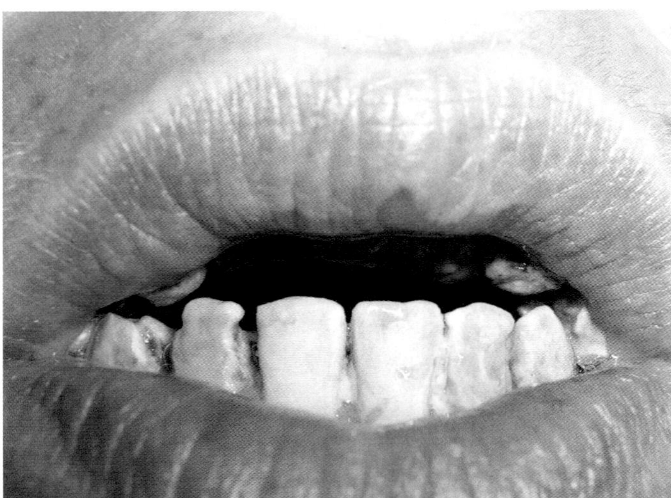

FIGURE 239-8 "Meth mouth" in a young woman actively using methamphetamine. (*Reproduced with permission from Richard P. Usatine, MD.*)

DIFFERENTIAL DIAGNOSIS

ACUTE METHAMPHETAMINE INTOXICATION

- Intoxication with other substances causing sympathetic stimulation and/or altered mental status (cocaine, ecstasy, phencyclidine [PCP], theophylline, aspirin, monoamine oxidase inhibitors, serotonin syndrome)
- Psychiatric disorders (bipolar disorder, panic attack, and schizophrenia)
- Hyperthyroidism and thyroid storm (see Chapter 227, Hyperthyroidism)

METHAMPHETAMINE-INDUCED SKIN LESIONS (METH MITES)

- Scabies—Burrows may be present; located on wrists, fingers, genital region, and spares face; very pruritic. Family members may be infected too (see Chapter 141, Scabies).
- Atopic dermatitis—Persistent pruritus (pruritus from meth stops after acute intoxication clears). In most cases there is a long history of the dermatitis before the meth use had begun (see Chapter 143, Atopic Dermatitis).
- Contact dermatitis is pruritic but is generally localized to the area in which the contact allergen has touched the skin. A good history should allow this to be differentiated from meth mites (see Chapter 144, Contact Dermatitis).
- Neurodermatitis and prurigo nodularis—Persistent complaints of severe pruritus. In many ways, these are similar to meth mites in that the stimulus to scratch is from the brain not just the skin. Absence of meth use should be present in these self-inflicted dermatoses to distinguish them from meth mites (see Chapter 147, Psychocutaneous Disorders).

MANAGEMENT

- Acute methamphetamine intoxication is treated with supportive measures. Sedation with haloperidol, droperidol, or benzodiazepines (diazepam and lorazepam) can be used for agitated patients. Methamphetamine-induced cardiac ischemia is treated with oxygen, nitrates, and β-blockers. Seizures and rhabdomyolysis are treated in the standard fashion.[14] SOR B
- There are no medications with proven efficacy for treatment of methamphetamine withdrawal. Mirtazapine and modafinil have shown some benefit in preliminary studies.[15] SOR C

Treatment of methamphetamine dependence and addiction is challenging. Inpatient detoxification may be required initially, followed by a long-term program of behavioral interventions. SOR C

- Refer patients to 12-step programs, which are valuable and free. Crystal Meth Anonymous is a 12-step program modeled on the 12 steps of Alcoholics Anonymous and the White Book of Narcotics Anonymous. If Crystal Meth Anonymous meetings are not available, any 12-step program can be of help in recovery and maintaining sobriety. SOR B
- The Matrix model, a behavioral treatment method initially developed for treatment of cocaine addiction, has been used successfully to treat methamphetamine addiction. It consists of a 16-week program, including group and individual therapy, relapse prevention, family involvement, participation in a 12-step program or other spiritual group, and weekly drug testing.[16] SOR C

In the context of outpatient behavioral treatment programs, providing small incentives for drug-free urine samples can help promote abstinence. One study found that 19% of incentivized patients achieved 12 weeks of continuous abstinence whereas only 5% of nonincentivized patients did so (number needed to treat [NNT] = 7.1) at a cost of only $2.42 per day per participant.[17] SOR B

- Although there currently are no Food and Drug Administration (FDA)-approved medications to help treat methamphetamine dependence, several medications under study have shown favorable early results, including modafinil, bupropion, and naltrexone. SOR B "Replacement" therapy using low-dose stimulants, similar to the way methadone and nicotine are used for opioid and nicotine dependence, respectively, has also shown some benefit.[18]
- Methamphetamine-related skin excoriation should heal without treatment if the picking behavior stops. However, postinflammatory hyperpigmentation may never resolve (see **Figure 239-6**). Antibiotic treatment with an antistaphylococcal agent, such as cephalexin or dicloxacillin, is indicated if the excoriations become infected. If methicillin-resistant *Staphylococcus aureus* (MRSA) is suspected, choose an antibiotic that covers MRSA (see Chapter 118, Impetigo).
- Referral for dental care is indicated for patients with gingivitis and dental caries caused by chronic methamphetamine use. Recommend daily use of a soft-bristled toothbrush and dental floss for treatment and prevention of oral pathology. SOR A Rinsing with a chlorhexidine-containing mouthwash may be a reasonable alternative for patients who find it too painful to floss. SOR C (see Chapter 35, Gingivitis and Periodontal Disease and Chapter 40, Adult Dental Caries).

FOLLOW-UP

- Methamphetamine users who have recently quit are at high risk of relapse. Close follow-up is indicated to identify relapses and to reinitiate treatment.
- Maintenance of abstinence can be aided by participation in an outpatient treatment program and 12-step programs.

- Methamphetamine-induced skin lesions should heal when the picking behavior ceases. Resolution is unlikely if methamphetamine abuse continues.

PATIENT EDUCATION

- Encourage patients to stop using methamphetamine. Offer referral to a treatment program in the community.
- Inform patients that methamphetamine use carries risks of heart attack, stroke, and death that can result from a single dose. There is no safe level of methamphetamine use.
- Counsel patients who have sex while using methamphetamine that this combination increases the likelihood of unsafe sexual practices and their risk of getting a sexually transmitted infection.
- Advise users who inject methamphetamine to use clean needles and to avoid sharing needles to decrease their risk of contracting hepatitis B, hepatitis C, and HIV.

PATIENT RESOURCES

- Crystal Meth Anonymous (12-step meetings)—**http://www.crystalmeth.org/.**
- Substance Abuse & Mental Health Services Administration (SAMHSA). *Substance Abuse Treatment Facility Locator*—**http://www.findtreatment.samhsa.gov/.**
- ADA Division of Communications; Journal of the American Dental Association; ADA Division of Scientific Affairs. For the dental patient methamphetamine use and oral health. *J Am Dent Assoc.* 2005;136(10):1491—**http://www.ada.org/sections/professionalResources/pdfs/patient_55.pdf.**
- PBS. *Frontline: the Meth Epidemic: How Meth Destroys the Body*—**http://www.pbs.org/wgbh/pages/frontline/meth/body/.**

PROVIDER RESOURCES

- National Institute on Drug Abuse—**http://www.nida.nih.gov/DrugPages/Methamphetamine.html.**
- American Society of Addiction Medicine: Research & Treatment—**http://www.asam.org/research-treatment/treatment.**

REFERENCES

1. United Nations Office of Drugs and Crime (UNODC). *2010 World Drug Report*. Vienna, Austria: UNODC; 2010. http://www.unodc.org/unodc/en/data-and-analysis/WDR-2010.html. Accessed April 3, 2012.
2. Monitoring the Future. *Trends in Lifetime Prevalence of Use of Various Drugs for Eight, Tenth and Twelfth Graders*. http://monitoringthe-future.org/data/11data/pr11t1.pdf. Accessed April 3, 2012.
3. Substance Abuse and Mental Health Services Administration, Drug Abuse Warning Network. *2009: National Estimates of Drug-Related Emergency Department Visits*. HHS Publication No. (SMA) 11-4659, DAWN Series D-35. Rockville, MD: Substance Abuse and Mental Health Services Administration; 2011.
4. Iritani BJ, Hallfors DD, Bauer DJ. Crystal methamphetamine use among young adults in the USA. *Addiction.* 2007;102:1102-1113.
5. Quest Diagnostics. *Press Release:* "Hawaii, Arkansas and Oklahoma Lead the Nation for Methamphetamine Use in the Workforce, Reveals Quest Diagnostics Drug Testing Index(TM): Five-year Data Suggest Methamphetamine's National Decline Has Halted and That the Drug's Stronghold May Be Moving Eastward." Madison, NJ: PRNewswire; Sept 2, 2011. http://ir.questdiagnostics.com/phoenix.zhtml?c=82068&p=irol-newsArticle_pf&ID=1603058&highlight=. Accessed April 3, 2012.
6. Lynn Police Department. *The Ingredients of Meth*. http://www.lynnpolice.org/ingredients_of_meth.htm. Accessed April 3, 2012.
7. Lineberry TW, Bostwick JM. Methamphetamine abuse: a perfect storm of complications. *Mayo Clin Proc.* 2006;81(1):77-84.
8. American Dental Association. *Methamphetamine Use (Meth Mouth)*. http://www.ada.org/2711.aspx. Accessed April 3, 2012.
9. Klasser G, Epstein J. Methamphetamine and its impact on dental care. *J Can Dent Assoc.* 2005;71(10):759-762.
10. Shaner JW, Kimmes N, Saini T, Edwards P. "Meth mouth": rampant caries in methamphetamine abusers. *AIDS Patient Care STDS.* 2006;20(3):146-150.
11. Rawson RA, Condon TP. Why do we need an Addiction supplement focused on methamphetamine? *Addiction.* 2007;102(suppl 1):1-4.
12. Cruickshank CC, KR Dyer. A review of the clinical pharmacology of methamphetamine. *Addiction.* 2009;104:1085-1099.
13. Gourlay DL, Heit HA, Caplan YH. Urine drug testing in clinical practice. California Academy of Family Physicians Monograph Edition 4, 2010. http://www.familydocs.org/files/UDTmono-graph _for_web.pdf. Accessed April 3, 2012.
14. Richard J. *Methamphetamine Toxicity*. http://emedicine.medscape.com/article/820918. Accessed April 3, 2012.
15. Pennay AE, Lee NK. Putting the call out for more research: the poor evidence base for treating methamphetamine withdrawal. *Drug Alcohol Rev.* 2011;30:216-222.
16. Rawson RA, Marinelli-Casey P, Anglin MD, et al. A multisite comparison of psychosocial approaches for the treatment of methamphetamine dependence. *Addiction.* 2004;99:708-717.
17. Petry NM, Peirce JM, Stitzer ML, et al. Effect of prize-based incentives on outcomes in stimulant abusers in outpatient psychosocial treatment programs: a National Drug Abuse Treatment Clinical Trials Network Study. *Arch Gen Psychiatry.* 2005;62(10):1148-1156.
18. Karila L, Weinstein W, Aubin HJ, et al. Pharmacological approaches to methamphetamine dependence: a focused review. *Br J Clin Pharmacol.* 2010;69(6):578-592.

240 COCAINE

Heidi Chumley, MD
Mindy A. Smith, MD, MS

PATIENT STORY

A 26-year-old man is brought into the emergency department in status epilepticus by his "friends," who promptly flee the scene. His seizures spontaneously cease, and he is noted to have an altered mental status. Intravenous (IV) access is obtained and he is stabilized. A urine toxicology screen is positive for cocaine and his creatinine phosphokinase is markedly elevated. He is admitted for cocaine-induced seizures and rhabdomyolysis. He survives the hospitalization and consents to a photograph of his eyes before discharge. **Figure 240-1** shows the bilateral subconjunctival hemorrhages that occurred during his seizures. The patient states that he understands the gravity of the -situation and will enter a drug rehabilitation program when he leaves the hospital.

INTRODUCTION

Cocaine use is common, and 5% to 6% of users develop dependence within the first year of use. Acutely intoxicated patients have increased heart rates, blood pressures, temperatures, and, initially, respiratory rates; mood changes, involuntary movements; and dilated pupils. Chronic addiction can be treated with a comprehensive program, although only one-third of patients will become and remain abstinent.

SYNONYMS

Cocaine is also called blow, C, coke, crack, flake, and snow.

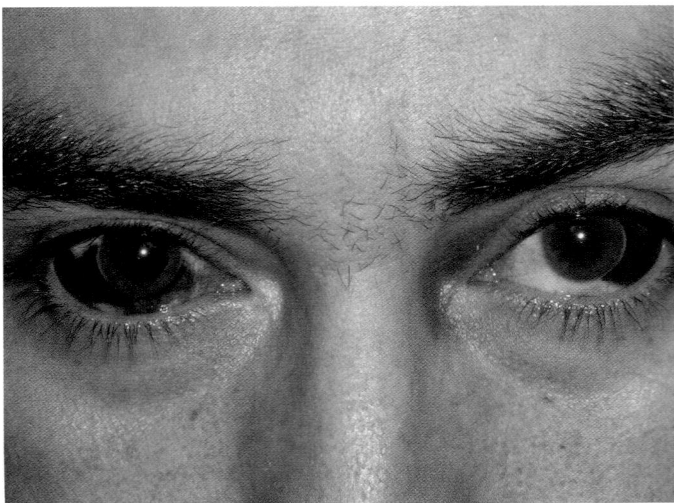

FIGURE 240-1 Bilateral subconjunctival hemorrhages after severe cocaine-induced seizures in a young man. This patient also developed rhabdomyolysis and was hospital zed. *(Reproduced with permission from Beau Willison, MD.)*

EPIDEMIOLOGY

- Based on the National Comorbidity Survey Replication (NCS-R) using interviews with a nationally representative sample of 9282 English-speaking respondents ages 18 years and older (conducted in 2001-2003), the cumulative incidence of cocaine use was 16%.[1]
- Similar numbers were reported from the National Survey on Drug Use and Health in 2005[2]:
  - Of Americans ages 12 years and older, 13.8% reported lifetime cocaine use in 2005.[2]
  - A total of 33.7 million Americans ages 12 years and older reported lifetime use of cocaine, and 7.9 million reported using crack cocaine.[2]
  - An estimated 2.4 million Americans reported current use of cocaine (682,000 of whom reported using crack).[2]
  - Of the estimated 860,000 new users of cocaine in 2005, most were age 18 years or older, with the average age of first use being 20 years.[2]
  - The percentage of youth ages 12 to 17 years reporting lifetime use of cocaine was 2.3%, and among young adults ages 18 to 25 years the rate was 15.1%.[2]
- For both male and female cocaine users, the estimated risk for developing cocaine dependence, based on data from the NCS-R, was 5% to 6% within the first year after first use.[3] Thereafter, the estimated risk decreased from the peak value, with a somewhat faster decline for females in the next 3 years after first use.
- Females may be more susceptible to crack/cocaine dependence; in a study of 152 individuals (37% female) in a residential substance-use treatment program, females evidenced greater use of crack/cocaine (current and lifetime heaviest) and were significantly more likely to show crack/cocaine dependence than males.[4]
- In one study, siblings of cocaine-dependent individuals had an elevated risk of developing cocaine dependence (relative risk [RR] = 1.71).[5]

ETIOLOGY AND PATHOPHYSIOLOGY

- Cocaine is a stimulant and local anesthetic that causes potent vasoconstriction.
- It produces its stimulant effects by causing increasing synaptic concentration of monoamine neurotransmitters (ie, dopamine, norepinephrine, and serotonin).[6]
- Similar to other local anesthetics, cocaine blocks the generation and conduction of electrical impulses in excitable tissues (eg, neurons and cardiac muscle) blocking the voltage-gated fast sodium channels in the cell membrane and abolishing the ability of the tissue to generate an action potential.[7]
- Effects are seen following oral, intranasal (as a powder [**Figure 240-2**]), IV, and inhalation administration (as crack cocaine [**Figure 240-3**], coca paste, and free base).

RISK FACTORS

- Family history/genetic predisposition.
- In a study of inner-city incarcerated male adolescents (23% of whom had used cocaine or crack in the month before arrest and 32% of whom had used cocaine at least once), current cocaine/crack users were more likely to have the following characteristics[8]:

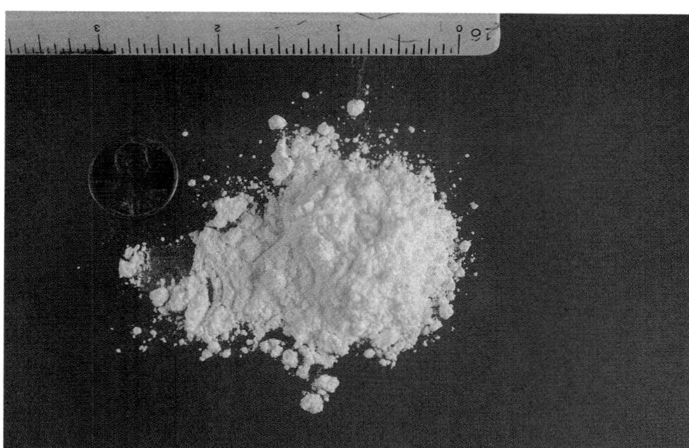

FIGURE 240-2 Cocaine in a powder form used for snorting and injecting. (*Reproduced with permission from the Drug Enforcement Agency.*)

- Alcohol, marijuana, and intranasal heroin use
- Multiple previous arrests
- To be out of school
- To be psychologically distressed
- To have been sexually molested as a child
- To have substance-abusing parents
- To have frequent sex with girls, to be gay or bisexual, and to engage in anal intercourse

• Among those who died from an accidental drug overdose in New York city, those dying from cocaine-only versus opiates were more likely to be male, black or Hispanic, have alcohol detected at autopsy, and to be of older age.[9]

DIAGNOSIS

CLINICAL FEATURES

• Acute effects occur within 3 to 5 minutes with intranasal administration (8-10 seconds with free base) and last approximately 1 hour, after which there is an abrupt disappearance of the effects.[6] When used IV or smoked as crack cocaine, the onset of action is immediate and the peak effect occurs 3 to 5 minutes later, lasting for 20 to 30 minutes.[7]
  - The acute effects include the following[6,7]:
    - Elevated heart rate, increased blood pressure, and usually increased temperature
    - Increased respiratory rate and/or dyspnea followed by decreased respiratory rate
    - Mood changes including enhanced mood/euphoria, hyperactivity, irritability and anxiety, excessive talking, and long periods without eating or sleeping
    - Involuntary movements (eg, tremors, chorea, and dystonic reactions)
  - Additional findings on physical examination can include the following:
    - Dilated pupils, nystagmus, and/or retinal hemorrhages.
    - Nasal septum perforation (**Figure 240-4**), epistaxis, and/or cerebrospinal fluid (CSF) rhinorrhea.
    - Wheezing, rales, and/or pneumothorax.
    - Absent bowel sounds (mesenteric ischemia) and/or right upper quadrant tenderness (hepatic necrosis).
    - Skin tracks from intravenous use (**Figure 240-5**).
    - Multiple areas of atrophic skin scars are from skin popping—injecting cocaine directly into the skin without finding a vein for intravenous injections (**Figure 240-6**).
  - Acute effects may be altered by concomitant use of other drugs or alcohol.

• Adverse effects of cocaine use can include the following[6]:
  - Respiratory depression that may result in death
  - Cardiac arrhythmias, chest pain, and myocardial infarction (MI)
  - Neurologic symptoms, including headache, tonic-clonic seizures, ischemic or hemorrhagic stroke, and subarachnoid hemorrhage
  - Myalgias and rhabdomyolysis
  - Severe pulmonary disease (eg, alveolar hemorrhage and pulmonary edema) and hepatic necrosis caused by crack cocaine
  - Exacerbation of existing hypertension, cardiac, and cerebrovascular disease
  - Recurrent diabetic ketoacidosis[10]

• Cutaneous vasculitis secondary to levamisole-adulterated cocaine has been reported many times in the literature.[11-15] This type of vasculitis

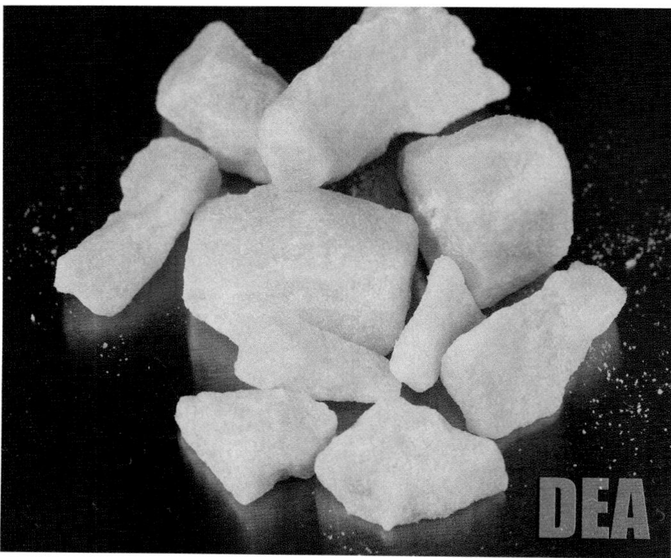

FIGURE 240-3 Crack cocaine used for smoking. (*Reproduced with permission from the Drug Enforcement Agency.*)

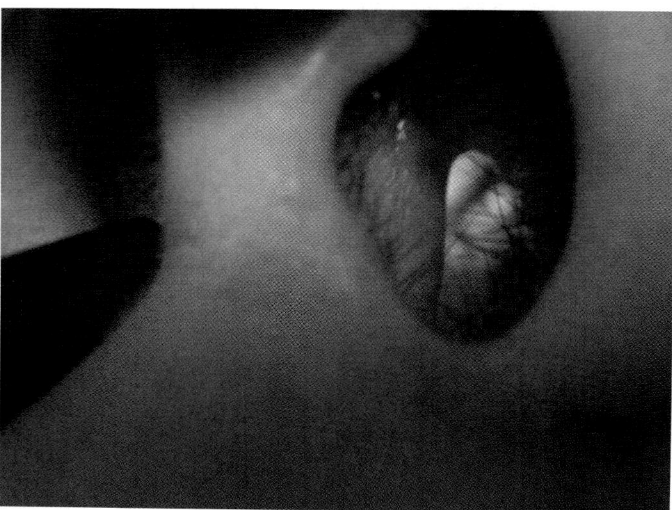

FIGURE 240-4 Shining a light through a hole in the nasal septum caused by 10 years of snorting cocaine. (*Reproduced with permission from Richard P. Usatine, MD.*)

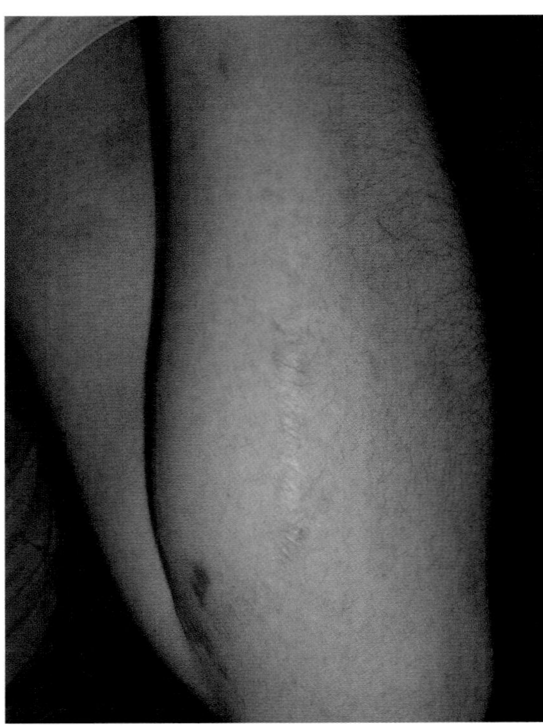

FIGURE 240-5 An injection track along the vein of a young woman in recovery from IV cocaine use and addiction. (*Reproduced with permission from Richard P. Usatine, MD.*)

presents with ear purpura (**Figure 240-7**), retiform (like a net) purpura (**Figure 240-8**) of the trunk or extremities, neutropenia, and positive tests for perinuclear antineutrophil cytoplasmic antibody (P-ANCA).[11] A 2010 US report found that more than 77% of seized cocaine in the United States is contaminated with levamisole.[13] This cutaneous vasculitis may also present on the nose or face (**Figure 240-9**).

- Chronic cocaine use is associated with decreased libido and impaired reproductive function.[1]

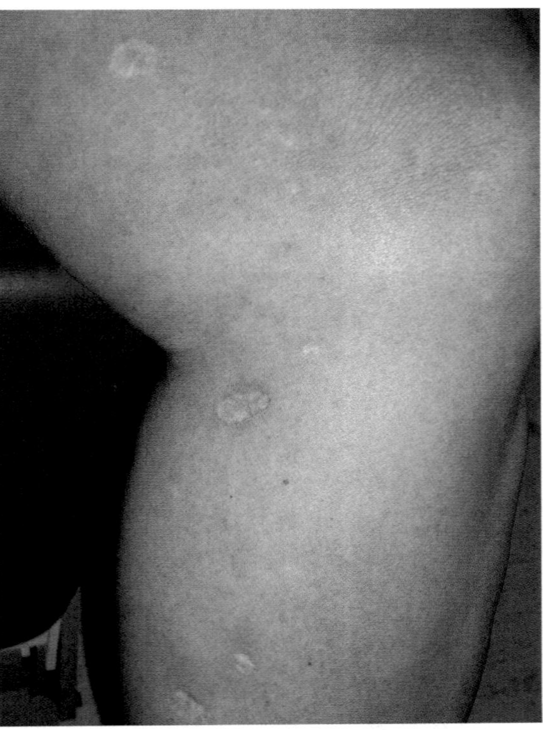

FIGURE 240-6 Multiple areas of atrophic skin scarring on the leg from skin popping cocaine. Note how the scars are depressed and relatively round or oval shaped. Some cocaine addicts inject the cocaine directly into the skin rather than look for a vein for intravenous injections. (*Reproduced with permission from Richard P. Usatine, MD.*)

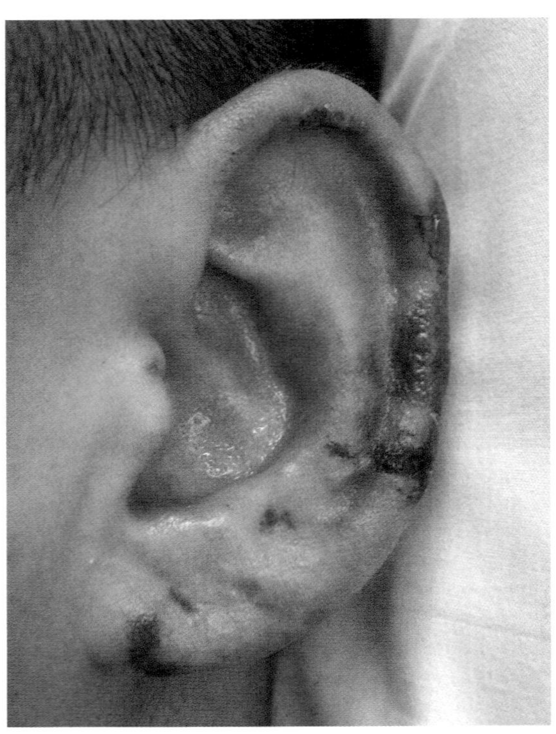

FIGURE 240-7 Cutaneous vasculitis of the ear caused by levamisole-adulterated cocaine. (*Reproduced with permission from Robert T. Gilson, MD.*)

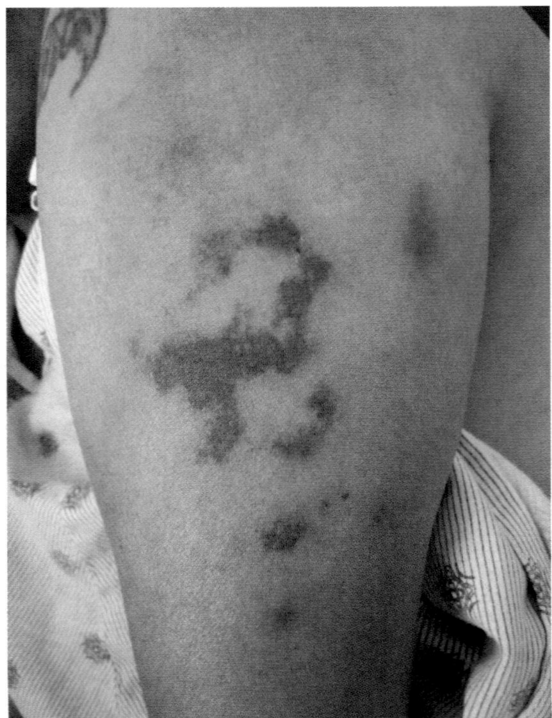

FIGURE 240-8 Cutaneous vasculitis in a retiform (net-like) pattern caused by the use of levamisole-adulterated cocaine. This is also called retiform purpura. (*Reproduced with permission from University of Texas Health Science Center San Antonio, Division of Dermatology.*)

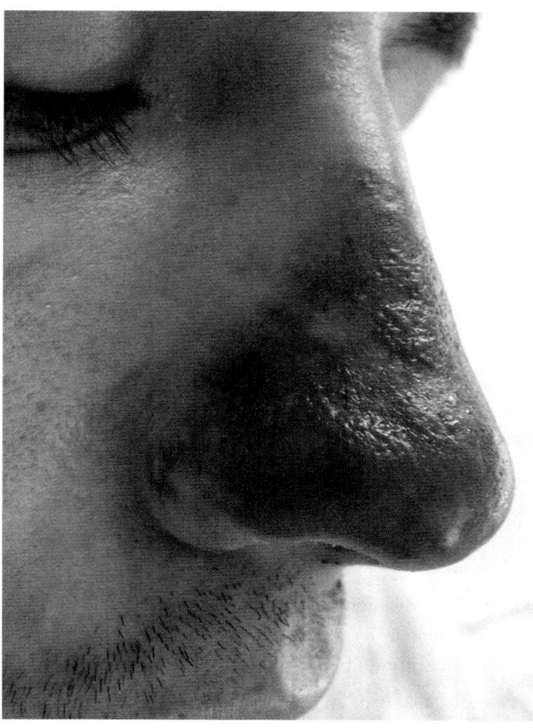

FIGURE 240-9 Cutaneous vasculitis of the nose secondary to the use of levamisole-adulterated cocaine. (*Reproduced with permission from Robert T. Gilson, MD.*)

- In men, cocaine can cause impotence and gynecomastia.
- In women, cocaine can cause galactorrhea, amenorrhea, and infertility.
- In pregnant women, crack cocaine is associated with an increase in placental abruption, miscarriage, and congenital malformation.

- Protracted use can cause paranoid ideation and visual and auditory hallucinations. Severe depression can follow recovery from cocaine intoxication (called "crashing").[1]
- Withdrawal from chronic cocaine use can cause depression, insomnia, and anorexia.

LABORATORY STUDIES

- Urine toxicology screen (using immunoassays) for commonly abused drugs (eg, cocaine, marijuana, and opiates) is the gold standard.
  - Cocaine may be detected in the urine for 24 hours after use and the metabolite of cocaine, benzoylecgonine, may be detected as long as 60 hours after a single use.[7]
  - In chronic cocaine users, benzoylecgonine may be detected for up to 22 days.[7]
  - A rapid urine test, OnTrak Testcup-5, was reported in a manufacturer-supported study to be accurate and reproducible for marijuana, cocaine, and heroin.[16]
- Saliva and hair tests are also available but may not be as accurate for all drugs of interest.
  - All injection-drug users should be screened for human immunodeficiency virus (HIV) (with consent) and hepatitides B and C.
  - If there is a history of multiple sexual partners, unsafe sex and/or sex for drugs, cocaine users should be screened for sexually transmitted diseases (STDs). This might include *Chlamydia*, gonorrhea, hepatitides B and C, HIV (with consent), and syphilis (**Figure 240-10**).

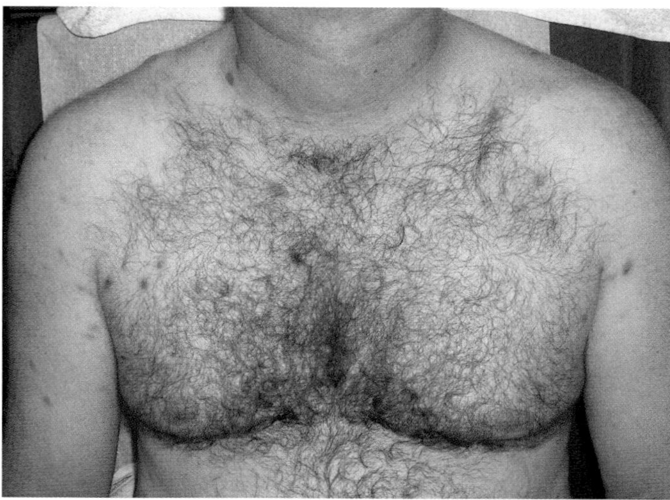

FIGURE 240-10 Secondary syphilis in a man who was involved in unsafe sex while addicted to cocaine. The papulonodular eruption is an unusual presentation of secondary syphilis that was diagnosed with a skin biopsy and confirmed with a rapid plasma reagin titer of 1:512. The specific treponemal blood test was also positive. (*Reproduced with permission from Richard P. Usatine, MD.*)

  - In an unconscious patient and in patients denying cocaine use, the following laboratory tests can be considered to rule out other diseases with similar symptoms[7]:
  - Serum glucose, magnesium, and phosphorus
  - Serum electrolytes
- Laboratory tests that can be completed to detect or monitor acute complications of cocaine overdose include the following[7]:
  - Arterial blood gas (respiratory acidosis or alkalosis)
  - Blood urea nitrogen (BUN) and/or creatinine (renal infarction)
  - Creatinine kinase (CK) (rhabdomyolysis) and isoenzyme of creatine kinase (CK-MB) (MI)
  - Liver function tests (liver necrosis)
  - Urine dipstick (rhabdomyolysis)

IMAGING AND OTHER TESTS

- Plain films of the abdomen (supine and upright) can be useful in the diagnosis of body packing or stuffing of cocaine (swallowing or inserting packets of cocaine into a body orifice), but false-negative results may occur. Serial abdominal roentgenograms may be useful in detecting the passage of drug packages.[7]
- A chest X-ray and head computed tomography (CT) can be considered for respiratory and neurologic symptoms, respectively.

DIFFERENTIAL DIAGNOSIS

- Adrenal hyperplasia or adenoma—Produces excess cortisol, causing signs and symptoms of Cushing syndrome, including hypertension and emotional changes (ranging from irritability to severe depression and psychosis). Distinguishing features are increased body weight with adipose deposition in the upper face ("moon" facies) and interscapular area ("buffalo" hump), hirsutism, violaceous cutaneous striae, and proximal myopathy. A 24-hour urine test for free cortisol or overnight dexamethasone suppression test is recommended for diagnosis.
- Hyperthyroidism—In addition to tachycardia and nervousness/agitation, patients can report fatigue, weight loss, and heat intolerance.

Exophthalmus and pretibial myxedema may be seen, and laboratory testing reveals a low or undetectable thyroid-stimulating hormone (TSH) and an elevated free thyroxin level (T_4) (see Chapter 227, Hyperthyroidism).

- Delirium—Defined as a state of confusion accompanied by agitation, hallucinations, tremor, and illusions, delirium can be caused by drug toxicity or withdrawal, seizure, head injury, systemic infections, metabolic disorders, or a chronic dementing condition. The history, physical examination, and laboratory tests (many noted above) can help to identify the etiology.
- Hypoglycemia—Low blood sugar most commonly caused by taking insulin or oral drugs used to treat diabetes mellitus. Symptoms include confusion, fatigue, seizures, and loss of consciousness. Autonomic responses to hypoglycemia include palpitations, sweating, tremor, and anxiety. Laboratory testing for serum glucose will document the condition, and symptoms resolve with administration of oral or IV glucose.
- Meningitis—Acute infection within the subarachnoid space presenting within hours or days with fever, headache, and stiff neck (more than 90% of patients); additional potential signs are change in mental status (eg, confusion and decreased consciousness), seizures, increased intracranial pressure, and stroke. The appearance of rash/petechiae can aid in the diagnosis (meningococcemia). Diagnosis is made with examination of the CSF following lumbar puncture (LP).
- Encephalitis—Acute infection of the central nervous system that involves the brain parenchyma usually caused by viruses. The clinical features include fever, altered level of consciousness, and focal (eg, aphasia, ataxia, hemiparesis, and involuntary movements) or diffuse (eg, agitation, hallucinations, and personality change) symptoms. Diagnosis is established with examination of the CSF following LP.

MANAGEMENT

MANAGEMENT OF ACUTE OVERDOSE

Acute overdose is a medical emergency best managed in the intensive care unit because of the hyperadrenergic state and seizures.

- Hyperthermia and severe psychomotor agitation are the most immediately life-threatening complications of cocaine poisoning.[7] Temperatures as high as 45.6°C (114°F) have been recorded. Rapid physical cooling with sponging, fans, ice baths, and cooling blankets can be used and gastric or peritoneal lavage with iced saline is considered if persistent.
- IV diazepam up to 0.5 mg/kg given over 8 hours is used to control psychomotor agitation and seizures.
  - Hypertension may also respond to benzodiazepines. β-Blockers should not be used in the setting of cocaine toxicity (except to control ventricular arrhythmia, as below) because they may result in unopposed alpha effects of cocaine.[7]
  - Avoid the use of neuroleptic agents because they can interfere with heat dissipation and, perhaps, lower the seizure threshold.[7]
  - Avoid physical restraints if possible. Benzodiazepines are safe to use as a pharmacologic restraint.[7]
- Propranolol (0.5-1 mg IV) can be used to control ventricular arrhythmia.
  - Perform defibrillation in all patients with pulseless ventricular tachycardia.[7]
  - Consider electrical cardioversion in all unstable patients.[7]
  - β-blockers should not be used in cocaine-induced cardiac ischemia.[17] Nitroglycerin may be used for cocaine-induced cardiac ischemia or infarct.[7]
  - Monitor for rhabdomyolysis and provide rapid fluid resuscitation as needed.[7]
  - Check a pregnancy test on women of childbearing years as 6% of emergency room patients may have an unrecognized pregnancy.[7]
- Administer activated charcoal to alert patients with oral ingestions of cocaine (ie, body stuffers and body packers) to reduce absorption. Whole-bowel irrigation may be used to reduce transit time in these patients.[7]
- Medical providers should be prepared to manage multiple drug effects, especially heroin.

MANAGEMENT OF CHRONIC ADDICTION

Cognitive-behavioral therapy is effective in the treatment of cocaine-dependent outpatients.[18]

- There is no current evidence supporting the clinical use of carbamazepine, antidepressants, dopamine agonists, disulfiram, mazindol, phenytoin, nimodipine, lithium, and NeuRecover-SA in the treatment of cocaine dependence.[19]
- Antidepressant medication exerts a modest beneficial effect for patients with combined depressive and substance-use disorders, but should be used as part of a program to directly target the addiction.[20]
- The cocaine vaccine elicits an immune response that binds cocaine, creating an immune complex that is too large to cross the blood-brain barrier. In early phase II trials, 57% of subjects remained abstinent at 6 months. The immunologic treatment of substance use disorders is an exciting new approach that needs further study.[21]

REFERRAL

Referral to specialists may be needed to assist patients with upper respiratory tract (eg, CSF rhinorrhea and nasal septum perforation) or ophthalmologic complications (eg, central retinal artery occlusion).

- Following withdrawal from chronic cocaine use, patients may benefit from individual, group, and/or family therapy and peer assistance.[6]

PROGNOSIS

Cocaine addiction is difficult to treat.

- Of patients enrolled in cocaine addiction programs, 42% do not complete treatment.[22]
- One-third of patients treated for cocaine addiction remain abstinent.[22] Some comprehensive therapy programs have demonstrated abstinence rates at 1 year of up to 58%.[23]
- Of 131 persons addicted to crack cocaine, 107 were able to be followed for 12-years: 43 (33%) were crack-free for at least 12 months, 22 (17%) continued to use, 13 (10%) were imprisoned, 2 (1.5%) were lost to follow-up, and 27 (20.5%) were deceased.[24]

FOLLOW-UP

- Patients and their families may need ongoing support, home health care, and physical and occupational therapy to address long-term neurologic and cardiovascular complications of cocaine including anoxic encephalopathy, stroke, intracerebral hemorrhage, congestive heart failure, and cardiomyopathy.

- Physicians should closely monitor and assist patients in managing depression, insomnia, and anorexia that may follow cessation of chronic cocaine use.[6]
- Among individuals leaving residential detoxification, chronic pain is a common problem and is associated independently with long-term substance use after detoxification; management of pain may improve long-term outcomes.[25]

PATIENT EDUCATION

- Encourage patients to quit cocaine use and offer assistance.
- Recommend 12-step programs including cocaine anonymous.
- Patients should be made aware of the potential complications associated with use of cocaine, including its powerful psychologically addictive properties.
- Instruct patients about seeking help in the emergency department for any of the following[26]:
  - A brisk nosebleed that does not stop after 10 minutes of direct pressure
  - Facial pain or headache with a fever
  - Severe chest pain, difficulty breathing, or shortness of breath
  - If pregnant, vaginal bleeding or premature labor pains
  - Significant swelling, pain, redness, and red lines leading from the injection site and accompanied by fever
  - Severe abdominal pain, persistent vomiting, and vomiting blood
  - If you think that one of your packets you have swallowed or stuffed in a body orifice (vagina and rectum) is leaking or has broken
- Instruct IV drug users who continue to use not to reuse or share needles or syringes; cleaning the skin before injection can also decrease risk of infection. Harm reduction programs exist that help addicts obtain and maintain clean needles and syringes.

PATIENT RESOURCES

- eMedicineHealth. *Cocaine Abuse*—**http://www.emedicinehealth.com/cocaine_abuse/article_em.htm.**
- The Substance Abuse and Mental Health Services Administration (SAMHSA) provides an online resource for locating drug and alcohol abuse treatment programs—**http://findtreatment.samhsa.gov/TreatmentLocator/faces/quickSearch.jspx.**
- The SAMHSA referral helpline in English and Spanish—**1-800-662-HELP.**
- National Institute on Drug Abuse. *Preventing Drug Abuse among Children and Adolescents (In Brief)* [for parents]—**http://www.drugabuse.gov/prevention/prevopen.html.**
- Cocaine Anonymous (CA). Meetings are free. "Hope, Faith and Courage: Stories from the Fellowship of Cocaine Anonymous" now has a new second volume to go with the first volume – both can be ordered online—**http://www.ca.org/.**

PROVIDER RESOURCES

- National Institute on Drug Abuse. *Cocaine*—**http://www.nida.nih.gov/drugpages/cocaine.html.**
- MedlinePlus. *Cocaine*—**http://www.nlm.nih.gov/medlineplus/cocaine.html.**
- U.S. Drug Enforcement Administration. *Cocaine*—**http://www.usdoj.gov/dea/concern/cocaine.html.**

REFERENCES

1. Degenhardt L, Chiu WT, Sampson N, et al. Epidemiological patterns of extra-medical drug use in the United States: evidence from the National Comorbidity Survey Replication, 2001-2003. *Drug Alcohol Depend.* 2007;90(2-3):210-223.
2. National Survey on Drug Use and Health. *Substance Abuse and Mental Health Services Administration.* http://www.samhsa.gov. Accessed May 14, 2012.
3. Wagner FA, Anthony JC. Male–female differences in the risk of progression from first use to dependence upon cannabis, cocaine, and alcohol. *Drug Alcohol Depend.* 2007;86(2-3): 191-198.
4. Lejuez CW, Bornovalova MA, Reynolds EK, et al. Risk factors in the relationship between gender and crack/cocaine. *Exp Clin Psychopharmacol.* 2007;15(2):165-175.
5. Bierut LJ, Dinwiddie SH, Begleiter H, et al. Familial transmission of substance dependence: alcohol, marijuana, cocaine, and habitual smoking: a report from the Collaborative Study on the Genetics of Alcoholism. *Arch Gen Psychiatry.* 1998;55(11):982-988.
6. Mendelson JH, Mello NK. Cocaine and other commonly abused drugs. In: Kasper DL, Braunwald E, Fauci AS, Hauser SL, Longo DL, Jameson JL, eds. *Harrison's Principles of Internal Medicine.* 16th ed. New York, NY: McGraw-Hill; 2005:2570-2573.
7. Burnett LB. *Cocaine Toxicity in Emergency Medicine Treatment and Management.* http://emedicine.medscape.com/article/813959, updated Mar 19, 2010. Accessed May 14, 2012.
8. Kang SY, Magura S, Shapiro JL. Correlates of cocaine/crack use among inner-city incarcerated adolescents. *Am J Drug Alcohol Abuse.* 1994;20(4):413-429.
9. Bernstein KT, Bucciarelli A, Piper TM, et al. Cocaine- and opiate-related fatal overdose in New York City, 1990-2000. *BMC Public Health.* 2007;7:31.
10. Nyenwe EA, Loganathan RS, Blum S, et al. Active use of cocaine: an independent risk factor for recurrent diabetic ketoacidosis in a city hospital. *Endocr Pract.* 2007;13(1):22-29.
11. Chung C, Tumeh PC, Birnbaum R, et al. Characteristic purpura of the ears, vasculitis, and neutropenia—a potential public health epidemic associated with levamisole-adulterated cocaine. *J Am Acad Dermatol.* 2011;65:722-725.
12. Gross RL, Brucker J, Bahce-Altuntas A, et al. A novel cutaneous vasculitis syndrome induced by levamisole-contaminated cocaine. *Clin Rheumatol.* 2011;30:1385-1392.
13. Gulati S, Donato AA. Lupus anticoagulant and ANCA associated thrombotic vasculopathy due to cocaine contaminated with levamisole: a case report and review of the literature. *J Thromb Thrombolysis.* 2012;34(1):7-10.
14. Jenkins J, Babu K, Hsu-Hung E, et al. ANCA-positive necrotizing vasculitis and thrombotic vasculopathy induced by levamisole-adulterated cocaine: a distinctive clinicopathologic presentation. *J Am Acad Dermatol.* 2011;65:e14-e16.
15. Larocque A, Hoffman RS. Levamisole in cocaine: unexpected news from an old acquaintance. *Clin Toxicol (Phila).* 2012;50: 231-241.
16. Yacoubian GS Jr, Wish ED, Choyka JD. A comparison of the OnTrak Testcup-5 to laboratory urinalysis among arrestees. *J Psychoactive Drugs.* 2002;34(3):325-329.

17. Sen A, Fairbairn T, Levy F. Best evidence topic report. Beta-blockers in cocaine induced acute coronary syndrome. *Emerg Med J.* 2006;23(5):401-402.
18. Carroll KM, Onken LS. Behavioral therapies for drug abuse. *Am J Psychiatry.* 2005;162(8):1452-1460.
19. de Lima MS, de Oliveira Soares BG, Reisser AA, Farrell M. Pharmacological treatment of cocaine dependence: a systematic review. *Addiction.* 2002;97(8):931-949.
20. Nunes EX, Levin FR. Treatment of depression in patients with alcohol or other drug dependence: a meta-analysis. *JAMA.* 2004;291(15):1887-1896.
21. Shorter D, Kosten TR. Novel pharmacotherapeutic treatments for cocaine addiction. *EMC Med.* 2001;9:119.
22. Dutra L, Stathopoulou G, Basden SL, et al. A meta-analytic review of psychosocial interventions for substance use disorders. *Am J Psychiatry.* 2008;165:179-187.
23. Secades-Villa R, García-Rodríguez O, García-Fernández G, et al. Community reinforcement approach plus vouchers among cocaine-dependent outpatients: twelve-month outcomes. *Psychol Addict Behav.* 2011;25(1):174-179.
24. Dias AC, Araujo MR, Laranjeira R. Evolution of drug use in a cohort of treated crack cocaine users. *Rev Saude Publica.* 2011;45(5):938-948.
25. Larson MJ, Paasche-Orlow M, Cheng DM, et al. Persistent pain is associated with substance use after detoxification: a prospective cohort analysis. *Addiction.* 2007;102(5):752-760.
26. Dryden-Edwards R. Cocaine Abuse. http://www.emedicinehealth.com/cocaine_abuse/article_em.htm. Accessed July 19, 2014.

241 INJECTION-DRUG USE

Heidi Chumley, MD
Richard P. Usatine, MD

PATIENT STORY

A 23-year-old woman is seen for her intake physical in a residential treatment program for women recovering from substance abuse. She has not injected heroin for 2 days now, but her tracks are still visible (**Figure 241-1**). Her parents were both addicted to heroin, and she admits to having been born addicted to heroin herself. She began using heroin on her own in her early teens and has been on and off heroin since that time. She acknowledges a history of physical and sexual abuse as a child. She has had many suicide attempts and has cut herself with a knife across her arm many times. She has traded sex for money to buy heroin. Her 2 children are in foster care after having been removed by Child Protective Services. She is an attractive young woman looking for help and is thankful to have been admitted to this program. She does not know whether she has acquired hepatitis B, hepatitis C, or HIV, but wants to be tested.

INTRODUCTION

Injection-drug use affects millions of people across the world. Combinations of genetic, environmental, and behavioral factors influence risk of drug use and addiction. People who inject drugs often have other medical and psychiatric diagnoses, as well as social, legal, and vocational problems. Comprehensive management includes acute treatment and continuing care. Relapse is common, but involvement in a treatment program improves outcomes.

EPIDEMIOLOGY

- An estimated 16 million people inject drugs worldwide, based on data from 148 countries. The largest numbers of injectors are in China, the United States, and Russia.[1]

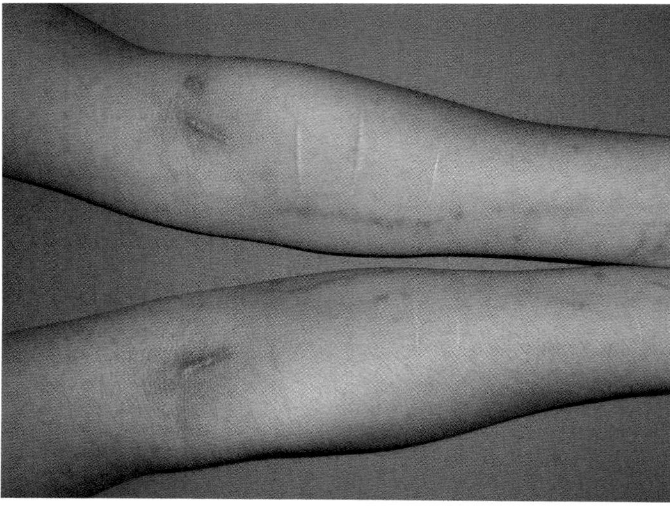

FIGURE 241-1 A 23-year-old woman with visible tracks on her arms from intravenous heroin use. She also has visible scars from self-mutilation with a knife. (*Reproduced with permission from Richard P. Usatine, MD.*)

- In the United States, injection-drug use among persons ages 15 to 29 years increased from 96 (1996) to 116 (2002) per 10,000 persons.[2]
- From 2000 to 2002, 1.5% of the US population older than the age of 12 years reported injection-drug use at any time; 0.19% reported injection-drug use within the last year—440,000 persons.[3]
- Prevalence was highest in persons ages 35 to 49 years (3.5%); higher in men than women (2.0% vs 1.0%); and higher in whites (1.7%) than African Americans (0.8%) or Hispanics (0.8%).[3]
- In 2002, the mean age of injection-drug users (IDUs) was 36 years compared to 21 years in 1979.[3]
- Needle sharing is common. In the previous 3 months, 46% of IDUs lent a person a used syringe[4] and 54% injected with a used syringe.[5]
- There were 27,8371-278,371 meant? substance-abuse treatment admissions for injection-drug use (14.2% of all admissions reported to Substance Abuse and Mental Health Services Administration's [SAMHSA] *Treatment Episode Data Set for 2009*).[6]
- The most commonly injected drug is heroin. Amphetamines, buprenorphine, benzodiazepines, cocaine, and barbiturates also are injected.[7]
- HIV prevalence among IDUs is estimated to be 20% to 40%.[1]
- The 2009 Monitoring the Future Survey showed that 2.5% of 12th-grade boys in the United States were using anabolic steroids (**Figure 241-2**).[8]
- Anabolic steroid abuse among athletes may range between 1% and 6%.[8]
- Some adolescents abuse steroids as part of a pattern of high-risk behaviors. These adolescents also take risks such as drinking and driving, carrying a gun, driving a motorcycle without a helmet, and abusing other illicit drugs.[8]

ETIOLOGY AND PATHOPHYSIOLOGY

- Drug use disorders are thought to be a result of combinations of multiple factors, including genetic, environmental, and individual risk-conferring behaviors.[9]
- Drug use alters the brain's structure and function. These changes persist after drug use stops.[10]

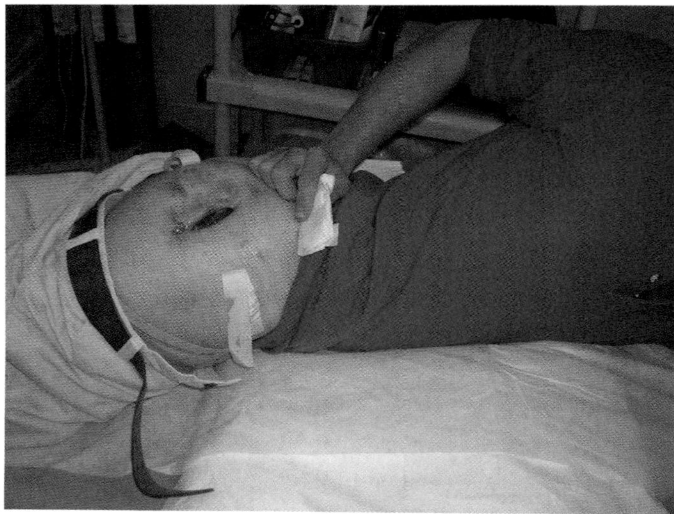

FIGURE 241-2 A high school athlete used injectable anabolic steroids for muscle building and developed a large abscess in his buttocks. This photograph was taken 2 months after the original abscess was drained and the wound is healing by secondary intention. (*Reproduced with permission from William Rodney, MD.*)

- Most injecting drug users inject drugs intravenously, but subcutaneous injection (skin-popping) also is common.[7]
- Injected, snorted, or smoked heroin causes an almost immediate "rush" or brief period of euphoria that wears off very quickly, terminating in a "crash." The user then experiences an intense craving to use more heroin to stop the crash and bring back the euphoria. The cycle of euphoria, crash, and craving—repeated several times a day—leads to a cycle of addiction.
- A heroin overdose can lead to death from respiratory depression, coma, and pulmonary edema. Death from the direct effects of cocaine is usually associated with cardiac dysrhythmias and conduction disturbances, leading to myocardial infarction (MI) and stroke.[7]
- Anabolic steroids can lead to early heart attacks, strokes, liver tumors, kidney failure, and serious psychiatric problems. In addition, because steroids are often injected, users who share needles or use nonsterile techniques when they inject steroids are at risk of contracting dangerous infections, such as HIV/AIDS and hepatitis B and hepatitis C (see **Figure 241-2**).[8]

RISK FACTORS

Family history

DIAGNOSIS

CLINICAL FEATURES

Heroin use produces the following clinical appearances:

- Pinpoint pupils and no response of pupils to light
- A rush of pleasurable feelings
- Cessation of physical pain
- Lethargy and drowsiness
- Slurred speech
- Shallow breathing
- Sweating
- Vomiting
- A drop in body temperature
- Sleepiness
- Loss of appetite

Cocaine (by injection) can produce the following signs, symptoms, and adverse effects:

- Dilated pupils
- Hyperactivity
- Euphoria
- Irritability and anxiety
- Excessive talking
- Depression or excessive sleeping
- Long periods without eating or sleeping
- Weight loss
- Dry mouth and nose
- Paranoia
- Cardiac—arrhythmias, chest pain, MI, and congestive heart failure (CHF)

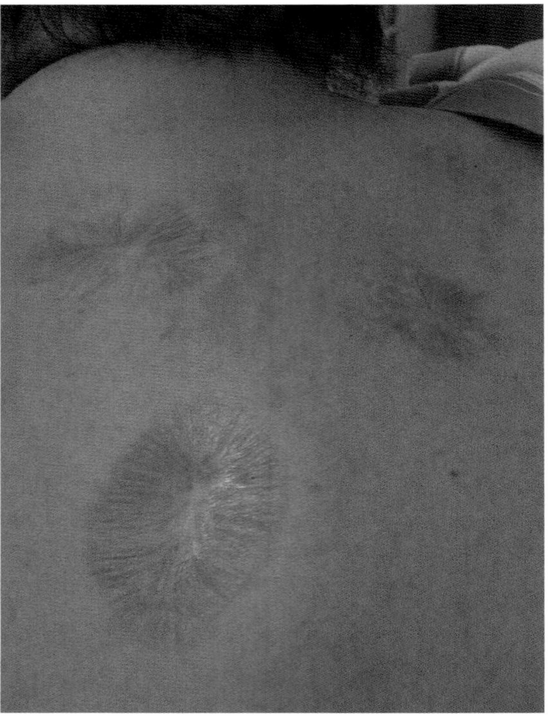

FIGURE 241-3 A 32-year-old woman with type 1 diabetes developed large abscesses all over her body secondary to injection of cocaine and heroin. Her back shows the large scars remaining after the healing of these abscesses. *(Reproduced with permission from Richard P. Usatine, MD.)*

- Strokes and seizures
- Respiratory failure

COMPLICATIONS OF INJECTING DRUG USE

- Local problems—Abscess (**Figures 241-2** and **241-3**; see Chapter 123, Abscess), cellulitis, septic thrombophlebitis, local induration, necrotizing fasciitis, gas gangrene, pyomyositis, mycotic aneurysm, compartmental syndromes, and foreign bodies (eg, broken needle parts) in local areas.[2]
    - IDUs are at higher risk of getting methicillin-resistant *Staphylococcus aureus* (MRSA) skin infections that the patient may think as spider bites (**Figure 241-4**).
    - Some IDUs give up trying to inject into their veins and put the cocaine directly into the skin. This causes local skin necrosis that produces round atrophic scars (**Figure 241-5**).
- IDUs are at risk for contracting systemic infections, including HIV and hepatitis B or hepatitis C.
    - Injecting drug users are at risk of endocarditis, osteomyelitis (**Figures 241-6** and **241-7**), and an abscess of the epidural region. These infections can lead to long hospitalizations for intravenous antibiotics. The endocarditis that occurs in IDUs involves the right-sided heart valves (see Chapter 47, Bacterial Endocarditis).[2] They are also at risk of septic emboli to the lungs, group A β-hemolytic streptococcal septicemia, septic arthritis, and candidal and other fungal infections.

LABORATORY TESTING

- All IDUs should be screened for HIV (with consent), hepatitis B, and hepatitis C.
- If there is a history of high-risk sexual behavior, screen for syphilis (rapid plasma reagin [RPR]), *Chlamydia*, and gonorrhea.

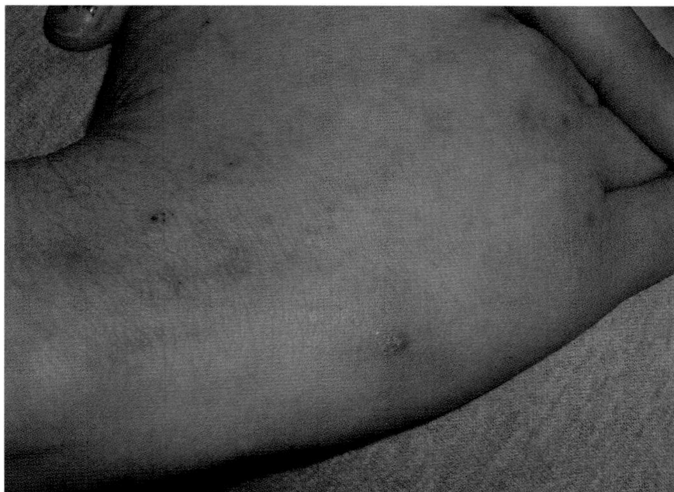

FIGURE 241-4 A young woman with methicillin-resistant *Staphylococcus aureus* (MRSA) infection from injection-drug use. Track visible on hand with pustule from MRSA. (*Reproduced with permission from Richard P. Usatine, MD.*)

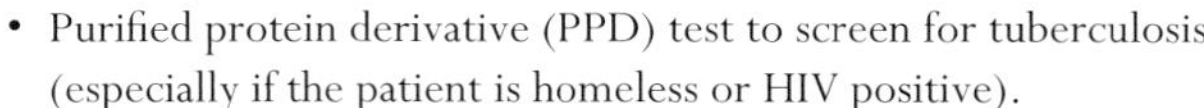

- Purified protein derivative (PPD) test to screen for tuberculosis (especially if the patient is homeless or HIV positive).
- Urine screen for common drugs of abuse may reveal other drugs not admitted to in the history.
- Electrocardiography (ECG) is warranted if there are any cardiac symptoms or if the physical examination reveals signs of cardiac disease.

DIFFERENTIAL DIAGNOSIS

Injection-drug use and dependence may be hidden problems. The differential diagnosis will differ based on the presenting complaints.

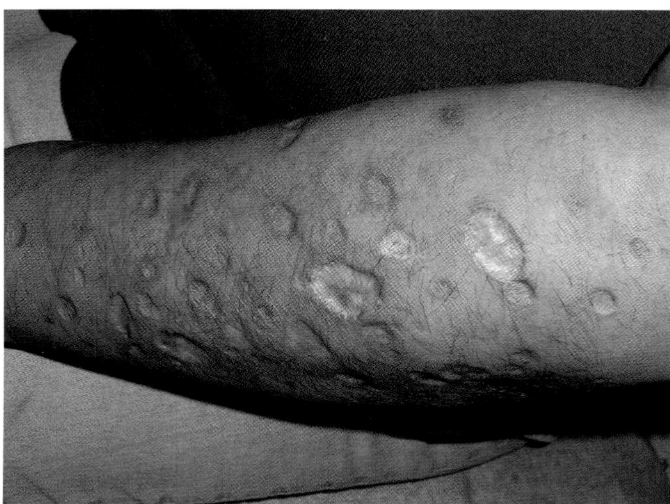

FIGURE 241-5 A young woman in residential treatment program with multiple scars from skin popping cocaine. She gave up trying to inject into her veins and put the cocaine directly into the skin. Note how the local skin necrosis caused round atrophic scars. (*Reproduced with permission from Richard P. Usatine, MD.*)

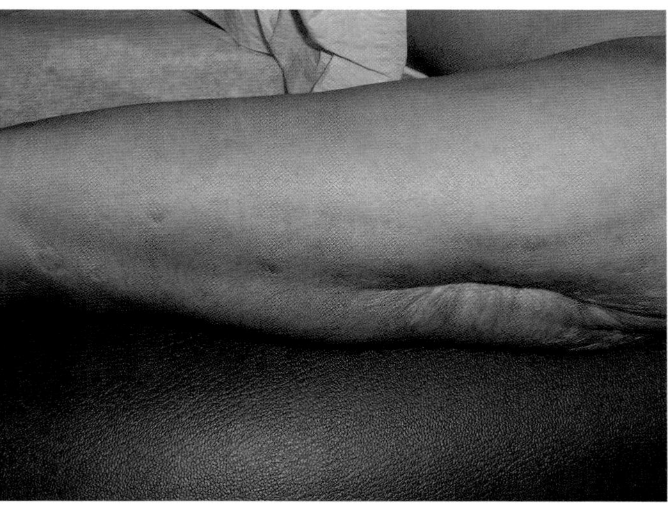

FIGURE 241-6 A 24-year-old woman with an 8-year history of injection-drug use. She has a large deep linear scar from osteomyelitis of the ulnar bone and smaller round scars from skin popping. A track is also visible above the deep scar. (*Reproduced with permission from Richard P. Usatine, MD.*)

MANAGEMENT

- Drug-abuse therapy is cost-effective. For example, 1 year of methadone maintenance therapy is approximately $4700 compared to 1 year of imprisonment, which costs $18,400.[10,11]
- Every $1 invested in addiction treatment saves $12 in health, legal, and theft costs.[10]

NONPHARMACOLOGIC

- Recognize addiction as a chronic illness that requires a comprehensive approach during the treatment phase (eg, residential/outpatient treatment) and continuing care (eg, drug-abuse monitoring, booster sessions, and reevaluation of treatment needs).[10]

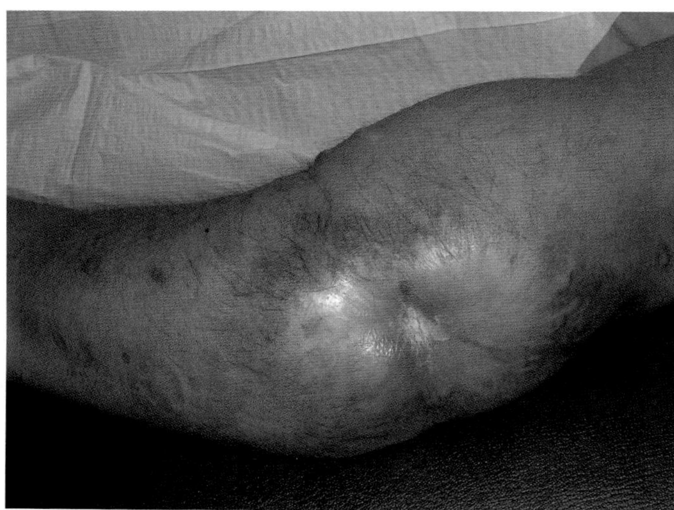

FIGURE 241-7 The other arm of the woman in **Figure 241-6** with deep scar from osteomyelitis secondary to injecting drugs that destroyed the bones in her left forearm. Her arm is deformed and poorly functional. (*Reproduced with permission from Richard P. Usatine, MD.*)

- Identify and address associated medical and psychiatric diagnoses, as well as social, legal, and work-related problems. Coexisting psychiatric illnesses are common.[10]
- For criminal justice-involved drug abusers and addicts, use this opportunity to engage individuals in treatment. Research supports the efficacy of combining criminal justice sanctions and drug-abuse treatment.[10]
- Test IDUs for HIV/AIDS, and hepatitis B and hepatitis C. Consider testing for tuberculosis and other infectious diseases as indicated.[10]
- Consider medically assisted detoxification to minimize withdrawal symptoms.
- Recommend an appropriate length of time for treatment. Most patients need at least 3 months to stop using drugs.[10]
- Encourage patients to engage in individual or group behavioral therapies and assist patients in finding programs that meet their individual needs.[10]
- Advise patients to join a self-help group, such as Narcotics Anonymous (NA) or Cocaine Anonymous (CA), which are based on the 12-step model. Most drug-addiction treatment programs encourage patients to participate in a self-help group during and after formal treatment.[6]

MEDICATIONS

- For opioid addiction, consider a methadone maintenance program.
  - Opioid replacement therapy reduces injecting drug use and thus reduces the mortality and morbidity associated with injecting drug use, including the transmission of HIV and hepatitis C virus (HCV).[7]
  - Opioid replacement combined with counseling, medical and psychiatric care, employment assistance, and family services is superior to opioid replacement alone.[10]
- Buprenorphine, a partial opioid agonist, is also used for opioid detoxification and for opioid replacement therapy.[7,10] In the United States, physicians who wish to prescribe buprenorphine must take a certification course.
- Naltrexone, a long-acting synthetic opioid antagonist, blocks opioid receptors, thereby preventing the effects of opioids. Treatment is initiated after patients have been opioid-free for several days to prevent a severe withdrawal.[10]
- Treating criminal justice-involved drug abusers and addicts—Drug abusers may come into contact with the criminal justice system earlier than with other health or social systems. Thus, the period of involvement with the criminal justice system may offer an opportunity to engage individuals in a treatment that can shorten a pattern of drug abuse and related crime. Research supports the efficacy of combining criminal justice sanctions and drug-abuse treatment.[11]
- Drug-abuse treatment is less expensive than alternatives, such as not treating addicts or incarcerating them. The average cost for 1 full year of methadone maintenance treatment is approximately $4700 per patient, whereas 1 full year of imprisonment costs approximately $18,400 per person. According to several conservative estimates, every $1 invested in addiction treatment programs yields up to $7 in savings, much of which results from reduced drug-related crime and criminal justice costs.[11] Although methadone maintenance is not as desirable as full abstinence, the comparative costs are in favor of drug treatment over incarceration.
- Recovery from drug addiction has 2 key components: treatment and continuing care. The clinical practices that make up the treatment phase (eg, residential/outpatient treatment) must be followed up by management of the disorder over time (eg, drug-abuse monitoring, booster sessions, and reevaluation of treatment needs).[11]
- Research shows that treatment must last, on average, at least 3 months to produce stable behavior change.[11] This accounts for the existence of 90-day residential treatment programs.
- A comprehensive assessment is the first step in the treatment process, and includes identifying individual strengths to facilitate treatment and recovery. In addition, drug abuse cannot be treated in isolation from related issues and potential threats, such as criminal behavior, mental health status, physical health, family functioning, employment status, homelessness, and HIV/AIDS.[11]
- Treatments that utilize cognitive behavioral therapies, residential treatment, contingency management, and medications have demonstrated effectiveness in reducing drug abuse and criminal behavior.[11]
- Medications are a key treatment component for drug abusers and can stabilize the brain and help return it to normal functioning. Methadone and buprenorphine are effective in helping individuals addicted to heroin or other opiates reduce their drug abuse. Naltrexone is also an effective medication for some opiate-addicted patients and those with concurrent alcohol dependence.[11]
- Family and friends can play critical roles in motivating individuals with drug problems to enter and stay in treatment. Family therapy is important, especially for adolescents. Involvement of a family member in an individual's treatment program can strengthen and extend the benefits of the program.[11]
- Buprenorphine (Subutex or, in combination with naloxone, Suboxone) is demonstrated to be a safe and acceptable addiction treatment. Congress passed the Drug Addiction Treatment Act (DATA 2000), permitting qualified physicians to prescribe narcotic medications (schedules III-V) for the treatment of opioid addiction. This legislation created a major paradigm shift by allowing access to opiate treatment in a medical setting rather than limiting it to specialized drug treatment clinics. Approximately 10,000 physicians have taken the training needed to prescribe these 2 medications, and nearly 7000 have registered as potential providers.
- Methadone and levo-α-acetyl methadol (LAAM) have more gradual onsets of action and longer half-lives than heroin. Patients stabilized on these medications do not experience the heroin rush. Both medications wear off much more slowly than heroin, so there is no sudden crash, and the brain and body are not exposed to the marked fluctuations seen with heroin use. Maintenance treatment with methadone or LAAM markedly reduces the desire for heroin.
- If an individual maintained on adequate, regular doses of methadone (once a day) or LAAM (several times per week) tries to take heroin, the euphoric effects of heroin will be significantly blocked. According to research, patients undergoing maintenance treatment do not suffer the medical abnormalities and behavioral destabilization that rapid fluctuations in drug levels cause in heroin addicts.

PREVENTION AND SCREENING

- The US Preventive Services Task Force concluded that there is insufficient evidence to screen for illicit drug use in adolescents, adults, or pregnant women, but advises clinicians to be alert for sign and symptoms of drug use.[12]

- Accurate and reliable office screening instruments include CRAFFT (adolescent drug use/misuse), and the ASSIST, CAGE-AID, and DAST (adults with drug misuse).[12]

PROGNOSIS

- Most patients who enter and remain in treatment stop injecting drugs and see improvements in their work, relationships, and psychological functioning.[10]
- Forty percent to 60% of patients relapse.[10]
- Drug injectors who do not enter treatment are up to 6 times more likely to become infected with HIV than are injectors who enter and remain in treatment. Drug users who enter and continue in treatment reduce activities that can spread disease, such as sharing injection equipment and engaging in unprotected sexual activity. Participation in treatment also presents opportunities for screening, counseling, and referral for additional services. The best drug-abuse treatment programs provide HIV counseling and offer HIV testing to their patients.[10]

FOLLOW-UP

Follow-up is important for the treatment of IDUs. Addiction is a chronic (and relapsing) condition and requires long-term follow-up. Your intervention and caring attitude can help the patient to overcome addiction and to live a sober and drug-free life. Do not give up on patients who relapse because it often takes more than one attempt before long-term cessation can be achieved. The frequency and intensity of follow-up depend on the substance, the addiction, and the patients and their complications.

PATIENT EDUCATION

- For patients who are not ready to stop their injecting drug use there are harm-reduction and counseling programs that can be helpful. Encourage patients to use clean and sterile needles and not to share their needles with anyone. Bleach can be used to clean and sterilize needles and prevent the spread of HIV and hepatitis.
- Refer continuing drug users to needle exchange programs that exist to help IDUs use clean needles and avoid infectious diseases. These programs can also be helpful if they give out condoms to encourage safe sex.
- Encourage patients to get help to become drug-free and abstinent. There is no safe level of injecting drug use.
- Explain to patients that addiction is a disease and not a failing of their moral character.
- Inform patients about the existing treatment programs in their community and offer them names and phone numbers so that they may get help.
- If your patient is not ready for help today, give the numbers and names for tomorrow.
- Speak about the value of 12-step programs including NA and CA because everyone can afford a 12-step program. There are 12-step programs in the community for everyone including nonsmokers and agnostics.

PATIENT RESOURCES

- Narcotics Anonymous. Provides information about meetings and literature in more than 40 different languages—**http://www.na.org/.**
- Cocaine Anonymous. Provides information about meetings and other resources—**http://www.ca.org/.**

PROVIDER RESOURCES

- OpioidRisk. *Substance Abuse Assessment Tools* (screening instruments for adults including the ASSIST, CAGE-AID, and DAST are available)—**http://www.opioidrisk.com/node/773.**
- The Center for Adolescent Substance Abuse Research. *The CRAFFT Screening Tool*—**http://www.ceasar-boston.org/clinicians/crafft.php.**
- The National Institute on Drug Abuse. *Medical Consequences of Drug Abuse*—**http://www.nida.nih.gov/consequences/.**
- Substance Abuse and Mental Health Services Administration. *Substance Abuse Treatment Facility Locator* (information on treatment programs in the United States)—**http://www.findtreatment.samhsa.gov.**

REFERENCES

1. Mathers BM, Degenhardt L, Phillips B, et al. Global epidemiology of injecting drug use and HIV among people who inject drugs: a systematic review. *Lancet.* 2008;372(9651):1733-1745.
2. Chatterjee A, Tempalski B, Pouget ER, et al. Changes in the prevalence of injection drug use among adolescents and young adults in large U.S. metropolitan areas. *AIDS Behav.* 2011;15(7):1570-1578.
3. Armstrong GL. Injection drug users in the United States, 1979-2002: an aging population. *Arch Intern Med.* 2007;167(2):166-173.
4. Golub ET, Strathdee SA, Bailey SL, et al; DUIT Study Team. Distributive syringe sharing among young adult injection drug users in five U.S. cities. *Drug Alcohol Depend.* 2007;91(suppl 1):S30-S38.
5. Bailey SL, Ouellet LJ, Mackesy-Amiti ME, et al. DUIT Study Team. Perceived risk, peer influences, and injection partner type predict receptive syringe sharing among young adult injection drug users in five U.S. cities. *Drug Alcohol Depend.* 2007;91(suppl 1):S18-S29.
6. Substance Abuse and Mental Health Services Administration. *Treatment Episode Data Set (TEDS). 1999-2009.* (National Admission to Substance Abuse Treatment Services, DASIS Series: S-56, HHS Publication No. 9SMA 11-4646.) Rockville, MD: Substance Abuse and Mental Health Services Administration; 2011.
7. Baciewicz GJ. *Injecting Drug Use.* Updated December 15, 2011. http://www.emedicine.com/med/topic586.htm. Accessed April 16, 2012.
8. Johnston LD, O'Malley PM, Bachman JG, Schulenberg JE. *Monitoring the Future: National Results on Adolescent Drug Use: Overview of Key*

Findings, 2009. (NIH Publication No. 10-7583). Bethesda, MD: National Institute on Drug Abuse.

9. Schulden JD, Thomas YF, Compton W. Substance abuse in the United States: findings from recent epidemiologic studies. *Curr Psychiatry Rep*. 2009;11(5):353-359.
10. National Institute on Drug Abuse. *Principles of Drug Addiction Treatment: A Research Based Guide*. 2nd ed. (NIH Publication No. 09-4180, revised April 2009.) Bethesda, MD: National Institutes of Health and U.S. Department of Health and Human Services; 2009.
11. *Principles of Drug Abuse Treatment for Criminal Justice Populations—A Research-Based Guide*. http://www.drugabuse.gov/drugpages/cj.html. Accessed May 6, 2012.
12. U.S. Preventive Services Task Force. *Screening for Illicit Drug Use*. http://www.uspreventiveservicestaskforce.org. Accessed April 16, 2012.

APPENDICES

Strength of Recommendation (SOR)	Definition
A	Recommendation based on consistent and good-quality patient-oriented evidence.*
B	Recommendation based on inconsistent or limited-quality patient-oriented evidence.*
C	Recommendation based on consensus, usual practice, opinion, disease-oriented evidence, or case series for studies of diagnosis, treatment, prevention, or screening.*

*See Appendix A on pages 1241-1244 for further information.

APPENDIX A INTERPRETING EVIDENCE-BASED MEDICINE

Mindy A. Smith, MD, MS

"Evidence-based medicine—is this something new?" asked my father, incredulously. "What were you practicing before?"

Like my father, our patients assume that we provide recommendations to them based on scientific evidence. The idea that there might not be relevant evidence or that we might not have access to that evidence has not even occurred to most of them. This is certainly not to imply that such evidence is the be-all and end-all of medical practice or that our patients would follow such recommendations blindly—rather, for me, it is a starting point from which to begin rational testing or outline a possible therapeutic plan.

The first time that I recall the term *evidence-based medicine* (EBM) being discussed was in the early 1990s.[1,2] It seemed that we would need to develop skills in evaluating the published literature and determining its quality, validity, and relevance to the care of our patients. As a teacher and researcher, I was intrigued by the challenges of critically appraising articles and teaching this newfound skill to others. As a clinician, however, I was most interested in answering clinical questions and doing so in a compressed time frame. I need rapid access to tools or sources that provided summary answers to those questions tagged to information about the quantity and quality of the evidence and the consistency of information across studies.

There seemed to be many systems for rating literature but few that met the needs of the busy practitioner trying to make sense of individual clinical trials and the hundreds of both evidence-based and consensus-based guidelines that seemed to spring up overnight. In 2004, the editors of the US family medicine and primary care journals and the Family Practice Inquiries Network published a paper on a unified taxonomy called *strength of recommendation* (SOR) taxonomy that seemed to fit the bill (**Figure A-1**).[3] This taxonomy made use of existing systems for judging study quality while incorporating the concept of patient-oriented (eg, mortality, morbidity, symptom improvement) rather than disease-oriented (eg, change in blood pressure, blood chemistry) outcomes as most relevant. SOR Ⓐ recommendation is one based on consistent, good-quality patient-oriented evidence; SOR Ⓑ is a recommendation based on inconsistent or limited-quality patient-oriented evidence; and SOR Ⓒ is a recommendation based on consensus, usual practice, opinion, disease-oriented evidence, or case series (**Figure A-1** and **A-2**).

In this book, we made a commitment to search for patient-oriented evidence to support the information that we provide in each of the chapter sections (ie, epidemiology, etiology and pathophysiology, risk factors, diagnosis, differential diagnosis, management, prevention, prognosis, and follow-up) and to provide a SOR rating for that evidence whenever possible. The bulleted format within these divisions would allow the practitioner to quickly find answers to their clinical questions while providing some direction about how confident we were that a recommendation had high-quality patient-oriented evidence to support it.

For example, a practitioner caring for a patient with severe chronic obstructive pulmonary disease (COPD) and frequent exacerbations who is already taking a combination long-acting β-agonist with an inhaled glucocorticoid asks, "What other options are available to reduce exacerbations?" This information can be found in the Management section of Chapter 56, Chronic Obstructive Pulmonary Disease, under Medications. Although the Global Initiative for Chronic Obstructive Lung Disease does not recommend mucolytics for routine use, authors of a Cochrane review, based on strong evidence SOR Ⓐ, concluded that these medications produce a small decrease in the frequency of exacerbations (0.5 fewer exacerbations/y) and in disability days.[4] Tiotropium (a long-acting anticholinergic) also reduces exacerbations and improves symptoms, but a recent meta-analysis concluded that mortality was increased with use of this medication SOR Ⓐ.[5] Theophylline also reduces exacerbations SOR Ⓑ but is associated with nausea. The physician armed with this information can discuss the options with this patient and explore potential benefits and risks. Particularly in difficult cases where there are multiple options, the clinician's experience and the patient preferences are important aspects of shared decision making. One definition of EBM is "The integration of best research evidence with clinical expertise and patient values."[6]

Several other concepts are used throughout the book that can assist practitioners in using evidence-based information and explaining that information to patients. Risk reductions from medical treatments are often presented in relative terms—the *relative risk reduction* (RRR) or the difference in the percentage of adverse outcomes between the intervention group and the control group divided by the percentage of adverse outcomes in the control group. These numbers are often large and use of them not only causes us to overestimate the importance of a treatment but misses its clinical relevance. A more meaningful term is the *absolute risk reduction* (ARR)—the risk difference between the 2 groups. This number can then be used to obtain a *number needed to treat* (NNT)—the number of patients that would need to be treated (over the same time as used in the treatment trial) to prevent 1 bad outcome or produce 1 good outcome. This is calculated as 100% divided by the ARR. NNT is more easily understood by us and our patients. See the NNT example in **Box A-1**.

In the above case, for example, the patient might ask how risky it could be to add tiotropium. As written in the chapter, the difference in death with use of this medication was 0.8% (2.4% vs 1.6% on placebo) making the number needed to harm (NNH) over 1 year to be equal to 124 (for every 124 patients treated, 1 additional death might occur in 1 year).

Another term that is used in this book is the *likelihood ratio* (LR). This number, based on the sensitivity and specificity of a diagnostic test, is used to determine the probability of a patient with a positive test (LR+) having the disease or the probability of the patient with a negative test (LR+) not having the disease in question. The LR is defined as the likelihood that a given test result would be expected in a patient with the target disorder compared to the likelihood that the same result would be expected in a patient without the target disorder.[6] The number obtained for the LR+ [sensitivity/(100 – specificity)] or the LR– [(100 – sensitivity)/specificity] can be multiplied by the pretest probability of disease to determine the posttest probability of disease. A nomogram (one can be found by visiting the website mentioned in Reference 6) can be used to more easily work with these numbers to convert a pretest probability into a posttest probability. A LR+ over 10 is considered strong evidence to rule in disease while a LR– of less than 0.1 is strong evidence to rule out disease.

We both are privileged and cursed with practicing medicine in an information-rich environment. We have designed our *Color Atlas* to link evidence to clinical recommendations so that we can provide our patients the best science available. When the evidence is lacking, we make that clear and encourage you to engage in frank and honest discussions that lead to the shared responsibility for decisions. Our patients are justified in expecting science along with humanism—can we give them anything less?

How recommendations are graded for strength, and underlying individual studies are rated for quality

In general, only key recommendations for readers require a grade of the "Strength of Recommendation." Recommendations should be based on the highest quality evidence available. For example, vitamin E was found in some cohort studies (level 2 study quality) to have a benefit for cardiovascular protection, but good-quality randomized trials (level 1) have not confirmed this effect. Therefore, it is preferable to base clinical recommendations in a manuscript on the level 1 studies.

Strength of recommendation	Definition
A	Recommendation based on consistent and good-quality patient-oriented evidence.*
B	Recommendation based on inconsistent or limited-quality patient-oriented evidence.*
C	Recommendation based on consensus, usual practice, opinion, disease-oriented evidence,* or case series for studies of diagnosis, treatment, prevention, or screening

Use the following scheme to determine whether a study measuring patient-oriented outcomes is of good or limited quality, and whether the results are consistent or inconsistent between studies.

	Type of Study		
Study quality	**Diagnosis**	**Treatment/prevention/ screening**	**Prognosis**
Level 1— good-quality patient-oriented evidence	Validated clinical decision rule SR/meta-analysis of high-quality studies High-quality diagnostic cohort study†	SR/meta-analysis of RCTs with consistent findings High-quality individual RCT‡ All-or-none study§	SR/meta-analysis of good-quality cohort studies Prospective cohort study with good follow-up
Level 2— limited-quality patient-oriented evidence	Unvalidated clinical decision rule SR/meta-analysis of lower-quality studies or studies with inconsistent findings Lower-quality diagnostic cohort study or diagnostic case-control study§	SR/meta-analysis lower-quality clinical trials or of studies with inconsistent findings Lower-quality clinical trial‡ or prospective cohort study Cohort study Case-control study	SR/meta-analysis of lower-quality cohort studies or with inconsistent results Retrospective cohort study with poor follow-up Case-control study Case series
Level 3— other evidence	Consensus guidelines, extrapolations from bench research, usual practice, opinion, other evidence disease-oriented evidence (intermediate or physiologic outcomes only), or case series for studies of diagnosis, treatment, prevention, or screening		

Consistency across studies

Consistent	Most studies found similar or at least coherent conclusions (coherence means that differences are explainable); ***or*** If high-quality and up-to-date systematic reviews or meta-analyses exist, they support the recommendation
Inconsistent	Considerable variation among study findings and lack of coherence; ***or*** If high-quality and up-to-date systematic reviews or meta-analyses exist, they do not find consistent evidence in favor of the recommendation

*Patient-oriented evidence measures outcomes that matter to patients: morbidity, mortality, symptom improvement, cost reduction, and quality of life. Disease-oriented evidence measures intermediate, physiologic, or surrogate end points that may or may not reflect improvements in patient outcomes (ie, blood pressure, blood chemistry, physiologic function, and pathologic findings).

† High-quality diagnostic cohort study: cohort design, adequate size, adequate spectrum of patients, blinding, and a consistent, well-defined reference standard.

‡ High-quality RCT: allocation concealed, blinding if possible, intention-to-treat analysis, adequate statistical power, adequate follow-up (greater than 80 percent).

§ In an all-or-none study, the treatment causes a dramatic change in outcomes, such as antibiotics for meningitis or surgery for appendicitis, which precludes study in a controlled trial.

SR, systematic review; RCT, randomized controlled trial

FIGURE A-1 *(Reproduced with permission from Ebell MH, Siwek J, Weiss BD, et al. Simplifying the language of evidence to improve patient care: strength of recommendation taxonomy (SORT).* J Fam Pract. 2004;53(2):110-120. Dowden Health Media.)

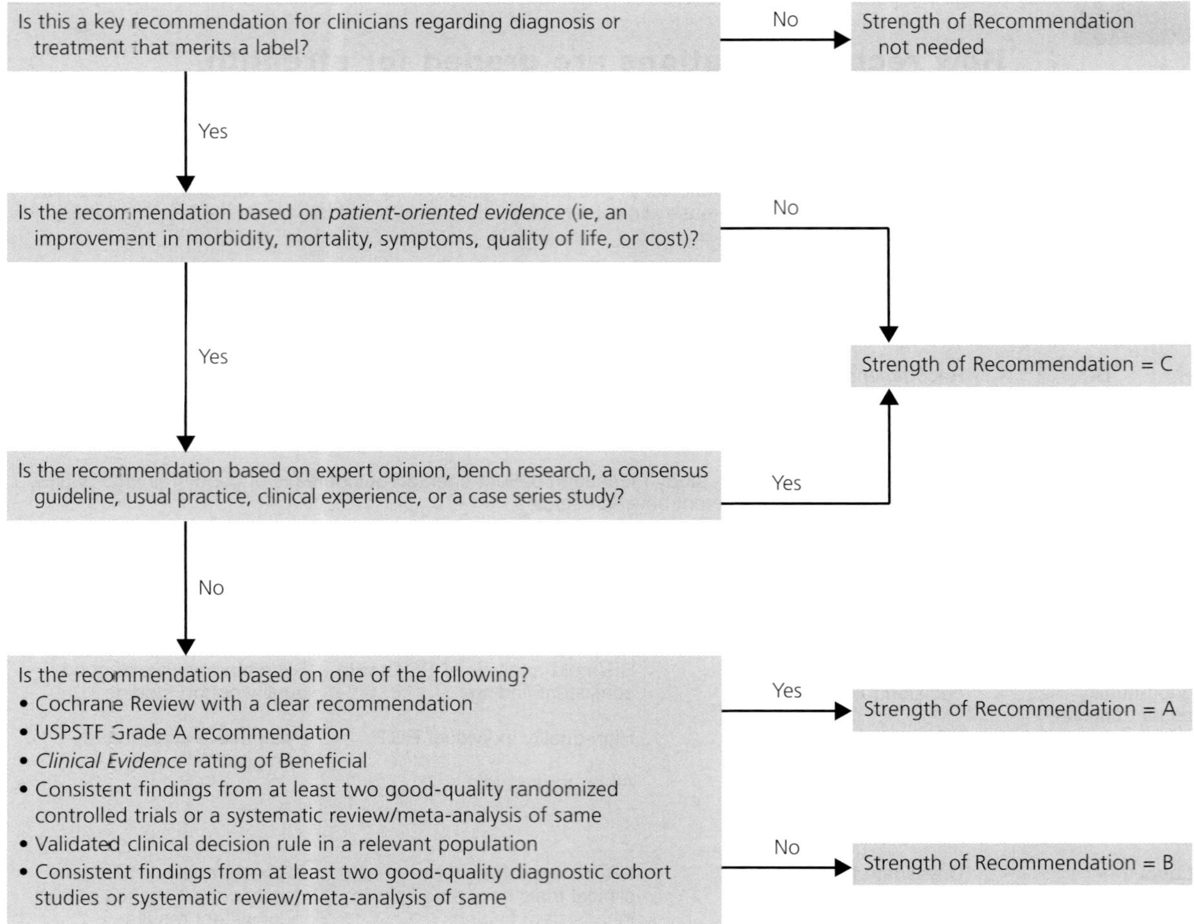

FIGURE A-2 Assigning a strength-of-recommendation grade based on a body of evidence. (USPSTF = US Preventive Services Task Force.) (*Reproduced with permission from Ebell MH, Siwek J, Weiss BD, et al. Simplifying the language of evidence to improve patient care: strength of recommendation taxonomy (SORT).* J Fam Pract. *2004;53(2):110-120.* Dowden Health Media.)

BOX A-1 NNT Example

If a new drug was released for the treatment of postherpetic neuralgia and a randomized controlled trial found that the 70% of the treated group reported significant pain control (based on the defined end point) and 20% of the placebo group reported significant pain control this would produce an absolute risk reduction (ARR) of 50%. In this case the NNT would be 100%/50% = 2. On average, only 2 patients would need to be treated for 1 patient to receive the defined pain control benefit. If the ARR was only 10% (30% of the intervention group and 20% of the control group benefitted), then the NNT = 10 or 10 patients would need treatment on average for 1 to receive benefit.

REFERENCES

1. Evidence-Based Medicine Working Group. Evidence-based medicine. A new approach to teaching the practice of medicine. *JAMA*. 1992;268:2420-2425.
2. Shaughnessy AF, Slawson DC, Bennett JH. Becoming an information master: a guidebook to the medical information jungle. *J Fam Pract*. 1994;39:489-499.
3. Ebell MA, Siwek J, Weiss BD, et al. Strength of Recommendation Taxonomy (SORT): a patient-centered approach to grading evidence in the medical literature. *J Fam Pract*. 2004 Feb; 53(2):111-120.
4. Poole P, Black PN. Mucolytic agents for chronic bronchitis or chronic obstructive pulmonary disease. *Cochrane Database Syst Rev*. 2010;(2):CD001287.
5. Singh S, Loke YK, Enright PL, Furberg CD. Mortality associated with tiotropium mist inhaler in patients with chronic obstructive pulmonary disease: systematic review and meta-analysis of randomised controlled trials. *BMJ*. 2011;342:d3215.
6. Center for Evidence-Based Medicine. http://www.cebm.net/category/ebm-resources/. Accessed July 19, 2014.

APPENDIX B GUIDE FOR THE USE OF TOPICAL AND INTRALESIONAL CORTICOSTEROIDS

TABLE B-1 Corticosteroid Potency Chart

Generic Name	Trade Name and Strength
Class 1—Superpotent	
Betamethasone dipropionate*	Diprolene ointment 0.05%
Diflorasone diacetate**	Psorcon ointment, 0.05%
Clobetasol propionate	Temovate cream, gel, ointment, shampoo, spray, or foam, 0.05%; also as Cormax, Clobex, Clarelux, Olux
Halobetasol propionate*	Ultravate cream/ointment, 0.05%
Class 2—Potent	
Amcinonide	Cyclocort cream/ointment/lotion, 0.1%
Betamethasone dipropionate	Diprosone ointment, 0.05%
Desoximetasone	Topicort cream 0.25%, gel 0.05%, and ointment 0.25%
Diflorasone diacetate**	Psorcon, ApexiCon ointment 0.05%
Fluocinonide	Lidex, Lidemol, Lyderm, Tiamol, Topactin, Topsyn, Vanos cream 0.05%, 0.1%/ointment/gel, 0.05%
Halcinonide	Halog cream/ointment/topical solution, 0.1%
Class 3—Upper mid-strength	
Betamethasone valerate*	Diprolene, Luxiq, Dermabet, Alphatrex, Diprolene AF, Diprolene Glycol, Diprosone, Valnac, BetaVal cream/lotion 0.05% or 0.1%, foam 0.12%
Diflorasone diacetate**	Psorcon, ApexiCon, ApexiCon E cream 0.05%
Mometasone furoate	Elocon cream/lotion/ointment, 0.1%
Triamcinolone acetonide	Kenalog topical, Pediaderm, Triacet, Trianex cream, 0.5%
Class 4—Mid-strength	
Desoximetasone	Topicort LP cream, 0.05%
Fluocinolone acetonide	Synalar-HP cream, 0.2%; Synalar ointment, 0.025%
Flurandrenolide	Cordran ointment, 0.05%
Triamcinolone acetonide	Aristocort, Kenalog ointments, 0.1%
Class 5—Lower mid-strength	
Betamethasone dipropionate	Diprosone lotion, 0.05%
Betamethasone valerate	Valisone cream, 0.1%; Betatrex 0.1%
Fluocinolone acetonide	Synalar cream, 0.025%
Flurandrenolide	Cordran cream, 0.05%
Hydrocortisone butyrate	Locoid cream, 0.1%
Hydrocortisone valerate	Westcort cream, 0.2%
Prednicarbate	Dermatop cream/ointment, 0.1%
Triamcinolone acetonide	Kenalog cream/lotion, 0.1%

(continued)

TABLE B-1 Corticosteroid Potency Chart (*Continued*)

Generic Name	Trade Name and Strength
Class 6—Mild	
Alclometasone dipropionate	Aclovate cream/ointment, 0.05%
Triamcinolone acetonide	Aristocort cream, 0.1%
Desonide	Desonate, DesOwen, Tridesilon, Verdeso cream/lotion/ointment 0.05%, foam 0.05%, gel, 0.05%, 0.05%
Fluocinolone acetonide	Synalar cream/solution, 0.01%; Capex shampoo, Dermasmooth, 0.01%
Betamethasone valerate	Valisone lotion, 0.1%
Class 7—Least potent	
Hydrocortisone	Hyton, Cortate, Unicort, other OTC cream/lotion/foam

*<12 years old, not recommended.
**Safety and efficacy not established in pediatric patients.

TABLE B-2 Common Side Effects of Topical Corticosteroids

Skin atrophy	Most common adverse effect
	Epidermal thinning may begin after only a few days
	Dermal thinning usually takes several weeks to develop
	Usually reversible within 2 mo after stopping the corticosteroid
Telangiectasia	Most often occurs on the face, neck, and upper chest
	Tends to decrease when steroid discontinued, but may be irreversible
Striae	Usually occur around flexures (groin, axillary, and inner thigh areas)
	Usually permanent, but may fade with time
Purpura	Frequently occurs after minimal trauma
	Attributed to loss of perivascular supporting tissue in the dermis
Hypopigmentation	Reversible upon discontinuing the corticosteroid
Acneform eruptions	Particularly common on the face, especially with the "potent" and "very potent" corticosteroids
	Usually reversible
Fine hair growth	Reversible upon discontinuation of the corticosteroid
Infections	May worsen viral, bacterial, or fungal skin infections
	May cause tinea incognito
Hypothalamic-pituitary-adrenal axis suppression	Rare with topicals
	>30 g/wk of "very potent" corticosteroids should be limited to 3-4 wk
	Children (>10 g/wk) and elderly are at higher risk because of thinner skin

TABLE B-3 Intralesional Steroids—Concentrations for Injection

Condition	Concentration of Triamcinolone Acetonide Solution (mg/cc)
Acne (**Figure B-1**)	2-2.5
Alopecia areata (**Figure B-2**)	5-10
Granuloma annulare	5-10
Psoriasis	5-10
Hypertrophic lichen planus	5-10
Prurigo nodularis	10
Hidradenitis suppurativa	10
Keloids and Hypertrophic Scars (**Figure B-3**)	10-40

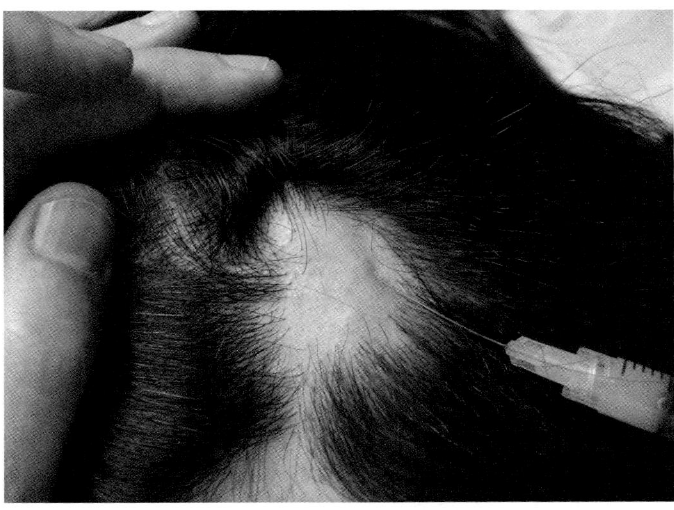

FIGURE B-2 Injecting alopecia areata with 5 mg/mL triamcinolone using a 27-gauge needle on a Luer-Lok syringe. (*Reproduced with permission from Richard P. Usatine, MD.*)

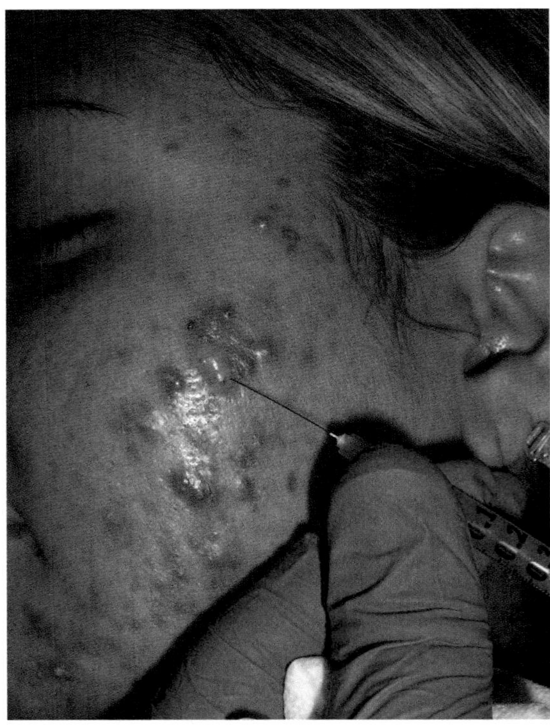

FIGURE B-1 Injecting painful cystic acne with 2 mg/mL triamcinolone using a 30-gauge needle. (*Reproduced with permission from Richard P. Usatine, MD.*)

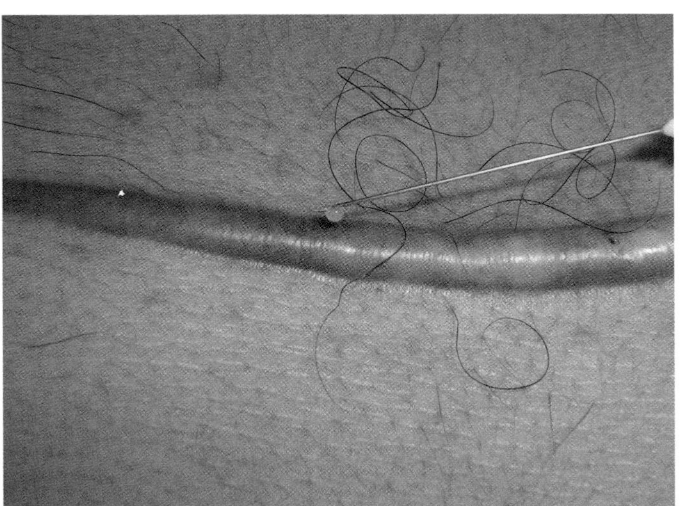

FIGURE B-3 Injecting a hypertrophic scar with 10 mg/mL triamcinolone using a 27-gauge needle on a Luer-Lok syringe. (*Reproduced with permission from Richard P. Usatine, MD.*)

APPENDIX C DERMOSCOPY

Ashfaq A. Marghoob, MD
Natalia Jaimes, MD
Richard P. Usatine, MD

Dermoscopy allows the clinician to visualize structures below the level of the stratum corneum. These structures are not routinely discernible without dermoscopy. The presence or absence of specific dermoscopic structures, their location and their distribution can assist the clinician in making a diagnosis or at least in narrowing the differential diagnosis.

The major goal of dermoscopy is to differentiate benign from malignant lesions on the skin so that one is less likely to miss a skin cancer (higher sensitivity) and less likely to perform unnecessary biopsies (higher specificity). Together, this will increase your diagnostic accuracy.

There are 3 major types of dermatoscopes:

1. Polarized
2. Nonpolarized
3. Hybrid, which combines a polarized mode with a nonpolarized mode in one dermatoscope

Because some structures are better seen under polarized light and others best seen without polarization is helpful to purchase a hybrid dermatoscope. Dermatoscopes are currently manufactured by 3Gen, Welch Allyn, Canfield, and Heine (**Figures C-1** and **C-2**). A number of dermatoscopes work well while attached to the iPhone for easy image capture and full screen images that can be shown to the patients.

Dermoscopic diagnosis is based on the 2-step dermoscopy algorithm described in **Figure C-3**.

Step 1 requires the observer to decide whether the lesion in question is of melanocytic origin (contains melanocytes and therefore could be a melanoma). If the lesion is deemed to be a melanocytic lesion then the observer proceeds to step 2. In this phase of the evaluation, the observer needs to decide whether the lesion is a benign nevus or a melanoma. However, if during step 1 analysis the lesion does not display any features of a melanocytic lesion then the observer needs to decide if the lesion possesses any criteria for a basal cell carcinoma, seborrheic keratosis, hemangioma, or dermatofibroma. If the lesion does not display any structures common to the aforementioned lesions then the lesion is considered nondescript or featureless. The index of suspicion needs to remain high for all featureless lesions as amelanotic melanoma can present as a completely structureless lesion. These featureless lesions sometimes do reveal blood vessels and, if present, their morphology can often help in narrowing the differential diagnosis.

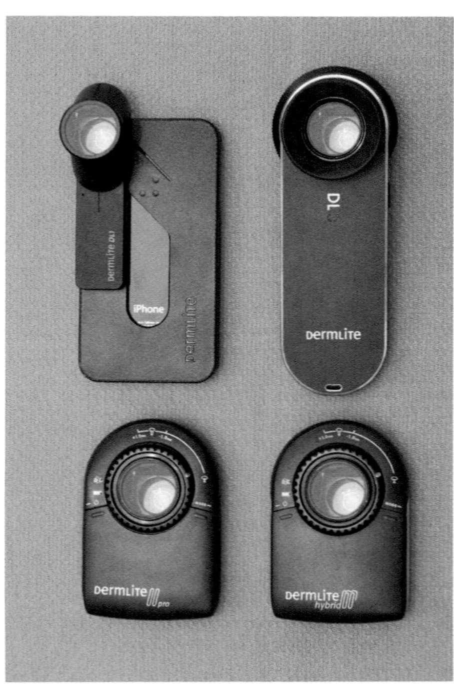

FIGURE C-1 An assortment of polarized and hybrid dermatoscopes from 3Gen. (*Reproduced with permission from Richard P. Usatine, MD and 3Gen, San Juan Capistrano, CA.*)

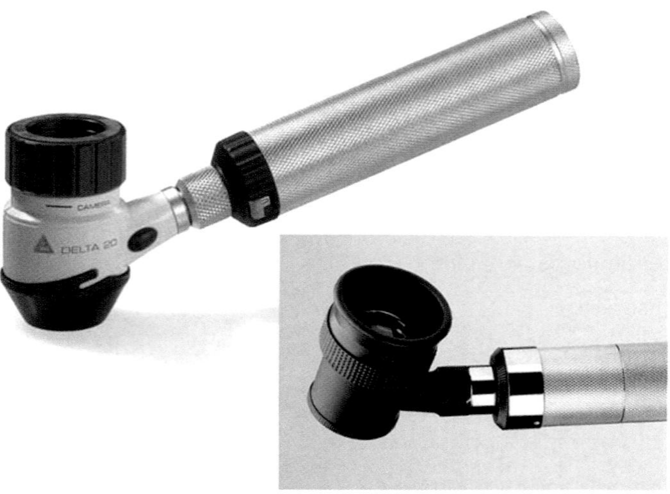

FIGURE C-2 Nonpolarized contact dermatoscopes from Heine and Welch-Allyn. (*Reproduced with permission from Heine, Herrsching, Germany, and Welch Allyn, Skaneateles Falls, NY.*)

STEP 1—LEVEL 1

A melanocytic lesion usually will display one of the following structures:

1. Pigment network (**Figure C-4**).
2. Negative network (**Figure C-5**).
3. Streaks (**Figure C-6**).

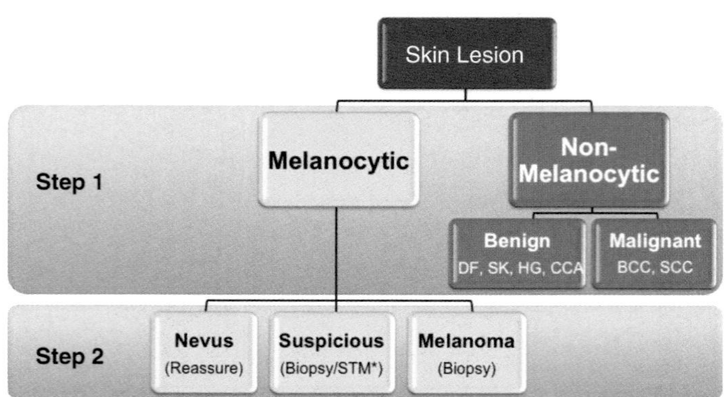

FIGURE C-3 Two-step diagnostic procedure requires separating all lesions into melanocytic or nonmelanocytic as step. BCC, basal cell carcinoma; CCA, clear-cell acanthoma; DF, dermatofibroma; HG, hemangioma; SCC, squamous cell carcinoma; SK, seborrheic keratosis; STM, Short term monitoring. *Never monitor palpable lesions.

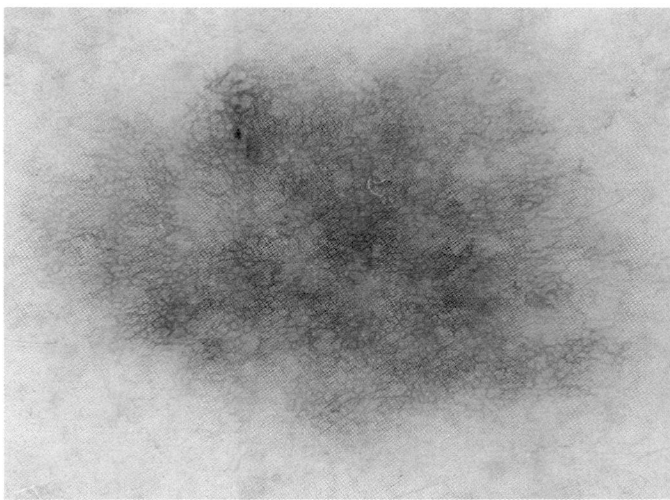

FIGURE C-4 Pigment network tells us this benign nevus is a melanocytic lesion in step 1 of the 2-step algorithm, that is, it contains melanocytes. (*Reproduced with permission from Ashfaq Marghoob, MD.*)

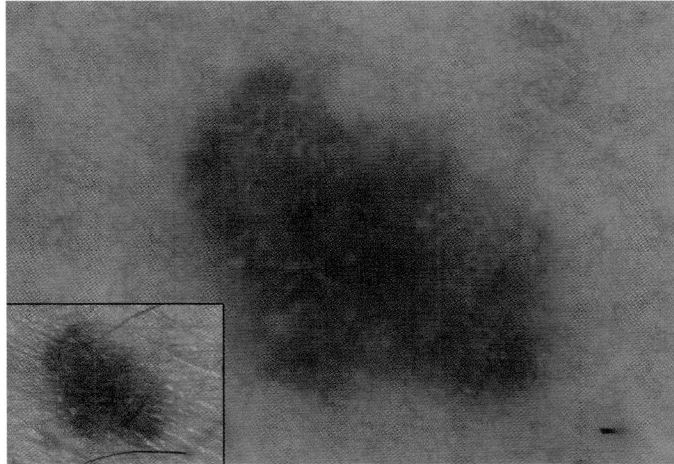

FIGURE C-5 Negative network informs us that this microinvasive melanoma is a melanocytic lesion. The negative network consists of dark, elongated, and curved globular structures surrounded by relative hypopigmentation. (*Reproduced with permission from Ashfaq Marghoob, MD.*)

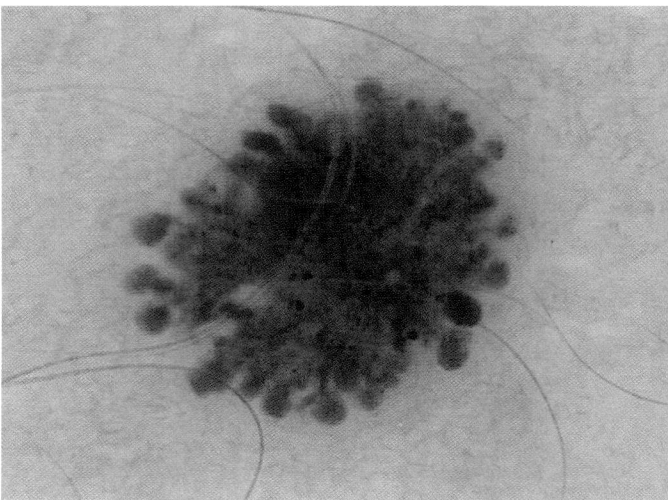

FIGURE C-6 Streaks of the pseudopod type inform us that this is a melanocytic lesion. The 360-degree symmetry is typical in a Spitz nevus. (*Reproduced with permission from Ashfaq Marghoob, MD.*)

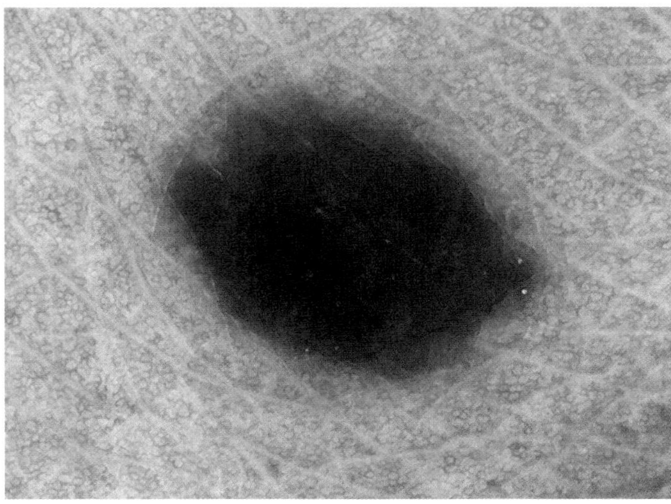

FIGURE C-7 Homogeneous blue pigmentation is a feature of a melanocytic lesion of the blue nevus type. (*Reproduced with permission from Richard P. Usatine, MD.*)

4. Homogeneous blue pigmentation (**Figure C-7**).
5. Aggregated globules (**Figure C-8**).
6. Pseudonetwork (facial skin) (**Figure C-9**).
7. Parallel pigment pattern (acral lesions) (**Figure C-10**).
8. There is one exception to including lesions with pigment network in the melanocytic category, that is, the dermatofibroma in which the pattern trumps the network (**Figure C-11**).

This lesion does not display any of the structures commonly seen in melanocytic lesions (ie, network, streaks, globules). It also does not have any features of a basal cell carcinoma, seborrheic keratosis, dermatofibroma, or hemangioma. Thus, this is a featureless lesion. However, it does display many irregular tortuous blood vessels, which may be a sign of neoangiogenesis. The possibility of melanoma needs to be entertained for such featureless lesion.

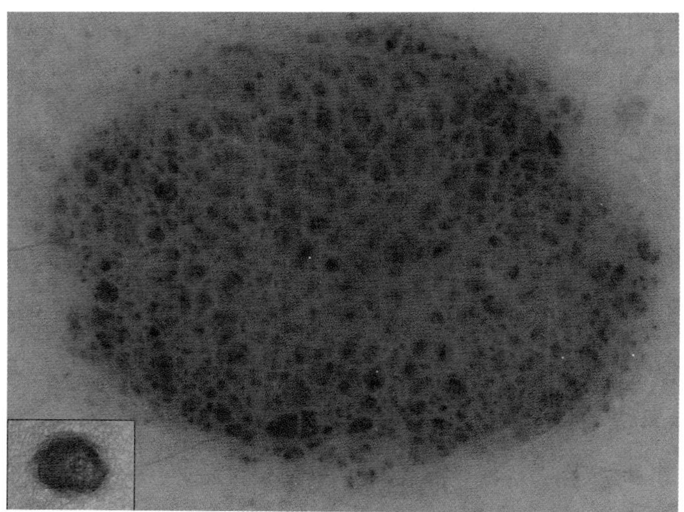

FIGURE C-8 Aggregated globules inform us that this benign nevus is melanocytic. (*Reproduced with permission from Ashfaq Marghoob, MD.*)

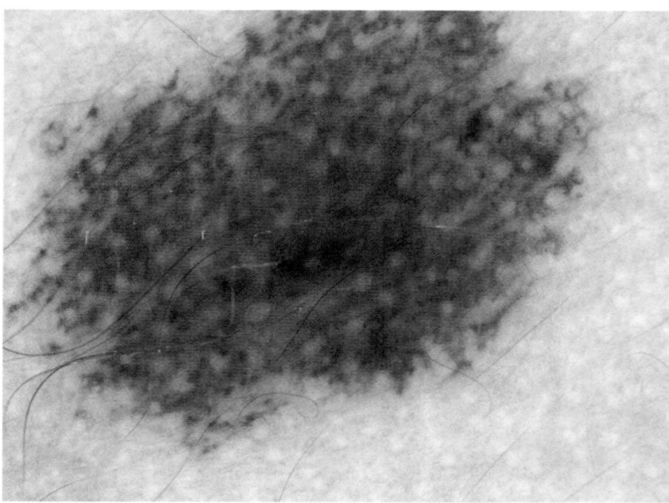

A

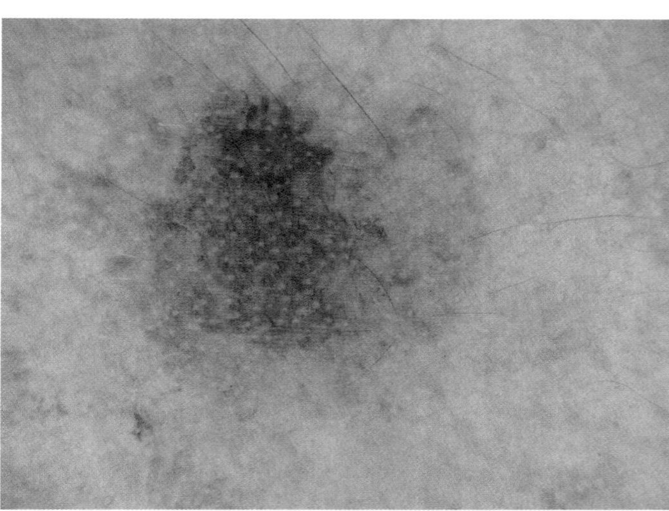

B

FIGURE C-9 Pseudonetwork is the net-like pattern made by white adnexal openings on the face within any pigmented lesion. **A.** Pseudonetwork pattern is seen on the face in this congenital nevus that is melanocytic. **B.** Although this solar lentigo also has a pseudonetwork pattern created by white adnexal openings it is not melanocytic. It does have a typical moth-eaten border found in solar lentigines and seborrheic keratoses. (*Reproduced with permission from Richard P. Usatine, MD.*)

STEP 2

If the lesion is deemed to be of melanocytic origin, then one needs to decide whether the lesion is a benign nevus or a melanoma.

Nevi tend to manifest one of the following 10 benign patterns (**Figure C-12**)

1. Diffuse reticular (**Figure C-13**)
2. Patchy reticular (**Figure C-14**)
3. Peripheral reticular with central hypopigmentation (**Figure C-15**)
4. Peripheral reticular with central hyperpigmentation (**Figure C-16**)
5. Homogeneous (**Figure C-17**)
6. Peripheral globules/starburst (**Figure C-18**)

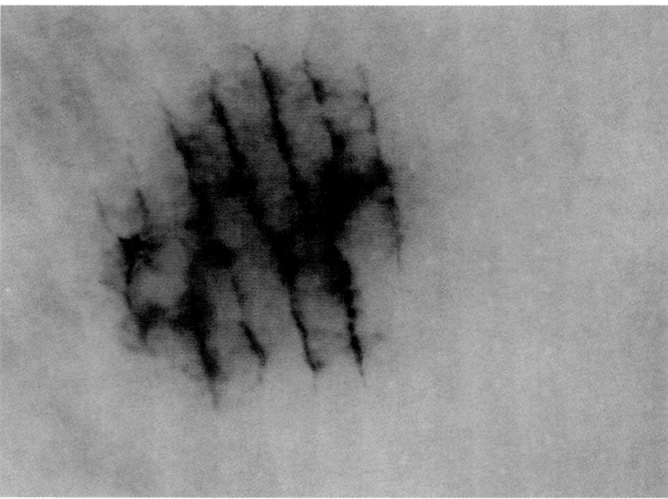

FIGURE C-10 Nevus on the sole of the foot showing parallel network pigment in the furrows (valleys) rather than the ridges. Note the white eccrine gland openings on the ridges which are wider than the furrows. (*Reproduced with permission from Richard P. Usatine, MD.*)

7. Peripheral reticular with central globules (**Figure C-19**)
8. Globular (**Figure C-20**)
9. Two-component (**Figure C-21**)
10. Symmetric multicomponent (note this pattern should be interpreted with caution and a biopsy is probably warranted for dermoscopic novices) (**Figure C-22**)

In contrast, melanomas tend to deviate from the benign pattern described earlier. Furthermore, the structures in a melanoma are often distributed in an asymmetric fashion. Most melanomas will also reveal one or more of the melanoma-specific structures (**Figure C-23**).

MELANOMA-SPECIFIC STRUCTURES

1. Atypical network (**Figure C-24**)
2. Streaks (pseudopods and radial streaming) (**Figure C-25**)
3. Negative pigment network (**Figure C-26**)

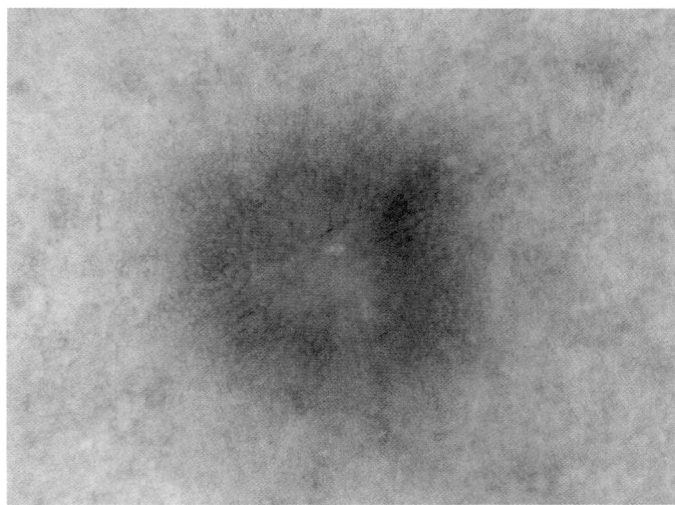

FIGURE C-11 Pattern trumps network in this dermatofibroma. Although this appears to have peripheral network, the central stellate scar makes this a dermatofibroma, which is not a melanocytic lesion. (*Reproduced with permission from Richard P. Usatine, MD.*)

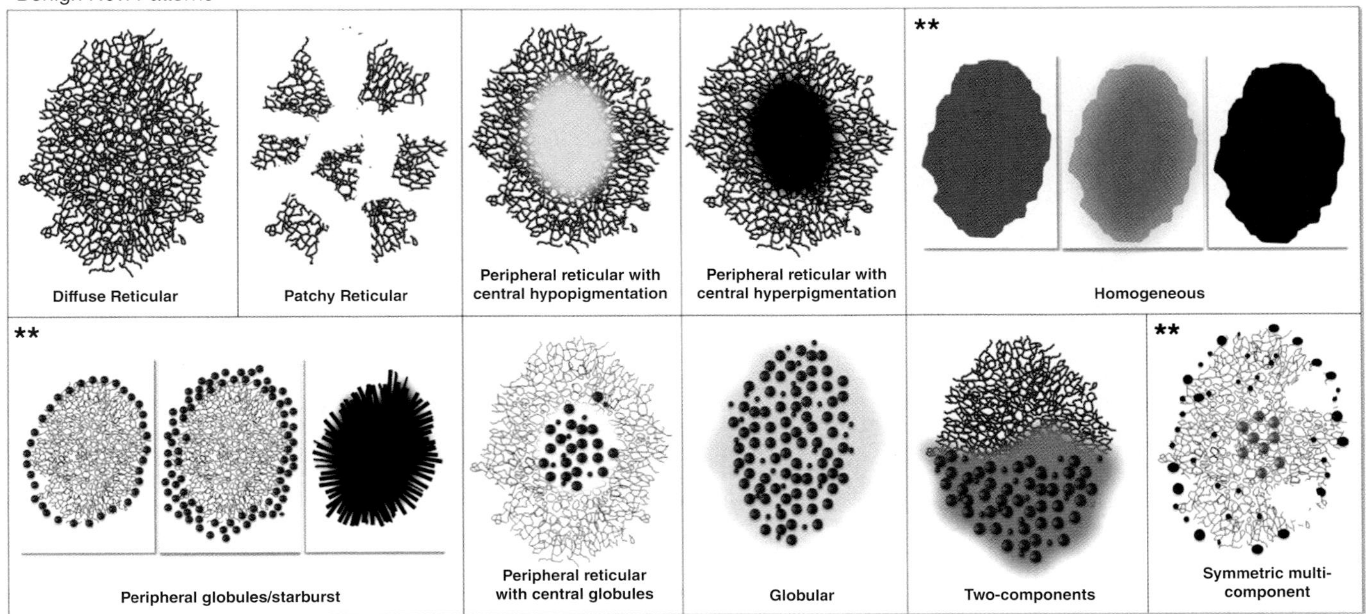

* Benign patterns encountered in many acquired nevi and dysplastic nevi. Blue nevi, some Spitz nevi and congenital melanocytic nevi can also manifest some of these patterns.
** N.B. to novices: Nevi with this pattern should be interpreted with caution.

FIGURE C-12 Step 2. Nevus vs. Melanoma. Benign nevi tend to adhere to 1 of 10 recurrent patterns. Melanoma is a melanocytic lesion that deviates from the 10 benign patterns. (*Concept and design by Natalia Jaimes, MD and Ashfaq A. Marghoob, MD*)

4. Shiny white lines (crystalline structures) (**Figure C-27**)
5. Atypical dots and or globules (**Figure C-28**)
4. Off-center blotch (**Figure C-29**)
5. Peripheral tan structureless areas (**Figure C-30**)
6. Blue-white veil overlying raised areas (**Figure C-31**)
7. Regression structures (blue-white veil overlying macular areas, scar-like areas, and/or peppering) (**Figure C-32**)
8. Atypical vascular structures (dotted vessels, serpentine vessels, polymorphous vessels, milky red areas, red globules, corkscrew vessels) (**Figure C-33**)

Note that melanoma on the soles or palms may present with a parallel ridge pattern (**Figure C-34**).

On the face melanoma may present with rhomboidal structures (**Figure C-35**).

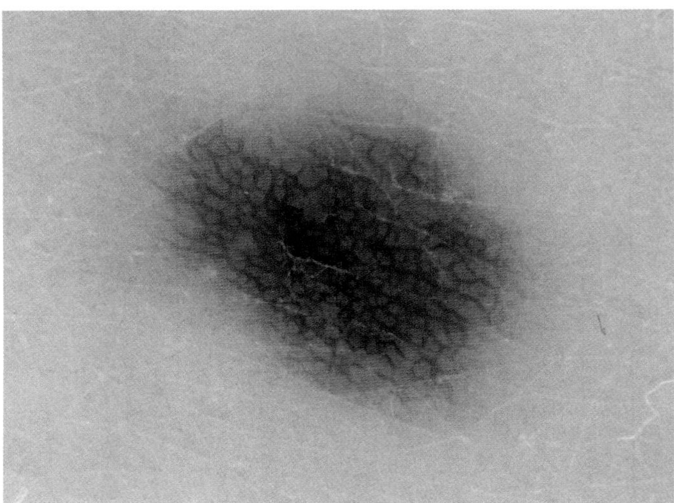

FIGURE C-13 Diffuse reticular pattern in a benign nevus. Note the regular line thickness and the fading of the lines at the periphery. (*Reproduced with permission from Richard P. Usatine, MD.*)

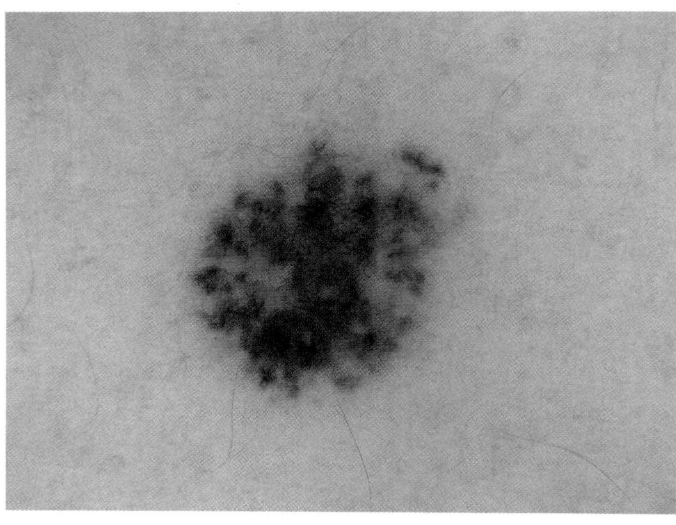

FIGURE C-14 Patchy reticular pattern in a benign nevus. (*Reproduced with permission from Richard P. Usatine, MD.*)

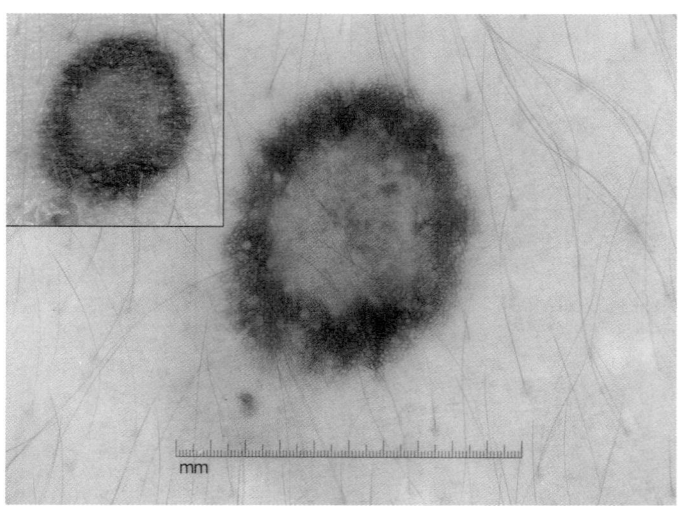

FIGURE C-15 Peripheral reticular pattern with central hypopigmentation in a benign nevus. (*Reproduced with permission from Ashfaq Marghoob, MD.*)

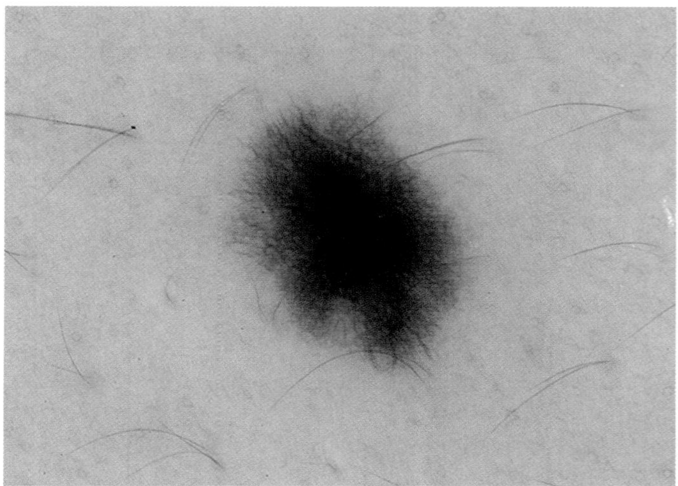

FIGURE C-16 Peripheral network with a central hyperpigmentation in this benign nevus. The central hyperpigmentation may also be called a typical blotch. (*Reproduced with permission from Ashfaq Marghoob, MD.*)

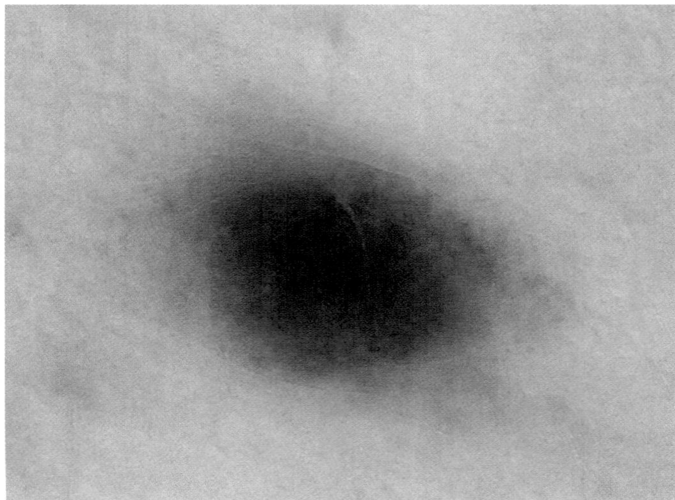

FIGURE C-17 Homogeneous pattern with a brown coloration in a benign nevus. The color may be brown, pink, or blue. (*Reproduced with permission from Richard P. Usatine. MD.*)

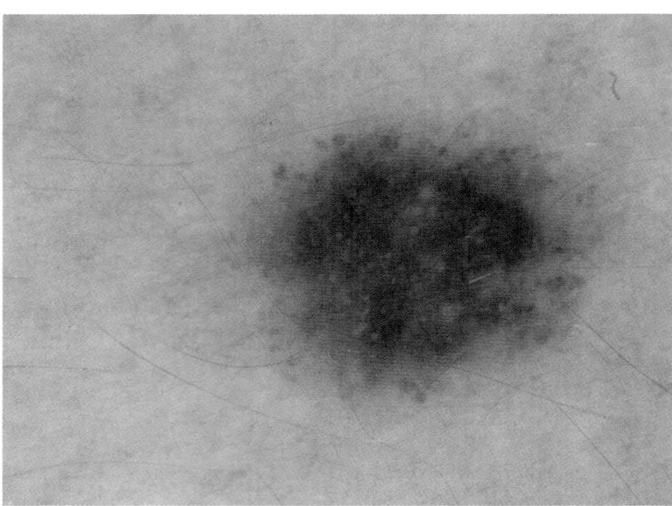

FIGURE C-18 Peripheral globules that are symmetrically placed are visible in this benign nevus. (*Reproduced with permission from Ashfaq Marghoob, MD.*)

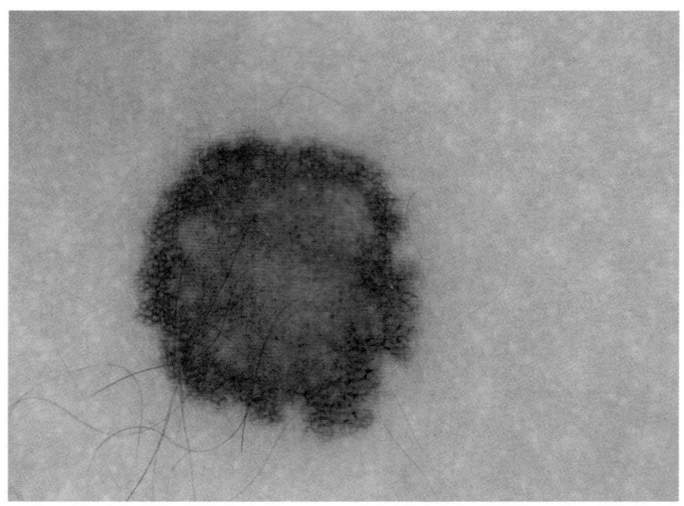

FIGURE C-19 Peripheral reticular pattern with central globules in this benign congenital nevus. (*Reproduced with permission from Richard P. Usatine, MD.*)

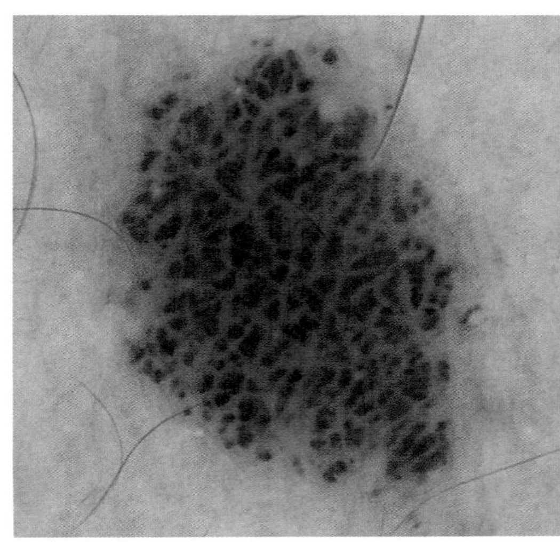

FIGURE C-20 Globular pattern in a benign nevus. Note these globules have a cobblestone pattern but other globules may be rounded. (*Reproduced with permission from Richard P. Usatine, MD.*)

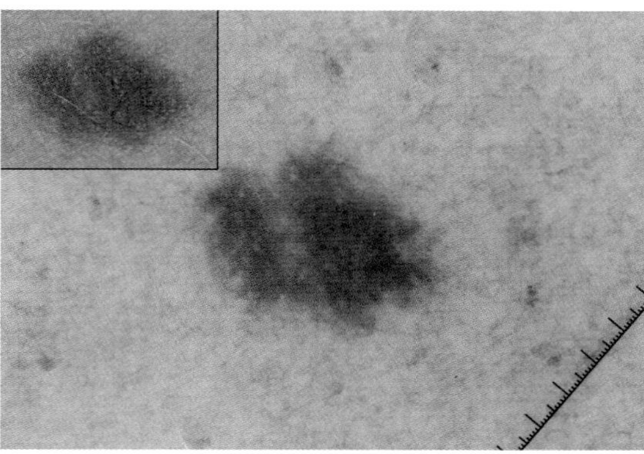

FIGURE C-21 Two-component pattern with globules on the right and a strictly reticular pattern on the left. (*Reproduced with permission from Ashfaq Marghoob, MD.*)

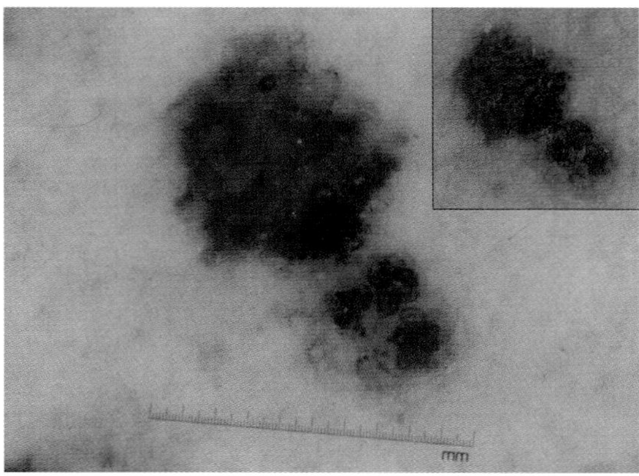

FIGURE C-22 Symmetric multicomponent pattern. Although this turned out to be a benign nevus, only the most experienced dermoscopist could afford to call this benign without a biopsy. (*Reproduced with permission from Ashfaq Marghoob, MD.*)

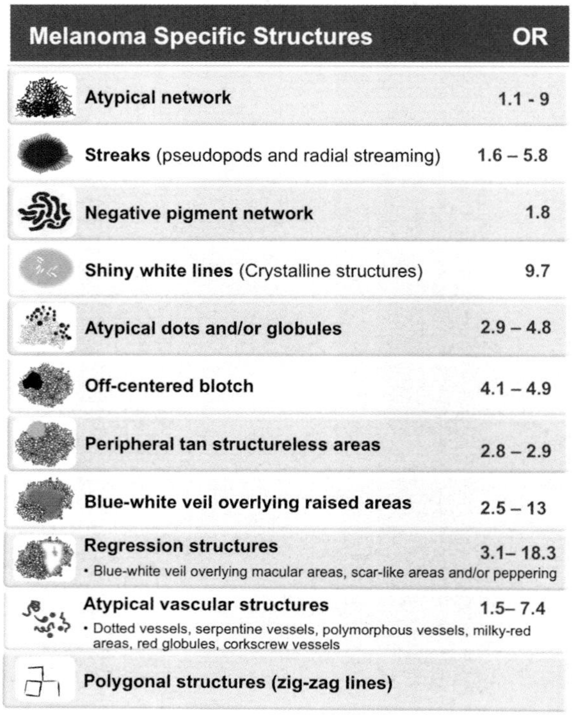

Melanoma Specific Structures	OR
Atypical network	1.1 - 9
Streaks (pseudopods and radial streaming)	1.6 – 5.8
Negative pigment network	1.8
Shiny white lines (Crystalline structures)	9.7
Atypical dots and/or globules	2.9 – 4.8
Off-centered blotch	4.1 – 4.9
Peripheral tan structureless areas	2.8 – 2.9
Blue-white veil overlying raised areas	2.5 – 13
Regression structures • Blue-white veil overlying macular areas, scar-like areas and/or peppering	3.1– 18.3
Atypical vascular structures • Dotted vessels, serpentine vessels, polymorphous vessels, milky-red areas, red globules, corkscrew vessels	1.5– 7.4
Polygonal structures (zig-zag lines)	

FIGURE C-23 Melanoma-specific structures and odds ratios that one of these structures predicts a diagnosis of melanoma.

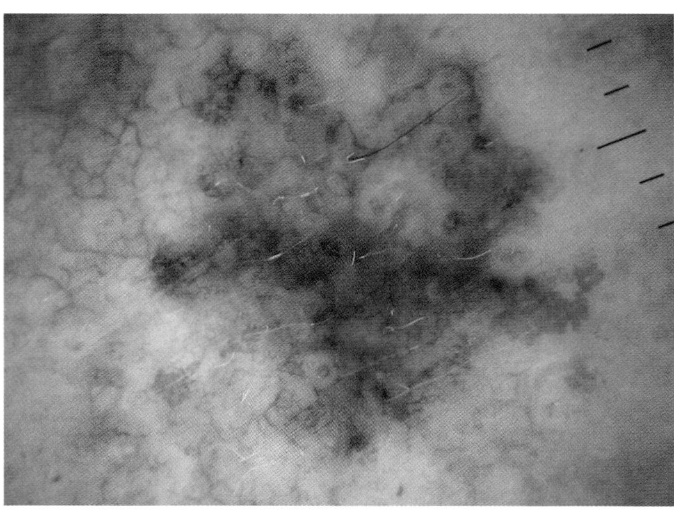

FIGURE C-24 Atypical network can be seen in this suspicious melanocytic lesion. (*Reproduced with permission from Richard P. Usatine, MD.*)

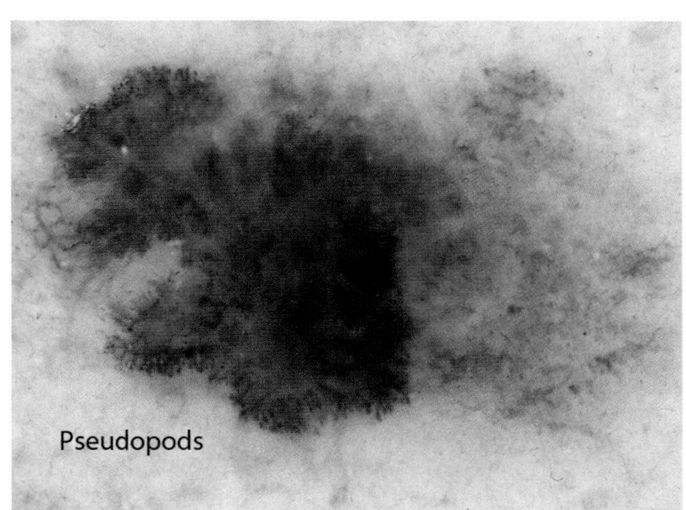

FIGURE C-25 Pseudopods can be seen in this melanoma. Pseudopods are streaks with radial streaming, a melanoma-specific structure. (*Copyright of Ashfaq Marghoob, MD.*)

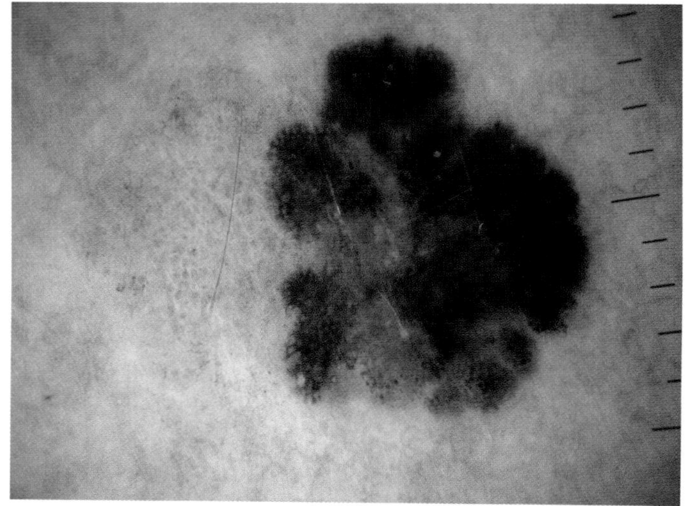

FIGURE C-26 Negative pigment network can be seen on the left side of this melanoma. (*Reproduced with permission from Richard P. Usatine, MD.*)

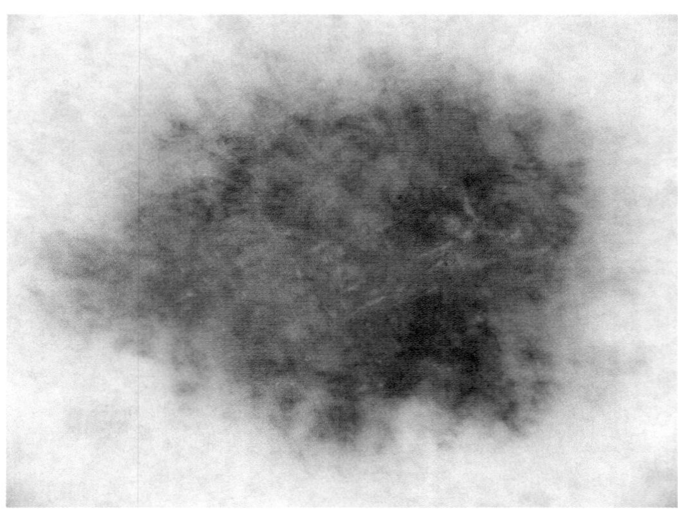

FIGURE C-27 Shiny white lines are visible in this melanoma. Shiny white lines are also called chrysalis or crystalline structures. (*Reproduced with permission from Ashfaq Marghoob, MD.*)

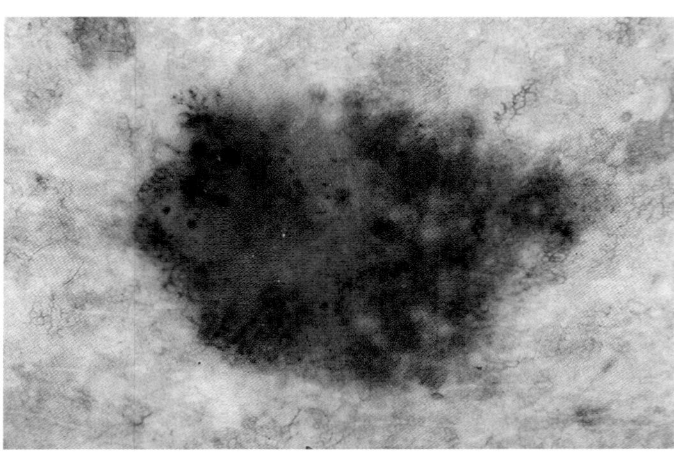

FIGURE C-28 Atypical dots and globules are seen in this melanoma. The dots and globules are peripheral and not symmetrically placed. A blue-white veil is also visible. (*Reproduced with permission from Ashfaq Marghoob, MD.*)

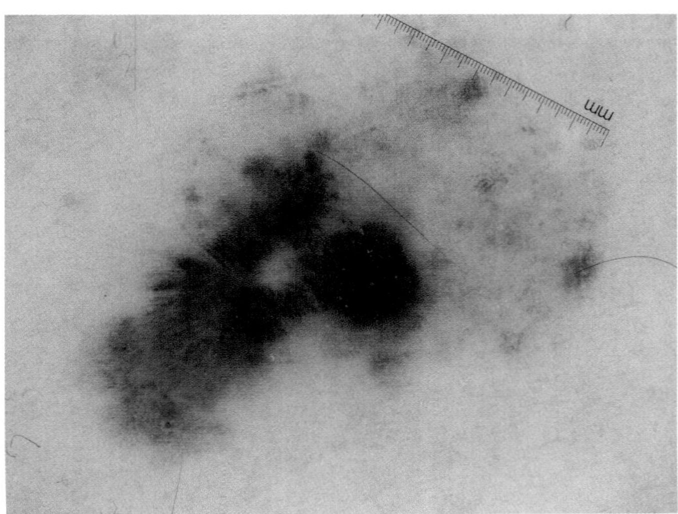

FIGURE C-29 Off-centered blotch in a melanoma. Note the blue-white veil, atypical globules, atypical network, and the peripheral tan structureless areas. (*Reproduced with permission from Ashfaq Marghoob, MD.*)

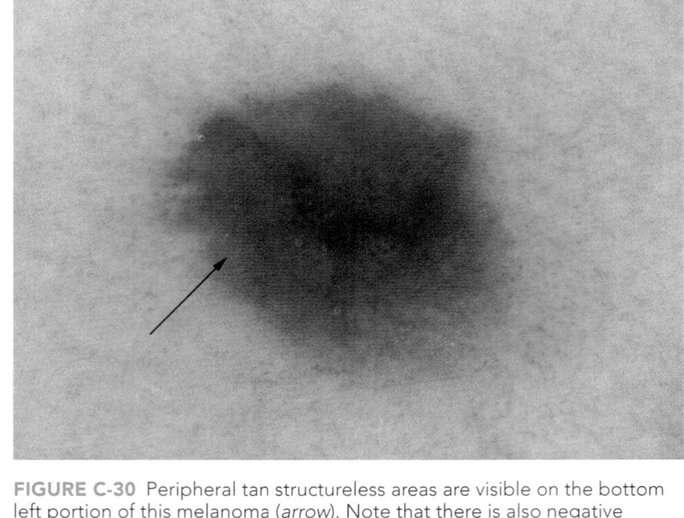

FIGURE C-30 Peripheral tan structureless areas are visible on the bottom left portion of this melanoma (*arrow*). Note that there is also negative network visible. (*Reproduced with permission from Ashfaq Marghoob, MD.*)

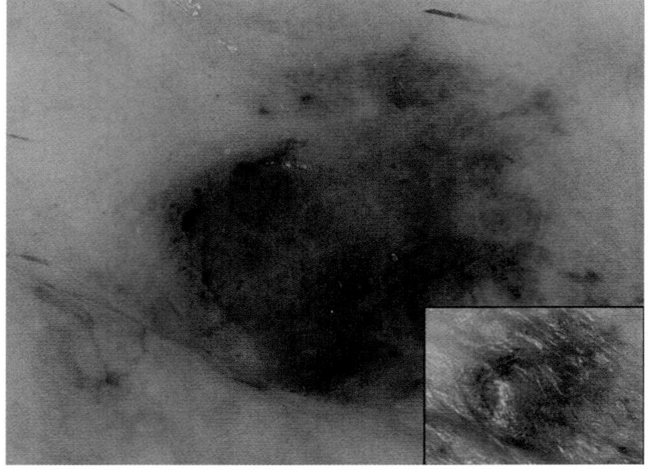

FIGURE C-31 Blue-white veil overlying raised area in a melanoma. (*Reproduced with permission from Ashfaq Marghoob, MD.*)

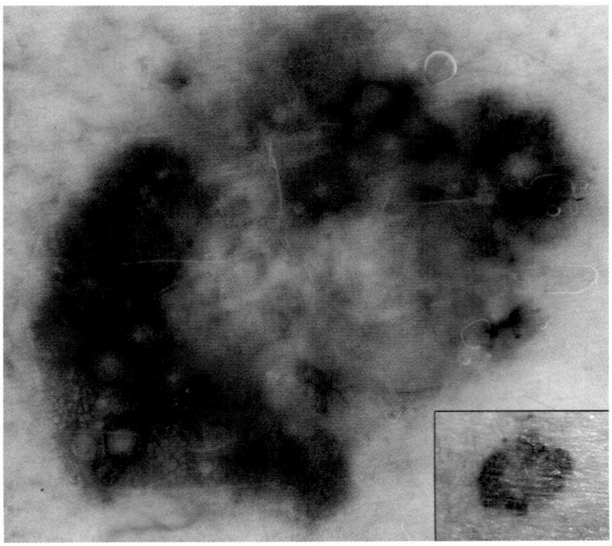

FIGURE C-32 Regression structures visible in this melanoma in situ. The regression structures consist of blue-white veil overlying macular areas and "peppering." (*Reproduced with permission from Richard P. Usatine, MD.*)

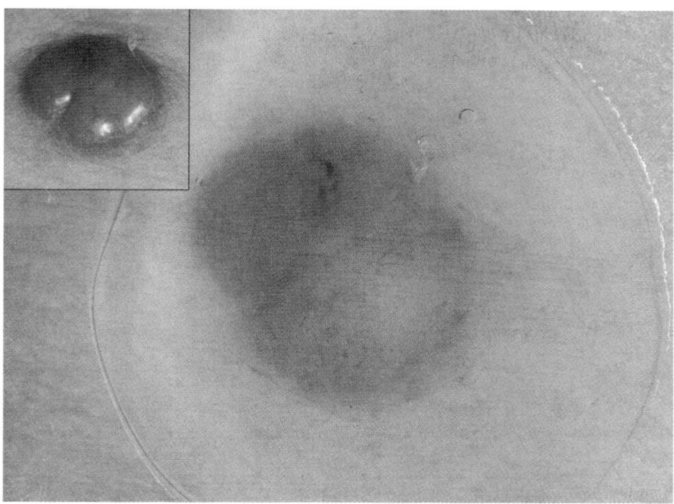

FIGURE C-33 Atypical vascular structures can be seen in this amelanotic nodular melanoma. Dotted and serpentine vessels are visible. (*Reproduced with permission from Ashfaq Marghoob, MD.*)

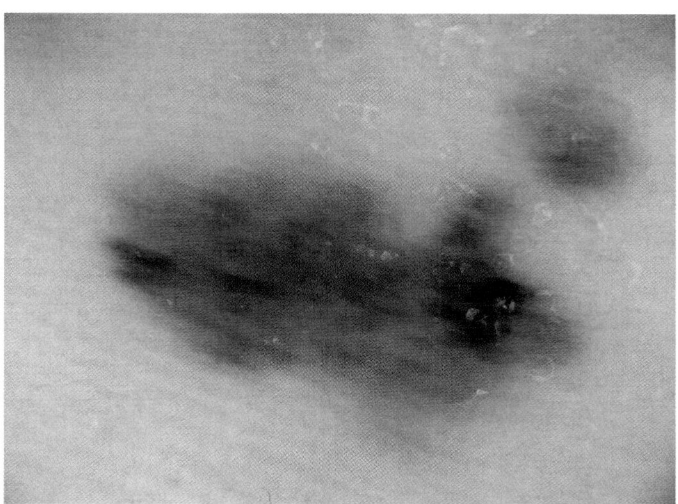

FIGURE C-34 Acrolentiginous melanoma on the foot with a parallel ridge pattern. (*Reproduced with permission from Richard P. Usatine, MD.*)

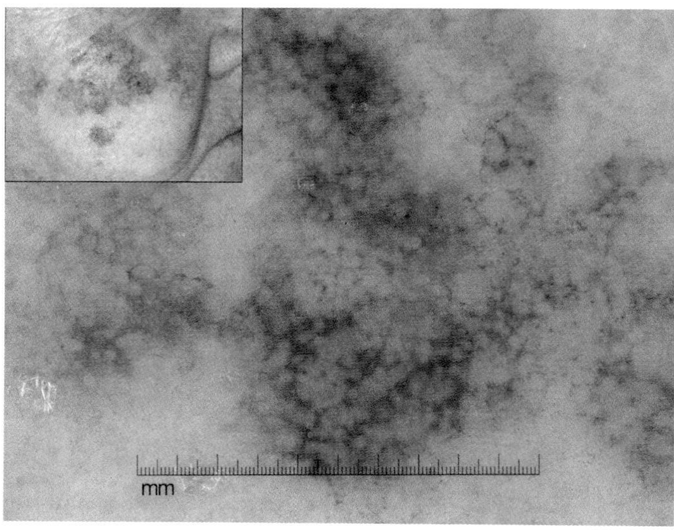

FIGURE C-35 Lentigo maligna on the face with rhomboidal structures. (*Reproduced with permission from Ashfaq Marghoob, MD.*)

The lesion adheres to one of the benign nevus patterns.	The lesion: 1) Adheres to one of the benign nevus patterns but also displays at least one of the melanoma specific structures. 2) Does not adhere to one of the benign nevus patterns and does not have any of the melanoma specific structures.	The lesion deviates from the benign nevus patterns and has at least one melanoma specific structure.
Nevus	**Indeterminate**	**Melanoma**

FIGURE C-36 Evaluating melanocytic lesions with dermoscopy. (*Concept and design by Natalia Jaimes, MD and Ashfaq A. Marghoob, MD*)

STEP 2 FOR MELANOCYTIC LESIONS

There are the following 3 possible pathways (**Figure C-36**):

1. The lesion adheres to one of the benign nevus patterns (see **Figures C-13** to **C-22**). Reassure the patient that the lesion is a benign nevus.
2. The lesion
   A. Adheres to one of the benign nevus patterns but also displays at least one of the melanoma-specific structures.
   B. Does not adhere to one of the benign nevus patterns and does not have any of the melanoma-specific structures.

   This is an indeterminate or suspicious lesion. The choices include perform a biopsy now or perform short-term mole monitoring with dermoscopic photographs and a 3-month follow-up. (Caveat: Do not monitor a raised lesion because a nodular melanoma can grow quickly with a worsened prognosis in a short time.)
3. The lesion deviates from the benign nevus patterns and has at least one melanoma-specific structure (see **Figures C-24** to **C-33**).

   Biopsy this lesion as a suspected melanoma (see Chapter 170, Melanoma).

STEP 1 FOR NONMELANOCYTIC TUMORS

If the lesion is not of melanocytic origin then one needs to look for structures seen in the following:

- Dermatofibromas
- Basal cell carcinomas
- Seborrheic keratoses
- Hemangiomas

DERMATOFIBROMA

a. Peripheral delicate fine network (**Figure C-37**)
b. Central scar-like area (see **Figure C-37**)
c. Blood vessels within the scar-like area (**Figure C-38**)
d. Ring-like globular structures (**Figure C-39**)

BASAL CELL CARCINOMA

a. Arborizing vessels (**Figure C-40**)
b. Spoke wheel-like structures/concentric structures (**Figure C-41**)
c. Leaf-like areas (**Figure C-42**)
d. Large blue-gray ovoid nest (see **Figure C-41**)
e. Multiple blue-gray globules (see **Figure C-42**)

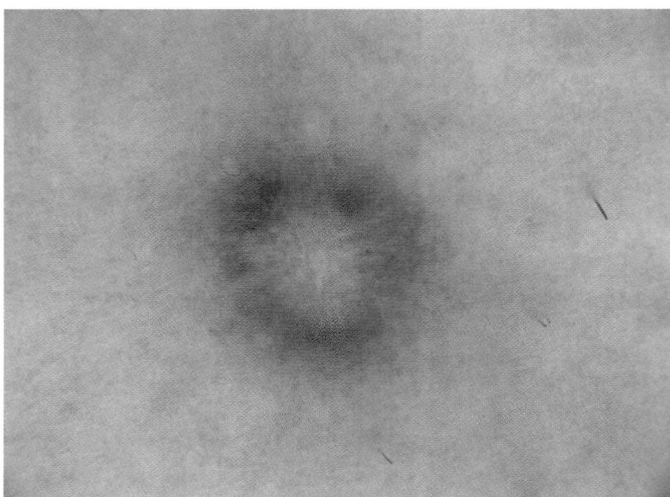

FIGURE C-37 Peripheral delicate fine network with a central scar-like area are visible in this typical dermatofibroma. (*Reproduced with permission from Richard P. Usatine, MD.*)

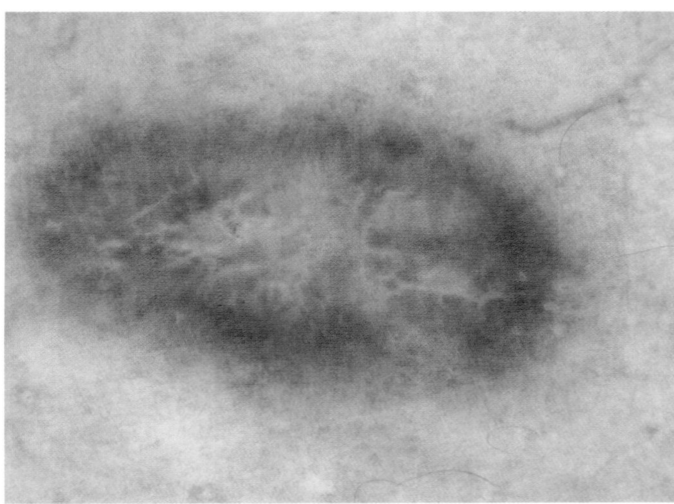

FIGURE C-38 Blood vessels are visible in the scar-like area of the dermatofibroma. (*Reproduced with permission from Richard P. Usatine, MD.*)

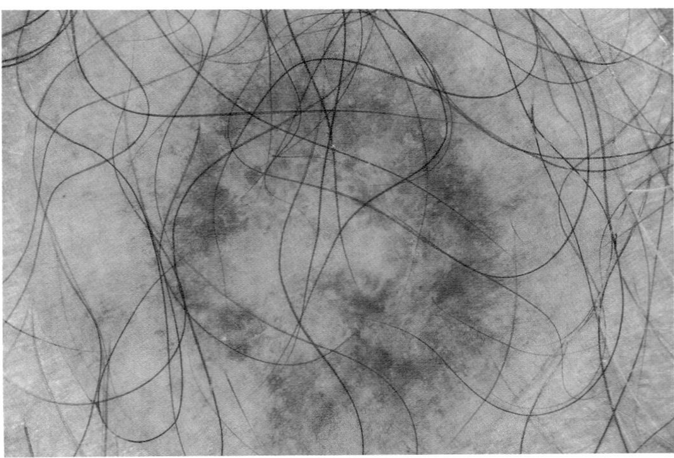

FIGURE C-39 Ring-like globular structures are visible in the central scar-like area of the dermatofibroma. (*Reproduced with permission from Ashfaq Marghoob, MD.*)

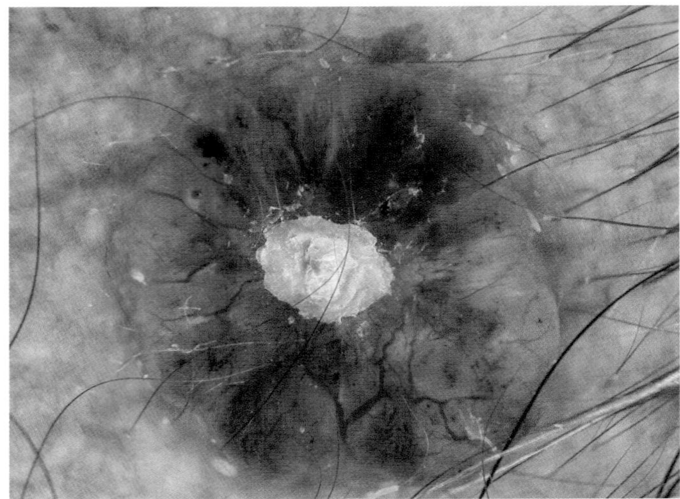

FIGURE C-40 Arborizing blood vessels like branching trees in a basal cell carcinoma. (*Reproduced with permission from Richard P. Usatine, MD.*)

f. Ulceration (**Figure C-43**)
g. Shiny white structures (crystalline structures) (see **Figure C-43**)

SEBORRHEIC KERATOSIS

a. Multiple (>2) milia-like cysts (**Figure C-44**)
b. Comedo-like openings (**Figure C-45**)
c. Gyri and sulci (fat finger-like structures) (**Figure C-46**) and cerebriform (**Figure C-47**)
d. Fingerprint-like structures (**Figure C-48**)
e. Moth-eaten borders (see **Figure C-48**)
f. Additional features: sharp demarcation, negative wobble sign (the lesion slides)

HEMANGIOMA

a. Red lacunae (**Figure C-49**)
b. Blue lacunae (**Figure C-50**)
c. Black lacunae = angiokeratoma (**Figure C-51**)

Note that dermoscopy can be helpful in detecting the scabies mite without having to scrape and use the microscope (**Figure C-52**; see Chapter 141, Scabies).

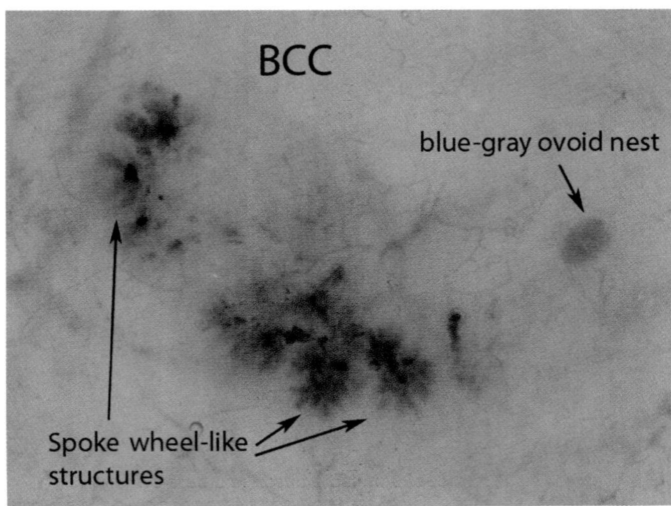

FIGURE C-41 Spoke wheel-like structures and isolated blue-gray ovoid nest on the left of this basal cell carcinoma. (*Reproduced with permission from Ashfaq Marghoob, MD.*)

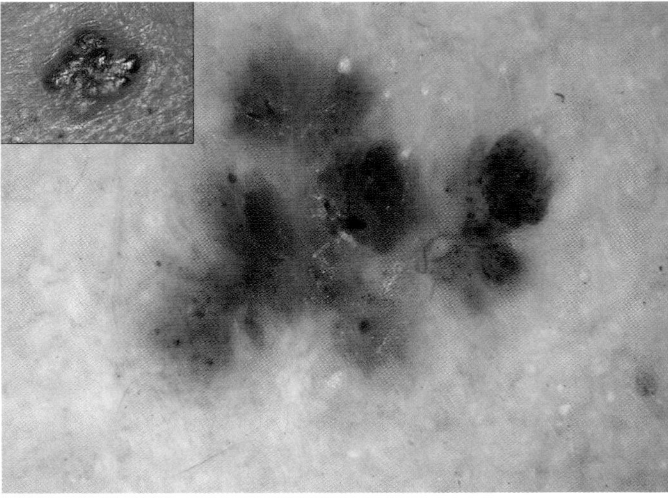

A

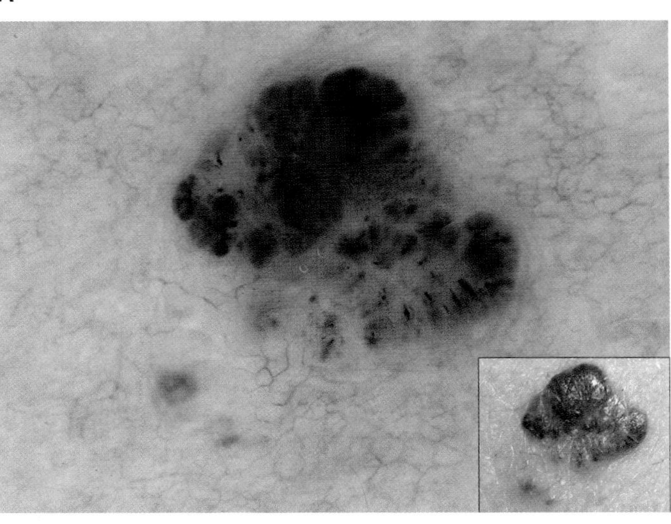

B

FIGURE C-42 A. Leaf-like structures in a pigmented basal cell carcinoma. B. Leaf-like structures and blue-gray ovoid nest in bottom left hand corner. (*Reproduced with permission from Richard P. Usatine, MD.*)

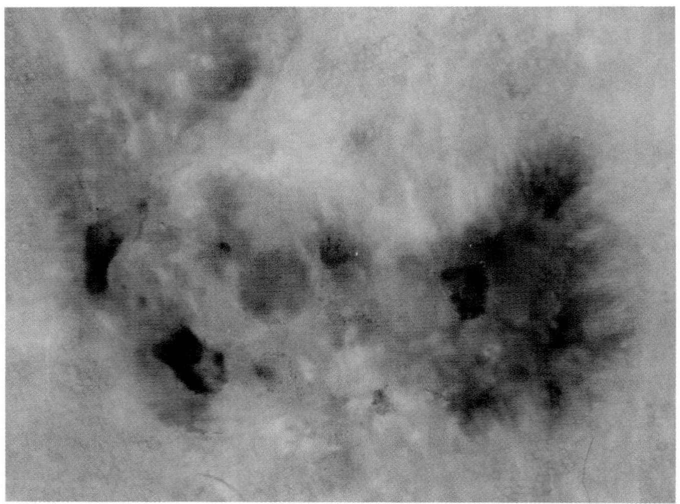

FIGURE C-43 Shiny white structures visible in this basal cell carcinoma. Also called chrystalline and chrysalis structures. (*Reproduced with permission from Ashfaq Marghoob, MD.*)

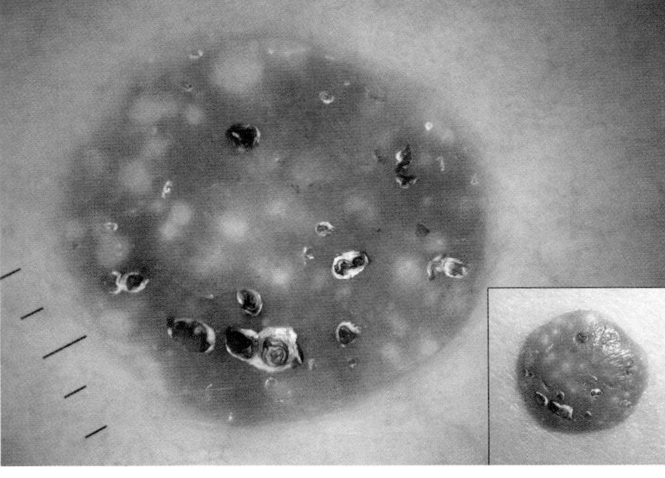

FIGURE C-44 Seborrheic keratosis with milia-like cysts and comedo-like openings. (*Reproduced with permission from Richard P. Usatine, MD.*)

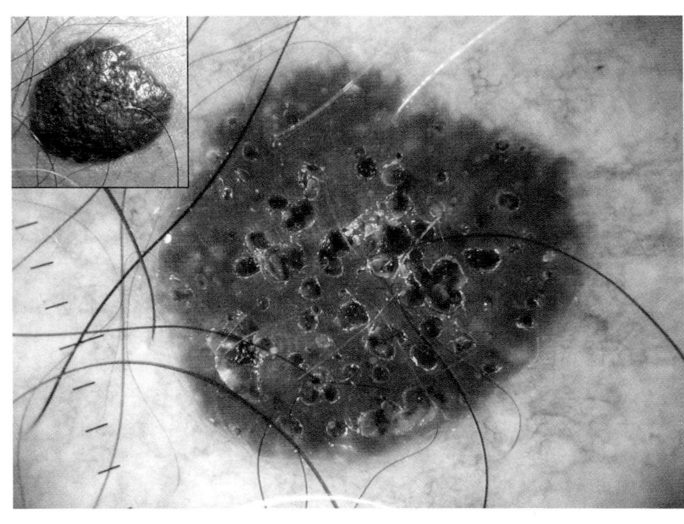

FIGURE C-45 Many comedone-like openings are visible in this seborrheic keratosis. (*Reproduced with permission from Richard P. Usatine, MD.*)

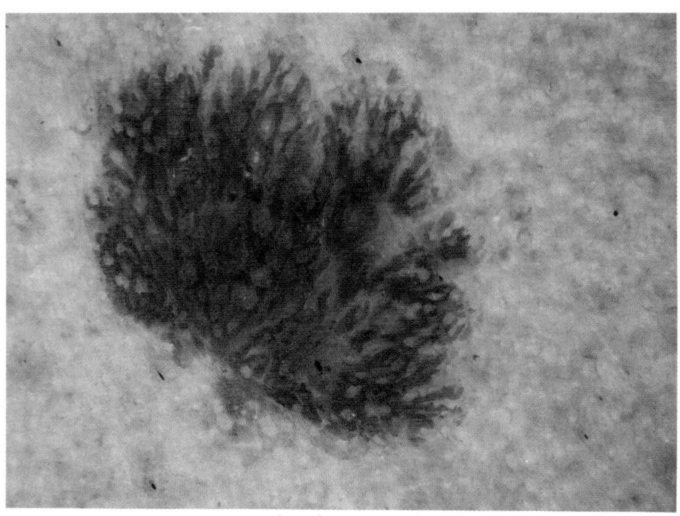

FIGURE C-46 Fat fingers are visible in this seborrheic keratosis. (*Reproduced with permission from Richard P. Usatine, MD.*)

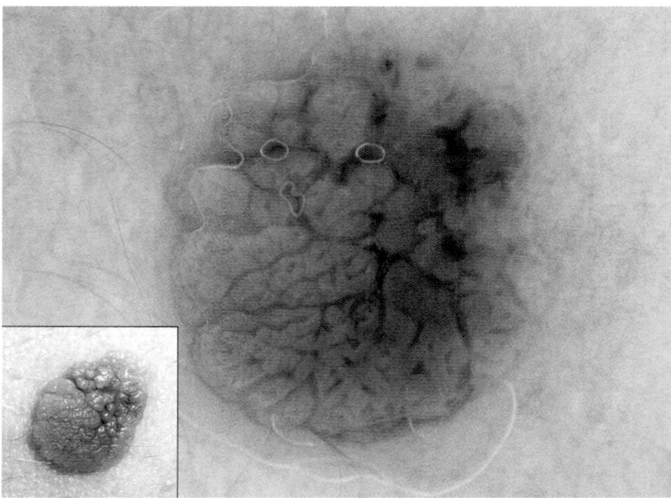

FIGURE C-47 Cerebriform seborrheic keratosis with gyri and sulci. (*Reproduced with permission from Richard P. Usatine, MD.*)

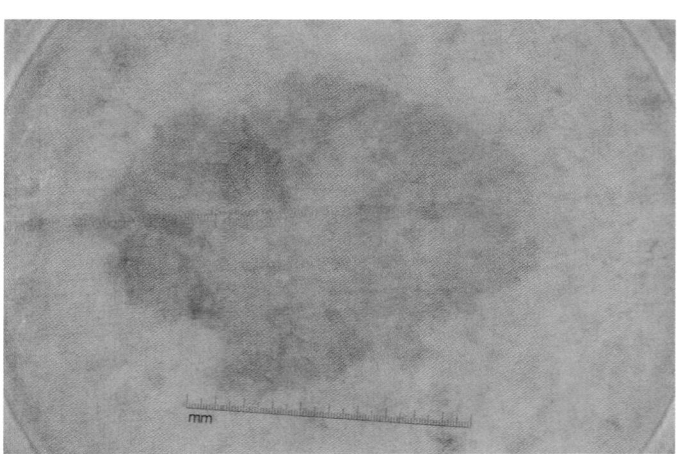

FIGURE C-48 Note the moth-eaten borders and fingerprint-like structures visible in this early seborrheic keratosis forming from any solar lentigo. (*Reproduced with permission from Ashfaq Marghoob, MD.*)

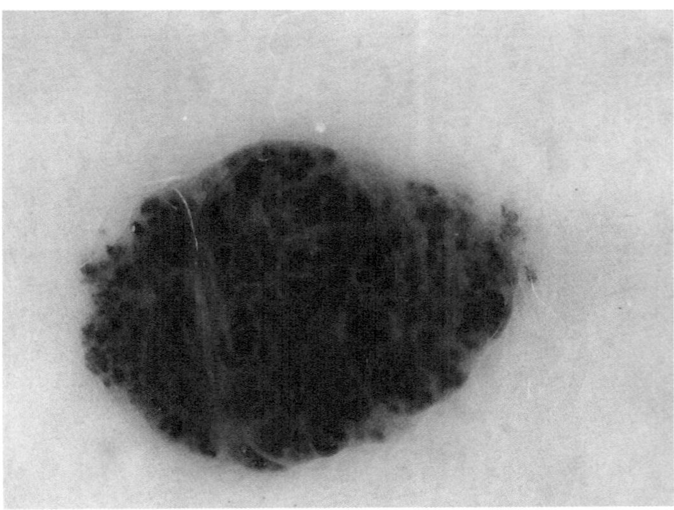

FIGURE C-49 Hemangioma showing red lacunae (lakes or lagoons of sharply demarcated vascular tissue). (*Reproduced with permission from Richard P. Usatine, MD.*)

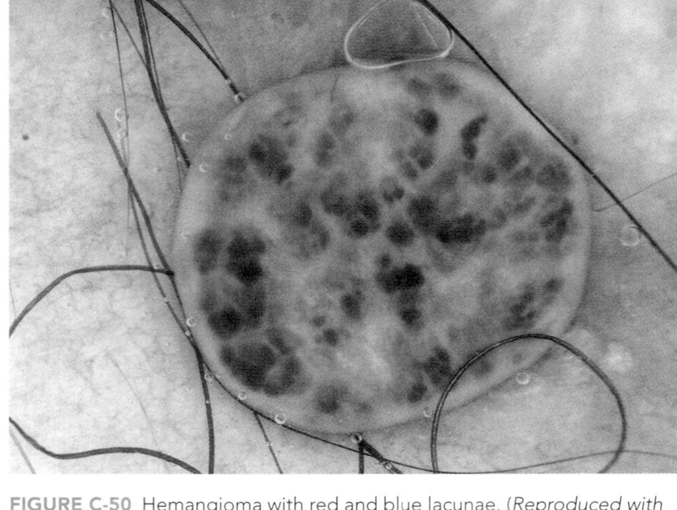

FIGURE C-50 Hemangioma with red and blue lacunae. (*Reproduced with permission from Ashfaq Marghoob, MD.*)

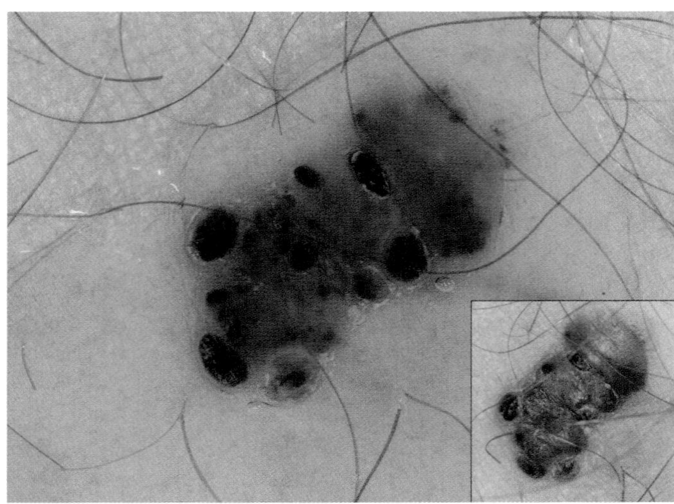

FIGURE C-51 Angiokeratoma showing purple and black lacunae. (*Reproduced with permission from Ashfaq Marghoob, MD.*)

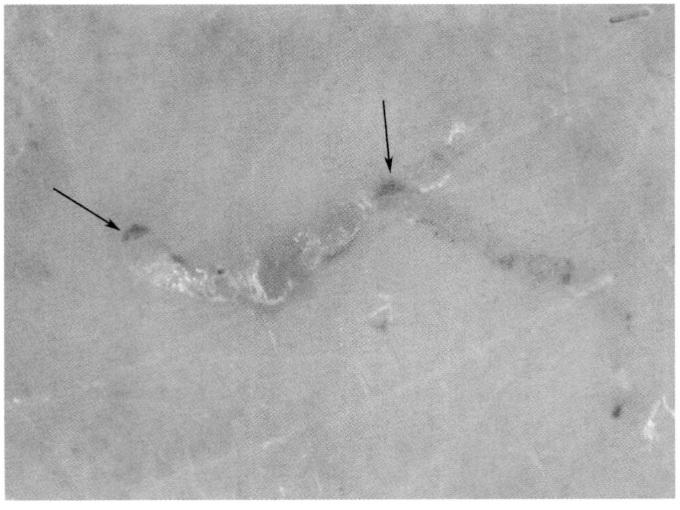

FIGURE C-52 Scabies mites (*arrows*) visible at the end of 2 intersecting burrows. The head and legs are most visible and resemble arrowheads pointing away from the burrows. (*Reproduced with permission from Richard P. Usatine, MD.*)

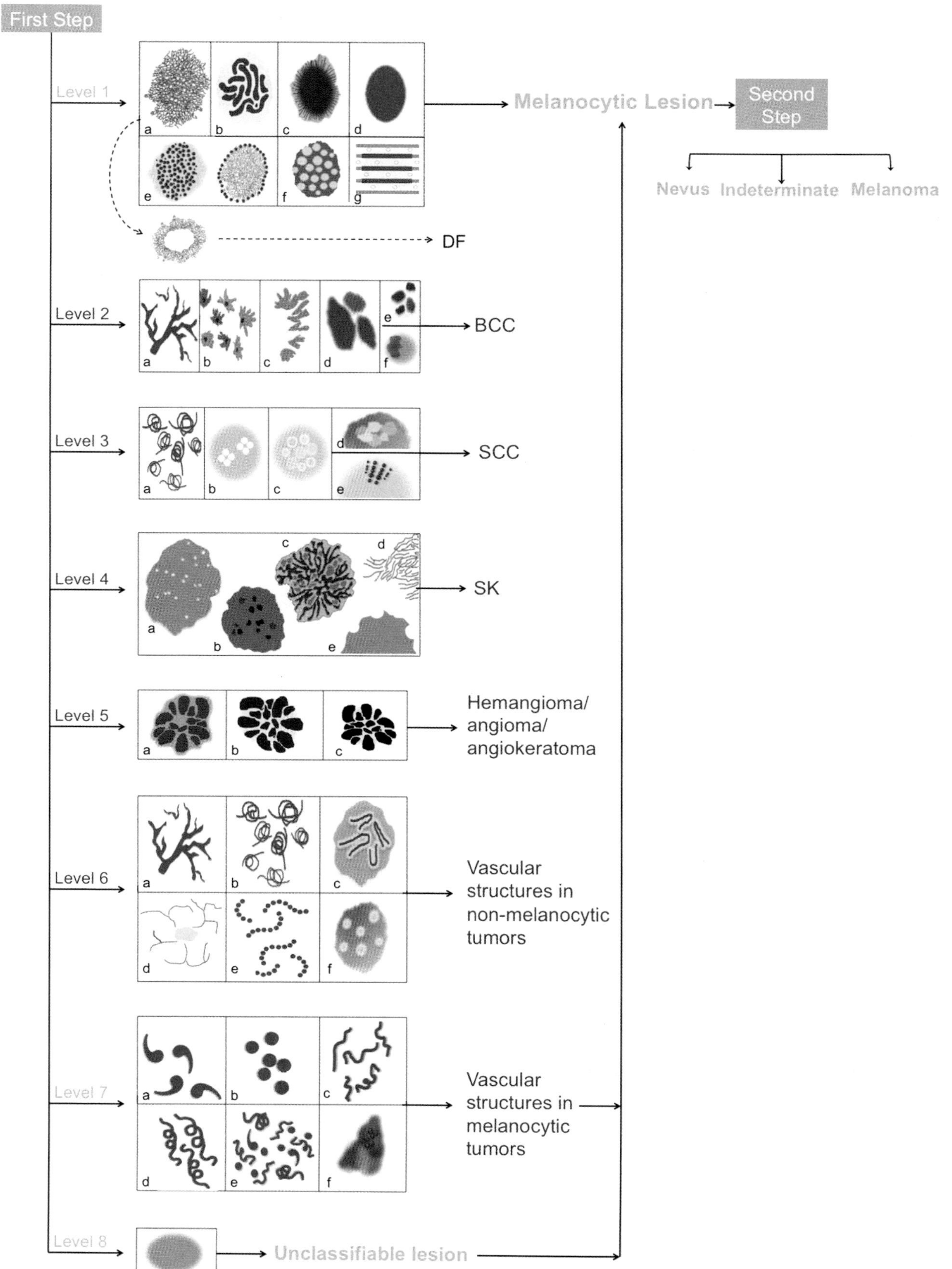

FIGURE C-53 Eight levels that are part of step 1 in the 2-step algorithm. (*Concept and design by Natalia Jaimes, MD and Ashfaq A. Marghoob, MD*)

Step 1: Melanocytic versus Non-melanocytic lesions							
Level 1: Melanocytic lesions	**Level 2: Basal cell carcinoma (BCC)**	**Level 3: Squamous cell carcinoma (SCC)**	**Level 4: Seborrheic keratosis (SK)**	**Level 5: Hemangioma / angioma/ angiokeratoma**	**Level 6: Blood vessels in non-melanocytic tumors***	**Level 7: Blood vessels in melanocytic tumors***	**Level 8: Unclassifiable lesions**
a. Pigment network* b. Negative network c. Streaks d. Homogeneous blue pigmentation e. Aggregated globules or peripheral rim of globules f. Pseudonetwork (Facial skin) g. Parallel pigment pattern (Acral lesions) * Exception to pigment network: Dermatofibroma (DF)	a. Arborizing vessels b. Spoke wheel-like structures / concentric structures c. Leaf-like areas d. Large blue-gray ovoid nests e. Multiple blue-gray globules f. Ulceration g. Additional clues: Shiny white structures	a. Focal glomerular vessels b. Rosettes c. Keratin pearls / White circles d. Yellow scale e. Brown dots/ globules aligned radially at the periphery	a. Multiple (>2) milia-like cysts b. Comedo-like opening c. Gyri and sulci (Fat finger-like structures) d. Fingerprint-like structures e. Moth-eaten borders f. Hairpin vessels with white halo g. Additional features: sharp demarcation; negative wobble sign: the lesion slides	a. Red lacunae b. Blue lacunae c. Black lacunae	**Morphology** a. Arborizing vessels b. Glomerular vessels c. Hairpin vessels with white halo **Arrangement** d. Crown e. Serpiginous or string of pearls f. "Strawberry" pattern g. Focal clusters at the periphery **Distribution** • Focal • Diffuse • Central • Peripheral • Random ***Usually seen in** a. BCC b. Squamous cell carcinoma (SCC) c. SK/ Keratoacanthom a d. Sebaceous hyperplasia (SH) e. Clear cell acanthoma (CCA) f. Actinic keratosis	**Morphology** a. Comma vessels b. Dotted vessels c. Serpentine vessels (linear irregular) d. Corkscrew vessels e. Polymorphou s vessels f. Milky-red area **Distribution** • Focal • Diffuse • Central • Peripheral • Random ***Usually in:** a. Intradermal nevi b – f .Melanoma	**None of the structures from levels 1 to 6 are noted**

FIGURE C-54 Explanation of the flow diagram in Figure C-53. (*Concept and design by Natalia Jaimes, MD and Ashfaq A. Marghoob, MD*)

VASCULAR STRUCTURES

Levels 5 and 6 (**Figures C-53 and C-54.**) in step 1 involve evaluating vascular structures in nonmelanocytic and melanocytic tumors. For further information about this more advanced steps see the resources below.

RESOURCES TO LEARN DERMOSCOPY

Dermoscopy. Website from Italy that includes a free dermoscopy tutorial—http://www.dermoscopy.org/

Free dermoscopy app—Dermoscopy: Two-Step Algorithm. iTunes and http://www.usatinemedia.com.

International Dermoscopy Society. http://www.dermoscopy-ids.org/.

Johr R, Stolz W. *Dermoscopy: An Illustrated Self-Assessment Guide*. New York, NY: McGraw-Hill; 2010, with an interactive app: see www.usatinemedia.com.

Malvehy J, Puig S, Braun RP, Marghoob AA, Kopf AW. *Handbook of Dermoscopy*. London, UK: Taylor & Francis; 2006.

Marghoob A, Braun R, Kopf A. *Interactive CD-ROM of Dermoscopy*. London, UK: Informa Healthcare; 2007.

Marghoob AA, Malvehy J, Braun R, eds. *Atlas of Dermoscopy*. 2nd ed. London, UK: Informa Healthcare; 2012.

Marghoob A, Usatine R. Dermoscopy. In: Usatine R, Pfenninger J, Stulberg D, Small R, eds. *Dermatologic and Cosmetic Procedures in Office Practice*. Philadelphia, PA: Elsevier; 2012.

Marghoob AA, Usatine RP, Jaimes N. Dermoscopy. In: Usatine R, Smith M, Mayeaux EJ, Chumley H. *Color Atlas of Family Medicine*. 2nd ed. New York, NY: McGraw-Hill; 2013

Marghoob AA, Usatine RP, Jaimes N. Dermoscopy for the family physician. *Am Fam Physician*. 2013 Oct 1;88(7):441-450.

Courses (all taught by the authors of this chapter) are as below:

American Dermoscopy Meeting is held yearly in the summer in a national park: http://www.americandermoscopy.com/.

Memorial Sloan-Kettering Cancer Center holds a yearly dermoscopy workshop each fall in New York City: http://www.mskcc.org/events/.

American Academy of Family Physicians (AAFP) yearly fall scientific assembly offers dermoscopy workshops: http://www.aafp.org/events/assembly.html.

AAFP sponsors a course on "Skin Problems and Diseases" that includes a dermoscopy workshop: http://www.aafp.org/cme/.

Note: In this index, the letters *b*, *f*, and *t* denote boxes, figures, and tables, respectively.

H

L

N

R